The Comparative Guide to American Hospitals

Volume 4

2/14

Fourth Edition

The Comparative Guide to American Hospitals

Volume 4: Western Region

4,834 Hospitals with Key Personnel and 67 Quality Measures Relating to Heart Attack, Heart Failure, Pneumonia, Stroke, Blood Clots, Childhood Asthma, Emergency Room Care, Surgical Care, Preventative Care, Medical Imaging and Patient Experience

A SEDGWICK PRESS Book

Grey House Publishing

PUBLISHER: Leslie Mackenzie
SENIOR EDITOR: David Garoogian
EDITORIAL DIRECTOR: Laura Mars
PRODUCTION MANAGER: Kristen Thatcher
MARKETING DIRECTOR: Jessica Moody

A Sedgewick Press Book
Grey House Publishing, Inc.
4919 Route 22
Amenia, NY 12501
518.789.8700
FAX 845.373.6390
www.greyhouse.com
e-mail: books @greyhouse.com

Fourth Edition

Printed in the Canada

Comparative guide to American hospitals. Vol. 4, Western region; [ed. David Garoogian]. — 4th ed. (2014)

4 v. ; cm.

Includes index.
"4,834 Hospitals with Key Personnel and 67 Quality Measures Relating to Heart Attack, Heart Failure, Pneumonia, Stroke, Blood Clots, Childhood Asthma, Emergency Room Care, Surgical Care, Preventative Care, Medical Imaging and Patient Experience."

1. Hospitals—United States—Directories. 2. Hospitals—United States—Periodicals. 3. Hospitals—Ratings—United States—Statistics—Periodicals. 4. Myocardial infarction—Hospitals—United States—Directories. 5. Heart failure—Hospitals—United States—Directories. 6. Pneumonia—Hospitals—United States—Directories. I. Garoogian, David.

RA977 .C66
610/.025

4-Volume Set ISBN: 978-1-61925-457-2
Volume 1 ISBN: 978-1-61925-458-9
Volume 2 ISBN: 978-1-61925-459-6
Volume 3 ISBN: 978-1-61925-460-2
Volume 4 ISBN: 978-1-61925-461-9

Table of Contents

Introduction

This is the fourth edition of *The Comparative Guide to American Hospitals*. It reports on how 4,834 hospitals—**141 more than last edition**—in America measure up when caring for patients with a number of specific conditions. The third edition reported on **Heart Attacks, Heart Failure, Pneumonia, Childhood Asthma, Surgical Care, Use of Medical Imaging**, and **Patients' Hospital Experiences**. This fourth edition includes new data on **Blood Clot Prevention and Treatment, Emergency Room Care, Preventative Care, Stroke,** and **Medicare Spending**. Also new are appendices on **Surgical Complication Rates** and **Best Hospitals by Category**.

This work is based on a Federal study (Hospital Compare) in which short-term acute care and critical access hospitals around the country voluntarily report on quality measures to receive an incentive payment established by the Medicare Prescription Drug, Improvement and Modernization Act of 2003. Each hospital in this edition is rated on 67 recognized quality measures—**18 more than last edition**—and is compared to both state and national averages.

In *The Comparative Guide to American Hospitals,* the data is organized, sorted and ranked by our editors. It is this organization and ranking that makes *The Comparative Guide to American Hospitals* a unique and valuable tool to the health care consumer. Data is presented in such a way as to inform and educate the user, who can then put the facts into a meaningful context as hospitals are evaluated state by state.

Due to the increased data, and the regional use of such data, this edition is again comprised of four regional volumes—**Eastern, Southern, Central** and **Western**. In addition to comprehensive **hospital rankings and profiles** for all states in the region, each volume includes four Appendices with additional information.

In addition to the data from Hospital Compare, each hospital profile in *The Comparative Guide to American Hospitals* is comprised of value-added data from Grey House's *Directory of Hospital Personnel*. This critical contact data includes fax numbers, web sites, email addresses, and number of beds plus 24,458 key contact names—**783 more names than last edition**. In addition, each state chapter includes **State Hospital Rankings**.

Section One: State Hospital Rankings & State Profiles

The first section of each regional volume of *The Comparative Guide to American Hospitals* is arranged alphabetically by state. Each state chapter starts with a ranking section, unique to Grey House, that ranks hospitals in that state on how often they meet each of the 67 accepted quality protocols. The quality measures ranked in *The Comparative Guide to American Hospitals* are based on accepted, effective treatments supported by the Centers for Medicare & Medical Services of the US Department of Health & Human Services and the Hospital Quality Alliance (HQA)—a public/private collaboration established to promote on hospital quality of care. HQA represents consumers, hospitals, doctors, employers, accrediting organizations and Federal agencies.

Following the ranking section, hospital profiles are listed first by city, then alpha within city. Profiles include name, address, phone, fax, web site, hospital type and ownership, number of beds, and whether the hospital provides emergency services. Further, each profile includes an average of five key medical contacts—representing not only the facility's top administration but also the physicians specifically responsible for the care of heart, pneumonia, and asthma patients, as well as surgical care. Again, these data points are unique to *The Comparative Guide to American Hospitals*, and complete the picture for health care consumers searching for quality care.

The remainder of each hospital profile examines the 67 quality measures in detail, comparing the hospital's score with both the state and national average: These measures include:

- **Timely and Effective Care:**
  - **Blood Clot Prevention and Treatment** *(NEW)* measures include anticoagulation overlap therapy, ICU venous thromboembolism prophylaxis, incidence of potentially preventable VTE, UFH with dosages/platelet count monitoring, venous thromboembolism prophylaxis, and warfarin therapy discharge instructions
  - **Chest Pain/Possible Heart Attack Care** measures include aspirin at arrival, median time to ECG, median time to transfer, and fibrinolytic medication timing
  - **Children's Asthma Care** measures include receiving systemic corticosteroids, receiving home management plan, and receiving reliever medication
  - **Emergency Department** *(NEW)* measures include admittance decision time, head CT results within 45 minutes of arrival, patients who left ER before being seen, time from ER arrival to admittance, time from ER arrival to discharge, time spent in ER before being evaluated, and time to pain medications for long-bone fractures
  - **Heart Attack Care** measures include aspirin given at discharge, statin prescribed at discharge, fibrinolytic medication timing, and percutaneous coronary intervention within 90 minutes of arrival
  - **Heart Failure Care** measures include angiotensin converting enzyme inhibitor or angiotensin receptor blocker for left ventricular systolic dysfunction, discharge instructions given, and evaluation of left ventricular systolic function
  - **Pneumonia Care** measures include appropriate initial antibiotic, and blood culture timing
  - **Pregnancy and Delivery Care** *(NEW)* measures include newborn deliveries scheduled early
  - **Preventive Care** *(NEW)* measures include immunization for influenza and immunization for pneumonia
  - **Stroke Care** *(NEW)* measures include anticoagulation therapy for atrial fibrillation, antithrombotic therapy timing, assessed for rehabilitation, discharged on antithrombotic therapy, discharged on statin medication, thrombolytic therapy timing, venous thromboembolism prophylaxis, and written stroke educational materials given
  - **Surgical Care** measures include appropriate venous thromboembolism prophylaxis within 24 hours, appropriate beta blocker usage, controlled postoperative blood glucose, perioperative temperature management *(NEW)*, prophylactic antibiotic timing, prophylactic antibiotic selection, prophylactic antibiotic stopped, and urinary catheter removal
- **Medicare Spending** *(NEW)* measures include Medicare spending per beneficiary
- **Use of Medical Imaging** measures include MRI for low back pain, cardiac imaging stress test before surgery *(NEW)*, follow-up mammogram/ultrasound, combination brain/sinus CT scan *(NEW)*, combination abdominal CT scan, and combination chest CT scan.
- **Survey of Patients' Hospital Experiences**
  HCAHPS (Hospital Consumer Assessment of Healthcare Providers and Systems) is a national, standardized survey of hospital patients. HCAHPS (pronounced "H-caps") was created to publicly report the patient's perspective of hospital care. The survey asks a random sample of recently discharged patients about important aspects of their hospital experience. The HCAHPS results allow consumers to make fair and objective comparisons between hospitals, and of individual hospitals to state and national benchmarks, on ten important measures of patients' perspectives of care:
  - How do patients rate the hospital overall?
  - How often did doctors communicate well with patients?
  - How often did nurses communicate well with patients?
  - How often did patients receive help quickly from hospital staff?
  - How often did staff explain about medicines before giving them to patients?
  - How often was patients' pain well controlled?
  - How often was the area around patients' rooms kept quiet at night?
  - How often were the patients' rooms and bathrooms kept clean?
  - Were patients given information about what to do during their recovery at home?
  - Would patients recommend the hospital to friends and family?

Section Two: Appendixes & Index

The second section of *The Comparative Guide to American Hospitals* includes:

- **Appendix A: 30-Day Death (Mortality) Rates** Unique to Grey House, this section takes data and organize it in a helpful, informative way for the reader. It lists hospitals nationwide that are "better" or "worse" than the national average, plus a State and National Summary of Hospital Mortality Rates.
- **Appendix B: 30-Day Readmission Rates** lists hospitals nationwide that are "better" or "worse" than the national average, plus a State and National Summary of Hospital Readmission Rates.
- **Appendix C: Surgical Complication Rates** lists hospitals nationwide that are "better" or "worse" than the national average, plus a State and National Summary of Hospital Readmission Rates. Surgical complications covered include:
    - A Wound That Splits Open After Surgery on the Abdomen or Pelvis
    - Accidental Cuts and Tears From Medical Treatment
    - Collapsed Lung Due to Medical Treatment
    - Deaths Among Patients With Serious Treatable Complications After Surgery
    - Rate of Complications for Hip/Knee Replacement Patients
    - Serious Blood Clots After Surgery
    - Serious Complications
- **Appendix D: Best Hospitals by Selected Category** lists best hospitals nationwide based on their average scores in 11 categories. The categories are:
    - Blood Clot Prevention and Treatment
    - Children's Asthma Care
    - Emergency Department Care
    - Heart Care
    - Pneumonia Care
    - Preventative Care
    - Stroke Care
    - Surgical Care
    - Patient's Hospital Experiences
    - Use of Medical Imaging
    - Lowest Medicare Spending per Beneficiary
- **Appendix E: Glossary** provides a list of 87 medical terms to make the best use possible of the data in this edition.
- **Regional Hospital Profile Index** lists hospitals included in each regional volume alphabetically, including city and state.
- **National Hospital Profile Index** lists all hospitals nationwide alphabetically, including volume number, city and state. Appears in Volume 4 only.

This completely revised fourth edition of *The Comparative Guide to American Hospitals* is a valuable guide for the entire medical community, with more hospitals, more criteria measures and more key executives than the last edition. It offers an indispensable snapshot of how hospitals measure up, not only to established "best practices," but also to each other.

We welcome your comments to this edition.

User's Guide

What is the *Comparative Guide to American Hospitals*?

The *Comparative Guide to American Hospitals* (CGAH) is based on a Federal study (Hospital Compare) in which short-term acute care and critical access hospitals around the country voluntarily report on quality measures to receive an incentive payment established by the Medicare Prescription Drug, Improvement and Modernization Act of 2003. Each hospital in this edition is rated on 67 recognized quality measures and is compared to both state and national averages. The measures are grouped into four major categories: Timely and Effective Care; Survey of Patients' Experiences; Use of Medical Imaging; and Medicare Spending Per Beneficiary.

Timely and Effective Care Measures (aka "Process of Care" Measures)

Process of care measures reported under the Hospital Inpatient Quality Reporting (IQR) and Outpatient Quality Reporting (OQR) programs show: 1) The percentage of hospital patients who receive treatments known to get the best results for certain common, serious medical conditions or surgical procedures; 2) How quickly hospitals treat patients who come to the hospital with certain medical emergencies. The measures only apply to patients for whom the recommended treatment would be appropriate. By law, any measures reported on the Hospital Compare website must reflect accepted standards of care, based on current scientific evidence. The measures are regularly reviewed and revised to ensure that they are up-to-date, and new measures and types of conditions and treatments are added over time. Process of care measures include:

- Blood Clot Prevention and Treatment
- Chest Pain/Possible Heart Attack Care
- Children's Asthma Care
- Emergency Department Care
- Heart Attack Care
- Heart Failure Care
- Pneumonia Care
- Pregnancy and Delivery Care
- Preventative Care
- Stroke Care
- Surgical Care Improvment Project

Where the Information Comes From
Measures of timely and effective care come from the data that hospitals get from medical records of their eligible patients, following standards for abstracting and reporting the information. Data submissions include auditing procedures and edit checks to assess whether data submitted are consistent with CMS's defined specifications. In addition, CMS validates the data submitted to provide assurance that the hospital, or its designated agent, can accurately abstract patient medical records and accurately submit data.

What Patients the Measures Apply To
The measures of timely and effective care apply to any adult patients treated at hospitals participating in the IQR and OQR programs for whom the recommended treatments would be appropriate, including Medicare patients, Medicare managed care patients, and non-Medicare patients. Hospitals with a large number of discharges may provide data from a sample of eligible Medicare and non-Medicare patients, based CMS sampling rules.

Risk Adjustment
The measures of timely and effective care do not require risk adjustment, because patients for whom the recommended treatment would not be appropriate are not included in the calculations.

Significance Testing
CMS does not perform tests of statistical significance in reporting the measures of timely and effective care. However, the smaller the sample size, the greater the difference in rates must be in order for that difference to be statistically meaningful. Large differences between individual hospitals' rates may be significant, but small differences between hospitals are usually not significant.

Reporting Period
These 50 measures are based on a reporting period of October 1, 2012 through September 30, 2013 except for the following: Emergency Department Care—Percentage of Patients Who Left the Emergency Department Before Being Seen—January 1, 2012 through December 31, 2012; Preventative Care—Patients Assessed and Given Influenza Vaccination—October 1, 2012 through March 31, 2013; All eight Stroke Care measures—January 1, 2013 through September 30, 2013; All six Blood Clot Prevention and Treatment measures—January 1, 2013 through September 30, 2013.

Survey of Patients' Experiences

The Centers for Medicare & Medicaid Services (CMS), along with the Agency for Healthcare Research and Quality (AHRQ), developed the HCAHPS (Hospital Consumer Assessment of Healthcare Providers and Systems) Survey, also known as Hospital CAHPS®, to provide a standardized survey instrument and data collection methodology for measuring patients' perspectives on hospital care. The HCAHPS Survey is administered to a random sample of patients continuously throughout the year. CMS cleans, adjusts and analyzes the data, then publicly reports the results.

Which Patients are Included
The HCAHPS survey is administered to a random sample of adult patients across medical conditions between 48 hours and six weeks after discharge; the survey is not restricted to Medicare beneficiaries.

Where the Information Comes From
All short-term, acute care, non-specialty hospitals are invited to participate in the HCAHPS Survey. Over 4,000 hospitals participate in HCAHPS. The goal is for each hospital to get at least 300 completed patient surveys per year. In general, the more patients that respond to the survey, the more the results shown on this website will reflect the experiences of all the patients who used that hospital. HCAHPS survey data must be collected by organizations that are trained by the federal government in HCAHPS data collection procedures. Data submitted to the HCAHPS data warehouse is cleaned, adjusted and analyzed by CMS, which calculates hospitals' HCAHPS scores and publicly reports them on the Hospital Compare website.

Adjusting Rates
Preparing the data for public reporting includes taking certain factors into account to ensure fair comparisons among hospitals. For example, the mix of patients can differ from one hospital to the next, and these differences in the patient mix can affect a hospital's HCAHPS results. Patient-mix adjustment takes these differences into account so that the survey results reported on this website are what would be expected for each hospital if all hospitals had a similar mix of patients.

Reporting Period
These 10 measures are based on a reporting period of October 1, 2012 through September 30, 2013.

Use of Medical Imaging

The six measures on the use of medical imaging show how often a hospital provides specific imaging tests for Medicare beneficiaries under circumstances where they may not be medically appropriate. Lower percentages suggest more efficient use of medical imaging. The purpose of reporting these measures is to reduce unnecessary exposure to contrast materials and/or radiation, to ensure adherence to evidence-based medicine and practice guidelines, and to prevent wasteful use of Medicare resources. The measures only apply to Medicare patients treated in hospital outpatient departments. It does not include tests performed in other ambulatory care settings or hospital inpatient settings.

What Patients are Included
Outpatient imaging efficiency measures apply only to Medicare beneficiaries enrolled in Original Medicare who were treated as outpatients in hospital facilities reimbursed through the Outpatient Prospective Payment System (OPPS). They do not include Medicare managed care patients, non-Medicare patients, or patients who were admitted to the hospital as inpatients.

Where the Information Comes From
CMS calculates imaging efficiency measures using data from claims that hospitals and physicians submit for Medicare beneficiaries enrolled in Original Medicare. The data are calculated only for hospitals paid through the Outpatient Prospective Payment System (OPPS). The measures are part of the Hospital Outpatient Quality Reporting Program (OQR).

Risk Adjustment
Outpatient imaging efficiency measures are not risk adjusted. However, measures specifications do not include cases where there were clear medical reasons for performing the tests.

Significance Testing
CMS does not perform tests of statistical significance in reporting the outpatient imaging efficiency measures. Large differences between hospitals' percentages may be significant, but small differences usually are not.

Reporting Period
These six measures are based on a reporting period of July 1, 2012 through June 30, 2013.

Medicare Spending per Beneficiary

The Medicare Spending per Beneficiary (MSPB) measure assesses Medicare Part A and Part B payments for services provided to a Medicare beneficiary during a spending-per-beneficiary episode that spans from three days prior to an inpatient hospital admission through 30 days after discharge. The payments included in this measure are price-standardized and risk-adjusted. Price standardization removes sources of variation that are due to geographic payment differences such as wage index and geographic practice cost differences, as well as indirect medical education (IME) or disproportionate share hospital (DSH) payments. Risk adjustment accounts for variation due to patient health status.

By measuring cost of care through this measure, CMS hopes to increase the transparency of care for consumers and recognize hospitals that are involved in the provision of high-quality care at lower cost to Medicare.

Reporting Period
This measure is based on a reporting period of January 1, 2012 through December 31, 2012.

Sample Entry

The listing below illustrates the kind of information that is or might be included in a Hospital Profile. Each numbered item of information is described in the paragraphs following the example.

1 ► **Cleveland Clinic**
9500 Euclid Avenue — Phone: 216-444-2200
Cleveland, OH 44195 — Fax: 216-445-7758
URL: www.clevelandclinic.org
Type: Acute Care Hospitals — Emergency Services: Yes
Ownership: Voluntary non-profit - Private — Beds: 1,113

2 ► **Key Personnel:**
CEO/President. . . . . Delos M Cosgrove, MD
Chief of Medical Staff. . . . . Marc Harrison, MD
Infection Control. . . . . David L Longworth, MD
Operating Room. . . . . Allan Siperstein, MD
Pediatric Ambulatory Care . . . . . . Robert Wyllie, MD
Quality Assurance . . . . J Michael Henderson, MD
Radiology. . . . . Gregory P Borkowski, MD

	Measure	Cases	This Hosp.	State Avg.	U.S. Avg.
3 ►					
4 ►	**Blood Clot Prevention and Treatment**				
	Anticoagulation Overlap Therapy[2]	400	98%	93%	93%
	ICU Venous Thromboembolism Prophylaxis[2]	84	98%	93%	92%
	Incidence of Potentially Preventable VTE[2]	168	2%	6%	10%
	UFH with Dosages/Platelet Monitoring[2]	444	100%	98%	97%
	Venous Thromboembolism Prophylaxis[2]	347	96%	88%	85%
	Warfarin Therapy Discharge Instructions[2]	237	89%	79%	75%
5 ►	**Chest Pain/Possible Heart Attack Care**				
	Aspirin Given Within 24 Hours of Arrival	190	96%	97%	96%
	Fibrinolytic Meds Within 30 Min. of Arrival[7]	-	-	44%	58%
	Median Time to ECG (minutes)	197	6	6	7
	Median Time to Transfer (minutes)[1]	-	-	58	60
6 ►	**Children's Asthma Care**				
	Received Home Management Plan of Care	74	99%	85%	88%
	Received Reliever Medication	75	100%	100%	100%
	Received Systemic Corticosteroids	74	100%	100%	100%
7 ►	**Emergency Department**				
	Admittance Decision Time (minutes)[2]	227	102	90	98%
	Head CT Results Within 45 Min. of Arrival	11	91%	63%	57%
	Patients Who Left ER Before Being Seen	82,229	2%	2%	2%
	Time from ER Arrival to Admit. (minutes)[2]	228	304	265	274
	Time from ER Arrival to Discharge (minutes)	294	131	128	134
	Time in ER Before Being Evaluated (minutes)	417	11	22	26
	Time to Pain Meds for Fractures (minutes)	194	46	54	57
8 ►	**Heart Attack Care**				
	Aspirin Given at Discharge	868	100%	99%	99%
	Fibrinolytic Meds Within 30 Min. of Arrival[7]	-	-	80%	54%
	PCI Within 90 Minutes of Arrival	13	92%	97%	96%
	Statin Prescribed at Discharge	834	100%	98%	98%
9 ►	**Heart Failure Care**				
	ACE Inhibitor or ARB for LVSD[2]	287	99%	97%	97%
	Discharge Instructions Given[2]	712	94%	96%	94%
	Evaluation of LVS Function[2]	858	100%	100%	99%
10 ►	**Medicare Spending**				
	Medicare Hospital Spending per Patient	-	0.99	1.01	0.98
11 ►	**Pneumonia Care**				
	Appropriate Initial Antibiotic Given	84	94%	96%	95%
	Blood Culture Timing	176	95%	98%	98%
12 ►	**Pregnancy and Delivery Care**				
	Newborn Deliveries Scheduled Early[1]	-	-	5%	6%

	Measure	Cases	This Hosp.	State Avg.	U.S. Avg.
13 ►	**Preventive Care**				
	Immunization for Influenza[2]	577	96%	93%	90%
	Immunization for Pneumonia[2]	747	95%	94%	92%
14 ►	**Stroke Care**				
	Anticoagulation Therapy for Atrial Fibrillation[2]	34	100%	95%	95%
	Antithrombotic Therapy Timing[2]	180	96%	98%	98%
	Assessed for Rehabilitation[2]	333	98%	98%	97%
	Discharged on Antithrombotic Therapy[2]	221	100%	99%	99%
	Discharged on Statin Medication[2]	152	99%	95%	94%
	Thrombolytic Therapy Timing[1,2]	-	-	65%	66%
	Venous Thromboembolism Prophylaxis[2]	349	100%	95%	94%
	Written Stroke Educational Materials Given[2]	125	98%	92%	88%
15 ►	**Surgical Care Improvement Project**				
	Appropriate Beta Blocker Usage[2]	356	99%	98%	98%
	Appropriate VTP Within 24 Hours[2]	447	99%	98%	98%
	Controlled Postoperative Blood Glucose[2]	253	96%	97%	97%
	Perioperative Temperature Management[2]	625	100%	100%	100%
	Prophylactic Antibiotic Selection[2]	570	99%	99%	99%
	Prophylactic Antibiotic Selection (Outpatient)	1,080	100%	98%	98%
	Prophylactic Antibiotic Stopped[2]	554	97%	98%	98%
	Prophylactic Antibiotic Timing[2]	570	99%	99%	99%
	Prophylactic Antibiotic Timing (Outpatient)	563	97%	97%	98%
	Urinary Catheter Removal[2]	381	98%	97%	97%
16 ►	**Survey of Patients' Hospital Experiences**				
	Area Around Room 'Always' Quiet at Night	300+	57%	58%	61%
	Doctors 'Always' Communicated Well	300+	82%	80%	82%
	Home Recovery Information Given	300+	90%	87%	85%
	Hospital Given 9 or 10 on 10 Point Scale	300+	84%	72%	71%
	Meds 'Always' Explained Before Given	300+	66%	64%	64%
	Nurses 'Always' Communicated Well	300+	83%	81%	79%
	Pain 'Always' Well Controlled	300+	72%	71%	71%
	Room and Bathroom 'Always' Clean	300+	78%	75%	73%
	Timely Help 'Always' Received	300+	68%	70%	68%
	Would Definitely Recommend Hospital	300+	87%	71%	71%
17 ►	**Use of Medical Imaging**				
	Cardiac Imaging Stress Test before Surgery	4,179	6.7%	5.4%	5.3%
	Combination Abdominal CT Scan	5,813	13.0%	7.1%	10.5%
	Combination Brain/Sinus CT Scan	2,131	1.7%	2.8%	2.7%
	Combination Chest CT Scan	6,539	0.1%	1.7%	2.7%
	Follow-up Mammogram/Ultrasound	9,962	9.3%	8.7%	8.8%
	Lumbar Spine MRI for Low Back Pain	661	31.9%	34.7%	37.2%

1▶ Hospital Name and Record Header: hospital name; street address; phone; fax; e-mail; URL; hospital type; ownership; emergency services (Yes/No); and number of beds.

2▶ Key Personnel: includes the names of key personnel primarily related to the conditions covered in this publication.

3▶ Hospital Compare Data: each profile contains data covering 67 measures contained in the Centers for Medicare & Medicaid Services Hospital Compare database. There are five columns:

Measure: the 67 quality measures reported.

There are 14 possible footnotes:

(1) The number of cases/patients is too few to report
This footnote is applied: when the number of cases/patients does not meet the required minimum amount for public reporting; when the number of cases/patients is too small to reliably tell how well a hospital is performing; and/or to protect personal health information.

(2) Data submitted were based on a sample of cases/patients
This footnote indicates that a hospital chose to submit data for a random sample of its cases/patients while following specific rules for how to select the patients.

(3) Results are based on a shorter time period than required
This footnote indicates that the hospital's results were based on data from less than the maximum possible time period generally used to collect data for a measure. See Reporting Periods for more information.

(4) Data suppressed by CMS (Centers for Medicare and Medicaid Services) for one or more quarters
The results for these measures were excluded for various reasons, such as data inaccuracies.

(5) Results are not available for this reporting period
This footnote is applied when the hospital does not have data to report.

(6) Fewer than 100 patients completed the HCAHPS survey.
This footnote is applied when the number of completed surveys the hospital or its vendor provided to CMS is less than 100. Use these scores with caution, as the number of surveys may be too low to reliably assess hospital performance.

(7) No cases met the criteria for this measure
This footnote is applied when a hospital did not have any cases meet the inclusion criteria for a measure.

(8) The lower limit of the confidence interval cannot be calculated
The lower limit of the confidence interval cannot be calculated if the number of observed infections equals zero.

(9) No data are available from the state/territory for this reporting period
This footnote is applied when: too few hospitals in a state/territory had data available; or no data was reported for this state/territory.

(10) The scores shown reflect fewer than 50 completed surveys.
This footnote is applied when the number of completed surveys the hospital or its vendor provided to CMS is less than 50. Use these scores with caution, as the number of surveys may be too low to reliably assess hospital performance.

(11) There were discrepancies in the data collection process
This footnote is applied when there have been deviations from data collection protocols. CMS is working to correct this situation.

(12) This measure does not apply to this hospital for this reporting period
This footnote is applied when: there were zero device days or procedures; the hospital does not have ICU locations; the hospital is a new member of the registry and didn't have an opportunity to submit any cases; or the hospital does not report this voluntary measure.

(13) Results cannot be calculated for this reporting period
This footnote is applied when: the number of predicted infections is less than 1; the number of observed MRSA or Clostridium difficile infections present on admission (community-onset prevalence) was above a pre-determined cut-point.

(14) The results for this state are combined with nearby states to protect confidentiality
This footnote is applied when a state has fewer than 10 hospitals in order to protect confidentiality. Results are combined as follows: 1) the District of Columbia and Delaware are combined; 2) Alaska and Washington are combined; 3) North Dakota and South Dakota are combined; and 4) New Hampshire and Vermont are combined. Hospitals located in Maryland and U.S. territories are excluded from the measure calculation.

Cases: the size of the data sample (number of patients) for each hospital and quality measure. In addition, the notation "0" is applied when a hospital provided care to patients with a condition, such as pneumonia, but the cases that the hospital submitted did not meet the specific criteria for being included in the calculation of the measure.

This Hospital: the performance rate that the hospital achieved for each quality measure. This value is expressed as a percentage of the sample size that was measured. The performance rate is calculated by dividing the numerator by the denominator. The denominator is the sum of all eligible cases (as defined in the measure specifications) submitted to the QIO Clinical Data Warehouse for the reporting period. The numerator is the sum of all eligible cases submitted for the same reporting period where the recommended care was provided.

State Average: the average rate for all hospitals reporting data in the state the hospital is located in.

U.S. Average: the average rate for all hospitals reporting nationwide.

Note: Beginning in December 2010, state and national averages for the process of care measures are calculated by summing the cases in the state or nation that "passed" the measure (Numerator) and dividing that sum by the number of cases in the state or national Denominator. For the national and state averages, a simple average was constructed where the numerator was the sum of all non-excluded hospitals' scores and the denominator was the total number of hospitals, each calculated at either the national or individual state level. For the process and survey measures, the national and state averages are calculated before excluding suppressed rates and are not recalculated using only published rates as was done prior to September 2009. Acute Care-VA Medical Centers are not included in the calculation of the national and state comparison rates.

The children's asthma care national and state averages are calculated differently. The average rate for all healthcare organizations in the nation that provide results for a measure. The average rate is calculated by dividing the total number of patients who had the recommended care provided for a measure by the total number of patients who met the inclusion and exclusion criteria for that measure in the nation for the timeframe being reported.

4▶ Blood Clot Prevention and Treatment

The measures listed below show how well hospitals are providing recommended care known to prevent or treat blood clots and how often blood clots occur that could have been prevented.

Anticoagulation Overlap Therapy

Patients with blood clots who got the recommended treatment, which includes using two different blood thinner medicines at the same time.
Patients who develop blood clots in their veins (also called venous thromboembolism, or VTE) need to get treatment that can break up the clots quickly and prevent others from forming. The recommended treatment is to first give a blood thinner that can get into the bloodstream quickly through an IV or injection (heparin), then give a slower-acting oral blood thinner medicine (warfarin), and continue giving both blood thinners for 5 days or until it is safe for the patient to transition off of the IV blood thinner and use only the oral blood thinner medicine. This measure shows the percentage of hospital patients who had a confirmed diagnosis of blood clot at hospital admission or during their hospital stay, and received both medicines for at least 5 days, or were discharged from the hospital on both kinds of medicine, unless their blood work showed they no longer needed it. *Higher percentages are better.*

ICU Venous Thromboembolism Prophylaxis

Patients who got treatment to prevent blood clots on the day of or day after being admitted to the intensive care unit (ICU).
Patients in the Intensive Care Unit (ICU) are at increased risk for developing blood clots in their veins (venous thromboembolism, or VTE), because they are in bed for a long period of time. These clots can break off and travel to other parts of the body, causing serious harm. Hospitals can prevent blood clots by routinely evaluating all patients for their risk of developing blood clots and using appropriate prevention and treatment procedures. Prevention can include compression stockings, blood thinners, and/or other medicines. This measure shows the percentage of ICU patients who received treatment to prevent blood clots: on the day of or day after arrival at the hospital; or on the day of or day after transfer to the ICU; or on the day of or day after having surgery. Patients who did not receive treatment may also be included in this measure, if they had paperwork in their chart to explain why. Reasons for not receiving treatment may include having a massive wound, actively bleeding, or having an allergy to blood thinners. *Higher percentages are better.*

Incidence of Potentially Preventable VTE
Patients who developed a blood clot while in the hospital who did not get treatment that could have prevented it.
Because hospital patients often have to stay in bed for long periods of time, all patients admitted to the hospital are at increased risk of developing blood clots in their veins (also called venous thromboembolism or VTE) that can break off and travel to other parts of the body, like the heart, brain, or lung. Hospitals can prevent blood clots by routinely evaluating patients for their risk of developing blood clots and using appropriate prevention and treatment procedures. Prevention can include compression stockings, blood thinners, and/or other medicines. This measure shows the percentage of patients who developed blood clots while in the hospital who did not receive preventative treatment beforehand. *Lower percentages are better.*

UFH with Dosages/Platelet Monitoring
Patients with blood clots who were treated with an intravenous blood thinner, and then were checked to determine if the blood thinner was putting the patient at an increased risk of bleeding.
Patients who have been diagnosed with a blood clot (also called venous thromboembolism, or VTE) are usually treated with a blood thinner such as IV heparin. Some patients may be prescribed a type of IV heparin called unfractionated heparin (UFH). Unfractionated heparin carries a higher risk of increased bleeding than a different type of IV heparin (called low molecular weight heparin). Risk for bleeding increases because blood thinners increase the time it takes your blood to clot. The most common signs of increased bleeding include unusual bruising, nosebleeds, and bleeding gums. Because of their higher risk of bleeding, patients getting unfractionated heparin should be given regular blood tests to determine if they are at an increased risk of bleeding from getting the medication. This measure shows the percentage of patients who developed a blood clot at admission or during their hospital stay, treated with unfractionated IV heparin who had their blood checked using recommended procedures. *Higher percentages are better.*

Venous Thromboembolism Prophylaxis
Patients who got treatment to prevent blood clots on the day of or day after hospital admission or surgery.
Because hospital patients often have to stay in bed for long periods of time, all patients admitted to the hospital are at increased risk of developing blood clots in their veins (also called venous thromboembolism, or VTE) that can break off and travel to other parts of the body, like the heart, brain, or lung. Hospitals can prevent blood clots by routinely evaluating patients for their risk of developing blood clots and using appropriate prevention and treatment procedures. Prevention can include compression stockings, blood thinners, and/or other medicines. This measure shows the percentage of patients who received treatment to prevent blood clots: on the day of or day after arrival at the hospital; or on the day of or day after having surgery. Patients who did not receive treatment may also be included in this measure, if they had paperwork in their chart to explain why. Reasons for not receiving treatment may include having a massive wound, actively bleeding, or having an allergy to blood thinners. *Higher percentages are better.*

Warfarin Therapy Discharge Instructions
Patients with blood clots who were discharged on a blood thinner medicine and received written instructions about that medicine.
Patients who develop blood clots (also called venous thromboembolism or VTE) will usually be given blood thinner medicines to take when they leave the hospital. Educating patients about how to take the medicine and its possible side effects can help prevent problems that could bring them back to the hospital. Before leaving the hospital, patients with a blood clot, who are taking a blood thinner medicine, and their caregiver should receive information about the following topics: Compliance (how to follow medication instructions); Diet (how to eat a healthy diet and avoid foods that interfere with blood thinners); Monitoring their blood thinner medicine; Adverse drug reactions (difficulty breathing, vomiting, nausea); When to call your health care provider (dizziness or weakness, a fall, bright red bleeding). This measure shows the percentage of patients diagnosed with a blood clot (either at admission or during their hospital stay) discharged from the hospital on blood thinners (anticoagulants or anticoagulant therapy or warfarin therapy) who received written educational instructions at hospital discharge. *Higher percentages are better.*

5▶ Chest Pain/Possible Heart Attack Care

Scientific evidence shows that the following measures represent the best practices for the treatment of chest pain/possible heart attack.

Aspirin Given Within 24 Hours of Arrival
Outpatients with chest pain or possible heart attack who got aspirin within 24 hours of arrival.
Blood clots can cause heart attacks. For many patients having a heart attack, taking aspirin soon after symptoms of a heart attack begin may help break up a clot and make the heart attack less severe. If patients have not taken aspirin themselves before going to the hospital, they should get aspirin when they arrive. Standards for care say that patients should get aspirin within 24 hours of arriving at the hospital. This measure tells what percent of patients got aspirin within this time period. *Higher percentages are better.*

Fibrinolytic Meds Within 30 Minutes of Arrival
Outpatients with chest pain or possible heart attack who got drugs to break up blood clots within 30 minutes of arrival.
Blood clots can cause heart attacks. Certain patients having a heart attack should get a "clot busting" drug to help break up the blood clots and improve blood flow to the heart. Standards for care say that a clot busting drug should be given within 30 minutes of arrival at the hospital. This measure tells the percent of patients who were given a clot busting drug within this time period. *Higher percentages are better.*

Average Time to ECG (minutes)
Average number of minutes before outpatients with chest pain or possible heart attack got an ECG.
"ECG" (sometimes called EKG) stands for electrocardiogram. An ECG is a test that can help doctors know whether patients are having a heart attack. Standards of care say that patients with chest pain or a possible heart attack should have an ECG upon arrival, preferably within 10 minutes. This measure shows the average number of minutes it takes before patients had an ECG (calculated as an arithmetic median). Sometimes patients get an ECG done before they get to the hospital (for example, by the ambulance staff). This is counted as "0 minutes." *Lower numbers are better.*

Average Time to Transfer (minutes)
Average number of minutes before outpatients with chest pain or possible heart attack who needed specialized care were transferred to another hospital.
If a hospital does not have the facilities to provide specialized heart attack care, it transfers patients with possible heart attack to another hospital that can give them this care. This measure shows how long it takes, on average, for hospitals to identify patients who need specialized heart attack care the hospital cannot provide and begin their transfer to another hospital. Specifically, it shows the average (arithmetic median) number of minutes it takes from the time patients arrive in the emergency department until they are transported to a different hospital. *Lower numbers are better.*

6▶ Children's Asthma Care

Scientific evidence shows that the following measures represent best practices for treating children with asthma.

Received Home Management Plan of Care
Children and their caregivers who received a home management plan of care document while hospitalized for asthma.
This measure shows the percentage of children with asthma and their caregivers who were given a home management plan of care document while hospitalized. Because asthma is a chronic condition, controlling a child's asthma symptoms at home will help reduce the risk of further attacks. Knowledge about the disease and its treatment is the key to good asthma control. Asthma that is not managed effectively may lead to more visits to the hospital. Medications can help prevent asthma symptoms and attacks from starting in the first place and can reduce how often attacks happen and severity of the attacks. It is important for children with asthma and their caregivers to know how to prevent asthma symptoms and attacks before they happen. The home management plan of care helps children with asthma and their caregivers develop a plan to manage the child's asthma symptoms and to know when to take action. It should address all of the following: arrangements for follow-up care; environmental control and control of other triggers; method and timing of rescue actions; use of controller medications; use of reliever medications. *Higher percentages are better.*

Received Reliever Medication
Children who received reliever medication while hospitalized for asthma.
National guidelines for treating children with asthma recommend using relievers in the severe phase and gradually cutting down the dosage of medications to provide control of asthma symptoms. Although there are guidelines for medication therapy for children with asthma, there is evidence that these guidelines are not being consistently followed. Using the appropriate medications will lower the risk of severe illness and/or death. This measure shows the percentage of children with asthma who were given reliever medication (like albuterol) while hospitalized. Relievers are medications that relax the bands of muscle surrounding the airways and make breathing easier. *Higher percentages are better.*

Received Systemic Corticosteroids
Children who received systemic corticosteroid medication (oral and IV medication that reduces inflammation and controls symptoms) while hospitalized for asthma.
Oral or IV steroid medications control severe asthma well. That is why they are important for hospital care. Unfortunately, they can cause serious side effects when used long-term. That is why they are mainly used for severe episodes or chronic severe asthma, which cannot be controlled with other medications (like inhaled or oral bronchodilators and anti-inflammatory medications). This measure shows the percentage of children with asthma who were given oral or IV steroid medications while hospitalized. These medications work in the body as a whole,

rather than just on the lungs. They help reduce inflammation and control allergic reactions. *Higher percentages are better.*

7▶ Emergency Department Care

Timely and effective care in hospital emergency departments is essential for good patient outcomes. Delays before receiving care in the emergency department can reduce the quality of care and increase risks and discomfort for patients with serious illnesses or injuries. Waiting times at different hospitals can vary widely, depending on the number of patients seen, staffing levels, efficiency, admitting procedures, or the availability of inpatient beds.

Admittance Decision Time (minutes)

For patients who had to be admitted to the hospital as an inpatient, average time patients spent in the emergency department, after the doctor decided to admit them as an inpatient before leaving the emergency department for their inpatient room.

Delays in transferring emergency department patients to an inpatient unit may be a sign that there's not enough staff or there's poor coordination among hospital departments. Long delays can also create more stress for patients and families. This measure shows the average (arithmetic median) time patients spent in the emergency department—from the time the doctor decided to admit them to the time they left the emergency department for an inpatient bed. *Lower numbers are better.*

Head CT Results Within 45 Minutes of Arrival

Percentage of patients who came to the emergency department with stroke symptoms who received brain scan results within 45 minutes of arrival.

People who suffer from strokes need to receive treatment immediately to lessen the amount of brain damage that occurs with any stroke. A scan of the brain must be taken to determine the type and severity of the stroke before treatment can be provided. Long waits may be a sign that the emergency department is understaffed or overcrowded and can lead to delayed diagnosis and treatment and may lead to further brain damage. Standards of care say that patients with stroke symptoms should receive brain scan results (to diagnose whether and how severely a stroke occurred) within 45 minutes of arriving at the emergency department. This measure shows the percentage of emergency department patients with stroke symptoms who received brain scan results within that time period. *Lower numbers are better.*

Patients Who Left ER Before Being Seen

Percentage of patients who left the emergency department before being seen.

Hospital emergency departments that have high percentages of patients who leave without being seen may not have the staff or resources to provide timely and effective emergency room care. Patients who leave the emergency department without being seen may be seriously ill, putting themselves at higher risk for poor health outcomes. This measure shows the percentage of all individuals who signed into an emergency department but left before being evaluated by a healthcare professional. *Lower numbers are better.*

Time from ER Arrival to Admittance (minutes)

For patients who had to be admitted to the hospital as an inpatient, average time patients spent in the emergency department, before they were admitted to the hospital as an inpatient.

Long stays in an emergency department before a patient is admitted may be a sign that the emergency department is understaffed or overcrowded. This may result in delays in treatment or lower quality care. This measure shows the average (arithmetic median) time patients spent in the emergency department—from the time they arrived to the time they left the emergency department for an inpatient bed. This number only includes patients who were admitted to the hospital as an inpatient. It does not include those people who went home. *Lower numbers are better.*

Time from ER Arrival to Discharge (minutes)

Average time patients spent in the emergency department before being sent home.

Long stays in the emergency department before a patient is sent home may be a sign that the emergency department is understaffed or overcrowded. This may result in delays in treatment, increased suffering for those who wait, and unpleasant treatment environments. This measure shows the average (arithmetic median) time in minutes that patients spent in the emergency department—from the time they arrived to the time they were sent home. It does not include patients who were later admitted to the hospital as inpatients, admitted for observation, transferred to another acute care hospital, or who left without being seen by a licensed provider. *Lower numbers are better.*

Time in ER Before Being Evaluated (minutes)

Average time patients spent in the emergency department before they were seen by a healthcare professional.

Delays in being seen by a healthcare provider may be a sign that the emergency department is understaffed or overcrowded. This may result in delays in treatment, lower quality care, and more stress for patients and families. For patients who were later sent home, this measure shows the average (arithmetic median) time in minutes spent in the emergency department—from the time they arrived until the time they were seen by a healthcare professional. It does not include patients who were admitted to the hospital, who died in the emergency department, or who left without being seen. *Lower numbers are better.*

Time to Pain Meds for Fractures (minutes)
Average time patients who came to the emergency department with broken bones had to wait before receiving pain medication.
Long waits before a patient is treated may be a sign that the emergency department is understaffed or overcrowded. For patients with broken bones, long waits without pain medication cause unnecessary suffering. For all patients 2 years and older who came to the emergency department with a broken arm or leg, this shows the average (arithmetic median) time they waited before receiving pain medication. *Lower numbers are better.*

8 ▶ Heart Attack Care

Scientific evidence shows that the following measures represent the best practices for the treatment of heart attack.

Aspirin Given at Discharge
Heart attack patients given aspirin at discharge.
Blood clots can block blood vessels. Aspirin can help prevent blood clots from forming or help dissolve blood clots that have formed. Following a heart attack, continued use of aspirin may help reduce the risk of another heart attack. Aspirin can have side effects like stomach inflammation, bleeding, or allergic reactions. Talk to your health care provider before using aspirin on a regular basis to make sure it's safe for you. This measure shows what percentage of patients were given aspirin upon leaving the hospital. *Higher percentages are better.*

Fibrinolytic Meds Within 30 Minutes of Arrival
Heart attack patients given fibrinolytic medication within 30 minutes of arrival.
The heart is a muscle that gets oxygen through blood vessels. Sometimes blood clots can block these blood vessels and the heart can't get enough oxygen. This can cause a heart attack. Fibrinolytic drugs are medicines that can help dissolve blood clots in blood vessels and improve blood flow to your heart. Standards for care say that patients should get them within 30 minutes of arrival at the hospital. This measure shows what percentage of patients got fibrinolytic drugs within this time period. *Higher percentages are better.*

PCI Within 90 Minutes of Arrival
Heart attack patients given PCI within 90 minutes of arrival.
The heart is a muscle that gets oxygen through blood vessels. Sometimes blood clots can block these blood vessels, and the heart cannot get enough oxygen. This can cause a heart attack. Percutaneous coronary interventions (PCI) are procedures that are among the most effective ways to open blocked blood vessels and help prevent further heart muscle damage. A PCI is performed by a doctor to open the blockage and increase blood flow in blocked blood vessels. Improving blood flow to your heart as quickly as possible lessens the damage to your heart muscle, and it also can increase your chances of surviving a heart attack. There are three procedures commonly described by the term PCI. These procedures all involve a catheter (a flexible tube) that is inserted, often through your leg, and guided through the blood vessels to the blockage. The three procedures are: angioplasty—a balloon is inflated to open the blood vessel; stenting—a small wire tube called a stent is placed in the blood vessel to hold it open; atherectomy—a blade or laser cuts through and removes the blockage. Standards for care say that patients should receive a PCI within 90 minutes of arriving at the hospital. This measure shows what percentage of patients got a PCI within this time period. *Higher percentages are better.*

Statin Prescribed at Discharge
Heart attack patients given a prescription for a statin at discharge.
Statins are drugs used to lower cholesterol. Cholesterol is a fat (also called a lipid) that your body needs to work properly. Cholesterol levels that are too high can increase your chance of getting heart disease, stroke, and other problems. For patients who have had one or more heart attacks and have high cholesterol, taking statins can lower the chance that they'll have another heart attack or die. This measure shows the percent of patients who had a heart attack who got a prescription for a statin upon leaving the hospital. Patients who shouldn't take statins aren't included in this measure. *Higher numbers are better.*

9 ▶ Heart Failure Care

Scientific evidence shows that the following measures represent the best practices for the treatment of heart failure.

ACE Inhibitor or ARB for LVSD
Heart failure patients given ACE inhibitor or ARB for left ventricular systolic dysfunction (LVSD).
ACE (angiotensin converting enzyme) inhibitors and ARBs (angiotensin receptor blockers) are medicines used to treat patients with heart failure and are particularly beneficial in those patients with decreased function of the left side of the heart. Early treatment with ACE inhibitors and ARBs in patients who have heart failure symptoms or decreased heart function after a heart attack can also reduce their risk of death from future heart attacks. ACE

inhibitors and ARBs work by limiting the effects of a hormone that narrows blood vessels, and may thus lower blood pressure and reduce the work the heart has to perform. Since the ways in which these two kinds of drugs work are different, your doctor will decide which drug is most appropriate for you. Standards for care say that if patients have a heart attack and/or heart failure, they should get a prescription for ACE inhibitors or ARBs if they have decreased heart function before leaving the hospital. *Higher percentages are better.*

Discharge Instructions Given
Heart failure patients given discharge instructions.
Heart failure is a chronic condition. It results in symptoms such as shortness of breath, dizziness, and fatigue. Before you leave the hospital, the staff at the hospital should provide you with information to help you manage the symptoms after you get home. The information should include your information about: activity level (what you can and can't do); diet (what you should, and shouldn't eat or drink); medications; your follow-up appointment; watching your daily weight; and what to do if your symptoms get worse. *Higher percentages are better.*

Evaluation of LVS Function
Heart failure patients given an evaluation of left ventricular systolic (LVS) function.
The proper treatment for heart failure depends on what area of your heart is affected. An important test is to check how your heart is pumping, called an "evaluation of the left ventricular systolic function." It can tell your health care provider whether the left side of your heart is pumping properly. Other ways to check on how your heart is pumping include: your medical history; a physical examination; listening to your heart sounds; and other tests as ordered by a physician (like an ECG (electrocardiogram), chest x-ray, blood work, and an echocardiogram) *Higher percentages are better.*

10 ▶ Medicare Spending

The Medicare Hospital Spending per Patient measure shows whether Medicare spends more, less, or about the same on an episode of care for a Medicare patient treated in a specific hospital compared to how much Medicare spends on an episode of care across all hospitals nationally. This measure includes any Medicare Part A and Part B payments made for services provided to a patient during an episode of care, which includes the 3 days prior to the hospital stay, during the stay, and during the 30 days after discharge from the hospital. This result is a ratio calculated by dividing the amount Medicare spends per patient for an episode of care initiated at this hospital by the median (or middle) amount Medicare spent per episode of care nationally.

- A ratio equal to the national average means that Medicare spends ABOUT THE SAME per patient for an episode of care initiated at this hospital as it does per episode of care across all hospitals nationally.
- A ratio that is more than the national average means that Medicare spends MORE per patient for an episode of care initiated at this hospital than it does per episode of care across all hospitals nationally.
- A ratio that is less than the national average means that Medicare spends LESS per patient for an episode of care initiated at this hospital than it does per episode of care across all hospitals nationally.

11 ▶ Pneumonia Care

Scientific evidence shows that the following measures represent the best practices for the treatment of community-acquired pneumonia.

Appropriate Initial Antibiotic Given
Pneumonia patients given the most appropriate initial antibiotic(s).
Pneumonia is a lung infection that is usually caused by bacteria or a virus. If pneumonia is caused by bacteria, hospitals will treat the infection with antibiotics. Different bacteria are treated with different antibiotics. *Higher percentages are better.*

Blood Culture Timing
Pneumonia patients whose initial emergency room blood culture was performed prior to the administration of the first hospital dose of antibiotics.
Different types of bacteria can cause pneumonia. A blood culture is a test that can help your health care provider identify which bacteria may have caused your pneumonia, and which antibiotic should be prescribed. A blood culture is not always needed, but for patients who are first seen in the hospital emergency department, it is important for the accuracy of the test that a blood culture be conducted before any antibiotics are started. It is also important to start antibiotics as soon as possible. *Higher percentages are better.*

12► Pregnancy and Delivery Care

Newborn Deliveries Scheduled Early

Percent of newborns whose deliveries were scheduled too early (1-3 weeks early), when a scheduled delivery was not medically necessary.

Guidelines developed by doctors and researchers say it's best to wait until the 39th completed week of pregnancy to deliver your baby because important fetal development takes place in your baby's brain and lungs during the last few weeks of pregnancy. Sometimes women go into early labor on their own, and early deliveries can't be prevented. Sometimes, doctors decide that inducing labor or delivering a baby early by C-section (called "elective delivery") is in the best interest of the mother and the baby. In these cases, early deliveries are medically necessary. However, doctors may also decide to induce labor or deliver babies by C-section early as a convenience to themselves or their patient. This practice is not recommended. Hospitals should work with doctors and patients to avoid early elective deliveries when they are not medically necessary. This measure shows the percent of pregnancy women who had elective deliveries 1-3 weeks early (either vaginally or by C-section) who early deliveries were not medically necessary. Higher numbers may indicate that hospitals aren't doing enough to discourage this unsafe practice. *Lower percentages are better.*

13► Preventive Care

Hospitals and other healthcare providers play a crucial role in promoting, providing and educating patients about preventive services and screenings and maintaining the health of their communities. Many diseases are preventable through immunizations, screenings, treatment, and lifestyle changes. The information below shows how well the hospitals you selected are providing preventive services.

Immunization for Influenza

Patients assessed and given influenza vaccination.

Influenza, or the "flu," is a respiratory illness that is caused by flu viruses and easily spread from person to person. There are over 200,000 hospitalizations from the flu on average every year. An average of 36,000 Americans die annually due to the flu and its complications. The best way to prevent the flu is to get a flu shot each year during the fall season. Because flu viruses change from year to year, it is important to get a flu shot each year. *Higher percentages are better.*

Immunization for Pneumonia

Patients assessed and given pneumonia vaccination.

Pneumonia is an infection of the lungs that is caused by bacteria or a virus and can spread from person to person. A cold or flu that gets worse can turn into pneumonia. Although antibiotics such as penicillin were once very effective at treating pneumonia, the disease has mutated (changed) so these treatments are not as effective. The best way to prevent pneumonia is to get a flu shot each year (as flu often leads to pneumonia) and frequently washing your hands. Those who are more at risk of getting pneumonia, such as young children, people over the age of 65, people with a chronic illness (such as heart or lung disease or diabetes), or people who have had pneumonia before, should get the pneumonia vaccine. Ask your doctor when the best time to be vaccinated is for you. *Higher percentages are better.*

14► Stroke Care

Scientific evidence shows that the following measures show some of the standards of stroke care that hospitals should follow, for adults who have had a stroke.

Anticoagulation Therapy for Atrial Fibrillation

Ischemic stroke patients with a type of irregular heartbeat who were given a prescription for a blood thinner at discharge.

Patients admitted with an ischemic stroke who have an irregular heartbeat (also called atrial fibrillation or atrial flutter) are at greater risk of having another stroke. Research suggests that medicine that thins the blood (called an anticoagulant) reduces the chance of another stroke in these patients. This measure shows the percentage of patients admitted with ischemic stroke and an irregular heartbeat (atrial fibrillation/atrial flutter) who were prescribed an anticoagulant before they were discharged from the hospital. *Higher percentages are better.*

Antithrombotic Therapy Timing

Ischemic stroke patients who received medicine known to prevent complications caused by blood clots within 2 days of arriving at the hospital.

Ischemic stroke patients should get medicine known to reduce death, disability and the risk of another stroke (known as Antithrombotic Therapy) while in the hospital. Research shows that hospitals should start this medicine within 2 days of arriving at the hospital to prevent and treat clots and reduce the risk of complications from the stroke. Serious complications caused by strokes include changes in thinking and memory; muscle, joint, and nerve problems; or difficulty swallowing or eating; or blood clots. This measure shows the percentage of patients admitted with an ischemic stroke who got antithrombotic therapy started within 2 days of arriving at the hospital. *Higher percentages are better.*

Assessed for Rehabilitation

Ischemic or hemorrhagic stroke patients who were evaluated for rehabilitation services.
Many ischemic stroke or hemorrhagic stroke patients will experience moderate or severe disability, including problems with physical, speech and mental functions. Stroke rehabilitation can help patients relearn those lost skills and regain independence. Once the stroke symptoms and related problems are under control, the hospital appropriate health care professionals should review the status of the patient and begin rehabilitation as soon as possible. Appropriate health care professionals include physicians, physical therapists, occupational therapists, speech and language therapists, and/or neuropsychologist. The earlier the patient starts rehabilitation, the better the recovery process. Patients who need stroke rehabilitation may begin while they are still at the hospital and continue in a rehabilitation setting that is right for the patient. These options include inpatient rehabilitation units (either stand-alone or part of a hospital/clinic), outpatient units (usually part of a hospital/clinic), nursing home, or home-based programs. This measure shows the percentage of patients admitted with an ischemic stroke or a hemorrhagic stroke who were evaluated for their need for rehabilitation services. *Higher percentages are better.*

Discharged on Antithrombotic Therapy

Ischemic stroke patients who received a prescription for medicine known to prevent complications caused by blood clots before discharge.
Patients admitted with an ischemic stroke are at risk for developing complications like another stroke even after discharge. These patients should get a prescription at discharge for a blood thinner that prevents complications like another stroke (called Antithrombotic Therapy.) Serious complications caused by strokes include changes in thinking and memory; muscle, joint, and nerve problems; or difficulty swallowing or eating; or blood clots. This measure shows the percentage of patients who were admitted with an ischemic stroke who were given a prescription for an antithrombotic before they were discharged from the hospital. *Higher percentages are better.*

Discharged on Statin Medication

Ischemic stroke patients needing medicine to lower cholesterol, who were given a prescription for this medicine before discharge.
Cholesterol is a fat (also called a lipid) that the body needs to work properly. Levels of bad cholesterol (LDL) that are too high can increase the chance of stroke, heart disease, and other problems. Medicines called statins can help lower LDL cholesterol levels. In patients with ischemic stroke who have high cholesterol, taking statins can help lower the chance of another stroke. This measure shows the percentage of patients admitted with an ischemic stroke who got a prescription for a statin before they were discharged from the hospital. Patients who shouldn't take statins are not included in this measure. *Higher percentages are better.*

Thrombolytic Therapy Timing

Ischemic stroke patients who got medicine to break up a blood clot within 3 hours after symptoms started.
Patients with ischemic stroke should get medicine called tissue plasminogen activator, or t-PA, to break up a blood clot within 3 hours after their symptoms start. T-PA is a kind of thrombolytic therapy. Research shows that hospitals that give t-PA within 3 hours after symptoms start can limit the damage and disability caused by an ischemic stroke. This measure shows the percentage of patients admitted with ischemic stroke who arrived in the emergency department (ED) within 2 hours of the onset of their symptoms and who got t-PA within three hours after the onset of their symptoms. *Higher percentages are better.*

Venous Thromboembolism Prophylaxis

Ischemic or hemorrhagic stroke patients who received treatment to keep blood clots from forming anywhere in the body within 2 days of arriving at the hospital.
Patients admitted to the hospital with ischemic stroke or hemorrhagic stroke are at increased risk of developing new blood clots in their veins that break off and travel to other parts of the body, like the brain or lung (also called venous thromboembolism). Research shows that hospitals should begin treatment to prevent new blood clots on the day of or day after these patients are arrived at the hospital. Treatment can include medicine, medical devices, or tightly fitting stockings designed to keep blood from clotting. This measure shows the percentage of patients admitted with an ischemic stroke or hemorrhagic stroke who either received treatment to prevent blood clots on the day of or day after arrival at the hospital or had paperwork in their chart to explain why they had not received this treatment. *Higher percentages are better.*

Written Stroke Educational Materials Given

Ischemic or hemorrhagic stroke patients or caregivers who received written educational materials about stroke care and prevention during the hospital stay.
Educating patients with ischemic stroke and hemorrhagic stroke and their caregivers about stroke care and prevention helps patients live healthier lives and reduces health care costs. During the hospital stay, hospital staff should give stroke patients and caregivers written information on: how to activate the hospital emergency system; the importance of doing follow-up after being released from the hospital; medicines prescribed at discharge;

what increases the chance of stroke; warning signs and symptoms of stroke. This measure shows the percentage of patients with an ischemic stroke or a hemorrhagic stroke or their caregivers who received written information about these topics during their hospital stay. *Higher percentages are better.*

15▶ Surgical Care Improvement Project

Scientific evidence shows that the following measures represent the best practices for preventing complications after certain surgeries: colon surgery, hip replacement, knee replacement, abdominal and vaginal hysterectomy, cardiac surgery- including coronary artery bypass grafts (CABG), and vascular surgery.

Appropriate Beta Blocker Usage
Surgery patients who were taking heart drugs called beta blockers before coming to the hospital, who were kept on the beta blockers during the period just before and after their surgery.
It is often standard procedure to stop taking usual medications for a while before and after surgery. But if patients who have been taking beta blockers suddenly stop taking them, they can have heart problems such as a fast heartbeat. For these patients, staying on beta blockers before and after surgery makes it less likely that they will have heart problems. This measure shows the percentage of patients who remained on beta blockers within this time period. *Higher percentages are better.*

Appropriate VTP Within 24 Hours
Patients who got treatment (venous thromboembolism prevention) at the right time (within 24 hours before or after their surgery) to help prevent blood clots after certain types of surgery.
Many factors influence a surgery patient's risk of developing a blood clot, including the type of surgery. When patients stay still for a long time after some types of surgery, they are more likely to develop a blood clot in the veins of the legs, thighs, or pelvis. A blood clot slows down the flow of blood, causing swelling, redness, and pain. A blood clot can also break off and travel to other parts of the body. If the blood clot gets into the lung, it is a serious problem that can sometimes cause death. Doctors can order treatments including blood-thinning medications, elastic support stockings, or mechanical air stockings that help with blood flow in the legs. These treatments need to be started at the right time, which is typically during the period that begins 24 hours before surgery and ends 24 hours after surgery. This measure shows the percentage of patients who received these treatments this time period. *Higher percentages are better.*

Controlled Postoperative Blood Glucose
Heart surgery patients whose blood sugar (blood glucose) is kept under good control in the days right after surgery.
Even if heart surgery patients do not have diabetes, keeping blood sugar under good control (200 mg/dL or less) after surgery lowers the risk of infection and other problems. This measure shows the percentage of patients who had their blood sugar kept under good control in the days right after surgery. *Higher percentages are better.*

Perioperative Temperature Management
Patients having surgery who were actively warmed in the operating room or whose body temperature was near normal by the end of surgery.
Hospitals can prevent surgical wound infections and other complications by keeping the patient's body temperature near normal during surgery. Medical research has shown that patients whose body temperatures drop during surgery have a greater risk of infection and their wounds may not heal as quickly. Standards of care say that patients should have their body temperature normal or near normal during the time period 30 minutes before the end of surgery to 15 minutes after anesthesia ended. This measure shows the percent of patients whose body temperature was normal or near normal within this time period. *Higher percentages are better.*

Prophylactic Antibiotic Selection
Surgery patients who were given the right kind of antibiotic to help prevent infection.
Surgical wound infections can be prevented. Medical research has shown that certain antibiotics work better to prevent wound infections for certain types of surgery. This measure shows the percentage of surgery patients who were given the right antibiotic during surgery. *Higher percentages are better.*

Prophylactic Antibiotic Selection (Outpatient)
Outpatients having surgery who got the right kind of antibiotic.
Hospitals can prevent surgical wound infections. Medical research has shown that certain antibiotics work better to prevent wound infections for certain types of surgery. Hospital staff should make sure patients get the antibiotic that works best for their type of surgery. This measure shows the percentage of patients who got the right antibiotic during surgery. *Higher percentages are better.*

Prophylactic Antibiotic Stopped
Surgery patients whose preventive antibiotics were stopped at the right time (within 24 hours after surgery).
Antibiotics are often given to patients before surgery to prevent infection. Taking these antibiotics for more than 24 hours after routine surgery is usually not necessary. Continuing the medication longer than necessary can in-

crease the risk of side effects such as stomach aches and serious types of diarrhea. Also, when antibiotics are used for too long, patients can develop resistance to them and the antibiotics won't work as well. This measure shows the percentage of patients who stopped getting preventive antibiotics within this time period. *Higher percentages are better.*

Prophylactic Antibiotic Timing
Surgery patients who were given an antibiotic at the right time (within one hour before surgery) to help prevent infection.
Surgical wound infections can be prevented. Medical research shows that surgery patients who get antibiotics within the hour before their surgery are less likely to get wound infections. Getting an antibiotic earlier, or after surgery begins, is not as effective. Hospital staff should make sure surgery patients get antibiotics at the right time. This measure shows the percentage of patients who got an antibiotic to prevent infection in this time period. *Higher percentages are better.*

Prophylactic Antibiotic Timing (Outpatient)
Outpatients having surgery who got an antibiotic at the right time (within one hour before surgery).
Hospitals can prevent surgical wound infections. Standards for care say that surgery patients who get antibiotics within an hour of their surgery are less likely to get wound infections. Getting an antibiotic earlier, or after surgery begins, is not as effective. This measure shows the percentage of patients who got an antibiotic in this time period. *Higher percentages are better.*

Urinary Catheter Removal
Surgery patients whose urinary catheters were removed on the first or second day after surgery.
Sometimes surgical patients need to have a urinary catheter, or thin tube, inserted into their bladder to help drain the urine. Catheters are usually attached to a bag that collects the urine. Surgery patients can develop infections when urinary catheters are left in place too long after surgery. Standards of care say that most surgery patients should have their urinary catheters removed within 2 days after surgery to help prevent infection. This measure shows the percent of surgery patients whose urinary catheters were removed on the first or second day after surgery. *Higher percentages are better.*

16► Survey of Patients' Hospital Experiences

The HCAHPS (Hospital Consumer Assessment of Healthcare Providers and Systems) Survey, also known as the CAHPS® Hospital Survey or Hospital CAHPS®, is a standardized survey instrument and data collection methodology that has been in use since 2006 to measure patients' perspectives of hospital care. A partnership of public and private organizations led by the Federal government, specifically the Centers for Medicare & Medicaid Services (CMS) and the Agency for Healthcare Research and Quality (AHRQ), created HCAHPS (pronounced "H-caps") to publicly report the patient's perspective of hospital care. The HCAHPS results posted on Hospital Compare allow consumers to make fair and objective comparisons between hospitals and with state and national averages, on important measures of patients' perspectives of care. For more on HCAHPS information, please visit the official HCAHPS website: www.hcahpsonline.org

The HCAHPS survey asks patients to give feedback about topics for which they are the best source of information. The survey asks patients to answer questions about their experiences in the hospital. To make sure the HCAHPS survey data is meaningful; patients only answer questions about topics with which they have experience. The HCAHPS survey asks patients to answer questions related to ten topics. The topics and questions are listed in the table below. Answers shown in italics are included in this publication.

Measure as it Appears in CGAH	HCAHPS Topic Text	HCAHPS Answer Description
Would Definitely Recommend Hospital	How do patients rate the hospital overall?	*Patients who gave a rating of 9 or 10 (high)*
		Patients who gave a rating of 7 or 8 (medium)
		Patients who gave a rating of 6 or lower (low)
Doctors 'Always' Communicated Well	How often did doctors communicate well with patients?	*Doctors always communicated well*
		Doctors usually communicated well
		Doctors sometimes or never communicated well
Nurses 'Always' Communicated Well	How often did nurses communicate well with patients?	*Nurses always communicated well*
		Nurses usually communicated well
		Nurses sometimes or never communicated well
Timely Help 'Always' Received	How often did patients receive help quickly from hospital staff?	*Patients always received help as soon as they wanted*
		Patients usually received help as soon as they wanted
		Patients sometimes or never received help as soon as they wanted

<table>
<tr><th>Measure as it Appears in CGAH</th><th>HCAHPS Topic Text</th><th>HCAHPS Answer Description</th></tr>
<tr><td rowspan="3">Meds 'Always' Explained Before Given</td><td rowspan="3">How often did staff explain about medicines before giving them to patients?</td><td>Staff always explained</td></tr>
<tr><td>Staff usually explained</td></tr>
<tr><td>Staff sometimes or never explained</td></tr>
<tr><td rowspan="3">Pain 'Always' Well Controlled</td><td rowspan="3">How often was patients' pain well controlled?</td><td>Pain was always well controlled</td></tr>
<tr><td>Pain was usually well controlled</td></tr>
<tr><td>Pain was sometimes or never well controlled</td></tr>
<tr><td rowspan="3">Area Around Room 'Always' Quiet at Night</td><td rowspan="3">How often was the area around patients' rooms kept quiet at night?</td><td>Always quiet at night</td></tr>
<tr><td>Usually quiet at night</td></tr>
<tr><td>Sometimes or never quiet at night</td></tr>
<tr><td rowspan="3">Room and Bathroom 'Always' Clean</td><td rowspan="3">How often were the patients' rooms and bathrooms kept clean?</td><td>Room was always clean</td></tr>
<tr><td>Room was usually clean</td></tr>
<tr><td>Room was sometimes or never clean</td></tr>
<tr><td rowspan="2">Home Recovery Information Given</td><td rowspan="2">Were patients given information about what to do during their recovery at home?</td><td>YES, staff did give patients this information</td></tr>
<tr><td>NO, staff did not give patients this information</td></tr>
<tr><td rowspan="3">Would Definitely Recommend Hospital</td><td rowspan="3">Would patients recommend the hospital to friends and family?</td><td>YES, patients would definitely recommend the hospital</td></tr>
<tr><td>YES, patients would probably recommend the hospital</td></tr>
<tr><td>NO, patients would not recommend the hospital (they probably would not or definitely would not recommend it)</td></tr>
</table>

17 ▸ Use of Medical Imaging

"Medical imaging" tests create images of various parts of the body to screen for or diagnose medical conditions. Examples of medical imaging include CT scans, MRIs, and mammograms.

Cardiac Imaging Stress Test before Surgery
Outpatients who got cardiac imaging stress tests before low-risk outpatient surgery.
A cardiac stress test measures the heart's ability to respond when it is stressed, and can be useful in evaluating a patient's surgical risk. Experts agree, however, that these tests are not necessary before most low-risk outpatient surgical procedures, such as colonoscopies, cataract surgery, biopsies, or endoscopies (using an instrument to look inside the body) because these procedures put very little stress on the heart. Patients with certain risk factors that increase the likelihood of having complications are not included in the measure. This measure shows the percentage of all cardiac stress tests done in a hospital outpatient imaging department (using echocardiograms, CT scans, and MRIs) for Medicare patients who were going to have certain low-risk outpatient surgical procedures. Hospital outpatient imaging departments that have higher percentages on this measure may be giving people more tests than they need. *Hospitals that are rated well will have lower percentages.* If a percentage is high, it may mean that the facility is doing unnecessary cardiac imaging before some low-risk surgeries.

Combination Abdominal CT Scan
Outpatient CT scans of the abdomen that were "combination" (double) scans.
A CT scan (also called a CAT scan) uses multiple X-rays to produce detailed pictures of the inside of the body (bones, organs, and other body parts). For some, a substance called "contrast" is put into the patient's body before the scan begins, which help make parts of the body stand out more clearly. Contrast can be either swallowed or injected into a vein. Risks of contrast include possible harm to the kidneys or allergic reactions. Contrast shouldn't be used if it isn't needed. "Combination" CT scan means that the patient gets two CT scans—one scan without contrast, followed by a second scan with contrast. Standards of quality care say that most patients who are getting a CT scan of the chest should be given a single CT scan rather than a "combination" CT scan. Although combination CT scans are appropriate for some parts of the body and for some medical conditions, combination scans are usually not appropriate for the chest. The range for these measures is from 0% to 100%. For hospitals with higher percentages, it may mean that the facility is routinely giving patients combination CT scans of the chest or abdomen when a single scan is all they need. Giving patients two scans when they only need one needlessly doubles their exposure to radiation: Radiation exposure from a single CT scan of the chest is about 350 times higher than for an ordinary chest X-ray. For combination CT scans, radiation exposure is 700 times higher than for a chest X-ray because the patient is given two scans. For a combination CT scan, radiation exposure is 22 times higher than for an X-ray of the abdomen because the patient is given two scans. Radiation exposure from a single CT scan of the abdomen is about 11 times higher than for an ordinary X-ray of the abdomen. When contrast is used, there are risks that can include possible harm to the kidneys or allergic reactions (especially if the contrast is injected). To avoid unnecessary risk, contrast should be used only when it is needed. If you need to have a CT scan of the chest or abdomen, feel free to ask your doctor these questions to determine

what's best for your medical condition: Do you need a single scan—either with or without contrast—or is a combination scan necessary? Is using contrast appropriate for your medical condition? *Hospitals that are rated well will have lower percentages.* If a percentage is high, it may mean that the facility is doing unnecessary double/combination scans.

Combination Brain/Sinus CT Scan
Outpatients with brain CT scans who got a sinus CT scan at the same time.
Brain CTs and sinus CTs can be important tools for diagnosing problems that may be causing severe headaches or chronic sinus infections, but they also expose patients to high levels of radiation. Brain CT scans cover large parts of the sinuses, so ordering both tests may be unnecessary. For patients with chronic sinusitis, a sinus CT is usually done first before deciding if a brain CT is also needed. Experts do not recommend doing both tests at once, unless patients have head injuries or tumors. Hospital outpatient imaging departments that have higher percentages on this measure may be giving people more tests than they need, exposing them to too much radiation. This measure shows the percentage of brain CT scans done in a hospital outpatient imaging department where a sinus CT scan was done at the same time on the same Medicare patient. It does not count cases where doctors had questions about complications due to injuries, cancer, or serious infections. *Hospitals that are rated well will have lower percentages.* If a percentage is high, it may mean that the facility is doing unnecessary scans.

Combination Chest CT Scan
Outpatient CT scans of the chest that were "combination" (double) scans.
A CT scan (also called a CAT scan) uses multiple X-rays to produce detailed pictures of the inside of the body (bones, organs, and other body parts). For some, a substance called "contrast" is put into the patient's body before the scan begins, which help make parts of the body stand out more clearly. Contrast can be either swallowed or injected into a vein. Risks of contrast include possible harm to the kidneys or allergic reactions. Contrast shouldn't be used if it isn't needed. "Combination" CT scan means that the patient gets two CT scans—one scan without contrast, followed by a second scan with contrast. Standards of quality care say that most patients who are getting a CT scan of the chest should be given a single CT scan rather than a "combination" CT scan. Although combination CT scans are appropriate for some parts of the body and for some medical conditions, combination scans are usually not appropriate for the chest. The range for these measures is from 0% to 100%. For hospitals with higher percentages, it may mean that the facility is routinely giving patients combination CT scans of the chest or abdomen when a single scan is all they need. Giving patients two scans when they only need one needlessly doubles their exposure to radiation. Radiation exposure from a single CT scan of the chest is about 350 times higher than for an ordinary chest X-ray. For combination CT scans, radiation exposure is 700 times higher than for a chest X-ray because the patient is given two scans. For a combination CT scan, radiation exposure is 22 times higher than for an X-ray of the abdomen because the patient is given two scans. Radiation exposure from a single CT scan of the abdomen is about 11 times higher than for an ordinary X-ray of the abdomen. When contrast is used, there are risks that can include possible harm to the kidneys or allergic reactions (especially if the contrast is injected). To avoid unnecessary risk, contrast should be used only when it is needed. If you need to have a CT scan of the chest or abdomen, feel free to ask your doctor these questions to determine what's best for your medical condition: Do you need a single scan - either with or without contrast - or is a combination scan necessary? Is using contrast appropriate for your medical condition? *Hospitals that are rated well will have lower percentages.* If a percentage is high, it may mean that the facility is doing unnecessary double/combination scans.

Follow-up Mammogram/Ultrasound
Outpatients who had a follow-up mammogram, ultrasound, or MRI of the breast within 45 days after a screening mammogram.
A screening mammogram is an X-ray of the breast to check for possible breast cancer before it can be detected by women or health care professionals. Although mammography is a good test, it is not perfect. Some women who do not have breast cancer will have an abnormal mammogram (even though they are cancer free), and some women with breast cancer will have a normal screening mammogram (their cancer is missed). Some women may be asked to come back for follow-up testing if there are signs of possible breast cancer. A follow-up visit usually means having more tests (mammograms, an ultrasound, and/or an MRI of the breast). The numbers of women asked to follow-up varies widely among mammography facilities in the United States. There are many reasons for differences in follow-up rates including poor technique (blurry X-rays that need to be repeated), a lack of skill or experience interpreting the screening mammograms, medical history of the woman undergoing screening, and whether a woman is being screened for the first time or has previously undergone mammography screening. The follow-up rates reported here for mammography facilities include follow-up exams performed on the same day as screening mammograms, as well as those performed up to 45 days later. Medical evidence suggests that there may be a problem if a facility has either a very low or very high rate of follow-ups. *Although values for a very low follow-up rate have not been established, a follow-up rate near zero may indicate a facility that misses signs of cancer. Follow-up rates around 9% are typical. Research has established that a follow-up rate above 14% is not appropriate, and may indicate a facility doing unnecessary follow up.* If you have a screening

mammogram and you are called back for additional testing, ask your doctor why and what this additional testing means in your case for how he or she makes an accurate diagnosis.

Lumbar Spine MRI for Low Back Pain

Outpatients with low back pain who had an MRI without trying recommended treatments first, such as physical therapy.

An MRI (magnetic resonance imaging) is a test that uses a powerful magnetic field and a computer to produce detailed pictures of the inside of the body (bones, organs, and other body parts). Although MRI scans can be helpful for diagnosing low back pain, they can also be used too much. Low back pain can improve or go away within six weeks and an MRI may not be needed. Standards of care say that most patients with low back pain should start with treatment such as physical therapy or chiropractic care, and have an MRI only if the treatment doesn't help. Finding out whether treatment helps or not before having an MRI can be a safe and effective way to avoid unnecessary stress, risk, or cost of doing an MRI. For patients with certain conditions, getting an MRI right away is appropriate care. Patients with these conditions are not included in this measure. If you have low back pain, you, your doctor, and the medical imaging facility staff can talk about the best time to do an MRI if you need one. Since MRIs use magnets rather than x-rays, there is no radiation risk. However, because the magnets attract some kinds of metal, it's important for the technician to know if there are any metal objects or implants inside your body, such as pacemakers, artificial joints, screws, stents, plates, or staples. Metal objects can pose serious risk to you during the MRI and interfere with the test. For some MRIs, a substance called "contrast" is injected before the test to make parts of the body stand out more clearly on the images. Risks of contrast include possible harm to the kidneys or allergic reactions. Contrast shouldn't be used if it isn't needed. Having the test can be stressful for some people. Patients must hold still for about 15 to 45 minutes while lying on a table that moves inside a large scanning machine. While images are being taken, the machine makes loud noises. *Hospitals that are rated well will have lower percentages.* If a percentage is high, it may mean that the facility is doing unnecessary MRIs for low back pain.

Blood Clot Prevention and Treatment

Anticoagulation Overlap Therapy

Hospital Name	City	Rate	Cases
Providence Alaska Medical Center[2]	Anchorage	98%	62

ICU Venous Thromboembolism Prophylaxis

Hospital Name	City	Rate	Cases
Alaska Regional Hospital[2]	Anchorage	98%	83
Central Peninsula General Hospital[2]	Soldotna	98%	51
Mat-Su Regional Medical Center[2]	Palmer	98%	53
Alaska Native Medical Center[2]	Anchorage	95%	66
Providence Alaska Medical Center[2]	Anchorage	93%	111
Bartlett Regional Hospital[2]	Juneau	92%	59
Fairbanks Memorial Hospital[2]	Fairbanks	82%	49
Mount Edgecumbe Hospital	Sitka	59%	51

Venous Thromboembolism Prophylaxis

Hospital Name	City	Rate	Cases
Mat-Su Regional Medical Center[2]	Palmer	98%	268
Alaska Native Medical Center[2]	Anchorage	94%	313
Central Peninsula General Hospital[2]	Soldotna	94%	136
Alaska Regional Hospital[2]	Anchorage	91%	243
Bartlett Regional Hospital[2]	Juneau	90%	117
Yukon Kuskokwim Delta Regional Hospital[2]	Bethel	90%	158
Providence Alaska Medical Center[2]	Anchorage	86%	308
Peacehealth Ketchikan Medical Center[2]	Ketchikan	81%	74
Fairbanks Memorial Hospital[2]	Fairbanks	69%	223
Mount Edgecumbe Hospital	Sitka	60%	214

Warfarin Therapy Discharge Instructions

Hospital Name	City	Rate	Cases
Providence Alaska Medical Center[2]	Anchorage	84%	50

Chest Pain/Possible Heart Attack Care

Aspirin Given Within 24 Hours of Arrival

Hospital Name	City	Rate	Cases
Central Peninsula General Hospital	Soldotna	99%	81

Average Time to ECG (minutes)

Hospital Name	City	Min.	Cases
Central Peninsula General Hospital	Soldotna	9	84

Children's Asthma Care

No hospitals met the 25 case threshold.

Emergency Department

Admittance Decision Time (minutes)

Hospital Name	City	Min.	Cases
Mount Edgecumbe Hospital	Sitka	25	77
Central Peninsula General Hospital[2]	Soldotna	92	280
Yukon Kuskokwim Delta Regional Hospital[2]	Bethel	97	223
Alaska Regional Hospital[2]	Anchorage	99	377
Alaska Native Medical Center[2]	Anchorage	106	400
Mat-Su Regional Medical Center[2]	Palmer	106	504
Fairbanks Memorial Hospital[2]	Fairbanks	122	358
Peacehealth Ketchikan Medical Center[2]	Ketchikan	155	275
Providence Alaska Medical Center[2]	Anchorage	280	499

Patients Who Left ER Before Being Seen

Hospital Name	City	Rate	Cases
Alaska Regional Hospital	Anchorage	0%	26028
Bartlett Regional Hospital	Juneau	0%	14481
Central Peninsula General Hospital	Soldotna	0%	15776
South Peninsula Hospital	Homer	0%	5075
Fairbanks Memorial Hospital	Fairbanks	1%	35332
Mat-Su Regional Medical Center	Palmer	1%	28557
Peacehealth Ketchikan Medical Center	Ketchikan	2%	9470
Providence Alaska Medical Center	Anchorage	2%	63947
Alaska Native Medical Center	Anchorage	7%	57496

Time from ER Arrival to Being Admitted (minutes)

Hospital Name	City	Min.	Cases
Mount Edgecumbe Hospital	Sitka	142	170
Mat-Su Regional Medical Center[2]	Palmer	244	560
Alaska Regional Hospital[2]	Anchorage	246	378
Peacehealth Ketchikan Medical Center[2]	Ketchikan	259	275
Fairbanks Memorial Hospital[2]	Fairbanks	268	372
Central Peninsula General Hospital[2]	Soldotna	291	303
Alaska Native Medical Center[2]	Anchorage	373	422
Providence Alaska Medical Center[2]	Anchorage	375	504
Yukon Kuskokwim Delta Regional Hospital[2]	Bethel	384	364

Time from ER Arrival to Discharge (minutes)

Hospital Name	City	Min.	Cases
Alaska Regional Hospital	Anchorage	100	414
Fairbanks Memorial Hospital	Fairbanks	122	321
South Peninsula Hospital[3]	Homer	122	26
Peacehealth Ketchikan Medical Center	Ketchikan	125	363
Mat-Su Regional Medical Center	Palmer	127	409
Providence Alaska Medical Center	Anchorage	134	375
Bartlett Regional Hospital	Juneau	139	389
Central Peninsula General Hospital	Soldotna	145	401
Alaska Native Medical Center	Anchorage	156	378

Time in ER Before Being Evaluated (minutes)

Hospital Name	City	Min.	Cases
South Peninsula Hospital[3]	Homer	8	32
Alaska Regional Hospital	Anchorage	17	436
Peacehealth Ketchikan Medical Center	Ketchikan	18	397
Providence Alaska Medical Center	Anchorage	20	277
Mat-Su Regional Medical Center	Palmer	21	410
Bartlett Regional Hospital	Juneau	28	246
Central Peninsula General Hospital	Soldotna	30	420
Alaska Native Medical Center	Anchorage	50	382

Time to Pain Meds for Bone Fractures (minutes)

Hospital Name	City	Min.	Cases
Fairbanks Memorial Hospital	Fairbanks	48	112
Central Peninsula General Hospital	Soldotna	50	80
Alaska Regional Hospital	Anchorage	54	57
Mat-Su Regional Medical Center	Palmer	54	196
Alaska Native Medical Center	Anchorage	58	138
Peacehealth Ketchikan Medical Center	Ketchikan	58	48
Bartlett Regional Hospital	Juneau	60	41
Providence Alaska Medical Center	Anchorage	66	191

Heart Attack Care

Aspirin Given at Discharge

Hospital Name	City	Rate	Cases
Alaska Regional Hospital	Anchorage	100%	143
Fairbanks Memorial Hospital	Fairbanks	100%	76
Mat-Su Regional Medical Center	Palmer	100%	76
Providence Alaska Medical Center	Anchorage	100%	364

PCI Within 90 Minutes of Arrival

Hospital Name	City	Rate	Cases
Providence Alaska Medical Center	Anchorage	93%	46

Statin Prescribed at Discharge

Hospital Name	City	Rate	Cases
Fairbanks Memorial Hospital	Fairbanks	100%	73
Mat-Su Regional Medical Center	Palmer	100%	66
Alaska Regional Hospital	Anchorage	99%	142
Providence Alaska Medical Center	Anchorage	99%	361

Heart Failure Care

ACE Inhibitor or ARB for LVSD

Hospital Name	City	Rate	Cases
Alaska Native Medical Center	Anchorage	100%	48
Alaska Regional Hospital	Anchorage	100%	28
Fairbanks Memorial Hospital	Fairbanks	100%	37
Mat-Su Regional Medical Center	Palmer	100%	26
Providence Alaska Medical Center	Anchorage	100%	144

Discharge Instructions Given

Hospital Name	City	Rate	Cases
Alaska Native Medical Center	Anchorage	100%	70
Providence Alaska Medical Center	Anchorage	100%	300
Mat-Su Regional Medical Center	Palmer	98%	62
Alaska Regional Hospital	Anchorage	97%	68
Fairbanks Memorial Hospital	Fairbanks	95%	73
Central Peninsula General Hospital	Soldotna	93%	29
Yukon Kuskokwim Delta Regional Hospital	Bethel	63%	38

Evaluation of LVS Function

Hospital Name	City	Rate	Cases
Alaska Native Medical Center	Anchorage	100%	73
Alaska Regional Hospital	Anchorage	100%	69
Central Peninsula General Hospital	Soldotna	100%	33
Fairbanks Memorial Hospital	Fairbanks	100%	73
Mat-Su Regional Medical Center	Palmer	100%	77
Providence Alaska Medical Center	Anchorage	100%	307
Yukon Kuskokwim Delta Regional Hospital	Bethel	97%	38

Medicare Spending

Medicare Spending per Patient (ratio)

Hospital Name	City	Ratio	Cases
Yukon Kuskokwim Delta Regional Hospital	Bethel	0.59	-
Mount Edgecumbe Hospital	Sitka	0.65	-
Fairbanks Memorial Hospital	Fairbanks	0.78	-
Alaska Native Medical Center	Anchorage	0.79	-
Mat-Su Regional Medical Center	Palmer	0.81	-
Bartlett Regional Hospital	Juneau	0.84	-
Alaska Regional Hospital	Anchorage	0.85	-
Providence Alaska Medical Center	Anchorage	0.85	-
Central Peninsula General Hospital	Soldotna	0.86	-

Pneumonia Care

Appropriate Initial Antibiotic Given

Hospital Name	City	Rate	Cases
Alaska Regional Hospital	Anchorage	100%	30
Central Peninsula General Hospital	Soldotna	100%	62
Mat-Su Regional Medical Center	Palmer	100%	89
Providence Alaska Medical Center	Anchorage	98%	160
Fairbanks Memorial Hospital	Fairbanks	92%	39
Alaska Native Medical Center	Anchorage	90%	104
Bartlett Regional Hospital	Juneau	88%	34
Yukon Kuskokwim Delta Regional Hospital	Bethel	86%	35

Blood Culture Timing

Hospital Name	City	Rate	Cases
Alaska Regional Hospital	Anchorage	100%	40
Bartlett Regional Hospital	Juneau	100%	39
Central Peninsula General Hospital	Soldotna	100%	86
Mat-Su Regional Medical Center	Palmer	100%	138
Providence Alaska Medical Center	Anchorage	100%	228
Fairbanks Memorial Hospital	Fairbanks	98%	82
Peacehealth Ketchikan Medical Center	Ketchikan	95%	42
Alaska Native Medical Center	Anchorage	94%	164
Yukon Kuskokwim Delta Regional Hospital	Bethel	87%	31

Pregnancy and Delivery Care

Newborns whose Deliveries were Scheduled Early

Hospital Name	City	Rate	Cases
Mat-Su Regional Medical Center[2]	Palmer	0%	36
Alaska Regional Hospital	Anchorage	2%	48
Providence Alaska Medical Center[2]	Anchorage	2%	46
Bartlett Regional Hospital	Juneau	4%	27

Preventive Care

Immunization for Influenza

Hospital Name	City	Rate	Cases
Mat-Su Regional Medical Center[2]	Palmer	99%	476
Central Peninsula General Hospital[2]	Soldotna	95%	263
Alaska Regional Hospital[2]	Anchorage	94%	527
Bartlett Regional Hospital[2]	Juneau	91%	276
Fairbanks Memorial Hospital[2]	Fairbanks	89%	461
Peacehealth Ketchikan Medical Center[2]	Ketchikan	82%	245
Mount Edgecumbe Hospital	Sitka	80%	319
Providence Alaska Medical Center[2]	Anchorage	80%	531
Alaska Native Medical Center[2]	Anchorage	65%	557
South Peninsula Hospital	Homer	62%	32
Yukon Kuskokwim Delta Regional Hospital[2]	Bethel	52%	279

Immunization for Pneumonia

Hospital Name	City	Rate	Cases
Mat-Su Regional Medical Center[2]	Palmer	100%	439
Central Peninsula General Hospital[2]	Soldotna	98%	233
Alaska Regional Hospital[2]	Anchorage	95%	541
Bartlett Regional Hospital[2]	Juneau	88%	222
Fairbanks Memorial Hospital[2]	Fairbanks	87%	345
Mount Edgecumbe Hospital	Sitka	87%	247
Providence Alaska Medical Center[2]	Anchorage	87%	467
Yukon Kuskokwim Delta Regional Hospital[2]	Bethel	87%	193
Peacehealth Ketchikan Medical Center[2]	Ketchikan	86%	207
Alaska Native Medical Center[2]	Anchorage	84%	352
South Peninsula Hospital[3]	Homer	72%	25

Stroke Care

Antithrombotic Therapy Timing

Hospital Name	City	Rate	Cases
Alaska Regional Hospital[2]	Anchorage	100%	38
Alaska Native Medical Center	Anchorage	98%	55
Providence Alaska Medical Center	Anchorage	98%	122

NOTE: Hospital profiles are in alphabetical order by state, then city, then hospital within the city; Rankings exclude hospitals with less than 25 cases except for patient surveys which excludes hospitals with less than 100 cases; (a) 100-299 cases; (1) The number of cases/patients is too few to report; (2) Data submitted were based on a sample of cases/patients; (3) Results are based on a shorter time period than required; (4) Data suppressed by CMS for one or more quarters; (5) Results are not available for this reporting period; (6) Fewer than 100 patients completed the HCAHPS survey; (7) No cases met the criteria for this measure; (8) The lower limit of the confidence interval cannot be calculated if the number of observed infections equals zero; (9) No data are available from the state/territory for this reporting period; (10) The scores shown reflect fewer than 50 completed surveys; (11) There were discrepancies in the data collection process; (12) This measure does not apply to this hospital for this reporting period; (13) Results cannot be calculated for this reporting period; (14) The results for this state are combined with nearby states to protect confidentiality; Please refer to the User's Guide for a full explanation of data.

Assessed for Rehabilitation

Hospital Name	City	Rate	Cases
Alaska Native Medical Center	Anchorage	100%	79
Alaska Regional Hospital[2]	Anchorage	100%	55
Mat-Su Regional Medical Center	Palmer	100%	26
Fairbanks Memorial Hospital	Fairbanks	97%	29
Providence Alaska Medical Center	Anchorage	94%	161

Discharged on Antithrombotic Therapy

Hospital Name	City	Rate	Cases
Alaska Native Medical Center	Anchorage	100%	64
Alaska Regional Hospital[2]	Anchorage	100%	43
Providence Alaska Medical Center	Anchorage	98%	138
Fairbanks Memorial Hospital	Fairbanks	97%	29

Discharged on Statin Medication

Hospital Name	City	Rate	Cases
Alaska Native Medical Center	Anchorage	100%	51
Alaska Regional Hospital[2]	Anchorage	93%	30
Providence Alaska Medical Center	Anchorage	93%	116

Venous Thromboembolism (VTE) Prophylaxis

Hospital Name	City	Rate	Cases
Mat-Su Regional Medical Center	Palmer	100%	25
Alaska Native Medical Center	Anchorage	98%	83
Alaska Regional Hospital[2]	Anchorage	97%	58
Providence Alaska Medical Center	Anchorage	92%	156
Fairbanks Memorial Hospital	Fairbanks	72%	25

Written Stroke Educational Materials Given

Hospital Name	City	Rate	Cases
Alaska Native Medical Center	Anchorage	100%	54
Providence Alaska Medical Center	Anchorage	97%	118
Alaska Regional Hospital[2]	Anchorage	82%	39

Surgical Care Improvement Project

Appropriate Beta Blocker Usage

Hospital Name	City	Rate	Cases
Central Peninsula General Hospital	Soldotna	100%	29
Alaska Regional Hospital[2]	Anchorage	97%	182
Mat-Su Regional Medical Center	Palmer	97%	70
Providence Alaska Medical Center[2]	Anchorage	97%	172
Alaska Native Medical Center[2]	Anchorage	95%	91
Fairbanks Memorial Hospital[2]	Fairbanks	94%	79
Bartlett Regional Hospital	Juneau	90%	30

Appropriate VTP Within 24 Hours

Hospital Name	City	Rate	Cases
Mat-Su Regional Medical Center	Palmer	100%	271
Alaska Regional Hospital[2]	Anchorage	99%	414
Central Peninsula General Hospital	Soldotna	99%	175
Providence Alaska Medical Center[2]	Anchorage	99%	338
Alaska Native Medical Center[2]	Anchorage	97%	373
Peacehealth Ketchikan Medical Center	Ketchikan	97%	77
Bartlett Regional Hospital	Juneau	96%	136
Fairbanks Memorial Hospital[2]	Fairbanks	94%	294
Mount Edgecumbe Hospital	Sitka	81%	27

Controlled Postoperative Blood Glucose

Hospital Name	City	Rate	Cases
Providence Alaska Medical Center[2]	Anchorage	98%	146
Alaska Regional Hospital[2]	Anchorage	89%	95

Perioperative Temperature Management

Hospital Name	City	Rate	Cases
Alaska Regional Hospital[2]	Anchorage	100%	515
Central Peninsula General Hospital	Soldotna	100%	198
Mat-Su Regional Medical Center	Palmer	100%	379
Peacehealth Ketchikan Medical Center	Ketchikan	100%	83
Providence Alaska Medical Center[2]	Anchorage	100%	437
South Peninsula Hospital	Homer	100%	29
Alaska Native Medical Center[2]	Anchorage	99%	432
Bartlett Regional Hospital	Juneau	99%	144
Fairbanks Memorial Hospital[2]	Fairbanks	99%	352
Mount Edgecumbe Hospital	Sitka	86%	28

Prophylactic Antibiotic Selection

Hospital Name	City	Rate	Cases
Bartlett Regional Hospital	Juneau	100%	95
Central Peninsula General Hospital	Soldotna	100%	144
Mat-Su Regional Medical Center	Palmer	100%	219
Peacehealth Ketchikan Medical Center	Ketchikan	100%	48
Alaska Native Medical Center[2]	Anchorage	99%	282
Alaska Regional Hospital[2]	Anchorage	99%	405
Fairbanks Memorial Hospital[2]	Fairbanks	99%	234
Providence Alaska Medical Center[2]	Anchorage	98%	439

Prophylactic Antibiotic Selection (Outpatient)

Hospital Name	City	Rate	Cases
Bartlett Regional Hospital	Juneau	100%	29
Mat-Su Regional Medical Center	Palmer	100%	49
Providence Alaska Medical Center	Anchorage	99%	512
Alaska Regional Hospital	Anchorage	98%	228
Fairbanks Memorial Hospital	Fairbanks	98%	125
Alaska Native Medical Center	Anchorage	94%	33

Prophylactic Antibiotic Stopped

Hospital Name	City	Rate	Cases
Alaska Native Medical Center[2]	Anchorage	100%	280
Bartlett Regional Hospital	Juneau	100%	95
Mat-Su Regional Medical Center	Palmer	100%	214
Alaska Regional Hospital[2]	Anchorage	99%	393
Central Peninsula General Hospital	Soldotna	99%	144
Fairbanks Memorial Hospital[2]	Fairbanks	98%	229
Peacehealth Ketchikan Medical Center	Ketchikan	98%	45
Providence Alaska Medical Center[2]	Anchorage	98%	427

Prophylactic Antibiotic Timing

Hospital Name	City	Rate	Cases
Alaska Regional Hospital[2]	Anchorage	100%	405
Mat-Su Regional Medical Center	Palmer	100%	219
Bartlett Regional Hospital	Juneau	99%	95
Central Peninsula General Hospital	Soldotna	99%	144
Alaska Native Medical Center[2]	Anchorage	98%	282
Fairbanks Memorial Hospital[2]	Fairbanks	98%	234
Providence Alaska Medical Center[2]	Anchorage	98%	441
Peacehealth Ketchikan Medical Center	Ketchikan	96%	48

Prophylactic Antibiotic Timing (Outpatient)

Hospital Name	City	Rate	Cases
Fairbanks Memorial Hospital	Fairbanks	98%	126
Alaska Regional Hospital	Anchorage	97%	232
Providence Alaska Medical Center	Anchorage	97%	516
Bartlett Regional Hospital	Juneau	96%	28
Mat-Su Regional Medical Center	Palmer	96%	51
Alaska Native Medical Center	Anchorage	86%	37

Urinary Catheter Removal

Hospital Name	City	Rate	Cases
Central Peninsula General Hospital	Soldotna	99%	146
Bartlett Regional Hospital	Juneau	98%	114
Mat-Su Regional Medical Center	Palmer	98%	116
Providence Alaska Medical Center[2]	Anchorage	98%	297
Alaska Native Medical Center[2]	Anchorage	97%	78
Alaska Regional Hospital[2]	Anchorage	97%	359
Peacehealth Ketchikan Medical Center	Ketchikan	96%	53
Fairbanks Memorial Hospital[2]	Fairbanks	95%	100

Survey of Patients' Hospital Experiences

Area Around Room 'Always' Quiet at Night

Hospital Name	City	Rate	Cases
Providence Kodiak Island Medical Center	Kodiak	72%	(a)
South Peninsula Hospital	Homer	69%	(a)
Peacehealth Ketchikan Medical Center	Ketchikan	64%	(a)
Bartlett Regional Hospital	Juneau	60%	300+
Mat-Su Regional Medical Center	Palmer	60%	300+
Alaska Regional Hospital	Anchorage	59%	300+
Fairbanks Memorial Hospital[11]	Fairbanks	59%	300+
Central Peninsula General Hospital	Soldotna	56%	300+
Providence Alaska Medical Center	Anchorage	55%	300+
Yukon Kuskokwim Delta Regional Hospital	Bethel	53%	(a)
Alaska Native Medical Center	Anchorage	51%	300+

Doctors 'Always' Communicated Well

Hospital Name	City	Rate	Cases
South Peninsula Hospital	Homer	87%	(a)
Peacehealth Ketchikan Medical Center	Ketchikan	86%	(a)
Providence Kodiak Island Medical Center	Kodiak	84%	(a)
Bartlett Regional Hospital	Juneau	82%	300+
Central Peninsula General Hospital	Soldotna	81%	300+
Fairbanks Memorial Hospital[11]	Fairbanks	80%	300+
Providence Alaska Medical Center	Anchorage	80%	300+
Mat-Su Regional Medical Center	Palmer	79%	300+
Alaska Regional Hospital	Anchorage	77%	300+
Alaska Native Medical Center	Anchorage	76%	300+
Yukon Kuskokwim Delta Regional Hospital	Bethel	75%	(a)

Home Recovery Information Given

Hospital Name	City	Rate	Cases
Fairbanks Memorial Hospital[11]	Fairbanks	91%	300+
South Peninsula Hospital	Homer	91%	(a)
Providence Kodiak Island Medical Center	Kodiak	90%	(a)
Peacehealth Ketchikan Medical Center	Ketchikan	89%	(a)
Central Peninsula General Hospital	Soldotna	88%	300+
Mat-Su Regional Medical Center	Palmer	88%	300+
Providence Alaska Medical Center	Anchorage	88%	300+
Alaska Native Medical Center	Anchorage	86%	300+
Alaska Regional Hospital	Anchorage	86%	300+
Bartlett Regional Hospital	Juneau	86%	300+
Yukon Kuskokwim Delta Regional Hospital	Bethel	77%	(a)

Hospital Given 9 or 10 on 10 Point Scale

Hospital Name	City	Rate	Cases
South Peninsula Hospital	Homer	80%	(a)
Providence Kodiak Island Medical Center	Kodiak	74%	(a)
Fairbanks Memorial Hospital[11]	Fairbanks	73%	300+
Providence Alaska Medical Center	Anchorage	73%	300+
Central Peninsula General Hospital	Soldotna	70%	300+
Mat-Su Regional Medical Center	Palmer	70%	300+
Peacehealth Ketchikan Medical Center	Ketchikan	67%	(a)
Alaska Native Medical Center	Anchorage	65%	300+
Alaska Regional Hospital	Anchorage	64%	300+
Bartlett Regional Hospital	Juneau	62%	300+
Yukon Kuskokwim Delta Regional Hospital	Bethel	49%	(a)

Meds 'Always' Explained Before Given

Hospital Name	City	Rate	Cases
Bartlett Regional Hospital	Juneau	69%	300+
Fairbanks Memorial Hospital[11]	Fairbanks	69%	300+
Central Peninsula General Hospital	Soldotna	68%	300+
Yukon Kuskokwim Delta Regional Hospital	Bethel	68%	(a)
South Peninsula Hospital	Homer	67%	(a)
Peacehealth Ketchikan Medical Center	Ketchikan	65%	(a)
Alaska Native Medical Center	Anchorage	64%	300+
Mat-Su Regional Medical Center	Palmer	64%	300+
Providence Kodiak Island Medical Center	Kodiak	63%	(a)
Alaska Regional Hospital	Anchorage	62%	300+
Providence Alaska Medical Center	Anchorage	61%	300+

Nurses 'Always' Communicated Well

Hospital Name	City	Rate	Cases
Providence Kodiak Island Medical Center	Kodiak	82%	(a)
South Peninsula Hospital	Homer	82%	(a)
Fairbanks Memorial Hospital[11]	Fairbanks	81%	300+
Peacehealth Ketchikan Medical Center	Ketchikan	80%	(a)
Central Peninsula General Hospital	Soldotna	78%	300+
Bartlett Regional Hospital	Juneau	77%	300+
Mat-Su Regional Medical Center	Palmer	77%	300+
Providence Alaska Medical Center	Anchorage	76%	300+
Alaska Native Medical Center	Anchorage	73%	300+
Alaska Regional Hospital	Anchorage	73%	300+
Yukon Kuskokwim Delta Regional Hospital	Bethel	69%	(a)

Pain 'Always' Well Controlled

Hospital Name	City	Rate	Cases
South Peninsula Hospital	Homer	74%	(a)
Peacehealth Ketchikan Medical Center	Ketchikan	73%	(a)
Fairbanks Memorial Hospital[11]	Fairbanks	72%	300+
Mat-Su Regional Medical Center	Palmer	69%	300+
Providence Alaska Medical Center	Anchorage	69%	300+
Alaska Regional Hospital	Anchorage	68%	300+
Bartlett Regional Hospital	Juneau	68%	300+
Central Peninsula General Hospital	Soldotna	66%	300+
Providence Kodiak Island Medical Center	Kodiak	66%	(a)
Alaska Native Medical Center	Anchorage	64%	300+
Yukon Kuskokwim Delta Regional Hospital	Bethel	60%	(a)

Room and Bathroom 'Always' Clean

Hospital Name	City	Rate	Cases
South Peninsula Hospital	Homer	83%	(a)
Providence Kodiak Island Medical Center	Kodiak	81%	(a)
Bartlett Regional Hospital	Juneau	75%	300+
Mat-Su Regional Medical Center	Palmer	75%	300+
Fairbanks Memorial Hospital[11]	Fairbanks	74%	300+
Central Peninsula General Hospital	Soldotna	73%	300+
Peacehealth Ketchikan Medical Center	Ketchikan	71%	(a)
Providence Alaska Medical Center	Anchorage	71%	300+
Alaska Regional Hospital	Anchorage	63%	300+
Yukon Kuskokwim Delta Regional Hospital	Bethel	63%	(a)
Alaska Native Medical Center	Anchorage	60%	300+

Timely Help 'Always' Received

Hospital Name	City	Rate	Cases
Providence Kodiak Island Medical Center	Kodiak	79%	(a)
Peacehealth Ketchikan Medical Center	Ketchikan	77%	(a)
Fairbanks Memorial Hospital[11]	Fairbanks	75%	300+
South Peninsula Hospital	Homer	74%	(a)
Bartlett Regional Hospital	Juneau	70%	300+
Central Peninsula General Hospital	Soldotna	65%	300+

NOTE: Hospital profiles are in alphabetical order by state, then city, then hospital within the city; Rankings exclude hospitals with less than 25 cases except for patient surveys which excludes hospitals with less than 100 cases; (a) 100-299 cases; (1) The number of cases/patients is too few to report; (2) Data submitted were based on a sample of cases/patients; (3) Results are based on a shorter time period than required; (4) Data suppressed by CMS for one or more quarters; (5) Results are not available for this reporting period; (6) Fewer than 100 patients completed the HCAHPS survey; (7) No cases met the criteria for this measure; (8) The lower limit of the confidence interval cannot be calculated if the number of observed infections equals zero; (9) No data are available from the state/territory for this reporting period; (10) The scores shown reflect fewer than 50 completed surveys; (11) There were discrepancies in the data collection process; (12) This measure does not apply to this hospital for this reporting period; (13) Results cannot be calculated for this reporting period; (14) The results for this state are combined with nearby states to protect confidentiality; Please refer to the User's Guide for a full explanation of data.

Hospital Name	City	Rate	Cases
Alaska Native Medical Center	Anchorage	64%	300+
Providence Alaska Medical Center	Anchorage	64%	300+
Yukon Kuskokwim Delta Regional Hospital	Bethel	64%	(a)
Alaska Regional Hospital	Anchorage	62%	300+
Mat-Su Regional Medical Center	Palmer	62%	300+

Would Definitely Recommend Hospital

Hospital Name	City	Rate	Cases
Providence Alaska Medical Center	Anchorage	79%	300+
South Peninsula Hospital	Homer	78%	(a)
Central Peninsula General Hospital	Soldotna	76%	300+
Providence Kodiak Island Medical Center	Kodiak	76%	(a)
Fairbanks Memorial Hospital[11]	Fairbanks	74%	300+
Mat-Su Regional Medical Center	Palmer	71%	300+
Peacehealth Ketchikan Medical Center	Ketchikan	71%	(a)
Alaska Native Medical Center	Anchorage	69%	300+
Bartlett Regional Hospital	Juneau	69%	300+
Alaska Regional Hospital	Anchorage	66%	300+
Yukon Kuskokwim Delta Regional Hospital	Bethel	49%	(a)

Use of Medical Imaging

Cardiac Imaging Stress Test before OP Surgery

Hospital Name	City	Rate	Cases
Bartlett Regional Hospital	Juneau	3.7%	54
Fairbanks Memorial Hospital	Fairbanks	4.1%	317
Central Peninsula General Hospital	Soldotna	5.0%	141
Peacehealth Ketchikan Medical Center	Ketchikan	5.8%	69
Providence Alaska Medical Center	Anchorage	5.8%	69

Combination Abdominal CT Scan

Hospital Name	City	Rate	Cases
South Peninsula Hospital	Homer	3.5%	201
Fairbanks Memorial Hospital	Fairbanks	5.5%	653
Central Peninsula General Hospital	Soldotna	6.4%	388
Providence Alaska Medical Center	Anchorage	6.4%	687
Bartlett Regional Hospital	Juneau	6.6%	196
Alaska Regional Hospital	Anchorage	6.8%	338
Mat-Su Regional Medical Center	Palmer	8.7%	423
Providence Kodiak Island Medical Center	Kodiak	9.5%	74
Peacehealth Ketchikan Medical Center	Ketchikan	11.4%	185

Combination Brain/Sinus CT Scan

Hospital Name	City	Rate	Cases
Bartlett Regional Hospital	Juneau	0.0%	122
Providence Kodiak Island Medical Center	Kodiak	0.0%	39
Alaska Regional Hospital	Anchorage	1.2%	171
Fairbanks Memorial Hospital	Fairbanks	1.3%	372
Providence Alaska Medical Center	Anchorage	1.9%	515

Combination Chest CT Scan

Hospital Name	City	Rate	Cases
Bartlett Regional Hospital	Juneau	0.0%	98
Central Peninsula General Hospital	Soldotna	0.0%	258
Peacehealth Ketchikan Medical Center	Ketchikan	0.0%	131
South Peninsula Hospital	Homer	0.0%	97
Alaska Regional Hospital	Anchorage	0.5%	191
Fairbanks Memorial Hospital	Fairbanks	0.5%	410
Providence Alaska Medical Center	Anchorage	0.8%	377
Mat-Su Regional Medical Center	Palmer	1.7%	172

Follow-up Mammogram/Ultrasound

A follow-up rate near zero may indicate missed cancer; a rate higher than 14% may mean there is unnecessary follow up.

Hospital Name	City	Rate	Cases
Peacehealth Ketchikan Medical Center	Ketchikan	5.2%	213
South Peninsula Hospital	Homer	6.9%	218
Alaska Regional Hospital	Anchorage	7.8%	281
Bartlett Regional Hospital	Juneau	8.0%	452
Fairbanks Memorial Hospital	Fairbanks	8.9%	671
Central Peninsula General Hospital	Soldotna	12.7%	599
Mat-Su Regional Medical Center	Palmer	13.5%	347
Providence Kodiak Island Medical Center	Kodiak	15.3%	98

Lumbar Spine MRI for Low Back Pain

Hospital Name	City	Rate	Cases
Mat-Su Regional Medical Center	Palmer	36.4%	55
Central Peninsula General Hospital	Soldotna	37.2%	137
Providence Alaska Medical Center	Anchorage	45.8%	48
Fairbanks Memorial Hospital	Fairbanks	47.4%	133
Peacehealth Ketchikan Medical Center	Ketchikan	50.0%	40

NOTE: Hospital profiles are in alphabetical order by state, then city, then hospital within the city; Rankings exclude hospitals with less than 25 cases except for patient surveys which excludes hospitals with less than 100 cases; (a) 100-299 cases; (1) The number of cases/patients is too few to report; (2) Data submitted were based on a sample of cases/patients; (3) Results are based on a shorter time period than required; (4) Data suppressed by CMS for one or more quarters; (5) Results are not available for this reporting period; (6) Fewer than 100 patients completed the HCAHPS survey; (7) No cases met the criteria for this measure; (8) The lower limit of the confidence interval cannot be calculated if the number of observed infections equals zero; (9) No data are available from the state/territory for this reporting period; (10) The scores shown reflect fewer than 50 completed surveys; (11) There were discrepancies in the data collection process; (12) This measure does not apply to this hospital for this reporting period; (13) Results cannot be calculated for this reporting period; (14) The results for this state are combined with nearby states to protect confidentiality; Please refer to the User's Guide for a full explanation of data.

Alaska Native Medical Center

4315 Diplomacy Dr
Anchorage, AK 99508
URL: www.anmc.org
Type: Acute Care Hospitals
Ownership: Government - Federal
Phone: 907-563-2662
Fax: 907-729-1984
Emergency Services: Yes
Beds: 150

Key Personnel:
Pediatric In-Patient Care .... Alice Faye Barthalemu
Operating Room.............. Kathy Belanger, RN
Infection Control.............. Carol Bromley
Quality Assurance .... Dawn Carman
Pediatric Ambulatory Care ...... Richard Mandsager
Cardiac Laboratory............ Matt Schenellbacher
Chief of Medical Staff.......... David Snyder, MD

Measure	Cases	This Hosp.	State Avg.	U.S. Avg.
Blood Clot Prevention and Treatment				
Anticoagulation Overlap Therapy[2]	11	100%	97%	93%
ICU Venous Thromboembolism Prophylaxis[2]	66	95%	90%	92%
Incidence of Potentially Preventable VTE[1,2]	-	-	17%	10%
UFH with Dosages/Platelet Monitoring[1,2]	-	-	98%	97%
Venous Thromboembolism Prophylaxis[2]	313	94%	86%	85%
Warfarin Therapy Discharge Instructions[2]	12	100%	80%	75%
Chest Pain/Possible Heart Attack Care				
Aspirin Given Within 24 Hours of Arrival[1,3]	-	-	99%	96%
Fibrinolytic Meds Within 30 Min. of Arrival[3,7]	-	-	92%	58%
Average Time to ECG (minutes)[1,3]	-	-	8	7
Average Time to Transfer (minutes)[3,7]	-	-	220	60
Children's Asthma Care				
Received Home Management Plan of Care	-	-	-	88%
Received Reliever Medication	-	-	-	100%
Received Systemic Corticosteroids	-	-	-	100%
Emergency Department				
Admittance Decision Time (minutes)[2]	400	106	118	98
Head CT Results Within 45 Min. of Arrival[3,7]	-	-	29%	57%
Patients Who Left ER Before Being Seen	57,496	7%	3%	2%
Time from ER Arrival to Admit. (minutes)[2]	422	373	287	274
Time from ER Arrival to Discharge (minutes)	378	156	132	134
Time in ER Before Being Evaluated (minutes)	382	50	24	26
Time to Pain Meds for Fractures (minutes)	138	58	57	57
Heart Attack Care				
Aspirin Given at Discharge	16	100%	100%	99%
Fibrinolytic Meds Within 30 Min. of Arrival[7]	-	-	75%	54%
PCI Within 90 Minutes of Arrival[7]	-	-	94%	96%
Statin Prescribed at Discharge	17	100%	99%	98%
Heart Failure Care				
ACE Inhibitor or ARB for LVSD	48	100%	99%	97%
Discharge Instructions Given	70	100%	94%	94%
Evaluation of LVS Function	73	100%	97%	99%
Medicare Spending				
Medicare Spending per Patient (ratio)	-	0.79	0.91	0.98
Pneumonia Care				
Appropriate Initial Antibiotic Given	104	90%	93%	95%
Blood Culture Timing	164	94%	97%	98%
Pregnancy and Delivery Care				
Newborn Deliveries Scheduled Early[2]	12	0%	2%	6%
Preventive Care				
Immunization for Influenza[2]	557	65%	83%	90%
Immunization for Pneumonia[2]	352	84%	90%	92%
Stroke Care				
Anticoagulation Therapy for Atrial Fibrillation[1]	-	-	80%	95%
Antithrombotic Therapy Timing	55	98%	99%	98%
Assessed for Rehabilitation	79	100%	97%	97%
Discharged on Antithrombotic Therapy	64	100%	98%	99%
Discharged on Statin Medication	51	100%	93%	94%
Thrombolytic Therapy Timing[1]	-	-	69%	66%
Venous Thromboembolism Prophylaxis	83	98%	93%	94%
Written Stroke Educational Materials Given	54	100%	92%	88%
Surgical Care Improvement Project				
Appropriate Beta Blocker Usage[2]	91	95%	96%	98%
Appropriate VTP Within 24 Hours[2]	373	97%	97%	98%
Controlled Postoperative Blood Glucose[2,7]	-	-	95%	97%
Perioperative Temperature Management[2]	432	99%	99%	100%
Prophylactic Antibiotic Selection[2]	282	99%	99%	99%
Prophylactic Antibiotic Selection (Outpatient)	33	94%	99%	98%
Prophylactic Antibiotic Stopped[2]	280	100%	99%	98%
Prophylactic Antibiotic Timing[2]	282	98%	99%	99%
Prophylactic Antibiotic Timing (Outpatient)	37	86%	97%	98%
Urinary Catheter Removal[2]	78	97%	97%	97%
Survey of Patients' Hospital Experiences				
Area Around Room 'Always' Quiet at Night	300+	51%	59%	61%
Doctors 'Always' Communicated Well	300+	76%	82%	82%
Home Recovery Information Given	300+	86%	87%	85%
Hospital Given 9 or 10 on 10 Point Scale	300+	65%	67%	71%
Meds 'Always' Explained Before Given	300+	64%	67%	64%
Nurses 'Always' Communicated Well	300+	73%	77%	79%
Pain 'Always' Well Controlled	300+	64%	68%	71%
Room and Bathroom 'Always' Clean	300+	60%	72%	73%
Timely Help 'Always' Received	300+	64%	71%	68%
Would Definitely Recommend Hospital	300+	69%	69%	71%
Use of Medical Imaging				
Cardiac Imaging Stress Test before Surgery[7]	-	-	4.5%	5.3%
Combination Abdominal CT Scan[7]	-	-	6.9%	10.5%
Combination Brain/Sinus CT Scan[7]	-	-	1.6%	2.7%
Combination Chest CT Scan[7]	-	-	0.8%	2.7%
Follow-up Mammogram/Ultrasound[7]	-	-	9.5%	8.8%
Lumbar Spine MRI for Low Back Pain[7]	-	-	44.4%	37.2%

Alaska Regional Hospital

2801 Debarr Road
Anchorage, AK 99508
URL: www.alaskaregional.com
Type: Acute Care Hospitals
Ownership: Proprietary
Phone: 907-276-1131
Fax: 907-264-1143
Emergency Services: Yes
Beds: 250

Key Personnel:
Chief of Medical Staff.......... David Cadogan, MD
Quality Assurance .... Rosemary Craig
Emergency Room .... Robin Richardson
CEO .... Julie Taylor

Measure	Cases	This Hosp.	State Avg.	U.S. Avg.
Blood Clot Prevention and Treatment				
Anticoagulation Overlap Therapy[2]	23	100%	97%	93%
ICU Venous Thromboembolism Prophylaxis[2]	83	98%	90%	92%
Incidence of Potentially Preventable VTE[2]	13	8%	17%	10%
UFH with Dosages/Platelet Monitoring[1,2]	-	-	98%	97%
Venous Thromboembolism Prophylaxis[2]	243	91%	86%	85%
Warfarin Therapy Discharge Instructions[2]	17	59%	80%	75%
Chest Pain/Possible Heart Attack Care				
Aspirin Given Within 24 Hours of Arrival[1,3]	-	-	99%	96%
Fibrinolytic Meds Within 30 Min. of Arrival[3,7]	-	-	92%	58%
Average Time to ECG (minutes)[1,3]	-	-	8	7
Average Time to Transfer (minutes)[3,7]	-	-	220	60
Children's Asthma Care				
Received Home Management Plan of Care	-	-	-	88%
Received Reliever Medication	-	-	-	100%
Received Systemic Corticosteroids	-	-	-	100%
Emergency Department				
Admittance Decision Time (minutes)[2]	377	99	118	98
Head CT Results Within 45 Min. of Arrival[3,7]	-	-	29%	57%
Patients Who Left ER Before Being Seen	26,028	0%	3%	2%
Time from ER Arrival to Admit. (minutes)[2]	378	246	287	274
Time from ER Arrival to Discharge (minutes)	414	100	132	134
Time in ER Before Being Evaluated (minutes)	436	17	24	26
Time to Pain Meds for Fractures (minutes)	57	54	57	57
Heart Attack Care				
Aspirin Given at Discharge	143	100%	100%	99%
Fibrinolytic Meds Within 30 Min. of Arrival[7]	-	-	75%	54%
PCI Within 90 Minutes of Arrival	16	94%	94%	96%
Statin Prescribed at Discharge	142	99%	99%	98%
Heart Failure Care				
ACE Inhibitor or ARB for LVSD	28	100%	99%	97%
Discharge Instructions Given	68	97%	94%	94%
Evaluation of LVS Function	69	100%	97%	99%
Medicare Spending				
Medicare Spending per Patient (ratio)	-	0.85	0.91	0.98
Pneumonia Care				
Appropriate Initial Antibiotic Given	30	100%	93%	95%
Blood Culture Timing	40	100%	97%	98%
Pregnancy and Delivery Care				
Newborn Deliveries Scheduled Early	48	2%	2%	6%
Preventive Care				
Immunization for Influenza[2]	527	94%	83%	90%
Immunization for Pneumonia[2]	541	95%	90%	92%
Stroke Care				
Anticoagulation Therapy for Atrial Fibrillation[1,2]	-	-	80%	95%
Antithrombotic Therapy Timing[2]	38	100%	99%	98%
Assessed for Rehabilitation[2]	55	100%	97%	97%
Discharged on Antithrombotic Therapy[2]	43	100%	98%	99%
Discharged on Statin Medication[2]	30	93%	93%	94%
Thrombolytic Therapy Timing[1,2]	-	-	69%	66%
Venous Thromboembolism Prophylaxis[2]	58	97%	93%	94%
Written Stroke Educational Materials Given[2]	39	82%	92%	88%
Surgical Care Improvement Project				
Appropriate Beta Blocker Usage[2]	182	97%	96%	98%
Appropriate VTP Within 24 Hours[2]	414	99%	97%	98%
Controlled Postoperative Blood Glucose[2]	95	89%	95%	97%
Perioperative Temperature Management[2]	515	100%	99%	100%
Prophylactic Antibiotic Selection[2]	405	99%	99%	99%
Prophylactic Antibiotic Selection (Outpatient)	228	98%	99%	98%
Prophylactic Antibiotic Stopped[2]	393	99%	99%	98%
Prophylactic Antibiotic Timing[2]	405	100%	99%	99%
Prophylactic Antibiotic Timing (Outpatient)	232	97%	97%	98%
Urinary Catheter Removal[2]	359	97%	97%	97%
Survey of Patients' Hospital Experiences				
Area Around Room 'Always' Quiet at Night	300+	59%	59%	61%
Doctors 'Always' Communicated Well	300+	77%	82%	82%
Home Recovery Information Given	300+	86%	87%	85%
Hospital Given 9 or 10 on 10 Point Scale	300+	64%	67%	71%
Meds 'Always' Explained Before Given	300+	62%	67%	64%
Nurses 'Always' Communicated Well	300+	73%	77%	79%
Pain 'Always' Well Controlled	300+	68%	68%	71%
Room and Bathroom 'Always' Clean	300+	63%	72%	73%
Timely Help 'Always' Received	300+	62%	71%	68%
Would Definitely Recommend Hospital	300+	66%	69%	71%
Use of Medical Imaging				
Cardiac Imaging Stress Test before Surgery[1]	-	-	4.5%	5.3%
Combination Abdominal CT Scan	338	6.8%	6.9%	10.5%
Combination Brain/Sinus CT Scan	171	1.2%	1.6%	2.7%
Combination Chest CT Scan	191	0.5%	0.8%	2.7%
Follow-up Mammogram/Ultrasound	281	7.8%	9.5%	8.8%
Lumbar Spine MRI for Low Back Pain[1]	-	-	44.4%	37.2%

Providence Alaska Medical Center

Box 196604
Anchorage, AK 99519
URL: www.providence.org
Type: Acute Care Hospitals
Ownership: Voluntary non-profit - Private
Phone: 907-261-3675
Fax: 907-261-3041
Emergency Services: Yes
Beds: 293

Key Personnel:
Radiology.................. Denise Farleigh, MD
Pediatric Ambulatory Care...... John Lyon, MD
Pediatric In-Patient Care .... John Lyon, MD
Quality Assurance .... Penny Meador
CEO/President............... Al Parrish
Operating Room.............. Diane Schack

Measure	Cases	This Hosp.	State Avg.	U.S. Avg.
Blood Clot Prevention and Treatment				
Anticoagulation Overlap Therapy[2]	62	98%	97%	93%
ICU Venous Thromboembolism Prophylaxis[2]	111	93%	90%	92%
Incidence of Potentially Preventable VTE[2]	20	25%	17%	10%
UFH with Dosages/Platelet Monitoring[2]	24	100%	98%	97%
Venous Thromboembolism Prophylaxis[2]	308	86%	86%	85%
Warfarin Therapy Discharge Instructions[2]	50	84%	80%	75%
Chest Pain/Possible Heart Attack Care				
Aspirin Given Within 24 Hours of Arrival[3,7]	-	-	99%	96%
Fibrinolytic Meds Within 30 Min. of Arrival[5]	-	-	92%	58%
Average Time to ECG (minutes)[3,7]	-	-	8	7
Average Time to Transfer (minutes)[5]	-	-	220	60
Children's Asthma Care				
Received Home Management Plan of Care	-	-	-	88%
Received Reliever Medication	-	-	-	100%
Received Systemic Corticosteroids	-	-	-	100%

NOTE: Hospital profiles are in alphabetical order by state, then city, then hospital within the city; Rankings exclude hospitals with less than 25 cases except for patient surveys which excludes hospitals with less than 100 cases; (a) 100-299 cases; (1) The number of cases/patients is too few to report; (2) Data submitted were based on a sample of cases/patients; (3) Results are based on a shorter time period than required; (4) Data suppressed by CMS for one or more quarters; (5) Results are not available for this reporting period; (6) Fewer than 100 patients completed the HCAHPS survey; (7) No cases met the criteria for this measure; (8) The lower limit of the confidence interval cannot be calculated if the number of observed infections equals zero; (9) No data are available from the state/territory for this reporting period; (10) The scores shown reflect fewer than 50 completed surveys; (11) There were discrepancies in the data collection process; (12) This measure does not apply to this hospital for this reporting period; (13) Results cannot be calculated for this reporting period; (14) The results for this state are combined with nearby states to protect confidentiality; Please refer to the User's Guide for a full explanation of data.

Measure	Cases	This Hosp.	State Avg.	U.S. Avg.
Emergency Department				
Admittance Decision Time (minutes)[2]	499	280	118	98
Head CT Results Within 45 Min. of Arrival	11	18%	29%	57%
Patients Who Left ER Before Being Seen	63,947	2%	3%	2%
Time from ER Arrival to Admit. (minutes)[2]	504	375	287	274
Time from ER Arrival to Discharge (minutes)	375	134	132	134
Time in ER Before Being Evaluated (minutes)	277	20	24	26
Time to Pain Meds for Fractures (minutes)	191	66	57	57
Heart Attack Care				
Aspirin Given at Discharge	364	100%	100%	99%
Fibrinolytic Meds Within 30 Min. of Arrival[7]	-	-	75%	54%
PCI Within 90 Minutes of Arrival	46	93%	94%	96%
Statin Prescribed at Discharge	361	99%	99%	98%
Heart Failure Care				
ACE Inhibitor or ARB for LVSD	144	100%	99%	97%
Discharge Instructions Given	300	100%	94%	94%
Evaluation of LVS Function	307	100%	97%	99%
Medicare Spending				
Medicare Spending per Patient (ratio)	-	0.85	0.91	0.98
Pneumonia Care				
Appropriate Initial Antibiotic Given	160	98%	93%	95%
Blood Culture Timing	228	100%	97%	98%
Pregnancy and Delivery Care				
Newborn Deliveries Scheduled Early[2]	46	2%	2%	6%
Preventive Care				
Immunization for Influenza[2]	531	80%	83%	90%
Immunization for Pneumonia[2]	467	87%	90%	92%
Stroke Care				
Anticoagulation Therapy for Atrial Fibrillation	19	63%	80%	95%
Antithrombotic Therapy Timing	122	98%	99%	98%
Assessed for Rehabilitation	161	94%	97%	97%
Discharged on Antithrombotic Therapy	138	98%	98%	99%
Discharged on Statin Medication	116	93%	93%	94%
Thrombolytic Therapy Timing	11	64%	69%	66%
Venous Thromboembolism Prophylaxis	156	92%	93%	94%
Written Stroke Educational Materials Given	118	97%	92%	88%
Surgical Care Improvement Project				
Appropriate Beta Blocker Usage[2]	172	97%	96%	98%
Appropriate VTP Within 24 Hours[2]	338	99%	97%	98%
Controlled Postoperative Blood Glucose[2]	146	98%	95%	97%
Perioperative Temperature Management[2]	437	100%	99%	100%
Prophylactic Antibiotic Selection[2]	439	98%	99%	99%
Prophylactic Antibiotic Selection (Outpatient)	512	99%	99%	98%
Prophylactic Antibiotic Stopped[2]	427	98%	99%	98%
Prophylactic Antibiotic Timing[2]	441	98%	99%	99%
Prophylactic Antibiotic Timing (Outpatient)	516	97%	97%	98%
Urinary Catheter Removal[2]	297	98%	97%	97%
Survey of Patients' Hospital Experiences				
Area Around Room 'Always' Quiet at Night	300+	55%	59%	61%
Doctors 'Always' Communicated Well	300+	80%	82%	82%
Home Recovery Information Given	300+	88%	87%	85%
Hospital Given 9 or 10 on 10 Point Scale	300+	73%	67%	71%
Meds 'Always' Explained Before Given	300+	61%	67%	64%
Nurses 'Always' Communicated Well	300+	76%	77%	79%
Pain 'Always' Well Controlled	300+	69%	68%	71%
Room and Bathroom 'Always' Clean	300+	71%	72%	73%
Timely Help 'Always' Received	300+	64%	71%	68%
Would Definitely Recommend Hospital	300+	79%	69%	71%
Use of Medical Imaging				
Cardiac Imaging Stress Test before Surgery	69	5.8%	4.5%	5.3%
Combination Abdominal CT Scan	687	6.4%	6.9%	10.5%
Combination Brain/Sinus CT Scan	515	1.9%	1.6%	2.7%
Combination Chest CT Scan	377	0.8%	0.8%	2.7%
Follow-up Mammogram/Ultrasound[7]	-	-	9.5%	8.8%
Lumbar Spine MRI for Low Back Pain	48	45.8%	44.4%	37.2%

Samuel Simmonds Memorial Hospital

PO Box 29
Barrow, AK 99723
Phone: 907-852-4611
Type: Critical Access Hospitals
Emergency Services: Yes
Ownership: Government - Federal

Measure	Cases	This Hosp.	State Avg.	U.S. Avg.
Blood Clot Prevention and Treatment				
Anticoagulation Overlap Therapy[5]	-	-	97%	93%
ICU Venous Thromboembolism Prophylaxis[5]	-	-	90%	92%
Incidence of Potentially Preventable VTE[5]	-	-	17%	10%
UFH with Dosages/Platelet Monitoring[5]	-	-	98%	97%
Venous Thromboembolism Prophylaxis[5]	-	-	86%	85%
Warfarin Therapy Discharge Instructions[5]	-	-	80%	75%
Chest Pain/Possible Heart Attack Care				
Aspirin Given Within 24 Hours of Arrival	-	-	99%	96%
Fibrinolytic Meds Within 30 Min. of Arrival	-	-	92%	58%
Average Time to ECG (minutes)	-	-	8	7
Average Time to Transfer (minutes)	-	-	220	60
Children's Asthma Care				
Received Home Management Plan of Care	-	-	-	88%
Received Reliever Medication	-	-	-	100%
Received Systemic Corticosteroids	-	-	-	100%
Emergency Department				
Admittance Decision Time (minutes)[5]	-	-	118	98
Head CT Results Within 45 Min. of Arrival	-	-	29%	57%
Patients Who Left ER Before Being Seen	-	-	3%	2%
Time from ER Arrival to Admit. (minutes)[5]	-	-	287	274
Time from ER Arrival to Discharge (minutes)	-	-	132	134
Time in ER Before Being Evaluated (minutes)	-	-	24	26
Time to Pain Meds for Fractures (minutes)	-	-	57	57
Heart Attack Care				
Aspirin Given at Discharge[5]	-	-	100%	99%
Fibrinolytic Meds Within 30 Min. of Arrival[5]	-	-	75%	54%
PCI Within 90 Minutes of Arrival[5]	-	-	94%	96%
Statin Prescribed at Discharge[5]	-	-	99%	98%
Heart Failure Care				
ACE Inhibitor or ARB for LVSD[3,7]	-	-	99%	97%
Discharge Instructions Given[1,3]	-	-	94%	94%
Evaluation of LVS Function[1,3]	-	-	97%	99%
Medicare Spending				
Medicare Spending per Patient (ratio)	-	-	0.91	0.98
Pneumonia Care				
Appropriate Initial Antibiotic Given[1,3]	-	-	93%	95%
Blood Culture Timing[1,3]	-	-	97%	98%
Pregnancy and Delivery Care				
Newborn Deliveries Scheduled Early[5]	-	-	2%	6%
Preventive Care				
Immunization for Influenza[5]	-	-	83%	90%
Immunization for Pneumonia[5]	-	-	90%	92%
Stroke Care				
Anticoagulation Therapy for Atrial Fibrillation[5]	-	-	80%	95%
Antithrombotic Therapy Timing[5]	-	-	99%	98%
Assessed for Rehabilitation[5]	-	-	97%	97%
Discharged on Antithrombotic Therapy[5]	-	-	98%	99%
Discharged on Statin Medication[5]	-	-	93%	94%
Thrombolytic Therapy Timing[5]	-	-	69%	66%
Venous Thromboembolism Prophylaxis[5]	-	-	93%	94%
Written Stroke Educational Materials Given[5]	-	-	92%	88%
Surgical Care Improvement Project				
Appropriate Beta Blocker Usage[5]	-	-	96%	98%
Appropriate VTP Within 24 Hours[5]	-	-	97%	98%
Controlled Postoperative Blood Glucose[5]	-	-	95%	97%
Perioperative Temperature Management[5]	-	-	99%	100%
Prophylactic Antibiotic Selection[5]	-	-	99%	99%
Prophylactic Antibiotic Selection (Outpatient)	-	-	99%	98%
Prophylactic Antibiotic Stopped[5]	-	-	99%	98%
Prophylactic Antibiotic Timing[5]	-	-	99%	99%
Prophylactic Antibiotic Timing (Outpatient)	-	-	97%	98%
Urinary Catheter Removal[5]	-	-	97%	97%
Survey of Patients' Hospital Experiences				
Area Around Room 'Always' Quiet at Night[5]	-	-	59%	61%
Doctors 'Always' Communicated Well[5]	-	-	82%	82%
Home Recovery Information Given[5]	-	-	87%	85%
Hospital Given 9 or 10 on 10 Point Scale[5]	-	-	67%	71%
Meds 'Always' Explained Before Given[5]	-	-	67%	64%
Nurses 'Always' Communicated Well[5]	-	-	77%	79%
Pain 'Always' Well Controlled[5]	-	-	68%	71%
Room and Bathroom 'Always' Clean[5]	-	-	72%	73%
Timely Help 'Always' Received[5]	-	-	71%	68%
Would Definitely Recommend Hospital[5]	-	-	69%	71%
Use of Medical Imaging				
Cardiac Imaging Stress Test before Surgery	-	-	4.5%	5.3%
Combination Abdominal CT Scan	-	-	6.9%	10.5%
Combination Brain/Sinus CT Scan	-	-	1.6%	2.7%
Combination Chest CT Scan	-	-	0.8%	2.7%
Follow-up Mammogram/Ultrasound	-	-	9.5%	8.8%
Lumbar Spine MRI for Low Back Pain	-	-	44.4%	37.2%

Yukon Kuskokwim Delta Regional Hospital

PO Box 287
Bethel, AK 99559
Phone: 907-543-6300
Fax: 907-543-6366
E-mail: info@ykhc.org
URL: www.ykhc.org
Type: Acute Care Hospitals
Emergency Services: Yes
Ownership: Government - Federal
Beds: 50

Key Personnel:
Operating Room. . . . . Ardean Selby
CEO/President. . . . . Dan Winkelman

Measure	Cases	This Hosp.	State Avg.	U.S. Avg.
Blood Clot Prevention and Treatment				
Anticoagulation Overlap Therapy[2,7]	-	-	97%	93%
ICU Venous Thromboembolism Prophylaxis[1,2]	-	-	90%	92%
Incidence of Potentially Preventable VTE[2,7]	-	-	17%	10%
UFH with Dosages/Platelet Monitoring[2,7]	-	-	98%	97%
Venous Thromboembolism Prophylaxis[2]	158	90%	86%	85%
Warfarin Therapy Discharge Instructions[2,7]	-	-	80%	75%
Chest Pain/Possible Heart Attack Care				
Aspirin Given Within 24 Hours of Arrival	-	-	99%	96%
Fibrinolytic Meds Within 30 Min. of Arrival	-	-	92%	58%
Average Time to ECG (minutes)	-	-	8	7
Average Time to Transfer (minutes)	-	-	220	60
Children's Asthma Care				
Received Home Management Plan of Care	-	-	-	88%
Received Reliever Medication	-	-	-	100%
Received Systemic Corticosteroids	-	-	-	100%
Emergency Department				
Admittance Decision Time (minutes)[2]	223	97	118	98
Head CT Results Within 45 Min. of Arrival	-	-	29%	57%
Patients Who Left ER Before Being Seen	-	-	3%	2%
Time from ER Arrival to Admit. (minutes)[2]	364	384	287	274
Time from ER Arrival to Discharge (minutes)	-	-	132	134
Time in ER Before Being Evaluated (minutes)	-	-	24	26
Time to Pain Meds for Fractures (minutes)	-	-	57	57
Heart Attack Care				
Aspirin Given at Discharge[5]	-	-	100%	99%
Fibrinolytic Meds Within 30 Min. of Arrival[5]	-	-	75%	54%
PCI Within 90 Minutes of Arrival[5]	-	-	94%	96%
Statin Prescribed at Discharge[5]	-	-	99%	98%
Heart Failure Care				
ACE Inhibitor or ARB for LVSD	16	100%	99%	97%
Discharge Instructions Given	38	63%	94%	94%
Evaluation of LVS Function	38	97%	97%	99%
Medicare Spending				
Medicare Spending per Patient (ratio)	-	0.59	0.91	0.98
Pneumonia Care				
Appropriate Initial Antibiotic Given	35	86%	93%	95%
Blood Culture Timing	31	87%	97%	98%
Pregnancy and Delivery Care				
Newborn Deliveries Scheduled Early	17	0%	2%	6%
Preventive Care				
Immunization for Influenza[2]	279	52%	83%	90%
Immunization for Pneumonia[2]	193	87%	90%	92%
Stroke Care				
Anticoagulation Therapy for Atrial Fibrillation[5]	-	-	80%	95%
Antithrombotic Therapy Timing[5]	-	-	99%	98%
Assessed for Rehabilitation[5]	-	-	97%	97%
Discharged on Antithrombotic Therapy[5]	-	-	98%	99%
Discharged on Statin Medication[5]	-	-	93%	94%
Thrombolytic Therapy Timing[5]	-	-	69%	66%
Venous Thromboembolism Prophylaxis[5]	-	-	93%	94%
Written Stroke Educational Materials Given[5]	-	-	92%	88%

NOTE: Hospital profiles are in alphabetical order by state, then city, then hospital within the city; Rankings exclude hospitals with less than 25 cases except for patient surveys which excludes hospitals with less than 100 cases; (a) 100-299 cases; (1) The number of cases/patients is too few to report; (2) Data submitted were based on a sample of cases/patients; (3) Results are based on a shorter time period than required; (4) Data suppressed by CMS for one or more quarters; (5) Results are not available for this reporting period; (6) Fewer than 100 patients completed the HCAHPS survey; (7) No cases met the criteria for this measure; (8) The lower limit of the confidence interval cannot be calculated if the number of observed infections equals zero; (9) No data are available from the state/territory for this reporting period; (10) The scores shown reflect fewer than 50 completed surveys; (11) There were discrepancies in the data collection process; (12) This measure does not apply to this hospital for this reporting period; (13) Results cannot be calculated for this reporting period; (14) The results for this state are combined with nearby states to protect confidentiality; Please refer to the User's Guide for a full explanation of data.

Measure	Cases	This Hosp.	State Avg.	U.S. Avg.
Surgical Care Improvement Project				
Appropriate Beta Blocker Usage[5]	-	-	96%	98%
Appropriate VTP Within 24 Hours[5]	-	-	97%	98%
Controlled Postoperative Blood Glucose[5]	-	-	95%	97%
Perioperative Temperature Management[5]	-	-	99%	100%
Prophylactic Antibiotic Selection[5]	-	-	99%	99%
Prophylactic Antibiotic Selection (Outpatient)	-	-	99%	98%
Prophylactic Antibiotic Stopped[5]	-	-	99%	98%
Prophylactic Antibiotic Timing[5]	-	-	99%	99%
Prophylactic Antibiotic Timing (Outpatient)	-	-	97%	98%
Urinary Catheter Removal[5]	-	-	97%	97%
Survey of Patients' Hospital Experiences				
Area Around Room 'Always' Quiet at Night	(a)	53%	59%	61%
Doctors 'Always' Communicated Well	(a)	75%	82%	82%
Home Recovery Information Given	(a)	77%	87%	85%
Hospital Given 9 or 10 on 10 Point Scale	(a)	49%	67%	71%
Meds 'Always' Explained Before Given	(a)	68%	67%	64%
Nurses 'Always' Communicated Well	(a)	69%	77%	79%
Pain 'Always' Well Controlled	(a)	60%	68%	71%
Room and Bathroom 'Always' Clean	(a)	63%	72%	73%
Timely Help 'Always' Received	(a)	64%	71%	68%
Would Definitely Recommend Hospital	(a)	49%	69%	71%
Use of Medical Imaging				
Cardiac Imaging Stress Test before Surgery	-	-	4.5%	5.3%
Combination Abdominal CT Scan	-	-	6.9%	10.5%
Combination Brain/Sinus CT Scan	-	-	1.6%	2.7%
Combination Chest CT Scan	-	-	0.8%	2.7%
Follow-up Mammogram/Ultrasound	-	-	9.5%	8.8%
Lumbar Spine MRI for Low Back Pain	-	-	44.4%	37.2%

Cordova Community Medical Center

PO Box 160 - 602 Chase Avenue
Cordova, AK 99574
Phone: 907-424-8000
Type: Critical Access Hospitals
Emergency Services: Yes
Ownership: Government - Local

Measure	Cases	This Hosp.	State Avg.	U.S. Avg.
Blood Clot Prevention and Treatment				
Anticoagulation Overlap Therapy[5]	-	-	97%	93%
ICU Venous Thromboembolism Prophylaxis[5]	-	-	90%	92%
Incidence of Potentially Preventable VTE[5]	-	-	17%	10%
UFH with Dosages/Platelet Monitoring[5]	-	-	98%	97%
Venous Thromboembolism Prophylaxis[5]	-	-	86%	85%
Warfarin Therapy Discharge Instructions[5]	-	-	80%	75%
Chest Pain/Possible Heart Attack Care				
Aspirin Given Within 24 Hours of Arrival	-	-	99%	96%
Fibrinolytic Meds Within 30 Min. of Arrival	-	-	92%	58%
Average Time to ECG (minutes)	-	-	8	7
Average Time to Transfer (minutes)	-	-	220	60
Children's Asthma Care				
Received Home Management Plan of Care	-	-	-	88%
Received Reliever Medication	-	-	-	100%
Received Systemic Corticosteroids	-	-	-	100%
Emergency Department				
Admittance Decision Time (minutes)[5]	-	-	118	98
Head CT Results Within 45 Min. of Arrival	-	-	29%	57%
Patients Who Left ER Before Being Seen	-	-	3%	2%
Time from ER Arrival to Admit. (minutes)[5]	-	-	287	274
Time from ER Arrival to Discharge (minutes)	-	-	132	134
Time in ER Before Being Evaluated (minutes)	-	-	24	26
Time to Pain Meds for Fractures (minutes)	-	-	57	57
Heart Attack Care				
Aspirin Given at Discharge[5]	-	-	100%	99%
Fibrinolytic Meds Within 30 Min. of Arrival[5]	-	-	75%	54%
PCI Within 90 Minutes of Arrival[5]	-	-	94%	96%
Statin Prescribed at Discharge[5]	-	-	99%	98%
Heart Failure Care				
ACE Inhibitor or ARB for LVSD[3,7]	-	-	99%	97%
Discharge Instructions Given[3,7]	-	-	94%	94%
Evaluation of LVS Function[3,7]	-	-	97%	99%
Medicare Spending				
Medicare Spending per Patient (ratio)	-	-	0.91	0.98
Pneumonia Care				
Appropriate Initial Antibiotic Given[5]	-	-	93%	95%
Blood Culture Timing[5]	-	-	97%	98%
Pregnancy and Delivery Care				
Newborn Deliveries Scheduled Early[5]	-	-	2%	6%
Preventive Care				
Immunization for Influenza[5]	-	-	83%	90%
Immunization for Pneumonia[5]	-	-	90%	92%
Stroke Care				
Anticoagulation Therapy for Atrial Fibrillation[5]	-	-	80%	95%
Antithrombotic Therapy Timing[5]	-	-	99%	98%
Assessed for Rehabilitation[5]	-	-	97%	97%
Discharged on Antithrombotic Therapy[5]	-	-	98%	99%
Discharged on Statin Medication[5]	-	-	93%	94%
Thrombolytic Therapy Timing[5]	-	-	69%	66%
Venous Thromboembolism Prophylaxis[5]	-	-	93%	94%
Written Stroke Educational Materials Given[5]	-	-	92%	88%
Surgical Care Improvement Project				
Appropriate Beta Blocker Usage[5]	-	-	96%	98%
Appropriate VTP Within 24 Hours[5]	-	-	97%	98%
Controlled Postoperative Blood Glucose[5]	-	-	95%	97%
Perioperative Temperature Management[5]	-	-	99%	100%
Prophylactic Antibiotic Selection[5]	-	-	99%	99%
Prophylactic Antibiotic Selection (Outpatient)	-	-	99%	98%
Prophylactic Antibiotic Stopped[5]	-	-	99%	98%
Prophylactic Antibiotic Timing[5]	-	-	99%	99%
Prophylactic Antibiotic Timing (Outpatient)	-	-	97%	98%
Urinary Catheter Removal[5]	-	-	97%	97%
Survey of Patients' Hospital Experiences				
Area Around Room 'Always' Quiet at Night[5]	-	-	59%	61%
Doctors 'Always' Communicated Well[5]	-	-	82%	82%
Home Recovery Information Given[5]	-	-	87%	85%
Hospital Given 9 or 10 on 10 Point Scale[5]	-	-	67%	71%
Meds 'Always' Explained Before Given[5]	-	-	67%	64%
Nurses 'Always' Communicated Well[5]	-	-	77%	79%
Pain 'Always' Well Controlled[5]	-	-	68%	71%
Room and Bathroom 'Always' Clean[5]	-	-	72%	73%
Timely Help 'Always' Received[5]	-	-	71%	68%
Would Definitely Recommend Hospital[5]	-	-	69%	71%
Use of Medical Imaging				
Cardiac Imaging Stress Test before Surgery	-	-	4.5%	5.3%
Combination Abdominal CT Scan	-	-	6.9%	10.5%
Combination Brain/Sinus CT Scan	-	-	1.6%	2.7%
Combination Chest CT Scan	-	-	0.8%	2.7%
Follow-up Mammogram/Ultrasound	-	-	9.5%	8.8%
Lumbar Spine MRI for Low Back Pain	-	-	44.4%	37.2%

Kanakanak Hospital

PO Box 130
Dillingham, AK 99576
Phone: 907-842-5201
Type: Critical Access Hospitals
Emergency Services: Yes
Ownership: Voluntary non-profit - Private

Measure	Cases	This Hosp.	State Avg.	U.S. Avg.
Blood Clot Prevention and Treatment				
Anticoagulation Overlap Therapy[5]	-	-	97%	93%
ICU Venous Thromboembolism Prophylaxis[5]	-	-	90%	92%
Incidence of Potentially Preventable VTE[5]	-	-	17%	10%
UFH with Dosages/Platelet Monitoring[5]	-	-	98%	97%
Venous Thromboembolism Prophylaxis[5]	-	-	86%	85%
Warfarin Therapy Discharge Instructions[5]	-	-	80%	75%
Chest Pain/Possible Heart Attack Care				
Aspirin Given Within 24 Hours of Arrival	-	-	99%	96%
Fibrinolytic Meds Within 30 Min. of Arrival	-	-	92%	58%
Average Time to ECG (minutes)	-	-	8	7
Average Time to Transfer (minutes)	-	-	220	60
Children's Asthma Care				
Received Home Management Plan of Care	-	-	-	88%
Received Reliever Medication	-	-	-	100%
Received Systemic Corticosteroids	-	-	-	100%
Emergency Department				
Admittance Decision Time (minutes)[5]	-	-	118	98
Head CT Results Within 45 Min. of Arrival	-	-	29%	57%
Patients Who Left ER Before Being Seen	-	-	3%	2%
Time from ER Arrival to Admit. (minutes)[5]	-	-	287	274
Time from ER Arrival to Discharge (minutes)	-	-	132	134
Time in ER Before Being Evaluated (minutes)	-	-	24	26
Time to Pain Meds for Fractures (minutes)	-	-	57	57
Heart Attack Care				
Aspirin Given at Discharge[5]	-	-	100%	99%
Fibrinolytic Meds Within 30 Min. of Arrival[5]	-	-	75%	54%
PCI Within 90 Minutes of Arrival[5]	-	-	94%	96%
Statin Prescribed at Discharge[5]	-	-	99%	98%
Heart Failure Care				
ACE Inhibitor or ARB for LVSD[3,7]	-	-	99%	97%
Discharge Instructions Given[1,3]	-	-	94%	94%
Evaluation of LVS Function[1,3]	-	-	97%	99%
Medicare Spending				
Medicare Spending per Patient (ratio)	-	-	0.91	0.98
Pneumonia Care				
Appropriate Initial Antibiotic Given[1,3]	-	-	93%	95%
Blood Culture Timing[1,3]	-	-	97%	98%
Pregnancy and Delivery Care				
Newborn Deliveries Scheduled Early[5]	-	-	2%	6%
Preventive Care				
Immunization for Influenza[5]	-	-	83%	90%
Immunization for Pneumonia[5]	-	-	90%	92%
Stroke Care				
Anticoagulation Therapy for Atrial Fibrillation[5]	-	-	80%	95%
Antithrombotic Therapy Timing[5]	-	-	99%	98%
Assessed for Rehabilitation[5]	-	-	97%	97%
Discharged on Antithrombotic Therapy[5]	-	-	98%	99%
Discharged on Statin Medication[5]	-	-	93%	94%
Thrombolytic Therapy Timing[5]	-	-	69%	66%
Venous Thromboembolism Prophylaxis[5]	-	-	93%	94%
Written Stroke Educational Materials Given[5]	-	-	92%	88%
Surgical Care Improvement Project				
Appropriate Beta Blocker Usage[5]	-	-	96%	98%
Appropriate VTP Within 24 Hours[5]	-	-	97%	98%
Controlled Postoperative Blood Glucose[5]	-	-	95%	97%
Perioperative Temperature Management[5]	-	-	99%	100%
Prophylactic Antibiotic Selection[5]	-	-	99%	99%
Prophylactic Antibiotic Selection (Outpatient)	-	-	99%	98%
Prophylactic Antibiotic Stopped[5]	-	-	99%	98%
Prophylactic Antibiotic Timing[5]	-	-	99%	99%
Prophylactic Antibiotic Timing (Outpatient)	-	-	97%	98%
Urinary Catheter Removal[5]	-	-	97%	97%
Survey of Patients' Hospital Experiences				
Area Around Room 'Always' Quiet at Night[5]	-	-	59%	61%
Doctors 'Always' Communicated Well[5]	-	-	82%	82%
Home Recovery Information Given[5]	-	-	87%	85%
Hospital Given 9 or 10 on 10 Point Scale[5]	-	-	67%	71%
Meds 'Always' Explained Before Given[5]	-	-	67%	64%
Nurses 'Always' Communicated Well[5]	-	-	77%	79%
Pain 'Always' Well Controlled[5]	-	-	68%	71%
Room and Bathroom 'Always' Clean[5]	-	-	72%	73%
Timely Help 'Always' Received[5]	-	-	71%	68%
Would Definitely Recommend Hospital[5]	-	-	69%	71%
Use of Medical Imaging				
Cardiac Imaging Stress Test before Surgery	-	-	4.5%	5.3%
Combination Abdominal CT Scan	-	-	6.9%	10.5%
Combination Brain/Sinus CT Scan	-	-	1.6%	2.7%
Combination Chest CT Scan	-	-	0.8%	2.7%
Follow-up Mammogram/Ultrasound	-	-	9.5%	8.8%
Lumbar Spine MRI for Low Back Pain	-	-	44.4%	37.2%

Fairbanks Memorial Hospital

1650 Cowles Street
Fairbanks, AK 99701
Phone: 907-452-8181
Fax: 907-458-5151
E-mail: lsmith@bannerhealth.com
URL: www.bannerhealth.com
Type: Acute Care Hospitals
Emergency Services: Yes
Ownership: Voluntary non-profit - Other
Beds: 152

Key Personnel:

Radiology. . . . . Paul Allan
Operating Room. . . . . Patt Cobb
Chief of Medical Staff . . . . Elizabeth Kohnen, MD
Pediatric Ambulatory Care . . . . . . Mary MacFarlane, MD
Pediatric In-Patient Care . . . . Mary MacFarlane, MD

NOTE: Hospital profiles are in alphabetical order by state, then city, then hospital within the city; Rankings exclude hospitals with less than 25 cases except for patient surveys which excludes hospitals with less than 100 cases; (a) 100-299 cases; (1) The number of cases/patients is too few to report; (2) Data submitted were based on a sample of cases/patients; (3) Results are based on a shorter time period than required; (4) Data suppressed by CMS for one or more quarters; (5) Results are not available for this reporting period; (6) Fewer than 100 patients completed the HCAHPS survey; (7) No cases met the criteria for this measure; (8) The lower limit of the confidence interval cannot be calculated if the number of observed infections equals zero; (9) No data are available from the state/territory for this reporting period; (10) The scores shown reflect fewer than 50 completed surveys; (11) There were discrepancies in the data collection process; (12) This measure does not apply to this hospital for this reporting period; (13) Results cannot be calculated for this reporting period; (14) The results for this state are combined with nearby states to protect confidentiality; Please refer to the User's Guide for a full explanation of data.

Emergency Room . . . . Carol Meyer
CEO . . . . Mike Powers
Quality Assurance . . . . Linda Smith

Measure	Cases	This Hosp.	State Avg.	U.S. Avg.
Blood Clot Prevention and Treatment				
Anticoagulation Overlap Therapy[1,2]	-	-	97%	93%
ICU Venous Thromboembolism Prophylaxis[2]	49	82%	90%	92%
Incidence of Potentially Preventable VTE[1,2]	-	-	17%	10%
UFH with Dosages/Platelet Monitoring[1,2]	-	-	98%	97%
Venous Thromboembolism Prophylaxis[2]	223	69%	86%	85%
Warfarin Therapy Discharge Instructions[2]	11	55%	80%	75%
Chest Pain/Possible Heart Attack Care				
Aspirin Given Within 24 Hours of Arrival[1,3]	-	-	99%	96%
Fibrinolytic Meds Within 30 Min. of Arrival[3,7]	-	-	92%	58%
Average Time to ECG (minutes)[1,3]	-	-	8	7
Average Time to Transfer (minutes)[1,3]	-	-	220	60
Children's Asthma Care				
Received Home Management Plan of Care	11	100%	-	88%
Received Reliever Medication	11	100%	-	100%
Received Systemic Corticosteroids	11	100%	-	100%
Emergency Department				
Admittance Decision Time (minutes)[2]	358	122	118	98
Head CT Results Within 45 Min. of Arrival[1]	-	-	29%	57%
Patients Who Left ER Before Being Seen	35,332	1%	3%	2%
Time from ER Arrival to Admit. (minutes)[2]	372	268	287	274
Time from ER Arrival to Discharge (minutes)	321	122	132	134
Time in ER Before Being Evaluated (minutes)	17	29	24	26
Time to Pain Meds for Fractures (minutes)	112	48	57	57
Heart Attack Care				
Aspirin Given at Discharge	76	100%	100%	99%
Fibrinolytic Meds Within 30 Min. of Arrival[7]	-	-	75%	54%
PCI Within 90 Minutes of Arrival	23	100%	94%	96%
Statin Prescribed at Discharge	73	100%	99%	98%
Heart Failure Care				
ACE Inhibitor or ARB for LVSD	37	100%	99%	97%
Discharge Instructions Given	73	95%	94%	94%
Evaluation of LVS Function	73	100%	97%	99%
Medicare Spending				
Medicare Spending per Patient (ratio)	-	0.78	0.91	0.98
Pneumonia Care				
Appropriate Initial Antibiotic Given	39	92%	93%	95%
Blood Culture Timing	82	98%	97%	98%
Pregnancy and Delivery Care				
Newborn Deliveries Scheduled Early[2]	23	0%	2%	6%
Preventive Care				
Immunization for Influenza[2]	461	89%	83%	90%
Immunization for Pneumonia[2]	345	87%	90%	92%
Stroke Care				
Anticoagulation Therapy for Atrial Fibrillation[1]	-	-	80%	95%
Antithrombotic Therapy Timing	22	100%	99%	98%
Assessed for Rehabilitation	29	97%	97%	97%
Discharged on Antithrombotic Therapy	29	97%	98%	99%
Discharged on Statin Medication	24	92%	93%	94%
Thrombolytic Therapy Timing[1]	-	-	69%	66%
Venous Thromboembolism Prophylaxis	25	72%	93%	94%
Written Stroke Educational Materials Given	23	61%	92%	88%
Surgical Care Improvement Project				
Appropriate Beta Blocker Usage[2]	79	94%	96%	98%
Appropriate VTP Within 24 Hours[2]	294	94%	97%	98%
Controlled Postoperative Blood Glucose[2,7]	-	-	95%	97%
Perioperative Temperature Management[2]	352	99%	99%	100%
Prophylactic Antibiotic Selection[2]	234	99%	99%	99%
Prophylactic Antibiotic Selection (Outpatient)	125	98%	99%	98%
Prophylactic Antibiotic Stopped[2]	229	98%	99%	98%
Prophylactic Antibiotic Timing[2]	234	98%	99%	99%
Prophylactic Antibiotic Timing (Outpatient)	126	98%	97%	98%
Urinary Catheter Removal[2]	100	95%	97%	97%
Survey of Patients' Hospital Experiences				
Area Around Room 'Always' Quiet at Night[11]	300+	59%	59%	61%
Doctors 'Always' Communicated Well[11]	300+	80%	82%	82%
Home Recovery Information Given[11]	300+	91%	87%	85%
Hospital Given 9 or 10 on 10 Point Scale[11]	300+	73%	67%	71%
Meds 'Always' Explained Before Given[11]	300+	69%	67%	64%
Nurses 'Always' Communicated Well[11]	300+	81%	77%	79%
Pain 'Always' Well Controlled[11]	300+	72%	68%	71%
Room and Bathroom 'Always' Clean[11]	300+	74%	72%	73%
Timely Help 'Always' Received[11]	300+	75%	71%	68%
Would Definitely Recommend Hospital[11]	300+	74%	69%	71%
Use of Medical Imaging				
Cardiac Imaging Stress Test before Surgery	317	4.1%	4.5%	5.3%
Combination Abdominal CT Scan	653	5.5%	6.9%	10.5%
Combination Brain/Sinus CT Scan	372	1.3%	1.6%	2.7%
Combination Chest CT Scan	410	0.5%	0.8%	2.7%
Follow-up Mammogram/Ultrasound	671	8.9%	9.5%	8.8%
Lumbar Spine MRI for Low Back Pain	133	47.4%	44.4%	37.2%

South Peninsula Hospital

4300 Bartlett St
Homer, AK 99603
URL: www.sphosp.com
Phone: 907-235-8101
Fax: 907-235-0253
Type: Critical Access Hospitals
Ownership: Voluntary non-profit - Private
Emergency Services: Yes
Beds: 40

Key Personnel:
Chief of Medical Staff. . . . . Rene Alvarez, MD
Operating Room. . . . . Rene Alvarez, RN
Quality Assurance . . . . Christine Anderson
Emergency Room . . . . Pam Fredrick, RN
CEO/President. . . . . Robert Letson
Infection Control. . . . . Donna Libal, RN
Radiology. . . . . William Roberts, MD
Anesthesiology. . . . . Larry Tripp, CRNA

Measure	Cases	This Hosp.	State Avg.	U.S. Avg.
Blood Clot Prevention and Treatment				
Anticoagulation Overlap Therapy[5]	-	-	97%	93%
ICU Venous Thromboembolism Prophylaxis[5]	-	-	90%	92%
Incidence of Potentially Preventable VTE[5]	-	-	17%	10%
UFH with Dosages/Platelet Monitoring[5]	-	-	98%	97%
Venous Thromboembolism Prophylaxis[5]	-	-	86%	85%
Warfarin Therapy Discharge Instructions[5]	-	-	80%	75%
Chest Pain/Possible Heart Attack Care				
Aspirin Given Within 24 Hours of Arrival[1,3]	-	-	99%	96%
Fibrinolytic Meds Within 30 Min. of Arrival[3,7]	-	-	92%	58%
Average Time to ECG (minutes)[1,3]	-	-	8	7
Average Time to Transfer (minutes)[1,3]	-	-	220	60
Children's Asthma Care				
Received Home Management Plan of Care	-	-	-	88%
Received Reliever Medication	-	-	-	100%
Received Systemic Corticosteroids	-	-	-	100%
Emergency Department				
Admittance Decision Time (minutes)[1,3]	-	-	118	98
Head CT Results Within 45 Min. of Arrival[1,3]	-	-	29%	57%
Patients Who Left ER Before Being Seen	5,075	0%	3%	2%
Time from ER Arrival to Admit. (minutes)[1,3]	-	-	287	274
Time from ER Arrival to Discharge (minutes)[3]	26	122	132	134
Time in ER Before Being Evaluated (minutes)[3]	32	8	24	26
Time to Pain Meds for Fractures (minutes)[1,3]	-	-	57	57
Heart Attack Care				
Aspirin Given at Discharge[3,7]	-	-	100%	99%
Fibrinolytic Meds Within 30 Min. of Arrival[3,7]	-	-	75%	54%
PCI Within 90 Minutes of Arrival[5]	-	-	94%	96%
Statin Prescribed at Discharge[3,7]	-	-	99%	98%
Heart Failure Care				
ACE Inhibitor or ARB for LVSD[1]	-	-	99%	97%
Discharge Instructions Given	17	94%	94%	94%
Evaluation of LVS Function	17	94%	97%	99%
Medicare Spending				
Medicare Spending per Patient (ratio)	-	-	0.91	0.98
Pneumonia Care				
Appropriate Initial Antibiotic Given	11	73%	93%	95%
Blood Culture Timing	11	100%	97%	98%
Pregnancy and Delivery Care				
Newborn Deliveries Scheduled Early[5]	-	-	2%	6%
Preventive Care				
Immunization for Influenza	32	62%	83%	90%
Immunization for Pneumonia[3]	25	72%	90%	92%
Stroke Care				
Anticoagulation Therapy for Atrial Fibrillation[5]	-	-	80%	95%
Antithrombotic Therapy Timing[5]	-	-	99%	98%
Assessed for Rehabilitation[5]	-	-	97%	97%
Discharged on Antithrombotic Therapy[5]	-	-	98%	99%
Discharged on Statin Medication[5]	-	-	93%	94%
Thrombolytic Therapy Timing[5]	-	-	69%	66%
Venous Thromboembolism Prophylaxis[5]	-	-	93%	94%
Written Stroke Educational Materials Given[5]	-	-	92%	88%
Surgical Care Improvement Project				
Appropriate Beta Blocker Usage[1]	-	-	96%	98%
Appropriate VTP Within 24 Hours	22	86%	97%	98%
Controlled Postoperative Blood Glucose[3,7]	-	-	95%	97%
Perioperative Temperature Management	29	100%	99%	100%
Prophylactic Antibiotic Selection	15	100%	99%	99%
Prophylactic Antibiotic Selection (Outpatient)[1,3]	-	-	99%	98%
Prophylactic Antibiotic Stopped	15	100%	99%	98%
Prophylactic Antibiotic Timing	15	100%	99%	99%
Prophylactic Antibiotic Timing (Outpatient)[1,3]	-	-	97%	98%
Urinary Catheter Removal	16	100%	97%	97%
Survey of Patients' Hospital Experiences				
Area Around Room 'Always' Quiet at Night	(a)	69%	59%	61%
Doctors 'Always' Communicated Well	(a)	87%	82%	82%
Home Recovery Information Given	(a)	91%	87%	85%
Hospital Given 9 or 10 on 10 Point Scale	(a)	80%	67%	71%
Meds 'Always' Explained Before Given	(a)	67%	67%	64%
Nurses 'Always' Communicated Well	(a)	82%	77%	79%
Pain 'Always' Well Controlled	(a)	74%	68%	71%
Room and Bathroom 'Always' Clean	(a)	83%	72%	73%
Timely Help 'Always' Received	(a)	74%	71%	68%
Would Definitely Recommend Hospital	(a)	78%	69%	71%
Use of Medical Imaging				
Cardiac Imaging Stress Test before Surgery[1]	-	-	4.5%	5.3%
Combination Abdominal CT Scan	201	3.5%	6.9%	10.5%
Combination Brain/Sinus CT Scan[1]	-	-	1.6%	2.7%
Combination Chest CT Scan	97	0.0%	0.8%	2.7%
Follow-up Mammogram/Ultrasound	218	6.9%	9.5%	8.8%
Lumbar Spine MRI for Low Back Pain[1]	-	-	44.4%	37.2%

Bartlett Regional Hospital

3260 Hospital Dr
Juneau, AK 99801
URL: www.bartletthospital.org
Phone: 907-796-8900
Fax: 907-796-8909
Type: Acute Care Hospitals
Ownership: Government - Local
Emergency Services: Yes
Beds: 55

Key Personnel:
CEO/President. . . . . Charles E. Bill
Operating Room. . . . . Pam A Gruchacz
Chief of Medical Staff. . . . . Deborah L Lessmeier
Quality Assurance . . . . Don Novotney
Radiology. . . . . William A Richey

Measure	Cases	This Hosp.	State Avg.	U.S. Avg.
Blood Clot Prevention and Treatment				
Anticoagulation Overlap Therapy[2]	11	100%	97%	93%
ICU Venous Thromboembolism Prophylaxis[2]	59	92%	90%	92%
Incidence of Potentially Preventable VTE[1,2]	-	-	17%	10%
UFH with Dosages/Platelet Monitoring[1,2]	-	-	98%	97%
Venous Thromboembolism Prophylaxis[2]	117	90%	86%	85%
Warfarin Therapy Discharge Instructions[2]	11	100%	80%	75%
Chest Pain/Possible Heart Attack Care				
Aspirin Given Within 24 Hours of Arrival	19	100%	99%	96%
Fibrinolytic Meds Within 30 Min. of Arrival[1]	-	-	92%	58%
Average Time to ECG (minutes)	20	4	8	7
Average Time to Transfer (minutes)[7]	-	-	220	60
Children's Asthma Care				
Received Home Management Plan of Care	-	-	-	88%
Received Reliever Medication	-	-	-	100%
Received Systemic Corticosteroids	-	-	-	100%
Emergency Department				
Admittance Decision Time (minutes)[2]	14	124	118	98
Head CT Results Within 45 Min. of Arrival[1]	-	-	29%	57%
Patients Who Left ER Before Being Seen	14,481	0%	3%	2%
Time from ER Arrival to Admit. (minutes)[2]	24	258	287	274
Time from ER Arrival to Discharge (minutes)	389	139	132	134

NOTE: Hospital profiles are in alphabetical order by state, then city, then hospital within the city; Rankings exclude hospitals with less than 25 cases except for patient surveys which excludes hospitals with less than 100 cases; (a) 100-299 cases; (1) The number of cases/patients is too few to report; (2) Data submitted were based on a sample of cases/patients; (3) Results are based on a shorter time period than required; (4) Data suppressed by CMS for one or more quarters; (5) Results are not available for this reporting period; (6) Fewer than 100 patients completed the HCAHPS survey; (7) No cases met the criteria for this measure; (8) The lower limit of the confidence interval cannot be calculated if the number of observed infections equals zero; (9) No data are available from the state/territory for this reporting period; (10) The scores shown reflect fewer than 50 completed surveys; (11) There were discrepancies in the data collection process; (12) This measure does not apply to this hospital for this reporting period; (13) Results cannot be calculated for this reporting period; (14) The results for this state are combined with nearby states to protect confidentiality; Please refer to the User's Guide for a full explanation of data.

Measure	Cases	This Hosp.	State Avg.	U.S. Avg.
Time in ER Before Being Evaluated (minutes)	246	28	24	26
Time to Pain Meds for Fractures (minutes)	41	60	57	57
Heart Attack Care				
Aspirin Given at Discharge[1,3]	-	-	100%	99%
Fibrinolytic Meds Within 30 Min. of Arrival[3,7]	-	-	75%	54%
PCI Within 90 Minutes of Arrival[3,7]	-	-	94%	96%
Statin Prescribed at Discharge[1,3]	-	-	99%	98%
Heart Failure Care				
ACE Inhibitor or ARB for LVSD	11	100%	99%	97%
Discharge Instructions Given	21	95%	94%	94%
Evaluation of LVS Function	21	100%	97%	99%
Medicare Spending				
Medicare Spending per Patient (ratio)	-	0.84	0.91	0.98
Pneumonia Care				
Appropriate Initial Antibiotic Given	34	88%	93%	95%
Blood Culture Timing	39	100%	97%	98%
Pregnancy and Delivery Care				
Newborn Deliveries Scheduled Early	27	4%	2%	6%
Preventive Care				
Immunization for Influenza[2]	276	91%	83%	90%
Immunization for Pneumonia[2]	222	88%	90%	92%
Stroke Care				
Anticoagulation Therapy for Atrial Fibrillation[1]	-	-	80%	95%
Antithrombotic Therapy Timing	13	100%	99%	98%
Assessed for Rehabilitation	19	100%	97%	97%
Discharged on Antithrombotic Therapy	18	100%	98%	99%
Discharged on Statin Medication[1]	-	-	93%	94%
Thrombolytic Therapy Timing[1]	-	-	69%	66%
Venous Thromboembolism Prophylaxis	14	86%	93%	94%
Written Stroke Educational Materials Given	17	100%	92%	88%
Surgical Care Improvement Project				
Appropriate Beta Blocker Usage	30	90%	96%	98%
Appropriate VTP Within 24 Hours	136	96%	97%	98%
Controlled Postoperative Blood Glucose[7]	-	-	95%	97%
Perioperative Temperature Management	144	99%	99%	100%
Prophylactic Antibiotic Selection	95	100%	99%	99%
Prophylactic Antibiotic Selection (Outpatient)	29	100%	99%	98%
Prophylactic Antibiotic Stopped	95	100%	99%	98%
Prophylactic Antibiotic Timing	95	99%	99%	99%
Prophylactic Antibiotic Timing (Outpatient)	28	96%	97%	98%
Urinary Catheter Removal	114	98%	97%	97%
Survey of Patients' Hospital Experiences				
Area Around Room 'Always' Quiet at Night	300+	60%	59%	61%
Doctors 'Always' Communicated Well	300+	82%	82%	82%
Home Recovery Information Given	300+	86%	87%	85%
Hospital Given 9 or 10 on 10 Point Scale	300+	62%	67%	71%
Meds 'Always' Explained Before Given	300+	69%	67%	64%
Nurses 'Always' Communicated Well	300+	77%	77%	79%
Pain 'Always' Well Controlled	300+	68%	68%	71%
Room and Bathroom 'Always' Clean	300+	75%	72%	73%
Timely Help 'Always' Received	300+	70%	71%	68%
Would Definitely Recommend Hospital	300+	69%	69%	71%
Use of Medical Imaging				
Cardiac Imaging Stress Test before Surgery	54	3.7%	4.5%	5.3%
Combination Abdominal CT Scan	196	6.6%	6.9%	10.5%
Combination Brain/Sinus CT Scan	122	0.0%	1.6%	2.7%
Combination Chest CT Scan	98	0.0%	0.8%	2.7%
Follow-up Mammogram/Ultrasound	452	8.0%	9.5%	8.8%
Lumbar Spine MRI for Low Back Pain[1]	-	-	44.4%	37.2%

Peacehealth Ketchikan Medical Center

3100 Tongass Avenue
Ketchikan, AK 99901
Phone: 907-225-5171
Fax: 907-228-8322
Type: Critical Access Hospitals
Emergency Services: Yes
Ownership: Voluntary non-profit - Church
Beds: 85

Key Personnel:
CEO/President. . . . . Patrick J Branco
Emergency Room . . . . Molly Hutsinpiller
Operating Room. . . . . Susan Leeman
Chief of Medical Staff . . . . Stacy Schultz, MD
Intensive Care Unit. . . . . Kathy Smith
Radiology. . . . . Frank Webb

Measure	Cases	This Hosp.	State Avg.	U.S. Avg.
Blood Clot Prevention and Treatment				
Anticoagulation Overlap Therapy[1,2]	-	-	97%	93%
ICU Venous Thromboembolism Prophylaxis[2]	17	82%	90%	92%
Incidence of Potentially Preventable VTE[1,2]	-	-	17%	10%
UFH with Dosages/Platelet Monitoring[1,2]	-	-	98%	97%
Venous Thromboembolism Prophylaxis[2]	74	81%	86%	85%
Warfarin Therapy Discharge Instructions[1,2]	-	-	80%	75%
Chest Pain/Possible Heart Attack Care				
Aspirin Given Within 24 Hours of Arrival	21	100%	99%	96%
Fibrinolytic Meds Within 30 Min. of Arrival[1]	-	-	92%	58%
Average Time to ECG (minutes)	20	6	8	7
Average Time to Transfer (minutes)[1]	-	-	220	60
Children's Asthma Care				
Received Home Management Plan of Care	-	-	-	88%
Received Reliever Medication	-	-	-	100%
Received Systemic Corticosteroids	-	-	-	100%
Emergency Department				
Admittance Decision Time (minutes)[2]	275	155	118	98
Head CT Results Within 45 Min. of Arrival[1]	-	-	29%	57%
Patients Who Left ER Before Being Seen	9,470	2%	3%	2%
Time from ER Arrival to Admit. (minutes)[2]	275	259	287	274
Time from ER Arrival to Discharge (minutes)	363	125	132	134
Time in ER Before Being Evaluated (minutes)	397	18	24	26
Time to Pain Meds for Fractures (minutes)	48	58	57	57
Heart Attack Care				
Aspirin Given at Discharge[1,3]	-	-	100%	99%
Fibrinolytic Meds Within 30 Min. of Arrival[1,3]	-	-	75%	54%
PCI Within 90 Minutes of Arrival[3,7]	-	-	94%	96%
Statin Prescribed at Discharge[1,3]	-	-	99%	98%
Heart Failure Care				
ACE Inhibitor or ARB for LVSD[1]	-	-	99%	97%
Discharge Instructions Given	12	83%	94%	94%
Evaluation of LVS Function	14	100%	97%	99%
Medicare Spending				
Medicare Spending per Patient (ratio)	-	-	0.91	0.98
Pneumonia Care				
Appropriate Initial Antibiotic Given	20	100%	93%	95%
Blood Culture Timing	42	95%	97%	98%
Pregnancy and Delivery Care				
Newborn Deliveries Scheduled Early	18	0%	2%	6%
Preventive Care				
Immunization for Influenza[2]	245	82%	83%	90%
Immunization for Pneumonia[2]	207	86%	90%	92%
Stroke Care				
Anticoagulation Therapy for Atrial Fibrillation[1]	-	-	80%	95%
Antithrombotic Therapy Timing	12	100%	99%	98%
Assessed for Rehabilitation	15	93%	97%	97%
Discharged on Antithrombotic Therapy	14	93%	98%	99%
Discharged on Statin Medication[1]	-	-	93%	94%
Thrombolytic Therapy Timing[7]	-	-	69%	66%
Venous Thromboembolism Prophylaxis	12	92%	93%	94%
Written Stroke Educational Materials Given	11	73%	92%	88%
Surgical Care Improvement Project				
Appropriate Beta Blocker Usage	18	89%	96%	98%
Appropriate VTP Within 24 Hours	77	97%	97%	98%
Controlled Postoperative Blood Glucose[7]	-	-	95%	97%
Perioperative Temperature Management	83	100%	99%	100%
Prophylactic Antibiotic Selection	48	100%	99%	99%
Prophylactic Antibiotic Selection (Outpatient)[3]	13	100%	99%	98%
Prophylactic Antibiotic Stopped	45	98%	99%	98%
Prophylactic Antibiotic Timing	48	96%	99%	99%
Prophylactic Antibiotic Timing (Outpatient)[1,3]	-	-	97%	98%
Urinary Catheter Removal	53	96%	97%	97%
Survey of Patients' Hospital Experiences				
Area Around Room 'Always' Quiet at Night	(a)	64%	59%	61%
Doctors 'Always' Communicated Well	(a)	86%	82%	82%
Home Recovery Information Given	(a)	89%	87%	85%
Hospital Given 9 or 10 on 10 Point Scale	(a)	67%	67%	71%
Meds 'Always' Explained Before Given	(a)	65%	67%	64%
Nurses 'Always' Communicated Well	(a)	80%	77%	79%
Pain 'Always' Well Controlled	(a)	73%	68%	71%
Room and Bathroom 'Always' Clean	(a)	71%	72%	73%
Timely Help 'Always' Received	(a)	77%	71%	68%
Would Definitely Recommend Hospital	(a)	71%	69%	71%
Use of Medical Imaging				
Cardiac Imaging Stress Test before Surgery	69	5.8%	4.5%	5.3%
Combination Abdominal CT Scan	185	11.4%	6.9%	10.5%
Combination Brain/Sinus CT Scan[1]	-	-	1.6%	2.7%
Combination Chest CT Scan	131	0.0%	0.8%	2.7%
Follow-up Mammogram/Ultrasound	213	5.2%	9.5%	8.8%
Lumbar Spine MRI for Low Back Pain	40	50.0%	44.4%	37.2%

Providence Kodiak Island Medical Center

1915 East Rezanof Drive
Kodiak, AK 99615
Phone: 907-486-9592
Fax: 907-486-2336
URL: www.providence.org
Type: Critical Access Hospitals
Emergency Services: Yes
Ownership: Voluntary non-profit - Private
Beds: 25

Key Personnel:
Anesthesiology. . . . . Marlene Brannen, CRNA
Quality Assurance . . . . Alice Coen, RN
Radiology. . . . . Carlos Rio, MD
Operating Room. . . . . Gene Robinson, RN
CEO/President. . . . . Don Rush
Chief of Medical Staff . . . . Steve Smith, MD
Emergency Room . . . . Steve Smith, MD

Measure	Cases	This Hosp.	State Avg.	U.S. Avg.
Blood Clot Prevention and Treatment				
Anticoagulation Overlap Therapy[5]	-	-	97%	93%
ICU Venous Thromboembolism Prophylaxis[5]	-	-	90%	92%
Incidence of Potentially Preventable VTE[5]	-	-	17%	10%
UFH with Dosages/Platelet Monitoring[5]	-	-	98%	97%
Venous Thromboembolism Prophylaxis[5]	-	-	86%	85%
Warfarin Therapy Discharge Instructions[5]	-	-	80%	75%
Chest Pain/Possible Heart Attack Care				
Aspirin Given Within 24 Hours of Arrival[1,3]	-	-	99%	96%
Fibrinolytic Meds Within 30 Min. of Arrival[5]	-	-	92%	58%
Average Time to ECG (minutes)[1,3]	-	-	8	7
Average Time to Transfer (minutes)[5]	-	-	220	60
Children's Asthma Care				
Received Home Management Plan of Care	-	-	-	88%
Received Reliever Medication	-	-	-	100%
Received Systemic Corticosteroids	-	-	-	100%
Emergency Department				
Admittance Decision Time (minutes)[5]	-	-	118	98
Head CT Results Within 45 Min. of Arrival[5]	-	-	29%	57%
Patients Who Left ER Before Being Seen[5]	-	-	3%	2%
Time from ER Arrival to Admit. (minutes)[5]	-	-	287	274
Time from ER Arrival to Discharge (minutes)[5]	-	-	132	134
Time in ER Before Being Evaluated (minutes)[5]	-	-	24	26
Time to Pain Meds for Fractures (minutes)[5]	-	-	57	57
Heart Attack Care				
Aspirin Given at Discharge[1,3]	-	-	100%	99%
Fibrinolytic Meds Within 30 Min. of Arrival[1,3]	-	-	75%	54%
PCI Within 90 Minutes of Arrival[3,7]	-	-	94%	96%
Statin Prescribed at Discharge[1,3]	-	-	99%	98%
Heart Failure Care				
ACE Inhibitor or ARB for LVSD[1]	-	-	99%	97%
Discharge Instructions Given	11	82%	94%	94%
Evaluation of LVS Function	12	92%	97%	99%
Medicare Spending				
Medicare Spending per Patient (ratio)	-	-	0.91	0.98
Pneumonia Care				
Appropriate Initial Antibiotic Given	20	90%	93%	95%
Blood Culture Timing	19	100%	97%	98%
Pregnancy and Delivery Care				
Newborn Deliveries Scheduled Early[5]	-	-	2%	6%
Preventive Care				
Immunization for Influenza[5]	-	-	83%	90%
Immunization for Pneumonia[5]	-	-	90%	92%
Stroke Care				
Anticoagulation Therapy for Atrial Fibrillation[5]	-	-	80%	95%
Antithrombotic Therapy Timing[5]	-	-	99%	98%
Assessed for Rehabilitation[5]	-	-	97%	97%
Discharged on Antithrombotic Therapy[5]	-	-	98%	99%
Discharged on Statin Medication[5]	-	-	93%	94%
Thrombolytic Therapy Timing[5]	-	-	69%	66%

NOTE: Hospital profiles are in alphabetical order by state, then city, then hospital within the city; Rankings exclude hospitals with less than 25 cases except for patient surveys which excludes hospitals with less than 100 cases; (a) 100-299 cases; (1) The number of cases/patients is too few to report; (2) Data submitted were based on a sample of cases/patients; (3) Results are based on a shorter time period than required; (4) Data suppressed by CMS for one or more quarters; (5) Results are not available for this reporting period; (6) Fewer than 100 patients completed the HCAHPS survey; (7) No cases met the criteria for this measure; (8) The lower limit of the confidence interval cannot be calculated if the number of observed infections equals zero; (9) No data are available from the state/territory for this reporting period; (10) The scores shown reflect fewer than 50 completed surveys; (11) There were discrepancies in the data collection process; (12) This measure does not apply to this hospital for this reporting period; (13) Results cannot be calculated for this reporting period; (14) The results for this state are combined with nearby states to protect confidentiality; Please refer to the User's Guide for a full explanation of data.

Measure	Cases	This Hosp.	State Avg.	U.S. Avg.
Venous Thromboembolism Prophylaxis[5]	-	-	93%	94%
Written Stroke Educational Materials Given[5]	-	-	92%	88%
Surgical Care Improvement Project				
Appropriate Beta Blocker Usage[7]	-	-	96%	98%
Appropriate VTP Within 24 Hours[1]	-	-	97%	98%
Controlled Postoperative Blood Glucose[7]	-	-	95%	97%
Perioperative Temperature Management[1]	-	-	99%	100%
Prophylactic Antibiotic Selection[1]	-	-	99%	99%
Prophylactic Antibiotic Selection (Outpatient)[1,3]	-	-	99%	98%
Prophylactic Antibiotic Stopped[1]	-	-	99%	98%
Prophylactic Antibiotic Timing[1]	-	-	99%	99%
Prophylactic Antibiotic Timing (Outpatient)[1,3]	-	-	97%	98%
Urinary Catheter Removal[1]	-	-	97%	97%
Survey of Patients' Hospital Experiences				
Area Around Room 'Always' Quiet at Night	(a)	72%	59%	61%
Doctors 'Always' Communicated Well	(a)	84%	82%	82%
Home Recovery Information Given	(a)	90%	87%	85%
Hospital Given 9 or 10 on 10 Point Scale	(a)	74%	67%	71%
Meds 'Always' Explained Before Given	(a)	63%	67%	64%
Nurses 'Always' Communicated Well	(a)	82%	77%	79%
Pain 'Always' Well Controlled	(a)	66%	68%	71%
Room and Bathroom 'Always' Clean	(a)	81%	72%	73%
Timely Help 'Always' Received	(a)	79%	71%	68%
Would Definitely Recommend Hospital	(a)	76%	69%	71%
Use of Medical Imaging				
Cardiac Imaging Stress Test before Surgery[7]	-	-	4.5%	5.3%
Combination Abdominal CT Scan	74	9.5%	6.9%	10.5%
Combination Brain/Sinus CT Scan	39	0.0%	1.6%	2.7%
Combination Chest CT Scan[1]	-	-	0.8%	2.7%
Follow-up Mammogram/Ultrasound	98	15.3%	9.5%	8.8%
Lumbar Spine MRI for Low Back Pain[1]	-	-	44.4%	37.2%

Norton Sound Regional Hospital

306 West 5th Avenue, PO Box 966
Nome, AK 99762
Phone: 907-443-3311
Fax: 907-443-3139
URL: www.nortonsoundhealth.org
Type: Critical Access Hospitals
Emergency Services: Yes
Ownership: Voluntary non-profit - Private
Beds: 30

Key Personnel:
Chief of Medical Staff.......... David Head
Quality Assurance .... Karla Homelrig
Ambulatory Care .... Louis Murphy
CEO/President................ Carol J Piscoya
Infection Control.............. Bridgett Watkins

Measure	Cases	This Hosp.	State Avg.	U.S. Avg.
Blood Clot Prevention and Treatment				
Anticoagulation Overlap Therapy[5]	-	-	97%	93%
ICU Venous Thromboembolism Prophylaxis[5]	-	-	90%	92%
Incidence of Potentially Preventable VTE[5]	-	-	17%	10%
UFH with Dosages/Platelet Monitoring[5]	-	-	98%	97%
Venous Thromboembolism Prophylaxis[5]	-	-	86%	85%
Warfarin Therapy Discharge Instructions[5]	-	-	80%	75%
Chest Pain/Possible Heart Attack Care				
Aspirin Given Within 24 Hours of Arrival	-	-	99%	96%
Fibrinolytic Meds Within 30 Min. of Arrival	-	-	92%	58%
Average Time to ECG (minutes)	-	-	8	7
Average Time to Transfer (minutes)	-	-	220	60
Children's Asthma Care				
Received Home Management Plan of Care	-	-	-	88%
Received Reliever Medication	-	-	-	100%
Received Systemic Corticosteroids	-	-	-	100%
Emergency Department				
Admittance Decision Time (minutes)[5]	-	-	118	98
Head CT Results Within 45 Min. of Arrival	-	-	29%	57%
Patients Who Left ER Before Being Seen	-	-	3%	2%
Time from ER Arrival to Admit. (minutes)[5]	-	-	287	274
Time from ER Arrival to Discharge (minutes)	-	-	132	134
Time in ER Before Being Evaluated (minutes)	-	-	24	26
Time to Pain Meds for Fractures (minutes)	-	-	57	57
Heart Attack Care				
Aspirin Given at Discharge[3,7]	-	-	100%	99%
Fibrinolytic Meds Within 30 Min. of Arrival[3,7]	-	-	75%	54%
PCI Within 90 Minutes of Arrival[3,7]	-	-	94%	96%
Statin Prescribed at Discharge[3,7]	-	-	99%	98%
Heart Failure Care				
ACE Inhibitor or ARB for LVSD[1,3]	-	-	99%	97%
Discharge Instructions Given[1,3]	-	-	94%	94%
Evaluation of LVS Function[1,3]	-	-	97%	99%
Medicare Spending				
Medicare Spending per Patient (ratio)	-	-	0.91	0.98
Pneumonia Care				
Appropriate Initial Antibiotic Given[1]	-	-	93%	95%
Blood Culture Timing[1]	-	-	97%	98%
Pregnancy and Delivery Care				
Newborn Deliveries Scheduled Early[5]	-	-	2%	6%
Preventive Care				
Immunization for Influenza[5]	-	-	83%	90%
Immunization for Pneumonia[5]	-	-	90%	92%
Stroke Care				
Anticoagulation Therapy for Atrial Fibrillation[5]	-	-	80%	95%
Antithrombotic Therapy Timing[5]	-	-	99%	98%
Assessed for Rehabilitation[5]	-	-	97%	97%
Discharged on Antithrombotic Therapy[5]	-	-	98%	99%
Discharged on Statin Medication[5]	-	-	93%	94%
Thrombolytic Therapy Timing[5]	-	-	69%	66%
Venous Thromboembolism Prophylaxis[5]	-	-	93%	94%
Written Stroke Educational Materials Given[5]	-	-	92%	88%
Surgical Care Improvement Project				
Appropriate Beta Blocker Usage[5]	-	-	96%	98%
Appropriate VTP Within 24 Hours[5]	-	-	97%	98%
Controlled Postoperative Blood Glucose[5]	-	-	95%	97%
Perioperative Temperature Management[5]	-	-	99%	100%
Prophylactic Antibiotic Selection[5]	-	-	99%	99%
Prophylactic Antibiotic Selection (Outpatient)	-	-	99%	98%
Prophylactic Antibiotic Stopped[5]	-	-	99%	98%
Prophylactic Antibiotic Timing[5]	-	-	99%	99%
Prophylactic Antibiotic Timing (Outpatient)	-	-	97%	98%
Urinary Catheter Removal[5]	-	-	97%	97%
Survey of Patients' Hospital Experiences				
Area Around Room 'Always' Quiet at Night[5]	-	-	59%	61%
Doctors 'Always' Communicated Well[5]	-	-	82%	82%
Home Recovery Information Given[5]	-	-	87%	85%
Hospital Given 9 or 10 on 10 Point Scale[5]	-	-	67%	71%
Meds 'Always' Explained Before Given[5]	-	-	67%	64%
Nurses 'Always' Communicated Well[5]	-	-	77%	79%
Pain 'Always' Well Controlled[5]	-	-	68%	71%
Room and Bathroom 'Always' Clean[5]	-	-	72%	73%
Timely Help 'Always' Received[5]	-	-	71%	68%
Would Definitely Recommend Hospital[5]	-	-	69%	71%
Use of Medical Imaging				
Cardiac Imaging Stress Test before Surgery	-	-	4.5%	5.3%
Combination Abdominal CT Scan	-	-	6.9%	10.5%
Combination Brain/Sinus CT Scan	-	-	1.6%	2.7%
Combination Chest CT Scan	-	-	0.8%	2.7%
Follow-up Mammogram/Ultrasound	-	-	9.5%	8.8%
Lumbar Spine MRI for Low Back Pain	-	-	44.4%	37.2%

Mat-Su Regional Medical Center

2500 South Woodworth Loop
Palmer, AK 99645
Phone: 907-746-8600
URL: www.matsuregional.com
Type: Acute Care Hospitals
Emergency Services: Yes
Ownership: Voluntary non-profit - Private

Measure	Cases	This Hosp.	State Avg.	U.S. Avg.
Blood Clot Prevention and Treatment				
Anticoagulation Overlap Therapy[2]	21	100%	97%	93%
ICU Venous Thromboembolism Prophylaxis[2]	53	98%	90%	92%
Incidence of Potentially Preventable VTE[1,2]	-	-	17%	10%
UFH with Dosages/Platelet Monitoring[1,2]	-	-	98%	97%
Venous Thromboembolism Prophylaxis[2]	268	98%	86%	85%
Warfarin Therapy Discharge Instructions[2]	15	87%	80%	75%
Chest Pain/Possible Heart Attack Care				
Aspirin Given Within 24 Hours of Arrival[1,3]	-	-	99%	96%
Fibrinolytic Meds Within 30 Min. of Arrival[5]	-	-	92%	58%
Average Time to ECG (minutes)[1,3]	-	-	8	7
Average Time to Transfer (minutes)[5]	-	-	220	60
Children's Asthma Care				
Received Home Management Plan of Care	-	-	-	88%
Received Reliever Medication	-	-	-	100%
Received Systemic Corticosteroids	-	-	-	100%
Emergency Department				
Admittance Decision Time (minutes)[2]	504	106	118	98
Head CT Results Within 45 Min. of Arrival[1]	-	-	29%	57%
Patients Who Left ER Before Being Seen	28,557	1%	3%	2%
Time from ER Arrival to Admit. (minutes)[2]	560	244	287	274
Time from ER Arrival to Discharge (minutes)	409	127	132	134
Time in ER Before Being Evaluated (minutes)	410	21	24	26
Time to Pain Meds for Fractures (minutes)	196	54	57	57
Heart Attack Care				
Aspirin Given at Discharge	76	100%	100%	99%
Fibrinolytic Meds Within 30 Min. of Arrival[7]	-	-	75%	54%
PCI Within 90 Minutes of Arrival	17	88%	94%	96%
Statin Prescribed at Discharge	66	100%	99%	98%
Heart Failure Care				
ACE Inhibitor or ARB for LVSD	26	100%	99%	97%
Discharge Instructions Given	62	98%	94%	94%
Evaluation of LVS Function	77	100%	97%	99%
Medicare Spending				
Medicare Spending per Patient (ratio)	-	0.81	0.91	0.98
Pneumonia Care				
Appropriate Initial Antibiotic Given	89	100%	93%	95%
Blood Culture Timing	138	100%	97%	98%
Pregnancy and Delivery Care				
Newborn Deliveries Scheduled Early[2]	36	0%	2%	6%
Preventive Care				
Immunization for Influenza[2]	476	99%	83%	90%
Immunization for Pneumonia[2]	439	100%	90%	92%
Stroke Care				
Anticoagulation Therapy for Atrial Fibrillation[1]	-	-	80%	95%
Antithrombotic Therapy Timing	23	100%	99%	98%
Assessed for Rehabilitation	26	100%	97%	97%
Discharged on Antithrombotic Therapy	23	100%	98%	99%
Discharged on Statin Medication	18	89%	93%	94%
Thrombolytic Therapy Timing[1]	-	-	69%	66%
Venous Thromboembolism Prophylaxis	25	100%	93%	94%
Written Stroke Educational Materials Given	18	100%	92%	88%
Surgical Care Improvement Project				
Appropriate Beta Blocker Usage	70	97%	96%	98%
Appropriate VTP Within 24 Hours	271	100%	97%	98%
Controlled Postoperative Blood Glucose[7]	-	-	95%	97%
Perioperative Temperature Management	379	100%	99%	100%
Prophylactic Antibiotic Selection	219	100%	99%	99%
Prophylactic Antibiotic Selection (Outpatient)	49	100%	99%	98%
Prophylactic Antibiotic Stopped	214	100%	99%	98%
Prophylactic Antibiotic Timing	219	100%	99%	99%
Prophylactic Antibiotic Timing (Outpatient)	51	96%	97%	98%
Urinary Catheter Removal	116	98%	97%	97%
Survey of Patients' Hospital Experiences				
Area Around Room 'Always' Quiet at Night	300+	60%	59%	61%
Doctors 'Always' Communicated Well	300+	79%	82%	82%
Home Recovery Information Given	300+	88%	87%	85%
Hospital Given 9 or 10 on 10 Point Scale	300+	70%	67%	71%
Meds 'Always' Explained Before Given	300+	64%	67%	64%
Nurses 'Always' Communicated Well	300+	77%	77%	79%
Pain 'Always' Well Controlled	300+	69%	68%	71%
Room and Bathroom 'Always' Clean	300+	75%	72%	73%
Timely Help 'Always' Received	300+	62%	71%	68%
Would Definitely Recommend Hospital	300+	71%	69%	71%
Use of Medical Imaging				
Cardiac Imaging Stress Test before Surgery[1]	-	-	4.5%	5.3%
Combination Abdominal CT Scan	423	8.7%	6.9%	10.5%
Combination Brain/Sinus CT Scan[1]	-	-	1.6%	2.7%
Combination Chest CT Scan	172	1.7%	0.8%	2.7%
Follow-up Mammogram/Ultrasound	347	13.5%	9.5%	8.8%
Lumbar Spine MRI for Low Back Pain	55	36.4%	44.4%	37.2%

NOTE: Hospital profiles are in alphabetical order by state, then city, then hospital within the city; Rankings exclude hospitals with less than 25 cases except for patient surveys which excludes hospitals with less than 100 cases; (a) 100-299 cases; (1) The number of cases/patients is too few to report; (2) Data submitted were based on a sample of cases/patients; (3) Results are based on a shorter time period than required; (4) Data suppressed by CMS for one or more quarters; (5) Results are not available for this reporting period; (6) Fewer than 100 patients completed the HCAHPS survey; (7) No cases met the criteria for this measure; (8) The lower limit of the confidence interval cannot be calculated if the number of observed infections equals zero; (9) No data are available from the state/territory for this reporting period; (10) The scores shown reflect fewer than 50 completed surveys; (11) There were discrepancies in the data collection process; (12) This measure does not apply to this hospital for this reporting period; (13) Results cannot be calculated for this reporting period; (14) The results for this state are combined with nearby states to protect confidentiality; Please refer to the User's Guide for a full explanation of data.

Petersburg Medical Center

PO Box 589
Petersburg, AK 99833
Phone: 907-772-4291
Type: Critical Access Hospitals
Emergency Services: Yes
Ownership: Government - Local

Measure	Cases	This Hosp.	State Avg.	U.S. Avg.
Blood Clot Prevention and Treatment				
Anticoagulation Overlap Therapy[5]	-	-	97%	93%
ICU Venous Thromboembolism Prophylaxis[5]	-	-	90%	92%
Incidence of Potentially Preventable VTE[5]	-	-	17%	10%
UFH with Dosages/Platelet Monitoring[5]	-	-	98%	97%
Venous Thromboembolism Prophylaxis[5]	-	-	86%	85%
Warfarin Therapy Discharge Instructions[5]	-	-	80%	75%
Chest Pain/Possible Heart Attack Care				
Aspirin Given Within 24 Hours of Arrival	-	-	99%	96%
Fibrinolytic Meds Within 30 Min. of Arrival	-	-	92%	58%
Average Time to ECG (minutes)	-	-	8	7
Average Time to Transfer (minutes)	-	-	220	60
Children's Asthma Care				
Received Home Management Plan of Care	-	-	-	88%
Received Reliever Medication	-	-	-	100%
Received Systemic Corticosteroids	-	-	-	100%
Emergency Department				
Admittance Decision Time (minutes)[5]	-	-	118	98
Head CT Results Within 45 Min. of Arrival	-	-	29%	57%
Patients Who Left ER Before Being Seen	-	-	3%	2%
Time from ER Arrival to Admit. (minutes)[5]	-	-	287	274
Time from ER Arrival to Discharge (minutes)	-	-	132	134
Time in ER Before Being Evaluated (minutes)	-	-	24	26
Time to Pain Meds for Fractures (minutes)	-	-	57	57
Heart Attack Care				
Aspirin Given at Discharge[1,3]	-	-	100%	99%
Fibrinolytic Meds Within 30 Min. of Arrival[3,7]	-	-	75%	54%
PCI Within 90 Minutes of Arrival[3,7]	-	-	94%	96%
Statin Prescribed at Discharge[1,3]	-	-	99%	98%
Heart Failure Care				
ACE Inhibitor or ARB for LVSD[3,7]	-	-	99%	97%
Discharge Instructions Given[1,3]	-	-	94%	94%
Evaluation of LVS Function[1,3]	-	-	97%	99%
Medicare Spending				
Medicare Spending per Patient (ratio)	-	-	0.91	0.98
Pneumonia Care				
Appropriate Initial Antibiotic Given[1,3]	-	-	93%	95%
Blood Culture Timing[1,3]	-	-	97%	98%
Pregnancy and Delivery Care				
Newborn Deliveries Scheduled Early[5]	-	-	2%	6%
Preventive Care				
Immunization for Influenza[5]	-	-	83%	90%
Immunization for Pneumonia[5]	-	-	90%	92%
Stroke Care				
Anticoagulation Therapy for Atrial Fibrillation[5]	-	-	80%	95%
Antithrombotic Therapy Timing[5]	-	-	99%	98%
Assessed for Rehabilitation[5]	-	-	97%	97%
Discharged on Antithrombotic Therapy[5]	-	-	98%	99%
Discharged on Statin Medication[5]	-	-	93%	94%
Thrombolytic Therapy Timing[5]	-	-	69%	66%
Venous Thromboembolism Prophylaxis[5]	-	-	93%	94%
Written Stroke Educational Materials Given[5]	-	-	92%	88%
Surgical Care Improvement Project				
Appropriate Beta Blocker Usage[5]	-	-	96%	98%
Appropriate VTP Within 24 Hours[5]	-	-	97%	98%
Controlled Postoperative Blood Glucose[5]	-	-	95%	97%
Perioperative Temperature Management[5]	-	-	99%	100%
Prophylactic Antibiotic Selection[5]	-	-	99%	99%
Prophylactic Antibiotic Selection (Outpatient)	-	-	99%	98%
Prophylactic Antibiotic Stopped[5]	-	-	99%	98%
Prophylactic Antibiotic Timing[5]	-	-	99%	99%
Prophylactic Antibiotic Timing (Outpatient)	-	-	97%	98%
Urinary Catheter Removal[5]	-	-	97%	97%
Survey of Patients' Hospital Experiences				
Area Around Room 'Always' Quiet at Night[10]	<100	51%	59%	61%
Doctors 'Always' Communicated Well[10]	<100	94%	82%	82%
Home Recovery Information Given[10]	<100	88%	87%	85%
Hospital Given 9 or 10 on 10 Point Scale[10]	<100	63%	67%	71%
Meds 'Always' Explained Before Given[10]	<100	80%	67%	64%
Nurses 'Always' Communicated Well[10]	<100	84%	77%	79%
Pain 'Always' Well Controlled[10]	<100	-	68%	71%
Room and Bathroom 'Always' Clean[10]	<100	71%	72%	73%
Timely Help 'Always' Received[10]	<100	96%	71%	68%
Would Definitely Recommend Hospital[10]	<100	60%	69%	71%
Use of Medical Imaging				
Cardiac Imaging Stress Test before Surgery	-	-	4.5%	5.3%
Combination Abdominal CT Scan	-	-	6.9%	10.5%
Combination Brain/Sinus CT Scan	-	-	1.6%	2.7%
Combination Chest CT Scan	-	-	0.8%	2.7%
Follow-up Mammogram/Ultrasound	-	-	9.5%	8.8%
Lumbar Spine MRI for Low Back Pain	-	-	44.4%	37.2%

Providence Seward Hospital

417 First Avenue, PO Box 365
Seward, AK 99664
Phone: 907-224-5205
Fax: 907-224-7248
URL: www.providence.org
Type: Critical Access Hospitals
Emergency Services: Yes
Ownership: Government - Local
Beds: 26

Key Personnel:

President/CEO. . . . . Rodney F. Hochman, MD
Quality Assurance . . . . Sandra Reese
Chief of Medical Staff. . . . . Michael Sullivan, MD

Measure	Cases	This Hosp.	State Avg.	U.S. Avg.
Blood Clot Prevention and Treatment				
Anticoagulation Overlap Therapy[5]	-	-	97%	93%
ICU Venous Thromboembolism Prophylaxis[5]	-	-	90%	92%
Incidence of Potentially Preventable VTE[5]	-	-	17%	10%
UFH with Dosages/Platelet Monitoring[5]	-	-	98%	97%
Venous Thromboembolism Prophylaxis[5]	-	-	86%	85%
Warfarin Therapy Discharge Instructions[5]	-	-	80%	75%
Chest Pain/Possible Heart Attack Care				
Aspirin Given Within 24 Hours of Arrival	-	-	99%	96%
Fibrinolytic Meds Within 30 Min. of Arrival	-	-	92%	58%
Average Time to ECG (minutes)	-	-	8	7
Average Time to Transfer (minutes)	-	-	220	60
Children's Asthma Care				
Received Home Management Plan of Care	-	-	-	88%
Received Reliever Medication	-	-	-	100%
Received Systemic Corticosteroids	-	-	-	100%
Emergency Department				
Admittance Decision Time (minutes)[5]	-	-	118	98
Head CT Results Within 45 Min. of Arrival	-	-	29%	57%
Patients Who Left ER Before Being Seen	-	-	3%	2%
Time from ER Arrival to Admit. (minutes)[5]	-	-	287	274
Time from ER Arrival to Discharge (minutes)	-	-	132	134
Time in ER Before Being Evaluated (minutes)	-	-	24	26
Time to Pain Meds for Fractures (minutes)	-	-	57	57
Heart Attack Care				
Aspirin Given at Discharge[1,3]	-	-	100%	99%
Fibrinolytic Meds Within 30 Min. of Arrival[3,7]	-	-	75%	54%
PCI Within 90 Minutes of Arrival[3,7]	-	-	94%	96%
Statin Prescribed at Discharge[1,3]	-	-	99%	98%
Heart Failure Care				
ACE Inhibitor or ARB for LVSD[3,7]	-	-	99%	97%
Discharge Instructions Given[1,3]	-	-	94%	94%
Evaluation of LVS Function[1,3]	-	-	97%	99%
Medicare Spending				
Medicare Spending per Patient (ratio)	-	-	0.91	0.98
Pneumonia Care				
Appropriate Initial Antibiotic Given[1,3]	-	-	93%	95%
Blood Culture Timing[1,3]	-	-	97%	98%
Pregnancy and Delivery Care				
Newborn Deliveries Scheduled Early[5]	-	-	2%	6%
Preventive Care				
Immunization for Influenza[5]	-	-	83%	90%
Immunization for Pneumonia[5]	-	-	90%	92%
Stroke Care				
Anticoagulation Therapy for Atrial Fibrillation[3,7]	-	-	80%	95%
Antithrombotic Therapy Timing[3,7]	-	-	99%	98%
Assessed for Rehabilitation[3,7]	-	-	97%	97%
Discharged on Antithrombotic Therapy[3,7]	-	-	98%	99%
Discharged on Statin Medication[3,7]	-	-	93%	94%
Thrombolytic Therapy Timing[3,7]	-	-	69%	66%
Venous Thromboembolism Prophylaxis[3,7]	-	-	93%	94%
Written Stroke Educational Materials Given[3,7]	-	-	92%	88%
Surgical Care Improvement Project				
Appropriate Beta Blocker Usage[5]	-	-	96%	98%
Appropriate VTP Within 24 Hours[5]	-	-	97%	98%
Controlled Postoperative Blood Glucose[5]	-	-	95%	97%
Perioperative Temperature Management[5]	-	-	99%	100%
Prophylactic Antibiotic Selection[5]	-	-	99%	99%
Prophylactic Antibiotic Selection (Outpatient)	-	-	99%	98%
Prophylactic Antibiotic Stopped[5]	-	-	99%	98%
Prophylactic Antibiotic Timing[5]	-	-	99%	99%
Prophylactic Antibiotic Timing (Outpatient)	-	-	97%	98%
Urinary Catheter Removal[5]	-	-	97%	97%
Survey of Patients' Hospital Experiences				
Area Around Room 'Always' Quiet at Night[5]	-	-	59%	61%
Doctors 'Always' Communicated Well[5]	-	-	82%	82%
Home Recovery Information Given[5]	-	-	87%	85%
Hospital Given 9 or 10 on 10 Point Scale[5]	-	-	67%	71%
Meds 'Always' Explained Before Given[5]	-	-	67%	64%
Nurses 'Always' Communicated Well[5]	-	-	77%	79%
Pain 'Always' Well Controlled[5]	-	-	68%	71%
Room and Bathroom 'Always' Clean[5]	-	-	72%	73%
Timely Help 'Always' Received[5]	-	-	71%	68%
Would Definitely Recommend Hospital[5]	-	-	69%	71%
Use of Medical Imaging				
Cardiac Imaging Stress Test before Surgery	-	-	4.5%	5.3%
Combination Abdominal CT Scan	-	-	6.9%	10.5%
Combination Brain/Sinus CT Scan	-	-	1.6%	2.7%
Combination Chest CT Scan	-	-	0.8%	2.7%
Follow-up Mammogram/Ultrasound	-	-	9.5%	8.8%
Lumbar Spine MRI for Low Back Pain	-	-	44.4%	37.2%

Mount Edgecumbe Hospital

222 Tongass Dr
Sitka, AK 99835
Phone: 907-966-2411
Fax: 907-966-8300
URL: www.searhc.org
Type: Acute Care Hospitals
Emergency Services: Yes
Ownership: Voluntary non-profit - Private
Beds: 78

Key Personnel:

Emergency Room . . . . Robert Carlson
Operating Room. . . . . Jeff Kroskopf
Radiology. . . . . Paul L Peter, MD
CEO/President. . . . . Frank Sutton
Quality Assurance . . . . Mary Therese Thompson

Measure	Cases	This Hosp.	State Avg.	U.S. Avg.
Blood Clot Prevention and Treatment				
Anticoagulation Overlap Therapy[7]	-	-	97%	93%
ICU Venous Thromboembolism Prophylaxis	51	59%	90%	92%
Incidence of Potentially Preventable VTE[7]	-	-	17%	10%
UFH with Dosages/Platelet Monitoring[7]	-	-	98%	97%
Venous Thromboembolism Prophylaxis	214	60%	86%	85%
Warfarin Therapy Discharge Instructions[7]	-	-	80%	75%
Chest Pain/Possible Heart Attack Care				
Aspirin Given Within 24 Hours of Arrival	-	-	99%	96%
Fibrinolytic Meds Within 30 Min. of Arrival	-	-	92%	58%
Average Time to ECG (minutes)	-	-	8	7
Average Time to Transfer (minutes)	-	-	220	60
Children's Asthma Care				
Received Home Management Plan of Care	-	-	-	88%
Received Reliever Medication	-	-	-	100%
Received Systemic Corticosteroids	-	-	-	100%
Emergency Department				
Admittance Decision Time (minutes)	77	25	118	98
Head CT Results Within 45 Min. of Arrival	-	-	29%	57%
Patients Who Left ER Before Being Seen	-	-	3%	2%
Time from ER Arrival to Admit. (minutes)	170	142	287	274
Time from ER Arrival to Discharge (minutes)	-	-	132	134
Time in ER Before Being Evaluated (minutes)	-	-	24	26
Time to Pain Meds for Fractures (minutes)	-	-	57	57

NOTE: Hospital profiles are in alphabetical order by state, then city, then hospital within the city; Rankings exclude hospitals with less than 25 cases except for patient surveys which excludes hospitals with less than 100 cases; (a) 100-299 cases; (1) The number of cases/patients is too few to report; (2) Data submitted were based on a sample of cases/patients; (3) Results are based on a shorter time period than required; (4) Data suppressed by CMS for one or more quarters; (5) Results are not available for this reporting period; (6) Fewer than 100 patients completed the HCAHPS survey; (7) No cases met the criteria for this measure; (8) The lower limit of the confidence interval cannot be calculated if the number of observed infections equals zero; (9) No data are available from the state/territory for this reporting period; (10) The scores shown reflect fewer than 50 completed surveys; (11) There were discrepancies in the data collection process; (12) This measure does not apply to this hospital for this reporting period; (13) Results cannot be calculated for this reporting period; (14) The results for this state are combined with nearby states to protect confidentiality; Please refer to the User's Guide for a full explanation of data.

Measure	Cases	This Hosp.	State Avg.	U.S. Avg.
Heart Attack Care				
Aspirin Given at Discharge[3,7]	-	-	100%	99%
Fibrinolytic Meds Within 30 Min. of Arrival[3,7]	-	-	75%	54%
PCI Within 90 Minutes of Arrival[3,7]	-	-	94%	96%
Statin Prescribed at Discharge[3,7]	-	-	99%	98%
Heart Failure Care				
ACE Inhibitor or ARB for LVSD[1,3]	-	-	99%	97%
Discharge Instructions Given[1,3]	-	-	94%	94%
Evaluation of LVS Function[1,3]	-	-	97%	99%
Medicare Spending				
Medicare Spending per Patient (ratio)	-	0.65	0.91	0.98
Pneumonia Care				
Appropriate Initial Antibiotic Given[1]	-	-	93%	95%
Blood Culture Timing[1]	-	-	97%	98%
Pregnancy and Delivery Care				
Newborn Deliveries Scheduled Early[1]	-	-	2%	6%
Preventive Care				
Immunization for Influenza	319	80%	83%	90%
Immunization for Pneumonia	247	87%	90%	92%
Stroke Care				
Anticoagulation Therapy for Atrial Fibrillation[7]	-	-	80%	95%
Antithrombotic Therapy Timing[1]	-	-	99%	98%
Assessed for Rehabilitation[1]	-	-	97%	97%
Discharged on Antithrombotic Therapy[1]	-	-	98%	99%
Discharged on Statin Medication[1]	-	-	93%	94%
Thrombolytic Therapy Timing[1]	-	-	69%	66%
Venous Thromboembolism Prophylaxis[1]	-	-	93%	94%
Written Stroke Educational Materials Given[1]	-	-	92%	88%
Surgical Care Improvement Project				
Appropriate Beta Blocker Usage[1]	-	-	96%	98%
Appropriate VTP Within 24 Hours	27	81%	97%	98%
Controlled Postoperative Blood Glucose[7]	-	-	95%	97%
Perioperative Temperature Management	28	86%	99%	100%
Prophylactic Antibiotic Selection[1]	-	-	99%	99%
Prophylactic Antibiotic Selection (Outpatient)	-	-	99%	98%
Prophylactic Antibiotic Stopped[1]	-	-	99%	98%
Prophylactic Antibiotic Timing[1]	-	-	99%	99%
Prophylactic Antibiotic Timing (Outpatient)	-	-	97%	98%
Urinary Catheter Removal[1]	-	-	97%	97%
Survey of Patients' Hospital Experiences				
Area Around Room 'Always' Quiet at Night[6]	<100	64%	59%	61%
Doctors 'Always' Communicated Well[6]	<100	81%	82%	82%
Home Recovery Information Given[6]	<100	84%	87%	85%
Hospital Given 9 or 10 on 10 Point Scale[6]	<100	62%	67%	71%
Meds 'Always' Explained Before Given[6]	<100	67%	67%	64%
Nurses 'Always' Communicated Well[6]	<100	72%	77%	79%
Pain 'Always' Well Controlled[6]	<100	68%	68%	71%
Room and Bathroom 'Always' Clean[6]	<100	73%	72%	73%
Timely Help 'Always' Received[6]	<100	75%	71%	68%
Would Definitely Recommend Hospital[6]	<100	54%	69%	71%
Use of Medical Imaging				
Cardiac Imaging Stress Test before Surgery	-	-	4.5%	5.3%
Combination Abdominal CT Scan	-	-	6.9%	10.5%
Combination Brain/Sinus CT Scan	-	-	1.6%	2.7%
Combination Chest CT Scan	-	-	0.8%	2.7%
Follow-up Mammogram/Ultrasound	-	-	9.5%	8.8%
Lumbar Spine MRI for Low Back Pain	-	-	44.4%	37.2%

Sitka Community Hospital

209 Moller Drive
Sitka, AK 99835
Phone: 907-747-3241
Fax: 907-747-1794
Type: Critical Access Hospitals
Emergency Services: Yes
Ownership: Government - Local
Beds: 27

Key Personnel:
Radiology. . . . . Ronda Anderson
Chief of Medical Staff . . . . Roger J Golub, MD

Measure	Cases	This Hosp.	State Avg.	U.S. Avg.
Blood Clot Prevention and Treatment				
Anticoagulation Overlap Therapy[5]	-	-	97%	93%
ICU Venous Thromboembolism Prophylaxis[5]	-	-	90%	92%
Incidence of Potentially Preventable VTE[5]	-	-	17%	10%
UFH with Dosages/Platelet Monitoring[5]	-	-	98%	97%
Venous Thromboembolism Prophylaxis[5]	-	-	86%	85%
Warfarin Therapy Discharge Instructions[5]	-	-	80%	75%
Chest Pain/Possible Heart Attack Care				
Aspirin Given Within 24 Hours of Arrival	-	-	99%	96%
Fibrinolytic Meds Within 30 Min. of Arrival	-	-	92%	58%
Average Time to ECG (minutes)	-	-	8	7
Average Time to Transfer (minutes)	-	-	220	60
Children's Asthma Care				
Received Home Management Plan of Care	-	-	-	88%
Received Reliever Medication	-	-	-	100%
Received Systemic Corticosteroids	-	-	-	100%
Emergency Department				
Admittance Decision Time (minutes)[5]	-	-	118	98
Head CT Results Within 45 Min. of Arrival	-	-	29%	57%
Patients Who Left ER Before Being Seen	-	-	3%	2%
Time from ER Arrival to Admit. (minutes)[5]	-	-	287	274
Time from ER Arrival to Discharge (minutes)	-	-	132	134
Time in ER Before Being Evaluated (minutes)	-	-	24	26
Time to Pain Meds for Fractures (minutes)	-	-	57	57
Heart Attack Care				
Aspirin Given at Discharge[3,7]	-	-	100%	99%
Fibrinolytic Meds Within 30 Min. of Arrival[3,7]	-	-	75%	54%
PCI Within 90 Minutes of Arrival[3,7]	-	-	94%	96%
Statin Prescribed at Discharge[3,7]	-	-	99%	98%
Heart Failure Care				
ACE Inhibitor or ARB for LVSD[3,7]	-	-	99%	97%
Discharge Instructions Given[1,3]	-	-	94%	94%
Evaluation of LVS Function[1,3]	-	-	97%	99%
Medicare Spending				
Medicare Spending per Patient (ratio)	-	-	0.91	0.98
Pneumonia Care				
Appropriate Initial Antibiotic Given[1,3]	-	-	93%	95%
Blood Culture Timing[3,7]	-	-	97%	98%
Pregnancy and Delivery Care				
Newborn Deliveries Scheduled Early[5]	-	-	2%	6%
Preventive Care				
Immunization for Influenza[5]	-	-	83%	90%
Immunization for Pneumonia[5]	-	-	90%	92%
Stroke Care				
Anticoagulation Therapy for Atrial Fibrillation[5]	-	-	80%	95%
Antithrombotic Therapy Timing[5]	-	-	99%	98%
Assessed for Rehabilitation[5]	-	-	97%	97%
Discharged on Antithrombotic Therapy[5]	-	-	98%	99%
Discharged on Statin Medication[5]	-	-	93%	94%
Thrombolytic Therapy Timing[5]	-	-	69%	66%
Venous Thromboembolism Prophylaxis[5]	-	-	93%	94%
Written Stroke Educational Materials Given[5]	-	-	92%	88%
Surgical Care Improvement Project				
Appropriate Beta Blocker Usage[3,7]	-	-	96%	98%
Appropriate VTP Within 24 Hours[1,3]	-	-	97%	98%
Controlled Postoperative Blood Glucose[3,7]	-	-	95%	97%
Perioperative Temperature Management[1,3]	-	-	99%	100%
Prophylactic Antibiotic Selection[3,7]	-	-	99%	99%
Prophylactic Antibiotic Selection (Outpatient)	-	-	99%	98%
Prophylactic Antibiotic Stopped[3,7]	-	-	99%	98%
Prophylactic Antibiotic Timing[3,7]	-	-	99%	99%
Prophylactic Antibiotic Timing (Outpatient)	-	-	97%	98%
Urinary Catheter Removal[1,3]	-	-	97%	97%
Survey of Patients' Hospital Experiences				
Area Around Room 'Always' Quiet at Night[5]	-	-	59%	61%
Doctors 'Always' Communicated Well[5]	-	-	82%	82%
Home Recovery Information Given[5]	-	-	87%	85%
Hospital Given 9 or 10 on 10 Point Scale[5]	-	-	67%	71%
Meds 'Always' Explained Before Given[5]	-	-	67%	64%
Nurses 'Always' Communicated Well[5]	-	-	77%	79%
Pain 'Always' Well Controlled[5]	-	-	68%	71%
Room and Bathroom 'Always' Clean[5]	-	-	72%	73%
Timely Help 'Always' Received[5]	-	-	71%	68%
Would Definitely Recommend Hospital[5]	-	-	69%	71%
Use of Medical Imaging				
Cardiac Imaging Stress Test before Surgery	-	-	4.5%	5.3%
Combination Abdominal CT Scan	-	-	6.9%	10.5%
Combination Brain/Sinus CT Scan	-	-	1.6%	2.7%
Combination Chest CT Scan	-	-	0.8%	2.7%
Follow-up Mammogram/Ultrasound	-	-	9.5%	8.8%
Lumbar Spine MRI for Low Back Pain	-	-	44.4%	37.2%

Central Peninsula General Hospital

250 Hospital Place
Soldotna, AK 99669
Phone: 907-262-4404
Fax: 907-714-4669
E-mail: bnichols@cpgh.org
URL: www.cpgh.org
Type: Acute Care Hospitals
Emergency Services: Yes
Ownership: Voluntary non-profit - Other
Beds: 49

Key Personnel:
Operating Room. . . . . Todd Boling, RN
CEO/President. . . . . Rick Davis
Emergency Room . . . . Teresa Ferguson, RN
Radiology. . . . . Jesse Kincaid, MD
Chief of Medical Staff . . . . Jan Krehel
Hemotology Center . . . . Kathy Lopeman
Infection Control. . . . . Ken Simmons, RN
Quality Assurance . . . . Alan Thye

Measure	Cases	This Hosp.	State Avg.	U.S. Avg.
Blood Clot Prevention and Treatment				
Anticoagulation Overlap Therapy[1,2]	-	-	97%	93%
ICU Venous Thromboembolism Prophylaxis[2]	51	98%	90%	92%
Incidence of Potentially Preventable VTE[1,2]	-	-	17%	10%
UFH with Dosages/Platelet Monitoring[2,7]	-	-	98%	97%
Venous Thromboembolism Prophylaxis[2]	136	94%	86%	85%
Warfarin Therapy Discharge Instructions[1,2]	-	-	80%	75%
Chest Pain/Possible Heart Attack Care				
Aspirin Given Within 24 Hours of Arrival	81	99%	99%	96%
Fibrinolytic Meds Within 30 Min. of Arrival	13	100%	92%	58%
Average Time to ECG (minutes)	84	9	8	7
Average Time to Transfer (minutes)[7]	-	-	220	60
Children's Asthma Care				
Received Home Management Plan of Care	-	-	-	88%
Received Reliever Medication	-	-	-	100%
Received Systemic Corticosteroids	-	-	-	100%
Emergency Department				
Admittance Decision Time (minutes)[2]	280	92	118	98
Head CT Results Within 45 Min. of Arrival[1]	-	-	29%	57%
Patients Who Left ER Before Being Seen	15,776	0%	3%	2%
Time from ER Arrival to Admit. (minutes)[2]	303	291	287	274
Time from ER Arrival to Discharge (minutes)	401	145	132	134
Time in ER Before Being Evaluated (minutes)	420	30	24	26
Time to Pain Meds for Fractures (minutes)	80	50	57	57
Heart Attack Care				
Aspirin Given at Discharge[1]	-	-	100%	99%
Fibrinolytic Meds Within 30 Min. of Arrival[7]	-	-	75%	54%
PCI Within 90 Minutes of Arrival[7]	-	-	94%	96%
Statin Prescribed at Discharge[1]	-	-	99%	98%
Heart Failure Care				
ACE Inhibitor or ARB for LVSD[1]	-	-	99%	97%
Discharge Instructions Given	29	93%	94%	94%
Evaluation of LVS Function	33	100%	97%	99%
Medicare Spending				
Medicare Spending per Patient (ratio)	-	0.86	0.91	0.98
Pneumonia Care				
Appropriate Initial Antibiotic Given	62	100%	93%	95%
Blood Culture Timing	86	100%	97%	98%
Pregnancy and Delivery Care				
Newborn Deliveries Scheduled Early	24	12%	2%	6%
Preventive Care				
Immunization for Influenza[2]	263	95%	83%	90%
Immunization for Pneumonia[2]	233	98%	90%	92%
Stroke Care				
Anticoagulation Therapy for Atrial Fibrillation[1]	-	-	80%	95%
Antithrombotic Therapy Timing	14	100%	99%	98%
Assessed for Rehabilitation	16	100%	97%	97%
Discharged on Antithrombotic Therapy	16	100%	98%	99%
Discharged on Statin Medication	12	83%	93%	94%
Thrombolytic Therapy Timing[1]	-	-	69%	66%
Venous Thromboembolism Prophylaxis	14	100%	93%	94%
Written Stroke Educational Materials Given	12	92%	92%	88%
Surgical Care Improvement Project				

NOTE: Hospital profiles are in alphabetical order by state, then city, then hospital within the city; Rankings exclude hospitals with less than 25 cases except for patient surveys which excludes hospitals with less than 100 cases; (a) 100-299 cases; (1) The number of cases/patients is too few to report; (2) Data submitted were based on a sample of cases/patients; (3) Results are based on a shorter time period than required; (4) Data suppressed by CMS for one or more quarters; (5) Results are not available for this reporting period; (6) Fewer than 100 patients completed the HCAHPS survey; (7) No cases met the criteria for this measure; (8) The lower limit of the confidence interval cannot be calculated if the number of observed infections equals zero; (9) No data are available from the state/territory for this reporting period; (10) The scores shown reflect fewer than 50 completed surveys; (11) There were discrepancies in the data collection process; (12) This measure does not apply to this hospital for this reporting period; (13) Results cannot be calculated for this reporting period; (14) The results for this state are combined with nearby states to protect confidentiality; Please refer to the User's Guide for a full explanation of data.

Measure	Cases	This Hosp.	State Avg.	U.S. Avg.
Appropriate Beta Blocker Usage	29	100%	96%	98%
Appropriate VTP Within 24 Hours	175	99%	97%	98%
Controlled Postoperative Blood Glucose[7]	-	-	95%	97%
Perioperative Temperature Management	198	100%	99%	100%
Prophylactic Antibiotic Selection	144	100%	99%	99%
Prophylactic Antibiotic Selection (Outpatient)[1,3]	-	-	99%	98%
Prophylactic Antibiotic Stopped	144	99%	99%	98%
Prophylactic Antibiotic Timing	144	99%	99%	99%
Prophylactic Antibiotic Timing (Outpatient)[1,3]	-	-	97%	98%
Urinary Catheter Removal	146	99%	97%	97%
Survey of Patients' Hospital Experiences				
Area Around Room 'Always' Quiet at Night	300+	56%	59%	61%
Doctors 'Always' Communicated Well	300+	81%	82%	82%
Home Recovery Information Given	300+	88%	87%	85%
Hospital Given 9 or 10 on 10 Point Scale	300+	70%	67%	71%
Meds 'Always' Explained Before Given	300+	68%	67%	64%
Nurses 'Always' Communicated Well	300+	78%	77%	79%
Pain 'Always' Well Controlled	300+	66%	68%	71%
Room and Bathroom 'Always' Clean	300+	73%	72%	73%
Timely Help 'Always' Received	300+	65%	71%	68%
Would Definitely Recommend Hospital	300+	76%	69%	71%
Use of Medical Imaging				
Cardiac Imaging Stress Test before Surgery	141	5.0%	4.5%	5.3%
Combination Abdominal CT Scan	388	6.4%	6.9%	10.5%
Combination Brain/Sinus CT Scan[1]	-	-	1.6%	2.7%
Combination Chest CT Scan	258	0.0%	0.8%	2.7%
Follow-up Mammogram/Ultrasound	599	12.7%	9.5%	8.8%
Lumbar Spine MRI for Low Back Pain	137	37.2%	44.4%	37.2%

Providence Valdez Medical Center

PO Box 550
Valdez, AK 99686
Phone: 907-835-2249
Type: Critical Access Hospitals
Emergency Services: Yes
Ownership: Government - Local

Measure	Cases	This Hosp.	State Avg.	U.S. Avg.
Blood Clot Prevention and Treatment				
Anticoagulation Overlap Therapy[5]	-	-	97%	93%
ICU Venous Thromboembolism Prophylaxis[5]	-	-	90%	92%
Incidence of Potentially Preventable VTE[5]	-	-	17%	10%
UFH with Dosages/Platelet Monitoring[5]	-	-	98%	97%
Venous Thromboembolism Prophylaxis[5]	-	-	86%	85%
Warfarin Therapy Discharge Instructions[5]	-	-	80%	75%
Chest Pain/Possible Heart Attack Care				
Aspirin Given Within 24 Hours of Arrival	-	-	99%	96%
Fibrinolytic Meds Within 30 Min. of Arrival	-	-	92%	58%
Average Time to ECG (minutes)	-	-	8	7
Average Time to Transfer (minutes)	-	-	220	60
Children's Asthma Care				
Received Home Management Plan of Care	-	-	-	88%
Received Reliever Medication	-	-	-	100%
Received Systemic Corticosteroids	-	-	-	100%
Emergency Department				
Admittance Decision Time (minutes)[5]	-	-	118	98
Head CT Results Within 45 Min. of Arrival	-	-	29%	57%
Patients Who Left ER Before Being Seen	-	-	3%	2%
Time from ER Arrival to Admit. (minutes)[5]	-	-	287	274
Time from ER Arrival to Discharge (minutes)	-	-	132	134
Time in ER Before Being Evaluated (minutes)	-	-	24	26
Time to Pain Meds for Fractures (minutes)	-	-	57	57
Heart Attack Care				
Aspirin Given at Discharge[1,3]	-	-	100%	99%
Fibrinolytic Meds Within 30 Min. of Arrival[1,3]	-	-	75%	54%
PCI Within 90 Minutes of Arrival[3,7]	-	-	94%	96%
Statin Prescribed at Discharge[1,3]	-	-	99%	98%
Heart Failure Care				
ACE Inhibitor or ARB for LVSD[1,3]	-	-	99%	97%
Discharge Instructions Given[1,3]	-	-	94%	94%
Evaluation of LVS Function[1,3]	-	-	97%	99%
Medicare Spending				
Medicare Spending per Patient (ratio)	-	-	0.91	0.98
Pneumonia Care				
Appropriate Initial Antibiotic Given[1,3]	-	-	93%	95%
Blood Culture Timing[3,7]	-	-	97%	98%
Pregnancy and Delivery Care				
Newborn Deliveries Scheduled Early[5]	-	-	2%	6%
Preventive Care				
Immunization for Influenza[5]	-	-	83%	90%
Immunization for Pneumonia[5]	-	-	90%	92%
Stroke Care				
Anticoagulation Therapy for Atrial Fibrillation[5]	-	-	80%	95%
Antithrombotic Therapy Timing[5]	-	-	99%	98%
Assessed for Rehabilitation[5]	-	-	97%	97%
Discharged on Antithrombotic Therapy[5]	-	-	98%	99%
Discharged on Statin Medication[5]	-	-	93%	94%
Thrombolytic Therapy Timing[5]	-	-	69%	66%
Venous Thromboembolism Prophylaxis[5]	-	-	93%	94%
Written Stroke Educational Materials Given[5]	-	-	92%	88%
Surgical Care Improvement Project				
Appropriate Beta Blocker Usage[5]	-	-	96%	98%
Appropriate VTP Within 24 Hours[5]	-	-	97%	98%
Controlled Postoperative Blood Glucose[5]	-	-	95%	97%
Perioperative Temperature Management[5]	-	-	99%	100%
Prophylactic Antibiotic Selection[5]	-	-	99%	99%
Prophylactic Antibiotic Selection (Outpatient)	-	-	99%	98%
Prophylactic Antibiotic Stopped[5]	-	-	99%	98%
Prophylactic Antibiotic Timing[5]	-	-	99%	99%
Prophylactic Antibiotic Timing (Outpatient)	-	-	97%	98%
Urinary Catheter Removal[5]	-	-	97%	97%
Survey of Patients' Hospital Experiences				
Area Around Room 'Always' Quiet at Night[5]	-	-	59%	61%
Doctors 'Always' Communicated Well[5]	-	-	82%	82%
Home Recovery Information Given[5]	-	-	87%	85%
Hospital Given 9 or 10 on 10 Point Scale[5]	-	-	67%	71%
Meds 'Always' Explained Before Given[5]	-	-	67%	64%
Nurses 'Always' Communicated Well[5]	-	-	77%	79%
Pain 'Always' Well Controlled[5]	-	-	68%	71%
Room and Bathroom 'Always' Clean[5]	-	-	72%	73%
Timely Help 'Always' Received[5]	-	-	71%	68%
Would Definitely Recommend Hospital[5]	-	-	69%	71%
Use of Medical Imaging				
Cardiac Imaging Stress Test before Surgery	-	-	4.5%	5.3%
Combination Abdominal CT Scan	-	-	6.9%	10.5%
Combination Brain/Sinus CT Scan	-	-	1.6%	2.7%
Combination Chest CT Scan	-	-	0.8%	2.7%
Follow-up Mammogram/Ultrasound	-	-	9.5%	8.8%
Lumbar Spine MRI for Low Back Pain	-	-	44.4%	37.2%

Wrangell Medical Center

310 Bennett Street PO Box 1081
Wrangell, AK 99929
Phone: 907-874-7000
Fax: 907-874-7100
E-mail: medavidson@wmemail.org
URL: www.wrangellmedicalcenter.com
Type: Critical Access Hospitals
Emergency Services: Yes
Ownership: Government - Local
Beds: 21

Key Personnel:
Operating Room. . . . . Deborah Aaron, RN
Quality Assurance . . . . Janet Buness, RN
CEO/President. . . . . Lynne Campbell
Radiology. . . . . Ann Kramer
Chief of Medical Staff . . . . Lynn Prysunka, MD

Measure	Cases	This Hosp.	State Avg.	U.S. Avg.
Blood Clot Prevention and Treatment				
Anticoagulation Overlap Therapy[5]	-	-	97%	93%
ICU Venous Thromboembolism Prophylaxis[5]	-	-	90%	92%
Incidence of Potentially Preventable VTE[5]	-	-	17%	10%
UFH with Dosages/Platelet Monitoring[5]	-	-	98%	97%
Venous Thromboembolism Prophylaxis[5]	-	-	86%	85%
Warfarin Therapy Discharge Instructions[5]	-	-	80%	75%
Chest Pain/Possible Heart Attack Care				
Aspirin Given Within 24 Hours of Arrival	-	-	99%	96%
Fibrinolytic Meds Within 30 Min. of Arrival	-	-	92%	58%
Average Time to ECG (minutes)	-	-	8	7
Average Time to Transfer (minutes)	-	-	220	60
Children's Asthma Care				
Received Home Management Plan of Care	-	-	-	88%
Received Reliever Medication	-	-	-	100%
Received Systemic Corticosteroids	-	-	-	100%
Emergency Department				
Admittance Decision Time (minutes)[5]	-	-	118	98
Head CT Results Within 45 Min. of Arrival	-	-	29%	57%
Patients Who Left ER Before Being Seen	-	-	3%	2%
Time from ER Arrival to Admit. (minutes)[5]	-	-	287	274
Time from ER Arrival to Discharge (minutes)	-	-	132	134
Time in ER Before Being Evaluated (minutes)	-	-	24	26
Time to Pain Meds for Fractures (minutes)	-	-	57	57
Heart Attack Care				
Aspirin Given at Discharge[3,7]	-	-	100%	99%
Fibrinolytic Meds Within 30 Min. of Arrival[3,7]	-	-	75%	54%
PCI Within 90 Minutes of Arrival[3,7]	-	-	94%	96%
Statin Prescribed at Discharge[3,7]	-	-	99%	98%
Heart Failure Care				
ACE Inhibitor or ARB for LVSD[3,7]	-	-	99%	97%
Discharge Instructions Given[1,3]	-	-	94%	94%
Evaluation of LVS Function[1,3]	-	-	97%	99%
Medicare Spending				
Medicare Spending per Patient (ratio)	-	-	0.91	0.98
Pneumonia Care				
Appropriate Initial Antibiotic Given[1,3]	-	-	93%	95%
Blood Culture Timing[1,3]	-	-	97%	98%
Pregnancy and Delivery Care				
Newborn Deliveries Scheduled Early[5]	-	-	2%	6%
Preventive Care				
Immunization for Influenza[5]	-	-	83%	90%
Immunization for Pneumonia[5]	-	-	90%	92%
Stroke Care				
Anticoagulation Therapy for Atrial Fibrillation[5]	-	-	80%	95%
Antithrombotic Therapy Timing[5]	-	-	99%	98%
Assessed for Rehabilitation[5]	-	-	97%	97%
Discharged on Antithrombotic Therapy[5]	-	-	98%	99%
Discharged on Statin Medication[5]	-	-	93%	94%
Thrombolytic Therapy Timing[5]	-	-	69%	66%
Venous Thromboembolism Prophylaxis[5]	-	-	93%	94%
Written Stroke Educational Materials Given[5]	-	-	92%	88%
Surgical Care Improvement Project				
Appropriate Beta Blocker Usage[5]	-	-	96%	98%
Appropriate VTP Within 24 Hours[5]	-	-	97%	98%
Controlled Postoperative Blood Glucose[5]	-	-	95%	97%
Perioperative Temperature Management[5]	-	-	99%	100%
Prophylactic Antibiotic Selection[5]	-	-	99%	99%
Prophylactic Antibiotic Selection (Outpatient)	-	-	99%	98%
Prophylactic Antibiotic Stopped[5]	-	-	99%	98%
Prophylactic Antibiotic Timing[5]	-	-	99%	99%
Prophylactic Antibiotic Timing (Outpatient)	-	-	97%	98%
Urinary Catheter Removal[5]	-	-	97%	97%
Survey of Patients' Hospital Experiences				
Area Around Room 'Always' Quiet at Night[5]	-	-	59%	61%
Doctors 'Always' Communicated Well[5]	-	-	82%	82%
Home Recovery Information Given[5]	-	-	87%	85%
Hospital Given 9 or 10 on 10 Point Scale[5]	-	-	67%	71%
Meds 'Always' Explained Before Given[5]	-	-	67%	64%
Nurses 'Always' Communicated Well[5]	-	-	77%	79%
Pain 'Always' Well Controlled[5]	-	-	68%	71%
Room and Bathroom 'Always' Clean[5]	-	-	72%	73%
Timely Help 'Always' Received[5]	-	-	71%	68%
Would Definitely Recommend Hospital[5]	-	-	69%	71%
Use of Medical Imaging				
Cardiac Imaging Stress Test before Surgery	-	-	4.5%	5.3%
Combination Abdominal CT Scan	-	-	6.9%	10.5%
Combination Brain/Sinus CT Scan	-	-	1.6%	2.7%
Combination Chest CT Scan	-	-	0.8%	2.7%
Follow-up Mammogram/Ultrasound	-	-	9.5%	8.8%
Lumbar Spine MRI for Low Back Pain	-	-	44.4%	37.2%

NOTE: Hospital profiles are in alphabetical order by state, then city, then hospital within the city; Rankings exclude hospitals with less than 25 cases except for patient surveys which excludes hospitals with less than 100 cases; (a) 100-299 cases; (1) The number of cases/patients is too few to report; (2) Data submitted were based on a sample of cases/patients; (3) Results are based on a shorter time period than required; (4) Data suppressed by CMS for one or more quarters; (5) Results are not available for this reporting period; (6) Fewer than 100 patients completed the HCAHPS survey; (7) No cases met the criteria for this measure; (8) The lower limit of the confidence interval cannot be calculated if the number of observed infections equals zero; (9) No data are available from the state/territory for this reporting period; (10) The scores shown reflect fewer than 50 completed surveys; (11) There were discrepancies in the data collection process; (12) This measure does not apply to this hospital for this reporting period; (13) Results cannot be calculated for this reporting period; (14) The results for this state are combined with nearby states to protect confidentiality; Please refer to the User's Guide for a full explanation of data.

Blood Clot Prevention and Treatment

Anticoagulation Overlap Therapy

Hospital Name	City	Rate	Cases
Carondelet Saint Marys Hospital[2]	Tucson	100%	100
Flagstaff Medical Center[2]	Flagstaff	100%	100
Northwest Medical Center[2]	Tucson	100%	138
Western Arizona Regional Medical Center[2]	Bullhead City	100%	50
Banner Estrella Medical Center[2]	Phoenix	99%	83
Chandler Regional Medical Center[2]	Chandler	99%	189
Tucson Medical Center[2]	Tucson	99%	178
Casa Grande Regional Medical Center[2]	Casa Grande	98%	57
Paradise Valley Hospital[2]	Phoenix	98%	45
Verde Valley Medical Center[2]	Cottonwood	98%	62
West Valley Hospital[2]	Goodyear	98%	58
John C Lincoln Deer Valley Hospital[2]	Phoenix	97%	124
Payson Regional Medical Center[2]	Payson	97%	29
Saint Joseph's Hospital & Medical Center[2]	Phoenix	97%	179
University of Arizona Medical Center[2]	Tucson	97%	39
Arrowhead Hospital[2]	Glendale	96%	76
Banner Gateway Medical Center[2]	Gilbert	96%	92
Banner Good Samaritan Medical Center[2]	Phoenix	96%	113
Havasu Regional Medical Center[2]	Lk Havasu City	96%	67
Oro Valley Hospital[2]	Oro Valley	96%	50
Phoenix Baptist Hospital[2]	Phoenix	96%	77
Banner Heart Hospital[2]	Mesa	95%	41
Banner Thunderbird Medical Center[2]	Glendale	95%	231
John C Lincoln North Mountain Hospital[2]	Phoenix	95%	184
Mayo Clinic Hospital[2]	Phoenix	95%	92
Mercy Gilbert Medical Center[2]	Gilbert	95%	138
Saint Luke's Medical Center[2]	Phoenix	95%	63
Banner Desert Medical Center[2]	Mesa	94%	168
Banner Baywood Medical Center[2]	Mesa	93%	209
Kingman Regional Medical Center[2]	Kingman	93%	82
Banner Boswell Medical Center[2]	Sun City	92%	180
Carondelet Saint Joseph's Hospital[2]	Tucson	92%	120
Maricopa Medical Center[2]	Phoenix	92%	65
Scottsdale Healthcare Osborn Med Ctr[2]	Scottsdale	91%	151
University of Arizona Medical Center[2]	Tucson	91%	156
Scottsdale Healthcare-Shea Med Ctr[2]	Scottsdale	90%	126
Sierra Vista Regional Health Center[2]	Sierra Vista	89%	38
Banner Del E Webb Medical Center[2]	Sun City West	88%	180
Summit Healthcare Regional Medical Center[2]	Show Low	87%	46
Yavapai Regional Medical Center - East[2]	Prescott Valley	86%	35
Scottsdale Hlthcare-Thompson Peak Hosp[2]	Scottsdale	82%	62
Yuma Regional Medical Center[2]	Yuma	77%	30
Yavapai Regional Medical Center[2]	Prescott	74%	106
Mountain Vista Medical Center[2]	Mesa	73%	93

ICU Venous Thromboembolism Prophylaxis

Hospital Name	City	Rate	Cases
Banner Gateway Medical Center[2]	Gilbert	100%	32
Casa Grande Regional Medical Center[2]	Casa Grande	100%	98
Chandler Regional Medical Center[2]	Chandler	100%	64
Havasu Regional Medical Center[2]	Lk Havasu City	100%	48
Payson Regional Medical Center[2]	Payson	100%	59
Arrowhead Hospital[2]	Glendale	99%	69
Flagstaff Medical Center[2]	Flagstaff	99%	152
Saint Joseph's Hospital & Medical Center[2]	Phoenix	99%	147
Western Arizona Regional Medical Center[2]	Bullhead City	99%	153
Fort Defiance Indian Hospital[2]	Fort Defiance	98%	55
John C Lincoln Deer Valley Hospital[2]	Phoenix	98%	90
Sierra Vista Regional Health Center[2]	Sierra Vista	98%	58
Banner Baywood Medical Center[2]	Mesa	97%	33
Carondelet Saint Marys Hospital[2]	Tucson	97%	106
Maryvale Hospital[2]	Phoenix	97%	93
Mercy Gilbert Medical Center[2]	Gilbert	97%	62
Phoenix Baptist Hospital[2]	Phoenix	97%	223
Scottsdale Healthcare Osborn Med Ctr[2]	Scottsdale	97%	119
Paradise Valley Hospital[2]	Phoenix	96%	73
Verde Valley Medical Center[2]	Cottonwood	96%	109
Banner Estrella Medical Center[2]	Phoenix	95%	76
Banner Good Samaritan Medical Center[2]	Phoenix	95%	114
Maricopa Medical Center[2]	Phoenix	95%	74
Mayo Clinic Hospital[2]	Phoenix	95%	40
Tuba City Reg Health Care Corporation[2]	Tuba City	95%	40
Tucson Medical Center[2]	Tucson	95%	43
Banner Desert Medical Center[2]	Mesa	94%	36
Valley View Medical Center[2]	Fort Mohave	94%	69
Scottsdale Hlthcare-Thompson Peak Hosp[2]	Scottsdale	93%	56
Chinle Comprehensive Health Care Facility[2]	Chinle	92%	53
University of Arizona Medical Center[2]	Tucson	92%	111
Yuma Regional Medical Center[2]	Yuma	92%	66
Banner Boswell Medical Center[2]	Sun City	91%	69
Carondelet Saint Joseph's Hospital[2]	Tucson	91%	112
Mount Graham Regional Medical Center[2]	Safford	91%	33
Northwest Medical Center[2]	Tucson	91%	90
John C Lincoln North Mountain Hospital[2]	Phoenix	90%	115
West Valley Hospital[2]	Goodyear	90%	68
Banner Thunderbird Medical Center[2]	Glendale	89%	66
University of Arizona Medical Center[2]	Tucson	89%	81
Banner Del E Webb Medical Center[2]	Sun City West	87%	54
Banner Heart Hospital[2]	Mesa	86%	135
Yavapai Regional Medical Center - East[2]	Prescott Valley	85%	53
Oro Valley Hospital[2]	Oro Valley	83%	47
Scottsdale Healthcare-Shea Med Ctr[2]	Scottsdale	83%	66
Kingman Regional Medical Center[2]	Kingman	79%	63
Saint Luke's Medical Center[2]	Phoenix	76%	121
Yavapai Regional Medical Center[2]	Prescott	76%	101
Mountain Vista Medical Center[2]	Mesa	72%	115
Summit Healthcare Regional Medical Center[2]	Show Low	71%	100

Incidence of Potentially Preventable VTE

Hospital Name	City	Rate	Cases
Tucson Medical Center[2]	Tucson	0%	36
Saint Joseph's Hospital & Medical Center[2]	Phoenix	2%	64
Banner Good Samaritan Medical Center[2]	Phoenix	3%	37
Banner Boswell Medical Center[2]	Sun City	7%	29
Maricopa Medical Center[2]	Phoenix	8%	26
Banner Baywood Medical Center[2]	Mesa	9%	33
Banner Desert Medical Center[2]	Mesa	10%	31
Banner Thunderbird Medical Center[2]	Glendale	10%	50
Scottsdale Healthcare Osborn Med Ctr[2]	Scottsdale	10%	30
University of Arizona Medical Center[2]	Tucson	10%	39
John C Lincoln North Mountain Hospital[2]	Phoenix	11%	45
Scottsdale Healthcare-Shea Med Ctr[2]	Scottsdale	12%	26
Banner Gateway Medical Center[2]	Gilbert	13%	31

UFH with Dosages/Platelet Count Monitoring

Hospital Name	City	Rate	Cases
Banner Baywood Medical Center[2]	Mesa	100%	207
Banner Boswell Medical Center[2]	Sun City	100%	85
Banner Del E Webb Medical Center[2]	Sun City West	100%	83
Banner Gateway Medical Center[2]	Gilbert	100%	43
Banner Good Samaritan Medical Center[2]	Phoenix	100%	68
Banner Heart Hospital[2]	Mesa	100%	40
Banner Thunderbird Medical Center[2]	Glendale	100%	125
Carondelet Saint Marys Hospital[2]	Tucson	100%	48
Casa Grande Regional Medical Center[2]	Casa Grande	100%	28
Chandler Regional Medical Center[2]	Chandler	100%	159
Flagstaff Medical Center[2]	Flagstaff	100%	58
John C Lincoln Deer Valley Hospital[2]	Phoenix	100%	38
John C Lincoln North Mountain Hospital[2]	Phoenix	100%	46
Maricopa Medical Center[2]	Phoenix	100%	31
Mayo Clinic Hospital[2]	Phoenix	100%	104
Mercy Gilbert Medical Center[2]	Gilbert	100%	120
Mountain Vista Medical Center[2]	Mesa	100%	90
Northwest Medical Center[2]	Tucson	100%	78
Oro Valley Hospital[2]	Oro Valley	100%	36
Saint Joseph's Hospital & Medical Center[2]	Phoenix	100%	97
Saint Luke's Medical Center[2]	Phoenix	100%	41
University of Arizona Medical Center[2]	Tucson	100%	139
University of Arizona Medical Center[2]	Tucson	100%	28
Phoenix Baptist Hospital[2]	Phoenix	99%	74
Arrowhead Hospital[2]	Glendale	98%	48
Scottsdale Healthcare-Shea Med Ctr[2]	Scottsdale	98%	46
Scottsdale Healthcare Osborn Med Ctr[2]	Scottsdale	98%	47
Banner Estrella Medical Center[2]	Phoenix	97%	32
West Valley Hospital[2]	Goodyear	97%	35
Banner Desert Medical Center[2]	Mesa	96%	110
Carondelet Saint Joseph's Hospital[2]	Tucson	91%	74
Tucson Medical Center[2]	Tucson	91%	94
Sierra Vista Regional Health Center[2]	Sierra Vista	84%	25
Kingman Regional Medical Center[2]	Kingman	24%	37

Venous Thromboembolism Prophylaxis

Hospital Name	City	Rate	Cases
Gilbert Hospital[2]	Gilbert	100%	106
Oasis Hospital[2]	Phoenix	100%	98
Western Arizona Regional Medical Center[2]	Bullhead City	100%	361
Havasu Regional Medical Center[2]	Lk Havasu City	99%	320
Mayo Clinic Hospital[2]	Phoenix	99%	324
Payson Regional Medical Center[2]	Payson	99%	238
The Surgical Hospital of Phoenix[2]	Phoenix	98%	41
Verde Valley Medical Center[2]	Cottonwood	98%	324
Flagstaff Medical Center[2]	Flagstaff	97%	309
Phoenix Indian Medical Center[2]	Phoenix	97%	150
Banner Gateway Medical Center[2]	Gilbert	96%	382
Casa Grande Regional Medical Center[2]	Casa Grande	95%	345
Chandler Regional Medical Center[2]	Chandler	95%	355
Fort Defiance Indian Hospital[2]	Fort Defiance	95%	103
Carondelet Holy Cross Hospital[2]	Nogales	94%	106
Carondelet Saint Marys Hospital[2]	Tucson	94%	340
Florence Hospital at Anthem[2]	Florence	94%	90
Maryvale Hospital[2]	Phoenix	94%	355
Oro Valley Hospital[2]	Oro Valley	94%	314
Paradise Valley Hospital[2]	Phoenix	94%	337
Whiteriver PHS Indian Hospital[2]	Whiteriver	94%	47
Saint Joseph's Hospital & Medical Center[2]	Phoenix	93%	267
Sierra Vista Regional Health Center[2]	Sierra Vista	93%	378
Banner Baywood Medical Center[2]	Mesa	91%	371
Mercy Gilbert Medical Center[2]	Gilbert	91%	339
Tuba City Reg Health Care Corporation[2]	Tuba City	91%	150
University of Arizona Medical Center[2]	Tucson	91%	281
Banner Heart Hospital[2]	Mesa	90%	296
Banner Ironwood Medical Center[2]	San Tan Valley	90%	129
John C Lincoln Deer Valley Hospital[2]	Phoenix	90%	296
Scottsdale Healthcare-Shea Med Ctr[2]	Scottsdale	90%	347
Tucson Medical Center[2]	Tucson	90%	312
Banner Good Samaritan Medical Center[2]	Phoenix	89%	283
Banner Thunderbird Medical Center[2]	Glendale	89%	345
Chinle Comprehensive Health Care Facility[2]	Chinle	89%	202
Scottsdale Healthcare Osborn Med Ctr[2]	Scottsdale	89%	317
Valley View Medical Center[2]	Fort Mohave	89%	198
West Valley Hospital[2]	Goodyear	89%	356
Scottsdale Hlthcare-Thompson Peak Hosp[2]	Scottsdale	87%	274
Banner Boswell Medical Center[2]	Sun City	86%	320
Banner Desert Medical Center[2]	Mesa	86%	359
Banner Estrella Medical Center[2]	Phoenix	86%	339
Maricopa Medical Center[2]	Phoenix	86%	368
Banner Del E Webb Medical Center[2]	Sun City West	85%	332
Phoenix Baptist Hospital[2]	Phoenix	85%	451
Northwest Medical Center[2]	Tucson	84%	361
Carondelet Saint Joseph's Hospital[2]	Tucson	82%	316
John C Lincoln North Mountain Hospital[2]	Phoenix	82%	316
University of Arizona Medical Center[2]	Tucson	82%	303
Yuma Regional Medical Center[2]	Yuma	81%	414
Summit Healthcare Regional Medical Center[2]	Show Low	80%	169
Yavapai Regional Medical Center - East[2]	Prescott Valley	78%	200
Saint Luke's Medical Center[2]	Phoenix	77%	389
Mount Graham Regional Medical Center[2]	Safford	75%	118
Arrowhead Hospital[2]	Glendale	74%	290
Kingman Regional Medical Center[2]	Kingman	74%	408
Yavapai Regional Medical Center[2]	Prescott	71%	301
Mountain Vista Medical Center[2]	Mesa	65%	327
San Carlos Indian Hospital[2]	San Carlos	7%	54

Warfarin Therapy Discharge Instructions

Hospital Name	City	Rate	Cases
Havasu Regional Medical Center[2]	Lk Havasu City	100%	59
Mercy Gilbert Medical Center[2]	Gilbert	100%	105
Western Arizona Regional Medical Center[2]	Bullhead City	100%	42
Chandler Regional Medical Center[2]	Chandler	99%	132
Mountain Vista Medical Center[2]	Mesa	99%	72
Carondelet Saint Marys Hospital[2]	Tucson	98%	81
Saint Luke's Medical Center[2]	Phoenix	98%	42
Casa Grande Regional Medical Center[2]	Casa Grande	96%	47
Saint Joseph's Hospital & Medical Center[2]	Phoenix	96%	129
Sierra Vista Regional Health Center[2]	Sierra Vista	96%	27
Verde Valley Medical Center[2]	Cottonwood	94%	47
Yavapai Regional Medical Center[2]	Prescott	94%	84
West Valley Hospital[2]	Goodyear	93%	41
Yavapai Regional Medical Center - East[2]	Prescott Valley	93%	27
Carondelet Saint Joseph's Hospital[2]	Tucson	92%	79
Northwest Medical Center[2]	Tucson	92%	104
Oro Valley Hospital[2]	Oro Valley	92%	50
John C Lincoln Deer Valley Hospital[2]	Phoenix	90%	97
Tucson Medical Center[2]	Tucson	90%	141
Flagstaff Medical Center[2]	Flagstaff	88%	78
Maricopa Medical Center[2]	Phoenix	85%	48
Mayo Clinic Hospital[2]	Phoenix	82%	72
Phoenix Baptist Hospital[2]	Phoenix	79%	57
Scottsdale Healthcare Osborn Med Ctr[2]	Scottsdale	77%	124
University of Arizona Medical Center[2]	Tucson	76%	34
Paradise Valley Hospital[2]	Phoenix	67%	36
Banner Gateway Medical Center[2]	Gilbert	62%	76
Banner Estrella Medical Center[2]	Phoenix	59%	70
Banner Del E Webb Medical Center[2]	Sun City West	58%	126
Banner Good Samaritan Medical Center[2]	Phoenix	58%	79
Banner Thunderbird Medical Center[2]	Glendale	57%	154
Banner Desert Medical Center[2]	Mesa	56%	134
Scottsdale Healthcare-Shea Med Ctr[2]	Scottsdale	56%	86
Banner Heart Hospital[2]	Mesa	53%	34
Banner Boswell Medical Center[2]	Sun City	51%	116
Banner Baywood Medical Center[2]	Mesa	48%	156
Summit Healthcare Regional Medical Center[2]	Show Low	47%	43
Scottsdale Hlthcare-Thompson Peak Hosp[2]	Scottsdale	46%	46
John C Lincoln North Mountain Hospital[2]	Phoenix	45%	126
Arrowhead Hospital[2]	Glendale	41%	58
University of Arizona Medical Center[2]	Tucson	40%	106
Kingman Regional Medical Center[2]	Kingman	25%	48

Chest Pain/Possible Heart Attack Care

Aspirin Given Within 24 Hours of Arrival

Hospital Name	City	Rate	Cases
Page Hospital	Page	100%	27
Payson Regional Medical Center	Payson	100%	64
West Valley Hospital	Goodyear	100%	36
Banner Baywood Medical Center	Mesa	99%	531

NOTE: Hospital profiles are in alphabetical order by state, then city, then hospital within the city; Rankings exclude hospitals with less than 25 cases except for patient surveys which excludes hospitals with less than 100 cases; (a) 100-299 cases; (1) The number of cases/patients is too few to report; (2) Data submitted were based on a sample of cases/patients; (3) Results are based on a shorter time period than required; (4) Data suppressed by CMS for one or more quarters; (5) Results are not available for this reporting period; (6) Fewer than 100 patients completed the HCAHPS survey; (7) No cases met the criteria for this measure; (8) The lower limit of the confidence interval cannot be calculated if the number of observed infections equals zero; (9) No data are available from the state/territory for this reporting period; (10) The scores shown reflect fewer than 50 completed surveys; (11) There were discrepancies in the data collection process; (12) This measure does not apply to this hospital for this reporting period; (13) Results cannot be calculated for this reporting period; (14) The results for this state are combined with nearby states to protect confidentiality; Please refer to the User's Guide for a full explanation of data.

Banner Ironwood Medical Center	San Tan Valley	99%	85
Banner Gateway Medical Center	Gilbert	98%	66
Yavapai Regional Medical Center - East	Prescott Valley	98%	108
Florence Hospital at Anthem[3]	Florence	97%	36
Sierra Vista Regional Health Center	Sierra Vista	97%	130
Summit Healthcare Regional Medical Center	Show Low	97%	69
White Mountain Regional Medical Center	Springerville	96%	26
Mount Graham Regional Medical Center	Safford	94%	72
University of Arizona Medical Center	Tucson	92%	38
Gilbert Hospital	Gilbert	89%	27

Average Time to ECG (minutes)

Hospital Name	City	Min.	Cases
West Valley Hospital	Goodyear	1	36
University of Arizona Medical Center	Tucson	2	38
Mount Graham Regional Medical Center	Safford	3	73
White Mountain Regional Medical Center	Springerville	3	25
Page Hospital	Page	4	28
Sierra Vista Regional Health Center	Sierra Vista	5	135
Banner Baywood Medical Center	Mesa	6	548
Banner Ironwood Medical Center	San Tan Valley	6	88
Florence Hospital at Anthem[3]	Florence	6	38
Payson Regional Medical Center	Payson	6	63
Summit Healthcare Regional Medical Center	Show Low	7	67
Gilbert Hospital	Gilbert	8	28
Yavapai Regional Medical Center - East	Prescott Valley	8	113
Banner Gateway Medical Center	Gilbert	10	69

Average Time to Transfer (minutes)

Hospital Name	City	Min.	Cases
Banner Baywood Medical Center	Mesa	38	48

Children's Asthma Care

Received Home Management Plan of Care

Hospital Name	City	Rate	Cases
University of Arizona Medical Center[2]	Tucson	96%	184
Banner Desert Medical Center[2]	Mesa	95%	271
Phoenix Children's Hospital[2]	Phoenix	91%	294

Received Reliever Medication

Hospital Name	City	Rate	Cases
Banner Desert Medical Center[2]	Mesa	100%	272
Phoenix Children's Hospital[2]	Phoenix	100%	294
University of Arizona Medical Center	Tucson	100%	184

Received Systemic Corticosteroids

Hospital Name	City	Rate	Cases
Banner Desert Medical Center[2]	Mesa	100%	269
Phoenix Children's Hospital[2]	Phoenix	100%	292
University of Arizona Medical Center	Tucson	99%	182

Emergency Department

Admittance Decision Time (minutes)

Hospital Name	City	Min.	Cases
Mount Graham Regional Medical Center[2]	Safford	49	251
Banner Ironwood Medical Center[2]	San Tan Valley	58	155
Chinle Comprehensive Health Care Facility[2]	Chinle	60	474
Fort Defiance Indian Hospital[2]	Fort Defiance	63	195
Banner Gateway Medical Center[2]	Gilbert	66	333
Florence Hospital at Anthem[2,3]	Florence	66	438
Banner Baywood Medical Center[2]	Mesa	67	809
Banner Del E Webb Medical Center[2]	Sun City West	67	604
John C Lincoln Deer Valley Hospital[2]	Phoenix	67	630
Gilbert Hospital[2]	Gilbert	68	340
John C Lincoln North Mountain Hospital[2]	Phoenix	69	259
Whiteriver PHS Indian Hospital[2,3]	Whiteriver	70	265
Banner Desert Medical Center[2]	Mesa	75	551
Valley View Medical Center[2]	Fort Mohave	76	468
Summit Healthcare Regional Medical Center[2]	Show Low	77	355
Tuba City Reg Health Care Corporation[2]	Tuba City	77	198
Western Arizona Regional Medical Center[2]	Bullhead City	78	1088
Banner Good Samaritan Medical Center[2]	Phoenix	79	289
Yavapai Regional Medical Center - East[2]	Prescott Valley	80	378
Banner Thunderbird Medical Center[2]	Glendale	82	609
Scottsdale Healthcare-Shea Med Ctr[2]	Scottsdale	83	405
Scottsdale Healthcare Osborn Med Ctr[2]	Scottsdale	83	741
Banner Boswell Medical Center[2]	Sun City	86	820
Casa Grande Regional Medical Center[2]	Casa Grande	88	616
Kingman Regional Medical Center[2]	Kingman	88	844
Maricopa Medical Center[2]	Phoenix	92	564
Scottsdale Hlthcare-Thompson Peak Hosp[2]	Scottsdale	92	573
Oro Valley Hospital[2]	Oro Valley	93	716
Paradise Valley Hospital[2]	Phoenix	96	718
Yuma Regional Medical Center[2]	Yuma	96	475
Mayo Clinic Hospital[2]	Phoenix	97	577
Tucson Medical Center[2]	Tucson	98	304
Yavapai Regional Medical Center[2]	Prescott	98	752
Maryvale Hospital[2]	Phoenix	99	854
University of Arizona Medical Center[2]	Tucson	100	443
Havasu Regional Medical Center[2]	Lk Havasu City	104	686
Mercy Gilbert Medical Center[2]	Gilbert	106	472
Banner Estrella Medical Center[2]	Phoenix	108	521
Phoenix Indian Medical Center[2]	Phoenix	108	351
Chandler Regional Medical Center[2]	Chandler	112	549
West Valley Hospital[2]	Goodyear	113	810
Arrowhead Hospital[2]	Glendale	114	498
Northwest Medical Center[2]	Tucson	120	411
Phoenix Baptist Hospital[2]	Phoenix	125	584
Payson Regional Medical Center[2]	Payson	135	469
Verde Valley Medical Center[2]	Cottonwood	136	430
Flagstaff Medical Center[2]	Flagstaff	138	457
Saint Luke's Medical Center[2]	Phoenix	148	562
Carondelet Saint Joseph's Hospital[2]	Tucson	165	497
Saint Joseph's Hospital & Medical Center[2]	Phoenix	174	374
Mountain Vista Medical Center[2]	Mesa	175	661
Carondelet Saint Marys Hospital[2]	Tucson	186	829
Sierra Vista Regional Health Center[2]	Sierra Vista	197	563
University of Arizona Medical Center[2]	Tucson	324	789

Head CT Results Within 45 Minutes of Arrival

Hospital Name	City	Rate	Cases
Sierra Vista Regional Health Center	Sierra Vista	89%	27
Arrowhead Hospital	Glendale	85%	26
Banner Del E Webb Medical Center	Sun City West	69%	32

Patients Who Left ER Before Being Seen

Hospital Name	City	Rate	Cases
Banner Ironwood Medical Center	San Tan Valley	0%	27671
Carondelet Holy Cross Hospital	Nogales	0%	6522
Chandler Regional Medical Center	Chandler	0%	63401
Florence Hospital at Anthem	Florence	0%	12018
Gilbert Hospital	Gilbert	0%	28106
Mercy Gilbert Medical Center	Gilbert	0%	44331
Mount Graham Regional Medical Center	Safford	0%	18516
Oasis Hospital	Phoenix	0%	47
Saint Joseph's Hospital & Medical Center	Phoenix	0%	84832
West Valley Hospital	Goodyear	0%	70277
Western Arizona Regional Medical Center	Bullhead City	0%	29206
Wickenburg Community Hospital	Wickenburg	0%	5458
Arrowhead Hospital	Glendale	1%	44904
Banner Baywood Medical Center	Mesa	1%	55856
Banner Boswell Medical Center	Sun City	1%	45485
Banner Del E Webb Medical Center	Sun City West	1%	59560
Banner Desert Medical Center	Mesa	1%	114812
Banner Gateway Medical Center	Gilbert	1%	51011
Carondelet Saint Marys Hospital	Tucson	1%	19158
Havasu Regional Medical Center	Lk Havasu City	1%	24869
Maricopa Medical Center	Phoenix	1%	55553
Mayo Clinic Hospital	Phoenix	1%	26143
Northwest Medical Center	Tucson	1%	58361
Oro Valley Hospital	Oro Valley	1%	21998
Page Hospital	Page	1%	8607
Paradise Valley Hospital	Phoenix	1%	35535
Payson Regional Medical Center	Payson	1%	13269
Phoenix Baptist Hospital	Phoenix	1%	62964
Saint Luke's Medical Center	Phoenix	1%	52242
Scottsdale Healthcare-Shea Med Ctr	Scottsdale	1%	46759
Scottsdale Hlthcare-Thompson Peak Hosp	Scottsdale	1%	19282
Scottsdale Healthcare Osborn Med Ctr	Scottsdale	1%	54141
Summit Healthcare Regional Medical Center	Show Low	1%	24421
Valley View Medical Center	Fort Mohave	1%	18724
Verde Valley Medical Center	Cottonwood	1%	30330
Yavapai Regional Medical Center	Prescott	1%	35850
Yavapai Regional Medical Center - East	Prescott Valley	1%	33917
Banner Good Samaritan Medical Center	Phoenix	2%	61587
Casa Grande Regional Medical Center	Casa Grande	2%	36816
Kingman Regional Medical Center	Kingman	2%	47689
Maryvale Hospital	Phoenix	2%	51019
Mountain Vista Medical Center	Mesa	2%	28190
Banner Estrella Medical Center	Phoenix	3%	95671
Banner Thunderbird Medical Center	Glendale	3%	95157
Carondelet Saint Joseph's Hospital	Tucson	3%	20576
Flagstaff Medical Center	Flagstaff	3%	39373
Sierra Vista Regional Health Center	Sierra Vista	3%	28832
Tucson Medical Center	Tucson	3%	87472
Yuma Regional Medical Center	Yuma	3%	70223
John C Lincoln Deer Valley Hospital	Phoenix	4%	75593
John C Lincoln North Mountain Hospital	Phoenix	4%	49527
University of Arizona Medical Center	Tucson	6%	78056
University of Arizona Medical Center	Tucson	8%	39281

Time from ER Arrival to Being Admitted (minutes)

Hospital Name	City	Min.	Cases
Scottsdale Healthcare-Shea Med Ctr[2]	Scottsdale	208	422
San Carlos Indian Hospital[2]	San Carlos	212	58
Scottsdale Healthcare Osborn Med Ctr[2]	Scottsdale	212	781
Banner Ironwood Medical Center[2]	San Tan Valley	219	182
Paradise Valley Hospital[2]	Phoenix	221	718
Valley View Medical Center[2]	Fort Mohave	229	469
Scottsdale Hlthcare-Thompson Peak Hosp[2]	Scottsdale	240	598
Florence Hospital at Anthem[2,3]	Florence	243	438
Banner Desert Medical Center[2]	Mesa	245	566
Casa Grande Regional Medical Center[2]	Casa Grande	246	633
Kingman Regional Medical Center[2]	Kingman	247	889
John C Lincoln North Mountain Hospital[2]	Phoenix	252	264
Mount Graham Regional Medical Center[2]	Safford	252	279
Oro Valley Hospital[2]	Oro Valley	252	725
Maryvale Hospital[2]	Phoenix	253	858
West Valley Hospital[2]	Goodyear	253	815
Gilbert Hospital[2]	Gilbert	257	340
Western Arizona Regional Medical Center[2]	Bullhead City	257	1089
Yavapai Regional Medical Center - East[2]	Prescott Valley	257	405
Havasu Regional Medical Center[2]	Lk Havasu City	262	687
Mercy Gilbert Medical Center[2]	Gilbert	268	480
Yavapai Regional Medical Center[2]	Prescott	269	806
Banner Baywood Medical Center[2]	Mesa	271	817
Banner Good Samaritan Medical Center[2]	Phoenix	271	305
Banner Gateway Medical Center[2]	Gilbert	275	337
Arrowhead Hospital[2]	Glendale	276	500
Summit Healthcare Regional Medical Center[2]	Show Low	281	371
John C Lincoln Deer Valley Hospital[2]	Phoenix	282	636
Banner Del E Webb Medical Center[2]	Sun City West	285	629
Carondelet Holy Cross Hospital[2]	Nogales	286	81
Chinle Comprehensive Health Care Facility[2]	Chinle	286	491
Banner Estrella Medical Center[2]	Phoenix	288	541
Chandler Regional Medical Center[2]	Chandler	290	552
Mayo Clinic Hospital[2]	Phoenix	290	580
Phoenix Baptist Hospital[2]	Phoenix	290	605
Tuba City Reg Health Care Corporation[2]	Tuba City	293	199
Tucson Medical Center[2]	Tucson	293	311
Banner Boswell Medical Center[2]	Sun City	294	834
Payson Regional Medical Center[2]	Payson	294	481
Flagstaff Medical Center[2]	Flagstaff	295	469
Fort Defiance Indian Hospital[2]	Fort Defiance	302	195
Banner Thunderbird Medical Center[2]	Glendale	309	621
Whiteriver PHS Indian Hospital[2,3]	Whiteriver	313	265
Verde Valley Medical Center[2]	Cottonwood	324	583
Northwest Medical Center[2]	Tucson	325	417
Yuma Regional Medical Center[2]	Yuma	327	482
Maricopa Medical Center[2]	Phoenix	353	587
Saint Luke's Medical Center[2]	Phoenix	353	589
Mountain Vista Medical Center[2]	Mesa	356	677
Saint Joseph's Hospital & Medical Center[2]	Phoenix	362	375
Sierra Vista Regional Health Center[2]	Sierra Vista	370	563
Carondelet Saint Marys Hospital[2]	Tucson	387	844
Carondelet Saint Joseph's Hospital[2]	Tucson	388	512
Phoenix Indian Medical Center[2]	Phoenix	445	368
University of Arizona Medical Center[2]	Tucson	480	464
University of Arizona Medical Center[2]	Tucson	531	790

Time from ER Arrival to Discharge (minutes)

Hospital Name	City	Min.	Cases
Valley View Medical Center	Fort Mohave	102	417
Paradise Valley Hospital	Phoenix	116	401
Mount Graham Regional Medical Center	Safford	121	332
West Valley Hospital	Goodyear	122	411
Maryvale Hospital	Phoenix	129	394
Florence Hospital at Anthem[3]	Florence	130	260
Gilbert Hospital	Gilbert	132	363
Kingman Regional Medical Center	Kingman	133	520
Payson Regional Medical Center	Payson	134	374
Yavapai Regional Medical Center - East	Prescott Valley	134	359
Havasu Regional Medical Center	Lk Havasu City	135	383
Verde Valley Medical Center	Cottonwood	135	373
John C Lincoln Deer Valley Hospital	Phoenix	137	362
Arrowhead Hospital	Glendale	142	398
Chandler Regional Medical Center	Chandler	144	376
Casa Grande Regional Medical Center	Casa Grande	147	365
Oro Valley Hospital	Oro Valley	149	387
Banner Ironwood Medical Center	San Tan Valley	150	340
Western Arizona Regional Medical Center	Bullhead City	152	372
Mercy Gilbert Medical Center	Gilbert	155	347
Phoenix Baptist Hospital	Phoenix	156	654
Sierra Vista Regional Health Center	Sierra Vista	159	397
Scottsdale Healthcare-Shea Med Ctr	Scottsdale	161	377
Summit Healthcare Regional Medical Center	Show Low	162	369
Flagstaff Medical Center	Flagstaff	164	378
Yavapai Regional Medical Center	Prescott	164	366
Saint Luke's Medical Center	Phoenix	166	445
Scottsdale Hlthcare-Thompson Peak Hosp	Scottsdale	166	377
Tucson Medical Center	Tucson	168	1540
Scottsdale Healthcare Osborn Med Ctr	Scottsdale	169	350
Mayo Clinic Hospital	Phoenix	176	438
Banner Good Samaritan Medical Center	Phoenix	177	328
Banner Estrella Medical Center	Phoenix	178	291
Yuma Regional Medical Center	Yuma	178	368
Saint Joseph's Hospital & Medical Center	Phoenix	180	367

NOTE: Hospital profiles are in alphabetical order by state, then city, then hospital within the city; Rankings exclude hospitals with less than 25 cases except for patient surveys which excludes hospitals with less than 100 cases; (a) 100-299 cases; (1) The number of cases/patients is too few to report; (2) Data submitted were based on a sample of cases/patients; (3) Results are based on a shorter time period than required; (4) Data suppressed by CMS for one or more quarters; (5) Results are not available for this reporting period; (6) Fewer than 100 patients completed the HCAHPS survey; (7) No cases met the criteria for this measure; (8) The lower limit of the confidence interval cannot be calculated if the number of observed infections equals zero; (9) No data are available from the state/territory for this reporting period; (10) The scores shown reflect fewer than 50 completed surveys; (11) There were discrepancies in the data collection process; (12) This measure does not apply to this hospital for this reporting period; (13) Results cannot be calculated for this reporting period; (14) The results for this state are combined with nearby states to protect confidentiality; Please refer to the User's Guide for a full explanation of data.

Hospital Name	City	Min.	Cases
Banner Del E Webb Medical Center	Sun City West	182	302
Northwest Medical Center	Tucson	187	376
Banner Baywood Medical Center	Mesa	189	306
Banner Desert Medical Center	Mesa	191	332
Carondelet Saint Marys Hospital	Tucson	191	348
Banner Gateway Medical Center	Gilbert	192	341
Maricopa Medical Center	Phoenix	193	355
John C Lincoln North Mountain Hospital	Phoenix	201	353
Banner Boswell Medical Center	Sun City	208	266
Mountain Vista Medical Center	Mesa	216	532
Banner Thunderbird Medical Center	Glendale	220	326
Carondelet Saint Joseph's Hospital	Tucson	228	365
University of Arizona Medical Center	Tucson	248	331
University of Arizona Medical Center	Tucson	268	361

Time in ER Before Being Evaluated (minutes)

Hospital Name	City	Min.	Cases
Gilbert Hospital	Gilbert	8	384
Mercy Gilbert Medical Center	Gilbert	8	390
Banner Ironwood Medical Center	San Tan Valley	10	404
Banner Del E Webb Medical Center	Sun City West	13	169
Florence Hospital at Anthem[3]	Florence	13	287
Mount Graham Regional Medical Center	Safford	13	472
Western Arizona Regional Medical Center	Bullhead City	13	421
Chandler Regional Medical Center	Chandler	15	408
Havasu Regional Medical Center	Lk Havasu City	15	443
Payson Regional Medical Center	Payson	15	419
Casa Grande Regional Medical Center	Casa Grande	16	410
Valley View Medical Center	Fort Mohave	16	443
Banner Baywood Medical Center	Mesa	17	390
Oro Valley Hospital	Oro Valley	19	419
Summit Healthcare Regional Medical Center	Show Low	19	402
Banner Good Samaritan Medical Center	Phoenix	21	382
Yavapai Regional Medical Center - East	Prescott Valley	22	402
Scottsdale Healthcare Osborn Med Ctr	Scottsdale	23	414
Banner Boswell Medical Center	Sun City	24	359
Scottsdale Hlthcare-Thompson Peak Hosp	Scottsdale	24	412
Paradise Valley Hospital	Phoenix	25	421
Yavapai Regional Medical Center	Prescott	25	410
Arrowhead Hospital	Glendale	26	414
Banner Desert Medical Center	Mesa	26	394
West Valley Hospital	Goodyear	26	430
Saint Joseph's Hospital & Medical Center	Phoenix	27	409
Scottsdale Healthcare-Shea Med Ctr	Scottsdale	27	421
Banner Gateway Medical Center	Gilbert	28	397
Carondelet Saint Marys Hospital	Tucson	28	410
Yuma Regional Medical Center	Yuma	28	381
Verde Valley Medical Center	Cottonwood	29	332
Banner Estrella Medical Center	Phoenix	30	393
Maryvale Hospital	Phoenix	30	420
Northwest Medical Center	Tucson	30	411
John C Lincoln Deer Valley Hospital	Phoenix	31	425
Phoenix Baptist Hospital	Phoenix	31	665
Maricopa Medical Center	Phoenix	33	422
Mayo Clinic Hospital	Phoenix	35	212
Banner Thunderbird Medical Center	Glendale	36	382
Flagstaff Medical Center	Flagstaff	40	410
Carondelet Saint Joseph's Hospital	Tucson	41	399
Tucson Medical Center	Tucson	42	1692
Kingman Regional Medical Center	Kingman	45	562
Sierra Vista Regional Health Center	Sierra Vista	48	432
Saint Luke's Medical Center	Phoenix	49	486
John C Lincoln North Mountain Hospital	Phoenix	57	386
Mountain Vista Medical Center	Mesa	65	619
University of Arizona Medical Center	Tucson	69	218
University of Arizona Medical Center	Tucson	73	384

Time to Pain Meds for Bone Fractures (minutes)

Hospital Name	City	Min.	Cases
Valley View Medical Center	Fort Mohave	27	49
John C Lincoln Deer Valley Hospital	Phoenix	29	174
Gilbert Hospital	Gilbert	32	85
Mercy Gilbert Medical Center	Gilbert	35	189
Florence Hospital at Anthem[3]	Florence	38	44
Banner Ironwood Medical Center	San Tan Valley	40	120
Banner Desert Medical Center	Mesa	42	411
West Valley Hospital	Goodyear	44	251
Flagstaff Medical Center	Flagstaff	46	127
Paradise Valley Hospital	Phoenix	46	110
Maryvale Hospital	Phoenix	47	157
Western Arizona Regional Medical Center	Bullhead City	47	172
Havasu Regional Medical Center	Lk Havasu City	48	99
Kingman Regional Medical Center	Kingman	49	107
Oro Valley Hospital	Oro Valley	50	93
Arrowhead Hospital	Glendale	54	160
Banner Del E Webb Medical Center	Sun City West	55	179
Mount Graham Regional Medical Center	Safford	55	54
Banner Thunderbird Medical Center	Glendale	56	233
Chandler Regional Medical Center	Chandler	56	268
Scottsdale Healthcare-Shea Med Ctr	Scottsdale	56	248
Summit Healthcare Regional Medical Center	Show Low	56	188
Yavapai Regional Medical Center - East	Prescott Valley	56	95
Banner Good Samaritan Medical Center	Phoenix	57	107
Yavapai Regional Medical Center	Prescott	57	121
Mayo Clinic Hospital	Phoenix	58	63
Scottsdale Hlthcare-Thompson Peak Hosp	Scottsdale	59	104
Scottsdale Healthcare Osborn Med Ctr	Scottsdale	59	131
Verde Valley Medical Center	Cottonwood	59	155
Banner Estrella Medical Center	Phoenix	62	278
Phoenix Baptist Hospital	Phoenix	63	129
Tucson Medical Center	Tucson	63	350
Banner Boswell Medical Center	Sun City	64	98
John C Lincoln North Mountain Hospital	Phoenix	66	76
Payson Regional Medical Center	Payson	66	72
Saint Joseph's Hospital & Medical Center	Phoenix	66	147
University of Arizona Medical Center	Tucson	66	201
Banner Baywood Medical Center	Mesa	67	127
Saint Luke's Medical Center	Phoenix	67	103
Yuma Regional Medical Center	Yuma	67	338
Casa Grande Regional Medical Center	Casa Grande	68	117
Maricopa Medical Center	Phoenix	69	180
Banner Gateway Medical Center	Gilbert	70	166
Northwest Medical Center	Tucson	73	187
Sierra Vista Regional Health Center	Sierra Vista	74	101
University of Arizona Medical Center	Tucson	75	135
Carondelet Saint Marys Hospital	Tucson	80	218
Mountain Vista Medical Center	Mesa	80	171
Carondelet Saint Joseph's Hospital	Tucson	105	238

Heart Attack Care

Aspirin Given at Discharge

Hospital Name	City	Rate	Cases
Arrowhead Hospital	Glendale	100%	150
Banner Boswell Medical Center[2]	Sun City	100%	273
Banner Del E Webb Medical Center[2]	Sun City West	100%	237
Banner Desert Medical Center[2]	Mesa	100%	263
Banner Estrella Medical Center[2]	Phoenix	100%	282
Banner Good Samaritan Medical Center[2]	Phoenix	100%	280
Banner Heart Hospital[2]	Mesa	100%	303
Banner Thunderbird Medical Center[2]	Glendale	100%	246
Carondelet Saint Marys Hospital	Tucson	100%	301
Casa Grande Regional Medical Center	Casa Grande	100%	85
John C Lincoln North Mountain Hospital	Phoenix	100%	144
Maryvale Hospital	Phoenix	100%	26
Mercy Gilbert Medical Center	Gilbert	100%	132
Northwest Medical Center	Tucson	100%	208
Oro Valley Hospital	Oro Valley	100%	73
Paradise Valley Hospital	Phoenix	100%	69
Phoenix Baptist Hospital	Phoenix	100%	241
Phoenix VA Medical Center	Phoenix	100%	29
Saint Joseph's Hospital & Medical Center	Phoenix	100%	202
Scottsdale Healthcare-Shea Med Ctr[2]	Scottsdale	100%	194
Scottsdale Hlthcare-Thompson Peak Hosp	Scottsdale	100%	68
Scottsdale Healthcare Osborn Med Ctr	Scottsdale	100%	145
Tucson Medical Center	Tucson	100%	453
University of Arizona Medical Center[2]	Tucson	100%	182
VA Southern Arizona Healthcare System	Tucson	100%	90
Valley View Medical Center[2]	Fort Mohave	100%	47
West Valley Hospital	Goodyear	100%	226
Western Arizona Regional Medical Center	Bullhead City	100%	151
Chandler Regional Medical Center[2]	Chandler	99%	332
Flagstaff Medical Center	Flagstaff	99%	181
Havasu Regional Medical Center	Lk Havasu City	99%	164
John C Lincoln Deer Valley Hospital	Phoenix	99%	195
Kingman Regional Medical Center[2]	Kingman	99%	156
University of Arizona Medical Center[2]	Tucson	99%	265
Verde Valley Medical Center	Cottonwood	99%	81
Carondelet Saint Joseph's Hospital[2]	Tucson	98%	174
Yavapai Regional Medical Center	Prescott	98%	341
Yuma Regional Medical Center	Yuma	98%	331
Maricopa Medical Center	Phoenix	97%	87
Mayo Clinic Hospital	Phoenix	97%	142
Saint Luke's Medical Center	Phoenix	97%	139
Summit Healthcare Regional Medical Center	Show Low	97%	78
Mountain Vista Medical Center	Mesa	94%	210
Sierra Vista Regional Health Center	Sierra Vista	91%	44

PCI Within 90 Minutes of Arrival

Hospital Name	City	Rate	Cases
Arrowhead Hospital	Glendale	100%	33
Carondelet Saint Joseph's Hospital[2]	Tucson	100%	41
Northwest Medical Center	Tucson	100%	36
Oro Valley Hospital	Oro Valley	100%	25
Paradise Valley Hospital	Phoenix	100%	27
Saint Joseph's Hospital & Medical Center	Phoenix	100%	39
Scottsdale Healthcare-Shea Med Ctr[2]	Scottsdale	100%	48
Scottsdale Healthcare Osborn Med Ctr	Scottsdale	100%	40
John C Lincoln Deer Valley Hospital	Phoenix	98%	41
Tucson Medical Center	Tucson	98%	56
West Valley Hospital	Goodyear	98%	58
Banner Boswell Medical Center[2]	Sun City	97%	35
Banner Estrella Medical Center[2]	Phoenix	97%	35
Banner Thunderbird Medical Center[2]	Glendale	97%	34
Banner Del E Webb Medical Center[2]	Sun City West	96%	47
Chandler Regional Medical Center[2]	Chandler	96%	55
John C Lincoln North Mountain Hospital	Phoenix	96%	26
Phoenix Baptist Hospital	Phoenix	96%	75
Mountain Vista Medical Center	Mesa	95%	38
Banner Desert Medical Center[2]	Mesa	93%	43
Verde Valley Medical Center	Cottonwood	93%	28
Carondelet Saint Marys Hospital	Tucson	92%	59
Havasu Regional Medical Center	Lk Havasu City	92%	37
Casa Grande Regional Medical Center	Casa Grande	90%	31
University of Arizona Medical Center[2]	Tucson	90%	29
Yavapai Regional Medical Center	Prescott	89%	44
Mercy Gilbert Medical Center	Gilbert	88%	34
Yuma Regional Medical Center	Yuma	87%	61
Kingman Regional Medical Center[2]	Kingman	84%	44
Flagstaff Medical Center	Flagstaff	81%	31

Statin Prescribed at Discharge

Hospital Name	City	Rate	Cases
Arrowhead Hospital	Glendale	100%	146
Banner Boswell Medical Center[2]	Sun City	100%	256
Banner Del E Webb Medical Center[2]	Sun City West	100%	228
Banner Desert Medical Center[2]	Mesa	100%	257
Banner Thunderbird Medical Center[2]	Glendale	100%	238
Carondelet Saint Marys Hospital	Tucson	100%	283
Flagstaff Medical Center	Flagstaff	100%	171
John C Lincoln Deer Valley Hospital	Phoenix	100%	191
Paradise Valley Hospital	Phoenix	100%	70
Phoenix Baptist Hospital	Phoenix	100%	237
Phoenix VA Medical Center	Phoenix	100%	30
Saint Joseph's Hospital & Medical Center	Phoenix	100%	200
Scottsdale Hlthcare-Thompson Peak Hosp	Scottsdale	100%	63
Summit Healthcare Regional Medical Center	Show Low	100%	75
Tucson Medical Center	Tucson	100%	421
University of Arizona Medical Center[2]	Tucson	100%	264
Valley View Medical Center[2]	Fort Mohave	100%	47
Banner Estrella Medical Center[2]	Phoenix	99%	271
Banner Heart Hospital[2]	Mesa	99%	293
Havasu Regional Medical Center	Lk Havasu City	99%	159
John C Lincoln North Mountain Hospital	Phoenix	99%	136
Northwest Medical Center	Tucson	99%	195
Scottsdale Healthcare-Shea Med Ctr[2]	Scottsdale	99%	187
Scottsdale Healthcare Osborn Med Ctr	Scottsdale	99%	143
University of Arizona Medical Center[2]	Tucson	99%	176
VA Southern Arizona Healthcare System	Tucson	99%	88
West Valley Hospital	Goodyear	99%	222
Carondelet Saint Joseph's Hospital[2]	Tucson	98%	166
Chandler Regional Medical Center[2]	Chandler	98%	327
Maricopa Medical Center	Phoenix	98%	87
Mayo Clinic Hospital	Phoenix	98%	135
Mercy Gilbert Medical Center	Gilbert	98%	129
Western Arizona Regional Medical Center	Bullhead City	98%	140
Yuma Regional Medical Center	Yuma	98%	317
Banner Good Samaritan Medical Center[2]	Phoenix	97%	264
Oro Valley Hospital	Oro Valley	97%	70
Verde Valley Medical Center	Cottonwood	97%	77
Yavapai Regional Medical Center	Prescott	95%	329
Casa Grande Regional Medical Center	Casa Grande	94%	81
Kingman Regional Medical Center[2]	Kingman	93%	152
Mountain Vista Medical Center	Mesa	91%	204
Saint Luke's Medical Center	Phoenix	89%	141
Sierra Vista Regional Health Center	Sierra Vista	72%	46

Heart Failure Care

ACE Inhibitor or ARB for LVSD

Hospital Name	City	Rate	Cases
Banner Boswell Medical Center[2]	Sun City	100%	68
Banner Del E Webb Medical Center[2]	Sun City West	100%	62
Banner Desert Medical Center[2]	Mesa	100%	114
Banner Gateway Medical Center	Gilbert	100%	31
Banner Heart Hospital[2]	Mesa	100%	122
Banner Thunderbird Medical Center[2]	Glendale	100%	90
Carondelet Saint Joseph's Hospital	Tucson	100%	56
Havasu Regional Medical Center	Lk Havasu City	100%	42
John C Lincoln North Mountain Hospital[2]	Phoenix	100%	103
Maryvale Hospital	Phoenix	100%	82
Mayo Clinic Hospital	Phoenix	100%	113
Northwest Medical Center	Tucson	100%	105
Paradise Valley Hospital	Phoenix	100%	44
Phoenix VA Medical Center	Phoenix	100%	85
Saint Joseph's Hospital & Medical Center[2]	Phoenix	100%	117
Scottsdale Healthcare-Shea Med Ctr[2]	Scottsdale	100%	78
Scottsdale Healthcare Osborn Med Ctr[2]	Scottsdale	100%	72
Tucson Medical Center[2]	Tucson	100%	80
University of Arizona Medical Center[2]	Tucson	100%	131

NOTE: Hospital profiles are in alphabetical order by state, then city, then hospital within the city; Rankings exclude hospitals with less than 25 cases except for patient surveys which excludes hospitals with less than 100 cases; (a) 100-299 cases; (1) The number of cases/patients is too few to report; (2) Data submitted were based on a sample of cases/patients; (3) Results are based on a shorter time period than required; (4) Data suppressed by CMS for one or more quarters; (5) Results are not available for this reporting period; (6) Fewer than 100 patients completed the HCAHPS survey; (7) No cases met the criteria for this measure; (8) The lower limit of the confidence interval cannot be calculated if the number of observed infections equals zero; (9) No data are available from the state/territory for this reporting period; (10) The scores shown reflect fewer than 50 completed surveys; (11) There were discrepancies in the data collection process; (12) This measure does not apply to this hospital for this reporting period; (13) Results cannot be calculated for this reporting period; (14) The results for this state are combined with nearby states to protect confidentiality; Please refer to the User's Guide for a full explanation of data.

Hospital Name	City	Rate	Cases
University of Arizona Medical Center	Tucson	100%	67
Western Arizona Regional Medical Center	Bullhead City	100%	54
Banner Estrella Medical Center[2]	Phoenix	99%	106
Banner Good Samaritan Medical Center[2]	Phoenix	99%	112
Carondelet Saint Marys Hospital[2]	Tucson	99%	102
John C Lincoln Deer Valley Hospital[2]	Phoenix	99%	88
Maricopa Medical Center[2]	Phoenix	99%	95
Mercy Gilbert Medical Center[2]	Gilbert	99%	79
VA Southern Arizona Healthcare System	Tucson	99%	80
Arrowhead Hospital	Glendale	98%	50
Banner Baywood Medical Center[2]	Mesa	98%	53
Chandler Regional Medical Center[2]	Chandler	98%	97
West Valley Hospital	Goodyear	98%	88
Yuma Regional Medical Center	Yuma	98%	170
Flagstaff Medical Center	Flagstaff	97%	62
Phoenix Baptist Hospital	Phoenix	97%	143
Casa Grande Regional Medical Center	Casa Grande	96%	49
Oro Valley Hospital	Oro Valley	96%	46
Kingman Regional Medical Center[2]	Kingman	94%	109
Tuba City Reg Health Care Corporation	Tuba City	94%	31
Yavapai Regional Medical Center	Prescott	94%	51
Mountain Vista Medical Center	Mesa	88%	91
Saint Luke's Medical Center	Phoenix	84%	67
Sierra Vista Regional Health Center	Sierra Vista	69%	35

Discharge Instructions Given

Hospital Name	City	Rate	Cases
Arrowhead Hospital	Glendale	100%	124
Casa Grande Regional Medical Center	Casa Grande	100%	110
Maryvale Hospital	Phoenix	100%	143
Mount Graham Regional Medical Center	Safford	100%	28
Paradise Valley Hospital	Phoenix	100%	79
Tucson Medical Center[2]	Tucson	100%	237
West Valley Hospital	Goodyear	100%	198
Yuma Regional Medical Center	Yuma	100%	365
Carondelet Saint Marys Hospital[2]	Tucson	99%	258
Chandler Regional Medical Center[2]	Chandler	99%	267
Flagstaff Medical Center	Flagstaff	99%	162
Havasu Regional Medical Center	Lk Havasu City	99%	152
Maricopa Medical Center[2]	Phoenix	99%	179
Phoenix Baptist Hospital	Phoenix	99%	315
University of Arizona Medical Center[2]	Tucson	99%	228
Valley View Medical Center[2]	Fort Mohave	99%	93
Verde Valley Medical Center	Cottonwood	99%	77
Banner Heart Hospital[2]	Mesa	98%	255
John C Lincoln North Mountain Hospital[2]	Phoenix	98%	216
Mayo Clinic Hospital	Phoenix	98%	265
Saint Joseph's Hospital & Medical Center[2]	Phoenix	98%	236
VA Northern Arizona Healthcare System	Prescott	98%	40
Western Arizona Regional Medical Center	Bullhead City	98%	253
Banner Boswell Medical Center[2]	Sun City	97%	232
Banner Desert Medical Center[2]	Mesa	97%	236
Banner Thunderbird Medical Center[2]	Glendale	97%	234
Sierra Vista Regional Health Center	Sierra Vista	97%	90
Banner Baywood Medical Center[2]	Mesa	96%	158
Banner Del E Webb Medical Center[2]	Sun City West	96%	202
Banner Estrella Medical Center[2]	Phoenix	96%	260
Banner Gateway Medical Center	Gilbert	96%	141
Banner Good Samaritan Medical Center[2]	Phoenix	96%	262
Mercy Gilbert Medical Center[2]	Gilbert	95%	220
Phoenix VA Medical Center	Phoenix	95%	201
Yavapai Regional Medical Center	Prescott	94%	115
Carondelet Saint Joseph's Hospital	Tucson	93%	189
John C Lincoln Deer Valley Hospital[2]	Phoenix	93%	208
Oro Valley Hospital	Oro Valley	93%	129
Cobre Valley Regional Medical Center	Globe	92%	50
Yavapai Regional Medical Center - East	Prescott Valley	90%	42
Northwest Medical Center	Tucson	89%	241
Payson Regional Medical Center	Payson	89%	27
Summit Healthcare Regional Medical Center	Show Low	89%	72
Mountain Vista Medical Center	Mesa	87%	188
University of Arizona Medical Center	Tucson	86%	130
Kingman Regional Medical Center[2]	Kingman	84%	238
Saint Luke's Medical Center	Phoenix	80%	120
Scottsdale Healthcare Osborn Med Ctr[2]	Scottsdale	76%	237
Scottsdale Healthcare-Shea Med Ctr[2]	Scottsdale	70%	243
VA Southern Arizona Healthcare System	Tucson	65%	179
Scottsdale Hlthcare-Thompson Peak Hosp	Scottsdale	64%	72
Tuba City Reg Health Care Corporation	Tuba City	60%	47
Chinle Comprehensive Health Care Facility[2]	Chinle	44%	25
Fort Defiance Indian Hospital[2]	Fort Defiance	35%	26

Evaluation of LVS Function

Hospital Name	City	Rate	Cases
Banner Baywood Medical Center[2]	Mesa	100%	204
Banner Boswell Medical Center[2]	Sun City	100%	285
Banner Del E Webb Medical Center[2]	Sun City West	100%	244
Banner Desert Medical Center[2]	Mesa	100%	288
Banner Estrella Medical Center[2]	Phoenix	100%	289
Banner Gateway Medical Center	Gilbert	100%	156
Banner Good Samaritan Medical Center[2]	Phoenix	100%	291
Banner Heart Hospital[2]	Mesa	100%	291
Banner Thunderbird Medical Center[2]	Glendale	100%	273
Carondelet Saint Joseph's Hospital	Tucson	100%	232
Carondelet Saint Marys Hospital[2]	Tucson	100%	292
Chandler Regional Medical Center[2]	Chandler	100%	298
Chinle Comprehensive Health Care Facility[2]	Chinle	100%	27
Cobre Valley Regional Medical Center	Globe	100%	68
Flagstaff Medical Center	Flagstaff	100%	178
Havasu Regional Medical Center	Lk Havasu City	100%	162
John C Lincoln Deer Valley Hospital[2]	Phoenix	100%	237
John C Lincoln North Mountain Hospital[2]	Phoenix	100%	251
Maryvale Hospital	Phoenix	100%	156
Mayo Clinic Hospital	Phoenix	100%	278
Mercy Gilbert Medical Center[2]	Gilbert	100%	252
Mount Graham Regional Medical Center	Safford	100%	28
Mountain Vista Medical Center	Mesa	100%	215
Northwest Medical Center	Tucson	100%	284
Oro Valley Hospital	Oro Valley	100%	138
Paradise Valley Hospital	Phoenix	100%	94
Payson Regional Medical Center	Payson	100%	33
Phoenix Baptist Hospital	Phoenix	100%	337
Phoenix VA Medical Center	Phoenix	100%	211
Saint Joseph's Hospital & Medical Center[2]	Phoenix	100%	258
Scottsdale Healthcare-Shea Med Ctr[2]	Scottsdale	100%	289
Scottsdale Hlthcare-Thompson Peak Hosp	Scottsdale	100%	87
Scottsdale Healthcare Osborn Med Ctr[2]	Scottsdale	100%	282
Tucson Medical Center[2]	Tucson	100%	273
University of Arizona Medical Center[2]	Tucson	100%	257
VA Northern Arizona Healthcare System	Prescott	100%	45
VA Southern Arizona Healthcare System	Tucson	100%	200
Valley View Medical Center[2]	Fort Mohave	100%	99
West Valley Hospital	Goodyear	100%	220
Arrowhead Hospital	Glendale	99%	144
Maricopa Medical Center[2]	Phoenix	99%	192
Saint Luke's Medical Center	Phoenix	99%	138
University of Arizona Medical Center	Tucson	99%	145
Verde Valley Medical Center	Cottonwood	99%	86
Western Arizona Regional Medical Center	Bullhead City	99%	278
Yuma Regional Medical Center	Yuma	99%	416
Kingman Regional Medical Center[2]	Kingman	98%	262
Yavapai Regional Medical Center - East	Prescott Valley	98%	47
Yavapai Regional Medical Center	Prescott	97%	132
Casa Grande Regional Medical Center	Casa Grande	96%	119
Sierra Vista Regional Health Center	Sierra Vista	96%	113
Tuba City Reg Health Care Corporation	Tuba City	94%	49
Summit Healthcare Regional Medical Center	Show Low	91%	82
Fort Defiance Indian Hospital[2]	Fort Defiance	82%	28

Medicare Spending

Medicare Spending per Patient (ratio)

Hospital Name	City	Ratio	Cases
Chinle Comprehensive Health Care Facility	Chinle	0.64	-
Whiteriver PHS Indian Hospital	Whiteriver	0.70	-
Fort Defiance Indian Hospital	Fort Defiance	0.72	-
Tuba City Reg Health Care Corporation	Tuba City	0.72	-
Phoenix Indian Medical Center	Phoenix	0.75	-
Mount Graham Regional Medical Center	Safford	0.84	-
Summit Healthcare Regional Medical Center	Show Low	0.85	-
Gilbert Hospital	Gilbert	0.87	-
Banner Ironwood Medical Center	San Tan Valley	0.88	-
Flagstaff Medical Center	Flagstaff	0.88	-
Havasu Regional Medical Center	Lk Havasu City	0.88	-
Western Arizona Regional Medical Center	Bullhead City	0.88	-
Valley View Medical Center	Fort Mohave	0.89	-
The Surgical Hospital of Phoenix	Phoenix	0.90	-
Kingman Regional Medical Center	Kingman	0.91	-
Maricopa Medical Center	Phoenix	0.91	-
Mayo Clinic Hospital	Phoenix	0.91	-
Payson Regional Medical Center	Payson	0.91	-
Sierra Vista Regional Health Center	Sierra Vista	0.92	-
Banner Estrella Medical Center	Phoenix	0.93	-
Oro Valley Hospital	Oro Valley	0.93	-
Arizona Spine & Joint Hospital	Mesa	0.94	-
Banner Boswell Medical Center	Sun City	0.94	-
Banner Heart Hospital	Mesa	0.94	-
Casa Grande Regional Medical Center	Casa Grande	0.94	-
Chandler Regional Medical Center	Chandler	0.95	-
Yavapai Regional Medical Center	Prescott	0.95	-
Banner Gateway Medical Center	Gilbert	0.96	-
Florence Hospital at Anthem	Florence	0.96	-
John C Lincoln Deer Valley Hospital	Phoenix	0.96	-
Carondelet Saint Marys Hospital	Tucson	0.97	-
John C Lincoln North Mountain Hospital	Phoenix	0.97	-
Maryvale Hospital	Phoenix	0.97	-
Oasis Hospital	Phoenix	0.97	-
Paradise Valley Hospital	Phoenix	0.97	-
Verde Valley Medical Center	Cottonwood	0.97	-
West Valley Hospital	Goodyear	0.97	-
Banner Baywood Medical Center	Mesa	0.98	-
Banner Del E Webb Medical Center	Sun City West	0.98	-
Banner Desert Medical Center	Mesa	0.98	-
Mercy Gilbert Medical Center	Gilbert	0.98	-
Phoenix Baptist Hospital	Phoenix	0.98	-
Scottsdale Hlthcare-Thompson Peak Hosp	Scottsdale	0.98	-
University of Arizona Medical Center	Tucson	0.98	-
University of Arizona Medical Center	Tucson	0.98	-
Banner Good Samaritan Medical Center	Phoenix	0.99	-
Banner Thunderbird Medical Center	Glendale	0.99	-
Tucson Medical Center	Tucson	0.99	-
Arrowhead Hospital	Glendale	1.00	-
Saint Joseph's Hospital & Medical Center	Phoenix	1.00	-
Yavapai Regional Medical Center - East	Prescott Valley	1.00	-
Yuma Regional Medical Center	Yuma	1.00	-
Carondelet Saint Joseph's Hospital	Tucson	1.01	-
Mountain Vista Medical Center	Mesa	1.01	-
Northwest Medical Center	Tucson	1.01	-
Saint Luke's Medical Center	Phoenix	1.01	-
Scottsdale Healthcare Osborn Med Ctr	Scottsdale	1.01	-
Scottsdale Healthcare-Shea Med Ctr	Scottsdale	1.03	-
Arizona Ortho & Surgical Spec Hosp	Chandler	1.04	-

Pneumonia Care

Appropriate Initial Antibiotic Given

Hospital Name	City	Rate	Cases
Arrowhead Hospital	Glendale	100%	223
Banner Boswell Medical Center[2]	Sun City	100%	83
Banner Del E Webb Medical Center[2]	Sun City West	100%	87
Banner Desert Medical Center[2]	Mesa	100%	93
Banner Good Samaritan Medical Center[2]	Phoenix	100%	81
Banner Ironwood Medical Center	San Tan Valley	100%	49
Flagstaff Medical Center[2]	Flagstaff	100%	104
Maryvale Hospital	Phoenix	100%	176
Saint Joseph's Hospital & Medical Center[2]	Phoenix	100%	61
Tucson Medical Center[2]	Tucson	100%	79
Banner Estrella Medical Center[2]	Phoenix	99%	91
Carondelet Saint Joseph's Hospital[2]	Tucson	99%	107
Chandler Regional Medical Center[2]	Chandler	99%	121
Cobre Valley Regional Medical Center	Globe	99%	75
Havasu Regional Medical Center	Lk Havasu City	99%	136
Oro Valley Hospital	Oro Valley	99%	88
Phoenix VA Medical Center	Phoenix	99%	71
West Valley Hospital	Goodyear	99%	268
Western Arizona Regional Medical Center	Bullhead City	99%	134
Yuma Regional Medical Center[2]	Yuma	99%	135
Banner Baywood Medical Center[2]	Mesa	98%	105
Banner Gateway Medical Center[2]	Gilbert	98%	88
Banner Thunderbird Medical Center[2]	Glendale	98%	85
Carondelet Saint Marys Hospital[2]	Tucson	98%	105
John C Lincoln North Mountain Hospital[2]	Phoenix	98%	60
Kingman Regional Medical Center[2]	Kingman	98%	244
Northwest Medical Center	Tucson	98%	257
Paradise Valley Hospital	Phoenix	98%	122
Payson Regional Medical Center	Payson	98%	64
Phoenix Indian Medical Center[2]	Phoenix	98%	55
Saint Luke's Medical Center	Phoenix	98%	98
John C Lincoln Deer Valley Hospital[2]	Phoenix	97%	115
Mercy Gilbert Medical Center[2]	Gilbert	97%	107
Phoenix Baptist Hospital	Phoenix	97%	159
Scottsdale Hlthcare-Thompson Peak Hosp[2]	Scottsdale	97%	90
Scottsdale Healthcare Osborn Med Ctr[2]	Scottsdale	97%	103
Mayo Clinic Hospital	Phoenix	96%	80
Scottsdale Healthcare-Shea Med Ctr[2]	Scottsdale	96%	103
Valley View Medical Center[2]	Fort Mohave	96%	47
Yavapai Regional Medical Center[2]	Prescott	96%	82
Casa Grande Regional Medical Center	Casa Grande	95%	180
Maricopa Medical Center[2]	Phoenix	94%	100
Mountain Vista Medical Center	Mesa	94%	272
Sierra Vista Regional Health Center	Sierra Vista	93%	89
University of Arizona Medical Center[2]	Tucson	93%	84
VA Northern Arizona Healthcare System	Prescott	93%	67
Verde Valley Medical Center	Cottonwood	93%	101
Florence Hospital at Anthem[3]	Florence	92%	25
Tuba City Reg Health Care Corporation	Tuba City	92%	38
VA Southern Arizona Healthcare System	Tucson	92%	62
Yavapai Regional Medical Center - East[2]	Prescott Valley	92%	102
Gilbert Hospital[2,3]	Gilbert	90%	40
Summit Healthcare Regional Medical Center	Show Low	90%	100
University of Arizona Medical Center[2]	Tucson	87%	55
Fort Defiance Indian Hospital	Fort Defiance	86%	76
Mount Graham Regional Medical Center	Safford	86%	49
Wickenburg Community Hospital	Wickenburg	85%	33
Chinle Comprehensive Health Care Facility[2]	Chinle	51%	47

Blood Culture Timing

Hospital Name	City	Rate	Cases
Chandler Regional Medical Center[2]	Chandler	100%	211
Maryvale Hospital	Phoenix	100%	294

NOTE: Hospital profiles are in alphabetical order by state, then city, then hospital within the city; Rankings exclude hospitals with less than 25 cases except for patient surveys which excludes hospitals with less than 100 cases; (a) 100-299 cases; (1) The number of cases/patients is too few to report; (2) Data submitted were based on a sample of cases/patients; (3) Results are based on a shorter time period than required; (4) Data suppressed by CMS for one or more quarters; (5) Results are not available for this reporting period; (6) Fewer than 100 patients completed the HCAHPS survey; (7) No cases met the criteria for this measure; (8) The lower limit of the confidence interval cannot be calculated if the number of observed infections equals zero; (9) No data are available from the state/territory for this reporting period; (10) The scores shown reflect fewer than 50 completed surveys; (11) There were discrepancies in the data collection process; (12) This measure does not apply to this hospital for this reporting period; (13) Results cannot be calculated for this reporting period; (14) The results for this state are combined with nearby states to protect confidentiality; Please refer to the User's Guide for a full explanation of data.

Hospital Name	City	Rate	Cases
Northwest Medical Center	Tucson	100%	288
Oro Valley Hospital	Oro Valley	100%	106
Paradise Valley Hospital	Phoenix	100%	205
Scottsdale Healthcare-Shea Med Ctr[2]	Scottsdale	100%	161
Scottsdale Hlthcare-Thompson Peak Hosp[2]	Scottsdale	100%	128
Scottsdale Healthcare Osborn Med Ctr[2]	Scottsdale	100%	176
Tucson Medical Center[2]	Tucson	100%	144
Valley View Medical Center[2]	Fort Mohave	100%	64
Arrowhead Hospital	Glendale	99%	324
Banner Baywood Medical Center[2]	Mesa	99%	131
Banner Del E Webb Medical Center[2]	Sun City West	99%	107
Banner Desert Medical Center[2]	Mesa	99%	91
Banner Estrella Medical Center[2]	Phoenix	99%	156
Banner Gateway Medical Center[2]	Gilbert	99%	141
Carondelet Saint Joseph's Hospital[2]	Tucson	99%	136
John C Lincoln Deer Valley Hospital[2]	Phoenix	99%	145
John C Lincoln North Mountain Hospital[2]	Phoenix	99%	134
Kingman Regional Medical Center[2]	Kingman	99%	452
Mayo Clinic Hospital	Phoenix	99%	165
VA Northern Arizona Healthcare System	Prescott	99%	82
West Valley Hospital	Goodyear	99%	375
Western Arizona Regional Medical Center	Bullhead City	99%	215
Banner Thunderbird Medical Center[2]	Glendale	98%	156
Carondelet Saint Marys Hospital[2]	Tucson	98%	116
Mercy Gilbert Medical Center[2]	Gilbert	98%	177
Payson Regional Medical Center	Payson	98%	87
Phoenix Baptist Hospital	Phoenix	98%	270
Phoenix VA Medical Center	Phoenix	98%	129
VA Southern Arizona Healthcare System	Tucson	98%	127
Banner Boswell Medical Center[2]	Sun City	97%	91
Banner Good Samaritan Medical Center[2]	Phoenix	97%	113
Havasu Regional Medical Center	Lk Havasu City	97%	213
Mountain Vista Medical Center	Mesa	97%	306
Saint Luke's Medical Center	Phoenix	97%	145
Sierra Vista Regional Health Center	Sierra Vista	97%	143
Verde Valley Medical Center	Cottonwood	97%	149
Yuma Regional Medical Center[2]	Yuma	97%	218
Banner Ironwood Medical Center	San Tan Valley	96%	57
Casa Grande Regional Medical Center	Casa Grande	96%	221
Mount Graham Regional Medical Center	Safford	96%	67
Saint Joseph's Hospital & Medical Center[2]	Phoenix	96%	159
Flagstaff Medical Center[2]	Flagstaff	95%	140
Yavapai Regional Medical Center[2]	Prescott	95%	125
Yavapai Regional Medical Center - East[2]	Prescott Valley	95%	166
Maricopa Medical Center[2]	Phoenix	94%	128
University of Arizona Medical Center[2]	Tucson	94%	136
University of Arizona Medical Center[2]	Tucson	94%	144
Cobre Valley Regional Medical Center	Globe	93%	104
Summit Healthcare Regional Medical Center	Show Low	92%	145
Fort Defiance Indian Hospital	Fort Defiance	89%	75
Benson Hospital	Benson	88%	33
Tuba City Reg Health Care Corporation	Tuba City	88%	57
Phoenix Indian Medical Center[2]	Phoenix	87%	61
Wickenburg Community Hospital	Wickenburg	87%	31
Chinle Comprehensive Health Care Facility[2]	Chinle	84%	69

Pregnancy and Delivery Care

Newborns whose Deliveries were Scheduled Early

Hospital Name	City	Rate	Cases
Chandler Regional Medical Center[2]	Chandler	0%	53
Fort Defiance Indian Hospital[2]	Fort Defiance	0%	43
Kingman Regional Medical Center[2]	Kingman	0%	58
Maricopa Medical Center[2]	Phoenix	0%	32
Maryvale Hospital[2]	Phoenix	0%	38
Mercy Gilbert Medical Center[2]	Gilbert	0%	62
Summit Healthcare Regional Medical Center	Show Low	0%	92
Banner Del E Webb Medical Center[2]	Sun City West	2%	45
Tucson Medical Center[2]	Tucson	2%	361
Verde Valley Medical Center[2]	Cottonwood	2%	43
Carondelet Holy Cross Hospital[2]	Nogales	3%	58
Mount Graham Regional Medical Center[2]	Safford	3%	76
Northwest Medical Center[2]	Tucson	3%	74
Phoenix Baptist Hospital[2]	Phoenix	3%	74
Sierra Vista Regional Health Center[2]	Sierra Vista	3%	34
Banner Desert Medical Center[2]	Mesa	4%	68
Flagstaff Medical Center[2]	Flagstaff	4%	28
Banner Estrella Medical Center[2]	Phoenix	5%	112
Banner Good Samaritan Medical Center[2]	Phoenix	5%	81
Carondelet Saint Joseph's Hospital[2]	Tucson	5%	40
University of Arizona Medical Center[2]	Tucson	6%	35
Arrowhead Hospital[2]	Glendale	7%	67
Saint Joseph's Hospital & Medical Center[2]	Phoenix	7%	94
West Valley Hospital[2]	Goodyear	7%	46
Banner Thunderbird Medical Center[2]	Glendale	8%	124
Paradise Valley Hospital[2]	Phoenix	8%	38
Saint Luke's Medical Center	Phoenix	9%	55
Scottsdale Healthcare-Shea Med Ctr[2]	Scottsdale	9%	99
Yuma Regional Medical Center[2]	Yuma	9%	57
Banner Gateway Medical Center[2]	Gilbert	11%	106
Tuba City Reg Health Care Corporation[2]	Tuba City	11%	28
Banner Ironwood Medical Center[2]	San Tan Valley	14%	36
Casa Grande Regional Medical Center	Casa Grande	14%	84
Banner Baywood Medical Center[2]	Mesa	15%	59
Havasu Regional Medical Center[2]	Lk Havasu City	16%	32
Chinle Comprehensive Health Care Facility[2]	Chinle	18%	77
Yavapai Regional Medical Center - East	Prescott Valley	22%	154
Mountain Vista Medical Center[2]	Mesa	26%	50
Valley View Medical Center[2]	Fort Mohave	33%	49

Preventive Care

Immunization for Influenza

Hospital Name	City	Rate	Cases
Arizona Ortho & Surgical Spec Hosp[2]	Chandler	100%	318
Arizona Spine & Joint Hospital	Mesa	100%	425
Western Arizona Regional Medical Center[2]	Bullhead City	100%	646
Banner Del E Webb Medical Center[2]	Sun City West	99%	542
Havasu Regional Medical Center[2]	Lk Havasu City	99%	548
Mercy Gilbert Medical Center[2]	Gilbert	99%	509
Paradise Valley Hospital[2]	Phoenix	99%	506
Banner Boswell Medical Center[2]	Sun City	98%	595
Banner Desert Medical Center[2]	Mesa	98%	492
Chandler Regional Medical Center[2]	Chandler	98%	553
John C Lincoln Deer Valley Hospital[2]	Phoenix	98%	628
Payson Regional Medical Center[2]	Payson	98%	302
Verde Valley Medical Center[2]	Cottonwood	98%	433
Banner Baywood Medical Center[2]	Mesa	97%	567
Flagstaff Medical Center[2]	Flagstaff	97%	540
Gilbert Hospital[2]	Gilbert	97%	290
Mountain Vista Medical Center[2]	Mesa	97%	704
West Valley Hospital[2]	Goodyear	97%	534
Arrowhead Hospital[2]	Glendale	96%	524
Oro Valley Hospital[2]	Oro Valley	96%	528
Banner Heart Hospital[2]	Mesa	95%	566
Mayo Clinic Hospital[2]	Phoenix	95%	696
Banner Estrella Medical Center[2]	Phoenix	94%	483
Banner Thunderbird Medical Center[2]	Glendale	94%	493
Carondelet Saint Marys Hospital[2]	Tucson	94%	624
Phoenix Baptist Hospital[2]	Phoenix	94%	774
Sierra Vista Regional Health Center[2]	Sierra Vista	94%	483
Tucson Medical Center[2]	Tucson	94%	483
Banner Good Samaritan Medical Center[2]	Phoenix	93%	490
John C Lincoln North Mountain Hospital[2]	Phoenix	93%	621
Saint Luke's Medical Center[2]	Phoenix	93%	766
Valley View Medical Center[2]	Fort Mohave	93%	326
Banner Ironwood Medical Center[2]	San Tan Valley	92%	233
Yuma Regional Medical Center[2]	Yuma	92%	509
Florence Hospital at Anthem[2,3]	Florence	91%	133
Saint Joseph's Hospital & Medical Center[2]	Phoenix	91%	513
Yavapai Regional Medical Center - East[2]	Prescott Valley	91%	385
Banner Gateway Medical Center[2]	Gilbert	90%	451
Maryvale Hospital[2]	Phoenix	90%	492
Yavapai Regional Medical Center[2]	Prescott	90%	621
Carondelet Saint Joseph's Hospital[2]	Tucson	89%	524
Kingman Regional Medical Center[2]	Kingman	89%	551
Northwest Medical Center[2]	Tucson	89%	666
Phoenix Indian Medical Center[2]	Phoenix	89%	296
Maricopa Medical Center[2]	Phoenix	88%	505
Mount Graham Regional Medical Center[2]	Safford	88%	347
University of Arizona Medical Center[2]	Tucson	87%	478
Casa Grande Regional Medical Center[2]	Casa Grande	85%	560
The Surgical Hospital of Phoenix[2]	Phoenix	83%	317
University of Arizona Medical Center[2]	Tucson	81%	521
Oasis Hospital[2]	Phoenix	80%	338
Scottsdale Hlthcare-Thompson Peak Hosp[2]	Scottsdale	78%	527
Scottsdale Healthcare Osborn Med Ctr[2]	Scottsdale	78%	590
VA Northern Arizona Healthcare System[2,3]	Prescott	77%	141
Carondelet Holy Cross Hospital[2]	Nogales	76%	192
Scottsdale Healthcare-Shea Med Ctr[2]	Scottsdale	75%	494
Chinle Comprehensive Health Care Facility[2]	Chinle	72%	293
Summit Healthcare Regional Medical Center[2]	Show Low	70%	379
Fort Defiance Indian Hospital[2]	Fort Defiance	60%	251
Tuba City Reg Health Care Corporation[2]	Tuba City	43%	258

Immunization for Pneumonia

Hospital Name	City	Rate	Cases
Arizona Spine & Joint Hospital[2]	Mesa	100%	497
Payson Regional Medical Center[2]	Payson	100%	436
Western Arizona Regional Medical Center[2]	Bullhead City	100%	984
Arrowhead Hospital[2]	Glendale	99%	486
Banner Del E Webb Medical Center[2]	Sun City West	99%	791
Havasu Regional Medical Center[2]	Lk Havasu City	99%	803
Maryvale Hospital[2]	Phoenix	99%	544
Paradise Valley Hospital[2]	Phoenix	99%	535
Verde Valley Medical Center[2]	Cottonwood	99%	552
Banner Boswell Medical Center[2]	Sun City	98%	1063
Flagstaff Medical Center[2]	Flagstaff	98%	546
John C Lincoln Deer Valley Hospital[2]	Phoenix	98%	729
Oro Valley Hospital[2]	Oro Valley	98%	806
Valley View Medical Center[2]	Fort Mohave	98%	374
West Valley Hospital[2]	Goodyear	98%	590
Banner Baywood Medical Center[2]	Mesa	97%	895
Phoenix Baptist Hospital[2]	Phoenix	97%	939
Banner Thunderbird Medical Center[2]	Glendale	96%	521
Chandler Regional Medical Center[2]	Chandler	96%	614
Gilbert Hospital[2]	Gilbert	96%	323
Mercy Gilbert Medical Center[2]	Gilbert	96%	522
Mountain Vista Medical Center[2]	Mesa	96%	852
Tucson Medical Center[2]	Tucson	96%	500
Banner Ironwood Medical Center[2]	San Tan Valley	95%	158
Banner Desert Medical Center[2]	Mesa	94%	468
Banner Estrella Medical Center[2]	Phoenix	94%	487
John C Lincoln North Mountain Hospital[2]	Phoenix	94%	821
Saint Luke's Medical Center[2]	Phoenix	94%	814
Yuma Regional Medical Center[2]	Yuma	94%	572
Arizona Ortho & Surgical Spec Hosp[2]	Chandler	93%	391
Banner Heart Hospital[2]	Mesa	93%	939
Sierra Vista Regional Health Center[2]	Sierra Vista	93%	566
Whiteriver PHS Indian Hospital[2,3]	Whiteriver	93%	124
Banner Gateway Medical Center[2]	Gilbert	92%	412
Banner Good Samaritan Medical Center[2]	Phoenix	92%	504
Carondelet Holy Cross Hospital[2]	Nogales	92%	79
Carondelet Saint Marys Hospital[2]	Tucson	92%	971
Florence Hospital at Anthem[2,3]	Florence	91%	250
Fort Defiance Indian Hospital[2]	Fort Defiance	91%	158
Kingman Regional Medical Center[2]	Kingman	91%	815
Mayo Clinic Hospital[2]	Phoenix	91%	883
Phoenix Indian Medical Center[2]	Phoenix	91%	272
Carondelet Saint Joseph's Hospital[2]	Tucson	90%	649
VA Northern Arizona Healthcare System[2,3]	Prescott	90%	347
Yavapai Regional Medical Center - East[2]	Prescott Valley	90%	401
Mount Graham Regional Medical Center[2]	Safford	89%	296
Northwest Medical Center[2]	Tucson	89%	777
Yavapai Regional Medical Center[2]	Prescott	89%	996
San Carlos Indian Hospital[2]	San Carlos	88%	49
Chinle Comprehensive Health Care Facility[2]	Chinle	87%	427
Maricopa Medical Center[2]	Phoenix	87%	306
The Surgical Hospital of Phoenix[2]	Phoenix	87%	326
University of Arizona Medical Center[2]	Tucson	86%	601
Casa Grande Regional Medical Center[2]	Casa Grande	85%	730
University of Arizona Medical Center[2]	Tucson	85%	513
Summit Healthcare Regional Medical Center[2]	Show Low	84%	395
Saint Joseph's Hospital & Medical Center[2]	Phoenix	83%	463
Tuba City Reg Health Care Corporation[2]	Tuba City	76%	210
Scottsdale Hlthcare-Thompson Peak Hosp[2]	Scottsdale	74%	694
Scottsdale Healthcare Osborn Med Ctr[2]	Scottsdale	73%	671
Oasis Hospital[2]	Phoenix	72%	439
Scottsdale Healthcare-Shea Med Ctr[2]	Scottsdale	68%	484

Stroke Care

Anticoagulation Therapy for Atrial Fibrillation

Hospital Name	City	Rate	Cases
Chandler Regional Medical Center	Chandler	100%	26
Mayo Clinic Hospital	Phoenix	100%	32
Scottsdale Healthcare Osborn Med Ctr	Scottsdale	100%	39
Tucson Medical Center	Tucson	100%	41
Saint Joseph's Hospital & Medical Center	Phoenix	96%	72
Carondelet Saint Joseph's Hospital	Tucson	94%	36
Banner Baywood Medical Center[2]	Mesa	93%	28

Antithrombotic Therapy Timing

Hospital Name	City	Rate	Cases
Banner Thunderbird Medical Center[2]	Glendale	100%	95
Chandler Regional Medical Center	Chandler	100%	144
Flagstaff Medical Center	Flagstaff	100%	68
Havasu Regional Medical Center	Lk Havasu City	100%	73
John C Lincoln North Mountain Hospital[2]	Phoenix	100%	82
Maryvale Hospital	Phoenix	100%	46
Scottsdale Healthcare-Shea Med Ctr	Scottsdale	100%	62
Scottsdale Healthcare Osborn Med Ctr	Scottsdale	100%	176
Summit Healthcare Regional Medical Center	Show Low	100%	39
University of Arizona Medical Center	Tucson	100%	106
Western Arizona Regional Medical Center	Bullhead City	100%	77
Yuma Regional Medical Center[2]	Yuma	100%	85
Banner Boswell Medical Center[2]	Sun City	99%	76
Banner Desert Medical Center[2]	Mesa	99%	87
Banner Estrella Medical Center[2]	Phoenix	99%	89
Saint Joseph's Hospital & Medical Center	Phoenix	99%	257
Arrowhead Hospital	Glendale	98%	92
Banner Baywood Medical Center[2]	Mesa	98%	121
Banner Del E Webb Medical Center[2]	Sun City West	98%	109
Banner Gateway Medical Center	Gilbert	98%	53
Banner Good Samaritan Medical Center[2]	Phoenix	98%	61
Carondelet Saint Marys Hospital	Tucson	98%	149
Mayo Clinic Hospital	Phoenix	98%	124
Northwest Medical Center	Tucson	98%	139
Oro Valley Hospital	Oro Valley	98%	56
Tucson Medical Center	Tucson	98%	150

NOTE: Hospital profiles are in alphabetical order by state, then city, then hospital within the city; Rankings exclude hospitals with less than 25 cases except for patient surveys which excludes hospitals with less than 100 cases; (a) 100-299 cases; (1) The number of cases/patients is too few to report; (2) Data submitted were based on a sample of cases/patients; (3) Results are based on a shorter time period than required; (4) Data suppressed by CMS for one or more quarters; (5) Results are not available for this reporting period; (6) Fewer than 100 patients completed the HCAHPS survey; (7) No cases met the criteria for this measure; (8) The lower limit of the confidence interval cannot be calculated if the number of observed infections equals zero; (9) No data are available from the state/territory for this reporting period; (10) The scores shown reflect fewer than 50 completed surveys; (11) There were discrepancies in the data collection process; (12) This measure does not apply to this hospital for this reporting period; (13) Results cannot be calculated for this reporting period; (14) The results for this state are combined with nearby states to protect confidentiality; Please refer to the User's Guide for a full explanation of data.

Hospital Name	City	Rate	Cases
Verde Valley Medical Center	Cottonwood	98%	48
West Valley Hospital	Goodyear	98%	91
Carondelet Saint Joseph's Hospital	Tucson	97%	172
John C Lincoln Deer Valley Hospital[2]	Phoenix	97%	93
Kingman Regional Medical Center[2]	Kingman	96%	56
Phoenix Baptist Hospital	Phoenix	96%	115
Yavapai Regional Medical Center	Prescott	96%	83
Yavapai Regional Medical Center - East	Prescott Valley	96%	25
Mercy Gilbert Medical Center	Gilbert	95%	94
Casa Grande Regional Medical Center	Casa Grande	94%	35
University of Arizona Medical Center	Tucson	94%	36
Mountain Vista Medical Center	Mesa	93%	123
Saint Luke's Medical Center	Phoenix	91%	34

Assessed for Rehabilitation

Hospital Name	City	Rate	Cases
Chandler Regional Medical Center	Chandler	100%	193
Flagstaff Medical Center	Flagstaff	100%	107
John C Lincoln Deer Valley Hospital[2]	Phoenix	100%	111
Northwest Medical Center	Tucson	100%	192
Tucson Medical Center	Tucson	100%	216
University of Arizona Medical Center	Tucson	100%	153
Yuma Regional Medical Center[2]	Yuma	100%	98
Banner Estrella Medical Center[2]	Phoenix	99%	112
Carondelet Saint Marys Hospital	Tucson	99%	188
John C Lincoln North Mountain Hospital[2]	Phoenix	99%	110
Mayo Clinic Hospital	Phoenix	99%	185
Mountain Vista Medical Center	Mesa	99%	139
Arrowhead Hospital	Glendale	98%	90
Maryvale Hospital	Phoenix	98%	46
Mercy Gilbert Medical Center	Gilbert	98%	126
Phoenix Baptist Hospital	Phoenix	98%	179
University of Arizona Medical Center	Tucson	98%	41
Verde Valley Medical Center	Cottonwood	98%	48
Western Arizona Regional Medical Center	Bullhead City	97%	74
Banner Boswell Medical Center[2]	Sun City	96%	99
Banner Del E Webb Medical Center[2]	Sun City West	96%	122
Banner Thunderbird Medical Center[2]	Glendale	96%	117
Havasu Regional Medical Center	Lk Havasu City	96%	74
Summit Healthcare Regional Medical Center	Show Low	96%	46
Banner Desert Medical Center[2]	Mesa	95%	107
Carondelet Saint Joseph's Hospital	Tucson	95%	235
Scottsdale Healthcare Osborn Med Ctr	Scottsdale	95%	234
Oro Valley Hospital	Oro Valley	94%	72
West Valley Hospital	Goodyear	94%	94
Banner Good Samaritan Medical Center[2]	Phoenix	92%	115
Saint Joseph's Hospital & Medical Center	Phoenix	92%	554
Banner Baywood Medical Center[2]	Mesa	91%	108
Kingman Regional Medical Center[2]	Kingman	91%	53
Banner Gateway Medical Center	Gilbert	90%	58
Yavapai Regional Medical Center	Prescott	88%	111
Yavapai Regional Medical Center - East	Prescott Valley	87%	30
Maricopa Medical Center	Phoenix	85%	39
Casa Grande Regional Medical Center	Casa Grande	83%	41
Scottsdale Healthcare-Shea Med Ctr	Scottsdale	83%	76
Saint Luke's Medical Center	Phoenix	82%	33
Scottsdale Hlthcare-Thompson Peak Hosp	Scottsdale	79%	34

Discharged on Antithrombotic Therapy

Hospital Name	City	Rate	Cases
Arrowhead Hospital	Glendale	100%	87
Banner Boswell Medical Center[2]	Sun City	100%	90
Banner Del E Webb Medical Center[2]	Sun City West	100%	120
Banner Estrella Medical Center[2]	Phoenix	100%	108
Banner Gateway Medical Center	Gilbert	100%	55
Carondelet Saint Marys Hospital	Tucson	100%	179
Flagstaff Medical Center	Flagstaff	100%	81
Havasu Regional Medical Center	Lk Havasu City	100%	72
John C Lincoln Deer Valley Hospital[2]	Phoenix	100%	108
John C Lincoln North Mountain Hospital[2]	Phoenix	100%	88
Maricopa Medical Center	Phoenix	100%	27
Oro Valley Hospital	Oro Valley	100%	71
Phoenix Baptist Hospital	Phoenix	100%	132
Scottsdale Hlthcare-Thompson Peak Hosp	Scottsdale	100%	32
Summit Healthcare Regional Medical Center	Show Low	100%	45
Tucson Medical Center	Tucson	100%	185
University of Arizona Medical Center	Tucson	100%	123
University of Arizona Medical Center	Tucson	100%	38
Verde Valley Medical Center	Cottonwood	100%	46
West Valley Hospital	Goodyear	100%	92
Western Arizona Regional Medical Center	Bullhead City	100%	73
Banner Baywood Medical Center[2]	Mesa	99%	105
Banner Desert Medical Center[2]	Mesa	99%	97
Banner Good Samaritan Medical Center[2]	Phoenix	99%	81
Banner Thunderbird Medical Center[2]	Glendale	99%	99
Carondelet Saint Joseph's Hospital	Tucson	99%	201
Chandler Regional Medical Center	Chandler	99%	172
Mercy Gilbert Medical Center	Gilbert	99%	110
Scottsdale Healthcare-Shea Med Ctr	Scottsdale	99%	70
Scottsdale Healthcare Osborn Med Ctr	Scottsdale	99%	202
Mayo Clinic Hospital	Phoenix	98%	160
Saint Joseph's Hospital & Medical Center	Phoenix	98%	325
Yavapai Regional Medical Center	Prescott	98%	101
Northwest Medical Center	Tucson	97%	179
Yavapai Regional Medical Center - East	Prescott Valley	97%	30
Kingman Regional Medical Center[2]	Kingman	96%	53
Maryvale Hospital	Phoenix	96%	46
Mountain Vista Medical Center	Mesa	96%	134
Yuma Regional Medical Center[2]	Yuma	96%	84
Saint Luke's Medical Center	Phoenix	94%	31
Casa Grande Regional Medical Center	Casa Grande	89%	38

Discharged on Statin Medication

Hospital Name	City	Rate	Cases
Banner Boswell Medical Center[2]	Sun City	100%	64
Banner Thunderbird Medical Center[2]	Glendale	100%	64
Carondelet Saint Marys Hospital	Tucson	100%	131
Havasu Regional Medical Center	Lk Havasu City	100%	49
John C Lincoln North Mountain Hospital[2]	Phoenix	100%	66
Verde Valley Medical Center	Cottonwood	100%	37
West Valley Hospital	Goodyear	100%	73
Mayo Clinic Hospital	Phoenix	99%	111
Mercy Gilbert Medical Center	Gilbert	99%	98
Northwest Medical Center	Tucson	99%	139
Phoenix Baptist Hospital	Phoenix	99%	101
Banner Estrella Medical Center[2]	Phoenix	98%	80
Tucson Medical Center	Tucson	98%	155
Banner Good Samaritan Medical Center[2]	Phoenix	97%	62
Saint Joseph's Hospital & Medical Center	Phoenix	97%	262
Flagstaff Medical Center	Flagstaff	96%	55
John C Lincoln Deer Valley Hospital[2]	Phoenix	96%	73
University of Arizona Medical Center	Tucson	96%	92
Arrowhead Hospital	Glendale	95%	65
Banner Del E Webb Medical Center[2]	Sun City West	95%	85
Chandler Regional Medical Center	Chandler	95%	131
Scottsdale Healthcare Osborn Med Ctr	Scottsdale	95%	153
Scottsdale Hlthcare-Thompson Peak Hosp	Scottsdale	94%	31
University of Arizona Medical Center	Tucson	94%	33
Banner Baywood Medical Center[2]	Mesa	93%	75
Carondelet Saint Joseph's Hospital	Tucson	93%	142
Western Arizona Regional Medical Center	Bullhead City	93%	58
Maryvale Hospital	Phoenix	91%	35
Oro Valley Hospital	Oro Valley	91%	58
Summit Healthcare Regional Medical Center	Show Low	91%	32
Banner Desert Medical Center[2]	Mesa	90%	73
Yuma Regional Medical Center[2]	Yuma	86%	69
Scottsdale Healthcare-Shea Med Ctr	Scottsdale	85%	66
Kingman Regional Medical Center[2]	Kingman	82%	38
Mountain Vista Medical Center	Mesa	81%	95
Banner Gateway Medical Center	Gilbert	76%	41
Yavapai Regional Medical Center	Prescott	74%	84
Casa Grande Regional Medical Center	Casa Grande	73%	33
Yavapai Regional Medical Center - East	Prescott Valley	69%	26
Saint Luke's Medical Center	Phoenix	68%	25

Thrombolytic Therapy Timing

Hospital Name	City	Rate	Cases
Carondelet Saint Marys Hospital	Tucson	100%	32
Saint Joseph's Hospital & Medical Center	Phoenix	97%	37
Northwest Medical Center	Tucson	88%	26
Scottsdale Healthcare Osborn Med Ctr	Scottsdale	86%	28

Venous Thromboembolism (VTE) Prophylaxis

Hospital Name	City	Rate	Cases
Flagstaff Medical Center	Flagstaff	100%	114
Havasu Regional Medical Center	Lk Havasu City	100%	75
Western Arizona Regional Medical Center	Bullhead City	100%	80
Scottsdale Healthcare Osborn Med Ctr	Scottsdale	99%	225
Tucson Medical Center	Tucson	99%	217
Arrowhead Hospital	Glendale	98%	97
Chandler Regional Medical Center	Chandler	98%	181
John C Lincoln North Mountain Hospital[2]	Phoenix	98%	116
Maryvale Hospital	Phoenix	98%	42
Verde Valley Medical Center	Cottonwood	98%	51
Banner Good Samaritan Medical Center[2]	Phoenix	97%	117
Northwest Medical Center	Tucson	97%	181
Saint Joseph's Hospital & Medical Center	Phoenix	97%	595
University of Arizona Medical Center	Tucson	97%	148
Mayo Clinic Hospital	Phoenix	96%	182
Mercy Gilbert Medical Center	Gilbert	96%	113
Banner Gateway Medical Center	Gilbert	95%	57
Banner Thunderbird Medical Center[2]	Glendale	95%	116
Carondelet Saint Marys Hospital	Tucson	95%	198
Maricopa Medical Center	Phoenix	95%	37
Banner Baywood Medical Center[2]	Mesa	91%	134
Banner Boswell Medical Center[2]	Sun City	91%	93
Banner Estrella Medical Center[2]	Phoenix	91%	105
Yuma Regional Medical Center[2]	Yuma	91%	94
Banner Del E Webb Medical Center[2]	Sun City West	90%	124
Casa Grande Regional Medical Center	Casa Grande	90%	40
Summit Healthcare Regional Medical Center	Show Low	90%	39
Banner Desert Medical Center[2]	Mesa	89%	105
John C Lincoln Deer Valley Hospital[2]	Phoenix	89%	97
West Valley Hospital	Goodyear	89%	101
Carondelet Saint Joseph's Hospital	Tucson	88%	249
Scottsdale Healthcare-Shea Med Ctr	Scottsdale	88%	59
Oro Valley Hospital	Oro Valley	87%	55
Phoenix Baptist Hospital	Phoenix	86%	201
University of Arizona Medical Center	Tucson	86%	43
Mountain Vista Medical Center	Mesa	80%	141
Saint Luke's Medical Center	Phoenix	72%	39
Yavapai Regional Medical Center	Prescott	71%	97
Kingman Regional Medical Center[2]	Kingman	67%	60
Yavapai Regional Medical Center - East	Prescott Valley	65%	26

Written Stroke Educational Materials Given

Hospital Name	City	Rate	Cases
Chandler Regional Medical Center	Chandler	100%	124
Havasu Regional Medical Center	Lk Havasu City	100%	47
John C Lincoln North Mountain Hospital[2]	Phoenix	100%	47
Maryvale Hospital	Phoenix	100%	28
Tucson Medical Center	Tucson	99%	112
West Valley Hospital	Goodyear	99%	69
Mountain Vista Medical Center	Mesa	98%	88
Western Arizona Regional Medical Center	Bullhead City	98%	52
Yuma Regional Medical Center[2]	Yuma	98%	60
Mercy Gilbert Medical Center	Gilbert	96%	73
Oro Valley Hospital	Oro Valley	96%	46
John C Lincoln Deer Valley Hospital[2]	Phoenix	95%	88
Mayo Clinic Hospital	Phoenix	95%	95
Scottsdale Healthcare Osborn Med Ctr	Scottsdale	95%	133
Northwest Medical Center	Tucson	94%	110
Phoenix Baptist Hospital	Phoenix	94%	109
Carondelet Saint Joseph's Hospital	Tucson	93%	115
Carondelet Saint Marys Hospital	Tucson	93%	104
Arrowhead Hospital	Glendale	90%	60
Banner Estrella Medical Center[2]	Phoenix	89%	74
University of Arizona Medical Center	Tucson	87%	84
Yavapai Regional Medical Center	Prescott	86%	56
Banner Boswell Medical Center[2]	Sun City	85%	53
Maricopa Medical Center	Phoenix	84%	31
Banner Del E Webb Medical Center[2]	Sun City West	82%	67
Banner Thunderbird Medical Center[2]	Glendale	81%	85
Flagstaff Medical Center	Flagstaff	77%	66
Summit Healthcare Regional Medical Center	Show Low	77%	35
Banner Desert Medical Center[2]	Mesa	76%	68
Saint Joseph's Hospital & Medical Center	Phoenix	72%	305
Casa Grande Regional Medical Center	Casa Grande	68%	31
Banner Baywood Medical Center[2]	Mesa	66%	61
Banner Good Samaritan Medical Center[2]	Phoenix	44%	73
Scottsdale Healthcare-Shea Med Ctr	Scottsdale	43%	47
Banner Gateway Medical Center	Gilbert	40%	45
Kingman Regional Medical Center[2]	Kingman	24%	38
University of Arizona Medical Center	Tucson	14%	28

Surgical Care Improvement Project

Appropriate Beta Blocker Usage

Hospital Name	City	Rate	Cases
Arizona Ortho & Surgical Spec Hosp[2]	Chandler	100%	54
Arizona Spine & Joint Hospital[2]	Mesa	100%	37
Arrowhead Hospital[2]	Glendale	100%	369
Banner Heart Hospital[2]	Mesa	100%	171
Flagstaff Medical Center[2]	Flagstaff	100%	123
Mount Graham Regional Medical Center	Safford	100%	30
Payson Regional Medical Center	Payson	100%	47
Scottsdale Healthcare-Shea Med Ctr[2]	Scottsdale	100%	202
Sierra Vista Regional Health Center	Sierra Vista	100%	45
Western Arizona Regional Medical Center	Bullhead City	100%	156
Banner Boswell Medical Center[2]	Sun City	99%	220
Banner Good Samaritan Medical Center[2]	Phoenix	99%	252
Banner Thunderbird Medical Center[2]	Glendale	99%	235
Carondelet Saint Joseph's Hospital[2]	Tucson	99%	141
Carondelet Saint Marys Hospital[2]	Tucson	99%	191
John C Lincoln North Mountain Hospital[2]	Phoenix	99%	185
Mayo Clinic Hospital[2]	Phoenix	99%	340
Phoenix VA Medical Center[2]	Phoenix	99%	133
Saint Joseph's Hospital & Medical Center[2]	Phoenix	99%	163
University of Arizona Medical Center[2]	Tucson	99%	150
Banner Gateway Medical Center[2]	Gilbert	98%	89
Chandler Regional Medical Center[2]	Chandler	98%	248
John C Lincoln Deer Valley Hospital[2]	Phoenix	98%	170
Northwest Medical Center	Tucson	98%	530
Paradise Valley Hospital[2]	Phoenix	98%	42
Phoenix Baptist Hospital[2]	Phoenix	98%	256
Saint Luke's Medical Center	Phoenix	98%	307
Banner Del E Webb Medical Center[2]	Sun City West	97%	127
Mercy Gilbert Medical Center[2]	Gilbert	97%	97
Oro Valley Hospital	Oro Valley	97%	251
Scottsdale Healthcare Osborn Med Ctr[2]	Scottsdale	97%	155

NOTE: Hospital profiles are in alphabetical order by state, then city, then hospital within the city; Rankings exclude hospitals with less than 25 cases except for patient surveys which excludes hospitals with less than 100 cases; (a) 100-299 cases; (1) The number of cases/patients is too few to report; (2) Data submitted were based on a sample of cases/patients; (3) Results are based on a shorter time period than required; (4) Data suppressed by CMS for one or more quarters; (5) Results are not available for this reporting period; (6) Fewer than 100 patients completed the HCAHPS survey; (7) No cases met the criteria for this measure; (8) The lower limit of the confidence interval cannot be calculated if the number of observed infections equals zero; (9) No data are available from the state/territory for this reporting period; (10) The scores shown reflect fewer than 50 completed surveys; (11) There were discrepancies in the data collection process; (12) This measure does not apply to this hospital for this reporting period; (13) Results cannot be calculated for this reporting period; (14) The results for this state are combined with nearby states to protect confidentiality; Please refer to the User's Guide for a full explanation of data.

Hospital Name	City	Rate	Cases
Tucson Medical Center[2]	Tucson	97%	244
VA Southern Arizona Healthcare System[2]	Tucson	97%	195
Banner Estrella Medical Center[2]	Phoenix	96%	129
Oasis Hospital[2]	Phoenix	96%	121
Verde Valley Medical Center[2]	Cottonwood	96%	113
Yuma Regional Medical Center[2]	Yuma	96%	272
Banner Desert Medical Center[2]	Mesa	95%	187
Havasu Regional Medical Center[2]	Lk Havasu City	95%	175
Scottsdale Hlthcare-Thompson Peak Hosp[2]	Scottsdale	95%	111
Summit Healthcare Regional Medical Center	Show Low	95%	79
West Valley Hospital[2]	Goodyear	95%	87
Banner Baywood Medical Center[2]	Mesa	94%	121
Kingman Regional Medical Center[2]	Kingman	94%	155
Mountain Vista Medical Center	Mesa	94%	228
Yavapai Regional Medical Center[2]	Prescott	94%	161
The Surgical Hospital of Phoenix[2]	Phoenix	92%	26
Valley View Medical Center[2]	Fort Mohave	92%	62
Yavapai Regional Medical Center - East[2]	Prescott Valley	89%	87
University of Arizona Medical Center	Tucson	85%	39
Casa Grande Regional Medical Center	Casa Grande	84%	140

Appropriate VTP Within 24 Hours

Hospital Name	City	Rate	Cases
Arizona Ortho & Surgical Spec Hosp[2]	Chandler	100%	249
Arizona Spine & Joint Hospital[2]	Mesa	100%	151
Arrowhead Hospital[2]	Glendale	100%	932
Banner Del E Webb Medical Center[2]	Sun City West	100%	336
Banner Ironwood Medical Center	San Tan Valley	100%	74
Carondelet Holy Cross Hospital	Nogales	100%	28
Mayo Clinic Hospital[2]	Phoenix	100%	950
Payson Regional Medical Center	Payson	100%	146
The Surgical Hospital of Phoenix[2]	Phoenix	100%	90
VA Southern Arizona Healthcare System[2]	Tucson	100%	356
Banner Thunderbird Medical Center[2]	Glendale	99%	352
Havasu Regional Medical Center[2]	Lk Havasu City	99%	355
John C Lincoln North Mountain Hospital[2]	Phoenix	99%	420
Mountain Vista Medical Center	Mesa	99%	556
Northwest Medical Center	Tucson	99%	1215
Paradise Valley Hospital[2]	Phoenix	99%	199
Scottsdale Healthcare-Shea Med Ctr[2]	Scottsdale	99%	393
Scottsdale Hlthcare-Thompson Peak Hosp[2]	Scottsdale	99%	450
Banner Baywood Medical Center[2]	Mesa	98%	337
Banner Boswell Medical Center[2]	Sun City	98%	324
Banner Gateway Medical Center[2]	Gilbert	98%	301
Banner Good Samaritan Medical Center[2]	Phoenix	98%	395
Carondelet Saint Joseph's Hospital[2]	Tucson	98%	446
Carondelet Saint Marys Hospital[2]	Tucson	98%	355
Chandler Regional Medical Center[2]	Chandler	98%	460
Flagstaff Medical Center[2]	Flagstaff	98%	402
John C Lincoln Deer Valley Hospital[2]	Phoenix	98%	390
Mercy Gilbert Medical Center[2]	Gilbert	98%	373
Oro Valley Hospital	Oro Valley	98%	930
Saint Joseph's Hospital & Medical Center[2]	Phoenix	98%	379
Scottsdale Healthcare Osborn Med Ctr[2]	Scottsdale	98%	340
Tucson Medical Center[2]	Tucson	98%	422
University of Arizona Medical Center[2]	Tucson	98%	315
Verde Valley Medical Center[2]	Cottonwood	98%	409
Banner Desert Medical Center[2]	Mesa	97%	359
Banner Estrella Medical Center[2]	Phoenix	97%	306
Kingman Regional Medical Center[2]	Kingman	97%	304
Maryvale Hospital[2]	Phoenix	97%	72
Oasis Hospital[2]	Phoenix	97%	569
Phoenix Baptist Hospital[2]	Phoenix	97%	367
Phoenix Indian Medical Center[2]	Phoenix	97%	76
Saint Luke's Medical Center	Phoenix	97%	793
West Valley Hospital[2]	Goodyear	97%	156
Western Arizona Regional Medical Center	Bullhead City	97%	257
Mount Graham Regional Medical Center	Safford	96%	103
Phoenix VA Medical Center[2]	Phoenix	96%	340
Summit Healthcare Regional Medical Center	Show Low	96%	281
Yavapai Regional Medical Center[2]	Prescott	96%	342
Banner Heart Hospital[2]	Mesa	95%	60
University of Arizona Medical Center	Tucson	95%	183
Yavapai Regional Medical Center - East[2]	Prescott Valley	95%	285
Casa Grande Regional Medical Center	Casa Grande	94%	461
Yuma Regional Medical Center[2]	Yuma	94%	662
Sierra Vista Regional Health Center	Sierra Vista	93%	167
Valley View Medical Center[2]	Fort Mohave	93%	137
Cobre Valley Regional Medical Center	Globe	92%	61
Maricopa Medical Center[2]	Phoenix	90%	208
Tuba City Reg Health Care Corporation[2]	Tuba City	90%	185

Controlled Postoperative Blood Glucose

Hospital Name	City	Rate	Cases
Banner Estrella Medical Center[2]	Phoenix	100%	58
Scottsdale Healthcare Osborn Med Ctr[2]	Scottsdale	100%	83
West Valley Hospital[2]	Goodyear	100%	65
Mayo Clinic Hospital[2]	Phoenix	99%	168
Phoenix Baptist Hospital[2]	Phoenix	99%	128
Saint Luke's Medical Center	Phoenix	99%	79
Scottsdale Healthcare-Shea Med Ctr[2]	Scottsdale	99%	144
Banner Boswell Medical Center[2]	Sun City	98%	160
Havasu Regional Medical Center[2]	Lk Havasu City	98%	119
Tucson Medical Center[2]	Tucson	98%	171
Flagstaff Medical Center[2]	Flagstaff	97%	141
John C Lincoln Deer Valley Hospital[2]	Phoenix	97%	79
John C Lincoln North Mountain Hospital[2]	Phoenix	97%	94
Northwest Medical Center	Tucson	97%	172
Banner Thunderbird Medical Center[2]	Glendale	96%	114
Carondelet Saint Marys Hospital[2]	Tucson	96%	139
Yuma Regional Medical Center[2]	Yuma	96%	126
Saint Joseph's Hospital & Medical Center[2]	Phoenix	95%	150
Arrowhead Hospital[2]	Glendale	94%	110
Kingman Regional Medical Center[2]	Kingman	94%	53
University of Arizona Medical Center[2]	Tucson	94%	114
Yavapai Regional Medical Center[2]	Prescott	93%	108
Banner Desert Medical Center[2]	Mesa	92%	118
Mountain Vista Medical Center	Mesa	92%	66
Banner Good Samaritan Medical Center[2]	Phoenix	90%	155
Banner Heart Hospital[2]	Mesa	90%	163
Chandler Regional Medical Center[2]	Chandler	89%	161
VA Southern Arizona Healthcare System[2]	Tucson	87%	103

Perioperative Temperature Management

Hospital Name	City	Rate	Cases
Arizona Ortho & Surgical Spec Hosp[2]	Chandler	100%	248
Arizona Spine & Joint Hospital[2]	Mesa	100%	180
Arrowhead Hospital[2]	Glendale	100%	1162
Banner Baywood Medical Center[2]	Mesa	100%	417
Banner Boswell Medical Center[2]	Sun City	100%	470
Banner Del E Webb Medical Center[2]	Sun City West	100%	445
Banner Desert Medical Center[2]	Mesa	100%	475
Banner Estrella Medical Center[2]	Phoenix	100%	410
Banner Gateway Medical Center[2]	Gilbert	100%	391
Banner Good Samaritan Medical Center[2]	Phoenix	100%	558
Banner Heart Hospital[2]	Mesa	100%	120
Banner Ironwood Medical Center	San Tan Valley	100%	95
Banner Thunderbird Medical Center[2]	Glendale	100%	533
Carondelet Holy Cross Hospital	Nogales	100%	39
Carondelet Saint Joseph's Hospital[2]	Tucson	100%	554
Carondelet Saint Marys Hospital[2]	Tucson	100%	537
Chandler Regional Medical Center[2]	Chandler	100%	554
Flagstaff Medical Center[2]	Flagstaff	100%	620
Fort Defiance Indian Hospital[3]	Fort Defiance	100%	25
Havasu Regional Medical Center[2]	Lk Havasu City	100%	424
John C Lincoln North Mountain Hospital[2]	Phoenix	100%	566
Kingman Regional Medical Center[2]	Kingman	100%	366
Maricopa Medical Center[2]	Phoenix	100%	260
Maryvale Hospital[2]	Phoenix	100%	85
Mayo Clinic Hospital[2]	Phoenix	100%	1160
Mercy Gilbert Medical Center[2]	Gilbert	100%	423
Mountain Vista Medical Center	Mesa	100%	667
Northwest Medical Center	Tucson	100%	1951
Oasis Hospital[2]	Phoenix	100%	637
Oro Valley Hospital	Oro Valley	100%	1046
Paradise Valley Hospital[2]	Phoenix	100%	244
Payson Regional Medical Center	Payson	100%	171
Phoenix Indian Medical Center[2]	Phoenix	100%	78
Phoenix VA Medical Center[2]	Phoenix	100%	392
Saint Joseph's Hospital & Medical Center[2]	Phoenix	100%	501
Saint Luke's Medical Center	Phoenix	100%	1174
Scottsdale Healthcare-Shea Med Ctr[2]	Scottsdale	100%	528
Scottsdale Hlthcare-Thompson Peak Hosp[2]	Scottsdale	100%	579
Scottsdale Healthcare Osborn Med Ctr[2]	Scottsdale	100%	482
Summit Healthcare Regional Medical Center	Show Low	100%	332
Tucson Medical Center[2]	Tucson	100%	565
Valley View Medical Center[2]	Fort Mohave	100%	162
Verde Valley Medical Center[2]	Cottonwood	100%	470
West Valley Hospital[2]	Goodyear	100%	228
Western Arizona Regional Medical Center	Bullhead City	100%	483
Yavapai Regional Medical Center[2]	Prescott	100%	384
Yavapai Regional Medical Center - East[2]	Prescott Valley	100%	348
Yuma Regional Medical Center[2]	Yuma	100%	908
Casa Grande Regional Medical Center	Casa Grande	99%	519
John C Lincoln Deer Valley Hospital[2]	Phoenix	99%	516
Mount Graham Regional Medical Center	Safford	99%	135
Phoenix Baptist Hospital[2]	Phoenix	99%	523
Tuba City Reg Health Care Corporation[2]	Tuba City	99%	214
VA Southern Arizona Healthcare System[2]	Tucson	99%	322
The Surgical Hospital of Phoenix[2]	Phoenix	98%	101
University of Arizona Medical Center[2]	Tucson	98%	432
Cobre Valley Regional Medical Center	Globe	97%	73
Sierra Vista Regional Health Center	Sierra Vista	97%	191
University of Arizona Medical Center	Tucson	97%	223

Prophylactic Antibiotic Selection

Hospital Name	City	Rate	Cases
Arizona Ortho & Surgical Spec Hosp[2]	Chandler	100%	206
Arizona Spine & Joint Hospital[2]	Mesa	100%	137
Arrowhead Hospital[2]	Glendale	100%	939
Banner Baywood Medical Center[2]	Mesa	100%	279
Banner Boswell Medical Center[2]	Sun City	100%	420
Banner Heart Hospital[2]	Mesa	100%	180
Banner Ironwood Medical Center	San Tan Valley	100%	67
Banner Thunderbird Medical Center[2]	Glendale	100%	396
Carondelet Holy Cross Hospital	Nogales	100%	36
Carondelet Saint Marys Hospital[2]	Tucson	100%	413
John C Lincoln Deer Valley Hospital[2]	Phoenix	100%	293
Oasis Hospital[2]	Phoenix	100%	418
Phoenix Baptist Hospital[2]	Phoenix	100%	413
Phoenix VA Medical Center	Phoenix	100%	257
Scottsdale Healthcare Osborn Med Ctr[2]	Scottsdale	100%	350
VA Southern Arizona Healthcare System	Tucson	100%	404
Yavapai Regional Medical Center[2]	Prescott	100%	297
Banner Del E Webb Medical Center[2]	Sun City West	99%	268
Banner Desert Medical Center[2]	Mesa	99%	437
Banner Estrella Medical Center[2]	Phoenix	99%	278
Banner Good Samaritan Medical Center[2]	Phoenix	99%	472
Casa Grande Regional Medical Center	Casa Grande	99%	353
Chandler Regional Medical Center[2]	Chandler	99%	479
Flagstaff Medical Center[2]	Flagstaff	99%	458
John C Lincoln North Mountain Hospital[2]	Phoenix	99%	385
Mayo Clinic Hospital[2]	Phoenix	99%	797
Mercy Gilbert Medical Center[2]	Gilbert	99%	243
Mount Graham Regional Medical Center	Safford	99%	87
Mountain Vista Medical Center	Mesa	99%	449
Northwest Medical Center	Tucson	99%	1372
Oro Valley Hospital	Oro Valley	99%	852
Paradise Valley Hospital[2]	Phoenix	99%	133
Payson Regional Medical Center	Payson	99%	111
Saint Luke's Medical Center	Phoenix	99%	846
Scottsdale Healthcare-Shea Med Ctr[2]	Scottsdale	99%	438
Scottsdale Hlthcare-Thompson Peak Hosp[2]	Scottsdale	99%	391
The Surgical Hospital of Phoenix[2]	Phoenix	99%	94
Tucson Medical Center[2]	Tucson	99%	521
Verde Valley Medical Center[2]	Cottonwood	99%	326
West Valley Hospital[2]	Goodyear	99%	148
Yavapai Regional Medical Center - East[2]	Prescott Valley	99%	258
Carondelet Saint Joseph's Hospital[2]	Tucson	98%	373
Saint Joseph's Hospital & Medical Center[2]	Phoenix	98%	381
University of Arizona Medical Center[2]	Tucson	98%	362
Banner Gateway Medical Center[2]	Gilbert	97%	236
Havasu Regional Medical Center[2]	Lk Havasu City	97%	392
Kingman Regional Medical Center[2]	Kingman	97%	260
Sierra Vista Regional Health Center	Sierra Vista	97%	127
University of Arizona Medical Center	Tucson	97%	123
Western Arizona Regional Medical Center	Bullhead City	97%	330
Yuma Regional Medical Center[2]	Yuma	97%	722
Cobre Valley Regional Medical Center	Globe	96%	48
Summit Healthcare Regional Medical Center	Show Low	96%	204
Maricopa Medical Center[2]	Phoenix	95%	123
Phoenix Indian Medical Center[2]	Phoenix	95%	37
Valley View Medical Center[2]	Fort Mohave	95%	118
Tuba City Reg Health Care Corporation[2]	Tuba City	93%	169

Prophylactic Antibiotic Selection (Outpatient)

Hospital Name	City	Rate	Cases
Arizona Ortho & Surgical Spec Hosp	Chandler	100%	39
Arizona Spine & Joint Hospital	Mesa	100%	37
Banner Desert Medical Center	Mesa	100%	638
Banner Good Samaritan Medical Center	Phoenix	100%	508
Banner Heart Hospital	Mesa	100%	524
John C Lincoln Deer Valley Hospital	Phoenix	100%	344
John C Lincoln North Mountain Hospital	Phoenix	100%	246
Paradise Valley Hospital	Phoenix	100%	231
Yavapai Regional Medical Center	Prescott	100%	218
Banner Del E Webb Medical Center	Sun City West	99%	365
Banner Estrella Medical Center	Phoenix	99%	341
Banner Thunderbird Medical Center	Glendale	99%	497
Carondelet Saint Joseph's Hospital	Tucson	99%	971
Carondelet Saint Marys Hospital	Tucson	99%	382
Flagstaff Medical Center	Flagstaff	99%	244
Havasu Regional Medical Center	Lk Havasu City	99%	262
Maricopa Medical Center	Phoenix	99%	67
Oasis Hospital	Phoenix	99%	269
Saint Joseph's Hospital & Medical Center	Phoenix	99%	504
Scottsdale Healthcare-Shea Med Ctr	Scottsdale	99%	752
Scottsdale Hlthcare-Thompson Peak Hosp	Scottsdale	99%	380
Scottsdale Healthcare Osborn Med Ctr	Scottsdale	99%	470
Tucson Medical Center	Tucson	99%	1024
Banner Boswell Medical Center	Sun City	98%	530
Chandler Regional Medical Center	Chandler	98%	496
Mayo Clinic Hospital	Phoenix	98%	886
Mercy Gilbert Medical Center	Gilbert	98%	359
Northwest Medical Center	Tucson	98%	763
Phoenix Baptist Hospital	Phoenix	98%	247
University of Arizona Medical Center	Tucson	98%	57
Verde Valley Medical Center	Cottonwood	98%	98
West Valley Hospital	Goodyear	98%	142
Arrowhead Hospital	Glendale	97%	506
Banner Baywood Medical Center	Mesa	97%	261

NOTE: Hospital profiles are in alphabetical order by state, then city, then hospital within the city; Rankings exclude hospitals with less than 25 cases except for patient surveys which excludes hospitals with less than 100 cases; (a) 100-299 cases; (1) The number of cases/patients is too few to report; (2) Data submitted were based on a sample of cases/patients; (3) Results are based on a shorter time period than required; (4) Data suppressed by CMS for one or more quarters; (5) Results are not available for this reporting period; (6) Fewer than 100 patients completed the HCAHPS survey; (7) No cases met the criteria for this measure; (8) The lower limit of the confidence interval cannot be calculated if the number of observed infections equals zero; (9) No data are available from the state/territory for this reporting period; (10) The scores shown reflect fewer than 50 completed surveys; (11) There were discrepancies in the data collection process; (12) This measure does not apply to this hospital for this reporting period; (13) Results cannot be calculated for this reporting period; (14) The results for this state are combined with nearby states to protect confidentiality; Please refer to the User's Guide for a full explanation of data.

Hospital Name	City	Rate	Cases
Banner Gateway Medical Center	Gilbert	97%	289
Kingman Regional Medical Center	Kingman	97%	131
Mountain Vista Medical Center	Mesa	97%	306
Oro Valley Hospital	Oro Valley	97%	117
Saint Luke's Medical Center	Phoenix	97%	137
The Surgical Hospital of Phoenix	Phoenix	97%	181
University of Arizona Medical Center	Tucson	97%	403
Western Arizona Regional Medical Center	Bullhead City	97%	61
Yavapai Regional Medical Center - East	Prescott Valley	97%	35
Valley View Medical Center	Fort Mohave	96%	165
Summit Healthcare Regional Medical Center	Show Low	95%	193
Casa Grande Regional Medical Center	Casa Grande	93%	29
Mount Graham Regional Medical Center	Safford	92%	71
Yuma Regional Medical Center	Yuma	91%	479
Sierra Vista Regional Health Center	Sierra Vista	90%	49

Prophylactic Antibiotic Stopped

Hospital Name	City	Rate	Cases
Arizona Ortho & Surgical Spec Hosp[2]	Chandler	100%	206
Arizona Spine & Joint Hospital[2]	Mesa	100%	136
Arrowhead Hospital[2]	Glendale	100%	899
Banner Del E Webb Medical Center[2]	Sun City West	100%	264
Carondelet Holy Cross Hospital	Nogales	100%	36
Carondelet Saint Marys Hospital[2]	Tucson	100%	399
Payson Regional Medical Center	Payson	100%	107
Scottsdale Hlthcare-Thompson Peak Hosp[2]	Scottsdale	100%	381
Banner Thunderbird Medical Center[2]	Glendale	99%	370
Chandler Regional Medical Center[2]	Chandler	99%	458
Flagstaff Medical Center[2]	Flagstaff	99%	444
Havasu Regional Medical Center[2]	Lk Havasu City	99%	378
John C Lincoln Deer Valley Hospital[2]	Phoenix	99%	278
Maricopa Medical Center[2]	Phoenix	99%	122
Mayo Clinic Hospital[2]	Phoenix	99%	769
Northwest Medical Center	Tucson	99%	1356
Oro Valley Hospital	Oro Valley	99%	846
Paradise Valley Hospital[2]	Phoenix	99%	125
Saint Luke's Medical Center	Phoenix	99%	827
Sierra Vista Regional Health Center	Sierra Vista	99%	126
Tucson Medical Center[2]	Tucson	99%	518
VA Southern Arizona Healthcare System	Tucson	99%	401
West Valley Hospital[2]	Goodyear	99%	135
Banner Boswell Medical Center[2]	Sun City	98%	403
Banner Estrella Medical Center[2]	Phoenix	98%	263
Banner Gateway Medical Center[2]	Gilbert	98%	231
Carondelet Saint Joseph's Hospital[2]	Tucson	98%	355
John C Lincoln North Mountain Hospital[2]	Phoenix	98%	370
Mercy Gilbert Medical Center[2]	Gilbert	98%	233
Oasis Hospital[2]	Phoenix	98%	417
Scottsdale Healthcare-Shea Med Ctr[2]	Scottsdale	98%	404
Scottsdale Healthcare Osborn Med Ctr[2]	Scottsdale	98%	336
The Surgical Hospital of Phoenix[2]	Phoenix	98%	93
Tuba City Reg Health Care Corporation[2]	Tuba City	98%	168
Yavapai Regional Medical Center - East[2]	Prescott Valley	98%	256
Banner Desert Medical Center[2]	Mesa	97%	421
Banner Heart Hospital[2]	Mesa	97%	170
Banner Ironwood Medical Center	San Tan Valley	97%	66
Mountain Vista Medical Center	Mesa	97%	430
Saint Joseph's Hospital & Medical Center[2]	Phoenix	97%	367
University of Arizona Medical Center[2]	Tucson	97%	358
Valley View Medical Center[2]	Fort Mohave	97%	117
Verde Valley Medical Center[2]	Cottonwood	97%	316
Western Arizona Regional Medical Center	Bullhead City	97%	326
Banner Baywood Medical Center[2]	Mesa	96%	268
Banner Good Samaritan Medical Center[2]	Phoenix	96%	453
Cobre Valley Regional Medical Center	Globe	96%	47
Phoenix Baptist Hospital[2]	Phoenix	96%	394
Phoenix VA Medical Center	Phoenix	96%	255
Yavapai Regional Medical Center[2]	Prescott	96%	284
Yuma Regional Medical Center[2]	Yuma	96%	714
Casa Grande Regional Medical Center	Casa Grande	95%	333
Mount Graham Regional Medical Center	Safford	95%	86
Phoenix Indian Medical Center[2]	Phoenix	95%	37
Kingman Regional Medical Center[2]	Kingman	94%	244
University of Arizona Medical Center	Tucson	94%	121
Summit Healthcare Regional Medical Center	Show Low	93%	196

Prophylactic Antibiotic Timing

Hospital Name	City	Rate	Cases
Arizona Ortho & Surgical Spec Hosp[2]	Chandler	100%	206
Arrowhead Hospital[2]	Glendale	100%	939
Banner Boswell Medical Center[2]	Sun City	100%	420
Banner Del E Webb Medical Center[2]	Sun City West	100%	268
Banner Gateway Medical Center[2]	Gilbert	100%	236
Banner Heart Hospital[2]	Mesa	100%	180
Banner Ironwood Medical Center	San Tan Valley	100%	67
Carondelet Holy Cross Hospital	Nogales	100%	36
Carondelet Saint Joseph's Hospital[2]	Tucson	100%	373
Carondelet Saint Marys Hospital[2]	Tucson	100%	414
Chandler Regional Medical Center[2]	Chandler	100%	479
John C Lincoln Deer Valley Hospital[2]	Phoenix	100%	293
Mercy Gilbert Medical Center[2]	Gilbert	100%	243
Northwest Medical Center	Tucson	100%	1373
Oro Valley Hospital	Oro Valley	100%	852
Phoenix Baptist Hospital[2]	Phoenix	100%	414
Saint Joseph's Hospital & Medical Center[2]	Phoenix	100%	380
Saint Luke's Medical Center	Phoenix	100%	846
Scottsdale Hlthcare-Thompson Peak Hosp[2]	Scottsdale	100%	391
Scottsdale Healthcare Osborn Med Ctr[2]	Scottsdale	100%	351
Tucson Medical Center[2]	Tucson	100%	521
Verde Valley Medical Center[2]	Cottonwood	100%	327
Yavapai Regional Medical Center[2]	Prescott	100%	297
Arizona Spine & Joint Hospital[2]	Mesa	99%	137
Banner Baywood Medical Center[2]	Mesa	99%	280
Banner Desert Medical Center[2]	Mesa	99%	438
Banner Estrella Medical Center[2]	Phoenix	99%	279
Banner Good Samaritan Medical Center[2]	Phoenix	99%	473
Banner Thunderbird Medical Center[2]	Glendale	99%	397
Casa Grande Regional Medical Center	Casa Grande	99%	353
Flagstaff Medical Center[2]	Flagstaff	99%	459
Havasu Regional Medical Center[2]	Lk Havasu City	99%	394
Kingman Regional Medical Center[2]	Kingman	99%	260
Mayo Clinic Hospital[2]	Phoenix	99%	797
Mountain Vista Medical Center	Mesa	99%	449
Oasis Hospital[2]	Phoenix	99%	418
Paradise Valley Hospital[2]	Phoenix	99%	133
Scottsdale Healthcare-Shea Med Ctr[2]	Scottsdale	99%	438
Summit Healthcare Regional Medical Center	Show Low	99%	204
The Surgical Hospital of Phoenix[2]	Phoenix	99%	94
West Valley Hospital[2]	Goodyear	99%	149
Yavapai Regional Medical Center - East[2]	Prescott Valley	99%	259
John C Lincoln North Mountain Hospital[2]	Phoenix	98%	387
University of Arizona Medical Center[2]	Tucson	98%	365
Western Arizona Regional Medical Center	Bullhead City	98%	330
Yuma Regional Medical Center[2]	Yuma	98%	723
Payson Regional Medical Center	Payson	97%	111
Phoenix Indian Medical Center[2]	Phoenix	97%	37
Phoenix VA Medical Center	Phoenix	97%	257
Valley View Medical Center[2]	Fort Mohave	97%	118
Cobre Valley Regional Medical Center	Globe	96%	48
Sierra Vista Regional Health Center	Sierra Vista	95%	127
VA Southern Arizona Healthcare System	Tucson	95%	409
Mount Graham Regional Medical Center	Safford	93%	87
University of Arizona Medical Center	Tucson	93%	123
Maricopa Medical Center[2]	Phoenix	92%	125
Tuba City Reg Health Care Corporation[2]	Tuba City	91%	170

Prophylactic Antibiotic Timing (Outpatient)

Hospital Name	City	Rate	Cases
Arizona Ortho & Surgical Spec Hosp	Chandler	100%	39
Arizona Spine & Joint Hospital	Mesa	100%	37
Banner Boswell Medical Center	Sun City	100%	531
Banner Desert Medical Center	Mesa	100%	638
Banner Heart Hospital	Mesa	100%	523
Banner Thunderbird Medical Center	Glendale	100%	497
Havasu Regional Medical Center	Lk Havasu City	100%	248
Saint Joseph's Hospital & Medical Center	Phoenix	100%	506
Valley View Medical Center	Fort Mohave	100%	165
Western Arizona Regional Medical Center	Bullhead City	100%	61
Yavapai Regional Medical Center - East	Prescott Valley	100%	35
Arrowhead Hospital	Glendale	99%	508
Banner Estrella Medical Center	Phoenix	99%	342
Banner Gateway Medical Center	Gilbert	99%	289
Carondelet Saint Joseph's Hospital	Tucson	99%	972
Carondelet Saint Marys Hospital	Tucson	99%	384
Chandler Regional Medical Center	Chandler	99%	497
Flagstaff Medical Center	Flagstaff	99%	245
John C Lincoln Deer Valley Hospital	Phoenix	99%	344
John C Lincoln North Mountain Hospital	Phoenix	99%	247
Mayo Clinic Hospital	Phoenix	99%	880
Mount Graham Regional Medical Center	Safford	99%	71
Mountain Vista Medical Center	Mesa	99%	305
Northwest Medical Center	Tucson	99%	767
Scottsdale Healthcare-Shea Med Ctr	Scottsdale	99%	752
Scottsdale Hlthcare-Thompson Peak Hosp	Scottsdale	99%	380
Tucson Medical Center	Tucson	99%	1027
Banner Baywood Medical Center	Mesa	98%	264
Banner Del E Webb Medical Center	Sun City West	98%	366
Banner Good Samaritan Medical Center	Phoenix	98%	504
Mercy Gilbert Medical Center	Gilbert	98%	361
Oasis Hospital	Phoenix	98%	269
Paradise Valley Hospital	Phoenix	98%	231
Scottsdale Healthcare Osborn Med Ctr	Scottsdale	98%	471
West Valley Hospital	Goodyear	98%	143
Yavapai Regional Medical Center	Prescott	98%	220
Casa Grande Regional Medical Center	Casa Grande	97%	29
Kingman Regional Medical Center	Kingman	97%	133
Saint Luke's Medical Center	Phoenix	97%	137
Summit Healthcare Regional Medical Center	Show Low	97%	196
The Surgical Hospital of Phoenix	Phoenix	97%	181
Oro Valley Hospital	Oro Valley	96%	122
Phoenix Baptist Hospital	Phoenix	96%	249
Sierra Vista Regional Health Center	Sierra Vista	96%	50
University of Arizona Medical Center	Tucson	95%	279
Yuma Regional Medical Center	Yuma	95%	496
Maricopa Medical Center	Phoenix	94%	70
Verde Valley Medical Center	Cottonwood	94%	103
University of Arizona Medical Center	Tucson	87%	54

Urinary Catheter Removal

Hospital Name	City	Rate	Cases
Arizona Ortho & Surgical Spec Hosp[2]	Chandler	100%	211
Arrowhead Hospital[2]	Glendale	100%	623
Banner Desert Medical Center[2]	Mesa	100%	218
Payson Regional Medical Center	Payson	100%	56
Phoenix VA Medical Center[2]	Phoenix	100%	162
The Surgical Hospital of Phoenix[2]	Phoenix	100%	60
Tucson Medical Center[2]	Tucson	100%	376
Western Arizona Regional Medical Center	Bullhead City	100%	236
Yavapai Regional Medical Center - East[2]	Prescott Valley	100%	244
Banner Boswell Medical Center[2]	Sun City	99%	233
Banner Del E Webb Medical Center[2]	Sun City West	99%	116
Banner Estrella Medical Center[2]	Phoenix	99%	190
Banner Gateway Medical Center[2]	Gilbert	99%	184
Banner Good Samaritan Medical Center[2]	Phoenix	99%	267
Banner Thunderbird Medical Center[2]	Glendale	99%	183
Flagstaff Medical Center[2]	Flagstaff	99%	396
Mayo Clinic Hospital[2]	Phoenix	99%	712
Paradise Valley Hospital[2]	Phoenix	99%	91
Saint Joseph's Hospital & Medical Center[2]	Phoenix	99%	343
Scottsdale Healthcare-Shea Med Ctr[2]	Scottsdale	99%	355
Scottsdale Hlthcare-Thompson Peak Hosp[2]	Scottsdale	99%	321
Verde Valley Medical Center[2]	Cottonwood	99%	243
Yavapai Regional Medical Center[2]	Prescott	99%	248
Arizona Spine & Joint Hospital[2]	Mesa	98%	103
Havasu Regional Medical Center[2]	Lk Havasu City	98%	378
John C Lincoln Deer Valley Hospital[2]	Phoenix	98%	306
Oro Valley Hospital	Oro Valley	98%	562
Phoenix Baptist Hospital[2]	Phoenix	98%	319
Valley View Medical Center[2]	Fort Mohave	98%	54
Banner Baywood Medical Center[2]	Mesa	97%	154
Banner Heart Hospital[2]	Mesa	97%	175
Carondelet Saint Joseph's Hospital[2]	Tucson	97%	307
Chandler Regional Medical Center[2]	Chandler	97%	342
John C Lincoln North Mountain Hospital[2]	Phoenix	97%	335
Mount Graham Regional Medical Center	Safford	97%	110
Northwest Medical Center	Tucson	97%	437
Scottsdale Healthcare Osborn Med Ctr[2]	Scottsdale	97%	302
VA Southern Arizona Healthcare System[2]	Tucson	97%	309
West Valley Hospital[2]	Goodyear	97%	120
Carondelet Saint Marys Hospital[2]	Tucson	96%	320
Oasis Hospital[2]	Phoenix	96%	435
Saint Luke's Medical Center	Phoenix	96%	298
University of Arizona Medical Center	Tucson	96%	103
Summit Healthcare Regional Medical Center	Show Low	95%	238
Tuba City Reg Health Care Corporation[2]	Tuba City	95%	130
University of Arizona Medical Center[2]	Tucson	93%	316
Mountain Vista Medical Center	Mesa	92%	265
Yuma Regional Medical Center[2]	Yuma	92%	653
Maricopa Medical Center[2]	Phoenix	91%	55
Kingman Regional Medical Center[2]	Kingman	90%	229
Mercy Gilbert Medical Center[2]	Gilbert	90%	187
Casa Grande Regional Medical Center	Casa Grande	89%	196
Sierra Vista Regional Health Center	Sierra Vista	89%	114

Survey of Patients' Hospital Experiences

Area Around Room 'Always' Quiet at Night

Hospital Name	City	Rate	Cases
The Surgical Hospital of Phoenix	Phoenix	78%	300+
Arizona Ortho & Surgical Spec Hosp	Chandler	76%	300+
Arizona Spine & Joint Hospital	Mesa	70%	300+
Banner Ironwood Medical Center[11]	San Tan Valley	70%	300+
Scottsdale Hlthcare-Thompson Peak Hosp	Scottsdale	70%	300+
Oasis Hospital	Phoenix	69%	300+
Wickenburg Community Hospital	Wickenburg	67%	(a)
Mercy Gilbert Medical Center	Gilbert	66%	300+
Banner Estrella Medical Center[11]	Phoenix	65%	300+
Gilbert Hospital	Gilbert	65%	(a)
Mayo Clinic Hospital[11]	Phoenix	65%	300+
Banner Gateway Medical Center[11]	Gilbert	63%	300+
Saint Luke's Medical Center	Phoenix	62%	300+
Flagstaff Medical Center	Flagstaff	61%	300+
Paradise Valley Hospital[11]	Phoenix	61%	300+
Page Hospital[11]	Page	60%	(a)
Payson Regional Medical Center	Payson	59%	300+
Saint Joseph's Hospital & Medical Center	Phoenix	59%	300+
Western Arizona Regional Medical Center	Bullhead City	59%	300+
Chandler Regional Medical Center	Chandler	58%	300+
Maryvale Hospital[11]	Phoenix	58%	300+
Mount Graham Regional Medical Center	Safford	58%	300+
Mountain Vista Medical Center	Mesa	58%	300+

NOTE: Hospital profiles are in alphabetical order by state, then city, then hospital within the city; Rankings exclude hospitals with less than 25 cases except for patient surveys which excludes hospitals with less than 100 cases; (a) 100-299 cases; (1) The number of cases/patients is too few to report; (2) Data submitted were based on a sample of cases/patients; (3) Results are based on a shorter time period than required; (4) Data suppressed by CMS for one or more quarters; (5) Results are not available for this reporting period; (6) Fewer than 100 patients completed the HCAHPS survey; (7) No cases met the criteria for this measure; (8) The lower limit of the confidence interval cannot be calculated if the number of observed infections equals zero; (9) No data are available from the state/territory for this reporting period; (10) The scores shown reflect fewer than 50 completed surveys; (11) There were discrepancies in the data collection process; (12) This measure does not apply to this hospital for this reporting period; (13) Results cannot be calculated for this reporting period; (14) The results for this state are combined with nearby states to protect confidentiality; Please refer to the User's Guide for a full explanation of data.

Hospital Name	City	Rate	Cases
Phoenix Baptist Hospital[11]	Phoenix	58%	300+
Yuma Regional Medical Center	Yuma	58%	300+
Kingman Regional Medical Center	Kingman	57%	300+
Scottsdale Healthcare-Shea Med Ctr	Scottsdale	57%	300+
Summit Healthcare Regional Medical Center	Show Low	57%	300+
Yavapai Regional Medical Center - East	Prescott Valley	57%	300+
Banner Thunderbird Medical Center[11]	Glendale	56%	300+
Phoenix Indian Medical Center	Phoenix	56%	300+
Valley View Medical Center	Fort Mohave	56%	300+
West Valley Hospital[11]	Goodyear	56%	300+
Banner Boswell Medical Center[11]	Sun City	55%	300+
Banner Desert Medical Center[11]	Mesa	55%	300+
Carondelet Holy Cross Hospital[11]	Nogales	55%	(a)
Carondelet Saint Marys Hospital[11]	Tucson	55%	300+
Tuba City Reg Health Care Corporation	Tuba City	55%	300+
Fort Defiance Indian Hospital	Fort Defiance	54%	(a)
John C Lincoln Deer Valley Hospital	Phoenix	54%	300+
Verde Valley Medical Center	Cottonwood	54%	300+
John C Lincoln North Mountain Hospital	Phoenix	53%	300+
Arrowhead Hospital[11]	Glendale	52%	300+
Banner Good Samaritan Medical Center[11]	Phoenix	52%	300+
Casa Grande Regional Medical Center	Casa Grande	52%	300+
Sierra Vista Regional Health Center	Sierra Vista	52%	300+
Banner Del E Webb Medical Center[11]	Sun City West	51%	300+
Banner Heart Hospital[11]	Mesa	51%	300+
Chinle Comprehensive Health Care Facility	Chinle	51%	(a)
Cobre Valley Regional Medical Center	Globe	51%	300+
Northwest Medical Center	Tucson	51%	300+
Oro Valley Hospital	Oro Valley	51%	300+
Tucson Medical Center	Tucson	51%	300+
Banner Baywood Medical Center[11]	Mesa	50%	300+
Havasu Regional Medical Center	Lk Havasu City	49%	300+
University of Arizona Medical Center	Tucson	49%	300+
Carondelet Saint Joseph's Hospital[11]	Tucson	48%	300+
Scottsdale Healthcare Osborn Med Ctr	Scottsdale	47%	300+
University of Arizona Medical Center	Tucson	44%	300+
Yavapai Regional Medical Center	Prescott	44%	300+
Maricopa Medical Center	Phoenix	41%	300+

Doctors 'Always' Communicated Well

Hospital Name	City	Rate	Cases
Arizona Ortho & Surgical Spec Hosp	Chandler	86%	300+
Mayo Clinic Hospital[11]	Phoenix	86%	300+
Page Hospital[11]	Page	84%	(a)
Banner Ironwood Medical Center[11]	San Tan Valley	83%	300+
Oasis Hospital	Phoenix	83%	300+
Arizona Spine & Joint Hospital	Mesa	82%	300+
Mount Graham Regional Medical Center	Safford	82%	300+
Phoenix Indian Medical Center	Phoenix	82%	300+
Wickenburg Community Hospital	Wickenburg	82%	(a)
Carondelet Saint Joseph's Hospital[11]	Tucson	81%	300+
Flagstaff Medical Center	Flagstaff	81%	300+
The Surgical Hospital of Phoenix	Phoenix	81%	300+
Banner Estrella Medical Center[11]	Phoenix	80%	300+
Banner Gateway Medical Center[11]	Gilbert	80%	300+
Banner Good Samaritan Medical Center[11]	Phoenix	80%	300+
Saint Luke's Medical Center	Phoenix	80%	300+
Verde Valley Medical Center	Cottonwood	80%	300+
Summit Healthcare Regional Medical Center	Show Low	79%	300+
Tucson Medical Center	Tucson	79%	300+
Yavapai Regional Medical Center - East	Prescott Valley	79%	300+
Banner Baywood Medical Center[11]	Mesa	78%	300+
Banner Desert Medical Center[11]	Mesa	78%	300+
Banner Thunderbird Medical Center[11]	Glendale	78%	300+
Carondelet Holy Cross Hospital[11]	Nogales	78%	(a)
Oro Valley Hospital	Oro Valley	78%	300+
Payson Regional Medical Center	Payson	78%	300+
Sierra Vista Regional Health Center	Sierra Vista	78%	300+
Arrowhead Hospital[11]	Glendale	77%	300+
Banner Boswell Medical Center[11]	Sun City	77%	300+
Banner Del E Webb Medical Center[11]	Sun City West	77%	300+
Carondelet Saint Marys Hospital[11]	Tucson	77%	300+
Cobre Valley Regional Medical Center	Globe	77%	300+
Northwest Medical Center	Tucson	77%	300+
Casa Grande Regional Medical Center	Casa Grande	76%	300+
Maryvale Hospital[11]	Phoenix	76%	300+
Mercy Gilbert Medical Center	Gilbert	76%	300+
Phoenix Baptist Hospital[11]	Phoenix	76%	300+
Saint Joseph's Hospital & Medical Center	Phoenix	76%	300+
Scottsdale Healthcare-Shea Med Ctr	Scottsdale	76%	300+
Scottsdale Hlthcare-Thompson Peak Hosp	Scottsdale	76%	300+
Yavapai Regional Medical Center	Prescott	76%	300+
Yuma Regional Medical Center	Yuma	76%	300+
Banner Heart Hospital[11]	Mesa	75%	300+
Paradise Valley Hospital[11]	Phoenix	75%	300+
Chandler Regional Medical Center	Chandler	74%	300+
John C Lincoln Deer Valley Hospital	Phoenix	74%	300+
John C Lincoln North Mountain Hospital	Phoenix	74%	300+
Maricopa Medical Center	Phoenix	74%	300+
West Valley Hospital[11]	Goodyear	74%	300+
Western Arizona Regional Medical Center	Bullhead City	74%	300+

Hospital Name	City	Rate	Cases
Gilbert Hospital	Gilbert	73%	(a)
Havasu Regional Medical Center	Lk Havasu City	73%	300+
University of Arizona Medical Center	Tucson	73%	300+
University of Arizona Medical Center	Tucson	73%	300+
Kingman Regional Medical Center	Kingman	72%	300+
Mountain Vista Medical Center	Mesa	72%	300+
Scottsdale Healthcare Osborn Med Ctr	Scottsdale	71%	300+
Tuba City Reg Health Care Corporation	Tuba City	71%	300+
Valley View Medical Center	Fort Mohave	71%	300+
Fort Defiance Indian Hospital	Fort Defiance	70%	(a)
Chinle Comprehensive Health Care Facility	Chinle	66%	(a)

Home Recovery Information Given

Hospital Name	City	Rate	Cases
Arizona Ortho & Surgical Spec Hosp	Chandler	92%	300+
Arizona Spine & Joint Hospital	Mesa	92%	300+
Oasis Hospital	Phoenix	91%	300+
Banner Boswell Medical Center[11]	Sun City	90%	300+
Banner Ironwood Medical Center[11]	San Tan Valley	90%	300+
Mayo Clinic Hospital[11]	Phoenix	90%	300+
Page Hospital[11]	Page	90%	(a)
Summit Healthcare Regional Medical Center	Show Low	90%	300+
Verde Valley Medical Center	Cottonwood	90%	300+
Banner Baywood Medical Center[11]	Mesa	89%	300+
Banner Desert Medical Center[11]	Mesa	89%	300+
Banner Gateway Medical Center[11]	Gilbert	89%	300+
Mount Graham Regional Medical Center	Safford	89%	300+
Banner Del E Webb Medical Center[11]	Sun City West	88%	300+
Banner Estrella Medical Center[11]	Phoenix	88%	300+
Banner Good Samaritan Medical Center[11]	Phoenix	88%	300+
Cobre Valley Regional Medical Center	Globe	88%	300+
Gilbert Hospital	Gilbert	88%	(a)
Oro Valley Hospital	Oro Valley	88%	300+
Payson Regional Medical Center	Payson	88%	300+
The Surgical Hospital of Phoenix	Phoenix	88%	300+
Yavapai Regional Medical Center - East	Prescott Valley	88%	300+
Arrowhead Hospital[11]	Glendale	87%	300+
Banner Heart Hospital[11]	Mesa	87%	300+
Banner Thunderbird Medical Center[11]	Glendale	87%	300+
Carondelet Saint Marys Hospital[11]	Tucson	87%	300+
Chandler Regional Medical Center	Chandler	87%	300+
Mercy Gilbert Medical Center	Gilbert	87%	300+
Northwest Medical Center	Tucson	87%	300+
Tucson Medical Center	Tucson	87%	300+
Flagstaff Medical Center	Flagstaff	86%	300+
Saint Luke's Medical Center	Phoenix	86%	300+
Carondelet Saint Joseph's Hospital[11]	Tucson	85%	300+
Casa Grande Regional Medical Center	Casa Grande	85%	300+
John C Lincoln Deer Valley Hospital	Phoenix	85%	300+
Kingman Regional Medical Center	Kingman	85%	300+
Havasu Regional Medical Center	Lk Havasu City	84%	300+
John C Lincoln North Mountain Hospital	Phoenix	84%	300+
Paradise Valley Hospital[11]	Phoenix	84%	300+
Saint Joseph's Hospital & Medical Center	Phoenix	84%	300+
Scottsdale Hlthcare-Thompson Peak Hosp	Scottsdale	84%	300+
Sierra Vista Regional Health Center	Sierra Vista	84%	300+
University of Arizona Medical Center	Tucson	84%	300+
Valley View Medical Center	Fort Mohave	84%	300+
West Valley Hospital[11]	Goodyear	84%	300+
Wickenburg Community Hospital	Wickenburg	84%	(a)
Yavapai Regional Medical Center	Prescott	84%	300+
Maryvale Hospital[11]	Phoenix	83%	300+
Phoenix Baptist Hospital[11]	Phoenix	83%	300+
Phoenix Indian Medical Center	Phoenix	83%	300+
Scottsdale Healthcare-Shea Med Ctr	Scottsdale	83%	300+
Western Arizona Regional Medical Center	Bullhead City	83%	300+
Maricopa Medical Center	Phoenix	82%	300+
Mountain Vista Medical Center	Mesa	82%	300+
Tuba City Reg Health Care Corporation	Tuba City	82%	300+
Yuma Regional Medical Center	Yuma	82%	300+
Carondelet Holy Cross Hospital[11]	Nogales	81%	(a)
Scottsdale Healthcare Osborn Med Ctr	Scottsdale	80%	300+
Fort Defiance Indian Hospital	Fort Defiance	78%	(a)
Chinle Comprehensive Health Care Facility	Chinle	77%	(a)
University of Arizona Medical Center	Tucson	76%	300+

Hospital Given 9 or 10 on 10 Point Scale

Hospital Name	City	Rate	Cases
Mayo Clinic Hospital[11]	Phoenix	91%	300+
Arizona Spine & Joint Hospital	Mesa	85%	300+
Arizona Ortho & Surgical Spec Hosp	Chandler	81%	300+
Oasis Hospital	Phoenix	81%	300+
The Surgical Hospital of Phoenix	Phoenix	81%	300+
Banner Ironwood Medical Center[11]	San Tan Valley	80%	300+
Banner Heart Hospital[11]	Mesa	78%	300+
Gilbert Hospital	Gilbert	78%	(a)
Mercy Gilbert Medical Center	Gilbert	78%	300+
Scottsdale Hlthcare-Thompson Peak Hosp	Scottsdale	78%	300+
Verde Valley Medical Center	Cottonwood	78%	300+
Banner Gateway Medical Center[11]	Gilbert	77%	300+
Flagstaff Medical Center	Flagstaff	76%	300+
Banner Estrella Medical Center[11]	Phoenix	75%	300+
Banner Good Samaritan Medical Center[11]	Phoenix	75%	300+
Yavapai Regional Medical Center - East	Prescott Valley	75%	300+
Banner Thunderbird Medical Center[11]	Glendale	74%	300+
Saint Joseph's Hospital & Medical Center	Phoenix	74%	300+
Summit Healthcare Regional Medical Center	Show Low	74%	300+
Banner Boswell Medical Center[11]	Sun City	73%	300+
Mount Graham Regional Medical Center	Safford	73%	300+
Page Hospital[11]	Page	73%	(a)
Oro Valley Hospital	Oro Valley	72%	300+
Scottsdale Healthcare-Shea Med Ctr	Scottsdale	72%	300+
Banner Desert Medical Center[11]	Mesa	71%	300+
Payson Regional Medical Center	Payson	71%	300+
Wickenburg Community Hospital	Wickenburg	71%	(a)
Banner Baywood Medical Center[11]	Mesa	70%	300+
Northwest Medical Center	Tucson	70%	300+
University of Arizona Medical Center	Tucson	70%	300+
Chandler Regional Medical Center	Chandler	69%	300+
John C Lincoln Deer Valley Hospital	Phoenix	69%	300+
Tucson Medical Center	Tucson	69%	300+
Arrowhead Hospital[11]	Glendale	68%	300+
Banner Del E Webb Medical Center[11]	Sun City West	68%	300+
Carondelet Saint Joseph's Hospital[11]	Tucson	68%	300+
Cobre Valley Regional Medical Center	Globe	68%	300+
John C Lincoln North Mountain Hospital	Phoenix	68%	300+
Paradise Valley Hospital[11]	Phoenix	68%	300+
Phoenix Baptist Hospital[11]	Phoenix	68%	300+
Saint Luke's Medical Center	Phoenix	68%	300+
Scottsdale Healthcare Osborn Med Ctr	Scottsdale	68%	300+
Yavapai Regional Medical Center	Prescott	68%	300+
Valley View Medical Center	Fort Mohave	67%	300+
Western Arizona Regional Medical Center	Bullhead City	67%	300+
Yuma Regional Medical Center	Yuma	67%	300+
Kingman Regional Medical Center	Kingman	65%	300+
Carondelet Holy Cross Hospital[11]	Nogales	64%	(a)
Carondelet Saint Marys Hospital[11]	Tucson	64%	300+
Maryvale Hospital[11]	Phoenix	64%	300+
West Valley Hospital[11]	Goodyear	64%	300+
Mountain Vista Medical Center	Mesa	63%	300+
Phoenix Indian Medical Center	Phoenix	63%	300+
Fort Defiance Indian Hospital	Fort Defiance	62%	(a)
Sierra Vista Regional Health Center	Sierra Vista	62%	300+
Casa Grande Regional Medical Center	Casa Grande	61%	300+
Maricopa Medical Center	Phoenix	60%	300+
University of Arizona Medical Center	Tucson	58%	300+
Havasu Regional Medical Center	Lk Havasu City	57%	300+
Tuba City Reg Health Care Corporation	Tuba City	52%	300+
Chinle Comprehensive Health Care Facility	Chinle	43%	(a)

Meds 'Always' Explained Before Given

Hospital Name	City	Rate	Cases
Arizona Spine & Joint Hospital	Mesa	75%	300+
Banner Ironwood Medical Center[11]	San Tan Valley	70%	300+
Mayo Clinic Hospital[11]	Phoenix	70%	300+
Arizona Ortho & Surgical Spec Hosp	Chandler	69%	300+
Oasis Hospital	Phoenix	69%	300+
Sierra Vista Regional Health Center	Sierra Vista	69%	300+
Page Hospital[11]	Page	68%	(a)
Phoenix Indian Medical Center	Phoenix	68%	300+
Gilbert Hospital	Gilbert	67%	(a)
Banner Heart Hospital[11]	Mesa	66%	300+
Saint Luke's Medical Center	Phoenix	66%	300+
Banner Baywood Medical Center[11]	Mesa	65%	300+
Banner Boswell Medical Center[11]	Sun City	65%	300+
Banner Estrella Medical Center[11]	Phoenix	65%	300+
Banner Good Samaritan Medical Center[11]	Phoenix	65%	300+
Carondelet Holy Cross Hospital[11]	Nogales	65%	(a)
The Surgical Hospital of Phoenix	Phoenix	65%	300+
Banner Thunderbird Medical Center[11]	Glendale	64%	300+
Carondelet Saint Joseph's Hospital[11]	Tucson	64%	300+
Flagstaff Medical Center	Flagstaff	64%	300+
John C Lincoln North Mountain Hospital	Phoenix	64%	300+
Western Arizona Regional Medical Center	Bullhead City	64%	300+
Wickenburg Community Hospital	Wickenburg	64%	(a)
Banner Desert Medical Center[11]	Mesa	63%	300+
Banner Gateway Medical Center[11]	Gilbert	63%	300+
Payson Regional Medical Center	Payson	63%	300+
Carondelet Saint Marys Hospital[11]	Tucson	62%	300+
Mercy Gilbert Medical Center	Gilbert	62%	300+
Summit Healthcare Regional Medical Center	Show Low	62%	300+
Tuba City Reg Health Care Corporation	Tuba City	62%	300+
Tucson Medical Center	Tucson	62%	300+
Yavapai Regional Medical Center	Prescott	62%	300+
Yuma Regional Medical Center	Yuma	62%	300+
Banner Del E Webb Medical Center[11]	Sun City West	61%	300+
Chinle Comprehensive Health Care Facility	Chinle	61%	(a)
Mount Graham Regional Medical Center	Safford	61%	300+
Saint Joseph's Hospital & Medical Center	Phoenix	61%	300+
Scottsdale Healthcare-Shea Med Ctr	Scottsdale	61%	300+
Scottsdale Hlthcare-Thompson Peak Hosp	Scottsdale	61%	300+

NOTE: Hospital profiles are in alphabetical order by state, then city, then hospital within the city; Rankings exclude hospitals with less than 25 cases except for patient surveys which excludes hospitals with less than 100 cases; (a) 100-299 cases; (1) The number of cases/patients is too few to report; (2) Data submitted were based on a sample of cases/patients; (3) Results are based on a shorter time period than required; (4) Data suppressed by CMS for one or more quarters; (5) Results are not available for this reporting period; (6) Fewer than 100 patients completed the HCAHPS survey; (7) No cases met the criteria for this measure; (8) The lower limit of the confidence interval cannot be calculated if the number of observed infections equals zero; (9) No data are available from the state/territory for this reporting period; (10) The scores shown reflect fewer than 50 completed surveys; (11) There were discrepancies in the data collection process; (12) This measure does not apply to this hospital for this reporting period; (13) Results cannot be calculated for this reporting period; (14) The results for this state are combined with nearby states to protect confidentiality; Please refer to the User's Guide for a full explanation of data.

Hospital Name	City	Rate	Cases
University of Arizona Medical Center	Tucson	61%	300+
Kingman Regional Medical Center	Kingman	60%	300+
Verde Valley Medical Center	Cottonwood	60%	300+
Casa Grande Regional Medical Center	Casa Grande	59%	300+
Chandler Regional Medical Center	Chandler	59%	300+
John C Lincoln Deer Valley Hospital	Phoenix	59%	300+
Maricopa Medical Center	Phoenix	59%	300+
Northwest Medical Center	Tucson	59%	300+
Oro Valley Hospital	Oro Valley	59%	300+
University of Arizona Medical Center	Tucson	59%	300+
West Valley Hospital[11]	Goodyear	59%	300+
Maryvale Hospital[11]	Phoenix	58%	300+
Phoenix Baptist Hospital[11]	Phoenix	58%	300+
Valley View Medical Center	Fort Mohave	58%	300+
Yavapai Regional Medical Center - East	Prescott Valley	58%	300+
Arrowhead Hospital[11]	Glendale	57%	300+
Cobre Valley Regional Medical Center	Globe	57%	300+
Mountain Vista Medical Center	Mesa	57%	300+
Fort Defiance Indian Hospital	Fort Defiance	56%	(a)
Paradise Valley Hospital[11]	Phoenix	56%	300+
Scottsdale Healthcare Osborn Med Ctr	Scottsdale	54%	300+
Havasu Regional Medical Center	Lk Havasu City	53%	300+

Nurses 'Always' Communicated Well

Hospital Name	City	Rate	Cases
Wickenburg Community Hospital	Wickenburg	88%	(a)
Arizona Ortho & Surgical Spec Hosp	Chandler	86%	300+
Mayo Clinic Hospital[11]	Phoenix	86%	300+
The Surgical Hospital of Phoenix	Phoenix	85%	300+
Arizona Spine & Joint Hospital	Mesa	84%	300+
Oasis Hospital	Phoenix	83%	300+
Banner Heart Hospital[11]	Mesa	81%	300+
Gilbert Hospital	Gilbert	81%	(a)
Page Hospital[11]	Page	81%	(a)
Verde Valley Medical Center	Cottonwood	81%	300+
Banner Boswell Medical Center[11]	Sun City	80%	300+
Banner Ironwood Medical Center[11]	San Tan Valley	80%	300+
Payson Regional Medical Center	Payson	80%	300+
Scottsdale Hlthcare-Thompson Peak Hosp	Scottsdale	80%	300+
Banner Good Samaritan Medical Center[11]	Phoenix	79%	300+
Banner Baywood Medical Center[11]	Mesa	78%	300+
Banner Estrella Medical Center[11]	Phoenix	78%	300+
Banner Gateway Medical Center[11]	Gilbert	78%	300+
Banner Thunderbird Medical Center[11]	Glendale	78%	300+
Flagstaff Medical Center	Flagstaff	78%	300+
Mount Graham Regional Medical Center	Safford	78%	300+
Sierra Vista Regional Health Center	Sierra Vista	78%	300+
Summit Healthcare Regional Medical Center	Show Low	78%	300+
Yavapai Regional Medical Center - East	Prescott Valley	78%	300+
Banner Del E Webb Medical Center[11]	Sun City West	76%	300+
Banner Desert Medical Center[11]	Mesa	76%	300+
Chandler Regional Medical Center	Chandler	76%	300+
Cobre Valley Regional Medical Center	Globe	76%	300+
Kingman Regional Medical Center	Kingman	76%	300+
Mercy Gilbert Medical Center	Gilbert	76%	300+
Northwest Medical Center	Tucson	76%	300+
Saint Luke's Medical Center	Phoenix	76%	300+
Scottsdale Healthcare-Shea Med Ctr	Scottsdale	76%	300+
Tucson Medical Center	Tucson	76%	300+
Western Arizona Regional Medical Center	Bullhead City	76%	300+
Arrowhead Hospital[11]	Glendale	75%	300+
John C Lincoln North Mountain Hospital	Phoenix	75%	300+
Oro Valley Hospital	Oro Valley	75%	300+
Phoenix Indian Medical Center	Phoenix	75%	300+
Saint Joseph's Hospital & Medical Center	Phoenix	75%	300+
Valley View Medical Center	Fort Mohave	75%	300+
Yavapai Regional Medical Center	Prescott	75%	300+
Yuma Regional Medical Center	Yuma	75%	300+
Carondelet Saint Marys Hospital[11]	Tucson	74%	300+
John C Lincoln Deer Valley Hospital	Phoenix	74%	300+
Paradise Valley Hospital[11]	Phoenix	74%	300+
Scottsdale Healthcare Osborn Med Ctr	Scottsdale	74%	300+
University of Arizona Medical Center	Tucson	74%	300+
West Valley Hospital[11]	Goodyear	74%	300+
Carondelet Holy Cross Hospital[11]	Nogales	73%	(a)
Carondelet Saint Joseph's Hospital[11]	Tucson	73%	300+
Casa Grande Regional Medical Center	Casa Grande	73%	300+
Phoenix Baptist Hospital[11]	Phoenix	73%	300+
Fort Defiance Indian Hospital	Fort Defiance	72%	(a)
Maricopa Medical Center	Phoenix	72%	300+
Maryvale Hospital[11]	Phoenix	72%	300+
Mountain Vista Medical Center	Mesa	71%	300+
University of Arizona Medical Center	Tucson	71%	300+
Havasu Regional Medical Center	Lk Havasu City	70%	300+
Tuba City Reg Health Care Corporation	Tuba City	65%	300+
Chinle Comprehensive Health Care Facility	Chinle	62%	(a)

Pain 'Always' Well Controlled

Hospital Name	City	Rate	Cases
Wickenburg Community Hospital	Wickenburg	84%	(a)
Mayo Clinic Hospital[11]	Phoenix	77%	300+
Phoenix Indian Medical Center	Phoenix	76%	300+
Banner Heart Hospital[11]	Mesa	75%	300+
Arizona Ortho & Surgical Spec Hosp	Chandler	74%	300+
Mount Graham Regional Medical Center	Safford	74%	300+
Page Hospital[11]	Page	74%	(a)
Scottsdale Hlthcare-Thompson Peak Hosp	Scottsdale	74%	300+
Banner Ironwood Medical Center[11]	San Tan Valley	73%	300+
Verde Valley Medical Center	Cottonwood	73%	300+
Banner Boswell Medical Center[11]	Sun City	72%	300+
Banner Good Samaritan Medical Center[11]	Phoenix	72%	300+
Carondelet Holy Cross Hospital[11]	Nogales	72%	(a)
Gilbert Hospital	Gilbert	72%	(a)
Payson Regional Medical Center	Payson	72%	300+
The Surgical Hospital of Phoenix	Phoenix	72%	300+
Arizona Spine & Joint Hospital	Mesa	71%	300+
Banner Estrella Medical Center[11]	Phoenix	71%	300+
Banner Gateway Medical Center[11]	Gilbert	71%	300+
Mercy Gilbert Medical Center	Gilbert	71%	300+
Saint Luke's Medical Center	Phoenix	71%	300+
Chandler Regional Medical Center	Chandler	70%	300+
Flagstaff Medical Center	Flagstaff	70%	300+
John C Lincoln North Mountain Hospital	Phoenix	70%	300+
Oasis Hospital	Phoenix	70%	300+
Paradise Valley Hospital[11]	Phoenix	70%	300+
Scottsdale Healthcare-Shea Med Ctr	Scottsdale	70%	300+
Banner Baywood Medical Center[11]	Mesa	69%	300+
Banner Del E Webb Medical Center[11]	Sun City West	69%	300+
Banner Desert Medical Center[11]	Mesa	69%	300+
Banner Thunderbird Medical Center[11]	Glendale	69%	300+
Casa Grande Regional Medical Center	Casa Grande	69%	300+
Northwest Medical Center	Tucson	69%	300+
Saint Joseph's Hospital & Medical Center	Phoenix	69%	300+
Sierra Vista Regional Health Center	Sierra Vista	69%	300+
Summit Healthcare Regional Medical Center	Show Low	69%	300+
Tucson Medical Center	Tucson	69%	300+
Valley View Medical Center	Fort Mohave	69%	300+
West Valley Hospital[11]	Goodyear	69%	300+
Western Arizona Regional Medical Center	Bullhead City	69%	300+
Yavapai Regional Medical Center - East	Prescott Valley	69%	300+
Arrowhead Hospital[11]	Glendale	68%	300+
Carondelet Saint Marys Hospital[11]	Tucson	68%	300+
Cobre Valley Regional Medical Center	Globe	68%	300+
Phoenix Baptist Hospital[11]	Phoenix	68%	300+
Scottsdale Healthcare Osborn Med Ctr	Scottsdale	68%	300+
Yuma Regional Medical Center	Yuma	68%	300+
John C Lincoln Deer Valley Hospital	Phoenix	67%	300+
Kingman Regional Medical Center	Kingman	67%	300+
Maricopa Medical Center	Phoenix	67%	300+
Maryvale Hospital[11]	Phoenix	67%	300+
Mountain Vista Medical Center	Mesa	67%	300+
Oro Valley Hospital	Oro Valley	67%	300+
University of Arizona Medical Center	Tucson	67%	300+
Fort Defiance Indian Hospital	Fort Defiance	65%	(a)
University of Arizona Medical Center	Tucson	65%	300+
Yavapai Regional Medical Center	Prescott	64%	300+
Carondelet Saint Joseph's Hospital[11]	Tucson	63%	300+
Havasu Regional Medical Center	Lk Havasu City	62%	300+
Chinle Comprehensive Health Care Facility	Chinle	58%	(a)
Tuba City Reg Health Care Corporation	Tuba City	56%	300+

Room and Bathroom 'Always' Clean

Hospital Name	City	Rate	Cases
Carondelet Holy Cross Hospital[11]	Nogales	84%	(a)
Gilbert Hospital	Gilbert	83%	(a)
Arizona Ortho & Surgical Spec Hosp	Chandler	82%	300+
Arizona Spine & Joint Hospital	Mesa	81%	300+
The Surgical Hospital of Phoenix	Phoenix	81%	300+
Wickenburg Community Hospital	Wickenburg	81%	(a)
Oasis Hospital	Phoenix	80%	300+
Mayo Clinic Hospital[11]	Phoenix	78%	300+
Valley View Medical Center	Fort Mohave	78%	300+
Verde Valley Medical Center	Cottonwood	76%	300+
Yavapai Regional Medical Center - East	Prescott Valley	76%	300+
Summit Healthcare Regional Medical Center	Show Low	75%	300+
Page Hospital[11]	Page	74%	(a)
Banner Ironwood Medical Center[11]	San Tan Valley	73%	300+
Cobre Valley Regional Medical Center	Globe	73%	300+
Scottsdale Hlthcare-Thompson Peak Hosp	Scottsdale	73%	300+
Mercy Gilbert Medical Center	Gilbert	72%	300+
Payson Regional Medical Center	Payson	72%	300+
Saint Joseph's Hospital & Medical Center	Phoenix	72%	300+
Banner Estrella Medical Center[11]	Phoenix	71%	300+
Banner Heart Hospital[11]	Mesa	71%	300+
Flagstaff Medical Center	Flagstaff	70%	300+
Kingman Regional Medical Center	Kingman	70%	300+
Phoenix Baptist Hospital[11]	Phoenix	70%	300+
Saint Luke's Medical Center	Phoenix	70%	300+
John C Lincoln North Mountain Hospital	Phoenix	69%	300+
Oro Valley Hospital	Oro Valley	69%	300+
Sierra Vista Regional Health Center	Sierra Vista	69%	300+
Western Arizona Regional Medical Center	Bullhead City	69%	300+
Banner Del E Webb Medical Center[11]	Sun City West	68%	300+
Chandler Regional Medical Center	Chandler	68%	300+
Fort Defiance Indian Hospital	Fort Defiance	68%	(a)
John C Lincoln Deer Valley Hospital	Phoenix	67%	300+
Maryvale Hospital[11]	Phoenix	67%	300+
Scottsdale Healthcare Osborn Med Ctr	Scottsdale	67%	300+
Yuma Regional Medical Center	Yuma	67%	300+
Arrowhead Hospital[11]	Glendale	66%	300+
Maricopa Medical Center	Phoenix	66%	300+
Mount Graham Regional Medical Center	Safford	66%	300+
Northwest Medical Center	Tucson	66%	300+
Paradise Valley Hospital[11]	Phoenix	66%	300+
Scottsdale Healthcare-Shea Med Ctr	Scottsdale	66%	300+
Banner Baywood Medical Center[11]	Mesa	65%	300+
Banner Boswell Medical Center[11]	Sun City	65%	300+
University of Arizona Medical Center	Tucson	65%	300+
Banner Thunderbird Medical Center[11]	Glendale	64%	300+
University of Arizona Medical Center	Tucson	64%	300+
Banner Desert Medical Center[11]	Mesa	63%	300+
Banner Good Samaritan Medical Center[11]	Phoenix	63%	300+
Mountain Vista Medical Center	Mesa	63%	300+
Phoenix Indian Medical Center	Phoenix	63%	300+
Tucson Medical Center	Tucson	62%	300+
Carondelet Saint Joseph's Hospital[11]	Tucson	61%	300+
Yavapai Regional Medical Center	Prescott	61%	300+
Carondelet Saint Marys Hospital[11]	Tucson	60%	300+
Casa Grande Regional Medical Center	Casa Grande	60%	300+
Havasu Regional Medical Center	Lk Havasu City	59%	300+
Tuba City Reg Health Care Corporation	Tuba City	59%	300+
West Valley Hospital[11]	Goodyear	59%	300+
Banner Gateway Medical Center[11]	Gilbert	58%	300+
Chinle Comprehensive Health Care Facility	Chinle	57%	(a)

Timely Help 'Always' Received

Hospital Name	City	Rate	Cases
Arizona Ortho & Surgical Spec Hosp	Chandler	82%	300+
The Surgical Hospital of Phoenix	Phoenix	81%	300+
Arizona Spine & Joint Hospital	Mesa	79%	300+
Mayo Clinic Hospital[11]	Phoenix	79%	300+
Page Hospital[11]	Page	77%	(a)
Oasis Hospital	Phoenix	75%	300+
Banner Heart Hospital[11]	Mesa	73%	300+
Banner Ironwood Medical Center[11]	San Tan Valley	73%	300+
Payson Regional Medical Center	Payson	73%	300+
Wickenburg Community Hospital	Wickenburg	71%	(a)
Banner Boswell Medical Center[11]	Sun City	70%	300+
Banner Good Samaritan Medical Center[11]	Phoenix	70%	300+
Flagstaff Medical Center	Flagstaff	70%	300+
Gilbert Hospital	Gilbert	70%	(a)
Verde Valley Medical Center	Cottonwood	70%	300+
Mount Graham Regional Medical Center	Safford	69%	300+
Phoenix Indian Medical Center	Phoenix	69%	300+
Scottsdale Hlthcare-Thompson Peak Hosp	Scottsdale	68%	300+
Carondelet Holy Cross Hospital[11]	Nogales	67%	(a)
Summit Healthcare Regional Medical Center	Show Low	67%	300+
Yavapai Regional Medical Center - East	Prescott Valley	67%	300+
Western Arizona Regional Medical Center	Bullhead City	66%	300+
Yavapai Regional Medical Center	Prescott	65%	300+
Arrowhead Hospital[11]	Glendale	64%	300+
Banner Estrella Medical Center[11]	Phoenix	64%	300+
Banner Gateway Medical Center[11]	Gilbert	64%	300+
Chandler Regional Medical Center	Chandler	64%	300+
Mercy Gilbert Medical Center	Gilbert	64%	300+
Northwest Medical Center	Tucson	64%	300+
Scottsdale Healthcare Osborn Med Ctr	Scottsdale	64%	300+
Sierra Vista Regional Health Center	Sierra Vista	64%	300+
Banner Desert Medical Center[11]	Mesa	63%	300+
Cobre Valley Regional Medical Center	Globe	63%	300+
Kingman Regional Medical Center	Kingman	63%	300+
Paradise Valley Hospital[11]	Phoenix	63%	300+
Scottsdale Healthcare-Shea Med Ctr	Scottsdale	63%	300+
Yuma Regional Medical Center	Yuma	63%	300+
Banner Baywood Medical Center[11]	Mesa	62%	300+
Banner Del E Webb Medical Center[11]	Sun City West	62%	300+
Banner Thunderbird Medical Center[11]	Glendale	61%	300+
Maricopa Medical Center	Phoenix	61%	300+
Oro Valley Hospital	Oro Valley	61%	300+
Phoenix Baptist Hospital[11]	Phoenix	61%	300+
Saint Luke's Medical Center	Phoenix	61%	300+
Valley View Medical Center	Fort Mohave	61%	300+
West Valley Hospital[11]	Goodyear	61%	300+
John C Lincoln Deer Valley Hospital	Phoenix	60%	300+
John C Lincoln North Mountain Hospital	Phoenix	60%	300+
Saint Joseph's Hospital & Medical Center	Phoenix	60%	300+
Tucson Medical Center	Tucson	60%	300+
Maryvale Hospital[11]	Phoenix	59%	300+
University of Arizona Medical Center	Tucson	59%	300+
Carondelet Saint Joseph's Hospital[11]	Tucson	58%	300+
Mountain Vista Medical Center	Mesa	58%	300+
Carondelet Saint Marys Hospital[11]	Tucson	57%	300+

NOTE: Hospital profiles are in alphabetical order by state, then city, then hospital within the city; Rankings exclude hospitals with less than 25 cases except for patient surveys which excludes hospitals with less than 100 cases; (a) 100-299 cases; (1) The number of cases/patients is too few to report; (2) Data submitted were based on a sample of cases/patients; (3) Results are based on a shorter time period than required; (4) Data suppressed by CMS for one or more quarters; (5) Results are not available for this reporting period; (6) Fewer than 100 patients completed the HCAHPS survey; (7) No cases met the criteria for this measure; (8) The lower limit of the confidence interval cannot be calculated if the number of observed infections equals zero; (9) No data are available from the state/territory for this reporting period; (10) The scores shown reflect fewer than 50 completed surveys; (11) There were discrepancies in the data collection process; (12) This measure does not apply to this hospital for this reporting period; (13) Results cannot be calculated for this reporting period; (14) The results for this state are combined with nearby states to protect confidentiality; Please refer to the User's Guide for a full explanation of data.

Chinle Comprehensive Health Care Facility	Chinle	57%	(a)
Fort Defiance Indian Hospital	Fort Defiance	56%	(a)
Casa Grande Regional Medical Center	Casa Grande	55%	300+
Tuba City Reg Health Care Corporation	Tuba City	53%	300+
Havasu Regional Medical Center	Lk Havasu City	52%	300+
University of Arizona Medical Center	Tucson	52%	300+

Would Definitely Recommend Hospital

Hospital Name	City	Rate	Cases
Mayo Clinic Hospital[11]	Phoenix	93%	300+
Arizona Spine & Joint Hospital	Mesa	87%	300+
Arizona Ortho & Surgical Spec Hosp	Chandler	85%	300+
Oasis Hospital	Phoenix	84%	300+
The Surgical Hospital of Phoenix	Phoenix	83%	300+
Banner Heart Hospital[11]	Mesa	82%	300+
Scottsdale Hlthcare-Thompson Peak Hosp	Scottsdale	82%	300+
Banner Gateway Medical Center[11]	Gilbert	80%	300+
Gilbert Hospital	Gilbert	80%	(a)
Mercy Gilbert Medical Center	Gilbert	80%	300+
Banner Ironwood Medical Center[11]	San Tan Valley	79%	300+
Banner Good Samaritan Medical Center[11]	Phoenix	77%	300+
Banner Thunderbird Medical Center[11]	Glendale	77%	300+
Flagstaff Medical Center	Flagstaff	77%	300+
Saint Joseph's Hospital & Medical Center	Phoenix	77%	300+
Summit Healthcare Regional Medical Center	Show Low	77%	300+
Yavapai Regional Medical Center - East	Prescott Valley	77%	300+
Banner Estrella Medical Center[11]	Phoenix	76%	300+
Oro Valley Hospital	Oro Valley	76%	300+
Banner Boswell Medical Center[11]	Sun City	75%	300+
Verde Valley Medical Center	Cottonwood	75%	300+
Banner Baywood Medical Center[11]	Mesa	74%	300+
Banner Desert Medical Center[11]	Mesa	74%	300+
Scottsdale Healthcare-Shea Med Ctr	Scottsdale	74%	300+
University of Arizona Medical Center	Tucson	74%	300+
Wickenburg Community Hospital	Wickenburg	74%	(a)
Tucson Medical Center	Tucson	73%	300+
Valley View Medical Center	Fort Mohave	73%	300+
Carondelet Saint Joseph's Hospital[11]	Tucson	72%	300+
John C Lincoln North Mountain Hospital	Phoenix	72%	300+
Northwest Medical Center	Tucson	72%	300+
Arrowhead Hospital[11]	Glendale	71%	300+
Banner Del E Webb Medical Center[11]	Sun City West	71%	300+
Chandler Regional Medical Center	Chandler	71%	300+
John C Lincoln Deer Valley Hospital	Phoenix	71%	300+
Mount Graham Regional Medical Center	Safford	71%	300+
Scottsdale Healthcare Osborn Med Ctr	Scottsdale	71%	300+
Western Arizona Regional Medical Center	Bullhead City	70%	300+
Page Hospital[11]	Page	69%	(a)
Yavapai Regional Medical Center	Prescott	68%	300+
Saint Luke's Medical Center	Phoenix	67%	300+
Kingman Regional Medical Center	Kingman	66%	300+
Payson Regional Medical Center	Payson	66%	300+
Phoenix Baptist Hospital[11]	Phoenix	66%	300+
Yuma Regional Medical Center	Yuma	66%	300+
Carondelet Saint Marys Hospital[11]	Tucson	65%	300+
Cobre Valley Regional Medical Center	Globe	65%	300+
Maricopa Medical Center	Phoenix	65%	300+
Paradise Valley Hospital[11]	Phoenix	65%	300+
Mountain Vista Medical Center	Mesa	64%	300+
West Valley Hospital[11]	Goodyear	64%	300+
University of Arizona Medical Center	Tucson	62%	300+
Sierra Vista Regional Health Center	Sierra Vista	61%	300+
Carondelet Holy Cross Hospital[11]	Nogales	59%	(a)
Casa Grande Regional Medical Center	Casa Grande	59%	300+
Phoenix Indian Medical Center	Phoenix	59%	300+
Maryvale Hospital[11]	Phoenix	58%	300+
Havasu Regional Medical Center	Lk Havasu City	57%	300+
Fort Defiance Indian Hospital	Fort Defiance	55%	(a)
Tuba City Reg Health Care Corporation	Tuba City	52%	300+
Chinle Comprehensive Health Care Facility	Chinle	35%	(a)

Use of Medical Imaging

Cardiac Imaging Stress Test before OP Surgery

Hospital Name	City	Rate	Cases
Phoenix Baptist Hospital	Phoenix	2.2%	134
Cobre Valley Regional Medical Center	Globe	2.3%	129
Havasu Regional Medical Center	Lk Havasu City	2.9%	410
West Valley Hospital	Goodyear	3.0%	66
White Mountain Regional Medical Center	Springerville	3.0%	67
Saint Joseph's Hospital & Medical Center	Phoenix	3.5%	170
Northwest Medical Center	Tucson	3.7%	925
Carondelet Saint Marys Hospital	Tucson	3.8%	186
Oro Valley Hospital	Oro Valley	4.0%	177
Payson Regional Medical Center	Payson	4.0%	274
Kingman Regional Medical Center	Kingman	4.1%	436
Banner Good Samaritan Medical Center	Phoenix	4.2%	166
Verde Valley Medical Center	Cottonwood	4.3%	374
Mercy Gilbert Medical Center	Gilbert	4.7%	169
Flagstaff Medical Center	Flagstaff	4.8%	145
Tucson Medical Center	Tucson	4.8%	311
Banner Del E Webb Medical Center	Sun City West	5.0%	200
John C Lincoln North Mountain Hospital	Phoenix	5.0%	80
Maricopa Medical Center	Phoenix	5.0%	60
Summit Healthcare Regional Medical Center	Show Low	5.0%	282
Carondelet Saint Joseph's Hospital	Tucson	5.3%	454
Casa Grande Regional Medical Center	Casa Grande	5.3%	114
Mount Graham Regional Medical Center	Safford	5.4%	112
Yavapai Regional Medical Center	Prescott	5.4%	277
Scottsdale Healthcare Osborn Med Ctr	Scottsdale	5.9%	188
Banner Thunderbird Medical Center	Glendale	6.1%	147
University of Arizona Medical Center	Tucson	6.1%	98
Arrowhead Hospital	Glendale	6.6%	76
Chandler Regional Medical Center	Chandler	6.7%	135
John C Lincoln Deer Valley Hospital	Phoenix	6.7%	120
Sierra Vista Regional Health Center	Sierra Vista	6.8%	133
Yavapai Regional Medical Center - East	Prescott Valley	7.3%	178
Banner Estrella Medical Center	Phoenix	7.5%	67
Banner Baywood Medical Center	Mesa	7.6%	264
Scottsdale Healthcare-Shea Med Ctr	Scottsdale	7.6%	381
Scottsdale Hlthcare-Thompson Peak Hosp	Scottsdale	7.8%	153
University of Arizona Medical Center	Tucson	7.9%	699
Banner Boswell Medical Center	Sun City	8.3%	120
Mayo Clinic Hospital	Phoenix	10.6%	912

Combination Abdominal CT Scan

Hospital Name	City	Rate	Cases
Maryvale Hospital	Phoenix	0.0%	117
Saint Luke's Medical Center	Phoenix	0.7%	140
Mercy Gilbert Medical Center	Gilbert	0.8%	723
Scottsdale Hlthcare-Thompson Peak Hosp	Scottsdale	0.8%	383
Scottsdale Healthcare Osborn Med Ctr	Scottsdale	1.4%	572
Banner Desert Medical Center	Mesa	1.5%	480
Phoenix Baptist Hospital	Phoenix	1.5%	201
Chandler Regional Medical Center	Chandler	1.6%	920
University of Arizona Medical Center	Tucson	1.7%	1292
University of Arizona Medical Center	Tucson	1.8%	275
Banner Baywood Medical Center	Mesa	1.9%	909
Scottsdale Healthcare-Shea Med Ctr	Scottsdale	2.1%	778
West Valley Hospital	Goodyear	2.3%	396
Flagstaff Medical Center	Flagstaff	2.6%	345
Mountain Vista Medical Center	Mesa	2.6%	422
Gilbert Hospital	Gilbert	2.7%	183
Paradise Valley Hospital	Phoenix	2.7%	257
Page Hospital	Page	2.9%	104
Banner Gateway Medical Center	Gilbert	3.0%	835
Banner Ironwood Medical Center	San Tan Valley	3.0%	237
Banner Boswell Medical Center	Sun City	3.4%	1051
Banner Estrella Medical Center	Phoenix	3.4%	597
Banner Thunderbird Medical Center	Glendale	3.5%	624
Arrowhead Hospital	Glendale	3.8%	425
Northwest Medical Center	Tucson	3.8%	711
Florence Hospital at Anthem	Florence	4.2%	119
Maricopa Medical Center	Phoenix	4.5%	243
Saint Joseph's Hospital & Medical Center	Phoenix	4.5%	510
Banner Del E Webb Medical Center	Sun City West	4.7%	1611
Carondelet Saint Joseph's Hospital	Tucson	4.8%	394
Verde Valley Medical Center	Cottonwood	4.8%	939
Tucson Medical Center	Tucson	5.5%	512
Carondelet Saint Marys Hospital	Tucson	5.8%	378
Mayo Clinic Hospital	Phoenix	6.0%	1190
Sage Memorial Hospital	Ganado	6.2%	65
White Mountain Regional Medical Center	Springerville	7.3%	82
Mount Graham Regional Medical Center	Safford	7.4%	376
John C Lincoln North Mountain Hospital	Phoenix	8.0%	846
Havasu Regional Medical Center	Lk Havasu City	9.4%	953
Carondelet Holy Cross Hospital	Nogales	10.9%	129
Oro Valley Hospital	Oro Valley	11.4%	700
Yavapai Regional Medical Center	Prescott	12.5%	806
Sierra Vista Regional Health Center	Sierra Vista	12.6%	421
Summit Healthcare Regional Medical Center	Show Low	12.9%	637
Yavapai Regional Medical Center - East	Prescott Valley	13.4%	686
John C Lincoln Deer Valley Hospital	Phoenix	13.9%	416
Kingman Regional Medical Center	Kingman	15.5%	1144
Banner Good Samaritan Medical Center	Phoenix	17.4%	621
Western Arizona Regional Medical Center	Bullhead City	17.7%	880
Wickenburg Community Hospital	Wickenburg	17.9%	347
Payson Regional Medical Center	Payson	19.0%	642
Valley View Medical Center	Fort Mohave	19.1%	721
Cobre Valley Regional Medical Center	Globe	25.9%	386
Casa Grande Regional Medical Center	Casa Grande	31.7%	715
Yuma Regional Medical Center	Yuma	48.4%	949

Combination Brain/Sinus CT Scan

Hospital Name	City	Rate	Cases
Northwest Medical Center	Tucson	1.1%	666
Oro Valley Hospital	Oro Valley	1.1%	523
Sierra Vista Regional Health Center	Sierra Vista	1.1%	436
Scottsdale Hlthcare-Thompson Peak Hosp	Scottsdale	1.3%	377
Banner Del E Webb Medical Center	Sun City West	1.8%	1359
Havasu Regional Medical Center	Lk Havasu City	1.8%	841
Banner Baywood Medical Center	Mesa	1.9%	1156
Mercy Gilbert Medical Center	Gilbert	2.0%	801
Saint Joseph's Hospital & Medical Center	Phoenix	2.1%	889
Yavapai Regional Medical Center - East	Prescott Valley	2.2%	681
Kingman Regional Medical Center	Kingman	2.3%	865
Scottsdale Healthcare Osborn Med Ctr	Scottsdale	2.3%	895
Verde Valley Medical Center	Cottonwood	2.3%	780
Yavapai Regional Medical Center	Prescott	2.5%	895
Chandler Regional Medical Center	Chandler	2.6%	1214
Banner Boswell Medical Center	Sun City	2.7%	1056
Mayo Clinic Hospital	Phoenix	2.7%	778
Banner Thunderbird Medical Center	Glendale	2.8%	603
Scottsdale Healthcare-Shea Med Ctr	Scottsdale	3.4%	804
Yuma Regional Medical Center	Yuma	3.4%	1565
Western Arizona Regional Medical Center	Bullhead City	3.7%	776
Summit Healthcare Regional Medical Center	Show Low	4.4%	617
John C Lincoln Deer Valley Hospital	Phoenix	4.5%	421
Tucson Medical Center	Tucson	4.5%	600
Banner Good Samaritan Medical Center	Phoenix	4.7%	423
Cobre Valley Regional Medical Center	Globe	4.7%	358
Banner Gateway Medical Center	Gilbert	4.9%	409
Paradise Valley Hospital	Phoenix	5.1%	254
Gilbert Hospital	Gilbert	5.6%	178
Payson Regional Medical Center	Payson	5.6%	586
John C Lincoln North Mountain Hospital	Phoenix	6.5%	709
Banner Desert Medical Center	Mesa	6.8%	676
University of Arizona Medical Center	Tucson	6.9%	391
University of Arizona Medical Center	Tucson	9.0%	812

Combination Chest CT Scan

Hospital Name	City	Rate	Cases
Maricopa Medical Center	Phoenix	0.0%	135
Sage Memorial Hospital	Ganado	0.0%	48
Scottsdale Hlthcare-Thompson Peak Hosp	Scottsdale	0.0%	78
Scottsdale Healthcare Osborn Med Ctr	Scottsdale	0.0%	134
Banner Boswell Medical Center	Sun City	0.2%	494
Chandler Regional Medical Center	Chandler	0.2%	666
Saint Joseph's Hospital & Medical Center	Phoenix	0.2%	469
University of Arizona Medical Center	Tucson	0.2%	1520
Verde Valley Medical Center	Cottonwood	0.2%	451
Banner Good Samaritan Medical Center	Phoenix	0.5%	383
Banner Baywood Medical Center	Mesa	0.7%	422
Mayo Clinic Hospital	Phoenix	0.7%	563
University of Arizona Medical Center	Tucson	0.7%	135
Banner Desert Medical Center	Mesa	0.8%	125
Banner Gateway Medical Center	Gilbert	0.8%	528
Mercy Gilbert Medical Center	Gilbert	0.8%	516
Scottsdale Healthcare-Shea Med Ctr	Scottsdale	0.8%	262
West Valley Hospital	Goodyear	1.0%	97
Banner Thunderbird Medical Center	Glendale	1.2%	171
Banner Ironwood Medical Center	San Tan Valley	1.3%	77
Carondelet Saint Joseph's Hospital	Tucson	1.6%	190
Mountain Vista Medical Center	Mesa	1.6%	123
Arrowhead Hospital	Glendale	1.8%	110
John C Lincoln North Mountain Hospital	Phoenix	1.9%	482
Page Hospital	Page	2.1%	47
Carondelet Saint Marys Hospital	Tucson	2.4%	83
Mount Graham Regional Medical Center	Safford	2.4%	292
Havasu Regional Medical Center	Lk Havasu City	2.5%	595
Carondelet Holy Cross Hospital	Nogales	3.2%	63
Paradise Valley Hospital	Phoenix	3.6%	56
Banner Estrella Medical Center	Phoenix	3.8%	133
Banner Del E Webb Medical Center	Sun City West	4.0%	569
John C Lincoln Deer Valley Hospital	Phoenix	4.8%	105
Oro Valley Hospital	Oro Valley	4.8%	289
Payson Regional Medical Center	Payson	5.0%	398
Northwest Medical Center	Tucson	5.8%	154
Tucson Medical Center	Tucson	7.0%	86
Phoenix Baptist Hospital	Phoenix	7.7%	78
Sierra Vista Regional Health Center	Sierra Vista	8.0%	512
Wickenburg Community Hospital	Wickenburg	9.0%	189
Yuma Regional Medical Center	Yuma	9.0%	580
Flagstaff Medical Center	Flagstaff	10.5%	209
Valley View Medical Center	Fort Mohave	11.3%	353
Kingman Regional Medical Center	Kingman	14.6%	783
Summit Healthcare Regional Medical Center	Show Low	14.6%	288
Yavapai Regional Medical Center	Prescott	14.6%	567
Yavapai Regional Medical Center - East	Prescott Valley	14.7%	375
White Mountain Regional Medical Center	Springerville	15.3%	72
Casa Grande Regional Medical Center	Casa Grande	21.1%	427
Western Arizona Regional Medical Center	Bullhead City	22.1%	411
Cobre Valley Regional Medical Center	Globe	39.4%	127

Follow-up Mammogram/Ultrasound

A follow-up rate near zero may indicate missed cancer; a rate higher than 14% may mean there is unnecessary follow up.

Hospital Name	City	Rate	Cases
Havasu Regional Medical Center	Lk Havasu City	2.1%	1770
Carondelet Holy Cross Hospital	Nogales	2.4%	82

NOTE: Hospital profiles are in alphabetical order by state, then city, then hospital within the city; Rankings exclude hospitals with less than 25 cases except for patient surveys which excludes hospitals with less than 100 cases; (a) 100-299 cases; (1) The number of cases/patients is too few to report; (2) Data submitted were based on a sample of cases/patients; (3) Results are based on a shorter time period than required; (4) Data suppressed by CMS for one or more quarters; (5) Results are not available for this reporting period; (6) Fewer than 100 patients completed the HCAHPS survey; (7) No cases met the criteria for this measure; (8) The lower limit of the confidence interval cannot be calculated if the number of observed infections equals zero; (9) No data are available from the state/territory for this reporting period; (10) The scores shown reflect fewer than 50 completed surveys; (11) There were discrepancies in the data collection process; (12) This measure does not apply to this hospital for this reporting period; (13) Results cannot be calculated for this reporting period; (14) The results for this state are combined with nearby states to protect confidentiality; Please refer to the User's Guide for a full explanation of data.

Banner Thunderbird Medical Center	Glendale	3.3%	182
Payson Regional Medical Center	Payson	3.7%	1146
Verde Valley Medical Center	Cottonwood	3.8%	2156
Mount Graham Regional Medical Center	Safford	3.9%	465
Valley View Medical Center	Fort Mohave	4.5%	770
Arrowhead Hospital	Glendale	5.5%	183
Western Arizona Regional Medical Center	Bullhead City	5.5%	995
Yavapai Regional Medical Center	Prescott	5.9%	524
Tucson Medical Center	Tucson	6.9%	683
Northwest Medical Center	Tucson	7.0%	1050
Oro Valley Hospital	Oro Valley	7.2%	1043
Yavapai Regional Medical Center - East	Prescott Valley	7.3%	1300
Summit Healthcare Regional Medical Center	Show Low	7.5%	949
Casa Grande Regional Medical Center	Casa Grande	7.6%	1085
Kingman Regional Medical Center	Kingman	8.1%	1610
Yuma Regional Medical Center	Yuma	8.2%	3292
Phoenix Baptist Hospital	Phoenix	8.4%	178
Banner Good Samaritan Medical Center	Phoenix	9.1%	320
Mountain Vista Medical Center	Mesa	9.6%	104
Banner Gateway Medical Center	Gilbert	9.8%	369
Sierra Vista Regional Health Center	Sierra Vista	9.9%	1012
Scottsdale Healthcare-Shea Med Ctr	Scottsdale	10.1%	562
Banner Del E Webb Medical Center	Sun City West	10.8%	4090
Maricopa Medical Center	Phoenix	12.1%	173
Wickenburg Community Hospital	Wickenburg	12.1%	455
Banner Boswell Medical Center	Sun City	13.0%	1233
John C Lincoln Deer Valley Hospital	Phoenix	14.0%	1741
Page Hospital	Page	14.6%	89
Banner Baywood Medical Center	Mesa	15.8%	967
Mercy Gilbert Medical Center	Gilbert	16.6%	241
Saint Joseph's Hospital & Medical Center	Phoenix	16.7%	270
Cobre Valley Regional Medical Center	Globe	16.8%	304
Chandler Regional Medical Center	Chandler	19.8%	450

Lumbar Spine MRI for Low Back Pain

Hospital Name	City	Rate	Cases
Kingman Regional Medical Center	Kingman	25.5%	110
Yavapai Regional Medical Center - East	Prescott Valley	25.8%	66
Flagstaff Medical Center	Flagstaff	32.0%	97
Verde Valley Medical Center	Cottonwood	32.7%	220
Banner Del E Webb Medical Center	Sun City West	34.3%	67
Summit Healthcare Regional Medical Center	Show Low	35.5%	76
Banner Boswell Medical Center	Sun City	36.4%	55
Havasu Regional Medical Center	Lk Havasu City	36.4%	129
Casa Grande Regional Medical Center	Casa Grande	37.0%	54
Mayo Clinic Hospital	Phoenix	38.3%	167
Sierra Vista Regional Health Center	Sierra Vista	38.3%	60
Saint Joseph's Hospital & Medical Center	Phoenix	39.1%	87
John C Lincoln North Mountain Hospital	Phoenix	39.2%	120
Yuma Regional Medical Center	Yuma	40.4%	198
Valley View Medical Center	Fort Mohave	40.9%	93
Payson Regional Medical Center	Payson	43.1%	116
University of Arizona Medical Center	Tucson	43.2%	95
Oro Valley Hospital	Oro Valley	45.6%	57

NOTE: Hospital profiles are in alphabetical order by state, then city, then hospital within the city; Rankings exclude hospitals with less than 25 cases except for patient surveys which excludes hospitals with less than 100 cases; (a) 100-299 cases; (1) The number of cases/patients is too few to report; (2) Data submitted were based on a sample of cases/patients; (3) Results are based on a shorter time period than required; (4) Data suppressed by CMS for one or more quarters; (5) Results are not available for this reporting period; (6) Fewer than 100 patients completed the HCAHPS survey; (7) No cases met the criteria for this measure; (8) The lower limit of the confidence interval cannot be calculated if the number of observed infections equals zero; (9) No data are available from the state/territory for this reporting period; (10) The scores shown reflect fewer than 50 completed surveys; (11) There were discrepancies in the data collection process; (12) This measure does not apply to this hospital for this reporting period; (13) Results cannot be calculated for this reporting period; (14) The results for this state are combined with nearby states to protect confidentiality; Please refer to the User's Guide for a full explanation of data.

Banner Goldfield Medical Center

2050 West Southern Avenue | Phone: 480-237-3200
Apache Junction, AZ 85120
Type: Acute Care Hospitals | Emergency Services: Yes
Ownership: Voluntary non-profit - Other

Measure	Cases	This Hosp.	State Avg.	U.S. Avg.
Blood Clot Prevention and Treatment				
Anticoagulation Overlap Therapy[5]	-	-	94%	93%
ICU Venous Thromboembolism Prophylaxis[5]	-	-	92%	92%
Incidence of Potentially Preventable VTE[5]	-	-	9%	10%
UFH with Dosages/Platelet Monitoring[5]	-	-	98%	97%
Venous Thromboembolism Prophylaxis[5]	-	-	88%	85%
Warfarin Therapy Discharge Instructions[5]	-	-	74%	75%
Chest Pain/Possible Heart Attack Care				
Aspirin Given Within 24 Hours of Arrival[5]	-	-	98%	96%
Fibrinolytic Meds Within 30 Min. of Arrival[5]	-	-	59%	58%
Average Time to ECG (minutes)[5]	-	-	6	7
Average Time to Transfer (minutes)[5]	-	-	48	60
Children's Asthma Care				
Received Home Management Plan of Care	-	-	-	88%
Received Reliever Medication	-	-	-	100%
Received Systemic Corticosteroids	-	-	-	100%
Emergency Department				
Admittance Decision Time (minutes)[5]	-	-	98	98
Head CT Results Within 45 Min. of Arrival[5]	-	-	64%	57%
Patients Who Left ER Before Being Seen[5]	-	-	2%	2%
Time from ER Arrival to Admit. (minutes)[5]	-	-	285	274
Time from ER Arrival to Discharge (minutes)[5]	-	-	162	134
Time in ER Before Being Evaluated (minutes)[5]	-	-	27	26
Time to Pain Meds for Fractures (minutes)[5]	-	-	58	57
Heart Attack Care				
Aspirin Given at Discharge[5]	-	-	99%	99%
Fibrinolytic Meds Within 30 Min. of Arrival[5]	-	-	67%	54%
PCI Within 90 Minutes of Arrival[5]	-	-	95%	96%
Statin Prescribed at Discharge[5]	-	-	98%	98%
Heart Failure Care				
ACE Inhibitor or ARB for LVSD[5]	-	-	98%	97%
Discharge Instructions Given[5]	-	-	94%	94%
Evaluation of LVS Function[5]	-	-	99%	99%
Medicare Spending				
Medicare Spending per Patient (ratio)	-	-	0.93	0.98
Pneumonia Care				
Appropriate Initial Antibiotic Given[5]	-	-	96%	95%
Blood Culture Timing[5]	-	-	97%	98%
Pregnancy and Delivery Care				
Newborn Deliveries Scheduled Early[5]	-	-	7%	6%
Preventive Care				
Immunization for Influenza[5]	-	-	91%	90%
Immunization for Pneumonia[5]	-	-	92%	92%
Stroke Care				
Anticoagulation Therapy for Atrial Fibrillation[5]	-	-	96%	95%
Antithrombotic Therapy Timing[5]	-	-	98%	98%
Assessed for Rehabilitation[5]	-	-	96%	97%
Discharged on Antithrombotic Therapy[5]	-	-	99%	99%
Discharged on Statin Medication[5]	-	-	94%	94%
Thrombolytic Therapy Timing[5]	-	-	81%	66%
Venous Thromboembolism Prophylaxis[5]	-	-	93%	94%
Written Stroke Educational Materials Given[5]	-	-	84%	88%
Surgical Care Improvement Project				
Appropriate Beta Blocker Usage[5]	-	-	97%	98%
Appropriate VTP Within 24 Hours[5]	-	-	98%	98%
Controlled Postoperative Blood Glucose[5]	-	-	96%	97%
Perioperative Temperature Management[5]	-	-	100%	100%
Prophylactic Antibiotic Selection[5]	-	-	99%	99%
Prophylactic Antibiotic Selection (Outpatient)[5]	-	-	98%	98%
Prophylactic Antibiotic Stopped[5]	-	-	98%	98%
Prophylactic Antibiotic Timing[5]	-	-	99%	99%
Prophylactic Antibiotic Timing (Outpatient)[5]	-	-	99%	98%
Urinary Catheter Removal[5]	-	-	97%	97%
Survey of Patients' Hospital Experiences				
Area Around Room 'Always' Quiet at Night[5]	-	-	57%	61%
Doctors 'Always' Communicated Well[5]	-	-	77%	82%
Home Recovery Information Given[5]	-	-	86%	85%
Hospital Given 9 or 10 on 10 Point Scale[5]	-	-	70%	71%
Meds 'Always' Explained Before Given[5]	-	-	62%	64%
Nurses 'Always' Communicated Well[5]	-	-	76%	79%
Pain 'Always' Well Controlled[5]	-	-	69%	71%
Room and Bathroom 'Always' Clean[5]	-	-	69%	73%
Timely Help 'Always' Received[5]	-	-	65%	68%
Would Definitely Recommend Hospital[5]	-	-	70%	71%
Use of Medical Imaging				
Cardiac Imaging Stress Test before Surgery[7]	-	-	5.8%	5.3%
Combination Abdominal CT Scan[7]	-	-	9.1%	10.5%
Combination Brain/Sinus CT Scan[7]	-	-	3.2%	2.7%
Combination Chest CT Scan[7]	-	-	5.5%	2.7%
Follow-up Mammogram/Ultrasound[7]	-	-	8.5%	8.8%
Lumbar Spine MRI for Low Back Pain[7]	-	-	37.4%	37.2%

Benson Hospital

450 South Ocotillo Street | Phone: 520-586-2261
Benson, AZ 85602 | Fax: 520-586-2265
URL: www.bensonhospital.org
Type: Critical Access Hospitals | Emergency Services: Yes
Ownership: Govt - Hospital Dist/Auth | Beds: 22

Key Personnel:
Emergency Room . . . . Mike Buenafe, MD
President . . . . Ann MacInnes Cook
Chief of Medical Staff . . . . Andrew Mayberry, MD
CEO . . . . Richard Polheber
Quality Assurance . . . . Shelley Seifert

Measure	Cases	This Hosp.	State Avg.	U.S. Avg.
Blood Clot Prevention and Treatment				
Anticoagulation Overlap Therapy[5]	-	-	94%	93%
ICU Venous Thromboembolism Prophylaxis[5]	-	-	92%	92%
Incidence of Potentially Preventable VTE[5]	-	-	9%	10%
UFH with Dosages/Platelet Monitoring[5]	-	-	98%	97%
Venous Thromboembolism Prophylaxis[5]	-	-	88%	85%
Warfarin Therapy Discharge Instructions[5]	-	-	74%	75%
Chest Pain/Possible Heart Attack Care				
Aspirin Given Within 24 Hours of Arrival	-	-	98%	96%
Fibrinolytic Meds Within 30 Min. of Arrival	-	-	59%	58%
Average Time to ECG (minutes)	-	-	6	7
Average Time to Transfer (minutes)	-	-	48	60
Children's Asthma Care				
Received Home Management Plan of Care	-	-	-	88%
Received Reliever Medication	-	-	-	100%
Received Systemic Corticosteroids	-	-	-	100%
Emergency Department				
Admittance Decision Time (minutes)[5]	-	-	98	98
Head CT Results Within 45 Min. of Arrival	-	-	64%	57%
Patients Who Left ER Before Being Seen	-	-	2%	2%
Time from ER Arrival to Admit. (minutes)[5]	-	-	285	274
Time from ER Arrival to Discharge (minutes)	-	-	162	134
Time in ER Before Being Evaluated (minutes)	-	-	27	26
Time to Pain Meds for Fractures (minutes)	-	-	58	57
Heart Attack Care				
Aspirin Given at Discharge[5]	-	-	99%	99%
Fibrinolytic Meds Within 30 Min. of Arrival[5]	-	-	67%	54%
PCI Within 90 Minutes of Arrival[5]	-	-	95%	96%
Statin Prescribed at Discharge[5]	-	-	98%	98%
Heart Failure Care				
ACE Inhibitor or ARB for LVSD[3,7]	-	-	98%	97%
Discharge Instructions Given[3,7]	-	-	94%	94%
Evaluation of LVS Function[3,7]	-	-	99%	99%
Medicare Spending				
Medicare Spending per Patient (ratio)	-	-	0.93	0.98
Pneumonia Care				
Appropriate Initial Antibiotic Given[7]	-	-	96%	95%
Blood Culture Timing	33	88%	97%	98%
Pregnancy and Delivery Care				
Newborn Deliveries Scheduled Early[5]	-	-	7%	6%
Preventive Care				
Immunization for Influenza[5]	-	-	91%	90%
Immunization for Pneumonia[5]	-	-	92%	92%
Stroke Care				
Anticoagulation Therapy for Atrial Fibrillation[5]	-	-	96%	95%
Antithrombotic Therapy Timing[5]	-	-	98%	98%
Assessed for Rehabilitation[5]	-	-	96%	97%
Discharged on Antithrombotic Therapy[5]	-	-	99%	99%
Discharged on Statin Medication[5]	-	-	94%	94%
Thrombolytic Therapy Timing[5]	-	-	81%	66%
Venous Thromboembolism Prophylaxis[5]	-	-	93%	94%
Written Stroke Educational Materials Given[5]	-	-	84%	88%
Surgical Care Improvement Project				
Appropriate Beta Blocker Usage[5]	-	-	97%	98%
Appropriate VTP Within 24 Hours[5]	-	-	98%	98%
Controlled Postoperative Blood Glucose[5]	-	-	96%	97%
Perioperative Temperature Management[5]	-	-	100%	100%
Prophylactic Antibiotic Selection[5]	-	-	99%	99%
Prophylactic Antibiotic Selection (Outpatient)	-	-	98%	98%
Prophylactic Antibiotic Stopped[5]	-	-	98%	98%
Prophylactic Antibiotic Timing[5]	-	-	99%	99%
Prophylactic Antibiotic Timing (Outpatient)	-	-	99%	98%
Urinary Catheter Removal[5]	-	-	97%	97%
Survey of Patients' Hospital Experiences				
Area Around Room 'Always' Quiet at Night[6]	<100	66%	57%	61%
Doctors 'Always' Communicated Well[6]	<100	89%	77%	82%
Home Recovery Information Given[6]	<100	88%	86%	85%
Hospital Given 9 or 10 on 10 Point Scale[6]	<100	75%	70%	71%
Meds 'Always' Explained Before Given[6]	<100	69%	62%	64%
Nurses 'Always' Communicated Well[6]	<100	85%	76%	79%
Pain 'Always' Well Controlled[6]	<100	68%	69%	71%
Room and Bathroom 'Always' Clean[6]	<100	77%	69%	73%
Timely Help 'Always' Received[6]	<100	68%	65%	68%
Would Definitely Recommend Hospital[6]	<100	81%	70%	71%
Use of Medical Imaging				
Cardiac Imaging Stress Test before Surgery	-	-	5.8%	5.3%
Combination Abdominal CT Scan	-	-	9.1%	10.5%
Combination Brain/Sinus CT Scan	-	-	3.2%	2.7%
Combination Chest CT Scan	-	-	5.5%	2.7%
Follow-up Mammogram/Ultrasound	-	-	8.5%	8.8%
Lumbar Spine MRI for Low Back Pain	-	-	37.4%	37.2%

Copper Queen Community Hospital

101 Cole Avenue | Phone: 520-432-5383
Bisbee, AZ 85603 | Fax: 520-432-8018
URL: www.cqch.org
Type: Critical Access Hospitals | Emergency Services: Yes
Ownership: Voluntary non-profit - Private | Beds: 28

Key Personnel:
Cardiac Laboratory. . . . . Sayed Avam
Chief of Medical Staff . . . . Peggy Avina, MD
CEO/President. . . . . James Dickson
Operating Room. . . . . Alberto Dominguez-Ve
Radiology. . . . . Donald Dupperret, MD
Quality Assurance . . . . Darla Francaviglia
Pediatric Ambulatory Care . . . . . . Stephen E Lindstrom, MD
Infection Control. . . . . Elizabeth Mitchell, RN

Measure	Cases	This Hosp.	State Avg.	U.S. Avg.
Blood Clot Prevention and Treatment				
Anticoagulation Overlap Therapy[5]	-	-	94%	93%
ICU Venous Thromboembolism Prophylaxis[5]	-	-	92%	92%
Incidence of Potentially Preventable VTE[5]	-	-	9%	10%
UFH with Dosages/Platelet Monitoring[5]	-	-	98%	97%
Venous Thromboembolism Prophylaxis[5]	-	-	88%	85%
Warfarin Therapy Discharge Instructions[5]	-	-	74%	75%
Chest Pain/Possible Heart Attack Care				
Aspirin Given Within 24 Hours of Arrival	-	-	98%	96%
Fibrinolytic Meds Within 30 Min. of Arrival	-	-	59%	58%
Average Time to ECG (minutes)	-	-	6	7
Average Time to Transfer (minutes)	-	-	48	60
Children's Asthma Care				
Received Home Management Plan of Care	-	-	-	88%
Received Reliever Medication	-	-	-	100%
Received Systemic Corticosteroids	-	-	-	100%
Emergency Department				
Admittance Decision Time (minutes)[5]	-	-	98	98
Head CT Results Within 45 Min. of Arrival	-	-	64%	57%
Patients Who Left ER Before Being Seen	-	-	2%	2%
Time from ER Arrival to Admit. (minutes)[5]	-	-	285	274

NOTE: Hospital profiles are in alphabetical order by state, then city, then hospital within the city; Rankings exclude hospitals with less than 25 cases except for patient surveys which excludes hospitals with less than 100 cases; (a) 100-299 cases; (1) The number of cases/patients is too few to report; (2) Data submitted were based on a sample of cases/patients; (3) Results are based on a shorter time period than required; (4) Data suppressed by CMS for one or more quarters; (5) Results are not available for this reporting period; (6) Fewer than 100 patients completed the HCAHPS survey; (7) No cases met the criteria for this measure; (8) The lower limit of the confidence interval cannot be calculated if the number of observed infections equals zero; (9) No data are available from the state/territory for this reporting period; (10) The scores shown reflect fewer than 50 completed surveys; (11) There were discrepancies in the data collection process; (12) This measure does not apply to this hospital for this reporting period; (13) Results cannot be calculated for this reporting period; (14) The results for this state are combined with nearby states to protect confidentiality; Please refer to the User's Guide for a full explanation of data.

Time from ER Arrival to Discharge (minutes)	-	-	162	134
Time in ER Before Being Evaluated (minutes)	-	-	27	26
Time to Pain Meds for Fractures (minutes)	-	-	58	57
Heart Attack Care				
Aspirin Given at Discharge[5]	-	-	99%	99%
Fibrinolytic Meds Within 30 Min. of Arrival[5]	-	-	67%	54%
PCI Within 90 Minutes of Arrival[5]	-	-	95%	96%
Statin Prescribed at Discharge[5]	-	-	98%	98%
Heart Failure Care				
ACE Inhibitor or ARB for LVSD[1,3]	-	-	98%	97%
Discharge Instructions Given[3,7]	-	-	94%	94%
Evaluation of LVS Function[1,3]	-	-	99%	99%
Medicare Spending				
Medicare Spending per Patient (ratio)	-	-	0.93	0.98
Pneumonia Care				
Appropriate Initial Antibiotic Given	18	89%	96%	95%
Blood Culture Timing	19	74%	97%	98%
Pregnancy and Delivery Care				
Newborn Deliveries Scheduled Early[5]	-	-	7%	6%
Preventive Care				
Immunization for Influenza[5]	-	-	91%	90%
Immunization for Pneumonia[5]	-	-	92%	92%
Stroke Care				
Anticoagulation Therapy for Atrial Fibrillation[5]	-	-	96%	95%
Antithrombotic Therapy Timing[5]	-	-	98%	98%
Assessed for Rehabilitation[5]	-	-	96%	97%
Discharged on Antithrombotic Therapy[5]	-	-	99%	99%
Discharged on Statin Medication[5]	-	-	94%	94%
Thrombolytic Therapy Timing[5]	-	-	81%	66%
Venous Thromboembolism Prophylaxis[5]	-	-	93%	94%
Written Stroke Educational Materials Given[5]	-	-	84%	88%
Surgical Care Improvement Project				
Appropriate Beta Blocker Usage[5]	-	-	97%	98%
Appropriate VTP Within 24 Hours[5]	-	-	98%	98%
Controlled Postoperative Blood Glucose[5]	-	-	96%	97%
Perioperative Temperature Management[5]	-	-	100%	100%
Prophylactic Antibiotic Selection[5]	-	-	99%	99%
Prophylactic Antibiotic Selection (Outpatient)	-	-	98%	98%
Prophylactic Antibiotic Stopped[5]	-	-	98%	98%
Prophylactic Antibiotic Timing[5]	-	-	99%	99%
Prophylactic Antibiotic Timing (Outpatient)	-	-	99%	98%
Urinary Catheter Removal[5]	-	-	97%	97%
Survey of Patients' Hospital Experiences				
Area Around Room 'Always' Quiet at Night[6]	<100	55%	57%	61%
Doctors 'Always' Communicated Well[6]	<100	88%	77%	82%
Home Recovery Information Given[6]	<100	83%	86%	85%
Hospital Given 9 or 10 on 10 Point Scale[6]	<100	70%	70%	71%
Meds 'Always' Explained Before Given[6]	<100	70%	62%	64%
Nurses 'Always' Communicated Well[6]	<100	83%	76%	79%
Pain 'Always' Well Controlled[6]	<100	63%	69%	71%
Room and Bathroom 'Always' Clean[6]	<100	78%	69%	73%
Timely Help 'Always' Received[6]	<100	66%	65%	68%
Would Definitely Recommend Hospital[6]	<100	78%	70%	71%
Use of Medical Imaging				
Cardiac Imaging Stress Test before Surgery	-	-	5.8%	5.3%
Combination Abdominal CT Scan	-	-	9.1%	10.5%
Combination Brain/Sinus CT Scan	-	-	3.2%	2.7%
Combination Chest CT Scan	-	-	5.5%	2.7%
Follow-up Mammogram/Ultrasound	-	-	8.5%	8.8%
Lumbar Spine MRI for Low Back Pain	-	-	37.4%	37.2%

Western Arizona Regional Medical Center

2735 Silver Creek Road
Bullhead City, AZ 86442
Phone: 928-763-2273
Fax: 928-704-6734
URL: www.warmc.com
Type: Acute Care Hospitals
Emergency Services: Yes
Ownership: Proprietary
Beds: 123

Key Personnel:
Pulmonary Disease . . . . Anees Arshad, MD
Pediatrics. . . . . Alan Barton, MD
Chief of Medical Staff . . . . Nathan Beneze
CEO/President. . . . . Lee Christenson
Operating Room. . . . . Ricky Knight
Radiology. . . . . Warren Mays
Quality Assurance . . . . Kathryn McMiller

Measure	Cases	This Hosp.	State Avg.	U.S. Avg.
Blood Clot Prevention and Treatment				
Anticoagulation Overlap Therapy[2]	50	100%	94%	93%
ICU Venous Thromboembolism Prophylaxis[2]	153	99%	92%	92%
Incidence of Potentially Preventable VTE[1,2]	-	-	9%	10%
UFH with Dosages/Platelet Monitoring[2]	14	100%	98%	97%
Venous Thromboembolism Prophylaxis[2]	361	100%	88%	85%
Warfarin Therapy Discharge Instructions[2]	42	100%	74%	75%
Chest Pain/Possible Heart Attack Care				
Aspirin Given Within 24 Hours of Arrival[1,3]	-	-	98%	96%
Fibrinolytic Meds Within 30 Min. of Arrival[3,7]	-	-	59%	58%
Average Time to ECG (minutes)[1,3]	-	-	6	7
Average Time to Transfer (minutes)[3,7]	-	-	48	60
Children's Asthma Care				
Received Home Management Plan of Care	-	-	-	88%
Received Reliever Medication	-	-	-	100%
Received Systemic Corticosteroids	-	-	-	100%
Emergency Department				
Admittance Decision Time (minutes)[2]	1,088	78	98	98
Head CT Results Within 45 Min. of Arrival	21	95%	64%	57%
Patients Who Left ER Before Being Seen	29,206	0%	2%	2%
Time from ER Arrival to Admit. (minutes)[2]	1,089	257	285	274
Time from ER Arrival to Discharge (minutes)	372	152	162	134
Time in ER Before Being Evaluated (minutes)	421	13	27	26
Time to Pain Meds for Fractures (minutes)	172	47	58	57
Heart Attack Care				
Aspirin Given at Discharge	151	100%	99%	99%
Fibrinolytic Meds Within 30 Min. of Arrival[1]	-	-	67%	54%
PCI Within 90 Minutes of Arrival	23	96%	95%	96%
Statin Prescribed at Discharge	140	98%	98%	98%
Heart Failure Care				
ACE Inhibitor or ARB for LVSD	54	100%	98%	97%
Discharge Instructions Given	253	98%	94%	94%
Evaluation of LVS Function	278	99%	99%	99%
Medicare Spending				
Medicare Spending per Patient (ratio)	-	0.88	0.93	0.98
Pneumonia Care				
Appropriate Initial Antibiotic Given	134	99%	96%	95%
Blood Culture Timing	215	99%	97%	98%
Pregnancy and Delivery Care				
Newborn Deliveries Scheduled Early[2]	14	0%	7%	6%
Preventive Care				
Immunization for Influenza[2]	646	100%	91%	90%
Immunization for Pneumonia[2]	984	100%	92%	92%
Stroke Care				
Anticoagulation Therapy for Atrial Fibrillation[1]	-	-	96%	95%
Antithrombotic Therapy Timing	77	100%	98%	98%
Assessed for Rehabilitation	74	97%	96%	97%
Discharged on Antithrombotic Therapy	73	100%	99%	99%
Discharged on Statin Medication	58	93%	94%	94%
Thrombolytic Therapy Timing[1]	-	-	81%	66%
Venous Thromboembolism Prophylaxis	80	100%	93%	94%
Written Stroke Educational Materials Given	52	98%	84%	88%
Surgical Care Improvement Project				
Appropriate Beta Blocker Usage	156	100%	97%	98%
Appropriate VTP Within 24 Hours	257	97%	98%	98%
Controlled Postoperative Blood Glucose[7]	-	-	96%	97%
Perioperative Temperature Management	483	100%	100%	100%
Prophylactic Antibiotic Selection	330	97%	99%	99%
Prophylactic Antibiotic Selection (Outpatient)	61	97%	98%	98%
Prophylactic Antibiotic Stopped	326	97%	98%	98%
Prophylactic Antibiotic Timing	330	98%	99%	99%
Prophylactic Antibiotic Timing (Outpatient)	61	100%	99%	98%
Urinary Catheter Removal	236	100%	97%	97%
Survey of Patients' Hospital Experiences				
Area Around Room 'Always' Quiet at Night	300+	59%	57%	61%
Doctors 'Always' Communicated Well	300+	74%	77%	82%
Home Recovery Information Given	300+	83%	86%	85%
Hospital Given 9 or 10 on 10 Point Scale	300+	67%	70%	71%
Meds 'Always' Explained Before Given	300+	64%	62%	64%
Nurses 'Always' Communicated Well	300+	76%	76%	79%
Pain 'Always' Well Controlled	300+	69%	69%	71%
Room and Bathroom 'Always' Clean	300+	69%	69%	73%
Timely Help 'Always' Received	300+	66%	65%	68%
Would Definitely Recommend Hospital	300+	70%	70%	71%
Use of Medical Imaging				
Cardiac Imaging Stress Test before Surgery[1]	-	-	5.8%	5.3%
Combination Abdominal CT Scan	880	17.7%	9.1%	10.5%
Combination Brain/Sinus CT Scan	776	3.7%	3.2%	2.7%
Combination Chest CT Scan	411	22.1%	5.5%	2.7%
Follow-up Mammogram/Ultrasound	995	5.5%	8.5%	8.8%
Lumbar Spine MRI for Low Back Pain[1]	-	-	37.4%	37.2%

Casa Grande Regional Medical Center

1800 East Florence Boulevard
Casa Grande, AZ 85222
Phone: 520-381-6453
Fax: 520-381-6435
URL: www.casagrandehospital.com
Type: Acute Care Hospitals
Emergency Services: Yes
Ownership: Voluntary non-profit - Other
Beds: 201

Key Personnel:
Operating Room. . . . . Joyce Bonenberger
CEO . . . . Rona Curphy
Quality Assurance . . . . Dolly Dempsey
Chief of Medical Staff . . . . Gilda Eakin
Infection Control. . . . . Mary Kay Johnson
Pediatric Ambulatory Care . . . . . . Robert Kull, MD
Pediatric In-Patient Care . . . . Robert Kull, MD
Radiology. . . . . Brian Zernich, MD

Measure	Cases	This Hosp.	State Avg.	U.S. Avg.
Blood Clot Prevention and Treatment				
Anticoagulation Overlap Therapy[2]	57	98%	94%	93%
ICU Venous Thromboembolism Prophylaxis[2]	98	100%	92%	92%
Incidence of Potentially Preventable VTE[1,2]	-	-	9%	10%
UFH with Dosages/Platelet Monitoring[2]	28	100%	98%	97%
Venous Thromboembolism Prophylaxis[2]	345	95%	88%	85%
Warfarin Therapy Discharge Instructions[2]	47	96%	74%	75%
Chest Pain/Possible Heart Attack Care				
Aspirin Given Within 24 Hours of Arrival[1,3]	-	-	98%	96%
Fibrinolytic Meds Within 30 Min. of Arrival[3,7]	-	-	59%	58%
Average Time to ECG (minutes)[1,3]	-	-	6	7
Average Time to Transfer (minutes)[3,7]	-	-	48	60
Children's Asthma Care				
Received Home Management Plan of Care	-	-	-	88%
Received Reliever Medication	-	-	-	100%
Received Systemic Corticosteroids	-	-	-	100%
Emergency Department				
Admittance Decision Time (minutes)[2]	616	88	98	98
Head CT Results Within 45 Min. of Arrival[1]	-	-	64%	57%
Patients Who Left ER Before Being Seen	36,816	2%	2%	2%
Time from ER Arrival to Admit. (minutes)[2]	633	246	285	274
Time from ER Arrival to Discharge (minutes)	365	147	162	134
Time in ER Before Being Evaluated (minutes)	410	16	27	26
Time to Pain Meds for Fractures (minutes)	117	68	58	57
Heart Attack Care				
Aspirin Given at Discharge	85	100%	99%	99%
Fibrinolytic Meds Within 30 Min. of Arrival[7]	-	-	67%	54%
PCI Within 90 Minutes of Arrival	31	90%	95%	96%
Statin Prescribed at Discharge	81	94%	98%	98%
Heart Failure Care				
ACE Inhibitor or ARB for LVSD	49	96%	98%	97%
Discharge Instructions Given	110	100%	94%	94%
Evaluation of LVS Function	119	96%	99%	99%
Medicare Spending				
Medicare Spending per Patient (ratio)	-	0.94	0.93	0.98
Pneumonia Care				
Appropriate Initial Antibiotic Given	180	95%	96%	95%
Blood Culture Timing	221	96%	97%	98%
Pregnancy and Delivery Care				
Newborn Deliveries Scheduled Early	84	14%	7%	6%
Preventive Care				
Immunization for Influenza[2]	560	85%	91%	90%
Immunization for Pneumonia[2]	730	85%	92%	92%
Stroke Care				
Anticoagulation Therapy for Atrial Fibrillation[1]	-	-	96%	95%
Antithrombotic Therapy Timing	35	94%	98%	98%
Assessed for Rehabilitation	41	83%	96%	97%

NOTE: Hospital profiles are in alphabetical order by state, then city, then hospital within the city; Rankings exclude hospitals with less than 25 cases except for patient surveys which excludes hospitals with less than 100 cases; (a) 100-299 cases; (1) The number of cases/patients is too few to report; (2) Data submitted were based on a sample of cases/patients; (3) Results are based on a shorter time period than required; (4) Data suppressed by CMS for one or more quarters; (5) Results are not available for this reporting period; (6) Fewer than 100 patients completed the HCAHPS survey; (7) No cases met the criteria for this measure; (8) The lower limit of the confidence interval cannot be calculated if the number of observed infections equals zero; (9) No data are available from the state/territory for this reporting period; (10) The scores shown reflect fewer than 50 completed surveys; (11) There were discrepancies in the data collection process; (12) This measure does not apply to this hospital for this reporting period; (13) Results cannot be calculated for this reporting period; (14) The results for this state are combined with nearby states to protect confidentiality; Please refer to the User's Guide for a full explanation of data.

Measure	Cases	This Hosp.	State Avg.	U.S. Avg.
Discharged on Antithrombotic Therapy	38	89%	99%	99%
Discharged on Statin Medication	33	73%	94%	94%
Thrombolytic Therapy Timing[1]	-	-	81%	66%
Venous Thromboembolism Prophylaxis	40	90%	93%	94%
Written Stroke Educational Materials Given	31	68%	84%	88%
Surgical Care Improvement Project				
Appropriate Beta Blocker Usage	140	84%	97%	98%
Appropriate VTP Within 24 Hours	461	94%	98%	98%
Controlled Postoperative Blood Glucose[7]	-	-	96%	97%
Perioperative Temperature Management	519	99%	100%	100%
Prophylactic Antibiotic Selection	353	99%	99%	99%
Prophylactic Antibiotic Selection (Outpatient)	29	93%	98%	98%
Prophylactic Antibiotic Stopped	333	95%	98%	98%
Prophylactic Antibiotic Timing	353	99%	99%	99%
Prophylactic Antibiotic Timing (Outpatient)	29	97%	99%	98%
Urinary Catheter Removal	196	89%	97%	97%
Survey of Patients' Hospital Experiences				
Area Around Room 'Always' Quiet at Night	300+	52%	57%	61%
Doctors 'Always' Communicated Well	300+	76%	77%	82%
Home Recovery Information Given	300+	85%	86%	85%
Hospital Given 9 or 10 on 10 Point Scale	300+	61%	70%	71%
Meds 'Always' Explained Before Given	300+	59%	62%	64%
Nurses 'Always' Communicated Well	300+	73%	76%	79%
Pain 'Always' Well Controlled	300+	69%	69%	71%
Room and Bathroom 'Always' Clean	300+	60%	69%	73%
Timely Help 'Always' Received	300+	55%	65%	68%
Would Definitely Recommend Hospital	300+	59%	70%	71%
Use of Medical Imaging				
Cardiac Imaging Stress Test before Surgery	114	5.3%	5.8%	5.3%
Combination Abdominal CT Scan	715	31.7%	9.1%	10.5%
Combination Brain/Sinus CT Scan[1]	-	-	3.2%	2.7%
Combination Chest CT Scan	427	21.1%	5.5%	2.7%
Follow-up Mammogram/Ultrasound	1,085	7.6%	8.5%	8.8%
Lumbar Spine MRI for Low Back Pain	54	37.0%	37.4%	37.2%

Arizona Orthopedic & Surgical Speciality Hospital

2905 West Warner Road
Chandler, AZ 85224
Phone: 480-603-9000
URL: www.azosh.com
Type: Acute Care Hospitals
Emergency Services: No
Ownership: Proprietary

Measure	Cases	This Hosp.	State Avg.	U.S. Avg.
Blood Clot Prevention and Treatment				
Anticoagulation Overlap Therapy[2,7]	-	-	94%	93%
ICU Venous Thromboembolism Prophylaxis[2,7]	-	-	92%	92%
Incidence of Potentially Preventable VTE[2,7]	-	-	9%	10%
UFH with Dosages/Platelet Monitoring[2,7]	-	-	98%	97%
Venous Thromboembolism Prophylaxis[2]	13	100%	88%	85%
Warfarin Therapy Discharge Instructions[2,7]	-	-	74%	75%
Chest Pain/Possible Heart Attack Care				
Aspirin Given Within 24 Hours of Arrival[5]	-	-	98%	96%
Fibrinolytic Meds Within 30 Min. of Arrival[5]	-	-	59%	58%
Average Time to ECG (minutes)[5]	-	-	6	7
Average Time to Transfer (minutes)[5]	-	-	48	60
Children's Asthma Care				
Received Home Management Plan of Care	-	-	-	88%
Received Reliever Medication	-	-	-	100%
Received Systemic Corticosteroids	-	-	-	100%
Emergency Department				
Admittance Decision Time (minutes)[2,7]	-	-	98	98
Head CT Results Within 45 Min. of Arrival[5]	-	-	64%	57%
Patients Who Left ER Before Being Seen[5]	-	-	2%	2%
Time from ER Arrival to Admit. (minutes)[2,7]	-	-	285	274
Time from ER Arrival to Discharge (minutes)[5]	-	-	162	134
Time in ER Before Being Evaluated (minutes)[5]	-	-	27	26
Time to Pain Meds for Fractures (minutes)[5]	-	-	58	57
Heart Attack Care				
Aspirin Given at Discharge[5]	-	-	99%	99%
Fibrinolytic Meds Within 30 Min. of Arrival[5]	-	-	67%	54%
PCI Within 90 Minutes of Arrival[5]	-	-	95%	96%
Statin Prescribed at Discharge[5]	-	-	98%	98%
Heart Failure Care				
ACE Inhibitor or ARB for LVSD[5]	-	-	98%	97%
Discharge Instructions Given[5]	-	-	94%	94%
Evaluation of LVS Function[5]	-	-	99%	99%
Medicare Spending				
Medicare Spending per Patient (ratio)	-	1.04	0.93	0.98
Pneumonia Care				
Appropriate Initial Antibiotic Given[5]	-	-	96%	95%
Blood Culture Timing[5]	-	-	97%	98%
Pregnancy and Delivery Care				
Newborn Deliveries Scheduled Early[7]	-	-	7%	6%
Preventive Care				
Immunization for Influenza[2]	318	100%	91%	90%
Immunization for Pneumonia[2]	391	93%	92%	92%
Stroke Care				
Anticoagulation Therapy for Atrial Fibrillation[5]	-	-	96%	95%
Antithrombotic Therapy Timing[5]	-	-	98%	98%
Assessed for Rehabilitation[5]	-	-	96%	97%
Discharged on Antithrombotic Therapy[5]	-	-	99%	99%
Discharged on Statin Medication[5]	-	-	94%	94%
Thrombolytic Therapy Timing[5]	-	-	81%	66%
Venous Thromboembolism Prophylaxis[5]	-	-	93%	94%
Written Stroke Educational Materials Given[5]	-	-	84%	88%
Surgical Care Improvement Project				
Appropriate Beta Blocker Usage[2]	54	100%	97%	98%
Appropriate VTP Within 24 Hours[2]	249	100%	98%	98%
Controlled Postoperative Blood Glucose[2,7]	-	-	96%	97%
Perioperative Temperature Management[2]	248	100%	100%	100%
Prophylactic Antibiotic Selection[2]	206	100%	99%	99%
Prophylactic Antibiotic Selection (Outpatient)	39	100%	98%	98%
Prophylactic Antibiotic Stopped[2]	206	100%	98%	98%
Prophylactic Antibiotic Timing[2]	206	100%	99%	99%
Prophylactic Antibiotic Timing (Outpatient)	39	100%	99%	98%
Urinary Catheter Removal[2]	211	100%	97%	97%
Survey of Patients' Hospital Experiences				
Area Around Room 'Always' Quiet at Night	300+	76%	57%	61%
Doctors 'Always' Communicated Well	300+	86%	77%	82%
Home Recovery Information Given	300+	92%	86%	85%
Hospital Given 9 or 10 on 10 Point Scale	300+	81%	70%	71%
Meds 'Always' Explained Before Given	300+	69%	62%	64%
Nurses 'Always' Communicated Well	300+	86%	76%	79%
Pain 'Always' Well Controlled	300+	74%	69%	71%
Room and Bathroom 'Always' Clean	300+	82%	69%	73%
Timely Help 'Always' Received	300+	82%	65%	68%
Would Definitely Recommend Hospital	300+	85%	70%	71%
Use of Medical Imaging				
Cardiac Imaging Stress Test before Surgery[7]	-	-	5.8%	5.3%
Combination Abdominal CT Scan[7]	-	-	9.1%	10.5%
Combination Brain/Sinus CT Scan[7]	-	-	3.2%	2.7%
Combination Chest CT Scan[7]	-	-	5.5%	2.7%
Follow-up Mammogram/Ultrasound[7]	-	-	8.5%	8.8%
Lumbar Spine MRI for Low Back Pain[1]	-	-	37.4%	37.2%

Chandler Regional Medical Center

1955 West Frye Road
Chandler, AZ 85224
Phone: 480-963-4561
Fax: 480-899-5548
URL: www.chandlerregional.com
Type: Acute Care Hospitals
Emergency Services: Yes
Ownership: Voluntary non-profit - Other
Beds: 210

Key Personnel:
President/CEO. . . . . Tim Bricker
Pediatric Ambulatory Care . . . . . . Stanley A Gering, MD
Pediatric In-Patient Care . . . . Stanley A Gering, MD
Chief of Medical Staff. . . . . Terry Happel, M.D., F.A.C.S.
Radiology. . . . . Martin H Lehman, MD
Operating Room. . . . . Jayne Mitton, RN
Quality Assurance . . . . Pat Ware, RN
Coronary Care. . . . . Nancy Wood, RN

Measure	Cases	This Hosp.	State Avg.	U.S. Avg.
Blood Clot Prevention and Treatment				
Anticoagulation Overlap Therapy[2]	189	99%	94%	93%
ICU Venous Thromboembolism Prophylaxis[2]	64	100%	92%	92%
Incidence of Potentially Preventable VTE[2]	21	0%	9%	10%
UFH with Dosages/Platelet Monitoring[2]	159	100%	98%	97%
Venous Thromboembolism Prophylaxis[2]	355	95%	88%	85%
Warfarin Therapy Discharge Instructions[2]	132	99%	74%	75%
Chest Pain/Possible Heart Attack Care				
Aspirin Given Within 24 Hours of Arrival	21	86%	98%	96%
Fibrinolytic Meds Within 30 Min. of Arrival[5]	-	-	59%	58%
Average Time to ECG (minutes)	21	11	6	7
Average Time to Transfer (minutes)[5]	-	-	48	60
Children's Asthma Care				
Received Home Management Plan of Care	-	-	-	88%
Received Reliever Medication	-	-	-	100%
Received Systemic Corticosteroids	-	-	-	100%
Emergency Department				
Admittance Decision Time (minutes)[2]	549	112	98	98
Head CT Results Within 45 Min. of Arrival	14	50%	64%	57%
Patients Who Left ER Before Being Seen	63,401	0%	2%	2%
Time from ER Arrival to Admit. (minutes)[2]	552	290	285	274
Time from ER Arrival to Discharge (minutes)	376	144	162	134
Time in ER Before Being Evaluated (minutes)	408	15	27	26
Time to Pain Meds for Fractures (minutes)	268	56	58	57
Heart Attack Care				
Aspirin Given at Discharge[2]	332	99%	99%	99%
Fibrinolytic Meds Within 30 Min. of Arrival[2,7]	-	-	67%	54%
PCI Within 90 Minutes of Arrival[2]	55	96%	95%	96%
Statin Prescribed at Discharge[2]	327	98%	98%	98%
Heart Failure Care				
ACE Inhibitor or ARB for LVSD[2]	97	98%	98%	97%
Discharge Instructions Given[2]	267	99%	94%	94%
Evaluation of LVS Function[2]	298	100%	99%	99%
Medicare Spending				
Medicare Spending per Patient (ratio)	-	0.95	0.93	0.98
Pneumonia Care				
Appropriate Initial Antibiotic Given[2]	121	99%	96%	95%
Blood Culture Timing[2]	211	100%	97%	98%
Pregnancy and Delivery Care				
Newborn Deliveries Scheduled Early[2]	53	0%	7%	6%
Preventive Care				
Immunization for Influenza[2]	553	98%	91%	90%
Immunization for Pneumonia[2]	614	96%	92%	92%
Stroke Care				
Anticoagulation Therapy for Atrial Fibrillation	26	100%	96%	95%
Antithrombotic Therapy Timing	144	100%	98%	98%
Assessed for Rehabilitation	193	100%	96%	97%
Discharged on Antithrombotic Therapy	172	99%	99%	99%
Discharged on Statin Medication	131	95%	94%	94%
Thrombolytic Therapy Timing	19	84%	81%	66%
Venous Thromboembolism Prophylaxis	181	98%	93%	94%
Written Stroke Educational Materials Given	124	100%	84%	88%
Surgical Care Improvement Project				
Appropriate Beta Blocker Usage[2]	248	98%	97%	98%
Appropriate VTP Within 24 Hours[2]	460	98%	98%	98%
Controlled Postoperative Blood Glucose[2]	161	89%	96%	97%
Perioperative Temperature Management[2]	554	100%	100%	100%
Prophylactic Antibiotic Selection[2]	479	99%	99%	99%
Prophylactic Antibiotic Selection (Outpatient)	496	98%	98%	98%
Prophylactic Antibiotic Stopped[2]	458	99%	98%	98%
Prophylactic Antibiotic Timing[2]	479	100%	99%	99%
Prophylactic Antibiotic Timing (Outpatient)	497	99%	99%	98%
Urinary Catheter Removal[2]	342	97%	97%	97%
Survey of Patients' Hospital Experiences				
Area Around Room 'Always' Quiet at Night	300+	58%	57%	61%
Doctors 'Always' Communicated Well	300+	74%	77%	82%
Home Recovery Information Given	300+	87%	86%	85%
Hospital Given 9 or 10 on 10 Point Scale	300+	69%	70%	71%
Meds 'Always' Explained Before Given	300+	59%	62%	64%
Nurses 'Always' Communicated Well	300+	76%	76%	79%
Pain 'Always' Well Controlled	300+	70%	69%	71%
Room and Bathroom 'Always' Clean	300+	68%	69%	73%
Timely Help 'Always' Received	300+	64%	65%	68%
Would Definitely Recommend Hospital	300+	71%	70%	71%
Use of Medical Imaging				
Cardiac Imaging Stress Test before Surgery	135	6.7%	5.8%	5.3%
Combination Abdominal CT Scan	920	1.6%	9.1%	10.5%
Combination Brain/Sinus CT Scan	1,214	2.6%	3.2%	2.7%

NOTE: Hospital profiles are in alphabetical order by state, then city, then hospital within the city; Rankings exclude hospitals with less than 25 cases except for patient surveys which excludes hospitals with less than 100 cases; (a) 100-299 cases; (1) The number of cases/patients is too few to report; (2) Data submitted were based on a sample of cases/patients; (3) Results are based on a shorter time period than required; (4) Data suppressed by CMS for one or more quarters; (5) Results are not available for this reporting period; (6) Fewer than 100 patients completed the HCAHPS survey; (7) No cases met the criteria for this measure; (8) The lower limit of the confidence interval cannot be calculated if the number of observed infections equals zero; (9) No data are available from the state/territory for this reporting period; (10) The scores shown reflect fewer than 50 completed surveys; (11) There were discrepancies in the data collection process; (12) This measure does not apply to this hospital for this reporting period; (13) Results cannot be calculated for this reporting period; (14) The results for this state are combined with nearby states to protect confidentiality; Please refer to the User's Guide for a full explanation of data.

Measure	Cases	This Hosp.	State Avg.	U.S. Avg.
Combination Chest CT Scan	666	0.2%	5.5%	2.7%
Follow-up Mammogram/Ultrasound	450	19.8%	8.5%	8.8%
Lumbar Spine MRI for Low Back Pain[1]	-	-	37.4%	37.2%

Chinle Comprehensive Health Care Facility

Us Hwy 191, Hospital Road
Chinle, AZ 86503
Phone: 928-674-7001
Fax: 928-674-7372
Type: Acute Care Hospitals
Emergency Services: No
Ownership: Government - Federal
Beds: 60

Key Personnel:
Emergency Room .... Deborah Levitt, MD
Pediatric Ambulatory Care ...... Andrew Reichert
Quality Assurance .... Marla Stewart
Chief of Medical Staff.......... Christian Thompson
CEO/President............... Ronald Tso
Operating Room.............. Laura Wartman, RN

Measure	Cases	This Hosp.	State Avg.	U.S. Avg.
Blood Clot Prevention and Treatment				
Anticoagulation Overlap Therapy[1,2]	-	-	94%	93%
ICU Venous Thromboembolism Prophylaxis[2]	53	92%	92%	92%
Incidence of Potentially Preventable VTE[2,7]	-	-	9%	10%
UFH with Dosages/Platelet Monitoring[1,2]	-	-	98%	97%
Venous Thromboembolism Prophylaxis[2]	202	89%	88%	85%
Warfarin Therapy Discharge Instructions[1,2]	-	-	74%	75%
Chest Pain/Possible Heart Attack Care				
Aspirin Given Within 24 Hours of Arrival	-	-	98%	96%
Fibrinolytic Meds Within 30 Min. of Arrival	-	-	59%	58%
Average Time to ECG (minutes)	-	-	6	7
Average Time to Transfer (minutes)	-	-	48	60
Children's Asthma Care				
Received Home Management Plan of Care	-	-	-	88%
Received Reliever Medication	-	-	-	100%
Received Systemic Corticosteroids	-	-	-	100%
Emergency Department				
Admittance Decision Time (minutes)[2]	474	60	98	98
Head CT Results Within 45 Min. of Arrival	-	-	64%	57%
Patients Who Left ER Before Being Seen	-	-	2%	2%
Time from ER Arrival to Admit. (minutes)[2]	491	286	285	274
Time from ER Arrival to Discharge (minutes)	-	-	162	134
Time in ER Before Being Evaluated (minutes)	-	-	27	26
Time to Pain Meds for Fractures (minutes)	-	-	58	57
Heart Attack Care				
Aspirin Given at Discharge[1,2]	-	-	99%	99%
Fibrinolytic Meds Within 30 Min. of Arrival[1,2]	-	-	67%	54%
PCI Within 90 Minutes of Arrival[2,3]	-	-	95%	96%
Statin Prescribed at Discharge[1,2]	-	-	98%	98%
Heart Failure Care				
ACE Inhibitor or ARB for LVSD[2]	13	92%	98%	97%
Discharge Instructions Given[2]	25	44%	94%	94%
Evaluation of LVS Function[2]	27	100%	99%	99%
Medicare Spending				
Medicare Spending per Patient (ratio)	-	0.64	0.93	0.98
Pneumonia Care				
Appropriate Initial Antibiotic Given[2]	47	51%	96%	95%
Blood Culture Timing[2]	69	84%	97%	98%
Pregnancy and Delivery Care				
Newborn Deliveries Scheduled Early[2]	77	18%	7%	6%
Preventive Care				
Immunization for Influenza[2]	293	72%	91%	90%
Immunization for Pneumonia[2]	427	87%	92%	92%
Stroke Care				
Anticoagulation Therapy for Atrial Fibrillation[1,2]	-	-	96%	95%
Antithrombotic Therapy Timing[2,3]	-	-	98%	98%
Assessed for Rehabilitation[1,2]	-	-	96%	97%
Discharged on Antithrombotic Therapy[1,2]	-	-	99%	99%
Discharged on Statin Medication[1,2]	-	-	94%	94%
Thrombolytic Therapy Timing[2,3]	-	-	81%	66%
Venous Thromboembolism Prophylaxis[2,3]	-	-	93%	94%
Written Stroke Educational Materials Given[1,2]	-	-	84%	88%
Surgical Care Improvement Project				
Appropriate Beta Blocker Usage[1,2]	-	-	97%	98%
Appropriate VTP Within 24 Hours[1,2]	-	-	98%	98%
Controlled Postoperative Blood Glucose[2,7]	-	-	96%	97%
Perioperative Temperature Management[2]	12	100%	100%	100%
Prophylactic Antibiotic Selection[2,7]	-	-	99%	99%
Prophylactic Antibiotic Selection (Outpatient)	-	-	98%	98%
Prophylactic Antibiotic Stopped[2,7]	-	-	98%	98%
Prophylactic Antibiotic Timing[2,7]	-	-	99%	99%
Prophylactic Antibiotic Timing (Outpatient)	-	-	99%	98%
Urinary Catheter Removal[1,2]	-	-	97%	97%
Survey of Patients' Hospital Experiences				
Area Around Room 'Always' Quiet at Night	(a)	51%	57%	61%
Doctors 'Always' Communicated Well	(a)	66%	77%	82%
Home Recovery Information Given	(a)	77%	86%	85%
Hospital Given 9 or 10 on 10 Point Scale	(a)	43%	70%	71%
Meds 'Always' Explained Before Given	(a)	61%	62%	64%
Nurses 'Always' Communicated Well	(a)	62%	76%	79%
Pain 'Always' Well Controlled	(a)	58%	69%	71%
Room and Bathroom 'Always' Clean	(a)	57%	69%	73%
Timely Help 'Always' Received	(a)	57%	65%	68%
Would Definitely Recommend Hospital	(a)	35%	70%	71%
Use of Medical Imaging				
Cardiac Imaging Stress Test before Surgery	-	-	5.8%	5.3%
Combination Abdominal CT Scan	-	-	9.1%	10.5%
Combination Brain/Sinus CT Scan	-	-	3.2%	2.7%
Combination Chest CT Scan	-	-	5.5%	2.7%
Follow-up Mammogram/Ultrasound	-	-	8.5%	8.8%
Lumbar Spine MRI for Low Back Pain	-	-	37.4%	37.2%

Verde Valley Medical Center

269 South Candy Lane
Cottonwood, AZ 86326
Phone: 928-639-6000
Fax: 928-639-6070
URL: www.nahealth.com/pp_vvmc/vvmc_about.htm
Type: Acute Care Hospitals
Emergency Services: Yes
Ownership: Voluntary non-profit - Private
Beds: 110

Key Personnel:
President/CEO............... Barbara Dember, M.H.A., F.A.C.H
Operating Room............. Blair Faulkner
Radiology................... Robert W Koepke
Quality Assurance .... Marion Polley

Measure	Cases	This Hosp.	State Avg.	U.S. Avg.
Blood Clot Prevention and Treatment				
Anticoagulation Overlap Therapy[2]	62	98%	94%	93%
ICU Venous Thromboembolism Prophylaxis[2]	109	96%	92%	92%
Incidence of Potentially Preventable VTE[1,2]	-	-	9%	10%
UFH with Dosages/Platelet Monitoring[2]	15	100%	98%	97%
Venous Thromboembolism Prophylaxis[2]	324	98%	88%	85%
Warfarin Therapy Discharge Instructions[2]	47	94%	74%	75%
Chest Pain/Possible Heart Attack Care				
Aspirin Given Within 24 Hours of Arrival[1]	-	-	98%	96%
Fibrinolytic Meds Within 30 Min. of Arrival[3,7]	-	-	59%	58%
Average Time to ECG (minutes)[1]	-	-	6	7
Average Time to Transfer (minutes)[3,7]	-	-	48	60
Children's Asthma Care				
Received Home Management Plan of Care	-	-	-	88%
Received Reliever Medication	-	-	-	100%
Received Systemic Corticosteroids	-	-	-	100%
Emergency Department				
Admittance Decision Time (minutes)[2]	430	136	98	98
Head CT Results Within 45 Min. of Arrival	21	38%	64%	57%
Patients Who Left ER Before Being Seen	30,330	1%	2%	2%
Time from ER Arrival to Admit. (minutes)[2]	583	324	285	274
Time from ER Arrival to Discharge (minutes)	373	135	162	134
Time in ER Before Being Evaluated (minutes)	332	29	27	26
Time to Pain Meds for Fractures (minutes)	155	59	58	57
Heart Attack Care				
Aspirin Given at Discharge	81	99%	99%	99%
Fibrinolytic Meds Within 30 Min. of Arrival[7]	-	-	67%	54%
PCI Within 90 Minutes of Arrival	28	93%	95%	96%
Statin Prescribed at Discharge	77	97%	98%	98%
Heart Failure Care				
ACE Inhibitor or ARB for LVSD	23	87%	98%	97%
Discharge Instructions Given	77	99%	94%	94%
Evaluation of LVS Function	86	99%	99%	99%
Medicare Spending				
Medicare Spending per Patient (ratio)	-	0.97	0.93	0.98
Pneumonia Care				
Appropriate Initial Antibiotic Given	101	93%	96%	95%
Blood Culture Timing	149	97%	97%	98%
Pregnancy and Delivery Care				
Newborn Deliveries Scheduled Early[2]	43	2%	7%	6%
Preventive Care				
Immunization for Influenza[2]	433	98%	91%	90%
Immunization for Pneumonia[2]	552	99%	92%	92%
Stroke Care				
Anticoagulation Therapy for Atrial Fibrillation[1]	-	-	96%	95%
Antithrombotic Therapy Timing	48	98%	98%	98%
Assessed for Rehabilitation	48	98%	96%	97%
Discharged on Antithrombotic Therapy	46	100%	99%	99%
Discharged on Statin Medication	37	100%	94%	94%
Thrombolytic Therapy Timing[1]	-	-	81%	66%
Venous Thromboembolism Prophylaxis	51	98%	93%	94%
Written Stroke Educational Materials Given	21	62%	84%	88%
Surgical Care Improvement Project				
Appropriate Beta Blocker Usage[2]	113	96%	97%	98%
Appropriate VTP Within 24 Hours[2]	409	98%	98%	98%
Controlled Postoperative Blood Glucose[2,7]	-	-	96%	97%
Perioperative Temperature Management[2]	470	100%	100%	100%
Prophylactic Antibiotic Selection[2]	326	99%	99%	99%
Prophylactic Antibiotic Selection (Outpatient)	98	98%	98%	98%
Prophylactic Antibiotic Stopped[2]	316	97%	98%	98%
Prophylactic Antibiotic Timing[2]	327	100%	99%	99%
Prophylactic Antibiotic Timing (Outpatient)	103	94%	99%	98%
Urinary Catheter Removal[2]	243	99%	97%	97%
Survey of Patients' Hospital Experiences				
Area Around Room 'Always' Quiet at Night	300+	54%	57%	61%
Doctors 'Always' Communicated Well	300+	80%	77%	82%
Home Recovery Information Given	300+	90%	86%	85%
Hospital Given 9 or 10 on 10 Point Scale	300+	78%	70%	71%
Meds 'Always' Explained Before Given	300+	60%	62%	64%
Nurses 'Always' Communicated Well	300+	81%	76%	79%
Pain 'Always' Well Controlled	300+	73%	69%	71%
Room and Bathroom 'Always' Clean	300+	76%	69%	73%
Timely Help 'Always' Received	300+	70%	65%	68%
Would Definitely Recommend Hospital	300+	75%	70%	71%
Use of Medical Imaging				
Cardiac Imaging Stress Test before Surgery	374	4.3%	5.8%	5.3%
Combination Abdominal CT Scan	939	4.8%	9.1%	10.5%
Combination Brain/Sinus CT Scan	780	2.3%	3.2%	2.7%
Combination Chest CT Scan	451	0.2%	5.5%	2.7%
Follow-up Mammogram/Ultrasound	2,156	3.8%	8.5%	8.8%
Lumbar Spine MRI for Low Back Pain	220	32.7%	37.4%	37.2%

Douglas Community Hospital

2174 West Oak Avenue
Douglas, AZ 85607
Phone: 520-364-7931
Fax: 520-364-2551
URL: www.samcdouglas.org
Type: Critical Access Hospitals
Emergency Services: No
Ownership: Voluntary non-profit - Private
Beds: 25

Key Personnel:
Quality Assurance .... Ann Benson
CEO/President............... Brian Bickel
Operating Room.............. Dr Alberto Dominguez
Infection Control............. Beth Spalsbury
Chief of Medical Staff.......... Christopher Spooner, MD
Emergency Room .... Edward Young

Measure	Cases	This Hosp.	State Avg.	U.S. Avg.
Blood Clot Prevention and Treatment				
Anticoagulation Overlap Therapy[5]	-	-	94%	93%
ICU Venous Thromboembolism Prophylaxis[5]	-	-	92%	92%
Incidence of Potentially Preventable VTE[5]	-	-	9%	10%
UFH with Dosages/Platelet Monitoring[5]	-	-	98%	97%
Venous Thromboembolism Prophylaxis[5]	-	-	88%	85%
Warfarin Therapy Discharge Instructions[5]	-	-	74%	75%
Chest Pain/Possible Heart Attack Care				
Aspirin Given Within 24 Hours of Arrival	-	-	98%	96%
Fibrinolytic Meds Within 30 Min. of Arrival	-	-	59%	58%
Average Time to ECG (minutes)	-	-	6	7
Average Time to Transfer (minutes)	-	-	48	60
Children's Asthma Care				
Received Home Management Plan of Care	-	-	-	88%

NOTE: Hospital profiles are in alphabetical order by state, then city, then hospital within the city; Rankings exclude hospitals with less than 25 cases except for patient surveys which excludes hospitals with less than 100 cases; (a) 100-299 cases; (1) The number of cases/patients is too few to report; (2) Data submitted were based on a sample of cases/patients; (3) Results are based on a shorter time period than required; (4) Data suppressed by CMS for one or more quarters; (5) Results are not available for this reporting period; (6) Fewer than 100 patients completed the HCAHPS survey; (7) No cases met the criteria for this measure; (8) The lower limit of the confidence interval cannot be calculated if the number of observed infections equals zero; (9) No data are available from the state/territory for this reporting period; (10) The scores shown reflect fewer than 50 completed surveys; (11) There were discrepancies in the data collection process; (12) This measure does not apply to this hospital for this reporting period; (13) Results cannot be calculated for this reporting period; (14) The results for this state are combined with nearby states to protect confidentiality; Please refer to the User's Guide for a full explanation of data.

Measure	Cases	This Hosp.	State Avg.	U.S. Avg.
Received Reliever Medication	-	-	-	100%
Received Systemic Corticosteroids	-	-	-	100%
Emergency Department				
Admittance Decision Time (minutes)[5]	-	-	98	98
Head CT Results Within 45 Min. of Arrival	-	-	64%	57%
Patients Who Left ER Before Being Seen	-	-	2%	2%
Time from ER Arrival to Admit. (minutes)[5]	-	-	285	274
Time from ER Arrival to Discharge (minutes)	-	-	162	134
Time in ER Before Being Evaluated (minutes)	-	-	27	26
Time to Pain Meds for Fractures (minutes)	-	-	58	57
Heart Attack Care				
Aspirin Given at Discharge[5]	-	-	99%	99%
Fibrinolytic Meds Within 30 Min. of Arrival[5]	-	-	67%	54%
PCI Within 90 Minutes of Arrival[5]	-	-	95%	96%
Statin Prescribed at Discharge[5]	-	-	98%	98%
Heart Failure Care				
ACE Inhibitor or ARB for LVSD[5]	-	-	98%	97%
Discharge Instructions Given[5]	-	-	94%	94%
Evaluation of LVS Function[5]	-	-	99%	99%
Medicare Spending				
Medicare Spending per Patient (ratio)	-	-	0.93	0.98
Pneumonia Care				
Appropriate Initial Antibiotic Given[3]	15	67%	96%	95%
Blood Culture Timing[3]	15	73%	97%	98%
Pregnancy and Delivery Care				
Newborn Deliveries Scheduled Early[5]	-	-	7%	6%
Preventive Care				
Immunization for Influenza[5]	-	-	91%	90%
Immunization for Pneumonia[5]	-	-	92%	92%
Stroke Care				
Anticoagulation Therapy for Atrial Fibrillation[5]	-	-	96%	95%
Antithrombotic Therapy Timing[5]	-	-	98%	98%
Assessed for Rehabilitation[5]	-	-	96%	97%
Discharged on Antithrombotic Therapy[5]	-	-	99%	99%
Discharged on Statin Medication[5]	-	-	94%	94%
Thrombolytic Therapy Timing[5]	-	-	81%	66%
Venous Thromboembolism Prophylaxis[5]	-	-	93%	94%
Written Stroke Educational Materials Given[5]	-	-	84%	88%
Surgical Care Improvement Project				
Appropriate Beta Blocker Usage[5]	-	-	97%	98%
Appropriate VTP Within 24 Hours[5]	-	-	98%	98%
Controlled Postoperative Blood Glucose[5]	-	-	96%	97%
Perioperative Temperature Management[5]	-	-	100%	100%
Prophylactic Antibiotic Selection[5]	-	-	99%	99%
Prophylactic Antibiotic Selection (Outpatient)	-	-	98%	98%
Prophylactic Antibiotic Stopped[5]	-	-	98%	98%
Prophylactic Antibiotic Timing[5]	-	-	99%	99%
Prophylactic Antibiotic Timing (Outpatient)	-	-	99%	98%
Urinary Catheter Removal[5]	-	-	97%	97%
Survey of Patients' Hospital Experiences				
Area Around Room 'Always' Quiet at Night[5]	-	-	57%	61%
Doctors 'Always' Communicated Well[5]	-	-	77%	82%
Home Recovery Information Given[5]	-	-	86%	85%
Hospital Given 9 or 10 on 10 Point Scale[5]	-	-	70%	71%
Meds 'Always' Explained Before Given[5]	-	-	62%	64%
Nurses 'Always' Communicated Well[5]	-	-	76%	79%
Pain 'Always' Well Controlled[5]	-	-	69%	71%
Room and Bathroom 'Always' Clean[5]	-	-	69%	73%
Timely Help 'Always' Received[5]	-	-	65%	68%
Would Definitely Recommend Hospital[5]	-	-	70%	71%
Use of Medical Imaging				
Cardiac Imaging Stress Test before Surgery	-	-	5.8%	5.3%
Combination Abdominal CT Scan	-	-	9.1%	10.5%
Combination Brain/Sinus CT Scan	-	-	3.2%	2.7%
Combination Chest CT Scan	-	-	5.5%	2.7%
Follow-up Mammogram/Ultrasound	-	-	8.5%	8.8%
Lumbar Spine MRI for Low Back Pain	-	-	37.4%	37.2%

Flagstaff Medical Center

1200 North Beaver Street — Phone: 928-773-2009
Flagstaff, AZ 86001 — Fax: 928-773-2579
URL: www.nahealth.com
Type: Acute Care Hospitals — Emergency Services: Yes
Ownership: Voluntary non-profit - Private — Beds: 238

Key Personnel:
Quality Assurance . . . . Debbie Candelaria
CEO/President. . . . . Stephen G Carlson
Emergency Room . . . . Sheila' O Connor
Chief of Medical Staff. . . . . Thomas Gaughan, MD

Measure	Cases	This Hosp.	State Avg.	U.S. Avg.
Blood Clot Prevention and Treatment				
Anticoagulation Overlap Therapy[2]	100	100%	94%	93%
ICU Venous Thromboembolism Prophylaxis[2]	152	99%	92%	92%
Incidence of Potentially Preventable VTE[1,2]	-	-	9%	10%
UFH with Dosages/Platelet Monitoring[2]	58	100%	98%	97%
Venous Thromboembolism Prophylaxis[2]	309	97%	88%	85%
Warfarin Therapy Discharge Instructions[2]	78	88%	74%	75%
Chest Pain/Possible Heart Attack Care				
Aspirin Given Within 24 Hours of Arrival[5]	-	-	98%	96%
Fibrinolytic Meds Within 30 Min. of Arrival[5]	-	-	59%	58%
Average Time to ECG (minutes)[5]	-	-	6	7
Average Time to Transfer (minutes)[5]	-	-	48	60
Children's Asthma Care				
Received Home Management Plan of Care	-	-	-	88%
Received Reliever Medication	-	-	-	100%
Received Systemic Corticosteroids	-	-	-	100%
Emergency Department				
Admittance Decision Time (minutes)[2]	457	138	98	98
Head CT Results Within 45 Min. of Arrival[1]	-	-	64%	57%
Patients Who Left ER Before Being Seen	39,373	3%	2%	2%
Time from ER Arrival to Admit. (minutes)[2]	469	295	285	274
Time from ER Arrival to Discharge (minutes)	378	164	162	134
Time in ER Before Being Evaluated (minutes)	410	40	27	26
Time to Pain Meds for Fractures (minutes)	127	46	58	57
Heart Attack Care				
Aspirin Given at Discharge	181	99%	99%	99%
Fibrinolytic Meds Within 30 Min. of Arrival[7]	-	-	67%	54%
PCI Within 90 Minutes of Arrival	31	81%	95%	96%
Statin Prescribed at Discharge	171	100%	98%	98%
Heart Failure Care				
ACE Inhibitor or ARB for LVSD	62	97%	98%	97%
Discharge Instructions Given	162	99%	94%	94%
Evaluation of LVS Function	178	100%	99%	99%
Medicare Spending				
Medicare Spending per Patient (ratio)	-	0.88	0.93	0.98
Pneumonia Care				
Appropriate Initial Antibiotic Given[2]	104	100%	96%	95%
Blood Culture Timing[2]	140	95%	97%	98%
Pregnancy and Delivery Care				
Newborn Deliveries Scheduled Early[2]	28	4%	7%	6%
Preventive Care				
Immunization for Influenza[2]	540	97%	91%	90%
Immunization for Pneumonia[2]	546	98%	92%	92%
Stroke Care				
Anticoagulation Therapy for Atrial Fibrillation[1]	-	-	96%	95%
Antithrombotic Therapy Timing	68	100%	98%	98%
Assessed for Rehabilitation	107	100%	96%	97%
Discharged on Antithrombotic Therapy	81	100%	99%	99%
Discharged on Statin Medication	55	96%	94%	94%
Thrombolytic Therapy Timing[1]	-	-	81%	66%
Venous Thromboembolism Prophylaxis	114	100%	93%	94%
Written Stroke Educational Materials Given	66	77%	84%	88%
Surgical Care Improvement Project				
Appropriate Beta Blocker Usage[2]	123	100%	97%	98%
Appropriate VTP Within 24 Hours[2]	402	98%	98%	98%
Controlled Postoperative Blood Glucose[2]	141	97%	96%	97%
Perioperative Temperature Management[2]	620	100%	100%	100%
Prophylactic Antibiotic Selection[2]	458	99%	99%	99%
Prophylactic Antibiotic Selection (Outpatient)	244	99%	98%	98%
Prophylactic Antibiotic Stopped[2]	444	99%	98%	98%
Prophylactic Antibiotic Timing[2]	459	99%	99%	99%
Prophylactic Antibiotic Timing (Outpatient)	245	99%	99%	98%
Urinary Catheter Removal[2]	396	99%	97%	97%
Survey of Patients' Hospital Experiences				
Area Around Room 'Always' Quiet at Night	300+	61%	57%	61%
Doctors 'Always' Communicated Well	300+	81%	77%	82%
Home Recovery Information Given	300+	86%	86%	85%
Hospital Given 9 or 10 on 10 Point Scale	300+	76%	70%	71%
Meds 'Always' Explained Before Given	300+	64%	62%	64%
Nurses 'Always' Communicated Well	300+	78%	76%	79%
Pain 'Always' Well Controlled	300+	70%	69%	71%
Room and Bathroom 'Always' Clean	300+	70%	69%	73%
Timely Help 'Always' Received	300+	70%	65%	68%
Would Definitely Recommend Hospital	300+	77%	70%	71%
Use of Medical Imaging				
Cardiac Imaging Stress Test before Surgery	145	4.8%	5.8%	5.3%
Combination Abdominal CT Scan	345	2.6%	9.1%	10.5%
Combination Brain/Sinus CT Scan[1]	-	-	3.2%	2.7%
Combination Chest CT Scan	209	10.5%	5.5%	2.7%
Follow-up Mammogram/Ultrasound[7]	-	-	8.5%	8.8%
Lumbar Spine MRI for Low Back Pain	97	32.0%	37.4%	37.2%

Florence Hospital at Anthem

4545 North Hunt Highway — Phone: 520-868-3333
Florence, AZ 85132
Type: Acute Care Hospitals — Emergency Services: Yes
Ownership: Proprietary

Measure	Cases	This Hosp.	State Avg.	U.S. Avg.
Blood Clot Prevention and Treatment				
Anticoagulation Overlap Therapy[1,2]	-	-	94%	93%
ICU Venous Thromboembolism Prophylaxis[2]	15	100%	92%	92%
Incidence of Potentially Preventable VTE[1,2]	-	-	9%	10%
UFH with Dosages/Platelet Monitoring[1,2]	-	-	98%	97%
Venous Thromboembolism Prophylaxis[2]	90	94%	88%	85%
Warfarin Therapy Discharge Instructions[1,2]	-	-	74%	75%
Chest Pain/Possible Heart Attack Care				
Aspirin Given Within 24 Hours of Arrival[3]	36	97%	98%	96%
Fibrinolytic Meds Within 30 Min. of Arrival[3,7]	-	-	59%	58%
Average Time to ECG (minutes)[3]	38	6	6	7
Average Time to Transfer (minutes)[3]	12	66	48	60
Children's Asthma Care				
Received Home Management Plan of Care	-	-	-	88%
Received Reliever Medication	-	-	-	100%
Received Systemic Corticosteroids	-	-	-	100%
Emergency Department				
Admittance Decision Time (minutes)[2,3]	438	66	98	98
Head CT Results Within 45 Min. of Arrival[3,7]	-	-	64%	57%
Patients Who Left ER Before Being Seen	12,018	0%	2%	2%
Time from ER Arrival to Admit. (minutes)[2,3]	438	243	285	274
Time from ER Arrival to Discharge (minutes)[3]	260	130	162	134
Time in ER Before Being Evaluated (minutes)[3]	287	13	27	26
Time to Pain Meds for Fractures (minutes)[3]	44	38	58	57
Heart Attack Care				
Aspirin Given at Discharge[5]	-	-	99%	99%
Fibrinolytic Meds Within 30 Min. of Arrival[5]	-	-	67%	54%
PCI Within 90 Minutes of Arrival[5]	-	-	95%	96%
Statin Prescribed at Discharge[5]	-	-	98%	98%
Heart Failure Care				
ACE Inhibitor or ARB for LVSD[1,3]	-	-	98%	97%
Discharge Instructions Given[3]	12	67%	94%	94%
Evaluation of LVS Function[3]	12	100%	99%	99%
Medicare Spending				
Medicare Spending per Patient (ratio)	-	0.96	0.93	0.98
Pneumonia Care				
Appropriate Initial Antibiotic Given[3]	25	92%	96%	95%
Blood Culture Timing[3]	22	86%	97%	98%
Pregnancy and Delivery Care				
Newborn Deliveries Scheduled Early[7]	-	-	7%	6%
Preventive Care				
Immunization for Influenza[2,3]	133	91%	91%	90%
Immunization for Pneumonia[2,3]	250	91%	92%	92%
Stroke Care				
Anticoagulation Therapy for Atrial Fibrillation[5]	-	-	96%	95%

NOTE: Hospital profiles are in alphabetical order by state, then city, then hospital within the city; Rankings exclude hospitals with less than 25 cases except for patient surveys which excludes hospitals with less than 100 cases; (a) 100-299 cases; (1) The number of cases/patients is too few to report; (2) Data submitted were based on a sample of cases/patients; (3) Results are based on a shorter time period than required; (4) Data suppressed by CMS for one or more quarters; (5) Results are not available for this reporting period; (6) Fewer than 100 patients completed the HCAHPS survey; (7) No cases met the criteria for this measure; (8) The lower limit of the confidence interval cannot be calculated if the number of observed infections equals zero; (9) No data are available from the state/territory for this reporting period; (10) The scores shown reflect fewer than 50 completed surveys; (11) There were discrepancies in the data collection process; (12) This measure does not apply to this hospital for this reporting period; (13) Results cannot be calculated for this reporting period; (14) The results for this state are combined with nearby states to protect confidentiality; Please refer to the User's Guide for a full explanation of data.

Measure	Cases	This Hosp.	State Avg.	U.S. Avg.
Antithrombotic Therapy Timing[5]	-	-	98%	98%
Assessed for Rehabilitation[5]	-	-	96%	97%
Discharged on Antithrombotic Therapy[5]	-	-	99%	99%
Discharged on Statin Medication[5]	-	-	94%	94%
Thrombolytic Therapy Timing[5]	-	-	81%	66%
Venous Thromboembolism Prophylaxis[5]	-	-	93%	94%
Written Stroke Educational Materials Given[5]	-	-	84%	88%
Surgical Care Improvement Project				
Appropriate Beta Blocker Usage[5]	-	-	97%	98%
Appropriate VTP Within 24 Hours[5]	-	-	98%	98%
Controlled Postoperative Blood Glucose[5]	-	-	96%	97%
Perioperative Temperature Management[5]	-	-	100%	100%
Prophylactic Antibiotic Selection[5]	-	-	99%	99%
Prophylactic Antibiotic Selection (Outpatient)[5]	-	-	98%	98%
Prophylactic Antibiotic Stopped[5]	-	-	98%	98%
Prophylactic Antibiotic Timing[5]	-	-	99%	99%
Prophylactic Antibiotic Timing (Outpatient)[5]	-	-	99%	98%
Urinary Catheter Removal[5]	-	-	97%	97%
Survey of Patients' Hospital Experiences				
Area Around Room 'Always' Quiet at Night[5]	-	-	57%	61%
Doctors 'Always' Communicated Well[5]	-	-	77%	82%
Home Recovery Information Given[5]	-	-	86%	85%
Hospital Given 9 or 10 on 10 Point Scale[5]	-	-	70%	71%
Meds 'Always' Explained Before Given[5]	-	-	62%	64%
Nurses 'Always' Communicated Well[5]	-	-	76%	79%
Pain 'Always' Well Controlled[5]	-	-	69%	71%
Room and Bathroom 'Always' Clean[5]	-	-	69%	73%
Timely Help 'Always' Received[5]	-	-	65%	68%
Would Definitely Recommend Hospital[5]	-	-	70%	71%
Use of Medical Imaging				
Cardiac Imaging Stress Test before Surgery[1]	-	-	5.8%	5.3%
Combination Abdominal CT Scan	119	4.2%	9.1%	10.5%
Combination Brain/Sinus CT Scan[1]	-	-	3.2%	2.7%
Combination Chest CT Scan[1]	-	-	5.5%	2.7%
Follow-up Mammogram/Ultrasound[7]	-	-	8.5%	8.8%
Lumbar Spine MRI for Low Back Pain[1]	-	-	37.4%	37.2%

Fort Defiance Indian Hospital

PO Box 649 Phone: 928-729-8000
Fort Defiance, AZ 86504 Fax: 928-871-7850
E-mail: cecelia.yazzie@fdih.his.gov
URL: www.home.navajo.his.gov
Type: Acute Care Hospitals Emergency Services: Yes
Ownership: Government - Federal Beds: 76

Key Personnel:
Cardiac Laboratory. . . . . David Downing
Pediatric Ambulatory Care . . . . . . Douglas Esposito, MD
Pediatric In-Patient Care . . . . . . Douglas Esposito, MD
CEO/President. . . . . Franklin R Freeland
Emergency Room . . . . Sherry Killingsworth, RN
Operating Room. . . . . Wilhelmina Matern, RN
Quality Assurance . . . . Velma Shirley-Manueli

Measure	Cases	This Hosp.	State Avg.	U.S. Avg.
Blood Clot Prevention and Treatment				
Anticoagulation Overlap Therapy[1,2]	-	-	94%	93%
ICU Venous Thromboembolism Prophylaxis[2]	55	98%	92%	92%
Incidence of Potentially Preventable VTE[1,2]	-	-	9%	10%
UFH with Dosages/Platelet Monitoring[2,7]	-	-	98%	97%
Venous Thromboembolism Prophylaxis[2]	103	95%	88%	85%
Warfarin Therapy Discharge Instructions[1,2]	-	-	74%	75%
Chest Pain/Possible Heart Attack Care				
Aspirin Given Within 24 Hours of Arrival	-	-	98%	96%
Fibrinolytic Meds Within 30 Min. of Arrival	-	-	59%	58%
Average Time to ECG (minutes)	-	-	6	7
Average Time to Transfer (minutes)	-	-	48	60
Children's Asthma Care				
Received Home Management Plan of Care	-	-	-	88%
Received Reliever Medication	-	-	-	100%
Received Systemic Corticosteroids	-	-	-	100%
Emergency Department				
Admittance Decision Time (minutes)[2]	195	63	98	98
Head CT Results Within 45 Min. of Arrival	-	-	64%	57%
Patients Who Left ER Before Being Seen	-	-	2%	2%
Time from ER Arrival to Admit. (minutes)[2]	195	302	285	274
Time from ER Arrival to Discharge (minutes)	-	-	162	134
Time in ER Before Being Evaluated (minutes)	-	-	27	26
Time to Pain Meds for Fractures (minutes)	-	-	58	57
Heart Attack Care				
Aspirin Given at Discharge[3,7]	-	-	99%	99%
Fibrinolytic Meds Within 30 Min. of Arrival[3,7]	-	-	67%	54%
PCI Within 90 Minutes of Arrival[3,7]	-	-	95%	96%
Statin Prescribed at Discharge[3,7]	-	-	98%	98%
Heart Failure Care				
ACE Inhibitor or ARB for LVSD[2]	13	100%	98%	97%
Discharge Instructions Given[2]	26	35%	94%	94%
Evaluation of LVS Function[2]	28	82%	99%	99%
Medicare Spending				
Medicare Spending per Patient (ratio)	-	0.72	0.93	0.98
Pneumonia Care				
Appropriate Initial Antibiotic Given	76	86%	96%	95%
Blood Culture Timing	75	89%	97%	98%
Pregnancy and Delivery Care				
Newborn Deliveries Scheduled Early[2]	43	0%	7%	6%
Preventive Care				
Immunization for Influenza[2]	251	60%	91%	90%
Immunization for Pneumonia[2]	158	91%	92%	92%
Stroke Care				
Anticoagulation Therapy for Atrial Fibrillation[5]	-	-	96%	95%
Antithrombotic Therapy Timing[5]	-	-	98%	98%
Assessed for Rehabilitation[5]	-	-	96%	97%
Discharged on Antithrombotic Therapy[5]	-	-	99%	99%
Discharged on Statin Medication[5]	-	-	94%	94%
Thrombolytic Therapy Timing[5]	-	-	81%	66%
Venous Thromboembolism Prophylaxis[5]	-	-	93%	94%
Written Stroke Educational Materials Given[5]	-	-	84%	88%
Surgical Care Improvement Project				
Appropriate Beta Blocker Usage[3,7]	-	-	97%	98%
Appropriate VTP Within 24 Hours[3,7]	-	-	98%	98%
Controlled Postoperative Blood Glucose[3,7]	-	-	96%	97%
Perioperative Temperature Management[3]	25	100%	100%	100%
Prophylactic Antibiotic Selection[1,3]	-	-	99%	99%
Prophylactic Antibiotic Selection (Outpatient)	-	-	98%	98%
Prophylactic Antibiotic Stopped[1,3]	-	-	98%	98%
Prophylactic Antibiotic Timing[1,3]	-	-	99%	99%
Prophylactic Antibiotic Timing (Outpatient)	-	-	99%	98%
Urinary Catheter Removal[1,3]	-	-	97%	97%
Survey of Patients' Hospital Experiences				
Area Around Room 'Always' Quiet at Night	(a)	54%	57%	61%
Doctors 'Always' Communicated Well	(a)	70%	77%	82%
Home Recovery Information Given	(a)	78%	86%	85%
Hospital Given 9 or 10 on 10 Point Scale	(a)	62%	70%	71%
Meds 'Always' Explained Before Given	(a)	56%	62%	64%
Nurses 'Always' Communicated Well	(a)	72%	76%	79%
Pain 'Always' Well Controlled	(a)	65%	69%	71%
Room and Bathroom 'Always' Clean	(a)	68%	69%	73%
Timely Help 'Always' Received	(a)	56%	65%	68%
Would Definitely Recommend Hospital	(a)	55%	70%	71%
Use of Medical Imaging				
Cardiac Imaging Stress Test before Surgery	-	-	5.8%	5.3%
Combination Abdominal CT Scan	-	-	9.1%	10.5%
Combination Brain/Sinus CT Scan	-	-	3.2%	2.7%
Combination Chest CT Scan	-	-	5.5%	2.7%
Follow-up Mammogram/Ultrasound	-	-	8.5%	8.8%
Lumbar Spine MRI for Low Back Pain	-	-	37.4%	37.2%

Valley View Medical Center

5330 South Highway 95 Phone: 928-788-2273
Fort Mohave, AZ 86426
URL: www.valleyviewmedicalcenter.net
Type: Acute Care Hospitals Emergency Services: Yes
Ownership: Proprietary Beds: 60

Key Personnel:
Chief of Medical Staff. . . . . Lanny R Copeland
CEO/President. . . . . Allen Peters

Measure	Cases	This Hosp.	State Avg.	U.S. Avg.
Blood Clot Prevention and Treatment				
Anticoagulation Overlap Therapy[2]	19	79%	94%	93%
ICU Venous Thromboembolism Prophylaxis[2]	69	94%	92%	92%
Incidence of Potentially Preventable VTE[2,7]	-	-	9%	10%
UFH with Dosages/Platelet Monitoring[1,2]	-	-	98%	97%
Venous Thromboembolism Prophylaxis[2]	198	89%	88%	85%
Warfarin Therapy Discharge Instructions[2]	18	100%	74%	75%
Chest Pain/Possible Heart Attack Care				
Aspirin Given Within 24 Hours of Arrival	11	91%	98%	96%
Fibrinolytic Meds Within 30 Min. of Arrival[7]	-	-	59%	58%
Average Time to ECG (minutes)	12	9	6	7
Average Time to Transfer (minutes)[1]	-	-	48	60
Children's Asthma Care				
Received Home Management Plan of Care	-	-	-	88%
Received Reliever Medication	-	-	-	100%
Received Systemic Corticosteroids	-	-	-	100%
Emergency Department				
Admittance Decision Time (minutes)[2]	468	76	98	98
Head CT Results Within 45 Min. of Arrival	15	67%	64%	57%
Patients Who Left ER Before Being Seen	18,724	1%	2%	2%
Time from ER Arrival to Admit. (minutes)[2]	469	229	285	274
Time from ER Arrival to Discharge (minutes)	417	102	162	134
Time in ER Before Being Evaluated (minutes)	443	16	27	26
Time to Pain Meds for Fractures (minutes)	49	27	58	57
Heart Attack Care				
Aspirin Given at Discharge[2]	47	100%	99%	99%
Fibrinolytic Meds Within 30 Min. of Arrival[2,7]	-	-	67%	54%
PCI Within 90 Minutes of Arrival[1,2]	-	-	95%	96%
Statin Prescribed at Discharge[2]	47	100%	98%	98%
Heart Failure Care				
ACE Inhibitor or ARB for LVSD[2]	22	100%	98%	97%
Discharge Instructions Given[2]	93	99%	94%	94%
Evaluation of LVS Function[2]	99	100%	99%	99%
Medicare Spending				
Medicare Spending per Patient (ratio)	-	0.89	0.93	0.98
Pneumonia Care				
Appropriate Initial Antibiotic Given[2]	47	96%	96%	95%
Blood Culture Timing[2]	64	100%	97%	98%
Pregnancy and Delivery Care				
Newborn Deliveries Scheduled Early[2]	49	33%	7%	6%
Preventive Care				
Immunization for Influenza[2]	326	93%	91%	90%
Immunization for Pneumonia[2]	374	98%	92%	92%
Stroke Care				
Anticoagulation Therapy for Atrial Fibrillation[1,2]	-	-	96%	95%
Antithrombotic Therapy Timing[2]	22	91%	98%	98%
Assessed for Rehabilitation[2]	20	100%	96%	97%
Discharged on Antithrombotic Therapy[2]	20	95%	99%	99%
Discharged on Statin Medication[2]	18	94%	94%	94%
Thrombolytic Therapy Timing[1,2]	-	-	81%	66%
Venous Thromboembolism Prophylaxis[2]	23	87%	93%	94%
Written Stroke Educational Materials Given[2]	16	94%	84%	88%
Surgical Care Improvement Project				
Appropriate Beta Blocker Usage[2]	62	92%	97%	98%
Appropriate VTP Within 24 Hours[2]	137	93%	98%	98%
Controlled Postoperative Blood Glucose[2,7]	-	-	96%	97%
Perioperative Temperature Management[2]	162	100%	100%	100%
Prophylactic Antibiotic Selection[2]	118	95%	99%	99%
Prophylactic Antibiotic Selection (Outpatient)	165	96%	98%	98%
Prophylactic Antibiotic Stopped[2]	117	97%	98%	98%
Prophylactic Antibiotic Timing[2]	118	97%	99%	99%
Prophylactic Antibiotic Timing (Outpatient)	165	100%	99%	98%
Urinary Catheter Removal[2]	54	98%	97%	97%
Survey of Patients' Hospital Experiences				
Area Around Room 'Always' Quiet at Night	300+	56%	57%	61%
Doctors 'Always' Communicated Well	300+	71%	77%	82%
Home Recovery Information Given	300+	84%	86%	85%
Hospital Given 9 or 10 on 10 Point Scale	300+	67%	70%	71%
Meds 'Always' Explained Before Given	300+	58%	62%	64%
Nurses 'Always' Communicated Well	300+	75%	76%	79%
Pain 'Always' Well Controlled	300+	69%	69%	71%
Room and Bathroom 'Always' Clean	300+	78%	69%	73%
Timely Help 'Always' Received	300+	61%	65%	68%
Would Definitely Recommend Hospital	300+	73%	70%	71%

NOTE: Hospital profiles are in alphabetical order by state, then city, then hospital within the city; Rankings exclude hospitals with less than 25 cases except for patient surveys which excludes hospitals with less than 100 cases; (a) 100-299 cases; (1) The number of cases/patients is too few to report; (2) Data submitted were based on a sample of cases/patients; (3) Results are based on a shorter time period than required; (4) Data suppressed by CMS for one or more quarters; (5) Results are not available for this reporting period; (6) Fewer than 100 patients completed the HCAHPS survey; (7) No cases met the criteria for this measure; (8) The lower limit of the confidence interval cannot be calculated if the number of observed infections equals zero; (9) No data are available from the state/territory for this reporting period; (10) The scores shown reflect fewer than 50 completed surveys; (11) There were discrepancies in the data collection process; (12) This measure does not apply to this hospital for this reporting period; (13) Results cannot be calculated for this reporting period; (14) The results for this state are combined with nearby states to protect confidentiality; Please refer to the User's Guide for a full explanation of data.

Use of Medical Imaging				
Cardiac Imaging Stress Test before Surgery[7]	-	-	5.8%	5.3%
Combination Abdominal CT Scan	721	19.1%	9.1%	10.5%
Combination Brain/Sinus CT Scan[1]	-	-	3.2%	2.7%
Combination Chest CT Scan	353	11.3%	5.5%	2.7%
Follow-up Mammogram/Ultrasound	770	4.5%	8.5%	8.8%
Lumbar Spine MRI for Low Back Pain	93	40.9%	37.4%	37.2%

Sage Memorial Hospital

State Route 264 South 191 Phone: 928-755-4559
Ganado, AZ 86505 Fax: 928-755-4557
URL: www.navajosage.org
Type: Critical Access Hospitals Emergency Services: No
Ownership: Voluntary non-profit - Private Beds: 45
Key Personnel:
Emergency Room . . . . Wanda Begay
Chief of Medical Staff . . . . Mohammed Illias
Quality Assurance . . . . Gloria Platero
CEO . . . . Ahmad R Razaghi

Measure	Cases	This Hosp.	State Avg.	U.S. Avg.
Blood Clot Prevention and Treatment				
Anticoagulation Overlap Therapy[5]	-	-	94%	93%
ICU Venous Thromboembolism Prophylaxis[5]	-	-	92%	92%
Incidence of Potentially Preventable VTE[5]	-	-	9%	10%
UFH with Dosages/Platelet Monitoring[5]	-	-	98%	97%
Venous Thromboembolism Prophylaxis[5]	-	-	88%	85%
Warfarin Therapy Discharge Instructions[5]	-	-	74%	75%
Chest Pain/Possible Heart Attack Care				
Aspirin Given Within 24 Hours of Arrival[5]	-	-	98%	96%
Fibrinolytic Meds Within 30 Min. of Arrival[5]	-	-	59%	58%
Average Time to ECG (minutes)[5]	-	-	6	7
Average Time to Transfer (minutes)[5]	-	-	48	60
Children's Asthma Care				
Received Home Management Plan of Care	-	-	-	88%
Received Reliever Medication	-	-	-	100%
Received Systemic Corticosteroids	-	-	-	100%
Emergency Department				
Admittance Decision Time (minutes)[5]	-	-	98	98
Head CT Results Within 45 Min. of Arrival[5]	-	-	64%	57%
Patients Who Left ER Before Being Seen[5]	-	-	2%	2%
Time from ER Arrival to Admit. (minutes)[5]	-	-	285	274
Time from ER Arrival to Discharge (minutes)[5]	-	-	162	134
Time in ER Before Being Evaluated (minutes)[5]	-	-	27	26
Time to Pain Meds for Fractures (minutes)[5]	-	-	58	57
Heart Attack Care				
Aspirin Given at Discharge[5]	-	-	99%	99%
Fibrinolytic Meds Within 30 Min. of Arrival[5]	-	-	67%	54%
PCI Within 90 Minutes of Arrival[5]	-	-	95%	96%
Statin Prescribed at Discharge[5]	-	-	98%	98%
Heart Failure Care				
ACE Inhibitor or ARB for LVSD[5]	-	-	98%	97%
Discharge Instructions Given[5]	-	-	94%	94%
Evaluation of LVS Function[5]	-	-	99%	99%
Medicare Spending				
Medicare Spending per Patient (ratio)	-	-	0.93	0.98
Pneumonia Care				
Appropriate Initial Antibiotic Given[2,3]	-	-	96%	95%
Blood Culture Timing[2,3]	-	-	97%	98%
Pregnancy and Delivery Care				
Newborn Deliveries Scheduled Early[5]	-	-	7%	6%
Preventive Care				
Immunization for Influenza[5]	-	-	91%	90%
Immunization for Pneumonia[5]	-	-	92%	92%
Stroke Care				
Anticoagulation Therapy for Atrial Fibrillation[5]	-	-	96%	95%
Antithrombotic Therapy Timing[5]	-	-	98%	98%
Assessed for Rehabilitation[5]	-	-	96%	97%
Discharged on Antithrombotic Therapy[5]	-	-	99%	99%
Discharged on Statin Medication[5]	-	-	94%	94%
Thrombolytic Therapy Timing[5]	-	-	81%	66%
Venous Thromboembolism Prophylaxis[5]	-	-	93%	94%
Written Stroke Educational Materials Given[5]	-	-	84%	88%
Surgical Care Improvement Project				
Appropriate Beta Blocker Usage[5]	-	-	97%	98%
Appropriate VTP Within 24 Hours[5]	-	-	98%	98%
Controlled Postoperative Blood Glucose[5]	-	-	96%	97%
Perioperative Temperature Management[5]	-	-	100%	100%
Prophylactic Antibiotic Selection[5]	-	-	99%	99%
Prophylactic Antibiotic Selection (Outpatient)[5]	-	-	98%	98%
Prophylactic Antibiotic Stopped[5]	-	-	98%	98%
Prophylactic Antibiotic Timing[5]	-	-	99%	99%
Prophylactic Antibiotic Timing (Outpatient)[5]	-	-	99%	98%
Urinary Catheter Removal[5]	-	-	97%	97%
Survey of Patients' Hospital Experiences				
Area Around Room 'Always' Quiet at Night[5]	-	-	57%	61%
Doctors 'Always' Communicated Well[5]	-	-	77%	82%
Home Recovery Information Given[5]	-	-	86%	85%
Hospital Given 9 or 10 on 10 Point Scale[5]	-	-	70%	71%
Meds 'Always' Explained Before Given[5]	-	-	62%	64%
Nurses 'Always' Communicated Well[5]	-	-	76%	79%
Pain 'Always' Well Controlled[5]	-	-	69%	71%
Room and Bathroom 'Always' Clean[5]	-	-	69%	73%
Timely Help 'Always' Received[5]	-	-	65%	68%
Would Definitely Recommend Hospital[5]	-	-	70%	71%
Use of Medical Imaging				
Cardiac Imaging Stress Test before Surgery[7]	-	-	5.8%	5.3%
Combination Abdominal CT Scan	65	6.2%	9.1%	10.5%
Combination Brain/Sinus CT Scan[1]	-	-	3.2%	2.7%
Combination Chest CT Scan	48	0.0%	5.5%	2.7%
Follow-up Mammogram/Ultrasound[7]	-	-	8.5%	8.8%
Lumbar Spine MRI for Low Back Pain[7]	-	-	37.4%	37.2%

Banner Gateway Medical Center

1900 North Higley Road Phone: 480-543-2000
Gilbert, AZ 85234
URL: www.healthgrades.com
Type: Acute Care Hospitals Emergency Services: Yes
Ownership: Voluntary non-profit - Other Beds: 168
Key Personnel:
Cardiology . . . . Marc Berkowitz, MD
Pulmonology . . . . William Peppo, DO
CEO . . . . Todd Werner

Measure	Cases	This Hosp.	State Avg.	U.S. Avg.
Blood Clot Prevention and Treatment				
Anticoagulation Overlap Therapy[2]	92	96%	94%	93%
ICU Venous Thromboembolism Prophylaxis[2]	32	100%	92%	92%
Incidence of Potentially Preventable VTE[2]	31	13%	9%	10%
UFH with Dosages/Platelet Monitoring[2]	43	100%	98%	97%
Venous Thromboembolism Prophylaxis[2]	382	96%	88%	85%
Warfarin Therapy Discharge Instructions[2]	76	62%	74%	75%
Chest Pain/Possible Heart Attack Care				
Aspirin Given Within 24 Hours of Arrival	66	98%	98%	96%
Fibrinolytic Meds Within 30 Min. of Arrival[7]	-	-	59%	58%
Average Time to ECG (minutes)	69	10	6	7
Average Time to Transfer (minutes)[1]	-	-	48	60
Children's Asthma Care				
Received Home Management Plan of Care	-	-	-	88%
Received Reliever Medication	-	-	-	100%
Received Systemic Corticosteroids	-	-	-	100%
Emergency Department				
Admittance Decision Time (minutes)[2]	333	66	98	98
Head CT Results Within 45 Min. of Arrival	13	62%	64%	57%
Patients Who Left ER Before Being Seen	51,011	1%	2%	2%
Time from ER Arrival to Admit. (minutes)[2]	337	275	285	274
Time from ER Arrival to Discharge (minutes)	341	192	162	134
Time in ER Before Being Evaluated (minutes)	397	28	27	26
Time to Pain Meds for Fractures (minutes)	166	70	58	57
Heart Attack Care				
Aspirin Given at Discharge[1]	-	-	99%	99%
Fibrinolytic Meds Within 30 Min. of Arrival[7]	-	-	67%	54%
PCI Within 90 Minutes of Arrival[7]	-	-	95%	96%
Statin Prescribed at Discharge[1]	-	-	98%	98%
Heart Failure Care				
ACE Inhibitor or ARB for LVSD	31	100%	98%	97%
Discharge Instructions Given	141	96%	94%	94%
Evaluation of LVS Function	156	100%	99%	99%
Medicare Spending				
Medicare Spending per Patient (ratio)	-	0.96	0.93	0.98
Pneumonia Care				
Appropriate Initial Antibiotic Given[2]	88	98%	96%	95%
Blood Culture Timing[2]	141	99%	97%	98%
Pregnancy and Delivery Care				
Newborn Deliveries Scheduled Early[2]	106	11%	7%	6%
Preventive Care				
Immunization for Influenza[2]	451	90%	91%	90%
Immunization for Pneumonia[2]	412	92%	92%	92%
Stroke Care				
Anticoagulation Therapy for Atrial Fibrillation[1]	-	-	96%	95%
Antithrombotic Therapy Timing	53	98%	98%	98%
Assessed for Rehabilitation	58	90%	96%	97%
Discharged on Antithrombotic Therapy	55	100%	99%	99%
Discharged on Statin Medication	41	76%	94%	94%
Thrombolytic Therapy Timing[1]	-	-	81%	66%
Venous Thromboembolism Prophylaxis	57	95%	93%	94%
Written Stroke Educational Materials Given	45	40%	84%	88%
Surgical Care Improvement Project				
Appropriate Beta Blocker Usage[2]	89	98%	97%	98%
Appropriate VTP Within 24 Hours[2]	301	98%	98%	98%
Controlled Postoperative Blood Glucose[2,7]	-	-	96%	97%
Perioperative Temperature Management[2]	391	100%	100%	100%
Prophylactic Antibiotic Selection[2]	236	97%	99%	99%
Prophylactic Antibiotic Selection (Outpatient)	289	97%	98%	98%
Prophylactic Antibiotic Stopped[2]	231	98%	98%	98%
Prophylactic Antibiotic Timing[2]	236	100%	99%	99%
Prophylactic Antibiotic Timing (Outpatient)	289	99%	99%	98%
Urinary Catheter Removal[2]	184	99%	97%	97%
Survey of Patients' Hospital Experiences				
Area Around Room 'Always' Quiet at Night[11]	300+	63%	57%	61%
Doctors 'Always' Communicated Well[11]	300+	80%	77%	82%
Home Recovery Information Given[11]	300+	89%	86%	85%
Hospital Given 9 or 10 on 10 Point Scale[11]	300+	77%	70%	71%
Meds 'Always' Explained Before Given[11]	300+	63%	62%	64%
Nurses 'Always' Communicated Well[11]	300+	78%	76%	79%
Pain 'Always' Well Controlled[11]	300+	71%	69%	71%
Room and Bathroom 'Always' Clean[11]	300+	58%	69%	73%
Timely Help 'Always' Received[11]	300+	64%	65%	68%
Would Definitely Recommend Hospital[11]	300+	80%	70%	71%
Use of Medical Imaging				
Cardiac Imaging Stress Test before Surgery[1]	-	-	5.8%	5.3%
Combination Abdominal CT Scan	835	3.0%	9.1%	10.5%
Combination Brain/Sinus CT Scan	409	4.9%	3.2%	2.7%
Combination Chest CT Scan	528	0.8%	5.5%	2.7%
Follow-up Mammogram/Ultrasound	369	9.8%	8.5%	8.8%
Lumbar Spine MRI for Low Back Pain[1]	-	-	37.4%	37.2%

Gilbert Hospital

5656 South Power Road Phone: 480-840-3715
Gilbert, AZ 85295
URL: www.gilberter.com/index.html
Type: Acute Care Hospitals Emergency Services: Yes
Ownership: Proprietary

Measure	Cases	This Hosp.	State Avg.	U.S. Avg.
Blood Clot Prevention and Treatment				
Anticoagulation Overlap Therapy[2]	21	86%	94%	93%
ICU Venous Thromboembolism Prophylaxis[1,2]	-	-	92%	92%
Incidence of Potentially Preventable VTE[2,7]	-	-	9%	10%
UFH with Dosages/Platelet Monitoring[1,2]	-	-	98%	97%
Venous Thromboembolism Prophylaxis[2]	106	100%	88%	85%
Warfarin Therapy Discharge Instructions[2]	20	100%	74%	75%
Chest Pain/Possible Heart Attack Care				
Aspirin Given Within 24 Hours of Arrival	27	89%	98%	96%
Fibrinolytic Meds Within 30 Min. of Arrival[7]	-	-	59%	58%
Average Time to ECG (minutes)	28	8	6	7
Average Time to Transfer (minutes)[1]	-	-	48	60
Children's Asthma Care				
Received Home Management Plan of Care	-	-	-	88%
Received Reliever Medication	-	-	-	100%
Received Systemic Corticosteroids	-	-	-	100%

NOTE: Hospital profiles are in alphabetical order by state, then city, then hospital within the city; Rankings exclude hospitals with less than 25 cases except for patient surveys which excludes hospitals with less than 100 cases; (a) 100-299 cases; (1) The number of cases/patients is too few to report; (2) Data submitted were based on a sample of cases/patients; (3) Results are based on a shorter time period than required; (4) Data suppressed by CMS for one or more quarters; (5) Results are not available for this reporting period; (6) Fewer than 100 patients completed the HCAHPS survey; (7) No cases met the criteria for this measure; (8) The lower limit of the confidence interval cannot be calculated if the number of observed infections equals zero; (9) No data are available from the state/territory for this reporting period; (10) The scores shown reflect fewer than 50 completed surveys; (11) There were discrepancies in the data collection process; (12) This measure does not apply to this hospital for this reporting period; (13) Results cannot be calculated for this reporting period; (14) The results for this state are combined with nearby states to protect confidentiality; Please refer to the User's Guide for a full explanation of data.

Measure	Cases	This Hosp.	State Avg.	U.S. Avg.
Emergency Department				
Admittance Decision Time (minutes)[2]	340	68	98	98
Head CT Results Within 45 Min. of Arrival[1]	-	-	64%	57%
Patients Who Left ER Before Being Seen	28,106	0%	2%	2%
Time from ER Arrival to Admit. (minutes)[2]	340	257	285	274
Time from ER Arrival to Discharge (minutes)	363	132	162	134
Time in ER Before Being Evaluated (minutes)	384	8	27	26
Time to Pain Meds for Fractures (minutes)	85	32	58	57
Heart Attack Care				
Aspirin Given at Discharge[5]	-	-	99%	99%
Fibrinolytic Meds Within 30 Min. of Arrival[5]	-	-	67%	54%
PCI Within 90 Minutes of Arrival[5]	-	-	95%	96%
Statin Prescribed at Discharge[5]	-	-	98%	98%
Heart Failure Care				
ACE Inhibitor or ARB for LVSD[3,7]	-	-	98%	97%
Discharge Instructions Given[1,3]	-	-	94%	94%
Evaluation of LVS Function[1,3]	-	-	99%	99%
Medicare Spending				
Medicare Spending per Patient (ratio)	-	0.87	0.93	0.98
Pneumonia Care				
Appropriate Initial Antibiotic Given[2,3]	40	90%	96%	95%
Blood Culture Timing[2,3]	18	89%	97%	98%
Pregnancy and Delivery Care				
Newborn Deliveries Scheduled Early[7]	-	-	7%	6%
Preventive Care				
Immunization for Influenza[2]	290	97%	91%	90%
Immunization for Pneumonia[2]	323	96%	92%	92%
Stroke Care				
Anticoagulation Therapy for Atrial Fibrillation[5]	-	-	96%	95%
Antithrombotic Therapy Timing[5]	-	-	98%	98%
Assessed for Rehabilitation[5]	-	-	96%	97%
Discharged on Antithrombotic Therapy[5]	-	-	99%	99%
Discharged on Statin Medication[5]	-	-	94%	94%
Thrombolytic Therapy Timing[5]	-	-	81%	66%
Venous Thromboembolism Prophylaxis[5]	-	-	93%	94%
Written Stroke Educational Materials Given[5]	-	-	84%	88%
Surgical Care Improvement Project				
Appropriate Beta Blocker Usage[5]	-	-	97%	98%
Appropriate VTP Within 24 Hours[5]	-	-	98%	98%
Controlled Postoperative Blood Glucose[5]	-	-	96%	97%
Perioperative Temperature Management[5]	-	-	100%	100%
Prophylactic Antibiotic Selection[5]	-	-	99%	99%
Prophylactic Antibiotic Selection (Outpatient)[5]	-	-	98%	98%
Prophylactic Antibiotic Stopped[5]	-	-	98%	98%
Prophylactic Antibiotic Timing[5]	-	-	99%	99%
Prophylactic Antibiotic Timing (Outpatient)[5]	-	-	99%	98%
Urinary Catheter Removal[5]	-	-	97%	97%
Survey of Patients' Hospital Experiences				
Area Around Room 'Always' Quiet at Night	(a)	65%	57%	61%
Doctors 'Always' Communicated Well	(a)	73%	77%	82%
Home Recovery Information Given	(a)	88%	86%	85%
Hospital Given 9 or 10 on 10 Point Scale	(a)	78%	70%	71%
Meds 'Always' Explained Before Given	(a)	67%	62%	64%
Nurses 'Always' Communicated Well	(a)	81%	76%	79%
Pain 'Always' Well Controlled	(a)	72%	69%	71%
Room and Bathroom 'Always' Clean	(a)	83%	69%	73%
Timely Help 'Always' Received	(a)	70%	65%	68%
Would Definitely Recommend Hospital	(a)	80%	70%	71%
Use of Medical Imaging				
Cardiac Imaging Stress Test before Surgery[1]	-	-	5.8%	5.3%
Combination Abdominal CT Scan	183	2.7%	9.1%	10.5%
Combination Brain/Sinus CT Scan	178	5.6%	3.2%	2.7%
Combination Chest CT Scan[1]	-	-	5.5%	2.7%
Follow-up Mammogram/Ultrasound[7]	-	-	8.5%	8.8%
Lumbar Spine MRI for Low Back Pain[1]	-	-	37.4%	37.2%

Mercy Gilbert Medical Center

3555 South Val Vista Drive — Phone: 480-728-8327
Gilbert, AZ 85296
URL: www.dignityhealth.org/mercygilbert
Type: Acute Care Hospitals — Emergency Services: Yes
Ownership: Voluntary non-profit - Church — Beds: 121

Key Personnel:
Intensive Care Unit. . . . . Karen Blancs
CEO/President. . . . . Tim Brecker
Operating Room. . . . . Abner Cruz
Emergency Room . . . . Victor Garcia
Pediatric In-Patient Care . . . . Deanna Grey
Quality Assurance . . . . Deb Heartman
Radiology. . . . . Ed Jones
Cardiac Laboratory. . . . . Jay Pockyarath

Measure	Cases	This Hosp.	State Avg.	U.S. Avg.
Blood Clot Prevention and Treatment				
Anticoagulation Overlap Therapy[2]	138	95%	94%	93%
ICU Venous Thromboembolism Prophylaxis[2]	62	97%	92%	92%
Incidence of Potentially Preventable VTE[2]	12	8%	9%	10%
UFH with Dosages/Platelet Monitoring[2]	120	100%	98%	97%
Venous Thromboembolism Prophylaxis[2]	339	91%	88%	85%
Warfarin Therapy Discharge Instructions[2]	105	100%	74%	75%
Chest Pain/Possible Heart Attack Care				
Aspirin Given Within 24 Hours of Arrival	13	100%	98%	96%
Fibrinolytic Meds Within 30 Min. of Arrival[3,7]	-	-	59%	58%
Average Time to ECG (minutes)	13	10	6	7
Average Time to Transfer (minutes)[1,3]	-	-	48	60
Children's Asthma Care				
Received Home Management Plan of Care	-	-	-	88%
Received Reliever Medication	-	-	-	100%
Received Systemic Corticosteroids	-	-	-	100%
Emergency Department				
Admittance Decision Time (minutes)[2]	472	106	98	98
Head CT Results Within 45 Min. of Arrival[1]	-	-	64%	57%
Patients Who Left ER Before Being Seen	44,331	0%	2%	2%
Time from ER Arrival to Admit. (minutes)[2]	480	268	285	274
Time from ER Arrival to Discharge (minutes)	347	155	162	134
Time in ER Before Being Evaluated (minutes)	390	8	27	26
Time to Pain Meds for Fractures (minutes)	189	35	58	57
Heart Attack Care				
Aspirin Given at Discharge	132	100%	99%	99%
Fibrinolytic Meds Within 30 Min. of Arrival[7]	-	-	67%	54%
PCI Within 90 Minutes of Arrival	34	88%	95%	96%
Statin Prescribed at Discharge	129	98%	98%	98%
Heart Failure Care				
ACE Inhibitor or ARB for LVSD[2]	79	99%	98%	97%
Discharge Instructions Given[2]	220	95%	94%	94%
Evaluation of LVS Function[2]	252	100%	99%	99%
Medicare Spending				
Medicare Spending per Patient (ratio)	-	0.98	0.93	0.98
Pneumonia Care				
Appropriate Initial Antibiotic Given[2]	107	97%	96%	95%
Blood Culture Timing[2]	177	98%	97%	98%
Pregnancy and Delivery Care				
Newborn Deliveries Scheduled Early[2]	62	0%	7%	6%
Preventive Care				
Immunization for Influenza[2]	509	99%	91%	90%
Immunization for Pneumonia[2]	522	96%	92%	92%
Stroke Care				
Anticoagulation Therapy for Atrial Fibrillation	14	100%	96%	95%
Antithrombotic Therapy Timing	94	95%	98%	98%
Assessed for Rehabilitation	126	98%	96%	97%
Discharged on Antithrombotic Therapy	110	99%	99%	99%
Discharged on Statin Medication	98	99%	94%	94%
Thrombolytic Therapy Timing	15	87%	81%	66%
Venous Thromboembolism Prophylaxis	113	96%	93%	94%
Written Stroke Educational Materials Given	73	96%	84%	88%
Surgical Care Improvement Project				
Appropriate Beta Blocker Usage[2]	97	97%	97%	98%
Appropriate VTP Within 24 Hours[2]	373	98%	98%	98%
Controlled Postoperative Blood Glucose[2,7]	-	-	96%	97%
Perioperative Temperature Management[2]	423	100%	100%	100%
Prophylactic Antibiotic Selection[2]	243	99%	99%	99%
Prophylactic Antibiotic Selection (Outpatient)	359	98%	98%	98%
Prophylactic Antibiotic Stopped[2]	233	98%	98%	98%
Prophylactic Antibiotic Timing[2]	243	100%	99%	99%
Prophylactic Antibiotic Timing (Outpatient)	361	98%	99%	98%
Urinary Catheter Removal[2]	187	90%	97%	97%
Survey of Patients' Hospital Experiences				
Area Around Room 'Always' Quiet at Night	300+	66%	57%	61%
Doctors 'Always' Communicated Well	300+	76%	77%	82%
Home Recovery Information Given	300+	87%	86%	85%
Hospital Given 9 or 10 on 10 Point Scale	300+	78%	70%	71%
Meds 'Always' Explained Before Given	300+	62%	62%	64%
Nurses 'Always' Communicated Well	300+	76%	76%	79%
Pain 'Always' Well Controlled	300+	71%	69%	71%
Room and Bathroom 'Always' Clean	300+	72%	69%	73%
Timely Help 'Always' Received	300+	64%	65%	68%
Would Definitely Recommend Hospital	300+	80%	70%	71%
Use of Medical Imaging				
Cardiac Imaging Stress Test before Surgery	169	4.7%	5.8%	5.3%
Combination Abdominal CT Scan	723	0.8%	9.1%	10.5%
Combination Brain/Sinus CT Scan	801	2.0%	3.2%	2.7%
Combination Chest CT Scan	516	0.8%	5.5%	2.7%
Follow-up Mammogram/Ultrasound	241	16.6%	8.5%	8.8%
Lumbar Spine MRI for Low Back Pain[1]	-	-	37.4%	37.2%

Arrowhead Hospital

18701 North 67th Avenue — Phone: 623-561-1000
Glendale, AZ 85308 — Fax: 623-561-7142
URL: www.arrowheadhospital.com
Type: Acute Care Hospitals — Emergency Services: Yes
Ownership: Proprietary — Beds: 115

Key Personnel:
Radiology. . . . . Ayad Agha
Chief of Medical Staff. . . . . Alan L Barnett
CEO/President. . . . . Jon Bartlett

Measure	Cases	This Hosp.	State Avg.	U.S. Avg.
Blood Clot Prevention and Treatment				
Anticoagulation Overlap Therapy[2]	76	96%	94%	93%
ICU Venous Thromboembolism Prophylaxis[2]	69	99%	92%	92%
Incidence of Potentially Preventable VTE[1,2]	-	-	9%	10%
UFH with Dosages/Platelet Monitoring[2]	48	98%	98%	97%
Venous Thromboembolism Prophylaxis[2]	290	74%	88%	85%
Warfarin Therapy Discharge Instructions[2]	58	41%	74%	75%
Chest Pain/Possible Heart Attack Care				
Aspirin Given Within 24 Hours of Arrival[1]	-	-	98%	96%
Fibrinolytic Meds Within 30 Min. of Arrival[5]	-	-	59%	58%
Average Time to ECG (minutes)[1]	-	-	6	7
Average Time to Transfer (minutes)[5]	-	-	48	60
Children's Asthma Care				
Received Home Management Plan of Care	-	-	-	88%
Received Reliever Medication	-	-	-	100%
Received Systemic Corticosteroids	-	-	-	100%
Emergency Department				
Admittance Decision Time (minutes)[2]	498	114	98	98
Head CT Results Within 45 Min. of Arrival	26	85%	64%	57%
Patients Who Left ER Before Being Seen	44,904	1%	2%	2%
Time from ER Arrival to Admit. (minutes)[2]	500	276	285	274
Time from ER Arrival to Discharge (minutes)	398	142	162	134
Time in ER Before Being Evaluated (minutes)	414	26	27	26
Time to Pain Meds for Fractures (minutes)	160	54	58	57
Heart Attack Care				
Aspirin Given at Discharge	150	100%	99%	99%
Fibrinolytic Meds Within 30 Min. of Arrival[7]	-	-	67%	54%
PCI Within 90 Minutes of Arrival	33	100%	95%	96%
Statin Prescribed at Discharge	146	100%	98%	98%
Heart Failure Care				
ACE Inhibitor or ARB for LVSD	50	98%	98%	97%
Discharge Instructions Given	124	100%	94%	94%
Evaluation of LVS Function	144	99%	99%	99%
Medicare Spending				
Medicare Spending per Patient (ratio)	-	1.00	0.93	0.98
Pneumonia Care				
Appropriate Initial Antibiotic Given	223	100%	96%	95%
Blood Culture Timing	324	99%	97%	98%
Pregnancy and Delivery Care				
Newborn Deliveries Scheduled Early[2]	67	7%	7%	6%
Preventive Care				
Immunization for Influenza[2]	524	96%	91%	90%
Immunization for Pneumonia[2]	486	99%	92%	92%
Stroke Care				
Anticoagulation Therapy for Atrial Fibrillation	11	100%	96%	95%

NOTE: Hospital profiles are in alphabetical order by state, then city, then hospital within the city; Rankings exclude hospitals with less than 25 cases except for patient surveys which excludes hospitals with less than 100 cases; (a) 100-299 cases; (1) The number of cases/patients is too few to report; (2) Data submitted were based on a sample of cases/patients; (3) Results are based on a shorter time period than required; (4) Data suppressed by CMS for one or more quarters; (5) Results are not available for this reporting period; (6) Fewer than 100 patients completed the HCAHPS survey; (7) No cases met the criteria for this measure; (8) The lower limit of the confidence interval cannot be calculated if the number of observed infections equals zero; (9) No data are available from the state/territory for this reporting period; (10) The scores shown reflect fewer than 50 completed surveys; (11) There were discrepancies in the data collection process; (12) This measure does not apply to this hospital for this reporting period; (13) Results cannot be calculated for this reporting period; (14) The results for this state are combined with nearby states to protect confidentiality; Please refer to the User's Guide for a full explanation of data.

Antithrombotic Therapy Timing	92	98%	98%	98%
Assessed for Rehabilitation	90	98%	96%	97%
Discharged on Antithrombotic Therapy	87	100%	99%	99%
Discharged on Statin Medication	65	95%	94%	94%
Thrombolytic Therapy Timing[1]	-	-	81%	66%
Venous Thromboembolism Prophylaxis	97	98%	93%	94%
Written Stroke Educational Materials Given	60	90%	84%	88%
Surgical Care Improvement Project				
Appropriate Beta Blocker Usage[2]	369	100%	97%	98%
Appropriate VTP Within 24 Hours[2]	932	100%	98%	98%
Controlled Postoperative Blood Glucose[2]	110	94%	96%	97%
Perioperative Temperature Management[2]	1,162	100%	100%	100%
Prophylactic Antibiotic Selection[2]	939	100%	99%	99%
Prophylactic Antibiotic Selection (Outpatient)	506	97%	98%	98%
Prophylactic Antibiotic Stopped[2]	899	100%	98%	98%
Prophylactic Antibiotic Timing[2]	939	100%	99%	99%
Prophylactic Antibiotic Timing (Outpatient)	508	99%	99%	98%
Urinary Catheter Removal[2]	623	100%	97%	97%
Survey of Patients' Hospital Experiences				
Area Around Room 'Always' Quiet at Night[11]	300+	52%	57%	61%
Doctors 'Always' Communicated Well[11]	300+	77%	77%	82%
Home Recovery Information Given[11]	300+	87%	86%	85%
Hospital Given 9 or 10 on 10 Point Scale[11]	300+	68%	70%	71%
Meds 'Always' Explained Before Given[11]	300+	57%	62%	64%
Nurses 'Always' Communicated Well[11]	300+	75%	76%	79%
Pain 'Always' Well Controlled[11]	300+	68%	69%	71%
Room and Bathroom 'Always' Clean[11]	300+	66%	69%	73%
Timely Help 'Always' Received[11]	300+	64%	65%	68%
Would Definitely Recommend Hospital[11]	300+	71%	70%	71%
Use of Medical Imaging				
Cardiac Imaging Stress Test before Surgery	76	6.6%	5.8%	5.3%
Combination Abdominal CT Scan	425	3.8%	9.1%	10.5%
Combination Brain/Sinus CT Scan[1]	-	-	3.2%	2.7%
Combination Chest CT Scan	110	1.8%	5.5%	2.7%
Follow-up Mammogram/Ultrasound	183	5.5%	8.5%	8.8%
Lumbar Spine MRI for Low Back Pain[1]	-	-	37.4%	37.2%

Banner Thunderbird Medical Center

5555 West Thunderbird Road
Glendale, AZ 85306
Phone: 602-588-5555
Fax: 602-865-5930
URL: www.bannerhealth.com
Type: Acute Care Hospitals
Emergency Services: Yes
Ownership: Govt - Hospital Dist/Auth
Beds: 409

Key Personnel:

CEO/President. . . . . Tom Dickson, FACHE
Emergency Room . . . . Amy Forsberg, RN
Chief of Medical Staff. . . . . Dr Kathryn Perkins, MD
Operating Room. . . . . Deb Roberts

Measure	Cases	This Hosp.	State Avg.	U.S. Avg.
Blood Clot Prevention and Treatment				
Anticoagulation Overlap Therapy[2]	231	95%	94%	93%
ICU Venous Thromboembolism Prophylaxis[2]	66	89%	92%	92%
Incidence of Potentially Preventable VTE[2]	50	10%	9%	10%
UFH with Dosages/Platelet Monitoring[2]	125	100%	98%	97%
Venous Thromboembolism Prophylaxis[2]	345	89%	88%	85%
Warfarin Therapy Discharge Instructions[2]	154	57%	74%	75%
Chest Pain/Possible Heart Attack Care				
Aspirin Given Within 24 Hours of Arrival[1,3]	-	-	98%	96%
Fibrinolytic Meds Within 30 Min. of Arrival[5]	-	-	59%	58%
Average Time to ECG (minutes)[1,3]	-	-	6	7
Average Time to Transfer (minutes)[5]	-	-	48	60
Children's Asthma Care				
Received Home Management Plan of Care	-	-	-	88%
Received Reliever Medication	-	-	-	100%
Received Systemic Corticosteroids	-	-	-	100%
Emergency Department				
Admittance Decision Time (minutes)[2]	609	82	98	98
Head CT Results Within 45 Min. of Arrival[1]	-	-	64%	57%
Patients Who Left ER Before Being Seen	95,157	3%	2%	2%
Time from ER Arrival to Admit. (minutes)[2]	621	309	285	274
Time from ER Arrival to Discharge (minutes)	326	220	162	134
Time in ER Before Being Evaluated (minutes)	382	36	27	26
Time to Pain Meds for Fractures (minutes)	233	56	58	57
Heart Attack Care				
Aspirin Given at Discharge[2]	246	100%	99%	99%
Fibrinolytic Meds Within 30 Min. of Arrival[2,7]	-	-	67%	54%
PCI Within 90 Minutes of Arrival[2]	34	97%	95%	96%
Statin Prescribed at Discharge[2]	238	100%	98%	98%
Heart Failure Care				
ACE Inhibitor or ARB for LVSD[2]	90	100%	98%	97%
Discharge Instructions Given[2]	234	97%	94%	94%
Evaluation of LVS Function[2]	273	100%	99%	99%
Medicare Spending				
Medicare Spending per Patient (ratio)	-	0.99	0.93	0.98
Pneumonia Care				
Appropriate Initial Antibiotic Given[2]	85	98%	96%	95%
Blood Culture Timing[2]	156	98%	97%	98%
Pregnancy and Delivery Care				
Newborn Deliveries Scheduled Early[2]	124	8%	7%	6%
Preventive Care				
Immunization for Influenza[2]	493	94%	91%	90%
Immunization for Pneumonia[2]	521	96%	92%	92%
Stroke Care				
Anticoagulation Therapy for Atrial Fibrillation[1,2]	-	-	96%	95%
Antithrombotic Therapy Timing[2]	95	100%	98%	98%
Assessed for Rehabilitation[2]	117	96%	96%	97%
Discharged on Antithrombotic Therapy[2]	99	99%	99%	99%
Discharged on Statin Medication[2]	64	100%	94%	94%
Thrombolytic Therapy Timing[2]	14	86%	81%	66%
Venous Thromboembolism Prophylaxis[2]	116	95%	93%	94%
Written Stroke Educational Materials Given[2]	85	81%	84%	88%
Surgical Care Improvement Project				
Appropriate Beta Blocker Usage[2]	235	99%	97%	98%
Appropriate VTP Within 24 Hours[2]	352	99%	98%	98%
Controlled Postoperative Blood Glucose[2]	114	96%	96%	97%
Perioperative Temperature Management[2]	533	100%	100%	100%
Prophylactic Antibiotic Selection[2]	396	100%	99%	99%
Prophylactic Antibiotic Selection (Outpatient)	497	99%	98%	98%
Prophylactic Antibiotic Stopped[2]	370	99%	98%	98%
Prophylactic Antibiotic Timing[2]	397	99%	99%	99%
Prophylactic Antibiotic Timing (Outpatient)	497	100%	99%	98%
Urinary Catheter Removal[2]	183	99%	97%	97%
Survey of Patients' Hospital Experiences				
Area Around Room 'Always' Quiet at Night[11]	300+	56%	57%	61%
Doctors 'Always' Communicated Well[11]	300+	78%	77%	82%
Home Recovery Information Given[11]	300+	87%	86%	85%
Hospital Given 9 or 10 on 10 Point Scale[11]	300+	74%	70%	71%
Meds 'Always' Explained Before Given[11]	300+	64%	62%	64%
Nurses 'Always' Communicated Well[11]	300+	78%	76%	79%
Pain 'Always' Well Controlled[11]	300+	69%	69%	71%
Room and Bathroom 'Always' Clean[11]	300+	64%	69%	73%
Timely Help 'Always' Received[11]	300+	61%	65%	68%
Would Definitely Recommend Hospital[11]	300+	77%	70%	71%
Use of Medical Imaging				
Cardiac Imaging Stress Test before Surgery	147	6.1%	5.8%	5.3%
Combination Abdominal CT Scan	624	3.5%	9.1%	10.5%
Combination Brain/Sinus CT Scan	603	2.8%	3.2%	2.7%
Combination Chest CT Scan	171	1.2%	5.5%	2.7%
Follow-up Mammogram/Ultrasound	182	3.3%	8.5%	8.8%
Lumbar Spine MRI for Low Back Pain[1]	-	-	37.4%	37.2%

Cobre Valley Regional Medical Center

5880 South Hospital Drive
Globe, AZ 85501
Phone: 928-425-3261
Fax: 928-425-7903
URL: www.cvchospital.com
Type: Critical Access Hospitals
Emergency Services: Yes
Ownership: Voluntary non-profit - Private
Beds: 49

Key Personnel:

Quality Assurance . . . . D Caldera
Radiology. . . . . James Collins
CEO/President. . . . . Jim Gingerich
Emergency Room . . . . Roberta Johnson, RN
Operating Room. . . . . Dana Miller, RN
Chief of Medical Staff. . . . . McClearen Ruesch

Measure	Cases	This Hosp.	State Avg.	U.S. Avg.
Blood Clot Prevention and Treatment				
Anticoagulation Overlap Therapy[5]	-	-	94%	93%
ICU Venous Thromboembolism Prophylaxis[5]	-	-	92%	92%
Incidence of Potentially Preventable VTE[5]	-	-	9%	10%
UFH with Dosages/Platelet Monitoring[5]	-	-	98%	97%
Venous Thromboembolism Prophylaxis[5]	-	-	88%	85%
Warfarin Therapy Discharge Instructions[5]	-	-	74%	75%
Chest Pain/Possible Heart Attack Care				
Aspirin Given Within 24 Hours of Arrival[5]	-	-	98%	96%
Fibrinolytic Meds Within 30 Min. of Arrival[5]	-	-	59%	58%
Average Time to ECG (minutes)[5]	-	-	6	7
Average Time to Transfer (minutes)[5]	-	-	48	60
Children's Asthma Care				
Received Home Management Plan of Care	-	-	-	88%
Received Reliever Medication	-	-	-	100%
Received Systemic Corticosteroids	-	-	-	100%
Emergency Department				
Admittance Decision Time (minutes)[5]	-	-	98	98
Head CT Results Within 45 Min. of Arrival[5]	-	-	64%	57%
Patients Who Left ER Before Being Seen[5]	-	-	2%	2%
Time from ER Arrival to Admit. (minutes)[5]	-	-	285	274
Time from ER Arrival to Discharge (minutes)[5]	-	-	162	134
Time in ER Before Being Evaluated (minutes)[5]	-	-	27	26
Time to Pain Meds for Fractures (minutes)[5]	-	-	58	57
Heart Attack Care				
Aspirin Given at Discharge[1]	-	-	99%	99%
Fibrinolytic Meds Within 30 Min. of Arrival[7]	-	-	67%	54%
PCI Within 90 Minutes of Arrival[7]	-	-	95%	96%
Statin Prescribed at Discharge[1]	-	-	98%	98%
Heart Failure Care				
ACE Inhibitor or ARB for LVSD[1]	-	-	98%	97%
Discharge Instructions Given	50	92%	94%	94%
Evaluation of LVS Function	68	100%	99%	99%
Medicare Spending				
Medicare Spending per Patient (ratio)	-	-	0.93	0.98
Pneumonia Care				
Appropriate Initial Antibiotic Given	75	99%	96%	95%
Blood Culture Timing	104	93%	97%	98%
Pregnancy and Delivery Care				
Newborn Deliveries Scheduled Early[5]	-	-	7%	6%
Preventive Care				
Immunization for Influenza[5]	-	-	91%	90%
Immunization for Pneumonia[5]	-	-	92%	92%
Stroke Care				
Anticoagulation Therapy for Atrial Fibrillation[5]	-	-	96%	95%
Antithrombotic Therapy Timing[5]	-	-	98%	98%
Assessed for Rehabilitation[5]	-	-	96%	97%
Discharged on Antithrombotic Therapy[5]	-	-	99%	99%
Discharged on Statin Medication[5]	-	-	94%	94%
Thrombolytic Therapy Timing[5]	-	-	81%	66%
Venous Thromboembolism Prophylaxis[5]	-	-	93%	94%
Written Stroke Educational Materials Given[5]	-	-	84%	88%
Surgical Care Improvement Project				
Appropriate Beta Blocker Usage	24	92%	97%	98%
Appropriate VTP Within 24 Hours	61	92%	98%	98%
Controlled Postoperative Blood Glucose[7]	-	-	96%	97%
Perioperative Temperature Management	73	97%	100%	100%
Prophylactic Antibiotic Selection	48	96%	99%	99%
Prophylactic Antibiotic Selection (Outpatient)[5]	-	-	98%	98%
Prophylactic Antibiotic Stopped	47	96%	98%	98%
Prophylactic Antibiotic Timing	48	96%	99%	99%
Prophylactic Antibiotic Timing (Outpatient)[5]	-	-	99%	98%
Urinary Catheter Removal	15	60%	97%	97%
Survey of Patients' Hospital Experiences				
Area Around Room 'Always' Quiet at Night	300+	51%	57%	61%
Doctors 'Always' Communicated Well	300+	77%	77%	82%
Home Recovery Information Given	300+	88%	86%	85%
Hospital Given 9 or 10 on 10 Point Scale	300+	68%	70%	71%
Meds 'Always' Explained Before Given	300+	57%	62%	64%
Nurses 'Always' Communicated Well	300+	76%	76%	79%
Pain 'Always' Well Controlled	300+	68%	69%	71%
Room and Bathroom 'Always' Clean	300+	73%	69%	73%
Timely Help 'Always' Received	300+	63%	65%	68%
Would Definitely Recommend Hospital	300+	65%	70%	71%

NOTE: Hospital profiles are in alphabetical order by state, then city, then hospital within the city; Rankings exclude hospitals with less than 25 cases except for patient surveys which excludes hospitals with less than 100 cases; (a) 100-299 cases; (1) The number of cases/patients is too few to report; (2) Data submitted were based on a sample of cases/patients; (3) Results are based on a shorter time period than required; (4) Data suppressed by CMS for one or more quarters; (5) Results are not available for this reporting period; (6) Fewer than 100 patients completed the HCAHPS survey; (7) No cases met the criteria for this measure; (8) The lower limit of the confidence interval cannot be calculated if the number of observed infections equals zero; (9) No data are available from the state/territory for this reporting period; (10) The scores shown reflect fewer than 50 completed surveys; (11) There were discrepancies in the data collection process; (12) This measure does not apply to this hospital for this reporting period; (13) Results cannot be calculated for this reporting period; (14) The results for this state are combined with nearby states to protect confidentiality; Please refer to the User's Guide for a full explanation of data.

Use of Medical Imaging				
Cardiac Imaging Stress Test before Surgery	129	2.3%	5.8%	5.3%
Combination Abdominal CT Scan	386	25.9%	9.1%	10.5%
Combination Brain/Sinus CT Scan	358	4.7%	3.2%	2.7%
Combination Chest CT Scan	127	39.4%	5.5%	2.7%
Follow-up Mammogram/Ultrasound	304	16.8%	8.5%	8.8%
Lumbar Spine MRI for Low Back Pain[1]	-	-	37.4%	37.2%

West Valley Hospital

13677 West Mcdowell Road | Phone: 623-882-1500
Goodyear, AZ 85395 | Fax: 623-848-5959
URL: www.wvhospital.com
Type: Acute Care Hospitals | Emergency Services: Yes
Ownership: Proprietary | Beds: 131

Key Personnel:
CEO/President. . . . . Jim Resendez

Measure	Cases	This Hosp.	State Avg.	U.S. Avg.
Blood Clot Prevention and Treatment				
Anticoagulation Overlap Therapy[2]	58	98%	94%	93%
ICU Venous Thromboembolism Prophylaxis[2]	68	90%	92%	92%
Incidence of Potentially Preventable VTE[2]	13	23%	9%	10%
UFH with Dosages/Platelet Monitoring[2]	35	97%	98%	97%
Venous Thromboembolism Prophylaxis[2]	356	89%	88%	85%
Warfarin Therapy Discharge Instructions[2]	41	93%	74%	75%
Chest Pain/Possible Heart Attack Care				
Aspirin Given Within 24 Hours of Arrival	36	100%	98%	96%
Fibrinolytic Meds Within 30 Min. of Arrival[3,7]	-	-	59%	58%
Average Time to ECG (minutes)	36	1	6	7
Average Time to Transfer (minutes)[3,7]	-	-	48	60
Children's Asthma Care				
Received Home Management Plan of Care	-	-	-	88%
Received Reliever Medication	-	-	-	100%
Received Systemic Corticosteroids	-	-	-	100%
Emergency Department				
Admittance Decision Time (minutes)[2]	810	113	98	98
Head CT Results Within 45 Min. of Arrival	17	94%	64%	57%
Patients Who Left ER Before Being Seen	70,277	0%	2%	2%
Time from ER Arrival to Admit. (minutes)[2]	815	253	285	274
Time from ER Arrival to Discharge (minutes)	411	122	162	134
Time in ER Before Being Evaluated (minutes)	430	26	27	26
Time to Pain Meds for Fractures (minutes)	251	44	58	57
Heart Attack Care				
Aspirin Given at Discharge	226	100%	99%	99%
Fibrinolytic Meds Within 30 Min. of Arrival[7]	-	-	67%	54%
PCI Within 90 Minutes of Arrival	58	98%	95%	96%
Statin Prescribed at Discharge	222	99%	98%	98%
Heart Failure Care				
ACE Inhibitor or ARB for LVSD	88	98%	98%	97%
Discharge Instructions Given	198	100%	94%	94%
Evaluation of LVS Function	220	100%	99%	99%
Medicare Spending				
Medicare Spending per Patient (ratio)	-	0.97	0.93	0.98
Pneumonia Care				
Appropriate Initial Antibiotic Given	268	99%	96%	95%
Blood Culture Timing	375	99%	97%	98%
Pregnancy and Delivery Care				
Newborn Deliveries Scheduled Early[2]	46	7%	7%	6%
Preventive Care				
Immunization for Influenza[2]	534	97%	91%	90%
Immunization for Pneumonia[2]	590	98%	92%	92%
Stroke Care				
Anticoagulation Therapy for Atrial Fibrillation[1]	-	-	96%	95%
Antithrombotic Therapy Timing	91	98%	98%	98%
Assessed for Rehabilitation	94	94%	96%	97%
Discharged on Antithrombotic Therapy	92	100%	99%	99%
Discharged on Statin Medication	73	100%	94%	94%
Thrombolytic Therapy Timing[1]	-	-	81%	66%
Venous Thromboembolism Prophylaxis	101	89%	93%	94%
Written Stroke Educational Materials Given	69	99%	84%	88%
Surgical Care Improvement Project				
Appropriate Beta Blocker Usage[2]	87	95%	97%	98%
Appropriate VTP Within 24 Hours[2]	156	97%	98%	98%
Controlled Postoperative Blood Glucose[2]	65	100%	96%	97%
Perioperative Temperature Management[2]	228	100%	100%	100%
Prophylactic Antibiotic Selection[2]	148	99%	99%	99%
Prophylactic Antibiotic Selection (Outpatient)	142	98%	98%	98%
Prophylactic Antibiotic Stopped[2]	135	99%	98%	98%
Prophylactic Antibiotic Timing[2]	149	99%	99%	99%
Prophylactic Antibiotic Timing (Outpatient)	143	98%	99%	98%
Urinary Catheter Removal[2]	120	97%	97%	97%
Survey of Patients' Hospital Experiences				
Area Around Room 'Always' Quiet at Night[11]	300+	56%	57%	61%
Doctors 'Always' Communicated Well[11]	300+	74%	77%	82%
Home Recovery Information Given[11]	300+	84%	86%	85%
Hospital Given 9 or 10 on 10 Point Scale[11]	300+	64%	70%	71%
Meds 'Always' Explained Before Given[11]	300+	59%	62%	64%
Nurses 'Always' Communicated Well[11]	300+	74%	76%	79%
Pain 'Always' Well Controlled[11]	300+	69%	69%	71%
Room and Bathroom 'Always' Clean[11]	300+	59%	69%	73%
Timely Help 'Always' Received[11]	300+	61%	65%	68%
Would Definitely Recommend Hospital[11]	300+	64%	70%	71%
Use of Medical Imaging				
Cardiac Imaging Stress Test before Surgery	66	3.0%	5.8%	5.3%
Combination Abdominal CT Scan	396	2.3%	9.1%	10.5%
Combination Brain/Sinus CT Scan[1]	-	-	3.2%	2.7%
Combination Chest CT Scan	97	1.0%	5.5%	2.7%
Follow-up Mammogram/Ultrasound[7]	-	-	8.5%	8.8%
Lumbar Spine MRI for Low Back Pain[1]	-	-	37.4%	37.2%

Kingman Regional Medical Center

3269 Stockton Hill Road | Phone: 928-757-2101
Kingman, AZ 86409 | Fax: 928-757-0604
URL: www.azkrmc.com
Type: Acute Care Hospitals | Emergency Services: Yes
Ownership: Govt - Hospital Dist/Auth | Beds: 213

Key Personnel:
Radiology. . . . . William R Burge, MD
Quality Assurance . . . . Karol Collison
Emergency Room . . . . Janet Gode
Pediatric Ambulatory Care . . . . . . Ahmad Saeed Khan, MD
Operating Room. . . . . M Azam Khan
CEO/President. . . . . Brian Turney

Measure	Cases	This Hosp.	State Avg.	U.S. Avg.
Blood Clot Prevention and Treatment				
Anticoagulation Overlap Therapy[2]	82	93%	94%	93%
ICU Venous Thromboembolism Prophylaxis[2]	63	79%	92%	92%
Incidence of Potentially Preventable VTE[1,2]	-	-	9%	10%
UFH with Dosages/Platelet Monitoring[2]	37	24%	98%	97%
Venous Thromboembolism Prophylaxis[2]	408	74%	88%	85%
Warfarin Therapy Discharge Instructions[2]	48	25%	74%	75%
Chest Pain/Possible Heart Attack Care				
Aspirin Given Within 24 Hours of Arrival[1,3]	-	-	98%	96%
Fibrinolytic Meds Within 30 Min. of Arrival[5]	-	-	59%	58%
Average Time to ECG (minutes)[1,3]	-	-	6	7
Average Time to Transfer (minutes)[5]	-	-	48	60
Children's Asthma Care				
Received Home Management Plan of Care	-	-	-	88%
Received Reliever Medication	-	-	-	100%
Received Systemic Corticosteroids	-	-	-	100%
Emergency Department				
Admittance Decision Time (minutes)[2]	844	88	98	98
Head CT Results Within 45 Min. of Arrival	15	87%	64%	57%
Patients Who Left ER Before Being Seen	47,689	2%	2%	2%
Time from ER Arrival to Admit. (minutes)[2]	889	247	285	274
Time from ER Arrival to Discharge (minutes)	520	133	162	134
Time in ER Before Being Evaluated (minutes)	562	45	27	26
Time to Pain Meds for Fractures (minutes)	107	49	58	57
Heart Attack Care				
Aspirin Given at Discharge[2]	156	99%	99%	99%
Fibrinolytic Meds Within 30 Min. of Arrival[2,7]	-	-	67%	54%
PCI Within 90 Minutes of Arrival[2]	44	84%	95%	96%
Statin Prescribed at Discharge[2]	152	93%	98%	98%
Heart Failure Care				
ACE Inhibitor or ARB for LVSD[2]	109	94%	98%	97%
Discharge Instructions Given[2]	238	84%	94%	94%
Evaluation of LVS Function[2]	262	98%	99%	99%
Medicare Spending				
Medicare Spending per Patient (ratio)	-	0.91	0.93	0.98
Pneumonia Care				
Appropriate Initial Antibiotic Given[2]	244	98%	96%	95%
Blood Culture Timing[2]	452	99%	97%	98%
Pregnancy and Delivery Care				
Newborn Deliveries Scheduled Early[2]	58	0%	7%	6%
Preventive Care				
Immunization for Influenza[2]	551	89%	91%	90%
Immunization for Pneumonia[2]	815	91%	92%	92%
Stroke Care				
Anticoagulation Therapy for Atrial Fibrillation[1,2]	-	-	96%	95%
Antithrombotic Therapy Timing[2]	56	96%	98%	98%
Assessed for Rehabilitation[2]	53	91%	96%	97%
Discharged on Antithrombotic Therapy[2]	53	96%	99%	99%
Discharged on Statin Medication[2]	38	82%	94%	94%
Thrombolytic Therapy Timing[1,2]	-	-	81%	66%
Venous Thromboembolism Prophylaxis[2]	60	67%	93%	94%
Written Stroke Educational Materials Given[2]	38	24%	84%	88%
Surgical Care Improvement Project				
Appropriate Beta Blocker Usage[2]	155	94%	97%	98%
Appropriate VTP Within 24 Hours[2]	304	97%	98%	98%
Controlled Postoperative Blood Glucose[2]	53	94%	96%	97%
Perioperative Temperature Management[2]	366	100%	100%	100%
Prophylactic Antibiotic Selection[2]	260	97%	99%	99%
Prophylactic Antibiotic Selection (Outpatient)	131	97%	98%	98%
Prophylactic Antibiotic Stopped[2]	244	94%	98%	98%
Prophylactic Antibiotic Timing[2]	260	99%	99%	99%
Prophylactic Antibiotic Timing (Outpatient)	133	97%	99%	98%
Urinary Catheter Removal[2]	229	90%	97%	97%
Survey of Patients' Hospital Experiences				
Area Around Room 'Always' Quiet at Night	300+	57%	57%	61%
Doctors 'Always' Communicated Well	300+	72%	77%	82%
Home Recovery Information Given	300+	85%	86%	85%
Hospital Given 9 or 10 on 10 Point Scale	300+	65%	70%	71%
Meds 'Always' Explained Before Given	300+	60%	62%	64%
Nurses 'Always' Communicated Well	300+	76%	76%	79%
Pain 'Always' Well Controlled	300+	67%	69%	71%
Room and Bathroom 'Always' Clean	300+	70%	69%	73%
Timely Help 'Always' Received	300+	63%	65%	68%
Would Definitely Recommend Hospital	300+	66%	70%	71%
Use of Medical Imaging				
Cardiac Imaging Stress Test before Surgery	436	4.1%	5.8%	5.3%
Combination Abdominal CT Scan	1,144	15.5%	9.1%	10.5%
Combination Brain/Sinus CT Scan	865	2.3%	3.2%	2.7%
Combination Chest CT Scan	783	14.6%	5.5%	2.7%
Follow-up Mammogram/Ultrasound	1,610	8.1%	8.5%	8.8%
Lumbar Spine MRI for Low Back Pain	110	25.5%	37.4%	37.2%

Havasu Regional Medical Center

101 Civic Center Lane | Phone: 928-855-8185
Lake Havasu City, AZ 86403 | Fax: 928-505-5744
URL: www.havasuregional.com
Type: Acute Care Hospitals | Emergency Services: Yes
Ownership: Proprietary | Beds: 138

Key Personnel:
Emergency Room . . . . Andrew Brenner
CEO . . . . Dana Ellerbe
Chief of Medical Staff. . . . . Douglas Hade
Operating Room. . . . . Nicholas Rizzo, RN
CEO/President. . . . . Dorothy Sawyer

Measure	Cases	This Hosp.	State Avg.	U.S. Avg.
Blood Clot Prevention and Treatment				
Anticoagulation Overlap Therapy[2]	67	96%	94%	93%
ICU Venous Thromboembolism Prophylaxis[2]	48	100%	92%	92%
Incidence of Potentially Preventable VTE[1,2]	-	-	9%	10%
UFH with Dosages/Platelet Monitoring[2]	11	100%	98%	97%
Venous Thromboembolism Prophylaxis[2]	320	99%	88%	85%
Warfarin Therapy Discharge Instructions[2]	59	100%	74%	75%
Chest Pain/Possible Heart Attack Care				
Aspirin Given Within 24 Hours of Arrival[1,3]	-	-	98%	96%
Fibrinolytic Meds Within 30 Min. of Arrival[3,7]	-	-	59%	58%
Average Time to ECG (minutes)[1,3]	-	-	6	7
Average Time to Transfer (minutes)[3,7]	-	-	48	60

NOTE: Hospital profiles are in alphabetical order by state, then city, then hospital within the city; Rankings exclude hospitals with less than 25 cases except for patient surveys which excludes hospitals with less than 100 cases; (a) 100-299 cases; (1) The number of cases/patients is too few to report; (2) Data submitted were based on a sample of cases/patients; (3) Results are based on a shorter time period than required; (4) Data suppressed by CMS for one or more quarters; (5) Results are not available for this reporting period; (6) Fewer than 100 patients completed the HCAHPS survey; (7) No cases met the criteria for this measure; (8) The lower limit of the confidence interval cannot be calculated if the number of observed infections equals zero; (9) No data are available from the state/territory for this reporting period; (10) The scores shown reflect fewer than 50 completed surveys; (11) There were discrepancies in the data collection process; (12) This measure does not apply to this hospital for this reporting period; (13) Results cannot be calculated for this reporting period; (14) The results for this state are combined with nearby states to protect confidentiality; Please refer to the User's Guide for a full explanation of data.

Measure	Cases	This Hosp.	State Avg.	U.S. Avg.
Children's Asthma Care				
Received Home Management Plan of Care	-	-	-	88%
Received Reliever Medication	-	-	-	100%
Received Systemic Corticosteroids	-	-	-	100%
Emergency Department				
Admittance Decision Time (minutes)[2]	686	104	98	98
Head CT Results Within 45 Min. of Arrival	23	78%	64%	57%
Patients Who Left ER Before Being Seen	24,869	1%	2%	2%
Time from ER Arrival to Admit. (minutes)[2]	687	262	285	274
Time from ER Arrival to Discharge (minutes)	383	135	162	134
Time in ER Before Being Evaluated (minutes)	443	15	27	26
Time to Pain Meds for Fractures (minutes)	99	48	58	57
Heart Attack Care				
Aspirin Given at Discharge	164	99%	99%	99%
Fibrinolytic Meds Within 30 Min. of Arrival[7]	-	-	67%	54%
PCI Within 90 Minutes of Arrival	37	92%	95%	96%
Statin Prescribed at Discharge	159	99%	98%	98%
Heart Failure Care				
ACE Inhibitor or ARB for LVSD	42	100%	98%	97%
Discharge Instructions Given	152	99%	94%	94%
Evaluation of LVS Function	162	100%	99%	99%
Medicare Spending				
Medicare Spending per Patient (ratio)	-	0.88	0.93	0.98
Pneumonia Care				
Appropriate Initial Antibiotic Given	136	99%	96%	95%
Blood Culture Timing	213	97%	97%	98%
Pregnancy and Delivery Care				
Newborn Deliveries Scheduled Early[2]	32	16%	7%	6%
Preventive Care				
Immunization for Influenza[2]	548	99%	91%	90%
Immunization for Pneumonia[2]	803	99%	92%	92%
Stroke Care				
Anticoagulation Therapy for Atrial Fibrillation[1]	-	-	96%	95%
Antithrombotic Therapy Timing	73	100%	98%	98%
Assessed for Rehabilitation	74	96%	96%	97%
Discharged on Antithrombotic Therapy	72	100%	99%	99%
Discharged on Statin Medication	49	100%	94%	94%
Thrombolytic Therapy Timing[7]	-	-	81%	66%
Venous Thromboembolism Prophylaxis	75	100%	93%	94%
Written Stroke Educational Materials Given	47	100%	84%	88%
Surgical Care Improvement Project				
Appropriate Beta Blocker Usage[2]	175	95%	97%	98%
Appropriate VTP Within 24 Hours[2]	355	99%	98%	98%
Controlled Postoperative Blood Glucose[2]	119	98%	96%	97%
Perioperative Temperature Management[2]	424	100%	100%	100%
Prophylactic Antibiotic Selection[2]	392	97%	99%	99%
Prophylactic Antibiotic Selection (Outpatient)	262	99%	98%	98%
Prophylactic Antibiotic Stopped[2]	378	99%	98%	98%
Prophylactic Antibiotic Timing[2]	394	99%	99%	99%
Prophylactic Antibiotic Timing (Outpatient)	248	100%	99%	98%
Urinary Catheter Removal[2]	378	98%	97%	97%
Survey of Patients' Hospital Experiences				
Area Around Room 'Always' Quiet at Night	300+	49%	57%	61%
Doctors 'Always' Communicated Well	300+	73%	77%	82%
Home Recovery Information Given	300+	84%	86%	85%
Hospital Given 9 or 10 on 10 Point Scale	300+	57%	70%	71%
Meds 'Always' Explained Before Given	300+	53%	62%	64%
Nurses 'Always' Communicated Well	300+	70%	76%	79%
Pain 'Always' Well Controlled	300+	62%	69%	71%
Room and Bathroom 'Always' Clean	300+	59%	69%	73%
Timely Help 'Always' Received	300+	52%	65%	68%
Would Definitely Recommend Hospital	300+	57%	70%	71%
Use of Medical Imaging				
Cardiac Imaging Stress Test before Surgery	410	2.9%	5.8%	5.3%
Combination Abdominal CT Scan	953	9.4%	9.1%	10.5%
Combination Brain/Sinus CT Scan	841	1.8%	3.2%	2.7%
Combination Chest CT Scan	595	2.5%	5.5%	2.7%
Follow-up Mammogram/Ultrasound	1,770	2.1%	8.5%	8.8%
Lumbar Spine MRI for Low Back Pain	129	36.4%	37.4%	37.2%

Arizona Spine & Joint Hospital

4620 East Baseline Road
Mesa, AZ 85206
Phone: 480-832-4770
Fax: 480-824-1269
E-mail: mail@azspineandjoint.com
URL: www.azspineandjoint.com
Type: Acute Care Hospitals
Emergency Services: No
Ownership: Proprietary
Beds: 18

Key Personnel:
CEO/President. . . . . Kristi McShay

Measure	Cases	This Hosp.	State Avg.	U.S. Avg.
Blood Clot Prevention and Treatment				
Anticoagulation Overlap Therapy[2,7]	-	-	94%	93%
ICU Venous Thromboembolism Prophylaxis[2,7]	-	-	92%	92%
Incidence of Potentially Preventable VTE[2,7]	-	-	9%	10%
UFH with Dosages/Platelet Monitoring[2,7]	-	-	98%	97%
Venous Thromboembolism Prophylaxis[2,7]	-	-	88%	85%
Warfarin Therapy Discharge Instructions[2,7]	-	-	74%	75%
Chest Pain/Possible Heart Attack Care				
Aspirin Given Within 24 Hours of Arrival[5]	-	-	98%	96%
Fibrinolytic Meds Within 30 Min. of Arrival[5]	-	-	59%	58%
Average Time to ECG (minutes)[5]	-	-	6	7
Average Time to Transfer (minutes)[5]	-	-	48	60
Children's Asthma Care				
Received Home Management Plan of Care	-	-	-	88%
Received Reliever Medication	-	-	-	100%
Received Systemic Corticosteroids	-	-	-	100%
Emergency Department				
Admittance Decision Time (minutes)[7]	-	-	98	98
Head CT Results Within 45 Min. of Arrival[5]	-	-	64%	57%
Patients Who Left ER Before Being Seen[1]	-	-	2%	2%
Time from ER Arrival to Admit. (minutes)[7]	-	-	285	274
Time from ER Arrival to Discharge (minutes)[5]	-	-	162	134
Time in ER Before Being Evaluated (minutes)[5]	-	-	27	26
Time to Pain Meds for Fractures (minutes)[5]	-	-	58	57
Heart Attack Care				
Aspirin Given at Discharge[5]	-	-	99%	99%
Fibrinolytic Meds Within 30 Min. of Arrival[5]	-	-	67%	54%
PCI Within 90 Minutes of Arrival[5]	-	-	95%	96%
Statin Prescribed at Discharge[5]	-	-	98%	98%
Heart Failure Care				
ACE Inhibitor or ARB for LVSD[5]	-	-	98%	97%
Discharge Instructions Given[5]	-	-	94%	94%
Evaluation of LVS Function[5]	-	-	99%	99%
Medicare Spending				
Medicare Spending per Patient (ratio)	-	0.94	0.93	0.98
Pneumonia Care				
Appropriate Initial Antibiotic Given[5]	-	-	96%	95%
Blood Culture Timing[5]	-	-	97%	98%
Pregnancy and Delivery Care				
Newborn Deliveries Scheduled Early[7]	-	-	7%	6%
Preventive Care				
Immunization for Influenza	425	100%	91%	90%
Immunization for Pneumonia[2]	497	100%	92%	92%
Stroke Care				
Anticoagulation Therapy for Atrial Fibrillation[5]	-	-	96%	95%
Antithrombotic Therapy Timing[5]	-	-	98%	98%
Assessed for Rehabilitation[5]	-	-	96%	97%
Discharged on Antithrombotic Therapy[5]	-	-	99%	99%
Discharged on Statin Medication[5]	-	-	94%	94%
Thrombolytic Therapy Timing[5]	-	-	81%	66%
Venous Thromboembolism Prophylaxis[5]	-	-	93%	94%
Written Stroke Educational Materials Given[5]	-	-	84%	88%
Surgical Care Improvement Project				
Appropriate Beta Blocker Usage[2]	37	100%	97%	98%
Appropriate VTP Within 24 Hours[2]	151	100%	98%	98%
Controlled Postoperative Blood Glucose[2,7]	-	-	96%	97%
Perioperative Temperature Management[2]	180	100%	100%	100%
Prophylactic Antibiotic Selection[2]	137	100%	99%	99%
Prophylactic Antibiotic Selection (Outpatient)	37	100%	98%	98%
Prophylactic Antibiotic Stopped[2]	136	100%	98%	98%
Prophylactic Antibiotic Timing[2]	137	99%	99%	99%
Prophylactic Antibiotic Timing (Outpatient)	37	100%	99%	98%
Urinary Catheter Removal[2]	103	98%	97%	97%
Survey of Patients' Hospital Experiences				
Area Around Room 'Always' Quiet at Night	300+	70%	57%	61%
Doctors 'Always' Communicated Well	300+	82%	77%	82%
Home Recovery Information Given	300+	92%	86%	85%
Hospital Given 9 or 10 on 10 Point Scale	300+	85%	70%	71%
Meds 'Always' Explained Before Given	300+	75%	62%	64%
Nurses 'Always' Communicated Well	300+	84%	76%	79%
Pain 'Always' Well Controlled	300+	71%	69%	71%
Room and Bathroom 'Always' Clean	300+	81%	69%	73%
Timely Help 'Always' Received	300+	79%	65%	68%
Would Definitely Recommend Hospital	300+	87%	70%	71%
Use of Medical Imaging				
Cardiac Imaging Stress Test before Surgery[7]	-	-	5.8%	5.3%
Combination Abdominal CT Scan[7]	-	-	9.1%	10.5%
Combination Brain/Sinus CT Scan[7]	-	-	3.2%	2.7%
Combination Chest CT Scan[7]	-	-	5.5%	2.7%
Follow-up Mammogram/Ultrasound[7]	-	-	8.5%	8.8%
Lumbar Spine MRI for Low Back Pain[7]	-	-	37.4%	37.2%

Banner Baywood Medical Center

6644 East Baywood Avenue
Mesa, AZ 85206
Phone: 480-321-2000
Fax: 480-981-4198
URL: www.bannerhealth.com
Type: Acute Care Hospitals
Emergency Services: No
Ownership: Voluntary non-profit - Private
Beds: 239

Key Personnel:
Quality Assurance . . . . Ellen Campbell
CEO/President. . . . . Don Evans
Operating Room. . . . . Chris Halowell
Chief of Medical Staff . . . . Larry Stratling

Measure	Cases	This Hosp.	State Avg.	U.S. Avg.
Blood Clot Prevention and Treatment				
Anticoagulation Overlap Therapy[2]	209	93%	94%	93%
ICU Venous Thromboembolism Prophylaxis[2]	33	97%	92%	92%
Incidence of Potentially Preventable VTE[2]	33	9%	9%	10%
UFH with Dosages/Platelet Monitoring[2]	207	100%	98%	97%
Venous Thromboembolism Prophylaxis[2]	371	91%	88%	85%
Warfarin Therapy Discharge Instructions[2]	156	48%	74%	75%
Chest Pain/Possible Heart Attack Care				
Aspirin Given Within 24 Hours of Arrival	531	99%	98%	96%
Fibrinolytic Meds Within 30 Min. of Arrival[1]	-	-	59%	58%
Average Time to ECG (minutes)	548	6	6	7
Average Time to Transfer (minutes)	48	38	48	60
Children's Asthma Care				
Received Home Management Plan of Care	-	-	-	88%
Received Reliever Medication	-	-	-	100%
Received Systemic Corticosteroids	-	-	-	100%
Emergency Department				
Admittance Decision Time (minutes)[2]	809	67	98	98
Head CT Results Within 45 Min. of Arrival	21	81%	64%	57%
Patients Who Left ER Before Being Seen	55,856	1%	2%	2%
Time from ER Arrival to Admit. (minutes)[2]	817	271	285	274
Time from ER Arrival to Discharge (minutes)	306	189	162	134
Time in ER Before Being Evaluated (minutes)	390	17	27	26
Time to Pain Meds for Fractures (minutes)	127	67	58	57
Heart Attack Care				
Aspirin Given at Discharge	11	100%	99%	99%
Fibrinolytic Meds Within 30 Min. of Arrival[7]	-	-	67%	54%
PCI Within 90 Minutes of Arrival[7]	-	-	95%	96%
Statin Prescribed at Discharge	11	91%	98%	98%
Heart Failure Care				
ACE Inhibitor or ARB for LVSD[2]	53	98%	98%	97%
Discharge Instructions Given[2]	158	96%	94%	94%
Evaluation of LVS Function[2]	204	100%	99%	99%
Medicare Spending				
Medicare Spending per Patient (ratio)	-	0.98	0.93	0.98
Pneumonia Care				
Appropriate Initial Antibiotic Given[2]	105	98%	96%	95%
Blood Culture Timing[2]	131	99%	97%	98%
Pregnancy and Delivery Care				
Newborn Deliveries Scheduled Early[2]	59	15%	7%	6%
Preventive Care				
Immunization for Influenza[2]	567	97%	91%	90%

NOTE: Hospital profiles are in alphabetical order by state, then city, then hospital within the city; Rankings exclude hospitals with less than 25 cases except for patient surveys which excludes hospitals with less than 100 cases; (a) 100-299 cases; (1) The number of cases/patients is too few to report; (2) Data submitted were based on a sample of cases/patients; (3) Results are based on a shorter time period than required; (4) Data suppressed by CMS for one or more quarters; (5) Results are not available for this reporting period; (6) Fewer than 100 patients completed the HCAHPS survey; (7) No cases met the criteria for this measure; (8) The lower limit of the confidence interval cannot be calculated if the number of observed infections equals zero; (9) No data are available from the state/territory for this reporting period; (10) The scores shown reflect fewer than 50 completed surveys; (11) There were discrepancies in the data collection process; (12) This measure does not apply to this hospital for this reporting period; (13) Results cannot be calculated for this reporting period; (14) The results for this state are combined with nearby states to protect confidentiality; Please refer to the User's Guide for a full explanation of data.

Measure	Cases	This Hosp.	State Avg.	U.S. Avg.
Immunization for Pneumonia[2]	895	97%	92%	92%
Stroke Care				
Anticoagulation Therapy for Atrial Fibrillation[2]	28	93%	96%	95%
Antithrombotic Therapy Timing[2]	121	98%	98%	98%
Assessed for Rehabilitation[2]	108	91%	96%	97%
Discharged on Antithrombotic Therapy[2]	105	99%	99%	99%
Discharged on Statin Medication[2]	75	93%	94%	94%
Thrombolytic Therapy Timing[1,2]	-	-	81%	66%
Venous Thromboembolism Prophylaxis[2]	134	91%	93%	94%
Written Stroke Educational Materials Given[2]	61	66%	84%	88%
Surgical Care Improvement Project				
Appropriate Beta Blocker Usage[2]	121	94%	97%	98%
Appropriate VTP Within 24 Hours[2]	337	98%	98%	98%
Controlled Postoperative Blood Glucose[2,7]	-	-	96%	97%
Perioperative Temperature Management[2]	417	100%	100%	100%
Prophylactic Antibiotic Selection[2]	279	100%	99%	99%
Prophylactic Antibiotic Selection (Outpatient)	261	97%	98%	98%
Prophylactic Antibiotic Stopped[2]	268	96%	98%	98%
Prophylactic Antibiotic Timing[2]	280	99%	99%	99%
Prophylactic Antibiotic Timing (Outpatient)	264	98%	99%	98%
Urinary Catheter Removal[2]	154	97%	97%	97%
Survey of Patients' Hospital Experiences				
Area Around Room 'Always' Quiet at Night[11]	300+	50%	57%	61%
Doctors 'Always' Communicated Well[11]	300+	78%	77%	82%
Home Recovery Information Given[11]	300+	89%	86%	85%
Hospital Given 9 or 10 on 10 Point Scale[11]	300+	70%	70%	71%
Meds 'Always' Explained Before Given[11]	300+	65%	62%	64%
Nurses 'Always' Communicated Well[11]	300+	78%	76%	79%
Pain 'Always' Well Controlled[11]	300+	69%	69%	71%
Room and Bathroom 'Always' Clean[11]	300+	65%	69%	73%
Timely Help 'Always' Received[11]	300+	62%	65%	68%
Would Definitely Recommend Hospital[11]	300+	74%	70%	71%
Use of Medical Imaging				
Cardiac Imaging Stress Test before Surgery	264	7.6%	5.8%	5.3%
Combination Abdominal CT Scan	909	1.9%	9.1%	10.5%
Combination Brain/Sinus CT Scan	1,156	1.9%	3.2%	2.7%
Combination Chest CT Scan	422	0.7%	5.5%	2.7%
Follow-up Mammogram/Ultrasound	967	15.8%	8.5%	8.8%
Lumbar Spine MRI for Low Back Pain[1]	-	-	37.4%	37.2%

Banner Desert Medical Center

1400 South Dobson Road
Mesa, AZ 85202
URL: www.bannerhealth.com
Phone: 480-412-3000
Fax: 480-835-8711
Type: Acute Care Hospitals
Emergency Services: Yes
Ownership: Voluntary non-profit - Private
Beds: 549

Key Personnel:

CEO . . . . Rob Gould
Chief of Medical Staff. . . . . Joseph Gutman, MD
Radiology. . . . . M Kornreich, MD
Pediatric In-Patient Care . . . . Jamed Leiferman
Infection Control. . . . . Patt Madson
Anesthesiology. . . . . Barry Miller
CEO/President. . . . . Bruce Pearson, FACHE
Operating Room. . . . . Susan Vitort

Measure	Cases	This Hosp.	State Avg.	U.S. Avg.
Blood Clot Prevention and Treatment				
Anticoagulation Overlap Therapy[2]	168	94%	94%	93%
ICU Venous Thromboembolism Prophylaxis[2]	36	94%	92%	92%
Incidence of Potentially Preventable VTE[2]	31	10%	9%	10%
UFH with Dosages/Platelet Monitoring[2]	110	96%	98%	97%
Venous Thromboembolism Prophylaxis[2]	359	86%	88%	85%
Warfarin Therapy Discharge Instructions[2]	134	56%	74%	75%
Chest Pain/Possible Heart Attack Care				
Aspirin Given Within 24 Hours of Arrival[1,3]	-	-	98%	96%
Fibrinolytic Meds Within 30 Min. of Arrival[3,7]	-	-	59%	58%
Average Time to ECG (minutes)[1,3]	-	-	6	7
Average Time to Transfer (minutes)[3,7]	-	-	48	60
Children's Asthma Care				
Received Home Management Plan of Care[2]	271	95%	-	88%
Received Reliever Medication[2]	272	100%	-	100%
Received Systemic Corticosteroids[2]	269	100%	-	100%
Emergency Department				
Admittance Decision Time (minutes)[2]	551	75	98	98
Head CT Results Within 45 Min. of Arrival	19	68%	64%	57%
Patients Who Left ER Before Being Seen	>100k	1%	2%	2%
Time from ER Arrival to Admit. (minutes)[2]	566	245	285	274
Time from ER Arrival to Discharge (minutes)	332	191	162	134
Time in ER Before Being Evaluated (minutes)	394	26	27	26
Time to Pain Meds for Fractures (minutes)	411	42	58	57
Heart Attack Care				
Aspirin Given at Discharge[2]	263	100%	99%	99%
Fibrinolytic Meds Within 30 Min. of Arrival[2,7]	-	-	67%	54%
PCI Within 90 Minutes of Arrival[2]	43	93%	95%	96%
Statin Prescribed at Discharge[2]	257	100%	98%	98%
Heart Failure Care				
ACE Inhibitor or ARB for LVSD[2]	114	100%	98%	97%
Discharge Instructions Given[2]	236	97%	94%	94%
Evaluation of LVS Function[2]	288	100%	99%	99%
Medicare Spending				
Medicare Spending per Patient (ratio)	-	0.98	0.93	0.98
Pneumonia Care				
Appropriate Initial Antibiotic Given[2]	93	100%	96%	95%
Blood Culture Timing[2]	91	99%	97%	98%
Pregnancy and Delivery Care				
Newborn Deliveries Scheduled Early[2]	68	4%	7%	6%
Preventive Care				
Immunization for Influenza[2]	492	98%	91%	90%
Immunization for Pneumonia[2]	468	94%	92%	92%
Stroke Care				
Anticoagulation Therapy for Atrial Fibrillation[2]	12	100%	96%	95%
Antithrombotic Therapy Timing[2]	87	99%	98%	98%
Assessed for Rehabilitation[2]	107	95%	96%	97%
Discharged on Antithrombotic Therapy[2]	97	99%	99%	99%
Discharged on Statin Medication[2]	73	90%	94%	94%
Thrombolytic Therapy Timing[2]	15	80%	81%	66%
Venous Thromboembolism Prophylaxis[2]	105	89%	93%	94%
Written Stroke Educational Materials Given[2]	68	76%	84%	88%
Surgical Care Improvement Project				
Appropriate Beta Blocker Usage[2]	187	95%	97%	98%
Appropriate VTP Within 24 Hours[2]	359	97%	98%	98%
Controlled Postoperative Blood Glucose[2]	118	92%	96%	97%
Perioperative Temperature Management[2]	475	100%	100%	100%
Prophylactic Antibiotic Selection[2]	437	99%	99%	99%
Prophylactic Antibiotic Selection (Outpatient)	638	100%	98%	98%
Prophylactic Antibiotic Stopped[2]	421	97%	98%	98%
Prophylactic Antibiotic Timing[2]	438	99%	99%	99%
Prophylactic Antibiotic Timing (Outpatient)	638	100%	99%	98%
Urinary Catheter Removal[2]	218	100%	97%	97%
Survey of Patients' Hospital Experiences				
Area Around Room 'Always' Quiet at Night[11]	300+	55%	57%	61%
Doctors 'Always' Communicated Well[11]	300+	78%	77%	82%
Home Recovery Information Given[11]	300+	89%	86%	85%
Hospital Given 9 or 10 on 10 Point Scale[11]	300+	71%	70%	71%
Meds 'Always' Explained Before Given[11]	300+	63%	62%	64%
Nurses 'Always' Communicated Well[11]	300+	76%	76%	79%
Pain 'Always' Well Controlled[11]	300+	69%	69%	71%
Room and Bathroom 'Always' Clean[11]	300+	63%	69%	73%
Timely Help 'Always' Received[11]	300+	63%	65%	68%
Would Definitely Recommend Hospital[11]	300+	74%	70%	71%
Use of Medical Imaging				
Cardiac Imaging Stress Test before Surgery[1]	-	-	5.8%	5.3%
Combination Abdominal CT Scan	480	1.5%	9.1%	10.5%
Combination Brain/Sinus CT Scan	676	6.8%	3.2%	2.7%
Combination Chest CT Scan	125	0.8%	5.5%	2.7%
Follow-up Mammogram/Ultrasound[7]	-	-	8.5%	8.8%
Lumbar Spine MRI for Low Back Pain[1]	-	-	37.4%	37.2%

Banner Heart Hospital

6750 East Baywood Avenue
Mesa, AZ 85206
URL: www.bannerhealth.com
Phone: 480-854-5050
Type: Acute Care Hospitals
Emergency Services: No
Ownership: Voluntary non-profit - Private

Key Personnel:

Operating Room. . . . . John Rajczyk
CEO . . . . Laura Robertson

Measure	Cases	This Hosp.	State Avg.	U.S. Avg.
Blood Clot Prevention and Treatment				
Anticoagulation Overlap Therapy[2]	41	95%	94%	93%
ICU Venous Thromboembolism Prophylaxis[2]	135	86%	92%	92%
Incidence of Potentially Preventable VTE[1,2]	-	-	9%	10%
UFH with Dosages/Platelet Monitoring[2]	40	100%	98%	97%
Venous Thromboembolism Prophylaxis[2]	296	90%	88%	85%
Warfarin Therapy Discharge Instructions[2]	34	53%	74%	75%
Chest Pain/Possible Heart Attack Care				
Aspirin Given Within 24 Hours of Arrival[5]	-	-	98%	96%
Fibrinolytic Meds Within 30 Min. of Arrival[5]	-	-	59%	58%
Average Time to ECG (minutes)[5]	-	-	6	7
Average Time to Transfer (minutes)[5]	-	-	48	60
Children's Asthma Care				
Received Home Management Plan of Care	-	-	-	88%
Received Reliever Medication	-	-	-	100%
Received Systemic Corticosteroids	-	-	-	100%
Emergency Department				
Admittance Decision Time (minutes)[2,7]	-	-	98	98
Head CT Results Within 45 Min. of Arrival[5]	-	-	64%	57%
Patients Who Left ER Before Being Seen[5]	-	-	2%	2%
Time from ER Arrival to Admit. (minutes)[2,7]	-	-	285	274
Time from ER Arrival to Discharge (minutes)[5]	-	-	162	134
Time in ER Before Being Evaluated (minutes)[5]	-	-	27	26
Time to Pain Meds for Fractures (minutes)[5]	-	-	58	57
Heart Attack Care				
Aspirin Given at Discharge[2]	303	100%	99%	99%
Fibrinolytic Meds Within 30 Min. of Arrival[2,7]	-	-	67%	54%
PCI Within 90 Minutes of Arrival[2,7]	-	-	95%	96%
Statin Prescribed at Discharge[2]	293	99%	98%	98%
Heart Failure Care				
ACE Inhibitor or ARB for LVSD[2]	122	100%	98%	97%
Discharge Instructions Given[2]	255	98%	94%	94%
Evaluation of LVS Function[2]	291	100%	99%	99%
Medicare Spending				
Medicare Spending per Patient (ratio)	-	0.94	0.93	0.98
Pneumonia Care				
Appropriate Initial Antibiotic Given[7]	-	-	96%	95%
Blood Culture Timing[7]	-	-	97%	98%
Pregnancy and Delivery Care				
Newborn Deliveries Scheduled Early[7]	-	-	7%	6%
Preventive Care				
Immunization for Influenza[2]	566	95%	91%	90%
Immunization for Pneumonia[2]	939	93%	92%	92%
Stroke Care				
Anticoagulation Therapy for Atrial Fibrillation[2,7]	-	-	96%	95%
Antithrombotic Therapy Timing[1,2]	-	-	98%	98%
Assessed for Rehabilitation[1,2]	-	-	96%	97%
Discharged on Antithrombotic Therapy[1,2]	-	-	99%	99%
Discharged on Statin Medication[1,2]	-	-	94%	94%
Thrombolytic Therapy Timing[2,7]	-	-	81%	66%
Venous Thromboembolism Prophylaxis[1,2]	-	-	93%	94%
Written Stroke Educational Materials Given[1,2]	-	-	84%	88%
Surgical Care Improvement Project				
Appropriate Beta Blocker Usage[2]	171	100%	97%	98%
Appropriate VTP Within 24 Hours[2]	60	95%	98%	98%
Controlled Postoperative Blood Glucose[2]	163	90%	96%	97%
Perioperative Temperature Management[2]	120	100%	100%	100%
Prophylactic Antibiotic Selection[2]	180	100%	99%	99%
Prophylactic Antibiotic Selection (Outpatient)	524	100%	98%	98%
Prophylactic Antibiotic Stopped[2]	170	97%	98%	98%
Prophylactic Antibiotic Timing[2]	180	100%	99%	99%
Prophylactic Antibiotic Timing (Outpatient)	523	100%	99%	98%
Urinary Catheter Removal[2]	175	97%	97%	97%
Survey of Patients' Hospital Experiences				
Area Around Room 'Always' Quiet at Night[11]	300+	51%	57%	61%
Doctors 'Always' Communicated Well[11]	300+	75%	77%	82%
Home Recovery Information Given[11]	300+	87%	86%	85%
Hospital Given 9 or 10 on 10 Point Scale[11]	300+	78%	70%	71%
Meds 'Always' Explained Before Given[11]	300+	66%	62%	64%
Nurses 'Always' Communicated Well[11]	300+	81%	76%	79%
Pain 'Always' Well Controlled[11]	300+	75%	69%	71%

NOTE: Hospital profiles are in alphabetical order by state, then city, then hospital within the city; Rankings exclude hospitals with less than 25 cases except for patient surveys which excludes hospitals with less than 100 cases; (a) 100-299 cases; (1) The number of cases/patients is too few to report; (2) Data submitted were based on a sample of cases/patients; (3) Results are based on a shorter time period than required; (4) Data suppressed by CMS for one or more quarters; (5) Results are not available for this reporting period; (6) Fewer than 100 patients completed the HCAHPS survey; (7) No cases met the criteria for this measure; (8) The lower limit of the confidence interval cannot be calculated if the number of observed infections equals zero; (9) No data are available from the state/territory for this reporting period; (10) The scores shown reflect fewer than 50 completed surveys; (11) There were discrepancies in the data collection process; (12) This measure does not apply to this hospital for this reporting period; (13) Results cannot be calculated for this reporting period; (14) The results for this state are combined with nearby states to protect confidentiality; Please refer to the User's Guide for a full explanation of data.

Room and Bathroom 'Always' Clean[11]	300+	71%	69%	73%
Timely Help 'Always' Received[11]	300+	73%	65%	68%
Would Definitely Recommend Hospital[11]	300+	82%	70%	71%
Use of Medical Imaging				
Cardiac Imaging Stress Test before Surgery[1]	-	-	5.8%	5.3%
Combination Abdominal CT Scan[1]	-	-	9.1%	10.5%
Combination Brain/Sinus CT Scan[1]	-	-	3.2%	2.7%
Combination Chest CT Scan[1]	-	-	5.5%	2.7%
Follow-up Mammogram/Ultrasound[7]	-	-	8.5%	8.8%
Lumbar Spine MRI for Low Back Pain[7]	-	-	37.4%	37.2%

Mountain Vista Medical Center

1301 South Crismon Road
Mesa, AZ 85209
Phone: 480-358-6100
URL: www.mvmedicalcenter.com
Type: Acute Care Hospitals
Emergency Services: Yes
Ownership: Proprietary
Beds: 178
Key Personnel:
CEO . . . . Tony Marinello

Measure	Cases	This Hosp.	State Avg.	U.S. Avg.
Blood Clot Prevention and Treatment				
Anticoagulation Overlap Therapy[2]	93	73%	94%	93%
ICU Venous Thromboembolism Prophylaxis[2]	115	72%	92%	92%
Incidence of Potentially Preventable VTE[2]	15	20%	9%	10%
UFH with Dosages/Platelet Monitoring[2]	90	100%	98%	97%
Venous Thromboembolism Prophylaxis[2]	327	65%	88%	85%
Warfarin Therapy Discharge Instructions[2]	72	99%	74%	75%
Chest Pain/Possible Heart Attack Care				
Aspirin Given Within 24 Hours of Arrival	13	100%	98%	96%
Fibrinolytic Meds Within 30 Min. of Arrival[3,7]	-	-	59%	58%
Average Time to ECG (minutes)	13	14	6	7
Average Time to Transfer (minutes)[3,7]	-	-	48	60
Children's Asthma Care				
Received Home Management Plan of Care	-	-	-	88%
Received Reliever Medication	-	-	-	100%
Received Systemic Corticosteroids	-	-	-	100%
Emergency Department				
Admittance Decision Time (minutes)[2]	661	175	98	98
Head CT Results Within 45 Min. of Arrival	23	96%	64%	57%
Patients Who Left ER Before Being Seen	28,190	2%	2%	2%
Time from ER Arrival to Admit. (minutes)[2]	677	356	285	274
Time from ER Arrival to Discharge (minutes)	532	216	162	134
Time in ER Before Being Evaluated (minutes)	619	65	27	26
Time to Pain Meds for Fractures (minutes)	171	80	58	57
Heart Attack Care				
Aspirin Given at Discharge	210	94%	99%	99%
Fibrinolytic Meds Within 30 Min. of Arrival[7]	-	-	67%	54%
PCI Within 90 Minutes of Arrival	38	95%	95%	96%
Statin Prescribed at Discharge	204	91%	98%	98%
Heart Failure Care				
ACE Inhibitor or ARB for LVSD	91	88%	98%	97%
Discharge Instructions Given	188	87%	94%	94%
Evaluation of LVS Function	215	100%	99%	99%
Medicare Spending				
Medicare Spending per Patient (ratio)	-	1.01	0.93	0.98
Pneumonia Care				
Appropriate Initial Antibiotic Given	272	94%	96%	95%
Blood Culture Timing	306	97%	97%	98%
Pregnancy and Delivery Care				
Newborn Deliveries Scheduled Early[2]	50	26%	7%	6%
Preventive Care				
Immunization for Influenza[2]	704	97%	91%	90%
Immunization for Pneumonia[2]	852	96%	92%	92%
Stroke Care				
Anticoagulation Therapy for Atrial Fibrillation	13	100%	96%	95%
Antithrombotic Therapy Timing	123	93%	98%	98%
Assessed for Rehabilitation	139	99%	96%	97%
Discharged on Antithrombotic Therapy	134	96%	99%	99%
Discharged on Statin Medication	95	81%	94%	94%
Thrombolytic Therapy Timing	23	70%	81%	66%
Venous Thromboembolism Prophylaxis	141	80%	93%	94%
Written Stroke Educational Materials Given	88	98%	84%	88%
Surgical Care Improvement Project				
Appropriate Beta Blocker Usage	228	94%	97%	98%
Appropriate VTP Within 24 Hours	556	99%	98%	98%
Controlled Postoperative Blood Glucose	66	92%	96%	97%
Perioperative Temperature Management	667	100%	100%	100%
Prophylactic Antibiotic Selection	449	99%	99%	99%
Prophylactic Antibiotic Selection (Outpatient)	306	97%	98%	98%
Prophylactic Antibiotic Stopped	430	97%	98%	98%
Prophylactic Antibiotic Timing	449	99%	99%	99%
Prophylactic Antibiotic Timing (Outpatient)	305	99%	99%	98%
Urinary Catheter Removal	265	92%	97%	97%
Survey of Patients' Hospital Experiences				
Area Around Room 'Always' Quiet at Night	300+	58%	57%	61%
Doctors 'Always' Communicated Well	300+	72%	77%	82%
Home Recovery Information Given	300+	82%	86%	85%
Hospital Given 9 or 10 on 10 Point Scale	300+	63%	70%	71%
Meds 'Always' Explained Before Given	300+	57%	62%	64%
Nurses 'Always' Communicated Well	300+	71%	76%	79%
Pain 'Always' Well Controlled	300+	67%	69%	71%
Room and Bathroom 'Always' Clean	300+	63%	69%	73%
Timely Help 'Always' Received	300+	58%	65%	68%
Would Definitely Recommend Hospital	300+	64%	70%	71%
Use of Medical Imaging				
Cardiac Imaging Stress Test before Surgery[1]	-	-	5.8%	5.3%
Combination Abdominal CT Scan	422	2.6%	9.1%	10.5%
Combination Brain/Sinus CT Scan[1]	-	-	3.2%	2.7%
Combination Chest CT Scan	123	1.6%	5.5%	2.7%
Follow-up Mammogram/Ultrasound	104	9.6%	8.5%	8.8%
Lumbar Spine MRI for Low Back Pain[1]	-	-	37.4%	37.2%

Carondelet Holy Cross Hospital

1171 West Target Range Road
Nogales, AZ 85621
Phone: 520-285-3000
Fax: 520-285-8015
URL: www.carondelet.org
Type: Critical Access Hospitals
Emergency Services: Yes
Ownership: Proprietary
Beds: 80
Key Personnel:
Cardiology . . . . David A Arzouman
Anesthesiology. . . . . Lynn Bianchi
Anesthesiology. . . . . Tony Borboa
Hemotology Center . . . . Robert Brooks
Cardiology . . . . Rehan Iftikhar
Hemotology Center . . . . Ali Madani
CEO/President. . . . . Richard Polheber

Measure	Cases	This Hosp.	State Avg.	U.S. Avg.
Blood Clot Prevention and Treatment				
Anticoagulation Overlap Therapy[1,2]	-	-	94%	93%
ICU Venous Thromboembolism Prophylaxis[2,7]	-	-	92%	92%
Incidence of Potentially Preventable VTE[2,7]	-	-	9%	10%
UFH with Dosages/Platelet Monitoring[2,7]	-	-	98%	97%
Venous Thromboembolism Prophylaxis[2]	106	94%	88%	85%
Warfarin Therapy Discharge Instructions[1,2]	-	-	74%	75%
Chest Pain/Possible Heart Attack Care				
Aspirin Given Within 24 Hours of Arrival[5]	-	-	98%	96%
Fibrinolytic Meds Within 30 Min. of Arrival[5]	-	-	59%	58%
Average Time to ECG (minutes)[5]	-	-	6	7
Average Time to Transfer (minutes)[5]	-	-	48	60
Children's Asthma Care				
Received Home Management Plan of Care	-	-	-	88%
Received Reliever Medication	-	-	-	100%
Received Systemic Corticosteroids	-	-	-	100%
Emergency Department				
Admittance Decision Time (minutes)[2]	21	187	98	98
Head CT Results Within 45 Min. of Arrival[5]	-	-	64%	57%
Patients Who Left ER Before Being Seen	6,522	0%	2%	2%
Time from ER Arrival to Admit. (minutes)[2]	81	286	285	274
Time from ER Arrival to Discharge (minutes)[5]	-	-	162	134
Time in ER Before Being Evaluated (minutes)[5]	-	-	27	26
Time to Pain Meds for Fractures (minutes)[5]	-	-	58	57
Heart Attack Care				
Aspirin Given at Discharge[5]	-	-	99%	99%
Fibrinolytic Meds Within 30 Min. of Arrival[5]	-	-	67%	54%
PCI Within 90 Minutes of Arrival[5]	-	-	95%	96%
Statin Prescribed at Discharge[5]	-	-	98%	98%
Heart Failure Care				
ACE Inhibitor or ARB for LVSD[1]	-	-	98%	97%
Discharge Instructions Given	12	100%	94%	94%
Evaluation of LVS Function[1]	-	-	99%	99%
Medicare Spending				
Medicare Spending per Patient (ratio)	-	-	0.93	0.98
Pneumonia Care				
Appropriate Initial Antibiotic Given	23	91%	96%	95%
Blood Culture Timing	16	94%	97%	98%
Pregnancy and Delivery Care				
Newborn Deliveries Scheduled Early[2]	58	3%	7%	6%
Preventive Care				
Immunization for Influenza[2]	192	76%	91%	90%
Immunization for Pneumonia[2]	79	92%	92%	92%
Stroke Care				
Anticoagulation Therapy for Atrial Fibrillation[5]	-	-	96%	95%
Antithrombotic Therapy Timing[5]	-	-	98%	98%
Assessed for Rehabilitation[5]	-	-	96%	97%
Discharged on Antithrombotic Therapy[5]	-	-	99%	99%
Discharged on Statin Medication[5]	-	-	94%	94%
Thrombolytic Therapy Timing[5]	-	-	81%	66%
Venous Thromboembolism Prophylaxis[5]	-	-	93%	94%
Written Stroke Educational Materials Given[5]	-	-	84%	88%
Surgical Care Improvement Project				
Appropriate Beta Blocker Usage[1]	-	-	97%	98%
Appropriate VTP Within 24 Hours	28	100%	98%	98%
Controlled Postoperative Blood Glucose[7]	-	-	96%	97%
Perioperative Temperature Management	39	100%	100%	100%
Prophylactic Antibiotic Selection	36	100%	99%	99%
Prophylactic Antibiotic Selection (Outpatient)[5]	-	-	98%	98%
Prophylactic Antibiotic Stopped	36	100%	98%	98%
Prophylactic Antibiotic Timing	36	100%	99%	99%
Prophylactic Antibiotic Timing (Outpatient)[5]	-	-	99%	98%
Urinary Catheter Removal[1]	-	-	97%	97%
Survey of Patients' Hospital Experiences				
Area Around Room 'Always' Quiet at Night[11]	(a)	55%	57%	61%
Doctors 'Always' Communicated Well[11]	(a)	78%	77%	82%
Home Recovery Information Given[11]	(a)	81%	86%	85%
Hospital Given 9 or 10 on 10 Point Scale[11]	(a)	64%	70%	71%
Meds 'Always' Explained Before Given[11]	(a)	65%	62%	64%
Nurses 'Always' Communicated Well[11]	(a)	73%	76%	79%
Pain 'Always' Well Controlled[11]	(a)	72%	69%	71%
Room and Bathroom 'Always' Clean[11]	(a)	84%	69%	73%
Timely Help 'Always' Received[11]	(a)	67%	65%	68%
Would Definitely Recommend Hospital[11]	(a)	59%	70%	71%
Use of Medical Imaging				
Cardiac Imaging Stress Test before Surgery[7]	-	-	5.8%	5.3%
Combination Abdominal CT Scan	129	10.9%	9.1%	10.5%
Combination Brain/Sinus CT Scan[1]	-	-	3.2%	2.7%
Combination Chest CT Scan	63	3.2%	5.5%	2.7%
Follow-up Mammogram/Ultrasound	82	2.4%	8.5%	8.8%
Lumbar Spine MRI for Low Back Pain[1]	-	-	37.4%	37.2%

Oro Valley Hospital

1551 East Tangerine Road
Oro Valley, AZ 85755
Phone: 520-901-3500
Fax: 520-901-3525
E-mail: nwmc.orovalley@triadhospitals.com
URL: www.nmcorovalley.com
Type: Acute Care Hospitals
Emergency Services: Yes
Ownership: Proprietary
Beds: 96
Key Personnel:
Chief of Medical Staff . . . . Robert Cobb, MD
CEO/President. . . . . Paul Kappelman
Intensive Care Unit. . . . . Randy Kesterson
Radiology. . . . . Todd Lessie
Emergency Room . . . . John Winter

Measure	Cases	This Hosp.	State Avg.	U.S. Avg.
Blood Clot Prevention and Treatment				
Anticoagulation Overlap Therapy[2]	50	96%	94%	93%
ICU Venous Thromboembolism Prophylaxis[2]	47	83%	92%	92%
Incidence of Potentially Preventable VTE[1,2]	-	-	9%	10%
UFH with Dosages/Platelet Monitoring[2]	36	100%	98%	97%
Venous Thromboembolism Prophylaxis[2]	314	94%	88%	85%
Warfarin Therapy Discharge Instructions[2]	50	92%	74%	75%
Chest Pain/Possible Heart Attack Care				

NOTE: Hospital profiles are in alphabetical order by state, then city, then hospital within the city; Rankings exclude hospitals with less than 25 cases except for patient surveys which excludes hospitals with less than 100 cases; (a) 100-299 cases; (1) The number of cases/patients is too few to report; (2) Data submitted were based on a sample of cases/patients; (3) Results are based on a shorter time period than required; (4) Data suppressed by CMS for one or more quarters; (5) Results are not available for this reporting period; (6) Fewer than 100 patients completed the HCAHPS survey; (7) No cases met the criteria for this measure; (8) The lower limit of the confidence interval cannot be calculated if the number of observed infections equals zero; (9) No data are available from the state/territory for this reporting period; (10) The scores shown reflect fewer than 50 completed surveys; (11) There were discrepancies in the data collection process; (12) This measure does not apply to this hospital for this reporting period; (13) Results cannot be calculated for this reporting period; (14) The results for this state are combined with nearby states to protect confidentiality; Please refer to the User's Guide for a full explanation of data.

Measure	Cases	This Hosp.	State Avg.	U.S. Avg.
Aspirin Given Within 24 Hours of Arrival[1,3]	-	-	98%	96%
Fibrinolytic Meds Within 30 Min. of Arrival[3,7]	-	-	59%	58%
Average Time to ECG (minutes)[1,3]	-	-	6	7
Average Time to Transfer (minutes)[3,7]	-	-	48	60
Children's Asthma Care				
Received Home Management Plan of Care	-	-	-	88%
Received Reliever Medication	-	-	-	100%
Received Systemic Corticosteroids	-	-	-	100%
Emergency Department				
Admittance Decision Time (minutes)[2]	716	93	98	98
Head CT Results Within 45 Min. of Arrival[1]	-	-	64%	57%
Patients Who Left ER Before Being Seen	21,998	1%	2%	2%
Time from ER Arrival to Admit. (minutes)[2]	725	252	285	274
Time from ER Arrival to Discharge (minutes)	387	149	162	134
Time in ER Before Being Evaluated (minutes)	419	19	27	26
Time to Pain Meds for Fractures (minutes)	93	50	58	57
Heart Attack Care				
Aspirin Given at Discharge	73	100%	99%	99%
Fibrinolytic Meds Within 30 Min. of Arrival[7]	-	-	67%	54%
PCI Within 90 Minutes of Arrival	25	100%	95%	96%
Statin Prescribed at Discharge	70	97%	98%	98%
Heart Failure Care				
ACE Inhibitor or ARB for LVSD	46	96%	98%	97%
Discharge Instructions Given	129	93%	94%	94%
Evaluation of LVS Function	138	100%	99%	99%
Medicare Spending				
Medicare Spending per Patient (ratio)	-	0.93	0.93	0.98
Pneumonia Care				
Appropriate Initial Antibiotic Given	88	99%	96%	95%
Blood Culture Timing	106	100%	97%	98%
Pregnancy and Delivery Care				
Newborn Deliveries Scheduled Early[7]	-	-	7%	6%
Preventive Care				
Immunization for Influenza[2]	528	96%	91%	90%
Immunization for Pneumonia[2]	806	98%	92%	92%
Stroke Care				
Anticoagulation Therapy for Atrial Fibrillation[1]	-	-	96%	95%
Antithrombotic Therapy Timing	56	98%	98%	98%
Assessed for Rehabilitation	72	94%	96%	97%
Discharged on Antithrombotic Therapy	71	100%	99%	99%
Discharged on Statin Medication	58	91%	94%	94%
Thrombolytic Therapy Timing[1]	-	-	81%	66%
Venous Thromboembolism Prophylaxis	55	87%	93%	94%
Written Stroke Educational Materials Given	46	96%	84%	88%
Surgical Care Improvement Project				
Appropriate Beta Blocker Usage	251	97%	97%	98%
Appropriate VTP Within 24 Hours	930	98%	98%	98%
Controlled Postoperative Blood Glucose[7]	-	-	96%	97%
Perioperative Temperature Management	1,046	100%	100%	100%
Prophylactic Antibiotic Selection	852	99%	99%	99%
Prophylactic Antibiotic Selection (Outpatient)	117	97%	98%	98%
Prophylactic Antibiotic Stopped	846	99%	98%	98%
Prophylactic Antibiotic Timing	852	100%	99%	99%
Prophylactic Antibiotic Timing (Outpatient)	122	96%	99%	98%
Urinary Catheter Removal	562	98%	97%	97%
Survey of Patients' Hospital Experiences				
Area Around Room 'Always' Quiet at Night	300+	51%	57%	61%
Doctors 'Always' Communicated Well	300+	78%	77%	82%
Home Recovery Information Given	300+	88%	86%	85%
Hospital Given 9 or 10 on 10 Point Scale	300+	72%	70%	71%
Meds 'Always' Explained Before Given	300+	59%	62%	64%
Nurses 'Always' Communicated Well	300+	75%	76%	79%
Pain 'Always' Well Controlled	300+	67%	69%	71%
Room and Bathroom 'Always' Clean	300+	69%	69%	73%
Timely Help 'Always' Received	300+	61%	65%	68%
Would Definitely Recommend Hospital	300+	76%	70%	71%
Use of Medical Imaging				
Cardiac Imaging Stress Test before Surgery	177	4.0%	5.8%	5.3%
Combination Abdominal CT Scan	700	11.4%	9.1%	10.5%
Combination Brain/Sinus CT Scan	523	1.1%	3.2%	2.7%
Combination Chest CT Scan	289	4.8%	5.5%	2.7%
Follow-up Mammogram/Ultrasound	1,043	7.2%	8.5%	8.8%
Lumbar Spine MRI for Low Back Pain	57	45.6%	37.4%	37.2%

Page Hospital

501 North Navajo Drive
Page, AZ 86040
Phone: 928-645-2424
Fax: 928-645-3549
Type: Critical Access Hospitals
Emergency Services: Yes
Ownership: Govt - Hospital Dist/Auth
Beds: 25

Key Personnel:
Emergency Room . . . . Elizabeth Faulk
CEO/President . . . . Sandy Haryasz
Operating Room. . . . . Polly Smith
Chief of Medical Staff . . . . Barbara Zimmerman

Measure	Cases	This Hosp.	State Avg.	U.S. Avg.
Blood Clot Prevention and Treatment				
Anticoagulation Overlap Therapy[5]	-	-	94%	93%
ICU Venous Thromboembolism Prophylaxis[5]	-	-	92%	92%
Incidence of Potentially Preventable VTE[5]	-	-	9%	10%
UFH with Dosages/Platelet Monitoring[5]	-	-	98%	97%
Venous Thromboembolism Prophylaxis[5]	-	-	88%	85%
Warfarin Therapy Discharge Instructions[5]	-	-	74%	75%
Chest Pain/Possible Heart Attack Care				
Aspirin Given Within 24 Hours of Arrival	27	100%	98%	96%
Fibrinolytic Meds Within 30 Min. of Arrival[1]	-	-	59%	58%
Average Time to ECG (minutes)	28	4	6	7
Average Time to Transfer (minutes)[1]	-	-	48	60
Children's Asthma Care				
Received Home Management Plan of Care	-	-	-	88%
Received Reliever Medication	-	-	-	100%
Received Systemic Corticosteroids	-	-	-	100%
Emergency Department				
Admittance Decision Time (minutes)[5]	-	-	98	98
Head CT Results Within 45 Min. of Arrival[5]	-	-	64%	57%
Patients Who Left ER Before Being Seen	8,607	1%	2%	2%
Time from ER Arrival to Admit. (minutes)[5]	-	-	285	274
Time from ER Arrival to Discharge (minutes)[5]	-	-	162	134
Time in ER Before Being Evaluated (minutes)[5]	-	-	27	26
Time to Pain Meds for Fractures (minutes)[5]	-	-	58	57
Heart Attack Care				
Aspirin Given at Discharge[1,3]	-	-	99%	99%
Fibrinolytic Meds Within 30 Min. of Arrival[3,7]	-	-	67%	54%
PCI Within 90 Minutes of Arrival[3,7]	-	-	95%	96%
Statin Prescribed at Discharge[3,7]	-	-	98%	98%
Heart Failure Care				
ACE Inhibitor or ARB for LVSD[1,3]	-	-	98%	97%
Discharge Instructions Given[1,3]	-	-	94%	94%
Evaluation of LVS Function[1,3]	-	-	99%	99%
Medicare Spending				
Medicare Spending per Patient (ratio)	-	-	0.93	0.98
Pneumonia Care				
Appropriate Initial Antibiotic Given	13	100%	96%	95%
Blood Culture Timing	16	100%	97%	98%
Pregnancy and Delivery Care				
Newborn Deliveries Scheduled Early[3,7]	-	-	7%	6%
Preventive Care				
Immunization for Influenza[5]	-	-	91%	90%
Immunization for Pneumonia[5]	-	-	92%	92%
Stroke Care				
Anticoagulation Therapy for Atrial Fibrillation[5]	-	-	96%	95%
Antithrombotic Therapy Timing[5]	-	-	98%	98%
Assessed for Rehabilitation[5]	-	-	96%	97%
Discharged on Antithrombotic Therapy[5]	-	-	99%	99%
Discharged on Statin Medication[5]	-	-	94%	94%
Thrombolytic Therapy Timing[5]	-	-	81%	66%
Venous Thromboembolism Prophylaxis[5]	-	-	93%	94%
Written Stroke Educational Materials Given[5]	-	-	84%	88%
Surgical Care Improvement Project				
Appropriate Beta Blocker Usage[3,7]	-	-	97%	98%
Appropriate VTP Within 24 Hours[1,3]	-	-	98%	98%
Controlled Postoperative Blood Glucose[3,7]	-	-	96%	97%
Perioperative Temperature Management[1,3]	-	-	100%	100%
Prophylactic Antibiotic Selection[1,3]	-	-	99%	99%
Prophylactic Antibiotic Selection (Outpatient)[1,3]	-	-	98%	98%
Prophylactic Antibiotic Stopped[1,3]	-	-	98%	98%
Prophylactic Antibiotic Timing[1,3]	-	-	99%	99%
Prophylactic Antibiotic Timing (Outpatient)[1,3]	-	-	99%	98%
Urinary Catheter Removal[1,3]	-	-	97%	97%
Survey of Patients' Hospital Experiences				
Area Around Room 'Always' Quiet at Night[11]	(a)	60%	57%	61%
Doctors 'Always' Communicated Well[11]	(a)	84%	77%	82%
Home Recovery Information Given[11]	(a)	90%	86%	85%
Hospital Given 9 or 10 on 10 Point Scale[11]	(a)	73%	70%	71%
Meds 'Always' Explained Before Given[11]	(a)	68%	62%	64%
Nurses 'Always' Communicated Well[11]	(a)	81%	76%	79%
Pain 'Always' Well Controlled[11]	(a)	74%	69%	71%
Room and Bathroom 'Always' Clean[11]	(a)	74%	69%	73%
Timely Help 'Always' Received[11]	(a)	77%	65%	68%
Would Definitely Recommend Hospital[11]	(a)	69%	70%	71%
Use of Medical Imaging				
Cardiac Imaging Stress Test before Surgery[1]	-	-	5.8%	5.3%
Combination Abdominal CT Scan	104	2.9%	9.1%	10.5%
Combination Brain/Sinus CT Scan[1]	-	-	3.2%	2.7%
Combination Chest CT Scan	47	2.1%	5.5%	2.7%
Follow-up Mammogram/Ultrasound	89	14.6%	8.5%	8.8%
Lumbar Spine MRI for Low Back Pain[1]	-	-	37.4%	37.2%

Payson Regional Medical Center

807 South Ponderosa Drive
Payson, AZ 85541
Phone: 928-474-3222
Fax: 928-472-1295
URL: www.paysonhospital.com
Type: Acute Care Hospitals
Emergency Services: Yes
Ownership: Voluntary non-profit - Other
Beds: 44

Key Personnel:
Operating Room. . . . . Mike McCleery
Emergency Room . . . . Kim Reger
Cardiac Laboratory. . . . . Kim Sleeper
Quality Assurance . . . . Lynn Sommars
Chief of Medical Staff . . . . John Vandruff
CEO/President. . . . . Chris Wolf

Measure	Cases	This Hosp.	State Avg.	U.S. Avg.
Blood Clot Prevention and Treatment				
Anticoagulation Overlap Therapy[2]	29	97%	94%	93%
ICU Venous Thromboembolism Prophylaxis[2]	59	100%	92%	92%
Incidence of Potentially Preventable VTE[1,2]	-	-	9%	10%
UFH with Dosages/Platelet Monitoring[1,2]	-	-	98%	97%
Venous Thromboembolism Prophylaxis[2]	238	99%	88%	85%
Warfarin Therapy Discharge Instructions[2]	17	94%	74%	75%
Chest Pain/Possible Heart Attack Care				
Aspirin Given Within 24 Hours of Arrival	64	100%	98%	96%
Fibrinolytic Meds Within 30 Min. of Arrival[1]	-	-	59%	58%
Average Time to ECG (minutes)	63	6	6	7
Average Time to Transfer (minutes)[1]	-	-	48	60
Children's Asthma Care				
Received Home Management Plan of Care	-	-	-	88%
Received Reliever Medication	-	-	-	100%
Received Systemic Corticosteroids	-	-	-	100%
Emergency Department				
Admittance Decision Time (minutes)[2]	469	135	98	98
Head CT Results Within 45 Min. of Arrival[1]	-	-	64%	57%
Patients Who Left ER Before Being Seen	13,269	1%	2%	2%
Time from ER Arrival to Admit. (minutes)[2]	481	294	285	274
Time from ER Arrival to Discharge (minutes)	374	134	162	134
Time in ER Before Being Evaluated (minutes)	419	15	27	26
Time to Pain Meds for Fractures (minutes)	72	66	58	57
Heart Attack Care				
Aspirin Given at Discharge[1]	-	-	99%	99%
Fibrinolytic Meds Within 30 Min. of Arrival[7]	-	-	67%	54%
PCI Within 90 Minutes of Arrival[7]	-	-	95%	96%
Statin Prescribed at Discharge[1]	-	-	98%	98%
Heart Failure Care				
ACE Inhibitor or ARB for LVSD[1]	-	-	98%	97%
Discharge Instructions Given	27	89%	94%	94%
Evaluation of LVS Function	33	100%	99%	99%
Medicare Spending				
Medicare Spending per Patient (ratio)	-	0.91	0.93	0.98
Pneumonia Care				
Appropriate Initial Antibiotic Given	64	98%	96%	95%
Blood Culture Timing	87	98%	97%	98%

NOTE: Hospital profiles are in alphabetical order by state, then city, then hospital within the city; Rankings exclude hospitals with less than 25 cases except for patient surveys which excludes hospitals with less than 100 cases; (a) 100-299 cases; (1) The number of cases/patients is too few to report; (2) Data submitted were based on a sample of cases/patients; (3) Results are based on a shorter time period than required; (4) Data suppressed by CMS for one or more quarters; (5) Results are not available for this reporting period; (6) Fewer than 100 patients completed the HCAHPS survey; (7) No cases met the criteria for this measure; (8) The lower limit of the confidence interval cannot be calculated if the number of observed infections equals zero; (9) No data are available from the state/territory for this reporting period; (10) The scores shown reflect fewer than 50 completed surveys; (11) There were discrepancies in the data collection process; (12) This measure does not apply to this hospital for this reporting period; (13) Results cannot be calculated for this reporting period; (14) The results for this state are combined with nearby states to protect confidentiality; Please refer to the User's Guide for a full explanation of data.

Pregnancy and Delivery Care				
Newborn Deliveries Scheduled Early[2]	20	0%	7%	6%
Preventive Care				
Immunization for Influenza[2]	302	98%	91%	90%
Immunization for Pneumonia[2]	436	100%	92%	92%
Stroke Care				
Anticoagulation Therapy for Atrial Fibrillation[1]	-	-	96%	95%
Antithrombotic Therapy Timing	15	100%	98%	98%
Assessed for Rehabilitation	16	94%	96%	97%
Discharged on Antithrombotic Therapy	16	100%	99%	99%
Discharged on Statin Medication	11	91%	94%	94%
Thrombolytic Therapy Timing[1]	-	-	81%	66%
Venous Thromboembolism Prophylaxis	15	93%	93%	94%
Written Stroke Educational Materials Given	13	92%	84%	88%
Surgical Care Improvement Project				
Appropriate Beta Blocker Usage	47	100%	97%	98%
Appropriate VTP Within 24 Hours	146	100%	98%	98%
Controlled Postoperative Blood Glucose[7]	-	-	96%	97%
Perioperative Temperature Management	171	100%	100%	100%
Prophylactic Antibiotic Selection	111	99%	99%	99%
Prophylactic Antibiotic Selection (Outpatient)	23	96%	98%	98%
Prophylactic Antibiotic Stopped	107	100%	98%	98%
Prophylactic Antibiotic Timing	111	97%	99%	99%
Prophylactic Antibiotic Timing (Outpatient)	23	100%	99%	98%
Urinary Catheter Removal	56	100%	97%	97%
Survey of Patients' Hospital Experiences				
Area Around Room 'Always' Quiet at Night	300+	59%	57%	61%
Doctors 'Always' Communicated Well	300+	78%	77%	82%
Home Recovery Information Given	300+	88%	86%	85%
Hospital Given 9 or 10 on 10 Point Scale	300+	71%	70%	71%
Meds 'Always' Explained Before Given	300+	63%	62%	64%
Nurses 'Always' Communicated Well	300+	80%	76%	79%
Pain 'Always' Well Controlled	300+	72%	69%	71%
Room and Bathroom 'Always' Clean	300+	72%	69%	73%
Timely Help 'Always' Received	300+	73%	65%	68%
Would Definitely Recommend Hospital	300+	66%	70%	71%
Use of Medical Imaging				
Cardiac Imaging Stress Test before Surgery	274	4.0%	5.8%	5.3%
Combination Abdominal CT Scan	642	19.0%	9.1%	10.5%
Combination Brain/Sinus CT Scan	586	5.6%	3.2%	2.7%
Combination Chest CT Scan	398	5.0%	5.5%	2.7%
Follow-up Mammogram/Ultrasound	1,146	3.7%	8.5%	8.8%
Lumbar Spine MRI for Low Back Pain	116	43.1%	37.4%	37.2%

Banner Estrella Medical Center

9201 West Thomas Road
Phoenix, AZ 85037
Phone: 623-327-4000
Fax: 623-327-7184
Type: Acute Care Hospitals
Emergency Services: Yes
Ownership: Voluntary non-profit - Private
Beds: 214

Key Personnel:
President/CEO. . . . . Peter S. Fine, FACHE

Measure	Cases	This Hosp.	State Avg.	U.S. Avg.
Blood Clot Prevention and Treatment				
Anticoagulation Overlap Therapy[2]	83	99%	94%	93%
ICU Venous Thromboembolism Prophylaxis[2]	76	95%	92%	92%
Incidence of Potentially Preventable VTE[2]	12	0%	9%	10%
UFH with Dosages/Platelet Monitoring[2]	32	97%	98%	97%
Venous Thromboembolism Prophylaxis[2]	339	86%	88%	85%
Warfarin Therapy Discharge Instructions[2]	70	59%	74%	75%
Chest Pain/Possible Heart Attack Care				
Aspirin Given Within 24 Hours of Arrival[1]	-	-	98%	96%
Fibrinolytic Meds Within 30 Min. of Arrival[3,7]	-	-	59%	58%
Average Time to ECG (minutes)[1]	-	-	6	7
Average Time to Transfer (minutes)[3,7]	-	-	48	60
Children's Asthma Care				
Received Home Management Plan of Care	-	-	-	88%
Received Reliever Medication	-	-	-	100%
Received Systemic Corticosteroids	-	-	-	100%
Emergency Department				
Admittance Decision Time (minutes)[2]	521	108	98	98
Head CT Results Within 45 Min. of Arrival	15	80%	64%	57%
Patients Who Left ER Before Being Seen	95,671	3%	2%	2%
Time from ER Arrival to Admit. (minutes)[2]	541	288	285	274
Time from ER Arrival to Discharge (minutes)	291	178	162	134
Time in ER Before Being Evaluated (minutes)	393	30	27	26
Time to Pain Meds for Fractures (minutes)	278	62	58	57
Heart Attack Care				
Aspirin Given at Discharge[2]	282	100%	99%	99%
Fibrinolytic Meds Within 30 Min. of Arrival[2,7]	-	-	67%	54%
PCI Within 90 Minutes of Arrival[2]	35	97%	95%	96%
Statin Prescribed at Discharge[2]	271	99%	98%	98%
Heart Failure Care				
ACE Inhibitor or ARB for LVSD[2]	106	99%	98%	97%
Discharge Instructions Given[2]	260	96%	94%	94%
Evaluation of LVS Function[2]	289	100%	99%	99%
Medicare Spending				
Medicare Spending per Patient (ratio)	-	0.93	0.93	0.98
Pneumonia Care				
Appropriate Initial Antibiotic Given[2]	91	99%	96%	95%
Blood Culture Timing[2]	156	99%	97%	98%
Pregnancy and Delivery Care				
Newborn Deliveries Scheduled Early[2]	112	5%	7%	6%
Preventive Care				
Immunization for Influenza[2]	483	94%	91%	90%
Immunization for Pneumonia[2]	487	94%	92%	92%
Stroke Care				
Anticoagulation Therapy for Atrial Fibrillation[1,2]	-	-	96%	95%
Antithrombotic Therapy Timing[2]	89	99%	98%	98%
Assessed for Rehabilitation[2]	112	99%	96%	97%
Discharged on Antithrombotic Therapy[2]	108	100%	99%	99%
Discharged on Statin Medication[2]	80	98%	94%	94%
Thrombolytic Therapy Timing[2]	14	86%	81%	66%
Venous Thromboembolism Prophylaxis[2]	105	91%	93%	94%
Written Stroke Educational Materials Given[2]	74	89%	84%	88%
Surgical Care Improvement Project				
Appropriate Beta Blocker Usage[2]	129	96%	97%	98%
Appropriate VTP Within 24 Hours[2]	306	97%	98%	98%
Controlled Postoperative Blood Glucose[2]	58	100%	96%	97%
Perioperative Temperature Management[2]	410	100%	100%	100%
Prophylactic Antibiotic Selection[2]	278	99%	99%	99%
Prophylactic Antibiotic Selection (Outpatient)	341	99%	98%	98%
Prophylactic Antibiotic Stopped[2]	263	98%	98%	98%
Prophylactic Antibiotic Timing[2]	279	99%	99%	99%
Prophylactic Antibiotic Timing (Outpatient)	342	99%	99%	98%
Urinary Catheter Removal[2]	190	99%	97%	97%
Survey of Patients' Hospital Experiences				
Area Around Room 'Always' Quiet at Night[11]	300+	65%	57%	61%
Doctors 'Always' Communicated Well[11]	300+	80%	77%	82%
Home Recovery Information Given[11]	300+	88%	86%	85%
Hospital Given 9 or 10 on 10 Point Scale[11]	300+	75%	70%	71%
Meds 'Always' Explained Before Given[11]	300+	65%	62%	64%
Nurses 'Always' Communicated Well[11]	300+	78%	76%	79%
Pain 'Always' Well Controlled[11]	300+	71%	69%	71%
Room and Bathroom 'Always' Clean[11]	300+	71%	69%	73%
Timely Help 'Always' Received[11]	300+	64%	65%	68%
Would Definitely Recommend Hospital[11]	300+	76%	70%	71%
Use of Medical Imaging				
Cardiac Imaging Stress Test before Surgery	67	7.5%	5.8%	5.3%
Combination Abdominal CT Scan	597	3.4%	9.1%	10.5%
Combination Brain/Sinus CT Scan[1]	-	-	3.2%	2.7%
Combination Chest CT Scan	133	3.8%	5.5%	2.7%
Follow-up Mammogram/Ultrasound[7]	-	-	8.5%	8.8%
Lumbar Spine MRI for Low Back Pain[1]	-	-	37.4%	37.2%

Banner Good Samaritan Medical Center

1111 East Mcdowell Road
Phoenix, AZ 85006
Phone: 602-239-2000
Fax: 602-239-3749
URL: www.bannerhealth.com
Type: Acute Care Hospitals
Emergency Services: Yes
Ownership: Voluntary non-profit - Other
Beds: 650

Key Personnel:
Pediatric Ambulatory Care . . . . . . Paul Charnetsky, MD
Pediatric In-Patient Care . . . . Paul Charnetsky, MD
Chief of Medical Staff. . . . . John Harlend, MD
Operating Room. . . . . Pat Menges, RN
Cardiac Laboratory. . . . . Beth Miller
CEO/President. . . . . Paul Mullings
CEO . . . . Steve Narang, MD
Infection Control. . . . . Beth Urndinski

Measure	Cases	This Hosp.	State Avg.	U.S. Avg.
Blood Clot Prevention and Treatment				
Anticoagulation Overlap Therapy[2]	113	96%	94%	93%
ICU Venous Thromboembolism Prophylaxis[2]	114	95%	92%	92%
Incidence of Potentially Preventable VTE[2]	37	3%	9%	10%
UFH with Dosages/Platelet Monitoring[2]	68	100%	98%	97%
Venous Thromboembolism Prophylaxis[2]	283	89%	88%	85%
Warfarin Therapy Discharge Instructions[2]	79	58%	74%	75%
Chest Pain/Possible Heart Attack Care				
Aspirin Given Within 24 Hours of Arrival[5]	-	-	98%	96%
Fibrinolytic Meds Within 30 Min. of Arrival[5]	-	-	59%	58%
Average Time to ECG (minutes)[5]	-	-	6	7
Average Time to Transfer (minutes)[5]	-	-	48	60
Children's Asthma Care				
Received Home Management Plan of Care	-	-	-	88%
Received Reliever Medication	-	-	-	100%
Received Systemic Corticosteroids	-	-	-	100%
Emergency Department				
Admittance Decision Time (minutes)[2]	289	79	98	98
Head CT Results Within 45 Min. of Arrival[1,3]	-	-	64%	57%
Patients Who Left ER Before Being Seen	61,587	2%	2%	2%
Time from ER Arrival to Admit. (minutes)[2]	305	271	285	274
Time from ER Arrival to Discharge (minutes)	328	177	162	134
Time in ER Before Being Evaluated (minutes)	382	21	27	26
Time to Pain Meds for Fractures (minutes)	107	57	58	57
Heart Attack Care				
Aspirin Given at Discharge[2]	280	100%	99%	99%
Fibrinolytic Meds Within 30 Min. of Arrival[2,7]	-	-	67%	54%
PCI Within 90 Minutes of Arrival[2]	23	91%	95%	96%
Statin Prescribed at Discharge[2]	264	97%	98%	98%
Heart Failure Care				
ACE Inhibitor or ARB for LVSD[2]	112	99%	98%	97%
Discharge Instructions Given[2]	262	96%	94%	94%
Evaluation of LVS Function[2]	291	100%	99%	99%
Medicare Spending				
Medicare Spending per Patient (ratio)	-	0.99	0.93	0.98
Pneumonia Care				
Appropriate Initial Antibiotic Given[2]	81	100%	96%	95%
Blood Culture Timing[2]	113	97%	97%	98%
Pregnancy and Delivery Care				
Newborn Deliveries Scheduled Early[2]	81	5%	7%	6%
Preventive Care				
Immunization for Influenza[2]	490	93%	91%	90%
Immunization for Pneumonia[2]	504	92%	92%	92%
Stroke Care				
Anticoagulation Therapy for Atrial Fibrillation[1,2]	-	-	96%	95%
Antithrombotic Therapy Timing[2]	61	98%	98%	98%
Assessed for Rehabilitation[2]	115	92%	96%	97%
Discharged on Antithrombotic Therapy[2]	81	99%	99%	99%
Discharged on Statin Medication[2]	62	97%	94%	94%
Thrombolytic Therapy Timing[1,2]	-	-	81%	66%
Venous Thromboembolism Prophylaxis[2]	117	97%	93%	94%
Written Stroke Educational Materials Given[2]	73	44%	84%	88%
Surgical Care Improvement Project				
Appropriate Beta Blocker Usage[2]	252	99%	97%	98%
Appropriate VTP Within 24 Hours[2]	395	98%	98%	98%
Controlled Postoperative Blood Glucose[2]	155	90%	96%	97%
Perioperative Temperature Management[2]	558	100%	100%	100%
Prophylactic Antibiotic Selection[2]	472	99%	99%	99%
Prophylactic Antibiotic Selection (Outpatient)	508	100%	98%	98%
Prophylactic Antibiotic Stopped[2]	453	96%	98%	98%
Prophylactic Antibiotic Timing[2]	473	99%	99%	99%
Prophylactic Antibiotic Timing (Outpatient)	504	98%	99%	98%
Urinary Catheter Removal[2]	267	99%	97%	97%
Survey of Patients' Hospital Experiences				
Area Around Room 'Always' Quiet at Night[11]	300+	52%	57%	61%
Doctors 'Always' Communicated Well[11]	300+	80%	77%	82%
Home Recovery Information Given[11]	300+	88%	86%	85%
Hospital Given 9 or 10 on 10 Point Scale[11]	300+	75%	70%	71%
Meds 'Always' Explained Before Given[11]	300+	65%	62%	64%

NOTE: Hospital profiles are in alphabetical order by state, then city, then hospital within the city; Rankings exclude hospitals with less than 25 cases except for patient surveys which excludes hospitals with less than 100 cases; (a) 100-299 cases; (1) The number of cases/patients is too few to report; (2) Data submitted were based on a sample of cases/patients; (3) Results are based on a shorter time period than required; (4) Data suppressed by CMS for one or more quarters; (5) Results are not available for this reporting period; (6) Fewer than 100 patients completed the HCAHPS survey; (7) No cases met the criteria for this measure; (8) The lower limit of the confidence interval cannot be calculated if the number of observed infections equals zero; (9) No data are available from the state/territory for this reporting period; (10) The scores shown reflect fewer than 50 completed surveys; (11) There were discrepancies in the data collection process; (12) This measure does not apply to this hospital for this reporting period; (13) Results cannot be calculated for this reporting period; (14) The results for this state are combined with nearby states to protect confidentiality; Please refer to the User's Guide for a full explanation of data.

Measure	Cases	This Hosp.	State Avg.	U.S. Avg.
Nurses 'Always' Communicated Well[11]	300+	79%	76%	79%
Pain 'Always' Well Controlled[11]	300+	72%	69%	71%
Room and Bathroom 'Always' Clean[11]	300+	63%	69%	73%
Timely Help 'Always' Received[11]	300+	70%	65%	68%
Would Definitely Recommend Hospital[11]	300+	77%	70%	71%
Use of Medical Imaging				
Cardiac Imaging Stress Test before Surgery	166	4.2%	5.8%	5.3%
Combination Abdominal CT Scan	621	17.4%	9.1%	10.5%
Combination Brain/Sinus CT Scan	423	4.7%	3.2%	2.7%
Combination Chest CT Scan	383	0.5%	5.5%	2.7%
Follow-up Mammogram/Ultrasound	320	9.1%	8.5%	8.8%
Lumbar Spine MRI for Low Back Pain[1]	-	-	37.4%	37.2%

John C Lincoln Deer Valley Hospital

19829 North 27th Avenue Phone: 623-879-5574
Phoenix, AZ 85027 Fax: 623-879-5400
URL: www.jcl.com
Type: Acute Care Hospitals Emergency Services: Yes
Ownership: Voluntary non-profit - Private Beds: 149
Key Personnel:
CEO/President. . . . . Dan C Coleman
Quality Assurance . . . . Susan Melker
Chief of Medical Staff. . . . . Clark York, DO

Measure	Cases	This Hosp.	State Avg.	U.S. Avg.
Blood Clot Prevention and Treatment				
Anticoagulation Overlap Therapy[2]	124	97%	94%	93%
ICU Venous Thromboembolism Prophylaxis[2]	90	98%	92%	92%
Incidence of Potentially Preventable VTE[2]	12	0%	9%	10%
UFH with Dosages/Platelet Monitoring[2]	38	100%	98%	97%
Venous Thromboembolism Prophylaxis[2]	296	90%	88%	85%
Warfarin Therapy Discharge Instructions[2]	97	90%	74%	75%
Chest Pain/Possible Heart Attack Care				
Aspirin Given Within 24 Hours of Arrival[1,3]	-	-	98%	96%
Fibrinolytic Meds Within 30 Min. of Arrival[3,7]	-	-	59%	58%
Average Time to ECG (minutes)[1,3]	-	-	6	7
Average Time to Transfer (minutes)[3,7]	-	-	48	60
Children's Asthma Care				
Received Home Management Plan of Care	-	-	-	88%
Received Reliever Medication	-	-	-	100%
Received Systemic Corticosteroids	-	-	-	100%
Emergency Department				
Admittance Decision Time (minutes)[2]	630	67	98	98
Head CT Results Within 45 Min. of Arrival[1]	-	-	64%	57%
Patients Who Left ER Before Being Seen	75,593	4%	2%	2%
Time from ER Arrival to Admit. (minutes)[2]	636	282	285	274
Time from ER Arrival to Discharge (minutes)	362	137	162	134
Time in ER Before Being Evaluated (minutes)	425	31	27	26
Time to Pain Meds for Fractures (minutes)	174	29	58	57
Heart Attack Care				
Aspirin Given at Discharge	195	99%	99%	99%
Fibrinolytic Meds Within 30 Min. of Arrival[7]	-	-	67%	54%
PCI Within 90 Minutes of Arrival	41	98%	95%	96%
Statin Prescribed at Discharge	191	100%	98%	98%
Heart Failure Care				
ACE Inhibitor or ARB for LVSD[2]	88	99%	98%	97%
Discharge Instructions Given[2]	208	93%	94%	94%
Evaluation of LVS Function[2]	237	100%	99%	99%
Medicare Spending				
Medicare Spending per Patient (ratio)	-	0.96	0.93	0.98
Pneumonia Care				
Appropriate Initial Antibiotic Given[2]	115	97%	96%	95%
Blood Culture Timing[2]	145	99%	97%	98%
Pregnancy and Delivery Care				
Newborn Deliveries Scheduled Early[7]	-	-	7%	6%
Preventive Care				
Immunization for Influenza[2]	628	98%	91%	90%
Immunization for Pneumonia[2]	729	98%	92%	92%
Stroke Care				
Anticoagulation Therapy for Atrial Fibrillation[2]	11	100%	96%	95%
Antithrombotic Therapy Timing[2]	93	97%	98%	98%
Assessed for Rehabilitation[2]	111	100%	96%	97%
Discharged on Antithrombotic Therapy[2]	108	100%	99%	99%
Discharged on Statin Medication[2]	73	96%	94%	94%
Thrombolytic Therapy Timing[1,2]	-	-	81%	66%
Venous Thromboembolism Prophylaxis[2]	97	89%	93%	94%
Written Stroke Educational Materials Given[2]	88	95%	84%	88%
Surgical Care Improvement Project				
Appropriate Beta Blocker Usage[2]	170	98%	97%	98%
Appropriate VTP Within 24 Hours[2]	390	98%	98%	98%
Controlled Postoperative Blood Glucose[2]	79	97%	96%	97%
Perioperative Temperature Management[2]	516	99%	100%	100%
Prophylactic Antibiotic Selection[2]	293	100%	99%	99%
Prophylactic Antibiotic Selection (Outpatient)	344	100%	98%	98%
Prophylactic Antibiotic Stopped[2]	278	99%	98%	98%
Prophylactic Antibiotic Timing[2]	293	100%	99%	99%
Prophylactic Antibiotic Timing (Outpatient)	344	99%	99%	98%
Urinary Catheter Removal[2]	306	98%	97%	97%
Survey of Patients' Hospital Experiences				
Area Around Room 'Always' Quiet at Night	300+	54%	57%	61%
Doctors 'Always' Communicated Well	300+	74%	77%	82%
Home Recovery Information Given	300+	85%	86%	85%
Hospital Given 9 or 10 on 10 Point Scale	300+	69%	70%	71%
Meds 'Always' Explained Before Given	300+	59%	62%	64%
Nurses 'Always' Communicated Well	300+	74%	76%	79%
Pain 'Always' Well Controlled	300+	67%	69%	71%
Room and Bathroom 'Always' Clean	300+	67%	69%	73%
Timely Help 'Always' Received	300+	60%	65%	68%
Would Definitely Recommend Hospital	300+	71%	70%	71%
Use of Medical Imaging				
Cardiac Imaging Stress Test before Surgery	120	6.7%	5.8%	5.3%
Combination Abdominal CT Scan	416	13.9%	9.1%	10.5%
Combination Brain/Sinus CT Scan	421	4.5%	3.2%	2.7%
Combination Chest CT Scan	105	4.8%	5.5%	2.7%
Follow-up Mammogram/Ultrasound	1,741	14.0%	8.5%	8.8%
Lumbar Spine MRI for Low Back Pain[1]	-	-	37.4%	37.2%

John C Lincoln North Mountain Hospital

250 East Dunlap Avenue Phone: 602-943-2381
Phoenix, AZ 85020 Fax: 602-944-9610
URL: www.jcl.com
Type: Acute Care Hospitals Emergency Services: Yes
Ownership: Proprietary Beds: 266
Key Personnel:
CEO/President. . . . . Maggi Griffin, RN, MS
Chief of Medical Staff. . . . . Tim Tracy

Measure	Cases	This Hosp.	State Avg.	U.S. Avg.
Blood Clot Prevention and Treatment				
Anticoagulation Overlap Therapy[2]	184	95%	94%	93%
ICU Venous Thromboembolism Prophylaxis[2]	115	90%	92%	92%
Incidence of Potentially Preventable VTE[2]	45	11%	9%	10%
UFH with Dosages/Platelet Monitoring[2]	46	100%	98%	97%
Venous Thromboembolism Prophylaxis[2]	316	82%	88%	85%
Warfarin Therapy Discharge Instructions[2]	126	45%	74%	75%
Chest Pain/Possible Heart Attack Care				
Aspirin Given Within 24 Hours of Arrival[1,3]	-	-	98%	96%
Fibrinolytic Meds Within 30 Min. of Arrival[5]	-	-	59%	58%
Average Time to ECG (minutes)[1,3]	-	-	6	7
Average Time to Transfer (minutes)[5]	-	-	48	60
Children's Asthma Care				
Received Home Management Plan of Care	-	-	-	88%
Received Reliever Medication	-	-	-	100%
Received Systemic Corticosteroids	-	-	-	100%
Emergency Department				
Admittance Decision Time (minutes)[2]	259	69	98	98
Head CT Results Within 45 Min. of Arrival[1]	-	-	64%	57%
Patients Who Left ER Before Being Seen	49,527	4%	2%	2%
Time from ER Arrival to Admit. (minutes)[2]	264	252	285	274
Time from ER Arrival to Discharge (minutes)	353	201	162	134
Time in ER Before Being Evaluated (minutes)	386	57	27	26
Time to Pain Meds for Fractures (minutes)	76	66	58	57
Heart Attack Care				
Aspirin Given at Discharge	144	100%	99%	99%
Fibrinolytic Meds Within 30 Min. of Arrival[7]	-	-	67%	54%
PCI Within 90 Minutes of Arrival	26	96%	95%	96%
Statin Prescribed at Discharge	136	99%	98%	98%
Heart Failure Care				
ACE Inhibitor or ARB for LVSD[2]	103	100%	98%	97%
Discharge Instructions Given[2]	216	98%	94%	94%
Evaluation of LVS Function[2]	251	100%	99%	99%
Medicare Spending				
Medicare Spending per Patient (ratio)	-	0.97	0.93	0.98
Pneumonia Care				
Appropriate Initial Antibiotic Given[2]	60	98%	96%	95%
Blood Culture Timing[2]	134	99%	97%	98%
Pregnancy and Delivery Care				
Newborn Deliveries Scheduled Early[7]	-	-	7%	6%
Preventive Care				
Immunization for Influenza[2]	621	93%	91%	90%
Immunization for Pneumonia[2]	821	94%	92%	92%
Stroke Care				
Anticoagulation Therapy for Atrial Fibrillation[2]	11	100%	96%	95%
Antithrombotic Therapy Timing[2]	82	100%	98%	98%
Assessed for Rehabilitation[2]	110	99%	96%	97%
Discharged on Antithrombotic Therapy[2]	88	100%	99%	99%
Discharged on Statin Medication[2]	66	100%	94%	94%
Thrombolytic Therapy Timing[2]	16	88%	81%	66%
Venous Thromboembolism Prophylaxis[2]	116	98%	93%	94%
Written Stroke Educational Materials Given[2]	47	100%	84%	88%
Surgical Care Improvement Project				
Appropriate Beta Blocker Usage[2]	185	99%	97%	98%
Appropriate VTP Within 24 Hours[2]	420	99%	98%	98%
Controlled Postoperative Blood Glucose[2]	94	97%	96%	97%
Perioperative Temperature Management[2]	566	100%	100%	100%
Prophylactic Antibiotic Selection[2]	385	99%	99%	99%
Prophylactic Antibiotic Selection (Outpatient)	246	100%	98%	98%
Prophylactic Antibiotic Stopped[2]	370	98%	98%	98%
Prophylactic Antibiotic Timing[2]	387	98%	99%	99%
Prophylactic Antibiotic Timing (Outpatient)	247	99%	99%	98%
Urinary Catheter Removal[2]	335	97%	97%	97%
Survey of Patients' Hospital Experiences				
Area Around Room 'Always' Quiet at Night	300+	53%	57%	61%
Doctors 'Always' Communicated Well	300+	74%	77%	82%
Home Recovery Information Given	300+	84%	86%	85%
Hospital Given 9 or 10 on 10 Point Scale	300+	68%	70%	71%
Meds 'Always' Explained Before Given	300+	64%	62%	64%
Nurses 'Always' Communicated Well	300+	75%	76%	79%
Pain 'Always' Well Controlled	300+	70%	69%	71%
Room and Bathroom 'Always' Clean	300+	69%	69%	73%
Timely Help 'Always' Received	300+	60%	65%	68%
Would Definitely Recommend Hospital	300+	72%	70%	71%
Use of Medical Imaging				
Cardiac Imaging Stress Test before Surgery	80	5.0%	5.8%	5.3%
Combination Abdominal CT Scan	846	8.0%	9.1%	10.5%
Combination Brain/Sinus CT Scan	709	6.5%	3.2%	2.7%
Combination Chest CT Scan	482	1.9%	5.5%	2.7%
Follow-up Mammogram/Ultrasound[1]	-	-	8.5%	8.8%
Lumbar Spine MRI for Low Back Pain	120	39.2%	37.4%	37.2%

Maricopa Medical Center

2601 East Roosevelt Street Phone: 602-344-5011
Phoenix, AZ 85008 Fax: 602-344-1132
E-mail: copanet@hcs.maricopa.gov
URL: www.mihs.org
Type: Acute Care Hospitals Emergency Services: Yes
Ownership: Government - Local Beds: 449
Key Personnel:
President . . . . Betsey Bayless
Chief of Medical Staff . . . . James Campbell Davis
Anesthesiology. . . . . Joseph Kryc, MD
Radiology. . . . . Petronio LeRona, MD
Infection Control. . . . . Rita Neibauer
Emergency Room . . . . Charles Pollack, MD
CEO/President. . . . . Steve Purves
Pediatric In-Patient Care . . . . Mary Rimsza, MD

Measure	Cases	This Hosp.	State Avg.	U.S. Avg.
Blood Clot Prevention and Treatment				
Anticoagulation Overlap Therapy[2]	65	92%	94%	93%
ICU Venous Thromboembolism Prophylaxis[2]	74	95%	92%	92%
Incidence of Potentially Preventable VTE[2]	26	8%	9%	10%
UFH with Dosages/Platelet Monitoring[2]	31	100%	98%	97%

NOTE: Hospital profiles are in alphabetical order by state, then city, then hospital within the city; Rankings exclude hospitals with less than 25 cases except for patient surveys which excludes hospitals with less than 100 cases; (a) 100-299 cases; (1) The number of cases/patients is too few to report; (2) Data submitted were based on a sample of cases/patients; (3) Results are based on a shorter time period than required; (4) Data suppressed by CMS for one or more quarters; (5) Results are not available for this reporting period; (6) Fewer than 100 patients completed the HCAHPS survey; (7) No cases met the criteria for this measure; (8) The lower limit of the confidence interval cannot be calculated if the number of observed infections equals zero; (9) No data are available from the state/territory for this reporting period; (10) The scores shown reflect fewer than 50 completed surveys; (11) There were discrepancies in the data collection process; (12) This measure does not apply to this hospital for this reporting period; (13) Results cannot be calculated for this reporting period; (14) The results for this state are combined with nearby states to protect confidentiality; Please refer to the User's Guide for a full explanation of data.

Measure	Cases	This Hosp.	State Avg.	U.S. Avg.
Venous Thromboembolism Prophylaxis[2]	368	86%	88%	85%
Warfarin Therapy Discharge Instructions[2]	48	85%	74%	75%
Chest Pain/Possible Heart Attack Care				
Aspirin Given Within 24 Hours of Arrival[1,3]	-	-	98%	96%
Fibrinolytic Meds Within 30 Min. of Arrival[3,7]	-	-	59%	58%
Average Time to ECG (minutes)[1,3]	-	-	6	7
Average Time to Transfer (minutes)[3,7]	-	-	48	60
Children's Asthma Care				
Received Home Management Plan of Care	-	-	-	88%
Received Reliever Medication	-	-	-	100%
Received Systemic Corticosteroids	-	-	-	100%
Emergency Department				
Admittance Decision Time (minutes)[2]	564	92	98	98
Head CT Results Within 45 Min. of Arrival[7]	-	-	64%	57%
Patients Who Left ER Before Being Seen	55,553	1%	2%	2%
Time from ER Arrival to Admit. (minutes)[2]	587	353	285	274
Time from ER Arrival to Discharge (minutes)	355	193	162	134
Time in ER Before Being Evaluated (minutes)	422	33	27	26
Time to Pain Meds for Fractures (minutes)	180	69	58	57
Heart Attack Care				
Aspirin Given at Discharge	87	97%	99%	99%
Fibrinolytic Meds Within 30 Min. of Arrival[7]	-	-	67%	54%
PCI Within 90 Minutes of Arrival	12	100%	95%	96%
Statin Prescribed at Discharge	87	98%	98%	98%
Heart Failure Care				
ACE Inhibitor or ARB for LVSD[2]	95	99%	98%	97%
Discharge Instructions Given[2]	179	99%	94%	94%
Evaluation of LVS Function[2]	192	99%	99%	99%
Medicare Spending				
Medicare Spending per Patient (ratio)	-	0.91	0.93	0.98
Pneumonia Care				
Appropriate Initial Antibiotic Given[2]	100	94%	96%	95%
Blood Culture Timing[2]	128	94%	97%	98%
Pregnancy and Delivery Care				
Newborn Deliveries Scheduled Early[2]	32	0%	7%	6%
Preventive Care				
Immunization for Influenza[2]	505	88%	91%	90%
Immunization for Pneumonia[2]	306	87%	92%	92%
Stroke Care				
Anticoagulation Therapy for Atrial Fibrillation[7]	-	-	96%	95%
Antithrombotic Therapy Timing	21	95%	98%	98%
Assessed for Rehabilitation	39	85%	96%	97%
Discharged on Antithrombotic Therapy	27	100%	99%	99%
Discharged on Statin Medication	23	87%	94%	94%
Thrombolytic Therapy Timing[7]	-	-	81%	66%
Venous Thromboembolism Prophylaxis	37	95%	93%	94%
Written Stroke Educational Materials Given	31	84%	84%	88%
Surgical Care Improvement Project				
Appropriate Beta Blocker Usage[2]	18	100%	97%	98%
Appropriate VTP Within 24 Hours[2]	208	90%	98%	98%
Controlled Postoperative Blood Glucose[1,2]	-	-	96%	97%
Perioperative Temperature Management[2]	260	100%	100%	100%
Prophylactic Antibiotic Selection[2]	123	95%	99%	99%
Prophylactic Antibiotic Selection (Outpatient)	67	99%	98%	98%
Prophylactic Antibiotic Stopped[2]	122	99%	98%	98%
Prophylactic Antibiotic Timing[2]	125	92%	99%	99%
Prophylactic Antibiotic Timing (Outpatient)	70	94%	99%	98%
Urinary Catheter Removal[2]	55	91%	97%	97%
Survey of Patients' Hospital Experiences				
Area Around Room 'Always' Quiet at Night	300+	41%	57%	61%
Doctors 'Always' Communicated Well	300+	74%	77%	82%
Home Recovery Information Given	300+	82%	86%	85%
Hospital Given 9 or 10 on 10 Point Scale	300+	60%	70%	71%
Meds 'Always' Explained Before Given	300+	59%	62%	64%
Nurses 'Always' Communicated Well	300+	72%	76%	79%
Pain 'Always' Well Controlled	300+	67%	69%	71%
Room and Bathroom 'Always' Clean	300+	66%	69%	73%
Timely Help 'Always' Received	300+	61%	65%	68%
Would Definitely Recommend Hospital	300+	65%	70%	71%
Use of Medical Imaging				
Cardiac Imaging Stress Test before Surgery	60	5.0%	5.8%	5.3%
Combination Abdominal CT Scan	243	4.5%	9.1%	10.5%
Combination Brain/Sinus CT Scan[1]	-	-	3.2%	2.7%
Combination Chest CT Scan	135	0.0%	5.5%	2.7%
Follow-up Mammogram/Ultrasound	173	12.1%	8.5%	8.8%
Lumbar Spine MRI for Low Back Pain[1]	-	-	37.4%	37.2%

Maryvale Hospital

5102 West Campbell Avenue
Phoenix, AZ 85031
Phone: 623-848-5000
Fax: 623-848-5553
URL: www.maryvalehospital.com
Type: Acute Care Hospitals
Emergency Services: Yes
Ownership: Proprietary
Beds: 239

Key Personnel:
Emergency Room . . . . Stacy Aragon
Quality Assurance . . . . Diane Fox
Cardiac Laboratory. . . . . Shane Jackson
CEO/President. . . . . Gregory Pizilla
Chief of Medical Staff . . . . Frederick Scott

Measure	Cases	This Hosp.	State Avg.	U.S. Avg.
Blood Clot Prevention and Treatment				
Anticoagulation Overlap Therapy[2]	24	100%	94%	93%
ICU Venous Thromboembolism Prophylaxis[2]	93	97%	92%	92%
Incidence of Potentially Preventable VTE[1,2]	-	-	9%	10%
UFH with Dosages/Platelet Monitoring[2]	20	100%	98%	97%
Venous Thromboembolism Prophylaxis[2]	355	94%	88%	85%
Warfarin Therapy Discharge Instructions[2]	19	95%	74%	75%
Chest Pain/Possible Heart Attack Care				
Aspirin Given Within 24 Hours of Arrival	22	95%	98%	96%
Fibrinolytic Meds Within 30 Min. of Arrival[3,7]	-	-	59%	58%
Average Time to ECG (minutes)	22	2	6	7
Average Time to Transfer (minutes)[1,3]	-	-	48	60
Children's Asthma Care				
Received Home Management Plan of Care	-	-	-	88%
Received Reliever Medication	-	-	-	100%
Received Systemic Corticosteroids	-	-	-	100%
Emergency Department				
Admittance Decision Time (minutes)[2]	854	99	98	98
Head CT Results Within 45 Min. of Arrival	24	62%	64%	57%
Patients Who Left ER Before Being Seen	51,019	2%	2%	2%
Time from ER Arrival to Admit. (minutes)[2]	858	253	285	274
Time from ER Arrival to Discharge (minutes)	394	129	162	134
Time in ER Before Being Evaluated (minutes)	420	30	27	26
Time to Pain Meds for Fractures (minutes)	157	47	58	57
Heart Attack Care				
Aspirin Given at Discharge	26	100%	99%	99%
Fibrinolytic Meds Within 30 Min. of Arrival[7]	-	-	67%	54%
PCI Within 90 Minutes of Arrival[1]	-	-	95%	96%
Statin Prescribed at Discharge	24	100%	98%	98%
Heart Failure Care				
ACE Inhibitor or ARB for LVSD	82	100%	98%	97%
Discharge Instructions Given	143	100%	94%	94%
Evaluation of LVS Function	156	100%	99%	99%
Medicare Spending				
Medicare Spending per Patient (ratio)	-	0.97	0.93	0.98
Pneumonia Care				
Appropriate Initial Antibiotic Given	176	100%	96%	95%
Blood Culture Timing	294	100%	97%	98%
Pregnancy and Delivery Care				
Newborn Deliveries Scheduled Early[2]	38	0%	7%	6%
Preventive Care				
Immunization for Influenza[2]	492	90%	91%	90%
Immunization for Pneumonia[2]	544	99%	92%	92%
Stroke Care				
Anticoagulation Therapy for Atrial Fibrillation[1]	-	-	96%	95%
Antithrombotic Therapy Timing	46	100%	98%	98%
Assessed for Rehabilitation	46	98%	96%	97%
Discharged on Antithrombotic Therapy	46	96%	99%	99%
Discharged on Statin Medication	35	91%	94%	94%
Thrombolytic Therapy Timing[1]	-	-	81%	66%
Venous Thromboembolism Prophylaxis	42	98%	93%	94%
Written Stroke Educational Materials Given	28	100%	84%	88%
Surgical Care Improvement Project				
Appropriate Beta Blocker Usage[1,2]	-	-	97%	98%
Appropriate VTP Within 24 Hours[2]	72	97%	98%	98%
Controlled Postoperative Blood Glucose[2,7]	-	-	96%	97%
Perioperative Temperature Management[2]	85	100%	100%	100%
Prophylactic Antibiotic Selection[2]	24	92%	99%	99%
Prophylactic Antibiotic Selection (Outpatient)[1,3]	-	-	98%	98%
Prophylactic Antibiotic Stopped[2]	24	96%	98%	98%
Prophylactic Antibiotic Timing[2]	24	100%	99%	99%
Prophylactic Antibiotic Timing (Outpatient)[1,3]	-	-	99%	98%
Urinary Catheter Removal[2]	24	100%	97%	97%
Survey of Patients' Hospital Experiences				
Area Around Room 'Always' Quiet at Night[11]	300+	58%	57%	61%
Doctors 'Always' Communicated Well[11]	300+	76%	77%	82%
Home Recovery Information Given[11]	300+	83%	86%	85%
Hospital Given 9 or 10 on 10 Point Scale[11]	300+	64%	70%	71%
Meds 'Always' Explained Before Given[11]	300+	58%	62%	64%
Nurses 'Always' Communicated Well[11]	300+	72%	76%	79%
Pain 'Always' Well Controlled[11]	300+	67%	69%	71%
Room and Bathroom 'Always' Clean[11]	300+	67%	69%	73%
Timely Help 'Always' Received[11]	300+	59%	65%	68%
Would Definitely Recommend Hospital[11]	300+	58%	70%	71%
Use of Medical Imaging				
Cardiac Imaging Stress Test before Surgery[1]	-	-	5.8%	5.3%
Combination Abdominal CT Scan	117	0.0%	9.1%	10.5%
Combination Brain/Sinus CT Scan[1]	-	-	3.2%	2.7%
Combination Chest CT Scan[1]	-	-	5.5%	2.7%
Follow-up Mammogram/Ultrasound[7]	-	-	8.5%	8.8%
Lumbar Spine MRI for Low Back Pain[7]	-	-	37.4%	37.2%

Mayo Clinic Hospital

5777 East Mayo Boulevard
Phoenix, AZ 85054
Phone: 480-342-2000
Fax: 480-342-1138
URL: www.mayoclinic.org
Type: Acute Care Hospitals
Emergency Services: Yes
Ownership: Voluntary non-profit - Private
Beds: 407

Key Personnel:
Hemotology Center . . . . Roberts H. Adams, MD
Anesthesiology. . . . . Ricky R. Arnold, MD
CEO/President. . . . . Denis Cortese, MD

Measure	Cases	This Hosp.	State Avg.	U.S. Avg.
Blood Clot Prevention and Treatment				
Anticoagulation Overlap Therapy[2]	92	95%	94%	93%
ICU Venous Thromboembolism Prophylaxis[2]	40	95%	92%	92%
Incidence of Potentially Preventable VTE[2]	17	0%	9%	10%
UFH with Dosages/Platelet Monitoring[2]	104	100%	98%	97%
Venous Thromboembolism Prophylaxis[2]	324	99%	88%	85%
Warfarin Therapy Discharge Instructions[2]	72	82%	74%	75%
Chest Pain/Possible Heart Attack Care				
Aspirin Given Within 24 Hours of Arrival[1,3]	-	-	98%	96%
Fibrinolytic Meds Within 30 Min. of Arrival[5]	-	-	59%	58%
Average Time to ECG (minutes)[1,3]	-	-	6	7
Average Time to Transfer (minutes)[5]	-	-	48	60
Children's Asthma Care				
Received Home Management Plan of Care	-	-	-	88%
Received Reliever Medication	-	-	-	100%
Received Systemic Corticosteroids	-	-	-	100%
Emergency Department				
Admittance Decision Time (minutes)[2]	577	97	98	98
Head CT Results Within 45 Min. of Arrival[1]	-	-	64%	57%
Patients Who Left ER Before Being Seen	26,143	1%	2%	2%
Time from ER Arrival to Admit. (minutes)[2]	580	290	285	274
Time from ER Arrival to Discharge (minutes)	438	176	162	134
Time in ER Before Being Evaluated (minutes)	212	35	27	26
Time to Pain Meds for Fractures (minutes)	63	58	58	57
Heart Attack Care				
Aspirin Given at Discharge	142	97%	99%	99%
Fibrinolytic Meds Within 30 Min. of Arrival[7]	-	-	67%	54%
PCI Within 90 Minutes of Arrival	15	100%	95%	96%
Statin Prescribed at Discharge	135	98%	98%	98%
Heart Failure Care				
ACE Inhibitor or ARB for LVSD	113	100%	98%	97%
Discharge Instructions Given	265	98%	94%	94%
Evaluation of LVS Function	278	100%	99%	99%
Medicare Spending				
Medicare Spending per Patient (ratio)	-	0.91	0.93	0.98
Pneumonia Care				

NOTE: Hospital profiles are in alphabetical order by state, then city, then hospital within the city; Rankings exclude hospitals with less than 25 cases except for patient surveys which excludes hospitals with less than 100 cases; (a) 100-299 cases; (1) The number of cases/patients is too few to report; (2) Data submitted were based on a sample of cases/patients; (3) Results are based on a shorter time period than required; (4) Data suppressed by CMS for one or more quarters; (5) Results are not available for this reporting period; (6) Fewer than 100 patients completed the HCAHPS survey; (7) No cases met the criteria for this measure; (8) The lower limit of the confidence interval cannot be calculated if the number of observed infections equals zero; (9) No data are available from the state/territory for this reporting period; (10) The scores shown reflect fewer than 50 completed surveys; (11) There were discrepancies in the data collection process; (12) This measure does not apply to this hospital for this reporting period; (13) Results cannot be calculated for this reporting period; (14) The results for this state are combined with nearby states to protect confidentiality; Please refer to the User's Guide for a full explanation of data.

Measure	Cases	This Hosp.	State Avg.	U.S. Avg.
Appropriate Initial Antibiotic Given	80	96%	96%	95%
Blood Culture Timing	165	99%	97%	98%
Pregnancy and Delivery Care				
Newborn Deliveries Scheduled Early[7]	-	-	7%	6%
Preventive Care				
Immunization for Influenza[2]	696	95%	91%	90%
Immunization for Pneumonia[2]	883	91%	92%	92%
Stroke Care				
Anticoagulation Therapy for Atrial Fibrillation	32	100%	96%	95%
Antithrombotic Therapy Timing	124	98%	98%	98%
Assessed for Rehabilitation	185	99%	96%	97%
Discharged on Antithrombotic Therapy	160	98%	99%	99%
Discharged on Statin Medication	111	99%	94%	94%
Thrombolytic Therapy Timing	23	100%	81%	66%
Venous Thromboembolism Prophylaxis	182	96%	93%	94%
Written Stroke Educational Materials Given	95	95%	84%	88%
Surgical Care Improvement Project				
Appropriate Beta Blocker Usage[2]	340	99%	97%	98%
Appropriate VTP Within 24 Hours[2]	950	100%	98%	98%
Controlled Postoperative Blood Glucose[2]	168	99%	96%	97%
Perioperative Temperature Management[2]	1,160	100%	100%	100%
Prophylactic Antibiotic Selection[2]	797	99%	99%	99%
Prophylactic Antibiotic Selection (Outpatient)	886	98%	98%	98%
Prophylactic Antibiotic Stopped[2]	769	99%	98%	98%
Prophylactic Antibiotic Timing[2]	797	99%	99%	99%
Prophylactic Antibiotic Timing (Outpatient)	880	99%	99%	98%
Urinary Catheter Removal[2]	712	99%	97%	97%
Survey of Patients' Hospital Experiences				
Area Around Room 'Always' Quiet at Night[11]	300+	65%	57%	61%
Doctors 'Always' Communicated Well[11]	300+	86%	77%	82%
Home Recovery Information Given[11]	300+	90%	86%	85%
Hospital Given 9 or 10 on 10 Point Scale[11]	300+	91%	70%	71%
Meds 'Always' Explained Before Given[11]	300+	70%	62%	64%
Nurses 'Always' Communicated Well[11]	300+	86%	76%	79%
Pain 'Always' Well Controlled[11]	300+	77%	69%	71%
Room and Bathroom 'Always' Clean[11]	300+	78%	69%	73%
Timely Help 'Always' Received[11]	300+	79%	65%	68%
Would Definitely Recommend Hospital[11]	300+	93%	70%	71%
Use of Medical Imaging				
Cardiac Imaging Stress Test before Surgery	912	10.6%	5.8%	5.3%
Combination Abdominal CT Scan	1,190	6.0%	9.1%	10.5%
Combination Brain/Sinus CT Scan	778	2.7%	3.2%	2.7%
Combination Chest CT Scan	563	0.7%	5.5%	2.7%
Follow-up Mammogram/Ultrasound[7]	-	-	8.5%	8.8%
Lumbar Spine MRI for Low Back Pain	167	38.3%	37.4%	37.2%

Oasis Hospital

750 North 40th Street
Phoenix, AZ 85008
Phone: 602-797-7700
Type: Acute Care Hospitals
Emergency Services: No
Ownership: Voluntary non-profit - Private

Measure	Cases	This Hosp.	State Avg.	U.S. Avg.
Blood Clot Prevention and Treatment				
Anticoagulation Overlap Therapy[1,2]	-	-	94%	93%
ICU Venous Thromboembolism Prophylaxis[1,2]	-	-	92%	92%
Incidence of Potentially Preventable VTE[1,2]	-	-	9%	10%
UFH with Dosages/Platelet Monitoring[1,2]	-	-	98%	97%
Venous Thromboembolism Prophylaxis[2]	98	100%	88%	85%
Warfarin Therapy Discharge Instructions[1,2]	-	-	74%	75%
Chest Pain/Possible Heart Attack Care				
Aspirin Given Within 24 Hours of Arrival[5]	-	-	98%	96%
Fibrinolytic Meds Within 30 Min. of Arrival[5]	-	-	59%	58%
Average Time to ECG (minutes)[5]	-	-	6	7
Average Time to Transfer (minutes)[5]	-	-	48	60
Children's Asthma Care				
Received Home Management Plan of Care	-	-	-	88%
Received Reliever Medication	-	-	-	100%
Received Systemic Corticosteroids	-	-	-	100%
Emergency Department				
Admittance Decision Time (minutes)[2,7]	-	-	98	98
Head CT Results Within 45 Min. of Arrival[5]	-	-	64%	57%
Patients Who Left ER Before Being Seen	47	0%	2%	2%
Time from ER Arrival to Admit. (minutes)[2,7]	-	-	285	274
Time from ER Arrival to Discharge (minutes)	19	40	162	134
Time in ER Before Being Evaluated (minutes)	17	15	27	26
Time to Pain Meds for Fractures (minutes)[5]	-	-	58	57
Heart Attack Care				
Aspirin Given at Discharge[5]	-	-	99%	99%
Fibrinolytic Meds Within 30 Min. of Arrival[5]	-	-	67%	54%
PCI Within 90 Minutes of Arrival[5]	-	-	95%	96%
Statin Prescribed at Discharge[5]	-	-	98%	98%
Heart Failure Care				
ACE Inhibitor or ARB for LVSD[5]	-	-	98%	97%
Discharge Instructions Given[5]	-	-	94%	94%
Evaluation of LVS Function[5]	-	-	99%	99%
Medicare Spending				
Medicare Spending per Patient (ratio)	-	0.97	0.93	0.98
Pneumonia Care				
Appropriate Initial Antibiotic Given[5]	-	-	96%	95%
Blood Culture Timing[5]	-	-	97%	98%
Pregnancy and Delivery Care				
Newborn Deliveries Scheduled Early[2,7]	-	-	7%	6%
Preventive Care				
Immunization for Influenza[2]	338	80%	91%	90%
Immunization for Pneumonia[2]	439	72%	92%	92%
Stroke Care				
Anticoagulation Therapy for Atrial Fibrillation[5]	-	-	96%	95%
Antithrombotic Therapy Timing[5]	-	-	98%	98%
Assessed for Rehabilitation[5]	-	-	96%	97%
Discharged on Antithrombotic Therapy[5]	-	-	99%	99%
Discharged on Statin Medication[5]	-	-	94%	94%
Thrombolytic Therapy Timing[5]	-	-	81%	66%
Venous Thromboembolism Prophylaxis[5]	-	-	93%	94%
Written Stroke Educational Materials Given[5]	-	-	84%	88%
Surgical Care Improvement Project				
Appropriate Beta Blocker Usage[2]	121	96%	97%	98%
Appropriate VTP Within 24 Hours[2]	569	97%	98%	98%
Controlled Postoperative Blood Glucose[2,7]	-	-	96%	97%
Perioperative Temperature Management[2]	637	100%	100%	100%
Prophylactic Antibiotic Selection[2]	418	100%	99%	99%
Prophylactic Antibiotic Selection (Outpatient)	269	99%	98%	98%
Prophylactic Antibiotic Stopped[2]	417	98%	98%	98%
Prophylactic Antibiotic Timing[2]	418	99%	99%	99%
Prophylactic Antibiotic Timing (Outpatient)	269	98%	99%	98%
Urinary Catheter Removal[2]	435	96%	97%	97%
Survey of Patients' Hospital Experiences				
Area Around Room 'Always' Quiet at Night	300+	69%	57%	61%
Doctors 'Always' Communicated Well	300+	83%	77%	82%
Home Recovery Information Given	300+	91%	86%	85%
Hospital Given 9 or 10 on 10 Point Scale	300+	81%	70%	71%
Meds 'Always' Explained Before Given	300+	69%	62%	64%
Nurses 'Always' Communicated Well	300+	83%	76%	79%
Pain 'Always' Well Controlled	300+	70%	69%	71%
Room and Bathroom 'Always' Clean	300+	80%	69%	73%
Timely Help 'Always' Received	300+	75%	65%	68%
Would Definitely Recommend Hospital	300+	84%	70%	71%
Use of Medical Imaging				
Cardiac Imaging Stress Test before Surgery[7]	-	-	5.8%	5.3%
Combination Abdominal CT Scan[7]	-	-	9.1%	10.5%
Combination Brain/Sinus CT Scan[7]	-	-	3.2%	2.7%
Combination Chest CT Scan[7]	-	-	5.5%	2.7%
Follow-up Mammogram/Ultrasound[7]	-	-	8.5%	8.8%
Lumbar Spine MRI for Low Back Pain[7]	-	-	37.4%	37.2%

Paradise Valley Hospital

3929 East Bell Road
Phoenix, AZ 85032
Phone: 602-923-5000
Fax: 602-923-5657
URL: www.paradisevalleyhospital.com
Type: Acute Care Hospitals
Emergency Services: Yes
Ownership: Proprietary
Beds: 140

Key Personnel:

Cardiology . . . . Genaro Fernandez, MD
Operating Room. . . . . Andy Fregley
Chief of Medical Staff. . . . . Dorothy Hairston, MD
CEO/President. . . . . John Harrington
Emergency Room . . . . Brian Helender
Quality Assurance . . . . Melody Milikich
President . . . . John Pressler
Chair/CEO . . . . Prem Reddy

Measure	Cases	This Hosp.	State Avg.	U.S. Avg.
Blood Clot Prevention and Treatment				
Anticoagulation Overlap Therapy[2]	45	98%	94%	93%
ICU Venous Thromboembolism Prophylaxis[2]	73	96%	92%	92%
Incidence of Potentially Preventable VTE[2]	13	15%	9%	10%
UFH with Dosages/Platelet Monitoring[2]	16	100%	98%	97%
Venous Thromboembolism Prophylaxis[2]	337	94%	88%	85%
Warfarin Therapy Discharge Instructions[2]	36	67%	74%	75%
Chest Pain/Possible Heart Attack Care				
Aspirin Given Within 24 Hours of Arrival[1,3]	-	-	98%	96%
Fibrinolytic Meds Within 30 Min. of Arrival[3,7]	-	-	59%	58%
Average Time to ECG (minutes)[1,3]	-	-	6	7
Average Time to Transfer (minutes)[3,7]	-	-	48	60
Children's Asthma Care				
Received Home Management Plan of Care	-	-	-	88%
Received Reliever Medication	-	-	-	100%
Received Systemic Corticosteroids	-	-	-	100%
Emergency Department				
Admittance Decision Time (minutes)[2]	718	96	98	98
Head CT Results Within 45 Min. of Arrival[1]	-	-	64%	57%
Patients Who Left ER Before Being Seen	35,535	1%	2%	2%
Time from ER Arrival to Admit. (minutes)[2]	718	221	285	274
Time from ER Arrival to Discharge (minutes)	401	116	162	134
Time in ER Before Being Evaluated (minutes)	421	25	27	26
Time to Pain Meds for Fractures (minutes)	110	46	58	57
Heart Attack Care				
Aspirin Given at Discharge	69	100%	99%	99%
Fibrinolytic Meds Within 30 Min. of Arrival[7]	-	-	67%	54%
PCI Within 90 Minutes of Arrival	27	100%	95%	96%
Statin Prescribed at Discharge	70	100%	98%	98%
Heart Failure Care				
ACE Inhibitor or ARB for LVSD	44	100%	98%	97%
Discharge Instructions Given	79	100%	94%	94%
Evaluation of LVS Function	94	100%	99%	99%
Medicare Spending				
Medicare Spending per Patient (ratio)	-	0.97	0.93	0.98
Pneumonia Care				
Appropriate Initial Antibiotic Given	122	98%	96%	95%
Blood Culture Timing	205	100%	97%	98%
Pregnancy and Delivery Care				
Newborn Deliveries Scheduled Early[2]	38	8%	7%	6%
Preventive Care				
Immunization for Influenza[2]	506	99%	91%	90%
Immunization for Pneumonia[2]	535	99%	92%	92%
Stroke Care				
Anticoagulation Therapy for Atrial Fibrillation[7]	-	-	96%	95%
Antithrombotic Therapy Timing[1]	-	-	98%	98%
Assessed for Rehabilitation[1]	-	-	96%	97%
Discharged on Antithrombotic Therapy[1]	-	-	99%	99%
Discharged on Statin Medication[1]	-	-	94%	94%
Thrombolytic Therapy Timing[1]	-	-	81%	66%
Venous Thromboembolism Prophylaxis[1]	-	-	93%	94%
Written Stroke Educational Materials Given[1]	-	-	84%	88%
Surgical Care Improvement Project				
Appropriate Beta Blocker Usage[2]	42	98%	97%	98%
Appropriate VTP Within 24 Hours[2]	199	99%	98%	98%
Controlled Postoperative Blood Glucose[2,7]	-	-	96%	97%
Perioperative Temperature Management[2]	244	100%	100%	100%
Prophylactic Antibiotic Selection[2]	133	99%	99%	99%
Prophylactic Antibiotic Selection (Outpatient)	231	100%	98%	98%
Prophylactic Antibiotic Stopped[2]	125	99%	98%	98%
Prophylactic Antibiotic Timing[2]	133	99%	99%	99%
Prophylactic Antibiotic Timing (Outpatient)	231	98%	99%	98%
Urinary Catheter Removal[2]	91	99%	97%	97%
Survey of Patients' Hospital Experiences				
Area Around Room 'Always' Quiet at Night[11]	300+	61%	57%	61%
Doctors 'Always' Communicated Well[11]	300+	75%	77%	82%
Home Recovery Information Given[11]	300+	84%	86%	85%
Hospital Given 9 or 10 on 10 Point Scale[11]	300+	68%	70%	71%
Meds 'Always' Explained Before Given[11]	300+	56%	62%	64%

NOTE: Hospital profiles are in alphabetical order by state, then city, then hospital within the city; Rankings exclude hospitals with less than 25 cases except for patient surveys which excludes hospitals with less than 100 cases; (a) 100-299 cases; (1) The number of cases/patients is too few to report; (2) Data submitted were based on a sample of cases/patients; (3) Results are based on a shorter time period than required; (4) Data suppressed by CMS for one or more quarters; (5) Results are not available for this reporting period; (6) Fewer than 100 patients completed the HCAHPS survey; (7) No cases met the criteria for this measure; (8) The lower limit of the confidence interval cannot be calculated if the number of observed infections equals zero; (9) No data are available from the state/territory for this reporting period; (10) The scores shown reflect fewer than 50 completed surveys; (11) There were discrepancies in the data collection process; (12) This measure does not apply to this hospital for this reporting period; (13) Results cannot be calculated for this reporting period; (14) The results for this state are combined with nearby states to protect confidentiality; Please refer to the User's Guide for a full explanation of data.

Measure	Cases	This Hosp.	State Avg.	U.S. Avg.
Nurses 'Always' Communicated Well[11]	300+	74%	76%	79%
Pain 'Always' Well Controlled[11]	300+	70%	69%	71%
Room and Bathroom 'Always' Clean[11]	300+	66%	69%	73%
Timely Help 'Always' Received[11]	300+	63%	65%	68%
Would Definitely Recommend Hospital[11]	300+	65%	70%	71%
Use of Medical Imaging				
Cardiac Imaging Stress Test before Surgery[1]	-	-	5.8%	5.3%
Combination Abdominal CT Scan	257	2.7%	9.1%	10.5%
Combination Brain/Sinus CT Scan	254	5.1%	3.2%	2.7%
Combination Chest CT Scan	56	3.6%	5.5%	2.7%
Follow-up Mammogram/Ultrasound[7]	-	-	8.5%	8.8%
Lumbar Spine MRI for Low Back Pain[1]	-	-	37.4%	37.2%

Phoenix Baptist Hospital

2000 West Bethany Home Road
Phoenix, AZ 85015
Phone: 602-249-0212
Fax: 602-246-5849
URL: www.phoenixbaptisthospital.com
Type: Acute Care Hospitals
Emergency Services: Yes
Ownership: Proprietary
Beds: 202

Key Personnel:
Quality Assurance .... Colleen Balak-Brinson
Operating Room.............. Collen Balak Brinson
Chief of Medical Staff.......... James Kennedy, MD
CEO/President............... Dennis Knox
Pediatric Ambulatory Care ...... Harold Magalnick, MD
Pediatric In-Patient Care .... Harold Magalnick, MD
Emergency Room .... Christiene Sinon

Measure	Cases	This Hosp.	State Avg.	U.S. Avg.
Blood Clot Prevention and Treatment				
Anticoagulation Overlap Therapy[2]	77	96%	94%	93%
ICU Venous Thromboembolism Prophylaxis[2]	223	97%	92%	92%
Incidence of Potentially Preventable VTE[2]	20	10%	9%	10%
UFH with Dosages/Platelet Monitoring[2]	74	99%	98%	97%
Venous Thromboembolism Prophylaxis[2]	451	85%	88%	85%
Warfarin Therapy Discharge Instructions[2]	57	79%	74%	75%
Chest Pain/Possible Heart Attack Care				
Aspirin Given Within 24 Hours of Arrival[1,3]	-	-	98%	96%
Fibrinolytic Meds Within 30 Min. of Arrival[3,7]	-	-	59%	58%
Average Time to ECG (minutes)[1,3]	-	-	6	7
Average Time to Transfer (minutes)[1,3]	-	-	48	60
Children's Asthma Care				
Received Home Management Plan of Care	-	-	-	88%
Received Reliever Medication	-	-	-	100%
Received Systemic Corticosteroids	-	-	-	100%
Emergency Department				
Admittance Decision Time (minutes)[2]	584	125	98	98
Head CT Results Within 45 Min. of Arrival[1]	-	-	64%	57%
Patients Who Left ER Before Being Seen	62,964	1%	2%	2%
Time from ER Arrival to Admit. (minutes)[2]	605	290	285	274
Time from ER Arrival to Discharge (minutes)	654	156	162	134
Time in ER Before Being Evaluated (minutes)	665	31	27	26
Time to Pain Meds for Fractures (minutes)	129	63	58	57
Heart Attack Care				
Aspirin Given at Discharge	241	100%	99%	99%
Fibrinolytic Meds Within 30 Min. of Arrival[7]	-	-	67%	54%
PCI Within 90 Minutes of Arrival	75	96%	95%	96%
Statin Prescribed at Discharge	237	100%	98%	98%
Heart Failure Care				
ACE Inhibitor or ARB for LVSD	143	97%	98%	97%
Discharge Instructions Given	315	99%	94%	94%
Evaluation of LVS Function	337	100%	99%	99%
Medicare Spending				
Medicare Spending per Patient (ratio)	-	0.98	0.93	0.98
Pneumonia Care				
Appropriate Initial Antibiotic Given	159	97%	96%	95%
Blood Culture Timing	270	98%	97%	98%
Pregnancy and Delivery Care				
Newborn Deliveries Scheduled Early[2]	74	3%	7%	6%
Preventive Care				
Immunization for Influenza[2]	774	94%	91%	90%
Immunization for Pneumonia[2]	939	97%	92%	92%
Stroke Care				
Anticoagulation Therapy for Atrial Fibrillation	22	95%	96%	95%
Antithrombotic Therapy Timing	115	96%	98%	98%
Assessed for Rehabilitation	179	98%	96%	97%
Discharged on Antithrombotic Therapy	132	100%	99%	99%
Discharged on Statin Medication	101	99%	94%	94%
Thrombolytic Therapy Timing[1]	-	-	81%	66%
Venous Thromboembolism Prophylaxis	201	86%	93%	94%
Written Stroke Educational Materials Given	109	94%	84%	88%
Surgical Care Improvement Project				
Appropriate Beta Blocker Usage[2]	256	98%	97%	98%
Appropriate VTP Within 24 Hours[2]	367	97%	98%	98%
Controlled Postoperative Blood Glucose[2]	128	99%	96%	97%
Perioperative Temperature Management[2]	523	99%	100%	100%
Prophylactic Antibiotic Selection[2]	413	100%	99%	99%
Prophylactic Antibiotic Selection (Outpatient)	247	98%	98%	98%
Prophylactic Antibiotic Stopped[2]	394	96%	98%	98%
Prophylactic Antibiotic Timing[2]	414	100%	99%	99%
Prophylactic Antibiotic Timing (Outpatient)	249	96%	99%	98%
Urinary Catheter Removal[2]	319	98%	97%	97%
Survey of Patients' Hospital Experiences				
Area Around Room 'Always' Quiet at Night[11]	300+	58%	57%	61%
Doctors 'Always' Communicated Well[11]	300+	76%	77%	82%
Home Recovery Information Given[11]	300+	83%	86%	85%
Hospital Given 9 or 10 on 10 Point Scale[11]	300+	68%	70%	71%
Meds 'Always' Explained Before Given[11]	300+	58%	62%	64%
Nurses 'Always' Communicated Well[11]	300+	73%	76%	79%
Pain 'Always' Well Controlled[11]	300+	68%	69%	71%
Room and Bathroom 'Always' Clean[11]	300+	70%	69%	73%
Timely Help 'Always' Received[11]	300+	61%	65%	68%
Would Definitely Recommend Hospital[11]	300+	66%	70%	71%
Use of Medical Imaging				
Cardiac Imaging Stress Test before Surgery	134	2.2%	5.8%	5.3%
Combination Abdominal CT Scan	201	1.5%	9.1%	10.5%
Combination Brain/Sinus CT Scan[1]	-	-	3.2%	2.7%
Combination Chest CT Scan	78	7.7%	5.5%	2.7%
Follow-up Mammogram/Ultrasound	178	8.4%	8.5%	8.8%
Lumbar Spine MRI for Low Back Pain[1]	-	-	37.4%	37.2%

Phoenix Children's Hospital

1919 East Thomas Road
Phoenix, AZ 85016
Phone: 602-933-0400
Fax: 602-546-5655
URL: www.phxchildrens.com
Type: Childrens
Emergency Services: Yes
Ownership: Voluntary non-profit - Private
Beds: 225

Key Personnel:
Pediatric Ambulatory Care ...... Ray Adelman, MD
Pediatric In-Patient Care .... Ray Adelman, MD
Radiology.................. Craig Barnes, MD
Quality Assurance .... Joyce Joyner
Emergency Room .... Craig Laser
President/CEO............... Robert Meyer
Chief of Medical Staff.......... Bruce Morgenstern, MD

Measure	Cases	This Hosp.	State Avg.	U.S. Avg.
Blood Clot Prevention and Treatment				
Anticoagulation Overlap Therapy[5]	-	-	94%	93%
ICU Venous Thromboembolism Prophylaxis[5]	-	-	92%	92%
Incidence of Potentially Preventable VTE[5]	-	-	9%	10%
UFH with Dosages/Platelet Monitoring[5]	-	-	98%	97%
Venous Thromboembolism Prophylaxis[5]	-	-	88%	85%
Warfarin Therapy Discharge Instructions[5]	-	-	74%	75%
Chest Pain/Possible Heart Attack Care				
Aspirin Given Within 24 Hours of Arrival	-	-	98%	96%
Fibrinolytic Meds Within 30 Min. of Arrival	-	-	59%	58%
Average Time to ECG (minutes)	-	-	6	7
Average Time to Transfer (minutes)	-	-	48	60
Children's Asthma Care				
Received Home Management Plan of Care[2]	294	91%	-	88%
Received Reliever Medication[2]	294	100%	-	100%
Received Systemic Corticosteroids[2]	292	100%	-	100%
Emergency Department				
Admittance Decision Time (minutes)[5]	-	-	98	98
Head CT Results Within 45 Min. of Arrival	-	-	64%	57%
Patients Who Left ER Before Being Seen	-	-	2%	2%
Time from ER Arrival to Admit. (minutes)[5]	-	-	285	274
Time from ER Arrival to Discharge (minutes)	-	-	162	134
Time in ER Before Being Evaluated (minutes)	-	-	27	26
Time to Pain Meds for Fractures (minutes)	-	-	58	57
Heart Attack Care				
Aspirin Given at Discharge[5]	-	-	99%	99%
Fibrinolytic Meds Within 30 Min. of Arrival[5]	-	-	67%	54%
PCI Within 90 Minutes of Arrival[5]	-	-	95%	96%
Statin Prescribed at Discharge[5]	-	-	98%	98%
Heart Failure Care				
ACE Inhibitor or ARB for LVSD[5]	-	-	98%	97%
Discharge Instructions Given[5]	-	-	94%	94%
Evaluation of LVS Function[5]	-	-	99%	99%
Medicare Spending				
Medicare Spending per Patient (ratio)	-	-	0.93	0.98
Pneumonia Care				
Appropriate Initial Antibiotic Given[5]	-	-	96%	95%
Blood Culture Timing[5]	-	-	97%	98%
Pregnancy and Delivery Care				
Newborn Deliveries Scheduled Early[5]	-	-	7%	6%
Preventive Care				
Immunization for Influenza[5]	-	-	91%	90%
Immunization for Pneumonia[5]	-	-	92%	92%
Stroke Care				
Anticoagulation Therapy for Atrial Fibrillation[5]	-	-	96%	95%
Antithrombotic Therapy Timing[5]	-	-	98%	98%
Assessed for Rehabilitation[5]	-	-	96%	97%
Discharged on Antithrombotic Therapy[5]	-	-	99%	99%
Discharged on Statin Medication[5]	-	-	94%	94%
Thrombolytic Therapy Timing[5]	-	-	81%	66%
Venous Thromboembolism Prophylaxis[5]	-	-	93%	94%
Written Stroke Educational Materials Given[5]	-	-	84%	88%
Surgical Care Improvement Project				
Appropriate Beta Blocker Usage[5]	-	-	97%	98%
Appropriate VTP Within 24 Hours[5]	-	-	98%	98%
Controlled Postoperative Blood Glucose[5]	-	-	96%	97%
Perioperative Temperature Management[5]	-	-	100%	100%
Prophylactic Antibiotic Selection[5]	-	-	99%	99%
Prophylactic Antibiotic Selection (Outpatient)	-	-	98%	98%
Prophylactic Antibiotic Stopped[5]	-	-	98%	98%
Prophylactic Antibiotic Timing[5]	-	-	99%	99%
Prophylactic Antibiotic Timing (Outpatient)	-	-	99%	98%
Urinary Catheter Removal[5]	-	-	97%	97%
Survey of Patients' Hospital Experiences				
Area Around Room 'Always' Quiet at Night[5]	-	-	57%	61%
Doctors 'Always' Communicated Well[5]	-	-	77%	82%
Home Recovery Information Given[5]	-	-	86%	85%
Hospital Given 9 or 10 on 10 Point Scale[5]	-	-	70%	71%
Meds 'Always' Explained Before Given[5]	-	-	62%	64%
Nurses 'Always' Communicated Well[5]	-	-	76%	79%
Pain 'Always' Well Controlled[5]	-	-	69%	71%
Room and Bathroom 'Always' Clean[5]	-	-	69%	73%
Timely Help 'Always' Received[5]	-	-	65%	68%
Would Definitely Recommend Hospital[5]	-	-	70%	71%
Use of Medical Imaging				
Cardiac Imaging Stress Test before Surgery	-	-	5.8%	5.3%
Combination Abdominal CT Scan	-	-	9.1%	10.5%
Combination Brain/Sinus CT Scan	-	-	3.2%	2.7%
Combination Chest CT Scan	-	-	5.5%	2.7%
Follow-up Mammogram/Ultrasound	-	-	8.5%	8.8%
Lumbar Spine MRI for Low Back Pain	-	-	37.4%	37.2%

Phoenix Indian Medical Center

4212 North 16th Street
Phoenix, AZ 85016
Phone: 602-263-1200
Fax: 602-263-1631
URL: www.ihs.gov
Type: Acute Care Hospitals
Emergency Services: No
Ownership: Government - Federal
Beds: 199

Key Personnel:
Operating Room.............. Patricia Gallagher, RN
Pediatric Ambulatory Care ...... Al Hargrave
Pediatric In-Patient Care .... Al Hargrave
Quality Assurance .... John Meeth

Measure	Cases	This Hosp.	State Avg.	U.S. Avg.
Blood Clot Prevention and Treatment				
Anticoagulation Overlap Therapy[2,7]	-	-	94%	93%

NOTE: Hospital profiles are in alphabetical order by state, then city, then hospital within the city; Rankings exclude hospitals with less than 25 cases except for patient surveys which excludes hospitals with less than 100 cases; (a) 100-299 cases; (1) The number of cases/patients is too few to report; (2) Data submitted were based on a sample of cases/patients; (3) Results are based on a shorter time period than required; (4) Data suppressed by CMS for one or more quarters; (5) Results are not available for this reporting period; (6) Fewer than 100 patients completed the HCAHPS survey; (7) No cases met the criteria for this measure; (8) The lower limit of the confidence interval cannot be calculated if the number of observed infections equals zero; (9) No data are available from the state/territory for this reporting period; (10) The scores shown reflect fewer than 50 completed surveys; (11) There were discrepancies in the data collection process; (12) This measure does not apply to this hospital for this reporting period; (13) Results cannot be calculated for this reporting period; (14) The results for this state are combined with nearby states to protect confidentiality; Please refer to the User's Guide for a full explanation of data.

Measure	Cases	This Hosp.	State Avg.	U.S. Avg.
ICU Venous Thromboembolism Prophylaxis[1,2]	-	-	92%	92%
Incidence of Potentially Preventable VTE[2,7]	-	-	9%	10%
UFH with Dosages/Platelet Monitoring[2,7]	-	-	98%	97%
Venous Thromboembolism Prophylaxis[2]	150	97%	88%	85%
Warfarin Therapy Discharge Instructions[2,7]	-	-	74%	75%
Chest Pain/Possible Heart Attack Care				
Aspirin Given Within 24 Hours of Arrival	-	-	98%	96%
Fibrinolytic Meds Within 30 Min. of Arrival	-	-	59%	58%
Average Time to ECG (minutes)	-	-	6	7
Average Time to Transfer (minutes)	-	-	48	60
Children's Asthma Care				
Received Home Management Plan of Care	-	-	-	88%
Received Reliever Medication	-	-	-	100%
Received Systemic Corticosteroids	-	-	-	100%
Emergency Department				
Admittance Decision Time (minutes)[2]	351	108	98	98
Head CT Results Within 45 Min. of Arrival	-	-	64%	57%
Patients Who Left ER Before Being Seen	-	-	2%	2%
Time from ER Arrival to Admit. (minutes)[2]	368	445	285	274
Time from ER Arrival to Discharge (minutes)	-	-	162	134
Time in ER Before Being Evaluated (minutes)	-	-	27	26
Time to Pain Meds for Fractures (minutes)	-	-	58	57
Heart Attack Care				
Aspirin Given at Discharge[5]	-	-	99%	99%
Fibrinolytic Meds Within 30 Min. of Arrival[5]	-	-	67%	54%
PCI Within 90 Minutes of Arrival[5]	-	-	95%	96%
Statin Prescribed at Discharge[5]	-	-	98%	98%
Heart Failure Care				
ACE Inhibitor or ARB for LVSD[5]	-	-	98%	97%
Discharge Instructions Given[5]	-	-	94%	94%
Evaluation of LVS Function[5]	-	-	99%	99%
Medicare Spending				
Medicare Spending per Patient (ratio)	-	0.75	0.93	0.98
Pneumonia Care				
Appropriate Initial Antibiotic Given[2]	55	98%	96%	95%
Blood Culture Timing[2]	61	87%	97%	98%
Pregnancy and Delivery Care				
Newborn Deliveries Scheduled Early[2]	11	0%	7%	6%
Preventive Care				
Immunization for Influenza[2]	296	89%	91%	90%
Immunization for Pneumonia[2]	272	91%	92%	92%
Stroke Care				
Anticoagulation Therapy for Atrial Fibrillation[5]	-	-	96%	95%
Antithrombotic Therapy Timing[5]	-	-	98%	98%
Assessed for Rehabilitation[5]	-	-	96%	97%
Discharged on Antithrombotic Therapy[5]	-	-	99%	99%
Discharged on Statin Medication[5]	-	-	94%	94%
Thrombolytic Therapy Timing[5]	-	-	81%	66%
Venous Thromboembolism Prophylaxis[5]	-	-	93%	94%
Written Stroke Educational Materials Given[5]	-	-	84%	88%
Surgical Care Improvement Project				
Appropriate Beta Blocker Usage[1,2]	-	-	97%	98%
Appropriate VTP Within 24 Hours[2]	76	97%	98%	98%
Controlled Postoperative Blood Glucose[2,7]	-	-	96%	97%
Perioperative Temperature Management[2]	78	100%	100%	100%
Prophylactic Antibiotic Selection[2]	37	95%	99%	99%
Prophylactic Antibiotic Selection (Outpatient)	-	-	98%	98%
Prophylactic Antibiotic Stopped[2]	37	95%	98%	98%
Prophylactic Antibiotic Timing[2]	37	97%	99%	99%
Prophylactic Antibiotic Timing (Outpatient)	-	-	99%	98%
Urinary Catheter Removal[1,2]	-	-	97%	97%
Survey of Patients' Hospital Experiences				
Area Around Room 'Always' Quiet at Night	300+	56%	57%	61%
Doctors 'Always' Communicated Well	300+	82%	77%	82%
Home Recovery Information Given	300+	83%	86%	85%
Hospital Given 9 or 10 on 10 Point Scale	300+	63%	70%	71%
Meds 'Always' Explained Before Given	300+	68%	62%	64%
Nurses 'Always' Communicated Well	300+	75%	76%	79%
Pain 'Always' Well Controlled	300+	76%	69%	71%
Room and Bathroom 'Always' Clean	300+	63%	69%	73%
Timely Help 'Always' Received	300+	69%	65%	68%
Would Definitely Recommend Hospital	300+	59%	70%	71%
Use of Medical Imaging				
Cardiac Imaging Stress Test before Surgery	-	-	5.8%	5.3%
Combination Abdominal CT Scan	-	-	9.1%	10.5%
Combination Brain/Sinus CT Scan	-	-	3.2%	2.7%
Combination Chest CT Scan	-	-	5.5%	2.7%
Follow-up Mammogram/Ultrasound	-	-	8.5%	8.8%
Lumbar Spine MRI for Low Back Pain	-	-	37.4%	37.2%

Phoenix VA Medical Center

650 E. Indian School Road
Phoenix, AZ 85012
Phone: 602-222-6444
Fax: 602-222-6489
URL: www.phoenix.med.va.gov
Type: Acute Care - VA
Emergency Services: No
Ownership: Government Federal
Key Personnel:
Chief of Medical Staff . . . . Raymond Chung, MD

Measure	Cases	This Hosp.	State Avg.	U.S. Avg.
Blood Clot Prevention and Treatment				
Anticoagulation Overlap Therapy	-	-	94%	93%
ICU Venous Thromboembolism Prophylaxis	-	-	92%	92%
Incidence of Potentially Preventable VTE	-	-	9%	10%
UFH with Dosages/Platelet Monitoring	-	-	98%	97%
Venous Thromboembolism Prophylaxis	-	-	88%	85%
Warfarin Therapy Discharge Instructions	-	-	74%	75%
Chest Pain/Possible Heart Attack Care				
Aspirin Given Within 24 Hours of Arrival	-	-	98%	96%
Fibrinolytic Meds Within 30 Min. of Arrival	-	-	59%	58%
Average Time to ECG (minutes)	-	-	6	7
Average Time to Transfer (minutes)	-	-	48	60
Children's Asthma Care				
Received Home Management Plan of Care	-	-	-	88%
Received Reliever Medication	-	-	-	100%
Received Systemic Corticosteroids	-	-	-	100%
Emergency Department				
Admittance Decision Time (minutes)	-	-	98	98
Head CT Results Within 45 Min. of Arrival	-	-	64%	57%
Patients Who Left ER Before Being Seen	-	-	2%	2%
Time from ER Arrival to Admit. (minutes)	-	-	285	274
Time from ER Arrival to Discharge (minutes)	-	-	162	134
Time in ER Before Being Evaluated (minutes)	-	-	27	26
Time to Pain Meds for Fractures (minutes)	-	-	58	57
Heart Attack Care				
Aspirin Given at Discharge	29	100%	99%	99%
Fibrinolytic Meds Within 30 Min. of Arrival[5]	-	-	67%	54%
PCI Within 90 Minutes of Arrival[5]	-	-	95%	96%
Statin Prescribed at Discharge	30	100%	98%	98%
Heart Failure Care				
ACE Inhibitor or ARB for LVSD	85	100%	98%	97%
Discharge Instructions Given	201	95%	94%	94%
Evaluation of LVS Function	211	100%	99%	99%
Medicare Spending				
Medicare Spending per Patient (ratio)	-	-	0.93	0.98
Pneumonia Care				
Appropriate Initial Antibiotic Given	71	99%	96%	95%
Blood Culture Timing	129	98%	97%	98%
Pregnancy and Delivery Care				
Newborn Deliveries Scheduled Early	-	-	7%	6%
Preventive Care				
Immunization for Influenza[5]	-	-	91%	90%
Immunization for Pneumonia[5]	-	-	92%	92%
Stroke Care				
Anticoagulation Therapy for Atrial Fibrillation	-	-	96%	95%
Antithrombotic Therapy Timing	-	-	98%	98%
Assessed for Rehabilitation	-	-	96%	97%
Discharged on Antithrombotic Therapy	-	-	99%	99%
Discharged on Statin Medication	-	-	94%	94%
Thrombolytic Therapy Timing	-	-	81%	66%
Venous Thromboembolism Prophylaxis	-	-	93%	94%
Written Stroke Educational Materials Given	-	-	84%	88%
Surgical Care Improvement Project				
Appropriate Beta Blocker Usage[2]	133	99%	97%	98%
Appropriate VTP Within 24 Hours[2]	340	96%	98%	98%
Controlled Postoperative Blood Glucose[5]	-	-	96%	97%
Perioperative Temperature Management[2]	392	100%	100%	100%
Prophylactic Antibiotic Selection	257	100%	99%	99%
Prophylactic Antibiotic Selection (Outpatient)	-	-	98%	98%
Prophylactic Antibiotic Stopped	255	96%	98%	98%
Prophylactic Antibiotic Timing	257	97%	99%	99%
Prophylactic Antibiotic Timing (Outpatient)	-	-	99%	98%
Urinary Catheter Removal[2]	162	100%	97%	97%
Survey of Patients' Hospital Experiences				
Area Around Room 'Always' Quiet at Night	-	-	57%	61%
Doctors 'Always' Communicated Well	-	-	77%	82%
Home Recovery Information Given	-	-	86%	85%
Hospital Given 9 or 10 on 10 Point Scale	-	-	70%	71%
Meds 'Always' Explained Before Given	-	-	62%	64%
Nurses 'Always' Communicated Well	-	-	76%	79%
Pain 'Always' Well Controlled	-	-	69%	71%
Room and Bathroom 'Always' Clean	-	-	69%	73%
Timely Help 'Always' Received	-	-	65%	68%
Would Definitely Recommend Hospital	-	-	70%	71%
Use of Medical Imaging				
Cardiac Imaging Stress Test before Surgery	-	-	5.8%	5.3%
Combination Abdominal CT Scan	-	-	9.1%	10.5%
Combination Brain/Sinus CT Scan	-	-	3.2%	2.7%
Combination Chest CT Scan	-	-	5.5%	2.7%
Follow-up Mammogram/Ultrasound	-	-	8.5%	8.8%
Lumbar Spine MRI for Low Back Pain	-	-	37.4%	37.2%

Saint Joseph's Hospital & Medical Center

350 West Thomas Road
Phoenix, AZ 85013
Phone: 602-406-3000
Fax: 602-406-7143
URL: www.stjosephs-phx.org
Type: Acute Care Hospitals
Emergency Services: Yes
Ownership: Voluntary non-profit - Church
Beds: 535
Key Personnel:
Chief of Medical Staff . . . . Edward Donahue, MD
Quality Assurance . . . . Charles P Francis
Pediatric In-Patient Care . . . . Gifford Loda
Pediatric Ambulatory Care . . . . . . Robert Pryor, MD
Anesthesiology. . . . . Elizabeth Shih
Emergency Room . . . . Julie Ward
CEO/President. . . . . Patty White
Patient Relations . . . . Patty White

Measure	Cases	This Hosp.	State Avg.	U.S. Avg.
Blood Clot Prevention and Treatment				
Anticoagulation Overlap Therapy[2]	179	97%	94%	93%
ICU Venous Thromboembolism Prophylaxis[2]	147	99%	92%	92%
Incidence of Potentially Preventable VTE[2]	64	2%	9%	10%
UFH with Dosages/Platelet Monitoring[2]	97	100%	98%	97%
Venous Thromboembolism Prophylaxis[2]	267	93%	88%	85%
Warfarin Therapy Discharge Instructions[2]	129	96%	74%	75%
Chest Pain/Possible Heart Attack Care				
Aspirin Given Within 24 Hours of Arrival[1,3]	-	-	98%	96%
Fibrinolytic Meds Within 30 Min. of Arrival[3,7]	-	-	59%	58%
Average Time to ECG (minutes)[1,3]	-	-	6	7
Average Time to Transfer (minutes)[3,7]	-	-	48	60
Children's Asthma Care				
Received Home Management Plan of Care	-	-	-	88%
Received Reliever Medication	-	-	-	100%
Received Systemic Corticosteroids	-	-	-	100%
Emergency Department				
Admittance Decision Time (minutes)[2]	374	174	98	98
Head CT Results Within 45 Min. of Arrival[1]	-	-	64%	57%
Patients Who Left ER Before Being Seen	84,832	0%	2%	2%
Time from ER Arrival to Admit. (minutes)[2]	375	362	285	274
Time from ER Arrival to Discharge (minutes)	367	180	162	134
Time in ER Before Being Evaluated (minutes)	409	27	27	26
Time to Pain Meds for Fractures (minutes)	147	66	58	57
Heart Attack Care				
Aspirin Given at Discharge	202	100%	99%	99%
Fibrinolytic Meds Within 30 Min. of Arrival[7]	-	-	67%	54%
PCI Within 90 Minutes of Arrival	39	100%	95%	96%
Statin Prescribed at Discharge	200	100%	98%	98%
Heart Failure Care				
ACE Inhibitor or ARB for LVSD[2]	117	100%	98%	97%
Discharge Instructions Given[2]	236	98%	94%	94%

NOTE: Hospital profiles are in alphabetical order by state, then city, then hospital within the city; Rankings exclude hospitals with less than 25 cases except for patient surveys which excludes hospitals with less than 100 cases; (a) 100-299 cases; (1) The number of cases/patients is too few to report; (2) Data submitted were based on a sample of cases/patients; (3) Results are based on a shorter time period than required; (4) Data suppressed by CMS for one or more quarters; (5) Results are not available for this reporting period; (6) Fewer than 100 patients completed the HCAHPS survey; (7) No cases met the criteria for this measure; (8) The lower limit of the confidence interval cannot be calculated if the number of observed infections equals zero; (9) No data are available from the state/territory for this reporting period; (10) The scores shown reflect fewer than 50 completed surveys; (11) There were discrepancies in the data collection process; (12) This measure does not apply to this hospital for this reporting period; (13) Results cannot be calculated for this reporting period; (14) The results for this state are combined with nearby states to protect confidentiality; Please refer to the User's Guide for a full explanation of data.

Measure	Cases	This Hosp.	State Avg.	U.S. Avg.
Evaluation of LVS Function[2]	258	100%	99%	99%
Medicare Spending				
Medicare Spending per Patient (ratio)	-	1.00	0.93	0.98
Pneumonia Care				
Appropriate Initial Antibiotic Given[2]	61	100%	96%	95%
Blood Culture Timing[2]	159	96%	97%	98%
Pregnancy and Delivery Care				
Newborn Deliveries Scheduled Early[2]	94	7%	7%	6%
Preventive Care				
Immunization for Influenza[2]	513	91%	91%	90%
Immunization for Pneumonia[2]	463	83%	92%	92%
Stroke Care				
Anticoagulation Therapy for Atrial Fibrillation	72	96%	96%	95%
Antithrombotic Therapy Timing	257	99%	98%	98%
Assessed for Rehabilitation	554	92%	96%	97%
Discharged on Antithrombotic Therapy	325	98%	99%	99%
Discharged on Statin Medication	262	97%	94%	94%
Thrombolytic Therapy Timing	37	97%	81%	66%
Venous Thromboembolism Prophylaxis	595	97%	93%	94%
Written Stroke Educational Materials Given	305	72%	84%	88%
Surgical Care Improvement Project				
Appropriate Beta Blocker Usage[2]	163	99%	97%	98%
Appropriate VTP Within 24 Hours[2]	379	98%	98%	98%
Controlled Postoperative Blood Glucose[2]	150	95%	96%	97%
Perioperative Temperature Management[2]	501	100%	100%	100%
Prophylactic Antibiotic Selection[2]	381	98%	99%	99%
Prophylactic Antibiotic Selection (Outpatient)	504	99%	98%	98%
Prophylactic Antibiotic Stopped[2]	367	97%	98%	98%
Prophylactic Antibiotic Timing[2]	380	100%	99%	99%
Prophylactic Antibiotic Timing (Outpatient)	506	100%	99%	98%
Urinary Catheter Removal[2]	343	99%	97%	97%
Survey of Patients' Hospital Experiences				
Area Around Room 'Always' Quiet at Night	300+	59%	57%	61%
Doctors 'Always' Communicated Well	300+	76%	77%	82%
Home Recovery Information Given	300+	84%	86%	85%
Hospital Given 9 or 10 on 10 Point Scale	300+	74%	70%	71%
Meds 'Always' Explained Before Given	300+	61%	62%	64%
Nurses 'Always' Communicated Well	300+	75%	76%	79%
Pain 'Always' Well Controlled	300+	69%	69%	71%
Room and Bathroom 'Always' Clean	300+	72%	69%	73%
Timely Help 'Always' Received	300+	60%	65%	68%
Would Definitely Recommend Hospital	300+	77%	70%	71%
Use of Medical Imaging				
Cardiac Imaging Stress Test before Surgery	170	3.5%	5.8%	5.3%
Combination Abdominal CT Scan	510	4.5%	9.1%	10.5%
Combination Brain/Sinus CT Scan	889	2.1%	3.2%	2.7%
Combination Chest CT Scan	469	0.2%	5.5%	2.7%
Follow-up Mammogram/Ultrasound	270	16.7%	8.5%	8.8%
Lumbar Spine MRI for Low Back Pain	87	39.1%	37.4%	37.2%

Saint Luke's Medical Center

1800 East Van Buren Street
Phoenix, AZ 85006
Phone: 602-251-8156
Fax: 602-251-8761
URL: www.stlukesmedcenter.com
Type: Acute Care Hospitals
Emergency Services: Yes
Ownership: Proprietary
Beds: 235

Key Personnel:
Radiology. . . . . Imtiaz Ahmed
Quality Assurance . . . . Ellen Campbell
CEO/President. . . . . Brent A Cope
Operating Room. . . . . John DeBarros
Patient Relations . . . . Deb Hartman
Chief of Medical Staff. . . . . Robert A Kearl, MD
Intensive Care Unit. . . . . Joesph Lotsko
Infection Control. . . . . Tery Thuoite

Measure	Cases	This Hosp.	State Avg.	U.S. Avg.
Blood Clot Prevention and Treatment				
Anticoagulation Overlap Therapy[2]	63	95%	94%	93%
ICU Venous Thromboembolism Prophylaxis[2]	121	76%	92%	92%
Incidence of Potentially Preventable VTE[2]	14	21%	9%	10%
UFH with Dosages/Platelet Monitoring[2]	41	100%	98%	97%
Venous Thromboembolism Prophylaxis[2]	389	77%	88%	85%
Warfarin Therapy Discharge Instructions[2]	42	98%	74%	75%
Chest Pain/Possible Heart Attack Care				
Aspirin Given Within 24 Hours of Arrival[1]	-	-	98%	96%
Fibrinolytic Meds Within 30 Min. of Arrival[5]	-	-	59%	58%
Average Time to ECG (minutes)[1]	-	-	6	7
Average Time to Transfer (minutes)[5]	-	-	48	60
Children's Asthma Care				
Received Home Management Plan of Care	-	-	-	88%
Received Reliever Medication	-	-	-	100%
Received Systemic Corticosteroids	-	-	-	100%
Emergency Department				
Admittance Decision Time (minutes)[2]	562	148	98	98
Head CT Results Within 45 Min. of Arrival[1]	-	-	64%	57%
Patients Who Left ER Before Being Seen	52,242	1%	2%	2%
Time from ER Arrival to Admit. (minutes)[2]	589	353	285	274
Time from ER Arrival to Discharge (minutes)	445	166	162	134
Time in ER Before Being Evaluated (minutes)	486	49	27	26
Time to Pain Meds for Fractures (minutes)	103	67	58	57
Heart Attack Care				
Aspirin Given at Discharge	139	97%	99%	99%
Fibrinolytic Meds Within 30 Min. of Arrival[7]	-	-	67%	54%
PCI Within 90 Minutes of Arrival[1]	-	-	95%	96%
Statin Prescribed at Discharge	141	89%	98%	98%
Heart Failure Care				
ACE Inhibitor or ARB for LVSD	67	84%	98%	97%
Discharge Instructions Given	120	80%	94%	94%
Evaluation of LVS Function	138	99%	99%	99%
Medicare Spending				
Medicare Spending per Patient (ratio)	-	1.01	0.93	0.98
Pneumonia Care				
Appropriate Initial Antibiotic Given	98	98%	96%	95%
Blood Culture Timing	145	97%	97%	98%
Pregnancy and Delivery Care				
Newborn Deliveries Scheduled Early	55	9%	7%	6%
Preventive Care				
Immunization for Influenza[2]	766	93%	91%	90%
Immunization for Pneumonia[2]	814	94%	92%	92%
Stroke Care				
Anticoagulation Therapy for Atrial Fibrillation[7]	-	-	96%	95%
Antithrombotic Therapy Timing	34	91%	98%	98%
Assessed for Rehabilitation	33	82%	96%	97%
Discharged on Antithrombotic Therapy	31	94%	99%	99%
Discharged on Statin Medication	25	68%	94%	94%
Thrombolytic Therapy Timing[1]	-	-	81%	66%
Venous Thromboembolism Prophylaxis	39	72%	93%	94%
Written Stroke Educational Materials Given	24	92%	84%	88%
Surgical Care Improvement Project				
Appropriate Beta Blocker Usage	307	98%	97%	98%
Appropriate VTP Within 24 Hours	793	97%	98%	98%
Controlled Postoperative Blood Glucose	79	99%	96%	97%
Perioperative Temperature Management	1,174	100%	100%	100%
Prophylactic Antibiotic Selection	846	99%	99%	99%
Prophylactic Antibiotic Selection (Outpatient)	137	97%	98%	98%
Prophylactic Antibiotic Stopped	827	99%	98%	98%
Prophylactic Antibiotic Timing	846	100%	99%	99%
Prophylactic Antibiotic Timing (Outpatient)	137	97%	99%	98%
Urinary Catheter Removal	298	96%	97%	97%
Survey of Patients' Hospital Experiences				
Area Around Room 'Always' Quiet at Night	300+	62%	57%	61%
Doctors 'Always' Communicated Well	300+	80%	77%	82%
Home Recovery Information Given	300+	86%	86%	85%
Hospital Given 9 or 10 on 10 Point Scale	300+	68%	70%	71%
Meds 'Always' Explained Before Given	300+	66%	62%	64%
Nurses 'Always' Communicated Well	300+	76%	76%	79%
Pain 'Always' Well Controlled	300+	71%	69%	71%
Room and Bathroom 'Always' Clean	300+	70%	69%	73%
Timely Help 'Always' Received	300+	61%	65%	68%
Would Definitely Recommend Hospital	300+	67%	70%	71%
Use of Medical Imaging				
Cardiac Imaging Stress Test before Surgery[1]	-	-	5.8%	5.3%
Combination Abdominal CT Scan	140	0.7%	9.1%	10.5%
Combination Brain/Sinus CT Scan[1]	-	-	3.2%	2.7%
Combination Chest CT Scan[1]	-	-	5.5%	2.7%
Follow-up Mammogram/Ultrasound[1]	-	-	8.5%	8.8%
Lumbar Spine MRI for Low Back Pain[1]	-	-	37.4%	37.2%

The Surgical Hospital of Phoenix

6501 North 19th Avenue
Phoenix, AZ 85015
Phone: 602-795-6020
Fax: 602-795-6022
E-mail: admin@sshaz.com
URL: www.sshaz.com
Type: Acute Care Hospitals
Emergency Services: No
Ownership: Proprietary
Beds: 27

Key Personnel:
Radiology. . . . . Richard Chesbrough, MD
Infection Control. . . . . Colleen Clarke, RN
CEO/President. . . . . Constance Harmsen, RN, MS
Operating Room. . . . . Rod Malone, RN
Anesthesiology. . . . . Jeffrey P. Serwin, D.O.
Chief of Medical Staff . . . . Marky Siegel, DO
Quality Assurance . . . . Jan Wilson, RN

Measure	Cases	This Hosp.	State Avg.	U.S. Avg.
Blood Clot Prevention and Treatment				
Anticoagulation Overlap Therapy[1,2]	-	-	94%	93%
ICU Venous Thromboembolism Prophylaxis[2,7]	-	-	92%	92%
Incidence of Potentially Preventable VTE[1,2]	-	-	9%	10%
UFH with Dosages/Platelet Monitoring[2,7]	-	-	98%	97%
Venous Thromboembolism Prophylaxis[2]	41	98%	88%	85%
Warfarin Therapy Discharge Instructions[1,2]	-	-	74%	75%
Chest Pain/Possible Heart Attack Care				
Aspirin Given Within 24 Hours of Arrival[5]	-	-	98%	96%
Fibrinolytic Meds Within 30 Min. of Arrival[5]	-	-	59%	58%
Average Time to ECG (minutes)[5]	-	-	6	7
Average Time to Transfer (minutes)[5]	-	-	48	60
Children's Asthma Care				
Received Home Management Plan of Care	-	-	-	88%
Received Reliever Medication	-	-	-	100%
Received Systemic Corticosteroids	-	-	-	100%
Emergency Department				
Admittance Decision Time (minutes)[2,7]	-	-	98	98
Head CT Results Within 45 Min. of Arrival[5]	-	-	64%	57%
Patients Who Left ER Before Being Seen[5]	-	-	2%	2%
Time from ER Arrival to Admit. (minutes)[2,7]	-	-	285	274
Time from ER Arrival to Discharge (minutes)[5]	-	-	162	134
Time in ER Before Being Evaluated (minutes)[5]	-	-	27	26
Time to Pain Meds for Fractures (minutes)[5]	-	-	58	57
Heart Attack Care				
Aspirin Given at Discharge[5]	-	-	99%	99%
Fibrinolytic Meds Within 30 Min. of Arrival[5]	-	-	67%	54%
PCI Within 90 Minutes of Arrival[5]	-	-	95%	96%
Statin Prescribed at Discharge[5]	-	-	98%	98%
Heart Failure Care				
ACE Inhibitor or ARB for LVSD[5]	-	-	98%	97%
Discharge Instructions Given[5]	-	-	94%	94%
Evaluation of LVS Function[5]	-	-	99%	99%
Medicare Spending				
Medicare Spending per Patient (ratio)	-	0.90	0.93	0.98
Pneumonia Care				
Appropriate Initial Antibiotic Given[5]	-	-	96%	95%
Blood Culture Timing[5]	-	-	97%	98%
Pregnancy and Delivery Care				
Newborn Deliveries Scheduled Early[2,7]	-	-	7%	6%
Preventive Care				
Immunization for Influenza[2]	317	83%	91%	90%
Immunization for Pneumonia[2]	326	87%	92%	92%
Stroke Care				
Anticoagulation Therapy for Atrial Fibrillation[5]	-	-	96%	95%
Antithrombotic Therapy Timing[5]	-	-	98%	98%
Assessed for Rehabilitation[5]	-	-	96%	97%
Discharged on Antithrombotic Therapy[5]	-	-	99%	99%
Discharged on Statin Medication[5]	-	-	94%	94%
Thrombolytic Therapy Timing[5]	-	-	81%	66%
Venous Thromboembolism Prophylaxis[5]	-	-	93%	94%
Written Stroke Educational Materials Given[5]	-	-	84%	88%
Surgical Care Improvement Project				
Appropriate Beta Blocker Usage[2]	26	92%	97%	98%
Appropriate VTP Within 24 Hours[2]	90	100%	98%	98%
Controlled Postoperative Blood Glucose[2,7]	-	-	96%	97%

NOTE: Hospital profiles are in alphabetical order by state, then city, then hospital within the city; Rankings exclude hospitals with less than 25 cases except for patient surveys which excludes hospitals with less than 100 cases; (a) 100-299 cases; (1) The number of cases/patients is too few to report; (2) Data submitted were based on a sample of cases/patients; (3) Results are based on a shorter time period than required; (4) Data suppressed by CMS for one or more quarters; (5) Results are not available for this reporting period; (6) Fewer than 100 patients completed the HCAHPS survey; (7) No cases met the criteria for this measure; (8) The lower limit of the confidence interval cannot be calculated if the number of observed infections equals zero; (9) No data are available from the state/territory for this reporting period; (10) The scores shown reflect fewer than 50 completed surveys; (11) There were discrepancies in the data collection process; (12) This measure does not apply to this hospital for this reporting period; (13) Results cannot be calculated for this reporting period; (14) The results for this state are combined with nearby states to protect confidentiality; Please refer to the User's Guide for a full explanation of data.

Measure	Cases	This Hosp.	State Avg.	U.S. Avg.
Perioperative Temperature Management[2]	101	98%	100%	100%
Prophylactic Antibiotic Selection[2]	94	99%	99%	99%
Prophylactic Antibiotic Selection (Outpatient)	181	97%	98%	98%
Prophylactic Antibiotic Stopped[2]	93	98%	98%	98%
Prophylactic Antibiotic Timing[2]	94	99%	99%	99%
Prophylactic Antibiotic Timing (Outpatient)	181	97%	99%	98%
Urinary Catheter Removal[2]	60	100%	97%	97%
Survey of Patients' Hospital Experiences				
Area Around Room 'Always' Quiet at Night	300+	78%	57%	61%
Doctors 'Always' Communicated Well	300+	81%	77%	82%
Home Recovery Information Given	300+	88%	86%	85%
Hospital Given 9 or 10 on 10 Point Scale	300+	81%	70%	71%
Meds 'Always' Explained Before Given	300+	65%	62%	64%
Nurses 'Always' Communicated Well	300+	85%	76%	79%
Pain 'Always' Well Controlled	300+	72%	69%	71%
Room and Bathroom 'Always' Clean	300+	81%	69%	73%
Timely Help 'Always' Received	300+	81%	65%	68%
Would Definitely Recommend Hospital	300+	83%	70%	71%
Use of Medical Imaging				
Cardiac Imaging Stress Test before Surgery[7]	-	-	5.8%	5.3%
Combination Abdominal CT Scan[1]	-	-	9.1%	10.5%
Combination Brain/Sinus CT Scan[1]	-	-	3.2%	2.7%
Combination Chest CT Scan[1]	-	-	5.5%	2.7%
Follow-up Mammogram/Ultrasound[7]	-	-	8.5%	8.8%
Lumbar Spine MRI for Low Back Pain[1]	-	-	37.4%	37.2%

Hopi Health Care Center

Highway 264, Milepost 388 | Phone: 928-737-6000
Polacca, AZ 86042
URL: www.ihs.gov/facilitiesservices/areaoffices/phoenix
Type: Critical Access Hospitals | Emergency Services: No
Ownership: Tribal | Beds: 15

Measure	Cases	This Hosp.	State Avg.	U.S. Avg.
Blood Clot Prevention and Treatment				
Anticoagulation Overlap Therapy[5]	-	-	94%	93%
ICU Venous Thromboembolism Prophylaxis[5]	-	-	92%	92%
Incidence of Potentially Preventable VTE[5]	-	-	9%	10%
UFH with Dosages/Platelet Monitoring[5]	-	-	98%	97%
Venous Thromboembolism Prophylaxis[5]	-	-	88%	85%
Warfarin Therapy Discharge Instructions[5]	-	-	74%	75%
Chest Pain/Possible Heart Attack Care				
Aspirin Given Within 24 Hours of Arrival	-	-	98%	96%
Fibrinolytic Meds Within 30 Min. of Arrival	-	-	59%	58%
Average Time to ECG (minutes)	-	-	6	7
Average Time to Transfer (minutes)	-	-	48	60
Children's Asthma Care				
Received Home Management Plan of Care	-	-	-	88%
Received Reliever Medication	-	-	-	100%
Received Systemic Corticosteroids	-	-	-	100%
Emergency Department				
Admittance Decision Time (minutes)[5]	-	-	98	98
Head CT Results Within 45 Min. of Arrival	-	-	64%	57%
Patients Who Left ER Before Being Seen	-	-	2%	2%
Time from ER Arrival to Admit. (minutes)[5]	-	-	285	274
Time from ER Arrival to Discharge (minutes)	-	-	162	134
Time in ER Before Being Evaluated (minutes)	-	-	27	26
Time to Pain Meds for Fractures (minutes)	-	-	58	57
Heart Attack Care				
Aspirin Given at Discharge[5]	-	-	99%	99%
Fibrinolytic Meds Within 30 Min. of Arrival[5]	-	-	67%	54%
PCI Within 90 Minutes of Arrival[5]	-	-	95%	96%
Statin Prescribed at Discharge[5]	-	-	98%	98%
Heart Failure Care				
ACE Inhibitor or ARB for LVSD[5]	-	-	98%	97%
Discharge Instructions Given[5]	-	-	94%	94%
Evaluation of LVS Function[5]	-	-	99%	99%
Medicare Spending				
Medicare Spending per Patient (ratio)	-	-	0.93	0.98
Pneumonia Care				
Appropriate Initial Antibiotic Given	21	81%	96%	95%
Blood Culture Timing	22	68%	97%	98%
Pregnancy and Delivery Care				
Newborn Deliveries Scheduled Early[5]	-	-	7%	6%
Preventive Care				
Immunization for Influenza[5]	-	-	91%	90%
Immunization for Pneumonia[5]	-	-	92%	92%
Stroke Care				
Anticoagulation Therapy for Atrial Fibrillation[5]	-	-	96%	95%
Antithrombotic Therapy Timing[5]	-	-	98%	98%
Assessed for Rehabilitation[5]	-	-	96%	97%
Discharged on Antithrombotic Therapy[5]	-	-	99%	99%
Discharged on Statin Medication[5]	-	-	94%	94%
Thrombolytic Therapy Timing[5]	-	-	81%	66%
Venous Thromboembolism Prophylaxis[5]	-	-	93%	94%
Written Stroke Educational Materials Given[5]	-	-	84%	88%
Surgical Care Improvement Project				
Appropriate Beta Blocker Usage[5]	-	-	97%	98%
Appropriate VTP Within 24 Hours[5]	-	-	98%	98%
Controlled Postoperative Blood Glucose[5]	-	-	96%	97%
Perioperative Temperature Management[5]	-	-	100%	100%
Prophylactic Antibiotic Selection[5]	-	-	99%	99%
Prophylactic Antibiotic Selection (Outpatient)	-	-	98%	98%
Prophylactic Antibiotic Stopped[5]	-	-	98%	98%
Prophylactic Antibiotic Timing[5]	-	-	99%	99%
Prophylactic Antibiotic Timing (Outpatient)	-	-	99%	98%
Urinary Catheter Removal[5]	-	-	97%	97%
Survey of Patients' Hospital Experiences				
Area Around Room 'Always' Quiet at Night[5]	-	-	57%	61%
Doctors 'Always' Communicated Well[5]	-	-	77%	82%
Home Recovery Information Given[5]	-	-	86%	85%
Hospital Given 9 or 10 on 10 Point Scale[5]	-	-	70%	71%
Meds 'Always' Explained Before Given[5]	-	-	62%	64%
Nurses 'Always' Communicated Well[5]	-	-	76%	79%
Pain 'Always' Well Controlled[5]	-	-	69%	71%
Room and Bathroom 'Always' Clean[5]	-	-	69%	73%
Timely Help 'Always' Received[5]	-	-	65%	68%
Would Definitely Recommend Hospital[5]	-	-	70%	71%
Use of Medical Imaging				
Cardiac Imaging Stress Test before Surgery	-	-	5.8%	5.3%
Combination Abdominal CT Scan	-	-	9.1%	10.5%
Combination Brain/Sinus CT Scan	-	-	3.2%	2.7%
Combination Chest CT Scan	-	-	5.5%	2.7%
Follow-up Mammogram/Ultrasound	-	-	8.5%	8.8%
Lumbar Spine MRI for Low Back Pain	-	-	37.4%	37.2%

VA Northern Arizona Healthcare System

500 Highway 89 North | Phone: 928-445-4860
Prescott, AZ 86313 | Fax: 928-776-6076
URL: www.va.gov/sta/guide/home.asp
Type: Acute Care - VA | Emergency Services: No
Ownership: Government Federal | Beds: 217

Key Personnel:
Quality Assurance . . . . James B McGuire
CEO/President. . . . . Patricia A McKlem
Chief of Medical Staff. . . . . Gary R Melvin, MD

Measure	Cases	This Hosp.	State Avg.	U.S. Avg.
Blood Clot Prevention and Treatment				
Anticoagulation Overlap Therapy	-	-	94%	93%
ICU Venous Thromboembolism Prophylaxis	-	-	92%	92%
Incidence of Potentially Preventable VTE	-	-	9%	10%
UFH with Dosages/Platelet Monitoring	-	-	98%	97%
Venous Thromboembolism Prophylaxis	-	-	88%	85%
Warfarin Therapy Discharge Instructions	-	-	74%	75%
Chest Pain/Possible Heart Attack Care				
Aspirin Given Within 24 Hours of Arrival	-	-	98%	96%
Fibrinolytic Meds Within 30 Min. of Arrival	-	-	59%	58%
Average Time to ECG (minutes)	-	-	6	7
Average Time to Transfer (minutes)	-	-	48	60
Children's Asthma Care				
Received Home Management Plan of Care	-	-	-	88%
Received Reliever Medication	-	-	-	100%
Received Systemic Corticosteroids	-	-	-	100%
Emergency Department				
Admittance Decision Time (minutes)	-	-	98	98
Head CT Results Within 45 Min. of Arrival	-	-	64%	57%
Patients Who Left ER Before Being Seen	-	-	2%	2%
Time from ER Arrival to Admit. (minutes)	-	-	285	274
Time from ER Arrival to Discharge (minutes)	-	-	162	134
Time in ER Before Being Evaluated (minutes)	-	-	27	26
Time to Pain Meds for Fractures (minutes)	-	-	58	57
Heart Attack Care				
Aspirin Given at Discharge[5]	-	-	99%	99%
Fibrinolytic Meds Within 30 Min. of Arrival[5]	-	-	67%	54%
PCI Within 90 Minutes of Arrival[5]	-	-	95%	96%
Statin Prescribed at Discharge[5]	-	-	98%	98%
Heart Failure Care				
ACE Inhibitor or ARB for LVSD[1]	11	82%	98%	97%
Discharge Instructions Given	40	98%	94%	94%
Evaluation of LVS Function	45	100%	99%	99%
Medicare Spending				
Medicare Spending per Patient (ratio)	-	-	0.93	0.98
Pneumonia Care				
Appropriate Initial Antibiotic Given	67	93%	96%	95%
Blood Culture Timing	82	99%	97%	98%
Pregnancy and Delivery Care				
Newborn Deliveries Scheduled Early	-	-	7%	6%
Preventive Care				
Immunization for Influenza[2,3]	141	77%	91%	90%
Immunization for Pneumonia[2,3]	347	90%	92%	92%
Stroke Care				
Anticoagulation Therapy for Atrial Fibrillation	-	-	96%	95%
Antithrombotic Therapy Timing	-	-	98%	98%
Assessed for Rehabilitation	-	-	96%	97%
Discharged on Antithrombotic Therapy	-	-	99%	99%
Discharged on Statin Medication	-	-	94%	94%
Thrombolytic Therapy Timing	-	-	81%	66%
Venous Thromboembolism Prophylaxis	-	-	93%	94%
Written Stroke Educational Materials Given	-	-	84%	88%
Surgical Care Improvement Project				
Appropriate Beta Blocker Usage[5]	-	-	97%	98%
Appropriate VTP Within 24 Hours[5]	-	-	98%	98%
Controlled Postoperative Blood Glucose[5]	-	-	96%	97%
Perioperative Temperature Management[5]	-	-	100%	100%
Prophylactic Antibiotic Selection[5]	-	-	99%	99%
Prophylactic Antibiotic Selection (Outpatient)	-	-	98%	98%
Prophylactic Antibiotic Stopped[5]	-	-	98%	98%
Prophylactic Antibiotic Timing[5]	-	-	99%	99%
Prophylactic Antibiotic Timing (Outpatient)	-	-	99%	98%
Urinary Catheter Removal[5]	-	-	97%	97%
Survey of Patients' Hospital Experiences				
Area Around Room 'Always' Quiet at Night	-	-	57%	61%
Doctors 'Always' Communicated Well	-	-	77%	82%
Home Recovery Information Given	-	-	86%	85%
Hospital Given 9 or 10 on 10 Point Scale	-	-	70%	71%
Meds 'Always' Explained Before Given	-	-	62%	64%
Nurses 'Always' Communicated Well	-	-	76%	79%
Pain 'Always' Well Controlled	-	-	69%	71%
Room and Bathroom 'Always' Clean	-	-	69%	73%
Timely Help 'Always' Received	-	-	65%	68%
Would Definitely Recommend Hospital	-	-	70%	71%
Use of Medical Imaging				
Cardiac Imaging Stress Test before Surgery	-	-	5.8%	5.3%
Combination Abdominal CT Scan	-	-	9.1%	10.5%
Combination Brain/Sinus CT Scan	-	-	3.2%	2.7%
Combination Chest CT Scan	-	-	5.5%	2.7%
Follow-up Mammogram/Ultrasound	-	-	8.5%	8.8%
Lumbar Spine MRI for Low Back Pain	-	-	37.4%	37.2%

Yavapai Regional Medical Center

1003 Willow Creek Road | Phone: 928-771-5676
Prescott, AZ 86301 | Fax: 928-771-5755
E-mail: webmaster@yrmc.org
URL: www.yrmc.org
Type: Acute Care Hospitals | Emergency Services: Yes
Ownership: Government - Local | Beds: 127

Key Personnel:
Radiology. . . . . David R Amstutz, MD
CEO/President. . . . . Timothy Barnett
Operating Room. . . . . Ruth Butts
Emergency Room . . . . Judy Denton

NOTE: Hospital profiles are in alphabetical order by state, then city, then hospital within the city; Rankings exclude hospitals with less than 25 cases except for patient surveys which excludes hospitals with less than 100 cases; (a) 100-299 cases; (1) The number of cases/patients is too few to report; (2) Data submitted were based on a sample of cases/patients; (3) Results are based on a shorter time period than required; (4) Data suppressed by CMS for one or more quarters; (5) Results are not available for this reporting period; (6) Fewer than 100 patients completed the HCAHPS survey; (7) No cases met the criteria for this measure; (8) The lower limit of the confidence interval cannot be calculated if the number of observed infections equals zero; (9) No data are available from the state/territory for this reporting period; (10) The scores shown reflect fewer than 50 completed surveys; (11) There were discrepancies in the data collection process; (12) This measure does not apply to this hospital for this reporting period; (13) Results cannot be calculated for this reporting period; (14) The results for this state are combined with nearby states to protect confidentiality; Please refer to the User's Guide for a full explanation of data.

Pediatric Ambulatory Care . . . . . . James Mick, MD
Pediatric In-Patient Care . . . . James Mick, MD
Chief of Medical Staff . . . . DJ Patel, MD
Quality Assurance . . . . Pat Trout

Measure	Cases	This Hosp.	State Avg.	U.S. Avg.
Blood Clot Prevention and Treatment				
Anticoagulation Overlap Therapy[2]	106	74%	94%	93%
ICU Venous Thromboembolism Prophylaxis[2]	101	76%	92%	92%
Incidence of Potentially Preventable VTE[1,2]	-	-	9%	10%
UFH with Dosages/Platelet Monitoring[2]	18	100%	98%	97%
Venous Thromboembolism Prophylaxis[2]	301	71%	88%	85%
Warfarin Therapy Discharge Instructions[2]	84	94%	74%	75%
Chest Pain/Possible Heart Attack Care				
Aspirin Given Within 24 Hours of Arrival[1]	-	-	98%	96%
Fibrinolytic Meds Within 30 Min. of Arrival[3,7]	-	-	59%	58%
Average Time to ECG (minutes)[1]	-	-	6	7
Average Time to Transfer (minutes)[3,7]	-	-	48	60
Children's Asthma Care				
Received Home Management Plan of Care	-	-	-	88%
Received Reliever Medication	-	-	-	100%
Received Systemic Corticosteroids	-	-	-	100%
Emergency Department				
Admittance Decision Time (minutes)[2]	752	98	98	98
Head CT Results Within 45 Min. of Arrival	20	35%	64%	57%
Patients Who Left ER Before Being Seen	35,850	1%	2%	2%
Time from ER Arrival to Admit. (minutes)[2]	806	269	285	274
Time from ER Arrival to Discharge (minutes)	366	164	162	134
Time in ER Before Being Evaluated (minutes)	410	25	27	26
Time to Pain Meds for Fractures (minutes)	121	57	58	57
Heart Attack Care				
Aspirin Given at Discharge	341	98%	99%	99%
Fibrinolytic Meds Within 30 Min. of Arrival[7]	-	-	67%	54%
PCI Within 90 Minutes of Arrival	44	89%	95%	96%
Statin Prescribed at Discharge	329	95%	98%	98%
Heart Failure Care				
ACE Inhibitor or ARB for LVSD	51	94%	98%	97%
Discharge Instructions Given	115	94%	94%	94%
Evaluation of LVS Function	132	97%	99%	99%
Medicare Spending				
Medicare Spending per Patient (ratio)	-	0.95	0.93	0.98
Pneumonia Care				
Appropriate Initial Antibiotic Given[2]	82	96%	96%	95%
Blood Culture Timing[2]	125	95%	97%	98%
Pregnancy and Delivery Care				
Newborn Deliveries Scheduled Early[7]	-	-	7%	6%
Preventive Care				
Immunization for Influenza[2]	621	90%	91%	90%
Immunization for Pneumonia[2]	996	89%	92%	92%
Stroke Care				
Anticoagulation Therapy for Atrial Fibrillation	22	95%	96%	95%
Antithrombotic Therapy Timing	83	96%	98%	98%
Assessed for Rehabilitation	111	88%	96%	97%
Discharged on Antithrombotic Therapy	101	98%	99%	99%
Discharged on Statin Medication	84	74%	94%	94%
Thrombolytic Therapy Timing	11	55%	81%	66%
Venous Thromboembolism Prophylaxis	97	71%	93%	94%
Written Stroke Educational Materials Given	56	86%	84%	88%
Surgical Care Improvement Project				
Appropriate Beta Blocker Usage[2]	161	94%	97%	98%
Appropriate VTP Within 24 Hours[2]	342	96%	98%	98%
Controlled Postoperative Blood Glucose[2]	108	93%	96%	97%
Perioperative Temperature Management[2]	384	100%	100%	100%
Prophylactic Antibiotic Selection[2]	297	100%	99%	99%
Prophylactic Antibiotic Selection (Outpatient)	218	100%	98%	98%
Prophylactic Antibiotic Stopped[2]	284	96%	98%	98%
Prophylactic Antibiotic Timing[2]	297	100%	99%	99%
Prophylactic Antibiotic Timing (Outpatient)	220	98%	99%	98%
Urinary Catheter Removal[2]	248	99%	97%	97%
Survey of Patients' Hospital Experiences				
Area Around Room 'Always' Quiet at Night	300+	44%	57%	61%
Doctors 'Always' Communicated Well	300+	76%	77%	82%
Home Recovery Information Given	300+	84%	86%	85%
Hospital Given 9 or 10 on 10 Point Scale	300+	68%	70%	71%
Meds 'Always' Explained Before Given	300+	62%	62%	64%
Nurses 'Always' Communicated Well	300+	75%	76%	79%
Pain 'Always' Well Controlled	300+	64%	69%	71%
Room and Bathroom 'Always' Clean	300+	61%	69%	73%
Timely Help 'Always' Received	300+	65%	65%	68%
Would Definitely Recommend Hospital	300+	68%	70%	71%
Use of Medical Imaging				
Cardiac Imaging Stress Test before Surgery	277	5.4%	5.8%	5.3%
Combination Abdominal CT Scan	806	12.5%	9.1%	10.5%
Combination Brain/Sinus CT Scan	895	2.5%	3.2%	2.7%
Combination Chest CT Scan	567	14.6%	5.5%	2.7%
Follow-up Mammogram/Ultrasound	524	5.9%	8.5%	8.8%
Lumbar Spine MRI for Low Back Pain[1]	-	-	37.4%	37.2%

Yavapai Regional Medical Center - East

7700 East Florentine Road
Prescott Valley, AZ 86314
Phone: 928-442-8165
E-mail: recruiter@yrmc.org
URL: www.yrmc.org/about/yrmceast.aspx
Type: Acute Care Hospitals
Emergency Services: Yes
Ownership: Voluntary non-profit - Private
Beds: 50

Key Personnel:
CEO/President. . . . . Tim Barnett

Measure	Cases	This Hosp.	State Avg.	U.S. Avg.
Blood Clot Prevention and Treatment				
Anticoagulation Overlap Therapy[2]	35	86%	94%	93%
ICU Venous Thromboembolism Prophylaxis[2]	53	85%	92%	92%
Incidence of Potentially Preventable VTE[1,2]	-	-	9%	10%
UFH with Dosages/Platelet Monitoring[1,2]	-	-	98%	97%
Venous Thromboembolism Prophylaxis[2]	200	78%	88%	85%
Warfarin Therapy Discharge Instructions[2]	27	93%	74%	75%
Chest Pain/Possible Heart Attack Care				
Aspirin Given Within 24 Hours of Arrival	108	98%	98%	96%
Fibrinolytic Meds Within 30 Min. of Arrival[7]	-	-	59%	58%
Average Time to ECG (minutes)	113	8	6	7
Average Time to Transfer (minutes)	24	42	48	60
Children's Asthma Care				
Received Home Management Plan of Care	-	-	-	88%
Received Reliever Medication	-	-	-	100%
Received Systemic Corticosteroids	-	-	-	100%
Emergency Department				
Admittance Decision Time (minutes)[2]	378	80	98	98
Head CT Results Within 45 Min. of Arrival	16	38%	64%	57%
Patients Who Left ER Before Being Seen	33,917	1%	2%	2%
Time from ER Arrival to Admit. (minutes)[2]	405	257	285	274
Time from ER Arrival to Discharge (minutes)	359	134	162	134
Time in ER Before Being Evaluated (minutes)	402	22	27	26
Time to Pain Meds for Fractures (minutes)	95	56	58	57
Heart Attack Care				
Aspirin Given at Discharge[1]	-	-	99%	99%
Fibrinolytic Meds Within 30 Min. of Arrival[7]	-	-	67%	54%
PCI Within 90 Minutes of Arrival[7]	-	-	95%	96%
Statin Prescribed at Discharge[1]	-	-	98%	98%
Heart Failure Care				
ACE Inhibitor or ARB for LVSD	16	94%	98%	97%
Discharge Instructions Given	42	90%	94%	94%
Evaluation of LVS Function	47	98%	99%	99%
Medicare Spending				
Medicare Spending per Patient (ratio)	-	1.00	0.93	0.98
Pneumonia Care				
Appropriate Initial Antibiotic Given[2]	102	92%	96%	95%
Blood Culture Timing[2]	166	95%	97%	98%
Pregnancy and Delivery Care				
Newborn Deliveries Scheduled Early	154	22%	7%	6%
Preventive Care				
Immunization for Influenza[2]	385	91%	91%	90%
Immunization for Pneumonia[2]	401	90%	92%	92%
Stroke Care				
Anticoagulation Therapy for Atrial Fibrillation[1]	-	-	96%	95%
Antithrombotic Therapy Timing	25	96%	98%	98%
Assessed for Rehabilitation	30	87%	96%	97%
Discharged on Antithrombotic Therapy	30	97%	99%	99%
Discharged on Statin Medication	26	69%	94%	94%
Thrombolytic Therapy Timing[7]	-	-	81%	66%
Venous Thromboembolism Prophylaxis	26	65%	93%	94%
Written Stroke Educational Materials Given	17	65%	84%	88%
Surgical Care Improvement Project				
Appropriate Beta Blocker Usage[2]	87	89%	97%	98%
Appropriate VTP Within 24 Hours[2]	285	95%	98%	98%
Controlled Postoperative Blood Glucose[2,7]	-	-	96%	97%
Perioperative Temperature Management[2]	348	100%	100%	100%
Prophylactic Antibiotic Selection[2]	258	99%	99%	99%
Prophylactic Antibiotic Selection (Outpatient)	35	97%	98%	98%
Prophylactic Antibiotic Stopped[2]	256	98%	98%	98%
Prophylactic Antibiotic Timing[2]	259	99%	99%	99%
Prophylactic Antibiotic Timing (Outpatient)	35	100%	99%	98%
Urinary Catheter Removal[2]	244	100%	97%	97%
Survey of Patients' Hospital Experiences				
Area Around Room 'Always' Quiet at Night	300+	57%	57%	61%
Doctors 'Always' Communicated Well	300+	79%	77%	82%
Home Recovery Information Given	300+	88%	86%	85%
Hospital Given 9 or 10 on 10 Point Scale	300+	75%	70%	71%
Meds 'Always' Explained Before Given	300+	58%	62%	64%
Nurses 'Always' Communicated Well	300+	78%	76%	79%
Pain 'Always' Well Controlled	300+	69%	69%	71%
Room and Bathroom 'Always' Clean	300+	76%	69%	73%
Timely Help 'Always' Received	300+	67%	65%	68%
Would Definitely Recommend Hospital	300+	77%	70%	71%
Use of Medical Imaging				
Cardiac Imaging Stress Test before Surgery	178	7.3%	5.8%	5.3%
Combination Abdominal CT Scan	686	13.4%	9.1%	10.5%
Combination Brain/Sinus CT Scan	681	2.2%	3.2%	2.7%
Combination Chest CT Scan	375	14.7%	5.5%	2.7%
Follow-up Mammogram/Ultrasound	1,300	7.3%	8.5%	8.8%
Lumbar Spine MRI for Low Back Pain	66	25.8%	37.4%	37.2%

Mount Graham Regional Medical Center

1600 South 20th Avenue
Safford, AZ 85546
Phone: 928-348-4000
Fax: 928-348-5701
URL: www.mtgraham.org
Type: Acute Care Hospitals
Emergency Services: Yes
Ownership: Govt - Hospital Dist/Auth
Beds: 59

Key Personnel:
Emergency Room . . . . Jason Branch, MD
Quality Assurance . . . . Jeannine Carpenter
Operating Room. . . . . Bart J Carter
Surgery . . . . Bart J. Carter, MD, FACS
Intensive Care Unit. . . . . Debbie Cherry
Chairman/CEO . . . . Caro Gaetje
CEO/President. . . . . Mark E. Marchetti
Chief of Medical Staff . . . . Mary Peters, MD

Measure	Cases	This Hosp.	State Avg.	U.S. Avg.
Blood Clot Prevention and Treatment				
Anticoagulation Overlap Therapy[2]	14	93%	94%	93%
ICU Venous Thromboembolism Prophylaxis[2]	33	91%	92%	92%
Incidence of Potentially Preventable VTE[2,7]	-	-	9%	10%
UFH with Dosages/Platelet Monitoring[1,2]	-	-	98%	97%
Venous Thromboembolism Prophylaxis[2]	118	75%	88%	85%
Warfarin Therapy Discharge Instructions[2]	12	100%	74%	75%
Chest Pain/Possible Heart Attack Care				
Aspirin Given Within 24 Hours of Arrival	72	94%	98%	96%
Fibrinolytic Meds Within 30 Min. of Arrival[1]	-	-	59%	58%
Average Time to ECG (minutes)	73	3	6	7
Average Time to Transfer (minutes)[1]	-	-	48	60
Children's Asthma Care				
Received Home Management Plan of Care	-	-	-	88%
Received Reliever Medication	-	-	-	100%
Received Systemic Corticosteroids	-	-	-	100%
Emergency Department				
Admittance Decision Time (minutes)[2]	251	49	98	98
Head CT Results Within 45 Min. of Arrival	14	57%	64%	57%
Patients Who Left ER Before Being Seen	18,516	0%	2%	2%
Time from ER Arrival to Admit. (minutes)[2]	279	252	285	274
Time from ER Arrival to Discharge (minutes)	332	121	162	134
Time in ER Before Being Evaluated (minutes)	472	13	27	26
Time to Pain Meds for Fractures (minutes)	54	55	58	57

NOTE: Hospital profiles are in alphabetical order by state, then city, then hospital within the city; Rankings exclude hospitals with less than 25 cases except for patient surveys which excludes hospitals with less than 100 cases; (a) 100-299 cases; (1) The number of cases/patients is too few to report; (2) Data submitted were based on a sample of cases/patients; (3) Results are based on a shorter time period than required; (4) Data suppressed by CMS for one or more quarters; (5) Results are not available for this reporting period; (6) Fewer than 100 patients completed the HCAHPS survey; (7) No cases met the criteria for this measure; (8) The lower limit of the confidence interval cannot be calculated if the number of observed infections equals zero; (9) No data are available from the state/territory for this reporting period; (10) The scores shown reflect fewer than 50 completed surveys; (11) There were discrepancies in the data collection process; (12) This measure does not apply to this hospital for this reporting period; (13) Results cannot be calculated for this reporting period; (14) The results for this state are combined with nearby states to protect confidentiality; Please refer to the User's Guide for a full explanation of data.

Measure	Cases	This Hosp.	State Avg.	U.S. Avg.
Heart Attack Care				
Aspirin Given at Discharge[1,3]	-	-	99%	99%
Fibrinolytic Meds Within 30 Min. of Arrival[3,7]	-	-	67%	54%
PCI Within 90 Minutes of Arrival[3,7]	-	-	95%	96%
Statin Prescribed at Discharge[1,3]	-	-	98%	98%
Heart Failure Care				
ACE Inhibitor or ARB for LVSD[1]	-	-	98%	97%
Discharge Instructions Given	28	100%	94%	94%
Evaluation of LVS Function	28	100%	99%	99%
Medicare Spending				
Medicare Spending per Patient (ratio)	-	0.84	0.93	0.98
Pneumonia Care				
Appropriate Initial Antibiotic Given	49	86%	96%	95%
Blood Culture Timing	67	96%	97%	98%
Pregnancy and Delivery Care				
Newborn Deliveries Scheduled Early[2]	76	3%	7%	6%
Preventive Care				
Immunization for Influenza[2]	347	88%	91%	90%
Immunization for Pneumonia[2]	296	89%	92%	92%
Stroke Care				
Anticoagulation Therapy for Atrial Fibrillation[1]	-	-	96%	95%
Antithrombotic Therapy Timing[1]	-	-	98%	98%
Assessed for Rehabilitation[1]	-	-	96%	97%
Discharged on Antithrombotic Therapy[1]	-	-	99%	99%
Discharged on Statin Medication[1]	-	-	94%	94%
Thrombolytic Therapy Timing[1]	-	-	81%	66%
Venous Thromboembolism Prophylaxis[1]	-	-	93%	94%
Written Stroke Educational Materials Given[1]	-	-	84%	88%
Surgical Care Improvement Project				
Appropriate Beta Blocker Usage	30	100%	97%	98%
Appropriate VTP Within 24 Hours	103	96%	98%	98%
Controlled Postoperative Blood Glucose[7]	-	-	96%	97%
Perioperative Temperature Management	135	99%	100%	100%
Prophylactic Antibiotic Selection	87	99%	99%	99%
Prophylactic Antibiotic Selection (Outpatient)	71	92%	98%	98%
Prophylactic Antibiotic Stopped	86	95%	98%	98%
Prophylactic Antibiotic Timing	87	93%	99%	99%
Prophylactic Antibiotic Timing (Outpatient)	71	99%	99%	98%
Urinary Catheter Removal	110	97%	97%	97%
Survey of Patients' Hospital Experiences				
Area Around Room 'Always' Quiet at Night	300+	58%	57%	61%
Doctors 'Always' Communicated Well	300+	82%	77%	82%
Home Recovery Information Given	300+	89%	86%	85%
Hospital Given 9 or 10 on 10 Point Scale	300+	73%	70%	71%
Meds 'Always' Explained Before Given	300+	61%	62%	64%
Nurses 'Always' Communicated Well	300+	78%	76%	79%
Pain 'Always' Well Controlled	300+	74%	69%	71%
Room and Bathroom 'Always' Clean	300+	66%	69%	73%
Timely Help 'Always' Received	300+	69%	65%	68%
Would Definitely Recommend Hospital	300+	71%	70%	71%
Use of Medical Imaging				
Cardiac Imaging Stress Test before Surgery	112	5.4%	5.8%	5.3%
Combination Abdominal CT Scan	376	7.4%	9.1%	10.5%
Combination Brain/Sinus CT Scan[1]	-	-	3.2%	2.7%
Combination Chest CT Scan	292	2.4%	5.5%	2.7%
Follow-up Mammogram/Ultrasound	465	3.9%	8.5%	8.8%
Lumbar Spine MRI for Low Back Pain[1]	-	-	37.4%	37.2%

San Carlos Indian Hospital

223 Cibecue Circle Road Phone: 928-475-7347
San Carlos, AZ 85550
URL: www.ihs.gov/facilitiesservices/areaoffices/phoenix
Type: Acute Care Hospitals Emergency Services: No
Ownership: Government - Federal Beds: 8
Key Personnel:
CEO/President. . . . . Yvette Roubideaux, MD

Measure	Cases	This Hosp.	State Avg.	U.S. Avg.
Blood Clot Prevention and Treatment				
Anticoagulation Overlap Therapy[2,7]	-	-	94%	93%
ICU Venous Thromboembolism Prophylaxis[2,7]	-	-	92%	92%
Incidence of Potentially Preventable VTE[2,7]	-	-	9%	10%
UFH with Dosages/Platelet Monitoring[2,7]	-	-	98%	97%
Venous Thromboembolism Prophylaxis[2]	54	7%	88%	85%
Warfarin Therapy Discharge Instructions[2,7]	-	-	74%	75%
Chest Pain/Possible Heart Attack Care				
Aspirin Given Within 24 Hours of Arrival[5]	-	-	98%	96%
Fibrinolytic Meds Within 30 Min. of Arrival[5]	-	-	59%	58%
Average Time to ECG (minutes)[5]	-	-	6	7
Average Time to Transfer (minutes)[5]	-	-	48	60
Children's Asthma Care				
Received Home Management Plan of Care	-	-	-	88%
Received Reliever Medication	-	-	-	100%
Received Systemic Corticosteroids	-	-	-	100%
Emergency Department				
Admittance Decision Time (minutes)[2,7]	-	-	98	98
Head CT Results Within 45 Min. of Arrival[5]	-	-	64%	57%
Patients Who Left ER Before Being Seen[5]	-	-	2%	2%
Time from ER Arrival to Admit. (minutes)[2]	58	212	285	274
Time from ER Arrival to Discharge (minutes)[5]	-	-	162	134
Time in ER Before Being Evaluated (minutes)[5]	-	-	27	26
Time to Pain Meds for Fractures (minutes)[5]	-	-	58	57
Heart Attack Care				
Aspirin Given at Discharge[5]	-	-	99%	99%
Fibrinolytic Meds Within 30 Min. of Arrival[5]	-	-	67%	54%
PCI Within 90 Minutes of Arrival[5]	-	-	95%	96%
Statin Prescribed at Discharge[5]	-	-	98%	98%
Heart Failure Care				
ACE Inhibitor or ARB for LVSD[5]	-	-	98%	97%
Discharge Instructions Given[5]	-	-	94%	94%
Evaluation of LVS Function[5]	-	-	99%	99%
Medicare Spending				
Medicare Spending per Patient (ratio)	-	-	0.93	0.98
Pneumonia Care				
Appropriate Initial Antibiotic Given[5]	-	-	96%	95%
Blood Culture Timing[5]	-	-	97%	98%
Pregnancy and Delivery Care				
Newborn Deliveries Scheduled Early[2,7]	-	-	7%	6%
Preventive Care				
Immunization for Influenza[2]	22	41%	91%	90%
Immunization for Pneumonia[2]	49	88%	92%	92%
Stroke Care				
Anticoagulation Therapy for Atrial Fibrillation[5]	-	-	96%	95%
Antithrombotic Therapy Timing[5]	-	-	98%	98%
Assessed for Rehabilitation[5]	-	-	96%	97%
Discharged on Antithrombotic Therapy[5]	-	-	99%	99%
Discharged on Statin Medication[5]	-	-	94%	94%
Thrombolytic Therapy Timing[5]	-	-	81%	66%
Venous Thromboembolism Prophylaxis[5]	-	-	93%	94%
Written Stroke Educational Materials Given[5]	-	-	84%	88%
Surgical Care Improvement Project				
Appropriate Beta Blocker Usage[5]	-	-	97%	98%
Appropriate VTP Within 24 Hours[5]	-	-	98%	98%
Controlled Postoperative Blood Glucose[5]	-	-	96%	97%
Perioperative Temperature Management[5]	-	-	100%	100%
Prophylactic Antibiotic Selection[5]	-	-	99%	99%
Prophylactic Antibiotic Selection (Outpatient)[5]	-	-	98%	98%
Prophylactic Antibiotic Stopped[5]	-	-	98%	98%
Prophylactic Antibiotic Timing[5]	-	-	99%	99%
Prophylactic Antibiotic Timing (Outpatient)[5]	-	-	99%	98%
Urinary Catheter Removal[5]	-	-	97%	97%
Survey of Patients' Hospital Experiences				
Area Around Room 'Always' Quiet at Night[6]	<100	76%	57%	61%
Doctors 'Always' Communicated Well[6]	<100	66%	77%	82%
Home Recovery Information Given[6]	<100	99%	86%	85%
Hospital Given 9 or 10 on 10 Point Scale[6]	<100	41%	70%	71%
Meds 'Always' Explained Before Given[6]	<100	51%	62%	64%
Nurses 'Always' Communicated Well[6]	<100	60%	76%	79%
Pain 'Always' Well Controlled[6]	<100	38%	69%	71%
Room and Bathroom 'Always' Clean[6]	<100	80%	69%	73%
Timely Help 'Always' Received[6]	<100	53%	65%	68%
Would Definitely Recommend Hospital[6]	<100	11%	70%	71%
Use of Medical Imaging				
Cardiac Imaging Stress Test before Surgery[7]	-	-	5.8%	5.3%
Combination Abdominal CT Scan[7]	-	-	9.1%	10.5%
Combination Brain/Sinus CT Scan[7]	-	-	3.2%	2.7%
Combination Chest CT Scan[7]	-	-	5.5%	2.7%
Follow-up Mammogram/Ultrasound[7]	-	-	8.5%	8.8%
Lumbar Spine MRI for Low Back Pain[7]	-	-	37.4%	37.2%

Banner Ironwood Medical Center

37000 North Gantzel Road Phone: 480-394-4030
San Tan Valley, AZ 85140
Type: Acute Care Hospitals Emergency Services: Yes
Ownership: Voluntary non-profit - Private

Measure	Cases	This Hosp.	State Avg.	U.S. Avg.
Blood Clot Prevention and Treatment				
Anticoagulation Overlap Therapy[2]	22	95%	94%	93%
ICU Venous Thromboembolism Prophylaxis[2]	21	95%	92%	92%
Incidence of Potentially Preventable VTE[1,2]	-	-	9%	10%
UFH with Dosages/Platelet Monitoring[1,2]	-	-	98%	97%
Venous Thromboembolism Prophylaxis[2]	129	90%	88%	85%
Warfarin Therapy Discharge Instructions[2]	21	62%	74%	75%
Chest Pain/Possible Heart Attack Care				
Aspirin Given Within 24 Hours of Arrival	85	99%	98%	96%
Fibrinolytic Meds Within 30 Min. of Arrival[7]	-	-	59%	58%
Average Time to ECG (minutes)	88	6	6	7
Average Time to Transfer (minutes)[1]	-	-	48	60
Children's Asthma Care				
Received Home Management Plan of Care	-	-	-	88%
Received Reliever Medication	-	-	-	100%
Received Systemic Corticosteroids	-	-	-	100%
Emergency Department				
Admittance Decision Time (minutes)[2]	155	58	98	98
Head CT Results Within 45 Min. of Arrival	13	69%	64%	57%
Patients Who Left ER Before Being Seen	27,671	0%	2%	2%
Time from ER Arrival to Admit. (minutes)[2]	182	219	285	274
Time from ER Arrival to Discharge (minutes)	340	150	162	134
Time in ER Before Being Evaluated (minutes)	404	10	27	26
Time to Pain Meds for Fractures (minutes)	120	40	58	57
Heart Attack Care				
Aspirin Given at Discharge[1,3]	-	-	99%	99%
Fibrinolytic Meds Within 30 Min. of Arrival[3,7]	-	-	67%	54%
PCI Within 90 Minutes of Arrival[3,7]	-	-	95%	96%
Statin Prescribed at Discharge[1,3]	-	-	98%	98%
Heart Failure Care				
ACE Inhibitor or ARB for LVSD[1]	-	-	98%	97%
Discharge Instructions Given	22	95%	94%	94%
Evaluation of LVS Function	22	100%	99%	99%
Medicare Spending				
Medicare Spending per Patient (ratio)	-	0.88	0.93	0.98
Pneumonia Care				
Appropriate Initial Antibiotic Given	49	100%	96%	95%
Blood Culture Timing	57	96%	97%	98%
Pregnancy and Delivery Care				
Newborn Deliveries Scheduled Early[2]	36	14%	7%	6%
Preventive Care				
Immunization for Influenza[2]	233	92%	91%	90%
Immunization for Pneumonia[2]	158	95%	92%	92%
Stroke Care				
Anticoagulation Therapy for Atrial Fibrillation[1,3]	-	-	96%	95%
Antithrombotic Therapy Timing[1,3]	-	-	98%	98%
Assessed for Rehabilitation[1,3]	-	-	96%	97%
Discharged on Antithrombotic Therapy[1,3]	-	-	99%	99%
Discharged on Statin Medication[1,3]	-	-	94%	94%
Thrombolytic Therapy Timing[3,7]	-	-	81%	66%
Venous Thromboembolism Prophylaxis[1,3]	-	-	93%	94%
Written Stroke Educational Materials Given[1,3]	-	-	84%	88%
Surgical Care Improvement Project				
Appropriate Beta Blocker Usage	14	93%	97%	98%
Appropriate VTP Within 24 Hours	74	100%	98%	98%
Controlled Postoperative Blood Glucose[7]	-	-	96%	97%
Perioperative Temperature Management	95	100%	100%	100%
Prophylactic Antibiotic Selection	67	100%	99%	99%
Prophylactic Antibiotic Selection (Outpatient)	19	100%	98%	98%
Prophylactic Antibiotic Stopped	66	97%	98%	98%
Prophylactic Antibiotic Timing	67	100%	99%	99%
Prophylactic Antibiotic Timing (Outpatient)	19	100%	99%	98%

NOTE: Hospital profiles are in alphabetical order by state, then city, then hospital within the city; Rankings exclude hospitals with less than 25 cases except for patient surveys which excludes hospitals with less than 100 cases; (a) 100-299 cases; (1) The number of cases/patients is too few to report; (2) Data submitted were based on a sample of cases/patients; (3) Results are based on a shorter time period than required; (4) Data suppressed by CMS for one or more quarters; (5) Results are not available for this reporting period; (6) Fewer than 100 patients completed the HCAHPS survey; (7) No cases met the criteria for this measure; (8) The lower limit of the confidence interval cannot be calculated if the number of observed infections equals zero; (9) No data are available from the state/territory for this reporting period; (10) The scores shown reflect fewer than 50 completed surveys; (11) There were discrepancies in the data collection process; (12) This measure does not apply to this hospital for this reporting period; (13) Results cannot be calculated for this reporting period; (14) The results for this state are combined with nearby states to protect confidentiality; Please refer to the User's Guide for a full explanation of data.

Urinary Catheter Removal	21	100%	97%	97%
Survey of Patients' Hospital Experiences				
Area Around Room 'Always' Quiet at Night[11]	300+	70%	57%	61%
Doctors 'Always' Communicated Well[11]	300+	83%	77%	82%
Home Recovery Information Given[11]	300+	90%	86%	85%
Hospital Given 9 or 10 on 10 Point Scale[11]	300+	80%	70%	71%
Meds 'Always' Explained Before Given[11]	300+	70%	62%	64%
Nurses 'Always' Communicated Well[11]	300+	80%	76%	79%
Pain 'Always' Well Controlled[11]	300+	73%	69%	71%
Room and Bathroom 'Always' Clean[11]	300+	73%	69%	73%
Timely Help 'Always' Received[11]	300+	73%	65%	68%
Would Definitely Recommend Hospital[11]	300+	79%	70%	71%
Use of Medical Imaging				
Cardiac Imaging Stress Test before Surgery[1]	-	-	5.8%	5.3%
Combination Abdominal CT Scan	237	3.0%	9.1%	10.5%
Combination Brain/Sinus CT Scan[1]	-	-	3.2%	2.7%
Combination Chest CT Scan	77	1.3%	5.5%	2.7%
Follow-up Mammogram/Ultrasound[7]	-	-	8.5%	8.8%
Lumbar Spine MRI for Low Back Pain[1]	-	-	37.4%	37.2%

Scottsdale Healthcare - Shea Medical Center

9003 East Shea Boulevard
Scottsdale, AZ 85260
Phone: 480-323-3009
Fax: 480-860-3510
URL: www.shc.org
Type: Acute Care Hospitals
Emergency Services: Yes
Ownership: Proprietary
Beds: 343

Key Personnel:

CEO .... Gary Baker
Chief of Medical Staff.......... James Burke, MD
Operating Room............... Michael Campbell
Quality Assurance .... Dennis Ettmueller
Pediatric Ambulatory Care ...... Ron Fischler, MD
Cardiac Laboratory............ Rob Gianguzzi
Radiology..................... Julie Hughes
Emergency Room .... Mary Kopp, RN

Measure	Cases	This Hosp.	State Avg.	U.S. Avg.
Blood Clot Prevention and Treatment				
Anticoagulation Overlap Therapy[2]	126	90%	94%	93%
ICU Venous Thromboembolism Prophylaxis[2]	66	83%	92%	92%
Incidence of Potentially Preventable VTE[2]	26	12%	9%	10%
UFH with Dosages/Platelet Monitoring[2]	46	98%	98%	97%
Venous Thromboembolism Prophylaxis[2]	347	90%	88%	85%
Warfarin Therapy Discharge Instructions[2]	86	56%	74%	75%
Chest Pain/Possible Heart Attack Care				
Aspirin Given Within 24 Hours of Arrival[1]	-	-	98%	96%
Fibrinolytic Meds Within 30 Min. of Arrival[3,7]	-	-	59%	58%
Average Time to ECG (minutes)[1]	-	-	6	7
Average Time to Transfer (minutes)[3,7]	-	-	48	60
Children's Asthma Care				
Received Home Management Plan of Care	-	-	-	88%
Received Reliever Medication	-	-	-	100%
Received Systemic Corticosteroids	-	-	-	100%
Emergency Department				
Admittance Decision Time (minutes)[2]	405	83	98	98
Head CT Results Within 45 Min. of Arrival[1]	-	-	64%	57%
Patients Who Left ER Before Being Seen	46,759	1%	2%	2%
Time from ER Arrival to Admit. (minutes)[2]	422	208	285	274
Time from ER Arrival to Discharge (minutes)	377	161	162	134
Time in ER Before Being Evaluated (minutes)	421	27	27	26
Time to Pain Meds for Fractures (minutes)	248	56	58	57
Heart Attack Care				
Aspirin Given at Discharge[2]	194	100%	99%	99%
Fibrinolytic Meds Within 30 Min. of Arrival[2,7]	-	-	67%	54%
PCI Within 90 Minutes of Arrival[2]	48	100%	95%	96%
Statin Prescribed at Discharge[2]	187	99%	98%	98%
Heart Failure Care				
ACE Inhibitor or ARB for LVSD[2]	78	100%	98%	97%
Discharge Instructions Given[2]	243	70%	94%	94%
Evaluation of LVS Function[2]	289	100%	99%	99%
Medicare Spending				
Medicare Spending per Patient (ratio)	-	1.03	0.93	0.98
Pneumonia Care				
Appropriate Initial Antibiotic Given[2]	103	96%	96%	95%
Blood Culture Timing[2]	161	100%	97%	98%
Pregnancy and Delivery Care				
Newborn Deliveries Scheduled Early[2]	99	9%	7%	6%
Preventive Care				
Immunization for Influenza[2]	494	75%	91%	90%
Immunization for Pneumonia[2]	484	68%	92%	92%
Stroke Care				
Anticoagulation Therapy for Atrial Fibrillation	11	100%	96%	95%
Antithrombotic Therapy Timing	62	100%	98%	98%
Assessed for Rehabilitation	76	83%	96%	97%
Discharged on Antithrombotic Therapy	70	99%	99%	99%
Discharged on Statin Medication	66	85%	94%	94%
Thrombolytic Therapy Timing[1]	-	-	81%	66%
Venous Thromboembolism Prophylaxis	59	88%	93%	94%
Written Stroke Educational Materials Given	47	43%	84%	88%
Surgical Care Improvement Project				
Appropriate Beta Blocker Usage[2]	202	100%	97%	98%
Appropriate VTP Within 24 Hours[2]	393	99%	98%	98%
Controlled Postoperative Blood Glucose[2]	144	99%	96%	97%
Perioperative Temperature Management[2]	528	100%	100%	100%
Prophylactic Antibiotic Selection[2]	438	99%	99%	99%
Prophylactic Antibiotic Selection (Outpatient)	752	99%	98%	98%
Prophylactic Antibiotic Stopped[2]	404	98%	98%	98%
Prophylactic Antibiotic Timing[2]	438	99%	99%	99%
Prophylactic Antibiotic Timing (Outpatient)	752	99%	99%	98%
Urinary Catheter Removal[2]	355	99%	97%	97%
Survey of Patients' Hospital Experiences				
Area Around Room 'Always' Quiet at Night	300+	57%	57%	61%
Doctors 'Always' Communicated Well	300+	76%	77%	82%
Home Recovery Information Given	300+	83%	86%	85%
Hospital Given 9 or 10 on 10 Point Scale	300+	72%	70%	71%
Meds 'Always' Explained Before Given	300+	61%	62%	64%
Nurses 'Always' Communicated Well	300+	76%	76%	79%
Pain 'Always' Well Controlled	300+	70%	69%	71%
Room and Bathroom 'Always' Clean	300+	66%	69%	73%
Timely Help 'Always' Received	300+	63%	65%	68%
Would Definitely Recommend Hospital	300+	74%	70%	71%
Use of Medical Imaging				
Cardiac Imaging Stress Test before Surgery	381	7.6%	5.8%	5.3%
Combination Abdominal CT Scan	778	2.1%	9.1%	10.5%
Combination Brain/Sinus CT Scan	804	3.4%	3.2%	2.7%
Combination Chest CT Scan	262	0.8%	5.5%	2.7%
Follow-up Mammogram/Ultrasound	562	10.1%	8.5%	8.8%
Lumbar Spine MRI for Low Back Pain[1]	-	-	37.4%	37.2%

Scottsdale Healthcare - Thompson Peak Hospital

7400 East Thompson Peak Parkway
Phone: 480-324-7004
Scottsdale, AZ 85255
URL: www.shc.org
Type: Acute Care Hospitals
Emergency Services: Yes
Ownership: Proprietary

Measure	Cases	This Hosp.	State Avg.	U.S. Avg.
Blood Clot Prevention and Treatment				
Anticoagulation Overlap Therapy[2]	62	82%	94%	93%
ICU Venous Thromboembolism Prophylaxis[2]	56	93%	92%	92%
Incidence of Potentially Preventable VTE[1,2]	-	-	9%	10%
UFH with Dosages/Platelet Monitoring[2]	16	94%	98%	97%
Venous Thromboembolism Prophylaxis[2]	274	87%	88%	85%
Warfarin Therapy Discharge Instructions[2]	46	46%	74%	75%
Chest Pain/Possible Heart Attack Care				
Aspirin Given Within 24 Hours of Arrival[1,3]	-	-	98%	96%
Fibrinolytic Meds Within 30 Min. of Arrival[3,7]	-	-	59%	58%
Average Time to ECG (minutes)[1,3]	-	-	6	7
Average Time to Transfer (minutes)[3,7]	-	-	48	60
Children's Asthma Care				
Received Home Management Plan of Care	-	-	-	88%
Received Reliever Medication	-	-	-	100%
Received Systemic Corticosteroids	-	-	-	100%
Emergency Department				
Admittance Decision Time (minutes)[2]	573	92	98	98
Head CT Results Within 45 Min. of Arrival[1]	-	-	64%	57%
Patients Who Left ER Before Being Seen	19,282	1%	2%	2%
Time from ER Arrival to Admit. (minutes)[2]	598	240	285	274
Time from ER Arrival to Discharge (minutes)	377	166	162	134
Time in ER Before Being Evaluated (minutes)	412	24	27	26
Time to Pain Meds for Fractures (minutes)	104	59	58	57
Heart Attack Care				
Aspirin Given at Discharge	68	100%	99%	99%
Fibrinolytic Meds Within 30 Min. of Arrival[7]	-	-	67%	54%
PCI Within 90 Minutes of Arrival	21	100%	95%	96%
Statin Prescribed at Discharge	63	100%	98%	98%
Heart Failure Care				
ACE Inhibitor or ARB for LVSD	16	100%	98%	97%
Discharge Instructions Given	72	64%	94%	94%
Evaluation of LVS Function	87	100%	99%	99%
Medicare Spending				
Medicare Spending per Patient (ratio)	-	0.98	0.93	0.98
Pneumonia Care				
Appropriate Initial Antibiotic Given[2]	90	97%	96%	95%
Blood Culture Timing[2]	128	100%	97%	98%
Pregnancy and Delivery Care				
Newborn Deliveries Scheduled Early[7]	-	-	7%	6%
Preventive Care				
Immunization for Influenza[2]	527	78%	91%	90%
Immunization for Pneumonia[2]	694	74%	92%	92%
Stroke Care				
Anticoagulation Therapy for Atrial Fibrillation[1]	-	-	96%	95%
Antithrombotic Therapy Timing	24	100%	98%	98%
Assessed for Rehabilitation	34	79%	96%	97%
Discharged on Antithrombotic Therapy	32	100%	99%	99%
Discharged on Statin Medication	31	94%	94%	94%
Thrombolytic Therapy Timing[1]	-	-	81%	66%
Venous Thromboembolism Prophylaxis	17	88%	93%	94%
Written Stroke Educational Materials Given	24	50%	84%	88%
Surgical Care Improvement Project				
Appropriate Beta Blocker Usage[2]	111	95%	97%	98%
Appropriate VTP Within 24 Hours[2]	450	99%	98%	98%
Controlled Postoperative Blood Glucose[2,7]	-	-	96%	97%
Perioperative Temperature Management[2]	579	100%	100%	100%
Prophylactic Antibiotic Selection[2]	391	99%	99%	99%
Prophylactic Antibiotic Selection (Outpatient)	380	99%	98%	98%
Prophylactic Antibiotic Stopped[2]	381	100%	98%	98%
Prophylactic Antibiotic Timing[2]	391	100%	99%	99%
Prophylactic Antibiotic Timing (Outpatient)	380	99%	99%	98%
Urinary Catheter Removal[2]	321	99%	97%	97%
Survey of Patients' Hospital Experiences				
Area Around Room 'Always' Quiet at Night	300+	70%	57%	61%
Doctors 'Always' Communicated Well	300+	76%	77%	82%
Home Recovery Information Given	300+	84%	86%	85%
Hospital Given 9 or 10 on 10 Point Scale	300+	78%	70%	71%
Meds 'Always' Explained Before Given	300+	61%	62%	64%
Nurses 'Always' Communicated Well	300+	80%	76%	79%
Pain 'Always' Well Controlled	300+	74%	69%	71%
Room and Bathroom 'Always' Clean	300+	73%	69%	73%
Timely Help 'Always' Received	300+	68%	65%	68%
Would Definitely Recommend Hospital	300+	82%	70%	71%
Use of Medical Imaging				
Cardiac Imaging Stress Test before Surgery	153	7.8%	5.8%	5.3%
Combination Abdominal CT Scan	383	0.8%	9.1%	10.5%
Combination Brain/Sinus CT Scan	377	1.3%	3.2%	2.7%
Combination Chest CT Scan	78	0.0%	5.5%	2.7%
Follow-up Mammogram/Ultrasound[7]	-	-	8.5%	8.8%
Lumbar Spine MRI for Low Back Pain[1]	-	-	37.4%	37.2%

Scottsdale Healthcare Osborn Medical Center

7400 East Osborn Road
Scottsdale, AZ 85251
Phone: 480-882-4000
Fax: 480-882-4989
URL: www.shc.org
Type: Acute Care Hospitals
Emergency Services: Yes
Ownership: Proprietary
Beds: 337

Key Personnel:

Patient Relations .... Gary E Baker
Operating Room.............. Mike Campbell, RN
Emergency Room .... Linda Ott, RN
CEO .... Bruce Pearson
CEO/President............... Thomas J Sadvary
Pediatric In-Patient Care .... Russelle Wallace, MD
Quality Assurance .... Debbie Weller

NOTE: Hospital profiles are in alphabetical order by state, then city, then hospital within the city; Rankings exclude hospitals with less than 25 cases except for patient surveys which excludes hospitals with less than 100 cases; (a) 100-299 cases; (1) The number of cases/patients is too few to report; (2) Data submitted were based on a sample of cases/patients; (3) Results are based on a shorter time period than required; (4) Data suppressed by CMS for one or more quarters; (5) Results are not available for this reporting period; (6) Fewer than 100 patients completed the HCAHPS survey; (7) No cases met the criteria for this measure; (8) The lower limit of the confidence interval cannot be calculated if the number of observed infections equals zero; (9) No data are available from the state/territory for this reporting period; (10) The scores shown reflect fewer than 50 completed surveys; (11) There were discrepancies in the data collection process; (12) This measure does not apply to this hospital for this reporting period; (13) Results cannot be calculated for this reporting period; (14) The results for this state are combined with nearby states to protect confidentiality; Please refer to the User's Guide for a full explanation of data.

Measure	Cases	This Hosp.	State Avg.	U.S. Avg.
Blood Clot Prevention and Treatment				
Anticoagulation Overlap Therapy[2]	151	91%	94%	93%
ICU Venous Thromboembolism Prophylaxis[2]	119	97%	92%	92%
Incidence of Potentially Preventable VTE[2]	30	10%	9%	10%
UFH with Dosages/Platelet Monitoring[2]	47	98%	98%	97%
Venous Thromboembolism Prophylaxis[2]	317	89%	88%	85%
Warfarin Therapy Discharge Instructions[2]	124	77%	74%	75%
Chest Pain/Possible Heart Attack Care				
Aspirin Given Within 24 Hours of Arrival[1]	-	-	98%	96%
Fibrinolytic Meds Within 30 Min. of Arrival[5]	-	-	59%	58%
Average Time to ECG (minutes)[1]	-	-	6	7
Average Time to Transfer (minutes)[5]	-	-	48	60
Children's Asthma Care				
Received Home Management Plan of Care	-	-	-	88%
Received Reliever Medication	-	-	-	100%
Received Systemic Corticosteroids	-	-	-	100%
Emergency Department				
Admittance Decision Time (minutes)[2]	741	83	98	98
Head CT Results Within 45 Min. of Arrival[1]	-	-	64%	57%
Patients Who Left ER Before Being Seen	54,141	1%	2%	2%
Time from ER Arrival to Admit. (minutes)[2]	781	212	285	274
Time from ER Arrival to Discharge (minutes)	350	169	162	134
Time in ER Before Being Evaluated (minutes)	414	23	27	26
Time to Pain Meds for Fractures (minutes)	131	59	58	57
Heart Attack Care				
Aspirin Given at Discharge	145	100%	99%	99%
Fibrinolytic Meds Within 30 Min. of Arrival[7]	-	-	67%	54%
PCI Within 90 Minutes of Arrival	40	100%	95%	96%
Statin Prescribed at Discharge	143	99%	98%	98%
Heart Failure Care				
ACE Inhibitor or ARB for LVSD[2]	72	100%	98%	97%
Discharge Instructions Given[2]	237	76%	94%	94%
Evaluation of LVS Function[2]	282	100%	99%	99%
Medicare Spending				
Medicare Spending per Patient (ratio)	-	1.01	0.93	0.98
Pneumonia Care				
Appropriate Initial Antibiotic Given[2]	103	97%	96%	95%
Blood Culture Timing[2]	176	100%	97%	98%
Pregnancy and Delivery Care				
Newborn Deliveries Scheduled Early[2]	24	4%	7%	6%
Preventive Care				
Immunization for Influenza[2]	590	78%	91%	90%
Immunization for Pneumonia[2]	671	73%	92%	92%
Stroke Care				
Anticoagulation Therapy for Atrial Fibrillation	39	100%	96%	95%
Antithrombotic Therapy Timing	176	100%	98%	98%
Assessed for Rehabilitation	234	95%	96%	97%
Discharged on Antithrombotic Therapy	202	99%	99%	99%
Discharged on Statin Medication	153	95%	94%	94%
Thrombolytic Therapy Timing	28	86%	81%	66%
Venous Thromboembolism Prophylaxis	225	99%	93%	94%
Written Stroke Educational Materials Given	133	95%	84%	88%
Surgical Care Improvement Project				
Appropriate Beta Blocker Usage[2]	155	97%	97%	98%
Appropriate VTP Within 24 Hours[2]	340	98%	98%	98%
Controlled Postoperative Blood Glucose[2]	83	100%	96%	97%
Perioperative Temperature Management[2]	482	100%	100%	100%
Prophylactic Antibiotic Selection[2]	350	100%	99%	99%
Prophylactic Antibiotic Selection (Outpatient)	470	99%	98%	98%
Prophylactic Antibiotic Stopped[2]	336	98%	98%	98%
Prophylactic Antibiotic Timing[2]	351	100%	99%	99%
Prophylactic Antibiotic Timing (Outpatient)	471	98%	99%	98%
Urinary Catheter Removal[2]	302	97%	97%	97%
Survey of Patients' Hospital Experiences				
Area Around Room 'Always' Quiet at Night	300+	47%	57%	61%
Doctors 'Always' Communicated Well	300+	71%	77%	82%
Home Recovery Information Given	300+	80%	86%	85%
Hospital Given 9 or 10 on 10 Point Scale	300+	68%	70%	71%
Meds 'Always' Explained Before Given	300+	54%	62%	64%
Nurses 'Always' Communicated Well	300+	74%	76%	79%
Pain 'Always' Well Controlled	300+	68%	69%	71%
Room and Bathroom 'Always' Clean	300+	67%	69%	73%
Timely Help 'Always' Received	300+	64%	65%	68%
Would Definitely Recommend Hospital	300+	71%	70%	71%
Use of Medical Imaging				
Cardiac Imaging Stress Test before Surgery	188	5.9%	5.8%	5.3%
Combination Abdominal CT Scan	572	1.4%	9.1%	10.5%
Combination Brain/Sinus CT Scan	895	2.3%	3.2%	2.7%
Combination Chest CT Scan	134	0.0%	5.5%	2.7%
Follow-up Mammogram/Ultrasound[7]	-	-	8.5%	8.8%
Lumbar Spine MRI for Low Back Pain[1]	-	-	37.4%	37.2%

Sells Indian Health Service Hospital

PO Box 548 Phone: 520-383-7200
Sells, AZ 85634 Fax: 520-383-7216
URL: www.ihs.gov
Type: Acute Care Hospitals Emergency Services: No
Ownership: Government - Federal Beds: 34

Key Personnel:
Emergency Room .... Jolene Ignacio, RN
CEO/President................ Priscilla Whitethorne
Chief of Medical Staff.......... Peter Zigler

Measure	Cases	This Hosp.	State Avg.	U.S. Avg.
Blood Clot Prevention and Treatment				
Anticoagulation Overlap Therapy[5]	-	-	94%	93%
ICU Venous Thromboembolism Prophylaxis[5]	-	-	92%	92%
Incidence of Potentially Preventable VTE[5]	-	-	9%	10%
UFH with Dosages/Platelet Monitoring[5]	-	-	98%	97%
Venous Thromboembolism Prophylaxis[5]	-	-	88%	85%
Warfarin Therapy Discharge Instructions[5]	-	-	74%	75%
Chest Pain/Possible Heart Attack Care				
Aspirin Given Within 24 Hours of Arrival	-	-	98%	96%
Fibrinolytic Meds Within 30 Min. of Arrival	-	-	59%	58%
Average Time to ECG (minutes)	-	-	6	7
Average Time to Transfer (minutes)	-	-	48	60
Children's Asthma Care				
Received Home Management Plan of Care	-	-	-	88%
Received Reliever Medication	-	-	-	100%
Received Systemic Corticosteroids	-	-	-	100%
Emergency Department				
Admittance Decision Time (minutes)[5]	-	-	98	98
Head CT Results Within 45 Min. of Arrival	-	-	64%	57%
Patients Who Left ER Before Being Seen	-	-	2%	2%
Time from ER Arrival to Admit. (minutes)[5]	-	-	285	274
Time from ER Arrival to Discharge (minutes)	-	-	162	134
Time in ER Before Being Evaluated (minutes)	-	-	27	26
Time to Pain Meds for Fractures (minutes)	-	-	58	57
Heart Attack Care				
Aspirin Given at Discharge[5]	-	-	99%	99%
Fibrinolytic Meds Within 30 Min. of Arrival[5]	-	-	67%	54%
PCI Within 90 Minutes of Arrival[5]	-	-	95%	96%
Statin Prescribed at Discharge[5]	-	-	98%	98%
Heart Failure Care				
ACE Inhibitor or ARB for LVSD[5]	-	-	98%	97%
Discharge Instructions Given[5]	-	-	94%	94%
Evaluation of LVS Function[5]	-	-	99%	99%
Medicare Spending				
Medicare Spending per Patient (ratio)[1]	-	-	0.93	0.98
Pneumonia Care				
Appropriate Initial Antibiotic Given	11	82%	96%	95%
Blood Culture Timing	12	83%	97%	98%
Pregnancy and Delivery Care				
Newborn Deliveries Scheduled Early[5]	-	-	7%	6%
Preventive Care				
Immunization for Influenza[5]	-	-	91%	90%
Immunization for Pneumonia[5]	-	-	92%	92%
Stroke Care				
Anticoagulation Therapy for Atrial Fibrillation[5]	-	-	96%	95%
Antithrombotic Therapy Timing[5]	-	-	98%	98%
Assessed for Rehabilitation[5]	-	-	96%	97%
Discharged on Antithrombotic Therapy[5]	-	-	99%	99%
Discharged on Statin Medication[5]	-	-	94%	94%
Thrombolytic Therapy Timing[5]	-	-	81%	66%
Venous Thromboembolism Prophylaxis[5]	-	-	93%	94%
Written Stroke Educational Materials Given[5]	-	-	84%	88%
Surgical Care Improvement Project				
Appropriate Beta Blocker Usage[5]	-	-	97%	98%
Appropriate VTP Within 24 Hours[5]	-	-	98%	98%
Controlled Postoperative Blood Glucose[5]	-	-	96%	97%
Perioperative Temperature Management[5]	-	-	100%	100%
Prophylactic Antibiotic Selection[5]	-	-	99%	99%
Prophylactic Antibiotic Selection (Outpatient)	-	-	98%	98%
Prophylactic Antibiotic Stopped[5]	-	-	98%	98%
Prophylactic Antibiotic Timing[5]	-	-	99%	99%
Prophylactic Antibiotic Timing (Outpatient)	-	-	99%	98%
Urinary Catheter Removal[5]	-	-	97%	97%
Survey of Patients' Hospital Experiences				
Area Around Room 'Always' Quiet at Night[5]	-	-	57%	61%
Doctors 'Always' Communicated Well[5]	-	-	77%	82%
Home Recovery Information Given[5]	-	-	86%	85%
Hospital Given 9 or 10 on 10 Point Scale[5]	-	-	70%	71%
Meds 'Always' Explained Before Given[5]	-	-	62%	64%
Nurses 'Always' Communicated Well[5]	-	-	76%	79%
Pain 'Always' Well Controlled[5]	-	-	69%	71%
Room and Bathroom 'Always' Clean[5]	-	-	69%	73%
Timely Help 'Always' Received[5]	-	-	65%	68%
Would Definitely Recommend Hospital[5]	-	-	70%	71%
Use of Medical Imaging				
Cardiac Imaging Stress Test before Surgery	-	-	5.8%	5.3%
Combination Abdominal CT Scan	-	-	9.1%	10.5%
Combination Brain/Sinus CT Scan	-	-	3.2%	2.7%
Combination Chest CT Scan	-	-	5.5%	2.7%
Follow-up Mammogram/Ultrasound	-	-	8.5%	8.8%
Lumbar Spine MRI for Low Back Pain	-	-	37.4%	37.2%

Summit Healthcare Regional Medical Center

2200 Show Low Lake Road Phone: 928-537-6399
Show Low, AZ 85901 Fax: 928-537-8839
URL: www.nrmc.org
Type: Acute Care Hospitals Emergency Services: Yes
Ownership: Proprietary

Key Personnel:
Chief of Medical Staff.......... Jones Cavanaugh
Operating Room............... Thia Ebert
CEO/President................ Kevin R Hawk
Emergency Room .... Shelley Jo Sackett
Intensive Care Unit............ Shelley Jo Sackett
Radiology.................... Tiffany Watson

Measure	Cases	This Hosp.	State Avg.	U.S. Avg.
Blood Clot Prevention and Treatment				
Anticoagulation Overlap Therapy[2]	46	87%	94%	93%
ICU Venous Thromboembolism Prophylaxis[2]	100	71%	92%	92%
Incidence of Potentially Preventable VTE[1,2]	-	-	9%	10%
UFH with Dosages/Platelet Monitoring[2]	24	100%	98%	97%
Venous Thromboembolism Prophylaxis[2]	169	80%	88%	85%
Warfarin Therapy Discharge Instructions[2]	43	47%	74%	75%
Chest Pain/Possible Heart Attack Care				
Aspirin Given Within 24 Hours of Arrival	69	97%	98%	96%
Fibrinolytic Meds Within 30 Min. of Arrival	12	42%	59%	58%
Average Time to ECG (minutes)	67	7	6	7
Average Time to Transfer (minutes)[1]	-	-	48	60
Children's Asthma Care				
Received Home Management Plan of Care	-	-	-	88%
Received Reliever Medication	-	-	-	100%
Received Systemic Corticosteroids	-	-	-	100%
Emergency Department				
Admittance Decision Time (minutes)[2]	355	77	98	98
Head CT Results Within 45 Min. of Arrival	19	42%	64%	57%
Patients Who Left ER Before Being Seen	24,421	1%	2%	2%
Time from ER Arrival to Admit. (minutes)[2]	371	281	285	274
Time from ER Arrival to Discharge (minutes)	369	162	162	134
Time in ER Before Being Evaluated (minutes)	402	19	27	26
Time to Pain Meds for Fractures (minutes)	188	56	58	57
Heart Attack Care				
Aspirin Given at Discharge	78	97%	99%	99%
Fibrinolytic Meds Within 30 Min. of Arrival[1]	-	-	67%	54%
PCI Within 90 Minutes of Arrival[1]	-	-	95%	96%
Statin Prescribed at Discharge	75	100%	98%	98%

NOTE: Hospital profiles are in alphabetical order by state, then city, then hospital within the city; Rankings exclude hospitals with less than 25 cases except for patient surveys which excludes hospitals with less than 100 cases; (a) 100-299 cases; (1) The number of cases/patients is too few to report; (2) Data submitted were based on a sample of cases/patients; (3) Results are based on a shorter time period than required; (4) Data suppressed by CMS for one or more quarters; (5) Results are not available for this reporting period; (6) Fewer than 100 patients completed the HCAHPS survey; (7) No cases met the criteria for this measure; (8) The lower limit of the confidence interval cannot be calculated if the number of observed infections equals zero; (9) No data are available from the state/territory for this reporting period; (10) The scores shown reflect fewer than 50 completed surveys; (11) There were discrepancies in the data collection process; (12) This measure does not apply to this hospital for this reporting period; (13) Results cannot be calculated for this reporting period; (14) The results for this state are combined with nearby states to protect confidentiality; Please refer to the User's Guide for a full explanation of data.

Measure	Cases	This Hosp.	State Avg.	U.S. Avg.
Heart Failure Care				
ACE Inhibitor or ARB for LVSD	23	100%	98%	97%
Discharge Instructions Given	72	89%	94%	94%
Evaluation of LVS Function	82	91%	99%	99%
Medicare Spending				
Medicare Spending per Patient (ratio)	-	0.85	0.93	0.98
Pneumonia Care				
Appropriate Initial Antibiotic Given	100	90%	96%	95%
Blood Culture Timing	145	92%	97%	98%
Pregnancy and Delivery Care				
Newborn Deliveries Scheduled Early	92	0%	7%	6%
Preventive Care				
Immunization for Influenza[2]	379	70%	91%	90%
Immunization for Pneumonia[2]	395	84%	92%	92%
Stroke Care				
Anticoagulation Therapy for Atrial Fibrillation[1]	-	-	96%	95%
Antithrombotic Therapy Timing	39	100%	98%	98%
Assessed for Rehabilitation	46	96%	96%	97%
Discharged on Antithrombotic Therapy	45	100%	99%	99%
Discharged on Statin Medication	32	91%	94%	94%
Thrombolytic Therapy Timing[1]	-	-	81%	66%
Venous Thromboembolism Prophylaxis	39	90%	93%	94%
Written Stroke Educational Materials Given	35	77%	84%	88%
Surgical Care Improvement Project				
Appropriate Beta Blocker Usage	79	95%	97%	98%
Appropriate VTP Within 24 Hours	281	96%	98%	98%
Controlled Postoperative Blood Glucose[7]	-	-	96%	97%
Perioperative Temperature Management	332	100%	100%	100%
Prophylactic Antibiotic Selection	204	96%	99%	99%
Prophylactic Antibiotic Selection (Outpatient)	193	95%	98%	98%
Prophylactic Antibiotic Stopped	196	93%	98%	98%
Prophylactic Antibiotic Timing	204	99%	99%	99%
Prophylactic Antibiotic Timing (Outpatient)	196	97%	99%	98%
Urinary Catheter Removal	238	95%	97%	97%
Survey of Patients' Hospital Experiences				
Area Around Room 'Always' Quiet at Night	300+	57%	57%	61%
Doctors 'Always' Communicated Well	300+	79%	77%	82%
Home Recovery Information Given	300+	90%	86%	85%
Hospital Given 9 or 10 on 10 Point Scale	300+	74%	70%	71%
Meds 'Always' Explained Before Given	300+	62%	62%	64%
Nurses 'Always' Communicated Well	300+	78%	76%	79%
Pain 'Always' Well Controlled	300+	69%	69%	71%
Room and Bathroom 'Always' Clean	300+	75%	69%	73%
Timely Help 'Always' Received	300+	67%	65%	68%
Would Definitely Recommend Hospital	300+	77%	70%	71%
Use of Medical Imaging				
Cardiac Imaging Stress Test before Surgery	282	5.0%	5.8%	5.3%
Combination Abdominal CT Scan	637	12.9%	9.1%	10.5%
Combination Brain/Sinus CT Scan	617	4.4%	3.2%	2.7%
Combination Chest CT Scan	288	14.6%	5.5%	2.7%
Follow-up Mammogram/Ultrasound	949	7.5%	8.5%	8.8%
Lumbar Spine MRI for Low Back Pain	76	35.5%	37.4%	37.2%

Sierra Vista Regional Health Center

300 El Camino Real Phone: 520-417-3001
Sierra Vista, AZ 85635 Fax: 520-458-2268
E-mail: admin@szch.com
URL: www.svch.com
Type: Acute Care Hospitals Emergency Services: Yes
Ownership: Voluntary non-profit - Other Beds: 86

Key Personnel:

Anesthesiology. . . . . John Cowan, MD
CEO/President. . . . . Margaret Hepburn
Operating Room. . . . . Jody Jenkins
Pediatric Ambulatory Care . . . . . . David W Leopold, DO
Pediatric In-Patient Care . . . . David W Leopold, DO
Chief of Medical Staff. . . . . Jaya Maddur
Radiology. . . . . Alan K Osumi, MD
Emergency Room . . . . Kimberly Riggs, MD

Measure	Cases	This Hosp.	State Avg.	U.S. Avg.
Blood Clot Prevention and Treatment				
Anticoagulation Overlap Therapy[2]	38	89%	94%	93%
ICU Venous Thromboembolism Prophylaxis[2]	58	98%	92%	92%
Incidence of Potentially Preventable VTE[1,2]	-	-	9%	10%
UFH with Dosages/Platelet Monitoring[2]	25	84%	98%	97%
Venous Thromboembolism Prophylaxis[2]	378	93%	88%	85%
Warfarin Therapy Discharge Instructions[2]	27	96%	74%	75%
Chest Pain/Possible Heart Attack Care				
Aspirin Given Within 24 Hours of Arrival	130	97%	98%	96%
Fibrinolytic Meds Within 30 Min. of Arrival[1]	-	-	59%	58%
Average Time to ECG (minutes)	135	5	6	7
Average Time to Transfer (minutes)[1]	-	-	48	60
Children's Asthma Care				
Received Home Management Plan of Care	-	-	-	88%
Received Reliever Medication	-	-	-	100%
Received Systemic Corticosteroids	-	-	-	100%
Emergency Department				
Admittance Decision Time (minutes)[2]	563	197	98	98
Head CT Results Within 45 Min. of Arrival	27	89%	64%	57%
Patients Who Left ER Before Being Seen	28,832	3%	2%	2%
Time from ER Arrival to Admit. (minutes)[2]	563	370	285	274
Time from ER Arrival to Discharge (minutes)	397	159	162	134
Time in ER Before Being Evaluated (minutes)	432	48	27	26
Time to Pain Meds for Fractures (minutes)	101	74	58	57
Heart Attack Care				
Aspirin Given at Discharge	44	91%	99%	99%
Fibrinolytic Meds Within 30 Min. of Arrival[7]	-	-	67%	54%
PCI Within 90 Minutes of Arrival[7]	-	-	95%	96%
Statin Prescribed at Discharge	46	72%	98%	98%
Heart Failure Care				
ACE Inhibitor or ARB for LVSD	35	69%	98%	97%
Discharge Instructions Given	90	97%	94%	94%
Evaluation of LVS Function	113	96%	99%	99%
Medicare Spending				
Medicare Spending per Patient (ratio)	-	0.92	0.93	0.98
Pneumonia Care				
Appropriate Initial Antibiotic Given	89	93%	96%	95%
Blood Culture Timing	143	97%	97%	98%
Pregnancy and Delivery Care				
Newborn Deliveries Scheduled Early[2]	34	3%	7%	6%
Preventive Care				
Immunization for Influenza[2]	483	94%	91%	90%
Immunization for Pneumonia[2]	566	93%	92%	92%
Stroke Care				
Anticoagulation Therapy for Atrial Fibrillation[1]	-	-	96%	95%
Antithrombotic Therapy Timing	22	95%	98%	98%
Assessed for Rehabilitation	23	91%	96%	97%
Discharged on Antithrombotic Therapy	23	100%	99%	99%
Discharged on Statin Medication	15	80%	94%	94%
Thrombolytic Therapy Timing[1]	-	-	81%	66%
Venous Thromboembolism Prophylaxis	23	91%	93%	94%
Written Stroke Educational Materials Given	14	71%	84%	88%
Surgical Care Improvement Project				
Appropriate Beta Blocker Usage	45	100%	97%	98%
Appropriate VTP Within 24 Hours	167	93%	98%	98%
Controlled Postoperative Blood Glucose[7]	-	-	96%	97%
Perioperative Temperature Management	191	97%	100%	100%
Prophylactic Antibiotic Selection	127	97%	99%	99%
Prophylactic Antibiotic Selection (Outpatient)	49	90%	98%	98%
Prophylactic Antibiotic Stopped	126	99%	98%	98%
Prophylactic Antibiotic Timing	127	95%	99%	99%
Prophylactic Antibiotic Timing (Outpatient)	50	96%	99%	98%
Urinary Catheter Removal	114	89%	97%	97%
Survey of Patients' Hospital Experiences				
Area Around Room 'Always' Quiet at Night	300+	52%	57%	61%
Doctors 'Always' Communicated Well	300+	78%	77%	82%
Home Recovery Information Given	300+	84%	86%	85%
Hospital Given 9 or 10 on 10 Point Scale	300+	62%	70%	71%
Meds 'Always' Explained Before Given	300+	69%	62%	64%
Nurses 'Always' Communicated Well	300+	78%	76%	79%
Pain 'Always' Well Controlled	300+	69%	69%	71%
Room and Bathroom 'Always' Clean	300+	69%	69%	73%
Timely Help 'Always' Received	300+	64%	65%	68%
Would Definitely Recommend Hospital	300+	61%	70%	71%
Use of Medical Imaging				
Cardiac Imaging Stress Test before Surgery	133	6.8%	5.8%	5.3%
Combination Abdominal CT Scan	421	12.6%	9.1%	10.5%
Combination Brain/Sinus CT Scan	436	1.1%	3.2%	2.7%
Combination Chest CT Scan	512	8.0%	5.5%	2.7%
Follow-up Mammogram/Ultrasound	1,012	9.9%	8.5%	8.8%
Lumbar Spine MRI for Low Back Pain	60	38.3%	37.4%	37.2%

White Mountain Regional Medical Center

118 South Mountain Avenue Phone: 928-333-4368
Springerville, AZ 85938 Fax: 928-333-4369
E-mail: info@wmrmc.com
URL: www.wmrmc.com
Type: Critical Access Hospitals Emergency Services: Yes
Ownership: Voluntary non-profit - Private Beds: 16

Key Personnel:

Infection Control. . . . . Jennifer Belisle
Quality Assurance . . . . Rogenia Dunn
Chief of Medical Staff. . . . . Scott Hamblin, MD
Cardiology . . . . Abdul Memon, MD
CEO . . . . Jim Robertson, FACHE
Pulmonology . . . . Carla Rotering, MD
Anesthesiology. . . . . Robert Shupak, MD

Measure	Cases	This Hosp.	State Avg.	U.S. Avg.
Blood Clot Prevention and Treatment				
Anticoagulation Overlap Therapy[5]	-	-	94%	93%
ICU Venous Thromboembolism Prophylaxis[5]	-	-	92%	92%
Incidence of Potentially Preventable VTE[5]	-	-	9%	10%
UFH with Dosages/Platelet Monitoring[5]	-	-	98%	97%
Venous Thromboembolism Prophylaxis[5]	-	-	88%	85%
Warfarin Therapy Discharge Instructions[5]	-	-	74%	75%
Chest Pain/Possible Heart Attack Care				
Aspirin Given Within 24 Hours of Arrival	26	96%	98%	96%
Fibrinolytic Meds Within 30 Min. of Arrival[1,3]	-	-	59%	58%
Average Time to ECG (minutes)	25	3	6	7
Average Time to Transfer (minutes)[1,3]	-	-	48	60
Children's Asthma Care				
Received Home Management Plan of Care	-	-	-	88%
Received Reliever Medication	-	-	-	100%
Received Systemic Corticosteroids	-	-	-	100%
Emergency Department				
Admittance Decision Time (minutes)[5]	-	-	98	98
Head CT Results Within 45 Min. of Arrival[5]	-	-	64%	57%
Patients Who Left ER Before Being Seen[5]	-	-	2%	2%
Time from ER Arrival to Admit. (minutes)[5]	-	-	285	274
Time from ER Arrival to Discharge (minutes)[5]	-	-	162	134
Time in ER Before Being Evaluated (minutes)[5]	-	-	27	26
Time to Pain Meds for Fractures (minutes)[5]	-	-	58	57
Heart Attack Care				
Aspirin Given at Discharge[5]	-	-	99%	99%
Fibrinolytic Meds Within 30 Min. of Arrival[5]	-	-	67%	54%
PCI Within 90 Minutes of Arrival[5]	-	-	95%	96%
Statin Prescribed at Discharge[5]	-	-	98%	98%
Heart Failure Care				
ACE Inhibitor or ARB for LVSD[3,7]	-	-	98%	97%
Discharge Instructions Given[1,3]	-	-	94%	94%
Evaluation of LVS Function[1,3]	-	-	99%	99%
Medicare Spending				
Medicare Spending per Patient (ratio)	-	-	0.93	0.98
Pneumonia Care				
Appropriate Initial Antibiotic Given[1]	-	-	96%	95%
Blood Culture Timing[1]	-	-	97%	98%
Pregnancy and Delivery Care				
Newborn Deliveries Scheduled Early[5]	-	-	7%	6%
Preventive Care				
Immunization for Influenza[5]	-	-	91%	90%
Immunization for Pneumonia[5]	-	-	92%	92%
Stroke Care				
Anticoagulation Therapy for Atrial Fibrillation[5]	-	-	96%	95%
Antithrombotic Therapy Timing[5]	-	-	98%	98%
Assessed for Rehabilitation[5]	-	-	96%	97%
Discharged on Antithrombotic Therapy[5]	-	-	99%	99%
Discharged on Statin Medication[5]	-	-	94%	94%
Thrombolytic Therapy Timing[5]	-	-	81%	66%
Venous Thromboembolism Prophylaxis[5]	-	-	93%	94%
Written Stroke Educational Materials Given[5]	-	-	84%	88%

NOTE: Hospital profiles are in alphabetical order by state, then city, then hospital within the city; Rankings exclude hospitals with less than 25 cases except for patient surveys which excludes hospitals with less than 100 cases; (a) 100-299 cases; (1) The number of cases/patients is too few to report; (2) Data submitted were based on a sample of cases/patients; (3) Results are based on a shorter time period than required; (4) Data suppressed by CMS for one or more quarters; (5) Results are not available for this reporting period; (6) Fewer than 100 patients completed the HCAHPS survey; (7) No cases met the criteria for this measure; (8) The lower limit of the confidence interval cannot be calculated if the number of observed infections equals zero; (9) No data are available from the state/territory for this reporting period; (10) The scores shown reflect fewer than 50 completed surveys; (11) There were discrepancies in the data collection process; (12) This measure does not apply to this hospital for this reporting period; (13) Results cannot be calculated for this reporting period; (14) The results for this state are combined with nearby states to protect confidentiality; Please refer to the User's Guide for a full explanation of data.

Measure	Cases	This Hosp.	State Avg.	U.S. Avg.
Surgical Care Improvement Project				
Appropriate Beta Blocker Usage[5]	-	-	97%	98%
Appropriate VTP Within 24 Hours[5]	-	-	98%	98%
Controlled Postoperative Blood Glucose[5]	-	-	96%	97%
Perioperative Temperature Management[5]	-	-	100%	100%
Prophylactic Antibiotic Selection[5]	-	-	99%	99%
Prophylactic Antibiotic Selection (Outpatient)[5]	-	-	98%	98%
Prophylactic Antibiotic Stopped[5]	-	-	98%	98%
Prophylactic Antibiotic Timing[5]	-	-	99%	99%
Prophylactic Antibiotic Timing (Outpatient)[5]	-	-	99%	98%
Urinary Catheter Removal[5]	-	-	97%	97%
Survey of Patients' Hospital Experiences				
Area Around Room 'Always' Quiet at Night[6]	<100	66%	57%	61%
Doctors 'Always' Communicated Well[6]	<100	84%	77%	82%
Home Recovery Information Given[6]	<100	88%	86%	85%
Hospital Given 9 or 10 on 10 Point Scale[6]	<100	77%	70%	71%
Meds 'Always' Explained Before Given[6]	<100	67%	62%	64%
Nurses 'Always' Communicated Well[6]	<100	75%	76%	79%
Pain 'Always' Well Controlled[6]	<100	61%	69%	71%
Room and Bathroom 'Always' Clean[6]	<100	79%	69%	73%
Timely Help 'Always' Received[6]	<100	73%	65%	68%
Would Definitely Recommend Hospital[6]	<100	74%	70%	71%
Use of Medical Imaging				
Cardiac Imaging Stress Test before Surgery	67	3.0%	5.8%	5.3%
Combination Abdominal CT Scan	82	7.3%	9.1%	10.5%
Combination Brain/Sinus CT Scan[1]	-	-	3.2%	2.7%
Combination Chest CT Scan	72	15.3%	5.5%	2.7%
Follow-up Mammogram/Ultrasound[7]	-	-	8.5%	8.8%
Lumbar Spine MRI for Low Back Pain[1]	-	-	37.4%	37.2%

Banner Boswell Medical Center

10401 West Thunderbird Boulevard Phone: 623-977-7211
Sun City, AZ 85351 Fax: 623-876-5795
URL: www.bannerhealth.com
Type: Acute Care Hospitals Emergency Services: Yes
Ownership: Voluntary non-profit - Other

Key Personnel:
Operating Room. . . . . Rita Borden
Radiology. . . . . Robert Charney
CEO/President. . . . . Peter S. Fine, FACHE
Chief of Medical Staff. . . . . John Hensing, MD
Quality Assurance . . . . John Kimball

Measure	Cases	This Hosp.	State Avg.	U.S. Avg.
Blood Clot Prevention and Treatment				
Anticoagulation Overlap Therapy[2]	180	92%	94%	93%
ICU Venous Thromboembolism Prophylaxis[2]	69	91%	92%	92%
Incidence of Potentially Preventable VTE[2]	29	7%	9%	10%
UFH with Dosages/Platelet Monitoring[2]	85	100%	98%	97%
Venous Thromboembolism Prophylaxis[2]	320	86%	88%	85%
Warfarin Therapy Discharge Instructions[2]	116	51%	74%	75%
Chest Pain/Possible Heart Attack Care				
Aspirin Given Within 24 Hours of Arrival[1,3]	-	-	98%	96%
Fibrinolytic Meds Within 30 Min. of Arrival[5]	-	-	59%	58%
Average Time to ECG (minutes)[1,3]	-	-	6	7
Average Time to Transfer (minutes)[5]	-	-	48	60
Children's Asthma Care				
Received Home Management Plan of Care	-	-	-	88%
Received Reliever Medication	-	-	-	100%
Received Systemic Corticosteroids	-	-	-	100%
Emergency Department				
Admittance Decision Time (minutes)[2]	820	86	98	98
Head CT Results Within 45 Min. of Arrival[1]	-	-	64%	57%
Patients Who Left ER Before Being Seen	45,485	1%	2%	2%
Time from ER Arrival to Admit. (minutes)[2]	834	294	285	274
Time from ER Arrival to Discharge (minutes)	266	208	162	134
Time in ER Before Being Evaluated (minutes)	359	24	27	26
Time to Pain Meds for Fractures (minutes)	98	64	58	57
Heart Attack Care				
Aspirin Given at Discharge[2]	273	100%	99%	99%
Fibrinolytic Meds Within 30 Min. of Arrival[2,7]	-	-	67%	54%
PCI Within 90 Minutes of Arrival[2]	35	97%	95%	96%
Statin Prescribed at Discharge[2]	256	100%	98%	98%
Heart Failure Care				
ACE Inhibitor or ARB for LVSD[2]	68	100%	98%	97%
Discharge Instructions Given[2]	232	97%	94%	94%
Evaluation of LVS Function[2]	285	100%	99%	99%
Medicare Spending				
Medicare Spending per Patient (ratio)	-	0.94	0.93	0.98
Pneumonia Care				
Appropriate Initial Antibiotic Given[2]	83	100%	96%	95%
Blood Culture Timing[2]	91	97%	97%	98%
Pregnancy and Delivery Care				
Newborn Deliveries Scheduled Early[7]	-	-	7%	6%
Preventive Care				
Immunization for Influenza[2]	595	98%	91%	90%
Immunization for Pneumonia[2]	1,063	98%	92%	92%
Stroke Care				
Anticoagulation Therapy for Atrial Fibrillation[2]	13	100%	96%	95%
Antithrombotic Therapy Timing[2]	76	99%	98%	98%
Assessed for Rehabilitation[2]	99	96%	96%	97%
Discharged on Antithrombotic Therapy[2]	90	100%	99%	99%
Discharged on Statin Medication[2]	64	100%	94%	94%
Thrombolytic Therapy Timing[2]	14	64%	81%	66%
Venous Thromboembolism Prophylaxis[2]	93	91%	93%	94%
Written Stroke Educational Materials Given[2]	53	85%	84%	88%
Surgical Care Improvement Project				
Appropriate Beta Blocker Usage[2]	220	99%	97%	98%
Appropriate VTP Within 24 Hours[2]	324	98%	98%	98%
Controlled Postoperative Blood Glucose[2]	160	98%	96%	97%
Perioperative Temperature Management[2]	470	100%	100%	100%
Prophylactic Antibiotic Selection[2]	420	100%	99%	99%
Prophylactic Antibiotic Selection (Outpatient)	530	98%	98%	98%
Prophylactic Antibiotic Stopped[2]	403	98%	98%	98%
Prophylactic Antibiotic Timing[2]	420	100%	99%	99%
Prophylactic Antibiotic Timing (Outpatient)	531	100%	99%	98%
Urinary Catheter Removal[2]	233	99%	97%	97%
Survey of Patients' Hospital Experiences				
Area Around Room 'Always' Quiet at Night[11]	300+	55%	57%	61%
Doctors 'Always' Communicated Well[11]	300+	77%	77%	82%
Home Recovery Information Given[11]	300+	90%	86%	85%
Hospital Given 9 or 10 on 10 Point Scale[11]	300+	73%	70%	71%
Meds 'Always' Explained Before Given[11]	300+	65%	62%	64%
Nurses 'Always' Communicated Well[11]	300+	80%	76%	79%
Pain 'Always' Well Controlled[11]	300+	72%	69%	71%
Room and Bathroom 'Always' Clean[11]	300+	65%	69%	73%
Timely Help 'Always' Received[11]	300+	70%	65%	68%
Would Definitely Recommend Hospital[11]	300+	75%	70%	71%
Use of Medical Imaging				
Cardiac Imaging Stress Test before Surgery	120	8.3%	5.8%	5.3%
Combination Abdominal CT Scan	1,051	3.4%	9.1%	10.5%
Combination Brain/Sinus CT Scan	1,056	2.7%	3.2%	2.7%
Combination Chest CT Scan	494	0.2%	5.5%	2.7%
Follow-up Mammogram/Ultrasound	1,233	13.0%	8.5%	8.8%
Lumbar Spine MRI for Low Back Pain	55	36.4%	37.4%	37.2%

Banner Del E Webb Medical Center

14502 West Meeker Boulevard Phone: 623-214-4000
Sun City West, AZ 85375 Fax: 623-214-4105
URL: www.sunhealth.org/delwebb
Type: Acute Care Hospitals Emergency Services: Yes
Ownership: Voluntary non-profit - Private Beds: 297

Key Personnel:
Chief of Medical Staff. . . . . Steven Charney, MD
CEO/President. . . . . Debbie Flores
Emergency Room . . . . Corlean Kuhl

Measure	Cases	This Hosp.	State Avg.	U.S. Avg.
Blood Clot Prevention and Treatment				
Anticoagulation Overlap Therapy[2]	180	88%	94%	93%
ICU Venous Thromboembolism Prophylaxis[2]	54	87%	92%	92%
Incidence of Potentially Preventable VTE[2]	15	0%	9%	10%
UFH with Dosages/Platelet Monitoring[2]	83	100%	98%	97%
Venous Thromboembolism Prophylaxis[2]	332	85%	88%	85%
Warfarin Therapy Discharge Instructions[2]	126	58%	74%	75%
Chest Pain/Possible Heart Attack Care				
Aspirin Given Within 24 Hours of Arrival[1]	-	-	98%	96%
Fibrinolytic Meds Within 30 Min. of Arrival[3,7]	-	-	59%	58%
Average Time to ECG (minutes)[1]	-	-	6	7
Average Time to Transfer (minutes)[3,7]	-	-	48	60
Children's Asthma Care				
Received Home Management Plan of Care	-	-	-	88%
Received Reliever Medication	-	-	-	100%
Received Systemic Corticosteroids	-	-	-	100%
Emergency Department				
Admittance Decision Time (minutes)[2]	604	67	98	98
Head CT Results Within 45 Min. of Arrival	32	69%	64%	57%
Patients Who Left ER Before Being Seen	59,560	1%	2%	2%
Time from ER Arrival to Admit. (minutes)[2]	629	285	285	274
Time from ER Arrival to Discharge (minutes)	302	182	162	134
Time in ER Before Being Evaluated (minutes)	169	13	27	26
Time to Pain Meds for Fractures (minutes)	179	55	58	57
Heart Attack Care				
Aspirin Given at Discharge[2]	237	100%	99%	99%
Fibrinolytic Meds Within 30 Min. of Arrival[2,7]	-	-	67%	54%
PCI Within 90 Minutes of Arrival[2]	47	96%	95%	96%
Statin Prescribed at Discharge[2]	228	100%	98%	98%
Heart Failure Care				
ACE Inhibitor or ARB for LVSD[2]	62	100%	98%	97%
Discharge Instructions Given[2]	202	96%	94%	94%
Evaluation of LVS Function[2]	244	100%	99%	99%
Medicare Spending				
Medicare Spending per Patient (ratio)	-	0.98	0.93	0.98
Pneumonia Care				
Appropriate Initial Antibiotic Given[2]	87	100%	96%	95%
Blood Culture Timing[2]	107	99%	97%	98%
Pregnancy and Delivery Care				
Newborn Deliveries Scheduled Early[2]	45	2%	7%	6%
Preventive Care				
Immunization for Influenza[2]	542	99%	91%	90%
Immunization for Pneumonia[2]	791	99%	92%	92%
Stroke Care				
Anticoagulation Therapy for Atrial Fibrillation[2]	23	87%	96%	95%
Antithrombotic Therapy Timing[2]	109	98%	98%	98%
Assessed for Rehabilitation[2]	122	96%	96%	97%
Discharged on Antithrombotic Therapy[2]	120	100%	99%	99%
Discharged on Statin Medication[2]	85	95%	94%	94%
Thrombolytic Therapy Timing[2]	15	100%	81%	66%
Venous Thromboembolism Prophylaxis[2]	124	90%	93%	94%
Written Stroke Educational Materials Given[2]	67	82%	84%	88%
Surgical Care Improvement Project				
Appropriate Beta Blocker Usage[2]	127	97%	97%	98%
Appropriate VTP Within 24 Hours[2]	336	100%	98%	98%
Controlled Postoperative Blood Glucose[2,7]	-	-	96%	97%
Perioperative Temperature Management[2]	445	100%	100%	100%
Prophylactic Antibiotic Selection[2]	268	99%	99%	99%
Prophylactic Antibiotic Selection (Outpatient)	365	99%	98%	98%
Prophylactic Antibiotic Stopped[2]	264	100%	98%	98%
Prophylactic Antibiotic Timing[2]	268	100%	99%	99%
Prophylactic Antibiotic Timing (Outpatient)	366	98%	99%	98%
Urinary Catheter Removal[2]	116	99%	97%	97%
Survey of Patients' Hospital Experiences				
Area Around Room 'Always' Quiet at Night[11]	300+	51%	57%	61%
Doctors 'Always' Communicated Well[11]	300+	77%	77%	82%
Home Recovery Information Given[11]	300+	88%	86%	85%
Hospital Given 9 or 10 on 10 Point Scale[11]	300+	68%	70%	71%
Meds 'Always' Explained Before Given[11]	300+	61%	62%	64%
Nurses 'Always' Communicated Well[11]	300+	76%	76%	79%
Pain 'Always' Well Controlled[11]	300+	69%	69%	71%
Room and Bathroom 'Always' Clean[11]	300+	68%	69%	73%
Timely Help 'Always' Received[11]	300+	62%	65%	68%
Would Definitely Recommend Hospital[11]	300+	71%	70%	71%
Use of Medical Imaging				
Cardiac Imaging Stress Test before Surgery	200	5.0%	5.8%	5.3%
Combination Abdominal CT Scan	1,611	4.7%	9.1%	10.5%
Combination Brain/Sinus CT Scan	1,359	1.8%	3.2%	2.7%
Combination Chest CT Scan	569	4.0%	5.5%	2.7%
Follow-up Mammogram/Ultrasound	4,090	10.8%	8.5%	8.8%
Lumbar Spine MRI for Low Back Pain	67	34.3%	37.4%	37.2%

NOTE: Hospital profiles are in alphabetical order by state, then city, then hospital within the city; Rankings exclude hospitals with less than 25 cases except for patient surveys which excludes hospitals with less than 100 cases; (a) 100-299 cases; (1) The number of cases/patients is too few to report; (2) Data submitted were based on a sample of cases/patients; (3) Results are based on a shorter time period than required; (4) Data suppressed by CMS for one or more quarters; (5) Results are not available for this reporting period; (6) Fewer than 100 patients completed the HCAHPS survey; (7) No cases met the criteria for this measure; (8) The lower limit of the confidence interval cannot be calculated if the number of observed infections equals zero; (9) No data are available from the state/territory for this reporting period; (10) The scores shown reflect fewer than 50 completed surveys; (11) There were discrepancies in the data collection process; (12) This measure does not apply to this hospital for this reporting period; (13) Results cannot be calculated for this reporting period; (14) The results for this state are combined with nearby states to protect confidentiality; Please refer to the User's Guide for a full explanation of data.

Tuba City Regional Health Care Corporation

PO Box 600 Phone: 928-283-2501
Tuba City, AZ 86045 Fax: 928-283-2516
E-mail: contacat@tcrhcc.org
URL: www.tcrhcc.org
Type: Acute Care Hospitals Emergency Services: No
Ownership: Voluntary non-profit - Other Beds: 65
Key Personnel:
Operating Room. . . . . Tori Davidson
CEO/President. . . . . Joseph T Engelken
Pediatric Ambulatory Care . . . . . . Steve Holve, MD
Pediatric In-Patient Care . . . . Steve Holve, MD
Surgery . . . . Dr. Thomas Peters
Quality Assurance . . . . Elida Vonloewe
Chief of Medical Staff. . . . . Steve Xolve

Measure	Cases	This Hosp.	State Avg.	U.S. Avg.
Blood Clot Prevention and Treatment				
Anticoagulation Overlap Therapy[1,2]	-	-	94%	93%
ICU Venous Thromboembolism Prophylaxis[2]	40	95%	92%	92%
Incidence of Potentially Preventable VTE[1,2]	-	-	9%	10%
UFH with Dosages/Platelet Monitoring[1,2]	-	-	98%	97%
Venous Thromboembolism Prophylaxis[2]	150	91%	88%	85%
Warfarin Therapy Discharge Instructions[1,2]	-	-	74%	75%
Chest Pain/Possible Heart Attack Care				
Aspirin Given Within 24 Hours of Arrival	-	-	98%	96%
Fibrinolytic Meds Within 30 Min. of Arrival	-	-	59%	58%
Average Time to ECG (minutes)	-	-	6	7
Average Time to Transfer (minutes)	-	-	48	60
Children's Asthma Care				
Received Home Management Plan of Care[1]	-	-	-	88%
Received Reliever Medication[1]	-	-	-	100%
Received Systemic Corticosteroids[1]	-	-	-	100%
Emergency Department				
Admittance Decision Time (minutes)[2]	198	77	98	98
Head CT Results Within 45 Min. of Arrival	-	-	64%	57%
Patients Who Left ER Before Being Seen	-	-	2%	2%
Time from ER Arrival to Admit. (minutes)[2]	199	293	285	274
Time from ER Arrival to Discharge (minutes)	-	-	162	134
Time in ER Before Being Evaluated (minutes)	-	-	27	26
Time to Pain Meds for Fractures (minutes)	-	-	58	57
Heart Attack Care				
Aspirin Given at Discharge[3,7]	-	-	99%	99%
Fibrinolytic Meds Within 30 Min. of Arrival[3,7]	-	-	67%	54%
PCI Within 90 Minutes of Arrival[3,7]	-	-	95%	96%
Statin Prescribed at Discharge[3,7]	-	-	98%	98%
Heart Failure Care				
ACE Inhibitor or ARB for LVSD	31	94%	98%	97%
Discharge Instructions Given	47	60%	94%	94%
Evaluation of LVS Function	49	94%	99%	99%
Medicare Spending				
Medicare Spending per Patient (ratio)	-	0.72	0.93	0.98
Pneumonia Care				
Appropriate Initial Antibiotic Given	38	92%	96%	95%
Blood Culture Timing	57	88%	97%	98%
Pregnancy and Delivery Care				
Newborn Deliveries Scheduled Early[2]	28	11%	7%	6%
Preventive Care				
Immunization for Influenza[2]	258	43%	91%	90%
Immunization for Pneumonia[2]	210	76%	92%	92%
Stroke Care				
Anticoagulation Therapy for Atrial Fibrillation[3,7]	-	-	96%	95%
Antithrombotic Therapy Timing[1,3]	-	-	98%	98%
Assessed for Rehabilitation[1,3]	-	-	96%	97%
Discharged on Antithrombotic Therapy[3,7]	-	-	99%	99%
Discharged on Statin Medication[1,3]	-	-	94%	94%
Thrombolytic Therapy Timing[3,7]	-	-	81%	66%
Venous Thromboembolism Prophylaxis[1,3]	-	-	93%	94%
Written Stroke Educational Materials Given[1,3]	-	-	84%	88%
Surgical Care Improvement Project				
Appropriate Beta Blocker Usage[2]	20	70%	97%	98%
Appropriate VTP Within 24 Hours[2]	185	90%	98%	98%
Controlled Postoperative Blood Glucose[2,7]	-	-	96%	97%
Perioperative Temperature Management[2]	214	99%	100%	100%
Prophylactic Antibiotic Selection[2]	169	93%	99%	99%
Prophylactic Antibiotic Selection (Outpatient)	-	-	98%	98%
Prophylactic Antibiotic Stopped[2]	168	98%	98%	98%
Prophylactic Antibiotic Timing[2]	170	91%	99%	99%
Prophylactic Antibiotic Timing (Outpatient)	-	-	99%	98%
Urinary Catheter Removal[2]	130	95%	97%	97%
Survey of Patients' Hospital Experiences				
Area Around Room 'Always' Quiet at Night	300+	55%	57%	61%
Doctors 'Always' Communicated Well	300+	71%	77%	82%
Home Recovery Information Given	300+	82%	86%	85%
Hospital Given 9 or 10 on 10 Point Scale	300+	52%	70%	71%
Meds 'Always' Explained Before Given	300+	62%	62%	64%
Nurses 'Always' Communicated Well	300+	65%	76%	79%
Pain 'Always' Well Controlled	300+	56%	69%	71%
Room and Bathroom 'Always' Clean	300+	59%	69%	73%
Timely Help 'Always' Received	300+	53%	65%	68%
Would Definitely Recommend Hospital	300+	52%	70%	71%
Use of Medical Imaging				
Cardiac Imaging Stress Test before Surgery	-	-	5.8%	5.3%
Combination Abdominal CT Scan	-	-	9.1%	10.5%
Combination Brain/Sinus CT Scan	-	-	3.2%	2.7%
Combination Chest CT Scan	-	-	5.5%	2.7%
Follow-up Mammogram/Ultrasound	-	-	8.5%	8.8%
Lumbar Spine MRI for Low Back Pain	-	-	37.4%	37.2%

Carondelet Saint Joseph's Hospital

350 North Wilmot Road Phone: 520-873-3000
Tucson, AZ 85711 Fax: 520-873-3921
URL: www.carondelet.org
Type: Acute Care Hospitals Emergency Services: Yes
Ownership: Voluntary non-profit - Other Beds: 471
Key Personnel:
Chief of Medical Staff. . . . . Donald Denmark, MD
CEO/President. . . . . Tony Fonze
Operating Room. . . . . Carol Martin
Emergency Room . . . . Karri Mcglone, RN
Radiology. . . . . Fred Swiderski

Measure	Cases	This Hosp.	State Avg.	U.S. Avg.
Blood Clot Prevention and Treatment				
Anticoagulation Overlap Therapy[2]	120	92%	94%	93%
ICU Venous Thromboembolism Prophylaxis[2]	112	91%	92%	92%
Incidence of Potentially Preventable VTE[2]	21	29%	9%	10%
UFH with Dosages/Platelet Monitoring[2]	74	91%	98%	97%
Venous Thromboembolism Prophylaxis[2]	316	82%	88%	85%
Warfarin Therapy Discharge Instructions[2]	79	92%	74%	75%
Chest Pain/Possible Heart Attack Care				
Aspirin Given Within 24 Hours of Arrival[5]	-	-	98%	96%
Fibrinolytic Meds Within 30 Min. of Arrival[5]	-	-	59%	58%
Average Time to ECG (minutes)[5]	-	-	6	7
Average Time to Transfer (minutes)[5]	-	-	48	60
Children's Asthma Care				
Received Home Management Plan of Care	-	-	-	88%
Received Reliever Medication	-	-	-	100%
Received Systemic Corticosteroids	-	-	-	100%
Emergency Department				
Admittance Decision Time (minutes)[2]	497	165	98	98
Head CT Results Within 45 Min. of Arrival[5]	-	-	64%	57%
Patients Who Left ER Before Being Seen	20,576	3%	2%	2%
Time from ER Arrival to Admit. (minutes)[2]	512	388	285	274
Time from ER Arrival to Discharge (minutes)	365	228	162	134
Time in ER Before Being Evaluated (minutes)	399	41	27	26
Time to Pain Meds for Fractures (minutes)	238	105	58	57
Heart Attack Care				
Aspirin Given at Discharge[2]	174	98%	99%	99%
Fibrinolytic Meds Within 30 Min. of Arrival[2,7]	-	-	67%	54%
PCI Within 90 Minutes of Arrival[2]	41	100%	95%	96%
Statin Prescribed at Discharge[2]	166	98%	98%	98%
Heart Failure Care				
ACE Inhibitor or ARB for LVSD	56	100%	98%	97%
Discharge Instructions Given	189	93%	94%	94%
Evaluation of LVS Function	232	100%	99%	99%
Medicare Spending				
Medicare Spending per Patient (ratio)	-	1.01	0.93	0.98
Pneumonia Care				
Appropriate Initial Antibiotic Given[2]	107	99%	96%	95%
Blood Culture Timing[2]	136	99%	97%	98%
Pregnancy and Delivery Care				
Newborn Deliveries Scheduled Early[2]	40	5%	7%	6%
Preventive Care				
Immunization for Influenza[2]	524	89%	91%	90%
Immunization for Pneumonia[2]	649	90%	92%	92%
Stroke Care				
Anticoagulation Therapy for Atrial Fibrillation	36	94%	96%	95%
Antithrombotic Therapy Timing	172	97%	98%	98%
Assessed for Rehabilitation	235	95%	96%	97%
Discharged on Antithrombotic Therapy	201	99%	99%	99%
Discharged on Statin Medication	142	93%	94%	94%
Thrombolytic Therapy Timing	16	100%	81%	66%
Venous Thromboembolism Prophylaxis	249	88%	93%	94%
Written Stroke Educational Materials Given	115	93%	84%	88%
Surgical Care Improvement Project				
Appropriate Beta Blocker Usage[2]	141	99%	97%	98%
Appropriate VTP Within 24 Hours[2]	446	98%	98%	98%
Controlled Postoperative Blood Glucose[2,7]	-	-	96%	97%
Perioperative Temperature Management[2]	554	100%	100%	100%
Prophylactic Antibiotic Selection[2]	373	98%	99%	99%
Prophylactic Antibiotic Selection (Outpatient)	971	99%	98%	98%
Prophylactic Antibiotic Stopped[2]	355	98%	98%	98%
Prophylactic Antibiotic Timing[2]	373	100%	99%	99%
Prophylactic Antibiotic Timing (Outpatient)	972	99%	99%	98%
Urinary Catheter Removal[2]	307	97%	97%	97%
Survey of Patients' Hospital Experiences				
Area Around Room 'Always' Quiet at Night[11]	300+	48%	57%	61%
Doctors 'Always' Communicated Well[11]	300+	81%	77%	82%
Home Recovery Information Given[11]	300+	85%	86%	85%
Hospital Given 9 or 10 on 10 Point Scale[11]	300+	68%	70%	71%
Meds 'Always' Explained Before Given[11]	300+	64%	62%	64%
Nurses 'Always' Communicated Well[11]	300+	73%	76%	79%
Pain 'Always' Well Controlled[11]	300+	63%	69%	71%
Room and Bathroom 'Always' Clean[11]	300+	61%	69%	73%
Timely Help 'Always' Received[11]	300+	58%	65%	68%
Would Definitely Recommend Hospital[11]	300+	72%	70%	71%
Use of Medical Imaging				
Cardiac Imaging Stress Test before Surgery	454	5.3%	5.8%	5.3%
Combination Abdominal CT Scan	394	4.8%	9.1%	10.5%
Combination Brain/Sinus CT Scan[1]	-	-	3.2%	2.7%
Combination Chest CT Scan	190	1.6%	5.5%	2.7%
Follow-up Mammogram/Ultrasound[7]	-	-	8.5%	8.8%
Lumbar Spine MRI for Low Back Pain[1]	-	-	37.4%	37.2%

Carondelet Saint Marys Hospital

1601 West Saint Mary's Road Phone: 520-872-3000
Tucson, AZ 85745 Fax: 520-872-6066
URL: www.carondelet.org
Type: Acute Care Hospitals Emergency Services: Yes
Ownership: Voluntary non-profit - Private Beds: 393
Key Personnel:
CEO/President. . . . . Amy Beiter, MD
Chief of Medical Staff. . . . . D Bowman
Emergency Room . . . . D McReynolds, MD

Measure	Cases	This Hosp.	State Avg.	U.S. Avg.
Blood Clot Prevention and Treatment				
Anticoagulation Overlap Therapy[2]	100	100%	94%	93%
ICU Venous Thromboembolism Prophylaxis[2]	106	97%	92%	92%
Incidence of Potentially Preventable VTE[2]	15	0%	9%	10%
UFH with Dosages/Platelet Monitoring[2]	48	100%	98%	97%
Venous Thromboembolism Prophylaxis[2]	340	94%	88%	85%
Warfarin Therapy Discharge Instructions[2]	81	98%	74%	75%
Chest Pain/Possible Heart Attack Care				
Aspirin Given Within 24 Hours of Arrival[5]	-	-	98%	96%
Fibrinolytic Meds Within 30 Min. of Arrival[5]	-	-	59%	58%
Average Time to ECG (minutes)[5]	-	-	6	7
Average Time to Transfer (minutes)[5]	-	-	48	60
Children's Asthma Care				
Received Home Management Plan of Care	-	-	-	88%
Received Reliever Medication	-	-	-	100%
Received Systemic Corticosteroids	-	-	-	100%

NOTE: Hospital profiles are in alphabetical order by state, then city, then hospital within the city; Rankings exclude hospitals with less than 25 cases except for patient surveys which excludes hospitals with less than 100 cases; (a) 100-299 cases; (1) The number of cases/patients is too few to report; (2) Data submitted were based on a sample of cases/patients; (3) Results are based on a shorter time period than required; (4) Data suppressed by CMS for one or more quarters; (5) Results are not available for this reporting period; (6) Fewer than 100 patients completed the HCAHPS survey; (7) No cases met the criteria for this measure; (8) The lower limit of the confidence interval cannot be calculated if the number of observed infections equals zero; (9) No data are available from the state/territory for this reporting period; (10) The scores shown reflect fewer than 50 completed surveys; (11) There were discrepancies in the data collection process; (12) This measure does not apply to this hospital for this reporting period; (13) Results cannot be calculated for this reporting period; (14) The results for this state are combined with nearby states to protect confidentiality; Please refer to the User's Guide for a full explanation of data.

Measure	Cases	This Hosp.	State Avg.	U.S. Avg.
Emergency Department				
Admittance Decision Time (minutes)[2]	829	186	98	98
Head CT Results Within 45 Min. of Arrival[3,7]	-	-	64%	57%
Patients Who Left ER Before Being Seen	19,158	1%	2%	2%
Time from ER Arrival to Admit. (minutes)[2]	844	387	285	274
Time from ER Arrival to Discharge (minutes)	348	191	162	134
Time in ER Before Being Evaluated (minutes)	410	28	27	26
Time to Pain Meds for Fractures (minutes)	218	80	58	57
Heart Attack Care				
Aspirin Given at Discharge	301	100%	99%	99%
Fibrinolytic Meds Within 30 Min. of Arrival[7]	-	-	67%	54%
PCI Within 90 Minutes of Arrival	59	92%	95%	96%
Statin Prescribed at Discharge	283	100%	98%	98%
Heart Failure Care				
ACE Inhibitor or ARB for LVSD[2]	102	99%	98%	97%
Discharge Instructions Given[2]	258	99%	94%	94%
Evaluation of LVS Function[2]	292	100%	99%	99%
Medicare Spending				
Medicare Spending per Patient (ratio)	-	0.97	0.93	0.98
Pneumonia Care				
Appropriate Initial Antibiotic Given[2]	105	98%	96%	95%
Blood Culture Timing[2]	116	98%	97%	98%
Pregnancy and Delivery Care				
Newborn Deliveries Scheduled Early[7]	-	-	7%	6%
Preventive Care				
Immunization for Influenza[2]	624	94%	91%	90%
Immunization for Pneumonia[2]	971	92%	92%	92%
Stroke Care				
Anticoagulation Therapy for Atrial Fibrillation	22	100%	96%	95%
Antithrombotic Therapy Timing	149	98%	98%	98%
Assessed for Rehabilitation	188	99%	96%	97%
Discharged on Antithrombotic Therapy	179	100%	99%	99%
Discharged on Statin Medication	131	100%	94%	94%
Thrombolytic Therapy Timing	32	100%	81%	66%
Venous Thromboembolism Prophylaxis	198	95%	93%	94%
Written Stroke Educational Materials Given	104	93%	84%	88%
Surgical Care Improvement Project				
Appropriate Beta Blocker Usage[2]	191	99%	97%	98%
Appropriate VTP Within 24 Hours[2]	355	98%	98%	98%
Controlled Postoperative Blood Glucose[2]	139	96%	96%	97%
Perioperative Temperature Management[2]	537	100%	100%	100%
Prophylactic Antibiotic Selection[2]	413	100%	99%	99%
Prophylactic Antibiotic Selection (Outpatient)	382	99%	98%	98%
Prophylactic Antibiotic Stopped[2]	399	100%	98%	98%
Prophylactic Antibiotic Timing[2]	414	100%	99%	99%
Prophylactic Antibiotic Timing (Outpatient)	384	99%	99%	98%
Urinary Catheter Removal[2]	320	96%	97%	97%
Survey of Patients' Hospital Experiences				
Area Around Room 'Always' Quiet at Night[11]	300+	55%	57%	61%
Doctors 'Always' Communicated Well[11]	300+	77%	77%	82%
Home Recovery Information Given[11]	300+	87%	86%	85%
Hospital Given 9 or 10 on 10 Point Scale[11]	300+	64%	70%	71%
Meds 'Always' Explained Before Given[11]	300+	62%	62%	64%
Nurses 'Always' Communicated Well[11]	300+	74%	76%	79%
Pain 'Always' Well Controlled[11]	300+	68%	69%	71%
Room and Bathroom 'Always' Clean[11]	300+	60%	69%	73%
Timely Help 'Always' Received[11]	300+	57%	65%	68%
Would Definitely Recommend Hospital[11]	300+	65%	70%	71%
Use of Medical Imaging				
Cardiac Imaging Stress Test before Surgery	186	3.8%	5.8%	5.3%
Combination Abdominal CT Scan	378	5.8%	9.1%	10.5%
Combination Brain/Sinus CT Scan[1]	-	-	3.2%	2.7%
Combination Chest CT Scan	83	2.4%	5.5%	2.7%
Follow-up Mammogram/Ultrasound[7]	-	-	8.5%	8.8%
Lumbar Spine MRI for Low Back Pain[1]	-	-	37.4%	37.2%

Northwest Medical Center

6200 North La Cholla Boulevard
Tucson, AZ 85741
Phone: 520-742-9000
Fax: 520-469-8101
URL: www.northwestmedicalcenter.com
Type: Acute Care Hospitals
Emergency Services: Yes
Ownership: Proprietary
Beds: 278

Key Personnel:

Chief of Medical Staff.......... Mitzi Barmatz, MD
CEO/President............... Jeff Comer
Emergency Room .... Katie Gleason
Infection Control.............. Melvin Morrow
Quality Assurance .... Annette Vince

Measure	Cases	This Hosp.	State Avg.	U.S. Avg.
Blood Clot Prevention and Treatment				
Anticoagulation Overlap Therapy[2]	138	100%	94%	93%
ICU Venous Thromboembolism Prophylaxis[2]	90	91%	92%	92%
Incidence of Potentially Preventable VTE[2]	16	6%	9%	10%
UFH with Dosages/Platelet Monitoring[2]	78	100%	98%	97%
Venous Thromboembolism Prophylaxis[2]	361	84%	88%	85%
Warfarin Therapy Discharge Instructions[2]	104	92%	74%	75%
Chest Pain/Possible Heart Attack Care				
Aspirin Given Within 24 Hours of Arrival[1,3]	-	-	98%	96%
Fibrinolytic Meds Within 30 Min. of Arrival[5]	-	-	59%	58%
Average Time to ECG (minutes)[1,3]	-	-	6	7
Average Time to Transfer (minutes)[5]	-	-	48	60
Children's Asthma Care				
Received Home Management Plan of Care	-	-	-	88%
Received Reliever Medication	-	-	-	100%
Received Systemic Corticosteroids	-	-	-	100%
Emergency Department				
Admittance Decision Time (minutes)[2]	411	120	98	98
Head CT Results Within 45 Min. of Arrival[1]	-	-	64%	57%
Patients Who Left ER Before Being Seen	58,361	1%	2%	2%
Time from ER Arrival to Admit. (minutes)[2]	417	325	285	274
Time from ER Arrival to Discharge (minutes)	376	187	162	134
Time in ER Before Being Evaluated (minutes)	411	30	27	26
Time to Pain Meds for Fractures (minutes)	187	73	58	57
Heart Attack Care				
Aspirin Given at Discharge	208	100%	99%	99%
Fibrinolytic Meds Within 30 Min. of Arrival[7]	-	-	67%	54%
PCI Within 90 Minutes of Arrival	36	100%	95%	96%
Statin Prescribed at Discharge	195	99%	98%	98%
Heart Failure Care				
ACE Inhibitor or ARB for LVSD	105	100%	98%	97%
Discharge Instructions Given	241	89%	94%	94%
Evaluation of LVS Function	284	100%	99%	99%
Medicare Spending				
Medicare Spending per Patient (ratio)	-	1.01	0.93	0.98
Pneumonia Care				
Appropriate Initial Antibiotic Given	257	98%	96%	95%
Blood Culture Timing	288	100%	97%	98%
Pregnancy and Delivery Care				
Newborn Deliveries Scheduled Early[2]	74	3%	7%	6%
Preventive Care				
Immunization for Influenza[2]	666	89%	91%	90%
Immunization for Pneumonia[2]	777	89%	92%	92%
Stroke Care				
Anticoagulation Therapy for Atrial Fibrillation	18	100%	96%	95%
Antithrombotic Therapy Timing	139	98%	98%	98%
Assessed for Rehabilitation	192	100%	96%	97%
Discharged on Antithrombotic Therapy	179	97%	99%	99%
Discharged on Statin Medication	139	99%	94%	94%
Thrombolytic Therapy Timing	26	88%	81%	66%
Venous Thromboembolism Prophylaxis	181	97%	93%	94%
Written Stroke Educational Materials Given	110	94%	84%	88%
Surgical Care Improvement Project				
Appropriate Beta Blocker Usage	530	98%	97%	98%
Appropriate VTP Within 24 Hours	1,215	99%	98%	98%
Controlled Postoperative Blood Glucose	172	97%	96%	97%
Perioperative Temperature Management	1,951	100%	100%	100%
Prophylactic Antibiotic Selection	1,372	99%	99%	99%
Prophylactic Antibiotic Selection (Outpatient)	763	98%	98%	98%
Prophylactic Antibiotic Stopped	1,356	99%	98%	98%
Prophylactic Antibiotic Timing	1,373	100%	99%	99%
Prophylactic Antibiotic Timing (Outpatient)	767	99%	99%	98%
Urinary Catheter Removal	437	97%	97%	97%
Survey of Patients' Hospital Experiences				
Area Around Room 'Always' Quiet at Night	300+	51%	57%	61%
Doctors 'Always' Communicated Well	300+	77%	77%	82%
Home Recovery Information Given	300+	87%	86%	85%
Hospital Given 9 or 10 on 10 Point Scale	300+	70%	70%	71%
Meds 'Always' Explained Before Given	300+	59%	62%	64%
Nurses 'Always' Communicated Well	300+	76%	76%	79%
Pain 'Always' Well Controlled	300+	69%	69%	71%
Room and Bathroom 'Always' Clean	300+	66%	69%	73%
Timely Help 'Always' Received	300+	64%	65%	68%
Would Definitely Recommend Hospital	300+	72%	70%	71%
Use of Medical Imaging				
Cardiac Imaging Stress Test before Surgery	925	3.7%	5.8%	5.3%
Combination Abdominal CT Scan	711	3.8%	9.1%	10.5%
Combination Brain/Sinus CT Scan	666	1.1%	3.2%	2.7%
Combination Chest CT Scan	154	5.8%	5.5%	2.7%
Follow-up Mammogram/Ultrasound	1,050	7.0%	8.5%	8.8%
Lumbar Spine MRI for Low Back Pain[1]	-	-	37.4%	37.2%

Tucson Medical Center

5301 East Grant Road
Tucson, AZ 85712
Phone: 520-327-5461
Fax: 520-324-2443
URL: www.tmcaz.com
Type: Acute Care Hospitals
Emergency Services: Yes
Ownership: Voluntary non-profit - Private
Beds: 609

Key Personnel:

CEO/President............... Frank Alcorez
Operating Room.............. Suzanne Filleul
Emergency Room .... Keith Kaback, MD
Quality Assurance .... Tom Monier
Chief of Medical Staff.......... Richard Rodriquez
Pediatric Ambulatory Care ...... Mark Wheeler
Pediatric In-Patient Care .... Mark Wheeler
Radiology.................. Edward Woolsey

Measure	Cases	This Hosp.	State Avg.	U.S. Avg.
Blood Clot Prevention and Treatment				
Anticoagulation Overlap Therapy[2]	178	99%	94%	93%
ICU Venous Thromboembolism Prophylaxis[2]	43	95%	92%	92%
Incidence of Potentially Preventable VTE[2]	36	0%	9%	10%
UFH with Dosages/Platelet Monitoring[2]	94	91%	98%	97%
Venous Thromboembolism Prophylaxis[2]	312	90%	88%	85%
Warfarin Therapy Discharge Instructions[2]	141	90%	74%	75%
Chest Pain/Possible Heart Attack Care				
Aspirin Given Within 24 Hours of Arrival[5]	-	-	98%	96%
Fibrinolytic Meds Within 30 Min. of Arrival[5]	-	-	59%	58%
Average Time to ECG (minutes)[5]	-	-	6	7
Average Time to Transfer (minutes)[5]	-	-	48	60
Children's Asthma Care				
Received Home Management Plan of Care	-	-	-	88%
Received Reliever Medication	-	-	-	100%
Received Systemic Corticosteroids	-	-	-	100%
Emergency Department				
Admittance Decision Time (minutes)[2]	304	98	98	98
Head CT Results Within 45 Min. of Arrival[1,3]	-	-	64%	57%
Patients Who Left ER Before Being Seen	87,472	3%	2%	2%
Time from ER Arrival to Admit. (minutes)[2]	311	293	285	274
Time from ER Arrival to Discharge (minutes)	1,540	168	162	134
Time in ER Before Being Evaluated (minutes)	1,692	42	27	26
Time to Pain Meds for Fractures (minutes)	350	63	58	57
Heart Attack Care				
Aspirin Given at Discharge	453	100%	99%	99%
Fibrinolytic Meds Within 30 Min. of Arrival[7]	-	-	67%	54%
PCI Within 90 Minutes of Arrival	56	98%	95%	96%
Statin Prescribed at Discharge	421	100%	98%	98%
Heart Failure Care				
ACE Inhibitor or ARB for LVSD[2]	80	100%	98%	97%
Discharge Instructions Given[2]	237	100%	94%	94%
Evaluation of LVS Function[2]	273	100%	99%	99%
Medicare Spending				
Medicare Spending per Patient (ratio)	-	0.99	0.93	0.98
Pneumonia Care				
Appropriate Initial Antibiotic Given[2]	79	100%	96%	95%
Blood Culture Timing[2]	144	100%	97%	98%
Pregnancy and Delivery Care				
Newborn Deliveries Scheduled Early[2]	361	2%	7%	6%
Preventive Care				
Immunization for Influenza[2]	483	94%	91%	90%
Immunization for Pneumonia[2]	500	96%	92%	92%

NOTE: Hospital profiles are in alphabetical order by state, then city, then hospital within the city; Rankings exclude hospitals with less than 25 cases except for patient surveys which excludes hospitals with less than 100 cases; (a) 100-299 cases; (1) The number of cases/patients is too few to report; (2) Data submitted were based on a sample of cases/patients; (3) Results are based on a shorter time period than required; (4) Data suppressed by CMS for one or more quarters; (5) Results are not available for this reporting period; (6) Fewer than 100 patients completed the HCAHPS survey; (7) No cases met the criteria for this measure; (8) The lower limit of the confidence interval cannot be calculated if the number of observed infections equals zero; (9) No data are available from the state/territory for this reporting period; (10) The scores shown reflect fewer than 50 completed surveys; (11) There were discrepancies in the data collection process; (12) This measure does not apply to this hospital for this reporting period; (13) Results cannot be calculated for this reporting period; (14) The results for this state are combined with nearby states to protect confidentiality; Please refer to the User's Guide for a full explanation of data.

Stroke Care				
Anticoagulation Therapy for Atrial Fibrillation	41	100%	96%	95%
Antithrombotic Therapy Timing	150	98%	98%	98%
Assessed for Rehabilitation	216	100%	96%	97%
Discharged on Antithrombotic Therapy	185	100%	99%	99%
Discharged on Statin Medication	155	98%	94%	94%
Thrombolytic Therapy Timing	23	96%	81%	66%
Venous Thromboembolism Prophylaxis	217	99%	93%	94%
Written Stroke Educational Materials Given	112	99%	84%	88%
Surgical Care Improvement Project				
Appropriate Beta Blocker Usage[2]	244	97%	97%	98%
Appropriate VTP Within 24 Hours[2]	422	98%	98%	98%
Controlled Postoperative Blood Glucose[2]	171	98%	96%	97%
Perioperative Temperature Management[2]	565	100%	100%	100%
Prophylactic Antibiotic Selection[2]	521	99%	99%	99%
Prophylactic Antibiotic Selection (Outpatient)	1,024	99%	98%	98%
Prophylactic Antibiotic Stopped[2]	518	99%	98%	98%
Prophylactic Antibiotic Timing[2]	521	100%	99%	99%
Prophylactic Antibiotic Timing (Outpatient)	1,027	99%	99%	98%
Urinary Catheter Removal[2]	376	100%	97%	97%
Survey of Patients' Hospital Experiences				
Area Around Room 'Always' Quiet at Night	300+	51%	57%	61%
Doctors 'Always' Communicated Well	300+	79%	77%	82%
Home Recovery Information Given	300+	87%	86%	85%
Hospital Given 9 or 10 on 10 Point Scale	300+	69%	70%	71%
Meds 'Always' Explained Before Given	300+	62%	62%	64%
Nurses 'Always' Communicated Well	300+	76%	76%	79%
Pain 'Always' Well Controlled	300+	69%	69%	71%
Room and Bathroom 'Always' Clean	300+	62%	69%	73%
Timely Help 'Always' Received	300+	60%	65%	68%
Would Definitely Recommend Hospital	300+	73%	70%	71%
Use of Medical Imaging				
Cardiac Imaging Stress Test before Surgery	311	4.8%	5.8%	5.3%
Combination Abdominal CT Scan	512	5.5%	9.1%	10.5%
Combination Brain/Sinus CT Scan	600	4.5%	3.2%	2.7%
Combination Chest CT Scan	86	7.0%	5.5%	2.7%
Follow-up Mammogram/Ultrasound	683	6.9%	8.5%	8.8%
Lumbar Spine MRI for Low Back Pain[1]	-	-	37.4%	37.2%

University of Arizona Medical Center

1501 North Campbell Avenue — Phone: 520-694-0111
Tucson, AZ 85724 — Fax: 520-694-4085
URL: www.azumc.com
Type: Acute Care Hospitals — Emergency Services: Yes
Ownership: Voluntary non-profit - Private — Beds: 365

Key Personnel:
Infection Control. . . . . Connie Clasby
Pediatric Ambulatory Care . . . . . . Fayez K Ghushan, MD
Pediatric In-Patient Care . . . . Fayez K Ghushan, MD
Chief of Medical Staff. . . . . Richard Lemen, MD
Quality Assurance . . . . Christina Melnykovych
Radiology. . . . . Theron Ovitt, MD
CEO/President. . . . . Gregory Pivirotto

Measure	Cases	This Hosp.	State Avg.	U.S. Avg.
Blood Clot Prevention and Treatment				
Anticoagulation Overlap Therapy[2]	156	91%	94%	93%
ICU Venous Thromboembolism Prophylaxis[2]	111	92%	92%	92%
Incidence of Potentially Preventable VTE[2]	39	10%	9%	10%
UFH with Dosages/Platelet Monitoring[2]	139	100%	98%	97%
Venous Thromboembolism Prophylaxis[2]	303	82%	88%	85%
Warfarin Therapy Discharge Instructions[2]	106	40%	74%	75%
Chest Pain/Possible Heart Attack Care				
Aspirin Given Within 24 Hours of Arrival[1,3]	-	-	98%	96%
Fibrinolytic Meds Within 30 Min. of Arrival[5]	-	-	59%	58%
Average Time to ECG (minutes)[1,3]	-	-	6	7
Average Time to Transfer (minutes)[5]	-	-	48	60
Children's Asthma Care				
Received Home Management Plan of Care[2]	184	96%	-	88%
Received Reliever Medication	184	100%	-	100%
Received Systemic Corticosteroids	182	99%	-	100%
Emergency Department				
Admittance Decision Time (minutes)[2]	443	100	98	98
Head CT Results Within 45 Min. of Arrival[1]	-	-	64%	57%
Patients Who Left ER Before Being Seen	78,056	6%	2%	2%
Time from ER Arrival to Admit. (minutes)[2]	464	480	285	274
Time from ER Arrival to Discharge (minutes)	331	248	162	134
Time in ER Before Being Evaluated (minutes)	218	69	27	26
Time to Pain Meds for Fractures (minutes)	201	66	58	57
Heart Attack Care				
Aspirin Given at Discharge[2]	265	99%	99%	99%
Fibrinolytic Meds Within 30 Min. of Arrival[2,7]	-	-	67%	54%
PCI Within 90 Minutes of Arrival[1,2]	-	-	95%	96%
Statin Prescribed at Discharge[2]	264	100%	98%	98%
Heart Failure Care				
ACE Inhibitor or ARB for LVSD[2]	131	100%	98%	97%
Discharge Instructions Given[2]	228	99%	94%	94%
Evaluation of LVS Function[2]	257	100%	99%	99%
Medicare Spending				
Medicare Spending per Patient (ratio)	-	0.98	0.93	0.98
Pneumonia Care				
Appropriate Initial Antibiotic Given[2]	55	87%	96%	95%
Blood Culture Timing[2]	136	94%	97%	98%
Pregnancy and Delivery Care				
Newborn Deliveries Scheduled Early[2]	35	6%	7%	6%
Preventive Care				
Immunization for Influenza[2]	521	81%	91%	90%
Immunization for Pneumonia[2]	513	85%	92%	92%
Stroke Care				
Anticoagulation Therapy for Atrial Fibrillation	19	100%	96%	95%
Antithrombotic Therapy Timing	106	100%	98%	98%
Assessed for Rehabilitation	153	100%	96%	97%
Discharged on Antithrombotic Therapy	123	100%	99%	99%
Discharged on Statin Medication	92	96%	94%	94%
Thrombolytic Therapy Timing	11	91%	81%	66%
Venous Thromboembolism Prophylaxis	148	97%	93%	94%
Written Stroke Educational Materials Given	84	87%	84%	88%
Surgical Care Improvement Project				
Appropriate Beta Blocker Usage[2]	150	99%	97%	98%
Appropriate VTP Within 24 Hours[2]	315	98%	98%	98%
Controlled Postoperative Blood Glucose[2]	114	94%	96%	97%
Perioperative Temperature Management[2]	432	98%	100%	100%
Prophylactic Antibiotic Selection[2]	362	98%	99%	99%
Prophylactic Antibiotic Selection (Outpatient)	403	97%	98%	98%
Prophylactic Antibiotic Stopped[2]	358	97%	98%	98%
Prophylactic Antibiotic Timing[2]	365	98%	99%	99%
Prophylactic Antibiotic Timing (Outpatient)	279	95%	99%	98%
Urinary Catheter Removal[2]	316	93%	97%	97%
Survey of Patients' Hospital Experiences				
Area Around Room 'Always' Quiet at Night	300+	49%	57%	61%
Doctors 'Always' Communicated Well	300+	73%	77%	82%
Home Recovery Information Given	300+	84%	86%	85%
Hospital Given 9 or 10 on 10 Point Scale	300+	70%	70%	71%
Meds 'Always' Explained Before Given	300+	61%	62%	64%
Nurses 'Always' Communicated Well	300+	74%	76%	79%
Pain 'Always' Well Controlled	300+	67%	69%	71%
Room and Bathroom 'Always' Clean	300+	64%	69%	73%
Timely Help 'Always' Received	300+	59%	65%	68%
Would Definitely Recommend Hospital	300+	74%	70%	71%
Use of Medical Imaging				
Cardiac Imaging Stress Test before Surgery	699	7.9%	5.8%	5.3%
Combination Abdominal CT Scan	1,292	1.7%	9.1%	10.5%
Combination Brain/Sinus CT Scan	812	9.0%	3.2%	2.7%
Combination Chest CT Scan	1,520	0.2%	5.5%	2.7%
Follow-up Mammogram/Ultrasound[7]	-	-	8.5%	8.8%
Lumbar Spine MRI for Low Back Pain	95	43.2%	37.4%	37.2%

University of Arizona Medical Center

2800 East Ajo Way — Phone: 520-294-4471
Tucson, AZ 85713 — Fax: 520-874-4280
Type: Acute Care Hospitals — Emergency Services: Yes
Ownership: Voluntary non-profit - Private — Beds: 190

Key Personnel:
CEO/President. . . . . Scott Floden
Chief of Medical Staff. . . . . Lupe Manriquez
Pediatric Ambulatory Care . . . . . . William Marshall, MD
Quality Assurance . . . . Sophiya Petrick, RN
Emergency Room . . . . Candy Simon

Measure	Cases	This Hosp.	State Avg.	U.S. Avg.
Blood Clot Prevention and Treatment				
Anticoagulation Overlap Therapy[2]	39	97%	94%	93%
ICU Venous Thromboembolism Prophylaxis[2]	81	89%	92%	92%
Incidence of Potentially Preventable VTE[1,2]	-	-	9%	10%
UFH with Dosages/Platelet Monitoring[2]	28	100%	98%	97%
Venous Thromboembolism Prophylaxis[2]	281	91%	88%	85%
Warfarin Therapy Discharge Instructions[2]	34	76%	74%	75%
Chest Pain/Possible Heart Attack Care				
Aspirin Given Within 24 Hours of Arrival	38	92%	98%	96%
Fibrinolytic Meds Within 30 Min. of Arrival[3,7]	-	-	59%	58%
Average Time to ECG (minutes)	38	2	6	7
Average Time to Transfer (minutes)[3,7]	-	-	48	60
Children's Asthma Care				
Received Home Management Plan of Care	-	-	-	88%
Received Reliever Medication	-	-	-	100%
Received Systemic Corticosteroids	-	-	-	100%
Emergency Department				
Admittance Decision Time (minutes)[2]	789	324	98	98
Head CT Results Within 45 Min. of Arrival[1]	-	-	64%	57%
Patients Who Left ER Before Being Seen	39,281	8%	2%	2%
Time from ER Arrival to Admit. (minutes)[2]	790	531	285	274
Time from ER Arrival to Discharge (minutes)	361	268	162	134
Time in ER Before Being Evaluated (minutes)	384	73	27	26
Time to Pain Meds for Fractures (minutes)	135	75	58	57
Heart Attack Care				
Aspirin Given at Discharge[2]	182	100%	99%	99%
Fibrinolytic Meds Within 30 Min. of Arrival[2,7]	-	-	67%	54%
PCI Within 90 Minutes of Arrival[2]	29	90%	95%	96%
Statin Prescribed at Discharge[2]	176	99%	98%	98%
Heart Failure Care				
ACE Inhibitor or ARB for LVSD	67	100%	98%	97%
Discharge Instructions Given	130	86%	94%	94%
Evaluation of LVS Function	145	99%	99%	99%
Medicare Spending				
Medicare Spending per Patient (ratio)	-	0.98	0.93	0.98
Pneumonia Care				
Appropriate Initial Antibiotic Given[2]	84	93%	96%	95%
Blood Culture Timing[2]	144	94%	97%	98%
Pregnancy and Delivery Care				
Newborn Deliveries Scheduled Early[7]	-	-	7%	6%
Preventive Care				
Immunization for Influenza[2]	478	87%	91%	90%
Immunization for Pneumonia[2]	601	86%	92%	92%
Stroke Care				
Anticoagulation Therapy for Atrial Fibrillation[1]	-	-	96%	95%
Antithrombotic Therapy Timing	36	94%	98%	98%
Assessed for Rehabilitation	41	98%	96%	97%
Discharged on Antithrombotic Therapy	38	100%	99%	99%
Discharged on Statin Medication	33	94%	94%	94%
Thrombolytic Therapy Timing[1]	-	-	81%	66%
Venous Thromboembolism Prophylaxis	43	86%	93%	94%
Written Stroke Educational Materials Given	28	14%	84%	88%
Surgical Care Improvement Project				
Appropriate Beta Blocker Usage	39	85%	97%	98%
Appropriate VTP Within 24 Hours	183	95%	98%	98%
Controlled Postoperative Blood Glucose[7]	-	-	96%	97%
Perioperative Temperature Management	223	97%	100%	100%
Prophylactic Antibiotic Selection	123	97%	99%	99%
Prophylactic Antibiotic Selection (Outpatient)	57	98%	98%	98%
Prophylactic Antibiotic Stopped	121	94%	98%	98%
Prophylactic Antibiotic Timing	123	93%	99%	99%
Prophylactic Antibiotic Timing (Outpatient)	54	87%	99%	98%
Urinary Catheter Removal	103	96%	97%	97%
Survey of Patients' Hospital Experiences				
Area Around Room 'Always' Quiet at Night	300+	44%	57%	61%
Doctors 'Always' Communicated Well	300+	73%	77%	82%
Home Recovery Information Given	300+	76%	86%	85%
Hospital Given 9 or 10 on 10 Point Scale	300+	58%	70%	71%
Meds 'Always' Explained Before Given	300+	59%	62%	64%
Nurses 'Always' Communicated Well	300+	71%	76%	79%
Pain 'Always' Well Controlled	300+	65%	69%	71%

NOTE: Hospital profiles are in alphabetical order by state, then city, then hospital within the city; Rankings exclude hospitals with less than 25 cases except for patient surveys which excludes hospitals with less than 100 cases; (a) 100-299 cases; (1) The number of cases/patients is too few to report; (2) Data submitted were based on a sample of cases/patients; (3) Results are based on a shorter time period than required; (4) Data suppressed by CMS for one or more quarters; (5) Results are not available for this reporting period; (6) Fewer than 100 patients completed the HCAHPS survey; (7) No cases met the criteria for this measure; (8) The lower limit of the confidence interval cannot be calculated if the number of observed infections equals zero; (9) No data are available from the state/territory for this reporting period; (10) The scores shown reflect fewer than 50 completed surveys; (11) There were discrepancies in the data collection process; (12) This measure does not apply to this hospital for this reporting period; (13) Results cannot be calculated for this reporting period; (14) The results for this state are combined with nearby states to protect confidentiality; Please refer to the User's Guide for a full explanation of data.

Room and Bathroom 'Always' Clean	300+	65%	69%	73%
Timely Help 'Always' Received	300+	52%	65%	68%
Would Definitely Recommend Hospital	300+	62%	70%	71%
Use of Medical Imaging				
Cardiac Imaging Stress Test before Surgery	98	6.1%	5.8%	5.3%
Combination Abdominal CT Scan	275	1.8%	9.1%	10.5%
Combination Brain/Sinus CT Scan	391	6.9%	3.2%	2.7%
Combination Chest CT Scan	135	0.7%	5.5%	2.7%
Follow-up Mammogram/Ultrasound[1]	-	-	8.5%	8.8%
Lumbar Spine MRI for Low Back Pain[1]	-	-	37.4%	37.2%

VA Southern Arizona Healthcare System

3601 South Sixth Avenue — Phone: 520-629-1821
Tucson, AZ 85723 — Fax: 520-629-1861
URL: www.va.gov/sta/guide/home.asp
Type: Acute Care - VA — Emergency Services: No
Ownership: Government Federal — Beds: 306

Key Personnel:
CEO/President. . . . . Jonathan H Gardner
Chief of Medical Staff. . . . . Fabia Kwiecinski, MD, FACP
Operating Room. . . . . Carmen Oberg, RN

Measure	Cases	This Hosp.	State Avg.	U.S. Avg.
Blood Clot Prevention and Treatment				
Anticoagulation Overlap Therapy	-	-	94%	93%
ICU Venous Thromboembolism Prophylaxis	-	-	92%	92%
Incidence of Potentially Preventable VTE	-	-	9%	10%
UFH with Dosages/Platelet Monitoring	-	-	98%	97%
Venous Thromboembolism Prophylaxis	-	-	88%	85%
Warfarin Therapy Discharge Instructions	-	-	74%	75%
Chest Pain/Possible Heart Attack Care				
Aspirin Given Within 24 Hours of Arrival	-	-	98%	96%
Fibrinolytic Meds Within 30 Min. of Arrival	-	-	59%	58%
Average Time to ECG (minutes)	-	-	6	7
Average Time to Transfer (minutes)	-	-	48	60
Children's Asthma Care				
Received Home Management Plan of Care	-	-	-	88%
Received Reliever Medication	-	-	-	100%
Received Systemic Corticosteroids	-	-	-	100%
Emergency Department				
Admittance Decision Time (minutes)	-	-	98	98
Head CT Results Within 45 Min. of Arrival	-	-	64%	57%
Patients Who Left ER Before Being Seen	-	-	2%	2%
Time from ER Arrival to Admit. (minutes)	-	-	285	274
Time from ER Arrival to Discharge (minutes)	-	-	162	134
Time in ER Before Being Evaluated (minutes)	-	-	27	26
Time to Pain Meds for Fractures (minutes)	-	-	58	57
Heart Attack Care				
Aspirin Given at Discharge	90	100%	99%	99%
Fibrinolytic Meds Within 30 Min. of Arrival[5]	-	-	67%	54%
PCI Within 90 Minutes of Arrival[1]	21	76%	95%	96%
Statin Prescribed at Discharge	88	99%	98%	98%
Heart Failure Care				
ACE Inhibitor or ARB for LVSD	80	99%	98%	97%
Discharge Instructions Given	179	65%	94%	94%
Evaluation of LVS Function	200	100%	99%	99%
Medicare Spending				
Medicare Spending per Patient (ratio)	-	-	0.93	0.98
Pneumonia Care				
Appropriate Initial Antibiotic Given	62	92%	96%	95%
Blood Culture Timing	127	98%	97%	98%
Pregnancy and Delivery Care				
Newborn Deliveries Scheduled Early	-	-	7%	6%
Preventive Care				
Immunization for Influenza[5]	-	-	91%	90%
Immunization for Pneumonia[5]	-	-	92%	92%
Stroke Care				
Anticoagulation Therapy for Atrial Fibrillation	-	-	96%	95%
Antithrombotic Therapy Timing	-	-	98%	98%
Assessed for Rehabilitation	-	-	96%	97%
Discharged on Antithrombotic Therapy	-	-	99%	99%
Discharged on Statin Medication	-	-	94%	94%
Thrombolytic Therapy Timing	-	-	81%	66%
Venous Thromboembolism Prophylaxis	-	-	93%	94%
Written Stroke Educational Materials Given	-	-	84%	88%
Surgical Care Improvement Project				
Appropriate Beta Blocker Usage[2]	195	97%	97%	98%
Appropriate VTP Within 24 Hours[2]	356	100%	98%	98%
Controlled Postoperative Blood Glucose[2]	103	87%	96%	97%
Perioperative Temperature Management[2]	322	99%	100%	100%
Prophylactic Antibiotic Selection	404	100%	99%	99%
Prophylactic Antibiotic Selection (Outpatient)	-	-	98%	98%
Prophylactic Antibiotic Stopped	401	99%	98%	98%
Prophylactic Antibiotic Timing	409	95%	99%	99%
Prophylactic Antibiotic Timing (Outpatient)	-	-	99%	98%
Urinary Catheter Removal[2]	309	97%	97%	97%
Survey of Patients' Hospital Experiences				
Area Around Room 'Always' Quiet at Night	-	-	57%	61%
Doctors 'Always' Communicated Well	-	-	77%	82%
Home Recovery Information Given	-	-	86%	85%
Hospital Given 9 or 10 on 10 Point Scale	-	-	70%	71%
Meds 'Always' Explained Before Given	-	-	62%	64%
Nurses 'Always' Communicated Well	-	-	76%	79%
Pain 'Always' Well Controlled	-	-	69%	71%
Room and Bathroom 'Always' Clean	-	-	69%	73%
Timely Help 'Always' Received	-	-	65%	68%
Would Definitely Recommend Hospital	-	-	70%	71%
Use of Medical Imaging				
Cardiac Imaging Stress Test before Surgery	-	-	5.8%	5.3%
Combination Abdominal CT Scan	-	-	9.1%	10.5%
Combination Brain/Sinus CT Scan	-	-	3.2%	2.7%
Combination Chest CT Scan	-	-	5.5%	2.7%
Follow-up Mammogram/Ultrasound	-	-	8.5%	8.8%
Lumbar Spine MRI for Low Back Pain	-	-	37.4%	37.2%

Whiteriver PHS Indian Hospital

200 West Hospital Drive — Phone: 928-338-4911
Whiteriver, AZ 85941
Type: Acute Care Hospitals — Emergency Services: No
Ownership: Government - Federal

Measure	Cases	This Hosp.	State Avg.	U.S. Avg.
Blood Clot Prevention and Treatment				
Anticoagulation Overlap Therapy[2,7]	-	-	94%	93%
ICU Venous Thromboembolism Prophylaxis[2,7]	-	-	92%	92%
Incidence of Potentially Preventable VTE[2,7]	-	-	9%	10%
UFH with Dosages/Platelet Monitoring[2,7]	-	-	98%	97%
Venous Thromboembolism Prophylaxis[2]	47	94%	88%	85%
Warfarin Therapy Discharge Instructions[2,7]	-	-	74%	75%
Chest Pain/Possible Heart Attack Care				
Aspirin Given Within 24 Hours of Arrival	-	-	98%	96%
Fibrinolytic Meds Within 30 Min. of Arrival	-	-	59%	58%
Average Time to ECG (minutes)	-	-	6	7
Average Time to Transfer (minutes)	-	-	48	60
Children's Asthma Care				
Received Home Management Plan of Care	-	-	-	88%
Received Reliever Medication	-	-	-	100%
Received Systemic Corticosteroids	-	-	-	100%
Emergency Department				
Admittance Decision Time (minutes)[2,3]	265	70	98	98
Head CT Results Within 45 Min. of Arrival	-	-	64%	57%
Patients Who Left ER Before Being Seen	-	-	2%	2%
Time from ER Arrival to Admit. (minutes)[2,3]	265	313	285	274
Time from ER Arrival to Discharge (minutes)	-	-	162	134
Time in ER Before Being Evaluated (minutes)	-	-	27	26
Time to Pain Meds for Fractures (minutes)	-	-	58	57
Heart Attack Care				
Aspirin Given at Discharge[5]	-	-	99%	99%
Fibrinolytic Meds Within 30 Min. of Arrival[5]	-	-	67%	54%
PCI Within 90 Minutes of Arrival[5]	-	-	95%	96%
Statin Prescribed at Discharge[5]	-	-	98%	98%
Heart Failure Care				
ACE Inhibitor or ARB for LVSD[5]	-	-	98%	97%
Discharge Instructions Given[5]	-	-	94%	94%
Evaluation of LVS Function[5]	-	-	99%	99%
Medicare Spending				
Medicare Spending per Patient (ratio)	-	0.70	0.93	0.98
Pneumonia Care				
Appropriate Initial Antibiotic Given[2,3]	-	-	96%	95%
Blood Culture Timing[2,3]	-	-	97%	98%
Pregnancy and Delivery Care				
Newborn Deliveries Scheduled Early[5]	-	-	7%	6%
Preventive Care				
Immunization for Influenza[2,3]	12	83%	91%	90%
Immunization for Pneumonia[2,3]	124	93%	92%	92%
Stroke Care				
Anticoagulation Therapy for Atrial Fibrillation[5]	-	-	96%	95%
Antithrombotic Therapy Timing[5]	-	-	98%	98%
Assessed for Rehabilitation[5]	-	-	96%	97%
Discharged on Antithrombotic Therapy[5]	-	-	99%	99%
Discharged on Statin Medication[5]	-	-	94%	94%
Thrombolytic Therapy Timing[5]	-	-	81%	66%
Venous Thromboembolism Prophylaxis[5]	-	-	93%	94%
Written Stroke Educational Materials Given[5]	-	-	84%	88%
Surgical Care Improvement Project				
Appropriate Beta Blocker Usage[5]	-	-	97%	98%
Appropriate VTP Within 24 Hours[5]	-	-	98%	98%
Controlled Postoperative Blood Glucose[5]	-	-	96%	97%
Perioperative Temperature Management[5]	-	-	100%	100%
Prophylactic Antibiotic Selection[5]	-	-	99%	99%
Prophylactic Antibiotic Selection (Outpatient)	-	-	98%	98%
Prophylactic Antibiotic Stopped[5]	-	-	98%	98%
Prophylactic Antibiotic Timing[5]	-	-	99%	99%
Prophylactic Antibiotic Timing (Outpatient)	-	-	99%	98%
Urinary Catheter Removal[5]	-	-	97%	97%
Survey of Patients' Hospital Experiences				
Area Around Room 'Always' Quiet at Night[5]	-	-	57%	61%
Doctors 'Always' Communicated Well[5]	-	-	77%	82%
Home Recovery Information Given[5]	-	-	86%	85%
Hospital Given 9 or 10 on 10 Point Scale[5]	-	-	70%	71%
Meds 'Always' Explained Before Given[5]	-	-	62%	64%
Nurses 'Always' Communicated Well[5]	-	-	76%	79%
Pain 'Always' Well Controlled[5]	-	-	69%	71%
Room and Bathroom 'Always' Clean[5]	-	-	69%	73%
Timely Help 'Always' Received[5]	-	-	65%	68%
Would Definitely Recommend Hospital[5]	-	-	70%	71%
Use of Medical Imaging				
Cardiac Imaging Stress Test before Surgery	-	-	5.8%	5.3%
Combination Abdominal CT Scan	-	-	9.1%	10.5%
Combination Brain/Sinus CT Scan	-	-	3.2%	2.7%
Combination Chest CT Scan	-	-	5.5%	2.7%
Follow-up Mammogram/Ultrasound	-	-	8.5%	8.8%
Lumbar Spine MRI for Low Back Pain	-	-	37.4%	37.2%

Wickenburg Community Hospital

520 Rose Lane — Phone: 928-684-5421
Wickenburg, AZ 85390 — Fax: 928-684-5081
URL: www.bannerhealth.com
Type: Critical Access Hospitals — Emergency Services: Yes
Ownership: Voluntary non-profit - Private — Beds: 80

Key Personnel:
Chief of Medical Staff . . . . Diego Cardenaf, MD
Operating Room. . . . . Carl Kubler
CEO/President. . . . . George Larson
Emergency Room . . . . Roger Wilder
Quality Assurance . . . . Roger Wilder

Measure	Cases	This Hosp.	State Avg.	U.S. Avg.
Blood Clot Prevention and Treatment				
Anticoagulation Overlap Therapy[5]	-	-	94%	93%
ICU Venous Thromboembolism Prophylaxis[5]	-	-	92%	92%
Incidence of Potentially Preventable VTE[5]	-	-	9%	10%
UFH with Dosages/Platelet Monitoring[5]	-	-	98%	97%
Venous Thromboembolism Prophylaxis[5]	-	-	88%	85%
Warfarin Therapy Discharge Instructions[5]	-	-	74%	75%
Chest Pain/Possible Heart Attack Care				
Aspirin Given Within 24 Hours of Arrival[5]	-	-	98%	96%
Fibrinolytic Meds Within 30 Min. of Arrival[5]	-	-	59%	58%
Average Time to ECG (minutes)[5]	-	-	6	7
Average Time to Transfer (minutes)[5]	-	-	48	60
Children's Asthma Care				

NOTE: Hospital profiles are in alphabetical order by state, then city, then hospital within the city; Rankings exclude hospitals with less than 25 cases except for patient surveys which excludes hospitals with less than 100 cases; (a) 100-299 cases; (1) The number of cases/patients is too few to report; (2) Data submitted were based on a sample of cases/patients; (3) Results are based on a shorter time period than required; (4) Data suppressed by CMS for one or more quarters; (5) Results are not available for this reporting period; (6) Fewer than 100 patients completed the HCAHPS survey; (7) No cases met the criteria for this measure; (8) The lower limit of the confidence interval cannot be calculated if the number of observed infections equals zero; (9) No data are available from the state/territory for this reporting period; (10) The scores shown reflect fewer than 50 completed surveys; (11) There were discrepancies in the data collection process; (12) This measure does not apply to this hospital for this reporting period; (13) Results cannot be calculated for this reporting period; (14) The results for this state are combined with nearby states to protect confidentiality; Please refer to the User's Guide for a full explanation of data.

Measure	Cases	This Hosp.	State Avg.	U.S. Avg.
Received Home Management Plan of Care	-	-	-	88%
Received Reliever Medication	-	-	-	100%
Received Systemic Corticosteroids	-	-	-	100%
Emergency Department				
Admittance Decision Time (minutes)[5]	-	-	98	98
Head CT Results Within 45 Min. of Arrival[5]	-	-	64%	57%
Patients Who Left ER Before Being Seen	5,458	0%	2%	2%
Time from ER Arrival to Admit. (minutes)[5]	-	-	285	274
Time from ER Arrival to Discharge (minutes)[5]	-	-	162	134
Time in ER Before Being Evaluated (minutes)[5]	-	-	27	26
Time to Pain Meds for Fractures (minutes)[5]	-	-	58	57
Heart Attack Care				
Aspirin Given at Discharge[3,7]	-	-	99%	99%
Fibrinolytic Meds Within 30 Min. of Arrival[3,7]	-	-	67%	54%
PCI Within 90 Minutes of Arrival[3,7]	-	-	95%	96%
Statin Prescribed at Discharge[3,7]	-	-	98%	98%
Heart Failure Care				
ACE Inhibitor or ARB for LVSD[1]	-	-	98%	97%
Discharge Instructions Given[1]	-	-	94%	94%
Evaluation of LVS Function[1]	-	-	99%	99%
Medicare Spending				
Medicare Spending per Patient (ratio)	-	-	0.93	0.98
Pneumonia Care				
Appropriate Initial Antibiotic Given	33	85%	96%	95%
Blood Culture Timing	31	87%	97%	98%
Pregnancy and Delivery Care				
Newborn Deliveries Scheduled Early[5]	-	-	7%	6%
Preventive Care				
Immunization for Influenza[5]	-	-	91%	90%
Immunization for Pneumonia[5]	-	-	92%	92%
Stroke Care				
Anticoagulation Therapy for Atrial Fibrillation[5]	-	-	96%	95%
Antithrombotic Therapy Timing[5]	-	-	98%	98%
Assessed for Rehabilitation[5]	-	-	96%	97%
Discharged on Antithrombotic Therapy[5]	-	-	99%	99%
Discharged on Statin Medication[5]	-	-	94%	94%
Thrombolytic Therapy Timing[5]	-	-	81%	66%
Venous Thromboembolism Prophylaxis[5]	-	-	93%	94%
Written Stroke Educational Materials Given[5]	-	-	84%	88%
Surgical Care Improvement Project				
Appropriate Beta Blocker Usage[5]	-	-	97%	98%
Appropriate VTP Within 24 Hours[5]	-	-	98%	98%
Controlled Postoperative Blood Glucose[5]	-	-	96%	97%
Perioperative Temperature Management[5]	-	-	100%	100%
Prophylactic Antibiotic Selection[5]	-	-	99%	99%
Prophylactic Antibiotic Selection (Outpatient)[5]	-	-	98%	98%
Prophylactic Antibiotic Stopped[5]	-	-	98%	98%
Prophylactic Antibiotic Timing[5]	-	-	99%	99%
Prophylactic Antibiotic Timing (Outpatient)[5]	-	-	99%	98%
Urinary Catheter Removal[5]	-	-	97%	97%
Survey of Patients' Hospital Experiences				
Area Around Room 'Always' Quiet at Night	(a)	67%	57%	61%
Doctors 'Always' Communicated Well	(a)	82%	77%	82%
Home Recovery Information Given	(a)	84%	86%	85%
Hospital Given 9 or 10 on 10 Point Scale	(a)	71%	70%	71%
Meds 'Always' Explained Before Given	(a)	64%	62%	64%
Nurses 'Always' Communicated Well	(a)	88%	76%	79%
Pain 'Always' Well Controlled	(a)	84%	69%	71%
Room and Bathroom 'Always' Clean	(a)	81%	69%	73%
Timely Help 'Always' Received	(a)	71%	65%	68%
Would Definitely Recommend Hospital	(a)	74%	70%	71%
Use of Medical Imaging				
Cardiac Imaging Stress Test before Surgery[1]	-	-	5.8%	5.3%
Combination Abdominal CT Scan	347	17.9%	9.1%	10.5%
Combination Brain/Sinus CT Scan[1]	-	-	3.2%	2.7%
Combination Chest CT Scan	189	9.0%	5.5%	2.7%
Follow-up Mammogram/Ultrasound	455	12.1%	8.5%	8.8%
Lumbar Spine MRI for Low Back Pain[1]	-	-	37.4%	37.2%

Northern Cochise Community Hospital

901 West Rex Allen Drive — Phone: 520-384-3541
Willcox, AZ 85643 — Fax: 520-384-9212
URL: www.ncch.com
Type: Critical Access Hospitals — Emergency Services: Yes
Ownership: Govt - Hospital Dist/Auth — Beds: 24

Key Personnel:
Emergency Room . . . . Pam Noland, RN
Quality Assurance . . . . Kim Schroeder
CEO/President. . . . . Harley Smith
Chief of Medical Staff. . . . . Henry Wedig, DO

Measure	Cases	This Hosp.	State Avg.	U.S. Avg.
Blood Clot Prevention and Treatment				
Anticoagulation Overlap Therapy[5]	-	-	94%	93%
ICU Venous Thromboembolism Prophylaxis[5]	-	-	92%	92%
Incidence of Potentially Preventable VTE[5]	-	-	9%	10%
UFH with Dosages/Platelet Monitoring[5]	-	-	98%	97%
Venous Thromboembolism Prophylaxis[5]	-	-	88%	85%
Warfarin Therapy Discharge Instructions[5]	-	-	74%	75%
Chest Pain/Possible Heart Attack Care				
Aspirin Given Within 24 Hours of Arrival	-	-	98%	96%
Fibrinolytic Meds Within 30 Min. of Arrival	-	-	59%	58%
Average Time to ECG (minutes)	-	-	6	7
Average Time to Transfer (minutes)	-	-	48	60
Children's Asthma Care				
Received Home Management Plan of Care	-	-	-	88%
Received Reliever Medication	-	-	-	100%
Received Systemic Corticosteroids	-	-	-	100%
Emergency Department				
Admittance Decision Time (minutes)[5]	-	-	98	98
Head CT Results Within 45 Min. of Arrival	-	-	64%	57%
Patients Who Left ER Before Being Seen	-	-	2%	2%
Time from ER Arrival to Admit. (minutes)[5]	-	-	285	274
Time from ER Arrival to Discharge (minutes)	-	-	162	134
Time in ER Before Being Evaluated (minutes)	-	-	27	26
Time to Pain Meds for Fractures (minutes)	-	-	58	57
Heart Attack Care				
Aspirin Given at Discharge[5]	-	-	99%	99%
Fibrinolytic Meds Within 30 Min. of Arrival[5]	-	-	67%	54%
PCI Within 90 Minutes of Arrival[5]	-	-	95%	96%
Statin Prescribed at Discharge[5]	-	-	98%	98%
Heart Failure Care				
ACE Inhibitor or ARB for LVSD[3,7]	-	-	98%	97%
Discharge Instructions Given[1,3]	-	-	94%	94%
Evaluation of LVS Function[1,3]	-	-	99%	99%
Medicare Spending				
Medicare Spending per Patient (ratio)	-	-	0.93	0.98
Pneumonia Care				
Appropriate Initial Antibiotic Given	21	90%	96%	95%
Blood Culture Timing	20	90%	97%	98%
Pregnancy and Delivery Care				
Newborn Deliveries Scheduled Early[5]	-	-	7%	6%
Preventive Care				
Immunization for Influenza[5]	-	-	91%	90%
Immunization for Pneumonia[5]	-	-	92%	92%
Stroke Care				
Anticoagulation Therapy for Atrial Fibrillation[5]	-	-	96%	95%
Antithrombotic Therapy Timing[5]	-	-	98%	98%
Assessed for Rehabilitation[5]	-	-	96%	97%
Discharged on Antithrombotic Therapy[5]	-	-	99%	99%
Discharged on Statin Medication[5]	-	-	94%	94%
Thrombolytic Therapy Timing[5]	-	-	81%	66%
Venous Thromboembolism Prophylaxis[5]	-	-	93%	94%
Written Stroke Educational Materials Given[5]	-	-	84%	88%
Surgical Care Improvement Project				
Appropriate Beta Blocker Usage[5]	-	-	97%	98%
Appropriate VTP Within 24 Hours[5]	-	-	98%	98%
Controlled Postoperative Blood Glucose[5]	-	-	96%	97%
Perioperative Temperature Management[5]	-	-	100%	100%
Prophylactic Antibiotic Selection[5]	-	-	99%	99%
Prophylactic Antibiotic Selection (Outpatient)	-	-	98%	98%
Prophylactic Antibiotic Stopped[5]	-	-	98%	98%
Prophylactic Antibiotic Timing[5]	-	-	99%	99%
Prophylactic Antibiotic Timing (Outpatient)	-	-	99%	98%
Urinary Catheter Removal[5]	-	-	97%	97%
Survey of Patients' Hospital Experiences				
Area Around Room 'Always' Quiet at Night[6]	<100	48%	57%	61%
Doctors 'Always' Communicated Well[6]	<100	79%	77%	82%
Home Recovery Information Given[6]	<100	78%	86%	85%
Hospital Given 9 or 10 on 10 Point Scale[6]	<100	63%	70%	71%
Meds 'Always' Explained Before Given[6]	<100	66%	62%	64%
Nurses 'Always' Communicated Well[6]	<100	78%	76%	79%
Pain 'Always' Well Controlled[6]	<100	73%	69%	71%
Room and Bathroom 'Always' Clean[6]	<100	68%	69%	73%
Timely Help 'Always' Received[6]	<100	71%	65%	68%
Would Definitely Recommend Hospital[6]	<100	64%	70%	71%
Use of Medical Imaging				
Cardiac Imaging Stress Test before Surgery	-	-	5.8%	5.3%
Combination Abdominal CT Scan	-	-	9.1%	10.5%
Combination Brain/Sinus CT Scan	-	-	3.2%	2.7%
Combination Chest CT Scan	-	-	5.5%	2.7%
Follow-up Mammogram/Ultrasound	-	-	8.5%	8.8%
Lumbar Spine MRI for Low Back Pain	-	-	37.4%	37.2%

Little Colorado Medical Center

1501 North Williamson Avenue — Phone: 928-289-4691
Winslow, AZ 86047 — Fax: 928-289-3855
Type: Critical Access Hospitals — Emergency Services: Yes
Ownership: Government - Local — Beds: 25

Key Personnel:
Emergency Room . . . . Daniel Bade
CEO/President. . . . . Jeff Hamblen
Infection Control. . . . . Marie Hancock
Chief of Medical Staff . . . . Perry Mitchell, MD
Anesthesiology. . . . . Bill Trimble
Quality Assurance . . . . Connie Walton
Pediatric Ambulatory Care . . . . . . Meriam Yu, MD
Pediatric In-Patient Care . . . . Meriam Yu, MD

Measure	Cases	This Hosp.	State Avg.	U.S. Avg.
Blood Clot Prevention and Treatment				
Anticoagulation Overlap Therapy[5]	-	-	94%	93%
ICU Venous Thromboembolism Prophylaxis[5]	-	-	92%	92%
Incidence of Potentially Preventable VTE[5]	-	-	9%	10%
UFH with Dosages/Platelet Monitoring[5]	-	-	98%	97%
Venous Thromboembolism Prophylaxis[5]	-	-	88%	85%
Warfarin Therapy Discharge Instructions[5]	-	-	74%	75%
Chest Pain/Possible Heart Attack Care				
Aspirin Given Within 24 Hours of Arrival	-	-	98%	96%
Fibrinolytic Meds Within 30 Min. of Arrival	-	-	59%	58%
Average Time to ECG (minutes)	-	-	6	7
Average Time to Transfer (minutes)	-	-	48	60
Children's Asthma Care				
Received Home Management Plan of Care	-	-	-	88%
Received Reliever Medication	-	-	-	100%
Received Systemic Corticosteroids	-	-	-	100%
Emergency Department				
Admittance Decision Time (minutes)[5]	-	-	98	98
Head CT Results Within 45 Min. of Arrival	-	-	64%	57%
Patients Who Left ER Before Being Seen	-	-	2%	2%
Time from ER Arrival to Admit. (minutes)[5]	-	-	285	274
Time from ER Arrival to Discharge (minutes)	-	-	162	134
Time in ER Before Being Evaluated (minutes)	-	-	27	26
Time to Pain Meds for Fractures (minutes)	-	-	58	57
Heart Attack Care				
Aspirin Given at Discharge[5]	-	-	99%	99%
Fibrinolytic Meds Within 30 Min. of Arrival[5]	-	-	67%	54%
PCI Within 90 Minutes of Arrival[5]	-	-	95%	96%
Statin Prescribed at Discharge[5]	-	-	98%	98%
Heart Failure Care				
ACE Inhibitor or ARB for LVSD[5]	-	-	98%	97%
Discharge Instructions Given[5]	-	-	94%	94%
Evaluation of LVS Function[5]	-	-	99%	99%
Medicare Spending				
Medicare Spending per Patient (ratio)	-	-	0.93	0.98
Pneumonia Care				
Appropriate Initial Antibiotic Given[5]	-	-	96%	95%
Blood Culture Timing[5]	-	-	97%	98%

NOTE: Hospital profiles are in alphabetical order by state, then city, then hospital within the city; Rankings exclude hospitals with less than 25 cases except for patient surveys which excludes hospitals with less than 100 cases; (a) 100-299 cases; (1) The number of cases/patients is too few to report; (2) Data submitted were based on a sample of cases/patients; (3) Results are based on a shorter time period than required; (4) Data suppressed by CMS for one or more quarters; (5) Results are not available for this reporting period; (6) Fewer than 100 patients completed the HCAHPS survey; (7) No cases met the criteria for this measure; (8) The lower limit of the confidence interval cannot be calculated if the number of observed infections equals zero; (9) No data are available from the state/territory for this reporting period; (10) The scores shown reflect fewer than 50 completed surveys; (11) There were discrepancies in the data collection process; (12) This measure does not apply to this hospital for this reporting period; (13) Results cannot be calculated for this reporting period; (14) The results for this state are combined with nearby states to protect confidentiality; Please refer to the User's Guide for a full explanation of data.

Measure	Cases	This Hosp.	State Avg.	U.S. Avg.
Pregnancy and Delivery Care				
Newborn Deliveries Scheduled Early[5]	-	-	7%	6%
Preventive Care				
Immunization for Influenza[5]	-	-	91%	90%
Immunization for Pneumonia[5]	-	-	92%	92%
Stroke Care				
Anticoagulation Therapy for Atrial Fibrillation[5]	-	-	96%	95%
Antithrombotic Therapy Timing[5]	-	-	98%	98%
Assessed for Rehabilitation[5]	-	-	96%	97%
Discharged on Antithrombotic Therapy[5]	-	-	99%	99%
Discharged on Statin Medication[5]	-	-	94%	94%
Thrombolytic Therapy Timing[5]	-	-	81%	66%
Venous Thromboembolism Prophylaxis[5]	-	-	93%	94%
Written Stroke Educational Materials Given[5]	-	-	84%	88%
Surgical Care Improvement Project				
Appropriate Beta Blocker Usage[5]	-	-	97%	98%
Appropriate VTP Within 24 Hours[5]	-	-	98%	98%
Controlled Postoperative Blood Glucose[5]	-	-	96%	97%
Perioperative Temperature Management[5]	-	-	100%	100%
Prophylactic Antibiotic Selection[5]	-	-	99%	99%
Prophylactic Antibiotic Selection (Outpatient)	-	-	98%	98%
Prophylactic Antibiotic Stopped[5]	-	-	98%	98%
Prophylactic Antibiotic Timing[5]	-	-	99%	99%
Prophylactic Antibiotic Timing (Outpatient)	-	-	99%	98%
Urinary Catheter Removal[5]	-	-	97%	97%
Survey of Patients' Hospital Experiences				
Area Around Room 'Always' Quiet at Night[5]	-	-	57%	61%
Doctors 'Always' Communicated Well[5]	-	-	77%	82%
Home Recovery Information Given[5]	-	-	86%	85%
Hospital Given 9 or 10 on 10 Point Scale[5]	-	-	70%	71%
Meds 'Always' Explained Before Given[5]	-	-	62%	64%
Nurses 'Always' Communicated Well[5]	-	-	76%	79%
Pain 'Always' Well Controlled[5]	-	-	69%	71%
Room and Bathroom 'Always' Clean[5]	-	-	69%	73%
Timely Help 'Always' Received[5]	-	-	65%	68%
Would Definitely Recommend Hospital[5]	-	-	70%	71%
Use of Medical Imaging				
Cardiac Imaging Stress Test before Surgery	-	-	5.8%	5.3%
Combination Abdominal CT Scan	-	-	9.1%	10.5%
Combination Brain/Sinus CT Scan	-	-	3.2%	2.7%
Combination Chest CT Scan	-	-	5.5%	2.7%
Follow-up Mammogram/Ultrasound	-	-	8.5%	8.8%
Lumbar Spine MRI for Low Back Pain	-	-	37.4%	37.2%

Yuma Regional Medical Center

2400 South Avenue A Phone: 928-336-7275
Yuma, AZ 85364 Fax: 928-336-7337
URL: www.yumaregional.org
Type: Acute Care Hospitals Emergency Services: Yes
Ownership: Voluntary non-profit - Private Beds: 279

Key Personnel:
Operating Room. . . . . Phyllis Abbott
Quality Assurance . . . . Deborah Aders
Cardiac Laboratory. . . . . Scott Bailey
Radiology. . . . . Frank Barby
Infection Control. . . . . Jo Doner
Intensive Care Unit. . . . . Karen Hardy
Chief of Medical Staff . . . . Louis K Miller
CEO/President. . . . . Pat Walz

Measure	Cases	This Hosp.	State Avg.	U.S. Avg.
Blood Clot Prevention and Treatment				
Anticoagulation Overlap Therapy[2]	30	77%	94%	93%
ICU Venous Thromboembolism Prophylaxis[2]	66	92%	92%	92%
Incidence of Potentially Preventable VTE[1,2]	-	-	9%	10%
UFH with Dosages/Platelet Monitoring[2]	11	100%	98%	97%
Venous Thromboembolism Prophylaxis[2]	414	81%	88%	85%
Warfarin Therapy Discharge Instructions[2]	17	100%	74%	75%
Chest Pain/Possible Heart Attack Care				
Aspirin Given Within 24 Hours of Arrival[1,3]	-	-	98%	96%
Fibrinolytic Meds Within 30 Min. of Arrival[5]	-	-	59%	58%
Average Time to ECG (minutes)[1,3]	-	-	6	7
Average Time to Transfer (minutes)[5]	-	-	48	60
Children's Asthma Care				
Received Home Management Plan of Care	-	-	-	88%
Received Reliever Medication	-	-	-	100%
Received Systemic Corticosteroids	-	-	-	100%
Emergency Department				
Admittance Decision Time (minutes)[2]	475	96	98	98
Head CT Results Within 45 Min. of Arrival	14	43%	64%	57%
Patients Who Left ER Before Being Seen	70,223	3%	2%	2%
Time from ER Arrival to Admit. (minutes)[2]	482	327	285	274
Time from ER Arrival to Discharge (minutes)	368	178	162	134
Time in ER Before Being Evaluated (minutes)	381	28	27	26
Time to Pain Meds for Fractures (minutes)	338	67	58	57
Heart Attack Care				
Aspirin Given at Discharge	331	98%	99%	99%
Fibrinolytic Meds Within 30 Min. of Arrival[7]	-	-	67%	54%
PCI Within 90 Minutes of Arrival	61	87%	95%	96%
Statin Prescribed at Discharge	317	98%	98%	98%
Heart Failure Care				
ACE Inhibitor or ARB for LVSD	170	98%	98%	97%
Discharge Instructions Given	365	100%	94%	94%
Evaluation of LVS Function	416	99%	99%	99%
Medicare Spending				
Medicare Spending per Patient (ratio)	-	1.00	0.93	0.98
Pneumonia Care				
Appropriate Initial Antibiotic Given[2]	135	99%	96%	95%
Blood Culture Timing[2]	218	97%	97%	98%
Pregnancy and Delivery Care				
Newborn Deliveries Scheduled Early[2]	57	9%	7%	6%
Preventive Care				
Immunization for Influenza[2]	509	92%	91%	90%
Immunization for Pneumonia[2]	572	94%	92%	92%
Stroke Care				
Anticoagulation Therapy for Atrial Fibrillation[2]	13	100%	96%	95%
Antithrombotic Therapy Timing[2]	85	100%	98%	98%
Assessed for Rehabilitation[2]	98	100%	96%	97%
Discharged on Antithrombotic Therapy[2]	84	96%	99%	99%
Discharged on Statin Medication[2]	69	86%	94%	94%
Thrombolytic Therapy Timing[1,2]	-	-	81%	66%
Venous Thromboembolism Prophylaxis[2]	94	91%	93%	94%
Written Stroke Educational Materials Given[2]	60	98%	84%	88%
Surgical Care Improvement Project				
Appropriate Beta Blocker Usage[2]	272	96%	97%	98%
Appropriate VTP Within 24 Hours[2]	662	94%	98%	98%
Controlled Postoperative Blood Glucose[2]	126	96%	96%	97%
Perioperative Temperature Management[2]	908	100%	100%	100%
Prophylactic Antibiotic Selection[2]	722	97%	99%	99%
Prophylactic Antibiotic Selection (Outpatient)	479	91%	98%	98%
Prophylactic Antibiotic Stopped[2]	714	96%	98%	98%
Prophylactic Antibiotic Timing[2]	723	98%	99%	99%
Prophylactic Antibiotic Timing (Outpatient)	496	95%	99%	98%
Urinary Catheter Removal[2]	653	92%	97%	97%
Survey of Patients' Hospital Experiences				
Area Around Room 'Always' Quiet at Night	300+	58%	57%	61%
Doctors 'Always' Communicated Well	300+	76%	77%	82%
Home Recovery Information Given	300+	82%	86%	85%
Hospital Given 9 or 10 on 10 Point Scale	300+	67%	70%	71%
Meds 'Always' Explained Before Given	300+	62%	62%	64%
Nurses 'Always' Communicated Well	300+	75%	76%	79%
Pain 'Always' Well Controlled	300+	68%	69%	71%
Room and Bathroom 'Always' Clean	300+	67%	69%	73%
Timely Help 'Always' Received	300+	63%	65%	68%
Would Definitely Recommend Hospital	300+	66%	70%	71%
Use of Medical Imaging				
Cardiac Imaging Stress Test before Surgery[1]	-	-	5.8%	5.3%
Combination Abdominal CT Scan	949	48.4%	9.1%	10.5%
Combination Brain/Sinus CT Scan	1,565	3.4%	3.2%	2.7%
Combination Chest CT Scan	580	9.0%	5.5%	2.7%
Follow-up Mammogram/Ultrasound	3,292	8.2%	8.5%	8.8%
Lumbar Spine MRI for Low Back Pain	198	40.4%	37.4%	37.2%

NOTE: Hospital profiles are in alphabetical order by state, then city, then hospital within the city; Rankings exclude hospitals with less than 25 cases except for patient surveys which excludes hospitals with less than 100 cases; (a) 100-299 cases; (1) The number of cases/patients is too few to report; (2) Data submitted were based on a sample of cases/patients; (3) Results are based on a shorter time period than required; (4) Data suppressed by CMS for one or more quarters; (5) Results are not available for this reporting period; (6) Fewer than 100 patients completed the HCAHPS survey; (7) No cases met the criteria for this measure; (8) The lower limit of the confidence interval cannot be calculated if the number of observed infections equals zero; (9) No data are available from the state/territory for this reporting period; (10) The scores shown reflect fewer than 50 completed surveys; (11) There were discrepancies in the data collection process; (12) This measure does not apply to this hospital for this reporting period; (13) Results cannot be calculated for this reporting period; (14) The results for this state are combined with nearby states to protect confidentiality; Please refer to the User's Guide for a full explanation of data.

Blood Clot Prevention and Treatment

Anticoagulation Overlap Therapy

Hospital Name	City	Rate	Cases
CA Pacific Med Ctr-Pacific Campus Hosp[2]	San Francisco	100%	80
Chino Valley Medical Center[2]	Chino	100%	28
Contra Costa Regional Medical Center[2]	Martinez	100%	40
Corona Regional Medical Center[2]	Corona	100%	33
Dameron Hospital[2]	Stockton	100%	47
Desert Valley Hospital[2]	Victorville	100%	59
Dominican Hospital[2]	Santa Cruz	100%	59
John Muir Medical Center - Concord Campus[2]	Concord	100%	49
Kaiser Foundation Hospital[2]	San Rafael	100%	34
Kaiser Fdn Hosp-Fremont/Hayward[2]	Hayward	100%	62
Kaiser Foundation Hospital - Fresno[2]	Fresno	100%	51
Kaiser Foundation Hospital - Manteca[2]	Manteca	100%	59
Kaiser Fdn Hosp-Oakland/Richmond[2]	Oakland	100%	82
Kaiser Foundation Hospital - Redwood City[2]	Redwood City	100%	56
Kaiser Foundation Hospital - Roseville[2]	Roseville	100%	93
Kaiser Fdn Hosp-San Francisco[2]	San Francisco	100%	54
Kaiser Foundation Hospital - San Jose[2]	San Jose	100%	68
Kaiser Foundation Hospital - Santa Clara[2]	Santa Clara	100%	61
Kaiser Foundation Hospital - Santa Rosa[2]	Santa Rosa	100%	44
Kaiser Fdn Hosp-S San Francisco[2]	S San Francisco	100%	37
Kaiser Foundation Hospital - Walnut Creek[2]	Walnut Creek	100%	103
Los Alamitos Medical Center[2]	Los Alamitos	100%	63
Marin General Hospital[2]	Greenbrae	100%	50
Marshall Medical Center[2]	Placerville	100%	49
Memorial Medical Center[2]	Modesto	100%	140
Mercy General Hospital[2]	Sacramento	100%	91
Mercy Hospital[2]	Bakersfield	100%	59
Mercy Hospital of Folsom[2]	Folsom	100%	47
Oroville Hospital[2]	Oroville	100%	54
Palomar Health Downtown Campus[2]	Escondido	100%	145
Pomona Valley Hospital Medical Center[2]	Pomona	100%	68
Prov Little Co of Mary Med Ctr Torrance[2]	Torrance	100%	96
Saint Johns Regional Medical Center[2]	Oxnard	100%	36
San Francisco General Hospital[2]	San Francisco	100%	65
San Leandro Hospital[2,3]	San Leandro	100%	26
Santa Monica-UCLA Med Ctr & Ortho Hosp[2]	Santa Monica	100%	60
Scripps Green Hospital[2]	La Jolla	100%	87
Scripps Memorial Hospital La Jolla[2]	La Jolla	100%	81
Shasta Regional Medical Center[2]	Redding	100%	65
Sonora Regional Medical Center[2]	Sonora	100%	53
Sutter Auburn Faith Hospital[2]	Auburn	100%	26
Torrance Memorial Medical Center[2]	Torrance	100%	85
Univ of CA Davis Med Ctr[2]	Sacramento	100%	163
Comm Hosp of the Monterey Peninsula[2]	Monterey	99%	77
Community Regional Medical Center[2]	Fresno	99%	151
El Camino Hospital[2]	Mountain View	99%	81
John Muir Med Ctr-Walnut Creek Campus[2]	Walnut Creek	99%	82
Kaiser Foundation Hospital - Antioch[2]	Antioch	99%	71
Kaiser Fdn Hosp S Sacramento[2]	Sacramento	99%	89
Methodist Hospital of Southern California[2]	Arcadia	99%	78
Orange Coast Memorial Medical Center[2]	Fountain Valley	99%	76
Riverside County Regional Medical Center[2]	Moreno Valley	99%	68
Scripps Memorial Hospital - Encinitas[2]	Encinitas	99%	89
UCSF Medical Center[2]	San Francisco	99%	71
Univ of California Irvine Med Ctr[2]	Orange	99%	99
Alta Bates Summit Medical Center[2]	Berkeley	98%	46
Centinela Hospital Medical Center[2]	Inglewood	98%	51
Kaiser Fdn Hosp-Panorama City[2]	Panorama City	98%	62
Kaiser Foundation Hospital - Sacramento[2]	Sacramento	98%	59
Kaiser Foundation Hospital - San Diego[2]	San Diego	98%	135
LAC/Harbor - UCLA Medical Center[2]	Torrance	98%	56
Lodi Memorial Hospital[2]	Lodi	98%	53
Marian Regional Medical Center[2]	Santa Maria	98%	43
O'Connor Hospital[2]	San Jose	98%	45
PIH Hospital - Downey[2]	Downey	98%	44
Queen of the Valley Medical Center[2]	Napa	98%	43
Saint Joseph Hospital[2]	Eureka	98%	40
Santa Clara Valley Medical Center[2]	San Jose	98%	57
Simi Valley Hosp & Health Care Svcs[2]	Simi Valley	98%	42
Valleycare Medical Center[2]	Pleasanton	98%	45
California Hosp Med Ctr Los Angeles[2]	Los Angeles	97%	63
Clovis Community Medical Center[2]	Clovis	97%	63
Eisenhower Medical Center[2]	Rancho Mirage	97%	86
Feather River Hospital[2]	Paradise	97%	38
Northridge Hospital Medical Center[2]	Northridge	97%	73
Saint Mary Medical Center[2]	Apple Valley	97%	115
Saint Vincent Medical Center[2]	Los Angeles	97%	29
Sutter General Hospital[2]	Sacramento	97%	132
Sutter Roseville Medical Center[2]	Roseville	97%	164
West Anaheim Medical Center[2]	Anaheim	97%	34
Alameda County Medical Center[2]	Oakland	96%	47
Eden Medical Center[2]	Castro Valley	96%	50
Kaiser Foundation Hospital & Rehab Center[2]	Vallejo	96%	50
Kaiser Foundation Hospital - Fontana[2]	Fontana	96%	209
Kaiser Fdn Hosp-Moreno Valley[2]	Moreno Valley	96%	26
Kaiser Fdn Hosp-Orange Co-Anaheim[2]	Anaheim	96%	163
Kaiser Foundation Hospital - West La[2]	Los Angeles	96%	56
LAC/Olive View - UCLA Medical Center[2]	Sylmar	96%	53
Santa Rosa Memorial Hospital[2]	Santa Rosa	96%	54
Stanford Hospital[2]	Stanford	96%	116
Sutter Medical Center of Santa Rosa[2]	Santa Rosa	96%	27
Alvarado Hospital Medical Center[2]	San Diego	95%	40
Cedars - Sinai Medical Center[2]	Los Angeles	95%	164
Good Samaritan Hospital[2]	San Jose	95%	93
Grossmont Hospital[2]	La Mesa	95%	135
Kaiser Foundation Hospital - Baldwin Park[2]	Baldwin Park	95%	63
Kaiser Foundation Hospital - South Bay[2]	Harbor City	95%	62
Providence Holy Cross Medical Center[2]	Mission Hills	95%	66
Saint Mary Medical Center[2]	Long Beach	95%	39
Santa Barbara Cottage Hospital[2]	Santa Barbara	95%	56
Sharp Memorial Hospital[2]	San Diego	95%	140
Southern California Hospital at Hollywood[2]	Hollywood	95%	37
Bakersfield Memorial Hospital[2]	Bakersfield	94%	65
Enloe Medical Center[2]	Chico	94%	98
Fountain Valley Reg Hosp & Med Ctr[2]	Fountain Valley	94%	51
Kaiser Foundation Hospital - Los Angeles[2]	Los Angeles	94%	103
Kaiser Foundation Hospital - Vacaville[2]	Vacaville	94%	36
Kaiser Fdn Hosp-Woodland Hills[2]	Woodland Hills	94%	72
Marina Del Rey Hospital[2]	Marina Del Rey	94%	52
Olympia Medical Center[2]	Los Angeles	94%	32
Tri - City Medical Center[2]	Oceanside	94%	103
West Hills Hospital & Medical Center[2]	West Hills	94%	48
Antelope Valley Hospital[2]	Lancaster	93%	115
Arrowhead Regional Medical Center[2]	Colton	93%	55
Doctors Medical Center - San Pablo[2]	San Pablo	93%	29
Mercy Medical Center - Redding[2]	Redding	93%	61
Scripps Mercy Hospital[2]	San Diego	93%	203
Seton Medical Center[2]	Daly City	93%	27
Univ of CA San Diego Med Ctr[2]	San Diego	93%	122
Ahmc Anaheim Regional Medical Center[2]	Anaheim	92%	59
Glendale Adventist Medical Center[2]	Glendale	92%	100
Kaiser Foundation Hospital - Downey[2]	Downey	92%	93
LAC+USC Medical Center[2]	Los Angeles	92%	65
Pomerado Hospital[2]	Poway	92%	48
Presbyterian Intercommunity Hospital[2]	Whittier	92%	106
Saint Jude Medical Center[2]	Fullerton	92%	78
Salinas Valley Memorial Hospital[2]	Salinas	92%	52
San Antonio Community Hospital[2]	Upland	92%	65
Sutter Delta Medical Center[2]	Antioch	92%	37
French Hospital Medical Center[2]	San Luis Obispo	91%	33
Hemet Valley Medical Center[2]	Hemet	91%	64
Kaiser Foundation Hospital - Riverside[2]	Riverside	91%	82
Loma Linda University Medical Center[2]	Loma Linda	91%	102
Mercy San Juan Medical Center[2]	Carmichael	91%	129
Mission Hospital Regional Medical Center[2]	Mission Viejo	91%	140
Providence Saint John's Health Center[2]	Santa Monica	91%	34
Saint Joseph's Medical Center of Stockton[2]	Stockton	91%	69
Garfield Medical Center[2]	Monterey Park	90%	29
Methodist Hospital of Sacramento[2]	Sacramento	90%	41
Sharp Chula Vista Medical Center[2]	Chula Vista	90%	69
White Memorial Medical Center[2]	Los Angeles	90%	39
Desert Regional Medical Center[2]	Palm Springs	88%	93
Lakewood Regional Medical Center[2]	Lakewood	88%	49
Mercy Medical Center[2]	Merced	88%	85
Saint Bernardine Medical Center[2]	San Bernardino	88%	67
Saint Francis Medical Center[2]	Lynwood	88%	82
Twin Cities Community Hospital[2]	Templeton	88%	49
Huntington Memorial Hospital[2]	Pasadena	87%	119
Loma Linda Univ Med Ctr-Murrieta[2]	Murrieta	87%	55
Doctors Medical Center[2]	Modesto	86%	129
Emanuel Medical Center[2]	Turlock	86%	43
Citrus Valley Medical Center - IC Campus[2]	Covina	85%	88
Mills - Peninsula Medical Center[2]	Burlingame	85%	92
Northbay Medical Center[2]	Fairfield	85%	61
San Joaquin Community Hospital[2]	Bakersfield	85%	98
Southwest Healthcare System[2]	Murrieta	85%	96
Sutter Tracy Community Hospital[2]	Tracy	85%	27
Washington Hospital[2]	Fremont	85%	60
Alta Bates Summit Medical Center[2]	Oakland	84%	51
Comm Mem Hosp San Buenaventura[2]	Ventura	84%	73
Redlands Community Hospital[2]	Redlands	84%	58
Saddleback Memorial Medical Center[2]	Laguna Hills	84%	88
Riverside Community Hospital[2]	Riverside	83%	112
Hollywood Presbyterian Medical Center[2]	Los Angeles	82%	33
Providence Tarzana Medical Center[2]	Tarzana	82%	68
Kaweah Delta Medical Center[2]	Visalia	81%	90
Los Angeles Community Hospital[2]	Los Angeles	81%	31
Regional Medical Center of San Jose[2]	San Jose	81%	52
Ronald Reagan UCLA Medical Center[2]	Los Angeles	81%	97
San Ramon Regional Medical Center[2]	San Ramon	81%	27
Hoag Memorial Hospital Presbyterian[2]	Newport Beach	80%	186
Los Robles Hospital & Medical Center[2]	Thousand Oaks	78%	68
Saint Joseph Hospital[2]	Orange	78%	50
Valley Presbyterian Hospital[2]	Van Nuys	78%	46
Sierra Nevada Memorial Hospital[2]	Grass Valley	76%	37
Palmdale Regional Medical Center[2]	Palmdale	75%	53
Bakersfield Heart Hospital[2]	Bakersfield	74%	31
Henry Mayo Newhall Memorial Hospital[2]	Valencia	74%	54
Victor Valley Global Medical Center[2]	Victorville	74%	34
Providence Saint Joseph Medical Center[2]	Burbank	72%	76
Saint Agnes Medical Center[2]	Fresno	71%	109
Long Beach Memorial Medical Center[2]	Long Beach	70%	100
Hi - Desert Medical Center[2]	Joshua Tree	67%	52
Glendale Mem Hosp & Health Ctr[2]	Glendale	64%	42
Adventist Medical Center[2]	Hanford	58%	55
El Centro Regional Medical Center[2]	El Centro	56%	34
Rideout Memorial Hospital[2]	Marysville	52%	81
Beverly Hospital[2]	Montebello	39%	41

ICU Venous Thromboembolism Prophylaxis

Hospital Name	City	Rate	Cases
CA Pacific Med Ctr-Davies Campus[2]	San Francisco	100%	79
Comm Hosp of the Monterey Peninsula[2]	Monterey	100%	41
Community Regional Medical Center[2]	Fresno	100%	40
Fallbrook Hospital[2]	Fallbrook	100%	34
French Hospital Medical Center[2]	San Luis Obispo	100%	90
Garfield Medical Center[2]	Monterey Park	100%	96
Huntington Beach Hospital[2]	Huntington Bch	100%	55
John Muir Medical Center - Concord Campus[2]	Concord	100%	75
Kaiser Foundation Hospital & Rehab Center[2]	Vallejo	100%	83
Kaiser Foundation Hospital - Antioch[2]	Antioch	100%	42
Kaiser Foundation Hospital - Downey[2]	Downey	100%	25
Kaiser Foundation Hospital - Fresno[2]	Fresno	100%	49
Kaiser Fdn Hosp-Oakland/Richmond[2]	Oakland	100%	45
Kaiser Foundation Hospital - Redwood City[2]	Redwood City	100%	77
Kaiser Foundation Hospital - Roseville[2]	Roseville	100%	86
Kaiser Fdn Hosp-S San Francisco[2]	S San Francisco	100%	69
Kern Medical Center[2]	Bakersfield	100%	39
Los Angeles Community Hospital[2]	Los Angeles	100%	43
Marin General Hospital[2]	Greenbrae	100%	45
Mercy General Hospital[2]	Sacramento	100%	130
Mercy Hospital[2]	Bakersfield	100%	81
Mercy Hospital of Folsom[2]	Folsom	100%	74
Mercy Medical Center - Redding[2]	Redding	100%	109
Northridge Hospital Medical Center[2]	Northridge	100%	85
Regional Medical Center of San Jose[2]	San Jose	100%	97
Saint Bernardine Medical Center[2]	San Bernardino	100%	113
Saint Joseph's Medical Center of Stockton[2]	Stockton	100%	118
Scripps Memorial Hospital - Encinitas[2]	Encinitas	100%	60
Torrance Memorial Medical Center[2]	Torrance	100%	69
Univ of California Irvine Med Ctr[2]	Orange	100%	104
Univ of CA San Diego Med Ctr[2]	San Diego	100%	75
Woodland Memorial Hospital[2]	Woodland	100%	71
Barstow Community Hospital[2]	Barstow	99%	68
California Hosp Med Ctr Los Angeles[2]	Los Angeles	99%	98
Cedars - Sinai Medical Center[2]	Los Angeles	99%	223
John Muir Med Ctr-Walnut Creek Campus[2]	Walnut Creek	99%	83
Kaiser Fdn Hosp S Sacramento[2]	Sacramento	99%	76
LAC+USC Medical Center[2]	Los Angeles	99%	159
LAC/Harbor - UCLA Medical Center[2]	Torrance	99%	75
Lodi Memorial Hospital[2]	Lodi	99%	74
Mercy Medical Center[2]	Merced	99%	75
Methodist Hospital of Sacramento[2]	Sacramento	99%	76
PIH Hospital - Downey[2]	Downey	99%	74
Presbyterian Intercommunity Hospital[2]	Whittier	99%	77
Saint Francis Memorial Hospital[2]	San Francisco	99%	177
Saint Johns Regional Medical Center[2]	Oxnard	99%	99
Saint Mary Medical Center[2]	Long Beach	99%	109
Saint Mary's Medical Center[2]	San Francisco	99%	123
Scripps Memorial Hospital La Jolla[2]	La Jolla	99%	125
Tri - City Medical Center[2]	Oceanside	99%	68
Western Medical Center Santa Ana[2]	Santa Ana	99%	145
Barton Memorial Hospital[2]	S Lake Tahoe	98%	45
Contra Costa Regional Medical Center[2]	Martinez	98%	41
Desert Regional Medical Center[2]	Palm Springs	98%	93
Desert Valley Hospital[2]	Victorville	98%	41
Eisenhower Medical Center[2]	Rancho Mirage	98%	44
El Camino Hospital[2]	Mountain View	98%	52
Huntington Memorial Hospital[2]	Pasadena	98%	40
Kaiser Fdn Hosp-Fremont/Hayward[2]	Hayward	98%	40
Kaiser Fdn Hosp-Moreno Valley[2]	Moreno Valley	98%	56
Kaiser Foundation Hospital - Sacramento[2]	Sacramento	98%	112
Kaiser Fdn Hosp-San Francisco[2]	San Francisco	98%	119
Kaiser Foundation Hospital - Santa Clara[2]	Santa Clara	98%	64
Kaiser Foundation Hospital - Santa Rosa[2]	Santa Rosa	98%	51
Kaiser Foundation Hospital - Vacaville[2]	Vacaville	98%	80
Kaweah Delta Medical Center[2]	Visalia	98%	57
Natividad Medical Center[2]	Salinas	98%	45
Novato Community Hospital[2]	Novato	98%	49
Pomona Valley Hospital Medical Center[2]	Pomona	98%	114
Salinas Valley Memorial Hospital[2]	Salinas	98%	51
Southwest Healthcare System[2]	Murrieta	98%	50
Sutter Auburn Faith Hospital[2]	Auburn	98%	64
Sutter Coast Hospital[2]	Crescent City	98%	80
Sutter Delta Medical Center[2]	Antioch	98%	63
Sutter Medical Center of Santa Rosa[2]	Santa Rosa	98%	112
Twin Cities Community Hospital[2]	Templeton	98%	49
Western Medical Center Hospital Anaheim[2]	Anaheim	98%	61

NOTE: Hospital profiles are in alphabetical order by state, then city, then hospital within the city; Rankings exclude hospitals with less than 25 cases except for patient surveys which excludes hospitals with less than 100 cases; (a) 100-299 cases; (1) The number of cases/patients is too few to report; (2) Data submitted were based on a sample of cases/patients; (3) Results are based on a shorter time period than required; (4) Data suppressed by CMS for one or more quarters; (5) Results are not available for this reporting period; (6) Fewer than 100 patients completed the HCAHPS survey; (7) No cases met the criteria for this measure; (8) The lower limit of the confidence interval cannot be calculated if the number of observed infections equals zero; (9) No data are available from the state/territory for this reporting period; (10) The scores shown reflect fewer than 50 completed surveys; (11) There were discrepancies in the data collection process; (12) This measure does not apply to this hospital for this reporting period; (13) Results cannot be calculated for this reporting period; (14) The results for this state are combined with nearby states to protect confidentiality; Please refer to the User's Guide for a full explanation of data.

Bakersfield Memorial Hospital[2]	Bakersfield	97%	67
CA Pacific Med Ctr-Pacific Campus Hosp[2]	San Francisco	97%	104
Centinela Hospital Medical Center[2]	Inglewood	97%	36
Chino Valley Medical Center[2]	Chino	97%	35
Feather River Hospital[2]	Paradise	97%	86
Garden Grove Hospital & Medical Center[2]	Garden Grove	97%	60
Good Samaritan Hospital[2]	San Jose	97%	87
Henry Mayo Newhall Memorial Hospital[2]	Valencia	97%	75
Hi - Desert Medical Center[2]	Joshua Tree	97%	38
Kaiser Foundation Hospital - Baldwin Park[2]	Baldwin Park	97%	38
Kaiser Foundation Hospital - Manteca[2]	Manteca	97%	110
Kaiser Foundation Hospital - South Bay[2]	Harbor City	97%	36
Kaiser Foundation Hospital - Walnut Creek[2]	Walnut Creek	97%	76
Kaiser Fdn Hosp-Woodland Hills[2]	Woodland Hills	97%	36
Mark Twain Medical Center[2]	San Andreas	97%	37
Orange Coast Memorial Medical Center[2]	Fountain Valley	97%	63
Palm Drive Hospital[2]	Sebastopol	97%	30
Palomar Health Downtown Campus[2]	Escondido	97%	38
Providence Holy Cross Medical Center[2]	Mission Hills	97%	73
Saint Helena Hospital - Clearlake[2]	Clearlake	97%	39
Saint Jude Medical Center[2]	Fullerton	97%	98
Saint Vincent Medical Center[2]	Los Angeles	97%	72
San Gabriel Valley Medical Center[2]	San Gabriel	97%	58
San Joaquin General Hospital[2]	French Camp	97%	91
Sierra Vista Regional Medical Center[2]	San Luis Obispo	97%	74
Sutter Tracy Community Hospital[2]	Tracy	97%	73
Alta Bates Summit Medical Center[2]	Berkeley	96%	56
Antelope Valley Hospital[2]	Lancaster	96%	80
Arrowhead Regional Medical Center[2]	Colton	96%	83
CA Pacific Med Ctr-St Luke's Campus[2]	San Francisco	96%	56
Corona Regional Medical Center[2]	Corona	96%	49
East Los Angeles Doctors Hospital[2]	Los Angeles	96%	50
Fairchild Medical Center[2]	Yreka	96%	117
Grossmont Hospital[2]	La Mesa	96%	69
Marshall Medical Center[2]	Placerville	96%	76
Mercy Medical Center - Mount Shasta[2]	Mount Shasta	96%	26
Prov Little Co of Mary Med Ctr Torrance[2]	Torrance	96%	70
Providence Tarzana Medical Center[2]	Tarzana	96%	67
Saint Johns Pleasant Valley Hospital[2]	Camarillo	96%	71
Santa Barbara Cottage Hospital[2]	Santa Barbara	96%	103
Santa Monica-UCLA Med Ctr & Ortho Hosp[2]	Santa Monica	96%	50
Santa Rosa Memorial Hospital[2]	Santa Rosa	96%	54
Sequoia Hospital[2]	Redwood City	96%	69
Shasta Regional Medical Center[2]	Redding	96%	72
Sonora Regional Medical Center[2]	Sonora	96%	52
Sutter Roseville Medical Center[2]	Roseville	96%	90
Watsonville Community Hospital[2]	Watsonville	96%	47
Ahmc Anaheim Regional Medical Center[2]	Anaheim	95%	99
Clovis Community Medical Center[2]	Clovis	95%	40
Doctors Medical Center[2]	Modesto	95%	104
Doctors Medical Center - San Pablo[2]	San Pablo	95%	96
Dominican Hospital[2]	Santa Cruz	95%	85
Eden Medical Center[2]	Castro Valley	95%	131
Kaiser Fdn Hosp-Panorama City[2]	Panorama City	95%	40
Keck Hospital of USC[2]	Los Angeles	95%	157
LAC/Olive View - UCLA Medical Center[2]	Sylmar	95%	43
Prov Little Co of Mary Med Ctr San Pedro[2]	San Pedro	95%	59
San Mateo Medical Center[2]	San Mateo	95%	43
Scripps Mercy Hospital[2]	San Diego	95%	65
Southern California Hospital at Hollywood[2]	Hollywood	95%	64
Stanford Hospital[2]	Stanford	95%	63
Sutter Amador Hospital[2]	Jackson	95%	57
Sutter Solano Medical Center[2]	Vallejo	95%	129
Ventura County Medical Center[2]	Ventura	95%	55
West Hills Hospital & Medical Center[2]	West Hills	95%	92
Community Hospital of Huntington Park[2]	Huntington Park	94%	53
Dameron Hospital[2]	Stockton	94%	106
Kaiser Foundation Hospital[2]	San Rafael	94%	63
Kaiser Fdn Hosp-Orange Co-Anaheim[2]	Anaheim	94%	33
Kaiser Foundation Hospital - San Jose[2]	San Jose	94%	67
Marian Regional Medical Center[2]	Santa Maria	94%	112
Memorial Hospital Los Banos	Los Banos	94%	35
Mission Community Hospital[2]	Panorama City	94%	63
Saint Mary Medical Center[2]	Apple Valley	94%	71
San Antonio Community Hospital[2]	Upland	94%	36
Sharp Chula Vista Medical Center[2]	Chula Vista	94%	104
Sutter General Hospital[2]	Sacramento	94%	111
Univ of CA Davis Med Ctr[2]	Sacramento	94%	86
West Anaheim Medical Center[2]	Anaheim	94%	77
Whittier Hospital Medical Center[2]	Whittier	94%	99
Hollywood Presbyterian Medical Center[2]	Los Angeles	93%	74
Kaiser Foundation Hospital - Los Angeles[2]	Los Angeles	93%	136
Mercy San Juan Medical Center[2]	Carmichael	93%	109
O'Connor Hospital[2]	San Jose	93%	82
Saddleback Memorial Medical Center[2]	Laguna Hills	93%	74
Saint Joseph Hospital[2]	Eureka	93%	41
Saint Joseph Hospital[2]	Orange	93%	74
Saint Rose Hospital[2]	Hayward	93%	54
San Joaquin Community Hospital[2]	Bakersfield	93%	86
Santa Clara Valley Medical Center[2]	San Jose	93%	55
Chapman Medical Center[2]	Orange	92%	60
Fresno Heart & Surgical Hospital[2]	Fresno	92%	26
Glendale Mem Hosp & Health Ctr[2]	Glendale	92%	93
Kaiser Foundation Hospital - Fontana[2]	Fontana	92%	65
Los Robles Hospital & Medical Center[2]	Thousand Oaks	92%	87
Mission Hospital Regional Medical Center[2]	Mission Viejo	92%	106
Northbay Medical Center[2]	Fairfield	92%	133
Sharp Memorial Hospital[2]	San Diego	92%	66
Alta Bates Summit Medical Center[2]	Oakland	91%	81
Community Hospital of San Bernardino[2]	San Bernardino	91%	100
Kaiser Foundation Hospital - West La[2]	Los Angeles	91%	53
Los Alamitos Medical Center[2]	Los Alamitos	91%	102
Mad River Community Hospital[2]	Arcata	91%	33
Methodist Hospital of Southern California[2]	Arcadia	91%	74
Rideout Memorial Hospital[2]	Marysville	91%	85
Riverside County Regional Medical Center[2]	Moreno Valley	91%	45
Sherman Oaks Hospital[2]	Sherman Oaks	91%	65
Sonoma Valley Hospital[2]	Sonoma	91%	44
Tulare Regional Medical Center[2]	Tulare	91%	67
Alvarado Hospital Medical Center[2]	San Diego	90%	72
Kaiser Foundation Hospital - Riverside[2]	Riverside	90%	51
Lakewood Regional Medical Center[2]	Lakewood	90%	116
Loma Linda University Medical Center[2]	Loma Linda	90%	101
Memorial Medical Center[2]	Modesto	90%	72
Monterey Park Hospital[2]	Monterey Park	90%	31
Riverside Community Hospital[2]	Riverside	90%	80
Ronald Reagan UCLA Medical Center[2]	Los Angeles	90%	115
Sutter Lakeside Hospital[2]	Lakeport	90%	39
El Centro Regional Medical Center[2]	El Centro	89%	75
Fountain Valley Reg Hosp & Med Ctr[2]	Fountain Valley	89%	79
Good Samaritan Hospital[2]	Los Angeles	89%	133
Hoag Memorial Hospital Presbyterian[2]	Newport Beach	89%	146
Memorial Hospital of Gardena[2]	Gardena	89%	64
Mills - Peninsula Medical Center[2]	Burlingame	89%	76
Adventist Medical Center[2]	Hanford	88%	94
Community Hospital of Long Beach[2]	Long Beach	88%	74
Loma Linda Univ Med Ctr-Murrieta[2]	Murrieta	88%	64
Olympia Medical Center[2]	Los Angeles	88%	49
Oroville Hospital[2]	Oroville	88%	26
Providence Saint Joseph Medical Center[2]	Burbank	88%	69
Scripps Green Hospital[2]	La Jolla	88%	86
Temple Community Hospital[2]	Los Angeles	88%	56
Valleycare Medical Center[2]	Pleasanton	88%	186
Marina Del Rey Hospital[2]	Marina Del Rey	87%	61
Placentia Linda Hospital[2]	Placentia	87%	53
Pomerado Hospital[2]	Poway	87%	71
Saint Agnes Medical Center[2]	Fresno	87%	71
San Gorgonio Memorial Hospital[2]	Banning	87%	71
Tri - City Regional Medical Center[2]	Hawaiian Grdns	87%	69
Comm Mem Hosp San Buenaventura[2]	Ventura	86%	73
Enloe Medical Center[2]	Chico	86%	78
Glendale Adventist Medical Center[2]	Glendale	86%	57
San Francisco General Hospital[2]	San Francisco	86%	49
Seton Medical Center[2]	Daly City	86%	105
Alhambra Hospital Medical Center[2]	Alhambra	85%	86
Montclair Hospital Medical Center[2]	Montclair	85%	48
Palmdale Regional Medical Center[2]	Palmdale	85%	84
USC Verdugo Hills Hospital[2]	Glendale	85%	27
Washington Hospital[2]	Fremont	85%	95
Alameda County Medical Center[2]	Oakland	84%	56
Long Beach Memorial Medical Center[2]	Long Beach	84%	69
Pacific Alliance Medical Center[2]	Los Angeles	84%	38
San Ramon Regional Medical Center[2]	San Ramon	84%	69
Simi Valley Hosp & Health Care Svcs[2]	Simi Valley	84%	64
UCSF Medical Center[2]	San Francisco	84%	87
White Memorial Medical Center[2]	Los Angeles	84%	55
Pioneers Memorial Healthcare District[2]	Brawley	82%	82
Queen of the Valley Medical Center[2]	Napa	82%	92
Redlands Community Hospital[2]	Redlands	82%	49
Hazel Hawkins Memorial Hospital[2]	Hollister	81%	84
Petaluma Valley Hospital[2]	Petaluma	81%	32
Hemet Valley Medical Center[2]	Hemet	80%	71
Providence Saint John's Health Center[2]	Santa Monica	80%	74
Saint Louise Regional Hospital[2]	Gilroy	80%	46
San Leandro Hospital[2,3]	San Leandro	80%	51
Sierra View District Hospital[2]	Porterville	80%	82
Frank R Howard Memorial Hospital[2]	Willits	79%	28
John F Kennedy Memorial Hospital[2]	Indio	78%	67
Paradise Valley Hospital[2]	National City	77%	62
Saint Francis Medical Center[2]	Lynwood	77%	73
Ukiah Valley Medical Center[2]	Ukiah	77%	47
Alameda Hospital[2]	Alameda	76%	58
Citrus Valley Medical Center - IC Campus[2]	Covina	76%	72
Parkview Comm Hosp Med Ctr[2]	Riverside	76%	38
Madera Community Hospital[2]	Madera	75%	59
Doctors Hospital of Manteca[2]	Manteca	74%	68
Greater El Monte Community Hospital[2]	South El Monte	74%	47
Tahoe Forest Hospital[2]	Truckee	74%	27
Saint Helena Hospital[2]	Saint Helena	73%	74
Beverly Hospital[2]	Montebello	72%	98
Foothill Presbyterian Hospital[2]	Glendora	72%	93
Sharp Coronado Hosp & Healthcare Ctr[2]	Coronado	72%	25
Valley Presbyterian Hospital[2]	Van Nuys	71%	68
San Dimas Community Hospital[2]	San Dimas	69%	45
Delano Regional Medical Center[2]	Delano	67%	30
Victor Valley Global Medical Center[2]	Victorville	63%	65
Coastal Communities Hospital[2]	Santa Ana	62%	50
Coast Plaza Hospital[2]	Norwalk	61%	41
Menifee Valley Medical Center[2]	Sun City	61%	61
Lompoc Valley Medical Center[2]	Lompoc	58%	53
Bakersfield Heart Hospital[2]	Bakersfield	56%	70
Palo Verde Hospital[2]	Blythe	56%	25
La Palma Intercommunity Hospital[2]	La Palma	52%	46
George L Mee Memorial Hospital[2]	King City	49%	55
Colusa Regional Medical Center[2]	Colusa	8%	25

Incidence of Potentially Preventable VTE

Hospital Name	City	Rate	Cases
Kaiser Foundation Hospital - Fontana[2]	Fontana	0%	25
Mills - Peninsula Medical Center[2]	Burlingame	0%	26
Saint Bernardine Medical Center[2]	San Bernardino	0%	29
Scripps Memorial Hospital La Jolla[2]	La Jolla	0%	51
Univ of California Irvine Med Ctr[2]	Orange	0%	67
Cedars - Sinai Medical Center[2]	Los Angeles	1%	85
Kaiser Foundation Hospital - Los Angeles[2]	Los Angeles	3%	31
Kaiser Fdn Hosp-Orange Co-Anaheim[2]	Anaheim	3%	33
Palomar Health Downtown Campus[2]	Escondido	3%	31
Kaiser Foundation Hospital - San Diego[2]	San Diego	4%	27
Scripps Mercy Hospital[2]	San Diego	4%	28
Univ of CA Davis Med Ctr[2]	Sacramento	4%	55
Stanford Hospital[2]	Stanford	5%	76
Mission Hospital Regional Medical Center[2]	Mission Viejo	6%	36
Univ of CA San Diego Med Ctr[2]	San Diego	6%	82
Community Regional Medical Center[2]	Fresno	8%	37
Keck Hospital of USC[2]	Los Angeles	9%	33
Sharp Memorial Hospital[2]	San Diego	9%	32
LAC+USC Medical Center[2]	Los Angeles	12%	25
Loma Linda University Medical Center[2]	Loma Linda	12%	41
San Francisco General Hospital[2]	San Francisco	12%	32
Doctors Medical Center[2]	Modesto	13%	39
Glendale Adventist Medical Center[2]	Glendale	16%	37
UCSF Medical Center[2]	San Francisco	20%	82
Ronald Reagan UCLA Medical Center[2]	Los Angeles	21%	42
Riverside Community Hospital[2]	Riverside	24%	25
Hoag Memorial Hospital Presbyterian[2]	Newport Beach	27%	37
Huntington Memorial Hospital[2]	Pasadena	31%	61
Long Beach Memorial Medical Center[2]	Long Beach	33%	42
Hemet Valley Medical Center[2]	Hemet	34%	29

UFH with Dosages/Platelet Count Monitoring

Hospital Name	City	Rate	Cases
Ahmc Anaheim Regional Medical Center[2]	Anaheim	100%	34
Alta Bates Summit Medical Center[2]	Oakland	100%	31
Arrowhead Regional Medical Center[2]	Colton	100%	44
California Hosp Med Ctr Los Angeles[2]	Los Angeles	100%	30
CA Pacific Med Ctr-Pacific Campus Hosp[2]	San Francisco	100%	37
Cedars - Sinai Medical Center[2]	Los Angeles	100%	218
Chino Valley Medical Center[2]	Chino	100%	43
Citrus Valley Medical Center - IC Campus[2]	Covina	100%	52
Comm Hosp of the Monterey Peninsula[2]	Monterey	100%	45
Community Regional Medical Center[2]	Fresno	100%	103
Dameron Hospital[2]	Stockton	100%	34
Doctors Medical Center[2]	Modesto	100%	102
Doctors Medical Center - San Pablo[2]	San Pablo	100%	26
Eisenhower Medical Center[2]	Rancho Mirage	100%	69
El Camino Hospital[2]	Mountain View	100%	30
Enloe Medical Center[2]	Chico	100%	44
Good Samaritan Hospital[2]	San Jose	100%	66
Grossmont Hospital[2]	La Mesa	100%	50
Hi - Desert Medical Center[2]	Joshua Tree	100%	52
John Muir Medical Center - Concord Campus[2]	Concord	100%	36
Kaiser Foundation Hospital & Rehab Center[2]	Vallejo	100%	40
Kaiser Foundation Hospital - Antioch[2]	Antioch	100%	29
Kaiser Foundation Hospital - Baldwin Park[2]	Baldwin Park	100%	29
Kaiser Foundation Hospital - Downey[2]	Downey	100%	46
Kaiser Fdn Hosp-Fremont/Hayward[2]	Hayward	100%	46
Kaiser Foundation Hospital - Los Angeles[2]	Los Angeles	100%	75
Kaiser Foundation Hospital - Manteca[2]	Manteca	100%	26
Kaiser Fdn Hosp-Oakland/Richmond[2]	Oakland	100%	45
Kaiser Fdn Hosp-Orange Co-Anaheim[2]	Anaheim	100%	108
Kaiser Foundation Hospital - Redwood City[2]	Redwood City	100%	37
Kaiser Foundation Hospital - Roseville[2]	Roseville	100%	62
Kaiser Foundation Hospital - Sacramento[2]	Sacramento	100%	33
Kaiser Foundation Hospital - San Diego[2]	San Diego	100%	96
Kaiser Fdn Hosp-San Francisco[2]	San Francisco	100%	43
Kaiser Foundation Hospital - San Jose[2]	San Jose	100%	47
Kaiser Foundation Hospital - Santa Clara[2]	Santa Clara	100%	47
Kaiser Foundation Hospital - Walnut Creek[2]	Walnut Creek	100%	37
Kaiser Fdn Hosp S Sacramento[2]	Sacramento	100%	52
Kaweah Delta Medical Center[2]	Visalia	100%	27
LAC+USC Medical Center[2]	Los Angeles	100%	66
LAC/Harbor - UCLA Medical Center[2]	Torrance	100%	60

NOTE: Hospital profiles are in alphabetical order by state, then city, then hospital within the city; Rankings exclude hospitals with less than 25 cases except for patient surveys which excludes hospitals with less than 100 cases; (a) 100-299 cases; (1) The number of cases/patients is too few to report; (2) Data submitted were based on a sample of cases/patients; (3) Results are based on a shorter time period than required; (4) Data suppressed by CMS for one or more quarters; (5) Results are not available for this reporting period; (6) Fewer than 100 patients completed the HCAHPS survey; (7) No cases met the criteria for this measure; (8) The lower limit of the confidence interval cannot be calculated if the number of observed infections equals zero; (9) No data are available from the state/territory for this reporting period; (10) The scores shown reflect fewer than 50 completed surveys; (11) There were discrepancies in the data collection process; (12) This measure does not apply to this hospital for this reporting period; (13) Results cannot be calculated for this reporting period; (14) The results for this state are combined with nearby states to protect confidentiality; Please refer to the User's Guide for a full explanation of data.

Hospital Name	City	Rate	Cases
Lakewood Regional Medical Center[2]	Lakewood	100%	26
Lodi Memorial Hospital[2]	Lodi	100%	31
Memorial Medical Center[2]	Modesto	100%	88
Mercy General Hospital[2]	Sacramento	100%	90
Mercy Hospital of Folsom[2]	Folsom	100%	26
Mercy Medical Center[2]	Merced	100%	54
Mercy Medical Center - Redding[2]	Redding	100%	25
Mercy San Juan Medical Center[2]	Carmichael	100%	82
Methodist Hospital of Southern California[2]	Arcadia	100%	28
Mills - Peninsula Medical Center[2]	Burlingame	100%	29
Mission Hospital Regional Medical Center[2]	Mission Viejo	100%	141
Northridge Hospital Medical Center[2]	Northridge	100%	52
Olympia Medical Center[2]	Los Angeles	100%	25
Palomar Health Downtown Campus[2]	Escondido	100%	80
Paradise Valley Hospital[2]	National City	100%	25
Presbyterian Intercommunity Hospital[2]	Whittier	100%	100
Riverside Community Hospital[2]	Riverside	100%	40
Saint Bernardine Medical Center[2]	San Bernardino	100%	83
Saint Francis Medical Center[2]	Lynwood	100%	30
Saint Joseph's Medical Center of Stockton[2]	Stockton	100%	81
Saint Jude Medical Center[2]	Fullerton	100%	37
Saint Mary Medical Center[2]	Long Beach	100%	25
Salinas Valley Memorial Hospital[2]	Salinas	100%	42
San Antonio Community Hospital[2]	Upland	100%	26
San Francisco General Hospital[2]	San Francisco	100%	47
Santa Clara Valley Medical Center[2]	San Jose	100%	39
Scripps Green Hospital[2]	La Jolla	100%	26
Scripps Memorial Hospital - Encinitas[2]	Encinitas	100%	30
Scripps Memorial Hospital La Jolla[2]	La Jolla	100%	31
Sharp Memorial Hospital[2]	San Diego	100%	33
Shasta Regional Medical Center[2]	Redding	100%	36
UCSF Medical Center[2]	San Francisco	100%	88
Univ of CA Davis Med Ctr[2]	Sacramento	100%	134
Univ of California Irvine Med Ctr[2]	Orange	100%	71
Univ of CA San Diego Med Ctr[2]	San Diego	100%	86
Valleycare Medical Center[2]	Pleasanton	100%	25
Washington Hospital[2]	Fremont	100%	34
Kaiser Foundation Hospital - Fontana[2]	Fontana	99%	153
Kaiser Foundation Hospital - Riverside[2]	Riverside	99%	73
Saddleback Memorial Medical Center[2]	Laguna Hills	99%	71
Regional Medical Center of San Jose[2]	San Jose	98%	47
Riverside County Regional Medical Center[2]	Moreno Valley	98%	57
Ronald Reagan UCLA Medical Center[2]	Los Angeles	98%	97
Scripps Mercy Hospital[2]	San Diego	98%	168
Stanford Hospital[2]	Stanford	98%	103
Sutter General Hospital[2]	Sacramento	98%	46
Comm Mem Hosp San Buenaventura[2]	Ventura	97%	29
Huntington Memorial Hospital[2]	Pasadena	97%	38
Orange Coast Memorial Medical Center[2]	Fountain Valley	97%	38
San Joaquin Community Hospital[2]	Bakersfield	97%	32
Sharp Chula Vista Medical Center[2]	Chula Vista	97%	67
Tri - City Medical Center[2]	Oceanside	97%	32
Alameda County Medical Center[2]	Oakland	96%	28
Kaiser Foundation Hospital - South Bay[2]	Harbor City	96%	46
Santa Barbara Cottage Hospital[2]	Santa Barbara	96%	25
Sutter Roseville Medical Center[2]	Roseville	96%	28
Glendale Adventist Medical Center[2]	Glendale	95%	40
LAC/Olive View - UCLA Medical Center[2]	Sylmar	95%	60
Antelope Valley Hospital[2]	Lancaster	94%	31
Dominican Hospital[2]	Santa Cruz	94%	31
Kaiser Foundation Hospital - West La[2]	Los Angeles	93%	45
Santa Monica-UCLA Med Ctr & Ortho Hosp[2]	Santa Monica	93%	58
Desert Regional Medical Center[2]	Palm Springs	92%	39
Providence Tarzana Medical Center[2]	Tarzana	92%	25
Keck Hospital of USC[2]	Los Angeles	90%	29
Providence Saint John's Health Center[2]	Santa Monica	90%	39
Loma Linda University Medical Center[2]	Loma Linda	87%	90
Rideout Memorial Hospital[2]	Marysville	77%	43
Long Beach Memorial Medical Center[2]	Long Beach	69%	64
Hoag Memorial Hospital Presbyterian[2]	Newport Beach	2%	177

Venous Thromboembolism Prophylaxis

Hospital Name	City	Rate	Cases
Barstow Community Hospital[2]	Barstow	100%	222
French Hospital Medical Center[2]	San Luis Obispo	100%	247
Garfield Medical Center[2]	Monterey Park	100%	286
Patients' Hospital of Redding	Redding	100%	86
Stanislaus Surgical Hospital[2]	Modesto	100%	47
Temple Community Hospital[2]	Los Angeles	100%	232
Woodland Memorial Hospital[2]	Woodland	100%	144
Kaiser Foundation Hospital - Antioch[2]	Antioch	99%	238
Kaiser Fdn Hosp-Oakland/Richmond[2]	Oakland	99%	314
Kaiser Foundation Hospital - Roseville[2]	Roseville	99%	232
Mercy Hospital[2]	Bakersfield	99%	341
Mercy Hospital of Folsom[2]	Folsom	99%	343
Natividad Medical Center[2]	Salinas	99%	272
PIH Hospital - Downey[2]	Downey	99%	312
Sutter Surgical Hospital - North Valley[2]	Yuba City	99%	111
Desert Valley Hospital[2]	Victorville	98%	377
Hoag Orthopedic Institute[2]	Irvine	98%	90
Kaiser Fdn Hosp-Moreno Valley[2]	Moreno Valley	98%	275
Kaiser Fdn Hosp-S San Francisco[2]	S San Francisco	98%	272
Kern Medical Center[2]	Bakersfield	98%	352
Saint Joseph's Medical Center of Stockton[2]	Stockton	98%	368
Saint Mary's Medical Center[2]	San Francisco	98%	321
Bakersfield Memorial Hospital[2]	Bakersfield	97%	320
Barton Memorial Hospital[2]	S Lake Tahoe	97%	148
Fallbrook Hospital[2]	Fallbrook	97%	152
Garden Grove Hospital & Medical Center[2]	Garden Grove	97%	355
Kaiser Foundation Hospital - Sacramento[2]	Sacramento	97%	272
Lodi Memorial Hospital[2]	Lodi	97%	403
Marin General Hospital[2]	Greenbrae	97%	354
Methodist Hospital of Sacramento[2]	Sacramento	97%	329
Saint Francis Memorial Hospital[2]	San Francisco	97%	236
Saint Mary Medical Center[2]	Long Beach	97%	318
Sierra Nevada Memorial Hospital[2]	Grass Valley	97%	350
Cedars - Sinai Medical Center[2]	Los Angeles	96%	1030
Chino Valley Medical Center[2]	Chino	96%	343
Community Hospital of Huntington Park[2]	Huntington Park	96%	358
Comm Hosp of the Monterey Peninsula[2]	Monterey	96%	351
Corona Regional Medical Center[2]	Corona	96%	397
East Los Angeles Doctors Hospital[2]	Los Angeles	96%	260
Kaiser Foundation Hospital - Baldwin Park[2]	Baldwin Park	96%	296
Kaiser Fdn Hosp-Fremont/Hayward[2]	Hayward	96%	276
Kaiser Fdn Hosp-San Francisco[2]	San Francisco	96%	267
Marshall Medical Center[2]	Placerville	96%	317
Mercy General Hospital[2]	Sacramento	96%	266
Mercy Medical Center[2]	Merced	96%	351
O'Connor Hospital[2]	San Jose	96%	321
Prov Little Co of Mary Med Ctr San Pedro[2]	San Pedro	96%	282
Saint Helena Hospital - Clearlake[2]	Clearlake	96%	94
Saint Johns Regional Medical Center[2]	Oxnard	96%	353
Shasta Regional Medical Center[2]	Redding	96%	356
Sutter Coast Hospital[2]	Crescent City	96%	133
Sutter Tracy Community Hospital[2]	Tracy	96%	238
Whittier Hospital Medical Center[2]	Whittier	96%	321
Centinela Hospital Medical Center[2]	Inglewood	95%	352
Contra Costa Regional Medical Center[2]	Martinez	95%	352
El Camino Hospital[2]	Mountain View	95%	274
Feather River Hospital[2]	Paradise	95%	348
Huntington Beach Hospital[2]	Huntington Bch	95%	292
John Muir Med Ctr-Walnut Creek Campus[2]	Walnut Creek	95%	311
Kaiser Foundation Hospital - Fresno[2]	Fresno	95%	326
Kaiser Fdn Hosp-Orange Co-Anaheim[2]	Anaheim	95%	328
Kaiser Foundation Hospital - Walnut Creek[2]	Walnut Creek	95%	307
Kaiser Fdn Hosp-Woodland Hills[2]	Woodland Hills	95%	309
Kaiser Fdn Hosp S Sacramento[2]	Sacramento	95%	269
LAC+USC Medical Center[2]	Los Angeles	95%	236
Palm Drive Hospital[2]	Sebastopol	95%	75
Salinas Valley Memorial Hospital[2]	Salinas	95%	352
Scripps Green Hospital[2]	La Jolla	95%	276
Univ of California Irvine Med Ctr[2]	Orange	95%	247
Watsonville Community Hospital[2]	Watsonville	95%	236
West Anaheim Medical Center[2]	Anaheim	95%	370
Dominican Hospital[2]	Santa Cruz	94%	317
John Muir Medical Center - Concord Campus[2]	Concord	94%	321
Marian Regional Medical Center[2]	Santa Maria	94%	419
Mercy Medical Center - Mount Shasta[2]	Mount Shasta	94%	87
Pacific Hospital of Long Beach[2,3]	Long Beach	94%	105
Providence Tarzana Medical Center[2]	Tarzana	94%	350
San Gabriel Valley Medical Center[2]	San Gabriel	94%	301
Scripps Memorial Hospital - Encinitas[2]	Encinitas	94%	332
Sonoma Valley Hospital[2]	Sonoma	94%	85
Arrowhead Regional Medical Center[2]	Colton	93%	307
Clovis Community Medical Center[2]	Clovis	93%	340
Kaiser Foundation Hospital - Redwood City[2]	Redwood City	93%	290
Kaiser Foundation Hospital - San Jose[2]	San Jose	93%	309
Kaiser Foundation Hospital - South Bay[2]	Harbor City	93%	286
Scripps Memorial Hospital La Jolla[2]	La Jolla	93%	265
Southern California Hospital at Hollywood[2]	Hollywood	93%	674
Sutter Maternity & Surgery Ctr	Santa Cruz	93%	72
Univ of CA San Diego Med Ctr[2]	San Diego	93%	311
West Hills Hospital & Medical Center[2]	West Hills	93%	318
Kaiser Foundation Hospital[2]	San Rafael	92%	251
Kaiser Foundation Hospital - Downey[2]	Downey	92%	303
Kaiser Foundation Hospital - Santa Rosa[2]	Santa Rosa	92%	306
Kaiser Foundation Hospital - Vacaville[2]	Vacaville	92%	321
Kaweah Delta Medical Center[2]	Visalia	92%	363
Monterey Park Hospital[2]	Monterey Park	92%	258
Presbyterian Intercommunity Hospital[2]	Whittier	92%	329
Prov Little Co of Mary Med Ctr Torrance[2]	Torrance	92%	328
Saint Joseph Hospital[2]	Orange	92%	299
Sequoia Hospital[2]	Redwood City	92%	309
Sierra Vista Regional Medical Center[2]	San Luis Obispo	92%	279
Sutter Solano Medical Center[2]	Vallejo	92%	277
Fairchild Medical Center[2]	Yreka	91%	502
Kaiser Foundation Hospital - Manteca[2]	Manteca	91%	247
LAC/Harbor - UCLA Medical Center[2]	Torrance	91%	308
Mercy Medical Center - Redding[2]	Redding	91%	273
Mercy San Juan Medical Center[2]	Carmichael	91%	276
Novato Community Hospital[2]	Novato	91%	135
Providence Holy Cross Medical Center[2]	Mission Hills	91%	318
Saint Joseph Hospital[2]	Eureka	91%	343
Sonora Regional Medical Center[2]	Sonora	91%	331
Dameron Hospital[2]	Stockton	90%	277
Kaiser Foundation Hospital - Los Angeles[2]	Los Angeles	90%	267
Kaiser Foundation Hospital - Santa Clara[2]	Santa Clara	90%	270
Mark Twain Medical Center[2]	San Andreas	90%	119
Northridge Hospital Medical Center[2]	Northridge	90%	322
Olympia Medical Center[2]	Los Angeles	90%	401
Providence Saint Joseph Medical Center[2]	Burbank	90%	309
Regional Medical Center of San Jose[2]	San Jose	90%	381
Riverside County Regional Medical Center[2]	Moreno Valley	90%	247
Santa Rosa Memorial Hospital[2]	Santa Rosa	90%	330
Sutter Medical Center of Santa Rosa[2]	Santa Rosa	90%	431
Alameda County Medical Center[2]	Oakland	89%	276
Emanuel Medical Center[2]	Turlock	89%	478
Enloe Medical Center[2]	Chico	89%	333
Kaiser Foundation Hospital - Fontana[2]	Fontana	89%	288
Memorial Hospital Los Banos	Los Banos	89%	272
Saint Bernardine Medical Center[2]	San Bernardino	89%	276
Saint Johns Pleasant Valley Hospital[2]	Camarillo	89%	262
Santa Monica-UCLA Med Ctr & Ortho Hosp[2]	Santa Monica	89%	351
Sutter Davis Hospital[2]	Davis	89%	153
California Hosp Med Ctr Los Angeles[2]	Los Angeles	88%	292
Kaiser Foundation Hospital & Rehab Center[2]	Vallejo	88%	320
Kaiser Foundation Hospital - San Diego[2]	San Diego	88%	361
Los Alamitos Medical Center[2]	Los Alamitos	88%	275
Saint Vincent Medical Center[2]	Los Angeles	88%	334
Sutter Auburn Faith Hospital[2]	Auburn	88%	276
Sutter Roseville Medical Center[2]	Roseville	88%	310
Chapman Medical Center[2]	Orange	87%	111
Community Hospital of San Bernardino[2]	San Bernardino	87%	333
Henry Mayo Newhall Memorial Hospital[2]	Valencia	87%	292
LAC/Olive View - UCLA Medical Center[2]	Sylmar	87%	304
Memorial Medical Center[2]	Modesto	87%	346
Northbay Medical Center[2]	Fairfield	87%	292
Tri - City Regional Medical Center[2]	Hawaiian Grdns	87%	285
Valleycare Medical Center[2]	Pleasanton	87%	796
Western Medical Center Santa Ana[2]	Santa Ana	87%	267
Ahmc Anaheim Regional Medical Center[2]	Anaheim	86%	354
Fresno Heart & Surgical Hospital[2]	Fresno	86%	256
Glendale Adventist Medical Center[2]	Glendale	86%	307
Los Angeles Community Hospital[2]	Los Angeles	86%	404
Mammoth Hospital	Mammoth Lakes	86%	182
Scripps Mercy Hospital[2]	San Diego	86%	361
Sutter General Hospital[2]	Sacramento	86%	276
Torrance Memorial Medical Center[2]	Torrance	86%	408
Alta Bates Summit Medical Center[2]	Berkeley	85%	345
Antelope Valley Hospital[2]	Lancaster	85%	303
CA Pacific Med Ctr-St Luke's Campus[2]	San Francisco	85%	218
Delano Regional Medical Center[2]	Delano	85%	229
Doctors Medical Center[2]	Modesto	85%	343
Kaiser Foundation Hospital - Riverside[2]	Riverside	85%	295
Mission Community Hospital[2]	Panorama City	85%	376
Oroville Hospital[2]	Oroville	85%	417
Palomar Health Downtown Campus[2]	Escondido	85%	329
Redlands Community Hospital[2]	Redlands	85%	300
Saint Mary Medical Center[2]	Apple Valley	85%	336
Santa Ynez Valley Cottage Hospital[2]	Solvang	85%	112
Twin Cities Community Hospital[2]	Templeton	85%	358
Univ of CA Davis Med Ctr[2]	Sacramento	85%	292
CA Pacific Med Ctr-Davies Campus[2]	San Francisco	84%	247
Kaiser Fdn Hosp-Panorama City[2]	Panorama City	84%	295
Los Robles Hospital & Medical Center[2]	Thousand Oaks	84%	336
Mission Hospital Regional Medical Center[2]	Mission Viejo	84%	258
Saint Elizabeth Community Hospital[2]	Red Bluff	84%	194
Santa Clara Valley Medical Center[2]	San Jose	84%	307
Seton Medical Center[2]	Daly City	84%	321
El Centro Regional Medical Center[2]	El Centro	83%	373
Grossmont Hospital[2]	La Mesa	83%	390
Lakewood Regional Medical Center[2]	Lakewood	83%	322
Ojai Valley Community Hospital[2]	Ojai	83%	77
Petaluma Valley Hospital[2]	Petaluma	83%	161
Placentia Linda Hospital[2]	Placentia	83%	289
San Gorgonio Memorial Hospital[2]	Banning	83%	313
San Joaquin General Hospital[2]	French Camp	83%	349
Sutter Lakeside Hospital[2]	Lakeport	83%	133
Tulare Regional Medical Center[2]	Tulare	83%	288
Ukiah Valley Medical Center[2]	Ukiah	83%	221
Memorial Hospital of Gardena[2]	Gardena	82%	368
Mills - Peninsula Medical Center[2]	Burlingame	82%	314
Pomona Valley Hospital Medical Center[2]	Pomona	82%	307
Riverside Community Hospital[2]	Riverside	82%	353
Saint Jude Medical Center[2]	Fullerton	82%	262
Sutter Delta Medical Center[2]	Antioch	82%	362
Tri - City Medical Center[2]	Oceanside	82%	297
Ventura County Medical Center[2]	Ventura	82%	301
Comm Mem Hosp San Buenaventura[2]	Ventura	81%	293
Community Regional Medical Center[2]	Fresno	81%	351
Desert Regional Medical Center[2]	Palm Springs	81%	285
Doctors Medical Center - San Pablo[2]	San Pablo	81%	345
Eden Medical Center[2]	Castro Valley	81%	420

NOTE: Hospital profiles are in alphabetical order by state, then city, then hospital within the city; Rankings exclude hospitals with less than 25 cases except for patient surveys which excludes hospitals with less than 100 cases; (a) 100-299 cases; (1) The number of cases/patients is too few to report; (2) Data submitted were based on a sample of cases/patients; (3) Results are based on a shorter time period than required; (4) Data suppressed by CMS for one or more quarters; (5) Results are not available for this reporting period; (6) Fewer than 100 patients completed the HCAHPS survey; (7) No cases met the criteria for this measure; (8) The lower limit of the confidence interval cannot be calculated if the number of observed infections equals zero; (9) No data are available from the state/territory for this reporting period; (10) The scores shown reflect fewer than 50 completed surveys; (11) There were discrepancies in the data collection process; (12) This measure does not apply to this hospital for this reporting period; (13) Results cannot be calculated for this reporting period; (14) The results for this state are combined with nearby states to protect confidentiality; Please refer to the User's Guide for a full explanation of data.

Ronald Reagan UCLA Medical Center[2]	Los Angeles	81%	285
Sharp Memorial Hospital[2]	San Diego	81%	332
Frank R Howard Memorial Hospital[2]	Willits	80%	94
Montclair Hospital Medical Center[2]	Montclair	80%	189
CA Pacific Med Ctr-Pacific Campus Hosp[2]	San Francisco	79%	245
Glendale Mem Hosp & Health Ctr[2]	Glendale	79%	363
Kaiser Foundation Hospital - West La[2]	Los Angeles	79%	290
Methodist Hospital of Southern California[2]	Arcadia	79%	339
San Antonio Community Hospital[2]	Upland	79%	303
San Francisco General Hospital[2]	San Francisco	79%	328
Santa Barbara Cottage Hospital[2]	Santa Barbara	79%	311
Greater El Monte Community Hospital[2]	South El Monte	78%	176
Keck Hospital of USC[2]	Los Angeles	78%	238
Alvarado Hospital Medical Center[2]	San Diego	77%	339
Good Samaritan Hospital[2]	Bakersfield	77%	111
Hoag Memorial Hospital Presbyterian[2]	Newport Beach	77%	416
Loma Linda University Medical Center[2]	Loma Linda	77%	298
Sharp Chula Vista Medical Center[2]	Chula Vista	77%	376
Simi Valley Hosp & Health Care Svcs[2]	Simi Valley	77%	312
Southwest Healthcare System[2]	Murrieta	77%	332
Sutter Amador Hospital[2]	Jackson	77%	180
Western Medical Center Hospital Anaheim[2]	Anaheim	77%	137
Sierra View District Hospital[2]	Porterville	76%	435
Eisenhower Medical Center[2]	Rancho Mirage	75%	332
Marina Del Rey Hospital[2]	Marina Del Rey	75%	317
San Dimas Community Hospital[2]	San Dimas	75%	249
Stanford Hospital[2]	Stanford	75%	314
Alta Bates Summit Medical Center[2]	Oakland	74%	325
Community Hospital of Long Beach[2]	Long Beach	74%	185
Goleta Valley Cottage Hospital[2]	Santa Barbara	74%	46
Loma Linda Univ Med Ctr-Murrieta[2]	Murrieta	74%	382
San Joaquin Community Hospital[2]	Bakersfield	74%	389
San Mateo Medical Center[2]	San Mateo	74%	237
USC Verdugo Hills Hospital[2]	Glendale	74%	322
Alhambra Hospital Medical Center[2]	Alhambra	73%	374
Mad River Community Hospital[2]	Arcata	73%	116
Providence Saint John's Health Center[2]	Santa Monica	73%	241
Saint Francis Medical Center[2]	Lynwood	73%	261
Bakersfield Heart Hospital[2]	Bakersfield	72%	311
Good Samaritan Hospital[2]	San Jose	72%	325
Pomerado Hospital[2]	Poway	72%	313
Saint Agnes Medical Center[2]	Fresno	72%	379
Saint Rose Hospital[2]	Hayward	72%	346
Adventist Medical Center - Reedley[2]	Reedley	71%	154
Orange Coast Memorial Medical Center[2]	Fountain Valley	71%	311
Saint Louise Regional Hospital[2]	Gilroy	71%	196
UCSF Medical Center[2]	San Francisco	71%	296
Encino Hospital Medical Center[2]	Encino	70%	171
Hi - Desert Medical Center[2]	Joshua Tree	70%	220
Hollywood Presbyterian Medical Center[2]	Los Angeles	70%	332
Tahoe Forest Hospital[2]	Truckee	69%	74
George L Mee Memorial Hospital[2]	King City	68%	190
Rideout Memorial Hospital[2]	Marysville	68%	503
East Valley Hospital Medical Center[2]	Glendora	67%	106
LAC/Rancho Los Amigos Ntl Rehab Ctr[2]	Downey	67%	419
John F Kennedy Memorial Hospital[2]	Indio	66%	283
Valley Presbyterian Hospital[2]	Van Nuys	66%	329
Fountain Valley Reg Hosp & Med Ctr[2]	Fountain Valley	65%	386
Saddleback Memorial Medical Center[2]	Laguna Hills	65%	324
Sharp Coronado Hosp & Healthcare Ctr[2]	Coronado	65%	88
Alameda Hospital[2]	Alameda	64%	238
Doctors Hospital of Manteca[2]	Manteca	64%	284
San Ramon Regional Medical Center[2]	San Ramon	64%	279
Saint Helena Hospital[2]	Saint Helena	63%	178
Sherman Oaks Hospital[2]	Sherman Oaks	63%	306
Madera Community Hospital[2]	Madera	62%	392
Pioneers Memorial Healthcare District[2]	Brawley	62%	303
Hazel Hawkins Memorial Hospital[2]	Hollister	61%	275
Queen of the Valley Medical Center[2]	Napa	61%	339
Huntington Memorial Hospital[2]	Pasadena	60%	291
San Leandro Hospital[2,3]	San Leandro	60%	166
Adventist Medical Center[2]	Hanford	59%	811
Paradise Valley Hospital[2]	National City	59%	370
Parkview Comm Hosp Med Ctr[2]	Riverside	59%	336
Coalinga Regional Medical Center	Coalinga	58%	111
Beverly Hospital[2]	Montebello	57%	327
Good Samaritan Hospital[2]	Los Angeles	56%	289
Palmdale Regional Medical Center[2]	Palmdale	55%	344
Citrus Valley Medical Center - IC Campus[2]	Covina	54%	260
Hemet Valley Medical Center[2]	Hemet	54%	315
Menifee Valley Medical Center[2]	Sun City	52%	293
White Memorial Medical Center[2]	Los Angeles	52%	298
Coastal Communities Hospital[2]	Santa Ana	51%	199
Pacific Alliance Medical Center[2]	Los Angeles	51%	380
Coast Plaza Hospital[2]	Norwalk	50%	310
Foothill Presbyterian Hospital[2]	Glendora	48%	288
Oak Valley District Hospital[2]	Oakdale	48%	104
Washington Hospital[2]	Fremont	48%	315
Long Beach Memorial Medical Center[2]	Long Beach	46%	309
Lompoc Valley Medical Center[2]	Lompoc	45%	204
Silver Lake Medical Center[2]	Los Angeles	43%	141
Chinese Hospital[2]	San Francisco	42%	219
La Palma Intercommunity Hospital[2]	La Palma	41%	296
Palo Verde Hospital[2]	Blythe	39%	90
Pacifica Hospital of the Valley[2]	Sun Valley	38%	220
Colusa Regional Medical Center[2]	Colusa	30%	207
Victor Valley Global Medical Center[2]	Victorville	30%	345
Doctors Hospital of West Covina	West Covina	27%	30
Bear Valley Community Hospital	Big Bear Lake	24%	82
Laguna Honda Hosp & Rehab Ctr	San Francisco	16%	64
Motion Picture & Television Hospital	Woodland Hills	12%	33
Sonoma Developmental Center[2]	Eldridge	3%	75

Warfarin Therapy Discharge Instructions

Hospital Name	City	Rate	Cases
Bakersfield Memorial Hospital[2]	Bakersfield	100%	44
Comm Hosp of the Monterey Peninsula[2]	Monterey	100%	52
Dameron Hospital[2]	Stockton	100%	36
Desert Valley Hospital[2]	Victorville	100%	55
Dominican Hospital[2]	Santa Cruz	100%	40
John Muir Medical Center - Concord Campus[2]	Concord	100%	34
Kaiser Fdn Hosp-Moreno Valley[2]	Moreno Valley	100%	25
Los Alamitos Medical Center[2]	Los Alamitos	100%	44
Los Robles Hospital & Medical Center[2]	Thousand Oaks	100%	47
Marin General Hospital[2]	Greenbrae	100%	34
Marshall Medical Center[2]	Placerville	100%	32
Mercy Hospital[2]	Bakersfield	100%	45
Mercy Medical Center - Redding[2]	Redding	100%	40
Methodist Hospital of Sacramento[2]	Sacramento	100%	28
Pomona Valley Hospital Medical Center[2]	Pomona	100%	45
Prov Little Co of Mary Med Ctr Torrance[2]	Torrance	100%	74
Regional Medical Center of San Jose[2]	San Jose	100%	39
Saint Bernardine Medical Center[2]	San Bernardino	100%	45
Saint Joseph's Medical Center of Stockton[2]	Stockton	100%	43
Scripps Green Hospital[2]	La Jolla	100%	83
Scripps Memorial Hospital - Encinitas[2]	Encinitas	100%	35
Scripps Memorial Hospital La Jolla[2]	La Jolla	100%	56
Shasta Regional Medical Center[2]	Redding	100%	50
Sonora Regional Medical Center[2]	Sonora	100%	43
Kaiser Foundation Hospital - Fontana[2]	Fontana	99%	190
Clovis Community Medical Center[2]	Clovis	98%	52
Doctors Medical Center[2]	Modesto	98%	90
John Muir Med Ctr-Walnut Creek Campus[2]	Walnut Creek	98%	54
Kaiser Foundation Hospital - South Bay[2]	Harbor City	98%	56
Riverside County Regional Medical Center[2]	Moreno Valley	98%	61
El Camino Hospital[2]	Mountain View	97%	68
Feather River Hospital[2]	Paradise	97%	29
Kaiser Foundation Hospital - Roseville[2]	Roseville	97%	86
Kaiser Foundation Hospital - San Diego[2]	San Diego	97%	107
Kaiser Fdn Hosp S Sacramento[2]	Sacramento	97%	74
Mercy General Hospital[2]	Sacramento	97%	70
Mercy Hospital of Folsom[2]	Folsom	97%	37
Oroville Hospital[2]	Oroville	97%	39
Palomar Health Downtown Campus[2]	Escondido	97%	119
PIH Hospital - Downey[2]	Downey	97%	33
Providence Saint John's Health Center[2]	Santa Monica	97%	30
Univ of California Irvine Med Ctr[2]	Orange	97%	75
Valleycare Medical Center[2]	Pleasanton	97%	35
Kaiser Foundation Hospital - Riverside[2]	Riverside	96%	76
Southwest Healthcare System[2]	Murrieta	96%	74
Tri - City Medical Center[2]	Oceanside	96%	79
Kaiser Foundation Hospital - Baldwin Park[2]	Baldwin Park	95%	65
Kaiser Fdn Hosp-Woodland Hills[2]	Woodland Hills	95%	65
Cedars - Sinai Medical Center[2]	Los Angeles	94%	101
Kaiser Foundation Hospital - Sacramento[2]	Sacramento	94%	47
LAC/Harbor - UCLA Medical Center[2]	Torrance	94%	54
Northridge Hospital Medical Center[2]	Northridge	94%	52
Centinela Hospital Medical Center[2]	Inglewood	93%	29
Kaiser Foundation Hospital - Redwood City[2]	Redwood City	93%	43
Palmdale Regional Medical Center[2]	Palmdale	93%	46
Saint Johns Regional Medical Center[2]	Oxnard	93%	30
Saint Joseph Hospital[2]	Eureka	93%	28
Sutter General Hospital[2]	Sacramento	93%	105
Community Regional Medical Center[2]	Fresno	92%	114
Enloe Medical Center[2]	Chico	92%	80
Kaiser Foundation Hospital - West La[2]	Los Angeles	92%	52
Santa Barbara Cottage Hospital[2]	Santa Barbara	92%	39
Twin Cities Community Hospital[2]	Templeton	92%	39
Adventist Medical Center[2]	Hanford	91%	47
Fountain Valley Reg Hosp & Med Ctr[2]	Fountain Valley	91%	33
Kaiser Foundation Hospital - Los Angeles[2]	Los Angeles	91%	80
Kaiser Fdn Hosp-Orange Co-Anaheim[2]	Anaheim	91%	143
Loma Linda Univ Med Ctr-Murrieta[2]	Murrieta	91%	32
Marian Regional Medical Center[2]	Santa Maria	91%	34
Memorial Medical Center[2]	Modesto	91%	97
Huntington Memorial Hospital[2]	Pasadena	90%	77
Northbay Medical Center[2]	Fairfield	90%	42
Salinas Valley Memorial Hospital[2]	Salinas	90%	31
Contra Costa Regional Medical Center[2]	Martinez	88%	32
Eisenhower Medical Center[2]	Rancho Mirage	88%	65
Sutter Roseville Medical Center[2]	Roseville	88%	117
Torrance Memorial Medical Center[2]	Torrance	88%	67
Providence Holy Cross Medical Center[2]	Mission Hills	86%	43
San Antonio Community Hospital[2]	Upland	86%	44
Good Samaritan Hospital[2]	San Jose	85%	67
Mercy San Juan Medical Center[2]	Carmichael	85%	98
Riverside Community Hospital[2]	Riverside	85%	67
Univ of CA Davis Med Ctr[2]	Sacramento	84%	118
West Hills Hospital & Medical Center[2]	West Hills	84%	32
Sharp Memorial Hospital[2]	San Diego	83%	110
Simi Valley Hosp & Health Care Svcs[2]	Simi Valley	83%	30
Citrus Valley Medical Center - IC Campus[2]	Covina	82%	60
Desert Regional Medical Center[2]	Palm Springs	82%	56
Kaiser Fdn Hosp-S San Francisco[2]	S San Francisco	82%	34
Kaiser Fdn Hosp-San Francisco[2]	San Francisco	80%	49
Ahmc Anaheim Regional Medical Center[2]	Anaheim	78%	41
Kaiser Fdn Hosp-Panorama City[2]	Panorama City	78%	51
Methodist Hospital of Southern California[2]	Arcadia	78%	46
Saint Mary Medical Center[2]	Apple Valley	77%	81
Saint Mary Medical Center[2]	Long Beach	77%	26
Kaiser Foundation Hospital - Manteca[2]	Manteca	76%	50
Lodi Memorial Hospital[2]	Lodi	76%	41
Kaiser Foundation Hospital - Walnut Creek[2]	Walnut Creek	75%	93
Kaiser Fdn Hosp-Oakland/Richmond[2]	Oakland	74%	70
LAC/Olive View - UCLA Medical Center[2]	Sylmar	74%	42
Sharp Chula Vista Medical Center[2]	Chula Vista	73%	51
Kaiser Foundation Hospital - Santa Clara[2]	Santa Clara	72%	58
Lakewood Regional Medical Center[2]	Lakewood	72%	29
Santa Clara Valley Medical Center[2]	San Jose	72%	50
California Hosp Med Ctr Los Angeles[2]	Los Angeles	71%	42
Glendale Adventist Medical Center[2]	Glendale	71%	59
Mercy Medical Center[2]	Merced	71%	51
Alta Bates Summit Medical Center[2]	Berkeley	70%	30
Antelope Valley Hospital[2]	Lancaster	70%	97
Henry Mayo Newhall Memorial Hospital[2]	Valencia	69%	35
San Francisco General Hospital[2]	San Francisco	69%	42
Grossmont Hospital[2]	La Mesa	68%	99
Kaiser Foundation Hospital - Antioch[2]	Antioch	68%	71
Kaiser Foundation Hospital - San Jose[2]	San Jose	68%	59
Hemet Valley Medical Center[2]	Hemet	67%	43
Providence Tarzana Medical Center[2]	Tarzana	67%	46
Mission Hospital Regional Medical Center[2]	Mission Viejo	66%	101
Queen of the Valley Medical Center[2]	Napa	66%	32
Kaiser Foundation Hospital & Rehab Center[2]	Vallejo	64%	53
Providence Saint Joseph Medical Center[2]	Burbank	64%	58
Santa Monica-UCLA Med Ctr & Ortho Hosp[2]	Santa Monica	64%	47
Kaiser Foundation Hospital - Santa Rosa[2]	Santa Rosa	63%	38
Kaiser Foundation Hospital - Fresno[2]	Fresno	62%	55
Kaiser Foundation Hospital - Downey[2]	Downey	60%	81
Kaiser Foundation Hospital - Vacaville[2]	Vacaville	60%	25
Saddleback Memorial Medical Center[2]	Laguna Hills	60%	62
Saint Joseph Hospital[2]	Orange	58%	40
Kaiser Fdn Hosp-Fremont/Hayward[2]	Hayward	57%	46
Pomerado Hospital[2]	Poway	57%	30
Presbyterian Intercommunity Hospital[2]	Whittier	57%	82
Kaweah Delta Medical Center[2]	Visalia	56%	72
LAC+USC Medical Center[2]	Los Angeles	56%	52
Ronald Reagan UCLA Medical Center[2]	Los Angeles	55%	76
Saint Agnes Medical Center[2]	Fresno	54%	82
Comm Mem Hosp San Buenaventura[2]	Ventura	53%	53
San Joaquin Community Hospital[2]	Bakersfield	51%	80
Alta Bates Summit Medical Center[2]	Oakland	50%	28
Saint Francis Medical Center[2]	Lynwood	50%	62
Stanford Hospital[2]	Stanford	48%	98
Sutter Delta Medical Center[2]	Antioch	48%	29
Loma Linda University Medical Center[2]	Loma Linda	46%	71
Washington Hospital[2]	Fremont	46%	35
Eden Medical Center[2]	Castro Valley	45%	31
Long Beach Memorial Medical Center[2]	Long Beach	44%	68
Santa Rosa Memorial Hospital[2]	Santa Rosa	43%	42
Emanuel Medical Center[2]	Turlock	40%	30
Hi - Desert Medical Center[2]	Joshua Tree	39%	46
Kaiser Foundation Hospital[2]	San Rafael	39%	33
O'Connor Hospital[2]	San Jose	38%	29
Saint Jude Medical Center[2]	Fullerton	34%	47
Mills - Peninsula Medical Center[2]	Burlingame	31%	65
Rideout Memorial Hospital[2]	Marysville	27%	67
Valley Presbyterian Hospital[2]	Van Nuys	27%	33
Orange Coast Memorial Medical Center[2]	Fountain Valley	22%	51
Victor Valley Global Medical Center[2]	Victorville	19%	31
Arrowhead Regional Medical Center[2]	Colton	15%	46
Scripps Mercy Hospital[2]	San Diego	10%	137
Sierra Nevada Memorial Hospital[2]	Grass Valley	10%	30
Hoag Memorial Hospital Presbyterian[2]	Newport Beach	9%	128
Redlands Community Hospital[2]	Redlands	5%	38
Univ of CA San Diego Med Ctr[2]	San Diego	4%	99
Glendale Mem Hosp & Health Ctr[2]	Glendale	3%	31
Marina Del Rey Hospital[2]	Marina Del Rey	3%	39
CA Pacific Med Ctr-Pacific Campus Hosp[2]	San Francisco	2%	65
Alameda County Medical Center[2]	Oakland	0%	39
UCSF Medical Center[2]	San Francisco	0%	63

NOTE: Hospital profiles are in alphabetical order by state, then city, then hospital within the city; Rankings exclude hospitals with less than 25 cases except for patient surveys which excludes hospitals with less than 100 cases; (a) 100-299 cases; (1) The number of cases/patients is too few to report; (2) Data submitted were based on a sample of cases/patients; (3) Results are based on a shorter time period than required; (4) Data suppressed by CMS for one or more quarters; (5) Results are not available for this reporting period; (6) Fewer than 100 patients completed the HCAHPS survey; (7) No cases met the criteria for this measure; (8) The lower limit of the confidence interval cannot be calculated if the number of observed infections equals zero; (9) No data are available from the state/territory for this reporting period; (10) The scores shown reflect fewer than 50 completed surveys; (11) There were discrepancies in the data collection process; (12) This measure does not apply to this hospital for this reporting period; (13) Results cannot be calculated for this reporting period; (14) The results for this state are combined with nearby states to protect confidentiality; Please refer to the User's Guide for a full explanation of data.

Chest Pain/Possible Heart Attack Care

Aspirin Given Within 24 Hours of Arrival

Hospital Name	City	Rate	Cases
Chino Valley Medical Center	Chino	100%	38
Community Hospital of San Bernardino	San Bernardino	100%	39
Eden Medical Center	Castro Valley	100%	29
El Centro Regional Medical Center[3]	El Centro	100%	49
Feather River Hospital	Paradise	100%	26
Foothill Presbyterian Hospital	Glendora	100%	41
Fountain Valley Reg Hosp & Med Ctr	Fountain Valley	100%	56
Garden Grove Hospital & Medical Center	Garden Grove	100%	49
Henry Mayo Newhall Memorial Hospital	Valencia	100%	145
John Muir Med Ctr-Walnut Creek Campus	Walnut Creek	100%	46
Lodi Memorial Hospital	Lodi	100%	32
Lompoc Valley Medical Center	Lompoc	100%	55
Los Robles Hospital & Medical Center	Thousand Oaks	100%	29
Marshall Medical Center	Placerville	100%	62
Memorial Hospital of Gardena	Gardena	100%	40
Mercy Medical Center - Mount Shasta	Mount Shasta	100%	34
Monterey Park Hospital	Monterey Park	100%	26
Petaluma Valley Hospital	Petaluma	100%	50
Pioneers Memorial Healthcare District	Brawley	100%	47
Placentia Linda Hospital	Placentia	100%	61
Pomerado Hospital	Poway	100%	37
Pomona Valley Hospital Medical Center	Pomona	100%	45
Presbyterian Intercommunity Hospital	Whittier	100%	42
Prov Little Co of Mary Med Ctr Torrance	Torrance	100%	70
Queen of the Valley Medical Center	Napa	100%	41
Saint Francis Memorial Hospital	San Francisco	100%	28
Saint Johns Pleasant Valley Hospital	Camarillo	100%	55
Saint Louise Regional Hospital	Gilroy	100%	34
San Gorgonio Memorial Hospital	Banning	100%	97
Sherman Oaks Hospital	Sherman Oaks	100%	29
Simi Valley Hosp & Health Care Svcs	Simi Valley	100%	78
Sonora Regional Medical Center	Sonora	100%	86
Southwest Healthcare System	Murrieta	100%	151
Sutter Auburn Faith Hospital	Auburn	100%	45
Sutter Davis Hospital	Davis	100%	51
Sutter Solano Medical Center	Vallejo	100%	32
Ukiah Valley Medical Center	Ukiah	100%	37
Whittier Hospital Medical Center	Whittier	100%	36
Woodland Memorial Hospital	Woodland	100%	47
Hi - Desert Medical Center	Joshua Tree	99%	70
Mercy Hospital	Bakersfield	99%	78
Scripps Memorial Hospital - Encinitas	Encinitas	99%	67
Sierra Nevada Memorial Hospital	Grass Valley	99%	134
Sutter Coast Hospital	Crescent City	99%	88
Alta Bates Summit Medical Center	Berkeley	98%	41
Citrus Valley Medical Center - IC Campus	Covina	98%	56
Corona Regional Medical Center	Corona	98%	50
Mercy Hospital of Folsom	Folsom	98%	85
Methodist Hospital of Sacramento	Sacramento	98%	91
Riverside County Regional Medical Center	Moreno Valley	98%	53
Saddleback Memorial Medical Center	Laguna Hills	98%	42
Saint Jude Medical Center	Fullerton	98%	44
Sharp Chula Vista Medical Center	Chula Vista	98%	46
Sutter Amador Hospital	Jackson	98%	111
Sutter General Hospital	Sacramento	98%	61
Twin Cities Community Hospital	Templeton	98%	66
Banner Lassen Medical Center	Susanville	97%	32
Community Hospital of Long Beach	Long Beach	97%	38
Marina Del Rey Hospital	Marina Del Rey	97%	29
Memorial Hospital Los Banos	Los Banos	97%	38
Parkview Comm Hosp Med Ctr[3]	Riverside	97%	31
Santa Ynez Valley Cottage Hospital	Solvang	97%	34
Scripps Mercy Hospital	San Diego	97%	37
Sierra Vista Regional Medical Center	San Luis Obispo	97%	29
Tri - City Medical Center	Oceanside	97%	73
Beverly Hospital	Montebello	96%	25
Community Hospital of Huntington Park	Huntington Park	96%	54
Grossmont Hospital	La Mesa	96%	28
LAC/Olive View - UCLA Medical Center	Sylmar	96%	28
Mad River Community Hospital	Arcata	96%	26
Menifee Valley Medical Center	Sun City	96%	27
Mercy Medical Center	Merced	96%	102
Saint Elizabeth Community Hospital	Red Bluff	96%	77
Sutter Lakeside Hospital	Lakeport	96%	69
Arrowhead Regional Medical Center	Colton	95%	42
Oak Valley District Hospital	Oakdale	95%	40
Oroville Hospital	Oroville	95%	40
San Mateo Medical Center	San Mateo	95%	40
Barton Memorial Hospital	S Lake Tahoe	94%	34
Hemet Valley Medical Center	Hemet	93%	46
Long Beach Memorial Medical Center	Long Beach	93%	29
Redlands Community Hospital	Redlands	93%	56
Saint Mary Medical Center	Apple Valley	93%	46
Saint Francis Medical Center	Lynwood	92%	59
Adventist Medical Center	Hanford	90%	96
Ahmc Anaheim Regional Medical Center	Anaheim	90%	30
Novato Community Hospital	Novato	90%	29
California Hosp Med Ctr Los Angeles	Los Angeles	89%	27
Hazel Hawkins Memorial Hospital	Hollister	89%	55
Seton Medical Center	Daly City	89%	27
Coalinga Regional Medical Center	Coalinga	88%	32
Delano Regional Medical Center	Delano	88%	41
Palo Verde Hospital	Blythe	88%	40
Goleta Valley Cottage Hospital	Santa Barbara	86%	37
Univ of California Irvine Med Ctr	Orange	83%	36
Bear Valley Community Hospital	Big Bear Lake	82%	60
Kern Valley Healthcare District	Lake Isabella	73%	48

Average Time to ECG (minutes)

Hospital Name	City	Min.	Cases
Henry Mayo Newhall Memorial Hospital	Valencia	0	147
Long Beach Memorial Medical Center	Long Beach	0	29
Menifee Valley Medical Center	Sun City	0	27
Pomona Valley Hospital Medical Center	Pomona	0	47
Saint Jude Medical Center	Fullerton	0	52
Tri - City Medical Center	Oceanside	0	78
Presbyterian Intercommunity Hospital	Whittier	2	42
Prov Little Co of Mary Med Ctr Torrance	Torrance	2	77
Sutter Auburn Faith Hospital	Auburn	2	44
Placentia Linda Hospital	Placentia	3	65
Riverside County Regional Medical Center	Moreno Valley	3	54
Ahmc Anaheim Regional Medical Center	Anaheim	4	36
Beverly Hospital	Montebello	4	28
Univ of California Irvine Med Ctr	Orange	4	36
El Centro Regional Medical Center[3]	El Centro	5	51
Fountain Valley Reg Hosp & Med Ctr	Fountain Valley	5	57
Grossmont Hospital	La Mesa	5	27
Mercy Hospital of Folsom	Folsom	5	85
Saddleback Memorial Medical Center	Laguna Hills	5	43
Saint Mary Medical Center	Apple Valley	5	47
Santa Ynez Valley Cottage Hospital	Solvang	5	35
Barton Memorial Hospital	S Lake Tahoe	6	39
Community Hospital of San Bernardino	San Bernardino	6	42
Hi - Desert Medical Center	Joshua Tree	6	71
Lodi Memorial Hospital	Lodi	6	33
Oak Valley District Hospital	Oakdale	6	42
Simi Valley Hosp & Health Care Svcs	Simi Valley	6	83
Sutter Coast Hospital	Crescent City	6	92
Sutter General Hospital	Sacramento	6	64
Twin Cities Community Hospital	Templeton	6	72
Queen of the Valley Medical Center	Napa	7	40
San Gorgonio Memorial Hospital	Banning	7	103
Southwest Healthcare System	Murrieta	7	156
Sutter Davis Hospital	Davis	7	51
Citrus Valley Medical Center - IC Campus	Covina	8	58
Delano Regional Medical Center	Delano	8	41
Foothill Presbyterian Hospital	Glendora	8	41
John Muir Med Ctr-Walnut Creek Campus	Walnut Creek	8	46
Los Robles Hospital & Medical Center	Thousand Oaks	8	32
Palo Verde Hospital	Blythe	8	38
USC Verdugo Hills Hospital	Glendale	8	26
Marshall Medical Center	Placerville	9	67
Pioneers Memorial Healthcare District	Brawley	9	48
Saint Johns Pleasant Valley Hospital	Camarillo	9	55
Sherman Oaks Hospital	Sherman Oaks	9	29
Hemet Valley Medical Center	Hemet	10	48
LAC/Olive View - UCLA Medical Center	Sylmar	10	30
Memorial Hospital Los Banos	Los Banos	10	40
Methodist Hospital of Sacramento	Sacramento	10	94
Petaluma Valley Hospital	Petaluma	10	53
Prov Little Co of Mary Med Ctr San Pedro[3]	San Pedro	10	25
Redlands Community Hospital	Redlands	10	58
Sutter Solano Medical Center	Vallejo	10	33
Whittier Hospital Medical Center	Whittier	10	33
Alta Bates Summit Medical Center	Berkeley	11	42
Arrowhead Regional Medical Center	Colton	11	42
Community Hospital of Long Beach	Long Beach	11	39
Mercy Medical Center	Merced	11	103
Saint Elizabeth Community Hospital	Red Bluff	11	79
Scripps Mercy Hospital	San Diego	11	34
Sharp Chula Vista Medical Center	Chula Vista	11	49
Sonora Regional Medical Center	Sonora	11	86
Banner Lassen Medical Center	Susanville	12	36
Corona Regional Medical Center	Corona	12	57
Goleta Valley Cottage Hospital	Santa Barbara	12	38
Mad River Community Hospital	Arcata	12	26
Marian Regional Medical Center[3]	Santa Maria	12	26
Novato Community Hospital	Novato	12	28
Saint Francis Medical Center	Lynwood	12	61
Woodland Memorial Hospital	Woodland	12	48
Coalinga Regional Medical Center	Coalinga	13	32
Sutter Amador Hospital	Jackson	13	120
Adventist Medical Center	Hanford	14	96
Bear Valley Community Hospital	Big Bear Lake	14	58
Chino Valley Medical Center	Chino	14	40
Feather River Hospital	Paradise	14	26
Garden Grove Hospital & Medical Center	Garden Grove	14	48
Lompoc Valley Medical Center	Lompoc	14	56
Pomerado Hospital	Poway	14	37
Scripps Memorial Hospital - Encinitas	Encinitas	14	72
Ukiah Valley Medical Center	Ukiah	14	40
Kern Valley Healthcare District	Lake Isabella	15	47
Monterey Park Hospital	Monterey Park	15	27
San Mateo Medical Center	San Mateo	15	43
Sierra Vista Regional Medical Center	San Luis Obispo	15	29
Sierra Nevada Memorial Hospital	Grass Valley	16	136
Eden Medical Center	Castro Valley	17	29
Oroville Hospital	Oroville	17	40
Saint Louise Regional Hospital	Gilroy	17	36
Marina Del Rey Hospital	Marina Del Rey	19	30
Mercy Hospital	Bakersfield	19	82
Mercy Medical Center - Mount Shasta	Mount Shasta	19	37
Sutter Lakeside Hospital	Lakeport	20	74
Memorial Hospital of Gardena	Gardena	22	42
Saint Francis Memorial Hospital	San Francisco	22	28
Seton Medical Center	Daly City	23	27
Parkview Comm Hosp Med Ctr[3]	Riverside	25	33
Community Hospital of Huntington Park	Huntington Park	28	54
Hazel Hawkins Memorial Hospital	Hollister	28	54
California Hosp Med Ctr Los Angeles	Los Angeles	29	27

Average Time to Transfer (minutes)

Hospital Name	City	Min.	Cases
Adventist Medical Center	Hanford	67	37
Southwest Healthcare System	Murrieta	67	39
Mercy Hospital	Bakersfield	72	25

Children's Asthma Care

Received Home Management Plan of Care

Hospital Name	City	Rate	Cases
Miller Children's Hospital	Long Beach	98%	468
UCSF Medical Center	San Francisco	97%	32
Lucile Salter Packard Children's Hosp[2]	Palo Alto	95%	147
Children's Hospital of Los Angeles[2]	Los Angeles	93%	237
El Centro Regional Medical Center	El Centro	92%	38
Saint Francis Medical Center	Lynwood	91%	53
CA Pacific Med Ctr-Pacific Campus Hosp	San Francisco	79%	73
Univ of CA Davis Med Ctr[2]	Sacramento	54%	132
Loma Linda University Medical Center	Loma Linda	52%	210

Received Reliever Medication

Hospital Name	City	Rate	Cases
CA Pacific Med Ctr-Pacific Campus Hosp	San Francisco	100%	74
Children's Hospital of Los Angeles[2]	Los Angeles	100%	237
El Centro Regional Medical Center	El Centro	100%	38
Loma Linda University Medical Center	Loma Linda	100%	211
Lucile Salter Packard Children's Hosp	Palo Alto	100%	147
Miller Children's Hospital	Long Beach	100%	469
Saint Francis Medical Center	Lynwood	100%	55
UCSF Medical Center	San Francisco	100%	32
Univ of CA Davis Med Ctr	Sacramento	98%	132

Received Systemic Corticosteroids

Hospital Name	City	Rate	Cases
CA Pacific Med Ctr-Pacific Campus Hosp	San Francisco	100%	74
Children's Hospital of Los Angeles[2]	Los Angeles	100%	236
El Centro Regional Medical Center	El Centro	100%	38
Lucile Salter Packard Children's Hosp	Palo Alto	100%	147
Miller Children's Hospital	Long Beach	100%	468
Saint Francis Medical Center	Lynwood	100%	55
UCSF Medical Center	San Francisco	100%	32
Univ of CA Davis Med Ctr	Sacramento	100%	131
Loma Linda University Medical Center	Loma Linda	99%	210

Emergency Department

Admittance Decision Time (minutes)

Hospital Name	City	Min.	Cases
Colusa Regional Medical Center[2]	Colusa	30	327
Delano Regional Medical Center[2]	Delano	32	303
Kaiser Fdn Hosp-San Francisco[2]	San Francisco	41	332
Kaiser Foundation Hospital - Vacaville[2]	Vacaville	41	627
Kaiser Fdn Hosp-S San Francisco[2]	S San Francisco	44	624
Alhambra Hospital Medical Center[2]	Alhambra	45	644
Kaiser Foundation Hospital - Santa Rosa[2]	Santa Rosa	45	509
Sonoma Valley Hospital[2]	Sonoma	45	168
Kaiser Foundation Hospital[2]	San Rafael	47	665
Kaiser Foundation Hospital - Sacramento[2]	Sacramento	47	667
Kaiser Foundation Hospital - Antioch[2]	Antioch	48	537
Kaiser Foundation Hospital - Manteca[2]	Manteca	48	440
Kaiser Foundation Hospital - Roseville[2]	Roseville	48	418
Encino Hospital Medical Center[2]	Encino	50	541
Kaiser Fdn Hosp-Fremont/Hayward[2]	Hayward	50	542
Kaiser Fdn Hosp-Oakland/Richmond[2]	Oakland	50	525
Kaiser Foundation Hospital - Redwood City[2]	Redwood City	50	426

NOTE: Hospital profiles are in alphabetical order by state, then city, then hospital within the city; Rankings exclude hospitals with less than 25 cases except for patient surveys which excludes hospitals with less than 100 cases; (a) 100-299 cases; (1) The number of cases/patients is too few to report; (2) Data submitted were based on a sample of cases/patients; (3) Results are based on a shorter time period than required; (4) Data suppressed by CMS for one or more quarters; (5) Results are not available for this reporting period; (6) Fewer than 100 patients completed the HCAHPS survey; (7) No cases met the criteria for this measure; (8) The lower limit of the confidence interval cannot be calculated if the number of observed infections equals zero; (9) No data are available from the state/territory for this reporting period; (10) The scores shown reflect fewer than 50 completed surveys; (11) There were discrepancies in the data collection process; (12) This measure does not apply to this hospital for this reporting period; (13) Results cannot be calculated for this reporting period; (14) The results for this state are combined with nearby states to protect confidentiality; Please refer to the User's Guide for a full explanation of data.

Kaiser Foundation Hospital - Santa Clara[2]	Santa Clara	51	428
Kaiser Foundation Hospital & Rehab Center[2]	Vallejo	52	494
Kaiser Foundation Hospital - Fresno[2]	Fresno	52	652
Kaiser Fdn Hosp S Sacramento[2]	Sacramento	53	565
Coalinga Regional Medical Center[2]	Coalinga	54	182
Kaiser Foundation Hospital - San Jose[2]	San Jose	57	507
Saint Mary's Medical Center[2]	San Francisco	57	459
Watsonville Community Hospital[2]	Watsonville	57	444
Sharp Coronado Hosp & Healthcare Ctr[2]	Coronado	58	319
Western Medical Center Santa Ana[2]	Santa Ana	58	113
Kaiser Foundation Hospital - Walnut Creek[2]	Walnut Creek	59	557
Fairchild Medical Center[2,3]	Yreka	60	216
Palo Verde Hospital[2]	Blythe	62	494
East Valley Hospital Medical Center[2]	Glendora	63	798
Chino Valley Medical Center[2]	Chino	65	974
Garfield Medical Center[2]	Monterey Park	65	457
Los Angeles Community Hospital[2]	Los Angeles	65	627
Monterey Park Hospital[2]	Monterey Park	65	395
Montclair Hospital Medical Center[2]	Montclair	66	527
Coast Plaza Hospital[2]	Norwalk	67	531
San Dimas Community Hospital[2]	San Dimas	67	593
Enloe Medical Center[2]	Chico	68	646
La Palma Intercommunity Hospital[2]	La Palma	68	466
Memorial Hospital Los Banos[2]	Los Banos	68	152
Paradise Valley Hospital[2]	National City	68	700
Mammoth Hospital[3]	Mammoth Lakes	69	182
Pacific Hospital of Long Beach[2,3]	Long Beach	69	129
Fallbrook Hospital[2]	Fallbrook	70	315
Mission Community Hospital[2]	Panorama City	71	316
Pacific Alliance Medical Center[2]	Los Angeles	71	99
Placentia Linda Hospital[2]	Placentia	71	604
Woodland Memorial Hospital[2]	Woodland	71	345
Kaiser Fdn Hosp-Moreno Valley[2]	Moreno Valley	72	441
Comm Hosp of the Monterey Peninsula[2]	Monterey	73	317
Ojai Valley Community Hospital[2]	Ojai	74	410
Sutter Davis Hospital[2]	Davis	74	261
Chinese Hospital[2]	San Francisco	75	454
Coastal Communities Hospital[2]	Santa Ana	75	274
Hoag Memorial Hospital Presbyterian[2]	Newport Beach	75	906
Sharp Memorial Hospital[2]	San Diego	75	443
Tri - City Regional Medical Center[2]	Hawaiian Grdns	75	366
Glendale Mem Hosp & Health Ctr[2]	Glendale	76	509
Kaiser Foundation Hospital - Baldwin Park[2]	Baldwin Park	76	434
Santa Ynez Valley Cottage Hospital	Solvang	77	175
French Hospital Medical Center[2]	San Luis Obispo	78	440
Kaiser Fdn Hosp-Orange Co-Anaheim[2]	Anaheim	78	402
Kaiser Foundation Hospital - South Bay[2]	Harbor City	78	372
Doctors Medical Center - San Pablo[2]	San Pablo	80	490
El Camino Hospital[2]	Mountain View	80	393
Huntington Beach Hospital[2]	Huntington Bch	80	632
Mark Twain Medical Center[2]	San Andreas	80	534
Mercy Hospital of Folsom[2]	Folsom	80	695
Kaiser Foundation Hospital - West La[2]	Los Angeles	81	449
Saint Louise Regional Hospital[2]	Gilroy	81	374
Orange Coast Memorial Medical Center[2]	Fountain Valley	82	636
USC Verdugo Hills Hospital[2]	Glendale	82	593
San Gabriel Valley Medical Center[2]	San Gabriel	84	472
Whittier Hospital Medical Center[2]	Whittier	84	372
Bear Valley Community Hospital	Big Bear Lake	85	52
Corcoran District Hospital[2,3]	Corcoran	85	37
Goleta Valley Cottage Hospital[2]	Santa Barbara	85	249
Greater El Monte Community Hospital[2]	South El Monte	85	417
Mercy General Hospital[2]	Sacramento	85	422
Ukiah Valley Medical Center[2]	Ukiah	85	456
Sierra Vista Regional Medical Center[2]	San Luis Obispo	86	475
Kaiser Fdn Hosp-Woodland Hills[2]	Woodland Hills	87	369
Saint Helena Hospital[2]	Saint Helena	88	135
Hazel Hawkins Memorial Hospital[2]	Hollister	89	470
San Ramon Regional Medical Center[2]	San Ramon	89	491
Ahmc Anaheim Regional Medical Center[2]	Anaheim	90	543
Kaiser Fdn Hosp-Panorama City[2]	Panorama City	92	505
Scripps Memorial Hospital - Encinitas[2]	Encinitas	92	481
Sutter Amador Hospital[2]	Jackson	92	390
Tri - City Medical Center[2]	Oceanside	92	563
CA Pacific Med Ctr-Pacific Campus Hosp[2]	San Francisco	95	296
Doctors Hospital of Manteca[2]	Manteca	95	425
Sutter Tracy Community Hospital[2]	Tracy	95	468
Kaiser Foundation Hospital - Fontana[2]	Fontana	96	445
Kaiser Foundation Hospital - San Diego[2]	San Diego	96	411
Sequoia Hospital[2]	Redwood City	96	452
Alvarado Hospital Medical Center[2]	San Diego	97	423
Kaiser Foundation Hospital - Riverside[2]	Riverside	97	298
Pacifica Hospital of the Valley[2]	Sun Valley	97	435
Marshall Medical Center[2]	Placerville	98	666
Santa Barbara Cottage Hospital[2]	Santa Barbara	99	525
Tahoe Forest Hospital[2]	Truckee	99	275
Community Hospital of Long Beach[2]	Long Beach	100	383
Mercy Medical Center - Mount Shasta[2]	Mount Shasta	100	321
Saint Agnes Medical Center[2]	Fresno	101	611
Saint Jude Medical Center[2]	Fullerton	101	485
George L Mee Memorial Hospital[2]	King City	102	92
Parkview Comm Hosp Med Ctr[2]	Riverside	102	218
Saint Vincent Medical Center[2]	Los Angeles	102	697
Tulare Regional Medical Center[2]	Tulare	104	360
Adventist Medical Center - Reedley[2]	Reedley	105	69
East Los Angeles Doctors Hospital[2]	Los Angeles	105	249
Kaweah Delta Medical Center[2]	Visalia	105	612
Mad River Community Hospital[2]	Arcata	105	305
Mission Hospital Regional Medical Center[2]	Mission Viejo	105	487
Olympia Medical Center[2]	Los Angeles	105	748
Sierra View District Hospital[2]	Porterville	105	668
Garden Grove Hospital & Medical Center[2]	Garden Grove	106	602
Mills - Peninsula Medical Center[2]	Burlingame	106	583
Saint Elizabeth Community Hospital[2]	Red Bluff	106	330
Scripps Memorial Hospital La Jolla[2]	La Jolla	106	349
Cedars - Sinai Medical Center[2]	Los Angeles	107	396
Lompoc Valley Medical Center[2]	Lompoc	107	259
Feather River Hospital[2]	Paradise	108	614
Sherman Oaks Hospital[2]	Sherman Oaks	110	654
Univ of California Irvine Med Ctr[2]	Orange	110	410
Western Medical Center Hospital Anaheim[2]	Anaheim	110	238
Novato Community Hospital[2]	Novato	111	327
Saint Rose Hospital[2]	Hayward	111	718
Alameda Hospital[2]	Alameda	112	450
Torrance Memorial Medical Center[2]	Torrance	112	828
Providence Saint Joseph Medical Center[2]	Burbank	113	524
Valleycare Medical Center[2]	Pleasanton	113	597
Eisenhower Medical Center[2]	Rancho Mirage	114	1240
CA Pacific Med Ctr-Davies Campus[2]	San Francisco	115	254
Northridge Hospital Medical Center[2]	Northridge	115	783
PIH Hospital - Downey[2]	Downey	115	259
Presbyterian Intercommunity Hospital[2]	Whittier	115	587
Community Hospital of Huntington Park[2]	Huntington Park	116	403
Kaiser Foundation Hospital - Downey[2]	Downey	116	389
Methodist Hospital of Southern California[2]	Arcadia	116	747
Simi Valley Hosp & Health Care Svcs[2]	Simi Valley	116	771
Dominican Hospital[2]	Santa Cruz	117	725
Queen of the Valley Medical Center[2]	Napa	117	691
Marian Regional Medical Center[2]	Santa Maria	118	765
Salinas Valley Memorial Hospital[2]	Salinas	119	555
Barstow Community Hospital[2]	Barstow	120	441
Huntington Memorial Hospital[2]	Pasadena	121	578
CA Pacific Med Ctr-St Luke's Campus[2]	San Francisco	123	342
Good Samaritan Hospital[2]	Los Angeles	125	381
Prov Little Co of Mary Med Ctr San Pedro[2]	San Pedro	126	703
Mercy Medical Center[2]	Merced	127	467
Redwood Memorial Hospital[2]	Fortuna	127	248
Sonora Regional Medical Center[2]	Sonora	129	446
Hi - Desert Medical Center[2]	Joshua Tree	130	432
Palm Drive Hospital[2]	Sebastopol	130	387
Citrus Valley Medical Center - IC Campus[2]	Covina	132	566
Lakewood Regional Medical Center[2]	Lakewood	132	990
Adventist Medical Center[2]	Hanford	133	1050
Alta Bates Summit Medical Center[2]	Berkeley	133	291
Centinela Hospital Medical Center[2]	Inglewood	133	1020
Lodi Memorial Hospital[2]	Lodi	133	759
Barton Memorial Hospital[2]	S Lake Tahoe	134	270
Shasta Regional Medical Center[2]	Redding	134	1033
Pomerado Hospital[2]	Poway	136	504
Beverly Hospital[2]	Montebello	138	732
Foothill Presbyterian Hospital[2]	Glendora	139	667
Seton Medical Center[2]	Daly City	139	790
Saint Mary Medical Center[2]	Long Beach	140	464
Emanuel Medical Center[2]	Turlock	141	883
Grossmont Hospital[2]	La Mesa	142	726
Long Beach Memorial Medical Center[2]	Long Beach	142	814
Marina Del Rey Hospital[2]	Marina Del Rey	142	536
Providence Holy Cross Medical Center[2]	Mission Hills	142	535
West Anaheim Medical Center[2]	Anaheim	142	1133
Fountain Valley Reg Hosp & Med Ctr[2]	Fountain Valley	143	597
John F Kennedy Memorial Hospital[2]	Indio	143	457
Los Alamitos Medical Center[2]	Los Alamitos	143	689
Mercy San Juan Medical Center[2]	Carmichael	143	686
Palomar Health Downtown Campus[2]	Escondido	143	519
Twin Cities Community Hospital[2]	Templeton	144	787
San Leandro Hospital[2,3]	San Leandro	145	224
Natividad Medical Center[2]	Salinas	146	362
Santa Rosa Memorial Hospital[2]	Santa Rosa	146	679
Scripps Mercy Hospital[2]	San Diego	146	581
Petaluma Valley Hospital[2]	Petaluma	147	339
Saint Francis Medical Center[2]	Lynwood	147	422
John Muir Medical Center - Concord Campus[2]	Concord	148	827
Saint Francis Memorial Hospital[2]	San Francisco	148	643
Memorial Medical Center[2]	Modesto	149	792
Eden Medical Center[2]	Castro Valley	150	913
Menifee Valley Medical Center[2]	Sun City	150	275
Sutter Medical Center of Santa Rosa[2]	Santa Rosa	150	337
Sutter Roseville Medical Center[2]	Roseville	150	705
Comm Mem Hosp San Buenaventura[2]	Ventura	151	445
Saint Joseph Hospital[2]	Orange	151	79
Sutter Auburn Faith Hospital[2]	Auburn	151	642
Valley Presbyterian Hospital[2]	Van Nuys	151	160
Dameron Hospital[2]	Stockton	152	531
Saddleback Memorial Medical Center[2]	Laguna Hills	152	657
Stanford Hospital[2]	Stanford	152	409
Alta Bates Summit Medical Center[2]	Oakland	154	848
Henry Mayo Newhall Memorial Hospital[2]	Valencia	158	770
California Hosp Med Ctr Los Angeles[2]	Los Angeles	159	557
Sierra Nevada Memorial Hospital[2]	Grass Valley	159	789
Southwest Healthcare System[2]	Murrieta	160	577
Sutter Delta Medical Center[2]	Antioch	160	704
Hemet Valley Medical Center[2]	Hemet	161	420
John Muir Med Ctr-Walnut Creek Campus[2]	Walnut Creek	161	591
Corona Regional Medical Center[2]	Corona	164	529
Sharp Chula Vista Medical Center[2]	Chula Vista	164	752
Los Robles Hospital & Medical Center[2]	Thousand Oaks	165	695
Marin General Hospital[2]	Greenbrae	165	525
Providence Tarzana Medical Center[2]	Tarzana	166	609
Northbay Medical Center[2]	Fairfield	167	722
San Antonio Community Hospital[2]	Upland	167	656
Oroville Hospital[2]	Oroville	168	996
Community Hospital of San Bernardino[2]	San Bernardino	170	226
Providence Saint John's Health Center[2]	Santa Monica	170	233
Sutter Lakeside Hospital[2]	Lakeport	170	189
Glendale Adventist Medical Center[2]	Glendale	171	695
Mercy Medical Center - Redding[2]	Redding	173	508
San Mateo Medical Center[2]	San Mateo	173	418
Chapman Medical Center[2]	Orange	175	161
Good Samaritan Hospital[2]	San Jose	175	555
O'Connor Hospital[2]	San Jose	175	455
Saint Johns Regional Medical Center[2]	Oxnard	178	463
Saint Joseph's Medical Center of Stockton[2]	Stockton	180	730
Saint Johns Pleasant Valley Hospital[2]	Camarillo	181	455
Desert Regional Medical Center[2]	Palm Springs	182	652
Victor Valley Global Medical Center[2]	Victorville	182	415
Sutter Coast Hospital[2]	Crescent City	184	153
San Joaquin General Hospital[2]	French Camp	185	482
Doctors Medical Center[2]	Modesto	186	579
Washington Hospital[2]	Fremont	188	470
Sutter General Hospital[2]	Sacramento	191	362
Methodist Hospital of Sacramento[2]	Sacramento	194	660
San Gorgonio Memorial Hospital[2]	Banning	195	331
LAC+USC Medical Center[2]	Los Angeles	198	687
Saint Joseph Hospital[2]	Eureka	200	294
Hollywood Presbyterian Medical Center[2]	Los Angeles	203	340
White Memorial Medical Center[2]	Los Angeles	212	478
Rideout Memorial Hospital[2]	Marysville	214	454
Contra Costa Regional Medical Center[2]	Martinez	217	467
UCSF Medical Center[2]	San Francisco	218	233
Mercy Hospital[2]	Bakersfield	224	665
Madera Community Hospital[2]	Madera	225	805
Santa Clara Valley Medical Center[2]	San Jose	227	545
LAC/Harbor - UCLA Medical Center[2]	Torrance	230	731
Pomona Valley Hospital Medical Center[2]	Pomona	233	337
Bakersfield Heart Hospital[2]	Bakersfield	235	510
Sutter Solano Medical Center[2]	Vallejo	236	646
Redlands Community Hospital[2]	Redlands	238	320
Kern Medical Center[2]	Bakersfield	242	107
San Francisco General Hospital[2]	San Francisco	242	730
El Centro Regional Medical Center[2]	El Centro	244	711
Desert Valley Hospital[2]	Victorville	246	877
Prov Little Co of Mary Med Ctr Torrance[2]	Torrance	247	727
Bakersfield Memorial Hospital[2]	Bakersfield	248	654
Pioneers Memorial Healthcare District[2]	Brawley	255	533
Saint Mary Medical Center[2]	Apple Valley	255	784
Regional Medical Center of San Jose[2]	San Jose	258	1138
Riverside Community Hospital[2]	Riverside	260	644
Ventura County Medical Center[2]	Ventura	260	526
Memorial Hospital of Gardena[2]	Gardena	262	786
Univ of CA Davis Med Ctr[2]	Sacramento	262	597
Kaiser Foundation Hospital - Los Angeles[2]	Los Angeles	265	351
West Hills Hospital & Medical Center[2]	West Hills	265	759
San Joaquin Community Hospital[2]	Bakersfield	276	604
Antelope Valley Hospital[2]	Lancaster	278	622
Univ of CA San Diego Med Ctr[2]	San Diego	287	494
LAC/Olive View - UCLA Medical Center[2]	Sylmar	291	833
Santa Monica-UCLA Med Ctr & Ortho Hosp[2]	Santa Monica	291	547
Ronald Reagan UCLA Medical Center[2]	Los Angeles	294	484
Loma Linda University Medical Center[2]	Loma Linda	295	505
San Bernardino Medical Center[2]	San Bernardino	300	445
Palmdale Regional Medical Center[2]	Palmdale	309	889
Loma Linda Univ Med Ctr-Murrieta[2]	Murrieta	312	1004
Clovis Community Medical Center[2]	Clovis	428	334
Arrowhead Regional Medical Center[2]	Colton	430	1047
Alameda County Medical Center[2]	Oakland	451	467
Community Regional Medical Center[2]	Fresno	462	657
Riverside County Regional Medical Center[2]	Moreno Valley	565	481

Head CT Results Within 45 Minutes of Arrival

Hospital Name	City	Rate	Cases
Paradise Valley Hospital	National City	89%	36
Methodist Hospital of Sacramento	Sacramento	87%	30
Mercy Hospital of Folsom	Folsom	82%	28

NOTE: Hospital profiles are in alphabetical order by state, then city, then hospital within the city; Rankings exclude hospitals with less than 25 cases except for patient surveys which excludes hospitals with less than 100 cases; (a) 100-299 cases; (1) The number of cases/patients is too few to report; (2) Data submitted were based on a sample of cases/patients; (3) Results are based on a shorter time period than required; (4) Data suppressed by CMS for one or more quarters; (5) Results are not available for this reporting period; (6) Fewer than 100 patients completed the HCAHPS survey; (7) No cases met the criteria for this measure; (8) The lower limit of the confidence interval cannot be calculated if the number of observed infections equals zero; (9) No data are available from the state/territory for this reporting period; (10) The scores shown reflect fewer than 50 completed surveys; (11) There were discrepancies in the data collection process; (12) This measure does not apply to this hospital for this reporting period; (13) Results cannot be calculated for this reporting period; (14) The results for this state are combined with nearby states to protect confidentiality; Please refer to the User's Guide for a full explanation of data.

Scripps Mercy Hospital	San Diego	79%	38
Corona Regional Medical Center	Corona	77%	47
San Gorgonio Memorial Hospital	Banning	77%	35
Presbyterian Intercommunity Hospital	Whittier	70%	30
Lakewood Regional Medical Center	Lakewood	62%	32
Northbay Medical Center	Fairfield	62%	50
John Muir Medical Center - Concord Campus	Concord	61%	38
Mercy Medical Center	Merced	54%	26
Sutter Lakeside Hospital	Lakeport	38%	32
Memorial Hospital Los Banos	Los Banos	27%	51
Adventist Medical Center	Hanford	26%	27
Emanuel Medical Center	Turlock	24%	29
Saint Mary Medical Center	Apple Valley	23%	31

Patients Who Left ER Before Being Seen

Hospital Name	City	Rate	Cases
Adventist Medical Center - Reedley	Reedley	0%	48835
Alameda Hospital	Alameda	0%	16815
Dameron Hospital	Stockton	0%	43601
East Valley Hospital Medical Center	Glendora	0%	4647
El Camino Hospital	Mountain View	0%	55528
Encino Hospital Medical Center	Encino	0%	9443
French Hospital Medical Center	San Luis Obispo	0%	16875
Glendale Adventist Medical Center	Glendale	0%	46146
Hi - Desert Medical Center	Joshua Tree	0%	22627
John Muir Med Ctr-Walnut Creek Campus	Walnut Creek	0%	47283
Los Robles Hospital & Medical Center	Thousand Oaks	0%	40563
Mark Twain Medical Center	San Andreas	0%	9398
Mercy Hospital of Folsom	Folsom	0%	33626
Mercy Medical Center - Mount Shasta	Mount Shasta	0%	8017
Olympia Medical Center	Los Angeles	0%	25247
Pioneers Memorial Healthcare District	Brawley	0%	43852
Pomerado Hospital	Poway	0%	20062
Pomona Valley Hospital Medical Center	Pomona	0%	81925
Saint Bernardine Medical Center	San Bernardino	0%	73545
Saint Helena Hospital	Saint Helena	0%	7446
Saint Johns Pleasant Valley Hospital	Camarillo	0%	19276
Saint Mary's Medical Center	San Francisco	0%	17503
Santa Ynez Valley Cottage Hospital	Solvang	0%	6696
Scripps Memorial Hospital La Jolla	La Jolla	0%	32328
Seton Medical Center	Daly City	0%	26323
Sierra Nevada Memorial Hospital	Grass Valley	0%	42386
Sierra Vista Regional Medical Center	San Luis Obispo	0%	21387
Simi Valley Hosp & Health Care Svcs	Simi Valley	0%	30155
Stanford Hospital	Stanford	0%	54101
Sutter Auburn Faith Hospital	Auburn	0%	245406
West Hills Hospital & Medical Center	West Hills	0%	39178
Adventist Medical Center	Hanford	1%	104919
Alhambra Hospital Medical Center	Alhambra	1%	13309
Bear Valley Community Hospital	Big Bear Lake	1%	10210
CA Pacific Med Ctr-Davies Campus	San Francisco	1%	14323
CA Pacific Med Ctr-Pacific Campus Hosp	San Francisco	1%	49007
Chinese Hospital	San Francisco	1%	6187
Chino Valley Medical Center	Chino	1%	38090
Clovis Community Medical Center	Clovis	1%	41189
Coalinga Regional Medical Center	Coalinga	1%	9187
Coastal Communities Hospital	Santa Ana	1%	21305
Colusa Regional Medical Center	Colusa	1%	6122
Community Hospital of San Bernardino	San Bernardino	1%	51113
Comm Mem Hosp San Buenaventura	Ventura	1%	40782
Desert Regional Medical Center	Palm Springs	1%	61648
Doctors Medical Center	Modesto	1%	85151
Doctors Medical Center - San Pablo	San Pablo	1%	90506
Eisenhower Medical Center	Rancho Mirage	1%	68057
Emanuel Medical Center	Turlock	1%	61364
Fountain Valley Reg Hosp & Med Ctr	Fountain Valley	1%	42133
Garden Grove Hospital & Medical Center	Garden Grove	1%	27212
Glendale Mem Hosp & Health Ctr	Glendale	1%	33067
Goleta Valley Cottage Hospital	Santa Barbara	1%	18694
Good Samaritan Hospital	San Jose	1%	44761
John Muir Medical Center - Concord Campus	Concord	1%	51705
Kaweah Delta Medical Center	Visalia	1%	85222
Kern Medical Center	Bakersfield	1%	35287
Long Beach Memorial Medical Center	Long Beach	1%	91800
Los Angeles Community Hospital	Los Angeles	1%	12230
Marian Regional Medical Center	Santa Maria	1%	61779
Marin General Hospital	Greenbrae	1%	35312
Mercy General Hospital	Sacramento	1%	41070
Mercy Hospital	Bakersfield	1%	72221
Mercy Medical Center	Merced	1%	65530
Mercy San Juan Medical Center	Carmichael	1%	69804
Methodist Hospital of Sacramento	Sacramento	1%	56353
Mills - Peninsula Medical Center	Burlingame	1%	47335
Mission Hospital Regional Medical Center	Mission Viejo	1%	56025
Natividad Medical Center	Salinas	1%	46413
Northridge Hospital Medical Center	Northridge	1%	58288
Oak Valley District Hospital	Oakdale	1%	19873
Ojai Valley Community Hospital	Ojai	1%	8106
Orange Coast Memorial Medical Center	Fountain Valley	1%	29129
Pacific Alliance Medical Center	Los Angeles	1%	11260
Palomar Health Downtown Campus	Escondido	1%	80208
Petaluma Valley Hospital	Petaluma	1%	17267
Placentia Linda Hospital	Placentia	1%	24718
Providence Holy Cross Medical Center	Mission Hills	1%	81982
Prov Little Co of Mary Med Ctr San Pedro	San Pedro	1%	37199
Queen of the Valley Medical Center	Napa	1%	29872
Redlands Community Hospital	Redlands	1%	44009
Rideout Memorial Hospital	Marysville	1%	50795
Riverside Community Hospital	Riverside	1%	81747
Saint Elizabeth Community Hospital	Red Bluff	1%	30472
Saint Francis Memorial Hospital	San Francisco	1%	33052
Saint Johns Regional Medical Center	Oxnard	1%	49229
Saint Joseph's Medical Center of Stockton	Stockton	1%	54159
Saint Vincent Medical Center	Los Angeles	1%	15175
Salinas Valley Memorial Hospital	Salinas	1%	43272
San Gabriel Valley Medical Center	San Gabriel	1%	25408
San Gorgonio Memorial Hospital	Banning	1%	34240
San Joaquin Community Hospital	Bakersfield	1%	71603
San Ramon Regional Medical Center	San Ramon	1%	16969
Santa Barbara Cottage Hospital	Santa Barbara	1%	44200
Santa Monica-UCLA Med Ctr & Ortho Hosp	Santa Monica	1%	41070
Scripps Memorial Hospital - Encinitas	Encinitas	1%	42460
Sequoia Hospital	Redwood City	1%	21019
Sharp Coronado Hosp & Healthcare Ctr	Coronado	1%	12134
Sharp Memorial Hospital	San Diego	1%	70523
Sherman Oaks Hospital	Sherman Oaks	1%	20962
Sonora Regional Medical Center	Sonora	1%	26725
Southwest Healthcare System	Murrieta	1%	79904
Sutter Amador Hospital	Jackson	1%	19025
Sutter Davis Hospital	Davis	1%	23208
Twin Cities Community Hospital	Templeton	1%	27524
Ukiah Valley Medical Center	Ukiah	1%	22200
USC Verdugo Hills Hospital	Glendale	1%	19058
Valleycare Medical Center	Pleasanton	1%	30229
Whittier Hospital Medical Center	Whittier	1%	26843
Woodland Memorial Hospital	Woodland	1%	21134
Bakersfield Memorial Hospital	Bakersfield	2%	75277
Banner Lassen Medical Center	Susanville	2%	10637
Barton Memorial Hospital	S Lake Tahoe	2%	19024
Beverly Hospital	Montebello	2%	34293
California Hosp Med Ctr Los Angeles	Los Angeles	2%	66747
Comm Hosp of the Monterey Peninsula	Monterey	2%	33170
Dominican Hospital	Santa Cruz	2%	42944
El Centro Regional Medical Center	El Centro	2%	39976
Fallbrook Hospital	Fallbrook	2%	11077
Feather River Hospital	Paradise	2%	23224
Foothill Presbyterian Hospital	Glendora	2%	30494
George L Mee Memorial Hospital	King City	2%	10141
Hazel Hawkins Memorial Hospital	Hollister	2%	16059
Hoag Memorial Hospital Presbyterian	Newport Beach	2%	68348
La Palma Intercommunity Hospital	La Palma	2%	15117
Lakewood Regional Medical Center	Lakewood	2%	45691
Loma Linda Univ Med Ctr-Murrieta	Murrieta	2%	34407
Madera Community Hospital	Madera	2%	44006
Marina Del Rey Hospital	Marina Del Rey	2%	22383
Marshall Medical Center	Placerville	2%	27700
Mercy Medical Center - Redding	Redding	2%	48804
Methodist Hospital of Southern California	Arcadia	2%	42996
Northbay Medical Center	Fairfield	2%	70630
Novato Community Hospital	Novato	2%	15015
O'Connor Hospital	San Jose	2%	54195
Pacific Hospital of Long Beach	Long Beach	2%	14435
Palo Verde Hospital	Blythe	2%	10459
Providence Saint John's Health Center	Santa Monica	2%	30372
Providence Saint Joseph Medical Center	Burbank	2%	63821
Providence Tarzana Medical Center	Tarzana	2%	34829
Regional Medical Center of San Jose	San Jose	2%	61126
Ronald Reagan UCLA Medical Center	Los Angeles	2%	46302
Saddleback Memorial Medical Center	Laguna Hills	2%	36683
Saint Jude Medical Center	Fullerton	2%	61664
Saint Mary Medical Center	Apple Valley	2%	81050
Saint Mary Medical Center	Long Beach	2%	55488
Saint Rose Hospital	Hayward	2%	35634
San Antonio Community Hospital	Upland	2%	74197
San Dimas Community Hospital	San Dimas	2%	15307
Scripps Mercy Hospital	San Diego	2%	110954
Sonoma Valley Hospital	Sonoma	2%	9492
Southern California Hospital at Hollywood	Hollywood	2%	25914
Sutter Coast Hospital	Crescent City	2%	21969
Sutter Roseville Medical Center	Roseville	2%	74081
Sutter Solano Medical Center	Vallejo	2%	39175
Tri - City Regional Medical Center	Hawaiian Grdns	2%	8548
Univ of CA San Diego Med Ctr	San Diego	2%	66694
Washington Hospital	Fremont	2%	12969
Watsonville Community Hospital	Watsonville	2%	27535
White Memorial Medical Center	Los Angeles	2%	52835
Alta Bates Summit Medical Center	Berkeley	3%	45109
Alta Bates Summit Medical Center	Oakland	3%	44877
Arrowhead Regional Medical Center	Colton	3%	114728
Cedars - Sinai Medical Center	Los Angeles	3%	87184
Chapman Medical Center	Orange	3%	9622
Coast Plaza Hospital	Norwalk	3%	13289
College Hospital Costa Mesa	Costa Mesa	3%	859
Corona Regional Medical Center	Corona	3%	43126
Delano Regional Medical Center	Delano	3%	22399
Eden Medical Center	Castro Valley	3%	51663
Enloe Medical Center	Chico	3%	45300
Garfield Medical Center	Monterey Park	3%	22974
Hemet Valley Medical Center	Hemet	3%	48911
Henry Mayo Newhall Memorial Hospital	Valencia	3%	49684
Huntington Beach Hospital	Huntington Bch	3%	17922
Lodi Memorial Hospital	Lodi	3%	31480
Lompoc Valley Medical Center	Lompoc	3%	20877
Los Alamitos Medical Center	Los Alamitos	3%	30503
Mad River Community Hospital	Arcata	3%	15811
Menifee Valley Medical Center	Sun City	3%	16930
Mission Community Hospital	Panorama City	3%	19964
Montclair Hospital Medical Center	Montclair	3%	21282
Monterey Park Hospital	Monterey Park	3%	11960
Palm Drive Hospital	Sebastopol	3%	7801
Parkview Comm Hosp Med Ctr	Riverside	3%	43901
Presbyterian Intercommunity Hospital	Whittier	3%	70349
Prov Little Co of Mary Med Ctr Torrance	Torrance	3%	66748
Saint Joseph Hospital	Eureka	3%	25913
Saint Joseph Hospital	Orange	3%	114560
Saint Louise Regional Hospital	Gilroy	3%	26450
Sharp Chula Vista Medical Center	Chula Vista	3%	36032
Shasta Regional Medical Center	Redding	3%	38956
Sierra View District Hospital	Porterville	3%	43805
Sutter Delta Medical Center	Antioch	3%	55628
Sutter General Hospital	Sacramento	3%	88048
Sutter Lakeside Hospital	Lakeport	3%	19157
Sutter Medical Center of Santa Rosa	Santa Rosa	3%	26618
Sutter Tracy Community Hospital	Tracy	3%	32559
Western Medical Center Santa Ana	Santa Ana	3%	25160
Ahmc Anaheim Regional Medical Center	Anaheim	4%	42172
Antelope Valley Hospital	Lancaster	4%	106300
Bakersfield Heart Hospital	Bakersfield	4%	12375
CA Pacific Med Ctr-St Luke's Campus	San Francisco	4%	27639
Community Hospital of Long Beach	Long Beach	4%	22721
Doctors Hospital of Manteca	Manteca	4%	337
East Los Angeles Doctors Hospital	Los Angeles	4%	14720
Greater El Monte Community Hospital	South El Monte	4%	18927
LAC+USC Medical Center	Los Angeles	4%	144742
Memorial Hospital Los Banos	Los Banos	4%	25285
Pacifica Hospital of the Valley	Sun Valley	4%	12756
PIH Hospital - Downey	Downey	4%	52385
San Joaquin General Hospital	French Camp	4%	39157
San Mateo Medical Center	San Mateo	4%	42570
Santa Clara Valley Medical Center	San Jose	4%	71611
Santa Rosa Memorial Hospital	Santa Rosa	4%	36961
Torrance Memorial Medical Center	Torrance	4%	16718
UCSF Medical Center	San Francisco	4%	38764
Univ of California Irvine Med Ctr	Orange	4%	32412
Valley Presbyterian Hospital	Van Nuys	4%	60812
Ventura County Medical Center	Ventura	4%	52387
West Anaheim Medical Center	Anaheim	4%	30450
Alvarado Hospital Medical Center	San Diego	5%	25779
Centinela Hospital Medical Center	Inglewood	5%	64464
Citrus Valley Medical Center - IC Campus	Covina	5%	80780
Community Hospital of Huntington Park	Huntington Park	5%	29131
Contra Costa Regional Medical Center	Martinez	5%	57154
Grossmont Hospital	La Mesa	5%	98314
Hollywood Presbyterian Medical Center	Los Angeles	5%	34944
Loma Linda University Medical Center	Loma Linda	5%	65307
Memorial Hospital of Gardena	Gardena	5%	28093
Memorial Medical Center	Modesto	5%	71043
Paradise Valley Hospital	National City	5%	34170
San Leandro Hospital	San Leandro	5%	9305
Tri - City Medical Center	Oceanside	5%	69898
Alameda County Medical Center	Oakland	6%	90132
Huntington Memorial Hospital	Pasadena	6%	60985
John F Kennedy Memorial Hospital	Indio	6%	35865
Kern Valley Healthcare District	Lake Isabella	6%	6989
Oroville Hospital	Oroville	6%	34910
Riverside County Regional Medical Center	Moreno Valley	6%	118328
Saint Francis Medical Center	Lynwood	6%	73135
Desert Valley Hospital	Victorville	7%	36887
Palmdale Regional Medical Center	Palmdale	7%	53219
Saint Agnes Medical Center	Fresno	7%	37349
Tulare Regional Medical Center	Tulare	7%	31590
Victor Valley Global Medical Center	Victorville	7%	35482
Western Medical Center Hospital Anaheim	Anaheim	7%	16963
LAC/Olive View - UCLA Medical Center	Sylmar	9%	64917
San Francisco General Hospital	San Francisco	9%	63335
LAC/Harbor - UCLA Medical Center	Torrance	10%	107978
Univ of CA Davis Med Ctr	Sacramento	10%	69293
Good Samaritan Hospital	Los Angeles	11%	32520
Community Regional Medical Center	Fresno	14%	114059
Barstow Community Hospital	Barstow	17%	25019

NOTE: Hospital profiles are in alphabetical order by state, then city, then hospital within the city; Rankings exclude hospitals with less than 25 cases except for patient surveys which excludes hospitals with less than 100 cases; (a) 100-299 cases; (1) The number of cases/patients is too few to report; (2) Data submitted were based on a sample of cases/patients; (3) Results are based on a shorter time period than required; (4) Data suppressed by CMS for one or more quarters; (5) Results are not available for this reporting period; (6) Fewer than 100 patients completed the HCAHPS survey; (7) No cases met the criteria for this measure; (8) The lower limit of the confidence interval cannot be calculated if the number of observed infections equals zero; (9) No data are available from the state/territory for this reporting period; (10) The scores shown reflect fewer than 50 completed surveys; (11) There were discrepancies in the data collection process; (12) This measure does not apply to this hospital for this reporting period; (13) Results cannot be calculated for this reporting period; (14) The results for this state are combined with nearby states to protect confidentiality; Please refer to the User's Guide for a full explanation of data.

Time from ER Arrival to Being Admitted (minutes)

Hospital Name	City	Min.	Cases
Pacifica Hospital of the Valley[2]	Sun Valley	103	445
Chino Valley Medical Center[2]	Chino	178	974
Encino Hospital Medical Center[2]	Encino	179	550
Colusa Regional Medical Center[2]	Colusa	190	383
Placentia Linda Hospital[2]	Placentia	206	606
Sharp Coronado Hosp & Healthcare Ctr[2]	Coronado	206	339
San Dimas Community Hospital[2]	San Dimas	209	617
Montclair Hospital Medical Center[2]	Montclair	210	528
Saint Helena Hospital[2]	Saint Helena	210	220
Sherman Oaks Hospital[2]	Sherman Oaks	211	655
Garfield Medical Center[2]	Monterey Park	214	461
Western Medical Center Santa Ana[2]	Santa Ana	216	990
Corcoran District Hospital[2,3]	Corcoran	217	40
French Hospital Medical Center[2]	San Luis Obispo	218	461
Los Angeles Community Hospital[2]	Los Angeles	220	697
Fairchild Medical Center[2,3]	Yreka	221	260
Mammoth Hospital[3]	Mammoth Lakes	226	184
Chinese Hospital[2]	San Francisco	227	465
Delano Regional Medical Center[2]	Delano	230	310
Goleta Valley Cottage Hospital[2]	Santa Barbara	230	249
Mills - Peninsula Medical Center[2]	Burlingame	230	585
Ojai Valley Community Hospital[2]	Ojai	231	474
Alhambra Hospital Medical Center[2]	Alhambra	232	654
Sequoia Hospital[2]	Redwood City	232	458
Sharp Memorial Hospital[2]	San Diego	232	459
Scripps Memorial Hospital La Jolla[2]	La Jolla	234	349
Pacific Alliance Medical Center[2]	Los Angeles	235	99
Ukiah Valley Medical Center[2]	Ukiah	236	463
Mission Community Hospital[2]	Panorama City	238	472
CA Pacific Med Ctr-Davies Campus[2]	San Francisco	239	254
Novato Community Hospital[2]	Novato	240	348
Comm Hosp of the Monterey Peninsula[2]	Monterey	241	317
Huntington Beach Hospital[2]	Huntington Bch	241	635
Ahmc Anaheim Regional Medical Center[2]	Anaheim	242	645
Tahoe Forest Hospital[2]	Truckee	242	280
Coast Plaza Hospital[2]	Norwalk	244	536
La Palma Intercommunity Hospital[2]	La Palma	245	537
CA Pacific Med Ctr-Pacific Campus Hosp[2]	San Francisco	246	297
Mark Twain Medical Center[2]	San Andreas	246	552
Kaiser Fdn Hosp-S San Francisco[2]	S San Francisco	247	624
Watsonville Community Hospital[2]	Watsonville	247	501
Saint Louise Regional Hospital[2]	Gilroy	248	376
Sierra Vista Regional Medical Center[2]	San Luis Obispo	248	475
Coastal Communities Hospital[2]	Santa Ana	249	278
Santa Ynez Valley Cottage Hospital	Solvang	252	175
Glendale Mem Hosp & Health Ctr[2]	Glendale	254	521
San Gabriel Valley Medical Center[2]	San Gabriel	255	472
Alameda Hospital[2]	Alameda	256	526
Seton Medical Center[2]	Daly City	257	790
Sonoma Valley Hospital[2]	Sonoma	257	269
Simi Valley Hosp & Health Care Svcs[2]	Simi Valley	259	772
Doctors Hospital of Manteca[2]	Manteca	260	430
Garden Grove Hospital & Medical Center[2]	Garden Grove	260	602
Saint Vincent Medical Center[2]	Los Angeles	263	703
Valleycare Medical Center[2]	Pleasanton	264	600
Kaiser Foundation Hospital - Redwood City[2]	Redwood City	265	432
San Ramon Regional Medical Center[2]	San Ramon	265	491
Tri - City Regional Medical Center[2]	Hawaiian Grdns	265	371
Mission Hospital Regional Medical Center[2]	Mission Viejo	266	500
Santa Barbara Cottage Hospital[2]	Santa Barbara	266	525
USC Verdugo Hills Hospital[2]	Glendale	267	593
CA Pacific Med Ctr-St Luke's Campus[2]	San Francisco	268	342
Kaiser Foundation Hospital[2]	San Rafael	269	666
Paradise Valley Hospital[2]	National City	270	701
Queen of the Valley Medical Center[2]	Napa	270	714
Saint Elizabeth Community Hospital[2]	Red Bluff	270	364
Saint Jude Medical Center[2]	Fullerton	270	516
Salinas Valley Memorial Hospital[2]	Salinas	271	570
Oak Valley District Hospital[2]	Oakdale	272	451
Orange Coast Memorial Medical Center[2]	Fountain Valley	272	636
Alvarado Hospital Medical Center[2]	San Diego	275	434
George L Mee Memorial Hospital[2]	King City	275	139
Hazel Hawkins Memorial Hospital[2]	Hollister	275	524
Marian Regional Medical Center[2]	Santa Maria	275	789
Hoag Memorial Hospital Presbyterian[2]	Newport Beach	276	917
Kaiser Fdn Hosp-San Francisco[2]	San Francisco	276	332
Prov Little Co of Mary Med Ctr San Pedro[2]	San Pedro	277	705
Twin Cities Community Hospital[2]	Templeton	277	787
Olympia Medical Center[2]	Los Angeles	278	816
Kaiser Foundation Hospital - Santa Rosa[2]	Santa Rosa	280	518
Monterey Park Hospital[2]	Monterey Park	280	397
Sutter Tracy Community Hospital[2]	Tracy	281	469
Fallbrook Hospital[2]	Fallbrook	282	317
Pacific Hospital of Long Beach[2,3]	Long Beach	283	138
Barstow Community Hospital[2]	Barstow	284	443
Barton Memorial Hospital[2]	S Lake Tahoe	284	272
El Camino Hospital[2]	Mountain View	284	393
East Valley Hospital Medical Center[2]	Glendora	285	796
Saint Mary's Medical Center[2]	San Francisco	285	674
Enloe Medical Center[2]	Chico	286	707
Kaiser Fdn Hosp-Fremont/Hayward[2]	Hayward	286	546
Methodist Hospital of Southern California[2]	Arcadia	286	751
Saint Rose Hospital[2]	Hayward	286	720
Palo Verde Hospital[2]	Blythe	289	517
Kaiser Foundation Hospital - Fresno[2]	Fresno	290	657
Memorial Hospital Los Banos[2]	Los Banos	290	161
Saint Mary Medical Center[2]	Long Beach	290	627
Woodland Memorial Hospital[2]	Woodland	290	345
Providence Tarzana Medical Center[2]	Tarzana	291	613
Kaiser Foundation Hospital - Roseville[2]	Roseville	292	420
Kaiser Foundation Hospital - Antioch[2]	Antioch	293	537
Mercy Medical Center - Mount Shasta[2]	Mount Shasta	294	321
Coalinga Regional Medical Center[2]	Coalinga	295	183
Providence Holy Cross Medical Center[2]	Mission Hills	295	553
Sutter Amador Hospital[2]	Jackson	295	401
Whittier Hospital Medical Center[2]	Whittier	295	386
Lompoc Valley Medical Center[2]	Lompoc	296	281
Parkview Comm Hosp Med Ctr[2]	Riverside	296	219
West Anaheim Medical Center[2]	Anaheim	296	1137
Feather River Hospital[2]	Paradise	297	717
Redwood Memorial Hospital[2]	Fortuna	297	274
Sonora Regional Medical Center[2]	Sonora	297	635
Pomerado Hospital[2]	Poway	298	508
Scripps Memorial Hospital - Encinitas[2]	Encinitas	299	485
Oroville Hospital[2]	Oroville	300	996
Sierra Nevada Memorial Hospital[2]	Grass Valley	300	824
Fountain Valley Reg Hosp & Med Ctr[2]	Fountain Valley	301	614
Good Samaritan Hospital[2]	San Jose	301	560
Kaiser Foundation Hospital - San Jose[2]	San Jose	301	512
Providence Saint Joseph Medical Center[2]	Burbank	301	531
Kaiser Fdn Hosp-Panorama City[2]	Panorama City	302	512
Sutter Davis Hospital[2]	Davis	304	270
John Muir Med Ctr-Walnut Creek Campus[2]	Walnut Creek	305	607
Kaweah Delta Medical Center[2]	Visalia	305	614
Adventist Medical Center[2]	Hanford	306	1547
Dominican Hospital[2]	Santa Cruz	306	742
Kaiser Foundation Hospital - Sacramento[2]	Sacramento	306	670
Tulare Regional Medical Center[2]	Tulare	306	372
Mercy General Hospital[2]	Sacramento	307	434
Mercy Hospital of Folsom[2]	Folsom	307	697
Cedars - Sinai Medical Center[2]	Los Angeles	310	396
Community Hospital of Long Beach[2]	Long Beach	310	438
Kaiser Fdn Hosp S Sacramento[2]	Sacramento	310	584
Lakewood Regional Medical Center[2]	Lakewood	310	993
Mad River Community Hospital[2]	Arcata	310	306
Saddleback Memorial Medical Center[2]	Laguna Hills	310	662
Palm Drive Hospital[2]	Sebastopol	312	403
Saint Francis Memorial Hospital[2]	San Francisco	314	649
Kaiser Foundation Hospital - Riverside[2]	Riverside	315	335
Kaiser Foundation Hospital - Baldwin Park[2]	Baldwin Park	317	444
Kaiser Foundation Hospital - South Bay[2]	Harbor City	318	403
Kaiser Foundation Hospital - Vacaville[2]	Vacaville	318	630
Providence Saint John's Health Center[2]	Santa Monica	318	237
Western Medical Center Hospital Anaheim[2]	Anaheim	318	249
Comm Mem Hosp San Buenaventura[2]	Ventura	319	461
Marin General Hospital[2]	Greenbrae	319	741
Marina Del Rey Hospital[2]	Marina Del Rey	319	542
Alta Bates Summit Medical Center[2]	Oakland	320	852
Eisenhower Medical Center[2]	Rancho Mirage	320	1246
Good Samaritan Hospital[2]	Los Angeles	320	383
Presbyterian Intercommunity Hospital[2]	Whittier	320	606
Valley Presbyterian Hospital[2]	Van Nuys	320	176
Bear Valley Community Hospital	Big Bear Lake	321	54
Los Alamitos Medical Center[2]	Los Alamitos	321	755
O'Connor Hospital[2]	San Jose	321	467
Sutter Auburn Faith Hospital[2]	Auburn	321	642
Los Robles Hospital & Medical Center[2]	Thousand Oaks	322	696
Shasta Regional Medical Center[2]	Redding	322	1033
Kaiser Fdn Hosp-Orange Co-Anaheim[2]	Anaheim	324	422
John Muir Medical Center - Concord Campus[2]	Concord	325	831
Saint Agnes Medical Center[2]	Fresno	325	620
Greater El Monte Community Hospital[2]	South El Monte	326	420
Saint Joseph Hospital[2]	Orange	326	88
Marshall Medical Center[2]	Placerville	328	692
Memorial Medical Center[2]	Modesto	328	807
Lodi Memorial Hospital[2]	Lodi	329	759
Northridge Hospital Medical Center[2]	Northridge	329	783
Santa Rosa Memorial Hospital[2]	Santa Rosa	329	682
Palomar Health Downtown Campus[2]	Escondido	330	522
Hi - Desert Medical Center[2]	Joshua Tree	331	437
Torrance Memorial Medical Center[2]	Torrance	331	829
Alta Bates Summit Medical Center[2]	Berkeley	332	294
Kaiser Fdn Hosp-Moreno Valley[2]	Moreno Valley	332	468
Kaiser Fdn Hosp-Oakland/Richmond[2]	Oakland	332	526
Dameron Hospital[2]	Stockton	333	531
Doctors Medical Center - San Pablo[2]	San Pablo	334	500
Saint Joseph Hospital[2]	Eureka	334	298
San Antonio Community Hospital[2]	Upland	334	656
Kaiser Foundation Hospital - Santa Clara[2]	Santa Clara	335	431
Adventist Medical Center - Reedley[2]	Reedley	336	139
Glendale Adventist Medical Center[2]	Glendale	336	695
Kaiser Fdn Hosp-Woodland Hills[2]	Woodland Hills	336	374
PIH Hospital - Downey[2]	Downey	337	411
Kaiser Foundation Hospital - Manteca[2]	Manteca	338	456
Sutter Coast Hospital[2]	Crescent City	338	392
Kaiser Foundation Hospital & Rehab Center[2]	Vallejo	340	502
Mercy San Juan Medical Center[2]	Carmichael	340	693
Eden Medical Center[2]	Castro Valley	341	991
Saint Johns Pleasant Valley Hospital[2]	Camarillo	343	461
Scripps Mercy Hospital[2]	San Diego	344	601
Sutter Medical Center of Santa Rosa[2]	Santa Rosa	346	349
Kaiser Foundation Hospital - Fontana[2]	Fontana	348	448
Stanford Hospital[2]	Stanford	348	414
Community Hospital of San Bernardino[2]	San Bernardino	349	237
Henry Mayo Newhall Memorial Hospital[2]	Valencia	349	809
San Gorgonio Memorial Hospital[2]	Banning	350	335
San Leandro Hospital[2,3]	San Leandro	350	237
Desert Regional Medical Center[2]	Palm Springs	352	663
Centinela Hospital Medical Center[2]	Inglewood	353	1021
Washington Hospital[2]	Fremont	353	472
Petaluma Valley Hospital[2]	Petaluma	354	341
Mercy Medical Center - Redding[2]	Redding	355	537
Saint Johns Regional Medical Center[2]	Oxnard	356	471
Sutter Delta Medical Center[2]	Antioch	358	736
Kaiser Foundation Hospital - Walnut Creek[2]	Walnut Creek	360	560
Sutter Roseville Medical Center[2]	Roseville	362	710
West Hills Hospital & Medical Center[2]	West Hills	362	759
Northbay Medical Center[2]	Fairfield	364	722
Tri - City Medical Center[2]	Oceanside	364	568
Kaiser Foundation Hospital - Downey[2]	Downey	365	419
Doctors Medical Center[2]	Modesto	372	598
Emanuel Medical Center[2]	Turlock	372	941
Univ of California Irvine Med Ctr[2]	Orange	372	465
Regional Medical Center of San Jose[2]	San Jose	373	1138
Chapman Medical Center[2]	Orange	374	200
Grossmont Hospital[2]	La Mesa	376	735
Kaiser Foundation Hospital - West La[2]	Los Angeles	377	450
Foothill Presbyterian Hospital[2]	Glendora	381	680
San Mateo Medical Center[2]	San Mateo	381	419
Citrus Valley Medical Center - IC Campus[2]	Covina	382	586
Community Hospital of Huntington Park[2]	Huntington Park	384	671
Huntington Memorial Hospital[2]	Pasadena	384	578
John F Kennedy Memorial Hospital[2]	Indio	386	561
Sierra View District Hospital[2]	Porterville	389	680
Sutter Lakeside Hospital[2]	Lakeport	389	337
Saint Joseph's Medical Center of Stockton[2]	Stockton	390	734
Ventura County Medical Center[2]	Ventura	390	529
Mercy Medical Center[2]	Merced	394	476
Natividad Medical Center[2]	Salinas	394	363
Rideout Memorial Hospital[2]	Marysville	396	459
Bakersfield Heart Hospital[2]	Bakersfield	397	525
Sharp Chula Vista Medical Center[2]	Chula Vista	398	784
California Hosp Med Ctr Los Angeles[2]	Los Angeles	400	558
Menifee Valley Medical Center[2]	Sun City	401	276
Hollywood Presbyterian Medical Center[2]	Los Angeles	405	375
Mercy Hospital[2]	Bakersfield	405	676
Long Beach Memorial Medical Center[2]	Long Beach	408	814
Santa Monica-UCLA Med Ctr & Ortho Hosp[2]	Santa Monica	409	547
Beverly Hospital[2]	Montebello	411	737
San Joaquin General Hospital[2]	French Camp	412	484
East Los Angeles Doctors Hospital[2]	Los Angeles	414	314
Southwest Healthcare System[2]	Murrieta	417	590
UCSF Medical Center[2]	San Francisco	417	233
Kaiser Foundation Hospital - San Diego[2]	San Diego	418	505
White Memorial Medical Center[2]	Los Angeles	418	494
Sutter Solano Medical Center[2]	Vallejo	423	649
Pioneers Memorial Healthcare District[2]	Brawley	427	540
Univ of CA San Diego Med Ctr[2]	San Diego	427	494
Corona Regional Medical Center[2]	Corona	428	616
Sutter General Hospital[2]	Sacramento	430	382
Bakersfield Memorial Hospital[2]	Bakersfield	435	703
Methodist Hospital of Sacramento[2]	Sacramento	444	661
San Joaquin Community Hospital[2]	Bakersfield	444	610
Pomona Valley Hospital Medical Center[2]	Pomona	446	356
Riverside Community Hospital[2]	Riverside	453	644
San Francisco General Hospital[2]	San Francisco	456	730
Saint Francis Medical Center[2]	Lynwood	462	423
Contra Costa Regional Medical Center[2]	Martinez	471	412
El Centro Regional Medical Center[2]	El Centro	471	711
Hemet Valley Medical Center[2]	Hemet	472	433
Prov Little Co of Mary Med Ctr Torrance[2]	Torrance	476	739
Redlands Community Hospital[2]	Redlands	479	379
Desert Valley Hospital[2]	Victorville	483	878
Madera Community Hospital[2]	Madera	487	807
Santa Clara Valley Medical Center[2]	San Jose	491	545
Saint Mary Medical Center[2]	Apple Valley	495	784
Victor Valley Global Medical Center[2]	Victorville	505	461
Memorial Hospital of Gardena[2]	Gardena	520	870
Saint Bernardine Medical Center[2]	San Bernardino	520	465
Ronald Reagan UCLA Medical Center[2]	Los Angeles	527	498

NOTE: Hospital profiles are in alphabetical order by state, then city, then hospital within the city; Rankings exclude hospitals with less than 25 cases except for patient surveys which excludes hospitals with less than 100 cases; (a) 100-299 cases; (1) The number of cases/patients is too few to report; (2) Data submitted were based on a sample of cases/patients; (3) Results are based on a shorter time period than required; (4) Data suppressed by CMS for one or more quarters; (5) Results are not available for this reporting period; (6) Fewer than 100 patients completed the HCAHPS survey; (7) No cases met the criteria for this measure; (8) The lower limit of the confidence interval cannot be calculated if the number of observed infections equals zero; (9) No data are available from the state/territory for this reporting period; (10) The scores shown reflect fewer than 50 completed surveys; (11) There were discrepancies in the data collection process; (12) This measure does not apply to this hospital for this reporting period; (13) Results cannot be calculated for this reporting period; (14) The results for this state are combined with nearby states to protect confidentiality; Please refer to the User's Guide for a full explanation of data.

Hospital Name	City	Min.	Cases
Loma Linda University Medical Center[2]	Loma Linda	528	514
Loma Linda Univ Med Ctr-Murrieta[2]	Murrieta	538	1034
Univ of CA Davis Med Ctr[2]	Sacramento	555	597
Kaiser Foundation Hospital - Los Angeles[2]	Los Angeles	557	356
Antelope Valley Hospital[2]	Lancaster	580	644
Palmdale Regional Medical Center[2]	Palmdale	604	970
Kern Medical Center[2]	Bakersfield	637	116
LAC/Harbor - UCLA Medical Center[2]	Torrance	637	799
LAC+USC Medical Center[2]	Los Angeles	652	693
LAC/Olive View - UCLA Medical Center[2]	Sylmar	678	833
Arrowhead Regional Medical Center[2]	Colton	680	1066
Alameda County Medical Center[2]	Oakland	782	486
Clovis Community Medical Center[2]	Clovis	782	336
Community Regional Medical Center[2]	Fresno	852	661
Riverside County Regional Medical Center[2]	Moreno Valley	905	489

Time from ER Arrival to Discharge (minutes)

Hospital Name	City	Min.	Cases
Corcoran District Hospital[3]	Corcoran	80	182
Encino Hospital Medical Center	Encino	88	495
Chino Valley Medical Center	Chino	89	415
Novato Community Hospital	Novato	90	359
Saint Bernardine Medical Center	San Bernardino	93	391
Placentia Linda Hospital	Placentia	97	467
San Gorgonio Memorial Hospital	Banning	98	372
George L Mee Memorial Hospital	King City	100	354
Coastal Communities Hospital	Santa Ana	105	345
Colusa Regional Medical Center	Colusa	105	464
Oak Valley District Hospital	Oakdale	106	453
Sharp Coronado Hosp & Healthcare Ctr	Coronado	106	380
Ojai Valley Community Hospital	Ojai	107	334
Sherman Oaks Hospital	Sherman Oaks	107	320
Goleta Valley Cottage Hospital	Santa Barbara	110	348
Marian Regional Medical Center	Santa Maria	110	591
Saint Helena Hospital	Saint Helena	113	360
Santa Ynez Valley Cottage Hospital	Solvang	113	364
Natividad Medical Center	Salinas	115	589
Sequoia Hospital	Redwood City	115	390
Sutter Amador Hospital	Jackson	115	378
Twin Cities Community Hospital	Templeton	115	481
French Hospital Medical Center	San Luis Obispo	116	382
Seton Medical Center	Daly City	116	601
Doctors Medical Center	Modesto	117	459
Woodland Memorial Hospital	Woodland	117	401
USC Verdugo Hills Hospital	Glendale	119	449
CA Pacific Med Ctr-Davies Campus	San Francisco	120	371
Coalinga Regional Medical Center	Coalinga	120	381
Memorial Hospital Los Banos	Los Banos	120	381
Emanuel Medical Center	Turlock	121	457
Mission Community Hospital	Panorama City	121	328
Chapman Medical Center	Orange	122	316
Mercy Medical Center	Merced	122	363
Sonoma Valley Hospital	Sonoma	124	360
Los Angeles Community Hospital	Los Angeles	125	336
Mad River Community Hospital	Arcata	125	280
Parkview Comm Hosp Med Ctr	Riverside	125	938
Providence Tarzana Medical Center	Tarzana	125	371
Saint Francis Memorial Hospital	San Francisco	125	341
Saint Mary Medical Center	Long Beach	126	370
Coast Plaza Hospital	Norwalk	127	343
Montclair Hospital Medical Center	Montclair	127	374
Saint Joseph Hospital	Eureka	127	359
Mills - Peninsula Medical Center	Burlingame	128	391
Valleycare Medical Center	Pleasanton	128	339
Doctors Hospital of Manteca	Manteca	129	469
Olympia Medical Center	Los Angeles	129	326
Tri - City Regional Medical Center	Hawaiian Grdns	129	305
Doctors Medical Center - San Pablo	San Pablo	130	265
Garfield Medical Center	Monterey Park	130	372
Palm Drive Hospital	Sebastopol	130	401
Saint Rose Hospital	Hayward	130	2026
Barton Memorial Hospital	S Lake Tahoe	131	349
El Camino Hospital	Mountain View	131	1193
Palo Verde Hospital	Blythe	131	371
Huntington Beach Hospital	Huntington Bch	132	343
Sutter Davis Hospital	Davis	132	392
Sierra Vista Regional Medical Center	San Luis Obispo	133	449
Community Hospital of Long Beach	Long Beach	134	322
Pacifica Hospital of the Valley[3]	Sun Valley	134	102
Prov Little Co of Mary Med Ctr San Pedro	San Pedro	134	383
Queen of the Valley Medical Center	Napa	134	394
Saint Johns Pleasant Valley Hospital	Camarillo	134	386
Sutter Solano Medical Center	Vallejo	134	375
San Dimas Community Hospital	San Dimas	135	377
Sutter Coast Hospital	Crescent City	135	350
Ahmc Anaheim Regional Medical Center	Anaheim	136	350
John Muir Medical Center - Concord Campus	Concord	136	432
Ukiah Valley Medical Center	Ukiah	136	346
Adventist Medical Center - Reedley	Reedley	137	366
O'Connor Hospital	San Jose	137	378
Saddleback Memorial Medical Center	Laguna Hills	137	338
Sierra Nevada Memorial Hospital	Grass Valley	137	363
Community Hospital of San Bernardino	San Bernardino	138	325
Barstow Community Hospital	Barstow	139	382
Saint Vincent Medical Center	Los Angeles	139	356
Alameda Hospital	Alameda	140	333
Chinese Hospital	San Francisco	140	973
Fallbrook Hospital	Fallbrook	140	420
Good Samaritan Hospital	San Jose	140	429
Saint Johns Regional Medical Center	Oxnard	140	414
West Hills Hospital & Medical Center	West Hills	141	468
Delano Regional Medical Center	Delano	142	344
John Muir Med Ctr-Walnut Creek Campus	Walnut Creek	142	384
Providence Saint John's Health Center	Santa Monica	142	486
Riverside Community Hospital	Riverside	142	412
Glendale Mem Hosp & Health Ctr	Glendale	143	373
Lakewood Regional Medical Center	Lakewood	143	451
Marin General Hospital	Greenbrae	143	413
Pacific Alliance Medical Center	Los Angeles	143	327
Adventist Medical Center	Hanford	144	875
Bear Valley Community Hospital	Big Bear Lake	144	390
CA Pacific Med Ctr-St Luke's Campus	San Francisco	144	355
Hi - Desert Medical Center	Joshua Tree	144	316
Lompoc Valley Medical Center	Lompoc	144	372
Pacific Hospital of Long Beach[3]	Long Beach	144	204
Pioneers Memorial Healthcare District	Brawley	144	400
Providence Holy Cross Medical Center	Mission Hills	144	359
San Gabriel Valley Medical Center	San Gabriel	144	369
Sutter Lakeside Hospital	Lakeport	145	355
Washington Hospital	Fremont	145	382
Henry Mayo Newhall Memorial Hospital	Valencia	146	364
La Palma Intercommunity Hospital	La Palma	146	740
Monterey Park Hospital	Monterey Park	146	331
Oroville Hospital	Oroville	146	390
Saint Elizabeth Community Hospital	Red Bluff	146	382
CA Pacific Med Ctr-Pacific Campus Hosp	San Francisco	148	378
Saint Louise Regional Hospital	Gilroy	148	378
Santa Monica-UCLA Med Ctr & Ortho Hosp	Santa Monica	148	410
East Valley Hospital Medical Center	Glendora	150	278
Orange Coast Memorial Medical Center	Fountain Valley	150	388
Shasta Regional Medical Center	Redding	151	409
Simi Valley Hosp & Health Care Svcs	Simi Valley	151	368
Mercy Hospital of Folsom	Folsom	152	376
Sutter Auburn Faith Hospital	Auburn	152	370
Mercy Hospital	Bakersfield	153	389
Saint Mary's Medical Center	San Francisco	153	365
Alhambra Hospital Medical Center	Alhambra	154	454
Dameron Hospital	Stockton	154	336
Sutter Delta Medical Center	Antioch	154	371
Salinas Valley Memorial Hospital	Salinas	155	384
Pomerado Hospital	Poway	156	358
Watsonville Community Hospital	Watsonville	157	355
Lodi Memorial Hospital	Lodi	158	365
Saint Jude Medical Center	Fullerton	158	328
San Ramon Regional Medical Center	San Ramon	158	394
Santa Barbara Cottage Hospital	Santa Barbara	158	357
Sutter Tracy Community Hospital	Tracy	158	402
Mercy General Hospital	Sacramento	159	358
Methodist Hospital of Sacramento	Sacramento	159	377
Northbay Medical Center	Fairfield	159	396
Sonora Regional Medical Center	Sonora	159	289
Garden Grove Hospital & Medical Center	Garden Grove	160	420
Petaluma Valley Hospital	Petaluma	160	342
Mercy Medical Center - Mount Shasta	Mount Shasta	161	368
Feather River Hospital	Paradise	163	355
Saint Joseph's Medical Center of Stockton	Stockton	163	385
Western Medical Center Hospital Anaheim	Anaheim	163	306
Comm Mem Hosp San Buenaventura	Ventura	164	366
Hazel Hawkins Memorial Hospital	Hollister	164	611
Hoag Memorial Hospital Presbyterian	Newport Beach	164	646
Regional Medical Center of San Jose	San Jose	164	450
Enloe Medical Center	Chico	165	388
Sutter Medical Center of Santa Rosa	Santa Rosa	165	377
Dominican Hospital	Santa Cruz	166	375
Mercy Medical Center - Redding	Redding	166	364
Desert Regional Medical Center	Palm Springs	167	361
El Centro Regional Medical Center	El Centro	167	423
Memorial Medical Center	Modesto	168	395
Northridge Hospital Medical Center	Northridge	168	397
Scripps Memorial Hospital - Encinitas	Encinitas	168	374
Tulare Regional Medical Center	Tulare	168	406
Fountain Valley Reg Hosp & Med Ctr	Fountain Valley	169	449
Alvarado Hospital Medical Center	San Diego	170	329
Marshall Medical Center	Placerville	170	371
Providence Saint Joseph Medical Center	Burbank	170	472
Victor Valley Global Medical Center	Victorville	170	342
Foothill Presbyterian Hospital	Glendora	171	380
Scripps Memorial Hospital La Jolla	La Jolla	171	363
Whittier Hospital Medical Center	Whittier	171	342
Bakersfield Heart Hospital	Bakersfield	174	347
Ventura County Medical Center[3]	Ventura	174	282
John F Kennedy Memorial Hospital	Indio	175	335
Los Alamitos Medical Center	Los Alamitos	176	357
Los Robles Hospital & Medical Center	Thousand Oaks	176	421
Santa Rosa Memorial Hospital	Santa Rosa	176	333
Sierra View District Hospital	Porterville	176	464
Western Medical Center Santa Ana	Santa Ana	176	310
Greater El Monte Community Hospital	South El Monte	177	320
Mission Hospital Regional Medical Center	Mission Viejo	177	339
Paradise Valley Hospital	National City	177	402
Southwest Healthcare System	Murrieta	177	413
Sutter General Hospital	Sacramento	177	359
Madera Community Hospital	Madera	178	542
Methodist Hospital of Southern California	Arcadia	180	394
Saint Joseph Hospital	Orange	180	220
San Leandro Hospital[3]	San Leandro	180	187
Sharp Memorial Hospital	San Diego	180	406
Bakersfield Memorial Hospital	Bakersfield	181	405
Pomona Valley Hospital Medical Center	Pomona	181	347
Contra Costa Regional Medical Center	Martinez	182	394
Glendale Adventist Medical Center	Glendale	182	352
Kaweah Delta Medical Center	Visalia	186	362
Marina Del Rey Hospital	Marina Del Rey	186	323
Palomar Health Downtown Campus	Escondido	186	361
West Anaheim Medical Center	Anaheim	187	334
Arrowhead Regional Medical Center	Colton	188	317
East Los Angeles Doctors Hospital	Los Angeles	188	294
Saint Mary Medical Center	Apple Valley	188	371
Sutter Roseville Medical Center	Roseville	188	379
Citrus Valley Medical Center - IC Campus	Covina	189	375
Corona Regional Medical Center	Corona	189	320
Memorial Hospital of Gardena	Gardena	190	336
Rideout Memorial Hospital	Marysville	190	830
Alta Bates Summit Medical Center	Berkeley	191	375
Valley Presbyterian Hospital	Van Nuys	191	355
Alta Bates Summit Medical Center	Oakland	193	379
San Mateo Medical Center	San Mateo	193	347
PIH Hospital - Downey	Downey	195	365
Mercy San Juan Medical Center	Carmichael	196	350
San Joaquin General Hospital	French Camp	196	359
Scripps Mercy Hospital	San Diego	197	363
Santa Clara Valley Medical Center	San Jose	199	340
Eden Medical Center	Castro Valley	200	557
Comm Hosp of the Monterey Peninsula	Monterey	202	195
Antelope Valley Hospital	Lancaster	204	459
California Hosp Med Ctr Los Angeles	Los Angeles	205	387
Cedars - Sinai Medical Center	Los Angeles	205	365
Eisenhower Medical Center	Rancho Mirage	205	387
Riverside County Regional Medical Center	Moreno Valley	205	313
Palmdale Regional Medical Center	Palmdale	208	379
Alameda County Medical Center	Oakland	210	337
Stanford Hospital	Stanford	210	363
Desert Valley Hospital	Victorville	212	350
Sharp Chula Vista Medical Center	Chula Vista	212	589
Community Hospital of Huntington Park	Huntington Park	218	429
Menifee Valley Medical Center	Sun City	218	319
Kern Medical Center	Bakersfield	220	359
Presbyterian Intercommunity Hospital	Whittier	220	385
Centinela Hospital Medical Center	Inglewood	221	417
San Antonio Community Hospital	Upland	221	343
Tri - City Medical Center	Oceanside	221	19168
Prov Little Co of Mary Med Ctr Torrance	Torrance	222	389
Redlands Community Hospital	Redlands	223	339
Torrance Memorial Medical Center	Torrance	223	1475
Saint Agnes Medical Center	Fresno	224	398
Clovis Community Medical Center	Clovis	227	343
Hollywood Presbyterian Medical Center	Los Angeles	227	307
San Joaquin Community Hospital	Bakersfield	228	332
Ronald Reagan UCLA Medical Center	Los Angeles	229	353
UCSF Medical Center	San Francisco	229	351
Hemet Valley Medical Center	Hemet	233	271
Grossmont Hospital	La Mesa	239	360
Beverly Hospital	Montebello	242	331
Univ of CA San Diego Med Ctr	San Diego	244	342
Loma Linda Univ Med Ctr-Murrieta	Murrieta	250	360
Long Beach Memorial Medical Center	Long Beach	251	354
White Memorial Medical Center	Los Angeles	259	367
San Francisco General Hospital	San Francisco	263	281
Univ of CA Davis Med Ctr	Sacramento	267	345
Huntington Memorial Hospital	Pasadena	270	362
Saint Francis Medical Center	Lynwood	275	399
Good Samaritan Hospital	Los Angeles	278	370
Univ of California Irvine Med Ctr	Orange	278	332
Community Regional Medical Center	Fresno	286	276
Loma Linda University Medical Center	Loma Linda	304	374
LAC/Harbor - UCLA Medical Center	Torrance	316	288
LAC+USC Medical Center	Los Angeles	369	290
LAC/Olive View - UCLA Medical Center	Sylmar	448	319

Time in ER Before Being Evaluated (minutes)

Hospital Name	City	Min.	Cases
Saint Bernardine Medical Center	San Bernardino	0	422
Saint Helena Hospital	Saint Helena	3	381

NOTE: Hospital profiles are in alphabetical order by state, then city, then hospital within the city; Rankings exclude hospitals with less than 25 cases except for patient surveys which excludes hospitals with less than 100 cases; (a) 100-299 cases; (1) The number of cases/patients is too few to report; (2) Data submitted were based on a sample of cases/patients; (3) Results are based on a shorter time period than required; (4) Data suppressed by CMS for one or more quarters; (5) Results are not available for this reporting period; (6) Fewer than 100 patients completed the HCAHPS survey; (7) No cases met the criteria for this measure; (8) The lower limit of the confidence interval cannot be calculated if the number of observed infections equals zero; (9) No data are available from the state/territory for this reporting period; (10) The scores shown reflect fewer than 50 completed surveys; (11) There were discrepancies in the data collection process; (12) This measure does not apply to this hospital for this reporting period; (13) Results cannot be calculated for this reporting period; (14) The results for this state are combined with nearby states to protect confidentiality; Please refer to the User's Guide for a full explanation of data.

Hollywood Presbyterian Medical Center	Los Angeles	4	341
Mercy Medical Center - Mount Shasta	Mount Shasta	4	402
Los Robles Hospital & Medical Center	Thousand Oaks	6	452
West Hills Hospital & Medical Center	West Hills	6	536
Good Samaritan Hospital	San Jose	7	455
Community Hospital of San Bernardino	San Bernardino	8	382
Mercy Hospital of Folsom	Folsom	8	380
Regional Medical Center of San Jose	San Jose	8	496
Long Beach Memorial Medical Center	Long Beach	9	380
Dameron Hospital	Stockton	10	384
French Hospital Medical Center	San Luis Obispo	10	405
Los Angeles Community Hospital	Los Angeles	10	345
Riverside Community Hospital	Riverside	10	437
Saint Mary Medical Center	Long Beach	10	398
Adventist Medical Center	Hanford	11	946
Pioneers Memorial Healthcare District	Brawley	11	425
Saint Francis Memorial Hospital	San Francisco	12	402
Simi Valley Hosp & Health Care Svcs	Simi Valley	12	408
Watsonville Community Hospital	Watsonville	12	381
East Valley Hospital Medical Center	Glendora	13	389
Kaweah Delta Medical Center	Visalia	13	405
Montclair Hospital Medical Center	Montclair	13	401
Bakersfield Memorial Hospital	Bakersfield	14	419
Delano Regional Medical Center	Delano	14	383
Fallbrook Hospital	Fallbrook	14	458
Glendale Mem Hosp & Health Ctr	Glendale	14	394
John F Kennedy Memorial Hospital	Indio	14	308
Mercy San Juan Medical Center	Carmichael	14	409
Placentia Linda Hospital	Placentia	14	498
Presbyterian Intercommunity Hospital	Whittier	14	421
Saint Mary's Medical Center	San Francisco	14	404
San Dimas Community Hospital	San Dimas	14	395
San Gorgonio Memorial Hospital	Banning	14	422
Sherman Oaks Hospital	Sherman Oaks	14	380
Sonoma Valley Hospital	Sonoma	14	44
Mercy General Hospital	Sacramento	15	408
Mercy Medical Center	Merced	15	398
Sierra Nevada Memorial Hospital	Grass Valley	15	405
Barstow Community Hospital	Barstow	16	412
Coalinga Regional Medical Center	Coalinga	16	475
Encino Hospital Medical Center	Encino	16	494
Henry Mayo Newhall Memorial Hospital	Valencia	16	407
John Muir Med Ctr-Walnut Creek Campus	Walnut Creek	16	432
Marian Regional Medical Center	Santa Maria	16	620
Saint Johns Pleasant Valley Hospital	Camarillo	16	406
Santa Ynez Valley Cottage Hospital	Solvang	16	384
Scripps Memorial Hospital La Jolla	La Jolla	16	405
Sequoia Hospital	Redwood City	16	401
Novato Community Hospital	Novato	17	358
Orange Coast Memorial Medical Center	Fountain Valley	17	419
Pomerado Hospital	Poway	17	392
Saint Elizabeth Community Hospital	Red Bluff	17	396
Bakersfield Heart Hospital	Bakersfield	18	290
Chino Valley Medical Center	Chino	18	437
Clovis Community Medical Center	Clovis	18	385
Dominican Hospital	Santa Cruz	18	417
El Centro Regional Medical Center	El Centro	18	449
Saint Joseph Hospital	Eureka	18	393
Sonora Regional Medical Center	Sonora	18	372
Doctors Medical Center	Modesto	19	498
El Camino Hospital	Mountain View	19	1263
Hi - Desert Medical Center	Joshua Tree	19	384
Mercy Hospital	Bakersfield	19	420
Methodist Hospital of Sacramento	Sacramento	19	425
Ojai Valley Community Hospital	Ojai	19	380
Rideout Memorial Hospital	Marysville	19	1095
Saint Johns Regional Medical Center	Oxnard	19	430
Saint Joseph's Medical Center of Stockton	Stockton	19	422
Valleycare Medical Center	Pleasanton	19	398
Woodland Memorial Hospital	Woodland	19	409
CA Pacific Med Ctr-Davies Campus	San Francisco	20	409
CA Pacific Med Ctr-Pacific Campus Hosp	San Francisco	20	413
George L Mee Memorial Hospital	King City	20	350
Olympia Medical Center	Los Angeles	20	372
Palo Verde Hospital	Blythe	20	421
Seton Medical Center	Daly City	20	634
Sutter Davis Hospital	Davis	20	418
Univ of CA San Diego Med Ctr	San Diego	20	383
Mercy Medical Center - Redding	Redding	21	405
Oak Valley District Hospital	Oakdale	21	481
Palomar Health Downtown Campus	Escondido	21	393
Prov Little Co of Mary Med Ctr San Pedro	San Pedro	21	408
Providence Tarzana Medical Center	Tarzana	21	383
San Joaquin Community Hospital	Bakersfield	21	377
Scripps Mercy Hospital	San Diego	21	400
Ukiah Valley Medical Center	Ukiah	21	143
Whittier Hospital Medical Center	Whittier	21	367
Beverly Hospital	Montebello	22	387
Coast Plaza Hospital	Norwalk	22	374
John Muir Medical Center - Concord Campus	Concord	22	475
Providence Saint John's Health Center	Santa Monica	22	458
Saddleback Memorial Medical Center	Laguna Hills	22	386
Scripps Memorial Hospital - Encinitas	Encinitas	22	404
Tri - City Regional Medical Center	Hawaiian Grdns	22	347
Bear Valley Community Hospital	Big Bear Lake	23	497
Marshall Medical Center	Placerville	23	404
Mills - Peninsula Medical Center	Burlingame	23	318
Mission Community Hospital	Panorama City	23	328
Northridge Hospital Medical Center	Northridge	23	428
O'Connor Hospital	San Jose	23	396
Washington Hospital	Fremont	23	426
Alhambra Hospital Medical Center	Alhambra	24	444
Barton Memorial Hospital	S Lake Tahoe	24	376
Petaluma Valley Hospital	Petaluma	24	317
Saint Louise Regional Hospital	Gilroy	24	413
Santa Monica-UCLA Med Ctr & Ortho Hosp	Santa Monica	24	430
Alameda Hospital	Alameda	25	357
Goleta Valley Cottage Hospital	Santa Barbara	25	392
Queen of the Valley Medical Center	Napa	25	388
San Gabriel Valley Medical Center	San Gabriel	25	413
Chinese Hospital	San Francisco	26	1043
Glendale Adventist Medical Center	Glendale	26	384
Natividad Medical Center	Salinas	26	637
Sharp Memorial Hospital	San Diego	26	385
Sierra Vista Regional Medical Center	San Luis Obispo	26	487
Southern California Hospital at Hollywood[3]	Hollywood	26	273
Methodist Hospital of Southern California	Arcadia	27	414
Sharp Coronado Hosp & Healthcare Ctr	Coronado	27	299
Stanford Hospital	Stanford	27	400
Twin Cities Community Hospital	Templeton	27	502
Chapman Medical Center	Orange	28	328
Coastal Communities Hospital	Santa Ana	28	366
Desert Regional Medical Center	Palm Springs	28	378
Emanuel Medical Center	Turlock	28	424
Pomona Valley Hospital Medical Center	Pomona	28	351
Redlands Community Hospital	Redlands	28	368
Sutter Delta Medical Center	Antioch	28	381
Ahmc Anaheim Regional Medical Center	Anaheim	29	377
California Hosp Med Ctr Los Angeles	Los Angeles	29	420
Feather River Hospital	Paradise	29	363
Marin General Hospital	Greenbrae	29	423
Saint Jude Medical Center	Fullerton	29	403
Sutter Coast Hospital	Crescent City	29	357
Adventist Medical Center - Reedley	Reedley	30	372
Colusa Regional Medical Center	Colusa	30	482
Corona Regional Medical Center	Corona	30	396
Garfield Medical Center	Monterey Park	30	402
Huntington Beach Hospital	Huntington Bch	30	386
Saint Rose Hospital	Hayward	30	2171
Western Medical Center Santa Ana	Santa Ana	30	84
Doctors Hospital of Manteca	Manteca	31	497
Doctors Medical Center - San Pablo	San Pablo	31	355
Garden Grove Hospital & Medical Center	Garden Grove	31	470
Mad River Community Hospital	Arcata	31	369
Memorial Hospital Los Banos	Los Banos	31	410
Northbay Medical Center	Fairfield	31	417
Providence Holy Cross Medical Center	Mission Hills	31	376
Sutter Roseville Medical Center	Roseville	31	385
Fountain Valley Reg Hosp & Med Ctr	Fountain Valley	32	493
La Palma Intercommunity Hospital	La Palma	32	750
San Ramon Regional Medical Center	San Ramon	32	413
Sutter Tracy Community Hospital	Tracy	32	422
White Memorial Medical Center	Los Angeles	32	397
Arrowhead Regional Medical Center	Colton	33	303
Comm Hosp of the Monterey Peninsula	Monterey	33	384
Palm Drive Hospital	Sebastopol	33	395
Santa Clara Valley Medical Center	San Jose	33	382
Southwest Healthcare System	Murrieta	33	423
Sutter Amador Hospital	Jackson	33	301
Sutter Auburn Faith Hospital	Auburn	33	407
Community Hospital of Long Beach	Long Beach	34	364
Corcoran District Hospital[3]	Corcoran	34	196
Hoag Memorial Hospital Presbyterian	Newport Beach	34	340
Memorial Medical Center	Modesto	34	412
Mission Hospital Regional Medical Center	Mission Viejo	34	383
Pacific Alliance Medical Center	Los Angeles	34	350
Saint Mary Medical Center	Apple Valley	34	403
Santa Rosa Memorial Hospital	Santa Rosa	34	314
UCSF Medical Center	San Francisco	34	383
Madera Community Hospital	Madera	35	606
Sutter Lakeside Hospital	Lakeport	35	357
Sutter Medical Center of Santa Rosa	Santa Rosa	35	359
CA Pacific Med Ctr-St Luke's Campus	San Francisco	36	411
Hazel Hawkins Memorial Hospital	Hollister	36	764
Victor Valley Global Medical Center	Victorville	36	366
Lompoc Valley Medical Center	Lompoc	37	349
Parkview Comm Hosp Med Ctr	Riverside	37	1293
Prov Little Co of Mary Med Ctr Torrance	Torrance	37	430
Enloe Medical Center	Chico	38	326
Providence Saint Joseph Medical Center	Burbank	38	514
Salinas Valley Memorial Hospital	Salinas	38	410
Santa Barbara Cottage Hospital	Santa Barbara	38	402
Univ of CA Davis Med Ctr	Sacramento	38	372
Saint Vincent Medical Center	Los Angeles	39	327
Sutter Solano Medical Center	Vallejo	39	408
Greater El Monte Community Hospital	South El Monte	40	356
Lodi Memorial Hospital	Lodi	40	405
Monterey Park Hospital	Monterey Park	40	389
San Francisco General Hospital	San Francisco	40	358
LAC+USC Medical Center	Los Angeles	42	324
Marina Del Rey Hospital	Marina Del Rey	42	382
Pacific Hospital of Long Beach[3]	Long Beach	42	149
Sutter General Hospital	Sacramento	42	403
USC Verdugo Hills Hospital	Glendale	42	393
Eisenhower Medical Center	Rancho Mirage	43	397
Los Alamitos Medical Center	Los Alamitos	43	381
Tri - City Medical Center	Oceanside	43	21797
Lakewood Regional Medical Center	Lakewood	44	475
Shasta Regional Medical Center	Redding	44	449
Sierra View District Hospital	Porterville	44	441
Alta Bates Summit Medical Center	Berkeley	46	384
Comm Mem Hosp San Buenaventura	Ventura	47	358
Western Medical Center Hospital Anaheim	Anaheim	48	353
Alta Bates Summit Medical Center	Oakland	49	381
Eden Medical Center	Castro Valley	49	591
Oroville Hospital	Oroville	49	397
Alvarado Hospital Medical Center	San Diego	50	198
Paradise Valley Hospital	National City	50	472
East Los Angeles Doctors Hospital	Los Angeles	51	371
San Antonio Community Hospital	Upland	51	389
Ronald Reagan UCLA Medical Center	Los Angeles	53	411
San Leandro Hospital[3]	San Leandro	53	200
West Anaheim Medical Center	Anaheim	53	391
San Mateo Medical Center	San Mateo	54	379
Menifee Valley Medical Center	Sun City	55	201
Pacifica Hospital of the Valley	Sun Valley	55	116
Centinela Hospital Medical Center	Inglewood	56	465
Good Samaritan Hospital	Los Angeles	56	406
Grossmont Hospital	La Mesa	56	355
Ventura County Medical Center[3]	Ventura	57	298
Contra Costa Regional Medical Center	Martinez	58	194
Desert Valley Hospital	Victorville	58	382
LAC/Harbor - UCLA Medical Center	Torrance	59	373
San Joaquin General Hospital	French Camp	59	335
Palmdale Regional Medical Center	Palmdale	60	405
Valley Presbyterian Hospital	Van Nuys	60	279
Cedars - Sinai Medical Center	Los Angeles	61	413
Saint Joseph Hospital	Orange	61	382
Citrus Valley Medical Center - IC Campus	Covina	62	313
Univ of California Irvine Med Ctr	Orange	64	376
Community Regional Medical Center	Fresno	65	345
Foothill Presbyterian Hospital	Glendora	69	289
Hemet Valley Medical Center	Hemet	70	209
Tulare Regional Medical Center	Tulare	70	398
Kern Medical Center	Bakersfield	71	377
Torrance Memorial Medical Center	Torrance	77	1552
Huntington Memorial Hospital	Pasadena	78	400
Riverside County Regional Medical Center	Moreno Valley	81	350
Saint Agnes Medical Center	Fresno	81	423
Community Hospital of Huntington Park	Huntington Park	82	462
Loma Linda Univ Med Ctr-Murrieta	Murrieta	82	291
Antelope Valley Hospital	Lancaster	84	472
PIH Hospital - Downey	Downey	90	354
Alameda County Medical Center	Oakland	95	399
Sharp Chula Vista Medical Center	Chula Vista	99	442
LAC/Olive View - UCLA Medical Center	Sylmar	101	371
Memorial Hospital of Gardena	Gardena	106	265
Saint Francis Medical Center	Lynwood	106	436
Loma Linda University Medical Center	Loma Linda	107	384

Time to Pain Meds for Bone Fractures (minutes)

Hospital Name	City	Min.	Cases
Santa Ynez Valley Cottage Hospital	Solvang	19	33
CA Pacific Med Ctr-Pacific Campus Hosp	San Francisco	28	172
Encino Hospital Medical Center	Encino	30	41
Foothill Presbyterian Hospital	Glendora	30	127
Sutter Davis Hospital	Davis	33	137
Goleta Valley Cottage Hospital	Santa Barbara	34	97
Novato Community Hospital	Novato	34	83
Scripps Memorial Hospital La Jolla	La Jolla	34	144
Saint Mary Medical Center	Long Beach	36	182
CA Pacific Med Ctr-Davies Campus	San Francisco	38	36
Coalinga Regional Medical Center	Coalinga	38	66
Coastal Communities Hospital	Santa Ana	38	76
Good Samaritan Hospital	San Jose	38	187
El Centro Regional Medical Center	El Centro	40	245
Placentia Linda Hospital	Placentia	40	181
Prov Little Co of Mary Med Ctr San Pedro	San Pedro	40	150
Sherman Oaks Hospital	Sherman Oaks	40	117
Glendale Mem Hosp & Health Ctr	Glendale	41	112
Simi Valley Hosp & Health Care Svcs	Simi Valley	41	90
Chino Valley Medical Center	Chino	42	197
Community Hospital of San Bernardino	San Bernardino	42	219

NOTE: Hospital profiles are in alphabetical order by state, then city, then hospital within the city; Rankings exclude hospitals with less than 25 cases except for patient surveys which excludes hospitals with less than 100 cases; (a) 100-299 cases; (1) The number of cases/patients is too few to report; (2) Data submitted were based on a sample of cases/patients; (3) Results are based on a shorter time period than required; (4) Data suppressed by CMS for one or more quarters; (5) Results are not available for this reporting period; (6) Fewer than 100 patients completed the HCAHPS survey; (7) No cases met the criteria for this measure; (8) The lower limit of the confidence interval cannot be calculated if the number of observed infections equals zero; (9) No data are available from the state/territory for this reporting period; (10) The scores shown reflect fewer than 50 completed surveys; (11) There were discrepancies in the data collection process; (12) This measure does not apply to this hospital for this reporting period; (13) Results cannot be calculated for this reporting period; (14) The results for this state are combined with nearby states to protect confidentiality; Please refer to the User's Guide for a full explanation of data.

French Hospital Medical Center	San Luis Obispo	42	66
Mercy San Juan Medical Center	Carmichael	42	198
Sharp Chula Vista Medical Center	Chula Vista	42	205
Henry Mayo Newhall Memorial Hospital	Valencia	43	243
Western Medical Center Santa Ana	Santa Ana	43	65
Alhambra Hospital Medical Center	Alhambra	44	42
Doctors Medical Center	Modesto	44	230
Emanuel Medical Center	Turlock	44	204
Methodist Hospital of Southern California	Arcadia	44	250
Pioneers Memorial Healthcare District	Brawley	44	179
Providence Holy Cross Medical Center	Mission Hills	44	240
Saint Bernardine Medical Center	San Bernardino	44	208
San Gorgonio Memorial Hospital	Banning	44	155
Scripps Mercy Hospital	San Diego	44	186
Sequoia Hospital	Redwood City	44	113
Marian Regional Medical Center	Santa Maria	45	260
Orange Coast Memorial Medical Center	Fountain Valley	45	85
Palo Verde Hospital	Blythe	45	34
Watsonville Community Hospital	Watsonville	45	44
West Hills Hospital & Medical Center	West Hills	45	171
Fallbrook Hospital	Fallbrook	46	46
George L Mee Memorial Hospital	King City	46	60
Natividad Medical Center	Salinas	46	147
Providence Tarzana Medical Center	Tarzana	46	137
Saint Helena Hospital	Saint Helena	46	45
Scripps Memorial Hospital - Encinitas	Encinitas	46	199
Sharp Coronado Hosp & Healthcare Ctr	Coronado	46	37
Ukiah Valley Medical Center	Ukiah	46	36
Saint Francis Memorial Hospital	San Francisco	47	50
Saint Johns Pleasant Valley Hospital	Camarillo	47	117
Saint Vincent Medical Center	Los Angeles	47	48
Los Alamitos Medical Center	Los Alamitos	48	224
Valleycare Medical Center	Pleasanton	48	217
Marshall Medical Center	Placerville	49	123
Colusa Regional Medical Center	Colusa	50	32
Delano Regional Medical Center	Delano	50	67
Hoag Memorial Hospital Presbyterian	Newport Beach	50	607
La Palma Intercommunity Hospital	La Palma	50	95
Saint Elizabeth Community Hospital	Red Bluff	50	164
Sharp Memorial Hospital	San Diego	50	163
Woodland Memorial Hospital	Woodland	50	114
Chapman Medical Center	Orange	51	35
Huntington Beach Hospital	Huntington Bch	51	99
Sutter Amador Hospital	Jackson	51	77
Ahmc Anaheim Regional Medical Center	Anaheim	52	149
Alameda Hospital	Alameda	52	35
Citrus Valley Medical Center - IC Campus	Covina	52	247
Hi - Desert Medical Center	Joshua Tree	52	48
Saddleback Memorial Medical Center	Laguna Hills	52	194
Saint Mary's Medical Center	San Francisco	52	80
Doctors Medical Center - San Pablo	San Pablo	53	159
Montclair Hospital Medical Center	Montclair	53	57
Pomerado Hospital	Poway	53	143
Saint Johns Regional Medical Center	Oxnard	53	212
Saint Jude Medical Center	Fullerton	53	341
Twin Cities Community Hospital	Templeton	53	152
Barton Memorial Hospital	S Lake Tahoe	54	133
Bear Valley Community Hospital	Big Bear Lake	54	230
Corona Regional Medical Center	Corona	54	309
Glendale Adventist Medical Center	Glendale	54	104
Marin General Hospital	Greenbrae	54	167
Mercy Hospital of Folsom	Folsom	54	170
Methodist Hospital of Sacramento	Sacramento	54	220
San Dimas Community Hospital	San Dimas	54	83
Santa Barbara Cottage Hospital	Santa Barbara	54	181
El Camino Hospital	Mountain View	55	345
Pacifica Hospital of the Valley	Sun Valley	55	42
Queen of the Valley Medical Center	Napa	55	154
Sutter Medical Center of Santa Rosa	Santa Rosa	55	60
Alta Bates Summit Medical Center	Berkeley	56	44
Monterey Park Hospital	Monterey Park	56	57
Santa Monica-UCLA Med Ctr & Ortho Hosp	Santa Monica	56	141
Sierra Vista Regional Medical Center	San Luis Obispo	56	151
Southern California Hospital at Hollywood[3]	Hollywood	56	71
Doctors Hospital of Manteca	Manteca	57	112
Mills - Peninsula Medical Center	Burlingame	57	159
Mission Community Hospital	Panorama City	57	38
Barstow Community Hospital	Barstow	58	58
John Muir Medical Center - Concord Campus	Concord	58	136
John Muir Med Ctr-Walnut Creek Campus	Walnut Creek	58	192
Memorial Hospital Los Banos	Los Banos	58	98
UCSF Medical Center	San Francisco	58	71
Northbay Medical Center	Fairfield	59	179
Providence Saint John's Health Center	Santa Monica	59	140
Riverside Community Hospital	Riverside	59	247
Ronald Reagan UCLA Medical Center	Los Angeles	59	104
Stanford Hospital	Stanford	59	326
Sutter Solano Medical Center	Vallejo	59	85
Grossmont Hospital	La Mesa	60	271
Lompoc Valley Medical Center	Lompoc	60	85
Mercy Medical Center - Mount Shasta	Mount Shasta	60	53
Sierra Nevada Memorial Hospital	Grass Valley	60	124
Sutter Auburn Faith Hospital	Auburn	60	143
Sutter Coast Hospital	Crescent City	60	92
Alta Bates Summit Medical Center	Oakland	61	37
California Hosp Med Ctr Los Angeles	Los Angeles	61	320
Palm Drive Hospital	Sebastopol	61	47
Saint Joseph's Medical Center of Stockton	Stockton	61	151
Saint Rose Hospital	Hayward	61	98
San Joaquin Community Hospital	Bakersfield	61	127
Adventist Medical Center	Hanford	62	207
Desert Regional Medical Center	Palm Springs	62	238
Garfield Medical Center	Monterey Park	62	138
Hollywood Presbyterian Medical Center	Los Angeles	62	86
Kaweah Delta Medical Center	Visalia	62	330
Lodi Memorial Hospital	Lodi	62	132
Mercy Medical Center - Redding	Redding	62	207
Northridge Hospital Medical Center	Northridge	62	198
Palomar Health Downtown Campus	Escondido	62	383
Presbyterian Intercommunity Hospital	Whittier	62	166
Seton Medical Center	Daly City	62	82
Washington Hospital	Fremont	62	172
Whittier Hospital Medical Center	Whittier	62	136
CA Pacific Med Ctr-St Luke's Campus	San Francisco	63	68
Clovis Community Medical Center	Clovis	63	145
LAC+USC Medical Center	Los Angeles	63	208
Mercy General Hospital	Sacramento	63	79
Sonoma Valley Hospital	Sonoma	63	61
Sutter Delta Medical Center	Antioch	63	174
Dameron Hospital	Stockton	64	121
Fountain Valley Reg Hosp & Med Ctr	Fountain Valley	64	158
O'Connor Hospital	San Jose	64	112
Pomona Valley Hospital Medical Center	Pomona	64	348
Southwest Healthcare System	Murrieta	64	382
Enloe Medical Center	Chico	65	109
Hazel Hawkins Memorial Hospital	Hollister	65	79
LAC/Harbor - UCLA Medical Center	Torrance	65	204
Madera Community Hospital	Madera	65	113
Petaluma Valley Hospital	Petaluma	65	87
Mission Hospital Regional Medical Center	Mission Viejo	66	124
San Gabriel Valley Medical Center	San Gabriel	66	114
Sutter Tracy Community Hospital	Tracy	66	173
Univ of CA San Diego Med Ctr	San Diego	66	94
Memorial Medical Center	Modesto	67	216
Oak Valley District Hospital	Oakdale	67	92
Sutter General Hospital	Sacramento	67	238
USC Verdugo Hills Hospital	Glendale	67	94
West Anaheim Medical Center	Anaheim	67	95
Adventist Medical Center - Reedley	Reedley	68	74
John F Kennedy Memorial Hospital	Indio	68	227
Lakewood Regional Medical Center	Lakewood	68	194
Saint Joseph Hospital	Eureka	68	118
San Ramon Regional Medical Center	San Ramon	68	148
Sutter Lakeside Hospital	Lakeport	68	120
Beverly Hospital	Montebello	69	145
Victor Valley Global Medical Center	Victorville	69	36
Saint Mary Medical Center	Apple Valley	70	208
Mad River Community Hospital	Arcata	72	85
San Francisco General Hospital	San Francisco	72	226
Torrance Memorial Medical Center	Torrance	72	276
Tulare Regional Medical Center	Tulare	72	124
Cedars - Sinai Medical Center	Los Angeles	73	219
Comm Hosp of the Monterey Peninsula	Monterey	73	77
Rideout Memorial Hospital	Marysville	73	254
Feather River Hospital	Paradise	74	46
Garden Grove Hospital & Medical Center	Garden Grove	74	122
Saint Louise Regional Hospital	Gilroy	74	51
Salinas Valley Memorial Hospital	Salinas	74	168
Tri - City Medical Center	Oceanside	74	204
Dominican Hospital	Santa Cruz	75	207
Los Robles Hospital & Medical Center	Thousand Oaks	75	219
Saint Joseph Hospital	Orange	75	302
Sonora Regional Medical Center	Sonora	75	145
Good Samaritan Hospital	Los Angeles	76	79
Long Beach Memorial Medical Center	Long Beach	76	39
Marina Del Rey Hospital	Marina Del Rey	76	126
San Antonio Community Hospital	Upland	76	64
Valley Presbyterian Hospital	Van Nuys	76	112
Greater El Monte Community Hospital	South El Monte	77	79
Kern Medical Center	Bakersfield	77	197
Mercy Hospital	Bakersfield	77	314
Regional Medical Center of San Jose	San Jose	77	191
Antelope Valley Hospital	Lancaster	78	246
Bakersfield Memorial Hospital	Bakersfield	78	239
East Los Angeles Doctors Hospital	Los Angeles	78	40
Shasta Regional Medical Center	Redding	78	174
Eisenhower Medical Center	Rancho Mirage	79	319
Sutter Roseville Medical Center	Roseville	79	334
Centinela Hospital Medical Center	Inglewood	80	235
Palmdale Regional Medical Center	Palmdale	82	224
Prov Little Co of Mary Med Ctr Torrance	Torrance	82	206
Mercy Medical Center	Merced	83	169
Ventura County Medical Center[3]	Ventura	83	183
Univ of California Irvine Med Ctr	Orange	84	66
Community Hospital of Long Beach	Long Beach	85	27
Eden Medical Center	Castro Valley	85	123
LAC/Olive View - UCLA Medical Center	Sylmar	85	78
Redlands Community Hospital	Redlands	85	191
Santa Rosa Memorial Hospital	Santa Rosa	85	125
Univ of CA Davis Med Ctr	Sacramento	85	231
Community Regional Medical Center	Fresno	88	306
PIH Hospital - Downey	Downey	88	156
Providence Saint Joseph Medical Center	Burbank	88	356
San Joaquin General Hospital	French Camp	88	124
Arrowhead Regional Medical Center	Colton	90	252
Comm Mem Hosp San Buenaventura	Ventura	91	37
Memorial Hospital of Gardena	Gardena	91	93
San Mateo Medical Center	San Mateo	91	81
Sierra View District Hospital	Porterville	93	86
Saint Agnes Medical Center	Fresno	94	180
Paradise Valley Hospital	National City	96	58
Desert Valley Hospital	Victorville	98	181
Loma Linda Univ Med Ctr-Murrieta	Murrieta	99	152
Oroville Hospital	Oroville	101	91
Contra Costa Regional Medical Center	Martinez	103	53
Coast Plaza Hospital	Norwalk	104	45
Santa Clara Valley Medical Center	San Jose	106	134
White Memorial Medical Center	Los Angeles	108	80
Riverside County Regional Medical Center	Moreno Valley	113	161
Alameda County Medical Center	Oakland	115	263
Community Hospital of Huntington Park	Huntington Park	123	221
Loma Linda University Medical Center	Loma Linda	124	174
Huntington Memorial Hospital	Pasadena	127	183
Hemet Valley Medical Center	Hemet	128	99
Saint Francis Medical Center	Lynwood	142	245
Western Medical Center Hospital Anaheim	Anaheim	143	31

Heart Attack Care

Aspirin Given at Discharge

Hospital Name	City	Rate	Cases
Ahmc Anaheim Regional Medical Center	Anaheim	100%	247
Alameda County Medical Center	Oakland	100%	99
Alta Bates Summit Medical Center	Oakland	100%	377
Alvarado Hospital Medical Center	San Diego	100%	87
CA Pacific Med Ctr-Pacific Campus Hosp	San Francisco	100%	199
Cedars - Sinai Medical Center	Los Angeles	100%	390
Centinela Hospital Medical Center[2]	Inglewood	100%	190
Clovis Community Medical Center[2]	Clovis	100%	50
Community Hospital of Huntington Park	Huntington Park	100%	26
Comm Mem Hosp San Buenaventura	Ventura	100%	219
Community Regional Medical Center[2]	Fresno	100%	513
Corona Regional Medical Center	Corona	100%	26
Desert Valley Hospital	Victorville	100%	152
Doctors Medical Center	Modesto	100%	312
Doctors Medical Center - San Pablo	San Pablo	100%	136
Eden Medical Center	Castro Valley	100%	43
El Camino Hospital	Mountain View	100%	192
Emanuel Medical Center	Turlock	100%	245
Enloe Medical Center	Chico	100%	295
Feather River Hospital	Paradise	100%	33
French Hospital Medical Center[2]	San Luis Obispo	100%	268
Fresno Heart & Surgical Hospital[2]	Fresno	100%	37
Garfield Medical Center[2]	Monterey Park	100%	196
Glendale Adventist Medical Center	Glendale	100%	329
Good Samaritan Hospital	Los Angeles	100%	238
Good Samaritan Hospital	San Jose	100%	198
Grossmont Hospital	La Mesa	100%	320
Henry Mayo Newhall Memorial Hospital	Valencia	100%	160
Hoag Memorial Hospital Presbyterian	Newport Beach	100%	346
John Muir Medical Center - Concord Campus	Concord	100%	322
John Muir Med Ctr-Walnut Creek Campus	Walnut Creek	100%	81
Kaiser Foundation Hospital	San Rafael	100%	43
Kaiser Foundation Hospital & Rehab Center	Vallejo	100%	146
Kaiser Foundation Hospital - Baldwin Park	Baldwin Park	100%	85
Kaiser Foundation Hospital - Downey	Downey	100%	97
Kaiser Foundation Hospital - Fontana	Fontana	100%	197
Kaiser Fdn Hosp-Fremont/Hayward	Hayward	100%	99
Kaiser Foundation Hospital - Fresno	Fresno	100%	77
Kaiser Foundation Hospital - Los Angeles[2]	Los Angeles	100%	733
Kaiser Foundation Hospital - Manteca	Manteca	100%	63
Kaiser Fdn Hosp-Moreno Valley	Moreno Valley	100%	32
Kaiser Fdn Hosp-Orange Co-Anaheim	Anaheim	100%	144
Kaiser Fdn Hosp-Panorama City	Panorama City	100%	57
Kaiser Foundation Hospital - Redwood City	Redwood City	100%	57
Kaiser Foundation Hospital - Sacramento	Sacramento	100%	79
Kaiser Foundation Hospital - San Diego	San Diego	100%	105
Kaiser Foundation Hospital - Santa Clara[2]	Santa Clara	100%	291
Kaiser Foundation Hospital - Santa Rosa	Santa Rosa	100%	51
Kaiser Foundation Hospital - South Bay	Harbor City	100%	54
Kaiser Fdn Hosp-S San Francisco	S San Francisco	100%	25
Kaiser Foundation Hospital - Vacaville	Vacaville	100%	65

NOTE: Hospital profiles are in alphabetical order by state, then city, then hospital within the city; Rankings exclude hospitals with less than 25 cases except for patient surveys which excludes hospitals with less than 100 cases; (a) 100-299 cases; (1) The number of cases/patients is too few to report; (2) Data submitted were based on a sample of cases/patients; (3) Results are based on a shorter time period than required; (4) Data suppressed by CMS for one or more quarters; (5) Results are not available for this reporting period; (6) Fewer than 100 patients completed the HCAHPS survey; (7) No cases met the criteria for this measure; (8) The lower limit of the confidence interval cannot be calculated if the number of observed infections equals zero; (9) No data are available from the state/territory for this reporting period; (10) The scores shown reflect fewer than 50 completed surveys; (11) There were discrepancies in the data collection process; (12) This measure does not apply to this hospital for this reporting period; (13) Results cannot be calculated for this reporting period; (14) The results for this state are combined with nearby states to protect confidentiality; Please refer to the User's Guide for a full explanation of data.

Kaiser Foundation Hospital - Walnut Creek	Walnut Creek	100%	204
Kaiser Foundation Hospital - West La	Los Angeles	100%	77
Kaiser Fdn Hosp-Woodland Hills	Woodland Hills	100%	93
Kaiser Fdn Hosp S Sacramento	Sacramento	100%	107
Keck Hospital of USC	Los Angeles	100%	55
La Palma Intercommunity Hospital	La Palma	100%	36
LAC+USC Medical Center	Los Angeles	100%	221
LAC/Olive View - UCLA Medical Center	Sylmar	100%	92
Loma Linda VA Medical Center	Loma Linda	100%	53
Los Robles Hospital & Medical Center	Thousand Oaks	100%	296
Marin General Hospital	Greenbrae	100%	176
Memorial Medical Center	Modesto	100%	352
Mercy General Hospital	Sacramento	100%	1112
Mercy Medical Center - Redding[2]	Redding	100%	234
Mercy San Juan Medical Center[2]	Carmichael	100%	241
Methodist Hospital of Southern California	Arcadia	100%	194
Mills - Peninsula Medical Center	Burlingame	100%	197
Northbay Medical Center	Fairfield	100%	202
Northridge Hospital Medical Center	Northridge	100%	237
Olympia Medical Center	Los Angeles	100%	34
Palmdale Regional Medical Center[2]	Palmdale	100%	198
Palo Alto VA Medical Center	Palo Alto	100%	59
Palomar Health Downtown Campus	Escondido	100%	398
Paradise Valley Hospital	National City	100%	30
Presbyterian Intercommunity Hospital[2]	Whittier	100%	252
Providence Holy Cross Medical Center	Mission Hills	100%	218
Prov Little Co of Mary Med Ctr Torrance	Torrance	100%	307
Providence Saint John's Health Center	Santa Monica	100%	124
Queen of the Valley Medical Center	Napa	100%	103
Riverside Community Hospital[2]	Riverside	100%	278
Riverside County Regional Medical Center	Moreno Valley	100%	36
Ronald Reagan UCLA Medical Center	Los Angeles	100%	185
Saint Bernardine Medical Center[2]	San Bernardino	100%	296
Saint Johns Regional Medical Center	Oxnard	100%	226
Saint Joseph's Medical Center of Stockton	Stockton	100%	326
Saint Jude Medical Center[2]	Fullerton	100%	263
Saint Mary Medical Center[2]	Apple Valley	100%	226
Saint Vincent Medical Center	Los Angeles	100%	134
Salinas Valley Memorial Hospital	Salinas	100%	202
San Francisco VA Medical Center	San Francisco	100%	39
San Gabriel Valley Medical Center	San Gabriel	100%	32
San Joaquin Community Hospital	Bakersfield	100%	253
San Joaquin General Hospital	French Camp	100%	43
San Ramon Regional Medical Center	San Ramon	100%	56
Santa Barbara Cottage Hospital	Santa Barbara	100%	230
Santa Clara Valley Medical Center	San Jose	100%	177
Santa Monica-UCLA Med Ctr & Ortho Hosp	Santa Monica	100%	150
Scripps Green Hospital	La Jolla	100%	195
Scripps Memorial Hospital - Encinitas	Encinitas	100%	155
Scripps Memorial Hospital La Jolla[2]	La Jolla	100%	269
Sequoia Hospital	Redwood City	100%	76
Seton Medical Center	Daly City	100%	138
Sharp Memorial Hospital	San Diego	100%	236
Sherman Oaks Hospital	Sherman Oaks	100%	65
Stanford Hospital	Stanford	100%	184
Sutter General Hospital	Sacramento	100%	436
Sutter Medical Center of Santa Rosa	Santa Rosa	100%	147
Sutter Tracy Community Hospital	Tracy	100%	30
Tri - City Medical Center[2]	Oceanside	100%	271
Tulare Regional Medical Center	Tulare	100%	26
UCSF Medical Center	San Francisco	100%	136
Univ of CA San Diego Med Ctr	San Diego	100%	266
VA Long Beach Healthcare System	Long Beach	100%	28
VA San Diego Healthcare System	San Diego	100%	79
Valleycare Medical Center	Pleasanton	100%	114
West Anaheim Medical Center	Anaheim	100%	129
Bakersfield Memorial Hospital[2]	Bakersfield	99%	292
Beverly Hospital	Montebello	99%	138
California Hosp Med Ctr Los Angeles	Los Angeles	99%	97
Dameron Hospital	Stockton	99%	261
Desert Regional Medical Center	Palm Springs	99%	363
Dominican Hospital[2]	Santa Cruz	99%	220
Glendale Mem Hosp & Health Ctr	Glendale	99%	172
John F Kennedy Memorial Hospital	Indio	99%	101
Kaiser Foundation Hospital - Antioch	Antioch	99%	89
Kaiser Fdn Hosp-Oakland/Richmond	Oakland	99%	80
Kaiser Foundation Hospital - Riverside	Riverside	99%	86
Kaiser Fdn Hosp-San Francisco[2]	San Francisco	99%	286
Kaiser Foundation Hospital - San Jose	San Jose	99%	116
LAC/Harbor - UCLA Medical Center[2]	Torrance	99%	237
Lakewood Regional Medical Center	Lakewood	99%	250
Long Beach Memorial Medical Center	Long Beach	99%	224
Los Alamitos Medical Center	Los Alamitos	99%	140
Mission Hospital Regional Medical Center	Mission Viejo	99%	250
O'Connor Hospital	San Jose	99%	170
PIH Hospital - Downey	Downey	99%	235
Providence Saint Joseph Medical Center	Burbank	99%	261
Providence Tarzana Medical Center	Tarzana	99%	122
Saddleback Memorial Medical Center	Laguna Hills	99%	245
Saint Joseph Hospital	Eureka	99%	168
Saint Mary Medical Center	Long Beach	99%	131
Saint Mary's Medical Center	San Francisco	99%	95
Saint Rose Hospital	Hayward	99%	135
San Antonio Community Hospital	Upland	99%	325
Santa Rosa Memorial Hospital	Santa Rosa	99%	219
Scripps Mercy Hospital	San Diego	99%	353
Sharp Chula Vista Medical Center	Chula Vista	99%	149
Shasta Regional Medical Center	Redding	99%	160
Southern California Hospital at Hollywood	Hollywood	99%	72
Sutter Delta Medical Center	Antioch	99%	121
Sutter Roseville Medical Center	Roseville	99%	234
Torrance Memorial Medical Center	Torrance	99%	341
Washington Hospital	Fremont	99%	224
West Hills Hospital & Medical Center	West Hills	99%	152
Western Medical Center Santa Ana	Santa Ana	99%	184
Antelope Valley Hospital	Lancaster	98%	284
Bakersfield Heart Hospital[2]	Bakersfield	98%	217
Citrus Valley Medical Center - IC Campus	Covina	98%	394
Comm Hosp of the Monterey Peninsula	Monterey	98%	117
Eisenhower Medical Center	Rancho Mirage	98%	376
Fountain Valley Reg Hosp & Med Ctr	Fountain Valley	98%	249
Hollywood Presbyterian Medical Center	Los Angeles	98%	159
Kaiser Foundation Hospital - Roseville[2]	Roseville	98%	216
Kaweah Delta Medical Center[2]	Visalia	98%	314
Loma Linda University Medical Center	Loma Linda	98%	445
Memorial Hospital of Gardena	Gardena	98%	41
Pomona Valley Hospital Medical Center[2]	Pomona	98%	243
Regional Medical Center of San Jose	San Jose	98%	235
Saint Agnes Medical Center	Fresno	98%	370
Saint Francis Medical Center	Lynwood	98%	111
Saint Joseph Hospital	Orange	98%	245
San Francisco General Hospital	San Francisco	98%	144
Southwest Healthcare System	Murrieta	98%	41
Univ of CA Davis Med Ctr[2]	Sacramento	98%	251
Univ of California Irvine Med Ctr	Orange	98%	123
VA Greater Los Angeles Healthcare System	W Los Angeles	98%	103
Valley Presbyterian Hospital	Van Nuys	98%	201
East Los Angeles Doctors Hospital	Los Angeles	97%	29
Huntington Memorial Hospital[2]	Pasadena	97%	211
Lodi Memorial Hospital	Lodi	97%	34
Madera Community Hospital[2]	Madera	97%	36
Marian Regional Medical Center	Santa Maria	97%	146
Pomerado Hospital	Poway	97%	33
Redlands Community Hospital	Redlands	97%	60
Rideout Memorial Hospital	Marysville	97%	230
Western Medical Center Hospital Anaheim	Anaheim	97%	70
White Memorial Medical Center	Los Angeles	97%	251
Arrowhead Regional Medical Center	Colton	95%	82
Menifee Valley Medical Center	Sun City	95%	37
Mercy Medical Center	Merced	95%	37
Orange Coast Memorial Medical Center	Fountain Valley	95%	133
Saint Helena Hospital	Saint Helena	95%	118
Los Angeles Community Hospital	Los Angeles	94%	84
Ventura County Medical Center	Ventura	94%	34
El Centro Regional Medical Center	El Centro	93%	42
San Gorgonio Memorial Hospital	Banning	93%	61
Sierra View District Hospital	Porterville	92%	36
USC Verdugo Hills Hospital	Glendale	92%	26
Loma Linda Univ Med Ctr-Murrieta[2]	Murrieta	89%	192
Hemet Valley Medical Center[2]	Hemet	84%	81

PCI Within 90 Minutes of Arrival

Hospital Name	City	Rate	Cases
CA Pacific Med Ctr-Pacific Campus Hosp	San Francisco	100%	30
Cedars - Sinai Medical Center	Los Angeles	100%	81
Doctors Medical Center	Modesto	100%	50
El Camino Hospital	Mountain View	100%	38
Fountain Valley Reg Hosp & Med Ctr	Fountain Valley	100%	43
French Hospital Medical Center[2]	San Luis Obispo	100%	36
Glendale Adventist Medical Center	Glendale	100%	45
Good Samaritan Hospital	San Jose	100%	51
Grossmont Hospital	La Mesa	100%	121
John Muir Medical Center - Concord Campus	Concord	100%	34
Kaiser Foundation Hospital & Rehab Center	Vallejo	100%	41
Kaiser Foundation Hospital - San Jose	San Jose	100%	55
Los Robles Hospital & Medical Center	Thousand Oaks	100%	64
Marin General Hospital	Greenbrae	100%	25
Memorial Medical Center	Modesto	100%	46
Methodist Hospital of Southern California	Arcadia	100%	49
Pomona Valley Hospital Medical Center[2]	Pomona	100%	53
Providence Holy Cross Medical Center	Mission Hills	100%	75
Prov Little Co of Mary Med Ctr Torrance	Torrance	100%	28
Providence Saint Joseph Medical Center	Burbank	100%	71
Queen of the Valley Medical Center	Napa	100%	28
Riverside Community Hospital[2]	Riverside	100%	57
Ronald Reagan UCLA Medical Center	Los Angeles	100%	35
Saddleback Memorial Medical Center	Laguna Hills	100%	55
Saint Joseph's Medical Center of Stockton	Stockton	100%	40
Saint Mary Medical Center[2]	Apple Valley	100%	34
Saint Rose Hospital	Hayward	100%	33
Salinas Valley Memorial Hospital	Salinas	100%	31
Scripps Memorial Hospital La Jolla[2]	La Jolla	100%	45
UCSF Medical Center	San Francisco	100%	26
Dominican Hospital[2]	Santa Cruz	99%	72
Kaiser Foundation Hospital - Roseville[2]	Roseville	99%	73
Saint Agnes Medical Center	Fresno	99%	77
Torrance Memorial Medical Center	Torrance	99%	71
Alta Bates Summit Medical Center	Oakland	98%	51
Citrus Valley Medical Center - IC Campus	Covina	98%	50
Kaiser Foundation Hospital - Walnut Creek	Walnut Creek	98%	44
Northbay Medical Center	Fairfield	98%	41
Regional Medical Center of San Jose	San Jose	98%	43
Sharp Chula Vista Medical Center	Chula Vista	98%	43
Tri - City Medical Center[2]	Oceanside	98%	62
Univ of CA San Diego Med Ctr	San Diego	98%	40
Valleycare Medical Center	Pleasanton	98%	45
Ahmc Anaheim Regional Medical Center	Anaheim	97%	31
Alameda County Medical Center	Oakland	97%	35
Good Samaritan Hospital	Los Angeles	97%	59
Hoag Memorial Hospital Presbyterian	Newport Beach	97%	101
Mills - Peninsula Medical Center	Burlingame	97%	35
Palmdale Regional Medical Center[2]	Palmdale	97%	32
Saint Johns Regional Medical Center	Oxnard	97%	31
Saint Jude Medical Center[2]	Fullerton	97%	67
Sutter Delta Medical Center	Antioch	97%	39
Antelope Valley Hospital	Lancaster	96%	49
Bakersfield Memorial Hospital[2]	Bakersfield	96%	27
Enloe Medical Center	Chico	96%	45
Lakewood Regional Medical Center	Lakewood	96%	51
Loma Linda University Medical Center	Loma Linda	96%	48
Mission Hospital Regional Medical Center	Mission Viejo	96%	51
Sharp Memorial Hospital	San Diego	96%	50
Comm Mem Hosp San Buenaventura	Ventura	95%	38
Long Beach Memorial Medical Center	Long Beach	95%	41
Palomar Health Downtown Campus	Escondido	95%	94
Rideout Memorial Hospital	Marysville	95%	55
Saint Joseph Hospital	Orange	95%	38
Santa Barbara Cottage Hospital	Santa Barbara	95%	39
Sutter Roseville Medical Center	Roseville	95%	63
Community Regional Medical Center[2]	Fresno	94%	68
Providence Saint John's Health Center	Santa Monica	94%	34
San Francisco General Hospital	San Francisco	94%	31
Scripps Mercy Hospital	San Diego	94%	69
John F Kennedy Memorial Hospital	Indio	93%	27
Los Alamitos Medical Center	Los Alamitos	93%	29
Marian Regional Medical Center	Santa Maria	93%	42
San Joaquin Community Hospital	Bakersfield	93%	46
Scripps Memorial Hospital - Encinitas	Encinitas	93%	29
Washington Hospital	Fremont	93%	28
West Anaheim Medical Center	Anaheim	93%	27
Desert Regional Medical Center	Palm Springs	92%	51
Emanuel Medical Center	Turlock	92%	52
Kaweah Delta Medical Center[2]	Visalia	92%	73
Santa Rosa Memorial Hospital	Santa Rosa	92%	48
Bakersfield Heart Hospital[2]	Bakersfield	91%	34
LAC+USC Medical Center	Los Angeles	91%	44
Mercy General Hospital	Sacramento	91%	88
San Antonio Community Hospital	Upland	91%	53
Glendale Mem Hosp & Health Ctr	Glendale	90%	30
Mercy Medical Center - Redding[2]	Redding	90%	29
Mercy San Juan Medical Center[2]	Carmichael	90%	69
Northridge Hospital Medical Center	Northridge	90%	31
Seton Medical Center	Daly City	90%	29
West Hills Hospital & Medical Center	West Hills	90%	42
White Memorial Medical Center	Los Angeles	90%	41
Eisenhower Medical Center	Rancho Mirage	89%	56
Stanford Hospital	Stanford	89%	27
Dameron Hospital	Stockton	88%	26
LAC/Harbor - UCLA Medical Center[2]	Torrance	86%	37
Univ of CA Davis Med Ctr[2]	Sacramento	86%	42
Valley Presbyterian Hospital	Van Nuys	86%	43
O'Connor Hospital	San Jose	85%	34
Huntington Memorial Hospital[2]	Pasadena	67%	36
Loma Linda Univ Med Ctr-Murrieta[2]	Murrieta	66%	29
Desert Valley Hospital	Victorville	65%	37

Statin Prescribed at Discharge

Hospital Name	City	Rate	Cases
Alameda County Medical Center	Oakland	100%	99
CA Pacific Med Ctr-Pacific Campus Hosp	San Francisco	100%	200
Cedars - Sinai Medical Center	Los Angeles	100%	377
Centinela Hospital Medical Center[2]	Inglewood	100%	158
Clovis Community Medical Center[2]	Clovis	100%	54
Desert Valley Hospital	Victorville	100%	150
Doctors Medical Center - San Pablo	San Pablo	100%	125
Eden Medical Center	Castro Valley	100%	39
El Camino Hospital	Mountain View	100%	179
Enloe Medical Center	Chico	100%	295
Glendale Adventist Medical Center	Glendale	100%	330
Good Samaritan Hospital	San Jose	100%	192
Grossmont Hospital	La Mesa	100%	297
John Muir Medical Center - Concord Campus	Concord	100%	314
Kaiser Foundation Hospital - Downey	Downey	100%	97

NOTE: Hospital profiles are in alphabetical order by state, then city, then hospital within the city; Rankings exclude hospitals with less than 25 cases except for patient surveys which excludes hospitals with less than 100 cases; (a) 100-299 cases; (1) The number of cases/patients is too few to report; (2) Data submitted were based on a sample of cases/patients; (3) Results are based on a shorter time period than required; (4) Data suppressed by CMS for one or more quarters; (5) Results are not available for this reporting period; (6) Fewer than 100 patients completed the HCAHPS survey; (7) No cases met the criteria for this measure; (8) The lower limit of the confidence interval cannot be calculated if the number of observed infections equals zero; (9) No data are available from the state/territory for this reporting period; (10) The scores shown reflect fewer than 50 completed surveys; (11) There were discrepancies in the data collection process; (12) This measure does not apply to this hospital for this reporting period; (13) Results cannot be calculated for this reporting period; (14) The results for this state are combined with nearby states to protect confidentiality; Please refer to the User's Guide for a full explanation of data.

Kaiser Fdn Hosp-Fremont/Hayward	Hayward	100%	108
Kaiser Foundation Hospital - Los Angeles[2]	Los Angeles	100%	715
Kaiser Foundation Hospital - Manteca	Manteca	100%	67
Kaiser Fdn Hosp-Moreno Valley	Moreno Valley	100%	31
Kaiser Fdn Hosp-Oakland/Richmond	Oakland	100%	83
Kaiser Fdn Hosp-Orange Co-Anaheim	Anaheim	100%	144
Kaiser Fdn Hosp-Panorama City	Panorama City	100%	63
Kaiser Foundation Hospital - Redwood City	Redwood City	100%	55
Kaiser Foundation Hospital - Riverside	Riverside	100%	87
Kaiser Foundation Hospital - Sacramento	Sacramento	100%	84
Kaiser Foundation Hospital - San Diego	San Diego	100%	108
Kaiser Fdn Hosp-San Francisco[2]	San Francisco	100%	281
Kaiser Foundation Hospital - Santa Clara[2]	Santa Clara	100%	287
Kaiser Foundation Hospital - Santa Rosa	Santa Rosa	100%	57
Kaiser Foundation Hospital - South Bay	Harbor City	100%	57
Kaiser Fdn Hosp-S San Francisco	S San Francisco	100%	26
Kaiser Foundation Hospital - Vacaville	Vacaville	100%	69
Kaiser Foundation Hospital - Walnut Creek	Walnut Creek	100%	200
Kaiser Foundation Hospital - West La	Los Angeles	100%	79
Kaiser Fdn Hosp-Woodland Hills	Woodland Hills	100%	93
Kaiser Fdn Hosp S Sacramento	Sacramento	100%	114
Keck Hospital of USC	Los Angeles	100%	56
La Palma Intercommunity Hospital	La Palma	100%	29
LAC+USC Medical Center	Los Angeles	100%	219
LAC/Olive View - UCLA Medical Center	Sylmar	100%	92
Loma Linda VA Medical Center	Loma Linda	100%	52
Los Alamitos Medical Center	Los Alamitos	100%	142
Los Robles Hospital & Medical Center	Thousand Oaks	100%	276
Mercy General Hospital	Sacramento	100%	1099
Mercy Medical Center - Redding[2]	Redding	100%	232
Methodist Hospital of Southern California	Arcadia	100%	195
Mills - Peninsula Medical Center	Burlingame	100%	199
Northridge Hospital Medical Center	Northridge	100%	237
Olympia Medical Center	Los Angeles	100%	27
Palomar Health Downtown Campus	Escondido	100%	378
Paradise Valley Hospital	National City	100%	31
Providence Holy Cross Medical Center	Mission Hills	100%	219
Prov Little Co of Mary Med Ctr Torrance	Torrance	100%	295
Providence Saint John's Health Center	Santa Monica	100%	122
Providence Tarzana Medical Center	Tarzana	100%	124
Riverside Community Hospital[2]	Riverside	100%	269
Riverside County Regional Medical Center	Moreno Valley	100%	36
Ronald Reagan UCLA Medical Center	Los Angeles	100%	182
Saint Joseph's Medical Center of Stockton	Stockton	100%	323
Saint Mary Medical Center[2]	Apple Valley	100%	235
Saint Mary's Medical Center	San Francisco	100%	97
Saint Vincent Medical Center	Los Angeles	100%	128
San Francisco VA Medical Center	San Francisco	100%	39
San Gabriel Valley Medical Center	San Gabriel	100%	34
San Joaquin Community Hospital	Bakersfield	100%	249
San Joaquin General Hospital	French Camp	100%	42
San Ramon Regional Medical Center	San Ramon	100%	54
Scripps Green Hospital	La Jolla	100%	176
Scripps Memorial Hospital - Encinitas	Encinitas	100%	139
Scripps Memorial Hospital La Jolla[2]	La Jolla	100%	260
Sequoia Hospital	Redwood City	100%	74
Sharp Memorial Hospital	San Diego	100%	236
Sherman Oaks Hospital	Sherman Oaks	100%	55
Sutter General Hospital	Sacramento	100%	416
Sutter Medical Center of Santa Rosa	Santa Rosa	100%	149
Sutter Roseville Medical Center	Roseville	100%	231
Sutter Tracy Community Hospital	Tracy	100%	28
Tri - City Medical Center[2]	Oceanside	100%	261
UCSF Medical Center	San Francisco	100%	135
Univ of California Irvine Med Ctr	Orange	100%	122
Univ of CA San Diego Med Ctr	San Diego	100%	263
VA Long Beach Healthcare System	Long Beach	100%	29
Valleycare Medical Center	Pleasanton	100%	115
West Anaheim Medical Center	Anaheim	100%	129
Ahmc Anaheim Regional Medical Center	Anaheim	99%	252
Alta Bates Summit Medical Center	Oakland	99%	376
California Hosp Med Ctr Los Angeles	Los Angeles	99%	88
Comm Mem Hosp San Buenaventura	Ventura	99%	214
Community Regional Medical Center[2]	Fresno	99%	529
Desert Regional Medical Center	Palm Springs	99%	354
Doctors Medical Center	Modesto	99%	321
Dominican Hospital[2]	Santa Cruz	99%	209
Garfield Medical Center[2]	Monterey Park	99%	199
Henry Mayo Newhall Memorial Hospital	Valencia	99%	157
Kaiser Foundation Hospital & Rehab Center	Vallejo	99%	142
Kaiser Foundation Hospital - Antioch	Antioch	99%	87
Kaiser Foundation Hospital - Baldwin Park	Baldwin Park	99%	89
Kaiser Foundation Hospital - Fontana	Fontana	99%	199
Kaiser Foundation Hospital - Fresno	Fresno	99%	74
Kaiser Foundation Hospital - Roseville[2]	Roseville	99%	217
Kaiser Foundation Hospital - San Jose	San Jose	99%	117
LAC/Harbor - UCLA Medical Center[2]	Torrance	99%	237
Lakewood Regional Medical Center	Lakewood	99%	252
Marian Regional Medical Center	Santa Maria	99%	135
Marin General Hospital	Greenbrae	99%	172
Memorial Medical Center	Modesto	99%	341
Mercy San Juan Medical Center[2]	Carmichael	99%	239
Northbay Medical Center	Fairfield	99%	199
O'Connor Hospital	San Jose	99%	166
Presbyterian Intercommunity Hospital[2]	Whittier	99%	259
Providence Saint Joseph Medical Center	Burbank	99%	257
Saint Bernardine Medical Center[2]	San Bernardino	99%	290
Saint Jude Medical Center[2]	Fullerton	99%	272
Saint Rose Hospital	Hayward	99%	130
Salinas Valley Memorial Hospital	Salinas	99%	192
Santa Barbara Cottage Hospital	Santa Barbara	99%	225
Santa Monica-UCLA Med Ctr & Ortho Hosp	Santa Monica	99%	147
Scripps Mercy Hospital	San Diego	99%	359
Sharp Chula Vista Medical Center	Chula Vista	99%	150
Shasta Regional Medical Center	Redding	99%	144
Stanford Hospital	Stanford	99%	179
VA San Diego Healthcare System	San Diego	99%	77
Washington Hospital	Fremont	99%	221
Antelope Valley Hospital	Lancaster	98%	281
Arrowhead Regional Medical Center	Colton	98%	82
Bakersfield Memorial Hospital[2]	Bakersfield	98%	287
Eisenhower Medical Center	Rancho Mirage	98%	364
El Centro Regional Medical Center	El Centro	98%	48
Emanuel Medical Center	Turlock	98%	237
Fountain Valley Reg Hosp & Med Ctr	Fountain Valley	98%	256
French Hospital Medical Center[2]	San Luis Obispo	98%	253
Glendale Mem Hosp & Health Ctr	Glendale	98%	176
Good Samaritan Hospital	Los Angeles	98%	236
Kaiser Foundation Hospital	San Rafael	98%	51
Long Beach Memorial Medical Center	Long Beach	98%	226
Palmdale Regional Medical Center[2]	Palmdale	98%	187
Palo Alto VA Medical Center	Palo Alto	98%	60
PIH Hospital - Downey	Downey	98%	243
Regional Medical Center of San Jose	San Jose	98%	235
Saint Francis Medical Center	Lynwood	98%	117
Saint Joseph Hospital	Eureka	98%	164
Santa Clara Valley Medical Center	San Jose	98%	178
Seton Medical Center	Daly City	98%	144
Southern California Hospital at Hollywood	Hollywood	98%	63
Torrance Memorial Medical Center	Torrance	98%	323
West Hills Hospital & Medical Center	West Hills	98%	156
White Memorial Medical Center	Los Angeles	98%	254
Beverly Hospital	Montebello	97%	143
Citrus Valley Medical Center - IC Campus	Covina	97%	400
Comm Hosp of the Monterey Peninsula	Monterey	97%	118
Dameron Hospital	Stockton	97%	266
Fresno Heart & Surgical Hospital[2]	Fresno	97%	35
Hoag Memorial Hospital Presbyterian	Newport Beach	97%	340
John Muir Med Ctr-Walnut Creek Campus	Walnut Creek	97%	76
Loma Linda University Medical Center	Loma Linda	97%	433
Queen of the Valley Medical Center	Napa	97%	105
Redlands Community Hospital	Redlands	97%	58
Rideout Memorial Hospital	Marysville	97%	216
Saint Agnes Medical Center	Fresno	97%	360
Saint Joseph Hospital	Orange	97%	245
San Antonio Community Hospital	Upland	97%	359
San Francisco General Hospital	San Francisco	97%	145
Santa Rosa Memorial Hospital	Santa Rosa	97%	210
Univ of CA Davis Med Ctr[2]	Sacramento	97%	251
VA Greater Los Angeles Healthcare System	W Los Angeles	97%	101
Ventura County Medical Center	Ventura	97%	34
Alvarado Hospital Medical Center	San Diego	96%	79
John F Kennedy Memorial Hospital	Indio	96%	101
Orange Coast Memorial Medical Center	Fountain Valley	96%	142
Pomona Valley Hospital Medical Center[2]	Pomona	96%	250
Saddleback Memorial Medical Center	Laguna Hills	96%	248
Saint Johns Regional Medical Center	Oxnard	96%	222
Saint Mary Medical Center	Long Beach	96%	134
Sutter Delta Medical Center	Antioch	96%	121
Western Medical Center Santa Ana	Santa Ana	96%	193
Whittier Hospital Medical Center	Whittier	96%	25
Bakersfield Heart Hospital[2]	Bakersfield	95%	206
Huntington Memorial Hospital[2]	Pasadena	95%	210
Kaweah Delta Medical Center[2]	Visalia	95%	310
Saint Helena Hospital	Saint Helena	95%	115
Southwest Healthcare System	Murrieta	95%	41
Valley Presbyterian Hospital	Van Nuys	95%	192
Hollywood Presbyterian Medical Center	Los Angeles	94%	158
Western Medical Center Hospital Anaheim	Anaheim	94%	66
Mission Hospital Regional Medical Center	Mission Viejo	93%	247
East Los Angeles Doctors Hospital	Los Angeles	92%	25
Feather River Hospital	Paradise	92%	26
Menifee Valley Medical Center	Sun City	92%	36
Lodi Memorial Hospital	Lodi	89%	36
Loma Linda Univ Med Ctr-Murrieta[2]	Murrieta	89%	186
Community Hospital of San Bernardino	San Bernardino	88%	25
Mercy Medical Center	Merced	86%	43
Pomerado Hospital	Poway	86%	28
Hemet Valley Medical Center[2]	Hemet	83%	78
Memorial Hospital of Gardena	Gardena	82%	44
Sierra View District Hospital	Porterville	81%	37
Madera Community Hospital[2]	Madera	75%	36
Los Angeles Community Hospital	Los Angeles	73%	84
San Gorgonio Memorial Hospital	Banning	68%	68

Heart Failure Care

ACE Inhibitor or ARB for LVSD

Hospital Name	City	Rate	Cases
Alameda County Medical Center	Oakland	100%	207
Alhambra Hospital Medical Center	Alhambra	100%	28
Cedars - Sinai Medical Center	Los Angeles	100%	299
Centinela Hospital Medical Center[2]	Inglewood	100%	126
Chino Valley Medical Center	Chino	100%	37
Community Hospital of San Bernardino	San Bernardino	100%	32
Comm Hosp of the Monterey Peninsula	Monterey	100%	76
Comm Mem Hosp San Buenaventura	Ventura	100%	81
Corona Regional Medical Center[2]	Corona	100%	58
Desert Valley Hospital[2]	Victorville	100%	114
Dominican Hospital[2]	Santa Cruz	100%	84
East Los Angeles Doctors Hospital	Los Angeles	100%	33
El Camino Hospital	Mountain View	100%	72
Emanuel Medical Center	Turlock	100%	90
Feather River Hospital	Paradise	100%	38
Foothill Presbyterian Hospital	Glendora	100%	38
French Hospital Medical Center	San Luis Obispo	100%	53
Fresno VA Med Ctr-VA Central CA	Fresno	100%	69
Garden Grove Hospital & Medical Center	Garden Grove	100%	28
Garfield Medical Center[2]	Monterey Park	100%	72
Good Samaritan Hospital	San Jose	100%	51
Grossmont Hospital	La Mesa	100%	255
Henry Mayo Newhall Memorial Hospital[2]	Valencia	100%	64
John F Kennedy Memorial Hospital	Indio	100%	37
John Muir Medical Center - Concord Campus	Concord	100%	60
Kaiser Foundation Hospital & Rehab Center	Vallejo	100%	49
Kaiser Foundation Hospital - Antioch	Antioch	100%	43
Kaiser Foundation Hospital - Baldwin Park	Baldwin Park	100%	124
Kaiser Foundation Hospital - Downey	Downey	100%	108
Kaiser Foundation Hospital - Fontana	Fontana	100%	212
Kaiser Fdn Hosp-Fremont/Hayward	Hayward	100%	76
Kaiser Foundation Hospital - Fresno[2]	Fresno	100%	71
Kaiser Foundation Hospital - Manteca	Manteca	100%	49
Kaiser Fdn Hosp-Moreno Valley	Moreno Valley	100%	52
Kaiser Fdn Hosp-Orange Co-Anaheim	Anaheim	100%	156
Kaiser Foundation Hospital - Redwood City	Redwood City	100%	27
Kaiser Foundation Hospital - Riverside	Riverside	100%	92
Kaiser Foundation Hospital - Roseville[2]	Roseville	100%	58
Kaiser Foundation Hospital - Sacramento	Sacramento	100%	57
Kaiser Fdn Hosp-San Francisco	San Francisco	100%	63
Kaiser Foundation Hospital - San Jose	San Jose	100%	49
Kaiser Foundation Hospital - Santa Clara[2]	Santa Clara	100%	76
Kaiser Foundation Hospital - Santa Rosa	Santa Rosa	100%	30
Kaiser Foundation Hospital - South Bay	Harbor City	100%	100
Kaiser Fdn Hosp-S San Francisco	S San Francisco	100%	38
Kaiser Foundation Hospital - Walnut Creek	Walnut Creek	100%	40
Kaiser Foundation Hospital - West La	Los Angeles	100%	102
Kaiser Fdn Hosp-Woodland Hills	Woodland Hills	100%	42
Kaiser Fdn Hosp S Sacramento[2]	Sacramento	100%	74
Keck Hospital of USC	Los Angeles	100%	37
La Palma Intercommunity Hospital	La Palma	100%	28
LAC+USC Medical Center	Los Angeles	100%	328
Lakewood Regional Medical Center	Lakewood	100%	108
Los Alamitos Medical Center	Los Alamitos	100%	87
Los Robles Hospital & Medical Center	Thousand Oaks	100%	80
Marin General Hospital[2]	Greenbrae	100%	41
Marina Del Rey Hospital	Marina Del Rey	100%	40
Marshall Medical Center	Placerville	100%	38
Memorial Medical Center[2]	Modesto	100%	70
Mercy Medical Center - Redding[2]	Redding	100%	127
Mercy San Juan Medical Center[2]	Carmichael	100%	99
Methodist Hospital of Southern California	Arcadia	100%	85
Mills - Peninsula Medical Center	Burlingame	100%	57
Mission Community Hospital	Panorama City	100%	26
Monterey Park Hospital	Monterey Park	100%	28
Olympia Medical Center	Los Angeles	100%	60
Palo Alto VA Medical Center	Palo Alto	100%	58
Paradise Valley Hospital	National City	100%	75
Pomona Valley Hospital Medical Center[2]	Pomona	100%	73
Providence Holy Cross Medical Center[2]	Mission Hills	100%	64
Prov Little Co of Mary Med Ctr Torrance[2]	Torrance	100%	113
Providence Saint John's Health Center	Santa Monica	100%	64
Riverside Community Hospital[2]	Riverside	100%	113
Riverside County Regional Medical Center[2]	Moreno Valley	100%	132
Saint Francis Medical Center	Lynwood	100%	231
Saint Francis Memorial Hospital	San Francisco	100%	36
Saint Johns Regional Medical Center	Oxnard	100%	52
Saint Rose Hospital	Hayward	100%	55
Saint Vincent Medical Center	Los Angeles	100%	108
Salinas Valley Memorial Hospital[2]	Salinas	100%	77
San Gabriel Valley Medical Center	San Gabriel	100%	46
San Joaquin General Hospital	French Camp	100%	93
San Leandro Hospital[3]	San Leandro	100%	25

NOTE: Hospital profiles are in alphabetical order by state, then city, then hospital within the city; Rankings exclude hospitals with less than 25 cases except for patient surveys which excludes hospitals with less than 100 cases; (a) 100-299 cases; (1) The number of cases/patients is too few to report; (2) Data submitted were based on a sample of cases/patients; (3) Results are based on a shorter time period than required; (4) Data suppressed by CMS for one or more quarters; (5) Results are not available for this reporting period; (6) Fewer than 100 patients completed the HCAHPS survey; (7) No cases met the criteria for this measure; (8) The lower limit of the confidence interval cannot be calculated if the number of observed infections equals zero; (9) No data are available from the state/territory for this reporting period; (10) The scores shown reflect fewer than 50 completed surveys; (11) There were discrepancies in the data collection process; (12) This measure does not apply to this hospital for this reporting period; (13) Results cannot be calculated for this reporting period; (14) The results for this state are combined with nearby states to protect confidentiality; Please refer to the User's Guide for a full explanation of data.

Hospital Name	City	Rate	Cases
San Mateo Medical Center	San Mateo	100%	44
Santa Clara Valley Medical Center[2]	San Jose	100%	119
Santa Monica-UCLA Med Ctr & Ortho Hosp[2]	Santa Monica	100%	54
Scripps Green Hospital	La Jolla	100%	90
Scripps Memorial Hospital - Encinitas	Encinitas	100%	58
Scripps Memorial Hospital La Jolla[2]	La Jolla	100%	91
Sequoia Hospital	Redwood City	100%	30
Sharp Chula Vista Medical Center	Chula Vista	100%	159
Sharp Memorial Hospital	San Diego	100%	148
Shasta Regional Medical Center	Redding	100%	95
Sutter General Hospital[2]	Sacramento	100%	108
Sutter Medical Center of Santa Rosa	Santa Rosa	100%	51
Sutter Roseville Medical Center[2]	Roseville	100%	84
Sutter Solano Medical Center	Vallejo	100%	55
Sutter Tracy Community Hospital	Tracy	100%	30
Temple Community Hospital	Los Angeles	100%	27
Tri - City Medical Center[2]	Oceanside	100%	65
Tulare Regional Medical Center	Tulare	100%	26
Twin Cities Community Hospital	Templeton	100%	30
UCSF Medical Center[2]	San Francisco	100%	65
Univ of California Irvine Med Ctr	Orange	100%	110
VA San Diego Healthcare System	San Diego	100%	87
West Anaheim Medical Center	Anaheim	100%	52
Whittier Hospital Medical Center	Whittier	100%	58
California Hosp Med Ctr Los Angeles	Los Angeles	99%	203
Citrus Valley Medical Center - IC Campus[2]	Covina	99%	88
Community Hospital of Huntington Park	Huntington Park	99%	67
Community Regional Medical Center[2]	Fresno	99%	398
Kaiser Foundation Hospital - Los Angeles	Los Angeles	99%	286
Kaiser Fdn Hosp-Oakland/Richmond[2]	Oakland	99%	114
Kaiser Foundation Hospital - San Diego	San Diego	99%	168
Long Beach Memorial Medical Center	Long Beach	99%	212
Memorial Hospital of Gardena	Gardena	99%	79
Mercy General Hospital	Sacramento	99%	164
Methodist Hospital of Sacramento[2]	Sacramento	99%	84
PIH Hospital - Downey	Downey	99%	135
Providence Saint Joseph Medical Center	Burbank	99%	139
Ronald Reagan UCLA Medical Center[2]	Los Angeles	99%	79
Saint Agnes Medical Center[2]	Fresno	99%	146
Saint Bernardine Medical Center[2]	San Bernardino	99%	119
Saint Joseph's Medical Center of Stockton[2]	Stockton	99%	145
Saint Mary's Medical Center	San Francisco	99%	69
San Joaquin Community Hospital	Bakersfield	99%	236
Southern California Hospital at Hollywood[2]	Hollywood	99%	75
Stanford Hospital	Stanford	99%	127
Torrance Memorial Medical Center	Torrance	99%	167
Washington Hospital	Fremont	99%	119
West Hills Hospital & Medical Center	West Hills	99%	68
Barstow Community Hospital	Barstow	98%	52
CA Pacific Med Ctr-Pacific Campus Hosp[2]	San Francisco	98%	65
Desert Regional Medical Center	Palm Springs	98%	162
Doctors Medical Center - San Pablo[2]	San Pablo	98%	119
Enloe Medical Center	Chico	98%	60
Glendale Adventist Medical Center	Glendale	98%	106
Hoag Memorial Hospital Presbyterian	Newport Beach	98%	86
John Muir Med Ctr-Walnut Creek Campus	Walnut Creek	98%	61
LAC/Olive View - UCLA Medical Center[2]	Sylmar	98%	130
Lodi Memorial Hospital[2]	Lodi	98%	104
O'Connor Hospital	San Jose	98%	66
Orange Coast Memorial Medical Center	Fountain Valley	98%	99
Palomar Health Downtown Campus	Escondido	98%	127
Queen of the Valley Medical Center	Napa	98%	61
Saddleback Memorial Medical Center	Laguna Hills	98%	109
Saint Joseph Hospital	Orange	98%	122
Scripps Mercy Hospital[2]	San Diego	98%	197
VA Northern California Healthcare System	Mather	98%	93
Valleycare Medical Center	Pleasanton	98%	51
Bakersfield Memorial Hospital[2]	Bakersfield	97%	99
Doctors Medical Center	Modesto	97%	144
Eden Medical Center	Castro Valley	97%	68
Good Samaritan Hospital[2]	Los Angeles	97%	102
Kaweah Delta Medical Center[2]	Visalia	97%	110
Loma Linda VA Medical Center	Loma Linda	97%	99
Marian Regional Medical Center	Santa Maria	97%	87
Northbay Medical Center	Fairfield	97%	117
Palmdale Regional Medical Center[2]	Palmdale	97%	110
Saint Louise Regional Hospital	Gilroy	97%	31
Saint Mary Medical Center[2]	Long Beach	97%	101
San Gorgonio Memorial Hospital	Banning	97%	38
Sierra Nevada Memorial Hospital	Grass Valley	97%	36
Sutter Delta Medical Center[2]	Antioch	97%	71
VA Greater Los Angeles Healthcare System	W Los Angeles	97%	116
Victor Valley Global Medical Center	Victorville	97%	58
White Memorial Medical Center	Los Angeles	97%	138
Alta Bates Summit Medical Center[2]	Oakland	96%	96
Antelope Valley Hospital	Lancaster	96%	141
Arrowhead Regional Medical Center[2]	Colton	96%	268
Glendale Mem Hosp & Health Ctr	Glendale	96%	121
Hollywood Presbyterian Medical Center[2]	Los Angeles	96%	78
Kaiser Fdn Hosp-Panorama City	Panorama City	96%	49
Kern Medical Center	Bakersfield	96%	56
LAC/Harbor - UCLA Medical Center[2]	Torrance	96%	144
Mark Twain Medical Center	San Andreas	96%	25
Pacific Alliance Medical Center	Los Angeles	96%	54
Petaluma Valley Hospital	Petaluma	96%	25
Prov Little Co of Mary Med Ctr San Pedro	San Pedro	96%	56
Saint Joseph Hospital	Eureka	96%	51
San Antonio Community Hospital	Upland	96%	133
San Francisco General Hospital[2]	San Francisco	96%	162
San Francisco VA Medical Center	San Francisco	96%	45
Sutter Coast Hospital	Crescent City	96%	27
Univ of CA San Diego Med Ctr[2]	San Diego	96%	101
Ahmc Anaheim Regional Medical Center	Anaheim	95%	133
Alta Bates Summit Medical Center[2]	Berkeley	95%	61
Clovis Community Medical Center[2]	Clovis	95%	58
Dameron Hospital	Stockton	95%	60
Fountain Valley Reg Hosp & Med Ctr	Fountain Valley	95%	107
Loma Linda University Medical Center[2]	Loma Linda	95%	127
Natividad Medical Center	Salinas	95%	38
Oroville Hospital	Oroville	95%	77
Pomerado Hospital	Poway	95%	41
Presbyterian Intercommunity Hospital[2]	Whittier	95%	84
Providence Tarzana Medical Center	Tarzana	95%	86
Saint Mary Medical Center[2]	Apple Valley	95%	110
Santa Barbara Cottage Hospital	Santa Barbara	95%	85
Santa Rosa Memorial Hospital	Santa Rosa	95%	83
Sierra View District Hospital	Porterville	95%	57
Mission Hospital Regional Medical Center	Mission Viejo	94%	78
Northridge Hospital Medical Center	Northridge	94%	122
Chinese Hospital	San Francisco	93%	30
Community Hospital of Long Beach	Long Beach	93%	30
Pioneers Memorial Healthcare District	Brawley	93%	58
Seton Medical Center	Daly City	93%	91
Southwest Healthcare System[2]	Murrieta	93%	76
Tri - City Regional Medical Center	Hawaiian Grdns	93%	28
Western Medical Center Santa Ana	Santa Ana	93%	41
Alvarado Hospital Medical Center	San Diego	92%	79
Contra Costa Regional Medical Center	Martinez	92%	85
Doctors Hospital of Manteca	Manteca	92%	48
Mercy Hospital	Bakersfield	92%	59
Parkview Comm Hosp Med Ctr[2]	Riverside	92%	48
Redlands Community Hospital	Redlands	92%	74
Saint Helena Hospital	Saint Helena	92%	38
VA Long Beach Healthcare System	Long Beach	92%	112
Bakersfield Heart Hospital[2]	Bakersfield	91%	79
Hi - Desert Medical Center	Joshua Tree	91%	43
Mercy Medical Center[2]	Merced	91%	95
Valley Presbyterian Hospital	Van Nuys	91%	107
Eisenhower Medical Center	Rancho Mirage	90%	202
Adventist Medical Center	Hanford	89%	138
Los Angeles Community Hospital[2]	Los Angeles	89%	91
Madera Community Hospital	Madera	89%	54
Regional Medical Center of San Jose	San Jose	89%	137
Univ of CA Davis Med Ctr[2]	Sacramento	89%	115
Beverly Hospital	Montebello	88%	81
Hemet Valley Medical Center[2]	Hemet	88%	112
Saint Elizabeth Community Hospital	Red Bluff	88%	26
El Centro Regional Medical Center	El Centro	87%	71
Menifee Valley Medical Center	Sun City	87%	45
Saint Jude Medical Center[2]	Fullerton	87%	123
Rideout Memorial Hospital	Marysville	85%	100
Ventura County Medical Center[2]	Ventura	85%	41
Huntington Memorial Hospital[2]	Pasadena	83%	111
Loma Linda Univ Med Ctr-Murrieta[2]	Murrieta	79%	111

Discharge Instructions Given

Hospital Name	City	Rate	Cases
Barstow Community Hospital	Barstow	100%	106
Cedars - Sinai Medical Center	Los Angeles	100%	901
Centinela Hospital Medical Center[2]	Inglewood	100%	230
Chino Valley Medical Center	Chino	100%	69
Community Hospital of Huntington Park	Huntington Park	100%	133
Community Hospital of San Bernardino	San Bernardino	100%	94
Dameron Hospital	Stockton	100%	149
Desert Valley Hospital[2]	Victorville	100%	276
Dominican Hospital[2]	Santa Cruz	100%	216
Encino Hospital Medical Center	Encino	100%	46
Garden Grove Hospital & Medical Center	Garden Grove	100%	66
Hollywood Presbyterian Medical Center[2]	Los Angeles	100%	202
Huntington Beach Hospital	Huntington Bch	100%	67
Kaiser Foundation Hospital & Rehab Center	Vallejo	100%	247
Kaiser Foundation Hospital - Antioch	Antioch	100%	209
Kaiser Foundation Hospital - Fontana	Fontana	100%	633
Kaiser Fdn Hosp-Fremont/Hayward	Hayward	100%	212
Kaiser Foundation Hospital - Fresno[2]	Fresno	100%	186
Kaiser Foundation Hospital - Manteca	Manteca	100%	179
Kaiser Fdn Hosp-Oakland/Richmond[2]	Oakland	100%	381
Kaiser Fdn Hosp-Orange Co-Anaheim	Anaheim	100%	418
Kaiser Fdn Hosp-Panorama City	Panorama City	100%	213
Kaiser Foundation Hospital - Redwood City	Redwood City	100%	91
Kaiser Foundation Hospital - Riverside	Riverside	100%	251
Kaiser Foundation Hospital - Roseville[2]	Roseville	100%	254
Kaiser Foundation Hospital - Sacramento	Sacramento	100%	156
Kaiser Foundation Hospital - San Diego	San Diego	100%	630
Kaiser Fdn Hosp-San Francisco	San Francisco	100%	245
Kaiser Foundation Hospital - San Jose	San Jose	100%	239
Kaiser Foundation Hospital - Santa Clara[2]	Santa Clara	100%	264
Kaiser Foundation Hospital - South Bay	Harbor City	100%	285
Kaiser Fdn Hosp-S San Francisco	S San Francisco	100%	187
Kaiser Foundation Hospital - Vacaville	Vacaville	100%	104
Kaiser Foundation Hospital - Walnut Creek	Walnut Creek	100%	232
Kaiser Fdn Hosp S Sacramento[2]	Sacramento	100%	283
Keck Hospital of USC	Los Angeles	100%	103
La Palma Intercommunity Hospital	La Palma	100%	84
Los Alamitos Medical Center	Los Alamitos	100%	223
Los Robles Hospital & Medical Center	Thousand Oaks	100%	228
Memorial Medical Center[2]	Modesto	100%	263
Methodist Hospital of Sacramento[2]	Sacramento	100%	245
Montclair Hospital Medical Center	Montclair	100%	51
Northridge Hospital Medical Center	Northridge	100%	284
Palomar Health Downtown Campus	Escondido	100%	436
Paradise Valley Hospital	National City	100%	209
Pioneers Memorial Healthcare District	Brawley	100%	140
Pomerado Hospital	Poway	100%	134
Prov Little Co of Mary Med Ctr Torrance[2]	Torrance	100%	257
Queen of the Valley Medical Center	Napa	100%	148
Riverside Community Hospital[2]	Riverside	100%	235
Riverside County Regional Medical Center[2]	Moreno Valley	100%	268
Saint Mary Medical Center[2]	Long Beach	100%	232
Saint Mary's Medical Center	San Francisco	100%	141
Saint Rose Hospital	Hayward	100%	188
San Antonio Community Hospital	Upland	100%	333
San Ramon Regional Medical Center	San Ramon	100%	50
Scripps Green Hospital	La Jolla	100%	223
Scripps Memorial Hospital La Jolla[2]	La Jolla	100%	214
Shasta Regional Medical Center	Redding	100%	245
Sherman Oaks Hospital	Sherman Oaks	100%	76
Silver Lake Medical Center	Los Angeles	100%	29
Sonora Regional Medical Center	Sonora	100%	87
Sutter Auburn Faith Hospital	Auburn	100%	59
Sutter Davis Hospital	Davis	100%	33
Sutter Lakeside Hospital	Lakeport	100%	40
Sutter Medical Center of Santa Rosa	Santa Rosa	100%	125
Sutter Solano Medical Center	Vallejo	100%	110
Temple Community Hospital	Los Angeles	100%	33
Tri - City Medical Center[2]	Oceanside	100%	205
Tulare Regional Medical Center	Tulare	100%	87
Twin Cities Community Hospital	Templeton	100%	93
USC Verdugo Hills Hospital	Glendale	100%	63
VA Northern California Healthcare System	Mather	100%	171
White Memorial Medical Center	Los Angeles	100%	288
Woodland Memorial Hospital	Woodland	100%	36
CA Pacific Med Ctr-St Luke's Campus	San Francisco	99%	97
Clovis Community Medical Center[2]	Clovis	99%	189
El Camino Hospital	Mountain View	99%	247
El Centro Regional Medical Center	El Centro	99%	196
Glendale Adventist Medical Center	Glendale	99%	335
Henry Mayo Newhall Memorial Hospital[2]	Valencia	99%	254
John Muir Medical Center - Concord Campus	Concord	99%	234
John Muir Med Ctr-Walnut Creek Campus	Walnut Creek	99%	234
Kaiser Foundation Hospital - Downey	Downey	99%	343
Kaiser Fdn Hosp-Moreno Valley	Moreno Valley	99%	115
Kaiser Foundation Hospital - West La	Los Angeles	99%	255
Marian Regional Medical Center	Santa Maria	99%	202
Mercy General Hospital	Sacramento	99%	383
Mercy San Juan Medical Center[2]	Carmichael	99%	256
Methodist Hospital of Southern California	Arcadia	99%	267
Mills - Peninsula Medical Center	Burlingame	99%	258
Palmdale Regional Medical Center[2]	Palmdale	99%	289
Presbyterian Intercommunity Hospital[2]	Whittier	99%	247
Providence Saint John's Health Center	Santa Monica	99%	145
Saint Louise Regional Hospital	Gilroy	99%	82
Salinas Valley Memorial Hospital[2]	Salinas	99%	213
San Gabriel Valley Medical Center	San Gabriel	99%	155
San Joaquin Community Hospital	Bakersfield	99%	505
Scripps Memorial Hospital - Encinitas	Encinitas	99%	199
Sierra View District Hospital	Porterville	99%	151
Stanford Hospital	Stanford	99%	292
Torrance Memorial Medical Center	Torrance	99%	405
VA Greater Los Angeles Healthcare System	W Los Angeles	99%	289
VA Long Beach Healthcare System	Long Beach	99%	230
VA San Diego Healthcare System	San Diego	99%	282
Washington Hospital	Fremont	99%	286
Watsonville Community Hospital	Watsonville	99%	71
West Anaheim Medical Center	Anaheim	99%	180
Whittier Hospital Medical Center	Whittier	99%	141
Adventist Medical Center	Hanford	98%	289
Community Regional Medical Center[2]	Fresno	98%	842
Desert Regional Medical Center	Palm Springs	98%	273
East Los Angeles Doctors Hospital	Los Angeles	98%	66
Good Samaritan Hospital	San Jose	98%	195
Hazel Hawkins Memorial Hospital[2]	Hollister	98%	43
John F Kennedy Memorial Hospital	Indio	98%	118

NOTE: Hospital profiles are in alphabetical order by state, then city, then hospital within the city; Rankings exclude hospitals with less than 25 cases except for patient surveys which excludes hospitals with less than 100 cases; (a) 100-299 cases; (1) The number of cases/patients is too few to report; (2) Data submitted were based on a sample of cases/patients; (3) Results are based on a shorter time period than required; (4) Data suppressed by CMS for one or more quarters; (5) Results are not available for this reporting period; (6) Fewer than 100 patients completed the HCAHPS survey; (7) No cases met the criteria for this measure; (8) The lower limit of the confidence interval cannot be calculated if the number of observed infections equals zero; (9) No data are available from the state/territory for this reporting period; (10) The scores shown reflect fewer than 50 completed surveys; (11) There were discrepancies in the data collection process; (12) This measure does not apply to this hospital for this reporting period; (13) Results cannot be calculated for this reporting period; (14) The results for this state are combined with nearby states to protect confidentiality; Please refer to the User's Guide for a full explanation of data.

Kaiser Foundation Hospital - Baldwin Park	Baldwin Park	98%	381
Kaiser Foundation Hospital - Los Angeles	Los Angeles	98%	533
Kaiser Foundation Hospital - Santa Rosa	Santa Rosa	98%	98
Kaiser Fdn Hosp-Woodland Hills	Woodland Hills	98%	247
LAC+USC Medical Center	Los Angeles	98%	618
Lakewood Regional Medical Center	Lakewood	98%	253
Long Beach Memorial Medical Center	Long Beach	98%	464
Mercy Hospital	Bakersfield	98%	143
O'Connor Hospital	San Jose	98%	234
Palo Alto VA Medical Center	Palo Alto	98%	154
Regional Medical Center of San Jose	San Jose	98%	407
Saint Elizabeth Community Hospital	Red Bluff	98%	63
Saint Francis Memorial Hospital	San Francisco	98%	108
Saint Johns Pleasant Valley Hospital	Camarillo	98%	81
Saint Joseph Hospital	Eureka	98%	135
Sierra Nevada Memorial Hospital	Grass Valley	98%	84
Sutter Amador Hospital	Jackson	98%	47
Sutter General Hospital[2]	Sacramento	98%	280
Sutter Roseville Medical Center[2]	Roseville	98%	225
Univ of California Irvine Med Ctr	Orange	98%	228
West Hills Hospital & Medical Center	West Hills	98%	147
CA Pacific Med Ctr-Pacific Campus Hosp[2]	San Francisco	97%	264
Enloe Medical Center	Chico	97%	175
French Hospital Medical Center	San Luis Obispo	97%	95
Fresno VA Med Ctr-VA Central CA	Fresno	97%	125
Kaiser Foundation Hospital	San Rafael	97%	104
Marin General Hospital[2]	Greenbrae	97%	147
Mercy Medical Center[2]	Merced	97%	240
Mercy Medical Center - Redding[2]	Redding	97%	229
Novato Community Hospital	Novato	97%	59
Oak Valley District Hospital	Oakdale	97%	32
Orange Coast Memorial Medical Center	Fountain Valley	97%	266
PIH Hospital - Downey	Downey	97%	291
Prov Little Co of Mary Med Ctr San Pedro	San Pedro	97%	116
Saint Agnes Medical Center[2]	Fresno	97%	362
San Francisco VA Medical Center	San Francisco	97%	147
Sharp Coronado Hosp & Healthcare Ctr	Coronado	97%	37
Sierra Vista Regional Medical Center	San Luis Obispo	97%	33
Simi Valley Hosp & Health Care Svcs	Simi Valley	97%	76
Sutter Tracy Community Hospital	Tracy	97%	76
Garfield Medical Center[2]	Monterey Park	96%	234
Grossmont Hospital	La Mesa	96%	619
Mad River Community Hospital	Arcata	96%	26
Mark Twain Medical Center	San Andreas	96%	48
Mercy Hospital of Folsom	Folsom	96%	103
Saint Bernardine Medical Center[2]	San Bernardino	96%	254
Saint Johns Regional Medical Center	Oxnard	96%	239
Saint Joseph's Medical Center of Stockton[2]	Stockton	96%	231
Saint Mary Medical Center[2]	Apple Valley	96%	240
San Dimas Community Hospital	San Dimas	96%	49
Scripps Mercy Hospital[2]	San Diego	96%	444
Sharp Chula Vista Medical Center	Chula Vista	96%	528
Sharp Memorial Hospital	San Diego	96%	448
Sutter Delta Medical Center[2]	Antioch	96%	237
Alhambra Hospital Medical Center	Alhambra	95%	78
Eisenhower Medical Center	Rancho Mirage	95%	436
Fallbrook Hospital	Fallbrook	95%	55
Los Angeles Community Hospital[2]	Los Angeles	95%	131
Marshall Medical Center	Placerville	95%	101
Pomona Valley Hospital Medical Center[2]	Pomona	95%	239
Saint Helena Hospital	Saint Helena	95%	100
San Joaquin General Hospital	French Camp	95%	153
Southern California Hospital at Hollywood[2]	Hollywood	95%	137
Valley Presbyterian Hospital	Van Nuys	95%	280
Western Medical Center Santa Ana	Santa Ana	95%	76
Chinese Hospital	San Francisco	94%	109
Coastal Communities Hospital	Santa Ana	94%	50
Fairchild Medical Center	Yreka	94%	32
Fountain Valley Reg Hosp & Med Ctr	Fountain Valley	94%	255
Frank R Howard Memorial Hospital	Willits	94%	35
Fresno Heart & Surgical Hospital[2]	Fresno	94%	78
Hoag Memorial Hospital Presbyterian	Newport Beach	94%	191
Kaweah Delta Medical Center[2]	Visalia	94%	261
LAC/Harbor - UCLA Medical Center[2]	Torrance	94%	280
Madera Community Hospital	Madera	94%	67
Northbay Medical Center	Fairfield	94%	245
Santa Clara Valley Medical Center[2]	San Jose	94%	266
Santa Rosa Memorial Hospital	Santa Rosa	94%	160
Corona Regional Medical Center[2]	Corona	93%	184
Doctors Medical Center	Modesto	93%	347
Redlands Community Hospital	Redlands	93%	162
Saint Joseph Hospital	Orange	93%	307
Sequoia Hospital	Redwood City	93%	150
UCSF Medical Center[2]	San Francisco	93%	219
Coast Plaza Hospital	Norwalk	92%	61
Comm Mem Hosp San Buenaventura	Ventura	92%	223
Eden Medical Center	Castro Valley	92%	235
Foothill Presbyterian Hospital	Glendora	92%	106
Placentia Linda Hospital	Placentia	92%	89
Saint Vincent Medical Center	Los Angeles	92%	263
San Mateo Medical Center	San Mateo	92%	83
Univ of CA Davis Med Ctr[2]	Sacramento	92%	274
Univ of CA San Diego Med Ctr[2]	San Diego	92%	242
Antelope Valley Hospital	Lancaster	91%	305
Arrowhead Regional Medical Center[2]	Colton	91%	506
Feather River Hospital	Paradise	91%	92
Monterey Park Hospital	Monterey Park	91%	91
Oroville Hospital	Oroville	91%	205
Providence Tarzana Medical Center	Tarzana	91%	233
Saint Jude Medical Center[2]	Fullerton	91%	249
San Gorgonio Memorial Hospital	Banning	91%	119
San Leandro Hospital[3]	San Leandro	91%	74
Bakersfield Memorial Hospital[2]	Bakersfield	90%	241
California Hosp Med Ctr Los Angeles	Los Angeles	90%	377
Comm Hosp of the Monterey Peninsula	Monterey	90%	169
Emanuel Medical Center	Turlock	90%	221
Lodi Memorial Hospital[2]	Lodi	90%	177
Petaluma Valley Hospital	Petaluma	90%	60
Providence Saint Joseph Medical Center	Burbank	90%	341
San Francisco General Hospital[2]	San Francisco	90%	254
Alameda Hospital	Alameda	89%	87
Doctors Hospital of Manteca	Manteca	89%	92
Huntington Memorial Hospital[2]	Pasadena	89%	218
Memorial Hospital of Gardena	Gardena	89%	184
Menifee Valley Medical Center	Sun City	89%	107
Olympia Medical Center	Los Angeles	89%	126
Pacific Hospital of Long Beach[3]	Long Beach	89%	28
Ahmc Anaheim Regional Medical Center	Anaheim	88%	332
Glendale Mem Hosp & Health Ctr	Glendale	88%	350
Redwood Memorial Hospital	Fortuna	88%	26
Southwest Healthcare System[2]	Murrieta	88%	221
Citrus Valley Medical Center - IC Campus[2]	Covina	87%	251
Doctors Medical Center - San Pablo[2]	San Pablo	87%	274
Kern Medical Center	Bakersfield	87%	103
LAC/Olive View - UCLA Medical Center[2]	Sylmar	87%	257
Ronald Reagan UCLA Medical Center[2]	Los Angeles	87%	250
Saddleback Memorial Medical Center	Laguna Hills	87%	359
Mission Hospital Regional Medical Center	Mission Viejo	86%	246
Pacific Alliance Medical Center	Los Angeles	86%	109
Santa Barbara Cottage Hospital	Santa Barbara	86%	232
Ukiah Valley Medical Center	Ukiah	86%	81
Valleycare Medical Center	Pleasanton	86%	150
Loma Linda VA Medical Center	Loma Linda	85%	194
Rideout Memorial Hospital	Marysville	85%	288
Tri - City Regional Medical Center	Hawaiian Grdns	85%	66
Bakersfield Heart Hospital[2]	Bakersfield	84%	255
Lompoc Valley Medical Center	Lompoc	84%	43
Sutter Coast Hospital	Crescent City	84%	68
Greater El Monte Community Hospital	South El Monte	83%	63
Providence Holy Cross Medical Center[2]	Mission Hills	83%	236
Alvarado Hospital Medical Center	San Diego	81%	118
Santa Monica-UCLA Med Ctr & Ortho Hosp[2]	Santa Monica	81%	215
Beverly Hospital	Montebello	80%	214
Hi - Desert Medical Center	Joshua Tree	80%	69
Mission Community Hospital	Panorama City	80%	108
Ventura County Medical Center[2]	Ventura	80%	119
Alta Bates Summit Medical Center[2]	Berkeley	79%	164
Saint Francis Medical Center	Lynwood	79%	441
Victor Valley Global Medical Center	Victorville	79%	151
Contra Costa Regional Medical Center	Martinez	78%	176
Barton Memorial Hospital	S Lake Tahoe	77%	43
Natividad Medical Center	Salinas	77%	83
Community Hospital of Long Beach	Long Beach	76%	51
Good Samaritan Hospital[2]	Los Angeles	76%	275
Hemet Valley Medical Center[2]	Hemet	76%	204
Loma Linda University Medical Center[2]	Loma Linda	76%	283
Parkview Comm Hosp Med Ctr[2]	Riverside	71%	157
Seton Medical Center	Daly City	70%	262
Alta Bates Summit Medical Center[2]	Oakland	69%	241
Delano Regional Medical Center	Delano	65%	46
Loma Linda Univ Med Ctr-Murrieta[2]	Murrieta	61%	238
Marina Del Rey Hospital	Marina Del Rey	61%	83
Pacifica Hospital of the Valley	Sun Valley	56%	54
Alameda County Medical Center	Oakland	39%	331

Evaluation of LVS Function

Hospital Name	City	Rate	Cases
Alameda County Medical Center	Oakland	100%	357
Alhambra Hospital Medical Center	Alhambra	100%	110
Alvarado Hospital Medical Center	San Diego	100%	176
Antelope Valley Hospital	Lancaster	100%	340
Bakersfield Heart Hospital[2]	Bakersfield	100%	296
Barstow Community Hospital	Barstow	100%	120
California Hosp Med Ctr Los Angeles	Los Angeles	100%	400
CA Pacific Med Ctr-Davies Campus	San Francisco	100%	28
CA Pacific Med Ctr-Pacific Campus Hosp[2]	San Francisco	100%	296
CA Pacific Med Ctr-St Luke's Campus	San Francisco	100%	105
Cedars - Sinai Medical Center	Los Angeles	100%	1032
Centinela Hospital Medical Center[2]	Inglewood	100%	268
Chino Valley Medical Center	Chino	100%	82
Citrus Valley Medical Center - IC Campus[2]	Covina	100%	304
Clovis Community Medical Center[2]	Clovis	100%	212
Community Hospital of Huntington Park	Huntington Park	100%	149
Comm Mem Hosp San Buenaventura	Ventura	100%	265
Community Regional Medical Center[2]	Fresno	100%	913
Dameron Hospital	Stockton	100%	187
Desert Regional Medical Center	Palm Springs	100%	366
Desert Valley Hospital[2]	Victorville	100%	288
Doctors Hospital of Manteca	Manteca	100%	114
Doctors Medical Center	Modesto	100%	394
Dominican Hospital[2]	Santa Cruz	100%	225
Eden Medical Center	Castro Valley	100%	297
Eisenhower Medical Center	Rancho Mirage	100%	543
El Camino Hospital	Mountain View	100%	323
Emanuel Medical Center	Turlock	100%	288
Encino Hospital Medical Center	Encino	100%	77
Enloe Medical Center	Chico	100%	225
Foothill Presbyterian Hospital	Glendora	100%	133
Frank R Howard Memorial Hospital	Willits	100%	39
Fresno Heart & Surgical Hospital[2]	Fresno	100%	87
Fresno VA Med Ctr-VA Central CA	Fresno	100%	141
Garden Grove Hospital & Medical Center	Garden Grove	100%	93
Garfield Medical Center[2]	Monterey Park	100%	271
Glendale Adventist Medical Center	Glendale	100%	402
Good Samaritan Hospital	San Jose	100%	249
Grossmont Hospital	La Mesa	100%	753
Henry Mayo Newhall Memorial Hospital[2]	Valencia	100%	299
Hoag Memorial Hospital Presbyterian	Newport Beach	100%	236
Huntington Beach Hospital	Huntington Bch	100%	87
Huntington Memorial Hospital[2]	Pasadena	100%	268
John Muir Medical Center - Concord Campus	Concord	100%	286
John Muir Med Ctr-Walnut Creek Campus	Walnut Creek	100%	307
Kaiser Foundation Hospital	San Rafael	100%	107
Kaiser Foundation Hospital & Rehab Center	Vallejo	100%	270
Kaiser Foundation Hospital - Antioch	Antioch	100%	228
Kaiser Foundation Hospital - Baldwin Park	Baldwin Park	100%	403
Kaiser Foundation Hospital - Downey	Downey	100%	363
Kaiser Foundation Hospital - Fontana	Fontana	100%	679
Kaiser Fdn Hosp-Fremont/Hayward	Hayward	100%	247
Kaiser Foundation Hospital - Fresno[2]	Fresno	100%	197
Kaiser Foundation Hospital - Los Angeles	Los Angeles	100%	566
Kaiser Foundation Hospital - Manteca	Manteca	100%	206
Kaiser Fdn Hosp-Moreno Valley	Moreno Valley	100%	125
Kaiser Fdn Hosp-Oakland/Richmond[2]	Oakland	100%	416
Kaiser Fdn Hosp-Orange Co-Anaheim	Anaheim	100%	451
Kaiser Fdn Hosp-Panorama City	Panorama City	100%	230
Kaiser Foundation Hospital - Redwood City	Redwood City	100%	106
Kaiser Foundation Hospital - Riverside	Riverside	100%	268
Kaiser Foundation Hospital - Roseville[2]	Roseville	100%	284
Kaiser Foundation Hospital - Sacramento	Sacramento	100%	180
Kaiser Foundation Hospital - San Diego	San Diego	100%	683
Kaiser Fdn Hosp-San Francisco	San Francisco	100%	265
Kaiser Foundation Hospital - San Jose	San Jose	100%	260
Kaiser Foundation Hospital - Santa Clara[2]	Santa Clara	100%	282
Kaiser Foundation Hospital - South Bay	Harbor City	100%	300
Kaiser Fdn Hosp-S San Francisco	S San Francisco	100%	198
Kaiser Foundation Hospital - Vacaville	Vacaville	100%	120
Kaiser Foundation Hospital - Walnut Creek	Walnut Creek	100%	263
Kaiser Foundation Hospital - West La	Los Angeles	100%	271
Kaiser Fdn Hosp-Woodland Hills	Woodland Hills	100%	264
Kaiser Fdn Hosp S Sacramento[2]	Sacramento	100%	308
Kaweah Delta Medical Center[2]	Visalia	100%	295
Keck Hospital of USC	Los Angeles	100%	116
La Palma Intercommunity Hospital	La Palma	100%	105
LAC+USC Medical Center	Los Angeles	100%	619
LAC/Harbor - UCLA Medical Center[2]	Torrance	100%	283
LAC/Olive View - UCLA Medical Center[2]	Sylmar	100%	260
Lakewood Regional Medical Center	Lakewood	100%	329
Lodi Memorial Hospital[2]	Lodi	100%	246
Loma Linda VA Medical Center	Loma Linda	100%	220
Long Beach Memorial Medical Center	Long Beach	100%	539
Los Alamitos Medical Center	Los Alamitos	100%	291
Los Robles Hospital & Medical Center	Thousand Oaks	100%	287
Marian Regional Medical Center	Santa Maria	100%	253
Marin General Hospital[2]	Greenbrae	100%	185
Mark Twain Medical Center	San Andreas	100%	55
Marshall Medical Center	Placerville	100%	134
Memorial Hospital of Gardena	Gardena	100%	218
Memorial Medical Center[2]	Modesto	100%	312
Mercy General Hospital	Sacramento	100%	444
Mercy Hospital	Bakersfield	100%	168
Mercy Hospital of Folsom	Folsom	100%	122
Mercy Medical Center - Redding[2]	Redding	100%	307
Mercy San Juan Medical Center[2]	Carmichael	100%	302
Methodist Hospital of Sacramento[2]	Sacramento	100%	274
Mills - Peninsula Medical Center	Burlingame	100%	299
Mission Community Hospital	Panorama City	100%	154
Montclair Hospital Medical Center	Montclair	100%	59
Monterey Park Hospital	Monterey Park	100%	102
Northbay Medical Center	Fairfield	100%	279
Northridge Hospital Medical Center	Northridge	100%	347
Novato Community Hospital	Novato	100%	72
O'Connor Hospital	San Jose	100%	300

NOTE: Hospital profiles are in alphabetical order by state, then city, then hospital within the city; Rankings exclude hospitals with less than 25 cases except for patient surveys which excludes hospitals with less than 100 cases; (a) 100-299 cases; (1) The number of cases/patients is too few to report; (2) Data submitted were based on a sample of cases/patients; (3) Results are based on a shorter time period than required; (4) Data suppressed by CMS for one or more quarters; (5) Results are not available for this reporting period; (6) Fewer than 100 patients completed the HCAHPS survey; (7) No cases met the criteria for this measure; (8) The lower limit of the confidence interval cannot be calculated if the number of observed infections equals zero; (9) No data are available from the state/territory for this reporting period; (10) The scores shown reflect fewer than 50 completed surveys; (11) There were discrepancies in the data collection process; (12) This measure does not apply to this hospital for this reporting period; (13) Results cannot be calculated for this reporting period; (14) The results for this state are combined with nearby states to protect confidentiality; Please refer to the User's Guide for a full explanation of data.

Oak Valley District Hospital	Oakdale	100%	36
Oroville Hospital	Oroville	100%	241
Palmdale Regional Medical Center[2]	Palmdale	100%	305
Palo Alto VA Medical Center	Palo Alto	100%	175
Paradise Valley Hospital	National City	100%	248
PIH Hospital - Downey	Downey	100%	368
Placentia Linda Hospital	Placentia	100%	114
Pomona Valley Hospital Medical Center[2]	Pomona	100%	307
Presbyterian Intercommunity Hospital[2]	Whittier	100%	305
Providence Holy Cross Medical Center[2]	Mission Hills	100%	281
Prov Little Co of Mary Med Ctr San Pedro	San Pedro	100%	136
Prov Little Co of Mary Med Ctr Torrance[2]	Torrance	100%	331
Providence Saint John's Health Center	Santa Monica	100%	186
Providence Tarzana Medical Center	Tarzana	100%	304
Queen of the Valley Medical Center	Napa	100%	213
Riverside Community Hospital[2]	Riverside	100%	290
Riverside County Regional Medical Center[2]	Moreno Valley	100%	278
Ronald Reagan UCLA Medical Center[2]	Los Angeles	100%	270
Saddleback Memorial Medical Center	Laguna Hills	100%	457
Saint Agnes Medical Center[2]	Fresno	100%	427
Saint Francis Medical Center	Lynwood	100%	509
Saint Helena Hospital	Saint Helena	100%	119
Saint Johns Pleasant Valley Hospital	Camarillo	100%	103
Saint Johns Regional Medical Center	Oxnard	100%	272
Saint Joseph Hospital	Eureka	100%	158
Saint Joseph Hospital	Orange	100%	368
Saint Joseph's Medical Center of Stockton[2]	Stockton	100%	314
Saint Louise Regional Hospital	Gilroy	100%	99
Saint Mary Medical Center[2]	Long Beach	100%	262
Saint Vincent Medical Center	Los Angeles	100%	310
Salinas Valley Memorial Hospital[2]	Salinas	100%	271
San Francisco General Hospital[2]	San Francisco	100%	266
San Joaquin Community Hospital	Bakersfield	100%	597
San Joaquin General Hospital	French Camp	100%	164
San Leandro Hospital[3]	San Leandro	100%	80
San Mateo Medical Center	San Mateo	100%	92
San Ramon Regional Medical Center	San Ramon	100%	64
Santa Barbara Cottage Hospital	Santa Barbara	100%	298
Santa Clara Valley Medical Center[2]	San Jose	100%	284
Santa Monica-UCLA Med Ctr & Ortho Hosp[2]	Santa Monica	100%	272
Scripps Green Hospital	La Jolla	100%	251
Scripps Memorial Hospital - Encinitas	Encinitas	100%	248
Scripps Memorial Hospital La Jolla[2]	La Jolla	100%	249
Scripps Mercy Hospital[2]	San Diego	100%	551
Sequoia Hospital	Redwood City	100%	179
Seton Medical Center	Daly City	100%	324
Sharp Chula Vista Medical Center	Chula Vista	100%	646
Sharp Coronado Hosp & Healthcare Ctr	Coronado	100%	48
Sharp Memorial Hospital	San Diego	100%	534
Shasta Regional Medical Center	Redding	100%	288
Sierra Vista Regional Medical Center	San Luis Obispo	100%	45
Silver Lake Medical Center	Los Angeles	100%	45
Simi Valley Hosp & Health Care Svcs	Simi Valley	100%	88
Sonoma Valley Hospital	Sonoma	100%	31
Stanford Hospital	Stanford	100%	326
Sutter Amador Hospital	Jackson	100%	56
Sutter Auburn Faith Hospital	Auburn	100%	83
Sutter Coast Hospital	Crescent City	100%	78
Sutter Davis Hospital	Davis	100%	37
Sutter Delta Medical Center[2]	Antioch	100%	264
Sutter General Hospital[2]	Sacramento	100%	317
Sutter Lakeside Hospital	Lakeport	100%	41
Sutter Medical Center of Santa Rosa	Santa Rosa	100%	137
Sutter Roseville Medical Center[2]	Roseville	100%	250
Sutter Solano Medical Center	Vallejo	100%	129
Temple Community Hospital	Los Angeles	100%	62
Torrance Memorial Medical Center	Torrance	100%	536
Tri - City Medical Center[2]	Oceanside	100%	259
Tulare Regional Medical Center	Tulare	100%	105
Twin Cities Community Hospital	Templeton	100%	110
UCSF Medical Center[2]	San Francisco	100%	238
Univ of CA Davis Med Ctr[2]	Sacramento	100%	289
Univ of California Irvine Med Ctr	Orange	100%	251
Univ of CA San Diego Med Ctr[2]	San Diego	100%	270
VA Greater Los Angeles Healthcare System	W Los Angeles	100%	320
VA Long Beach Healthcare System	Long Beach	100%	243
VA Northern California Healthcare System	Mather	100%	205
VA San Diego Healthcare System	San Diego	100%	293
Valleycare Medical Center	Pleasanton	100%	197
Washington Hospital	Fremont	100%	354
Watsonville Community Hospital	Watsonville	100%	93
West Anaheim Medical Center	Anaheim	100%	234
Western Medical Center Hospital Anaheim	Anaheim	100%	26
Whittier Hospital Medical Center	Whittier	100%	187
Woodland Memorial Hospital	Woodland	100%	50
Ahmc Anaheim Regional Medical Center	Anaheim	99%	409
Alameda Hospital	Alameda	99%	115
Alta Bates Summit Medical Center[2]	Oakland	99%	300
Arrowhead Regional Medical Center[2]	Colton	99%	523
Bakersfield Memorial Hospital[2]	Bakersfield	99%	288
Beverly Hospital	Montebello	99%	286
Chinese Hospital	San Francisco	99%	116
Community Hospital of San Bernardino	San Bernardino	99%	95
Comm Hosp of the Monterey Peninsula	Monterey	99%	206
Contra Costa Regional Medical Center	Martinez	99%	193
Corona Regional Medical Center[2]	Corona	99%	250
Doctors Medical Center - San Pablo[2]	San Pablo	99%	325
East Los Angeles Doctors Hospital	Los Angeles	99%	84
Feather River Hospital	Paradise	99%	111
Fountain Valley Reg Hosp & Med Ctr	Fountain Valley	99%	318
French Hospital Medical Center	San Luis Obispo	99%	118
Good Samaritan Hospital[2]	Los Angeles	99%	347
Greater El Monte Community Hospital	South El Monte	99%	76
Kaiser Foundation Hospital - Santa Rosa	Santa Rosa	99%	112
Loma Linda University Medical Center[2]	Loma Linda	99%	316
Mercy Medical Center[2]	Merced	99%	287
Methodist Hospital of Southern California	Arcadia	99%	380
Mission Hospital Regional Medical Center	Mission Viejo	99%	297
Natividad Medical Center	Salinas	99%	91
Olympia Medical Center	Los Angeles	99%	180
Orange Coast Memorial Medical Center	Fountain Valley	99%	322
Pacific Alliance Medical Center	Los Angeles	99%	136
Palomar Health Downtown Campus	Escondido	99%	547
Petaluma Valley Hospital	Petaluma	99%	74
Providence Saint Joseph Medical Center	Burbank	99%	419
Saint Bernardine Medical Center[2]	San Bernardino	99%	288
Saint Francis Memorial Hospital	San Francisco	99%	123
Saint Jude Medical Center[2]	Fullerton	99%	336
Saint Mary Medical Center[2]	Apple Valley	99%	262
Saint Rose Hospital	Hayward	99%	229
San Dimas Community Hospital	San Dimas	99%	80
San Francisco VA Medical Center	San Francisco	99%	157
San Gabriel Valley Medical Center	San Gabriel	99%	234
Sierra Nevada Memorial Hospital	Grass Valley	99%	114
Sonora Regional Medical Center	Sonora	99%	97
Southern California Hospital at Hollywood[2]	Hollywood	99%	220
Southwest Healthcare System[2]	Murrieta	99%	258
Sutter Tracy Community Hospital	Tracy	99%	95
Tri - City Regional Medical Center	Hawaiian Grdns	99%	92
Ukiah Valley Medical Center	Ukiah	99%	90
West Hills Hospital & Medical Center	West Hills	99%	196
Alta Bates Summit Medical Center[2]	Berkeley	98%	223
Barton Memorial Hospital	S Lake Tahoe	98%	45
Glendale Mem Hosp & Health Ctr	Glendale	98%	411
Hazel Hawkins Memorial Hospital[2]	Hollister	98%	57
John F Kennedy Memorial Hospital	Indio	98%	132
Kern Medical Center	Bakersfield	98%	106
Lompoc Valley Medical Center	Lompoc	98%	46
Marina Del Rey Hospital	Marina Del Rey	98%	110
Pacific Hospital of Long Beach[3]	Long Beach	98%	45
Pomerado Hospital	Poway	98%	173
Redlands Community Hospital	Redlands	98%	212
Regional Medical Center of San Jose	San Jose	98%	501
Saint Mary's Medical Center	San Francisco	98%	185
San Antonio Community Hospital	Upland	98%	397
Santa Rosa Memorial Hospital	Santa Rosa	98%	223
Sherman Oaks Hospital	Sherman Oaks	98%	104
Ventura County Medical Center[2]	Ventura	98%	138
Western Medical Center Santa Ana	Santa Ana	98%	84
White Memorial Medical Center	Los Angeles	98%	332
Coastal Communities Hospital	Santa Ana	97%	61
Pioneers Memorial Healthcare District	Brawley	97%	148
Redwood Memorial Hospital	Fortuna	97%	30
Saint Elizabeth Community Hospital	Red Bluff	97%	77
Valley Presbyterian Hospital	Van Nuys	97%	349
Adventist Medical Center	Hanford	96%	325
Los Angeles Community Hospital[2]	Los Angeles	96%	194
Mad River Community Hospital	Arcata	96%	28
San Gorgonio Memorial Hospital	Banning	96%	151
Community Hospital of Long Beach	Long Beach	95%	76
Fallbrook Hospital	Fallbrook	95%	64
Hemet Valley Medical Center[2]	Hemet	95%	270
Parkview Comm Hosp Med Ctr[2]	Riverside	95%	214
Sierra View District Hospital	Porterville	95%	170
Hollywood Presbyterian Medical Center[2]	Los Angeles	94%	252
Loma Linda Univ Med Ctr-Murrieta[2]	Murrieta	94%	254
Madera Community Hospital	Madera	94%	94
Rideout Memorial Hospital	Marysville	94%	336
USC Verdugo Hills Hospital	Glendale	94%	87
Coast Plaza Hospital	Norwalk	93%	75
El Centro Regional Medical Center	El Centro	93%	214
Fairchild Medical Center	Yreka	93%	27
Menifee Valley Medical Center	Sun City	93%	131
Hi - Desert Medical Center	Joshua Tree	92%	96
Victor Valley Global Medical Center	Victorville	92%	154
Delano Regional Medical Center	Delano	89%	55
Pacifica Hospital of the Valley	Sun Valley	71%	73
Colusa Regional Medical Center	Colusa	52%	27

Medicare Spending

Medicare Spending per Patient (ratio)

Hospital Name	City	Ratio	Cases
Laguna Honda Hosp & Rehab Ctr	San Francisco	0.62	-
Sonoma Developmental Center	Eldridge	0.70	-
Kaiser Foundation Hospital - Fresno	Fresno	0.71	-
Kaiser Foundation Hospital - San Diego	San Diego	0.73	-
Kaiser Fdn Hosp-San Francisco	San Francisco	0.73	-
Kaiser Fdn Hosp-S San Francisco	S San Francisco	0.73	-
Kaiser Foundation Hospital - Antioch	Antioch	0.74	-
Kaiser Foundation Hospital - Vacaville	Vacaville	0.74	-
Kaiser Foundation Hospital - South Bay	Harbor City	0.76	-
Coalinga Regional Medical Center	Coalinga	0.78	-
Kaiser Foundation Hospital - Baldwin Park	Baldwin Park	0.78	-
Kaiser Foundation Hospital - Manteca	Manteca	0.78	-
Patients' Hospital of Redding	Redding	0.78	-
Kaiser Foundation Hospital & Rehab Center	Vallejo	0.79	-
Kaiser Foundation Hospital - Downey	Downey	0.79	-
Kaiser Fdn Hosp-Oakland/Richmond	Oakland	0.80	-
Kaiser Fdn Hosp-Panorama City	Panorama City	0.80	-
Kaiser Foundation Hospital - Walnut Creek	Walnut Creek	0.80	-
Corcoran District Hospital	Corcoran	0.81	-
Kaiser Fdn Hosp-Fremont/Hayward	Hayward	0.81	-
Kaiser Foundation Hospital - Redwood City	Redwood City	0.81	-
Kaiser Foundation Hospital - Riverside	Riverside	0.81	-
Kaiser Foundation Hospital - Santa Clara	Santa Clara	0.81	-
Motion Picture & Television Hospital	Woodland Hills	0.81	-
Sutter Coast Hospital	Crescent City	0.81	-
Kaiser Fdn Hosp-Woodland Hills	Woodland Hills	0.82	-
Sharp Coronado Hosp & Healthcare Ctr	Coronado	0.82	-
Kaiser Fdn Hosp-Orange Co-Anaheim	Anaheim	0.84	-
Kaiser Fdn Hosp S Sacramento	Sacramento	0.84	-
Saint Helena Hospital	Saint Helena	0.84	-
Contra Costa Regional Medical Center	Martinez	0.85	-
Sonora Regional Medical Center	Sonora	0.85	-
Sutter Davis Hospital	Davis	0.85	-
Fresno Surgical Hospital	Fresno	0.86	-
Kaiser Foundation Hospital - Fontana	Fontana	0.86	-
Kaiser Foundation Hospital - Santa Rosa	Santa Rosa	0.86	-
Kaiser Foundation Hospital - West La	Los Angeles	0.86	-
LAC/Olive View - UCLA Medical Center	Sylmar	0.86	-
Barton Memorial Hospital	S Lake Tahoe	0.87	-
Hi - Desert Medical Center	Joshua Tree	0.87	-
Kaiser Foundation Hospital - Los Angeles	Los Angeles	0.87	-
Kaiser Foundation Hospital - Sacramento	Sacramento	0.87	-
Kaiser Foundation Hospital - San Jose	San Jose	0.87	-
Lompoc Valley Medical Center	Lompoc	0.87	-
Menlo Park Surgical Hospital	Menlo Park	0.87	-
Ojai Valley Community Hospital	Ojai	0.87	-
Sonoma Valley Hospital	Sonoma	0.87	-
George L Mee Memorial Hospital	King City	0.88	-
Kaiser Foundation Hospital - Roseville	Roseville	0.88	-
Marshall Medical Center	Placerville	0.88	-
Methodist Hospital of Sacramento	Sacramento	0.88	-
Mills - Peninsula Medical Center	Burlingame	0.88	-
Oroville Hospital	Oroville	0.88	-
Ukiah Valley Medical Center	Ukiah	0.88	-
Desert Valley Hospital	Victorville	0.89	-
Doctors Hospital of West Covina	West Covina	0.89	-
El Centro Regional Medical Center	El Centro	0.89	-
Kern Medical Center	Bakersfield	0.89	-
LAC/Harbor - UCLA Medical Center	Torrance	0.89	-
Riverside County Regional Medical Center	Moreno Valley	0.89	-
Sutter Amador Hospital	Jackson	0.89	-
Barstow Community Hospital	Barstow	0.90	-
CA Pacific Med Ctr-Pacific Campus Hosp	San Francisco	0.90	-
CA Pacific Med Ctr-St Luke's Campus	San Francisco	0.90	-
Feather River Hospital	Paradise	0.90	-
Good Samaritan Hospital	Bakersfield	0.90	-
Hazel Hawkins Memorial Hospital	Hollister	0.90	-
San Mateo Medical Center	San Mateo	0.90	-
Univ of CA Davis Med Ctr	Sacramento	0.90	-
Community Hospital of Huntington Park	Huntington Park	0.91	-
Delano Regional Medical Center	Delano	0.91	-
Mad River Community Hospital	Arcata	0.91	-
Saint Elizabeth Community Hospital	Red Bluff	0.91	-
Sutter Maternity & Surgery Ctr	Santa Cruz	0.91	-
Bear Valley Community Hospital	Big Bear Lake	0.92	-
Fallbrook Hospital	Fallbrook	0.92	-
Palo Verde Hospital	Blythe	0.92	-
San Francisco General Hospital	San Francisco	0.92	-
Shasta Regional Medical Center	Redding	0.92	-
Sutter Surgical Hospital - North Valley	Yuba City	0.92	-
Ventura County Medical Center	Ventura	0.92	-
Watsonville Community Hospital	Watsonville	0.92	-
Adventist Medical Center	Hanford	0.93	-
Memorial Hospital Los Banos	Los Banos	0.93	-
Mercy Hospital of Folsom	Folsom	0.93	-
Oak Valley District Hospital	Oakdale	0.93	-
Queen of the Valley Medical Center	Napa	0.93	-

NOTE: Hospital profiles are in alphabetical order by state, then city, then hospital within the city; Rankings exclude hospitals with less than 25 cases except for patient surveys which excludes hospitals with less than 100 cases; (a) 100-299 cases; (1) The number of cases/patients is too few to report; (2) Data submitted were based on a sample of cases/patients; (3) Results are based on a shorter time period than required; (4) Data suppressed by CMS for one or more quarters; (5) Results are not available for this reporting period; (6) Fewer than 100 patients completed the HCAHPS survey; (7) No cases met the criteria for this measure; (8) The lower limit of the confidence interval cannot be calculated if the number of observed infections equals zero; (9) No data are available from the state/territory for this reporting period; (10) The scores shown reflect fewer than 50 completed surveys; (11) There were discrepancies in the data collection process; (12) This measure does not apply to this hospital for this reporting period; (13) Results cannot be calculated for this reporting period; (14) The results for this state are combined with nearby states to protect confidentiality; Please refer to the User's Guide for a full explanation of data.

Rideout Memorial Hospital	Marysville	0.93	-
Saint Joseph Hospital	Eureka	0.93	-
Sierra Nevada Memorial Hospital	Grass Valley	0.93	-
Sierra View District Hospital	Porterville	0.93	-
Stanislaus Surgical Hospital	Modesto	0.93	-
Sutter General Hospital	Sacramento	0.93	-
Woodland Memorial Hospital	Woodland	0.93	-
Chinese Hospital	San Francisco	0.94	-
Comm Mem Hosp San Buenaventura	Ventura	0.94	-
Goleta Valley Cottage Hospital	Santa Barbara	0.94	-
LAC+USC Medical Center	Los Angeles	0.94	-
Marian Regional Medical Center	Santa Maria	0.94	-
Mercy General Hospital	Sacramento	0.94	-
Natividad Medical Center	Salinas	0.94	-
Palm Drive Hospital	Sebastopol	0.94	-
Pioneers Memorial Healthcare District	Brawley	0.94	-
Santa Barbara Cottage Hospital	Santa Barbara	0.94	-
Sutter Auburn Faith Hospital	Auburn	0.94	-
Sutter Roseville Medical Center	Roseville	0.94	-
Alameda Hospital	Alameda	0.95	-
Bakersfield Heart Hospital	Bakersfield	0.95	-
Chino Valley Medical Center	Chino	0.95	-
Doctors Medical Center - San Pablo	San Pablo	0.95	-
Emanuel Medical Center	Turlock	0.95	-
Loma Linda Univ Med Ctr-Murrieta	Murrieta	0.95	-
Mercy Medical Center	Merced	0.95	-
Mercy San Juan Medical Center	Carmichael	0.95	-
Petaluma Valley Hospital	Petaluma	0.95	-
Pomerado Hospital	Poway	0.95	-
Saint Mary's Medical Center	San Francisco	0.95	-
Scripps Green Hospital	La Jolla	0.95	-
Sutter Delta Medical Center	Antioch	0.95	-
Comm Hosp of the Monterey Peninsula	Monterey	0.96	-
Doctors Hospital of Manteca	Manteca	0.96	-
Doctors Medical Center	Modesto	0.96	-
Enloe Medical Center	Chico	0.96	-
French Hospital Medical Center	San Luis Obispo	0.96	-
Hoag Orthopedic Institute	Irvine	0.96	-
Kaweah Delta Medical Center	Visalia	0.96	-
Loma Linda University Medical Center	Loma Linda	0.96	-
Monterey Park Hospital	Monterey Park	0.96	-
Redlands Community Hospital	Redlands	0.96	-
Saint Mary Medical Center	Apple Valley	0.96	-
Sequoia Hospital	Redwood City	0.96	-
Tulare Regional Medical Center	Tulare	0.96	-
Washington Hospital	Fremont	0.96	-
Alta Bates Summit Medical Center	Berkeley	0.97	-
Arrowhead Regional Medical Center	Colton	0.97	-
Colusa Regional Medical Center	Colusa	0.97	-
Memorial Medical Center	Modesto	0.97	-
Providence Saint John's Health Center	Santa Monica	0.97	-
Santa Clara Valley Medical Center	San Jose	0.97	-
Santa Rosa Memorial Hospital	Santa Rosa	0.97	-
Sutter Tracy Community Hospital	Tracy	0.97	-
UCSF Medical Center	San Francisco	0.97	-
Univ of CA San Diego Med Ctr	San Diego	0.97	-
Good Samaritan Hospital	Los Angeles	0.98	-
Huntington Memorial Hospital	Pasadena	0.98	-
John F Kennedy Memorial Hospital	Indio	0.98	-
Menifee Valley Medical Center	Sun City	0.98	-
Mercy Medical Center - Redding	Redding	0.98	-
Northbay Medical Center	Fairfield	0.98	-
O'Connor Hospital	San Jose	0.98	-
Regional Medical Center of San Jose	San Jose	0.98	-
Ronald Reagan UCLA Medical Center	Los Angeles	0.98	-
Saddleback Memorial Medical Center	Laguna Hills	0.98	-
Saint Johns Pleasant Valley Hospital	Camarillo	0.98	-
Saint Louise Regional Hospital	Gilroy	0.98	-
Salinas Valley Memorial Hospital	Salinas	0.98	-
Sharp Chula Vista Medical Center	Chula Vista	0.98	-
Torrance Memorial Medical Center	Torrance	0.98	-
Twin Cities Community Hospital	Templeton	0.98	-
Valleycare Medical Center	Pleasanton	0.98	-
Victor Valley Global Medical Center	Victorville	0.98	-
Adventist Medical Center - Reedley	Reedley	0.99	-
Alta Bates Summit Medical Center	Oakland	0.99	-
CA Pacific Med Ctr-Davies Campus	San Francisco	0.99	-
Community Regional Medical Center	Fresno	0.99	-
Desert Regional Medical Center	Palm Springs	0.99	-
Dominican Hospital	Santa Cruz	0.99	-
Eden Medical Center	Castro Valley	0.99	-
Eisenhower Medical Center	Rancho Mirage	0.99	-
Fresno Heart & Surgical Hospital	Fresno	0.99	-
Kaiser Fdn Hosp-Moreno Valley	Moreno Valley	0.99	-
Keck Hospital of USC	Los Angeles	0.99	-
Los Robles Hospital & Medical Center	Thousand Oaks	0.99	-
Mission Hospital Regional Medical Center	Mission Viejo	0.99	-
Palmdale Regional Medical Center	Palmdale	0.99	-
Saint Johns Regional Medical Center	Oxnard	0.99	-
San Joaquin General Hospital	French Camp	0.99	-
Southwest Healthcare System	Murrieta	0.99	-
Stanford Hospital	Stanford	0.99	-
Sutter Medical Center of Santa Rosa	Santa Rosa	0.99	-
California Hosp Med Ctr Los Angeles	Los Angeles	1.00	-
Clovis Community Medical Center	Clovis	1.00	-
El Camino Hospital	Mountain View	1.00	-
Hemet Valley Medical Center	Hemet	1.00	-
John Muir Medical Center - Concord Campus	Concord	1.00	-
Novato Community Hospital	Novato	1.00	-
Prov Little Co of Mary Med Ctr San Pedro	San Pedro	1.00	-
Saint Agnes Medical Center	Fresno	1.00	-
Saint Joseph Hospital	Orange	1.00	-
Seton Medical Center	Daly City	1.00	-
Sharp Memorial Hospital	San Diego	1.00	-
Sierra Vista Regional Medical Center	San Luis Obispo	1.00	-
Centinela Hospital Medical Center	Inglewood	1.01	-
Grossmont Hospital	La Mesa	1.01	-
Kaiser Foundation Hospital	San Rafael	1.01	-
Madera Community Hospital	Madera	1.01	-
Marina Del Rey Hospital	Marina Del Rey	1.01	-
Presbyterian Intercommunity Hospital	Whittier	1.01	-
Prov Little Co of Mary Med Ctr Torrance	Torrance	1.01	-
Saint Joseph's Medical Center of Stockton	Stockton	1.01	-
San Joaquin Community Hospital	Bakersfield	1.01	-
San Ramon Regional Medical Center	San Ramon	1.01	-
Santa Monica-UCLA Med Ctr & Ortho Hosp	Santa Monica	1.01	-
Alameda County Medical Center	Oakland	1.02	-
Cedars - Sinai Medical Center	Los Angeles	1.02	-
Community Hospital of San Bernardino	San Bernardino	1.02	-
Dameron Hospital	Stockton	1.02	-
Good Samaritan Hospital	San Jose	1.02	-
Marin General Hospital	Greenbrae	1.02	-
Orange Coast Memorial Medical Center	Fountain Valley	1.02	-
Palomar Health Downtown Campus	Escondido	1.02	-
Providence Saint Joseph Medical Center	Burbank	1.02	-
Providence Tarzana Medical Center	Tarzana	1.02	-
San Gorgonio Memorial Hospital	Banning	1.02	-
Scripps Memorial Hospital - Encinitas	Encinitas	1.02	-
Simi Valley Hosp & Health Care Svcs	Simi Valley	1.02	-
Sutter Solano Medical Center	Vallejo	1.02	-
Univ of California Irvine Med Ctr	Orange	1.02	-
Antelope Valley Hospital	Lancaster	1.03	-
Henry Mayo Newhall Memorial Hospital	Valencia	1.03	-
Hoag Memorial Hospital Presbyterian	Newport Beach	1.03	-
Bakersfield Memorial Hospital	Bakersfield	1.04	-
Methodist Hospital of Southern California	Arcadia	1.04	-
Northridge Hospital Medical Center	Northridge	1.04	-
Saint Vincent Medical Center	Los Angeles	1.04	-
San Antonio Community Hospital	Upland	1.04	-
Scripps Memorial Hospital La Jolla	La Jolla	1.04	-
Scripps Mercy Hospital	San Diego	1.04	-
Tri - City Medical Center	Oceanside	1.04	-
East Los Angeles Doctors Hospital	Los Angeles	1.05	-
Encino Hospital Medical Center	Encino	1.05	-
Glendale Mem Hosp & Health Ctr	Glendale	1.05	-
John Muir Med Ctr-Walnut Creek Campus	Walnut Creek	1.05	-
Long Beach Memorial Medical Center	Long Beach	1.05	-
Mercy Hospital	Bakersfield	1.05	-
Providence Holy Cross Medical Center	Mission Hills	1.05	-
Riverside Community Hospital	Riverside	1.05	-
Saint Bernardine Medical Center	San Bernardino	1.05	-
Saint Jude Medical Center	Fullerton	1.05	-
Saint Rose Hospital	Hayward	1.05	-
Corona Regional Medical Center	Corona	1.06	-
Glendale Adventist Medical Center	Glendale	1.06	-
Alvarado Hospital Medical Center	San Diego	1.07	-
Los Alamitos Medical Center	Los Alamitos	1.07	-
Pacific Alliance Medical Center	Los Angeles	1.07	-
Placentia Linda Hospital	Placentia	1.07	-
Saint Francis Medical Center	Lynwood	1.07	-
College Hospital Costa Mesa	Costa Mesa	1.08	-
Lodi Memorial Hospital	Lodi	1.08	-
Saint Francis Memorial Hospital	San Francisco	1.08	-
Sherman Oaks Hospital	Sherman Oaks	1.08	-
USC Verdugo Hills Hospital	Glendale	1.08	-
Western Medical Center Santa Ana	Santa Ana	1.08	-
White Memorial Medical Center	Los Angeles	1.08	-
Ahmc Anaheim Regional Medical Center	Anaheim	1.09	-
Beverly Hospital	Montebello	1.09	-
Chapman Medical Center	Orange	1.09	-
Montclair Hospital Medical Center	Montclair	1.09	-
PIH Hospital - Downey	Downey	1.09	-
Pomona Valley Hospital Medical Center	Pomona	1.09	-
West Anaheim Medical Center	Anaheim	1.09	-
Garfield Medical Center	Monterey Park	1.10	-
Valley Presbyterian Hospital	Van Nuys	1.10	-
West Hills Hospital & Medical Center	West Hills	1.10	-
Citrus Valley Medical Center - IC Campus	Covina	1.11	-
Foothill Presbyterian Hospital	Glendora	1.11	-
Hollywood Presbyterian Medical Center	Los Angeles	1.11	-
Huntington Beach Hospital	Huntington Bch	1.11	-
Pacifica Hospital of the Valley	Sun Valley	1.11	-
Fountain Valley Reg Hosp & Med Ctr	Fountain Valley	1.12	-
Garden Grove Hospital & Medical Center	Garden Grove	1.12	-
Olympia Medical Center	Los Angeles	1.12	-
La Palma Intercommunity Hospital	La Palma	1.13	-
Lakewood Regional Medical Center	Lakewood	1.13	-
Paradise Valley Hospital	National City	1.13	-
Parkview Comm Hosp Med Ctr	Riverside	1.13	-
Mission Community Hospital	Panorama City	1.14	-
San Gabriel Valley Medical Center	San Gabriel	1.14	-
Saint Mary Medical Center	Long Beach	1.15	-
San Dimas Community Hospital	San Dimas	1.15	-
Western Medical Center Hospital Anaheim	Anaheim	1.15	-
Community Hospital of Long Beach	Long Beach	1.16	-
Coast Plaza Hospital	Norwalk	1.19	-
Alhambra Hospital Medical Center	Alhambra	1.20	-
LAC/Rancho Los Amigos Ntl Rehab Ctr	Downey	1.22	-
Greater El Monte Community Hospital	South El Monte	1.23	-
Southern California Hospital at Hollywood	Hollywood	1.26	-
Coastal Communities Hospital	Santa Ana	1.28	-
Memorial Hospital of Gardena	Gardena	1.30	-
Tri - City Regional Medical Center	Hawaiian Grdns	1.30	-
Whittier Hospital Medical Center	Whittier	1.30	-
Los Angeles Community Hospital	Los Angeles	1.31	-
Silver Lake Medical Center	Los Angeles	1.33	-
Temple Community Hospital	Los Angeles	1.38	-
East Valley Hospital Medical Center	Glendora	1.54	-

Pneumonia Care

Appropriate Initial Antibiotic Given

Hospital Name	City	Rate	Cases
CA Pacific Med Ctr-Davies Campus	San Francisco	100%	27
CA Pacific Med Ctr-Pacific Campus Hosp[2]	San Francisco	100%	77
CA Pacific Med Ctr-St Luke's Campus[2]	San Francisco	100%	57
Centinela Hospital Medical Center[2]	Inglewood	100%	50
Chapman Medical Center	Orange	100%	31
Coastal Communities Hospital	Santa Ana	100%	46
Dominican Hospital[2]	Santa Cruz	100%	107
El Camino Hospital[2]	Mountain View	100%	142
Encino Hospital Medical Center	Encino	100%	25
Fresno VA Med Ctr-VA Central CA	Fresno	100%	52
Garden Grove Hospital & Medical Center	Garden Grove	100%	72
Garfield Medical Center[2]	Monterey Park	100%	71
Greater El Monte Community Hospital[2]	South El Monte	100%	31
Henry Mayo Newhall Memorial Hospital[2]	Valencia	100%	96
Huntington Beach Hospital[2]	Huntington Bch	100%	38
Kaiser Foundation Hospital[2]	San Rafael	100%	60
Kaiser Foundation Hospital - Antioch[2]	Antioch	100%	78
Kaiser Foundation Hospital - Baldwin Park[2]	Baldwin Park	100%	95
Kaiser Foundation Hospital - Fresno[2]	Fresno	100%	84
Kaiser Foundation Hospital - Manteca[2]	Manteca	100%	61
Kaiser Fdn Hosp-Orange Co-Anaheim[2]	Anaheim	100%	110
Kaiser Foundation Hospital - Riverside[2]	Riverside	100%	85
Kaiser Foundation Hospital - Roseville[2]	Roseville	100%	87
Kaiser Foundation Hospital - San Jose[2]	San Jose	100%	80
Kaiser Foundation Hospital - Santa Clara[2]	Santa Clara	100%	64
Kaiser Foundation Hospital - South Bay[2]	Harbor City	100%	68
Kaiser Fdn Hosp-S San Francisco[2]	S San Francisco	100%	88
Kaiser Foundation Hospital - Walnut Creek[2]	Walnut Creek	100%	73
Kaiser Fdn Hosp S Sacramento[2]	Sacramento	100%	84
La Palma Intercommunity Hospital	La Palma	100%	53
Loma Linda VA Medical Center	Loma Linda	100%	43
Marin General Hospital[2]	Greenbrae	100%	74
Memorial Hospital Los Banos	Los Banos	100%	26
Memorial Medical Center[2]	Modesto	100%	90
Mercy General Hospital	Sacramento	100%	141
Palomar Health Downtown Campus	Escondido	100%	303
Paradise Valley Hospital	National City	100%	106
Pioneers Memorial Healthcare District	Brawley	100%	98
Queen of the Valley Medical Center	Napa	100%	66
Regional Medical Center of San Jose[2]	San Jose	100%	98
Saint Helena Hospital - Clearlake	Clearlake	100%	57
Saint Louise Regional Hospital	Gilroy	100%	52
Saint Mary Medical Center[2]	Long Beach	100%	62
Santa Clara Valley Medical Center[2]	San Jose	100%	52
Scripps Memorial Hospital - Encinitas[2]	Encinitas	100%	85
Scripps Mercy Hospital[2]	San Diego	100%	68
Sharp Coronado Hosp & Healthcare Ctr	Coronado	100%	26
Shasta Regional Medical Center	Redding	100%	142
Sutter Medical Center of Santa Rosa[2]	Santa Rosa	100%	44
Sutter Tracy Community Hospital	Tracy	100%	54
Univ of CA Davis Med Ctr[2]	Sacramento	100%	55
VA San Diego Healthcare System	San Diego	100%	59
Alhambra Hospital Medical Center	Alhambra	99%	68
Alvarado Hospital Medical Center[2]	San Diego	99%	73
Cedars - Sinai Medical Center	Los Angeles	99%	243
Clovis Community Medical Center[2]	Clovis	99%	91
Community Hospital of Huntington Park	Huntington Park	99%	85
Corona Regional Medical Center[2]	Corona	99%	71
Desert Regional Medical Center[2]	Palm Springs	99%	126

NOTE: Hospital profiles are in alphabetical order by state, then city, then hospital within the city; Rankings exclude hospitals with less than 25 cases except for patient surveys which excludes hospitals with less than 100 cases; (a) 100-299 cases; (1) The number of cases/patients is too few to report; (2) Data submitted were based on a sample of cases/patients; (3) Results are based on a shorter time period than required; (4) Data suppressed by CMS for one or more quarters; (5) Results are not available for this reporting period; (6) Fewer than 100 patients completed the HCAHPS survey; (7) No cases met the criteria for this measure; (8) The lower limit of the confidence interval cannot be calculated if the number of observed infections equals zero; (9) No data are available from the state/territory for this reporting period; (10) The scores shown reflect fewer than 50 completed surveys; (11) There were discrepancies in the data collection process; (12) This measure does not apply to this hospital for this reporting period; (13) Results cannot be calculated for this reporting period; (14) The results for this state are combined with nearby states to protect confidentiality; Please refer to the User's Guide for a full explanation of data.

Hospital Name	City	Rate	Cases
Desert Valley Hospital[2]	Victorville	99%	76
Eden Medical Center[2]	Castro Valley	99%	80
Eisenhower Medical Center	Rancho Mirage	99%	328
John Muir Medical Center - Concord Campus[2]	Concord	99%	119
Kaiser Foundation Hospital - Fontana[2]	Fontana	99%	105
Kaiser Fdn Hosp-Moreno Valley[2]	Moreno Valley	99%	86
Kaiser Fdn Hosp-Panorama City[2]	Panorama City	99%	69
Kaiser Fdn Hosp-San Francisco[2]	San Francisco	99%	107
Kaiser Foundation Hospital - Santa Rosa[2]	Santa Rosa	99%	90
Kaiser Fdn Hosp-Woodland Hills[2]	Woodland Hills	99%	80
Los Robles Hospital & Medical Center	Thousand Oaks	99%	125
Marian Regional Medical Center	Santa Maria	99%	186
Mercy Hospital of Folsom[2]	Folsom	99%	103
Methodist Hospital of Sacramento[2]	Sacramento	99%	87
Northridge Hospital Medical Center	Northridge	99%	161
Presbyterian Intercommunity Hospital[2]	Whittier	99%	79
Redlands Community Hospital[2]	Redlands	99%	75
Riverside Community Hospital[2]	Riverside	99%	81
Saint Johns Regional Medical Center	Oxnard	99%	134
Saint Joseph Hospital	Eureka	99%	85
Saint Joseph Hospital	Orange	99%	168
Saint Mary's Medical Center	San Francisco	99%	120
San Antonio Community Hospital[2]	Upland	99%	77
San Francisco General Hospital[2]	San Francisco	99%	74
San Joaquin General Hospital	French Camp	99%	90
San Ramon Regional Medical Center	San Ramon	99%	70
Scripps Green Hospital	La Jolla	99%	120
Seton Medical Center	Daly City	99%	101
Sharp Memorial Hospital	San Diego	99%	274
Sonora Regional Medical Center	Sonora	99%	136
Sutter Amador Hospital[2]	Jackson	99%	97
Sutter Auburn Faith Hospital[2]	Auburn	99%	69
Sutter Coast Hospital	Crescent City	99%	104
Sutter General Hospital[2]	Sacramento	99%	79
Tulare Regional Medical Center	Tulare	99%	107
Twin Cities Community Hospital	Templeton	99%	122
West Anaheim Medical Center[2]	Anaheim	99%	80
Alta Bates Summit Medical Center[2]	Oakland	98%	94
Dameron Hospital	Stockton	98%	96
Delano Regional Medical Center	Delano	98%	50
Doctors Medical Center[2]	Modesto	98%	220
East Los Angeles Doctors Hospital	Los Angeles	98%	49
Fountain Valley Reg Hosp & Med Ctr[2]	Fountain Valley	98%	127
French Hospital Medical Center[2]	San Luis Obispo	98%	64
Kaiser Foundation Hospital & Rehab Center[2]	Vallejo	98%	93
Kaiser Foundation Hospital - Los Angeles[2]	Los Angeles	98%	58
Kaiser Fdn Hosp-Oakland/Richmond[2]	Oakland	98%	60
Kaiser Foundation Hospital - San Diego[2]	San Diego	98%	47
Kaiser Foundation Hospital - Vacaville[2]	Vacaville	98%	113
LAC+USC Medical Center	Los Angeles	98%	194
Long Beach Memorial Medical Center[2]	Long Beach	98%	109
Mercy San Juan Medical Center[2]	Carmichael	98%	62
Methodist Hospital of Southern California	Arcadia	98%	230
Pomerado Hospital	Poway	98%	129
Pomona Valley Hospital Medical Center[2]	Pomona	98%	65
Providence Holy Cross Medical Center[2]	Mission Hills	98%	55
Providence Saint John's Health Center	Santa Monica	98%	108
Providence Tarzana Medical Center	Tarzana	98%	130
Riverside County Regional Medical Center[2]	Moreno Valley	98%	55
Saint Elizabeth Community Hospital[2]	Red Bluff	98%	88
Saint Francis Memorial Hospital[2]	San Francisco	98%	80
Saint Mary Medical Center[2]	Apple Valley	98%	84
Saint Rose Hospital	Hayward	98%	54
San Francisco VA Medical Center	San Francisco	98%	41
Scripps Memorial Hospital La Jolla[2]	La Jolla	98%	87
Sierra Nevada Memorial Hospital[2]	Grass Valley	98%	110
Sierra Vista Regional Medical Center	San Luis Obispo	98%	43
Stanford Hospital	Stanford	98%	126
Sutter Davis Hospital[2]	Davis	98%	55
Sutter Delta Medical Center[2]	Antioch	98%	121
Sutter Lakeside Hospital	Lakeport	98%	54
UCSF Medical Center[2]	San Francisco	98%	53
USC Verdugo Hills Hospital[2]	Glendale	98%	56
Washington Hospital[2]	Fremont	98%	86
West Hills Hospital & Medical Center[2]	West Hills	98%	61
Whittier Hospital Medical Center	Whittier	98%	92
Bakersfield Memorial Hospital[2]	Bakersfield	97%	64
Barstow Community Hospital	Barstow	97%	35
California Hosp Med Ctr Los Angeles[2]	Los Angeles	97%	111
Chinese Hospital	San Francisco	97%	78
Citrus Valley Medical Center - IC Campus[2]	Covina	97%	99
Community Hospital of Long Beach	Long Beach	97%	60
Comm Mem Hosp San Buenaventura	Ventura	97%	177
Community Regional Medical Center[2]	Fresno	97%	153
Doctors Medical Center - San Pablo[2]	San Pablo	97%	70
Fallbrook Hospital	Fallbrook	97%	30
Good Samaritan Hospital[2]	San Jose	97%	118
Grossmont Hospital	La Mesa	97%	282
John Muir Med Ctr-Walnut Creek Campus[2]	Walnut Creek	97%	108
Kaiser Fdn Hosp-Fremont/Hayward[2]	Hayward	97%	71
Kaiser Foundation Hospital - Redwood City[2]	Redwood City	97%	67
Kaiser Foundation Hospital - Sacramento[2]	Sacramento	97%	62
Kaiser Foundation Hospital - West La[2]	Los Angeles	97%	65
LAC/Olive View - UCLA Medical Center[2]	Sylmar	97%	39
Lakewood Regional Medical Center[2]	Lakewood	97%	90
Lodi Memorial Hospital[2]	Lodi	97%	111
Memorial Hospital of Gardena	Gardena	97%	88
Mills - Peninsula Medical Center[2]	Burlingame	97%	116
Mission Community Hospital	Panorama City	97%	59
Novato Community Hospital	Novato	97%	38
O'Connor Hospital	San Jose	97%	153
Orange Coast Memorial Medical Center	Fountain Valley	97%	91
Saint Agnes Medical Center[2]	Fresno	97%	153
Saint Francis Medical Center	Lynwood	97%	104
Saint Vincent Medical Center	Los Angeles	97%	100
San Gorgonio Memorial Hospital	Banning	97%	98
Santa Monica-UCLA Med Ctr & Ortho Hosp[2]	Santa Monica	97%	58
Santa Rosa Memorial Hospital	Santa Rosa	97%	111
Southwest Healthcare System[2]	Murrieta	97%	87
Sutter Roseville Medical Center[2]	Roseville	97%	90
Sutter Solano Medical Center[2]	Vallejo	97%	76
Tri - City Medical Center[2]	Oceanside	97%	65
Ukiah Valley Medical Center	Ukiah	97%	89
Univ of California Irvine Med Ctr	Orange	97%	33
Watsonville Community Hospital	Watsonville	97%	87
Adventist Medical Center[2]	Hanford	96%	170
Ahmc Anaheim Regional Medical Center	Anaheim	96%	161
Chino Valley Medical Center	Chino	96%	51
Comm Hosp of the Monterey Peninsula[2]	Monterey	96%	139
Fairchild Medical Center	Yreka	96%	69
Glendale Adventist Medical Center	Glendale	96%	221
Los Angeles Community Hospital[2]	Los Angeles	96%	25
Marshall Medical Center[2]	Placerville	96%	103
Mercy Hospital[2]	Bakersfield	96%	79
Mercy Medical Center - Redding[2]	Redding	96%	95
Mission Hospital Regional Medical Center	Mission Viejo	96%	188
Placentia Linda Hospital[2]	Placentia	96%	83
Providence Saint Joseph Medical Center[2]	Burbank	96%	144
Redwood Memorial Hospital	Fortuna	96%	27
Saddleback Memorial Medical Center	Laguna Hills	96%	203
Saint Joseph's Medical Center of Stockton[2]	Stockton	96%	85
Saint Jude Medical Center[2]	Fullerton	96%	102
San Gabriel Valley Medical Center[2]	San Gabriel	96%	49
San Mateo Medical Center	San Mateo	96%	53
Sharp Chula Vista Medical Center	Chula Vista	96%	248
Southern California Hospital at Hollywood[2]	Hollywood	96%	78
VA Greater Los Angeles Healthcare System	W Los Angeles	96%	50
VA Long Beach Healthcare System	Long Beach	96%	53
Victor Valley Global Medical Center[2]	Victorville	96%	56
Western Medical Center Hospital Anaheim	Anaheim	96%	28
Western Medical Center Santa Ana	Santa Ana	96%	53
Emanuel Medical Center	Turlock	95%	259
Enloe Medical Center	Chico	95%	185
Feather River Hospital	Paradise	95%	146
Foothill Presbyterian Hospital	Glendora	95%	84
John F Kennedy Memorial Hospital[2]	Indio	95%	81
Kaiser Foundation Hospital - Downey[2]	Downey	95%	74
Kaweah Delta Medical Center[2]	Visalia	95%	78
Kern Medical Center	Bakersfield	95%	44
Los Alamitos Medical Center	Los Alamitos	95%	155
Menifee Valley Medical Center[2]	Sun City	95%	66
Mercy Medical Center[2]	Merced	95%	76
Montclair Hospital Medical Center	Montclair	95%	41
Monterey Park Hospital[2]	Monterey Park	95%	39
Northbay Medical Center	Fairfield	95%	129
Palm Drive Hospital	Sebastopol	95%	39
Palmdale Regional Medical Center[2]	Palmdale	95%	110
Petaluma Valley Hospital	Petaluma	95%	58
PIH Hospital - Downey	Downey	95%	127
Prov Little Co of Mary Med Ctr San Pedro	San Pedro	95%	106
Rideout Memorial Hospital[2]	Marysville	95%	138
Saint Bernardine Medical Center[2]	San Bernardino	95%	59
San Joaquin Community Hospital	Bakersfield	95%	194
Simi Valley Hosp & Health Care Svcs	Simi Valley	95%	76
Woodland Memorial Hospital[2]	Woodland	95%	57
Adventist Medical Center - Reedley	Reedley	94%	34
Alameda Hospital[2]	Alameda	94%	52
Community Hospital of San Bernardino[2]	San Bernardino	94%	52
Contra Costa Regional Medical Center[2]	Martinez	94%	70
Doctors Hospital of Manteca	Manteca	94%	62
Hemet Valley Medical Center[2]	Hemet	94%	64
Hi - Desert Medical Center	Joshua Tree	94%	98
Hoag Memorial Hospital Presbyterian[2]	Newport Beach	94%	120
Sequoia Hospital[2]	Redwood City	94%	81
Sherman Oaks Hospital	Sherman Oaks	94%	65
Torrance Memorial Medical Center[2]	Torrance	94%	77
Alta Bates Summit Medical Center[2]	Berkeley	93%	95
Bakersfield Heart Hospital[2]	Bakersfield	93%	68
Good Samaritan Hospital[2]	Los Angeles	93%	81
Parkview Comm Hosp Med Ctr[2]	Riverside	93%	150
Prov Little Co of Mary Med Ctr Torrance[2]	Torrance	93%	89
Salinas Valley Memorial Hospital[2]	Salinas	93%	76
San Dimas Community Hospital[2]	San Dimas	93%	45
Sonoma Valley Hospital	Sonoma	93%	29
Valley Presbyterian Hospital[2]	Van Nuys	93%	81
Valleycare Medical Center	Pleasanton	93%	157
White Memorial Medical Center	Los Angeles	93%	102
Alameda County Medical Center	Oakland	92%	84
Barton Memorial Hospital	S Lake Tahoe	92%	48
Beverly Hospital[2]	Montebello	92%	83
Glendale Mem Hosp & Health Ctr	Glendale	92%	120
Mark Twain Medical Center	San Andreas	92%	39
Oak Valley District Hospital	Oakdale	92%	40
Saint Johns Pleasant Valley Hospital	Camarillo	92%	66
Santa Barbara Cottage Hospital	Santa Barbara	92%	144
Tri - City Regional Medical Center	Hawaiian Grdns	92%	25
Antelope Valley Hospital[2]	Lancaster	91%	111
Arrowhead Regional Medical Center[2]	Colton	91%	151
Madera Community Hospital	Madera	91%	64
Oroville Hospital[2]	Oroville	91%	151
Pacific Alliance Medical Center[2]	Los Angeles	91%	32
Sierra View District Hospital	Porterville	91%	152
Ventura County Medical Center[2]	Ventura	91%	99
Hollywood Presbyterian Medical Center[2]	Los Angeles	90%	58
Lompoc Valley Medical Center	Lompoc	90%	70
Marina Del Rey Hospital	Marina Del Rey	90%	70
Natividad Medical Center	Salinas	90%	40
Univ of CA San Diego Med Ctr[2]	San Diego	90%	40
Hazel Hawkins Memorial Hospital[2]	Hollister	89%	44
Loma Linda University Medical Center[2]	Loma Linda	89%	37
Mad River Community Hospital	Arcata	89%	53
Mercy Medical Center - Mount Shasta	Mount Shasta	89%	27
VA Northern California Healthcare System	Mather	89%	65
Banner Lassen Medical Center[2]	Susanville	88%	33
Bear Valley Community Hospital	Big Bear Lake	88%	25
LAC/Harbor - UCLA Medical Center[2]	Torrance	88%	74
Ojai Valley Community Hospital	Ojai	88%	26
Palo Alto VA Medical Center	Palo Alto	88%	57
El Centro Regional Medical Center	El Centro	86%	135
Coast Plaza Hospital	Norwalk	84%	49
Healdsburg District Hospital	Healdsburg	84%	32
Loma Linda Univ Med Ctr-Murrieta[2]	Murrieta	84%	119
Huntington Memorial Hospital[2]	Pasadena	80%	89
Kern Valley Healthcare District	Lake Isabella	76%	50
Palo Verde Hospital[2]	Blythe	76%	25
Colusa Regional Medical Center	Colusa	71%	28
Good Samaritan Hospital	Bakersfield	67%	27

Blood Culture Timing

Hospital Name	City	Rate	Cases
Ahmc Anaheim Regional Medical Center	Anaheim	100%	289
Beverly Hospital[2]	Montebello	100%	177
CA Pacific Med Ctr-Pacific Campus Hosp[2]	San Francisco	100%	161
CA Pacific Med Ctr-St Luke's Campus[2]	San Francisco	100%	87
Centinela Hospital Medical Center[2]	Inglewood	100%	99
Dameron Hospital	Stockton	100%	179
Doctors Medical Center[2]	Modesto	100%	344
Dominican Hospital[2]	Santa Cruz	100%	170
El Camino Hospital[2]	Mountain View	100%	229
Encino Hospital Medical Center	Encino	100%	63
Frank R Howard Memorial Hospital	Willits	100%	29
Garden Grove Hospital & Medical Center	Garden Grove	100%	169
Glendale Adventist Medical Center	Glendale	100%	497
Good Samaritan Hospital[2]	San Jose	100%	179
Huntington Beach Hospital[2]	Huntington Bch	100%	120
Kaiser Fdn Hosp-Oakland/Richmond[2]	Oakland	100%	119
Kaiser Fdn Hosp-Orange Co-Anaheim[2]	Anaheim	100%	184
Kaiser Foundation Hospital - San Jose[2]	San Jose	100%	135
Kaiser Foundation Hospital - Santa Clara[2]	Santa Clara	100%	128
Loma Linda University Medical Center[2]	Loma Linda	100%	96
Los Alamitos Medical Center	Los Alamitos	100%	176
Marin General Hospital[2]	Greenbrae	100%	193
Memorial Hospital Los Banos	Los Banos	100%	45
Mercy General Hospital	Sacramento	100%	228
Montclair Hospital Medical Center	Montclair	100%	116
Monterey Park Hospital[2]	Monterey Park	100%	59
Northridge Hospital Medical Center	Northridge	100%	301
Novato Community Hospital	Novato	100%	85
Pacific Alliance Medical Center[2]	Los Angeles	100%	58
Placentia Linda Hospital[2]	Placentia	100%	132
Pomona Valley Hospital Medical Center[2]	Pomona	100%	143
Providence Saint John's Health Center	Santa Monica	100%	193
Regional Medical Center of San Jose[2]	San Jose	100%	136
Riverside Community Hospital[2]	Riverside	100%	137
Ronald Reagan UCLA Medical Center[2]	Los Angeles	100%	61
Saint Helena Hospital	Saint Helena	100%	26
Saint Joseph Hospital	Orange	100%	316
Saint Louise Regional Hospital	Gilroy	100%	91
Saint Mary's Medical Center	San Francisco	100%	232
San Ramon Regional Medical Center	San Ramon	100%	108
Santa Monica-UCLA Med Ctr & Ortho Hosp[2]	Santa Monica	100%	100
Scripps Memorial Hospital La Jolla[2]	La Jolla	100%	156
Scripps Mercy Hospital[2]	San Diego	100%	136

NOTE: Hospital profiles are in alphabetical order by state, then city, then hospital within the city; Rankings exclude hospitals with less than 25 cases except for patient surveys which excludes hospitals with less than 100 cases; (a) 100-299 cases; (1) The number of cases/patients is too few to report; (2) Data submitted were based on a sample of cases/patients; (3) Results are based on a shorter time period than required; (4) Data suppressed by CMS for one or more quarters; (5) Results are not available for this reporting period; (6) Fewer than 100 patients completed the HCAHPS survey; (7) No cases met the criteria for this measure; (8) The lower limit of the confidence interval cannot be calculated if the number of observed infections equals zero; (9) No data are available from the state/territory for this reporting period; (10) The scores shown reflect fewer than 50 completed surveys; (11) There were discrepancies in the data collection process; (12) This measure does not apply to this hospital for this reporting period; (13) Results cannot be calculated for this reporting period; (14) The results for this state are combined with nearby states to protect confidentiality; Please refer to the User's Guide for a full explanation of data.

Hospital Name	City	Rate	Cases
Sharp Coronado Hosp & Healthcare Ctr	Coronado	100%	37
Sharp Memorial Hospital	San Diego	100%	401
Shasta Regional Medical Center	Redding	100%	212
Stanford Hospital	Stanford	100%	319
Sutter Auburn Faith Hospital[2]	Auburn	100%	131
Sutter Medical Center of Santa Rosa[2]	Santa Rosa	100%	98
Twin Cities Community Hospital	Templeton	100%	131
Ukiah Valley Medical Center	Ukiah	100%	120
VA Northern California Healthcare System	Mather	100%	48
Valleycare Medical Center	Pleasanton	100%	205
West Anaheim Medical Center[2]	Anaheim	100%	169
West Hills Hospital & Medical Center[2]	West Hills	100%	155
Western Medical Center Hospital Anaheim	Anaheim	100%	50
Woodland Memorial Hospital[2]	Woodland	100%	114
Alvarado Hospital Medical Center[2]	San Diego	99%	136
Barton Memorial Hospital	S Lake Tahoe	99%	83
Cedars - Sinai Medical Center	Los Angeles	99%	392
Citrus Valley Medical Center - IC Campus[2]	Covina	99%	199
Coastal Communities Hospital	Santa Ana	99%	93
Emanuel Medical Center	Turlock	99%	332
Fountain Valley Reg Hosp & Med Ctr[2]	Fountain Valley	99%	171
French Hospital Medical Center[2]	San Luis Obispo	99%	104
Fresno VA Med Ctr-VA Central CA	Fresno	99%	99
Grossmont Hospital	La Mesa	99%	519
Henry Mayo Newhall Memorial Hospital[2]	Valencia	99%	169
Hoag Memorial Hospital Presbyterian[2]	Newport Beach	99%	231
Hollywood Presbyterian Medical Center[2]	Los Angeles	99%	155
Kaiser Foundation Hospital - Downey[2]	Downey	99%	161
Kaiser Foundation Hospital - Fontana[2]	Fontana	99%	176
Kaiser Fdn Hosp-Fremont/Hayward[2]	Hayward	99%	148
Kaiser Fdn Hosp-Moreno Valley[2]	Moreno Valley	99%	117
Kaiser Fdn Hosp-Panorama City[2]	Panorama City	99%	156
Kaiser Foundation Hospital - Redwood City[2]	Redwood City	99%	133
Kaiser Foundation Hospital - Roseville[2]	Roseville	99%	127
Kaiser Foundation Hospital - San Diego[2]	San Diego	99%	152
Kaiser Foundation Hospital - South Bay[2]	Harbor City	99%	156
Kaiser Foundation Hospital - Vacaville[2]	Vacaville	99%	146
La Palma Intercommunity Hospital	La Palma	99%	156
Lakewood Regional Medical Center[2]	Lakewood	99%	159
Long Beach Memorial Medical Center[2]	Long Beach	99%	204
Los Robles Hospital & Medical Center	Thousand Oaks	99%	228
Madera Community Hospital	Madera	99%	76
Marian Regional Medical Center	Santa Maria	99%	280
Marshall Medical Center[2]	Placerville	99%	167
Memorial Medical Center[2]	Modesto	99%	164
Menifee Valley Medical Center[2]	Sun City	99%	93
Mercy Hospital of Folsom[2]	Folsom	99%	169
Methodist Hospital of Southern California	Arcadia	99%	353
Mills - Peninsula Medical Center[2]	Burlingame	99%	160
O'Connor Hospital	San Jose	99%	247
Olympia Medical Center[2]	Los Angeles	99%	136
Palomar Health Downtown Campus	Escondido	99%	358
Providence Holy Cross Medical Center[2]	Mission Hills	99%	131
Providence Saint Joseph Medical Center[2]	Burbank	99%	229
Providence Tarzana Medical Center	Tarzana	99%	370
Queen of the Valley Medical Center	Napa	99%	136
Saint Bernardine Medical Center[2]	San Bernardino	99%	125
Saint Francis Memorial Hospital[2]	San Francisco	99%	165
Saint Vincent Medical Center	Los Angeles	99%	197
San Gabriel Valley Medical Center[2]	San Gabriel	99%	162
Scripps Memorial Hospital - Encinitas[2]	Encinitas	99%	171
Sequoia Hospital[2]	Redwood City	99%	114
Seton Medical Center	Daly City	99%	184
Sharp Chula Vista Medical Center	Chula Vista	99%	402
Sherman Oaks Hospital	Sherman Oaks	99%	147
Simi Valley Hosp & Health Care Svcs	Simi Valley	99%	125
Sonora Regional Medical Center	Sonora	99%	197
Sutter Amador Hospital[2]	Jackson	99%	149
Sutter Davis Hospital[2]	Davis	99%	96
Sutter Lakeside Hospital	Lakeport	99%	96
Sutter Tracy Community Hospital	Tracy	99%	99
Univ of CA Davis Med Ctr[2]	Sacramento	99%	134
VA San Diego Healthcare System	San Diego	99%	150
Alameda Hospital[2]	Alameda	98%	120
Alta Bates Summit Medical Center[2]	Berkeley	98%	150
Alta Bates Summit Medical Center[2]	Oakland	98%	164
Barstow Community Hospital	Barstow	98%	62
California Hosp Med Ctr Los Angeles[2]	Los Angeles	98%	175
CA Pacific Med Ctr-Davies Campus	San Francisco	98%	52
Chapman Medical Center	Orange	98%	59
Community Hospital of Huntington Park	Huntington Park	98%	62
Corona Regional Medical Center[2]	Corona	98%	159
Desert Regional Medical Center[2]	Palm Springs	98%	167
Eden Medical Center[2]	Castro Valley	98%	214
Eisenhower Medical Center	Rancho Mirage	98%	492
Feather River Hospital	Paradise	98%	265
Foothill Presbyterian Hospital	Glendora	98%	145
Garfield Medical Center[2]	Monterey Park	98%	130
Greater El Monte Community Hospital[2]	South El Monte	98%	110
John F Kennedy Memorial Hospital[2]	Indio	98%	148
John Muir Med Ctr-Walnut Creek Campus[2]	Walnut Creek	98%	124
Kaiser Foundation Hospital - Antioch[2]	Antioch	98%	154
Kaiser Foundation Hospital - Baldwin Park[2]	Baldwin Park	98%	172
Kaiser Foundation Hospital - Riverside[2]	Riverside	98%	111
Kaiser Foundation Hospital - Sacramento[2]	Sacramento	98%	132
Kaiser Fdn Hosp-San Francisco[2]	San Francisco	98%	161
Kaiser Fdn Hosp-S San Francisco[2]	S San Francisco	98%	127
Kaiser Foundation Hospital - Walnut Creek[2]	Walnut Creek	98%	150
Kaiser Fdn Hosp-Woodland Hills[2]	Woodland Hills	98%	128
Kaweah Delta Medical Center[2]	Visalia	98%	161
LAC+USC Medical Center	Los Angeles	98%	358
Loma Linda VA Medical Center	Loma Linda	98%	160
Mercy Hospital[2]	Bakersfield	98%	180
Palo Alto VA Medical Center	Palo Alto	98%	123
Paradise Valley Hospital	National City	98%	257
Petaluma Valley Hospital	Petaluma	98%	88
Presbyterian Intercommunity Hospital[2]	Whittier	98%	169
Prov Little Co of Mary Med Ctr Torrance[2]	Torrance	98%	191
Redlands Community Hospital[2]	Redlands	98%	132
Saddleback Memorial Medical Center	Laguna Hills	98%	331
Saint Agnes Medical Center[2]	Fresno	98%	187
Saint Joseph Hospital	Eureka	98%	114
Saint Joseph's Medical Center of Stockton[2]	Stockton	98%	158
Saint Rose Hospital	Hayward	98%	107
Salinas Valley Memorial Hospital[2]	Salinas	98%	131
San Francisco VA Medical Center	San Francisco	98%	90
San Gorgonio Memorial Hospital	Banning	98%	176
Santa Barbara Cottage Hospital	Santa Barbara	98%	252
Santa Clara Valley Medical Center[2]	San Jose	98%	124
Sierra Vista Regional Medical Center	San Luis Obispo	98%	46
Sonoma Valley Hospital	Sonoma	98%	47
Sutter Coast Hospital	Crescent City	98%	182
Sutter General Hospital[2]	Sacramento	98%	163
Univ of California Irvine Med Ctr	Orange	98%	122
VA Greater Los Angeles Healthcare System	W Los Angeles	98%	101
Watsonville Community Hospital	Watsonville	98%	120
Whittier Hospital Medical Center	Whittier	98%	204
Alhambra Hospital Medical Center	Alhambra	97%	245
Chino Valley Medical Center	Chino	97%	76
Coast Plaza Hospital	Norwalk	97%	139
Community Hospital of San Bernardino[2]	San Bernardino	97%	119
Comm Hosp of the Monterey Peninsula[2]	Monterey	97%	239
Delano Regional Medical Center	Delano	97%	60
Doctors Medical Center - San Pablo[2]	San Pablo	97%	151
East Los Angeles Doctors Hospital	Los Angeles	97%	77
Glendale Mem Hosp & Health Ctr	Glendale	97%	256
Hemet Valley Medical Center[2]	Hemet	97%	115
John Muir Medical Center - Concord Campus[2]	Concord	97%	152
Kaiser Foundation Hospital - Manteca[2]	Manteca	97%	119
Lodi Memorial Hospital[2]	Lodi	97%	204
Mark Twain Medical Center	San Andreas	97%	69
Memorial Hospital of Gardena	Gardena	97%	231
Mercy Medical Center - Redding[2]	Redding	97%	122
Mission Hospital Regional Medical Center	Mission Viejo	97%	319
Ojai Valley Community Hospital	Ojai	97%	35
Orange Coast Memorial Medical Center	Fountain Valley	97%	153
Prov Little Co of Mary Med Ctr San Pedro	San Pedro	97%	198
Rideout Memorial Hospital[2]	Marysville	97%	152
Saint Helena Hospital - Clearlake	Clearlake	97%	67
Saint Jude Medical Center[2]	Fullerton	97%	190
Saint Mary Medical Center[2]	Apple Valley	97%	138
Saint Mary Medical Center[2]	Long Beach	97%	152
San Dimas Community Hospital[2]	San Dimas	97%	120
San Joaquin Community Hospital	Bakersfield	97%	375
San Joaquin General Hospital	French Camp	97%	171
Santa Rosa Memorial Hospital	Santa Rosa	97%	169
Sierra Nevada Memorial Hospital[2]	Grass Valley	97%	160
Sierra View District Hospital	Porterville	97%	200
Southwest Healthcare System[2]	Murrieta	97%	143
Sutter Delta Medical Center[2]	Antioch	97%	175
Sutter Roseville Medical Center[2]	Roseville	97%	157
Tri - City Regional Medical Center	Hawaiian Grdns	97%	116
Tulare Regional Medical Center	Tulare	97%	148
USC Verdugo Hills Hospital[2]	Glendale	97%	133
VA Long Beach Healthcare System	Long Beach	97%	118
Washington Hospital[2]	Fremont	97%	136
Western Medical Center Santa Ana	Santa Ana	97%	119
Antelope Valley Hospital[2]	Lancaster	96%	148
Bakersfield Heart Hospital[2]	Bakersfield	96%	145
Bakersfield Memorial Hospital[2]	Bakersfield	96%	120
Desert Valley Hospital[2]	Victorville	96%	114
Doctors Hospital of Manteca	Manteca	96%	70
East Valley Hospital Medical Center	Glendora	96%	99
Enloe Medical Center	Chico	96%	315
Kaiser Foundation Hospital - Santa Rosa[2]	Santa Rosa	96%	139
Mad River Community Hospital	Arcata	96%	68
Methodist Hospital of Sacramento[2]	Sacramento	96%	138
Northbay Medical Center	Fairfield	96%	229
Palm Drive Hospital	Sebastopol	96%	47
Pioneers Memorial Healthcare District	Brawley	96%	143
Pomerado Hospital	Poway	96%	169
Redwood Memorial Hospital	Fortuna	96%	50
Saint Elizabeth Community Hospital[2]	Red Bluff	96%	94
Saint Francis Medical Center	Lynwood	96%	187
Saint Johns Pleasant Valley Hospital	Camarillo	96%	150
Saint Johns Regional Medical Center	Oxnard	96%	248
Southern California Hospital at Hollywood[2]	Hollywood	96%	167
Sutter Solano Medical Center[2]	Vallejo	96%	130
Torrance Memorial Medical Center[2]	Torrance	96%	140
Univ of CA San Diego Med Ctr[2]	San Diego	96%	136
White Memorial Medical Center	Los Angeles	96%	249
Adventist Medical Center[2]	Hanford	95%	261
Arrowhead Regional Medical Center[2]	Colton	95%	264
Chinese Hospital	San Francisco	95%	108
Clovis Community Medical Center[2]	Clovis	95%	76
Community Hospital of Long Beach	Long Beach	95%	206
Comm Mem Hosp San Buenaventura	Ventura	95%	242
Community Regional Medical Center[2]	Fresno	95%	388
Fairchild Medical Center	Yreka	95%	75
Huntington Memorial Hospital[2]	Pasadena	95%	133
Kaiser Foundation Hospital[2]	San Rafael	95%	110
Kaiser Foundation Hospital & Rehab Center[2]	Vallejo	95%	152
Kaiser Foundation Hospital - Los Angeles[2]	Los Angeles	95%	158
Kaiser Fdn Hosp S Sacramento[2]	Sacramento	95%	132
Los Angeles Community Hospital[2]	Los Angeles	95%	61
Mercy Medical Center[2]	Merced	95%	172
Mercy San Juan Medical Center[2]	Carmichael	95%	111
Oroville Hospital[2]	Oroville	95%	250
Riverside County Regional Medical Center[2]	Moreno Valley	95%	97
San Antonio Community Hospital[2]	Upland	95%	161
San Mateo Medical Center	San Mateo	95%	66
Tri - City Medical Center[2]	Oceanside	95%	147
Ventura County Medical Center[2]	Ventura	95%	167
Banner Lassen Medical Center[2]	Susanville	94%	33
Contra Costa Regional Medical Center[2]	Martinez	94%	72
Good Samaritan Hospital[2]	Los Angeles	94%	157
Healdsburg District Hospital	Healdsburg	94%	35
Kaiser Foundation Hospital - West La[2]	Los Angeles	94%	118
Lompoc Valley Medical Center	Lompoc	94%	100
Palmdale Regional Medical Center[2]	Palmdale	94%	95
Parkview Comm Hosp Med Ctr[2]	Riverside	94%	317
PIH Hospital - Downey	Downey	94%	260
UCSF Medical Center[2]	San Francisco	94%	121
Valley Presbyterian Hospital[2]	Van Nuys	94%	189
Adventist Medical Center - Reedley	Reedley	93%	43
Fallbrook Hospital	Fallbrook	93%	46
Goleta Valley Cottage Hospital	Santa Barbara	93%	29
Kaiser Foundation Hospital - Fresno[2]	Fresno	93%	138
LAC/Harbor - UCLA Medical Center[2]	Torrance	93%	96
LAC/Olive View - UCLA Medical Center[2]	Sylmar	93%	73
Marina Del Rey Hospital	Marina Del Rey	93%	94
Oak Valley District Hospital	Oakdale	93%	43
El Centro Regional Medical Center	El Centro	92%	202
Mercy Medical Center - Mount Shasta	Mount Shasta	92%	37
Pacific Hospital of Long Beach[3]	Long Beach	92%	91
Victor Valley Global Medical Center[2]	Victorville	92%	103
Kern Valley Healthcare District	Lake Isabella	91%	55
Mission Community Hospital	Panorama City	91%	175
Natividad Medical Center	Salinas	91%	64
Pacifica Hospital of the Valley	Sun Valley	91%	53
Kern Medical Center	Bakersfield	90%	69
Alameda County Medical Center	Oakland	86%	162
Hazel Hawkins Memorial Hospital[2]	Hollister	85%	60
Hi - Desert Medical Center	Joshua Tree	84%	148
San Francisco General Hospital[2]	San Francisco	84%	143
Loma Linda Univ Med Ctr-Murrieta[2]	Murrieta	82%	141
Colusa Regional Medical Center	Colusa	81%	27
Palo Verde Hospital[2]	Blythe	77%	30

Pregnancy and Delivery Care

Newborns whose Deliveries were Scheduled Early

Hospital Name	City	Rate	Cases
Antelope Valley Hospital[2]	Lancaster	0%	98
Barstow Community Hospital[2]	Barstow	0%	26
Barton Memorial Hospital[2]	S Lake Tahoe	0%	27
CA Pacific Med Ctr-Pacific Campus Hosp	San Francisco	0%	222
CA Pacific Med Ctr-St Luke's Campus	San Francisco	0%	60
Citrus Valley Medical Center - IC Campus	Covina	0%	474
Clovis Community Medical Center[2]	Clovis	0%	62
Coastal Communities Hospital[2]	Santa Ana	0%	25
Comm Hosp of the Monterey Peninsula[2]	Monterey	0%	27
Doctors Hospital of Manteca[2]	Manteca	0%	33
Eden Medical Center	Castro Valley	0%	80
Enloe Medical Center[2]	Chico	0%	25
Feather River Hospital[2]	Paradise	0%	29
French Hospital Medical Center	San Luis Obispo	0%	30
Good Samaritan Hospital[2]	San Jose	0%	49
Henry Mayo Newhall Memorial Hospital	Valencia	0%	268
Kaiser Foundation Hospital & Rehab Center[2]	Vallejo	0%	32
Kaiser Foundation Hospital - Baldwin Park	Baldwin Park	0%	209
Kaiser Fdn Hosp-Fremont/Hayward[2]	Hayward	0%	39

NOTE: Hospital profiles are in alphabetical order by state, then city, then hospital within the city; Rankings exclude hospitals with less than 25 cases except for patient surveys which excludes hospitals with less than 100 cases; (a) 100-299 cases; (1) The number of cases/patients is too few to report; (2) Data submitted were based on a sample of cases/patients; (3) Results are based on a shorter time period than required; (4) Data suppressed by CMS for one or more quarters; (5) Results are not available for this reporting period; (6) Fewer than 100 patients completed the HCAHPS survey; (7) No cases met the criteria for this measure; (8) The lower limit of the confidence interval cannot be calculated if the number of observed infections equals zero; (9) No data are available from the state/territory for this reporting period; (10) The scores shown reflect fewer than 50 completed surveys; (11) There were discrepancies in the data collection process; (12) This measure does not apply to this hospital for this reporting period; (13) Results cannot be calculated for this reporting period; (14) The results for this state are combined with nearby states to protect confidentiality; Please refer to the User's Guide for a full explanation of data.

Kaiser Foundation Hospital - Los Angeles	Los Angeles	0%	201
Kaiser Fdn Hosp-Moreno Valley[2]	Moreno Valley	0%	93
Kaiser Fdn Hosp-Orange Co-Anaheim	Anaheim	0%	554
Kaiser Fdn Hosp-Panorama City[2]	Panorama City	0%	132
Kaiser Foundation Hospital - Redwood City[2]	Redwood City	0%	27
Kaiser Foundation Hospital - Riverside	Riverside	0%	237
Kaiser Fdn Hosp-San Francisco[2]	San Francisco	0%	26
Kaiser Foundation Hospital - San Jose[2]	San Jose	0%	25
Kaiser Foundation Hospital - Walnut Creek[2]	Walnut Creek	0%	41
Kaiser Fdn Hosp S Sacramento[2]	Sacramento	0%	30
La Palma Intercommunity Hospital	La Palma	0%	60
Lodi Memorial Hospital[2]	Lodi	0%	31
Los Alamitos Medical Center[2]	Los Alamitos	0%	36
Los Robles Hospital & Medical Center[2]	Thousand Oaks	0%	45
Marian Regional Medical Center[2]	Santa Maria	0%	53
Memorial Hospital Los Banos	Los Banos	0%	99
Mercy Hospital[2]	Bakersfield	0%	44
Mercy San Juan Medical Center[2]	Carmichael	0%	35
Northridge Hospital Medical Center[2]	Northridge	0%	52
Palo Verde Hospital[2]	Blythe	0%	48
Paradise Valley Hospital	National City	0%	88
PIH Hospital - Downey[2]	Downey	0%	66
Pomerado Hospital[2]	Poway	0%	28
Presbyterian Intercommunity Hospital[2]	Whittier	0%	101
Regional Medical Center of San Jose[2]	San Jose	0%	50
Rideout Memorial Hospital[2]	Marysville	0%	64
Riverside Community Hospital[2]	Riverside	0%	73
Riverside County Regional Medical Center[2]	Moreno Valley	0%	36
Saddleback Memorial Medical Center[2]	Laguna Hills	0%	29
Saint Agnes Medical Center[2]	Fresno	0%	115
Saint Joseph's Medical Center of Stockton[2]	Stockton	0%	72
Saint Jude Medical Center[2]	Fullerton	0%	47
Saint Louise Regional Hospital[2]	Gilroy	0%	40
Saint Rose Hospital[2]	Hayward	0%	62
San Dimas Community Hospital[2]	San Dimas	0%	35
San Joaquin General Hospital[2]	French Camp	0%	34
Scripps Memorial Hospital - Encinitas[2]	Encinitas	0%	35
Scripps Mercy Hospital[2]	San Diego	0%	81
Sutter Coast Hospital	Crescent City	0%	45
Sutter Davis Hospital	Davis	0%	112
Sutter Medical Center of Santa Rosa	Santa Rosa	0%	61
Sutter Solano Medical Center	Vallejo	0%	82
Sutter Tracy Community Hospital	Tracy	0%	39
Torrance Memorial Medical Center[2]	Torrance	0%	54
Watsonville Community Hospital[2]	Watsonville	0%	32
Whittier Hospital Medical Center[2]	Whittier	0%	33
Cedars - Sinai Medical Center[2]	Los Angeles	1%	107
Community Regional Medical Center[2]	Fresno	1%	81
Dameron Hospital	Stockton	1%	90
Fountain Valley Reg Hosp & Med Ctr[2]	Fountain Valley	1%	68
Kaiser Foundation Hospital - Downey	Downey	1%	464
Kaiser Fdn Hosp-Woodland Hills[2]	Woodland Hills	1%	143
Memorial Medical Center	Modesto	1%	135
Northbay Medical Center	Fairfield	1%	107
Pomona Valley Hospital Medical Center[2]	Pomona	1%	76
Saint Joseph Hospital[2]	Orange	1%	99
San Joaquin Community Hospital[2]	Bakersfield	1%	94
Sutter General Hospital	Sacramento	1%	398
Sutter Roseville Medical Center	Roseville	1%	240
White Memorial Medical Center[2]	Los Angeles	1%	72
Alta Bates Summit Medical Center	Berkeley	2%	492
California Hosp Med Ctr Los Angeles[2]	Los Angeles	2%	83
Community Hospital of San Bernardino[2]	San Bernardino	2%	44
Fallbrook Hospital[2]	Fallbrook	2%	42
Garfield Medical Center[2]	Monterey Park	2%	102
Good Samaritan Hospital[2]	Los Angeles	2%	92
Kaiser Foundation Hospital - Fontana	Fontana	2%	315
Kaiser Foundation Hospital - Roseville[2]	Roseville	2%	54
Kaiser Foundation Hospital - South Bay[2]	Harbor City	2%	181
Loma Linda University Medical Center[2]	Loma Linda	2%	45
Methodist Hospital of Southern California[2]	Arcadia	2%	217
Mills - Peninsula Medical Center	Burlingame	2%	154
Montclair Hospital Medical Center[2]	Montclair	2%	48
Pacific Alliance Medical Center[2]	Los Angeles	2%	91
Prov Little Co of Mary Med Ctr Torrance[2]	Torrance	2%	84
Saint Bernardine Medical Center[2]	San Bernardino	2%	47
Salinas Valley Memorial Hospital[2]	Salinas	2%	304
San Antonio Community Hospital[2]	Upland	2%	46
Santa Clara Valley Medical Center[2]	San Jose	2%	54
Sharp Memorial Hospital	San Diego	2%	876
Sutter Maternity & Surgery Ctr	Santa Cruz	2%	43
USC Verdugo Hills Hospital[2]	Glendale	2%	45
Valley Presbyterian Hospital[2]	Van Nuys	2%	116
Washington Hospital	Fremont	2%	183
Western Medical Center Santa Ana[2]	Santa Ana	2%	247
Bakersfield Memorial Hospital[2]	Bakersfield	3%	118
Centinela Hospital Medical Center[2]	Inglewood	3%	30
Emanuel Medical Center[2]	Turlock	3%	36
Grossmont Hospital	La Mesa	3%	374
Kaiser Foundation Hospital - San Diego	San Diego	3%	345
Kaiser Foundation Hospital - Santa Clara[2]	Santa Clara	3%	35
Marshall Medical Center	Placerville	3%	77
Monterey Park Hospital[2]	Monterey Park	3%	29
Natividad Medical Center[2]	Salinas	3%	35
Orange Coast Memorial Medical Center[2]	Fountain Valley	3%	37
Prov Little Co of Mary Med Ctr San Pedro[2]	San Pedro	3%	162
Saint Mary Medical Center[2]	Long Beach	3%	63
Sequoia Hospital[2]	Redwood City	3%	29
Sutter Delta Medical Center	Antioch	3%	88
Western Medical Center Hospital Anaheim[2]	Anaheim	3%	105
Ahmc Anaheim Regional Medical Center	Anaheim	4%	186
Corona Regional Medical Center[2]	Corona	4%	45
Desert Valley Hospital[2]	Victorville	4%	49
El Centro Regional Medical Center[2]	El Centro	4%	28
Glendale Mem Hosp & Health Ctr[2]	Glendale	4%	68
Kaiser Foundation Hospital - Fresno[2]	Fresno	4%	27
Kaiser Foundation Hospital - West La	Los Angeles	4%	157
Scripps Memorial Hospital La Jolla[2]	La Jolla	4%	72
Simi Valley Hosp & Health Care Svcs[2]	Simi Valley	4%	26
Southwest Healthcare System[2]	Murrieta	4%	75
Tri - City Medical Center	Oceanside	4%	178
UCSF Medical Center	San Francisco	4%	69
Ukiah Valley Medical Center[2]	Ukiah	4%	26
Desert Regional Medical Center[2]	Palm Springs	5%	60
Garden Grove Hospital & Medical Center[2]	Garden Grove	5%	42
Greater El Monte Community Hospital[2]	South El Monte	5%	43
Hoag Memorial Hospital Presbyterian[2]	Newport Beach	5%	99
Kern Medical Center[2]	Bakersfield	5%	44
Mercy General Hospital[2]	Sacramento	5%	39
Saint Francis Medical Center[2]	Lynwood	5%	108
Doctors Medical Center[2]	Modesto	6%	70
East Los Angeles Doctors Hospital[2]	Los Angeles	6%	86
El Camino Hospital[2]	Mountain View	6%	430
Madera Community Hospital	Madera	6%	310
Mercy Medical Center[2]	Merced	6%	64
Providence Holy Cross Medical Center[2]	Mission Hills	6%	67
Redlands Community Hospital	Redlands	6%	342
Santa Barbara Cottage Hospital	Santa Barbara	6%	155
Sharp Chula Vista Medical Center	Chula Vista	6%	361
Twin Cities Community Hospital[2]	Templeton	6%	31
Foothill Presbyterian Hospital	Glendora	7%	115
Saint Joseph Hospital	Eureka	7%	42
Saint Mary Medical Center	Apple Valley	7%	336
San Gorgonio Memorial Hospital[2]	Banning	7%	55
Mission Hospital Regional Medical Center[2]	Mission Viejo	8%	61
Parkview Comm Hosp Med Ctr	Riverside	8%	179
Comm Mem Hosp San Buenaventura	Ventura	9%	209
Methodist Hospital of Sacramento[2]	Sacramento	9%	35
O'Connor Hospital[2]	San Jose	9%	67
Providence Tarzana Medical Center[2]	Tarzana	9%	69
Tulare Regional Medical Center[2]	Tulare	9%	56
Adventist Medical Center[2]	Hanford	10%	51
Central Valley General Hospital[2]	Hanford	10%	48
Lompoc Valley Medical Center[2]	Lompoc	10%	49
Beverly Hospital[2]	Montebello	11%	57
Saint Johns Regional Medical Center[2]	Oxnard	11%	54
Hollywood Presbyterian Medical Center[2]	Los Angeles	12%	108
Huntington Memorial Hospital[2]	Pasadena	12%	65
John F Kennedy Memorial Hospital[2]	Indio	12%	64
Palomar Health Downtown Campus[2]	Escondido	12%	64
Arrowhead Regional Medical Center[2]	Colton	13%	174
Mercy Medical Center - Redding[2]	Redding	13%	39
Pioneers Memorial Healthcare District[2]	Brawley	13%	55
Providence Saint Joseph Medical Center[2]	Burbank	13%	123
Sierra Nevada Memorial Hospital	Grass Valley	13%	30
Sierra View District Hospital[2]	Porterville	14%	51
John Muir Med Ctr-Walnut Creek Campus[2]	Walnut Creek	15%	53
Loma Linda Univ Med Ctr-Murrieta[2]	Murrieta	15%	66
Pacifica Hospital of the Valley[2]	Sun Valley	15%	139
Delano Regional Medical Center[2]	Delano	16%	49
San Gabriel Valley Medical Center[2]	San Gabriel	17%	452
Adventist Medical Center - Reedley[2]	Reedley	18%	40
Glendale Adventist Medical Center	Glendale	21%	376
Kaweah Delta Medical Center	Visalia	21%	448
Victor Valley Global Medical Center[2]	Victorville	21%	48
Oroville Hospital	Oroville	29%	38
LAC/Harbor - UCLA Medical Center[2]	Torrance	39%	33
Memorial Hospital of Gardena	Gardena	77%	218

Preventive Care

Immunization for Influenza

Hospital Name	City	Rate	Cases
Barstow Community Hospital[2]	Barstow	100%	296
Centinela Hospital Medical Center[2]	Inglewood	100%	530
Community Hospital of Huntington Park[2]	Huntington Park	100%	410
Encino Hospital Medical Center[2]	Encino	100%	290
Garden Grove Hospital & Medical Center[2]	Garden Grove	100%	440
Huntington Beach Hospital[2]	Huntington Bch	100%	323
Memorial Hospital Los Banos[2]	Los Banos	100%	210
Mills - Peninsula Medical Center[2]	Burlingame	100%	527
Scripps Green Hospital[2]	La Jolla	100%	631
Sherman Oaks Hospital[2]	Sherman Oaks	100%	365
Sonoma Developmental Center	Eldridge	100%	62
Temple Community Hospital[2]	Los Angeles	100%	295
West Anaheim Medical Center[2]	Anaheim	100%	569
Ahmc Anaheim Regional Medical Center[2]	Anaheim	99%	540
Chino Valley Medical Center[2]	Chino	99%	542
Doctors Medical Center[2]	Modesto	99%	536
El Camino Hospital[2]	Mountain View	99%	471
Grossmont Hospital[2]	La Mesa	99%	511
Hoag Orthopedic Institute[2]	Irvine	99%	409
La Palma Intercommunity Hospital[2]	La Palma	99%	327
Los Alamitos Medical Center[2]	Los Alamitos	99%	555
Memorial Medical Center[2]	Modesto	99%	557
Mercy General Hospital[2]	Sacramento	99%	547
Methodist Hospital of Sacramento[2]	Sacramento	99%	511
Olympia Medical Center[2]	Los Angeles	99%	548
Palm Drive Hospital[2]	Sebastopol	99%	327
Placentia Linda Hospital[2]	Placentia	99%	417
San Joaquin Community Hospital[2]	Bakersfield	99%	527
Sutter Coast Hospital[2]	Crescent City	99%	267
Sutter Davis Hospital[2]	Davis	99%	332
Sutter Tracy Community Hospital[2]	Tracy	99%	361
Twin Cities Community Hospital[2]	Templeton	99%	542
Watsonville Community Hospital[2]	Watsonville	99%	505
West Hills Hospital & Medical Center[2]	West Hills	99%	540
Clovis Community Medical Center[2]	Clovis	98%	442
Feather River Hospital[2]	Paradise	98%	527
French Hospital Medical Center[2]	San Luis Obispo	98%	455
Henry Mayo Newhall Memorial Hospital[2]	Valencia	98%	557
Kaiser Foundation Hospital - South Bay[2]	Harbor City	98%	515
Long Beach Memorial Medical Center[2]	Long Beach	98%	583
Mercy Hospital[2]	Bakersfield	98%	526
Mercy Hospital of Folsom[2]	Folsom	98%	573
Mercy Medical Center - Redding[2]	Redding	98%	516
Montclair Hospital Medical Center[2]	Montclair	98%	382
Novato Community Hospital[2]	Novato	98%	299
Prov Little Co of Mary Med Ctr Torrance[2]	Torrance	98%	543
Saint Francis Memorial Hospital[2]	San Francisco	98%	432
Sharp Chula Vista Medical Center[2]	Chula Vista	98%	656
Sharp Coronado Hosp & Healthcare Ctr[2]	Coronado	98%	461
Silver Lake Medical Center[2]	Los Angeles	98%	612
Stanford Hospital[2]	Stanford	98%	613
Sutter Amador Hospital[2]	Jackson	98%	270
Sutter Solano Medical Center[2]	Vallejo	98%	493
Antelope Valley Hospital[2]	Lancaster	97%	580
Chapman Medical Center[2]	Orange	97%	291
Coastal Communities Hospital[2]	Santa Ana	97%	375
Community Hospital of San Bernardino[2]	San Bernardino	97%	467
Desert Valley Hospital[2]	Victorville	97%	543
Emanuel Medical Center[2]	Turlock	97%	599
Fountain Valley Reg Hosp & Med Ctr[2]	Fountain Valley	97%	546
Garfield Medical Center[2]	Monterey Park	97%	481
Good Samaritan Hospital[2]	San Jose	97%	513
Kaiser Fdn Hosp-Moreno Valley[2]	Moreno Valley	97%	410
Kaiser Fdn Hosp-Panorama City[2]	Panorama City	97%	506
Kaiser Fdn Hosp-San Francisco[2]	San Francisco	97%	505
Kaiser Fdn Hosp-S San Francisco[2]	S San Francisco	97%	547
Marshall Medical Center[2]	Placerville	97%	523
PIH Hospital - Downey[2]	Downey	97%	556
Presbyterian Intercommunity Hospital[2]	Whittier	97%	661
Saint Mary Medical Center[2]	Apple Valley	97%	500
Saint Mary Medical Center[2]	Long Beach	97%	475
Scripps Memorial Hospital La Jolla[2]	La Jolla	97%	497
Sequoia Hospital[2]	Redwood City	97%	486
Sharp Memorial Hospital[2]	San Diego	97%	532
Sonora Regional Medical Center[2]	Sonora	97%	450
Sutter Lakeside Hospital[2]	Lakeport	97%	270
Barton Memorial Hospital[2]	S Lake Tahoe	96%	256
California Hosp Med Ctr Los Angeles[2]	Los Angeles	96%	485
Community Hospital of Long Beach[2]	Long Beach	96%	404
Dameron Hospital[2]	Stockton	96%	480
Glendale Adventist Medical Center[2]	Glendale	96%	516
Good Samaritan Hospital[2]	Los Angeles	96%	450
Kaiser Fdn Hosp-Orange Co-Anaheim[2]	Anaheim	96%	501
Kaiser Fdn Hosp-Woodland Hills[2]	Woodland Hills	96%	514
Lodi Memorial Hospital[2]	Lodi	96%	532
Mercy Medical Center[2]	Merced	96%	465
Mission Hospital Regional Medical Center[2]	Mission Viejo	96%	534
Saint Mary's Medical Center[2]	San Francisco	96%	474
Saint Vincent Medical Center[2]	Los Angeles	96%	593
Shasta Regional Medical Center[2]	Redding	96%	594
Sierra Vista Regional Medical Center[2]	San Luis Obispo	96%	490
Simi Valley Hosp & Health Care Svcs[2]	Simi Valley	96%	504
Sutter Roseville Medical Center[2]	Roseville	96%	524
Valleycare Medical Center[2]	Pleasanton	96%	661
Woodland Memorial Hospital[2]	Woodland	96%	323
Alvarado Hospital Medical Center[2]	San Diego	95%	631
CA Pacific Med Ctr-Davies Campus[2]	San Francisco	95%	327
Cedars - Sinai Medical Center[2]	Los Angeles	95%	519
Kaiser Foundation Hospital - Riverside[2]	Riverside	95%	497

NOTE: Hospital profiles are in alphabetical order by state, then city, then hospital within the city; Rankings exclude hospitals with less than 25 cases except for patient surveys which excludes hospitals with less than 100 cases; (a) 100-299 cases; (1) The number of cases/patients is too few to report; (2) Data submitted were based on a sample of cases/patients; (3) Results are based on a shorter time period than required; (4) Data suppressed by CMS for one or more quarters; (5) Results are not available for this reporting period; (6) Fewer than 100 patients completed the HCAHPS survey; (7) No cases met the criteria for this measure; (8) The lower limit of the confidence interval cannot be calculated if the number of observed infections equals zero; (9) No data are available from the state/territory for this reporting period; (10) The scores shown reflect fewer than 50 completed surveys; (11) There were discrepancies in the data collection process; (12) This measure does not apply to this hospital for this reporting period; (13) Results cannot be calculated for this reporting period; (14) The results for this state are combined with nearby states to protect confidentiality; Please refer to the User's Guide for a full explanation of data.

Kaiser Foundation Hospital - Walnut Creek[2]	Walnut Creek	95%	477
Madera Community Hospital[2]	Madera	95%	817
Menifee Valley Medical Center[2]	Sun City	95%	315
Northridge Hospital Medical Center[2]	Northridge	95%	543
Pacific Hospital of Long Beach[2]	Long Beach	95%	589
Queen of the Valley Medical Center[2]	Napa	95%	570
Riverside Community Hospital[2]	Riverside	95%	551
Saint Bernardine Medical Center[2]	San Bernardino	95%	553
San Dimas Community Hospital[2]	San Dimas	95%	388
Sutter Auburn Faith Hospital[2]	Auburn	95%	404
Torrance Memorial Medical Center[2]	Torrance	95%	697
Alhambra Hospital Medical Center[2]	Alhambra	94%	429
Bakersfield Memorial Hospital[2]	Bakersfield	94%	472
Corona Regional Medical Center[2]	Corona	94%	505
Desert Regional Medical Center[2]	Palm Springs	94%	545
Fallbrook Hospital[2]	Fallbrook	94%	279
Kaiser Foundation Hospital - Fresno[2]	Fresno	94%	519
Kaiser Foundation Hospital - Redwood City[2]	Redwood City	94%	500
Kaiser Foundation Hospital - Roseville[2]	Roseville	94%	469
Kaiser Foundation Hospital - Santa Clara[2]	Santa Clara	94%	504
Kaweah Delta Medical Center[2]	Visalia	94%	513
Los Robles Hospital & Medical Center[2]	Thousand Oaks	94%	591
Mercy San Juan Medical Center[2]	Carmichael	94%	561
Patients' Hospital of Redding	Redding	94%	117
Providence Saint Joseph Medical Center[2]	Burbank	94%	559
Santa Ynez Valley Cottage Hospital	Solvang	94%	112
Scripps Memorial Hospital - Encinitas[2]	Encinitas	94%	507
Scripps Mercy Hospital[2]	San Diego	94%	537
Sierra View District Hospital[2]	Porterville	94%	553
Washington Hospital[2]	Fremont	94%	527
Whittier Hospital Medical Center[2]	Whittier	94%	448
Alameda Hospital[2]	Alameda	93%	289
Bakersfield Heart Hospital[2]	Bakersfield	93%	374
CA Pacific Med Ctr-Pacific Campus Hosp[2]	San Francisco	93%	481
Comm Hosp of the Monterey Peninsula[2]	Monterey	93%	636
Enloe Medical Center[2]	Chico	93%	507
Good Samaritan Hospital[2]	Bakersfield	93%	307
John Muir Medical Center - Concord Campus[2]	Concord	93%	612
Kaiser Foundation Hospital & Rehab Center[2]	Vallejo	93%	481
Kaiser Foundation Hospital - Baldwin Park[2]	Baldwin Park	93%	494
Kaiser Foundation Hospital - Vacaville[2]	Vacaville	93%	383
Marian Regional Medical Center[2]	Santa Maria	93%	488
O'Connor Hospital[2]	San Jose	93%	457
Regional Medical Center of San Jose[2]	San Jose	93%	574
Riverside County Regional Medical Center[2]	Moreno Valley	93%	533
Stanislaus Surgical Hospital[2]	Modesto	93%	304
Arrowhead Regional Medical Center[2]	Colton	92%	593
Hemet Valley Medical Center[2]	Hemet	92%	532
Kaiser Fdn Hosp-Fremont/Hayward[2]	Hayward	92%	497
Kaiser Foundation Hospital - Sacramento[2]	Sacramento	92%	616
Kaiser Foundation Hospital - San Diego[2]	San Diego	92%	493
Kaiser Fdn Hosp S Sacramento[2]	Sacramento	92%	490
Methodist Hospital of Southern California[2]	Arcadia	92%	558
Pomona Valley Hospital Medical Center[2]	Pomona	92%	461
Providence Tarzana Medical Center[2]	Tarzana	92%	479
Saint Francis Medical Center[2]	Lynwood	92%	459
Saint Rose Hospital[2]	Hayward	92%	507
Sonoma Valley Hospital[2]	Sonoma	92%	286
Sutter General Hospital[2]	Sacramento	92%	502
Sutter Surgical Hospital - North Valley	Yuba City	92%	253
Ventura County Medical Center[2]	Ventura	92%	461
Kaiser Foundation Hospital[2]	San Rafael	91%	442
Kaiser Foundation Hospital - Downey[2]	Downey	91%	508
Oak Valley District Hospital[2]	Oakdale	91%	269
Pacific Alliance Medical Center[2]	Los Angeles	91%	448
Paradise Valley Hospital[2]	National City	91%	512
Saddleback Memorial Medical Center[2]	Laguna Hills	91%	520
Saint Joseph's Medical Center of Stockton[2]	Stockton	91%	515
San Gorgonio Memorial Hospital[2]	Banning	91%	294
Sierra Nevada Memorial Hospital[2]	Grass Valley	91%	511
Southwest Healthcare System[2]	Murrieta	91%	493
Tri - City Regional Medical Center[2]	Hawaiian Grdns	91%	305
USC Verdugo Hills Hospital[2]	Glendale	91%	464
Western Medical Center Santa Ana[2]	Santa Ana	91%	1101
Alta Bates Summit Medical Center[2]	Oakland	90%	616
John F Kennedy Memorial Hospital[2]	Indio	90%	493
John Muir Med Ctr-Walnut Creek Campus[2]	Walnut Creek	90%	528
Kaiser Foundation Hospital - Santa Rosa[2]	Santa Rosa	90%	466
Mark Twain Medical Center[2]	San Andreas	90%	298
Northbay Medical Center[2]	Fairfield	90%	542
Prov Little Co of Mary Med Ctr San Pedro[2]	San Pedro	90%	507
Saint Louise Regional Hospital[2]	Gilroy	90%	296
Sutter Medical Center of Santa Rosa[2]	Santa Rosa	90%	499
Univ of CA San Diego Med Ctr[2]	San Diego	90%	527
Western Medical Center Hospital Anaheim[2]	Anaheim	90%	362
Adventist Medical Center[2]	Hanford	89%	1061
Doctors Hospital of Manteca[2]	Manteca	89%	414
Fresno Surgical Hospital[2]	Fresno	89%	346
Glendale Mem Hosp & Health Ctr[2]	Glendale	89%	497
Goleta Valley Cottage Hospital[2]	Santa Barbara	89%	321
Kaiser Fdn Hosp-Oakland/Richmond[2]	Oakland	89%	524
LAC/Olive View - UCLA Medical Center[2]	Sylmar	89%	565
Lakewood Regional Medical Center[2]	Lakewood	89%	623
Loma Linda University Medical Center[2]	Loma Linda	89%	531
Loma Linda Univ Med Ctr-Murrieta[2]	Murrieta	89%	707
Ojai Valley Community Hospital[2]	Ojai	89%	264
Saint Elizabeth Community Hospital[2]	Red Bluff	89%	302
Salinas Valley Memorial Hospital[2]	Salinas	89%	513
Sutter Delta Medical Center[2]	Antioch	89%	520
Alta Bates Summit Medical Center[2]	Berkeley	88%	448
Kaiser Foundation Hospital - Antioch[2]	Antioch	88%	516
Kaiser Foundation Hospital - Fontana[2]	Fontana	88%	510
Kaiser Foundation Hospital - Manteca[2]	Manteca	88%	467
Keck Hospital of USC[2]	Los Angeles	88%	571
LAC/Harbor - UCLA Medical Center[2]	Torrance	88%	558
Marina Del Rey Hospital[2]	Marina Del Rey	88%	434
Redlands Community Hospital[2]	Redlands	88%	472
Saint Agnes Medical Center[2]	Fresno	88%	538
Southern California Hospital at Hollywood[2]	Hollywood	88%	591
Doctors Medical Center - San Pablo[2]	San Pablo	87%	592
Foothill Presbyterian Hospital[2]	Glendora	87%	489
Huntington Memorial Hospital[2]	Pasadena	87%	512
Sutter Maternity & Surgery Ctr[2]	Santa Cruz	87%	190
Tahoe Forest Hospital[2]	Truckee	87%	290
Citrus Valley Medical Center - IC Campus[2]	Covina	86%	484
Kaiser Foundation Hospital - San Jose[2]	San Jose	86%	497
Lompoc Valley Medical Center[2]	Lompoc	86%	256
Marin General Hospital[2]	Greenbrae	86%	544
Monterey Park Hospital[2]	Monterey Park	86%	439
Oroville Hospital[2]	Oroville	86%	509
Parkview Comm Hosp Med Ctr[2]	Riverside	86%	462
Santa Clara Valley Medical Center[2]	San Jose	86%	470
Victor Valley Global Medical Center[2]	Victorville	86%	524
CA Pacific Med Ctr-St Luke's Campus[2]	San Francisco	85%	378
Corcoran District Hospital[2]	Corcoran	85%	189
San Antonio Community Hospital[2]	Upland	85%	545
Univ of California Irvine Med Ctr[2]	Orange	85%	560
College Hospital Costa Mesa[2]	Costa Mesa	84%	308
Dominican Hospital[2]	Santa Cruz	84%	528
Rideout Memorial Hospital[2]	Marysville	84%	506
Saint Joseph Hospital[2]	Eureka	84%	533
Univ of CA Davis Med Ctr[2]	Sacramento	84%	529
Community Regional Medical Center[2]	Fresno	83%	485
Hi - Desert Medical Center[2]	Joshua Tree	83%	287
Laguna Honda Hosp & Rehab Ctr	San Francisco	83%	47
Saint Johns Pleasant Valley Hospital[2]	Camarillo	83%	294
Beverly Hospital[2]	Montebello	82%	537
Eisenhower Medical Center[2]	Rancho Mirage	82%	932
Hoag Memorial Hospital Presbyterian[2]	Newport Beach	82%	860
LAC+USC Medical Center[2]	Los Angeles	82%	513
Orange Coast Memorial Medical Center[2]	Fountain Valley	82%	512
Providence Holy Cross Medical Center[2]	Mission Hills	82%	500
Saint Joseph Hospital[2]	Orange	82%	461
Tri - City Medical Center[2]	Oceanside	82%	505
Adventist Medical Center - Reedley[2]	Reedley	81%	235
Comm Mem Hosp San Buenaventura[2]	Ventura	81%	485
East Valley Hospital Medical Center[2]	Glendora	81%	802
Los Angeles Community Hospital[2]	Los Angeles	81%	549
Santa Monica-UCLA Med Ctr & Ortho Hosp[2]	Santa Monica	81%	539
Hazel Hawkins Memorial Hospital[2]	Hollister	80%	299
Kaiser Foundation Hospital - Los Angeles[2]	Los Angeles	80%	530
Mission Community Hospital[2]	Panorama City	80%	439
Redwood Memorial Hospital[2]	Fortuna	78%	243
Bear Valley Community Hospital	Big Bear Lake	77%	69
Chinese Hospital[2]	San Francisco	77%	281
Kaiser Foundation Hospital - West La[2]	Los Angeles	77%	535
Palmdale Regional Medical Center[2]	Palmdale	77%	614
Pomerado Hospital[2]	Poway	77%	484
Doctors Hospital of West Covina	West Covina	76%	58
Memorial Hospital of Gardena[2]	Gardena	76%	646
Petaluma Valley Hospital[2]	Petaluma	76%	263
Saint Jude Medical Center[2]	Fullerton	75%	511
San Francisco General Hospital[2]	San Francisco	75%	524
Santa Rosa Memorial Hospital[2]	Santa Rosa	75%	527
Eden Medical Center[2]	Castro Valley	74%	857
El Centro Regional Medical Center[2]	El Centro	74%	499
John C Fremont Healthcare District[3]	Mariposa	74%	27
UCSF Medical Center[2]	San Francisco	74%	529
Providence Saint John's Health Center[2]	Santa Monica	73%	515
Ronald Reagan UCLA Medical Center[2]	Los Angeles	73%	509
Santa Barbara Cottage Hospital[2]	Santa Barbara	73%	542
Colusa Regional Medical Center[2]	Colusa	70%	283
San Mateo Medical Center[2]	San Mateo	70%	332
Seton Medical Center[2]	Daly City	70%	531
Ukiah Valley Medical Center[2]	Ukiah	70%	361
Alameda County Medical Center[2]	Oakland	69%	548
Fresno Heart & Surgical Hospital[2]	Fresno	69%	315
San Ramon Regional Medical Center[2]	San Ramon	69%	482
Tulare Regional Medical Center[2]	Tulare	69%	392
Coast Plaza Hospital[2]	Norwalk	68%	305
Delano Regional Medical Center[2]	Delano	68%	287
Greater El Monte Community Hospital[2]	South El Monte	67%	375
Hollywood Presbyterian Medical Center[2]	Los Angeles	67%	542
San Joaquin General Hospital[2]	French Camp	67%	457
Pioneers Memorial Healthcare District[2]	Brawley	65%	460
Palomar Health Downtown Campus[2]	Escondido	63%	504
Valley Presbyterian Hospital[2]	Van Nuys	63%	596
San Gabriel Valley Medical Center[2]	San Gabriel	62%	454
Kern Medical Center[2]	Bakersfield	61%	439
Mad River Community Hospital[2]	Arcata	61%	222
Natividad Medical Center[2]	Salinas	60%	438
Saint Johns Regional Medical Center[2]	Oxnard	60%	491
Coalinga Regional Medical Center[2]	Coalinga	59%	165
White Memorial Medical Center[2]	Los Angeles	57%	530
Central Valley General Hospital[2]	Hanford	56%	243
Saint Helena Hospital[2]	Saint Helena	55%	524
Kern Valley Healthcare District[3]	Lake Isabella	54%	116
Menlo Park Surgical Hospital	Menlo Park	53%	149
George L Mee Memorial Hospital[2]	King City	50%	216
LAC/Rancho Los Amigos Ntl Rehab Ctr[2]	Downey	50%	368
Mercy Medical Center - Mount Shasta[2]	Mount Shasta	48%	256
Contra Costa Regional Medical Center[2]	Martinez	43%	543
East Los Angeles Doctors Hospital[2]	Los Angeles	43%	374
Motion Picture & Television Hospital	Woodland Hills	43%	94
Palo Verde Hospital[2]	Blythe	23%	295
Pacifica Hospital of the Valley[2]	Sun Valley	16%	496

Immunization for Pneumonia

Hospital Name	City	Rate	Cases
Barstow Community Hospital[2]	Barstow	100%	357
Centinela Hospital Medical Center[2]	Inglewood	100%	754
Encino Hospital Medical Center[2]	Encino	100%	455
Garden Grove Hospital & Medical Center[2]	Garden Grove	100%	443
Henry Mayo Newhall Memorial Hospital[2]	Valencia	100%	628
Huntington Beach Hospital[2]	Huntington Bch	100%	413
La Palma Intercommunity Hospital[2]	La Palma	100%	465
Memorial Hospital Los Banos[2]	Los Banos	100%	117
Memorial Medical Center[2]	Modesto	100%	720
Mills - Peninsula Medical Center[2]	Burlingame	100%	648
Sherman Oaks Hospital[2]	Sherman Oaks	100%	499
Sonoma Developmental Center	Eldridge	100%	55
Temple Community Hospital[2]	Los Angeles	100%	419
West Anaheim Medical Center[2]	Anaheim	100%	818
Ahmc Anaheim Regional Medical Center[2]	Anaheim	99%	664
Chino Valley Medical Center[2]	Chino	99%	620
Dameron Hospital[2]	Stockton	99%	542
Desert Valley Hospital[2]	Victorville	99%	735
El Camino Hospital[2]	Mountain View	99%	448
Fallbrook Hospital[2]	Fallbrook	99%	317
French Hospital Medical Center[2]	San Luis Obispo	99%	551
Grossmont Hospital[2]	La Mesa	99%	561
Kaiser Fdn Hosp-S San Francisco[2]	S San Francisco	99%	793
Los Alamitos Medical Center[2]	Los Alamitos	99%	731
Olympia Medical Center[2]	Los Angeles	99%	783
Placentia Linda Hospital[2]	Placentia	99%	550
Scripps Green Hospital[2]	La Jolla	99%	918
Stanford Hospital[2]	Stanford	99%	722
Sutter Coast Hospital[2]	Crescent City	99%	335
Sutter Solano Medical Center[2]	Vallejo	99%	574
Watsonville Community Hospital[2]	Watsonville	99%	433
Kaiser Fdn Hosp-Moreno Valley[2]	Moreno Valley	98%	426
Kaiser Foundation Hospital - Roseville[2]	Roseville	98%	445
Kaiser Fdn Hosp-San Francisco[2]	San Francisco	98%	536
Kaiser Foundation Hospital - South Bay[2]	Harbor City	98%	598
Kaiser Fdn Hosp-Woodland Hills[2]	Woodland Hills	98%	639
Long Beach Memorial Medical Center[2]	Long Beach	98%	721
Mercy General Hospital[2]	Sacramento	98%	706
Mercy Hospital[2]	Bakersfield	98%	471
Montclair Hospital Medical Center[2]	Montclair	98%	342
Novato Community Hospital[2]	Novato	98%	463
PIH Hospital - Downey[2]	Downey	98%	714
Prov Little Co of Mary Med Ctr Torrance[2]	Torrance	98%	595
San Joaquin Community Hospital[2]	Bakersfield	98%	551
Scripps Memorial Hospital - Encinitas[2]	Encinitas	98%	522
Scripps Memorial Hospital La Jolla[2]	La Jolla	98%	440
Shasta Regional Medical Center[2]	Redding	98%	881
Sierra Vista Regional Medical Center[2]	San Luis Obispo	98%	402
Sutter Amador Hospital[2]	Jackson	98%	329
Sutter Lakeside Hospital[2]	Lakeport	98%	292
Sutter Roseville Medical Center[2]	Roseville	98%	539
Sutter Tracy Community Hospital[2]	Tracy	98%	398
Twin Cities Community Hospital[2]	Templeton	98%	611
West Hills Hospital & Medical Center[2]	West Hills	98%	679
Alvarado Hospital Medical Center[2]	San Diego	97%	902
Antelope Valley Hospital[2]	Lancaster	97%	490
Bakersfield Memorial Hospital[2]	Bakersfield	97%	452
Community Hospital of San Bernardino[2]	San Bernardino	97%	387
Fairchild Medical Center[2,3]	Yreka	97%	230
Feather River Hospital[2]	Paradise	97%	604
Kaiser Foundation Hospital - Fresno[2]	Fresno	97%	698
Kaiser Fdn Hosp-Panorama City[2]	Panorama City	97%	602
Kaiser Foundation Hospital - Redwood City[2]	Redwood City	97%	570
Kaweah Delta Medical Center[2]	Visalia	97%	529

NOTE: Hospital profiles are in alphabetical order by state, then city, then hospital within the city; Rankings exclude hospitals with less than 25 cases except for patient surveys which excludes hospitals with less than 100 cases; (a) 100-299 cases; (1) The number of cases/patients is too few to report; (2) Data submitted were based on a sample of cases/patients; (3) Results are based on a shorter time period than required; (4) Data suppressed by CMS for one or more quarters; (5) Results are not available for this reporting period; (6) Fewer than 100 patients completed the HCAHPS survey; (7) No cases met the criteria for this measure; (8) The lower limit of the confidence interval cannot be calculated if the number of observed infections equals zero; (9) No data are available from the state/territory for this reporting period; (10) The scores shown reflect fewer than 50 completed surveys; (11) There were discrepancies in the data collection process; (12) This measure does not apply to this hospital for this reporting period; (13) Results cannot be calculated for this reporting period; (14) The results for this state are combined with nearby states to protect confidentiality; Please refer to the User's Guide for a full explanation of data.

Hospital Name	City	Rate	Cases
Lodi Memorial Hospital[2]	Lodi	97%	652
Madera Community Hospital[2]	Madera	97%	773
Mercy Medical Center[2]	Merced	97%	516
Oak Valley District Hospital[2]	Oakdale	97%	336
Presbyterian Intercommunity Hospital[2]	Whittier	97%	725
Riverside Community Hospital[2]	Riverside	97%	600
Saint Mary Medical Center[2]	Apple Valley	97%	603
Saint Mary's Medical Center[2]	San Francisco	97%	692
Saint Vincent Medical Center[2]	Los Angeles	97%	935
Salinas Valley Memorial Hospital[2]	Salinas	97%	555
San Dimas Community Hospital[2]	San Dimas	97%	440
Sharp Coronado Hosp & Healthcare Ctr[2]	Coronado	97%	538
Silver Lake Medical Center[2]	Los Angeles	97%	735
Sonora Regional Medical Center[2]	Sonora	97%	552
USC Verdugo Hills Hospital[2]	Glendale	97%	583
Whittier Hospital Medical Center[2]	Whittier	97%	376
Alhambra Hospital Medical Center[2]	Alhambra	96%	667
Cedars - Sinai Medical Center[2]	Los Angeles	96%	548
Clovis Community Medical Center[2]	Clovis	96%	384
Community Hospital of Long Beach[2]	Long Beach	96%	415
Desert Regional Medical Center[2]	Palm Springs	96%	559
Emanuel Medical Center[2]	Turlock	96%	693
Fountain Valley Reg Hosp & Med Ctr[2]	Fountain Valley	96%	557
Garfield Medical Center[2]	Monterey Park	96%	453
Good Samaritan Hospital[2]	San Jose	96%	488
Greater El Monte Community Hospital[2]	South El Monte	96%	259
Hi - Desert Medical Center[2]	Joshua Tree	96%	398
Kaiser Foundation Hospital[2]	San Rafael	96%	691
Kaiser Fdn Hosp-Oakland/Richmond[2]	Oakland	96%	590
Kaiser Foundation Hospital - Sacramento[2]	Sacramento	96%	844
Kaiser Foundation Hospital - Vacaville[2]	Vacaville	96%	572
Kaiser Foundation Hospital - Walnut Creek[2]	Walnut Creek	96%	534
Loma Linda Univ Med Ctr-Murrieta[2]	Murrieta	96%	843
Marshall Medical Center[2]	Placerville	96%	673
Methodist Hospital of Sacramento[2]	Sacramento	96%	596
Northridge Hospital Medical Center[2]	Northridge	96%	557
Pomona Valley Hospital Medical Center[2]	Pomona	96%	346
Providence Tarzana Medical Center[2]	Tarzana	96%	558
Queen of the Valley Medical Center[2]	Napa	96%	695
Saint Francis Memorial Hospital[2]	San Francisco	96%	495
Sharp Chula Vista Medical Center[2]	Chula Vista	96%	688
Sierra Nevada Memorial Hospital[2]	Grass Valley	96%	656
Sutter Davis Hospital[2]	Davis	96%	252
Woodland Memorial Hospital[2]	Woodland	96%	301
Barton Memorial Hospital[2]	S Lake Tahoe	95%	236
Beverly Hospital[2]	Montebello	95%	613
Doctors Medical Center[2]	Modesto	95%	511
Glendale Mem Hosp & Health Ctr[2]	Glendale	95%	617
Kaiser Foundation Hospital - Antioch[2]	Antioch	95%	624
Kaiser Foundation Hospital - Baldwin Park[2]	Baldwin Park	95%	552
Kaiser Foundation Hospital - Downey[2]	Downey	95%	497
Kaiser Foundation Hospital - Riverside[2]	Riverside	95%	516
Kaiser Foundation Hospital - San Diego[2]	San Diego	95%	533
Mercy Medical Center - Redding[2]	Redding	95%	605
Northbay Medical Center[2]	Fairfield	95%	641
O'Connor Hospital[2]	San Jose	95%	433
Palm Drive Hospital[2]	Sebastopol	95%	473
Regional Medical Center of San Jose[2]	San Jose	95%	875
Saint Joseph's Medical Center of Stockton[2]	Stockton	95%	641
Santa Ynez Valley Cottage Hospital	Solvang	95%	169
Sequoia Hospital[2]	Redwood City	95%	536
Sharp Memorial Hospital[2]	San Diego	95%	417
Simi Valley Hosp & Health Care Svcs[2]	Simi Valley	95%	555
Stanislaus Surgical Hospital[2]	Modesto	95%	337
Sutter Auburn Faith Hospital[2]	Auburn	95%	606
Alameda Hospital[2]	Alameda	94%	453
Arrowhead Regional Medical Center[2]	Colton	94%	1289
California Hosp Med Ctr Los Angeles[2]	Los Angeles	94%	366
Community Hospital of Huntington Park[2]	Huntington Park	94%	449
Corona Regional Medical Center[2]	Corona	94%	539
Doctors Hospital of Manteca[2]	Manteca	94%	462
Goleta Valley Cottage Hospital[2]	Santa Barbara	94%	382
Hoag Orthopedic Institute[2]	Irvine	94%	575
Kaiser Fdn Hosp-Fremont/Hayward[2]	Hayward	94%	569
Kaiser Foundation Hospital - Santa Clara[2]	Santa Clara	94%	562
Kaiser Fdn Hosp S Sacramento[2]	Sacramento	94%	588
Los Robles Hospital & Medical Center[2]	Thousand Oaks	94%	686
Prov Little Co of Mary Med Ctr San Pedro[2]	San Pedro	94%	562
San Gorgonio Memorial Hospital[2]	Banning	94%	433
Scripps Mercy Hospital[2]	San Diego	94%	615
Sutter General Hospital[2]	Sacramento	94%	473
Torrance Memorial Medical Center[2]	Torrance	94%	829
Victor Valley Global Medical Center[2]	Victorville	94%	423
CA Pacific Med Ctr-St Luke's Campus[2]	San Francisco	93%	360
Chinese Hospital[2]	San Francisco	93%	519
East Valley Hospital Medical Center[2]	Glendora	93%	859
Enloe Medical Center[2]	Chico	93%	646
Good Samaritan Hospital[2]	Los Angeles	93%	430
Kaiser Foundation Hospital & Rehab Center[2]	Vallejo	93%	592
Kaiser Foundation Hospital - Manteca[2]	Manteca	93%	495
Kaiser Foundation Hospital - San Jose[2]	San Jose	93%	597
Kaiser Foundation Hospital - Santa Rosa[2]	Santa Rosa	93%	530
Mercy Hospital of Folsom[2]	Folsom	93%	593
Pacific Alliance Medical Center[2]	Los Angeles	93%	366
Paradise Valley Hospital[2]	National City	93%	658
Providence Saint Joseph Medical Center[2]	Burbank	93%	604
Redlands Community Hospital[2]	Redlands	93%	520
Saint Bernardine Medical Center[2]	San Bernardino	93%	705
Saint Mary Medical Center[2]	Long Beach	93%	439
Sierra View District Hospital[2]	Porterville	93%	528
Valleycare Medical Center[2]	Pleasanton	93%	721
College Hospital Costa Mesa[2]	Costa Mesa	92%	87
Glendale Adventist Medical Center[2]	Glendale	92%	615
Good Samaritan Hospital[2]	Bakersfield	92%	420
John F Kennedy Memorial Hospital[2]	Indio	92%	431
Kaiser Fdn Hosp-Orange Co-Anaheim[2]	Anaheim	92%	508
Laguna Honda Hosp & Rehab Ctr	San Francisco	92%	61
Marian Regional Medical Center[2]	Santa Maria	92%	665
Memorial Hospital of Gardena[2]	Gardena	92%	700
Monterey Park Hospital[2]	Monterey Park	92%	411
Providence Holy Cross Medical Center[2]	Mission Hills	92%	548
Sutter Delta Medical Center[2]	Antioch	92%	636
Univ of CA Davis Med Ctr[2]	Sacramento	92%	507
Bakersfield Heart Hospital[2]	Bakersfield	91%	695
John Muir Medical Center - Concord Campus[2]	Concord	91%	891
Mercy San Juan Medical Center[2]	Carmichael	91%	632
Methodist Hospital of Southern California[2]	Arcadia	91%	713
Mission Hospital Regional Medical Center[2]	Mission Viejo	91%	551
Pacific Hospital of Long Beach[2,3]	Long Beach	91%	368
Patients' Hospital of Redding	Redding	91%	96
Riverside County Regional Medical Center[2]	Moreno Valley	91%	352
San Antonio Community Hospital[2]	Upland	91%	589
Sutter Surgical Hospital - North Valley	Yuba City	91%	316
Chapman Medical Center[2]	Orange	90%	273
Coastal Communities Hospital[2]	Santa Ana	90%	284
Delano Regional Medical Center[2]	Delano	90%	242
Kaiser Foundation Hospital - Fontana[2]	Fontana	90%	508
Saint Francis Medical Center[2]	Lynwood	90%	335
San Gabriel Valley Medical Center[2]	San Gabriel	90%	462
Washington Hospital[2]	Fremont	90%	663
CA Pacific Med Ctr-Davies Campus[2]	San Francisco	89%	328
Foothill Presbyterian Hospital[2]	Glendora	89%	557
Menifee Valley Medical Center[2]	Sun City	89%	494
Redwood Memorial Hospital[2]	Fortuna	89%	251
Saint Johns Pleasant Valley Hospital[2]	Camarillo	89%	443
Saint Louise Regional Hospital[2]	Gilroy	89%	320
Tri - City Regional Medical Center[2]	Hawaiian Grdns	89%	414
CA Pacific Med Ctr-Pacific Campus Hosp[2]	San Francisco	88%	440
Corcoran District Hospital[2,3]	Corcoran	88%	95
Doctors Hospital of West Covina	West Covina	88%	49
Doctors Medical Center - San Pablo[2]	San Pablo	88%	905
El Centro Regional Medical Center[2]	El Centro	88%	546
John Muir Med Ctr-Walnut Creek Campus[2]	Walnut Creek	88%	568
Kaiser Foundation Hospital - Los Angeles[2]	Los Angeles	88%	552
Mark Twain Medical Center[2]	San Andreas	88%	482
Saddleback Memorial Medical Center[2]	Laguna Hills	88%	648
Saint Agnes Medical Center[2]	Fresno	88%	690
Saint Rose Hospital[2]	Hayward	88%	659
Sonoma Valley Hospital[2]	Sonoma	88%	348
Southwest Healthcare System[2]	Murrieta	88%	504
Sutter Maternity & Surgery Ctr[2]	Santa Cruz	88%	78
Sutter Medical Center of Santa Rosa[2]	Santa Rosa	88%	474
Western Medical Center Hospital Anaheim[2]	Anaheim	88%	200
Comm Hosp of the Monterey Peninsula[2]	Monterey	87%	756
Kaiser Foundation Hospital - West La[2]	Los Angeles	87%	612
Orange Coast Memorial Medical Center[2]	Fountain Valley	87%	575
Saint Joseph Hospital[2]	Eureka	87%	686
Santa Monica-UCLA Med Ctr & Ortho Hosp[2]	Santa Monica	87%	604
Southern California Hospital at Hollywood[2]	Hollywood	87%	983
Western Medical Center Santa Ana[2]	Santa Ana	87%	832
Adventist Medical Center[2]	Hanford	86%	1306
LAC+USC Medical Center[2]	Los Angeles	86%	288
LAC/Harbor - UCLA Medical Center[2]	Torrance	86%	428
Lakewood Regional Medical Center[2]	Lakewood	86%	919
Lompoc Valley Medical Center[2]	Lompoc	86%	250
Marina Del Rey Hospital[2]	Marina Del Rey	86%	526
Ojai Valley Community Hospital[2]	Ojai	86%	403
Fresno Surgical Hospital[2]	Fresno	85%	445
Hemet Valley Medical Center[2]	Hemet	85%	703
John C Fremont Healthcare District[3]	Mariposa	85%	78
Rideout Memorial Hospital[2]	Marysville	85%	844
Saint Elizabeth Community Hospital[2]	Red Bluff	85%	335
Saint Johns Regional Medical Center[2]	Oxnard	85%	485
Tahoe Forest Hospital[2]	Truckee	85%	225
Tri - City Medical Center[2]	Oceanside	85%	545
Citrus Valley Medical Center - IC Campus[2]	Covina	84%	503
Community Regional Medical Center[2]	Fresno	84%	493
Loma Linda University Medical Center[2]	Loma Linda	84%	406
Marin General Hospital[2]	Greenbrae	84%	626
Natividad Medical Center[2]	Salinas	84%	262
Petaluma Valley Hospital[2]	Petaluma	84%	291
Saint Joseph Hospital[2]	Orange	84%	444
Saint Jude Medical Center[2]	Fullerton	84%	689
LAC/Olive View - UCLA Medical Center[2]	Sylmar	83%	501
Mad River Community Hospital[2]	Arcata	83%	193
Oroville Hospital[2]	Oroville	83%	978
San Leandro Hospital[2,3]	San Leandro	83%	242
Univ of California Irvine Med Ctr[2]	Orange	83%	478
Comm Mem Hosp San Buenaventura[2]	Ventura	82%	532
Huntington Memorial Hospital[2]	Pasadena	82%	541
Keck Hospital of USC[2]	Los Angeles	82%	675
Los Angeles Community Hospital[2]	Los Angeles	82%	720
Santa Rosa Memorial Hospital[2]	Santa Rosa	82%	605
Tulare Regional Medical Center[2]	Tulare	82%	316
Univ of CA San Diego Med Ctr[2]	San Diego	82%	535
Eisenhower Medical Center[2]	Rancho Mirage	81%	1308
Hazel Hawkins Memorial Hospital[2]	Hollister	81%	399
Hollywood Presbyterian Medical Center[2]	Los Angeles	81%	467
Pomerado Hospital[2]	Poway	81%	530
San Joaquin General Hospital[2]	French Camp	80%	367
Eden Medical Center[2]	Castro Valley	79%	894
Hoag Memorial Hospital Presbyterian[2]	Newport Beach	79%	732
San Francisco General Hospital[2]	San Francisco	79%	476
San Ramon Regional Medical Center[2]	San Ramon	79%	451
Seton Medical Center[2]	Daly City	79%	785
Alta Bates Summit Medical Center[2]	Berkeley	78%	326
Dominican Hospital[2]	Santa Cruz	78%	628
Mission Community Hospital[2]	Panorama City	78%	689
Palomar Health Downtown Campus[2]	Escondido	78%	542
Santa Barbara Cottage Hospital[2]	Santa Barbara	78%	535
Colusa Regional Medical Center[2]	Colusa	77%	278
Pioneers Memorial Healthcare District[2]	Brawley	77%	364
UCSF Medical Center[2]	San Francisco	77%	408
Ukiah Valley Medical Center[2]	Ukiah	76%	402
Menlo Park Surgical Hospital	Menlo Park	75%	93
Parkview Comm Hosp Med Ctr[2]	Riverside	75%	461
Ronald Reagan UCLA Medical Center[2]	Los Angeles	75%	457
Valley Presbyterian Hospital[2]	Van Nuys	75%	457
White Memorial Medical Center[2]	Los Angeles	74%	638
Providence Saint John's Health Center[2]	Santa Monica	73%	608
San Mateo Medical Center[2]	San Mateo	73%	290
Adventist Medical Center - Reedley[2]	Reedley	72%	130
Alameda County Medical Center[2]	Oakland	72%	408
Alta Bates Summit Medical Center[2]	Oakland	72%	952
Mercy Medical Center - Mount Shasta[2]	Mount Shasta	72%	249
Palmdale Regional Medical Center[2]	Palmdale	72%	820
East Los Angeles Doctors Hospital[2]	Los Angeles	70%	322
Kern Valley Healthcare District[3]	Lake Isabella	70%	344
Santa Clara Valley Medical Center[2]	San Jose	70%	411
Ventura County Medical Center[2]	Ventura	69%	384
Coalinga Regional Medical Center[2]	Coalinga	68%	203
Coast Plaza Hospital[2]	Norwalk	65%	353
Bear Valley Community Hospital	Big Bear Lake	63%	95
Fresno Heart & Surgical Hospital[2]	Fresno	63%	409
Contra Costa Regional Medical Center[2]	Martinez	62%	462
George L Mee Memorial Hospital[2]	King City	60%	128
Saint Helena Hospital[2]	Saint Helena	59%	604
Kern Medical Center[2]	Bakersfield	56%	213
Motion Picture & Television Hospital	Woodland Hills	54%	116
LAC/Rancho Los Amigos Ntl Rehab Ctr[2]	Downey	52%	364
Palo Verde Hospital[2]	Blythe	31%	346
Pacifica Hospital of the Valley[2]	Sun Valley	13%	419

Stroke Care

Anticoagulation Therapy for Atrial Fibrillation

Hospital Name	City	Rate	Cases
CA Pacific Med Ctr-Davies Campus	San Francisco	100%	47
CA Pacific Med Ctr-Pacific Campus Hosp	San Francisco	100%	30
Comm Hosp of the Monterey Peninsula	Monterey	100%	27
Eden Medical Center	Castro Valley	100%	31
Eisenhower Medical Center	Rancho Mirage	100%	46
Glendale Adventist Medical Center	Glendale	100%	29
Grossmont Hospital	La Mesa	100%	41
Kaiser Foundation Hospital[2]	San Rafael	100%	26
Methodist Hospital of Southern California	Arcadia	100%	26
Mills - Peninsula Medical Center	Burlingame	100%	45
Presbyterian Intercommunity Hospital[2]	Whittier	100%	28
Providence Saint Joseph Medical Center	Burbank	100%	41
Saint Joseph Hospital	Orange	100%	35
San Antonio Community Hospital	Upland	100%	26
Scripps Memorial Hospital La Jolla	La Jolla	100%	27
Scripps Mercy Hospital	San Diego	100%	50
Torrance Memorial Medical Center	Torrance	100%	36
Tri - City Medical Center	Oceanside	100%	38
Univ of California Irvine Med Ctr	Orange	100%	30
Univ of CA San Diego Med Ctr	San Diego	100%	26
John Muir Med Ctr-Walnut Creek Campus	Walnut Creek	98%	43
Mercy San Juan Medical Center	Carmichael	98%	41
Saint Jude Medical Center	Fullerton	98%	40
Stanford Hospital	Stanford	98%	46
Desert Regional Medical Center	Palm Springs	97%	37

NOTE: Hospital profiles are in alphabetical order by state, then city, then hospital within the city; Rankings exclude hospitals with less than 25 cases except for patient surveys which excludes hospitals with less than 100 cases; (a) 100-299 cases; (1) The number of cases/patients is too few to report; (2) Data submitted were based on a sample of cases/patients; (3) Results are based on a shorter time period than required; (4) Data suppressed by CMS for one or more quarters; (5) Results are not available for this reporting period; (6) Fewer than 100 patients completed the HCAHPS survey; (7) No cases met the criteria for this measure; (8) The lower limit of the confidence interval cannot be calculated if the number of observed infections equals zero; (9) No data are available from the state/territory for this reporting period; (10) The scores shown reflect fewer than 50 completed surveys; (11) There were discrepancies in the data collection process; (12) This measure does not apply to this hospital for this reporting period; (13) Results cannot be calculated for this reporting period; (14) The results for this state are combined with nearby states to protect confidentiality; Please refer to the User's Guide for a full explanation of data.

Hospital Name	City	Rate	Cases
Enloe Medical Center	Chico	97%	36
Providence Holy Cross Medical Center	Mission Hills	97%	30
Sharp Memorial Hospital	San Diego	97%	35
Washington Hospital	Fremont	97%	30
Cedars - Sinai Medical Center	Los Angeles	96%	49
Hoag Memorial Hospital Presbyterian	Newport Beach	96%	67
Kaiser Foundation Hospital - Walnut Creek[2]	Walnut Creek	96%	26
Santa Barbara Cottage Hospital	Santa Barbara	96%	50
Huntington Memorial Hospital	Pasadena	94%	33
Mission Hospital Regional Medical Center	Mission Viejo	94%	33
Saddleback Memorial Medical Center	Laguna Hills	94%	34
Northridge Hospital Medical Center	Northridge	93%	27
Sutter Roseville Medical Center	Roseville	93%	27
Community Regional Medical Center[2]	Fresno	92%	39
Sharp Chula Vista Medical Center	Chula Vista	90%	29
Saint Agnes Medical Center[2]	Fresno	88%	25
Hemet Valley Medical Center[2]	Hemet	85%	26
Comm Mem Hosp San Buenaventura	Ventura	82%	38
Prov Little Co of Mary Med Ctr Torrance	Torrance	80%	25

Antithrombotic Therapy Timing

Hospital Name	City	Rate	Cases
CA Pacific Med Ctr-Davies Campus	San Francisco	100%	71
CA Pacific Med Ctr-Pacific Campus Hosp	San Francisco	100%	98
Cedars - Sinai Medical Center	Los Angeles	100%	269
Centinela Hospital Medical Center[2]	Inglewood	100%	93
Comm Hosp of the Monterey Peninsula	Monterey	100%	111
Contra Costa Regional Medical Center	Martinez	100%	42
Corona Regional Medical Center	Corona	100%	39
Dameron Hospital	Stockton	100%	57
Desert Valley Hospital	Victorville	100%	85
Eden Medical Center	Castro Valley	100%	143
El Camino Hospital	Mountain View	100%	97
Emanuel Medical Center	Turlock	100%	49
Feather River Hospital	Paradise	100%	59
Foothill Presbyterian Hospital	Glendora	100%	34
French Hospital Medical Center	San Luis Obispo	100%	35
Garden Grove Hospital & Medical Center	Garden Grove	100%	25
Glendale Adventist Medical Center	Glendale	100%	133
Good Samaritan Hospital[2]	San Jose	100%	78
Hoag Memorial Hospital Presbyterian	Newport Beach	100%	256
Hollywood Presbyterian Medical Center	Los Angeles	100%	83
Kaiser Foundation Hospital - Antioch[2]	Antioch	100%	64
Kaiser Foundation Hospital - Baldwin Park[2]	Baldwin Park	100%	94
Kaiser Foundation Hospital - Downey[2]	Downey	100%	92
Kaiser Foundation Hospital - Fontana[2]	Fontana	100%	58
Kaiser Foundation Hospital - Los Angeles[2]	Los Angeles	100%	40
Kaiser Foundation Hospital - Manteca[2]	Manteca	100%	54
Kaiser Foundation Hospital - Redwood City[2]	Redwood City	100%	43
Kaiser Foundation Hospital - Sacramento[2]	Sacramento	100%	44
Kaiser Foundation Hospital - San Diego[2]	San Diego	100%	66
Kaiser Foundation Hospital - San Jose[2]	San Jose	100%	77
Kaiser Foundation Hospital - Santa Clara[2]	Santa Clara	100%	75
Kaiser Fdn Hosp-S San Francisco[2]	S San Francisco	100%	76
Kaiser Foundation Hospital - Vacaville	Vacaville	100%	54
Kaiser Foundation Hospital - Walnut Creek[2]	Walnut Creek	100%	87
Kaiser Fdn Hosp S Sacramento[2]	Sacramento	100%	72
Keck Hospital of USC[2]	Los Angeles	100%	42
LAC/Harbor - UCLA Medical Center[2]	Torrance	100%	97
Lodi Memorial Hospital	Lodi	100%	38
Loma Linda Univ Med Ctr-Murrieta	Murrieta	100%	46
Los Alamitos Medical Center	Los Alamitos	100%	88
Marin General Hospital	Greenbrae	100%	95
Marshall Medical Center	Placerville	100%	64
Memorial Hospital of Gardena	Gardena	100%	32
Memorial Medical Center	Modesto	100%	147
Mercy Hospital	Bakersfield	100%	97
Mercy Hospital of Folsom	Folsom	100%	35
Mercy San Juan Medical Center	Carmichael	100%	227
Methodist Hospital of Sacramento	Sacramento	100%	136
Methodist Hospital of Southern California	Arcadia	100%	179
Northridge Hospital Medical Center	Northridge	100%	119
Orange Coast Memorial Medical Center	Fountain Valley	100%	47
Oroville Hospital[2]	Oroville	100%	60
Parkview Comm Hosp Med Ctr	Riverside	100%	71
Placentia Linda Hospital	Placentia	100%	25
Redlands Community Hospital	Redlands	100%	105
Regional Medical Center of San Jose[2]	San Jose	100%	88
Riverside County Regional Medical Center	Moreno Valley	100%	103
Saint Francis Memorial Hospital	San Francisco	100%	56
Saint Johns Regional Medical Center	Oxnard	100%	88
Saint Joseph Hospital	Eureka	100%	55
Saint Joseph Hospital	Orange	100%	129
Saint Mary Medical Center	Apple Valley	100%	142
Saint Mary's Medical Center	San Francisco	100%	53
Salinas Valley Memorial Hospital[2]	Salinas	100%	112
San Francisco General Hospital[2]	San Francisco	100%	56
San Gabriel Valley Medical Center	San Gabriel	100%	38
San Gorgonio Memorial Hospital	Banning	100%	27
San Ramon Regional Medical Center	San Ramon	100%	42
Santa Monica-UCLA Med Ctr & Ortho Hosp	Santa Monica	100%	62
Scripps Green Hospital	La Jolla	100%	36
Scripps Memorial Hospital La Jolla	La Jolla	100%	100
Sequoia Hospital	Redwood City	100%	45
Shasta Regional Medical Center	Redding	100%	76
Sierra Nevada Memorial Hospital	Grass Valley	100%	49
Sonora Regional Medical Center	Sonora	100%	55
Sutter Amador Hospital	Jackson	100%	28
Sutter Auburn Faith Hospital	Auburn	100%	46
Sutter Coast Hospital	Crescent City	100%	30
Sutter General Hospital	Sacramento	100%	207
Sutter Lakeside Hospital	Lakeport	100%	25
Sutter Medical Center of Santa Rosa	Santa Rosa	100%	36
Temple Community Hospital	Los Angeles	100%	52
Twin Cities Community Hospital	Templeton	100%	54
Univ of CA San Diego Med Ctr	San Diego	100%	129
Ventura County Medical Center	Ventura	100%	35
Watsonville Community Hospital	Watsonville	100%	45
Alameda County Medical Center	Oakland	99%	69
Arrowhead Regional Medical Center	Colton	99%	163
Bakersfield Memorial Hospital	Bakersfield	99%	127
California Hosp Med Ctr Los Angeles	Los Angeles	99%	124
Citrus Valley Medical Center - IC Campus	Covina	99%	184
Clovis Community Medical Center[2]	Clovis	99%	75
Dominican Hospital	Santa Cruz	99%	75
Eisenhower Medical Center	Rancho Mirage	99%	295
Fountain Valley Reg Hosp & Med Ctr	Fountain Valley	99%	170
Kaiser Foundation Hospital[2]	San Rafael	99%	77
Kaiser Foundation Hospital - Fresno[2]	Fresno	99%	78
Kaiser Fdn Hosp-Panorama City[2]	Panorama City	99%	84
Kaiser Foundation Hospital - Riverside[2]	Riverside	99%	69
Kaiser Foundation Hospital - South Bay[2]	Harbor City	99%	80
Kaiser Foundation Hospital - West La[2]	Los Angeles	99%	88
Kaiser Fdn Hosp-Woodland Hills[2]	Woodland Hills	99%	73
Kaweah Delta Medical Center[2]	Visalia	99%	74
Los Robles Hospital & Medical Center[2]	Thousand Oaks	99%	70
Mercy General Hospital	Sacramento	99%	149
Mercy Medical Center - Redding	Redding	99%	99
Mills - Peninsula Medical Center	Burlingame	99%	123
Northbay Medical Center	Fairfield	99%	90
O'Connor Hospital[2]	San Jose	99%	67
Palomar Health Downtown Campus[2]	Escondido	99%	70
PIH Hospital - Downey	Downey	99%	82
Presbyterian Intercommunity Hospital[2]	Whittier	99%	140
Providence Saint Joseph Medical Center	Burbank	99%	178
Saint Bernardine Medical Center	San Bernardino	99%	82
San Joaquin Community Hospital[2]	Bakersfield	99%	77
Scripps Memorial Hospital - Encinitas	Encinitas	99%	88
Scripps Mercy Hospital	San Diego	99%	265
Seton Medical Center[2]	Daly City	99%	69
Torrance Memorial Medical Center	Torrance	99%	183
Tri - City Medical Center	Oceanside	99%	108
West Hills Hospital & Medical Center[2]	West Hills	99%	73
White Memorial Medical Center	Los Angeles	99%	134
Alta Bates Summit Medical Center	Oakland	98%	164
Barstow Community Hospital	Barstow	98%	41
Desert Regional Medical Center	Palm Springs	98%	168
Doctors Medical Center	Modesto	98%	184
Doctors Medical Center - San Pablo	San Pablo	98%	99
Garfield Medical Center	Monterey Park	98%	124
John Muir Medical Center - Concord Campus	Concord	98%	83
John Muir Med Ctr-Walnut Creek Campus	Walnut Creek	98%	128
Kaiser Foundation Hospital & Rehab Center[2]	Vallejo	98%	96
Kaiser Fdn Hosp-Moreno Valley	Moreno Valley	98%	50
Kaiser Fdn Hosp-Orange Co-Anaheim[2]	Anaheim	98%	61
LAC/Olive View - UCLA Medical Center	Sylmar	98%	64
Marian Regional Medical Center	Santa Maria	98%	91
Pomerado Hospital[2]	Poway	98%	61
Pomona Valley Hospital Medical Center[2]	Pomona	98%	102
Prov Little Co of Mary Med Ctr San Pedro	San Pedro	98%	47
Prov Little Co of Mary Med Ctr Torrance	Torrance	98%	162
Providence Saint John's Health Center	Santa Monica	98%	54
Ronald Reagan UCLA Medical Center[2]	Los Angeles	98%	45
Saddleback Memorial Medical Center	Laguna Hills	98%	161
Saint Johns Pleasant Valley Hospital	Camarillo	98%	46
Saint Jude Medical Center	Fullerton	98%	168
Saint Mary Medical Center	Long Beach	98%	62
San Antonio Community Hospital	Upland	98%	123
San Joaquin General Hospital	French Camp	98%	59
Sharp Memorial Hospital	San Diego	98%	191
Sierra View District Hospital	Porterville	98%	57
Simi Valley Hosp & Health Care Svcs	Simi Valley	98%	48
Southern California Hospital at Hollywood	Hollywood	98%	42
Sutter Solano Medical Center	Vallejo	98%	62
UCSF Medical Center[2]	San Francisco	98%	46
Valleycare Medical Center	Pleasanton	98%	48
Alhambra Hospital Medical Center	Alhambra	97%	35
Alta Bates Summit Medical Center	Berkeley	97%	118
Community Regional Medical Center[2]	Fresno	97%	314
Doctors Hospital of Manteca	Manteca	97%	30
Enloe Medical Center	Chico	97%	155
Grossmont Hospital	La Mesa	97%	319
Hemet Valley Medical Center[2]	Hemet	97%	88
Henry Mayo Newhall Memorial Hospital	Valencia	97%	112
Kaiser Foundation Hospital - Roseville[2]	Roseville	97%	75
Kaiser Fdn Hosp-San Francisco[2]	San Francisco	97%	77
Mercy Medical Center	Merced	97%	107
Olympia Medical Center	Los Angeles	97%	32
Saint Vincent Medical Center	Los Angeles	97%	66
Sharp Chula Vista Medical Center	Chula Vista	97%	161
Sierra Vista Regional Medical Center	San Luis Obispo	97%	30
Southwest Healthcare System[2]	Murrieta	97%	103
Sutter Delta Medical Center	Antioch	97%	58
Sutter Roseville Medical Center	Roseville	97%	172
Valley Presbyterian Hospital	Van Nuys	97%	86
Whittier Hospital Medical Center	Whittier	97%	34
Antelope Valley Hospital	Lancaster	96%	142
Glendale Mem Hosp & Health Ctr	Glendale	96%	52
Good Samaritan Hospital[2]	Los Angeles	96%	79
Kaiser Fdn Hosp-Fremont/Hayward[2]	Hayward	96%	70
Kaiser Fdn Hosp-Oakland/Richmond[2]	Oakland	96%	94
Loma Linda University Medical Center[2]	Loma Linda	96%	134
Long Beach Memorial Medical Center[2]	Long Beach	96%	71
Menifee Valley Medical Center	Sun City	96%	52
Mission Community Hospital	Panorama City	96%	27
Mission Hospital Regional Medical Center	Mission Viejo	96%	139
Pioneers Memorial Healthcare District	Brawley	96%	45
Saint Agnes Medical Center[2]	Fresno	96%	121
Santa Barbara Cottage Hospital	Santa Barbara	96%	197
Stanford Hospital	Stanford	96%	119
El Centro Regional Medical Center[2]	El Centro	95%	94
LAC/Rancho Los Amigos Ntl Rehab Ctr[2]	Downey	95%	87
Lakewood Regional Medical Center	Lakewood	95%	146
Rideout Memorial Hospital	Marysville	95%	129
Riverside Community Hospital[2]	Riverside	95%	84
Saint Francis Medical Center[2]	Lynwood	95%	76
Saint Joseph's Medical Center of Stockton[2]	Stockton	95%	94
Santa Rosa Memorial Hospital[2]	Santa Rosa	95%	87
Ukiah Valley Medical Center	Ukiah	95%	38
Univ of CA Davis Med Ctr[2]	Sacramento	95%	64
Ahmc Anaheim Regional Medical Center	Anaheim	94%	85
Bakersfield Heart Hospital	Bakersfield	94%	36
Chinese Hospital	San Francisco	94%	36
Huntington Memorial Hospital	Pasadena	94%	189
LAC+USC Medical Center[2]	Los Angeles	94%	50
Providence Holy Cross Medical Center	Mission Hills	94%	139
Providence Tarzana Medical Center	Tarzana	94%	81
Univ of California Irvine Med Ctr	Orange	94%	138
Washington Hospital	Fremont	94%	127
West Anaheim Medical Center	Anaheim	94%	35
USC Verdugo Hills Hospital	Glendale	93%	41
Adventist Medical Center	Hanford	92%	80
Alvarado Hospital Medical Center	San Diego	92%	51
Comm Mem Hosp San Buenaventura	Ventura	92%	92
Kaiser Foundation Hospital - Santa Rosa[2]	Santa Rosa	92%	53
Palmdale Regional Medical Center	Palmdale	92%	62
Santa Clara Valley Medical Center[2]	San Jose	92%	77
Western Medical Center Santa Ana	Santa Ana	92%	77
Alameda Hospital	Alameda	91%	34
Queen of the Valley Medical Center	Napa	91%	45
Paradise Valley Hospital	National City	89%	44
Saint Louise Regional Hospital[2]	Gilroy	87%	31
Pacific Alliance Medical Center	Los Angeles	85%	48
Beverly Hospital	Montebello	84%	86
La Palma Intercommunity Hospital	La Palma	83%	29
Hi - Desert Medical Center	Joshua Tree	80%	25
Tulare Regional Medical Center	Tulare	80%	25
Victor Valley Global Medical Center	Victorville	80%	46
Los Angeles Community Hospital	Los Angeles	70%	30

Assessed for Rehabilitation

Hospital Name	City	Rate	Cases
Alhambra Hospital Medical Center	Alhambra	100%	45
Barstow Community Hospital	Barstow	100%	42
CA Pacific Med Ctr-Davies Campus	San Francisco	100%	213
CA Pacific Med Ctr-Pacific Campus Hosp	San Francisco	100%	169
Cedars - Sinai Medical Center	Los Angeles	100%	438
Community Regional Medical Center[2]	Fresno	100%	423
Dameron Hospital	Stockton	100%	61
Desert Valley Hospital	Victorville	100%	94
Dominican Hospital	Santa Cruz	100%	112
Eden Medical Center	Castro Valley	100%	261
French Hospital Medical Center	San Luis Obispo	100%	36
Garden Grove Hospital & Medical Center	Garden Grove	100%	34
Garfield Medical Center	Monterey Park	100%	193
Glendale Adventist Medical Center	Glendale	100%	197
Good Samaritan Hospital[2]	San Jose	100%	120
Grossmont Hospital	La Mesa	100%	402
Hoag Memorial Hospital Presbyterian	Newport Beach	100%	372
Hollywood Presbyterian Medical Center	Los Angeles	100%	112
Kaiser Foundation Hospital[2]	San Rafael	100%	105
Kaiser Foundation Hospital & Rehab Center[2]	Vallejo	100%	120
Kaiser Foundation Hospital - Antioch[2]	Antioch	100%	101

NOTE: Hospital profiles are in alphabetical order by state, then city, then hospital within the city; Rankings exclude hospitals with less than 25 cases except for patient surveys which excludes hospitals with less than 100 cases; (a) 100-299 cases; (1) The number of cases/patients is too few to report; (2) Data submitted were based on a sample of cases/patients; (3) Results are based on a shorter time period than required; (4) Data suppressed by CMS for one or more quarters; (5) Results are not available for this reporting period; (6) Fewer than 100 patients completed the HCAHPS survey; (7) No cases met the criteria for this measure; (8) The lower limit of the confidence interval cannot be calculated if the number of observed infections equals zero; (9) No data are available from the state/territory for this reporting period; (10) The scores shown reflect fewer than 50 completed surveys; (11) There were discrepancies in the data collection process; (12) This measure does not apply to this hospital for this reporting period; (13) Results cannot be calculated for this reporting period; (14) The results for this state are combined with nearby states to protect confidentiality; Please refer to the User's Guide for a full explanation of data.

Hospital Name	City	Rate	Cases
Kaiser Foundation Hospital - Baldwin Park[2]	Baldwin Park	100%	113
Kaiser Fdn Hosp-Orange Co-Anaheim[2]	Anaheim	100%	105
Kaiser Fdn Hosp-Panorama City[2]	Panorama City	100%	98
Kaiser Foundation Hospital - Redwood City[2]	Redwood City	100%	111
Kaiser Foundation Hospital - South Bay[2]	Harbor City	100%	93
Kaiser Fdn Hosp-S San Francisco[2]	S San Francisco	100%	83
Kaiser Foundation Hospital - Vacaville	Vacaville	100%	65
Kaiser Fdn Hosp-Woodland Hills[2]	Woodland Hills	100%	90
Kaiser Fdn Hosp S Sacramento[2]	Sacramento	100%	124
Lodi Memorial Hospital	Lodi	100%	41
Marin General Hospital	Greenbrae	100%	98
Marshall Medical Center	Placerville	100%	72
Memorial Medical Center	Modesto	100%	205
Mercy Hospital	Bakersfield	100%	120
Mercy Hospital of Folsom	Folsom	100%	43
Methodist Hospital of Southern California	Arcadia	100%	224
Mills - Peninsula Medical Center	Burlingame	100%	162
O'Connor Hospital[2]	San Jose	100%	83
Oroville Hospital[2]	Oroville	100%	61
Palmdale Regional Medical Center	Palmdale	100%	72
Placentia Linda Hospital	Placentia	100%	32
Pomerado Hospital[2]	Poway	100%	59
Pomona Valley Hospital Medical Center[2]	Pomona	100%	146
Saint Johns Regional Medical Center	Oxnard	100%	118
Saint Joseph Hospital	Orange	100%	195
Saint Jude Medical Center	Fullerton	100%	252
Saint Mary Medical Center	Long Beach	100%	83
Saint Mary's Medical Center	San Francisco	100%	59
Salinas Valley Memorial Hospital[2]	Salinas	100%	120
San Gabriel Valley Medical Center	San Gabriel	100%	49
San Joaquin General Hospital	French Camp	100%	92
San Ramon Regional Medical Center	San Ramon	100%	67
Scripps Green Hospital	La Jolla	100%	114
Scripps Memorial Hospital - Encinitas	Encinitas	100%	131
Scripps Memorial Hospital La Jolla	La Jolla	100%	165
Scripps Mercy Hospital	San Diego	100%	325
Shasta Regional Medical Center	Redding	100%	93
Sierra Nevada Memorial Hospital	Grass Valley	100%	51
Sonora Regional Medical Center	Sonora	100%	59
Sutter Auburn Faith Hospital	Auburn	100%	61
Sutter Coast Hospital	Crescent City	100%	38
Sutter Davis Hospital	Davis	100%	27
Sutter Lakeside Hospital	Lakeport	100%	26
Sutter Medical Center of Santa Rosa	Santa Rosa	100%	43
Sutter Solano Medical Center	Vallejo	100%	57
Temple Community Hospital	Los Angeles	100%	60
Tri - City Medical Center	Oceanside	100%	209
Univ of CA Davis Med Ctr[2]	Sacramento	100%	96
Ventura County Medical Center	Ventura	100%	49
Washington Hospital	Fremont	100%	164
Alta Bates Summit Medical Center	Oakland	99%	177
Antelope Valley Hospital	Lancaster	99%	185
Comm Hosp of the Monterey Peninsula	Monterey	99%	148
Doctors Medical Center - San Pablo	San Pablo	99%	105
El Camino Hospital	Mountain View	99%	152
Fountain Valley Reg Hosp & Med Ctr	Fountain Valley	99%	214
Huntington Memorial Hospital	Pasadena	99%	239
John Muir Medical Center - Concord Campus	Concord	99%	125
John Muir Med Ctr-Walnut Creek Campus	Walnut Creek	99%	253
Kaiser Foundation Hospital - Fresno[2]	Fresno	99%	108
Kaiser Foundation Hospital - Roseville[2]	Roseville	99%	124
Kaiser Foundation Hospital - San Diego[2]	San Diego	99%	120
Kaiser Fdn Hosp-San Francisco[2]	San Francisco	99%	109
Kaiser Foundation Hospital - San Jose[2]	San Jose	99%	121
Kaiser Foundation Hospital - Santa Clara[2]	Santa Clara	99%	134
Kaiser Foundation Hospital - Santa Rosa[2]	Santa Rosa	99%	85
Los Alamitos Medical Center	Los Alamitos	99%	141
Los Robles Hospital & Medical Center[2]	Thousand Oaks	99%	86
Mercy Medical Center	Merced	99%	106
Mercy Medical Center - Redding	Redding	99%	152
Mercy San Juan Medical Center	Carmichael	99%	378
Methodist Hospital of Sacramento	Sacramento	99%	144
Mission Hospital Regional Medical Center	Mission Viejo	99%	218
Palomar Health Downtown Campus[2]	Escondido	99%	98
Presbyterian Intercommunity Hospital[2]	Whittier	99%	197
Providence Saint Joseph Medical Center	Burbank	99%	250
Redlands Community Hospital	Redlands	99%	119
Regional Medical Center of San Jose[2]	San Jose	99%	118
Riverside County Regional Medical Center	Moreno Valley	99%	119
San Antonio Community Hospital	Upland	99%	199
Santa Monica-UCLA Med Ctr & Ortho Hosp	Santa Monica	99%	70
Seton Medical Center[2]	Daly City	99%	91
Sharp Chula Vista Medical Center	Chula Vista	99%	193
Sharp Memorial Hospital	San Diego	99%	296
Sutter Roseville Medical Center	Roseville	99%	198
Torrance Memorial Medical Center	Torrance	99%	265
Univ of CA San Diego Med Ctr	San Diego	99%	188
White Memorial Medical Center	Los Angeles	99%	187
Alameda Hospital	Alameda	98%	44
Alta Bates Summit Medical Center	Berkeley	98%	190
Alvarado Hospital Medical Center	San Diego	98%	63
California Hosp Med Ctr Los Angeles	Los Angeles	98%	149
Centinela Hospital Medical Center[2]	Inglewood	98%	94
Citrus Valley Medical Center - IC Campus	Covina	98%	255
Corona Regional Medical Center	Corona	98%	56
Doctors Medical Center	Modesto	98%	218
Kaiser Fdn Hosp-Moreno Valley	Moreno Valley	98%	49
Kaiser Foundation Hospital - Sacramento[2]	Sacramento	98%	122
Kaiser Foundation Hospital - Walnut Creek[2]	Walnut Creek	98%	118
Kaiser Foundation Hospital - West La[2]	Los Angeles	98%	120
Keck Hospital of USC[2]	Los Angeles	98%	136
Loma Linda University Medical Center[2]	Loma Linda	98%	211
Mercy General Hospital	Sacramento	98%	240
Northbay Medical Center	Fairfield	98%	97
Prov Little Co of Mary Med Ctr Torrance	Torrance	98%	241
Queen of the Valley Medical Center	Napa	98%	64
Saint Agnes Medical Center[2]	Fresno	98%	142
Saint Johns Pleasant Valley Hospital	Camarillo	98%	50
San Francisco General Hospital[2]	San Francisco	98%	86
Sequoia Hospital	Redwood City	98%	65
Stanford Hospital	Stanford	98%	289
Sutter Amador Hospital	Jackson	98%	40
UCSF Medical Center[2]	San Francisco	98%	128
Watsonville Community Hospital	Watsonville	98%	48
Arrowhead Regional Medical Center	Colton	97%	216
Bakersfield Memorial Hospital	Bakersfield	97%	156
Chinese Hospital	San Francisco	97%	36
Clovis Community Medical Center[2]	Clovis	97%	90
Comm Mem Hosp San Buenaventura	Ventura	97%	131
Desert Regional Medical Center	Palm Springs	97%	310
Doctors Hospital of Manteca	Manteca	97%	32
Eisenhower Medical Center	Rancho Mirage	97%	408
Enloe Medical Center	Chico	97%	203
Kaiser Foundation Hospital - Fontana[2]	Fontana	97%	105
Kaiser Fdn Hosp-Fremont/Hayward[2]	Hayward	97%	100
Kaiser Foundation Hospital - Los Angeles[2]	Los Angeles	97%	115
Kaiser Foundation Hospital - Manteca[2]	Manteca	97%	63
Kaiser Fdn Hosp-Oakland/Richmond[2]	Oakland	97%	128
Lakewood Regional Medical Center	Lakewood	97%	175
Marian Regional Medical Center	Santa Maria	97%	119
Northridge Hospital Medical Center	Northridge	97%	150
Prov Little Co of Mary Med Ctr San Pedro	San Pedro	97%	62
Saint Francis Memorial Hospital	San Francisco	97%	60
Saint Joseph's Medical Center of Stockton[2]	Stockton	97%	100
Saint Louise Regional Hospital[2]	Gilroy	97%	38
Saint Rose Hospital	Hayward	97%	32
Saint Vincent Medical Center	Los Angeles	97%	68
Simi Valley Hosp & Health Care Svcs	Simi Valley	97%	60
Sutter General Hospital	Sacramento	97%	273
Univ of California Irvine Med Ctr	Orange	97%	252
West Anaheim Medical Center	Anaheim	97%	32
Ahmc Anaheim Regional Medical Center	Anaheim	96%	102
Chino Valley Medical Center	Chino	96%	26
El Centro Regional Medical Center[2]	El Centro	96%	92
Henry Mayo Newhall Memorial Hospital	Valencia	96%	136
Marina Del Rey Hospital	Marina Del Rey	96%	25
Orange Coast Memorial Medical Center	Fountain Valley	96%	74
PIH Hospital - Downey	Downey	96%	106
Saddleback Memorial Medical Center	Laguna Hills	96%	184
Saint Joseph Hospital	Eureka	96%	69
San Dimas Community Hospital	San Dimas	96%	25
San Joaquin Community Hospital[2]	Bakersfield	96%	109
Santa Barbara Cottage Hospital	Santa Barbara	96%	335
Sierra Vista Regional Medical Center	San Luis Obispo	96%	69
Southwest Healthcare System[2]	Murrieta	96%	116
Adventist Medical Center	Hanford	95%	88
Feather River Hospital	Paradise	95%	56
Kaiser Foundation Hospital - Riverside[2]	Riverside	95%	91
Long Beach Memorial Medical Center[2]	Long Beach	95%	104
Olympia Medical Center	Los Angeles	95%	40
Providence Holy Cross Medical Center	Mission Hills	95%	172
Providence Tarzana Medical Center	Tarzana	95%	93
Riverside Community Hospital[2]	Riverside	95%	106
Santa Clara Valley Medical Center[2]	San Jose	95%	109
Santa Rosa Memorial Hospital[2]	Santa Rosa	95%	130
Valleycare Medical Center	Pleasanton	95%	41
Western Medical Center Santa Ana	Santa Ana	95%	115
Whittier Hospital Medical Center	Whittier	95%	42
Good Samaritan Hospital[2]	Los Angeles	94%	83
Kaiser Foundation Hospital - Downey[2]	Downey	94%	109
Woodland Memorial Hospital	Woodland	94%	32
Bakersfield Heart Hospital	Bakersfield	93%	43
LAC/Rancho Los Amigos Ntl Rehab Ctr[2]	Downey	93%	122
Memorial Hospital of Gardena	Gardena	93%	30
Pacific Alliance Medical Center	Los Angeles	93%	58
San Gorgonio Memorial Hospital	Banning	93%	28
West Hills Hospital & Medical Center[2]	West Hills	93%	89
Foothill Presbyterian Hospital	Glendora	92%	39
Twin Cities Community Hospital	Templeton	92%	64
Saint Bernardine Medical Center	San Bernardino	91%	100
Ukiah Valley Medical Center	Ukiah	91%	43
Emanuel Medical Center	Turlock	90%	52
Saint Mary Medical Center	Apple Valley	90%	141
Sutter Delta Medical Center	Antioch	90%	63
Valley Presbyterian Hospital	Van Nuys	90%	110
Glendale Mem Hosp & Health Ctr	Glendale	89%	57
Ronald Reagan UCLA Medical Center[2]	Los Angeles	89%	92
Menifee Valley Medical Center	Sun City	88%	50
Rideout Memorial Hospital	Marysville	88%	145
Southern California Hospital at Hollywood	Hollywood	88%	49
USC Verdugo Hills Hospital	Glendale	88%	48
Alameda County Medical Center	Oakland	87%	92
LAC+USC Medical Center[2]	Los Angeles	87%	76
Providence Saint John's Health Center	Santa Monica	87%	60
Contra Costa Regional Medical Center	Martinez	86%	43
Kaweah Delta Medical Center[2]	Visalia	86%	87
LAC/Olive View - UCLA Medical Center	Sylmar	86%	73
Saint Elizabeth Community Hospital	Red Bluff	86%	28
La Palma Intercommunity Hospital	La Palma	84%	31
Parkview Comm Hosp Med Ctr	Riverside	84%	75
Pioneers Memorial Healthcare District	Brawley	84%	51
Mission Community Hospital	Panorama City	83%	29
Sierra View District Hospital	Porterville	83%	54
Los Angeles Community Hospital	Los Angeles	81%	53
Saint Francis Medical Center[2]	Lynwood	81%	97
Beverly Hospital	Montebello	80%	82
Hemet Valley Medical Center[2]	Hemet	80%	94
Monterey Park Hospital	Monterey Park	80%	25
Paradise Valley Hospital	National City	79%	53
Hi - Desert Medical Center	Joshua Tree	78%	27
LAC/Harbor - UCLA Medical Center[2]	Torrance	77%	115
Victor Valley Global Medical Center	Victorville	77%	47
Tulare Regional Medical Center	Tulare	76%	25
Loma Linda Univ Med Ctr-Murrieta	Murrieta	66%	83
John F Kennedy Memorial Hospital	Indio	64%	25

Discharged on Antithrombotic Therapy

Hospital Name	City	Rate	Cases
Alameda Hospital	Alameda	100%	39
Alhambra Hospital Medical Center	Alhambra	100%	37
Barstow Community Hospital	Barstow	100%	42
CA Pacific Med Ctr-Davies Campus	San Francisco	100%	147
CA Pacific Med Ctr-Pacific Campus Hosp	San Francisco	100%	131
Cedars - Sinai Medical Center	Los Angeles	100%	321
Centinela Hospital Medical Center[2]	Inglewood	100%	84
Chino Valley Medical Center	Chino	100%	25
Comm Hosp of the Monterey Peninsula	Monterey	100%	137
Dameron Hospital	Stockton	100%	58
Desert Regional Medical Center	Palm Springs	100%	230
Desert Valley Hospital	Victorville	100%	84
Doctors Hospital of Manteca	Manteca	100%	28
Doctors Medical Center - San Pablo	San Pablo	100%	101
Dominican Hospital	Santa Cruz	100%	94
Eisenhower Medical Center	Rancho Mirage	100%	369
El Camino Hospital	Mountain View	100%	128
Emanuel Medical Center	Turlock	100%	48
Enloe Medical Center	Chico	100%	184
Feather River Hospital	Paradise	100%	55
Fountain Valley Reg Hosp & Med Ctr	Fountain Valley	100%	183
French Hospital Medical Center	San Luis Obispo	100%	36
Garden Grove Hospital & Medical Center	Garden Grove	100%	29
Garfield Medical Center	Monterey Park	100%	147
Glendale Adventist Medical Center	Glendale	100%	152
Glendale Mem Hosp & Health Ctr	Glendale	100%	52
Good Samaritan Hospital[2]	San Jose	100%	95
Grossmont Hospital	La Mesa	100%	340
Henry Mayo Newhall Memorial Hospital	Valencia	100%	122
Kaiser Foundation Hospital - Baldwin Park[2]	Baldwin Park	100%	108
Kaiser Foundation Hospital - Downey[2]	Downey	100%	90
Kaiser Foundation Hospital - Fontana[2]	Fontana	100%	77
Kaiser Fdn Hosp-Panorama City[2]	Panorama City	100%	90
Kaiser Foundation Hospital - Redwood City[2]	Redwood City	100%	50
Kaiser Foundation Hospital - Riverside[2]	Riverside	100%	83
Kaiser Foundation Hospital - Roseville[2]	Roseville	100%	117
Kaiser Foundation Hospital - San Diego[2]	San Diego	100%	96
Kaiser Foundation Hospital - Santa Rosa[2]	Santa Rosa	100%	69
Kaiser Foundation Hospital - South Bay[2]	Harbor City	100%	82
Kaiser Fdn Hosp-S San Francisco[2]	S San Francisco	100%	68
Kaiser Fdn Hosp-Woodland Hills[2]	Woodland Hills	100%	85
Keck Hospital of USC[2]	Los Angeles	100%	65
LAC+USC Medical Center[2]	Los Angeles	100%	46
LAC/Olive View - UCLA Medical Center	Sylmar	100%	66
Lodi Memorial Hospital	Lodi	100%	38
Los Alamitos Medical Center	Los Alamitos	100%	122
Los Robles Hospital & Medical Center[2]	Thousand Oaks	100%	78
Marin General Hospital	Greenbrae	100%	94
Marshall Medical Center	Placerville	100%	69
Memorial Hospital of Gardena	Gardena	100%	30
Memorial Medical Center	Modesto	100%	162
Mercy Hospital	Bakersfield	100%	106
Mercy Hospital of Folsom	Folsom	100%	40
Methodist Hospital of Sacramento	Sacramento	100%	132
Methodist Hospital of Southern California	Arcadia	100%	194

NOTE: Hospital profiles are in alphabetical order by state, then city, then hospital within the city; Rankings exclude hospitals with less than 25 cases except for patient surveys which excludes hospitals with less than 100 cases; (a) 100-299 cases; (1) The number of cases/patients is too few to report; (2) Data submitted were based on a sample of cases/patients; (3) Results are based on a shorter time period than required; (4) Data suppressed by CMS for one or more quarters; (5) Results are not available for this reporting period; (6) Fewer than 100 patients completed the HCAHPS survey; (7) No cases met the criteria for this measure; (8) The lower limit of the confidence interval cannot be calculated if the number of observed infections equals zero; (9) No data are available from the state/territory for this reporting period; (10) The scores shown reflect fewer than 50 completed surveys; (11) There were discrepancies in the data collection process; (12) This measure does not apply to this hospital for this reporting period; (13) Results cannot be calculated for this reporting period; (14) The results for this state are combined with nearby states to protect confidentiality; Please refer to the User's Guide for a full explanation of data.

Mills - Peninsula Medical Center	Burlingame	100%	139
Northbay Medical Center	Fairfield	100%	93
Northridge Hospital Medical Center	Northridge	100%	129
PIH Hospital - Downey	Downey	100%	87
Pomona Valley Hospital Medical Center[2]	Pomona	100%	118
Prov Little Co of Mary Med Ctr San Pedro	San Pedro	100%	56
Providence Saint Joseph Medical Center	Burbank	100%	213
Providence Tarzana Medical Center	Tarzana	100%	84
Queen of the Valley Medical Center	Napa	100%	56
Ronald Reagan UCLA Medical Center[2]	Los Angeles	100%	62
Saint Johns Regional Medical Center	Oxnard	100%	86
Saint Joseph Hospital	Eureka	100%	63
Saint Jude Medical Center	Fullerton	100%	201
Saint Mary Medical Center	Apple Valley	100%	129
Saint Mary's Medical Center	San Francisco	100%	56
Saint Rose Hospital	Hayward	100%	26
Salinas Valley Memorial Hospital[2]	Salinas	100%	112
San Gabriel Valley Medical Center	San Gabriel	100%	40
San Ramon Regional Medical Center	San Ramon	100%	61
Santa Barbara Cottage Hospital	Santa Barbara	100%	239
Santa Monica-UCLA Med Ctr & Ortho Hosp	Santa Monica	100%	69
Scripps Green Hospital	La Jolla	100%	70
Scripps Memorial Hospital - Encinitas	Encinitas	100%	110
Scripps Memorial Hospital La Jolla	La Jolla	100%	124
Scripps Mercy Hospital	San Diego	100%	288
Seton Medical Center[2]	Daly City	100%	75
Shasta Regional Medical Center	Redding	100%	92
Sierra Nevada Memorial Hospital	Grass Valley	100%	49
Sonora Regional Medical Center	Sonora	100%	56
Southern California Hospital at Hollywood	Hollywood	100%	33
Stanford Hospital	Stanford	100%	180
Sutter Amador Hospital	Jackson	100%	38
Sutter Auburn Faith Hospital	Auburn	100%	58
Sutter Coast Hospital	Crescent City	100%	37
Sutter Davis Hospital	Davis	100%	25
Sutter General Hospital	Sacramento	100%	223
Sutter Medical Center of Santa Rosa	Santa Rosa	100%	41
Sutter Roseville Medical Center	Roseville	100%	172
Sutter Solano Medical Center	Vallejo	100%	53
Temple Community Hospital	Los Angeles	100%	54
Torrance Memorial Medical Center	Torrance	100%	230
UCSF Medical Center[2]	San Francisco	100%	62
Univ of CA Davis Med Ctr[2]	Sacramento	100%	76
Univ of CA San Diego Med Ctr	San Diego	100%	148
Ventura County Medical Center	Ventura	100%	39
Watsonville Community Hospital	Watsonville	100%	45
West Hills Hospital & Medical Center[2]	West Hills	100%	73
Western Medical Center Santa Ana	Santa Ana	100%	75
White Memorial Medical Center	Los Angeles	100%	153
Whittier Hospital Medical Center	Whittier	100%	33
Woodland Memorial Hospital	Woodland	100%	29
Alameda County Medical Center	Oakland	99%	72
Alta Bates Summit Medical Center	Berkeley	99%	138
Alta Bates Summit Medical Center	Oakland	99%	161
Antelope Valley Hospital	Lancaster	99%	157
Bakersfield Memorial Hospital	Bakersfield	99%	136
Clovis Community Medical Center[2]	Clovis	99%	78
Community Regional Medical Center[2]	Fresno	99%	315
Doctors Medical Center	Modesto	99%	181
Eden Medical Center	Castro Valley	99%	173
Hoag Memorial Hospital Presbyterian	Newport Beach	99%	308
Hollywood Presbyterian Medical Center	Los Angeles	99%	90
John Muir Medical Center - Concord Campus	Concord	99%	119
John Muir Med Ctr-Walnut Creek Campus	Walnut Creek	99%	167
Kaiser Foundation Hospital[2]	San Rafael	99%	96
Kaiser Fdn Hosp-Oakland/Richmond[2]	Oakland	99%	116
Kaiser Fdn Hosp-Orange Co-Anaheim[2]	Anaheim	99%	84
Kaiser Foundation Hospital - San Jose[2]	San Jose	99%	102
Kaiser Foundation Hospital - Walnut Creek[2]	Walnut Creek	99%	102
Kaiser Foundation Hospital - West La[2]	Los Angeles	99%	105
Kaiser Fdn Hosp S Sacramento[2]	Sacramento	99%	111
Kaweah Delta Medical Center[2]	Visalia	99%	83
LAC/Harbor - UCLA Medical Center[2]	Torrance	99%	96
Marian Regional Medical Center	Santa Maria	99%	107
Mercy San Juan Medical Center	Carmichael	99%	270
Mission Hospital Regional Medical Center	Mission Viejo	99%	165
Palomar Health Downtown Campus[2]	Escondido	99%	86
Providence Holy Cross Medical Center	Mission Hills	99%	150
Prov Little Co of Mary Med Ctr Torrance	Torrance	99%	203
Regional Medical Center of San Jose[2]	San Jose	99%	91
Rideout Memorial Hospital	Marysville	99%	128
Riverside County Regional Medical Center	Moreno Valley	99%	104
Saddleback Memorial Medical Center	Laguna Hills	99%	168
Saint Bernardine Medical Center	San Bernardino	99%	81
Saint Francis Medical Center[2]	Lynwood	99%	79
Saint Joseph Hospital	Orange	99%	163
Saint Mary Medical Center	Long Beach	99%	70
San Joaquin General Hospital	French Camp	99%	75
Sharp Chula Vista Medical Center	Chula Vista	99%	175
Sharp Memorial Hospital	San Diego	99%	234
Tri - City Medical Center	Oceanside	99%	167
Ahmc Anaheim Regional Medical Center	Anaheim	98%	94
Arrowhead Regional Medical Center	Colton	98%	162
Contra Costa Regional Medical Center	Martinez	98%	41
Corona Regional Medical Center	Corona	98%	49
Huntington Memorial Hospital	Pasadena	98%	196
Kaiser Foundation Hospital - Fresno[2]	Fresno	98%	92
Kaiser Foundation Hospital - Los Angeles[2]	Los Angeles	98%	62
Kaiser Foundation Hospital - Manteca[2]	Manteca	98%	58
Kaiser Fdn Hosp-Moreno Valley	Moreno Valley	98%	46
Kaiser Foundation Hospital - Sacramento[2]	Sacramento	98%	61
Kaiser Foundation Hospital - Santa Clara[2]	Santa Clara	98%	115
Menifee Valley Medical Center	Sun City	98%	48
Mercy General Hospital	Sacramento	98%	194
Mercy Medical Center	Merced	98%	99
Mercy Medical Center - Redding	Redding	98%	123
O'Connor Hospital[2]	San Jose	98%	65
Orange Coast Memorial Medical Center	Fountain Valley	98%	60
Oroville Hospital[2]	Oroville	98%	58
Pomerado Hospital[2]	Poway	98%	58
Presbyterian Intercommunity Hospital[2]	Whittier	98%	164
Providence Saint John's Health Center	Santa Monica	98%	43
Redlands Community Hospital	Redlands	98%	110
Saint Agnes Medical Center[2]	Fresno	98%	133
Saint Johns Pleasant Valley Hospital	Camarillo	98%	47
Saint Joseph's Medical Center of Stockton[2]	Stockton	98%	88
Saint Vincent Medical Center	Los Angeles	98%	62
San Antonio Community Hospital	Upland	98%	149
San Francisco General Hospital[2]	San Francisco	98%	61
San Joaquin Community Hospital[2]	Bakersfield	98%	91
Santa Rosa Memorial Hospital[2]	Santa Rosa	98%	108
Sequoia Hospital	Redwood City	98%	62
Sierra Vista Regional Medical Center	San Luis Obispo	98%	44
Southwest Healthcare System[2]	Murrieta	98%	102
Univ of California Irvine Med Ctr	Orange	98%	164
Valley Presbyterian Hospital	Van Nuys	98%	94
Valleycare Medical Center	Pleasanton	98%	41
California Hosp Med Ctr Los Angeles	Los Angeles	97%	119
Citrus Valley Medical Center - IC Campus	Covina	97%	220
Comm Mem Hosp San Buenaventura	Ventura	97%	109
Foothill Presbyterian Hospital	Glendora	97%	34
Kaiser Foundation Hospital - Antioch[2]	Antioch	97%	91
Loma Linda University Medical Center[2]	Loma Linda	97%	138
Olympia Medical Center	Los Angeles	97%	32
Riverside Community Hospital[2]	Riverside	97%	87
Santa Clara Valley Medical Center[2]	San Jose	97%	89
Sutter Delta Medical Center	Antioch	97%	60
Kaiser Fdn Hosp-San Francisco[2]	San Francisco	96%	94
Lakewood Regional Medical Center	Lakewood	96%	145
Loma Linda Univ Med Ctr-Murrieta	Murrieta	96%	71
Long Beach Memorial Medical Center[2]	Long Beach	96%	77
Saint Elizabeth Community Hospital	Red Bluff	96%	28
Saint Francis Memorial Hospital	San Francisco	96%	52
San Gorgonio Memorial Hospital	Banning	96%	25
Sierra View District Hospital	Porterville	96%	50
Simi Valley Hosp & Health Care Svcs	Simi Valley	96%	52
Victor Valley Global Medical Center	Victorville	96%	46
Washington Hospital	Fremont	96%	134
West Anaheim Medical Center	Anaheim	96%	28
Adventist Medical Center	Hanford	95%	82
Alvarado Hospital Medical Center	San Diego	95%	56
Bakersfield Heart Hospital	Bakersfield	95%	41
Good Samaritan Hospital[2]	Los Angeles	95%	80
LAC/Rancho Los Amigos Ntl Rehab Ctr[2]	Downey	95%	110
Ukiah Valley Medical Center	Ukiah	95%	40
Chinese Hospital	San Francisco	94%	34
Kaiser Fdn Hosp-Fremont/Hayward[2]	Hayward	94%	84
Kaiser Foundation Hospital - Vacaville	Vacaville	94%	62
El Centro Regional Medical Center[2]	El Centro	93%	87
Paradise Valley Hospital	National City	93%	44
Placentia Linda Hospital	Placentia	93%	30
Twin Cities Community Hospital	Templeton	93%	59
Hi - Desert Medical Center	Joshua Tree	92%	26
Kaiser Foundation Hospital & Rehab Center[2]	Vallejo	92%	106
Mission Community Hospital	Panorama City	92%	26
Parkview Comm Hosp Med Ctr	Riverside	92%	72
Beverly Hospital	Montebello	91%	79
Hemet Valley Medical Center[2]	Hemet	91%	92
USC Verdugo Hills Hospital	Glendale	91%	43
Pioneers Memorial Healthcare District	Brawley	90%	48
Pacific Alliance Medical Center	Los Angeles	89%	53
La Palma Intercommunity Hospital	La Palma	88%	26
Saint Louise Regional Hospital[2]	Gilroy	88%	33
Palmdale Regional Medical Center	Palmdale	86%	63
Los Angeles Community Hospital	Los Angeles	72%	25

Discharged on Statin Medication

Hospital Name	City	Rate	Cases
Alameda County Medical Center	Oakland	100%	65
CA Pacific Med Ctr-Davies Campus	San Francisco	100%	113
CA Pacific Med Ctr-Pacific Campus Hosp	San Francisco	100%	100
Contra Costa Regional Medical Center	Martinez	100%	31
Desert Valley Hospital	Victorville	100%	59
Feather River Hospital	Paradise	100%	34
French Hospital Medical Center	San Luis Obispo	100%	26
Good Samaritan Hospital[2]	San Jose	100%	76
Kaiser Foundation Hospital - Baldwin Park[2]	Baldwin Park	100%	88
Kaiser Foundation Hospital - Downey[2]	Downey	100%	75
Kaiser Foundation Hospital - Fontana[2]	Fontana	100%	73
Kaiser Foundation Hospital - Los Angeles[2]	Los Angeles	100%	55
Kaiser Foundation Hospital - Redwood City[2]	Redwood City	100%	36
Kaiser Foundation Hospital - Roseville[2]	Roseville	100%	97
Kaiser Foundation Hospital - San Diego[2]	San Diego	100%	79
Kaiser Foundation Hospital - Santa Clara[2]	Santa Clara	100%	91
Kaiser Foundation Hospital - Santa Rosa[2]	Santa Rosa	100%	67
Kaiser Foundation Hospital - South Bay[2]	Harbor City	100%	72
Kaiser Fdn Hosp-S San Francisco[2]	S San Francisco	100%	56
LAC/Olive View - UCLA Medical Center	Sylmar	100%	61
Los Alamitos Medical Center	Los Alamitos	100%	86
Marin General Hospital	Greenbrae	100%	61
Marshall Medical Center	Placerville	100%	55
Mercy Hospital	Bakersfield	100%	75
Methodist Hospital of Southern California	Arcadia	100%	160
Mills - Peninsula Medical Center	Burlingame	100%	105
Oroville Hospital[2]	Oroville	100%	40
Riverside County Regional Medical Center	Moreno Valley	100%	76
Saint Mary's Medical Center	San Francisco	100%	51
Salinas Valley Memorial Hospital[2]	Salinas	100%	81
San Gabriel Valley Medical Center	San Gabriel	100%	26
San Ramon Regional Medical Center	San Ramon	100%	49
Santa Monica-UCLA Med Ctr & Ortho Hosp	Santa Monica	100%	50
Scripps Memorial Hospital - Encinitas	Encinitas	100%	76
Scripps Memorial Hospital La Jolla	La Jolla	100%	86
Seton Medical Center[2]	Daly City	100%	57
Shasta Regional Medical Center	Redding	100%	63
Sierra Nevada Memorial Hospital	Grass Valley	100%	38
Sutter Auburn Faith Hospital	Auburn	100%	44
Sutter Coast Hospital	Crescent City	100%	25
Temple Community Hospital	Los Angeles	100%	38
Univ of CA Davis Med Ctr[2]	Sacramento	100%	57
Doctors Medical Center - San Pablo	San Pablo	99%	76
Dominican Hospital	Santa Cruz	99%	71
Eden Medical Center	Castro Valley	99%	140
Enloe Medical Center	Chico	99%	139
Fountain Valley Reg Hosp & Med Ctr	Fountain Valley	99%	142
Grossmont Hospital	La Mesa	99%	261
Hoag Memorial Hospital Presbyterian	Newport Beach	99%	253
John Muir Medical Center - Concord Campus	Concord	99%	89
Kaiser Foundation Hospital[2]	San Rafael	99%	78
Kaiser Fdn Hosp-Oakland/Richmond[2]	Oakland	99%	89
Kaiser Fdn Hosp-Orange Co-Anaheim[2]	Anaheim	99%	73
Kaiser Fdn Hosp-Panorama City[2]	Panorama City	99%	77
Kaiser Foundation Hospital - San Jose[2]	San Jose	99%	85
Kaiser Foundation Hospital - Walnut Creek[2]	Walnut Creek	99%	85
Kaiser Fdn Hosp S Sacramento[2]	Sacramento	99%	82
Methodist Hospital of Sacramento	Sacramento	99%	107
Palomar Health Downtown Campus[2]	Escondido	99%	69
Pomona Valley Hospital Medical Center[2]	Pomona	99%	95
Regional Medical Center of San Jose[2]	San Jose	99%	69
San Joaquin Community Hospital[2]	Bakersfield	99%	69
Sharp Chula Vista Medical Center	Chula Vista	99%	116
Sutter Roseville Medical Center	Roseville	99%	141
White Memorial Medical Center	Los Angeles	99%	123
Alta Bates Summit Medical Center	Berkeley	98%	91
Antelope Valley Hospital	Lancaster	98%	124
Comm Hosp of the Monterey Peninsula	Monterey	98%	104
Community Regional Medical Center[2]	Fresno	98%	261
Doctors Medical Center	Modesto	98%	146
Garfield Medical Center	Monterey Park	98%	112
Glendale Adventist Medical Center	Glendale	98%	130
Kaiser Foundation Hospital - Manteca[2]	Manteca	98%	52
Kaiser Fdn Hosp-Moreno Valley	Moreno Valley	98%	41
Keck Hospital of USC[2]	Los Angeles	98%	64
Los Robles Hospital & Medical Center[2]	Thousand Oaks	98%	61
Memorial Medical Center	Modesto	98%	132
Northridge Hospital Medical Center	Northridge	98%	102
O'Connor Hospital[2]	San Jose	98%	52
Presbyterian Intercommunity Hospital[2]	Whittier	98%	130
Saint Joseph Hospital	Orange	98%	123
Saint Jude Medical Center	Fullerton	98%	164
Saint Mary Medical Center	Long Beach	98%	61
Saint Vincent Medical Center	Los Angeles	98%	48
San Joaquin General Hospital	French Camp	98%	52
Scripps Green Hospital	La Jolla	98%	58
Torrance Memorial Medical Center	Torrance	98%	189
UCSF Medical Center[2]	San Francisco	98%	50
Univ of California Irvine Med Ctr	Orange	98%	131
Univ of CA San Diego Med Ctr	San Diego	98%	101
Bakersfield Memorial Hospital	Bakersfield	97%	112
Barstow Community Hospital	Barstow	97%	33
Comm Mem Hosp San Buenaventura	Ventura	97%	86
Desert Regional Medical Center	Palm Springs	97%	157
Eisenhower Medical Center	Rancho Mirage	97%	264

NOTE: Hospital profiles are in alphabetical order by state, then city, then hospital within the city; Rankings exclude hospitals with less than 25 cases except for patient surveys which excludes hospitals with less than 100 cases; (a) 100-299 cases; (1) The number of cases/patients is too few to report; (2) Data submitted were based on a sample of cases/patients; (3) Results are based on a shorter time period than required; (4) Data suppressed by CMS for one or more quarters; (5) Results are not available for this reporting period; (6) Fewer than 100 patients completed the HCAHPS survey; (7) No cases met the criteria for this measure; (8) The lower limit of the confidence interval cannot be calculated if the number of observed infections equals zero; (9) No data are available from the state/territory for this reporting period; (10) The scores shown reflect fewer than 50 completed surveys; (11) There were discrepancies in the data collection process; (12) This measure does not apply to this hospital for this reporting period; (13) Results cannot be calculated for this reporting period; (14) The results for this state are combined with nearby states to protect confidentiality; Please refer to the User's Guide for a full explanation of data.

Hospital Name	City	Rate	Cases
Kaiser Fdn Hosp-Fremont/Hayward[2]	Hayward	97%	68
Kaiser Foundation Hospital - Fresno[2]	Fresno	97%	75
Kaiser Fdn Hosp-Woodland Hills[2]	Woodland Hills	97%	74
Loma Linda University Medical Center[2]	Loma Linda	97%	103
Mercy Hospital of Folsom	Folsom	97%	32
Providence Holy Cross Medical Center	Mission Hills	97%	124
Providence Saint Joseph Medical Center	Burbank	97%	158
Scripps Mercy Hospital	San Diego	97%	227
Stanford Hospital	Stanford	97%	150
Sutter Medical Center of Santa Rosa	Santa Rosa	97%	31
Watsonville Community Hospital	Watsonville	97%	39
West Hills Hospital & Medical Center[2]	West Hills	97%	58
Whittier Hospital Medical Center	Whittier	97%	31
Ahmc Anaheim Regional Medical Center	Anaheim	96%	75
Arrowhead Regional Medical Center	Colton	96%	142
Kaiser Foundation Hospital - Antioch[2]	Antioch	96%	78
Kaiser Foundation Hospital - Sacramento[2]	Sacramento	96%	50
Kaiser Foundation Hospital - West La[2]	Los Angeles	96%	103
LAC/Harbor - UCLA Medical Center[2]	Torrance	96%	82
Mercy General Hospital	Sacramento	96%	151
Northbay Medical Center	Fairfield	96%	77
Placentia Linda Hospital	Placentia	96%	27
Prov Little Co of Mary Med Ctr San Pedro	San Pedro	96%	45
Saint Joseph's Medical Center of Stockton[2]	Stockton	96%	72
Saint Mary Medical Center	Apple Valley	96%	98
San Francisco General Hospital[2]	San Francisco	96%	47
Sequoia Hospital	Redwood City	96%	56
Sonora Regional Medical Center	Sonora	96%	47
Sutter Delta Medical Center	Antioch	96%	49
Sutter General Hospital	Sacramento	96%	170
Sutter Solano Medical Center	Vallejo	96%	46
Tri - City Medical Center	Oceanside	96%	123
Emanuel Medical Center	Turlock	95%	42
John Muir Med Ctr-Walnut Creek Campus	Walnut Creek	95%	120
Kaiser Foundation Hospital - Riverside[2]	Riverside	95%	66
Providence Tarzana Medical Center	Tarzana	95%	73
Santa Clara Valley Medical Center[2]	San Jose	95%	77
Cedars - Sinai Medical Center	Los Angeles	94%	235
Henry Mayo Newhall Memorial Hospital	Valencia	94%	103
Kaiser Fdn Hosp-San Francisco[2]	San Francisco	94%	82
LAC+USC Medical Center[2]	Los Angeles	94%	36
Mercy San Juan Medical Center	Carmichael	94%	188
PIH Hospital - Downey	Downey	94%	72
Riverside Community Hospital[2]	Riverside	94%	72
San Antonio Community Hospital	Upland	94%	121
Sharp Memorial Hospital	San Diego	94%	161
Southern California Hospital at Hollywood	Hollywood	94%	35
Alameda Hospital	Alameda	93%	29
Bakersfield Heart Hospital	Bakersfield	93%	30
El Camino Hospital	Mountain View	93%	102
Hollywood Presbyterian Medical Center	Los Angeles	93%	72
Mercy Medical Center - Redding	Redding	93%	91
Pomerado Hospital[2]	Poway	93%	44
Alta Bates Summit Medical Center	Oakland	92%	122
Glendale Mem Hosp & Health Ctr	Glendale	92%	49
Kaiser Foundation Hospital & Rehab Center[2]	Vallejo	92%	88
Prov Little Co of Mary Med Ctr Torrance	Torrance	92%	166
Redlands Community Hospital	Redlands	92%	90
Saint Francis Memorial Hospital	San Francisco	92%	39
Washington Hospital	Fremont	92%	107
Western Medical Center Santa Ana	Santa Ana	92%	59
Clovis Community Medical Center[2]	Clovis	91%	69
Dameron Hospital	Stockton	91%	47
Queen of the Valley Medical Center	Napa	91%	44
Ronald Reagan UCLA Medical Center[2]	Los Angeles	91%	58
Saint Agnes Medical Center[2]	Fresno	91%	96
Santa Barbara Cottage Hospital	Santa Barbara	91%	171
Simi Valley Hosp & Health Care Svcs	Simi Valley	91%	44
Citrus Valley Medical Center - IC Campus	Covina	90%	171
Lakewood Regional Medical Center	Lakewood	90%	109
Long Beach Memorial Medical Center[2]	Long Beach	90%	62
Marian Regional Medical Center	Santa Maria	90%	91
Saint Johns Regional Medical Center	Oxnard	90%	67
Twin Cities Community Hospital	Templeton	90%	48
California Hosp Med Ctr Los Angeles	Los Angeles	89%	95
Huntington Memorial Hospital	Pasadena	89%	151
Alvarado Hospital Medical Center	San Diego	88%	42
Kaiser Foundation Hospital - Vacaville	Vacaville	88%	42
Santa Rosa Memorial Hospital[2]	Santa Rosa	88%	77
Centinela Hospital Medical Center[2]	Inglewood	87%	62
Mission Hospital Regional Medical Center	Mission Viejo	87%	137
Sierra Vista Regional Medical Center	San Luis Obispo	87%	38
Southwest Healthcare System[2]	Murrieta	87%	95
Adventist Medical Center	Hanford	86%	78
LAC/Rancho Los Amigos Ntl Rehab Ctr[2]	Downey	86%	71
Saddleback Memorial Medical Center	Laguna Hills	86%	120
Valleycare Medical Center	Pleasanton	86%	28
Palmdale Regional Medical Center	Palmdale	85%	52
Pioneers Memorial Healthcare District	Brawley	85%	40
Providence Saint John's Health Center	Santa Monica	85%	39
Saint Bernardine Medical Center	San Bernardino	85%	66
Saint Rose Hospital	Hayward	85%	27
El Centro Regional Medical Center[2]	El Centro	84%	86
Lodi Memorial Hospital	Lodi	84%	32
Loma Linda Univ Med Ctr-Murrieta	Murrieta	84%	61
Los Angeles Community Hospital	Los Angeles	84%	38
Saint Joseph Hospital	Eureka	83%	52
Valley Presbyterian Hospital	Van Nuys	83%	66
Corona Regional Medical Center	Corona	82%	34
Mercy Medical Center	Merced	82%	84
Saint Louise Regional Hospital[2]	Gilroy	82%	28
Chinese Hospital	San Francisco	81%	32
Orange Coast Memorial Medical Center	Fountain Valley	81%	52
Victor Valley Global Medical Center	Victorville	81%	36
Saint Johns Pleasant Valley Hospital	Camarillo	80%	41
Ukiah Valley Medical Center	Ukiah	80%	35
Foothill Presbyterian Hospital	Glendora	78%	27
Kaweah Delta Medical Center[2]	Visalia	78%	64
Parkview Comm Hosp Med Ctr	Riverside	78%	60
Beverly Hospital	Montebello	77%	70
Good Samaritan Hospital[2]	Los Angeles	77%	60
Memorial Hospital of Gardena	Gardena	77%	26
Pacific Alliance Medical Center	Los Angeles	76%	46
Rideout Memorial Hospital	Marysville	76%	98
Menifee Valley Medical Center	Sun City	74%	46
Paradise Valley Hospital	National City	72%	39
USC Verdugo Hills Hospital	Glendale	71%	34
Saint Francis Medical Center[2]	Lynwood	69%	70
Alhambra Hospital Medical Center	Alhambra	59%	29
Hemet Valley Medical Center[2]	Hemet	59%	87
Sierra View District Hospital	Porterville	56%	39
Saint Elizabeth Community Hospital	Red Bluff	44%	27

Thrombolytic Therapy Timing

Hospital Name	City	Rate	Cases
Cedars - Sinai Medical Center	Los Angeles	100%	28
Saint Jude Medical Center	Fullerton	100%	57
Scripps Memorial Hospital La Jolla	La Jolla	100%	28
White Memorial Medical Center	Los Angeles	100%	30
Grossmont Hospital	La Mesa	98%	40
Enloe Medical Center	Chico	97%	31
John Muir Medical Center - Concord Campus	Concord	96%	27
San Antonio Community Hospital	Upland	96%	26
Scripps Mercy Hospital	San Diego	96%	27
Tri - City Medical Center	Oceanside	94%	53
Eisenhower Medical Center	Rancho Mirage	93%	27
Hoag Memorial Hospital Presbyterian	Newport Beach	93%	27
Providence Saint Joseph Medical Center	Burbank	93%	29
Eden Medical Center	Castro Valley	83%	29
Sharp Memorial Hospital	San Diego	78%	27
Mercy General Hospital	Sacramento	60%	30
Mercy San Juan Medical Center	Carmichael	58%	60
Adventist Medical Center	Hanford	8%	26
El Centro Regional Medical Center[2]	El Centro	2%	41
Palmdale Regional Medical Center	Palmdale	2%	43
Loma Linda Univ Med Ctr-Murrieta	Murrieta	0%	26

Venous Thromboembolism (VTE) Prophylaxis

Hospital Name	City	Rate	Cases
CA Pacific Med Ctr-Davies Campus	San Francisco	100%	246
CA Pacific Med Ctr-Pacific Campus Hosp	San Francisco	100%	158
Chino Valley Medical Center	Chino	100%	25
Clovis Community Medical Center[2]	Clovis	100%	93
French Hospital Medical Center	San Luis Obispo	100%	34
Garfield Medical Center	Monterey Park	100%	207
Henry Mayo Newhall Memorial Hospital	Valencia	100%	146
Huntington Beach Hospital	Huntington Bch	100%	25
Kaiser Fdn Hosp-Moreno Valley	Moreno Valley	100%	42
Kaiser Fdn Hosp-Orange Co-Anaheim[2]	Anaheim	100%	98
Kaiser Fdn Hosp-Panorama City[2]	Panorama City	100%	94
Kaiser Foundation Hospital - Roseville[2]	Roseville	100%	87
Kaiser Foundation Hospital - Sacramento[2]	Sacramento	100%	117
Kaiser Fdn Hosp-San Francisco[2]	San Francisco	100%	96
Kaiser Foundation Hospital - South Bay[2]	Harbor City	100%	65
Kaiser Fdn Hosp-S San Francisco[2]	S San Francisco	100%	96
Kaiser Foundation Hospital - Vacaville	Vacaville	100%	56
Kaiser Fdn Hosp-Woodland Hills[2]	Woodland Hills	100%	83
Kaiser Fdn Hosp S Sacramento[2]	Sacramento	100%	86
Keck Hospital of USC[2]	Los Angeles	100%	152
Los Alamitos Medical Center	Los Alamitos	100%	134
Marin General Hospital	Greenbrae	100%	105
Marshall Medical Center	Placerville	100%	64
Mercy Hospital	Bakersfield	100%	126
Methodist Hospital of Southern California	Arcadia	100%	239
PIH Hospital - Downey	Downey	100%	101
Saint Joseph Hospital	Orange	100%	174
Saint Mary Medical Center	Long Beach	100%	93
Saint Mary's Medical Center	San Francisco	100%	57
Salinas Valley Memorial Hospital[2]	Salinas	100%	126
San Gabriel Valley Medical Center	San Gabriel	100%	48
San Ramon Regional Medical Center	San Ramon	100%	67
Shasta Regional Medical Center	Redding	100%	88
Sierra Nevada Memorial Hospital	Grass Valley	100%	49
Sutter Auburn Faith Hospital	Auburn	100%	50
Sutter Coast Hospital	Crescent City	100%	32
Sutter Medical Center of Santa Rosa	Santa Rosa	100%	40
Temple Community Hospital	Los Angeles	100%	63
Univ of California Irvine Med Ctr	Orange	100%	286
Bakersfield Memorial Hospital	Bakersfield	99%	160
Cedars - Sinai Medical Center	Los Angeles	99%	477
Comm Hosp of the Monterey Peninsula	Monterey	99%	144
Desert Regional Medical Center	Palm Springs	99%	294
Enloe Medical Center	Chico	99%	211
Glendale Adventist Medical Center	Glendale	99%	197
Kaiser Fdn Hosp-Fremont/Hayward[2]	Hayward	99%	97
Kaiser Foundation Hospital - Fresno[2]	Fresno	99%	90
Kaiser Foundation Hospital - Los Angeles[2]	Los Angeles	99%	118
Kaiser Foundation Hospital - Redwood City[2]	Redwood City	99%	128
Kaiser Foundation Hospital - Riverside[2]	Riverside	99%	69
Kaiser Foundation Hospital - San Diego[2]	San Diego	99%	86
Kaiser Foundation Hospital - Santa Clara[2]	Santa Clara	99%	104
Mercy Medical Center	Merced	99%	117
Methodist Hospital of Sacramento	Sacramento	99%	148
Mills - Peninsula Medical Center	Burlingame	99%	166
Northridge Hospital Medical Center	Northridge	99%	161
O'Connor Hospital[2]	San Jose	99%	85
Regional Medical Center of San Jose[2]	San Jose	99%	128
Saint Francis Memorial Hospital	San Francisco	99%	76
Saint Jude Medical Center	Fullerton	99%	273
Saint Vincent Medical Center	Los Angeles	99%	73
San Antonio Community Hospital	Upland	99%	190
Santa Rosa Memorial Hospital[2]	Santa Rosa	99%	141
Scripps Green Hospital	La Jolla	99%	102
Scripps Memorial Hospital La Jolla	La Jolla	99%	181
Sierra Vista Regional Medical Center	San Luis Obispo	99%	74
Stanford Hospital	Stanford	99%	287
Sutter Roseville Medical Center	Roseville	99%	223
Torrance Memorial Medical Center	Torrance	99%	241
Tri - City Medical Center	Oceanside	99%	207
Univ of CA San Diego Med Ctr	San Diego	99%	179
Western Medical Center Santa Ana	Santa Ana	99%	143
White Memorial Medical Center	Los Angeles	99%	207
Antelope Valley Hospital	Lancaster	98%	195
Barstow Community Hospital	Barstow	98%	43
Corona Regional Medical Center	Corona	98%	53
Desert Valley Hospital	Victorville	98%	93
Doctors Medical Center	Modesto	98%	239
Dominican Hospital	Santa Cruz	98%	104
Feather River Hospital	Paradise	98%	61
Good Samaritan Hospital[2]	San Jose	98%	121
Kaiser Foundation Hospital & Rehab Center[2]	Vallejo	98%	96
Kaiser Foundation Hospital - Baldwin Park[2]	Baldwin Park	98%	87
Kaiser Foundation Hospital - Downey[2]	Downey	98%	97
Kaiser Foundation Hospital - West La[2]	Los Angeles	98%	99
Lodi Memorial Hospital	Lodi	98%	43
Providence Saint Joseph Medical Center	Burbank	98%	271
Riverside County Regional Medical Center	Moreno Valley	98%	125
Scripps Memorial Hospital - Encinitas	Encinitas	98%	130
Sharp Memorial Hospital	San Diego	98%	280
Sonora Regional Medical Center	Sonora	98%	58
Sutter Solano Medical Center	Vallejo	98%	64
Ventura County Medical Center	Ventura	98%	48
California Hosp Med Ctr Los Angeles	Los Angeles	97%	177
Centinela Hospital Medical Center[2]	Inglewood	97%	115
Community Regional Medical Center[2]	Fresno	97%	475
Eden Medical Center	Castro Valley	97%	300
Grossmont Hospital	La Mesa	97%	425
Hollywood Presbyterian Medical Center	Los Angeles	97%	115
John Muir Med Ctr-Walnut Creek Campus	Walnut Creek	97%	291
Kaiser Foundation Hospital - Antioch[2]	Antioch	97%	90
Kaiser Fdn Hosp-Oakland/Richmond[2]	Oakland	97%	118
LAC+USC Medical Center[2]	Los Angeles	97%	113
Mercy General Hospital	Sacramento	97%	232
Mercy Hospital of Folsom	Folsom	97%	39
Mercy Medical Center - Redding	Redding	97%	158
Mercy San Juan Medical Center	Carmichael	97%	411
Monterey Park Hospital	Monterey Park	97%	29
Providence Holy Cross Medical Center	Mission Hills	97%	178
Southern California Hospital at Hollywood	Hollywood	97%	58
Sutter Amador Hospital	Jackson	97%	32
John Muir Medical Center - Concord Campus	Concord	96%	117
Kaweah Delta Medical Center[2]	Visalia	96%	83
Marian Regional Medical Center	Santa Maria	96%	109
Northbay Medical Center	Fairfield	96%	104
Prov Little Co of Mary Med Ctr San Pedro	San Pedro	96%	53
Saint Mary Medical Center	Apple Valley	96%	154
Santa Barbara Cottage Hospital	Santa Barbara	96%	364
Sonoma Valley Hospital	Sonoma	96%	26
Watsonville Community Hospital	Watsonville	96%	47
Eisenhower Medical Center	Rancho Mirage	95%	369
El Camino Hospital	Mountain View	95%	143
Hoag Memorial Hospital Presbyterian	Newport Beach	95%	327

NOTE: Hospital profiles are in alphabetical order by state, then city, then hospital within the city; Rankings exclude hospitals with less than 25 cases except for patient surveys which excludes hospitals with less than 100 cases; (a) 100-299 cases; (1) The number of cases/patients is too few to report; (2) Data submitted were based on a sample of cases/patients; (3) Results are based on a shorter time period than required; (4) Data suppressed by CMS for one or more quarters; (5) Results are not available for this reporting period; (6) Fewer than 100 patients completed the HCAHPS survey; (7) No cases met the criteria for this measure; (8) The lower limit of the confidence interval cannot be calculated if the number of observed infections equals zero; (9) No data are available from the state/territory for this reporting period; (10) The scores shown reflect fewer than 50 completed surveys; (11) There were discrepancies in the data collection process; (12) This measure does not apply to this hospital for this reporting period; (13) Results cannot be calculated for this reporting period; (14) The results for this state are combined with nearby states to protect confidentiality; Please refer to the User's Guide for a full explanation of data.

Kaiser Foundation Hospital - Walnut Creek[2]	Walnut Creek	95%	99
Los Robles Hospital & Medical Center[2]	Thousand Oaks	95%	88
Mission Hospital Regional Medical Center	Mission Viejo	95%	226
Saint Joseph's Medical Center of Stockton[2]	Stockton	95%	112
Sequoia Hospital	Redwood City	95%	57
Sharp Chula Vista Medical Center	Chula Vista	95%	211
Twin Cities Community Hospital	Templeton	95%	58
UCSF Medical Center[2]	San Francisco	95%	149
Univ of CA Davis Med Ctr[2]	Sacramento	95%	92
West Anaheim Medical Center	Anaheim	95%	39
West Hills Hospital & Medical Center[2]	West Hills	95%	92
Whittier Hospital Medical Center	Whittier	95%	44
Alta Bates Summit Medical Center	Berkeley	94%	195
Garden Grove Hospital & Medical Center	Garden Grove	94%	32
Kaiser Foundation Hospital[2]	San Rafael	94%	93
Kaiser Foundation Hospital - Manteca[2]	Manteca	94%	47
Kaiser Foundation Hospital - San Jose[2]	San Jose	94%	94
Kaiser Foundation Hospital - Santa Rosa[2]	Santa Rosa	94%	81
Lakewood Regional Medical Center	Lakewood	94%	191
Mission Community Hospital	Panorama City	94%	32
Pomona Valley Hospital Medical Center[2]	Pomona	94%	144
Presbyterian Intercommunity Hospital[2]	Whittier	94%	190
Prov Little Co of Mary Med Ctr Torrance	Torrance	94%	224
Saddleback Memorial Medical Center	Laguna Hills	94%	194
Scripps Mercy Hospital	San Diego	94%	333
Simi Valley Hosp & Health Care Svcs	Simi Valley	94%	63
Sutter General Hospital	Sacramento	94%	270
Kaiser Foundation Hospital - Fontana[2]	Fontana	93%	90
Oroville Hospital[2]	Oroville	93%	68
Palomar Health Downtown Campus[2]	Escondido	93%	99
Saint Joseph Hospital	Eureka	93%	61
Alameda Hospital	Alameda	92%	51
Alta Bates Summit Medical Center	Oakland	92%	198
Dameron Hospital	Stockton	92%	62
Doctors Medical Center - San Pablo	San Pablo	92%	103
Fountain Valley Reg Hosp & Med Ctr	Fountain Valley	92%	225
LAC/Rancho Los Amigos Ntl Rehab Ctr[2]	Downey	92%	100
Providence Tarzana Medical Center	Tarzana	92%	93
Saint Johns Regional Medical Center	Oxnard	92%	126
San Francisco General Hospital[2]	San Francisco	92%	103
San Joaquin Community Hospital[2]	Bakersfield	92%	113
San Joaquin General Hospital	French Camp	92%	85
Santa Monica-UCLA Med Ctr & Ortho Hosp	Santa Monica	92%	66
Sutter Lakeside Hospital	Lakeport	92%	25
Washington Hospital	Fremont	92%	174
Ahmc Anaheim Regional Medical Center	Anaheim	91%	101
Loma Linda University Medical Center[2]	Loma Linda	91%	242
Memorial Medical Center	Modesto	91%	207
Seton Medical Center[2]	Daly City	91%	99
Contra Costa Regional Medical Center	Martinez	90%	42
Huntington Memorial Hospital	Pasadena	90%	258
Saint Agnes Medical Center[2]	Fresno	90%	139
Saint Bernardine Medical Center	San Bernardino	90%	102
Emanuel Medical Center	Turlock	89%	56
Los Angeles Community Hospital	Los Angeles	89%	55
Sutter Delta Medical Center	Antioch	89%	65
Arrowhead Regional Medical Center	Colton	88%	240
Memorial Hospital of Gardena	Gardena	88%	32
Pomerado Hospital[2]	Poway	87%	62
Glendale Mem Hosp & Health Ctr	Glendale	86%	58
Southwest Healthcare System[2]	Murrieta	86%	119
Valley Presbyterian Hospital	Van Nuys	86%	117
Alameda County Medical Center	Oakland	85%	93
Citrus Valley Medical Center - IC Campus	Covina	85%	238
Doctors Hospital of Manteca	Manteca	85%	34
Orange Coast Memorial Medical Center	Fountain Valley	84%	63
Riverside Community Hospital[2]	Riverside	84%	114
Saint Johns Pleasant Valley Hospital	Camarillo	84%	51
Sierra View District Hospital	Porterville	84%	58
Loma Linda Univ Med Ctr-Murrieta	Murrieta	83%	70
Santa Clara Valley Medical Center[2]	San Jose	83%	99
Olympia Medical Center	Los Angeles	82%	45
Queen of the Valley Medical Center	Napa	82%	73
Redlands Community Hospital	Redlands	82%	121
Alhambra Hospital Medical Center	Alhambra	81%	43
Good Samaritan Hospital[2]	Los Angeles	81%	91
Palmdale Regional Medical Center	Palmdale	81%	70
Placentia Linda Hospital	Placentia	81%	26
Saint Louise Regional Hospital[2]	Gilroy	81%	42
Adventist Medical Center	Hanford	80%	85
Bakersfield Heart Hospital	Bakersfield	80%	40
LAC/Harbor - UCLA Medical Center[2]	Torrance	80%	128
LAC/Olive View - UCLA Medical Center	Sylmar	80%	75
Ukiah Valley Medical Center	Ukiah	80%	46
Alvarado Hospital Medical Center	San Diego	79%	66
Foothill Presbyterian Hospital	Glendora	79%	39
Long Beach Memorial Medical Center[2]	Long Beach	79%	113
Providence Saint John's Health Center	Santa Monica	79%	71
Comm Mem Hosp San Buenaventura	Ventura	78%	119
Rideout Memorial Hospital	Marysville	78%	152
Ronald Reagan UCLA Medical Center[2]	Los Angeles	77%	88
Saint Rose Hospital	Hayward	76%	29
Valleycare Medical Center	Pleasanton	76%	45
El Centro Regional Medical Center[2]	El Centro	74%	99
Hi - Desert Medical Center	Joshua Tree	73%	26
Pioneers Memorial Healthcare District	Brawley	73%	51
Parkview Comm Hosp Med Ctr	Riverside	71%	75
Saint Francis Medical Center[2]	Lynwood	68%	111
Hemet Valley Medical Center[2]	Hemet	67%	96
San Gorgonio Memorial Hospital	Banning	66%	29
Paradise Valley Hospital	National City	63%	51
Beverly Hospital	Montebello	60%	93
Menifee Valley Medical Center	Sun City	57%	53
Pacific Alliance Medical Center	Los Angeles	56%	54
San Dimas Community Hospital	San Dimas	54%	26
Victor Valley Global Medical Center	Victorville	49%	51
USC Verdugo Hills Hospital	Glendale	47%	49
Chinese Hospital	San Francisco	44%	39
La Palma Intercommunity Hospital	La Palma	42%	31

Written Stroke Educational Materials Given

Hospital Name	City	Rate	Cases
Barstow Community Hospital	Barstow	100%	29
Cedars - Sinai Medical Center	Los Angeles	100%	197
Dameron Hospital	Stockton	100%	32
Garfield Medical Center	Monterey Park	100%	61
Glendale Adventist Medical Center	Glendale	100%	98
Hoag Memorial Hospital Presbyterian	Newport Beach	100%	227
Hollywood Presbyterian Medical Center	Los Angeles	100%	54
Kaiser Foundation Hospital - Antioch[2]	Antioch	100%	54
Kaiser Fdn Hosp-Fremont/Hayward[2]	Hayward	100%	44
Kaiser Foundation Hospital - Redwood City[2]	Redwood City	100%	75
Kaiser Foundation Hospital - San Diego[2]	San Diego	100%	78
Kaiser Foundation Hospital - Santa Clara[2]	Santa Clara	100%	92
Kaiser Foundation Hospital - South Bay[2]	Harbor City	100%	52
Kaiser Fdn Hosp-S San Francisco[2]	S San Francisco	100%	46
Kaiser Fdn Hosp-Woodland Hills[2]	Woodland Hills	100%	66
Long Beach Memorial Medical Center[2]	Long Beach	100%	46
Los Alamitos Medical Center	Los Alamitos	100%	77
Los Robles Hospital & Medical Center[2]	Thousand Oaks	100%	45
Mercy Hospital	Bakersfield	100%	72
Mercy Hospital of Folsom	Folsom	100%	32
Methodist Hospital of Sacramento	Sacramento	100%	106
Mills - Peninsula Medical Center	Burlingame	100%	102
O'Connor Hospital[2]	San Jose	100%	47
Orange Coast Memorial Medical Center	Fountain Valley	100%	50
Oroville Hospital[2]	Oroville	100%	40
Palomar Health Downtown Campus[2]	Escondido	100%	56
Riverside Community Hospital[2]	Riverside	100%	45
Riverside County Regional Medical Center	Moreno Valley	100%	88
Saint Joseph Hospital	Orange	100%	100
Saint Mary's Medical Center	San Francisco	100%	30
Salinas Valley Memorial Hospital[2]	Salinas	100%	54
San Gabriel Valley Medical Center	San Gabriel	100%	26
San Joaquin Community Hospital[2]	Bakersfield	100%	63
San Ramon Regional Medical Center	San Ramon	100%	39
Scripps Memorial Hospital - Encinitas	Encinitas	100%	71
Scripps Memorial Hospital La Jolla	La Jolla	100%	92
Scripps Mercy Hospital	San Diego	100%	173
Shasta Regional Medical Center	Redding	100%	60
Sierra Nevada Memorial Hospital	Grass Valley	100%	26
Sonora Regional Medical Center	Sonora	100%	35
Sutter Auburn Faith Hospital	Auburn	100%	31
Temple Community Hospital	Los Angeles	100%	30
Tri - City Medical Center	Oceanside	100%	103
Ventura County Medical Center	Ventura	100%	43
West Hills Hospital & Medical Center[2]	West Hills	100%	52
White Memorial Medical Center	Los Angeles	100%	81
Bakersfield Memorial Hospital	Bakersfield	99%	79
El Camino Hospital	Mountain View	99%	70
Good Samaritan Hospital[2]	San Jose	99%	70
Kaiser Foundation Hospital[2]	San Rafael	99%	70
Kaiser Fdn Hosp-Oakland/Richmond[2]	Oakland	99%	69
Kaiser Fdn Hosp-Orange Co-Anaheim[2]	Anaheim	99%	75
Kaiser Foundation Hospital - San Jose[2]	San Jose	99%	81
Kaiser Fdn Hosp S Sacramento[2]	Sacramento	99%	78
Methodist Hospital of Southern California	Arcadia	99%	120
San Antonio Community Hospital	Upland	99%	88
Scripps Green Hospital	La Jolla	99%	70
Comm Hosp of the Monterey Peninsula	Monterey	98%	94
Community Regional Medical Center[2]	Fresno	98%	255
Doctors Medical Center	Modesto	98%	130
Kaiser Foundation Hospital - Baldwin Park[2]	Baldwin Park	98%	80
Marshall Medical Center	Placerville	98%	42
Regional Medical Center of San Jose[2]	San Jose	98%	52
Saint Mary Medical Center	Apple Valley	98%	98
San Joaquin General Hospital	French Camp	98%	63
CA Pacific Med Ctr-Davies Campus	San Francisco	97%	91
Clovis Community Medical Center[2]	Clovis	97%	60
Doctors Medical Center - San Pablo	San Pablo	97%	59
Eisenhower Medical Center	Rancho Mirage	97%	221
Grossmont Hospital	La Mesa	97%	238
Kaiser Fdn Hosp-Panorama City[2]	Panorama City	97%	65
Kaiser Foundation Hospital - Riverside[2]	Riverside	97%	62
Kaiser Foundation Hospital - Roseville[2]	Roseville	97%	73
Kaiser Foundation Hospital - Walnut Creek[2]	Walnut Creek	97%	61
Mercy San Juan Medical Center	Carmichael	97%	205
Pomona Valley Hospital Medical Center[2]	Pomona	97%	75
Presbyterian Intercommunity Hospital[2]	Whittier	97%	103
Saint Jude Medical Center	Fullerton	97%	113
Saint Vincent Medical Center	Los Angeles	97%	33
Sutter Medical Center of Santa Rosa	Santa Rosa	97%	32
Torrance Memorial Medical Center	Torrance	97%	141
Kaiser Foundation Hospital & Rehab Center[2]	Vallejo	96%	80
Kaiser Foundation Hospital - Fresno[2]	Fresno	96%	71
Kaiser Fdn Hosp-San Francisco[2]	San Francisco	96%	71
Saint Francis Memorial Hospital	San Francisco	96%	25
Sharp Memorial Hospital	San Diego	96%	159
Watsonville Community Hospital	Watsonville	96%	27
Antelope Valley Hospital	Lancaster	95%	117
CA Pacific Med Ctr-Pacific Campus Hosp	San Francisco	95%	93
Desert Regional Medical Center	Palm Springs	95%	164
Dominican Hospital	Santa Cruz	95%	41
Fountain Valley Reg Hosp & Med Ctr	Fountain Valley	95%	108
Kaiser Foundation Hospital - Downey[2]	Downey	95%	77
Kaiser Foundation Hospital - Sacramento[2]	Sacramento	95%	81
Saint Mary Medical Center	Long Beach	95%	37
Arrowhead Regional Medical Center	Colton	94%	158
Henry Mayo Newhall Memorial Hospital	Valencia	94%	81
Kaiser Foundation Hospital - West La[2]	Los Angeles	94%	71
Saint Johns Regional Medical Center	Oxnard	94%	63
Sierra Vista Regional Medical Center	San Luis Obispo	94%	32
Stanford Hospital	Stanford	94%	163
Citrus Valley Medical Center - IC Campus	Covina	93%	138
Kaiser Foundation Hospital - Vacaville	Vacaville	93%	45
Lakewood Regional Medical Center	Lakewood	93%	86
Mercy Medical Center - Redding	Redding	93%	89
Northridge Hospital Medical Center	Northridge	93%	87
Providence Saint Joseph Medical Center	Burbank	93%	150
Saddleback Memorial Medical Center	Laguna Hills	93%	86
Saint Joseph's Medical Center of Stockton[2]	Stockton	93%	45
Santa Barbara Cottage Hospital	Santa Barbara	93%	168
Sutter Amador Hospital	Jackson	93%	28
Sutter Roseville Medical Center	Roseville	93%	104
Sutter Solano Medical Center	Vallejo	93%	29
Univ of CA San Diego Med Ctr	San Diego	93%	121
Enloe Medical Center	Chico	92%	87
John Muir Medical Center - Concord Campus	Concord	92%	77
Kaiser Foundation Hospital - Manteca[2]	Manteca	92%	36
LAC/Rancho Los Amigos Ntl Rehab Ctr[2]	Downey	92%	62
Mercy General Hospital	Sacramento	92%	125
Providence Saint John's Health Center	Santa Monica	92%	36
Kaiser Foundation Hospital - Fontana[2]	Fontana	91%	64
Pomerado Hospital[2]	Poway	91%	34
Santa Rosa Memorial Hospital[2]	Santa Rosa	91%	70
Sharp Chula Vista Medical Center	Chula Vista	91%	102
Southwest Healthcare System[2]	Murrieta	91%	74
California Hosp Med Ctr Los Angeles	Los Angeles	90%	72
Kaiser Foundation Hospital - Santa Rosa[2]	Santa Rosa	90%	41
Prov Little Co of Mary Med Ctr Torrance	Torrance	90%	106
Redlands Community Hospital	Redlands	90%	58
Seton Medical Center[2]	Daly City	90%	50
Sutter General Hospital	Sacramento	90%	174
Whittier Hospital Medical Center	Whittier	90%	29
Contra Costa Regional Medical Center	Martinez	89%	36
Rideout Memorial Hospital	Marysville	89%	87
San Francisco General Hospital[2]	San Francisco	89%	45
Marin General Hospital	Greenbrae	88%	51
Ronald Reagan UCLA Medical Center[2]	Los Angeles	88%	52
Valley Presbyterian Hospital	Van Nuys	88%	60
Memorial Medical Center	Modesto	87%	117
Saint Agnes Medical Center[2]	Fresno	87%	77
Western Medical Center Santa Ana	Santa Ana	87%	55
PIH Hospital - Downey	Downey	86%	66
Huntington Memorial Hospital	Pasadena	85%	131
Centinela Hospital Medical Center[2]	Inglewood	84%	56
Kaiser Fdn Hosp-Moreno Valley	Moreno Valley	84%	32
Northbay Medical Center	Fairfield	84%	69
Sequoia Hospital	Redwood City	84%	37
Alta Bates Summit Medical Center	Oakland	83%	75
John Muir Med Ctr-Walnut Creek Campus	Walnut Creek	83%	119
Kaiser Foundation Hospital - Los Angeles[2]	Los Angeles	83%	81
Mercy Medical Center	Merced	82%	50
Simi Valley Hosp & Health Care Svcs	Simi Valley	82%	38
Ahmc Anaheim Regional Medical Center	Anaheim	81%	62
Kaweah Delta Medical Center[2]	Visalia	81%	47
Saint Johns Pleasant Valley Hospital	Camarillo	81%	27
Good Samaritan Hospital[2]	Los Angeles	80%	40
Washington Hospital	Fremont	80%	89
Feather River Hospital	Paradise	79%	34
Twin Cities Community Hospital	Templeton	79%	39
Keck Hospital of USC[2]	Los Angeles	77%	69
Providence Tarzana Medical Center	Tarzana	77%	53

NOTE: Hospital profiles are in alphabetical order by state, then city, then hospital within the city; Rankings exclude hospitals with less than 25 cases except for patient surveys which excludes hospitals with less than 100 cases; (a) 100-299 cases; (1) The number of cases/patients is too few to report; (2) Data submitted were based on a sample of cases/patients; (3) Results are based on a shorter time period than required; (4) Data suppressed by CMS for one or more quarters; (5) Results are not available for this reporting period; (6) Fewer than 100 patients completed the HCAHPS survey; (7) No cases met the criteria for this measure; (8) The lower limit of the confidence interval cannot be calculated if the number of observed infections equals zero; (9) No data are available from the state/territory for this reporting period; (10) The scores shown reflect fewer than 50 completed surveys; (11) There were discrepancies in the data collection process; (12) This measure does not apply to this hospital for this reporting period; (13) Results cannot be calculated for this reporting period; (14) The results for this state are combined with nearby states to protect confidentiality; Please refer to the User's Guide for a full explanation of data.

Hospital Name	City	Rate	Cases
Santa Clara Valley Medical Center[2]	San Jose	77%	86
Sierra View District Hospital	Porterville	77%	30
UCSF Medical Center[2]	San Francisco	77%	61
Palmdale Regional Medical Center	Palmdale	76%	55
Adventist Medical Center	Hanford	75%	60
Alvarado Hospital Medical Center	San Diego	74%	38
Mission Hospital Regional Medical Center	Mission Viejo	74%	111
Univ of California Irvine Med Ctr	Orange	74%	136
Saint Joseph Hospital	Eureka	72%	46
Emanuel Medical Center	Turlock	70%	33
Pacific Alliance Medical Center	Los Angeles	70%	30
Providence Holy Cross Medical Center	Mission Hills	67%	94
Santa Monica-UCLA Med Ctr & Ortho Hosp	Santa Monica	66%	35
Loma Linda University Medical Center[2]	Loma Linda	65%	124
Eden Medical Center	Castro Valley	64%	118
Alta Bates Summit Medical Center	Berkeley	63%	71
Univ of CA Davis Med Ctr[2]	Sacramento	63%	65
Bakersfield Heart Hospital	Bakersfield	62%	32
Desert Valley Hospital	Victorville	61%	85
Marian Regional Medical Center	Santa Maria	60%	62
Glendale Mem Hosp & Health Ctr	Glendale	58%	36
Paradise Valley Hospital	National City	58%	26
Beverly Hospital	Montebello	57%	44
Comm Mem Hosp San Buenaventura	Ventura	57%	88
Victor Valley Global Medical Center	Victorville	52%	40
LAC/Harbor - UCLA Medical Center[2]	Torrance	48%	85
Sutter Delta Medical Center	Antioch	45%	44
Hemet Valley Medical Center[2]	Hemet	42%	48
Corona Regional Medical Center	Corona	41%	29
Saint Francis Medical Center[2]	Lynwood	38%	56
Loma Linda Univ Med Ctr-Murrieta	Murrieta	37%	60
Parkview Comm Hosp Med Ctr	Riverside	26%	39
Saint Bernardine Medical Center	San Bernardino	22%	63
LAC/Olive View - UCLA Medical Center	Sylmar	20%	65
Pioneers Memorial Healthcare District	Brawley	14%	28
LAC+USC Medical Center[2]	Los Angeles	4%	47
El Centro Regional Medical Center[2]	El Centro	2%	63
Alameda County Medical Center	Oakland	0%	41

Surgical Care Improvement Project

Appropriate Beta Blocker Usage

Hospital Name	City	Rate	Cases
Community Regional Medical Center[2]	Fresno	100%	491
Corona Regional Medical Center[2]	Corona	100%	43
Desert Valley Hospital[2]	Victorville	100%	39
Doctors Medical Center[2]	Modesto	100%	353
Emanuel Medical Center	Turlock	100%	105
Frank R Howard Memorial Hospital	Willits	100%	45
Fresno Heart & Surgical Hospital[2]	Fresno	100%	225
Fresno VA Med Ctr-VA Central CA[2]	Fresno	100%	29
Garden Grove Hospital & Medical Center	Garden Grove	100%	31
John Muir Medical Center - Concord Campus[2]	Concord	100%	250
John Muir Med Ctr-Walnut Creek Campus[2]	Walnut Creek	100%	100
Kaiser Foundation Hospital[2]	San Rafael	100%	96
Kaiser Foundation Hospital - Antioch[2]	Antioch	100%	124
Kaiser Fdn Hosp-Fremont/Hayward[2]	Hayward	100%	164
Kaiser Foundation Hospital - Manteca[2]	Manteca	100%	139
Kaiser Fdn Hosp-Oakland/Richmond[2]	Oakland	100%	98
Kaiser Fdn Hosp-Panorama City[2]	Panorama City	100%	128
Kaiser Foundation Hospital - Redwood City[2]	Redwood City	100%	109
Kaiser Foundation Hospital - Santa Clara[2]	Santa Clara	100%	260
Kaiser Foundation Hospital - South Bay[2]	Harbor City	100%	128
Kaiser Foundation Hospital - Vacaville[2]	Vacaville	100%	107
Kaiser Foundation Hospital - Walnut Creek[2]	Walnut Creek	100%	152
Loma Linda VA Medical Center[2]	Loma Linda	100%	129
Marin General Hospital[2]	Greenbrae	100%	119
Mark Twain Medical Center[2]	San Andreas	100%	27
Marshall Medical Center[2]	Placerville	100%	87
Memorial Medical Center[2]	Modesto	100%	218
Mercy Hospital of Folsom[2]	Folsom	100%	79
Providence Holy Cross Medical Center[2]	Mission Hills	100%	181
Providence Saint John's Health Center[2]	Santa Monica	100%	113
Providence Saint Joseph Medical Center[2]	Burbank	100%	149
Ronald Reagan UCLA Medical Center[2]	Los Angeles	100%	146
Saint Francis Memorial Hospital[2]	San Francisco	100%	54
Saint Joseph's Medical Center of Stockton[2]	Stockton	100%	218
Salinas Valley Memorial Hospital[2]	Salinas	100%	137
San Antonio Community Hospital[2]	Upland	100%	229
San Francisco General Hospital[2]	San Francisco	100%	56
Santa Monica-UCLA Med Ctr & Ortho Hosp[2]	Santa Monica	100%	80
Scripps Memorial Hospital - Encinitas[2]	Encinitas	100%	90
Scripps Memorial Hospital La Jolla[2]	La Jolla	100%	251
Scripps Mercy Hospital[2]	San Diego	100%	249
Sierra View District Hospital	Porterville	100%	37
Sierra Vista Regional Medical Center	San Luis Obispo	100%	96
Sonora Regional Medical Center	Sonora	100%	100
Southwest Healthcare System[2]	Murrieta	100%	113
Stanford Hospital[2]	Stanford	100%	220
Sutter Davis Hospital[2]	Davis	100%	44
Sutter General Hospital[2]	Sacramento	100%	299
Sutter Maternity & Surgery Ctr	Santa Cruz	100%	44
Sutter Surgical Hospital - North Valley	Yuba City	100%	57
USC Verdugo Hills Hospital[2]	Glendale	100%	44
VA Long Beach Healthcare System[2]	Long Beach	100%	81
VA Northern California Healthcare System[2]	Mather	100%	59
VA San Diego Healthcare System[2]	San Diego	100%	182
Valleycare Medical Center	Pleasanton	100%	206
Watsonville Community Hospital	Watsonville	100%	45
West Anaheim Medical Center	Anaheim	100%	28
Woodland Memorial Hospital[2]	Woodland	100%	54
Dameron Hospital	Stockton	99%	190
Dominican Hospital[2]	Santa Cruz	99%	121
El Camino Hospital[2]	Mountain View	99%	344
Fallbrook Hospital	Fallbrook	99%	84
Garfield Medical Center[2]	Monterey Park	99%	86
Grossmont Hospital[2]	La Mesa	99%	379
Hoag Orthopedic Institute[2]	Irvine	99%	165
John F Kennedy Memorial Hospital[2]	Indio	99%	143
Kaiser Foundation Hospital & Rehab Center[2]	Vallejo	99%	144
Kaiser Foundation Hospital - Baldwin Park[2]	Baldwin Park	99%	136
Kaiser Foundation Hospital - Fontana[2]	Fontana	99%	128
Kaiser Fdn Hosp-Orange Co-Anaheim[2]	Anaheim	99%	174
Kaiser Foundation Hospital - Roseville[2]	Roseville	99%	124
Kaiser Foundation Hospital - San Diego[2]	San Diego	99%	134
Kaiser Fdn Hosp-San Francisco[2]	San Francisco	99%	283
Kaiser Foundation Hospital - San Jose[2]	San Jose	99%	126
Kaiser Fdn Hosp-Woodland Hills[2]	Woodland Hills	99%	117
Kaiser Fdn Hosp S Sacramento[2]	Sacramento	99%	110
LAC/Harbor - UCLA Medical Center[2]	Torrance	99%	133
Long Beach Memorial Medical Center[2]	Long Beach	99%	246
Los Alamitos Medical Center[2]	Los Alamitos	99%	152
Mercy Hospital[2]	Bakersfield	99%	98
Palmdale Regional Medical Center[2]	Palmdale	99%	69
Prov Little Co of Mary Med Ctr Torrance[2]	Torrance	99%	148
Providence Tarzana Medical Center[2]	Tarzana	99%	143
Redlands Community Hospital[2]	Redlands	99%	280
Riverside Community Hospital[2]	Riverside	99%	225
Saint Helena Hospital	Saint Helena	99%	298
Saint Mary Medical Center	Apple Valley	99%	237
Saint Vincent Medical Center[2]	Los Angeles	99%	217
Scripps Green Hospital[2]	La Jolla	99%	183
Sharp Coronado Hosp & Healthcare Ctr	Coronado	99%	327
Sharp Memorial Hospital[2]	San Diego	99%	476
Shasta Regional Medical Center	Redding	99%	144
Sutter Auburn Faith Hospital[2]	Auburn	99%	95
Sutter Medical Center of Santa Rosa[2]	Santa Rosa	99%	131
Torrance Memorial Medical Center[2]	Torrance	99%	237
Tri - City Medical Center[2]	Oceanside	99%	154
UCSF Medical Center[2]	San Francisco	99%	139
Univ of CA Davis Med Ctr[2]	Sacramento	99%	153
Washington Hospital[2]	Fremont	99%	167
West Hills Hospital & Medical Center[2]	West Hills	99%	114
Alta Bates Summit Medical Center[2]	Oakland	98%	236
CA Pacific Med Ctr-Pacific Campus Hosp[2]	San Francisco	98%	200
Cedars - Sinai Medical Center	Los Angeles	98%	1081
Centinela Hospital Medical Center[2]	Inglewood	98%	42
Desert Regional Medical Center[2]	Palm Springs	98%	160
Doctors Medical Center - San Pablo[2]	San Pablo	98%	65
Eden Medical Center[2]	Castro Valley	98%	113
Eisenhower Medical Center	Rancho Mirage	98%	488
Feather River Hospital[2]	Paradise	98%	92
Fountain Valley Reg Hosp & Med Ctr[2]	Fountain Valley	98%	198
French Hospital Medical Center[2]	San Luis Obispo	98%	156
Glendale Adventist Medical Center[2]	Glendale	98%	305
Glendale Mem Hosp & Health Ctr[2]	Glendale	98%	218
Good Samaritan Hospital[2]	San Jose	98%	212
Hoag Memorial Hospital Presbyterian[2]	Newport Beach	98%	247
Kaiser Foundation Hospital - Downey[2]	Downey	98%	132
Kaiser Foundation Hospital - Fresno[2]	Fresno	98%	160
Kaiser Foundation Hospital - Los Angeles[2]	Los Angeles	98%	261
Kaiser Foundation Hospital - Sacramento[2]	Sacramento	98%	122
Kaiser Foundation Hospital - Santa Rosa[2]	Santa Rosa	98%	131
Kaiser Foundation Hospital - West La[2]	Los Angeles	98%	129
Lodi Memorial Hospital[2]	Lodi	98%	86
Loma Linda University Medical Center[2]	Loma Linda	98%	250
Los Robles Hospital & Medical Center[2]	Thousand Oaks	98%	187
Mercy Medical Center - Redding[2]	Redding	98%	189
Methodist Hospital of Sacramento[2]	Sacramento	98%	63
Mills - Peninsula Medical Center[2]	Burlingame	98%	164
Northbay Medical Center	Fairfield	98%	119
O'Connor Hospital[2]	San Jose	98%	174
Olympia Medical Center	Los Angeles	98%	42
Orange Coast Memorial Medical Center[2]	Fountain Valley	98%	205
Placentia Linda Hospital[2]	Placentia	98%	131
Pomona Valley Hospital Medical Center[2]	Pomona	98%	191
Presbyterian Intercommunity Hospital[2]	Whittier	98%	134
Prov Little Co of Mary Med Ctr San Pedro[2]	San Pedro	98%	42
Queen of the Valley Medical Center[2]	Napa	98%	125
Riverside County Regional Medical Center[2]	Moreno Valley	98%	49
Saddleback Memorial Medical Center[2]	Laguna Hills	98%	126
Saint Johns Pleasant Valley Hospital[2]	Camarillo	98%	59
Saint Johns Regional Medical Center[2]	Oxnard	98%	176
Saint Joseph Hospital[2]	Orange	98%	175
Saint Mary's Medical Center[2]	San Francisco	98%	81
San Francisco VA Medical Center[2]	San Francisco	98%	216
San Gabriel Valley Medical Center[2]	San Gabriel	98%	52
San Joaquin Community Hospital[2]	Bakersfield	98%	247
Santa Rosa Memorial Hospital[2]	Santa Rosa	98%	87
Sequoia Hospital[2]	Redwood City	98%	155
Stanislaus Surgical Hospital[2]	Modesto	98%	41
Sutter Solano Medical Center[2]	Vallejo	98%	110
Sutter Tracy Community Hospital	Tracy	98%	45
Twin Cities Community Hospital	Templeton	98%	109
Univ of California Irvine Med Ctr[2]	Orange	98%	131
Univ of CA San Diego Med Ctr[2]	San Diego	98%	168
Bakersfield Memorial Hospital[2]	Bakersfield	97%	255
Citrus Valley Medical Center - IC Campus[2]	Covina	97%	252
Comm Hosp of the Monterey Peninsula	Monterey	97%	322
Doctors Hospital of Manteca	Manteca	97%	35
Good Samaritan Hospital[2]	Los Angeles	97%	180
Huntington Memorial Hospital[2]	Pasadena	97%	152
Kaiser Foundation Hospital - Riverside[2]	Riverside	97%	106
Kaiser Fdn Hosp-S San Francisco[2]	S San Francisco	97%	156
Keck Hospital of USC[2]	Los Angeles	97%	255
Marian Regional Medical Center[2]	Santa Maria	97%	179
Mercy General Hospital[2]	Sacramento	97%	242
Mercy Medical Center[2]	Merced	97%	124
Northridge Hospital Medical Center[2]	Northridge	97%	234
Rideout Memorial Hospital[2]	Marysville	97%	144
Saint Louise Regional Hospital[2]	Gilroy	97%	29
Saint Rose Hospital[2]	Hayward	97%	79
San Dimas Community Hospital[2]	San Dimas	97%	59
San Gorgonio Memorial Hospital	Banning	97%	72
San Ramon Regional Medical Center[2]	San Ramon	97%	64
Antelope Valley Hospital[2]	Lancaster	96%	189
Clovis Community Medical Center[2]	Clovis	96%	114
Enloe Medical Center[2]	Chico	96%	219
Henry Mayo Newhall Memorial Hospital[2]	Valencia	96%	107
Kaweah Delta Medical Center[2]	Visalia	96%	200
LAC+USC Medical Center[2]	Los Angeles	96%	153
Lakewood Regional Medical Center[2]	Lakewood	96%	192
Mission Community Hospital	Panorama City	96%	26
Mission Hospital Regional Medical Center[2]	Mission Viejo	96%	139
Palomar Health Downtown Campus[2]	Escondido	96%	83
Santa Barbara Cottage Hospital[2]	Santa Barbara	96%	110
Sharp Chula Vista Medical Center[2]	Chula Vista	96%	161
Southern California Hospital at Hollywood	Hollywood	96%	25
Western Medical Center Hospital Anaheim	Anaheim	96%	51
Barton Memorial Hospital	S Lake Tahoe	95%	40
California Hosp Med Ctr Los Angeles[2]	Los Angeles	95%	64
Chapman Medical Center	Orange	95%	39
Foothill Presbyterian Hospital[2]	Glendora	95%	65
Fresno Surgical Hospital[2]	Fresno	95%	111
Mercy San Juan Medical Center[2]	Carmichael	95%	237
Pacific Alliance Medical Center[2]	Los Angeles	95%	41
Saint Agnes Medical Center[2]	Fresno	95%	259
Santa Clara Valley Medical Center[2]	San Jose	95%	154
Sutter Delta Medical Center[2]	Antioch	95%	59
VA Greater Los Angeles Healthcare System[2]	W Los Angeles	95%	172
Alta Bates Summit Medical Center[2]	Berkeley	94%	89
Arrowhead Regional Medical Center	Colton	94%	79
Bakersfield Heart Hospital[2]	Bakersfield	94%	87
CA Pacific Med Ctr-St Luke's Campus[2]	San Francisco	94%	34
Madera Community Hospital	Madera	94%	31
Palo Alto VA Medical Center[2]	Palo Alto	94%	163
Regional Medical Center of San Jose[2]	San Jose	94%	118
San Mateo Medical Center	San Mateo	94%	36
Sutter Roseville Medical Center[2]	Roseville	94%	117
White Memorial Medical Center[2]	Los Angeles	94%	181
Alvarado Hospital Medical Center	San Diego	93%	145
Comm Mem Hosp San Buenaventura[2]	Ventura	93%	152
Goleta Valley Cottage Hospital[2]	Santa Barbara	93%	56
Methodist Hospital of Southern California[2]	Arcadia	93%	145
Novato Community Hospital	Novato	93%	29
Saint Mary Medical Center[2]	Long Beach	93%	55
Sutter Lakeside Hospital	Lakeport	93%	42
Ahmc Anaheim Regional Medical Center[2]	Anaheim	92%	142
Oroville Hospital[2]	Oroville	92%	79
Saint Bernardine Medical Center[2]	San Bernardino	92%	210
Saint Jude Medical Center[2]	Fullerton	92%	126
Sierra Nevada Memorial Hospital[2]	Grass Valley	92%	64
Ukiah Valley Medical Center	Ukiah	92%	26
Ventura County Medical Center[2]	Ventura	92%	53
Loma Linda Univ Med Ctr-Murrieta[2]	Murrieta	91%	147
Parkview Comm Hosp Med Ctr[2]	Riverside	91%	110
Saint Francis Medical Center[2]	Lynwood	91%	78
Victor Valley Global Medical Center[2]	Victorville	91%	67
Beverly Hospital	Montebello	90%	78
Menifee Valley Medical Center[2]	Sun City	90%	70
Mercy Medical Center - Mount Shasta[2]	Mount Shasta	90%	40
PIH Hospital - Downey[2]	Downey	90%	156

NOTE: Hospital profiles are in alphabetical order by state, then city, then hospital within the city; Rankings exclude hospitals with less than 25 cases except for patient surveys which excludes hospitals with less than 100 cases; (a) 100-299 cases; (1) The number of cases/patients is too few to report; (2) Data submitted were based on a sample of cases/patients; (3) Results are based on a shorter time period than required; (4) Data suppressed by CMS for one or more quarters; (5) Results are not available for this reporting period; (6) Fewer than 100 patients completed the HCAHPS survey; (7) No cases met the criteria for this measure; (8) The lower limit of the confidence interval cannot be calculated if the number of observed infections equals zero; (9) No data are available from the state/territory for this reporting period; (10) The scores shown reflect fewer than 50 completed surveys; (11) There were discrepancies in the data collection process; (12) This measure does not apply to this hospital for this reporting period; (13) Results cannot be calculated for this reporting period; (14) The results for this state are combined with nearby states to protect confidentiality; Please refer to the User's Guide for a full explanation of data.

Seton Medical Center[2]	Daly City	90%	93
Valley Presbyterian Hospital[2]	Van Nuys	90%	154
Western Medical Center Santa Ana	Santa Ana	90%	82
Palm Drive Hospital[2]	Sebastopol	88%	26
Saint Joseph Hospital[2]	Eureka	88%	97
Whittier Hospital Medical Center	Whittier	88%	40
Alameda County Medical Center	Oakland	87%	38
Marina Del Rey Hospital[2]	Marina Del Rey	87%	46
Simi Valley Hosp & Health Care Svcs[2]	Simi Valley	87%	67
Alameda Hospital	Alameda	86%	35
Hi - Desert Medical Center	Joshua Tree	86%	28
Saint Elizabeth Community Hospital[2]	Red Bluff	86%	37
Kern Medical Center[2]	Bakersfield	85%	26
Tahoe Forest Hospital	Truckee	85%	33
Lompoc Valley Medical Center	Lompoc	83%	41
Adventist Medical Center[2]	Hanford	82%	65
Hemet Valley Medical Center[2]	Hemet	82%	66
Pomerado Hospital[2]	Poway	82%	57
San Joaquin General Hospital	French Camp	81%	48
Pioneers Memorial Healthcare District	Brawley	77%	30
Hollywood Presbyterian Medical Center[2]	Los Angeles	75%	40
El Centro Regional Medical Center[2]	El Centro	67%	52
Chinese Hospital	San Francisco	60%	42
LAC/Rancho Los Amigos Ntl Rehab Ctr[2]	Downey	37%	35

Appropriate VTP Within 24 Hours

Hospital Name	City	Rate	Cases
California Hosp Med Ctr Los Angeles[2]	Los Angeles	100%	349
Chino Valley Medical Center	Chino	100%	40
Dameron Hospital	Stockton	100%	610
Desert Valley Hospital[2]	Victorville	100%	153
East Los Angeles Doctors Hospital	Los Angeles	100%	53
Garden Grove Hospital & Medical Center	Garden Grove	100%	154
Garfield Medical Center[2]	Monterey Park	100%	225
Huntington Beach Hospital	Huntington Bch	100%	34
Kaiser Foundation Hospital[2]	San Rafael	100%	343
Kaiser Foundation Hospital - Antioch[2]	Antioch	100%	381
Kaiser Foundation Hospital - Baldwin Park[2]	Baldwin Park	100%	378
Kaiser Foundation Hospital - Fontana[2]	Fontana	100%	372
Kaiser Fdn Hosp-Fremont/Hayward[2]	Hayward	100%	429
Kaiser Foundation Hospital - Fresno[2]	Fresno	100%	334
Kaiser Foundation Hospital - Los Angeles[2]	Los Angeles	100%	425
Kaiser Foundation Hospital - Manteca[2]	Manteca	100%	358
Kaiser Fdn Hosp-Moreno Valley[2]	Moreno Valley	100%	102
Kaiser Fdn Hosp-Orange Co-Anaheim[2]	Anaheim	100%	497
Kaiser Fdn Hosp-Panorama City[2]	Panorama City	100%	378
Kaiser Foundation Hospital - Redwood City[2]	Redwood City	100%	350
Kaiser Foundation Hospital - Roseville[2]	Roseville	100%	373
Kaiser Foundation Hospital - Sacramento[2]	Sacramento	100%	423
Kaiser Foundation Hospital - San Diego[2]	San Diego	100%	358
Kaiser Foundation Hospital - San Jose[2]	San Jose	100%	374
Kaiser Foundation Hospital - Santa Clara[2]	Santa Clara	100%	350
Kaiser Foundation Hospital - Santa Rosa[2]	Santa Rosa	100%	368
Kaiser Foundation Hospital - South Bay[2]	Harbor City	100%	379
Kaiser Foundation Hospital - Vacaville[2]	Vacaville	100%	289
Kaiser Foundation Hospital - West La[2]	Los Angeles	100%	303
Kaiser Fdn Hosp-Woodland Hills[2]	Woodland Hills	100%	318
La Palma Intercommunity Hospital	La Palma	100%	42
Memorial Medical Center[2]	Modesto	100%	446
Mercy Medical Center - Mount Shasta[2]	Mount Shasta	100%	66
Mills - Peninsula Medical Center[2]	Burlingame	100%	426
Mission Community Hospital	Panorama City	100%	137
Montclair Hospital Medical Center	Montclair	100%	27
Oak Valley District Hospital	Oakdale	100%	34
Paradise Valley Hospital	National City	100%	65
Patients' Hospital of Redding	Redding	100%	47
Placentia Linda Hospital[2]	Placentia	100%	475
Prov Little Co of Mary Med Ctr Torrance[2]	Torrance	100%	447
Providence Saint John's Health Center[2]	Santa Monica	100%	347
Riverside Community Hospital[2]	Riverside	100%	460
Ronald Reagan UCLA Medical Center[2]	Los Angeles	100%	290
Saint Mary Medical Center	Apple Valley	100%	515
Saint Mary Medical Center[2]	Long Beach	100%	160
Salinas Valley Memorial Hospital[2]	Salinas	100%	322
San Gabriel Valley Medical Center[2]	San Gabriel	100%	277
Santa Monica-UCLA Med Ctr & Ortho Hosp[2]	Santa Monica	100%	279
Scripps Green Hospital[2]	La Jolla	100%	438
Sherman Oaks Hospital	Sherman Oaks	100%	107
Sutter Maternity & Surgery Ctr	Santa Cruz	100%	224
Sutter Tracy Community Hospital	Tracy	100%	147
Temple Community Hospital	Los Angeles	100%	40
UCSF Medical Center[2]	San Francisco	100%	403
VA San Diego Healthcare System[2]	San Diego	100%	260
West Anaheim Medical Center	Anaheim	100%	95
Woodland Memorial Hospital[2]	Woodland	100%	219
Alta Bates Summit Medical Center[2]	Berkeley	99%	406
Antelope Valley Hospital[2]	Lancaster	99%	719
Bakersfield Memorial Hospital[2]	Bakersfield	99%	434
Barton Memorial Hospital	S Lake Tahoe	99%	225
Centinela Hospital Medical Center[2]	Inglewood	99%	144
Community Hospital of San Bernardino[2]	San Bernardino	99%	107
Doctors Medical Center[2]	Modesto	99%	736
Dominican Hospital[2]	Santa Cruz	99%	382
Eden Medical Center[2]	Castro Valley	99%	394
El Camino Hospital[2]	Mountain View	99%	912
Fallbrook Hospital	Fallbrook	99%	307
Feather River Hospital[2]	Paradise	99%	296
French Hospital Medical Center[2]	San Luis Obispo	99%	297
Fresno Surgical Hospital[2]	Fresno	99%	324
Good Samaritan Hospital[2]	San Jose	99%	470
Grossmont Hospital[2]	La Mesa	99%	818
Hoag Orthopedic Institute[2]	Irvine	99%	576
John F Kennedy Memorial Hospital[2]	Indio	99%	604
John Muir Medical Center - Concord Campus[2]	Concord	99%	344
Kaiser Foundation Hospital & Rehab Center[2]	Vallejo	99%	342
Kaiser Foundation Hospital - Downey[2]	Downey	99%	349
Kaiser Foundation Hospital - Riverside[2]	Riverside	99%	398
Kaiser Fdn Hosp-San Francisco[2]	San Francisco	99%	379
Kaiser Fdn Hosp-S San Francisco[2]	S San Francisco	99%	351
Kaiser Foundation Hospital - Walnut Creek[2]	Walnut Creek	99%	391
Keck Hospital of USC[2]	Los Angeles	99%	582
LAC/Olive View - UCLA Medical Center[2]	Sylmar	99%	192
Loma Linda University Medical Center[2]	Loma Linda	99%	427
Loma Linda VA Medical Center[2]	Loma Linda	99%	321
Los Alamitos Medical Center[2]	Los Alamitos	99%	639
Los Robles Hospital & Medical Center[2]	Thousand Oaks	99%	451
Marin General Hospital[2]	Greenbrae	99%	336
Mark Twain Medical Center[2]	San Andreas	99%	79
Marshall Medical Center[2]	Placerville	99%	287
Mercy General Hospital[2]	Sacramento	99%	390
Mercy Hospital[2]	Bakersfield	99%	416
Mercy Hospital of Folsom[2]	Folsom	99%	364
Mercy Medical Center[2]	Merced	99%	436
Mercy San Juan Medical Center[2]	Carmichael	99%	440
Monterey Park Hospital[2]	Monterey Park	99%	92
Novato Community Hospital	Novato	99%	141
Olympia Medical Center	Los Angeles	99%	173
Orange Coast Memorial Medical Center[2]	Fountain Valley	99%	555
Oroville Hospital[2]	Oroville	99%	288
Pacific Hospital of Long Beach[3]	Long Beach	99%	70
Palo Alto VA Medical Center[2]	Palo Alto	99%	395
Palomar Health Downtown Campus[2]	Escondido	99%	335
Pomona Valley Hospital Medical Center[2]	Pomona	99%	355
Presbyterian Intercommunity Hospital[2]	Whittier	99%	362
Providence Holy Cross Medical Center[2]	Mission Hills	99%	321
Providence Saint Joseph Medical Center[2]	Burbank	99%	307
Providence Tarzana Medical Center[2]	Tarzana	99%	281
Redlands Community Hospital[2]	Redlands	99%	921
Riverside County Regional Medical Center[2]	Moreno Valley	99%	273
Saddleback Memorial Medical Center[2]	Laguna Hills	99%	289
Saint Francis Memorial Hospital[2]	San Francisco	99%	255
Saint Vincent Medical Center[2]	Los Angeles	99%	597
San Francisco General Hospital[2]	San Francisco	99%	244
San Francisco VA Medical Center[2]	San Francisco	99%	339
San Gorgonio Memorial Hospital	Banning	99%	96
San Joaquin Community Hospital[2]	Bakersfield	99%	579
San Mateo Medical Center	San Mateo	99%	152
Scripps Memorial Hospital - Encinitas[2]	Encinitas	99%	404
Scripps Memorial Hospital La Jolla[2]	La Jolla	99%	479
Sequoia Hospital[2]	Redwood City	99%	339
Sharp Coronado Hosp & Healthcare Ctr	Coronado	99%	1216
Sharp Memorial Hospital[2]	San Diego	99%	1341
Shasta Regional Medical Center	Redding	99%	453
Sonoma Valley Hospital	Sonoma	99%	124
Sonora Regional Medical Center	Sonora	99%	359
Stanford Hospital[2]	Stanford	99%	590
Stanislaus Surgical Hospital[2]	Modesto	99%	179
Sutter Coast Hospital	Crescent City	99%	67
Sutter Lakeside Hospital	Lakeport	99%	165
Sutter Medical Center of Santa Rosa[2]	Santa Rosa	99%	327
Sutter Solano Medical Center[2]	Vallejo	99%	340
Torrance Memorial Medical Center[2]	Torrance	99%	775
Twin Cities Community Hospital	Templeton	99%	484
VA Greater Los Angeles Healthcare System[2]	W Los Angeles	99%	257
VA Long Beach Healthcare System[2]	Long Beach	99%	243
Watsonville Community Hospital	Watsonville	99%	198
West Hills Hospital & Medical Center[2]	West Hills	99%	343
Ahmc Anaheim Regional Medical Center[2]	Anaheim	98%	300
Alameda County Medical Center	Oakland	98%	363
Barstow Community Hospital	Barstow	98%	57
CA Pacific Med Ctr-Pacific Campus Hosp[2]	San Francisco	98%	452
Cedars - Sinai Medical Center	Los Angeles	98%	3322
Chapman Medical Center	Orange	98%	116
Community Hospital of Huntington Park	Huntington Park	98%	40
Comm Hosp of the Monterey Peninsula	Monterey	98%	820
Contra Costa Regional Medical Center[2]	Martinez	98%	140
Corona Regional Medical Center[2]	Corona	98%	189
Doctors Hospital of Manteca	Manteca	98%	118
Doctors Hospital of West Covina	West Covina	98%	54
Eisenhower Medical Center	Rancho Mirage	98%	1383
Enloe Medical Center[2]	Chico	98%	656
Fresno Heart & Surgical Hospital[2]	Fresno	98%	229
Glendale Adventist Medical Center[2]	Glendale	98%	583
Goleta Valley Cottage Hospital[2]	Santa Barbara	98%	297
Good Samaritan Hospital[2]	Los Angeles	98%	439
Henry Mayo Newhall Memorial Hospital[2]	Valencia	98%	314
Huntington Memorial Hospital[2]	Pasadena	98%	331
Kaiser Fdn Hosp-Oakland/Richmond[2]	Oakland	98%	389
Kaiser Fdn Hosp S Sacramento[2]	Sacramento	98%	322
LAC+USC Medical Center[2]	Los Angeles	98%	517
LAC/Harbor - UCLA Medical Center[2]	Torrance	98%	285
LAC/Rancho Los Amigos Ntl Rehab Ctr[2]	Downey	98%	206
Mercy Medical Center - Redding[2]	Redding	98%	399
Northern Inyo Hospital	Bishop	98%	51
O'Connor Hospital[2]	San Jose	98%	495
Ojai Valley Community Hospital	Ojai	98%	41
Pacific Alliance Medical Center[2]	Los Angeles	98%	190
Pomerado Hospital[2]	Poway	98%	279
Saint Francis Medical Center[2]	Lynwood	98%	250
Saint Johns Pleasant Valley Hospital[2]	Camarillo	98%	254
Saint Johns Regional Medical Center[2]	Oxnard	98%	381
Saint Joseph's Medical Center of Stockton[2]	Stockton	98%	338
Saint Jude Medical Center[2]	Fullerton	98%	390
Saint Mary's Medical Center[2]	San Francisco	98%	304
Santa Clara Valley Medical Center[2]	San Jose	98%	282
Scripps Mercy Hospital[2]	San Diego	98%	420
Sharp Chula Vista Medical Center[2]	Chula Vista	98%	305
Sierra Nevada Memorial Hospital[2]	Grass Valley	98%	266
Sierra View District Hospital	Porterville	98%	256
Sierra Vista Regional Medical Center	San Luis Obispo	98%	388
Southern California Hospital at Hollywood	Hollywood	98%	83
Southwest Healthcare System[2]	Murrieta	98%	440
Sutter Davis Hospital[2]	Davis	98%	181
Sutter Delta Medical Center[2]	Antioch	98%	193
Sutter General Hospital[2]	Sacramento	98%	429
Sutter Roseville Medical Center[2]	Roseville	98%	404
Sutter Surgical Hospital - North Valley	Yuba City	98%	280
Univ of California Irvine Med Ctr[2]	Orange	98%	335
Univ of CA San Diego Med Ctr[2]	San Diego	98%	324
Valley Presbyterian Hospital[2]	Van Nuys	98%	560
Valleycare Medical Center	Pleasanton	98%	537
Washington Hospital[2]	Fremont	98%	321
White Memorial Medical Center[2]	Los Angeles	98%	450
Whittier Hospital Medical Center	Whittier	98%	179
Alta Bates Summit Medical Center[2]	Oakland	97%	386
Arrowhead Regional Medical Center	Colton	97%	628
Citrus Valley Medical Center - IC Campus[2]	Covina	97%	675
Clovis Community Medical Center[2]	Clovis	97%	612
Coastal Communities Hospital	Santa Ana	97%	148
Comm Mem Hosp San Buenaventura[2]	Ventura	97%	300
Community Regional Medical Center[2]	Fresno	97%	1302
Delano Regional Medical Center[2]	Delano	97%	131
Hollywood Presbyterian Medical Center[2]	Los Angeles	97%	275
John Muir Med Ctr-Walnut Creek Campus[2]	Walnut Creek	97%	437
Mammoth Hospital	Mammoth Lakes	97%	60
Marina Del Rey Hospital[2]	Marina Del Rey	97%	179
Methodist Hospital of Sacramento[2]	Sacramento	97%	323
Northridge Hospital Medical Center[2]	Northridge	97%	728
Palmdale Regional Medical Center[2]	Palmdale	97%	364
Saint Elizabeth Community Hospital[2]	Red Bluff	97%	146
Saint Joseph Hospital[2]	Orange	97%	304
San Joaquin General Hospital	French Camp	97%	279
Santa Barbara Cottage Hospital[2]	Santa Barbara	97%	400
Seton Medical Center[2]	Daly City	97%	245
Sutter Auburn Faith Hospital[2]	Auburn	97%	322
Univ of CA Davis Med Ctr[2]	Sacramento	97%	337
Alameda Hospital	Alameda	96%	95
CA Pacific Med Ctr-Davies Campus[2]	San Francisco	96%	94
Desert Regional Medical Center[2]	Palm Springs	96%	321
Fountain Valley Reg Hosp & Med Ctr[2]	Fountain Valley	96%	452
Frank R Howard Memorial Hospital	Willits	96%	246
Glendale Mem Hosp & Health Ctr[2]	Glendale	96%	354
Hoag Memorial Hospital Presbyterian[2]	Newport Beach	96%	477
Kaweah Delta Medical Center[2]	Visalia	96%	425
Lakewood Regional Medical Center[2]	Lakewood	96%	405
Lodi Memorial Hospital[2]	Lodi	96%	261
Marian Regional Medical Center[2]	Santa Maria	96%	453
Memorial Hospital of Gardena	Gardena	96%	98
Mendocino Coast District Hospital	Fort Bragg	96%	54
Methodist Hospital of Southern California[2]	Arcadia	96%	445
Northbay Medical Center	Fairfield	96%	308
PIH Hospital - Downey[2]	Downey	96%	465
Saint Bernardine Medical Center[2]	San Bernardino	96%	409
Saint Rose Hospital[2]	Hayward	96%	257
San Ramon Regional Medical Center[2]	San Ramon	96%	213
Tri - City Medical Center[2]	Oceanside	96%	315
Tri - City Regional Medical Center	Hawaiian Grdns	96%	136
Tulare Regional Medical Center	Tulare	96%	109
USC Verdugo Hills Hospital[2]	Glendale	96%	272
Alhambra Hospital Medical Center	Alhambra	95%	137
Beverly Hospital	Montebello	95%	283
CA Pacific Med Ctr-St Luke's Campus[2]	San Francisco	95%	152
Emanuel Medical Center	Turlock	95%	304

NOTE: Hospital profiles are in alphabetical order by state, then city, then hospital within the city; Rankings exclude hospitals with less than 25 cases except for patient surveys which excludes hospitals with less than 100 cases; (a) 100-299 cases; (1) The number of cases/patients is too few to report; (2) Data submitted were based on a sample of cases/patients; (3) Results are based on a shorter time period than required; (4) Data suppressed by CMS for one or more quarters; (5) Results are not available for this reporting period; (6) Fewer than 100 patients completed the HCAHPS survey; (7) No cases met the criteria for this measure; (8) The lower limit of the confidence interval cannot be calculated if the number of observed infections equals zero; (9) No data are available from the state/territory for this reporting period; (10) The scores shown reflect fewer than 50 completed surveys; (11) There were discrepancies in the data collection process; (12) This measure does not apply to this hospital for this reporting period; (13) Results cannot be calculated for this reporting period; (14) The results for this state are combined with nearby states to protect confidentiality; Please refer to the User's Guide for a full explanation of data.

Foothill Presbyterian Hospital[2]	Glendora	95%	239
Fresno VA Med Ctr-VA Central CA[2]	Fresno	95%	59
Hazel Hawkins Memorial Hospital	Hollister	95%	62
Long Beach Memorial Medical Center[2]	Long Beach	95%	375
Los Angeles Community Hospital[2]	Los Angeles	95%	60
Menifee Valley Medical Center[2]	Sun City	95%	167
Mission Hospital Regional Medical Center[2]	Mission Viejo	95%	316
Palm Drive Hospital[2]	Sebastopol	95%	129
Queen of the Valley Medical Center[2]	Napa	95%	243
San Antonio Community Hospital[2]	Upland	95%	352
San Dimas Community Hospital[2]	San Dimas	95%	194
Tahoe Forest Hospital	Truckee	95%	177
Ventura County Medical Center[2]	Ventura	95%	404
Bakersfield Heart Hospital[2]	Bakersfield	94%	51
Fairchild Medical Center	Yreka	94%	134
Healdsburg District Hospital	Healdsburg	94%	90
Loma Linda Univ Med Ctr-Murrieta[2]	Murrieta	94%	450
Petaluma Valley Hospital[2]	Petaluma	94%	124
Prov Little Co of Mary Med Ctr San Pedro[2]	San Pedro	94%	200
Saint Joseph Hospital[2]	Eureka	94%	272
Simi Valley Hosp & Health Care Svcs[2]	Simi Valley	94%	266
VA Northern California Healthcare System[2]	Mather	94%	116
Alvarado Hospital Medical Center	San Diego	93%	237
Santa Rosa Memorial Hospital[2]	Santa Rosa	93%	263
Chinese Hospital	San Francisco	92%	115
Doctors Medical Center - San Pablo[2]	San Pablo	92%	186
Hi - Desert Medical Center	Joshua Tree	92%	106
Rideout Memorial Hospital[2]	Marysville	92%	297
Saint Agnes Medical Center[2]	Fresno	92%	547
Saint Louise Regional Hospital[2]	Gilroy	92%	109
Sutter Amador Hospital[2]	Jackson	92%	103
Western Medical Center Santa Ana	Santa Ana	92%	303
Adventist Medical Center[2]	Hanford	91%	307
Natividad Medical Center	Salinas	91%	134
Saint Helena Hospital	Saint Helena	91%	159
Ukiah Valley Medical Center	Ukiah	91%	162
Victor Valley Global Medical Center[2]	Victorville	91%	265
Hemet Valley Medical Center[2]	Hemet	90%	293
Parkview Comm Hosp Med Ctr[2]	Riverside	90%	493
Pioneers Memorial Healthcare District	Brawley	90%	144
Kern Medical Center[2]	Bakersfield	89%	321
Regional Medical Center of San Jose[2]	San Jose	89%	259
Western Medical Center Hospital Anaheim	Anaheim	88%	67
Community Hospital of Long Beach	Long Beach	87%	47
El Centro Regional Medical Center[2]	El Centro	87%	245
Mad River Community Hospital[2]	Arcata	87%	45
Lompoc Valley Medical Center	Lompoc	84%	139
Coast Plaza Hospital	Norwalk	81%	27
George L Mee Memorial Hospital	King City	81%	27
Greater El Monte Community Hospital	South El Monte	81%	42
Saint Helena Hospital - Clearlake	Clearlake	81%	37
Madera Community Hospital	Madera	80%	164
Pacifica Hospital of the Valley	Sun Valley	73%	52

Controlled Postoperative Blood Glucose

Hospital Name	City	Rate	Cases
California Hosp Med Ctr Los Angeles[2]	Los Angeles	100%	26
Comm Mem Hosp San Buenaventura[2]	Ventura	100%	101
Emanuel Medical Center	Turlock	100%	39
Fountain Valley Reg Hosp & Med Ctr[2]	Fountain Valley	100%	103
Grossmont Hospital[2]	La Mesa	100%	170
Hoag Memorial Hospital Presbyterian[2]	Newport Beach	100%	200
LAC/Harbor - UCLA Medical Center[2]	Torrance	100%	102
Providence Saint John's Health Center[2]	Santa Monica	100%	83
Providence Saint Joseph Medical Center[2]	Burbank	100%	86
Saint Agnes Medical Center[2]	Fresno	100%	182
Saint Jude Medical Center[2]	Fullerton	100%	98
San Ramon Regional Medical Center[2]	San Ramon	100%	31
Scripps Green Hospital[2]	La Jolla	100%	113
Scripps Mercy Hospital[2]	San Diego	100%	144
Shasta Regional Medical Center	Redding	100%	83
White Memorial Medical Center[2]	Los Angeles	100%	50
Citrus Valley Medical Center - IC Campus[2]	Covina	99%	136
Comm Hosp of the Monterey Peninsula	Monterey	99%	169
Glendale Adventist Medical Center[2]	Glendale	99%	99
Good Samaritan Hospital[2]	San Jose	99%	131
Mercy Medical Center - Redding[2]	Redding	99%	152
Regional Medical Center of San Jose[2]	San Jose	99%	76
Saint Mary Medical Center	Apple Valley	99%	125
San Francisco VA Medical Center[2]	San Francisco	99%	71
Scripps Memorial Hospital La Jolla[2]	La Jolla	99%	204
Sharp Chula Vista Medical Center[2]	Chula Vista	99%	121
Sharp Memorial Hospital[2]	San Diego	99%	253
Sutter General Hospital[2]	Sacramento	99%	191
Torrance Memorial Medical Center[2]	Torrance	99%	89
Univ of California Irvine Med Ctr[2]	Orange	99%	71
Univ of CA San Diego Med Ctr[2]	San Diego	99%	138
VA San Diego Healthcare System[2]	San Diego	99%	85
Ahmc Anaheim Regional Medical Center[2]	Anaheim	98%	111
CA Pacific Med Ctr-Pacific Campus Hosp[2]	San Francisco	98%	145
Doctors Medical Center[2]	Modesto	98%	207
Eisenhower Medical Center	Rancho Mirage	98%	214
John Muir Medical Center - Concord Campus[2]	Concord	98%	153
Kaiser Fdn Hosp-San Francisco[2]	San Francisco	98%	173
Keck Hospital of USC[2]	Los Angeles	98%	168
Long Beach Memorial Medical Center[2]	Long Beach	98%	131
Memorial Medical Center[2]	Modesto	98%	129
Mercy General Hospital[2]	Sacramento	98%	228
Mercy San Juan Medical Center[2]	Carmichael	98%	123
O'Connor Hospital[2]	San Jose	98%	46
Rideout Memorial Hospital[2]	Marysville	98%	101
Saint Bernardine Medical Center[2]	San Bernardino	98%	192
Saint Joseph's Medical Center of Stockton[2]	Stockton	98%	181
Salinas Valley Memorial Hospital[2]	Salinas	98%	104
Alta Bates Summit Medical Center[2]	Oakland	97%	186
Desert Regional Medical Center[2]	Palm Springs	97%	130
El Camino Hospital[2]	Mountain View	97%	150
French Hospital Medical Center[2]	San Luis Obispo	97%	143
Good Samaritan Hospital[2]	Los Angeles	97%	128
Kaiser Foundation Hospital - Los Angeles[2]	Los Angeles	97%	227
Kaweah Delta Medical Center[2]	Visalia	97%	124
Los Robles Hospital & Medical Center[2]	Thousand Oaks	97%	118
Marin General Hospital[2]	Greenbrae	97%	61
Mills - Peninsula Medical Center[2]	Burlingame	97%	87
Pomona Valley Hospital Medical Center[2]	Pomona	97%	112
Providence Tarzana Medical Center[2]	Tarzana	97%	69
Queen of the Valley Medical Center[2]	Napa	97%	67
Riverside Community Hospital[2]	Riverside	97%	152
San Antonio Community Hospital[2]	Upland	97%	117
San Joaquin Community Hospital[2]	Bakersfield	97%	75
Sequoia Hospital[2]	Redwood City	97%	136
Bakersfield Heart Hospital[2]	Bakersfield	96%	97
Beverly Hospital	Montebello	96%	25
Cedars - Sinai Medical Center	Los Angeles	96%	470
Centinela Hospital Medical Center[2]	Inglewood	96%	26
Dominican Hospital[2]	Santa Cruz	96%	93
Kaiser Foundation Hospital - Santa Clara[2]	Santa Clara	96%	174
Methodist Hospital of Southern California[2]	Arcadia	96%	50
Northridge Hospital Medical Center[2]	Northridge	96%	77
Presbyterian Intercommunity Hospital[2]	Whittier	96%	109
Prov Little Co of Mary Med Ctr Torrance[2]	Torrance	96%	102
Ronald Reagan UCLA Medical Center[2]	Los Angeles	96%	110
Saddleback Memorial Medical Center[2]	Laguna Hills	96%	83
Sutter Medical Center of Santa Rosa[2]	Santa Rosa	96%	111
Tri - City Medical Center[2]	Oceanside	96%	94
UCSF Medical Center[2]	San Francisco	96%	91
West Hills Hospital & Medical Center[2]	West Hills	96%	56
Western Medical Center Hospital Anaheim	Anaheim	96%	57
Bakersfield Memorial Hospital[2]	Bakersfield	95%	182
Enloe Medical Center[2]	Chico	95%	134
Providence Holy Cross Medical Center[2]	Mission Hills	95%	78
Saint Joseph Hospital[2]	Eureka	95%	40
Saint Joseph Hospital[2]	Orange	95%	125
Saint Mary Medical Center[2]	Long Beach	95%	39
Santa Barbara Cottage Hospital[2]	Santa Barbara	95%	159
Stanford Hospital[2]	Stanford	95%	175
Fresno Heart & Surgical Hospital[2]	Fresno	94%	197
Garfield Medical Center[2]	Monterey Park	94%	89
Huntington Memorial Hospital[2]	Pasadena	94%	123
Saint Vincent Medical Center[2]	Los Angeles	94%	78
VA Greater Los Angeles Healthcare System[2]	W Los Angeles	94%	106
Valley Presbyterian Hospital[2]	Van Nuys	94%	47
Washington Hospital[2]	Fremont	94%	116
Glendale Mem Hosp & Health Ctr[2]	Glendale	93%	134
Lakewood Regional Medical Center[2]	Lakewood	93%	97
Loma Linda University Medical Center[2]	Loma Linda	93%	134
Northbay Medical Center	Fairfield	93%	46
Saint Helena Hospital	Saint Helena	93%	105
Saint Johns Regional Medical Center[2]	Oxnard	93%	102
Santa Clara Valley Medical Center[2]	San Jose	93%	102
Univ of CA Davis Med Ctr[2]	Sacramento	93%	98
Mission Hospital Regional Medical Center[2]	Mission Viejo	92%	103
Orange Coast Memorial Medical Center[2]	Fountain Valley	92%	98
Saint Mary's Medical Center[2]	San Francisco	92%	25
Santa Rosa Memorial Hospital[2]	Santa Rosa	92%	89
Valleycare Medical Center	Pleasanton	92%	38
LAC+USC Medical Center[2]	Los Angeles	91%	169
Saint Francis Medical Center[2]	Lynwood	91%	35
Palo Alto VA Medical Center[2]	Palo Alto	90%	58
Seton Medical Center[2]	Daly City	90%	52
Hollywood Presbyterian Medical Center[2]	Los Angeles	89%	36
Loma Linda Univ Med Ctr-Murrieta[2]	Murrieta	89%	81
Marian Regional Medical Center[2]	Santa Maria	89%	84
West Anaheim Medical Center	Anaheim	88%	26
Palomar Health Downtown Campus[2]	Escondido	86%	59
Community Regional Medical Center[2]	Fresno	85%	247
PIH Hospital - Downey[2]	Downey	85%	48
Western Medical Center Santa Ana	Santa Ana	81%	79
Alvarado Hospital Medical Center	San Diego	80%	50

Perioperative Temperature Management

Hospital Name	City	Rate	Cases
Adventist Medical Center[2]	Hanford	100%	399
Ahmc Anaheim Regional Medical Center[2]	Anaheim	100%	351
Alameda County Medical Center	Oakland	100%	435
Alameda Hospital	Alameda	100%	103
Alhambra Hospital Medical Center	Alhambra	100%	140
Alta Bates Summit Medical Center[2]	Berkeley	100%	469
Alta Bates Summit Medical Center[2]	Oakland	100%	447
Antelope Valley Hospital[2]	Lancaster	100%	887
Arrowhead Regional Medical Center	Colton	100%	731
Bakersfield Heart Hospital[2]	Bakersfield	100%	157
Bakersfield Memorial Hospital[2]	Bakersfield	100%	596
Barstow Community Hospital	Barstow	100%	66
Barton Memorial Hospital	S Lake Tahoe	100%	245
Beverly Hospital	Montebello	100%	311
California Hosp Med Ctr Los Angeles[2]	Los Angeles	100%	422
CA Pacific Med Ctr-Davies Campus[2]	San Francisco	100%	108
CA Pacific Med Ctr-Pacific Campus Hosp[2]	San Francisco	100%	551
CA Pacific Med Ctr-St Luke's Campus[2]	San Francisco	100%	178
Cedars - Sinai Medical Center	Los Angeles	100%	4224
Centinela Hospital Medical Center[2]	Inglewood	100%	166
Chapman Medical Center	Orange	100%	131
Chinese Hospital	San Francisco	100%	127
Chino Valley Medical Center	Chino	100%	44
Citrus Valley Medical Center - IC Campus[2]	Covina	100%	775
Clovis Community Medical Center[2]	Clovis	100%	721
Community Hospital of Huntington Park	Huntington Park	100%	45
Community Hospital of Long Beach	Long Beach	100%	54
Comm Hosp of the Monterey Peninsula	Monterey	100%	966
Comm Mem Hosp San Buenaventura[2]	Ventura	100%	385
Community Regional Medical Center[2]	Fresno	100%	1878
Contra Costa Regional Medical Center[2]	Martinez	100%	147
Corona Regional Medical Center[2]	Corona	100%	235
Dameron Hospital	Stockton	100%	658
Delano Regional Medical Center[2]	Delano	100%	142
Desert Regional Medical Center[2]	Palm Springs	100%	508
Desert Valley Hospital[2]	Victorville	100%	198
Doctors Hospital of Manteca	Manteca	100%	153
Doctors Hospital of West Covina	West Covina	100%	54
Doctors Medical Center[2]	Modesto	100%	874
Doctors Medical Center - San Pablo[2]	San Pablo	100%	206
Dominican Hospital[2]	Santa Cruz	100%	505
East Los Angeles Doctors Hospital	Los Angeles	100%	57
Eden Medical Center[2]	Castro Valley	100%	463
Eisenhower Medical Center	Rancho Mirage	100%	1634
El Camino Hospital[2]	Mountain View	100%	1121
Emanuel Medical Center	Turlock	100%	424
Enloe Medical Center[2]	Chico	100%	828
Fairchild Medical Center	Yreka	100%	164
Feather River Hospital[2]	Paradise	100%	360
Foothill Presbyterian Hospital[2]	Glendora	100%	273
Fountain Valley Reg Hosp & Med Ctr[2]	Fountain Valley	100%	513
Frank R Howard Memorial Hospital	Willits	100%	266
French Hospital Medical Center[2]	San Luis Obispo	100%	390
Garden Grove Hospital & Medical Center	Garden Grove	100%	179
Garfield Medical Center[2]	Monterey Park	100%	348
George L Mee Memorial Hospital	King City	100%	33
Glendale Adventist Medical Center[2]	Glendale	100%	718
Glendale Mem Hosp & Health Ctr[2]	Glendale	100%	406
Goleta Valley Cottage Hospital[2]	Santa Barbara	100%	317
Good Samaritan Hospital[2]	Los Angeles	100%	549
Good Samaritan Hospital[2]	San Jose	100%	557
Grossmont Hospital[2]	La Mesa	100%	984
Hazel Hawkins Memorial Hospital	Hollister	100%	97
Henry Mayo Newhall Memorial Hospital[2]	Valencia	100%	460
Hoag Memorial Hospital Presbyterian[2]	Newport Beach	100%	616
Hoag Orthopedic Institute[2]	Irvine	100%	667
Hollywood Presbyterian Medical Center[2]	Los Angeles	100%	340
Huntington Beach Hospital	Huntington Bch	100%	41
Huntington Memorial Hospital[2]	Pasadena	100%	421
John F Kennedy Memorial Hospital[2]	Indio	100%	669
John Muir Medical Center - Concord Campus[2]	Concord	100%	448
John Muir Med Ctr-Walnut Creek Campus[2]	Walnut Creek	100%	483
Kaiser Foundation Hospital[2]	San Rafael	100%	396
Kaiser Foundation Hospital & Rehab Center[2]	Vallejo	100%	427
Kaiser Foundation Hospital - Antioch[2]	Antioch	100%	461
Kaiser Foundation Hospital - Baldwin Park[2]	Baldwin Park	100%	477
Kaiser Foundation Hospital - Downey[2]	Downey	100%	464
Kaiser Fdn Hosp-Fremont/Hayward[2]	Hayward	100%	512
Kaiser Foundation Hospital - Fresno[2]	Fresno	100%	395
Kaiser Foundation Hospital - Los Angeles[2]	Los Angeles	100%	516
Kaiser Foundation Hospital - Manteca[2]	Manteca	100%	481
Kaiser Fdn Hosp-Moreno Valley[2]	Moreno Valley	100%	115
Kaiser Fdn Hosp-Oakland/Richmond[2]	Oakland	100%	494
Kaiser Fdn Hosp-Orange Co-Anaheim[2]	Anaheim	100%	623
Kaiser Fdn Hosp-Panorama City[2]	Panorama City	100%	461
Kaiser Foundation Hospital - Redwood City[2]	Redwood City	100%	381
Kaiser Foundation Hospital - Riverside[2]	Riverside	100%	448
Kaiser Foundation Hospital - Roseville[2]	Roseville	100%	477

NOTE: Hospital profiles are in alphabetical order by state, then city, then hospital within the city; Rankings exclude hospitals with less than 25 cases except for patient surveys which excludes hospitals with less than 100 cases; (a) 100-299 cases; (1) The number of cases/patients is too few to report; (2) Data submitted were based on a sample of cases/patients; (3) Results are based on a shorter time period than required; (4) Data suppressed by CMS for one or more quarters; (5) Results are not available for this reporting period; (6) Fewer than 100 patients completed the HCAHPS survey; (7) No cases met the criteria for this measure; (8) The lower limit of the confidence interval cannot be calculated if the number of observed infections equals zero; (9) No data are available from the state/territory for this reporting period; (10) The scores shown reflect fewer than 50 completed surveys; (11) There were discrepancies in the data collection process; (12) This measure does not apply to this hospital for this reporting period; (13) Results cannot be calculated for this reporting period; (14) The results for this state are combined with nearby states to protect confidentiality; Please refer to the User's Guide for a full explanation of data.

Hospital Name	City	Rate	Cases
Kaiser Foundation Hospital - Sacramento[2]	Sacramento	100%	487
Kaiser Foundation Hospital - San Diego[2]	San Diego	100%	469
Kaiser Fdn Hosp-San Francisco[2]	San Francisco	100%	487
Kaiser Foundation Hospital - San Jose[2]	San Jose	100%	459
Kaiser Foundation Hospital - Santa Clara[2]	Santa Clara	100%	519
Kaiser Foundation Hospital - Santa Rosa[2]	Santa Rosa	100%	437
Kaiser Foundation Hospital - South Bay[2]	Harbor City	100%	447
Kaiser Fdn Hosp-S San Francisco[2]	S San Francisco	100%	382
Kaiser Foundation Hospital - Vacaville[2]	Vacaville	100%	325
Kaiser Foundation Hospital - Walnut Creek[2]	Walnut Creek	100%	456
Kaiser Foundation Hospital - West La[2]	Los Angeles	100%	434
Kaiser Fdn Hosp-Woodland Hills[2]	Woodland Hills	100%	443
Kaweah Delta Medical Center[2]	Visalia	100%	526
Keck Hospital of USC[2]	Los Angeles	100%	868
Kern Medical Center[2]	Bakersfield	100%	353
La Palma Intercommunity Hospital	La Palma	100%	56
LAC+USC Medical Center[2]	Los Angeles	100%	683
LAC/Harbor - UCLA Medical Center[2]	Torrance	100%	354
LAC/Olive View - UCLA Medical Center[2]	Sylmar	100%	218
LAC/Rancho Los Amigos Ntl Rehab Ctr[2]	Downey	100%	217
Lakewood Regional Medical Center[2]	Lakewood	100%	447
Lodi Memorial Hospital[2]	Lodi	100%	290
Loma Linda Univ Med Ctr-Murrieta[2]	Murrieta	100%	496
Loma Linda VA Medical Center[2]	Loma Linda	100%	368
Los Alamitos Medical Center[2]	Los Alamitos	100%	730
Los Angeles Community Hospital[2]	Los Angeles	100%	69
Los Robles Hospital & Medical Center[2]	Thousand Oaks	100%	587
Mad River Community Hospital[2]	Arcata	100%	52
Mammoth Hospital	Mammoth Lakes	100%	71
Marian Regional Medical Center[2]	Santa Maria	100%	558
Marin General Hospital[2]	Greenbrae	100%	473
Mark Twain Medical Center[2]	San Andreas	100%	88
Marshall Medical Center[2]	Placerville	100%	329
Memorial Hospital Los Banos	Los Banos	100%	25
Memorial Hospital of Gardena	Gardena	100%	106
Memorial Medical Center[2]	Modesto	100%	562
Mercy General Hospital[2]	Sacramento	100%	531
Mercy Hospital[2]	Bakersfield	100%	488
Mercy Hospital of Folsom[2]	Folsom	100%	455
Mercy Medical Center[2]	Merced	100%	481
Mercy Medical Center - Mount Shasta[2]	Mount Shasta	100%	142
Mercy Medical Center - Redding[2]	Redding	100%	644
Mercy San Juan Medical Center[2]	Carmichael	100%	581
Methodist Hospital of Sacramento[2]	Sacramento	100%	444
Methodist Hospital of Southern California[2]	Arcadia	100%	546
Mills - Peninsula Medical Center[2]	Burlingame	100%	521
Mission Community Hospital	Panorama City	100%	190
Montclair Hospital Medical Center	Montclair	100%	31
Monterey Park Hospital[2]	Monterey Park	100%	113
Northbay Medical Center	Fairfield	100%	394
Northern Inyo Hospital	Bishop	100%	65
Northridge Hospital Medical Center[2]	Northridge	100%	827
Novato Community Hospital	Novato	100%	156
O'Connor Hospital[2]	San Jose	100%	614
Oak Valley District Hospital	Oakdale	100%	39
Ojai Valley Community Hospital	Ojai	100%	45
Olympia Medical Center	Los Angeles	100%	195
Pacific Alliance Medical Center[2]	Los Angeles	100%	216
Pacific Hospital of Long Beach[3]	Long Beach	100%	71
Palm Drive Hospital[2]	Sebastopol	100%	138
Palmdale Regional Medical Center[2]	Palmdale	100%	402
Palo Alto VA Medical Center[2]	Palo Alto	100%	441
Palomar Health Downtown Campus[2]	Escondido	100%	418
Paradise Valley Hospital	National City	100%	71
Patients' Hospital of Redding	Redding	100%	51
PIH Hospital - Downey[2]	Downey	100%	509
Pioneers Memorial Healthcare District	Brawley	100%	162
Placentia Linda Hospital[2]	Placentia	100%	509
Pomerado Hospital[2]	Poway	100%	338
Pomona Valley Hospital Medical Center[2]	Pomona	100%	423
Presbyterian Intercommunity Hospital[2]	Whittier	100%	408
Providence Holy Cross Medical Center[2]	Mission Hills	100%	401
Prov Little Co of Mary Med Ctr San Pedro[2]	San Pedro	100%	246
Prov Little Co of Mary Med Ctr Torrance[2]	Torrance	100%	551
Providence Saint John's Health Center[2]	Santa Monica	100%	408
Providence Saint Joseph Medical Center[2]	Burbank	100%	447
Providence Tarzana Medical Center[2]	Tarzana	100%	384
Queen of the Valley Medical Center[2]	Napa	100%	353
Redlands Community Hospital[2]	Redlands	100%	1085
Regional Medical Center of San Jose[2]	San Jose	100%	297
Riverside Community Hospital[2]	Riverside	100%	568
Riverside County Regional Medical Center[2]	Moreno Valley	100%	315
Ronald Reagan UCLA Medical Center[2]	Los Angeles	100%	387
Saddleback Memorial Medical Center[2]	Laguna Hills	100%	378
Saint Bernardine Medical Center[2]	San Bernardino	100%	451
Saint Elizabeth Community Hospital[2]	Red Bluff	100%	237
Saint Francis Medical Center[2]	Lynwood	100%	284
Saint Francis Memorial Hospital[2]	San Francisco	100%	299
Saint Helena Hospital	Saint Helena	100%	1096
Saint Helena Hospital - Clearlake	Clearlake	100%	54
Saint Johns Pleasant Valley Hospital[2]	Camarillo	100%	268
Saint Johns Regional Medical Center[2]	Oxnard	100%	508
Saint Joseph Hospital[2]	Eureka	100%	443
Saint Joseph Hospital[2]	Orange	100%	553
Saint Joseph's Medical Center of Stockton[2]	Stockton	100%	565
Saint Jude Medical Center[2]	Fullerton	100%	481
Saint Louise Regional Hospital[2]	Gilroy	100%	140
Saint Mary Medical Center	Apple Valley	100%	721
Saint Mary Medical Center[2]	Long Beach	100%	182
Saint Mary's Medical Center[2]	San Francisco	100%	351
Saint Rose Hospital[2]	Hayward	100%	286
Saint Vincent Medical Center[2]	Los Angeles	100%	653
Salinas Valley Memorial Hospital[2]	Salinas	100%	400
San Antonio Community Hospital[2]	Upland	100%	422
San Dimas Community Hospital[2]	San Dimas	100%	223
San Francisco General Hospital[2]	San Francisco	100%	292
San Francisco VA Medical Center[2]	San Francisco	100%	388
San Gabriel Valley Medical Center[2]	San Gabriel	100%	308
San Gorgonio Memorial Hospital	Banning	100%	236
San Joaquin Community Hospital[2]	Bakersfield	100%	775
San Joaquin General Hospital	French Camp	100%	325
San Leandro Hospital[3]	San Leandro	100%	28
San Mateo Medical Center	San Mateo	100%	165
San Ramon Regional Medical Center[2]	San Ramon	100%	240
Santa Clara Valley Medical Center[2]	San Jose	100%	328
Santa Monica-UCLA Med Ctr & Ortho Hosp[2]	Santa Monica	100%	350
Santa Rosa Memorial Hospital[2]	Santa Rosa	100%	336
Scripps Green Hospital[2]	La Jolla	100%	598
Scripps Memorial Hospital - Encinitas[2]	Encinitas	100%	488
Scripps Memorial Hospital La Jolla[2]	La Jolla	100%	624
Scripps Mercy Hospital[2]	San Diego	100%	529
Sequoia Hospital[2]	Redwood City	100%	437
Seton Medical Center[2]	Daly City	100%	324
Sharp Chula Vista Medical Center[2]	Chula Vista	100%	429
Sharp Coronado Hosp & Healthcare Ctr	Coronado	100%	1325
Sharp Memorial Hospital[2]	San Diego	100%	1500
Shasta Regional Medical Center	Redding	100%	546
Sherman Oaks Hospital	Sherman Oaks	100%	114
Sierra Nevada Memorial Hospital[2]	Grass Valley	100%	305
Sierra View District Hospital	Porterville	100%	271
Sierra Vista Regional Medical Center	San Luis Obispo	100%	460
Silver Lake Medical Center	Los Angeles	100%	30
Sonoma Valley Hospital	Sonoma	100%	139
Sonora Regional Medical Center	Sonora	100%	471
Southern California Hospital at Hollywood	Hollywood	100%	109
Southwest Healthcare System[2]	Murrieta	100%	517
Stanford Hospital[2]	Stanford	100%	705
Stanislaus Surgical Hospital[2]	Modesto	100%	204
Sutter Amador Hospital[2]	Jackson	100%	116
Sutter Auburn Faith Hospital[2]	Auburn	100%	392
Sutter Coast Hospital	Crescent City	100%	75
Sutter Davis Hospital[2]	Davis	100%	224
Sutter Delta Medical Center[2]	Antioch	100%	215
Sutter General Hospital[2]	Sacramento	100%	632
Sutter Lakeside Hospital	Lakeport	100%	199
Sutter Maternity & Surgery Ctr	Santa Cruz	100%	261
Sutter Medical Center of Santa Rosa[2]	Santa Rosa	100%	497
Sutter Roseville Medical Center[2]	Roseville	100%	525
Sutter Solano Medical Center[2]	Vallejo	100%	364
Sutter Surgical Hospital - North Valley	Yuba City	100%	320
Sutter Tracy Community Hospital	Tracy	100%	194
Tahoe Forest Hospital	Truckee	100%	218
Temple Community Hospital	Los Angeles	100%	43
Torrance Memorial Medical Center[2]	Torrance	100%	915
Tri - City Medical Center[2]	Oceanside	100%	390
Twin Cities Community Hospital	Templeton	100%	539
Ukiah Valley Medical Center	Ukiah	100%	190
Univ of CA Davis Med Ctr[2]	Sacramento	100%	466
Univ of California Irvine Med Ctr[2]	Orange	100%	429
USC Verdugo Hills Hospital[2]	Glendale	100%	319
VA Greater Los Angeles Healthcare System[2]	W Los Angeles	100%	316
VA Long Beach Healthcare System[2]	Long Beach	100%	261
VA San Diego Healthcare System[2]	San Diego	100%	419
Valley Presbyterian Hospital[2]	Van Nuys	100%	622
Valleycare Medical Center	Pleasanton	100%	666
Victor Valley Global Medical Center[2]	Victorville	100%	340
Washington Hospital[2]	Fremont	100%	475
Watsonville Community Hospital	Watsonville	100%	249
West Anaheim Medical Center	Anaheim	100%	107
West Hills Hospital & Medical Center[2]	West Hills	100%	401
Western Medical Center Hospital Anaheim	Anaheim	100%	81
White Memorial Medical Center[2]	Los Angeles	100%	527
Whittier Hospital Medical Center	Whittier	100%	197
Woodland Memorial Hospital[2]	Woodland	100%	257
Alvarado Hospital Medical Center	San Diego	99%	301
Coastal Communities Hospital	Santa Ana	99%	164
Community Hospital of San Bernardino[2]	San Bernardino	99%	132
Fallbrook Hospital	Fallbrook	99%	335
Fresno Heart & Surgical Hospital[2]	Fresno	99%	502
Fresno Surgical Hospital[2]	Fresno	99%	540
Healdsburg District Hospital	Healdsburg	99%	91
Hemet Valley Medical Center[2]	Hemet	99%	338
Hi - Desert Medical Center	Joshua Tree	99%	125
Kaiser Foundation Hospital - Fontana[2]	Fontana	99%	442
Kaiser Fdn Hosp S Sacramento[2]	Sacramento	99%	467
Lompoc Valley Medical Center	Lompoc	99%	162
Long Beach Memorial Medical Center[2]	Long Beach	99%	563
Orange Coast Memorial Medical Center[2]	Fountain Valley	99%	632
Oroville Hospital[2]	Oroville	99%	350
Parkview Comm Hosp Med Ctr[2]	Riverside	99%	530
Petaluma Valley Hospital[2]	Petaluma	99%	141
Rideout Memorial Hospital[2]	Marysville	99%	359
Saint Agnes Medical Center[2]	Fresno	99%	728
Santa Barbara Cottage Hospital[2]	Santa Barbara	99%	548
Simi Valley Hosp & Health Care Svcs[2]	Simi Valley	99%	322
Tri - City Regional Medical Center	Hawaiian Grdns	99%	156
Tulare Regional Medical Center	Tulare	99%	129
Univ of CA San Diego Med Ctr[2]	San Diego	99%	470
Western Medical Center Santa Ana	Santa Ana	99%	346
Greater El Monte Community Hospital	South El Monte	98%	52
Loma Linda University Medical Center[2]	Loma Linda	98%	635
Madera Community Hospital	Madera	98%	183
Menifee Valley Medical Center[2]	Sun City	98%	189
Mission Hospital Regional Medical Center[2]	Mission Viejo	98%	411
Natividad Medical Center	Salinas	98%	163
UCSF Medical Center[2]	San Francisco	98%	533
VA Northern California Healthcare System[2]	Mather	98%	162
Ventura County Medical Center[2]	Ventura	98%	497
El Centro Regional Medical Center[2]	El Centro	97%	300
Coast Plaza Hospital	Norwalk	95%	38
Fresno VA Med Ctr-VA Central CA[2]	Fresno	95%	66
Palo Verde Hospital[2]	Blythe	93%	29
Mendocino Coast District Hospital	Fort Bragg	92%	62
Marina Del Rey Hospital[2]	Marina Del Rey	90%	201
Pacifica Hospital of the Valley	Sun Valley	85%	62

Prophylactic Antibiotic Selection

Hospital Name	City	Rate	Cases
Alameda Hospital	Alameda	100%	56
Alta Bates Summit Medical Center[2]	Oakland	100%	454
Bakersfield Memorial Hospital[2]	Bakersfield	100%	533
Barton Memorial Hospital	S Lake Tahoe	100%	183
California Hosp Med Ctr Los Angeles[2]	Los Angeles	100%	256
CA Pacific Med Ctr-Pacific Campus Hosp[2]	San Francisco	100%	496
Centinela Hospital Medical Center[2]	Inglewood	100%	75
Clovis Community Medical Center[2]	Clovis	100%	341
Dameron Hospital	Stockton	100%	522
Doctors Medical Center[2]	Modesto	100%	767
El Camino Hospital[2]	Mountain View	100%	885
Enloe Medical Center[2]	Chico	100%	683
Fresno Surgical Hospital[2]	Fresno	100%	468
Garden Grove Hospital & Medical Center	Garden Grove	100%	88
Glendale Adventist Medical Center[2]	Glendale	100%	609
Goleta Valley Cottage Hospital[2]	Santa Barbara	100%	237
Good Samaritan Hospital[2]	San Jose	100%	470
Hoag Memorial Hospital Presbyterian[2]	Newport Beach	100%	412
Hoag Orthopedic Institute[2]	Irvine	100%	535
John F Kennedy Memorial Hospital[2]	Indio	100%	540
John Muir Medical Center - Concord Campus[2]	Concord	100%	436
Kaiser Foundation Hospital[2]	San Rafael	100%	264
Kaiser Foundation Hospital - Baldwin Park[2]	Baldwin Park	100%	325
Kaiser Foundation Hospital - Downey[2]	Downey	100%	313
Kaiser Foundation Hospital - Fontana[2]	Fontana	100%	284
Kaiser Fdn Hosp-Fremont/Hayward[2]	Hayward	100%	319
Kaiser Foundation Hospital - Fresno[2]	Fresno	100%	250
Kaiser Foundation Hospital - Manteca[2]	Manteca	100%	325
Kaiser Fdn Hosp-Moreno Valley[2]	Moreno Valley	100%	81
Kaiser Fdn Hosp-Oakland/Richmond[2]	Oakland	100%	329
Kaiser Fdn Hosp-Orange Co-Anaheim[2]	Anaheim	100%	382
Kaiser Fdn Hosp-Panorama City[2]	Panorama City	100%	310
Kaiser Foundation Hospital - Redwood City[2]	Redwood City	100%	233
Kaiser Foundation Hospital - Roseville[2]	Roseville	100%	316
Kaiser Foundation Hospital - San Diego[2]	San Diego	100%	271
Kaiser Foundation Hospital - San Jose[2]	San Jose	100%	314
Kaiser Foundation Hospital - Santa Clara[2]	Santa Clara	100%	487
Kaiser Foundation Hospital - Santa Rosa[2]	Santa Rosa	100%	283
Kaiser Foundation Hospital - South Bay[2]	Harbor City	100%	278
Kaiser Fdn Hosp-S San Francisco[2]	S San Francisco	100%	250
Kaiser Foundation Hospital - West La[2]	Los Angeles	100%	244
Kaiser Fdn Hosp-Woodland Hills[2]	Woodland Hills	100%	290
Loma Linda University Medical Center[2]	Loma Linda	100%	441
Los Robles Hospital & Medical Center[2]	Thousand Oaks	100%	460
Marian Regional Medical Center[2]	Santa Maria	100%	445
Marin General Hospital[2]	Greenbrae	100%	329
Mark Twain Medical Center[2]	San Andreas	100%	52
Marshall Medical Center[2]	Placerville	100%	235
Memorial Medical Center[2]	Modesto	100%	442
Mercy Hospital[2]	Bakersfield	100%	319
Mercy Hospital of Folsom[2]	Folsom	100%	299
Mercy Medical Center - Mount Shasta[2]	Mount Shasta	100%	105
Monterey Park Hospital[2]	Monterey Park	100%	45
Northern Inyo Hospital	Bishop	100%	47
Ojai Valley Community Hospital	Ojai	100%	28

NOTE: Hospital profiles are in alphabetical order by state, then city, then hospital within the city; Rankings exclude hospitals with less than 25 cases except for patient surveys which excludes hospitals with less than 100 cases; (a) 100-299 cases; (1) The number of cases/patients is too few to report; (2) Data submitted were based on a sample of cases/patients; (3) Results are based on a shorter time period than required; (4) Data suppressed by CMS for one or more quarters; (5) Results are not available for this reporting period; (6) Fewer than 100 patients completed the HCAHPS survey; (7) No cases met the criteria for this measure; (8) The lower limit of the confidence interval cannot be calculated if the number of observed infections equals zero; (9) No data are available from the state/territory for this reporting period; (10) The scores shown reflect fewer than 50 completed surveys; (11) There were discrepancies in the data collection process; (12) This measure does not apply to this hospital for this reporting period; (13) Results cannot be calculated for this reporting period; (14) The results for this state are combined with nearby states to protect confidentiality; Please refer to the User's Guide for a full explanation of data.

Hospital Name	City	Rate	Cases
Olympia Medical Center	Los Angeles	100%	105
Pacific Alliance Medical Center[2]	Los Angeles	100%	136
Pacific Hospital of Long Beach[3]	Long Beach	100%	56
Palm Drive Hospital[2]	Sebastopol	100%	116
Palo Alto VA Medical Center	Palo Alto	100%	396
Patients' Hospital of Redding	Redding	100%	45
Placentia Linda Hospital[2]	Placentia	100%	407
Pomerado Hospital[2]	Poway	100%	219
Pomona Valley Hospital Medical Center[2]	Pomona	100%	388
Prov Little Co of Mary Med Ctr Torrance[2]	Torrance	100%	411
Providence Saint Joseph Medical Center[2]	Burbank	100%	321
Riverside Community Hospital[2]	Riverside	100%	502
Ronald Reagan UCLA Medical Center[2]	Los Angeles	100%	269
Saint Francis Memorial Hospital[2]	San Francisco	100%	211
Saint Joseph Hospital[2]	Orange	100%	398
Saint Mary Medical Center[2]	Long Beach	100%	106
Salinas Valley Memorial Hospital[2]	Salinas	100%	380
San Antonio Community Hospital[2]	Upland	100%	387
San Francisco VA Medical Center	San Francisco	100%	315
Scripps Green Hospital[2]	La Jolla	100%	435
Scripps Memorial Hospital - Encinitas[2]	Encinitas	100%	319
Scripps Memorial Hospital La Jolla[2]	La Jolla	100%	587
Sequoia Hospital[2]	Redwood City	100%	408
Sharp Coronado Hosp & Healthcare Ctr	Coronado	100%	1227
Sharp Memorial Hospital[2]	San Diego	100%	1418
Shasta Regional Medical Center	Redding	100%	418
Sierra Nevada Memorial Hospital[2]	Grass Valley	100%	205
Sierra Vista Regional Medical Center	San Luis Obispo	100%	240
Sutter Auburn Faith Hospital[2]	Auburn	100%	250
Sutter Coast Hospital	Crescent City	100%	33
Sutter Davis Hospital[2]	Davis	100%	137
Sutter Lakeside Hospital	Lakeport	100%	135
Sutter Medical Center of Santa Rosa[2]	Santa Rosa	100%	340
Sutter Roseville Medical Center[2]	Roseville	100%	353
Sutter Solano Medical Center[2]	Vallejo	100%	212
Sutter Tracy Community Hospital	Tracy	100%	150
Torrance Memorial Medical Center[2]	Torrance	100%	617
VA Greater Los Angeles Healthcare System	W Los Angeles	100%	279
VA Long Beach Healthcare System	Long Beach	100%	141
VA Northern California Healthcare System	Mather	100%	50
VA San Diego Healthcare System	San Diego	100%	259
Washington Hospital[2]	Fremont	100%	399
Watsonville Community Hospital	Watsonville	100%	102
West Anaheim Medical Center	Anaheim	100%	54
White Memorial Medical Center[2]	Los Angeles	100%	373
Ahmc Anaheim Regional Medical Center[2]	Anaheim	99%	314
Alta Bates Summit Medical Center[2]	Berkeley	99%	329
Antelope Valley Hospital[2]	Lancaster	99%	679
Bakersfield Heart Hospital[2]	Bakersfield	99%	195
CA Pacific Med Ctr-St Luke's Campus[2]	San Francisco	99%	98
Cedars - Sinai Medical Center	Los Angeles	99%	2288
Chapman Medical Center	Orange	99%	85
Chinese Hospital	San Francisco	99%	87
Citrus Valley Medical Center - IC Campus[2]	Covina	99%	649
Comm Hosp of the Monterey Peninsula	Monterey	99%	783
Community Regional Medical Center[2]	Fresno	99%	905
Delano Regional Medical Center[2]	Delano	99%	76
Desert Regional Medical Center[2]	Palm Springs	99%	444
Doctors Hospital of Manteca	Manteca	99%	99
Dominican Hospital[2]	Santa Cruz	99%	394
Eisenhower Medical Center	Rancho Mirage	99%	1161
El Centro Regional Medical Center[2]	El Centro	99%	161
Fallbrook Hospital	Fallbrook	99%	274
Fountain Valley Reg Hosp & Med Ctr[2]	Fountain Valley	99%	463
Frank R Howard Memorial Hospital	Willits	99%	211
French Hospital Medical Center[2]	San Luis Obispo	99%	407
Glendale Mem Hosp & Health Ctr[2]	Glendale	99%	385
Grossmont Hospital[2]	La Mesa	99%	854
Healdsburg District Hospital	Healdsburg	99%	83
John Muir Med Ctr-Walnut Creek Campus[2]	Walnut Creek	99%	329
Kaiser Foundation Hospital & Rehab Center[2]	Vallejo	99%	283
Kaiser Foundation Hospital - Riverside[2]	Riverside	99%	264
Kaiser Foundation Hospital - Sacramento[2]	Sacramento	99%	324
Kaiser Fdn Hosp-San Francisco[2]	San Francisco	99%	488
Kaiser Foundation Hospital - Vacaville[2]	Vacaville	99%	195
Kaiser Foundation Hospital - Walnut Creek[2]	Walnut Creek	99%	294
Kaiser Fdn Hosp S Sacramento[2]	Sacramento	99%	313
Kaweah Delta Medical Center[2]	Visalia	99%	487
Keck Hospital of USC[2]	Los Angeles	99%	455
LAC/Harbor - UCLA Medical Center[2]	Torrance	99%	309
Lodi Memorial Hospital[2]	Lodi	99%	157
Loma Linda VA Medical Center	Loma Linda	99%	241
Los Alamitos Medical Center[2]	Los Alamitos	99%	549
Marina Del Rey Hospital[2]	Marina Del Rey	99%	120
Mercy General Hospital[2]	Sacramento	99%	585
Mercy Medical Center - Redding[2]	Redding	99%	502
Mills - Peninsula Medical Center[2]	Burlingame	99%	411
Mission Hospital Regional Medical Center[2]	Mission Viejo	99%	344
Northridge Hospital Medical Center[2]	Northridge	99%	672
O'Connor Hospital[2]	San Jose	99%	478
Palomar Health Downtown Campus[2]	Escondido	99%	320
Petaluma Valley Hospital[2]	Petaluma	99%	96
PIH Hospital - Downey[2]	Downey	99%	315
Providence Holy Cross Medical Center[2]	Mission Hills	99%	317
Prov Little Co of Mary Med Ctr San Pedro[2]	San Pedro	99%	134
Providence Saint John's Health Center[2]	Santa Monica	99%	367
Queen of the Valley Medical Center[2]	Napa	99%	231
Redlands Community Hospital[2]	Redlands	99%	867
Rideout Memorial Hospital[2]	Marysville	99%	249
Saddleback Memorial Medical Center[2]	Laguna Hills	99%	289
Saint Agnes Medical Center[2]	Fresno	99%	506
Saint Bernardine Medical Center[2]	San Bernardino	99%	477
Saint Elizabeth Community Hospital[2]	Red Bluff	99%	149
Saint Francis Medical Center[2]	Lynwood	99%	182
Saint Helena Hospital	Saint Helena	99%	1000
Saint Johns Pleasant Valley Hospital[2]	Camarillo	99%	179
Saint Johns Regional Medical Center[2]	Oxnard	99%	367
Saint Joseph's Medical Center of Stockton[2]	Stockton	99%	460
Saint Jude Medical Center[2]	Fullerton	99%	408
Saint Vincent Medical Center[2]	Los Angeles	99%	576
San Dimas Community Hospital[2]	San Dimas	99%	172
San Francisco General Hospital[2]	San Francisco	99%	190
San Gorgonio Memorial Hospital	Banning	99%	166
San Joaquin Community Hospital[2]	Bakersfield	99%	653
San Mateo Medical Center	San Mateo	99%	100
San Ramon Regional Medical Center[2]	San Ramon	99%	168
Scripps Mercy Hospital[2]	San Diego	99%	466
Sharp Chula Vista Medical Center[2]	Chula Vista	99%	361
Sherman Oaks Hospital	Sherman Oaks	99%	76
Sierra View District Hospital	Porterville	99%	187
Sonoma Valley Hospital	Sonoma	99%	96
Sonora Regional Medical Center	Sonora	99%	361
Stanford Hospital[2]	Stanford	99%	588
Stanislaus Surgical Hospital[2]	Modesto	99%	178
Sutter General Hospital[2]	Sacramento	99%	592
Sutter Surgical Hospital - North Valley	Yuba City	99%	271
Tahoe Forest Hospital	Truckee	99%	170
Tri - City Medical Center[2]	Oceanside	99%	351
Twin Cities Community Hospital	Templeton	99%	393
UCSF Medical Center[2]	San Francisco	99%	354
Univ of CA Davis Med Ctr[2]	Sacramento	99%	350
Univ of CA San Diego Med Ctr[2]	San Diego	99%	372
Valley Presbyterian Hospital[2]	Van Nuys	99%	466
Valleycare Medical Center	Pleasanton	99%	562
Ventura County Medical Center[2]	Ventura	99%	258
Victor Valley Global Medical Center[2]	Victorville	99%	220
West Hills Hospital & Medical Center[2]	West Hills	99%	305
Alhambra Hospital Medical Center	Alhambra	98%	80
Alvarado Hospital Medical Center	San Diego	98%	209
Arrowhead Regional Medical Center	Colton	98%	277
Beverly Hospital	Montebello	98%	208
Coastal Communities Hospital	Santa Ana	98%	90
Doctors Hospital of West Covina	West Covina	98%	44
Eden Medical Center[2]	Castro Valley	98%	250
Emanuel Medical Center	Turlock	98%	323
Garfield Medical Center[2]	Monterey Park	98%	227
Good Samaritan Hospital[2]	Los Angeles	98%	366
Hazel Hawkins Memorial Hospital	Hollister	98%	64
Huntington Memorial Hospital[2]	Pasadena	98%	373
Kaiser Foundation Hospital - Antioch[2]	Antioch	98%	312
Kaiser Foundation Hospital - Los Angeles[2]	Los Angeles	98%	532
LAC+USC Medical Center[2]	Los Angeles	98%	582
LAC/Olive View - UCLA Medical Center[2]	Sylmar	98%	116
LAC/Rancho Los Amigos Ntl Rehab Ctr[2]	Downey	98%	176
Long Beach Memorial Medical Center[2]	Long Beach	98%	462
Mercy Medical Center[2]	Merced	98%	318
Mercy San Juan Medical Center[2]	Carmichael	98%	526
Northbay Medical Center	Fairfield	98%	224
Novato Community Hospital	Novato	98%	115
Orange Coast Memorial Medical Center[2]	Fountain Valley	98%	482
Oroville Hospital[2]	Oroville	98%	225
Palmdale Regional Medical Center[2]	Palmdale	98%	255
Presbyterian Intercommunity Hospital[2]	Whittier	98%	356
Providence Tarzana Medical Center[2]	Tarzana	98%	270
Regional Medical Center of San Jose[2]	San Jose	98%	209
Riverside County Regional Medical Center[2]	Moreno Valley	98%	200
Saint Joseph Hospital[2]	Eureka	98%	341
Saint Mary's Medical Center[2]	San Francisco	98%	249
Saint Rose Hospital[2]	Hayward	98%	186
San Joaquin General Hospital	French Camp	98%	150
Santa Barbara Cottage Hospital[2]	Santa Barbara	98%	534
Santa Clara Valley Medical Center[2]	San Jose	98%	309
Santa Monica-UCLA Med Ctr & Ortho Hosp[2]	Santa Monica	98%	221
Seton Medical Center[2]	Daly City	98%	205
Southern California Hospital at Hollywood	Hollywood	98%	58
Sutter Maternity & Surgery Ctr	Santa Cruz	98%	190
Ukiah Valley Medical Center	Ukiah	98%	114
USC Verdugo Hills Hospital[2]	Glendale	98%	243
Comm Mem Hosp San Buenaventura[2]	Ventura	97%	356
Doctors Medical Center - San Pablo[2]	San Pablo	97%	117
Fairchild Medical Center	Yreka	97%	129
Feather River Hospital[2]	Paradise	97%	243
Fresno Heart & Surgical Hospital[2]	Fresno	97%	291
Hi - Desert Medical Center	Joshua Tree	97%	74
Hollywood Presbyterian Medical Center[2]	Los Angeles	97%	182
Lakewood Regional Medical Center[2]	Lakewood	97%	395
Loma Linda Univ Med Ctr-Murrieta[2]	Murrieta	97%	402
Memorial Hospital of Gardena	Gardena	97%	38
Methodist Hospital of Southern California[2]	Arcadia	97%	372
Pacifica Hospital of the Valley	Sun Valley	97%	30
Parkview Comm Hosp Med Ctr[2]	Riverside	97%	420
San Gabriel Valley Medical Center[2]	San Gabriel	97%	184
Santa Rosa Memorial Hospital[2]	Santa Rosa	97%	265
Southwest Healthcare System[2]	Murrieta	97%	329
Sutter Amador Hospital[2]	Jackson	97%	71
Sutter Delta Medical Center[2]	Antioch	97%	100
Univ of California Irvine Med Ctr[2]	Orange	97%	346
Woodland Memorial Hospital[2]	Woodland	97%	178
Community Hospital of San Bernardino[2]	San Bernardino	96%	56
Corona Regional Medical Center[2]	Corona	96%	134
Desert Valley Hospital[2]	Victorville	96%	98
Lompoc Valley Medical Center	Lompoc	96%	114
Mammoth Hospital	Mammoth Lakes	96%	49
Mendocino Coast District Hospital	Fort Bragg	96%	56
Menifee Valley Medical Center[2]	Sun City	96%	131
Methodist Hospital of Sacramento[2]	Sacramento	96%	304
Mission Community Hospital	Panorama City	96%	101
Natividad Medical Center	Salinas	96%	76
Pioneers Memorial Healthcare District	Brawley	96%	123
Saint Mary Medical Center	Apple Valley	96%	413
Simi Valley Hosp & Health Care Svcs[2]	Simi Valley	96%	193
Western Medical Center Hospital Anaheim	Anaheim	96%	95
Whittier Hospital Medical Center	Whittier	96%	103
Adventist Medical Center[2]	Hanford	95%	283
Foothill Presbyterian Hospital[2]	Glendora	95%	153
Hemet Valley Medical Center[2]	Hemet	95%	212
Henry Mayo Newhall Memorial Hospital[2]	Valencia	95%	294
Western Medical Center Santa Ana	Santa Ana	95%	207
Alameda County Medical Center	Oakland	94%	178
Saint Louise Regional Hospital[2]	Gilroy	94%	85
Tulare Regional Medical Center	Tulare	94%	52
Contra Costa Regional Medical Center[2]	Martinez	93%	58
Los Angeles Community Hospital[2]	Los Angeles	93%	27
Kern Medical Center[2]	Bakersfield	92%	224
Tri - City Regional Medical Center	Hawaiian Grdns	89%	91
Madera Community Hospital	Madera	87%	129

Prophylactic Antibiotic Selection (Outpatient)

Hospital Name	City	Rate	Cases
Bakersfield Heart Hospital	Bakersfield	100%	226
Barstow Community Hospital	Barstow	100%	35
Community Regional Medical Center	Fresno	100%	406
Corona Regional Medical Center	Corona	100%	57
Doctors Hospital of Manteca	Manteca	100%	41
El Camino Hospital	Mountain View	100%	650
Hoag Orthopedic Institute	Irvine	100%	224
John Muir Medical Center - Concord Campus	Concord	100%	252
Marina Del Rey Hospital	Marina Del Rey	100%	116
Memorial Medical Center	Modesto	100%	146
Menifee Valley Medical Center	Sun City	100%	30
Mercy Medical Center - Mount Shasta	Mount Shasta	100%	37
Northbay Medical Center	Fairfield	100%	170
Petaluma Valley Hospital	Petaluma	100%	40
PIH Hospital - Downey	Downey	100%	73
Saint Elizabeth Community Hospital	Red Bluff	100%	79
Saint Johns Pleasant Valley Hospital	Camarillo	100%	36
Saint Mary Medical Center	Long Beach	100%	96
Saint Rose Hospital	Hayward	100%	31
Salinas Valley Memorial Hospital	Salinas	100%	183
San Francisco General Hospital	San Francisco	100%	50
San Leandro Hospital[3]	San Leandro	100%	35
San Mateo Medical Center	San Mateo	100%	97
Scripps Green Hospital	La Jolla	100%	413
Scripps Memorial Hospital La Jolla	La Jolla	100%	564
Sharp Chula Vista Medical Center	Chula Vista	100%	205
Sierra Nevada Memorial Hospital	Grass Valley	100%	31
Sonoma Valley Hospital	Sonoma	100%	30
Southern California Hospital at Hollywood[3]	Hollywood	100%	76
Sutter Lakeside Hospital	Lakeport	100%	58
Sutter Tracy Community Hospital	Tracy	100%	91
Temple Community Hospital	Los Angeles	100%	33
Valley Presbyterian Hospital	Van Nuys	100%	89
Woodland Memorial Hospital	Woodland	100%	67
Arrowhead Regional Medical Center	Colton	99%	179
Barton Memorial Hospital	S Lake Tahoe	99%	87
California Hosp Med Ctr Los Angeles	Los Angeles	99%	105
CA Pacific Med Ctr-Davies Campus	San Francisco	99%	148
CA Pacific Med Ctr-Pacific Campus Hosp	San Francisco	99%	359
Citrus Valley Medical Center - IC Campus	Covina	99%	298
Dameron Hospital	Stockton	99%	116
Dominican Hospital	Santa Cruz	99%	126
Eden Medical Center	Castro Valley	99%	169
LAC+USC Medical Center	Los Angeles	99%	205

NOTE: Hospital profiles are in alphabetical order by state, then city, then hospital within the city; Rankings exclude hospitals with less than 25 cases except for patient surveys which excludes hospitals with less than 100 cases; (a) 100-299 cases; (1) The number of cases/patients is too few to report; (2) Data submitted were based on a sample of cases/patients; (3) Results are based on a shorter time period than required; (4) Data suppressed by CMS for one or more quarters; (5) Results are not available for this reporting period; (6) Fewer than 100 patients completed the HCAHPS survey; (7) No cases met the criteria for this measure; (8) The lower limit of the confidence interval cannot be calculated if the number of observed infections equals zero; (9) No data are available from the state/territory for this reporting period; (10) The scores shown reflect fewer than 50 completed surveys; (11) There were discrepancies in the data collection process; (12) This measure does not apply to this hospital for this reporting period; (13) Results cannot be calculated for this reporting period; (14) The results for this state are combined with nearby states to protect confidentiality; Please refer to the User's Guide for a full explanation of data.

Hospital Name	City	Rate	Cases
LAC/Olive View - UCLA Medical Center	Sylmar	99%	204
Lodi Memorial Hospital	Lodi	99%	282
Los Alamitos Medical Center	Los Alamitos	99%	138
Marian Regional Medical Center	Santa Maria	99%	316
Marin General Hospital	Greenbrae	99%	205
Marshall Medical Center	Placerville	99%	163
Mercy General Hospital	Sacramento	99%	394
Mercy Hospital	Bakersfield	99%	177
Mercy San Juan Medical Center	Carmichael	99%	126
Mills - Peninsula Medical Center	Burlingame	99%	175
Northridge Hospital Medical Center	Northridge	99%	178
Pioneers Memorial Healthcare District	Brawley	99%	136
Prov Little Co of Mary Med Ctr Torrance	Torrance	99%	289
Providence Saint Joseph Medical Center	Burbank	99%	364
Saint Bernardine Medical Center	San Bernardino	99%	152
Saint Joseph Hospital	Eureka	99%	241
Saint Joseph Hospital	Orange	99%	609
San Ramon Regional Medical Center	San Ramon	99%	194
Santa Barbara Cottage Hospital	Santa Barbara	99%	632
Santa Monica-UCLA Med Ctr & Ortho Hosp	Santa Monica	99%	208
Scripps Memorial Hospital - Encinitas	Encinitas	99%	264
Sequoia Hospital	Redwood City	99%	274
Seton Medical Center	Daly City	99%	135
Sharp Memorial Hospital	San Diego	99%	577
Shasta Regional Medical Center	Redding	99%	218
Southwest Healthcare System	Murrieta	99%	162
Stanislaus Surgical Hospital	Modesto	99%	93
Sutter General Hospital	Sacramento	99%	467
Sutter Medical Center of Santa Rosa	Santa Rosa	99%	144
Torrance Memorial Medical Center	Torrance	99%	380
UCSF Medical Center	San Francisco	99%	802
Univ of CA San Diego Med Ctr	San Diego	99%	349
USC Verdugo Hills Hospital	Glendale	99%	124
Washington Hospital	Fremont	99%	150
Alta Bates Summit Medical Center	Oakland	98%	301
Alvarado Hospital Medical Center	San Diego	98%	101
Antelope Valley Hospital	Lancaster	98%	124
Desert Regional Medical Center	Palm Springs	98%	189
Enloe Medical Center	Chico	98%	292
Fountain Valley Reg Hosp & Med Ctr	Fountain Valley	98%	267
Fresno Heart & Surgical Hospital	Fresno	98%	285
Hoag Memorial Hospital Presbyterian	Newport Beach	98%	729
John F Kennedy Memorial Hospital	Indio	98%	50
Los Robles Hospital & Medical Center	Thousand Oaks	98%	243
Mercy Medical Center - Redding	Redding	98%	448
Mission Hospital Regional Medical Center	Mission Viejo	98%	364
Patients' Hospital of Redding	Redding	98%	44
Presbyterian Intercommunity Hospital	Whittier	98%	234
Queen of the Valley Medical Center	Napa	98%	229
Redlands Community Hospital	Redlands	98%	475
Regional Medical Center of San Jose	San Jose	98%	133
Riverside County Regional Medical Center	Moreno Valley	98%	100
Saddleback Memorial Medical Center	Laguna Hills	98%	502
Saint Johns Regional Medical Center	Oxnard	98%	163
Saint Joseph's Medical Center of Stockton	Stockton	98%	248
Saint Jude Medical Center	Fullerton	98%	533
San Joaquin Community Hospital	Bakersfield	98%	260
San Joaquin General Hospital	French Camp	98%	40
Stanford Hospital	Stanford	98%	691
Sutter Roseville Medical Center	Roseville	98%	241
Sutter Surgical Hospital - North Valley	Yuba City	98%	47
Tri - City Medical Center	Oceanside	98%	342
Tulare Regional Medical Center	Tulare	98%	112
Univ of CA Davis Med Ctr	Sacramento	98%	470
Univ of California Irvine Med Ctr	Orange	98%	347
Valleycare Medical Center	Pleasanton	98%	166
Watsonville Community Hospital	Watsonville	98%	53
Alta Bates Summit Medical Center	Berkeley	97%	77
Bakersfield Memorial Hospital	Bakersfield	97%	497
CA Pacific Med Ctr-St Luke's Campus	San Francisco	97%	31
Cedars - Sinai Medical Center	Los Angeles	97%	859
Community Hospital of San Bernardino	San Bernardino	97%	29
Eisenhower Medical Center	Rancho Mirage	97%	496
Garfield Medical Center	Monterey Park	97%	304
Good Samaritan Hospital	Los Angeles	97%	214
Hemet Valley Medical Center	Hemet	97%	116
Kaweah Delta Medical Center	Visalia	97%	320
LAC/Harbor - UCLA Medical Center	Torrance	97%	69
Loma Linda Univ Med Ctr-Murrieta	Murrieta	97%	146
Long Beach Memorial Medical Center	Long Beach	97%	242
Olympia Medical Center	Los Angeles	97%	34
Palmdale Regional Medical Center	Palmdale	97%	68
Providence Holy Cross Medical Center	Mission Hills	97%	138
Rideout Memorial Hospital	Marysville	97%	167
Saint Mary's Medical Center	San Francisco	97%	99
Sutter Maternity & Surgery Ctr	Santa Cruz	97%	117
Sutter Solano Medical Center	Vallejo	97%	92
Twin Cities Community Hospital	Templeton	97%	68
Western Medical Center Hospital Anaheim	Anaheim	97%	38
Western Medical Center Santa Ana	Santa Ana	97%	79
Ahmc Anaheim Regional Medical Center	Anaheim	96%	255
Comm Hosp of the Monterey Peninsula	Monterey	96%	175
Foothill Presbyterian Hospital	Glendora	96%	73
French Hospital Medical Center	San Luis Obispo	96%	169
Huntington Memorial Hospital	Pasadena	96%	230
John Muir Med Ctr-Walnut Creek Campus	Walnut Creek	96%	260
Keck Hospital of USC	Los Angeles	96%	363
Memorial Hospital of Gardena	Gardena	96%	28
Mercy Medical Center	Merced	96%	131
Orange Coast Memorial Medical Center	Fountain Valley	96%	326
Placentia Linda Hospital	Placentia	96%	76
Riverside Community Hospital	Riverside	96%	455
Saint Mary Medical Center	Apple Valley	96%	157
San Antonio Community Hospital	Upland	96%	369
Santa Rosa Memorial Hospital	Santa Rosa	96%	363
Sierra View District Hospital	Porterville	96%	126
Sierra Vista Regional Medical Center	San Luis Obispo	96%	28
Simi Valley Hosp & Health Care Svcs	Simi Valley	96%	50
West Hills Hospital & Medical Center	West Hills	96%	136
White Memorial Medical Center	Los Angeles	96%	211
Centinela Hospital Medical Center	Inglewood	95%	57
Clovis Community Medical Center	Clovis	95%	341
Doctors Medical Center	Modesto	95%	483
Glendale Mem Hosp & Health Ctr	Glendale	95%	164
Good Samaritan Hospital	San Jose	95%	439
Henry Mayo Newhall Memorial Hospital	Valencia	95%	63
Paradise Valley Hospital	National City	95%	57
Pomona Valley Hospital Medical Center	Pomona	95%	306
Ronald Reagan UCLA Medical Center	Los Angeles	95%	299
Saint Agnes Medical Center	Fresno	95%	398
Santa Clara Valley Medical Center	San Jose	95%	288
Scripps Mercy Hospital	San Diego	95%	485
Sonora Regional Medical Center	Sonora	95%	133
Sutter Delta Medical Center	Antioch	95%	56
Whittier Hospital Medical Center	Whittier	95%	42
Grossmont Hospital	La Mesa	94%	311
Kern Medical Center	Bakersfield	94%	169
Mission Community Hospital	Panorama City	94%	65
Comm Mem Hosp San Buenaventura	Ventura	93%	406
El Centro Regional Medical Center	El Centro	93%	137
Emanuel Medical Center	Turlock	93%	84
Feather River Hospital	Paradise	93%	85
Glendale Adventist Medical Center	Glendale	93%	115
Memorial Hospital Los Banos	Los Banos	93%	55
Methodist Hospital of Southern California	Arcadia	93%	222
Parkview Comm Hosp Med Ctr	Riverside	93%	30
Sutter Auburn Faith Hospital	Auburn	93%	57
Ukiah Valley Medical Center	Ukiah	93%	46
Coastal Communities Hospital	Santa Ana	92%	26
Delano Regional Medical Center	Delano	92%	25
Fresno Surgical Hospital	Fresno	92%	89
Hollywood Presbyterian Medical Center	Los Angeles	92%	59
Monterey Park Hospital	Monterey Park	92%	89
Palomar Health Downtown Campus	Escondido	92%	252
Providence Saint John's Health Center	Santa Monica	92%	311
Saint Francis Medical Center	Lynwood	92%	115
Beverly Hospital	Montebello	91%	90
Lakewood Regional Medical Center	Lakewood	91%	251
Providence Tarzana Medical Center	Tarzana	90%	292
Saint Louise Regional Hospital	Gilroy	90%	59
San Gabriel Valley Medical Center	San Gabriel	90%	52
Sutter Davis Hospital	Davis	89%	37
Saint Vincent Medical Center	Los Angeles	87%	212
Prov Little Co of Mary Med Ctr San Pedro	San Pedro	86%	44
Goleta Valley Cottage Hospital	Santa Barbara	85%	33
Loma Linda University Medical Center	Loma Linda	85%	436
Adventist Medical Center	Hanford	84%	74
Alhambra Hospital Medical Center	Alhambra	83%	47
O'Connor Hospital	San Jose	81%	150
Saint Helena Hospital	Saint Helena	80%	184
Doctors Medical Center - San Pablo	San Pablo	74%	107
Pomerado Hospital	Poway	70%	69
Alameda County Medical Center[3]	Oakland	64%	33

Prophylactic Antibiotic Stopped

Hospital Name	City	Rate	Cases
Alameda County Medical Center	Oakland	100%	178
CA Pacific Med Ctr-Pacific Campus Hosp[2]	San Francisco	100%	477
Centinela Hospital Medical Center[2]	Inglewood	100%	75
Community Hospital of San Bernardino[2]	San Bernardino	100%	55
Dameron Hospital	Stockton	100%	522
Desert Valley Hospital[2]	Victorville	100%	67
Fairchild Medical Center	Yreka	100%	129
Foothill Presbyterian Hospital[2]	Glendora	100%	133
French Hospital Medical Center[2]	San Luis Obispo	100%	401
Garden Grove Hospital & Medical Center	Garden Grove	100%	88
Kaiser Foundation Hospital & Rehab Center[2]	Vallejo	100%	283
Kaiser Fdn Hosp-Fremont/Hayward[2]	Hayward	100%	313
Kaiser Foundation Hospital - Fresno[2]	Fresno	100%	250
Kaiser Foundation Hospital - Manteca[2]	Manteca	100%	319
Kaiser Fdn Hosp-Moreno Valley[2]	Moreno Valley	100%	80
Kaiser Fdn Hosp-Oakland/Richmond[2]	Oakland	100%	322
Kaiser Fdn Hosp-Orange Co-Anaheim[2]	Anaheim	100%	368
Kaiser Foundation Hospital - Redwood City[2]	Redwood City	100%	230
Kaiser Foundation Hospital - Roseville[2]	Roseville	100%	316
Kaiser Foundation Hospital - Sacramento[2]	Sacramento	100%	322
Kaiser Foundation Hospital - San Diego[2]	San Diego	100%	257
Kaiser Foundation Hospital - San Jose[2]	San Jose	100%	314
Kaiser Foundation Hospital - Santa Clara[2]	Santa Clara	100%	486
Kaiser Foundation Hospital - South Bay[2]	Harbor City	100%	272
Kaiser Fdn Hosp-S San Francisco[2]	S San Francisco	100%	247
Kaiser Foundation Hospital - Vacaville[2]	Vacaville	100%	195
Kaiser Fdn Hosp-Woodland Hills[2]	Woodland Hills	100%	283
Kaiser Fdn Hosp S Sacramento[2]	Sacramento	100%	310
LAC/Olive View - UCLA Medical Center[2]	Sylmar	100%	116
LAC/Rancho Los Amigos Ntl Rehab Ctr[2]	Downey	100%	174
Mark Twain Medical Center[2]	San Andreas	100%	51
Memorial Medical Center[2]	Modesto	100%	419
Mendocino Coast District Hospital	Fort Bragg	100%	54
Mercy General Hospital[2]	Sacramento	100%	566
Mercy Medical Center - Mount Shasta[2]	Mount Shasta	100%	105
Methodist Hospital of Sacramento[2]	Sacramento	100%	304
Novato Community Hospital	Novato	100%	115
Olympia Medical Center	Los Angeles	100%	97
Patients' Hospital of Redding	Redding	100%	45
Saint Francis Memorial Hospital[2]	San Francisco	100%	207
Saint Johns Regional Medical Center[2]	Oxnard	100%	339
Scripps Memorial Hospital - Encinitas[2]	Encinitas	100%	301
Sharp Coronado Hosp & Healthcare Ctr	Coronado	100%	1220
Sherman Oaks Hospital	Sherman Oaks	100%	76
Sierra Vista Regional Medical Center	San Luis Obispo	100%	240
Sutter Coast Hospital	Crescent City	100%	32
Sutter General Hospital[2]	Sacramento	100%	581
Sutter Surgical Hospital - North Valley	Yuba City	100%	269
VA Long Beach Healthcare System	Long Beach	100%	140
Ventura County Medical Center[2]	Ventura	100%	250
Watsonville Community Hospital	Watsonville	100%	101
Woodland Memorial Hospital[2]	Woodland	100%	177
Alta Bates Summit Medical Center[2]	Oakland	99%	441
Barton Memorial Hospital	S Lake Tahoe	99%	180
Chapman Medical Center	Orange	99%	84
Chinese Hospital	San Francisco	99%	81
Doctors Medical Center[2]	Modesto	99%	693
Eden Medical Center[2]	Castro Valley	99%	240
Fallbrook Hospital	Fallbrook	99%	271
Fresno Surgical Hospital[2]	Fresno	99%	467
Garfield Medical Center[2]	Monterey Park	99%	192
Glendale Mem Hosp & Health Ctr[2]	Glendale	99%	364
Good Samaritan Hospital[2]	San Jose	99%	459
Grossmont Hospital[2]	La Mesa	99%	832
Henry Mayo Newhall Memorial Hospital[2]	Valencia	99%	282
Hoag Memorial Hospital Presbyterian[2]	Newport Beach	99%	401
Hoag Orthopedic Institute[2]	Irvine	99%	528
John Muir Medical Center - Concord Campus[2]	Concord	99%	417
Kaiser Foundation Hospital[2]	San Rafael	99%	259
Kaiser Foundation Hospital - Antioch[2]	Antioch	99%	306
Kaiser Foundation Hospital - Fontana[2]	Fontana	99%	277
Kaiser Foundation Hospital - Los Angeles[2]	Los Angeles	99%	523
Kaiser Fdn Hosp-Panorama City[2]	Panorama City	99%	307
Kaiser Foundation Hospital - West La[2]	Los Angeles	99%	240
Loma Linda VA Medical Center	Loma Linda	99%	228
Long Beach Memorial Medical Center[2]	Long Beach	99%	423
Los Alamitos Medical Center[2]	Los Alamitos	99%	520
Los Robles Hospital & Medical Center[2]	Thousand Oaks	99%	446
Marian Regional Medical Center[2]	Santa Maria	99%	441
Marin General Hospital[2]	Greenbrae	99%	329
Marshall Medical Center[2]	Placerville	99%	225
Mercy Hospital of Folsom[2]	Folsom	99%	289
Northbay Medical Center	Fairfield	99%	212
O'Connor Hospital[2]	San Jose	99%	454
Palm Drive Hospital[2]	Sebastopol	99%	115
Palomar Health Downtown Campus[2]	Escondido	99%	314
Pomerado Hospital[2]	Poway	99%	217
Providence Holy Cross Medical Center[2]	Mission Hills	99%	279
Prov Little Co of Mary Med Ctr Torrance[2]	Torrance	99%	390
Providence Saint John's Health Center[2]	Santa Monica	99%	334
Providence Saint Joseph Medical Center[2]	Burbank	99%	303
Riverside Community Hospital[2]	Riverside	99%	470
Saddleback Memorial Medical Center[2]	Laguna Hills	99%	273
Saint Helena Hospital	Saint Helena	99%	993
Saint Johns Pleasant Valley Hospital[2]	Camarillo	99%	157
Saint Jude Medical Center[2]	Fullerton	99%	398
Saint Mary Medical Center[2]	Long Beach	99%	102
Saint Mary's Medical Center[2]	San Francisco	99%	247
Saint Vincent Medical Center[2]	Los Angeles	99%	568
Salinas Valley Memorial Hospital[2]	Salinas	99%	376
San Joaquin Community Hospital[2]	Bakersfield	99%	616
San Joaquin General Hospital	French Camp	99%	148
San Mateo Medical Center	San Mateo	99%	98
Santa Monica-UCLA Med Ctr & Ortho Hosp[2]	Santa Monica	99%	211
Scripps Green Hospital[2]	La Jolla	99%	425
Scripps Memorial Hospital La Jolla[2]	La Jolla	99%	548
Scripps Mercy Hospital[2]	San Diego	99%	453

NOTE: Hospital profiles are in alphabetical order by state, then city, then hospital within the city; Rankings exclude hospitals with less than 25 cases except for patient surveys which excludes hospitals with less than 100 cases; (a) 100-299 cases; (1) The number of cases/patients is too few to report; (2) Data submitted were based on a sample of cases/patients; (3) Results are based on a shorter time period than required; (4) Data suppressed by CMS for one or more quarters; (5) Results are not available for this reporting period; (6) Fewer than 100 patients completed the HCAHPS survey; (7) No cases met the criteria for this measure; (8) The lower limit of the confidence interval cannot be calculated if the number of observed infections equals zero; (9) No data are available from the state/territory for this reporting period; (10) The scores shown reflect fewer than 50 completed surveys; (11) There were discrepancies in the data collection process; (12) This measure does not apply to this hospital for this reporting period; (13) Results cannot be calculated for this reporting period; (14) The results for this state are combined with nearby states to protect confidentiality; Please refer to the User's Guide for a full explanation of data.

Hospital Name	City	Rate	Cases
Seton Medical Center[2]	Daly City	99%	196
Sharp Memorial Hospital[2]	San Diego	99%	1371
Shasta Regional Medical Center	Redding	99%	410
Sonoma Valley Hospital	Sonoma	99%	93
Sonora Regional Medical Center	Sonora	99%	350
Stanford Hospital[2]	Stanford	99%	564
Sutter Davis Hospital[2]	Davis	99%	137
Sutter Maternity & Surgery Ctr	Santa Cruz	99%	188
Sutter Medical Center of Santa Rosa[2]	Santa Rosa	99%	331
Sutter Solano Medical Center[2]	Vallejo	99%	202
Sutter Tracy Community Hospital	Tracy	99%	144
Torrance Memorial Medical Center[2]	Torrance	99%	585
Tri - City Medical Center[2]	Oceanside	99%	328
Twin Cities Community Hospital	Templeton	99%	384
Univ of California Irvine Med Ctr[2]	Orange	99%	329
VA San Diego Healthcare System	San Diego	99%	256
Valleycare Medical Center	Pleasanton	99%	552
West Hills Hospital & Medical Center[2]	West Hills	99%	300
Bakersfield Memorial Hospital[2]	Bakersfield	98%	506
California Hosp Med Ctr Los Angeles[2]	Los Angeles	98%	246
Coastal Communities Hospital	Santa Ana	98%	88
Comm Hosp of the Monterey Peninsula	Monterey	98%	761
Comm Mem Hosp San Buenaventura[2]	Ventura	98%	347
Contra Costa Regional Medical Center[2]	Martinez	98%	58
Desert Regional Medical Center[2]	Palm Springs	98%	443
Doctors Hospital of Manteca	Manteca	98%	93
Dominican Hospital[2]	Santa Cruz	98%	392
Eisenhower Medical Center	Rancho Mirage	98%	1146
El Camino Hospital[2]	Mountain View	98%	859
Emanuel Medical Center	Turlock	98%	317
Enloe Medical Center[2]	Chico	98%	639
Feather River Hospital[2]	Paradise	98%	237
Frank R Howard Memorial Hospital	Willits	98%	208
Goleta Valley Cottage Hospital[2]	Santa Barbara	98%	230
John Muir Med Ctr-Walnut Creek Campus[2]	Walnut Creek	98%	314
Kaiser Foundation Hospital - Baldwin Park[2]	Baldwin Park	98%	317
Kaiser Foundation Hospital - Downey[2]	Downey	98%	294
Kaiser Foundation Hospital - Riverside[2]	Riverside	98%	251
Kaiser Foundation Hospital - Santa Rosa[2]	Santa Rosa	98%	275
Kaiser Foundation Hospital - Walnut Creek[2]	Walnut Creek	98%	288
Mercy Hospital[2]	Bakersfield	98%	316
Mercy Medical Center[2]	Merced	98%	314
Monterey Park Hospital[2]	Monterey Park	98%	43
Northridge Hospital Medical Center[2]	Northridge	98%	642
Orange Coast Memorial Medical Center[2]	Fountain Valley	98%	453
Oroville Hospital[2]	Oroville	98%	223
Pacific Alliance Medical Center[2]	Los Angeles	98%	134
Palmdale Regional Medical Center[2]	Palmdale	98%	250
Palo Alto VA Medical Center	Palo Alto	98%	392
Placentia Linda Hospital[2]	Placentia	98%	400
Pomona Valley Hospital Medical Center[2]	Pomona	98%	371
Presbyterian Intercommunity Hospital[2]	Whittier	98%	339
Providence Tarzana Medical Center[2]	Tarzana	98%	253
Queen of the Valley Medical Center[2]	Napa	98%	224
Rideout Memorial Hospital[2]	Marysville	98%	236
Ronald Reagan UCLA Medical Center[2]	Los Angeles	98%	241
Saint Joseph Hospital[2]	Eureka	98%	332
Saint Joseph Hospital[2]	Orange	98%	377
Saint Joseph's Medical Center of Stockton[2]	Stockton	98%	448
San Dimas Community Hospital[2]	San Dimas	98%	167
San Gorgonio Memorial Hospital	Banning	98%	162
San Ramon Regional Medical Center[2]	San Ramon	98%	162
Santa Rosa Memorial Hospital[2]	Santa Rosa	98%	261
Sequoia Hospital[2]	Redwood City	98%	393
Sierra View District Hospital	Porterville	98%	174
Southern California Hospital at Hollywood	Hollywood	98%	47
Southwest Healthcare System[2]	Murrieta	98%	317
Sutter Auburn Faith Hospital[2]	Auburn	98%	245
Sutter Roseville Medical Center[2]	Roseville	98%	347
Univ of CA Davis Med Ctr[2]	Sacramento	98%	334
USC Verdugo Hills Hospital[2]	Glendale	98%	243
Washington Hospital[2]	Fremont	98%	393
White Memorial Medical Center[2]	Los Angeles	98%	354
Antelope Valley Hospital[2]	Lancaster	97%	646
CA Pacific Med Ctr-St Luke's Campus[2]	San Francisco	97%	91
Cedars - Sinai Medical Center	Los Angeles	97%	2150
Community Regional Medical Center[2]	Fresno	97%	894
Corona Regional Medical Center[2]	Corona	97%	132
El Centro Regional Medical Center[2]	El Centro	97%	159
Fresno Heart & Surgical Hospital[2]	Fresno	97%	284
Kaiser Fdn Hosp-San Francisco[2]	San Francisco	97%	471
LAC/Harbor - UCLA Medical Center[2]	Torrance	97%	294
Loma Linda University Medical Center[2]	Loma Linda	97%	432
Mercy Medical Center - Redding[2]	Redding	97%	495
Mercy San Juan Medical Center[2]	Carmichael	97%	513
Mills - Peninsula Medical Center[2]	Burlingame	97%	406
Mission Hospital Regional Medical Center[2]	Mission Viejo	97%	328
Redlands Community Hospital[2]	Redlands	97%	852
Riverside County Regional Medical Center[2]	Moreno Valley	97%	183
Saint Agnes Medical Center[2]	Fresno	97%	490
Saint Francis Medical Center[2]	Lynwood	97%	154
Saint Louise Regional Hospital[2]	Gilroy	97%	79
Saint Mary Medical Center	Apple Valley	97%	382
San Francisco VA Medical Center	San Francisco	97%	309
San Gabriel Valley Medical Center[2]	San Gabriel	97%	170
Sharp Chula Vista Medical Center[2]	Chula Vista	97%	349
Sierra Nevada Memorial Hospital[2]	Grass Valley	97%	201
Stanislaus Surgical Hospital[2]	Modesto	97%	178
Sutter Amador Hospital[2]	Jackson	97%	71
UCSF Medical Center[2]	San Francisco	97%	343
West Anaheim Medical Center	Anaheim	97%	39
Alhambra Hospital Medical Center	Alhambra	96%	78
Alta Bates Summit Medical Center[2]	Berkeley	96%	322
Alvarado Hospital Medical Center	San Diego	96%	202
Arrowhead Regional Medical Center	Colton	96%	267
Bakersfield Heart Hospital[2]	Bakersfield	96%	192
Clovis Community Medical Center[2]	Clovis	96%	333
Delano Regional Medical Center[2]	Delano	96%	72
Hollywood Presbyterian Medical Center[2]	Los Angeles	96%	167
Huntington Memorial Hospital[2]	Pasadena	96%	359
LAC+USC Medical Center[2]	Los Angeles	96%	574
Madera Community Hospital	Madera	96%	128
PIH Hospital - Downey[2]	Downey	96%	297
Saint Bernardine Medical Center[2]	San Bernardino	96%	466
Saint Rose Hospital[2]	Hayward	96%	179
San Antonio Community Hospital[2]	Upland	96%	368
San Francisco General Hospital[2]	San Francisco	96%	190
Santa Barbara Cottage Hospital[2]	Santa Barbara	96%	524
Sutter Lakeside Hospital	Lakeport	96%	130
Tulare Regional Medical Center	Tulare	96%	49
Univ of CA San Diego Med Ctr[2]	San Diego	96%	348
Ahmc Anaheim Regional Medical Center[2]	Anaheim	95%	300
Citrus Valley Medical Center - IC Campus[2]	Covina	95%	598
Doctors Medical Center - San Pablo[2]	San Pablo	95%	113
Fountain Valley Reg Hosp & Med Ctr[2]	Fountain Valley	95%	415
Glendale Adventist Medical Center[2]	Glendale	95%	590
Good Samaritan Hospital[2]	Los Angeles	95%	353
Hazel Hawkins Memorial Hospital	Hollister	95%	62
Healdsburg District Hospital	Healdsburg	95%	83
Keck Hospital of USC[2]	Los Angeles	95%	432
Lodi Memorial Hospital[2]	Lodi	95%	153
Natividad Medical Center	Salinas	95%	75
Petaluma Valley Hospital[2]	Petaluma	95%	92
Saint Elizabeth Community Hospital[2]	Red Bluff	95%	147
Sutter Delta Medical Center[2]	Antioch	95%	94
VA Greater Los Angeles Healthcare System	W Los Angeles	95%	262
Alameda Hospital	Alameda	94%	53
Beverly Hospital	Montebello	94%	204
Hi - Desert Medical Center	Joshua Tree	94%	72
Memorial Hospital of Gardena	Gardena	94%	34
Methodist Hospital of Southern California[2]	Arcadia	94%	350
Parkview Comm Hosp Med Ctr[2]	Riverside	94%	419
Prov Little Co of Mary Med Ctr San Pedro[2]	San Pedro	94%	131
Simi Valley Hosp & Health Care Svcs[2]	Simi Valley	94%	187
Tahoe Forest Hospital	Truckee	94%	167
Marina Del Rey Hospital[2]	Marina Del Rey	93%	110
Ojai Valley Community Hospital	Ojai	93%	27
Pacific Hospital of Long Beach[3]	Long Beach	93%	55
Western Medical Center Hospital Anaheim	Anaheim	93%	87
Adventist Medical Center[2]	Hanford	92%	280
Kaweah Delta Medical Center[2]	Visalia	92%	468
Lakewood Regional Medical Center[2]	Lakewood	92%	360
Pioneers Memorial Healthcare District	Brawley	92%	122
Regional Medical Center of San Jose[2]	San Jose	92%	197
Santa Clara Valley Medical Center[2]	San Jose	92%	292
Whittier Hospital Medical Center	Whittier	92%	100
Mission Community Hospital	Panorama City	91%	94
Northern Inyo Hospital	Bishop	91%	44
Ukiah Valley Medical Center	Ukiah	91%	113
Hemet Valley Medical Center[2]	Hemet	90%	205
Valley Presbyterian Hospital[2]	Van Nuys	90%	454
Victor Valley Global Medical Center[2]	Victorville	90%	215
John F Kennedy Memorial Hospital[2]	Indio	89%	528
Tri - City Regional Medical Center	Hawaiian Grdns	89%	89
Western Medical Center Santa Ana	Santa Ana	88%	204
VA Northern California Healthcare System	Mather	87%	47
Doctors Hospital of West Covina	West Covina	84%	45
Menifee Valley Medical Center[2]	Sun City	83%	121
Mammoth Hospital	Mammoth Lakes	82%	49
Loma Linda Univ Med Ctr-Murrieta[2]	Murrieta	81%	398
Lompoc Valley Medical Center	Lompoc	73%	113
Kern Medical Center[2]	Bakersfield	63%	219
Pacifica Hospital of the Valley	Sun Valley	62%	29

Prophylactic Antibiotic Timing

Hospital Name	City	Rate	Cases
Alhambra Hospital Medical Center	Alhambra	100%	80
Barton Memorial Hospital	S Lake Tahoe	100%	183
Beverly Hospital	Montebello	100%	208
CA Pacific Med Ctr-Pacific Campus Hosp[2]	San Francisco	100%	497
Cedars - Sinai Medical Center	Los Angeles	100%	2289
Centinela Hospital Medical Center[2]	Inglewood	100%	75
Corona Regional Medical Center[2]	Corona	100%	134
Delano Regional Medical Center[2]	Delano	100%	76
Desert Valley Hospital[2]	Victorville	100%	98
Doctors Hospital of Manteca	Manteca	100%	99
Dominican Hospital[2]	Santa Cruz	100%	394
Eden Medical Center[2]	Castro Valley	100%	251
El Camino Hospital[2]	Mountain View	100%	889
French Hospital Medical Center[2]	San Luis Obispo	100%	407
Garden Grove Hospital & Medical Center	Garden Grove	100%	88
Garfield Medical Center[2]	Monterey Park	100%	227
Glendale Adventist Medical Center[2]	Glendale	100%	610
Grossmont Hospital[2]	La Mesa	100%	853
Hazel Hawkins Memorial Hospital	Hollister	100%	64
Hoag Orthopedic Institute[2]	Irvine	100%	535
John Muir Medical Center - Concord Campus[2]	Concord	100%	436
John Muir Med Ctr-Walnut Creek Campus[2]	Walnut Creek	100%	329
Kaiser Foundation Hospital[2]	San Rafael	100%	264
Kaiser Foundation Hospital - Fontana[2]	Fontana	100%	283
Kaiser Foundation Hospital - Fresno[2]	Fresno	100%	250
Kaiser Foundation Hospital - Manteca[2]	Manteca	100%	326
Kaiser Fdn Hosp-Moreno Valley[2]	Moreno Valley	100%	81
Kaiser Fdn Hosp-Oakland/Richmond[2]	Oakland	100%	329
Kaiser Fdn Hosp-Orange Co-Anaheim[2]	Anaheim	100%	382
Kaiser Fdn Hosp-Panorama City[2]	Panorama City	100%	310
Kaiser Foundation Hospital - Redwood City[2]	Redwood City	100%	233
Kaiser Foundation Hospital - Riverside[2]	Riverside	100%	264
Kaiser Foundation Hospital - Sacramento[2]	Sacramento	100%	324
Kaiser Foundation Hospital - San Jose[2]	San Jose	100%	314
Kaiser Foundation Hospital - Santa Clara[2]	Santa Clara	100%	487
Kaiser Fdn Hosp-S San Francisco[2]	S San Francisco	100%	250
Kaiser Foundation Hospital - West La[2]	Los Angeles	100%	244
Los Robles Hospital & Medical Center[2]	Thousand Oaks	100%	461
Marin General Hospital[2]	Greenbrae	100%	329
Marina Del Rey Hospital[2]	Marina Del Rey	100%	120
Mark Twain Medical Center[2]	San Andreas	100%	52
Marshall Medical Center[2]	Placerville	100%	235
Memorial Medical Center[2]	Modesto	100%	444
Mercy General Hospital[2]	Sacramento	100%	585
Methodist Hospital of Sacramento[2]	Sacramento	100%	304
Methodist Hospital of Southern California[2]	Arcadia	100%	372
Novato Community Hospital	Novato	100%	115
O'Connor Hospital[2]	San Jose	100%	479
Olympia Medical Center	Los Angeles	100%	105
Patients' Hospital of Redding	Redding	100%	45
PIH Hospital - Downey[2]	Downey	100%	315
Pomona Valley Hospital Medical Center[2]	Pomona	100%	388
Presbyterian Intercommunity Hospital[2]	Whittier	100%	357
Prov Little Co of Mary Med Ctr Torrance[2]	Torrance	100%	411
Providence Saint Joseph Medical Center[2]	Burbank	100%	321
Rideout Memorial Hospital[2]	Marysville	100%	251
Riverside Community Hospital[2]	Riverside	100%	503
Saint Agnes Medical Center[2]	Fresno	100%	507
Saint Francis Memorial Hospital[2]	San Francisco	100%	211
Saint Helena Hospital	Saint Helena	100%	1000
Saint Johns Pleasant Valley Hospital[2]	Camarillo	100%	179
Saint Joseph's Medical Center of Stockton[2]	Stockton	100%	461
Salinas Valley Memorial Hospital[2]	Salinas	100%	380
San Francisco VA Medical Center	San Francisco	100%	315
Santa Monica-UCLA Med Ctr & Ortho Hosp[2]	Santa Monica	100%	222
Scripps Green Hospital[2]	La Jolla	100%	435
Scripps Memorial Hospital - Encinitas[2]	Encinitas	100%	319
Scripps Memorial Hospital La Jolla[2]	La Jolla	100%	588
Sharp Chula Vista Medical Center[2]	Chula Vista	100%	362
Sharp Coronado Hosp & Healthcare Ctr	Coronado	100%	1229
Sharp Memorial Hospital[2]	San Diego	100%	1417
Sherman Oaks Hospital	Sherman Oaks	100%	76
Sierra View District Hospital	Porterville	100%	187
Southern California Hospital at Hollywood	Hollywood	100%	58
Sutter Amador Hospital[2]	Jackson	100%	71
Sutter Lakeside Hospital	Lakeport	100%	135
Sutter Medical Center of Santa Rosa[2]	Santa Rosa	100%	340
Sutter Solano Medical Center[2]	Vallejo	100%	212
Sutter Surgical Hospital - North Valley	Yuba City	100%	271
Sutter Tracy Community Hospital	Tracy	100%	150
Torrance Memorial Medical Center[2]	Torrance	100%	617
Tri - City Medical Center[2]	Oceanside	100%	352
Twin Cities Community Hospital	Templeton	100%	393
Univ of California Irvine Med Ctr[2]	Orange	100%	346
USC Verdugo Hills Hospital[2]	Glendale	100%	243
VA Long Beach Healthcare System	Long Beach	100%	142
VA San Diego Healthcare System	San Diego	100%	259
Washington Hospital[2]	Fremont	100%	399
Watsonville Community Hospital	Watsonville	100%	102
West Hills Hospital & Medical Center[2]	West Hills	100%	305
Western Medical Center Hospital Anaheim	Anaheim	100%	95
Woodland Memorial Hospital[2]	Woodland	100%	178
Ahmc Anaheim Regional Medical Center[2]	Anaheim	99%	314
Alta Bates Summit Medical Center[2]	Oakland	99%	457
Alvarado Hospital Medical Center	San Diego	99%	209
Antelope Valley Hospital[2]	Lancaster	99%	679
Arrowhead Regional Medical Center	Colton	99%	277

NOTE: Hospital profiles are in alphabetical order by state, then city, then hospital within the city; Rankings exclude hospitals with less than 25 cases except for patient surveys which excludes hospitals with less than 100 cases; (a) 100-299 cases; (1) The number of cases/patients is too few to report; (2) Data submitted were based on a sample of cases/patients; (3) Results are based on a shorter time period than required; (4) Data suppressed by CMS for one or more quarters; (5) Results are not available for this reporting period; (6) Fewer than 100 patients completed the HCAHPS survey; (7) No cases met the criteria for this measure; (8) The lower limit of the confidence interval cannot be calculated if the number of observed infections equals zero; (9) No data are available from the state/territory for this reporting period; (10) The scores shown reflect fewer than 50 completed surveys; (11) There were discrepancies in the data collection process; (12) This measure does not apply to this hospital for this reporting period; (13) Results cannot be calculated for this reporting period; (14) The results for this state are combined with nearby states to protect confidentiality; Please refer to the User's Guide for a full explanation of data.

Bakersfield Heart Hospital[2]	Bakersfield	99%	195
California Hosp Med Ctr Los Angeles[2]	Los Angeles	99%	256
CA Pacific Med Ctr-St Luke's Campus[2]	San Francisco	99%	98
Chapman Medical Center	Orange	99%	85
Citrus Valley Medical Center - IC Campus[2]	Covina	99%	649
Comm Hosp of the Monterey Peninsula	Monterey	99%	788
Dameron Hospital	Stockton	99%	522
Desert Regional Medical Center[2]	Palm Springs	99%	446
Doctors Medical Center[2]	Modesto	99%	768
Eisenhower Medical Center	Rancho Mirage	99%	1163
Feather River Hospital[2]	Paradise	99%	243
Fountain Valley Reg Hosp & Med Ctr[2]	Fountain Valley	99%	464
Frank R Howard Memorial Hospital	Willits	99%	211
Fresno Heart & Surgical Hospital[2]	Fresno	99%	291
Fresno Surgical Hospital[2]	Fresno	99%	468
Good Samaritan Hospital[2]	San Jose	99%	470
Henry Mayo Newhall Memorial Hospital[2]	Valencia	99%	297
Hoag Memorial Hospital Presbyterian[2]	Newport Beach	99%	415
Hollywood Presbyterian Medical Center[2]	Los Angeles	99%	183
John F Kennedy Memorial Hospital[2]	Indio	99%	540
Kaiser Foundation Hospital & Rehab Center[2]	Vallejo	99%	283
Kaiser Foundation Hospital - Antioch[2]	Antioch	99%	313
Kaiser Foundation Hospital - Baldwin Park[2]	Baldwin Park	99%	325
Kaiser Fdn Hosp-Fremont/Hayward[2]	Hayward	99%	319
Kaiser Foundation Hospital - Los Angeles[2]	Los Angeles	99%	532
Kaiser Foundation Hospital - Roseville[2]	Roseville	99%	317
Kaiser Foundation Hospital - San Diego[2]	San Diego	99%	271
Kaiser Fdn Hosp-San Francisco[2]	San Francisco	99%	488
Kaiser Foundation Hospital - Santa Rosa[2]	Santa Rosa	99%	283
Kaiser Foundation Hospital - South Bay[2]	Harbor City	99%	278
Kaiser Foundation Hospital - Walnut Creek[2]	Walnut Creek	99%	294
Kaiser Fdn Hosp-Woodland Hills[2]	Woodland Hills	99%	290
Keck Hospital of USC[2]	Los Angeles	99%	455
LAC/Harbor - UCLA Medical Center[2]	Torrance	99%	312
LAC/Olive View - UCLA Medical Center[2]	Sylmar	99%	116
Lakewood Regional Medical Center[2]	Lakewood	99%	395
Lodi Memorial Hospital[2]	Lodi	99%	157
Loma Linda VA Medical Center	Loma Linda	99%	242
Long Beach Memorial Medical Center[2]	Long Beach	99%	461
Marian Regional Medical Center[2]	Santa Maria	99%	445
Mercy Hospital of Folsom[2]	Folsom	99%	299
Mercy Medical Center[2]	Merced	99%	319
Mercy Medical Center - Redding[2]	Redding	99%	506
Mercy San Juan Medical Center[2]	Carmichael	99%	526
Mills - Peninsula Medical Center[2]	Burlingame	99%	411
Northbay Medical Center	Fairfield	99%	224
Pioneers Memorial Healthcare District	Brawley	99%	123
Placentia Linda Hospital[2]	Placentia	99%	407
Pomerado Hospital[2]	Poway	99%	219
Providence Holy Cross Medical Center[2]	Mission Hills	99%	319
Providence Saint John's Health Center[2]	Santa Monica	99%	372
Providence Tarzana Medical Center[2]	Tarzana	99%	270
Queen of the Valley Medical Center[2]	Napa	99%	231
Redlands Community Hospital[2]	Redlands	99%	868
Regional Medical Center of San Jose[2]	San Jose	99%	209
Ronald Reagan UCLA Medical Center[2]	Los Angeles	99%	269
Saddleback Memorial Medical Center[2]	Laguna Hills	99%	290
Saint Bernardine Medical Center[2]	San Bernardino	99%	478
Saint Johns Regional Medical Center[2]	Oxnard	99%	367
Saint Joseph Hospital[2]	Eureka	99%	344
Saint Joseph Hospital[2]	Orange	99%	398
Saint Louise Regional Hospital[2]	Gilroy	99%	85
Saint Mary Medical Center[2]	Long Beach	99%	106
Saint Mary's Medical Center[2]	San Francisco	99%	249
Saint Rose Hospital[2]	Hayward	99%	186
Saint Vincent Medical Center[2]	Los Angeles	99%	578
San Francisco General Hospital[2]	San Francisco	99%	190
San Gabriel Valley Medical Center[2]	San Gabriel	99%	184
San Joaquin Community Hospital[2]	Bakersfield	99%	654
San Mateo Medical Center	San Mateo	99%	100
San Ramon Regional Medical Center[2]	San Ramon	99%	168
Santa Barbara Cottage Hospital[2]	Santa Barbara	99%	535
Santa Clara Valley Medical Center[2]	San Jose	99%	310
Scripps Mercy Hospital[2]	San Diego	99%	466
Shasta Regional Medical Center	Redding	99%	418
Sierra Nevada Memorial Hospital[2]	Grass Valley	99%	205
Sierra Vista Regional Medical Center	San Luis Obispo	99%	240
Simi Valley Hosp & Health Care Svcs[2]	Simi Valley	99%	193
Sonoma Valley Hospital	Sonoma	99%	96
Sonora Regional Medical Center	Sonora	99%	363
Southwest Healthcare System[2]	Murrieta	99%	329
Stanford Hospital[2]	Stanford	99%	588
Sutter Auburn Faith Hospital[2]	Auburn	99%	250
Sutter Davis Hospital[2]	Davis	99%	137
Sutter General Hospital[2]	Sacramento	99%	593
Sutter Maternity & Surgery Ctr	Santa Cruz	99%	190
Sutter Roseville Medical Center[2]	Roseville	99%	353
Victor Valley Global Medical Center[2]	Victorville	99%	222
Whittier Hospital Medical Center	Whittier	99%	103
Alameda Hospital	Alameda	98%	57
Alta Bates Summit Medical Center[2]	Berkeley	98%	329
Bakersfield Memorial Hospital[2]	Bakersfield	98%	533
Chinese Hospital	San Francisco	98%	87
Clovis Community Medical Center[2]	Clovis	98%	343
Coastal Communities Hospital	Santa Ana	98%	90
Community Hospital of San Bernardino[2]	San Bernardino	98%	57
Comm Mem Hosp San Buenaventura[2]	Ventura	98%	357
Emanuel Medical Center	Turlock	98%	323
Enloe Medical Center[2]	Chico	98%	683
Fallbrook Hospital	Fallbrook	98%	274
Foothill Presbyterian Hospital[2]	Glendora	98%	153
Good Samaritan Hospital[2]	Los Angeles	98%	366
Hemet Valley Medical Center[2]	Hemet	98%	212
Huntington Memorial Hospital[2]	Pasadena	98%	374
Kaiser Fdn Hosp S Sacramento[2]	Sacramento	98%	313
Kaweah Delta Medical Center[2]	Visalia	98%	491
LAC+USC Medical Center[2]	Los Angeles	98%	583
Los Alamitos Medical Center[2]	Los Alamitos	98%	549
Mercy Hospital[2]	Bakersfield	98%	320
Monterey Park Hospital[2]	Monterey Park	98%	45
Northridge Hospital Medical Center[2]	Northridge	98%	671
Orange Coast Memorial Medical Center[2]	Fountain Valley	98%	482
Pacific Hospital of Long Beach[3]	Long Beach	98%	56
Palmdale Regional Medical Center[2]	Palmdale	98%	257
Palo Alto VA Medical Center	Palo Alto	98%	396
Palomar Health Downtown Campus[2]	Escondido	98%	321
Prov Little Co of Mary Med Ctr San Pedro[2]	San Pedro	98%	134
Riverside County Regional Medical Center[2]	Moreno Valley	98%	199
Saint Francis Medical Center[2]	Lynwood	98%	182
Saint Jude Medical Center[2]	Fullerton	98%	409
Saint Mary Medical Center	Apple Valley	98%	416
San Antonio Community Hospital[2]	Upland	98%	388
San Gorgonio Memorial Hospital	Banning	98%	168
Santa Rosa Memorial Hospital[2]	Santa Rosa	98%	265
Sequoia Hospital[2]	Redwood City	98%	408
Seton Medical Center[2]	Daly City	98%	206
Tahoe Forest Hospital	Truckee	98%	170
Univ of CA Davis Med Ctr[2]	Sacramento	98%	351
Univ of CA San Diego Med Ctr[2]	San Diego	98%	371
Valleycare Medical Center	Pleasanton	98%	562
West Anaheim Medical Center	Anaheim	98%	54
Community Regional Medical Center[2]	Fresno	97%	906
Doctors Medical Center - San Pablo[2]	San Pablo	97%	117
Fairchild Medical Center	Yreka	97%	129
Goleta Valley Cottage Hospital[2]	Santa Barbara	97%	237
Kaiser Foundation Hospital - Downey[2]	Downey	97%	314
Kaiser Foundation Hospital - Vacaville[2]	Vacaville	97%	195
LAC/Rancho Los Amigos Ntl Rehab Ctr[2]	Downey	97%	176
Lompoc Valley Medical Center	Lompoc	97%	114
Memorial Hospital of Gardena	Gardena	97%	38
Ojai Valley Community Hospital	Ojai	97%	29
Pacific Alliance Medical Center[2]	Los Angeles	97%	137
Petaluma Valley Hospital[2]	Petaluma	97%	97
Saint Elizabeth Community Hospital[2]	Red Bluff	97%	149
San Dimas Community Hospital[2]	San Dimas	97%	172
San Joaquin General Hospital	French Camp	97%	150
UCSF Medical Center[2]	San Francisco	97%	355
VA Greater Los Angeles Healthcare System	W Los Angeles	97%	279
White Memorial Medical Center[2]	Los Angeles	97%	374
Adventist Medical Center[2]	Hanford	96%	284
Glendale Mem Hosp & Health Ctr[2]	Glendale	96%	386
Kern Medical Center[2]	Bakersfield	96%	225
Mercy Medical Center - Mount Shasta[2]	Mount Shasta	96%	105
Mission Hospital Regional Medical Center[2]	Mission Viejo	96%	346
Oak Valley District Hospital	Oakdale	96%	25
Parkview Comm Hosp Med Ctr[2]	Riverside	96%	423
VA Northern California Healthcare System	Mather	96%	50
Ventura County Medical Center[2]	Ventura	96%	260
Western Medical Center Santa Ana	Santa Ana	96%	208
Madera Community Hospital	Madera	95%	129
Stanislaus Surgical Hospital[2]	Modesto	95%	178
Sutter Delta Medical Center[2]	Antioch	95%	101
Tri - City Regional Medical Center	Hawaiian Grdns	95%	91
Healdsburg District Hospital	Healdsburg	94%	83
Natividad Medical Center	Salinas	94%	78
Palm Drive Hospital[2]	Sebastopol	94%	116
Sutter Coast Hospital	Crescent City	94%	33
Ukiah Valley Medical Center	Ukiah	94%	115
Alameda County Medical Center	Oakland	93%	179
Loma Linda University Medical Center[2]	Loma Linda	93%	450
Los Angeles Community Hospital[2]	Los Angeles	93%	27
Mission Community Hospital	Panorama City	93%	101
Valley Presbyterian Hospital[2]	Van Nuys	93%	467
Contra Costa Regional Medical Center[2]	Martinez	92%	62
Hi - Desert Medical Center	Joshua Tree	92%	74
Mammoth Hospital	Mammoth Lakes	92%	49
Oroville Hospital[2]	Oroville	92%	225
Tulare Regional Medical Center	Tulare	92%	52
Mendocino Coast District Hospital	Fort Bragg	91%	56
Menifee Valley Medical Center[2]	Sun City	91%	133
El Centro Regional Medical Center[2]	El Centro	90%	162
Loma Linda Univ Med Ctr-Murrieta[2]	Murrieta	90%	406
Doctors Hospital of West Covina	West Covina	89%	45
Pacifica Hospital of the Valley	Sun Valley	83%	30
Northern Inyo Hospital	Bishop	79%	48

Prophylactic Antibiotic Timing (Outpatient)

Hospital Name	City	Rate	Cases
Ahmc Anaheim Regional Medical Center	Anaheim	100%	251
Alhambra Hospital Medical Center	Alhambra	100%	47
California Hosp Med Ctr Los Angeles	Los Angeles	100%	105
Doctors Hospital of Manteca	Manteca	100%	41
Dominican Hospital	Santa Cruz	100%	126
French Hospital Medical Center	San Luis Obispo	100%	169
Fresno Surgical Hospital	Fresno	100%	89
Hoag Orthopedic Institute	Irvine	100%	224
John Muir Med Ctr-Walnut Creek Campus	Walnut Creek	100%	261
Lodi Memorial Hospital	Lodi	100%	282
Los Alamitos Medical Center	Los Alamitos	100%	138
Marina Del Rey Hospital	Marina Del Rey	100%	116
Marshall Medical Center	Placerville	100%	163
Olympia Medical Center	Los Angeles	100%	34
Patients' Hospital of Redding	Redding	100%	44
Placentia Linda Hospital	Placentia	100%	76
Prov Little Co of Mary Med Ctr Torrance	Torrance	100%	289
Queen of the Valley Medical Center	Napa	100%	212
Saint Johns Pleasant Valley Hospital	Camarillo	100%	36
Saint Louise Regional Hospital	Gilroy	100%	59
San Gabriel Valley Medical Center	San Gabriel	100%	52
San Leandro Hospital[3]	San Leandro	100%	35
Scripps Green Hospital	La Jolla	100%	413
Scripps Memorial Hospital - Encinitas	Encinitas	100%	264
Scripps Memorial Hospital La Jolla	La Jolla	100%	564
Sequoia Hospital	Redwood City	100%	274
Sharp Memorial Hospital	San Diego	100%	577
Shasta Regional Medical Center	Redding	100%	218
Southern California Hospital at Hollywood[3]	Hollywood	100%	76
Sutter Davis Hospital	Davis	100%	37
Sutter General Hospital	Sacramento	100%	469
Sutter Tracy Community Hospital	Tracy	100%	91
Temple Community Hospital	Los Angeles	100%	32
Tri - City Medical Center	Oceanside	100%	336
Ukiah Valley Medical Center	Ukiah	100%	46
Univ of CA Davis Med Ctr	Sacramento	100%	235
Western Medical Center Hospital Anaheim	Anaheim	100%	38
Alta Bates Summit Medical Center	Oakland	99%	291
Dameron Hospital	Stockton	99%	116
Desert Regional Medical Center	Palm Springs	99%	190
Doctors Medical Center	Modesto	99%	484
Eden Medical Center	Castro Valley	99%	169
Foothill Presbyterian Hospital	Glendora	99%	72
Garfield Medical Center	Monterey Park	99%	306
Hoag Memorial Hospital Presbyterian	Newport Beach	99%	730
Los Robles Hospital & Medical Center	Thousand Oaks	99%	245
Mercy General Hospital	Sacramento	99%	395
Mercy Hospital	Bakersfield	99%	177
Mercy Medical Center - Redding	Redding	99%	448
Mercy San Juan Medical Center	Carmichael	99%	126
Providence Saint Joseph Medical Center	Burbank	99%	365
Providence Tarzana Medical Center	Tarzana	99%	292
Redlands Community Hospital	Redlands	99%	475
Regional Medical Center of San Jose	San Jose	99%	135
Saint Elizabeth Community Hospital	Red Bluff	99%	79
Saint Joseph's Medical Center of Stockton	Stockton	99%	249
Saint Jude Medical Center	Fullerton	99%	537
Salinas Valley Memorial Hospital	Salinas	99%	184
San Ramon Regional Medical Center	San Ramon	99%	195
Santa Rosa Memorial Hospital	Santa Rosa	99%	361
Southwest Healthcare System	Murrieta	99%	163
Sutter Medical Center of Santa Rosa	Santa Rosa	99%	122
Sutter Roseville Medical Center	Roseville	99%	242
Sutter Solano Medical Center	Vallejo	99%	93
USC Verdugo Hills Hospital	Glendale	99%	125
Valleycare Medical Center	Pleasanton	99%	167
White Memorial Medical Center	Los Angeles	99%	211
Bakersfield Memorial Hospital	Bakersfield	98%	500
Centinela Hospital Medical Center	Inglewood	98%	58
Clovis Community Medical Center	Clovis	98%	348
Comm Hosp of the Monterey Peninsula	Monterey	98%	176
El Camino Hospital	Mountain View	98%	653
Grossmont Hospital	La Mesa	98%	313
John Muir Medical Center - Concord Campus	Concord	98%	253
LAC+USC Medical Center	Los Angeles	98%	127
LAC/Olive View - UCLA Medical Center	Sylmar	98%	46
Long Beach Memorial Medical Center	Long Beach	98%	242
Marian Regional Medical Center	Santa Maria	98%	317
Marin General Hospital	Greenbrae	98%	204
Memorial Hospital Los Banos	Los Banos	98%	56
Mercy Medical Center	Merced	98%	132
Monterey Park Hospital	Monterey Park	98%	90
Riverside Community Hospital	Riverside	98%	459
Saddleback Memorial Medical Center	Laguna Hills	98%	503
Saint Mary Medical Center	Apple Valley	98%	160

NOTE: Hospital profiles are in alphabetical order by state, then city, then hospital within the city; Rankings exclude hospitals with less than 25 cases except for patient surveys which excludes hospitals with less than 100 cases; (a) 100-299 cases; (1) The number of cases/patients is too few to report; (2) Data submitted were based on a sample of cases/patients; (3) Results are based on a shorter time period than required; (4) Data suppressed by CMS for one or more quarters; (5) Results are not available for this reporting period; (6) Fewer than 100 patients completed the HCAHPS survey; (7) No cases met the criteria for this measure; (8) The lower limit of the confidence interval cannot be calculated if the number of observed infections equals zero; (9) No data are available from the state/territory for this reporting period; (10) The scores shown reflect fewer than 50 completed surveys; (11) There were discrepancies in the data collection process; (12) This measure does not apply to this hospital for this reporting period; (13) Results cannot be calculated for this reporting period; (14) The results for this state are combined with nearby states to protect confidentiality; Please refer to the User's Guide for a full explanation of data.

Saint Mary Medical Center	Long Beach	98%	97
San Joaquin Community Hospital	Bakersfield	98%	262
Santa Barbara Cottage Hospital	Santa Barbara	98%	634
Santa Clara Valley Medical Center	San Jose	98%	121
Sharp Chula Vista Medical Center	Chula Vista	98%	206
Sierra View District Hospital	Porterville	98%	128
Sonora Regional Medical Center	Sonora	98%	134
Sutter Maternity & Surgery Ctr	Santa Cruz	98%	118
Sutter Surgical Hospital - North Valley	Yuba City	98%	47
Tulare Regional Medical Center	Tulare	98%	114
West Hills Hospital & Medical Center	West Hills	98%	138
Alvarado Hospital Medical Center	San Diego	97%	102
Bakersfield Heart Hospital	Bakersfield	97%	226
Barstow Community Hospital	Barstow	97%	35
CA Pacific Med Ctr-Pacific Campus Hosp	San Francisco	97%	363
Cedars - Sinai Medical Center	Los Angeles	97%	808
Citrus Valley Medical Center - IC Campus	Covina	97%	302
Comm Mem Hosp San Buenaventura	Ventura	97%	397
Enloe Medical Center	Chico	97%	295
Fountain Valley Reg Hosp & Med Ctr	Fountain Valley	97%	268
Fresno Heart & Surgical Hospital	Fresno	97%	285
Good Samaritan Hospital	Los Angeles	97%	217
Henry Mayo Newhall Memorial Hospital	Valencia	97%	64
Huntington Memorial Hospital	Pasadena	97%	234
LAC/Harbor - UCLA Medical Center	Torrance	97%	71
Lakewood Regional Medical Center	Lakewood	97%	259
Memorial Medical Center	Modesto	97%	147
Menifee Valley Medical Center	Sun City	97%	31
Mills - Peninsula Medical Center	Burlingame	97%	179
Northridge Hospital Medical Center	Northridge	97%	172
PIH Hospital - Downey	Downey	97%	74
Saint Agnes Medical Center	Fresno	97%	401
Saint Bernardine Medical Center	San Bernardino	97%	155
Saint Joseph Hospital	Eureka	97%	248
Saint Joseph Hospital	Orange	97%	612
Saint Mary's Medical Center	San Francisco	97%	100
San Antonio Community Hospital	Upland	97%	370
Sierra Vista Regional Medical Center	San Luis Obispo	97%	29
Stanford Hospital	Stanford	97%	637
Sutter Lakeside Hospital	Lakeport	97%	59
Torrance Memorial Medical Center	Torrance	97%	386
UCSF Medical Center	San Francisco	97%	479
Univ of California Irvine Med Ctr	Orange	97%	266
Univ of CA San Diego Med Ctr	San Diego	97%	241
Alta Bates Summit Medical Center	Berkeley	96%	79
Antelope Valley Hospital	Lancaster	96%	126
Arrowhead Regional Medical Center	Colton	96%	142
Barton Memorial Hospital	S Lake Tahoe	96%	89
Eisenhower Medical Center	Rancho Mirage	96%	499
Glendale Adventist Medical Center	Glendale	96%	116
Glendale Mem Hosp & Health Ctr	Glendale	96%	164
John F Kennedy Memorial Hospital	Indio	96%	52
Kaweah Delta Medical Center	Visalia	96%	322
Memorial Hospital of Gardena	Gardena	96%	28
Methodist Hospital of Southern California	Arcadia	96%	224
Northbay Medical Center	Fairfield	96%	170
Paradise Valley Hospital	National City	96%	57
Pomona Valley Hospital Medical Center	Pomona	96%	309
Rideout Memorial Hospital	Marysville	96%	170
Saint Vincent Medical Center	Los Angeles	96%	211
Santa Monica-UCLA Med Ctr & Ortho Hosp	Santa Monica	96%	211
Simi Valley Hosp & Health Care Svcs	Simi Valley	96%	50
Sutter Auburn Faith Hospital	Auburn	96%	56
Twin Cities Community Hospital	Templeton	96%	70
Washington Hospital	Fremont	96%	153
Corona Regional Medical Center	Corona	95%	59
Doctors Medical Center - San Pablo	San Pablo	95%	106
Good Samaritan Hospital	San Jose	95%	440
Hemet Valley Medical Center	Hemet	95%	118
Keck Hospital of USC	Los Angeles	95%	370
Mission Community Hospital	Panorama City	95%	66
Mission Hospital Regional Medical Center	Mission Viejo	95%	347
Petaluma Valley Hospital	Petaluma	95%	41
Presbyterian Intercommunity Hospital	Whittier	95%	241
Providence Saint John's Health Center	Santa Monica	95%	299
Seton Medical Center	Daly City	95%	137
Watsonville Community Hospital	Watsonville	95%	55
Community Regional Medical Center	Fresno	94%	413
Kern Medical Center	Bakersfield	94%	170
Mercy Medical Center - Mount Shasta	Mount Shasta	94%	32
O'Connor Hospital	San Jose	94%	151
Orange Coast Memorial Medical Center	Fountain Valley	94%	268
Providence Holy Cross Medical Center	Mission Hills	94%	143
Prov Little Co of Mary Med Ctr San Pedro	San Pedro	94%	47
Saint Rose Hospital	Hayward	94%	33
Scripps Mercy Hospital	San Diego	94%	501
Western Medical Center Santa Ana	Santa Ana	94%	81
Beverly Hospital	Montebello	93%	91
CA Pacific Med Ctr-Davies Campus	San Francisco	93%	153
Hollywood Presbyterian Medical Center	Los Angeles	93%	60
Loma Linda University Medical Center	Loma Linda	93%	434
Ronald Reagan UCLA Medical Center	Los Angeles	93%	302
Saint Johns Regional Medical Center	Oxnard	93%	165
Sonoma Valley Hospital	Sonoma	93%	30
Sutter Delta Medical Center	Antioch	93%	55
Whittier Hospital Medical Center	Whittier	93%	43
Woodland Memorial Hospital	Woodland	93%	72
Feather River Hospital	Paradise	92%	85
Saint Helena Hospital	Saint Helena	92%	155
San Mateo Medical Center	San Mateo	92%	66
Stanislaus Surgical Hospital	Modesto	92%	100
Palmdale Regional Medical Center	Palmdale	91%	74
Sierra Nevada Memorial Hospital	Grass Valley	91%	34
Riverside County Regional Medical Center	Moreno Valley	90%	41
San Joaquin General Hospital	French Camp	90%	41
Valley Presbyterian Hospital	Van Nuys	90%	98
Goleta Valley Cottage Hospital	Santa Barbara	89%	28
Pioneers Memorial Healthcare District	Brawley	89%	142
CA Pacific Med Ctr-St Luke's Campus	San Francisco	88%	33
Palomar Health Downtown Campus	Escondido	88%	258
Delano Regional Medical Center	Delano	86%	29
Emanuel Medical Center	Turlock	86%	88
Community Hospital of San Bernardino	San Bernardino	84%	31
Loma Linda Univ Med Ctr-Murrieta	Murrieta	84%	148
Pomerado Hospital	Poway	84%	69
Coastal Communities Hospital	Santa Ana	83%	29
Parkview Comm Hosp Med Ctr	Riverside	82%	33
Saint Francis Medical Center	Lynwood	82%	125
Adventist Medical Center	Hanford	80%	86
Oroville Hospital	Oroville	70%	30
Alameda County Medical Center[3]	Oakland	62%	34
El Centro Regional Medical Center	El Centro	52%	165
Contra Costa Regional Medical Center	Martinez	43%	28

Urinary Catheter Removal

Hospital Name	City	Rate	Cases
Barstow Community Hospital	Barstow	100%	27
Barton Memorial Hospital	S Lake Tahoe	100%	207
Dameron Hospital	Stockton	100%	544
Dominican Hospital[2]	Santa Cruz	100%	288
Fallbrook Hospital	Fallbrook	100%	228
Fresno Heart & Surgical Hospital[2]	Fresno	100%	356
Garfield Medical Center[2]	Monterey Park	100%	114
Good Samaritan Hospital[2]	Los Angeles	100%	417
Healdsburg District Hospital	Healdsburg	100%	85
Hoag Orthopedic Institute[2]	Irvine	100%	586
Kaiser Foundation Hospital[2]	San Rafael	100%	325
Kaiser Foundation Hospital - Antioch[2]	Antioch	100%	301
Kaiser Foundation Hospital - Fontana[2]	Fontana	100%	274
Kaiser Fdn Hosp-Fremont/Hayward[2]	Hayward	100%	345
Kaiser Foundation Hospital - Los Angeles[2]	Los Angeles	100%	433
Kaiser Fdn Hosp-Moreno Valley[2]	Moreno Valley	100%	71
Kaiser Fdn Hosp-Oakland/Richmond[2]	Oakland	100%	274
Kaiser Foundation Hospital - Redwood City[2]	Redwood City	100%	307
Kaiser Foundation Hospital - Roseville[2]	Roseville	100%	323
Kaiser Foundation Hospital - Sacramento[2]	Sacramento	100%	284
Kaiser Foundation Hospital - San Diego[2]	San Diego	100%	311
Kaiser Fdn Hosp-San Francisco[2]	San Francisco	100%	445
Kaiser Foundation Hospital - San Jose[2]	San Jose	100%	290
Kaiser Foundation Hospital - Santa Clara[2]	Santa Clara	100%	346
Kaiser Foundation Hospital - Santa Rosa[2]	Santa Rosa	100%	368
Kaiser Foundation Hospital - South Bay[2]	Harbor City	100%	286
Kaiser Fdn Hosp-S San Francisco[2]	S San Francisco	100%	284
Kaiser Foundation Hospital - Vacaville[2]	Vacaville	100%	267
Kaiser Foundation Hospital - West La[2]	Los Angeles	100%	280
Kaiser Fdn Hosp-Woodland Hills[2]	Woodland Hills	100%	255
LAC/Rancho Los Amigos Ntl Rehab Ctr[2]	Downey	100%	159
Mercy General Hospital[2]	Sacramento	100%	350
Methodist Hospital of Sacramento[2]	Sacramento	100%	56
Palmdale Regional Medical Center[2]	Palmdale	100%	109
Palo Alto VA Medical Center[2]	Palo Alto	100%	272
Paradise Valley Hospital	National City	100%	27
Pomona Valley Hospital Medical Center[2]	Pomona	100%	327
Prov Little Co of Mary Med Ctr Torrance[2]	Torrance	100%	351
Providence Saint John's Health Center[2]	Santa Monica	100%	269
Ronald Reagan UCLA Medical Center[2]	Los Angeles	100%	258
Saint Francis Memorial Hospital[2]	San Francisco	100%	222
Saint Vincent Medical Center[2]	Los Angeles	100%	496
Salinas Valley Memorial Hospital[2]	Salinas	100%	284
San Gabriel Valley Medical Center[2]	San Gabriel	100%	154
Santa Monica-UCLA Med Ctr & Ortho Hosp[2]	Santa Monica	100%	211
Scripps Green Hospital[2]	La Jolla	100%	390
Scripps Memorial Hospital - Encinitas[2]	Encinitas	100%	303
Sharp Coronado Hosp & Healthcare Ctr	Coronado	100%	1256
Southern California Hospital at Hollywood	Hollywood	100%	52
Stanford Hospital[2]	Stanford	100%	458
Sutter Davis Hospital[2]	Davis	100%	142
Sutter General Hospital[2]	Sacramento	100%	544
Sutter Maternity & Surgery Ctr	Santa Cruz	100%	163
Sutter Solano Medical Center[2]	Vallejo	100%	249
Sutter Tracy Community Hospital	Tracy	100%	126
Temple Community Hospital	Los Angeles	100%	35
VA Long Beach Healthcare System[2]	Long Beach	100%	163
VA San Diego Healthcare System[2]	San Diego	100%	288
Watsonville Community Hospital	Watsonville	100%	61
West Hills Hospital & Medical Center[2]	West Hills	100%	274
Western Medical Center Hospital Anaheim	Anaheim	100%	41
Woodland Memorial Hospital[2]	Woodland	100%	128
Centinela Hospital Medical Center[2]	Inglewood	99%	81
Citrus Valley Medical Center - IC Campus[2]	Covina	99%	577
Clovis Community Medical Center[2]	Clovis	99%	163
Desert Valley Hospital[2]	Victorville	99%	94
Doctors Medical Center[2]	Modesto	99%	485
El Camino Hospital[2]	Mountain View	99%	709
Emanuel Medical Center	Turlock	99%	184
Feather River Hospital[2]	Paradise	99%	214
French Hospital Medical Center[2]	San Luis Obispo	99%	350
Fresno Surgical Hospital[2]	Fresno	99%	310
Goleta Valley Cottage Hospital[2]	Santa Barbara	99%	295
Good Samaritan Hospital[2]	San Jose	99%	347
Grossmont Hospital[2]	La Mesa	99%	830
John F Kennedy Memorial Hospital[2]	Indio	99%	569
Kaiser Foundation Hospital & Rehab Center[2]	Vallejo	99%	304
Kaiser Foundation Hospital - Downey[2]	Downey	99%	253
Kaiser Foundation Hospital - Fresno[2]	Fresno	99%	314
Kaiser Foundation Hospital - Manteca[2]	Manteca	99%	302
Kaiser Fdn Hosp-Orange Co-Anaheim[2]	Anaheim	99%	378
Kaiser Fdn Hosp-Panorama City[2]	Panorama City	99%	145
Kaiser Foundation Hospital - Riverside[2]	Riverside	99%	265
Kaiser Foundation Hospital - Walnut Creek[2]	Walnut Creek	99%	291
Lodi Memorial Hospital[2]	Lodi	99%	191
Los Alamitos Medical Center[2]	Los Alamitos	99%	444
Marin General Hospital[2]	Greenbrae	99%	213
Memorial Medical Center[2]	Modesto	99%	327
Mercy Hospital[2]	Bakersfield	99%	242
Mercy Medical Center[2]	Merced	99%	274
Mercy Medical Center - Mount Shasta[2]	Mount Shasta	99%	102
Mills - Peninsula Medical Center[2]	Burlingame	99%	358
Northbay Medical Center	Fairfield	99%	298
Northridge Hospital Medical Center[2]	Northridge	99%	634
Placentia Linda Hospital[2]	Placentia	99%	360
Providence Holy Cross Medical Center[2]	Mission Hills	99%	274
Prov Little Co of Mary Med Ctr San Pedro[2]	San Pedro	99%	126
Providence Saint Joseph Medical Center[2]	Burbank	99%	298
Providence Tarzana Medical Center[2]	Tarzana	99%	205
Redlands Community Hospital[2]	Redlands	99%	621
Riverside Community Hospital[2]	Riverside	99%	337
Riverside County Regional Medical Center[2]	Moreno Valley	99%	155
Saint Elizabeth Community Hospital[2]	Red Bluff	99%	122
Saint Joseph Hospital[2]	Orange	99%	332
Saint Jude Medical Center[2]	Fullerton	99%	285
Saint Mary Medical Center[2]	Long Beach	99%	98
Saint Mary's Medical Center[2]	San Francisco	99%	109
San Dimas Community Hospital[2]	San Dimas	99%	157
San Francisco General Hospital[2]	San Francisco	99%	150
San Mateo Medical Center	San Mateo	99%	92
San Ramon Regional Medical Center[2]	San Ramon	99%	154
Scripps Memorial Hospital La Jolla[2]	La Jolla	99%	438
Scripps Mercy Hospital[2]	San Diego	99%	422
Sharp Chula Vista Medical Center[2]	Chula Vista	99%	286
Sharp Memorial Hospital[2]	San Diego	99%	1245
Sierra View District Hospital	Porterville	99%	141
Sonora Regional Medical Center	Sonora	99%	320
Sutter Medical Center of Santa Rosa[2]	Santa Rosa	99%	343
Torrance Memorial Medical Center[2]	Torrance	99%	551
VA Greater Los Angeles Healthcare System[2]	W Los Angeles	99%	255
Beverly Hospital	Montebello	98%	141
CA Pacific Med Ctr-Pacific Campus Hosp[2]	San Francisco	98%	454
Community Regional Medical Center[2]	Fresno	98%	591
Enloe Medical Center[2]	Chico	98%	560
Fairchild Medical Center	Yreka	98%	93
Hollywood Presbyterian Medical Center[2]	Los Angeles	98%	182
John Muir Med Ctr-Walnut Creek Campus[2]	Walnut Creek	98%	297
Kaiser Foundation Hospital - Baldwin Park[2]	Baldwin Park	98%	292
Kaiser Fdn Hosp S Sacramento[2]	Sacramento	98%	241
Keck Hospital of USC[2]	Los Angeles	98%	449
LAC/Harbor - UCLA Medical Center[2]	Torrance	98%	181
LAC/Olive View - UCLA Medical Center[2]	Sylmar	98%	57
Los Robles Hospital & Medical Center[2]	Thousand Oaks	98%	425
Marian Regional Medical Center[2]	Santa Maria	98%	391
Mercy Hospital of Folsom[2]	Folsom	98%	113
Olympia Medical Center	Los Angeles	98%	110
Pacific Hospital of Long Beach[3]	Long Beach	98%	56
Petaluma Valley Hospital[2]	Petaluma	98%	112
Presbyterian Intercommunity Hospital[2]	Whittier	98%	327
Queen of the Valley Medical Center[2]	Napa	98%	253
Saint Johns Regional Medical Center[2]	Oxnard	98%	312
Saint Joseph's Medical Center of Stockton[2]	Stockton	98%	263
Saint Mary Medical Center	Apple Valley	98%	365
Saint Rose Hospital[2]	Hayward	98%	210
San Joaquin Community Hospital[2]	Bakersfield	98%	423
Sequoia Hospital[2]	Redwood City	98%	407
Seton Medical Center[2]	Daly City	98%	200

NOTE: Hospital profiles are in alphabetical order by state, then city, then hospital within the city; Rankings exclude hospitals with less than 25 cases except for patient surveys which excludes hospitals with less than 100 cases; (a) 100-299 cases; (1) The number of cases/patients is too few to report; (2) Data submitted were based on a sample of cases/patients; (3) Results are based on a shorter time period than required; (4) Data suppressed by CMS for one or more quarters; (5) Results are not available for this reporting period; (6) Fewer than 100 patients completed the HCAHPS survey; (7) No cases met the criteria for this measure; (8) The lower limit of the confidence interval cannot be calculated if the number of observed infections equals zero; (9) No data are available from the state/territory for this reporting period; (10) The scores shown reflect fewer than 50 completed surveys; (11) There were discrepancies in the data collection process; (12) This measure does not apply to this hospital for this reporting period; (13) Results cannot be calculated for this reporting period; (14) The results for this state are combined with nearby states to protect confidentiality; Please refer to the User's Guide for a full explanation of data.

Shasta Regional Medical Center	Redding	98%	412
Sherman Oaks Hospital	Sherman Oaks	98%	54
Sonoma Valley Hospital	Sonoma	98%	108
Stanislaus Surgical Hospital[2]	Modesto	98%	50
Sutter Auburn Faith Hospital[2]	Auburn	98%	262
Sutter Lakeside Hospital	Lakeport	98%	83
Sutter Surgical Hospital - North Valley	Yuba City	98%	236
Tri - City Medical Center[2]	Oceanside	98%	264
Tulare Regional Medical Center	Tulare	98%	43
Univ of CA Davis Med Ctr[2]	Sacramento	98%	250
Univ of CA San Diego Med Ctr[2]	San Diego	98%	316
VA Northern California Healthcare System[2]	Mather	98%	56
Valleycare Medical Center	Pleasanton	98%	452
West Anaheim Medical Center	Anaheim	98%	59
Whittier Hospital Medical Center	Whittier	98%	59
Antelope Valley Hospital[2]	Lancaster	97%	489
Bakersfield Memorial Hospital[2]	Bakersfield	97%	377
California Hosp Med Ctr Los Angeles[2]	Los Angeles	97%	222
Cedars - Sinai Medical Center	Los Angeles	97%	2661
Chapman Medical Center	Orange	97%	89
Community Hospital of San Bernardino[2]	San Bernardino	97%	29
Comm Mem Hosp San Buenaventura[2]	Ventura	97%	297
Glendale Adventist Medical Center[2]	Glendale	97%	487
Glendale Mem Hosp & Health Ctr[2]	Glendale	97%	289
Henry Mayo Newhall Memorial Hospital[2]	Valencia	97%	209
John Muir Medical Center - Concord Campus[2]	Concord	97%	375
Kern Medical Center[2]	Bakersfield	97%	156
LAC+USC Medical Center[2]	Los Angeles	97%	243
Lakewood Regional Medical Center[2]	Lakewood	97%	367
Long Beach Memorial Medical Center[2]	Long Beach	97%	362
Marina Del Rey Hospital[2]	Marina Del Rey	97%	120
Memorial Hospital of Gardena	Gardena	97%	29
Mercy Medical Center - Redding[2]	Redding	97%	458
Monterey Park Hospital[2]	Monterey Park	97%	36
Novato Community Hospital	Novato	97%	119
Ojai Valley Community Hospital	Ojai	97%	34
Rideout Memorial Hospital[2]	Marysville	97%	174
San Francisco VA Medical Center[2]	San Francisco	97%	338
Sierra Vista Regional Medical Center	San Luis Obispo	97%	284
Southwest Healthcare System[2]	Murrieta	97%	280
Twin Cities Community Hospital	Templeton	97%	327
Univ of California Irvine Med Ctr[2]	Orange	97%	243
Washington Hospital[2]	Fremont	97%	340
White Memorial Medical Center[2]	Los Angeles	97%	357
Alta Bates Summit Medical Center[2]	Oakland	96%	306
CA Pacific Med Ctr-St Luke's Campus[2]	San Francisco	96%	89
Community Hospital of Long Beach	Long Beach	96%	27
Desert Regional Medical Center[2]	Palm Springs	96%	291
Doctors Hospital of Manteca	Manteca	96%	79
Eisenhower Medical Center	Rancho Mirage	96%	1307
Loma Linda VA Medical Center[2]	Loma Linda	96%	72
Marshall Medical Center[2]	Placerville	96%	226
Mercy San Juan Medical Center[2]	Carmichael	96%	291
Mission Community Hospital	Panorama City	96%	72
Mission Hospital Regional Medical Center[2]	Mission Viejo	96%	358
Pacific Alliance Medical Center[2]	Los Angeles	96%	81
Saint Louise Regional Hospital[2]	Gilroy	96%	81
San Antonio Community Hospital[2]	Upland	96%	300
Santa Barbara Cottage Hospital[2]	Santa Barbara	96%	406
Santa Clara Valley Medical Center[2]	San Jose	96%	218
USC Verdugo Hills Hospital[2]	Glendale	96%	141
Ahmc Anaheim Regional Medical Center[2]	Anaheim	95%	234
Alameda County Medical Center	Oakland	95%	170
Comm Hosp of the Monterey Peninsula	Monterey	95%	470
Doctors Medical Center - San Pablo[2]	San Pablo	95%	155
Fountain Valley Reg Hosp & Med Ctr[2]	Fountain Valley	95%	282
Hoag Memorial Hospital Presbyterian[2]	Newport Beach	95%	434
Huntington Memorial Hospital[2]	Pasadena	95%	331
Palm Drive Hospital[2]	Sebastopol	95%	44
Palomar Health Downtown Campus[2]	Escondido	95%	253
PIH Hospital - Downey[2]	Downey	95%	131
Saddleback Memorial Medical Center[2]	Laguna Hills	95%	309
Saint Francis Medical Center[2]	Lynwood	95%	104
Saint Helena Hospital	Saint Helena	95%	193
Santa Rosa Memorial Hospital[2]	Santa Rosa	95%	272
Sierra Nevada Memorial Hospital[2]	Grass Valley	95%	96
Sutter Roseville Medical Center[2]	Roseville	95%	304
Tri - City Regional Medical Center	Hawaiian Grdns	95%	37
Ventura County Medical Center[2]	Ventura	95%	245
Alvarado Hospital Medical Center	San Diego	94%	232
CA Pacific Med Ctr-Davies Campus[2]	San Francisco	94%	63
Eden Medical Center[2]	Castro Valley	94%	253
Frank R Howard Memorial Hospital	Willits	94%	36
Loma Linda University Medical Center[2]	Loma Linda	94%	280
Mammoth Hospital	Mammoth Lakes	94%	52
Mark Twain Medical Center[2]	San Andreas	94%	32
Menifee Valley Medical Center[2]	Sun City	94%	106
Parkview Comm Hosp Med Ctr[2]	Riverside	94%	387
Saint Bernardine Medical Center[2]	San Bernardino	94%	314
Tahoe Forest Hospital	Truckee	94%	158
Ukiah Valley Medical Center	Ukiah	94%	109
Adventist Medical Center[2]	Hanford	93%	199
Arrowhead Regional Medical Center	Colton	93%	223
Mendocino Coast District Hospital	Fort Bragg	93%	55
Northern Inyo Hospital	Bishop	93%	43
Orange Coast Memorial Medical Center[2]	Fountain Valley	93%	264
Pomerado Hospital[2]	Poway	93%	172
Saint Agnes Medical Center[2]	Fresno	93%	440
Sutter Amador Hospital[2]	Jackson	93%	55
Sutter Coast Hospital	Crescent City	93%	27
Delano Regional Medical Center[2]	Delano	92%	49
Kaweah Delta Medical Center[2]	Visalia	92%	281
Methodist Hospital of Southern California[2]	Arcadia	92%	355
O'Connor Hospital[2]	San Jose	92%	119
San Joaquin General Hospital	French Camp	92%	119
UCSF Medical Center[2]	San Francisco	92%	368
Natividad Medical Center	Salinas	91%	68
Regional Medical Center of San Jose[2]	San Jose	91%	194
Valley Presbyterian Hospital[2]	Van Nuys	91%	434
Alhambra Hospital Medical Center	Alhambra	90%	86
Corona Regional Medical Center[2]	Corona	90%	77
Sutter Delta Medical Center[2]	Antioch	90%	97
Saint Johns Pleasant Valley Hospital[2]	Camarillo	89%	152
Alameda Hospital	Alameda	88%	41
Alta Bates Summit Medical Center[2]	Berkeley	88%	94
Bakersfield Heart Hospital[2]	Bakersfield	88%	118
Contra Costa Regional Medical Center[2]	Martinez	88%	52
Foothill Presbyterian Hospital[2]	Glendora	88%	123
Fresno VA Med Ctr-VA Central CA[2]	Fresno	88%	40
Victor Valley Global Medical Center[2]	Victorville	88%	165
Saint Joseph Hospital[2]	Eureka	87%	211
Hi - Desert Medical Center	Joshua Tree	86%	88
Madera Community Hospital	Madera	86%	79
Oroville Hospital[2]	Oroville	86%	177
Simi Valley Hosp & Health Care Svcs[2]	Simi Valley	86%	169
Loma Linda Univ Med Ctr-Murrieta[2]	Murrieta	85%	336
Pioneers Memorial Healthcare District	Brawley	85%	108
Chinese Hospital	San Francisco	82%	78
Hemet Valley Medical Center[2]	Hemet	79%	165
Western Medical Center Santa Ana	Santa Ana	76%	136
Lompoc Valley Medical Center	Lompoc	74%	101
Hazel Hawkins Memorial Hospital	Hollister	71%	42
El Centro Regional Medical Center[2]	El Centro	42%	77

Survey of Patients' Hospital Experiences

Area Around Room 'Always' Quiet at Night

Hospital Name	City	Rate	Cases
Menlo Park Surgical Hospital	Menlo Park	95%	(a)
Patients' Hospital of Redding	Redding	90%	(a)
Fresno Surgical Hospital	Fresno	78%	300+
Fresno Heart & Surgical Hospital	Fresno	77%	300+
Sutter Surgical Hospital - North Valley	Yuba City	77%	(a)
Stanislaus Surgical Hospital	Modesto	75%	300+
Loma Linda Univ Med Ctr-Murrieta	Murrieta	74%	300+
Sutter Maternity & Surgery Ctr	Santa Cruz	73%	300+
Hoag Orthopedic Institute	Irvine	71%	300+
Sharp Coronado Hosp & Healthcare Ctr	Coronado	71%	300+
Olympia Medical Center	Los Angeles	70%	300+
Palmdale Regional Medical Center	Palmdale	70%	300+
Temple Community Hospital	Los Angeles	67%	(a)
Palo Verde Hospital	Blythe	66%	(a)
Sharp Memorial Hospital	San Diego	66%	300+
Banner Lassen Medical Center[11]	Susanville	65%	(a)
City of Hope Helford Clinical Res Hosp	Duarte	65%	300+
Colusa Regional Medical Center	Colusa	65%	(a)
Good Samaritan Hospital	Bakersfield	65%	(a)
Novato Community Hospital	Novato	64%	300+
Pacific Hospital of Long Beach	Long Beach	64%	300+
Kaiser Fdn Hosp-Orange Co-Anaheim	Anaheim	62%	300+
Marian Regional Medical Center	Santa Maria	62%	300+
Northern Inyo Hospital	Bishop	62%	(a)
Sutter Davis Hospital	Davis	62%	300+
Tahoe Forest Hospital	Truckee	62%	(a)
Barstow Community Hospital	Barstow	61%	300+
Kaiser Fdn Hosp-Panorama City	Panorama City	61%	300+
Memorial Hospital Los Banos	Los Banos	61%	(a)
Mills - Peninsula Medical Center	Burlingame	61%	300+
Sutter Amador Hospital	Jackson	61%	300+
Univ of California Irvine Med Ctr	Orange	61%	300+
Clovis Community Medical Center	Clovis	60%	300+
Eden Medical Center	Castro Valley	60%	300+
Kaiser Foundation Hospital - West La	Los Angeles	60%	300+
Santa Barbara Cottage Hospital	Santa Barbara	60%	300+
Seton Medical Center	Daly City	60%	300+
Hi - Desert Medical Center	Joshua Tree	59%	300+
John Muir Med Ctr-Walnut Creek Campus	Walnut Creek	59%	300+
Kaiser Foundation Hospital - Downey	Downey	59%	300+
Ojai Valley Community Hospital	Ojai	59%	(a)
Saint Agnes Medical Center	Fresno	59%	300+
Saint Francis Medical Center	Lynwood	59%	300+
Sutter Coast Hospital	Crescent City	59%	300+
Sutter Solano Medical Center	Vallejo	59%	300+
Eisenhower Medical Center	Rancho Mirage	58%	300+
Glendale Adventist Medical Center	Glendale	58%	300+
Huntington Memorial Hospital	Pasadena	58%	300+
Kaiser Foundation Hospital - Los Angeles	Los Angeles	58%	300+
Kaiser Foundation Hospital - Manteca	Manteca	58%	300+
Mark Twain Medical Center	San Andreas	58%	(a)
Mendocino Coast District Hospital	Fort Bragg	58%	(a)
Mercy Medical Center	Merced	58%	300+
Mercy Medical Center - Mount Shasta	Mount Shasta	58%	(a)
Presbyterian Intercommunity Hospital	Whittier	58%	300+
Providence Saint John's Health Center	Santa Monica	58%	300+
Saint Helena Hospital	Saint Helena	58%	300+
Saint Joseph Hospital	Orange	58%	300+
Central Valley General Hospital	Hanford	57%	300+
El Camino Hospital	Mountain View	57%	300+
John Muir Medical Center - Concord Campus	Concord	57%	300+
Kaiser Foundation Hospital - Baldwin Park	Baldwin Park	57%	300+
Montclair Hospital Medical Center[11]	Montclair	57%	(a)
Redlands Community Hospital	Redlands	57%	300+
Ronald Reagan UCLA Medical Center	Los Angeles	57%	300+
Saint Bernardine Medical Center	San Bernardino	57%	300+
Santa Monica-UCLA Med Ctr & Ortho Hosp	Santa Monica	57%	300+
Scripps Green Hospital	La Jolla	57%	300+
Sutter Tracy Community Hospital	Tracy	57%	300+
Cedars - Sinai Medical Center	Los Angeles	56%	300+
Community Hospital of San Bernardino	San Bernardino	56%	300+
Kaiser Foundation Hospital - Antioch	Antioch	56%	300+
Keck Hospital of USC	Los Angeles	56%	300+
Palomar Health Downtown Campus	Escondido	56%	300+
Providence Saint Joseph Medical Center	Burbank	56%	300+
Simi Valley Hosp & Health Care Svcs	Simi Valley	56%	300+
Univ of CA San Diego Med Ctr	San Diego	56%	300+
White Memorial Medical Center	Los Angeles	56%	300+
Comm Hosp of the Monterey Peninsula	Monterey	55%	300+
Desert Valley Hospital	Victorville	55%	300+
Hoag Memorial Hospital Presbyterian	Newport Beach	55%	300+
Hollywood Presbyterian Medical Center	Los Angeles	55%	300+
Kaiser Foundation Hospital - Fontana	Fontana	55%	300+
Kaiser Foundation Hospital - Santa Clara	Santa Clara	55%	300+
Kaiser Foundation Hospital - Santa Rosa	Santa Rosa	55%	300+
Kaiser Foundation Hospital - Vacaville	Vacaville	55%	300+
La Palma Intercommunity Hospital	La Palma	55%	(a)
Mammoth Hospital	Mammoth Lakes	55%	(a)
Paradise Valley Hospital[11]	National City	55%	(a)
Saint Johns Regional Medical Center	Oxnard	55%	300+
Saint Rose Hospital	Hayward	55%	300+
Sutter Lakeside Hospital	Lakeport	55%	300+
Sutter Roseville Medical Center	Roseville	55%	300+
UCSF Medical Center	San Francisco	55%	300+
Alvarado Hospital Medical Center	San Diego	54%	300+
Enloe Medical Center	Chico	54%	300+
Kaiser Foundation Hospital & Rehab Center	Vallejo	54%	300+
Kaiser Foundation Hospital - South Bay	Harbor City	54%	300+
Lakewood Regional Medical Center	Lakewood	54%	300+
O'Connor Hospital	San Jose	54%	300+
Petaluma Valley Hospital	Petaluma	54%	300+
Arrowhead Regional Medical Center	Colton	53%	300+
Barton Memorial Hospital	S Lake Tahoe	53%	300+
Chapman Medical Center	Orange	53%	300+
Doctors Hospital of Manteca	Manteca	53%	300+
Fairchild Medical Center	Yreka	53%	300+
Kaweah Delta Medical Center	Visalia	53%	300+
Lodi Memorial Hospital	Lodi	53%	300+
Mission Hospital Regional Medical Center	Mission Viejo	53%	300+
Prov Little Co of Mary Med Ctr Torrance	Torrance	53%	300+
Redwood Memorial Hospital	Fortuna	53%	300+
Saint Mary Medical Center	Long Beach	53%	300+
San Dimas Community Hospital[11]	San Dimas	53%	300+
San Joaquin Community Hospital	Bakersfield	53%	300+
San Leandro Hospital	San Leandro	53%	(a)
Scripps Memorial Hospital La Jolla	La Jolla	53%	300+
Sierra View District Hospital	Porterville	53%	300+
Adventist Medical Center	Hanford	52%	300+
Chino Valley Medical Center[11]	Chino	52%	300+
Glendale Mem Hosp & Health Ctr	Glendale	52%	300+
Goleta Valley Cottage Hospital	Santa Barbara	52%	300+
Kaiser Fdn Hosp-Moreno Valley	Moreno Valley	52%	300+
Kaiser Foundation Hospital - Roseville	Roseville	52%	300+
Kaiser Fdn Hosp-San Francisco	San Francisco	52%	300+
LAC+USC Medical Center[11]	Los Angeles	52%	300+
Lompoc Valley Medical Center	Lompoc	52%	300+
Los Robles Hospital & Medical Center	Thousand Oaks	52%	300+
Placentia Linda Hospital	Placentia	52%	300+
Saint Helena Hospital - Clearlake	Clearlake	52%	(a)
San Ramon Regional Medical Center	San Ramon	52%	300+
Tri - City Regional Medical Center	Hawaiian Grdns	52%	300+
Watsonville Community Hospital	Watsonville	52%	300+
Adventist Medical Center - Reedley	Reedley	51%	(a)
Bakersfield Memorial Hospital	Bakersfield	51%	300+

NOTE: Hospital profiles are in alphabetical order by state, then city, then hospital within the city; Rankings exclude hospitals with less than 25 cases except for patient surveys which excludes hospitals with less than 100 cases; (a) 100-299 cases; (1) The number of cases/patients is too few to report; (2) Data submitted were based on a sample of cases/patients; (3) Results are based on a shorter time period than required; (4) Data suppressed by CMS for one or more quarters; (5) Results are not available for this reporting period; (6) Fewer than 100 patients completed the HCAHPS survey; (7) No cases met the criteria for this measure; (8) The lower limit of the confidence interval cannot be calculated if the number of observed infections equals zero; (9) No data are available from the state/territory for this reporting period; (10) The scores shown reflect fewer than 50 completed surveys; (11) There were discrepancies in the data collection process; (12) This measure does not apply to this hospital for this reporting period; (13) Results cannot be calculated for this reporting period; (14) The results for this state are combined with nearby states to protect confidentiality; Please refer to the User's Guide for a full explanation of data.

Hospital Name	City	Rate	Cases
Centinela Hospital Medical Center[11]	Inglewood	51%	300+
Citrus Valley Medical Center - IC Campus	Covina	51%	300+
Foothill Presbyterian Hospital	Glendora	51%	300+
Good Samaritan Hospital	Los Angeles	51%	300+
Kaiser Foundation Hospital - Fresno	Fresno	51%	300+
Kaiser Fdn Hosp-Woodland Hills	Woodland Hills	51%	300+
LAC/Rancho Los Amigos Ntl Rehab Ctr	Downey	51%	300+
Memorial Medical Center	Modesto	51%	300+
Pacifica Hospital of the Valley	Sun Valley	51%	(a)
Palm Drive Hospital	Sebastopol	51%	(a)
Pomona Valley Hospital Medical Center	Pomona	51%	300+
Saint Vincent Medical Center	Los Angeles	51%	300+
Sharp Chula Vista Medical Center	Chula Vista	51%	300+
Silver Lake Medical Center	Los Angeles	51%	(a)
Bakersfield Heart Hospital	Bakersfield	50%	300+
California Hosp Med Ctr Los Angeles	Los Angeles	50%	300+
Fallbrook Hospital	Fallbrook	50%	300+
Greater El Monte Community Hospital	South El Monte	50%	300+
Grossmont Hospital	La Mesa	50%	300+
Healdsburg District Hospital	Healdsburg	50%	(a)
Loma Linda University Medical Center	Loma Linda	50%	300+
Menifee Valley Medical Center	Sun City	50%	300+
Methodist Hospital of Southern California	Arcadia	50%	300+
Orange Coast Memorial Medical Center	Fountain Valley	50%	300+
Pioneers Memorial Healthcare District	Brawley	50%	300+
Shasta Regional Medical Center[11]	Redding	50%	300+
Sierra Nevada Memorial Hospital	Grass Valley	50%	300+
Sonoma Valley Hospital	Sonoma	50%	(a)
Southwest Healthcare System	Murrieta	50%	300+
Sutter Auburn Faith Hospital	Auburn	50%	300+
Torrance Memorial Medical Center	Torrance	50%	300+
Twin Cities Community Hospital	Templeton	50%	300+
Victor Valley Global Medical Center	Victorville	50%	300+
Ahmc Anaheim Regional Medical Center	Anaheim	49%	300+
CA Pacific Med Ctr-St Luke's Campus	San Francisco	49%	300+
Community Hospital of Huntington Park	Huntington Park	49%	300+
Desert Regional Medical Center	Palm Springs	49%	300+
George L Mee Memorial Hospital	King City	49%	(a)
Good Samaritan Hospital	San Jose	49%	300+
Kaiser Fdn Hosp S Sacramento	Sacramento	49%	300+
Long Beach Memorial Medical Center	Long Beach	49%	300+
Memorial Hospital of Gardena	Gardena	49%	300+
Mercy General Hospital	Sacramento	49%	300+
Mercy Hospital of Folsom	Folsom	49%	300+
Methodist Hospital of Sacramento	Sacramento	49%	300+
Prov Little Co of Mary Med Ctr San Pedro	San Pedro	49%	300+
Regional Medical Center of San Jose	San Jose	49%	300+
Scripps Memorial Hospital - Encinitas	Encinitas	49%	300+
Sherman Oaks Hospital[11]	Sherman Oaks	49%	(a)
Southern California Hospital at Hollywood	Hollywood	49%	300+
Sutter Delta Medical Center	Antioch	49%	(a)
Sutter General Hospital	Sacramento	49%	300+
West Anaheim Medical Center	Anaheim	49%	300+
Woodland Memorial Hospital	Woodland	49%	(a)
Alhambra Hospital Medical Center	Alhambra	48%	300+
Dameron Hospital	Stockton	48%	300+
Hazel Hawkins Memorial Hospital	Hollister	48%	300+
Monterey Park Hospital	Monterey Park	48%	300+
Saint Joseph's Medical Center of Stockton	Stockton	48%	300+
Saint Jude Medical Center	Fullerton	48%	300+
Scripps Mercy Hospital	San Diego	48%	300+
Sierra Vista Regional Medical Center	San Luis Obispo	48%	300+
Valleycare Medical Center	Pleasanton	48%	300+
Washington Hospital	Fremont	48%	300+
Kaiser Fdn Hosp-Fremont/Hayward	Hayward	47%	300+
Kaiser Foundation Hospital - San Jose	San Jose	47%	300+
Marshall Medical Center	Placerville	47%	300+
Mercy San Juan Medical Center	Carmichael	47%	300+
Northbay Medical Center	Fairfield	47%	300+
Pomerado Hospital	Poway	47%	300+
Riverside County Regional Medical Center	Moreno Valley	47%	300+
Saint Elizabeth Community Hospital	Red Bluff	47%	300+
Valley Presbyterian Hospital	Van Nuys	47%	300+
Comm Mem Hosp San Buenaventura	Ventura	46%	300+
Delano Regional Medical Center	Delano	46%	300+
El Centro Regional Medical Center	El Centro	46%	(a)
Garden Grove Hospital & Medical Center[11]	Garden Grove	46%	300+
Kaiser Foundation Hospital - Redwood City	Redwood City	46%	300+
Natividad Medical Center	Salinas	46%	300+
Sonora Regional Medical Center	Sonora	46%	300+
Univ of CA Davis Med Ctr	Sacramento	46%	300+
Whittier Hospital Medical Center	Whittier	46%	300+
Antelope Valley Hospital	Lancaster	45%	300+
Community Regional Medical Center	Fresno	45%	300+
French Hospital Medical Center	San Luis Obispo	45%	300+
Kaiser Foundation Hospital - San Diego	San Diego	45%	300+
Kaiser Fdn Hosp-S San Francisco	S San Francisco	45%	300+
Mad River Community Hospital	Arcata	45%	300+
Marin General Hospital	Greenbrae	45%	300+
Marina Del Rey Hospital	Marina Del Rey	45%	300+
Mission Community Hospital	Panorama City	45%	300+
Northridge Hospital Medical Center	Northridge	45%	300+
Providence Holy Cross Medical Center	Mission Hills	45%	300+
Saint Joseph Hospital	Eureka	45%	300+
Tulare Regional Medical Center	Tulare	45%	300+
USC Verdugo Hills Hospital	Glendale	45%	300+
Beverly Hospital	Montebello	44%	300+
East Los Angeles Doctors Hospital	Los Angeles	44%	300+
Henry Mayo Newhall Memorial Hospital	Valencia	44%	300+
Kaiser Foundation Hospital - Riverside	Riverside	44%	300+
Saddleback Memorial Medical Center	Laguna Hills	44%	300+
Saint Francis Memorial Hospital	San Francisco	44%	300+
San Gabriel Valley Medical Center	San Gabriel	44%	300+
San Mateo Medical Center	San Mateo	44%	300+
West Hills Hospital & Medical Center	West Hills	44%	300+
Alta Bates Summit Medical Center	Berkeley	43%	300+
Alta Bates Summit Medical Center	Oakland	43%	300+
Community Hospital of Long Beach	Long Beach	43%	300+
Doctors Medical Center	Modesto	43%	300+
Fountain Valley Reg Hosp & Med Ctr	Fountain Valley	43%	300+
John F Kennedy Memorial Hospital	Indio	43%	300+
Saint Johns Pleasant Valley Hospital	Camarillo	43%	300+
San Antonio Community Hospital	Upland	43%	300+
San Joaquin General Hospital	French Camp	43%	300+
Santa Rosa Memorial Hospital	Santa Rosa	43%	300+
Sequoia Hospital	Redwood City	43%	300+
Tri - City Medical Center	Oceanside	43%	300+
CA Pacific Med Ctr-Davies Campus	San Francisco	42%	300+
Huntington Beach Hospital	Huntington Bch	42%	(a)
Mercy Hospital	Bakersfield	42%	300+
Oak Valley District Hospital	Oakdale	42%	(a)
PIH Hospital - Downey	Downey	42%	300+
Queen of the Valley Medical Center	Napa	42%	300+
Saint Louise Regional Hospital	Gilroy	42%	300+
Ventura County Medical Center	Ventura	42%	300+
Western Medical Center Santa Ana	Santa Ana	42%	300+
Corona Regional Medical Center	Corona	41%	300+
Frank R Howard Memorial Hospital	Willits	41%	300+
Kaiser Foundation Hospital - Sacramento	Sacramento	41%	300+
Saint Mary Medical Center	Apple Valley	41%	300+
Salinas Valley Memorial Hospital	Salinas	41%	300+
San Gorgonio Memorial Hospital	Banning	41%	300+
Sutter Medical Center of Santa Rosa	Santa Rosa	41%	300+
Western Medical Center Hospital Anaheim	Anaheim	41%	300+
Chinese Hospital	San Francisco	40%	300+
Emanuel Medical Center	Turlock	40%	300+
Kaiser Fdn Hosp-Oakland/Richmond	Oakland	40%	300+
Kaiser Foundation Hospital - Walnut Creek	Walnut Creek	40%	300+
LAC/Harbor - UCLA Medical Center	Torrance	40%	300+
Madera Community Hospital	Madera	40%	300+
Mercy Medical Center - Redding	Redding	40%	300+
Pacific Alliance Medical Center	Los Angeles	40%	300+
Alameda County Medical Center	Oakland	39%	300+
Coast Plaza Hospital	Norwalk	39%	300+
Coastal Communities Hospital	Santa Ana	39%	300+
Feather River Hospital	Paradise	39%	300+
Kaiser Foundation Hospital	San Rafael	39%	300+
Providence Tarzana Medical Center	Tarzana	39%	300+
Rideout Memorial Hospital	Marysville	39%	300+
Stanford Hospital	Stanford	39%	300+
Ukiah Valley Medical Center	Ukiah	39%	300+
Doctors Medical Center - San Pablo	San Pablo	38%	300+
Oroville Hospital	Oroville	38%	300+
Riverside Community Hospital	Riverside	38%	300+
Saint Mary's Medical Center	San Francisco	38%	300+
Santa Clara Valley Medical Center	San Jose	38%	300+
CA Pacific Med Ctr-Pacific Campus Hosp	San Francisco	37%	300+
Garfield Medical Center	Monterey Park	37%	300+
Kern Medical Center	Bakersfield	37%	300+
LAC/Olive View - UCLA Medical Center	Sylmar	37%	300+
Los Angeles Community Hospital	Los Angeles	37%	300+
Alameda Hospital	Alameda	35%	300+
Hemet Valley Medical Center	Hemet	35%	300+
Parkview Comm Hosp Med Ctr	Riverside	35%	300+
San Francisco General Hospital	San Francisco	35%	(a)
Contra Costa Regional Medical Center	Martinez	34%	300+
Dominican Hospital	Santa Cruz	34%	300+
Los Alamitos Medical Center	Los Alamitos	33%	300+

Doctors 'Always' Communicated Well

Hospital Name	City	Rate	Cases
Menlo Park Surgical Hospital	Menlo Park	89%	(a)
Patients' Hospital of Redding	Redding	89%	(a)
Colusa Regional Medical Center	Colusa	87%	(a)
Hoag Orthopedic Institute	Irvine	87%	300+
City of Hope Helford Clinical Res Hosp	Duarte	86%	300+
Scripps Green Hospital	La Jolla	86%	300+
Frank R Howard Memorial Hospital	Willits	85%	300+
Fresno Surgical Hospital	Fresno	85%	300+
Healdsburg District Hospital	Healdsburg	85%	(a)
Mammoth Hospital	Mammoth Lakes	85%	(a)
Stanford Hospital	Stanford	85%	300+
Sutter Davis Hospital	Davis	85%	300+
Sutter Surgical Hospital - North Valley	Yuba City	85%	(a)
Banner Lassen Medical Center[11]	Susanville	84%	(a)
Doctors Hospital of Manteca	Manteca	84%	300+
Goleta Valley Cottage Hospital	Santa Barbara	84%	300+
Good Samaritan Hospital	Bakersfield	84%	(a)
Ojai Valley Community Hospital	Ojai	84%	(a)
Sharp Coronado Hosp & Healthcare Ctr	Coronado	84%	300+
Stanislaus Surgical Hospital	Modesto	84%	300+
Sutter Auburn Faith Hospital	Auburn	84%	300+
Fresno Heart & Surgical Hospital	Fresno	83%	300+
Kaiser Foundation Hospital	San Rafael	83%	300+
Kaiser Foundation Hospital - Antioch	Antioch	83%	300+
Kaiser Foundation Hospital - Baldwin Park	Baldwin Park	83%	300+
Kaiser Fdn Hosp-Orange Co-Anaheim	Anaheim	83%	300+
Kaiser Foundation Hospital - Sacramento	Sacramento	83%	300+
Kaiser Foundation Hospital - South Bay	Harbor City	83%	300+
Kaiser Foundation Hospital - West La	Los Angeles	83%	300+
Kaiser Fdn Hosp S Sacramento	Sacramento	83%	300+
Keck Hospital of USC	Los Angeles	83%	300+
Northern Inyo Hospital	Bishop	83%	(a)
Novato Community Hospital	Novato	83%	300+
Placentia Linda Hospital	Placentia	83%	300+
Pomerado Hospital	Poway	83%	300+
Sierra Vista Regional Medical Center	San Luis Obispo	83%	300+
Chapman Medical Center	Orange	82%	300+
Coastal Communities Hospital	Santa Ana	82%	300+
Huntington Memorial Hospital	Pasadena	82%	300+
Kaiser Foundation Hospital - Fontana	Fontana	82%	300+
Kaiser Foundation Hospital - Fresno	Fresno	82%	300+
Kaiser Foundation Hospital - Redwood City	Redwood City	82%	300+
Kaiser Foundation Hospital - Santa Clara	Santa Clara	82%	300+
Kaiser Fdn Hosp-S San Francisco	S San Francisco	82%	300+
Kaiser Fdn Hosp-Woodland Hills	Woodland Hills	82%	300+
Loma Linda Univ Med Ctr-Murrieta	Murrieta	82%	300+
Mercy Medical Center - Mount Shasta	Mount Shasta	82%	(a)
Scripps Memorial Hospital La Jolla	La Jolla	82%	300+
Sequoia Hospital	Redwood City	82%	300+
Sharp Memorial Hospital	San Diego	82%	300+
Sutter Medical Center of Santa Rosa	Santa Rosa	82%	300+
Temple Community Hospital	Los Angeles	82%	(a)
Twin Cities Community Hospital	Templeton	82%	300+
Valleycare Medical Center	Pleasanton	82%	300+
White Memorial Medical Center	Los Angeles	82%	300+
Woodland Memorial Hospital	Woodland	82%	(a)
Clovis Community Medical Center	Clovis	81%	300+
Comm Mem Hosp San Buenaventura	Ventura	81%	300+
French Hospital Medical Center	San Luis Obispo	81%	300+
Hoag Memorial Hospital Presbyterian	Newport Beach	81%	300+
John Muir Medical Center - Concord Campus	Concord	81%	300+
Kaiser Foundation Hospital - Downey	Downey	81%	300+
Kaiser Fdn Hosp-Panorama City	Panorama City	81%	300+
Kaiser Foundation Hospital - Riverside	Riverside	81%	300+
Kaiser Foundation Hospital - Roseville	Roseville	81%	300+
Kaiser Foundation Hospital - San Diego	San Diego	81%	300+
Kaiser Fdn Hosp-San Francisco	San Francisco	81%	300+
Kaiser Foundation Hospital - San Jose	San Jose	81%	300+
LAC/Harbor - UCLA Medical Center	Torrance	81%	300+
LAC/Rancho Los Amigos Ntl Rehab Ctr	Downey	81%	300+
Los Alamitos Medical Center	Los Alamitos	81%	300+
Mills - Peninsula Medical Center	Burlingame	81%	300+
Palm Drive Hospital	Sebastopol	81%	(a)
Saint Elizabeth Community Hospital	Red Bluff	81%	300+
San Ramon Regional Medical Center	San Ramon	81%	300+
Sutter General Hospital	Sacramento	81%	300+
Sutter Lakeside Hospital	Lakeport	81%	300+
Sutter Tracy Community Hospital	Tracy	81%	300+
Tahoe Forest Hospital	Truckee	81%	(a)
UCSF Medical Center	San Francisco	81%	300+
USC Verdugo Hills Hospital	Glendale	81%	300+
Western Medical Center Hospital Anaheim	Anaheim	81%	300+
Western Medical Center Santa Ana	Santa Ana	81%	300+
CA Pacific Med Ctr-Davies Campus	San Francisco	80%	300+
Comm Hosp of the Monterey Peninsula	Monterey	80%	300+
Doctors Medical Center	Modesto	80%	300+
Enloe Medical Center	Chico	80%	300+
Kaiser Foundation Hospital & Rehab Center	Vallejo	80%	300+
Kaiser Fdn Hosp-Fremont/Hayward	Hayward	80%	300+
Kaiser Foundation Hospital - Los Angeles	Los Angeles	80%	300+
Kaiser Foundation Hospital - Manteca	Manteca	80%	300+
Kaiser Fdn Hosp-Moreno Valley	Moreno Valley	80%	300+
Kaiser Foundation Hospital - Santa Rosa	Santa Rosa	80%	300+
Kaiser Foundation Hospital - Vacaville	Vacaville	80%	300+
LAC/Olive View - UCLA Medical Center	Sylmar	80%	300+
Lakewood Regional Medical Center	Lakewood	80%	300+
Memorial Hospital Los Banos	Los Banos	80%	(a)
Mercy General Hospital	Sacramento	80%	300+
Mercy Hospital of Folsom	Folsom	80%	300+
Methodist Hospital of Southern California	Arcadia	80%	300+
Olympia Medical Center	Los Angeles	80%	300+
Presbyterian Intercommunity Hospital	Whittier	80%	300+

NOTE: Hospital profiles are in alphabetical order by state, then city, then hospital within the city; Rankings exclude hospitals with less than 25 cases except for patient surveys which excludes hospitals with less than 100 cases; (a) 100-299 cases; (1) The number of cases/patients is too few to report; (2) Data submitted were based on a sample of cases/patients; (3) Results are based on a shorter time period than required; (4) Data suppressed by CMS for one or more quarters; (5) Results are not available for this reporting period; (6) Fewer than 100 patients completed the HCAHPS survey; (7) No cases met the criteria for this measure; (8) The lower limit of the confidence interval cannot be calculated if the number of observed infections equals zero; (9) No data are available from the state/territory for this reporting period; (10) The scores shown reflect fewer than 50 completed surveys; (11) There were discrepancies in the data collection process; (12) This measure does not apply to this hospital for this reporting period; (13) Results cannot be calculated for this reporting period; (14) The results for this state are combined with nearby states to protect confidentiality; Please refer to the User's Guide for a full explanation of data.

Hospital Name	City	Rate	Cases
Prov Little Co of Mary Med Ctr San Pedro	San Pedro	80%	300+
Prov Little Co of Mary Med Ctr Torrance	Torrance	80%	300+
Providence Saint Joseph Medical Center	Burbank	80%	300+
Providence Tarzana Medical Center	Tarzana	80%	300+
Redlands Community Hospital	Redlands	80%	300+
Saint Helena Hospital	Saint Helena	80%	300+
Santa Barbara Cottage Hospital	Santa Barbara	80%	300+
Sutter Coast Hospital	Crescent City	80%	300+
Sutter Delta Medical Center	Antioch	80%	(a)
Ukiah Valley Medical Center	Ukiah	80%	300+
Univ of California Irvine Med Ctr	Orange	80%	300+
Univ of CA San Diego Med Ctr	San Diego	80%	300+
Barton Memorial Hospital	S Lake Tahoe	79%	300+
Cedars - Sinai Medical Center	Los Angeles	79%	300+
Eden Medical Center	Castro Valley	79%	300+
Eisenhower Medical Center	Rancho Mirage	79%	300+
Fallbrook Hospital	Fallbrook	79%	300+
Glendale Adventist Medical Center	Glendale	79%	300+
Kaiser Foundation Hospital - Walnut Creek	Walnut Creek	79%	300+
Memorial Medical Center	Modesto	79%	300+
Mission Hospital Regional Medical Center	Mission Viejo	79%	300+
Natividad Medical Center	Salinas	79%	300+
Northbay Medical Center	Fairfield	79%	300+
O'Connor Hospital	San Jose	79%	300+
Palo Verde Hospital	Blythe	79%	(a)
Queen of the Valley Medical Center	Napa	79%	300+
Riverside County Regional Medical Center	Moreno Valley	79%	300+
Saddleback Memorial Medical Center	Laguna Hills	79%	300+
Saint Agnes Medical Center	Fresno	79%	300+
Saint Joseph Hospital	Orange	79%	300+
Salinas Valley Memorial Hospital	Salinas	79%	300+
San Leandro Hospital	San Leandro	79%	(a)
Scripps Memorial Hospital - Encinitas	Encinitas	79%	300+
Scripps Mercy Hospital	San Diego	79%	300+
Sierra View District Hospital	Porterville	79%	300+
Sonoma Valley Hospital	Sonoma	79%	(a)
Sutter Maternity & Surgery Ctr	Santa Cruz	79%	300+
Univ of CA Davis Med Ctr	Sacramento	79%	300+
Ventura County Medical Center	Ventura	79%	300+
Washington Hospital	Fremont	79%	300+
Watsonville Community Hospital	Watsonville	79%	300+
Adventist Medical Center - Reedley	Reedley	78%	(a)
Barstow Community Hospital	Barstow	78%	300+
Community Regional Medical Center	Fresno	78%	300+
Dameron Hospital	Stockton	78%	300+
Desert Regional Medical Center	Palm Springs	78%	300+
El Camino Hospital	Mountain View	78%	300+
Foothill Presbyterian Hospital	Glendora	78%	300+
Good Samaritan Hospital	San Jose	78%	300+
John Muir Med Ctr-Walnut Creek Campus	Walnut Creek	78%	300+
Kaiser Fdn Hosp-Oakland/Richmond	Oakland	78%	300+
Loma Linda University Medical Center	Loma Linda	78%	300+
Long Beach Memorial Medical Center	Long Beach	78%	300+
Marshall Medical Center	Placerville	78%	300+
Mercy San Juan Medical Center	Carmichael	78%	300+
Orange Coast Memorial Medical Center	Fountain Valley	78%	300+
Palomar Health Downtown Campus	Escondido	78%	300+
Providence Holy Cross Medical Center	Mission Hills	78%	300+
Providence Saint John's Health Center	Santa Monica	78%	300+
Redwood Memorial Hospital	Fortuna	78%	300+
Saint Helena Hospital - Clearlake	Clearlake	78%	(a)
Saint Johns Pleasant Valley Hospital	Camarillo	78%	300+
Saint Louise Regional Hospital	Gilroy	78%	300+
Saint Rose Hospital	Hayward	78%	300+
Saint Vincent Medical Center	Los Angeles	78%	300+
San Antonio Community Hospital	Upland	78%	300+
Seton Medical Center	Daly City	78%	300+
Sharp Chula Vista Medical Center	Chula Vista	78%	300+
Sutter Amador Hospital	Jackson	78%	300+
Sutter Roseville Medical Center	Roseville	78%	300+
Sutter Solano Medical Center	Vallejo	78%	300+
Torrance Memorial Medical Center	Torrance	78%	300+
Chino Valley Medical Center[11]	Chino	77%	300+
Dominican Hospital	Santa Cruz	77%	300+
Fairchild Medical Center	Yreka	77%	300+
George L Mee Memorial Hospital	King City	77%	(a)
Glendale Mem Hosp & Health Ctr	Glendale	77%	300+
Grossmont Hospital	La Mesa	77%	300+
John F Kennedy Memorial Hospital	Indio	77%	300+
Lompoc Valley Medical Center	Lompoc	77%	300+
Marin General Hospital	Greenbrae	77%	300+
Mark Twain Medical Center	San Andreas	77%	(a)
Oak Valley District Hospital	Oakdale	77%	(a)
Pacific Hospital of Long Beach	Long Beach	77%	300+
Palmdale Regional Medical Center	Palmdale	77%	300+
Petaluma Valley Hospital	Petaluma	77%	300+
Ronald Reagan UCLA Medical Center	Los Angeles	77%	300+
San Joaquin Community Hospital	Bakersfield	77%	300+
Santa Monica-UCLA Med Ctr & Ortho Hosp	Santa Monica	77%	300+
Sonora Regional Medical Center	Sonora	77%	300+
Tri - City Medical Center	Oceanside	77%	300+
Tri - City Regional Medical Center	Hawaiian Grdns	77%	300+
Alameda County Medical Center	Oakland	76%	300+
Alta Bates Summit Medical Center	Oakland	76%	300+
Alvarado Hospital Medical Center	San Diego	76%	300+
Arrowhead Regional Medical Center	Colton	76%	300+
CA Pacific Med Ctr-Pacific Campus Hosp	San Francisco	76%	300+
CA Pacific Med Ctr-St Luke's Campus	San Francisco	76%	300+
Citrus Valley Medical Center - IC Campus	Covina	76%	300+
Contra Costa Regional Medical Center	Martinez	76%	300+
Delano Regional Medical Center	Delano	76%	300+
East Los Angeles Doctors Hospital	Los Angeles	76%	300+
Feather River Hospital	Paradise	76%	300+
Good Samaritan Hospital	Los Angeles	76%	300+
Hazel Hawkins Memorial Hospital	Hollister	76%	300+
LAC+USC Medical Center[11]	Los Angeles	76%	300+
Lodi Memorial Hospital	Lodi	76%	300+
Marian Regional Medical Center	Santa Maria	76%	300+
Mercy Medical Center - Redding	Redding	76%	300+
Pacifica Hospital of the Valley	Sun Valley	76%	(a)
Saint Bernardine Medical Center	San Bernardino	76%	300+
Saint Jude Medical Center	Fullerton	76%	300+
Saint Mary's Medical Center	San Francisco	76%	300+
San Gorgonio Memorial Hospital	Banning	76%	300+
Santa Clara Valley Medical Center	San Jose	76%	300+
Shasta Regional Medical Center[11]	Redding	76%	300+
Simi Valley Hosp & Health Care Svcs	Simi Valley	76%	300+
Antelope Valley Hospital	Lancaster	75%	300+
Centinela Hospital Medical Center[11]	Inglewood	75%	300+
Coast Plaza Hospital	Norwalk	75%	300+
Henry Mayo Newhall Memorial Hospital	Valencia	75%	300+
Kaweah Delta Medical Center	Visalia	75%	300+
Los Robles Hospital & Medical Center	Thousand Oaks	75%	300+
Marina Del Rey Hospital	Marina Del Rey	75%	300+
Mendocino Coast District Hospital	Fort Bragg	75%	(a)
Mercy Medical Center	Merced	75%	300+
Methodist Hospital of Sacramento	Sacramento	75%	300+
Saint Johns Regional Medical Center	Oxnard	75%	300+
Saint Joseph's Medical Center of Stockton	Stockton	75%	300+
San Dimas Community Hospital[11]	San Dimas	75%	300+
San Mateo Medical Center	San Mateo	75%	300+
Tulare Regional Medical Center	Tulare	75%	300+
West Hills Hospital & Medical Center	West Hills	75%	300+
Adventist Medical Center	Hanford	74%	300+
Alameda Hospital	Alameda	74%	300+
Alta Bates Summit Medical Center	Berkeley	74%	300+
Central Valley General Hospital	Hanford	74%	300+
Community Hospital of Huntington Park	Huntington Park	74%	300+
Desert Valley Hospital	Victorville	74%	300+
Fountain Valley Reg Hosp & Med Ctr	Fountain Valley	74%	300+
Hi - Desert Medical Center	Joshua Tree	74%	300+
Mad River Community Hospital	Arcata	74%	300+
Madera Community Hospital	Madera	74%	300+
Northridge Hospital Medical Center	Northridge	74%	300+
Paradise Valley Hospital[11]	National City	74%	(a)
PIH Hospital - Downey	Downey	74%	300+
Riverside Community Hospital	Riverside	74%	300+
Saint Francis Memorial Hospital	San Francisco	74%	300+
Saint Mary Medical Center	Long Beach	74%	300+
San Joaquin General Hospital	French Camp	74%	300+
Santa Rosa Memorial Hospital	Santa Rosa	74%	300+
Sierra Nevada Memorial Hospital	Grass Valley	74%	300+
Southwest Healthcare System	Murrieta	74%	300+
Valley Presbyterian Hospital	Van Nuys	74%	300+
Victor Valley Global Medical Center	Victorville	74%	300+
Whittier Hospital Medical Center	Whittier	74%	300+
Bakersfield Memorial Hospital	Bakersfield	73%	300+
Menifee Valley Medical Center	Sun City	73%	300+
Ahmc Anaheim Regional Medical Center	Anaheim	72%	300+
California Hosp Med Ctr Los Angeles	Los Angeles	72%	300+
Corona Regional Medical Center	Corona	72%	300+
Doctors Medical Center - San Pablo	San Pablo	72%	300+
Garden Grove Hospital & Medical Center[11]	Garden Grove	72%	300+
Kern Medical Center	Bakersfield	72%	300+
Memorial Hospital of Gardena	Gardena	72%	300+
Montclair Hospital Medical Center[11]	Montclair	72%	(a)
Pomona Valley Hospital Medical Center	Pomona	72%	300+
Saint Mary Medical Center	Apple Valley	72%	300+
Beverly Hospital	Montebello	71%	300+
Hollywood Presbyterian Medical Center	Los Angeles	71%	300+
Pioneers Memorial Healthcare District	Brawley	71%	300+
Regional Medical Center of San Jose	San Jose	71%	300+
Rideout Memorial Hospital	Marysville	71%	300+
Saint Francis Medical Center	Lynwood	71%	300+
Saint Joseph Hospital	Eureka	71%	300+
Bakersfield Heart Hospital	Bakersfield	70%	300+
El Centro Regional Medical Center	El Centro	70%	(a)
Greater El Monte Community Hospital	South El Monte	70%	300+
Mercy Hospital	Bakersfield	70%	300+
Mission Community Hospital	Panorama City	70%	300+
Pacific Alliance Medical Center	Los Angeles	70%	300+
Parkview Comm Hosp Med Ctr	Riverside	70%	300+
San Gabriel Valley Medical Center	San Gabriel	70%	300+
Chinese Hospital	San Francisco	69%	300+
Hemet Valley Medical Center	Hemet	69%	300+
La Palma Intercommunity Hospital	La Palma	69%	(a)
Monterey Park Hospital	Monterey Park	69%	300+
Sherman Oaks Hospital[11]	Sherman Oaks	69%	(a)
Community Hospital of Long Beach	Long Beach	68%	300+
Emanuel Medical Center	Turlock	68%	300+
Silver Lake Medical Center	Los Angeles	68%	(a)
Southern California Hospital at Hollywood	Hollywood	68%	300+
Garfield Medical Center	Monterey Park	67%	300+
West Anaheim Medical Center	Anaheim	67%	300+
Community Hospital of San Bernardino	San Bernardino	66%	300+
Oroville Hospital	Oroville	66%	300+
Alhambra Hospital Medical Center	Alhambra	65%	300+
Los Angeles Community Hospital	Los Angeles	65%	300+
San Francisco General Hospital	San Francisco	65%	(a)
Huntington Beach Hospital	Huntington Bch	63%	(a)

Home Recovery Information Given

Hospital Name	City	Rate	Cases
Patients' Hospital of Redding	Redding	93%	(a)
Sharp Coronado Hosp & Healthcare Ctr	Coronado	93%	300+
Hoag Orthopedic Institute	Irvine	92%	300+
Banner Lassen Medical Center[11]	Susanville	91%	(a)
Barton Memorial Hospital	S Lake Tahoe	91%	300+
Fresno Surgical Hospital	Fresno	91%	300+
City of Hope Helford Clinical Res Hosp	Duarte	90%	300+
Northern Inyo Hospital	Bishop	90%	(a)
Frank R Howard Memorial Hospital	Willits	89%	300+
Goleta Valley Cottage Hospital	Santa Barbara	89%	300+
Mammoth Hospital	Mammoth Lakes	89%	(a)
Mercy Medical Center - Mount Shasta	Mount Shasta	89%	(a)
Saint Helena Hospital	Saint Helena	89%	300+
Sutter Davis Hospital	Davis	89%	300+
Enloe Medical Center	Chico	88%	300+
Fresno Heart & Surgical Hospital	Fresno	88%	300+
George L Mee Memorial Hospital	King City	88%	(a)
Healdsburg District Hospital	Healdsburg	88%	(a)
Kaiser Foundation Hospital	San Rafael	88%	300+
Kaiser Foundation Hospital - Antioch	Antioch	88%	300+
Kaiser Fdn Hosp-Orange Co-Anaheim	Anaheim	88%	300+
Kaiser Foundation Hospital - Sacramento	Sacramento	88%	300+
Mendocino Coast District Hospital	Fort Bragg	88%	(a)
Methodist Hospital of Sacramento	Sacramento	88%	300+
Sierra Vista Regional Medical Center	San Luis Obispo	88%	300+
Stanislaus Surgical Hospital	Modesto	88%	300+
Sutter Coast Hospital	Crescent City	88%	300+
Sutter Surgical Hospital - North Valley	Yuba City	88%	(a)
UCSF Medical Center	San Francisco	88%	300+
Ukiah Valley Medical Center	Ukiah	88%	300+
Comm Hosp of the Monterey Peninsula	Monterey	87%	300+
Doctors Medical Center	Modesto	87%	300+
Feather River Hospital	Paradise	87%	300+
Glendale Adventist Medical Center	Glendale	87%	300+
Kaiser Foundation Hospital - Baldwin Park	Baldwin Park	87%	300+
Kaiser Foundation Hospital - Fontana	Fontana	87%	300+
Kaiser Foundation Hospital - Fresno	Fresno	87%	300+
Kaiser Foundation Hospital - Redwood City	Redwood City	87%	300+
Kaiser Foundation Hospital - San Diego	San Diego	87%	300+
Kaiser Foundation Hospital - San Jose	San Jose	87%	300+
Kaiser Foundation Hospital - Santa Clara	Santa Clara	87%	300+
Kaiser Foundation Hospital - Santa Rosa	Santa Rosa	87%	300+
Kaiser Foundation Hospital - South Bay	Harbor City	87%	300+
Kaiser Fdn Hosp S Sacramento	Sacramento	87%	300+
LAC/Rancho Los Amigos Ntl Rehab Ctr	Downey	87%	300+
Mad River Community Hospital	Arcata	87%	300+
Menlo Park Surgical Hospital	Menlo Park	87%	(a)
Placentia Linda Hospital	Placentia	87%	300+
Saint Johns Pleasant Valley Hospital	Camarillo	87%	300+
Sharp Chula Vista Medical Center	Chula Vista	87%	300+
Sharp Memorial Hospital	San Diego	87%	300+
Sierra Nevada Memorial Hospital	Grass Valley	87%	300+
Sonora Regional Medical Center	Sonora	87%	300+
Stanford Hospital	Stanford	87%	300+
Sutter General Hospital	Sacramento	87%	300+
Sutter Maternity & Surgery Ctr	Santa Cruz	87%	300+
Twin Cities Community Hospital	Templeton	87%	300+
Univ of CA Davis Med Ctr	Sacramento	87%	300+
Valleycare Medical Center	Pleasanton	87%	300+
Barstow Community Hospital	Barstow	86%	300+
Community Regional Medical Center	Fresno	86%	300+
Hi - Desert Medical Center	Joshua Tree	86%	300+
John Muir Medical Center - Concord Campus	Concord	86%	300+
Kaiser Foundation Hospital & Rehab Center	Vallejo	86%	300+
Kaiser Foundation Hospital - Los Angeles	Los Angeles	86%	300+
Kaiser Fdn Hosp-Moreno Valley	Moreno Valley	86%	300+
Kaiser Foundation Hospital - Roseville	Roseville	86%	300+
Kaiser Fdn Hosp-San Francisco	San Francisco	86%	300+
Kaiser Fdn Hosp-S San Francisco	S San Francisco	86%	300+
Kaiser Foundation Hospital - Vacaville	Vacaville	86%	300+

NOTE: Hospital profiles are in alphabetical order by state, then city, then hospital within the city; Rankings exclude hospitals with less than 25 cases except for patient surveys which excludes hospitals with less than 100 cases; (a) 100-299 cases; (1) The number of cases/patients is too few to report; (2) Data submitted were based on a sample of cases/patients; (3) Results are based on a shorter time period than required; (4) Data suppressed by CMS for one or more quarters; (5) Results are not available for this reporting period; (6) Fewer than 100 patients completed the HCAHPS survey; (7) No cases met the criteria for this measure; (8) The lower limit of the confidence interval cannot be calculated if the number of observed infections equals zero; (9) No data are available from the state/territory for this reporting period; (10) The scores shown reflect fewer than 50 completed surveys; (11) There were discrepancies in the data collection process; (12) This measure does not apply to this hospital for this reporting period; (13) Results cannot be calculated for this reporting period; (14) The results for this state are combined with nearby states to protect confidentiality; Please refer to the User's Guide for a full explanation of data.

Loma Linda Univ Med Ctr-Murrieta	Murrieta	86%	300+
Marshall Medical Center	Placerville	86%	300+
Mercy General Hospital	Sacramento	86%	300+
Mercy Hospital of Folsom	Folsom	86%	300+
Natividad Medical Center	Salinas	86%	300+
Northbay Medical Center	Fairfield	86%	300+
Novato Community Hospital	Novato	86%	300+
Ojai Valley Community Hospital	Ojai	86%	(a)
Palmdale Regional Medical Center	Palmdale	86%	300+
Redlands Community Hospital	Redlands	86%	300+
Redwood Memorial Hospital	Fortuna	86%	300+
Saint Jude Medical Center	Fullerton	86%	300+
San Francisco General Hospital	San Francisco	86%	(a)
Scripps Green Hospital	La Jolla	86%	300+
Sonoma Valley Hospital	Sonoma	86%	(a)
Sutter Amador Hospital	Jackson	86%	300+
Sutter Lakeside Hospital	Lakeport	86%	300+
Tahoe Forest Hospital	Truckee	86%	(a)
Univ of California Irvine Med Ctr	Orange	86%	300+
Univ of CA San Diego Med Ctr	San Diego	86%	300+
Washington Hospital	Fremont	86%	300+
Woodland Memorial Hospital	Woodland	86%	(a)
Alhambra Hospital Medical Center	Alhambra	85%	300+
Contra Costa Regional Medical Center	Martinez	85%	300+
Doctors Hospital of Manteca	Manteca	85%	300+
El Centro Regional Medical Center	El Centro	85%	(a)
Fairchild Medical Center	Yreka	85%	300+
French Hospital Medical Center	San Luis Obispo	85%	300+
Grossmont Hospital	La Mesa	85%	300+
Hoag Memorial Hospital Presbyterian	Newport Beach	85%	300+
Kaiser Foundation Hospital - Downey	Downey	85%	300+
Kaiser Foundation Hospital - Manteca	Manteca	85%	300+
Kaiser Fdn Hosp-Panorama City	Panorama City	85%	300+
Kaiser Foundation Hospital - Riverside	Riverside	85%	300+
Kaiser Foundation Hospital - Walnut Creek	Walnut Creek	85%	300+
Kaiser Foundation Hospital - West La	Los Angeles	85%	300+
Kaiser Fdn Hosp-Woodland Hills	Woodland Hills	85%	300+
Loma Linda University Medical Center	Loma Linda	85%	300+
Madera Community Hospital	Madera	85%	300+
Marian Regional Medical Center	Santa Maria	85%	300+
Memorial Hospital Los Banos	Los Banos	85%	(a)
Memorial Medical Center	Modesto	85%	300+
Mercy Medical Center - Redding	Redding	85%	300+
Mercy San Juan Medical Center	Carmichael	85%	300+
Palm Drive Hospital	Sebastopol	85%	(a)
Ronald Reagan UCLA Medical Center	Los Angeles	85%	300+
Saint Agnes Medical Center	Fresno	85%	300+
Saint Elizabeth Community Hospital	Red Bluff	85%	300+
Saint Joseph Hospital	Orange	85%	300+
Saint Mary's Medical Center	San Francisco	85%	300+
Salinas Valley Memorial Hospital	Salinas	85%	300+
San Antonio Community Hospital	Upland	85%	300+
Seton Medical Center	Daly City	85%	300+
Shasta Regional Medical Center[11]	Redding	85%	300+
Sutter Auburn Faith Hospital	Auburn	85%	300+
Sutter Medical Center of Santa Rosa	Santa Rosa	85%	300+
Sutter Roseville Medical Center	Roseville	85%	300+
Adventist Medical Center	Hanford	84%	300+
Alvarado Hospital Medical Center	San Diego	84%	300+
Cedars - Sinai Medical Center	Los Angeles	84%	300+
Clovis Community Medical Center	Clovis	84%	300+
Colusa Regional Medical Center	Colusa	84%	(a)
Corona Regional Medical Center	Corona	84%	300+
Dameron Hospital	Stockton	84%	300+
Dominican Hospital	Santa Cruz	84%	300+
Eisenhower Medical Center	Rancho Mirage	84%	300+
El Camino Hospital	Mountain View	84%	300+
Foothill Presbyterian Hospital	Glendora	84%	300+
Hazel Hawkins Memorial Hospital	Hollister	84%	300+
Huntington Memorial Hospital	Pasadena	84%	300+
Kaiser Fdn Hosp-Oakland/Richmond	Oakland	84%	300+
Keck Hospital of USC	Los Angeles	84%	300+
Lodi Memorial Hospital	Lodi	84%	300+
Mercy Medical Center	Merced	84%	300+
Mills - Peninsula Medical Center	Burlingame	84%	300+
Palo Verde Hospital	Blythe	84%	(a)
Petaluma Valley Hospital	Petaluma	84%	300+
Providence Holy Cross Medical Center	Mission Hills	84%	300+
Queen of the Valley Medical Center	Napa	84%	300+
Saddleback Memorial Medical Center	Laguna Hills	84%	300+
Saint Helena Hospital - Clearlake	Clearlake	84%	(a)
Saint Johns Regional Medical Center	Oxnard	84%	300+
Saint Mary Medical Center	Long Beach	84%	300+
Scripps Memorial Hospital - Encinitas	Encinitas	84%	300+
Sutter Tracy Community Hospital	Tracy	84%	300+
Torrance Memorial Medical Center	Torrance	84%	300+
White Memorial Medical Center	Los Angeles	84%	300+
Bakersfield Memorial Hospital	Bakersfield	83%	300+
Chapman Medical Center	Orange	83%	300+
Chinese Hospital	San Francisco	83%	300+
Chino Valley Medical Center[11]	Chino	83%	300+
Desert Regional Medical Center	Palm Springs	83%	300+
Fallbrook Hospital	Fallbrook	83%	300+
Good Samaritan Hospital	Bakersfield	83%	(a)
Good Samaritan Hospital	Los Angeles	83%	300+
John F Kennedy Memorial Hospital	Indio	83%	300+
Kaiser Fdn Hosp-Fremont/Hayward	Hayward	83%	300+
Lompoc Valley Medical Center	Lompoc	83%	300+
Los Alamitos Medical Center	Los Alamitos	83%	300+
Los Robles Hospital & Medical Center	Thousand Oaks	83%	300+
Mark Twain Medical Center	San Andreas	83%	(a)
Montclair Hospital Medical Center[11]	Montclair	83%	(a)
O'Connor Hospital	San Jose	83%	300+
Pacific Hospital of Long Beach	Long Beach	83%	300+
Presbyterian Intercommunity Hospital	Whittier	83%	300+
Prov Little Co of Mary Med Ctr Torrance	Torrance	83%	300+
Providence Saint John's Health Center	Santa Monica	83%	300+
Providence Saint Joseph Medical Center	Burbank	83%	300+
Riverside Community Hospital	Riverside	83%	300+
Saint Francis Memorial Hospital	San Francisco	83%	300+
Saint Joseph Hospital	Eureka	83%	300+
Saint Rose Hospital	Hayward	83%	300+
Saint Vincent Medical Center	Los Angeles	83%	300+
San Ramon Regional Medical Center	San Ramon	83%	300+
Santa Barbara Cottage Hospital	Santa Barbara	83%	300+
Santa Rosa Memorial Hospital	Santa Rosa	83%	300+
Scripps Memorial Hospital La Jolla	La Jolla	83%	300+
Scripps Mercy Hospital	San Diego	83%	300+
Sierra View District Hospital	Porterville	83%	300+
Simi Valley Hosp & Health Care Svcs	Simi Valley	83%	300+
Southwest Healthcare System	Murrieta	83%	300+
Sutter Solano Medical Center	Vallejo	83%	300+
Tri - City Medical Center	Oceanside	83%	300+
Comm Mem Hosp San Buenaventura	Ventura	82%	300+
Garden Grove Hospital & Medical Center[11]	Garden Grove	82%	300+
Garfield Medical Center	Monterey Park	82%	300+
Glendale Mem Hosp & Health Ctr	Glendale	82%	300+
Henry Mayo Newhall Memorial Hospital	Valencia	82%	300+
Marin General Hospital	Greenbrae	82%	300+
Mission Hospital Regional Medical Center	Mission Viejo	82%	300+
Northridge Hospital Medical Center	Northridge	82%	300+
Oak Valley District Hospital	Oakdale	82%	(a)
Orange Coast Memorial Medical Center	Fountain Valley	82%	300+
Paradise Valley Hospital[11]	National City	82%	(a)
Pioneers Memorial Healthcare District	Brawley	82%	300+
Riverside County Regional Medical Center	Moreno Valley	82%	300+
Saint Francis Medical Center	Lynwood	82%	300+
San Dimas Community Hospital[11]	San Dimas	82%	300+
San Gorgonio Memorial Hospital	Banning	82%	300+
San Joaquin Community Hospital	Bakersfield	82%	300+
Sequoia Hospital	Redwood City	82%	300+
Sutter Delta Medical Center	Antioch	82%	(a)
Watsonville Community Hospital	Watsonville	82%	300+
West Anaheim Medical Center	Anaheim	82%	300+
West Hills Hospital & Medical Center	West Hills	82%	300+
Ahmc Anaheim Regional Medical Center	Anaheim	81%	300+
Antelope Valley Hospital	Lancaster	81%	300+
CA Pacific Med Ctr-Pacific Campus Hosp	San Francisco	81%	300+
CA Pacific Med Ctr-St Luke's Campus	San Francisco	81%	300+
Eden Medical Center	Castro Valley	81%	300+
Good Samaritan Hospital	San Jose	81%	300+
Hollywood Presbyterian Medical Center	Los Angeles	81%	300+
John Muir Med Ctr-Walnut Creek Campus	Walnut Creek	81%	300+
Kaweah Delta Medical Center	Visalia	81%	300+
La Palma Intercommunity Hospital	La Palma	81%	(a)
LAC/Olive View - UCLA Medical Center	Sylmar	81%	300+
Lakewood Regional Medical Center	Lakewood	81%	300+
Long Beach Memorial Medical Center	Long Beach	81%	300+
Olympia Medical Center	Los Angeles	81%	300+
Palomar Health Downtown Campus	Escondido	81%	300+
Parkview Comm Hosp Med Ctr	Riverside	81%	300+
Pomerado Hospital	Poway	81%	300+
Pomona Valley Hospital Medical Center	Pomona	81%	300+
Prov Little Co of Mary Med Ctr San Pedro	San Pedro	81%	300+
Saint Bernardine Medical Center	San Bernardino	81%	300+
Saint Joseph's Medical Center of Stockton	Stockton	81%	300+
Saint Louise Regional Hospital	Gilroy	81%	300+
Saint Mary Medical Center	Apple Valley	81%	300+
Victor Valley Global Medical Center	Victorville	81%	300+
Western Medical Center Hospital Anaheim	Anaheim	81%	300+
Western Medical Center Santa Ana	Santa Ana	81%	300+
Whittier Hospital Medical Center	Whittier	81%	300+
Alameda County Medical Center	Oakland	80%	300+
Alta Bates Summit Medical Center	Berkeley	80%	300+
Beverly Hospital	Montebello	80%	300+
CA Pacific Med Ctr-Davies Campus	San Francisco	80%	300+
Centinela Hospital Medical Center[11]	Inglewood	80%	300+
Citrus Valley Medical Center - IC Campus	Covina	80%	300+
Community Hospital of San Bernardino	San Bernardino	80%	300+
Delano Regional Medical Center	Delano	80%	300+
Fountain Valley Reg Hosp & Med Ctr	Fountain Valley	80%	300+
LAC+USC Medical Center[11]	Los Angeles	80%	300+
LAC/Harbor - UCLA Medical Center	Torrance	80%	300+
Mercy Hospital	Bakersfield	80%	300+
Monterey Park Hospital	Monterey Park	80%	300+
Pacific Alliance Medical Center	Los Angeles	80%	300+
San Joaquin General Hospital	French Camp	80%	300+
San Leandro Hospital	San Leandro	80%	(a)
Tri - City Regional Medical Center	Hawaiian Grdns	80%	300+
Adventist Medical Center - Reedley	Reedley	79%	(a)
Alameda Hospital	Alameda	79%	300+
Alta Bates Summit Medical Center	Oakland	79%	300+
Arrowhead Regional Medical Center	Colton	79%	300+
East Los Angeles Doctors Hospital	Los Angeles	79%	300+
Emanuel Medical Center	Turlock	79%	300+
Greater El Monte Community Hospital	South El Monte	79%	300+
Kern Medical Center	Bakersfield	79%	300+
Menifee Valley Medical Center	Sun City	79%	300+
Methodist Hospital of Southern California	Arcadia	79%	300+
Providence Tarzana Medical Center	Tarzana	79%	300+
Regional Medical Center of San Jose	San Jose	79%	300+
Santa Monica-UCLA Med Ctr & Ortho Hosp	Santa Monica	79%	300+
Sherman Oaks Hospital[11]	Sherman Oaks	79%	(a)
Temple Community Hospital	Los Angeles	79%	(a)
Valley Presbyterian Hospital	Van Nuys	79%	300+
Bakersfield Heart Hospital	Bakersfield	78%	300+
Coastal Communities Hospital	Santa Ana	78%	300+
Desert Valley Hospital	Victorville	78%	300+
San Gabriel Valley Medical Center	San Gabriel	78%	300+
San Mateo Medical Center	San Mateo	78%	300+
USC Verdugo Hills Hospital	Glendale	78%	300+
California Hosp Med Ctr Los Angeles	Los Angeles	77%	300+
Coast Plaza Hospital	Norwalk	77%	300+
Marina Del Rey Hospital	Marina Del Rey	77%	300+
PIH Hospital - Downey	Downey	77%	300+
Santa Clara Valley Medical Center	San Jose	77%	300+
Ventura County Medical Center	Ventura	77%	300+
Central Valley General Hospital	Hanford	76%	300+
Oroville Hospital	Oroville	76%	300+
Tulare Regional Medical Center	Tulare	76%	300+
Hemet Valley Medical Center	Hemet	75%	300+
Memorial Hospital of Gardena	Gardena	75%	300+
Mission Community Hospital	Panorama City	75%	300+
Southern California Hospital at Hollywood	Hollywood	75%	300+
Community Hospital of Huntington Park	Huntington Park	74%	300+
Doctors Medical Center - San Pablo	San Pablo	74%	300+
Huntington Beach Hospital	Huntington Bch	74%	(a)
Rideout Memorial Hospital	Marysville	74%	300+
Pacifica Hospital of the Valley	Sun Valley	73%	(a)
Silver Lake Medical Center	Los Angeles	71%	(a)
Los Angeles Community Hospital	Los Angeles	69%	300+
Community Hospital of Long Beach	Long Beach	67%	300+

Hospital Given 9 or 10 on 10 Point Scale

Hospital Name	City	Rate	Cases
Patients' Hospital of Redding	Redding	95%	(a)
Hoag Orthopedic Institute	Irvine	90%	300+
Menlo Park Surgical Hospital	Menlo Park	88%	(a)
Sutter Maternity & Surgery Ctr	Santa Cruz	88%	300+
Sutter Surgical Hospital - North Valley	Yuba City	88%	(a)
Fresno Heart & Surgical Hospital	Fresno	86%	300+
Stanislaus Surgical Hospital	Modesto	86%	300+
Sutter Davis Hospital	Davis	86%	300+
City of Hope Helford Clinical Res Hosp	Duarte	85%	300+
Fresno Surgical Hospital	Fresno	85%	300+
Sharp Memorial Hospital	San Diego	85%	300+
Kaiser Fdn Hosp-Orange Co-Anaheim	Anaheim	84%	300+
Novato Community Hospital	Novato	84%	300+
Tahoe Forest Hospital	Truckee	83%	(a)
Comm Hosp of the Monterey Peninsula	Monterey	82%	300+
Hoag Memorial Hospital Presbyterian	Newport Beach	82%	300+
Huntington Memorial Hospital	Pasadena	82%	300+
Santa Barbara Cottage Hospital	Santa Barbara	82%	300+
Kaiser Foundation Hospital - Vacaville	Vacaville	81%	300+
Mills - Peninsula Medical Center	Burlingame	81%	300+
Presbyterian Intercommunity Hospital	Whittier	81%	300+
Scripps Green Hospital	La Jolla	81%	300+
Sharp Coronado Hosp & Healthcare Ctr	Coronado	81%	300+
Healdsburg District Hospital	Healdsburg	80%	(a)
John Muir Medical Center - Concord Campus	Concord	80%	300+
John Muir Med Ctr-Walnut Creek Campus	Walnut Creek	80%	300+
Mammoth Hospital	Mammoth Lakes	80%	(a)
Saint Joseph Hospital	Orange	80%	300+
Kaiser Foundation Hospital - Manteca	Manteca	79%	300+
Kaiser Foundation Hospital - Santa Clara	Santa Clara	79%	300+
Kaiser Fdn Hosp-Woodland Hills	Woodland Hills	79%	300+
LAC/Rancho Los Amigos Ntl Rehab Ctr	Downey	79%	300+
Loma Linda Univ Med Ctr-Murrieta	Murrieta	79%	300+
Saint Helena Hospital	Saint Helena	79%	300+
Stanford Hospital	Stanford	79%	300+
Banner Lassen Medical Center[11]	Susanville	78%	(a)
Cedars - Sinai Medical Center	Los Angeles	78%	300+
Enloe Medical Center	Chico	78%	300+

NOTE: Hospital profiles are in alphabetical order by state, then city, then hospital within the city; Rankings exclude hospitals with less than 25 cases except for patient surveys which excludes hospitals with less than 100 cases; (a) 100-299 cases; (1) The number of cases/patients is too few to report; (2) Data submitted were based on a sample of cases/patients; (3) Results are based on a shorter time period than required; (4) Data suppressed by CMS for one or more quarters; (5) Results are not available for this reporting period; (6) Fewer than 100 patients completed the HCAHPS survey; (7) No cases met the criteria for this measure; (8) The lower limit of the confidence interval cannot be calculated if the number of observed infections equals zero; (9) No data are available from the state/territory for this reporting period; (10) The scores shown reflect fewer than 50 completed surveys; (11) There were discrepancies in the data collection process; (12) This measure does not apply to this hospital for this reporting period; (13) Results cannot be calculated for this reporting period; (14) The results for this state are combined with nearby states to protect confidentiality; Please refer to the User's Guide for a full explanation of data.

Frank R Howard Memorial Hospital	Willits	78%	300+
Goleta Valley Cottage Hospital	Santa Barbara	78%	300+
Kaiser Foundation Hospital - Downey	Downey	78%	300+
Kaiser Foundation Hospital - Fontana	Fontana	78%	300+
Kaiser Fdn Hosp-Panorama City	Panorama City	78%	300+
Kaiser Foundation Hospital - Roseville	Roseville	78%	300+
Kaiser Foundation Hospital - Santa Rosa	Santa Rosa	78%	300+
Mercy Medical Center - Mount Shasta	Mount Shasta	78%	(a)
Redlands Community Hospital	Redlands	78%	300+
UCSF Medical Center	San Francisco	78%	300+
Univ of California Irvine Med Ctr	Orange	78%	300+
Clovis Community Medical Center	Clovis	77%	300+
Eisenhower Medical Center	Rancho Mirage	77%	300+
Kaiser Foundation Hospital - Antioch	Antioch	77%	300+
Kaiser Foundation Hospital - Baldwin Park	Baldwin Park	77%	300+
Kaiser Foundation Hospital - Fresno	Fresno	77%	300+
Kaiser Foundation Hospital - Los Angeles	Los Angeles	77%	300+
Keck Hospital of USC	Los Angeles	77%	300+
Ronald Reagan UCLA Medical Center	Los Angeles	77%	300+
Saint Jude Medical Center	Fullerton	77%	300+
Sutter Tracy Community Hospital	Tracy	77%	300+
Valleycare Medical Center	Pleasanton	77%	300+
White Memorial Medical Center	Los Angeles	77%	300+
Kaiser Foundation Hospital - South Bay	Harbor City	76%	300+
Mission Hospital Regional Medical Center	Mission Viejo	76%	300+
Palomar Health Downtown Campus	Escondido	76%	300+
Prov Little Co of Mary Med Ctr Torrance	Torrance	76%	300+
Providence Saint Joseph Medical Center	Burbank	76%	300+
Scripps Memorial Hospital La Jolla	La Jolla	76%	300+
Desert Regional Medical Center	Palm Springs	75%	300+
Feather River Hospital	Paradise	75%	300+
French Hospital Medical Center	San Luis Obispo	75%	300+
Marshall Medical Center	Placerville	75%	300+
Methodist Hospital of Southern California	Arcadia	75%	300+
Palmdale Regional Medical Center	Palmdale	75%	300+
Placentia Linda Hospital	Placentia	75%	300+
Providence Holy Cross Medical Center	Mission Hills	75%	300+
Sutter Auburn Faith Hospital	Auburn	75%	300+
Sutter Roseville Medical Center	Roseville	75%	300+
Torrance Memorial Medical Center	Torrance	75%	300+
Bakersfield Heart Hospital	Bakersfield	74%	300+
Kaiser Foundation Hospital - Riverside	Riverside	74%	300+
Kaiser Fdn Hosp-San Francisco	San Francisco	74%	300+
Kaiser Foundation Hospital - West La	Los Angeles	74%	300+
Marian Regional Medical Center	Santa Maria	74%	300+
Memorial Hospital Los Banos	Los Banos	74%	(a)
San Ramon Regional Medical Center	San Ramon	74%	300+
El Camino Hospital	Mountain View	73%	300+
Kaiser Foundation Hospital	San Rafael	73%	300+
Kaiser Fdn Hosp-S San Francisco	S San Francisco	73%	300+
Kaiser Fdn Hosp S Sacramento	Sacramento	73%	300+
Natividad Medical Center	Salinas	73%	300+
Northern Inyo Hospital	Bishop	73%	(a)
Queen of the Valley Medical Center	Napa	73%	300+
Santa Monica-UCLA Med Ctr & Ortho Hosp	Santa Monica	73%	300+
Sharp Chula Vista Medical Center	Chula Vista	73%	300+
Sierra Vista Regional Medical Center	San Luis Obispo	73%	300+
George L Mee Memorial Hospital	King City	72%	(a)
Kaiser Foundation Hospital & Rehab Center	Vallejo	72%	300+
LAC+USC Medical Center[11]	Los Angeles	72%	300+
Long Beach Memorial Medical Center	Long Beach	72%	300+
Memorial Medical Center	Modesto	72%	300+
Prov Little Co of Mary Med Ctr San Pedro	San Pedro	72%	300+
Saint Mary Medical Center	Long Beach	72%	300+
Watsonville Community Hospital	Watsonville	72%	300+
Barton Memorial Hospital	S Lake Tahoe	71%	300+
Doctors Medical Center	Modesto	71%	300+
Foothill Presbyterian Hospital	Glendora	71%	300+
Grossmont Hospital	La Mesa	71%	300+
Hi - Desert Medical Center	Joshua Tree	71%	300+
Kaiser Foundation Hospital - San Diego	San Diego	71%	300+
Lodi Memorial Hospital	Lodi	71%	300+
Loma Linda University Medical Center	Loma Linda	71%	300+
Saint Agnes Medical Center	Fresno	71%	300+
San Antonio Community Hospital	Upland	71%	300+
Scripps Memorial Hospital - Encinitas	Encinitas	71%	300+
Citrus Valley Medical Center - IC Campus	Covina	70%	300+
Eden Medical Center	Castro Valley	70%	300+
Mercy Hospital of Folsom	Folsom	70%	300+
Ojai Valley Community Hospital	Ojai	70%	(a)
Palm Drive Hospital	Sebastopol	70%	(a)
Providence Saint John's Health Center	Santa Monica	70%	300+
Redwood Memorial Hospital	Fortuna	70%	300+
Saint Bernardine Medical Center	San Bernardino	70%	300+
Simi Valley Hosp & Health Care Svcs	Simi Valley	70%	300+
Univ of CA Davis Med Ctr	Sacramento	70%	300+
Univ of CA San Diego Med Ctr	San Diego	70%	300+
Chino Valley Medical Center[11]	Chino	69%	300+
Doctors Hospital of Manteca	Manteca	69%	300+
Kaiser Fdn Hosp-Moreno Valley	Moreno Valley	69%	300+
Kaiser Foundation Hospital - Sacramento	Sacramento	69%	300+
Los Robles Hospital & Medical Center	Thousand Oaks	69%	300+
Pioneers Memorial Healthcare District	Brawley	69%	300+
Saint Francis Medical Center	Lynwood	69%	300+
Saint Johns Pleasant Valley Hospital	Camarillo	69%	300+
Saint Johns Regional Medical Center	Oxnard	69%	300+
Saint Vincent Medical Center	Los Angeles	69%	300+
Sutter Amador Hospital	Jackson	69%	300+
Sutter Medical Center of Santa Rosa	Santa Rosa	69%	300+
Twin Cities Community Hospital	Templeton	69%	300+
USC Verdugo Hills Hospital	Glendale	69%	300+
Woodland Memorial Hospital	Woodland	69%	(a)
Barstow Community Hospital	Barstow	68%	300+
Coastal Communities Hospital	Santa Ana	68%	300+
Good Samaritan Hospital	Los Angeles	68%	300+
Kaiser Foundation Hospital - Redwood City	Redwood City	68%	300+
Kaiser Foundation Hospital - San Jose	San Jose	68%	300+
Mercy General Hospital	Sacramento	68%	300+
Orange Coast Memorial Medical Center	Fountain Valley	68%	300+
Petaluma Valley Hospital	Petaluma	68%	300+
Saddleback Memorial Medical Center	Laguna Hills	68%	300+
Sutter General Hospital	Sacramento	68%	300+
Ukiah Valley Medical Center	Ukiah	68%	300+
Western Medical Center Hospital Anaheim	Anaheim	68%	300+
Western Medical Center Santa Ana	Santa Ana	68%	300+
Arrowhead Regional Medical Center	Colton	67%	300+
Bakersfield Memorial Hospital	Bakersfield	67%	300+
Community Regional Medical Center	Fresno	67%	300+
Dameron Hospital	Stockton	67%	300+
Glendale Adventist Medical Center	Glendale	67%	300+
LAC/Olive View - UCLA Medical Center	Sylmar	67%	300+
Northbay Medical Center	Fairfield	67%	300+
O'Connor Hospital	San Jose	67%	300+
Olympia Medical Center	Los Angeles	67%	300+
Pomerado Hospital	Poway	67%	300+
Saint Elizabeth Community Hospital	Red Bluff	67%	300+
Saint Mary's Medical Center	San Francisco	67%	300+
Salinas Valley Memorial Hospital	Salinas	67%	300+
CA Pacific Med Ctr-Pacific Campus Hosp	San Francisco	66%	300+
Colusa Regional Medical Center	Colusa	66%	(a)
Comm Mem Hosp San Buenaventura	Ventura	66%	300+
Hazel Hawkins Memorial Hospital	Hollister	66%	300+
Henry Mayo Newhall Memorial Hospital	Valencia	66%	300+
Kaiser Fdn Hosp-Fremont/Hayward	Hayward	66%	300+
Kaiser Foundation Hospital - Walnut Creek	Walnut Creek	66%	300+
Mercy San Juan Medical Center	Carmichael	66%	300+
Montclair Hospital Medical Center[11]	Montclair	66%	(a)
Monterey Park Hospital	Monterey Park	66%	300+
Pacific Hospital of Long Beach	Long Beach	66%	300+
Pomona Valley Hospital Medical Center	Pomona	66%	300+
Saint Francis Memorial Hospital	San Francisco	66%	300+
San Joaquin Community Hospital	Bakersfield	66%	300+
Scripps Mercy Hospital	San Diego	66%	300+
Shasta Regional Medical Center[11]	Redding	66%	300+
Sonora Regional Medical Center	Sonora	66%	300+
Sutter Lakeside Hospital	Lakeport	66%	300+
CA Pacific Med Ctr-Davies Campus	San Francisco	65%	300+
Fallbrook Hospital	Fallbrook	65%	300+
Lompoc Valley Medical Center	Lompoc	65%	300+
Mad River Community Hospital	Arcata	65%	300+
Marin General Hospital	Greenbrae	65%	300+
Mercy Medical Center	Merced	65%	300+
Mercy Medical Center - Redding	Redding	65%	300+
Methodist Hospital of Sacramento	Sacramento	65%	300+
Paradise Valley Hospital[11]	National City	65%	(a)
San Dimas Community Hospital[11]	San Dimas	65%	300+
Sequoia Hospital	Redwood City	65%	300+
Seton Medical Center	Daly City	65%	300+
Sutter Solano Medical Center	Vallejo	65%	300+
Washington Hospital	Fremont	65%	300+
Adventist Medical Center	Hanford	64%	300+
Community Hospital of San Bernardino	San Bernardino	64%	300+
Good Samaritan Hospital	San Jose	64%	300+
John F Kennedy Memorial Hospital	Indio	64%	300+
Kaweah Delta Medical Center	Visalia	64%	300+
Mark Twain Medical Center	San Andreas	64%	(a)
Saint Joseph's Medical Center of Stockton	Stockton	64%	300+
Saint Mary Medical Center	Apple Valley	64%	300+
Saint Rose Hospital	Hayward	64%	300+
Sierra Nevada Memorial Hospital	Grass Valley	64%	300+
Sutter Coast Hospital	Crescent City	64%	300+
Ventura County Medical Center	Ventura	64%	300+
Delano Regional Medical Center	Delano	63%	300+
Desert Valley Hospital	Victorville	63%	300+
Glendale Mem Hosp & Health Ctr	Glendale	63%	300+
Los Alamitos Medical Center	Los Alamitos	63%	300+
Santa Rosa Memorial Hospital	Santa Rosa	63%	300+
Sierra View District Hospital	Porterville	63%	300+
Sonoma Valley Hospital	Sonoma	63%	(a)
Ahmc Anaheim Regional Medical Center	Anaheim	62%	300+
Antelope Valley Hospital	Lancaster	62%	300+
California Hosp Med Ctr Los Angeles	Los Angeles	62%	300+
Contra Costa Regional Medical Center	Martinez	62%	300+
East Los Angeles Doctors Hospital	Los Angeles	62%	300+
Good Samaritan Hospital	Bakersfield	62%	(a)
Northridge Hospital Medical Center	Northridge	62%	300+
Oak Valley District Hospital	Oakdale	62%	(a)
Saint Louise Regional Hospital	Gilroy	62%	300+
Southwest Healthcare System	Murrieta	62%	300+
Valley Presbyterian Hospital	Van Nuys	62%	300+
Alameda County Medical Center	Oakland	61%	300+
Alhambra Hospital Medical Center	Alhambra	61%	300+
Alvarado Hospital Medical Center	San Diego	61%	300+
Chapman Medical Center	Orange	61%	300+
Garden Grove Hospital & Medical Center[11]	Garden Grove	61%	300+
Lakewood Regional Medical Center	Lakewood	61%	300+
Mercy Hospital	Bakersfield	61%	300+
Riverside County Regional Medical Center	Moreno Valley	61%	300+
San Mateo Medical Center	San Mateo	61%	300+
Adventist Medical Center - Reedley	Reedley	60%	(a)
Centinela Hospital Medical Center[11]	Inglewood	60%	300+
Dominican Hospital	Santa Cruz	60%	300+
El Centro Regional Medical Center	El Centro	60%	(a)
Hollywood Presbyterian Medical Center	Los Angeles	60%	300+
Kaiser Fdn Hosp-Oakland/Richmond	Oakland	60%	300+
Pacifica Hospital of the Valley	Sun Valley	60%	(a)
San Joaquin General Hospital	French Camp	60%	300+
Beverly Hospital	Montebello	59%	300+
Community Hospital of Huntington Park	Huntington Park	59%	300+
LAC/Harbor - UCLA Medical Center	Torrance	59%	300+
Menifee Valley Medical Center	Sun City	59%	300+
Saint Helena Hospital - Clearlake	Clearlake	59%	(a)
Santa Clara Valley Medical Center	San Jose	59%	300+
Tri - City Medical Center	Oceanside	59%	300+
Whittier Hospital Medical Center	Whittier	59%	300+
Alta Bates Summit Medical Center	Berkeley	58%	300+
CA Pacific Med Ctr-St Luke's Campus	San Francisco	58%	300+
Fairchild Medical Center	Yreka	58%	300+
Mendocino Coast District Hospital	Fort Bragg	58%	(a)
Pacific Alliance Medical Center	Los Angeles	58%	300+
San Francisco General Hospital	San Francisco	58%	(a)
San Leandro Hospital	San Leandro	58%	(a)
Emanuel Medical Center	Turlock	57%	300+
Fountain Valley Reg Hosp & Med Ctr	Fountain Valley	57%	300+
Providence Tarzana Medical Center	Tarzana	57%	300+
Regional Medical Center of San Jose	San Jose	57%	300+
Riverside Community Hospital	Riverside	57%	300+
Saint Joseph Hospital	Eureka	57%	300+
Sutter Delta Medical Center	Antioch	57%	(a)
PIH Hospital - Downey	Downey	56%	300+
San Gorgonio Memorial Hospital	Banning	56%	300+
Victor Valley Global Medical Center	Victorville	56%	300+
West Anaheim Medical Center	Anaheim	56%	300+
West Hills Hospital & Medical Center	West Hills	56%	300+
Alameda Hospital	Alameda	55%	300+
Alta Bates Summit Medical Center	Oakland	55%	300+
Coast Plaza Hospital	Norwalk	55%	300+
Corona Regional Medical Center	Corona	55%	300+
Garfield Medical Center	Monterey Park	55%	300+
Kern Medical Center	Bakersfield	55%	300+
Marina Del Rey Hospital	Marina Del Rey	55%	300+
Temple Community Hospital	Los Angeles	55%	(a)
Tri - City Regional Medical Center	Hawaiian Grdns	55%	300+
Tulare Regional Medical Center	Tulare	55%	300+
Central Valley General Hospital	Hanford	54%	300+
Mission Community Hospital	Panorama City	54%	300+
Sherman Oaks Hospital[11]	Sherman Oaks	54%	(a)
Silver Lake Medical Center	Los Angeles	54%	(a)
Community Hospital of Long Beach	Long Beach	53%	300+
La Palma Intercommunity Hospital	La Palma	53%	(a)
Madera Community Hospital	Madera	53%	300+
Memorial Hospital of Gardena	Gardena	53%	300+
San Gabriel Valley Medical Center	San Gabriel	53%	300+
Greater El Monte Community Hospital	South El Monte	51%	300+
Palo Verde Hospital	Blythe	51%	(a)
Southern California Hospital at Hollywood	Hollywood	51%	300+
Oroville Hospital	Oroville	50%	300+
Huntington Beach Hospital	Huntington Bch	49%	(a)
Parkview Comm Hosp Med Ctr	Riverside	49%	300+
Doctors Medical Center - San Pablo	San Pablo	48%	300+
Chinese Hospital	San Francisco	44%	300+
Los Angeles Community Hospital	Los Angeles	44%	300+
Rideout Memorial Hospital	Marysville	44%	300+
Hemet Valley Medical Center	Hemet	42%	300+

Meds 'Always' Explained Before Given

Hospital Name	City	Rate	Cases
Patients' Hospital of Redding	Redding	84%	(a)
Mercy Medical Center - Mount Shasta	Mount Shasta	77%	(a)
Menlo Park Surgical Hospital	Menlo Park	75%	(a)
Sutter Surgical Hospital - North Valley	Yuba City	75%	(a)
Hoag Orthopedic Institute	Irvine	74%	300+
Sutter Davis Hospital	Davis	73%	300+

NOTE: Hospital profiles are in alphabetical order by state, then city, then hospital within the city; Rankings exclude hospitals with less than 25 cases except for patient surveys which excludes hospitals with less than 100 cases; (a) 100-299 cases; (1) The number of cases/patients is too few to report; (2) Data submitted were based on a sample of cases/patients; (3) Results are based on a shorter time period than required; (4) Data suppressed by CMS for one or more quarters; (5) Results are not available for this reporting period; (6) Fewer than 100 patients completed the HCAHPS survey; (7) No cases met the criteria for this measure; (8) The lower limit of the confidence interval cannot be calculated if the number of observed infections equals zero; (9) No data are available from the state/territory for this reporting period; (10) The scores shown reflect fewer than 50 completed surveys; (11) There were discrepancies in the data collection process; (12) This measure does not apply to this hospital for this reporting period; (13) Results cannot be calculated for this reporting period; (14) The results for this state are combined with nearby states to protect confidentiality; Please refer to the User's Guide for a full explanation of data.

Banner Lassen Medical Center[11]	Susanville	72%	(a)
Fresno Surgical Hospital	Fresno	72%	300+
Healdsburg District Hospital	Healdsburg	72%	(a)
Sharp Coronado Hosp & Healthcare Ctr	Coronado	72%	300+
Placentia Linda Hospital	Placentia	71%	300+
Stanislaus Surgical Hospital	Modesto	71%	300+
Colusa Regional Medical Center	Colusa	69%	(a)
Doctors Medical Center	Modesto	69%	300+
Frank R Howard Memorial Hospital	Willits	69%	300+
Saint Helena Hospital	Saint Helena	69%	300+
City of Hope Helford Clinical Res Hosp	Duarte	68%	300+
Fresno Heart & Surgical Hospital	Fresno	68%	300+
Glendale Adventist Medical Center	Glendale	68%	300+
Northern Inyo Hospital	Bishop	68%	(a)
Sierra Vista Regional Medical Center	San Luis Obispo	68%	300+
Sutter Maternity & Surgery Ctr	Santa Cruz	68%	300+
Woodland Memorial Hospital	Woodland	68%	(a)
Enloe Medical Center	Chico	67%	300+
George L Mee Memorial Hospital	King City	67%	(a)
Marian Regional Medical Center	Santa Maria	67%	300+
Palo Verde Hospital	Blythe	67%	(a)
Scripps Green Hospital	La Jolla	67%	300+
Sharp Memorial Hospital	San Diego	67%	300+
Twin Cities Community Hospital	Templeton	67%	300+
UCSF Medical Center	San Francisco	67%	300+
Community Hospital of San Bernardino	San Bernardino	66%	300+
Comm Hosp of the Monterey Peninsula	Monterey	66%	300+
Community Regional Medical Center	Fresno	66%	300+
French Hospital Medical Center	San Luis Obispo	66%	300+
Huntington Memorial Hospital	Pasadena	66%	300+
Kaiser Foundation Hospital - Vacaville	Vacaville	66%	300+
Mammoth Hospital	Mammoth Lakes	66%	(a)
Natividad Medical Center	Salinas	66%	300+
Palm Drive Hospital	Sebastopol	66%	(a)
Sierra View District Hospital	Porterville	66%	300+
Sutter Auburn Faith Hospital	Auburn	66%	300+
Tahoe Forest Hospital	Truckee	66%	(a)
Goleta Valley Cottage Hospital	Santa Barbara	65%	300+
Good Samaritan Hospital	Bakersfield	65%	(a)
Kaiser Foundation Hospital - Baldwin Park	Baldwin Park	65%	300+
Kaiser Fdn Hosp-Orange Co-Anaheim	Anaheim	65%	300+
Kaiser Foundation Hospital - Santa Clara	Santa Clara	65%	300+
Kaiser Foundation Hospital - Santa Rosa	Santa Rosa	65%	300+
Kaiser Fdn Hosp-S San Francisco	S San Francisco	65%	300+
Kaiser Foundation Hospital - West La	Los Angeles	65%	300+
Kaiser Fdn Hosp-Woodland Hills	Woodland Hills	65%	300+
Palmdale Regional Medical Center	Palmdale	65%	300+
Paradise Valley Hospital[11]	National City	65%	(a)
San Ramon Regional Medical Center	San Ramon	65%	300+
Santa Barbara Cottage Hospital	Santa Barbara	65%	300+
Scripps Memorial Hospital La Jolla	La Jolla	65%	300+
Sharp Chula Vista Medical Center	Chula Vista	65%	300+
Sutter Medical Center of Santa Rosa	Santa Rosa	65%	300+
Sutter Tracy Community Hospital	Tracy	65%	300+
USC Verdugo Hills Hospital	Glendale	65%	300+
Barton Memorial Hospital	S Lake Tahoe	64%	300+
Coastal Communities Hospital	Santa Ana	64%	300+
Desert Regional Medical Center	Palm Springs	64%	300+
Doctors Hospital of Manteca	Manteca	64%	300+
Kaiser Foundation Hospital - Fontana	Fontana	64%	300+
Kaiser Foundation Hospital - Riverside	Riverside	64%	300+
Kaiser Foundation Hospital - San Diego	San Diego	64%	300+
Kaiser Fdn Hosp-San Francisco	San Francisco	64%	300+
Kaiser Fdn Hosp S Sacramento	Sacramento	64%	300+
LAC/Rancho Los Amigos Ntl Rehab Ctr	Downey	64%	300+
Marshall Medical Center	Placerville	64%	300+
Northbay Medical Center	Fairfield	64%	300+
Novato Community Hospital	Novato	64%	300+
Ojai Valley Community Hospital	Ojai	64%	(a)
Petaluma Valley Hospital	Petaluma	64%	300+
Stanford Hospital	Stanford	64%	300+
Temple Community Hospital	Los Angeles	64%	(a)
Ukiah Valley Medical Center	Ukiah	64%	300+
Univ of California Irvine Med Ctr	Orange	64%	300+
Valleycare Medical Center	Pleasanton	64%	300+
Barstow Community Hospital	Barstow	63%	300+
Chapman Medical Center	Orange	63%	300+
Clovis Community Medical Center	Clovis	63%	300+
Dameron Hospital	Stockton	63%	300+
Eisenhower Medical Center	Rancho Mirage	63%	300+
Fairchild Medical Center	Yreka	63%	300+
Fallbrook Hospital	Fallbrook	63%	300+
John Muir Medical Center - Concord Campus	Concord	63%	300+
Kaiser Foundation Hospital	San Rafael	63%	300+
Kaiser Foundation Hospital - Fresno	Fresno	63%	300+
Kaiser Foundation Hospital - Manteca	Manteca	63%	300+
Kaiser Foundation Hospital - Roseville	Roseville	63%	300+
Memorial Hospital Los Banos	Los Banos	63%	(a)
Memorial Medical Center	Modesto	63%	300+
Mercy General Hospital	Sacramento	63%	300+
Methodist Hospital of Sacramento	Sacramento	63%	300+

Pomerado Hospital	Poway	63%	300+
Presbyterian Intercommunity Hospital	Whittier	63%	300+
Prov Little Co of Mary Med Ctr San Pedro	San Pedro	63%	300+
Prov Little Co of Mary Med Ctr Torrance	Torrance	63%	300+
Redlands Community Hospital	Redlands	63%	300+
Saint Elizabeth Community Hospital	Red Bluff	63%	300+
Saint Mary's Medical Center	San Francisco	63%	300+
San Leandro Hospital	San Leandro	63%	(a)
Scripps Mercy Hospital	San Diego	63%	300+
Sonoma Valley Hospital	Sonoma	63%	(a)
Tulare Regional Medical Center	Tulare	63%	300+
Univ of CA Davis Med Ctr	Sacramento	63%	300+
Western Medical Center Santa Ana	Santa Ana	63%	300+
Contra Costa Regional Medical Center	Martinez	62%	300+
El Centro Regional Medical Center	El Centro	62%	(a)
Feather River Hospital	Paradise	62%	300+
Garfield Medical Center	Monterey Park	62%	300+
Grossmont Hospital	La Mesa	62%	300+
Hoag Memorial Hospital Presbyterian	Newport Beach	62%	300+
John F Kennedy Memorial Hospital	Indio	62%	300+
Kaiser Foundation Hospital & Rehab Center	Vallejo	62%	300+
Kaiser Foundation Hospital - Downey	Downey	62%	300+
Kaiser Fdn Hosp-Panorama City	Panorama City	62%	300+
Kaiser Foundation Hospital - Redwood City	Redwood City	62%	300+
Kaiser Foundation Hospital - Sacramento	Sacramento	62%	300+
Kaiser Foundation Hospital - South Bay	Harbor City	62%	300+
Mad River Community Hospital	Arcata	62%	300+
Mercy San Juan Medical Center	Carmichael	62%	300+
Methodist Hospital of Southern California	Arcadia	62%	300+
Mills - Peninsula Medical Center	Burlingame	62%	300+
Palomar Health Downtown Campus	Escondido	62%	300+
Pioneers Memorial Healthcare District	Brawley	62%	300+
Redwood Memorial Hospital	Fortuna	62%	300+
Saint Joseph Hospital	Orange	62%	300+
San Antonio Community Hospital	Upland	62%	300+
Scripps Memorial Hospital - Encinitas	Encinitas	62%	300+
Sierra Nevada Memorial Hospital	Grass Valley	62%	300+
Sonora Regional Medical Center	Sonora	62%	300+
Sutter General Hospital	Sacramento	62%	300+
Sutter Lakeside Hospital	Lakeport	62%	300+
Torrance Memorial Medical Center	Torrance	62%	300+
Tri - City Medical Center	Oceanside	62%	300+
Univ of CA San Diego Med Ctr	San Diego	62%	300+
Washington Hospital	Fremont	62%	300+
White Memorial Medical Center	Los Angeles	62%	300+
Adventist Medical Center - Reedley	Reedley	61%	(a)
Arrowhead Regional Medical Center	Colton	61%	300+
CA Pacific Med Ctr-Davies Campus	San Francisco	61%	300+
Comm Mem Hosp San Buenaventura	Ventura	61%	300+
Hazel Hawkins Memorial Hospital	Hollister	61%	300+
John Muir Med Ctr-Walnut Creek Campus	Walnut Creek	61%	300+
Kaiser Foundation Hospital - Antioch	Antioch	61%	300+
Kaiser Fdn Hosp-Fremont/Hayward	Hayward	61%	300+
Kaiser Foundation Hospital - Los Angeles	Los Angeles	61%	300+
Kaiser Foundation Hospital - San Jose	San Jose	61%	300+
Keck Hospital of USC	Los Angeles	61%	300+
LAC/Olive View - UCLA Medical Center	Sylmar	61%	300+
Mercy Hospital of Folsom	Folsom	61%	300+
Mercy Medical Center	Merced	61%	300+
Montclair Hospital Medical Center[11]	Montclair	61%	(a)
Orange Coast Memorial Medical Center	Fountain Valley	61%	300+
Pacific Hospital of Long Beach	Long Beach	61%	300+
Providence Saint Joseph Medical Center	Burbank	61%	300+
Saint Bernardine Medical Center	San Bernardino	61%	300+
Saint Helena Hospital - Clearlake	Clearlake	61%	(a)
Saint Johns Pleasant Valley Hospital	Camarillo	61%	300+
Saint Johns Regional Medical Center	Oxnard	61%	300+
Saint Louise Regional Hospital	Gilroy	61%	300+
Salinas Valley Memorial Hospital	Salinas	61%	300+
San Joaquin Community Hospital	Bakersfield	61%	300+
Simi Valley Hosp & Health Care Svcs	Simi Valley	61%	300+
Sutter Amador Hospital	Jackson	61%	300+
Sutter Coast Hospital	Crescent City	61%	300+
Sutter Roseville Medical Center	Roseville	61%	300+
Sutter Solano Medical Center	Vallejo	61%	300+
Victor Valley Global Medical Center	Victorville	61%	300+
Watsonville Community Hospital	Watsonville	61%	300+
Western Medical Center Hospital Anaheim	Anaheim	61%	300+
El Camino Hospital	Mountain View	60%	300+
Foothill Presbyterian Hospital	Glendora	60%	300+
Glendale Mem Hosp & Health Ctr	Glendale	60%	300+
Henry Mayo Newhall Memorial Hospital	Valencia	60%	300+
Loma Linda University Medical Center	Loma Linda	60%	300+
Long Beach Memorial Medical Center	Long Beach	60%	300+
Mark Twain Medical Center	San Andreas	60%	(a)
Mendocino Coast District Hospital	Fort Bragg	60%	(a)
Northridge Hospital Medical Center	Northridge	60%	300+
Queen of the Valley Medical Center	Napa	60%	300+
Ronald Reagan UCLA Medical Center	Los Angeles	60%	300+
Saint Mary Medical Center	Long Beach	60%	300+
San Joaquin General Hospital	French Camp	60%	300+

Santa Monica-UCLA Med Ctr & Ortho Hosp	Santa Monica	60%	300+
Shasta Regional Medical Center[11]	Redding	60%	300+
Ahmc Anaheim Regional Medical Center	Anaheim	59%	300+
Bakersfield Memorial Hospital	Bakersfield	59%	300+
Centinela Hospital Medical Center[11]	Inglewood	59%	300+
Coast Plaza Hospital	Norwalk	59%	300+
Hi - Desert Medical Center	Joshua Tree	59%	300+
Kaiser Fdn Hosp-Moreno Valley	Moreno Valley	59%	300+
Loma Linda Univ Med Ctr-Murrieta	Murrieta	59%	300+
Mercy Medical Center - Redding	Redding	59%	300+
Mission Hospital Regional Medical Center	Mission Viejo	59%	300+
Olympia Medical Center	Los Angeles	59%	300+
Saddleback Memorial Medical Center	Laguna Hills	59%	300+
Whittier Hospital Medical Center	Whittier	59%	300+
Antelope Valley Hospital	Lancaster	58%	300+
CA Pacific Med Ctr-St Luke's Campus	San Francisco	58%	300+
Cedars - Sinai Medical Center	Los Angeles	58%	300+
Citrus Valley Medical Center - IC Campus	Covina	58%	300+
Community Hospital of Huntington Park	Huntington Park	58%	300+
Delano Regional Medical Center	Delano	58%	300+
Kaweah Delta Medical Center	Visalia	58%	300+
Lakewood Regional Medical Center	Lakewood	58%	300+
Lompoc Valley Medical Center	Lompoc	58%	300+
Madera Community Hospital	Madera	58%	300+
Providence Holy Cross Medical Center	Mission Hills	58%	300+
Saint Joseph's Medical Center of Stockton	Stockton	58%	300+
Saint Jude Medical Center	Fullerton	58%	300+
Southwest Healthcare System	Murrieta	58%	300+
Adventist Medical Center	Hanford	57%	300+
Bakersfield Heart Hospital	Bakersfield	57%	300+
CA Pacific Med Ctr-Pacific Campus Hosp	San Francisco	57%	300+
Chino Valley Medical Center[11]	Chino	57%	300+
Corona Regional Medical Center	Corona	57%	300+
Dominican Hospital	Santa Cruz	57%	300+
Emanuel Medical Center	Turlock	57%	300+
Kaiser Foundation Hospital - Walnut Creek	Walnut Creek	57%	300+
Lodi Memorial Hospital	Lodi	57%	300+
Los Alamitos Medical Center	Los Alamitos	57%	300+
PIH Hospital - Downey	Downey	57%	300+
Saint Francis Memorial Hospital	San Francisco	57%	300+
Saint Rose Hospital	Hayward	57%	300+
Saint Vincent Medical Center	Los Angeles	57%	300+
San Mateo Medical Center	San Mateo	57%	300+
Santa Clara Valley Medical Center	San Jose	57%	300+
Santa Rosa Memorial Hospital	Santa Rosa	57%	300+
Tri - City Regional Medical Center	Hawaiian Grdns	57%	300+
Ventura County Medical Center	Ventura	57%	300+
Central Valley General Hospital	Hanford	56%	300+
Chinese Hospital	San Francisco	56%	300+
East Los Angeles Doctors Hospital	Los Angeles	56%	300+
Kaiser Fdn Hosp-Oakland/Richmond	Oakland	56%	300+
La Palma Intercommunity Hospital	La Palma	56%	(a)
LAC/Harbor - UCLA Medical Center	Torrance	56%	300+
Mercy Hospital	Bakersfield	56%	300+
Monterey Park Hospital	Monterey Park	56%	300+
O'Connor Hospital	San Jose	56%	300+
Riverside County Regional Medical Center	Moreno Valley	56%	300+
Saint Agnes Medical Center	Fresno	56%	300+
Saint Francis Medical Center	Lynwood	56%	300+
Saint Joseph Hospital	Eureka	56%	300+
Saint Mary Medical Center	Apple Valley	56%	300+
Sequoia Hospital	Redwood City	56%	300+
Seton Medical Center	Daly City	56%	300+
Sherman Oaks Hospital[11]	Sherman Oaks	56%	(a)
Valley Presbyterian Hospital	Van Nuys	56%	300+
Alameda County Medical Center	Oakland	55%	300+
California Hosp Med Ctr Los Angeles	Los Angeles	55%	300+
Eden Medical Center	Castro Valley	55%	300+
Good Samaritan Hospital	Los Angeles	55%	300+
LAC+USC Medical Center[11]	Los Angeles	55%	300+
Marin General Hospital	Greenbrae	55%	300+
Marina Del Rey Hospital	Marina Del Rey	55%	300+
Menifee Valley Medical Center	Sun City	55%	300+
Pacifica Hospital of the Valley	Sun Valley	55%	(a)
Pomona Valley Hospital Medical Center	Pomona	55%	300+
Providence Saint John's Health Center	Santa Monica	55%	300+
Sutter Delta Medical Center	Antioch	55%	(a)
Alameda Hospital	Alameda	54%	300+
Alvarado Hospital Medical Center	San Diego	54%	300+
Doctors Medical Center - San Pablo	San Pablo	54%	300+
Fountain Valley Reg Hosp & Med Ctr	Fountain Valley	54%	300+
Los Robles Hospital & Medical Center	Thousand Oaks	54%	300+
Oroville Hospital	Oroville	54%	300+
Pacific Alliance Medical Center	Los Angeles	54%	300+
Providence Tarzana Medical Center	Tarzana	54%	300+
Regional Medical Center of San Jose	San Jose	54%	300+
Riverside Community Hospital	Riverside	54%	300+
San Gorgonio Memorial Hospital	Banning	54%	300+
Alhambra Hospital Medical Center	Alhambra	53%	300+
Alta Bates Summit Medical Center	Berkeley	53%	300+
Desert Valley Hospital	Victorville	53%	300+

NOTE: Hospital profiles are in alphabetical order by state, then city, then hospital within the city; Rankings exclude hospitals with less than 25 cases except for patient surveys which excludes hospitals with less than 100 cases; (a) 100-299 cases; (1) The number of cases/patients is too few to report; (2) Data submitted were based on a sample of cases/patients; (3) Results are based on a shorter time period than required; (4) Data suppressed by CMS for one or more quarters; (5) Results are not available for this reporting period; (6) Fewer than 100 patients completed the HCAHPS survey; (7) No cases met the criteria for this measure; (8) The lower limit of the confidence interval cannot be calculated if the number of observed infections equals zero; (9) No data are available from the state/territory for this reporting period; (10) The scores shown reflect fewer than 50 completed surveys; (11) There were discrepancies in the data collection process; (12) This measure does not apply to this hospital for this reporting period; (13) Results cannot be calculated for this reporting period; (14) The results for this state are combined with nearby states to protect confidentiality; Please refer to the User's Guide for a full explanation of data.

Hollywood Presbyterian Medical Center	Los Angeles	53%	300+
Kern Medical Center	Bakersfield	53%	300+
San Dimas Community Hospital[11]	San Dimas	53%	300+
San Gabriel Valley Medical Center	San Gabriel	53%	300+
West Hills Hospital & Medical Center	West Hills	53%	300+
Alta Bates Summit Medical Center	Oakland	52%	300+
Community Hospital of Long Beach	Long Beach	52%	300+
Oak Valley District Hospital	Oakdale	52%	(a)
Beverly Hospital	Montebello	51%	300+
Good Samaritan Hospital	San Jose	51%	300+
Parkview Comm Hosp Med Ctr	Riverside	51%	300+
Rideout Memorial Hospital	Marysville	51%	300+
Garden Grove Hospital & Medical Center[11]	Garden Grove	50%	300+
Greater El Monte Community Hospital	South El Monte	50%	300+
Huntington Beach Hospital	Huntington Bch	50%	(a)
Hemet Valley Medical Center	Hemet	49%	300+
San Francisco General Hospital	San Francisco	49%	(a)
Southern California Hospital at Hollywood	Hollywood	49%	300+
West Anaheim Medical Center	Anaheim	49%	300+
Memorial Hospital of Gardena	Gardena	48%	300+
Mission Community Hospital	Panorama City	48%	300+
Los Angeles Community Hospital	Los Angeles	45%	300+
Silver Lake Medical Center	Los Angeles	43%	(a)

Nurses 'Always' Communicated Well

Hospital Name	City	Rate	Cases
Patients' Hospital of Redding	Redding	94%	(a)
Hoag Orthopedic Institute	Irvine	88%	300+
Stanislaus Surgical Hospital	Modesto	88%	300+
Fresno Surgical Hospital	Fresno	87%	300+
Ojai Valley Community Hospital	Ojai	87%	(a)
Sutter Surgical Hospital - North Valley	Yuba City	87%	(a)
Sharp Coronado Hosp & Healthcare Ctr	Coronado	86%	300+
Sutter Davis Hospital	Davis	86%	300+
Tahoe Forest Hospital	Truckee	85%	(a)
Fresno Heart & Surgical Hospital	Fresno	84%	300+
Menlo Park Surgical Hospital	Menlo Park	84%	(a)
Banner Lassen Medical Center[11]	Susanville	83%	(a)
Frank R Howard Memorial Hospital	Willits	83%	300+
Goleta Valley Cottage Hospital	Santa Barbara	83%	300+
Saint Helena Hospital	Saint Helena	83%	300+
Sharp Memorial Hospital	San Diego	83%	300+
Sutter Maternity & Surgery Ctr	Santa Cruz	83%	300+
City of Hope Helford Clinical Res Hosp	Duarte	82%	300+
Colusa Regional Medical Center	Colusa	82%	(a)
Healdsburg District Hospital	Healdsburg	82%	(a)
Northern Inyo Hospital	Bishop	82%	(a)
Novato Community Hospital	Novato	82%	300+
Stanford Hospital	Stanford	82%	300+
Huntington Memorial Hospital	Pasadena	81%	300+
Marshall Medical Center	Placerville	81%	300+
Mercy Medical Center - Mount Shasta	Mount Shasta	81%	(a)
Placentia Linda Hospital	Placentia	81%	300+
Scripps Memorial Hospital La Jolla	La Jolla	81%	300+
Sierra Vista Regional Medical Center	San Luis Obispo	81%	300+
Sutter Medical Center of Santa Rosa	Santa Rosa	81%	300+
Valleycare Medical Center	Pleasanton	81%	300+
Enloe Medical Center	Chico	80%	300+
French Hospital Medical Center	San Luis Obispo	80%	300+
John Muir Medical Center - Concord Campus	Concord	80%	300+
Mammoth Hospital	Mammoth Lakes	80%	(a)
Memorial Hospital Los Banos	Los Banos	80%	(a)
Santa Barbara Cottage Hospital	Santa Barbara	80%	300+
Scripps Green Hospital	La Jolla	80%	300+
Sharp Chula Vista Medical Center	Chula Vista	80%	300+
Sutter Amador Hospital	Jackson	80%	300+
Sutter Coast Hospital	Crescent City	80%	300+
Sutter Tracy Community Hospital	Tracy	80%	300+
Twin Cities Community Hospital	Templeton	80%	300+
UCSF Medical Center	San Francisco	80%	300+
Kaiser Foundation Hospital - Santa Clara	Santa Clara	79%	300+
Kaiser Fdn Hosp-Woodland Hills	Woodland Hills	79%	300+
Palm Drive Hospital	Sebastopol	79%	(a)
Palo Verde Hospital	Blythe	79%	(a)
Sutter Auburn Faith Hospital	Auburn	79%	300+
White Memorial Medical Center	Los Angeles	79%	300+
Comm Mem Hosp San Buenaventura	Ventura	78%	300+
Feather River Hospital	Paradise	78%	300+
George L Mee Memorial Hospital	King City	78%	(a)
Glendale Adventist Medical Center	Glendale	78%	300+
Grossmont Hospital	La Mesa	78%	300+
Hoag Memorial Hospital Presbyterian	Newport Beach	78%	300+
Kaiser Foundation Hospital - Fresno	Fresno	78%	300+
Kaiser Fdn Hosp-Orange Co-Anaheim	Anaheim	78%	300+
Kaiser Fdn Hosp-S San Francisco	S San Francisco	78%	300+
Kaiser Foundation Hospital - Vacaville	Vacaville	78%	300+
LAC/Rancho Los Amigos Ntl Rehab Ctr	Downey	78%	300+
Loma Linda Univ Med Ctr-Murrieta	Murrieta	78%	300+
Memorial Medical Center	Modesto	78%	300+
Northbay Medical Center	Fairfield	78%	300+
Presbyterian Intercommunity Hospital	Whittier	78%	300+
Prov Little Co of Mary Med Ctr San Pedro	San Pedro	78%	300+
San Ramon Regional Medical Center	San Ramon	78%	300+
Scripps Memorial Hospital - Encinitas	Encinitas	78%	300+
Sutter General Hospital	Sacramento	78%	300+
Ukiah Valley Medical Center	Ukiah	78%	300+
Cedars - Sinai Medical Center	Los Angeles	77%	300+
Comm Hosp of the Monterey Peninsula	Monterey	77%	300+
Desert Regional Medical Center	Palm Springs	77%	300+
Doctors Medical Center	Modesto	77%	300+
Eisenhower Medical Center	Rancho Mirage	77%	300+
John Muir Med Ctr-Walnut Creek Campus	Walnut Creek	77%	300+
Kaiser Foundation Hospital - Fontana	Fontana	77%	300+
Kaiser Foundation Hospital - Los Angeles	Los Angeles	77%	300+
Kaiser Foundation Hospital - Manteca	Manteca	77%	300+
Kaiser Foundation Hospital - San Diego	San Diego	77%	300+
Kaiser Fdn Hosp-San Francisco	San Francisco	77%	300+
Kaiser Foundation Hospital - Santa Rosa	Santa Rosa	77%	300+
Kaiser Foundation Hospital - West La	Los Angeles	77%	300+
Kaweah Delta Medical Center	Visalia	77%	300+
Keck Hospital of USC	Los Angeles	77%	300+
Lodi Memorial Hospital	Lodi	77%	300+
Mad River Community Hospital	Arcata	77%	300+
Mercy General Hospital	Sacramento	77%	300+
Mills - Peninsula Medical Center	Burlingame	77%	300+
Petaluma Valley Hospital	Petaluma	77%	300+
Prov Little Co of Mary Med Ctr Torrance	Torrance	77%	300+
Providence Saint Joseph Medical Center	Burbank	77%	300+
Redlands Community Hospital	Redlands	77%	300+
Saint Johns Pleasant Valley Hospital	Camarillo	77%	300+
Saint Joseph Hospital	Orange	77%	300+
San Antonio Community Hospital	Upland	77%	300+
Sonora Regional Medical Center	Sonora	77%	300+
Torrance Memorial Medical Center	Torrance	77%	300+
USC Verdugo Hills Hospital	Glendale	77%	300+
Barton Memorial Hospital	S Lake Tahoe	76%	300+
Clovis Community Medical Center	Clovis	76%	300+
El Camino Hospital	Mountain View	76%	300+
Foothill Presbyterian Hospital	Glendora	76%	300+
Hazel Hawkins Memorial Hospital	Hollister	76%	300+
Hi - Desert Medical Center	Joshua Tree	76%	300+
Kaiser Foundation Hospital - Baldwin Park	Baldwin Park	76%	300+
Kaiser Foundation Hospital - Downey	Downey	76%	300+
Kaiser Foundation Hospital - Roseville	Roseville	76%	300+
Kaiser Foundation Hospital - Sacramento	Sacramento	76%	300+
Kaiser Foundation Hospital - South Bay	Harbor City	76%	300+
Mendocino Coast District Hospital	Fort Bragg	76%	(a)
Mission Hospital Regional Medical Center	Mission Viejo	76%	300+
Palmdale Regional Medical Center	Palmdale	76%	300+
Providence Holy Cross Medical Center	Mission Hills	76%	300+
Redwood Memorial Hospital	Fortuna	76%	300+
Saint Louise Regional Hospital	Gilroy	76%	300+
Shasta Regional Medical Center[11]	Redding	76%	300+
Sierra View District Hospital	Porterville	76%	300+
Sonoma Valley Hospital	Sonoma	76%	(a)
Sutter Lakeside Hospital	Lakeport	76%	300+
Sutter Roseville Medical Center	Roseville	76%	300+
Sutter Solano Medical Center	Vallejo	76%	300+
Univ of CA San Diego Med Ctr	San Diego	76%	300+
Western Medical Center Santa Ana	Santa Ana	76%	300+
Woodland Memorial Hospital	Woodland	76%	(a)
Arrowhead Regional Medical Center	Colton	75%	300+
Barstow Community Hospital	Barstow	75%	300+
Dameron Hospital	Stockton	75%	300+
Doctors Hospital of Manteca	Manteca	75%	300+
Henry Mayo Newhall Memorial Hospital	Valencia	75%	300+
Kaiser Foundation Hospital	San Rafael	75%	300+
Kaiser Foundation Hospital - Antioch	Antioch	75%	300+
Kaiser Foundation Hospital - Redwood City	Redwood City	75%	300+
Kaiser Fdn Hosp S Sacramento	Sacramento	75%	300+
Long Beach Memorial Medical Center	Long Beach	75%	300+
Marian Regional Medical Center	Santa Maria	75%	300+
Olympia Medical Center	Los Angeles	75%	300+
Palomar Health Downtown Campus	Escondido	75%	300+
Pomerado Hospital	Poway	75%	300+
Saddleback Memorial Medical Center	Laguna Hills	75%	300+
Saint Agnes Medical Center	Fresno	75%	300+
Saint Elizabeth Community Hospital	Red Bluff	75%	300+
Saint Helena Hospital - Clearlake	Clearlake	75%	(a)
Sierra Nevada Memorial Hospital	Grass Valley	75%	300+
Tri - City Medical Center	Oceanside	75%	300+
Univ of CA Davis Med Ctr	Sacramento	75%	300+
Univ of California Irvine Med Ctr	Orange	75%	300+
Watsonville Community Hospital	Watsonville	75%	300+
Western Medical Center Hospital Anaheim	Anaheim	75%	300+
Coastal Communities Hospital	Santa Ana	74%	300+
Fairchild Medical Center	Yreka	74%	300+
Fallbrook Hospital	Fallbrook	74%	300+
Kaiser Foundation Hospital & Rehab Center	Vallejo	74%	300+
Kaiser Fdn Hosp-Moreno Valley	Moreno Valley	74%	300+
Kaiser Fdn Hosp-Panorama City	Panorama City	74%	300+
Kaiser Foundation Hospital - Riverside	Riverside	74%	300+
Loma Linda University Medical Center	Loma Linda	74%	300+
Methodist Hospital of Southern California	Arcadia	74%	300+
Natividad Medical Center	Salinas	74%	300+
Orange Coast Memorial Medical Center	Fountain Valley	74%	300+
Pacific Hospital of Long Beach	Long Beach	74%	300+
Paradise Valley Hospital[11]	National City	74%	(a)
Pioneers Memorial Healthcare District	Brawley	74%	300+
Queen of the Valley Medical Center	Napa	74%	300+
Saint Bernardine Medical Center	San Bernardino	74%	300+
San Dimas Community Hospital[11]	San Dimas	74%	300+
San Gorgonio Memorial Hospital	Banning	74%	300+
Scripps Mercy Hospital	San Diego	74%	300+
Seton Medical Center	Daly City	74%	300+
Sutter Delta Medical Center	Antioch	74%	(a)
Washington Hospital	Fremont	74%	300+
Antelope Valley Hospital	Lancaster	73%	300+
CA Pacific Med Ctr-Pacific Campus Hosp	San Francisco	73%	300+
Chapman Medical Center	Orange	73%	300+
Citrus Valley Medical Center - IC Campus	Covina	73%	300+
Delano Regional Medical Center	Delano	73%	300+
Eden Medical Center	Castro Valley	73%	300+
John F Kennedy Memorial Hospital	Indio	73%	300+
Kaiser Fdn Hosp-Fremont/Hayward	Hayward	73%	300+
Kaiser Foundation Hospital - San Jose	San Jose	73%	300+
Lakewood Regional Medical Center	Lakewood	73%	300+
Los Alamitos Medical Center	Los Alamitos	73%	300+
Madera Community Hospital	Madera	73%	300+
Mark Twain Medical Center	San Andreas	73%	(a)
Mercy Hospital of Folsom	Folsom	73%	300+
Mercy Medical Center	Merced	73%	300+
Mercy Medical Center - Redding	Redding	73%	300+
Mercy San Juan Medical Center	Carmichael	73%	300+
Methodist Hospital of Sacramento	Sacramento	73%	300+
O'Connor Hospital	San Jose	73%	300+
Saint Mary Medical Center	Long Beach	73%	300+
Salinas Valley Memorial Hospital	Salinas	73%	300+
San Joaquin Community Hospital	Bakersfield	73%	300+
Temple Community Hospital	Los Angeles	73%	(a)
Adventist Medical Center - Reedley	Reedley	72%	(a)
Bakersfield Heart Hospital	Bakersfield	72%	300+
Bakersfield Memorial Hospital	Bakersfield	72%	300+
CA Pacific Med Ctr-Davies Campus	San Francisco	72%	300+
Chino Valley Medical Center[11]	Chino	72%	300+
Community Regional Medical Center	Fresno	72%	300+
Desert Valley Hospital	Victorville	72%	300+
Good Samaritan Hospital	Los Angeles	72%	300+
Lompoc Valley Medical Center	Lompoc	72%	300+
Los Robles Hospital & Medical Center	Thousand Oaks	72%	300+
Montclair Hospital Medical Center[11]	Montclair	72%	(a)
Pacifica Hospital of the Valley	Sun Valley	72%	(a)
Ronald Reagan UCLA Medical Center	Los Angeles	72%	300+
Saint Johns Regional Medical Center	Oxnard	72%	300+
Saint Jude Medical Center	Fullerton	72%	300+
Saint Mary's Medical Center	San Francisco	72%	300+
Saint Vincent Medical Center	Los Angeles	72%	300+
Santa Rosa Memorial Hospital	Santa Rosa	72%	300+
Community Hospital of Huntington Park	Huntington Park	71%	300+
Dominican Hospital	Santa Cruz	71%	300+
Glendale Mem Hosp & Health Ctr	Glendale	71%	300+
Good Samaritan Hospital	San Jose	71%	300+
Kaiser Foundation Hospital - Walnut Creek	Walnut Creek	71%	300+
LAC/Harbor - UCLA Medical Center	Torrance	71%	300+
LAC/Olive View - UCLA Medical Center	Sylmar	71%	300+
Menifee Valley Medical Center	Sun City	71%	300+
Oak Valley District Hospital	Oakdale	71%	(a)
Pomona Valley Hospital Medical Center	Pomona	71%	300+
Saint Joseph's Medical Center of Stockton	Stockton	71%	300+
Saint Rose Hospital	Hayward	71%	300+
San Leandro Hospital	San Leandro	71%	(a)
Santa Monica-UCLA Med Ctr & Ortho Hosp	Santa Monica	71%	300+
Simi Valley Hosp & Health Care Svcs	Simi Valley	71%	300+
Ventura County Medical Center	Ventura	71%	300+
Victor Valley Global Medical Center	Victorville	71%	300+
Adventist Medical Center	Hanford	70%	300+
Ahmc Anaheim Regional Medical Center	Anaheim	70%	300+
CA Pacific Med Ctr-St Luke's Campus	San Francisco	70%	300+
Community Hospital of San Bernardino	San Bernardino	70%	300+
Good Samaritan Hospital	Bakersfield	70%	(a)
Marin General Hospital	Greenbrae	70%	300+
Northridge Hospital Medical Center	Northridge	70%	300+
Oroville Hospital	Oroville	70%	300+
Saint Francis Medical Center	Lynwood	70%	300+
Saint Mary Medical Center	Apple Valley	70%	300+
Sequoia Hospital	Redwood City	70%	300+
Southwest Healthcare System	Murrieta	70%	300+
Tulare Regional Medical Center	Tulare	70%	300+
Whittier Hospital Medical Center	Whittier	70%	300+
Alta Bates Summit Medical Center	Oakland	69%	300+
Alvarado Hospital Medical Center	San Diego	69%	300+
Centinela Hospital Medical Center[11]	Inglewood	69%	300+
Central Valley General Hospital	Hanford	69%	300+

NOTE: Hospital profiles are in alphabetical order by state, then city, then hospital within the city; Rankings exclude hospitals with less than 25 cases except for patient surveys which excludes hospitals with less than 100 cases; (a) 100-299 cases; (1) The number of cases/patients is too few to report; (2) Data submitted were based on a sample of cases/patients; (3) Results are based on a shorter time period than required; (4) Data suppressed by CMS for one or more quarters; (5) Results are not available for this reporting period; (6) Fewer than 100 patients completed the HCAHPS survey; (7) No cases met the criteria for this measure; (8) The lower limit of the confidence interval cannot be calculated if the number of observed infections equals zero; (9) No data are available from the state/territory for this reporting period; (10) The scores shown reflect fewer than 50 completed surveys; (11) There were discrepancies in the data collection process; (12) This measure does not apply to this hospital for this reporting period; (13) Results cannot be calculated for this reporting period; (14) The results for this state are combined with nearby states to protect confidentiality; Please refer to the User's Guide for a full explanation of data.

Hospital Name	City	Rate	Cases
Corona Regional Medical Center	Corona	69%	300+
East Los Angeles Doctors Hospital	Los Angeles	69%	300+
El Centro Regional Medical Center	El Centro	69%	(a)
Emanuel Medical Center	Turlock	69%	300+
La Palma Intercommunity Hospital	La Palma	69%	(a)
LAC+USC Medical Center[11]	Los Angeles	69%	300+
Marina Del Rey Hospital	Marina Del Rey	69%	300+
Mercy Hospital	Bakersfield	69%	300+
Pacific Alliance Medical Center	Los Angeles	69%	300+
Providence Saint John's Health Center	Santa Monica	69%	300+
Riverside Community Hospital	Riverside	69%	300+
Riverside County Regional Medical Center	Moreno Valley	69%	300+
San Mateo Medical Center	San Mateo	69%	300+
Valley Presbyterian Hospital	Van Nuys	69%	300+
Coast Plaza Hospital	Norwalk	68%	300+
Contra Costa Regional Medical Center	Martinez	68%	300+
Fountain Valley Reg Hosp & Med Ctr	Fountain Valley	68%	300+
Kaiser Fdn Hosp-Oakland/Richmond	Oakland	68%	300+
Monterey Park Hospital	Monterey Park	68%	300+
Providence Tarzana Medical Center	Tarzana	68%	300+
San Joaquin General Hospital	French Camp	68%	300+
Santa Clara Valley Medical Center	San Jose	68%	300+
Tri - City Regional Medical Center	Hawaiian Grdns	68%	300+
Beverly Hospital	Montebello	67%	300+
California Hosp Med Ctr Los Angeles	Los Angeles	67%	300+
Community Hospital of Long Beach	Long Beach	67%	300+
Garfield Medical Center	Monterey Park	67%	300+
Kern Medical Center	Bakersfield	67%	300+
PIH Hospital - Downey	Downey	67%	300+
Alameda Hospital	Alameda	66%	300+
Alta Bates Summit Medical Center	Berkeley	66%	300+
Doctors Medical Center - San Pablo	San Pablo	66%	300+
Memorial Hospital of Gardena	Gardena	66%	300+
Parkview Comm Hosp Med Ctr	Riverside	66%	300+
Saint Francis Memorial Hospital	San Francisco	66%	300+
Saint Joseph Hospital	Eureka	66%	300+
West Anaheim Medical Center	Anaheim	66%	300+
Alameda County Medical Center	Oakland	65%	300+
Garden Grove Hospital & Medical Center[11]	Garden Grove	65%	300+
Hollywood Presbyterian Medical Center	Los Angeles	65%	300+
Regional Medical Center of San Jose	San Jose	65%	300+
Rideout Memorial Hospital	Marysville	65%	300+
San Gabriel Valley Medical Center	San Gabriel	64%	300+
Sherman Oaks Hospital[11]	Sherman Oaks	64%	(a)
West Hills Hospital & Medical Center	West Hills	64%	300+
Alhambra Hospital Medical Center	Alhambra	63%	300+
Chinese Hospital	San Francisco	63%	300+
Hemet Valley Medical Center	Hemet	63%	300+
Huntington Beach Hospital	Huntington Bch	63%	(a)
Mission Community Hospital	Panorama City	62%	300+
San Francisco General Hospital	San Francisco	62%	(a)
Southern California Hospital at Hollywood	Hollywood	62%	300+
Greater El Monte Community Hospital	South El Monte	61%	300+
Los Angeles Community Hospital	Los Angeles	61%	300+
Silver Lake Medical Center	Los Angeles	61%	(a)

Pain 'Always' Well Controlled

Hospital Name	City	Rate	Cases
Patients' Hospital of Redding	Redding	82%	(a)
Menlo Park Surgical Hospital	Menlo Park	81%	(a)
Stanislaus Surgical Hospital	Modesto	79%	300+
Fresno Heart & Surgical Hospital	Fresno	78%	300+
Healdsburg District Hospital	Healdsburg	78%	(a)
Hoag Orthopedic Institute	Irvine	78%	300+
Northern Inyo Hospital	Bishop	78%	(a)
Fresno Surgical Hospital	Fresno	77%	300+
Sharp Coronado Hosp & Healthcare Ctr	Coronado	77%	300+
Sutter Surgical Hospital - North Valley	Yuba City	77%	(a)
Banner Lassen Medical Center[11]	Susanville	76%	(a)
Kaiser Foundation Hospital - Fresno	Fresno	76%	300+
Mills - Peninsula Medical Center	Burlingame	76%	300+
Novato Community Hospital	Novato	76%	300+
Placentia Linda Hospital	Placentia	76%	300+
Saint Helena Hospital	Saint Helena	76%	300+
Scripps Memorial Hospital La Jolla	La Jolla	76%	300+
Sharp Memorial Hospital	San Diego	76%	300+
Sutter Davis Hospital	Davis	76%	300+
City of Hope Helford Clinical Res Hosp	Duarte	75%	300+
Huntington Memorial Hospital	Pasadena	75%	300+
Ojai Valley Community Hospital	Ojai	75%	(a)
Scripps Green Hospital	La Jolla	75%	300+
Sutter Medical Center of Santa Rosa	Santa Rosa	75%	300+
Comm Hosp of the Monterey Peninsula	Monterey	74%	300+
French Hospital Medical Center	San Luis Obispo	74%	300+
Goleta Valley Cottage Hospital	Santa Barbara	74%	300+
Kaiser Foundation Hospital - Santa Rosa	Santa Rosa	74%	300+
Kaiser Fdn Hosp-Woodland Hills	Woodland Hills	74%	300+
Marshall Medical Center	Placerville	74%	300+
Memorial Hospital Los Banos	Los Banos	74%	(a)
Mercy Medical Center - Mount Shasta	Mount Shasta	74%	(a)
Presbyterian Intercommunity Hospital	Whittier	74%	300+
Prov Little Co of Mary Med Ctr San Pedro	San Pedro	74%	300+
Santa Barbara Cottage Hospital	Santa Barbara	74%	300+
Sharp Chula Vista Medical Center	Chula Vista	74%	300+
Sutter Coast Hospital	Crescent City	74%	300+
Sutter Maternity & Surgery Ctr	Santa Cruz	74%	300+
White Memorial Medical Center	Los Angeles	74%	300+
Woodland Memorial Hospital	Woodland	74%	(a)
Frank R Howard Memorial Hospital	Willits	73%	300+
Kaiser Foundation Hospital - Baldwin Park	Baldwin Park	73%	300+
Kaiser Foundation Hospital - Manteca	Manteca	73%	300+
Kaiser Fdn Hosp-Orange Co-Anaheim	Anaheim	73%	300+
Kaiser Foundation Hospital - Roseville	Roseville	73%	300+
Kaiser Foundation Hospital - Sacramento	Sacramento	73%	300+
Kaiser Fdn Hosp-San Francisco	San Francisco	73%	300+
Kaiser Foundation Hospital - Santa Clara	Santa Clara	73%	300+
Kaiser Fdn Hosp-S San Francisco	S San Francisco	73%	300+
Kaiser Foundation Hospital - West La	Los Angeles	73%	300+
Palmdale Regional Medical Center	Palmdale	73%	300+
Palo Verde Hospital	Blythe	73%	(a)
Providence Holy Cross Medical Center	Mission Hills	73%	300+
Sierra Vista Regional Medical Center	San Luis Obispo	73%	300+
Sutter Amador Hospital	Jackson	73%	300+
Sutter Auburn Faith Hospital	Auburn	73%	300+
Sutter Delta Medical Center	Antioch	73%	(a)
Sutter Tracy Community Hospital	Tracy	73%	300+
Valleycare Medical Center	Pleasanton	73%	300+
Western Medical Center Santa Ana	Santa Ana	73%	300+
Chapman Medical Center	Orange	72%	(a)
Comm Mem Hosp San Buenaventura	Ventura	72%	300+
Enloe Medical Center	Chico	72%	300+
Hoag Memorial Hospital Presbyterian	Newport Beach	72%	300+
John Muir Med Ctr-Walnut Creek Campus	Walnut Creek	72%	300+
Kaiser Foundation Hospital	San Rafael	72%	300+
Kaiser Foundation Hospital - Los Angeles	Los Angeles	72%	300+
Kaiser Foundation Hospital - Redwood City	Redwood City	72%	300+
Kaiser Foundation Hospital - San Diego	San Diego	72%	300+
Kaiser Foundation Hospital - South Bay	Harbor City	72%	300+
Kaiser Foundation Hospital - Vacaville	Vacaville	72%	300+
LAC/Rancho Los Amigos Ntl Rehab Ctr	Downey	72%	300+
Memorial Medical Center	Modesto	72%	300+
Mendocino Coast District Hospital	Fort Bragg	72%	(a)
Prov Little Co of Mary Med Ctr Torrance	Torrance	72%	300+
Providence Saint Joseph Medical Center	Burbank	72%	300+
Sierra Nevada Memorial Hospital	Grass Valley	72%	300+
Sonoma Valley Hospital	Sonoma	72%	(a)
Tahoe Forest Hospital	Truckee	72%	(a)
Watsonville Community Hospital	Watsonville	72%	300+
Western Medical Center Hospital Anaheim	Anaheim	72%	300+
Barton Memorial Hospital	S Lake Tahoe	71%	300+
Clovis Community Medical Center	Clovis	71%	300+
Eisenhower Medical Center	Rancho Mirage	71%	300+
El Camino Hospital	Mountain View	71%	300+
George L Mee Memorial Hospital	King City	71%	(a)
Glendale Adventist Medical Center	Glendale	71%	300+
Kaiser Foundation Hospital - Fontana	Fontana	71%	300+
Kaiser Fdn Hosp-Moreno Valley	Moreno Valley	71%	300+
Kaiser Foundation Hospital - Riverside	Riverside	71%	300+
Kaiser Foundation Hospital - San Jose	San Jose	71%	300+
Kaiser Fdn Hosp S Sacramento	Sacramento	71%	300+
Los Alamitos Medical Center	Los Alamitos	71%	300+
Mission Hospital Regional Medical Center	Mission Viejo	71%	300+
Northbay Medical Center	Fairfield	71%	300+
Pacifica Hospital of the Valley	Sun Valley	71%	(a)
Petaluma Valley Hospital	Petaluma	71%	300+
Pomerado Hospital	Poway	71%	300+
Redlands Community Hospital	Redlands	71%	300+
Scripps Memorial Hospital - Encinitas	Encinitas	71%	300+
Twin Cities Community Hospital	Templeton	71%	300+
Ukiah Valley Medical Center	Ukiah	71%	300+
Barstow Community Hospital	Barstow	70%	300+
Colusa Regional Medical Center	Colusa	70%	(a)
Dameron Hospital	Stockton	70%	300+
Doctors Hospital of Manteca	Manteca	70%	300+
Doctors Medical Center	Modesto	70%	300+
Foothill Presbyterian Hospital	Glendora	70%	300+
Grossmont Hospital	La Mesa	70%	300+
Hazel Hawkins Memorial Hospital	Hollister	70%	300+
John Muir Medical Center - Concord Campus	Concord	70%	300+
Kaiser Foundation Hospital - Antioch	Antioch	70%	300+
Kaiser Foundation Hospital - Downey	Downey	70%	300+
Kaiser Fdn Hosp-Fremont/Hayward	Hayward	70%	300+
Kaiser Fdn Hosp-Panorama City	Panorama City	70%	300+
Keck Hospital of USC	Los Angeles	70%	300+
Loma Linda Univ Med Ctr-Murrieta	Murrieta	70%	300+
Mad River Community Hospital	Arcata	70%	300+
Mammoth Hospital	Mammoth Lakes	70%	(a)
Mark Twain Medical Center	San Andreas	70%	(a)
Pacific Hospital of Long Beach	Long Beach	70%	300+
Palm Drive Hospital	Sebastopol	70%	(a)
Saddleback Memorial Medical Center	Laguna Hills	70%	300+
Saint Johns Pleasant Valley Hospital	Camarillo	70%	300+
Saint Joseph Hospital	Orange	70%	300+
Saint Louise Regional Hospital	Gilroy	70%	300+
Salinas Valley Memorial Hospital	Salinas	70%	300+
San Antonio Community Hospital	Upland	70%	300+
Sierra View District Hospital	Porterville	70%	300+
Stanford Hospital	Stanford	70%	300+
Sutter General Hospital	Sacramento	70%	300+
Sutter Lakeside Hospital	Lakeport	70%	300+
Sutter Roseville Medical Center	Roseville	70%	300+
Torrance Memorial Medical Center	Torrance	70%	300+
Univ of CA San Diego Med Ctr	San Diego	70%	300+
USC Verdugo Hills Hospital	Glendale	70%	300+
Antelope Valley Hospital	Lancaster	69%	300+
Arrowhead Regional Medical Center	Colton	69%	300+
CA Pacific Med Ctr-St Luke's Campus	San Francisco	69%	300+
Cedars - Sinai Medical Center	Los Angeles	69%	300+
Chino Valley Medical Center[11]	Chino	69%	300+
Coastal Communities Hospital	Santa Ana	69%	300+
Community Regional Medical Center	Fresno	69%	300+
Corona Regional Medical Center	Corona	69%	300+
Desert Regional Medical Center	Palm Springs	69%	300+
Fallbrook Hospital	Fallbrook	69%	300+
Henry Mayo Newhall Memorial Hospital	Valencia	69%	300+
Kaiser Foundation Hospital & Rehab Center	Vallejo	69%	300+
Kaiser Foundation Hospital - Walnut Creek	Walnut Creek	69%	300+
Mercy General Hospital	Sacramento	69%	300+
Mercy San Juan Medical Center	Carmichael	69%	300+
Olympia Medical Center	Los Angeles	69%	300+
Queen of the Valley Medical Center	Napa	69%	300+
Redwood Memorial Hospital	Fortuna	69%	300+
Saint Agnes Medical Center	Fresno	69%	300+
Saint Bernardine Medical Center	San Bernardino	69%	300+
Saint Elizabeth Community Hospital	Red Bluff	69%	300+
San Joaquin Community Hospital	Bakersfield	69%	300+
San Leandro Hospital	San Leandro	69%	(a)
San Ramon Regional Medical Center	San Ramon	69%	300+
Scripps Mercy Hospital	San Diego	69%	300+
Shasta Regional Medical Center[11]	Redding	69%	300+
Sutter Solano Medical Center	Vallejo	69%	300+
Univ of CA Davis Med Ctr	Sacramento	69%	300+
Univ of California Irvine Med Ctr	Orange	69%	300+
Valley Presbyterian Hospital	Van Nuys	69%	300+
Bakersfield Heart Hospital	Bakersfield	68%	300+
CA Pacific Med Ctr-Pacific Campus Hosp	San Francisco	68%	300+
Citrus Valley Medical Center - IC Campus	Covina	68%	300+
Feather River Hospital	Paradise	68%	300+
Glendale Mem Hosp & Health Ctr	Glendale	68%	300+
Kaweah Delta Medical Center	Visalia	68%	300+
LAC/Olive View - UCLA Medical Center	Sylmar	68%	300+
Long Beach Memorial Medical Center	Long Beach	68%	300+
Orange Coast Memorial Medical Center	Fountain Valley	68%	300+
Oroville Hospital	Oroville	68%	300+
Palomar Health Downtown Campus	Escondido	68%	300+
Pioneers Memorial Healthcare District	Brawley	68%	300+
San Joaquin General Hospital	French Camp	68%	300+
Santa Rosa Memorial Hospital	Santa Rosa	68%	300+
Sonora Regional Medical Center	Sonora	68%	300+
Tri - City Regional Medical Center	Hawaiian Grdns	68%	300+
Washington Hospital	Fremont	68%	300+
Adventist Medical Center - Reedley	Reedley	67%	(a)
Bakersfield Memorial Hospital	Bakersfield	67%	300+
Community Hospital of Huntington Park	Huntington Park	67%	300+
El Centro Regional Medical Center	El Centro	67%	(a)
Good Samaritan Hospital	Bakersfield	67%	(a)
Good Samaritan Hospital	San Jose	67%	300+
Hi - Desert Medical Center	Joshua Tree	67%	300+
John F Kennedy Memorial Hospital	Indio	67%	300+
Lodi Memorial Hospital	Lodi	67%	300+
Marian Regional Medical Center	Santa Maria	67%	300+
Mercy Medical Center	Merced	67%	300+
Methodist Hospital of Southern California	Arcadia	67%	300+
Natividad Medical Center	Salinas	67%	300+
Saint Helena Hospital - Clearlake	Clearlake	67%	(a)
Saint Joseph's Medical Center of Stockton	Stockton	67%	300+
Saint Mary's Medical Center	San Francisco	67%	300+
Whittier Hospital Medical Center	Whittier	67%	300+
Desert Valley Hospital	Victorville	66%	300+
Dominican Hospital	Santa Cruz	66%	300+
Eden Medical Center	Castro Valley	66%	300+
Kaiser Fdn Hosp-Oakland/Richmond	Oakland	66%	300+
LAC+USC Medical Center[11]	Los Angeles	66%	300+
LAC/Harbor - UCLA Medical Center	Torrance	66%	300+
Lompoc Valley Medical Center	Lompoc	66%	300+
Los Robles Hospital & Medical Center	Thousand Oaks	66%	300+
Marina Del Rey Hospital	Marina Del Rey	66%	300+
O'Connor Hospital	San Jose	66%	300+
Riverside Community Hospital	Riverside	66%	300+
Ronald Reagan UCLA Medical Center	Los Angeles	66%	300+
Saint Johns Regional Medical Center	Oxnard	66%	300+
Saint Jude Medical Center	Fullerton	66%	300+
Saint Mary Medical Center	Apple Valley	66%	300+

NOTE: Hospital profiles are in alphabetical order by state, then city, then hospital within the city; Rankings exclude hospitals with less than 25 cases except for patient surveys which excludes hospitals with less than 100 cases; (a) 100-299 cases; (1) The number of cases/patients is too few to report; (2) Data submitted were based on a sample of cases/patients; (3) Results are based on a shorter time period than required; (4) Data suppressed by CMS for one or more quarters; (5) Results are not available for this reporting period; (6) Fewer than 100 patients completed the HCAHPS survey; (7) No cases met the criteria for this measure; (8) The lower limit of the confidence interval cannot be calculated if the number of observed infections equals zero; (9) No data are available from the state/territory for this reporting period; (10) The scores shown reflect fewer than 50 completed surveys; (11) There were discrepancies in the data collection process; (12) This measure does not apply to this hospital for this reporting period; (13) Results cannot be calculated for this reporting period; (14) The results for this state are combined with nearby states to protect confidentiality; Please refer to the User's Guide for a full explanation of data.

Hospital Name	City	Rate	Cases
Saint Rose Hospital	Hayward	66%	300+
Saint Vincent Medical Center	Los Angeles	66%	300+
San Dimas Community Hospital[11]	San Dimas	66%	300+
San Gorgonio Memorial Hospital	Banning	66%	300+
Santa Monica-UCLA Med Ctr & Ortho Hosp	Santa Monica	66%	300+
Simi Valley Hosp & Health Care Svcs	Simi Valley	66%	300+
Southwest Healthcare System	Murrieta	66%	300+
UCSF Medical Center	San Francisco	66%	300+
Ahmc Anaheim Regional Medical Center	Anaheim	65%	300+
Alta Bates Summit Medical Center	Berkeley	65%	300+
CA Pacific Med Ctr-Davies Campus	San Francisco	65%	300+
Delano Regional Medical Center	Delano	65%	300+
East Los Angeles Doctors Hospital	Los Angeles	65%	300+
Fairchild Medical Center	Yreka	65%	300+
Good Samaritan Hospital	Los Angeles	65%	300+
Lakewood Regional Medical Center	Lakewood	65%	300+
Loma Linda University Medical Center	Loma Linda	65%	300+
Marin General Hospital	Greenbrae	65%	300+
Memorial Hospital of Gardena	Gardena	65%	300+
Mercy Hospital	Bakersfield	65%	300+
Mercy Hospital of Folsom	Folsom	65%	300+
Mercy Medical Center - Redding	Redding	65%	300+
Methodist Hospital of Sacramento	Sacramento	65%	300+
Northridge Hospital Medical Center	Northridge	65%	300+
Providence Saint John's Health Center	Santa Monica	65%	300+
Saint Joseph Hospital	Eureka	65%	300+
Saint Mary Medical Center	Long Beach	65%	300+
Santa Clara Valley Medical Center	San Jose	65%	300+
Sequoia Hospital	Redwood City	65%	300+
Seton Medical Center	Daly City	65%	300+
Adventist Medical Center	Hanford	64%	300+
Alameda County Medical Center	Oakland	64%	300+
Alta Bates Summit Medical Center	Oakland	64%	300+
Community Hospital of San Bernardino	San Bernardino	64%	300+
Fountain Valley Reg Hosp & Med Ctr	Fountain Valley	64%	300+
Montclair Hospital Medical Center[11]	Montclair	64%	(a)
Parkview Comm Hosp Med Ctr	Riverside	64%	300+
Riverside County Regional Medical Center	Moreno Valley	64%	300+
Saint Francis Medical Center	Lynwood	64%	300+
San Mateo Medical Center	San Mateo	64%	300+
Tri - City Medical Center	Oceanside	64%	300+
Tulare Regional Medical Center	Tulare	64%	300+
Ventura County Medical Center	Ventura	64%	300+
West Hills Hospital & Medical Center	West Hills	64%	300+
Coast Plaza Hospital	Norwalk	63%	300+
Contra Costa Regional Medical Center	Martinez	63%	300+
Alameda Hospital	Alameda	62%	300+
Alvarado Hospital Medical Center	San Diego	62%	300+
Central Valley General Hospital	Hanford	62%	300+
Community Hospital of Long Beach	Long Beach	62%	300+
Emanuel Medical Center	Turlock	62%	300+
Garden Grove Hospital & Medical Center[11]	Garden Grove	62%	300+
Menifee Valley Medical Center	Sun City	62%	300+
Monterey Park Hospital	Monterey Park	62%	300+
Pacific Alliance Medical Center	Los Angeles	62%	300+
Paradise Valley Hospital[11]	National City	62%	(a)
Pomona Valley Hospital Medical Center	Pomona	62%	300+
Providence Tarzana Medical Center	Tarzana	62%	300+
Regional Medical Center of San Jose	San Jose	62%	300+
Saint Francis Memorial Hospital	San Francisco	62%	300+
Beverly Hospital	Montebello	61%	300+
California Hosp Med Ctr Los Angeles	Los Angeles	61%	300+
Centinela Hospital Medical Center[11]	Inglewood	61%	300+
Doctors Medical Center - San Pablo	San Pablo	61%	300+
PIH Hospital - Downey	Downey	61%	300+
Temple Community Hospital	Los Angeles	61%	(a)
Victor Valley Global Medical Center	Victorville	61%	300+
Hollywood Presbyterian Medical Center	Los Angeles	60%	300+
Kern Medical Center	Bakersfield	60%	300+
Madera Community Hospital	Madera	60%	300+
Alhambra Hospital Medical Center	Alhambra	59%	300+
Garfield Medical Center	Monterey Park	59%	300+
Oak Valley District Hospital	Oakdale	59%	(a)
Rideout Memorial Hospital	Marysville	59%	300+
San Gabriel Valley Medical Center	San Gabriel	59%	300+
West Anaheim Medical Center	Anaheim	59%	300+
La Palma Intercommunity Hospital	La Palma	58%	(a)
Mission Community Hospital	Panorama City	58%	300+
Greater El Monte Community Hospital	South El Monte	57%	300+
Hemet Valley Medical Center	Hemet	57%	300+
San Francisco General Hospital	San Francisco	57%	(a)
Sherman Oaks Hospital[11]	Sherman Oaks	57%	(a)
Southern California Hospital at Hollywood	Hollywood	57%	300+
Los Angeles Community Hospital	Los Angeles	56%	300+
Chinese Hospital	San Francisco	50%	300+
Huntington Beach Hospital	Huntington Bch	50%	(a)
Silver Lake Medical Center	Los Angeles	49%	(a)

Room and Bathroom 'Always' Clean

Hospital Name	City	Rate	Cases
Patients' Hospital of Redding	Redding	90%	(a)
Healdsburg District Hospital	Healdsburg	89%	(a)
Menlo Park Surgical Hospital	Menlo Park	89%	(a)
Stanislaus Surgical Hospital	Modesto	88%	300+
Sutter Surgical Hospital - North Valley	Yuba City	87%	(a)
Tahoe Forest Hospital	Truckee	86%	(a)
Memorial Hospital Los Banos	Los Banos	85%	(a)
Fresno Surgical Hospital	Fresno	84%	300+
Comm Hosp of the Monterey Peninsula	Monterey	83%	300+
Hoag Orthopedic Institute	Irvine	83%	300+
Sharp Coronado Hosp & Healthcare Ctr	Coronado	83%	300+
Northern Inyo Hospital	Bishop	82%	(a)
Sutter Amador Hospital	Jackson	82%	300+
Frank R Howard Memorial Hospital	Willits	81%	300+
Petaluma Valley Hospital	Petaluma	81%	300+
Barton Memorial Hospital	S Lake Tahoe	80%	300+
Colusa Regional Medical Center	Colusa	80%	(a)
Fresno Heart & Surgical Hospital	Fresno	80%	300+
John Muir Medical Center - Concord Campus	Concord	80%	300+
Ojai Valley Community Hospital	Ojai	80%	(a)
Sutter Maternity & Surgery Ctr	Santa Cruz	80%	300+
George L Mee Memorial Hospital	King City	79%	(a)
Goleta Valley Cottage Hospital	Santa Barbara	79%	300+
Kaiser Fdn Hosp-Panorama City	Panorama City	79%	300+
Mercy Medical Center - Mount Shasta	Mount Shasta	79%	(a)
Pacific Hospital of Long Beach	Long Beach	79%	300+
Prov Little Co of Mary Med Ctr San Pedro	San Pedro	79%	300+
Saint Helena Hospital	Saint Helena	79%	300+
Sutter Auburn Faith Hospital	Auburn	79%	300+
Sutter Davis Hospital	Davis	79%	300+
Kaiser Foundation Hospital - Manteca	Manteca	78%	300+
Kaiser Fdn Hosp-Orange Co-Anaheim	Anaheim	78%	300+
Marian Regional Medical Center	Santa Maria	78%	300+
Barstow Community Hospital	Barstow	77%	300+
Kaiser Foundation Hospital - Vacaville	Vacaville	77%	300+
Madera Community Hospital	Madera	77%	300+
Monterey Park Hospital	Monterey Park	77%	300+
Novato Community Hospital	Novato	77%	300+
Palmdale Regional Medical Center	Palmdale	77%	300+
Saint Mary Medical Center	Long Beach	77%	300+
Sharp Chula Vista Medical Center	Chula Vista	77%	300+
Sharp Memorial Hospital	San Diego	77%	300+
John Muir Med Ctr-Walnut Creek Campus	Walnut Creek	76%	300+
Kaiser Fdn Hosp-Woodland Hills	Woodland Hills	76%	300+
Lompoc Valley Medical Center	Lompoc	76%	300+
Palomar Health Downtown Campus	Escondido	76%	300+
Santa Barbara Cottage Hospital	Santa Barbara	76%	300+
Sonora Regional Medical Center	Sonora	76%	300+
Sutter Tracy Community Hospital	Tracy	76%	300+
USC Verdugo Hills Hospital	Glendale	76%	300+
Clovis Community Medical Center	Clovis	75%	300+
Enloe Medical Center	Chico	75%	300+
Fairchild Medical Center	Yreka	75%	300+
Feather River Hospital	Paradise	75%	300+
Kaiser Foundation Hospital - Antioch	Antioch	75%	300+
Kaiser Foundation Hospital - Downey	Downey	75%	300+
Kaiser Foundation Hospital - Riverside	Riverside	75%	300+
Kaiser Foundation Hospital - Santa Rosa	Santa Rosa	75%	300+
Marshall Medical Center	Placerville	75%	300+
Memorial Medical Center	Modesto	75%	300+
Methodist Hospital of Southern California	Arcadia	75%	300+
Palm Drive Hospital	Sebastopol	75%	(a)
Palo Verde Hospital	Blythe	75%	(a)
Placentia Linda Hospital	Placentia	75%	300+
Redlands Community Hospital	Redlands	75%	300+
Saint Louise Regional Hospital	Gilroy	75%	300+
Simi Valley Hosp & Health Care Svcs	Simi Valley	75%	300+
Univ of California Irvine Med Ctr	Orange	75%	300+
Whittier Hospital Medical Center	Whittier	75%	300+
East Los Angeles Doctors Hospital	Los Angeles	74%	300+
Eden Medical Center	Castro Valley	74%	300+
Hoag Memorial Hospital Presbyterian	Newport Beach	74%	300+
LAC/Rancho Los Amigos Ntl Rehab Ctr	Downey	74%	300+
Mad River Community Hospital	Arcata	74%	300+
Mills - Peninsula Medical Center	Burlingame	74%	300+
Montclair Hospital Medical Center[11]	Montclair	74%	(a)
Redwood Memorial Hospital	Fortuna	74%	300+
Scripps Green Hospital	La Jolla	74%	300+
Bakersfield Heart Hospital	Bakersfield	73%	300+
City of Hope Helford Clinical Res Hosp	Duarte	73%	300+
Coastal Communities Hospital	Santa Ana	73%	300+
Dameron Hospital	Stockton	73%	300+
Eisenhower Medical Center	Rancho Mirage	73%	300+
Hi - Desert Medical Center	Joshua Tree	73%	300+
Kaiser Foundation Hospital - Baldwin Park	Baldwin Park	73%	300+
Kaiser Foundation Hospital - Fontana	Fontana	73%	300+
Kaiser Foundation Hospital - Fresno	Fresno	73%	300+
Kaiser Foundation Hospital - Los Angeles	Los Angeles	73%	300+
Kaiser Foundation Hospital - Roseville	Roseville	73%	300+
Kaiser Foundation Hospital - Santa Clara	Santa Clara	73%	300+
Oak Valley District Hospital	Oakdale	73%	(a)
Pacifica Hospital of the Valley	Sun Valley	73%	(a)
Pomona Valley Hospital Medical Center	Pomona	73%	300+
Presbyterian Intercommunity Hospital	Whittier	73%	300+
Saddleback Memorial Medical Center	Laguna Hills	73%	300+
Seton Medical Center	Daly City	73%	300+
Woodland Memorial Hospital	Woodland	73%	(a)
Bakersfield Memorial Hospital	Bakersfield	72%	300+
Central Valley General Hospital	Hanford	72%	300+
Delano Regional Medical Center	Delano	72%	300+
Hazel Hawkins Memorial Hospital	Hollister	72%	300+
Kaiser Foundation Hospital - Redwood City	Redwood City	72%	300+
Kaiser Foundation Hospital - San Diego	San Diego	72%	300+
Kaiser Fdn Hosp-S San Francisco	S San Francisco	72%	300+
Kaiser Foundation Hospital - West La	Los Angeles	72%	300+
Lodi Memorial Hospital	Lodi	72%	300+
Mark Twain Medical Center	San Andreas	72%	(a)
Mercy Hospital of Folsom	Folsom	72%	300+
PIH Hospital - Downey	Downey	72%	300+
Providence Saint Joseph Medical Center	Burbank	72%	300+
Ronald Reagan UCLA Medical Center	Los Angeles	72%	300+
Saint Elizabeth Community Hospital	Red Bluff	72%	300+
Scripps Memorial Hospital - Encinitas	Encinitas	72%	300+
Stanford Hospital	Stanford	72%	300+
Sutter Solano Medical Center	Vallejo	72%	300+
Temple Community Hospital	Los Angeles	72%	(a)
Torrance Memorial Medical Center	Torrance	72%	300+
UCSF Medical Center	San Francisco	72%	300+
Univ of CA San Diego Med Ctr	San Diego	72%	300+
Washington Hospital	Fremont	72%	300+
Western Medical Center Hospital Anaheim	Anaheim	72%	300+
Adventist Medical Center	Hanford	71%	300+
Banner Lassen Medical Center[11]	Susanville	71%	(a)
Chapman Medical Center	Orange	71%	300+
Chino Valley Medical Center[11]	Chino	71%	300+
El Centro Regional Medical Center	El Centro	71%	(a)
Foothill Presbyterian Hospital	Glendora	71%	300+
Good Samaritan Hospital	Los Angeles	71%	300+
Kaiser Foundation Hospital - Sacramento	Sacramento	71%	300+
La Palma Intercommunity Hospital	La Palma	71%	(a)
Mission Community Hospital	Panorama City	71%	300+
Northbay Medical Center	Fairfield	71%	300+
Orange Coast Memorial Medical Center	Fountain Valley	71%	300+
Prov Little Co of Mary Med Ctr Torrance	Torrance	71%	300+
Saint Johns Pleasant Valley Hospital	Camarillo	71%	300+
Saint Jude Medical Center	Fullerton	71%	300+
Saint Mary's Medical Center	San Francisco	71%	300+
Scripps Memorial Hospital La Jolla	La Jolla	71%	300+
Silver Lake Medical Center	Los Angeles	71%	(a)
Sutter General Hospital	Sacramento	71%	300+
Sutter Lakeside Hospital	Lakeport	71%	300+
Twin Cities Community Hospital	Templeton	71%	300+
White Memorial Medical Center	Los Angeles	71%	300+
Beverly Hospital	Montebello	70%	300+
Cedars - Sinai Medical Center	Los Angeles	70%	300+
Grossmont Hospital	La Mesa	70%	300+
Huntington Memorial Hospital	Pasadena	70%	300+
Kaiser Fdn Hosp-Fremont/Hayward	Hayward	70%	300+
Kaiser Fdn Hosp-Moreno Valley	Moreno Valley	70%	300+
Kaiser Foundation Hospital - South Bay	Harbor City	70%	300+
Kaiser Fdn Hosp S Sacramento	Sacramento	70%	300+
Mercy Medical Center	Merced	70%	300+
Northridge Hospital Medical Center	Northridge	70%	300+
Pioneers Memorial Healthcare District	Brawley	70%	300+
Providence Holy Cross Medical Center	Mission Hills	70%	300+
Saint Johns Regional Medical Center	Oxnard	70%	300+
Saint Joseph Hospital	Orange	70%	300+
San Dimas Community Hospital[11]	San Dimas	70%	300+
San Gorgonio Memorial Hospital	Banning	70%	300+
San Ramon Regional Medical Center	San Ramon	70%	300+
Santa Monica-UCLA Med Ctr & Ortho Hosp	Santa Monica	70%	300+
Santa Rosa Memorial Hospital	Santa Rosa	70%	300+
Sierra Nevada Memorial Hospital	Grass Valley	70%	300+
Sierra View District Hospital	Porterville	70%	300+
Sutter Medical Center of Santa Rosa	Santa Rosa	70%	300+
Sutter Roseville Medical Center	Roseville	70%	300+
Ukiah Valley Medical Center	Ukiah	70%	300+
Western Medical Center Santa Ana	Santa Ana	70%	300+
Community Hospital of Huntington Park	Huntington Park	69%	300+
Desert Regional Medical Center	Palm Springs	69%	300+
El Camino Hospital	Mountain View	69%	300+
French Hospital Medical Center	San Luis Obispo	69%	300+
Garfield Medical Center	Monterey Park	69%	300+
Good Samaritan Hospital	Bakersfield	69%	(a)
Kaiser Foundation Hospital	San Rafael	69%	300+
Kaiser Foundation Hospital - San Jose	San Jose	69%	300+
Keck Hospital of USC	Los Angeles	69%	300+
Long Beach Memorial Medical Center	Long Beach	69%	300+
Menifee Valley Medical Center	Sun City	69%	300+
Mercy San Juan Medical Center	Carmichael	69%	300+
Mission Hospital Regional Medical Center	Mission Viejo	69%	300+
Olympia Medical Center	Los Angeles	69%	300+
Paradise Valley Hospital[11]	National City	69%	(a)

NOTE: Hospital profiles are in alphabetical order by state, then city, then hospital within the city; Rankings exclude hospitals with less than 25 cases except for patient surveys which excludes hospitals with less than 100 cases; (a) 100-299 cases; (1) The number of cases/patients is too few to report; (2) Data submitted were based on a sample of cases/patients; (3) Results are based on a shorter time period than required; (4) Data suppressed by CMS for one or more quarters; (5) Results are not available for this reporting period; (6) Fewer than 100 patients completed the HCAHPS survey; (7) No cases met the criteria for this measure; (8) The lower limit of the confidence interval cannot be calculated if the number of observed infections equals zero; (9) No data are available from the state/territory for this reporting period; (10) The scores shown reflect fewer than 50 completed surveys; (11) There were discrepancies in the data collection process; (12) This measure does not apply to this hospital for this reporting period; (13) Results cannot be calculated for this reporting period; (14) The results for this state are combined with nearby states to protect confidentiality; Please refer to the User's Guide for a full explanation of data.

Saint Vincent Medical Center	Los Angeles	69%	300+
San Joaquin General Hospital	French Camp	69%	300+
Sonoma Valley Hospital	Sonoma	69%	(a)
Valleycare Medical Center	Pleasanton	69%	300+
Ventura County Medical Center	Ventura	69%	300+
Ahmc Anaheim Regional Medical Center	Anaheim	68%	300+
Alhambra Hospital Medical Center	Alhambra	68%	300+
CA Pacific Med Ctr-Pacific Campus Hosp	San Francisco	68%	300+
Comm Mem Hosp San Buenaventura	Ventura	68%	300+
Community Regional Medical Center	Fresno	68%	300+
Fountain Valley Reg Hosp & Med Ctr	Fountain Valley	68%	300+
Kaiser Foundation Hospital & Rehab Center	Vallejo	68%	300+
Kaiser Fdn Hosp-San Francisco	San Francisco	68%	300+
Lakewood Regional Medical Center	Lakewood	68%	300+
Los Robles Hospital & Medical Center	Thousand Oaks	68%	300+
Mendocino Coast District Hospital	Fort Bragg	68%	(a)
Mercy General Hospital	Sacramento	68%	300+
Mercy Medical Center - Redding	Redding	68%	300+
Natividad Medical Center	Salinas	68%	300+
Queen of the Valley Medical Center	Napa	68%	300+
Saint Agnes Medical Center	Fresno	68%	300+
Saint Rose Hospital	Hayward	68%	300+
Sequoia Hospital	Redwood City	68%	300+
Sutter Delta Medical Center	Antioch	68%	(a)
CA Pacific Med Ctr-Davies Campus	San Francisco	67%	300+
CA Pacific Med Ctr-St Luke's Campus	San Francisco	67%	300+
Citrus Valley Medical Center - IC Campus	Covina	67%	300+
Community Hospital of San Bernardino	San Bernardino	67%	300+
Doctors Medical Center	Modesto	67%	300+
John F Kennedy Memorial Hospital	Indio	67%	300+
Kaiser Foundation Hospital - Walnut Creek	Walnut Creek	67%	300+
Mammoth Hospital	Mammoth Lakes	67%	(a)
Methodist Hospital of Sacramento	Sacramento	67%	300+
Providence Saint John's Health Center	Santa Monica	67%	300+
Saint Francis Medical Center	Lynwood	67%	300+
Salinas Valley Memorial Hospital	Salinas	67%	300+
Sherman Oaks Hospital[11]	Sherman Oaks	67%	(a)
Sutter Coast Hospital	Crescent City	67%	300+
Victor Valley Global Medical Center	Victorville	67%	300+
Watsonville Community Hospital	Watsonville	67%	300+
Arrowhead Regional Medical Center	Colton	66%	300+
Desert Valley Hospital	Victorville	66%	300+
Doctors Hospital of Manteca	Manteca	66%	300+
Emanuel Medical Center	Turlock	66%	300+
Glendale Adventist Medical Center	Glendale	66%	300+
Glendale Mem Hosp & Health Ctr	Glendale	66%	300+
Henry Mayo Newhall Memorial Hospital	Valencia	66%	300+
Kaweah Delta Medical Center	Visalia	66%	300+
Loma Linda Univ Med Ctr-Murrieta	Murrieta	66%	300+
O'Connor Hospital	San Jose	66%	300+
Saint Joseph Hospital	Eureka	66%	300+
San Antonio Community Hospital	Upland	66%	300+
Scripps Mercy Hospital	San Diego	66%	300+
Shasta Regional Medical Center[11]	Redding	66%	300+
Southwest Healthcare System	Murrieta	66%	300+
Tri - City Medical Center	Oceanside	66%	300+
Tri - City Regional Medical Center	Hawaiian Grdns	66%	300+
West Anaheim Medical Center	Anaheim	66%	300+
Adventist Medical Center - Reedley	Reedley	65%	(a)
Alvarado Hospital Medical Center	San Diego	65%	300+
Antelope Valley Hospital	Lancaster	65%	300+
Community Hospital of Long Beach	Long Beach	65%	300+
LAC+USC Medical Center[11]	Los Angeles	65%	300+
LAC/Olive View - UCLA Medical Center	Sylmar	65%	300+
Loma Linda University Medical Center	Loma Linda	65%	300+
Pacific Alliance Medical Center	Los Angeles	65%	300+
Saint Bernardine Medical Center	San Bernardino	65%	300+
San Mateo Medical Center	San Mateo	65%	300+
Alameda Hospital	Alameda	64%	300+
Centinela Hospital Medical Center[11]	Inglewood	64%	300+
Garden Grove Hospital & Medical Center[11]	Garden Grove	64%	300+
Huntington Beach Hospital	Huntington Bch	64%	(a)
Memorial Hospital of Gardena	Gardena	64%	300+
Oroville Hospital	Oroville	64%	300+
Parkview Comm Hosp Med Ctr	Riverside	64%	300+
Saint Francis Memorial Hospital	San Francisco	64%	300+
Saint Joseph's Medical Center of Stockton	Stockton	64%	300+
San Joaquin Community Hospital	Bakersfield	64%	300+
Valley Presbyterian Hospital	Van Nuys	64%	300+
Fallbrook Hospital	Fallbrook	63%	300+
Good Samaritan Hospital	San Jose	63%	300+
Mercy Hospital	Bakersfield	63%	300+
San Gabriel Valley Medical Center	San Gabriel	63%	300+
California Hosp Med Ctr Los Angeles	Los Angeles	62%	300+
Chinese Hospital	San Francisco	62%	300+
Corona Regional Medical Center	Corona	62%	300+
Dominican Hospital	Santa Cruz	62%	300+
Greater El Monte Community Hospital	South El Monte	62%	300+
Kaiser Fdn Hosp-Oakland/Richmond	Oakland	62%	300+
Los Alamitos Medical Center	Los Alamitos	62%	300+
Marina Del Rey Hospital	Marina Del Rey	62%	300+
Providence Tarzana Medical Center	Tarzana	62%	300+
Regional Medical Center of San Jose	San Jose	62%	300+
Sierra Vista Regional Medical Center	San Luis Obispo	62%	300+
Coast Plaza Hospital	Norwalk	61%	300+
Contra Costa Regional Medical Center	Martinez	61%	300+
Doctors Medical Center - San Pablo	San Pablo	61%	300+
Hollywood Presbyterian Medical Center	Los Angeles	61%	300+
Pomerado Hospital	Poway	61%	300+
Riverside Community Hospital	Riverside	61%	300+
Saint Helena Hospital - Clearlake	Clearlake	61%	(a)
Saint Mary Medical Center	Apple Valley	61%	300+
Southern California Hospital at Hollywood	Hollywood	61%	300+
Tulare Regional Medical Center	Tulare	61%	300+
Kern Medical Center	Bakersfield	60%	300+
Rideout Memorial Hospital	Marysville	60%	300+
LAC/Harbor - UCLA Medical Center	Torrance	59%	300+
Santa Clara Valley Medical Center	San Jose	59%	300+
Univ of CA Davis Med Ctr	Sacramento	59%	300+
San Leandro Hospital	San Leandro	58%	(a)
Hemet Valley Medical Center	Hemet	56%	300+
Marin General Hospital	Greenbrae	56%	300+
West Hills Hospital & Medical Center	West Hills	56%	300+
Alta Bates Summit Medical Center	Berkeley	55%	300+
San Francisco General Hospital	San Francisco	55%	(a)
Los Angeles Community Hospital	Los Angeles	54%	300+
Riverside County Regional Medical Center	Moreno Valley	54%	300+
Alta Bates Summit Medical Center	Oakland	53%	300+
Alameda County Medical Center	Oakland	52%	300+

Timely Help 'Always' Received

Hospital Name	City	Rate	Cases
Patients' Hospital of Redding	Redding	93%	(a)
Menlo Park Surgical Hospital	Menlo Park	88%	(a)
Stanislaus Surgical Hospital	Modesto	85%	300+
Sutter Surgical Hospital - North Valley	Yuba City	85%	(a)
Fresno Surgical Hospital	Fresno	84%	300+
Mammoth Hospital	Mammoth Lakes	81%	(a)
Hoag Orthopedic Institute	Irvine	80%	300+
Mercy Medical Center - Mount Shasta	Mount Shasta	78%	(a)
Sharp Coronado Hosp & Healthcare Ctr	Coronado	78%	300+
Goleta Valley Cottage Hospital	Santa Barbara	77%	300+
Colusa Regional Medical Center	Colusa	76%	(a)
Northern Inyo Hospital	Bishop	75%	(a)
Ojai Valley Community Hospital	Ojai	75%	(a)
Sutter Maternity & Surgery Ctr	Santa Cruz	75%	300+
Banner Lassen Medical Center[11]	Susanville	74%	(a)
Frank R Howard Memorial Hospital	Willits	74%	(a)
Fresno Heart & Surgical Hospital	Fresno	73%	300+
Novato Community Hospital	Novato	73%	300+
Sutter Davis Hospital	Davis	73%	300+
Tahoe Forest Hospital	Truckee	73%	(a)
Valleycare Medical Center	Pleasanton	72%	300+
Healdsburg District Hospital	Healdsburg	71%	(a)
Kaiser Fdn Hosp-Woodland Hills	Woodland Hills	71%	300+
Memorial Hospital Los Banos	Los Banos	71%	(a)
Sharp Memorial Hospital	San Diego	71%	300+
French Hospital Medical Center	San Luis Obispo	70%	300+
Kaiser Foundation Hospital - Los Angeles	Los Angeles	70%	300+
Mendocino Coast District Hospital	Fort Bragg	70%	(a)
Petaluma Valley Hospital	Petaluma	70%	300+
Pomerado Hospital	Poway	70%	300+
Saint Helena Hospital	Saint Helena	70%	300+
Sierra Vista Regional Medical Center	San Luis Obispo	70%	300+
Twin Cities Community Hospital	Templeton	70%	300+
Barton Memorial Hospital	S Lake Tahoe	69%	300+
Kaiser Foundation Hospital - Manteca	Manteca	69%	300+
Kaiser Fdn Hosp-Orange Co-Anaheim	Anaheim	69%	300+
Mad River Community Hospital	Arcata	69%	300+
Palm Drive Hospital	Sebastopol	69%	(a)
Temple Community Hospital	Los Angeles	69%	(a)
George L Mee Memorial Hospital	King City	68%	(a)
Kaiser Foundation Hospital	San Rafael	68%	300+
Kaiser Foundation Hospital - Sacramento	Sacramento	68%	300+
Marshall Medical Center	Placerville	68%	300+
Placentia Linda Hospital	Placentia	68%	300+
Sharp Chula Vista Medical Center	Chula Vista	68%	300+
Stanford Hospital	Stanford	68%	300+
Sutter Coast Hospital	Crescent City	68%	300+
Sutter Lakeside Hospital	Lakeport	68%	300+
Sutter Roseville Medical Center	Roseville	68%	300+
USC Verdugo Hills Hospital	Glendale	68%	300+
Enloe Medical Center	Chico	67%	300+
Huntington Memorial Hospital	Pasadena	67%	300+
Kaiser Fdn Hosp-Moreno Valley	Moreno Valley	67%	300+
Kaiser Fdn Hosp-San Francisco	San Francisco	67%	300+
Kaiser Foundation Hospital - Santa Clara	Santa Clara	67%	300+
Kaiser Fdn Hosp-S San Francisco	S San Francisco	67%	300+
Pacific Hospital of Long Beach	Long Beach	67%	300+
Saint Helena Hospital - Clearlake	Clearlake	67%	(a)
San Ramon Regional Medical Center	San Ramon	67%	300+
Scripps Green Hospital	La Jolla	67%	300+
Sonoma Valley Hospital	Sonoma	67%	(a)
Sonora Regional Medical Center	Sonora	67%	300+
Sutter Amador Hospital	Jackson	67%	300+
Comm Hosp of the Monterey Peninsula	Monterey	66%	300+
Desert Regional Medical Center	Palm Springs	66%	300+
John Muir Medical Center - Concord Campus	Concord	66%	300+
Kaiser Foundation Hospital - Fontana	Fontana	66%	300+
Kaiser Foundation Hospital - Redwood City	Redwood City	66%	300+
Kaiser Foundation Hospital - San Diego	San Diego	66%	300+
Kaiser Foundation Hospital - South Bay	Harbor City	66%	300+
Kaiser Foundation Hospital - Vacaville	Vacaville	66%	300+
Prov Little Co of Mary Med Ctr San Pedro	San Pedro	66%	300+
Hazel Hawkins Memorial Hospital	Hollister	65%	300+
Kaiser Foundation Hospital - Fresno	Fresno	65%	300+
Lompoc Valley Medical Center	Lompoc	65%	300+
Northbay Medical Center	Fairfield	65%	300+
Palo Verde Hospital	Blythe	65%	(a)
Providence Holy Cross Medical Center	Mission Hills	65%	300+
Redlands Community Hospital	Redlands	65%	300+
Redwood Memorial Hospital	Fortuna	65%	300+
Scripps Memorial Hospital La Jolla	La Jolla	65%	300+
Sutter Medical Center of Santa Rosa	Santa Rosa	65%	300+
Sutter Tracy Community Hospital	Tracy	65%	300+
Univ of California Irvine Med Ctr	Orange	65%	300+
Woodland Memorial Hospital	Woodland	65%	(a)
Bakersfield Heart Hospital	Bakersfield	64%	300+
CA Pacific Med Ctr-Pacific Campus Hosp	San Francisco	64%	300+
Chinese Hospital	San Francisco	64%	300+
Clovis Community Medical Center	Clovis	64%	300+
Comm Mem Hosp San Buenaventura	Ventura	64%	300+
Hi - Desert Medical Center	Joshua Tree	64%	300+
Kaiser Foundation Hospital - Antioch	Antioch	64%	300+
Kaiser Foundation Hospital - Baldwin Park	Baldwin Park	64%	300+
Kaiser Foundation Hospital - Downey	Downey	64%	300+
Kaiser Foundation Hospital - Riverside	Riverside	64%	300+
Kaiser Foundation Hospital - Santa Rosa	Santa Rosa	64%	300+
Kaiser Foundation Hospital - West La	Los Angeles	64%	300+
LAC/Rancho Los Amigos Ntl Rehab Ctr	Downey	64%	300+
Mark Twain Medical Center	San Andreas	64%	(a)
Palmdale Regional Medical Center	Palmdale	64%	300+
Providence Saint Joseph Medical Center	Burbank	64%	300+
Sierra View District Hospital	Porterville	64%	300+
Ukiah Valley Medical Center	Ukiah	64%	300+
Univ of CA San Diego Med Ctr	San Diego	64%	300+
Ahmc Anaheim Regional Medical Center	Anaheim	63%	300+
Dameron Hospital	Stockton	63%	300+
Eisenhower Medical Center	Rancho Mirage	63%	300+
Feather River Hospital	Paradise	63%	300+
Kaiser Foundation Hospital & Rehab Center	Vallejo	63%	300+
Kaiser Fdn Hosp-Fremont/Hayward	Hayward	63%	300+
Kaiser Fdn Hosp-Panorama City	Panorama City	63%	300+
Kaiser Foundation Hospital - Roseville	Roseville	63%	300+
Kaiser Fdn Hosp S Sacramento	Sacramento	63%	300+
Memorial Medical Center	Modesto	63%	300+
Mercy General Hospital	Sacramento	63%	300+
Palomar Health Downtown Campus	Escondido	63%	300+
Presbyterian Intercommunity Hospital	Whittier	63%	300+
Saint Elizabeth Community Hospital	Red Bluff	63%	300+
San Gorgonio Memorial Hospital	Banning	63%	300+
Santa Barbara Cottage Hospital	Santa Barbara	63%	300+
Scripps Memorial Hospital - Encinitas	Encinitas	63%	300+
Sierra Nevada Memorial Hospital	Grass Valley	63%	300+
Sutter Auburn Faith Hospital	Auburn	63%	300+
Tri - City Medical Center	Oceanside	63%	300+
UCSF Medical Center	San Francisco	63%	300+
White Memorial Medical Center	Los Angeles	63%	300+
Barstow Community Hospital	Barstow	62%	300+
El Camino Hospital	Mountain View	62%	300+
Glendale Adventist Medical Center	Glendale	62%	300+
Henry Mayo Newhall Memorial Hospital	Valencia	62%	300+
Lakewood Regional Medical Center	Lakewood	62%	300+
Saint Joseph Hospital	Orange	62%	300+
Seton Medical Center	Daly City	62%	300+
Simi Valley Hosp & Health Care Svcs	Simi Valley	62%	300+
Cedars - Sinai Medical Center	Los Angeles	61%	300+
City of Hope Helford Clinical Res Hosp	Duarte	61%	300+
Desert Valley Hospital	Victorville	61%	300+
Doctors Hospital of Manteca	Manteca	61%	300+
Eden Medical Center	Castro Valley	61%	300+
Fairchild Medical Center	Yreka	61%	300+
Foothill Presbyterian Hospital	Glendora	61%	300+
Good Samaritan Hospital	Bakersfield	61%	(a)
Grossmont Hospital	La Mesa	61%	300+
Hoag Memorial Hospital Presbyterian	Newport Beach	61%	300+
John Muir Med Ctr-Walnut Creek Campus	Walnut Creek	61%	300+
Kaweah Delta Medical Center	Visalia	61%	300+
Ronald Reagan UCLA Medical Center	Los Angeles	61%	300+
Saint Agnes Medical Center	Fresno	61%	300+
Saint Vincent Medical Center	Los Angeles	61%	300+
Santa Rosa Memorial Hospital	Santa Rosa	61%	300+
Shasta Regional Medical Center[11]	Redding	61%	300+

NOTE: Hospital profiles are in alphabetical order by state, then city, then hospital within the city; Rankings exclude hospitals with less than 25 cases except for patient surveys which excludes hospitals with less than 100 cases; (a) 100-299 cases; (1) The number of cases/patients is too few to report; (2) Data submitted were based on a sample of cases/patients; (3) Results are based on a shorter time period than required; (4) Data suppressed by CMS for one or more quarters; (5) Results are not available for this reporting period; (6) Fewer than 100 patients completed the HCAHPS survey; (7) No cases met the criteria for this measure; (8) The lower limit of the confidence interval cannot be calculated if the number of observed infections equals zero; (9) No data are available from the state/territory for this reporting period; (10) The scores shown reflect fewer than 50 completed surveys; (11) There were discrepancies in the data collection process; (12) This measure does not apply to this hospital for this reporting period; (13) Results cannot be calculated for this reporting period; (14) The results for this state are combined with nearby states to protect confidentiality; Please refer to the User's Guide for a full explanation of data.

Sutter Solano Medical Center	Vallejo	61%	300+
Univ of CA Davis Med Ctr	Sacramento	61%	300+
Washington Hospital	Fremont	61%	300+
Watsonville Community Hospital	Watsonville	61%	300+
Western Medical Center Santa Ana	Santa Ana	61%	300+
Coast Plaza Hospital	Norwalk	60%	300+
Coastal Communities Hospital	Santa Ana	60%	300+
Community Hospital of Huntington Park	Huntington Park	60%	300+
Doctors Medical Center	Modesto	60%	300+
Kaiser Foundation Hospital - San Jose	San Jose	60%	300+
Keck Hospital of USC	Los Angeles	60%	300+
Loma Linda University Medical Center	Loma Linda	60%	300+
Loma Linda Univ Med Ctr-Murrieta	Murrieta	60%	300+
Los Alamitos Medical Center	Los Alamitos	60%	300+
Marina Del Rey Hospital	Marina Del Rey	60%	300+
Mercy Hospital of Folsom	Folsom	60%	300+
Methodist Hospital of Sacramento	Sacramento	60%	300+
Mills - Peninsula Medical Center	Burlingame	60%	300+
Mission Hospital Regional Medical Center	Mission Viejo	60%	300+
Olympia Medical Center	Los Angeles	60%	300+
Orange Coast Memorial Medical Center	Fountain Valley	60%	300+
Paradise Valley Hospital[11]	National City	60%	(a)
Santa Monica-UCLA Med Ctr & Ortho Hosp	Santa Monica	60%	300+
Sutter Delta Medical Center	Antioch	60%	(a)
Torrance Memorial Medical Center	Torrance	60%	300+
Western Medical Center Hospital Anaheim	Anaheim	60%	300+
Adventist Medical Center - Reedley	Reedley	59%	(a)
Antelope Valley Hospital	Lancaster	59%	300+
CA Pacific Med Ctr-St Luke's Campus	San Francisco	59%	300+
Chino Valley Medical Center[11]	Chino	59%	300+
East Los Angeles Doctors Hospital	Los Angeles	59%	300+
Fallbrook Hospital	Fallbrook	59%	300+
Garfield Medical Center	Monterey Park	59%	300+
John F Kennedy Memorial Hospital	Indio	59%	300+
Kaiser Fdn Hosp-Oakland/Richmond	Oakland	59%	300+
Marian Regional Medical Center	Santa Maria	59%	300+
Menifee Valley Medical Center	Sun City	59%	300+
Mercy San Juan Medical Center	Carmichael	59%	300+
Montclair Hospital Medical Center[11]	Montclair	59%	(a)
Natividad Medical Center	Salinas	59%	300+
O'Connor Hospital	San Jose	59%	300+
Pacifica Hospital of the Valley	Sun Valley	59%	(a)
Pioneers Memorial Healthcare District	Brawley	59%	300+
Prov Little Co of Mary Med Ctr Torrance	Torrance	59%	300+
Saint Francis Medical Center	Lynwood	59%	300+
Saint Johns Pleasant Valley Hospital	Camarillo	59%	300+
Saint Jude Medical Center	Fullerton	59%	300+
Saint Mary's Medical Center	San Francisco	59%	300+
Sutter General Hospital	Sacramento	59%	300+
Tri - City Regional Medical Center	Hawaiian Grdns	59%	300+
Adventist Medical Center	Hanford	58%	300+
Arrowhead Regional Medical Center	Colton	58%	300+
Citrus Valley Medical Center - IC Campus	Covina	58%	300+
Glendale Mem Hosp & Health Ctr	Glendale	58%	300+
Kaiser Foundation Hospital - Walnut Creek	Walnut Creek	58%	300+
La Palma Intercommunity Hospital	La Palma	58%	(a)
Lodi Memorial Hospital	Lodi	58%	300+
Queen of the Valley Medical Center	Napa	58%	300+
Saddleback Memorial Medical Center	Laguna Hills	58%	300+
Saint Bernardine Medical Center	San Bernardino	58%	300+
Saint Louise Regional Hospital	Gilroy	58%	300+
Saint Mary Medical Center	Long Beach	58%	300+
San Antonio Community Hospital	Upland	58%	300+
San Dimas Community Hospital[11]	San Dimas	58%	300+
San Joaquin Community Hospital	Bakersfield	58%	300+
Scripps Mercy Hospital	San Diego	58%	300+
Whittier Hospital Medical Center	Whittier	58%	300+
Alhambra Hospital Medical Center	Alhambra	57%	300+
Alvarado Hospital Medical Center	San Diego	57%	300+
Community Regional Medical Center	Fresno	57%	300+
Delano Regional Medical Center	Delano	57%	300+
El Centro Regional Medical Center	El Centro	57%	(a)
Good Samaritan Hospital	Los Angeles	57%	300+
LAC+USC Medical Center[11]	Los Angeles	57%	300+
Long Beach Memorial Medical Center	Long Beach	57%	300+
Marin General Hospital	Greenbrae	57%	300+
Hollywood Presbyterian Medical Center	Los Angeles	56%	300+
LAC/Olive View - UCLA Medical Center	Sylmar	56%	300+
Madera Community Hospital	Madera	56%	300+
Mercy Medical Center - Redding	Redding	56%	300+
Methodist Hospital of Southern California	Arcadia	56%	300+
Saint Joseph's Medical Center of Stockton	Stockton	56%	300+
Salinas Valley Memorial Hospital	Salinas	56%	300+
Southwest Healthcare System	Murrieta	56%	300+
Bakersfield Memorial Hospital	Bakersfield	55%	300+
Chapman Medical Center	Orange	55%	300+
Dominican Hospital	Santa Cruz	55%	300+
Mercy Medical Center	Merced	55%	300+
Oroville Hospital	Oroville	55%	300+
Pacific Alliance Medical Center	Los Angeles	55%	300+
Parkview Comm Hosp Med Ctr	Riverside	55%	300+
Pomona Valley Hospital Medical Center	Pomona	55%	300+
San Leandro Hospital	San Leandro	55%	(a)
Central Valley General Hospital	Hanford	54%	300+
Garden Grove Hospital & Medical Center[11]	Garden Grove	54%	300+
LAC/Harbor - UCLA Medical Center	Torrance	54%	300+
Mission Community Hospital	Panorama City	54%	300+
Monterey Park Hospital	Monterey Park	54%	300+
Regional Medical Center of San Jose	San Jose	54%	300+
Ventura County Medical Center	Ventura	54%	300+
Contra Costa Regional Medical Center	Martinez	53%	300+
Los Robles Hospital & Medical Center	Thousand Oaks	53%	300+
Memorial Hospital of Gardena	Gardena	53%	300+
Mercy Hospital	Bakersfield	53%	300+
Oak Valley District Hospital	Oakdale	53%	(a)
PIH Hospital - Downey	Downey	53%	300+
Saint Francis Memorial Hospital	San Francisco	53%	300+
Saint Rose Hospital	Hayward	53%	300+
Valley Presbyterian Hospital	Van Nuys	53%	300+
Alameda County Medical Center	Oakland	52%	300+
Centinela Hospital Medical Center[11]	Inglewood	52%	300+
Community Hospital of Long Beach	Long Beach	52%	300+
Community Hospital of San Bernardino	San Bernardino	52%	300+
Emanuel Medical Center	Turlock	52%	300+
Good Samaritan Hospital	San Jose	52%	300+
Providence Tarzana Medical Center	Tarzana	52%	300+
Riverside County Regional Medical Center	Moreno Valley	52%	300+
Saint Johns Regional Medical Center	Oxnard	52%	300+
Saint Mary Medical Center	Apple Valley	52%	300+
San Gabriel Valley Medical Center	San Gabriel	52%	300+
San Mateo Medical Center	San Mateo	52%	300+
Victor Valley Global Medical Center	Victorville	52%	300+
Alameda Hospital	Alameda	51%	300+
Beverly Hospital	Montebello	51%	300+
California Hosp Med Ctr Los Angeles	Los Angeles	51%	300+
Corona Regional Medical Center	Corona	51%	300+
Fountain Valley Reg Hosp & Med Ctr	Fountain Valley	51%	300+
Greater El Monte Community Hospital	South El Monte	51%	300+
Northridge Hospital Medical Center	Northridge	51%	300+
Tulare Regional Medical Center	Tulare	51%	300+
Doctors Medical Center - San Pablo	San Pablo	50%	300+
Kern Medical Center	Bakersfield	50%	300+
Providence Saint John's Health Center	Santa Monica	50%	300+
Riverside Community Hospital	Riverside	50%	300+
West Anaheim Medical Center	Anaheim	50%	300+
Alta Bates Summit Medical Center	Oakland	49%	300+
Huntington Beach Hospital	Huntington Bch	49%	(a)
Saint Joseph Hospital	Eureka	49%	300+
Santa Clara Valley Medical Center	San Jose	49%	300+
CA Pacific Med Ctr-Davies Campus	San Francisco	48%	300+
Rideout Memorial Hospital	Marysville	48%	300+
San Francisco General Hospital	San Francisco	48%	(a)
Sequoia Hospital	Redwood City	48%	300+
Southern California Hospital at Hollywood	Hollywood	47%	300+
West Hills Hospital & Medical Center	West Hills	47%	300+
Alta Bates Summit Medical Center	Berkeley	46%	300+
Hemet Valley Medical Center	Hemet	46%	300+
Sherman Oaks Hospital[11]	Sherman Oaks	46%	(a)
Los Angeles Community Hospital	Los Angeles	45%	300+
San Joaquin General Hospital	French Camp	45%	300+
Silver Lake Medical Center	Los Angeles	36%	(a)

Would Definitely Recommend Hospital

Hospital Name	City	Rate	Cases
Patients' Hospital of Redding	Redding	96%	(a)
Sutter Surgical Hospital - North Valley	Yuba City	93%	(a)
Hoag Orthopedic Institute	Irvine	92%	300+
City of Hope Helford Clinical Res Hosp	Duarte	91%	300+
Sutter Maternity & Surgery Ctr	Santa Cruz	91%	300+
Fresno Surgical Hospital	Fresno	89%	300+
Novato Community Hospital	Novato	88%	300+
Stanislaus Surgical Hospital	Modesto	88%	300+
Fresno Heart & Surgical Hospital	Fresno	87%	300+
Huntington Memorial Hospital	Pasadena	87%	300+
Santa Barbara Cottage Hospital	Santa Barbara	87%	300+
Hoag Memorial Hospital Presbyterian	Newport Beach	86%	300+
Menlo Park Surgical Hospital	Menlo Park	86%	(a)
Sharp Memorial Hospital	San Diego	86%	300+
Sutter Davis Hospital	Davis	86%	300+
Tahoe Forest Hospital	Truckee	86%	(a)
John Muir Medical Center - Concord Campus	Concord	85%	300+
Mills - Peninsula Medical Center	Burlingame	85%	300+
Scripps Green Hospital	La Jolla	85%	300+
Sharp Coronado Hosp & Healthcare Ctr	Coronado	85%	300+
Stanford Hospital	Stanford	85%	300+
Comm Hosp of the Monterey Peninsula	Monterey	84%	300+
Goleta Valley Cottage Hospital	Santa Barbara	84%	300+
John Muir Med Ctr-Walnut Creek Campus	Walnut Creek	84%	300+
Kaiser Fdn Hosp-Orange Co-Anaheim	Anaheim	84%	300+
Eisenhower Medical Center	Rancho Mirage	83%	300+
Healdsburg District Hospital	Healdsburg	83%	(a)
Loma Linda Univ Med Ctr-Murrieta	Murrieta	83%	300+
Saint Helena Hospital	Saint Helena	83%	300+
El Camino Hospital	Mountain View	82%	300+
French Hospital Medical Center	San Luis Obispo	82%	300+
Kaiser Foundation Hospital - Vacaville	Vacaville	82%	300+
Keck Hospital of USC	Los Angeles	82%	300+
Presbyterian Intercommunity Hospital	Whittier	82%	300+
Saint Joseph Hospital	Orange	82%	300+
UCSF Medical Center	San Francisco	82%	300+
Kaiser Foundation Hospital - Antioch	Antioch	81%	300+
Kaiser Foundation Hospital - Roseville	Roseville	81%	300+
Kaiser Foundation Hospital - Santa Clara	Santa Clara	81%	300+
Kaiser Foundation Hospital - Santa Rosa	Santa Rosa	81%	300+
LAC/Rancho Los Amigos Ntl Rehab Ctr	Downey	81%	300+
Mission Hospital Regional Medical Center	Mission Viejo	81%	300+
Saint Jude Medical Center	Fullerton	81%	300+
Univ of California Irvine Med Ctr	Orange	81%	300+
Valleycare Medical Center	Pleasanton	81%	300+
Frank R Howard Memorial Hospital	Willits	80%	300+
Kaiser Foundation Hospital - Downey	Downey	80%	300+
Kaiser Foundation Hospital - Fresno	Fresno	80%	300+
Mercy Medical Center - Mount Shasta	Mount Shasta	80%	(a)
Northern Inyo Hospital	Bishop	80%	(a)
Prov Little Co of Mary Med Ctr Torrance	Torrance	80%	300+
Providence Saint Joseph Medical Center	Burbank	80%	300+
Scripps Memorial Hospital La Jolla	La Jolla	80%	300+
Sierra Vista Regional Medical Center	San Luis Obispo	80%	300+
Cedars - Sinai Medical Center	Los Angeles	79%	300+
Clovis Community Medical Center	Clovis	79%	300+
Kaiser Foundation Hospital - Los Angeles	Los Angeles	79%	300+
Kaiser Foundation Hospital - Manteca	Manteca	79%	300+
Kaiser Fdn Hosp-Panorama City	Panorama City	79%	300+
Kaiser Fdn Hosp-Woodland Hills	Woodland Hills	79%	300+
Mammoth Hospital	Mammoth Lakes	79%	(a)
Memorial Medical Center	Modesto	79%	300+
Palm Drive Hospital	Sebastopol	79%	(a)
Palomar Health Downtown Campus	Escondido	79%	300+
Providence Holy Cross Medical Center	Mission Hills	79%	300+
Ronald Reagan UCLA Medical Center	Los Angeles	79%	300+
Sutter Roseville Medical Center	Roseville	79%	300+
Sutter Tracy Community Hospital	Tracy	79%	300+
Torrance Memorial Medical Center	Torrance	79%	300+
White Memorial Medical Center	Los Angeles	79%	300+
Bakersfield Heart Hospital	Bakersfield	78%	300+
Enloe Medical Center	Chico	78%	300+
Feather River Hospital	Paradise	78%	300+
Kaiser Foundation Hospital - Fontana	Fontana	78%	300+
Long Beach Memorial Medical Center	Long Beach	78%	300+
Methodist Hospital of Southern California	Arcadia	78%	300+
Redlands Community Hospital	Redlands	78%	300+
San Ramon Regional Medical Center	San Ramon	78%	300+
Univ of CA San Diego Med Ctr	San Diego	78%	300+
Kaiser Foundation Hospital	San Rafael	77%	300+
Kaiser Foundation Hospital - Baldwin Park	Baldwin Park	77%	300+
Kaiser Fdn Hosp-San Francisco	San Francisco	77%	300+
Providence Saint John's Health Center	Santa Monica	77%	300+
Santa Monica-UCLA Med Ctr & Ortho Hosp	Santa Monica	77%	300+
Scripps Memorial Hospital - Encinitas	Encinitas	77%	300+
Sharp Chula Vista Medical Center	Chula Vista	77%	300+
Sutter Auburn Faith Hospital	Auburn	77%	300+
Desert Regional Medical Center	Palm Springs	76%	300+
Eden Medical Center	Castro Valley	76%	300+
Kaiser Fdn Hosp-S San Francisco	S San Francisco	76%	300+
Loma Linda University Medical Center	Loma Linda	76%	300+
Palmdale Regional Medical Center	Palmdale	76%	300+
Pioneers Memorial Healthcare District	Brawley	76%	300+
Placentia Linda Hospital	Placentia	76%	300+
Queen of the Valley Medical Center	Napa	76%	300+
San Antonio Community Hospital	Upland	76%	300+
Grossmont Hospital	La Mesa	75%	300+
Kaiser Foundation Hospital & Rehab Center	Vallejo	75%	300+
Kaiser Foundation Hospital - Riverside	Riverside	75%	300+
Kaiser Foundation Hospital - South Bay	Harbor City	75%	300+
Kaiser Fdn Hosp S Sacramento	Sacramento	75%	300+
Marian Regional Medical Center	Santa Maria	75%	300+
Prov Little Co of Mary Med Ctr San Pedro	San Pedro	75%	300+
Univ of CA Davis Med Ctr	Sacramento	75%	300+
Woodland Memorial Hospital	Woodland	75%	(a)
Banner Lassen Medical Center[11]	Susanville	74%	(a)
CA Pacific Med Ctr-Pacific Campus Hosp	San Francisco	74%	300+
Doctors Medical Center	Modesto	74%	300+
Foothill Presbyterian Hospital	Glendora	74%	300+
Kaiser Foundation Hospital - West La	Los Angeles	74%	300+
Marshall Medical Center	Placerville	74%	300+
Mercy Medical Center - Redding	Redding	74%	300+
Ojai Valley Community Hospital	Ojai	74%	(a)
Kaiser Foundation Hospital - Redwood City	Redwood City	73%	300+
Kaiser Foundation Hospital - San Diego	San Diego	73%	300+
LAC+USC Medical Center[11]	Los Angeles	73%	300+
LAC/Olive View - UCLA Medical Center	Sylmar	73%	300+
Redwood Memorial Hospital	Fortuna	73%	300+
Saint Agnes Medical Center	Fresno	73%	300+

NOTE: Hospital profiles are in alphabetical order by state, then city, then hospital within the city; Rankings exclude hospitals with less than 25 cases except for patient surveys which excludes hospitals with less than 100 cases; (a) 100-299 cases; (1) The number of cases/patients is too few to report; (2) Data submitted were based on a sample of cases/patients; (3) Results are based on a shorter time period than required; (4) Data suppressed by CMS for one or more quarters; (5) Results are not available for this reporting period; (6) Fewer than 100 patients completed the HCAHPS survey; (7) No cases met the criteria for this measure; (8) The lower limit of the confidence interval cannot be calculated if the number of observed infections equals zero; (9) No data are available from the state/territory for this reporting period; (10) The scores shown reflect fewer than 50 completed surveys; (11) There were discrepancies in the data collection process; (12) This measure does not apply to this hospital for this reporting period; (13) Results cannot be calculated for this reporting period; (14) The results for this state are combined with nearby states to protect confidentiality; Please refer to the User's Guide for a full explanation of data.

Saint Vincent Medical Center	Los Angeles	73%	300+
USC Verdugo Hills Hospital	Glendale	73%	300+
Washington Hospital	Fremont	73%	300+
Comm Mem Hosp San Buenaventura	Ventura	72%	300+
Glendale Adventist Medical Center	Glendale	72%	300+
Good Samaritan Hospital	Los Angeles	72%	300+
Kaiser Foundation Hospital - Sacramento	Sacramento	72%	300+
Mad River Community Hospital	Arcata	72%	300+
O'Connor Hospital	San Jose	72%	300+
Pomerado Hospital	Poway	72%	300+
Seton Medical Center	Daly City	72%	300+
Shasta Regional Medical Center[11]	Redding	72%	300+
Sutter Amador Hospital	Jackson	72%	300+
Sutter General Hospital	Sacramento	72%	300+
Bakersfield Memorial Hospital	Bakersfield	71%	300+
Barton Memorial Hospital	S Lake Tahoe	71%	300+
Doctors Hospital of Manteca	Manteca	71%	300+
Kaiser Foundation Hospital - San Jose	San Jose	71%	300+
Kaiser Foundation Hospital - Walnut Creek	Walnut Creek	71%	300+
Los Robles Hospital & Medical Center	Thousand Oaks	71%	300+
Mercy Hospital of Folsom	Folsom	71%	300+
Natividad Medical Center	Salinas	71%	300+
Orange Coast Memorial Medical Center	Fountain Valley	71%	300+
Petaluma Valley Hospital	Petaluma	71%	300+
Saddleback Memorial Medical Center	Laguna Hills	71%	300+
Saint Bernardine Medical Center	San Bernardino	71%	300+
Saint Mary Medical Center	Long Beach	71%	300+
Salinas Valley Memorial Hospital	Salinas	71%	300+
Sequoia Hospital	Redwood City	71%	300+
Sutter Medical Center of Santa Rosa	Santa Rosa	71%	300+
Twin Cities Community Hospital	Templeton	71%	300+
Alta Bates Summit Medical Center	Berkeley	70%	300+
Good Samaritan Hospital	San Jose	70%	300+
Kaiser Fdn Hosp-Moreno Valley	Moreno Valley	70%	300+
Marin General Hospital	Greenbrae	70%	300+
Memorial Hospital Los Banos	Los Banos	70%	(a)
Mercy General Hospital	Sacramento	70%	300+
Olympia Medical Center	Los Angeles	70%	300+
Saint Johns Pleasant Valley Hospital	Camarillo	70%	300+
Saint Johns Regional Medical Center	Oxnard	70%	300+
San Joaquin Community Hospital	Bakersfield	70%	300+
Santa Rosa Memorial Hospital	Santa Rosa	70%	300+
Ukiah Valley Medical Center	Ukiah	70%	300+
CA Pacific Med Ctr-Davies Campus	San Francisco	69%	300+
Kaiser Fdn Hosp-Fremont/Hayward	Hayward	69%	300+
Kaweah Delta Medical Center	Visalia	69%	300+
Lodi Memorial Hospital	Lodi	69%	300+
Pacific Hospital of Long Beach	Long Beach	69%	300+
Saint Elizabeth Community Hospital	Red Bluff	69%	300+
Saint Mary Medical Center	Apple Valley	69%	300+
Saint Mary's Medical Center	San Francisco	69%	300+
Scripps Mercy Hospital	San Diego	69%	300+
Simi Valley Hosp & Health Care Svcs	Simi Valley	69%	300+
Chino Valley Medical Center[11]	Chino	68%	300+
Saint Francis Memorial Hospital	San Francisco	68%	300+
Saint Joseph's Medical Center of Stockton	Stockton	68%	300+
Sutter Lakeside Hospital	Lakeport	68%	300+
Sutter Solano Medical Center	Vallejo	68%	300+
Arrowhead Regional Medical Center	Colton	67%	300+
CA Pacific Med Ctr-St Luke's Campus	San Francisco	67%	300+
Citrus Valley Medical Center - IC Campus	Covina	67%	300+
Community Regional Medical Center	Fresno	67%	300+
Dameron Hospital	Stockton	67%	300+
Mercy San Juan Medical Center	Carmichael	67%	300+
Montclair Hospital Medical Center[11]	Montclair	67%	(a)
Northbay Medical Center	Fairfield	67%	300+
Oak Valley District Hospital	Oakdale	67%	(a)
Sonoma Valley Hospital	Sonoma	67%	(a)
Sonora Regional Medical Center	Sonora	67%	300+
Alameda Hospital	Alameda	66%	300+
Barstow Community Hospital	Barstow	66%	300+
Chapman Medical Center	Orange	66%	300+
Saint Francis Medical Center	Lynwood	66%	300+
Saint Louise Regional Hospital	Gilroy	66%	300+
Saint Rose Hospital	Hayward	66%	300+
San Dimas Community Hospital[11]	San Dimas	66%	300+
Sierra Nevada Memorial Hospital	Grass Valley	66%	300+
Ventura County Medical Center	Ventura	66%	300+
George L Mee Memorial Hospital	King City	65%	(a)
Glendale Mem Hosp & Health Ctr	Glendale	65%	300+
Henry Mayo Newhall Memorial Hospital	Valencia	65%	300+
Kaiser Fdn Hosp-Oakland/Richmond	Oakland	65%	300+
Lakewood Regional Medical Center	Lakewood	65%	300+
Lompoc Valley Medical Center	Lompoc	65%	300+
Los Alamitos Medical Center	Los Alamitos	65%	300+
Mendocino Coast District Hospital	Fort Bragg	65%	(a)
Mercy Hospital	Bakersfield	65%	300+
Methodist Hospital of Sacramento	Sacramento	65%	300+
Northridge Hospital Medical Center	Northridge	65%	300+
San Leandro Hospital	San Leandro	65%	(a)
Sutter Coast Hospital	Crescent City	65%	300+
Tri - City Medical Center	Oceanside	65%	300+
Western Medical Center Santa Ana	Santa Ana	65%	300+
Coastal Communities Hospital	Santa Ana	64%	300+
Desert Valley Hospital	Victorville	64%	300+
Dominican Hospital	Santa Cruz	64%	300+
Hi - Desert Medical Center	Joshua Tree	64%	300+
LAC/Harbor - UCLA Medical Center	Torrance	64%	300+
Monterey Park Hospital	Monterey Park	64%	300+
San Mateo Medical Center	San Mateo	64%	300+
Southwest Healthcare System	Murrieta	64%	300+
Valley Presbyterian Hospital	Van Nuys	64%	300+
Western Medical Center Hospital Anaheim	Anaheim	64%	300+
Ahmc Anaheim Regional Medical Center	Anaheim	63%	300+
Alta Bates Summit Medical Center	Oakland	63%	300+
California Hosp Med Ctr Los Angeles	Los Angeles	63%	300+
Contra Costa Regional Medical Center	Martinez	63%	300+
Fallbrook Hospital	Fallbrook	63%	300+
La Palma Intercommunity Hospital	La Palma	63%	(a)
Mercy Medical Center	Merced	63%	300+
San Joaquin General Hospital	French Camp	63%	300+
Alvarado Hospital Medical Center	San Diego	62%	300+
Community Hospital of San Bernardino	San Bernardino	62%	300+
Garden Grove Hospital & Medical Center[11]	Garden Grove	62%	300+
Saint Joseph Hospital	Eureka	62%	300+
Watsonville Community Hospital	Watsonville	62%	300+
Alameda County Medical Center	Oakland	61%	300+
Colusa Regional Medical Center	Colusa	61%	(a)
Fountain Valley Reg Hosp & Med Ctr	Fountain Valley	61%	300+
Paradise Valley Hospital[11]	National City	61%	(a)
Providence Tarzana Medical Center	Tarzana	61%	300+
West Hills Hospital & Medical Center	West Hills	61%	300+
Adventist Medical Center	Hanford	60%	300+
Adventist Medical Center - Reedley	Reedley	60%	(a)
Alhambra Hospital Medical Center	Alhambra	60%	300+
Antelope Valley Hospital	Lancaster	60%	300+
Hollywood Presbyterian Medical Center	Los Angeles	60%	300+
Mark Twain Medical Center	San Andreas	60%	(a)
Menifee Valley Medical Center	Sun City	60%	300+
Pomona Valley Hospital Medical Center	Pomona	60%	300+
Riverside Community Hospital	Riverside	60%	300+
Riverside County Regional Medical Center	Moreno Valley	60%	300+
Sutter Delta Medical Center	Antioch	60%	(a)
Beverly Hospital	Montebello	59%	300+
Centinela Hospital Medical Center[11]	Inglewood	59%	300+
Community Hospital of Huntington Park	Huntington Park	59%	300+
El Centro Regional Medical Center	El Centro	59%	(a)
Hazel Hawkins Memorial Hospital	Hollister	59%	300+
John F Kennedy Memorial Hospital	Indio	59%	300+
Saint Helena Hospital - Clearlake	Clearlake	59%	(a)
Tri - City Regional Medical Center	Hawaiian Grdns	59%	300+
Emanuel Medical Center	Turlock	58%	300+
Fairchild Medical Center	Yreka	58%	300+
Marina Del Rey Hospital	Marina Del Rey	58%	300+
San Francisco General Hospital	San Francisco	58%	(a)
San Gorgonio Memorial Hospital	Banning	58%	300+
West Anaheim Medical Center	Anaheim	58%	300+
Whittier Hospital Medical Center	Whittier	58%	300+
Good Samaritan Hospital	Bakersfield	57%	(a)
Pacific Alliance Medical Center	Los Angeles	57%	300+
Pacifica Hospital of the Valley	Sun Valley	57%	(a)
Garfield Medical Center	Monterey Park	56%	300+
PIH Hospital - Downey	Downey	56%	300+
Regional Medical Center of San Jose	San Jose	56%	300+
Sierra View District Hospital	Porterville	56%	300+
Community Hospital of Long Beach	Long Beach	55%	300+
East Los Angeles Doctors Hospital	Los Angeles	55%	300+
San Gabriel Valley Medical Center	San Gabriel	55%	300+
Temple Community Hospital	Los Angeles	55%	(a)
Corona Regional Medical Center	Corona	54%	300+
Delano Regional Medical Center	Delano	54%	300+
Victor Valley Global Medical Center	Victorville	54%	300+
Central Valley General Hospital	Hanford	53%	300+
Huntington Beach Hospital	Huntington Bch	53%	(a)
Santa Clara Valley Medical Center	San Jose	53%	300+
Silver Lake Medical Center	Los Angeles	53%	(a)
Tulare Regional Medical Center	Tulare	53%	300+
Madera Community Hospital	Madera	52%	300+
Mission Community Hospital	Panorama City	52%	300+
Coast Plaza Hospital	Norwalk	51%	300+
Parkview Comm Hosp Med Ctr	Riverside	50%	300+
Doctors Medical Center - San Pablo	San Pablo	49%	300+
Greater El Monte Community Hospital	South El Monte	49%	300+
Kern Medical Center	Bakersfield	49%	300+
Southern California Hospital at Hollywood	Hollywood	49%	300+
Chinese Hospital	San Francisco	47%	300+
Memorial Hospital of Gardena	Gardena	47%	300+
Palo Verde Hospital	Blythe	46%	(a)
Rideout Memorial Hospital	Marysville	46%	300+
Oroville Hospital	Oroville	45%	300+
Sherman Oaks Hospital[11]	Sherman Oaks	45%	(a)
Los Angeles Community Hospital	Los Angeles	42%	300+
Hemet Valley Medical Center	Hemet	41%	300+

Use of Medical Imaging

Cardiac Imaging Stress Test before OP Surgery

Hospital Name	City	Rate	Cases
Alameda County Medical Center	Oakland	0.0%	62
Saint Elizabeth Community Hospital	Red Bluff	0.0%	59
Watsonville Community Hospital	Watsonville	0.0%	51
Alameda Hospital	Alameda	1.2%	85
Contra Costa Regional Medical Center	Martinez	1.4%	69
Doctors Medical Center - San Pablo	San Pablo	1.6%	61
San Mateo Medical Center	San Mateo	1.7%	60
Santa Clara Valley Medical Center	San Jose	1.7%	573
PIH Hospital - Downey	Downey	1.8%	110
Rideout Memorial Hospital	Marysville	1.8%	449
Bakersfield Heart Hospital	Bakersfield	1.9%	54
Kaweah Delta Medical Center	Visalia	1.9%	469
Emanuel Medical Center	Turlock	2.0%	245
Saint Joseph's Medical Center of Stockton	Stockton	2.0%	50
Eden Medical Center	Castro Valley	2.2%	46
Enloe Medical Center	Chico	2.2%	230
Sonoma Valley Hospital	Sonoma	2.2%	139
Salinas Valley Memorial Hospital	Salinas	2.3%	389
Marin General Hospital	Greenbrae	2.6%	1449
Sutter Delta Medical Center	Antioch	2.6%	115
Mercy Medical Center - Mount Shasta	Mount Shasta	2.7%	149
Community Regional Medical Center	Fresno	2.9%	241
Redlands Community Hospital	Redlands	2.9%	103
Ukiah Valley Medical Center	Ukiah	2.9%	346
Natividad Medical Center	Salinas	3.0%	99
Sierra Nevada Memorial Hospital	Grass Valley	3.0%	703
Alta Bates Summit Medical Center	Berkeley	3.1%	127
Comm Hosp of the Monterey Peninsula	Monterey	3.1%	352
Dameron Hospital	Stockton	3.1%	127
Pomerado Hospital	Poway	3.1%	130
Saint Helena Hospital	Saint Helena	3.1%	227
Saint Joseph Hospital	Eureka	3.1%	229
Santa Rosa Memorial Hospital	Santa Rosa	3.1%	229
Shasta Regional Medical Center	Redding	3.1%	65
Doctors Medical Center	Modesto	3.3%	1280
Mercy Hospital of Folsom	Folsom	3.3%	180
Arrowhead Regional Medical Center	Colton	3.4%	118
Sutter Davis Hospital	Davis	3.4%	146
Lodi Memorial Hospital	Lodi	3.5%	202
Los Robles Hospital & Medical Center	Thousand Oaks	3.6%	111
Saint Francis Memorial Hospital	San Francisco	3.6%	84
San Joaquin General Hospital	French Camp	3.6%	112
Tri - City Medical Center	Oceanside	3.6%	531
Mercy Medical Center - Redding	Redding	3.7%	134
Saint Francis Medical Center	Lynwood	3.7%	81
Sharp Chula Vista Medical Center	Chula Vista	3.7%	135
Orange Coast Memorial Medical Center	Fountain Valley	3.8%	80
Sutter Amador Hospital	Jackson	3.8%	604
John F Kennedy Memorial Hospital	Indio	3.9%	77
Saint Mary Medical Center	Apple Valley	3.9%	282
Sutter Solano Medical Center	Vallejo	3.9%	152
Desert Valley Hospital	Victorville	4.0%	50
Huntington Memorial Hospital	Pasadena	4.0%	200
Mercy San Juan Medical Center	Carmichael	4.0%	521
Regional Medical Center of San Jose	San Jose	4.0%	253
Northbay Medical Center	Fairfield	4.1%	344
Sonora Regional Medical Center	Sonora	4.1%	533
Sutter Roseville Medical Center	Roseville	4.1%	269
Valley Presbyterian Hospital	Van Nuys	4.1%	123
Marina Del Rey Hospital	Marina Del Rey	4.2%	72
Memorial Medical Center	Modesto	4.2%	308
Santa Barbara Cottage Hospital	Santa Barbara	4.2%	192
Scripps Memorial Hospital La Jolla	La Jolla	4.2%	118
CA Pacific Med Ctr-St Luke's Campus	San Francisco	4.3%	211
Presbyterian Intercommunity Hospital	Whittier	4.4%	386
Alta Bates Summit Medical Center	Oakland	4.5%	201
Mills - Peninsula Medical Center	Burlingame	4.5%	381
O'Connor Hospital	San Jose	4.5%	156
Sutter General Hospital	Sacramento	4.5%	177
Methodist Hospital of Sacramento	Sacramento	4.6%	240
Palomar Health Downtown Campus	Escondido	4.6%	240
UCSF Medical Center	San Francisco	4.6%	697
Seton Medical Center	Daly City	4.7%	316
Chinese Hospital	San Francisco	4.8%	293
Prov Little Co of Mary Med Ctr Torrance	Torrance	4.9%	672
Sharp Memorial Hospital	San Diego	4.9%	267
Feather River Hospital	Paradise	5.0%	424
Glendale Mem Hosp & Health Ctr	Glendale	5.0%	180
Comm Mem Hosp San Buenaventura	Ventura	5.1%	254
Loma Linda University Medical Center	Loma Linda	5.1%	765
Ronald Reagan UCLA Medical Center	Los Angeles	5.1%	350
Valleycare Medical Center	Pleasanton	5.1%	353
Barton Memorial Hospital	S Lake Tahoe	5.2%	210
Long Beach Memorial Medical Center	Long Beach	5.2%	268

NOTE: Hospital profiles are in alphabetical order by state, then city, then hospital within the city; Rankings exclude hospitals with less than 25 cases except for patient surveys which excludes hospitals with less than 100 cases; (a) 100-299 cases; (1) The number of cases/patients is too few to report; (2) Data submitted were based on a sample of cases/patients; (3) Results are based on a shorter time period than required; (4) Data suppressed by CMS for one or more quarters; (5) Results are not available for this reporting period; (6) Fewer than 100 patients completed the HCAHPS survey; (7) No cases met the criteria for this measure; (8) The lower limit of the confidence interval cannot be calculated if the number of observed infections equals zero; (9) No data are available from the state/territory for this reporting period; (10) The scores shown reflect fewer than 50 completed surveys; (11) There were discrepancies in the data collection process; (12) This measure does not apply to this hospital for this reporting period; (13) Results cannot be calculated for this reporting period; (14) The results for this state are combined with nearby states to protect confidentiality; Please refer to the User's Guide for a full explanation of data.

Mission Hospital Regional Medical Center	Mission Viejo	5.2%	252
Providence Tarzana Medical Center	Tarzana	5.2%	310
Queen of the Valley Medical Center	Napa	5.2%	77
CA Pacific Med Ctr-Pacific Campus Hosp	San Francisco	5.3%	609
El Centro Regional Medical Center	El Centro	5.3%	94
Mercy General Hospital	Sacramento	5.3%	342
Saint Jude Medical Center	Fullerton	5.3%	282
Sutter Lakeside Hospital	Lakeport	5.3%	133
Grossmont Hospital	La Mesa	5.4%	241
Mission Community Hospital	Panorama City	5.4%	56
Saint Agnes Medical Center	Fresno	5.4%	297
Good Samaritan Hospital	San Jose	5.5%	55
Antelope Valley Hospital	Lancaster	5.6%	126
Dominican Hospital	Santa Cruz	5.6%	162
Marshall Medical Center	Placerville	5.6%	604
Saddleback Memorial Medical Center	Laguna Hills	5.6%	231
Torrance Memorial Medical Center	Torrance	5.6%	682
California Hosp Med Ctr Los Angeles	Los Angeles	5.7%	87
Good Samaritan Hospital	Los Angeles	5.7%	227
Univ of CA San Diego Med Ctr	San Diego	5.7%	898
White Memorial Medical Center	Los Angeles	5.8%	86
Scripps Mercy Hospital	San Diego	5.9%	221
Sutter Auburn Faith Hospital	Auburn	5.9%	204
Lompoc Valley Medical Center	Lompoc	6.0%	133
Mark Twain Medical Center	San Andreas	6.0%	117
Providence Saint Joseph Medical Center	Burbank	6.0%	233
Eisenhower Medical Center	Rancho Mirage	6.1%	1150
Lakewood Regional Medical Center	Lakewood	6.1%	179
San Joaquin Community Hospital	Bakersfield	6.1%	277
Sherman Oaks Hospital	Sherman Oaks	6.1%	66
Oroville Hospital	Oroville	6.2%	291
Saint Mary Medical Center	Long Beach	6.2%	226
Citrus Valley Medical Center - IC Campus	Covina	6.3%	287
Univ of California Irvine Med Ctr	Orange	6.3%	381
Woodland Memorial Hospital	Woodland	6.3%	63
Saint Bernardine Medical Center	San Bernardino	6.4%	251
Saint Vincent Medical Center	Los Angeles	6.4%	265
Hemet Valley Medical Center	Hemet	6.5%	153
John Muir Med Ctr-Walnut Creek Campus	Walnut Creek	6.6%	305
Marian Regional Medical Center	Santa Maria	6.6%	334
Methodist Hospital of Southern California	Arcadia	6.6%	227
Providence Holy Cross Medical Center	Mission Hills	6.7%	180
Saint Johns Pleasant Valley Hospital	Camarillo	6.7%	89
Saint Joseph Hospital	Orange	6.7%	300
Ventura County Medical Center	Ventura	6.8%	190
West Hills Hospital & Medical Center	West Hills	6.8%	222
Centinela Hospital Medical Center	Inglewood	6.9%	130
Stanford Hospital	Stanford	6.9%	1107
Scripps Green Hospital	La Jolla	7.0%	388
Glendale Adventist Medical Center	Glendale	7.1%	310
Hollywood Presbyterian Medical Center	Los Angeles	7.1%	155
Pomona Valley Hospital Medical Center	Pomona	7.2%	111
Prov Little Co of Mary Med Ctr San Pedro	San Pedro	7.4%	122
Desert Regional Medical Center	Palm Springs	7.5%	292
Northridge Hospital Medical Center	Northridge	7.5%	293
Saint Mary's Medical Center	San Francisco	7.5%	147
Washington Hospital	Fremont	7.5%	362
Fountain Valley Reg Hosp & Med Ctr	Fountain Valley	7.7%	417
Cedars - Sinai Medical Center	Los Angeles	7.8%	1288
Univ of CA Davis Med Ctr	Sacramento	7.8%	680
Saint Rose Hospital	Hayward	7.9%	89
Providence Saint John's Health Center	Santa Monica	8.0%	176
John Muir Medical Center - Concord Campus	Concord	8.1%	209
Alvarado Hospital Medical Center	San Diego	8.2%	159
Hoag Memorial Hospital Presbyterian	Newport Beach	8.3%	494
Henry Mayo Newhall Memorial Hospital	Valencia	8.4%	226
Loma Linda Univ Med Ctr-Murrieta	Murrieta	8.4%	83
Doctors Hospital of Manteca	Manteca	8.8%	102
Saint Johns Regional Medical Center	Oxnard	9.0%	311
San Antonio Community Hospital	Upland	9.0%	144
Southwest Healthcare System	Murrieta	9.2%	65
Corona Regional Medical Center	Corona	9.3%	216
Scripps Memorial Hospital - Encinitas	Encinitas	9.3%	150
Riverside Community Hospital	Riverside	9.7%	165
Keck Hospital of USC	Los Angeles	10.2%	825
Los Alamitos Medical Center	Los Alamitos	10.8%	93
Bakersfield Memorial Hospital	Bakersfield	11.3%	80
San Ramon Regional Medical Center	San Ramon	11.3%	133

Combination Abdominal CT Scan

Hospital Name	City	Rate	Cases
Community Hospital of Long Beach	Long Beach	0.0%	124
Dameron Hospital	Stockton	0.0%	309
Memorial Hospital of Gardena	Gardena	0.0%	208
Montclair Hospital Medical Center	Montclair	0.0%	80
Sutter Roseville Medical Center	Roseville	0.0%	721
Henry Mayo Newhall Memorial Hospital	Valencia	0.2%	407
John Muir Medical Center - Concord Campus	Concord	0.2%	418
Methodist Hospital of Southern California	Arcadia	0.2%	498
Sutter General Hospital	Sacramento	0.3%	585
Salinas Valley Memorial Hospital	Salinas	0.4%	478
Enloe Medical Center	Chico	0.5%	613
Northbay Medical Center	Fairfield	0.5%	580
Saint Johns Regional Medical Center	Oxnard	0.5%	596
Beverly Hospital	Montebello	0.6%	336
LAC+USC Medical Center	Los Angeles	0.6%	155
Mercy Medical Center - Redding	Redding	0.6%	695
West Hills Hospital & Medical Center	West Hills	0.6%	347
Memorial Medical Center	Modesto	0.7%	668
Sharp Chula Vista Medical Center	Chula Vista	0.7%	586
Bakersfield Heart Hospital	Bakersfield	0.8%	121
Huntington Memorial Hospital	Pasadena	0.9%	437
Mercy San Juan Medical Center	Carmichael	0.9%	703
Shasta Regional Medical Center	Redding	0.9%	452
Oak Valley District Hospital	Oakdale	1.0%	198
San Dimas Community Hospital	San Dimas	1.0%	101
Antelope Valley Hospital	Lancaster	1.1%	476
Mercy General Hospital	Sacramento	1.1%	542
Palomar Health Downtown Campus	Escondido	1.1%	717
San Leandro Hospital	San Leandro	1.1%	93
Sharp Memorial Hospital	San Diego	1.1%	1075
Sherman Oaks Hospital	Sherman Oaks	1.1%	174
Tri - City Regional Medical Center	Hawaiian Grdns	1.2%	84
Emanuel Medical Center	Turlock	1.3%	375
Encino Hospital Medical Center	Encino	1.3%	75
Doctors Medical Center	Modesto	1.4%	366
East Los Angeles Doctors Hospital	Los Angeles	1.4%	71
John F Kennedy Memorial Hospital	Indio	1.5%	272
Mercy Hospital of Folsom	Folsom	1.5%	405
Methodist Hospital of Sacramento	Sacramento	1.5%	656
Northridge Hospital Medical Center	Northridge	1.5%	589
Palmdale Regional Medical Center	Palmdale	1.7%	461
Regional Medical Center of San Jose	San Jose	1.7%	752
Chapman Medical Center	Orange	1.8%	56
Lakewood Regional Medical Center	Lakewood	1.8%	445
O'Connor Hospital	San Jose	1.8%	870
Petaluma Valley Hospital	Petaluma	1.9%	319
San Joaquin General Hospital	French Camp	1.9%	260
Pomerado Hospital	Poway	2.0%	456
Seneca District Hospital	Chester	2.1%	48
Dominican Hospital	Santa Cruz	2.2%	542
Eastern Plumas Hospital - Portola Campus	Portola	2.3%	129
Huntington Beach Hospital	Huntington Bch	2.3%	87
Tulare Regional Medical Center	Tulare	2.3%	482
Bakersfield Memorial Hospital	Bakersfield	2.4%	335
LAC/Olive View - UCLA Medical Center	Sylmar	2.4%	84
Community Hospital of Huntington Park	Huntington Park	2.5%	119
Saint Joseph's Medical Center of Stockton	Stockton	2.6%	873
Santa Rosa Memorial Hospital	Santa Rosa	2.6%	651
Palm Drive Hospital	Sebastopol	2.7%	187
Centinela Hospital Medical Center	Inglewood	2.8%	506
Comm Hosp of the Monterey Peninsula	Monterey	2.8%	2025
Rideout Memorial Hospital	Marysville	2.8%	578
Cedars - Sinai Medical Center	Los Angeles	2.9%	3768
Sutter Medical Center of Santa Rosa	Santa Rosa	2.9%	209
CA Pacific Med Ctr-St Luke's Campus	San Francisco	3.0%	301
Prov Little Co of Mary Med Ctr Torrance	Torrance	3.0%	1108
Sutter Delta Medical Center	Antioch	3.0%	338
Hi - Desert Medical Center	Joshua Tree	3.1%	360
Mercy Hospital	Bakersfield	3.1%	521
Santa Barbara Cottage Hospital	Santa Barbara	3.1%	670
Western Medical Center Santa Ana	Santa Ana	3.1%	130
Memorial Hospital Los Banos	Los Banos	3.2%	309
Mercy Medical Center	Merced	3.2%	774
Scripps Memorial Hospital - Encinitas	Encinitas	3.2%	815
Sutter Lakeside Hospital	Lakeport	3.2%	621
Saint Johns Pleasant Valley Hospital	Camarillo	3.4%	440
Sutter Davis Hospital	Davis	3.4%	175
George L Mee Memorial Hospital	King City	3.5%	85
Pacific Hospital of Long Beach	Long Beach	3.5%	115
Saint Mary Medical Center	Apple Valley	3.5%	621
Community Regional Medical Center	Fresno	3.6%	890
Mark Twain Medical Center	San Andreas	3.6%	274
Pioneers Memorial Healthcare District	Brawley	3.6%	749
Saint Rose Hospital	Hayward	3.6%	332
Paradise Valley Hospital	National City	3.7%	218
Saint Agnes Medical Center	Fresno	3.7%	1629
Healdsburg District Hospital	Healdsburg	3.9%	259
Saint Francis Memorial Hospital	San Francisco	3.9%	259
Victor Valley Global Medical Center	Victorville	3.9%	155
Chinese Hospital	San Francisco	4.0%	353
Fountain Valley Reg Hosp & Med Ctr	Fountain Valley	4.0%	506
Goleta Valley Cottage Hospital	Santa Barbara	4.1%	219
Good Samaritan Hospital	San Jose	4.1%	762
Southwest Healthcare System	Murrieta	4.1%	654
Loma Linda Univ Med Ctr-Murrieta	Murrieta	4.2%	672
Providence Saint John's Health Center	Santa Monica	4.2%	568
Watsonville Community Hospital	Watsonville	4.2%	283
California Hosp Med Ctr Los Angeles	Los Angeles	4.4%	341
Scripps Mercy Hospital	San Diego	4.4%	1453
Arrowhead Regional Medical Center	Colton	4.5%	441
Sutter Auburn Faith Hospital	Auburn	4.5%	333
Alameda Hospital	Alameda	4.6%	175
Doctors Medical Center - San Pablo	San Pablo	4.6%	369
Mills - Peninsula Medical Center	Burlingame	4.6%	1190
Sutter Tracy Community Hospital	Tracy	4.6%	474
Novato Community Hospital	Novato	4.7%	364
Los Angeles Community Hospital	Los Angeles	4.8%	63
Eden Medical Center	Castro Valley	4.9%	649
Providence Holy Cross Medical Center	Mission Hills	4.9%	1027
Washington Hospital	Fremont	4.9%	874
Alta Bates Summit Medical Center	Berkeley	5.0%	323
Coast Plaza Hospital	Norwalk	5.0%	101
Tri - City Medical Center	Oceanside	5.1%	894
Grossmont Hospital	La Mesa	5.2%	1295
Saint Elizabeth Community Hospital	Red Bluff	5.2%	755
Sutter Amador Hospital	Jackson	5.2%	555
USC Verdugo Hills Hospital	Glendale	5.2%	251
Twin Cities Community Hospital	Templeton	5.4%	405
Alvarado Hospital Medical Center	San Diego	5.5%	291
Prov Little Co of Mary Med Ctr San Pedro	San Pedro	5.5%	400
San Gabriel Valley Medical Center	San Gabriel	5.5%	235
Marin General Hospital	Greenbrae	5.6%	799
Banner Lassen Medical Center	Susanville	5.7%	193
Olympia Medical Center	Los Angeles	5.7%	157
Saint Helena Hospital	Saint Helena	5.7%	265
San Mateo Medical Center	San Mateo	5.7%	123
El Centro Regional Medical Center	El Centro	5.8%	920
John Muir Med Ctr-Walnut Creek Campus	Walnut Creek	5.8%	570
Lodi Memorial Hospital	Lodi	5.8%	815
Queen of the Valley Medical Center	Napa	5.8%	553
Mission Community Hospital	Panorama City	5.9%	202
Valley Presbyterian Hospital	Van Nuys	5.9%	444
West Anaheim Medical Center	Anaheim	5.9%	204
Contra Costa Regional Medical Center	Martinez	6.0%	315
Glendale Mem Hosp & Health Ctr	Glendale	6.1%	657
Univ of California Irvine Med Ctr	Orange	6.1%	1422
Woodland Memorial Hospital	Woodland	6.3%	272
Barstow Community Hospital	Barstow	6.4%	251
Mad River Community Hospital	Arcata	6.5%	246
Providence Tarzana Medical Center	Tarzana	6.5%	445
Sutter Solano Medical Center	Vallejo	6.6%	301
Saint Mary's Medical Center	San Francisco	6.7%	360
Sequoia Hospital	Redwood City	6.9%	432
Sonora Regional Medical Center	Sonora	6.9%	859
Good Samaritan Hospital	Los Angeles	7.0%	230
Desert Regional Medical Center	Palm Springs	7.2%	822
Scripps Memorial Hospital La Jolla	La Jolla	7.2%	723
Desert Valley Hospital	Victorville	7.4%	216
Sharp Coronado Hosp & Healthcare Ctr	Coronado	7.4%	189
Madera Community Hospital	Madera	7.5%	345
San Gorgonio Memorial Hospital	Banning	7.5%	187
Stanford Hospital	Stanford	7.6%	2654
Colusa Regional Medical Center	Colusa	7.7%	130
Clovis Community Medical Center	Clovis	8.0%	578
Redlands Community Hospital	Redlands	8.2%	414
Ukiah Valley Medical Center	Ukiah	8.2%	488
Sonoma Valley Hospital	Sonoma	8.3%	265
Barton Memorial Hospital	S Lake Tahoe	8.7%	300
Doctors Hospital of Manteca	Manteca	8.7%	393
El Camino Hospital	Mountain View	8.7%	878
Saint Louise Regional Hospital	Gilroy	8.7%	335
Saint Mary Medical Center	Long Beach	8.7%	380
Natividad Medical Center	Salinas	8.8%	147
Providence Saint Joseph Medical Center	Burbank	8.8%	1006
Marian Regional Medical Center	Santa Maria	8.9%	1390
PIH Hospital - Downey	Downey	8.9%	372
Ahmc Anaheim Regional Medical Center	Anaheim	9.0%	378
Placentia Linda Hospital	Placentia	9.2%	380
Pomona Valley Hospital Medical Center	Pomona	9.2%	857
Fresno Heart & Surgical Hospital	Fresno	9.4%	127
Bear Valley Community Hospital	Big Bear Lake	9.6%	135
La Palma Intercommunity Hospital	La Palma	9.6%	157
Univ of CA San Diego Med Ctr	San Diego	9.7%	2173
Long Beach Memorial Medical Center	Long Beach	10.1%	789
Alta Bates Summit Medical Center	Oakland	10.2%	678
San Francisco General Hospital	San Francisco	10.2%	628
San Ramon Regional Medical Center	San Ramon	10.4%	327
Saint Joseph Hospital	Orange	11.1%	879
Kern Valley Healthcare District	Lake Isabella	11.4%	175
Palo Verde Hospital	Blythe	11.7%	171
Trinity Hospital	Weaverville	11.7%	137
Hoag Memorial Hospital Presbyterian	Newport Beach	11.8%	3530
Los Alamitos Medical Center	Los Alamitos	11.8%	709
Valleycare Medical Center	Pleasanton	11.9%	539
Sierra Vista Regional Medical Center	San Luis Obispo	12.0%	275
Community Hospital of San Bernardino	San Bernardino	12.2%	213
Hollywood Presbyterian Medical Center	Los Angeles	12.3%	579
Torrance Memorial Medical Center	Torrance	12.7%	1462
Kern Medical Center	Bakersfield	12.8%	117
Oroville Hospital	Oroville	12.9%	564
Chino Valley Medical Center	Chino	13.0%	115
Riverside County Regional Medical Center	Moreno Valley	13.0%	215

NOTE: Hospital profiles are in alphabetical order by state, then city, then hospital within the city; Rankings exclude hospitals with less than 25 cases except for patient surveys which excludes hospitals with less than 100 cases; (a) 100-299 cases; (1) The number of cases/patients is too few to report; (2) Data submitted were based on a sample of cases/patients; (3) Results are based on a shorter time period than required; (4) Data suppressed by CMS for one or more quarters; (5) Results are not available for this reporting period; (6) Fewer than 100 patients completed the HCAHPS survey; (7) No cases met the criteria for this measure; (8) The lower limit of the confidence interval cannot be calculated if the number of observed infections equals zero; (9) No data are available from the state/territory for this reporting period; (10) The scores shown reflect fewer than 50 completed surveys; (11) There were discrepancies in the data collection process; (12) This measure does not apply to this hospital for this reporting period; (13) Results cannot be calculated for this reporting period; (14) The results for this state are combined with nearby states to protect confidentiality; Please refer to the User's Guide for a full explanation of data.

Marshall Medical Center	Placerville	13.4%	790
Pacific Alliance Medical Center	Los Angeles	13.7%	190
Alhambra Hospital Medical Center	Alhambra	13.9%	144
Univ of CA Davis Med Ctr	Sacramento	13.9%	2010
Feather River Hospital	Paradise	14.1%	681
San Antonio Community Hospital	Upland	14.3%	1016
Santa Ynez Valley Cottage Hospital	Solvang	14.3%	349
Coalinga Regional Medical Center	Coalinga	14.4%	97
Simi Valley Hosp & Health Care Svcs	Simi Valley	14.7%	566
Sutter Coast Hospital	Crescent City	14.7%	443
Parkview Comm Hosp Med Ctr	Riverside	14.8%	310
Comm Mem Hosp San Buenaventura	Ventura	14.9%	582
Riverside Community Hospital	Riverside	15.0%	702
Sierra Nevada Memorial Hospital	Grass Valley	15.0%	924
Alameda County Medical Center	Oakland	15.1%	271
Scripps Green Hospital	La Jolla	15.4%	934
Saint Joseph Hospital	Eureka	15.6%	802
Foothill Presbyterian Hospital	Glendora	15.8%	253
Ojai Valley Community Hospital	Ojai	16.1%	161
Saint Bernardine Medical Center	San Bernardino	16.1%	602
Saint Francis Medical Center	Lynwood	16.1%	411
CA Pacific Med Ctr-Davies Campus	San Francisco	16.5%	310
Ventura County Medical Center	Ventura	16.7%	245
CA Pacific Med Ctr-Pacific Campus Hosp	San Francisco	16.9%	1362
Corona Regional Medical Center	Corona	17.5%	411
Mission Hospital Regional Medical Center	Mission Viejo	17.7%	1308
Whittier Hospital Medical Center	Whittier	18.9%	159
UCSF Medical Center	San Francisco	19.8%	2186
Seton Medical Center	Daly City	20.1%	597
Citrus Valley Medical Center - IC Campus	Covina	20.2%	568
Fallbrook Hospital	Fallbrook	20.3%	153
Glendale Adventist Medical Center	Glendale	20.4%	876
Garden Grove Hospital & Medical Center	Garden Grove	20.7%	164
LAC/Harbor - UCLA Medical Center	Torrance	21.1%	133
Santa Clara Valley Medical Center	San Jose	21.4%	1024
Motion Picture & Television Hospital	Woodland Hills	22.2%	81
French Hospital Medical Center	San Luis Obispo	22.4%	419
Garfield Medical Center	Monterey Park	22.4%	85
Marina Del Rey Hospital	Marina Del Rey	22.6%	217
Adventist Medical Center - Reedley	Reedley	23.2%	177
White Memorial Medical Center	Los Angeles	23.2%	444
Saddleback Memorial Medical Center	Laguna Hills	23.6%	860
Sierra View District Hospital	Porterville	24.0%	642
Kaweah Delta Medical Center	Visalia	25.9%	1336
Adventist Medical Center	Hanford	28.8%	1179
Orange Coast Memorial Medical Center	Fountain Valley	30.6%	507
Delano Regional Medical Center	Delano	31.4%	296
Loma Linda University Medical Center	Loma Linda	34.5%	1549
Menifee Valley Medical Center	Sun City	36.2%	105
Presbyterian Intercommunity Hospital	Whittier	36.9%	880
Los Robles Hospital & Medical Center	Thousand Oaks	37.0%	784
San Joaquin Community Hospital	Bakersfield	39.7%	1255
Santa Monica-UCLA Med Ctr & Ortho Hosp	Santa Monica	39.9%	424
Saint Jude Medical Center	Fullerton	40.2%	1588
Lompoc Valley Medical Center	Lompoc	40.4%	537
Hemet Valley Medical Center	Hemet	44.7%	217
Hazel Hawkins Memorial Hospital	Hollister	45.7%	317
Eisenhower Medical Center	Rancho Mirage	49.7%	1272
Saint Vincent Medical Center	Los Angeles	56.6%	495
Keck Hospital of USC	Los Angeles	59.9%	791
Stanislaus Surgical Hospital	Modesto	61.2%	49
Monterey Park Hospital	Monterey Park	61.9%	226
Mercy Medical Center - Mount Shasta	Mount Shasta	69.2%	260
Ronald Reagan UCLA Medical Center	Los Angeles	72.0%	1161
Biggs Gridley Memorial Hospital	Gridley	79.0%	281

Combination Brain/Sinus CT Scan

Hospital Name	City	Rate	Cases
Coastal Communities Hospital	Santa Ana	0.0%	93
Corcoran District Hospital	Corcoran	0.0%	43
San Mateo Medical Center	San Mateo	0.0%	102
Silver Lake Medical Center	Los Angeles	0.0%	37
CA Pacific Med Ctr-Pacific Campus Hosp	San Francisco	0.2%	541
Fountain Valley Reg Hosp & Med Ctr	Fountain Valley	0.2%	572
Lakewood Regional Medical Center	Lakewood	0.2%	579
Mills - Peninsula Medical Center	Burlingame	0.2%	666
PIH Hospital - Downey	Downey	0.2%	575
Comm Hosp of the Monterey Peninsula	Monterey	0.3%	980
Watsonville Community Hospital	Watsonville	0.3%	371
Monterey Park Hospital	Monterey Park	0.4%	225
Saint Joseph Hospital	Orange	0.4%	729
Kern Valley Healthcare District	Lake Isabella	0.5%	201
Pomona Valley Hospital Medical Center	Pomona	0.5%	919
Saint Mary Medical Center	Apple Valley	0.5%	580
Simi Valley Hosp & Health Care Svcs	Simi Valley	0.5%	426
Chinese Hospital	San Francisco	0.6%	361
Corona Regional Medical Center	Corona	0.8%	488
Doctors Medical Center	Modesto	0.8%	605
Marshall Medical Center	Placerville	0.8%	597
Regional Medical Center of San Jose	San Jose	0.8%	916
Torrance Memorial Medical Center	Torrance	0.8%	873
Twin Cities Community Hospital	Templeton	0.8%	513
Good Samaritan Hospital	San Jose	0.9%	701
Marian Regional Medical Center	Santa Maria	0.9%	1498
Presbyterian Intercommunity Hospital	Whittier	0.9%	794
Alameda Hospital	Alameda	1.0%	208
Comm Mem Hosp San Buenaventura	Ventura	1.0%	613
Dominican Hospital	Santa Cruz	1.0%	795
Garfield Medical Center	Monterey Park	1.0%	194
Saint Rose Hospital	Hayward	1.0%	387
Sierra Vista Regional Medical Center	San Luis Obispo	1.0%	304
Tri - City Medical Center	Oceanside	1.0%	966
Ahmc Anaheim Regional Medical Center	Anaheim	1.1%	376
Hoag Memorial Hospital Presbyterian	Newport Beach	1.1%	1845
Redlands Community Hospital	Redlands	1.1%	437
UCSF Medical Center	San Francisco	1.1%	560
Washington Hospital	Fremont	1.1%	964
Long Beach Memorial Medical Center	Long Beach	1.2%	695
Pioneers Memorial Healthcare District	Brawley	1.2%	592
Queen of the Valley Medical Center	Napa	1.2%	490
Saint Joseph Hospital	Eureka	1.2%	497
San Gorgonio Memorial Hospital	Banning	1.2%	345
Sharp Chula Vista Medical Center	Chula Vista	1.2%	846
Sutter Lakeside Hospital	Lakeport	1.2%	515
Cedars - Sinai Medical Center	Los Angeles	1.3%	1431
Mercy General Hospital	Sacramento	1.3%	716
Novato Community Hospital	Novato	1.3%	313
Sutter Delta Medical Center	Antioch	1.3%	447
Citrus Valley Medical Center - IC Campus	Covina	1.4%	641
El Camino Hospital	Mountain View	1.4%	987
Memorial Hospital Los Banos	Los Banos	1.4%	349
Orange Coast Memorial Medical Center	Fountain Valley	1.4%	360
Paradise Valley Hospital	National City	1.4%	444
Sequoia Hospital	Redwood City	1.4%	440
Doctors Medical Center - San Pablo	San Pablo	1.5%	475
Los Alamitos Medical Center	Los Alamitos	1.5%	599
Prov Little Co of Mary Med Ctr San Pedro	San Pedro	1.5%	409
Saint Agnes Medical Center	Fresno	1.5%	1754
Sonora Regional Medical Center	Sonora	1.5%	729
White Memorial Medical Center	Los Angeles	1.5%	671
Kaweah Delta Medical Center	Visalia	1.6%	1349
Saint Jude Medical Center	Fullerton	1.6%	1436
San Antonio Community Hospital	Upland	1.6%	924
Seton Medical Center	Daly City	1.6%	382
Antelope Valley Hospital	Lancaster	1.7%	589
Bakersfield Memorial Hospital	Bakersfield	1.7%	646
Clovis Community Medical Center	Clovis	1.7%	516
Feather River Hospital	Paradise	1.7%	755
Madera Community Hospital	Madera	1.7%	411
Memorial Medical Center	Modesto	1.7%	785
Sutter Auburn Faith Hospital	Auburn	1.7%	356
West Hills Hospital & Medical Center	West Hills	1.7%	594
French Hospital Medical Center	San Luis Obispo	1.8%	487
O'Connor Hospital	San Jose	1.8%	764
Saint Bernardine Medical Center	San Bernardino	1.8%	607
Santa Rosa Memorial Hospital	Santa Rosa	1.8%	768
El Centro Regional Medical Center	El Centro	1.9%	977
John Muir Medical Center - Concord Campus	Concord	1.9%	673
Saint Johns Regional Medical Center	Oxnard	1.9%	824
Saint Mary Medical Center	Long Beach	1.9%	413
Sutter Coast Hospital	Crescent City	1.9%	486
Valleycare Medical Center	Pleasanton	1.9%	428
Desert Regional Medical Center	Palm Springs	2.0%	609
Enloe Medical Center	Chico	2.0%	748
Loma Linda Univ Med Ctr-Murrieta	Murrieta	2.0%	489
Mercy Medical Center	Merced	2.0%	940
Scripps Memorial Hospital La Jolla	La Jolla	2.0%	736
Sutter General Hospital	Sacramento	2.0%	703
Hemet Valley Medical Center	Hemet	2.1%	561
Lodi Memorial Hospital	Lodi	2.1%	848
Providence Saint Joseph Medical Center	Burbank	2.1%	906
Univ of California Irvine Med Ctr	Orange	2.1%	565
Valley Presbyterian Hospital	Van Nuys	2.1%	561
Alvarado Hospital Medical Center	San Diego	2.2%	418
Centinela Hospital Medical Center	Inglewood	2.2%	668
Huntington Memorial Hospital	Pasadena	2.2%	729
Prov Little Co of Mary Med Ctr Torrance	Torrance	2.2%	1127
Ronald Reagan UCLA Medical Center	Los Angeles	2.2%	497
Sierra Nevada Memorial Hospital	Grass Valley	2.2%	742
Sierra View District Hospital	Porterville	2.2%	732
Alta Bates Summit Medical Center	Oakland	2.3%	730
Community Regional Medical Center	Fresno	2.3%	1080
Emanuel Medical Center	Turlock	2.3%	572
Glendale Mem Hosp & Health Ctr	Glendale	2.3%	522
Grossmont Hospital	La Mesa	2.3%	1653
Marin General Hospital	Greenbrae	2.3%	697
Methodist Hospital of Sacramento	Sacramento	2.3%	800
Riverside Community Hospital	Riverside	2.3%	650
Salinas Valley Memorial Hospital	Salinas	2.3%	665
Sutter Roseville Medical Center	Roseville	2.3%	981
Eisenhower Medical Center	Rancho Mirage	2.4%	1210
Methodist Hospital of Southern California	Arcadia	2.4%	804
Saint Johns Pleasant Valley Hospital	Camarillo	2.4%	507
Adventist Medical Center	Hanford	2.5%	1098
Eden Medical Center	Castro Valley	2.5%	842
Northbay Medical Center	Fairfield	2.5%	1023
Saint Joseph's Medical Center of Stockton	Stockton	2.5%	994
Santa Clara Valley Medical Center	San Jose	2.5%	967
Pomerado Hospital	Poway	2.7%	629
Mercy San Juan Medical Center	Carmichael	2.8%	1084
Scripps Memorial Hospital - Encinitas	Encinitas	2.8%	971
John Muir Med Ctr-Walnut Creek Campus	Walnut Creek	2.9%	836
Univ of CA Davis Med Ctr	Sacramento	2.9%	1049
San Joaquin Community Hospital	Bakersfield	3.0%	973
Los Robles Hospital & Medical Center	Thousand Oaks	3.1%	751
Rideout Memorial Hospital	Marysville	3.1%	1021
Loma Linda University Medical Center	Loma Linda	3.2%	770
Providence Tarzana Medical Center	Tarzana	3.2%	651
Mercy Medical Center - Redding	Redding	3.3%	960
Saddleback Memorial Medical Center	Laguna Hills	3.3%	841
Southwest Healthcare System	Murrieta	3.3%	759
Univ of CA San Diego Med Ctr	San Diego	3.3%	823
Mission Hospital Regional Medical Center	Mission Viejo	3.4%	1242
Sharp Memorial Hospital	San Diego	3.5%	1309
Stanford Hospital	Stanford	3.5%	972
Providence Holy Cross Medical Center	Mission Hills	3.6%	974
Palomar Health Downtown Campus	Escondido	3.7%	1109
Saint Elizabeth Community Hospital	Red Bluff	3.8%	606
Glendale Adventist Medical Center	Glendale	4.0%	880
Hollywood Presbyterian Medical Center	Los Angeles	4.0%	619
Shasta Regional Medical Center	Redding	4.0%	474
Good Samaritan Hospital	Los Angeles	4.1%	537
Scripps Mercy Hospital	San Diego	4.2%	1717
Mercy Hospital	Bakersfield	4.3%	903
Henry Mayo Newhall Memorial Hospital	Valencia	4.4%	458
Marina Del Rey Hospital	Marina Del Rey	4.4%	321
Alta Bates Summit Medical Center	Berkeley	4.5%	403
Oroville Hospital	Oroville	4.5%	550
Saint Vincent Medical Center	Los Angeles	4.7%	422
Western Medical Center Santa Ana	Santa Ana	5.0%	301
Sutter Solano Medical Center	Vallejo	5.2%	268
Banner Lassen Medical Center	Susanville	5.3%	228
California Hosp Med Ctr Los Angeles	Los Angeles	5.3%	437
Northridge Hospital Medical Center	Northridge	5.3%	760
San Francisco General Hospital	San Francisco	5.9%	424
Pacific Hospital of Long Beach	Long Beach	6.3%	191
Colusa Regional Medical Center	Colusa	6.5%	139
Fallbrook Hospital	Fallbrook	7.4%	188
Palo Verde Hospital	Blythe	7.9%	152
Ukiah Valley Medical Center	Ukiah	8.0%	338
East Valley Hospital Medical Center	Glendora	11.4%	44

Combination Chest CT Scan

Hospital Name	City	Rate	Cases
Alameda Hospital	Alameda	0.0%	90
Alvarado Hospital Medical Center	San Diego	0.0%	96
Bakersfield Heart Hospital	Bakersfield	0.0%	50
Bakersfield Memorial Hospital	Bakersfield	0.0%	170
Banner Lassen Medical Center	Susanville	0.0%	91
Beverly Hospital	Montebello	0.0%	161
CA Pacific Med Ctr-Davies Campus	San Francisco	0.0%	185
CA Pacific Med Ctr-St Luke's Campus	San Francisco	0.0%	115
Chinese Hospital	San Francisco	0.0%	239
Colusa Regional Medical Center	Colusa	0.0%	62
Comm Hosp of the Monterey Peninsula	Monterey	0.0%	1535
Dameron Hospital	Stockton	0.0%	101
Desert Valley Hospital	Victorville	0.0%	85
Doctors Hospital of Manteca	Manteca	0.0%	134
Doctors Medical Center	Modesto	0.0%	79
Doctors Medical Center - San Pablo	San Pablo	0.0%	191
Dominican Hospital	Santa Cruz	0.0%	255
Eastern Plumas Hospital - Portola Campus	Portola	0.0%	47
Emanuel Medical Center	Turlock	0.0%	103
Enloe Medical Center	Chico	0.0%	81
George L Mee Memorial Hospital	King City	0.0%	46
Good Samaritan Hospital	San Jose	0.0%	387
Healdsburg District Hospital	Healdsburg	0.0%	107
John Muir Med Ctr-Walnut Creek Campus	Walnut Creek	0.0%	134
Kern Medical Center	Bakersfield	0.0%	50
LAC+USC Medical Center	Los Angeles	0.0%	110
Los Robles Hospital & Medical Center	Thousand Oaks	0.0%	238
Menifee Valley Medical Center	Sun City	0.0%	51
Mercy General Hospital	Sacramento	0.0%	95
Mercy Medical Center - Mount Shasta	Mount Shasta	0.0%	141
Mercy San Juan Medical Center	Carmichael	0.0%	147
Methodist Hospital of Sacramento	Sacramento	0.0%	115
Methodist Hospital of Southern California	Arcadia	0.0%	199
Monterey Park Hospital	Monterey Park	0.0%	85
Northbay Medical Center	Fairfield	0.0%	144
O'Connor Hospital	San Jose	0.0%	304
Oak Valley District Hospital	Oakdale	0.0%	95
Ojai Valley Community Hospital	Ojai	0.0%	77
Palomar Health Downtown Campus	Escondido	0.0%	150

NOTE: Hospital profiles are in alphabetical order by state, then city, then hospital within the city; Rankings exclude hospitals with less than 25 cases except for patient surveys which excludes hospitals with less than 100 cases; (a) 100-299 cases; (1) The number of cases/patients is too few to report; (2) Data submitted were based on a sample of cases/patients; (3) Results are based on a shorter time period than required; (4) Data suppressed by CMS for one or more quarters; (5) Results are not available for this reporting period; (6) Fewer than 100 patients completed the HCAHPS survey; (7) No cases met the criteria for this measure; (8) The lower limit of the confidence interval cannot be calculated if the number of observed infections equals zero; (9) No data are available from the state/territory for this reporting period; (10) The scores shown reflect fewer than 50 completed surveys; (11) There were discrepancies in the data collection process; (12) This measure does not apply to this hospital for this reporting period; (13) Results cannot be calculated for this reporting period; (14) The results for this state are combined with nearby states to protect confidentiality; Please refer to the User's Guide for a full explanation of data.

Paradise Valley Hospital	National City	0.0%	210
Petaluma Valley Hospital	Petaluma	0.0%	193
PIH Hospital - Downey	Downey	0.0%	154
Pomerado Hospital	Poway	0.0%	126
Pomona Valley Hospital Medical Center	Pomona	0.0%	332
Redlands Community Hospital	Redlands	0.0%	214
Regional Medical Center of San Jose	San Jose	0.0%	259
Saint Agnes Medical Center	Fresno	0.0%	774
Saint Johns Regional Medical Center	Oxnard	0.0%	101
Saint Joseph Hospital	Orange	0.0%	696
Saint Mary's Medical Center	San Francisco	0.0%	192
Salinas Valley Memorial Hospital	Salinas	0.0%	96
San Ramon Regional Medical Center	San Ramon	0.0%	148
Sharp Coronado Hosp & Healthcare Ctr	Coronado	0.0%	116
Simi Valley Hosp & Health Care Svcs	Simi Valley	0.0%	210
Sonoma Valley Hospital	Sonoma	0.0%	145
Sutter Davis Hospital	Davis	0.0%	85
Sutter Delta Medical Center	Antioch	0.0%	92
Sutter Roseville Medical Center	Roseville	0.0%	279
Tri - City Medical Center	Oceanside	0.0%	415
USC Verdugo Hills Hospital	Glendale	0.0%	125
Valley Presbyterian Hospital	Van Nuys	0.0%	91
Valleycare Medical Center	Pleasanton	0.0%	290
West Hills Hospital & Medical Center	West Hills	0.0%	80
Western Medical Center Santa Ana	Santa Ana	0.0%	45
Woodland Memorial Hospital	Woodland	0.0%	158
Santa Barbara Cottage Hospital	Santa Barbara	0.1%	905
Torrance Memorial Medical Center	Torrance	0.1%	966
Alta Bates Summit Medical Center	Oakland	0.2%	502
Cedars - Sinai Medical Center	Los Angeles	0.2%	4979
Keck Hospital of USC	Los Angeles	0.2%	938
Queen of the Valley Medical Center	Napa	0.2%	490
San Francisco General Hospital	San Francisco	0.2%	455
Sonora Regional Medical Center	Sonora	0.2%	406
Stanford Hospital	Stanford	0.2%	3376
Univ of CA Davis Med Ctr	Sacramento	0.2%	2093
Univ of CA San Diego Med Ctr	San Diego	0.2%	2241
CA Pacific Med Ctr-Pacific Campus Hosp	San Francisco	0.3%	1175
Desert Regional Medical Center	Palm Springs	0.3%	338
Glendale Mem Hosp & Health Ctr	Glendale	0.3%	363
Arrowhead Regional Medical Center	Colton	0.4%	241
Marin General Hospital	Greenbrae	0.4%	714
Saint Helena Hospital	Saint Helena	0.4%	235
UCSF Medical Center	San Francisco	0.4%	2875
Ahmc Anaheim Regional Medical Center	Anaheim	0.5%	208
Glendale Adventist Medical Center	Glendale	0.5%	418
Lodi Memorial Hospital	Lodi	0.5%	407
Los Alamitos Medical Center	Los Alamitos	0.5%	429
Rideout Memorial Hospital	Marysville	0.5%	394
Saint Johns Pleasant Valley Hospital	Camarillo	0.5%	209
White Memorial Medical Center	Los Angeles	0.5%	202
Community Regional Medical Center	Fresno	0.6%	356
Scripps Memorial Hospital - Encinitas	Encinitas	0.6%	350
Mercy Medical Center - Redding	Redding	0.7%	148
Saint Francis Medical Center	Lynwood	0.7%	139
Santa Ynez Valley Cottage Hospital	Solvang	0.7%	272
Sutter Solano Medical Center	Vallejo	0.7%	134
El Camino Hospital	Mountain View	0.8%	394
Mills - Peninsula Medical Center	Burlingame	0.8%	824
Scripps Green Hospital	La Jolla	0.8%	922
Eden Medical Center	Castro Valley	0.9%	226
Goleta Valley Cottage Hospital	Santa Barbara	0.9%	111
Mercy Medical Center	Merced	0.9%	445
Oroville Hospital	Oroville	0.9%	425
Sutter Lakeside Hospital	Lakeport	0.9%	336
Biggs Gridley Memorial Hospital	Gridley	1.0%	104
Prov Little Co of Mary Med Ctr Torrance	Torrance	1.0%	304
Saint Francis Memorial Hospital	San Francisco	1.0%	102
Fountain Valley Reg Hosp & Med Ctr	Fountain Valley	1.1%	180
Lakewood Regional Medical Center	Lakewood	1.1%	188
Long Beach Memorial Medical Center	Long Beach	1.1%	435
Marshall Medical Center	Placerville	1.1%	370
Palmdale Regional Medical Center	Palmdale	1.1%	88
Presbyterian Intercommunity Hospital	Whittier	1.1%	623
San Antonio Community Hospital	Upland	1.1%	624
San Gabriel Valley Medical Center	San Gabriel	1.1%	89
Marian Regional Medical Center	Santa Maria	1.2%	594
Providence Tarzana Medical Center	Tarzana	1.2%	169
Scripps Mercy Hospital	San Diego	1.2%	726
Sutter General Hospital	Sacramento	1.2%	250
Henry Mayo Newhall Memorial Hospital	Valencia	1.3%	78
Palm Drive Hospital	Sebastopol	1.3%	75
San Joaquin General Hospital	French Camp	1.3%	77
Sequoia Hospital	Redwood City	1.4%	431
Kaweah Delta Medical Center	Visalia	1.5%	618
Hazel Hawkins Memorial Hospital	Hollister	1.6%	182
Huntington Memorial Hospital	Pasadena	1.6%	122
LAC/Olive View - UCLA Medical Center	Sylmar	1.6%	63
Prov Little Co of Mary Med Ctr San Pedro	San Pedro	1.6%	125
Saint Louise Regional Hospital	Gilroy	1.6%	129
Sutter Amador Hospital	Jackson	1.6%	374
San Joaquin Community Hospital	Bakersfield	1.7%	634
Sutter Auburn Faith Hospital	Auburn	1.7%	242
California Hosp Med Ctr Los Angeles	Los Angeles	1.8%	55
Hemet Valley Medical Center	Hemet	1.8%	113
Memorial Medical Center	Modesto	1.8%	227
Scripps Memorial Hospital La Jolla	La Jolla	1.8%	387
Watsonville Community Hospital	Watsonville	1.8%	110
Sutter Medical Center of Santa Rosa	Santa Rosa	1.9%	108
Saint Joseph's Medical Center of Stockton	Stockton	2.0%	349
Saint Jude Medical Center	Fullerton	2.0%	1144
Univ of California Irvine Med Ctr	Orange	2.0%	1176
Santa Rosa Memorial Hospital	Santa Rosa	2.1%	189
Clovis Community Medical Center	Clovis	2.2%	136
Northridge Hospital Medical Center	Northridge	2.2%	272
Mission Hospital Regional Medical Center	Mission Viejo	2.3%	910
Novato Community Hospital	Novato	2.3%	256
Providence Saint John's Health Center	Santa Monica	2.3%	222
Lompoc Valley Medical Center	Lompoc	2.4%	371
Saddleback Memorial Medical Center	Laguna Hills	2.4%	458
Memorial Hospital Los Banos	Los Banos	2.5%	120
Olympia Medical Center	Los Angeles	2.5%	81
Placentia Linda Hospital	Placentia	2.5%	118
Santa Clara Valley Medical Center	San Jose	2.6%	609
Mark Twain Medical Center	San Andreas	2.7%	112
Sutter Tracy Community Hospital	Tracy	2.8%	181
Ventura County Medical Center	Ventura	2.8%	108
Saint Joseph Hospital	Eureka	2.9%	516
Barton Memorial Hospital	S Lake Tahoe	3.0%	230
Mercy Hospital	Bakersfield	3.2%	189
Saint Rose Hospital	Hayward	3.2%	157
Ukiah Valley Medical Center	Ukiah	3.2%	217
El Centro Regional Medical Center	El Centro	3.3%	389
Citrus Valley Medical Center - IC Campus	Covina	3.4%	236
Kern Valley Healthcare District	Lake Isabella	3.4%	58
Antelope Valley Hospital	Lancaster	3.5%	57
West Anaheim Medical Center	Anaheim	3.5%	86
John F Kennedy Memorial Hospital	Indio	3.6%	56
Saint Elizabeth Community Hospital	Red Bluff	3.6%	280
Contra Costa Regional Medical Center	Martinez	3.7%	189
Grossmont Hospital	La Mesa	3.7%	429
Pacific Hospital of Long Beach	Long Beach	3.8%	53
Whittier Hospital Medical Center	Whittier	3.8%	52
Providence Holy Cross Medical Center	Mission Hills	3.9%	361
Ronald Reagan UCLA Medical Center	Los Angeles	3.9%	1445
Sharp Chula Vista Medical Center	Chula Vista	4.0%	124
Pioneers Memorial Healthcare District	Brawley	4.1%	296
Tulare Regional Medical Center	Tulare	4.4%	158
Feather River Hospital	Paradise	4.5%	471
Good Samaritan Hospital	Los Angeles	4.5%	67
Saint Mary Medical Center	Apple Valley	4.7%	149
Sharp Memorial Hospital	San Diego	4.8%	435
Loma Linda Univ Med Ctr-Murrieta	Murrieta	4.9%	267
Washington Hospital	Fremont	5.1%	547
Madera Community Hospital	Madera	5.2%	155
Seton Medical Center	Daly City	5.4%	429
Foothill Presbyterian Hospital	Glendora	5.6%	72
Providence Saint Joseph Medical Center	Burbank	5.7%	574
Southwest Healthcare System	Murrieta	5.9%	186
Sierra Vista Regional Medical Center	San Luis Obispo	6.0%	133
Corona Regional Medical Center	Corona	6.2%	162
Hoag Memorial Hospital Presbyterian	Newport Beach	6.2%	2596
Barstow Community Hospital	Barstow	6.3%	111
Hi - Desert Medical Center	Joshua Tree	6.3%	175
Sierra Nevada Memorial Hospital	Grass Valley	6.5%	430
LAC/Harbor - UCLA Medical Center	Torrance	6.7%	90
San Mateo Medical Center	San Mateo	6.8%	73
Orange Coast Memorial Medical Center	Fountain Valley	7.0%	302
Hollywood Presbyterian Medical Center	Los Angeles	7.1%	184
Saint Vincent Medical Center	Los Angeles	7.2%	263
Loma Linda University Medical Center	Loma Linda	7.8%	934
Eisenhower Medical Center	Rancho Mirage	8.3%	84
Mad River Community Hospital	Arcata	8.3%	108
Alameda County Medical Center	Oakland	8.9%	192
Fresno Heart & Surgical Hospital	Fresno	9.5%	84
Bear Valley Community Hospital	Big Bear Lake	10.0%	80
French Hospital Medical Center	San Luis Obispo	10.2%	205
Centinela Hospital Medical Center	Inglewood	10.3%	97
Sutter Coast Hospital	Crescent City	10.4%	164
Saint Mary Medical Center	Long Beach	10.5%	209
Trinity Hospital	Weaverville	11.0%	73
Santa Monica-UCLA Med Ctr & Ortho Hosp	Santa Monica	13.0%	247
Riverside Community Hospital	Riverside	13.4%	299
Riverside County Regional Medical Center	Moreno Valley	15.4%	91
Fallbrook Hospital	Fallbrook	15.6%	90
Parkview Comm Hosp Med Ctr	Riverside	15.8%	101
Comm Mem Hosp San Buenaventura	Ventura	21.8%	188
Saint Bernardine Medical Center	San Bernardino	22.4%	170
Delano Regional Medical Center	Delano	24.6%	130
Palo Verde Hospital	Blythe	32.5%	83
Sierra View District Hospital	Porterville	32.9%	353
Adventist Medical Center	Hanford	35.5%	625

Follow-up Mammogram/Ultrasound

A follow-up rate near zero may indicate missed cancer; a rate higher than 14% may mean there is unnecessary follow up.

Hospital Name	City	Rate	Cases
Palo Verde Hospital	Blythe	1.2%	85
Chinese Hospital	San Francisco	1.8%	735
Mission Community Hospital	Panorama City	2.1%	140
Northridge Hospital Medical Center	Northridge	2.2%	1378
Tri - City Regional Medical Center	Hawaiian Grdns	2.2%	93
Saint Vincent Medical Center	Los Angeles	2.4%	503
Saint Rose Hospital	Hayward	2.5%	636
Delano Regional Medical Center	Delano	2.6%	345
San Dimas Community Hospital	San Dimas	2.6%	77
La Palma Intercommunity Hospital	La Palma	2.8%	141
Hollywood Presbyterian Medical Center	Los Angeles	3.1%	517
USC Verdugo Hills Hospital	Glendale	3.1%	1012
CA Pacific Med Ctr-St Luke's Campus	San Francisco	3.2%	896
Healdsburg District Hospital	Healdsburg	3.5%	480
Pacific Hospital of Long Beach	Long Beach	3.5%	113
Watsonville Community Hospital	Watsonville	3.6%	1032
Garfield Medical Center	Monterey Park	3.7%	54
Regional Medical Center of San Jose	San Jose	3.8%	504
Los Alamitos Medical Center	Los Alamitos	4.0%	1542
Mammoth Hospital	Mammoth Lakes	4.5%	89
CA Pacific Med Ctr-Pacific Campus Hosp	San Francisco	4.6%	3984
George L Mee Memorial Hospital	King City	4.6%	217
Whittier Hospital Medical Center	Whittier	4.6%	130
Comm Hosp of the Monterey Peninsula	Monterey	4.7%	3735
Pomona Valley Hospital Medical Center	Pomona	4.7%	1575
Providence Tarzana Medical Center	Tarzana	4.7%	3123
San Francisco General Hospital	San Francisco	4.7%	950
San Ramon Regional Medical Center	San Ramon	4.7%	815
Alameda County Medical Center	Oakland	4.8%	251
Community Hospital of San Bernardino	San Bernardino	4.8%	104
Contra Costa Regional Medical Center	Martinez	4.8%	914
Santa Ynez Valley Cottage Hospital	Solvang	4.8%	454
Saint Jude Medical Center	Fullerton	5.0%	3217
Goleta Valley Cottage Hospital	Santa Barbara	5.1%	631
Mad River Community Hospital	Arcata	5.1%	565
Saint Elizabeth Community Hospital	Red Bluff	5.1%	568
Santa Clara Valley Medical Center	San Jose	5.1%	673
Arrowhead Regional Medical Center	Colton	5.2%	403
Southwest Healthcare System	Murrieta	5.2%	211
Sutter Coast Hospital	Crescent City	5.2%	615
Saint Mary Medical Center	Apple Valley	5.3%	246
Sonoma Valley Hospital	Sonoma	5.3%	800
Ronald Reagan UCLA Medical Center	Los Angeles	5.4%	2061
Santa Barbara Cottage Hospital	Santa Barbara	5.4%	184
Sutter Tracy Community Hospital	Tracy	5.4%	858
Emanuel Medical Center	Turlock	5.5%	1324
Mercy Medical Center - Mount Shasta	Mount Shasta	5.5%	510
Doctors Hospital of Manteca	Manteca	5.6%	869
Mercy Medical Center	Merced	5.6%	765
Ukiah Valley Medical Center	Ukiah	5.6%	1338
Ventura County Medical Center	Ventura	5.6%	305
Alta Bates Summit Medical Center	Oakland	5.7%	2650
Citrus Valley Medical Center - IC Campus	Covina	5.7%	1109
Henry Mayo Newhall Memorial Hospital	Valencia	5.8%	1336
Lompoc Valley Medical Center	Lompoc	5.8%	891
Riverside County Regional Medical Center	Moreno Valley	5.8%	104
Sierra Nevada Memorial Hospital	Grass Valley	5.8%	2353
California Hosp Med Ctr Los Angeles	Los Angeles	5.9%	270
Monterey Park Hospital	Monterey Park	5.9%	204
Sequoia Hospital	Redwood City	5.9%	943
Sutter Solano Medical Center	Vallejo	5.9%	461
Doctors Medical Center - San Pablo	San Pablo	6.0%	911
Saint Francis Medical Center	Lynwood	6.0%	504
Alta Bates Summit Medical Center	Berkeley	6.1%	3676
El Centro Regional Medical Center	El Centro	6.1%	1157
Fallbrook Hospital	Fallbrook	6.1%	245
Marshall Medical Center	Placerville	6.1%	1877
Novato Community Hospital	Novato	6.1%	1134
Prov Little Co of Mary Med Ctr Torrance	Torrance	6.1%	2231
Scripps Mercy Hospital	San Diego	6.1%	1642
Tri - City Medical Center	Oceanside	6.2%	1716
San Gorgonio Memorial Hospital	Banning	6.3%	253
Sutter Lakeside Hospital	Lakeport	6.3%	902
UCSF Medical Center	San Francisco	6.3%	2361
O'Connor Hospital	San Jose	6.4%	590
Eden Medical Center	Castro Valley	6.5%	1003
Oak Valley District Hospital	Oakdale	6.5%	356
Parkview Comm Hosp Med Ctr	Riverside	6.5%	230
Redlands Community Hospital	Redlands	6.5%	417
Saint Joseph's Medical Center of Stockton	Stockton	6.5%	1722
Hazel Hawkins Memorial Hospital	Hollister	6.7%	628
Motion Picture & Television Hospital	Woodland Hills	6.7%	627
John Muir Med Ctr-Walnut Creek Campus	Walnut Creek	6.8%	4759
Seton Medical Center	Daly City	6.8%	1250
West Anaheim Medical Center	Anaheim	6.8%	73
Glendale Mem Hosp & Health Ctr	Glendale	6.9%	1829

NOTE: Hospital profiles are in alphabetical order by state, then city, then hospital within the city; Rankings exclude hospitals with less than 25 cases except for patient surveys which excludes hospitals with less than 100 cases; (a) 100-299 cases; (1) The number of cases/patients is too few to report; (2) Data submitted were based on a sample of cases/patients; (3) Results are based on a shorter time period than required; (4) Data suppressed by CMS for one or more quarters; (5) Results are not available for this reporting period; (6) Fewer than 100 patients completed the HCAHPS survey; (7) No cases met the criteria for this measure; (8) The lower limit of the confidence interval cannot be calculated if the number of observed infections equals zero; (9) No data are available from the state/territory for this reporting period; (10) The scores shown reflect fewer than 50 completed surveys; (11) There were discrepancies in the data collection process; (12) This measure does not apply to this hospital for this reporting period; (13) Results cannot be calculated for this reporting period; (14) The results for this state are combined with nearby states to protect confidentiality; Please refer to the User's Guide for a full explanation of data.

Mercy Hospital	Bakersfield	6.9%	202
Stanford Hospital	Stanford	7.0%	1127
Banner Lassen Medical Center	Susanville	7.1%	367
Long Beach Memorial Medical Center	Long Beach	7.2%	3590
Providence Saint John's Health Center	Santa Monica	7.3%	689
Saint Joseph Hospital	Eureka	7.3%	1735
Saint Mary's Medical Center	San Francisco	7.3%	628
Beverly Hospital	Montebello	7.4%	704
Marin General Hospital	Greenbrae	7.4%	3034
Mark Twain Medical Center	San Andreas	7.4%	688
Saint Joseph Hospital	Orange	7.5%	550
Sierra Vista Regional Medical Center	San Luis Obispo	7.5%	371
Univ of CA Davis Med Ctr	Sacramento	7.5%	3031
Adventist Medical Center - Reedley	Reedley	7.6%	393
Hi - Desert Medical Center	Joshua Tree	7.6%	471
Hoag Memorial Hospital Presbyterian	Newport Beach	7.6%	5357
Kaweah Delta Medical Center	Visalia	7.7%	1260
Tulare Regional Medical Center	Tulare	7.7%	726
Victor Valley Global Medical Center	Victorville	7.7%	156
Coastal Communities Hospital	Santa Ana	7.8%	77
French Hospital Medical Center	San Luis Obispo	7.8%	474
Marian Regional Medical Center	Santa Maria	7.8%	2985
Orange Coast Memorial Medical Center	Fountain Valley	7.8%	741
Providence Holy Cross Medical Center	Mission Hills	7.8%	606
Sharp Memorial Hospital	San Diego	7.8%	1636
Centinela Hospital Medical Center	Inglewood	7.9%	466
Sutter Delta Medical Center	Antioch	7.9%	520
Washington Hospital	Fremont	7.9%	1633
Memorial Hospital Los Banos	Los Banos	8.0%	263
Saint Helena Hospital	Saint Helena	8.0%	413
Scripps Memorial Hospital La Jolla	La Jolla	8.0%	1985
Barton Memorial Hospital	S Lake Tahoe	8.1%	533
Saint Louise Regional Hospital	Gilroy	8.3%	506
Bear Valley Community Hospital	Big Bear Lake	8.4%	107
El Camino Hospital	Mountain View	8.5%	1323
John Muir Medical Center - Concord Campus	Concord	8.5%	998
Pacific Alliance Medical Center	Los Angeles	8.5%	213
Cedars - Sinai Medical Center	Los Angeles	8.6%	3298
Ojai Valley Community Hospital	Ojai	8.6%	304
Saint Mary Medical Center	Long Beach	8.7%	527
Kern Medical Center	Bakersfield	8.8%	68
Seneca District Hospital	Chester	8.8%	125
Valleycare Medical Center	Pleasanton	8.8%	1293
Eisenhower Medical Center	Rancho Mirage	8.9%	6860
San Joaquin General Hospital	French Camp	8.9%	225
Sutter Amador Hospital	Jackson	8.9%	966
Torrance Memorial Medical Center	Torrance	8.9%	5028
Saint Johns Pleasant Valley Hospital	Camarillo	9.0%	933
Sierra View District Hospital	Porterville	9.0%	1463
Olympia Medical Center	Los Angeles	9.1%	88
San Mateo Medical Center	San Mateo	9.1%	263
West Hills Hospital & Medical Center	West Hills	9.1%	1465
Univ of CA San Diego Med Ctr	San Diego	9.3%	1370
Colusa Regional Medical Center	Colusa	9.4%	191
White Memorial Medical Center	Los Angeles	9.4%	902
Sonora Regional Medical Center	Sonora	9.5%	2401
Ahmc Anaheim Regional Medical Center	Anaheim	9.7%	1009
Saint Francis Memorial Hospital	San Francisco	9.7%	269
Clovis Community Medical Center	Clovis	9.8%	1429
Saint Agnes Medical Center	Fresno	9.9%	3126
Univ of California Irvine Med Ctr	Orange	10.0%	663
Glendale Adventist Medical Center	Glendale	10.1%	1031
Loma Linda Univ Med Ctr-Murrieta	Murrieta	10.3%	117
Methodist Hospital of Southern California	Arcadia	10.4%	106
Sharp Coronado Hosp & Healthcare Ctr	Coronado	10.4%	490
Community Regional Medical Center	Fresno	10.5%	829
Scripps Green Hospital	La Jolla	10.6%	1124
Fountain Valley Reg Hosp & Med Ctr	Fountain Valley	10.7%	674
Palm Drive Hospital	Sebastopol	10.7%	299
Presbyterian Intercommunity Hospital	Whittier	10.7%	1576
Corona Regional Medical Center	Corona	10.8%	526
PIH Hospital - Downey	Downey	10.9%	700
Salinas Valley Memorial Hospital	Salinas	11.2%	3007
Simi Valley Hosp & Health Care Svcs	Simi Valley	11.2%	1025
Alameda Hospital	Alameda	11.3%	283
Natividad Medical Center	Salinas	11.3%	213
Providence Saint Joseph Medical Center	Burbank	11.3%	2238
Saint Bernardine Medical Center	San Bernardino	11.3%	247
Biggs Gridley Memorial Hospital	Gridley	11.4%	193
Los Robles Hospital & Medical Center	Thousand Oaks	11.4%	79
San Gabriel Valley Medical Center	San Gabriel	11.4%	132
Scripps Memorial Hospital - Encinitas	Encinitas	11.4%	581
Prov Little Co of Mary Med Ctr San Pedro	San Pedro	12.0%	669
San Antonio Community Hospital	Upland	12.1%	1645
Loma Linda University Medical Center	Loma Linda	12.4%	1407
Coalinga Regional Medical Center	Coalinga	12.5%	112
Eastern Plumas Hospital - Portola Campus	Portola	12.6%	159
Madera Community Hospital	Madera	12.7%	772
Riverside Community Hospital	Riverside	13.0%	637
Pomerado Hospital	Poway	13.1%	662
Pioneers Memorial Healthcare District	Brawley	13.2%	333
Saddleback Memorial Medical Center	Laguna Hills	13.4%	2640
Desert Regional Medical Center	Palm Springs	13.5%	1373
Mission Hospital Regional Medical Center	Mission Viejo	13.7%	2774
Feather River Hospital	Paradise	13.8%	1884
Queen of the Valley Medical Center	Napa	13.8%	1684
Placentia Linda Hospital	Placentia	13.9%	309
Barstow Community Hospital	Barstow	14.0%	178
Good Samaritan Hospital	San Jose	14.1%	2867
Petaluma Valley Hospital	Petaluma	14.8%	813
San Joaquin Community Hospital	Bakersfield	15.2%	1574
Lakewood Regional Medical Center	Lakewood	15.7%	389
Menifee Valley Medical Center	Sun City	15.9%	126
Adventist Medical Center	Hanford	16.0%	1403
Mills - Peninsula Medical Center	Burlingame	16.7%	3877
Foothill Presbyterian Hospital	Glendora	17.2%	116
Oroville Hospital	Oroville	18.0%	1427
Marina Del Rey Hospital	Marina Del Rey	19.0%	84
Stanislaus Surgical Hospital	Modesto	19.1%	157
Sutter Auburn Faith Hospital	Auburn	19.4%	484
Rideout Memorial Hospital	Marysville	21.6%	162

Lumbar Spine MRI for Low Back Pain

Hospital Name	City	Rate	Cases
Centinela Hospital Medical Center	Inglewood	16.7%	72
Saint Jude Medical Center	Fullerton	25.5%	231
Saint Johns Pleasant Valley Hospital	Camarillo	26.1%	92
Oroville Hospital	Oroville	26.8%	112
Ronald Reagan UCLA Medical Center	Los Angeles	27.1%	144
Scripps Mercy Hospital	San Diego	27.4%	175
Pomona Valley Hospital Medical Center	Pomona	27.7%	112
Queen of the Valley Medical Center	Napa	27.7%	188
Scripps Memorial Hospital La Jolla	La Jolla	27.7%	65
White Memorial Medical Center	Los Angeles	28.1%	121
Saint Mary's Medical Center	San Francisco	28.5%	172
Sonora Regional Medical Center	Sonora	28.5%	277
Sierra View District Hospital	Porterville	28.6%	105
Mission Hospital Regional Medical Center	Mission Viejo	29.0%	155
Providence Saint John's Health Center	Santa Monica	29.4%	68
Novato Community Hospital	Novato	29.8%	57
Providence Saint Joseph Medical Center	Burbank	30.0%	140
Madera Community Hospital	Madera	30.1%	73
Simi Valley Hosp & Health Care Svcs	Simi Valley	30.2%	53
Univ of CA Davis Med Ctr	Sacramento	30.2%	331
UCSF Medical Center	San Francisco	30.3%	238
Saint Vincent Medical Center	Los Angeles	30.4%	69
USC Verdugo Hills Hospital	Glendale	30.4%	69
Saint Joseph Hospital	Orange	30.5%	59
Santa Barbara Cottage Hospital	Santa Barbara	30.6%	108
Sutter Lakeside Hospital	Lakeport	30.6%	85
Ukiah Valley Medical Center	Ukiah	30.6%	98
Feather River Hospital	Paradise	30.8%	159
Scripps Green Hospital	La Jolla	31.8%	157
Marian Regional Medical Center	Santa Maria	31.9%	141
Scripps Memorial Hospital - Encinitas	Encinitas	31.9%	119
Marina Del Rey Hospital	Marina Del Rey	32.0%	50
Santa Monica-UCLA Med Ctr & Ortho Hosp	Santa Monica	33.0%	103
Adventist Medical Center	Hanford	33.1%	142
El Camino Hospital	Mountain View	33.3%	60
Mercy Medical Center - Mount Shasta	Mount Shasta	33.3%	72
O'Connor Hospital	San Jose	33.3%	87
Tri - City Medical Center	Oceanside	33.3%	69
Keck Hospital of USC	Los Angeles	33.6%	122
Sutter Coast Hospital	Crescent City	33.7%	83
Prov Little Co of Mary Med Ctr Torrance	Torrance	33.8%	68
Univ of California Irvine Med Ctr	Orange	34.2%	79
San Antonio Community Hospital	Upland	34.3%	70
Providence Holy Cross Medical Center	Mission Hills	34.6%	81
Valleycare Medical Center	Pleasanton	34.8%	66
Cedars - Sinai Medical Center	Los Angeles	34.9%	524
Saint Joseph Hospital	Eureka	35.3%	272
Stanford Hospital	Stanford	35.3%	317
Torrance Memorial Medical Center	Torrance	35.3%	190
Hoag Memorial Hospital Presbyterian	Newport Beach	35.5%	259
San Joaquin Community Hospital	Bakersfield	35.7%	230
Lompoc Valley Medical Center	Lompoc	35.8%	81
Comm Mem Hosp San Buenaventura	Ventura	36.0%	50
Kaweah Delta Medical Center	Visalia	36.3%	171
Univ of CA San Diego Med Ctr	San Diego	36.3%	146
Glendale Mem Hosp & Health Ctr	Glendale	36.4%	55
Saint Agnes Medical Center	Fresno	36.6%	82
Comm Hosp of the Monterey Peninsula	Monterey	36.7%	384
Glendale Adventist Medical Center	Glendale	36.9%	176
Santa Clara Valley Medical Center	San Jose	36.9%	65
Presbyterian Intercommunity Hospital	Whittier	37.4%	155
Sierra Nevada Memorial Hospital	Grass Valley	37.9%	203
Loma Linda University Medical Center	Loma Linda	38.1%	155
Saint Joseph's Medical Center of Stockton	Stockton	38.2%	55
El Centro Regional Medical Center	El Centro	38.6%	44
Marshall Medical Center	Placerville	38.6%	132
Grossmont Hospital	La Mesa	38.7%	62
Mills - Peninsula Medical Center	Burlingame	38.7%	199
Placentia Linda Hospital	Placentia	39.5%	43
Sonoma Valley Hospital	Sonoma	39.7%	58
Doctors Hospital of Manteca	Manteca	39.8%	103
Eden Medical Center	Castro Valley	40.0%	40
Tulare Regional Medical Center	Tulare	40.4%	47
CA Pacific Med Ctr-Davies Campus	San Francisco	40.5%	42
Sutter Amador Hospital	Jackson	40.6%	101
John Muir Med Ctr-Walnut Creek Campus	Walnut Creek	40.7%	54
Mark Twain Medical Center	San Andreas	40.7%	54
Santa Ynez Valley Cottage Hospital	Solvang	41.0%	39
Barton Memorial Hospital	S Lake Tahoe	41.7%	60
Loma Linda Univ Med Ctr-Murrieta	Murrieta	42.0%	50
Saint Elizabeth Community Hospital	Red Bluff	42.1%	114
Pioneers Memorial Healthcare District	Brawley	42.9%	42
Prov Little Co of Mary Med Ctr San Pedro	San Pedro	42.9%	63
Seton Medical Center	Daly City	43.2%	81
Desert Regional Medical Center	Palm Springs	44.4%	45
Rideout Memorial Hospital	Marysville	44.7%	38
Banner Lassen Medical Center	Susanville	47.6%	42

NOTE: Hospital profiles are in alphabetical order by state, then city, then hospital within the city; Rankings exclude hospitals with less than 25 cases except for patient surveys which excludes hospitals with less than 100 cases; (a) 100-299 cases; (1) The number of cases/patients is too few to report; (2) Data submitted were based on a sample of cases/patients; (3) Results are based on a shorter time period than required; (4) Data suppressed by CMS for one or more quarters; (5) Results are not available for this reporting period; (6) Fewer than 100 patients completed the HCAHPS survey; (7) No cases met the criteria for this measure; (8) The lower limit of the confidence interval cannot be calculated if the number of observed infections equals zero; (9) No data are available from the state/territory for this reporting period; (10) The scores shown reflect fewer than 50 completed surveys; (11) There were discrepancies in the data collection process; (12) This measure does not apply to this hospital for this reporting period; (13) Results cannot be calculated for this reporting period; (14) The results for this state are combined with nearby states to protect confidentiality; Please refer to the User's Guide for a full explanation of data.

Alameda Hospital

2070 Clinton Ave
Alameda, CA 94501
Phone: 510-522-3700
Fax: 510-814-4005
E-mail: communityrelations@alamedahospital.org
URL: www.alamedahospital.org

Type: Acute Care Hospitals
Emergency Services: Yes
Ownership: Voluntary non-profit - Private
Beds: 135

Key Personnel:
Radiology. . . . . Ravi Alagappan, MD
Operating Room. . . . . Roberto Celada, RN
Quality Assurance . . . . Janet Dike, RN
CEO/President. . . . . Stuart Jed
Emergency Room . . . . Cindy Lambdin, RN
President . . . . J. Michael McCormick
Chief of Medical Staff. . . . . Eric Otani, MD
CEO . . . . Deborah E. Stebbins

Measure	Cases	This Hosp.	State Avg.	U.S. Avg.
Blood Clot Prevention and Treatment				
Anticoagulation Overlap Therapy[2]	15	93%	92%	93%
ICU Venous Thromboembolism Prophylaxis[2]	58	76%	92%	92%
Incidence of Potentially Preventable VTE[1,2]	-	-	11%	10%
UFH with Dosages/Platelet Monitoring[1,2]	-	-	96%	97%
Venous Thromboembolism Prophylaxis[2]	238	64%	83%	85%
Warfarin Therapy Discharge Instructions[2]	12	75%	75%	75%
Chest Pain/Possible Heart Attack Care				
Aspirin Given Within 24 Hours of Arrival[1,3]	-	-	97%	96%
Fibrinolytic Meds Within 30 Min. of Arrival[3,7]	-	-	62%	58%
Average Time to ECG (minutes)[1,3]	-	-	9	7
Average Time to Transfer (minutes)[1,3]	-	-	62	60
Children's Asthma Care				
Received Home Management Plan of Care	-	-	88%	88%
Received Reliever Medication	-	-	100%	100%
Received Systemic Corticosteroids	-	-	100%	100%
Emergency Department				
Admittance Decision Time (minutes)[2]	450	112	125	98
Head CT Results Within 45 Min. of Arrival[1]	-	-	55%	57%
Patients Who Left ER Before Being Seen	16,815	0%	3%	2%
Time from ER Arrival to Admit. (minutes)[2]	526	256	323	274
Time from ER Arrival to Discharge (minutes)	333	140	168	134
Time in ER Before Being Evaluated (minutes)	357	25	29	26
Time to Pain Meds for Fractures (minutes)	35	52	62	57
Heart Attack Care				
Aspirin Given at Discharge	11	100%	99%	99%
Fibrinolytic Meds Within 30 Min. of Arrival[7]	-	-	73%	54%
PCI Within 90 Minutes of Arrival[7]	-	-	95%	96%
Statin Prescribed at Discharge	13	92%	98%	98%
Heart Failure Care				
ACE Inhibitor or ARB for LVSD	24	100%	97%	97%
Discharge Instructions Given	87	89%	94%	94%
Evaluation of LVS Function	115	99%	99%	99%
Medicare Spending				
Medicare Spending per Patient (ratio)	-	0.95	0.98	0.98
Pneumonia Care				
Appropriate Initial Antibiotic Given[2]	52	94%	97%	95%
Blood Culture Timing[2]	120	98%	98%	98%
Pregnancy and Delivery Care				
Newborn Deliveries Scheduled Early[7]	-	-	5%	6%
Preventive Care				
Immunization for Influenza[2]	289	93%	89%	90%
Immunization for Pneumonia[2]	453	94%	90%	92%
Stroke Care				
Anticoagulation Therapy for Atrial Fibrillation	13	85%	95%	95%
Antithrombotic Therapy Timing	34	91%	98%	98%
Assessed for Rehabilitation	44	98%	97%	97%
Discharged on Antithrombotic Therapy	39	100%	99%	99%
Discharged on Statin Medication	29	93%	94%	94%
Thrombolytic Therapy Timing[1]	-	-	72%	66%
Venous Thromboembolism Prophylaxis	51	92%	94%	94%
Written Stroke Educational Materials Given	22	91%	87%	88%
Surgical Care Improvement Project				
Appropriate Beta Blocker Usage	35	86%	97%	98%
Appropriate VTP Within 24 Hours	95	96%	98%	98%
Controlled Postoperative Blood Glucose[7]	-	-	96%	97%
Perioperative Temperature Management	103	100%	100%	100%
Prophylactic Antibiotic Selection	56	100%	99%	99%
Prophylactic Antibiotic Selection (Outpatient)[1]	-	-	97%	98%
Prophylactic Antibiotic Stopped	53	94%	98%	98%
Prophylactic Antibiotic Timing	57	98%	99%	99%
Prophylactic Antibiotic Timing (Outpatient)[1]	-	-	97%	98%
Urinary Catheter Removal	41	88%	97%	97%
Survey of Patients' Hospital Experiences				
Area Around Room 'Always' Quiet at Night	300+	35%	51%	61%
Doctors 'Always' Communicated Well	300+	74%	78%	82%
Home Recovery Information Given	300+	79%	83%	85%
Hospital Given 9 or 10 on 10 Point Scale	300+	55%	68%	71%
Meds 'Always' Explained Before Given	300+	54%	61%	64%
Nurses 'Always' Communicated Well	300+	66%	74%	79%
Pain 'Always' Well Controlled	300+	62%	68%	71%
Room and Bathroom 'Always' Clean	300+	64%	70%	73%
Timely Help 'Always' Received	300+	51%	62%	68%
Would Definitely Recommend Hospital	300+	66%	70%	71%
Use of Medical Imaging				
Cardiac Imaging Stress Test before Surgery	85	1.2%	5.2%	5.3%
Combination Abdominal CT Scan	175	4.6%	13.4%	10.5%
Combination Brain/Sinus CT Scan	208	1.0%	2.2%	2.7%
Combination Chest CT Scan	90	0.0%	2.3%	2.7%
Follow-up Mammogram/Ultrasound	283	11.3%	8.2%	8.8%
Lumbar Spine MRI for Low Back Pain[1]	-	-	34.2%	37.2%

Alhambra Hospital Medical Center

100 S Raymond Ave
Alhambra, CA 91801
Phone: 626-570-1606
Fax: 626-570-8825
E-mail: info@alhambrahospital.com
URL: www.alhambrahospital.com

Type: Acute Care Hospitals
Emergency Services: Yes
Ownership: Proprietary
Beds: 144

Key Personnel:
Operating Room. . . . . Cheng-Hsiung Chen
CEO/President. . . . . Lee Fuyenaga
CEO . . . . Iris Lai
Chief of Medical Staff. . . . . Tommy Lu, MD
Quality Assurance . . . . Eleanor Martinez, RN

Measure	Cases	This Hosp.	State Avg.	U.S. Avg.
Blood Clot Prevention and Treatment				
Anticoagulation Overlap Therapy[2]	13	77%	92%	93%
ICU Venous Thromboembolism Prophylaxis[2]	86	85%	92%	92%
Incidence of Potentially Preventable VTE[1,2]	-	-	11%	10%
UFH with Dosages/Platelet Monitoring[1,2]	-	-	96%	97%
Venous Thromboembolism Prophylaxis[2]	374	73%	83%	85%
Warfarin Therapy Discharge Instructions[1,2]	-	-	75%	75%
Chest Pain/Possible Heart Attack Care				
Aspirin Given Within 24 Hours of Arrival[3]	23	100%	97%	96%
Fibrinolytic Meds Within 30 Min. of Arrival[3,7]	-	-	62%	58%
Average Time to ECG (minutes)[3]	22	6	9	7
Average Time to Transfer (minutes)[1,3]	-	-	62	60
Children's Asthma Care				
Received Home Management Plan of Care	-	-	88%	88%
Received Reliever Medication	-	-	100%	100%
Received Systemic Corticosteroids	-	-	100%	100%
Emergency Department				
Admittance Decision Time (minutes)[2]	644	45	125	98
Head CT Results Within 45 Min. of Arrival[1]	-	-	55%	57%
Patients Who Left ER Before Being Seen	13,309	1%	3%	2%
Time from ER Arrival to Admit. (minutes)[2]	654	232	323	274
Time from ER Arrival to Discharge (minutes)	454	154	168	134
Time in ER Before Being Evaluated (minutes)	444	24	29	26
Time to Pain Meds for Fractures (minutes)	42	44	62	57
Heart Attack Care				
Aspirin Given at Discharge	12	100%	99%	99%
Fibrinolytic Meds Within 30 Min. of Arrival[7]	-	-	73%	54%
PCI Within 90 Minutes of Arrival[7]	-	-	95%	96%
Statin Prescribed at Discharge	11	91%	98%	98%
Heart Failure Care				
ACE Inhibitor or ARB for LVSD	28	100%	97%	97%
Discharge Instructions Given	78	95%	94%	94%
Evaluation of LVS Function	110	100%	99%	99%
Medicare Spending				
Medicare Spending per Patient (ratio)	-	1.20	0.98	0.98
Pneumonia Care				
Appropriate Initial Antibiotic Given	68	99%	97%	95%
Blood Culture Timing	245	97%	98%	98%
Pregnancy and Delivery Care				
Newborn Deliveries Scheduled Early[7]	-	-	5%	6%
Preventive Care				
Immunization for Influenza[2]	429	94%	89%	90%
Immunization for Pneumonia[2]	667	96%	90%	92%
Stroke Care				
Anticoagulation Therapy for Atrial Fibrillation[1]	-	-	95%	95%
Antithrombotic Therapy Timing	35	97%	98%	98%
Assessed for Rehabilitation	45	100%	97%	97%
Discharged on Antithrombotic Therapy	37	100%	99%	99%
Discharged on Statin Medication	29	59%	94%	94%
Thrombolytic Therapy Timing[1]	-	-	72%	66%
Venous Thromboembolism Prophylaxis	43	81%	94%	94%
Written Stroke Educational Materials Given	14	100%	87%	88%
Surgical Care Improvement Project				
Appropriate Beta Blocker Usage	17	82%	97%	98%
Appropriate VTP Within 24 Hours	137	95%	98%	98%
Controlled Postoperative Blood Glucose[7]	-	-	96%	97%
Perioperative Temperature Management	140	100%	100%	100%
Prophylactic Antibiotic Selection	80	98%	99%	99%
Prophylactic Antibiotic Selection (Outpatient)	47	83%	97%	98%
Prophylactic Antibiotic Stopped	78	96%	98%	98%
Prophylactic Antibiotic Timing	80	100%	99%	99%
Prophylactic Antibiotic Timing (Outpatient)	47	100%	97%	98%
Urinary Catheter Removal	86	90%	97%	97%
Survey of Patients' Hospital Experiences				
Area Around Room 'Always' Quiet at Night	300+	48%	51%	61%
Doctors 'Always' Communicated Well	300+	65%	78%	82%
Home Recovery Information Given	300+	85%	83%	85%
Hospital Given 9 or 10 on 10 Point Scale	300+	61%	68%	71%
Meds 'Always' Explained Before Given	300+	53%	61%	64%
Nurses 'Always' Communicated Well	300+	63%	74%	79%
Pain 'Always' Well Controlled	300+	59%	68%	71%
Room and Bathroom 'Always' Clean	300+	68%	70%	73%
Timely Help 'Always' Received	300+	57%	62%	68%
Would Definitely Recommend Hospital	300+	60%	70%	71%
Use of Medical Imaging				
Cardiac Imaging Stress Test before Surgery[1]	-	-	5.2%	5.3%
Combination Abdominal CT Scan	144	13.9%	13.4%	10.5%
Combination Brain/Sinus CT Scan[1]	-	-	2.2%	2.7%
Combination Chest CT Scan[1]	-	-	2.3%	2.7%
Follow-up Mammogram/Ultrasound[7]	-	-	8.2%	8.8%
Lumbar Spine MRI for Low Back Pain[1]	-	-	34.2%	37.2%

Modoc Medical Center

228 W Mcdowell Ave
Alturas, CA 96101
Phone: 530-233-5131

Type: Critical Access Hospitals
Emergency Services: Yes
Ownership: Govt - Hospital Dist/Auth

Measure	Cases	This Hosp.	State Avg.	U.S. Avg.
Blood Clot Prevention and Treatment				
Anticoagulation Overlap Therapy[5]	-	-	92%	93%
ICU Venous Thromboembolism Prophylaxis[5]	-	-	92%	92%
Incidence of Potentially Preventable VTE[5]	-	-	11%	10%
UFH with Dosages/Platelet Monitoring[5]	-	-	96%	97%
Venous Thromboembolism Prophylaxis[5]	-	-	83%	85%
Warfarin Therapy Discharge Instructions[5]	-	-	75%	75%
Chest Pain/Possible Heart Attack Care				
Aspirin Given Within 24 Hours of Arrival	-	-	97%	96%
Fibrinolytic Meds Within 30 Min. of Arrival	-	-	62%	58%
Average Time to ECG (minutes)	-	-	9	7
Average Time to Transfer (minutes)	-	-	62	60
Children's Asthma Care				
Received Home Management Plan of Care	-	-	88%	88%
Received Reliever Medication	-	-	100%	100%
Received Systemic Corticosteroids	-	-	100%	100%
Emergency Department				
Admittance Decision Time (minutes)[5]	-	-	125	98
Head CT Results Within 45 Min. of Arrival	-	-	55%	57%

NOTE: Hospital profiles are in alphabetical order by state, then city, then hospital within the city; Rankings exclude hospitals with less than 25 cases except for patient surveys which excludes hospitals with less than 100 cases; (a) 100-299 cases; (1) The number of cases/patients is too few to report; (2) Data submitted were based on a sample of cases/patients; (3) Results are based on a shorter time period than required; (4) Data suppressed by CMS for one or more quarters; (5) Results are not available for this reporting period; (6) Fewer than 100 patients completed the HCAHPS survey; (7) No cases met the criteria for this measure; (8) The lower limit of the confidence interval cannot be calculated if the number of observed infections equals zero; (9) No data are available from the state/territory for this reporting period; (10) The scores shown reflect fewer than 50 completed surveys; (11) There were discrepancies in the data collection process; (12) This measure does not apply to this hospital for this reporting period; (13) Results cannot be calculated for this reporting period; (14) The results for this state are combined with nearby states to protect confidentiality; Please refer to the User's Guide for a full explanation of data.

Measure	Cases	This Hosp.	State Avg.	U.S. Avg.
Patients Who Left ER Before Being Seen	-	-	3%	2%
Time from ER Arrival to Admit. (minutes)[5]	-	-	323	274
Time from ER Arrival to Discharge (minutes)	-	-	168	134
Time in ER Before Being Evaluated (minutes)	-	-	29	26
Time to Pain Meds for Fractures (minutes)	-	-	62	57
Heart Attack Care				
Aspirin Given at Discharge[5]	-	-	99%	99%
Fibrinolytic Meds Within 30 Min. of Arrival[5]	-	-	73%	54%
PCI Within 90 Minutes of Arrival[5]	-	-	95%	96%
Statin Prescribed at Discharge[5]	-	-	98%	98%
Heart Failure Care				
ACE Inhibitor or ARB for LVSD[5]	-	-	97%	97%
Discharge Instructions Given[5]	-	-	94%	94%
Evaluation of LVS Function[5]	-	-	99%	99%
Medicare Spending				
Medicare Spending per Patient (ratio)	-	-	0.98	0.98
Pneumonia Care				
Appropriate Initial Antibiotic Given[5]	-	-	97%	95%
Blood Culture Timing[5]	-	-	98%	98%
Pregnancy and Delivery Care				
Newborn Deliveries Scheduled Early[5]	-	-	5%	6%
Preventive Care				
Immunization for Influenza[5]	-	-	89%	90%
Immunization for Pneumonia[5]	-	-	90%	92%
Stroke Care				
Anticoagulation Therapy for Atrial Fibrillation[5]	-	-	95%	95%
Antithrombotic Therapy Timing[5]	-	-	98%	98%
Assessed for Rehabilitation[5]	-	-	97%	97%
Discharged on Antithrombotic Therapy[5]	-	-	99%	99%
Discharged on Statin Medication[5]	-	-	94%	94%
Thrombolytic Therapy Timing[5]	-	-	72%	66%
Venous Thromboembolism Prophylaxis[5]	-	-	94%	94%
Written Stroke Educational Materials Given[5]	-	-	87%	88%
Surgical Care Improvement Project				
Appropriate Beta Blocker Usage[5]	-	-	97%	98%
Appropriate VTP Within 24 Hours[5]	-	-	98%	98%
Controlled Postoperative Blood Glucose[5]	-	-	96%	97%
Perioperative Temperature Management[5]	-	-	100%	100%
Prophylactic Antibiotic Selection[5]	-	-	99%	99%
Prophylactic Antibiotic Selection (Outpatient)	-	-	97%	98%
Prophylactic Antibiotic Stopped[5]	-	-	98%	98%
Prophylactic Antibiotic Timing[5]	-	-	99%	99%
Prophylactic Antibiotic Timing (Outpatient)	-	-	97%	98%
Urinary Catheter Removal[5]	-	-	97%	97%
Survey of Patients' Hospital Experiences				
Area Around Room 'Always' Quiet at Night[10]	<100	48%	51%	61%
Doctors 'Always' Communicated Well[10]	<100	91%	78%	82%
Home Recovery Information Given[10]	<100	81%	83%	85%
Hospital Given 9 or 10 on 10 Point Scale[10]	<100	69%	68%	71%
Meds 'Always' Explained Before Given[10]	<100	68%	61%	64%
Nurses 'Always' Communicated Well[10]	<100	80%	74%	79%
Pain 'Always' Well Controlled[10]	<100	74%	68%	71%
Room and Bathroom 'Always' Clean[10]	<100	84%	70%	73%
Timely Help 'Always' Received[10]	<100	87%	62%	68%
Would Definitely Recommend Hospital[10]	<100	59%	70%	71%
Use of Medical Imaging				
Cardiac Imaging Stress Test before Surgery	-	-	5.2%	5.3%
Combination Abdominal CT Scan	-	-	13.4%	10.5%
Combination Brain/Sinus CT Scan	-	-	2.2%	2.7%
Combination Chest CT Scan	-	-	2.3%	2.7%
Follow-up Mammogram/Ultrasound	-	-	8.2%	8.8%
Lumbar Spine MRI for Low Back Pain	-	-	34.2%	37.2%

Ahmc Anaheim Regional Medical Center

1111 W La Palma Avenue
Anaheim, CA 92801
Phone: 714-774-1450
Fax: 714-999-6027
URL: www.memorialcare.org/anaheim
Type: Acute Care Hospitals
Emergency Services: Yes
Ownership: Voluntary non-profit - Private
Beds: 223

Key Personnel:
Cardiac Laboratory. . . . . Abdulehan Y Abu Qare
Hemotology Center . . . . Kambiz Afrasiabi, MD
Patient Relations . . . . Angela E Azar
Radiology. . . . . Edward C Callaway, MD
Pediatric In-Patient Care . . . . . . Samara Cardenas, MD
Infection Control. . . . . Jeff Duroche
CEO . . . . Patrick Petre

Measure	Cases	This Hosp.	State Avg.	U.S. Avg.
Blood Clot Prevention and Treatment				
Anticoagulation Overlap Therapy[2]	59	92%	92%	93%
ICU Venous Thromboembolism Prophylaxis[2]	99	95%	92%	92%
Incidence of Potentially Preventable VTE[2]	16	6%	11%	10%
UFH with Dosages/Platelet Monitoring[2]	34	100%	96%	97%
Venous Thromboembolism Prophylaxis[2]	354	86%	83%	85%
Warfarin Therapy Discharge Instructions[2]	41	78%	75%	75%
Chest Pain/Possible Heart Attack Care				
Aspirin Given Within 24 Hours of Arrival	30	90%	97%	96%
Fibrinolytic Meds Within 30 Min. of Arrival[5]	-	-	62%	58%
Average Time to ECG (minutes)	36	4	9	7
Average Time to Transfer (minutes)[5]	-	-	62	60
Children's Asthma Care				
Received Home Management Plan of Care	-	-	88%	88%
Received Reliever Medication	-	-	100%	100%
Received Systemic Corticosteroids	-	-	100%	100%
Emergency Department				
Admittance Decision Time (minutes)[2]	543	90	125	98
Head CT Results Within 45 Min. of Arrival[1]	-	-	55%	57%
Patients Who Left ER Before Being Seen	42,172	4%	3%	2%
Time from ER Arrival to Admit. (minutes)[2]	645	242	323	274
Time from ER Arrival to Discharge (minutes)	350	136	168	134
Time in ER Before Being Evaluated (minutes)	377	29	29	26
Time to Pain Meds for Fractures (minutes)	149	52	62	57
Heart Attack Care				
Aspirin Given at Discharge	247	100%	99%	99%
Fibrinolytic Meds Within 30 Min. of Arrival[7]	-	-	73%	54%
PCI Within 90 Minutes of Arrival	31	97%	95%	96%
Statin Prescribed at Discharge	252	99%	98%	98%
Heart Failure Care				
ACE Inhibitor or ARB for LVSD	133	95%	97%	97%
Discharge Instructions Given	332	88%	94%	94%
Evaluation of LVS Function	409	99%	99%	99%
Medicare Spending				
Medicare Spending per Patient (ratio)	-	1.09	0.98	0.98
Pneumonia Care				
Appropriate Initial Antibiotic Given	161	96%	97%	95%
Blood Culture Timing	289	100%	98%	98%
Pregnancy and Delivery Care				
Newborn Deliveries Scheduled Early	186	4%	5%	6%
Preventive Care				
Immunization for Influenza[2]	540	99%	89%	90%
Immunization for Pneumonia[2]	664	99%	90%	92%
Stroke Care				
Anticoagulation Therapy for Atrial Fibrillation	12	100%	95%	95%
Antithrombotic Therapy Timing	85	94%	98%	98%
Assessed for Rehabilitation	102	96%	97%	97%
Discharged on Antithrombotic Therapy	94	98%	99%	99%
Discharged on Statin Medication	75	96%	94%	94%
Thrombolytic Therapy Timing[1]	-	-	72%	66%
Venous Thromboembolism Prophylaxis	101	91%	94%	94%
Written Stroke Educational Materials Given	62	81%	87%	88%
Surgical Care Improvement Project				
Appropriate Beta Blocker Usage[2]	142	92%	97%	98%
Appropriate VTP Within 24 Hours[2]	300	98%	98%	98%
Controlled Postoperative Blood Glucose[2]	111	98%	96%	97%
Perioperative Temperature Management[2]	351	100%	100%	100%
Prophylactic Antibiotic Selection[2]	314	99%	99%	99%
Prophylactic Antibiotic Selection (Outpatient)	255	96%	97%	98%
Prophylactic Antibiotic Stopped[2]	300	95%	98%	98%
Prophylactic Antibiotic Timing[2]	314	99%	99%	99%
Prophylactic Antibiotic Timing (Outpatient)	251	100%	97%	98%
Urinary Catheter Removal[2]	234	95%	97%	97%
Survey of Patients' Hospital Experiences				
Area Around Room 'Always' Quiet at Night	300+	49%	51%	61%
Doctors 'Always' Communicated Well	300+	72%	78%	82%
Home Recovery Information Given	300+	81%	83%	85%
Hospital Given 9 or 10 on 10 Point Scale	300+	62%	68%	71%
Meds 'Always' Explained Before Given	300+	59%	61%	64%
Nurses 'Always' Communicated Well	300+	70%	74%	79%
Pain 'Always' Well Controlled	300+	65%	68%	71%
Room and Bathroom 'Always' Clean	300+	68%	70%	73%
Timely Help 'Always' Received	300+	63%	62%	68%
Would Definitely Recommend Hospital	300+	63%	70%	71%
Use of Medical Imaging				
Cardiac Imaging Stress Test before Surgery[1]	-	-	5.2%	5.3%
Combination Abdominal CT Scan	378	9.0%	13.4%	10.5%
Combination Brain/Sinus CT Scan	376	1.1%	2.2%	2.7%
Combination Chest CT Scan	208	0.5%	2.3%	2.7%
Follow-up Mammogram/Ultrasound	1,009	9.7%	8.2%	8.8%
Lumbar Spine MRI for Low Back Pain[1]	-	-	34.2%	37.2%

Kaiser Foundation Hospital - Orange Co-Anaheim

3440 E La Palma Avenue
Anaheim, CA 92806
Phone: 714-644-2000
Fax: 714-279-5590
URL: www.healthy.kaiserpermanente.org
Type: Acute Care Hospitals
Emergency Services: Yes
Ownership: Voluntary non-profit - Other
Beds: 200

Key Personnel:
Emergency Room . . . . Robert Becker, MD
Anesthesiology. . . . . James DeFontes, MD
Chief of Medical Staff . . . . Edward Ellison, MD
Intensive Care Unit. . . . . Denise Giambalvo, RN
CEO/President. . . . . Janice Head
Operating Room. . . . . Shiela Smith, RN
Cardiac Laboratory. . . . . Kerry Tepoinsly
Quality Assurance . . . . Sharon Valli

Measure	Cases	This Hosp.	State Avg.	U.S. Avg.
Blood Clot Prevention and Treatment				
Anticoagulation Overlap Therapy[2]	163	96%	92%	93%
ICU Venous Thromboembolism Prophylaxis[2]	33	94%	92%	92%
Incidence of Potentially Preventable VTE[2]	33	3%	11%	10%
UFH with Dosages/Platelet Monitoring[2]	108	100%	96%	97%
Venous Thromboembolism Prophylaxis[2]	328	95%	83%	85%
Warfarin Therapy Discharge Instructions[2]	143	91%	75%	75%
Chest Pain/Possible Heart Attack Care				
Aspirin Given Within 24 Hours of Arrival	-	-	97%	96%
Fibrinolytic Meds Within 30 Min. of Arrival	-	-	62%	58%
Average Time to ECG (minutes)	-	-	9	7
Average Time to Transfer (minutes)	-	-	62	60
Children's Asthma Care				
Received Home Management Plan of Care	-	-	88%	88%
Received Reliever Medication	-	-	100%	100%
Received Systemic Corticosteroids	-	-	100%	100%
Emergency Department				
Admittance Decision Time (minutes)[2]	402	78	125	98
Head CT Results Within 45 Min. of Arrival	-	-	55%	57%
Patients Who Left ER Before Being Seen	-	-	3%	2%
Time from ER Arrival to Admit. (minutes)[2]	422	324	323	274
Time from ER Arrival to Discharge (minutes)	-	-	168	134
Time in ER Before Being Evaluated (minutes)	-	-	29	26
Time to Pain Meds for Fractures (minutes)	-	-	62	57
Heart Attack Care				
Aspirin Given at Discharge	144	100%	99%	99%
Fibrinolytic Meds Within 30 Min. of Arrival[1]	-	-	73%	54%
PCI Within 90 Minutes of Arrival[7]	-	-	95%	96%
Statin Prescribed at Discharge	144	100%	98%	98%
Heart Failure Care				
ACE Inhibitor or ARB for LVSD	156	100%	97%	97%
Discharge Instructions Given	418	100%	94%	94%
Evaluation of LVS Function	451	100%	99%	99%
Medicare Spending				
Medicare Spending per Patient (ratio)	-	0.84	0.98	0.98
Pneumonia Care				
Appropriate Initial Antibiotic Given[2]	110	100%	97%	95%
Blood Culture Timing[2]	184	100%	98%	98%
Pregnancy and Delivery Care				
Newborn Deliveries Scheduled Early	554	0%	5%	6%
Preventive Care				
Immunization for Influenza[2]	501	96%	89%	90%
Immunization for Pneumonia[2]	508	92%	90%	92%
Stroke Care				
Anticoagulation Therapy for Atrial Fibrillation[2]	14	86%	95%	95%

NOTE: Hospital profiles are in alphabetical order by state, then city, then hospital within the city; Rankings exclude hospitals with less than 25 cases except for patient surveys which excludes hospitals with less than 100 cases; (a) 100-299 cases; (1) The number of cases/patients is too few to report; (2) Data submitted were based on a sample of cases/patients; (3) Results are based on a shorter time period than required; (4) Data suppressed by CMS for one or more quarters; (5) Results are not available for this reporting period; (6) Fewer than 100 patients completed the HCAHPS survey; (7) No cases met the criteria for this measure; (8) The lower limit of the confidence interval cannot be calculated if the number of observed infections equals zero; (9) No data are available from the state/territory for this reporting period; (10) The scores shown reflect fewer than 50 completed surveys; (11) There were discrepancies in the data collection process; (12) This measure does not apply to this hospital for this reporting period; (13) Results cannot be calculated for this reporting period; (14) The results for this state are combined with nearby states to protect confidentiality; Please refer to the User's Guide for a full explanation of data.

Measure	Cases	This Hosp.	State Avg.	U.S. Avg.
Antithrombotic Therapy Timing[2]	61	98%	98%	98%
Assessed for Rehabilitation[2]	105	100%	97%	97%
Discharged on Antithrombotic Therapy[2]	84	99%	99%	99%
Discharged on Statin Medication[2]	73	99%	94%	94%
Thrombolytic Therapy Timing[1,2]	-	-	72%	66%
Venous Thromboembolism Prophylaxis[2]	98	100%	94%	94%
Written Stroke Educational Materials Given[2]	75	99%	87%	88%
Surgical Care Improvement Project				
Appropriate Beta Blocker Usage[2]	174	99%	97%	98%
Appropriate VTP Within 24 Hours[2]	497	100%	98%	98%
Controlled Postoperative Blood Glucose[2,7]	-	-	96%	97%
Perioperative Temperature Management[2]	623	100%	100%	100%
Prophylactic Antibiotic Selection[2]	382	100%	99%	99%
Prophylactic Antibiotic Selection (Outpatient)	-	-	97%	98%
Prophylactic Antibiotic Stopped[2]	368	100%	98%	98%
Prophylactic Antibiotic Timing[2]	382	100%	99%	99%
Prophylactic Antibiotic Timing (Outpatient)	-	-	97%	98%
Urinary Catheter Removal[2]	378	99%	97%	97%
Survey of Patients' Hospital Experiences				
Area Around Room 'Always' Quiet at Night	300+	62%	51%	61%
Doctors 'Always' Communicated Well	300+	83%	78%	82%
Home Recovery Information Given	300+	88%	83%	85%
Hospital Given 9 or 10 on 10 Point Scale	300+	84%	68%	71%
Meds 'Always' Explained Before Given	300+	65%	61%	64%
Nurses 'Always' Communicated Well	300+	78%	74%	79%
Pain 'Always' Well Controlled	300+	73%	68%	71%
Room and Bathroom 'Always' Clean	300+	78%	70%	73%
Timely Help 'Always' Received	300+	69%	62%	68%
Would Definitely Recommend Hospital	300+	84%	70%	71%
Use of Medical Imaging				
Cardiac Imaging Stress Test before Surgery	-	-	5.2%	5.3%
Combination Abdominal CT Scan	-	-	13.4%	10.5%
Combination Brain/Sinus CT Scan	-	-	2.2%	2.7%
Combination Chest CT Scan	-	-	2.3%	2.7%
Follow-up Mammogram/Ultrasound	-	-	8.2%	8.8%
Lumbar Spine MRI for Low Back Pain	-	-	34.2%	37.2%
Time to Pain Meds for Fractures (minutes)	95	67	62	57
Heart Attack Care				
Aspirin Given at Discharge	129	100%	99%	99%
Fibrinolytic Meds Within 30 Min. of Arrival[7]	-	-	73%	54%
PCI Within 90 Minutes of Arrival	27	93%	95%	96%
Statin Prescribed at Discharge	129	100%	98%	98%
Heart Failure Care				
ACE Inhibitor or ARB for LVSD	52	100%	97%	97%
Discharge Instructions Given	180	99%	94%	94%
Evaluation of LVS Function	234	100%	99%	99%
Medicare Spending				
Medicare Spending per Patient (ratio)	-	1.09	0.98	0.98
Pneumonia Care				
Appropriate Initial Antibiotic Given[2]	80	99%	97%	95%
Blood Culture Timing[2]	169	100%	98%	98%
Pregnancy and Delivery Care				
Newborn Deliveries Scheduled Early[7]	-	-	5%	6%
Preventive Care				
Immunization for Influenza[2]	569	100%	89%	90%
Immunization for Pneumonia[2]	818	100%	90%	92%

West Anaheim Medical Center

3033 W Orange Avenue
Anaheim, CA 92804
Phone: 714-827-3000
Fax: 714-229-4052
E-mail: info@westanaheimmedctr.com
URL: www.wamc.phcs.us
Type: Acute Care Hospitals
Emergency Services: Yes
Ownership: Proprietary
Beds: 219

Key Personnel:
Chief of Medical Staff . . . . Hassan Alkhouli, MD
Emergency Room . . . . George Baskevitch, MD
CEO . . . . Virg Narbutas
Ambulatory Care . . . . Fred Shalom, MD

Measure	Cases	This Hosp.	State Avg.	U.S. Avg.
Blood Clot Prevention and Treatment				
Anticoagulation Overlap Therapy[2]	34	97%	92%	93%
ICU Venous Thromboembolism Prophylaxis[2]	77	94%	92%	92%
Incidence of Potentially Preventable VTE[1,2]	-	-	11%	10%
UFH with Dosages/Platelet Monitoring[2]	11	100%	96%	97%
Venous Thromboembolism Prophylaxis[2]	370	95%	83%	85%
Warfarin Therapy Discharge Instructions[2]	18	89%	75%	75%
Chest Pain/Possible Heart Attack Care				
Aspirin Given Within 24 Hours of Arrival	11	100%	97%	96%
Fibrinolytic Meds Within 30 Min. of Arrival[3,7]	-	-	62%	58%
Average Time to ECG (minutes)	11	0	9	7
Average Time to Transfer (minutes)[3,7]	-	-	62	60
Children's Asthma Care				
Received Home Management Plan of Care	-	-	88%	88%
Received Reliever Medication	-	-	100%	100%
Received Systemic Corticosteroids	-	-	100%	100%
Emergency Department				
Admittance Decision Time (minutes)[2]	1,133	142	125	98
Head CT Results Within 45 Min. of Arrival[1]	-	-	55%	57%
Patients Who Left ER Before Being Seen	30,450	4%	3%	2%
Time from ER Arrival to Admit. (minutes)[2]	1,137	296	323	274
Time from ER Arrival to Discharge (minutes)	334	187	168	134
Time in ER Before Being Evaluated (minutes)	391	53	29	26
Stroke Care				
Anticoagulation Therapy for Atrial Fibrillation[1]	-	-	95%	95%
Antithrombotic Therapy Timing	35	94%	98%	98%
Assessed for Rehabilitation	32	97%	97%	97%
Discharged on Antithrombotic Therapy	28	96%	99%	99%
Discharged on Statin Medication	20	90%	94%	94%
Thrombolytic Therapy Timing[1]	-	-	72%	66%
Venous Thromboembolism Prophylaxis	39	95%	94%	94%
Written Stroke Educational Materials Given	16	100%	87%	88%
Surgical Care Improvement Project				
Appropriate Beta Blocker Usage	28	100%	97%	98%
Appropriate VTP Within 24 Hours	95	100%	98%	98%
Controlled Postoperative Blood Glucose	26	88%	96%	97%
Perioperative Temperature Management	107	100%	100%	100%
Prophylactic Antibiotic Selection	54	100%	99%	99%
Prophylactic Antibiotic Selection (Outpatient)	12	100%	97%	98%
Prophylactic Antibiotic Stopped	39	97%	98%	98%
Prophylactic Antibiotic Timing	54	98%	99%	99%
Prophylactic Antibiotic Timing (Outpatient)	13	92%	97%	98%
Urinary Catheter Removal	59	98%	97%	97%
Survey of Patients' Hospital Experiences				
Area Around Room 'Always' Quiet at Night	300+	49%	51%	61%
Doctors 'Always' Communicated Well	300+	67%	78%	82%
Home Recovery Information Given	300+	82%	83%	85%
Hospital Given 9 or 10 on 10 Point Scale	300+	56%	68%	71%
Meds 'Always' Explained Before Given	300+	49%	61%	64%
Nurses 'Always' Communicated Well	300+	66%	74%	79%
Pain 'Always' Well Controlled	300+	59%	68%	71%
Room and Bathroom 'Always' Clean	300+	66%	70%	73%
Timely Help 'Always' Received	300+	50%	62%	68%
Would Definitely Recommend Hospital	300+	58%	70%	71%
Use of Medical Imaging				
Cardiac Imaging Stress Test before Surgery[1]	-	-	5.2%	5.3%
Combination Abdominal CT Scan	204	5.9%	13.4%	10.5%
Combination Brain/Sinus CT Scan[1]	-	-	2.2%	2.7%
Combination Chest CT Scan	86	3.5%	2.3%	2.7%
Follow-up Mammogram/Ultrasound	73	6.8%	8.2%	8.8%
Lumbar Spine MRI for Low Back Pain[1]	-	-	34.2%	37.2%

Western Medical Center Hospital Anaheim

1025 S Anaheim Blvd
Anaheim, CA 92805
Phone: 714-533-6220
Fax: 714-563-2839
URL: www.westernmedanaheim.com
Type: Acute Care Hospitals
Emergency Services: Yes
Ownership: Proprietary
Beds: 188

Key Personnel:
Radiology. . . . . Andrew William Bauer
Operating Room. . . . . Gayle Cantrall
Emergency Room . . . . Mary Groell, RN
Quality Assurance . . . . Pam Helmes
CEO/President. . . . . Josh D Luke PhD
Chief of Medical Staff. . . . . Jayanti Patel
Pediatric Ambulatory Care . . . . . Patrick Walsh, MD
Pediatric In-Patient Care . . . . Patrick Walsh, MD

Measure	Cases	This Hosp.	State Avg.	U.S. Avg.
Blood Clot Prevention and Treatment				
Anticoagulation Overlap Therapy[1,2]	-	-	92%	93%
ICU Venous Thromboembolism Prophylaxis[2]	61	98%	92%	92%
Incidence of Potentially Preventable VTE[1,2]	-	-	11%	10%
UFH with Dosages/Platelet Monitoring[1,2]	-	-	96%	97%
Venous Thromboembolism Prophylaxis[2]	137	77%	83%	85%
Warfarin Therapy Discharge Instructions[1,2]	-	-	75%	75%
Chest Pain/Possible Heart Attack Care				
Aspirin Given Within 24 Hours of Arrival[3,7]	-	-	97%	96%
Fibrinolytic Meds Within 30 Min. of Arrival[5]	-	-	62%	58%
Average Time to ECG (minutes)[3,7]	-	-	9	7
Average Time to Transfer (minutes)[5]	-	-	62	60
Children's Asthma Care				
Received Home Management Plan of Care	-	-	88%	88%
Received Reliever Medication	-	-	100%	100%
Received Systemic Corticosteroids	-	-	100%	100%
Emergency Department				
Admittance Decision Time (minutes)[2]	238	110	125	98
Head CT Results Within 45 Min. of Arrival[3,7]	-	-	55%	57%
Patients Who Left ER Before Being Seen	16,963	7%	3%	2%
Time from ER Arrival to Admit. (minutes)[2]	249	318	323	274
Time from ER Arrival to Discharge (minutes)	306	163	168	134
Time in ER Before Being Evaluated (minutes)	353	48	29	26
Time to Pain Meds for Fractures (minutes)	31	143	62	57
Heart Attack Care				
Aspirin Given at Discharge	70	97%	99%	99%
Fibrinolytic Meds Within 30 Min. of Arrival[7]	-	-	73%	54%
PCI Within 90 Minutes of Arrival[1]	-	-	95%	96%
Statin Prescribed at Discharge	66	94%	98%	98%
Heart Failure Care				
ACE Inhibitor or ARB for LVSD[1]	-	-	97%	97%
Discharge Instructions Given	22	95%	94%	94%
Evaluation of LVS Function	26	100%	99%	99%
Medicare Spending				
Medicare Spending per Patient (ratio)	-	1.15	0.98	0.98
Pneumonia Care				
Appropriate Initial Antibiotic Given	28	96%	97%	95%
Blood Culture Timing	50	100%	98%	98%
Pregnancy and Delivery Care				
Newborn Deliveries Scheduled Early[2]	105	3%	5%	6%
Preventive Care				
Immunization for Influenza[2]	362	90%	89%	90%
Immunization for Pneumonia[2]	200	88%	90%	92%
Stroke Care				
Anticoagulation Therapy for Atrial Fibrillation[7]	-	-	95%	95%
Antithrombotic Therapy Timing[1]	-	-	98%	98%
Assessed for Rehabilitation[1]	-	-	97%	97%
Discharged on Antithrombotic Therapy[1]	-	-	99%	99%
Discharged on Statin Medication[1]	-	-	94%	94%
Thrombolytic Therapy Timing[7]	-	-	72%	66%
Venous Thromboembolism Prophylaxis[1]	-	-	94%	94%
Written Stroke Educational Materials Given[1]	-	-	87%	88%
Surgical Care Improvement Project				
Appropriate Beta Blocker Usage	51	96%	97%	98%
Appropriate VTP Within 24 Hours	67	88%	98%	98%
Controlled Postoperative Blood Glucose	57	96%	96%	97%
Perioperative Temperature Management	81	100%	100%	100%
Prophylactic Antibiotic Selection	95	96%	99%	99%
Prophylactic Antibiotic Selection (Outpatient)	38	97%	97%	98%
Prophylactic Antibiotic Stopped	87	93%	98%	98%
Prophylactic Antibiotic Timing	95	100%	99%	99%
Prophylactic Antibiotic Timing (Outpatient)	38	100%	97%	98%
Urinary Catheter Removal	41	100%	97%	97%
Survey of Patients' Hospital Experiences				
Area Around Room 'Always' Quiet at Night	300+	41%	51%	61%
Doctors 'Always' Communicated Well	300+	81%	78%	82%
Home Recovery Information Given	300+	81%	83%	85%
Hospital Given 9 or 10 on 10 Point Scale	300+	68%	68%	71%
Meds 'Always' Explained Before Given	300+	61%	61%	64%
Nurses 'Always' Communicated Well	300+	75%	74%	79%
Pain 'Always' Well Controlled	300+	72%	68%	71%

NOTE: Hospital profiles are in alphabetical order by state, then city, then hospital within the city; Rankings exclude hospitals with less than 25 cases except for patient surveys which excludes hospitals with less than 100 cases; (a) 100-299 cases; (1) The number of cases/patients is too few to report; (2) Data submitted were based on a sample of cases/patients; (3) Results are based on a shorter time period than required; (4) Data suppressed by CMS for one or more quarters; (5) Results are not available for this reporting period; (6) Fewer than 100 patients completed the HCAHPS survey; (7) No cases met the criteria for this measure; (8) The lower limit of the confidence interval cannot be calculated if the number of observed infections equals zero; (9) No data are available from the state/territory for this reporting period; (10) The scores shown reflect fewer than 50 completed surveys; (11) There were discrepancies in the data collection process; (12) This measure does not apply to this hospital for this reporting period; (13) Results cannot be calculated for this reporting period; (14) The results for this state are combined with nearby states to protect confidentiality; Please refer to the User's Guide for a full explanation of data.

Measure	Cases	This Hosp.	State Avg.	U.S. Avg.
Room and Bathroom 'Always' Clean	300+	72%	70%	73%
Timely Help 'Always' Received	300+	60%	62%	68%
Would Definitely Recommend Hospital	300+	64%	70%	71%
Use of Medical Imaging				
Cardiac Imaging Stress Test before Surgery[1]	-	-	5.2%	5.3%
Combination Abdominal CT Scan[1]	-	-	13.4%	10.5%
Combination Brain/Sinus CT Scan[1]	-	-	2.2%	2.7%
Combination Chest CT Scan[1]	-	-	2.3%	2.7%
Follow-up Mammogram/Ultrasound[7]	-	-	8.2%	8.8%
Lumbar Spine MRI for Low Back Pain[7]	-	-	34.2%	37.2%

Kaiser Foundation Hospital - Antioch

4501 Sand Creek Road
Antioch, CA 94531
Phone: 925-813-6500
URL: www.kaiserpermanente.org
Type: Acute Care Hospitals
Emergency Services: Yes
Ownership: Voluntary non-profit - Private

Measure	Cases	This Hosp.	State Avg.	U.S. Avg.
Blood Clot Prevention and Treatment				
Anticoagulation Overlap Therapy[2]	71	99%	92%	93%
ICU Venous Thromboembolism Prophylaxis[2]	42	100%	92%	92%
Incidence of Potentially Preventable VTE[1,2]	-	-	11%	10%
UFH with Dosages/Platelet Monitoring[2]	29	100%	96%	97%
Venous Thromboembolism Prophylaxis[2]	238	99%	83%	85%
Warfarin Therapy Discharge Instructions[2]	71	68%	75%	75%
Chest Pain/Possible Heart Attack Care				
Aspirin Given Within 24 Hours of Arrival	-	-	97%	96%
Fibrinolytic Meds Within 30 Min. of Arrival	-	-	62%	58%
Average Time to ECG (minutes)	-	-	9	7
Average Time to Transfer (minutes)	-	-	62	60
Children's Asthma Care				
Received Home Management Plan of Care	-	-	88%	88%
Received Reliever Medication	-	-	100%	100%
Received Systemic Corticosteroids	-	-	100%	100%
Emergency Department				
Admittance Decision Time (minutes)[2]	537	48	125	98
Head CT Results Within 45 Min. of Arrival	-	-	55%	57%
Patients Who Left ER Before Being Seen	-	-	3%	2%
Time from ER Arrival to Admit. (minutes)[2]	537	293	323	274
Time from ER Arrival to Discharge (minutes)	-	-	168	134
Time in ER Before Being Evaluated (minutes)	-	-	29	26
Time to Pain Meds for Fractures (minutes)	-	-	62	57
Heart Attack Care				
Aspirin Given at Discharge	89	99%	99%	99%
Fibrinolytic Meds Within 30 Min. of Arrival[7]	-	-	73%	54%
PCI Within 90 Minutes of Arrival[7]	-	-	95%	96%
Statin Prescribed at Discharge	87	99%	98%	98%
Heart Failure Care				
ACE Inhibitor or ARB for LVSD	43	100%	97%	97%
Discharge Instructions Given	209	100%	94%	94%
Evaluation of LVS Function	228	100%	99%	99%
Medicare Spending				
Medicare Spending per Patient (ratio)	-	0.74	0.98	0.98
Pneumonia Care				
Appropriate Initial Antibiotic Given[2]	78	100%	97%	95%
Blood Culture Timing[2]	154	98%	98%	98%
Pregnancy and Delivery Care				
Newborn Deliveries Scheduled Early[2]	21	0%	5%	6%
Preventive Care				
Immunization for Influenza[2]	516	88%	89%	90%
Immunization for Pneumonia[2]	624	95%	90%	92%
Stroke Care				
Anticoagulation Therapy for Atrial Fibrillation[2]	19	89%	95%	95%
Antithrombotic Therapy Timing[2]	64	100%	98%	98%
Assessed for Rehabilitation[2]	101	100%	97%	97%
Discharged on Antithrombotic Therapy[2]	91	97%	99%	99%
Discharged on Statin Medication[2]	78	96%	94%	94%
Thrombolytic Therapy Timing[2]	12	100%	72%	66%
Venous Thromboembolism Prophylaxis[2]	90	97%	94%	94%
Written Stroke Educational Materials Given[2]	54	100%	87%	88%
Surgical Care Improvement Project				
Appropriate Beta Blocker Usage[2]	124	100%	97%	98%
Appropriate VTP Within 24 Hours[2]	381	100%	98%	98%
Controlled Postoperative Blood Glucose[2,7]	-	-	96%	97%
Perioperative Temperature Management[2]	461	100%	100%	100%
Prophylactic Antibiotic Selection[2]	312	98%	99%	99%
Prophylactic Antibiotic Selection (Outpatient)	-	-	97%	98%
Prophylactic Antibiotic Stopped[2]	306	99%	98%	98%
Prophylactic Antibiotic Timing[2]	313	99%	99%	99%
Prophylactic Antibiotic Timing (Outpatient)	-	-	97%	98%
Urinary Catheter Removal[2]	301	100%	97%	97%
Survey of Patients' Hospital Experiences				
Area Around Room 'Always' Quiet at Night	300+	56%	51%	61%
Doctors 'Always' Communicated Well	300+	83%	78%	82%
Home Recovery Information Given	300+	88%	83%	85%
Hospital Given 9 or 10 on 10 Point Scale	300+	77%	68%	71%
Meds 'Always' Explained Before Given	300+	61%	61%	64%
Nurses 'Always' Communicated Well	300+	75%	74%	79%
Pain 'Always' Well Controlled	300+	70%	68%	71%
Room and Bathroom 'Always' Clean	300+	75%	70%	73%
Timely Help 'Always' Received	300+	64%	62%	68%
Would Definitely Recommend Hospital	300+	81%	70%	71%
Use of Medical Imaging				
Cardiac Imaging Stress Test before Surgery	-	-	5.2%	5.3%
Combination Abdominal CT Scan	-	-	13.4%	10.5%
Combination Brain/Sinus CT Scan	-	-	2.2%	2.7%
Combination Chest CT Scan	-	-	2.3%	2.7%
Follow-up Mammogram/Ultrasound	-	-	8.2%	8.8%
Lumbar Spine MRI for Low Back Pain	-	-	34.2%	37.2%

Sutter Delta Medical Center

3901 Lone Tree Way
Antioch, CA 94509
Phone: 925-779-7200
Fax: 925-779-7276
E-mail: monfort@sutterdelta.org
URL: www.sutterdelta.org
Type: Acute Care Hospitals
Emergency Services: Yes
Ownership: Voluntary non-profit - Private
Beds: 111

Key Personnel:

Radiology. . . . . Richard B Baxter, MD
Pediatric Ambulatory Care . . . . . . Lance Gershen, MD
Pediatric In-Patient Care . . . . Lance Gershen, MD
CEO/President. . . . . Linda Horn
Emergency Room . . . . Allison Mielicke
Chief of Medical Staff. . . . . Sanjay Ray, MD

Measure	Cases	This Hosp.	State Avg.	U.S. Avg.
Blood Clot Prevention and Treatment				
Anticoagulation Overlap Therapy[2]	37	92%	92%	93%
ICU Venous Thromboembolism Prophylaxis[2]	63	98%	92%	92%
Incidence of Potentially Preventable VTE[1,2]	-	-	11%	10%
UFH with Dosages/Platelet Monitoring[2]	17	100%	96%	97%
Venous Thromboembolism Prophylaxis[2]	362	82%	83%	85%
Warfarin Therapy Discharge Instructions[2]	29	48%	75%	75%
Chest Pain/Possible Heart Attack Care				
Aspirin Given Within 24 Hours of Arrival[1]	-	-	97%	96%
Fibrinolytic Meds Within 30 Min. of Arrival[3,7]	-	-	62%	58%
Average Time to ECG (minutes)[1]	-	-	9	7
Average Time to Transfer (minutes)[1,3]	-	-	62	60
Children's Asthma Care				
Received Home Management Plan of Care	-	-	88%	88%
Received Reliever Medication	-	-	100%	100%
Received Systemic Corticosteroids	-	-	100%	100%
Emergency Department				
Admittance Decision Time (minutes)[2]	704	160	125	98
Head CT Results Within 45 Min. of Arrival[1]	-	-	55%	57%
Patients Who Left ER Before Being Seen	55,628	3%	3%	2%
Time from ER Arrival to Admit. (minutes)[2]	736	358	323	274
Time from ER Arrival to Discharge (minutes)	371	154	168	134
Time in ER Before Being Evaluated (minutes)	381	28	29	26
Time to Pain Meds for Fractures (minutes)	174	63	62	57
Heart Attack Care				
Aspirin Given at Discharge	121	99%	99%	99%
Fibrinolytic Meds Within 30 Min. of Arrival[7]	-	-	73%	54%
PCI Within 90 Minutes of Arrival	39	97%	95%	96%
Statin Prescribed at Discharge	121	96%	98%	98%
Heart Failure Care				
ACE Inhibitor or ARB for LVSD[2]	71	97%	97%	97%
Discharge Instructions Given[2]	237	96%	94%	94%
Evaluation of LVS Function[2]	264	100%	99%	99%
Medicare Spending				
Medicare Spending per Patient (ratio)	-	0.95	0.98	0.98
Pneumonia Care				
Appropriate Initial Antibiotic Given[2]	121	98%	97%	95%
Blood Culture Timing[2]	175	97%	98%	98%
Pregnancy and Delivery Care				
Newborn Deliveries Scheduled Early	88	3%	5%	6%
Preventive Care				
Immunization for Influenza[2]	520	89%	89%	90%
Immunization for Pneumonia[2]	636	92%	90%	92%
Stroke Care				
Anticoagulation Therapy for Atrial Fibrillation	11	91%	95%	95%
Antithrombotic Therapy Timing	58	97%	98%	98%
Assessed for Rehabilitation	63	90%	97%	97%
Discharged on Antithrombotic Therapy	60	97%	99%	99%
Discharged on Statin Medication	49	96%	94%	94%
Thrombolytic Therapy Timing[1]	-	-	72%	66%
Venous Thromboembolism Prophylaxis	65	89%	94%	94%
Written Stroke Educational Materials Given	44	45%	87%	88%
Surgical Care Improvement Project				
Appropriate Beta Blocker Usage[2]	59	95%	97%	98%
Appropriate VTP Within 24 Hours[2]	193	98%	98%	98%
Controlled Postoperative Blood Glucose[2,7]	-	-	96%	97%
Perioperative Temperature Management[2]	215	100%	100%	100%
Prophylactic Antibiotic Selection[2]	100	97%	99%	99%
Prophylactic Antibiotic Selection (Outpatient)	56	95%	97%	98%
Prophylactic Antibiotic Stopped[2]	94	95%	98%	98%
Prophylactic Antibiotic Timing[2]	101	95%	99%	99%
Prophylactic Antibiotic Timing (Outpatient)	55	93%	97%	98%
Urinary Catheter Removal[2]	97	90%	97%	97%
Survey of Patients' Hospital Experiences				
Area Around Room 'Always' Quiet at Night	(a)	49%	51%	61%
Doctors 'Always' Communicated Well	(a)	80%	78%	82%
Home Recovery Information Given	(a)	82%	83%	85%
Hospital Given 9 or 10 on 10 Point Scale	(a)	57%	68%	71%
Meds 'Always' Explained Before Given	(a)	55%	61%	64%
Nurses 'Always' Communicated Well	(a)	74%	74%	79%
Pain 'Always' Well Controlled	(a)	73%	68%	71%
Room and Bathroom 'Always' Clean	(a)	68%	70%	73%
Timely Help 'Always' Received	(a)	60%	62%	68%
Would Definitely Recommend Hospital	(a)	60%	70%	71%
Use of Medical Imaging				
Cardiac Imaging Stress Test before Surgery	115	2.6%	5.2%	5.3%
Combination Abdominal CT Scan	338	3.0%	13.4%	10.5%
Combination Brain/Sinus CT Scan	447	1.3%	2.2%	2.7%
Combination Chest CT Scan	92	0.0%	2.3%	2.7%
Follow-up Mammogram/Ultrasound	520	7.9%	8.2%	8.8%
Lumbar Spine MRI for Low Back Pain[1]	-	-	34.2%	37.2%

Saint Mary Medical Center

18300 Highway 18
Apple Valley, CA 92307
Phone: 760-242-2311
Fax: 760-242-9750
URL: www.stmaryapplevalley.com
Type: Acute Care Hospitals
Emergency Services: Yes
Ownership: Voluntary non-profit - Private
Beds: 186

Key Personnel:

Chief of Medical Staff. . . . . Nanda Biswas, MD
President/CEO. . . . . Alan H. Garrett
Emergency Room . . . . Rick Smith

Measure	Cases	This Hosp.	State Avg.	U.S. Avg.
Blood Clot Prevention and Treatment				
Anticoagulation Overlap Therapy[2]	115	97%	92%	93%
ICU Venous Thromboembolism Prophylaxis[2]	71	94%	92%	92%
Incidence of Potentially Preventable VTE[2]	19	11%	11%	10%
UFH with Dosages/Platelet Monitoring[2]	24	100%	96%	97%
Venous Thromboembolism Prophylaxis[2]	336	85%	83%	85%
Warfarin Therapy Discharge Instructions[2]	81	77%	75%	75%
Chest Pain/Possible Heart Attack Care				
Aspirin Given Within 24 Hours of Arrival	46	93%	97%	96%
Fibrinolytic Meds Within 30 Min. of Arrival[3,7]	-	-	62%	58%
Average Time to ECG (minutes)	47	5	9	7

NOTE: Hospital profiles are in alphabetical order by state, then city, then hospital within the city; Rankings exclude hospitals with less than 25 cases except for patient surveys which excludes hospitals with less than 100 cases; (a) 100-299 cases; (1) The number of cases/patients is too few to report; (2) Data submitted were based on a sample of cases/patients; (3) Results are based on a shorter time period than required; (4) Data suppressed by CMS for one or more quarters; (5) Results are not available for this reporting period; (6) Fewer than 100 patients completed the HCAHPS survey; (7) No cases met the criteria for this measure; (8) The lower limit of the confidence interval cannot be calculated if the number of observed infections equals zero; (9) No data are available from the state/territory for this reporting period; (10) The scores shown reflect fewer than 50 completed surveys; (11) There were discrepancies in the data collection process; (12) This measure does not apply to this hospital for this reporting period; (13) Results cannot be calculated for this reporting period; (14) The results for this state are combined with nearby states to protect confidentiality; Please refer to the User's Guide for a full explanation of data.

Measure	Cases	This Hosp.	State Avg.	U.S. Avg.
Average Time to Transfer (minutes)[3,7]	-	-	62	60
Children's Asthma Care				
Received Home Management Plan of Care	-	-	88%	88%
Received Reliever Medication	-	-	100%	100%
Received Systemic Corticosteroids	-	-	100%	100%
Emergency Department				
Admittance Decision Time (minutes)[2]	784	255	125	98
Head CT Results Within 45 Min. of Arrival	31	23%	55%	57%
Patients Who Left ER Before Being Seen	81,050	2%	3%	2%
Time from ER Arrival to Admit. (minutes)[2]	784	495	323	274
Time from ER Arrival to Discharge (minutes)	371	188	168	134
Time in ER Before Being Evaluated (minutes)	403	34	29	26
Time to Pain Meds for Fractures (minutes)	208	70	62	57
Heart Attack Care				
Aspirin Given at Discharge[2]	226	100%	99%	99%
Fibrinolytic Meds Within 30 Min. of Arrival[2,7]	-	-	73%	54%
PCI Within 90 Minutes of Arrival[2]	34	100%	95%	96%
Statin Prescribed at Discharge[2]	235	100%	98%	98%
Heart Failure Care				
ACE Inhibitor or ARB for LVSD[2]	110	95%	97%	97%
Discharge Instructions Given[2]	240	96%	94%	94%
Evaluation of LVS Function[2]	262	99%	99%	99%
Medicare Spending				
Medicare Spending per Patient (ratio)	-	0.96	0.98	0.98
Pneumonia Care				
Appropriate Initial Antibiotic Given[2]	84	98%	97%	95%
Blood Culture Timing[2]	138	97%	98%	98%
Pregnancy and Delivery Care				
Newborn Deliveries Scheduled Early	336	7%	5%	6%
Preventive Care				
Immunization for Influenza[2]	500	97%	89%	90%
Immunization for Pneumonia[2]	603	97%	90%	92%
Stroke Care				
Anticoagulation Therapy for Atrial Fibrillation	12	100%	95%	95%
Antithrombotic Therapy Timing	142	100%	98%	98%
Assessed for Rehabilitation	141	90%	97%	97%
Discharged on Antithrombotic Therapy	129	100%	99%	99%
Discharged on Statin Medication	98	96%	94%	94%
Thrombolytic Therapy Timing[1]	-	-	72%	66%
Venous Thromboembolism Prophylaxis	154	96%	94%	94%
Written Stroke Educational Materials Given	98	98%	87%	88%
Surgical Care Improvement Project				
Appropriate Beta Blocker Usage	237	99%	97%	98%
Appropriate VTP Within 24 Hours	515	100%	98%	98%
Controlled Postoperative Blood Glucose	125	99%	96%	97%
Perioperative Temperature Management	721	100%	100%	100%
Prophylactic Antibiotic Selection	413	96%	99%	99%
Prophylactic Antibiotic Selection (Outpatient)	157	96%	97%	98%
Prophylactic Antibiotic Stopped	382	97%	98%	98%
Prophylactic Antibiotic Timing	416	98%	99%	99%
Prophylactic Antibiotic Timing (Outpatient)	160	98%	97%	98%
Urinary Catheter Removal	365	98%	97%	97%
Survey of Patients' Hospital Experiences				
Area Around Room 'Always' Quiet at Night	300+	41%	51%	61%
Doctors 'Always' Communicated Well	300+	72%	78%	82%
Home Recovery Information Given	300+	81%	83%	85%
Hospital Given 9 or 10 on 10 Point Scale	300+	64%	68%	71%
Meds 'Always' Explained Before Given	300+	56%	61%	64%
Nurses 'Always' Communicated Well	300+	70%	74%	79%
Pain 'Always' Well Controlled	300+	66%	68%	71%
Room and Bathroom 'Always' Clean	300+	61%	70%	73%
Timely Help 'Always' Received	300+	52%	62%	68%
Would Definitely Recommend Hospital	300+	69%	70%	71%
Use of Medical Imaging				
Cardiac Imaging Stress Test before Surgery	282	3.9%	5.2%	5.3%
Combination Abdominal CT Scan	621	3.5%	13.4%	10.5%
Combination Brain/Sinus CT Scan	580	0.5%	2.2%	2.7%
Combination Chest CT Scan	149	4.7%	2.3%	2.7%
Follow-up Mammogram/Ultrasound	246	5.3%	8.2%	8.8%
Lumbar Spine MRI for Low Back Pain[1]	-	-	34.2%	37.2%

Methodist Hospital of Southern California

300 W Huntington Dr
Arcadia, CA 91006
E-mail: info@methodisthospital.org
URL: www.methodisthospital.org
Type: Acute Care Hospitals
Ownership: Voluntary non-profit - Church
Phone: 626-445-4441
Fax: 626-574-3767
Emergency Services: Yes
Beds: 460

Key Personnel:
CEO/President. . . . . Dan F. Ausman
Chief of Medical Staff . . . . B.S. Chandrasekhar, MD
Quality Assurance . . . . Claire Hanks
Intensive Care Unit. . . . . Delia Jervis, RN
Infection Control. . . . . Pauline Lopez, RN
Radiology. . . . . Joseph Lussier
Pediatric Ambulatory Care . . . . . . Hargurmeet Sandhu, MD
Pediatric In-Patient Care . . . . Hargurmeet Sandhu, MD

Measure	Cases	This Hosp.	State Avg.	U.S. Avg.
Blood Clot Prevention and Treatment				
Anticoagulation Overlap Therapy[2]	78	99%	92%	93%
ICU Venous Thromboembolism Prophylaxis[2]	74	91%	92%	92%
Incidence of Potentially Preventable VTE[1,2]	-	-	11%	10%
UFH with Dosages/Platelet Monitoring[2]	28	100%	96%	97%
Venous Thromboembolism Prophylaxis[2]	339	79%	83%	85%
Warfarin Therapy Discharge Instructions[2]	46	78%	75%	75%
Chest Pain/Possible Heart Attack Care				
Aspirin Given Within 24 Hours of Arrival[1]	-	-	97%	96%
Fibrinolytic Meds Within 30 Min. of Arrival[3,7]	-	-	62%	58%
Average Time to ECG (minutes)[1]	-	-	9	7
Average Time to Transfer (minutes)[3,7]	-	-	62	60
Children's Asthma Care				
Received Home Management Plan of Care	-	-	88%	88%
Received Reliever Medication	-	-	100%	100%
Received Systemic Corticosteroids	-	-	100%	100%
Emergency Department				
Admittance Decision Time (minutes)[2]	747	116	125	98
Head CT Results Within 45 Min. of Arrival	11	45%	55%	57%
Patients Who Left ER Before Being Seen	42,996	2%	3%	2%
Time from ER Arrival to Admit. (minutes)[2]	751	286	323	274
Time from ER Arrival to Discharge (minutes)	394	180	168	134
Time in ER Before Being Evaluated (minutes)	414	27	29	26
Time to Pain Meds for Fractures (minutes)	250	44	62	57
Heart Attack Care				
Aspirin Given at Discharge	194	100%	99%	99%
Fibrinolytic Meds Within 30 Min. of Arrival[7]	-	-	73%	54%
PCI Within 90 Minutes of Arrival	49	100%	95%	96%
Statin Prescribed at Discharge	195	100%	98%	98%
Heart Failure Care				
ACE Inhibitor or ARB for LVSD	85	100%	97%	97%
Discharge Instructions Given	267	99%	94%	94%
Evaluation of LVS Function	380	99%	99%	99%
Medicare Spending				
Medicare Spending per Patient (ratio)	-	1.04	0.98	0.98
Pneumonia Care				
Appropriate Initial Antibiotic Given	230	98%	97%	95%
Blood Culture Timing	353	99%	98%	98%
Pregnancy and Delivery Care				
Newborn Deliveries Scheduled Early[2]	217	2%	5%	6%
Preventive Care				
Immunization for Influenza[2]	558	92%	89%	90%
Immunization for Pneumonia[2]	713	91%	90%	92%
Stroke Care				
Anticoagulation Therapy for Atrial Fibrillation	26	100%	95%	95%
Antithrombotic Therapy Timing	179	100%	98%	98%
Assessed for Rehabilitation	224	100%	97%	97%
Discharged on Antithrombotic Therapy	194	100%	99%	99%
Discharged on Statin Medication	160	100%	94%	94%
Thrombolytic Therapy Timing	24	96%	72%	66%
Venous Thromboembolism Prophylaxis	239	100%	94%	94%
Written Stroke Educational Materials Given	120	99%	87%	88%
Surgical Care Improvement Project				
Appropriate Beta Blocker Usage[2]	145	93%	97%	98%
Appropriate VTP Within 24 Hours[2]	445	96%	98%	98%
Controlled Postoperative Blood Glucose[2]	50	96%	96%	97%
Perioperative Temperature Management[2]	546	100%	100%	100%
Prophylactic Antibiotic Selection[2]	372	97%	99%	99%
Prophylactic Antibiotic Selection (Outpatient)	222	93%	97%	98%
Prophylactic Antibiotic Stopped[2]	350	94%	98%	98%
Prophylactic Antibiotic Timing[2]	372	100%	99%	99%
Prophylactic Antibiotic Timing (Outpatient)	224	96%	97%	98%
Urinary Catheter Removal[2]	355	92%	97%	97%
Survey of Patients' Hospital Experiences				
Area Around Room 'Always' Quiet at Night	300+	50%	51%	61%
Doctors 'Always' Communicated Well	300+	80%	78%	82%
Home Recovery Information Given	300+	79%	83%	85%
Hospital Given 9 or 10 on 10 Point Scale	300+	75%	68%	71%
Meds 'Always' Explained Before Given	300+	62%	61%	64%
Nurses 'Always' Communicated Well	300+	74%	74%	79%
Pain 'Always' Well Controlled	300+	67%	68%	71%
Room and Bathroom 'Always' Clean	300+	75%	70%	73%
Timely Help 'Always' Received	300+	56%	62%	68%
Would Definitely Recommend Hospital	300+	78%	70%	71%
Use of Medical Imaging				
Cardiac Imaging Stress Test before Surgery	227	6.6%	5.2%	5.3%
Combination Abdominal CT Scan	498	0.2%	13.4%	10.5%
Combination Brain/Sinus CT Scan	804	2.4%	2.2%	2.7%
Combination Chest CT Scan	199	0.0%	2.3%	2.7%
Follow-up Mammogram/Ultrasound	106	10.4%	8.2%	8.8%
Lumbar Spine MRI for Low Back Pain[1]	-	-	34.2%	37.2%

Mad River Community Hospital

3800 Janes Rd
Arcata, CA 95521
E-mail: mrch@madriverhospital.com
URL: www.madriverhospital.com
Type: Acute Care Hospitals
Ownership: Proprietary
Phone: 707-822-3621
Fax: 707-822-6311
Emergency Services: No
Beds: 78

Key Personnel:
Hemotology Center . . . . Renee Blumenthal
Quality Assurance . . . . Steve Engle
Chief of Medical Staff . . . . Gary Garcia
Anesthesiology. . . . . Sara Isaacson
Emergency Room . . . . Donna Iverson
CEO/President. . . . . Douglas Shaw
Infection Control. . . . . Ken ifer Terpening

Measure	Cases	This Hosp.	State Avg.	U.S. Avg.
Blood Clot Prevention and Treatment				
Anticoagulation Overlap Therapy[1,2]	-	-	92%	93%
ICU Venous Thromboembolism Prophylaxis[2]	33	91%	92%	92%
Incidence of Potentially Preventable VTE[2,7]	-	-	11%	10%
UFH with Dosages/Platelet Monitoring[1,2]	-	-	96%	97%
Venous Thromboembolism Prophylaxis[2]	116	73%	83%	85%
Warfarin Therapy Discharge Instructions[1,2]	-	-	75%	75%
Chest Pain/Possible Heart Attack Care				
Aspirin Given Within 24 Hours of Arrival	26	96%	97%	96%
Fibrinolytic Meds Within 30 Min. of Arrival[1]	-	-	62%	58%
Average Time to ECG (minutes)	26	12	9	7
Average Time to Transfer (minutes)[1]	-	-	62	60
Children's Asthma Care				
Received Home Management Plan of Care	-	-	88%	88%
Received Reliever Medication	-	-	100%	100%
Received Systemic Corticosteroids	-	-	100%	100%
Emergency Department				
Admittance Decision Time (minutes)[2]	305	105	125	98
Head CT Results Within 45 Min. of Arrival[1]	-	-	55%	57%
Patients Who Left ER Before Being Seen	15,811	3%	3%	2%
Time from ER Arrival to Admit. (minutes)[2]	306	310	323	274
Time from ER Arrival to Discharge (minutes)	280	125	168	134
Time in ER Before Being Evaluated (minutes)	369	31	29	26
Time to Pain Meds for Fractures (minutes)	85	72	62	57
Heart Attack Care				
Aspirin Given at Discharge[1]	-	-	99%	99%
Fibrinolytic Meds Within 30 Min. of Arrival[7]	-	-	73%	54%
PCI Within 90 Minutes of Arrival[7]	-	-	95%	96%
Statin Prescribed at Discharge[1]	-	-	98%	98%
Heart Failure Care				
ACE Inhibitor or ARB for LVSD	14	86%	97%	97%
Discharge Instructions Given	26	96%	94%	94%
Evaluation of LVS Function	28	96%	99%	99%

NOTE: Hospital profiles are in alphabetical order by state, then city, then hospital within the city; Rankings exclude hospitals with less than 25 cases except for patient surveys which excludes hospitals with less than 100 cases; (a) 100-299 cases; (1) The number of cases/patients is too few to report; (2) Data submitted were based on a sample of cases/patients; (3) Results are based on a shorter time period than required; (4) Data suppressed by CMS for one or more quarters; (5) Results are not available for this reporting period; (6) Fewer than 100 patients completed the HCAHPS survey; (7) No cases met the criteria for this measure; (8) The lower limit of the confidence interval cannot be calculated if the number of observed infections equals zero; (9) No data are available from the state/territory for this reporting period; (10) The scores shown reflect fewer than 50 completed surveys; (11) There were discrepancies in the data collection process; (12) This measure does not apply to this hospital for this reporting period; (13) Results cannot be calculated for this reporting period; (14) The results for this state are combined with nearby states to protect confidentiality; Please refer to the User's Guide for a full explanation of data.

Measure	Cases	This Hosp.	State Avg.	U.S. Avg.
Medicare Spending				
Medicare Spending per Patient (ratio)	-	0.91	0.98	0.98
Pneumonia Care				
Appropriate Initial Antibiotic Given	53	89%	97%	95%
Blood Culture Timing	68	96%	98%	98%
Pregnancy and Delivery Care				
Newborn Deliveries Scheduled Early[2]	14	0%	5%	6%
Preventive Care				
Immunization for Influenza[2]	222	61%	89%	90%
Immunization for Pneumonia[2]	193	83%	90%	92%
Stroke Care				
Anticoagulation Therapy for Atrial Fibrillation[7]	-	-	95%	95%
Antithrombotic Therapy Timing[1]	-	-	98%	98%
Assessed for Rehabilitation	13	92%	97%	97%
Discharged on Antithrombotic Therapy	11	91%	99%	99%
Discharged on Statin Medication[1]	-	-	94%	94%
Thrombolytic Therapy Timing[1]	-	-	72%	66%
Venous Thromboembolism Prophylaxis	17	76%	94%	94%
Written Stroke Educational Materials Given[1]	-	-	87%	88%
Surgical Care Improvement Project				
Appropriate Beta Blocker Usage[1,2]	-	-	97%	98%
Appropriate VTP Within 24 Hours[2]	45	87%	98%	98%
Controlled Postoperative Blood Glucose[2,7]	-	-	96%	97%
Perioperative Temperature Management[2]	52	100%	100%	100%
Prophylactic Antibiotic Selection[2]	23	83%	99%	99%
Prophylactic Antibiotic Selection (Outpatient)[1,3]	-	-	97%	98%
Prophylactic Antibiotic Stopped[2]	23	96%	98%	98%
Prophylactic Antibiotic Timing[2]	23	96%	99%	99%
Prophylactic Antibiotic Timing (Outpatient)[1,3]	-	-	97%	98%
Urinary Catheter Removal[2]	16	81%	97%	97%
Survey of Patients' Hospital Experiences				
Area Around Room 'Always' Quiet at Night	300+	45%	51%	61%
Doctors 'Always' Communicated Well	300+	74%	78%	82%
Home Recovery Information Given	300+	87%	83%	85%
Hospital Given 9 or 10 on 10 Point Scale	300+	65%	68%	71%
Meds 'Always' Explained Before Given	300+	62%	61%	64%
Nurses 'Always' Communicated Well	300+	77%	74%	79%
Pain 'Always' Well Controlled	300+	70%	68%	71%
Room and Bathroom 'Always' Clean	300+	74%	70%	73%
Timely Help 'Always' Received	300+	69%	62%	68%
Would Definitely Recommend Hospital	300+	72%	70%	71%
Use of Medical Imaging				
Cardiac Imaging Stress Test before Surgery[1]	-	-	5.2%	5.3%
Combination Abdominal CT Scan	246	6.5%	13.4%	10.5%
Combination Brain/Sinus CT Scan[1]	-	-	2.2%	2.7%
Combination Chest CT Scan	108	8.3%	2.3%	2.7%
Follow-up Mammogram/Ultrasound	565	5.1%	8.2%	8.8%
Lumbar Spine MRI for Low Back Pain[1]	-	-	34.2%	37.2%

Sutter Auburn Faith Hospital

11815 Education Street
Auburn, CA 95603
URL: www.sutterauburnfaith.org
Phone: 530-888-4500
Fax: 530-889-6054
Type: Acute Care Hospitals
Emergency Services: Yes
Ownership: Voluntary non-profit - Other
Beds: 110

Key Personnel:
President . . . . James Conforti
Administrator . . . . Patrick Fry
CEO . . . . Christopher Johnson
Radiology. . . . . Vartan Malian
Emergency Room . . . . Lisa Ralston
Operating Room. . . . . Debbie Roberston
Quality Assurance . . . . Kathie Wolf

Measure	Cases	This Hosp.	State Avg.	U.S. Avg.
Blood Clot Prevention and Treatment				
Anticoagulation Overlap Therapy[2]	26	100%	92%	93%
ICU Venous Thromboembolism Prophylaxis[2]	64	98%	92%	92%
Incidence of Potentially Preventable VTE[1,2]	-	-	11%	10%
UFH with Dosages/Platelet Monitoring[1,2]	-	-	96%	97%
Venous Thromboembolism Prophylaxis[2]	276	88%	83%	85%
Warfarin Therapy Discharge Instructions[2]	16	100%	75%	75%
Chest Pain/Possible Heart Attack Care				
Aspirin Given Within 24 Hours of Arrival	45	100%	97%	96%
Fibrinolytic Meds Within 30 Min. of Arrival[7]	-	-	62%	58%
Average Time to ECG (minutes)	44	2	9	7
Average Time to Transfer (minutes)	11	43	62	60
Children's Asthma Care				
Received Home Management Plan of Care	-	-	88%	88%
Received Reliever Medication	-	-	100%	100%
Received Systemic Corticosteroids	-	-	100%	100%
Emergency Department				
Admittance Decision Time (minutes)[2]	642	151	125	98
Head CT Results Within 45 Min. of Arrival[1]	-	-	55%	57%
Patients Who Left ER Before Being Seen	>100k	0%	3%	2%
Time from ER Arrival to Admit. (minutes)[2]	642	321	323	274
Time from ER Arrival to Discharge (minutes)	370	152	168	134
Time in ER Before Being Evaluated (minutes)	407	33	29	26
Time to Pain Meds for Fractures (minutes)	143	60	62	57
Heart Attack Care				
Aspirin Given at Discharge	18	100%	99%	99%
Fibrinolytic Meds Within 30 Min. of Arrival[7]	-	-	73%	54%
PCI Within 90 Minutes of Arrival[7]	-	-	95%	96%
Statin Prescribed at Discharge	19	100%	98%	98%
Heart Failure Care				
ACE Inhibitor or ARB for LVSD	20	100%	97%	97%
Discharge Instructions Given	59	100%	94%	94%
Evaluation of LVS Function	83	100%	99%	99%
Medicare Spending				
Medicare Spending per Patient (ratio)	-	0.94	0.98	0.98
Pneumonia Care				
Appropriate Initial Antibiotic Given[2]	69	99%	97%	95%
Blood Culture Timing[2]	131	100%	98%	98%
Pregnancy and Delivery Care				
Newborn Deliveries Scheduled Early[7]	-	-	5%	6%
Preventive Care				
Immunization for Influenza[2]	404	95%	89%	90%
Immunization for Pneumonia[2]	606	95%	90%	92%
Stroke Care				
Anticoagulation Therapy for Atrial Fibrillation	12	92%	95%	95%
Antithrombotic Therapy Timing	46	100%	98%	98%
Assessed for Rehabilitation	61	100%	97%	97%
Discharged on Antithrombotic Therapy	58	100%	99%	99%
Discharged on Statin Medication	44	100%	94%	94%
Thrombolytic Therapy Timing[1]	-	-	72%	66%
Venous Thromboembolism Prophylaxis	50	100%	94%	94%
Written Stroke Educational Materials Given	31	100%	87%	88%
Surgical Care Improvement Project				
Appropriate Beta Blocker Usage[2]	95	99%	97%	98%
Appropriate VTP Within 24 Hours[2]	322	97%	98%	98%
Controlled Postoperative Blood Glucose[2,7]	-	-	96%	97%
Perioperative Temperature Management[2]	392	100%	100%	100%
Prophylactic Antibiotic Selection[2]	250	100%	99%	99%
Prophylactic Antibiotic Selection (Outpatient)	57	93%	97%	98%
Prophylactic Antibiotic Stopped[2]	245	98%	98%	98%
Prophylactic Antibiotic Timing[2]	250	99%	99%	99%
Prophylactic Antibiotic Timing (Outpatient)	56	96%	97%	98%
Urinary Catheter Removal[2]	262	98%	97%	97%
Survey of Patients' Hospital Experiences				
Area Around Room 'Always' Quiet at Night	300+	50%	51%	61%
Doctors 'Always' Communicated Well	300+	84%	78%	82%
Home Recovery Information Given	300+	85%	83%	85%
Hospital Given 9 or 10 on 10 Point Scale	300+	75%	68%	71%
Meds 'Always' Explained Before Given	300+	66%	61%	64%
Nurses 'Always' Communicated Well	300+	79%	74%	79%
Pain 'Always' Well Controlled	300+	73%	68%	71%
Room and Bathroom 'Always' Clean	300+	79%	70%	73%
Timely Help 'Always' Received	300+	63%	62%	68%
Would Definitely Recommend Hospital	300+	77%	70%	71%
Use of Medical Imaging				
Cardiac Imaging Stress Test before Surgery	204	5.9%	5.2%	5.3%
Combination Abdominal CT Scan	333	4.5%	13.4%	10.5%
Combination Brain/Sinus CT Scan	356	1.7%	2.2%	2.7%
Combination Chest CT Scan	242	1.7%	2.3%	2.7%
Follow-up Mammogram/Ultrasound	484	19.4%	8.2%	8.8%
Lumbar Spine MRI for Low Back Pain[1]	-	-	34.2%	37.2%

Catalina Island Medical Center

100 Falls Canyon Road
Avalon, CA 90704
Phone: 310-510-0700
Fax: 310-510-2938
Type: Critical Access Hospitals
Emergency Services: No
Ownership: Voluntary non-profit - Church
Beds: 12

Key Personnel:
Infection Control. . . . . Judy Alft, RN
CEO . . . . John Friel
Quality Assurance . . . . Doreen Macktah, RN
Chief of Medical Staff . . . . Doreen Macktal, MD

Measure	Cases	This Hosp.	State Avg.	U.S. Avg.
Blood Clot Prevention and Treatment				
Anticoagulation Overlap Therapy[5]	-	-	92%	93%
ICU Venous Thromboembolism Prophylaxis[5]	-	-	92%	92%
Incidence of Potentially Preventable VTE[5]	-	-	11%	10%
UFH with Dosages/Platelet Monitoring[5]	-	-	96%	97%
Venous Thromboembolism Prophylaxis[5]	-	-	83%	85%
Warfarin Therapy Discharge Instructions[5]	-	-	75%	75%
Chest Pain/Possible Heart Attack Care				
Aspirin Given Within 24 Hours of Arrival	-	-	97%	96%
Fibrinolytic Meds Within 30 Min. of Arrival	-	-	62%	58%
Average Time to ECG (minutes)	-	-	9	7
Average Time to Transfer (minutes)	-	-	62	60
Children's Asthma Care				
Received Home Management Plan of Care	-	-	88%	88%
Received Reliever Medication	-	-	100%	100%
Received Systemic Corticosteroids	-	-	100%	100%
Emergency Department				
Admittance Decision Time (minutes)[5]	-	-	125	98
Head CT Results Within 45 Min. of Arrival	-	-	55%	57%
Patients Who Left ER Before Being Seen	-	-	3%	2%
Time from ER Arrival to Admit. (minutes)[5]	-	-	323	274
Time from ER Arrival to Discharge (minutes)	-	-	168	134
Time in ER Before Being Evaluated (minutes)	-	-	29	26
Time to Pain Meds for Fractures (minutes)	-	-	62	57
Heart Attack Care				
Aspirin Given at Discharge[5]	-	-	99%	99%
Fibrinolytic Meds Within 30 Min. of Arrival[5]	-	-	73%	54%
PCI Within 90 Minutes of Arrival[5]	-	-	95%	96%
Statin Prescribed at Discharge[5]	-	-	98%	98%
Heart Failure Care				
ACE Inhibitor or ARB for LVSD[5]	-	-	97%	97%
Discharge Instructions Given[5]	-	-	94%	94%
Evaluation of LVS Function[5]	-	-	99%	99%
Medicare Spending				
Medicare Spending per Patient (ratio)	-	-	0.98	0.98
Pneumonia Care				
Appropriate Initial Antibiotic Given[2,3]	-	-	97%	95%
Blood Culture Timing[2,3]	-	-	98%	98%
Pregnancy and Delivery Care				
Newborn Deliveries Scheduled Early[5]	-	-	5%	6%
Preventive Care				
Immunization for Influenza[5]	-	-	89%	90%
Immunization for Pneumonia[5]	-	-	90%	92%
Stroke Care				
Anticoagulation Therapy for Atrial Fibrillation[5]	-	-	95%	95%
Antithrombotic Therapy Timing[5]	-	-	98%	98%
Assessed for Rehabilitation[5]	-	-	97%	97%
Discharged on Antithrombotic Therapy[5]	-	-	99%	99%
Discharged on Statin Medication[5]	-	-	94%	94%
Thrombolytic Therapy Timing[5]	-	-	72%	66%
Venous Thromboembolism Prophylaxis[5]	-	-	94%	94%
Written Stroke Educational Materials Given[5]	-	-	87%	88%
Surgical Care Improvement Project				
Appropriate Beta Blocker Usage[5]	-	-	97%	98%
Appropriate VTP Within 24 Hours[5]	-	-	98%	98%
Controlled Postoperative Blood Glucose[5]	-	-	96%	97%
Perioperative Temperature Management[5]	-	-	100%	100%
Prophylactic Antibiotic Selection[5]	-	-	99%	99%
Prophylactic Antibiotic Selection (Outpatient)	-	-	97%	98%
Prophylactic Antibiotic Stopped[5]	-	-	98%	98%
Prophylactic Antibiotic Timing[5]	-	-	99%	99%
Prophylactic Antibiotic Timing (Outpatient)	-	-	97%	98%

NOTE: Hospital profiles are in alphabetical order by state, then city, then hospital within the city; Rankings exclude hospitals with less than 25 cases except for patient surveys which excludes hospitals with less than 100 cases; (a) 100-299 cases; (1) The number of cases/patients is too few to report; (2) Data submitted were based on a sample of cases/patients; (3) Results are based on a shorter time period than required; (4) Data suppressed by CMS for one or more quarters; (5) Results are not available for this reporting period; (6) Fewer than 100 patients completed the HCAHPS survey; (7) No cases met the criteria for this measure; (8) The lower limit of the confidence interval cannot be calculated if the number of observed infections equals zero; (9) No data are available from the state/territory for this reporting period; (10) The scores shown reflect fewer than 50 completed surveys; (11) There were discrepancies in the data collection process; (12) This measure does not apply to this hospital for this reporting period; (13) Results cannot be calculated for this reporting period; (14) The results for this state are combined with nearby states to protect confidentiality; Please refer to the User's Guide for a full explanation of data.

Measure	Cases	This Hosp.	State Avg.	U.S. Avg.
Urinary Catheter Removal[5]	-	-	97%	97%
Survey of Patients' Hospital Experiences				
Area Around Room 'Always' Quiet at Night[5]	-	-	51%	61%
Doctors 'Always' Communicated Well[5]	-	-	78%	82%
Home Recovery Information Given[5]	-	-	83%	85%
Hospital Given 9 or 10 on 10 Point Scale[5]	-	-	68%	71%
Meds 'Always' Explained Before Given[5]	-	-	61%	64%
Nurses 'Always' Communicated Well[5]	-	-	74%	79%
Pain 'Always' Well Controlled[5]	-	-	68%	71%
Room and Bathroom 'Always' Clean[5]	-	-	70%	73%
Timely Help 'Always' Received[5]	-	-	62%	68%
Would Definitely Recommend Hospital[5]	-	-	70%	71%
Use of Medical Imaging				
Cardiac Imaging Stress Test before Surgery	-	-	5.2%	5.3%
Combination Abdominal CT Scan	-	-	13.4%	10.5%
Combination Brain/Sinus CT Scan	-	-	2.2%	2.7%
Combination Chest CT Scan	-	-	2.3%	2.7%
Follow-up Mammogram/Ultrasound	-	-	8.2%	8.8%
Lumbar Spine MRI for Low Back Pain	-	-	34.2%	37.2%

Bakersfield Heart Hospital

3001 Sillect Avenue Phone: 661-316-6000
Bakersfield, CA 93308
URL: www.bakersfieldhearthospital.com
Type: Acute Care Hospitals Emergency Services: Yes
Ownership: Proprietary Beds: 47
Key Personnel:
CEO/President. . . . . Randall H Rolfe

Measure	Cases	This Hosp.	State Avg.	U.S. Avg.
Blood Clot Prevention and Treatment				
Anticoagulation Overlap Therapy[2]	31	74%	92%	93%
ICU Venous Thromboembolism Prophylaxis[2]	70	56%	92%	92%
Incidence of Potentially Preventable VTE[1,2]	-	-	11%	10%
UFH with Dosages/Platelet Monitoring[2]	14	0%	96%	97%
Venous Thromboembolism Prophylaxis[2]	311	72%	83%	85%
Warfarin Therapy Discharge Instructions[2]	24	58%	75%	75%
Chest Pain/Possible Heart Attack Care				
Aspirin Given Within 24 Hours of Arrival[3]	15	93%	97%	96%
Fibrinolytic Meds Within 30 Min. of Arrival[3,7]	-	-	62%	58%
Average Time to ECG (minutes)[3]	15	7	9	7
Average Time to Transfer (minutes)[3,7]	-	-	62	60
Children's Asthma Care				
Received Home Management Plan of Care	-	-	88%	88%
Received Reliever Medication	-	-	100%	100%
Received Systemic Corticosteroids	-	-	100%	100%
Emergency Department				
Admittance Decision Time (minutes)[2]	510	235	125	98
Head CT Results Within 45 Min. of Arrival[1]	-	-	55%	57%
Patients Who Left ER Before Being Seen	12,375	4%	3%	2%
Time from ER Arrival to Admit. (minutes)[2]	525	397	323	274
Time from ER Arrival to Discharge (minutes)	347	174	168	134
Time in ER Before Being Evaluated (minutes)	290	18	29	26
Time to Pain Meds for Fractures (minutes)	20	64	62	57
Heart Attack Care				
Aspirin Given at Discharge[2]	217	98%	99%	99%
Fibrinolytic Meds Within 30 Min. of Arrival[2,7]	-	-	73%	54%
PCI Within 90 Minutes of Arrival[2]	34	91%	95%	96%
Statin Prescribed at Discharge[2]	206	95%	98%	98%
Heart Failure Care				
ACE Inhibitor or ARB for LVSD[2]	79	91%	97%	97%
Discharge Instructions Given[2]	255	84%	94%	94%
Evaluation of LVS Function[2]	296	100%	99%	99%
Medicare Spending				
Medicare Spending per Patient (ratio)	-	0.95	0.98	0.98
Pneumonia Care				
Appropriate Initial Antibiotic Given[2]	68	93%	97%	95%
Blood Culture Timing[2]	145	96%	98%	98%
Pregnancy and Delivery Care				
Newborn Deliveries Scheduled Early[7]	-	-	5%	6%
Preventive Care				
Immunization for Influenza[2]	374	93%	89%	90%
Immunization for Pneumonia[2]	695	91%	90%	92%
Stroke Care				
Anticoagulation Therapy for Atrial Fibrillation[1]	-	-	95%	95%
Antithrombotic Therapy Timing	36	94%	98%	98%
Assessed for Rehabilitation	43	93%	97%	97%
Discharged on Antithrombotic Therapy	41	95%	99%	99%
Discharged on Statin Medication	30	93%	94%	94%
Thrombolytic Therapy Timing[1]	-	-	72%	66%
Venous Thromboembolism Prophylaxis	40	80%	94%	94%
Written Stroke Educational Materials Given	32	62%	87%	88%
Surgical Care Improvement Project				
Appropriate Beta Blocker Usage[2]	87	94%	97%	98%
Appropriate VTP Within 24 Hours[2]	51	94%	98%	98%
Controlled Postoperative Blood Glucose[2]	97	96%	96%	97%
Perioperative Temperature Management[2]	157	100%	100%	100%
Prophylactic Antibiotic Selection[2]	195	99%	99%	99%
Prophylactic Antibiotic Selection (Outpatient)	226	100%	97%	98%
Prophylactic Antibiotic Stopped[2]	192	96%	98%	98%
Prophylactic Antibiotic Timing[2]	195	99%	99%	99%
Prophylactic Antibiotic Timing (Outpatient)	226	97%	97%	98%
Urinary Catheter Removal[2]	118	88%	97%	97%
Survey of Patients' Hospital Experiences				
Area Around Room 'Always' Quiet at Night	300+	50%	51%	61%
Doctors 'Always' Communicated Well	300+	70%	78%	82%
Home Recovery Information Given	300+	78%	83%	85%
Hospital Given 9 or 10 on 10 Point Scale	300+	74%	68%	71%
Meds 'Always' Explained Before Given	300+	57%	61%	64%
Nurses 'Always' Communicated Well	300+	72%	74%	79%
Pain 'Always' Well Controlled	300+	68%	68%	71%
Room and Bathroom 'Always' Clean	300+	73%	70%	73%
Timely Help 'Always' Received	300+	64%	62%	68%
Would Definitely Recommend Hospital	300+	78%	70%	71%
Use of Medical Imaging				
Cardiac Imaging Stress Test before Surgery	54	1.9%	5.2%	5.3%
Combination Abdominal CT Scan	121	0.8%	13.4%	10.5%
Combination Brain/Sinus CT Scan[1]	-	-	2.2%	2.7%
Combination Chest CT Scan	50	0.0%	2.3%	2.7%
Follow-up Mammogram/Ultrasound[7]	-	-	8.2%	8.8%
Lumbar Spine MRI for Low Back Pain[1]	-	-	34.2%	37.2%

Bakersfield Memorial Hospital

420 34th Saint Box 1888 Phone: 661-327-1792
Bakersfield, CA 93301 Fax: 661-326-0706
URL: www.bakersfieldmemorial.org
Type: Acute Care Hospitals Emergency Services: Yes
Ownership: Voluntary non-profit - Private Beds: 355
Key Personnel:
Quality Assurance . . . . Karen Barnes
Anesthesiology. . . . . Kamalnath Lyer, MD
Chief of Medical Staff. . . . . Robert Marshall, MD
Intensive Care Unit. . . . . Terri Totzke, RN
CEO/President. . . . . Jon Van Boening
Pediatric Ambulatory Care . . . . . . Susan Walker, MD
Pediatric In-Patient Care . . . . Susan Walker, MD

Measure	Cases	This Hosp.	State Avg.	U.S. Avg.
Blood Clot Prevention and Treatment				
Anticoagulation Overlap Therapy[2]	65	94%	92%	93%
ICU Venous Thromboembolism Prophylaxis[2]	67	97%	92%	92%
Incidence of Potentially Preventable VTE[1,2]	-	-	11%	10%
UFH with Dosages/Platelet Monitoring[2]	16	100%	96%	97%
Venous Thromboembolism Prophylaxis[2]	320	97%	83%	85%
Warfarin Therapy Discharge Instructions[2]	44	100%	75%	75%
Chest Pain/Possible Heart Attack Care				
Aspirin Given Within 24 Hours of Arrival[1]	-	-	97%	96%
Fibrinolytic Meds Within 30 Min. of Arrival[5]	-	-	62%	58%
Average Time to ECG (minutes)[1]	-	-	9	7
Average Time to Transfer (minutes)[5]	-	-	62	60
Children's Asthma Care				
Received Home Management Plan of Care	-	-	88%	88%
Received Reliever Medication	-	-	100%	100%
Received Systemic Corticosteroids	-	-	100%	100%
Emergency Department				
Admittance Decision Time (minutes)[2]	654	248	125	98
Head CT Results Within 45 Min. of Arrival[1]	-	-	55%	57%
Patients Who Left ER Before Being Seen	75,277	2%	3%	2%
Time from ER Arrival to Admit. (minutes)[2]	703	435	323	274
Time from ER Arrival to Discharge (minutes)	405	181	168	134
Time in ER Before Being Evaluated (minutes)	419	14	29	26
Time to Pain Meds for Fractures (minutes)	239	78	62	57
Heart Attack Care				
Aspirin Given at Discharge[2]	292	99%	99%	99%
Fibrinolytic Meds Within 30 Min. of Arrival[2,7]	-	-	73%	54%
PCI Within 90 Minutes of Arrival[2]	27	96%	95%	96%
Statin Prescribed at Discharge[2]	287	98%	98%	98%
Heart Failure Care				
ACE Inhibitor or ARB for LVSD[2]	99	97%	97%	97%
Discharge Instructions Given[2]	241	90%	94%	94%
Evaluation of LVS Function[2]	288	99%	99%	99%
Medicare Spending				
Medicare Spending per Patient (ratio)	-	1.04	0.98	0.98
Pneumonia Care				
Appropriate Initial Antibiotic Given[2]	64	97%	97%	95%
Blood Culture Timing[2]	120	96%	98%	98%
Pregnancy and Delivery Care				
Newborn Deliveries Scheduled Early[2]	118	3%	5%	6%
Preventive Care				
Immunization for Influenza[2]	472	94%	89%	90%
Immunization for Pneumonia[2]	452	97%	90%	92%
Stroke Care				
Anticoagulation Therapy for Atrial Fibrillation	19	79%	95%	95%
Antithrombotic Therapy Timing	127	99%	98%	98%
Assessed for Rehabilitation	156	97%	97%	97%
Discharged on Antithrombotic Therapy	136	99%	99%	99%
Discharged on Statin Medication	112	97%	94%	94%
Thrombolytic Therapy Timing[1]	-	-	72%	66%
Venous Thromboembolism Prophylaxis	160	99%	94%	94%
Written Stroke Educational Materials Given	79	99%	87%	88%
Surgical Care Improvement Project				
Appropriate Beta Blocker Usage[2]	255	97%	97%	98%
Appropriate VTP Within 24 Hours[2]	434	99%	98%	98%
Controlled Postoperative Blood Glucose[2]	182	95%	96%	97%
Perioperative Temperature Management[2]	596	100%	100%	100%
Prophylactic Antibiotic Selection[2]	533	100%	99%	99%
Prophylactic Antibiotic Selection (Outpatient)	497	97%	97%	98%
Prophylactic Antibiotic Stopped[2]	506	98%	98%	98%
Prophylactic Antibiotic Timing[2]	533	98%	99%	99%
Prophylactic Antibiotic Timing (Outpatient)	500	98%	97%	98%
Urinary Catheter Removal[2]	377	97%	97%	97%
Survey of Patients' Hospital Experiences				
Area Around Room 'Always' Quiet at Night	300+	51%	51%	61%
Doctors 'Always' Communicated Well	300+	73%	78%	82%
Home Recovery Information Given	300+	83%	83%	85%
Hospital Given 9 or 10 on 10 Point Scale	300+	67%	68%	71%
Meds 'Always' Explained Before Given	300+	59%	61%	64%
Nurses 'Always' Communicated Well	300+	72%	74%	79%
Pain 'Always' Well Controlled	300+	67%	68%	71%
Room and Bathroom 'Always' Clean	300+	72%	70%	73%
Timely Help 'Always' Received	300+	55%	62%	68%
Would Definitely Recommend Hospital	300+	71%	70%	71%
Use of Medical Imaging				
Cardiac Imaging Stress Test before Surgery	80	11.3%	5.2%	5.3%
Combination Abdominal CT Scan	335	2.4%	13.4%	10.5%
Combination Brain/Sinus CT Scan	646	1.7%	2.2%	2.7%
Combination Chest CT Scan	170	0.0%	2.3%	2.7%
Follow-up Mammogram/Ultrasound[7]	-	-	8.2%	8.8%
Lumbar Spine MRI for Low Back Pain[1]	-	-	34.2%	37.2%

Good Samaritan Hospital

901 Olive Drive Phone: 661-399-4461
Bakersfield, CA 93308 Fax: 661-399-4224
Type: Acute Care Hospitals Emergency Services: No
Ownership: Proprietary Beds: 64
Key Personnel:
Chief of Medical Staff. . . . . Ronnie Claiborne
Cardiac Laboratory. . . . . D Estoso, MD
Infection Control. . . . . Linda Head, RN
Operating Room. . . . . Edgare Sangueza
CEO/President. . . . . James Theiring
Anesthesiology. . . . . David Wu

NOTE: Hospital profiles are in alphabetical order by state, then city, then hospital within the city; Rankings exclude hospitals with less than 25 cases except for patient surveys which excludes hospitals with less than 100 cases; (a) 100-299 cases; (1) The number of cases/patients is too few to report; (2) Data submitted were based on a sample of cases/patients; (3) Results are based on a shorter time period than required; (4) Data suppressed by CMS for one or more quarters; (5) Results are not available for this reporting period; (6) Fewer than 100 patients completed the HCAHPS survey; (7) No cases met the criteria for this measure; (8) The lower limit of the confidence interval cannot be calculated if the number of observed infections equals zero; (9) No data are available from the state/territory for this reporting period; (10) The scores shown reflect fewer than 50 completed surveys; (11) There were discrepancies in the data collection process; (12) This measure does not apply to this hospital for this reporting period; (13) Results cannot be calculated for this reporting period; (14) The results for this state are combined with nearby states to protect confidentiality; Please refer to the User's Guide for a full explanation of data.

Measure	Cases	This Hosp.	State Avg.	U.S. Avg.
Blood Clot Prevention and Treatment				
Anticoagulation Overlap Therapy[2,7]	-	-	92%	93%
ICU Venous Thromboembolism Prophylaxis[2,7]	-	-	92%	92%
Incidence of Potentially Preventable VTE[2,7]	-	-	11%	10%
UFH with Dosages/Platelet Monitoring[2,7]	-	-	96%	97%
Venous Thromboembolism Prophylaxis[2]	111	77%	83%	85%
Warfarin Therapy Discharge Instructions[2,7]	-	-	75%	75%
Chest Pain/Possible Heart Attack Care				
Aspirin Given Within 24 Hours of Arrival[5]	-	-	97%	96%
Fibrinolytic Meds Within 30 Min. of Arrival[5]	-	-	62%	58%
Average Time to ECG (minutes)[5]	-	-	9	7
Average Time to Transfer (minutes)[5]	-	-	62	60
Children's Asthma Care				
Received Home Management Plan of Care	-	-	88%	88%
Received Reliever Medication	-	-	100%	100%
Received Systemic Corticosteroids	-	-	100%	100%
Emergency Department				
Admittance Decision Time (minutes)[2,7]	-	-	125	98
Head CT Results Within 45 Min. of Arrival[5]	-	-	55%	57%
Patients Who Left ER Before Being Seen[5]	-	-	3%	2%
Time from ER Arrival to Admit. (minutes)[2,7]	-	-	323	274
Time from ER Arrival to Discharge (minutes)[5]	-	-	168	134
Time in ER Before Being Evaluated (minutes)[5]	-	-	29	26
Time to Pain Meds for Fractures (minutes)[5]	-	-	62	57
Heart Attack Care				
Aspirin Given at Discharge[5]	-	-	99%	99%
Fibrinolytic Meds Within 30 Min. of Arrival[5]	-	-	73%	54%
PCI Within 90 Minutes of Arrival[5]	-	-	95%	96%
Statin Prescribed at Discharge[5]	-	-	98%	98%
Heart Failure Care				
ACE Inhibitor or ARB for LVSD[1]	-	-	97%	97%
Discharge Instructions Given	21	95%	94%	94%
Evaluation of LVS Function	20	50%	99%	99%
Medicare Spending				
Medicare Spending per Patient (ratio)	-	0.90	0.98	0.98
Pneumonia Care				
Appropriate Initial Antibiotic Given	27	67%	97%	95%
Blood Culture Timing[1]	-	-	98%	98%
Pregnancy and Delivery Care				
Newborn Deliveries Scheduled Early[7]	-	-	5%	6%
Preventive Care				
Immunization for Influenza[2]	307	93%	89%	90%
Immunization for Pneumonia[2]	420	92%	90%	92%
Stroke Care				
Anticoagulation Therapy for Atrial Fibrillation[5]	-	-	95%	95%
Antithrombotic Therapy Timing[5]	-	-	98%	98%
Assessed for Rehabilitation[5]	-	-	97%	97%
Discharged on Antithrombotic Therapy[5]	-	-	99%	99%
Discharged on Statin Medication[5]	-	-	94%	94%
Thrombolytic Therapy Timing[5]	-	-	72%	66%
Venous Thromboembolism Prophylaxis[5]	-	-	94%	94%
Written Stroke Educational Materials Given[5]	-	-	87%	88%
Surgical Care Improvement Project				
Appropriate Beta Blocker Usage[3,7]	-	-	97%	98%
Appropriate VTP Within 24 Hours[3,7]	-	-	98%	98%
Controlled Postoperative Blood Glucose[3,7]	-	-	96%	97%
Perioperative Temperature Management[1,3]	-	-	100%	100%
Prophylactic Antibiotic Selection[3,7]	-	-	99%	99%
Prophylactic Antibiotic Selection (Outpatient)[5]	-	-	97%	98%
Prophylactic Antibiotic Stopped[3,7]	-	-	98%	98%
Prophylactic Antibiotic Timing[3,7]	-	-	99%	99%
Prophylactic Antibiotic Timing (Outpatient)[5]	-	-	97%	98%
Urinary Catheter Removal[3,7]	-	-	97%	97%
Survey of Patients' Hospital Experiences				
Area Around Room 'Always' Quiet at Night	(a)	65%	51%	61%
Doctors 'Always' Communicated Well	(a)	84%	78%	82%
Home Recovery Information Given	(a)	83%	83%	85%
Hospital Given 9 or 10 on 10 Point Scale	(a)	62%	68%	71%
Meds 'Always' Explained Before Given	(a)	65%	61%	64%
Nurses 'Always' Communicated Well	(a)	70%	74%	79%
Pain 'Always' Well Controlled	(a)	67%	68%	71%
Room and Bathroom 'Always' Clean	(a)	69%	70%	73%
Timely Help 'Always' Received	(a)	61%	62%	68%
Would Definitely Recommend Hospital	(a)	57%	70%	71%
Use of Medical Imaging				
Cardiac Imaging Stress Test before Surgery[7]	-	-	5.2%	5.3%
Combination Abdominal CT Scan[1]	-	-	13.4%	10.5%
Combination Brain/Sinus CT Scan[1]	-	-	2.2%	2.7%
Combination Chest CT Scan[1]	-	-	2.3%	2.7%
Follow-up Mammogram/Ultrasound[7]	-	-	8.2%	8.8%
Lumbar Spine MRI for Low Back Pain[7]	-	-	34.2%	37.2%

Kern Medical Center

1700 Mount Vernon Avenue
Bakersfield, CA 93306
Phone: 661-326-2000
Fax: 661-862-7630
E-mail: ewaldm@kernmedctr.com
URL: www.kernmedicalcenter.com
Type: Acute Care Hospitals
Emergency Services: Yes
Ownership: Voluntary non-profit - Other
Beds: 243

Key Personnel:
Pediatric Ambulatory Care . . . . . . Navin Amin, MD
Pediatric In-Patient Care . . . . Navin Amin, MD
Chief of Medical Staff . . . . Shehla Baqi
Emergency Room . . . . Christopher Bradburn
CEO/President . . . . Peter K Bryan
Operating Room . . . . Daniel D'Amico
Quality Assurance . . . . Anne Hollingsead

Measure	Cases	This Hosp.	State Avg.	U.S. Avg.
Blood Clot Prevention and Treatment				
Anticoagulation Overlap Therapy[2]	21	86%	92%	93%
ICU Venous Thromboembolism Prophylaxis[2]	39	100%	92%	92%
Incidence of Potentially Preventable VTE[2]	12	8%	11%	10%
UFH with Dosages/Platelet Monitoring[2]	12	100%	96%	97%
Venous Thromboembolism Prophylaxis[2]	352	98%	83%	85%
Warfarin Therapy Discharge Instructions[2]	20	80%	75%	75%
Chest Pain/Possible Heart Attack Care				
Aspirin Given Within 24 Hours of Arrival[5]	-	-	97%	96%
Fibrinolytic Meds Within 30 Min. of Arrival[5]	-	-	62%	58%
Average Time to ECG (minutes)[5]	-	-	9	7
Average Time to Transfer (minutes)[5]	-	-	62	60
Children's Asthma Care				
Received Home Management Plan of Care	-	-	88%	88%
Received Reliever Medication	-	-	100%	100%
Received Systemic Corticosteroids	-	-	100%	100%
Emergency Department				
Admittance Decision Time (minutes)[2]	107	242	125	98
Head CT Results Within 45 Min. of Arrival[1,3]	-	-	55%	57%
Patients Who Left ER Before Being Seen	35,287	1%	3%	2%
Time from ER Arrival to Admit. (minutes)[2]	116	637	323	274
Time from ER Arrival to Discharge (minutes)	359	220	168	134
Time in ER Before Being Evaluated (minutes)	377	71	29	26
Time to Pain Meds for Fractures (minutes)	197	77	62	57
Heart Attack Care				
Aspirin Given at Discharge[1,3]	-	-	99%	99%
Fibrinolytic Meds Within 30 Min. of Arrival[3,7]	-	-	73%	54%
PCI Within 90 Minutes of Arrival[3,7]	-	-	95%	96%
Statin Prescribed at Discharge[1,3]	-	-	98%	98%
Heart Failure Care				
ACE Inhibitor or ARB for LVSD	56	96%	97%	97%
Discharge Instructions Given	103	87%	94%	94%
Evaluation of LVS Function	106	98%	99%	99%
Medicare Spending				
Medicare Spending per Patient (ratio)	-	0.89	0.98	0.98
Pneumonia Care				
Appropriate Initial Antibiotic Given	44	95%	97%	95%
Blood Culture Timing	69	90%	98%	98%
Pregnancy and Delivery Care				
Newborn Deliveries Scheduled Early[2]	44	5%	5%	6%
Preventive Care				
Immunization for Influenza[2]	439	61%	89%	90%
Immunization for Pneumonia[2]	213	56%	90%	92%
Stroke Care				
Anticoagulation Therapy for Atrial Fibrillation[1]	-	-	95%	95%
Antithrombotic Therapy Timing	18	78%	98%	98%
Assessed for Rehabilitation	22	68%	97%	97%
Discharged on Antithrombotic Therapy	18	72%	99%	99%
Discharged on Statin Medication	15	73%	94%	94%
Thrombolytic Therapy Timing[1]	-	-	72%	66%
Venous Thromboembolism Prophylaxis	24	79%	94%	94%
Written Stroke Educational Materials Given	20	60%	87%	88%
Surgical Care Improvement Project				
Appropriate Beta Blocker Usage[2]	26	85%	97%	98%
Appropriate VTP Within 24 Hours[2]	321	89%	98%	98%
Controlled Postoperative Blood Glucose[1,2]	-	-	96%	97%
Perioperative Temperature Management[2]	353	100%	100%	100%
Prophylactic Antibiotic Selection[2]	224	92%	99%	99%
Prophylactic Antibiotic Selection (Outpatient)	169	94%	97%	98%
Prophylactic Antibiotic Stopped[2]	219	63%	98%	98%
Prophylactic Antibiotic Timing[2]	225	96%	99%	99%
Prophylactic Antibiotic Timing (Outpatient)	170	94%	97%	98%
Urinary Catheter Removal[2]	156	97%	97%	97%
Survey of Patients' Hospital Experiences				
Area Around Room 'Always' Quiet at Night	300+	37%	51%	61%
Doctors 'Always' Communicated Well	300+	72%	78%	82%
Home Recovery Information Given	300+	79%	83%	85%
Hospital Given 9 or 10 on 10 Point Scale	300+	55%	68%	71%
Meds 'Always' Explained Before Given	300+	53%	61%	64%
Nurses 'Always' Communicated Well	300+	67%	74%	79%
Pain 'Always' Well Controlled	300+	60%	68%	71%
Room and Bathroom 'Always' Clean	300+	60%	70%	73%
Timely Help 'Always' Received	300+	50%	62%	68%
Would Definitely Recommend Hospital	300+	49%	70%	71%
Use of Medical Imaging				
Cardiac Imaging Stress Test before Surgery[1]	-	-	5.2%	5.3%
Combination Abdominal CT Scan	117	12.8%	13.4%	10.5%
Combination Brain/Sinus CT Scan[1]	-	-	2.2%	2.7%
Combination Chest CT Scan	50	0.0%	2.3%	2.7%
Follow-up Mammogram/Ultrasound	68	8.8%	8.2%	8.8%
Lumbar Spine MRI for Low Back Pain[1]	-	-	34.2%	37.2%

Mercy Hospital

2215 Truxtun Avenue
Bakersfield, CA 93301
Phone: 661-632-5000
Fax: 661-322-8543
URL: www.mercybakersfield.org
Type: Acute Care Hospitals
Emergency Services: Yes
Ownership: Voluntary non-profit - Other
Beds: 260

Key Personnel:
Quality Assurance . . . . Patti Carroll
CEO/President . . . . Russell Judd
Chief of Medical Staff . . . . Dr Mitesh Patel
Radiology . . . . Bradley Snyder

Measure	Cases	This Hosp.	State Avg.	U.S. Avg.
Blood Clot Prevention and Treatment				
Anticoagulation Overlap Therapy[2]	59	100%	92%	93%
ICU Venous Thromboembolism Prophylaxis[2]	81	100%	92%	92%
Incidence of Potentially Preventable VTE[1,2]	-	-	11%	10%
UFH with Dosages/Platelet Monitoring[2]	14	100%	96%	97%
Venous Thromboembolism Prophylaxis[2]	341	99%	83%	85%
Warfarin Therapy Discharge Instructions[2]	45	100%	75%	75%
Chest Pain/Possible Heart Attack Care				
Aspirin Given Within 24 Hours of Arrival	78	99%	97%	96%
Fibrinolytic Meds Within 30 Min. of Arrival[7]	-	-	62%	58%
Average Time to ECG (minutes)	82	19	9	7
Average Time to Transfer (minutes)	25	72	62	60
Children's Asthma Care				
Received Home Management Plan of Care	-	-	88%	88%
Received Reliever Medication	-	-	100%	100%
Received Systemic Corticosteroids	-	-	100%	100%
Emergency Department				
Admittance Decision Time (minutes)[2]	665	224	125	98
Head CT Results Within 45 Min. of Arrival[1]	-	-	55%	57%
Patients Who Left ER Before Being Seen	72,221	1%	3%	2%
Time from ER Arrival to Admit. (minutes)[2]	676	405	323	274
Time from ER Arrival to Discharge (minutes)	389	153	168	134
Time in ER Before Being Evaluated (minutes)	420	19	29	26
Time to Pain Meds for Fractures (minutes)	314	77	62	57
Heart Attack Care				
Aspirin Given at Discharge	18	100%	99%	99%

NOTE: Hospital profiles are in alphabetical order by state, then city, then hospital within the city; Rankings exclude hospitals with less than 25 cases except for patient surveys which excludes hospitals with less than 100 cases; (a) 100-299 cases; (1) The number of cases/patients is too few to report; (2) Data submitted were based on a sample of cases/patients; (3) Results are based on a shorter time period than required; (4) Data suppressed by CMS for one or more quarters; (5) Results are not available for this reporting period; (6) Fewer than 100 patients completed the HCAHPS survey; (7) No cases met the criteria for this measure; (8) The lower limit of the confidence interval cannot be calculated if the number of observed infections equals zero; (9) No data are available from the state/territory for this reporting period; (10) The scores shown reflect fewer than 50 completed surveys; (11) There were discrepancies in the data collection process; (12) This measure does not apply to this hospital for this reporting period; (13) Results cannot be calculated for this reporting period; (14) The results for this state are combined with nearby states to protect confidentiality; Please refer to the User's Guide for a full explanation of data.

Measure	Cases	This Hosp.	State Avg.	U.S. Avg.
Fibrinolytic Meds Within 30 Min. of Arrival[7]	-	-	73%	54%
PCI Within 90 Minutes of Arrival[7]	-	-	95%	96%
Statin Prescribed at Discharge	19	100%	98%	98%
Heart Failure Care				
ACE Inhibitor or ARB for LVSD	59	92%	97%	97%
Discharge Instructions Given	143	98%	94%	94%
Evaluation of LVS Function	168	100%	99%	99%
Medicare Spending				
Medicare Spending per Patient (ratio)	-	1.05	0.98	0.98
Pneumonia Care				
Appropriate Initial Antibiotic Given[2]	79	96%	97%	95%
Blood Culture Timing[2]	180	98%	98%	98%
Pregnancy and Delivery Care				
Newborn Deliveries Scheduled Early[2]	44	0%	5%	6%
Preventive Care				
Immunization for Influenza[2]	526	98%	89%	90%
Immunization for Pneumonia[2]	471	98%	90%	92%
Stroke Care				
Anticoagulation Therapy for Atrial Fibrillation	13	100%	95%	95%
Antithrombotic Therapy Timing	97	100%	98%	98%
Assessed for Rehabilitation	120	100%	97%	97%
Discharged on Antithrombotic Therapy	106	100%	99%	99%
Discharged on Statin Medication	75	100%	94%	94%
Thrombolytic Therapy Timing[1]	-	-	72%	66%
Venous Thromboembolism Prophylaxis	126	100%	94%	94%
Written Stroke Educational Materials Given[2]	72	100%	87%	88%
Surgical Care Improvement Project				
Appropriate Beta Blocker Usage[2]	98	99%	97%	98%
Appropriate VTP Within 24 Hours[2]	416	99%	98%	98%
Controlled Postoperative Blood Glucose[2,7]	-	-	96%	97%
Perioperative Temperature Management[2]	488	100%	100%	100%
Prophylactic Antibiotic Selection[2]	319	100%	99%	99%
Prophylactic Antibiotic Selection (Outpatient)	177	99%	97%	98%
Prophylactic Antibiotic Stopped[2]	316	98%	98%	98%
Prophylactic Antibiotic Timing[2]	320	98%	99%	99%
Prophylactic Antibiotic Timing (Outpatient)	177	99%	97%	98%
Urinary Catheter Removal[2]	242	99%	97%	97%
Survey of Patients' Hospital Experiences				
Area Around Room 'Always' Quiet at Night	300+	42%	51%	61%
Doctors 'Always' Communicated Well	300+	70%	78%	82%
Home Recovery Information Given	300+	80%	83%	85%
Hospital Given 9 or 10 on 10 Point Scale	300+	61%	68%	71%
Meds 'Always' Explained Before Given	300+	56%	61%	64%
Nurses 'Always' Communicated Well	300+	69%	74%	79%
Pain 'Always' Well Controlled	300+	65%	68%	71%
Room and Bathroom 'Always' Clean	300+	63%	70%	73%
Timely Help 'Always' Received	300+	53%	62%	68%
Would Definitely Recommend Hospital	300+	65%	70%	71%
Use of Medical Imaging				
Cardiac Imaging Stress Test before Surgery[1]	-	-	5.2%	5.3%
Combination Abdominal CT Scan	521	3.1%	13.4%	10.5%
Combination Brain/Sinus CT Scan	903	4.3%	2.2%	2.7%
Combination Chest CT Scan	189	3.2%	2.3%	2.7%
Follow-up Mammogram/Ultrasound	202	6.9%	8.2%	8.8%
Lumbar Spine MRI for Low Back Pain[1]	-	-	34.2%	37.2%

San Joaquin Community Hospital

2615 Chester Avenue
Bakersfield, CA 93301
Phone: 661-395-3000
Fax: 661-324-5162
URL: www.sanjoaquinhospital.org
Type: Acute Care Hospitals
Emergency Services: Yes
Ownership: Voluntary non-profit - Private
Beds: 252

Key Personnel:
Chief of Medical Staff . . . . Donald Cornforth, MD
President/CEO. . . . . Douglas Duffield
Ambulatory Care . . . . Sam Itani
Operating Room. . . . . Rick Knapp
Emergency Room . . . . Jackie Laws
Quality Assurance . . . . Martha Samora
Pediatric Ambulatory Care . . . . . . Margaret White

Measure	Cases	This Hosp.	State Avg.	U.S. Avg.
Blood Clot Prevention and Treatment				
Anticoagulation Overlap Therapy[2]	98	85%	92%	93%
ICU Venous Thromboembolism Prophylaxis[2]	86	93%	92%	92%
Incidence of Potentially Preventable VTE[2]	24	8%	11%	10%
UFH with Dosages/Platelet Monitoring[2]	32	97%	96%	97%
Venous Thromboembolism Prophylaxis[2]	389	74%	83%	85%
Warfarin Therapy Discharge Instructions[2]	80	51%	75%	75%
Chest Pain/Possible Heart Attack Care				
Aspirin Given Within 24 Hours of Arrival[1]	-	-	97%	96%
Fibrinolytic Meds Within 30 Min. of Arrival[5]	-	-	62%	58%
Average Time to ECG (minutes)[1]	-	-	9	7
Average Time to Transfer (minutes)[5]	-	-	62	60
Children's Asthma Care				
Received Home Management Plan of Care	-	-	88%	88%
Received Reliever Medication	-	-	100%	100%
Received Systemic Corticosteroids	-	-	100%	100%
Emergency Department				
Admittance Decision Time (minutes)[2]	604	276	125	98
Head CT Results Within 45 Min. of Arrival[1]	-	-	55%	57%
Patients Who Left ER Before Being Seen	71,603	1%	3%	2%
Time from ER Arrival to Admit. (minutes)[2]	610	444	323	274
Time from ER Arrival to Discharge (minutes)	332	228	168	134
Time in ER Before Being Evaluated (minutes)	377	21	29	26
Time to Pain Meds for Fractures (minutes)	127	61	62	57
Heart Attack Care				
Aspirin Given at Discharge	253	100%	99%	99%
Fibrinolytic Meds Within 30 Min. of Arrival[7]	-	-	73%	54%
PCI Within 90 Minutes of Arrival	46	93%	95%	96%
Statin Prescribed at Discharge	249	100%	98%	98%
Heart Failure Care				
ACE Inhibitor or ARB for LVSD	236	99%	97%	97%
Discharge Instructions Given	505	99%	94%	94%
Evaluation of LVS Function	597	100%	99%	99%
Medicare Spending				
Medicare Spending per Patient (ratio)	-	1.01	0.98	0.98
Pneumonia Care				
Appropriate Initial Antibiotic Given	194	95%	97%	95%
Blood Culture Timing	375	97%	98%	98%
Pregnancy and Delivery Care				
Newborn Deliveries Scheduled Early[2]	94	1%	5%	6%
Preventive Care				
Immunization for Influenza[2]	527	99%	89%	90%
Immunization for Pneumonia[2]	551	98%	90%	92%
Stroke Care				
Anticoagulation Therapy for Atrial Fibrillation[1,2]	-	-	95%	95%
Antithrombotic Therapy Timing[2]	77	99%	98%	98%
Assessed for Rehabilitation[2]	109	96%	97%	97%
Discharged on Antithrombotic Therapy[2]	91	98%	99%	99%
Discharged on Statin Medication[2]	69	99%	94%	94%
Thrombolytic Therapy Timing[1,2]	-	-	72%	66%
Venous Thromboembolism Prophylaxis[2]	113	92%	94%	94%
Written Stroke Educational Materials Given[2]	63	100%	87%	88%
Surgical Care Improvement Project				
Appropriate Beta Blocker Usage[2]	247	98%	97%	98%
Appropriate VTP Within 24 Hours[2]	579	99%	98%	98%
Controlled Postoperative Blood Glucose[2]	75	97%	96%	97%
Perioperative Temperature Management[2]	775	100%	100%	100%
Prophylactic Antibiotic Selection[2]	653	99%	99%	99%
Prophylactic Antibiotic Selection (Outpatient)	260	98%	97%	98%
Prophylactic Antibiotic Stopped[2]	616	99%	98%	98%
Prophylactic Antibiotic Timing[2]	654	99%	99%	99%
Prophylactic Antibiotic Timing (Outpatient)	262	98%	97%	98%
Urinary Catheter Removal[2]	423	98%	97%	97%
Survey of Patients' Hospital Experiences				
Area Around Room 'Always' Quiet at Night	300+	53%	51%	61%
Doctors 'Always' Communicated Well	300+	77%	78%	82%
Home Recovery Information Given	300+	82%	83%	85%
Hospital Given 9 or 10 on 10 Point Scale	300+	66%	68%	71%
Meds 'Always' Explained Before Given	300+	61%	61%	64%
Nurses 'Always' Communicated Well	300+	73%	74%	79%
Pain 'Always' Well Controlled	300+	69%	68%	71%
Room and Bathroom 'Always' Clean	300+	64%	70%	73%
Timely Help 'Always' Received	300+	58%	62%	68%
Would Definitely Recommend Hospital	300+	70%	70%	71%
Use of Medical Imaging				
Cardiac Imaging Stress Test before Surgery	277	6.1%	5.2%	5.3%
Combination Abdominal CT Scan	1,255	39.7%	13.4%	10.5%
Combination Brain/Sinus CT Scan	973	3.0%	2.2%	2.7%
Combination Chest CT Scan	634	1.7%	2.3%	2.7%
Follow-up Mammogram/Ultrasound	1,574	15.2%	8.2%	8.8%
Lumbar Spine MRI for Low Back Pain	230	35.7%	34.2%	37.2%

Kaiser Foundation Hospital - Baldwin Park

1011 Baldwin Park Blvd
Baldwin Park, CA 91706
Phone: 626-851-1011
Type: Acute Care Hospitals
Emergency Services: Yes
Ownership: Voluntary non-profit - Other
Beds: 222

Measure	Cases	This Hosp.	State Avg.	U.S. Avg.
Blood Clot Prevention and Treatment				
Anticoagulation Overlap Therapy[2]	63	95%	92%	93%
ICU Venous Thromboembolism Prophylaxis[2]	38	97%	92%	92%
Incidence of Potentially Preventable VTE[1,2]	-	-	11%	10%
UFH with Dosages/Platelet Monitoring[2]	29	100%	96%	97%
Venous Thromboembolism Prophylaxis[2]	296	96%	83%	85%
Warfarin Therapy Discharge Instructions[2]	65	95%	75%	75%
Chest Pain/Possible Heart Attack Care				
Aspirin Given Within 24 Hours of Arrival	-	-	97%	96%
Fibrinolytic Meds Within 30 Min. of Arrival	-	-	62%	58%
Average Time to ECG (minutes)	-	-	9	7
Average Time to Transfer (minutes)	-	-	62	60
Children's Asthma Care				
Received Home Management Plan of Care	-	-	88%	88%
Received Reliever Medication	-	-	100%	100%
Received Systemic Corticosteroids	-	-	100%	100%
Emergency Department				
Admittance Decision Time (minutes)[2]	434	76	125	98
Head CT Results Within 45 Min. of Arrival	-	-	55%	57%
Patients Who Left ER Before Being Seen	-	-	3%	2%
Time from ER Arrival to Admit. (minutes)[2]	444	317	323	274
Time from ER Arrival to Discharge (minutes)	-	-	168	134
Time in ER Before Being Evaluated (minutes)	-	-	29	26
Time to Pain Meds for Fractures (minutes)	-	-	62	57
Heart Attack Care				
Aspirin Given at Discharge	85	100%	99%	99%
Fibrinolytic Meds Within 30 Min. of Arrival[1]	-	-	73%	54%
PCI Within 90 Minutes of Arrival[7]	-	-	95%	96%
Statin Prescribed at Discharge	89	99%	98%	98%
Heart Failure Care				
ACE Inhibitor or ARB for LVSD	124	100%	97%	97%
Discharge Instructions Given	381	98%	94%	94%
Evaluation of LVS Function	403	100%	99%	99%
Medicare Spending				
Medicare Spending per Patient (ratio)	-	0.78	0.98	0.98
Pneumonia Care				
Appropriate Initial Antibiotic Given[2]	95	100%	97%	95%
Blood Culture Timing[2]	172	98%	98%	98%
Pregnancy and Delivery Care				
Newborn Deliveries Scheduled Early	209	0%	5%	6%
Preventive Care				
Immunization for Influenza[2]	494	93%	89%	90%
Immunization for Pneumonia[2]	552	95%	90%	92%
Stroke Care				
Anticoagulation Therapy for Atrial Fibrillation[2]	13	92%	95%	95%
Antithrombotic Therapy Timing[2]	94	100%	98%	98%
Assessed for Rehabilitation[2]	113	100%	97%	97%
Discharged on Antithrombotic Therapy[2]	108	100%	99%	99%
Discharged on Statin Medication[2]	88	100%	94%	94%
Thrombolytic Therapy Timing[1,2]	-	-	72%	66%
Venous Thromboembolism Prophylaxis[2]	87	98%	94%	94%
Written Stroke Educational Materials Given[2]	80	98%	87%	88%
Surgical Care Improvement Project				
Appropriate Beta Blocker Usage[2]	136	99%	97%	98%
Appropriate VTP Within 24 Hours[2]	378	100%	98%	98%
Controlled Postoperative Blood Glucose[2,7]	-	-	96%	97%
Perioperative Temperature Management[2]	477	100%	100%	100%
Prophylactic Antibiotic Selection[2]	325	100%	99%	99%
Prophylactic Antibiotic Selection (Outpatient)	-	-	97%	98%

NOTE: Hospital profiles are in alphabetical order by state, then city, then hospital within the city; Rankings exclude hospitals with less than 25 cases except for patient surveys which excludes hospitals with less than 100 cases; (a) 100-299 cases; (1) The number of cases/patients is too few to report; (2) Data submitted were based on a sample of cases/patients; (3) Results are based on a shorter time period than required; (4) Data suppressed by CMS for one or more quarters; (5) Results are not available for this reporting period; (6) Fewer than 100 patients completed the HCAHPS survey; (7) No cases met the criteria for this measure; (8) The lower limit of the confidence interval cannot be calculated if the number of observed infections equals zero; (9) No data are available from the state/territory for this reporting period; (10) The scores shown reflect fewer than 50 completed surveys; (11) There were discrepancies in the data collection process; (12) This measure does not apply to this hospital for this reporting period; (13) Results cannot be calculated for this reporting period; (14) The results for this state are combined with nearby states to protect confidentiality; Please refer to the User's Guide for a full explanation of data.

Measure	Cases	This Hosp.	State Avg.	U.S. Avg.
Prophylactic Antibiotic Stopped[2]	317	98%	98%	98%
Prophylactic Antibiotic Timing[2]	325	99%	99%	99%
Prophylactic Antibiotic Timing (Outpatient)	-	-	97%	98%
Urinary Catheter Removal[2]	292	98%	97%	97%
Survey of Patients' Hospital Experiences				
Area Around Room 'Always' Quiet at Night	300+	57%	51%	61%
Doctors 'Always' Communicated Well	300+	83%	78%	82%
Home Recovery Information Given	300+	87%	83%	85%
Hospital Given 9 or 10 on 10 Point Scale	300+	77%	68%	71%
Meds 'Always' Explained Before Given	300+	65%	61%	64%
Nurses 'Always' Communicated Well	300+	76%	74%	79%
Pain 'Always' Well Controlled	300+	73%	68%	71%
Room and Bathroom 'Always' Clean	300+	73%	70%	73%
Timely Help 'Always' Received	300+	64%	62%	68%
Would Definitely Recommend Hospital	300+	77%	70%	71%
Use of Medical Imaging				
Cardiac Imaging Stress Test before Surgery	-	-	5.2%	5.3%
Combination Abdominal CT Scan	-	-	13.4%	10.5%
Combination Brain/Sinus CT Scan	-	-	2.2%	2.7%
Combination Chest CT Scan	-	-	2.3%	2.7%
Follow-up Mammogram/Ultrasound	-	-	8.2%	8.8%
Lumbar Spine MRI for Low Back Pain	-	-	34.2%	37.2%

San Gorgonio Memorial Hospital

600 North Highland Springs Avenue
Banning, CA 92220
E-mail: info@sgmh.org
URL: www.sgmh.org
Phone: 951-769-2101
Fax: 951-845-2836
Type: Acute Care Hospitals
Ownership: Govt - Hospital Dist/Auth
Emergency Services: Yes
Beds: 77

Key Personnel:

Anesthesiology. . . . . Devin F Borna
Anesthesiology. . . . . Farzad Farrohki
Cardiology . . . . John H Marais, MD
Cardiology . . . . Kaustubh Patankar, MD
Cardiology . . . . Shadi A Quasquas, RN
CEO/President. . . . . Mark Turner

Measure	Cases	This Hosp.	State Avg.	U.S. Avg.
Blood Clot Prevention and Treatment				
Anticoagulation Overlap Therapy[2]	24	100%	92%	93%
ICU Venous Thromboembolism Prophylaxis[2]	71	87%	92%	92%
Incidence of Potentially Preventable VTE[1,2]	-	-	11%	10%
UFH with Dosages/Platelet Monitoring[1,2]	-	-	96%	97%
Venous Thromboembolism Prophylaxis[2]	313	83%	83%	85%
Warfarin Therapy Discharge Instructions[2]	19	68%	75%	75%
Chest Pain/Possible Heart Attack Care				
Aspirin Given Within 24 Hours of Arrival	97	100%	97%	96%
Fibrinolytic Meds Within 30 Min. of Arrival[7]	-	-	62%	58%
Average Time to ECG (minutes)	103	7	9	7
Average Time to Transfer (minutes)[7]	-	-	62	60
Children's Asthma Care				
Received Home Management Plan of Care	-	-	88%	88%
Received Reliever Medication	-	-	100%	100%
Received Systemic Corticosteroids	-	-	100%	100%
Emergency Department				
Admittance Decision Time (minutes)[2]	331	195	125	98
Head CT Results Within 45 Min. of Arrival	35	77%	55%	57%
Patients Who Left ER Before Being Seen	34,240	1%	3%	2%
Time from ER Arrival to Admit. (minutes)[2]	335	350	323	274
Time from ER Arrival to Discharge (minutes)	372	98	168	134
Time in ER Before Being Evaluated (minutes)	422	14	29	26
Time to Pain Meds for Fractures (minutes)	155	44	62	57
Heart Attack Care				
Aspirin Given at Discharge	61	93%	99%	99%
Fibrinolytic Meds Within 30 Min. of Arrival[7]	-	-	73%	54%
PCI Within 90 Minutes of Arrival[7]	-	-	95%	96%
Statin Prescribed at Discharge	68	68%	98%	98%
Heart Failure Care				
ACE Inhibitor or ARB for LVSD	38	97%	97%	97%
Discharge Instructions Given	119	91%	94%	94%
Evaluation of LVS Function	151	96%	99%	99%
Medicare Spending				
Medicare Spending per Patient (ratio)	-	1.02	0.98	0.98
Pneumonia Care				
Appropriate Initial Antibiotic Given	98	97%	97%	95%
Blood Culture Timing	176	98%	98%	98%
Pregnancy and Delivery Care				
Newborn Deliveries Scheduled Early[2]	55	7%	5%	6%
Preventive Care				
Immunization for Influenza[2]	294	91%	89%	90%
Immunization for Pneumonia[2]	433	94%	90%	92%
Stroke Care				
Anticoagulation Therapy for Atrial Fibrillation[1]	-	-	95%	95%
Antithrombotic Therapy Timing	27	100%	98%	98%
Assessed for Rehabilitation	28	93%	97%	97%
Discharged on Antithrombotic Therapy	25	96%	99%	99%
Discharged on Statin Medication	24	54%	94%	94%
Thrombolytic Therapy Timing[1]	-	-	72%	66%
Venous Thromboembolism Prophylaxis	29	66%	94%	94%
Written Stroke Educational Materials Given	12	58%	87%	88%
Surgical Care Improvement Project				
Appropriate Beta Blocker Usage	72	97%	97%	98%
Appropriate VTP Within 24 Hours	96	99%	98%	98%
Controlled Postoperative Blood Glucose[7]	-	-	96%	97%
Perioperative Temperature Management	236	100%	100%	100%
Prophylactic Antibiotic Selection	166	99%	99%	99%
Prophylactic Antibiotic Selection (Outpatient)	20	100%	97%	98%
Prophylactic Antibiotic Stopped	162	98%	98%	98%
Prophylactic Antibiotic Timing	168	98%	99%	99%
Prophylactic Antibiotic Timing (Outpatient)	20	100%	97%	98%
Urinary Catheter Removal	19	74%	97%	97%
Survey of Patients' Hospital Experiences				
Area Around Room 'Always' Quiet at Night	300+	41%	51%	61%
Doctors 'Always' Communicated Well	300+	76%	78%	82%
Home Recovery Information Given	300+	82%	83%	85%
Hospital Given 9 or 10 on 10 Point Scale	300+	56%	68%	71%
Meds 'Always' Explained Before Given	300+	54%	61%	64%
Nurses 'Always' Communicated Well	300+	74%	74%	79%
Pain 'Always' Well Controlled	300+	66%	68%	71%
Room and Bathroom 'Always' Clean	300+	70%	70%	73%
Timely Help 'Always' Received	300+	63%	62%	68%
Would Definitely Recommend Hospital	300+	58%	70%	71%
Use of Medical Imaging				
Cardiac Imaging Stress Test before Surgery[1]	-	-	5.2%	5.3%
Combination Abdominal CT Scan	187	7.5%	13.4%	10.5%
Combination Brain/Sinus CT Scan	345	1.2%	2.2%	2.7%
Combination Chest CT Scan[1]	-	-	2.3%	2.7%
Follow-up Mammogram/Ultrasound	253	6.3%	8.2%	8.8%
Lumbar Spine MRI for Low Back Pain[7]	-	-	34.2%	37.2%

Barstow Community Hospital

820 E Mountain View Street
Barstow, CA 92311
URL: www.barstowhospital.com
Phone: 760-256-1761
Fax: 760-957-3359
Type: Acute Care Hospitals
Ownership: Proprietary
Emergency Services: Yes
Beds: 56

Key Personnel:

Pediatric Ambulatory Care . . . . . . Donald Case, MD
Pediatric In-Patient Care . . . . Donald Case, MD
Quality Assurance . . . . Dave Grant
CEO/President. . . . . Randall Hempling
Chief of Medical Staff. . . . . Alberta Olegario, MD
Radiology. . . . . Robert Rippner, MD
Operating Room. . . . . Joy Zane, RN

Measure	Cases	This Hosp.	State Avg.	U.S. Avg.
Blood Clot Prevention and Treatment				
Anticoagulation Overlap Therapy[2]	11	100%	92%	93%
ICU Venous Thromboembolism Prophylaxis[2]	68	99%	92%	92%
Incidence of Potentially Preventable VTE[1,2]	-	-	11%	10%
UFH with Dosages/Platelet Monitoring[1,2]	-	-	96%	97%
Venous Thromboembolism Prophylaxis[2]	222	100%	83%	85%
Warfarin Therapy Discharge Instructions[1,2]	-	-	75%	75%
Chest Pain/Possible Heart Attack Care				
Aspirin Given Within 24 Hours of Arrival	15	100%	97%	96%
Fibrinolytic Meds Within 30 Min. of Arrival[7]	-	-	62%	58%
Average Time to ECG (minutes)	15	5	9	7
Average Time to Transfer (minutes)[1]	-	-	62	60
Children's Asthma Care				
Received Home Management Plan of Care	-	-	88%	88%
Received Reliever Medication	-	-	100%	100%
Received Systemic Corticosteroids	-	-	100%	100%
Emergency Department				
Admittance Decision Time (minutes)[2]	441	120	125	98
Head CT Results Within 45 Min. of Arrival[1]	-	-	55%	57%
Patients Who Left ER Before Being Seen	25,019	17%	3%	2%
Time from ER Arrival to Admit. (minutes)[2]	443	284	323	274
Time from ER Arrival to Discharge (minutes)	382	139	168	134
Time in ER Before Being Evaluated (minutes)	412	16	29	26
Time to Pain Meds for Fractures (minutes)	58	58	62	57
Heart Attack Care				
Aspirin Given at Discharge	14	100%	99%	99%
Fibrinolytic Meds Within 30 Min. of Arrival[7]	-	-	73%	54%
PCI Within 90 Minutes of Arrival[7]	-	-	95%	96%
Statin Prescribed at Discharge	14	100%	98%	98%
Heart Failure Care				
ACE Inhibitor or ARB for LVSD	52	98%	97%	97%
Discharge Instructions Given	106	100%	94%	94%
Evaluation of LVS Function	120	100%	99%	99%
Medicare Spending				
Medicare Spending per Patient (ratio)	-	0.90	0.98	0.98
Pneumonia Care				
Appropriate Initial Antibiotic Given	35	97%	97%	95%
Blood Culture Timing	62	98%	98%	98%
Pregnancy and Delivery Care				
Newborn Deliveries Scheduled Early[2]	26	0%	5%	6%
Preventive Care				
Immunization for Influenza[2]	296	100%	89%	90%
Immunization for Pneumonia[2]	357	100%	90%	92%
Stroke Care				
Anticoagulation Therapy for Atrial Fibrillation[1]	-	-	95%	95%
Antithrombotic Therapy Timing	41	98%	98%	98%
Assessed for Rehabilitation	42	100%	97%	97%
Discharged on Antithrombotic Therapy	42	100%	99%	99%
Discharged on Statin Medication	33	97%	94%	94%
Thrombolytic Therapy Timing[1]	-	-	72%	66%
Venous Thromboembolism Prophylaxis	43	98%	94%	94%
Written Stroke Educational Materials Given	29	100%	87%	88%
Surgical Care Improvement Project				
Appropriate Beta Blocker Usage	18	94%	97%	98%
Appropriate VTP Within 24 Hours	57	98%	98%	98%
Controlled Postoperative Blood Glucose[7]	-	-	96%	97%
Perioperative Temperature Management	66	100%	100%	100%
Prophylactic Antibiotic Selection	23	96%	99%	99%
Prophylactic Antibiotic Selection (Outpatient)	35	100%	97%	98%
Prophylactic Antibiotic Stopped	20	100%	98%	98%
Prophylactic Antibiotic Timing	23	100%	99%	99%
Prophylactic Antibiotic Timing (Outpatient)	35	97%	97%	98%
Urinary Catheter Removal	27	100%	97%	97%
Survey of Patients' Hospital Experiences				
Area Around Room 'Always' Quiet at Night	300+	61%	51%	61%
Doctors 'Always' Communicated Well	300+	78%	78%	82%
Home Recovery Information Given	300+	86%	83%	85%
Hospital Given 9 or 10 on 10 Point Scale	300+	68%	68%	71%
Meds 'Always' Explained Before Given	300+	63%	61%	64%
Nurses 'Always' Communicated Well	300+	75%	74%	79%
Pain 'Always' Well Controlled	300+	70%	68%	71%
Room and Bathroom 'Always' Clean	300+	77%	70%	73%
Timely Help 'Always' Received	300+	62%	62%	68%
Would Definitely Recommend Hospital	300+	66%	70%	71%
Use of Medical Imaging				
Cardiac Imaging Stress Test before Surgery[1]	-	-	5.2%	5.3%
Combination Abdominal CT Scan	251	6.4%	13.4%	10.5%
Combination Brain/Sinus CT Scan[1]	-	-	2.2%	2.7%
Combination Chest CT Scan	111	6.3%	2.3%	2.7%
Follow-up Mammogram/Ultrasound	178	14.0%	8.2%	8.8%
Lumbar Spine MRI for Low Back Pain[1]	-	-	34.2%	37.2%

NOTE: Hospital profiles are in alphabetical order by state, then city, then hospital within the city; Rankings exclude hospitals with less than 25 cases except for patient surveys which excludes hospitals with less than 100 cases; (a) 100-299 cases; (1) The number of cases/patients is too few to report; (2) Data submitted were based on a sample of cases/patients; (3) Results are based on a shorter time period than required; (4) Data suppressed by CMS for one or more quarters; (5) Results are not available for this reporting period; (6) Fewer than 100 patients completed the HCAHPS survey; (7) No cases met the criteria for this measure; (8) The lower limit of the confidence interval cannot be calculated if the number of observed infections equals zero; (9) No data are available from the state/territory for this reporting period; (10) The scores shown reflect fewer than 50 completed surveys; (11) There were discrepancies in the data collection process; (12) This measure does not apply to this hospital for this reporting period; (13) Results cannot be calculated for this reporting period; (14) The results for this state are combined with nearby states to protect confidentiality; Please refer to the User's Guide for a full explanation of data.

Alta Bates Summit Medical Center

2450 Ashby Ave | Phone: 510-204-4444
Berkeley, CA 94705 | Fax: 510-204-5203
URL: www.altabates.com
Type: Acute Care Hospitals | Emergency Services: Yes
Ownership: Voluntary non-profit - Private | Beds: 551

Key Personnel:
Chief of Medical Staff.......... Janet Arnesty
Radiology.................. John Bokelman
CEO/President.............. Warren J Kirk

Measure	Cases	This Hosp.	State Avg.	U.S. Avg.
Blood Clot Prevention and Treatment				
Anticoagulation Overlap Therapy[2]	46	98%	92%	93%
ICU Venous Thromboembolism Prophylaxis[2]	56	96%	92%	92%
Incidence of Potentially Preventable VTE[2]	14	36%	11%	10%
UFH with Dosages/Platelet Monitoring[1,2]	-	-	96%	97%
Venous Thromboembolism Prophylaxis[2]	345	85%	83%	85%
Warfarin Therapy Discharge Instructions[2]	30	70%	75%	75%
Chest Pain/Possible Heart Attack Care				
Aspirin Given Within 24 Hours of Arrival	41	98%	97%	96%
Fibrinolytic Meds Within 30 Min. of Arrival[7]	-	-	62%	58%
Average Time to ECG (minutes)	42	11	9	7
Average Time to Transfer (minutes)	17	61	62	60
Children's Asthma Care				
Received Home Management Plan of Care	-	-	88%	88%
Received Reliever Medication	-	-	100%	100%
Received Systemic Corticosteroids	-	-	100%	100%
Emergency Department				
Admittance Decision Time (minutes)[2]	291	133	125	98
Head CT Results Within 45 Min. of Arrival[1]	-	-	55%	57%
Patients Who Left ER Before Being Seen	45,109	3%	3%	2%
Time from ER Arrival to Admit. (minutes)[2]	294	332	323	274
Time from ER Arrival to Discharge (minutes)	375	191	168	134
Time in ER Before Being Evaluated (minutes)	384	46	29	26
Time to Pain Meds for Fractures (minutes)	44	56	62	57
Heart Attack Care				
Aspirin Given at Discharge	18	100%	99%	99%
Fibrinolytic Meds Within 30 Min. of Arrival[7]	-	-	73%	54%
PCI Within 90 Minutes of Arrival[7]	-	-	95%	96%
Statin Prescribed at Discharge	19	89%	98%	98%
Heart Failure Care				
ACE Inhibitor or ARB for LVSD[2]	61	95%	97%	97%
Discharge Instructions Given[2]	164	79%	94%	94%
Evaluation of LVS Function[2]	223	98%	99%	99%
Medicare Spending				
Medicare Spending per Patient (ratio)	-	0.97	0.98	0.98
Pneumonia Care				
Appropriate Initial Antibiotic Given[2]	95	93%	97%	95%
Blood Culture Timing[2]	150	98%	98%	98%
Pregnancy and Delivery Care				
Newborn Deliveries Scheduled Early	492	2%	5%	6%
Preventive Care				
Immunization for Influenza[2]	448	88%	89%	90%
Immunization for Pneumonia[2]	326	78%	90%	92%
Stroke Care				
Anticoagulation Therapy for Atrial Fibrillation	14	86%	95%	95%
Antithrombotic Therapy Timing	118	97%	98%	98%
Assessed for Rehabilitation	190	98%	97%	97%
Discharged on Antithrombotic Therapy	138	99%	99%	99%
Discharged on Statin Medication	91	98%	94%	94%
Thrombolytic Therapy Timing	12	92%	72%	66%
Venous Thromboembolism Prophylaxis	195	94%	94%	94%
Written Stroke Educational Materials Given	71	63%	87%	88%
Surgical Care Improvement Project				
Appropriate Beta Blocker Usage[2]	89	94%	97%	98%
Appropriate VTP Within 24 Hours[2]	406	99%	98%	98%
Controlled Postoperative Blood Glucose[2,7]	-	-	96%	97%
Perioperative Temperature Management[2]	469	100%	100%	100%
Prophylactic Antibiotic Selection[2]	329	99%	99%	99%
Prophylactic Antibiotic Selection (Outpatient)	77	97%	97%	98%
Prophylactic Antibiotic Stopped[2]	322	96%	98%	98%
Prophylactic Antibiotic Timing[2]	329	98%	99%	99%
Prophylactic Antibiotic Timing (Outpatient)	79	96%	97%	98%
Urinary Catheter Removal[2]	94	88%	97%	97%
Survey of Patients' Hospital Experiences				
Area Around Room 'Always' Quiet at Night	300+	43%	51%	61%
Doctors 'Always' Communicated Well	300+	74%	78%	82%
Home Recovery Information Given	300+	80%	83%	85%
Hospital Given 9 or 10 on 10 Point Scale	300+	58%	68%	71%
Meds 'Always' Explained Before Given	300+	53%	61%	64%
Nurses 'Always' Communicated Well	300+	66%	74%	79%
Pain 'Always' Well Controlled	300+	65%	68%	71%
Room and Bathroom 'Always' Clean	300+	55%	70%	73%
Timely Help 'Always' Received	300+	46%	62%	68%
Would Definitely Recommend Hospital	300+	70%	70%	71%
Use of Medical Imaging				
Cardiac Imaging Stress Test before Surgery	127	3.1%	5.2%	5.3%
Combination Abdominal CT Scan	323	5.0%	13.4%	10.5%
Combination Brain/Sinus CT Scan	403	4.5%	2.2%	2.7%
Combination Chest CT Scan[1]	-	-	2.3%	2.7%
Follow-up Mammogram/Ultrasound	3,676	6.1%	8.2%	8.8%
Lumbar Spine MRI for Low Back Pain[1]	-	-	34.2%	37.2%

Bear Valley Community Hospital

41870 Garstin Dr | Phone: 909-866-6501
Big Bear Lake, CA 92315 | Fax: 909-878-8282
E-mail: garstin@excite.com
URL: www.bvchd.com
Type: Acute Care Hospitals | Emergency Services: Yes
Ownership: Govt - Hospital Dist/Auth | Beds: 30

Key Personnel:
Anesthesiology.............. Dion Babaldon, CRNA
Emergency Room .... Chris Fagan, MD
Infection Control............ Ann Haggard, RN
Quality Assurance .... Armaleen Hunter
Chief of Medical Staff.......... Michael Norman, DO
Radiology.................. Scott Rogers, MD
President.................. Kevin Shanley
Operating Room.............. John Sharp

Measure	Cases	This Hosp.	State Avg.	U.S. Avg.
Blood Clot Prevention and Treatment				
Anticoagulation Overlap Therapy[1]	-	-	92%	93%
ICU Venous Thromboembolism Prophylaxis[7]	-	-	92%	92%
Incidence of Potentially Preventable VTE[7]	-	-	11%	10%
UFH with Dosages/Platelet Monitoring[7]	-	-	96%	97%
Venous Thromboembolism Prophylaxis	82	24%	83%	85%
Warfarin Therapy Discharge Instructions[1]	-	-	75%	75%
Chest Pain/Possible Heart Attack Care				
Aspirin Given Within 24 Hours of Arrival	60	82%	97%	96%
Fibrinolytic Meds Within 30 Min. of Arrival[1]	-	-	62%	58%
Average Time to ECG (minutes)	58	14	9	7
Average Time to Transfer (minutes)[1]	-	-	62	60
Children's Asthma Care				
Received Home Management Plan of Care	-	-	88%	88%
Received Reliever Medication	-	-	100%	100%
Received Systemic Corticosteroids	-	-	100%	100%
Emergency Department				
Admittance Decision Time (minutes)	52	85	125	98
Head CT Results Within 45 Min. of Arrival[1,3]	-	-	55%	57%
Patients Who Left ER Before Being Seen	10,210	1%	3%	2%
Time from ER Arrival to Admit. (minutes)	54	321	323	274
Time from ER Arrival to Discharge (minutes)	390	144	168	134
Time in ER Before Being Evaluated (minutes)	497	23	29	26
Time to Pain Meds for Fractures (minutes)	230	54	62	57
Heart Attack Care				
Aspirin Given at Discharge[5]	-	-	99%	99%
Fibrinolytic Meds Within 30 Min. of Arrival[5]	-	-	73%	54%
PCI Within 90 Minutes of Arrival[5]	-	-	95%	96%
Statin Prescribed at Discharge[5]	-	-	98%	98%
Heart Failure Care				
ACE Inhibitor or ARB for LVSD[7]	-	-	97%	97%
Discharge Instructions Given[1]	-	-	94%	94%
Evaluation of LVS Function[1]	-	-	99%	99%
Medicare Spending				
Medicare Spending per Patient (ratio)	-	0.92	0.98	0.98
Pneumonia Care				
Appropriate Initial Antibiotic Given	25	88%	97%	95%
Blood Culture Timing	19	95%	98%	98%
Pregnancy and Delivery Care				
Newborn Deliveries Scheduled Early[7]	-	-	5%	6%
Preventive Care				
Immunization for Influenza	69	77%	89%	90%
Immunization for Pneumonia	95	63%	90%	92%
Stroke Care				
Anticoagulation Therapy for Atrial Fibrillation[3,7]	-	-	95%	95%
Antithrombotic Therapy Timing[3,7]	-	-	98%	98%
Assessed for Rehabilitation[3,7]	-	-	97%	97%
Discharged on Antithrombotic Therapy[3,7]	-	-	99%	99%
Discharged on Statin Medication[3,7]	-	-	94%	94%
Thrombolytic Therapy Timing[3,7]	-	-	72%	66%
Venous Thromboembolism Prophylaxis[3,7]	-	-	94%	94%
Written Stroke Educational Materials Given[3,7]	-	-	87%	88%
Surgical Care Improvement Project				
Appropriate Beta Blocker Usage[5]	-	-	97%	98%
Appropriate VTP Within 24 Hours[5]	-	-	98%	98%
Controlled Postoperative Blood Glucose[5]	-	-	96%	97%
Perioperative Temperature Management[5]	-	-	100%	100%
Prophylactic Antibiotic Selection[5]	-	-	99%	99%
Prophylactic Antibiotic Selection (Outpatient)[5]	-	-	97%	98%
Prophylactic Antibiotic Stopped[5]	-	-	98%	98%
Prophylactic Antibiotic Timing[5]	-	-	99%	99%
Prophylactic Antibiotic Timing (Outpatient)[5]	-	-	97%	98%
Urinary Catheter Removal[5]	-	-	97%	97%
Survey of Patients' Hospital Experiences				
Area Around Room 'Always' Quiet at Night[10]	<100	65%	51%	61%
Doctors 'Always' Communicated Well[10]	<100	78%	78%	82%
Home Recovery Information Given[10]	<100	88%	83%	85%
Hospital Given 9 or 10 on 10 Point Scale[10]	<100	84%	68%	71%
Meds 'Always' Explained Before Given[10]	<100	61%	61%	64%
Nurses 'Always' Communicated Well[10]	<100	85%	74%	79%
Pain 'Always' Well Controlled[10]	<100	73%	68%	71%
Room and Bathroom 'Always' Clean[10]	<100	74%	70%	73%
Timely Help 'Always' Received[10]	<100	85%	62%	68%
Would Definitely Recommend Hospital[10]	<100	76%	70%	71%
Use of Medical Imaging				
Cardiac Imaging Stress Test before Surgery[7]	-	-	5.2%	5.3%
Combination Abdominal CT Scan	135	9.6%	13.4%	10.5%
Combination Brain/Sinus CT Scan[1]	-	-	2.2%	2.7%
Combination Chest CT Scan	80	10.0%	2.3%	2.7%
Follow-up Mammogram/Ultrasound	107	8.4%	8.2%	8.8%
Lumbar Spine MRI for Low Back Pain[7]	-	-	34.2%	37.2%

Northern Inyo Hospital

150 Pioneer Lane | Phone: 760-873-5811
Bishop, CA 93514 | Fax: 760-872-2768
URL: www.nih.org
Type: Critical Access Hospitals | Emergency Services: Yes
Ownership: Govt - Hospital Dist/Auth | Beds: 32

Key Personnel:
Emergency Room .... Helena Black, MD
Chief of Medical Staff.......... Michael Dillon, MD
President.................. M.C. Hubbard
Radiology.................. John W Nesson

Measure	Cases	This Hosp.	State Avg.	U.S. Avg.
Blood Clot Prevention and Treatment				
Anticoagulation Overlap Therapy[5]	-	-	92%	93%
ICU Venous Thromboembolism Prophylaxis[5]	-	-	92%	92%
Incidence of Potentially Preventable VTE[5]	-	-	11%	10%
UFH with Dosages/Platelet Monitoring[5]	-	-	96%	97%
Venous Thromboembolism Prophylaxis[5]	-	-	83%	85%
Warfarin Therapy Discharge Instructions[5]	-	-	75%	75%
Chest Pain/Possible Heart Attack Care				
Aspirin Given Within 24 Hours of Arrival	-	-	97%	96%
Fibrinolytic Meds Within 30 Min. of Arrival	-	-	62%	58%
Average Time to ECG (minutes)	-	-	9	7
Average Time to Transfer (minutes)	-	-	62	60
Children's Asthma Care				
Received Home Management Plan of Care	-	-	88%	88%
Received Reliever Medication	-	-	100%	100%
Received Systemic Corticosteroids	-	-	100%	100%

NOTE: Hospital profiles are in alphabetical order by state, then city, then hospital within the city; Rankings exclude hospitals with less than 25 cases except for patient surveys which excludes hospitals with less than 100 cases; (a) 100-299 cases; (1) The number of cases/patients is too few to report; (2) Data submitted were based on a sample of cases/patients; (3) Results are based on a shorter time period than required; (4) Data suppressed by CMS for one or more quarters; (5) Results are not available for this reporting period; (6) Fewer than 100 patients completed the HCAHPS survey; (7) No cases met the criteria for this measure; (8) The lower limit of the confidence interval cannot be calculated if the number of observed infections equals zero; (9) No data are available from the state/territory for this reporting period; (10) The scores shown reflect fewer than 50 completed surveys; (11) There were discrepancies in the data collection process; (12) This measure does not apply to this hospital for this reporting period; (13) Results cannot be calculated for this reporting period; (14) The results for this state are combined with nearby states to protect confidentiality; Please refer to the User's Guide for a full explanation of data.

Measure	Cases	This Hosp.	State Avg.	U.S. Avg.
Emergency Department				
Admittance Decision Time (minutes)[5]	-	-	125	98
Head CT Results Within 45 Min. of Arrival	-	-	55%	57%
Patients Who Left ER Before Being Seen	-	-	3%	2%
Time from ER Arrival to Admit. (minutes)[5]	-	-	323	274
Time from ER Arrival to Discharge (minutes)	-	-	168	134
Time in ER Before Being Evaluated (minutes)	-	-	29	26
Time to Pain Meds for Fractures (minutes)	-	-	62	57
Heart Attack Care				
Aspirin Given at Discharge[1]	-	-	99%	99%
Fibrinolytic Meds Within 30 Min. of Arrival[7]	-	-	73%	54%
PCI Within 90 Minutes of Arrival[7]	-	-	95%	96%
Statin Prescribed at Discharge[1]	-	-	98%	98%
Heart Failure Care				
ACE Inhibitor or ARB for LVSD[1]	-	-	97%	97%
Discharge Instructions Given[1]	-	-	94%	94%
Evaluation of LVS Function[1]	-	-	99%	99%
Medicare Spending				
Medicare Spending per Patient (ratio)	-	-	0.98	0.98
Pneumonia Care				
Appropriate Initial Antibiotic Given[1]	-	-	97%	95%
Blood Culture Timing[1]	-	-	98%	98%
Pregnancy and Delivery Care				
Newborn Deliveries Scheduled Early[5]	-	-	5%	6%
Preventive Care				
Immunization for Influenza[5]	-	-	89%	90%
Immunization for Pneumonia[5]	-	-	90%	92%
Stroke Care				
Anticoagulation Therapy for Atrial Fibrillation[5]	-	-	95%	95%
Antithrombotic Therapy Timing[5]	-	-	98%	98%
Assessed for Rehabilitation[5]	-	-	97%	97%
Discharged on Antithrombotic Therapy[5]	-	-	99%	99%
Discharged on Statin Medication[5]	-	-	94%	94%
Thrombolytic Therapy Timing[5]	-	-	72%	66%
Venous Thromboembolism Prophylaxis[5]	-	-	94%	94%
Written Stroke Educational Materials Given[5]	-	-	87%	88%
Surgical Care Improvement Project				
Appropriate Beta Blocker Usage	11	91%	97%	98%
Appropriate VTP Within 24 Hours	51	98%	98%	98%
Controlled Postoperative Blood Glucose[7]	-	-	96%	97%
Perioperative Temperature Management	65	100%	100%	100%
Prophylactic Antibiotic Selection	47	100%	99%	99%
Prophylactic Antibiotic Selection (Outpatient)	-	-	97%	98%
Prophylactic Antibiotic Stopped	44	91%	98%	98%
Prophylactic Antibiotic Timing	48	79%	99%	99%
Prophylactic Antibiotic Timing (Outpatient)	-	-	97%	98%
Urinary Catheter Removal	43	93%	97%	97%
Survey of Patients' Hospital Experiences				
Area Around Room 'Always' Quiet at Night	(a)	62%	51%	61%
Doctors 'Always' Communicated Well	(a)	83%	78%	82%
Home Recovery Information Given	(a)	90%	83%	85%
Hospital Given 9 or 10 on 10 Point Scale	(a)	73%	68%	71%
Meds 'Always' Explained Before Given	(a)	68%	61%	64%
Nurses 'Always' Communicated Well	(a)	82%	74%	79%
Pain 'Always' Well Controlled	(a)	78%	68%	71%
Room and Bathroom 'Always' Clean	(a)	82%	70%	73%
Timely Help 'Always' Received	(a)	75%	62%	68%
Would Definitely Recommend Hospital	(a)	80%	70%	71%
Use of Medical Imaging				
Cardiac Imaging Stress Test before Surgery	-	-	5.2%	5.3%
Combination Abdominal CT Scan	-	-	13.4%	10.5%
Combination Brain/Sinus CT Scan	-	-	2.2%	2.7%
Combination Chest CT Scan	-	-	2.3%	2.7%
Follow-up Mammogram/Ultrasound	-	-	8.2%	8.8%
Lumbar Spine MRI for Low Back Pain	-	-	34.2%	37.2%

Palo Verde Hospital

250 North First Street — Phone: 760-922-4115
Blythe, CA 92225 — Fax: 760-921-5201
URL: www.paloverdehospital.org
Type: Acute Care Hospitals — Emergency Services: Yes
Ownership: Government - Federal — Beds: 51

Key Personnel:
CEO . . . . Sandra Anaya
Intensive Care Unit. . . . . Andrea Barrera
Radiology. . . . . Cecil Bowen
CEO/President. . . . . Jim Carney
Infection Control . . . . Leida Meek
Emergency Room . . . . Roseanne Pahnka
President . . . . Trina Sartin

Measure	Cases	This Hosp.	State Avg.	U.S. Avg.
Blood Clot Prevention and Treatment				
Anticoagulation Overlap Therapy[1,2]	-	-	92%	93%
ICU Venous Thromboembolism Prophylaxis[2]	25	56%	92%	92%
Incidence of Potentially Preventable VTE[1,2]	-	-	11%	10%
UFH with Dosages/Platelet Monitoring[1,2]	-	-	96%	97%
Venous Thromboembolism Prophylaxis[2]	90	39%	83%	85%
Warfarin Therapy Discharge Instructions[1,2]	-	-	75%	75%
Chest Pain/Possible Heart Attack Care				
Aspirin Given Within 24 Hours of Arrival	40	88%	97%	96%
Fibrinolytic Meds Within 30 Min. of Arrival[1,3]	-	-	62%	58%
Average Time to ECG (minutes)	38	8	9	7
Average Time to Transfer (minutes)[1,3]	-	-	62	60
Children's Asthma Care				
Received Home Management Plan of Care	-	-	88%	88%
Received Reliever Medication	-	-	100%	100%
Received Systemic Corticosteroids	-	-	100%	100%
Emergency Department				
Admittance Decision Time (minutes)[2]	494	62	125	98
Head CT Results Within 45 Min. of Arrival[1]	-	-	55%	57%
Patients Who Left ER Before Being Seen	10,459	2%	3%	2%
Time from ER Arrival to Admit. (minutes)[2]	517	289	323	274
Time from ER Arrival to Discharge (minutes)	371	131	168	134
Time in ER Before Being Evaluated (minutes)	421	20	29	26
Time to Pain Meds for Fractures (minutes)	34	45	62	57
Heart Attack Care				
Aspirin Given at Discharge[1,3]	-	-	99%	99%
Fibrinolytic Meds Within 30 Min. of Arrival[3,7]	-	-	73%	54%
PCI Within 90 Minutes of Arrival[3,7]	-	-	95%	96%
Statin Prescribed at Discharge[1,3]	-	-	98%	98%
Heart Failure Care				
ACE Inhibitor or ARB for LVSD[3,7]	-	-	97%	97%
Discharge Instructions Given[1,3]	-	-	94%	94%
Evaluation of LVS Function[1,3]	-	-	99%	99%
Medicare Spending				
Medicare Spending per Patient (ratio)	-	0.92	0.98	0.98
Pneumonia Care				
Appropriate Initial Antibiotic Given[2]	25	76%	97%	95%
Blood Culture Timing[2]	30	77%	98%	98%
Pregnancy and Delivery Care				
Newborn Deliveries Scheduled Early[2]	48	0%	5%	6%
Preventive Care				
Immunization for Influenza[2]	295	23%	89%	90%
Immunization for Pneumonia[2]	346	31%	90%	92%
Stroke Care				
Anticoagulation Therapy for Atrial Fibrillation[5]	-	-	95%	95%
Antithrombotic Therapy Timing[5]	-	-	98%	98%
Assessed for Rehabilitation[5]	-	-	97%	97%
Discharged on Antithrombotic Therapy[5]	-	-	99%	99%
Discharged on Statin Medication[5]	-	-	94%	94%
Thrombolytic Therapy Timing[5]	-	-	72%	66%
Venous Thromboembolism Prophylaxis[5]	-	-	94%	94%
Written Stroke Educational Materials Given[5]	-	-	87%	88%
Surgical Care Improvement Project				
Appropriate Beta Blocker Usage[1,2]	-	-	97%	98%
Appropriate VTP Within 24 Hours[2]	23	57%	98%	98%
Controlled Postoperative Blood Glucose[2,7]	-	-	96%	97%
Perioperative Temperature Management[2]	29	93%	100%	100%
Prophylactic Antibiotic Selection[1,2]	-	-	99%	99%
Prophylactic Antibiotic Selection (Outpatient)[5]	-	-	97%	98%
Prophylactic Antibiotic Stopped[1,2]	-	-	98%	98%
Prophylactic Antibiotic Timing[1,2]	-	-	99%	99%
Prophylactic Antibiotic Timing (Outpatient)[5]	-	-	97%	98%
Urinary Catheter Removal[1,2]	-	-	97%	97%
Survey of Patients' Hospital Experiences				
Area Around Room 'Always' Quiet at Night	(a)	66%	51%	61%
Doctors 'Always' Communicated Well	(a)	79%	78%	82%
Home Recovery Information Given	(a)	84%	83%	85%
Hospital Given 9 or 10 on 10 Point Scale	(a)	51%	68%	71%
Meds 'Always' Explained Before Given	(a)	67%	61%	64%
Nurses 'Always' Communicated Well	(a)	79%	74%	79%
Pain 'Always' Well Controlled	(a)	73%	68%	71%
Room and Bathroom 'Always' Clean	(a)	75%	70%	73%
Timely Help 'Always' Received	(a)	65%	62%	68%
Would Definitely Recommend Hospital	(a)	46%	70%	71%
Use of Medical Imaging				
Cardiac Imaging Stress Test before Surgery[7]	-	-	5.2%	5.3%
Combination Abdominal CT Scan	171	11.7%	13.4%	10.5%
Combination Brain/Sinus CT Scan	152	7.9%	2.2%	2.7%
Combination Chest CT Scan	83	32.5%	2.3%	2.7%
Follow-up Mammogram/Ultrasound	85	1.2%	8.2%	8.8%
Lumbar Spine MRI for Low Back Pain[1]	-	-	34.2%	37.2%

Pioneers Memorial Healthcare District

207 West Legion Road — Phone: 760-351-3333
Brawley, CA 92227 — Fax: 760-344-4401
URL: www.pmhd.org
Type: Acute Care Hospitals — Emergency Services: Yes
Ownership: Govt - Hospital Dist/Auth — Beds: 99

Key Personnel:
Operating Room. . . . . Cedric Bautista, RN
Emergency Room . . . . Michael Berger
Anesthesiology. . . . . Devendra Kapoor, MD
Chief of Medical Staff . . . . Arthur Mejia
CEO/President. . . . . Richard L Mendoza
Infection Control. . . . . Kathleen Messerschmidt, BSN
Quality Assurance . . . . Susana Sanchez, RN
Intensive Care Unit. . . . . Sal Vargis, RN

Measure	Cases	This Hosp.	State Avg.	U.S. Avg.
Blood Clot Prevention and Treatment				
Anticoagulation Overlap Therapy[2]	13	62%	92%	93%
ICU Venous Thromboembolism Prophylaxis[2]	82	82%	92%	92%
Incidence of Potentially Preventable VTE[1,2]	-	-	11%	10%
UFH with Dosages/Platelet Monitoring[1,2]	-	-	96%	97%
Venous Thromboembolism Prophylaxis[2]	303	62%	83%	85%
Warfarin Therapy Discharge Instructions[2]	11	100%	75%	75%
Chest Pain/Possible Heart Attack Care				
Aspirin Given Within 24 Hours of Arrival	47	100%	97%	96%
Fibrinolytic Meds Within 30 Min. of Arrival[1]	-	-	62%	58%
Average Time to ECG (minutes)	48	9	9	7
Average Time to Transfer (minutes)[1]	-	-	62	60
Children's Asthma Care				
Received Home Management Plan of Care	-	-	88%	88%
Received Reliever Medication	-	-	100%	100%
Received Systemic Corticosteroids	-	-	100%	100%
Emergency Department				
Admittance Decision Time (minutes)[2]	533	255	125	98
Head CT Results Within 45 Min. of Arrival	13	0%	55%	57%
Patients Who Left ER Before Being Seen	43,852	0%	3%	2%
Time from ER Arrival to Admit. (minutes)[2]	540	427	323	274
Time from ER Arrival to Discharge (minutes)	400	144	168	134
Time in ER Before Being Evaluated (minutes)	425	11	29	26
Time to Pain Meds for Fractures (minutes)	179	44	62	57
Heart Attack Care				
Aspirin Given at Discharge	13	100%	99%	99%
Fibrinolytic Meds Within 30 Min. of Arrival[7]	-	-	73%	54%
PCI Within 90 Minutes of Arrival[7]	-	-	95%	96%
Statin Prescribed at Discharge	12	83%	98%	98%
Heart Failure Care				
ACE Inhibitor or ARB for LVSD	58	93%	97%	97%
Discharge Instructions Given	140	100%	94%	94%
Evaluation of LVS Function	148	97%	99%	99%
Medicare Spending				
Medicare Spending per Patient (ratio)	-	0.94	0.98	0.98
Pneumonia Care				
Appropriate Initial Antibiotic Given	98	100%	97%	95%
Blood Culture Timing	143	96%	98%	98%
Pregnancy and Delivery Care				
Newborn Deliveries Scheduled Early[2]	55	13%	5%	6%
Preventive Care				
Immunization for Influenza[2]	460	65%	89%	90%

NOTE: Hospital profiles are in alphabetical order by state, then city, then hospital within the city; Rankings exclude hospitals with less than 25 cases except for patient surveys which excludes hospitals with less than 100 cases; (a) 100-299 cases; (1) The number of cases/patients is too few to report; (2) Data submitted were based on a sample of cases/patients; (3) Results are based on a shorter time period than required; (4) Data suppressed by CMS for one or more quarters; (5) Results are not available for this reporting period; (6) Fewer than 100 patients completed the HCAHPS survey; (7) No cases met the criteria for this measure; (8) The lower limit of the confidence interval cannot be calculated if the number of observed infections equals zero; (9) No data are available from the state/territory for this reporting period; (10) The scores shown reflect fewer than 50 completed surveys; (11) There were discrepancies in the data collection process; (12) This measure does not apply to this hospital for this reporting period; (13) Results cannot be calculated for this reporting period; (14) The results for this state are combined with nearby states to protect confidentiality; Please refer to the User's Guide for a full explanation of data.

Immunization for Pneumonia[2]	364	77%	90%	92%
Stroke Care				
Anticoagulation Therapy for Atrial Fibrillation[1]	-	-	95%	95%
Antithrombotic Therapy Timing	45	96%	98%	98%
Assessed for Rehabilitation	51	84%	97%	97%
Discharged on Antithrombotic Therapy	48	90%	99%	99%
Discharged on Statin Medication	40	85%	94%	94%
Thrombolytic Therapy Timing	22	14%	72%	66%
Venous Thromboembolism Prophylaxis	51	73%	94%	94%
Written Stroke Educational Materials Given	28	14%	87%	88%
Surgical Care Improvement Project				
Appropriate Beta Blocker Usage	30	77%	97%	98%
Appropriate VTP Within 24 Hours	144	90%	98%	98%
Controlled Postoperative Blood Glucose[7]	-	-	96%	97%
Perioperative Temperature Management	162	100%	100%	100%
Prophylactic Antibiotic Selection	123	96%	99%	99%
Prophylactic Antibiotic Selection (Outpatient)	136	99%	97%	98%
Prophylactic Antibiotic Stopped	122	92%	98%	98%
Prophylactic Antibiotic Timing	123	99%	99%	99%
Prophylactic Antibiotic Timing (Outpatient)	142	89%	97%	98%
Urinary Catheter Removal	108	85%	97%	97%
Survey of Patients' Hospital Experiences				
Area Around Room 'Always' Quiet at Night	300+	50%	51%	61%
Doctors 'Always' Communicated Well	300+	71%	78%	82%
Home Recovery Information Given	300+	82%	83%	85%
Hospital Given 9 or 10 on 10 Point Scale	300+	69%	68%	71%
Meds 'Always' Explained Before Given	300+	62%	61%	64%
Nurses 'Always' Communicated Well	300+	74%	74%	79%
Pain 'Always' Well Controlled	300+	68%	68%	71%
Room and Bathroom 'Always' Clean	300+	70%	70%	73%
Timely Help 'Always' Received	300+	59%	62%	68%
Would Definitely Recommend Hospital	300+	76%	70%	71%
Use of Medical Imaging				
Cardiac Imaging Stress Test before Surgery[1]	-	-	5.2%	5.3%
Combination Abdominal CT Scan	749	3.6%	13.4%	10.5%
Combination Brain/Sinus CT Scan	592	1.2%	2.2%	2.7%
Combination Chest CT Scan	296	4.1%	2.3%	2.7%
Follow-up Mammogram/Ultrasound	333	13.2%	8.2%	8.8%
Lumbar Spine MRI for Low Back Pain	42	42.9%	34.2%	37.2%

Providence Saint Joseph Medical Center

501 South Buena Vista Phone: 818-843-5111
Burbank, CA 91505
URL: www.providence.org/losangeles
Type: Acute Care Hospitals Emergency Services: Yes
Ownership: Voluntary non-profit - Church Beds: 431
Key Personnel:
CEO/President. . . . . Michael Rembis
Chief of Medical Staff. . . . . Nicholas Testa, MD, FAECP

Measure	Cases	This Hosp.	State Avg.	U.S. Avg.
Blood Clot Prevention and Treatment				
Anticoagulation Overlap Therapy[2]	76	72%	92%	93%
ICU Venous Thromboembolism Prophylaxis[2]	69	88%	92%	92%
Incidence of Potentially Preventable VTE[2]	19	5%	11%	10%
UFH with Dosages/Platelet Monitoring[2]	23	100%	96%	97%
Venous Thromboembolism Prophylaxis[2]	309	90%	83%	85%
Warfarin Therapy Discharge Instructions[2]	58	64%	75%	75%
Chest Pain/Possible Heart Attack Care				
Aspirin Given Within 24 Hours of Arrival	20	100%	97%	96%
Fibrinolytic Meds Within 30 Min. of Arrival[5]	-	-	62%	58%
Average Time to ECG (minutes)	22	0	9	7
Average Time to Transfer (minutes)[5]	-	-	62	60
Children's Asthma Care				
Received Home Management Plan of Care	-	-	88%	88%
Received Reliever Medication	-	-	100%	100%
Received Systemic Corticosteroids	-	-	100%	100%
Emergency Department				
Admittance Decision Time (minutes)[2]	524	113	125	98
Head CT Results Within 45 Min. of Arrival[1]	-	-	55%	57%
Patients Who Left ER Before Being Seen	63,821	2%	3%	2%
Time from ER Arrival to Admit. (minutes)[2]	531	301	323	274
Time from ER Arrival to Discharge (minutes)	472	170	168	134
Time in ER Before Being Evaluated (minutes)	514	38	29	26
Time to Pain Meds for Fractures (minutes)	356	88	62	57
Heart Attack Care				
Aspirin Given at Discharge	261	99%	99%	99%
Fibrinolytic Meds Within 30 Min. of Arrival[7]	-	-	73%	54%
PCI Within 90 Minutes of Arrival	71	100%	95%	96%
Statin Prescribed at Discharge	257	99%	98%	98%
Heart Failure Care				
ACE Inhibitor or ARB for LVSD	139	99%	97%	97%
Discharge Instructions Given	341	90%	94%	94%
Evaluation of LVS Function	419	99%	99%	99%
Medicare Spending				
Medicare Spending per Patient (ratio)	-	1.02	0.98	0.98
Pneumonia Care				
Appropriate Initial Antibiotic Given[2]	144	96%	97%	95%
Blood Culture Timing[2]	229	99%	98%	98%
Pregnancy and Delivery Care				
Newborn Deliveries Scheduled Early[2]	123	13%	5%	6%
Preventive Care				
Immunization for Influenza[2]	559	94%	89%	90%
Immunization for Pneumonia[2]	604	93%	90%	92%
Stroke Care				
Anticoagulation Therapy for Atrial Fibrillation	41	100%	95%	95%
Antithrombotic Therapy Timing	178	99%	98%	98%
Assessed for Rehabilitation	250	99%	97%	97%
Discharged on Antithrombotic Therapy	213	100%	99%	99%
Discharged on Statin Medication	158	97%	94%	94%
Thrombolytic Therapy Timing	29	93%	72%	66%
Venous Thromboembolism Prophylaxis	271	98%	94%	94%
Written Stroke Educational Materials Given	150	93%	87%	88%
Surgical Care Improvement Project				
Appropriate Beta Blocker Usage[2]	149	100%	97%	98%
Appropriate VTP Within 24 Hours[2]	307	99%	98%	98%
Controlled Postoperative Blood Glucose[2]	86	100%	96%	97%
Perioperative Temperature Management[2]	447	100%	100%	100%
Prophylactic Antibiotic Selection[2]	321	100%	99%	99%
Prophylactic Antibiotic Selection (Outpatient)	364	99%	97%	98%
Prophylactic Antibiotic Stopped[2]	303	99%	98%	98%
Prophylactic Antibiotic Timing[2]	321	100%	99%	99%
Prophylactic Antibiotic Timing (Outpatient)	365	99%	97%	98%
Urinary Catheter Removal[2]	298	99%	97%	97%
Survey of Patients' Hospital Experiences				
Area Around Room 'Always' Quiet at Night	300+	56%	51%	61%
Doctors 'Always' Communicated Well	300+	80%	78%	82%
Home Recovery Information Given	300+	83%	83%	85%
Hospital Given 9 or 10 on 10 Point Scale	300+	76%	68%	71%
Meds 'Always' Explained Before Given	300+	61%	61%	64%
Nurses 'Always' Communicated Well	300+	77%	74%	79%
Pain 'Always' Well Controlled	300+	72%	68%	71%
Room and Bathroom 'Always' Clean	300+	72%	70%	73%
Timely Help 'Always' Received	300+	64%	62%	68%
Would Definitely Recommend Hospital	300+	80%	70%	71%
Use of Medical Imaging				
Cardiac Imaging Stress Test before Surgery	233	6.0%	5.2%	5.3%
Combination Abdominal CT Scan	1,006	8.8%	13.4%	10.5%
Combination Brain/Sinus CT Scan	906	2.1%	2.2%	2.7%
Combination Chest CT Scan	574	5.7%	2.3%	2.7%
Follow-up Mammogram/Ultrasound	2,238	11.3%	8.2%	8.8%
Lumbar Spine MRI for Low Back Pain	140	30.0%	34.2%	37.2%

Mills - Peninsula Medical Center

1501 Trousdale Drive Phone: 650-696-5270
Burlingame, CA 94010
URL: www.mills-peninsula.org
Type: Acute Care Hospitals Emergency Services: Yes
Ownership: Voluntary non-profit - Private
Key Personnel:
CEO . . . . Janet Wagner

Measure	Cases	This Hosp.	State Avg.	U.S. Avg.
Blood Clot Prevention and Treatment				
Anticoagulation Overlap Therapy[2]	92	85%	92%	93%
ICU Venous Thromboembolism Prophylaxis[2]	76	89%	92%	92%
Incidence of Potentially Preventable VTE[2]	26	0%	11%	10%
UFH with Dosages/Platelet Monitoring[2]	29	100%	96%	97%
Venous Thromboembolism Prophylaxis[2]	314	82%	83%	85%
Warfarin Therapy Discharge Instructions[2]	65	31%	75%	75%
Chest Pain/Possible Heart Attack Care				
Aspirin Given Within 24 Hours of Arrival[5]	-	-	97%	96%
Fibrinolytic Meds Within 30 Min. of Arrival[5]	-	-	62%	58%
Average Time to ECG (minutes)[5]	-	-	9	7
Average Time to Transfer (minutes)[5]	-	-	62	60
Children's Asthma Care				
Received Home Management Plan of Care	-	-	88%	88%
Received Reliever Medication	-	-	100%	100%
Received Systemic Corticosteroids	-	-	100%	100%
Emergency Department				
Admittance Decision Time (minutes)[2]	583	106	125	98
Head CT Results Within 45 Min. of Arrival[1]	-	-	55%	57%
Patients Who Left ER Before Being Seen	47,335	1%	3%	2%
Time from ER Arrival to Admit. (minutes)[2]	585	230	323	274
Time from ER Arrival to Discharge (minutes)	391	128	168	134
Time in ER Before Being Evaluated (minutes)	318	23	29	26
Time to Pain Meds for Fractures (minutes)	159	57	62	57
Heart Attack Care				
Aspirin Given at Discharge	197	100%	99%	99%
Fibrinolytic Meds Within 30 Min. of Arrival[7]	-	-	73%	54%
PCI Within 90 Minutes of Arrival	35	97%	95%	96%
Statin Prescribed at Discharge	199	100%	98%	98%
Heart Failure Care				
ACE Inhibitor or ARB for LVSD	57	100%	97%	97%
Discharge Instructions Given	258	99%	94%	94%
Evaluation of LVS Function	299	100%	99%	99%
Medicare Spending				
Medicare Spending per Patient (ratio)	-	0.88	0.98	0.98
Pneumonia Care				
Appropriate Initial Antibiotic Given[2]	116	97%	97%	95%
Blood Culture Timing[2]	160	99%	98%	98%
Pregnancy and Delivery Care				
Newborn Deliveries Scheduled Early	154	2%	5%	6%
Preventive Care				
Immunization for Influenza[2]	527	100%	89%	90%
Immunization for Pneumonia[2]	648	100%	90%	92%
Stroke Care				
Anticoagulation Therapy for Atrial Fibrillation	45	100%	95%	95%
Antithrombotic Therapy Timing	123	99%	98%	98%
Assessed for Rehabilitation	162	100%	97%	97%
Discharged on Antithrombotic Therapy	139	100%	99%	99%
Discharged on Statin Medication	105	100%	94%	94%
Thrombolytic Therapy Timing	20	85%	72%	66%
Venous Thromboembolism Prophylaxis	166	99%	94%	94%
Written Stroke Educational Materials Given	102	100%	87%	88%
Surgical Care Improvement Project				
Appropriate Beta Blocker Usage[2]	164	98%	97%	98%
Appropriate VTP Within 24 Hours[2]	426	100%	98%	98%
Controlled Postoperative Blood Glucose[2]	87	97%	96%	97%
Perioperative Temperature Management[2]	521	100%	100%	100%
Prophylactic Antibiotic Selection[2]	411	99%	99%	99%
Prophylactic Antibiotic Selection (Outpatient)	175	99%	97%	98%
Prophylactic Antibiotic Stopped[2]	406	97%	98%	98%
Prophylactic Antibiotic Timing[2]	411	99%	99%	99%
Prophylactic Antibiotic Timing (Outpatient)	179	97%	97%	98%
Urinary Catheter Removal[2]	358	99%	97%	97%
Survey of Patients' Hospital Experiences				
Area Around Room 'Always' Quiet at Night	300+	61%	51%	61%
Doctors 'Always' Communicated Well	300+	81%	78%	82%
Home Recovery Information Given	300+	84%	83%	85%
Hospital Given 9 or 10 on 10 Point Scale	300+	81%	68%	71%
Meds 'Always' Explained Before Given	300+	62%	61%	64%
Nurses 'Always' Communicated Well	300+	77%	74%	79%
Pain 'Always' Well Controlled	300+	76%	68%	71%
Room and Bathroom 'Always' Clean	300+	74%	70%	73%
Timely Help 'Always' Received	300+	60%	62%	68%
Would Definitely Recommend Hospital	300+	85%	70%	71%
Use of Medical Imaging				
Cardiac Imaging Stress Test before Surgery	381	4.5%	5.2%	5.3%
Combination Abdominal CT Scan	1,190	4.6%	13.4%	10.5%

NOTE: Hospital profiles are in alphabetical order by state, then city, then hospital within the city; Rankings exclude hospitals with less than 25 cases except for patient surveys which excludes hospitals with less than 100 cases; (a) 100-299 cases; (1) The number of cases/patients is too few to report; (2) Data submitted were based on a sample of cases/patients; (3) Results are based on a shorter time period than required; (4) Data suppressed by CMS for one or more quarters; (5) Results are not available for this reporting period; (6) Fewer than 100 patients completed the HCAHPS survey; (7) No cases met the criteria for this measure; (8) The lower limit of the confidence interval cannot be calculated if the number of observed infections equals zero; (9) No data are available from the state/territory for this reporting period; (10) The scores shown reflect fewer than 50 completed surveys; (11) There were discrepancies in the data collection process; (12) This measure does not apply to this hospital for this reporting period; (13) Results cannot be calculated for this reporting period; (14) The results for this state are combined with nearby states to protect confidentiality; Please refer to the User's Guide for a full explanation of data.

Measure	Cases	This Hosp.	State Avg.	U.S. Avg.
Combination Brain/Sinus CT Scan	666	0.2%	2.2%	2.7%
Combination Chest CT Scan	824	0.8%	2.3%	2.7%
Follow-up Mammogram/Ultrasound	3,877	16.7%	8.2%	8.8%
Lumbar Spine MRI for Low Back Pain	199	38.7%	34.2%	37.2%

Saint Johns Pleasant Valley Hospital

2309 Antonio Ave Phone: 805-389-5800
Camarillo, CA 93010 Fax: 805-383-7450
URL: www.stjohnshealth.org
Type: Acute Care Hospitals Emergency Services: Yes
Ownership: Voluntary non-profit - Church Beds: 187
Key Personnel:
Radiology. . . . . Steven Berrett
Chief of Medical Staff . . . . George Bo-Linn, MD
CEO/President. . . . . Sally Crain
Patient Relations . . . . Charles P Francis
Emergency Room . . . . Becky Hansen
Operating Room. . . . . Karen O'Connell
Quality Assurance . . . . Ballow Pat

Measure	Cases	This Hosp.	State Avg.	U.S. Avg.
Blood Clot Prevention and Treatment				
Anticoagulation Overlap Therapy[2]	21	95%	92%	93%
ICU Venous Thromboembolism Prophylaxis[2]	71	96%	92%	92%
Incidence of Potentially Preventable VTE[1,2]	-	-	11%	10%
UFH with Dosages/Platelet Monitoring[2]	15	100%	96%	97%
Venous Thromboembolism Prophylaxis[2]	262	89%	83%	85%
Warfarin Therapy Discharge Instructions[2]	12	100%	75%	75%
Chest Pain/Possible Heart Attack Care				
Aspirin Given Within 24 Hours of Arrival	55	100%	97%	96%
Fibrinolytic Meds Within 30 Min. of Arrival[7]	-	-	62%	58%
Average Time to ECG (minutes)	55	9	9	7
Average Time to Transfer (minutes)	14	34	62	60
Children's Asthma Care				
Received Home Management Plan of Care	-	-	88%	88%
Received Reliever Medication	-	-	100%	100%
Received Systemic Corticosteroids	-	-	100%	100%
Emergency Department				
Admittance Decision Time (minutes)[2]	455	181	125	98
Head CT Results Within 45 Min. of Arrival[1]	-	-	55%	57%
Patients Who Left ER Before Being Seen	19,276	0%	3%	2%
Time from ER Arrival to Admit. (minutes)[2]	461	343	323	274
Time from ER Arrival to Discharge (minutes)	386	134	168	134
Time in ER Before Being Evaluated (minutes)	406	16	29	26
Time to Pain Meds for Fractures (minutes)	117	47	62	57
Heart Attack Care				
Aspirin Given at Discharge[1]	-	-	99%	99%
Fibrinolytic Meds Within 30 Min. of Arrival[7]	-	-	73%	54%
PCI Within 90 Minutes of Arrival[7]	-	-	95%	96%
Statin Prescribed at Discharge[1]	-	-	98%	98%
Heart Failure Care				
ACE Inhibitor or ARB for LVSD	15	100%	97%	97%
Discharge Instructions Given	81	98%	94%	94%
Evaluation of LVS Function	103	100%	99%	99%
Medicare Spending				
Medicare Spending per Patient (ratio)	-	0.98	0.98	0.98
Pneumonia Care				
Appropriate Initial Antibiotic Given	66	92%	97%	95%
Blood Culture Timing	150	96%	98%	98%
Pregnancy and Delivery Care				
Newborn Deliveries Scheduled Early[7]	-	-	5%	6%
Preventive Care				
Immunization for Influenza[2]	294	83%	89%	90%
Immunization for Pneumonia[2]	443	89%	90%	92%
Stroke Care				
Anticoagulation Therapy for Atrial Fibrillation[1]	-	-	95%	95%
Antithrombotic Therapy Timing	46	98%	98%	98%
Assessed for Rehabilitation	50	98%	97%	97%
Discharged on Antithrombotic Therapy	47	98%	99%	99%
Discharged on Statin Medication	41	80%	94%	94%
Thrombolytic Therapy Timing[1]	-	-	72%	66%
Venous Thromboembolism Prophylaxis	51	84%	94%	94%
Written Stroke Educational Materials Given	27	81%	87%	88%
Surgical Care Improvement Project				
Appropriate Beta Blocker Usage[2]	59	98%	97%	98%
Appropriate VTP Within 24 Hours[2]	254	98%	98%	98%
Controlled Postoperative Blood Glucose[2,7]	-	-	96%	97%
Perioperative Temperature Management[2]	268	100%	100%	100%
Prophylactic Antibiotic Selection[2]	179	99%	99%	99%
Prophylactic Antibiotic Selection (Outpatient)	36	100%	97%	98%
Prophylactic Antibiotic Stopped[2]	157	99%	98%	98%
Prophylactic Antibiotic Timing[2]	179	100%	99%	99%
Prophylactic Antibiotic Timing (Outpatient)	36	100%	97%	98%
Urinary Catheter Removal[2]	152	89%	97%	97%
Survey of Patients' Hospital Experiences				
Area Around Room 'Always' Quiet at Night	300+	43%	51%	61%
Doctors 'Always' Communicated Well	300+	78%	78%	82%
Home Recovery Information Given	300+	87%	83%	85%
Hospital Given 9 or 10 on 10 Point Scale	300+	69%	68%	71%
Meds 'Always' Explained Before Given	300+	61%	61%	64%
Nurses 'Always' Communicated Well	300+	77%	74%	79%
Pain 'Always' Well Controlled	300+	70%	68%	71%
Room and Bathroom 'Always' Clean	300+	71%	70%	73%
Timely Help 'Always' Received	300+	59%	62%	68%
Would Definitely Recommend Hospital	300+	70%	70%	71%
Use of Medical Imaging				
Cardiac Imaging Stress Test before Surgery	89	6.7%	5.2%	5.3%
Combination Abdominal CT Scan	440	3.4%	13.4%	10.5%
Combination Brain/Sinus CT Scan	507	2.4%	2.2%	2.7%
Combination Chest CT Scan	209	0.5%	2.3%	2.7%
Follow-up Mammogram/Ultrasound	933	9.0%	8.2%	8.8%
Lumbar Spine MRI for Low Back Pain	92	26.1%	34.2%	37.2%

Mercy San Juan Medical Center

6501 Coyle Ave Phone: 916-537-5000
Carmichael, CA 95608 Fax: 916-537-5111
E-mail: bgaron@chw.edu
URL: www.mercysanjuan.org
Type: Acute Care Hospitals Emergency Services: Yes
Ownership: Voluntary non-profit - Other Beds: 260
Key Personnel:
Emergency Room . . . . Rogeren Lloydugh, RN
Pediatric In-Patient Care . . . . Maureen McGinlry
Infection Control. . . . . Jane Nelson
Radiology. . . . . Ed Oliyarrs
Chief of Medical Staff. . . . . Kuldip Sandhu, MD
Operating Room. . . . . Jeannette Smith
CEO/President. . . . . Michael J Uboldi
Ambulatory Care . . . . Irmgrad Webster, RN

Measure	Cases	This Hosp.	State Avg.	U.S. Avg.
Blood Clot Prevention and Treatment				
Anticoagulation Overlap Therapy[2]	129	91%	92%	93%
ICU Venous Thromboembolism Prophylaxis[2]	109	93%	92%	92%
Incidence of Potentially Preventable VTE[2]	15	0%	11%	10%
UFH with Dosages/Platelet Monitoring[2]	82	100%	96%	97%
Venous Thromboembolism Prophylaxis[2]	276	91%	83%	85%
Warfarin Therapy Discharge Instructions[2]	98	85%	75%	75%
Chest Pain/Possible Heart Attack Care				
Aspirin Given Within 24 Hours of Arrival[1]	-	-	97%	96%
Fibrinolytic Meds Within 30 Min. of Arrival[3,7]	-	-	62%	58%
Average Time to ECG (minutes)[1]	-	-	9	7
Average Time to Transfer (minutes)[3,7]	-	-	62	60
Children's Asthma Care				
Received Home Management Plan of Care	-	-	88%	88%
Received Reliever Medication	-	-	100%	100%
Received Systemic Corticosteroids	-	-	100%	100%
Emergency Department				
Admittance Decision Time (minutes)[2]	686	143	125	98
Head CT Results Within 45 Min. of Arrival[1]	-	-	55%	57%
Patients Who Left ER Before Being Seen	69,804	1%	3%	2%
Time from ER Arrival to Admit. (minutes)[2]	693	340	323	274
Time from ER Arrival to Discharge (minutes)	350	196	168	134
Time in ER Before Being Evaluated (minutes)	409	14	29	26
Time to Pain Meds for Fractures (minutes)	198	42	62	57
Heart Attack Care				
Aspirin Given at Discharge[2]	241	100%	99%	99%
Fibrinolytic Meds Within 30 Min. of Arrival[1,2]	-	-	73%	54%
PCI Within 90 Minutes of Arrival[2]	69	90%	95%	96%
Statin Prescribed at Discharge[2]	239	99%	98%	98%
Heart Failure Care				
ACE Inhibitor or ARB for LVSD[2]	99	100%	97%	97%
Discharge Instructions Given[2]	256	99%	94%	94%
Evaluation of LVS Function[2]	302	100%	99%	99%
Medicare Spending				
Medicare Spending per Patient (ratio)	-	0.95	0.98	0.98
Pneumonia Care				
Appropriate Initial Antibiotic Given[2]	62	98%	97%	95%
Blood Culture Timing[2]	111	95%	98%	98%
Pregnancy and Delivery Care				
Newborn Deliveries Scheduled Early[2]	35	0%	5%	6%
Preventive Care				
Immunization for Influenza[2]	561	94%	89%	90%
Immunization for Pneumonia[2]	632	91%	90%	92%
Stroke Care				
Anticoagulation Therapy for Atrial Fibrillation	41	98%	95%	95%
Antithrombotic Therapy Timing	227	100%	98%	98%
Assessed for Rehabilitation	378	99%	97%	97%
Discharged on Antithrombotic Therapy	270	99%	99%	99%
Discharged on Statin Medication	188	94%	94%	94%
Thrombolytic Therapy Timing	60	58%	72%	66%
Venous Thromboembolism Prophylaxis	411	97%	94%	94%
Written Stroke Educational Materials Given	205	97%	87%	88%
Surgical Care Improvement Project				
Appropriate Beta Blocker Usage[2]	237	95%	97%	98%
Appropriate VTP Within 24 Hours[2]	440	99%	98%	98%
Controlled Postoperative Blood Glucose[2]	123	98%	96%	97%
Perioperative Temperature Management[2]	581	100%	100%	100%
Prophylactic Antibiotic Selection[2]	526	98%	99%	99%
Prophylactic Antibiotic Selection (Outpatient)	126	99%	97%	98%
Prophylactic Antibiotic Stopped[2]	513	97%	98%	98%
Prophylactic Antibiotic Timing[2]	526	99%	99%	99%
Prophylactic Antibiotic Timing (Outpatient)	126	99%	97%	98%
Urinary Catheter Removal[2]	291	96%	97%	97%
Survey of Patients' Hospital Experiences				
Area Around Room 'Always' Quiet at Night	300+	47%	51%	61%
Doctors 'Always' Communicated Well	300+	78%	78%	82%
Home Recovery Information Given	300+	85%	83%	85%
Hospital Given 9 or 10 on 10 Point Scale	300+	66%	68%	71%
Meds 'Always' Explained Before Given	300+	62%	61%	64%
Nurses 'Always' Communicated Well	300+	73%	74%	79%
Pain 'Always' Well Controlled	300+	69%	68%	71%
Room and Bathroom 'Always' Clean	300+	69%	70%	73%
Timely Help 'Always' Received	300+	59%	62%	68%
Would Definitely Recommend Hospital	300+	67%	70%	71%
Use of Medical Imaging				
Cardiac Imaging Stress Test before Surgery	521	4.0%	5.2%	5.3%
Combination Abdominal CT Scan	703	0.9%	13.4%	10.5%
Combination Brain/Sinus CT Scan	1,084	2.8%	2.2%	2.7%
Combination Chest CT Scan	147	0.0%	2.3%	2.7%
Follow-up Mammogram/Ultrasound[7]	-	-	8.2%	8.8%
Lumbar Spine MRI for Low Back Pain[1]	-	-	34.2%	37.2%

Eden Medical Center

20103 Lake Chabot Road Phone: 510-537-1234
Castro Valley, CA 94546
URL: www.edenmedcenter.org
Type: Acute Care Hospitals Emergency Services: Yes
Ownership: Voluntary non-profit - Other Beds: 302
Key Personnel:
CEO/President. . . . . George Bischalaney

Measure	Cases	This Hosp.	State Avg.	U.S. Avg.
Blood Clot Prevention and Treatment				
Anticoagulation Overlap Therapy[2]	50	96%	92%	93%
ICU Venous Thromboembolism Prophylaxis[2]	131	95%	92%	92%
Incidence of Potentially Preventable VTE[2]	15	20%	11%	10%
UFH with Dosages/Platelet Monitoring[2]	24	100%	96%	97%
Venous Thromboembolism Prophylaxis[2]	420	81%	83%	85%
Warfarin Therapy Discharge Instructions[2]	31	45%	75%	75%
Chest Pain/Possible Heart Attack Care				
Aspirin Given Within 24 Hours of Arrival	29	100%	97%	96%
Fibrinolytic Meds Within 30 Min. of Arrival[7]	-	-	62%	58%
Average Time to ECG (minutes)	29	17	9	7

NOTE: Hospital profiles are in alphabetical order by state, then city, then hospital within the city; Rankings exclude hospitals with less than 25 cases except for patient surveys which excludes hospitals with less than 100 cases; (a) 100-299 cases; (1) The number of cases/patients is too few to report; (2) Data submitted were based on a sample of cases/patients; (3) Results are based on a shorter time period than required; (4) Data suppressed by CMS for one or more quarters; (5) Results are not available for this reporting period; (6) Fewer than 100 patients completed the HCAHPS survey; (7) No cases met the criteria for this measure; (8) The lower limit of the confidence interval cannot be calculated if the number of observed infections equals zero; (9) No data are available from the state/territory for this reporting period; (10) The scores shown reflect fewer than 50 completed surveys; (11) There were discrepancies in the data collection process; (12) This measure does not apply to this hospital for this reporting period; (13) Results cannot be calculated for this reporting period; (14) The results for this state are combined with nearby states to protect confidentiality; Please refer to the User's Guide for a full explanation of data.

Measure	Cases	This Hosp.	State Avg.	U.S. Avg.
Average Time to Transfer (minutes)	13	77	62	60
Children's Asthma Care				
Received Home Management Plan of Care	-	-	88%	88%
Received Reliever Medication	-	-	100%	100%
Received Systemic Corticosteroids	-	-	100%	100%
Emergency Department				
Admittance Decision Time (minutes)[2]	913	150	125	98
Head CT Results Within 45 Min. of Arrival[1]	-	-	55%	57%
Patients Who Left ER Before Being Seen	51,663	3%	3%	2%
Time from ER Arrival to Admit. (minutes)[2]	991	341	323	274
Time from ER Arrival to Discharge (minutes)[1]	557	200	168	134
Time in ER Before Being Evaluated (minutes)	591	49	29	26
Time to Pain Meds for Fractures (minutes)	123	85	62	57
Heart Attack Care				
Aspirin Given at Discharge	43	100%	99%	99%
Fibrinolytic Meds Within 30 Min. of Arrival[7]	-	-	73%	54%
PCI Within 90 Minutes of Arrival[7]	-	-	95%	96%
Statin Prescribed at Discharge	39	100%	98%	98%
Heart Failure Care				
ACE Inhibitor or ARB for LVSD	68	97%	97%	97%
Discharge Instructions Given	235	92%	94%	94%
Evaluation of LVS Function	297	100%	99%	99%
Medicare Spending				
Medicare Spending per Patient (ratio)	-	0.99	0.98	0.98
Pneumonia Care				
Appropriate Initial Antibiotic Given[2]	80	99%	97%	95%
Blood Culture Timing[2]	214	98%	98%	98%
Pregnancy and Delivery Care				
Newborn Deliveries Scheduled Early	80	0%	5%	6%
Preventive Care				
Immunization for Influenza[2]	857	74%	89%	90%
Immunization for Pneumonia[2]	894	79%	90%	92%
Stroke Care				
Anticoagulation Therapy for Atrial Fibrillation	31	100%	95%	95%
Antithrombotic Therapy Timing	143	100%	98%	98%
Assessed for Rehabilitation	261	100%	97%	97%
Discharged on Antithrombotic Therapy	173	99%	99%	99%
Discharged on Statin Medication	140	99%	94%	94%
Thrombolytic Therapy Timing	29	83%	72%	66%
Venous Thromboembolism Prophylaxis	300	97%	94%	94%
Written Stroke Educational Materials Given	118	64%	87%	88%
Surgical Care Improvement Project				
Appropriate Beta Blocker Usage[2]	113	98%	97%	98%
Appropriate VTP Within 24 Hours[2]	394	99%	98%	98%
Controlled Postoperative Blood Glucose[2,7]	-	-	96%	97%
Perioperative Temperature Management[2]	463	100%	100%	100%
Prophylactic Antibiotic Selection[2]	250	98%	99%	99%
Prophylactic Antibiotic Selection (Outpatient)	169	99%	97%	98%
Prophylactic Antibiotic Stopped[2]	240	99%	98%	98%
Prophylactic Antibiotic Timing[2]	251	100%	99%	99%
Prophylactic Antibiotic Timing (Outpatient)	169	99%	97%	98%
Urinary Catheter Removal[2]	253	94%	97%	97%
Survey of Patients' Hospital Experiences				
Area Around Room 'Always' Quiet at Night	300+	60%	51%	61%
Doctors 'Always' Communicated Well	300+	79%	78%	82%
Home Recovery Information Given	300+	81%	83%	85%
Hospital Given 9 or 10 on 10 Point Scale	300+	70%	68%	71%
Meds 'Always' Explained Before Given	300+	55%	61%	64%
Nurses 'Always' Communicated Well	300+	73%	74%	79%
Pain 'Always' Well Controlled	300+	66%	68%	71%
Room and Bathroom 'Always' Clean	300+	74%	70%	73%
Timely Help 'Always' Received	300+	61%	62%	68%
Would Definitely Recommend Hospital	300+	76%	70%	71%
Use of Medical Imaging				
Cardiac Imaging Stress Test before Surgery	46	2.2%	5.2%	5.3%
Combination Abdominal CT Scan	649	4.9%	13.4%	10.5%
Combination Brain/Sinus CT Scan	842	2.5%	2.2%	2.7%
Combination Chest CT Scan	226	0.9%	2.3%	2.7%
Follow-up Mammogram/Ultrasound	1,003	6.5%	8.2%	8.8%
Lumbar Spine MRI for Low Back Pain	40	40.0%	34.2%	37.2%

Surprise Valley Community Hospital

741 North Main Street
Cedarville, CA 96104
Type: Critical Access Hospitals
Ownership: Govt - Hospital Dist/Auth
Phone: 530-279-6111
Fax: 530-279-2680
Emergency Services: Yes
Beds: 26

Key Personnel:
President . . . . Jason Diven
Quality Assurance . . . . Janet Hill

Measure	Cases	This Hosp.	State Avg.	U.S. Avg.
Blood Clot Prevention and Treatment				
Anticoagulation Overlap Therapy[5]	-	-	92%	93%
ICU Venous Thromboembolism Prophylaxis[5]	-	-	92%	92%
Incidence of Potentially Preventable VTE[5]	-	-	11%	10%
UFH with Dosages/Platelet Monitoring[5]	-	-	96%	97%
Venous Thromboembolism Prophylaxis[5]	-	-	83%	85%
Warfarin Therapy Discharge Instructions[5]	-	-	75%	75%
Chest Pain/Possible Heart Attack Care				
Aspirin Given Within 24 Hours of Arrival	-	-	97%	96%
Fibrinolytic Meds Within 30 Min. of Arrival	-	-	62%	58%
Average Time to ECG (minutes)	-	-	9	7
Average Time to Transfer (minutes)	-	-	62	60
Children's Asthma Care				
Received Home Management Plan of Care	-	-	88%	88%
Received Reliever Medication	-	-	100%	100%
Received Systemic Corticosteroids	-	-	100%	100%
Emergency Department				
Admittance Decision Time (minutes)[5]	-	-	125	98
Head CT Results Within 45 Min. of Arrival	-	-	55%	57%
Patients Who Left ER Before Being Seen	-	-	3%	2%
Time from ER Arrival to Admit. (minutes)[5]	-	-	323	274
Time from ER Arrival to Discharge (minutes)	-	-	168	134
Time in ER Before Being Evaluated (minutes)	-	-	29	26
Time to Pain Meds for Fractures (minutes)	-	-	62	57
Heart Attack Care				
Aspirin Given at Discharge[5]	-	-	99%	99%
Fibrinolytic Meds Within 30 Min. of Arrival[5]	-	-	73%	54%
PCI Within 90 Minutes of Arrival[5]	-	-	95%	96%
Statin Prescribed at Discharge[5]	-	-	98%	98%
Heart Failure Care				
ACE Inhibitor or ARB for LVSD[3,7]	-	-	97%	97%
Discharge Instructions Given[3,7]	-	-	94%	94%
Evaluation of LVS Function[3,7]	-	-	99%	99%
Medicare Spending				
Medicare Spending per Patient (ratio)	-	-	0.98	0.98
Pneumonia Care				
Appropriate Initial Antibiotic Given[5]	-	-	97%	95%
Blood Culture Timing[5]	-	-	98%	98%
Pregnancy and Delivery Care				
Newborn Deliveries Scheduled Early[5]	-	-	5%	6%
Preventive Care				
Immunization for Influenza[5]	-	-	89%	90%
Immunization for Pneumonia[5]	-	-	90%	92%
Stroke Care				
Anticoagulation Therapy for Atrial Fibrillation[5]	-	-	95%	95%
Antithrombotic Therapy Timing[5]	-	-	98%	98%
Assessed for Rehabilitation[5]	-	-	97%	97%
Discharged on Antithrombotic Therapy[5]	-	-	99%	99%
Discharged on Statin Medication[5]	-	-	94%	94%
Thrombolytic Therapy Timing[5]	-	-	72%	66%
Venous Thromboembolism Prophylaxis[5]	-	-	94%	94%
Written Stroke Educational Materials Given[5]	-	-	87%	88%
Surgical Care Improvement Project				
Appropriate Beta Blocker Usage[5]	-	-	97%	98%
Appropriate VTP Within 24 Hours[5]	-	-	98%	98%
Controlled Postoperative Blood Glucose[5]	-	-	96%	97%
Perioperative Temperature Management[5]	-	-	100%	100%
Prophylactic Antibiotic Selection[5]	-	-	99%	99%
Prophylactic Antibiotic Selection (Outpatient)	-	-	97%	98%
Prophylactic Antibiotic Stopped[5]	-	-	98%	98%
Prophylactic Antibiotic Timing[5]	-	-	99%	99%
Prophylactic Antibiotic Timing (Outpatient)	-	-	97%	98%
Urinary Catheter Removal[5]	-	-	97%	97%
Survey of Patients' Hospital Experiences				
Area Around Room 'Always' Quiet at Night[5]	-	-	51%	61%
Doctors 'Always' Communicated Well[5]	-	-	78%	82%
Home Recovery Information Given[5]	-	-	83%	85%
Hospital Given 9 or 10 on 10 Point Scale[5]	-	-	68%	71%
Meds 'Always' Explained Before Given[5]	-	-	61%	64%
Nurses 'Always' Communicated Well[5]	-	-	74%	79%
Pain 'Always' Well Controlled[5]	-	-	68%	71%
Room and Bathroom 'Always' Clean[5]	-	-	70%	73%
Timely Help 'Always' Received[5]	-	-	62%	68%
Would Definitely Recommend Hospital[5]	-	-	70%	71%
Use of Medical Imaging				
Cardiac Imaging Stress Test before Surgery	-	-	5.2%	5.3%
Combination Abdominal CT Scan	-	-	13.4%	10.5%
Combination Brain/Sinus CT Scan	-	-	2.2%	2.7%
Combination Chest CT Scan	-	-	2.3%	2.7%
Follow-up Mammogram/Ultrasound	-	-	8.2%	8.8%
Lumbar Spine MRI for Low Back Pain	-	-	34.2%	37.2%

Seneca District Hospital

130 Brentwood Drive
Chester, CA 96020
URL: www.senecahospital.org
Type: Critical Access Hospitals
Ownership: Govt - Hospital Dist/Auth
Phone: 530-258-2121
Fax: 530-258-3836
Emergency Services: Yes
Beds: 26

Key Personnel:
Quality Assurance . . . . Bernard Hietpas
CEO . . . . Linda Wagner, RN, MSN, MHA, F
Chief of Medical Staff . . . . Chris Ward, MD

Measure	Cases	This Hosp.	State Avg.	U.S. Avg.
Blood Clot Prevention and Treatment				
Anticoagulation Overlap Therapy[5]	-	-	92%	93%
ICU Venous Thromboembolism Prophylaxis[5]	-	-	92%	92%
Incidence of Potentially Preventable VTE[5]	-	-	11%	10%
UFH with Dosages/Platelet Monitoring[5]	-	-	96%	97%
Venous Thromboembolism Prophylaxis[5]	-	-	83%	85%
Warfarin Therapy Discharge Instructions[5]	-	-	75%	75%
Chest Pain/Possible Heart Attack Care				
Aspirin Given Within 24 Hours of Arrival[5]	-	-	97%	96%
Fibrinolytic Meds Within 30 Min. of Arrival[5]	-	-	62%	58%
Average Time to ECG (minutes)[5]	-	-	9	7
Average Time to Transfer (minutes)[5]	-	-	62	60
Children's Asthma Care				
Received Home Management Plan of Care	-	-	88%	88%
Received Reliever Medication	-	-	100%	100%
Received Systemic Corticosteroids	-	-	100%	100%
Emergency Department				
Admittance Decision Time (minutes)[5]	-	-	125	98
Head CT Results Within 45 Min. of Arrival[5]	-	-	55%	57%
Patients Who Left ER Before Being Seen[5]	-	-	3%	2%
Time from ER Arrival to Admit. (minutes)[5]	-	-	323	274
Time from ER Arrival to Discharge (minutes)[3,7]	-	-	168	134
Time in ER Before Being Evaluated (minutes)[1,3]	-	-	29	26
Time to Pain Meds for Fractures (minutes)[5]	-	-	62	57
Heart Attack Care				
Aspirin Given at Discharge[5]	-	-	99%	99%
Fibrinolytic Meds Within 30 Min. of Arrival[5]	-	-	73%	54%
PCI Within 90 Minutes of Arrival[5]	-	-	95%	96%
Statin Prescribed at Discharge[5]	-	-	98%	98%
Heart Failure Care				
ACE Inhibitor or ARB for LVSD[5]	-	-	97%	97%
Discharge Instructions Given[5]	-	-	94%	94%
Evaluation of LVS Function[5]	-	-	99%	99%
Medicare Spending				
Medicare Spending per Patient (ratio)	-	-	0.98	0.98
Pneumonia Care				
Appropriate Initial Antibiotic Given[3,7]	-	-	97%	95%
Blood Culture Timing[3,7]	-	-	98%	98%
Pregnancy and Delivery Care				
Newborn Deliveries Scheduled Early[5]	-	-	5%	6%
Preventive Care				
Immunization for Influenza[5]	-	-	89%	90%
Immunization for Pneumonia[5]	-	-	90%	92%

NOTE: Hospital profiles are in alphabetical order by state, then city, then hospital within the city; Rankings exclude hospitals with less than 25 cases except for patient surveys which excludes hospitals with less than 100 cases; (a) 100-299 cases; (1) The number of cases/patients is too few to report; (2) Data submitted were based on a sample of cases/patients; (3) Results are based on a shorter time period than required; (4) Data suppressed by CMS for one or more quarters; (5) Results are not available for this reporting period; (6) Fewer than 100 patients completed the HCAHPS survey; (7) No cases met the criteria for this measure; (8) The lower limit of the confidence interval cannot be calculated if the number of observed infections equals zero; (9) No data are available from the state/territory for this reporting period; (10) The scores shown reflect fewer than 50 completed surveys; (11) There were discrepancies in the data collection process; (12) This measure does not apply to this hospital for this reporting period; (13) Results cannot be calculated for this reporting period; (14) The results for this state are combined with nearby states to protect confidentiality; Please refer to the User's Guide for a full explanation of data.

Stroke Care				
Anticoagulation Therapy for Atrial Fibrillation[5]	-	-	95%	95%
Antithrombotic Therapy Timing[5]	-	-	98%	98%
Assessed for Rehabilitation[5]	-	-	97%	97%
Discharged on Antithrombotic Therapy[5]	-	-	99%	99%
Discharged on Statin Medication[5]	-	-	94%	94%
Thrombolytic Therapy Timing[5]	-	-	72%	66%
Venous Thromboembolism Prophylaxis[5]	-	-	94%	94%
Written Stroke Educational Materials Given[5]	-	-	87%	88%
Surgical Care Improvement Project				
Appropriate Beta Blocker Usage[5]	-	-	97%	98%
Appropriate VTP Within 24 Hours[5]	-	-	98%	98%
Controlled Postoperative Blood Glucose[5]	-	-	96%	97%
Perioperative Temperature Management[5]	-	-	100%	100%
Prophylactic Antibiotic Selection[5]	-	-	99%	99%
Prophylactic Antibiotic Selection (Outpatient)[5]	-	-	97%	98%
Prophylactic Antibiotic Stopped[5]	-	-	98%	98%
Prophylactic Antibiotic Timing[5]	-	-	99%	99%
Prophylactic Antibiotic Timing (Outpatient)[5]	-	-	97%	98%
Urinary Catheter Removal[5]	-	-	97%	97%
Survey of Patients' Hospital Experiences				
Area Around Room 'Always' Quiet at Night[5]	-	-	51%	61%
Doctors 'Always' Communicated Well[5]	-	-	78%	82%
Home Recovery Information Given[5]	-	-	83%	85%
Hospital Given 9 or 10 on 10 Point Scale[5]	-	-	68%	71%
Meds 'Always' Explained Before Given[5]	-	-	61%	64%
Nurses 'Always' Communicated Well[5]	-	-	74%	79%
Pain 'Always' Well Controlled[5]	-	-	68%	71%
Room and Bathroom 'Always' Clean[5]	-	-	70%	73%
Timely Help 'Always' Received[5]	-	-	62%	68%
Would Definitely Recommend Hospital[5]	-	-	70%	71%
Use of Medical Imaging				
Cardiac Imaging Stress Test before Surgery[7]	-	-	5.2%	5.3%
Combination Abdominal CT Scan	48	2.1%	13.4%	10.5%
Combination Brain/Sinus CT Scan[1]	-	-	2.2%	2.7%
Combination Chest CT Scan[1]	-	-	2.3%	2.7%
Follow-up Mammogram/Ultrasound	125	8.8%	8.2%	8.8%
Lumbar Spine MRI for Low Back Pain[1]	-	-	34.2%	37.2%

Enloe Medical Center

1531 Esplanade Phone: 530-332-7300
Chico, CA 95926 Fax: 530-899-2026
URL: www.enloe.org
Type: Acute Care Hospitals Emergency Services: Yes
Ownership: Voluntary non-profit - Private Beds: 369

Key Personnel:
Quality Assurance .... George Fribance
Operating Room.............. Ann Marie Johansen
Chair/CEO.................. Eric Larrabee
Radiology.................... Dail Lodge
Pediatric Ambulatory Care ...... Jill Mark, RN
Pediatric In-Patient Care .... Jill Mark, RN
Chief of Medical Staff.......... Bonnie Perry
Infection Control.............. Alivia Strawn, RN

Measure	Cases	This Hosp.	State Avg.	U.S. Avg.
Blood Clot Prevention and Treatment				
Anticoagulation Overlap Therapy[2]	98	94%	92%	93%
ICU Venous Thromboembolism Prophylaxis[2]	78	86%	92%	92%
Incidence of Potentially Preventable VTE[1,2]	-	-	11%	10%
UFH with Dosages/Platelet Monitoring[2]	44	100%	96%	97%
Venous Thromboembolism Prophylaxis[2]	333	89%	83%	85%
Warfarin Therapy Discharge Instructions[2]	80	92%	75%	75%
Chest Pain/Possible Heart Attack Care				
Aspirin Given Within 24 Hours of Arrival[5]	-	-	97%	96%
Fibrinolytic Meds Within 30 Min. of Arrival[5]	-	-	62%	58%
Average Time to ECG (minutes)[5]	-	-	9	7
Average Time to Transfer (minutes)[5]	-	-	62	60
Children's Asthma Care				
Received Home Management Plan of Care	-	-	88%	88%
Received Reliever Medication	-	-	100%	100%
Received Systemic Corticosteroids	-	-	100%	100%
Emergency Department				
Admittance Decision Time (minutes)[2]	646	68	125	98
Head CT Results Within 45 Min. of Arrival[1]	-	-	55%	57%
Patients Who Left ER Before Being Seen	45,300	3%	3%	2%
Time from ER Arrival to Admit. (minutes)[2]	707	286	323	274
Time from ER Arrival to Discharge (minutes)	388	165	168	134
Time in ER Before Being Evaluated (minutes)	326	38	29	26
Time to Pain Meds for Fractures (minutes)	109	65	62	57
Heart Attack Care				
Aspirin Given at Discharge	295	100%	99%	99%
Fibrinolytic Meds Within 30 Min. of Arrival[7]	-	-	73%	54%
PCI Within 90 Minutes of Arrival	45	96%	95%	96%
Statin Prescribed at Discharge	295	100%	98%	98%
Heart Failure Care				
ACE Inhibitor or ARB for LVSD	60	98%	97%	97%
Discharge Instructions Given	175	97%	94%	94%
Evaluation of LVS Function	225	100%	99%	99%
Medicare Spending				
Medicare Spending per Patient (ratio)	-	0.96	0.98	0.98
Pneumonia Care				
Appropriate Initial Antibiotic Given	185	95%	97%	95%
Blood Culture Timing	315	96%	98%	98%
Pregnancy and Delivery Care				
Newborn Deliveries Scheduled Early[2]	25	0%	5%	6%
Preventive Care				
Immunization for Influenza[2]	507	93%	89%	90%
Immunization for Pneumonia[2]	646	93%	90%	92%
Stroke Care				
Anticoagulation Therapy for Atrial Fibrillation	36	97%	95%	95%
Antithrombotic Therapy Timing	155	97%	98%	98%
Assessed for Rehabilitation	203	97%	97%	97%
Discharged on Antithrombotic Therapy	184	100%	99%	99%
Discharged on Statin Medication	139	99%	94%	94%
Thrombolytic Therapy Timing	31	97%	72%	66%
Venous Thromboembolism Prophylaxis	211	99%	94%	94%
Written Stroke Educational Materials Given	87	92%	87%	88%
Surgical Care Improvement Project				
Appropriate Beta Blocker Usage[2]	219	96%	97%	98%
Appropriate VTP Within 24 Hours[2]	656	98%	98%	98%
Controlled Postoperative Blood Glucose[2]	134	95%	96%	97%
Perioperative Temperature Management[2]	828	100%	100%	100%
Prophylactic Antibiotic Selection[2]	683	100%	99%	99%
Prophylactic Antibiotic Selection (Outpatient)	292	98%	97%	98%
Prophylactic Antibiotic Stopped[2]	639	98%	98%	98%
Prophylactic Antibiotic Timing[2]	683	98%	99%	99%
Prophylactic Antibiotic Timing (Outpatient)	295	97%	97%	98%
Urinary Catheter Removal[2]	560	98%	97%	97%
Survey of Patients' Hospital Experiences				
Area Around Room 'Always' Quiet at Night	300+	54%	51%	61%
Doctors 'Always' Communicated Well	300+	80%	78%	82%
Home Recovery Information Given	300+	88%	83%	85%
Hospital Given 9 or 10 on 10 Point Scale	300+	78%	68%	71%
Meds 'Always' Explained Before Given	300+	67%	61%	64%
Nurses 'Always' Communicated Well	300+	80%	74%	79%
Pain 'Always' Well Controlled	300+	72%	68%	71%
Room and Bathroom 'Always' Clean	300+	75%	70%	73%
Timely Help 'Always' Received	300+	67%	62%	68%
Would Definitely Recommend Hospital	300+	78%	70%	71%
Use of Medical Imaging				
Cardiac Imaging Stress Test before Surgery	230	2.2%	5.2%	5.3%
Combination Abdominal CT Scan	613	0.5%	13.4%	10.5%
Combination Brain/Sinus CT Scan	748	2.0%	2.2%	2.7%
Combination Chest CT Scan	81	0.0%	2.3%	2.7%
Follow-up Mammogram/Ultrasound[7]	-	-	8.2%	8.8%
Lumbar Spine MRI for Low Back Pain[1]	-	-	34.2%	37.2%

Chino Valley Medical Center

5451 Walnut Ave Phone: 909-627-6111
Chino, CA 91710 Fax: 909-464-8882
URL: www.cvmc.com
Type: Acute Care Hospitals Emergency Services: Yes
Ownership: Proprietary Beds: 126

Key Personnel:
Quality Assurance .... Pat Becker
Chief of Medical Staff.......... James M. Lally, DO, MMM
Infection Control.............. Jeanine Martin
CEO/President................ Prem Reddy, MD, FACC, FCCP
Operating Room.............. Rosemary Rundle, RN
Pediatric In-Patient Care .... Myrna Saludares, MD
Radiology.................... Dave Symonds

Measure	Cases	This Hosp.	State Avg.	U.S. Avg.
Blood Clot Prevention and Treatment				
Anticoagulation Overlap Therapy[2]	28	100%	92%	93%
ICU Venous Thromboembolism Prophylaxis[2]	35	97%	92%	92%
Incidence of Potentially Preventable VTE[2,7]	-	-	11%	10%
UFH with Dosages/Platelet Monitoring[2]	43	100%	96%	97%
Venous Thromboembolism Prophylaxis[2]	343	96%	83%	85%
Warfarin Therapy Discharge Instructions[2]	19	84%	75%	75%
Chest Pain/Possible Heart Attack Care				
Aspirin Given Within 24 Hours of Arrival	38	100%	97%	96%
Fibrinolytic Meds Within 30 Min. of Arrival[7]	-	-	62%	58%
Average Time to ECG (minutes)	40	14	9	7
Average Time to Transfer (minutes)[1]	-	-	62	60
Children's Asthma Care				
Received Home Management Plan of Care	-	-	88%	88%
Received Reliever Medication	-	-	100%	100%
Received Systemic Corticosteroids	-	-	100%	100%
Emergency Department				
Admittance Decision Time (minutes)[2]	974	65	125	98
Head CT Results Within 45 Min. of Arrival[1]	-	-	55%	57%
Patients Who Left ER Before Being Seen	38,090	1%	3%	2%
Time from ER Arrival to Admit. (minutes)[2]	974	178	323	274
Time from ER Arrival to Discharge (minutes)	415	89	168	134
Time in ER Before Being Evaluated (minutes)	437	18	29	26
Time to Pain Meds for Fractures (minutes)	197	42	62	57
Heart Attack Care				
Aspirin Given at Discharge[1]	-	-	99%	99%
Fibrinolytic Meds Within 30 Min. of Arrival[7]	-	-	73%	54%
PCI Within 90 Minutes of Arrival[7]	-	-	95%	96%
Statin Prescribed at Discharge[1]	-	-	98%	98%
Heart Failure Care				
ACE Inhibitor or ARB for LVSD	37	100%	97%	97%
Discharge Instructions Given	69	100%	94%	94%
Evaluation of LVS Function	82	100%	99%	99%
Medicare Spending				
Medicare Spending per Patient (ratio)	-	0.95	0.98	0.98
Pneumonia Care				
Appropriate Initial Antibiotic Given	51	96%	97%	95%
Blood Culture Timing	76	97%	98%	98%
Pregnancy and Delivery Care				
Newborn Deliveries Scheduled Early[7]	-	-	5%	6%
Preventive Care				
Immunization for Influenza[2]	542	99%	89%	90%
Immunization for Pneumonia[2]	620	99%	90%	92%
Stroke Care				
Anticoagulation Therapy for Atrial Fibrillation[1]	-	-	95%	95%
Antithrombotic Therapy Timing	21	95%	98%	98%
Assessed for Rehabilitation	26	96%	97%	97%
Discharged on Antithrombotic Therapy	25	100%	99%	99%
Discharged on Statin Medication	18	100%	94%	94%
Thrombolytic Therapy Timing[7]	-	-	72%	66%
Venous Thromboembolism Prophylaxis	25	100%	94%	94%
Written Stroke Educational Materials Given	22	73%	87%	88%
Surgical Care Improvement Project				
Appropriate Beta Blocker Usage[1]	-	-	97%	98%
Appropriate VTP Within 24 Hours	40	100%	98%	98%
Controlled Postoperative Blood Glucose[7]	-	-	96%	97%
Perioperative Temperature Management	44	100%	100%	100%
Prophylactic Antibiotic Selection	12	100%	99%	99%
Prophylactic Antibiotic Selection (Outpatient)[1,3]	-	-	97%	98%
Prophylactic Antibiotic Stopped	12	92%	98%	98%
Prophylactic Antibiotic Timing	12	100%	99%	99%
Prophylactic Antibiotic Timing (Outpatient)[1,3]	-	-	97%	98%
Urinary Catheter Removal	17	88%	97%	97%
Survey of Patients' Hospital Experiences				
Area Around Room 'Always' Quiet at Night[11]	300+	52%	51%	61%
Doctors 'Always' Communicated Well[11]	300+	77%	78%	82%
Home Recovery Information Given[11]	300+	83%	83%	85%
Hospital Given 9 or 10 on 10 Point Scale[11]	300+	69%	68%	71%
Meds 'Always' Explained Before Given[11]	300+	57%	61%	64%

NOTE: Hospital profiles are in alphabetical order by state, then city, then hospital within the city; Rankings exclude hospitals with less than 25 cases except for patient surveys which excludes hospitals with less than 100 cases; (a) 100-299 cases; (1) The number of cases/patients is too few to report; (2) Data submitted were based on a sample of cases/patients; (3) Results are based on a shorter time period than required; (4) Data suppressed by CMS for one or more quarters; (5) Results are not available for this reporting period; (6) Fewer than 100 patients completed the HCAHPS survey; (7) No cases met the criteria for this measure; (8) The lower limit of the confidence interval cannot be calculated if the number of observed infections equals zero; (9) No data are available from the state/territory for this reporting period; (10) The scores shown reflect fewer than 50 completed surveys; (11) There were discrepancies in the data collection process; (12) This measure does not apply to this hospital for this reporting period; (13) Results cannot be calculated for this reporting period; (14) The results for this state are combined with nearby states to protect confidentiality; Please refer to the User's Guide for a full explanation of data.

Measure	Cases	This Hosp.	State Avg.	U.S. Avg.
Nurses 'Always' Communicated Well[11]	300+	72%	74%	79%
Pain 'Always' Well Controlled[11]	300+	69%	68%	71%
Room and Bathroom 'Always' Clean[11]	300+	71%	70%	73%
Timely Help 'Always' Received[11]	300+	59%	62%	68%
Would Definitely Recommend Hospital[11]	300+	68%	70%	71%
Use of Medical Imaging				
Cardiac Imaging Stress Test before Surgery[1]	-	-	5.2%	5.3%
Combination Abdominal CT Scan	115	13.0%	13.4%	10.5%
Combination Brain/Sinus CT Scan[1]	-	-	2.2%	2.7%
Combination Chest CT Scan[1]	-	-	2.3%	2.7%
Follow-up Mammogram/Ultrasound[1]	-	-	8.2%	8.8%
Lumbar Spine MRI for Low Back Pain[7]	-	-	34.2%	37.2%

Sharp Chula Vista Medical Center

751 Medical Center Court
Chula Vista, CA 91911
Phone: 619-502-5800
Fax: 619-482-3535
E-mail: info@sharp.com
URL: www.sharp.com
Type: Acute Care Hospitals
Emergency Services: Yes
Ownership: Proprietary
Beds: 343

Key Personnel:
CEO/President. . . . . Christopher L Boyd
Cardiac Laboratory. . . . . Daniel Copin, MD
Radiology. . . . . Jeffrey Liebesman
Infection Control. . . . . Linda Riley
Operating Room. . . . . Karen Simpson
Chief of Medical Staff. . . . . Seung-Yi T Song, MD

Measure	Cases	This Hosp.	State Avg.	U.S. Avg.
Blood Clot Prevention and Treatment				
Anticoagulation Overlap Therapy[2]	69	90%	92%	93%
ICU Venous Thromboembolism Prophylaxis[2]	104	94%	92%	92%
Incidence of Potentially Preventable VTE[2]	20	10%	11%	10%
UFH with Dosages/Platelet Monitoring[2]	67	97%	96%	97%
Venous Thromboembolism Prophylaxis[2]	376	77%	83%	85%
Warfarin Therapy Discharge Instructions[2]	51	73%	75%	75%
Chest Pain/Possible Heart Attack Care				
Aspirin Given Within 24 Hours of Arrival	46	98%	97%	96%
Fibrinolytic Meds Within 30 Min. of Arrival[3,7]	-	-	62%	58%
Average Time to ECG (minutes)	49	11	9	7
Average Time to Transfer (minutes)[3,7]	-	-	62	60
Children's Asthma Care				
Received Home Management Plan of Care	-	-	88%	88%
Received Reliever Medication	-	-	100%	100%
Received Systemic Corticosteroids	-	-	100%	100%
Emergency Department				
Admittance Decision Time (minutes)[2]	752	164	125	98
Head CT Results Within 45 Min. of Arrival[1]	-	-	55%	57%
Patients Who Left ER Before Being Seen	36,032	3%	3%	2%
Time from ER Arrival to Admit. (minutes)[2]	784	398	323	274
Time from ER Arrival to Discharge (minutes)	589	212	168	134
Time in ER Before Being Evaluated (minutes)	442	99	29	26
Time to Pain Meds for Fractures (minutes)	205	42	62	57
Heart Attack Care				
Aspirin Given at Discharge	149	99%	99%	99%
Fibrinolytic Meds Within 30 Min. of Arrival[7]	-	-	73%	54%
PCI Within 90 Minutes of Arrival	43	98%	95%	96%
Statin Prescribed at Discharge	150	99%	98%	98%
Heart Failure Care				
ACE Inhibitor or ARB for LVSD	159	100%	97%	97%
Discharge Instructions Given	528	96%	94%	94%
Evaluation of LVS Function	646	100%	99%	99%
Medicare Spending				
Medicare Spending per Patient (ratio)	-	0.98	0.98	0.98
Pneumonia Care				
Appropriate Initial Antibiotic Given	248	96%	97%	95%
Blood Culture Timing	402	99%	98%	98%
Pregnancy and Delivery Care				
Newborn Deliveries Scheduled Early	361	6%	5%	6%
Preventive Care				
Immunization for Influenza[2]	656	98%	89%	90%
Immunization for Pneumonia[2]	688	96%	90%	92%
Stroke Care				
Anticoagulation Therapy for Atrial Fibrillation	29	90%	95%	95%
Antithrombotic Therapy Timing	161	97%	98%	98%
Assessed for Rehabilitation	193	99%	97%	97%
Discharged on Antithrombotic Therapy	175	99%	99%	99%
Discharged on Statin Medication	116	99%	94%	94%
Thrombolytic Therapy Timing	21	90%	72%	66%
Venous Thromboembolism Prophylaxis	211	95%	94%	94%
Written Stroke Educational Materials Given	102	91%	87%	88%
Surgical Care Improvement Project				
Appropriate Beta Blocker Usage[2]	161	96%	97%	98%
Appropriate VTP Within 24 Hours[2]	305	98%	98%	98%
Controlled Postoperative Blood Glucose[2]	121	99%	96%	97%
Perioperative Temperature Management[2]	429	100%	100%	100%
Prophylactic Antibiotic Selection[2]	361	99%	99%	99%
Prophylactic Antibiotic Selection (Outpatient)	205	100%	97%	98%
Prophylactic Antibiotic Stopped[2]	349	97%	98%	98%
Prophylactic Antibiotic Timing[2]	362	100%	99%	99%
Prophylactic Antibiotic Timing (Outpatient)	206	98%	97%	98%
Urinary Catheter Removal[2]	286	99%	97%	97%
Survey of Patients' Hospital Experiences				
Area Around Room 'Always' Quiet at Night	300+	51%	51%	61%
Doctors 'Always' Communicated Well	300+	78%	78%	82%
Home Recovery Information Given	300+	87%	83%	85%
Hospital Given 9 or 10 on 10 Point Scale	300+	73%	68%	71%
Meds 'Always' Explained Before Given	300+	65%	61%	64%
Nurses 'Always' Communicated Well	300+	80%	74%	79%
Pain 'Always' Well Controlled	300+	74%	68%	71%
Room and Bathroom 'Always' Clean	300+	77%	70%	73%
Timely Help 'Always' Received	300+	68%	62%	68%
Would Definitely Recommend Hospital	300+	77%	70%	71%
Use of Medical Imaging				
Cardiac Imaging Stress Test before Surgery	135	3.7%	5.2%	5.3%
Combination Abdominal CT Scan	586	0.7%	13.4%	10.5%
Combination Brain/Sinus CT Scan	846	1.2%	2.2%	2.7%
Combination Chest CT Scan	124	4.0%	2.3%	2.7%
Follow-up Mammogram/Ultrasound[7]	-	-	8.2%	8.8%
Lumbar Spine MRI for Low Back Pain[1]	-	-	34.2%	37.2%

Saint Helena Hospital - Clearlake

15630 18th Ave - Hwy 53
Clearlake, CA 95422
Phone: 707-994-6486
Fax: 707-995-3516
URL: www.redbudhospital.org
Type: Critical Access Hospitals
Emergency Services: Yes
Ownership: Voluntary non-profit - Church
Beds: 32

Key Personnel:
Operating Room. . . . . Arthur Bikangaga, RN
Radiology. . . . . Jerrold I Grayson
Quality Assurance . . . . Cindy Hiday
Coronary Care . . . . Ilona Horton
Infection Control. . . . . Maureen Milligan
Chief of Medical Staff. . . . . Steve Shepper
CEO/President. . . . . Jennifer Swenson

Measure	Cases	This Hosp.	State Avg.	U.S. Avg.
Blood Clot Prevention and Treatment				
Anticoagulation Overlap Therapy[2]	11	100%	92%	93%
ICU Venous Thromboembolism Prophylaxis[2]	39	97%	92%	92%
Incidence of Potentially Preventable VTE[1,2]	-	-	11%	10%
UFH with Dosages/Platelet Monitoring[2,7]	-	-	96%	97%
Venous Thromboembolism Prophylaxis[2]	94	96%	83%	85%
Warfarin Therapy Discharge Instructions[1,2]	-	-	75%	75%
Chest Pain/Possible Heart Attack Care				
Aspirin Given Within 24 Hours of Arrival	-	-	97%	96%
Fibrinolytic Meds Within 30 Min. of Arrival	-	-	62%	58%
Average Time to ECG (minutes)	-	-	9	7
Average Time to Transfer (minutes)	-	-	62	60
Children's Asthma Care				
Received Home Management Plan of Care	-	-	88%	88%
Received Reliever Medication	-	-	100%	100%
Received Systemic Corticosteroids	-	-	100%	100%
Emergency Department				
Admittance Decision Time (minutes)[5]	-	-	125	98
Head CT Results Within 45 Min. of Arrival	-	-	55%	57%
Patients Who Left ER Before Being Seen	-	-	3%	2%
Time from ER Arrival to Admit. (minutes)[5]	-	-	323	274
Time from ER Arrival to Discharge (minutes)	-	-	168	134
Time in ER Before Being Evaluated (minutes)	-	-	29	26
Time to Pain Meds for Fractures (minutes)	-	-	62	57
Heart Attack Care				
Aspirin Given at Discharge[1]	-	-	99%	99%
Fibrinolytic Meds Within 30 Min. of Arrival[7]	-	-	73%	54%
PCI Within 90 Minutes of Arrival[7]	-	-	95%	96%
Statin Prescribed at Discharge[1]	-	-	98%	98%
Heart Failure Care				
ACE Inhibitor or ARB for LVSD[1]	-	-	97%	97%
Discharge Instructions Given	22	95%	94%	94%
Evaluation of LVS Function	24	100%	99%	99%
Medicare Spending				
Medicare Spending per Patient (ratio)	-	-	0.98	0.98
Pneumonia Care				
Appropriate Initial Antibiotic Given	57	100%	97%	95%
Blood Culture Timing	67	97%	98%	98%
Pregnancy and Delivery Care				
Newborn Deliveries Scheduled Early[5]	-	-	5%	6%
Preventive Care				
Immunization for Influenza[5]	-	-	89%	90%
Immunization for Pneumonia[5]	-	-	90%	92%
Stroke Care				
Anticoagulation Therapy for Atrial Fibrillation[3,7]	-	-	95%	95%
Antithrombotic Therapy Timing[1,3]	-	-	98%	98%
Assessed for Rehabilitation[1,3]	-	-	97%	97%
Discharged on Antithrombotic Therapy[1,3]	-	-	99%	99%
Discharged on Statin Medication[1,3]	-	-	94%	94%
Thrombolytic Therapy Timing[3,7]	-	-	72%	66%
Venous Thromboembolism Prophylaxis[1,3]	-	-	94%	94%
Written Stroke Educational Materials Given[3,7]	-	-	87%	88%
Surgical Care Improvement Project				
Appropriate Beta Blocker Usage	11	100%	97%	98%
Appropriate VTP Within 24 Hours	37	81%	98%	98%
Controlled Postoperative Blood Glucose[7]	-	-	96%	97%
Perioperative Temperature Management	54	100%	100%	100%
Prophylactic Antibiotic Selection	22	91%	99%	99%
Prophylactic Antibiotic Selection (Outpatient)	-	-	97%	98%
Prophylactic Antibiotic Stopped	21	100%	98%	98%
Prophylactic Antibiotic Timing	22	95%	99%	99%
Prophylactic Antibiotic Timing (Outpatient)	-	-	97%	98%
Urinary Catheter Removal	17	76%	97%	97%
Survey of Patients' Hospital Experiences				
Area Around Room 'Always' Quiet at Night	(a)	52%	51%	61%
Doctors 'Always' Communicated Well	(a)	78%	78%	82%
Home Recovery Information Given	(a)	84%	83%	85%
Hospital Given 9 or 10 on 10 Point Scale	(a)	59%	68%	71%
Meds 'Always' Explained Before Given	(a)	61%	61%	64%
Nurses 'Always' Communicated Well	(a)	75%	74%	79%
Pain 'Always' Well Controlled	(a)	67%	68%	71%
Room and Bathroom 'Always' Clean	(a)	61%	70%	73%
Timely Help 'Always' Received	(a)	67%	62%	68%
Would Definitely Recommend Hospital	(a)	59%	70%	71%
Use of Medical Imaging				
Cardiac Imaging Stress Test before Surgery	-	-	5.2%	5.3%
Combination Abdominal CT Scan	-	-	13.4%	10.5%
Combination Brain/Sinus CT Scan	-	-	2.2%	2.7%
Combination Chest CT Scan	-	-	2.3%	2.7%
Follow-up Mammogram/Ultrasound	-	-	8.2%	8.8%
Lumbar Spine MRI for Low Back Pain	-	-	34.2%	37.2%

Clovis Community Medical Center

2755 Herndon Ave
Clovis, CA 93611
Phone: 559-324-4000
Fax: 559-459-3851
URL: www.communitymedical.org
Type: Acute Care Hospitals
Emergency Services: Yes
Ownership: Voluntary non-profit - Private
Beds: 109

Key Personnel:
Operating Room. . . . . Kathryn C Amirikia
CEO . . . . Craig Castro
Emergency Room . . . . Kan Coon
President/CEO. . . . . Tim A. Joslin
Radiology. . . . . Brent L Kane
Cardiac Laboratory. . . . . Cindy McCoy
Quality Assurance . . . . Colleen Strom
CEO . . . . Craig Wagoner

NOTE: Hospital profiles are in alphabetical order by state, then city, then hospital within the city; Rankings exclude hospitals with less than 25 cases except for patient surveys which excludes hospitals with less than 100 cases; (a) 100-299 cases; (1) The number of cases/patients is too few to report; (2) Data submitted were based on a sample of cases/patients; (3) Results are based on a shorter time period than required; (4) Data suppressed by CMS for one or more quarters; (5) Results are not available for this reporting period; (6) Fewer than 100 patients completed the HCAHPS survey; (7) No cases met the criteria for this measure; (8) The lower limit of the confidence interval cannot be calculated if the number of observed infections equals zero; (9) No data are available from the state/territory for this reporting period; (10) The scores shown reflect fewer than 50 completed surveys; (11) There were discrepancies in the data collection process; (12) This measure does not apply to this hospital for this reporting period; (13) Results cannot be calculated for this reporting period; (14) The results for this state are combined with nearby states to protect confidentiality; Please refer to the User's Guide for a full explanation of data.

Measure	Cases	This Hosp.	State Avg.	U.S. Avg.
Blood Clot Prevention and Treatment				
Anticoagulation Overlap Therapy[2]	63	97%	92%	93%
ICU Venous Thromboembolism Prophylaxis[2]	40	95%	92%	92%
Incidence of Potentially Preventable VTE[1,2]	-	-	11%	10%
UFH with Dosages/Platelet Monitoring[2]	23	100%	96%	97%
Venous Thromboembolism Prophylaxis[2]	340	93%	83%	85%
Warfarin Therapy Discharge Instructions[2]	52	98%	75%	75%
Chest Pain/Possible Heart Attack Care				
Aspirin Given Within 24 Hours of Arrival[1,3]	-	-	97%	96%
Fibrinolytic Meds Within 30 Min. of Arrival[3,7]	-	-	62%	58%
Average Time to ECG (minutes)[1,3]	-	-	9	7
Average Time to Transfer (minutes)[3,7]	-	-	62	60
Children's Asthma Care				
Received Home Management Plan of Care	-	-	88%	88%
Received Reliever Medication	-	-	100%	100%
Received Systemic Corticosteroids	-	-	100%	100%
Emergency Department				
Admittance Decision Time (minutes)[2]	334	428	125	98
Head CT Results Within 45 Min. of Arrival[1]	-	-	55%	57%
Patients Who Left ER Before Being Seen	41,189	1%	3%	2%
Time from ER Arrival to Admit. (minutes)[2]	336	782	323	274
Time from ER Arrival to Discharge (minutes)	343	227	168	134
Time in ER Before Being Evaluated (minutes)	385	18	29	26
Time to Pain Meds for Fractures (minutes)	145	63	62	57
Heart Attack Care				
Aspirin Given at Discharge[2]	50	100%	99%	99%
Fibrinolytic Meds Within 30 Min. of Arrival[2,7]	-	-	73%	54%
PCI Within 90 Minutes of Arrival[1,2]	-	-	95%	96%
Statin Prescribed at Discharge[2]	54	100%	98%	98%
Heart Failure Care				
ACE Inhibitor or ARB for LVSD[2]	58	95%	97%	97%
Discharge Instructions Given[2]	189	99%	94%	94%
Evaluation of LVS Function[2]	212	100%	99%	99%
Medicare Spending				
Medicare Spending per Patient (ratio)	-	1.00	0.98	0.98
Pneumonia Care				
Appropriate Initial Antibiotic Given[2]	91	99%	97%	95%
Blood Culture Timing[2]	76	95%	98%	98%
Pregnancy and Delivery Care				
Newborn Deliveries Scheduled Early[2]	62	0%	5%	6%
Preventive Care				
Immunization for Influenza[2]	442	98%	89%	90%
Immunization for Pneumonia[2]	384	96%	90%	92%
Stroke Care				
Anticoagulation Therapy for Atrial Fibrillation[1,2]	-	-	95%	95%
Antithrombotic Therapy Timing[2]	75	99%	98%	98%
Assessed for Rehabilitation[2]	90	97%	97%	97%
Discharged on Antithrombotic Therapy[2]	78	99%	99%	99%
Discharged on Statin Medication[2]	69	91%	94%	94%
Thrombolytic Therapy Timing[1,2]	-	-	72%	66%
Venous Thromboembolism Prophylaxis[2]	93	100%	94%	94%
Written Stroke Educational Materials Given[2]	60	97%	87%	88%
Surgical Care Improvement Project				
Appropriate Beta Blocker Usage[2]	114	96%	97%	98%
Appropriate VTP Within 24 Hours[2]	612	97%	98%	98%
Controlled Postoperative Blood Glucose[2,7]	-	-	96%	97%
Perioperative Temperature Management[2]	721	100%	100%	100%
Prophylactic Antibiotic Selection[2]	341	100%	99%	99%
Prophylactic Antibiotic Selection (Outpatient)	341	95%	97%	98%
Prophylactic Antibiotic Stopped[2]	333	96%	98%	98%
Prophylactic Antibiotic Timing[2]	343	98%	99%	99%
Prophylactic Antibiotic Timing (Outpatient)	348	98%	97%	98%
Urinary Catheter Removal[2]	163	99%	97%	97%
Survey of Patients' Hospital Experiences				
Area Around Room 'Always' Quiet at Night	300+	60%	51%	61%
Doctors 'Always' Communicated Well	300+	81%	78%	82%
Home Recovery Information Given	300+	84%	83%	85%
Hospital Given 9 or 10 on 10 Point Scale	300+	77%	68%	71%
Meds 'Always' Explained Before Given	300+	63%	61%	64%
Nurses 'Always' Communicated Well	300+	76%	74%	79%
Pain 'Always' Well Controlled	300+	71%	68%	71%
Room and Bathroom 'Always' Clean	300+	75%	70%	73%
Timely Help 'Always' Received	300+	64%	62%	68%
Would Definitely Recommend Hospital	300+	79%	70%	71%
Use of Medical Imaging				
Cardiac Imaging Stress Test before Surgery[1]	-	-	5.2%	5.3%
Combination Abdominal CT Scan	578	8.0%	13.4%	10.5%
Combination Brain/Sinus CT Scan	516	1.7%	2.2%	2.7%
Combination Chest CT Scan	136	2.2%	2.3%	2.7%
Follow-up Mammogram/Ultrasound	1,429	9.8%	8.2%	8.8%
Lumbar Spine MRI for Low Back Pain[1]	-	-	34.2%	37.2%

Coalinga Regional Medical Center

1191 Phelps Avenue
Coalinga, CA 93210
Phone: 559-935-6400
Fax: 559-935-6596
E-mail: admincrmc@onemain.com
URL: www.coalingamedicalcenter.com
Type: Acute Care Hospitals
Emergency Services: Yes
Ownership: Govt - Hospital Dist/Auth
Beds: 78

Key Personnel:
Infection Control. . . . . Lori Bryan, RN, DON
CEO/President. . . . . Sharon Spurgeon
Operating Room. . . . . Nina Williams
Chief of Medical Staff. . . . . H J Zwang, MD

Measure	Cases	This Hosp.	State Avg.	U.S. Avg.
Blood Clot Prevention and Treatment				
Anticoagulation Overlap Therapy[1]	-	-	92%	93%
ICU Venous Thromboembolism Prophylaxis[7]	-	-	92%	92%
Incidence of Potentially Preventable VTE[7]	-	-	11%	10%
UFH with Dosages/Platelet Monitoring[7]	-	-	96%	97%
Venous Thromboembolism Prophylaxis	111	58%	83%	85%
Warfarin Therapy Discharge Instructions[1]	-	-	75%	75%
Chest Pain/Possible Heart Attack Care				
Aspirin Given Within 24 Hours of Arrival	32	88%	97%	96%
Fibrinolytic Meds Within 30 Min. of Arrival[1]	-	-	62%	58%
Average Time to ECG (minutes)	32	13	9	7
Average Time to Transfer (minutes)[1]	-	-	62	60
Children's Asthma Care				
Received Home Management Plan of Care	-	-	88%	88%
Received Reliever Medication	-	-	100%	100%
Received Systemic Corticosteroids	-	-	100%	100%
Emergency Department				
Admittance Decision Time (minutes)[2]	182	54	125	98
Head CT Results Within 45 Min. of Arrival[1]	-	-	55%	57%
Patients Who Left ER Before Being Seen	9,187	1%	3%	2%
Time from ER Arrival to Admit. (minutes)[2]	183	295	323	274
Time from ER Arrival to Discharge (minutes)	381	120	168	134
Time in ER Before Being Evaluated (minutes)	475	16	29	26
Time to Pain Meds for Fractures (minutes)	66	38	62	57
Heart Attack Care				
Aspirin Given at Discharge[1,3]	-	-	99%	99%
Fibrinolytic Meds Within 30 Min. of Arrival[3,7]	-	-	73%	54%
PCI Within 90 Minutes of Arrival[3,7]	-	-	95%	96%
Statin Prescribed at Discharge[1,3]	-	-	98%	98%
Heart Failure Care				
ACE Inhibitor or ARB for LVSD[1]	-	-	97%	97%
Discharge Instructions Given	20	65%	94%	94%
Evaluation of LVS Function	22	36%	99%	99%
Medicare Spending				
Medicare Spending per Patient (ratio)	-	0.78	0.98	0.98
Pneumonia Care				
Appropriate Initial Antibiotic Given[1]	-	-	97%	95%
Blood Culture Timing	12	67%	98%	98%
Pregnancy and Delivery Care				
Newborn Deliveries Scheduled Early[7]	-	-	5%	6%
Preventive Care				
Immunization for Influenza[2]	165	59%	89%	90%
Immunization for Pneumonia[2]	203	68%	90%	92%
Stroke Care				
Anticoagulation Therapy for Atrial Fibrillation[3,7]	-	-	95%	95%
Antithrombotic Therapy Timing[1,3]	-	-	98%	98%
Assessed for Rehabilitation[1,3]	-	-	97%	97%
Discharged on Antithrombotic Therapy[1,3]	-	-	99%	99%
Discharged on Statin Medication[1,3]	-	-	94%	94%
Thrombolytic Therapy Timing[1,3]	-	-	72%	66%
Venous Thromboembolism Prophylaxis[1,3]	-	-	94%	94%
Written Stroke Educational Materials Given[1,3]	-	-	87%	88%
Surgical Care Improvement Project				
Appropriate Beta Blocker Usage[5]	-	-	97%	98%
Appropriate VTP Within 24 Hours[5]	-	-	98%	98%
Controlled Postoperative Blood Glucose[5]	-	-	96%	97%
Perioperative Temperature Management[5]	-	-	100%	100%
Prophylactic Antibiotic Selection[5]	-	-	99%	99%
Prophylactic Antibiotic Selection (Outpatient)[5]	-	-	97%	98%
Prophylactic Antibiotic Stopped[5]	-	-	98%	98%
Prophylactic Antibiotic Timing[5]	-	-	99%	99%
Prophylactic Antibiotic Timing (Outpatient)[5]	-	-	97%	98%
Urinary Catheter Removal[5]	-	-	97%	97%
Survey of Patients' Hospital Experiences				
Area Around Room 'Always' Quiet at Night[10]	<100	71%	51%	61%
Doctors 'Always' Communicated Well[10]	<100	87%	78%	82%
Home Recovery Information Given[10]	<100	90%	83%	85%
Hospital Given 9 or 10 on 10 Point Scale[10]	<100	58%	68%	71%
Meds 'Always' Explained Before Given[10]	<100	72%	61%	64%
Nurses 'Always' Communicated Well[10]	<100	90%	74%	79%
Pain 'Always' Well Controlled[10]	<100	83%	68%	71%
Room and Bathroom 'Always' Clean[10]	<100	93%	70%	73%
Timely Help 'Always' Received[10]	<100	82%	62%	68%
Would Definitely Recommend Hospital[10]	<100	74%	70%	71%
Use of Medical Imaging				
Cardiac Imaging Stress Test before Surgery[7]	-	-	5.2%	5.3%
Combination Abdominal CT Scan	97	14.4%	13.4%	10.5%
Combination Brain/Sinus CT Scan[1]	-	-	2.2%	2.7%
Combination Chest CT Scan[1]	-	-	2.3%	2.7%
Follow-up Mammogram/Ultrasound	112	12.5%	8.2%	8.8%
Lumbar Spine MRI for Low Back Pain[1]	-	-	34.2%	37.2%

Arrowhead Regional Medical Center

400 North Pepper Avenue
Colton, CA 92324
Phone: 909-580-1000
Fax: 909-580-1388
URL: www.arrowheadmedcenter.org
Type: Acute Care Hospitals
Emergency Services: Yes
Ownership: Government - Local
Beds: 373

Key Personnel:
Chief of Medical Staff . . . . Dev Gnanadev, MD
Infection Control. . . . . Kuo-Liang Huang
Cardiac Laboratory. . . . . Aslam Mohammed, MD
Radiology. . . . . Fred Orr, MD
CEO/President. . . . . Patrick Petre
Quality Assurance . . . . Joycen Wiegand
Pediatric Ambulatory Care . . . . . . Webster Wong, MD

Measure	Cases	This Hosp.	State Avg.	U.S. Avg.
Blood Clot Prevention and Treatment				
Anticoagulation Overlap Therapy[2]	55	93%	92%	93%
ICU Venous Thromboembolism Prophylaxis[2]	83	96%	92%	92%
Incidence of Potentially Preventable VTE[1,2]	-	-	11%	10%
UFH with Dosages/Platelet Monitoring[2]	44	100%	96%	97%
Venous Thromboembolism Prophylaxis[2]	307	93%	83%	85%
Warfarin Therapy Discharge Instructions[2]	46	15%	75%	75%
Chest Pain/Possible Heart Attack Care				
Aspirin Given Within 24 Hours of Arrival	42	95%	97%	96%
Fibrinolytic Meds Within 30 Min. of Arrival[7]	-	-	62%	58%
Average Time to ECG (minutes)	42	11	9	7
Average Time to Transfer (minutes)	20	46	62	60
Children's Asthma Care				
Received Home Management Plan of Care	-	-	88%	88%
Received Reliever Medication	-	-	100%	100%
Received Systemic Corticosteroids	-	-	100%	100%
Emergency Department				
Admittance Decision Time (minutes)[2]	1,047	430	125	98
Head CT Results Within 45 Min. of Arrival	14	100%	55%	57%
Patients Who Left ER Before Being Seen	>100k	3%	3%	2%
Time from ER Arrival to Admit. (minutes)[2]	1,066	680	323	274
Time from ER Arrival to Discharge (minutes)	317	188	168	134
Time in ER Before Being Evaluated (minutes)	303	33	29	26
Time to Pain Meds for Fractures (minutes)	252	90	62	57
Heart Attack Care				
Aspirin Given at Discharge	82	95%	99%	99%
Fibrinolytic Meds Within 30 Min. of Arrival[7]	-	-	73%	54%

NOTE: Hospital profiles are in alphabetical order by state, then city, then hospital within the city; Rankings exclude hospitals with less than 25 cases except for patient surveys which excludes hospitals with less than 100 cases; (a) 100-299 cases; (1) The number of cases/patients is too few to report; (2) Data submitted were based on a sample of cases/patients; (3) Results are based on a shorter time period than required; (4) Data suppressed by CMS for one or more quarters; (5) Results are not available for this reporting period; (6) Fewer than 100 patients completed the HCAHPS survey; (7) No cases met the criteria for this measure; (8) The lower limit of the confidence interval cannot be calculated if the number of observed infections equals zero; (9) No data are available from the state/territory for this reporting period; (10) The scores shown reflect fewer than 50 completed surveys; (11) There were discrepancies in the data collection process; (12) This measure does not apply to this hospital for this reporting period; (13) Results cannot be calculated for this reporting period; (14) The results for this state are combined with nearby states to protect confidentiality; Please refer to the User's Guide for a full explanation of data.

PCI Within 90 Minutes of Arrival[1]	-	-	95%	96%
Statin Prescribed at Discharge	82	98%	98%	98%
Heart Failure Care				
ACE Inhibitor or ARB for LVSD[2]	268	96%	97%	97%
Discharge Instructions Given[2]	506	91%	94%	94%
Evaluation of LVS Function[2]	523	99%	99%	99%
Medicare Spending				
Medicare Spending per Patient (ratio)	-	0.97	0.98	0.98
Pneumonia Care				
Appropriate Initial Antibiotic Given[2]	151	91%	97%	95%
Blood Culture Timing[2]	264	95%	98%	98%
Pregnancy and Delivery Care				
Newborn Deliveries Scheduled Early[2]	174	13%	5%	6%
Preventive Care				
Immunization for Influenza[2]	593	92%	89%	90%
Immunization for Pneumonia[2]	1,289	94%	90%	92%
Stroke Care				
Anticoagulation Therapy for Atrial Fibrillation	12	100%	95%	95%
Antithrombotic Therapy Timing	163	99%	98%	98%
Assessed for Rehabilitation	216	97%	97%	97%
Discharged on Antithrombotic Therapy	162	98%	99%	99%
Discharged on Statin Medication	142	96%	94%	94%
Thrombolytic Therapy Timing[1]	-	-	72%	66%
Venous Thromboembolism Prophylaxis	240	88%	94%	94%
Written Stroke Educational Materials Given	158	94%	87%	88%
Surgical Care Improvement Project				
Appropriate Beta Blocker Usage	79	94%	97%	98%
Appropriate VTP Within 24 Hours	628	97%	98%	98%
Controlled Postoperative Blood Glucose[1]	-	-	96%	97%
Perioperative Temperature Management	731	100%	100%	100%
Prophylactic Antibiotic Selection	277	98%	99%	99%
Prophylactic Antibiotic Selection (Outpatient)	179	99%	97%	98%
Prophylactic Antibiotic Stopped	267	96%	98%	98%
Prophylactic Antibiotic Timing	277	99%	99%	99%
Prophylactic Antibiotic Timing (Outpatient)	142	96%	97%	98%
Urinary Catheter Removal	223	93%	97%	97%
Survey of Patients' Hospital Experiences				
Area Around Room 'Always' Quiet at Night	300+	53%	51%	61%
Doctors 'Always' Communicated Well	300+	76%	78%	82%
Home Recovery Information Given	300+	79%	83%	85%
Hospital Given 9 or 10 on 10 Point Scale	300+	67%	68%	71%
Meds 'Always' Explained Before Given	300+	61%	61%	64%
Nurses 'Always' Communicated Well	300+	75%	74%	79%
Pain 'Always' Well Controlled	300+	69%	68%	71%
Room and Bathroom 'Always' Clean	300+	66%	70%	73%
Timely Help 'Always' Received	300+	58%	62%	68%
Would Definitely Recommend Hospital	300+	67%	70%	71%
Use of Medical Imaging				
Cardiac Imaging Stress Test before Surgery	118	3.4%	5.2%	5.3%
Combination Abdominal CT Scan	441	4.5%	13.4%	10.5%
Combination Brain/Sinus CT Scan[1]	-	-	2.2%	2.7%
Combination Chest CT Scan	241	0.4%	2.3%	2.7%
Follow-up Mammogram/Ultrasound	403	5.2%	8.2%	8.8%
Lumbar Spine MRI for Low Back Pain[1]	-	-	34.2%	37.2%

Colusa Regional Medical Center

199 East Webster St
Colusa, CA 95932
Phone: 530-458-5821
Fax: 530-458-3210
URL: www.colusamedicalcenter.org
Type: Acute Care Hospitals
Emergency Services: Yes
Ownership: Voluntary non-profit - Other
Beds: 48

Key Personnel:
Radiology. . . . . Dale Bass
Chief of Medical Staff. . . . . Julian Delgado, MD
Intensive Care Unit. . . . . Christine Gregory, RN
Infection Control. . . . . Katherine Hughes, RN
Quality Assurance . . . . Katherine Hughes, RN
CEO/President. . . . . Dale Kirby
Emergency Room . . . . Samuel Medrano, MD
Operating Room. . . . . Irene Parnell, RN

Measure	Cases	This Hosp.	State Avg.	U.S. Avg.
Blood Clot Prevention and Treatment				
Anticoagulation Overlap Therapy[1,2]	-	-	92%	93%
ICU Venous Thromboembolism Prophylaxis[2]	25	8%	92%	92%
Incidence of Potentially Preventable VTE[2,7]	-	-	11%	10%
UFH with Dosages/Platelet Monitoring[2,7]	-	-	96%	97%
Venous Thromboembolism Prophylaxis[2]	207	30%	83%	85%
Warfarin Therapy Discharge Instructions[1,2]	-	-	75%	75%
Chest Pain/Possible Heart Attack Care				
Aspirin Given Within 24 Hours of Arrival	17	94%	97%	96%
Fibrinolytic Meds Within 30 Min. of Arrival[7]	-	-	62%	58%
Average Time to ECG (minutes)	17	19	9	7
Average Time to Transfer (minutes)[1]	-	-	62	60
Children's Asthma Care				
Received Home Management Plan of Care	-	-	88%	88%
Received Reliever Medication	-	-	100%	100%
Received Systemic Corticosteroids	-	-	100%	100%
Emergency Department				
Admittance Decision Time (minutes)[2]	327	30	125	98
Head CT Results Within 45 Min. of Arrival[1]	-	-	55%	57%
Patients Who Left ER Before Being Seen	6,122	1%	3%	2%
Time from ER Arrival to Admit. (minutes)[2]	383	190	323	274
Time from ER Arrival to Discharge (minutes)	464	105	168	134
Time in ER Before Being Evaluated (minutes)	482	30	29	26
Time to Pain Meds for Fractures (minutes)	32	50	62	57
Heart Attack Care				
Aspirin Given at Discharge[1]	-	-	99%	99%
Fibrinolytic Meds Within 30 Min. of Arrival[7]	-	-	73%	54%
PCI Within 90 Minutes of Arrival[7]	-	-	95%	96%
Statin Prescribed at Discharge[1]	-	-	98%	98%
Heart Failure Care				
ACE Inhibitor or ARB for LVSD[1]	-	-	97%	97%
Discharge Instructions Given	24	67%	94%	94%
Evaluation of LVS Function	27	52%	99%	99%
Medicare Spending				
Medicare Spending per Patient (ratio)	-	0.97	0.98	0.98
Pneumonia Care				
Appropriate Initial Antibiotic Given	28	71%	97%	95%
Blood Culture Timing	27	81%	98%	98%
Pregnancy and Delivery Care				
Newborn Deliveries Scheduled Early[1]	-	-	5%	6%
Preventive Care				
Immunization for Influenza[2]	283	70%	89%	90%
Immunization for Pneumonia[2]	278	77%	90%	92%
Stroke Care				
Anticoagulation Therapy for Atrial Fibrillation[7]	-	-	95%	95%
Antithrombotic Therapy Timing[7]	-	-	98%	98%
Assessed for Rehabilitation[1]	-	-	97%	97%
Discharged on Antithrombotic Therapy[1]	-	-	99%	99%
Discharged on Statin Medication[1]	-	-	94%	94%
Thrombolytic Therapy Timing[1]	-	-	72%	66%
Venous Thromboembolism Prophylaxis[1]	-	-	94%	94%
Written Stroke Educational Materials Given[1]	-	-	87%	88%
Surgical Care Improvement Project				
Appropriate Beta Blocker Usage[1]	-	-	97%	98%
Appropriate VTP Within 24 Hours	15	60%	98%	98%
Controlled Postoperative Blood Glucose[7]	-	-	96%	97%
Perioperative Temperature Management	16	100%	100%	100%
Prophylactic Antibiotic Selection[1]	-	-	99%	99%
Prophylactic Antibiotic Selection (Outpatient)[1,3]	-	-	97%	98%
Prophylactic Antibiotic Stopped[1]	-	-	98%	98%
Prophylactic Antibiotic Timing[1]	-	-	99%	99%
Prophylactic Antibiotic Timing (Outpatient)[1,3]	-	-	97%	98%
Urinary Catheter Removal[1]	-	-	97%	97%
Survey of Patients' Hospital Experiences				
Area Around Room 'Always' Quiet at Night	(a)	65%	51%	61%
Doctors 'Always' Communicated Well	(a)	87%	78%	82%
Home Recovery Information Given	(a)	84%	83%	85%
Hospital Given 9 or 10 on 10 Point Scale	(a)	66%	68%	71%
Meds 'Always' Explained Before Given	(a)	69%	61%	64%
Nurses 'Always' Communicated Well	(a)	82%	74%	79%
Pain 'Always' Well Controlled	(a)	70%	68%	71%
Room and Bathroom 'Always' Clean	(a)	80%	70%	73%
Timely Help 'Always' Received	(a)	76%	62%	68%
Would Definitely Recommend Hospital	(a)	61%	70%	71%
Use of Medical Imaging				
Cardiac Imaging Stress Test before Surgery[1]	-	-	5.2%	5.3%
Combination Abdominal CT Scan	130	7.7%	13.4%	10.5%
Combination Brain/Sinus CT Scan	139	6.5%	2.2%	2.7%
Combination Chest CT Scan	62	0.0%	2.3%	2.7%
Follow-up Mammogram/Ultrasound	191	9.4%	8.2%	8.8%
Lumbar Spine MRI for Low Back Pain[1]	-	-	34.2%	37.2%

John Muir Medical Center - Concord Campus

2540 East St
Concord, CA 94520
Phone: 925-674-2002
Fax: 925-674-2009
URL: www.johnmuirhealth.com
Type: Acute Care Hospitals
Emergency Services: Yes
Ownership: Voluntary non-profit - Private
Beds: 267

Key Personnel:
Chief of Medical Staff. . . . . David Birdsall, MD
Pediatric Ambulatory Care . . . . . . Alan Burckin, MD
Operating Room. . . . . Karen Herrick
Emergency Room . . . . Kathy Hester, RN
Quality Assurance . . . . Carol Johnstone
Radiology. . . . . Robert Schick, MD
CEO/President. . . . . Michael S. Thomas

Measure	Cases	This Hosp.	State Avg.	U.S. Avg.
Blood Clot Prevention and Treatment				
Anticoagulation Overlap Therapy[2]	49	100%	92%	93%
ICU Venous Thromboembolism Prophylaxis[2]	75	100%	92%	92%
Incidence of Potentially Preventable VTE[1,2]	-	-	11%	10%
UFH with Dosages/Platelet Monitoring[2]	36	100%	96%	97%
Venous Thromboembolism Prophylaxis[2]	321	94%	83%	85%
Warfarin Therapy Discharge Instructions[2]	34	100%	75%	75%
Chest Pain/Possible Heart Attack Care				
Aspirin Given Within 24 Hours of Arrival[1]	-	-	97%	96%
Fibrinolytic Meds Within 30 Min. of Arrival[3,7]	-	-	62%	58%
Average Time to ECG (minutes)[1]	-	-	9	7
Average Time to Transfer (minutes)[3,7]	-	-	62	60
Children's Asthma Care				
Received Home Management Plan of Care	-	-	88%	88%
Received Reliever Medication	-	-	100%	100%
Received Systemic Corticosteroids	-	-	100%	100%
Emergency Department				
Admittance Decision Time (minutes)[2]	827	148	125	98
Head CT Results Within 45 Min. of Arrival	38	61%	55%	57%
Patients Who Left ER Before Being Seen	51,705	1%	3%	2%
Time from ER Arrival to Admit. (minutes)[2]	831	325	323	274
Time from ER Arrival to Discharge (minutes)	432	136	168	134
Time in ER Before Being Evaluated (minutes)	475	22	29	26
Time to Pain Meds for Fractures (minutes)	136	58	62	57
Heart Attack Care				
Aspirin Given at Discharge	322	100%	99%	99%
Fibrinolytic Meds Within 30 Min. of Arrival[7]	-	-	73%	54%
PCI Within 90 Minutes of Arrival	34	100%	95%	96%
Statin Prescribed at Discharge	314	100%	98%	98%
Heart Failure Care				
ACE Inhibitor or ARB for LVSD	60	100%	97%	97%
Discharge Instructions Given	234	99%	94%	94%
Evaluation of LVS Function	286	100%	99%	99%
Medicare Spending				
Medicare Spending per Patient (ratio)	-	1.00	0.98	0.98
Pneumonia Care				
Appropriate Initial Antibiotic Given[2]	119	99%	97%	95%
Blood Culture Timing[2]	152	97%	98%	98%
Pregnancy and Delivery Care				
Newborn Deliveries Scheduled Early[7]	-	-	5%	6%
Preventive Care				
Immunization for Influenza[2]	612	93%	89%	90%
Immunization for Pneumonia[2]	891	91%	90%	92%
Stroke Care				
Anticoagulation Therapy for Atrial Fibrillation	23	100%	95%	95%
Antithrombotic Therapy Timing	83	98%	98%	98%
Assessed for Rehabilitation	125	99%	97%	97%
Discharged on Antithrombotic Therapy	119	99%	99%	99%
Discharged on Statin Medication	89	99%	94%	94%
Thrombolytic Therapy Timing	27	96%	72%	66%
Venous Thromboembolism Prophylaxis	117	96%	94%	94%
Written Stroke Educational Materials Given	77	92%	87%	88%

NOTE: Hospital profiles are in alphabetical order by state, then city, then hospital within the city; Rankings exclude hospitals with less than 25 cases except for patient surveys which excludes hospitals with less than 100 cases; (a) 100-299 cases; (1) The number of cases/patients is too few to report; (2) Data submitted were based on a sample of cases/patients; (3) Results are based on a shorter time period than required; (4) Data suppressed by CMS for one or more quarters; (5) Results are not available for this reporting period; (6) Fewer than 100 patients completed the HCAHPS survey; (7) No cases met the criteria for this measure; (8) The lower limit of the confidence interval cannot be calculated if the number of observed infections equals zero; (9) No data are available from the state/territory for this reporting period; (10) The scores shown reflect fewer than 50 completed surveys; (11) There were discrepancies in the data collection process; (12) This measure does not apply to this hospital for this reporting period; (13) Results cannot be calculated for this reporting period; (14) The results for this state are combined with nearby states to protect confidentiality; Please refer to the User's Guide for a full explanation of data.

Measure	Cases	This Hosp.	State Avg.	U.S. Avg.
Surgical Care Improvement Project				
Appropriate Beta Blocker Usage[2]	250	100%	97%	98%
Appropriate VTP Within 24 Hours[2]	344	99%	98%	98%
Controlled Postoperative Blood Glucose[2]	153	98%	96%	97%
Perioperative Temperature Management[2]	448	100%	100%	100%
Prophylactic Antibiotic Selection[2]	436	100%	99%	99%
Prophylactic Antibiotic Selection (Outpatient)	252	100%	97%	98%
Prophylactic Antibiotic Stopped[2]	417	99%	98%	98%
Prophylactic Antibiotic Timing[2]	436	100%	99%	99%
Prophylactic Antibiotic Timing (Outpatient)	253	98%	97%	98%
Urinary Catheter Removal[2]	375	97%	97%	97%
Survey of Patients' Hospital Experiences				
Area Around Room 'Always' Quiet at Night	300+	57%	51%	61%
Doctors 'Always' Communicated Well	300+	81%	78%	82%
Home Recovery Information Given	300+	86%	83%	85%
Hospital Given 9 or 10 on 10 Point Scale	300+	80%	68%	71%
Meds 'Always' Explained Before Given	300+	63%	61%	64%
Nurses 'Always' Communicated Well	300+	80%	74%	79%
Pain 'Always' Well Controlled	300+	70%	68%	71%
Room and Bathroom 'Always' Clean	300+	80%	70%	73%
Timely Help 'Always' Received	300+	66%	62%	68%
Would Definitely Recommend Hospital	300+	85%	70%	71%
Use of Medical Imaging				
Cardiac Imaging Stress Test before Surgery	209	8.1%	5.2%	5.3%
Combination Abdominal CT Scan	418	0.2%	13.4%	10.5%
Combination Brain/Sinus CT Scan	673	1.9%	2.2%	2.7%
Combination Chest CT Scan[1]	-	-	2.3%	2.7%
Follow-up Mammogram/Ultrasound	998	8.5%	8.2%	8.8%
Lumbar Spine MRI for Low Back Pain[1]	-	-	34.2%	37.2%

Corcoran District Hospital

1310 Hanna Ave
Corcoran, CA 93212
Phone: 559-992-5051
Fax: 559-992-3972
Type: Acute Care Hospitals
Emergency Services: No
Ownership: Government - State
Beds: 32

Key Personnel:

Anesthesiology. . . . . Wynn Allan
CEO . . . . Jonathan Brenn
Operating Room. . . . . Susan Fairchild, RN
Chief of Medical Staff. . . . . Ravi Kumar, MD
Emergency Room . . . . Thomas Lambert, MD
Quality Assurance . . . . Marleen Samrt
Infection Control. . . . . Judy Wofford

Measure	Cases	This Hosp.	State Avg.	U.S. Avg.
Blood Clot Prevention and Treatment				
Anticoagulation Overlap Therapy[3,7]	-	-	92%	93%
ICU Venous Thromboembolism Prophylaxis[1,3]	-	-	92%	92%
Incidence of Potentially Preventable VTE[3,7]	-	-	11%	10%
UFH with Dosages/Platelet Monitoring[3,7]	-	-	96%	97%
Venous Thromboembolism Prophylaxis[3]	22	9%	83%	85%
Warfarin Therapy Discharge Instructions[3,7]	-	-	75%	75%
Chest Pain/Possible Heart Attack Care				
Aspirin Given Within 24 Hours of Arrival[5]	-	-	97%	96%
Fibrinolytic Meds Within 30 Min. of Arrival[5]	-	-	62%	58%
Average Time to ECG (minutes)[5]	-	-	9	7
Average Time to Transfer (minutes)[5]	-	-	62	60
Children's Asthma Care				
Received Home Management Plan of Care	-	-	88%	88%
Received Reliever Medication	-	-	100%	100%
Received Systemic Corticosteroids	-	-	100%	100%
Emergency Department				
Admittance Decision Time (minutes)[2,3]	37	85	125	98
Head CT Results Within 45 Min. of Arrival[5]	-	-	55%	57%
Patients Who Left ER Before Being Seen[5]	-	-	3%	2%
Time from ER Arrival to Admit. (minutes)[2,3]	40	217	323	274
Time from ER Arrival to Discharge (minutes)[3]	182	80	168	134
Time in ER Before Being Evaluated (minutes)[3]	196	34	29	26
Time to Pain Meds for Fractures (minutes)[5]	-	-	62	57
Heart Attack Care				
Aspirin Given at Discharge[5]	-	-	99%	99%
Fibrinolytic Meds Within 30 Min. of Arrival[5]	-	-	73%	54%
PCI Within 90 Minutes of Arrival[5]	-	-	95%	96%
Statin Prescribed at Discharge[5]	-	-	98%	98%
Heart Failure Care				
ACE Inhibitor or ARB for LVSD[1,2]	-	-	97%	97%
Discharge Instructions Given[1,2]	-	-	94%	94%
Evaluation of LVS Function[1,2]	-	-	99%	99%
Medicare Spending				
Medicare Spending per Patient (ratio)	-	0.81	0.98	0.98
Pneumonia Care				
Appropriate Initial Antibiotic Given[1,2]	-	-	97%	95%
Blood Culture Timing[1,2]	-	-	98%	98%
Pregnancy and Delivery Care				
Newborn Deliveries Scheduled Early[3,7]	-	-	5%	6%
Preventive Care				
Immunization for Influenza[2]	189	85%	89%	90%
Immunization for Pneumonia[2,3]	95	88%	90%	92%
Stroke Care				
Anticoagulation Therapy for Atrial Fibrillation[5]	-	-	95%	95%
Antithrombotic Therapy Timing[5]	-	-	98%	98%
Assessed for Rehabilitation[5]	-	-	97%	97%
Discharged on Antithrombotic Therapy[5]	-	-	99%	99%
Discharged on Statin Medication[5]	-	-	94%	94%
Thrombolytic Therapy Timing[5]	-	-	72%	66%
Venous Thromboembolism Prophylaxis[5]	-	-	94%	94%
Written Stroke Educational Materials Given[5]	-	-	87%	88%
Surgical Care Improvement Project				
Appropriate Beta Blocker Usage[5]	-	-	97%	98%
Appropriate VTP Within 24 Hours[5]	-	-	98%	98%
Controlled Postoperative Blood Glucose[5]	-	-	96%	97%
Perioperative Temperature Management[5]	-	-	100%	100%
Prophylactic Antibiotic Selection[5]	-	-	99%	99%
Prophylactic Antibiotic Selection (Outpatient)[5]	-	-	97%	98%
Prophylactic Antibiotic Stopped[5]	-	-	98%	98%
Prophylactic Antibiotic Timing[5]	-	-	99%	99%
Prophylactic Antibiotic Timing (Outpatient)[5]	-	-	97%	98%
Urinary Catheter Removal[5]	-	-	97%	97%
Survey of Patients' Hospital Experiences				
Area Around Room 'Always' Quiet at Night[10]	<100	53%	51%	61%
Doctors 'Always' Communicated Well[10]	<100	78%	78%	82%
Home Recovery Information Given[10]	<100	77%	83%	85%
Hospital Given 9 or 10 on 10 Point Scale[10]	<100	62%	68%	71%
Meds 'Always' Explained Before Given[10]	<100	61%	61%	64%
Nurses 'Always' Communicated Well[10]	<100	75%	74%	79%
Pain 'Always' Well Controlled[10]	<100	69%	68%	71%
Room and Bathroom 'Always' Clean[10]	<100	64%	70%	73%
Timely Help 'Always' Received[10]	<100	70%	62%	68%
Would Definitely Recommend Hospital[10]	<100	45%	70%	71%
Use of Medical Imaging				
Cardiac Imaging Stress Test before Surgery[7]	-	-	5.2%	5.3%
Combination Abdominal CT Scan[1]	-	-	13.4%	10.5%
Combination Brain/Sinus CT Scan	43	0.0%	2.2%	2.7%
Combination Chest CT Scan[1]	-	-	2.3%	2.7%
Follow-up Mammogram/Ultrasound[7]	-	-	8.2%	8.8%
Lumbar Spine MRI for Low Back Pain[7]	-	-	34.2%	37.2%

Corona Regional Medical Center

800 South Main Street
Corona, CA 92882
Phone: 951-737-4343
Fax: 951-736-6334
URL: www.coronaregional.com
Type: Acute Care Hospitals
Emergency Services: Yes
Ownership: Proprietary
Beds: 228

Key Personnel:

Emergency Room . . . . Nancy Bakewell
Pediatric Ambulatory Care . . . . . . Steven Deterville, MD
Pediatric In-Patient Care . . . . . . Steven Deterville, MD
Chief of Medical Staff. . . . . Anoop Maheshwari, MD
Quality Assurance . . . . Avelina Ortiz
Operating Room. . . . . Gisella Sandy
CEO . . . . Mark Uffer
Radiology. . . . . Jeffrey Wasserman

Measure	Cases	This Hosp.	State Avg.	U.S. Avg.
Blood Clot Prevention and Treatment				
Anticoagulation Overlap Therapy[2]	33	100%	92%	93%
ICU Venous Thromboembolism Prophylaxis[2]	49	96%	92%	92%
Incidence of Potentially Preventable VTE[1,2]	-	-	11%	10%
UFH with Dosages/Platelet Monitoring[1,2]	-	-	96%	97%
Venous Thromboembolism Prophylaxis[2]	397	96%	83%	85%
Warfarin Therapy Discharge Instructions[2]	23	87%	75%	75%
Chest Pain/Possible Heart Attack Care				
Aspirin Given Within 24 Hours of Arrival	50	98%	97%	96%
Fibrinolytic Meds Within 30 Min. of Arrival[7]	-	-	62%	58%
Average Time to ECG (minutes)	57	12	9	7
Average Time to Transfer (minutes)[1]	-	-	62	60
Children's Asthma Care				
Received Home Management Plan of Care	-	-	88%	88%
Received Reliever Medication	-	-	100%	100%
Received Systemic Corticosteroids	-	-	100%	100%
Emergency Department				
Admittance Decision Time (minutes)[2]	529	164	125	98
Head CT Results Within 45 Min. of Arrival	47	77%	55%	57%
Patients Who Left ER Before Being Seen	43,126	3%	3%	2%
Time from ER Arrival to Admit. (minutes)[2]	616	428	323	274
Time from ER Arrival to Discharge (minutes)	320	189	168	134
Time in ER Before Being Evaluated (minutes)	396	30	29	26
Time to Pain Meds for Fractures (minutes)	309	54	62	57
Heart Attack Care				
Aspirin Given at Discharge	26	100%	99%	99%
Fibrinolytic Meds Within 30 Min. of Arrival[7]	-	-	73%	54%
PCI Within 90 Minutes of Arrival[7]	-	-	95%	96%
Statin Prescribed at Discharge	23	100%	98%	98%
Heart Failure Care				
ACE Inhibitor or ARB for LVSD[2]	58	100%	97%	97%
Discharge Instructions Given[2]	184	93%	94%	94%
Evaluation of LVS Function[2]	250	99%	99%	99%
Medicare Spending				
Medicare Spending per Patient (ratio)	-	1.06	0.98	0.98
Pneumonia Care				
Appropriate Initial Antibiotic Given[2]	71	99%	97%	95%
Blood Culture Timing[2]	159	98%	98%	98%
Pregnancy and Delivery Care				
Newborn Deliveries Scheduled Early[2]	45	4%	5%	6%
Preventive Care				
Immunization for Influenza[2]	505	94%	89%	90%
Immunization for Pneumonia[2]	539	94%	90%	92%
Stroke Care				
Anticoagulation Therapy for Atrial Fibrillation[1]	-	-	95%	95%
Antithrombotic Therapy Timing	39	100%	98%	98%
Assessed for Rehabilitation	56	98%	97%	97%
Discharged on Antithrombotic Therapy	49	98%	99%	99%
Discharged on Statin Medication	34	82%	94%	94%
Thrombolytic Therapy Timing	13	0%	72%	66%
Venous Thromboembolism Prophylaxis	53	98%	94%	94%
Written Stroke Educational Materials Given	29	41%	87%	88%
Surgical Care Improvement Project				
Appropriate Beta Blocker Usage[2]	43	100%	97%	98%
Appropriate VTP Within 24 Hours[2]	189	98%	98%	98%
Controlled Postoperative Blood Glucose[2,7]	-	-	96%	97%
Perioperative Temperature Management[2]	235	100%	100%	100%
Prophylactic Antibiotic Selection[2]	134	96%	99%	99%
Prophylactic Antibiotic Selection (Outpatient)	57	100%	97%	98%
Prophylactic Antibiotic Stopped[2]	132	97%	98%	98%
Prophylactic Antibiotic Timing[2]	134	100%	99%	99%
Prophylactic Antibiotic Timing (Outpatient)	59	95%	97%	98%
Urinary Catheter Removal[2]	77	90%	97%	97%
Survey of Patients' Hospital Experiences				
Area Around Room 'Always' Quiet at Night	300+	41%	51%	61%
Doctors 'Always' Communicated Well	300+	72%	78%	82%
Home Recovery Information Given	300+	84%	83%	85%
Hospital Given 9 or 10 on 10 Point Scale	300+	55%	68%	71%
Meds 'Always' Explained Before Given	300+	57%	61%	64%
Nurses 'Always' Communicated Well	300+	69%	74%	79%
Pain 'Always' Well Controlled	300+	69%	68%	71%
Room and Bathroom 'Always' Clean	300+	62%	70%	73%
Timely Help 'Always' Received	300+	51%	62%	68%
Would Definitely Recommend Hospital	300+	54%	70%	71%
Use of Medical Imaging				
Cardiac Imaging Stress Test before Surgery	216	9.3%	5.2%	5.3%
Combination Abdominal CT Scan	411	17.5%	13.4%	10.5%
Combination Brain/Sinus CT Scan	488	0.8%	2.2%	2.7%

NOTE: Hospital profiles are in alphabetical order by state, then city, then hospital within the city; Rankings exclude hospitals with less than 25 cases except for patient surveys which excludes hospitals with less than 100 cases; (a) 100-299 cases; (1) The number of cases/patients is too few to report; (2) Data submitted were based on a sample of cases/patients; (3) Results are based on a shorter time period than required; (4) Data suppressed by CMS for one or more quarters; (5) Results are not available for this reporting period; (6) Fewer than 100 patients completed the HCAHPS survey; (7) No cases met the criteria for this measure; (8) The lower limit of the confidence interval cannot be calculated if the number of observed infections equals zero; (9) No data are available from the state/territory for this reporting period; (10) The scores shown reflect fewer than 50 completed surveys; (11) There were discrepancies in the data collection process; (12) This measure does not apply to this hospital for this reporting period; (13) Results cannot be calculated for this reporting period; (14) The results for this state are combined with nearby states to protect confidentiality; Please refer to the User's Guide for a full explanation of data.

Combination Chest CT Scan	162	6.2%	2.3%	2.7%
Follow-up Mammogram/Ultrasound	526	10.8%	8.2%	8.8%
Lumbar Spine MRI for Low Back Pain[1]	-	-	34.2%	37.2%

Sharp Coronado Hospital & Healthcare Center

250 Prospect Place
Coronado, CA 92118
URL: www.sharp.com/coronado
Type: Acute Care Hospitals
Ownership: Voluntary non-profit - Other

Phone: 619-435-6251
Fax: 619-522-3777
Emergency Services: Yes
Beds: 204

Key Personnel:
Radiology. . . . . Gregg Alzate
Cardiac Laboratory. . . . . Ray Daniels
Emergency Room . . . . Katy Green
CEO/President. . . . . Marcia K Hall
Chief of Medical Staff . . . . Matthew Horn, MD
Ambulatory Care . . . . Pat Pine
Operating Room. . . . . Pat Pine
Patient Relations . . . . Harriet Sangrey

Measure	Cases	This Hosp.	State Avg.	U.S. Avg.
Blood Clot Prevention and Treatment				
Anticoagulation Overlap Therapy[1,2]	-	-	92%	93%
ICU Venous Thromboembolism Prophylaxis[2]	25	72%	92%	92%
Incidence of Potentially Preventable VTE[1,2]	-	-	11%	10%
UFH with Dosages/Platelet Monitoring[1,2]	-	-	96%	97%
Venous Thromboembolism Prophylaxis[2]	88	65%	83%	85%
Warfarin Therapy Discharge Instructions[1,2]	-	-	75%	75%
Chest Pain/Possible Heart Attack Care				
Aspirin Given Within 24 Hours of Arrival[1,3]	-	-	97%	96%
Fibrinolytic Meds Within 30 Min. of Arrival[3,7]	-	-	62%	58%
Average Time to ECG (minutes)[1,3]	-	-	9	7
Average Time to Transfer (minutes)[1,3]	-	-	62	60
Children's Asthma Care				
Received Home Management Plan of Care	-	-	88%	88%
Received Reliever Medication	-	-	100%	100%
Received Systemic Corticosteroids	-	-	100%	100%
Emergency Department				
Admittance Decision Time (minutes)[2]	319	58	125	98
Head CT Results Within 45 Min. of Arrival[1]	-	-	55%	57%
Patients Who Left ER Before Being Seen	12,134	1%	3%	2%
Time from ER Arrival to Admit. (minutes)[2]	339	206	323	274
Time from ER Arrival to Discharge (minutes)	380	106	168	134
Time in ER Before Being Evaluated (minutes)	299	27	29	26
Time to Pain Meds for Fractures (minutes)	37	46	62	57
Heart Attack Care				
Aspirin Given at Discharge[1,3]	-	-	99%	99%
Fibrinolytic Meds Within 30 Min. of Arrival[3,7]	-	-	73%	54%
PCI Within 90 Minutes of Arrival[3,7]	-	-	95%	96%
Statin Prescribed at Discharge[1,3]	-	-	98%	98%
Heart Failure Care				
ACE Inhibitor or ARB for LVSD[1]	-	-	97%	97%
Discharge Instructions Given	37	97%	94%	94%
Evaluation of LVS Function	48	100%	99%	99%
Medicare Spending				
Medicare Spending per Patient (ratio)	-	0.82	0.98	0.98
Pneumonia Care				
Appropriate Initial Antibiotic Given	26	100%	97%	95%
Blood Culture Timing	37	100%	98%	98%
Pregnancy and Delivery Care				
Newborn Deliveries Scheduled Early[7]	-	-	5%	6%
Preventive Care				
Immunization for Influenza[2]	461	98%	89%	90%
Immunization for Pneumonia[2]	538	97%	90%	92%
Stroke Care				
Anticoagulation Therapy for Atrial Fibrillation[1]	-	-	95%	95%
Antithrombotic Therapy Timing	13	100%	98%	98%
Assessed for Rehabilitation	13	85%	97%	97%
Discharged on Antithrombotic Therapy	13	100%	99%	99%
Discharged on Statin Medication[1]	-	-	94%	94%
Thrombolytic Therapy Timing[1]	-	-	72%	66%
Venous Thromboembolism Prophylaxis	13	92%	94%	94%
Written Stroke Educational Materials Given[1]	-	-	87%	88%
Surgical Care Improvement Project				
Appropriate Beta Blocker Usage	327	99%	97%	98%
Appropriate VTP Within 24 Hours	1,216	99%	98%	98%
Controlled Postoperative Blood Glucose[7]	-	-	96%	97%
Perioperative Temperature Management	1,325	100%	100%	100%
Prophylactic Antibiotic Selection	1,227	100%	99%	99%
Prophylactic Antibiotic Selection (Outpatient)	16	100%	97%	98%
Prophylactic Antibiotic Stopped	1,220	100%	98%	98%
Prophylactic Antibiotic Timing	1,229	100%	99%	99%
Prophylactic Antibiotic Timing (Outpatient)	16	94%	97%	98%
Urinary Catheter Removal	1,256	100%	97%	97%
Survey of Patients' Hospital Experiences				
Area Around Room 'Always' Quiet at Night	300+	71%	51%	61%
Doctors 'Always' Communicated Well	300+	84%	78%	82%
Home Recovery Information Given	300+	93%	83%	85%
Hospital Given 9 or 10 on 10 Point Scale	300+	81%	68%	71%
Meds 'Always' Explained Before Given	300+	72%	61%	64%
Nurses 'Always' Communicated Well	300+	86%	74%	79%
Pain 'Always' Well Controlled	300+	77%	68%	71%
Room and Bathroom 'Always' Clean	300+	83%	70%	73%
Timely Help 'Always' Received	300+	78%	62%	68%
Would Definitely Recommend Hospital	300+	85%	70%	71%
Use of Medical Imaging				
Cardiac Imaging Stress Test before Surgery[1]	-	-	5.2%	5.3%
Combination Abdominal CT Scan	189	7.4%	13.4%	10.5%
Combination Brain/Sinus CT Scan[1]	-	-	2.2%	2.7%
Combination Chest CT Scan	116	0.0%	2.3%	2.7%
Follow-up Mammogram/Ultrasound	490	10.4%	8.2%	8.8%
Lumbar Spine MRI for Low Back Pain[1]	-	-	34.2%	37.2%

College Hospital Costa Mesa

301 Victoria Street
Costa Mesa, CA 92627
URL: www.collegehospitals.com
Type: Acute Care Hospitals
Ownership: Proprietary

Phone: 949-642-2734
Fax: 949-574-3695
Emergency Services: No
Beds: 125

Key Personnel:
Operating Room. . . . . Diana Christensen
Quality Assurance . . . . Ann Foster
CEO/President. . . . . Wayne Lingenfelter
Chief of Medical Staff . . . . Michael Schwartz
CEO . . . . Susan L. Taylor

Measure	Cases	This Hosp.	State Avg.	U.S. Avg.
Blood Clot Prevention and Treatment				
Anticoagulation Overlap Therapy[2,7]	-	-	92%	93%
ICU Venous Thromboembolism Prophylaxis[2,7]	-	-	92%	92%
Incidence of Potentially Preventable VTE[2,7]	-	-	11%	10%
UFH with Dosages/Platelet Monitoring[2,7]	-	-	96%	97%
Venous Thromboembolism Prophylaxis[2]	12	0%	83%	85%
Warfarin Therapy Discharge Instructions[2,7]	-	-	75%	75%
Chest Pain/Possible Heart Attack Care				
Aspirin Given Within 24 Hours of Arrival[5]	-	-	97%	96%
Fibrinolytic Meds Within 30 Min. of Arrival[5]	-	-	62%	58%
Average Time to ECG (minutes)[5]	-	-	9	7
Average Time to Transfer (minutes)[5]	-	-	62	60
Children's Asthma Care				
Received Home Management Plan of Care	-	-	88%	88%
Received Reliever Medication	-	-	100%	100%
Received Systemic Corticosteroids	-	-	100%	100%
Emergency Department				
Admittance Decision Time (minutes)[2,7]	-	-	125	98
Head CT Results Within 45 Min. of Arrival[5]	-	-	55%	57%
Patients Who Left ER Before Being Seen	859	3%	3%	2%
Time from ER Arrival to Admit. (minutes)[2,7]	-	-	323	274
Time from ER Arrival to Discharge (minutes)[5]	-	-	168	134
Time in ER Before Being Evaluated (minutes)[5]	-	-	29	26
Time to Pain Meds for Fractures (minutes)[5]	-	-	62	57
Heart Attack Care				
Aspirin Given at Discharge[5]	-	-	99%	99%
Fibrinolytic Meds Within 30 Min. of Arrival[5]	-	-	73%	54%
PCI Within 90 Minutes of Arrival[5]	-	-	95%	96%
Statin Prescribed at Discharge[5]	-	-	98%	98%
Heart Failure Care				
ACE Inhibitor or ARB for LVSD[5]	-	-	97%	97%
Discharge Instructions Given[5]	-	-	94%	94%
Evaluation of LVS Function[5]	-	-	99%	99%
Medicare Spending				
Medicare Spending per Patient (ratio)	-	1.08	0.98	0.98
Pneumonia Care				
Appropriate Initial Antibiotic Given[5]	-	-	97%	95%
Blood Culture Timing[5]	-	-	98%	98%
Pregnancy and Delivery Care				
Newborn Deliveries Scheduled Early[7]	-	-	5%	6%
Preventive Care				
Immunization for Influenza[2]	308	84%	89%	90%
Immunization for Pneumonia[2]	87	92%	90%	92%
Stroke Care				
Anticoagulation Therapy for Atrial Fibrillation[5]	-	-	95%	95%
Antithrombotic Therapy Timing[5]	-	-	98%	98%
Assessed for Rehabilitation[5]	-	-	97%	97%
Discharged on Antithrombotic Therapy[5]	-	-	99%	99%
Discharged on Statin Medication[5]	-	-	94%	94%
Thrombolytic Therapy Timing[5]	-	-	72%	66%
Venous Thromboembolism Prophylaxis[5]	-	-	94%	94%
Written Stroke Educational Materials Given[5]	-	-	87%	88%
Surgical Care Improvement Project				
Appropriate Beta Blocker Usage[5]	-	-	97%	98%
Appropriate VTP Within 24 Hours[5]	-	-	98%	98%
Controlled Postoperative Blood Glucose[5]	-	-	96%	97%
Perioperative Temperature Management[5]	-	-	100%	100%
Prophylactic Antibiotic Selection[5]	-	-	99%	99%
Prophylactic Antibiotic Selection (Outpatient)[5]	-	-	97%	98%
Prophylactic Antibiotic Stopped[5]	-	-	98%	98%
Prophylactic Antibiotic Timing[5]	-	-	99%	99%
Prophylactic Antibiotic Timing (Outpatient)[5]	-	-	97%	98%
Urinary Catheter Removal[5]	-	-	97%	97%
Survey of Patients' Hospital Experiences				
Area Around Room 'Always' Quiet at Night[10]	<100	44%	51%	61%
Doctors 'Always' Communicated Well[10]	<100	57%	78%	82%
Home Recovery Information Given[10]	<100	81%	83%	85%
Hospital Given 9 or 10 on 10 Point Scale[10]	<100	54%	68%	71%
Meds 'Always' Explained Before Given[10]	<100	73%	61%	64%
Nurses 'Always' Communicated Well[10]	<100	77%	74%	79%
Pain 'Always' Well Controlled[10]	<100	49%	68%	71%
Room and Bathroom 'Always' Clean[10]	<100	51%	70%	73%
Timely Help 'Always' Received[10]	<100	34%	62%	68%
Would Definitely Recommend Hospital[10]	<100	52%	70%	71%
Use of Medical Imaging				
Cardiac Imaging Stress Test before Surgery[7]	-	-	5.2%	5.3%
Combination Abdominal CT Scan[7]	-	-	13.4%	10.5%
Combination Brain/Sinus CT Scan[7]	-	-	2.2%	2.7%
Combination Chest CT Scan[7]	-	-	2.3%	2.7%
Follow-up Mammogram/Ultrasound[7]	-	-	8.2%	8.8%
Lumbar Spine MRI for Low Back Pain[7]	-	-	34.2%	37.2%

Citrus Valley Medical Center - IC Campus

210 W San Bernardino Road
Covina, CA 91723
URL: www.cvhp.org
Type: Acute Care Hospitals
Ownership: Proprietary

Phone: 626-814-2468
Fax: 626-814-2428
Emergency Services: Yes
Beds: 252

Key Personnel:
Chief of Medical Staff . . . . Pavelijit Bindra, MD MBA
Quality Assurance . . . . Rosemary Butler, RN
President/CEO. . . . . Robert Curry
Operating Room. . . . . Jenny Drennan, RN
Pediatric Ambulatory Care . . . . . . Mary Hanes, MD
Pediatric In-Patient Care . . . . Mary Hanes, MD
Radiology. . . . . David Underwood, MD
CEO . . . . Joe Zanetta, JD

Measure	Cases	This Hosp.	State Avg.	U.S. Avg.
Blood Clot Prevention and Treatment				
Anticoagulation Overlap Therapy[2]	88	85%	92%	93%
ICU Venous Thromboembolism Prophylaxis[2]	72	76%	92%	92%
Incidence of Potentially Preventable VTE[2]	22	41%	11%	10%
UFH with Dosages/Platelet Monitoring[2]	52	100%	96%	97%
Venous Thromboembolism Prophylaxis[2]	260	54%	83%	85%
Warfarin Therapy Discharge Instructions[2]	60	82%	75%	75%
Chest Pain/Possible Heart Attack Care				

NOTE: Hospital profiles are in alphabetical order by state, then city, then hospital within the city; Rankings exclude hospitals with less than 25 cases except for patient surveys which excludes hospitals with less than 100 cases; (a) 100-299 cases; (1) The number of cases/patients is too few to report; (2) Data submitted were based on a sample of cases/patients; (3) Results are based on a shorter time period than required; (4) Data suppressed by CMS for one or more quarters; (5) Results are not available for this reporting period; (6) Fewer than 100 patients completed the HCAHPS survey; (7) No cases met the criteria for this measure; (8) The lower limit of the confidence interval cannot be calculated if the number of observed infections equals zero; (9) No data are available from the state/territory for this reporting period; (10) The scores shown reflect fewer than 50 completed surveys; (11) There were discrepancies in the data collection process; (12) This measure does not apply to this hospital for this reporting period; (13) Results cannot be calculated for this reporting period; (14) The results for this state are combined with nearby states to protect confidentiality; Please refer to the User's Guide for a full explanation of data.

Measure	Cases	This Hosp.	State Avg.	U.S. Avg.
Aspirin Given Within 24 Hours of Arrival	56	98%	97%	96%
Fibrinolytic Meds Within 30 Min. of Arrival[7]	-	-	62%	58%
Average Time to ECG (minutes)	58	8	9	7
Average Time to Transfer (minutes)	13	40	62	60
Children's Asthma Care				
Received Home Management Plan of Care	-	-	88%	88%
Received Reliever Medication	-	-	100%	100%
Received Systemic Corticosteroids	-	-	100%	100%
Emergency Department				
Admittance Decision Time (minutes)[2]	566	132	125	98
Head CT Results Within 45 Min. of Arrival	12	50%	55%	57%
Patients Who Left ER Before Being Seen	80,780	5%	3%	2%
Time from ER Arrival to Admit. (minutes)[2]	586	382	323	274
Time from ER Arrival to Discharge (minutes)	375	189	168	134
Time in ER Before Being Evaluated (minutes)	313	62	29	26
Time to Pain Meds for Fractures (minutes)	247	52	62	57
Heart Attack Care				
Aspirin Given at Discharge	394	98%	99%	99%
Fibrinolytic Meds Within 30 Min. of Arrival[7]	-	-	73%	54%
PCI Within 90 Minutes of Arrival	50	98%	95%	96%
Statin Prescribed at Discharge	400	97%	98%	98%
Heart Failure Care				
ACE Inhibitor or ARB for LVSD[2]	88	99%	97%	97%
Discharge Instructions Given[2]	251	87%	94%	94%
Evaluation of LVS Function[2]	304	100%	99%	99%
Medicare Spending				
Medicare Spending per Patient (ratio)	-	1.11	0.98	0.98
Pneumonia Care				
Appropriate Initial Antibiotic Given[2]	99	97%	97%	95%
Blood Culture Timing[2]	199	99%	98%	98%
Pregnancy and Delivery Care				
Newborn Deliveries Scheduled Early	474	0%	5%	6%
Preventive Care				
Immunization for Influenza[2]	484	86%	89%	90%
Immunization for Pneumonia[2]	503	84%	90%	92%
Stroke Care				
Anticoagulation Therapy for Atrial Fibrillation	19	95%	95%	95%
Antithrombotic Therapy Timing	184	99%	98%	98%
Assessed for Rehabilitation	255	98%	97%	97%
Discharged on Antithrombotic Therapy	220	97%	99%	99%
Discharged on Statin Medication	171	90%	94%	94%
Thrombolytic Therapy Timing	14	100%	72%	66%
Venous Thromboembolism Prophylaxis	238	85%	94%	94%
Written Stroke Educational Materials Given	138	93%	87%	88%
Surgical Care Improvement Project				
Appropriate Beta Blocker Usage[2]	252	97%	97%	98%
Appropriate VTP Within 24 Hours[2]	675	97%	98%	98%
Controlled Postoperative Blood Glucose[2]	136	99%	96%	97%
Perioperative Temperature Management[2]	775	100%	100%	100%
Prophylactic Antibiotic Selection[2]	649	99%	99%	99%
Prophylactic Antibiotic Selection (Outpatient)	298	99%	97%	98%
Prophylactic Antibiotic Stopped[2]	598	95%	98%	98%
Prophylactic Antibiotic Timing[2]	649	99%	99%	99%
Prophylactic Antibiotic Timing (Outpatient)	302	97%	97%	98%
Urinary Catheter Removal[2]	577	99%	97%	97%
Survey of Patients' Hospital Experiences				
Area Around Room 'Always' Quiet at Night	300+	51%	51%	61%
Doctors 'Always' Communicated Well	300+	76%	78%	82%
Home Recovery Information Given	300+	80%	83%	85%
Hospital Given 9 or 10 on 10 Point Scale	300+	70%	68%	71%
Meds 'Always' Explained Before Given	300+	58%	61%	64%
Nurses 'Always' Communicated Well	300+	73%	74%	79%
Pain 'Always' Well Controlled	300+	68%	68%	71%
Room and Bathroom 'Always' Clean	300+	67%	70%	73%
Timely Help 'Always' Received	300+	58%	62%	68%
Would Definitely Recommend Hospital	300+	67%	70%	71%
Use of Medical Imaging				
Cardiac Imaging Stress Test before Surgery	287	6.3%	5.2%	5.3%
Combination Abdominal CT Scan	568	20.2%	13.4%	10.5%
Combination Brain/Sinus CT Scan	641	1.4%	2.2%	2.7%
Combination Chest CT Scan	236	3.4%	2.3%	2.7%
Follow-up Mammogram/Ultrasound	1,109	5.7%	8.2%	8.8%
Lumbar Spine MRI for Low Back Pain[1]	-	-	34.2%	37.2%

Sutter Coast Hospital

800 E Washington Blvd — Phone: 707-464-8880
Crescent City, CA 95531 — Fax: 707-464-8941
E-mail: suttercoast@sutterhealth.org
URL: www.suttercoast.org
Type: Acute Care Hospitals — Emergency Services: Yes
Ownership: Govt - Hospital Dist/Auth — Beds: 49

Key Personnel:
Radiology. . . . . Edward Cafala
Quality Assurance . . . . Toni Drisey
Chief of Medical Staff . . . . Gregory Higgins, MD
CEO/President. . . . . John E Menaugh

Measure	Cases	This Hosp.	State Avg.	U.S. Avg.
Blood Clot Prevention and Treatment				
Anticoagulation Overlap Therapy[2]	12	92%	92%	93%
ICU Venous Thromboembolism Prophylaxis[2]	80	98%	92%	92%
Incidence of Potentially Preventable VTE[1,2]	-	-	11%	10%
UFH with Dosages/Platelet Monitoring[1,2]	-	-	96%	97%
Venous Thromboembolism Prophylaxis[2]	133	96%	83%	85%
Warfarin Therapy Discharge Instructions[2]	14	93%	75%	75%
Chest Pain/Possible Heart Attack Care				
Aspirin Given Within 24 Hours of Arrival	88	99%	97%	96%
Fibrinolytic Meds Within 30 Min. of Arrival	11	73%	62%	58%
Average Time to ECG (minutes)	92	6	9	7
Average Time to Transfer (minutes)[1]	-	-	62	60
Children's Asthma Care				
Received Home Management Plan of Care	-	-	88%	88%
Received Reliever Medication	-	-	100%	100%
Received Systemic Corticosteroids	-	-	100%	100%
Emergency Department				
Admittance Decision Time (minutes)[2]	153	184	125	98
Head CT Results Within 45 Min. of Arrival[1]	-	-	55%	57%
Patients Who Left ER Before Being Seen	21,969	2%	3%	2%
Time from ER Arrival to Admit. (minutes)[2]	392	338	323	274
Time from ER Arrival to Discharge (minutes)	350	135	168	134
Time in ER Before Being Evaluated (minutes)	357	29	29	26
Time to Pain Meds for Fractures (minutes)	92	60	62	57
Heart Attack Care				
Aspirin Given at Discharge	13	100%	99%	99%
Fibrinolytic Meds Within 30 Min. of Arrival[7]	-	-	73%	54%
PCI Within 90 Minutes of Arrival[7]	-	-	95%	96%
Statin Prescribed at Discharge	14	86%	98%	98%
Heart Failure Care				
ACE Inhibitor or ARB for LVSD	27	96%	97%	97%
Discharge Instructions Given	68	84%	94%	94%
Evaluation of LVS Function	78	100%	99%	99%
Medicare Spending				
Medicare Spending per Patient (ratio)	-	0.81	0.98	0.98
Pneumonia Care				
Appropriate Initial Antibiotic Given	104	99%	97%	95%
Blood Culture Timing	182	98%	98%	98%
Pregnancy and Delivery Care				
Newborn Deliveries Scheduled Early	45	0%	5%	6%
Preventive Care				
Immunization for Influenza[2]	267	99%	89%	90%
Immunization for Pneumonia[2]	335	99%	90%	92%
Stroke Care				
Anticoagulation Therapy for Atrial Fibrillation[1]	-	-	95%	95%
Antithrombotic Therapy Timing	30	100%	98%	98%
Assessed for Rehabilitation	38	100%	97%	97%
Discharged on Antithrombotic Therapy	37	100%	99%	99%
Discharged on Statin Medication	25	100%	94%	94%
Thrombolytic Therapy Timing[1]	-	-	72%	66%
Venous Thromboembolism Prophylaxis	32	100%	94%	94%
Written Stroke Educational Materials Given	22	91%	87%	88%
Surgical Care Improvement Project				
Appropriate Beta Blocker Usage	14	100%	97%	98%
Appropriate VTP Within 24 Hours	67	99%	98%	98%
Controlled Postoperative Blood Glucose[7]	-	-	96%	97%
Perioperative Temperature Management	75	100%	100%	100%
Prophylactic Antibiotic Selection	33	100%	99%	99%
Prophylactic Antibiotic Selection (Outpatient)	24	100%	97%	98%
Prophylactic Antibiotic Stopped	32	100%	98%	98%
Prophylactic Antibiotic Timing	33	94%	99%	99%
Prophylactic Antibiotic Timing (Outpatient)	24	100%	97%	98%
Urinary Catheter Removal	27	93%	97%	97%
Survey of Patients' Hospital Experiences				
Area Around Room 'Always' Quiet at Night	300+	59%	51%	61%
Doctors 'Always' Communicated Well	300+	80%	78%	82%
Home Recovery Information Given	300+	88%	83%	85%
Hospital Given 9 or 10 on 10 Point Scale	300+	64%	68%	71%
Meds 'Always' Explained Before Given	300+	61%	61%	64%
Nurses 'Always' Communicated Well	300+	80%	74%	79%
Pain 'Always' Well Controlled	300+	74%	68%	71%
Room and Bathroom 'Always' Clean	300+	67%	70%	73%
Timely Help 'Always' Received	300+	68%	62%	68%
Would Definitely Recommend Hospital	300+	65%	70%	71%
Use of Medical Imaging				
Cardiac Imaging Stress Test before Surgery[1]	-	-	5.2%	5.3%
Combination Abdominal CT Scan	443	14.7%	13.4%	10.5%
Combination Brain/Sinus CT Scan	486	1.9%	2.2%	2.7%
Combination Chest CT Scan	164	10.4%	2.3%	2.7%
Follow-up Mammogram/Ultrasound	615	5.2%	8.2%	8.8%
Lumbar Spine MRI for Low Back Pain	83	33.7%	34.2%	37.2%

Seton Medical Center

1900 Sullivan Avenue — Phone: 650-992-4000
Daly City, CA 94015 — Fax: 650-991-6025
URL: www.setonmedicalcenter.org
Type: Acute Care Hospitals — Emergency Services: Yes
Ownership: Voluntary non-profit - Church — Beds: 357

Key Personnel:
Quality Assurance . . . . Geri Allen
Operating Room. . . . . BJ Clark
Chief of Medical Staff . . . . Robert Dunlap, MD
Infection Control. . . . . Robert Grisnak
Radiology. . . . . Ron Krause
CEO/President. . . . . John Williams
Pediatric Ambulatory Care . . . . . . Robert Zaglin, MD
Pediatric In-Patient Care . . . . Robert Zaglin, MD

Measure	Cases	This Hosp.	State Avg.	U.S. Avg.
Blood Clot Prevention and Treatment				
Anticoagulation Overlap Therapy[2]	27	93%	92%	93%
ICU Venous Thromboembolism Prophylaxis[2]	105	86%	92%	92%
Incidence of Potentially Preventable VTE[2]	12	0%	11%	10%
UFH with Dosages/Platelet Monitoring[2]	24	100%	96%	97%
Venous Thromboembolism Prophylaxis[2]	321	84%	83%	85%
Warfarin Therapy Discharge Instructions[1,2]	-	-	75%	75%
Chest Pain/Possible Heart Attack Care				
Aspirin Given Within 24 Hours of Arrival	27	89%	97%	96%
Fibrinolytic Meds Within 30 Min. of Arrival[3,7]	-	-	62%	58%
Average Time to ECG (minutes)	27	23	9	7
Average Time to Transfer (minutes)[1,3]	-	-	62	60
Children's Asthma Care				
Received Home Management Plan of Care	-	-	88%	88%
Received Reliever Medication	-	-	100%	100%
Received Systemic Corticosteroids	-	-	100%	100%
Emergency Department				
Admittance Decision Time (minutes)[2]	790	139	125	98
Head CT Results Within 45 Min. of Arrival[1]	-	-	55%	57%
Patients Who Left ER Before Being Seen	26,323	0%	3%	2%
Time from ER Arrival to Admit. (minutes)[2]	790	257	323	274
Time from ER Arrival to Discharge (minutes)	601	116	168	134
Time in ER Before Being Evaluated (minutes)	634	20	29	26
Time to Pain Meds for Fractures (minutes)	82	62	62	57
Heart Attack Care				
Aspirin Given at Discharge	138	100%	99%	99%
Fibrinolytic Meds Within 30 Min. of Arrival[7]	-	-	73%	54%
PCI Within 90 Minutes of Arrival	29	90%	95%	96%
Statin Prescribed at Discharge	144	98%	98%	98%
Heart Failure Care				
ACE Inhibitor or ARB for LVSD	91	93%	97%	97%
Discharge Instructions Given	262	70%	94%	94%
Evaluation of LVS Function	324	100%	99%	99%
Medicare Spending				
Medicare Spending per Patient (ratio)	-	1.00	0.98	0.98

NOTE: Hospital profiles are in alphabetical order by state, then city, then hospital within the city; Rankings exclude hospitals with less than 25 cases except for patient surveys which excludes hospitals with less than 100 cases; (a) 100-299 cases; (1) The number of cases/patients is too few to report; (2) Data submitted were based on a sample of cases/patients; (3) Results are based on a shorter time period than required; (4) Data suppressed by CMS for one or more quarters; (5) Results are not available for this reporting period; (6) Fewer than 100 patients completed the HCAHPS survey; (7) No cases met the criteria for this measure; (8) The lower limit of the confidence interval cannot be calculated if the number of observed infections equals zero; (9) No data are available from the state/territory for this reporting period; (10) The scores shown reflect fewer than 50 completed surveys; (11) There were discrepancies in the data collection process; (12) This measure does not apply to this hospital for this reporting period; (13) Results cannot be calculated for this reporting period; (14) The results for this state are combined with nearby states to protect confidentiality; Please refer to the User's Guide for a full explanation of data.

Measure	Cases	This Hosp.	State Avg.	U.S. Avg.
Pneumonia Care				
Appropriate Initial Antibiotic Given	101	99%	97%	95%
Blood Culture Timing	184	99%	98%	98%
Pregnancy and Delivery Care				
Newborn Deliveries Scheduled Early[2]	19	5%	5%	6%
Preventive Care				
Immunization for Influenza[2]	531	70%	89%	90%
Immunization for Pneumonia[2]	785	79%	90%	92%
Stroke Care				
Anticoagulation Therapy for Atrial Fibrillation[2]	18	100%	95%	95%
Antithrombotic Therapy Timing[2]	69	99%	98%	98%
Assessed for Rehabilitation[2]	91	99%	97%	97%
Discharged on Antithrombotic Therapy[2]	75	100%	99%	99%
Discharged on Statin Medication[2]	57	100%	94%	94%
Thrombolytic Therapy Timing[1,2]	-	-	72%	66%
Venous Thromboembolism Prophylaxis[2]	99	91%	94%	94%
Written Stroke Educational Materials Given[2]	50	90%	87%	88%
Surgical Care Improvement Project				
Appropriate Beta Blocker Usage[2]	93	90%	97%	98%
Appropriate VTP Within 24 Hours[2]	245	97%	98%	98%
Controlled Postoperative Blood Glucose[2]	52	90%	96%	97%
Perioperative Temperature Management[2]	324	100%	100%	100%
Prophylactic Antibiotic Selection[2]	205	98%	99%	99%
Prophylactic Antibiotic Selection (Outpatient)	135	99%	97%	98%
Prophylactic Antibiotic Stopped[2]	196	99%	98%	98%
Prophylactic Antibiotic Timing[2]	206	98%	99%	99%
Prophylactic Antibiotic Timing (Outpatient)	137	95%	97%	98%
Urinary Catheter Removal[2]	200	98%	97%	97%
Survey of Patients' Hospital Experiences				
Area Around Room 'Always' Quiet at Night	300+	60%	51%	61%
Doctors 'Always' Communicated Well	300+	78%	78%	82%
Home Recovery Information Given	300+	85%	83%	85%
Hospital Given 9 or 10 on 10 Point Scale	300+	65%	68%	71%
Meds 'Always' Explained Before Given	300+	56%	61%	64%
Nurses 'Always' Communicated Well	300+	74%	74%	79%
Pain 'Always' Well Controlled	300+	65%	68%	71%
Room and Bathroom 'Always' Clean	300+	73%	70%	73%
Timely Help 'Always' Received	300+	62%	62%	68%
Would Definitely Recommend Hospital	300+	72%	70%	71%
Use of Medical Imaging				
Cardiac Imaging Stress Test before Surgery	316	4.7%	5.2%	5.3%
Combination Abdominal CT Scan	597	20.1%	13.4%	10.5%
Combination Brain/Sinus CT Scan	382	1.6%	2.2%	2.7%
Combination Chest CT Scan	429	5.4%	2.3%	2.7%
Follow-up Mammogram/Ultrasound	1,250	6.8%	8.2%	8.8%
Lumbar Spine MRI for Low Back Pain	81	43.2%	34.2%	37.2%

Sutter Davis Hospital

2000 Sutter Place
Davis, CA 95616
Phone: 530-756-6440
Fax: 530-757-5779
URL: www.sutterdavis.org
Type: Acute Care Hospitals
Emergency Services: Yes
Ownership: Proprietary
Beds: 48

Key Personnel:

Radiology. Regan K Asher
Chief of Medical Staff. . . . . Stuart G Bostrom, MD
CEO/President. . . . . Sarah Krevans

Measure	Cases	This Hosp.	State Avg.	U.S. Avg.
Blood Clot Prevention and Treatment				
Anticoagulation Overlap Therapy[1,2]	-	-	92%	93%
ICU Venous Thromboembolism Prophylaxis[2]	21	95%	92%	92%
Incidence of Potentially Preventable VTE[1,2]	-	-	11%	10%
UFH with Dosages/Platelet Monitoring[1,2]	-	-	96%	97%
Venous Thromboembolism Prophylaxis[2]	153	89%	83%	85%
Warfarin Therapy Discharge Instructions[1,2]	-	-	75%	75%
Chest Pain/Possible Heart Attack Care				
Aspirin Given Within 24 Hours of Arrival	51	100%	97%	96%
Fibrinolytic Meds Within 30 Min. of Arrival[1]	-	-	62%	58%
Average Time to ECG (minutes)	51	7	9	7
Average Time to Transfer (minutes)[7]	-	-	62	60
Children's Asthma Care				
Received Home Management Plan of Care	-	-	88%	88%
Received Reliever Medication	-	-	100%	100%
Received Systemic Corticosteroids	-	-	100%	100%
Emergency Department				
Admittance Decision Time (minutes)[2]	261	74	125	98
Head CT Results Within 45 Min. of Arrival	14	79%	55%	57%
Patients Who Left ER Before Being Seen	23,208	1%	3%	2%
Time from ER Arrival to Admit. (minutes)[2]	270	304	323	274
Time from ER Arrival to Discharge (minutes)	392	132	168	134
Time in ER Before Being Evaluated (minutes)	418	20	29	26
Time to Pain Meds for Fractures (minutes)	137	33	62	57
Heart Attack Care				
Aspirin Given at Discharge[1,3]	-	-	99%	99%
Fibrinolytic Meds Within 30 Min. of Arrival[3,7]	-	-	73%	54%
PCI Within 90 Minutes of Arrival[3,7]	-	-	95%	96%
Statin Prescribed at Discharge[1,3]	-	-	98%	98%
Heart Failure Care				
ACE Inhibitor or ARB for LVSD	18	94%	97%	97%
Discharge Instructions Given	33	100%	94%	94%
Evaluation of LVS Function	37	100%	99%	99%
Medicare Spending				
Medicare Spending per Patient (ratio)	-	0.85	0.98	0.98
Pneumonia Care				
Appropriate Initial Antibiotic Given[2]	55	98%	97%	95%
Blood Culture Timing[2]	96	99%	98%	98%
Pregnancy and Delivery Care				
Newborn Deliveries Scheduled Early	112	0%	5%	6%
Preventive Care				
Immunization for Influenza[2]	332	99%	89%	90%
Immunization for Pneumonia[2]	252	96%	90%	92%
Stroke Care				
Anticoagulation Therapy for Atrial Fibrillation[1]	-	-	95%	95%
Antithrombotic Therapy Timing	17	100%	98%	98%
Assessed for Rehabilitation	27	100%	97%	97%
Discharged on Antithrombotic Therapy	25	100%	99%	99%
Discharged on Statin Medication	15	100%	94%	94%
Thrombolytic Therapy Timing[7]	-	-	72%	66%
Venous Thromboembolism Prophylaxis	16	100%	94%	94%
Written Stroke Educational Materials Given	17	100%	87%	88%
Surgical Care Improvement Project				
Appropriate Beta Blocker Usage[2]	44	100%	97%	98%
Appropriate VTP Within 24 Hours[2]	181	98%	98%	98%
Controlled Postoperative Blood Glucose[2,7]	-	-	96%	97%
Perioperative Temperature Management[2]	224	100%	100%	100%
Prophylactic Antibiotic Selection[2]	137	100%	99%	99%
Prophylactic Antibiotic Selection (Outpatient)	37	89%	97%	98%
Prophylactic Antibiotic Stopped[2]	137	99%	98%	98%
Prophylactic Antibiotic Timing[2]	137	99%	99%	99%
Prophylactic Antibiotic Timing (Outpatient)	37	100%	97%	98%
Urinary Catheter Removal[2]	142	100%	97%	97%
Survey of Patients' Hospital Experiences				
Area Around Room 'Always' Quiet at Night	300+	62%	51%	61%
Doctors 'Always' Communicated Well	300+	85%	78%	82%
Home Recovery Information Given	300+	89%	83%	85%
Hospital Given 9 or 10 on 10 Point Scale	300+	86%	68%	71%
Meds 'Always' Explained Before Given	300+	73%	61%	64%
Nurses 'Always' Communicated Well	300+	86%	74%	79%
Pain 'Always' Well Controlled	300+	76%	68%	71%
Room and Bathroom 'Always' Clean	300+	79%	70%	73%
Timely Help 'Always' Received	300+	73%	62%	68%
Would Definitely Recommend Hospital	300+	86%	70%	71%
Use of Medical Imaging				
Cardiac Imaging Stress Test before Surgery	146	3.4%	5.2%	5.3%
Combination Abdominal CT Scan	175	3.4%	13.4%	10.5%
Combination Brain/Sinus CT Scan[1]	-	-	2.2%	2.7%
Combination Chest CT Scan	85	0.0%	2.3%	2.7%
Follow-up Mammogram/Ultrasound[7]	-	-	8.2%	8.8%
Lumbar Spine MRI for Low Back Pain[1]	-	-	34.2%	37.2%

Delano Regional Medical Center

1401 Garces Highway
Delano, CA 93215
Phone: 661-725-4800
Fax: 661-721-5355
URL: www.drmc.com
Type: Acute Care Hospitals
Emergency Services: Yes
Ownership: Proprietary
Beds: 156

Key Personnel:

Quality Assurance . . . . Debbie Anderson
Chief of Medical Staff. . . . . Radhey Bansel
Radiology. . . . . Donald E Cornforth
Emergency Room . . . . Barbara Faller
President . . . . Bahram Ghaffari

Measure	Cases	This Hosp.	State Avg.	U.S. Avg.
Blood Clot Prevention and Treatment				
Anticoagulation Overlap Therapy[1,2]	-	-	92%	93%
ICU Venous Thromboembolism Prophylaxis[2]	30	67%	92%	92%
Incidence of Potentially Preventable VTE[2,7]	-	-	11%	10%
UFH with Dosages/Platelet Monitoring[1,2]	-	-	96%	97%
Venous Thromboembolism Prophylaxis[2]	229	85%	83%	85%
Warfarin Therapy Discharge Instructions[1,2]	-	-	75%	75%
Chest Pain/Possible Heart Attack Care				
Aspirin Given Within 24 Hours of Arrival	41	88%	97%	96%
Fibrinolytic Meds Within 30 Min. of Arrival[1]	-	-	62%	58%
Average Time to ECG (minutes)	41	8	9	7
Average Time to Transfer (minutes)[1]	-	-	62	60
Children's Asthma Care				
Received Home Management Plan of Care	-	-	88%	88%
Received Reliever Medication	-	-	100%	100%
Received Systemic Corticosteroids	-	-	100%	100%
Emergency Department				
Admittance Decision Time (minutes)[2]	303	32	125	98
Head CT Results Within 45 Min. of Arrival[1]	-	-	55%	57%
Patients Who Left ER Before Being Seen	22,399	3%	3%	2%
Time from ER Arrival to Admit. (minutes)[2]	310	230	323	274
Time from ER Arrival to Discharge (minutes)	344	142	168	134
Time in ER Before Being Evaluated (minutes)	383	14	29	26
Time to Pain Meds for Fractures (minutes)	67	50	62	57
Heart Attack Care				
Aspirin Given at Discharge[1]	-	-	99%	99%
Fibrinolytic Meds Within 30 Min. of Arrival[7]	-	-	73%	54%
PCI Within 90 Minutes of Arrival[7]	-	-	95%	96%
Statin Prescribed at Discharge[1]	-	-	98%	98%
Heart Failure Care				
ACE Inhibitor or ARB for LVSD	19	95%	97%	97%
Discharge Instructions Given	46	65%	94%	94%
Evaluation of LVS Function	55	89%	99%	99%
Medicare Spending				
Medicare Spending per Patient (ratio)	-	0.91	0.98	0.98
Pneumonia Care				
Appropriate Initial Antibiotic Given	50	98%	97%	95%
Blood Culture Timing	60	97%	98%	98%
Pregnancy and Delivery Care				
Newborn Deliveries Scheduled Early[2]	49	16%	5%	6%
Preventive Care				
Immunization for Influenza[2]	287	68%	89%	90%
Immunization for Pneumonia[2]	242	90%	90%	92%
Stroke Care				
Anticoagulation Therapy for Atrial Fibrillation[7]	-	-	95%	95%
Antithrombotic Therapy Timing[1]	-	-	98%	98%
Assessed for Rehabilitation[1]	-	-	97%	97%
Discharged on Antithrombotic Therapy[1]	-	-	99%	99%
Discharged on Statin Medication[1]	-	-	94%	94%
Thrombolytic Therapy Timing[7]	-	-	72%	66%
Venous Thromboembolism Prophylaxis[1]	-	-	94%	94%
Written Stroke Educational Materials Given[1]	-	-	87%	88%
Surgical Care Improvement Project				
Appropriate Beta Blocker Usage[2]	22	77%	97%	98%
Appropriate VTP Within 24 Hours[2]	131	97%	98%	98%
Controlled Postoperative Blood Glucose[2,7]	-	-	96%	97%
Perioperative Temperature Management[2]	142	100%	100%	100%
Prophylactic Antibiotic Selection[2]	76	99%	99%	99%
Prophylactic Antibiotic Selection (Outpatient)	25	92%	97%	98%
Prophylactic Antibiotic Stopped[2]	72	96%	98%	98%

NOTE: Hospital profiles are in alphabetical order by state, then city, then hospital within the city; Rankings exclude hospitals with less than 25 cases except for patient surveys which excludes hospitals with less than 100 cases; (a) 100-299 cases; (1) The number of cases/patients is too few to report; (2) Data submitted were based on a sample of cases/patients; (3) Results are based on a shorter time period than required; (4) Data suppressed by CMS for one or more quarters; (5) Results are not available for this reporting period; (6) Fewer than 100 patients completed the HCAHPS survey; (7) No cases met the criteria for this measure; (8) The lower limit of the confidence interval cannot be calculated if the number of observed infections equals zero; (9) No data are available from the state/territory for this reporting period; (10) The scores shown reflect fewer than 50 completed surveys; (11) There were discrepancies in the data collection process; (12) This measure does not apply to this hospital for this reporting period; (13) Results cannot be calculated for this reporting period; (14) The results for this state are combined with nearby states to protect confidentiality; Please refer to the User's Guide for a full explanation of data.

Measure	Cases	This Hosp.	State Avg.	U.S. Avg.
Prophylactic Antibiotic Timing[2]	76	100%	99%	99%
Prophylactic Antibiotic Timing (Outpatient)	29	86%	97%	98%
Urinary Catheter Removal[2]	49	92%	97%	97%
Survey of Patients' Hospital Experiences				
Area Around Room 'Always' Quiet at Night	300+	46%	51%	61%
Doctors 'Always' Communicated Well	300+	76%	78%	82%
Home Recovery Information Given	300+	80%	83%	85%
Hospital Given 9 or 10 on 10 Point Scale	300+	63%	68%	71%
Meds 'Always' Explained Before Given	300+	58%	61%	64%
Nurses 'Always' Communicated Well	300+	73%	74%	79%
Pain 'Always' Well Controlled	300+	65%	68%	71%
Room and Bathroom 'Always' Clean	300+	72%	70%	73%
Timely Help 'Always' Received	300+	57%	62%	68%
Would Definitely Recommend Hospital	300+	54%	70%	71%
Use of Medical Imaging				
Cardiac Imaging Stress Test before Surgery[7]	-	-	5.2%	5.3%
Combination Abdominal CT Scan	296	31.4%	13.4%	10.5%
Combination Brain/Sinus CT Scan[1]	-	-	2.2%	2.7%
Combination Chest CT Scan	130	24.6%	2.3%	2.7%
Follow-up Mammogram/Ultrasound	345	2.6%	8.2%	8.8%
Lumbar Spine MRI for Low Back Pain[1]	-	-	34.2%	37.2%

Kaiser Foundation Hospital - Downey

9333 Imperial Highway
Downey, CA 90242
Phone: 562-461-6007
URL: www.kaiserpermanente.org
Type: Acute Care Hospitals
Emergency Services: Yes
Ownership: Voluntary non-profit - Other

Measure	Cases	This Hosp.	State Avg.	U.S. Avg.
Blood Clot Prevention and Treatment				
Anticoagulation Overlap Therapy[2]	93	92%	92%	93%
ICU Venous Thromboembolism Prophylaxis[2]	25	100%	92%	92%
Incidence of Potentially Preventable VTE[2]	19	5%	11%	10%
UFH with Dosages/Platelet Monitoring[2]	46	100%	96%	97%
Venous Thromboembolism Prophylaxis[2]	303	92%	83%	85%
Warfarin Therapy Discharge Instructions[2]	81	60%	75%	75%
Chest Pain/Possible Heart Attack Care				
Aspirin Given Within 24 Hours of Arrival	-	-	97%	96%
Fibrinolytic Meds Within 30 Min. of Arrival	-	-	62%	58%
Average Time to ECG (minutes)	-	-	9	7
Average Time to Transfer (minutes)	-	-	62	60
Children's Asthma Care				
Received Home Management Plan of Care	-	-	88%	88%
Received Reliever Medication	-	-	100%	100%
Received Systemic Corticosteroids	-	-	100%	100%
Emergency Department				
Admittance Decision Time (minutes)[2]	389	116	125	98
Head CT Results Within 45 Min. of Arrival	-	-	55%	57%
Patients Who Left ER Before Being Seen	-	-	3%	2%
Time from ER Arrival to Admit. (minutes)[2]	419	365	323	274
Time from ER Arrival to Discharge (minutes)	-	-	168	134
Time in ER Before Being Evaluated (minutes)	-	-	29	26
Time to Pain Meds for Fractures (minutes)	-	-	62	57
Heart Attack Care				
Aspirin Given at Discharge	97	100%	99%	99%
Fibrinolytic Meds Within 30 Min. of Arrival[1]	-	-	73%	54%
PCI Within 90 Minutes of Arrival[7]	-	-	95%	96%
Statin Prescribed at Discharge	97	100%	98%	98%
Heart Failure Care				
ACE Inhibitor or ARB for LVSD	108	100%	97%	97%
Discharge Instructions Given	343	99%	94%	94%
Evaluation of LVS Function	363	100%	99%	99%
Medicare Spending				
Medicare Spending per Patient (ratio)	-	0.79	0.98	0.98
Pneumonia Care				
Appropriate Initial Antibiotic Given[2]	74	95%	97%	95%
Blood Culture Timing[2]	161	99%	98%	98%
Pregnancy and Delivery Care				
Newborn Deliveries Scheduled Early	464	1%	5%	6%
Preventive Care				
Immunization for Influenza[2]	508	91%	89%	90%
Immunization for Pneumonia[2]	497	95%	90%	92%
Stroke Care				
Anticoagulation Therapy for Atrial Fibrillation[1,2]	-	-	95%	95%
Antithrombotic Therapy Timing[2]	92	100%	98%	98%
Assessed for Rehabilitation[2]	109	94%	97%	97%
Discharged on Antithrombotic Therapy[2]	90	100%	99%	99%
Discharged on Statin Medication[2]	75	100%	94%	94%
Thrombolytic Therapy Timing[2,7]	-	-	72%	66%
Venous Thromboembolism Prophylaxis[2]	97	98%	94%	94%
Written Stroke Educational Materials Given[2]	77	95%	87%	88%
Surgical Care Improvement Project				
Appropriate Beta Blocker Usage[2]	132	98%	97%	98%
Appropriate VTP Within 24 Hours[2]	349	99%	98%	98%
Controlled Postoperative Blood Glucose[2,7]	-	-	96%	97%
Perioperative Temperature Management[2]	464	100%	100%	100%
Prophylactic Antibiotic Selection[2]	313	100%	99%	99%
Prophylactic Antibiotic Selection (Outpatient)	-	-	97%	98%
Prophylactic Antibiotic Stopped[2]	294	98%	98%	98%
Prophylactic Antibiotic Timing[2]	314	97%	99%	99%
Prophylactic Antibiotic Timing (Outpatient)	-	-	97%	98%
Urinary Catheter Removal[2]	253	99%	97%	97%
Survey of Patients' Hospital Experiences				
Area Around Room 'Always' Quiet at Night	300+	59%	51%	61%
Doctors 'Always' Communicated Well	300+	81%	78%	82%
Home Recovery Information Given	300+	85%	83%	85%
Hospital Given 9 or 10 on 10 Point Scale	300+	78%	68%	71%
Meds 'Always' Explained Before Given	300+	62%	61%	64%
Nurses 'Always' Communicated Well	300+	76%	74%	79%
Pain 'Always' Well Controlled	300+	70%	68%	71%
Room and Bathroom 'Always' Clean	300+	75%	70%	73%
Timely Help 'Always' Received	300+	64%	62%	68%
Would Definitely Recommend Hospital	300+	80%	70%	71%
Use of Medical Imaging				
Cardiac Imaging Stress Test before Surgery	-	-	5.2%	5.3%
Combination Abdominal CT Scan	-	-	13.4%	10.5%
Combination Brain/Sinus CT Scan	-	-	2.2%	2.7%
Combination Chest CT Scan	-	-	2.3%	2.7%
Follow-up Mammogram/Ultrasound	-	-	8.2%	8.8%
Lumbar Spine MRI for Low Back Pain	-	-	34.2%	37.2%

LAC/Rancho Los Amigos National Rehab Center

7601 East Imperial Highway
Downey, CA 90242
Phone: 562-401-7022
Fax: 562-803-3486
URL: www.rancho.org
Type: Acute Care Hospitals
Emergency Services: No
Ownership: Government - Local
Beds: 395

Key Personnel:
Pediatric Ambulatory Care . . . . . . Irene Gilgoff, MD
Pediatric In-Patient Care . . . . Irene Gilgoff, MD
Quality Assurance . . . . Maria Heckman
Chief of Medical Staff. . . . . Mindy Lipson Aisen, MD
CEO/President. . . . . Jorge Orozco, PT
Infection Control . . . . Francisco Sapico, MD
Operating Room. . . . . Alvin Shon, RN
Cardiac Laboratory. . . . . D Svlachcac, MD

Measure	Cases	This Hosp.	State Avg.	U.S. Avg.
Blood Clot Prevention and Treatment				
Anticoagulation Overlap Therapy[2]	11	27%	92%	93%
ICU Venous Thromboembolism Prophylaxis[1,2]	-	-	92%	92%
Incidence of Potentially Preventable VTE[1,2]	-	-	11%	10%
UFH with Dosages/Platelet Monitoring[1,2]	-	-	96%	97%
Venous Thromboembolism Prophylaxis[2]	419	67%	83%	85%
Warfarin Therapy Discharge Instructions[1,2]	-	-	75%	75%
Chest Pain/Possible Heart Attack Care				
Aspirin Given Within 24 Hours of Arrival[5]	-	-	97%	96%
Fibrinolytic Meds Within 30 Min. of Arrival[5]	-	-	62%	58%
Average Time to ECG (minutes)[5]	-	-	9	7
Average Time to Transfer (minutes)[5]	-	-	62	60
Children's Asthma Care				
Received Home Management Plan of Care	-	-	88%	88%
Received Reliever Medication	-	-	100%	100%
Received Systemic Corticosteroids	-	-	100%	100%
Emergency Department				
Admittance Decision Time (minutes)[2,7]	-	-	125	98
Head CT Results Within 45 Min. of Arrival[5]	-	-	55%	57%
Patients Who Left ER Before Being Seen[5]	-	-	3%	2%
Time from ER Arrival to Admit. (minutes)[2,7]	-	-	323	274
Time from ER Arrival to Discharge (minutes)[5]	-	-	168	134
Time in ER Before Being Evaluated (minutes)[5]	-	-	29	26
Time to Pain Meds for Fractures (minutes)[5]	-	-	62	57
Heart Attack Care				
Aspirin Given at Discharge[1]	-	-	99%	99%
Fibrinolytic Meds Within 30 Min. of Arrival[7]	-	-	73%	54%
PCI Within 90 Minutes of Arrival[7]	-	-	95%	96%
Statin Prescribed at Discharge[1]	-	-	98%	98%
Heart Failure Care				
ACE Inhibitor or ARB for LVSD[1,3]	-	-	97%	97%
Discharge Instructions Given[1,3]	-	-	94%	94%
Evaluation of LVS Function[1,3]	-	-	99%	99%
Medicare Spending				
Medicare Spending per Patient (ratio)	-	1.22	0.98	0.98
Pneumonia Care				
Appropriate Initial Antibiotic Given[7]	-	-	97%	95%
Blood Culture Timing[7]	-	-	98%	98%
Pregnancy and Delivery Care				
Newborn Deliveries Scheduled Early[7]	-	-	5%	6%
Preventive Care				
Immunization for Influenza[2]	368	50%	89%	90%
Immunization for Pneumonia[2]	364	52%	90%	92%
Stroke Care				
Anticoagulation Therapy for Atrial Fibrillation[1,2]	-	-	95%	95%
Antithrombotic Therapy Timing[2]	87	95%	98%	98%
Assessed for Rehabilitation[2]	122	93%	97%	97%
Discharged on Antithrombotic Therapy[2]	110	95%	99%	99%
Discharged on Statin Medication[2]	71	86%	94%	94%
Thrombolytic Therapy Timing[2,7]	-	-	72%	66%
Venous Thromboembolism Prophylaxis[2]	100	92%	94%	94%
Written Stroke Educational Materials Given[2]	62	92%	87%	88%
Surgical Care Improvement Project				
Appropriate Beta Blocker Usage[2]	35	37%	97%	98%
Appropriate VTP Within 24 Hours[2]	206	98%	98%	98%
Controlled Postoperative Blood Glucose[2,7]	-	-	96%	97%
Perioperative Temperature Management[2]	217	100%	100%	100%
Prophylactic Antibiotic Selection[2]	176	98%	99%	99%
Prophylactic Antibiotic Selection (Outpatient)[5]	-	-	97%	98%
Prophylactic Antibiotic Stopped[2]	174	100%	98%	98%
Prophylactic Antibiotic Timing[2]	176	97%	99%	99%
Prophylactic Antibiotic Timing (Outpatient)[5]	-	-	97%	98%
Urinary Catheter Removal[2]	159	100%	97%	97%
Survey of Patients' Hospital Experiences				
Area Around Room 'Always' Quiet at Night	300+	51%	51%	61%
Doctors 'Always' Communicated Well	300+	81%	78%	82%
Home Recovery Information Given	300+	87%	83%	85%
Hospital Given 9 or 10 on 10 Point Scale	300+	79%	68%	71%
Meds 'Always' Explained Before Given	300+	64%	61%	64%
Nurses 'Always' Communicated Well	300+	78%	74%	79%
Pain 'Always' Well Controlled	300+	72%	68%	71%
Room and Bathroom 'Always' Clean	300+	74%	70%	73%
Timely Help 'Always' Received	300+	64%	62%	68%
Would Definitely Recommend Hospital	300+	81%	70%	71%
Use of Medical Imaging				
Cardiac Imaging Stress Test before Surgery[1]	-	-	5.2%	5.3%
Combination Abdominal CT Scan[1]	-	-	13.4%	10.5%
Combination Brain/Sinus CT Scan[1]	-	-	2.2%	2.7%
Combination Chest CT Scan[1]	-	-	2.3%	2.7%
Follow-up Mammogram/Ultrasound[7]	-	-	8.2%	8.8%
Lumbar Spine MRI for Low Back Pain[7]	-	-	34.2%	37.2%

PIH Hospital - Downey

11500 Brookshire Avenue
Downey, CA 90241
Phone: 526-904-5000
Fax: 562-904-5309
URL: www.drmci.org
Type: Acute Care Hospitals
Emergency Services: Yes
Ownership: Voluntary non-profit - Private
Beds: 199

Key Personnel:
Administrator . . . . Peggy Chulack
Emergency Room . . . . Richard Guess, MD
Chief of Medical Staff . . . . Rosalio Lopez, MD
Quality Assurance . . . . Connie Meinke
Operating Room. . . . . Bill Stein

NOTE: Hospital profiles are in alphabetical order by state, then city, then hospital within the city; Rankings exclude hospitals with less than 25 cases except for patient surveys which excludes hospitals with less than 100 cases; (a) 100-299 cases; (1) The number of cases/patients is too few to report; (2) Data submitted were based on a sample of cases/patients; (3) Results are based on a shorter time period than required; (4) Data suppressed by CMS for one or more quarters; (5) Results are not available for this reporting period; (6) Fewer than 100 patients completed the HCAHPS survey; (7) No cases met the criteria for this measure; (8) The lower limit of the confidence interval cannot be calculated if the number of observed infections equals zero; (9) No data are available from the state/territory for this reporting period; (10) The scores shown reflect fewer than 50 completed surveys; (11) There were discrepancies in the data collection process; (12) This measure does not apply to this hospital for this reporting period; (13) Results cannot be calculated for this reporting period; (14) The results for this state are combined with nearby states to protect confidentiality; Please refer to the User's Guide for a full explanation of data.

Infection Control . . . . Mary Stevens
President/CEO . . . . Jim West

Measure	Cases	This Hosp.	State Avg.	U.S. Avg.
Blood Clot Prevention and Treatment				
Anticoagulation Overlap Therapy[2]	44	98%	92%	93%
ICU Venous Thromboembolism Prophylaxis[2]	74	99%	92%	92%
Incidence of Potentially Preventable VTE[1,2]	-	-	11%	10%
UFH with Dosages/Platelet Monitoring[2]	24	100%	96%	97%
Venous Thromboembolism Prophylaxis[2]	312	99%	83%	85%
Warfarin Therapy Discharge Instructions[2]	33	97%	75%	75%
Chest Pain/Possible Heart Attack Care				
Aspirin Given Within 24 Hours of Arrival[1]	-	-	97%	96%
Fibrinolytic Meds Within 30 Min. of Arrival[5]	-	-	62%	58%
Average Time to ECG (minutes)[1]	-	-	9	7
Average Time to Transfer (minutes)[5]	-	-	62	60
Children's Asthma Care				
Received Home Management Plan of Care	-	-	88%	88%
Received Reliever Medication	-	-	100%	100%
Received Systemic Corticosteroids	-	-	100%	100%
Emergency Department				
Admittance Decision Time (minutes)[2]	259	115	125	98
Head CT Results Within 45 Min. of Arrival[7]	-	-	55%	57%
Patients Who Left ER Before Being Seen	52,385	4%	3%	2%
Time from ER Arrival to Admit. (minutes)[2]	411	337	323	274
Time from ER Arrival to Discharge (minutes)	365	195	168	134
Time in ER Before Being Evaluated (minutes)	354	90	29	26
Time to Pain Meds for Fractures (minutes)	156	88	62	57
Heart Attack Care				
Aspirin Given at Discharge	235	99%	99%	99%
Fibrinolytic Meds Within 30 Min. of Arrival[1]	-	-	73%	54%
PCI Within 90 Minutes of Arrival	22	23%	95%	96%
Statin Prescribed at Discharge	243	98%	98%	98%
Heart Failure Care				
ACE Inhibitor or ARB for LVSD	135	99%	97%	97%
Discharge Instructions Given	291	97%	94%	94%
Evaluation of LVS Function	368	100%	99%	99%
Medicare Spending				
Medicare Spending per Patient (ratio)	-	1.09	0.98	0.98
Pneumonia Care				
Appropriate Initial Antibiotic Given	127	95%	97%	95%
Blood Culture Timing	260	94%	98%	98%
Pregnancy and Delivery Care				
Newborn Deliveries Scheduled Early[2]	66	0%	5%	6%
Preventive Care				
Immunization for Influenza[2]	556	97%	89%	90%
Immunization for Pneumonia[2]	714	98%	90%	92%
Stroke Care				
Anticoagulation Therapy for Atrial Fibrillation[1]	-	-	95%	95%
Antithrombotic Therapy Timing	82	99%	98%	98%
Assessed for Rehabilitation	106	96%	97%	97%
Discharged on Antithrombotic Therapy	87	100%	99%	99%
Discharged on Statin Medication	72	94%	94%	94%
Thrombolytic Therapy Timing[1]	-	-	72%	66%
Venous Thromboembolism Prophylaxis	101	100%	94%	94%
Written Stroke Educational Materials Given	66	86%	87%	88%
Surgical Care Improvement Project				
Appropriate Beta Blocker Usage[2]	156	90%	97%	98%
Appropriate VTP Within 24 Hours[2]	465	96%	98%	98%
Controlled Postoperative Blood Glucose[2]	48	85%	96%	97%
Perioperative Temperature Management[2]	509	100%	100%	100%
Prophylactic Antibiotic Selection[2]	315	99%	99%	99%
Prophylactic Antibiotic Selection (Outpatient)	73	100%	97%	98%
Prophylactic Antibiotic Stopped[2]	297	96%	98%	98%
Prophylactic Antibiotic Timing[2]	315	100%	99%	99%
Prophylactic Antibiotic Timing (Outpatient)	74	97%	97%	98%
Urinary Catheter Removal[2]	131	95%	97%	97%
Survey of Patients' Hospital Experiences				
Area Around Room 'Always' Quiet at Night	300+	42%	51%	61%
Doctors 'Always' Communicated Well	300+	74%	78%	82%
Home Recovery Information Given	300+	77%	83%	85%
Hospital Given 9 or 10 on 10 Point Scale	300+	56%	68%	71%
Meds 'Always' Explained Before Given	300+	57%	61%	64%
Nurses 'Always' Communicated Well	300+	67%	74%	79%
Pain 'Always' Well Controlled	300+	61%	68%	71%
Room and Bathroom 'Always' Clean	300+	72%	70%	73%
Timely Help 'Always' Received	300+	53%	62%	68%
Would Definitely Recommend Hospital	300+	56%	70%	71%
Use of Medical Imaging				
Cardiac Imaging Stress Test before Surgery	110	1.8%	5.2%	5.3%
Combination Abdominal CT Scan	372	8.9%	13.4%	10.5%
Combination Brain/Sinus CT Scan	575	0.2%	2.2%	2.7%
Combination Chest CT Scan	154	0.0%	2.3%	2.7%
Follow-up Mammogram/Ultrasound	700	10.9%	8.2%	8.8%
Lumbar Spine MRI for Low Back Pain[1]	-	-	34.2%	37.2%

City of Hope Helford Clinical Research Hospital

1500 E Duarte Road — Phone: 626-359-8111
Duarte, CA 91010
Type: Acute Care Hospitals — Emergency Services: No
Ownership: Voluntary non-profit - Other

Measure	Cases	This Hosp.	State Avg.	U.S. Avg.
Blood Clot Prevention and Treatment				
Anticoagulation Overlap Therapy[5]	-	-	92%	93%
ICU Venous Thromboembolism Prophylaxis[5]	-	-	92%	92%
Incidence of Potentially Preventable VTE[5]	-	-	11%	10%
UFH with Dosages/Platelet Monitoring[5]	-	-	96%	97%
Venous Thromboembolism Prophylaxis[5]	-	-	83%	85%
Warfarin Therapy Discharge Instructions[5]	-	-	75%	75%
Chest Pain/Possible Heart Attack Care				
Aspirin Given Within 24 Hours of Arrival	-	-	97%	96%
Fibrinolytic Meds Within 30 Min. of Arrival	-	-	62%	58%
Average Time to ECG (minutes)	-	-	9	7
Average Time to Transfer (minutes)	-	-	62	60
Children's Asthma Care				
Received Home Management Plan of Care	-	-	88%	88%
Received Reliever Medication	-	-	100%	100%
Received Systemic Corticosteroids	-	-	100%	100%
Emergency Department				
Admittance Decision Time (minutes)[5]	-	-	125	98
Head CT Results Within 45 Min. of Arrival	-	-	55%	57%
Patients Who Left ER Before Being Seen	-	-	3%	2%
Time from ER Arrival to Admit. (minutes)[5]	-	-	323	274
Time from ER Arrival to Discharge (minutes)	-	-	168	134
Time in ER Before Being Evaluated (minutes)	-	-	29	26
Time to Pain Meds for Fractures (minutes)	-	-	62	57
Heart Attack Care				
Aspirin Given at Discharge[5]	-	-	99%	99%
Fibrinolytic Meds Within 30 Min. of Arrival[5]	-	-	73%	54%
PCI Within 90 Minutes of Arrival[5]	-	-	95%	96%
Statin Prescribed at Discharge[5]	-	-	98%	98%
Heart Failure Care				
ACE Inhibitor or ARB for LVSD[5]	-	-	97%	97%
Discharge Instructions Given[5]	-	-	94%	94%
Evaluation of LVS Function[5]	-	-	99%	99%
Medicare Spending				
Medicare Spending per Patient (ratio)	-	-	0.98	0.98
Pneumonia Care				
Appropriate Initial Antibiotic Given[5]	-	-	97%	95%
Blood Culture Timing[5]	-	-	98%	98%
Pregnancy and Delivery Care				
Newborn Deliveries Scheduled Early[5]	-	-	5%	6%
Preventive Care				
Immunization for Influenza[5]	-	-	89%	90%
Immunization for Pneumonia[5]	-	-	90%	92%
Stroke Care				
Anticoagulation Therapy for Atrial Fibrillation[5]	-	-	95%	95%
Antithrombotic Therapy Timing[5]	-	-	98%	98%
Assessed for Rehabilitation[5]	-	-	97%	97%
Discharged on Antithrombotic Therapy[5]	-	-	99%	99%
Discharged on Statin Medication[5]	-	-	94%	94%
Thrombolytic Therapy Timing[5]	-	-	72%	66%
Venous Thromboembolism Prophylaxis[5]	-	-	94%	94%
Written Stroke Educational Materials Given[5]	-	-	87%	88%
Surgical Care Improvement Project				
Appropriate Beta Blocker Usage[5]	-	-	97%	98%
Appropriate VTP Within 24 Hours[5]	-	-	98%	98%
Controlled Postoperative Blood Glucose[5]	-	-	96%	97%
Perioperative Temperature Management[5]	-	-	100%	100%
Prophylactic Antibiotic Selection[5]	-	-	99%	99%
Prophylactic Antibiotic Selection (Outpatient)	-	-	97%	98%
Prophylactic Antibiotic Stopped[5]	-	-	98%	98%
Prophylactic Antibiotic Timing[5]	-	-	99%	99%
Prophylactic Antibiotic Timing (Outpatient)	-	-	97%	98%
Urinary Catheter Removal[5]	-	-	97%	97%
Survey of Patients' Hospital Experiences				
Area Around Room 'Always' Quiet at Night	300+	65%	51%	61%
Doctors 'Always' Communicated Well	300+	86%	78%	82%
Home Recovery Information Given	300+	90%	83%	85%
Hospital Given 9 or 10 on 10 Point Scale	300+	85%	68%	71%
Meds 'Always' Explained Before Given	300+	68%	61%	64%
Nurses 'Always' Communicated Well	300+	82%	74%	79%
Pain 'Always' Well Controlled	300+	75%	68%	71%
Room and Bathroom 'Always' Clean	300+	73%	70%	73%
Timely Help 'Always' Received	300+	61%	62%	68%
Would Definitely Recommend Hospital	300+	91%	70%	71%
Use of Medical Imaging				
Cardiac Imaging Stress Test before Surgery	-	-	5.2%	5.3%
Combination Abdominal CT Scan	-	-	13.4%	10.5%
Combination Brain/Sinus CT Scan	-	-	2.2%	2.7%
Combination Chest CT Scan	-	-	2.3%	2.7%
Follow-up Mammogram/Ultrasound	-	-	8.2%	8.8%
Lumbar Spine MRI for Low Back Pain	-	-	34.2%	37.2%

El Centro Regional Medical Center

1415 Ross Avenue — Phone: 760-339-7100
El Centro, CA 92243 — Fax: 760-339-7363
E-mail: wecare@ecrmc.org
URL: www.ecrmc.org
Type: Acute Care Hospitals — Emergency Services: Yes
Ownership: Government - Local — Beds: 165

Key Personnel:

CEO/President. . . . . David R Green
Chief of Medical Staff . . . . Leslie Mukau, MD
Anesthesiology. . . . . Servando Rodriguez, MD
Cardiac Laboratory. . . . . Randy Steffen
Operating Room. . . . . Karen Timmerman, RN
Pediatric Ambulatory Care . . . . . . LuzElva Tristan, MD
Quality Assurance . . . . Kathy Valvi
Emergency Room . . . . Tomas Virgen, RN

Measure	Cases	This Hosp.	State Avg.	U.S. Avg.
Blood Clot Prevention and Treatment				
Anticoagulation Overlap Therapy[2]	34	56%	92%	93%
ICU Venous Thromboembolism Prophylaxis[2]	75	89%	92%	92%
Incidence of Potentially Preventable VTE[1,2]	-	-	11%	10%
UFH with Dosages/Platelet Monitoring[2]	18	100%	96%	97%
Venous Thromboembolism Prophylaxis[2]	373	83%	83%	85%
Warfarin Therapy Discharge Instructions[2]	20	85%	75%	75%
Chest Pain/Possible Heart Attack Care				
Aspirin Given Within 24 Hours of Arrival[3]	49	100%	97%	96%
Fibrinolytic Meds Within 30 Min. of Arrival[1,3]	-	-	62%	58%
Average Time to ECG (minutes)[3]	51	5	9	7
Average Time to Transfer (minutes)[3,7]	-	-	62	60
Children's Asthma Care				
Received Home Management Plan of Care	38	92%	88%	88%
Received Reliever Medication	38	100%	100%	100%
Received Systemic Corticosteroids	38	100%	100%	100%
Emergency Department				
Admittance Decision Time (minutes)[2]	711	244	125	98
Head CT Results Within 45 Min. of Arrival	24	38%	55%	57%
Patients Who Left ER Before Being Seen	39,976	2%	3%	2%
Time from ER Arrival to Admit. (minutes)[2]	711	471	323	274
Time from ER Arrival to Discharge (minutes)	423	167	168	134
Time in ER Before Being Evaluated (minutes)	449	18	29	26
Time to Pain Meds for Fractures (minutes)	245	40	62	57
Heart Attack Care				
Aspirin Given at Discharge	42	93%	99%	99%
Fibrinolytic Meds Within 30 Min. of Arrival[1]	-	-	73%	54%
PCI Within 90 Minutes of Arrival[7]	-	-	95%	96%

NOTE: Hospital profiles are in alphabetical order by state, then city, then hospital within the city; Rankings exclude hospitals with less than 25 cases except for patient surveys which excludes hospitals with less than 100 cases; (a) 100-299 cases; (1) The number of cases/patients is too few to report; (2) Data submitted were based on a sample of cases/patients; (3) Results are based on a shorter time period than required; (4) Data suppressed by CMS for one or more quarters; (5) Results are not available for this reporting period; (6) Fewer than 100 patients completed the HCAHPS survey; (7) No cases met the criteria for this measure; (8) The lower limit of the confidence interval cannot be calculated if the number of observed infections equals zero; (9) No data are available from the state/territory for this reporting period; (10) The scores shown reflect fewer than 50 completed surveys; (11) There were discrepancies in the data collection process; (12) This measure does not apply to this hospital for this reporting period; (13) Results cannot be calculated for this reporting period; (14) The results for this state are combined with nearby states to protect confidentiality; Please refer to the User's Guide for a full explanation of data.

Measure	Cases	This Hosp.	State Avg.	U.S. Avg.
Statin Prescribed at Discharge	48	98%	98%	98%
Heart Failure Care				
ACE Inhibitor or ARB for LVSD	71	87%	97%	97%
Discharge Instructions Given	196	99%	94%	94%
Evaluation of LVS Function	214	93%	99%	99%
Medicare Spending				
Medicare Spending per Patient (ratio)	-	0.89	0.98	0.98
Pneumonia Care				
Appropriate Initial Antibiotic Given	135	86%	97%	95%
Blood Culture Timing	202	92%	98%	98%
Pregnancy and Delivery Care				
Newborn Deliveries Scheduled Early[2]	28	4%	5%	6%
Preventive Care				
Immunization for Influenza[2]	499	74%	89%	90%
Immunization for Pneumonia[2]	546	88%	90%	92%
Stroke Care				
Anticoagulation Therapy for Atrial Fibrillation[2]	16	75%	95%	95%
Antithrombotic Therapy Timing[2]	94	95%	98%	98%
Assessed for Rehabilitation[2]	92	96%	97%	97%
Discharged on Antithrombotic Therapy[2]	87	93%	99%	99%
Discharged on Statin Medication[2]	86	84%	94%	94%
Thrombolytic Therapy Timing[2]	41	2%	72%	66%
Venous Thromboembolism Prophylaxis[2]	99	74%	94%	94%
Written Stroke Educational Materials Given[2]	63	2%	87%	88%
Surgical Care Improvement Project				
Appropriate Beta Blocker Usage[2]	52	67%	97%	98%
Appropriate VTP Within 24 Hours[2]	245	87%	98%	98%
Controlled Postoperative Blood Glucose[2,7]	-	-	96%	97%
Perioperative Temperature Management[2]	300	97%	100%	100%
Prophylactic Antibiotic Selection[2]	161	99%	99%	99%
Prophylactic Antibiotic Selection (Outpatient)	137	93%	97%	98%
Prophylactic Antibiotic Stopped[2]	159	97%	98%	98%
Prophylactic Antibiotic Timing[2]	162	90%	99%	99%
Prophylactic Antibiotic Timing (Outpatient)	165	52%	97%	98%
Urinary Catheter Removal[2]	77	42%	97%	97%
Survey of Patients' Hospital Experiences				
Area Around Room 'Always' Quiet at Night	(a)	46%	51%	61%
Doctors 'Always' Communicated Well	(a)	70%	78%	82%
Home Recovery Information Given	(a)	85%	83%	85%
Hospital Given 9 or 10 on 10 Point Scale	(a)	60%	68%	71%
Meds 'Always' Explained Before Given	(a)	62%	61%	64%
Nurses 'Always' Communicated Well	(a)	69%	74%	79%
Pain 'Always' Well Controlled	(a)	67%	68%	71%
Room and Bathroom 'Always' Clean	(a)	71%	70%	73%
Timely Help 'Always' Received	(a)	57%	62%	68%
Would Definitely Recommend Hospital	(a)	59%	70%	71%
Use of Medical Imaging				
Cardiac Imaging Stress Test before Surgery	94	5.3%	5.2%	5.3%
Combination Abdominal CT Scan	920	5.8%	13.4%	10.5%
Combination Brain/Sinus CT Scan	977	1.9%	2.2%	2.7%
Combination Chest CT Scan	389	3.3%	2.3%	2.7%
Follow-up Mammogram/Ultrasound	1,157	6.1%	8.2%	8.8%
Lumbar Spine MRI for Low Back Pain	44	38.6%	34.2%	37.2%

Sonoma Developmental Center

PO Box 1493 Phone: 707-938-6393
Eldridge, CA 95431 Fax: 707-938-3605
URL: www.dds.ca.gov/sonoma/index.cfm
Type: Acute Care Hospitals Emergency Services: No
Ownership: Government - Federal Beds: 1,421
Key Personnel:
Chief of Medical Staff.......... Judith Bjorndal
Quality Assurance .... Karen Faria
Emergency Room .... David Grey
Radiology.................... Ted Hansen

Measure	Cases	This Hosp.	State Avg.	U.S. Avg.
Blood Clot Prevention and Treatment				
Anticoagulation Overlap Therapy[2,7]	-	-	92%	93%
ICU Venous Thromboembolism Prophylaxis[2,7]	-	-	92%	92%
Incidence of Potentially Preventable VTE[2,7]	-	-	11%	10%
UFH with Dosages/Platelet Monitoring[2,7]	-	-	96%	97%
Venous Thromboembolism Prophylaxis[2]	75	3%	83%	85%
Warfarin Therapy Discharge Instructions[2,7]	-	-	75%	75%
Chest Pain/Possible Heart Attack Care				
Aspirin Given Within 24 Hours of Arrival[5]	-	-	97%	96%
Fibrinolytic Meds Within 30 Min. of Arrival[5]	-	-	62%	58%
Average Time to ECG (minutes)[5]	-	-	9	7
Average Time to Transfer (minutes)[5]	-	-	62	60
Children's Asthma Care				
Received Home Management Plan of Care	-	-	88%	88%
Received Reliever Medication	-	-	100%	100%
Received Systemic Corticosteroids	-	-	100%	100%
Emergency Department				
Admittance Decision Time (minutes)[7]	-	-	125	98
Head CT Results Within 45 Min. of Arrival[5]	-	-	55%	57%
Patients Who Left ER Before Being Seen[5]	-	-	3%	2%
Time from ER Arrival to Admit. (minutes)[7]	-	-	323	274
Time from ER Arrival to Discharge (minutes)[5]	-	-	168	134
Time in ER Before Being Evaluated (minutes)[5]	-	-	29	26
Time to Pain Meds for Fractures (minutes)[5]	-	-	62	57
Heart Attack Care				
Aspirin Given at Discharge[5]	-	-	99%	99%
Fibrinolytic Meds Within 30 Min. of Arrival[5]	-	-	73%	54%
PCI Within 90 Minutes of Arrival[5]	-	-	95%	96%
Statin Prescribed at Discharge[5]	-	-	98%	98%
Heart Failure Care				
ACE Inhibitor or ARB for LVSD[5]	-	-	97%	97%
Discharge Instructions Given[5]	-	-	94%	94%
Evaluation of LVS Function[5]	-	-	99%	99%
Medicare Spending				
Medicare Spending per Patient (ratio)	-	0.70	0.98	0.98
Pneumonia Care				
Appropriate Initial Antibiotic Given[3,7]	-	-	97%	95%
Blood Culture Timing[3,7]	-	-	98%	98%
Pregnancy and Delivery Care				
Newborn Deliveries Scheduled Early[7]	-	-	5%	6%
Preventive Care				
Immunization for Influenza	62	100%	89%	90%
Immunization for Pneumonia	55	100%	90%	92%
Stroke Care				
Anticoagulation Therapy for Atrial Fibrillation[5]	-	-	95%	95%
Antithrombotic Therapy Timing[5]	-	-	98%	98%
Assessed for Rehabilitation[5]	-	-	97%	97%
Discharged on Antithrombotic Therapy[5]	-	-	99%	99%
Discharged on Statin Medication[5]	-	-	94%	94%
Thrombolytic Therapy Timing[5]	-	-	72%	66%
Venous Thromboembolism Prophylaxis[5]	-	-	94%	94%
Written Stroke Educational Materials Given[5]	-	-	87%	88%
Surgical Care Improvement Project				
Appropriate Beta Blocker Usage[5]	-	-	97%	98%
Appropriate VTP Within 24 Hours[5]	-	-	98%	98%
Controlled Postoperative Blood Glucose[5]	-	-	96%	97%
Perioperative Temperature Management[5]	-	-	100%	100%
Prophylactic Antibiotic Selection[5]	-	-	99%	99%
Prophylactic Antibiotic Selection (Outpatient)[5]	-	-	97%	98%
Prophylactic Antibiotic Stopped[5]	-	-	98%	98%
Prophylactic Antibiotic Timing[5]	-	-	99%	99%
Prophylactic Antibiotic Timing (Outpatient)[5]	-	-	97%	98%
Urinary Catheter Removal[5]	-	-	97%	97%
Survey of Patients' Hospital Experiences				
Area Around Room 'Always' Quiet at Night[1]	-	-	51%	61%
Doctors 'Always' Communicated Well[1]	-	-	78%	82%
Home Recovery Information Given[1]	-	-	83%	85%
Hospital Given 9 or 10 on 10 Point Scale[1]	-	-	68%	71%
Meds 'Always' Explained Before Given[1]	-	-	61%	64%
Nurses 'Always' Communicated Well[1]	-	-	74%	79%
Pain 'Always' Well Controlled[1]	-	-	68%	71%
Room and Bathroom 'Always' Clean[1]	-	-	70%	73%
Timely Help 'Always' Received[1]	-	-	62%	68%
Would Definitely Recommend Hospital[1]	-	-	70%	71%
Use of Medical Imaging				
Cardiac Imaging Stress Test before Surgery[7]	-	-	5.2%	5.3%
Combination Abdominal CT Scan[1]	-	-	13.4%	10.5%
Combination Brain/Sinus CT Scan[7]	-	-	2.2%	2.7%
Combination Chest CT Scan[7]	-	-	2.3%	2.7%
Follow-up Mammogram/Ultrasound[7]	-	-	8.2%	8.8%
Lumbar Spine MRI for Low Back Pain[7]	-	-	34.2%	37.2%

Scripps Memorial Hospital - Encinitas

354 Santa Fe Drive Phone: 760-753-6501
Encinitas, CA 92024 Fax: 760-633-7356
URL: www.scripps.org
Type: Acute Care Hospitals Emergency Services: Yes
Ownership: Voluntary non-profit - Private Beds: 140
Key Personnel:
CEO/President............... Chris Van Gorder
Cardiology.................. James Heywood, MD
Quality Assurance .... Ana Jackson
Chief of Medical Staff.......... James LaBelle, MD
Operating Room.............. Dio Sumagaysay
Radiology.................. Paul Sylvan, MD
Emergency Room .... Jan Zachary

Measure	Cases	This Hosp.	State Avg.	U.S. Avg.
Blood Clot Prevention and Treatment				
Anticoagulation Overlap Therapy[2]	89	99%	92%	93%
ICU Venous Thromboembolism Prophylaxis[2]	60	100%	92%	92%
Incidence of Potentially Preventable VTE[1,2]	-	-	11%	10%
UFH with Dosages/Platelet Monitoring[2]	30	100%	96%	97%
Venous Thromboembolism Prophylaxis[2]	332	94%	83%	85%
Warfarin Therapy Discharge Instructions[2]	35	100%	75%	75%
Chest Pain/Possible Heart Attack Care				
Aspirin Given Within 24 Hours of Arrival	67	99%	97%	96%
Fibrinolytic Meds Within 30 Min. of Arrival[3,7]	-	-	62%	58%
Average Time to ECG (minutes)	72	14	9	7
Average Time to Transfer (minutes)[3,7]	-	-	62	60
Children's Asthma Care				
Received Home Management Plan of Care	-	-	88%	88%
Received Reliever Medication	-	-	100%	100%
Received Systemic Corticosteroids	-	-	100%	100%
Emergency Department				
Admittance Decision Time (minutes)[2]	481	92	125	98
Head CT Results Within 45 Min. of Arrival[1]	-	-	55%	57%
Patients Who Left ER Before Being Seen	42,460	1%	3%	2%
Time from ER Arrival to Admit. (minutes)[2]	485	299	323	274
Time from ER Arrival to Discharge (minutes)	374	168	168	134
Time in ER Before Being Evaluated (minutes)	404	22	29	26
Time to Pain Meds for Fractures (minutes)	199	46	62	57
Heart Attack Care				
Aspirin Given at Discharge	155	100%	99%	99%
Fibrinolytic Meds Within 30 Min. of Arrival[7]	-	-	73%	54%
PCI Within 90 Minutes of Arrival	29	93%	95%	96%
Statin Prescribed at Discharge	139	100%	98%	98%
Heart Failure Care				
ACE Inhibitor or ARB for LVSD	58	100%	97%	97%
Discharge Instructions Given	199	99%	94%	94%
Evaluation of LVS Function	248	100%	99%	99%
Medicare Spending				
Medicare Spending per Patient (ratio)	-	1.02	0.98	0.98
Pneumonia Care				
Appropriate Initial Antibiotic Given[2]	85	100%	97%	95%
Blood Culture Timing[2]	171	99%	98%	98%
Pregnancy and Delivery Care				
Newborn Deliveries Scheduled Early[2]	35	0%	5%	6%
Preventive Care				
Immunization for Influenza[2]	507	94%	89%	90%
Immunization for Pneumonia[2]	522	98%	90%	92%
Stroke Care				
Anticoagulation Therapy for Atrial Fibrillation	23	100%	95%	95%
Antithrombotic Therapy Timing	88	99%	98%	98%
Assessed for Rehabilitation	131	100%	97%	97%
Discharged on Antithrombotic Therapy	110	100%	99%	99%
Discharged on Statin Medication	76	100%	94%	94%
Thrombolytic Therapy Timing	14	100%	72%	66%
Venous Thromboembolism Prophylaxis	130	98%	94%	94%
Written Stroke Educational Materials Given	71	100%	87%	88%
Surgical Care Improvement Project				
Appropriate Beta Blocker Usage[2]	90	100%	97%	98%
Appropriate VTP Within 24 Hours[2]	404	99%	98%	98%
Controlled Postoperative Blood Glucose[2,7]	-	-	96%	97%

NOTE: Hospital profiles are in alphabetical order by state, then city, then hospital within the city; Rankings exclude hospitals with less than 25 cases except for patient surveys which excludes hospitals with less than 100 cases; (a) 100-299 cases; (1) The number of cases/patients is too few to report; (2) Data submitted were based on a sample of cases/patients; (3) Results are based on a shorter time period than required; (4) Data suppressed by CMS for one or more quarters; (5) Results are not available for this reporting period; (6) Fewer than 100 patients completed the HCAHPS survey; (7) No cases met the criteria for this measure; (8) The lower limit of the confidence interval cannot be calculated if the number of observed infections equals zero; (9) No data are available from the state/territory for this reporting period; (10) The scores shown reflect fewer than 50 completed surveys; (11) There were discrepancies in the data collection process; (12) This measure does not apply to this hospital for this reporting period; (13) Results cannot be calculated for this reporting period; (14) The results for this state are combined with nearby states to protect confidentiality; Please refer to the User's Guide for a full explanation of data.

Perioperative Temperature Management[2]	488	100%	100%	100%
Prophylactic Antibiotic Selection[2]	319	100%	99%	99%
Prophylactic Antibiotic Selection (Outpatient)	264	99%	97%	98%
Prophylactic Antibiotic Stopped[2]	301	100%	98%	98%
Prophylactic Antibiotic Timing[2]	319	100%	99%	99%
Prophylactic Antibiotic Timing (Outpatient)	264	100%	97%	98%
Urinary Catheter Removal[2]	303	100%	97%	97%
Survey of Patients' Hospital Experiences				
Area Around Room 'Always' Quiet at Night	300+	49%	51%	61%
Doctors 'Always' Communicated Well	300+	79%	78%	82%
Home Recovery Information Given	300+	84%	83%	85%
Hospital Given 9 or 10 on 10 Point Scale	300+	71%	68%	71%
Meds 'Always' Explained Before Given	300+	62%	61%	64%
Nurses 'Always' Communicated Well	300+	78%	74%	79%
Pain 'Always' Well Controlled	300+	71%	68%	71%
Room and Bathroom 'Always' Clean	300+	72%	70%	73%
Timely Help 'Always' Received	300+	63%	62%	68%
Would Definitely Recommend Hospital	300+	77%	70%	71%
Use of Medical Imaging				
Cardiac Imaging Stress Test before Surgery	150	9.3%	5.2%	5.3%
Combination Abdominal CT Scan	815	3.2%	13.4%	10.5%
Combination Brain/Sinus CT Scan	971	2.8%	2.2%	2.7%
Combination Chest CT Scan	350	0.6%	2.3%	2.7%
Follow-up Mammogram/Ultrasound	581	11.4%	8.2%	8.8%
Lumbar Spine MRI for Low Back Pain	119	31.9%	34.2%	37.2%

Encino Hospital Medical Center

16237 Ventura Blvd — Phone: 818-995-5000
Encino, CA 91436 — Fax: 818-907-8630
E-mail: etrmcpublicrelations@tenethealth.com
URL: www.encino-tarzana.com
Type: Acute Care Hospitals — Emergency Services: Yes
Ownership: Proprietary — Beds: 151

Key Personnel:
Operating Room. . . . . Monica Angelbello
Chair/CEO . . . . Sandeep Bhatia, MD
Patient Relations . . . . Barbara Gardener
Quality Assurance . . . . Sharon Gross
Infection Control. . . . . Hala Mashed
CEO/President. . . . . Dr. Prem Reddy
Chief of Medical Staff . . . . J. Nathan Rubin, MD
Intensive Care Unit. . . . . Brenda Scott Manzur

Measure	Cases	This Hosp.	State Avg.	U.S. Avg.
Blood Clot Prevention and Treatment				
Anticoagulation Overlap Therapy[1,2]	-	-	92%	93%
ICU Venous Thromboembolism Prophylaxis[2]	18	94%	92%	92%
Incidence of Potentially Preventable VTE[1,2]	-	-	11%	10%
UFH with Dosages/Platelet Monitoring[1,2]	-	-	96%	97%
Venous Thromboembolism Prophylaxis[2]	171	70%	83%	85%
Warfarin Therapy Discharge Instructions[1,2]	-	-	75%	75%
Chest Pain/Possible Heart Attack Care				
Aspirin Given Within 24 Hours of Arrival[1]	-	-	97%	96%
Fibrinolytic Meds Within 30 Min. of Arrival[5]	-	-	62%	58%
Average Time to ECG (minutes)[1]	-	-	9	7
Average Time to Transfer (minutes)[5]	-	-	62	60
Children's Asthma Care				
Received Home Management Plan of Care	-	-	88%	88%
Received Reliever Medication	-	-	100%	100%
Received Systemic Corticosteroids	-	-	100%	100%
Emergency Department				
Admittance Decision Time (minutes)[2]	541	50	125	98
Head CT Results Within 45 Min. of Arrival[3,7]	-	-	55%	57%
Patients Who Left ER Before Being Seen	9,443	0%	3%	2%
Time from ER Arrival to Admit. (minutes)[2]	550	179	323	274
Time from ER Arrival to Discharge (minutes)	495	88	168	134
Time in ER Before Being Evaluated (minutes)	494	16	29	26
Time to Pain Meds for Fractures (minutes)	41	30	62	57
Heart Attack Care				
Aspirin Given at Discharge	23	100%	99%	99%
Fibrinolytic Meds Within 30 Min. of Arrival[7]	-	-	73%	54%
PCI Within 90 Minutes of Arrival[7]	-	-	95%	96%
Statin Prescribed at Discharge	19	100%	98%	98%
Heart Failure Care				
ACE Inhibitor or ARB for LVSD	16	100%	97%	97%
Discharge Instructions Given	46	100%	94%	94%
Evaluation of LVS Function	77	100%	99%	99%
Medicare Spending				
Medicare Spending per Patient (ratio)	-	1.05	0.98	0.98
Pneumonia Care				
Appropriate Initial Antibiotic Given	25	100%	97%	95%
Blood Culture Timing	63	100%	98%	98%
Pregnancy and Delivery Care				
Newborn Deliveries Scheduled Early[7]	-	-	5%	6%
Preventive Care				
Immunization for Influenza[2]	290	100%	89%	90%
Immunization for Pneumonia[2]	455	100%	90%	92%
Stroke Care				
Anticoagulation Therapy for Atrial Fibrillation[1]	-	-	95%	95%
Antithrombotic Therapy Timing[1]	-	-	98%	98%
Assessed for Rehabilitation	12	92%	97%	97%
Discharged on Antithrombotic Therapy	11	100%	99%	99%
Discharged on Statin Medication[1]	-	-	94%	94%
Thrombolytic Therapy Timing[7]	-	-	72%	66%
Venous Thromboembolism Prophylaxis[1]	-	-	94%	94%
Written Stroke Educational Materials Given[1]	-	-	87%	88%
Surgical Care Improvement Project				
Appropriate Beta Blocker Usage[1]	-	-	97%	98%
Appropriate VTP Within 24 Hours	12	100%	98%	98%
Controlled Postoperative Blood Glucose[7]	-	-	96%	97%
Perioperative Temperature Management	14	100%	100%	100%
Prophylactic Antibiotic Selection[1]	-	-	99%	99%
Prophylactic Antibiotic Selection (Outpatient)[1,3]	-	-	97%	98%
Prophylactic Antibiotic Stopped[1]	-	-	98%	98%
Prophylactic Antibiotic Timing[1]	-	-	99%	99%
Prophylactic Antibiotic Timing (Outpatient)[1,3]	-	-	97%	98%
Urinary Catheter Removal[1]	-	-	97%	97%
Survey of Patients' Hospital Experiences				
Area Around Room 'Always' Quiet at Night[6,11]	<100	48%	51%	61%
Doctors 'Always' Communicated Well[6,11]	<100	75%	78%	82%
Home Recovery Information Given[6,11]	<100	79%	83%	85%
Hospital Given 9 or 10 on 10 Point Scale[6,11]	<100	58%	68%	71%
Meds 'Always' Explained Before Given[6,11]	<100	43%	61%	64%
Nurses 'Always' Communicated Well[6,11]	<100	60%	74%	79%
Pain 'Always' Well Controlled[6,11]	<100	53%	68%	71%
Room and Bathroom 'Always' Clean[6,11]	<100	62%	70%	73%
Timely Help 'Always' Received[6,11]	<100	58%	62%	68%
Would Definitely Recommend Hospital[6,11]	<100	61%	70%	71%
Use of Medical Imaging				
Cardiac Imaging Stress Test before Surgery[1]	-	-	5.2%	5.3%
Combination Abdominal CT Scan	75	1.3%	13.4%	10.5%
Combination Brain/Sinus CT Scan[1]	-	-	2.2%	2.7%
Combination Chest CT Scan[1]	-	-	2.3%	2.7%
Follow-up Mammogram/Ultrasound[7]	-	-	8.2%	8.8%
Lumbar Spine MRI for Low Back Pain[7]	-	-	34.2%	37.2%

Palomar Health Downtown Campus

555 E Valley Parkway — Phone: 760-739-3000
Escondido, CA 92025 — Fax: 760-739-3108
E-mail: tlc@pph.org
URL: www.pph.org
Type: Acute Care Hospitals — Emergency Services: Yes
Ownership: Govt - Hospital Dist/Auth — Beds: 332

Key Personnel:
Quality Assurance . . . . Janie Frincke
CEO/President. . . . . Robert A. Hemker
Pediatric Ambulatory Care . . . . . . Marshall Littman, MD
Pediatric In-Patient Care . . . . Marshall Littman, MD
Infection Control. . . . . Lina Mendenhall
Coronary Care . . . . Lorrie Shoemaker, RN
Radiology. . . . . Earl Shultz, MD
Chief of Medical Staff . . . . Charles Smith, MD

Measure	Cases	This Hosp.	State Avg.	U.S. Avg.
Blood Clot Prevention and Treatment				
Anticoagulation Overlap Therapy[2]	145	100%	92%	93%
ICU Venous Thromboembolism Prophylaxis[2]	38	97%	92%	92%
Incidence of Potentially Preventable VTE[2]	31	3%	11%	10%
UFH with Dosages/Platelet Monitoring[2]	80	100%	96%	97%
Venous Thromboembolism Prophylaxis[2]	329	85%	83%	85%
Warfarin Therapy Discharge Instructions[2]	119	97%	75%	75%
Chest Pain/Possible Heart Attack Care				
Aspirin Given Within 24 Hours of Arrival[5]	-	-	97%	96%
Fibrinolytic Meds Within 30 Min. of Arrival[5]	-	-	62%	58%
Average Time to ECG (minutes)[5]	-	-	9	7
Average Time to Transfer (minutes)[5]	-	-	62	60
Children's Asthma Care				
Received Home Management Plan of Care	-	-	88%	88%
Received Reliever Medication	-	-	100%	100%
Received Systemic Corticosteroids	-	-	100%	100%
Emergency Department				
Admittance Decision Time (minutes)[2]	519	143	125	98
Head CT Results Within 45 Min. of Arrival[1]	-	-	55%	57%
Patients Who Left ER Before Being Seen	80,208	1%	3%	2%
Time from ER Arrival to Admit. (minutes)[2]	522	330	323	274
Time from ER Arrival to Discharge (minutes)	361	186	168	134
Time in ER Before Being Evaluated (minutes)	393	21	29	26
Time to Pain Meds for Fractures (minutes)	383	62	62	57
Heart Attack Care				
Aspirin Given at Discharge	398	100%	99%	99%
Fibrinolytic Meds Within 30 Min. of Arrival[1]	-	-	73%	54%
PCI Within 90 Minutes of Arrival	94	95%	95%	96%
Statin Prescribed at Discharge	378	100%	98%	98%
Heart Failure Care				
ACE Inhibitor or ARB for LVSD	127	98%	97%	97%
Discharge Instructions Given	436	100%	94%	94%
Evaluation of LVS Function	547	99%	99%	99%
Medicare Spending				
Medicare Spending per Patient (ratio)	-	1.02	0.98	0.98
Pneumonia Care				
Appropriate Initial Antibiotic Given	303	100%	97%	95%
Blood Culture Timing	358	99%	98%	98%
Pregnancy and Delivery Care				
Newborn Deliveries Scheduled Early[2]	64	12%	5%	6%
Preventive Care				
Immunization for Influenza[2]	504	63%	89%	90%
Immunization for Pneumonia[2]	542	78%	90%	92%
Stroke Care				
Anticoagulation Therapy for Atrial Fibrillation[2]	19	100%	95%	95%
Antithrombotic Therapy Timing[2]	70	99%	98%	98%
Assessed for Rehabilitation[2]	98	99%	97%	97%
Discharged on Antithrombotic Therapy[2]	86	99%	99%	99%
Discharged on Statin Medication[2]	69	99%	94%	94%
Thrombolytic Therapy Timing[2]	20	50%	72%	66%
Venous Thromboembolism Prophylaxis[2]	99	93%	94%	94%
Written Stroke Educational Materials Given[2]	56	100%	87%	88%
Surgical Care Improvement Project				
Appropriate Beta Blocker Usage[2]	83	96%	97%	98%
Appropriate VTP Within 24 Hours[2]	335	99%	98%	98%
Controlled Postoperative Blood Glucose[2]	59	86%	96%	97%
Perioperative Temperature Management[2]	418	100%	100%	100%
Prophylactic Antibiotic Selection[2]	320	99%	99%	99%
Prophylactic Antibiotic Selection (Outpatient)	252	92%	97%	98%
Prophylactic Antibiotic Stopped[2]	314	99%	98%	98%
Prophylactic Antibiotic Timing[2]	321	98%	99%	99%
Prophylactic Antibiotic Timing (Outpatient)	258	88%	97%	98%
Urinary Catheter Removal[2]	253	95%	97%	97%
Survey of Patients' Hospital Experiences				
Area Around Room 'Always' Quiet at Night	300+	56%	51%	61%
Doctors 'Always' Communicated Well	300+	78%	78%	82%
Home Recovery Information Given	300+	81%	83%	85%
Hospital Given 9 or 10 on 10 Point Scale	300+	76%	68%	71%
Meds 'Always' Explained Before Given	300+	62%	61%	64%
Nurses 'Always' Communicated Well	300+	75%	74%	79%
Pain 'Always' Well Controlled	300+	68%	68%	71%
Room and Bathroom 'Always' Clean	300+	76%	70%	73%
Timely Help 'Always' Received	300+	63%	62%	68%
Would Definitely Recommend Hospital	300+	79%	70%	71%
Use of Medical Imaging				
Cardiac Imaging Stress Test before Surgery	240	4.6%	5.2%	5.3%
Combination Abdominal CT Scan	717	1.1%	13.4%	10.5%
Combination Brain/Sinus CT Scan	1,109	3.7%	2.2%	2.7%

NOTE: Hospital profiles are in alphabetical order by state, then city, then hospital within the city; Rankings exclude hospitals with less than 25 cases except for patient surveys which excludes hospitals with less than 100 cases; (a) 100-299 cases; (1) The number of cases/patients is too few to report; (2) Data submitted were based on a sample of cases/patients; (3) Results are based on a shorter time period than required; (4) Data suppressed by CMS for one or more quarters; (5) Results are not available for this reporting period; (6) Fewer than 100 patients completed the HCAHPS survey; (7) No cases met the criteria for this measure; (8) The lower limit of the confidence interval cannot be calculated if the number of observed infections equals zero; (9) No data are available from the state/territory for this reporting period; (10) The scores shown reflect fewer than 50 completed surveys; (11) There were discrepancies in the data collection process; (12) This measure does not apply to this hospital for this reporting period; (13) Results cannot be calculated for this reporting period; (14) The results for this state are combined with nearby states to protect confidentiality; Please refer to the User's Guide for a full explanation of data.

Combination Chest CT Scan	150	0.0%	2.3%	2.7%
Follow-up Mammogram/Ultrasound[7]	-	-	8.2%	8.8%
Lumbar Spine MRI for Low Back Pain[1]	-	-	34.2%	37.2%

Saint Joseph Hospital

2700 Dolbeer St — Phone: 707-445-8121
Eureka, CA 95501 — Fax: 707-269-3897
URL: www.stjosepheureka.org
Type: Acute Care Hospitals — Emergency Services: Yes
Ownership: Voluntary non-profit - Private — Beds: 189

Measure	Cases	This Hosp.	State Avg.	U.S. Avg.
Blood Clot Prevention and Treatment				
Anticoagulation Overlap Therapy[2]	40	98%	92%	93%
ICU Venous Thromboembolism Prophylaxis[2]	41	93%	92%	92%
Incidence of Potentially Preventable VTE[1,2]	-	-	11%	10%
UFH with Dosages/Platelet Monitoring[2]	18	100%	96%	97%
Venous Thromboembolism Prophylaxis[2]	343	91%	83%	85%
Warfarin Therapy Discharge Instructions[2]	28	93%	75%	75%
Chest Pain/Possible Heart Attack Care				
Aspirin Given Within 24 Hours of Arrival[5]	-	-	97%	96%
Fibrinolytic Meds Within 30 Min. of Arrival[5]	-	-	62%	58%
Average Time to ECG (minutes)[5]	-	-	9	7
Average Time to Transfer (minutes)[5]	-	-	62	60
Children's Asthma Care				
Received Home Management Plan of Care	-	-	88%	88%
Received Reliever Medication	-	-	100%	100%
Received Systemic Corticosteroids	-	-	100%	100%
Emergency Department				
Admittance Decision Time (minutes)[2]	294	200	125	98
Head CT Results Within 45 Min. of Arrival[1]	-	-	55%	57%
Patients Who Left ER Before Being Seen	25,913	3%	3%	2%
Time from ER Arrival to Admit. (minutes)[2]	298	334	323	274
Time from ER Arrival to Discharge (minutes)	359	127	168	134
Time in ER Before Being Evaluated (minutes)	393	18	29	26
Time to Pain Meds for Fractures (minutes)	118	68	62	57
Heart Attack Care				
Aspirin Given at Discharge	168	99%	99%	99%
Fibrinolytic Meds Within 30 Min. of Arrival[7]	-	-	73%	54%
PCI Within 90 Minutes of Arrival	22	86%	95%	96%
Statin Prescribed at Discharge	164	98%	98%	98%
Heart Failure Care				
ACE Inhibitor or ARB for LVSD	51	96%	97%	97%
Discharge Instructions Given	135	98%	94%	94%
Evaluation of LVS Function	158	100%	99%	99%
Medicare Spending				
Medicare Spending per Patient (ratio)	-	0.93	0.98	0.98
Pneumonia Care				
Appropriate Initial Antibiotic Given	85	99%	97%	95%
Blood Culture Timing	114	98%	98%	98%
Pregnancy and Delivery Care				
Newborn Deliveries Scheduled Early	42	7%	5%	6%
Preventive Care				
Immunization for Influenza[2]	533	84%	89%	90%
Immunization for Pneumonia[2]	686	87%	90%	92%
Stroke Care				
Anticoagulation Therapy for Atrial Fibrillation[1]	-	-	95%	95%
Antithrombotic Therapy Timing	55	100%	98%	98%
Assessed for Rehabilitation	69	96%	97%	97%
Discharged on Antithrombotic Therapy	63	100%	99%	99%
Discharged on Statin Medication	52	83%	94%	94%
Thrombolytic Therapy Timing[1]	-	-	72%	66%
Venous Thromboembolism Prophylaxis	61	93%	94%	94%
Written Stroke Educational Materials Given	46	72%	87%	88%
Surgical Care Improvement Project				
Appropriate Beta Blocker Usage[2]	97	88%	97%	98%
Appropriate VTP Within 24 Hours[2]	272	94%	98%	98%
Controlled Postoperative Blood Glucose[2]	40	95%	96%	97%
Perioperative Temperature Management[2]	443	100%	100%	100%
Prophylactic Antibiotic Selection[2]	341	98%	99%	99%
Prophylactic Antibiotic Selection (Outpatient)	241	99%	97%	98%
Prophylactic Antibiotic Stopped[2]	332	98%	98%	98%
Prophylactic Antibiotic Timing[2]	344	99%	99%	99%
Prophylactic Antibiotic Timing (Outpatient)	248	97%	97%	98%
Urinary Catheter Removal[2]	211	87%	97%	97%
Survey of Patients' Hospital Experiences				
Area Around Room 'Always' Quiet at Night	300+	45%	51%	61%
Doctors 'Always' Communicated Well	300+	71%	78%	82%
Home Recovery Information Given	300+	83%	83%	85%
Hospital Given 9 or 10 on 10 Point Scale	300+	57%	68%	71%
Meds 'Always' Explained Before Given	300+	56%	61%	64%
Nurses 'Always' Communicated Well	300+	66%	74%	79%
Pain 'Always' Well Controlled	300+	65%	68%	71%
Room and Bathroom 'Always' Clean	300+	66%	70%	73%
Timely Help 'Always' Received	300+	49%	62%	68%
Would Definitely Recommend Hospital	300+	62%	70%	71%
Use of Medical Imaging				
Cardiac Imaging Stress Test before Surgery	229	3.1%	5.2%	5.3%
Combination Abdominal CT Scan	802	15.6%	13.4%	10.5%
Combination Brain/Sinus CT Scan	497	1.2%	2.2%	2.7%
Combination Chest CT Scan	516	2.9%	2.3%	2.7%
Follow-up Mammogram/Ultrasound	1,735	7.3%	8.2%	8.8%
Lumbar Spine MRI for Low Back Pain	272	35.3%	34.2%	37.2%

Northbay Medical Center

1200 B Gale Wilson Blvd — Phone: 707-646-5000
Fairfield, CA 94533 — Fax: 707-426-5287
URL: www.northbay.org
Type: Acute Care Hospitals — Emergency Services: Yes
Ownership: Voluntary non-profit - Other — Beds: 132

Key Personnel:
Chief of Medical Staff.......... Teresa Auyeung
Emergency Room .... Ed Ballerine
Operating Room............. Coletta Ciccarelli
CEO/President.............. Gary Passama
Quality Assurance .... Linda Pryor

Measure	Cases	This Hosp.	State Avg.	U.S. Avg.
Blood Clot Prevention and Treatment				
Anticoagulation Overlap Therapy[2]	61	85%	92%	93%
ICU Venous Thromboembolism Prophylaxis[2]	133	92%	92%	92%
Incidence of Potentially Preventable VTE[1,2]	-	-	11%	10%
UFH with Dosages/Platelet Monitoring[2]	13	100%	96%	97%
Venous Thromboembolism Prophylaxis[2]	292	87%	83%	85%
Warfarin Therapy Discharge Instructions[2]	42	90%	75%	75%
Chest Pain/Possible Heart Attack Care				
Aspirin Given Within 24 Hours of Arrival	12	100%	97%	96%
Fibrinolytic Meds Within 30 Min. of Arrival[3,7]	-	-	62%	58%
Average Time to ECG (minutes)	12	2	9	7
Average Time to Transfer (minutes)[1,3]	-	-	62	60
Children's Asthma Care				
Received Home Management Plan of Care	-	-	88%	88%
Received Reliever Medication	-	-	100%	100%
Received Systemic Corticosteroids	-	-	100%	100%
Emergency Department				
Admittance Decision Time (minutes)[2]	722	167	125	98
Head CT Results Within 45 Min. of Arrival	50	62%	55%	57%
Patients Who Left ER Before Being Seen	70,630	2%	3%	2%
Time from ER Arrival to Admit. (minutes)[2]	722	364	323	274
Time from ER Arrival to Discharge (minutes)	396	159	168	134
Time in ER Before Being Evaluated (minutes)	417	31	29	26
Time to Pain Meds for Fractures (minutes)	179	59	62	57
Heart Attack Care				
Aspirin Given at Discharge	202	100%	99%	99%
Fibrinolytic Meds Within 30 Min. of Arrival[7]	-	-	73%	54%
PCI Within 90 Minutes of Arrival	41	98%	95%	96%
Statin Prescribed at Discharge	199	99%	98%	98%
Heart Failure Care				
ACE Inhibitor or ARB for LVSD	117	97%	97%	97%
Discharge Instructions Given	245	94%	94%	94%
Evaluation of LVS Function	279	100%	99%	99%
Medicare Spending				
Medicare Spending per Patient (ratio)	-	0.98	0.98	0.98
Pneumonia Care				
Appropriate Initial Antibiotic Given	129	95%	97%	95%
Blood Culture Timing	229	96%	98%	98%
Pregnancy and Delivery Care				
Newborn Deliveries Scheduled Early	107	1%	5%	6%
Preventive Care				
Immunization for Influenza[2]	542	90%	89%	90%
Immunization for Pneumonia[2]	641	95%	90%	92%
Stroke Care				
Anticoagulation Therapy for Atrial Fibrillation	18	94%	95%	95%
Antithrombotic Therapy Timing	90	99%	98%	98%
Assessed for Rehabilitation	97	98%	97%	97%
Discharged on Antithrombotic Therapy	93	100%	99%	99%
Discharged on Statin Medication	77	96%	94%	94%
Thrombolytic Therapy Timing	12	58%	72%	66%
Venous Thromboembolism Prophylaxis	104	96%	94%	94%
Written Stroke Educational Materials Given	69	84%	87%	88%
Surgical Care Improvement Project				
Appropriate Beta Blocker Usage	119	98%	97%	98%
Appropriate VTP Within 24 Hours	308	96%	98%	98%
Controlled Postoperative Blood Glucose	46	93%	96%	97%
Perioperative Temperature Management	394	100%	100%	100%
Prophylactic Antibiotic Selection	224	98%	99%	99%
Prophylactic Antibiotic Selection (Outpatient)	170	100%	97%	98%
Prophylactic Antibiotic Stopped	212	99%	98%	98%
Prophylactic Antibiotic Timing	224	99%	99%	99%
Prophylactic Antibiotic Timing (Outpatient)	170	96%	97%	98%
Urinary Catheter Removal	298	99%	97%	97%
Survey of Patients' Hospital Experiences				
Area Around Room 'Always' Quiet at Night	300+	47%	51%	61%
Doctors 'Always' Communicated Well	300+	79%	78%	82%
Home Recovery Information Given	300+	86%	83%	85%
Hospital Given 9 or 10 on 10 Point Scale	300+	67%	68%	71%
Meds 'Always' Explained Before Given	300+	64%	61%	64%
Nurses 'Always' Communicated Well	300+	78%	74%	79%
Pain 'Always' Well Controlled	300+	71%	68%	71%
Room and Bathroom 'Always' Clean	300+	71%	70%	73%
Timely Help 'Always' Received	300+	65%	62%	68%
Would Definitely Recommend Hospital	300+	67%	70%	71%
Use of Medical Imaging				
Cardiac Imaging Stress Test before Surgery	344	4.1%	5.2%	5.3%
Combination Abdominal CT Scan	580	0.5%	13.4%	10.5%
Combination Brain/Sinus CT Scan	1,023	2.5%	2.2%	2.7%
Combination Chest CT Scan	144	0.0%	2.3%	2.7%
Follow-up Mammogram/Ultrasound[7]	-	-	8.2%	8.8%
Lumbar Spine MRI for Low Back Pain[1]	-	-	34.2%	37.2%

Mayers Memorial Hospital

43563 Hwy 299 East — Phone: 530-336-5511
Fall River Mills, CA 96028 — Fax: 530-336-5755
E-mail: mmhl@shasta.com
URL: www.mayersmemorial.com
Type: Critical Access Hospitals — Emergency Services: Yes
Ownership: Govt - Hospital Dist/Auth — Beds: 121

Key Personnel:
President.................. Allen Albaugh
CEO/President.............. Katharine Ann Campbell
Operating Room............. Brenda Dahle
Quality Assurance .... Carolyn Lease, RN
Administrator .... Matt Rees
Infection Control.............. Terry Sampson
Chief of Medical Staff.......... Steven Scharps, MD

Measure	Cases	This Hosp.	State Avg.	U.S. Avg.
Blood Clot Prevention and Treatment				
Anticoagulation Overlap Therapy[5]	-	-	92%	93%
ICU Venous Thromboembolism Prophylaxis[5]	-	-	92%	92%
Incidence of Potentially Preventable VTE[5]	-	-	11%	10%
UFH with Dosages/Platelet Monitoring[5]	-	-	96%	97%
Venous Thromboembolism Prophylaxis[5]	-	-	83%	85%
Warfarin Therapy Discharge Instructions[5]	-	-	75%	75%
Chest Pain/Possible Heart Attack Care				
Aspirin Given Within 24 Hours of Arrival	-	-	97%	96%
Fibrinolytic Meds Within 30 Min. of Arrival	-	-	62%	58%
Average Time to ECG (minutes)	-	-	9	7
Average Time to Transfer (minutes)	-	-	62	60
Children's Asthma Care				
Received Home Management Plan of Care	-	-	88%	88%
Received Reliever Medication	-	-	100%	100%
Received Systemic Corticosteroids	-	-	100%	100%

NOTE: Hospital profiles are in alphabetical order by state, then city, then hospital within the city; Rankings exclude hospitals with less than 25 cases except for patient surveys which excludes hospitals with less than 100 cases; (a) 100-299 cases; (1) The number of cases/patients is too few to report; (2) Data submitted were based on a sample of cases/patients; (3) Results are based on a shorter time period than required; (4) Data suppressed by CMS for one or more quarters; (5) Results are not available for this reporting period; (6) Fewer than 100 patients completed the HCAHPS survey; (7) No cases met the criteria for this measure; (8) The lower limit of the confidence interval cannot be calculated if the number of observed infections equals zero; (9) No data are available from the state/territory for this reporting period; (10) The scores shown reflect fewer than 50 completed surveys; (11) There were discrepancies in the data collection process; (12) This measure does not apply to this hospital for this reporting period; (13) Results cannot be calculated for this reporting period; (14) The results for this state are combined with nearby states to protect confidentiality; Please refer to the User's Guide for a full explanation of data.

Emergency Department				
Admittance Decision Time (minutes)[5]	-	-	125	98
Head CT Results Within 45 Min. of Arrival	-	-	55%	57%
Patients Who Left ER Before Being Seen	-	-	3%	2%
Time from ER Arrival to Admit. (minutes)[5]	-	-	323	274
Time from ER Arrival to Discharge (minutes)	-	-	168	134
Time in ER Before Being Evaluated (minutes)	-	-	29	26
Time to Pain Meds for Fractures (minutes)	-	-	62	57
Heart Attack Care				
Aspirin Given at Discharge[5]	-	-	99%	99%
Fibrinolytic Meds Within 30 Min. of Arrival[5]	-	-	73%	54%
PCI Within 90 Minutes of Arrival[5]	-	-	95%	96%
Statin Prescribed at Discharge[5]	-	-	98%	98%
Heart Failure Care				
ACE Inhibitor or ARB for LVSD[1,2]	-	-	97%	97%
Discharge Instructions Given[1,2]	-	-	94%	94%
Evaluation of LVS Function[1,2]	-	-	99%	99%
Medicare Spending				
Medicare Spending per Patient (ratio)	-	-	0.98	0.98
Pneumonia Care				
Appropriate Initial Antibiotic Given[1,2]	-	-	97%	95%
Blood Culture Timing[1,2]	-	-	98%	98%
Pregnancy and Delivery Care				
Newborn Deliveries Scheduled Early[5]	-	-	5%	6%
Preventive Care				
Immunization for Influenza[5]	-	-	89%	90%
Immunization for Pneumonia[5]	-	-	90%	92%
Stroke Care				
Anticoagulation Therapy for Atrial Fibrillation[5]	-	-	95%	95%
Antithrombotic Therapy Timing[5]	-	-	98%	98%
Assessed for Rehabilitation[5]	-	-	97%	97%
Discharged on Antithrombotic Therapy[5]	-	-	99%	99%
Discharged on Statin Medication[5]	-	-	94%	94%
Thrombolytic Therapy Timing[5]	-	-	72%	66%
Venous Thromboembolism Prophylaxis[5]	-	-	94%	94%
Written Stroke Educational Materials Given[5]	-	-	87%	88%
Surgical Care Improvement Project				
Appropriate Beta Blocker Usage[5]	-	-	97%	98%
Appropriate VTP Within 24 Hours[5]	-	-	98%	98%
Controlled Postoperative Blood Glucose[5]	-	-	96%	97%
Perioperative Temperature Management[5]	-	-	100%	100%
Prophylactic Antibiotic Selection[5]	-	-	99%	99%
Prophylactic Antibiotic Selection (Outpatient)	-	-	97%	98%
Prophylactic Antibiotic Stopped[5]	-	-	98%	98%
Prophylactic Antibiotic Timing[5]	-	-	99%	99%
Prophylactic Antibiotic Timing (Outpatient)	-	-	97%	98%
Urinary Catheter Removal[5]	-	-	97%	97%
Survey of Patients' Hospital Experiences				
Area Around Room 'Always' Quiet at Night[5]	-	-	51%	61%
Doctors 'Always' Communicated Well[5]	-	-	78%	82%
Home Recovery Information Given[5]	-	-	83%	85%
Hospital Given 9 or 10 on 10 Point Scale[5]	-	-	68%	71%
Meds 'Always' Explained Before Given[5]	-	-	61%	64%
Nurses 'Always' Communicated Well[5]	-	-	74%	79%
Pain 'Always' Well Controlled[5]	-	-	68%	71%
Room and Bathroom 'Always' Clean[5]	-	-	70%	73%
Timely Help 'Always' Received[5]	-	-	62%	68%
Would Definitely Recommend Hospital[5]	-	-	70%	71%
Use of Medical Imaging				
Cardiac Imaging Stress Test before Surgery	-	-	5.2%	5.3%
Combination Abdominal CT Scan	-	-	13.4%	10.5%
Combination Brain/Sinus CT Scan	-	-	2.2%	2.7%
Combination Chest CT Scan	-	-	2.3%	2.7%
Follow-up Mammogram/Ultrasound	-	-	8.2%	8.8%
Lumbar Spine MRI for Low Back Pain	-	-	34.2%	37.2%

Fallbrook Hospital

624 E Elder St — Phone: 760-728-1191
Fallbrook, CA 92028 — Fax: 760-723-6214
URL: www.fallbrook.com
Type: Acute Care Hospitals — Emergency Services: Yes
Ownership: Govt - Hospital Dist/Auth — Beds: 146
Key Personnel:
Chief of Medical Staff . . . . Anthony Bianchi
Quality Assurance . . . . Sharon Jensen
CEO/President. . . . . Larry W Payton
Operating Room. . . . . Betsy Rogers

Measure	Cases	This Hosp.	State Avg.	U.S. Avg.
Blood Clot Prevention and Treatment				
Anticoagulation Overlap Therapy[1,2]	-	-	92%	93%
ICU Venous Thromboembolism Prophylaxis[2]	34	100%	92%	92%
Incidence of Potentially Preventable VTE[2,7]	-	-	11%	10%
UFH with Dosages/Platelet Monitoring[1,2]	-	-	96%	97%
Venous Thromboembolism Prophylaxis[2]	152	97%	83%	85%
Warfarin Therapy Discharge Instructions[1,2]	-	-	75%	75%
Chest Pain/Possible Heart Attack Care				
Aspirin Given Within 24 Hours of Arrival[1]	-	-	97%	96%
Fibrinolytic Meds Within 30 Min. of Arrival[3,7]	-	-	62%	58%
Average Time to ECG (minutes)[1]	-	-	9	7
Average Time to Transfer (minutes)[1,3]	-	-	62	60
Children's Asthma Care				
Received Home Management Plan of Care	-	-	88%	88%
Received Reliever Medication	-	-	100%	100%
Received Systemic Corticosteroids	-	-	100%	100%
Emergency Department				
Admittance Decision Time (minutes)[2]	315	70	125	98
Head CT Results Within 45 Min. of Arrival[7]	-	-	55%	57%
Patients Who Left ER Before Being Seen	11,077	2%	3%	2%
Time from ER Arrival to Admit. (minutes)[2]	317	282	323	274
Time from ER Arrival to Discharge (minutes)	420	140	168	134
Time in ER Before Being Evaluated (minutes)	458	14	29	26
Time to Pain Meds for Fractures (minutes)	46	46	62	57
Heart Attack Care				
Aspirin Given at Discharge[1]	-	-	99%	99%
Fibrinolytic Meds Within 30 Min. of Arrival[7]	-	-	73%	54%
PCI Within 90 Minutes of Arrival[7]	-	-	95%	96%
Statin Prescribed at Discharge[1]	-	-	98%	98%
Heart Failure Care				
ACE Inhibitor or ARB for LVSD	18	100%	97%	97%
Discharge Instructions Given	55	95%	94%	94%
Evaluation of LVS Function	64	95%	99%	99%
Medicare Spending				
Medicare Spending per Patient (ratio)	-	0.92	0.98	0.98
Pneumonia Care				
Appropriate Initial Antibiotic Given	30	97%	97%	95%
Blood Culture Timing	46	93%	98%	98%
Pregnancy and Delivery Care				
Newborn Deliveries Scheduled Early[2]	42	2%	5%	6%
Preventive Care				
Immunization for Influenza[2]	279	94%	89%	90%
Immunization for Pneumonia[2]	317	99%	90%	92%
Stroke Care				
Anticoagulation Therapy for Atrial Fibrillation[1]	-	-	95%	95%
Antithrombotic Therapy Timing	11	100%	98%	98%
Assessed for Rehabilitation	14	100%	97%	97%
Discharged on Antithrombotic Therapy	14	100%	99%	99%
Discharged on Statin Medication[1]	-	-	94%	94%
Thrombolytic Therapy Timing[1]	-	-	72%	66%
Venous Thromboembolism Prophylaxis	12	92%	94%	94%
Written Stroke Educational Materials Given[1]	-	-	87%	88%
Surgical Care Improvement Project				
Appropriate Beta Blocker Usage	84	99%	97%	98%
Appropriate VTP Within 24 Hours	307	99%	98%	98%
Controlled Postoperative Blood Glucose[7]	-	-	96%	97%
Perioperative Temperature Management	335	99%	100%	100%
Prophylactic Antibiotic Selection	274	99%	99%	99%
Prophylactic Antibiotic Selection (Outpatient)	15	93%	97%	98%
Prophylactic Antibiotic Stopped	271	99%	98%	98%
Prophylactic Antibiotic Timing	274	98%	99%	99%
Prophylactic Antibiotic Timing (Outpatient)	15	100%	97%	98%
Urinary Catheter Removal	228	100%	97%	97%
Survey of Patients' Hospital Experiences				
Area Around Room 'Always' Quiet at Night	300+	50%	51%	61%
Doctors 'Always' Communicated Well	300+	79%	78%	82%
Home Recovery Information Given	300+	83%	83%	85%
Hospital Given 9 or 10 on 10 Point Scale	300+	65%	68%	71%
Meds 'Always' Explained Before Given	300+	63%	61%	64%
Nurses 'Always' Communicated Well	300+	74%	74%	79%
Pain 'Always' Well Controlled	300+	69%	68%	71%
Room and Bathroom 'Always' Clean	300+	63%	70%	73%
Timely Help 'Always' Received	300+	59%	62%	68%
Would Definitely Recommend Hospital	300+	63%	70%	71%
Use of Medical Imaging				
Cardiac Imaging Stress Test before Surgery[1]	-	-	5.2%	5.3%
Combination Abdominal CT Scan	153	20.3%	13.4%	10.5%
Combination Brain/Sinus CT Scan	188	7.4%	2.2%	2.7%
Combination Chest CT Scan	90	15.6%	2.3%	2.7%
Follow-up Mammogram/Ultrasound	245	6.1%	8.2%	8.8%
Lumbar Spine MRI for Low Back Pain[1]	-	-	34.2%	37.2%

Mercy Hospital of Folsom

1650 Creekside Drive — Phone: 916-983-7400
Folsom, CA 95630 — Fax: 916-983-7406
URL: www.mercyfolsom.org
Type: Acute Care Hospitals — Emergency Services: Yes
Ownership: Voluntary non-profit - Private — Beds: 85
Key Personnel:
Chief of Medical Staff . . . . Terence A Degan
Radiology. . . . . Brian D Fellmeth
CEO/President. . . . . Donald C Hudson
Operating Room. . . . . Craig Simmons

Measure	Cases	This Hosp.	State Avg.	U.S. Avg.
Blood Clot Prevention and Treatment				
Anticoagulation Overlap Therapy[2]	47	100%	92%	93%
ICU Venous Thromboembolism Prophylaxis[2]	74	100%	92%	92%
Incidence of Potentially Preventable VTE[1,2]	-	-	11%	10%
UFH with Dosages/Platelet Monitoring[2]	26	100%	96%	97%
Venous Thromboembolism Prophylaxis[2]	343	99%	83%	85%
Warfarin Therapy Discharge Instructions[2]	37	97%	75%	75%
Chest Pain/Possible Heart Attack Care				
Aspirin Given Within 24 Hours of Arrival	85	98%	97%	96%
Fibrinolytic Meds Within 30 Min. of Arrival[1]	-	-	62%	58%
Average Time to ECG (minutes)	85	5	9	7
Average Time to Transfer (minutes)[1]	-	-	62	60
Children's Asthma Care				
Received Home Management Plan of Care	-	-	88%	88%
Received Reliever Medication	-	-	100%	100%
Received Systemic Corticosteroids	-	-	100%	100%
Emergency Department				
Admittance Decision Time (minutes)[2]	695	80	125	98
Head CT Results Within 45 Min. of Arrival	28	82%	55%	57%
Patients Who Left ER Before Being Seen	33,626	0%	3%	2%
Time from ER Arrival to Admit. (minutes)[2]	697	307	323	274
Time from ER Arrival to Discharge (minutes)	376	152	168	134
Time in ER Before Being Evaluated (minutes)	380	8	29	26
Time to Pain Meds for Fractures (minutes)	170	54	62	57
Heart Attack Care				
Aspirin Given at Discharge[1]	-	-	99%	99%
Fibrinolytic Meds Within 30 Min. of Arrival[7]	-	-	73%	54%
PCI Within 90 Minutes of Arrival[7]	-	-	95%	96%
Statin Prescribed at Discharge[1]	-	-	98%	98%
Heart Failure Care				
ACE Inhibitor or ARB for LVSD	20	100%	97%	97%
Discharge Instructions Given	103	96%	94%	94%
Evaluation of LVS Function	122	100%	99%	99%
Medicare Spending				
Medicare Spending per Patient (ratio)	-	0.93	0.98	0.98
Pneumonia Care				
Appropriate Initial Antibiotic Given[2]	103	99%	97%	95%
Blood Culture Timing[2]	169	99%	98%	98%
Pregnancy and Delivery Care				
Newborn Deliveries Scheduled Early[2]	18	6%	5%	6%
Preventive Care				
Immunization for Influenza[2]	573	98%	89%	90%
Immunization for Pneumonia[2]	593	93%	90%	92%
Stroke Care				
Anticoagulation Therapy for Atrial Fibrillation[1]	-	-	95%	95%
Antithrombotic Therapy Timing	35	100%	98%	98%
Assessed for Rehabilitation	43	100%	97%	97%

NOTE: Hospital profiles are in alphabetical order by state, then city, then hospital within the city; Rankings exclude hospitals with less than 25 cases except for patient surveys which excludes hospitals with less than 100 cases; (a) 100-299 cases; (1) The number of cases/patients is too few to report; (2) Data submitted were based on a sample of cases/patients; (3) Results are based on a shorter time period than required; (4) Data suppressed by CMS for one or more quarters; (5) Results are not available for this reporting period; (6) Fewer than 100 patients completed the HCAHPS survey; (7) No cases met the criteria for this measure; (8) The lower limit of the confidence interval cannot be calculated if the number of observed infections equals zero; (9) No data are available from the state/territory for this reporting period; (10) The scores shown reflect fewer than 50 completed surveys; (11) There were discrepancies in the data collection process; (12) This measure does not apply to this hospital for this reporting period; (13) Results cannot be calculated for this reporting period; (14) The results for this state are combined with nearby states to protect confidentiality; Please refer to the User's Guide for a full explanation of data.

Measure	Cases	This Hosp.	State Avg.	U.S. Avg.
Discharged on Antithrombotic Therapy	40	100%	99%	99%
Discharged on Statin Medication	32	97%	94%	94%
Thrombolytic Therapy Timing[1]	-	-	72%	66%
Venous Thromboembolism Prophylaxis	39	97%	94%	94%
Written Stroke Educational Materials Given	32	100%	87%	88%
Surgical Care Improvement Project				
Appropriate Beta Blocker Usage[2]	79	100%	97%	98%
Appropriate VTP Within 24 Hours[2]	364	99%	98%	98%
Controlled Postoperative Blood Glucose[2,7]	-	-	96%	97%
Perioperative Temperature Management[2]	455	100%	100%	100%
Prophylactic Antibiotic Selection[2]	299	100%	99%	99%
Prophylactic Antibiotic Selection (Outpatient)	21	100%	97%	98%
Prophylactic Antibiotic Stopped[2]	289	99%	98%	98%
Prophylactic Antibiotic Timing[2]	299	99%	99%	99%
Prophylactic Antibiotic Timing (Outpatient)	21	95%	97%	98%
Urinary Catheter Removal[2]	113	98%	97%	97%
Survey of Patients' Hospital Experiences				
Area Around Room 'Always' Quiet at Night	300+	49%	51%	61%
Doctors 'Always' Communicated Well	300+	80%	78%	82%
Home Recovery Information Given	300+	86%	83%	85%
Hospital Given 9 or 10 on 10 Point Scale	300+	70%	68%	71%
Meds 'Always' Explained Before Given	300+	61%	61%	64%
Nurses 'Always' Communicated Well	300+	73%	74%	79%
Pain 'Always' Well Controlled	300+	65%	68%	71%
Room and Bathroom 'Always' Clean	300+	72%	70%	73%
Timely Help 'Always' Received	300+	60%	62%	68%
Would Definitely Recommend Hospital	300+	71%	70%	71%
Use of Medical Imaging				
Cardiac Imaging Stress Test before Surgery	180	3.3%	5.2%	5.3%
Combination Abdominal CT Scan	405	1.5%	13.4%	10.5%
Combination Brain/Sinus CT Scan[1]	-	-	2.2%	2.7%
Combination Chest CT Scan[1]	-	-	2.3%	2.7%
Follow-up Mammogram/Ultrasound[7]	-	-	8.2%	8.8%
Lumbar Spine MRI for Low Back Pain[7]	-	-	34.2%	37.2%

Kaiser Foundation Hospital - Fontana

9961 Sierra Ave
Fontana, CA 92335
Phone: 909-427-5500
Fax: 909-427-7359
URL: www.kaiserpermanente.com
Type: Acute Care Hospitals
Emergency Services: Yes
Ownership: Voluntary non-profit - Private
Beds: 444
Key Personnel:
Pediatric Ambulatory Care . . . . . . Edward Curry, MD
Pediatric In-Patient Care . . . . Edward Curry, MD
Radiology. Johan D'Abreo, MD
Coronary Care . . . . Diane Kehler - Bird
Infection Control. . . . . Mike Lynd
Quality Assurance . . . . Ahmad Mohammad
Operating Room. . . . . Mary Ty, RN

Measure	Cases	This Hosp.	State Avg.	U.S. Avg.
Blood Clot Prevention and Treatment				
Anticoagulation Overlap Therapy[2]	209	96%	92%	93%
ICU Venous Thromboembolism Prophylaxis[2]	65	92%	92%	92%
Incidence of Potentially Preventable VTE[2]	25	0%	11%	10%
UFH with Dosages/Platelet Monitoring[2]	153	99%	96%	97%
Venous Thromboembolism Prophylaxis[2]	288	89%	83%	85%
Warfarin Therapy Discharge Instructions[2]	190	99%	75%	75%
Chest Pain/Possible Heart Attack Care				
Aspirin Given Within 24 Hours of Arrival	-	-	97%	96%
Fibrinolytic Meds Within 30 Min. of Arrival	-	-	62%	58%
Average Time to ECG (minutes)	-	-	9	7
Average Time to Transfer (minutes)	-	-	62	60
Children's Asthma Care				
Received Home Management Plan of Care	-	-	88%	88%
Received Reliever Medication	-	-	100%	100%
Received Systemic Corticosteroids	-	-	100%	100%
Emergency Department				
Admittance Decision Time (minutes)[2]	445	96	125	98
Head CT Results Within 45 Min. of Arrival	-	-	55%	57%
Patients Who Left ER Before Being Seen	-	-	3%	2%
Time from ER Arrival to Admit. (minutes)[2]	448	348	323	274
Time from ER Arrival to Discharge (minutes)	-	-	168	134
Time in ER Before Being Evaluated (minutes)	-	-	29	26
Time to Pain Meds for Fractures (minutes)	-	-	62	57
Heart Attack Care				
Aspirin Given at Discharge	197	100%	99%	99%
Fibrinolytic Meds Within 30 Min. of Arrival[7]	-	-	73%	54%
PCI Within 90 Minutes of Arrival[7]	-	-	95%	96%
Statin Prescribed at Discharge	199	99%	98%	98%
Heart Failure Care				
ACE Inhibitor or ARB for LVSD	212	100%	97%	97%
Discharge Instructions Given	633	100%	94%	94%
Evaluation of LVS Function	679	100%	99%	99%
Medicare Spending				
Medicare Spending per Patient (ratio)	-	0.86	0.98	0.98
Pneumonia Care				
Appropriate Initial Antibiotic Given[2]	105	99%	97%	95%
Blood Culture Timing[2]	176	99%	98%	98%
Pregnancy and Delivery Care				
Newborn Deliveries Scheduled Early	315	2%	5%	6%
Preventive Care				
Immunization for Influenza[2]	510	88%	89%	90%
Immunization for Pneumonia[2]	508	90%	90%	92%
Stroke Care				
Anticoagulation Therapy for Atrial Fibrillation[1,2]	-	-	95%	95%
Antithrombotic Therapy Timing[2]	58	100%	98%	98%
Assessed for Rehabilitation[2]	105	97%	97%	97%
Discharged on Antithrombotic Therapy[2]	77	100%	99%	99%
Discharged on Statin Medication[2]	73	100%	94%	94%
Thrombolytic Therapy Timing[1,2]	-	-	72%	66%
Venous Thromboembolism Prophylaxis[2]	90	93%	94%	94%
Written Stroke Educational Materials Given[2]	64	91%	87%	88%
Surgical Care Improvement Project				
Appropriate Beta Blocker Usage[2]	128	99%	97%	98%
Appropriate VTP Within 24 Hours[2]	372	100%	98%	98%
Controlled Postoperative Blood Glucose[2,7]	-	-	96%	97%
Perioperative Temperature Management[2]	442	99%	100%	100%
Prophylactic Antibiotic Selection[2]	284	100%	99%	99%
Prophylactic Antibiotic Selection (Outpatient)	-	-	97%	98%
Prophylactic Antibiotic Stopped[2]	277	99%	98%	98%
Prophylactic Antibiotic Timing[2]	283	100%	99%	99%
Prophylactic Antibiotic Timing (Outpatient)	-	-	97%	98%
Urinary Catheter Removal[2]	274	100%	97%	97%
Survey of Patients' Hospital Experiences				
Area Around Room 'Always' Quiet at Night	300+	55%	51%	61%
Doctors 'Always' Communicated Well	300+	82%	78%	82%
Home Recovery Information Given	300+	87%	83%	85%
Hospital Given 9 or 10 on 10 Point Scale	300+	78%	68%	71%
Meds 'Always' Explained Before Given	300+	64%	61%	64%
Nurses 'Always' Communicated Well	300+	77%	74%	79%
Pain 'Always' Well Controlled	300+	71%	68%	71%
Room and Bathroom 'Always' Clean	300+	73%	70%	73%
Timely Help 'Always' Received	300+	66%	62%	68%
Would Definitely Recommend Hospital	300+	78%	70%	71%
Use of Medical Imaging				
Cardiac Imaging Stress Test before Surgery	-	-	5.2%	5.3%
Combination Abdominal CT Scan	-	-	13.4%	10.5%
Combination Brain/Sinus CT Scan	-	-	2.2%	2.7%
Combination Chest CT Scan	-	-	2.3%	2.7%
Follow-up Mammogram/Ultrasound	-	-	8.2%	8.8%
Lumbar Spine MRI for Low Back Pain	-	-	34.2%	37.2%

Mendocino Coast District Hospital

700 River Dr
Fort Bragg, CA 95437
Phone: 707-961-1234
Fax: 707-961-4781
E-mail: info@mcdh.org
URL: www.mcdh.org
Type: Critical Access Hospitals
Emergency Services: Yes
Ownership: Govt - Hospital Dist/Auth
Beds: 25
Key Personnel:
CEO . . . . Wayne Allen
Pulmonology . . . . Randall Boberg
Radiology. . . . . Helena Coello
Emergency Room . . . . Jeff Diehl
Patient Relations . . . . Carol Hance
Operating Room. . . . . Robin Modder, DO
Chief of Medical Staff. . . . . Pam Seale, DPM

Measure	Cases	This Hosp.	State Avg.	U.S. Avg.
Blood Clot Prevention and Treatment				
Anticoagulation Overlap Therapy[5]	-	-	92%	93%
ICU Venous Thromboembolism Prophylaxis[5]	-	-	92%	92%
Incidence of Potentially Preventable VTE[5]	-	-	11%	10%
UFH with Dosages/Platelet Monitoring[5]	-	-	96%	97%
Venous Thromboembolism Prophylaxis[5]	-	-	83%	85%
Warfarin Therapy Discharge Instructions[5]	-	-	75%	75%
Chest Pain/Possible Heart Attack Care				
Aspirin Given Within 24 Hours of Arrival	-	-	97%	96%
Fibrinolytic Meds Within 30 Min. of Arrival	-	-	62%	58%
Average Time to ECG (minutes)	-	-	9	7
Average Time to Transfer (minutes)	-	-	62	60
Children's Asthma Care				
Received Home Management Plan of Care	-	-	88%	88%
Received Reliever Medication	-	-	100%	100%
Received Systemic Corticosteroids	-	-	100%	100%
Emergency Department				
Admittance Decision Time (minutes)[5]	-	-	125	98
Head CT Results Within 45 Min. of Arrival	-	-	55%	57%
Patients Who Left ER Before Being Seen	-	-	3%	2%
Time from ER Arrival to Admit. (minutes)[5]	-	-	323	274
Time from ER Arrival to Discharge (minutes)	-	-	168	134
Time in ER Before Being Evaluated (minutes)	-	-	29	26
Time to Pain Meds for Fractures (minutes)	-	-	62	57
Heart Attack Care				
Aspirin Given at Discharge[1,3]	-	-	99%	99%
Fibrinolytic Meds Within 30 Min. of Arrival[3,7]	-	-	73%	54%
PCI Within 90 Minutes of Arrival[3,7]	-	-	95%	96%
Statin Prescribed at Discharge[3,7]	-	-	98%	98%
Heart Failure Care				
ACE Inhibitor or ARB for LVSD[1]	-	-	97%	97%
Discharge Instructions Given[1]	-	-	94%	94%
Evaluation of LVS Function	12	58%	99%	99%
Medicare Spending				
Medicare Spending per Patient (ratio)	-	-	0.98	0.98
Pneumonia Care				
Appropriate Initial Antibiotic Given	17	76%	97%	95%
Blood Culture Timing	24	79%	98%	98%
Pregnancy and Delivery Care				
Newborn Deliveries Scheduled Early[5]	-	-	5%	6%
Preventive Care				
Immunization for Influenza[5]	-	-	89%	90%
Immunization for Pneumonia[5]	-	-	90%	92%
Stroke Care				
Anticoagulation Therapy for Atrial Fibrillation[5]	-	-	95%	95%
Antithrombotic Therapy Timing[5]	-	-	98%	98%
Assessed for Rehabilitation[5]	-	-	97%	97%
Discharged on Antithrombotic Therapy[5]	-	-	99%	99%
Discharged on Statin Medication[5]	-	-	94%	94%
Thrombolytic Therapy Timing[5]	-	-	72%	66%
Venous Thromboembolism Prophylaxis[5]	-	-	94%	94%
Written Stroke Educational Materials Given[5]	-	-	87%	88%
Surgical Care Improvement Project				
Appropriate Beta Blocker Usage[1]	-	-	97%	98%
Appropriate VTP Within 24 Hours	54	96%	98%	98%
Controlled Postoperative Blood Glucose[3,7]	-	-	96%	97%
Perioperative Temperature Management	62	92%	100%	100%
Prophylactic Antibiotic Selection	56	96%	99%	99%
Prophylactic Antibiotic Selection (Outpatient)	-	-	97%	98%
Prophylactic Antibiotic Stopped	54	100%	98%	98%
Prophylactic Antibiotic Timing	56	91%	99%	99%
Prophylactic Antibiotic Timing (Outpatient)	-	-	97%	98%
Urinary Catheter Removal	55	93%	97%	97%
Survey of Patients' Hospital Experiences				
Area Around Room 'Always' Quiet at Night	(a)	58%	51%	61%
Doctors 'Always' Communicated Well	(a)	75%	78%	82%
Home Recovery Information Given	(a)	88%	83%	85%
Hospital Given 9 or 10 on 10 Point Scale	(a)	58%	68%	71%
Meds 'Always' Explained Before Given	(a)	60%	61%	64%
Nurses 'Always' Communicated Well	(a)	76%	74%	79%
Pain 'Always' Well Controlled	(a)	72%	68%	71%
Room and Bathroom 'Always' Clean	(a)	68%	70%	73%

NOTE: Hospital profiles are in alphabetical order by state, then city, then hospital within the city; Rankings exclude hospitals with less than 25 cases except for patient surveys which excludes hospitals with less than 100 cases; (a) 100-299 cases; (1) The number of cases/patients is too few to report; (2) Data submitted were based on a sample of cases/patients; (3) Results are based on a shorter time period than required; (4) Data suppressed by CMS for one or more quarters; (5) Results are not available for this reporting period; (6) Fewer than 100 patients completed the HCAHPS survey; (7) No cases met the criteria for this measure; (8) The lower limit of the confidence interval cannot be calculated if the number of observed infections equals zero; (9) No data are available from the state/territory for this reporting period; (10) The scores shown reflect fewer than 50 completed surveys; (11) There were discrepancies in the data collection process; (12) This measure does not apply to this hospital for this reporting period; (13) Results cannot be calculated for this reporting period; (14) The results for this state are combined with nearby states to protect confidentiality; Please refer to the User's Guide for a full explanation of data.

Measure	Cases	This Hosp.	State Avg.	U.S. Avg.
Timely Help 'Always' Received	(a)	70%	62%	68%
Would Definitely Recommend Hospital	(a)	65%	70%	71%
Use of Medical Imaging				
Cardiac Imaging Stress Test before Surgery	-	-	5.2%	5.3%
Combination Abdominal CT Scan	-	-	13.4%	10.5%
Combination Brain/Sinus CT Scan	-	-	2.2%	2.7%
Combination Chest CT Scan	-	-	2.3%	2.7%
Follow-up Mammogram/Ultrasound	-	-	8.2%	8.8%
Lumbar Spine MRI for Low Back Pain	-	-	34.2%	37.2%

Redwood Memorial Hospital

3300 Renner Drive
Fortuna, CA 95540
Phone: 707-445-8121
Fax: 707-725-7212
URL: www.redwoodmemorial.org
Type: Critical Access Hospitals
Emergency Services: Yes
Ownership: Voluntary non-profit - Private
Beds: 25

Key Personnel:
CEO/President. . . . . Joe Mark
President . . . . David O'Brien, M.D.
Quality Assurance . . . . Ann Warner, RN

Measure	Cases	This Hosp.	State Avg.	U.S. Avg.
Blood Clot Prevention and Treatment				
Anticoagulation Overlap Therapy[5]	-	-	92%	93%
ICU Venous Thromboembolism Prophylaxis[5]	-	-	92%	92%
Incidence of Potentially Preventable VTE[5]	-	-	11%	10%
UFH with Dosages/Platelet Monitoring[5]	-	-	96%	97%
Venous Thromboembolism Prophylaxis[5]	-	-	83%	85%
Warfarin Therapy Discharge Instructions[5]	-	-	75%	75%
Chest Pain/Possible Heart Attack Care				
Aspirin Given Within 24 Hours of Arrival	-	-	97%	96%
Fibrinolytic Meds Within 30 Min. of Arrival	-	-	62%	58%
Average Time to ECG (minutes)	-	-	9	7
Average Time to Transfer (minutes)	-	-	62	60
Children's Asthma Care				
Received Home Management Plan of Care	-	-	88%	88%
Received Reliever Medication	-	-	100%	100%
Received Systemic Corticosteroids	-	-	100%	100%
Emergency Department				
Admittance Decision Time (minutes)[2]	248	127	125	98
Head CT Results Within 45 Min. of Arrival	-	-	55%	57%
Patients Who Left ER Before Being Seen	-	-	3%	2%
Time from ER Arrival to Admit. (minutes)[2]	274	297	323	274
Time from ER Arrival to Discharge (minutes)	-	-	168	134
Time in ER Before Being Evaluated (minutes)	-	-	29	26
Time to Pain Meds for Fractures (minutes)	-	-	62	57
Heart Attack Care				
Aspirin Given at Discharge[1]	-	-	99%	99%
Fibrinolytic Meds Within 30 Min. of Arrival[7]	-	-	73%	54%
PCI Within 90 Minutes of Arrival[7]	-	-	95%	96%
Statin Prescribed at Discharge[1]	-	-	98%	98%
Heart Failure Care				
ACE Inhibitor or ARB for LVSD[1]	-	-	97%	97%
Discharge Instructions Given	26	88%	94%	94%
Evaluation of LVS Function	30	97%	99%	99%
Medicare Spending				
Medicare Spending per Patient (ratio)	-	-	0.98	0.98
Pneumonia Care				
Appropriate Initial Antibiotic Given	27	96%	97%	95%
Blood Culture Timing	50	96%	98%	98%
Pregnancy and Delivery Care				
Newborn Deliveries Scheduled Early[5]	-	-	5%	6%
Preventive Care				
Immunization for Influenza[2]	243	78%	89%	90%
Immunization for Pneumonia[2]	251	89%	90%	92%
Stroke Care				
Anticoagulation Therapy for Atrial Fibrillation[5]	-	-	95%	95%
Antithrombotic Therapy Timing[5]	-	-	98%	98%
Assessed for Rehabilitation[5]	-	-	97%	97%
Discharged on Antithrombotic Therapy[5]	-	-	99%	99%
Discharged on Statin Medication[5]	-	-	94%	94%
Thrombolytic Therapy Timing[5]	-	-	72%	66%
Venous Thromboembolism Prophylaxis[5]	-	-	94%	94%
Written Stroke Educational Materials Given[5]	-	-	87%	88%
Surgical Care Improvement Project				
Appropriate Beta Blocker Usage[5]	-	-	97%	98%
Appropriate VTP Within 24 Hours[5]	-	-	98%	98%
Controlled Postoperative Blood Glucose[5]	-	-	96%	97%
Perioperative Temperature Management[5]	-	-	100%	100%
Prophylactic Antibiotic Selection[5]	-	-	99%	99%
Prophylactic Antibiotic Selection (Outpatient)	-	-	97%	98%
Prophylactic Antibiotic Stopped[5]	-	-	98%	98%
Prophylactic Antibiotic Timing[5]	-	-	99%	99%
Prophylactic Antibiotic Timing (Outpatient)	-	-	97%	98%
Urinary Catheter Removal[5]	-	-	97%	97%
Survey of Patients' Hospital Experiences				
Area Around Room 'Always' Quiet at Night	300+	53%	51%	61%
Doctors 'Always' Communicated Well	300+	78%	78%	82%
Home Recovery Information Given	300+	86%	83%	85%
Hospital Given 9 or 10 on 10 Point Scale	300+	70%	68%	71%
Meds 'Always' Explained Before Given	300+	62%	61%	64%
Nurses 'Always' Communicated Well	300+	76%	74%	79%
Pain 'Always' Well Controlled	300+	69%	68%	71%
Room and Bathroom 'Always' Clean	300+	74%	70%	73%
Timely Help 'Always' Received	300+	65%	62%	68%
Would Definitely Recommend Hospital	300+	73%	70%	71%
Use of Medical Imaging				
Cardiac Imaging Stress Test before Surgery	-	-	5.2%	5.3%
Combination Abdominal CT Scan	-	-	13.4%	10.5%
Combination Brain/Sinus CT Scan	-	-	2.2%	2.7%
Combination Chest CT Scan	-	-	2.3%	2.7%
Follow-up Mammogram/Ultrasound	-	-	8.2%	8.8%
Lumbar Spine MRI for Low Back Pain	-	-	34.2%	37.2%

Fountain Valley Regional Hospital & Medical Center

17100 Euclid Street
Fountain Valley, CA 92708
Phone: 714-966-7200
Fax: 714-966-8039
URL: www.fountainvalleyhospital.com
Type: Acute Care Hospitals
Emergency Services: Yes
Ownership: Proprietary
Beds: 413

Key Personnel:
CEO/President. . . . . B. Joseph Badalian
Emergency Room . . . . Cess Canson
Infection Control. . . . . Barbara Goss
Radiology. . . . . Bob McKewen
Operating Room. . . . . Mary Meola
Cardiac Laboratory. . . . . Lynn Redwater
Quality Assurance . . . . Barbara Silverstone

Measure	Cases	This Hosp.	State Avg.	U.S. Avg.
Blood Clot Prevention and Treatment				
Anticoagulation Overlap Therapy[2]	51	94%	92%	93%
ICU Venous Thromboembolism Prophylaxis[2]	79	89%	92%	92%
Incidence of Potentially Preventable VTE[2]	17	0%	11%	10%
UFH with Dosages/Platelet Monitoring[2]	19	100%	96%	97%
Venous Thromboembolism Prophylaxis[2]	386	65%	83%	85%
Warfarin Therapy Discharge Instructions[2]	33	91%	75%	75%
Chest Pain/Possible Heart Attack Care				
Aspirin Given Within 24 Hours of Arrival	56	100%	97%	96%
Fibrinolytic Meds Within 30 Min. of Arrival[3,7]	-	-	62%	58%
Average Time to ECG (minutes)	57	5	9	7
Average Time to Transfer (minutes)[3,7]	-	-	62	60
Children's Asthma Care				
Received Home Management Plan of Care	-	-	88%	88%
Received Reliever Medication	-	-	100%	100%
Received Systemic Corticosteroids	-	-	100%	100%
Emergency Department				
Admittance Decision Time (minutes)[2]	597	143	125	98
Head CT Results Within 45 Min. of Arrival[1]	-	-	55%	57%
Patients Who Left ER Before Being Seen	42,133	1%	3%	2%
Time from ER Arrival to Admit. (minutes)[2]	614	301	323	274
Time from ER Arrival to Discharge (minutes)	449	169	168	134
Time in ER Before Being Evaluated (minutes)	493	32	29	26
Time to Pain Meds for Fractures (minutes)	158	64	62	57
Heart Attack Care				
Aspirin Given at Discharge	249	98%	99%	99%
Fibrinolytic Meds Within 30 Min. of Arrival[7]	-	-	73%	54%
PCI Within 90 Minutes of Arrival	43	100%	95%	96%
Statin Prescribed at Discharge	256	98%	98%	98%
Heart Failure Care				
ACE Inhibitor or ARB for LVSD	107	95%	97%	97%
Discharge Instructions Given	255	94%	94%	94%
Evaluation of LVS Function	318	99%	99%	99%
Medicare Spending				
Medicare Spending per Patient (ratio)	-	1.12	0.98	0.98
Pneumonia Care				
Appropriate Initial Antibiotic Given[2]	127	98%	97%	95%
Blood Culture Timing[2]	171	99%	98%	98%
Pregnancy and Delivery Care				
Newborn Deliveries Scheduled Early[2]	68	1%	5%	6%
Preventive Care				
Immunization for Influenza[2]	546	97%	89%	90%
Immunization for Pneumonia[2]	557	96%	90%	92%
Stroke Care				
Anticoagulation Therapy for Atrial Fibrillation	19	95%	95%	95%
Antithrombotic Therapy Timing	170	99%	98%	98%
Assessed for Rehabilitation	214	99%	97%	97%
Discharged on Antithrombotic Therapy	183	100%	99%	99%
Discharged on Statin Medication	142	99%	94%	94%
Thrombolytic Therapy Timing	23	100%	72%	66%
Venous Thromboembolism Prophylaxis	225	92%	94%	94%
Written Stroke Educational Materials Given	108	95%	87%	88%
Surgical Care Improvement Project				
Appropriate Beta Blocker Usage[2]	198	98%	97%	98%
Appropriate VTP Within 24 Hours[2]	452	96%	98%	98%
Controlled Postoperative Blood Glucose[2]	103	100%	96%	97%
Perioperative Temperature Management[2]	513	100%	100%	100%
Prophylactic Antibiotic Selection[2]	463	99%	99%	99%
Prophylactic Antibiotic Selection (Outpatient)	267	98%	97%	98%
Prophylactic Antibiotic Stopped[2]	415	95%	98%	98%
Prophylactic Antibiotic Timing[2]	464	99%	99%	99%
Prophylactic Antibiotic Timing (Outpatient)	268	97%	97%	98%
Urinary Catheter Removal[2]	282	95%	97%	97%
Survey of Patients' Hospital Experiences				
Area Around Room 'Always' Quiet at Night	300+	43%	51%	61%
Doctors 'Always' Communicated Well	300+	74%	78%	82%
Home Recovery Information Given	300+	80%	83%	85%
Hospital Given 9 or 10 on 10 Point Scale	300+	57%	68%	71%
Meds 'Always' Explained Before Given	300+	54%	61%	64%
Nurses 'Always' Communicated Well	300+	68%	74%	79%
Pain 'Always' Well Controlled	300+	64%	68%	71%
Room and Bathroom 'Always' Clean	300+	68%	70%	73%
Timely Help 'Always' Received	300+	51%	62%	68%
Would Definitely Recommend Hospital	300+	61%	70%	71%
Use of Medical Imaging				
Cardiac Imaging Stress Test before Surgery	417	7.7%	5.2%	5.3%
Combination Abdominal CT Scan	506	4.0%	13.4%	10.5%
Combination Brain/Sinus CT Scan	572	0.2%	2.2%	2.7%
Combination Chest CT Scan	180	1.1%	2.3%	2.7%
Follow-up Mammogram/Ultrasound	674	10.7%	8.2%	8.8%
Lumbar Spine MRI for Low Back Pain[1]	-	-	34.2%	37.2%

Orange Coast Memorial Medical Center

9920 Talbert Avenue
Fountain Valley, CA 92708
Phone: 714-378-7406
Fax: 714-378-7474
Type: Acute Care Hospitals
Emergency Services: Yes
Ownership: Proprietary
Beds: 230

Key Personnel:
Operating Room. . . . . Reginald G Abraham
Pediatric Ambulatory Care . . . . . . N Kent
Pediatric In-Patient Care . . . . N Kent
CEO/President. . . . . Marcia Mauker
Radiology. . . . . Stuart A Souders
Emergency Room . . . . Dale Vital

Measure	Cases	This Hosp.	State Avg.	U.S. Avg.
Blood Clot Prevention and Treatment				
Anticoagulation Overlap Therapy[2]	76	99%	92%	93%
ICU Venous Thromboembolism Prophylaxis[2]	63	97%	92%	92%
Incidence of Potentially Preventable VTE[2]	13	15%	11%	10%
UFH with Dosages/Platelet Monitoring[2]	38	97%	96%	97%
Venous Thromboembolism Prophylaxis[2]	311	71%	83%	85%
Warfarin Therapy Discharge Instructions[2]	51	22%	75%	75%
Chest Pain/Possible Heart Attack Care				

NOTE: Hospital profiles are in alphabetical order by state, then city, then hospital within the city; Rankings exclude hospitals with less than 25 cases except for patient surveys which excludes hospitals with less than 100 cases; (a) 100-299 cases; (1) The number of cases/patients is too few to report; (2) Data submitted were based on a sample of cases/patients; (3) Results are based on a shorter time period than required; (4) Data suppressed by CMS for one or more quarters; (5) Results are not available for this reporting period; (6) Fewer than 100 patients completed the HCAHPS survey; (7) No cases met the criteria for this measure; (8) The lower limit of the confidence interval cannot be calculated if the number of observed infections equals zero; (9) No data are available from the state/territory for this reporting period; (10) The scores shown reflect fewer than 50 completed surveys; (11) There were discrepancies in the data collection process; (12) This measure does not apply to this hospital for this reporting period; (13) Results cannot be calculated for this reporting period; (14) The results for this state are combined with nearby states to protect confidentiality; Please refer to the User's Guide for a full explanation of data.

Measure	Cases	This Hosp.	State Avg.	U.S. Avg.
Aspirin Given Within 24 Hours of Arrival	20	95%	97%	96%
Fibrinolytic Meds Within 30 Min. of Arrival[5]	-	-	62%	58%
Average Time to ECG (minutes)	23	12	9	7
Average Time to Transfer (minutes)[5]	-	-	62	60
Children's Asthma Care				
Received Home Management Plan of Care	-	-	88%	88%
Received Reliever Medication	-	-	100%	100%
Received Systemic Corticosteroids	-	-	100%	100%
Emergency Department				
Admittance Decision Time (minutes)[2]	636	82	125	98
Head CT Results Within 45 Min. of Arrival[1]	-	-	55%	57%
Patients Who Left ER Before Being Seen	29,129	1%	3%	2%
Time from ER Arrival to Admit. (minutes)[2]	636	272	323	274
Time from ER Arrival to Discharge (minutes)	388	150	168	134
Time in ER Before Being Evaluated (minutes)	419	17	29	26
Time to Pain Meds for Fractures (minutes)	85	45	62	57
Heart Attack Care				
Aspirin Given at Discharge	133	95%	99%	99%
Fibrinolytic Meds Within 30 Min. of Arrival[7]	-	-	73%	54%
PCI Within 90 Minutes of Arrival	20	90%	95%	96%
Statin Prescribed at Discharge	142	96%	98%	98%
Heart Failure Care				
ACE Inhibitor or ARB for LVSD	99	98%	97%	97%
Discharge Instructions Given	266	97%	94%	94%
Evaluation of LVS Function	322	99%	99%	99%
Medicare Spending				
Medicare Spending per Patient (ratio)	-	1.02	0.98	0.98
Pneumonia Care				
Appropriate Initial Antibiotic Given	91	97%	97%	95%
Blood Culture Timing	153	97%	98%	98%
Pregnancy and Delivery Care				
Newborn Deliveries Scheduled Early[2]	37	3%	5%	6%
Preventive Care				
Immunization for Influenza[2]	512	82%	89%	90%
Immunization for Pneumonia[2]	575	87%	90%	92%
Stroke Care				
Anticoagulation Therapy for Atrial Fibrillation[1]	-	-	95%	95%
Antithrombotic Therapy Timing	47	100%	98%	98%
Assessed for Rehabilitation	74	96%	97%	97%
Discharged on Antithrombotic Therapy	60	98%	99%	99%
Discharged on Statin Medication	52	81%	94%	94%
Thrombolytic Therapy Timing[7]	-	-	72%	66%
Venous Thromboembolism Prophylaxis	63	84%	94%	94%
Written Stroke Educational Materials Given	50	100%	87%	88%
Surgical Care Improvement Project				
Appropriate Beta Blocker Usage[2]	205	98%	97%	98%
Appropriate VTP Within 24 Hours[2]	555	99%	98%	98%
Controlled Postoperative Blood Glucose[2]	98	92%	96%	97%
Perioperative Temperature Management[2]	632	99%	100%	100%
Prophylactic Antibiotic Selection[2]	482	98%	99%	99%
Prophylactic Antibiotic Selection (Outpatient)	326	96%	97%	98%
Prophylactic Antibiotic Stopped[2]	453	98%	98%	98%
Prophylactic Antibiotic Timing[2]	482	98%	99%	99%
Prophylactic Antibiotic Timing (Outpatient)	268	94%	97%	98%
Urinary Catheter Removal[2]	264	93%	97%	97%
Survey of Patients' Hospital Experiences				
Area Around Room 'Always' Quiet at Night	300+	50%	51%	61%
Doctors 'Always' Communicated Well	300+	78%	78%	82%
Home Recovery Information Given	300+	82%	83%	85%
Hospital Given 9 or 10 on 10 Point Scale	300+	68%	68%	71%
Meds 'Always' Explained Before Given	300+	61%	61%	64%
Nurses 'Always' Communicated Well	300+	74%	74%	79%
Pain 'Always' Well Controlled	300+	68%	68%	71%
Room and Bathroom 'Always' Clean	300+	71%	70%	73%
Timely Help 'Always' Received	300+	60%	62%	68%
Would Definitely Recommend Hospital	300+	71%	70%	71%
Use of Medical Imaging				
Cardiac Imaging Stress Test before Surgery	80	3.8%	5.2%	5.3%
Combination Abdominal CT Scan	507	30.6%	13.4%	10.5%
Combination Brain/Sinus CT Scan	360	1.4%	2.2%	2.7%
Combination Chest CT Scan	302	7.0%	2.3%	2.7%
Follow-up Mammogram/Ultrasound	741	7.8%	8.2%	8.8%
Lumbar Spine MRI for Low Back Pain[1]	-	-	34.2%	37.2%

Washington Hospital

2000 Mowry Ave
Fremont, CA 94538
URL: www.whhs.com
Phone: 510-797-1111
Fax: 510-791-3496
Type: Acute Care Hospitals
Ownership: Govt - Hospital Dist/Auth
Emergency Services: Yes
Beds: 337

Key Personnel:
Emergency Room . . . . Brenda Brennan, RN
CEO/President. . . . . Nancy Farber
Quality Assurance . . . . Kris LaVoy, RN
Radiology. . . . . Bruce Nixon
Operating Room. . . . . Toppy Ryan
Chief of Medical Staff . . . . Ahmed Sadiq
Pediatric Ambulatory Care . . . . . . Tina Scobel
Pediatric In-Patient Care . . . . Tina Scobel

Measure	Cases	This Hosp.	State Avg.	U.S. Avg.
Blood Clot Prevention and Treatment				
Anticoagulation Overlap Therapy[2]	60	85%	92%	93%
ICU Venous Thromboembolism Prophylaxis[2]	95	85%	92%	92%
Incidence of Potentially Preventable VTE[2]	12	8%	11%	10%
UFH with Dosages/Platelet Monitoring[2]	34	100%	96%	97%
Venous Thromboembolism Prophylaxis[2]	315	48%	83%	85%
Warfarin Therapy Discharge Instructions[2]	35	46%	75%	75%
Chest Pain/Possible Heart Attack Care				
Aspirin Given Within 24 Hours of Arrival[5]	-	-	97%	96%
Fibrinolytic Meds Within 30 Min. of Arrival[5]	-	-	62%	58%
Average Time to ECG (minutes)[5]	-	-	9	7
Average Time to Transfer (minutes)[5]	-	-	62	60
Children's Asthma Care				
Received Home Management Plan of Care	-	-	88%	88%
Received Reliever Medication	-	-	100%	100%
Received Systemic Corticosteroids	-	-	100%	100%
Emergency Department				
Admittance Decision Time (minutes)[2]	470	188	125	98
Head CT Results Within 45 Min. of Arrival[1]	-	-	55%	57%
Patients Who Left ER Before Being Seen	12,969	2%	3%	2%
Time from ER Arrival to Admit. (minutes)[2]	472	353	323	274
Time from ER Arrival to Discharge (minutes)	382	145	168	134
Time in ER Before Being Evaluated (minutes)	426	23	29	26
Time to Pain Meds for Fractures (minutes)	172	62	62	57
Heart Attack Care				
Aspirin Given at Discharge	224	99%	99%	99%
Fibrinolytic Meds Within 30 Min. of Arrival[7]	-	-	73%	54%
PCI Within 90 Minutes of Arrival	28	93%	95%	96%
Statin Prescribed at Discharge	221	99%	98%	98%
Heart Failure Care				
ACE Inhibitor or ARB for LVSD	119	99%	97%	97%
Discharge Instructions Given	286	99%	94%	94%
Evaluation of LVS Function	354	100%	99%	99%
Medicare Spending				
Medicare Spending per Patient (ratio)	-	0.96	0.98	0.98
Pneumonia Care				
Appropriate Initial Antibiotic Given[2]	86	98%	97%	95%
Blood Culture Timing[2]	136	97%	98%	98%
Pregnancy and Delivery Care				
Newborn Deliveries Scheduled Early	183	2%	5%	6%
Preventive Care				
Immunization for Influenza[2]	527	94%	89%	90%
Immunization for Pneumonia[2]	663	90%	90%	92%
Stroke Care				
Anticoagulation Therapy for Atrial Fibrillation	30	97%	95%	95%
Antithrombotic Therapy Timing	127	94%	98%	98%
Assessed for Rehabilitation	164	100%	97%	97%
Discharged on Antithrombotic Therapy	134	96%	99%	99%
Discharged on Statin Medication	107	92%	94%	94%
Thrombolytic Therapy Timing	13	62%	72%	66%
Venous Thromboembolism Prophylaxis	174	92%	94%	94%
Written Stroke Educational Materials Given	89	80%	87%	88%
Surgical Care Improvement Project				
Appropriate Beta Blocker Usage[2]	167	99%	97%	98%
Appropriate VTP Within 24 Hours[2]	321	98%	98%	98%
Controlled Postoperative Blood Glucose[2]	116	94%	96%	97%
Perioperative Temperature Management[2]	475	100%	100%	100%
Prophylactic Antibiotic Selection[2]	399	100%	99%	99%
Prophylactic Antibiotic Selection (Outpatient)	150	99%	97%	98%
Prophylactic Antibiotic Stopped[2]	393	98%	98%	98%
Prophylactic Antibiotic Timing[2]	399	100%	99%	99%
Prophylactic Antibiotic Timing (Outpatient)	153	96%	97%	98%
Urinary Catheter Removal[2]	340	97%	97%	97%
Survey of Patients' Hospital Experiences				
Area Around Room 'Always' Quiet at Night	300+	48%	51%	61%
Doctors 'Always' Communicated Well	300+	79%	78%	82%
Home Recovery Information Given	300+	86%	83%	85%
Hospital Given 9 or 10 on 10 Point Scale	300+	65%	68%	71%
Meds 'Always' Explained Before Given	300+	62%	61%	64%
Nurses 'Always' Communicated Well	300+	74%	74%	79%
Pain 'Always' Well Controlled	300+	68%	68%	71%
Room and Bathroom 'Always' Clean	300+	72%	70%	73%
Timely Help 'Always' Received	300+	61%	62%	68%
Would Definitely Recommend Hospital	300+	73%	70%	71%
Use of Medical Imaging				
Cardiac Imaging Stress Test before Surgery	362	7.5%	5.2%	5.3%
Combination Abdominal CT Scan	874	4.9%	13.4%	10.5%
Combination Brain/Sinus CT Scan	964	1.1%	2.2%	2.7%
Combination Chest CT Scan	547	5.1%	2.3%	2.7%
Follow-up Mammogram/Ultrasound	1,633	7.9%	8.2%	8.8%
Lumbar Spine MRI for Low Back Pain[1]	-	-	34.2%	37.2%

San Joaquin General Hospital

500 W Hospital Road
French Camp, CA 95231
URL: www.sjgeneralhospital.com
Phone: 209-468-6000
Type: Acute Care Hospitals
Ownership: Government - Local
Emergency Services: Yes
Beds: 234

Key Personnel:
CEO/President. . . . . Kenneth B Cohen
Quality Assurance . . . . Donna Haight
Chief of Medical Staff . . . . Shital Hubli, MD
Operating Room. . . . . Jeff Medina, RN

Measure	Cases	This Hosp.	State Avg.	U.S. Avg.
Blood Clot Prevention and Treatment				
Anticoagulation Overlap Therapy[2]	23	96%	92%	93%
ICU Venous Thromboembolism Prophylaxis[2]	91	97%	92%	92%
Incidence of Potentially Preventable VTE[1,2]	-	-	11%	10%
UFH with Dosages/Platelet Monitoring[2]	18	100%	96%	97%
Venous Thromboembolism Prophylaxis[2]	349	83%	83%	85%
Warfarin Therapy Discharge Instructions[2]	17	29%	75%	75%
Chest Pain/Possible Heart Attack Care				
Aspirin Given Within 24 Hours of Arrival[1,3]	-	-	97%	96%
Fibrinolytic Meds Within 30 Min. of Arrival[1,3]	-	-	62%	58%
Average Time to ECG (minutes)[1,3]	-	-	9	7
Average Time to Transfer (minutes)[3,7]	-	-	62	60
Children's Asthma Care				
Received Home Management Plan of Care	-	-	88%	88%
Received Reliever Medication	-	-	100%	100%
Received Systemic Corticosteroids	-	-	100%	100%
Emergency Department				
Admittance Decision Time (minutes)[2]	482	185	125	98
Head CT Results Within 45 Min. of Arrival[1]	-	-	55%	57%
Patients Who Left ER Before Being Seen	39,157	4%	3%	2%
Time from ER Arrival to Admit. (minutes)[2]	484	412	323	274
Time from ER Arrival to Discharge (minutes)	359	196	168	134
Time in ER Before Being Evaluated (minutes)	335	59	29	26
Time to Pain Meds for Fractures (minutes)	124	88	62	57
Heart Attack Care				
Aspirin Given at Discharge	43	100%	99%	99%
Fibrinolytic Meds Within 30 Min. of Arrival[1]	-	-	73%	54%
PCI Within 90 Minutes of Arrival[7]	-	-	95%	96%
Statin Prescribed at Discharge	42	100%	98%	98%
Heart Failure Care				
ACE Inhibitor or ARB for LVSD	93	100%	97%	97%
Discharge Instructions Given	153	95%	94%	94%
Evaluation of LVS Function	164	100%	99%	99%
Medicare Spending				
Medicare Spending per Patient (ratio)	-	0.99	0.98	0.98

NOTE: Hospital profiles are in alphabetical order by state, then city, then hospital within the city; Rankings exclude hospitals with less than 25 cases except for patient surveys which excludes hospitals with less than 100 cases; (a) 100-299 cases; (1) The number of cases/patients is too few to report; (2) Data submitted were based on a sample of cases/patients; (3) Results are based on a shorter time period than required; (4) Data suppressed by CMS for one or more quarters; (5) Results are not available for this reporting period; (6) Fewer than 100 patients completed the HCAHPS survey; (7) No cases met the criteria for this measure; (8) The lower limit of the confidence interval cannot be calculated if the number of observed infections equals zero; (9) No data are available from the state/territory for this reporting period; (10) The scores shown reflect fewer than 50 completed surveys; (11) There were discrepancies in the data collection process; (12) This measure does not apply to this hospital for this reporting period; (13) Results cannot be calculated for this reporting period; (14) The results for this state are combined with nearby states to protect confidentiality; Please refer to the User's Guide for a full explanation of data.

Measure	Cases	This Hosp.	State Avg.	U.S. Avg.
Pneumonia Care				
Appropriate Initial Antibiotic Given	90	99%	97%	95%
Blood Culture Timing	171	97%	98%	98%
Pregnancy and Delivery Care				
Newborn Deliveries Scheduled Early[2]	34	0%	5%	6%
Preventive Care				
Immunization for Influenza[2]	457	67%	89%	90%
Immunization for Pneumonia[2]	367	80%	90%	92%
Stroke Care				
Anticoagulation Therapy for Atrial Fibrillation[1]	-	-	95%	95%
Antithrombotic Therapy Timing	59	98%	98%	98%
Assessed for Rehabilitation	92	100%	97%	97%
Discharged on Antithrombotic Therapy	75	99%	99%	99%
Discharged on Statin Medication	52	98%	94%	94%
Thrombolytic Therapy Timing	13	85%	72%	66%
Venous Thromboembolism Prophylaxis	85	92%	94%	94%
Written Stroke Educational Materials Given	63	98%	87%	88%
Surgical Care Improvement Project				
Appropriate Beta Blocker Usage	48	81%	97%	98%
Appropriate VTP Within 24 Hours	279	97%	98%	98%
Controlled Postoperative Blood Glucose[7]	-	-	96%	97%
Perioperative Temperature Management	325	100%	100%	100%
Prophylactic Antibiotic Selection	150	98%	99%	99%
Prophylactic Antibiotic Selection (Outpatient)	40	98%	97%	98%
Prophylactic Antibiotic Stopped	148	99%	98%	98%
Prophylactic Antibiotic Timing	150	97%	99%	99%
Prophylactic Antibiotic Timing (Outpatient)	41	90%	97%	98%
Urinary Catheter Removal	119	92%	97%	97%
Survey of Patients' Hospital Experiences				
Area Around Room 'Always' Quiet at Night	300+	43%	51%	61%
Doctors 'Always' Communicated Well	300+	74%	78%	82%
Home Recovery Information Given	300+	80%	83%	85%
Hospital Given 9 or 10 on 10 Point Scale	300+	60%	68%	71%
Meds 'Always' Explained Before Given	300+	60%	61%	64%
Nurses 'Always' Communicated Well	300+	68%	74%	79%
Pain 'Always' Well Controlled	300+	68%	68%	71%
Room and Bathroom 'Always' Clean	300+	69%	70%	73%
Timely Help 'Always' Received	300+	45%	62%	68%
Would Definitely Recommend Hospital	300+	63%	70%	71%
Use of Medical Imaging				
Cardiac Imaging Stress Test before Surgery	112	3.6%	5.2%	5.3%
Combination Abdominal CT Scan	260	1.9%	13.4%	10.5%
Combination Brain/Sinus CT Scan[1]	-	-	2.2%	2.7%
Combination Chest CT Scan	77	1.3%	2.3%	2.7%
Follow-up Mammogram/Ultrasound	225	8.9%	8.2%	8.8%
Lumbar Spine MRI for Low Back Pain[7]	-	-	34.2%	37.2%

Community Regional Medical Center

2823 Fresno Street
Fresno, CA 93715
Phone: 559-459-6000
Fax: 559-459-2450
URL: www.communitymedical.org
Type: Acute Care Hospitals
Emergency Services: Yes
Ownership: Voluntary non-profit - Private
Beds: 452

Key Personnel:
Chair/CEO................. Florence Dunn
CEO/President.............. Tim A Joslin
Quality Assurance .... Colleen Strom
Chief of Medical Staff.......... Thomas Utecht, MD

Measure	Cases	This Hosp.	State Avg.	U.S. Avg.
Blood Clot Prevention and Treatment				
Anticoagulation Overlap Therapy[2]	151	99%	92%	93%
ICU Venous Thromboembolism Prophylaxis[2]	40	100%	92%	92%
Incidence of Potentially Preventable VTE[2]	37	8%	11%	10%
UFH with Dosages/Platelet Monitoring[2]	103	100%	96%	97%
Venous Thromboembolism Prophylaxis[2]	351	81%	83%	85%
Warfarin Therapy Discharge Instructions[2]	114	92%	75%	75%
Chest Pain/Possible Heart Attack Care				
Aspirin Given Within 24 Hours of Arrival[3]	12	75%	97%	96%
Fibrinolytic Meds Within 30 Min. of Arrival[5]	-	-	62%	58%
Average Time to ECG (minutes)[3]	12	12	9	7
Average Time to Transfer (minutes)[5]	-	-	62	60
Children's Asthma Care				
Received Home Management Plan of Care	-	-	88%	88%
Received Reliever Medication	-	-	100%	100%
Received Systemic Corticosteroids	-	-	100%	100%
Emergency Department				
Admittance Decision Time (minutes)[2]	657	462	125	98
Head CT Results Within 45 Min. of Arrival[1]	-	-	55%	57%
Patients Who Left ER Before Being Seen	>100k	14%	3%	2%
Time from ER Arrival to Admit. (minutes)[2]	661	852	323	274
Time from ER Arrival to Discharge (minutes)	276	286	168	134
Time in ER Before Being Evaluated (minutes)	345	65	29	26
Time to Pain Meds for Fractures (minutes)	306	88	62	57
Heart Attack Care				
Aspirin Given at Discharge[2]	513	100%	99%	99%
Fibrinolytic Meds Within 30 Min. of Arrival[2,7]	-	-	73%	54%
PCI Within 90 Minutes of Arrival[2]	68	94%	95%	96%
Statin Prescribed at Discharge[2]	529	99%	98%	98%
Heart Failure Care				
ACE Inhibitor or ARB for LVSD[2]	398	99%	97%	97%
Discharge Instructions Given[2]	842	98%	94%	94%
Evaluation of LVS Function[2]	913	100%	99%	99%
Medicare Spending				
Medicare Spending per Patient (ratio)	-	0.99	0.98	0.98
Pneumonia Care				
Appropriate Initial Antibiotic Given[2]	153	97%	97%	95%
Blood Culture Timing[2]	388	95%	98%	98%
Pregnancy and Delivery Care				
Newborn Deliveries Scheduled Early[2]	81	1%	5%	6%
Preventive Care				
Immunization for Influenza[2]	485	83%	89%	90%
Immunization for Pneumonia[2]	493	84%	90%	92%
Stroke Care				
Anticoagulation Therapy for Atrial Fibrillation[2]	39	92%	95%	95%
Antithrombotic Therapy Timing[2]	314	97%	98%	98%
Assessed for Rehabilitation[2]	423	100%	97%	97%
Discharged on Antithrombotic Therapy[2]	315	99%	99%	99%
Discharged on Statin Medication[2]	261	98%	94%	94%
Thrombolytic Therapy Timing[2]	19	74%	72%	66%
Venous Thromboembolism Prophylaxis[2]	475	97%	94%	94%
Written Stroke Educational Materials Given[2]	255	98%	87%	88%
Surgical Care Improvement Project				
Appropriate Beta Blocker Usage[2]	491	100%	97%	98%
Appropriate VTP Within 24 Hours[2]	1,302	97%	98%	98%
Controlled Postoperative Blood Glucose[2]	247	85%	96%	97%
Perioperative Temperature Management[2]	1,878	100%	100%	100%
Prophylactic Antibiotic Selection[2]	905	99%	99%	99%
Prophylactic Antibiotic Selection (Outpatient)	406	100%	97%	98%
Prophylactic Antibiotic Stopped[2]	894	97%	98%	98%
Prophylactic Antibiotic Timing[2]	906	97%	99%	99%
Prophylactic Antibiotic Timing (Outpatient)	413	94%	97%	98%
Urinary Catheter Removal[2]	591	98%	97%	97%
Survey of Patients' Hospital Experiences				
Area Around Room 'Always' Quiet at Night	300+	45%	51%	61%
Doctors 'Always' Communicated Well	300+	78%	78%	82%
Home Recovery Information Given	300+	86%	83%	85%
Hospital Given 9 or 10 on 10 Point Scale	300+	67%	68%	71%
Meds 'Always' Explained Before Given	300+	66%	61%	64%
Nurses 'Always' Communicated Well	300+	72%	74%	79%
Pain 'Always' Well Controlled	300+	69%	68%	71%
Room and Bathroom 'Always' Clean	300+	68%	70%	73%
Timely Help 'Always' Received	300+	57%	62%	68%
Would Definitely Recommend Hospital	300+	67%	70%	71%
Use of Medical Imaging				
Cardiac Imaging Stress Test before Surgery	241	2.9%	5.2%	5.3%
Combination Abdominal CT Scan	890	3.6%	13.4%	10.5%
Combination Brain/Sinus CT Scan	1,080	2.3%	2.2%	2.7%
Combination Chest CT Scan	356	0.6%	2.3%	2.7%
Follow-up Mammogram/Ultrasound	829	10.5%	8.2%	8.8%
Lumbar Spine MRI for Low Back Pain[1]	-	-	34.2%	37.2%

Fresno Heart & Surgical Hospital

15 East Audubon Drive
Fresno, CA 93720
Phone: 559-433-8000
Fax: 559-433-8125
URL: www.fresnoheart.com
Type: Acute Care Hospitals
Emergency Services: No
Ownership: Voluntary non-profit - Private
Beds: 66

Key Personnel:
CEO/President............... Wanda Holderman
Chief of Medical Staff.......... Bipin Joshi
Operating Room.............. Debi Stephen-Lesser, RN

Measure	Cases	This Hosp.	State Avg.	U.S. Avg.
Blood Clot Prevention and Treatment				
Anticoagulation Overlap Therapy[2]	11	100%	92%	93%
ICU Venous Thromboembolism Prophylaxis[2]	26	92%	92%	92%
Incidence of Potentially Preventable VTE[1,2]	-	-	11%	10%
UFH with Dosages/Platelet Monitoring[1,2]	-	-	96%	97%
Venous Thromboembolism Prophylaxis[2]	256	86%	83%	85%
Warfarin Therapy Discharge Instructions[2]	11	73%	75%	75%
Chest Pain/Possible Heart Attack Care				
Aspirin Given Within 24 Hours of Arrival[5]	-	-	97%	96%
Fibrinolytic Meds Within 30 Min. of Arrival[5]	-	-	62%	58%
Average Time to ECG (minutes)[5]	-	-	9	7
Average Time to Transfer (minutes)[5]	-	-	62	60
Children's Asthma Care				
Received Home Management Plan of Care	-	-	88%	88%
Received Reliever Medication	-	-	100%	100%
Received Systemic Corticosteroids	-	-	100%	100%
Emergency Department				
Admittance Decision Time (minutes)[2,7]	-	-	125	98
Head CT Results Within 45 Min. of Arrival[5]	-	-	55%	57%
Patients Who Left ER Before Being Seen[5]	-	-	3%	2%
Time from ER Arrival to Admit. (minutes)[2,7]	-	-	323	274
Time from ER Arrival to Discharge (minutes)[5]	-	-	168	134
Time in ER Before Being Evaluated (minutes)[5]	-	-	29	26
Time to Pain Meds for Fractures (minutes)[5]	-	-	62	57
Heart Attack Care				
Aspirin Given at Discharge[2]	37	100%	99%	99%
Fibrinolytic Meds Within 30 Min. of Arrival[2,7]	-	-	73%	54%
PCI Within 90 Minutes of Arrival[2,7]	-	-	95%	96%
Statin Prescribed at Discharge[2]	35	97%	98%	98%
Heart Failure Care				
ACE Inhibitor or ARB for LVSD[2]	15	100%	97%	97%
Discharge Instructions Given[2]	78	94%	94%	94%
Evaluation of LVS Function[2]	87	100%	99%	99%
Medicare Spending				
Medicare Spending per Patient (ratio)	-	0.99	0.98	0.98
Pneumonia Care				
Appropriate Initial Antibiotic Given[1,2]	-	-	97%	95%
Blood Culture Timing[1,2]	-	-	98%	98%
Pregnancy and Delivery Care				
Newborn Deliveries Scheduled Early[7]	-	-	5%	6%
Preventive Care				
Immunization for Influenza[2]	315	69%	89%	90%
Immunization for Pneumonia[2]	409	63%	90%	92%
Stroke Care				
Anticoagulation Therapy for Atrial Fibrillation[2,7]	-	-	95%	95%
Antithrombotic Therapy Timing[2,7]	-	-	98%	98%
Assessed for Rehabilitation[1,2]	-	-	97%	97%
Discharged on Antithrombotic Therapy[2,7]	-	-	99%	99%
Discharged on Statin Medication[1,2]	-	-	94%	94%
Thrombolytic Therapy Timing[2,7]	-	-	72%	66%
Venous Thromboembolism Prophylaxis[2,7]	-	-	94%	94%
Written Stroke Educational Materials Given[1,2]	-	-	87%	88%
Surgical Care Improvement Project				
Appropriate Beta Blocker Usage[2]	225	100%	97%	98%
Appropriate VTP Within 24 Hours[2]	229	98%	98%	98%
Controlled Postoperative Blood Glucose[2]	197	94%	96%	97%
Perioperative Temperature Management[2]	502	99%	100%	100%
Prophylactic Antibiotic Selection[2]	291	97%	99%	99%
Prophylactic Antibiotic Selection (Outpatient)	285	98%	97%	98%
Prophylactic Antibiotic Stopped[2]	284	97%	98%	98%
Prophylactic Antibiotic Timing[2]	291	99%	99%	99%
Prophylactic Antibiotic Timing (Outpatient)	285	97%	97%	98%

NOTE: Hospital profiles are in alphabetical order by state, then city, then hospital within the city; Rankings exclude hospitals with less than 25 cases except for patient surveys which excludes hospitals with less than 100 cases; (a) 100-299 cases; (1) The number of cases/patients is too few to report; (2) Data submitted were based on a sample of cases/patients; (3) Results are based on a shorter time period than required; (4) Data suppressed by CMS for one or more quarters; (5) Results are not available for this reporting period; (6) Fewer than 100 patients completed the HCAHPS survey; (7) No cases met the criteria for this measure; (8) The lower limit of the confidence interval cannot be calculated if the number of observed infections equals zero; (9) No data are available from the state/territory for this reporting period; (10) The scores shown reflect fewer than 50 completed surveys; (11) There were discrepancies in the data collection process; (12) This measure does not apply to this hospital for this reporting period; (13) Results cannot be calculated for this reporting period; (14) The results for this state are combined with nearby states to protect confidentiality; Please refer to the User's Guide for a full explanation of data.

Measure	Cases	This Hosp.	State Avg.	U.S. Avg.
Urinary Catheter Removal[2]	356	100%	97%	97%
Survey of Patients' Hospital Experiences				
Area Around Room 'Always' Quiet at Night	300+	77%	51%	61%
Doctors 'Always' Communicated Well	300+	83%	78%	82%
Home Recovery Information Given	300+	88%	83%	85%
Hospital Given 9 or 10 on 10 Point Scale	300+	86%	68%	71%
Meds 'Always' Explained Before Given	300+	68%	61%	64%
Nurses 'Always' Communicated Well	300+	84%	74%	79%
Pain 'Always' Well Controlled	300+	78%	68%	71%
Room and Bathroom 'Always' Clean	300+	80%	70%	73%
Timely Help 'Always' Received	300+	73%	62%	68%
Would Definitely Recommend Hospital	300+	87%	70%	71%
Use of Medical Imaging				
Cardiac Imaging Stress Test before Surgery[1]	-	-	5.2%	5.3%
Combination Abdominal CT Scan	127	9.4%	13.4%	10.5%
Combination Brain/Sinus CT Scan[1]	-	-	2.2%	2.7%
Combination Chest CT Scan	84	9.5%	2.3%	2.7%
Follow-up Mammogram/Ultrasound[7]	-	-	8.2%	8.8%
Lumbar Spine MRI for Low Back Pain[7]	-	-	34.2%	37.2%

Fresno Surgical Hospital

6125 North Fresno St | Phone: 559-431-8000
Fresno, CA 93710 | Fax: 559-431-8242
URL: www.fresnosurgerycenter.com
Type: Acute Care Hospitals | Emergency Services: No
Ownership: Proprietary

Key Personnel:
Radiology. . . . . Sadri Akin
Chief of Medical Staff . . . . Harry Joe, MD
Quality Assurance . . . . Kelli Johnston, RN, MHN

Measure	Cases	This Hosp.	State Avg.	U.S. Avg.
Blood Clot Prevention and Treatment				
Anticoagulation Overlap Therapy[2,7]	-	-	92%	93%
ICU Venous Thromboembolism Prophylaxis[2,7]	-	-	92%	92%
Incidence of Potentially Preventable VTE[2,7]	-	-	11%	10%
UFH with Dosages/Platelet Monitoring[2,7]	-	-	96%	97%
Venous Thromboembolism Prophylaxis[1,2]	-	-	83%	85%
Warfarin Therapy Discharge Instructions[2,7]	-	-	75%	75%
Chest Pain/Possible Heart Attack Care				
Aspirin Given Within 24 Hours of Arrival[5]	-	-	97%	96%
Fibrinolytic Meds Within 30 Min. of Arrival[5]	-	-	62%	58%
Average Time to ECG (minutes)[5]	-	-	9	7
Average Time to Transfer (minutes)[5]	-	-	62	60
Children's Asthma Care				
Received Home Management Plan of Care	-	-	88%	88%
Received Reliever Medication	-	-	100%	100%
Received Systemic Corticosteroids	-	-	100%	100%
Emergency Department				
Admittance Decision Time (minutes)[2,7]	-	-	125	98
Head CT Results Within 45 Min. of Arrival[5]	-	-	55%	57%
Patients Who Left ER Before Being Seen[5]	-	-	3%	2%
Time from ER Arrival to Admit. (minutes)[2,7]	-	-	323	274
Time from ER Arrival to Discharge (minutes)[5]	-	-	168	134
Time in ER Before Being Evaluated (minutes)[5]	-	-	29	26
Time to Pain Meds for Fractures (minutes)[5]	-	-	62	57
Heart Attack Care				
Aspirin Given at Discharge[5]	-	-	99%	99%
Fibrinolytic Meds Within 30 Min. of Arrival[5]	-	-	73%	54%
PCI Within 90 Minutes of Arrival[5]	-	-	95%	96%
Statin Prescribed at Discharge[5]	-	-	98%	98%
Heart Failure Care				
ACE Inhibitor or ARB for LVSD[5]	-	-	97%	97%
Discharge Instructions Given[5]	-	-	94%	94%
Evaluation of LVS Function[5]	-	-	99%	99%
Medicare Spending				
Medicare Spending per Patient (ratio)	-	0.86	0.98	0.98
Pneumonia Care				
Appropriate Initial Antibiotic Given[5]	-	-	97%	95%
Blood Culture Timing[5]	-	-	98%	98%
Pregnancy and Delivery Care				
Newborn Deliveries Scheduled Early[7]	-	-	5%	6%
Preventive Care				
Immunization for Influenza[2]	346	89%	89%	90%
Immunization for Pneumonia[2]	445	85%	90%	92%
Stroke Care				
Anticoagulation Therapy for Atrial Fibrillation[5]	-	-	95%	95%
Antithrombotic Therapy Timing[5]	-	-	98%	98%
Assessed for Rehabilitation[5]	-	-	97%	97%
Discharged on Antithrombotic Therapy[5]	-	-	99%	99%
Discharged on Statin Medication[5]	-	-	94%	94%
Thrombolytic Therapy Timing[5]	-	-	72%	66%
Venous Thromboembolism Prophylaxis[5]	-	-	94%	94%
Written Stroke Educational Materials Given[5]	-	-	87%	88%
Surgical Care Improvement Project				
Appropriate Beta Blocker Usage[2]	111	95%	97%	98%
Appropriate VTP Within 24 Hours[2]	324	99%	98%	98%
Controlled Postoperative Blood Glucose[2,7]	-	-	96%	97%
Perioperative Temperature Management[2]	540	99%	100%	100%
Prophylactic Antibiotic Selection[2]	468	100%	99%	99%
Prophylactic Antibiotic Selection (Outpatient)	89	92%	97%	98%
Prophylactic Antibiotic Stopped[2]	467	99%	98%	98%
Prophylactic Antibiotic Timing[2]	468	99%	99%	99%
Prophylactic Antibiotic Timing (Outpatient)	89	100%	97%	98%
Urinary Catheter Removal[2]	310	99%	97%	97%
Survey of Patients' Hospital Experiences				
Area Around Room 'Always' Quiet at Night	300+	78%	51%	61%
Doctors 'Always' Communicated Well	300+	85%	78%	82%
Home Recovery Information Given	300+	91%	83%	85%
Hospital Given 9 or 10 on 10 Point Scale	300+	85%	68%	71%
Meds 'Always' Explained Before Given	300+	72%	61%	64%
Nurses 'Always' Communicated Well	300+	87%	74%	79%
Pain 'Always' Well Controlled	300+	77%	68%	71%
Room and Bathroom 'Always' Clean	300+	84%	70%	73%
Timely Help 'Always' Received	300+	84%	62%	68%
Would Definitely Recommend Hospital	300+	89%	70%	71%
Use of Medical Imaging				
Cardiac Imaging Stress Test before Surgery[7]	-	-	5.2%	5.3%
Combination Abdominal CT Scan[7]	-	-	13.4%	10.5%
Combination Brain/Sinus CT Scan[7]	-	-	2.2%	2.7%
Combination Chest CT Scan[7]	-	-	2.3%	2.7%
Follow-up Mammogram/Ultrasound[7]	-	-	8.2%	8.8%
Lumbar Spine MRI for Low Back Pain[7]	-	-	34.2%	37.2%

Fresno VA Medical Center - VA Central California

2615 E. Clinton Avenue | Phone: 559-228-5338
Fresno, CA 93703 | Fax: 559-228-6903
URL: www1.va.gov/directory/guide
Type: Acute Care - VA | Emergency Services: No
Ownership: Government Federal | Beds: 157

Key Personnel:
Intensive Care Unit. . . . . Rhonda Eisenzimmer
Operating Room. . . . . Mike Enquist
Anesthesiology. . . . . Michael Gattey, MD
Chief of Medical Staff . . . . Paul Goebel, MD
Infection Control . . . . William Hamilton
CEO/President. . . . . Alan S Perry
Quality Assurance . . . . Jack Shantz, RN
Ambulatory Care . . . . Don Taylor, MD

Measure	Cases	This Hosp.	State Avg.	U.S. Avg.
Blood Clot Prevention and Treatment				
Anticoagulation Overlap Therapy	-	-	92%	93%
ICU Venous Thromboembolism Prophylaxis	-	-	92%	92%
Incidence of Potentially Preventable VTE	-	-	11%	10%
UFH with Dosages/Platelet Monitoring	-	-	96%	97%
Venous Thromboembolism Prophylaxis	-	-	83%	85%
Warfarin Therapy Discharge Instructions	-	-	75%	75%
Chest Pain/Possible Heart Attack Care				
Aspirin Given Within 24 Hours of Arrival	-	-	97%	96%
Fibrinolytic Meds Within 30 Min. of Arrival	-	-	62%	58%
Average Time to ECG (minutes)	-	-	9	7
Average Time to Transfer (minutes)	-	-	62	60
Children's Asthma Care				
Received Home Management Plan of Care	-	-	88%	88%
Received Reliever Medication	-	-	100%	100%
Received Systemic Corticosteroids	-	-	100%	100%
Emergency Department				
Admittance Decision Time (minutes)	-	-	125	98
Head CT Results Within 45 Min. of Arrival	-	-	55%	57%
Patients Who Left ER Before Being Seen	-	-	3%	2%
Time from ER Arrival to Admit. (minutes)	-	-	323	274
Time from ER Arrival to Discharge (minutes)	-	-	168	134
Time in ER Before Being Evaluated (minutes)	-	-	29	26
Time to Pain Meds for Fractures (minutes)	-	-	62	57
Heart Attack Care				
Aspirin Given at Discharge[1]	13	100%	99%	99%
Fibrinolytic Meds Within 30 Min. of Arrival[5]	-	-	73%	54%
PCI Within 90 Minutes of Arrival[5]	-	-	95%	96%
Statin Prescribed at Discharge[1]	12	100%	98%	98%
Heart Failure Care				
ACE Inhibitor or ARB for LVSD	69	100%	97%	97%
Discharge Instructions Given	125	97%	94%	94%
Evaluation of LVS Function	141	100%	99%	99%
Medicare Spending				
Medicare Spending per Patient (ratio)	-	-	0.98	0.98
Pneumonia Care				
Appropriate Initial Antibiotic Given	52	100%	97%	95%
Blood Culture Timing	99	99%	98%	98%
Pregnancy and Delivery Care				
Newborn Deliveries Scheduled Early	-	-	5%	6%
Preventive Care				
Immunization for Influenza[5]	-	-	89%	90%
Immunization for Pneumonia[5]	-	-	90%	92%
Stroke Care				
Anticoagulation Therapy for Atrial Fibrillation	-	-	95%	95%
Antithrombotic Therapy Timing	-	-	98%	98%
Assessed for Rehabilitation	-	-	97%	97%
Discharged on Antithrombotic Therapy	-	-	99%	99%
Discharged on Statin Medication	-	-	94%	94%
Thrombolytic Therapy Timing	-	-	72%	66%
Venous Thromboembolism Prophylaxis	-	-	94%	94%
Written Stroke Educational Materials Given	-	-	87%	88%
Surgical Care Improvement Project				
Appropriate Beta Blocker Usage[2]	29	100%	97%	98%
Appropriate VTP Within 24 Hours[2]	59	95%	98%	98%
Controlled Postoperative Blood Glucose[5]	-	-	96%	97%
Perioperative Temperature Management[2]	66	95%	100%	100%
Prophylactic Antibiotic Selection[1]	21	95%	99%	99%
Prophylactic Antibiotic Selection (Outpatient)	-	-	97%	98%
Prophylactic Antibiotic Stopped[1]	18	78%	98%	98%
Prophylactic Antibiotic Timing[1]	21	86%	99%	99%
Prophylactic Antibiotic Timing (Outpatient)	-	-	97%	98%
Urinary Catheter Removal[2]	40	88%	97%	97%
Survey of Patients' Hospital Experiences				
Area Around Room 'Always' Quiet at Night	-	-	51%	61%
Doctors 'Always' Communicated Well	-	-	78%	82%
Home Recovery Information Given	-	-	83%	85%
Hospital Given 9 or 10 on 10 Point Scale	-	-	68%	71%
Meds 'Always' Explained Before Given	-	-	61%	64%
Nurses 'Always' Communicated Well	-	-	74%	79%
Pain 'Always' Well Controlled	-	-	68%	71%
Room and Bathroom 'Always' Clean	-	-	70%	73%
Timely Help 'Always' Received	-	-	62%	68%
Would Definitely Recommend Hospital	-	-	70%	71%
Use of Medical Imaging				
Cardiac Imaging Stress Test before Surgery	-	-	5.2%	5.3%
Combination Abdominal CT Scan	-	-	13.4%	10.5%
Combination Brain/Sinus CT Scan	-	-	2.2%	2.7%
Combination Chest CT Scan	-	-	2.3%	2.7%
Follow-up Mammogram/Ultrasound	-	-	8.2%	8.8%
Lumbar Spine MRI for Low Back Pain	-	-	34.2%	37.2%

Kaiser Foundation Hospital - Fresno

7300 North Fresno St | Phone: 559-448-4500
Fresno, CA 93720
URL: www.kaiserpermanente.org
Type: Acute Care Hospitals | Emergency Services: Yes
Ownership: Voluntary non-profit - Private | Beds: 169

Measure	Cases	This Hosp.	State Avg.	U.S. Avg.
Blood Clot Prevention and Treatment				

NOTE: Hospital profiles are in alphabetical order by state, then city, then hospital within the city; Rankings exclude hospitals with less than 25 cases except for patient surveys which excludes hospitals with less than 100 cases; (a) 100-299 cases; (1) The number of cases/patients is too few to report; (2) Data submitted were based on a sample of cases/patients; (3) Results are based on a shorter time period than required; (4) Data suppressed by CMS for one or more quarters; (5) Results are not available for this reporting period; (6) Fewer than 100 patients completed the HCAHPS survey; (7) No cases met the criteria for this measure; (8) The lower limit of the confidence interval cannot be calculated if the number of observed infections equals zero; (9) No data are available from the state/territory for this reporting period; (10) The scores shown reflect fewer than 50 completed surveys; (11) There were discrepancies in the data collection process; (12) This measure does not apply to this hospital for this reporting period; (13) Results cannot be calculated for this reporting period; (14) The results for this state are combined with nearby states to protect confidentiality; Please refer to the User's Guide for a full explanation of data.

Measure	Cases	This Hosp.	State Avg.	U.S. Avg.
Anticoagulation Overlap Therapy[2]	51	100%	92%	93%
ICU Venous Thromboembolism Prophylaxis[2]	49	100%	92%	92%
Incidence of Potentially Preventable VTE[1,2]	-	-	11%	10%
UFH with Dosages/Platelet Monitoring[2]	11	100%	96%	97%
Venous Thromboembolism Prophylaxis[2]	326	95%	83%	85%
Warfarin Therapy Discharge Instructions[2]	55	62%	75%	75%
Chest Pain/Possible Heart Attack Care				
Aspirin Given Within 24 Hours of Arrival	-	-	97%	96%
Fibrinolytic Meds Within 30 Min. of Arrival	-	-	62%	58%
Average Time to ECG (minutes)	-	-	9	7
Average Time to Transfer (minutes)	-	-	62	60
Children's Asthma Care				
Received Home Management Plan of Care	-	-	88%	88%
Received Reliever Medication	-	-	100%	100%
Received Systemic Corticosteroids	-	-	100%	100%
Emergency Department				
Admittance Decision Time (minutes)[2]	652	52	125	98
Head CT Results Within 45 Min. of Arrival	-	-	55%	57%
Patients Who Left ER Before Being Seen	-	-	3%	2%
Time from ER Arrival to Admit. (minutes)[2]	657	290	323	274
Time from ER Arrival to Discharge (minutes)	-	-	168	134
Time in ER Before Being Evaluated (minutes)	-	-	29	26
Time to Pain Meds for Fractures (minutes)	-	-	62	57
Heart Attack Care				
Aspirin Given at Discharge	77	100%	99%	99%
Fibrinolytic Meds Within 30 Min. of Arrival[7]	-	-	73%	54%
PCI Within 90 Minutes of Arrival[7]	-	-	95%	96%
Statin Prescribed at Discharge	74	99%	98%	98%
Heart Failure Care				
ACE Inhibitor or ARB for LVSD[2]	71	100%	97%	97%
Discharge Instructions Given[2]	186	100%	94%	94%
Evaluation of LVS Function[2]	197	100%	99%	99%
Medicare Spending				
Medicare Spending per Patient (ratio)	-	0.71	0.98	0.98
Pneumonia Care				
Appropriate Initial Antibiotic Given[2]	84	100%	97%	95%
Blood Culture Timing[2]	138	93%	98%	98%
Pregnancy and Delivery Care				
Newborn Deliveries Scheduled Early[2]	27	4%	5%	6%
Preventive Care				
Immunization for Influenza[2]	519	94%	89%	90%
Immunization for Pneumonia[2]	698	97%	90%	92%
Stroke Care				
Anticoagulation Therapy for Atrial Fibrillation[2]	15	73%	95%	95%
Antithrombotic Therapy Timing[2]	78	99%	98%	98%
Assessed for Rehabilitation[2]	108	99%	97%	97%
Discharged on Antithrombotic Therapy[2]	92	98%	99%	99%
Discharged on Statin Medication[2]	75	97%	94%	94%
Thrombolytic Therapy Timing[1,2]	-	-	72%	66%
Venous Thromboembolism Prophylaxis[2]	90	99%	94%	94%
Written Stroke Educational Materials Given[2]	71	96%	87%	88%
Surgical Care Improvement Project				
Appropriate Beta Blocker Usage[2]	160	98%	97%	98%
Appropriate VTP Within 24 Hours[2]	334	100%	98%	98%
Controlled Postoperative Blood Glucose[2,7]	-	-	96%	97%
Perioperative Temperature Management[2]	395	100%	100%	100%
Prophylactic Antibiotic Selection[2]	250	100%	99%	99%
Prophylactic Antibiotic Selection (Outpatient)	-	-	97%	98%
Prophylactic Antibiotic Stopped[2]	250	100%	98%	98%
Prophylactic Antibiotic Timing[2]	250	100%	99%	99%
Prophylactic Antibiotic Timing (Outpatient)	-	-	97%	98%
Urinary Catheter Removal[2]	314	99%	97%	97%
Survey of Patients' Hospital Experiences				
Area Around Room 'Always' Quiet at Night	300+	51%	51%	61%
Doctors 'Always' Communicated Well	300+	82%	78%	82%
Home Recovery Information Given	300+	87%	83%	85%
Hospital Given 9 or 10 on 10 Point Scale	300+	77%	68%	71%
Meds 'Always' Explained Before Given	300+	63%	61%	64%
Nurses 'Always' Communicated Well	300+	78%	74%	79%
Pain 'Always' Well Controlled	300+	76%	68%	71%
Room and Bathroom 'Always' Clean	300+	73%	70%	73%
Timely Help 'Always' Received	300+	65%	62%	68%
Would Definitely Recommend Hospital	300+	80%	70%	71%
Use of Medical Imaging				
Cardiac Imaging Stress Test before Surgery	-	-	5.2%	5.3%
Combination Abdominal CT Scan	-	-	13.4%	10.5%
Combination Brain/Sinus CT Scan	-	-	2.2%	2.7%
Combination Chest CT Scan	-	-	2.3%	2.7%
Follow-up Mammogram/Ultrasound	-	-	8.2%	8.8%
Lumbar Spine MRI for Low Back Pain	-	-	34.2%	37.2%

Saint Agnes Medical Center

1303 E Herndon Ave
Fresno, CA 93710
Phone: 559-450-3000
URL: www.samc.com
Type: Acute Care Hospitals
Ownership: Voluntary non-profit - Church
Emergency Services: Yes
Beds: 330

Measure	Cases	This Hosp.	State Avg.	U.S. Avg.
Blood Clot Prevention and Treatment				
Anticoagulation Overlap Therapy[2]	109	71%	92%	93%
ICU Venous Thromboembolism Prophylaxis[2]	71	87%	92%	92%
Incidence of Potentially Preventable VTE[2]	11	27%	11%	10%
UFH with Dosages/Platelet Monitoring[2]	15	73%	96%	97%
Venous Thromboembolism Prophylaxis[2]	379	72%	83%	85%
Warfarin Therapy Discharge Instructions[2]	82	54%	75%	75%
Chest Pain/Possible Heart Attack Care				
Aspirin Given Within 24 Hours of Arrival[1,3]	-	-	97%	96%
Fibrinolytic Meds Within 30 Min. of Arrival[5]	-	-	62%	58%
Average Time to ECG (minutes)[1,3]	-	-	9	7
Average Time to Transfer (minutes)[5]	-	-	62	60
Children's Asthma Care				
Received Home Management Plan of Care	-	-	88%	88%
Received Reliever Medication	-	-	100%	100%
Received Systemic Corticosteroids	-	-	100%	100%
Emergency Department				
Admittance Decision Time (minutes)[2]	611	101	125	98
Head CT Results Within 45 Min. of Arrival	24	29%	55%	57%
Patients Who Left ER Before Being Seen	37,349	7%	3%	2%
Time from ER Arrival to Admit. (minutes)[2]	620	325	323	274
Time from ER Arrival to Discharge (minutes)	398	224	168	134
Time in ER Before Being Evaluated (minutes)	423	81	29	26
Time to Pain Meds for Fractures (minutes)	180	94	62	57
Heart Attack Care				
Aspirin Given at Discharge	370	98%	99%	99%
Fibrinolytic Meds Within 30 Min. of Arrival[7]	-	-	73%	54%
PCI Within 90 Minutes of Arrival	77	99%	95%	96%
Statin Prescribed at Discharge	360	97%	98%	98%
Heart Failure Care				
ACE Inhibitor or ARB for LVSD[2]	146	99%	97%	97%
Discharge Instructions Given[2]	362	97%	94%	94%
Evaluation of LVS Function[2]	427	100%	99%	99%
Medicare Spending				
Medicare Spending per Patient (ratio)	-	1.00	0.98	0.98
Pneumonia Care				
Appropriate Initial Antibiotic Given[2]	153	97%	97%	95%
Blood Culture Timing[2]	187	98%	98%	98%
Pregnancy and Delivery Care				
Newborn Deliveries Scheduled Early[2]	115	0%	5%	6%
Preventive Care				
Immunization for Influenza[2]	538	88%	89%	90%
Immunization for Pneumonia[2]	690	88%	90%	92%
Stroke Care				
Anticoagulation Therapy for Atrial Fibrillation[2]	25	88%	95%	95%
Antithrombotic Therapy Timing[2]	121	96%	98%	98%
Assessed for Rehabilitation[2]	142	98%	97%	97%
Discharged on Antithrombotic Therapy[2]	133	98%	99%	99%
Discharged on Statin Medication[2]	96	91%	94%	94%
Thrombolytic Therapy Timing[1,2]	-	-	72%	66%
Venous Thromboembolism Prophylaxis[2]	139	90%	94%	94%
Written Stroke Educational Materials Given[2]	77	87%	87%	88%
Surgical Care Improvement Project				
Appropriate Beta Blocker Usage[2]	259	95%	97%	98%
Appropriate VTP Within 24 Hours[2]	547	92%	98%	98%
Controlled Postoperative Blood Glucose[2]	182	100%	96%	97%
Perioperative Temperature Management[2]	728	99%	100%	100%
Prophylactic Antibiotic Selection[2]	506	99%	99%	99%
Prophylactic Antibiotic Selection (Outpatient)	398	95%	97%	98%
Prophylactic Antibiotic Stopped[2]	490	97%	98%	98%
Prophylactic Antibiotic Timing[2]	507	100%	99%	99%
Prophylactic Antibiotic Timing (Outpatient)	401	97%	97%	98%
Urinary Catheter Removal[2]	440	93%	97%	97%
Survey of Patients' Hospital Experiences				
Area Around Room 'Always' Quiet at Night	300+	59%	51%	61%
Doctors 'Always' Communicated Well	300+	79%	78%	82%
Home Recovery Information Given	300+	85%	83%	85%
Hospital Given 9 or 10 on 10 Point Scale	300+	71%	68%	71%
Meds 'Always' Explained Before Given	300+	56%	61%	64%
Nurses 'Always' Communicated Well	300+	75%	74%	79%
Pain 'Always' Well Controlled	300+	69%	68%	71%
Room and Bathroom 'Always' Clean	300+	68%	70%	73%
Timely Help 'Always' Received	300+	61%	62%	68%
Would Definitely Recommend Hospital	300+	73%	70%	71%
Use of Medical Imaging				
Cardiac Imaging Stress Test before Surgery	297	5.4%	5.2%	5.3%
Combination Abdominal CT Scan	1,629	3.7%	13.4%	10.5%
Combination Brain/Sinus CT Scan	1,754	1.5%	2.2%	2.7%
Combination Chest CT Scan	774	0.0%	2.3%	2.7%
Follow-up Mammogram/Ultrasound	3,126	9.9%	8.2%	8.8%
Lumbar Spine MRI for Low Back Pain	82	36.6%	34.2%	37.2%

Saint Jude Medical Center

101 E Valencia Mesa Drive
Fullerton, CA 92835
Phone: 714-992-3000
Fax: 714-992-3029
URL: www.stjudemedicalcenter.org
Type: Acute Care Hospitals
Ownership: Voluntary non-profit - Church
Emergency Services: Yes
Beds: 347

Key Personnel:

Operating Room. . . . . Deborah Butler, RN
Pediatric Ambulatory Care . . . . . . Dan Chiles, MD
Pediatric In-Patient Care . . . . Dan Chiles, MD
CEO/President. . . . . Robert J Fraschetti
Emergency Room . . . . Janet Magnani, RN
Radiology. . . . . Robert Morten, MD
Chief of Medical Staff . . . . Mark Song
Quality Assurance . . . . Pat Wardell

Measure	Cases	This Hosp.	State Avg.	U.S. Avg.
Blood Clot Prevention and Treatment				
Anticoagulation Overlap Therapy[2]	78	92%	92%	93%
ICU Venous Thromboembolism Prophylaxis[2]	98	97%	92%	92%
Incidence of Potentially Preventable VTE[1,2]	-	-	11%	10%
UFH with Dosages/Platelet Monitoring[2]	37	100%	96%	97%
Venous Thromboembolism Prophylaxis[2]	262	82%	83%	85%
Warfarin Therapy Discharge Instructions[2]	47	34%	75%	75%
Chest Pain/Possible Heart Attack Care				
Aspirin Given Within 24 Hours of Arrival	44	98%	97%	96%
Fibrinolytic Meds Within 30 Min. of Arrival[3,7]	-	-	62%	58%
Average Time to ECG (minutes)	52	0	9	7
Average Time to Transfer (minutes)[3,7]	-	-	62	60
Children's Asthma Care				
Received Home Management Plan of Care	-	-	88%	88%
Received Reliever Medication	-	-	100%	100%
Received Systemic Corticosteroids	-	-	100%	100%
Emergency Department				
Admittance Decision Time (minutes)[2]	485	101	125	98
Head CT Results Within 45 Min. of Arrival	19	79%	55%	57%
Patients Who Left ER Before Being Seen	61,664	2%	3%	2%
Time from ER Arrival to Admit. (minutes)[2]	516	270	323	274
Time from ER Arrival to Discharge (minutes)	328	158	168	134
Time in ER Before Being Evaluated (minutes)	403	29	29	26
Time to Pain Meds for Fractures (minutes)	341	53	62	57
Heart Attack Care				
Aspirin Given at Discharge[2]	263	100%	99%	99%
Fibrinolytic Meds Within 30 Min. of Arrival[2,7]	-	-	73%	54%
PCI Within 90 Minutes of Arrival[2]	67	97%	95%	96%
Statin Prescribed at Discharge[2]	272	99%	98%	98%
Heart Failure Care				
ACE Inhibitor or ARB for LVSD[2]	123	87%	97%	97%
Discharge Instructions Given[2]	249	91%	94%	94%

NOTE: Hospital profiles are in alphabetical order by state, then city, then hospital within the city; Rankings exclude hospitals with less than 25 cases except for patient surveys which excludes hospitals with less than 100 cases; (a) 100-299 cases; (1) The number of cases/patients is too few to report; (2) Data submitted were based on a sample of cases/patients; (3) Results are based on a shorter time period than required; (4) Data suppressed by CMS for one or more quarters; (5) Results are not available for this reporting period; (6) Fewer than 100 patients completed the HCAHPS survey; (7) No cases met the criteria for this measure; (8) The lower limit of the confidence interval cannot be calculated if the number of observed infections equals zero; (9) No data are available from the state/territory for this reporting period; (10) The scores shown reflect fewer than 50 completed surveys; (11) There were discrepancies in the data collection process; (12) This measure does not apply to this hospital for this reporting period; (13) Results cannot be calculated for this reporting period; (14) The results for this state are combined with nearby states to protect confidentiality; Please refer to the User's Guide for a full explanation of data.

Evaluation of LVS Function[2]	336	99%	99%	99%
Medicare Spending				
Medicare Spending per Patient (ratio)	-	1.05	0.98	0.98
Pneumonia Care				
Appropriate Initial Antibiotic Given[2]	102	96%	97%	95%
Blood Culture Timing[2]	190	97%	98%	98%
Pregnancy and Delivery Care				
Newborn Deliveries Scheduled Early[2]	47	0%	5%	6%
Preventive Care				
Immunization for Influenza[2]	511	75%	89%	90%
Immunization for Pneumonia[2]	689	84%	90%	92%
Stroke Care				
Anticoagulation Therapy for Atrial Fibrillation	40	98%	95%	95%
Antithrombotic Therapy Timing	168	98%	98%	98%
Assessed for Rehabilitation	252	100%	97%	97%
Discharged on Antithrombotic Therapy	201	100%	99%	99%
Discharged on Statin Medication	164	98%	94%	94%
Thrombolytic Therapy Timing	57	100%	72%	66%
Venous Thromboembolism Prophylaxis	273	99%	94%	94%
Written Stroke Educational Materials Given	113	97%	87%	88%
Surgical Care Improvement Project				
Appropriate Beta Blocker Usage[2]	126	92%	97%	98%
Appropriate VTP Within 24 Hours[2]	390	98%	98%	98%
Controlled Postoperative Blood Glucose[2]	98	100%	96%	97%
Perioperative Temperature Management[2]	481	100%	100%	100%
Prophylactic Antibiotic Selection[2]	408	99%	99%	99%
Prophylactic Antibiotic Selection (Outpatient)	533	98%	97%	98%
Prophylactic Antibiotic Stopped[2]	398	99%	98%	98%
Prophylactic Antibiotic Timing[2]	409	98%	99%	99%
Prophylactic Antibiotic Timing (Outpatient)	537	99%	97%	98%
Urinary Catheter Removal[2]	285	99%	97%	97%
Survey of Patients' Hospital Experiences				
Area Around Room 'Always' Quiet at Night	300+	48%	51%	61%
Doctors 'Always' Communicated Well	300+	76%	78%	82%
Home Recovery Information Given	300+	86%	83%	85%
Hospital Given 9 or 10 on 10 Point Scale	300+	77%	68%	71%
Meds 'Always' Explained Before Given	300+	58%	61%	64%
Nurses 'Always' Communicated Well	300+	72%	74%	79%
Pain 'Always' Well Controlled	300+	66%	68%	71%
Room and Bathroom 'Always' Clean	300+	71%	70%	73%
Timely Help 'Always' Received	300+	59%	62%	68%
Would Definitely Recommend Hospital	300+	81%	70%	71%
Use of Medical Imaging				
Cardiac Imaging Stress Test before Surgery	282	5.3%	5.2%	5.3%
Combination Abdominal CT Scan	1,588	40.2%	13.4%	10.5%
Combination Brain/Sinus CT Scan	1,436	1.6%	2.2%	2.7%
Combination Chest CT Scan	1,144	2.0%	2.3%	2.7%
Follow-up Mammogram/Ultrasound	3,217	5.0%	8.2%	8.8%
Lumbar Spine MRI for Low Back Pain	231	25.5%	34.2%	37.2%

Jerold Phelps Community Hospital

733 Cedar St
Garberville, CA 95542
Phone: 707-923-3921
Fax: 707-923-9352
E-mail: shchadmin@asis.com
URL: www.shchd.org
Type: Critical Access Hospitals
Emergency Services: Yes
Ownership: Govt - Hospital Dist/Auth
Beds: 9

Key Personnel:

Quality Assurance . . . . Kari Barker, RN
Chief of Medical Staff . . . . Jerold Phelps
President . . . . Barbara Truitt

Measure	Cases	This Hosp.	State Avg.	U.S. Avg.
Blood Clot Prevention and Treatment				
Anticoagulation Overlap Therapy[5]	-	-	92%	93%
ICU Venous Thromboembolism Prophylaxis[5]	-	-	92%	92%
Incidence of Potentially Preventable VTE[5]	-	-	11%	10%
UFH with Dosages/Platelet Monitoring[5]	-	-	96%	97%
Venous Thromboembolism Prophylaxis[5]	-	-	83%	85%
Warfarin Therapy Discharge Instructions[5]	-	-	75%	75%
Chest Pain/Possible Heart Attack Care				
Aspirin Given Within 24 Hours of Arrival	-	-	97%	96%
Fibrinolytic Meds Within 30 Min. of Arrival	-	-	62%	58%
Average Time to ECG (minutes)	-	-	9	7
Average Time to Transfer (minutes)	-	-	62	60
Children's Asthma Care				
Received Home Management Plan of Care	-	-	88%	88%
Received Reliever Medication	-	-	100%	100%
Received Systemic Corticosteroids	-	-	100%	100%
Emergency Department				
Admittance Decision Time (minutes)[5]	-	-	125	98
Head CT Results Within 45 Min. of Arrival	-	-	55%	57%
Patients Who Left ER Before Being Seen	-	-	3%	2%
Time from ER Arrival to Admit. (minutes)[5]	-	-	323	274
Time from ER Arrival to Discharge (minutes)	-	-	168	134
Time in ER Before Being Evaluated (minutes)	-	-	29	26
Time to Pain Meds for Fractures (minutes)	-	-	62	57
Heart Attack Care				
Aspirin Given at Discharge[5]	-	-	99%	99%
Fibrinolytic Meds Within 30 Min. of Arrival[5]	-	-	73%	54%
PCI Within 90 Minutes of Arrival[5]	-	-	95%	96%
Statin Prescribed at Discharge[5]	-	-	98%	98%
Heart Failure Care				
ACE Inhibitor or ARB for LVSD[5]	-	-	97%	97%
Discharge Instructions Given[5]	-	-	94%	94%
Evaluation of LVS Function[5]	-	-	99%	99%
Medicare Spending				
Medicare Spending per Patient (ratio)	-	-	0.98	0.98
Pneumonia Care				
Appropriate Initial Antibiotic Given[5]	-	-	97%	95%
Blood Culture Timing[5]	-	-	98%	98%
Pregnancy and Delivery Care				
Newborn Deliveries Scheduled Early[5]	-	-	5%	6%
Preventive Care				
Immunization for Influenza[5]	-	-	89%	90%
Immunization for Pneumonia[5]	-	-	90%	92%
Stroke Care				
Anticoagulation Therapy for Atrial Fibrillation[5]	-	-	95%	95%
Antithrombotic Therapy Timing[5]	-	-	98%	98%
Assessed for Rehabilitation[5]	-	-	97%	97%
Discharged on Antithrombotic Therapy[5]	-	-	99%	99%
Discharged on Statin Medication[5]	-	-	94%	94%
Thrombolytic Therapy Timing[5]	-	-	72%	66%
Venous Thromboembolism Prophylaxis[5]	-	-	94%	94%
Written Stroke Educational Materials Given[5]	-	-	87%	88%
Surgical Care Improvement Project				
Appropriate Beta Blocker Usage[5]	-	-	97%	98%
Appropriate VTP Within 24 Hours[5]	-	-	98%	98%
Controlled Postoperative Blood Glucose[5]	-	-	96%	97%
Perioperative Temperature Management[5]	-	-	100%	100%
Prophylactic Antibiotic Selection[5]	-	-	99%	99%
Prophylactic Antibiotic Selection (Outpatient)	-	-	97%	98%
Prophylactic Antibiotic Stopped[5]	-	-	98%	98%
Prophylactic Antibiotic Timing[5]	-	-	99%	99%
Prophylactic Antibiotic Timing (Outpatient)	-	-	97%	98%
Urinary Catheter Removal[5]	-	-	97%	97%
Survey of Patients' Hospital Experiences				
Area Around Room 'Always' Quiet at Night[5]	-	-	51%	61%
Doctors 'Always' Communicated Well[5]	-	-	78%	82%
Home Recovery Information Given[5]	-	-	83%	85%
Hospital Given 9 or 10 on 10 Point Scale[5]	-	-	68%	71%
Meds 'Always' Explained Before Given[5]	-	-	61%	64%
Nurses 'Always' Communicated Well[5]	-	-	74%	79%
Pain 'Always' Well Controlled[5]	-	-	68%	71%
Room and Bathroom 'Always' Clean[5]	-	-	70%	73%
Timely Help 'Always' Received[5]	-	-	62%	68%
Would Definitely Recommend Hospital[5]	-	-	70%	71%
Use of Medical Imaging				
Cardiac Imaging Stress Test before Surgery	-	-	5.2%	5.3%
Combination Abdominal CT Scan	-	-	13.4%	10.5%
Combination Brain/Sinus CT Scan	-	-	2.2%	2.7%
Combination Chest CT Scan	-	-	2.3%	2.7%
Follow-up Mammogram/Ultrasound	-	-	8.2%	8.8%
Lumbar Spine MRI for Low Back Pain	-	-	34.2%	37.2%

Garden Grove Hospital & Medical Center

12601 Garden Grove Blvd
Garden Grove, CA 92843
Phone: 714-537-5160
Fax: 714-741-3332
URL: www.gardengrovehospital.com
Type: Acute Care Hospitals
Emergency Services: Yes
Ownership: Proprietary
Beds: 167

Key Personnel:

Cardiac Laboratory. . . . . Ed Barrus
Infection Control. . . . . Jose Cartagener
CEO/President. . . . . Maxine Cooper
Chief of Medical Staff . . . . H. Joseph Khan, MD
Operating Room. . . . . Andrea Meh
Quality Assurance . . . . Corine Morales
Pediatric Ambulatory Care . . . . . . Jacob Sweidan, MD
Pediatric In-Patient Care . . . . Jacob Sweidan, MD

Measure	Cases	This Hosp.	State Avg.	U.S. Avg.
Blood Clot Prevention and Treatment				
Anticoagulation Overlap Therapy[2]	21	100%	92%	93%
ICU Venous Thromboembolism Prophylaxis[2]	60	97%	92%	92%
Incidence of Potentially Preventable VTE[2,7]	-	-	11%	10%
UFH with Dosages/Platelet Monitoring[1,2]	-	-	96%	97%
Venous Thromboembolism Prophylaxis[2]	355	97%	83%	85%
Warfarin Therapy Discharge Instructions[2]	11	100%	75%	75%
Chest Pain/Possible Heart Attack Care				
Aspirin Given Within 24 Hours of Arrival	49	100%	97%	96%
Fibrinolytic Meds Within 30 Min. of Arrival[7]	-	-	62%	58%
Average Time to ECG (minutes)	48	14	9	7
Average Time to Transfer (minutes)[1]	-	-	62	60
Children's Asthma Care				
Received Home Management Plan of Care	-	-	88%	88%
Received Reliever Medication	-	-	100%	100%
Received Systemic Corticosteroids	-	-	100%	100%
Emergency Department				
Admittance Decision Time (minutes)[2]	602	106	125	98
Head CT Results Within 45 Min. of Arrival[1]	-	-	55%	57%
Patients Who Left ER Before Being Seen	27,212	1%	3%	2%
Time from ER Arrival to Admit. (minutes)[2]	602	260	323	274
Time from ER Arrival to Discharge (minutes)	420	160	168	134
Time in ER Before Being Evaluated (minutes)	470	31	29	26
Time to Pain Meds for Fractures (minutes)	122	74	62	57
Heart Attack Care				
Aspirin Given at Discharge	20	100%	99%	99%
Fibrinolytic Meds Within 30 Min. of Arrival[7]	-	-	73%	54%
PCI Within 90 Minutes of Arrival[7]	-	-	95%	96%
Statin Prescribed at Discharge	15	100%	98%	98%
Heart Failure Care				
ACE Inhibitor or ARB for LVSD	28	100%	97%	97%
Discharge Instructions Given	66	100%	94%	94%
Evaluation of LVS Function	93	100%	99%	99%
Medicare Spending				
Medicare Spending per Patient (ratio)	-	1.12	0.98	0.98
Pneumonia Care				
Appropriate Initial Antibiotic Given	72	100%	97%	95%
Blood Culture Timing	169	100%	98%	98%
Pregnancy and Delivery Care				
Newborn Deliveries Scheduled Early[2]	42	5%	5%	6%
Preventive Care				
Immunization for Influenza[2]	440	100%	89%	90%
Immunization for Pneumonia[2]	443	100%	90%	92%
Stroke Care				
Anticoagulation Therapy for Atrial Fibrillation[1]	-	-	95%	95%
Antithrombotic Therapy Timing	25	100%	98%	98%
Assessed for Rehabilitation	34	100%	97%	97%
Discharged on Antithrombotic Therapy	29	100%	99%	99%
Discharged on Statin Medication	15	100%	94%	94%
Thrombolytic Therapy Timing[7]	-	-	72%	66%
Venous Thromboembolism Prophylaxis	32	94%	94%	94%
Written Stroke Educational Materials Given	21	100%	87%	88%
Surgical Care Improvement Project				
Appropriate Beta Blocker Usage	31	100%	97%	98%
Appropriate VTP Within 24 Hours	154	100%	98%	98%
Controlled Postoperative Blood Glucose[7]	-	-	96%	97%
Perioperative Temperature Management	179	100%	100%	100%
Prophylactic Antibiotic Selection	88	100%	99%	99%

NOTE: Hospital profiles are in alphabetical order by state, then city, then hospital within the city; Rankings exclude hospitals with less than 25 cases except for patient surveys which excludes hospitals with less than 100 cases; (a) 100-299 cases; (1) The number of cases/patients is too few to report; (2) Data submitted were based on a sample of cases/patients; (3) Results are based on a shorter time period than required; (4) Data suppressed by CMS for one or more quarters; (5) Results are not available for this reporting period; (6) Fewer than 100 patients completed the HCAHPS survey; (7) No cases met the criteria for this measure; (8) The lower limit of the confidence interval cannot be calculated if the number of observed infections equals zero; (9) No data are available from the state/territory for this reporting period; (10) The scores shown reflect fewer than 50 completed surveys; (11) There were discrepancies in the data collection process; (12) This measure does not apply to this hospital for this reporting period; (13) Results cannot be calculated for this reporting period; (14) The results for this state are combined with nearby states to protect confidentiality; Please refer to the User's Guide for a full explanation of data.

Measure	Cases	This Hosp.	State Avg.	U.S. Avg.
Prophylactic Antibiotic Selection (Outpatient)	24	100%	97%	98%
Prophylactic Antibiotic Stopped	88	100%	98%	98%
Prophylactic Antibiotic Timing	88	100%	99%	99%
Prophylactic Antibiotic Timing (Outpatient)	24	96%	97%	98%
Urinary Catheter Removal	21	100%	97%	97%
Survey of Patients' Hospital Experiences				
Area Around Room 'Always' Quiet at Night[11]	300+	46%	51%	61%
Doctors 'Always' Communicated Well[11]	300+	72%	78%	82%
Home Recovery Information Given[11]	300+	82%	83%	85%
Hospital Given 9 or 10 on 10 Point Scale[11]	300+	61%	68%	71%
Meds 'Always' Explained Before Given[11]	300+	50%	61%	64%
Nurses 'Always' Communicated Well[11]	300+	65%	74%	79%
Pain 'Always' Well Controlled[11]	300+	62%	68%	71%
Room and Bathroom 'Always' Clean[11]	300+	64%	70%	73%
Timely Help 'Always' Received[11]	300+	54%	62%	68%
Would Definitely Recommend Hospital[11]	300+	62%	70%	71%
Use of Medical Imaging				
Cardiac Imaging Stress Test before Surgery[1]	-	-	5.2%	5.3%
Combination Abdominal CT Scan	164	20.7%	13.4%	10.5%
Combination Brain/Sinus CT Scan[1]	-	-	2.2%	2.7%
Combination Chest CT Scan[1]	-	-	2.3%	2.7%
Follow-up Mammogram/Ultrasound[7]	-	-	8.2%	8.8%
Lumbar Spine MRI for Low Back Pain[7]	-	-	34.2%	37.2%

Memorial Hospital of Gardena

1145 W Redondo Beach Blvd
Gardena, CA 90247
URL: www.avantihospitals.com
Type: Acute Care Hospitals
Ownership: Proprietary

Phone: 310-532-4200
Fax: 310-538-6680
Emergency Services: Yes
Beds: 180

Key Personnel:
Chief of Medical Staff. . . . . Alfonso Bayz
Emergency Room . . . . Sammy Chan
Operating Room. . . . . Arthur Fox
Radiology. . . . . Matthew Lotysch, MD
Quality Assurance . . . . Judy McLaren
CEO/President. . . . . Edward Mirzabegian

Measure	Cases	This Hosp.	State Avg.	U.S. Avg.
Blood Clot Prevention and Treatment				
Anticoagulation Overlap Therapy[2]	17	59%	92%	93%
ICU Venous Thromboembolism Prophylaxis[2]	64	89%	92%	92%
Incidence of Potentially Preventable VTE[1,2]	-	-	11%	10%
UFH with Dosages/Platelet Monitoring[1,2]	-	-	96%	97%
Venous Thromboembolism Prophylaxis[2]	368	82%	83%	85%
Warfarin Therapy Discharge Instructions[1,2]	-	-	75%	75%
Chest Pain/Possible Heart Attack Care				
Aspirin Given Within 24 Hours of Arrival	40	100%	97%	96%
Fibrinolytic Meds Within 30 Min. of Arrival[7]	-	-	62%	58%
Average Time to ECG (minutes)	42	22	9	7
Average Time to Transfer (minutes)[1]	-	-	62	60
Children's Asthma Care				
Received Home Management Plan of Care	-	-	88%	88%
Received Reliever Medication	-	-	100%	100%
Received Systemic Corticosteroids	-	-	100%	100%
Emergency Department				
Admittance Decision Time (minutes)[2]	786	262	125	98
Head CT Results Within 45 Min. of Arrival[1]	-	-	55%	57%
Patients Who Left ER Before Being Seen	28,093	5%	3%	2%
Time from ER Arrival to Admit. (minutes)[2]	870	520	323	274
Time from ER Arrival to Discharge (minutes)	336	190	168	134
Time in ER Before Being Evaluated (minutes)	265	106	29	26
Time to Pain Meds for Fractures (minutes)	93	91	62	57
Heart Attack Care				
Aspirin Given at Discharge	41	98%	99%	99%
Fibrinolytic Meds Within 30 Min. of Arrival[7]	-	-	73%	54%
PCI Within 90 Minutes of Arrival[7]	-	-	95%	96%
Statin Prescribed at Discharge	44	82%	98%	98%
Heart Failure Care				
ACE Inhibitor or ARB for LVSD	79	99%	97%	97%
Discharge Instructions Given	184	89%	94%	94%
Evaluation of LVS Function	218	100%	99%	99%
Medicare Spending				
Medicare Spending per Patient (ratio)	-	1.30	0.98	0.98
Pneumonia Care				
Appropriate Initial Antibiotic Given	88	97%	97%	95%
Blood Culture Timing	231	97%	98%	98%
Pregnancy and Delivery Care				
Newborn Deliveries Scheduled Early	218	77%	5%	6%
Preventive Care				
Immunization for Influenza[2]	646	76%	89%	90%
Immunization for Pneumonia[2]	700	92%	90%	92%
Stroke Care				
Anticoagulation Therapy for Atrial Fibrillation[1]	-	-	95%	95%
Antithrombotic Therapy Timing	32	100%	98%	98%
Assessed for Rehabilitation	30	93%	97%	97%
Discharged on Antithrombotic Therapy	30	100%	99%	99%
Discharged on Statin Medication	26	77%	94%	94%
Thrombolytic Therapy Timing[1]	-	-	72%	66%
Venous Thromboembolism Prophylaxis	32	88%	94%	94%
Written Stroke Educational Materials Given	15	73%	87%	88%
Surgical Care Improvement Project				
Appropriate Beta Blocker Usage	12	92%	97%	98%
Appropriate VTP Within 24 Hours	98	96%	98%	98%
Controlled Postoperative Blood Glucose[7]	-	-	96%	97%
Perioperative Temperature Management	106	100%	100%	100%
Prophylactic Antibiotic Selection	38	97%	99%	99%
Prophylactic Antibiotic Selection (Outpatient)	28	96%	97%	98%
Prophylactic Antibiotic Stopped	34	94%	98%	98%
Prophylactic Antibiotic Timing	38	97%	99%	99%
Prophylactic Antibiotic Timing (Outpatient)	28	96%	97%	98%
Urinary Catheter Removal	29	97%	97%	97%
Survey of Patients' Hospital Experiences				
Area Around Room 'Always' Quiet at Night	300+	49%	51%	61%
Doctors 'Always' Communicated Well	300+	72%	78%	82%
Home Recovery Information Given	300+	75%	83%	85%
Hospital Given 9 or 10 on 10 Point Scale	300+	53%	68%	71%
Meds 'Always' Explained Before Given	300+	48%	61%	64%
Nurses 'Always' Communicated Well	300+	66%	74%	79%
Pain 'Always' Well Controlled	300+	65%	68%	71%
Room and Bathroom 'Always' Clean	300+	64%	70%	73%
Timely Help 'Always' Received	300+	53%	62%	68%
Would Definitely Recommend Hospital	300+	47%	70%	71%
Use of Medical Imaging				
Cardiac Imaging Stress Test before Surgery[1]	-	-	5.2%	5.3%
Combination Abdominal CT Scan	208	0.0%	13.4%	10.5%
Combination Brain/Sinus CT Scan[1]	-	-	2.2%	2.7%
Combination Chest CT Scan[1]	-	-	2.3%	2.7%
Follow-up Mammogram/Ultrasound[7]	-	-	8.2%	8.8%
Lumbar Spine MRI for Low Back Pain[1]	-	-	34.2%	37.2%

Saint Louise Regional Hospital

9400 No Name Uno
Gilroy, CA 95020
URL: www.saintlouiseregionalhospital.org
Type: Acute Care Hospitals
Ownership: Voluntary non-profit - Church

Phone: 408-848-2000
Fax: 408-842-2155
Emergency Services: Yes
Beds: 93

Key Personnel:
CEO/President. . . . . Joanne Allen
Radiology. . . . . David Board
Quality Assurance . . . . Marilouise Salsiccia
Operating Room. . . . . Patty Seheld, RN
Chief of Medical Staff. . . . . Jumnah Thanapathy

Measure	Cases	This Hosp.	State Avg.	U.S. Avg.
Blood Clot Prevention and Treatment				
Anticoagulation Overlap Therapy[1,2]	-	-	92%	93%
ICU Venous Thromboembolism Prophylaxis[2]	46	80%	92%	92%
Incidence of Potentially Preventable VTE[1,2]	-	-	11%	10%
UFH with Dosages/Platelet Monitoring[1,2]	-	-	96%	97%
Venous Thromboembolism Prophylaxis[2]	196	71%	83%	85%
Warfarin Therapy Discharge Instructions[1,2]	-	-	75%	75%
Chest Pain/Possible Heart Attack Care				
Aspirin Given Within 24 Hours of Arrival	34	100%	97%	96%
Fibrinolytic Meds Within 30 Min. of Arrival[1]	-	-	62%	58%
Average Time to ECG (minutes)	36	17	9	7
Average Time to Transfer (minutes)[1]	-	-	62	60
Children's Asthma Care				
Received Home Management Plan of Care	-	-	88%	88%
Received Reliever Medication	-	-	100%	100%
Received Systemic Corticosteroids	-	-	100%	100%
Emergency Department				
Admittance Decision Time (minutes)[2]	374	81	125	98
Head CT Results Within 45 Min. of Arrival	19	53%	55%	57%
Patients Who Left ER Before Being Seen	26,450	3%	3%	2%
Time from ER Arrival to Admit. (minutes)[2]	376	248	323	274
Time from ER Arrival to Discharge (minutes)	378	148	168	134
Time in ER Before Being Evaluated (minutes)	413	24	29	26
Time to Pain Meds for Fractures (minutes)	51	74	62	57
Heart Attack Care				
Aspirin Given at Discharge	13	100%	99%	99%
Fibrinolytic Meds Within 30 Min. of Arrival[7]	-	-	73%	54%
PCI Within 90 Minutes of Arrival[7]	-	-	95%	96%
Statin Prescribed at Discharge	12	100%	98%	98%
Heart Failure Care				
ACE Inhibitor or ARB for LVSD	31	97%	97%	97%
Discharge Instructions Given	82	99%	94%	94%
Evaluation of LVS Function	99	100%	99%	99%
Medicare Spending				
Medicare Spending per Patient (ratio)	-	0.98	0.98	0.98
Pneumonia Care				
Appropriate Initial Antibiotic Given	52	100%	97%	95%
Blood Culture Timing	91	100%	98%	98%
Pregnancy and Delivery Care				
Newborn Deliveries Scheduled Early[2]	40	0%	5%	6%
Preventive Care				
Immunization for Influenza[2]	296	90%	89%	90%
Immunization for Pneumonia[2]	320	89%	90%	92%
Stroke Care				
Anticoagulation Therapy for Atrial Fibrillation[1,2]	-	-	95%	95%
Antithrombotic Therapy Timing[2]	31	87%	98%	98%
Assessed for Rehabilitation[2]	38	97%	97%	97%
Discharged on Antithrombotic Therapy[2]	33	88%	99%	99%
Discharged on Statin Medication[2]	28	82%	94%	94%
Thrombolytic Therapy Timing[1,2]	-	-	72%	66%
Venous Thromboembolism Prophylaxis[2]	42	81%	94%	94%
Written Stroke Educational Materials Given[2]	22	73%	87%	88%
Surgical Care Improvement Project				
Appropriate Beta Blocker Usage[2]	29	97%	97%	98%
Appropriate VTP Within 24 Hours[2]	109	92%	98%	98%
Controlled Postoperative Blood Glucose[2,7]	-	-	96%	97%
Perioperative Temperature Management[2]	140	100%	100%	100%
Prophylactic Antibiotic Selection[2]	85	94%	99%	99%
Prophylactic Antibiotic Selection (Outpatient)	59	90%	97%	98%
Prophylactic Antibiotic Stopped[2]	79	97%	98%	98%
Prophylactic Antibiotic Timing[2]	85	99%	99%	99%
Prophylactic Antibiotic Timing (Outpatient)	59	100%	97%	98%
Urinary Catheter Removal[2]	81	96%	97%	97%
Survey of Patients' Hospital Experiences				
Area Around Room 'Always' Quiet at Night	300+	42%	51%	61%
Doctors 'Always' Communicated Well	300+	78%	78%	82%
Home Recovery Information Given	300+	81%	83%	85%
Hospital Given 9 or 10 on 10 Point Scale	300+	62%	68%	71%
Meds 'Always' Explained Before Given	300+	61%	61%	64%
Nurses 'Always' Communicated Well	300+	76%	74%	79%
Pain 'Always' Well Controlled	300+	70%	68%	71%
Room and Bathroom 'Always' Clean	300+	75%	70%	73%
Timely Help 'Always' Received	300+	58%	62%	68%
Would Definitely Recommend Hospital	300+	66%	70%	71%
Use of Medical Imaging				
Cardiac Imaging Stress Test before Surgery[7]	-	-	5.2%	5.3%
Combination Abdominal CT Scan	335	8.7%	13.4%	10.5%
Combination Brain/Sinus CT Scan[1]	-	-	2.2%	2.7%
Combination Chest CT Scan	129	1.6%	2.3%	2.7%
Follow-up Mammogram/Ultrasound	506	8.3%	8.2%	8.8%
Lumbar Spine MRI for Low Back Pain[1]	-	-	34.2%	37.2%

NOTE: Hospital profiles are in alphabetical order by state, then city, then hospital within the city; Rankings exclude hospitals with less than 25 cases except for patient surveys which excludes hospitals with less than 100 cases; (a) 100-299 cases; (1) The number of cases/patients is too few to report; (2) Data submitted were based on a sample of cases/patients; (3) Results are based on a shorter time period than required; (4) Data suppressed by CMS for one or more quarters; (5) Results are not available for this reporting period; (6) Fewer than 100 patients completed the HCAHPS survey; (7) No cases met the criteria for this measure; (8) The lower limit of the confidence interval cannot be calculated if the number of observed infections equals zero; (9) No data are available from the state/territory for this reporting period; (10) The scores shown reflect fewer than 50 completed surveys; (11) There were discrepancies in the data collection process; (12) This measure does not apply to this hospital for this reporting period; (13) Results cannot be calculated for this reporting period; (14) The results for this state are combined with nearby states to protect confidentiality; Please refer to the User's Guide for a full explanation of data.

Glendale Adventist Medical Center

1509 E Wilson Terrace Phone: 818-409-8202
Glendale, CA 91206 Fax: 818-546-5600
URL: www.glendaleadventist.com
Type: Acute Care Hospitals Emergency Services: Yes
Ownership: Voluntary non-profit - Church Beds: 448

Key Personnel:
Chief of Medical Staff.......... Carl B Ermshar, MD
Infection Control.............. Michelle Garcia
Quality Assurance .... Ellen Hooker
Cardiac Laboratory............ Robert Marchuck
Radiology.................... Robert McKay, MD
CEO/President............... Kevin A. Roberts, FACHE

Measure	Cases	This Hosp.	State Avg.	U.S. Avg.
Blood Clot Prevention and Treatment				
Anticoagulation Overlap Therapy[2]	100	92%	92%	93%
ICU Venous Thromboembolism Prophylaxis[2]	57	86%	92%	92%
Incidence of Potentially Preventable VTE[2]	37	16%	11%	10%
UFH with Dosages/Platelet Monitoring[2]	40	95%	96%	97%
Venous Thromboembolism Prophylaxis[2]	307	86%	83%	85%
Warfarin Therapy Discharge Instructions[2]	59	71%	75%	75%
Chest Pain/Possible Heart Attack Care				
Aspirin Given Within 24 Hours of Arrival	20	100%	97%	96%
Fibrinolytic Meds Within 30 Min. of Arrival[5]	-	-	62%	58%
Average Time to ECG (minutes)	21	5	9	7
Average Time to Transfer (minutes)[5]	-	-	62	60
Children's Asthma Care				
Received Home Management Plan of Care	-	-	88%	88%
Received Reliever Medication	-	-	100%	100%
Received Systemic Corticosteroids	-	-	100%	100%
Emergency Department				
Admittance Decision Time (minutes)[2]	695	171	125	98
Head CT Results Within 45 Min. of Arrival[1]	-	-	55%	57%
Patients Who Left ER Before Being Seen	46,146	0%	3%	2%
Time from ER Arrival to Admit. (minutes)[2]	695	336	323	274
Time from ER Arrival to Discharge (minutes)	352	182	168	134
Time in ER Before Being Evaluated (minutes)	384	26	29	26
Time to Pain Meds for Fractures (minutes)	104	54	62	57
Heart Attack Care				
Aspirin Given at Discharge	329	100%	99%	99%
Fibrinolytic Meds Within 30 Min. of Arrival[7]	-	-	73%	54%
PCI Within 90 Minutes of Arrival	45	100%	95%	96%
Statin Prescribed at Discharge	330	100%	98%	98%
Heart Failure Care				
ACE Inhibitor or ARB for LVSD	106	98%	97%	97%
Discharge Instructions Given	335	99%	94%	94%
Evaluation of LVS Function	402	100%	99%	99%
Medicare Spending				
Medicare Spending per Patient (ratio)	-	1.06	0.98	0.98
Pneumonia Care				
Appropriate Initial Antibiotic Given	221	96%	97%	95%
Blood Culture Timing	497	100%	98%	98%
Pregnancy and Delivery Care				
Newborn Deliveries Scheduled Early	376	21%	5%	6%
Preventive Care				
Immunization for Influenza[2]	516	96%	89%	90%
Immunization for Pneumonia[2]	615	92%	90%	92%
Stroke Care				
Anticoagulation Therapy for Atrial Fibrillation	29	100%	95%	95%
Antithrombotic Therapy Timing	133	100%	98%	98%
Assessed for Rehabilitation	197	100%	97%	97%
Discharged on Antithrombotic Therapy	152	100%	99%	99%
Discharged on Statin Medication	130	98%	94%	94%
Thrombolytic Therapy Timing	21	100%	72%	66%
Venous Thromboembolism Prophylaxis	197	99%	94%	94%
Written Stroke Educational Materials Given	98	100%	87%	88%
Surgical Care Improvement Project				
Appropriate Beta Blocker Usage[2]	305	98%	97%	98%
Appropriate VTP Within 24 Hours[2]	583	98%	98%	98%
Controlled Postoperative Blood Glucose[2]	99	99%	96%	97%
Perioperative Temperature Management[2]	718	100%	100%	100%
Prophylactic Antibiotic Selection[2]	609	100%	99%	99%
Prophylactic Antibiotic Selection (Outpatient)	115	93%	97%	98%
Prophylactic Antibiotic Stopped[2]	590	95%	98%	98%
Prophylactic Antibiotic Timing[2]	610	100%	99%	99%
Prophylactic Antibiotic Timing (Outpatient)	116	96%	97%	98%
Urinary Catheter Removal[2]	487	97%	97%	97%
Survey of Patients' Hospital Experiences				
Area Around Room 'Always' Quiet at Night	300+	58%	51%	61%
Doctors 'Always' Communicated Well	300+	79%	78%	82%
Home Recovery Information Given	300+	87%	83%	85%
Hospital Given 9 or 10 on 10 Point Scale	300+	67%	68%	71%
Meds 'Always' Explained Before Given	300+	68%	61%	64%
Nurses 'Always' Communicated Well	300+	78%	74%	79%
Pain 'Always' Well Controlled	300+	71%	68%	71%
Room and Bathroom 'Always' Clean	300+	66%	70%	73%
Timely Help 'Always' Received	300+	62%	62%	68%
Would Definitely Recommend Hospital	300+	72%	70%	71%
Use of Medical Imaging				
Cardiac Imaging Stress Test before Surgery	310	7.1%	5.2%	5.3%
Combination Abdominal CT Scan	876	20.4%	13.4%	10.5%
Combination Brain/Sinus CT Scan	880	4.0%	2.2%	2.7%
Combination Chest CT Scan	418	0.5%	2.3%	2.7%
Follow-up Mammogram/Ultrasound	1,031	10.1%	8.2%	8.8%
Lumbar Spine MRI for Low Back Pain	176	36.9%	34.2%	37.2%

Glendale Memorial Hospital & Health Center

1420 S Central Ave Phone: 818-502-1900
Glendale, CA 91204 Fax: 818-409-7688
URL: www.glendalememorialhospital.org
Type: Acute Care Hospitals Emergency Services: Yes
Ownership: Voluntary non-profit - Private Beds: 334

Key Personnel:
Emergency Room .... Michael Agron, MD
Infection Control............ Kaye Baymiller, RN
Quality Assurance .... Donna Hansen, RN
Operating Room............. Davis Kaymel, RN
CEO/President.............. Mark Meyers
Cardiac Laboratory........... Santo S Polito, MD
Patient Relations .... Rhoda Vincent, RN
Hemotology Center .... Lois Winston, PhD

Measure	Cases	This Hosp.	State Avg.	U.S. Avg.
Blood Clot Prevention and Treatment				
Anticoagulation Overlap Therapy[2]	42	64%	92%	93%
ICU Venous Thromboembolism Prophylaxis[2]	93	92%	92%	92%
Incidence of Potentially Preventable VTE[1,2]	-	-	11%	10%
UFH with Dosages/Platelet Monitoring[2]	15	100%	96%	97%
Venous Thromboembolism Prophylaxis[2]	363	79%	83%	85%
Warfarin Therapy Discharge Instructions[2]	31	3%	75%	75%
Chest Pain/Possible Heart Attack Care				
Aspirin Given Within 24 Hours of Arrival	12	92%	97%	96%
Fibrinolytic Meds Within 30 Min. of Arrival[5]	-	-	62%	58%
Average Time to ECG (minutes)	13	4	9	7
Average Time to Transfer (minutes)[5]	-	-	62	60
Children's Asthma Care				
Received Home Management Plan of Care	-	-	88%	88%
Received Reliever Medication	-	-	100%	100%
Received Systemic Corticosteroids	-	-	100%	100%
Emergency Department				
Admittance Decision Time (minutes)[2]	509	76	125	98
Head CT Results Within 45 Min. of Arrival[1,3]	-	-	55%	57%
Patients Who Left ER Before Being Seen	33,067	1%	3%	2%
Time from ER Arrival to Admit. (minutes)[2]	521	254	323	274
Time from ER Arrival to Discharge (minutes)	373	143	168	134
Time in ER Before Being Evaluated (minutes)	394	14	29	26
Time to Pain Meds for Fractures (minutes)	112	41	62	57
Heart Attack Care				
Aspirin Given at Discharge	172	99%	99%	99%
Fibrinolytic Meds Within 30 Min. of Arrival[7]	-	-	73%	54%
PCI Within 90 Minutes of Arrival	30	90%	95%	96%
Statin Prescribed at Discharge	176	98%	98%	98%
Heart Failure Care				
ACE Inhibitor or ARB for LVSD	121	96%	97%	97%
Discharge Instructions Given	350	88%	94%	94%
Evaluation of LVS Function	411	98%	99%	99%
Medicare Spending				
Medicare Spending per Patient (ratio)	-	1.05	0.98	0.98
Pneumonia Care				
Appropriate Initial Antibiotic Given	120	92%	97%	95%
Blood Culture Timing	256	97%	98%	98%
Pregnancy and Delivery Care				
Newborn Deliveries Scheduled Early[2]	68	4%	5%	6%
Preventive Care				
Immunization for Influenza[2]	497	89%	89%	90%
Immunization for Pneumonia[2]	617	95%	90%	92%
Stroke Care				
Anticoagulation Therapy for Atrial Fibrillation[1]	-	-	95%	95%
Antithrombotic Therapy Timing	52	96%	98%	98%
Assessed for Rehabilitation	57	89%	97%	97%
Discharged on Antithrombotic Therapy	52	100%	99%	99%
Discharged on Statin Medication	49	92%	94%	94%
Thrombolytic Therapy Timing[1]	-	-	72%	66%
Venous Thromboembolism Prophylaxis	58	86%	94%	94%
Written Stroke Educational Materials Given	36	58%	87%	88%
Surgical Care Improvement Project				
Appropriate Beta Blocker Usage[2]	218	98%	97%	98%
Appropriate VTP Within 24 Hours[2]	354	96%	98%	98%
Controlled Postoperative Blood Glucose[2]	134	93%	96%	97%
Perioperative Temperature Management[2]	406	100%	100%	100%
Prophylactic Antibiotic Selection[2]	385	99%	99%	99%
Prophylactic Antibiotic Selection (Outpatient)	164	95%	97%	98%
Prophylactic Antibiotic Stopped[2]	364	99%	98%	98%
Prophylactic Antibiotic Timing[2]	386	96%	99%	99%
Prophylactic Antibiotic Timing (Outpatient)	164	96%	97%	98%
Urinary Catheter Removal[2]	289	97%	97%	97%
Survey of Patients' Hospital Experiences				
Area Around Room 'Always' Quiet at Night	300+	52%	51%	61%
Doctors 'Always' Communicated Well	300+	77%	78%	82%
Home Recovery Information Given	300+	82%	83%	85%
Hospital Given 9 or 10 on 10 Point Scale	300+	63%	68%	71%
Meds 'Always' Explained Before Given	300+	60%	61%	64%
Nurses 'Always' Communicated Well	300+	71%	74%	79%
Pain 'Always' Well Controlled	300+	68%	68%	71%
Room and Bathroom 'Always' Clean	300+	66%	70%	73%
Timely Help 'Always' Received	300+	58%	62%	68%
Would Definitely Recommend Hospital	300+	65%	70%	71%
Use of Medical Imaging				
Cardiac Imaging Stress Test before Surgery	180	5.0%	5.2%	5.3%
Combination Abdominal CT Scan	657	6.1%	13.4%	10.5%
Combination Brain/Sinus CT Scan	522	2.3%	2.2%	2.7%
Combination Chest CT Scan	363	0.3%	2.3%	2.7%
Follow-up Mammogram/Ultrasound	1,829	6.9%	8.2%	8.8%
Lumbar Spine MRI for Low Back Pain	55	36.4%	34.2%	37.2%

USC Verdugo Hills Hospital

1812 Verdugo Blvd Phone: 818-790-7100
Glendale, CA 91209 Fax: 818-952-3597
URL: www.verdugohillshospital.org
Type: Acute Care Hospitals Emergency Services: Yes
Ownership: Voluntary non-profit - Private Beds: 158

Key Personnel:
Quality Assurance .... David Greer
Chief of Medical Staff.......... Steven L Hartford, MD
Chair/CEO.................. Thomas E. Jackiewicz
CEO/President............... Leonard Labbella
Radiology................... George Rappard
Emergency Room .... Kevin Traber, RN

Measure	Cases	This Hosp.	State Avg.	U.S. Avg.
Blood Clot Prevention and Treatment				
Anticoagulation Overlap Therapy[2]	13	100%	92%	93%
ICU Venous Thromboembolism Prophylaxis[2]	27	85%	92%	92%
Incidence of Potentially Preventable VTE[2,7]	-	-	11%	10%
UFH with Dosages/Platelet Monitoring[1,2]	-	-	96%	97%
Venous Thromboembolism Prophylaxis[2]	322	74%	83%	85%
Warfarin Therapy Discharge Instructions[1,2]	-	-	75%	75%
Chest Pain/Possible Heart Attack Care				
Aspirin Given Within 24 Hours of Arrival	23	87%	97%	96%
Fibrinolytic Meds Within 30 Min. of Arrival[7]	-	-	62%	58%
Average Time to ECG (minutes)	26	8	9	7
Average Time to Transfer (minutes)[1]	-	-	62	60
Children's Asthma Care				
Received Home Management Plan of Care	-	-	88%	88%

NOTE: Hospital profiles are in alphabetical order by state, then city, then hospital within the city; Rankings exclude hospitals with less than 25 cases except for patient surveys which excludes hospitals with less than 100 cases; (a) 100-299 cases; (1) The number of cases/patients is too few to report; (2) Data submitted were based on a sample of cases/patients; (3) Results are based on a shorter time period than required; (4) Data suppressed by CMS for one or more quarters; (5) Results are not available for this reporting period; (6) Fewer than 100 patients completed the HCAHPS survey; (7) No cases met the criteria for this measure; (8) The lower limit of the confidence interval cannot be calculated if the number of observed infections equals zero; (9) No data are available from the state/territory for this reporting period; (10) The scores shown reflect fewer than 50 completed surveys; (11) There were discrepancies in the data collection process; (12) This measure does not apply to this hospital for this reporting period; (13) Results cannot be calculated for this reporting period; (14) The results for this state are combined with nearby states to protect confidentiality; Please refer to the User's Guide for a full explanation of data.

Measure	Cases	This Hosp.	State Avg.	U.S. Avg.
Received Reliever Medication	-	-	100%	100%
Received Systemic Corticosteroids	-	-	100%	100%
Emergency Department				
Admittance Decision Time (minutes)[2]	593	82	125	98
Head CT Results Within 45 Min. of Arrival[1]	-	-	55%	57%
Patients Who Left ER Before Being Seen	19,058	1%	3%	2%
Time from ER Arrival to Admit. (minutes)[2]	593	267	323	274
Time from ER Arrival to Discharge (minutes)	449	119	168	134
Time in ER Before Being Evaluated (minutes)	393	42	29	26
Time to Pain Meds for Fractures (minutes)	94	67	62	57
Heart Attack Care				
Aspirin Given at Discharge	26	92%	99%	99%
Fibrinolytic Meds Within 30 Min. of Arrival[7]	-	-	73%	54%
PCI Within 90 Minutes of Arrival[7]	-	-	95%	96%
Statin Prescribed at Discharge	24	88%	98%	98%
Heart Failure Care				
ACE Inhibitor or ARB for LVSD	17	94%	97%	97%
Discharge Instructions Given	63	100%	94%	94%
Evaluation of LVS Function	87	94%	99%	99%
Medicare Spending				
Medicare Spending per Patient (ratio)	-	1.08	0.98	0.98
Pneumonia Care				
Appropriate Initial Antibiotic Given[2]	56	98%	97%	95%
Blood Culture Timing[2]	133	97%	98%	98%
Pregnancy and Delivery Care				
Newborn Deliveries Scheduled Early[2]	45	2%	5%	6%
Preventive Care				
Immunization for Influenza[2]	464	91%	89%	90%
Immunization for Pneumonia[2]	583	97%	90%	92%
Stroke Care				
Anticoagulation Therapy for Atrial Fibrillation[1]	-	-	95%	95%
Antithrombotic Therapy Timing	41	93%	98%	98%
Assessed for Rehabilitation	48	88%	97%	97%
Discharged on Antithrombotic Therapy	43	91%	99%	99%
Discharged on Statin Medication	34	71%	94%	94%
Thrombolytic Therapy Timing[1]	-	-	72%	66%
Venous Thromboembolism Prophylaxis	49	47%	94%	94%
Written Stroke Educational Materials Given	16	62%	87%	88%
Surgical Care Improvement Project				
Appropriate Beta Blocker Usage[2]	44	100%	97%	98%
Appropriate VTP Within 24 Hours[2]	272	96%	98%	98%
Controlled Postoperative Blood Glucose[2,7]	-	-	96%	97%
Perioperative Temperature Management[2]	319	100%	100%	100%
Prophylactic Antibiotic Selection[2]	243	98%	99%	99%
Prophylactic Antibiotic Selection (Outpatient)	124	99%	97%	98%
Prophylactic Antibiotic Stopped[2]	243	98%	98%	98%
Prophylactic Antibiotic Timing[2]	243	100%	99%	99%
Prophylactic Antibiotic Timing (Outpatient)	125	99%	97%	98%
Urinary Catheter Removal[2]	141	96%	97%	97%
Survey of Patients' Hospital Experiences				
Area Around Room 'Always' Quiet at Night	300+	45%	51%	61%
Doctors 'Always' Communicated Well	300+	81%	78%	82%
Home Recovery Information Given	300+	78%	83%	85%
Hospital Given 9 or 10 on 10 Point Scale	300+	69%	68%	71%
Meds 'Always' Explained Before Given	300+	65%	61%	64%
Nurses 'Always' Communicated Well	300+	77%	74%	79%
Pain 'Always' Well Controlled	300+	70%	68%	71%
Room and Bathroom 'Always' Clean	300+	76%	70%	73%
Timely Help 'Always' Received	300+	68%	62%	68%
Would Definitely Recommend Hospital	300+	73%	70%	71%
Use of Medical Imaging				
Cardiac Imaging Stress Test before Surgery[1]	-	-	5.2%	5.3%
Combination Abdominal CT Scan	251	5.2%	13.4%	10.5%
Combination Brain/Sinus CT Scan[1]	-	-	2.2%	2.7%
Combination Chest CT Scan	125	0.0%	2.3%	2.7%
Follow-up Mammogram/Ultrasound	1,012	3.1%	8.2%	8.8%
Lumbar Spine MRI for Low Back Pain	69	30.4%	34.2%	37.2%

East Valley Hospital Medical Center

150 West Route 66 Phone: 626-335-0231
Glendora, CA 91740 Fax: 626-852-5022
URL: www.eastvalleyhospital.org
Type: Acute Care Hospitals Emergency Services: Yes
Ownership: Voluntary non-profit - Private Beds: 128

Key Personnel:
CEO/President. . . . . C Joseph Chang
Patient Relations . . . . Marge Chick
Chief of Medical Staff . . . . Marc Domaguing, MD
Quality Assurance . . . . Shirley Lewis
Emergency Room . . . . Richard MacDonald, RN
Intensive Care Unit. . . . . Richard MacDonald, RN
Infection Control. . . . . Milad Shokair
Operating Room. . . . . Madeline Talah

Measure	Cases	This Hosp.	State Avg.	U.S. Avg.
Blood Clot Prevention and Treatment				
Anticoagulation Overlap Therapy[2]	11	91%	92%	93%
ICU Venous Thromboembolism Prophylaxis[2]	16	75%	92%	92%
Incidence of Potentially Preventable VTE[1,2]	-	-	11%	10%
UFH with Dosages/Platelet Monitoring[1,2]	-	-	96%	97%
Venous Thromboembolism Prophylaxis[2]	106	67%	83%	85%
Warfarin Therapy Discharge Instructions[1,2]	-	-	75%	75%
Chest Pain/Possible Heart Attack Care				
Aspirin Given Within 24 Hours of Arrival[1,3]	-	-	97%	96%
Fibrinolytic Meds Within 30 Min. of Arrival[3,7]	-	-	62%	58%
Average Time to ECG (minutes)[1,3]	-	-	9	7
Average Time to Transfer (minutes)[1,3]	-	-	62	60
Children's Asthma Care				
Received Home Management Plan of Care	-	-	88%	88%
Received Reliever Medication	-	-	100%	100%
Received Systemic Corticosteroids	-	-	100%	100%
Emergency Department				
Admittance Decision Time (minutes)[2]	798	63	125	98
Head CT Results Within 45 Min. of Arrival[3,7]	-	-	55%	57%
Patients Who Left ER Before Being Seen	4,647	0%	3%	2%
Time from ER Arrival to Admit. (minutes)[2]	796	285	323	274
Time from ER Arrival to Discharge (minutes)	278	150	168	134
Time in ER Before Being Evaluated (minutes)	389	13	29	26
Time to Pain Meds for Fractures (minutes)[1]	-	-	62	57
Heart Attack Care				
Aspirin Given at Discharge	13	100%	99%	99%
Fibrinolytic Meds Within 30 Min. of Arrival[7]	-	-	73%	54%
PCI Within 90 Minutes of Arrival[7]	-	-	95%	96%
Statin Prescribed at Discharge	12	92%	98%	98%
Heart Failure Care				
ACE Inhibitor or ARB for LVSD[1]	-	-	97%	97%
Discharge Instructions Given[1]	-	-	94%	94%
Evaluation of LVS Function	14	100%	99%	99%
Medicare Spending				
Medicare Spending per Patient (ratio)	-	1.54	0.98	0.98
Pneumonia Care				
Appropriate Initial Antibiotic Given[1]	-	-	97%	95%
Blood Culture Timing	99	96%	98%	98%
Pregnancy and Delivery Care				
Newborn Deliveries Scheduled Early	18	6%	5%	6%
Preventive Care				
Immunization for Influenza[2]	802	81%	89%	90%
Immunization for Pneumonia[2]	859	93%	90%	92%
Stroke Care				
Anticoagulation Therapy for Atrial Fibrillation[7]	-	-	95%	95%
Antithrombotic Therapy Timing[1]	-	-	98%	98%
Assessed for Rehabilitation[1]	-	-	97%	97%
Discharged on Antithrombotic Therapy[1]	-	-	99%	99%
Discharged on Statin Medication[1]	-	-	94%	94%
Thrombolytic Therapy Timing[7]	-	-	72%	66%
Venous Thromboembolism Prophylaxis[1]	-	-	94%	94%
Written Stroke Educational Materials Given[1]	-	-	87%	88%
Surgical Care Improvement Project				
Appropriate Beta Blocker Usage[1]	-	-	97%	98%
Appropriate VTP Within 24 Hours	11	91%	98%	98%
Controlled Postoperative Blood Glucose[7]	-	-	96%	97%
Perioperative Temperature Management	12	100%	100%	100%
Prophylactic Antibiotic Selection[1]	-	-	99%	99%
Prophylactic Antibiotic Selection (Outpatient)[1,3]	-	-	97%	98%
Prophylactic Antibiotic Stopped[1]	-	-	98%	98%
Prophylactic Antibiotic Timing[1]	-	-	99%	99%
Prophylactic Antibiotic Timing (Outpatient)[1,3]	-	-	97%	98%
Urinary Catheter Removal[1]	-	-	97%	97%
Survey of Patients' Hospital Experiences				
Area Around Room 'Always' Quiet at Night[6]	<100	58%	51%	61%
Doctors 'Always' Communicated Well[6]	<100	73%	78%	82%
Home Recovery Information Given[6]	<100	79%	83%	85%
Hospital Given 9 or 10 on 10 Point Scale[6]	<100	48%	68%	71%
Meds 'Always' Explained Before Given[6]	<100	55%	61%	64%
Nurses 'Always' Communicated Well[6]	<100	69%	74%	79%
Pain 'Always' Well Controlled[6]	<100	69%	68%	71%
Room and Bathroom 'Always' Clean[6]	<100	70%	70%	73%
Timely Help 'Always' Received[6]	<100	67%	62%	68%
Would Definitely Recommend Hospital[6]	<100	47%	70%	71%
Use of Medical Imaging				
Cardiac Imaging Stress Test before Surgery[7]	-	-	5.2%	5.3%
Combination Abdominal CT Scan[1]	-	-	13.4%	10.5%
Combination Brain/Sinus CT Scan	44	11.4%	2.2%	2.7%
Combination Chest CT Scan[1]	-	-	2.3%	2.7%
Follow-up Mammogram/Ultrasound[7]	-	-	8.2%	8.8%
Lumbar Spine MRI for Low Back Pain[7]	-	-	34.2%	37.2%

Foothill Presbyterian Hospital

250 S Grand Ave Phone: 626-963-8411
Glendora, CA 91740 Fax: 626-814-2428
URL: www.cvhp.org
Type: Acute Care Hospitals Emergency Services: Yes
Ownership: Voluntary non-profit - Private Beds: 106

Key Personnel:
Chief of Medical Staff . . . . Ihsan Hikimah', MD
Operating Room. . . . . Mary Mosesson
Pediatric Ambulatory Care . . . . . . P Patel, MD
Pediatric In-Patient Care . . . . P Patel, MD
Radiology. . . . . Uri M Zisblatt

Measure	Cases	This Hosp.	State Avg.	U.S. Avg.
Blood Clot Prevention and Treatment				
Anticoagulation Overlap Therapy[2]	23	83%	92%	93%
ICU Venous Thromboembolism Prophylaxis[2]	93	72%	92%	92%
Incidence of Potentially Preventable VTE[1,2]	-	-	11%	10%
UFH with Dosages/Platelet Monitoring[2]	14	93%	96%	97%
Venous Thromboembolism Prophylaxis[2]	288	48%	83%	85%
Warfarin Therapy Discharge Instructions[2]	15	73%	75%	75%
Chest Pain/Possible Heart Attack Care				
Aspirin Given Within 24 Hours of Arrival	41	100%	97%	96%
Fibrinolytic Meds Within 30 Min. of Arrival[7]	-	-	62%	58%
Average Time to ECG (minutes)	41	8	9	7
Average Time to Transfer (minutes)	12	40	62	60
Children's Asthma Care				
Received Home Management Plan of Care	-	-	88%	88%
Received Reliever Medication	-	-	100%	100%
Received Systemic Corticosteroids	-	-	100%	100%
Emergency Department				
Admittance Decision Time (minutes)[2]	667	139	125	98
Head CT Results Within 45 Min. of Arrival[1]	-	-	55%	57%
Patients Who Left ER Before Being Seen	30,494	2%	3%	2%
Time from ER Arrival to Admit. (minutes)[2]	680	381	323	274
Time from ER Arrival to Discharge (minutes)	380	171	168	134
Time in ER Before Being Evaluated (minutes)	289	69	29	26
Time to Pain Meds for Fractures (minutes)	127	30	62	57
Heart Attack Care				
Aspirin Given at Discharge	11	100%	99%	99%
Fibrinolytic Meds Within 30 Min. of Arrival[7]	-	-	73%	54%
PCI Within 90 Minutes of Arrival[7]	-	-	95%	96%
Statin Prescribed at Discharge[1]	-	-	98%	98%
Heart Failure Care				
ACE Inhibitor or ARB for LVSD	38	100%	97%	97%
Discharge Instructions Given	106	92%	94%	94%
Evaluation of LVS Function	133	100%	99%	99%
Medicare Spending				
Medicare Spending per Patient (ratio)	-	1.11	0.98	0.98
Pneumonia Care				

NOTE: Hospital profiles are in alphabetical order by state, then city, then hospital within the city; Rankings exclude hospitals with less than 25 cases except for patient surveys which excludes hospitals with less than 100 cases; (a) 100-299 cases; (1) The number of cases/patients is too few to report; (2) Data submitted were based on a sample of cases/patients; (3) Results are based on a shorter time period than required; (4) Data suppressed by CMS for one or more quarters; (5) Results are not available for this reporting period; (6) Fewer than 100 patients completed the HCAHPS survey; (7) No cases met the criteria for this measure; (8) The lower limit of the confidence interval cannot be calculated if the number of observed infections equals zero; (9) No data are available from the state/territory for this reporting period; (10) The scores shown reflect fewer than 50 completed surveys; (11) There were discrepancies in the data collection process; (12) This measure does not apply to this hospital for this reporting period; (13) Results cannot be calculated for this reporting period; (14) The results for this state are combined with nearby states to protect confidentiality; Please refer to the User's Guide for a full explanation of data.

Measure	Cases	This Hosp.	State Avg.	U.S. Avg.
Appropriate Initial Antibiotic Given	84	95%	97%	95%
Blood Culture Timing	145	98%	98%	98%
Pregnancy and Delivery Care				
Newborn Deliveries Scheduled Early	115	7%	5%	6%
Preventive Care				
Immunization for Influenza[2]	489	87%	89%	90%
Immunization for Pneumonia[2]	557	89%	90%	92%
Stroke Care				
Anticoagulation Therapy for Atrial Fibrillation[1]	-	-	95%	95%
Antithrombotic Therapy Timing	34	100%	98%	98%
Assessed for Rehabilitation	39	92%	97%	97%
Discharged on Antithrombotic Therapy	34	97%	99%	99%
Discharged on Statin Medication	27	78%	94%	94%
Thrombolytic Therapy Timing[1]	-	-	72%	66%
Venous Thromboembolism Prophylaxis	39	79%	94%	94%
Written Stroke Educational Materials Given	20	90%	87%	88%
Surgical Care Improvement Project				
Appropriate Beta Blocker Usage[2]	65	95%	97%	98%
Appropriate VTP Within 24 Hours[2]	239	95%	98%	98%
Controlled Postoperative Blood Glucose[2,7]	-	-	96%	97%
Perioperative Temperature Management[2]	273	100%	100%	100%
Prophylactic Antibiotic Selection[2]	153	95%	99%	99%
Prophylactic Antibiotic Selection (Outpatient)	73	96%	97%	98%
Prophylactic Antibiotic Stopped[2]	133	100%	98%	98%
Prophylactic Antibiotic Timing[2]	153	98%	99%	99%
Prophylactic Antibiotic Timing (Outpatient)	72	99%	97%	98%
Urinary Catheter Removal[2]	123	88%	97%	97%
Survey of Patients' Hospital Experiences				
Area Around Room 'Always' Quiet at Night	300+	51%	51%	61%
Doctors 'Always' Communicated Well	300+	78%	78%	82%
Home Recovery Information Given	300+	84%	83%	85%
Hospital Given 9 or 10 on 10 Point Scale	300+	71%	68%	71%
Meds 'Always' Explained Before Given	300+	60%	61%	64%
Nurses 'Always' Communicated Well	300+	76%	74%	79%
Pain 'Always' Well Controlled	300+	70%	68%	71%
Room and Bathroom 'Always' Clean	300+	71%	70%	73%
Timely Help 'Always' Received	300+	61%	62%	68%
Would Definitely Recommend Hospital	300+	74%	70%	71%
Use of Medical Imaging				
Cardiac Imaging Stress Test before Surgery[1]	-	-	5.2%	5.3%
Combination Abdominal CT Scan	253	15.8%	13.4%	10.5%
Combination Brain/Sinus CT Scan[1]	-	-	2.2%	2.7%
Combination Chest CT Scan	72	5.6%	2.3%	2.7%
Follow-up Mammogram/Ultrasound	116	17.2%	8.2%	8.8%
Lumbar Spine MRI for Low Back Pain[7]	-	-	34.2%	37.2%

Sierra Nevada Memorial Hospital

155 Glasson Way Phone: 530-274-6000
Grass Valley, CA 95945 Fax: 530-274-6614
E-mail: info@snmh.org
URL: www.snmh.org
Type: Acute Care Hospitals Emergency Services: Yes
Ownership: Voluntary non-profit - Other Beds: 75

Key Personnel:
Operating Room. . . . . Thomas M Boyle
Emergency Room . . . . Joseph Britton
Chief of Medical Staff . . . . Robert Lowe
CEO/President. . . . . Katherine A Medeiros
Radiology. . . . . Mark F Richey

Measure	Cases	This Hosp.	State Avg.	U.S. Avg.
Blood Clot Prevention and Treatment				
Anticoagulation Overlap Therapy[2]	37	76%	92%	93%
ICU Venous Thromboembolism Prophylaxis[2]	23	91%	92%	92%
Incidence of Potentially Preventable VTE[1,2]	-	-	11%	10%
UFH with Dosages/Platelet Monitoring[1,2]	-	-	96%	97%
Venous Thromboembolism Prophylaxis[2]	350	97%	83%	85%
Warfarin Therapy Discharge Instructions[2]	30	10%	75%	75%
Chest Pain/Possible Heart Attack Care				
Aspirin Given Within 24 Hours of Arrival	134	99%	97%	96%
Fibrinolytic Meds Within 30 Min. of Arrival	17	76%	62%	58%
Average Time to ECG (minutes)	136	16	9	7
Average Time to Transfer (minutes)[1]	-	-	62	60
Children's Asthma Care				
Received Home Management Plan of Care	-	-	88%	88%
Received Reliever Medication	-	-	100%	100%
Received Systemic Corticosteroids	-	-	100%	100%
Emergency Department				
Admittance Decision Time (minutes)[2]	789	159	125	98
Head CT Results Within 45 Min. of Arrival	12	75%	55%	57%
Patients Who Left ER Before Being Seen	42,386	0%	3%	2%
Time from ER Arrival to Admit. (minutes)[2]	824	300	323	274
Time from ER Arrival to Discharge (minutes)	363	137	168	134
Time in ER Before Being Evaluated (minutes)	405	15	29	26
Time to Pain Meds for Fractures (minutes)	124	60	62	57
Heart Attack Care				
Aspirin Given at Discharge	24	100%	99%	99%
Fibrinolytic Meds Within 30 Min. of Arrival[1]	-	-	73%	54%
PCI Within 90 Minutes of Arrival[7]	-	-	95%	96%
Statin Prescribed at Discharge	23	96%	98%	98%
Heart Failure Care				
ACE Inhibitor or ARB for LVSD	36	97%	97%	97%
Discharge Instructions Given	84	98%	94%	94%
Evaluation of LVS Function	114	99%	99%	99%
Medicare Spending				
Medicare Spending per Patient (ratio)	-	0.93	0.98	0.98
Pneumonia Care				
Appropriate Initial Antibiotic Given[2]	110	98%	97%	95%
Blood Culture Timing[2]	160	97%	98%	98%
Pregnancy and Delivery Care				
Newborn Deliveries Scheduled Early	30	13%	5%	6%
Preventive Care				
Immunization for Influenza[2]	511	91%	89%	90%
Immunization for Pneumonia[2]	656	96%	90%	92%
Stroke Care				
Anticoagulation Therapy for Atrial Fibrillation	11	100%	95%	95%
Antithrombotic Therapy Timing	49	100%	98%	98%
Assessed for Rehabilitation	51	100%	97%	97%
Discharged on Antithrombotic Therapy	49	100%	99%	99%
Discharged on Statin Medication	38	100%	94%	94%
Thrombolytic Therapy Timing[1]	-	-	72%	66%
Venous Thromboembolism Prophylaxis	49	100%	94%	94%
Written Stroke Educational Materials Given	26	100%	87%	88%
Surgical Care Improvement Project				
Appropriate Beta Blocker Usage[2]	64	92%	97%	98%
Appropriate VTP Within 24 Hours[2]	266	98%	98%	98%
Controlled Postoperative Blood Glucose[2,7]	-	-	96%	97%
Perioperative Temperature Management[2]	305	100%	100%	100%
Prophylactic Antibiotic Selection[2]	205	100%	99%	99%
Prophylactic Antibiotic Selection (Outpatient)	31	100%	97%	98%
Prophylactic Antibiotic Stopped[2]	201	97%	98%	98%
Prophylactic Antibiotic Timing[2]	205	99%	99%	99%
Prophylactic Antibiotic Timing (Outpatient)	34	91%	97%	98%
Urinary Catheter Removal[2]	96	95%	97%	97%
Survey of Patients' Hospital Experiences				
Area Around Room 'Always' Quiet at Night	300+	50%	51%	61%
Doctors 'Always' Communicated Well	300+	74%	78%	82%
Home Recovery Information Given	300+	87%	83%	85%
Hospital Given 9 or 10 on 10 Point Scale	300+	64%	68%	71%
Meds 'Always' Explained Before Given	300+	62%	61%	64%
Nurses 'Always' Communicated Well	300+	75%	74%	79%
Pain 'Always' Well Controlled	300+	72%	68%	71%
Room and Bathroom 'Always' Clean	300+	70%	70%	73%
Timely Help 'Always' Received	300+	63%	62%	68%
Would Definitely Recommend Hospital	300+	66%	70%	71%
Use of Medical Imaging				
Cardiac Imaging Stress Test before Surgery	703	3.0%	5.2%	5.3%
Combination Abdominal CT Scan	924	15.0%	13.4%	10.5%
Combination Brain/Sinus CT Scan	742	2.2%	2.2%	2.7%
Combination Chest CT Scan	430	6.5%	2.3%	2.7%
Follow-up Mammogram/Ultrasound	2,353	5.8%	8.2%	8.8%
Lumbar Spine MRI for Low Back Pain	203	37.9%	34.2%	37.2%

Marin General Hospital

250 Bon Air Road, PO Box 8010 Phone: 415-925-7900
Greenbrae, CA 94904 Fax: 415-925-7518
URL: www.maringeneral.com
Type: Acute Care Hospitals Emergency Services: Yes
Ownership: Government - Local Beds: 235

Key Personnel:
Radiology. . . . . Stephen I Abedon
Quality Assurance . . . . Denise Adams
Emergency Room . . . . Mark S Bason-Mitchell, MD
CEO/President. . . . . David Bradley
Intensive Care Unit. . . . . Mark Kobe
Anesthesiology. . . . . Paul Ulrich, MD
Chief of Medical Staff . . . . Gerald Wilner, MD

Measure	Cases	This Hosp.	State Avg.	U.S. Avg.
Blood Clot Prevention and Treatment				
Anticoagulation Overlap Therapy[2]	50	100%	92%	93%
ICU Venous Thromboembolism Prophylaxis[2]	45	100%	92%	92%
Incidence of Potentially Preventable VTE[2]	12	0%	11%	10%
UFH with Dosages/Platelet Monitoring[2]	18	100%	96%	97%
Venous Thromboembolism Prophylaxis[2]	354	97%	83%	85%
Warfarin Therapy Discharge Instructions[2]	34	100%	75%	75%
Chest Pain/Possible Heart Attack Care				
Aspirin Given Within 24 Hours of Arrival[5]	-	-	97%	96%
Fibrinolytic Meds Within 30 Min. of Arrival[5]	-	-	62%	58%
Average Time to ECG (minutes)[5]	-	-	9	7
Average Time to Transfer (minutes)[5]	-	-	62	60
Children's Asthma Care				
Received Home Management Plan of Care	-	-	88%	88%
Received Reliever Medication	-	-	100%	100%
Received Systemic Corticosteroids	-	-	100%	100%
Emergency Department				
Admittance Decision Time (minutes)[2]	525	165	125	98
Head CT Results Within 45 Min. of Arrival[1,3]	-	-	55%	57%
Patients Who Left ER Before Being Seen	35,312	1%	3%	2%
Time from ER Arrival to Admit. (minutes)[2]	741	319	323	274
Time from ER Arrival to Discharge (minutes)	413	143	168	134
Time in ER Before Being Evaluated (minutes)	423	29	29	26
Time to Pain Meds for Fractures (minutes)	167	54	62	57
Heart Attack Care				
Aspirin Given at Discharge	176	100%	99%	99%
Fibrinolytic Meds Within 30 Min. of Arrival[7]	-	-	73%	54%
PCI Within 90 Minutes of Arrival	25	100%	95%	96%
Statin Prescribed at Discharge	172	99%	98%	98%
Heart Failure Care				
ACE Inhibitor or ARB for LVSD[2]	41	100%	97%	97%
Discharge Instructions Given[2]	147	97%	94%	94%
Evaluation of LVS Function[2]	185	100%	99%	99%
Medicare Spending				
Medicare Spending per Patient (ratio)	-	1.02	0.98	0.98
Pneumonia Care				
Appropriate Initial Antibiotic Given[2]	74	100%	97%	95%
Blood Culture Timing[2]	193	100%	98%	98%
Pregnancy and Delivery Care				
Newborn Deliveries Scheduled Early[2]	14	0%	5%	6%
Preventive Care				
Immunization for Influenza[2]	544	86%	89%	90%
Immunization for Pneumonia[2]	626	84%	90%	92%
Stroke Care				
Anticoagulation Therapy for Atrial Fibrillation	20	100%	95%	95%
Antithrombotic Therapy Timing	95	100%	98%	98%
Assessed for Rehabilitation	98	100%	97%	97%
Discharged on Antithrombotic Therapy	94	100%	99%	99%
Discharged on Statin Medication	61	100%	94%	94%
Thrombolytic Therapy Timing[1]	-	-	72%	66%
Venous Thromboembolism Prophylaxis	105	100%	94%	94%
Written Stroke Educational Materials Given	51	88%	87%	88%
Surgical Care Improvement Project				
Appropriate Beta Blocker Usage[2]	119	100%	97%	98%
Appropriate VTP Within 24 Hours[2]	336	99%	98%	98%
Controlled Postoperative Blood Glucose[2]	61	97%	96%	97%
Perioperative Temperature Management[2]	473	100%	100%	100%
Prophylactic Antibiotic Selection[2]	329	100%	99%	99%
Prophylactic Antibiotic Selection (Outpatient)	205	99%	97%	98%

NOTE: Hospital profiles are in alphabetical order by state, then city, then hospital within the city; Rankings exclude hospitals with less than 25 cases except for patient surveys which excludes hospitals with less than 100 cases; (a) 100-299 cases; (1) The number of cases/patients is too few to report; (2) Data submitted were based on a sample of cases/patients; (3) Results are based on a shorter time period than required; (4) Data suppressed by CMS for one or more quarters; (5) Results are not available for this reporting period; (6) Fewer than 100 patients completed the HCAHPS survey; (7) No cases met the criteria for this measure; (8) The lower limit of the confidence interval cannot be calculated if the number of observed infections equals zero; (9) No data are available from the state/territory for this reporting period; (10) The scores shown reflect fewer than 50 completed surveys; (11) There were discrepancies in the data collection process; (12) This measure does not apply to this hospital for this reporting period; (13) Results cannot be calculated for this reporting period; (14) The results for this state are combined with nearby states to protect confidentiality; Please refer to the User's Guide for a full explanation of data.

Prophylactic Antibiotic Stopped[2]	329	99%	98%	98%
Prophylactic Antibiotic Timing[2]	329	100%	99%	99%
Prophylactic Antibiotic Timing (Outpatient)	204	98%	97%	98%
Urinary Catheter Removal[2]	213	99%	97%	97%
Survey of Patients' Hospital Experiences				
Area Around Room 'Always' Quiet at Night	300+	45%	51%	61%
Doctors 'Always' Communicated Well	300+	77%	78%	82%
Home Recovery Information Given	300+	82%	83%	85%
Hospital Given 9 or 10 on 10 Point Scale	300+	65%	68%	71%
Meds 'Always' Explained Before Given	300+	55%	61%	64%
Nurses 'Always' Communicated Well	300+	70%	74%	79%
Pain 'Always' Well Controlled	300+	65%	68%	71%
Room and Bathroom 'Always' Clean	300+	56%	70%	73%
Timely Help 'Always' Received	300+	57%	62%	68%
Would Definitely Recommend Hospital	300+	70%	70%	71%
Use of Medical Imaging				
Cardiac Imaging Stress Test before Surgery	1,449	2.6%	5.2%	5.3%
Combination Abdominal CT Scan	799	5.6%	13.4%	10.5%
Combination Brain/Sinus CT Scan	697	2.3%	2.2%	2.7%
Combination Chest CT Scan	714	0.4%	2.3%	2.7%
Follow-up Mammogram/Ultrasound	3,034	7.4%	8.2%	8.8%
Lumbar Spine MRI for Low Back Pain[1]	-	-	34.2%	37.2%

Biggs Gridley Memorial Hospital

240 Spruce Street Phone: 530-846-5671
Gridley, CA 95948
URL: www.bgmh.us.com
Type: Critical Access Hospitals Emergency Services: Yes
Ownership: Voluntary non-profit - Private Beds: 45

Key Personnel:
Intensive Care Unit. . . . . Vickie Addison, RN
Quality Assurance . . . . Jay Croy
Chair/CEO . . . . John T. Harris
Emergency Room . . . . Mike Houser, RN
Chief of Medical Staff. . . . . Raymond Rurez, MD
Operating Room. . . . . Raub Slack
CEO/President. . . . . David L Yarbrough, CEO

Measure	Cases	This Hosp.	State Avg.	U.S. Avg.
Blood Clot Prevention and Treatment				
Anticoagulation Overlap Therapy[5]	-	-	92%	93%
ICU Venous Thromboembolism Prophylaxis[5]	-	-	92%	92%
Incidence of Potentially Preventable VTE[5]	-	-	11%	10%
UFH with Dosages/Platelet Monitoring[5]	-	-	96%	97%
Venous Thromboembolism Prophylaxis[5]	-	-	83%	85%
Warfarin Therapy Discharge Instructions[5]	-	-	75%	75%
Chest Pain/Possible Heart Attack Care				
Aspirin Given Within 24 Hours of Arrival[5]	-	-	97%	96%
Fibrinolytic Meds Within 30 Min. of Arrival[5]	-	-	62%	58%
Average Time to ECG (minutes)[5]	-	-	9	7
Average Time to Transfer (minutes)[5]	-	-	62	60
Children's Asthma Care				
Received Home Management Plan of Care	-	-	88%	88%
Received Reliever Medication	-	-	100%	100%
Received Systemic Corticosteroids	-	-	100%	100%
Emergency Department				
Admittance Decision Time (minutes)[5]	-	-	125	98
Head CT Results Within 45 Min. of Arrival[5]	-	-	55%	57%
Patients Who Left ER Before Being Seen[5]	-	-	3%	2%
Time from ER Arrival to Admit. (minutes)[5]	-	-	323	274
Time from ER Arrival to Discharge (minutes)[3]	19	205	168	134
Time in ER Before Being Evaluated (minutes)[3]	19	3	29	26
Time to Pain Meds for Fractures (minutes)[5]	-	-	62	57
Heart Attack Care				
Aspirin Given at Discharge[5]	-	-	99%	99%
Fibrinolytic Meds Within 30 Min. of Arrival[5]	-	-	73%	54%
PCI Within 90 Minutes of Arrival[5]	-	-	95%	96%
Statin Prescribed at Discharge[5]	-	-	98%	98%
Heart Failure Care				
ACE Inhibitor or ARB for LVSD[1,3]	-	-	97%	97%
Discharge Instructions Given[1,3]	-	-	94%	94%
Evaluation of LVS Function[3]	13	31%	99%	99%
Medicare Spending				
Medicare Spending per Patient (ratio)	-	-	0.98	0.98
Pneumonia Care				
Appropriate Initial Antibiotic Given[1,3]	-	-	97%	95%
Blood Culture Timing[1,3]	-	-	98%	98%
Pregnancy and Delivery Care				
Newborn Deliveries Scheduled Early[5]	-	-	5%	6%
Preventive Care				
Immunization for Influenza[5]	-	-	89%	90%
Immunization for Pneumonia[5]	-	-	90%	92%
Stroke Care				
Anticoagulation Therapy for Atrial Fibrillation[5]	-	-	95%	95%
Antithrombotic Therapy Timing[5]	-	-	98%	98%
Assessed for Rehabilitation[5]	-	-	97%	97%
Discharged on Antithrombotic Therapy[5]	-	-	99%	99%
Discharged on Statin Medication[5]	-	-	94%	94%
Thrombolytic Therapy Timing[5]	-	-	72%	66%
Venous Thromboembolism Prophylaxis[5]	-	-	94%	94%
Written Stroke Educational Materials Given[5]	-	-	87%	88%
Surgical Care Improvement Project				
Appropriate Beta Blocker Usage[5]	-	-	97%	98%
Appropriate VTP Within 24 Hours[5]	-	-	98%	98%
Controlled Postoperative Blood Glucose[5]	-	-	96%	97%
Perioperative Temperature Management[5]	-	-	100%	100%
Prophylactic Antibiotic Selection[5]	-	-	99%	99%
Prophylactic Antibiotic Selection (Outpatient)[5]	-	-	97%	98%
Prophylactic Antibiotic Stopped[5]	-	-	98%	98%
Prophylactic Antibiotic Timing[5]	-	-	99%	99%
Prophylactic Antibiotic Timing (Outpatient)[5]	-	-	97%	98%
Urinary Catheter Removal[5]	-	-	97%	97%
Survey of Patients' Hospital Experiences				
Area Around Room 'Always' Quiet at Night[5]	-	-	51%	61%
Doctors 'Always' Communicated Well[5]	-	-	78%	82%
Home Recovery Information Given[5]	-	-	83%	85%
Hospital Given 9 or 10 on 10 Point Scale[5]	-	-	68%	71%
Meds 'Always' Explained Before Given[5]	-	-	61%	64%
Nurses 'Always' Communicated Well[5]	-	-	74%	79%
Pain 'Always' Well Controlled[5]	-	-	68%	71%
Room and Bathroom 'Always' Clean[5]	-	-	70%	73%
Timely Help 'Always' Received[5]	-	-	62%	68%
Would Definitely Recommend Hospital[5]	-	-	70%	71%
Use of Medical Imaging				
Cardiac Imaging Stress Test before Surgery[7]	-	-	5.2%	5.3%
Combination Abdominal CT Scan	281	79.0%	13.4%	10.5%
Combination Brain/Sinus CT Scan[1]	-	-	2.2%	2.7%
Combination Chest CT Scan	104	1.0%	2.3%	2.7%
Follow-up Mammogram/Ultrasound	193	11.4%	8.2%	8.8%
Lumbar Spine MRI for Low Back Pain[1]	-	-	34.2%	37.2%

Adventist Medical Center

115 Mall Drive Phone: 559-582-9000
Hanford, CA 93230 Fax: 559-584-7401
URL: www.hanfordhealth.com
Type: Acute Care Hospitals Emergency Services: Yes
Ownership: Voluntary non-profit - Church Beds: 60

Key Personnel:
Radiology. . . . . Muhammad Chaudhri
Quality Assurance . . . . Brandy Gass, RN
Chief of Medical Staff. . . . . MR Goodman, MD
Operating Room. . . . . Marilyn Harris, RN
Patient Relations . . . . Carol Hasselbrack
Emergency Room . . . . Trini Juarez
CEO/President. . . . . Scott Reiner

Measure	Cases	This Hosp.	State Avg.	U.S. Avg.
Blood Clot Prevention and Treatment				
Anticoagulation Overlap Therapy[2]	55	58%	92%	93%
ICU Venous Thromboembolism Prophylaxis[2]	94	88%	92%	92%
Incidence of Potentially Preventable VTE[1,2]	-	-	11%	10%
UFH with Dosages/Platelet Monitoring[1,2]	-	-	96%	97%
Venous Thromboembolism Prophylaxis[2]	811	59%	83%	85%
Warfarin Therapy Discharge Instructions[2]	47	91%	75%	75%
Chest Pain/Possible Heart Attack Care				
Aspirin Given Within 24 Hours of Arrival	96	90%	97%	96%
Fibrinolytic Meds Within 30 Min. of Arrival[7]	-	-	62%	58%
Average Time to ECG (minutes)	96	14	9	7
Average Time to Transfer (minutes)	37	67	62	60
Children's Asthma Care				
Received Home Management Plan of Care	-	-	88%	88%
Received Reliever Medication	-	-	100%	100%
Received Systemic Corticosteroids	-	-	100%	100%
Emergency Department				
Admittance Decision Time (minutes)[2]	1,050	133	125	98
Head CT Results Within 45 Min. of Arrival	27	26%	55%	57%
Patients Who Left ER Before Being Seen	>100k	1%	3%	2%
Time from ER Arrival to Admit. (minutes)[2]	1,547	306	323	274
Time from ER Arrival to Discharge (minutes)	875	144	168	134
Time in ER Before Being Evaluated (minutes)	946	11	29	26
Time to Pain Meds for Fractures (minutes)	207	62	62	57
Heart Attack Care				
Aspirin Given at Discharge	24	92%	99%	99%
Fibrinolytic Meds Within 30 Min. of Arrival[7]	-	-	73%	54%
PCI Within 90 Minutes of Arrival[7]	-	-	95%	96%
Statin Prescribed at Discharge	23	87%	98%	98%
Heart Failure Care				
ACE Inhibitor or ARB for LVSD	138	89%	97%	97%
Discharge Instructions Given	289	98%	94%	94%
Evaluation of LVS Function	325	96%	99%	99%
Medicare Spending				
Medicare Spending per Patient (ratio)	-	0.93	0.98	0.98
Pneumonia Care				
Appropriate Initial Antibiotic Given[2]	170	96%	97%	95%
Blood Culture Timing[2]	261	95%	98%	98%
Pregnancy and Delivery Care				
Newborn Deliveries Scheduled Early[2]	51	10%	5%	6%
Preventive Care				
Immunization for Influenza[2]	1,061	89%	89%	90%
Immunization for Pneumonia[2]	1,306	86%	90%	92%
Stroke Care				
Anticoagulation Therapy for Atrial Fibrillation	12	100%	95%	95%
Antithrombotic Therapy Timing	80	92%	98%	98%
Assessed for Rehabilitation	88	95%	97%	97%
Discharged on Antithrombotic Therapy	82	95%	99%	99%
Discharged on Statin Medication	78	86%	94%	94%
Thrombolytic Therapy Timing	26	8%	72%	66%
Venous Thromboembolism Prophylaxis	85	80%	94%	94%
Written Stroke Educational Materials Given	60	75%	87%	88%
Surgical Care Improvement Project				
Appropriate Beta Blocker Usage[2]	65	82%	97%	98%
Appropriate VTP Within 24 Hours[2]	307	91%	98%	98%
Controlled Postoperative Blood Glucose[2,7]	-	-	96%	97%
Perioperative Temperature Management[2]	399	100%	100%	100%
Prophylactic Antibiotic Selection[2]	283	95%	99%	99%
Prophylactic Antibiotic Selection (Outpatient)	74	84%	97%	98%
Prophylactic Antibiotic Stopped[2]	280	92%	98%	98%
Prophylactic Antibiotic Timing[2]	284	96%	99%	99%
Prophylactic Antibiotic Timing (Outpatient)	86	80%	97%	98%
Urinary Catheter Removal[2]	199	93%	97%	97%
Survey of Patients' Hospital Experiences				
Area Around Room 'Always' Quiet at Night	300+	52%	51%	61%
Doctors 'Always' Communicated Well	300+	74%	78%	82%
Home Recovery Information Given	300+	84%	83%	85%
Hospital Given 9 or 10 on 10 Point Scale	300+	64%	68%	71%
Meds 'Always' Explained Before Given	300+	57%	61%	64%
Nurses 'Always' Communicated Well	300+	70%	74%	79%
Pain 'Always' Well Controlled	300+	64%	68%	71%
Room and Bathroom 'Always' Clean	300+	71%	70%	73%
Timely Help 'Always' Received	300+	58%	62%	68%
Would Definitely Recommend Hospital	300+	60%	70%	71%
Use of Medical Imaging				
Cardiac Imaging Stress Test before Surgery[1]	-	-	5.2%	5.3%
Combination Abdominal CT Scan	1,179	28.8%	13.4%	10.5%
Combination Brain/Sinus CT Scan	1,098	2.5%	2.2%	2.7%
Combination Chest CT Scan	625	35.5%	2.3%	2.7%
Follow-up Mammogram/Ultrasound	1,403	16.0%	8.2%	8.8%
Lumbar Spine MRI for Low Back Pain	142	33.1%	34.2%	37.2%

NOTE: Hospital profiles are in alphabetical order by state, then city, then hospital within the city; Rankings exclude hospitals with less than 25 cases except for patient surveys which excludes hospitals with less than 100 cases; (a) 100-299 cases; (1) The number of cases/patients is too few to report; (2) Data submitted were based on a sample of cases/patients; (3) Results are based on a shorter time period than required; (4) Data suppressed by CMS for one or more quarters; (5) Results are not available for this reporting period; (6) Fewer than 100 patients completed the HCAHPS survey; (7) No cases met the criteria for this measure; (8) The lower limit of the confidence interval cannot be calculated if the number of observed infections equals zero; (9) No data are available from the state/territory for this reporting period; (10) The scores shown reflect fewer than 50 completed surveys; (11) There were discrepancies in the data collection process; (12) This measure does not apply to this hospital for this reporting period; (13) Results cannot be calculated for this reporting period; (14) The results for this state are combined with nearby states to protect confidentiality; Please refer to the User's Guide for a full explanation of data.

Central Valley General Hospital

1025 N Douty St | Phone: 559-583-2100
Hanford, CA 93230 | Fax: 559-583-2225
URL: www.hanfordhealth.com
Type: Acute Care Hospitals | Emergency Services: Yes
Ownership: Voluntary non-profit - Church | Beds: 49

Key Personnel:

Cardiac Laboratory. . . . . Anita Anivigate
Radiology. . . . . Muhammad Chaudhri
Chief of Medical Staff . . . . Charles Craft
Quality Assurance . . . . Brandy Gass
Infection Control . . . . Kathy Palusko
CEO/President. . . . . Rick Rawson
Operating Room. . . . . Marylyn Reiber, MD

Measure	Cases	This Hosp.	State Avg.	U.S. Avg.
Blood Clot Prevention and Treatment				
Anticoagulation Overlap Therapy[7]	-	-	92%	93%
ICU Venous Thromboembolism Prophylaxis[7]	-	-	92%	92%
Incidence of Potentially Preventable VTE[7]	-	-	11%	10%
UFH with Dosages/Platelet Monitoring[7]	-	-	96%	97%
Venous Thromboembolism Prophylaxis[1]	-	-	83%	85%
Warfarin Therapy Discharge Instructions[7]	-	-	75%	75%
Chest Pain/Possible Heart Attack Care				
Aspirin Given Within 24 Hours of Arrival	-	-	97%	96%
Fibrinolytic Meds Within 30 Min. of Arrival	-	-	62%	58%
Average Time to ECG (minutes)	-	-	9	7
Average Time to Transfer (minutes)	-	-	62	60
Children's Asthma Care				
Received Home Management Plan of Care	-	-	88%	88%
Received Reliever Medication	-	-	100%	100%
Received Systemic Corticosteroids	-	-	100%	100%
Emergency Department				
Admittance Decision Time (minutes)[2,7]	-	-	125	98
Head CT Results Within 45 Min. of Arrival	-	-	55%	57%
Patients Who Left ER Before Being Seen	-	-	3%	2%
Time from ER Arrival to Admit. (minutes)[2,7]	-	-	323	274
Time from ER Arrival to Discharge (minutes)	-	-	168	134
Time in ER Before Being Evaluated (minutes)	-	-	29	26
Time to Pain Meds for Fractures (minutes)	-	-	62	57
Heart Attack Care				
Aspirin Given at Discharge[5]	-	-	99%	99%
Fibrinolytic Meds Within 30 Min. of Arrival[5]	-	-	73%	54%
PCI Within 90 Minutes of Arrival[5]	-	-	95%	96%
Statin Prescribed at Discharge[5]	-	-	98%	98%
Heart Failure Care				
ACE Inhibitor or ARB for LVSD[5]	-	-	97%	97%
Discharge Instructions Given[5]	-	-	94%	94%
Evaluation of LVS Function[5]	-	-	99%	99%
Medicare Spending				
Medicare Spending per Patient (ratio)[1]	-	-	0.98	0.98
Pneumonia Care				
Appropriate Initial Antibiotic Given[5]	-	-	97%	95%
Blood Culture Timing[5]	-	-	98%	98%
Pregnancy and Delivery Care				
Newborn Deliveries Scheduled Early[2]	48	10%	5%	6%
Preventive Care				
Immunization for Influenza[2]	243	56%	89%	90%
Immunization for Pneumonia[2]	20	15%	90%	92%
Stroke Care				
Anticoagulation Therapy for Atrial Fibrillation[5]	-	-	95%	95%
Antithrombotic Therapy Timing[5]	-	-	98%	98%
Assessed for Rehabilitation[5]	-	-	97%	97%
Discharged on Antithrombotic Therapy[5]	-	-	99%	99%
Discharged on Statin Medication[5]	-	-	94%	94%
Thrombolytic Therapy Timing[5]	-	-	72%	66%
Venous Thromboembolism Prophylaxis[5]	-	-	94%	94%
Written Stroke Educational Materials Given[5]	-	-	87%	88%
Surgical Care Improvement Project				
Appropriate Beta Blocker Usage[5]	-	-	97%	98%
Appropriate VTP Within 24 Hours[5]	-	-	98%	98%
Controlled Postoperative Blood Glucose[5]	-	-	96%	97%
Perioperative Temperature Management[5]	-	-	100%	100%
Prophylactic Antibiotic Selection[5]	-	-	99%	99%
Prophylactic Antibiotic Selection (Outpatient)	-	-	97%	98%
Prophylactic Antibiotic Stopped[5]	-	-	98%	98%
Prophylactic Antibiotic Timing[5]	-	-	99%	99%
Prophylactic Antibiotic Timing (Outpatient)	-	-	97%	98%
Urinary Catheter Removal[5]	-	-	97%	97%
Survey of Patients' Hospital Experiences				
Area Around Room 'Always' Quiet at Night	300+	57%	51%	61%
Doctors 'Always' Communicated Well	300+	74%	78%	82%
Home Recovery Information Given	300+	76%	83%	85%
Hospital Given 9 or 10 on 10 Point Scale	300+	54%	68%	71%
Meds 'Always' Explained Before Given	300+	56%	61%	64%
Nurses 'Always' Communicated Well	300+	69%	74%	79%
Pain 'Always' Well Controlled	300+	62%	68%	71%
Room and Bathroom 'Always' Clean	300+	72%	70%	73%
Timely Help 'Always' Received	300+	54%	62%	68%
Would Definitely Recommend Hospital	300+	53%	70%	71%
Use of Medical Imaging				
Cardiac Imaging Stress Test before Surgery	-	-	5.2%	5.3%
Combination Abdominal CT Scan	-	-	13.4%	10.5%
Combination Brain/Sinus CT Scan	-	-	2.2%	2.7%
Combination Chest CT Scan	-	-	2.3%	2.7%
Follow-up Mammogram/Ultrasound	-	-	8.2%	8.8%
Lumbar Spine MRI for Low Back Pain	-	-	34.2%	37.2%

Kaiser Foundation Hospital - South Bay

25825 South Vermont Avenue | Phone: 310-517-6441
Harbor City, CA 90710 | Fax: 310-517-3424
URL: www.kaiserpermanente.org
Type: Acute Care Hospitals | Emergency Services: Yes
Ownership: Voluntary non-profit - Other | Beds: 251

Key Personnel:

Operating Room. . . . . Mary Lou Carnahan
Pediatric Ambulatory Care . . . . . . Barbara Carnes, MD
CEO/President. . . . . George Halvorson
Quality Assurance . . . . Genny Hulbrook
Chief of Medical Staff. . . . . Randel King, MD
Radiology. . . . . Augusto Salceda, MD

Measure	Cases	This Hosp.	State Avg.	U.S. Avg.
Blood Clot Prevention and Treatment				
Anticoagulation Overlap Therapy[2]	62	95%	92%	93%
ICU Venous Thromboembolism Prophylaxis[2]	36	97%	92%	92%
Incidence of Potentially Preventable VTE[2]	11	27%	11%	10%
UFH with Dosages/Platelet Monitoring[2]	46	96%	96%	97%
Venous Thromboembolism Prophylaxis[2]	286	93%	83%	85%
Warfarin Therapy Discharge Instructions[2]	56	98%	75%	75%
Chest Pain/Possible Heart Attack Care				
Aspirin Given Within 24 Hours of Arrival	-	-	97%	96%
Fibrinolytic Meds Within 30 Min. of Arrival	-	-	62%	58%
Average Time to ECG (minutes)	-	-	9	7
Average Time to Transfer (minutes)	-	-	62	60
Children's Asthma Care				
Received Home Management Plan of Care	-	-	88%	88%
Received Reliever Medication	-	-	100%	100%
Received Systemic Corticosteroids	-	-	100%	100%
Emergency Department				
Admittance Decision Time (minutes)[2]	372	78	125	98
Head CT Results Within 45 Min. of Arrival	-	-	55%	57%
Patients Who Left ER Before Being Seen	-	-	3%	2%
Time from ER Arrival to Admit. (minutes)[2]	403	318	323	274
Time from ER Arrival to Discharge (minutes)	-	-	168	134
Time in ER Before Being Evaluated (minutes)	-	-	29	26
Time to Pain Meds for Fractures (minutes)	-	-	62	57
Heart Attack Care				
Aspirin Given at Discharge	54	100%	99%	99%
Fibrinolytic Meds Within 30 Min. of Arrival[1]	-	-	73%	54%
PCI Within 90 Minutes of Arrival[7]	-	-	95%	96%
Statin Prescribed at Discharge	57	100%	98%	98%
Heart Failure Care				
ACE Inhibitor or ARB for LVSD	100	100%	97%	97%
Discharge Instructions Given	285	100%	94%	94%
Evaluation of LVS Function	300	100%	99%	99%
Medicare Spending				
Medicare Spending per Patient (ratio)	-	0.76	0.98	0.98
Pneumonia Care				
Appropriate Initial Antibiotic Given[2]	68	100%	97%	95%
Blood Culture Timing[2]	156	99%	98%	98%
Pregnancy and Delivery Care				
Newborn Deliveries Scheduled Early[2]	181	2%	5%	6%
Preventive Care				
Immunization for Influenza[2]	515	98%	89%	90%
Immunization for Pneumonia[2]	598	98%	90%	92%
Stroke Care				
Anticoagulation Therapy for Atrial Fibrillation[1,2]	-	-	95%	95%
Antithrombotic Therapy Timing[2]	80	99%	98%	98%
Assessed for Rehabilitation[2]	93	100%	97%	97%
Discharged on Antithrombotic Therapy[2]	82	100%	99%	99%
Discharged on Statin Medication[2]	72	100%	94%	94%
Thrombolytic Therapy Timing[1,2]	-	-	72%	66%
Venous Thromboembolism Prophylaxis[2]	65	100%	94%	94%
Written Stroke Educational Materials Given[2]	52	100%	87%	88%
Surgical Care Improvement Project				
Appropriate Beta Blocker Usage[2]	128	100%	97%	98%
Appropriate VTP Within 24 Hours[2]	379	100%	98%	98%
Controlled Postoperative Blood Glucose[2,7]	-	-	96%	97%
Perioperative Temperature Management[2]	447	100%	100%	100%
Prophylactic Antibiotic Selection[2]	278	100%	99%	99%
Prophylactic Antibiotic Selection (Outpatient)	-	-	97%	98%
Prophylactic Antibiotic Stopped[2]	272	100%	98%	98%
Prophylactic Antibiotic Timing[2]	278	99%	99%	99%
Prophylactic Antibiotic Timing (Outpatient)	-	-	97%	98%
Urinary Catheter Removal[2]	286	100%	97%	97%
Survey of Patients' Hospital Experiences				
Area Around Room 'Always' Quiet at Night	300+	54%	51%	61%
Doctors 'Always' Communicated Well	300+	83%	78%	82%
Home Recovery Information Given	300+	87%	83%	85%
Hospital Given 9 or 10 on 10 Point Scale	300+	76%	68%	71%
Meds 'Always' Explained Before Given	300+	62%	61%	64%
Nurses 'Always' Communicated Well	300+	76%	74%	79%
Pain 'Always' Well Controlled	300+	72%	68%	71%
Room and Bathroom 'Always' Clean	300+	70%	70%	73%
Timely Help 'Always' Received	300+	66%	62%	68%
Would Definitely Recommend Hospital	300+	75%	70%	71%
Use of Medical Imaging				
Cardiac Imaging Stress Test before Surgery	-	-	5.2%	5.3%
Combination Abdominal CT Scan	-	-	13.4%	10.5%
Combination Brain/Sinus CT Scan	-	-	2.2%	2.7%
Combination Chest CT Scan	-	-	2.3%	2.7%
Follow-up Mammogram/Ultrasound	-	-	8.2%	8.8%
Lumbar Spine MRI for Low Back Pain	-	-	34.2%	37.2%

Tri - City Regional Medical Center

21530 S Pioneer Blvd | Phone: 562-860-0401
Hawaiian Gardens, CA 90716 | Fax: 562-924-5871
URL: www.tri-cityrmc.org
Type: Acute Care Hospitals | Emergency Services: Yes
Ownership: Govt - Hospital Dist/Auth | Beds: 137

Measure	Cases	This Hosp.	State Avg.	U.S. Avg.
Blood Clot Prevention and Treatment				
Anticoagulation Overlap Therapy[1,2]	-	-	92%	93%
ICU Venous Thromboembolism Prophylaxis[2]	69	87%	92%	92%
Incidence of Potentially Preventable VTE[1,2]	-	-	11%	10%
UFH with Dosages/Platelet Monitoring[1,2]	-	-	96%	97%
Venous Thromboembolism Prophylaxis[2]	285	87%	83%	85%
Warfarin Therapy Discharge Instructions[1,2]	-	-	75%	75%
Chest Pain/Possible Heart Attack Care				
Aspirin Given Within 24 Hours of Arrival[1,3]	-	-	97%	96%
Fibrinolytic Meds Within 30 Min. of Arrival[5]	-	-	62%	58%
Average Time to ECG (minutes)[1,3]	-	-	9	7
Average Time to Transfer (minutes)[5]	-	-	62	60
Children's Asthma Care				
Received Home Management Plan of Care	-	-	88%	88%
Received Reliever Medication	-	-	100%	100%
Received Systemic Corticosteroids	-	-	100%	100%
Emergency Department				
Admittance Decision Time (minutes)[2]	366	75	125	98
Head CT Results Within 45 Min. of Arrival[1,3]	-	-	55%	57%
Patients Who Left ER Before Being Seen	8,548	2%	3%	2%

NOTE: Hospital profiles are in alphabetical order by state, then city, then hospital within the city; Rankings exclude hospitals with less than 25 cases except for patient surveys which excludes hospitals with less than 100 cases; (a) 100-299 cases; (1) The number of cases/patients is too few to report; (2) Data submitted were based on a sample of cases/patients; (3) Results are based on a shorter time period than required; (4) Data suppressed by CMS for one or more quarters; (5) Results are not available for this reporting period; (6) Fewer than 100 patients completed the HCAHPS survey; (7) No cases met the criteria for this measure; (8) The lower limit of the confidence interval cannot be calculated if the number of observed infections equals zero; (9) No data are available from the state/territory for this reporting period; (10) The scores shown reflect fewer than 50 completed surveys; (11) There were discrepancies in the data collection process; (12) This measure does not apply to this hospital for this reporting period; (13) Results cannot be calculated for this reporting period; (14) The results for this state are combined with nearby states to protect confidentiality; Please refer to the User's Guide for a full explanation of data.

Measure	Cases	This Hosp.	State Avg.	U.S. Avg.
Time from ER Arrival to Admit. (minutes)[2]	371	265	323	274
Time from ER Arrival to Discharge (minutes)	305	129	168	134
Time in ER Before Being Evaluated (minutes)	347	22	29	26
Time to Pain Meds for Fractures (minutes)	16	34	62	57
Heart Attack Care				
Aspirin Given at Discharge[1]	-	-	99%	99%
Fibrinolytic Meds Within 30 Min. of Arrival[7]	-	-	73%	54%
PCI Within 90 Minutes of Arrival[7]	-	-	95%	96%
Statin Prescribed at Discharge[1]	-	-	98%	98%
Heart Failure Care				
ACE Inhibitor or ARB for LVSD	28	93%	97%	97%
Discharge Instructions Given	66	85%	94%	94%
Evaluation of LVS Function	92	99%	99%	99%
Medicare Spending				
Medicare Spending per Patient (ratio)	-	1.30	0.98	0.98
Pneumonia Care				
Appropriate Initial Antibiotic Given	25	92%	97%	95%
Blood Culture Timing	116	97%	98%	98%
Pregnancy and Delivery Care				
Newborn Deliveries Scheduled Early[7]	-	-	5%	6%
Preventive Care				
Immunization for Influenza[2]	305	91%	89%	90%
Immunization for Pneumonia[2]	414	89%	90%	92%
Stroke Care				
Anticoagulation Therapy for Atrial Fibrillation[1]	-	-	95%	95%
Antithrombotic Therapy Timing[1]	-	-	98%	98%
Assessed for Rehabilitation	13	77%	97%	97%
Discharged on Antithrombotic Therapy	11	91%	99%	99%
Discharged on Statin Medication[1]	-	-	94%	94%
Thrombolytic Therapy Timing[7]	-	-	72%	66%
Venous Thromboembolism Prophylaxis	13	92%	94%	94%
Written Stroke Educational Materials Given[1]	-	-	87%	88%
Surgical Care Improvement Project				
Appropriate Beta Blocker Usage	20	80%	97%	98%
Appropriate VTP Within 24 Hours	136	96%	98%	98%
Controlled Postoperative Blood Glucose[7]	-	-	96%	97%
Perioperative Temperature Management	156	99%	100%	100%
Prophylactic Antibiotic Selection	91	89%	99%	99%
Prophylactic Antibiotic Selection (Outpatient)[1]	-	-	97%	98%
Prophylactic Antibiotic Stopped	89	89%	98%	98%
Prophylactic Antibiotic Timing	91	95%	99%	99%
Prophylactic Antibiotic Timing (Outpatient)	14	64%	97%	98%
Urinary Catheter Removal	37	95%	97%	97%
Survey of Patients' Hospital Experiences				
Area Around Room 'Always' Quiet at Night	300+	52%	51%	61%
Doctors 'Always' Communicated Well	300+	77%	78%	82%
Home Recovery Information Given	300+	80%	83%	85%
Hospital Given 9 or 10 on 10 Point Scale	300+	55%	68%	71%
Meds 'Always' Explained Before Given	300+	57%	61%	64%
Nurses 'Always' Communicated Well	300+	68%	74%	79%
Pain 'Always' Well Controlled	300+	68%	68%	71%
Room and Bathroom 'Always' Clean	300+	66%	70%	73%
Timely Help 'Always' Received	300+	59%	62%	68%
Would Definitely Recommend Hospital	300+	59%	70%	71%
Use of Medical Imaging				
Cardiac Imaging Stress Test before Surgery[1]	-	-	5.2%	5.3%
Combination Abdominal CT Scan	84	1.2%	13.4%	10.5%
Combination Brain/Sinus CT Scan[1]	-	-	2.2%	2.7%
Combination Chest CT Scan[1]	-	-	2.3%	2.7%
Follow-up Mammogram/Ultrasound	93	2.2%	8.2%	8.8%
Lumbar Spine MRI for Low Back Pain[1]	-	-	34.2%	37.2%

Kaiser Foundation Hospital - Fremont/Hayward

27400 Hesperian Blvd
Hayward, CA 94545
Phone: 510-784-4000
Fax: 510-784-2791
URL: www.kaiserpermanente.org
Type: Acute Care Hospitals
Emergency Services: Yes
Ownership: Voluntary non-profit - Other
Beds: 234

Key Personnel:

Operating Room. . . . . Michelle Clark
Quality Assurance . . . . Cathy Crisfield
Patient Relations . . . . Sal Esparza
Coronary Care . . . . Robert Heller, MD
Pediatric Ambulatory Care . . . . . . Arndt Herz, MD
Chief of Medical Staff . . . . Anabel Andarson Imberg
Emergency Room . . . . Terri Pillow-Noriega

Measure	Cases	This Hosp.	State Avg.	U.S. Avg.
Blood Clot Prevention and Treatment				
Anticoagulation Overlap Therapy[2]	62	100%	92%	93%
ICU Venous Thromboembolism Prophylaxis[2]	40	98%	92%	92%
Incidence of Potentially Preventable VTE[1,2]	-	-	11%	10%
UFH with Dosages/Platelet Monitoring[2]	46	100%	96%	97%
Venous Thromboembolism Prophylaxis[2]	276	96%	83%	85%
Warfarin Therapy Discharge Instructions[2]	46	57%	75%	75%
Chest Pain/Possible Heart Attack Care				
Aspirin Given Within 24 Hours of Arrival	-	-	97%	96%
Fibrinolytic Meds Within 30 Min. of Arrival	-	-	62%	58%
Average Time to ECG (minutes)	-	-	9	7
Average Time to Transfer (minutes)	-	-	62	60
Children's Asthma Care				
Received Home Management Plan of Care	-	-	88%	88%
Received Reliever Medication	-	-	100%	100%
Received Systemic Corticosteroids	-	-	100%	100%
Emergency Department				
Admittance Decision Time (minutes)[2]	542	50	125	98
Head CT Results Within 45 Min. of Arrival	-	-	55%	57%
Patients Who Left ER Before Being Seen	-	-	3%	2%
Time from ER Arrival to Admit. (minutes)[2]	546	286	323	274
Time from ER Arrival to Discharge (minutes)	-	-	168	134
Time in ER Before Being Evaluated (minutes)	-	-	29	26
Time to Pain Meds for Fractures (minutes)	-	-	62	57
Heart Attack Care				
Aspirin Given at Discharge	99	100%	99%	99%
Fibrinolytic Meds Within 30 Min. of Arrival[7]	-	-	73%	54%
PCI Within 90 Minutes of Arrival	23	96%	95%	96%
Statin Prescribed at Discharge	108	100%	98%	98%
Heart Failure Care				
ACE Inhibitor or ARB for LVSD	76	100%	97%	97%
Discharge Instructions Given	212	100%	94%	94%
Evaluation of LVS Function	247	100%	99%	99%
Medicare Spending				
Medicare Spending per Patient (ratio)	-	0.81	0.98	0.98
Pneumonia Care				
Appropriate Initial Antibiotic Given[2]	71	97%	97%	95%
Blood Culture Timing[2]	148	99%	98%	98%
Pregnancy and Delivery Care				
Newborn Deliveries Scheduled Early[2]	39	0%	5%	6%
Preventive Care				
Immunization for Influenza[2]	497	92%	89%	90%
Immunization for Pneumonia[2]	569	94%	90%	92%
Stroke Care				
Anticoagulation Therapy for Atrial Fibrillation[1,2]	-	-	95%	95%
Antithrombotic Therapy Timing[2]	70	96%	98%	98%
Assessed for Rehabilitation[2]	100	97%	97%	97%
Discharged on Antithrombotic Therapy[2]	84	94%	99%	99%
Discharged on Statin Medication[2]	68	97%	94%	94%
Thrombolytic Therapy Timing[2]	13	100%	72%	66%
Venous Thromboembolism Prophylaxis[2]	97	99%	94%	94%
Written Stroke Educational Materials Given[2]	44	100%	87%	88%
Surgical Care Improvement Project				
Appropriate Beta Blocker Usage[2]	164	100%	97%	98%
Appropriate VTP Within 24 Hours[2]	429	100%	98%	98%
Controlled Postoperative Blood Glucose[2,7]	-	-	96%	97%
Perioperative Temperature Management[2]	512	100%	100%	100%
Prophylactic Antibiotic Selection[2]	319	100%	99%	99%
Prophylactic Antibiotic Selection (Outpatient)	-	-	97%	98%
Prophylactic Antibiotic Stopped[2]	313	100%	98%	98%
Prophylactic Antibiotic Timing[2]	319	99%	99%	99%
Prophylactic Antibiotic Timing (Outpatient)	-	-	97%	98%
Urinary Catheter Removal[2]	345	100%	97%	97%
Survey of Patients' Hospital Experiences				
Area Around Room 'Always' Quiet at Night	300+	47%	51%	61%
Doctors 'Always' Communicated Well	300+	80%	78%	82%
Home Recovery Information Given	300+	83%	83%	85%
Hospital Given 9 or 10 on 10 Point Scale	300+	66%	68%	71%
Meds 'Always' Explained Before Given	300+	61%	61%	64%
Nurses 'Always' Communicated Well	300+	73%	74%	79%
Pain 'Always' Well Controlled	300+	70%	68%	71%
Room and Bathroom 'Always' Clean	300+	70%	70%	73%
Timely Help 'Always' Received	300+	63%	62%	68%
Would Definitely Recommend Hospital	300+	69%	70%	71%
Use of Medical Imaging				
Cardiac Imaging Stress Test before Surgery	-	-	5.2%	5.3%
Combination Abdominal CT Scan	-	-	13.4%	10.5%
Combination Brain/Sinus CT Scan	-	-	2.2%	2.7%
Combination Chest CT Scan	-	-	2.3%	2.7%
Follow-up Mammogram/Ultrasound	-	-	8.2%	8.8%
Lumbar Spine MRI for Low Back Pain	-	-	34.2%	37.2%

Saint Rose Hospital

27200 Calaroga Ave
Hayward, CA 94545
Phone: 510-782-6200
Fax: 510-264-4076
URL: www.strosehospital.org
Type: Acute Care Hospitals
Emergency Services: Yes
Ownership: Voluntary non-profit - Church
Beds: 175

Key Personnel:

Quality Assurance . . . . Carol Ann Lemmon
Chief of Medical Staff . . . . Vasiliki Economou, MD
Emergency Room . . . . Patrick Evangelista
CEO/President. . . . . Lex Reddy

Measure	Cases	This Hosp.	State Avg.	U.S. Avg.
Blood Clot Prevention and Treatment				
Anticoagulation Overlap Therapy[2]	19	100%	92%	93%
ICU Venous Thromboembolism Prophylaxis[2]	54	93%	92%	92%
Incidence of Potentially Preventable VTE[1,2]	-	-	11%	10%
UFH with Dosages/Platelet Monitoring[1,2]	-	-	96%	97%
Venous Thromboembolism Prophylaxis[2]	346	72%	83%	85%
Warfarin Therapy Discharge Instructions[2]	12	100%	75%	75%
Chest Pain/Possible Heart Attack Care				
Aspirin Given Within 24 Hours of Arrival[1,3]	-	-	97%	96%
Fibrinolytic Meds Within 30 Min. of Arrival[5]	-	-	62%	58%
Average Time to ECG (minutes)[1,3]	-	-	9	7
Average Time to Transfer (minutes)[5]	-	-	62	60
Children's Asthma Care				
Received Home Management Plan of Care	-	-	88%	88%
Received Reliever Medication	-	-	100%	100%
Received Systemic Corticosteroids	-	-	100%	100%
Emergency Department				
Admittance Decision Time (minutes)[2]	718	111	125	98
Head CT Results Within 45 Min. of Arrival[1]	-	-	55%	57%
Patients Who Left ER Before Being Seen	35,634	2%	3%	2%
Time from ER Arrival to Admit. (minutes)[2]	720	286	323	274
Time from ER Arrival to Discharge (minutes)	2,026	130	168	134
Time in ER Before Being Evaluated (minutes)	2,171	30	29	26
Time to Pain Meds for Fractures (minutes)	98	61	62	57
Heart Attack Care				
Aspirin Given at Discharge	135	99%	99%	99%
Fibrinolytic Meds Within 30 Min. of Arrival[7]	-	-	73%	54%
PCI Within 90 Minutes of Arrival	33	100%	95%	96%
Statin Prescribed at Discharge	130	99%	98%	98%
Heart Failure Care				
ACE Inhibitor or ARB for LVSD	55	100%	97%	97%
Discharge Instructions Given	188	100%	94%	94%
Evaluation of LVS Function	229	99%	99%	99%
Medicare Spending				
Medicare Spending per Patient (ratio)	-	1.05	0.98	0.98
Pneumonia Care				
Appropriate Initial Antibiotic Given	54	98%	97%	95%
Blood Culture Timing	107	98%	98%	98%
Pregnancy and Delivery Care				
Newborn Deliveries Scheduled Early[2]	62	0%	5%	6%
Preventive Care				
Immunization for Influenza[2]	507	92%	89%	90%
Immunization for Pneumonia[2]	659	88%	90%	92%
Stroke Care				
Anticoagulation Therapy for Atrial Fibrillation[1]	-	-	95%	95%
Antithrombotic Therapy Timing	20	100%	98%	98%
Assessed for Rehabilitation	32	97%	97%	97%
Discharged on Antithrombotic Therapy	26	100%	99%	99%

NOTE: Hospital profiles are in alphabetical order by state, then city, then hospital within the city; Rankings exclude hospitals with less than 25 cases except for patient surveys which excludes hospitals with less than 100 cases; (a) 100-299 cases; (1) The number of cases/patients is too few to report; (2) Data submitted were based on a sample of cases/patients; (3) Results are based on a shorter time period than required; (4) Data suppressed by CMS for one or more quarters; (5) Results are not available for this reporting period; (6) Fewer than 100 patients completed the HCAHPS survey; (7) No cases met the criteria for this measure; (8) The lower limit of the confidence interval cannot be calculated if the number of observed infections equals zero; (9) No data are available from the state/territory for this reporting period; (10) The scores shown reflect fewer than 50 completed surveys; (11) There were discrepancies in the data collection process; (12) This measure does not apply to this hospital for this reporting period; (13) Results cannot be calculated for this reporting period; (14) The results for this state are combined with nearby states to protect confidentiality; Please refer to the User's Guide for a full explanation of data.

Measure	Cases	This Hosp.	State Avg.	U.S. Avg.
Discharged on Statin Medication	27	85%	94%	94%
Thrombolytic Therapy Timing[1]	-	-	72%	66%
Venous Thromboembolism Prophylaxis	29	76%	94%	94%
Written Stroke Educational Materials Given	17	35%	87%	88%
Surgical Care Improvement Project				
Appropriate Beta Blocker Usage[2]	79	97%	97%	98%
Appropriate VTP Within 24 Hours[2]	257	96%	98%	98%
Controlled Postoperative Blood Glucose[2,7]	-	-	96%	97%
Perioperative Temperature Management[2]	286	100%	100%	100%
Prophylactic Antibiotic Selection[2]	186	98%	99%	99%
Prophylactic Antibiotic Selection (Outpatient)	31	100%	97%	98%
Prophylactic Antibiotic Stopped[2]	179	96%	98%	98%
Prophylactic Antibiotic Timing[2]	186	99%	99%	99%
Prophylactic Antibiotic Timing (Outpatient)	33	94%	97%	98%
Urinary Catheter Removal[2]	210	98%	97%	97%
Survey of Patients' Hospital Experiences				
Area Around Room 'Always' Quiet at Night	300+	55%	51%	61%
Doctors 'Always' Communicated Well	300+	78%	78%	82%
Home Recovery Information Given	300+	83%	83%	85%
Hospital Given 9 or 10 on 10 Point Scale	300+	64%	68%	71%
Meds 'Always' Explained Before Given	300+	57%	61%	64%
Nurses 'Always' Communicated Well	300+	71%	74%	79%
Pain 'Always' Well Controlled	300+	66%	68%	71%
Room and Bathroom 'Always' Clean	300+	68%	70%	73%
Timely Help 'Always' Received	300+	53%	62%	68%
Would Definitely Recommend Hospital	300+	66%	70%	71%
Use of Medical Imaging				
Cardiac Imaging Stress Test before Surgery	89	7.9%	5.2%	5.3%
Combination Abdominal CT Scan	332	3.6%	13.4%	10.5%
Combination Brain/Sinus CT Scan	387	1.0%	2.2%	2.7%
Combination Chest CT Scan	157	3.2%	2.3%	2.7%
Follow-up Mammogram/Ultrasound	636	2.5%	8.2%	8.8%
Lumbar Spine MRI for Low Back Pain[1]	-	-	34.2%	37.2%

Healdsburg District Hospital

1375 University Avenue
Healdsburg, CA 95448
URL: www.h-g-h.org
Phone: 707-431-6500
Fax: 707-431-6588

Type: Critical Access Hospitals
Ownership: Govt - Hospital Dist/Auth
Emergency Services: Yes
Beds: 43

Key Personnel:

Chief of Medical Staff.......... William Bowden, DO
Infection Control.............. Mary Daniels
Quality Assurance .... Linda Easterbrook
Chairman/CEO .... William D. Esselstein
Operating Room............... Sharon Hughes
Anesthesiology............... Donald Loarie, MD
Emergency Room .... Walter Maack, MD
CEO/President............... Nancy Schmid

Measure	Cases	This Hosp.	State Avg.	U.S. Avg.
Blood Clot Prevention and Treatment				
Anticoagulation Overlap Therapy[5]	-	-	92%	93%
ICU Venous Thromboembolism Prophylaxis[5]	-	-	92%	92%
Incidence of Potentially Preventable VTE[5]	-	-	11%	10%
UFH with Dosages/Platelet Monitoring[5]	-	-	96%	97%
Venous Thromboembolism Prophylaxis[5]	-	-	83%	85%
Warfarin Therapy Discharge Instructions[5]	-	-	75%	75%
Chest Pain/Possible Heart Attack Care				
Aspirin Given Within 24 Hours of Arrival[5]	-	-	97%	96%
Fibrinolytic Meds Within 30 Min. of Arrival[5]	-	-	62%	58%
Average Time to ECG (minutes)[5]	-	-	9	7
Average Time to Transfer (minutes)[5]	-	-	62	60
Children's Asthma Care				
Received Home Management Plan of Care	-	-	88%	88%
Received Reliever Medication	-	-	100%	100%
Received Systemic Corticosteroids	-	-	100%	100%
Emergency Department				
Admittance Decision Time (minutes)[5]	-	-	125	98
Head CT Results Within 45 Min. of Arrival[5]	-	-	55%	57%
Patients Who Left ER Before Being Seen[5]	-	-	3%	2%
Time from ER Arrival to Admit. (minutes)[5]	-	-	323	274
Time from ER Arrival to Discharge (minutes)[5]	-	-	168	134
Time in ER Before Being Evaluated (minutes)[5]	-	-	29	26
Time to Pain Meds for Fractures (minutes)[5]	-	-	62	57
Heart Attack Care				
Aspirin Given at Discharge[1,3]	-	-	99%	99%
Fibrinolytic Meds Within 30 Min. of Arrival[3,7]	-	-	73%	54%
PCI Within 90 Minutes of Arrival[3,7]	-	-	95%	96%
Statin Prescribed at Discharge[1,3]	-	-	98%	98%
Heart Failure Care				
ACE Inhibitor or ARB for LVSD[1]	-	-	97%	97%
Discharge Instructions Given	13	54%	94%	94%
Evaluation of LVS Function	17	94%	99%	99%
Medicare Spending				
Medicare Spending per Patient (ratio)	-	-	0.98	0.98
Pneumonia Care				
Appropriate Initial Antibiotic Given	32	84%	97%	95%
Blood Culture Timing	35	94%	98%	98%
Pregnancy and Delivery Care				
Newborn Deliveries Scheduled Early[5]	-	-	5%	6%
Preventive Care				
Immunization for Influenza[5]	-	-	89%	90%
Immunization for Pneumonia[5]	-	-	90%	92%
Stroke Care				
Anticoagulation Therapy for Atrial Fibrillation[3,7]	-	-	95%	95%
Antithrombotic Therapy Timing[1,3]	-	-	98%	98%
Assessed for Rehabilitation[3]	11	91%	97%	97%
Discharged on Antithrombotic Therapy[1,3]	-	-	99%	99%
Discharged on Statin Medication[1,3]	-	-	94%	94%
Thrombolytic Therapy Timing[1,3]	-	-	72%	66%
Venous Thromboembolism Prophylaxis[1,3]	-	-	94%	94%
Written Stroke Educational Materials Given[1,3]	-	-	87%	88%
Surgical Care Improvement Project				
Appropriate Beta Blocker Usage	16	81%	97%	98%
Appropriate VTP Within 24 Hours	90	94%	98%	98%
Controlled Postoperative Blood Glucose[7]	-	-	96%	97%
Perioperative Temperature Management	91	99%	100%	100%
Prophylactic Antibiotic Selection	83	99%	99%	99%
Prophylactic Antibiotic Selection (Outpatient)[5]	-	-	97%	98%
Prophylactic Antibiotic Stopped	83	95%	98%	98%
Prophylactic Antibiotic Timing	83	94%	99%	99%
Prophylactic Antibiotic Timing (Outpatient)[5]	-	-	97%	98%
Urinary Catheter Removal	85	100%	97%	97%
Survey of Patients' Hospital Experiences				
Area Around Room 'Always' Quiet at Night	(a)	50%	51%	61%
Doctors 'Always' Communicated Well	(a)	85%	78%	82%
Home Recovery Information Given	(a)	88%	83%	85%
Hospital Given 9 or 10 on 10 Point Scale	(a)	80%	68%	71%
Meds 'Always' Explained Before Given	(a)	72%	61%	64%
Nurses 'Always' Communicated Well	(a)	82%	74%	79%
Pain 'Always' Well Controlled	(a)	78%	68%	71%
Room and Bathroom 'Always' Clean	(a)	89%	70%	73%
Timely Help 'Always' Received	(a)	71%	62%	68%
Would Definitely Recommend Hospital	(a)	83%	70%	71%
Use of Medical Imaging				
Cardiac Imaging Stress Test before Surgery[7]	-	-	5.2%	5.3%
Combination Abdominal CT Scan	259	3.9%	13.4%	10.5%
Combination Brain/Sinus CT Scan[1]	-	-	2.2%	2.7%
Combination Chest CT Scan	107	0.0%	2.3%	2.7%
Follow-up Mammogram/Ultrasound	480	3.5%	8.2%	8.8%
Lumbar Spine MRI for Low Back Pain[1]	-	-	34.2%	37.2%

Hemet Valley Medical Center

1117 East Devonshire
Hemet, CA 92543
E-mail: info@valleyhealthsystem.com
URL: www.valleyhealthsystem.com/hemmain
Phone: 951-652-2811
Fax: 951-766-6415

Type: Acute Care Hospitals
Ownership: Government - State
Emergency Services: Yes
Beds: 240

Key Personnel:

Chief of Medical Staff.......... Leslee B Cochrane
Radiology.................... Thavinsakdi Viravath

Measure	Cases	This Hosp.	State Avg.	U.S. Avg.
Blood Clot Prevention and Treatment				
Anticoagulation Overlap Therapy[2]	64	91%	92%	93%
ICU Venous Thromboembolism Prophylaxis[2]	71	80%	92%	92%
Incidence of Potentially Preventable VTE[2]	29	34%	11%	10%
UFH with Dosages/Platelet Monitoring[1,2]	-	-	96%	97%
Venous Thromboembolism Prophylaxis[2]	315	54%	83%	85%
Warfarin Therapy Discharge Instructions[2]	43	67%	75%	75%
Chest Pain/Possible Heart Attack Care				
Aspirin Given Within 24 Hours of Arrival	46	93%	97%	96%
Fibrinolytic Meds Within 30 Min. of Arrival[7]	-	-	62%	58%
Average Time to ECG (minutes)	48	10	9	7
Average Time to Transfer (minutes)	14	76	62	60
Children's Asthma Care				
Received Home Management Plan of Care	-	-	88%	88%
Received Reliever Medication	-	-	100%	100%
Received Systemic Corticosteroids	-	-	100%	100%
Emergency Department				
Admittance Decision Time (minutes)[2]	420	161	125	98
Head CT Results Within 45 Min. of Arrival[1]	-	-	55%	57%
Patients Who Left ER Before Being Seen	48,911	3%	3%	2%
Time from ER Arrival to Admit. (minutes)[2]	433	472	323	274
Time from ER Arrival to Discharge (minutes)	271	233	168	134
Time in ER Before Being Evaluated (minutes)	209	70	29	26
Time to Pain Meds for Fractures (minutes)	99	128	62	57
Heart Attack Care				
Aspirin Given at Discharge[2]	81	84%	99%	99%
Fibrinolytic Meds Within 30 Min. of Arrival[2,7]	-	-	73%	54%
PCI Within 90 Minutes of Arrival[2,7]	-	-	95%	96%
Statin Prescribed at Discharge[2]	78	83%	98%	98%
Heart Failure Care				
ACE Inhibitor or ARB for LVSD[2]	112	88%	97%	97%
Discharge Instructions Given[2]	204	76%	94%	94%
Evaluation of LVS Function[2]	270	95%	99%	99%
Medicare Spending				
Medicare Spending per Patient (ratio)	-	1.00	0.98	0.98
Pneumonia Care				
Appropriate Initial Antibiotic Given[2]	64	94%	97%	95%
Blood Culture Timing[2]	115	97%	98%	98%
Pregnancy and Delivery Care				
Newborn Deliveries Scheduled Early[2]	22	5%	5%	6%
Preventive Care				
Immunization for Influenza[2]	532	92%	89%	90%
Immunization for Pneumonia[2]	703	85%	90%	92%
Stroke Care				
Anticoagulation Therapy for Atrial Fibrillation[2]	26	85%	95%	95%
Antithrombotic Therapy Timing[2]	88	97%	98%	98%
Assessed for Rehabilitation[2]	94	80%	97%	97%
Discharged on Antithrombotic Therapy[2]	92	91%	99%	99%
Discharged on Statin Medication[2]	87	59%	94%	94%
Thrombolytic Therapy Timing[1,2]	-	-	72%	66%
Venous Thromboembolism Prophylaxis[2]	96	67%	94%	94%
Written Stroke Educational Materials Given[2]	48	42%	87%	88%
Surgical Care Improvement Project				
Appropriate Beta Blocker Usage[2]	66	82%	97%	98%
Appropriate VTP Within 24 Hours[2]	293	90%	98%	98%
Controlled Postoperative Blood Glucose[2,7]	-	-	96%	97%
Perioperative Temperature Management[2]	338	99%	100%	100%
Prophylactic Antibiotic Selection[2]	212	95%	99%	99%
Prophylactic Antibiotic Selection (Outpatient)	116	97%	97%	98%
Prophylactic Antibiotic Stopped[2]	205	90%	98%	98%
Prophylactic Antibiotic Timing[2]	212	98%	99%	99%
Prophylactic Antibiotic Timing (Outpatient)	118	95%	97%	98%
Urinary Catheter Removal[2]	165	79%	97%	97%
Survey of Patients' Hospital Experiences				
Area Around Room 'Always' Quiet at Night	300+	35%	51%	61%
Doctors 'Always' Communicated Well	300+	69%	78%	82%
Home Recovery Information Given	300+	75%	83%	85%
Hospital Given 9 or 10 on 10 Point Scale	300+	42%	68%	71%
Meds 'Always' Explained Before Given	300+	49%	61%	64%
Nurses 'Always' Communicated Well	300+	63%	74%	79%
Pain 'Always' Well Controlled	300+	57%	68%	71%
Room and Bathroom 'Always' Clean	300+	56%	70%	73%
Timely Help 'Always' Received	300+	46%	62%	68%
Would Definitely Recommend Hospital	300+	41%	70%	71%
Use of Medical Imaging				
Cardiac Imaging Stress Test before Surgery	153	6.5%	5.2%	5.3%

NOTE: Hospital profiles are in alphabetical order by state, then city, then hospital within the city; Rankings exclude hospitals with less than 25 cases except for patient surveys which excludes hospitals with less than 100 cases; (a) 100-299 cases; (1) The number of cases/patients is too few to report; (2) Data submitted were based on a sample of cases/patients; (3) Results are based on a shorter time period than required; (4) Data suppressed by CMS for one or more quarters; (5) Results are not available for this reporting period; (6) Fewer than 100 patients completed the HCAHPS survey; (7) No cases met the criteria for this measure; (8) The lower limit of the confidence interval cannot be calculated if the number of observed infections equals zero; (9) No data are available from the state/territory for this reporting period; (10) The scores shown reflect fewer than 50 completed surveys; (11) There were discrepancies in the data collection process; (12) This measure does not apply to this hospital for this reporting period; (13) Results cannot be calculated for this reporting period; (14) The results for this state are combined with nearby states to protect confidentiality; Please refer to the User's Guide for a full explanation of data.

Measure	Cases	This Hosp.	State Avg.	U.S. Avg.
Combination Abdominal CT Scan	217	44.7%	13.4%	10.5%
Combination Brain/Sinus CT Scan	561	2.1%	2.2%	2.7%
Combination Chest CT Scan	113	1.8%	2.3%	2.7%
Follow-up Mammogram/Ultrasound[7]	-	-	8.2%	8.8%
Lumbar Spine MRI for Low Back Pain[7]	-	-	34.2%	37.2%

Hazel Hawkins Memorial Hospital

911 Sunset Drive Phone: 831-637-5711
Hollister, CA 95023 Fax: 831-636-2668
E-mail: fvalent@hazelhawkins.com
URL: www.hazelhawkins.com
Type: Acute Care Hospitals Emergency Services: No
Ownership: Govt - Hospital Dist/Auth Beds: 101

Key Personnel:
Quality Assurance . . . . Linda Anderson, RN
Emergency Room . . . . Marian Anderson, RN
Operating Room. . . . . Leonard Caputo, RN
Chief of Medical Staff. . . . . Leonard Catuto, MD
Radiology. . . . . Garth Harley, MD
President . . . . Gordon A. Machado
Pediatric Ambulatory Care . . . . . . B Yager, MD
Pediatric In-Patient Care . . . . B Yager, MD

Measure	Cases	This Hosp.	State Avg.	U.S. Avg.
Blood Clot Prevention and Treatment				
Anticoagulation Overlap Therapy[2]	14	86%	92%	93%
ICU Venous Thromboembolism Prophylaxis[2]	84	81%	92%	92%
Incidence of Potentially Preventable VTE[2,7]	-	-	11%	10%
UFH with Dosages/Platelet Monitoring[1,2]	-	-	96%	97%
Venous Thromboembolism Prophylaxis[2]	275	61%	83%	85%
Warfarin Therapy Discharge Instructions[2]	12	67%	75%	75%
Chest Pain/Possible Heart Attack Care				
Aspirin Given Within 24 Hours of Arrival	55	89%	97%	96%
Fibrinolytic Meds Within 30 Min. of Arrival[1]	-	-	62%	58%
Average Time to ECG (minutes)	54	28	9	7
Average Time to Transfer (minutes)[1]	-	-	62	60
Children's Asthma Care				
Received Home Management Plan of Care	-	-	88%	88%
Received Reliever Medication	-	-	100%	100%
Received Systemic Corticosteroids	-	-	100%	100%
Emergency Department				
Admittance Decision Time (minutes)[2]	470	89	125	98
Head CT Results Within 45 Min. of Arrival	20	15%	55%	57%
Patients Who Left ER Before Being Seen	16,059	2%	3%	2%
Time from ER Arrival to Admit. (minutes)[2]	524	275	323	274
Time from ER Arrival to Discharge (minutes)	611	164	168	134
Time in ER Before Being Evaluated (minutes)	764	36	29	26
Time to Pain Meds for Fractures (minutes)	79	65	62	57
Heart Attack Care				
Aspirin Given at Discharge	19	95%	99%	99%
Fibrinolytic Meds Within 30 Min. of Arrival[7]	-	-	73%	54%
PCI Within 90 Minutes of Arrival[7]	-	-	95%	96%
Statin Prescribed at Discharge	16	75%	98%	98%
Heart Failure Care				
ACE Inhibitor or ARB for LVSD[2]	17	100%	97%	97%
Discharge Instructions Given[2]	43	98%	94%	94%
Evaluation of LVS Function[2]	57	98%	99%	99%
Medicare Spending				
Medicare Spending per Patient (ratio)	-	0.90	0.98	0.98
Pneumonia Care				
Appropriate Initial Antibiotic Given[2]	44	89%	97%	95%
Blood Culture Timing[2]	60	85%	98%	98%
Pregnancy and Delivery Care				
Newborn Deliveries Scheduled Early[2]	13	8%	5%	6%
Preventive Care				
Immunization for Influenza[2]	299	80%	89%	90%
Immunization for Pneumonia[2]	399	81%	90%	92%
Stroke Care				
Anticoagulation Therapy for Atrial Fibrillation[1,2]	-	-	95%	95%
Antithrombotic Therapy Timing[2]	12	92%	98%	98%
Assessed for Rehabilitation[2]	11	100%	97%	97%
Discharged on Antithrombotic Therapy[2]	11	100%	99%	99%
Discharged on Statin Medication[1,2]	-	-	94%	94%
Thrombolytic Therapy Timing[1,2]	-	-	72%	66%
Venous Thromboembolism Prophylaxis[2]	13	85%	94%	94%
Written Stroke Educational Materials Given[1,2]	-	-	87%	88%
Surgical Care Improvement Project				
Appropriate Beta Blocker Usage	22	73%	97%	98%
Appropriate VTP Within 24 Hours	62	95%	98%	98%
Controlled Postoperative Blood Glucose[7]	-	-	96%	97%
Perioperative Temperature Management	97	100%	100%	100%
Prophylactic Antibiotic Selection	64	98%	99%	99%
Prophylactic Antibiotic Selection (Outpatient)[1,3]	-	-	97%	98%
Prophylactic Antibiotic Stopped	62	95%	98%	98%
Prophylactic Antibiotic Timing	64	100%	99%	99%
Prophylactic Antibiotic Timing (Outpatient)[1,3]	-	-	97%	98%
Urinary Catheter Removal	42	71%	97%	97%
Survey of Patients' Hospital Experiences				
Area Around Room 'Always' Quiet at Night	300+	48%	51%	61%
Doctors 'Always' Communicated Well	300+	76%	78%	82%
Home Recovery Information Given	300+	84%	83%	85%
Hospital Given 9 or 10 on 10 Point Scale	300+	66%	68%	71%
Meds 'Always' Explained Before Given	300+	61%	61%	64%
Nurses 'Always' Communicated Well	300+	76%	74%	79%
Pain 'Always' Well Controlled	300+	70%	68%	71%
Room and Bathroom 'Always' Clean	300+	72%	70%	73%
Timely Help 'Always' Received	300+	65%	62%	68%
Would Definitely Recommend Hospital	300+	59%	70%	71%
Use of Medical Imaging				
Cardiac Imaging Stress Test before Surgery[1]	-	-	5.2%	5.3%
Combination Abdominal CT Scan	317	45.7%	13.4%	10.5%
Combination Brain/Sinus CT Scan[1]	-	-	2.2%	2.7%
Combination Chest CT Scan	182	1.6%	2.3%	2.7%
Follow-up Mammogram/Ultrasound	628	6.7%	8.2%	8.8%
Lumbar Spine MRI for Low Back Pain[1]	-	-	34.2%	37.2%

Southern California Hospital at Hollywood

6245 De Longpre Ave Phone: 323-462-2271
Hollywood, CA 90028 Fax: 323-461-9278
Type: Acute Care Hospitals Emergency Services: Yes
Ownership: Voluntary non-profit - Other Beds: 160

Key Personnel:
Operating Room. . . . . Romy Anderson
CEO/President. . . . . Angelita Andrian
Quality Assurance . . . . Jeanne McKeehan
Chief of Medical Staff. . . . . Vence Rubio, MD

Measure	Cases	This Hosp.	State Avg.	U.S. Avg.
Blood Clot Prevention and Treatment				
Anticoagulation Overlap Therapy[2]	37	95%	92%	93%
ICU Venous Thromboembolism Prophylaxis[2]	64	95%	92%	92%
Incidence of Potentially Preventable VTE[2]	24	0%	11%	10%
UFH with Dosages/Platelet Monitoring[2]	20	95%	96%	97%
Venous Thromboembolism Prophylaxis[2]	674	93%	83%	85%
Warfarin Therapy Discharge Instructions[2]	12	83%	75%	75%
Chest Pain/Possible Heart Attack Care				
Aspirin Given Within 24 Hours of Arrival[1,3]	-	-	97%	96%
Fibrinolytic Meds Within 30 Min. of Arrival[3,7]	-	-	62%	58%
Average Time to ECG (minutes)[1,3]	-	-	9	7
Average Time to Transfer (minutes)[3,7]	-	-	62	60
Children's Asthma Care				
Received Home Management Plan of Care	-	-	88%	88%
Received Reliever Medication	-	-	100%	100%
Received Systemic Corticosteroids	-	-	100%	100%
Emergency Department				
Admittance Decision Time (minutes)[2,7]	-	-	125	98
Head CT Results Within 45 Min. of Arrival[3,7]	-	-	55%	57%
Patients Who Left ER Before Being Seen	25,914	2%	3%	2%
Time from ER Arrival to Admit. (minutes)[2,7]	-	-	323	274
Time from ER Arrival to Discharge (minutes)[3,7]	-	-	168	134
Time in ER Before Being Evaluated (minutes)[3]	273	26	29	26
Time to Pain Meds for Fractures (minutes)[3]	71	56	62	57
Heart Attack Care				
Aspirin Given at Discharge	72	99%	99%	99%
Fibrinolytic Meds Within 30 Min. of Arrival[7]	-	-	73%	54%
PCI Within 90 Minutes of Arrival[7]	-	-	95%	96%
Statin Prescribed at Discharge	63	98%	98%	98%
Heart Failure Care				
ACE Inhibitor or ARB for LVSD[2]	75	99%	97%	97%
Discharge Instructions Given[2]	137	95%	94%	94%
Evaluation of LVS Function[2]	220	99%	99%	99%
Medicare Spending				
Medicare Spending per Patient (ratio)	-	1.26	0.98	0.98
Pneumonia Care				
Appropriate Initial Antibiotic Given[2]	78	96%	97%	95%
Blood Culture Timing[2]	167	96%	98%	98%
Pregnancy and Delivery Care				
Newborn Deliveries Scheduled Early[2,7]	-	-	5%	6%
Preventive Care				
Immunization for Influenza[2]	591	88%	89%	90%
Immunization for Pneumonia[2]	983	87%	90%	92%
Stroke Care				
Anticoagulation Therapy for Atrial Fibrillation[1]	-	-	95%	95%
Antithrombotic Therapy Timing	42	98%	98%	98%
Assessed for Rehabilitation	49	88%	97%	97%
Discharged on Antithrombotic Therapy	33	100%	99%	99%
Discharged on Statin Medication	35	94%	94%	94%
Thrombolytic Therapy Timing[7]	-	-	72%	66%
Venous Thromboembolism Prophylaxis	58	97%	94%	94%
Written Stroke Educational Materials Given	21	90%	87%	88%
Surgical Care Improvement Project				
Appropriate Beta Blocker Usage	25	96%	97%	98%
Appropriate VTP Within 24 Hours	83	98%	98%	98%
Controlled Postoperative Blood Glucose[7]	-	-	96%	97%
Perioperative Temperature Management	109	100%	100%	100%
Prophylactic Antibiotic Selection	58	98%	99%	99%
Prophylactic Antibiotic Selection (Outpatient)[3]	76	100%	97%	98%
Prophylactic Antibiotic Stopped	47	98%	98%	98%
Prophylactic Antibiotic Timing	58	100%	99%	99%
Prophylactic Antibiotic Timing (Outpatient)[3]	76	100%	97%	98%
Urinary Catheter Removal	52	100%	97%	97%
Survey of Patients' Hospital Experiences				
Area Around Room 'Always' Quiet at Night	300+	49%	51%	61%
Doctors 'Always' Communicated Well	300+	68%	78%	82%
Home Recovery Information Given	300+	75%	83%	85%
Hospital Given 9 or 10 on 10 Point Scale	300+	51%	68%	71%
Meds 'Always' Explained Before Given	300+	49%	61%	64%
Nurses 'Always' Communicated Well	300+	62%	74%	79%
Pain 'Always' Well Controlled	300+	57%	68%	71%
Room and Bathroom 'Always' Clean	300+	61%	70%	73%
Timely Help 'Always' Received	300+	47%	62%	68%
Would Definitely Recommend Hospital	300+	49%	70%	71%
Use of Medical Imaging				
Cardiac Imaging Stress Test before Surgery[1]	-	-	5.2%	5.3%
Combination Abdominal CT Scan[1]	-	-	13.4%	10.5%
Combination Brain/Sinus CT Scan[1]	-	-	2.2%	2.7%
Combination Chest CT Scan[1]	-	-	2.3%	2.7%
Follow-up Mammogram/Ultrasound[7]	-	-	8.2%	8.8%
Lumbar Spine MRI for Low Back Pain[1]	-	-	34.2%	37.2%

Huntington Beach Hospital

17772 Beach Blvd Phone: 714-843-5000
Huntington Beach, CA 92647 Fax: 714-843-5038
URL: www.hbhospital.com
Type: Acute Care Hospitals Emergency Services: Yes
Ownership: Proprietary Beds: 135

Key Personnel:
Chairman/CEO . . . . Hassan Alkhouli, MD
CEO/President. . . . . Mary Botticella
Chief of Medical Staff. . . . . Joseph Nassir, MD
Operating Room. . . . . Sandra Stallone

Measure	Cases	This Hosp.	State Avg.	U.S. Avg.
Blood Clot Prevention and Treatment				
Anticoagulation Overlap Therapy[1,2]	-	-	92%	93%
ICU Venous Thromboembolism Prophylaxis[2]	55	100%	92%	92%
Incidence of Potentially Preventable VTE[2,7]	-	-	11%	10%
UFH with Dosages/Platelet Monitoring[1,2]	-	-	96%	97%
Venous Thromboembolism Prophylaxis[2]	292	95%	83%	85%
Warfarin Therapy Discharge Instructions[1,2]	-	-	75%	75%
Chest Pain/Possible Heart Attack Care				
Aspirin Given Within 24 Hours of Arrival	19	100%	97%	96%
Fibrinolytic Meds Within 30 Min. of Arrival[7]	-	-	62%	58%

NOTE: Hospital profiles are in alphabetical order by state, then city, then hospital within the city; Rankings exclude hospitals with less than 25 cases except for patient surveys which excludes hospitals with less than 100 cases; (a) 100-299 cases; (1) The number of cases/patients is too few to report; (2) Data submitted were based on a sample of cases/patients; (3) Results are based on a shorter time period than required; (4) Data suppressed by CMS for one or more quarters; (5) Results are not available for this reporting period; (6) Fewer than 100 patients completed the HCAHPS survey; (7) No cases met the criteria for this measure; (8) The lower limit of the confidence interval cannot be calculated if the number of observed infections equals zero; (9) No data are available from the state/territory for this reporting period; (10) The scores shown reflect fewer than 50 completed surveys; (11) There were discrepancies in the data collection process; (12) This measure does not apply to this hospital for this reporting period; (13) Results cannot be calculated for this reporting period; (14) The results for this state are combined with nearby states to protect confidentiality; Please refer to the User's Guide for a full explanation of data.

Measure	Cases	This Hosp.	State Avg.	U.S. Avg.
Average Time to ECG (minutes)	19	9	9	7
Average Time to Transfer (minutes)[1]	-	-	62	60
Children's Asthma Care				
Received Home Management Plan of Care	-	-	88%	88%
Received Reliever Medication	-	-	100%	100%
Received Systemic Corticosteroids	-	-	100%	100%
Emergency Department				
Admittance Decision Time (minutes)[2]	632	80	125	98
Head CT Results Within 45 Min. of Arrival[7]	-	-	55%	57%
Patients Who Left ER Before Being Seen	17,922	3%	3%	2%
Time from ER Arrival to Admit. (minutes)[2]	635	241	323	274
Time from ER Arrival to Discharge (minutes)	343	132	168	134
Time in ER Before Being Evaluated (minutes)	386	30	29	26
Time to Pain Meds for Fractures (minutes)	99	51	62	57
Heart Attack Care				
Aspirin Given at Discharge	12	100%	99%	99%
Fibrinolytic Meds Within 30 Min. of Arrival[7]	-	-	73%	54%
PCI Within 90 Minutes of Arrival[7]	-	-	95%	96%
Statin Prescribed at Discharge[1]	-	-	98%	98%
Heart Failure Care				
ACE Inhibitor or ARB for LVSD	13	100%	97%	97%
Discharge Instructions Given	67	100%	94%	94%
Evaluation of LVS Function	87	100%	99%	99%
Medicare Spending				
Medicare Spending per Patient (ratio)	-	1.11	0.98	0.98
Pneumonia Care				
Appropriate Initial Antibiotic Given[2]	38	100%	97%	95%
Blood Culture Timing[2]	120	100%	98%	98%
Pregnancy and Delivery Care				
Newborn Deliveries Scheduled Early[7]	-	-	5%	6%
Preventive Care				
Immunization for Influenza[2]	323	100%	89%	90%
Immunization for Pneumonia[2]	413	100%	90%	92%
Stroke Care				
Anticoagulation Therapy for Atrial Fibrillation[1]	-	-	95%	95%
Antithrombotic Therapy Timing	21	100%	98%	98%
Assessed for Rehabilitation	22	100%	97%	97%
Discharged on Antithrombotic Therapy	18	100%	99%	99%
Discharged on Statin Medication	13	100%	94%	94%
Thrombolytic Therapy Timing[7]	-	-	72%	66%
Venous Thromboembolism Prophylaxis	25	100%	94%	94%
Written Stroke Educational Materials Given	12	100%	87%	88%
Surgical Care Improvement Project				
Appropriate Beta Blocker Usage[1]	-	-	97%	98%
Appropriate VTP Within 24 Hours	34	100%	98%	98%
Controlled Postoperative Blood Glucose[7]	-	-	96%	97%
Perioperative Temperature Management	41	100%	100%	100%
Prophylactic Antibiotic Selection[1]	-	-	99%	99%
Prophylactic Antibiotic Selection (Outpatient)[1,3]	-	-	97%	98%
Prophylactic Antibiotic Stopped[1]	-	-	98%	98%
Prophylactic Antibiotic Timing[1]	-	-	99%	99%
Prophylactic Antibiotic Timing (Outpatient)[1,3]	-	-	97%	98%
Urinary Catheter Removal	12	100%	97%	97%
Survey of Patients' Hospital Experiences				
Area Around Room 'Always' Quiet at Night	(a)	42%	51%	61%
Doctors 'Always' Communicated Well	(a)	63%	78%	82%
Home Recovery Information Given	(a)	74%	83%	85%
Hospital Given 9 or 10 on 10 Point Scale	(a)	49%	68%	71%
Meds 'Always' Explained Before Given	(a)	50%	61%	64%
Nurses 'Always' Communicated Well	(a)	63%	74%	79%
Pain 'Always' Well Controlled	(a)	50%	68%	71%
Room and Bathroom 'Always' Clean	(a)	64%	70%	73%
Timely Help 'Always' Received	(a)	49%	62%	68%
Would Definitely Recommend Hospital	(a)	53%	70%	71%
Use of Medical Imaging				
Cardiac Imaging Stress Test before Surgery[1]	-	-	5.2%	5.3%
Combination Abdominal CT Scan	87	2.3%	13.4%	10.5%
Combination Brain/Sinus CT Scan[1]	-	-	2.2%	2.7%
Combination Chest CT Scan[1]	-	-	2.3%	2.7%
Follow-up Mammogram/Ultrasound[7]	-	-	8.2%	8.8%
Lumbar Spine MRI for Low Back Pain[7]	-	-	34.2%	37.2%

Community Hospital of Huntington Park

2623 E Slauson Ave
Huntington Park, CA 90255
Phone: 323-583-1931
Fax: 323-582-8179
Type: Acute Care Hospitals
Emergency Services: Yes
Ownership: Voluntary non-profit - Private
Beds: 81

Key Personnel:

CEO/President. . . . . Charles Martinez
Pediatric Ambulatory Care . . . . . . Pau Nguyen, MD
Pediatric In-Patient Care . . . . Pau Nguyen, MD
Quality Assurance . . . . Rick Paige, RN
Operating Room. . . . . Marla Pruznick
Chief of Medical Staff. . . . . Jesus Ramirez
Coronary Care . . . . Daniel Suarez

Measure	Cases	This Hosp.	State Avg.	U.S. Avg.
Blood Clot Prevention and Treatment				
Anticoagulation Overlap Therapy[2]	12	100%	92%	93%
ICU Venous Thromboembolism Prophylaxis[2]	53	94%	92%	92%
Incidence of Potentially Preventable VTE[1,2]	-	-	11%	10%
UFH with Dosages/Platelet Monitoring[1,2]	-	-	96%	97%
Venous Thromboembolism Prophylaxis[2]	358	96%	83%	85%
Warfarin Therapy Discharge Instructions[1,2]	-	-	75%	75%
Chest Pain/Possible Heart Attack Care				
Aspirin Given Within 24 Hours of Arrival	54	96%	97%	96%
Fibrinolytic Meds Within 30 Min. of Arrival[7]	-	-	62%	58%
Average Time to ECG (minutes)	54	28	9	7
Average Time to Transfer (minutes)[1]	-	-	62	60
Children's Asthma Care				
Received Home Management Plan of Care	-	-	88%	88%
Received Reliever Medication	-	-	100%	100%
Received Systemic Corticosteroids	-	-	100%	100%
Emergency Department				
Admittance Decision Time (minutes)[2]	403	116	125	98
Head CT Results Within 45 Min. of Arrival[1]	-	-	55%	57%
Patients Who Left ER Before Being Seen	29,131	5%	3%	2%
Time from ER Arrival to Admit. (minutes)[2]	671	384	323	274
Time from ER Arrival to Discharge (minutes)	429	218	168	134
Time in ER Before Being Evaluated (minutes)	462	82	29	26
Time to Pain Meds for Fractures (minutes)	221	123	62	57
Heart Attack Care				
Aspirin Given at Discharge	26	100%	99%	99%
Fibrinolytic Meds Within 30 Min. of Arrival[7]	-	-	73%	54%
PCI Within 90 Minutes of Arrival[7]	-	-	95%	96%
Statin Prescribed at Discharge	20	95%	98%	98%
Heart Failure Care				
ACE Inhibitor or ARB for LVSD	67	99%	97%	97%
Discharge Instructions Given	133	100%	94%	94%
Evaluation of LVS Function	149	100%	99%	99%
Medicare Spending				
Medicare Spending per Patient (ratio)	-	0.91	0.98	0.98
Pneumonia Care				
Appropriate Initial Antibiotic Given	85	99%	97%	95%
Blood Culture Timing	62	98%	98%	98%
Pregnancy and Delivery Care				
Newborn Deliveries Scheduled Early[7]	-	-	5%	6%
Preventive Care				
Immunization for Influenza[2]	410	100%	89%	90%
Immunization for Pneumonia[2]	449	94%	90%	92%
Stroke Care				
Anticoagulation Therapy for Atrial Fibrillation[7]	-	-	95%	95%
Antithrombotic Therapy Timing	13	85%	98%	98%
Assessed for Rehabilitation[1]	-	-	97%	97%
Discharged on Antithrombotic Therapy[1]	-	-	99%	99%
Discharged on Statin Medication[1]	-	-	94%	94%
Thrombolytic Therapy Timing[7]	-	-	72%	66%
Venous Thromboembolism Prophylaxis	15	93%	94%	94%
Written Stroke Educational Materials Given[1]	-	-	87%	88%
Surgical Care Improvement Project				
Appropriate Beta Blocker Usage[1]	-	-	97%	98%
Appropriate VTP Within 24 Hours	40	98%	98%	98%
Controlled Postoperative Blood Glucose[7]	-	-	96%	97%
Perioperative Temperature Management	45	100%	100%	100%
Prophylactic Antibiotic Selection[1]	-	-	99%	99%
Prophylactic Antibiotic Selection (Outpatient)[3,7]	-	-	97%	98%
Prophylactic Antibiotic Stopped[1]	-	-	98%	98%
Prophylactic Antibiotic Timing[1]	-	-	99%	99%
Prophylactic Antibiotic Timing (Outpatient)[1,3]	-	-	97%	98%
Urinary Catheter Removal	13	69%	97%	97%
Survey of Patients' Hospital Experiences				
Area Around Room 'Always' Quiet at Night	300+	49%	51%	61%
Doctors 'Always' Communicated Well	300+	74%	78%	82%
Home Recovery Information Given	300+	74%	83%	85%
Hospital Given 9 or 10 on 10 Point Scale	300+	59%	68%	71%
Meds 'Always' Explained Before Given	300+	58%	61%	64%
Nurses 'Always' Communicated Well	300+	71%	74%	79%
Pain 'Always' Well Controlled	300+	67%	68%	71%
Room and Bathroom 'Always' Clean	300+	69%	70%	73%
Timely Help 'Always' Received	300+	60%	62%	68%
Would Definitely Recommend Hospital	300+	59%	70%	71%
Use of Medical Imaging				
Cardiac Imaging Stress Test before Surgery[1]	-	-	5.2%	5.3%
Combination Abdominal CT Scan	119	2.5%	13.4%	10.5%
Combination Brain/Sinus CT Scan[1]	-	-	2.2%	2.7%
Combination Chest CT Scan[1]	-	-	2.3%	2.7%
Follow-up Mammogram/Ultrasound[7]	-	-	8.2%	8.8%
Lumbar Spine MRI for Low Back Pain[7]	-	-	34.2%	37.2%

John F Kennedy Memorial Hospital

47-111 Monroe Street
Indio, CA 92201
Phone: 760-347-6191
Fax: 760-775-8014
URL: www.jfkmemorialhosp.com
Type: Acute Care Hospitals
Emergency Services: Yes
Ownership: Proprietary
Beds: 145

Key Personnel:

CEO/President. . . . . Stan Adams
Chief of Medical Staff. . . . . Dr Jennifer Daley
Quality Assurance . . . . Patricia Fuller
CEO . . . . Gary Honts
Emergency Room . . . . Reiner Jakel
Radiology. . . . . Theodore Masek
Operating Room. . . . . Karen Timmerman, RN

Measure	Cases	This Hosp.	State Avg.	U.S. Avg.
Blood Clot Prevention and Treatment				
Anticoagulation Overlap Therapy[2]	22	68%	92%	93%
ICU Venous Thromboembolism Prophylaxis[2]	67	78%	92%	92%
Incidence of Potentially Preventable VTE[1,2]	-	-	11%	10%
UFH with Dosages/Platelet Monitoring[2]	11	91%	96%	97%
Venous Thromboembolism Prophylaxis[2]	283	66%	83%	85%
Warfarin Therapy Discharge Instructions[2]	15	60%	75%	75%
Chest Pain/Possible Heart Attack Care				
Aspirin Given Within 24 Hours of Arrival[1]	-	-	97%	96%
Fibrinolytic Meds Within 30 Min. of Arrival[3,7]	-	-	62%	58%
Average Time to ECG (minutes)[1]	-	-	9	7
Average Time to Transfer (minutes)[1,3]	-	-	62	60
Children's Asthma Care				
Received Home Management Plan of Care	-	-	88%	88%
Received Reliever Medication	-	-	100%	100%
Received Systemic Corticosteroids	-	-	100%	100%
Emergency Department				
Admittance Decision Time (minutes)[2]	457	143	125	98
Head CT Results Within 45 Min. of Arrival	21	14%	55%	57%
Patients Who Left ER Before Being Seen	35,865	6%	3%	2%
Time from ER Arrival to Admit. (minutes)[2]	561	386	323	274
Time from ER Arrival to Discharge (minutes)	335	175	168	134
Time in ER Before Being Evaluated (minutes)	308	14	29	26
Time to Pain Meds for Fractures (minutes)	227	68	62	57
Heart Attack Care				
Aspirin Given at Discharge	101	99%	99%	99%
Fibrinolytic Meds Within 30 Min. of Arrival[7]	-	-	73%	54%
PCI Within 90 Minutes of Arrival	27	93%	95%	96%
Statin Prescribed at Discharge	101	96%	98%	98%
Heart Failure Care				
ACE Inhibitor or ARB for LVSD	37	100%	97%	97%
Discharge Instructions Given	118	98%	94%	94%
Evaluation of LVS Function	132	98%	99%	99%
Medicare Spending				
Medicare Spending per Patient (ratio)	-	0.98	0.98	0.98
Pneumonia Care				
Appropriate Initial Antibiotic Given[2]	81	95%	97%	95%

NOTE: Hospital profiles are in alphabetical order by state, then city, then hospital within the city; Rankings exclude hospitals with less than 25 cases except for patient surveys which excludes hospitals with less than 100 cases; (a) 100-299 cases; (1) The number of cases/patients is too few to report; (2) Data submitted were based on a sample of cases/patients; (3) Results are based on a shorter time period than required; (4) Data suppressed by CMS for one or more quarters; (5) Results are not available for this reporting period; (6) Fewer than 100 patients completed the HCAHPS survey; (7) No cases met the criteria for this measure; (8) The lower limit of the confidence interval cannot be calculated if the number of observed infections equals zero; (9) No data are available from the state/territory for this reporting period; (10) The scores shown reflect fewer than 50 completed surveys; (11) There were discrepancies in the data collection process; (12) This measure does not apply to this hospital for this reporting period; (13) Results cannot be calculated for this reporting period; (14) The results for this state are combined with nearby states to protect confidentiality; Please refer to the User's Guide for a full explanation of data.

Measure	Cases	This Hosp.	State Avg.	U.S. Avg.
Blood Culture Timing[2]	148	98%	98%	98%
Pregnancy and Delivery Care				
Newborn Deliveries Scheduled Early[2]	64	12%	5%	6%
Preventive Care				
Immunization for Influenza[2]	493	90%	89%	90%
Immunization for Pneumonia[2]	431	92%	90%	92%
Stroke Care				
Anticoagulation Therapy for Atrial Fibrillation[1]	-	-	95%	95%
Antithrombotic Therapy Timing	19	58%	98%	98%
Assessed for Rehabilitation	25	64%	97%	97%
Discharged on Antithrombotic Therapy	24	75%	99%	99%
Discharged on Statin Medication	19	58%	94%	94%
Thrombolytic Therapy Timing[1]	-	-	72%	66%
Venous Thromboembolism Prophylaxis	19	63%	94%	94%
Written Stroke Educational Materials Given	14	64%	87%	88%
Surgical Care Improvement Project				
Appropriate Beta Blocker Usage[2]	143	99%	97%	98%
Appropriate VTP Within 24 Hours[2]	604	99%	98%	98%
Controlled Postoperative Blood Glucose[2,7]	-	-	96%	97%
Perioperative Temperature Management[2]	669	100%	100%	100%
Prophylactic Antibiotic Selection[2]	540	100%	99%	99%
Prophylactic Antibiotic Selection (Outpatient)	50	98%	97%	98%
Prophylactic Antibiotic Stopped[2]	528	89%	98%	98%
Prophylactic Antibiotic Timing[2]	540	99%	99%	99%
Prophylactic Antibiotic Timing (Outpatient)	52	96%	97%	98%
Urinary Catheter Removal[2]	569	99%	97%	97%
Survey of Patients' Hospital Experiences				
Area Around Room 'Always' Quiet at Night	300+	43%	51%	61%
Doctors 'Always' Communicated Well	300+	77%	78%	82%
Home Recovery Information Given	300+	83%	83%	85%
Hospital Given 9 or 10 on 10 Point Scale	300+	64%	68%	71%
Meds 'Always' Explained Before Given	300+	62%	61%	64%
Nurses 'Always' Communicated Well	300+	73%	74%	79%
Pain 'Always' Well Controlled	300+	67%	68%	71%
Room and Bathroom 'Always' Clean	300+	67%	70%	73%
Timely Help 'Always' Received	300+	59%	62%	68%
Would Definitely Recommend Hospital	300+	59%	70%	71%
Use of Medical Imaging				
Cardiac Imaging Stress Test before Surgery	77	3.9%	5.2%	5.3%
Combination Abdominal CT Scan	272	1.5%	13.4%	10.5%
Combination Brain/Sinus CT Scan[1]	-	-	2.2%	2.7%
Combination Chest CT Scan	56	3.6%	2.3%	2.7%
Follow-up Mammogram/Ultrasound[7]	-	-	8.2%	8.8%
Lumbar Spine MRI for Low Back Pain[1]	-	-	34.2%	37.2%

Centinela Hospital Medical Center

555 East Hardy Street Phone: 310-673-4660
Inglewood, CA 90301 Fax: 310-674-9604
URL: www.centinelafreeman.com
Type: Acute Care Hospitals Emergency Services: Yes
Ownership: Proprietary Beds: 400

Key Personnel:
Infection Control. . . . . Geri Braddock, RN
CEO/President. . . . . Linda Bradley
Chief of Medical Staff . . . . Rama Chandran, MD
Intensive Care Unit. . . . . Kathy Frengel
Emergency Room . . . . Jan Hartfield
Radiology. . . . . Paul Marino, MD
Quality Assurance . . . . Sherry Pilkvist, RN

Measure	Cases	This Hosp.	State Avg.	U.S. Avg.
Blood Clot Prevention and Treatment				
Anticoagulation Overlap Therapy[2]	51	98%	92%	93%
ICU Venous Thromboembolism Prophylaxis[2]	36	97%	92%	92%
Incidence of Potentially Preventable VTE[2]	22	0%	11%	10%
UFH with Dosages/Platelet Monitoring[2]	23	100%	96%	97%
Venous Thromboembolism Prophylaxis[2]	352	95%	83%	85%
Warfarin Therapy Discharge Instructions[2]	29	93%	75%	75%
Chest Pain/Possible Heart Attack Care				
Aspirin Given Within 24 Hours of Arrival	17	100%	97%	96%
Fibrinolytic Meds Within 30 Min. of Arrival[3,7]	-	-	62%	58%
Average Time to ECG (minutes)	18	20	9	7
Average Time to Transfer (minutes)[3,7]	-	-	62	60
Children's Asthma Care				
Received Home Management Plan of Care	-	-	88%	88%
Received Reliever Medication	-	-	100%	100%
Received Systemic Corticosteroids	-	-	100%	100%
Emergency Department				
Admittance Decision Time (minutes)[2]	1,020	133	125	98
Head CT Results Within 45 Min. of Arrival[1]	-	-	55%	57%
Patients Who Left ER Before Being Seen	64,464	5%	3%	2%
Time from ER Arrival to Admit. (minutes)[2]	1,021	353	323	274
Time from ER Arrival to Discharge (minutes)	417	221	168	134
Time in ER Before Being Evaluated (minutes)	465	56	29	26
Time to Pain Meds for Fractures (minutes)	235	80	62	57
Heart Attack Care				
Aspirin Given at Discharge[2]	190	100%	99%	99%
Fibrinolytic Meds Within 30 Min. of Arrival[2,7]	-	-	73%	54%
PCI Within 90 Minutes of Arrival[2,7]	-	-	95%	96%
Statin Prescribed at Discharge[2]	158	100%	98%	98%
Heart Failure Care				
ACE Inhibitor or ARB for LVSD[2]	126	100%	97%	97%
Discharge Instructions Given[2]	230	100%	94%	94%
Evaluation of LVS Function[2]	268	100%	99%	99%
Medicare Spending				
Medicare Spending per Patient (ratio)	-	1.01	0.98	0.98
Pneumonia Care				
Appropriate Initial Antibiotic Given[2]	50	100%	97%	95%
Blood Culture Timing[2]	99	100%	98%	98%
Pregnancy and Delivery Care				
Newborn Deliveries Scheduled Early[2]	30	3%	5%	6%
Preventive Care				
Immunization for Influenza[2]	530	100%	89%	90%
Immunization for Pneumonia[2]	754	100%	90%	92%
Stroke Care				
Anticoagulation Therapy for Atrial Fibrillation[1,2]	-	-	95%	95%
Antithrombotic Therapy Timing[2]	93	100%	98%	98%
Assessed for Rehabilitation[2]	94	98%	97%	97%
Discharged on Antithrombotic Therapy[2]	84	100%	99%	99%
Discharged on Statin Medication[2]	62	87%	94%	94%
Thrombolytic Therapy Timing[2,7]	-	-	72%	66%
Venous Thromboembolism Prophylaxis[2]	115	97%	94%	94%
Written Stroke Educational Materials Given[2]	56	84%	87%	88%
Surgical Care Improvement Project				
Appropriate Beta Blocker Usage[2]	42	98%	97%	98%
Appropriate VTP Within 24 Hours[2]	144	99%	98%	98%
Controlled Postoperative Blood Glucose[2]	26	96%	96%	97%
Perioperative Temperature Management[2]	166	100%	100%	100%
Prophylactic Antibiotic Selection[2]	75	100%	99%	99%
Prophylactic Antibiotic Selection (Outpatient)	57	95%	97%	98%
Prophylactic Antibiotic Stopped[2]	75	100%	98%	98%
Prophylactic Antibiotic Timing[2]	75	100%	99%	99%
Prophylactic Antibiotic Timing (Outpatient)	58	98%	97%	98%
Urinary Catheter Removal[2]	81	99%	97%	97%
Survey of Patients' Hospital Experiences				
Area Around Room 'Always' Quiet at Night[11]	300+	51%	51%	61%
Doctors 'Always' Communicated Well[11]	300+	75%	78%	82%
Home Recovery Information Given[11]	300+	80%	83%	85%
Hospital Given 9 or 10 on 10 Point Scale[11]	300+	60%	68%	71%
Meds 'Always' Explained Before Given[11]	300+	59%	61%	64%
Nurses 'Always' Communicated Well[11]	300+	69%	74%	79%
Pain 'Always' Well Controlled[11]	300+	61%	68%	71%
Room and Bathroom 'Always' Clean[11]	300+	64%	70%	73%
Timely Help 'Always' Received[11]	300+	52%	62%	68%
Would Definitely Recommend Hospital[11]	300+	59%	70%	71%
Use of Medical Imaging				
Cardiac Imaging Stress Test before Surgery	130	6.9%	5.2%	5.3%
Combination Abdominal CT Scan	506	2.8%	13.4%	10.5%
Combination Brain/Sinus CT Scan	668	2.2%	2.2%	2.7%
Combination Chest CT Scan	97	10.3%	2.3%	2.7%
Follow-up Mammogram/Ultrasound	466	7.9%	8.2%	8.8%
Lumbar Spine MRI for Low Back Pain	72	16.7%	34.2%	37.2%

Hoag Orthopedic Institute

16250 Sand Canyon Avenue Phone: 949-727-5000
Irvine, CA 92618
URL: www.orthopedichospital.com
Type: Acute Care Hospitals Emergency Services: No
Ownership: Proprietary

Measure	Cases	This Hosp.	State Avg.	U.S. Avg.
Blood Clot Prevention and Treatment				
Anticoagulation Overlap Therapy[1,2]	-	-	92%	93%
ICU Venous Thromboembolism Prophylaxis[2,7]	-	-	92%	92%
Incidence of Potentially Preventable VTE[1,2]	-	-	11%	10%
UFH with Dosages/Platelet Monitoring[2,7]	-	-	96%	97%
Venous Thromboembolism Prophylaxis[2]	90	98%	83%	85%
Warfarin Therapy Discharge Instructions[1,2]	-	-	75%	75%
Chest Pain/Possible Heart Attack Care				
Aspirin Given Within 24 Hours of Arrival[5]	-	-	97%	96%
Fibrinolytic Meds Within 30 Min. of Arrival[5]	-	-	62%	58%
Average Time to ECG (minutes)[5]	-	-	9	7
Average Time to Transfer (minutes)[5]	-	-	62	60
Children's Asthma Care				
Received Home Management Plan of Care	-	-	88%	88%
Received Reliever Medication	-	-	100%	100%
Received Systemic Corticosteroids	-	-	100%	100%
Emergency Department				
Admittance Decision Time (minutes)[2,7]	-	-	125	98
Head CT Results Within 45 Min. of Arrival[5]	-	-	55%	57%
Patients Who Left ER Before Being Seen[5]	-	-	3%	2%
Time from ER Arrival to Admit. (minutes)[2,7]	-	-	323	274
Time from ER Arrival to Discharge (minutes)[5]	-	-	168	134
Time in ER Before Being Evaluated (minutes)[5]	-	-	29	26
Time to Pain Meds for Fractures (minutes)[5]	-	-	62	57
Heart Attack Care				
Aspirin Given at Discharge[5]	-	-	99%	99%
Fibrinolytic Meds Within 30 Min. of Arrival[5]	-	-	73%	54%
PCI Within 90 Minutes of Arrival[5]	-	-	95%	96%
Statin Prescribed at Discharge[5]	-	-	98%	98%
Heart Failure Care				
ACE Inhibitor or ARB for LVSD[5]	-	-	97%	97%
Discharge Instructions Given[5]	-	-	94%	94%
Evaluation of LVS Function[5]	-	-	99%	99%
Medicare Spending				
Medicare Spending per Patient (ratio)	-	0.96	0.98	0.98
Pneumonia Care				
Appropriate Initial Antibiotic Given[5]	-	-	97%	95%
Blood Culture Timing[5]	-	-	98%	98%
Pregnancy and Delivery Care				
Newborn Deliveries Scheduled Early[7]	-	-	5%	6%
Preventive Care				
Immunization for Influenza[2]	409	99%	89%	90%
Immunization for Pneumonia[2]	575	94%	90%	92%
Stroke Care				
Anticoagulation Therapy for Atrial Fibrillation[5]	-	-	95%	95%
Antithrombotic Therapy Timing[5]	-	-	98%	98%
Assessed for Rehabilitation[5]	-	-	97%	97%
Discharged on Antithrombotic Therapy[5]	-	-	99%	99%
Discharged on Statin Medication[5]	-	-	94%	94%
Thrombolytic Therapy Timing[5]	-	-	72%	66%
Venous Thromboembolism Prophylaxis[5]	-	-	94%	94%
Written Stroke Educational Materials Given[5]	-	-	87%	88%
Surgical Care Improvement Project				
Appropriate Beta Blocker Usage[2]	165	99%	97%	98%
Appropriate VTP Within 24 Hours[2]	576	99%	98%	98%
Controlled Postoperative Blood Glucose[2,7]	-	-	96%	97%
Perioperative Temperature Management[2]	667	100%	100%	100%
Prophylactic Antibiotic Selection[2]	535	100%	99%	99%
Prophylactic Antibiotic Selection (Outpatient)	224	100%	97%	98%
Prophylactic Antibiotic Stopped[2]	528	99%	98%	98%
Prophylactic Antibiotic Timing[2]	535	100%	99%	99%
Prophylactic Antibiotic Timing (Outpatient)	224	100%	97%	98%
Urinary Catheter Removal[2]	586	100%	97%	97%
Survey of Patients' Hospital Experiences				
Area Around Room 'Always' Quiet at Night	300+	71%	51%	61%

NOTE: Hospital profiles are in alphabetical order by state, then city, then hospital within the city; Rankings exclude hospitals with less than 25 cases except for patient surveys which excludes hospitals with less than 100 cases; (a) 100-299 cases; (1) The number of cases/patients is too few to report; (2) Data submitted were based on a sample of cases/patients; (3) Results are based on a shorter time period than required; (4) Data suppressed by CMS for one or more quarters; (5) Results are not available for this reporting period; (6) Fewer than 100 patients completed the HCAHPS survey; (7) No cases met the criteria for this measure; (8) The lower limit of the confidence interval cannot be calculated if the number of observed infections equals zero; (9) No data are available from the state/territory for this reporting period; (10) The scores shown reflect fewer than 50 completed surveys; (11) There were discrepancies in the data collection process; (12) This measure does not apply to this hospital for this reporting period; (13) Results cannot be calculated for this reporting period; (14) The results for this state are combined with nearby states to protect confidentiality; Please refer to the User's Guide for a full explanation of data.

Measure	Cases	This Hosp.	State Avg.	U.S. Avg.
Doctors 'Always' Communicated Well	300+	87%	78%	82%
Home Recovery Information Given	300+	92%	83%	85%
Hospital Given 9 or 10 on 10 Point Scale	300+	90%	68%	71%
Meds 'Always' Explained Before Given	300+	74%	61%	64%
Nurses 'Always' Communicated Well	300+	88%	74%	79%
Pain 'Always' Well Controlled	300+	78%	68%	71%
Room and Bathroom 'Always' Clean	300+	83%	70%	73%
Timely Help 'Always' Received	300+	80%	62%	68%
Would Definitely Recommend Hospital	300+	92%	70%	71%
Use of Medical Imaging				
Cardiac Imaging Stress Test before Surgery[7]	-	-	5.2%	5.3%
Combination Abdominal CT Scan[7]	-	-	13.4%	10.5%
Combination Brain/Sinus CT Scan[1]	-	-	2.2%	2.7%
Combination Chest CT Scan[7]	-	-	2.3%	2.7%
Follow-up Mammogram/Ultrasound[7]	-	-	8.2%	8.8%
Lumbar Spine MRI for Low Back Pain[7]	-	-	34.2%	37.2%

Sutter Amador Hospital

200 Mission Blvd
Jackson, CA 95642
Phone: 209-223-7500
Fax: 209-223-7509
E-mail: boetzej@sutterhealth.org
URL: www.sutteramador.org
Type: Acute Care Hospitals
Emergency Services: Yes
Ownership: Government - Local
Beds: 66

Key Personnel:
Chief of Medical Staff. . . . . Thomas Bowhay
Quality Assurance . . . . Catherine Furtado
Operating Room. . . . . Jim Jeffery, RN
CEO/President. . . . . Anne Platt

Measure	Cases	This Hosp.	State Avg.	U.S. Avg.
Blood Clot Prevention and Treatment				
Anticoagulation Overlap Therapy[2]	21	90%	92%	93%
ICU Venous Thromboembolism Prophylaxis[2]	57	95%	92%	92%
Incidence of Potentially Preventable VTE[1,2]	-	-	11%	10%
UFH with Dosages/Platelet Monitoring[1,2]	-	-	96%	97%
Venous Thromboembolism Prophylaxis[2]	180	77%	83%	85%
Warfarin Therapy Discharge Instructions[2]	16	56%	75%	75%
Chest Pain/Possible Heart Attack Care				
Aspirin Given Within 24 Hours of Arrival	111	98%	97%	96%
Fibrinolytic Meds Within 30 Min. of Arrival[1]	-	-	62%	58%
Average Time to ECG (minutes)	120	13	9	7
Average Time to Transfer (minutes)[7]	-	-	62	60
Children's Asthma Care				
Received Home Management Plan of Care	-	-	88%	88%
Received Reliever Medication	-	-	100%	100%
Received Systemic Corticosteroids	-	-	100%	100%
Emergency Department				
Admittance Decision Time (minutes)[2]	390	92	125	98
Head CT Results Within 45 Min. of Arrival[7]	-	-	55%	57%
Patients Who Left ER Before Being Seen	19,025	1%	3%	2%
Time from ER Arrival to Admit. (minutes)[2]	401	295	323	274
Time from ER Arrival to Discharge (minutes)	378	115	168	134
Time in ER Before Being Evaluated (minutes)	301	33	29	26
Time to Pain Meds for Fractures (minutes)	77	51	62	57
Heart Attack Care				
Aspirin Given at Discharge[1]	-	-	99%	99%
Fibrinolytic Meds Within 30 Min. of Arrival[7]	-	-	73%	54%
PCI Within 90 Minutes of Arrival[7]	-	-	95%	96%
Statin Prescribed at Discharge[1]	-	-	98%	98%
Heart Failure Care				
ACE Inhibitor or ARB for LVSD[1]	-	-	97%	97%
Discharge Instructions Given	47	98%	94%	94%
Evaluation of LVS Function	56	100%	99%	99%
Medicare Spending				
Medicare Spending per Patient (ratio)	-	0.89	0.98	0.98
Pneumonia Care				
Appropriate Initial Antibiotic Given[2]	97	99%	97%	95%
Blood Culture Timing[2]	149	99%	98%	98%
Pregnancy and Delivery Care				
Newborn Deliveries Scheduled Early	12	0%	5%	6%
Preventive Care				
Immunization for Influenza[2]	270	98%	89%	90%
Immunization for Pneumonia[2]	329	98%	90%	92%
Stroke Care				
Anticoagulation Therapy for Atrial Fibrillation[1]	-	-	95%	95%
Antithrombotic Therapy Timing	26	100%	98%	98%
Assessed for Rehabilitation	40	98%	97%	97%
Discharged on Antithrombotic Therapy	38	100%	99%	99%
Discharged on Statin Medication	23	96%	94%	94%
Thrombolytic Therapy Timing[1]	-	-	72%	66%
Venous Thromboembolism Prophylaxis	32	97%	94%	94%
Written Stroke Educational Materials Given	28	93%	87%	88%
Surgical Care Improvement Project				
Appropriate Beta Blocker Usage[2]	19	95%	97%	98%
Appropriate VTP Within 24 Hours[2]	103	92%	98%	98%
Controlled Postoperative Blood Glucose[2,7]	-	-	96%	97%
Perioperative Temperature Management[2]	116	100%	100%	100%
Prophylactic Antibiotic Selection[2]	71	97%	99%	99%
Prophylactic Antibiotic Selection (Outpatient)[1,3]	-	-	97%	98%
Prophylactic Antibiotic Stopped[2]	71	97%	98%	98%
Prophylactic Antibiotic Timing[2]	71	100%	99%	99%
Prophylactic Antibiotic Timing (Outpatient)[1,3]	-	-	97%	98%
Urinary Catheter Removal[2]	55	93%	97%	97%
Survey of Patients' Hospital Experiences				
Area Around Room 'Always' Quiet at Night	300+	61%	51%	61%
Doctors 'Always' Communicated Well	300+	78%	78%	82%
Home Recovery Information Given	300+	86%	83%	85%
Hospital Given 9 or 10 on 10 Point Scale	300+	69%	68%	71%
Meds 'Always' Explained Before Given	300+	61%	61%	64%
Nurses 'Always' Communicated Well	300+	80%	74%	79%
Pain 'Always' Well Controlled	300+	73%	68%	71%
Room and Bathroom 'Always' Clean	300+	82%	70%	73%
Timely Help 'Always' Received	300+	67%	62%	68%
Would Definitely Recommend Hospital	300+	72%	70%	71%
Use of Medical Imaging				
Cardiac Imaging Stress Test before Surgery	604	3.8%	5.2%	5.3%
Combination Abdominal CT Scan	555	5.2%	13.4%	10.5%
Combination Brain/Sinus CT Scan[1]	-	-	2.2%	2.7%
Combination Chest CT Scan	374	1.6%	2.3%	2.7%
Follow-up Mammogram/Ultrasound	966	8.9%	8.2%	8.8%
Lumbar Spine MRI for Low Back Pain	101	40.6%	34.2%	37.2%

Hi - Desert Medical Center

6601 White Feather Road
Joshua Tree, CA 92252
Phone: 760-366-6285
Fax: 760-366-6136
E-mail: admin@hdmc.org
URL: www.hdmc.org
Type: Acute Care Hospitals
Emergency Services: Yes
Ownership: Govt - Hospital Dist/Auth
Beds: 181

Key Personnel:
Patient Relations . . . . Jackie Combs
Chief of Medical Staff. . . . . Rui DaSilva
Operating Room. . . . . Renato Guzman
Emergency Room . . . . Donna Johnson
Quality Assurance . . . . Avelina Ortiz
CEO . . . . Robert Tyk
Infection Control. . . . . Peggy Ventura

Measure	Cases	This Hosp.	State Avg.	U.S. Avg.
Blood Clot Prevention and Treatment				
Anticoagulation Overlap Therapy[2]	52	67%	92%	93%
ICU Venous Thromboembolism Prophylaxis[2]	38	97%	92%	92%
Incidence of Potentially Preventable VTE[2]	11	64%	11%	10%
UFH with Dosages/Platelet Monitoring[2]	52	100%	96%	97%
Venous Thromboembolism Prophylaxis[2]	220	70%	83%	85%
Warfarin Therapy Discharge Instructions[2]	46	39%	75%	75%
Chest Pain/Possible Heart Attack Care				
Aspirin Given Within 24 Hours of Arrival	70	99%	97%	96%
Fibrinolytic Meds Within 30 Min. of Arrival[7]	-	-	62%	58%
Average Time to ECG (minutes)	71	6	9	7
Average Time to Transfer (minutes)[1]	-	-	62	60
Children's Asthma Care				
Received Home Management Plan of Care	-	-	88%	88%
Received Reliever Medication	-	-	100%	100%
Received Systemic Corticosteroids	-	-	100%	100%
Emergency Department				
Admittance Decision Time (minutes)[2]	432	130	125	98
Head CT Results Within 45 Min. of Arrival[1]	-	-	55%	57%
Patients Who Left ER Before Being Seen	22,627	0%	3%	2%
Time from ER Arrival to Admit. (minutes)[2]	437	331	323	274
Time from ER Arrival to Discharge (minutes)	316	144	168	134
Time in ER Before Being Evaluated (minutes)	384	19	29	26
Time to Pain Meds for Fractures (minutes)	48	52	62	57
Heart Attack Care				
Aspirin Given at Discharge[1]	-	-	99%	99%
Fibrinolytic Meds Within 30 Min. of Arrival[7]	-	-	73%	54%
PCI Within 90 Minutes of Arrival[7]	-	-	95%	96%
Statin Prescribed at Discharge[1]	-	-	98%	98%
Heart Failure Care				
ACE Inhibitor or ARB for LVSD	43	91%	97%	97%
Discharge Instructions Given	69	80%	94%	94%
Evaluation of LVS Function	96	92%	99%	99%
Medicare Spending				
Medicare Spending per Patient (ratio)	-	0.87	0.98	0.98
Pneumonia Care				
Appropriate Initial Antibiotic Given	98	94%	97%	95%
Blood Culture Timing	148	84%	98%	98%
Pregnancy and Delivery Care				
Newborn Deliveries Scheduled Early	21	10%	5%	6%
Preventive Care				
Immunization for Influenza[2]	287	83%	89%	90%
Immunization for Pneumonia[2]	398	96%	90%	92%
Stroke Care				
Anticoagulation Therapy for Atrial Fibrillation[1]	-	-	95%	95%
Antithrombotic Therapy Timing	25	80%	98%	98%
Assessed for Rehabilitation	27	78%	97%	97%
Discharged on Antithrombotic Therapy	26	92%	99%	99%
Discharged on Statin Medication	22	55%	94%	94%
Thrombolytic Therapy Timing[1]	-	-	72%	66%
Venous Thromboembolism Prophylaxis	26	73%	94%	94%
Written Stroke Educational Materials Given	19	21%	87%	88%
Surgical Care Improvement Project				
Appropriate Beta Blocker Usage	28	86%	97%	98%
Appropriate VTP Within 24 Hours	106	92%	98%	98%
Controlled Postoperative Blood Glucose[7]	-	-	96%	97%
Perioperative Temperature Management	125	99%	100%	100%
Prophylactic Antibiotic Selection	74	97%	99%	99%
Prophylactic Antibiotic Selection (Outpatient)[1,3]	-	-	97%	98%
Prophylactic Antibiotic Stopped	72	94%	98%	98%
Prophylactic Antibiotic Timing	74	92%	99%	99%
Prophylactic Antibiotic Timing (Outpatient)[1,3]	-	-	97%	98%
Urinary Catheter Removal	88	86%	97%	97%
Survey of Patients' Hospital Experiences				
Area Around Room 'Always' Quiet at Night	300+	59%	51%	61%
Doctors 'Always' Communicated Well	300+	74%	78%	82%
Home Recovery Information Given	300+	86%	83%	85%
Hospital Given 9 or 10 on 10 Point Scale	300+	71%	68%	71%
Meds 'Always' Explained Before Given	300+	59%	61%	64%
Nurses 'Always' Communicated Well	300+	76%	74%	79%
Pain 'Always' Well Controlled	300+	67%	68%	71%
Room and Bathroom 'Always' Clean	300+	73%	70%	73%
Timely Help 'Always' Received	300+	64%	62%	68%
Would Definitely Recommend Hospital	300+	64%	70%	71%
Use of Medical Imaging				
Cardiac Imaging Stress Test before Surgery[7]	-	-	5.2%	5.3%
Combination Abdominal CT Scan	360	3.1%	13.4%	10.5%
Combination Brain/Sinus CT Scan[1]	-	-	2.2%	2.7%
Combination Chest CT Scan	175	6.3%	2.3%	2.7%
Follow-up Mammogram/Ultrasound	471	7.6%	8.2%	8.8%
Lumbar Spine MRI for Low Back Pain[1]	-	-	34.2%	37.2%

George L Mee Memorial Hospital

300 Canal Street
King City, CA 93930
Phone: 831-385-6000
Fax: 831-385-7171
E-mail: info@meememorial.com
URL: www.meememorial.com
Type: Acute Care Hospitals
Emergency Services: Yes
Ownership: Voluntary non-profit - Other
Beds: 123

Key Personnel:
Cardiac Laboratory. . . . . Jerilyn Adler
Radiology. . . . . Michael Basse
Emergency Room . . . . Carlos Bayardo
CEO/President. . . . . Walt Beck
Operating Room. . . . . Margaret Johnson, RN

NOTE: Hospital profiles are in alphabetical order by state, then city, then hospital within the city; Rankings exclude hospitals with less than 25 cases except for patient surveys which excludes hospitals with less than 100 cases; (a) 100-299 cases; (1) The number of cases/patients is too few to report; (2) Data submitted were based on a sample of cases/patients; (3) Results are based on a shorter time period than required; (4) Data suppressed by CMS for one or more quarters; (5) Results are not available for this reporting period; (6) Fewer than 100 patients completed the HCAHPS survey; (7) No cases met the criteria for this measure; (8) The lower limit of the confidence interval cannot be calculated if the number of observed infections equals zero; (9) No data are available from the state/territory for this reporting period; (10) The scores shown reflect fewer than 50 completed surveys; (11) There were discrepancies in the data collection process; (12) This measure does not apply to this hospital for this reporting period; (13) Results cannot be calculated for this reporting period; (14) The results for this state are combined with nearby states to protect confidentiality; Please refer to the User's Guide for a full explanation of data.

Quality Assurance . . . . Denise Miller, RN
CEO . . . . Lex T. Smith, FACHE
Chief of Medical Staff . . . . Christina Zaro

Measure	Cases	This Hosp.	State Avg.	U.S. Avg.
Blood Clot Prevention and Treatment				
Anticoagulation Overlap Therapy[1,2]	-	-	92%	93%
ICU Venous Thromboembolism Prophylaxis[2]	55	49%	92%	92%
Incidence of Potentially Preventable VTE[1,2]	-	-	11%	10%
UFH with Dosages/Platelet Monitoring[1,2]	-	-	96%	97%
Venous Thromboembolism Prophylaxis[2]	190	68%	83%	85%
Warfarin Therapy Discharge Instructions[1,2]	-	-	75%	75%
Chest Pain/Possible Heart Attack Care				
Aspirin Given Within 24 Hours of Arrival	15	100%	97%	96%
Fibrinolytic Meds Within 30 Min. of Arrival[7]	-	-	62%	58%
Average Time to ECG (minutes)	17	15	9	7
Average Time to Transfer (minutes)[1]	-	-	62	60
Children's Asthma Care				
Received Home Management Plan of Care	-	-	88%	88%
Received Reliever Medication	-	-	100%	100%
Received Systemic Corticosteroids	-	-	100%	100%
Emergency Department				
Admittance Decision Time (minutes)[2]	92	102	125	98
Head CT Results Within 45 Min. of Arrival[1]	-	-	55%	57%
Patients Who Left ER Before Being Seen	10,141	2%	3%	2%
Time from ER Arrival to Admit. (minutes)[2]	139	275	323	274
Time from ER Arrival to Discharge (minutes)	354	100	168	134
Time in ER Before Being Evaluated (minutes)	350	20	29	26
Time to Pain Meds for Fractures (minutes)	60	46	62	57
Heart Attack Care				
Aspirin Given at Discharge[5]	-	-	99%	99%
Fibrinolytic Meds Within 30 Min. of Arrival[5]	-	-	73%	54%
PCI Within 90 Minutes of Arrival[5]	-	-	95%	96%
Statin Prescribed at Discharge[5]	-	-	98%	98%
Heart Failure Care				
ACE Inhibitor or ARB for LVSD[1]	-	-	97%	97%
Discharge Instructions Given	14	0%	94%	94%
Evaluation of LVS Function	17	88%	99%	99%
Medicare Spending				
Medicare Spending per Patient (ratio)	-	0.88	0.98	0.98
Pneumonia Care				
Appropriate Initial Antibiotic Given	20	80%	97%	95%
Blood Culture Timing	18	83%	98%	98%
Pregnancy and Delivery Care				
Newborn Deliveries Scheduled Early[2]	24	4%	5%	6%
Preventive Care				
Immunization for Influenza[2]	216	50%	89%	90%
Immunization for Pneumonia[2]	128	60%	90%	92%
Stroke Care				
Anticoagulation Therapy for Atrial Fibrillation[3,7]	-	-	95%	95%
Antithrombotic Therapy Timing[1,3]	-	-	98%	98%
Assessed for Rehabilitation[1,3]	-	-	97%	97%
Discharged on Antithrombotic Therapy[1,3]	-	-	99%	99%
Discharged on Statin Medication[1,3]	-	-	94%	94%
Thrombolytic Therapy Timing[3,7]	-	-	72%	66%
Venous Thromboembolism Prophylaxis[1,3]	-	-	94%	94%
Written Stroke Educational Materials Given[1,3]	-	-	87%	88%
Surgical Care Improvement Project				
Appropriate Beta Blocker Usage[1]	-	-	97%	98%
Appropriate VTP Within 24 Hours	27	81%	98%	98%
Controlled Postoperative Blood Glucose[7]	-	-	96%	97%
Perioperative Temperature Management	33	100%	100%	100%
Prophylactic Antibiotic Selection	20	85%	99%	99%
Prophylactic Antibiotic Selection (Outpatient)[1,3]	-	-	97%	98%
Prophylactic Antibiotic Stopped	20	100%	98%	98%
Prophylactic Antibiotic Timing	20	95%	99%	99%
Prophylactic Antibiotic Timing (Outpatient)[1,3]	-	-	97%	98%
Urinary Catheter Removal	17	76%	97%	97%
Survey of Patients' Hospital Experiences				
Area Around Room 'Always' Quiet at Night	(a)	49%	51%	61%
Doctors 'Always' Communicated Well	(a)	77%	78%	82%
Home Recovery Information Given	(a)	88%	83%	85%
Hospital Given 9 or 10 on 10 Point Scale	(a)	72%	68%	71%
Meds 'Always' Explained Before Given	(a)	67%	61%	64%
Nurses 'Always' Communicated Well	(a)	78%	74%	79%
Pain 'Always' Well Controlled	(a)	71%	68%	71%
Room and Bathroom 'Always' Clean	(a)	79%	70%	73%
Timely Help 'Always' Received	(a)	68%	62%	68%
Would Definitely Recommend Hospital	(a)	65%	70%	71%
Use of Medical Imaging				
Cardiac Imaging Stress Test before Surgery[7]	-	-	5.2%	5.3%
Combination Abdominal CT Scan	85	3.5%	13.4%	10.5%
Combination Brain/Sinus CT Scan[1]	-	-	2.2%	2.7%
Combination Chest CT Scan	46	0.0%	2.3%	2.7%
Follow-up Mammogram/Ultrasound	217	4.6%	8.2%	8.8%
Lumbar Spine MRI for Low Back Pain[1]	-	-	34.2%	37.2%

Scripps Green Hospital

10666 North Torrey Pines Road
La Jolla, CA 92037
Phone: 858-554-3600
Fax: 858-554-3170
URL: www.scrippshealth.org
Type: Acute Care Hospitals
Emergency Services: No
Ownership: Voluntary non-profit - Private
Beds: 173
Key Personnel:
Chief of Medical Staff . . . . A Brent Eastman, MD
Radiology . . . . Walter Goff
CEO/President . . . . Chris Van Gorder
Operating Room . . . . Barbara Keto-Reed
Quality Assurance . . . . June Komar

Measure	Cases	This Hosp.	State Avg.	U.S. Avg.
Blood Clot Prevention and Treatment				
Anticoagulation Overlap Therapy[2]	87	100%	92%	93%
ICU Venous Thromboembolism Prophylaxis[2]	86	88%	92%	92%
Incidence of Potentially Preventable VTE[2]	22	0%	11%	10%
UFH with Dosages/Platelet Monitoring[2]	26	100%	96%	97%
Venous Thromboembolism Prophylaxis[2]	276	95%	83%	85%
Warfarin Therapy Discharge Instructions[2]	83	100%	75%	75%
Chest Pain/Possible Heart Attack Care				
Aspirin Given Within 24 Hours of Arrival[5]	-	-	97%	96%
Fibrinolytic Meds Within 30 Min. of Arrival[5]	-	-	62%	58%
Average Time to ECG (minutes)[5]	-	-	9	7
Average Time to Transfer (minutes)[5]	-	-	62	60
Children's Asthma Care				
Received Home Management Plan of Care	-	-	88%	88%
Received Reliever Medication	-	-	100%	100%
Received Systemic Corticosteroids	-	-	100%	100%
Emergency Department				
Admittance Decision Time (minutes)[2,7]	-	-	125	98
Head CT Results Within 45 Min. of Arrival[5]	-	-	55%	57%
Patients Who Left ER Before Being Seen[5]	-	-	3%	2%
Time from ER Arrival to Admit. (minutes)[2,7]	-	-	323	274
Time from ER Arrival to Discharge (minutes)[5]	-	-	168	134
Time in ER Before Being Evaluated (minutes)[5]	-	-	29	26
Time to Pain Meds for Fractures (minutes)[5]	-	-	62	57
Heart Attack Care				
Aspirin Given at Discharge	195	100%	99%	99%
Fibrinolytic Meds Within 30 Min. of Arrival[7]	-	-	73%	54%
PCI Within 90 Minutes of Arrival	19	100%	95%	96%
Statin Prescribed at Discharge	176	100%	98%	98%
Heart Failure Care				
ACE Inhibitor or ARB for LVSD	90	100%	97%	97%
Discharge Instructions Given	223	100%	94%	94%
Evaluation of LVS Function	251	100%	99%	99%
Medicare Spending				
Medicare Spending per Patient (ratio)	-	0.95	0.98	0.98
Pneumonia Care				
Appropriate Initial Antibiotic Given	120	99%	97%	95%
Blood Culture Timing[7]	-	-	98%	98%
Pregnancy and Delivery Care				
Newborn Deliveries Scheduled Early[7]	-	-	5%	6%
Preventive Care				
Immunization for Influenza[2]	631	100%	89%	90%
Immunization for Pneumonia[2]	918	99%	90%	92%
Stroke Care				
Anticoagulation Therapy for Atrial Fibrillation	13	100%	95%	95%
Antithrombotic Therapy Timing	36	100%	98%	98%
Assessed for Rehabilitation	114	100%	97%	97%
Discharged on Antithrombotic Therapy	70	100%	99%	99%
Discharged on Statin Medication	58	98%	94%	94%
Thrombolytic Therapy Timing[7]	-	-	72%	66%
Venous Thromboembolism Prophylaxis	102	99%	94%	94%
Written Stroke Educational Materials Given	70	99%	87%	88%
Surgical Care Improvement Project				
Appropriate Beta Blocker Usage[2]	183	99%	97%	98%
Appropriate VTP Within 24 Hours[2]	438	100%	98%	98%
Controlled Postoperative Blood Glucose[2]	113	100%	96%	97%
Perioperative Temperature Management[2]	598	100%	100%	100%
Prophylactic Antibiotic Selection[2]	435	100%	99%	99%
Prophylactic Antibiotic Selection (Outpatient)	413	100%	97%	98%
Prophylactic Antibiotic Stopped[2]	425	99%	98%	98%
Prophylactic Antibiotic Timing[2]	435	100%	99%	99%
Prophylactic Antibiotic Timing (Outpatient)	413	100%	97%	98%
Urinary Catheter Removal[2]	390	100%	97%	97%
Survey of Patients' Hospital Experiences				
Area Around Room 'Always' Quiet at Night	300+	57%	51%	61%
Doctors 'Always' Communicated Well	300+	86%	78%	82%
Home Recovery Information Given	300+	86%	83%	85%
Hospital Given 9 or 10 on 10 Point Scale	300+	81%	68%	71%
Meds 'Always' Explained Before Given	300+	67%	61%	64%
Nurses 'Always' Communicated Well	300+	80%	74%	79%
Pain 'Always' Well Controlled	300+	75%	68%	71%
Room and Bathroom 'Always' Clean	300+	74%	70%	73%
Timely Help 'Always' Received	300+	67%	62%	68%
Would Definitely Recommend Hospital	300+	85%	70%	71%
Use of Medical Imaging				
Cardiac Imaging Stress Test before Surgery	388	7.0%	5.2%	5.3%
Combination Abdominal CT Scan	934	15.4%	13.4%	10.5%
Combination Brain/Sinus CT Scan[1]	-	-	2.2%	2.7%
Combination Chest CT Scan	922	0.8%	2.3%	2.7%
Follow-up Mammogram/Ultrasound	1,124	10.6%	8.2%	8.8%
Lumbar Spine MRI for Low Back Pain	157	31.8%	34.2%	37.2%

Scripps Memorial Hospital La Jolla

9888 Genesee Avenue
La Jolla, CA 92037
Phone: 858-626-4123
Fax: 858-678-6900
URL: www.scrippshealth.org
Type: Acute Care Hospitals
Emergency Services: Yes
Ownership: Voluntary non-profit - Other
Beds: 293
Key Personnel:
Operating Room . . . . Phyllis Abbott, RN
Intensive Care Unit . . . . Linda Hodges, RN
Quality Assurance . . . . June Komar
Emergency Room . . . . Duane Kusler, RN
Chief of Medical Staff . . . . James LaBelle, MD
Infection Control . . . . Stephanie Meyers, RN
CEO/President . . . . Chris Van Gorder, FACHE

Measure	Cases	This Hosp.	State Avg.	U.S. Avg.
Blood Clot Prevention and Treatment				
Anticoagulation Overlap Therapy[2]	81	100%	92%	93%
ICU Venous Thromboembolism Prophylaxis[2]	125	99%	92%	92%
Incidence of Potentially Preventable VTE[2]	51	0%	11%	10%
UFH with Dosages/Platelet Monitoring[2]	31	100%	96%	97%
Venous Thromboembolism Prophylaxis[2]	265	93%	83%	85%
Warfarin Therapy Discharge Instructions[2]	56	100%	75%	75%
Chest Pain/Possible Heart Attack Care				
Aspirin Given Within 24 Hours of Arrival	17	100%	97%	96%
Fibrinolytic Meds Within 30 Min. of Arrival[3,7]	-	-	62%	58%
Average Time to ECG (minutes)	20	12	9	7
Average Time to Transfer (minutes)[3,7]	-	-	62	60
Children's Asthma Care				
Received Home Management Plan of Care	-	-	88%	88%
Received Reliever Medication	-	-	100%	100%
Received Systemic Corticosteroids	-	-	100%	100%
Emergency Department				
Admittance Decision Time (minutes)[2]	349	106	125	98
Head CT Results Within 45 Min. of Arrival[1]	-	-	55%	57%
Patients Who Left ER Before Being Seen	32,328	0%	3%	2%
Time from ER Arrival to Admit. (minutes)[2]	349	234	323	274
Time from ER Arrival to Discharge (minutes)	363	171	168	134
Time in ER Before Being Evaluated (minutes)	405	16	29	26
Time to Pain Meds for Fractures (minutes)	144	34	62	57

NOTE: Hospital profiles are in alphabetical order by state, then city, then hospital within the city; Rankings exclude hospitals with less than 25 cases except for patient surveys which excludes hospitals with less than 100 cases; (a) 100-299 cases; (1) The number of cases/patients is too few to report; (2) Data submitted were based on a sample of cases/patients; (3) Results are based on a shorter time period than required; (4) Data suppressed by CMS for one or more quarters; (5) Results are not available for this reporting period; (6) Fewer than 100 patients completed the HCAHPS survey; (7) No cases met the criteria for this measure; (8) The lower limit of the confidence interval cannot be calculated if the number of observed infections equals zero; (9) No data are available from the state/territory for this reporting period; (10) The scores shown reflect fewer than 50 completed surveys; (11) There were discrepancies in the data collection process; (12) This measure does not apply to this hospital for this reporting period; (13) Results cannot be calculated for this reporting period; (14) The results for this state are combined with nearby states to protect confidentiality; Please refer to the User's Guide for a full explanation of data.

Heart Attack Care				
Aspirin Given at Discharge[2]	269	100%	99%	99%
Fibrinolytic Meds Within 30 Min. of Arrival[1,2]	-	-	73%	54%
PCI Within 90 Minutes of Arrival[2]	45	100%	95%	96%
Statin Prescribed at Discharge[2]	260	100%	98%	98%
Heart Failure Care				
ACE Inhibitor or ARB for LVSD[2]	91	100%	97%	97%
Discharge Instructions Given[2]	214	100%	94%	94%
Evaluation of LVS Function[2]	249	100%	99%	99%
Medicare Spending				
Medicare Spending per Patient (ratio)	-	1.04	0.98	0.98
Pneumonia Care				
Appropriate Initial Antibiotic Given[2]	87	98%	97%	95%
Blood Culture Timing[2]	156	100%	98%	98%
Pregnancy and Delivery Care				
Newborn Deliveries Scheduled Early[2]	72	4%	5%	6%
Preventive Care				
Immunization for Influenza[2]	497	97%	89%	90%
Immunization for Pneumonia[2]	440	98%	90%	92%
Stroke Care				
Anticoagulation Therapy for Atrial Fibrillation	27	100%	95%	95%
Antithrombotic Therapy Timing	100	100%	98%	98%
Assessed for Rehabilitation	165	100%	97%	97%
Discharged on Antithrombotic Therapy	124	100%	99%	99%
Discharged on Statin Medication	86	100%	94%	94%
Thrombolytic Therapy Timing	28	100%	72%	66%
Venous Thromboembolism Prophylaxis	181	99%	94%	94%
Written Stroke Educational Materials Given	92	100%	87%	88%
Surgical Care Improvement Project				
Appropriate Beta Blocker Usage[2]	251	100%	97%	98%
Appropriate VTP Within 24 Hours[2]	479	99%	98%	98%
Controlled Postoperative Blood Glucose[2]	204	99%	96%	97%
Perioperative Temperature Management[2]	624	100%	100%	100%
Prophylactic Antibiotic Selection[2]	587	100%	99%	99%
Prophylactic Antibiotic Selection (Outpatient)	564	100%	97%	98%
Prophylactic Antibiotic Stopped[2]	548	99%	98%	98%
Prophylactic Antibiotic Timing[2]	588	100%	99%	99%
Prophylactic Antibiotic Timing (Outpatient)	564	100%	97%	98%
Urinary Catheter Removal[2]	438	99%	97%	97%
Survey of Patients' Hospital Experiences				
Area Around Room 'Always' Quiet at Night	300+	53%	51%	61%
Doctors 'Always' Communicated Well	300+	82%	78%	82%
Home Recovery Information Given	300+	83%	83%	85%
Hospital Given 9 or 10 on 10 Point Scale	300+	76%	68%	71%
Meds 'Always' Explained Before Given	300+	65%	61%	64%
Nurses 'Always' Communicated Well	300+	81%	74%	79%
Pain 'Always' Well Controlled	300+	76%	68%	71%
Room and Bathroom 'Always' Clean	300+	71%	70%	73%
Timely Help 'Always' Received	300+	65%	62%	68%
Would Definitely Recommend Hospital	300+	80%	70%	71%
Use of Medical Imaging				
Cardiac Imaging Stress Test before Surgery	118	4.2%	5.2%	5.3%
Combination Abdominal CT Scan	723	7.2%	13.4%	10.5%
Combination Brain/Sinus CT Scan	736	2.0%	2.2%	2.7%
Combination Chest CT Scan	387	1.8%	2.3%	2.7%
Follow-up Mammogram/Ultrasound	1,985	8.0%	8.2%	8.8%
Lumbar Spine MRI for Low Back Pain	65	27.7%	34.2%	37.2%

Grossmont Hospital

5555 Grossmont Center Drive Box 58
La Mesa, CA 91942
Phone: 619-465-0711
Fax: 619-740-4255
URL: www.sharp.com
Type: Acute Care Hospitals
Emergency Services: Yes
Ownership: Govt - Hospital Dist/Auth
Beds: 536

Key Personnel:

Quality Assurance . . . . Karen Bernstein
Chief of Medical Staff. . . . . Margret Elizando
Emergency Room . . . . Dale Fox
Anesthesiology. . . . . Christopher Glazener
CEO/President. . . . . Barry Jantz
Operating Room. . . . . Susie Werner

Measure	Cases	This Hosp.	State Avg.	U.S. Avg.
Blood Clot Prevention and Treatment				
Anticoagulation Overlap Therapy[2]	135	95%	92%	93%
ICU Venous Thromboembolism Prophylaxis[2]	69	96%	92%	92%
Incidence of Potentially Preventable VTE[2]	21	29%	11%	10%
UFH with Dosages/Platelet Monitoring[2]	50	100%	96%	97%
Venous Thromboembolism Prophylaxis[2]	390	83%	83%	85%
Warfarin Therapy Discharge Instructions[2]	99	68%	75%	75%
Chest Pain/Possible Heart Attack Care				
Aspirin Given Within 24 Hours of Arrival	28	96%	97%	96%
Fibrinolytic Meds Within 30 Min. of Arrival[3,7]	-	-	62%	58%
Average Time to ECG (minutes)	27	5	9	7
Average Time to Transfer (minutes)[1,3]	-	-	62	60
Children's Asthma Care				
Received Home Management Plan of Care	-	-	88%	88%
Received Reliever Medication	-	-	100%	100%
Received Systemic Corticosteroids	-	-	100%	100%
Emergency Department				
Admittance Decision Time (minutes)[2]	726	142	125	98
Head CT Results Within 45 Min. of Arrival[1]	-	-	55%	57%
Patients Who Left ER Before Being Seen	98,314	5%	3%	2%
Time from ER Arrival to Admit. (minutes)[2]	735	376	323	274
Time from ER Arrival to Discharge (minutes)	360	239	168	134
Time in ER Before Being Evaluated (minutes)	355	56	29	26
Time to Pain Meds for Fractures (minutes)	271	60	62	57
Heart Attack Care				
Aspirin Given at Discharge	320	100%	99%	99%
Fibrinolytic Meds Within 30 Min. of Arrival[7]	-	-	73%	54%
PCI Within 90 Minutes of Arrival	121	100%	95%	96%
Statin Prescribed at Discharge	297	100%	98%	98%
Heart Failure Care				
ACE Inhibitor or ARB for LVSD	255	100%	97%	97%
Discharge Instructions Given	619	96%	94%	94%
Evaluation of LVS Function	753	100%	99%	99%
Medicare Spending				
Medicare Spending per Patient (ratio)	-	1.01	0.98	0.98
Pneumonia Care				
Appropriate Initial Antibiotic Given	282	97%	97%	95%
Blood Culture Timing	519	99%	98%	98%
Pregnancy and Delivery Care				
Newborn Deliveries Scheduled Early	374	3%	5%	6%
Preventive Care				
Immunization for Influenza[2]	511	99%	89%	90%
Immunization for Pneumonia[2]	561	99%	90%	92%
Stroke Care				
Anticoagulation Therapy for Atrial Fibrillation	41	100%	95%	95%
Antithrombotic Therapy Timing	319	97%	98%	98%
Assessed for Rehabilitation	402	100%	97%	97%
Discharged on Antithrombotic Therapy	340	100%	99%	99%
Discharged on Statin Medication	261	99%	94%	94%
Thrombolytic Therapy Timing	40	98%	72%	66%
Venous Thromboembolism Prophylaxis	425	97%	94%	94%
Written Stroke Educational Materials Given	238	97%	87%	88%
Surgical Care Improvement Project				
Appropriate Beta Blocker Usage[2]	379	99%	97%	98%
Appropriate VTP Within 24 Hours[2]	818	99%	98%	98%
Controlled Postoperative Blood Glucose[2]	170	100%	96%	97%
Perioperative Temperature Management[2]	984	100%	100%	100%
Prophylactic Antibiotic Selection[2]	854	99%	99%	99%
Prophylactic Antibiotic Selection (Outpatient)	311	94%	97%	98%
Prophylactic Antibiotic Stopped[2]	832	99%	98%	98%
Prophylactic Antibiotic Timing[2]	853	100%	99%	99%
Prophylactic Antibiotic Timing (Outpatient)	313	98%	97%	98%
Urinary Catheter Removal[2]	830	99%	97%	97%
Survey of Patients' Hospital Experiences				
Area Around Room 'Always' Quiet at Night	300+	50%	51%	61%
Doctors 'Always' Communicated Well	300+	77%	78%	82%
Home Recovery Information Given	300+	85%	83%	85%
Hospital Given 9 or 10 on 10 Point Scale	300+	71%	68%	71%
Meds 'Always' Explained Before Given	300+	62%	61%	64%
Nurses 'Always' Communicated Well	300+	78%	74%	79%
Pain 'Always' Well Controlled	300+	70%	68%	71%
Room and Bathroom 'Always' Clean	300+	70%	70%	73%
Timely Help 'Always' Received	300+	61%	62%	68%
Would Definitely Recommend Hospital	300+	75%	70%	71%
Use of Medical Imaging				
Cardiac Imaging Stress Test before Surgery	241	5.4%	5.2%	5.3%
Combination Abdominal CT Scan	1,295	5.2%	13.4%	10.5%
Combination Brain/Sinus CT Scan	1,653	2.3%	2.2%	2.7%
Combination Chest CT Scan	429	3.7%	2.3%	2.7%
Follow-up Mammogram/Ultrasound[7]	-	-	8.2%	8.8%
Lumbar Spine MRI for Low Back Pain	62	38.7%	34.2%	37.2%

La Palma Intercommunity Hospital

7901 Walker Street
La Palma, CA 90623
Phone: 714-670-7400
Fax: 714-670-6004
URL: www.lapalmaintercommunityhospital.com
Type: Acute Care Hospitals
Emergency Services: Yes
Ownership: Proprietary
Beds: 139

Key Personnel:

Operating Room. . . . . Colleen Belanger
Hemotology Center . . . . Veena Charu, MD
Intensive Care Unit. . . . . H Fatemi, MD
Pediatric Ambulatory Care . . . . . . L Hansen, MD
Pediatric In-Patient Care . . . . L Hansen, MD
CEO . . . . Virg Narbutas
Chief of Medical Staff. . . . . Sami Shoukair, MD
Quality Assurance . . . . P Smith, RN

Measure	Cases	This Hosp.	State Avg.	U.S. Avg.
Blood Clot Prevention and Treatment				
Anticoagulation Overlap Therapy[1,2]	-	-	92%	93%
ICU Venous Thromboembolism Prophylaxis[2]	46	52%	92%	92%
Incidence of Potentially Preventable VTE[2,7]	-	-	11%	10%
UFH with Dosages/Platelet Monitoring[1,2]	-	-	96%	97%
Venous Thromboembolism Prophylaxis[2]	296	41%	83%	85%
Warfarin Therapy Discharge Instructions[1,2]	-	-	75%	75%
Chest Pain/Possible Heart Attack Care				
Aspirin Given Within 24 Hours of Arrival	14	100%	97%	96%
Fibrinolytic Meds Within 30 Min. of Arrival[7]	-	-	62%	58%
Average Time to ECG (minutes)	17	5	9	7
Average Time to Transfer (minutes)[7]	-	-	62	60
Children's Asthma Care				
Received Home Management Plan of Care	-	-	88%	88%
Received Reliever Medication	-	-	100%	100%
Received Systemic Corticosteroids	-	-	100%	100%
Emergency Department				
Admittance Decision Time (minutes)[2]	466	68	125	98
Head CT Results Within 45 Min. of Arrival[1]	-	-	55%	57%
Patients Who Left ER Before Being Seen	15,117	2%	3%	2%
Time from ER Arrival to Admit. (minutes)[2]	537	245	323	274
Time from ER Arrival to Discharge (minutes)	740	146	168	134
Time in ER Before Being Evaluated (minutes)	750	32	29	26
Time to Pain Meds for Fractures (minutes)	95	50	62	57
Heart Attack Care				
Aspirin Given at Discharge	36	100%	99%	99%
Fibrinolytic Meds Within 30 Min. of Arrival[7]	-	-	73%	54%
PCI Within 90 Minutes of Arrival[7]	-	-	95%	96%
Statin Prescribed at Discharge	29	100%	98%	98%
Heart Failure Care				
ACE Inhibitor or ARB for LVSD	28	100%	97%	97%
Discharge Instructions Given	84	100%	94%	94%
Evaluation of LVS Function	105	100%	99%	99%
Medicare Spending				
Medicare Spending per Patient (ratio)	-	1.13	0.98	0.98
Pneumonia Care				
Appropriate Initial Antibiotic Given	53	100%	97%	95%
Blood Culture Timing	156	99%	98%	98%
Pregnancy and Delivery Care				
Newborn Deliveries Scheduled Early	60	0%	5%	6%
Preventive Care				
Immunization for Influenza[2]	327	99%	89%	90%
Immunization for Pneumonia[2]	465	100%	90%	92%
Stroke Care				
Anticoagulation Therapy for Atrial Fibrillation[1]	-	-	95%	95%
Antithrombotic Therapy Timing	29	83%	98%	98%
Assessed for Rehabilitation	31	84%	97%	97%
Discharged on Antithrombotic Therapy	26	88%	99%	99%
Discharged on Statin Medication	20	65%	94%	94%
Thrombolytic Therapy Timing	12	0%	72%	66%

NOTE: Hospital profiles are in alphabetical order by state, then city, then hospital within the city; Rankings exclude hospitals with less than 25 cases except for patient surveys which excludes hospitals with less than 100 cases; (a) 100-299 cases; (1) The number of cases/patients is too few to report; (2) Data submitted were based on a sample of cases/patients; (3) Results are based on a shorter time period than required; (4) Data suppressed by CMS for one or more quarters; (5) Results are not available for this reporting period; (6) Fewer than 100 patients completed the HCAHPS survey; (7) No cases met the criteria for this measure; (8) The lower limit of the confidence interval cannot be calculated if the number of observed infections equals zero; (9) No data are available from the state/territory for this reporting period; (10) The scores shown reflect fewer than 50 completed surveys; (11) There were discrepancies in the data collection process; (12) This measure does not apply to this hospital for this reporting period; (13) Results cannot be calculated for this reporting period; (14) The results for this state are combined with nearby states to protect confidentiality; Please refer to the User's Guide for a full explanation of data.

Measure	Cases	This Hosp.	State Avg.	U.S. Avg.
Venous Thromboembolism Prophylaxis	31	42%	94%	94%
Written Stroke Educational Materials Given	18	28%	87%	88%
Surgical Care Improvement Project				
Appropriate Beta Blocker Usage[1]	-	-	97%	98%
Appropriate VTP Within 24 Hours	42	100%	98%	98%
Controlled Postoperative Blood Glucose[7]	-	-	96%	97%
Perioperative Temperature Management	56	100%	100%	100%
Prophylactic Antibiotic Selection	14	100%	99%	99%
Prophylactic Antibiotic Selection (Outpatient)[1]	-	-	97%	98%
Prophylactic Antibiotic Stopped	14	100%	98%	98%
Prophylactic Antibiotic Timing	14	100%	99%	99%
Prophylactic Antibiotic Timing (Outpatient)[1]	-	-	97%	98%
Urinary Catheter Removal	23	100%	97%	97%
Survey of Patients' Hospital Experiences				
Area Around Room 'Always' Quiet at Night	(a)	55%	51%	61%
Doctors 'Always' Communicated Well	(a)	69%	78%	82%
Home Recovery Information Given	(a)	81%	83%	85%
Hospital Given 9 or 10 on 10 Point Scale	(a)	53%	68%	71%
Meds 'Always' Explained Before Given	(a)	56%	61%	64%
Nurses 'Always' Communicated Well	(a)	69%	74%	79%
Pain 'Always' Well Controlled	(a)	58%	68%	71%
Room and Bathroom 'Always' Clean	(a)	71%	70%	73%
Timely Help 'Always' Received	(a)	58%	62%	68%
Would Definitely Recommend Hospital	(a)	63%	70%	71%
Use of Medical Imaging				
Cardiac Imaging Stress Test before Surgery[1]	-	-	5.2%	5.3%
Combination Abdominal CT Scan	157	9.6%	13.4%	10.5%
Combination Brain/Sinus CT Scan[1]	-	-	2.2%	2.7%
Combination Chest CT Scan[1]	-	-	2.3%	2.7%
Follow-up Mammogram/Ultrasound	141	2.8%	8.2%	8.8%
Lumbar Spine MRI for Low Back Pain[1]	-	-	34.2%	37.2%

Saddleback Memorial Medical Center

24451 Health Center Drive
Laguna Hills, CA 92653
Phone: 949-837-4500
Fax: 949-452-3549
URL: www.memorialcare.org/saddleback
Type: Acute Care Hospitals
Emergency Services: Yes
Ownership: Voluntary non-profit - Private
Beds: 325
Key Personnel:
CEO/President . . . . Barry Arbuckle, PhD
Chief of Medical Staff . . . . David Lagrew

Measure	Cases	This Hosp.	State Avg.	U.S. Avg.
Blood Clot Prevention and Treatment				
Anticoagulation Overlap Therapy[2]	88	84%	92%	93%
ICU Venous Thromboembolism Prophylaxis[2]	74	93%	92%	92%
Incidence of Potentially Preventable VTE[2]	17	12%	11%	10%
UFH with Dosages/Platelet Monitoring[2]	71	99%	96%	97%
Venous Thromboembolism Prophylaxis[2]	324	65%	83%	85%
Warfarin Therapy Discharge Instructions[2]	62	60%	75%	75%
Chest Pain/Possible Heart Attack Care				
Aspirin Given Within 24 Hours of Arrival	42	98%	97%	96%
Fibrinolytic Meds Within 30 Min. of Arrival[3,7]	-	-	62%	58%
Average Time to ECG (minutes)	43	5	9	7
Average Time to Transfer (minutes)[1,3]	-	-	62	60
Children's Asthma Care				
Received Home Management Plan of Care	-	-	88%	88%
Received Reliever Medication	-	-	100%	100%
Received Systemic Corticosteroids	-	-	100%	100%
Emergency Department				
Admittance Decision Time (minutes)[2]	657	152	125	98
Head CT Results Within 45 Min. of Arrival	24	58%	55%	57%
Patients Who Left ER Before Being Seen	36,683	2%	3%	2%
Time from ER Arrival to Admit. (minutes)[2]	662	310	323	274
Time from ER Arrival to Discharge (minutes)	338	137	168	134
Time in ER Before Being Evaluated (minutes)	386	22	29	26
Time to Pain Meds for Fractures (minutes)	194	52	62	57
Heart Attack Care				
Aspirin Given at Discharge	245	99%	99%	99%
Fibrinolytic Meds Within 30 Min. of Arrival[7]	-	-	73%	54%
PCI Within 90 Minutes of Arrival	55	100%	95%	96%
Statin Prescribed at Discharge	248	96%	98%	98%
Heart Failure Care				
ACE Inhibitor or ARB for LVSD	109	98%	97%	97%
Discharge Instructions Given	359	87%	94%	94%
Evaluation of LVS Function	457	100%	99%	99%
Medicare Spending				
Medicare Spending per Patient (ratio)	-	0.98	0.98	0.98
Pneumonia Care				
Appropriate Initial Antibiotic Given	203	96%	97%	95%
Blood Culture Timing	331	98%	98%	98%
Pregnancy and Delivery Care				
Newborn Deliveries Scheduled Early[2]	29	0%	5%	6%
Preventive Care				
Immunization for Influenza[2]	520	91%	89%	90%
Immunization for Pneumonia[2]	648	88%	90%	92%
Stroke Care				
Anticoagulation Therapy for Atrial Fibrillation	34	94%	95%	95%
Antithrombotic Therapy Timing	161	98%	98%	98%
Assessed for Rehabilitation	184	96%	97%	97%
Discharged on Antithrombotic Therapy	168	99%	99%	99%
Discharged on Statin Medication	120	86%	94%	94%
Thrombolytic Therapy Timing	12	67%	72%	66%
Venous Thromboembolism Prophylaxis	194	94%	94%	94%
Written Stroke Educational Materials Given	86	93%	87%	88%
Surgical Care Improvement Project				
Appropriate Beta Blocker Usage[2]	126	98%	97%	98%
Appropriate VTP Within 24 Hours[2]	289	99%	98%	98%
Controlled Postoperative Blood Glucose[2]	83	96%	96%	97%
Perioperative Temperature Management[2]	378	100%	100%	100%
Prophylactic Antibiotic Selection[2]	289	99%	99%	99%
Prophylactic Antibiotic Selection (Outpatient)	502	98%	97%	98%
Prophylactic Antibiotic Stopped[2]	273	99%	98%	98%
Prophylactic Antibiotic Timing[2]	290	99%	99%	99%
Prophylactic Antibiotic Timing (Outpatient)	503	98%	97%	98%
Urinary Catheter Removal[2]	309	95%	97%	97%
Survey of Patients' Hospital Experiences				
Area Around Room 'Always' Quiet at Night	300+	44%	51%	61%
Doctors 'Always' Communicated Well	300+	79%	78%	82%
Home Recovery Information Given	300+	84%	83%	85%
Hospital Given 9 or 10 on 10 Point Scale	300+	68%	68%	71%
Meds 'Always' Explained Before Given	300+	59%	61%	64%
Nurses 'Always' Communicated Well	300+	75%	74%	79%
Pain 'Always' Well Controlled	300+	70%	68%	71%
Room and Bathroom 'Always' Clean	300+	73%	70%	73%
Timely Help 'Always' Received	300+	58%	62%	68%
Would Definitely Recommend Hospital	300+	71%	70%	71%
Use of Medical Imaging				
Cardiac Imaging Stress Test before Surgery	231	5.6%	5.2%	5.3%
Combination Abdominal CT Scan	860	23.6%	13.4%	10.5%
Combination Brain/Sinus CT Scan	841	3.3%	2.2%	2.7%
Combination Chest CT Scan	458	2.4%	2.3%	2.7%
Follow-up Mammogram/Ultrasound	2,640	13.4%	8.2%	8.8%
Lumbar Spine MRI for Low Back Pain[1]	-	-	34.2%	37.2%

Mountains Community Hospital

29101 Hospital Road
Lake Arrowhead, CA 92352
Phone: 909-336-3651
Fax: 909-336-1179
URL: www.mchcares.com
Type: Critical Access Hospitals
Emergency Services: Yes
Ownership: Govt - Hospital Dist/Auth
Beds: 37
Key Personnel:
President . . . . Kieth Burkart, OD
Quality Assurance . . . . Charles Harrison
Patient Relations . . . . Susan Lowell
Emergency Room . . . . Terri Montgomery
Operating Room. . . . . Terri Montgomery, RN
Infection Control. . . . . Riitta Speer
Anesthesiology. . . . . John Wild, CRNA

Measure	Cases	This Hosp.	State Avg.	U.S. Avg.
Blood Clot Prevention and Treatment				
Anticoagulation Overlap Therapy[5]	-	-	92%	93%
ICU Venous Thromboembolism Prophylaxis[5]	-	-	92%	92%
Incidence of Potentially Preventable VTE[5]	-	-	11%	10%
UFH with Dosages/Platelet Monitoring[5]	-	-	96%	97%
Venous Thromboembolism Prophylaxis[5]	-	-	83%	85%
Warfarin Therapy Discharge Instructions[5]	-	-	75%	75%
Chest Pain/Possible Heart Attack Care				
Aspirin Given Within 24 Hours of Arrival	-	-	97%	96%
Fibrinolytic Meds Within 30 Min. of Arrival	-	-	62%	58%
Average Time to ECG (minutes)	-	-	9	7
Average Time to Transfer (minutes)	-	-	62	60
Children's Asthma Care				
Received Home Management Plan of Care	-	-	88%	88%
Received Reliever Medication	-	-	100%	100%
Received Systemic Corticosteroids	-	-	100%	100%
Emergency Department				
Admittance Decision Time (minutes)[5]	-	-	125	98
Head CT Results Within 45 Min. of Arrival	-	-	55%	57%
Patients Who Left ER Before Being Seen	-	-	3%	2%
Time from ER Arrival to Admit. (minutes)[5]	-	-	323	274
Time from ER Arrival to Discharge (minutes)	-	-	168	134
Time in ER Before Being Evaluated (minutes)	-	-	29	26
Time to Pain Meds for Fractures (minutes)	-	-	62	57
Heart Attack Care				
Aspirin Given at Discharge[5]	-	-	99%	99%
Fibrinolytic Meds Within 30 Min. of Arrival[5]	-	-	73%	54%
PCI Within 90 Minutes of Arrival[5]	-	-	95%	96%
Statin Prescribed at Discharge[5]	-	-	98%	98%
Heart Failure Care				
ACE Inhibitor or ARB for LVSD[5]	-	-	97%	97%
Discharge Instructions Given[5]	-	-	94%	94%
Evaluation of LVS Function[5]	-	-	99%	99%
Medicare Spending				
Medicare Spending per Patient (ratio)	-	-	0.98	0.98
Pneumonia Care				
Appropriate Initial Antibiotic Given[3,7]	-	-	97%	95%
Blood Culture Timing[3,7]	-	-	98%	98%
Pregnancy and Delivery Care				
Newborn Deliveries Scheduled Early[5]	-	-	5%	6%
Preventive Care				
Immunization for Influenza[5]	-	-	89%	90%
Immunization for Pneumonia[5]	-	-	90%	92%
Stroke Care				
Anticoagulation Therapy for Atrial Fibrillation[5]	-	-	95%	95%
Antithrombotic Therapy Timing[5]	-	-	98%	98%
Assessed for Rehabilitation[5]	-	-	97%	97%
Discharged on Antithrombotic Therapy[5]	-	-	99%	99%
Discharged on Statin Medication[5]	-	-	94%	94%
Thrombolytic Therapy Timing[5]	-	-	72%	66%
Venous Thromboembolism Prophylaxis[5]	-	-	94%	94%
Written Stroke Educational Materials Given[5]	-	-	87%	88%
Surgical Care Improvement Project				
Appropriate Beta Blocker Usage[5]	-	-	97%	98%
Appropriate VTP Within 24 Hours[5]	-	-	98%	98%
Controlled Postoperative Blood Glucose[5]	-	-	96%	97%
Perioperative Temperature Management[5]	-	-	100%	100%
Prophylactic Antibiotic Selection[5]	-	-	99%	99%
Prophylactic Antibiotic Selection (Outpatient)	-	-	97%	98%
Prophylactic Antibiotic Stopped[5]	-	-	98%	98%
Prophylactic Antibiotic Timing[5]	-	-	99%	99%
Prophylactic Antibiotic Timing (Outpatient)	-	-	97%	98%
Urinary Catheter Removal[5]	-	-	97%	97%
Survey of Patients' Hospital Experiences				
Area Around Room 'Always' Quiet at Night[5]	-	-	51%	61%
Doctors 'Always' Communicated Well[5]	-	-	78%	82%
Home Recovery Information Given[5]	-	-	83%	85%
Hospital Given 9 or 10 on 10 Point Scale[5]	-	-	68%	71%
Meds 'Always' Explained Before Given[5]	-	-	61%	64%
Nurses 'Always' Communicated Well[5]	-	-	74%	79%
Pain 'Always' Well Controlled[5]	-	-	68%	71%
Room and Bathroom 'Always' Clean[5]	-	-	70%	73%
Timely Help 'Always' Received[5]	-	-	62%	68%
Would Definitely Recommend Hospital[5]	-	-	70%	71%
Use of Medical Imaging				
Cardiac Imaging Stress Test before Surgery	-	-	5.2%	5.3%
Combination Abdominal CT Scan	-	-	13.4%	10.5%
Combination Brain/Sinus CT Scan	-	-	2.2%	2.7%
Combination Chest CT Scan	-	-	2.3%	2.7%
Follow-up Mammogram/Ultrasound	-	-	8.2%	8.8%

NOTE: Hospital profiles are in alphabetical order by state, then city, then hospital within the city; Rankings exclude hospitals with less than 25 cases except for patient surveys which excludes hospitals with less than 100 cases; (a) 100-299 cases; (1) The number of cases/patients is too few to report; (2) Data submitted were based on a sample of cases/patients; (3) Results are based on a shorter time period than required; (4) Data suppressed by CMS for one or more quarters; (5) Results are not available for this reporting period; (6) Fewer than 100 patients completed the HCAHPS survey; (7) No cases met the criteria for this measure; (8) The lower limit of the confidence interval cannot be calculated if the number of observed infections equals zero; (9) No data are available from the state/territory for this reporting period; (10) The scores shown reflect fewer than 50 completed surveys; (11) There were discrepancies in the data collection process; (12) This measure does not apply to this hospital for this reporting period; (13) Results cannot be calculated for this reporting period; (14) The results for this state are combined with nearby states to protect confidentiality; Please refer to the User's Guide for a full explanation of data.

Measure	Cases	This Hosp.	State Avg.	U.S. Avg.
Lumbar Spine MRI for Low Back Pain	-	-	34.2%	37.2%

Kern Valley Healthcare District

6412 Laurel Ave
Lake Isabella, CA 93240
Phone: 760-379-2681
Fax: 760-379-0066
E-mail: michelerosato@kvhd.org
URL: www.kvhd.org
Type: Critical Access Hospitals
Emergency Services: Yes
Ownership: Govt - Hospital Dist/Auth
Beds: 101

Key Personnel:
Infection Control. . . . . Carol Bradshaw
Operating Room. . . . . Mary Completo
Chief of Medical Staff . . . . Gary Finstad, MD
Intensive Care Unit. . . . . Gary Finstad, MD
Radiology. . . . . Eleanor Fraser, MD
Quality Assurance . . . . Judy Littrell
CEO/President. . . . . Pamela Ott

Measure	Cases	This Hosp.	State Avg.	U.S. Avg.
Blood Clot Prevention and Treatment				
Anticoagulation Overlap Therapy[5]	-	-	92%	93%
ICU Venous Thromboembolism Prophylaxis[5]	-	-	92%	92%
Incidence of Potentially Preventable VTE[5]	-	-	11%	10%
UFH with Dosages/Platelet Monitoring[5]	-	-	96%	97%
Venous Thromboembolism Prophylaxis[5]	-	-	83%	85%
Warfarin Therapy Discharge Instructions[5]	-	-	75%	75%
Chest Pain/Possible Heart Attack Care				
Aspirin Given Within 24 Hours of Arrival	48	73%	97%	96%
Fibrinolytic Meds Within 30 Min. of Arrival[1]	-	-	62%	58%
Average Time to ECG (minutes)	47	15	9	7
Average Time to Transfer (minutes)[1]	-	-	62	60
Children's Asthma Care				
Received Home Management Plan of Care	-	-	88%	88%
Received Reliever Medication	-	-	100%	100%
Received Systemic Corticosteroids	-	-	100%	100%
Emergency Department				
Admittance Decision Time (minutes)[5]	-	-	125	98
Head CT Results Within 45 Min. of Arrival[5]	-	-	55%	57%
Patients Who Left ER Before Being Seen	6,989	6%	3%	2%
Time from ER Arrival to Admit. (minutes)[5]	-	-	323	274
Time from ER Arrival to Discharge (minutes)[5]	-	-	168	134
Time in ER Before Being Evaluated (minutes)[5]	-	-	29	26
Time to Pain Meds for Fractures (minutes)[5]	-	-	62	57
Heart Attack Care				
Aspirin Given at Discharge[5]	-	-	99%	99%
Fibrinolytic Meds Within 30 Min. of Arrival[5]	-	-	73%	54%
PCI Within 90 Minutes of Arrival[5]	-	-	95%	96%
Statin Prescribed at Discharge[5]	-	-	98%	98%
Heart Failure Care				
ACE Inhibitor or ARB for LVSD[1]	-	-	97%	97%
Discharge Instructions Given	14	21%	94%	94%
Evaluation of LVS Function	21	38%	99%	99%
Medicare Spending				
Medicare Spending per Patient (ratio)	-	-	0.98	0.98
Pneumonia Care				
Appropriate Initial Antibiotic Given	50	76%	97%	95%
Blood Culture Timing	55	91%	98%	98%
Pregnancy and Delivery Care				
Newborn Deliveries Scheduled Early[3,7]	-	-	5%	6%
Preventive Care				
Immunization for Influenza[3]	116	54%	89%	90%
Immunization for Pneumonia[3]	344	70%	90%	92%
Stroke Care				
Anticoagulation Therapy for Atrial Fibrillation[5]	-	-	95%	95%
Antithrombotic Therapy Timing[5]	-	-	98%	98%
Assessed for Rehabilitation[5]	-	-	97%	97%
Discharged on Antithrombotic Therapy[5]	-	-	99%	99%
Discharged on Statin Medication[5]	-	-	94%	94%
Thrombolytic Therapy Timing[5]	-	-	72%	66%
Venous Thromboembolism Prophylaxis[5]	-	-	94%	94%
Written Stroke Educational Materials Given[5]	-	-	87%	88%
Surgical Care Improvement Project				
Appropriate Beta Blocker Usage[3,7]	-	-	97%	98%
Appropriate VTP Within 24 Hours[3,7]	-	-	98%	98%
Controlled Postoperative Blood Glucose[5]	-	-	96%	97%
Perioperative Temperature Management[1,3]	-	-	100%	100%
Prophylactic Antibiotic Selection[3,7]	-	-	99%	99%
Prophylactic Antibiotic Selection (Outpatient)[5]	-	-	97%	98%
Prophylactic Antibiotic Stopped[3,7]	-	-	98%	98%
Prophylactic Antibiotic Timing[3,7]	-	-	99%	99%
Prophylactic Antibiotic Timing (Outpatient)[5]	-	-	97%	98%
Urinary Catheter Removal[3,7]	-	-	97%	97%
Survey of Patients' Hospital Experiences				
Area Around Room 'Always' Quiet at Night[5]	-	-	51%	61%
Doctors 'Always' Communicated Well[5]	-	-	78%	82%
Home Recovery Information Given[5]	-	-	83%	85%
Hospital Given 9 or 10 on 10 Point Scale[5]	-	-	68%	71%
Meds 'Always' Explained Before Given[5]	-	-	61%	64%
Nurses 'Always' Communicated Well[5]	-	-	74%	79%
Pain 'Always' Well Controlled[5]	-	-	68%	71%
Room and Bathroom 'Always' Clean[5]	-	-	70%	73%
Timely Help 'Always' Received[5]	-	-	62%	68%
Would Definitely Recommend Hospital[5]	-	-	70%	71%
Use of Medical Imaging				
Cardiac Imaging Stress Test before Surgery[7]	-	-	5.2%	5.3%
Combination Abdominal CT Scan	175	11.4%	13.4%	10.5%
Combination Brain/Sinus CT Scan	201	0.5%	2.2%	2.7%
Combination Chest CT Scan	58	3.4%	2.3%	2.7%
Follow-up Mammogram/Ultrasound[7]	-	-	8.2%	8.8%
Lumbar Spine MRI for Low Back Pain[7]	-	-	34.2%	37.2%

Sutter Lakeside Hospital

5176 Hill Road East
Lakeport, CA 95453
Phone: 707-262-5000
Fax: 707-262-5003
URL: www.sutterlakeside.org
Type: Critical Access Hospitals
Emergency Services: Yes
Ownership: Voluntary non-profit - Private
Beds: 25

Key Personnel:
Quality Assurance . . . . Elsie Cramer
Intensive Care Unit. . . . . John Gorbened, RNO
Emergency Room . . . . John Gorberko, RN
Operating Room. . . . . Patricia Mahaffey, RN
Infection Control. . . . . Susan Meyers, RN
CEO/President. . . . . Siri Nelson, CAO
Cardiac Laboratory. . . . . Donald Pifer
Radiology. . . . . Vivek Reddy

Measure	Cases	This Hosp.	State Avg.	U.S. Avg.
Blood Clot Prevention and Treatment				
Anticoagulation Overlap Therapy[1,2]	-	-	92%	93%
ICU Venous Thromboembolism Prophylaxis[2]	39	90%	92%	92%
Incidence of Potentially Preventable VTE[1,2]	-	-	11%	10%
UFH with Dosages/Platelet Monitoring[2,7]	-	-	96%	97%
Venous Thromboembolism Prophylaxis[2]	133	83%	83%	85%
Warfarin Therapy Discharge Instructions[1,2]	-	-	75%	75%
Chest Pain/Possible Heart Attack Care				
Aspirin Given Within 24 Hours of Arrival	69	96%	97%	96%
Fibrinolytic Meds Within 30 Min. of Arrival[1]	-	-	62%	58%
Average Time to ECG (minutes)	74	20	9	7
Average Time to Transfer (minutes)[1]	-	-	62	60
Children's Asthma Care				
Received Home Management Plan of Care	-	-	88%	88%
Received Reliever Medication	-	-	100%	100%
Received Systemic Corticosteroids	-	-	100%	100%
Emergency Department				
Admittance Decision Time (minutes)[2]	189	170	125	98
Head CT Results Within 45 Min. of Arrival	32	38%	55%	57%
Patients Who Left ER Before Being Seen	19,157	3%	3%	2%
Time from ER Arrival to Admit. (minutes)[2]	337	389	323	274
Time from ER Arrival to Discharge (minutes)	355	145	168	134
Time in ER Before Being Evaluated (minutes)	357	35	29	26
Time to Pain Meds for Fractures (minutes)	120	68	62	57
Heart Attack Care				
Aspirin Given at Discharge[1]	-	-	99%	99%
Fibrinolytic Meds Within 30 Min. of Arrival[7]	-	-	73%	54%
PCI Within 90 Minutes of Arrival[7]	-	-	95%	96%
Statin Prescribed at Discharge[1]	-	-	98%	98%
Heart Failure Care				
ACE Inhibitor or ARB for LVSD	21	100%	97%	97%
Discharge Instructions Given	35	100%	94%	94%
Evaluation of LVS Function	41	100%	99%	99%
Medicare Spending				
Medicare Spending per Patient (ratio)	-	-	0.98	0.98
Pneumonia Care				
Appropriate Initial Antibiotic Given	54	98%	97%	95%
Blood Culture Timing	96	99%	98%	98%
Pregnancy and Delivery Care				
Newborn Deliveries Scheduled Early[3]	24	0%	5%	6%
Preventive Care				
Immunization for Influenza[2]	270	97%	89%	90%
Immunization for Pneumonia[2]	292	98%	90%	92%
Stroke Care				
Anticoagulation Therapy for Atrial Fibrillation[1]	-	-	95%	95%
Antithrombotic Therapy Timing	25	100%	98%	98%
Assessed for Rehabilitation	26	100%	97%	97%
Discharged on Antithrombotic Therapy	24	100%	99%	99%
Discharged on Statin Medication	21	67%	94%	94%
Thrombolytic Therapy Timing[1]	-	-	72%	66%
Venous Thromboembolism Prophylaxis	25	92%	94%	94%
Written Stroke Educational Materials Given	15	67%	87%	88%
Surgical Care Improvement Project				
Appropriate Beta Blocker Usage	42	93%	97%	98%
Appropriate VTP Within 24 Hours	165	99%	98%	98%
Controlled Postoperative Blood Glucose[7]	-	-	96%	97%
Perioperative Temperature Management	199	100%	100%	100%
Prophylactic Antibiotic Selection	135	100%	99%	99%
Prophylactic Antibiotic Selection (Outpatient)	58	100%	97%	98%
Prophylactic Antibiotic Stopped	130	96%	98%	98%
Prophylactic Antibiotic Timing	135	100%	99%	99%
Prophylactic Antibiotic Timing (Outpatient)	59	97%	97%	98%
Urinary Catheter Removal	83	98%	97%	97%
Survey of Patients' Hospital Experiences				
Area Around Room 'Always' Quiet at Night	300+	55%	51%	61%
Doctors 'Always' Communicated Well	300+	81%	78%	82%
Home Recovery Information Given	300+	86%	83%	85%
Hospital Given 9 or 10 on 10 Point Scale	300+	66%	68%	71%
Meds 'Always' Explained Before Given	300+	62%	61%	64%
Nurses 'Always' Communicated Well	300+	76%	74%	79%
Pain 'Always' Well Controlled	300+	70%	68%	71%
Room and Bathroom 'Always' Clean	300+	71%	70%	73%
Timely Help 'Always' Received	300+	68%	62%	68%
Would Definitely Recommend Hospital	300+	68%	70%	71%
Use of Medical Imaging				
Cardiac Imaging Stress Test before Surgery	133	5.3%	5.2%	5.3%
Combination Abdominal CT Scan	621	3.2%	13.4%	10.5%
Combination Brain/Sinus CT Scan	515	1.2%	2.2%	2.7%
Combination Chest CT Scan	336	0.9%	2.3%	2.7%
Follow-up Mammogram/Ultrasound	902	6.3%	8.2%	8.8%
Lumbar Spine MRI for Low Back Pain	85	30.6%	34.2%	37.2%

Lakewood Regional Medical Center

3700 E South St
Lakewood, CA 90712
Phone: 562-602-6751
Fax: 562-602-0083
URL: www.lakewoodregional.com
Type: Acute Care Hospitals
Emergency Services: Yes
Ownership: Proprietary
Beds: 161

Key Personnel:
Coronary Care . . . . Joel Epstien, MD
Chief of Medical Staff . . . . Rodger Epstien, MD
Infection Control. . . . . Stuart Finklestein, MD
Anesthesiology. . . . . Danilo Jaravata, MD
CEO/President. . . . . Mark D Korth
Radiology. . . . . Sven Rose
Cardiac Laboratory. . . . . Miguel Sanmarco, MD

Measure	Cases	This Hosp.	State Avg.	U.S. Avg.
Blood Clot Prevention and Treatment				
Anticoagulation Overlap Therapy[2]	49	88%	92%	93%
ICU Venous Thromboembolism Prophylaxis[2]	116	90%	92%	92%
Incidence of Potentially Preventable VTE[2]	11	0%	11%	10%
UFH with Dosages/Platelet Monitoring[2]	26	100%	96%	97%
Venous Thromboembolism Prophylaxis[2]	322	83%	83%	85%
Warfarin Therapy Discharge Instructions[2]	29	72%	75%	75%
Chest Pain/Possible Heart Attack Care				
Aspirin Given Within 24 Hours of Arrival	15	93%	97%	96%

NOTE: Hospital profiles are in alphabetical order by state, then city, then hospital within the city; Rankings exclude hospitals with less than 25 cases except for patient surveys which excludes hospitals with less than 100 cases; (a) 100-299 cases; (1) The number of cases/patients is too few to report; (2) Data submitted were based on a sample of cases/patients; (3) Results are based on a shorter time period than required; (4) Data suppressed by CMS for one or more quarters; (5) Results are not available for this reporting period; (6) Fewer than 100 patients completed the HCAHPS survey; (7) No cases met the criteria for this measure; (8) The lower limit of the confidence interval cannot be calculated if the number of observed infections equals zero; (9) No data are available from the state/territory for this reporting period; (10) The scores shown reflect fewer than 50 completed surveys; (11) There were discrepancies in the data collection process; (12) This measure does not apply to this hospital for this reporting period; (13) Results cannot be calculated for this reporting period; (14) The results for this state are combined with nearby states to protect confidentiality; Please refer to the User's Guide for a full explanation of data.

Fibrinolytic Meds Within 30 Min. of Arrival[5]	-	-	62%	58%
Average Time to ECG (minutes)	16	14	9	7
Average Time to Transfer (minutes)[5]	-	-	62	60
Children's Asthma Care				
Received Home Management Plan of Care	-	-	88%	88%
Received Reliever Medication	-	-	100%	100%
Received Systemic Corticosteroids	-	-	100%	100%
Emergency Department				
Admittance Decision Time (minutes)[2]	990	132	125	98
Head CT Results Within 45 Min. of Arrival	32	62%	55%	57%
Patients Who Left ER Before Being Seen	45,691	2%	3%	2%
Time from ER Arrival to Admit. (minutes)[2]	993	310	323	274
Time from ER Arrival to Discharge (minutes)	451	143	168	134
Time in ER Before Being Evaluated (minutes)	475	44	29	26
Time to Pain Meds for Fractures (minutes)	194	68	62	57
Heart Attack Care				
Aspirin Given at Discharge	250	99%	99%	99%
Fibrinolytic Meds Within 30 Min. of Arrival[7]	-	-	73%	54%
PCI Within 90 Minutes of Arrival	51	96%	95%	96%
Statin Prescribed at Discharge	252	99%	98%	98%
Heart Failure Care				
ACE Inhibitor or ARB for LVSD	108	100%	97%	97%
Discharge Instructions Given	253	98%	94%	94%
Evaluation of LVS Function	329	100%	99%	99%
Medicare Spending				
Medicare Spending per Patient (ratio)	-	1.13	0.98	0.98
Pneumonia Care				
Appropriate Initial Antibiotic Given[2]	90	97%	97%	95%
Blood Culture Timing[2]	159	99%	98%	98%
Pregnancy and Delivery Care				
Newborn Deliveries Scheduled Early[7]	-	-	5%	6%
Preventive Care				
Immunization for Influenza[2]	623	89%	89%	90%
Immunization for Pneumonia[2]	919	86%	90%	92%
Stroke Care				
Anticoagulation Therapy for Atrial Fibrillation	20	95%	95%	95%
Antithrombotic Therapy Timing	146	95%	98%	98%
Assessed for Rehabilitation	175	97%	97%	97%
Discharged on Antithrombotic Therapy	145	96%	99%	99%
Discharged on Statin Medication	109	90%	94%	94%
Thrombolytic Therapy Timing	14	43%	72%	66%
Venous Thromboembolism Prophylaxis	191	94%	94%	94%
Written Stroke Educational Materials Given	86	93%	87%	88%
Surgical Care Improvement Project				
Appropriate Beta Blocker Usage[2]	192	96%	97%	98%
Appropriate VTP Within 24 Hours[2]	405	96%	98%	98%
Controlled Postoperative Blood Glucose[2]	97	93%	96%	97%
Perioperative Temperature Management[2]	447	100%	100%	100%
Prophylactic Antibiotic Selection[2]	395	97%	99%	99%
Prophylactic Antibiotic Selection (Outpatient)	251	91%	97%	98%
Prophylactic Antibiotic Stopped[2]	360	92%	98%	98%
Prophylactic Antibiotic Timing[2]	395	99%	99%	99%
Prophylactic Antibiotic Timing (Outpatient)	259	97%	97%	98%
Urinary Catheter Removal[2]	367	97%	97%	97%
Survey of Patients' Hospital Experiences				
Area Around Room 'Always' Quiet at Night	300+	54%	51%	61%
Doctors 'Always' Communicated Well	300+	80%	78%	82%
Home Recovery Information Given	300+	81%	83%	85%
Hospital Given 9 or 10 on 10 Point Scale	300+	61%	68%	71%
Meds 'Always' Explained Before Given	300+	58%	61%	64%
Nurses 'Always' Communicated Well	300+	73%	74%	79%
Pain 'Always' Well Controlled	300+	65%	68%	71%
Room and Bathroom 'Always' Clean	300+	68%	70%	73%
Timely Help 'Always' Received	300+	62%	62%	68%
Would Definitely Recommend Hospital	300+	65%	70%	71%
Use of Medical Imaging				
Cardiac Imaging Stress Test before Surgery	179	6.1%	5.2%	5.3%
Combination Abdominal CT Scan	445	1.8%	13.4%	10.5%
Combination Brain/Sinus CT Scan	579	0.2%	2.2%	2.7%
Combination Chest CT Scan	188	1.1%	2.3%	2.7%
Follow-up Mammogram/Ultrasound	389	15.7%	8.2%	8.8%
Lumbar Spine MRI for Low Back Pain[1]	-	-	34.2%	37.2%

Antelope Valley Hospital

1600 W Ave J
Lancaster, CA 93534
Phone: 661-949-5000
URL: www.avhospital.org
Type: Acute Care Hospitals
Emergency Services: Yes
Ownership: Govt - Hospital Dist/Auth
Beds: 378

Key Personnel:
Coronary Care . . . . Brenda Burns
Intensive Care Unit. . . . . Brenda Burns
Quality Assurance . . . . Bonnie Daniel
Chair/CEO . . . . Abdallah S. Farrukh, MD
CEO/President. . . . . Dennis M. Knox, FACHE
Chief of Medical Staff . . . . Radha Krishnan, MD
Emergency Room . . . . John Lynn, MD
Radiology. . . . . Alberto Pernudi

Measure	Cases	This Hosp.	State Avg.	U.S. Avg.
Blood Clot Prevention and Treatment				
Anticoagulation Overlap Therapy[2]	115	93%	92%	93%
ICU Venous Thromboembolism Prophylaxis[2]	80	96%	92%	92%
Incidence of Potentially Preventable VTE[2]	16	25%	11%	10%
UFH with Dosages/Platelet Monitoring[2]	31	94%	96%	97%
Venous Thromboembolism Prophylaxis[2]	303	85%	83%	85%
Warfarin Therapy Discharge Instructions[2]	97	70%	75%	75%
Chest Pain/Possible Heart Attack Care				
Aspirin Given Within 24 Hours of Arrival[1,3]	-	-	97%	96%
Fibrinolytic Meds Within 30 Min. of Arrival[3,7]	-	-	62%	58%
Average Time to ECG (minutes)[1,3]	-	-	9	7
Average Time to Transfer (minutes)[1,3]	-	-	62	60
Children's Asthma Care				
Received Home Management Plan of Care	-	-	88%	88%
Received Reliever Medication	-	-	100%	100%
Received Systemic Corticosteroids	-	-	100%	100%
Emergency Department				
Admittance Decision Time (minutes)[2]	622	278	125	98
Head CT Results Within 45 Min. of Arrival[1]	-	-	55%	57%
Patients Who Left ER Before Being Seen	>100k	4%	3%	2%
Time from ER Arrival to Admit. (minutes)[2]	644	580	323	274
Time from ER Arrival to Discharge (minutes)	459	204	168	134
Time in ER Before Being Evaluated (minutes)	472	84	29	26
Time to Pain Meds for Fractures (minutes)	246	78	62	57
Heart Attack Care				
Aspirin Given at Discharge	284	98%	99%	99%
Fibrinolytic Meds Within 30 Min. of Arrival[1]	-	-	73%	54%
PCI Within 90 Minutes of Arrival	49	96%	95%	96%
Statin Prescribed at Discharge	281	98%	98%	98%
Heart Failure Care				
ACE Inhibitor or ARB for LVSD	141	96%	97%	97%
Discharge Instructions Given	305	91%	94%	94%
Evaluation of LVS Function	340	100%	99%	99%
Medicare Spending				
Medicare Spending per Patient (ratio)	-	1.03	0.98	0.98
Pneumonia Care				
Appropriate Initial Antibiotic Given[2]	111	91%	97%	95%
Blood Culture Timing[2]	148	96%	98%	98%
Pregnancy and Delivery Care				
Newborn Deliveries Scheduled Early[2]	98	0%	5%	6%
Preventive Care				
Immunization for Influenza[2]	580	97%	89%	90%
Immunization for Pneumonia[2]	490	97%	90%	92%
Stroke Care				
Anticoagulation Therapy for Atrial Fibrillation	19	100%	95%	95%
Antithrombotic Therapy Timing	142	96%	98%	98%
Assessed for Rehabilitation	185	99%	97%	97%
Discharged on Antithrombotic Therapy	157	99%	99%	99%
Discharged on Statin Medication	124	98%	94%	94%
Thrombolytic Therapy Timing	13	85%	72%	66%
Venous Thromboembolism Prophylaxis	195	98%	94%	94%
Written Stroke Educational Materials Given	117	95%	87%	88%
Surgical Care Improvement Project				
Appropriate Beta Blocker Usage[2]	189	96%	97%	98%
Appropriate VTP Within 24 Hours[2]	719	99%	98%	98%
Controlled Postoperative Blood Glucose[2]	19	95%	96%	97%
Perioperative Temperature Management[2]	887	100%	100%	100%
Prophylactic Antibiotic Selection[2]	679	99%	99%	99%
Prophylactic Antibiotic Selection (Outpatient)	124	98%	97%	98%
Prophylactic Antibiotic Stopped[2]	646	97%	98%	98%
Prophylactic Antibiotic Timing[2]	679	99%	99%	99%
Prophylactic Antibiotic Timing (Outpatient)	126	96%	97%	98%
Urinary Catheter Removal[2]	489	97%	97%	97%
Survey of Patients' Hospital Experiences				
Area Around Room 'Always' Quiet at Night	300+	45%	51%	61%
Doctors 'Always' Communicated Well	300+	75%	78%	82%
Home Recovery Information Given	300+	81%	83%	85%
Hospital Given 9 or 10 on 10 Point Scale	300+	62%	68%	71%
Meds 'Always' Explained Before Given	300+	58%	61%	64%
Nurses 'Always' Communicated Well	300+	73%	74%	79%
Pain 'Always' Well Controlled	300+	69%	68%	71%
Room and Bathroom 'Always' Clean	300+	65%	70%	73%
Timely Help 'Always' Received	300+	59%	62%	68%
Would Definitely Recommend Hospital	300+	60%	70%	71%
Use of Medical Imaging				
Cardiac Imaging Stress Test before Surgery	126	5.6%	5.2%	5.3%
Combination Abdominal CT Scan	476	1.1%	13.4%	10.5%
Combination Brain/Sinus CT Scan	589	1.7%	2.2%	2.7%
Combination Chest CT Scan	57	3.5%	2.3%	2.7%
Follow-up Mammogram/Ultrasound[7]	-	-	8.2%	8.8%
Lumbar Spine MRI for Low Back Pain[1]	-	-	34.2%	37.2%

Lodi Memorial Hospital

975 S Fairmont Avenue
Lodi, CA 95240
Phone: 209-334-3411
Fax: 209-368-3745
URL: www.lodihealth.org
Type: Acute Care Hospitals
Emergency Services: Yes
Ownership: Voluntary non-profit - Other
Beds: 181

Key Personnel:
Operating Room. . . . . Debbie Aspling
Chief of Medical Staff . . . . Mary Brown, MD
Radiology. . . . . Susan Gootnick
CEO/President. . . . . Joseph Harrington
Pediatric Ambulatory Care . . . . . . Roy Ishii, MD
Pediatric In-Patient Care . . . . Roy Ishii, MD
Cardiac Laboratory. . . . . Willis Marvolf
Quality Assurance . . . . Ken Wood

Measure	Cases	This Hosp.	State Avg.	U.S. Avg.
Blood Clot Prevention and Treatment				
Anticoagulation Overlap Therapy[2]	53	98%	92%	93%
ICU Venous Thromboembolism Prophylaxis[2]	74	99%	92%	92%
Incidence of Potentially Preventable VTE[1,2]	-	-	11%	10%
UFH with Dosages/Platelet Monitoring[2]	31	100%	96%	97%
Venous Thromboembolism Prophylaxis[2]	403	97%	83%	85%
Warfarin Therapy Discharge Instructions[2]	41	76%	75%	75%
Chest Pain/Possible Heart Attack Care				
Aspirin Given Within 24 Hours of Arrival	32	100%	97%	96%
Fibrinolytic Meds Within 30 Min. of Arrival[1]	-	-	62%	58%
Average Time to ECG (minutes)	33	6	9	7
Average Time to Transfer (minutes)[1]	-	-	62	60
Children's Asthma Care				
Received Home Management Plan of Care	-	-	88%	88%
Received Reliever Medication	-	-	100%	100%
Received Systemic Corticosteroids	-	-	100%	100%
Emergency Department				
Admittance Decision Time (minutes)[2]	759	133	125	98
Head CT Results Within 45 Min. of Arrival	23	70%	55%	57%
Patients Who Left ER Before Being Seen	31,480	3%	3%	2%
Time from ER Arrival to Admit. (minutes)[2]	759	329	323	274
Time from ER Arrival to Discharge (minutes)	365	158	168	134
Time in ER Before Being Evaluated (minutes)	405	40	29	26
Time to Pain Meds for Fractures (minutes)	132	62	62	57
Heart Attack Care				
Aspirin Given at Discharge	34	97%	99%	99%
Fibrinolytic Meds Within 30 Min. of Arrival[1]	-	-	73%	54%
PCI Within 90 Minutes of Arrival[7]	-	-	95%	96%
Statin Prescribed at Discharge	36	89%	98%	98%
Heart Failure Care				
ACE Inhibitor or ARB for LVSD[2]	104	98%	97%	97%
Discharge Instructions Given[2]	177	90%	94%	94%
Evaluation of LVS Function[2]	246	100%	99%	99%
Medicare Spending				

NOTE: Hospital profiles are in alphabetical order by state, then city, then hospital within the city; Rankings exclude hospitals with less than 25 cases except for patient surveys which excludes hospitals with less than 100 cases; (a) 100-299 cases; (1) The number of cases/patients is too few to report; (2) Data submitted were based on a sample of cases/patients; (3) Results are based on a shorter time period than required; (4) Data suppressed by CMS for one or more quarters; (5) Results are not available for this reporting period; (6) Fewer than 100 patients completed the HCAHPS survey; (7) No cases met the criteria for this measure; (8) The lower limit of the confidence interval cannot be calculated if the number of observed infections equals zero; (9) No data are available from the state/territory for this reporting period; (10) The scores shown reflect fewer than 50 completed surveys; (11) There were discrepancies in the data collection process; (12) This measure does not apply to this hospital for this reporting period; (13) Results cannot be calculated for this reporting period; (14) The results for this state are combined with nearby states to protect confidentiality; Please refer to the User's Guide for a full explanation of data.

Measure	Cases	This Hosp.	State Avg.	U.S. Avg.
Medicare Spending per Patient (ratio)	-	1.08	0.98	0.98
Pneumonia Care				
Appropriate Initial Antibiotic Given[2]	111	97%	97%	95%
Blood Culture Timing[2]	204	97%	98%	98%
Pregnancy and Delivery Care				
Newborn Deliveries Scheduled Early[2]	31	0%	5%	6%
Preventive Care				
Immunization for Influenza[2]	532	96%	89%	90%
Immunization for Pneumonia[2]	652	97%	90%	92%
Stroke Care				
Anticoagulation Therapy for Atrial Fibrillation[1]	-	-	95%	95%
Antithrombotic Therapy Timing	38	100%	98%	98%
Assessed for Rehabilitation	41	100%	97%	97%
Discharged on Antithrombotic Therapy	38	100%	99%	99%
Discharged on Statin Medication	32	84%	94%	94%
Thrombolytic Therapy Timing[1]	-	-	72%	66%
Venous Thromboembolism Prophylaxis	43	98%	94%	94%
Written Stroke Educational Materials Given	12	25%	87%	88%
Surgical Care Improvement Project				
Appropriate Beta Blocker Usage[2]	86	98%	97%	98%
Appropriate VTP Within 24 Hours[2]	261	96%	98%	98%
Controlled Postoperative Blood Glucose[2,7]	-	-	96%	97%
Perioperative Temperature Management[2]	290	100%	100%	100%
Prophylactic Antibiotic Selection[2]	157	99%	99%	99%
Prophylactic Antibiotic Selection (Outpatient)	282	99%	97%	98%
Prophylactic Antibiotic Stopped[2]	153	95%	98%	98%
Prophylactic Antibiotic Timing[2]	157	99%	99%	99%
Prophylactic Antibiotic Timing (Outpatient)	282	100%	97%	98%
Urinary Catheter Removal[2]	191	99%	97%	97%
Survey of Patients' Hospital Experiences				
Area Around Room 'Always' Quiet at Night	300+	53%	51%	61%
Doctors 'Always' Communicated Well	300+	76%	78%	82%
Home Recovery Information Given	300+	84%	83%	85%
Hospital Given 9 or 10 on 10 Point Scale	300+	71%	68%	71%
Meds 'Always' Explained Before Given	300+	57%	61%	64%
Nurses 'Always' Communicated Well	300+	77%	74%	79%
Pain 'Always' Well Controlled	300+	67%	68%	71%
Room and Bathroom 'Always' Clean	300+	72%	70%	73%
Timely Help 'Always' Received	300+	58%	62%	68%
Would Definitely Recommend Hospital	300+	69%	70%	71%
Use of Medical Imaging				
Cardiac Imaging Stress Test before Surgery	202	3.5%	5.2%	5.3%
Combination Abdominal CT Scan	815	5.8%	13.4%	10.5%
Combination Brain/Sinus CT Scan	848	2.1%	2.2%	2.7%
Combination Chest CT Scan	407	0.5%	2.3%	2.7%
Follow-up Mammogram/Ultrasound[7]	-	-	8.2%	8.8%
Lumbar Spine MRI for Low Back Pain[7]	-	-	34.2%	37.2%

Loma Linda University Medical Center

11234 Anderson St — Phone: 909-558-4000
Loma Linda, CA 92354 — Fax: 909-558-4058
URL: www.llumc.edu
Type: Acute Care Hospitals — Emergency Services: Yes
Ownership: Voluntary non-profit - Private — Beds: 724

Key Personnel:
Operating Room. . . . . Ahmed M Abou-Zamzam
Radiology. . . . . Phiroze Billimo, MD
CEO/President. . . . . Richard H. Hart, MD, DrPH
Quality Assurance . . . . Mark L Hubbard
Pediatric Ambulatory Care . . . . . . John W Mace, MD

Measure	Cases	This Hosp.	State Avg.	U.S. Avg.
Blood Clot Prevention and Treatment				
Anticoagulation Overlap Therapy[2]	102	91%	92%	93%
ICU Venous Thromboembolism Prophylaxis[2]	101	90%	92%	92%
Incidence of Potentially Preventable VTE[2]	41	12%	11%	10%
UFH with Dosages/Platelet Monitoring[2]	90	87%	96%	97%
Venous Thromboembolism Prophylaxis[2]	298	77%	83%	85%
Warfarin Therapy Discharge Instructions[2]	71	46%	75%	75%
Chest Pain/Possible Heart Attack Care				
Aspirin Given Within 24 Hours of Arrival	16	100%	97%	96%
Fibrinolytic Meds Within 30 Min. of Arrival[3,7]	-	-	62%	58%
Average Time to ECG (minutes)	16	4	9	7
Average Time to Transfer (minutes)[3,7]	-	-	62	60
Children's Asthma Care				
Received Home Management Plan of Care	210	52%	88%	88%
Received Reliever Medication	211	100%	100%	100%
Received Systemic Corticosteroids	210	99%	100%	100%
Emergency Department				
Admittance Decision Time (minutes)[2]	505	295	125	98
Head CT Results Within 45 Min. of Arrival[1]	-	-	55%	57%
Patients Who Left ER Before Being Seen	65,307	5%	3%	2%
Time from ER Arrival to Admit. (minutes)[2]	514	528	323	274
Time from ER Arrival to Discharge (minutes)	374	304	168	134
Time in ER Before Being Evaluated (minutes)	384	107	29	26
Time to Pain Meds for Fractures (minutes)	174	124	62	57
Heart Attack Care				
Aspirin Given at Discharge	445	98%	99%	99%
Fibrinolytic Meds Within 30 Min. of Arrival[1]	-	-	73%	54%
PCI Within 90 Minutes of Arrival	48	96%	95%	96%
Statin Prescribed at Discharge	433	97%	98%	98%
Heart Failure Care				
ACE Inhibitor or ARB for LVSD[2]	127	95%	97%	97%
Discharge Instructions Given[2]	283	76%	94%	94%
Evaluation of LVS Function[2]	316	99%	99%	99%
Medicare Spending				
Medicare Spending per Patient (ratio)	-	0.96	0.98	0.98
Pneumonia Care				
Appropriate Initial Antibiotic Given[2]	37	89%	97%	95%
Blood Culture Timing[2]	96	100%	98%	98%
Pregnancy and Delivery Care				
Newborn Deliveries Scheduled Early[2]	45	2%	5%	6%
Preventive Care				
Immunization for Influenza[2]	531	89%	89%	90%
Immunization for Pneumonia[2]	406	84%	90%	92%
Stroke Care				
Anticoagulation Therapy for Atrial Fibrillation[2]	21	90%	95%	95%
Antithrombotic Therapy Timing[2]	134	96%	98%	98%
Assessed for Rehabilitation[2]	211	98%	97%	97%
Discharged on Antithrombotic Therapy[2]	138	97%	99%	99%
Discharged on Statin Medication[2]	103	97%	94%	94%
Thrombolytic Therapy Timing[2]	14	71%	72%	66%
Venous Thromboembolism Prophylaxis[2]	242	91%	94%	94%
Written Stroke Educational Materials Given[2]	124	65%	87%	88%
Surgical Care Improvement Project				
Appropriate Beta Blocker Usage[2]	250	98%	97%	98%
Appropriate VTP Within 24 Hours[2]	427	99%	98%	98%
Controlled Postoperative Blood Glucose[2]	134	93%	96%	97%
Perioperative Temperature Management[2]	635	98%	100%	100%
Prophylactic Antibiotic Selection[2]	441	100%	99%	99%
Prophylactic Antibiotic Selection (Outpatient)	436	85%	97%	98%
Prophylactic Antibiotic Stopped[2]	432	97%	98%	98%
Prophylactic Antibiotic Timing[2]	450	93%	99%	99%
Prophylactic Antibiotic Timing (Outpatient)	434	93%	97%	98%
Urinary Catheter Removal[2]	280	94%	97%	97%
Survey of Patients' Hospital Experiences				
Area Around Room 'Always' Quiet at Night	300+	50%	51%	61%
Doctors 'Always' Communicated Well	300+	78%	78%	82%
Home Recovery Information Given	300+	85%	83%	85%
Hospital Given 9 or 10 on 10 Point Scale	300+	71%	68%	71%
Meds 'Always' Explained Before Given	300+	60%	61%	64%
Nurses 'Always' Communicated Well	300+	74%	74%	79%
Pain 'Always' Well Controlled	300+	65%	68%	71%
Room and Bathroom 'Always' Clean	300+	65%	70%	73%
Timely Help 'Always' Received	300+	60%	62%	68%
Would Definitely Recommend Hospital	300+	76%	70%	71%
Use of Medical Imaging				
Cardiac Imaging Stress Test before Surgery	765	5.1%	5.2%	5.3%
Combination Abdominal CT Scan	1,549	34.5%	13.4%	10.5%
Combination Brain/Sinus CT Scan	770	3.2%	2.2%	2.7%
Combination Chest CT Scan	934	7.8%	2.3%	2.7%
Follow-up Mammogram/Ultrasound	1,407	12.4%	8.2%	8.8%
Lumbar Spine MRI for Low Back Pain	155	38.1%	34.2%	37.2%

Loma Linda VA Medical Center

11201 Benton Street — Phone: 909-825-7084
Loma Linda, CA 92357 — Fax: 909-422-3106
E-mail: vets@lom.med.va.gov
URL: www.lom.med.va.gov
Type: Acute Care - VA — Emergency Services: No
Ownership: Government Federal — Beds: 203

Key Personnel:
Operating Room. . . . . Elva Abogado
Administrator . . . . Shane M. Elliott, MBA
Chief of Medical Staff . . . . Dwight C Evans, MD
Quality Assurance . . . . Sandy Hinshaw
Anesthesiology. . . . . Wayne Jacobsen, MD
Emergency Room . . . . Ofelia Willis

Measure	Cases	This Hosp.	State Avg.	U.S. Avg.
Blood Clot Prevention and Treatment				
Anticoagulation Overlap Therapy	-	-	92%	93%
ICU Venous Thromboembolism Prophylaxis	-	-	92%	92%
Incidence of Potentially Preventable VTE	-	-	11%	10%
UFH with Dosages/Platelet Monitoring	-	-	96%	97%
Venous Thromboembolism Prophylaxis	-	-	83%	85%
Warfarin Therapy Discharge Instructions	-	-	75%	75%
Chest Pain/Possible Heart Attack Care				
Aspirin Given Within 24 Hours of Arrival	-	-	97%	96%
Fibrinolytic Meds Within 30 Min. of Arrival	-	-	62%	58%
Average Time to ECG (minutes)	-	-	9	7
Average Time to Transfer (minutes)	-	-	62	60
Children's Asthma Care				
Received Home Management Plan of Care	-	-	88%	88%
Received Reliever Medication	-	-	100%	100%
Received Systemic Corticosteroids	-	-	100%	100%
Emergency Department				
Admittance Decision Time (minutes)	-	-	125	98
Head CT Results Within 45 Min. of Arrival	-	-	55%	57%
Patients Who Left ER Before Being Seen	-	-	3%	2%
Time from ER Arrival to Admit. (minutes)	-	-	323	274
Time from ER Arrival to Discharge (minutes)	-	-	168	134
Time in ER Before Being Evaluated (minutes)	-	-	29	26
Time to Pain Meds for Fractures (minutes)	-	-	62	57
Heart Attack Care				
Aspirin Given at Discharge	53	100%	99%	99%
Fibrinolytic Meds Within 30 Min. of Arrival[5]	-	-	73%	54%
PCI Within 90 Minutes of Arrival[5]	-	-	95%	96%
Statin Prescribed at Discharge	52	100%	98%	98%
Heart Failure Care				
ACE Inhibitor or ARB for LVSD	99	97%	97%	97%
Discharge Instructions Given	194	85%	94%	94%
Evaluation of LVS Function	220	100%	99%	99%
Medicare Spending				
Medicare Spending per Patient (ratio)	-	-	0.98	0.98
Pneumonia Care				
Appropriate Initial Antibiotic Given	43	100%	97%	95%
Blood Culture Timing	160	98%	98%	98%
Pregnancy and Delivery Care				
Newborn Deliveries Scheduled Early	-	-	5%	6%
Preventive Care				
Immunization for Influenza[5]	-	-	89%	90%
Immunization for Pneumonia[5]	-	-	90%	92%
Stroke Care				
Anticoagulation Therapy for Atrial Fibrillation	-	-	95%	95%
Antithrombotic Therapy Timing	-	-	98%	98%
Assessed for Rehabilitation	-	-	97%	97%
Discharged on Antithrombotic Therapy	-	-	99%	99%
Discharged on Statin Medication	-	-	94%	94%
Thrombolytic Therapy Timing	-	-	72%	66%
Venous Thromboembolism Prophylaxis	-	-	94%	94%
Written Stroke Educational Materials Given	-	-	87%	88%
Surgical Care Improvement Project				
Appropriate Beta Blocker Usage[2]	129	100%	97%	98%
Appropriate VTP Within 24 Hours[2]	321	99%	98%	98%
Controlled Postoperative Blood Glucose[5]	-	-	96%	97%
Perioperative Temperature Management[2]	368	100%	100%	100%
Prophylactic Antibiotic Selection	241	99%	99%	99%
Prophylactic Antibiotic Selection (Outpatient)	-	-	97%	98%

NOTE: Hospital profiles are in alphabetical order by state, then city, then hospital within the city; Rankings exclude hospitals with less than 25 cases except for patient surveys which excludes hospitals with less than 100 cases; (a) 100-299 cases; (1) The number of cases/patients is too few to report; (2) Data submitted were based on a sample of cases/patients; (3) Results are based on a shorter time period than required; (4) Data suppressed by CMS for one or more quarters; (5) Results are not available for this reporting period; (6) Fewer than 100 patients completed the HCAHPS survey; (7) No cases met the criteria for this measure; (8) The lower limit of the confidence interval cannot be calculated if the number of observed infections equals zero; (9) No data are available from the state/territory for this reporting period; (10) The scores shown reflect fewer than 50 completed surveys; (11) There were discrepancies in the data collection process; (12) This measure does not apply to this hospital for this reporting period; (13) Results cannot be calculated for this reporting period; (14) The results for this state are combined with nearby states to protect confidentiality; Please refer to the User's Guide for a full explanation of data.

Measure	Cases	This Hosp.	State Avg.	U.S. Avg.
Prophylactic Antibiotic Stopped	228	99%	98%	98%
Prophylactic Antibiotic Timing	242	99%	99%	99%
Prophylactic Antibiotic Timing (Outpatient)	-	-	97%	98%
Urinary Catheter Removal[2]	72	96%	97%	97%
Survey of Patients' Hospital Experiences				
Area Around Room 'Always' Quiet at Night	-	-	51%	61%
Doctors 'Always' Communicated Well	-	-	78%	82%
Home Recovery Information Given	-	-	83%	85%
Hospital Given 9 or 10 on 10 Point Scale	-	-	68%	71%
Meds 'Always' Explained Before Given	-	-	61%	64%
Nurses 'Always' Communicated Well	-	-	74%	79%
Pain 'Always' Well Controlled	-	-	68%	71%
Room and Bathroom 'Always' Clean	-	-	70%	73%
Timely Help 'Always' Received	-	-	62%	68%
Would Definitely Recommend Hospital	-	-	70%	71%
Use of Medical Imaging				
Cardiac Imaging Stress Test before Surgery	-	-	5.2%	5.3%
Combination Abdominal CT Scan	-	-	13.4%	10.5%
Combination Brain/Sinus CT Scan	-	-	2.2%	2.7%
Combination Chest CT Scan	-	-	2.3%	2.7%
Follow-up Mammogram/Ultrasound	-	-	8.2%	8.8%
Lumbar Spine MRI for Low Back Pain	-	-	34.2%	37.2%

Lompoc Valley Medical Center

1515 E Ocean Avenue
Lompoc, CA 93436
Phone: 805-737-3300
Fax: 805-735-8591
E-mail: webmaster@lompochospital.org
URL: www.lompochospital.org
Type: Acute Care Hospitals
Emergency Services: Yes
Ownership: Govt - Hospital Dist/Auth
Beds: 170

Key Personnel:
Chief of Medical Staff.......... Rollin Bailey, MD
Cardiac Laboratory............ Larry Coughlin
Quality Assurance .... Linda Everly, RN
Operating Room.............. Judy Monroe
CEO/President................ Jim Raggio
President.................... Frank M. Signorelli
Emergency Room .... Glenn Wollman, MD

Measure	Cases	This Hosp.	State Avg.	U.S. Avg.
Blood Clot Prevention and Treatment				
Anticoagulation Overlap Therapy[2]	16	75%	92%	93%
ICU Venous Thromboembolism Prophylaxis[2]	53	58%	92%	92%
Incidence of Potentially Preventable VTE[1,2]	-	-	11%	10%
UFH with Dosages/Platelet Monitoring[1,2]	-	-	96%	97%
Venous Thromboembolism Prophylaxis[2]	204	45%	83%	85%
Warfarin Therapy Discharge Instructions[2]	12	8%	75%	75%
Chest Pain/Possible Heart Attack Care				
Aspirin Given Within 24 Hours of Arrival	55	100%	97%	96%
Fibrinolytic Meds Within 30 Min. of Arrival[7]	-	-	62%	58%
Average Time to ECG (minutes)	56	14	9	7
Average Time to Transfer (minutes)	15	60	62	60
Children's Asthma Care				
Received Home Management Plan of Care	-	-	88%	88%
Received Reliever Medication	-	-	100%	100%
Received Systemic Corticosteroids	-	-	100%	100%
Emergency Department				
Admittance Decision Time (minutes)[2]	259	107	125	98
Head CT Results Within 45 Min. of Arrival	13	31%	55%	57%
Patients Who Left ER Before Being Seen	20,877	3%	3%	2%
Time from ER Arrival to Admit. (minutes)[2]	281	296	323	274
Time from ER Arrival to Discharge (minutes)	372	144	168	134
Time in ER Before Being Evaluated (minutes)	349	37	29	26
Time to Pain Meds for Fractures (minutes)	85	60	62	57
Heart Attack Care				
Aspirin Given at Discharge[1]	-	-	99%	99%
Fibrinolytic Meds Within 30 Min. of Arrival[7]	-	-	73%	54%
PCI Within 90 Minutes of Arrival[7]	-	-	95%	96%
Statin Prescribed at Discharge[1]	-	-	98%	98%
Heart Failure Care				
ACE Inhibitor or ARB for LVSD	19	89%	97%	97%
Discharge Instructions Given	43	84%	94%	94%
Evaluation of LVS Function	46	98%	99%	99%
Medicare Spending				
Medicare Spending per Patient (ratio)	-	0.87	0.98	0.98
Pneumonia Care				
Appropriate Initial Antibiotic Given	70	90%	97%	95%
Blood Culture Timing	100	94%	98%	98%
Pregnancy and Delivery Care				
Newborn Deliveries Scheduled Early[2]	49	10%	5%	6%
Preventive Care				
Immunization for Influenza[2]	256	86%	89%	90%
Immunization for Pneumonia[2]	250	86%	90%	92%
Stroke Care				
Anticoagulation Therapy for Atrial Fibrillation[1]	-	-	95%	95%
Antithrombotic Therapy Timing	20	95%	98%	98%
Assessed for Rehabilitation	17	100%	97%	97%
Discharged on Antithrombotic Therapy	17	82%	99%	99%
Discharged on Statin Medication	16	50%	94%	94%
Thrombolytic Therapy Timing[1]	-	-	72%	66%
Venous Thromboembolism Prophylaxis	22	41%	94%	94%
Written Stroke Educational Materials Given[1]	-	-	87%	88%
Surgical Care Improvement Project				
Appropriate Beta Blocker Usage	41	83%	97%	98%
Appropriate VTP Within 24 Hours	139	84%	98%	98%
Controlled Postoperative Blood Glucose[7]	-	-	96%	97%
Perioperative Temperature Management	162	99%	100%	100%
Prophylactic Antibiotic Selection	114	96%	99%	99%
Prophylactic Antibiotic Selection (Outpatient)	11	91%	97%	98%
Prophylactic Antibiotic Stopped	113	73%	98%	98%
Prophylactic Antibiotic Timing	114	97%	99%	99%
Prophylactic Antibiotic Timing (Outpatient)	11	100%	97%	98%
Urinary Catheter Removal	101	74%	97%	97%
Survey of Patients' Hospital Experiences				
Area Around Room 'Always' Quiet at Night	300+	52%	51%	61%
Doctors 'Always' Communicated Well	300+	77%	78%	82%
Home Recovery Information Given	300+	83%	83%	85%
Hospital Given 9 or 10 on 10 Point Scale	300+	65%	68%	71%
Meds 'Always' Explained Before Given	300+	58%	61%	64%
Nurses 'Always' Communicated Well	300+	72%	74%	79%
Pain 'Always' Well Controlled	300+	66%	68%	71%
Room and Bathroom 'Always' Clean	300+	76%	70%	73%
Timely Help 'Always' Received	300+	65%	62%	68%
Would Definitely Recommend Hospital	300+	65%	70%	71%
Use of Medical Imaging				
Cardiac Imaging Stress Test before Surgery	133	6.0%	5.2%	5.3%
Combination Abdominal CT Scan	537	40.4%	13.4%	10.5%
Combination Brain/Sinus CT Scan[1]	-	-	2.2%	2.7%
Combination Chest CT Scan	371	2.4%	2.3%	2.7%
Follow-up Mammogram/Ultrasound	891	5.8%	8.2%	8.8%
Lumbar Spine MRI for Low Back Pain	81	35.8%	34.2%	37.2%

Southern Inyo Hospital

501 East Locust Street
Lone Pine, CA 93545
Phone: 760-876-5501
Fax: 760-876-4388
URL: www.sihd.org
Type: Critical Access Hospitals
Emergency Services: Yes
Ownership: Govt - Hospital Dist/Auth
Beds: 37

Key Personnel:
Chief of Medical Staff.......... David Barabe, MD
CEO/President................ Lee Barron
Emergency Room .... Sandy Manning

Measure	Cases	This Hosp.	State Avg.	U.S. Avg.
Blood Clot Prevention and Treatment				
Anticoagulation Overlap Therapy[5]	-	-	92%	93%
ICU Venous Thromboembolism Prophylaxis[5]	-	-	92%	92%
Incidence of Potentially Preventable VTE[5]	-	-	11%	10%
UFH with Dosages/Platelet Monitoring[5]	-	-	96%	97%
Venous Thromboembolism Prophylaxis[5]	-	-	83%	85%
Warfarin Therapy Discharge Instructions[5]	-	-	75%	75%
Chest Pain/Possible Heart Attack Care				
Aspirin Given Within 24 Hours of Arrival[5]	-	-	97%	96%
Fibrinolytic Meds Within 30 Min. of Arrival[5]	-	-	62%	58%
Average Time to ECG (minutes)[5]	-	-	9	7
Average Time to Transfer (minutes)[5]	-	-	62	60
Children's Asthma Care				
Received Home Management Plan of Care	-	-	88%	88%
Received Reliever Medication	-	-	100%	100%
Received Systemic Corticosteroids	-	-	100%	100%
Emergency Department				
Admittance Decision Time (minutes)[5]	-	-	125	98
Head CT Results Within 45 Min. of Arrival[5]	-	-	55%	57%
Patients Who Left ER Before Being Seen[5]	-	-	3%	2%
Time from ER Arrival to Admit. (minutes)[5]	-	-	323	274
Time from ER Arrival to Discharge (minutes)[3]	24	106	168	134
Time in ER Before Being Evaluated (minutes)[3]	24	18	29	26
Time to Pain Meds for Fractures (minutes)[5]	-	-	62	57
Heart Attack Care				
Aspirin Given at Discharge[5]	-	-	99%	99%
Fibrinolytic Meds Within 30 Min. of Arrival[5]	-	-	73%	54%
PCI Within 90 Minutes of Arrival[5]	-	-	95%	96%
Statin Prescribed at Discharge[5]	-	-	98%	98%
Heart Failure Care				
ACE Inhibitor or ARB for LVSD[5]	-	-	97%	97%
Discharge Instructions Given[5]	-	-	94%	94%
Evaluation of LVS Function[5]	-	-	99%	99%
Medicare Spending				
Medicare Spending per Patient (ratio)		-	0.98	0.98
Pneumonia Care				
Appropriate Initial Antibiotic Given[1,3]	-	-	97%	95%
Blood Culture Timing[3,7]	-	-	98%	98%
Pregnancy and Delivery Care				
Newborn Deliveries Scheduled Early[5]	-	-	5%	6%
Preventive Care				
Immunization for Influenza[5]	-	-	89%	90%
Immunization for Pneumonia[5]	-	-	90%	92%
Stroke Care				
Anticoagulation Therapy for Atrial Fibrillation[5]	-	-	95%	95%
Antithrombotic Therapy Timing[5]	-	-	98%	98%
Assessed for Rehabilitation[5]	-	-	97%	97%
Discharged on Antithrombotic Therapy[5]	-	-	99%	99%
Discharged on Statin Medication[5]	-	-	94%	94%
Thrombolytic Therapy Timing[5]	-	-	72%	66%
Venous Thromboembolism Prophylaxis[5]	-	-	94%	94%
Written Stroke Educational Materials Given[5]	-	-	87%	88%
Surgical Care Improvement Project				
Appropriate Beta Blocker Usage[5]	-	-	97%	98%
Appropriate VTP Within 24 Hours[5]	-	-	98%	98%
Controlled Postoperative Blood Glucose[5]	-	-	96%	97%
Perioperative Temperature Management[5]	-	-	100%	100%
Prophylactic Antibiotic Selection[5]	-	-	99%	99%
Prophylactic Antibiotic Selection (Outpatient)[5]	-	-	97%	98%
Prophylactic Antibiotic Stopped[5]	-	-	98%	98%
Prophylactic Antibiotic Timing[5]	-	-	99%	99%
Prophylactic Antibiotic Timing (Outpatient)[5]	-	-	97%	98%
Urinary Catheter Removal[5]	-	-	97%	97%
Survey of Patients' Hospital Experiences				
Area Around Room 'Always' Quiet at Night[5]	-	-	51%	61%
Doctors 'Always' Communicated Well[5]	-	-	78%	82%
Home Recovery Information Given[5]	-	-	83%	85%
Hospital Given 9 or 10 on 10 Point Scale[5]	-	-	68%	71%
Meds 'Always' Explained Before Given[5]	-	-	61%	64%
Nurses 'Always' Communicated Well[5]	-	-	74%	79%
Pain 'Always' Well Controlled[5]	-	-	68%	71%
Room and Bathroom 'Always' Clean[5]	-	-	70%	73%
Timely Help 'Always' Received[5]	-	-	62%	68%
Would Definitely Recommend Hospital[5]	-	-	70%	71%
Use of Medical Imaging				
Cardiac Imaging Stress Test before Surgery[7]	-	-	5.2%	5.3%
Combination Abdominal CT Scan[1]	-	-	13.4%	10.5%
Combination Brain/Sinus CT Scan[1]	-	-	2.2%	2.7%
Combination Chest CT Scan[1]	-	-	2.3%	2.7%
Follow-up Mammogram/Ultrasound[7]	-	-	8.2%	8.8%
Lumbar Spine MRI for Low Back Pain[7]	-	-	34.2%	37.2%

NOTE: Hospital profiles are in alphabetical order by state, then city, then hospital within the city; Rankings exclude hospitals with less than 25 cases except for patient surveys which excludes hospitals with less than 100 cases; (a) 100-299 cases; (1) The number of cases/patients is too few to report; (2) Data submitted were based on a sample of cases/patients; (3) Results are based on a shorter time period than required; (4) Data suppressed by CMS for one or more quarters; (5) Results are not available for this reporting period; (6) Fewer than 100 patients completed the HCAHPS survey; (7) No cases met the criteria for this measure; (8) The lower limit of the confidence interval cannot be calculated if the number of observed infections equals zero; (9) No data are available from the state/territory for this reporting period; (10) The scores shown reflect fewer than 50 completed surveys; (11) There were discrepancies in the data collection process; (12) This measure does not apply to this hospital for this reporting period; (13) Results cannot be calculated for this reporting period; (14) The results for this state are combined with nearby states to protect confidentiality; Please refer to the User's Guide for a full explanation of data.

Community Hospital of Long Beach

1720 Termino Avenue Phone: 562-494-0600
Long Beach, CA 90804 Fax: 562-498-4434
URL: www.chlb.org
Type: Acute Care Hospitals Emergency Services: Yes
Ownership: Voluntary non-profit - Private Beds: 256

Key Personnel:
Operating Room. . . . . Lester Asch, RN
Radiology. . . . . William L Bernstein
CEO/President. . . . . Ray Jankowski, MD
Chief of Medical Staff. . . . . Andrew Manos, DO
Infection Control. . . . . Bill Reeder
Quality Assurance . . . . Pauline Ward

Measure	Cases	This Hosp.	State Avg.	U.S. Avg.
Blood Clot Prevention and Treatment				
Anticoagulation Overlap Therapy[2]	13	85%	92%	93%
ICU Venous Thromboembolism Prophylaxis[2]	74	88%	92%	92%
Incidence of Potentially Preventable VTE[1,2]	-	-	11%	10%
UFH with Dosages/Platelet Monitoring[1,2]	-	-	96%	97%
Venous Thromboembolism Prophylaxis[2]	185	74%	83%	85%
Warfarin Therapy Discharge Instructions[1,2]	-	-	75%	75%
Chest Pain/Possible Heart Attack Care				
Aspirin Given Within 24 Hours of Arrival	38	97%	97%	96%
Fibrinolytic Meds Within 30 Min. of Arrival[3,7]	-	-	62%	58%
Average Time to ECG (minutes)	39	11	9	7
Average Time to Transfer (minutes)[1,3]	-	-	62	60
Children's Asthma Care				
Received Home Management Plan of Care	-	-	88%	88%
Received Reliever Medication	-	-	100%	100%
Received Systemic Corticosteroids	-	-	100%	100%
Emergency Department				
Admittance Decision Time (minutes)[2]	383	100	125	98
Head CT Results Within 45 Min. of Arrival[1,3]	-	-	55%	57%
Patients Who Left ER Before Being Seen	22,721	4%	3%	2%
Time from ER Arrival to Admit. (minutes)[2]	438	310	323	274
Time from ER Arrival to Discharge (minutes)	322	134	168	134
Time in ER Before Being Evaluated (minutes)	364	34	29	26
Time to Pain Meds for Fractures (minutes)	27	85	62	57
Heart Attack Care				
Aspirin Given at Discharge	22	86%	99%	99%
Fibrinolytic Meds Within 30 Min. of Arrival[7]	-	-	73%	54%
PCI Within 90 Minutes of Arrival[7]	-	-	95%	96%
Statin Prescribed at Discharge	17	88%	98%	98%
Heart Failure Care				
ACE Inhibitor or ARB for LVSD	30	93%	97%	97%
Discharge Instructions Given	51	76%	94%	94%
Evaluation of LVS Function	76	95%	99%	99%
Medicare Spending				
Medicare Spending per Patient (ratio)	-	1.16	0.98	0.98
Pneumonia Care				
Appropriate Initial Antibiotic Given	60	97%	97%	95%
Blood Culture Timing	206	95%	98%	98%
Pregnancy and Delivery Care				
Newborn Deliveries Scheduled Early[2,7]	-	-	5%	6%
Preventive Care				
Immunization for Influenza[2]	404	96%	89%	90%
Immunization for Pneumonia[2]	415	96%	90%	92%
Stroke Care				
Anticoagulation Therapy for Atrial Fibrillation[1]	-	-	95%	95%
Antithrombotic Therapy Timing	20	95%	98%	98%
Assessed for Rehabilitation	23	91%	97%	97%
Discharged on Antithrombotic Therapy	20	95%	99%	99%
Discharged on Statin Medication	17	59%	94%	94%
Thrombolytic Therapy Timing[7]	-	-	72%	66%
Venous Thromboembolism Prophylaxis	22	73%	94%	94%
Written Stroke Educational Materials Given[1]	-	-	87%	88%
Surgical Care Improvement Project				
Appropriate Beta Blocker Usage	11	82%	97%	98%
Appropriate VTP Within 24 Hours	47	87%	98%	98%
Controlled Postoperative Blood Glucose[7]	-	-	96%	97%
Perioperative Temperature Management	54	100%	100%	100%
Prophylactic Antibiotic Selection	18	100%	99%	99%
Prophylactic Antibiotic Selection (Outpatient)[7]	-	-	97%	98%
Prophylactic Antibiotic Stopped	16	88%	98%	98%
Prophylactic Antibiotic Timing	18	100%	99%	99%
Prophylactic Antibiotic Timing (Outpatient)[1]	-	-	97%	98%
Urinary Catheter Removal	27	96%	97%	97%
Survey of Patients' Hospital Experiences				
Area Around Room 'Always' Quiet at Night	300+	43%	51%	61%
Doctors 'Always' Communicated Well	300+	68%	78%	82%
Home Recovery Information Given	300+	67%	83%	85%
Hospital Given 9 or 10 on 10 Point Scale	300+	53%	68%	71%
Meds 'Always' Explained Before Given	300+	52%	61%	64%
Nurses 'Always' Communicated Well	300+	67%	74%	79%
Pain 'Always' Well Controlled	300+	62%	68%	71%
Room and Bathroom 'Always' Clean	300+	65%	70%	73%
Timely Help 'Always' Received	300+	52%	62%	68%
Would Definitely Recommend Hospital	300+	55%	70%	71%
Use of Medical Imaging				
Cardiac Imaging Stress Test before Surgery[1]	-	-	5.2%	5.3%
Combination Abdominal CT Scan	124	0.0%	13.4%	10.5%
Combination Brain/Sinus CT Scan[1]	-	-	2.2%	2.7%
Combination Chest CT Scan[1]	-	-	2.3%	2.7%
Follow-up Mammogram/Ultrasound[7]	-	-	8.2%	8.8%
Lumbar Spine MRI for Low Back Pain[1]	-	-	34.2%	37.2%

Long Beach Memorial Medical Center

2801 Atlantic Ave Phone: 562-933-2000
Long Beach, CA 90806 Fax: 562-933-1299
URL: www.memorialcare.com/long_beach
Type: Acute Care Hospitals Emergency Services: Yes
Ownership: Voluntary non-profit - Other Beds: 716

Key Personnel:
CEO/President. . . . . Barry Arbuckle, PhD
Radiology. . . . . Paul Berger, MD
Coronary Care . . . . John Messenger, MD
Quality Assurance . . . . John Metcalfe
Chief of Medical Staff. . . . . Gainer Pillsbury Jr, MD
Infection Control. . . . . Harriett Pitt
Pediatric Ambulatory Care . . . . . . Harris Stutman, MD
Pediatric In-Patient Care . . . . Harris Stutman, MD

Measure	Cases	This Hosp.	State Avg.	U.S. Avg.
Blood Clot Prevention and Treatment				
Anticoagulation Overlap Therapy[2]	100	70%	92%	93%
ICU Venous Thromboembolism Prophylaxis[2]	69	84%	92%	92%
Incidence of Potentially Preventable VTE[2]	42	33%	11%	10%
UFH with Dosages/Platelet Monitoring[2]	64	69%	96%	97%
Venous Thromboembolism Prophylaxis[2]	309	46%	83%	85%
Warfarin Therapy Discharge Instructions[2]	68	44%	75%	75%
Chest Pain/Possible Heart Attack Care				
Aspirin Given Within 24 Hours of Arrival	29	93%	97%	96%
Fibrinolytic Meds Within 30 Min. of Arrival[5]	-	-	62%	58%
Average Time to ECG (minutes)	29	0	9	7
Average Time to Transfer (minutes)[5]	-	-	62	60
Children's Asthma Care				
Received Home Management Plan of Care	-	-	88%	88%
Received Reliever Medication	-	-	100%	100%
Received Systemic Corticosteroids	-	-	100%	100%
Emergency Department				
Admittance Decision Time (minutes)[2]	814	142	125	98
Head CT Results Within 45 Min. of Arrival[1,3]	-	-	55%	57%
Patients Who Left ER Before Being Seen	91,800	1%	3%	2%
Time from ER Arrival to Admit. (minutes)[2]	814	408	323	274
Time from ER Arrival to Discharge (minutes)	354	251	168	134
Time in ER Before Being Evaluated (minutes)	380	9	29	26
Time to Pain Meds for Fractures (minutes)	39	76	62	57
Heart Attack Care				
Aspirin Given at Discharge	224	99%	99%	99%
Fibrinolytic Meds Within 30 Min. of Arrival[7]	-	-	73%	54%
PCI Within 90 Minutes of Arrival	41	95%	95%	96%
Statin Prescribed at Discharge	226	98%	98%	98%
Heart Failure Care				
ACE Inhibitor or ARB for LVSD	212	99%	97%	97%
Discharge Instructions Given	464	98%	94%	94%
Evaluation of LVS Function	539	100%	99%	99%
Medicare Spending				
Medicare Spending per Patient (ratio)	-	1.05	0.98	0.98
Pneumonia Care				
Appropriate Initial Antibiotic Given[2]	109	98%	97%	95%
Blood Culture Timing[2]	204	99%	98%	98%
Pregnancy and Delivery Care				
Newborn Deliveries Scheduled Early[7]	-	-	5%	6%
Preventive Care				
Immunization for Influenza[2]	583	98%	89%	90%
Immunization for Pneumonia[2]	721	98%	90%	92%
Stroke Care				
Anticoagulation Therapy for Atrial Fibrillation[1,2]	-	-	95%	95%
Antithrombotic Therapy Timing[2]	71	96%	98%	98%
Assessed for Rehabilitation[2]	104	95%	97%	97%
Discharged on Antithrombotic Therapy[2]	77	96%	99%	99%
Discharged on Statin Medication[2]	62	90%	94%	94%
Thrombolytic Therapy Timing[1,2]	-	-	72%	66%
Venous Thromboembolism Prophylaxis[2]	113	79%	94%	94%
Written Stroke Educational Materials Given[2]	46	100%	87%	88%
Surgical Care Improvement Project				
Appropriate Beta Blocker Usage[2]	246	99%	97%	98%
Appropriate VTP Within 24 Hours[2]	375	95%	98%	98%
Controlled Postoperative Blood Glucose[2]	131	98%	96%	97%
Perioperative Temperature Management[2]	563	99%	100%	100%
Prophylactic Antibiotic Selection[2]	462	98%	99%	99%
Prophylactic Antibiotic Selection (Outpatient)	242	97%	97%	98%
Prophylactic Antibiotic Stopped[2]	423	99%	98%	98%
Prophylactic Antibiotic Timing[2]	461	99%	99%	99%
Prophylactic Antibiotic Timing (Outpatient)	242	98%	97%	98%
Urinary Catheter Removal[2]	362	97%	97%	97%
Survey of Patients' Hospital Experiences				
Area Around Room 'Always' Quiet at Night	300+	49%	51%	61%
Doctors 'Always' Communicated Well	300+	78%	78%	82%
Home Recovery Information Given	300+	81%	83%	85%
Hospital Given 9 or 10 on 10 Point Scale	300+	72%	68%	71%
Meds 'Always' Explained Before Given	300+	60%	61%	64%
Nurses 'Always' Communicated Well	300+	75%	74%	79%
Pain 'Always' Well Controlled	300+	68%	68%	71%
Room and Bathroom 'Always' Clean	300+	69%	70%	73%
Timely Help 'Always' Received	300+	57%	62%	68%
Would Definitely Recommend Hospital	300+	78%	70%	71%
Use of Medical Imaging				
Cardiac Imaging Stress Test before Surgery	268	5.2%	5.2%	5.3%
Combination Abdominal CT Scan	789	10.1%	13.4%	10.5%
Combination Brain/Sinus CT Scan	695	1.2%	2.2%	2.7%
Combination Chest CT Scan	435	1.1%	2.3%	2.7%
Follow-up Mammogram/Ultrasound	3,590	7.2%	8.2%	8.8%
Lumbar Spine MRI for Low Back Pain[1]	-	-	34.2%	37.2%

Miller Children's Hospital

2801 Atlantic Avenue Phone: 562-933-8001
Long Beach, CA 90806
URL: www.millerchildrenshospitallb.org
Type: Childrens Emergency Services: Yes
Ownership: Voluntary non-profit - Other

Key Personnel:
CEO . . . . Diana Hendel

Measure	Cases	This Hosp.	State Avg.	U.S. Avg.
Blood Clot Prevention and Treatment				
Anticoagulation Overlap Therapy[5]	-	-	92%	93%
ICU Venous Thromboembolism Prophylaxis[5]	-	-	92%	92%
Incidence of Potentially Preventable VTE[5]	-	-	11%	10%
UFH with Dosages/Platelet Monitoring[5]	-	-	96%	97%
Venous Thromboembolism Prophylaxis[5]	-	-	83%	85%
Warfarin Therapy Discharge Instructions[5]	-	-	75%	75%
Chest Pain/Possible Heart Attack Care				
Aspirin Given Within 24 Hours of Arrival	-	-	97%	96%
Fibrinolytic Meds Within 30 Min. of Arrival	-	-	62%	58%
Average Time to ECG (minutes)	-	-	9	7
Average Time to Transfer (minutes)	-	-	62	60
Children's Asthma Care				
Received Home Management Plan of Care	468	98%	88%	88%
Received Reliever Medication	469	100%	100%	100%
Received Systemic Corticosteroids	468	100%	100%	100%
Emergency Department				
Admittance Decision Time (minutes)[5]	-	-	125	98

NOTE: Hospital profiles are in alphabetical order by state, then city, then hospital within the city; Rankings exclude hospitals with less than 25 cases except for patient surveys which excludes hospitals with less than 100 cases; (a) 100-299 cases; (1) The number of cases/patients is too few to report; (2) Data submitted were based on a sample of cases/patients; (3) Results are based on a shorter time period than required; (4) Data suppressed by CMS for one or more quarters; (5) Results are not available for this reporting period; (6) Fewer than 100 patients completed the HCAHPS survey; (7) No cases met the criteria for this measure; (8) The lower limit of the confidence interval cannot be calculated if the number of observed infections equals zero; (9) No data are available from the state/territory for this reporting period; (10) The scores shown reflect fewer than 50 completed surveys; (11) There were discrepancies in the data collection process; (12) This measure does not apply to this hospital for this reporting period; (13) Results cannot be calculated for this reporting period; (14) The results for this state are combined with nearby states to protect confidentiality; Please refer to the User's Guide for a full explanation of data.

Measure	Cases	This Hosp.	State Avg.	U.S. Avg.
Head CT Results Within 45 Min. of Arrival	-	-	55%	57%
Patients Who Left ER Before Being Seen	-	-	3%	2%
Time from ER Arrival to Admit. (minutes)[5]	-	-	323	274
Time from ER Arrival to Discharge (minutes)	-	-	168	134
Time in ER Before Being Evaluated (minutes)	-	-	29	26
Time to Pain Meds for Fractures (minutes)	-	-	62	57
Heart Attack Care				
Aspirin Given at Discharge[5]	-	-	99%	99%
Fibrinolytic Meds Within 30 Min. of Arrival[5]	-	-	73%	54%
PCI Within 90 Minutes of Arrival[5]	-	-	95%	96%
Statin Prescribed at Discharge[5]	-	-	98%	98%
Heart Failure Care				
ACE Inhibitor or ARB for LVSD[5]	-	-	97%	97%
Discharge Instructions Given[5]	-	-	94%	94%
Evaluation of LVS Function[5]	-	-	99%	99%
Medicare Spending				
Medicare Spending per Patient (ratio)	-	-	0.98	0.98
Pneumonia Care				
Appropriate Initial Antibiotic Given[5]	-	-	97%	95%
Blood Culture Timing[5]	-	-	98%	98%
Pregnancy and Delivery Care				
Newborn Deliveries Scheduled Early[5]	-	-	5%	6%
Preventive Care				
Immunization for Influenza[5]	-	-	89%	90%
Immunization for Pneumonia[5]	-	-	90%	92%
Stroke Care				
Anticoagulation Therapy for Atrial Fibrillation[5]	-	-	95%	95%
Antithrombotic Therapy Timing[5]	-	-	98%	98%
Assessed for Rehabilitation[5]	-	-	97%	97%
Discharged on Antithrombotic Therapy[5]	-	-	99%	99%
Discharged on Statin Medication[5]	-	-	94%	94%
Thrombolytic Therapy Timing[5]	-	-	72%	66%
Venous Thromboembolism Prophylaxis[5]	-	-	94%	94%
Written Stroke Educational Materials Given[5]	-	-	87%	88%
Surgical Care Improvement Project				
Appropriate Beta Blocker Usage[5]	-	-	97%	98%
Appropriate VTP Within 24 Hours[5]	-	-	98%	98%
Controlled Postoperative Blood Glucose[5]	-	-	96%	97%
Perioperative Temperature Management[5]	-	-	100%	100%
Prophylactic Antibiotic Selection[5]	-	-	99%	99%
Prophylactic Antibiotic Selection (Outpatient)	-	-	97%	98%
Prophylactic Antibiotic Stopped[5]	-	-	98%	98%
Prophylactic Antibiotic Timing[5]	-	-	99%	99%
Prophylactic Antibiotic Timing (Outpatient)	-	-	97%	98%
Urinary Catheter Removal[5]	-	-	97%	97%
Survey of Patients' Hospital Experiences				
Area Around Room 'Always' Quiet at Night[5]	-	-	51%	61%
Doctors 'Always' Communicated Well[5]	-	-	78%	82%
Home Recovery Information Given[5]	-	-	83%	85%
Hospital Given 9 or 10 on 10 Point Scale[5]	-	-	68%	71%
Meds 'Always' Explained Before Given[5]	-	-	61%	64%
Nurses 'Always' Communicated Well[5]	-	-	74%	79%
Pain 'Always' Well Controlled[5]	-	-	68%	71%
Room and Bathroom 'Always' Clean[5]	-	-	70%	73%
Timely Help 'Always' Received[5]	-	-	62%	68%
Would Definitely Recommend Hospital[5]	-	-	70%	71%
Use of Medical Imaging				
Cardiac Imaging Stress Test before Surgery	-	-	5.2%	5.3%
Combination Abdominal CT Scan	-	-	13.4%	10.5%
Combination Brain/Sinus CT Scan	-	-	2.2%	2.7%
Combination Chest CT Scan	-	-	2.3%	2.7%
Follow-up Mammogram/Ultrasound	-	-	8.2%	8.8%
Lumbar Spine MRI for Low Back Pain	-	-	34.2%	37.2%

Pacific Hospital of Long Beach

2776 Pacific Ave
Long Beach, CA 90806
URL: www.phlb.org
Phone: 562-595-1911
Fax: 562-492-1363
Type: Acute Care Hospitals
Ownership: Proprietary
Emergency Services: Yes
Beds: 184

Key Personnel:
Radiology. William L Bernstein, MD
Emergency Room . . . . Theresa Cesiro, RN
Intensive Care Unit. . . . . Theresa Cesiro, MD
Operating Room. . . . . Franklin Horowitz
Patient Relations . . . . Kevin Kimbrough
Quality Assurance . . . . Karen Scott, RN
Infection Control. . . . . Alfonso Torres-Cook
Chief of Medical Staff . . . . Luke Watson, MD

Measure	Cases	This Hosp.	State Avg.	U.S. Avg.
Blood Clot Prevention and Treatment				
Anticoagulation Overlap Therapy[1,2]	-	-	92%	93%
ICU Venous Thromboembolism Prophylaxis[2,3]	19	89%	92%	92%
Incidence of Potentially Preventable VTE[1,2]	-	-	11%	10%
UFH with Dosages/Platelet Monitoring[1,2]	-	-	96%	97%
Venous Thromboembolism Prophylaxis[2,3]	105	94%	83%	85%
Warfarin Therapy Discharge Instructions[1,2]	-	-	75%	75%
Chest Pain/Possible Heart Attack Care				
Aspirin Given Within 24 Hours of Arrival[1,3]	-	-	97%	96%
Fibrinolytic Meds Within 30 Min. of Arrival[5]	-	-	62%	58%
Average Time to ECG (minutes)[1,3]	-	-	9	7
Average Time to Transfer (minutes)[5]	-	-	62	60
Children's Asthma Care				
Received Home Management Plan of Care	-	-	88%	88%
Received Reliever Medication	-	-	100%	100%
Received Systemic Corticosteroids	-	-	100%	100%
Emergency Department				
Admittance Decision Time (minutes)[2,3]	129	69	125	98
Head CT Results Within 45 Min. of Arrival[1,3]	-	-	55%	57%
Patients Who Left ER Before Being Seen	14,435	2%	3%	2%
Time from ER Arrival to Admit. (minutes)[2,3]	138	283	323	274
Time from ER Arrival to Discharge (minutes)[3]	204	144	168	134
Time in ER Before Being Evaluated (minutes)[3]	149	42	29	26
Time to Pain Meds for Fractures (minutes)[1,3]	-	-	62	57
Heart Attack Care				
Aspirin Given at Discharge[1,3]	-	-	99%	99%
Fibrinolytic Meds Within 30 Min. of Arrival[3,7]	-	-	73%	54%
PCI Within 90 Minutes of Arrival[3,7]	-	-	95%	96%
Statin Prescribed at Discharge[1,3]	-	-	98%	98%
Heart Failure Care				
ACE Inhibitor or ARB for LVSD[3]	18	100%	97%	97%
Discharge Instructions Given[3]	28	89%	94%	94%
Evaluation of LVS Function[3]	45	98%	99%	99%
Medicare Spending				
Medicare Spending per Patient (ratio)	-	-	0.98	0.98
Pneumonia Care				
Appropriate Initial Antibiotic Given[3]	22	100%	97%	95%
Blood Culture Timing[3]	91	92%	98%	98%
Pregnancy and Delivery Care				
Newborn Deliveries Scheduled Early[2,3]	17	6%	5%	6%
Preventive Care				
Immunization for Influenza[2]	589	95%	89%	90%
Immunization for Pneumonia[2,3]	368	91%	90%	92%
Stroke Care				
Anticoagulation Therapy for Atrial Fibrillation[3,7]	-	-	95%	95%
Antithrombotic Therapy Timing[1,3]	-	-	98%	98%
Assessed for Rehabilitation[1,3]	-	-	97%	97%
Discharged on Antithrombotic Therapy[1,3]	-	-	99%	99%
Discharged on Statin Medication[1,3]	-	-	94%	94%
Thrombolytic Therapy Timing[3,7]	-	-	72%	66%
Venous Thromboembolism Prophylaxis[1,3]	-	-	94%	94%
Written Stroke Educational Materials Given[1,3]	-	-	87%	88%
Surgical Care Improvement Project				
Appropriate Beta Blocker Usage[3]	15	100%	97%	98%
Appropriate VTP Within 24 Hours[3]	70	99%	98%	98%
Controlled Postoperative Blood Glucose[3,7]	-	-	96%	97%
Perioperative Temperature Management[3]	71	100%	100%	100%
Prophylactic Antibiotic Selection[3]	56	100%	99%	99%
Prophylactic Antibiotic Selection (Outpatient)[1,3]	-	-	97%	98%
Prophylactic Antibiotic Stopped[3]	55	93%	98%	98%
Prophylactic Antibiotic Timing[3]	56	98%	99%	99%
Prophylactic Antibiotic Timing (Outpatient)[1,3]	-	-	97%	98%
Urinary Catheter Removal[3]	56	98%	97%	97%
Survey of Patients' Hospital Experiences				
Area Around Room 'Always' Quiet at Night	300+	64%	51%	61%
Doctors 'Always' Communicated Well	300+	77%	78%	82%
Home Recovery Information Given	300+	83%	83%	85%
Hospital Given 9 or 10 on 10 Point Scale	300+	66%	68%	71%
Meds 'Always' Explained Before Given	300+	61%	61%	64%
Nurses 'Always' Communicated Well	300+	74%	74%	79%
Pain 'Always' Well Controlled	300+	70%	68%	71%
Room and Bathroom 'Always' Clean	300+	79%	70%	73%
Timely Help 'Always' Received	300+	67%	62%	68%
Would Definitely Recommend Hospital	300+	69%	70%	71%
Use of Medical Imaging				
Cardiac Imaging Stress Test before Surgery[1]	-	-	5.2%	5.3%
Combination Abdominal CT Scan	115	3.5%	13.4%	10.5%
Combination Brain/Sinus CT Scan	191	6.3%	2.2%	2.7%
Combination Chest CT Scan	53	3.8%	2.3%	2.7%
Follow-up Mammogram/Ultrasound	113	3.5%	8.2%	8.8%
Lumbar Spine MRI for Low Back Pain[1]	-	-	34.2%	37.2%

Saint Mary Medical Center

1050 Linden Ave
Long Beach, CA 90813
URL: www.stmarymedicalcenter.org
Phone: 562-491-9000
Fax: 562-436-6378
Type: Acute Care Hospitals
Ownership: Voluntary non-profit - Church
Emergency Services: Yes
Beds: 389

Key Personnel:
Operating Room. . . . . Gayle Cantrall, RN
Cardiac Laboratory. . . . . Pam Fair, RN
Intensive Care Unit. . . . . Pam Fair, RN
CEO/President. . . . . Drew Gagner
Chief of Medical Staff . . . . Merrill Knopf, MD
Quality Assurance . . . . Jane Nakagawa
Infection Control. . . . . Jerry Pennington, RN
Emergency Room . . . . Stephen Shea, MD

Measure	Cases	This Hosp.	State Avg.	U.S. Avg.
Blood Clot Prevention and Treatment				
Anticoagulation Overlap Therapy[2]	39	95%	92%	93%
ICU Venous Thromboembolism Prophylaxis[2]	109	99%	92%	92%
Incidence of Potentially Preventable VTE[1,2]	-	-	11%	10%
UFH with Dosages/Platelet Monitoring[2]	25	100%	96%	97%
Venous Thromboembolism Prophylaxis[2]	318	97%	83%	85%
Warfarin Therapy Discharge Instructions[2]	26	77%	75%	75%
Chest Pain/Possible Heart Attack Care				
Aspirin Given Within 24 Hours of Arrival	22	82%	97%	96%
Fibrinolytic Meds Within 30 Min. of Arrival[3,7]	-	-	62%	58%
Average Time to ECG (minutes)	23	12	9	7
Average Time to Transfer (minutes)[3,7]	-	-	62	60
Children's Asthma Care				
Received Home Management Plan of Care	-	-	88%	88%
Received Reliever Medication	-	-	100%	100%
Received Systemic Corticosteroids	-	-	100%	100%
Emergency Department				
Admittance Decision Time (minutes)[2]	464	140	125	98
Head CT Results Within 45 Min. of Arrival[1]	-	-	55%	57%
Patients Who Left ER Before Being Seen	55,488	2%	3%	2%
Time from ER Arrival to Admit. (minutes)[2]	627	290	323	274
Time from ER Arrival to Discharge (minutes)	370	126	168	134
Time in ER Before Being Evaluated (minutes)	398	10	29	26
Time to Pain Meds for Fractures (minutes)	182	36	62	57
Heart Attack Care				
Aspirin Given at Discharge	131	99%	99%	99%
Fibrinolytic Meds Within 30 Min. of Arrival[1]	-	-	73%	54%
PCI Within 90 Minutes of Arrival	18	100%	95%	96%
Statin Prescribed at Discharge	134	96%	98%	98%
Heart Failure Care				
ACE Inhibitor or ARB for LVSD[2]	101	97%	97%	97%
Discharge Instructions Given[2]	232	100%	94%	94%
Evaluation of LVS Function[2]	262	100%	99%	99%
Medicare Spending				
Medicare Spending per Patient (ratio)	-	1.15	0.98	0.98
Pneumonia Care				
Appropriate Initial Antibiotic Given[2]	62	100%	97%	95%
Blood Culture Timing[2]	152	97%	98%	98%
Pregnancy and Delivery Care				
Newborn Deliveries Scheduled Early[2]	63	3%	5%	6%
Preventive Care				
Immunization for Influenza[2]	475	97%	89%	90%

NOTE: Hospital profiles are in alphabetical order by state, then city, then hospital within the city; Rankings exclude hospitals with less than 25 cases except for patient surveys which excludes hospitals with less than 100 cases; (a) 100-299 cases; (1) The number of cases/patients is too few to report; (2) Data submitted were based on a sample of cases/patients; (3) Results are based on a shorter time period than required; (4) Data suppressed by CMS for one or more quarters; (5) Results are not available for this reporting period; (6) Fewer than 100 patients completed the HCAHPS survey; (7) No cases met the criteria for this measure; (8) The lower limit of the confidence interval cannot be calculated if the number of observed infections equals zero; (9) No data are available from the state/territory for this reporting period; (10) The scores shown reflect fewer than 50 completed surveys; (11) There were discrepancies in the data collection process; (12) This measure does not apply to this hospital for this reporting period; (13) Results cannot be calculated for this reporting period; (14) The results for this state are combined with nearby states to protect confidentiality; Please refer to the User's Guide for a full explanation of data.

Measure	Cases	This Hosp.	State Avg.	U.S. Avg.
Immunization for Pneumonia[2]	439	93%	90%	92%
Stroke Care				
Anticoagulation Therapy for Atrial Fibrillation[1]	-	-	95%	95%
Antithrombotic Therapy Timing	62	98%	98%	98%
Assessed for Rehabilitation	83	100%	97%	97%
Discharged on Antithrombotic Therapy	70	99%	99%	99%
Discharged on Statin Medication	61	98%	94%	94%
Thrombolytic Therapy Timing[1]	-	-	72%	66%
Venous Thromboembolism Prophylaxis	93	100%	94%	94%
Written Stroke Educational Materials Given	37	95%	87%	88%
Surgical Care Improvement Project				
Appropriate Beta Blocker Usage[2]	55	93%	97%	98%
Appropriate VTP Within 24 Hours[2]	160	100%	98%	98%
Controlled Postoperative Blood Glucose[2]	39	95%	96%	97%
Perioperative Temperature Management[2]	182	100%	100%	100%
Prophylactic Antibiotic Selection[2]	106	100%	99%	99%
Prophylactic Antibiotic Selection (Outpatient)	96	100%	97%	98%
Prophylactic Antibiotic Stopped[2]	102	99%	98%	98%
Prophylactic Antibiotic Timing[2]	106	99%	99%	99%
Prophylactic Antibiotic Timing (Outpatient)	97	98%	97%	98%
Urinary Catheter Removal[2]	98	99%	97%	97%
Survey of Patients' Hospital Experiences				
Area Around Room 'Always' Quiet at Night	300+	53%	51%	61%
Doctors 'Always' Communicated Well	300+	74%	78%	82%
Home Recovery Information Given	300+	84%	83%	85%
Hospital Given 9 or 10 on 10 Point Scale	300+	72%	68%	71%
Meds 'Always' Explained Before Given	300+	60%	61%	64%
Nurses 'Always' Communicated Well	300+	73%	74%	79%
Pain 'Always' Well Controlled	300+	65%	68%	71%
Room and Bathroom 'Always' Clean	300+	77%	70%	73%
Timely Help 'Always' Received	300+	58%	62%	68%
Would Definitely Recommend Hospital	300+	71%	70%	71%
Use of Medical Imaging				
Cardiac Imaging Stress Test before Surgery	226	6.2%	5.2%	5.3%
Combination Abdominal CT Scan	380	8.7%	13.4%	10.5%
Combination Brain/Sinus CT Scan	413	1.9%	2.2%	2.7%
Combination Chest CT Scan	209	10.5%	2.3%	2.7%
Follow-up Mammogram/Ultrasound	527	8.7%	8.2%	8.8%
Lumbar Spine MRI for Low Back Pain[1]	-	-	34.2%	37.2%

VA Long Beach Healthcare System

5901 E. Seventh Street
Long Beach, CA 90822
Phone: 562-826-8000
Fax: 562-826-5549
URL: www.longbeach.va.gov
Type: Acute Care - VA
Emergency Services: No
Ownership: Government Federal
Beds: 237

Key Personnel:
Intensive Care Unit. . . . . Suzanne Chretian, RN
CEO/President. . . . . Isabel Duff, MS
Emergency Room . . . . Susan A Hopp, MD
Operating Room. . . . . Usha Parashar, RN
Quality Assurance . . . . Eileen Potvin, RN
Chief of Medical Staff. . . . . Sandor Szabo, MD PhD
Radiology. . . . . Thavinsakdi Viravathana, MD
Anesthesiology. . . . . David H Wong, MD

Measure	Cases	This Hosp.	State Avg.	U.S. Avg.
Blood Clot Prevention and Treatment				
Anticoagulation Overlap Therapy	-	-	92%	93%
ICU Venous Thromboembolism Prophylaxis	-	-	92%	92%
Incidence of Potentially Preventable VTE	-	-	11%	10%
UFH with Dosages/Platelet Monitoring	-	-	96%	97%
Venous Thromboembolism Prophylaxis	-	-	83%	85%
Warfarin Therapy Discharge Instructions	-	-	75%	75%
Chest Pain/Possible Heart Attack Care				
Aspirin Given Within 24 Hours of Arrival	-	-	97%	96%
Fibrinolytic Meds Within 30 Min. of Arrival	-	-	62%	58%
Average Time to ECG (minutes)	-	-	9	7
Average Time to Transfer (minutes)	-	-	62	60
Children's Asthma Care				
Received Home Management Plan of Care	-	-	88%	88%
Received Reliever Medication	-	-	100%	100%
Received Systemic Corticosteroids	-	-	100%	100%
Emergency Department				
Admittance Decision Time (minutes)	-	-	125	98
Head CT Results Within 45 Min. of Arrival	-	-	55%	57%
Patients Who Left ER Before Being Seen	-	-	3%	2%
Time from ER Arrival to Admit. (minutes)	-	-	323	274
Time from ER Arrival to Discharge (minutes)	-	-	168	134
Time in ER Before Being Evaluated (minutes)	-	-	29	26
Time to Pain Meds for Fractures (minutes)	-	-	62	57
Heart Attack Care				
Aspirin Given at Discharge	28	100%	99%	99%
Fibrinolytic Meds Within 30 Min. of Arrival[5]	-	-	73%	54%
PCI Within 90 Minutes of Arrival[5]	-	-	95%	96%
Statin Prescribed at Discharge	29	100%	98%	98%
Heart Failure Care				
ACE Inhibitor or ARB for LVSD	112	92%	97%	97%
Discharge Instructions Given	230	99%	94%	94%
Evaluation of LVS Function	243	100%	99%	99%
Medicare Spending				
Medicare Spending per Patient (ratio)	-	-	0.98	0.98
Pneumonia Care				
Appropriate Initial Antibiotic Given	53	96%	97%	95%
Blood Culture Timing	118	97%	98%	98%
Pregnancy and Delivery Care				
Newborn Deliveries Scheduled Early	-	-	5%	6%
Preventive Care				
Immunization for Influenza[5]	-	-	89%	90%
Immunization for Pneumonia[5]	-	-	90%	92%
Stroke Care				
Anticoagulation Therapy for Atrial Fibrillation	-	-	95%	95%
Antithrombotic Therapy Timing	-	-	98%	98%
Assessed for Rehabilitation	-	-	97%	97%
Discharged on Antithrombotic Therapy	-	-	99%	99%
Discharged on Statin Medication	-	-	94%	94%
Thrombolytic Therapy Timing	-	-	72%	66%
Venous Thromboembolism Prophylaxis	-	-	94%	94%
Written Stroke Educational Materials Given	-	-	87%	88%
Surgical Care Improvement Project				
Appropriate Beta Blocker Usage[2]	81	100%	97%	98%
Appropriate VTP Within 24 Hours[2]	243	99%	98%	98%
Controlled Postoperative Blood Glucose[5]	-	-	96%	97%
Perioperative Temperature Management[2]	261	100%	100%	100%
Prophylactic Antibiotic Selection	141	100%	99%	99%
Prophylactic Antibiotic Selection (Outpatient)	-	-	97%	98%
Prophylactic Antibiotic Stopped	140	100%	98%	98%
Prophylactic Antibiotic Timing	142	100%	99%	99%
Prophylactic Antibiotic Timing (Outpatient)	-	-	97%	98%
Urinary Catheter Removal[2]	163	100%	97%	97%
Survey of Patients' Hospital Experiences				
Area Around Room 'Always' Quiet at Night	-	-	51%	61%
Doctors 'Always' Communicated Well	-	-	78%	82%
Home Recovery Information Given	-	-	83%	85%
Hospital Given 9 or 10 on 10 Point Scale	-	-	68%	71%
Meds 'Always' Explained Before Given	-	-	61%	64%
Nurses 'Always' Communicated Well	-	-	74%	79%
Pain 'Always' Well Controlled	-	-	68%	71%
Room and Bathroom 'Always' Clean	-	-	70%	73%
Timely Help 'Always' Received	-	-	62%	68%
Would Definitely Recommend Hospital	-	-	70%	71%
Use of Medical Imaging				
Cardiac Imaging Stress Test before Surgery	-	-	5.2%	5.3%
Combination Abdominal CT Scan	-	-	13.4%	10.5%
Combination Brain/Sinus CT Scan	-	-	2.2%	2.7%
Combination Chest CT Scan	-	-	2.3%	2.7%
Follow-up Mammogram/Ultrasound	-	-	8.2%	8.8%
Lumbar Spine MRI for Low Back Pain	-	-	34.2%	37.2%

Los Alamitos Medical Center

3751 Katella Avenue
Los Alamitos, CA 90720
Phone: 562-799-3220
Fax: 562-493-2812
URL: www.losalamitosmedctr.com
Type: Acute Care Hospitals
Emergency Services: Yes
Ownership: Proprietary
Beds: 167

Key Personnel:
Infection Control. . . . . Joan Blake
Chief of Medical Staff. . . . . Dr Jennifer Daley
CEO/President. . . . . Michele Finney
Quality Assurance . . . . Lorraine Lpes
Radiology. . . . . Karen Ragland, MD
Surgery . . . . Imad Shbeeb, MD
Pediatric Ambulatory Care . . . . . . Nasir Tejani, MD
Pediatric In-Patient Care . . . . Nasir Tejani, MD

Measure	Cases	This Hosp.	State Avg.	U.S. Avg.
Blood Clot Prevention and Treatment				
Anticoagulation Overlap Therapy[2]	63	100%	92%	93%
ICU Venous Thromboembolism Prophylaxis[2]	102	91%	92%	92%
Incidence of Potentially Preventable VTE[2]	11	9%	11%	10%
UFH with Dosages/Platelet Monitoring[2]	21	100%	96%	97%
Venous Thromboembolism Prophylaxis[2]	275	88%	83%	85%
Warfarin Therapy Discharge Instructions[2]	44	100%	75%	75%
Chest Pain/Possible Heart Attack Care				
Aspirin Given Within 24 Hours of Arrival	11	100%	97%	96%
Fibrinolytic Meds Within 30 Min. of Arrival[3,7]	-	-	62%	58%
Average Time to ECG (minutes)	11	10	9	7
Average Time to Transfer (minutes)[3,7]	-	-	62	60
Children's Asthma Care				
Received Home Management Plan of Care	-	-	88%	88%
Received Reliever Medication	-	-	100%	100%
Received Systemic Corticosteroids	-	-	100%	100%
Emergency Department				
Admittance Decision Time (minutes)[2]	689	143	125	98
Head CT Results Within 45 Min. of Arrival	23	100%	55%	57%
Patients Who Left ER Before Being Seen	30,503	3%	3%	2%
Time from ER Arrival to Admit. (minutes)[2]	755	321	323	274
Time from ER Arrival to Discharge (minutes)	357	176	168	134
Time in ER Before Being Evaluated (minutes)	381	43	29	26
Time to Pain Meds for Fractures (minutes)	224	48	62	57
Heart Attack Care				
Aspirin Given at Discharge	140	99%	99%	99%
Fibrinolytic Meds Within 30 Min. of Arrival[7]	-	-	73%	54%
PCI Within 90 Minutes of Arrival	29	93%	95%	96%
Statin Prescribed at Discharge	142	100%	98%	98%
Heart Failure Care				
ACE Inhibitor or ARB for LVSD	87	100%	97%	97%
Discharge Instructions Given	223	100%	94%	94%
Evaluation of LVS Function	291	100%	99%	99%
Medicare Spending				
Medicare Spending per Patient (ratio)	-	1.07	0.98	0.98
Pneumonia Care				
Appropriate Initial Antibiotic Given	155	95%	97%	95%
Blood Culture Timing	176	100%	98%	98%
Pregnancy and Delivery Care				
Newborn Deliveries Scheduled Early[2]	36	0%	5%	6%
Preventive Care				
Immunization for Influenza[2]	555	99%	89%	90%
Immunization for Pneumonia[2]	731	99%	90%	92%
Stroke Care				
Anticoagulation Therapy for Atrial Fibrillation	22	100%	95%	95%
Antithrombotic Therapy Timing	88	100%	98%	98%
Assessed for Rehabilitation	141	99%	97%	97%
Discharged on Antithrombotic Therapy	122	100%	99%	99%
Discharged on Statin Medication	86	100%	94%	94%
Thrombolytic Therapy Timing	11	91%	72%	66%
Venous Thromboembolism Prophylaxis	134	100%	94%	94%
Written Stroke Educational Materials Given	77	100%	87%	88%
Surgical Care Improvement Project				
Appropriate Beta Blocker Usage[2]	152	99%	97%	98%
Appropriate VTP Within 24 Hours[2]	639	99%	98%	98%
Controlled Postoperative Blood Glucose[2,7]	-	-	96%	97%
Perioperative Temperature Management[2]	730	100%	100%	100%
Prophylactic Antibiotic Selection[2]	549	99%	99%	99%
Prophylactic Antibiotic Selection (Outpatient)	138	99%	97%	98%
Prophylactic Antibiotic Stopped[2]	520	99%	98%	98%
Prophylactic Antibiotic Timing[2]	549	98%	99%	99%
Prophylactic Antibiotic Timing (Outpatient)	138	100%	97%	98%
Urinary Catheter Removal[2]	444	99%	97%	97%
Survey of Patients' Hospital Experiences				
Area Around Room 'Always' Quiet at Night	300+	33%	51%	61%
Doctors 'Always' Communicated Well	300+	81%	78%	82%

NOTE: Hospital profiles are in alphabetical order by state, then city, then hospital within the city; Rankings exclude hospitals with less than 25 cases except for patient surveys which excludes hospitals with less than 100 cases; (a) 100-299 cases; (1) The number of cases/patients is too few to report; (2) Data submitted were based on a sample of cases/patients; (3) Results are based on a shorter time period than required; (4) Data suppressed by CMS for one or more quarters; (5) Results are not available for this reporting period; (6) Fewer than 100 patients completed the HCAHPS survey; (7) No cases met the criteria for this measure; (8) The lower limit of the confidence interval cannot be calculated if the number of observed infections equals zero; (9) No data are available from the state/territory for this reporting period; (10) The scores shown reflect fewer than 50 completed surveys; (11) There were discrepancies in the data collection process; (12) This measure does not apply to this hospital for this reporting period; (13) Results cannot be calculated for this reporting period; (14) The results for this state are combined with nearby states to protect confidentiality; Please refer to the User's Guide for a full explanation of data.

Measure	Cases	This Hosp.	State Avg.	U.S. Avg.
Home Recovery Information Given	300+	83%	83%	85%
Hospital Given 9 or 10 on 10 Point Scale	300+	63%	68%	71%
Meds 'Always' Explained Before Given	300+	57%	61%	64%
Nurses 'Always' Communicated Well	300+	73%	74%	79%
Pain 'Always' Well Controlled	300+	71%	68%	71%
Room and Bathroom 'Always' Clean	300+	62%	70%	73%
Timely Help 'Always' Received	300+	60%	62%	68%
Would Definitely Recommend Hospital	300+	65%	70%	71%
Use of Medical Imaging				
Cardiac Imaging Stress Test before Surgery	93	10.8%	5.2%	5.3%
Combination Abdominal CT Scan	709	11.8%	13.4%	10.5%
Combination Brain/Sinus CT Scan	599	1.5%	2.2%	2.7%
Combination Chest CT Scan	429	0.5%	2.3%	2.7%
Follow-up Mammogram/Ultrasound	1,542	4.0%	8.2%	8.8%
Lumbar Spine MRI for Low Back Pain[1]	-	-	34.2%	37.2%

California Hospital Medical Center Los Angeles

1401 South Grand Avenue — Phone: 213-748-2411
Los Angeles, CA 90015 — Fax: 213-742-5913
URL: www.chmcla.org
Type: Acute Care Hospitals — Emergency Services: Yes
Ownership: Voluntary non-profit - Other — Beds: 313

Key Personnel:
Cardiac Laboratory. . . . . Phil Fairchild
Chief of Medical Staff . . . . Bruce A Greenfield, MD
Quality Assurance . . . . Karen Horlick
Pediatric Ambulatory Care . . . . . . Michael Lem, MD
Pediatric In-Patient Care . . . . Michael Lem, MD
Emergency Room . . . . Robert Swan

Measure	Cases	This Hosp.	State Avg.	U.S. Avg.
Blood Clot Prevention and Treatment				
Anticoagulation Overlap Therapy[2]	63	97%	92%	93%
ICU Venous Thromboembolism Prophylaxis[2]	98	99%	92%	92%
Incidence of Potentially Preventable VTE[2]	12	8%	11%	10%
UFH with Dosages/Platelet Monitoring[2]	30	100%	96%	97%
Venous Thromboembolism Prophylaxis[2]	292	88%	83%	85%
Warfarin Therapy Discharge Instructions[2]	42	71%	75%	75%
Chest Pain/Possible Heart Attack Care				
Aspirin Given Within 24 Hours of Arrival	27	89%	97%	96%
Fibrinolytic Meds Within 30 Min. of Arrival[3,7]	-	-	62%	58%
Average Time to ECG (minutes)	27	29	9	7
Average Time to Transfer (minutes)[3,7]	-	-	62	60
Children's Asthma Care				
Received Home Management Plan of Care	-	-	88%	88%
Received Reliever Medication	-	-	100%	100%
Received Systemic Corticosteroids	-	-	100%	100%
Emergency Department				
Admittance Decision Time (minutes)[2]	557	159	125	98
Head CT Results Within 45 Min. of Arrival[1]	-	-	55%	57%
Patients Who Left ER Before Being Seen	66,747	2%	3%	2%
Time from ER Arrival to Admit. (minutes)[2]	558	400	323	274
Time from ER Arrival to Discharge (minutes)	387	205	168	134
Time in ER Before Being Evaluated (minutes)	420	29	29	26
Time to Pain Meds for Fractures (minutes)	320	61	62	57
Heart Attack Care				
Aspirin Given at Discharge	97	99%	99%	99%
Fibrinolytic Meds Within 30 Min. of Arrival[7]	-	-	73%	54%
PCI Within 90 Minutes of Arrival	21	52%	95%	96%
Statin Prescribed at Discharge	88	99%	98%	98%
Heart Failure Care				
ACE Inhibitor or ARB for LVSD	203	99%	97%	97%
Discharge Instructions Given	377	90%	94%	94%
Evaluation of LVS Function	400	100%	99%	99%
Medicare Spending				
Medicare Spending per Patient (ratio)	-	1.00	0.98	0.98
Pneumonia Care				
Appropriate Initial Antibiotic Given[2]	111	97%	97%	95%
Blood Culture Timing[2]	175	98%	98%	98%
Pregnancy and Delivery Care				
Newborn Deliveries Scheduled Early[2]	83	2%	5%	6%
Preventive Care				
Immunization for Influenza[2]	485	96%	89%	90%
Immunization for Pneumonia[2]	366	94%	90%	92%
Stroke Care				
Anticoagulation Therapy for Atrial Fibrillation[1]	-	-	95%	95%
Antithrombotic Therapy Timing	124	99%	98%	98%
Assessed for Rehabilitation	149	98%	97%	97%
Discharged on Antithrombotic Therapy	119	97%	99%	99%
Discharged on Statin Medication	95	89%	94%	94%
Thrombolytic Therapy Timing	18	94%	72%	66%
Venous Thromboembolism Prophylaxis	177	97%	94%	94%
Written Stroke Educational Materials Given	72	90%	87%	88%
Surgical Care Improvement Project				
Appropriate Beta Blocker Usage[2]	64	95%	97%	98%
Appropriate VTP Within 24 Hours[2]	349	100%	98%	98%
Controlled Postoperative Blood Glucose[2]	26	100%	96%	97%
Perioperative Temperature Management[2]	422	100%	100%	100%
Prophylactic Antibiotic Selection[2]	256	100%	99%	99%
Prophylactic Antibiotic Selection (Outpatient)	105	99%	97%	98%
Prophylactic Antibiotic Stopped[2]	246	98%	98%	98%
Prophylactic Antibiotic Timing[2]	256	99%	99%	99%
Prophylactic Antibiotic Timing (Outpatient)	105	100%	97%	98%
Urinary Catheter Removal[2]	222	97%	97%	97%
Survey of Patients' Hospital Experiences				
Area Around Room 'Always' Quiet at Night	300+	50%	51%	61%
Doctors 'Always' Communicated Well	300+	72%	78%	82%
Home Recovery Information Given	300+	77%	83%	85%
Hospital Given 9 or 10 on 10 Point Scale	300+	62%	68%	71%
Meds 'Always' Explained Before Given	300+	55%	61%	64%
Nurses 'Always' Communicated Well	300+	67%	74%	79%
Pain 'Always' Well Controlled	300+	61%	68%	71%
Room and Bathroom 'Always' Clean	300+	62%	70%	73%
Timely Help 'Always' Received	300+	51%	62%	68%
Would Definitely Recommend Hospital	300+	63%	70%	71%
Use of Medical Imaging				
Cardiac Imaging Stress Test before Surgery	87	5.7%	5.2%	5.3%
Combination Abdominal CT Scan	341	4.4%	13.4%	10.5%
Combination Brain/Sinus CT Scan	437	5.3%	2.2%	2.7%
Combination Chest CT Scan	55	1.8%	2.3%	2.7%
Follow-up Mammogram/Ultrasound	270	5.9%	8.2%	8.8%
Lumbar Spine MRI for Low Back Pain[1]	-	-	34.2%	37.2%

Cedars - Sinai Medical Center

8700 Beverly Blvd — Phone: 310-423-5000
Los Angeles, CA 90048 — Fax: 310-423-0470
URL: www.cedars-sinai.edu
Type: Acute Care Hospitals — Emergency Services: Yes
Ownership: Voluntary non-profit - Other — Beds: 930

Key Personnel:
Operating Room. . . . . Bruce L Gewertz, MD
Chair/CEO . . . . Vera S. Guerin
Chief of Medical Staff. . . . . Michael Langberg, MD
Cardiac Laboratory. . . . . Eduardo Marbian, MD, PhD
Hemotology Center . . . . Steven Piantadosi, MD, PhD
CEO/President. . . . . Thomas M Priselac
Radiology. . . . . Howard M Sandler, MD
Pediatric Ambulatory Care . . . . . . Charles F Simmons, Jr, MD

Measure	Cases	This Hosp.	State Avg.	U.S. Avg.
Blood Clot Prevention and Treatment				
Anticoagulation Overlap Therapy[2]	164	95%	92%	93%
ICU Venous Thromboembolism Prophylaxis[2]	223	99%	92%	92%
Incidence of Potentially Preventable VTE[2]	85	1%	11%	10%
UFH with Dosages/Platelet Monitoring[2]	218	100%	96%	97%
Venous Thromboembolism Prophylaxis[2]	1,030	96%	83%	85%
Warfarin Therapy Discharge Instructions[2]	101	94%	75%	75%
Chest Pain/Possible Heart Attack Care				
Aspirin Given Within 24 Hours of Arrival[5]	-	-	97%	96%
Fibrinolytic Meds Within 30 Min. of Arrival[5]	-	-	62%	58%
Average Time to ECG (minutes)[5]	-	-	9	7
Average Time to Transfer (minutes)[5]	-	-	62	60
Children's Asthma Care				
Received Home Management Plan of Care	-	-	88%	88%
Received Reliever Medication	-	-	100%	100%
Received Systemic Corticosteroids	-	-	100%	100%
Emergency Department				
Admittance Decision Time (minutes)[2]	396	107	125	98
Head CT Results Within 45 Min. of Arrival[1]	-	-	55%	57%
Patients Who Left ER Before Being Seen	87,184	3%	3%	2%
Time from ER Arrival to Admit. (minutes)[2]	396	310	323	274
Time from ER Arrival to Discharge (minutes)	365	205	168	134
Time in ER Before Being Evaluated (minutes)	413	61	29	26
Time to Pain Meds for Fractures (minutes)	219	73	62	57
Heart Attack Care				
Aspirin Given at Discharge	390	100%	99%	99%
Fibrinolytic Meds Within 30 Min. of Arrival[7]	-	-	73%	54%
PCI Within 90 Minutes of Arrival	81	100%	95%	96%
Statin Prescribed at Discharge	377	100%	98%	98%
Heart Failure Care				
ACE Inhibitor or ARB for LVSD	299	100%	97%	97%
Discharge Instructions Given	901	100%	94%	94%
Evaluation of LVS Function	1,032	100%	99%	99%
Medicare Spending				
Medicare Spending per Patient (ratio)	-	1.02	0.98	0.98
Pneumonia Care				
Appropriate Initial Antibiotic Given	243	99%	97%	95%
Blood Culture Timing	392	99%	98%	98%
Pregnancy and Delivery Care				
Newborn Deliveries Scheduled Early[2]	107	1%	5%	6%
Preventive Care				
Immunization for Influenza[2]	519	95%	89%	90%
Immunization for Pneumonia[2]	548	96%	90%	92%
Stroke Care				
Anticoagulation Therapy for Atrial Fibrillation	49	96%	95%	95%
Antithrombotic Therapy Timing	269	100%	98%	98%
Assessed for Rehabilitation	438	100%	97%	97%
Discharged on Antithrombotic Therapy	321	100%	99%	99%
Discharged on Statin Medication	235	94%	94%	94%
Thrombolytic Therapy Timing	28	100%	72%	66%
Venous Thromboembolism Prophylaxis	477	99%	94%	94%
Written Stroke Educational Materials Given	197	100%	87%	88%
Surgical Care Improvement Project				
Appropriate Beta Blocker Usage	1,081	98%	97%	98%
Appropriate VTP Within 24 Hours	3,322	98%	98%	98%
Controlled Postoperative Blood Glucose	470	96%	96%	97%
Perioperative Temperature Management	4,224	100%	100%	100%
Prophylactic Antibiotic Selection	2,288	99%	99%	99%
Prophylactic Antibiotic Selection (Outpatient)	859	97%	97%	98%
Prophylactic Antibiotic Stopped	2,150	97%	98%	98%
Prophylactic Antibiotic Timing	2,289	100%	99%	99%
Prophylactic Antibiotic Timing (Outpatient)	808	97%	97%	98%
Urinary Catheter Removal	2,661	97%	97%	97%
Survey of Patients' Hospital Experiences				
Area Around Room 'Always' Quiet at Night	300+	56%	51%	61%
Doctors 'Always' Communicated Well	300+	79%	78%	82%
Home Recovery Information Given	300+	84%	83%	85%
Hospital Given 9 or 10 on 10 Point Scale	300+	78%	68%	71%
Meds 'Always' Explained Before Given	300+	58%	61%	64%
Nurses 'Always' Communicated Well	300+	77%	74%	79%
Pain 'Always' Well Controlled	300+	69%	68%	71%
Room and Bathroom 'Always' Clean	300+	70%	70%	73%
Timely Help 'Always' Received	300+	61%	62%	68%
Would Definitely Recommend Hospital	300+	79%	70%	71%
Use of Medical Imaging				
Cardiac Imaging Stress Test before Surgery	1,288	7.8%	5.2%	5.3%
Combination Abdominal CT Scan	3,768	2.9%	13.4%	10.5%
Combination Brain/Sinus CT Scan	1,431	1.3%	2.2%	2.7%
Combination Chest CT Scan	4,979	0.2%	2.3%	2.7%
Follow-up Mammogram/Ultrasound	3,298	8.6%	8.2%	8.8%
Lumbar Spine MRI for Low Back Pain	524	34.9%	34.2%	37.2%

Children's Hospital of Los Angeles

4650 Sunset Blvd — Phone: 323-669-2164
Los Angeles, CA 90027 — Fax: 323-663-1645
URL: www.chla.org
Type: Childrens — Emergency Services: Yes
Ownership: Voluntary non-profit - Private — Beds: 286

Key Personnel:
CEO/President. . . . . Richard D Cordova
Surgery . . . . Henri R Ford, MD, MHA
Chief of Medical Staff. . . . . Carl Grushkin, MD
Infection Control. . . . . Marysia Meylan
Operating Room. . . . . Beryl Muniz

NOTE: Hospital profiles are in alphabetical order by state, then city, then hospital within the city; Rankings exclude hospitals with less than 25 cases except for patient surveys which excludes hospitals with less than 100 cases; (a) 100-299 cases; (1) The number of cases/patients is too few to report; (2) Data submitted were based on a sample of cases/patients; (3) Results are based on a shorter time period than required; (4) Data suppressed by CMS for one or more quarters; (5) Results are not available for this reporting period; (6) Fewer than 100 patients completed the HCAHPS survey; (7) No cases met the criteria for this measure; (8) The lower limit of the confidence interval cannot be calculated if the number of observed infections equals zero; (9) No data are available from the state/territory for this reporting period; (10) The scores shown reflect fewer than 50 completed surveys; (11) There were discrepancies in the data collection process; (12) This measure does not apply to this hospital for this reporting period; (13) Results cannot be calculated for this reporting period; (14) The results for this state are combined with nearby states to protect confidentiality; Please refer to the User's Guide for a full explanation of data.

Radiology. . . . . Marvin D. Nelson, Jr., MD, MBA, FACR
Pediatric In-Patient Care . . . . D. Brent Polk, MD
Quality Assurance . . . . Karen Prommer

Measure	Cases	This Hosp.	State Avg.	U.S. Avg.
Blood Clot Prevention and Treatment				
Anticoagulation Overlap Therapy[5]	-	-	92%	93%
ICU Venous Thromboembolism Prophylaxis[5]	-	-	92%	92%
Incidence of Potentially Preventable VTE[5]	-	-	11%	10%
UFH with Dosages/Platelet Monitoring[5]	-	-	96%	97%
Venous Thromboembolism Prophylaxis[5]	-	-	83%	85%
Warfarin Therapy Discharge Instructions[5]	-	-	75%	75%
Chest Pain/Possible Heart Attack Care				
Aspirin Given Within 24 Hours of Arrival	-	-	97%	96%
Fibrinolytic Meds Within 30 Min. of Arrival	-	-	62%	58%
Average Time to ECG (minutes)	-	-	9	7
Average Time to Transfer (minutes)	-	-	62	60
Children's Asthma Care				
Received Home Management Plan of Care[2]	237	93%	88%	88%
Received Reliever Medication[2]	237	100%	100%	100%
Received Systemic Corticosteroids[2]	236	100%	100%	100%
Emergency Department				
Admittance Decision Time (minutes)[5]	-	-	125	98
Head CT Results Within 45 Min. of Arrival	-	-	55%	57%
Patients Who Left ER Before Being Seen	-	-	3%	2%
Time from ER Arrival to Admit. (minutes)[5]	-	-	323	274
Time from ER Arrival to Discharge (minutes)	-	-	168	134
Time in ER Before Being Evaluated (minutes)	-	-	29	26
Time to Pain Meds for Fractures (minutes)	-	-	62	57
Heart Attack Care				
Aspirin Given at Discharge[5]	-	-	99%	99%
Fibrinolytic Meds Within 30 Min. of Arrival[5]	-	-	73%	54%
PCI Within 90 Minutes of Arrival[5]	-	-	95%	96%
Statin Prescribed at Discharge[5]	-	-	98%	98%
Heart Failure Care				
ACE Inhibitor or ARB for LVSD[5]	-	-	97%	97%
Discharge Instructions Given[5]	-	-	94%	94%
Evaluation of LVS Function[5]	-	-	99%	99%
Medicare Spending				
Medicare Spending per Patient (ratio)	-	-	0.98	0.98
Pneumonia Care				
Appropriate Initial Antibiotic Given[5]	-	-	97%	95%
Blood Culture Timing[5]	-	-	98%	98%
Pregnancy and Delivery Care				
Newborn Deliveries Scheduled Early[5]	-	-	5%	6%
Preventive Care				
Immunization for Influenza[5]	-	-	89%	90%
Immunization for Pneumonia[5]	-	-	90%	92%
Stroke Care				
Anticoagulation Therapy for Atrial Fibrillation[5]	-	-	95%	95%
Antithrombotic Therapy Timing[5]	-	-	98%	98%
Assessed for Rehabilitation[5]	-	-	97%	97%
Discharged on Antithrombotic Therapy[5]	-	-	99%	99%
Discharged on Statin Medication[5]	-	-	94%	94%
Thrombolytic Therapy Timing[5]	-	-	72%	66%
Venous Thromboembolism Prophylaxis[5]	-	-	94%	94%
Written Stroke Educational Materials Given[5]	-	-	87%	88%
Surgical Care Improvement Project				
Appropriate Beta Blocker Usage[5]	-	-	97%	98%
Appropriate VTP Within 24 Hours[5]	-	-	98%	98%
Controlled Postoperative Blood Glucose[5]	-	-	96%	97%
Perioperative Temperature Management[5]	-	-	100%	100%
Prophylactic Antibiotic Selection[5]	-	-	99%	99%
Prophylactic Antibiotic Selection (Outpatient)	-	-	97%	98%
Prophylactic Antibiotic Stopped[5]	-	-	98%	98%
Prophylactic Antibiotic Timing[5]	-	-	99%	99%
Prophylactic Antibiotic Timing (Outpatient)	-	-	97%	98%
Urinary Catheter Removal[5]	-	-	97%	97%
Survey of Patients' Hospital Experiences				
Area Around Room 'Always' Quiet at Night[5]	-	-	51%	61%
Doctors 'Always' Communicated Well[5]	-	-	78%	82%
Home Recovery Information Given[5]	-	-	83%	85%
Hospital Given 9 or 10 on 10 Point Scale[5]	-	-	68%	71%
Meds 'Always' Explained Before Given[5]	-	-	61%	64%
Nurses 'Always' Communicated Well[5]	-	-	74%	79%
Pain 'Always' Well Controlled[5]	-	-	68%	71%
Room and Bathroom 'Always' Clean[5]	-	-	70%	73%
Timely Help 'Always' Received[5]	-	-	62%	68%
Would Definitely Recommend Hospital[5]	-	-	70%	71%
Use of Medical Imaging				
Cardiac Imaging Stress Test before Surgery	-	-	5.2%	5.3%
Combination Abdominal CT Scan	-	-	13.4%	10.5%
Combination Brain/Sinus CT Scan	-	-	2.2%	2.7%
Combination Chest CT Scan	-	-	2.3%	2.7%
Follow-up Mammogram/Ultrasound	-	-	8.2%	8.8%
Lumbar Spine MRI for Low Back Pain	-	-	34.2%	37.2%

East Los Angeles Doctors Hospital

4060 Whittier Blvd
Los Angeles, CA 90023
Phone: 323-268-5514
Fax: 323-266-1256
Type: Acute Care Hospitals
Ownership: Proprietary
Emergency Services: Yes
Beds: 127

Key Personnel:
Radiology. . . . . Carleton A Allen
Chief of Medical Staff . . . . Masad Arbid, MD
Infection Control. . . . . Barbara Edmonds
Operating Room. . . . . Anita Esteban, RN
Quality Assurance . . . . Hector Hernandez
Pediatric Ambulatory Care . . . . . . T Jeyaranian, MD
Pediatric In-Patient Care . . . . T Jeyaranian, MD
CEO . . . . Araceli Lonergan

Measure	Cases	This Hosp.	State Avg.	U.S. Avg.
Blood Clot Prevention and Treatment				
Anticoagulation Overlap Therapy[1,2]	-	-	92%	93%
ICU Venous Thromboembolism Prophylaxis[2]	50	96%	92%	92%
Incidence of Potentially Preventable VTE[1,2]	-	-	11%	10%
UFH with Dosages/Platelet Monitoring[1,2]	-	-	96%	97%
Venous Thromboembolism Prophylaxis[2]	260	96%	83%	85%
Warfarin Therapy Discharge Instructions[1,2]	-	-	75%	75%
Chest Pain/Possible Heart Attack Care				
Aspirin Given Within 24 Hours of Arrival	15	100%	97%	96%
Fibrinolytic Meds Within 30 Min. of Arrival[3,7]	-	-	62%	58%
Average Time to ECG (minutes)	14	28	9	7
Average Time to Transfer (minutes)[1,3]	-	-	62	60
Children's Asthma Care				
Received Home Management Plan of Care	-	-	88%	88%
Received Reliever Medication	-	-	100%	100%
Received Systemic Corticosteroids	-	-	100%	100%
Emergency Department				
Admittance Decision Time (minutes)[2]	249	105	125	98
Head CT Results Within 45 Min. of Arrival[3,7]	-	-	55%	57%
Patients Who Left ER Before Being Seen	14,720	4%	3%	2%
Time from ER Arrival to Admit. (minutes)[2]	314	414	323	274
Time from ER Arrival to Discharge (minutes)	294	188	168	134
Time in ER Before Being Evaluated (minutes)	371	51	29	26
Time to Pain Meds for Fractures (minutes)	40	78	62	57
Heart Attack Care				
Aspirin Given at Discharge	29	97%	99%	99%
Fibrinolytic Meds Within 30 Min. of Arrival[7]	-	-	73%	54%
PCI Within 90 Minutes of Arrival[7]	-	-	95%	96%
Statin Prescribed at Discharge	25	92%	98%	98%
Heart Failure Care				
ACE Inhibitor or ARB for LVSD	33	100%	97%	97%
Discharge Instructions Given	66	98%	94%	94%
Evaluation of LVS Function	84	99%	99%	99%
Medicare Spending				
Medicare Spending per Patient (ratio)	-	1.05	0.98	0.98
Pneumonia Care				
Appropriate Initial Antibiotic Given	49	98%	97%	95%
Blood Culture Timing	77	97%	98%	98%
Pregnancy and Delivery Care				
Newborn Deliveries Scheduled Early[2]	86	6%	5%	6%
Preventive Care				
Immunization for Influenza[2]	374	43%	89%	90%
Immunization for Pneumonia[2]	322	70%	90%	92%
Stroke Care				
Anticoagulation Therapy for Atrial Fibrillation[7]	-	-	95%	95%
Antithrombotic Therapy Timing	12	83%	98%	98%
Assessed for Rehabilitation[1]	-	-	97%	97%
Discharged on Antithrombotic Therapy[1]	-	-	99%	99%
Discharged on Statin Medication[1]	-	-	94%	94%
Thrombolytic Therapy Timing[1]	-	-	72%	66%
Venous Thromboembolism Prophylaxis	12	100%	94%	94%
Written Stroke Educational Materials Given[1]	-	-	87%	88%
Surgical Care Improvement Project				
Appropriate Beta Blocker Usage[1]	-	-	97%	98%
Appropriate VTP Within 24 Hours	53	100%	98%	98%
Controlled Postoperative Blood Glucose[7]	-	-	96%	97%
Perioperative Temperature Management	57	100%	100%	100%
Prophylactic Antibiotic Selection	20	95%	99%	99%
Prophylactic Antibiotic Selection (Outpatient)[1]	-	-	97%	98%
Prophylactic Antibiotic Stopped	19	89%	98%	98%
Prophylactic Antibiotic Timing	20	75%	99%	99%
Prophylactic Antibiotic Timing (Outpatient)[1]	-	-	97%	98%
Urinary Catheter Removal	15	80%	97%	97%
Survey of Patients' Hospital Experiences				
Area Around Room 'Always' Quiet at Night	300+	44%	51%	61%
Doctors 'Always' Communicated Well	300+	76%	78%	82%
Home Recovery Information Given	300+	79%	83%	85%
Hospital Given 9 or 10 on 10 Point Scale	300+	62%	68%	71%
Meds 'Always' Explained Before Given	300+	56%	61%	64%
Nurses 'Always' Communicated Well	300+	69%	74%	79%
Pain 'Always' Well Controlled	300+	65%	68%	71%
Room and Bathroom 'Always' Clean	300+	74%	70%	73%
Timely Help 'Always' Received	300+	59%	62%	68%
Would Definitely Recommend Hospital	300+	55%	70%	71%
Use of Medical Imaging				
Cardiac Imaging Stress Test before Surgery[7]	-	-	5.2%	5.3%
Combination Abdominal CT Scan	71	1.4%	13.4%	10.5%
Combination Brain/Sinus CT Scan[1]	-	-	2.2%	2.7%
Combination Chest CT Scan[1]	-	-	2.3%	2.7%
Follow-up Mammogram/Ultrasound[7]	-	-	8.2%	8.8%
Lumbar Spine MRI for Low Back Pain[7]	-	-	34.2%	37.2%

Good Samaritan Hospital

1225 Wilshire Boulevard
Los Angeles, CA 90017
Phone: 213-977-2121
Fax: 213-482-2770
E-mail: info@goodsam.org
URL: www.goodsam.org
Type: Acute Care Hospitals
Ownership: Proprietary
Emergency Services: Yes
Beds: 408

Key Personnel:
Emergency Room . . . . Philip Fagan, MD
Radiology. . . . . Richard Gritz
CEO/President. . . . . Andrew B Leeka
Chief of Medical Staff . . . . Thomas Shook, MD

Measure	Cases	This Hosp.	State Avg.	U.S. Avg.
Blood Clot Prevention and Treatment				
Anticoagulation Overlap Therapy[2]	22	91%	92%	93%
ICU Venous Thromboembolism Prophylaxis[2]	133	89%	92%	92%
Incidence of Potentially Preventable VTE[2]	12	8%	11%	10%
UFH with Dosages/Platelet Monitoring[2]	11	100%	96%	97%
Venous Thromboembolism Prophylaxis[2]	289	56%	83%	85%
Warfarin Therapy Discharge Instructions[2]	13	85%	75%	75%
Chest Pain/Possible Heart Attack Care				
Aspirin Given Within 24 Hours of Arrival	22	95%	97%	96%
Fibrinolytic Meds Within 30 Min. of Arrival[5]	-	-	62%	58%
Average Time to ECG (minutes)	23	0	9	7
Average Time to Transfer (minutes)[5]	-	-	62	60
Children's Asthma Care				
Received Home Management Plan of Care	-	-	88%	88%
Received Reliever Medication	-	-	100%	100%
Received Systemic Corticosteroids	-	-	100%	100%
Emergency Department				
Admittance Decision Time (minutes)[2]	381	125	125	98
Head CT Results Within 45 Min. of Arrival[1]	-	-	55%	57%
Patients Who Left ER Before Being Seen	32,520	11%	3%	2%
Time from ER Arrival to Admit. (minutes)[2]	383	320	323	274
Time from ER Arrival to Discharge (minutes)	370	278	168	134

NOTE: Hospital profiles are in alphabetical order by state, then city, then hospital within the city; Rankings exclude hospitals with less than 25 cases except for patient surveys which excludes hospitals with less than 100 cases; (a) 100-299 cases; (1) The number of cases/patients is too few to report; (2) Data submitted were based on a sample of cases/patients; (3) Results are based on a shorter time period than required; (4) Data suppressed by CMS for one or more quarters; (5) Results are not available for this reporting period; (6) Fewer than 100 patients completed the HCAHPS survey; (7) No cases met the criteria for this measure; (8) The lower limit of the confidence interval cannot be calculated if the number of observed infections equals zero; (9) No data are available from the state/territory for this reporting period; (10) The scores shown reflect fewer than 50 completed surveys; (11) There were discrepancies in the data collection process; (12) This measure does not apply to this hospital for this reporting period; (13) Results cannot be calculated for this reporting period; (14) The results for this state are combined with nearby states to protect confidentiality; Please refer to the User's Guide for a full explanation of data.

Time in ER Before Being Evaluated (minutes)	406	56	29	26
Time to Pain Meds for Fractures (minutes)	79	76	62	57
Heart Attack Care				
Aspirin Given at Discharge	238	100%	99%	99%
Fibrinolytic Meds Within 30 Min. of Arrival[7]	-	-	73%	54%
PCI Within 90 Minutes of Arrival	59	97%	95%	96%
Statin Prescribed at Discharge	236	98%	98%	98%
Heart Failure Care				
ACE Inhibitor or ARB for LVSD[2]	102	97%	97%	97%
Discharge Instructions Given[2]	275	76%	94%	94%
Evaluation of LVS Function[2]	347	99%	99%	99%
Medicare Spending				
Medicare Spending per Patient (ratio)	-	0.98	0.98	0.98
Pneumonia Care				
Appropriate Initial Antibiotic Given[2]	81	93%	97%	95%
Blood Culture Timing[2]	157	94%	98%	98%
Pregnancy and Delivery Care				
Newborn Deliveries Scheduled Early[2]	92	2%	5%	6%
Preventive Care				
Immunization for Influenza[2]	450	96%	89%	90%
Immunization for Pneumonia[2]	430	93%	90%	92%
Stroke Care				
Anticoagulation Therapy for Atrial Fibrillation[2]	11	91%	95%	95%
Antithrombotic Therapy Timing[2]	79	96%	98%	98%
Assessed for Rehabilitation[2]	83	94%	97%	97%
Discharged on Antithrombotic Therapy[2]	80	95%	99%	99%
Discharged on Statin Medication[2]	60	77%	94%	94%
Thrombolytic Therapy Timing[1,2]	-	-	72%	66%
Venous Thromboembolism Prophylaxis[2]	91	81%	94%	94%
Written Stroke Educational Materials Given[2]	40	80%	87%	88%
Surgical Care Improvement Project				
Appropriate Beta Blocker Usage[2]	180	97%	97%	98%
Appropriate VTP Within 24 Hours[2]	439	98%	98%	98%
Controlled Postoperative Blood Glucose[2]	128	97%	96%	97%
Perioperative Temperature Management[2]	549	100%	100%	100%
Prophylactic Antibiotic Selection[2]	366	98%	99%	99%
Prophylactic Antibiotic Selection (Outpatient)	214	97%	97%	98%
Prophylactic Antibiotic Stopped[2]	353	95%	98%	98%
Prophylactic Antibiotic Timing[2]	366	98%	99%	99%
Prophylactic Antibiotic Timing (Outpatient)	217	97%	97%	98%
Urinary Catheter Removal[2]	417	100%	97%	97%
Survey of Patients' Hospital Experiences				
Area Around Room 'Always' Quiet at Night	300+	51%	51%	61%
Doctors 'Always' Communicated Well	300+	76%	78%	82%
Home Recovery Information Given	300+	83%	83%	85%
Hospital Given 9 or 10 on 10 Point Scale	300+	68%	68%	71%
Meds 'Always' Explained Before Given	300+	55%	61%	64%
Nurses 'Always' Communicated Well	300+	72%	74%	79%
Pain 'Always' Well Controlled	300+	65%	68%	71%
Room and Bathroom 'Always' Clean	300+	71%	70%	73%
Timely Help 'Always' Received	300+	57%	62%	68%
Would Definitely Recommend Hospital	300+	72%	70%	71%
Use of Medical Imaging				
Cardiac Imaging Stress Test before Surgery	227	5.7%	5.2%	5.3%
Combination Abdominal CT Scan	230	7.0%	13.4%	10.5%
Combination Brain/Sinus CT Scan	537	4.1%	2.2%	2.7%
Combination Chest CT Scan	67	4.5%	2.3%	2.7%
Follow-up Mammogram/Ultrasound[7]	-	-	8.2%	8.8%
Lumbar Spine MRI for Low Back Pain[1]	-	-	34.2%	37.2%

Hollywood Presbyterian Medical Center

1300 N Vermont Ave
Los Angeles, CA 90028
Phone: 213-413-3000
Fax: 323-644-4411
E-mail: doris.stanley@tenethealthc.com
URL: www.qahpmc.com
Type: Acute Care Hospitals
Emergency Services: Yes
Ownership: Proprietary
Beds: 434

Key Personnel:

Operating Room. . . . . Lee Craig
Cardiac Laboratory. . . . . Rose Gumadi
Radiology. . . . . Rebecca Hatcher
CEO/President. . . . . Jeff Nelson
Patient Relations . . . . Doris Stanley
Emergency Room . . . . Julie Tatico
Intensive Care Unit. . . . . Cynthia Tugo

Measure	Cases	This Hosp.	State Avg.	U.S. Avg.
Blood Clot Prevention and Treatment				
Anticoagulation Overlap Therapy[2]	33	82%	92%	93%
ICU Venous Thromboembolism Prophylaxis[2]	74	93%	92%	92%
Incidence of Potentially Preventable VTE[1,2]	-	-	11%	10%
UFH with Dosages/Platelet Monitoring[2]	14	100%	96%	97%
Venous Thromboembolism Prophylaxis[2]	332	70%	83%	85%
Warfarin Therapy Discharge Instructions[2]	22	95%	75%	75%
Chest Pain/Possible Heart Attack Care				
Aspirin Given Within 24 Hours of Arrival[1]	-	-	97%	96%
Fibrinolytic Meds Within 30 Min. of Arrival[3,7]	-	-	62%	58%
Average Time to ECG (minutes)[1]	-	-	9	7
Average Time to Transfer (minutes)[3,7]	-	-	62	60
Children's Asthma Care				
Received Home Management Plan of Care	-	-	88%	88%
Received Reliever Medication	-	-	100%	100%
Received Systemic Corticosteroids	-	-	100%	100%
Emergency Department				
Admittance Decision Time (minutes)[2]	340	203	125	98
Head CT Results Within 45 Min. of Arrival[1]	-	-	55%	57%
Patients Who Left ER Before Being Seen	34,944	5%	3%	2%
Time from ER Arrival to Admit. (minutes)[2]	375	405	323	274
Time from ER Arrival to Discharge (minutes)	307	227	168	134
Time in ER Before Being Evaluated (minutes)	341	4	29	26
Time to Pain Meds for Fractures (minutes)	86	62	62	57
Heart Attack Care				
Aspirin Given at Discharge	159	98%	99%	99%
Fibrinolytic Meds Within 30 Min. of Arrival[7]	-	-	73%	54%
PCI Within 90 Minutes of Arrival	21	100%	95%	96%
Statin Prescribed at Discharge	158	94%	98%	98%
Heart Failure Care				
ACE Inhibitor or ARB for LVSD[2]	78	96%	97%	97%
Discharge Instructions Given[2]	202	100%	94%	94%
Evaluation of LVS Function[2]	252	94%	99%	99%
Medicare Spending				
Medicare Spending per Patient (ratio)	-	1.11	0.98	0.98
Pneumonia Care				
Appropriate Initial Antibiotic Given[2]	58	90%	97%	95%
Blood Culture Timing[2]	155	99%	98%	98%
Pregnancy and Delivery Care				
Newborn Deliveries Scheduled Early[2]	108	12%	5%	6%
Preventive Care				
Immunization for Influenza[2]	542	67%	89%	90%
Immunization for Pneumonia[2]	467	81%	90%	92%
Stroke Care				
Anticoagulation Therapy for Atrial Fibrillation	14	100%	95%	95%
Antithrombotic Therapy Timing	83	100%	98%	98%
Assessed for Rehabilitation	112	100%	97%	97%
Discharged on Antithrombotic Therapy	90	99%	99%	99%
Discharged on Statin Medication	72	93%	94%	94%
Thrombolytic Therapy Timing[1]	-	-	72%	66%
Venous Thromboembolism Prophylaxis	115	97%	94%	94%
Written Stroke Educational Materials Given	54	100%	87%	88%
Surgical Care Improvement Project				
Appropriate Beta Blocker Usage[2]	40	75%	97%	98%
Appropriate VTP Within 24 Hours[2]	275	97%	98%	98%
Controlled Postoperative Blood Glucose[2]	36	89%	96%	97%
Perioperative Temperature Management[2]	340	100%	100%	100%
Prophylactic Antibiotic Selection[2]	182	97%	99%	99%
Prophylactic Antibiotic Selection (Outpatient)	59	92%	97%	98%
Prophylactic Antibiotic Stopped[2]	167	96%	98%	98%
Prophylactic Antibiotic Timing[2]	183	99%	99%	99%
Prophylactic Antibiotic Timing (Outpatient)	60	93%	97%	98%
Urinary Catheter Removal[2]	182	98%	97%	97%
Survey of Patients' Hospital Experiences				
Area Around Room 'Always' Quiet at Night	300+	55%	51%	61%
Doctors 'Always' Communicated Well	300+	71%	78%	82%
Home Recovery Information Given	300+	81%	83%	85%
Hospital Given 9 or 10 on 10 Point Scale	300+	60%	68%	71%
Meds 'Always' Explained Before Given	300+	53%	61%	64%
Nurses 'Always' Communicated Well	300+	65%	74%	79%
Pain 'Always' Well Controlled	300+	60%	68%	71%
Room and Bathroom 'Always' Clean	300+	61%	70%	73%
Timely Help 'Always' Received	300+	56%	62%	68%
Would Definitely Recommend Hospital	300+	60%	70%	71%
Use of Medical Imaging				
Cardiac Imaging Stress Test before Surgery	155	7.1%	5.2%	5.3%
Combination Abdominal CT Scan	579	12.3%	13.4%	10.5%
Combination Brain/Sinus CT Scan	619	4.0%	2.2%	2.7%
Combination Chest CT Scan	184	7.1%	2.3%	2.7%
Follow-up Mammogram/Ultrasound	517	3.1%	8.2%	8.8%
Lumbar Spine MRI for Low Back Pain[1]	-	-	34.2%	37.2%

Kaiser Foundation Hospital - Los Angeles

4867 Sunset Blvd
Phone: 323-783-4011
Los Angeles, CA 90027
Fax: 323-783-7946
URL: www.kaiserpermanente.org
Type: Acute Care Hospitals
Emergency Services: Yes
Ownership: Voluntary non-profit - Other
Beds: 737

Key Personnel:

CEO/President. . . . . Anthony Armada
Quality Assurance . . . . Carolyn Godfrey, RN
Pediatric Ambulatory Care . . . . . . Ron Rosengart, MD
Pediatric In-Patient Care . . . . Ron Rosengart, MD
Infection Control. . . . . Joel Ruskin, MD
Radiology. . . . . Morley Slote, MD
Chief of Medical Staff . . . . Maureen Spell, MD
Operating Room. . . . . Margaret Spies, RN

Measure	Cases	This Hosp.	State Avg.	U.S. Avg.
Blood Clot Prevention and Treatment				
Anticoagulation Overlap Therapy[2]	103	94%	92%	93%
ICU Venous Thromboembolism Prophylaxis[2]	136	93%	92%	92%
Incidence of Potentially Preventable VTE[2]	31	3%	11%	10%
UFH with Dosages/Platelet Monitoring[2]	75	100%	96%	97%
Venous Thromboembolism Prophylaxis[2]	267	90%	83%	85%
Warfarin Therapy Discharge Instructions[2]	80	91%	75%	75%
Chest Pain/Possible Heart Attack Care				
Aspirin Given Within 24 Hours of Arrival	-	-	97%	96%
Fibrinolytic Meds Within 30 Min. of Arrival	-	-	62%	58%
Average Time to ECG (minutes)	-	-	9	7
Average Time to Transfer (minutes)	-	-	62	60
Children's Asthma Care				
Received Home Management Plan of Care	-	-	88%	88%
Received Reliever Medication	-	-	100%	100%
Received Systemic Corticosteroids	-	-	100%	100%
Emergency Department				
Admittance Decision Time (minutes)[2]	351	265	125	98
Head CT Results Within 45 Min. of Arrival	-	-	55%	57%
Patients Who Left ER Before Being Seen	-	-	3%	2%
Time from ER Arrival to Admit. (minutes)[2]	356	557	323	274
Time from ER Arrival to Discharge (minutes)	-	-	168	134
Time in ER Before Being Evaluated (minutes)	-	-	29	26
Time to Pain Meds for Fractures (minutes)	-	-	62	57
Heart Attack Care				
Aspirin Given at Discharge[2]	733	100%	99%	99%
Fibrinolytic Meds Within 30 Min. of Arrival[2,7]	-	-	73%	54%
PCI Within 90 Minutes of Arrival[1,2]	-	-	95%	96%
Statin Prescribed at Discharge[2]	715	100%	98%	98%
Heart Failure Care				
ACE Inhibitor or ARB for LVSD	286	99%	97%	97%
Discharge Instructions Given	533	98%	94%	94%
Evaluation of LVS Function	566	100%	99%	99%
Medicare Spending				
Medicare Spending per Patient (ratio)	-	0.87	0.98	0.98
Pneumonia Care				
Appropriate Initial Antibiotic Given[2]	58	98%	97%	95%
Blood Culture Timing[2]	158	95%	98%	98%
Pregnancy and Delivery Care				
Newborn Deliveries Scheduled Early	201	0%	5%	6%
Preventive Care				
Immunization for Influenza[2]	530	80%	89%	90%
Immunization for Pneumonia[2]	552	88%	90%	92%
Stroke Care				
Anticoagulation Therapy for Atrial Fibrillation[1,2]	-	-	95%	95%
Antithrombotic Therapy Timing[2]	40	100%	98%	98%
Assessed for Rehabilitation[2]	115	97%	97%	97%

NOTE: Hospital profiles are in alphabetical order by state, then city, then hospital within the city; Rankings exclude hospitals with less than 25 cases except for patient surveys which excludes hospitals with less than 100 cases; (a) 100-299 cases; (1) The number of cases/patients is too few to report; (2) Data submitted were based on a sample of cases/patients; (3) Results are based on a shorter time period than required; (4) Data suppressed by CMS for one or more quarters; (5) Results are not available for this reporting period; (6) Fewer than 100 patients completed the HCAHPS survey; (7) No cases met the criteria for this measure; (8) The lower limit of the confidence interval cannot be calculated if the number of observed infections equals zero; (9) No data are available from the state/territory for this reporting period; (10) The scores shown reflect fewer than 50 completed surveys; (11) There were discrepancies in the data collection process; (12) This measure does not apply to this hospital for this reporting period; (13) Results cannot be calculated for this reporting period; (14) The results for this state are combined with nearby states to protect confidentiality; Please refer to the User's Guide for a full explanation of data.

Discharged on Antithrombotic Therapy[2]	62	98%	99%	99%
Discharged on Statin Medication[2]	55	100%	94%	94%
Thrombolytic Therapy Timing[1,2]	-	-	72%	66%
Venous Thromboembolism Prophylaxis[2]	118	99%	94%	94%
Written Stroke Educational Materials Given[2]	81	83%	87%	88%
Surgical Care Improvement Project				
Appropriate Beta Blocker Usage[2]	261	98%	97%	98%
Appropriate VTP Within 24 Hours[2]	425	100%	98%	98%
Controlled Postoperative Blood Glucose[2]	227	97%	96%	97%
Perioperative Temperature Management[2]	516	100%	100%	100%
Prophylactic Antibiotic Selection[2]	532	98%	99%	99%
Prophylactic Antibiotic Selection (Outpatient)	-	-	97%	98%
Prophylactic Antibiotic Stopped[2]	523	99%	98%	98%
Prophylactic Antibiotic Timing[2]	532	99%	99%	99%
Prophylactic Antibiotic Timing (Outpatient)	-	-	97%	98%
Urinary Catheter Removal[2]	433	100%	97%	97%
Survey of Patients' Hospital Experiences				
Area Around Room 'Always' Quiet at Night	300+	58%	51%	61%
Doctors 'Always' Communicated Well	300+	80%	78%	82%
Home Recovery Information Given	300+	86%	83%	85%
Hospital Given 9 or 10 on 10 Point Scale	300+	77%	68%	71%
Meds 'Always' Explained Before Given	300+	61%	61%	64%
Nurses 'Always' Communicated Well	300+	77%	74%	79%
Pain 'Always' Well Controlled	300+	72%	68%	71%
Room and Bathroom 'Always' Clean	300+	73%	70%	73%
Timely Help 'Always' Received	300+	70%	62%	68%
Would Definitely Recommend Hospital	300+	79%	70%	71%
Use of Medical Imaging				
Cardiac Imaging Stress Test before Surgery	-	-	5.2%	5.3%
Combination Abdominal CT Scan	-	-	13.4%	10.5%
Combination Brain/Sinus CT Scan	-	-	2.2%	2.7%
Combination Chest CT Scan	-	-	2.3%	2.7%
Follow-up Mammogram/Ultrasound	-	-	8.2%	8.8%
Lumbar Spine MRI for Low Back Pain	-	-	34.2%	37.2%

Kaiser Foundation Hospital - West La

6041 Cadillac Ave
Los Angeles, CA 90034
Phone: 213-857-2201
Fax: 323-857-4051
URL: www.kaiserpermanente.org
Type: Acute Care Hospitals
Emergency Services: Yes
Ownership: Voluntary non-profit - Private
Beds: 306

Key Personnel:
Radiology. . . . . Curt Anderson, DA
Emergency Room . . . . Robert Becker, MD
Anesthesiology. . . . . James DeFontes, MD
Chief of Medical Staff. . . . . Edward Ellison, MD
Intensive Care Unit. . . . . Denise Giambalvo, RN
CEO/President. . . . . Janice Head
Operating Room. . . . . Shiela Smith, DA
Quality Assurance . . . . Carmen Thorpe

Measure	Cases	This Hosp.	State Avg.	U.S. Avg.
Blood Clot Prevention and Treatment				
Anticoagulation Overlap Therapy[2]	56	96%	92%	93%
ICU Venous Thromboembolism Prophylaxis[2]	53	91%	92%	92%
Incidence of Potentially Preventable VTE[1,2]	-	-	11%	10%
UFH with Dosages/Platelet Monitoring[2]	45	93%	96%	97%
Venous Thromboembolism Prophylaxis[2]	290	79%	83%	85%
Warfarin Therapy Discharge Instructions[2]	52	92%	75%	75%
Chest Pain/Possible Heart Attack Care				
Aspirin Given Within 24 Hours of Arrival	-	-	97%	96%
Fibrinolytic Meds Within 30 Min. of Arrival	-	-	62%	58%
Average Time to ECG (minutes)	-	-	9	7
Average Time to Transfer (minutes)	-	-	62	60
Children's Asthma Care				
Received Home Management Plan of Care	-	-	88%	88%
Received Reliever Medication	-	-	100%	100%
Received Systemic Corticosteroids	-	-	100%	100%
Emergency Department				
Admittance Decision Time (minutes)[2]	449	81	125	98
Head CT Results Within 45 Min. of Arrival	-	-	55%	57%
Patients Who Left ER Before Being Seen	-	-	3%	2%
Time from ER Arrival to Admit. (minutes)[2]	450	377	323	274
Time from ER Arrival to Discharge (minutes)	-	-	168	134
Time in ER Before Being Evaluated (minutes)	-	-	29	26
Time to Pain Meds for Fractures (minutes)	-	-	62	57
Heart Attack Care				
Aspirin Given at Discharge	77	100%	99%	99%
Fibrinolytic Meds Within 30 Min. of Arrival[1]	-	-	73%	54%
PCI Within 90 Minutes of Arrival[7]	-	-	95%	96%
Statin Prescribed at Discharge	79	100%	98%	98%
Heart Failure Care				
ACE Inhibitor or ARB for LVSD	102	100%	97%	97%
Discharge Instructions Given	255	99%	94%	94%
Evaluation of LVS Function	271	100%	99%	99%
Medicare Spending				
Medicare Spending per Patient (ratio)	-	0.86	0.98	0.98
Pneumonia Care				
Appropriate Initial Antibiotic Given[2]	65	97%	97%	95%
Blood Culture Timing[2]	118	94%	98%	98%
Pregnancy and Delivery Care				
Newborn Deliveries Scheduled Early	157	4%	5%	6%
Preventive Care				
Immunization for Influenza[2]	535	77%	89%	90%
Immunization for Pneumonia[2]	612	87%	90%	92%
Stroke Care				
Anticoagulation Therapy for Atrial Fibrillation[2]	20	70%	95%	95%
Antithrombotic Therapy Timing[2]	88	99%	98%	98%
Assessed for Rehabilitation[2]	120	98%	97%	97%
Discharged on Antithrombotic Therapy[2]	105	99%	99%	99%
Discharged on Statin Medication[2]	103	96%	94%	94%
Thrombolytic Therapy Timing[2,7]	-	-	72%	66%
Venous Thromboembolism Prophylaxis[2]	99	98%	94%	94%
Written Stroke Educational Materials Given[2]	71	94%	87%	88%
Surgical Care Improvement Project				
Appropriate Beta Blocker Usage[2]	129	98%	97%	98%
Appropriate VTP Within 24 Hours[2]	303	100%	98%	98%
Controlled Postoperative Blood Glucose[2,7]	-	-	96%	97%
Perioperative Temperature Management[2]	434	100%	100%	100%
Prophylactic Antibiotic Selection[2]	244	100%	99%	99%
Prophylactic Antibiotic Selection (Outpatient)	-	-	97%	98%
Prophylactic Antibiotic Stopped[2]	240	99%	98%	98%
Prophylactic Antibiotic Timing[2]	244	100%	99%	99%
Prophylactic Antibiotic Timing (Outpatient)	-	-	97%	98%
Urinary Catheter Removal[2]	280	100%	97%	97%
Survey of Patients' Hospital Experiences				
Area Around Room 'Always' Quiet at Night	300+	60%	51%	61%
Doctors 'Always' Communicated Well	300+	83%	78%	82%
Home Recovery Information Given	300+	85%	83%	85%
Hospital Given 9 or 10 on 10 Point Scale	300+	74%	68%	71%
Meds 'Always' Explained Before Given	300+	65%	61%	64%
Nurses 'Always' Communicated Well	300+	77%	74%	79%
Pain 'Always' Well Controlled	300+	73%	68%	71%
Room and Bathroom 'Always' Clean	300+	72%	70%	73%
Timely Help 'Always' Received	300+	64%	62%	68%
Would Definitely Recommend Hospital	300+	74%	70%	71%
Use of Medical Imaging				
Cardiac Imaging Stress Test before Surgery	-	-	5.2%	5.3%
Combination Abdominal CT Scan	-	-	13.4%	10.5%
Combination Brain/Sinus CT Scan	-	-	2.2%	2.7%
Combination Chest CT Scan	-	-	2.3%	2.7%
Follow-up Mammogram/Ultrasound	-	-	8.2%	8.8%
Lumbar Spine MRI for Low Back Pain	-	-	34.2%	37.2%

Keck Hospital of USC

1500 San Pablo St
Los Angeles, CA 90033
Phone: 323-442-8656
Fax: 323-442-8672
URL: www.uscuh.com
Type: Acute Care Hospitals
Emergency Services: No
Ownership: Voluntary non-profit - Other
Beds: 411

Key Personnel:
Chief of Medical Staff. . . . . Mohamed El-Shahawy
CEO/President. . . . . Scott Evans, MHA, PharmD

Measure	Cases	This Hosp.	State Avg.	U.S. Avg.
Blood Clot Prevention and Treatment				
Anticoagulation Overlap Therapy[2]	21	76%	92%	93%
ICU Venous Thromboembolism Prophylaxis[2]	157	95%	92%	92%
Incidence of Potentially Preventable VTE[2]	33	9%	11%	10%
UFH with Dosages/Platelet Monitoring[2]	29	90%	96%	97%
Venous Thromboembolism Prophylaxis[2]	238	78%	83%	85%
Warfarin Therapy Discharge Instructions[2]	11	9%	75%	75%
Chest Pain/Possible Heart Attack Care				
Aspirin Given Within 24 Hours of Arrival[5]	-	-	97%	96%
Fibrinolytic Meds Within 30 Min. of Arrival[5]	-	-	62%	58%
Average Time to ECG (minutes)[5]	-	-	9	7
Average Time to Transfer (minutes)[5]	-	-	62	60
Children's Asthma Care				
Received Home Management Plan of Care	-	-	88%	88%
Received Reliever Medication	-	-	100%	100%
Received Systemic Corticosteroids	-	-	100%	100%
Emergency Department				
Admittance Decision Time (minutes)[2,7]	-	-	125	98
Head CT Results Within 45 Min. of Arrival[5]	-	-	55%	57%
Patients Who Left ER Before Being Seen[5]	-	-	3%	2%
Time from ER Arrival to Admit. (minutes)[2,7]	-	-	323	274
Time from ER Arrival to Discharge (minutes)[5]	-	-	168	134
Time in ER Before Being Evaluated (minutes)[5]	-	-	29	26
Time to Pain Meds for Fractures (minutes)[5]	-	-	62	57
Heart Attack Care				
Aspirin Given at Discharge	55	100%	99%	99%
Fibrinolytic Meds Within 30 Min. of Arrival[1]	-	-	73%	54%
PCI Within 90 Minutes of Arrival[7]	-	-	95%	96%
Statin Prescribed at Discharge	56	100%	98%	98%
Heart Failure Care				
ACE Inhibitor or ARB for LVSD	37	100%	97%	97%
Discharge Instructions Given	103	100%	94%	94%
Evaluation of LVS Function	116	100%	99%	99%
Medicare Spending				
Medicare Spending per Patient (ratio)	-	0.99	0.98	0.98
Pneumonia Care				
Appropriate Initial Antibiotic Given[1]	-	-	97%	95%
Blood Culture Timing[7]	-	-	98%	98%
Pregnancy and Delivery Care				
Newborn Deliveries Scheduled Early[7]	-	-	5%	6%
Preventive Care				
Immunization for Influenza[2]	571	88%	89%	90%
Immunization for Pneumonia[2]	675	82%	90%	92%
Stroke Care				
Anticoagulation Therapy for Atrial Fibrillation[2]	19	95%	95%	95%
Antithrombotic Therapy Timing[2]	42	100%	98%	98%
Assessed for Rehabilitation[2]	136	98%	97%	97%
Discharged on Antithrombotic Therapy[2]	65	100%	99%	99%
Discharged on Statin Medication[2]	64	98%	94%	94%
Thrombolytic Therapy Timing[2,7]	-	-	72%	66%
Venous Thromboembolism Prophylaxis[2]	152	100%	94%	94%
Written Stroke Educational Materials Given[2]	69	77%	87%	88%
Surgical Care Improvement Project				
Appropriate Beta Blocker Usage[2]	255	97%	97%	98%
Appropriate VTP Within 24 Hours[2]	582	99%	98%	98%
Controlled Postoperative Blood Glucose[2]	168	98%	96%	97%
Perioperative Temperature Management[2]	868	100%	100%	100%
Prophylactic Antibiotic Selection[2]	455	99%	99%	99%
Prophylactic Antibiotic Selection (Outpatient)	363	96%	97%	98%
Prophylactic Antibiotic Stopped[2]	432	95%	98%	98%
Prophylactic Antibiotic Timing[2]	455	99%	99%	99%
Prophylactic Antibiotic Timing (Outpatient)	370	95%	97%	98%
Urinary Catheter Removal[2]	449	98%	97%	97%
Survey of Patients' Hospital Experiences				
Area Around Room 'Always' Quiet at Night	300+	56%	51%	61%
Doctors 'Always' Communicated Well	300+	83%	78%	82%
Home Recovery Information Given	300+	84%	83%	85%
Hospital Given 9 or 10 on 10 Point Scale	300+	77%	68%	71%
Meds 'Always' Explained Before Given	300+	61%	61%	64%
Nurses 'Always' Communicated Well	300+	77%	74%	79%
Pain 'Always' Well Controlled	300+	70%	68%	71%
Room and Bathroom 'Always' Clean	300+	69%	70%	73%
Timely Help 'Always' Received	300+	60%	62%	68%
Would Definitely Recommend Hospital	300+	82%	70%	71%
Use of Medical Imaging				
Cardiac Imaging Stress Test before Surgery	825	10.2%	5.2%	5.3%

NOTE: Hospital profiles are in alphabetical order by state, then city, then hospital within the city; Rankings exclude hospitals with less than 25 cases except for patient surveys which excludes hospitals with less than 100 cases; (a) 100-299 cases; (1) The number of cases/patients is too few to report; (2) Data submitted were based on a sample of cases/patients; (3) Results are based on a shorter time period than required; (4) Data suppressed by CMS for one or more quarters; (5) Results are not available for this reporting period; (6) Fewer than 100 patients completed the HCAHPS survey; (7) No cases met the criteria for this measure; (8) The lower limit of the confidence interval cannot be calculated if the number of observed infections equals zero; (9) No data are available from the state/territory for this reporting period; (10) The scores shown reflect fewer than 50 completed surveys; (11) There were discrepancies in the data collection process; (12) This measure does not apply to this hospital for this reporting period; (13) Results cannot be calculated for this reporting period; (14) The results for this state are combined with nearby states to protect confidentiality; Please refer to the User's Guide for a full explanation of data.

Combination Abdominal CT Scan	791	59.9%	13.4%	10.5%
Combination Brain/Sinus CT Scan[1]	-	-	2.2%	2.7%
Combination Chest CT Scan	938	0.2%	2.3%	2.7%
Follow-up Mammogram/Ultrasound[1]	-	-	8.2%	8.8%
Lumbar Spine MRI for Low Back Pain	122	33.6%	34.2%	37.2%

LAC+USC Medical Center

1200 N State St, Room C2k100 Phone: 323-226-2800
Los Angeles, CA 90033 Fax: 323-226-6518
E-mail: webinformatics@ladhs.org
URL: www.ladhs.org/wps/portal/lacuschomepage
Type: Acute Care Hospitals Emergency Services: Yes
Ownership: Government - Local Beds: 1,395

Key Personnel:
Emergency Room . . . . Gail Anderson, MD
Quality Assurance . . . . Janet Baker
CEO/President. . . . . Pete Delgado
Intensive Care Unit. . . . . Steve Giannotta, MD
Radiology. . . . . James Halls, MD
Chief of Medical Staff . . . . Philip Lamb, M.B., B.S.
Pediatric In-Patient Care . . . . Lawrence Opas, MD
Anesthesiology. . . . . Vladimir Zelman

Measure	Cases	This Hosp.	State Avg.	U.S. Avg.
Blood Clot Prevention and Treatment				
Anticoagulation Overlap Therapy[2]	65	92%	92%	93%
ICU Venous Thromboembolism Prophylaxis[2]	159	99%	92%	92%
Incidence of Potentially Preventable VTE[2]	25	12%	11%	10%
UFH with Dosages/Platelet Monitoring[2]	66	100%	96%	97%
Venous Thromboembolism Prophylaxis[2]	236	95%	83%	85%
Warfarin Therapy Discharge Instructions[2]	52	56%	75%	75%
Chest Pain/Possible Heart Attack Care				
Aspirin Given Within 24 Hours of Arrival[1]	-	-	97%	96%
Fibrinolytic Meds Within 30 Min. of Arrival[3,7]	-	-	62%	58%
Average Time to ECG (minutes)[1]	-	-	9	7
Average Time to Transfer (minutes)[3,7]	-	-	62	60
Children's Asthma Care				
Received Home Management Plan of Care	-	-	88%	88%
Received Reliever Medication	-	-	100%	100%
Received Systemic Corticosteroids	-	-	100%	100%
Emergency Department				
Admittance Decision Time (minutes)[2]	687	198	125	98
Head CT Results Within 45 Min. of Arrival[1]	-	-	55%	57%
Patients Who Left ER Before Being Seen	>100k	4%	3%	2%
Time from ER Arrival to Admit. (minutes)[2]	693	652	323	274
Time from ER Arrival to Discharge (minutes)	290	369	168	134
Time in ER Before Being Evaluated (minutes)	324	42	29	26
Time to Pain Meds for Fractures (minutes)	208	63	62	57
Heart Attack Care				
Aspirin Given at Discharge	221	100%	99%	99%
Fibrinolytic Meds Within 30 Min. of Arrival[7]	-	-	73%	54%
PCI Within 90 Minutes of Arrival	44	91%	95%	96%
Statin Prescribed at Discharge	219	100%	98%	98%
Heart Failure Care				
ACE Inhibitor or ARB for LVSD	328	100%	97%	97%
Discharge Instructions Given	618	98%	94%	94%
Evaluation of LVS Function	619	100%	99%	99%
Medicare Spending				
Medicare Spending per Patient (ratio)	-	0.94	0.98	0.98
Pneumonia Care				
Appropriate Initial Antibiotic Given	194	98%	97%	95%
Blood Culture Timing	358	98%	98%	98%
Pregnancy and Delivery Care				
Newborn Deliveries Scheduled Early[2]	20	15%	5%	6%
Preventive Care				
Immunization for Influenza[2]	513	82%	89%	90%
Immunization for Pneumonia[2]	288	86%	90%	92%
Stroke Care				
Anticoagulation Therapy for Atrial Fibrillation[1,2]	-	-	95%	95%
Antithrombotic Therapy Timing[2]	50	94%	98%	98%
Assessed for Rehabilitation[2]	76	87%	97%	97%
Discharged on Antithrombotic Therapy[2]	46	100%	99%	99%
Discharged on Statin Medication[2]	36	94%	94%	94%
Thrombolytic Therapy Timing[1,2]	-	-	72%	66%
Venous Thromboembolism Prophylaxis[2]	113	97%	94%	94%
Written Stroke Educational Materials Given[2]	47	4%	87%	88%
Surgical Care Improvement Project				
Appropriate Beta Blocker Usage[2]	153	96%	97%	98%
Appropriate VTP Within 24 Hours[2]	517	98%	98%	98%
Controlled Postoperative Blood Glucose[2]	169	91%	96%	97%
Perioperative Temperature Management[2]	683	100%	100%	100%
Prophylactic Antibiotic Selection[2]	582	98%	99%	99%
Prophylactic Antibiotic Selection (Outpatient)[2]	205	99%	97%	98%
Prophylactic Antibiotic Stopped[2]	574	96%	98%	98%
Prophylactic Antibiotic Timing[2]	583	98%	99%	99%
Prophylactic Antibiotic Timing (Outpatient)	127	98%	97%	98%
Urinary Catheter Removal[2]	243	97%	97%	97%
Survey of Patients' Hospital Experiences				
Area Around Room 'Always' Quiet at Night[11]	300+	52%	51%	61%
Doctors 'Always' Communicated Well[11]	300+	76%	78%	82%
Home Recovery Information Given[11]	300+	80%	83%	85%
Hospital Given 9 or 10 on 10 Point Scale[11]	300+	72%	68%	71%
Meds 'Always' Explained Before Given[11]	300+	55%	61%	64%
Nurses 'Always' Communicated Well[11]	300+	69%	74%	79%
Pain 'Always' Well Controlled[11]	300+	66%	68%	71%
Room and Bathroom 'Always' Clean[11]	300+	65%	70%	73%
Timely Help 'Always' Received[11]	300+	57%	62%	68%
Would Definitely Recommend Hospital[11]	300+	73%	70%	71%
Use of Medical Imaging				
Cardiac Imaging Stress Test before Surgery[1]	-	-	5.2%	5.3%
Combination Abdominal CT Scan	155	0.6%	13.4%	10.5%
Combination Brain/Sinus CT Scan[1]	-	-	2.2%	2.7%
Combination Chest CT Scan	110	0.0%	2.3%	2.7%
Follow-up Mammogram/Ultrasound[7]	-	-	8.2%	8.8%
Lumbar Spine MRI for Low Back Pain[1]	-	-	34.2%	37.2%

Los Angeles Community Hospital

4081 E Olympic Blvd Phone: 323-267-0477
Los Angeles, CA 90023
URL: www.altacorp.com
Type: Acute Care Hospitals Emergency Services: Yes
Ownership: Proprietary

Key Personnel:
Anesthesiology. . . . . Serafin Ariola
Radiology. . . . . Clive Negatani

Measure	Cases	This Hosp.	State Avg.	U.S. Avg.
Blood Clot Prevention and Treatment				
Anticoagulation Overlap Therapy[2]	31	81%	92%	93%
ICU Venous Thromboembolism Prophylaxis[2]	43	100%	92%	92%
Incidence of Potentially Preventable VTE[1,2]	-	-	11%	10%
UFH with Dosages/Platelet Monitoring[2]	18	100%	96%	97%
Venous Thromboembolism Prophylaxis[2]	404	86%	83%	85%
Warfarin Therapy Discharge Instructions[2]	12	50%	75%	75%
Chest Pain/Possible Heart Attack Care				
Aspirin Given Within 24 Hours of Arrival[1,3]	-	-	97%	96%
Fibrinolytic Meds Within 30 Min. of Arrival[3,7]	-	-	62%	58%
Average Time to ECG (minutes)[1,3]	-	-	9	7
Average Time to Transfer (minutes)[1,3]	-	-	62	60
Children's Asthma Care				
Received Home Management Plan of Care	-	-	88%	88%
Received Reliever Medication	-	-	100%	100%
Received Systemic Corticosteroids	-	-	100%	100%
Emergency Department				
Admittance Decision Time (minutes)[2]	627	65	125	98
Head CT Results Within 45 Min. of Arrival[1,3]	-	-	55%	57%
Patients Who Left ER Before Being Seen	12,230	1%	3%	2%
Time from ER Arrival to Admit. (minutes)[2]	697	220	323	274
Time from ER Arrival to Discharge (minutes)	336	125	168	134
Time in ER Before Being Evaluated (minutes)	345	10	29	26
Time to Pain Meds for Fractures (minutes)	22	53	62	57
Heart Attack Care				
Aspirin Given at Discharge	84	94%	99%	99%
Fibrinolytic Meds Within 30 Min. of Arrival[7]	-	-	73%	54%
PCI Within 90 Minutes of Arrival[7]	-	-	95%	96%
Statin Prescribed at Discharge	84	73%	98%	98%
Heart Failure Care				
ACE Inhibitor or ARB for LVSD[2]	91	89%	97%	97%
Discharge Instructions Given[2]	131	95%	94%	94%
Evaluation of LVS Function[2]	194	96%	99%	99%
Medicare Spending				
Medicare Spending per Patient (ratio)	-	1.31	0.98	0.98
Pneumonia Care				
Appropriate Initial Antibiotic Given[2]	25	96%	97%	95%
Blood Culture Timing[2]	61	95%	98%	98%
Pregnancy and Delivery Care				
Newborn Deliveries Scheduled Early[2]	23	39%	5%	6%
Preventive Care				
Immunization for Influenza[2]	549	81%	89%	90%
Immunization for Pneumonia[2]	720	82%	90%	92%
Stroke Care				
Anticoagulation Therapy for Atrial Fibrillation[1]	-	-	95%	95%
Antithrombotic Therapy Timing	30	70%	98%	98%
Assessed for Rehabilitation	53	81%	97%	97%
Discharged on Antithrombotic Therapy	25	72%	99%	99%
Discharged on Statin Medication	38	84%	94%	94%
Thrombolytic Therapy Timing	15	0%	72%	66%
Venous Thromboembolism Prophylaxis	55	89%	94%	94%
Written Stroke Educational Materials Given	19	42%	87%	88%
Surgical Care Improvement Project				
Appropriate Beta Blocker Usage[2]	16	94%	97%	98%
Appropriate VTP Within 24 Hours[2]	60	95%	98%	98%
Controlled Postoperative Blood Glucose[2,7]	-	-	96%	97%
Perioperative Temperature Management[2]	69	100%	100%	100%
Prophylactic Antibiotic Selection[2]	27	93%	99%	99%
Prophylactic Antibiotic Selection (Outpatient)[1,3]	-	-	97%	98%
Prophylactic Antibiotic Stopped[2]	17	88%	98%	98%
Prophylactic Antibiotic Timing[2]	27	93%	99%	99%
Prophylactic Antibiotic Timing (Outpatient)[1,3]	-	-	97%	98%
Urinary Catheter Removal[2]	20	90%	97%	97%
Survey of Patients' Hospital Experiences				
Area Around Room 'Always' Quiet at Night	300+	37%	51%	61%
Doctors 'Always' Communicated Well	300+	65%	78%	82%
Home Recovery Information Given	300+	69%	83%	85%
Hospital Given 9 or 10 on 10 Point Scale	300+	44%	68%	71%
Meds 'Always' Explained Before Given	300+	45%	61%	64%
Nurses 'Always' Communicated Well	300+	61%	74%	79%
Pain 'Always' Well Controlled	300+	56%	68%	71%
Room and Bathroom 'Always' Clean	300+	54%	70%	73%
Timely Help 'Always' Received	300+	45%	62%	68%
Would Definitely Recommend Hospital	300+	42%	70%	71%
Use of Medical Imaging				
Cardiac Imaging Stress Test before Surgery[1]	-	-	5.2%	5.3%
Combination Abdominal CT Scan	63	4.8%	13.4%	10.5%
Combination Brain/Sinus CT Scan[1]	-	-	2.2%	2.7%
Combination Chest CT Scan[1]	-	-	2.3%	2.7%
Follow-up Mammogram/Ultrasound[7]	-	-	8.2%	8.8%
Lumbar Spine MRI for Low Back Pain[7]	-	-	34.2%	37.2%

Miracle Mile Medical Center

6000 San Vicente Blvd Phone: 323-930-1040
Los Angeles, CA 90036
Type: Acute Care Hospitals Emergency Services: No
Ownership: Proprietary

Key Personnel:
CEO/President. . . . . Jack Lahidjani
Chief of Medical Staff . . . . Gil Tepper, MD, FACS

Measure	Cases	This Hosp.	State Avg.	U.S. Avg.
Blood Clot Prevention and Treatment				
Anticoagulation Overlap Therapy[3,7]	-	-	92%	93%
ICU Venous Thromboembolism Prophylaxis[3,7]	-	-	92%	92%
Incidence of Potentially Preventable VTE[3,7]	-	-	11%	10%
UFH with Dosages/Platelet Monitoring[3,7]	-	-	96%	97%
Venous Thromboembolism Prophylaxis[1,3]	-	-	83%	85%
Warfarin Therapy Discharge Instructions[3,7]	-	-	75%	75%
Chest Pain/Possible Heart Attack Care				
Aspirin Given Within 24 Hours of Arrival[5]	-	-	97%	96%
Fibrinolytic Meds Within 30 Min. of Arrival[5]	-	-	62%	58%
Average Time to ECG (minutes)[5]	-	-	9	7
Average Time to Transfer (minutes)[5]	-	-	62	60
Children's Asthma Care				
Received Home Management Plan of Care	-	-	88%	88%

NOTE: Hospital profiles are in alphabetical order by state, then city, then hospital within the city; Rankings exclude hospitals with less than 25 cases except for patient surveys which excludes hospitals with less than 100 cases; (a) 100-299 cases; (1) The number of cases/patients is too few to report; (2) Data submitted were based on a sample of cases/patients; (3) Results are based on a shorter time period than required; (4) Data suppressed by CMS for one or more quarters; (5) Results are not available for this reporting period; (6) Fewer than 100 patients completed the HCAHPS survey; (7) No cases met the criteria for this measure; (8) The lower limit of the confidence interval cannot be calculated if the number of observed infections equals zero; (9) No data are available from the state/territory for this reporting period; (10) The scores shown reflect fewer than 50 completed surveys; (11) There were discrepancies in the data collection process; (12) This measure does not apply to this hospital for this reporting period; (13) Results cannot be calculated for this reporting period; (14) The results for this state are combined with nearby states to protect confidentiality; Please refer to the User's Guide for a full explanation of data.

Measure	Cases	This Hosp.	State Avg.	U.S. Avg.
Received Reliever Medication	-	-	100%	100%
Received Systemic Corticosteroids	-	-	100%	100%
Emergency Department				
Admittance Decision Time (minutes)[3,7]	-	-	125	98
Head CT Results Within 45 Min. of Arrival[5]	-	-	55%	57%
Patients Who Left ER Before Being Seen[5]	-	-	3%	2%
Time from ER Arrival to Admit. (minutes)[3,7]	-	-	323	274
Time from ER Arrival to Discharge (minutes)[5]	-	-	168	134
Time in ER Before Being Evaluated (minutes)[5]	-	-	29	26
Time to Pain Meds for Fractures (minutes)[5]	-	-	62	57
Heart Attack Care				
Aspirin Given at Discharge[5]	-	-	99%	99%
Fibrinolytic Meds Within 30 Min. of Arrival[5]	-	-	73%	54%
PCI Within 90 Minutes of Arrival[5]	-	-	95%	96%
Statin Prescribed at Discharge[5]	-	-	98%	98%
Heart Failure Care				
ACE Inhibitor or ARB for LVSD[5]	-	-	97%	97%
Discharge Instructions Given[5]	-	-	94%	94%
Evaluation of LVS Function[5]	-	-	99%	99%
Medicare Spending				
Medicare Spending per Patient (ratio)[1]	-	-	0.98	0.98
Pneumonia Care				
Appropriate Initial Antibiotic Given[5]	-	-	97%	95%
Blood Culture Timing[5]	-	-	98%	98%
Pregnancy and Delivery Care				
Newborn Deliveries Scheduled Early[2,7]	-	-	5%	6%
Preventive Care				
Immunization for Influenza[5]	-	-	89%	90%
Immunization for Pneumonia[1,3]	-	-	90%	92%
Stroke Care				
Anticoagulation Therapy for Atrial Fibrillation[5]	-	-	95%	95%
Antithrombotic Therapy Timing[5]	-	-	98%	98%
Assessed for Rehabilitation[5]	-	-	97%	97%
Discharged on Antithrombotic Therapy[5]	-	-	99%	99%
Discharged on Statin Medication[5]	-	-	94%	94%
Thrombolytic Therapy Timing[5]	-	-	72%	66%
Venous Thromboembolism Prophylaxis[5]	-	-	94%	94%
Written Stroke Educational Materials Given[5]	-	-	87%	88%
Surgical Care Improvement Project				
Appropriate Beta Blocker Usage[5]	-	-	97%	98%
Appropriate VTP Within 24 Hours[5]	-	-	98%	98%
Controlled Postoperative Blood Glucose[5]	-	-	96%	97%
Perioperative Temperature Management[5]	-	-	100%	100%
Prophylactic Antibiotic Selection[5]	-	-	99%	99%
Prophylactic Antibiotic Selection (Outpatient)[5]	-	-	97%	98%
Prophylactic Antibiotic Stopped[5]	-	-	98%	98%
Prophylactic Antibiotic Timing[5]	-	-	99%	99%
Prophylactic Antibiotic Timing (Outpatient)[5]	-	-	97%	98%
Urinary Catheter Removal[5]	-	-	97%	97%
Survey of Patients' Hospital Experiences				
Area Around Room 'Always' Quiet at Night[6]	<100	78%	51%	61%
Doctors 'Always' Communicated Well[6]	<100	87%	78%	82%
Home Recovery Information Given[6]	<100	83%	83%	85%
Hospital Given 9 or 10 on 10 Point Scale[6]	<100	82%	68%	71%
Meds 'Always' Explained Before Given[6]	<100	65%	61%	64%
Nurses 'Always' Communicated Well[6]	<100	86%	74%	79%
Pain 'Always' Well Controlled[6]	<100	85%	68%	71%
Room and Bathroom 'Always' Clean[6]	<100	89%	70%	73%
Timely Help 'Always' Received[6]	<100	84%	62%	68%
Would Definitely Recommend Hospital[6]	<100	81%	70%	71%
Use of Medical Imaging				
Cardiac Imaging Stress Test before Surgery[7]	-	-	5.2%	5.3%
Combination Abdominal CT Scan[7]	-	-	13.4%	10.5%
Combination Brain/Sinus CT Scan[7]	-	-	2.2%	2.7%
Combination Chest CT Scan[7]	-	-	2.3%	2.7%
Follow-up Mammogram/Ultrasound[7]	-	-	8.2%	8.8%
Lumbar Spine MRI for Low Back Pain[1]	-	-	34.2%	37.2%

Olympia Medical Center

5900 West Olympic Boulevard
Los Angeles, CA 90036
URL: www.olympiamc.com
Type: Acute Care Hospitals
Ownership: Proprietary
Phone: 310-657-5900
Fax: 323-932-5163
Emergency Services: Yes
Beds: 204

Key Personnel:
CEO . . . . John A. Calderone

Measure	Cases	This Hosp.	State Avg.	U.S. Avg.
Blood Clot Prevention and Treatment				
Anticoagulation Overlap Therapy[2]	32	94%	92%	93%
ICU Venous Thromboembolism Prophylaxis[2]	49	88%	92%	92%
Incidence of Potentially Preventable VTE[2]	14	14%	11%	10%
UFH with Dosages/Platelet Monitoring[2]	25	100%	96%	97%
Venous Thromboembolism Prophylaxis[2]	401	90%	83%	85%
Warfarin Therapy Discharge Instructions[2]	14	64%	75%	75%
Chest Pain/Possible Heart Attack Care				
Aspirin Given Within 24 Hours of Arrival	20	100%	97%	96%
Fibrinolytic Meds Within 30 Min. of Arrival[3,7]	-	-	62%	58%
Average Time to ECG (minutes)	20	10	9	7
Average Time to Transfer (minutes)[1,3]	-	-	62	60
Children's Asthma Care				
Received Home Management Plan of Care	-	-	88%	88%
Received Reliever Medication	-	-	100%	100%
Received Systemic Corticosteroids	-	-	100%	100%
Emergency Department				
Admittance Decision Time (minutes)[2]	748	105	125	98
Head CT Results Within 45 Min. of Arrival[1]	-	-	55%	57%
Patients Who Left ER Before Being Seen	25,247	0%	3%	2%
Time from ER Arrival to Admit. (minutes)[2]	816	278	323	274
Time from ER Arrival to Discharge (minutes)	326	129	168	134
Time in ER Before Being Evaluated (minutes)	372	20	29	26
Time to Pain Meds for Fractures (minutes)	20	46	62	57
Heart Attack Care				
Aspirin Given at Discharge	34	100%	99%	99%
Fibrinolytic Meds Within 30 Min. of Arrival[7]	-	-	73%	54%
PCI Within 90 Minutes of Arrival[7]	-	-	95%	96%
Statin Prescribed at Discharge	27	100%	98%	98%
Heart Failure Care				
ACE Inhibitor or ARB for LVSD	60	100%	97%	97%
Discharge Instructions Given	126	89%	94%	94%
Evaluation of LVS Function	180	99%	99%	99%
Medicare Spending				
Medicare Spending per Patient (ratio)	-	1.12	0.98	0.98
Pneumonia Care				
Appropriate Initial Antibiotic Given[2]	24	100%	97%	95%
Blood Culture Timing[2]	136	99%	98%	98%
Pregnancy and Delivery Care				
Newborn Deliveries Scheduled Early[7]	-	-	5%	6%
Preventive Care				
Immunization for Influenza[2]	548	99%	89%	90%
Immunization for Pneumonia[2]	783	99%	90%	92%
Stroke Care				
Anticoagulation Therapy for Atrial Fibrillation[1]	-	-	95%	95%
Antithrombotic Therapy Timing	32	97%	98%	98%
Assessed for Rehabilitation	40	95%	97%	97%
Discharged on Antithrombotic Therapy	32	97%	99%	99%
Discharged on Statin Medication	21	95%	94%	94%
Thrombolytic Therapy Timing[1]	-	-	72%	66%
Venous Thromboembolism Prophylaxis	45	82%	94%	94%
Written Stroke Educational Materials Given	19	79%	87%	88%
Surgical Care Improvement Project				
Appropriate Beta Blocker Usage	42	98%	97%	98%
Appropriate VTP Within 24 Hours	173	99%	98%	98%
Controlled Postoperative Blood Glucose[7]	-	-	96%	97%
Perioperative Temperature Management	195	100%	100%	100%
Prophylactic Antibiotic Selection	105	100%	99%	99%
Prophylactic Antibiotic Selection (Outpatient)	34	97%	97%	98%
Prophylactic Antibiotic Stopped	97	100%	98%	98%
Prophylactic Antibiotic Timing	105	100%	99%	99%
Prophylactic Antibiotic Timing (Outpatient)	34	100%	97%	98%
Urinary Catheter Removal	110	98%	97%	97%
Survey of Patients' Hospital Experiences				
Area Around Room 'Always' Quiet at Night	300+	70%	51%	61%
Doctors 'Always' Communicated Well	300+	80%	78%	82%
Home Recovery Information Given	300+	81%	83%	85%
Hospital Given 9 or 10 on 10 Point Scale	300+	67%	68%	71%
Meds 'Always' Explained Before Given	300+	59%	61%	64%
Nurses 'Always' Communicated Well	300+	75%	74%	79%
Pain 'Always' Well Controlled	300+	69%	68%	71%
Room and Bathroom 'Always' Clean	300+	69%	70%	73%
Timely Help 'Always' Received	300+	60%	62%	68%
Would Definitely Recommend Hospital	300+	70%	70%	71%
Use of Medical Imaging				
Cardiac Imaging Stress Test before Surgery[1]	-	-	5.2%	5.3%
Combination Abdominal CT Scan	157	5.7%	13.4%	10.5%
Combination Brain/Sinus CT Scan[1]	-	-	2.2%	2.7%
Combination Chest CT Scan	81	2.5%	2.3%	2.7%
Follow-up Mammogram/Ultrasound	88	9.1%	8.2%	8.8%
Lumbar Spine MRI for Low Back Pain[1]	-	-	34.2%	37.2%

Pacific Alliance Medical Center

531 W College St
Los Angeles, CA 90012
URL: www.pamc.net
Type: Acute Care Hospitals
Ownership: Proprietary
Phone: 213-624-8411
Fax: 213-626-3107
Emergency Services: No
Beds: 122

Key Personnel:
Emergency Room . . . . Ruby Blak
CEO/President. . . . . John R Edwards
Chief of Medical Staff . . . . Martha Maleon
Cardiac Laboratory. . . . . Micheal McCarthy

Measure	Cases	This Hosp.	State Avg.	U.S. Avg.
Blood Clot Prevention and Treatment				
Anticoagulation Overlap Therapy[2]	16	69%	92%	93%
ICU Venous Thromboembolism Prophylaxis[2]	38	84%	92%	92%
Incidence of Potentially Preventable VTE[1,2]	-	-	11%	10%
UFH with Dosages/Platelet Monitoring[1,2]	-	-	96%	97%
Venous Thromboembolism Prophylaxis[2]	380	51%	83%	85%
Warfarin Therapy Discharge Instructions[2]	13	54%	75%	75%
Chest Pain/Possible Heart Attack Care				
Aspirin Given Within 24 Hours of Arrival[1]	-	-	97%	96%
Fibrinolytic Meds Within 30 Min. of Arrival[3,7]	-	-	62%	58%
Average Time to ECG (minutes)[1]	-	-	9	7
Average Time to Transfer (minutes)[3,7]	-	-	62	60
Children's Asthma Care				
Received Home Management Plan of Care	-	-	88%	88%
Received Reliever Medication	-	-	100%	100%
Received Systemic Corticosteroids	-	-	100%	100%
Emergency Department				
Admittance Decision Time (minutes)[2]	99	71	125	98
Head CT Results Within 45 Min. of Arrival[7]	-	-	55%	57%
Patients Who Left ER Before Being Seen	11,260	1%	3%	2%
Time from ER Arrival to Admit. (minutes)[2]	99	235	323	274
Time from ER Arrival to Discharge (minutes)	327	143	168	134
Time in ER Before Being Evaluated (minutes)	350	34	29	26
Time to Pain Meds for Fractures (minutes)	16	76	62	57
Heart Attack Care				
Aspirin Given at Discharge[1]	-	-	99%	99%
Fibrinolytic Meds Within 30 Min. of Arrival[7]	-	-	73%	54%
PCI Within 90 Minutes of Arrival[7]	-	-	95%	96%
Statin Prescribed at Discharge[1]	-	-	98%	98%
Heart Failure Care				
ACE Inhibitor or ARB for LVSD	54	96%	97%	97%
Discharge Instructions Given	109	86%	94%	94%
Evaluation of LVS Function	136	99%	99%	99%
Medicare Spending				
Medicare Spending per Patient (ratio)	-	1.07	0.98	0.98
Pneumonia Care				
Appropriate Initial Antibiotic Given[2]	32	91%	97%	95%
Blood Culture Timing[2]	58	100%	98%	98%
Pregnancy and Delivery Care				
Newborn Deliveries Scheduled Early[2]	91	2%	5%	6%
Preventive Care				
Immunization for Influenza[2]	448	91%	89%	90%
Immunization for Pneumonia[2]	366	93%	90%	92%

NOTE: Hospital profiles are in alphabetical order by state, then city, then hospital within the city; Rankings exclude hospitals with less than 25 cases except for patient surveys which excludes hospitals with less than 100 cases; (a) 100-299 cases; (1) The number of cases/patients is too few to report; (2) Data submitted were based on a sample of cases/patients; (3) Results are based on a shorter time period than required; (4) Data suppressed by CMS for one or more quarters; (5) Results are not available for this reporting period; (6) Fewer than 100 patients completed the HCAHPS survey; (7) No cases met the criteria for this measure; (8) The lower limit of the confidence interval cannot be calculated if the number of observed infections equals zero; (9) No data are available from the state/territory for this reporting period; (10) The scores shown reflect fewer than 50 completed surveys; (11) There were discrepancies in the data collection process; (12) This measure does not apply to this hospital for this reporting period; (13) Results cannot be calculated for this reporting period; (14) The results for this state are combined with nearby states to protect confidentiality; Please refer to the User's Guide for a full explanation of data.

Stroke Care				
Anticoagulation Therapy for Atrial Fibrillation[1]	-	-	95%	95%
Antithrombotic Therapy Timing	48	85%	98%	98%
Assessed for Rehabilitation	58	93%	97%	97%
Discharged on Antithrombotic Therapy	53	89%	99%	99%
Discharged on Statin Medication	46	76%	94%	94%
Thrombolytic Therapy Timing[1]	-	-	72%	66%
Venous Thromboembolism Prophylaxis	54	56%	94%	94%
Written Stroke Educational Materials Given	30	70%	87%	88%
Surgical Care Improvement Project				
Appropriate Beta Blocker Usage[2]	41	95%	97%	98%
Appropriate VTP Within 24 Hours[2]	190	98%	98%	98%
Controlled Postoperative Blood Glucose[2,7]	-	-	96%	97%
Perioperative Temperature Management[2]	216	100%	100%	100%
Prophylactic Antibiotic Selection[2]	136	100%	99%	99%
Prophylactic Antibiotic Selection (Outpatient)	13	92%	97%	98%
Prophylactic Antibiotic Stopped[2]	134	98%	98%	98%
Prophylactic Antibiotic Timing[2]	137	97%	99%	99%
Prophylactic Antibiotic Timing (Outpatient)	13	92%	97%	98%
Urinary Catheter Removal[2]	81	96%	97%	97%
Survey of Patients' Hospital Experiences				
Area Around Room 'Always' Quiet at Night	300+	40%	51%	61%
Doctors 'Always' Communicated Well	300+	70%	78%	82%
Home Recovery Information Given	300+	80%	83%	85%
Hospital Given 9 or 10 on 10 Point Scale	300+	58%	68%	71%
Meds 'Always' Explained Before Given	300+	54%	61%	64%
Nurses 'Always' Communicated Well	300+	69%	74%	79%
Pain 'Always' Well Controlled	300+	62%	68%	71%
Room and Bathroom 'Always' Clean	300+	65%	70%	73%
Timely Help 'Always' Received	300+	55%	62%	68%
Would Definitely Recommend Hospital	300+	57%	70%	71%
Use of Medical Imaging				
Cardiac Imaging Stress Test before Surgery[1]	-	-	5.2%	5.3%
Combination Abdominal CT Scan	190	13.7%	13.4%	10.5%
Combination Brain/Sinus CT Scan[1]	-	-	2.2%	2.7%
Combination Chest CT Scan[1]	-	-	2.3%	2.7%
Follow-up Mammogram/Ultrasound	213	8.5%	8.2%	8.8%
Lumbar Spine MRI for Low Back Pain[1]	-	-	34.2%	37.2%

Ronald Reagan UCLA Medical Center

757 Westwood Plaza Phone: 310-825-6301
Los Angeles, CA 90095
URL: www.uclahealth.org
Type: Acute Care Hospitals Emergency Services: Yes
Ownership: Government - State Beds: 581
Key Personnel:
Emergency Room .... Marshall T Morgan

Measure	Cases	This Hosp.	State Avg.	U.S. Avg.
Blood Clot Prevention and Treatment				
Anticoagulation Overlap Therapy[2]	97	81%	92%	93%
ICU Venous Thromboembolism Prophylaxis[2]	115	90%	92%	92%
Incidence of Potentially Preventable VTE[2]	42	21%	11%	10%
UFH with Dosages/Platelet Monitoring[2]	97	98%	96%	97%
Venous Thromboembolism Prophylaxis[2]	285	81%	83%	85%
Warfarin Therapy Discharge Instructions[2]	76	55%	75%	75%
Chest Pain/Possible Heart Attack Care				
Aspirin Given Within 24 Hours of Arrival[1,3]	-	-	97%	96%
Fibrinolytic Meds Within 30 Min. of Arrival[5]	-	-	62%	58%
Average Time to ECG (minutes)[1,3]	-	-	9	7
Average Time to Transfer (minutes)[5]	-	-	62	60
Children's Asthma Care				
Received Home Management Plan of Care	-	-	88%	88%
Received Reliever Medication	-	-	100%	100%
Received Systemic Corticosteroids	-	-	100%	100%
Emergency Department				
Admittance Decision Time (minutes)[2]	484	294	125	98
Head CT Results Within 45 Min. of Arrival[5]	-	-	55%	57%
Patients Who Left ER Before Being Seen	46,302	2%	3%	2%
Time from ER Arrival to Admit. (minutes)[2]	498	527	323	274
Time from ER Arrival to Discharge (minutes)	353	229	168	134
Time in ER Before Being Evaluated (minutes)	411	53	29	26
Time to Pain Meds for Fractures (minutes)	104	59	62	57
Heart Attack Care				
Aspirin Given at Discharge	185	100%	99%	99%
Fibrinolytic Meds Within 30 Min. of Arrival[7]	-	-	73%	54%
PCI Within 90 Minutes of Arrival	35	100%	95%	96%
Statin Prescribed at Discharge	182	100%	98%	98%
Heart Failure Care				
ACE Inhibitor or ARB for LVSD[2]	79	99%	97%	97%
Discharge Instructions Given[2]	250	87%	94%	94%
Evaluation of LVS Function[2]	270	100%	99%	99%
Medicare Spending				
Medicare Spending per Patient (ratio)	-	0.98	0.98	0.98
Pneumonia Care				
Appropriate Initial Antibiotic Given[2]	24	96%	97%	95%
Blood Culture Timing[2]	61	100%	98%	98%
Pregnancy and Delivery Care				
Newborn Deliveries Scheduled Early[2]	12	0%	5%	6%
Preventive Care				
Immunization for Influenza[2]	509	73%	89%	90%
Immunization for Pneumonia[2]	457	75%	90%	92%
Stroke Care				
Anticoagulation Therapy for Atrial Fibrillation[2]	15	87%	95%	95%
Antithrombotic Therapy Timing[2]	45	98%	98%	98%
Assessed for Rehabilitation[2]	92	89%	97%	97%
Discharged on Antithrombotic Therapy[2]	62	100%	99%	99%
Discharged on Statin Medication[2]	58	91%	94%	94%
Thrombolytic Therapy Timing[2]	15	53%	72%	66%
Venous Thromboembolism Prophylaxis[2]	88	77%	94%	94%
Written Stroke Educational Materials Given[2]	52	88%	87%	88%
Surgical Care Improvement Project				
Appropriate Beta Blocker Usage[2]	146	100%	97%	98%
Appropriate VTP Within 24 Hours[2]	290	100%	98%	98%
Controlled Postoperative Blood Glucose[2]	110	96%	96%	97%
Perioperative Temperature Management[2]	387	100%	100%	100%
Prophylactic Antibiotic Selection[2]	269	100%	99%	99%
Prophylactic Antibiotic Selection (Outpatient)	299	95%	97%	98%
Prophylactic Antibiotic Stopped[2]	241	98%	98%	98%
Prophylactic Antibiotic Timing[2]	269	99%	99%	99%
Prophylactic Antibiotic Timing (Outpatient)	302	93%	97%	98%
Urinary Catheter Removal[2]	258	100%	97%	97%
Survey of Patients' Hospital Experiences				
Area Around Room 'Always' Quiet at Night	300+	57%	51%	61%
Doctors 'Always' Communicated Well	300+	77%	78%	82%
Home Recovery Information Given	300+	85%	83%	85%
Hospital Given 9 or 10 on 10 Point Scale	300+	77%	68%	71%
Meds 'Always' Explained Before Given	300+	60%	61%	64%
Nurses 'Always' Communicated Well	300+	72%	74%	79%
Pain 'Always' Well Controlled	300+	66%	68%	71%
Room and Bathroom 'Always' Clean	300+	72%	70%	73%
Timely Help 'Always' Received	300+	61%	62%	68%
Would Definitely Recommend Hospital	300+	79%	70%	71%
Use of Medical Imaging				
Cardiac Imaging Stress Test before Surgery	350	5.1%	5.2%	5.3%
Combination Abdominal CT Scan	1,161	72.0%	13.4%	10.5%
Combination Brain/Sinus CT Scan	497	2.2%	2.2%	2.7%
Combination Chest CT Scan	1,445	3.9%	2.3%	2.7%
Follow-up Mammogram/Ultrasound	2,061	5.4%	8.2%	8.8%
Lumbar Spine MRI for Low Back Pain	144	27.1%	34.2%	37.2%

Saint Vincent Medical Center

2131 W 3rd St Phone: 213-484-7111
Los Angeles, CA 90057 Fax: 213-353-0325
URL: www.stvincent.dochs.org
Type: Acute Care Hospitals Emergency Services: Yes
Ownership: Voluntary non-profit - Church Beds: 131
Key Personnel:
Emergency Room .... Kevin Chamas
Chief of Medical Staff.......... Ronald Fishbach
Pediatric In-Patient Care .... Robin Gaylord
Intensive Care Unit............ Sandy Klatt
Ambulatory Care .... Portia Moore
Patient Relations .... Jody Spector

Measure	Cases	This Hosp.	State Avg.	U.S. Avg.
Blood Clot Prevention and Treatment				
Anticoagulation Overlap Therapy[2]	29	97%	92%	93%
ICU Venous Thromboembolism Prophylaxis[2]	72	97%	92%	92%
Incidence of Potentially Preventable VTE[1,2]	-	-	11%	10%
UFH with Dosages/Platelet Monitoring[2]	17	94%	96%	97%
Venous Thromboembolism Prophylaxis[2]	334	88%	83%	85%
Warfarin Therapy Discharge Instructions[2]	22	82%	75%	75%
Chest Pain/Possible Heart Attack Care				
Aspirin Given Within 24 Hours of Arrival[1,3]	-	-	97%	96%
Fibrinolytic Meds Within 30 Min. of Arrival[3,7]	-	-	62%	58%
Average Time to ECG (minutes)[1,3]	-	-	9	7
Average Time to Transfer (minutes)[3,7]	-	-	62	60
Children's Asthma Care				
Received Home Management Plan of Care	-	-	88%	88%
Received Reliever Medication	-	-	100%	100%
Received Systemic Corticosteroids	-	-	100%	100%
Emergency Department				
Admittance Decision Time (minutes)[2]	697	102	125	98
Head CT Results Within 45 Min. of Arrival[3,7]	-	-	55%	57%
Patients Who Left ER Before Being Seen	15,175	1%	3%	2%
Time from ER Arrival to Admit. (minutes)[2]	703	263	323	274
Time from ER Arrival to Discharge (minutes)	356	139	168	134
Time in ER Before Being Evaluated (minutes)	327	39	29	26
Time to Pain Meds for Fractures (minutes)	48	47	62	57
Heart Attack Care				
Aspirin Given at Discharge	134	100%	99%	99%
Fibrinolytic Meds Within 30 Min. of Arrival[7]	-	-	73%	54%
PCI Within 90 Minutes of Arrival[1]	-	-	95%	96%
Statin Prescribed at Discharge	128	100%	98%	98%
Heart Failure Care				
ACE Inhibitor or ARB for LVSD	108	100%	97%	97%
Discharge Instructions Given	263	92%	94%	94%
Evaluation of LVS Function	310	100%	99%	99%
Medicare Spending				
Medicare Spending per Patient (ratio)	-	1.04	0.98	0.98
Pneumonia Care				
Appropriate Initial Antibiotic Given	100	97%	97%	95%
Blood Culture Timing	197	99%	98%	98%
Pregnancy and Delivery Care				
Newborn Deliveries Scheduled Early[7]	-	-	5%	6%
Preventive Care				
Immunization for Influenza[2]	593	96%	89%	90%
Immunization for Pneumonia[2]	935	97%	90%	92%
Stroke Care				
Anticoagulation Therapy for Atrial Fibrillation	11	100%	95%	95%
Antithrombotic Therapy Timing	66	97%	98%	98%
Assessed for Rehabilitation	68	97%	97%	97%
Discharged on Antithrombotic Therapy	62	98%	99%	99%
Discharged on Statin Medication	48	98%	94%	94%
Thrombolytic Therapy Timing[1]	-	-	72%	66%
Venous Thromboembolism Prophylaxis	73	99%	94%	94%
Written Stroke Educational Materials Given	33	97%	87%	88%
Surgical Care Improvement Project				
Appropriate Beta Blocker Usage[2]	217	99%	97%	98%
Appropriate VTP Within 24 Hours[2]	597	99%	98%	98%
Controlled Postoperative Blood Glucose[2]	78	94%	96%	97%
Perioperative Temperature Management[2]	653	100%	100%	100%
Prophylactic Antibiotic Selection[2]	576	99%	99%	99%
Prophylactic Antibiotic Selection (Outpatient)	212	87%	97%	98%
Prophylactic Antibiotic Stopped[2]	568	99%	98%	98%
Prophylactic Antibiotic Timing[2]	578	99%	99%	99%
Prophylactic Antibiotic Timing (Outpatient)	211	96%	97%	98%
Urinary Catheter Removal[2]	496	100%	97%	97%
Survey of Patients' Hospital Experiences				
Area Around Room 'Always' Quiet at Night	300+	51%	51%	61%
Doctors 'Always' Communicated Well	300+	78%	78%	82%
Home Recovery Information Given	300+	83%	83%	85%
Hospital Given 9 or 10 on 10 Point Scale	300+	69%	68%	71%
Meds 'Always' Explained Before Given	300+	57%	61%	64%
Nurses 'Always' Communicated Well	300+	72%	74%	79%
Pain 'Always' Well Controlled	300+	66%	68%	71%
Room and Bathroom 'Always' Clean	300+	69%	70%	73%
Timely Help 'Always' Received	300+	61%	62%	68%
Would Definitely Recommend Hospital	300+	73%	70%	71%
Use of Medical Imaging				

NOTE: Hospital profiles are in alphabetical order by state, then city, then hospital within the city; Rankings exclude hospitals with less than 25 cases except for patient surveys which excludes hospitals with less than 100 cases; (a) 100-299 cases; (1) The number of cases/patients is too few to report; (2) Data submitted were based on a sample of cases/patients; (3) Results are based on a shorter time period than required; (4) Data suppressed by CMS for one or more quarters; (5) Results are not available for this reporting period; (6) Fewer than 100 patients completed the HCAHPS survey; (7) No cases met the criteria for this measure; (8) The lower limit of the confidence interval cannot be calculated if the number of observed infections equals zero; (9) No data are available from the state/territory for this reporting period; (10) The scores shown reflect fewer than 50 completed surveys; (11) There were discrepancies in the data collection process; (12) This measure does not apply to this hospital for this reporting period; (13) Results cannot be calculated for this reporting period; (14) The results for this state are combined with nearby states to protect confidentiality; Please refer to the User's Guide for a full explanation of data.

Measure	Cases	This Hosp.	State Avg.	U.S. Avg.
Cardiac Imaging Stress Test before Surgery	265	6.4%	5.2%	5.3%
Combination Abdominal CT Scan	495	56.6%	13.4%	10.5%
Combination Brain/Sinus CT Scan	422	4.7%	2.2%	2.7%
Combination Chest CT Scan	263	7.2%	2.3%	2.7%
Follow-up Mammogram/Ultrasound	503	2.4%	8.2%	8.8%
Lumbar Spine MRI for Low Back Pain	69	30.4%	34.2%	37.2%

Silver Lake Medical Center

1711 West Temple Street
Phone: 213-989-6123
Los Angeles, CA 90026
Type: Acute Care Hospitals
Emergency Services: No
Ownership: Proprietary

Measure	Cases	This Hosp.	State Avg.	U.S. Avg.
Blood Clot Prevention and Treatment				
Anticoagulation Overlap Therapy[1,2]	-	-	92%	93%
ICU Venous Thromboembolism Prophylaxis[2]	11	82%	92%	92%
Incidence of Potentially Preventable VTE[1,2]	-	-	11%	10%
UFH with Dosages/Platelet Monitoring[1,2]	-	-	96%	97%
Venous Thromboembolism Prophylaxis[2]	141	43%	83%	85%
Warfarin Therapy Discharge Instructions[1,2]	-	-	75%	75%
Chest Pain/Possible Heart Attack Care				
Aspirin Given Within 24 Hours of Arrival[5]	-	-	97%	96%
Fibrinolytic Meds Within 30 Min. of Arrival[5]	-	-	62%	58%
Average Time to ECG (minutes)[5]	-	-	9	7
Average Time to Transfer (minutes)[5]	-	-	62	60
Children's Asthma Care				
Received Home Management Plan of Care	-	-	88%	88%
Received Reliever Medication	-	-	100%	100%
Received Systemic Corticosteroids	-	-	100%	100%
Emergency Department				
Admittance Decision Time (minutes)[2,7]	-	-	125	98
Head CT Results Within 45 Min. of Arrival[5]	-	-	55%	57%
Patients Who Left ER Before Being Seen[5]	-	-	3%	2%
Time from ER Arrival to Admit. (minutes)[2,7]	-	-	323	274
Time from ER Arrival to Discharge (minutes)[5]	-	-	168	134
Time in ER Before Being Evaluated (minutes)[5]	-	-	29	26
Time to Pain Meds for Fractures (minutes)[5]	-	-	62	57
Heart Attack Care				
Aspirin Given at Discharge[1,3]	-	-	99%	99%
Fibrinolytic Meds Within 30 Min. of Arrival[3,7]	-	-	73%	54%
PCI Within 90 Minutes of Arrival[3,7]	-	-	95%	96%
Statin Prescribed at Discharge[1,3]	-	-	98%	98%
Heart Failure Care				
ACE Inhibitor or ARB for LVSD[1]	-	-	97%	97%
Discharge Instructions Given	29	100%	94%	94%
Evaluation of LVS Function	45	100%	99%	99%
Medicare Spending				
Medicare Spending per Patient (ratio)	-	1.33	0.98	0.98
Pneumonia Care				
Appropriate Initial Antibiotic Given[1]	-	-	97%	95%
Blood Culture Timing[7]	-	-	98%	98%
Pregnancy and Delivery Care				
Newborn Deliveries Scheduled Early[7]	-	-	5%	6%
Preventive Care				
Immunization for Influenza[2]	612	98%	89%	90%
Immunization for Pneumonia[2]	735	97%	90%	92%
Stroke Care				
Anticoagulation Therapy for Atrial Fibrillation[1]	-	-	95%	95%
Antithrombotic Therapy Timing[1]	-	-	98%	98%
Assessed for Rehabilitation[1]	-	-	97%	97%
Discharged on Antithrombotic Therapy[1]	-	-	99%	99%
Discharged on Statin Medication[1]	-	-	94%	94%
Thrombolytic Therapy Timing[7]	-	-	72%	66%
Venous Thromboembolism Prophylaxis[1]	-	-	94%	94%
Written Stroke Educational Materials Given[1]	-	-	87%	88%
Surgical Care Improvement Project				
Appropriate Beta Blocker Usage[1]	-	-	97%	98%
Appropriate VTP Within 24 Hours	19	95%	98%	98%
Controlled Postoperative Blood Glucose[7]	-	-	96%	97%
Perioperative Temperature Management	30	100%	100%	100%
Prophylactic Antibiotic Selection[1]	-	-	99%	99%
Prophylactic Antibiotic Selection (Outpatient)[1]	-	-	97%	98%
Prophylactic Antibiotic Stopped[1]	-	-	98%	98%
Prophylactic Antibiotic Timing[1]	-	-	99%	99%
Prophylactic Antibiotic Timing (Outpatient)[1]	-	-	97%	98%
Urinary Catheter Removal	15	100%	97%	97%
Survey of Patients' Hospital Experiences				
Area Around Room 'Always' Quiet at Night	(a)	51%	51%	61%
Doctors 'Always' Communicated Well	(a)	68%	78%	82%
Home Recovery Information Given	(a)	71%	83%	85%
Hospital Given 9 or 10 on 10 Point Scale	(a)	54%	68%	71%
Meds 'Always' Explained Before Given	(a)	43%	61%	64%
Nurses 'Always' Communicated Well	(a)	61%	74%	79%
Pain 'Always' Well Controlled	(a)	49%	68%	71%
Room and Bathroom 'Always' Clean	(a)	71%	70%	73%
Timely Help 'Always' Received	(a)	36%	62%	68%
Would Definitely Recommend Hospital	(a)	53%	70%	71%
Use of Medical Imaging				
Cardiac Imaging Stress Test before Surgery[7]	-	-	5.2%	5.3%
Combination Abdominal CT Scan[1]	-	-	13.4%	10.5%
Combination Brain/Sinus CT Scan	37	0.0%	2.2%	2.7%
Combination Chest CT Scan[1]	-	-	2.3%	2.7%
Follow-up Mammogram/Ultrasound[7]	-	-	8.2%	8.8%
Lumbar Spine MRI for Low Back Pain[7]	-	-	34.2%	37.2%

Temple Community Hospital

235 N Hoover St
Phone: 213-382-7252
Los Angeles, CA 90004
Fax: 213-389-4559
URL: www.templecommunityhospital.com
Type: Acute Care Hospitals
Emergency Services: No
Ownership: Proprietary
Beds: 170

Key Personnel:

Radiology. . . . . Jimmy Chanbonpi
Intensive Care Unit. . . . . Sonja Hernandez
Anesthesiology. . . . . Keith Jackson
Chief of Medical Staff. . . . . I Y Kim
Infection Control. . . . . Terry McCabe
Operating Room. . . . . Cynthia Milo, RN
CEO/President. . . . . Herbert Needman
Quality Assurance . . . . Annika Nowlin

Measure	Cases	This Hosp.	State Avg.	U.S. Avg.
Blood Clot Prevention and Treatment				
Anticoagulation Overlap Therapy[1,2]	-	-	92%	93%
ICU Venous Thromboembolism Prophylaxis[2]	56	88%	92%	92%
Incidence of Potentially Preventable VTE[1,2]	-	-	11%	10%
UFH with Dosages/Platelet Monitoring[1,2]	-	-	96%	97%
Venous Thromboembolism Prophylaxis[2]	232	100%	83%	85%
Warfarin Therapy Discharge Instructions[1,2]	-	-	75%	75%
Chest Pain/Possible Heart Attack Care				
Aspirin Given Within 24 Hours of Arrival[5]	-	-	97%	96%
Fibrinolytic Meds Within 30 Min. of Arrival[5]	-	-	62%	58%
Average Time to ECG (minutes)[5]	-	-	9	7
Average Time to Transfer (minutes)[5]	-	-	62	60
Children's Asthma Care				
Received Home Management Plan of Care	-	-	88%	88%
Received Reliever Medication	-	-	100%	100%
Received Systemic Corticosteroids	-	-	100%	100%
Emergency Department				
Admittance Decision Time (minutes)[2,7]	-	-	125	98
Head CT Results Within 45 Min. of Arrival[5]	-	-	55%	57%
Patients Who Left ER Before Being Seen[5]	-	-	3%	2%
Time from ER Arrival to Admit. (minutes)[2,7]	-	-	323	274
Time from ER Arrival to Discharge (minutes)[5]	-	-	168	134
Time in ER Before Being Evaluated (minutes)[5]	-	-	29	26
Time to Pain Meds for Fractures (minutes)[5]	-	-	62	57
Heart Attack Care				
Aspirin Given at Discharge	13	100%	99%	99%
Fibrinolytic Meds Within 30 Min. of Arrival[7]	-	-	73%	54%
PCI Within 90 Minutes of Arrival[7]	-	-	95%	96%
Statin Prescribed at Discharge	13	100%	98%	98%
Heart Failure Care				
ACE Inhibitor or ARB for LVSD	27	100%	97%	97%
Discharge Instructions Given	33	100%	94%	94%
Evaluation of LVS Function	62	100%	99%	99%
Medicare Spending				
Medicare Spending per Patient (ratio)	-	1.38	0.98	0.98
Pneumonia Care				
Appropriate Initial Antibiotic Given[1]	-	-	97%	95%
Blood Culture Timing[7]	-	-	98%	98%
Pregnancy and Delivery Care				
Newborn Deliveries Scheduled Early[7]	-	-	5%	6%
Preventive Care				
Immunization for Influenza[2]	295	100%	89%	90%
Immunization for Pneumonia[2]	419	100%	90%	92%
Stroke Care				
Anticoagulation Therapy for Atrial Fibrillation[1]	-	-	95%	95%
Antithrombotic Therapy Timing	52	100%	98%	98%
Assessed for Rehabilitation	60	100%	97%	97%
Discharged on Antithrombotic Therapy	54	100%	99%	99%
Discharged on Statin Medication	38	100%	94%	94%
Thrombolytic Therapy Timing[7]	-	-	72%	66%
Venous Thromboembolism Prophylaxis	63	100%	94%	94%
Written Stroke Educational Materials Given	30	100%	87%	88%
Surgical Care Improvement Project				
Appropriate Beta Blocker Usage[1]	-	-	97%	98%
Appropriate VTP Within 24 Hours	40	100%	98%	98%
Controlled Postoperative Blood Glucose[7]	-	-	96%	97%
Perioperative Temperature Management	43	100%	100%	100%
Prophylactic Antibiotic Selection	17	94%	99%	99%
Prophylactic Antibiotic Selection (Outpatient)	33	100%	97%	98%
Prophylactic Antibiotic Stopped	15	100%	98%	98%
Prophylactic Antibiotic Timing	17	100%	99%	99%
Prophylactic Antibiotic Timing (Outpatient)	32	100%	97%	98%
Urinary Catheter Removal	35	100%	97%	97%
Survey of Patients' Hospital Experiences				
Area Around Room 'Always' Quiet at Night	(a)	67%	51%	61%
Doctors 'Always' Communicated Well	(a)	82%	78%	82%
Home Recovery Information Given	(a)	79%	83%	85%
Hospital Given 9 or 10 on 10 Point Scale	(a)	55%	68%	71%
Meds 'Always' Explained Before Given	(a)	64%	61%	64%
Nurses 'Always' Communicated Well	(a)	73%	74%	79%
Pain 'Always' Well Controlled	(a)	61%	68%	71%
Room and Bathroom 'Always' Clean	(a)	72%	70%	73%
Timely Help 'Always' Received	(a)	69%	62%	68%
Would Definitely Recommend Hospital	(a)	55%	70%	71%
Use of Medical Imaging				
Cardiac Imaging Stress Test before Surgery[1]	-	-	5.2%	5.3%
Combination Abdominal CT Scan[1]	-	-	13.4%	10.5%
Combination Brain/Sinus CT Scan[1]	-	-	2.2%	2.7%
Combination Chest CT Scan[1]	-	-	2.3%	2.7%
Follow-up Mammogram/Ultrasound[7]	-	-	8.2%	8.8%
Lumbar Spine MRI for Low Back Pain[7]	-	-	34.2%	37.2%

USC Kenneth Norris Jr Cancer Hospital

1441 Eastlake Ave
Phone: 323-865-3000
Los Angeles, CA 90089
Fax: 323-865-3868
Type: Acute Care Hospitals
Emergency Services: No
Ownership: Voluntary non-profit - Other
Beds: 60

Key Personnel:

Infection Control. . . . . Victor Farez
CEO/President. . . . . Trevor Fetter
Cardiac Laboratory. . . . . Marvyn Kalman
Quality Assurance . . . . Tavone Dalebou Richardson
Radiology. . . . . Oscar Streeter, MD

Measure	Cases	This Hosp.	State Avg.	U.S. Avg.
Blood Clot Prevention and Treatment				
Anticoagulation Overlap Therapy[5]	-	-	92%	93%
ICU Venous Thromboembolism Prophylaxis[5]	-	-	92%	92%
Incidence of Potentially Preventable VTE[5]	-	-	11%	10%
UFH with Dosages/Platelet Monitoring[5]	-	-	96%	97%
Venous Thromboembolism Prophylaxis[5]	-	-	83%	85%
Warfarin Therapy Discharge Instructions[5]	-	-	75%	75%
Chest Pain/Possible Heart Attack Care				
Aspirin Given Within 24 Hours of Arrival	-	-	97%	96%
Fibrinolytic Meds Within 30 Min. of Arrival	-	-	62%	58%
Average Time to ECG (minutes)	-	-	9	7
Average Time to Transfer (minutes)	-	-	62	60
Children's Asthma Care				
Received Home Management Plan of Care	-	-	88%	88%

NOTE: Hospital profiles are in alphabetical order by state, then city, then hospital within the city; Rankings exclude hospitals with less than 25 cases except for patient surveys which excludes hospitals with less than 100 cases; (a) 100-299 cases; (1) The number of cases/patients is too few to report; (2) Data submitted were based on a sample of cases/patients; (3) Results are based on a shorter time period than required; (4) Data suppressed by CMS for one or more quarters; (5) Results are not available for this reporting period; (6) Fewer than 100 patients completed the HCAHPS survey; (7) No cases met the criteria for this measure; (8) The lower limit of the confidence interval cannot be calculated if the number of observed infections equals zero; (9) No data are available from the state/territory for this reporting period; (10) The scores shown reflect fewer than 50 completed surveys; (11) There were discrepancies in the data collection process; (12) This measure does not apply to this hospital for this reporting period; (13) Results cannot be calculated for this reporting period; (14) The results for this state are combined with nearby states to protect confidentiality; Please refer to the User's Guide for a full explanation of data.

Received Reliever Medication	-	-	100%	100%
Received Systemic Corticosteroids	-	-	100%	100%
Emergency Department				
Admittance Decision Time (minutes)[5]	-	-	125	98
Head CT Results Within 45 Min. of Arrival	-	-	55%	57%
Patients Who Left ER Before Being Seen	-	-	3%	2%
Time from ER Arrival to Admit. (minutes)[5]	-	-	323	274
Time from ER Arrival to Discharge (minutes)	-	-	168	134
Time in ER Before Being Evaluated (minutes)	-	-	29	26
Time to Pain Meds for Fractures (minutes)	-	-	62	57
Heart Attack Care				
Aspirin Given at Discharge[5]	-	-	99%	99%
Fibrinolytic Meds Within 30 Min. of Arrival[5]	-	-	73%	54%
PCI Within 90 Minutes of Arrival[5]	-	-	95%	96%
Statin Prescribed at Discharge[5]	-	-	98%	98%
Heart Failure Care				
ACE Inhibitor or ARB for LVSD[5]	-	-	97%	97%
Discharge Instructions Given[5]	-	-	94%	94%
Evaluation of LVS Function[5]	-	-	99%	99%
Medicare Spending				
Medicare Spending per Patient (ratio)	-	-	0.98	0.98
Pneumonia Care				
Appropriate Initial Antibiotic Given[5]	-	-	97%	95%
Blood Culture Timing[5]	-	-	98%	98%
Pregnancy and Delivery Care				
Newborn Deliveries Scheduled Early[5]	-	-	5%	6%
Preventive Care				
Immunization for Influenza[5]	-	-	89%	90%
Immunization for Pneumonia[5]	-	-	90%	92%
Stroke Care				
Anticoagulation Therapy for Atrial Fibrillation[5]	-	-	95%	95%
Antithrombotic Therapy Timing[5]	-	-	98%	98%
Assessed for Rehabilitation[5]	-	-	97%	97%
Discharged on Antithrombotic Therapy[5]	-	-	99%	99%
Discharged on Statin Medication[5]	-	-	94%	94%
Thrombolytic Therapy Timing[5]	-	-	72%	66%
Venous Thromboembolism Prophylaxis[5]	-	-	94%	94%
Written Stroke Educational Materials Given[5]	-	-	87%	88%
Surgical Care Improvement Project				
Appropriate Beta Blocker Usage[5]	-	-	97%	98%
Appropriate VTP Within 24 Hours[5]	-	-	98%	98%
Controlled Postoperative Blood Glucose[5]	-	-	96%	97%
Perioperative Temperature Management[5]	-	-	100%	100%
Prophylactic Antibiotic Selection[5]	-	-	99%	99%
Prophylactic Antibiotic Selection (Outpatient)	-	-	97%	98%
Prophylactic Antibiotic Stopped[5]	-	-	98%	98%
Prophylactic Antibiotic Timing[5]	-	-	99%	99%
Prophylactic Antibiotic Timing (Outpatient)	-	-	97%	98%
Urinary Catheter Removal[5]	-	-	97%	97%
Survey of Patients' Hospital Experiences				
Area Around Room 'Always' Quiet at Night[5]	-	-	51%	61%
Doctors 'Always' Communicated Well[5]	-	-	78%	82%
Home Recovery Information Given[5]	-	-	83%	85%
Hospital Given 9 or 10 on 10 Point Scale[5]	-	-	68%	71%
Meds 'Always' Explained Before Given[5]	-	-	61%	64%
Nurses 'Always' Communicated Well[5]	-	-	74%	79%
Pain 'Always' Well Controlled[5]	-	-	68%	71%
Room and Bathroom 'Always' Clean[5]	-	-	70%	73%
Timely Help 'Always' Received[5]	-	-	62%	68%
Would Definitely Recommend Hospital[5]	-	-	70%	71%
Use of Medical Imaging				
Cardiac Imaging Stress Test before Surgery	-	-	5.2%	5.3%
Combination Abdominal CT Scan	-	-	13.4%	10.5%
Combination Brain/Sinus CT Scan	-	-	2.2%	2.7%
Combination Chest CT Scan	-	-	2.3%	2.7%
Follow-up Mammogram/Ultrasound	-	-	8.2%	8.8%
Lumbar Spine MRI for Low Back Pain	-	-	34.2%	37.2%

White Memorial Medical Center

1720 E Cesar Avenue Phone: 323-268-5000
Los Angeles, CA 90033 Fax: 323-881-8605
URL: www.whitememorial.com
Type: Acute Care Hospitals Emergency Services: Yes
Ownership: Voluntary non-profit - Church Beds: 369

Key Personnel:
Infection Control. . . . . Rebecca Berberian
Pediatric In-Patient Care . . . . Anne Marie Floyd
Coronary Care . . . . Diane Freeman
Pediatric Ambulatory Care . . . . . . Anthony Hirsch, MD
Chief of Medical Staff. . . . . Brian D Johnston, MD
Quality Assurance . . . . Sue LaPisto
Radiology. . . . . Michael Neglio, MD
CEO/President. . . . . Beth D Zachary, FACHE

Measure	Cases	This Hosp.	State Avg.	U.S. Avg.
Blood Clot Prevention and Treatment				
Anticoagulation Overlap Therapy[2]	39	90%	92%	93%
ICU Venous Thromboembolism Prophylaxis[2]	55	84%	92%	92%
Incidence of Potentially Preventable VTE[2]	18	44%	11%	10%
UFH with Dosages/Platelet Monitoring[2]	23	100%	96%	97%
Venous Thromboembolism Prophylaxis[2]	298	52%	83%	85%
Warfarin Therapy Discharge Instructions[2]	24	100%	75%	75%
Chest Pain/Possible Heart Attack Care				
Aspirin Given Within 24 Hours of Arrival	12	100%	97%	96%
Fibrinolytic Meds Within 30 Min. of Arrival[3,7]	-	-	62%	58%
Average Time to ECG (minutes)	13	9	9	7
Average Time to Transfer (minutes)[3,7]	-	-	62	60
Children's Asthma Care				
Received Home Management Plan of Care	-	-	88%	88%
Received Reliever Medication	-	-	100%	100%
Received Systemic Corticosteroids	-	-	100%	100%
Emergency Department				
Admittance Decision Time (minutes)[2]	478	212	125	98
Head CT Results Within 45 Min. of Arrival	15	87%	55%	57%
Patients Who Left ER Before Being Seen	52,835	2%	3%	2%
Time from ER Arrival to Admit. (minutes)[2]	494	418	323	274
Time from ER Arrival to Discharge (minutes)	367	259	168	134
Time in ER Before Being Evaluated (minutes)	397	32	29	26
Time to Pain Meds for Fractures (minutes)	80	108	62	57
Heart Attack Care				
Aspirin Given at Discharge	251	97%	99%	99%
Fibrinolytic Meds Within 30 Min. of Arrival[7]	-	-	73%	54%
PCI Within 90 Minutes of Arrival	41	90%	95%	96%
Statin Prescribed at Discharge	254	98%	98%	98%
Heart Failure Care				
ACE Inhibitor or ARB for LVSD	138	97%	97%	97%
Discharge Instructions Given	288	100%	94%	94%
Evaluation of LVS Function	332	98%	99%	99%
Medicare Spending				
Medicare Spending per Patient (ratio)	-	1.08	0.98	0.98
Pneumonia Care				
Appropriate Initial Antibiotic Given	102	93%	97%	95%
Blood Culture Timing	249	96%	98%	98%
Pregnancy and Delivery Care				
Newborn Deliveries Scheduled Early[2]	72	1%	5%	6%
Preventive Care				
Immunization for Influenza[2]	530	57%	89%	90%
Immunization for Pneumonia[2]	638	74%	90%	92%
Stroke Care				
Anticoagulation Therapy for Atrial Fibrillation	17	100%	95%	95%
Antithrombotic Therapy Timing	134	99%	98%	98%
Assessed for Rehabilitation	187	99%	97%	97%
Discharged on Antithrombotic Therapy	153	100%	99%	99%
Discharged on Statin Medication	123	99%	94%	94%
Thrombolytic Therapy Timing	30	100%	72%	66%
Venous Thromboembolism Prophylaxis	207	99%	94%	94%
Written Stroke Educational Materials Given	81	100%	87%	88%
Surgical Care Improvement Project				
Appropriate Beta Blocker Usage[2]	181	94%	97%	98%
Appropriate VTP Within 24 Hours[2]	450	98%	98%	98%
Controlled Postoperative Blood Glucose[2]	50	100%	96%	97%
Perioperative Temperature Management[2]	527	100%	100%	100%
Prophylactic Antibiotic Selection[2]	373	100%	99%	99%
Prophylactic Antibiotic Selection (Outpatient)	211	96%	97%	98%
Prophylactic Antibiotic Stopped[2]	354	98%	98%	98%
Prophylactic Antibiotic Timing[2]	374	97%	99%	99%
Prophylactic Antibiotic Timing (Outpatient)	211	99%	97%	98%
Urinary Catheter Removal[2]	357	97%	97%	97%
Survey of Patients' Hospital Experiences				
Area Around Room 'Always' Quiet at Night	300+	56%	51%	61%
Doctors 'Always' Communicated Well	300+	82%	78%	82%
Home Recovery Information Given	300+	84%	83%	85%
Hospital Given 9 or 10 on 10 Point Scale	300+	77%	68%	71%
Meds 'Always' Explained Before Given	300+	62%	61%	64%
Nurses 'Always' Communicated Well	300+	79%	74%	79%
Pain 'Always' Well Controlled	300+	74%	68%	71%
Room and Bathroom 'Always' Clean	300+	71%	70%	73%
Timely Help 'Always' Received	300+	63%	62%	68%
Would Definitely Recommend Hospital	300+	79%	70%	71%
Use of Medical Imaging				
Cardiac Imaging Stress Test before Surgery	86	5.8%	5.2%	5.3%
Combination Abdominal CT Scan	444	23.2%	13.4%	10.5%
Combination Brain/Sinus CT Scan	671	1.5%	2.2%	2.7%
Combination Chest CT Scan	202	0.5%	2.3%	2.7%
Follow-up Mammogram/Ultrasound	902	9.4%	8.2%	8.8%
Lumbar Spine MRI for Low Back Pain	121	28.1%	34.2%	37.2%

Memorial Hospital Los Banos

520 West I St Phone: 209-826-0591
Los Banos, CA 93635 Fax: 209-826-1943
E-mail: mhalosbanos@sutterhealth.org
URL: www.memoriallosbanos.org
Type: Acute Care Hospitals Emergency Services: Yes
Ownership: Voluntary non-profit - Private Beds: 48

Key Personnel:
Operating Room. . . . . Francisco A Alonso, RN
Coronary Care . . . . Susan Benson, RN
Radiology. . . . . David Board
Chief of Medical Staff. . . . . Daniel Hardy, MD
CEO/President. . . . . Richard S Liszewski
Quality Assurance . . . . Shari Lock, RN
Infection Control. . . . . Carolyn Nazabal, RN
Pediatric In-Patient Care . . . . Misty Warthy, RN

Measure	Cases	This Hosp.	State Avg.	U.S. Avg.
Blood Clot Prevention and Treatment				
Anticoagulation Overlap Therapy[1]	-	-	92%	93%
ICU Venous Thromboembolism Prophylaxis	35	94%	92%	92%
Incidence of Potentially Preventable VTE[7]	-	-	11%	10%
UFH with Dosages/Platelet Monitoring[1]	-	-	96%	97%
Venous Thromboembolism Prophylaxis	272	89%	83%	85%
Warfarin Therapy Discharge Instructions[1]	-	-	75%	75%
Chest Pain/Possible Heart Attack Care				
Aspirin Given Within 24 Hours of Arrival	38	97%	97%	96%
Fibrinolytic Meds Within 30 Min. of Arrival[1,3]	-	-	62%	58%
Average Time to ECG (minutes)	40	10	9	7
Average Time to Transfer (minutes)[1,3]	-	-	62	60
Children's Asthma Care				
Received Home Management Plan of Care	-	-	88%	88%
Received Reliever Medication	-	-	100%	100%
Received Systemic Corticosteroids	-	-	100%	100%
Emergency Department				
Admittance Decision Time (minutes)[2]	152	68	125	98
Head CT Results Within 45 Min. of Arrival	51	27%	55%	57%
Patients Who Left ER Before Being Seen	25,285	4%	3%	2%
Time from ER Arrival to Admit. (minutes)[2]	161	290	323	274
Time from ER Arrival to Discharge (minutes)	381	120	168	134
Time in ER Before Being Evaluated (minutes)	410	31	29	26
Time to Pain Meds for Fractures (minutes)	98	58	62	57
Heart Attack Care				
Aspirin Given at Discharge[3,7]	-	-	99%	99%
Fibrinolytic Meds Within 30 Min. of Arrival[3,7]	-	-	73%	54%
PCI Within 90 Minutes of Arrival[3,7]	-	-	95%	96%
Statin Prescribed at Discharge[3,7]	-	-	98%	98%
Heart Failure Care				
ACE Inhibitor or ARB for LVSD[1,3]	-	-	97%	97%
Discharge Instructions Given[3]	13	100%	94%	94%
Evaluation of LVS Function[3]	18	100%	99%	99%

NOTE: Hospital profiles are in alphabetical order by state, then city, then hospital within the city; Rankings exclude hospitals with less than 25 cases except for patient surveys which excludes hospitals with less than 100 cases; (a) 100-299 cases; (1) The number of cases/patients is too few to report; (2) Data submitted were based on a sample of cases/patients; (3) Results are based on a shorter time period than required; (4) Data suppressed by CMS for one or more quarters; (5) Results are not available for this reporting period; (6) Fewer than 100 patients completed the HCAHPS survey; (7) No cases met the criteria for this measure; (8) The lower limit of the confidence interval cannot be calculated if the number of observed infections equals zero; (9) No data are available from the state/territory for this reporting period; (10) The scores shown reflect fewer than 50 completed surveys; (11) There were discrepancies in the data collection process; (12) This measure does not apply to this hospital for this reporting period; (13) Results cannot be calculated for this reporting period; (14) The results for this state are combined with nearby states to protect confidentiality; Please refer to the User's Guide for a full explanation of data.

Measure	Cases	This Hosp.	State Avg.	U.S. Avg.
Medicare Spending				
Medicare Spending per Patient (ratio)	-	0.93	0.98	0.98
Pneumonia Care				
Appropriate Initial Antibiotic Given	26	100%	97%	95%
Blood Culture Timing	45	100%	98%	98%
Pregnancy and Delivery Care				
Newborn Deliveries Scheduled Early	99	0%	5%	6%
Preventive Care				
Immunization for Influenza[2]	210	100%	89%	90%
Immunization for Pneumonia[2]	117	100%	90%	92%
Stroke Care				
Anticoagulation Therapy for Atrial Fibrillation[7]	-	-	95%	95%
Antithrombotic Therapy Timing[7]	-	-	98%	98%
Assessed for Rehabilitation[1]	-	-	97%	97%
Discharged on Antithrombotic Therapy[7]	-	-	99%	99%
Discharged on Statin Medication[1]	-	-	94%	94%
Thrombolytic Therapy Timing[7]	-	-	72%	66%
Venous Thromboembolism Prophylaxis[1]	-	-	94%	94%
Written Stroke Educational Materials Given[7]	-	-	87%	88%
Surgical Care Improvement Project				
Appropriate Beta Blocker Usage[1]	-	-	97%	98%
Appropriate VTP Within 24 Hours	16	100%	98%	98%
Controlled Postoperative Blood Glucose[7]	-	-	96%	97%
Perioperative Temperature Management	25	100%	100%	100%
Prophylactic Antibiotic Selection	12	100%	99%	99%
Prophylactic Antibiotic Selection (Outpatient)	55	93%	97%	98%
Prophylactic Antibiotic Stopped	11	100%	98%	98%
Prophylactic Antibiotic Timing	12	100%	99%	99%
Prophylactic Antibiotic Timing (Outpatient)	56	98%	97%	98%
Urinary Catheter Removal[1]	-	-	97%	97%
Survey of Patients' Hospital Experiences				
Area Around Room 'Always' Quiet at Night	(a)	61%	51%	61%
Doctors 'Always' Communicated Well	(a)	80%	78%	82%
Home Recovery Information Given	(a)	85%	83%	85%
Hospital Given 9 or 10 on 10 Point Scale	(a)	74%	68%	71%
Meds 'Always' Explained Before Given	(a)	63%	61%	64%
Nurses 'Always' Communicated Well	(a)	80%	74%	79%
Pain 'Always' Well Controlled	(a)	74%	68%	71%
Room and Bathroom 'Always' Clean	(a)	85%	70%	73%
Timely Help 'Always' Received	(a)	71%	62%	68%
Would Definitely Recommend Hospital	(a)	70%	70%	71%
Use of Medical Imaging				
Cardiac Imaging Stress Test before Surgery[1]	-	-	5.2%	5.3%
Combination Abdominal CT Scan	309	3.2%	13.4%	10.5%
Combination Brain/Sinus CT Scan	349	1.4%	2.2%	2.7%
Combination Chest CT Scan	120	2.5%	2.3%	2.7%
Follow-up Mammogram/Ultrasound	263	8.0%	8.2%	8.8%
Lumbar Spine MRI for Low Back Pain[1]	-	-	34.2%	37.2%

Saint Francis Medical Center

3630 East Imperial Highway
Lynwood, CA 90262
Phone: 310-900-8900
Fax: 310-604-0864
URL: www.stfrancis.dochs.org
Type: Acute Care Hospitals
Emergency Services: Yes
Ownership: Voluntary non-profit - Church
Beds: 328

Key Personnel:

Quality Assurance . . . . Marsha Chan
Operating Room. . . . . Karen Karnott
CEO/President. . . . . Gerald Kozai
Pediatric Ambulatory Care . . . . . . Andy Moosa
Pediatric In-Patient Care . . . . Andy Moosa
Radiology. . . . . Dan Schimmel
Chief of Medical Staff. . . . . Jose Stiwak
Infection Control. . . . . Ana Torres

Measure	Cases	This Hosp.	State Avg.	U.S. Avg.
Blood Clot Prevention and Treatment				
Anticoagulation Overlap Therapy[2]	82	88%	92%	93%
ICU Venous Thromboembolism Prophylaxis[2]	73	77%	92%	92%
Incidence of Potentially Preventable VTE[2]	22	9%	11%	10%
UFH with Dosages/Platelet Monitoring[2]	30	100%	96%	97%
Venous Thromboembolism Prophylaxis[2]	261	73%	83%	85%
Warfarin Therapy Discharge Instructions[2]	62	50%	75%	75%
Chest Pain/Possible Heart Attack Care				
Aspirin Given Within 24 Hours of Arrival	59	92%	97%	96%
Fibrinolytic Meds Within 30 Min. of Arrival[7]	-	-	62%	58%
Average Time to ECG (minutes)	61	12	9	7
Average Time to Transfer (minutes)[1]	-	-	62	60
Children's Asthma Care				
Received Home Management Plan of Care	53	91%	88%	88%
Received Reliever Medication	55	100%	100%	100%
Received Systemic Corticosteroids	55	100%	100%	100%
Emergency Department				
Admittance Decision Time (minutes)[2]	422	147	125	98
Head CT Results Within 45 Min. of Arrival[1]	-	-	55%	57%
Patients Who Left ER Before Being Seen	73,135	6%	3%	2%
Time from ER Arrival to Admit. (minutes)[2]	423	462	323	274
Time from ER Arrival to Discharge (minutes)	399	275	168	134
Time in ER Before Being Evaluated (minutes)	436	106	29	26
Time to Pain Meds for Fractures (minutes)	245	142	62	57
Heart Attack Care				
Aspirin Given at Discharge	111	98%	99%	99%
Fibrinolytic Meds Within 30 Min. of Arrival[7]	-	-	73%	54%
PCI Within 90 Minutes of Arrival[7]	-	-	95%	96%
Statin Prescribed at Discharge	117	98%	98%	98%
Heart Failure Care				
ACE Inhibitor or ARB for LVSD	231	100%	97%	97%
Discharge Instructions Given	441	79%	94%	94%
Evaluation of LVS Function	509	100%	99%	99%
Medicare Spending				
Medicare Spending per Patient (ratio)	-	1.07	0.98	0.98
Pneumonia Care				
Appropriate Initial Antibiotic Given	104	97%	97%	95%
Blood Culture Timing	187	96%	98%	98%
Pregnancy and Delivery Care				
Newborn Deliveries Scheduled Early[2]	108	5%	5%	6%
Preventive Care				
Immunization for Influenza[2]	459	92%	89%	90%
Immunization for Pneumonia[2]	335	90%	90%	92%
Stroke Care				
Anticoagulation Therapy for Atrial Fibrillation[1,2]	-	-	95%	95%
Antithrombotic Therapy Timing[2]	76	95%	98%	98%
Assessed for Rehabilitation[2]	97	81%	97%	97%
Discharged on Antithrombotic Therapy[2]	79	99%	99%	99%
Discharged on Statin Medication[2]	70	69%	94%	94%
Thrombolytic Therapy Timing[1,2]	-	-	72%	66%
Venous Thromboembolism Prophylaxis[2]	111	68%	94%	94%
Written Stroke Educational Materials Given[2]	56	38%	87%	88%
Surgical Care Improvement Project				
Appropriate Beta Blocker Usage[2]	78	91%	97%	98%
Appropriate VTP Within 24 Hours[2]	250	98%	98%	98%
Controlled Postoperative Blood Glucose[2]	35	91%	96%	97%
Perioperative Temperature Management[2]	284	100%	100%	100%
Prophylactic Antibiotic Selection[2]	182	99%	99%	99%
Prophylactic Antibiotic Selection (Outpatient)	115	92%	97%	98%
Prophylactic Antibiotic Stopped[2]	154	97%	98%	98%
Prophylactic Antibiotic Timing[2]	182	98%	99%	99%
Prophylactic Antibiotic Timing (Outpatient)	125	82%	97%	98%
Urinary Catheter Removal[2]	104	95%	97%	97%
Survey of Patients' Hospital Experiences				
Area Around Room 'Always' Quiet at Night	300+	59%	51%	61%
Doctors 'Always' Communicated Well	300+	71%	78%	82%
Home Recovery Information Given	300+	82%	83%	85%
Hospital Given 9 or 10 on 10 Point Scale	300+	69%	68%	71%
Meds 'Always' Explained Before Given	300+	56%	61%	64%
Nurses 'Always' Communicated Well	300+	70%	74%	79%
Pain 'Always' Well Controlled	300+	64%	68%	71%
Room and Bathroom 'Always' Clean	300+	67%	70%	73%
Timely Help 'Always' Received	300+	59%	62%	68%
Would Definitely Recommend Hospital	300+	66%	70%	71%
Use of Medical Imaging				
Cardiac Imaging Stress Test before Surgery	81	3.7%	5.2%	5.3%
Combination Abdominal CT Scan	411	16.1%	13.4%	10.5%
Combination Brain/Sinus CT Scan[1]	-	-	2.2%	2.7%
Combination Chest CT Scan	139	0.7%	2.3%	2.7%
Follow-up Mammogram/Ultrasound	504	6.0%	8.2%	8.8%
Lumbar Spine MRI for Low Back Pain[1]	-	-	34.2%	37.2%

Madera Community Hospital

1250 E Almond Ave
Madera, CA 93637
Phone: 559-675-5555
Fax: 559-675-5509
E-mail: rkelley@maderahospital.org
URL: www.maderahospital.org
Type: Acute Care Hospitals
Emergency Services: Yes
Ownership: Voluntary non-profit - Other
Beds: 106

Key Personnel:

Operating Room. . . . . Muhammad Anwar, RN
Intensive Care Unit. . . . . Pat Ash
Patient Relations . . . . Mary Farrell
CEO/President. . . . . John W Frye, JR
Chief of Medical Staff . . . . Todd Spencer
Radiology. . . . . Todd Spencer
Quality Assurance . . . . Bettie Timmons
Emergency Room . . . . Robert Toman

Measure	Cases	This Hosp.	State Avg.	U.S. Avg.
Blood Clot Prevention and Treatment				
Anticoagulation Overlap Therapy[2]	18	50%	92%	93%
ICU Venous Thromboembolism Prophylaxis[2]	59	75%	92%	92%
Incidence of Potentially Preventable VTE[1,2]	-	-	11%	10%
UFH with Dosages/Platelet Monitoring[2]	11	100%	96%	97%
Venous Thromboembolism Prophylaxis[2]	392	62%	83%	85%
Warfarin Therapy Discharge Instructions[2]	18	100%	75%	75%
Chest Pain/Possible Heart Attack Care				
Aspirin Given Within 24 Hours of Arrival	20	100%	97%	96%
Fibrinolytic Meds Within 30 Min. of Arrival[3,7]	-	-	62%	58%
Average Time to ECG (minutes)	20	20	9	7
Average Time to Transfer (minutes)[1,3]	-	-	62	60
Children's Asthma Care				
Received Home Management Plan of Care	-	-	88%	88%
Received Reliever Medication	-	-	100%	100%
Received Systemic Corticosteroids	-	-	100%	100%
Emergency Department				
Admittance Decision Time (minutes)[2]	805	225	125	98
Head CT Results Within 45 Min. of Arrival[1]	-	-	55%	57%
Patients Who Left ER Before Being Seen	44,006	2%	3%	2%
Time from ER Arrival to Admit. (minutes)[2]	807	487	323	274
Time from ER Arrival to Discharge (minutes)	542	178	168	134
Time in ER Before Being Evaluated (minutes)	606	35	29	26
Time to Pain Meds for Fractures (minutes)	113	65	62	57
Heart Attack Care				
Aspirin Given at Discharge[2]	36	97%	99%	99%
Fibrinolytic Meds Within 30 Min. of Arrival[2,7]	-	-	73%	54%
PCI Within 90 Minutes of Arrival[2,7]	-	-	95%	96%
Statin Prescribed at Discharge[2]	36	75%	98%	98%
Heart Failure Care				
ACE Inhibitor or ARB for LVSD	54	89%	97%	97%
Discharge Instructions Given	67	94%	94%	94%
Evaluation of LVS Function	94	94%	99%	99%
Medicare Spending				
Medicare Spending per Patient (ratio)	-	1.01	0.98	0.98
Pneumonia Care				
Appropriate Initial Antibiotic Given	64	91%	97%	95%
Blood Culture Timing	76	99%	98%	98%
Pregnancy and Delivery Care				
Newborn Deliveries Scheduled Early	310	6%	5%	6%
Preventive Care				
Immunization for Influenza[2]	817	95%	89%	90%
Immunization for Pneumonia[2]	773	97%	90%	92%
Stroke Care				
Anticoagulation Therapy for Atrial Fibrillation[1,2]	-	-	95%	95%
Antithrombotic Therapy Timing[2]	16	69%	98%	98%
Assessed for Rehabilitation[2]	15	87%	97%	97%
Discharged on Antithrombotic Therapy[2]	13	69%	99%	99%
Discharged on Statin Medication[2]	14	86%	94%	94%
Thrombolytic Therapy Timing[1,2]	-	-	72%	66%
Venous Thromboembolism Prophylaxis[2]	16	44%	94%	94%
Written Stroke Educational Materials Given[1,2]	-	-	87%	88%
Surgical Care Improvement Project				
Appropriate Beta Blocker Usage	31	94%	97%	98%
Appropriate VTP Within 24 Hours	164	80%	98%	98%
Controlled Postoperative Blood Glucose[7]	-	-	96%	97%
Perioperative Temperature Management	183	98%	100%	100%

NOTE: Hospital profiles are in alphabetical order by state, then city, then hospital within the city; Rankings exclude hospitals with less than 25 cases except for patient surveys which excludes hospitals with less than 100 cases; (a) 100-299 cases; (1) The number of cases/patients is too few to report; (2) Data submitted were based on a sample of cases/patients; (3) Results are based on a shorter time period than required; (4) Data suppressed by CMS for one or more quarters; (5) Results are not available for this reporting period; (6) Fewer than 100 patients completed the HCAHPS survey; (7) No cases met the criteria for this measure; (8) The lower limit of the confidence interval cannot be calculated if the number of observed infections equals zero; (9) No data are available from the state/territory for this reporting period; (10) The scores shown reflect fewer than 50 completed surveys; (11) There were discrepancies in the data collection process; (12) This measure does not apply to this hospital for this reporting period; (13) Results cannot be calculated for this reporting period; (14) The results for this state are combined with nearby states to protect confidentiality; Please refer to the User's Guide for a full explanation of data.

Measure	Cases	This Hosp.	State Avg.	U.S. Avg.
Prophylactic Antibiotic Selection	129	87%	99%	99%
Prophylactic Antibiotic Selection (Outpatient)	22	100%	97%	98%
Prophylactic Antibiotic Stopped	128	96%	98%	98%
Prophylactic Antibiotic Timing	129	95%	99%	99%
Prophylactic Antibiotic Timing (Outpatient)	23	83%	97%	98%
Urinary Catheter Removal	79	86%	97%	97%
Survey of Patients' Hospital Experiences				
Area Around Room 'Always' Quiet at Night	300+	40%	51%	61%
Doctors 'Always' Communicated Well	300+	74%	78%	82%
Home Recovery Information Given	300+	85%	83%	85%
Hospital Given 9 or 10 on 10 Point Scale	300+	53%	68%	71%
Meds 'Always' Explained Before Given	300+	58%	61%	64%
Nurses 'Always' Communicated Well	300+	73%	74%	79%
Pain 'Always' Well Controlled	300+	60%	68%	71%
Room and Bathroom 'Always' Clean	300+	77%	70%	73%
Timely Help 'Always' Received	300+	56%	62%	68%
Would Definitely Recommend Hospital	300+	52%	70%	71%
Use of Medical Imaging				
Cardiac Imaging Stress Test before Surgery[1]	-	-	5.2%	5.3%
Combination Abdominal CT Scan	345	7.5%	13.4%	10.5%
Combination Brain/Sinus CT Scan	411	1.7%	2.2%	2.7%
Combination Chest CT Scan	155	5.2%	2.3%	2.7%
Follow-up Mammogram/Ultrasound	772	12.7%	8.2%	8.8%
Lumbar Spine MRI for Low Back Pain	73	30.1%	34.2%	37.2%

Mammoth Hospital

85 Sierra Park Road PO Box 660 Phone: 760-934-3311
Mammoth Lakes, CA 93546
Type: Critical Access Hospitals Emergency Services: Yes
Ownership: Govt - Hospital Dist/Auth

Measure	Cases	This Hosp.	State Avg.	U.S. Avg.
Blood Clot Prevention and Treatment				
Anticoagulation Overlap Therapy[1]	-	-	92%	93%
ICU Venous Thromboembolism Prophylaxis	13	100%	92%	92%
Incidence of Potentially Preventable VTE[1]	-	-	11%	10%
UFH with Dosages/Platelet Monitoring[1]	-	-	96%	97%
Venous Thromboembolism Prophylaxis	182	86%	83%	85%
Warfarin Therapy Discharge Instructions[1]	-	-	75%	75%
Chest Pain/Possible Heart Attack Care				
Aspirin Given Within 24 Hours of Arrival[5]	-	-	97%	96%
Fibrinolytic Meds Within 30 Min. of Arrival[5]	-	-	62%	58%
Average Time to ECG (minutes)[5]	-	-	9	7
Average Time to Transfer (minutes)[5]	-	-	62	60
Children's Asthma Care				
Received Home Management Plan of Care	-	-	88%	88%
Received Reliever Medication	-	-	100%	100%
Received Systemic Corticosteroids	-	-	100%	100%
Emergency Department				
Admittance Decision Time (minutes)[3]	182	69	125	98
Head CT Results Within 45 Min. of Arrival[5]	-	-	55%	57%
Patients Who Left ER Before Being Seen[5]	-	-	3%	2%
Time from ER Arrival to Admit. (minutes)[3]	184	226	323	274
Time from ER Arrival to Discharge (minutes)[5]	-	-	168	134
Time in ER Before Being Evaluated (minutes)[5]	-	-	29	26
Time to Pain Meds for Fractures (minutes)[5]	-	-	62	57
Heart Attack Care				
Aspirin Given at Discharge[5]	-	-	99%	99%
Fibrinolytic Meds Within 30 Min. of Arrival[5]	-	-	73%	54%
PCI Within 90 Minutes of Arrival[5]	-	-	95%	96%
Statin Prescribed at Discharge[5]	-	-	98%	98%
Heart Failure Care				
ACE Inhibitor or ARB for LVSD[3,7]	-	-	97%	97%
Discharge Instructions Given[1,3]	-	-	94%	94%
Evaluation of LVS Function[1,3]	-	-	99%	99%
Medicare Spending				
Medicare Spending per Patient (ratio)	-	-	0.98	0.98
Pneumonia Care				
Appropriate Initial Antibiotic Given[1]	-	-	97%	95%
Blood Culture Timing[1]	-	-	98%	98%
Pregnancy and Delivery Care				
Newborn Deliveries Scheduled Early[5]	-	-	5%	6%
Preventive Care				
Immunization for Influenza[1,3]	-	-	89%	90%
Immunization for Pneumonia[3,7]	-	-	90%	92%
Stroke Care				
Anticoagulation Therapy for Atrial Fibrillation[3,7]	-	-	95%	95%
Antithrombotic Therapy Timing[3,7]	-	-	98%	98%
Assessed for Rehabilitation[1,3]	-	-	97%	97%
Discharged on Antithrombotic Therapy[1,3]	-	-	99%	99%
Discharged on Statin Medication[1,3]	-	-	94%	94%
Thrombolytic Therapy Timing[3,7]	-	-	72%	66%
Venous Thromboembolism Prophylaxis[3,7]	-	-	94%	94%
Written Stroke Educational Materials Given[1,3]	-	-	87%	88%
Surgical Care Improvement Project				
Appropriate Beta Blocker Usage	11	27%	97%	98%
Appropriate VTP Within 24 Hours	60	97%	98%	98%
Controlled Postoperative Blood Glucose[7]	-	-	96%	97%
Perioperative Temperature Management	71	100%	100%	100%
Prophylactic Antibiotic Selection	49	96%	99%	99%
Prophylactic Antibiotic Selection (Outpatient)[5]	-	-	97%	98%
Prophylactic Antibiotic Stopped	49	82%	98%	98%
Prophylactic Antibiotic Timing	49	92%	99%	99%
Prophylactic Antibiotic Timing (Outpatient)[5]	-	-	97%	98%
Urinary Catheter Removal	52	94%	97%	97%
Survey of Patients' Hospital Experiences				
Area Around Room 'Always' Quiet at Night	(a)	55%	51%	61%
Doctors 'Always' Communicated Well	(a)	85%	78%	82%
Home Recovery Information Given	(a)	89%	83%	85%
Hospital Given 9 or 10 on 10 Point Scale	(a)	80%	68%	71%
Meds 'Always' Explained Before Given	(a)	66%	61%	64%
Nurses 'Always' Communicated Well	(a)	80%	74%	79%
Pain 'Always' Well Controlled	(a)	70%	68%	71%
Room and Bathroom 'Always' Clean	(a)	67%	70%	73%
Timely Help 'Always' Received	(a)	81%	62%	68%
Would Definitely Recommend Hospital	(a)	79%	70%	71%
Use of Medical Imaging				
Cardiac Imaging Stress Test before Surgery[7]	-	-	5.2%	5.3%
Combination Abdominal CT Scan[1]	-	-	13.4%	10.5%
Combination Brain/Sinus CT Scan[1]	-	-	2.2%	2.7%
Combination Chest CT Scan[1]	-	-	2.3%	2.7%
Follow-up Mammogram/Ultrasound	89	4.5%	8.2%	8.8%
Lumbar Spine MRI for Low Back Pain[1]	-	-	34.2%	37.2%

Doctors Hospital of Manteca

1205 E North St Phone: 209-823-3111
Manteca, CA 95336 Fax: 209-239-8329
E-mail: gregg.bixel@tenethelp.com
URL: www.doctorsmanteca.com
Type: Acute Care Hospitals Emergency Services: Yes
Ownership: Proprietary Beds: 73

Key Personnel:
Chief of Medical Staff. . . . . Michael Davis, MD
Emergency Room . . . . Susan Pepe, RN
Radiology. . . . . Richard Porzio
CEO . . . . Nicholas Tejeda, MHA,FACHE
Quality Assurance . . . . Judy Vasquez
Operating Room. . . . . Jerry Weiner, RN

Measure	Cases	This Hosp.	State Avg.	U.S. Avg.
Blood Clot Prevention and Treatment				
Anticoagulation Overlap Therapy[2]	22	82%	92%	93%
ICU Venous Thromboembolism Prophylaxis[2]	68	74%	92%	92%
Incidence of Potentially Preventable VTE[1,2]	-	-	11%	10%
UFH with Dosages/Platelet Monitoring[2]	11	100%	96%	97%
Venous Thromboembolism Prophylaxis[2]	284	64%	83%	85%
Warfarin Therapy Discharge Instructions[2]	16	100%	75%	75%
Chest Pain/Possible Heart Attack Care				
Aspirin Given Within 24 Hours of Arrival	11	100%	97%	96%
Fibrinolytic Meds Within 30 Min. of Arrival[1]	-	-	62%	58%
Average Time to ECG (minutes)	12	6	9	7
Average Time to Transfer (minutes)[1]	-	-	62	60
Children's Asthma Care				
Received Home Management Plan of Care	-	-	88%	88%
Received Reliever Medication	-	-	100%	100%
Received Systemic Corticosteroids	-	-	100%	100%
Emergency Department				
Admittance Decision Time (minutes)[2]	425	95	125	98
Head CT Results Within 45 Min. of Arrival[1]	-	-	55%	57%
Patients Who Left ER Before Being Seen	337	4%	3%	2%
Time from ER Arrival to Admit. (minutes)[2]	430	260	323	274
Time from ER Arrival to Discharge (minutes)	469	129	168	134
Time in ER Before Being Evaluated (minutes)	497	31	29	26
Time to Pain Meds for Fractures (minutes)	112	57	62	57
Heart Attack Care				
Aspirin Given at Discharge[1]	-	-	99%	99%
Fibrinolytic Meds Within 30 Min. of Arrival[1]	-	-	73%	54%
PCI Within 90 Minutes of Arrival[7]	-	-	95%	96%
Statin Prescribed at Discharge[1]	-	-	98%	98%
Heart Failure Care				
ACE Inhibitor or ARB for LVSD	48	92%	97%	97%
Discharge Instructions Given	92	89%	94%	94%
Evaluation of LVS Function	114	100%	99%	99%
Medicare Spending				
Medicare Spending per Patient (ratio)	-	0.96	0.98	0.98
Pneumonia Care				
Appropriate Initial Antibiotic Given	62	94%	97%	95%
Blood Culture Timing	70	96%	98%	98%
Pregnancy and Delivery Care				
Newborn Deliveries Scheduled Early[2]	33	0%	5%	6%
Preventive Care				
Immunization for Influenza[2]	414	89%	89%	90%
Immunization for Pneumonia[2]	462	94%	90%	92%
Stroke Care				
Anticoagulation Therapy for Atrial Fibrillation[1]	-	-	95%	95%
Antithrombotic Therapy Timing	30	97%	98%	98%
Assessed for Rehabilitation	32	97%	97%	97%
Discharged on Antithrombotic Therapy	28	100%	99%	99%
Discharged on Statin Medication	20	80%	94%	94%
Thrombolytic Therapy Timing[1]	-	-	72%	66%
Venous Thromboembolism Prophylaxis	34	85%	94%	94%
Written Stroke Educational Materials Given	17	47%	87%	88%
Surgical Care Improvement Project				
Appropriate Beta Blocker Usage	35	97%	97%	98%
Appropriate VTP Within 24 Hours	118	98%	98%	98%
Controlled Postoperative Blood Glucose[7]	-	-	96%	97%
Perioperative Temperature Management	153	100%	100%	100%
Prophylactic Antibiotic Selection	99	99%	99%	99%
Prophylactic Antibiotic Selection (Outpatient)	41	100%	97%	98%
Prophylactic Antibiotic Stopped	93	98%	98%	98%
Prophylactic Antibiotic Timing	99	100%	99%	99%
Prophylactic Antibiotic Timing (Outpatient)	41	100%	97%	98%
Urinary Catheter Removal	79	96%	97%	97%
Survey of Patients' Hospital Experiences				
Area Around Room 'Always' Quiet at Night	300+	53%	51%	61%
Doctors 'Always' Communicated Well	300+	84%	78%	82%
Home Recovery Information Given	300+	85%	83%	85%
Hospital Given 9 or 10 on 10 Point Scale	300+	69%	68%	71%
Meds 'Always' Explained Before Given	300+	64%	61%	64%
Nurses 'Always' Communicated Well	300+	75%	74%	79%
Pain 'Always' Well Controlled	300+	70%	68%	71%
Room and Bathroom 'Always' Clean	300+	66%	70%	73%
Timely Help 'Always' Received	300+	61%	62%	68%
Would Definitely Recommend Hospital	300+	71%	70%	71%
Use of Medical Imaging				
Cardiac Imaging Stress Test before Surgery	102	8.8%	5.2%	5.3%
Combination Abdominal CT Scan	393	8.7%	13.4%	10.5%
Combination Brain/Sinus CT Scan[1]	-	-	2.2%	2.7%
Combination Chest CT Scan	134	0.0%	2.3%	2.7%
Follow-up Mammogram/Ultrasound	869	5.6%	8.2%	8.8%
Lumbar Spine MRI for Low Back Pain	103	39.8%	34.2%	37.2%

Kaiser Foundation Hospital - Manteca

1777 West Yosemite Ave Phone: 209-825-3700
Manteca, CA 95337
URL: www.healthy.kaiserpermanente.org
Type: Acute Care Hospitals Emergency Services: Yes
Ownership: Voluntary non-profit - Private Beds: 61

Measure	Cases	This Hosp.	State Avg.	U.S. Avg.
Blood Clot Prevention and Treatment				

NOTE: Hospital profiles are in alphabetical order by state, then city, then hospital within the city; Rankings exclude hospitals with less than 25 cases except for patient surveys which excludes hospitals with less than 100 cases; (a) 100-299 cases; (1) The number of cases/patients is too few to report; (2) Data submitted were based on a sample of cases/patients; (3) Results are based on a shorter time period than required; (4) Data suppressed by CMS for one or more quarters; (5) Results are not available for this reporting period; (6) Fewer than 100 patients completed the HCAHPS survey; (7) No cases met the criteria for this measure; (8) The lower limit of the confidence interval cannot be calculated if the number of observed infections equals zero; (9) No data are available from the state/territory for this reporting period; (10) The scores shown reflect fewer than 50 completed surveys; (11) There were discrepancies in the data collection process; (12) This measure does not apply to this hospital for this reporting period; (13) Results cannot be calculated for this reporting period; (14) The results for this state are combined with nearby states to protect confidentiality; Please refer to the User's Guide for a full explanation of data.

Measure	Cases	This Hosp.	State Avg.	U.S. Avg.
Anticoagulation Overlap Therapy[2]	59	100%	92%	93%
ICU Venous Thromboembolism Prophylaxis[2]	110	97%	92%	92%
Incidence of Potentially Preventable VTE[2]	15	13%	11%	10%
UFH with Dosages/Platelet Monitoring[2]	26	100%	96%	97%
Venous Thromboembolism Prophylaxis[2]	247	91%	83%	85%
Warfarin Therapy Discharge Instructions[2]	50	76%	75%	75%
Chest Pain/Possible Heart Attack Care				
Aspirin Given Within 24 Hours of Arrival	-	-	97%	96%
Fibrinolytic Meds Within 30 Min. of Arrival	-	-	62%	58%
Average Time to ECG (minutes)	-	-	9	7
Average Time to Transfer (minutes)	-	-	62	60
Children's Asthma Care				
Received Home Management Plan of Care	-	-	88%	88%
Received Reliever Medication	-	-	100%	100%
Received Systemic Corticosteroids	-	-	100%	100%
Emergency Department				
Admittance Decision Time (minutes)[2]	440	48	125	98
Head CT Results Within 45 Min. of Arrival	-	-	55%	57%
Patients Who Left ER Before Being Seen	-	-	3%	2%
Time from ER Arrival to Admit. (minutes)[2]	456	338	323	274
Time from ER Arrival to Discharge (minutes)	-	-	168	134
Time in ER Before Being Evaluated (minutes)	-	-	29	26
Time to Pain Meds for Fractures (minutes)	-	-	62	57
Heart Attack Care				
Aspirin Given at Discharge	63	100%	99%	99%
Fibrinolytic Meds Within 30 Min. of Arrival[7]	-	-	73%	54%
PCI Within 90 Minutes of Arrival[7]	-	-	95%	96%
Statin Prescribed at Discharge	67	100%	98%	98%
Heart Failure Care				
ACE Inhibitor or ARB for LVSD	49	100%	97%	97%
Discharge Instructions Given	179	100%	94%	94%
Evaluation of LVS Function	206	100%	99%	99%
Medicare Spending				
Medicare Spending per Patient (ratio)	-	0.78	0.98	0.98
Pneumonia Care				
Appropriate Initial Antibiotic Given[2]	61	100%	97%	95%
Blood Culture Timing[2]	119	97%	98%	98%
Pregnancy and Delivery Care				
Newborn Deliveries Scheduled Early[2]	23	0%	5%	6%
Preventive Care				
Immunization for Influenza[2]	467	88%	89%	90%
Immunization for Pneumonia[2]	495	93%	90%	92%
Stroke Care				
Anticoagulation Therapy for Atrial Fibrillation[1,2]	-	-	95%	95%
Antithrombotic Therapy Timing[2]	54	100%	98%	98%
Assessed for Rehabilitation[2]	63	97%	97%	97%
Discharged on Antithrombotic Therapy[2]	58	98%	99%	99%
Discharged on Statin Medication[2]	52	98%	94%	94%
Thrombolytic Therapy Timing[1,2]	-	-	72%	66%
Venous Thromboembolism Prophylaxis[2]	47	94%	94%	94%
Written Stroke Educational Materials Given[2]	36	92%	87%	88%
Surgical Care Improvement Project				
Appropriate Beta Blocker Usage[2]	139	100%	97%	98%
Appropriate VTP Within 24 Hours[2]	358	100%	98%	98%
Controlled Postoperative Blood Glucose[2,7]	-	-	96%	97%
Perioperative Temperature Management[2]	481	100%	100%	100%
Prophylactic Antibiotic Selection[2]	325	100%	99%	99%
Prophylactic Antibiotic Selection (Outpatient)	-	-	97%	98%
Prophylactic Antibiotic Stopped[2]	319	100%	98%	98%
Prophylactic Antibiotic Timing[2]	326	100%	99%	99%
Prophylactic Antibiotic Timing (Outpatient)	-	-	97%	98%
Urinary Catheter Removal[2]	302	99%	97%	97%
Survey of Patients' Hospital Experiences				
Area Around Room 'Always' Quiet at Night	300+	58%	51%	61%
Doctors 'Always' Communicated Well	300+	80%	78%	82%
Home Recovery Information Given	300+	85%	83%	85%
Hospital Given 9 or 10 on 10 Point Scale	300+	79%	68%	71%
Meds 'Always' Explained Before Given	300+	63%	61%	64%
Nurses 'Always' Communicated Well	300+	77%	74%	79%
Pain 'Always' Well Controlled	300+	73%	68%	71%
Room and Bathroom 'Always' Clean	300+	78%	70%	73%
Timely Help 'Always' Received	300+	69%	62%	68%
Would Definitely Recommend Hospital	300+	79%	70%	71%
Use of Medical Imaging				
Cardiac Imaging Stress Test before Surgery	-	-	5.2%	5.3%
Combination Abdominal CT Scan	-	-	13.4%	10.5%
Combination Brain/Sinus CT Scan	-	-	2.2%	2.7%
Combination Chest CT Scan	-	-	2.3%	2.7%
Follow-up Mammogram/Ultrasound	-	-	8.2%	8.8%
Lumbar Spine MRI for Low Back Pain	-	-	34.2%	37.2%

Marina Del Rey Hospital

4650 Lincoln Blvd — Phone: 310-823-8911
Marina Del Rey, CA 90291
Type: Acute Care Hospitals — Emergency Services: Yes
Ownership: Proprietary

Measure	Cases	This Hosp.	State Avg.	U.S. Avg.
Blood Clot Prevention and Treatment				
Anticoagulation Overlap Therapy[2]	52	94%	92%	93%
ICU Venous Thromboembolism Prophylaxis[2]	61	87%	92%	92%
Incidence of Potentially Preventable VTE[2]	11	0%	11%	10%
UFH with Dosages/Platelet Monitoring[1,2]	-	-	96%	97%
Venous Thromboembolism Prophylaxis[2]	317	75%	83%	85%
Warfarin Therapy Discharge Instructions[2]	39	3%	75%	75%
Chest Pain/Possible Heart Attack Care				
Aspirin Given Within 24 Hours of Arrival	29	97%	97%	96%
Fibrinolytic Meds Within 30 Min. of Arrival[7]	-	-	62%	58%
Average Time to ECG (minutes)	30	19	9	7
Average Time to Transfer (minutes)[1]	-	-	62	60
Children's Asthma Care				
Received Home Management Plan of Care	-	-	88%	88%
Received Reliever Medication	-	-	100%	100%
Received Systemic Corticosteroids	-	-	100%	100%
Emergency Department				
Admittance Decision Time (minutes)[2]	536	142	125	98
Head CT Results Within 45 Min. of Arrival[1]	-	-	55%	57%
Patients Who Left ER Before Being Seen	22,383	2%	3%	2%
Time from ER Arrival to Admit. (minutes)[2]	542	319	323	274
Time from ER Arrival to Discharge (minutes)	323	186	168	134
Time in ER Before Being Evaluated (minutes)	382	42	29	26
Time to Pain Meds for Fractures (minutes)	126	76	62	57
Heart Attack Care				
Aspirin Given at Discharge	15	93%	99%	99%
Fibrinolytic Meds Within 30 Min. of Arrival[7]	-	-	73%	54%
PCI Within 90 Minutes of Arrival[7]	-	-	95%	96%
Statin Prescribed at Discharge	16	94%	98%	98%
Heart Failure Care				
ACE Inhibitor or ARB for LVSD	40	100%	97%	97%
Discharge Instructions Given	83	61%	94%	94%
Evaluation of LVS Function	110	98%	99%	99%
Medicare Spending				
Medicare Spending per Patient (ratio)	-	1.01	0.98	0.98
Pneumonia Care				
Appropriate Initial Antibiotic Given	70	90%	97%	95%
Blood Culture Timing	94	93%	98%	98%
Pregnancy and Delivery Care				
Newborn Deliveries Scheduled Early[2,7]	-	-	5%	6%
Preventive Care				
Immunization for Influenza[2]	434	88%	89%	90%
Immunization for Pneumonia[2]	526	86%	90%	92%
Stroke Care				
Anticoagulation Therapy for Atrial Fibrillation[1]	-	-	95%	95%
Antithrombotic Therapy Timing	19	79%	98%	98%
Assessed for Rehabilitation	25	96%	97%	97%
Discharged on Antithrombotic Therapy	23	96%	99%	99%
Discharged on Statin Medication	18	50%	94%	94%
Thrombolytic Therapy Timing[1]	-	-	72%	66%
Venous Thromboembolism Prophylaxis	23	61%	94%	94%
Written Stroke Educational Materials Given	12	0%	87%	88%
Surgical Care Improvement Project				
Appropriate Beta Blocker Usage[2]	46	87%	97%	98%
Appropriate VTP Within 24 Hours[2]	179	97%	98%	98%
Controlled Postoperative Blood Glucose[2,7]	-	-	96%	97%
Perioperative Temperature Management[2]	201	90%	100%	100%
Prophylactic Antibiotic Selection[2]	120	99%	99%	99%
Prophylactic Antibiotic Selection (Outpatient)	116	100%	97%	98%
Prophylactic Antibiotic Stopped[2]	110	93%	98%	98%
Prophylactic Antibiotic Timing[2]	120	100%	99%	99%
Prophylactic Antibiotic Timing (Outpatient)	116	100%	97%	98%
Urinary Catheter Removal[2]	120	97%	97%	97%
Survey of Patients' Hospital Experiences				
Area Around Room 'Always' Quiet at Night	300+	45%	51%	61%
Doctors 'Always' Communicated Well	300+	75%	78%	82%
Home Recovery Information Given	300+	77%	83%	85%
Hospital Given 9 or 10 on 10 Point Scale	300+	55%	68%	71%
Meds 'Always' Explained Before Given	300+	55%	61%	64%
Nurses 'Always' Communicated Well	300+	69%	74%	79%
Pain 'Always' Well Controlled	300+	66%	68%	71%
Room and Bathroom 'Always' Clean	300+	62%	70%	73%
Timely Help 'Always' Received	300+	60%	62%	68%
Would Definitely Recommend Hospital	300+	58%	70%	71%
Use of Medical Imaging				
Cardiac Imaging Stress Test before Surgery	72	4.2%	5.2%	5.3%
Combination Abdominal CT Scan	217	22.6%	13.4%	10.5%
Combination Brain/Sinus CT Scan	321	4.4%	2.2%	2.7%
Combination Chest CT Scan[1]	-	-	2.3%	2.7%
Follow-up Mammogram/Ultrasound	84	19.0%	8.2%	8.8%
Lumbar Spine MRI for Low Back Pain	50	32.0%	34.2%	37.2%

John C Fremont Healthcare District

5189 Hospital Road — Phone: 209-966-3631
Mariposa, CA 95338 — Fax: 209-966-3776
E-mail: jcfadm@jcf-hospital.com
URL: www.jcf-hospitasl.com
Type: Critical Access Hospitals — Emergency Services: Yes
Ownership: Govt - Hospital Dist/Auth — Beds: 34

Key Personnel:
CEO/President. . . . . Charles E Bill, CEO
Infection Control. . . . . Evon Kruse, RN
Chief of Medical Staff. . . . . Stephan J Lee, MD
Quality Assurance . . . . Jean Potter, RHIT
Operating Room. . . . . Maureen Spacke, RN
Radiology. . . . . Mark A Wagner, DO
Emergency Room . . . . Nanette Wardle, RN

Measure	Cases	This Hosp.	State Avg.	U.S. Avg.
Blood Clot Prevention and Treatment				
Anticoagulation Overlap Therapy[5]	-	-	92%	93%
ICU Venous Thromboembolism Prophylaxis[5]	-	-	92%	92%
Incidence of Potentially Preventable VTE[5]	-	-	11%	10%
UFH with Dosages/Platelet Monitoring[5]	-	-	96%	97%
Venous Thromboembolism Prophylaxis[5]	-	-	83%	85%
Warfarin Therapy Discharge Instructions[5]	-	-	75%	75%
Chest Pain/Possible Heart Attack Care				
Aspirin Given Within 24 Hours of Arrival	-	-	97%	96%
Fibrinolytic Meds Within 30 Min. of Arrival	-	-	62%	58%
Average Time to ECG (minutes)	-	-	9	7
Average Time to Transfer (minutes)	-	-	62	60
Children's Asthma Care				
Received Home Management Plan of Care	-	-	88%	88%
Received Reliever Medication	-	-	100%	100%
Received Systemic Corticosteroids	-	-	100%	100%
Emergency Department				
Admittance Decision Time (minutes)[5]	-	-	125	98
Head CT Results Within 45 Min. of Arrival	-	-	55%	57%
Patients Who Left ER Before Being Seen	-	-	3%	2%
Time from ER Arrival to Admit. (minutes)[5]	-	-	323	274
Time from ER Arrival to Discharge (minutes)	-	-	168	134
Time in ER Before Being Evaluated (minutes)	-	-	29	26
Time to Pain Meds for Fractures (minutes)	-	-	62	57
Heart Attack Care				
Aspirin Given at Discharge[5]	-	-	99%	99%
Fibrinolytic Meds Within 30 Min. of Arrival[5]	-	-	73%	54%
PCI Within 90 Minutes of Arrival[5]	-	-	95%	96%
Statin Prescribed at Discharge[5]	-	-	98%	98%
Heart Failure Care				
ACE Inhibitor or ARB for LVSD[1,3]	-	-	97%	97%
Discharge Instructions Given[1,3]	-	-	94%	94%
Evaluation of LVS Function[1,3]	-	-	99%	99%

NOTE: Hospital profiles are in alphabetical order by state, then city, then hospital within the city; Rankings exclude hospitals with less than 25 cases except for patient surveys which excludes hospitals with less than 100 cases; (a) 100-299 cases; (1) The number of cases/patients is too few to report; (2) Data submitted were based on a sample of cases/patients; (3) Results are based on a shorter time period than required; (4) Data suppressed by CMS for one or more quarters; (5) Results are not available for this reporting period; (6) Fewer than 100 patients completed the HCAHPS survey; (7) No cases met the criteria for this measure; (8) The lower limit of the confidence interval cannot be calculated if the number of observed infections equals zero; (9) No data are available from the state/territory for this reporting period; (10) The scores shown reflect fewer than 50 completed surveys; (11) There were discrepancies in the data collection process; (12) This measure does not apply to this hospital for this reporting period; (13) Results cannot be calculated for this reporting period; (14) The results for this state are combined with nearby states to protect confidentiality; Please refer to the User's Guide for a full explanation of data.

Measure	Cases	This Hosp.	State Avg.	U.S. Avg.
Medicare Spending				
Medicare Spending per Patient (ratio)	-	-	0.98	0.98
Pneumonia Care				
Appropriate Initial Antibiotic Given	15	93%	97%	95%
Blood Culture Timing	18	94%	98%	98%
Pregnancy and Delivery Care				
Newborn Deliveries Scheduled Early[5]	-	-	5%	6%
Preventive Care				
Immunization for Influenza[3]	27	74%	89%	90%
Immunization for Pneumonia[3]	78	85%	90%	92%
Stroke Care				
Anticoagulation Therapy for Atrial Fibrillation[5]	-	-	95%	95%
Antithrombotic Therapy Timing[5]	-	-	98%	98%
Assessed for Rehabilitation[5]	-	-	97%	97%
Discharged on Antithrombotic Therapy[5]	-	-	99%	99%
Discharged on Statin Medication[5]	-	-	94%	94%
Thrombolytic Therapy Timing[5]	-	-	72%	66%
Venous Thromboembolism Prophylaxis[5]	-	-	94%	94%
Written Stroke Educational Materials Given[5]	-	-	87%	88%
Surgical Care Improvement Project				
Appropriate Beta Blocker Usage[5]	-	-	97%	98%
Appropriate VTP Within 24 Hours[5]	-	-	98%	98%
Controlled Postoperative Blood Glucose[5]	-	-	96%	97%
Perioperative Temperature Management[5]	-	-	100%	100%
Prophylactic Antibiotic Selection[5]	-	-	99%	99%
Prophylactic Antibiotic Selection (Outpatient)	-	-	97%	98%
Prophylactic Antibiotic Stopped[5]	-	-	98%	98%
Prophylactic Antibiotic Timing[5]	-	-	99%	99%
Prophylactic Antibiotic Timing (Outpatient)	-	-	97%	98%
Urinary Catheter Removal[5]	-	-	97%	97%
Survey of Patients' Hospital Experiences				
Area Around Room 'Always' Quiet at Night[10]	<100	59%	51%	61%
Doctors 'Always' Communicated Well[10]	<100	74%	78%	82%
Home Recovery Information Given[10]	<100	91%	83%	85%
Hospital Given 9 or 10 on 10 Point Scale[10]	<100	57%	68%	71%
Meds 'Always' Explained Before Given[10]	<100	77%	61%	64%
Nurses 'Always' Communicated Well[10]	<100	77%	74%	79%
Pain 'Always' Well Controlled[10]	<100	76%	68%	71%
Room and Bathroom 'Always' Clean[10]	<100	69%	70%	73%
Timely Help 'Always' Received[10]	<100	72%	62%	68%
Would Definitely Recommend Hospital[10]	<100	79%	70%	71%
Use of Medical Imaging				
Cardiac Imaging Stress Test before Surgery	-	-	5.2%	5.3%
Combination Abdominal CT Scan	-	-	13.4%	10.5%
Combination Brain/Sinus CT Scan	-	-	2.2%	2.7%
Combination Chest CT Scan	-	-	2.3%	2.7%
Follow-up Mammogram/Ultrasound	-	-	8.2%	8.8%
Lumbar Spine MRI for Low Back Pain	-	-	34.2%	37.2%

Contra Costa Regional Medical Center

2500 Alhambra Ave
Martinez, CA 94553
Phone: 925-370-5000
Fax: 925-370-5138
URL: www.cchealth.org/medical-center
Type: Acute Care Hospitals
Emergency Services: Yes
Ownership: Government - Local
Beds: 166

Measure	Cases	This Hosp.	State Avg.	U.S. Avg.
Blood Clot Prevention and Treatment				
Anticoagulation Overlap Therapy[2]	40	100%	92%	93%
ICU Venous Thromboembolism Prophylaxis[2]	41	98%	92%	92%
Incidence of Potentially Preventable VTE[1,2]	-	-	11%	10%
UFH with Dosages/Platelet Monitoring[1,2]	-	-	96%	97%
Venous Thromboembolism Prophylaxis[2]	352	95%	83%	85%
Warfarin Therapy Discharge Instructions[2]	32	88%	75%	75%
Chest Pain/Possible Heart Attack Care				
Aspirin Given Within 24 Hours of Arrival[1,3]	-	-	97%	96%
Fibrinolytic Meds Within 30 Min. of Arrival[3,7]	-	-	62%	58%
Average Time to ECG (minutes)[1,3]	-	-	9	7
Average Time to Transfer (minutes)[1,3]	-	-	62	60
Children's Asthma Care				
Received Home Management Plan of Care	-	-	88%	88%
Received Reliever Medication	-	-	100%	100%
Received Systemic Corticosteroids	-	-	100%	100%
Emergency Department				
Admittance Decision Time (minutes)[2]	467	217	125	98
Head CT Results Within 45 Min. of Arrival[1]	-	-	55%	57%
Patients Who Left ER Before Being Seen	57,154	5%	3%	2%
Time from ER Arrival to Admit. (minutes)[2]	412	471	323	274
Time from ER Arrival to Discharge (minutes)	394	182	168	134
Time in ER Before Being Evaluated (minutes)	194	58	29	26
Time to Pain Meds for Fractures (minutes)	53	103	62	57
Heart Attack Care				
Aspirin Given at Discharge	21	100%	99%	99%
Fibrinolytic Meds Within 30 Min. of Arrival[7]	-	-	73%	54%
PCI Within 90 Minutes of Arrival[7]	-	-	95%	96%
Statin Prescribed at Discharge	21	95%	98%	98%
Heart Failure Care				
ACE Inhibitor or ARB for LVSD	85	92%	97%	97%
Discharge Instructions Given	176	78%	94%	94%
Evaluation of LVS Function	193	99%	99%	99%
Medicare Spending				
Medicare Spending per Patient (ratio)	-	0.85	0.98	0.98
Pneumonia Care				
Appropriate Initial Antibiotic Given[2]	70	94%	97%	95%
Blood Culture Timing[2]	72	94%	98%	98%
Pregnancy and Delivery Care				
Newborn Deliveries Scheduled Early[2]	24	17%	5%	6%
Preventive Care				
Immunization for Influenza[2]	543	43%	89%	90%
Immunization for Pneumonia[2]	462	62%	90%	92%
Stroke Care				
Anticoagulation Therapy for Atrial Fibrillation[1]	-	-	95%	95%
Antithrombotic Therapy Timing	42	100%	98%	98%
Assessed for Rehabilitation	43	86%	97%	97%
Discharged on Antithrombotic Therapy	41	98%	99%	99%
Discharged on Statin Medication	31	100%	94%	94%
Thrombolytic Therapy Timing[1]	-	-	72%	66%
Venous Thromboembolism Prophylaxis	42	90%	94%	94%
Written Stroke Educational Materials Given	36	89%	87%	88%
Surgical Care Improvement Project				
Appropriate Beta Blocker Usage[2]	12	67%	97%	98%
Appropriate VTP Within 24 Hours[2]	140	98%	98%	98%
Controlled Postoperative Blood Glucose[2,7]	-	-	96%	97%
Perioperative Temperature Management[2]	147	100%	100%	100%
Prophylactic Antibiotic Selection[2]	58	93%	99%	99%
Prophylactic Antibiotic Selection (Outpatient)	24	62%	97%	98%
Prophylactic Antibiotic Stopped[2]	58	98%	98%	98%
Prophylactic Antibiotic Timing[2]	62	92%	99%	99%
Prophylactic Antibiotic Timing (Outpatient)	28	43%	97%	98%
Urinary Catheter Removal[2]	52	88%	97%	97%
Survey of Patients' Hospital Experiences				
Area Around Room 'Always' Quiet at Night	300+	34%	51%	61%
Doctors 'Always' Communicated Well	300+	76%	78%	82%
Home Recovery Information Given	300+	85%	83%	85%
Hospital Given 9 or 10 on 10 Point Scale	300+	62%	68%	71%
Meds 'Always' Explained Before Given	300+	62%	61%	64%
Nurses 'Always' Communicated Well	300+	68%	74%	79%
Pain 'Always' Well Controlled	300+	63%	68%	71%
Room and Bathroom 'Always' Clean	300+	61%	70%	73%
Timely Help 'Always' Received	300+	53%	62%	68%
Would Definitely Recommend Hospital	300+	63%	70%	71%
Use of Medical Imaging				
Cardiac Imaging Stress Test before Surgery	69	1.4%	5.2%	5.3%
Combination Abdominal CT Scan	315	6.0%	13.4%	10.5%
Combination Brain/Sinus CT Scan[1]	-	-	2.2%	2.7%
Combination Chest CT Scan	189	3.7%	2.3%	2.7%
Follow-up Mammogram/Ultrasound	914	4.8%	8.2%	8.8%
Lumbar Spine MRI for Low Back Pain[1]	-	-	34.2%	37.2%

Rideout Memorial Hospital

726 4th St
Marysville, CA 95901
Phone: 530-749-4300
Fax: 530-751-4226
URL: www.frhg.org
Type: Acute Care Hospitals
Emergency Services: Yes
Ownership: Voluntary non-profit - Other
Beds: 164

Key Personnel:
Chief of Medical Staff . . . . Michael Fahey, MD
CEO/President . . . . Theresa Hamilton
Operating Room . . . . Richard Lewis
Radiology . . . . Philip Shelton
Quality Assurance . . . . Judy Wilbur
Chairman/CEO . . . . John Wright

Measure	Cases	This Hosp.	State Avg.	U.S. Avg.
Blood Clot Prevention and Treatment				
Anticoagulation Overlap Therapy[2]	81	52%	92%	93%
ICU Venous Thromboembolism Prophylaxis[2]	85	91%	92%	92%
Incidence of Potentially Preventable VTE[2]	13	23%	11%	10%
UFH with Dosages/Platelet Monitoring[2]	43	77%	96%	97%
Venous Thromboembolism Prophylaxis[2]	503	68%	83%	85%
Warfarin Therapy Discharge Instructions[2]	67	27%	75%	75%
Chest Pain/Possible Heart Attack Care				
Aspirin Given Within 24 Hours of Arrival[1]	-	-	97%	96%
Fibrinolytic Meds Within 30 Min. of Arrival[5]	-	-	62%	58%
Average Time to ECG (minutes)[1]	-	-	9	7
Average Time to Transfer (minutes)[5]	-	-	62	60
Children's Asthma Care				
Received Home Management Plan of Care	-	-	88%	88%
Received Reliever Medication	-	-	100%	100%
Received Systemic Corticosteroids	-	-	100%	100%
Emergency Department				
Admittance Decision Time (minutes)[2]	454	214	125	98
Head CT Results Within 45 Min. of Arrival[1]	-	-	55%	57%
Patients Who Left ER Before Being Seen	50,795	1%	3%	2%
Time from ER Arrival to Admit. (minutes)[2]	459	396	323	274
Time from ER Arrival to Discharge (minutes)	830	190	168	134
Time in ER Before Being Evaluated (minutes)	1,095	19	29	26
Time to Pain Meds for Fractures (minutes)	254	73	62	57
Heart Attack Care				
Aspirin Given at Discharge	230	97%	99%	99%
Fibrinolytic Meds Within 30 Min. of Arrival[1]	-	-	73%	54%
PCI Within 90 Minutes of Arrival	55	95%	95%	96%
Statin Prescribed at Discharge	216	97%	98%	98%
Heart Failure Care				
ACE Inhibitor or ARB for LVSD	100	85%	97%	97%
Discharge Instructions Given	288	85%	94%	94%
Evaluation of LVS Function	336	94%	99%	99%
Medicare Spending				
Medicare Spending per Patient (ratio)	-	0.93	0.98	0.98
Pneumonia Care				
Appropriate Initial Antibiotic Given[2]	138	95%	97%	95%
Blood Culture Timing[2]	152	97%	98%	98%
Pregnancy and Delivery Care				
Newborn Deliveries Scheduled Early[2]	64	0%	5%	6%
Preventive Care				
Immunization for Influenza[2]	506	84%	89%	90%
Immunization for Pneumonia[2]	844	85%	90%	92%
Stroke Care				
Anticoagulation Therapy for Atrial Fibrillation	21	86%	95%	95%
Antithrombotic Therapy Timing	129	95%	98%	98%
Assessed for Rehabilitation	145	88%	97%	97%
Discharged on Antithrombotic Therapy	128	99%	99%	99%
Discharged on Statin Medication	98	76%	94%	94%
Thrombolytic Therapy Timing	16	31%	72%	66%
Venous Thromboembolism Prophylaxis	152	78%	94%	94%
Written Stroke Educational Materials Given	87	89%	87%	88%
Surgical Care Improvement Project				
Appropriate Beta Blocker Usage[2]	144	97%	97%	98%
Appropriate VTP Within 24 Hours[2]	297	92%	98%	98%
Controlled Postoperative Blood Glucose[2]	101	98%	96%	97%
Perioperative Temperature Management[2]	359	99%	100%	100%
Prophylactic Antibiotic Selection[2]	249	99%	99%	99%
Prophylactic Antibiotic Selection (Outpatient)	167	97%	97%	98%
Prophylactic Antibiotic Stopped[2]	236	98%	98%	98%
Prophylactic Antibiotic Timing[2]	251	100%	99%	99%
Prophylactic Antibiotic Timing (Outpatient)	170	96%	97%	98%
Urinary Catheter Removal[2]	174	97%	97%	97%
Survey of Patients' Hospital Experiences				
Area Around Room 'Always' Quiet at Night	300+	39%	51%	61%
Doctors 'Always' Communicated Well	300+	71%	78%	82%

NOTE: Hospital profiles are in alphabetical order by state, then city, then hospital within the city; Rankings exclude hospitals with less than 25 cases except for patient surveys which excludes hospitals with less than 100 cases; (a) 100-299 cases; (1) The number of cases/patients is too few to report; (2) Data submitted were based on a sample of cases/patients; (3) Results are based on a shorter time period than required; (4) Data suppressed by CMS for one or more quarters; (5) Results are not available for this reporting period; (6) Fewer than 100 patients completed the HCAHPS survey; (7) No cases met the criteria for this measure; (8) The lower limit of the confidence interval cannot be calculated if the number of observed infections equals zero; (9) No data are available from the state/territory for this reporting period; (10) The scores shown reflect fewer than 50 completed surveys; (11) There were discrepancies in the data collection process; (12) This measure does not apply to this hospital for this reporting period; (13) Results cannot be calculated for this reporting period; (14) The results for this state are combined with nearby states to protect confidentiality; Please refer to the User's Guide for a full explanation of data.

Home Recovery Information Given	300+	74%	83%	85%
Hospital Given 9 or 10 on 10 Point Scale	300+	44%	68%	71%
Meds 'Always' Explained Before Given	300+	51%	61%	64%
Nurses 'Always' Communicated Well	300+	65%	74%	79%
Pain 'Always' Well Controlled	300+	59%	68%	71%
Room and Bathroom 'Always' Clean	300+	60%	70%	73%
Timely Help 'Always' Received	300+	48%	62%	68%
Would Definitely Recommend Hospital	300+	46%	70%	71%
Use of Medical Imaging				
Cardiac Imaging Stress Test before Surgery	449	1.8%	5.2%	5.3%
Combination Abdominal CT Scan	578	2.8%	13.4%	10.5%
Combination Brain/Sinus CT Scan	1,021	3.1%	2.2%	2.7%
Combination Chest CT Scan	394	0.5%	2.3%	2.7%
Follow-up Mammogram/Ultrasound	162	21.6%	8.2%	8.8%
Lumbar Spine MRI for Low Back Pain	38	44.7%	34.2%	37.2%

VA Northern California Healthcare System

10535 Hospital Way
Mather, CA 95655
Phone: 800-382-8387
URL: www.northerncalifornia.va.gov
Type: Acute Care - VA
Emergency Services: No
Ownership: Government Federal

Measure	Cases	This Hosp.	State Avg.	U.S. Avg.
Blood Clot Prevention and Treatment				
Anticoagulation Overlap Therapy	-	-	92%	93%
ICU Venous Thromboembolism Prophylaxis	-	-	92%	92%
Incidence of Potentially Preventable VTE	-	-	11%	10%
UFH with Dosages/Platelet Monitoring	-	-	96%	97%
Venous Thromboembolism Prophylaxis	-	-	83%	85%
Warfarin Therapy Discharge Instructions	-	-	75%	75%
Chest Pain/Possible Heart Attack Care				
Aspirin Given Within 24 Hours of Arrival	-	-	97%	96%
Fibrinolytic Meds Within 30 Min. of Arrival	-	-	62%	58%
Average Time to ECG (minutes)	-	-	9	7
Average Time to Transfer (minutes)	-	-	62	60
Children's Asthma Care				
Received Home Management Plan of Care	-	-	88%	88%
Received Reliever Medication	-	-	100%	100%
Received Systemic Corticosteroids	-	-	100%	100%
Emergency Department				
Admittance Decision Time (minutes)	-	-	125	98
Head CT Results Within 45 Min. of Arrival	-	-	55%	57%
Patients Who Left ER Before Being Seen	-	-	3%	2%
Time from ER Arrival to Admit. (minutes)	-	-	323	274
Time from ER Arrival to Discharge (minutes)	-	-	168	134
Time in ER Before Being Evaluated (minutes)	-	-	29	26
Time to Pain Meds for Fractures (minutes)	-	-	62	57
Heart Attack Care				
Aspirin Given at Discharge[1]	19	95%	99%	99%
Fibrinolytic Meds Within 30 Min. of Arrival[5]	-	-	73%	54%
PCI Within 90 Minutes of Arrival[5]	-	-	95%	96%
Statin Prescribed at Discharge[1]	22	91%	98%	98%
Heart Failure Care				
ACE Inhibitor or ARB for LVSD	93	98%	97%	97%
Discharge Instructions Given	171	100%	94%	94%
Evaluation of LVS Function	205	100%	99%	99%
Medicare Spending				
Medicare Spending per Patient (ratio)	-	-	0.98	0.98
Pneumonia Care				
Appropriate Initial Antibiotic Given	65	89%	97%	95%
Blood Culture Timing	48	100%	98%	98%
Pregnancy and Delivery Care				
Newborn Deliveries Scheduled Early	-	-	5%	6%
Preventive Care				
Immunization for Influenza[5]	-	-	89%	90%
Immunization for Pneumonia[5]	-	-	90%	92%
Stroke Care				
Anticoagulation Therapy for Atrial Fibrillation	-	-	95%	95%
Antithrombotic Therapy Timing	-	-	98%	98%
Assessed for Rehabilitation	-	-	97%	97%
Discharged on Antithrombotic Therapy	-	-	99%	99%
Discharged on Statin Medication	-	-	94%	94%
Thrombolytic Therapy Timing	-	-	72%	66%
Venous Thromboembolism Prophylaxis	-	-	94%	94%
Written Stroke Educational Materials Given	-	-	87%	88%
Surgical Care Improvement Project				
Appropriate Beta Blocker Usage[2]	59	100%	97%	98%
Appropriate VTP Within 24 Hours[2]	116	94%	98%	98%
Controlled Postoperative Blood Glucose[5]	-	-	96%	97%
Perioperative Temperature Management[2]	162	98%	100%	100%
Prophylactic Antibiotic Selection	50	100%	99%	99%
Prophylactic Antibiotic Selection (Outpatient)	-	-	97%	98%
Prophylactic Antibiotic Stopped	47	87%	98%	98%
Prophylactic Antibiotic Timing	50	96%	99%	99%
Prophylactic Antibiotic Timing (Outpatient)	-	-	97%	98%
Urinary Catheter Removal[2]	56	98%	97%	97%
Survey of Patients' Hospital Experiences				
Area Around Room 'Always' Quiet at Night	-	-	51%	61%
Doctors 'Always' Communicated Well	-	-	78%	82%
Home Recovery Information Given	-	-	83%	85%
Hospital Given 9 or 10 on 10 Point Scale	-	-	68%	71%
Meds 'Always' Explained Before Given	-	-	61%	64%
Nurses 'Always' Communicated Well	-	-	74%	79%
Pain 'Always' Well Controlled	-	-	68%	71%
Room and Bathroom 'Always' Clean	-	-	70%	73%
Timely Help 'Always' Received	-	-	62%	68%
Would Definitely Recommend Hospital	-	-	70%	71%
Use of Medical Imaging				
Cardiac Imaging Stress Test before Surgery	-	-	5.2%	5.3%
Combination Abdominal CT Scan	-	-	13.4%	10.5%
Combination Brain/Sinus CT Scan	-	-	2.2%	2.7%
Combination Chest CT Scan	-	-	2.3%	2.7%
Follow-up Mammogram/Ultrasound	-	-	8.2%	8.8%
Lumbar Spine MRI for Low Back Pain	-	-	34.2%	37.2%

Menlo Park Surgical Hospital

570 Willow Road
Menlo Park, CA 94025
Phone: 650-324-8500
URL: www.pamf.org/mpsh
Type: Acute Care Hospitals
Emergency Services: No
Ownership: Voluntary non-profit - Private
Beds: 16
Key Personnel:
CEO . . . . Kathi Palange

Measure	Cases	This Hosp.	State Avg.	U.S. Avg.
Blood Clot Prevention and Treatment				
Anticoagulation Overlap Therapy[7]	-	-	92%	93%
ICU Venous Thromboembolism Prophylaxis[7]	-	-	92%	92%
Incidence of Potentially Preventable VTE[7]	-	-	11%	10%
UFH with Dosages/Platelet Monitoring[7]	-	-	96%	97%
Venous Thromboembolism Prophylaxis[1]	-	-	83%	85%
Warfarin Therapy Discharge Instructions[7]	-	-	75%	75%
Chest Pain/Possible Heart Attack Care				
Aspirin Given Within 24 Hours of Arrival[5]	-	-	97%	96%
Fibrinolytic Meds Within 30 Min. of Arrival[5]	-	-	62%	58%
Average Time to ECG (minutes)[5]	-	-	9	7
Average Time to Transfer (minutes)[5]	-	-	62	60
Children's Asthma Care				
Received Home Management Plan of Care	-	-	88%	88%
Received Reliever Medication	-	-	100%	100%
Received Systemic Corticosteroids	-	-	100%	100%
Emergency Department				
Admittance Decision Time (minutes)[7]	-	-	125	98
Head CT Results Within 45 Min. of Arrival[5]	-	-	55%	57%
Patients Who Left ER Before Being Seen[5]	-	-	3%	2%
Time from ER Arrival to Admit. (minutes)[7]	-	-	323	274
Time from ER Arrival to Discharge (minutes)[5]	-	-	168	134
Time in ER Before Being Evaluated (minutes)[5]	-	-	29	26
Time to Pain Meds for Fractures (minutes)[5]	-	-	62	57
Heart Attack Care				
Aspirin Given at Discharge[5]	-	-	99%	99%
Fibrinolytic Meds Within 30 Min. of Arrival[5]	-	-	73%	54%
PCI Within 90 Minutes of Arrival[5]	-	-	95%	96%
Statin Prescribed at Discharge[5]	-	-	98%	98%
Heart Failure Care				
ACE Inhibitor or ARB for LVSD[5]	-	-	97%	97%
Discharge Instructions Given[5]	-	-	94%	94%
Evaluation of LVS Function[5]	-	-	99%	99%
Medicare Spending				
Medicare Spending per Patient (ratio)	-	0.87	0.98	0.98
Pneumonia Care				
Appropriate Initial Antibiotic Given[5]	-	-	97%	95%
Blood Culture Timing[5]	-	-	98%	98%
Pregnancy and Delivery Care				
Newborn Deliveries Scheduled Early[7]	-	-	5%	6%
Preventive Care				
Immunization for Influenza	149	53%	89%	90%
Immunization for Pneumonia	93	75%	90%	92%
Stroke Care				
Anticoagulation Therapy for Atrial Fibrillation[5]	-	-	95%	95%
Antithrombotic Therapy Timing[5]	-	-	98%	98%
Assessed for Rehabilitation[5]	-	-	97%	97%
Discharged on Antithrombotic Therapy[5]	-	-	99%	99%
Discharged on Statin Medication[5]	-	-	94%	94%
Thrombolytic Therapy Timing[5]	-	-	72%	66%
Venous Thromboembolism Prophylaxis[5]	-	-	94%	94%
Written Stroke Educational Materials Given[5]	-	-	87%	88%
Surgical Care Improvement Project				
Appropriate Beta Blocker Usage[7]	-	-	97%	98%
Appropriate VTP Within 24 Hours[1]	-	-	98%	98%
Controlled Postoperative Blood Glucose[7]	-	-	96%	97%
Perioperative Temperature Management[1]	-	-	100%	100%
Prophylactic Antibiotic Selection[1]	-	-	99%	99%
Prophylactic Antibiotic Selection (Outpatient)[1]	-	-	97%	98%
Prophylactic Antibiotic Stopped[1]	-	-	98%	98%
Prophylactic Antibiotic Timing[1]	-	-	99%	99%
Prophylactic Antibiotic Timing (Outpatient)[1]	-	-	97%	98%
Urinary Catheter Removal[1]	-	-	97%	97%
Survey of Patients' Hospital Experiences				
Area Around Room 'Always' Quiet at Night	(a)	95%	51%	61%
Doctors 'Always' Communicated Well	(a)	89%	78%	82%
Home Recovery Information Given	(a)	87%	83%	85%
Hospital Given 9 or 10 on 10 Point Scale	(a)	88%	68%	71%
Meds 'Always' Explained Before Given	(a)	75%	61%	64%
Nurses 'Always' Communicated Well	(a)	84%	74%	79%
Pain 'Always' Well Controlled	(a)	81%	68%	71%
Room and Bathroom 'Always' Clean	(a)	89%	70%	73%
Timely Help 'Always' Received	(a)	88%	62%	68%
Would Definitely Recommend Hospital	(a)	86%	70%	71%
Use of Medical Imaging				
Cardiac Imaging Stress Test before Surgery[7]	-	-	5.2%	5.3%
Combination Abdominal CT Scan[7]	-	-	13.4%	10.5%
Combination Brain/Sinus CT Scan[7]	-	-	2.2%	2.7%
Combination Chest CT Scan[7]	-	-	2.3%	2.7%
Follow-up Mammogram/Ultrasound[7]	-	-	8.2%	8.8%
Lumbar Spine MRI for Low Back Pain[7]	-	-	34.2%	37.2%

Mercy Medical Center

333 Mercy Avenue
Merced, CA 95340
Phone: 209-564-5000
Fax: 209-385-7062
URL: www.mercymercedcares.org
Type: Acute Care Hospitals
Emergency Services: Yes
Ownership: Voluntary non-profit - Private
Beds: 174
Key Personnel:
Radiology. . . . . Dean Batten, MD
Quality Assurance . . . . Doreen Faiello Burnett
Chief of Medical Staff . . . . Lynn Cooman
CEO/President. . . . . David S Dunham
Cardiac Laboratory. . . . . Jerry Parker

Measure	Cases	This Hosp.	State Avg.	U.S. Avg.
Blood Clot Prevention and Treatment				
Anticoagulation Overlap Therapy[2]	85	88%	92%	93%
ICU Venous Thromboembolism Prophylaxis[2]	75	99%	92%	92%
Incidence of Potentially Preventable VTE[2]	11	9%	11%	10%
UFH with Dosages/Platelet Monitoring[2]	54	100%	96%	97%
Venous Thromboembolism Prophylaxis[2]	351	96%	83%	85%
Warfarin Therapy Discharge Instructions[2]	51	71%	75%	75%
Chest Pain/Possible Heart Attack Care				
Aspirin Given Within 24 Hours of Arrival	102	96%	97%	96%

NOTE: Hospital profiles are in alphabetical order by state, then city, then hospital within the city; Rankings exclude hospitals with less than 25 cases except for patient surveys which excludes hospitals with less than 100 cases; (a) 100-299 cases; (1) The number of cases/patients is too few to report; (2) Data submitted were based on a sample of cases/patients; (3) Results are based on a shorter time period than required; (4) Data suppressed by CMS for one or more quarters; (5) Results are not available for this reporting period; (6) Fewer than 100 patients completed the HCAHPS survey; (7) No cases met the criteria for this measure; (8) The lower limit of the confidence interval cannot be calculated if the number of observed infections equals zero; (9) No data are available from the state/territory for this reporting period; (10) The scores shown reflect fewer than 50 completed surveys; (11) There were discrepancies in the data collection process; (12) This measure does not apply to this hospital for this reporting period; (13) Results cannot be calculated for this reporting period; (14) The results for this state are combined with nearby states to protect confidentiality; Please refer to the User's Guide for a full explanation of data.

Measure	Cases	This Hosp.	State Avg.	U.S. Avg.
Fibrinolytic Meds Within 30 Min. of Arrival[1]	-	-	62%	58%
Average Time to ECG (minutes)	103	11	9	7
Average Time to Transfer (minutes)[1]	-	-	62	60
Children's Asthma Care				
Received Home Management Plan of Care	-	-	88%	88%
Received Reliever Medication	-	-	100%	100%
Received Systemic Corticosteroids	-	-	100%	100%
Emergency Department				
Admittance Decision Time (minutes)[2]	467	127	125	98
Head CT Results Within 45 Min. of Arrival	26	54%	55%	57%
Patients Who Left ER Before Being Seen	65,530	1%	3%	2%
Time from ER Arrival to Admit. (minutes)[2]	476	394	323	274
Time from ER Arrival to Discharge (minutes)	363	122	168	134
Time in ER Before Being Evaluated (minutes)	398	15	29	26
Time to Pain Meds for Fractures (minutes)	169	83	62	57
Heart Attack Care				
Aspirin Given at Discharge	37	95%	99%	99%
Fibrinolytic Meds Within 30 Min. of Arrival[1]	-	-	73%	54%
PCI Within 90 Minutes of Arrival[7]	-	-	95%	96%
Statin Prescribed at Discharge	43	86%	98%	98%
Heart Failure Care				
ACE Inhibitor or ARB for LVSD[2]	95	91%	97%	97%
Discharge Instructions Given[2]	240	97%	94%	94%
Evaluation of LVS Function[2]	287	99%	99%	99%
Medicare Spending				
Medicare Spending per Patient (ratio)	-	0.95	0.98	0.98
Pneumonia Care				
Appropriate Initial Antibiotic Given[2]	76	95%	97%	95%
Blood Culture Timing[2]	172	95%	98%	98%
Pregnancy and Delivery Care				
Newborn Deliveries Scheduled Early[2]	64	6%	5%	6%
Preventive Care				
Immunization for Influenza[2]	465	96%	89%	90%
Immunization for Pneumonia[2]	516	97%	90%	92%
Stroke Care				
Anticoagulation Therapy for Atrial Fibrillation	21	90%	95%	95%
Antithrombotic Therapy Timing	107	97%	98%	98%
Assessed for Rehabilitation	106	99%	97%	97%
Discharged on Antithrombotic Therapy	99	98%	99%	99%
Discharged on Statin Medication	84	82%	94%	94%
Thrombolytic Therapy Timing[1]	-	-	72%	66%
Venous Thromboembolism Prophylaxis	117	99%	94%	94%
Written Stroke Educational Materials Given	50	82%	87%	88%
Surgical Care Improvement Project				
Appropriate Beta Blocker Usage[2]	124	97%	97%	98%
Appropriate VTP Within 24 Hours[2]	436	99%	98%	98%
Controlled Postoperative Blood Glucose[2,7]	-	-	96%	97%
Perioperative Temperature Management[2]	481	100%	100%	100%
Prophylactic Antibiotic Selection[2]	318	98%	99%	99%
Prophylactic Antibiotic Selection (Outpatient)	131	96%	97%	98%
Prophylactic Antibiotic Stopped[2]	314	98%	98%	98%
Prophylactic Antibiotic Timing[2]	319	99%	99%	99%
Prophylactic Antibiotic Timing (Outpatient)	132	98%	97%	98%
Urinary Catheter Removal[2]	274	99%	97%	97%
Survey of Patients' Hospital Experiences				
Area Around Room 'Always' Quiet at Night	300+	58%	51%	61%
Doctors 'Always' Communicated Well	300+	75%	78%	82%
Home Recovery Information Given	300+	84%	83%	85%
Hospital Given 9 or 10 on 10 Point Scale	300+	65%	68%	71%
Meds 'Always' Explained Before Given	300+	61%	61%	64%
Nurses 'Always' Communicated Well	300+	73%	74%	79%
Pain 'Always' Well Controlled	300+	67%	68%	71%
Room and Bathroom 'Always' Clean	300+	70%	70%	73%
Timely Help 'Always' Received	300+	55%	62%	68%
Would Definitely Recommend Hospital	300+	63%	70%	71%
Use of Medical Imaging				
Cardiac Imaging Stress Test before Surgery[1]	-	-	5.2%	5.3%
Combination Abdominal CT Scan	774	3.2%	13.4%	10.5%
Combination Brain/Sinus CT Scan	940	2.0%	2.2%	2.7%
Combination Chest CT Scan	445	0.9%	2.3%	2.7%
Follow-up Mammogram/Ultrasound	765	5.6%	8.2%	8.8%
Lumbar Spine MRI for Low Back Pain[1]	-	-	34.2%	37.2%

Providence Holy Cross Medical Center

15031 Rinaldi St
Mission Hills, CA 91346
Phone: 818-365-8051
Fax: 818-898-4569
URL: www.providence.org
Type: Acute Care Hospitals
Emergency Services: Yes
Ownership: Voluntary non-profit - Church
Beds: 257

Key Personnel:
Operating Room. . . . . Missy Blackstock, RN
President/CEO. . . . . Rodney F. Hochman, MD
Quality Assurance . . . . Jean-Marie Kane
Chief of Medical Staff. . . . . Reza Nahed, MD

Measure	Cases	This Hosp.	State Avg.	U.S. Avg.
Blood Clot Prevention and Treatment				
Anticoagulation Overlap Therapy[2]	66	95%	92%	93%
ICU Venous Thromboembolism Prophylaxis[2]	73	97%	92%	92%
Incidence of Potentially Preventable VTE[2]	20	5%	11%	10%
UFH with Dosages/Platelet Monitoring[2]	24	92%	96%	97%
Venous Thromboembolism Prophylaxis[2]	318	91%	83%	85%
Warfarin Therapy Discharge Instructions[2]	43	86%	75%	75%
Chest Pain/Possible Heart Attack Care				
Aspirin Given Within 24 Hours of Arrival[3]	11	100%	97%	96%
Fibrinolytic Meds Within 30 Min. of Arrival[5]	-	-	62%	58%
Average Time to ECG (minutes)[3]	12	0	9	7
Average Time to Transfer (minutes)[5]	-	-	62	60
Children's Asthma Care				
Received Home Management Plan of Care	-	-	88%	88%
Received Reliever Medication	-	-	100%	100%
Received Systemic Corticosteroids	-	-	100%	100%
Emergency Department				
Admittance Decision Time (minutes)[2]	535	142	125	98
Head CT Results Within 45 Min. of Arrival	13	77%	55%	57%
Patients Who Left ER Before Being Seen	81,982	1%	3%	2%
Time from ER Arrival to Admit. (minutes)[2]	553	295	323	274
Time from ER Arrival to Discharge (minutes)	359	144	168	134
Time in ER Before Being Evaluated (minutes)	376	31	29	26
Time to Pain Meds for Fractures (minutes)	240	44	62	57
Heart Attack Care				
Aspirin Given at Discharge	218	100%	99%	99%
Fibrinolytic Meds Within 30 Min. of Arrival[7]	-	-	73%	54%
PCI Within 90 Minutes of Arrival	75	100%	95%	96%
Statin Prescribed at Discharge	219	100%	98%	98%
Heart Failure Care				
ACE Inhibitor or ARB for LVSD[2]	64	100%	97%	97%
Discharge Instructions Given[2]	236	83%	94%	94%
Evaluation of LVS Function[2]	281	100%	99%	99%
Medicare Spending				
Medicare Spending per Patient (ratio)	-	1.05	0.98	0.98
Pneumonia Care				
Appropriate Initial Antibiotic Given[2]	55	98%	97%	95%
Blood Culture Timing[2]	131	99%	98%	98%
Pregnancy and Delivery Care				
Newborn Deliveries Scheduled Early[2]	67	6%	5%	6%
Preventive Care				
Immunization for Influenza[2]	500	82%	89%	90%
Immunization for Pneumonia[2]	548	92%	90%	92%
Stroke Care				
Anticoagulation Therapy for Atrial Fibrillation	30	97%	95%	95%
Antithrombotic Therapy Timing	139	94%	98%	98%
Assessed for Rehabilitation	172	95%	97%	97%
Discharged on Antithrombotic Therapy	150	99%	99%	99%
Discharged on Statin Medication	124	97%	94%	94%
Thrombolytic Therapy Timing[1]	-	-	72%	66%
Venous Thromboembolism Prophylaxis	178	97%	94%	94%
Written Stroke Educational Materials Given	94	67%	87%	88%
Surgical Care Improvement Project				
Appropriate Beta Blocker Usage[2]	181	100%	97%	98%
Appropriate VTP Within 24 Hours[2]	321	99%	98%	98%
Controlled Postoperative Blood Glucose[2]	78	95%	96%	97%
Perioperative Temperature Management[2]	401	100%	100%	100%
Prophylactic Antibiotic Selection[2]	317	99%	99%	99%
Prophylactic Antibiotic Selection (Outpatient)	138	97%	97%	98%
Prophylactic Antibiotic Stopped[2]	279	99%	98%	98%
Prophylactic Antibiotic Timing[2]	319	99%	99%	99%
Prophylactic Antibiotic Timing (Outpatient)	143	94%	97%	98%
Urinary Catheter Removal[2]	274	99%	97%	97%
Survey of Patients' Hospital Experiences				
Area Around Room 'Always' Quiet at Night	300+	45%	51%	61%
Doctors 'Always' Communicated Well	300+	78%	78%	82%
Home Recovery Information Given	300+	84%	83%	85%
Hospital Given 9 or 10 on 10 Point Scale	300+	75%	68%	71%
Meds 'Always' Explained Before Given	300+	58%	61%	64%
Nurses 'Always' Communicated Well	300+	76%	74%	79%
Pain 'Always' Well Controlled	300+	73%	68%	71%
Room and Bathroom 'Always' Clean	300+	70%	70%	73%
Timely Help 'Always' Received	300+	65%	62%	68%
Would Definitely Recommend Hospital	300+	79%	70%	71%
Use of Medical Imaging				
Cardiac Imaging Stress Test before Surgery	180	6.7%	5.2%	5.3%
Combination Abdominal CT Scan	1,027	4.9%	13.4%	10.5%
Combination Brain/Sinus CT Scan	974	3.6%	2.2%	2.7%
Combination Chest CT Scan	361	3.9%	2.3%	2.7%
Follow-up Mammogram/Ultrasound	606	7.8%	8.2%	8.8%
Lumbar Spine MRI for Low Back Pain	81	34.6%	34.2%	37.2%

Mission Hospital Regional Medical Center

27700 Medical Center Rd
Mission Viejo, CA 92691
Phone: 949-364-1400
Fax: 818-904-3529
URL: www.mission4health.com
Type: Acute Care Hospitals
Emergency Services: Yes
Ownership: Voluntary non-profit - Private
Beds: 331

Key Personnel:
Quality Assurance . . . . Micheal Beck
Radiology. . . . . Brian J Bigoni
CEO/President. . . . . Kenneth McFarland
Chief of Medical Staff. . . . . Linda Sieglen, MD, MMM

Measure	Cases	This Hosp.	State Avg.	U.S. Avg.
Blood Clot Prevention and Treatment				
Anticoagulation Overlap Therapy[2]	140	91%	92%	93%
ICU Venous Thromboembolism Prophylaxis[2]	106	92%	92%	92%
Incidence of Potentially Preventable VTE[2]	36	6%	11%	10%
UFH with Dosages/Platelet Monitoring[2]	141	100%	96%	97%
Venous Thromboembolism Prophylaxis[2]	258	84%	83%	85%
Warfarin Therapy Discharge Instructions[2]	101	66%	75%	75%
Chest Pain/Possible Heart Attack Care				
Aspirin Given Within 24 Hours of Arrival	21	95%	97%	96%
Fibrinolytic Meds Within 30 Min. of Arrival[3,7]	-	-	62%	58%
Average Time to ECG (minutes)	21	3	9	7
Average Time to Transfer (minutes)[3,7]	-	-	62	60
Children's Asthma Care				
Received Home Management Plan of Care	-	-	88%	88%
Received Reliever Medication	-	-	100%	100%
Received Systemic Corticosteroids	-	-	100%	100%
Emergency Department				
Admittance Decision Time (minutes)[2]	487	105	125	98
Head CT Results Within 45 Min. of Arrival[1]	-	-	55%	57%
Patients Who Left ER Before Being Seen	56,025	1%	3%	2%
Time from ER Arrival to Admit. (minutes)[2]	500	266	323	274
Time from ER Arrival to Discharge (minutes)	339	177	168	134
Time in ER Before Being Evaluated (minutes)	383	34	29	26
Time to Pain Meds for Fractures (minutes)	124	66	62	57
Heart Attack Care				
Aspirin Given at Discharge	250	99%	99%	99%
Fibrinolytic Meds Within 30 Min. of Arrival[7]	-	-	73%	54%
PCI Within 90 Minutes of Arrival	51	96%	95%	96%
Statin Prescribed at Discharge	247	93%	98%	98%
Heart Failure Care				
ACE Inhibitor or ARB for LVSD	78	94%	97%	97%
Discharge Instructions Given	246	86%	94%	94%
Evaluation of LVS Function	297	99%	99%	99%
Medicare Spending				
Medicare Spending per Patient (ratio)	-	0.99	0.98	0.98
Pneumonia Care				
Appropriate Initial Antibiotic Given	188	96%	97%	95%
Blood Culture Timing	319	97%	98%	98%
Pregnancy and Delivery Care				
Newborn Deliveries Scheduled Early[2]	61	8%	5%	6%

NOTE: Hospital profiles are in alphabetical order by state, then city, then hospital within the city; Rankings exclude hospitals with less than 25 cases except for patient surveys which excludes hospitals with less than 100 cases; (a) 100-299 cases; (1) The number of cases/patients is too few to report; (2) Data submitted were based on a sample of cases/patients; (3) Results are based on a shorter time period than required; (4) Data suppressed by CMS for one or more quarters; (5) Results are not available for this reporting period; (6) Fewer than 100 patients completed the HCAHPS survey; (7) No cases met the criteria for this measure; (8) The lower limit of the confidence interval cannot be calculated if the number of observed infections equals zero; (9) No data are available from the state/territory for this reporting period; (10) The scores shown reflect fewer than 50 completed surveys; (11) There were discrepancies in the data collection process; (12) This measure does not apply to this hospital for this reporting period; (13) Results cannot be calculated for this reporting period; (14) The results for this state are combined with nearby states to protect confidentiality; Please refer to the User's Guide for a full explanation of data.

Measure	Cases	This Hosp.	State Avg.	U.S. Avg.
Preventive Care				
Immunization for Influenza[2]	534	96%	89%	90%
Immunization for Pneumonia[2]	551	91%	90%	92%
Stroke Care				
Anticoagulation Therapy for Atrial Fibrillation	33	94%	95%	95%
Antithrombotic Therapy Timing	139	96%	98%	98%
Assessed for Rehabilitation	218	99%	97%	97%
Discharged on Antithrombotic Therapy	165	99%	99%	99%
Discharged on Statin Medication	137	87%	94%	94%
Thrombolytic Therapy Timing	21	67%	72%	66%
Venous Thromboembolism Prophylaxis	226	95%	94%	94%
Written Stroke Educational Materials Given	111	74%	87%	88%
Surgical Care Improvement Project				
Appropriate Beta Blocker Usage[2]	139	96%	97%	98%
Appropriate VTP Within 24 Hours[2]	316	95%	98%	98%
Controlled Postoperative Blood Glucose[2]	103	92%	96%	97%
Perioperative Temperature Management[2]	411	98%	100%	100%
Prophylactic Antibiotic Selection[2]	344	99%	99%	99%
Prophylactic Antibiotic Selection (Outpatient)	364	98%	97%	98%
Prophylactic Antibiotic Stopped[2]	328	97%	98%	98%
Prophylactic Antibiotic Timing[2]	346	96%	99%	99%
Prophylactic Antibiotic Timing (Outpatient)	347	95%	97%	98%
Urinary Catheter Removal[2]	358	96%	97%	97%
Survey of Patients' Hospital Experiences				
Area Around Room 'Always' Quiet at Night	300+	53%	51%	61%
Doctors 'Always' Communicated Well	300+	79%	78%	82%
Home Recovery Information Given	300+	82%	83%	85%
Hospital Given 9 or 10 on 10 Point Scale	300+	76%	68%	71%
Meds 'Always' Explained Before Given	300+	59%	61%	64%
Nurses 'Always' Communicated Well	300+	76%	74%	79%
Pain 'Always' Well Controlled	300+	71%	68%	71%
Room and Bathroom 'Always' Clean	300+	69%	70%	73%
Timely Help 'Always' Received	300+	60%	62%	68%
Would Definitely Recommend Hospital	300+	81%	70%	71%
Use of Medical Imaging				
Cardiac Imaging Stress Test before Surgery	252	5.2%	5.2%	5.3%
Combination Abdominal CT Scan	1,308	17.7%	13.4%	10.5%
Combination Brain/Sinus CT Scan	1,242	3.4%	2.2%	2.7%
Combination Chest CT Scan	910	2.3%	2.3%	2.7%
Follow-up Mammogram/Ultrasound	2,774	13.7%	8.2%	8.8%
Lumbar Spine MRI for Low Back Pain	155	29.0%	34.2%	37.2%

Doctors Medical Center

1441 Florida Avenue
Modesto, CA 95350
Phone: 209-578-1211
Fax: 209-576-3680
E-mail: catherine.larson@tenethealth.com
URL: www.dmc-modesto.com
Type: Acute Care Hospitals
Emergency Services: Yes
Ownership: Proprietary
Beds: 456

Key Personnel:
Radiology. . . . . Roberta Edge
Operating Room. . . . . Syd Fuentes
CEO/President. . . . . Warren J. Kirk
Quality Assurance . . . . Jay Krishnasuiamy
Emergency Room . . . . Laura List

Measure	Cases	This Hosp.	State Avg.	U.S. Avg.
Blood Clot Prevention and Treatment				
Anticoagulation Overlap Therapy[2]	129	86%	92%	93%
ICU Venous Thromboembolism Prophylaxis[2]	104	95%	92%	92%
Incidence of Potentially Preventable VTE[2]	39	13%	11%	10%
UFH with Dosages/Platelet Monitoring[2]	102	100%	96%	97%
Venous Thromboembolism Prophylaxis[2]	343	85%	83%	85%
Warfarin Therapy Discharge Instructions[2]	90	98%	75%	75%
Chest Pain/Possible Heart Attack Care				
Aspirin Given Within 24 Hours of Arrival[1,3]	-	-	97%	96%
Fibrinolytic Meds Within 30 Min. of Arrival[5]	-	-	62%	58%
Average Time to ECG (minutes)[1,3]	-	-	9	7
Average Time to Transfer (minutes)[5]	-	-	62	60
Children's Asthma Care				
Received Home Management Plan of Care	-	-	88%	88%
Received Reliever Medication	-	-	100%	100%
Received Systemic Corticosteroids	-	-	100%	100%
Emergency Department				
Admittance Decision Time (minutes)[2]	579	186	125	98
Head CT Results Within 45 Min. of Arrival[1]	-	-	55%	57%
Patients Who Left ER Before Being Seen	85,151	1%	3%	2%
Time from ER Arrival to Admit. (minutes)[2]	598	372	323	274
Time from ER Arrival to Discharge (minutes)	459	117	168	134
Time in ER Before Being Evaluated (minutes)	498	19	29	26
Time to Pain Meds for Fractures (minutes)	230	44	62	57
Heart Attack Care				
Aspirin Given at Discharge	312	100%	99%	99%
Fibrinolytic Meds Within 30 Min. of Arrival[1]	-	-	73%	54%
PCI Within 90 Minutes of Arrival	50	100%	95%	96%
Statin Prescribed at Discharge	321	99%	98%	98%
Heart Failure Care				
ACE Inhibitor or ARB for LVSD	144	97%	97%	97%
Discharge Instructions Given	347	93%	94%	94%
Evaluation of LVS Function	394	100%	99%	99%
Medicare Spending				
Medicare Spending per Patient (ratio)	-	0.96	0.98	0.98
Pneumonia Care				
Appropriate Initial Antibiotic Given[2]	220	98%	97%	95%
Blood Culture Timing[2]	344	100%	98%	98%
Pregnancy and Delivery Care				
Newborn Deliveries Scheduled Early[2]	70	6%	5%	6%
Preventive Care				
Immunization for Influenza[2]	536	99%	89%	90%
Immunization for Pneumonia[2]	511	95%	90%	92%
Stroke Care				
Anticoagulation Therapy for Atrial Fibrillation	18	89%	95%	95%
Antithrombotic Therapy Timing	184	98%	98%	98%
Assessed for Rehabilitation	218	98%	97%	97%
Discharged on Antithrombotic Therapy	181	99%	99%	99%
Discharged on Statin Medication	146	98%	94%	94%
Thrombolytic Therapy Timing[1]	-	-	72%	66%
Venous Thromboembolism Prophylaxis	239	98%	94%	94%
Written Stroke Educational Materials Given	130	98%	87%	88%
Surgical Care Improvement Project				
Appropriate Beta Blocker Usage[2]	353	100%	97%	98%
Appropriate VTP Within 24 Hours[2]	736	99%	98%	98%
Controlled Postoperative Blood Glucose[2]	207	98%	96%	97%
Perioperative Temperature Management[2]	874	100%	100%	100%
Prophylactic Antibiotic Selection[2]	767	100%	99%	99%
Prophylactic Antibiotic Selection (Outpatient)	483	95%	97%	98%
Prophylactic Antibiotic Stopped[2]	693	99%	98%	98%
Prophylactic Antibiotic Timing[2]	768	99%	99%	99%
Prophylactic Antibiotic Timing (Outpatient)	484	99%	97%	98%
Urinary Catheter Removal[2]	485	99%	97%	97%
Survey of Patients' Hospital Experiences				
Area Around Room 'Always' Quiet at Night	300+	43%	51%	61%
Doctors 'Always' Communicated Well	300+	80%	78%	82%
Home Recovery Information Given	300+	87%	83%	85%
Hospital Given 9 or 10 on 10 Point Scale	300+	71%	68%	71%
Meds 'Always' Explained Before Given	300+	69%	61%	64%
Nurses 'Always' Communicated Well	300+	77%	74%	79%
Pain 'Always' Well Controlled	300+	70%	68%	71%
Room and Bathroom 'Always' Clean	300+	67%	70%	73%
Timely Help 'Always' Received	300+	60%	62%	68%
Would Definitely Recommend Hospital	300+	74%	70%	71%
Use of Medical Imaging				
Cardiac Imaging Stress Test before Surgery	1,280	3.3%	5.2%	5.3%
Combination Abdominal CT Scan	366	1.4%	13.4%	10.5%
Combination Brain/Sinus CT Scan	605	0.8%	2.2%	2.7%
Combination Chest CT Scan	79	0.0%	2.3%	2.7%
Follow-up Mammogram/Ultrasound[7]	-	-	8.2%	8.8%
Lumbar Spine MRI for Low Back Pain[1]	-	-	34.2%	37.2%

Memorial Medical Center

1700 Coffee Rd
Modesto, CA 95355
Phone: 209-526-4500
Fax: 209-576-7385
URL: www.memorialmedicalcenter.org
Type: Acute Care Hospitals
Emergency Services: Yes
Ownership: Voluntary non-profit - Private
Beds: 112

Key Personnel:
Quality Assurance . . . . Ruth Ann Burris
CEO . . . . Daryn J. Kumar
Chief of Medical Staff. . . . . Jeremy Mesches
Administrator . . . . Nikhil Singal

Measure	Cases	This Hosp.	State Avg.	U.S. Avg.
Blood Clot Prevention and Treatment				
Anticoagulation Overlap Therapy[2]	140	100%	92%	93%
ICU Venous Thromboembolism Prophylaxis[2]	72	90%	92%	92%
Incidence of Potentially Preventable VTE[2]	15	0%	11%	10%
UFH with Dosages/Platelet Monitoring[2]	88	100%	96%	97%
Venous Thromboembolism Prophylaxis[2]	346	87%	83%	85%
Warfarin Therapy Discharge Instructions[2]	97	91%	75%	75%
Chest Pain/Possible Heart Attack Care				
Aspirin Given Within 24 Hours of Arrival[1,3]	-	-	97%	96%
Fibrinolytic Meds Within 30 Min. of Arrival[5]	-	-	62%	58%
Average Time to ECG (minutes)[1,3]	-	-	9	7
Average Time to Transfer (minutes)[5]	-	-	62	60
Children's Asthma Care				
Received Home Management Plan of Care	-	-	88%	88%
Received Reliever Medication	-	-	100%	100%
Received Systemic Corticosteroids	-	-	100%	100%
Emergency Department				
Admittance Decision Time (minutes)[2]	792	149	125	98
Head CT Results Within 45 Min. of Arrival	12	67%	55%	57%
Patients Who Left ER Before Being Seen	71,043	5%	3%	2%
Time from ER Arrival to Admit. (minutes)[2]	807	328	323	274
Time from ER Arrival to Discharge (minutes)	395	168	168	134
Time in ER Before Being Evaluated (minutes)	412	34	29	26
Time to Pain Meds for Fractures (minutes)	216	67	62	57
Heart Attack Care				
Aspirin Given at Discharge	352	100%	99%	99%
Fibrinolytic Meds Within 30 Min. of Arrival[7]	-	-	73%	54%
PCI Within 90 Minutes of Arrival	46	100%	95%	96%
Statin Prescribed at Discharge	341	99%	98%	98%
Heart Failure Care				
ACE Inhibitor or ARB for LVSD[2]	70	100%	97%	97%
Discharge Instructions Given[2]	263	100%	94%	94%
Evaluation of LVS Function[2]	312	100%	99%	99%
Medicare Spending				
Medicare Spending per Patient (ratio)	-	0.97	0.98	0.98
Pneumonia Care				
Appropriate Initial Antibiotic Given[2]	90	100%	97%	95%
Blood Culture Timing[2]	164	99%	98%	98%
Pregnancy and Delivery Care				
Newborn Deliveries Scheduled Early	135	1%	5%	6%
Preventive Care				
Immunization for Influenza[2]	557	99%	89%	90%
Immunization for Pneumonia[2]	720	100%	90%	92%
Stroke Care				
Anticoagulation Therapy for Atrial Fibrillation	22	100%	95%	95%
Antithrombotic Therapy Timing	147	100%	98%	98%
Assessed for Rehabilitation	205	100%	97%	97%
Discharged on Antithrombotic Therapy	162	100%	99%	99%
Discharged on Statin Medication	132	98%	94%	94%
Thrombolytic Therapy Timing[1]	-	-	72%	66%
Venous Thromboembolism Prophylaxis	207	91%	94%	94%
Written Stroke Educational Materials Given	117	87%	87%	88%
Surgical Care Improvement Project				
Appropriate Beta Blocker Usage[2]	218	100%	97%	98%
Appropriate VTP Within 24 Hours[2]	446	100%	98%	98%
Controlled Postoperative Blood Glucose[2]	129	98%	96%	97%
Perioperative Temperature Management[2]	562	100%	100%	100%
Prophylactic Antibiotic Selection[2]	442	100%	99%	99%
Prophylactic Antibiotic Selection (Outpatient)	146	100%	97%	98%
Prophylactic Antibiotic Stopped[2]	419	100%	98%	98%
Prophylactic Antibiotic Timing[2]	444	100%	99%	99%
Prophylactic Antibiotic Timing (Outpatient)	147	97%	97%	98%
Urinary Catheter Removal[2]	327	99%	97%	97%
Survey of Patients' Hospital Experiences				
Area Around Room 'Always' Quiet at Night	300+	51%	51%	61%
Doctors 'Always' Communicated Well	300+	79%	78%	82%
Home Recovery Information Given	300+	85%	83%	85%
Hospital Given 9 or 10 on 10 Point Scale	300+	72%	68%	71%
Meds 'Always' Explained Before Given	300+	63%	61%	64%

NOTE: Hospital profiles are in alphabetical order by state, then city, then hospital within the city; Rankings exclude hospitals with less than 25 cases except for patient surveys which excludes hospitals with less than 100 cases; (a) 100-299 cases; (1) The number of cases/patients is too few to report; (2) Data submitted were based on a sample of cases/patients; (3) Results are based on a shorter time period than required; (4) Data suppressed by CMS for one or more quarters; (5) Results are not available for this reporting period; (6) Fewer than 100 patients completed the HCAHPS survey; (7) No cases met the criteria for this measure; (8) The lower limit of the confidence interval cannot be calculated if the number of observed infections equals zero; (9) No data are available from the state/territory for this reporting period; (10) The scores shown reflect fewer than 50 completed surveys; (11) There were discrepancies in the data collection process; (12) This measure does not apply to this hospital for this reporting period; (13) Results cannot be calculated for this reporting period; (14) The results for this state are combined with nearby states to protect confidentiality; Please refer to the User's Guide for a full explanation of data.

Nurses 'Always' Communicated Well	300+	78%	74%	79%
Pain 'Always' Well Controlled	300+	72%	68%	71%
Room and Bathroom 'Always' Clean	300+	75%	70%	73%
Timely Help 'Always' Received	300+	63%	62%	68%
Would Definitely Recommend Hospital	300+	79%	70%	71%
Use of Medical Imaging				
Cardiac Imaging Stress Test before Surgery	308	4.2%	5.2%	5.3%
Combination Abdominal CT Scan	668	0.7%	13.4%	10.5%
Combination Brain/Sinus CT Scan	785	1.7%	2.2%	2.7%
Combination Chest CT Scan	227	1.8%	2.3%	2.7%
Follow-up Mammogram/Ultrasound[7]	-	-	8.2%	8.8%
Lumbar Spine MRI for Low Back Pain[1]	-	-	34.2%	37.2%

Stanislaus Surgical Hospital

1421 Oakdale Road Phone: 209-572-2700
Modesto, CA 95355
URL: www.stanislaussurgical.com
Type: Acute Care Hospitals Emergency Services: No
Ownership: Proprietary
Key Personnel:
Radiology. . . . . Serge Djukic
CEO . . . . Douglas V. Johnson

Measure	Cases	This Hosp.	State Avg.	U.S. Avg.
Blood Clot Prevention and Treatment				
Anticoagulation Overlap Therapy[2,7]	-	-	92%	93%
ICU Venous Thromboembolism Prophylaxis[2,7]	-	-	92%	92%
Incidence of Potentially Preventable VTE[2,7]	-	-	11%	10%
UFH with Dosages/Platelet Monitoring[2,7]	-	-	96%	97%
Venous Thromboembolism Prophylaxis[2]	47	100%	83%	85%
Warfarin Therapy Discharge Instructions[2,7]	-	-	75%	75%
Chest Pain/Possible Heart Attack Care				
Aspirin Given Within 24 Hours of Arrival[5]	-	-	97%	96%
Fibrinolytic Meds Within 30 Min. of Arrival[5]	-	-	62%	58%
Average Time to ECG (minutes)[5]	-	-	9	7
Average Time to Transfer (minutes)[5]	-	-	62	60
Children's Asthma Care				
Received Home Management Plan of Care	-	-	88%	88%
Received Reliever Medication	-	-	100%	100%
Received Systemic Corticosteroids	-	-	100%	100%
Emergency Department				
Admittance Decision Time (minutes)[2,7]	-	-	125	98
Head CT Results Within 45 Min. of Arrival[5]	-	-	55%	57%
Patients Who Left ER Before Being Seen[5]	-	-	3%	2%
Time from ER Arrival to Admit. (minutes)[2,7]	-	-	323	274
Time from ER Arrival to Discharge (minutes)[5]	-	-	168	134
Time in ER Before Being Evaluated (minutes)[5]	-	-	29	26
Time to Pain Meds for Fractures (minutes)[5]	-	-	62	57
Heart Attack Care				
Aspirin Given at Discharge[5]	-	-	99%	99%
Fibrinolytic Meds Within 30 Min. of Arrival[5]	-	-	73%	54%
PCI Within 90 Minutes of Arrival[5]	-	-	95%	96%
Statin Prescribed at Discharge[5]	-	-	98%	98%
Heart Failure Care				
ACE Inhibitor or ARB for LVSD[5]	-	-	97%	97%
Discharge Instructions Given[5]	-	-	94%	94%
Evaluation of LVS Function[5]	-	-	99%	99%
Medicare Spending				
Medicare Spending per Patient (ratio)	-	0.93	0.98	0.98
Pneumonia Care				
Appropriate Initial Antibiotic Given[5]	-	-	97%	95%
Blood Culture Timing[5]	-	-	98%	98%
Pregnancy and Delivery Care				
Newborn Deliveries Scheduled Early[2,7]	-	-	5%	6%
Preventive Care				
Immunization for Influenza[2]	304	93%	89%	90%
Immunization for Pneumonia[2]	337	95%	90%	92%
Stroke Care				
Anticoagulation Therapy for Atrial Fibrillation[5]	-	-	95%	95%
Antithrombotic Therapy Timing[5]	-	-	98%	98%
Assessed for Rehabilitation[5]	-	-	97%	97%
Discharged on Antithrombotic Therapy[5]	-	-	99%	99%
Discharged on Statin Medication[5]	-	-	94%	94%
Thrombolytic Therapy Timing[5]	-	-	72%	66%
Venous Thromboembolism Prophylaxis[5]	-	-	94%	94%
Written Stroke Educational Materials Given[5]	-	-	87%	88%
Surgical Care Improvement Project				
Appropriate Beta Blocker Usage[2]	41	98%	97%	98%
Appropriate VTP Within 24 Hours[2]	179	99%	98%	98%
Controlled Postoperative Blood Glucose[2,7]	-	-	96%	97%
Perioperative Temperature Management[2]	204	100%	100%	100%
Prophylactic Antibiotic Selection[2]	178	99%	99%	99%
Prophylactic Antibiotic Selection (Outpatient)	93	99%	97%	98%
Prophylactic Antibiotic Stopped[2]	178	97%	98%	98%
Prophylactic Antibiotic Timing[2]	178	95%	99%	99%
Prophylactic Antibiotic Timing (Outpatient)	100	92%	97%	98%
Urinary Catheter Removal[2]	50	98%	97%	97%
Survey of Patients' Hospital Experiences				
Area Around Room 'Always' Quiet at Night	300+	75%	51%	61%
Doctors 'Always' Communicated Well	300+	84%	78%	82%
Home Recovery Information Given	300+	88%	83%	85%
Hospital Given 9 or 10 on 10 Point Scale	300+	86%	68%	71%
Meds 'Always' Explained Before Given	300+	71%	61%	64%
Nurses 'Always' Communicated Well	300+	88%	74%	79%
Pain 'Always' Well Controlled	300+	79%	68%	71%
Room and Bathroom 'Always' Clean	300+	88%	70%	73%
Timely Help 'Always' Received	300+	85%	62%	68%
Would Definitely Recommend Hospital	300+	88%	70%	71%
Use of Medical Imaging				
Cardiac Imaging Stress Test before Surgery[7]	-	-	5.2%	5.3%
Combination Abdominal CT Scan	49	61.2%	13.4%	10.5%
Combination Brain/Sinus CT Scan[1]	-	-	2.2%	2.7%
Combination Chest CT Scan[1]	-	-	2.3%	2.7%
Follow-up Mammogram/Ultrasound	157	19.1%	8.2%	8.8%
Lumbar Spine MRI for Low Back Pain[1]	-	-	34.2%	37.2%

Montclair Hospital Medical Center

5000 San Bernardino St Phone: 909-625-8300
Montclair, CA 91763 Fax: 909-626-4777
URL: www.dhmcm.com
Type: Acute Care Hospitals Emergency Services: Yes
Ownership: Voluntary non-profit - Private Beds: 102
Key Personnel:
Radiology. . . . . Bienvenido R Alona
Emergency Room . . . . Nini Dyogi, RN
Pediatric In-Patient Care . . . . Bharati Ghosh, MD
Chief of Medical Staff. . . . . Joseph Hourany, MD
Intensive Care Unit. . . . . J Frank Hsu, MD
Quality Assurance . . . . Gary Lai, MD
CEO/President. . . . . Lex Reddy
Operating Room. . . . . Deepak Sheth, MD

Measure	Cases	This Hosp.	State Avg.	U.S. Avg.
Blood Clot Prevention and Treatment				
Anticoagulation Overlap Therapy[1,2]	-	-	92%	93%
ICU Venous Thromboembolism Prophylaxis[2]	48	85%	92%	92%
Incidence of Potentially Preventable VTE[2,7]	-	-	11%	10%
UFH with Dosages/Platelet Monitoring[1,2]	-	-	96%	97%
Venous Thromboembolism Prophylaxis[2]	189	80%	83%	85%
Warfarin Therapy Discharge Instructions[1,2]	-	-	75%	75%
Chest Pain/Possible Heart Attack Care				
Aspirin Given Within 24 Hours of Arrival[1]	-	-	97%	96%
Fibrinolytic Meds Within 30 Min. of Arrival[7]	-	-	62%	58%
Average Time to ECG (minutes)[1]	-	-	9	7
Average Time to Transfer (minutes)[1]	-	-	62	60
Children's Asthma Care				
Received Home Management Plan of Care	-	-	88%	88%
Received Reliever Medication	-	-	100%	100%
Received Systemic Corticosteroids	-	-	100%	100%
Emergency Department				
Admittance Decision Time (minutes)[2]	527	66	125	98
Head CT Results Within 45 Min. of Arrival[1,3]	-	-	55%	57%
Patients Who Left ER Before Being Seen	21,282	3%	3%	2%
Time from ER Arrival to Admit. (minutes)[2]	528	210	323	274
Time from ER Arrival to Discharge (minutes)	374	127	168	134
Time in ER Before Being Evaluated (minutes)	401	13	29	26
Time to Pain Meds for Fractures (minutes)	57	53	62	57
Heart Attack Care				
Aspirin Given at Discharge	17	100%	99%	99%
Fibrinolytic Meds Within 30 Min. of Arrival[7]	-	-	73%	54%
PCI Within 90 Minutes of Arrival[7]	-	-	95%	96%
Statin Prescribed at Discharge	13	100%	98%	98%
Heart Failure Care				
ACE Inhibitor or ARB for LVSD	17	100%	97%	97%
Discharge Instructions Given	51	100%	94%	94%
Evaluation of LVS Function	59	100%	99%	99%
Medicare Spending				
Medicare Spending per Patient (ratio)	-	1.09	0.98	0.98
Pneumonia Care				
Appropriate Initial Antibiotic Given	41	95%	97%	95%
Blood Culture Timing	116	100%	98%	98%
Pregnancy and Delivery Care				
Newborn Deliveries Scheduled Early[2]	48	2%	5%	6%
Preventive Care				
Immunization for Influenza[2]	382	98%	89%	90%
Immunization for Pneumonia[2]	342	98%	90%	92%
Stroke Care				
Anticoagulation Therapy for Atrial Fibrillation[7]	-	-	95%	95%
Antithrombotic Therapy Timing[1]	-	-	98%	98%
Assessed for Rehabilitation[1]	-	-	97%	97%
Discharged on Antithrombotic Therapy[1]	-	-	99%	99%
Discharged on Statin Medication[1]	-	-	94%	94%
Thrombolytic Therapy Timing[7]	-	-	72%	66%
Venous Thromboembolism Prophylaxis[1]	-	-	94%	94%
Written Stroke Educational Materials Given[1]	-	-	87%	88%
Surgical Care Improvement Project				
Appropriate Beta Blocker Usage[1]	-	-	97%	98%
Appropriate VTP Within 24 Hours	27	100%	98%	98%
Controlled Postoperative Blood Glucose[7]	-	-	96%	97%
Perioperative Temperature Management	31	100%	100%	100%
Prophylactic Antibiotic Selection[1]	-	-	99%	99%
Prophylactic Antibiotic Selection (Outpatient)[1,3]	-	-	97%	98%
Prophylactic Antibiotic Stopped[1]	-	-	98%	98%
Prophylactic Antibiotic Timing[1]	-	-	99%	99%
Prophylactic Antibiotic Timing (Outpatient)[1,3]	-	-	97%	98%
Urinary Catheter Removal[1]	-	-	97%	97%
Survey of Patients' Hospital Experiences				
Area Around Room 'Always' Quiet at Night[11]	(a)	57%	51%	61%
Doctors 'Always' Communicated Well[11]	(a)	72%	78%	82%
Home Recovery Information Given[11]	(a)	83%	83%	85%
Hospital Given 9 or 10 on 10 Point Scale[11]	(a)	66%	68%	71%
Meds 'Always' Explained Before Given[11]	(a)	61%	61%	64%
Nurses 'Always' Communicated Well[11]	(a)	72%	74%	79%
Pain 'Always' Well Controlled[11]	(a)	64%	68%	71%
Room and Bathroom 'Always' Clean[11]	(a)	74%	70%	73%
Timely Help 'Always' Received[11]	(a)	59%	62%	68%
Would Definitely Recommend Hospital[11]	(a)	67%	70%	71%
Use of Medical Imaging				
Cardiac Imaging Stress Test before Surgery[7]	-	-	5.2%	5.3%
Combination Abdominal CT Scan	80	0.0%	13.4%	10.5%
Combination Brain/Sinus CT Scan[1]	-	-	2.2%	2.7%
Combination Chest CT Scan[1]	-	-	2.3%	2.7%
Follow-up Mammogram/Ultrasound[7]	-	-	8.2%	8.8%
Lumbar Spine MRI for Low Back Pain[7]	-	-	34.2%	37.2%

Beverly Hospital

309 W Beverly Blvd Phone: 323-726-1222
Montebello, CA 90640 Fax: 323-837-3481
URL: www.beverly.org
Type: Acute Care Hospitals Emergency Services: Yes
Ownership: Voluntary non-profit - Private Beds: 223
Key Personnel:
Pediatric In-Patient Care . . . . Marcia Batzloff, RN
Radiology. . . . . Stephen Greenberg
Coronary Care . . . . Ruth Johnson, RN
CEO/President. . . . . Gary V Kiff
Chief of Medical Staff. . . . . Jackson Ma
Operating Room. . . . . Lynda Mansfield, RN
Quality Assurance . . . . Carol Poore

Measure	Cases	This Hosp.	State Avg.	U.S. Avg.
Blood Clot Prevention and Treatment				
Anticoagulation Overlap Therapy[2]	41	39%	92%	93%
ICU Venous Thromboembolism Prophylaxis[2]	98	72%	92%	92%

NOTE: Hospital profiles are in alphabetical order by state, then city, then hospital within the city; Rankings exclude hospitals with less than 25 cases except for patient surveys which excludes hospitals with less than 100 cases; (a) 100-299 cases; (1) The number of cases/patients is too few to report; (2) Data submitted were based on a sample of cases/patients; (3) Results are based on a shorter time period than required; (4) Data suppressed by CMS for one or more quarters; (5) Results are not available for this reporting period; (6) Fewer than 100 patients completed the HCAHPS survey; (7) No cases met the criteria for this measure; (8) The lower limit of the confidence interval cannot be calculated if the number of observed infections equals zero; (9) No data are available from the state/territory for this reporting period; (10) The scores shown reflect fewer than 50 completed surveys; (11) There were discrepancies in the data collection process; (12) This measure does not apply to this hospital for this reporting period; (13) Results cannot be calculated for this reporting period; (14) The results for this state are combined with nearby states to protect confidentiality; Please refer to the User's Guide for a full explanation of data.

Incidence of Potentially Preventable VTE[1,2]	-	-	11%	10%
UFH with Dosages/Platelet Monitoring[2]	20	100%	96%	97%
Venous Thromboembolism Prophylaxis[2]	327	57%	83%	85%
Warfarin Therapy Discharge Instructions[2]	24	96%	75%	75%
Chest Pain/Possible Heart Attack Care				
Aspirin Given Within 24 Hours of Arrival	25	96%	97%	96%
Fibrinolytic Meds Within 30 Min. of Arrival[3,7]	-	-	62%	58%
Average Time to ECG (minutes)	28	4	9	7
Average Time to Transfer (minutes)[3,7]	-	-	62	60
Children's Asthma Care				
Received Home Management Plan of Care	-	-	88%	88%
Received Reliever Medication	-	-	100%	100%
Received Systemic Corticosteroids	-	-	100%	100%
Emergency Department				
Admittance Decision Time (minutes)[2]	732	138	125	98
Head CT Results Within 45 Min. of Arrival[1]	-	-	55%	57%
Patients Who Left ER Before Being Seen	34,293	2%	3%	2%
Time from ER Arrival to Admit. (minutes)[2]	737	411	323	274
Time from ER Arrival to Discharge (minutes)	331	242	168	134
Time in ER Before Being Evaluated (minutes)	387	22	29	26
Time to Pain Meds for Fractures (minutes)	145	69	62	57
Heart Attack Care				
Aspirin Given at Discharge	138	99%	99%	99%
Fibrinolytic Meds Within 30 Min. of Arrival[7]	-	-	73%	54%
PCI Within 90 Minutes of Arrival	22	77%	95%	96%
Statin Prescribed at Discharge	143	97%	98%	98%
Heart Failure Care				
ACE Inhibitor or ARB for LVSD	81	88%	97%	97%
Discharge Instructions Given	214	80%	94%	94%
Evaluation of LVS Function	286	99%	99%	99%
Medicare Spending				
Medicare Spending per Patient (ratio)	-	1.09	0.98	0.98
Pneumonia Care				
Appropriate Initial Antibiotic Given[2]	83	92%	97%	95%
Blood Culture Timing[2]	177	100%	98%	98%
Pregnancy and Delivery Care				
Newborn Deliveries Scheduled Early[2]	57	11%	5%	6%
Preventive Care				
Immunization for Influenza[2]	537	82%	89%	90%
Immunization for Pneumonia[2]	613	95%	90%	92%
Stroke Care				
Anticoagulation Therapy for Atrial Fibrillation	13	62%	95%	95%
Antithrombotic Therapy Timing	86	84%	98%	98%
Assessed for Rehabilitation	82	80%	97%	97%
Discharged on Antithrombotic Therapy	79	91%	99%	99%
Discharged on Statin Medication	70	77%	94%	94%
Thrombolytic Therapy Timing[1]	-	-	72%	66%
Venous Thromboembolism Prophylaxis	93	60%	94%	94%
Written Stroke Educational Materials Given	44	57%	87%	88%
Surgical Care Improvement Project				
Appropriate Beta Blocker Usage	78	90%	97%	98%
Appropriate VTP Within 24 Hours	283	95%	98%	98%
Controlled Postoperative Blood Glucose	25	96%	96%	97%
Perioperative Temperature Management	311	100%	100%	100%
Prophylactic Antibiotic Selection	208	98%	99%	99%
Prophylactic Antibiotic Selection (Outpatient)	90	91%	97%	98%
Prophylactic Antibiotic Stopped	204	94%	98%	98%
Prophylactic Antibiotic Timing	208	100%	99%	99%
Prophylactic Antibiotic Timing (Outpatient)	91	93%	97%	98%
Urinary Catheter Removal	141	98%	97%	97%
Survey of Patients' Hospital Experiences				
Area Around Room 'Always' Quiet at Night	300+	44%	51%	61%
Doctors 'Always' Communicated Well	300+	71%	78%	82%
Home Recovery Information Given	300+	80%	83%	85%
Hospital Given 9 or 10 on 10 Point Scale	300+	59%	68%	71%
Meds 'Always' Explained Before Given	300+	51%	61%	64%
Nurses 'Always' Communicated Well	300+	67%	74%	79%
Pain 'Always' Well Controlled	300+	61%	68%	71%
Room and Bathroom 'Always' Clean	300+	70%	70%	73%
Timely Help 'Always' Received	300+	51%	62%	68%
Would Definitely Recommend Hospital	300+	59%	70%	71%
Use of Medical Imaging				
Cardiac Imaging Stress Test before Surgery[1]	-	-	5.2%	5.3%
Combination Abdominal CT Scan	336	0.6%	13.4%	10.5%
Combination Brain/Sinus CT Scan[1]	-	-	2.2%	2.7%
Combination Chest CT Scan	161	0.0%	2.3%	2.7%
Follow-up Mammogram/Ultrasound	704	7.4%	8.2%	8.8%
Lumbar Spine MRI for Low Back Pain[1]	-	-	34.2%	37.2%

Community Hospital of the Monterey Peninsula

23625 W R Holman Highway
Monterey, CA 93940
Phone: 831-624-5311
Fax: 831-624-0497
E-mail: information@chomp.org
URL: www.chomp.org
Type: Acute Care Hospitals
Emergency Services: Yes
Ownership: Voluntary non-profit - Private
Beds: 205

Key Personnel:

Cardiac Laboratory. . . . . Mike Barber, RN
CEO/President. . . . . Steven J Packer, MD
Emergency Room . . . . Jodi Schaffer, RN

Measure	Cases	This Hosp.	State Avg.	U.S. Avg.
Blood Clot Prevention and Treatment				
Anticoagulation Overlap Therapy[2]	77	99%	92%	93%
ICU Venous Thromboembolism Prophylaxis[2]	41	100%	92%	92%
Incidence of Potentially Preventable VTE[1,2]	-	-	11%	10%
UFH with Dosages/Platelet Monitoring[2]	45	100%	96%	97%
Venous Thromboembolism Prophylaxis[2]	351	96%	83%	85%
Warfarin Therapy Discharge Instructions[2]	52	100%	75%	75%
Chest Pain/Possible Heart Attack Care				
Aspirin Given Within 24 Hours of Arrival[1,3]	-	-	97%	96%
Fibrinolytic Meds Within 30 Min. of Arrival[3,7]	-	-	62%	58%
Average Time to ECG (minutes)[1,3]	-	-	9	7
Average Time to Transfer (minutes)[3,7]	-	-	62	60
Children's Asthma Care				
Received Home Management Plan of Care	-	-	88%	88%
Received Reliever Medication	-	-	100%	100%
Received Systemic Corticosteroids	-	-	100%	100%
Emergency Department				
Admittance Decision Time (minutes)[2]	317	73	125	98
Head CT Results Within 45 Min. of Arrival[1]	-	-	55%	57%
Patients Who Left ER Before Being Seen	33,170	2%	3%	2%
Time from ER Arrival to Admit. (minutes)[2]	317	241	323	274
Time from ER Arrival to Discharge (minutes)	195	202	168	134
Time in ER Before Being Evaluated (minutes)	384	33	29	26
Time to Pain Meds for Fractures (minutes)	77	73	62	57
Heart Attack Care				
Aspirin Given at Discharge	117	98%	99%	99%
Fibrinolytic Meds Within 30 Min. of Arrival[7]	-	-	73%	54%
PCI Within 90 Minutes of Arrival	24	96%	95%	96%
Statin Prescribed at Discharge	118	97%	98%	98%
Heart Failure Care				
ACE Inhibitor or ARB for LVSD	76	100%	97%	97%
Discharge Instructions Given	169	90%	94%	94%
Evaluation of LVS Function	206	99%	99%	99%
Medicare Spending				
Medicare Spending per Patient (ratio)	-	0.96	0.98	0.98
Pneumonia Care				
Appropriate Initial Antibiotic Given[2]	139	96%	97%	95%
Blood Culture Timing[2]	239	97%	98%	98%
Pregnancy and Delivery Care				
Newborn Deliveries Scheduled Early[2]	27	0%	5%	6%
Preventive Care				
Immunization for Influenza[2]	636	93%	89%	90%
Immunization for Pneumonia[2]	756	87%	90%	92%
Stroke Care				
Anticoagulation Therapy for Atrial Fibrillation	27	100%	95%	95%
Antithrombotic Therapy Timing	111	100%	98%	98%
Assessed for Rehabilitation	148	99%	97%	97%
Discharged on Antithrombotic Therapy	137	100%	99%	99%
Discharged on Statin Medication	104	98%	94%	94%
Thrombolytic Therapy Timing	15	100%	72%	66%
Venous Thromboembolism Prophylaxis	144	99%	94%	94%
Written Stroke Educational Materials Given	94	98%	87%	88%
Surgical Care Improvement Project				
Appropriate Beta Blocker Usage	322	97%	97%	98%
Appropriate VTP Within 24 Hours	820	98%	98%	98%
Controlled Postoperative Blood Glucose	169	99%	96%	97%
Perioperative Temperature Management	966	100%	100%	100%
Prophylactic Antibiotic Selection	783	99%	99%	99%
Prophylactic Antibiotic Selection (Outpatient)	175	96%	97%	98%
Prophylactic Antibiotic Stopped	761	98%	98%	98%
Prophylactic Antibiotic Timing	788	99%	99%	99%
Prophylactic Antibiotic Timing (Outpatient)	176	98%	97%	98%
Urinary Catheter Removal	470	95%	97%	97%
Survey of Patients' Hospital Experiences				
Area Around Room 'Always' Quiet at Night	300+	55%	51%	61%
Doctors 'Always' Communicated Well	300+	80%	78%	82%
Home Recovery Information Given	300+	87%	83%	85%
Hospital Given 9 or 10 on 10 Point Scale	300+	82%	68%	71%
Meds 'Always' Explained Before Given	300+	66%	61%	64%
Nurses 'Always' Communicated Well	300+	77%	74%	79%
Pain 'Always' Well Controlled	300+	74%	68%	71%
Room and Bathroom 'Always' Clean	300+	83%	70%	73%
Timely Help 'Always' Received	300+	66%	62%	68%
Would Definitely Recommend Hospital	300+	84%	70%	71%
Use of Medical Imaging				
Cardiac Imaging Stress Test before Surgery	352	3.1%	5.2%	5.3%
Combination Abdominal CT Scan	2,025	2.8%	13.4%	10.5%
Combination Brain/Sinus CT Scan	980	0.3%	2.2%	2.7%
Combination Chest CT Scan	1,535	0.0%	2.3%	2.7%
Follow-up Mammogram/Ultrasound	3,735	4.7%	8.2%	8.8%
Lumbar Spine MRI for Low Back Pain	384	36.7%	34.2%	37.2%

Garfield Medical Center

525 N Garfield Ave
Monterey Park, CA 91754
Phone: 626-573-2222
Fax: 626-571-8972
URL: www.garfieldmedicalcenter.com
Type: Acute Care Hospitals
Emergency Services: Yes
Ownership: Proprietary
Beds: 210

Key Personnel:

CEO . . . . David Batista
Quality Assurance . . . . Ruth Honig
Chief of Medical Staff . . . . Tim Ker
Patient Relations . . . . Gilbert Lopez
Intensive Care Unit. . . . . Simon Marcus
Infection Control. . . . . Alicia Pettles
Operating Room. . . . . Un Hee Song
Radiology. . . . . Alan Turner

Measure	Cases	This Hosp.	State Avg.	U.S. Avg.
Blood Clot Prevention and Treatment				
Anticoagulation Overlap Therapy[2]	29	90%	92%	93%
ICU Venous Thromboembolism Prophylaxis[2]	96	100%	92%	92%
Incidence of Potentially Preventable VTE[1,2]	-	-	11%	10%
UFH with Dosages/Platelet Monitoring[2]	18	100%	96%	97%
Venous Thromboembolism Prophylaxis[2]	286	100%	83%	85%
Warfarin Therapy Discharge Instructions[2]	19	100%	75%	75%
Chest Pain/Possible Heart Attack Care				
Aspirin Given Within 24 Hours of Arrival	11	100%	97%	96%
Fibrinolytic Meds Within 30 Min. of Arrival[5]	-	-	62%	58%
Average Time to ECG (minutes)	11	0	9	7
Average Time to Transfer (minutes)[5]	-	-	62	60
Children's Asthma Care				
Received Home Management Plan of Care	-	-	88%	88%
Received Reliever Medication	-	-	100%	100%
Received Systemic Corticosteroids	-	-	100%	100%
Emergency Department				
Admittance Decision Time (minutes)[2]	457	65	125	98
Head CT Results Within 45 Min. of Arrival[1]	-	-	55%	57%
Patients Who Left ER Before Being Seen	22,974	3%	3%	2%
Time from ER Arrival to Admit. (minutes)[2]	461	214	323	274
Time from ER Arrival to Discharge (minutes)	372	130	168	134
Time in ER Before Being Evaluated (minutes)	402	30	29	26
Time to Pain Meds for Fractures (minutes)	138	62	62	57
Heart Attack Care				
Aspirin Given at Discharge[2]	196	100%	99%	99%
Fibrinolytic Meds Within 30 Min. of Arrival[2,7]	-	-	73%	54%
PCI Within 90 Minutes of Arrival[2]	24	92%	95%	96%
Statin Prescribed at Discharge[2]	199	99%	98%	98%
Heart Failure Care				

NOTE: Hospital profiles are in alphabetical order by state, then city, then hospital within the city; Rankings exclude hospitals with less than 25 cases except for patient surveys which excludes hospitals with less than 100 cases; (a) 100-299 cases; (1) The number of cases/patients is too few to report; (2) Data submitted were based on a sample of cases/patients; (3) Results are based on a shorter time period than required; (4) Data suppressed by CMS for one or more quarters; (5) Results are not available for this reporting period; (6) Fewer than 100 patients completed the HCAHPS survey; (7) No cases met the criteria for this measure; (8) The lower limit of the confidence interval cannot be calculated if the number of observed infections equals zero; (9) No data are available from the state/territory for this reporting period; (10) The scores shown reflect fewer than 50 completed surveys; (11) There were discrepancies in the data collection process; (12) This measure does not apply to this hospital for this reporting period; (13) Results cannot be calculated for this reporting period; (14) The results for this state are combined with nearby states to protect confidentiality; Please refer to the User's Guide for a full explanation of data.

Measure	Cases	This Hosp.	State Avg.	U.S. Avg.
ACE Inhibitor or ARB for LVSD[2]	72	100%	97%	97%
Discharge Instructions Given[2]	234	96%	94%	94%
Evaluation of LVS Function[2]	271	100%	99%	99%
Medicare Spending				
Medicare Spending per Patient (ratio)	-	1.10	0.98	0.98
Pneumonia Care				
Appropriate Initial Antibiotic Given[2]	71	100%	97%	95%
Blood Culture Timing[2]	130	98%	98%	98%
Pregnancy and Delivery Care				
Newborn Deliveries Scheduled Early[2]	102	2%	5%	6%
Preventive Care				
Immunization for Influenza[2]	481	97%	89%	90%
Immunization for Pneumonia[2]	453	96%	90%	92%
Stroke Care				
Anticoagulation Therapy for Atrial Fibrillation	17	100%	95%	95%
Antithrombotic Therapy Timing	124	98%	98%	98%
Assessed for Rehabilitation	193	100%	97%	97%
Discharged on Antithrombotic Therapy	147	100%	99%	99%
Discharged on Statin Medication	112	98%	94%	94%
Thrombolytic Therapy Timing	19	100%	72%	66%
Venous Thromboembolism Prophylaxis	207	100%	94%	94%
Written Stroke Educational Materials Given	61	100%	87%	88%
Surgical Care Improvement Project				
Appropriate Beta Blocker Usage[2]	86	99%	97%	98%
Appropriate VTP Within 24 Hours[2]	225	100%	98%	98%
Controlled Postoperative Blood Glucose[2]	89	94%	96%	97%
Perioperative Temperature Management[2]	348	100%	100%	100%
Prophylactic Antibiotic Selection[2]	227	98%	99%	99%
Prophylactic Antibiotic Selection (Outpatient)	304	97%	97%	98%
Prophylactic Antibiotic Stopped[2]	192	99%	98%	98%
Prophylactic Antibiotic Timing[2]	227	100%	99%	99%
Prophylactic Antibiotic Timing (Outpatient)	306	99%	97%	98%
Urinary Catheter Removal[2]	114	100%	97%	97%
Survey of Patients' Hospital Experiences				
Area Around Room 'Always' Quiet at Night	300+	37%	51%	61%
Doctors 'Always' Communicated Well	300+	67%	78%	82%
Home Recovery Information Given	300+	82%	83%	85%
Hospital Given 9 or 10 on 10 Point Scale	300+	55%	68%	71%
Meds 'Always' Explained Before Given	300+	62%	61%	64%
Nurses 'Always' Communicated Well	300+	67%	74%	79%
Pain 'Always' Well Controlled	300+	59%	68%	71%
Room and Bathroom 'Always' Clean	300+	69%	70%	73%
Timely Help 'Always' Received	300+	59%	62%	68%
Would Definitely Recommend Hospital	300+	56%	70%	71%
Use of Medical Imaging				
Cardiac Imaging Stress Test before Surgery[1]	-	-	5.2%	5.3%
Combination Abdominal CT Scan	85	22.4%	13.4%	10.5%
Combination Brain/Sinus CT Scan	194	1.0%	2.2%	2.7%
Combination Chest CT Scan[1]	-	-	2.3%	2.7%
Follow-up Mammogram/Ultrasound	54	3.7%	8.2%	8.8%
Lumbar Spine MRI for Low Back Pain[1]	-	-	34.2%	37.2%

Monterey Park Hospital

900 S Atlantic Blvd
Monterey Park, CA 91754
Phone: 626-570-9000
Fax: 626-281-4719
URL: www.montereyparkhosp.com
Type: Acute Care Hospitals
Emergency Services: Yes
Ownership: Proprietary
Beds: 101

Key Personnel:

Operating Room. . . . . Bert Basconcillo, RN
Coronary Care . . . . Jeanie Cervantes, RN
Pediatric Ambulatory Care . . . . . . Michelle Connors, RN
Pediatric In-Patient Care . . . . Michelle Connors, RN
CEO/President. . . . . Robert M Dubbs
Radiology. . . . . Michael Fischer, MD
Quality Assurance . . . . Dan Price
Infection Control. . . . . Sheila Segura

Measure	Cases	This Hosp.	State Avg.	U.S. Avg.
Blood Clot Prevention and Treatment				
Anticoagulation Overlap Therapy[1,2]	-	-	92%	93%
ICU Venous Thromboembolism Prophylaxis[2]	31	90%	92%	92%
Incidence of Potentially Preventable VTE[1,2]	-	-	11%	10%
UFH with Dosages/Platelet Monitoring[1,2]	-	-	96%	97%
Venous Thromboembolism Prophylaxis[2]	258	92%	83%	85%
Warfarin Therapy Discharge Instructions[1,2]	-	-	75%	75%
Chest Pain/Possible Heart Attack Care				
Aspirin Given Within 24 Hours of Arrival	26	100%	97%	96%
Fibrinolytic Meds Within 30 Min. of Arrival[7]	-	-	62%	58%
Average Time to ECG (minutes)	27	15	9	7
Average Time to Transfer (minutes)[1]	-	-	62	60
Children's Asthma Care				
Received Home Management Plan of Care	-	-	88%	88%
Received Reliever Medication	-	-	100%	100%
Received Systemic Corticosteroids	-	-	100%	100%
Emergency Department				
Admittance Decision Time (minutes)[2]	395	65	125	98
Head CT Results Within 45 Min. of Arrival[3,7]	-	-	55%	57%
Patients Who Left ER Before Being Seen	11,960	3%	3%	2%
Time from ER Arrival to Admit. (minutes)[2]	397	280	323	274
Time from ER Arrival to Discharge (minutes)	331	146	168	134
Time in ER Before Being Evaluated (minutes)	389	40	29	26
Time to Pain Meds for Fractures (minutes)	57	56	62	57
Heart Attack Care				
Aspirin Given at Discharge[1]	-	-	99%	99%
Fibrinolytic Meds Within 30 Min. of Arrival[7]	-	-	73%	54%
PCI Within 90 Minutes of Arrival[7]	-	-	95%	96%
Statin Prescribed at Discharge[1]	-	-	98%	98%
Heart Failure Care				
ACE Inhibitor or ARB for LVSD	28	100%	97%	97%
Discharge Instructions Given	91	91%	94%	94%
Evaluation of LVS Function	102	100%	99%	99%
Medicare Spending				
Medicare Spending per Patient (ratio)	-	0.96	0.98	0.98
Pneumonia Care				
Appropriate Initial Antibiotic Given[2]	39	95%	97%	95%
Blood Culture Timing[2]	59	100%	98%	98%
Pregnancy and Delivery Care				
Newborn Deliveries Scheduled Early[2]	29	3%	5%	6%
Preventive Care				
Immunization for Influenza[2]	439	86%	89%	90%
Immunization for Pneumonia[2]	411	92%	90%	92%
Stroke Care				
Anticoagulation Therapy for Atrial Fibrillation[1]	-	-	95%	95%
Antithrombotic Therapy Timing	24	100%	98%	98%
Assessed for Rehabilitation	25	80%	97%	97%
Discharged on Antithrombotic Therapy	22	95%	99%	99%
Discharged on Statin Medication	19	100%	94%	94%
Thrombolytic Therapy Timing[1]	-	-	72%	66%
Venous Thromboembolism Prophylaxis	29	97%	94%	94%
Written Stroke Educational Materials Given	20	60%	87%	88%
Surgical Care Improvement Project				
Appropriate Beta Blocker Usage[2]	15	100%	97%	98%
Appropriate VTP Within 24 Hours[2]	92	99%	98%	98%
Controlled Postoperative Blood Glucose[2,7]	-	-	96%	97%
Perioperative Temperature Management[2]	113	100%	100%	100%
Prophylactic Antibiotic Selection[2]	45	100%	99%	99%
Prophylactic Antibiotic Selection (Outpatient)	89	92%	97%	98%
Prophylactic Antibiotic Stopped[2]	43	98%	98%	98%
Prophylactic Antibiotic Timing[2]	45	98%	99%	99%
Prophylactic Antibiotic Timing (Outpatient)	90	98%	97%	98%
Urinary Catheter Removal[2]	36	97%	97%	97%
Survey of Patients' Hospital Experiences				
Area Around Room 'Always' Quiet at Night	300+	48%	51%	61%
Doctors 'Always' Communicated Well	300+	69%	78%	82%
Home Recovery Information Given	300+	80%	83%	85%
Hospital Given 9 or 10 on 10 Point Scale	300+	66%	68%	71%
Meds 'Always' Explained Before Given	300+	56%	61%	64%
Nurses 'Always' Communicated Well	300+	68%	74%	79%
Pain 'Always' Well Controlled	300+	62%	68%	71%
Room and Bathroom 'Always' Clean	300+	77%	70%	73%
Timely Help 'Always' Received	300+	54%	62%	68%
Would Definitely Recommend Hospital	300+	64%	70%	71%
Use of Medical Imaging				
Cardiac Imaging Stress Test before Surgery[1]	-	-	5.2%	5.3%
Combination Abdominal CT Scan	226	61.9%	13.4%	10.5%
Combination Brain/Sinus CT Scan	225	0.4%	2.2%	2.7%
Combination Chest CT Scan	85	0.0%	2.3%	2.7%
Follow-up Mammogram/Ultrasound	204	5.9%	8.2%	8.8%
Lumbar Spine MRI for Low Back Pain[1]	-	-	34.2%	37.2%

Kaiser Foundation Hospital - Moreno Valley

27300 Iris Avenue
Phone: 951-243-0811
Moreno Valley, CA 92555
Type: Acute Care Hospitals
Emergency Services: Yes
Ownership: Govt - Hospital Dist/Auth

Key Personnel:

Radiology. . . . . Allan Cortez
CEO/President. . . . . Barbara Patton

Measure	Cases	This Hosp.	State Avg.	U.S. Avg.
Blood Clot Prevention and Treatment				
Anticoagulation Overlap Therapy[2]	26	96%	92%	93%
ICU Venous Thromboembolism Prophylaxis[2]	56	98%	92%	92%
Incidence of Potentially Preventable VTE[2,7]	-	-	11%	10%
UFH with Dosages/Platelet Monitoring[2]	14	100%	96%	97%
Venous Thromboembolism Prophylaxis[2]	275	98%	83%	85%
Warfarin Therapy Discharge Instructions[2]	25	100%	75%	75%
Chest Pain/Possible Heart Attack Care				
Aspirin Given Within 24 Hours of Arrival	-	-	97%	96%
Fibrinolytic Meds Within 30 Min. of Arrival	-	-	62%	58%
Average Time to ECG (minutes)	-	-	9	7
Average Time to Transfer (minutes)	-	-	62	60
Children's Asthma Care				
Received Home Management Plan of Care	-	-	88%	88%
Received Reliever Medication	-	-	100%	100%
Received Systemic Corticosteroids	-	-	100%	100%
Emergency Department				
Admittance Decision Time (minutes)[2]	441	72	125	98
Head CT Results Within 45 Min. of Arrival	-	-	55%	57%
Patients Who Left ER Before Being Seen	-	-	3%	2%
Time from ER Arrival to Admit. (minutes)[2]	468	332	323	274
Time from ER Arrival to Discharge (minutes)	-	-	168	134
Time in ER Before Being Evaluated (minutes)	-	-	29	26
Time to Pain Meds for Fractures (minutes)	-	-	62	57
Heart Attack Care				
Aspirin Given at Discharge	32	100%	99%	99%
Fibrinolytic Meds Within 30 Min. of Arrival[7]	-	-	73%	54%
PCI Within 90 Minutes of Arrival[7]	-	-	95%	96%
Statin Prescribed at Discharge	31	100%	98%	98%
Heart Failure Care				
ACE Inhibitor or ARB for LVSD	52	100%	97%	97%
Discharge Instructions Given	115	99%	94%	94%
Evaluation of LVS Function	125	100%	99%	99%
Medicare Spending				
Medicare Spending per Patient (ratio)	-	0.99	0.98	0.98
Pneumonia Care				
Appropriate Initial Antibiotic Given[2]	86	99%	97%	95%
Blood Culture Timing[2]	117	99%	98%	98%
Pregnancy and Delivery Care				
Newborn Deliveries Scheduled Early[2]	93	0%	5%	6%
Preventive Care				
Immunization for Influenza[2]	410	97%	89%	90%
Immunization for Pneumonia[2]	426	98%	90%	92%
Stroke Care				
Anticoagulation Therapy for Atrial Fibrillation[1]	-	-	95%	95%
Antithrombotic Therapy Timing	50	98%	98%	98%
Assessed for Rehabilitation	49	98%	97%	97%
Discharged on Antithrombotic Therapy	46	98%	99%	99%
Discharged on Statin Medication	41	98%	94%	94%
Thrombolytic Therapy Timing[7]	-	-	72%	66%
Venous Thromboembolism Prophylaxis	42	100%	94%	94%
Written Stroke Educational Materials Given	32	84%	87%	88%
Surgical Care Improvement Project				
Appropriate Beta Blocker Usage[2]	12	100%	97%	98%
Appropriate VTP Within 24 Hours[2]	102	100%	98%	98%
Controlled Postoperative Blood Glucose[2,7]	-	-	96%	97%
Perioperative Temperature Management[2]	115	100%	100%	100%
Prophylactic Antibiotic Selection[2]	81	100%	99%	99%
Prophylactic Antibiotic Selection (Outpatient)	-	-	97%	98%
Prophylactic Antibiotic Stopped[2]	80	100%	98%	98%

NOTE: Hospital profiles are in alphabetical order by state, then city, then hospital within the city; Rankings exclude hospitals with less than 25 cases except for patient surveys which excludes hospitals with less than 100 cases; (a) 100-299 cases; (1) The number of cases/patients is too few to report; (2) Data submitted were based on a sample of cases/patients; (3) Results are based on a shorter time period than required; (4) Data suppressed by CMS for one or more quarters; (5) Results are not available for this reporting period; (6) Fewer than 100 patients completed the HCAHPS survey; (7) No cases met the criteria for this measure; (8) The lower limit of the confidence interval cannot be calculated if the number of observed infections equals zero; (9) No data are available from the state/territory for this reporting period; (10) The scores shown reflect fewer than 50 completed surveys; (11) There were discrepancies in the data collection process; (12) This measure does not apply to this hospital for this reporting period; (13) Results cannot be calculated for this reporting period; (14) The results for this state are combined with nearby states to protect confidentiality; Please refer to the User's Guide for a full explanation of data.

Measure	Cases	This Hosp.	State Avg.	U.S. Avg.
Prophylactic Antibiotic Timing[2]	81	100%	99%	99%
Prophylactic Antibiotic Timing (Outpatient)	-	-	97%	98%
Urinary Catheter Removal[2]	71	100%	97%	97%
Survey of Patients' Hospital Experiences				
Area Around Room 'Always' Quiet at Night	300+	52%	51%	61%
Doctors 'Always' Communicated Well	300+	80%	78%	82%
Home Recovery Information Given	300+	86%	83%	85%
Hospital Given 9 or 10 on 10 Point Scale	300+	69%	68%	71%
Meds 'Always' Explained Before Given	300+	59%	61%	64%
Nurses 'Always' Communicated Well	300+	74%	74%	79%
Pain 'Always' Well Controlled	300+	71%	68%	71%
Room and Bathroom 'Always' Clean	300+	70%	70%	73%
Timely Help 'Always' Received	300+	67%	62%	68%
Would Definitely Recommend Hospital	300+	70%	70%	71%
Use of Medical Imaging				
Cardiac Imaging Stress Test before Surgery	-	-	5.2%	5.3%
Combination Abdominal CT Scan	-	-	13.4%	10.5%
Combination Brain/Sinus CT Scan	-	-	2.2%	2.7%
Combination Chest CT Scan	-	-	2.3%	2.7%
Follow-up Mammogram/Ultrasound	-	-	8.2%	8.8%
Lumbar Spine MRI for Low Back Pain	-	-	34.2%	37.2%

Riverside County Regional Medical Center

26520 Cactus Avenue — Phone: 951-486-4000
Moreno Valley, CA 92555
URL: www.rcrmc.org
Type: Acute Care Hospitals — Emergency Services: Yes
Ownership: Government - Local — Beds: 362
Key Personnel:
CEO/President. . . . . Lowell Johnson
Chief of Medical Staff . . . . Arnold Tabuenca

Measure	Cases	This Hosp.	State Avg.	U.S. Avg.
Blood Clot Prevention and Treatment				
Anticoagulation Overlap Therapy[2]	68	99%	92%	93%
ICU Venous Thromboembolism Prophylaxis[2]	45	91%	92%	92%
Incidence of Potentially Preventable VTE[2]	12	0%	11%	10%
UFH with Dosages/Platelet Monitoring[2]	57	98%	96%	97%
Venous Thromboembolism Prophylaxis[2]	247	90%	83%	85%
Warfarin Therapy Discharge Instructions[2]	61	98%	75%	75%
Chest Pain/Possible Heart Attack Care				
Aspirin Given Within 24 Hours of Arrival	53	98%	97%	96%
Fibrinolytic Meds Within 30 Min. of Arrival[7]	-	-	62%	58%
Average Time to ECG (minutes)	54	3	9	7
Average Time to Transfer (minutes)	22	50	62	60
Children's Asthma Care				
Received Home Management Plan of Care	-	-	88%	88%
Received Reliever Medication	-	-	100%	100%
Received Systemic Corticosteroids	-	-	100%	100%
Emergency Department				
Admittance Decision Time (minutes)[2]	481	565	125	98
Head CT Results Within 45 Min. of Arrival[1]	-	-	55%	57%
Patients Who Left ER Before Being Seen	>100k	6%	3%	2%
Time from ER Arrival to Admit. (minutes)[2]	489	905	323	274
Time from ER Arrival to Discharge (minutes)	313	205	168	134
Time in ER Before Being Evaluated (minutes)	350	81	29	26
Time to Pain Meds for Fractures (minutes)	161	113	62	57
Heart Attack Care				
Aspirin Given at Discharge	36	100%	99%	99%
Fibrinolytic Meds Within 30 Min. of Arrival[7]	-	-	73%	54%
PCI Within 90 Minutes of Arrival[7]	-	-	95%	96%
Statin Prescribed at Discharge	36	100%	98%	98%
Heart Failure Care				
ACE Inhibitor or ARB for LVSD[2]	132	100%	97%	97%
Discharge Instructions Given[2]	268	100%	94%	94%
Evaluation of LVS Function[2]	278	100%	99%	99%
Medicare Spending				
Medicare Spending per Patient (ratio)	-	0.89	0.98	0.98
Pneumonia Care				
Appropriate Initial Antibiotic Given[2]	55	98%	97%	95%
Blood Culture Timing[2]	97	95%	98%	98%
Pregnancy and Delivery Care				
Newborn Deliveries Scheduled Early[2]	36	0%	5%	6%
Preventive Care				
Immunization for Influenza[2]	533	93%	89%	90%
Immunization for Pneumonia[2]	352	91%	90%	92%
Stroke Care				
Anticoagulation Therapy for Atrial Fibrillation[1]	-	-	95%	95%
Antithrombotic Therapy Timing	103	100%	98%	98%
Assessed for Rehabilitation	119	99%	97%	97%
Discharged on Antithrombotic Therapy	104	99%	99%	99%
Discharged on Statin Medication	76	100%	94%	94%
Thrombolytic Therapy Timing[1]	-	-	72%	66%
Venous Thromboembolism Prophylaxis	125	98%	94%	94%
Written Stroke Educational Materials Given	88	100%	87%	88%
Surgical Care Improvement Project				
Appropriate Beta Blocker Usage[2]	49	98%	97%	98%
Appropriate VTP Within 24 Hours[2]	273	99%	98%	98%
Controlled Postoperative Blood Glucose[2,7]	-	-	96%	97%
Perioperative Temperature Management[2]	315	100%	100%	100%
Prophylactic Antibiotic Selection[2]	200	98%	99%	99%
Prophylactic Antibiotic Selection (Outpatient)	100	98%	97%	98%
Prophylactic Antibiotic Stopped[2]	183	97%	98%	98%
Prophylactic Antibiotic Timing[2]	199	98%	99%	99%
Prophylactic Antibiotic Timing (Outpatient)	41	90%	97%	98%
Urinary Catheter Removal[2]	155	99%	97%	97%
Survey of Patients' Hospital Experiences				
Area Around Room 'Always' Quiet at Night	300+	47%	51%	61%
Doctors 'Always' Communicated Well	300+	79%	78%	82%
Home Recovery Information Given	300+	82%	83%	85%
Hospital Given 9 or 10 on 10 Point Scale	300+	61%	68%	71%
Meds 'Always' Explained Before Given	300+	56%	61%	64%
Nurses 'Always' Communicated Well	300+	69%	74%	79%
Pain 'Always' Well Controlled	300+	64%	68%	71%
Room and Bathroom 'Always' Clean	300+	54%	70%	73%
Timely Help 'Always' Received	300+	52%	62%	68%
Would Definitely Recommend Hospital	300+	60%	70%	71%
Use of Medical Imaging				
Cardiac Imaging Stress Test before Surgery[1]	-	-	5.2%	5.3%
Combination Abdominal CT Scan	215	13.0%	13.4%	10.5%
Combination Brain/Sinus CT Scan[1]	-	-	2.2%	2.7%
Combination Chest CT Scan	91	15.4%	2.3%	2.7%
Follow-up Mammogram/Ultrasound	104	5.8%	8.2%	8.8%
Lumbar Spine MRI for Low Back Pain[1]	-	-	34.2%	37.2%

Mercy Medical Center - Mount Shasta

914 Pine Street — Phone: 530-926-6111
Mount Shasta, CA 96067 — Fax: 530-926-0517
URL: www.mercymtshasta.org
Type: Critical Access Hospitals — Emergency Services: Yes
Ownership: Voluntary non-profit - Other — Beds: 80
Key Personnel:
Radiology. . . . . Rebecca L Dyson
Quality Assurance . . . . Charles P Francis
Operating Room. . . . . Larry Hand, RN
Emergency Room . . . . Thomas Morris, RN
Infection Control. . . . . Sharon Piva, RN
CEO/President. . . . . Kenneth Platou
Chief of Medical Staff. . . . . Robert Wiebe, MD
Intensive Care Unit. . . . . Ola Winte

Measure	Cases	This Hosp.	State Avg.	U.S. Avg.
Blood Clot Prevention and Treatment				
Anticoagulation Overlap Therapy[1,2]	-	-	92%	93%
ICU Venous Thromboembolism Prophylaxis[2]	26	96%	92%	92%
Incidence of Potentially Preventable VTE[2,7]	-	-	11%	10%
UFH with Dosages/Platelet Monitoring[2,7]	-	-	96%	97%
Venous Thromboembolism Prophylaxis[2]	87	94%	83%	85%
Warfarin Therapy Discharge Instructions[1,2]	-	-	75%	75%
Chest Pain/Possible Heart Attack Care				
Aspirin Given Within 24 Hours of Arrival	34	100%	97%	96%
Fibrinolytic Meds Within 30 Min. of Arrival[1]	-	-	62%	58%
Average Time to ECG (minutes)	37	19	9	7
Average Time to Transfer (minutes)[1]	-	-	62	60
Children's Asthma Care				
Received Home Management Plan of Care	-	-	88%	88%
Received Reliever Medication	-	-	100%	100%
Received Systemic Corticosteroids	-	-	100%	100%
Emergency Department				
Admittance Decision Time (minutes)[2]	321	100	125	98
Head CT Results Within 45 Min. of Arrival[1,3]	-	-	55%	57%
Patients Who Left ER Before Being Seen	8,017	0%	3%	2%
Time from ER Arrival to Admit. (minutes)[2]	321	294	323	274
Time from ER Arrival to Discharge (minutes)	368	161	168	134
Time in ER Before Being Evaluated (minutes)	402	4	29	26
Time to Pain Meds for Fractures (minutes)	53	60	62	57
Heart Attack Care				
Aspirin Given at Discharge[1,3]	-	-	99%	99%
Fibrinolytic Meds Within 30 Min. of Arrival[3,7]	-	-	73%	54%
PCI Within 90 Minutes of Arrival[3,7]	-	-	95%	96%
Statin Prescribed at Discharge[1,3]	-	-	98%	98%
Heart Failure Care				
ACE Inhibitor or ARB for LVSD[1]	-	-	97%	97%
Discharge Instructions Given	21	100%	94%	94%
Evaluation of LVS Function	21	100%	99%	99%
Medicare Spending				
Medicare Spending per Patient (ratio)	-	-	0.98	0.98
Pneumonia Care				
Appropriate Initial Antibiotic Given	27	89%	97%	95%
Blood Culture Timing	37	92%	98%	98%
Pregnancy and Delivery Care				
Newborn Deliveries Scheduled Early[1]	-	-	5%	6%
Preventive Care				
Immunization for Influenza[2]	256	48%	89%	90%
Immunization for Pneumonia[2]	249	72%	90%	92%
Stroke Care				
Anticoagulation Therapy for Atrial Fibrillation[1]	-	-	95%	95%
Antithrombotic Therapy Timing[1]	-	-	98%	98%
Assessed for Rehabilitation	12	100%	97%	97%
Discharged on Antithrombotic Therapy[1]	-	-	99%	99%
Discharged on Statin Medication[1]	-	-	94%	94%
Thrombolytic Therapy Timing[1]	-	-	72%	66%
Venous Thromboembolism Prophylaxis[1]	-	-	94%	94%
Written Stroke Educational Materials Given[1]	-	-	87%	88%
Surgical Care Improvement Project				
Appropriate Beta Blocker Usage[2]	40	90%	97%	98%
Appropriate VTP Within 24 Hours[2]	66	100%	98%	98%
Controlled Postoperative Blood Glucose[2,7]	-	-	96%	97%
Perioperative Temperature Management[2]	142	100%	100%	100%
Prophylactic Antibiotic Selection[2]	105	100%	99%	99%
Prophylactic Antibiotic Selection (Outpatient)	37	100%	97%	98%
Prophylactic Antibiotic Stopped[2]	105	100%	98%	98%
Prophylactic Antibiotic Timing[2]	105	96%	99%	99%
Prophylactic Antibiotic Timing (Outpatient)	32	94%	97%	98%
Urinary Catheter Removal[2]	102	99%	97%	97%
Survey of Patients' Hospital Experiences				
Area Around Room 'Always' Quiet at Night	(a)	58%	51%	61%
Doctors 'Always' Communicated Well	(a)	82%	78%	82%
Home Recovery Information Given	(a)	89%	83%	85%
Hospital Given 9 or 10 on 10 Point Scale	(a)	78%	68%	71%
Meds 'Always' Explained Before Given	(a)	77%	61%	64%
Nurses 'Always' Communicated Well	(a)	81%	74%	79%
Pain 'Always' Well Controlled	(a)	74%	68%	71%
Room and Bathroom 'Always' Clean	(a)	79%	70%	73%
Timely Help 'Always' Received	(a)	78%	62%	68%
Would Definitely Recommend Hospital	(a)	80%	70%	71%
Use of Medical Imaging				
Cardiac Imaging Stress Test before Surgery	149	2.7%	5.2%	5.3%
Combination Abdominal CT Scan	260	69.2%	13.4%	10.5%
Combination Brain/Sinus CT Scan[1]	-	-	2.2%	2.7%
Combination Chest CT Scan	141	0.0%	2.3%	2.7%
Follow-up Mammogram/Ultrasound	510	5.5%	8.2%	8.8%
Lumbar Spine MRI for Low Back Pain	72	33.3%	34.2%	37.2%

El Camino Hospital

2500 Grant Road — Phone: 650-940-7000
Mountain View, CA 94040 — Fax: 650-988-8100
URL: www.elcaminohospital.org
Type: Acute Care Hospitals — Emergency Services: Yes
Ownership: Govt - Hospital Dist/Auth — Beds: 395
Key Personnel:
Emergency Room . . . . Robert Burnett
Radiology. . . . . Samuel Dawn

NOTE: Hospital profiles are in alphabetical order by state, then city, then hospital within the city; Rankings exclude hospitals with less than 25 cases except for patient surveys which excludes hospitals with less than 100 cases; (a) 100-299 cases; (1) The number of cases/patients is too few to report; (2) Data submitted were based on a sample of cases/patients; (3) Results are based on a shorter time period than required; (4) Data suppressed by CMS for one or more quarters; (5) Results are not available for this reporting period; (6) Fewer than 100 patients completed the HCAHPS survey; (7) No cases met the criteria for this measure; (8) The lower limit of the confidence interval cannot be calculated if the number of observed infections equals zero; (9) No data are available from the state/territory for this reporting period; (10) The scores shown reflect fewer than 50 completed surveys; (11) There were discrepancies in the data collection process; (12) This measure does not apply to this hospital for this reporting period; (13) Results cannot be calculated for this reporting period; (14) The results for this state are combined with nearby states to protect confidentiality; Please refer to the User's Guide for a full explanation of data.

Chief of Medical Staff . . . . Eric Pifer, MD
Patient Relations . . . . Diana Russell, MSN, RN
CEO/President. . . . . Tomi Ryba

Measure	Cases	This Hosp.	State Avg.	U.S. Avg.
Blood Clot Prevention and Treatment				
Anticoagulation Overlap Therapy[2]	81	99%	92%	93%
ICU Venous Thromboembolism Prophylaxis[2]	52	98%	92%	92%
Incidence of Potentially Preventable VTE[2]	16	12%	11%	10%
UFH with Dosages/Platelet Monitoring[2]	30	100%	96%	97%
Venous Thromboembolism Prophylaxis[2]	274	95%	83%	85%
Warfarin Therapy Discharge Instructions[2]	68	97%	75%	75%
Chest Pain/Possible Heart Attack Care				
Aspirin Given Within 24 Hours of Arrival[1]	-	-	97%	96%
Fibrinolytic Meds Within 30 Min. of Arrival[7]	-	-	62%	58%
Average Time to ECG (minutes)[1]	-	-	9	7
Average Time to Transfer (minutes)[7]	-	-	62	60
Children's Asthma Care				
Received Home Management Plan of Care	-	-	88%	88%
Received Reliever Medication	-	-	100%	100%
Received Systemic Corticosteroids	-	-	100%	100%
Emergency Department				
Admittance Decision Time (minutes)[2]	393	80	125	98
Head CT Results Within 45 Min. of Arrival	17	29%	55%	57%
Patients Who Left ER Before Being Seen	55,528	0%	3%	2%
Time from ER Arrival to Admit. (minutes)[2]	393	284	323	274
Time from ER Arrival to Discharge (minutes)	1,193	131	168	134
Time in ER Before Being Evaluated (minutes)	1,263	19	29	26
Time to Pain Meds for Fractures (minutes)	345	55	62	57
Heart Attack Care				
Aspirin Given at Discharge	192	100%	99%	99%
Fibrinolytic Meds Within 30 Min. of Arrival[7]	-	-	73%	54%
PCI Within 90 Minutes of Arrival	38	100%	95%	96%
Statin Prescribed at Discharge	179	100%	98%	98%
Heart Failure Care				
ACE Inhibitor or ARB for LVSD	72	100%	97%	97%
Discharge Instructions Given	247	99%	94%	94%
Evaluation of LVS Function	323	100%	99%	99%
Medicare Spending				
Medicare Spending per Patient (ratio)	-	1.00	0.98	0.98
Pneumonia Care				
Appropriate Initial Antibiotic Given[2]	142	100%	97%	95%
Blood Culture Timing[2]	229	100%	98%	98%
Pregnancy and Delivery Care				
Newborn Deliveries Scheduled Early[2]	430	6%	5%	6%
Preventive Care				
Immunization for Influenza[2]	471	99%	89%	90%
Immunization for Pneumonia[2]	448	99%	90%	92%
Stroke Care				
Anticoagulation Therapy for Atrial Fibrillation	24	100%	95%	95%
Antithrombotic Therapy Timing	97	100%	98%	98%
Assessed for Rehabilitation	152	99%	97%	97%
Discharged on Antithrombotic Therapy	128	100%	99%	99%
Discharged on Statin Medication	102	93%	94%	94%
Thrombolytic Therapy Timing	23	96%	72%	66%
Venous Thromboembolism Prophylaxis	143	95%	94%	94%
Written Stroke Educational Materials Given	70	99%	87%	88%
Surgical Care Improvement Project				
Appropriate Beta Blocker Usage[2]	344	99%	97%	98%
Appropriate VTP Within 24 Hours[2]	912	99%	98%	98%
Controlled Postoperative Blood Glucose[2]	150	97%	96%	97%
Perioperative Temperature Management[2]	1,121	100%	100%	100%
Prophylactic Antibiotic Selection[2]	885	100%	99%	99%
Prophylactic Antibiotic Selection (Outpatient)	650	100%	97%	98%
Prophylactic Antibiotic Stopped[2]	859	98%	98%	98%
Prophylactic Antibiotic Timing[2]	889	100%	99%	99%
Prophylactic Antibiotic Timing (Outpatient)	653	98%	97%	98%
Urinary Catheter Removal[2]	709	99%	97%	97%
Survey of Patients' Hospital Experiences				
Area Around Room 'Always' Quiet at Night	300+	57%	51%	61%
Doctors 'Always' Communicated Well	300+	78%	78%	82%
Home Recovery Information Given	300+	84%	83%	85%
Hospital Given 9 or 10 on 10 Point Scale	300+	73%	68%	71%
Meds 'Always' Explained Before Given	300+	60%	61%	64%
Nurses 'Always' Communicated Well	300+	76%	74%	79%
Pain 'Always' Well Controlled	300+	71%	68%	71%
Room and Bathroom 'Always' Clean	300+	69%	70%	73%
Timely Help 'Always' Received	300+	62%	62%	68%
Would Definitely Recommend Hospital	300+	82%	70%	71%
Use of Medical Imaging				
Cardiac Imaging Stress Test before Surgery[1]	-	-	5.2%	5.3%
Combination Abdominal CT Scan	878	8.7%	13.4%	10.5%
Combination Brain/Sinus CT Scan	987	1.4%	2.2%	2.7%
Combination Chest CT Scan	394	0.8%	2.3%	2.7%
Follow-up Mammogram/Ultrasound	1,323	8.5%	8.2%	8.8%
Lumbar Spine MRI for Low Back Pain	60	33.3%	34.2%	37.2%

Loma Linda University Medical Center - Murrieta

28062 Baxter Road Phone: 951-290-4000
Murrieta, CA 92563
Type: Acute Care Hospitals Emergency Services: Yes
Ownership: Proprietary

Measure	Cases	This Hosp.	State Avg.	U.S. Avg.
Blood Clot Prevention and Treatment				
Anticoagulation Overlap Therapy[2]	55	87%	92%	93%
ICU Venous Thromboembolism Prophylaxis[2]	64	88%	92%	92%
Incidence of Potentially Preventable VTE[1,2]	-	-	11%	10%
UFH with Dosages/Platelet Monitoring[2]	20	90%	96%	97%
Venous Thromboembolism Prophylaxis[2]	382	74%	83%	85%
Warfarin Therapy Discharge Instructions[2]	32	91%	75%	75%
Chest Pain/Possible Heart Attack Care				
Aspirin Given Within 24 Hours of Arrival	13	100%	97%	96%
Fibrinolytic Meds Within 30 Min. of Arrival[3,7]	-	-	62%	58%
Average Time to ECG (minutes)	17	10	9	7
Average Time to Transfer (minutes)[1,3]	-	-	62	60
Children's Asthma Care				
Received Home Management Plan of Care	-	-	88%	88%
Received Reliever Medication	-	-	100%	100%
Received Systemic Corticosteroids	-	-	100%	100%
Emergency Department				
Admittance Decision Time (minutes)[2]	1,004	312	125	98
Head CT Results Within 45 Min. of Arrival	16	75%	55%	57%
Patients Who Left ER Before Being Seen	34,407	2%	3%	2%
Time from ER Arrival to Admit. (minutes)[2]	1,034	538	323	274
Time from ER Arrival to Discharge (minutes)	360	250	168	134
Time in ER Before Being Evaluated (minutes)	291	82	29	26
Time to Pain Meds for Fractures (minutes)	152	99	62	57
Heart Attack Care				
Aspirin Given at Discharge[2]	192	89%	99%	99%
Fibrinolytic Meds Within 30 Min. of Arrival[2,7]	-	-	73%	54%
PCI Within 90 Minutes of Arrival[2]	29	66%	95%	96%
Statin Prescribed at Discharge[2]	186	89%	98%	98%
Heart Failure Care				
ACE Inhibitor or ARB for LVSD[2]	111	79%	97%	97%
Discharge Instructions Given[2]	238	61%	94%	94%
Evaluation of LVS Function[2]	254	94%	99%	99%
Medicare Spending				
Medicare Spending per Patient (ratio)	-	0.95	0.98	0.98
Pneumonia Care				
Appropriate Initial Antibiotic Given[2]	119	84%	97%	95%
Blood Culture Timing[2]	141	82%	98%	98%
Pregnancy and Delivery Care				
Newborn Deliveries Scheduled Early[2]	66	15%	5%	6%
Preventive Care				
Immunization for Influenza[2]	707	89%	89%	90%
Immunization for Pneumonia[2]	843	96%	90%	92%
Stroke Care				
Anticoagulation Therapy for Atrial Fibrillation[1]	-	-	95%	95%
Antithrombotic Therapy Timing	46	100%	98%	98%
Assessed for Rehabilitation	83	66%	97%	97%
Discharged on Antithrombotic Therapy	71	96%	99%	99%
Discharged on Statin Medication	61	84%	94%	94%
Thrombolytic Therapy Timing	26	0%	72%	66%
Venous Thromboembolism Prophylaxis	70	83%	94%	94%
Written Stroke Educational Materials Given	60	37%	87%	88%
Surgical Care Improvement Project				
Appropriate Beta Blocker Usage[2]	147	91%	97%	98%
Appropriate VTP Within 24 Hours[2]	450	94%	98%	98%
Controlled Postoperative Blood Glucose[2]	81	89%	96%	97%
Perioperative Temperature Management[2]	496	100%	100%	100%
Prophylactic Antibiotic Selection[2]	402	97%	99%	99%
Prophylactic Antibiotic Selection (Outpatient)	146	97%	97%	98%
Prophylactic Antibiotic Stopped[2]	398	81%	98%	98%
Prophylactic Antibiotic Timing[2]	406	90%	99%	99%
Prophylactic Antibiotic Timing (Outpatient)	148	84%	97%	98%
Urinary Catheter Removal[2]	336	85%	97%	97%
Survey of Patients' Hospital Experiences				
Area Around Room 'Always' Quiet at Night	300+	74%	51%	61%
Doctors 'Always' Communicated Well	300+	82%	78%	82%
Home Recovery Information Given	300+	86%	83%	85%
Hospital Given 9 or 10 on 10 Point Scale	300+	79%	68%	71%
Meds 'Always' Explained Before Given	300+	59%	61%	64%
Nurses 'Always' Communicated Well	300+	78%	74%	79%
Pain 'Always' Well Controlled	300+	70%	68%	71%
Room and Bathroom 'Always' Clean	300+	66%	70%	73%
Timely Help 'Always' Received	300+	60%	62%	68%
Would Definitely Recommend Hospital	300+	83%	70%	71%
Use of Medical Imaging				
Cardiac Imaging Stress Test before Surgery	83	8.4%	5.2%	5.3%
Combination Abdominal CT Scan	672	4.2%	13.4%	10.5%
Combination Brain/Sinus CT Scan	489	2.0%	2.2%	2.7%
Combination Chest CT Scan	267	4.9%	2.3%	2.7%
Follow-up Mammogram/Ultrasound	117	10.3%	8.2%	8.8%
Lumbar Spine MRI for Low Back Pain	50	42.0%	34.2%	37.2%

Southwest Healthcare System

25500 Medical Center Drive Phone: 951-696-6000
Murrieta, CA 92562 Fax: 951-698-7721
URL: www.ivmc-rsmc.com
Type: Acute Care Hospitals Emergency Services: Yes
Ownership: Proprietary Beds: 96
Key Personnel:
Chief of Medical Staff . . . . Michael Basch, MD
CEO/President. . . . . Dennis Knox

Measure	Cases	This Hosp.	State Avg.	U.S. Avg.
Blood Clot Prevention and Treatment				
Anticoagulation Overlap Therapy[2]	96	85%	92%	93%
ICU Venous Thromboembolism Prophylaxis[2]	50	98%	92%	92%
Incidence of Potentially Preventable VTE[1,2]	-	-	11%	10%
UFH with Dosages/Platelet Monitoring[2]	17	88%	96%	97%
Venous Thromboembolism Prophylaxis[2]	332	77%	83%	85%
Warfarin Therapy Discharge Instructions[2]	74	96%	75%	75%
Chest Pain/Possible Heart Attack Care				
Aspirin Given Within 24 Hours of Arrival	151	100%	97%	96%
Fibrinolytic Meds Within 30 Min. of Arrival[7]	-	-	62%	58%
Average Time to ECG (minutes)	156	7	9	7
Average Time to Transfer (minutes)	39	67	62	60
Children's Asthma Care				
Received Home Management Plan of Care	-	-	88%	88%
Received Reliever Medication	-	-	100%	100%
Received Systemic Corticosteroids	-	-	100%	100%
Emergency Department				
Admittance Decision Time (minutes)[2]	577	160	125	98
Head CT Results Within 45 Min. of Arrival	16	38%	55%	57%
Patients Who Left ER Before Being Seen	79,904	1%	3%	2%
Time from ER Arrival to Admit. (minutes)[2]	590	417	323	274
Time from ER Arrival to Discharge (minutes)	413	177	168	134
Time in ER Before Being Evaluated (minutes)	423	33	29	26
Time to Pain Meds for Fractures (minutes)	382	64	62	57
Heart Attack Care				
Aspirin Given at Discharge	41	98%	99%	99%
Fibrinolytic Meds Within 30 Min. of Arrival[7]	-	-	73%	54%
PCI Within 90 Minutes of Arrival[7]	-	-	95%	96%
Statin Prescribed at Discharge	41	95%	98%	98%
Heart Failure Care				
ACE Inhibitor or ARB for LVSD[2]	76	93%	97%	97%
Discharge Instructions Given[2]	221	88%	94%	94%
Evaluation of LVS Function[2]	258	99%	99%	99%

NOTE: Hospital profiles are in alphabetical order by state, then city, then hospital within the city; Rankings exclude hospitals with less than 25 cases except for patient surveys which excludes hospitals with less than 100 cases; (a) 100-299 cases; (1) The number of cases/patients is too few to report; (2) Data submitted were based on a sample of cases/patients; (3) Results are based on a shorter time period than required; (4) Data suppressed by CMS for one or more quarters; (5) Results are not available for this reporting period; (6) Fewer than 100 patients completed the HCAHPS survey; (7) No cases met the criteria for this measure; (8) The lower limit of the confidence interval cannot be calculated if the number of observed infections equals zero; (9) No data are available from the state/territory for this reporting period; (10) The scores shown reflect fewer than 50 completed surveys; (11) There were discrepancies in the data collection process; (12) This measure does not apply to this hospital for this reporting period; (13) Results cannot be calculated for this reporting period; (14) The results for this state are combined with nearby states to protect confidentiality; Please refer to the User's Guide for a full explanation of data.

Measure	Cases	This Hosp.	State Avg.	U.S. Avg.
Medicare Spending				
Medicare Spending per Patient (ratio)	-	0.99	0.98	0.98
Pneumonia Care				
Appropriate Initial Antibiotic Given[2]	87	97%	97%	95%
Blood Culture Timing[2]	143	97%	98%	98%
Pregnancy and Delivery Care				
Newborn Deliveries Scheduled Early[2]	75	4%	5%	6%
Preventive Care				
Immunization for Influenza[2]	493	91%	89%	90%
Immunization for Pneumonia[2]	504	88%	90%	92%
Stroke Care				
Anticoagulation Therapy for Atrial Fibrillation[2]	14	93%	95%	95%
Antithrombotic Therapy Timing[2]	103	97%	98%	98%
Assessed for Rehabilitation[2]	116	96%	97%	97%
Discharged on Antithrombotic Therapy[2]	102	98%	99%	99%
Discharged on Statin Medication[2]	95	87%	94%	94%
Thrombolytic Therapy Timing[1,2]	-	-	72%	66%
Venous Thromboembolism Prophylaxis[2]	119	86%	94%	94%
Written Stroke Educational Materials Given[2]	74	91%	87%	88%
Surgical Care Improvement Project				
Appropriate Beta Blocker Usage[2]	113	100%	97%	98%
Appropriate VTP Within 24 Hours[2]	440	98%	98%	98%
Controlled Postoperative Blood Glucose[2,7]	-	-	96%	97%
Perioperative Temperature Management[2]	517	100%	100%	100%
Prophylactic Antibiotic Selection[2]	329	97%	99%	99%
Prophylactic Antibiotic Selection (Outpatient)	162	99%	97%	98%
Prophylactic Antibiotic Stopped[2]	317	98%	98%	98%
Prophylactic Antibiotic Timing[2]	329	99%	99%	99%
Prophylactic Antibiotic Timing (Outpatient)	163	99%	97%	98%
Urinary Catheter Removal[2]	280	97%	97%	97%
Survey of Patients' Hospital Experiences				
Area Around Room 'Always' Quiet at Night	300+	50%	51%	61%
Doctors 'Always' Communicated Well	300+	74%	78%	82%
Home Recovery Information Given	300+	83%	83%	85%
Hospital Given 9 or 10 on 10 Point Scale	300+	62%	68%	71%
Meds 'Always' Explained Before Given	300+	58%	61%	64%
Nurses 'Always' Communicated Well	300+	70%	74%	79%
Pain 'Always' Well Controlled	300+	66%	68%	71%
Room and Bathroom 'Always' Clean	300+	66%	70%	73%
Timely Help 'Always' Received	300+	56%	62%	68%
Would Definitely Recommend Hospital	300+	64%	70%	71%
Use of Medical Imaging				
Cardiac Imaging Stress Test before Surgery	65	9.2%	5.2%	5.3%
Combination Abdominal CT Scan	654	4.1%	13.4%	10.5%
Combination Brain/Sinus CT Scan	759	3.3%	2.2%	2.7%
Combination Chest CT Scan	186	5.9%	2.3%	2.7%
Follow-up Mammogram/Ultrasound	211	5.2%	8.2%	8.8%
Lumbar Spine MRI for Low Back Pain[1]	-	-	34.2%	37.2%

Queen of the Valley Medical Center

1000 Trancas St
Napa, CA 94558
Phone: 707-252-4411
Fax: 707-257-7221
URL: www.thequeen.org
Type: Acute Care Hospitals
Emergency Services: Yes
Ownership: Voluntary non-profit - Church
Beds: 166

Key Personnel:
Radiology. . . . . Daniel H Bunnell
Chair/CEO . . . . Francis J. Collin, Jr
Quality Assurance . . . . Patty Gray
CEO/President. . . . . Walt Micken
Chief of Medical Staff . . . . Vincent Morgese
Patient Relations . . . . Suki Stanton

Measure	Cases	This Hosp.	State Avg.	U.S. Avg.
Blood Clot Prevention and Treatment				
Anticoagulation Overlap Therapy[2]	43	98%	92%	93%
ICU Venous Thromboembolism Prophylaxis[2]	92	82%	92%	92%
Incidence of Potentially Preventable VTE[1,2]	-	-	11%	10%
UFH with Dosages/Platelet Monitoring[1,2]	-	-	96%	97%
Venous Thromboembolism Prophylaxis[2]	339	61%	83%	85%
Warfarin Therapy Discharge Instructions[2]	32	66%	75%	75%
Chest Pain/Possible Heart Attack Care				
Aspirin Given Within 24 Hours of Arrival	41	100%	97%	96%
Fibrinolytic Meds Within 30 Min. of Arrival[3,7]	-	-	62%	58%
Average Time to ECG (minutes)	40	7	9	7
Average Time to Transfer (minutes)[3,7]	-	-	62	60
Children's Asthma Care				
Received Home Management Plan of Care	-	-	88%	88%
Received Reliever Medication	-	-	100%	100%
Received Systemic Corticosteroids	-	-	100%	100%
Emergency Department				
Admittance Decision Time (minutes)[2]	691	117	125	98
Head CT Results Within 45 Min. of Arrival	11	18%	55%	57%
Patients Who Left ER Before Being Seen	29,872	1%	3%	2%
Time from ER Arrival to Admit. (minutes)[2]	714	270	323	274
Time from ER Arrival to Discharge (minutes)	394	134	168	134
Time in ER Before Being Evaluated (minutes)	388	25	29	26
Time to Pain Meds for Fractures (minutes)	154	55	62	57
Heart Attack Care				
Aspirin Given at Discharge	103	100%	99%	99%
Fibrinolytic Meds Within 30 Min. of Arrival[7]	-	-	73%	54%
PCI Within 90 Minutes of Arrival	28	100%	95%	96%
Statin Prescribed at Discharge	105	97%	98%	98%
Heart Failure Care				
ACE Inhibitor or ARB for LVSD	61	98%	97%	97%
Discharge Instructions Given	148	100%	94%	94%
Evaluation of LVS Function	213	100%	99%	99%
Medicare Spending				
Medicare Spending per Patient (ratio)	-	0.93	0.98	0.98
Pneumonia Care				
Appropriate Initial Antibiotic Given	66	100%	97%	95%
Blood Culture Timing	136	99%	98%	98%
Pregnancy and Delivery Care				
Newborn Deliveries Scheduled Early[2]	22	5%	5%	6%
Preventive Care				
Immunization for Influenza[2]	570	95%	89%	90%
Immunization for Pneumonia[2]	695	96%	90%	92%
Stroke Care				
Anticoagulation Therapy for Atrial Fibrillation	13	92%	95%	95%
Antithrombotic Therapy Timing	45	91%	98%	98%
Assessed for Rehabilitation	64	98%	97%	97%
Discharged on Antithrombotic Therapy	56	100%	99%	99%
Discharged on Statin Medication	44	91%	94%	94%
Thrombolytic Therapy Timing	14	79%	72%	66%
Venous Thromboembolism Prophylaxis	73	82%	94%	94%
Written Stroke Educational Materials Given	24	92%	87%	88%
Surgical Care Improvement Project				
Appropriate Beta Blocker Usage[2]	125	98%	97%	98%
Appropriate VTP Within 24 Hours[2]	243	95%	98%	98%
Controlled Postoperative Blood Glucose[2]	67	97%	96%	97%
Perioperative Temperature Management[2]	353	100%	100%	100%
Prophylactic Antibiotic Selection[2]	231	99%	99%	99%
Prophylactic Antibiotic Selection (Outpatient)	229	98%	97%	98%
Prophylactic Antibiotic Stopped[2]	224	98%	98%	98%
Prophylactic Antibiotic Timing[2]	231	99%	99%	99%
Prophylactic Antibiotic Timing (Outpatient)	212	100%	97%	98%
Urinary Catheter Removal[2]	253	98%	97%	97%
Survey of Patients' Hospital Experiences				
Area Around Room 'Always' Quiet at Night	300+	42%	51%	61%
Doctors 'Always' Communicated Well	300+	79%	78%	82%
Home Recovery Information Given	300+	84%	83%	85%
Hospital Given 9 or 10 on 10 Point Scale	300+	73%	68%	71%
Meds 'Always' Explained Before Given	300+	60%	61%	64%
Nurses 'Always' Communicated Well	300+	74%	74%	79%
Pain 'Always' Well Controlled	300+	69%	68%	71%
Room and Bathroom 'Always' Clean	300+	68%	70%	73%
Timely Help 'Always' Received	300+	58%	62%	68%
Would Definitely Recommend Hospital	300+	76%	70%	71%
Use of Medical Imaging				
Cardiac Imaging Stress Test before Surgery	77	5.2%	5.2%	5.3%
Combination Abdominal CT Scan	553	5.8%	13.4%	10.5%
Combination Brain/Sinus CT Scan	490	1.2%	2.2%	2.7%
Combination Chest CT Scan	490	0.2%	2.3%	2.7%
Follow-up Mammogram/Ultrasound	1,684	13.8%	8.2%	8.8%
Lumbar Spine MRI for Low Back Pain	188	27.7%	34.2%	37.2%

Paradise Valley Hospital

2400 East 4th St
National City, CA 91950
Phone: 619-470-4321
Fax: 619-470-4124
URL: www.paradisevalleyhospital.org
Type: Acute Care Hospitals
Emergency Services: Yes
Ownership: Voluntary non-profit - Church
Beds: 301

Key Personnel:
Pediatric In-Patient Care . . . . Ahmed Bailony, MD
Quality Assurance . . . . Barbara Baynton
Pediatric Ambulatory Care . . . . . . Blanca Fresno, MD
Chief of Medical Staff. . . . . Dorothy Hairston, MD
Radiology. . . . . John Holden, MD
CEO/President. . . . . Luis Leon
Infection Control. . . . . Jerome Robinson, MD
Operating Room. . . . . Jeanne Wilson

Measure	Cases	This Hosp.	State Avg.	U.S. Avg.
Blood Clot Prevention and Treatment				
Anticoagulation Overlap Therapy[2]	22	100%	92%	93%
ICU Venous Thromboembolism Prophylaxis[2]	62	77%	92%	92%
Incidence of Potentially Preventable VTE[1,2]	-	-	11%	10%
UFH with Dosages/Platelet Monitoring[2]	25	100%	96%	97%
Venous Thromboembolism Prophylaxis[2]	370	59%	83%	85%
Warfarin Therapy Discharge Instructions[2]	11	91%	75%	75%
Chest Pain/Possible Heart Attack Care				
Aspirin Given Within 24 Hours of Arrival[1]	-	-	97%	96%
Fibrinolytic Meds Within 30 Min. of Arrival[7]	-	-	62%	58%
Average Time to ECG (minutes)[1]	-	-	9	7
Average Time to Transfer (minutes)[1]	-	-	62	60
Children's Asthma Care				
Received Home Management Plan of Care	-	-	88%	88%
Received Reliever Medication	-	-	100%	100%
Received Systemic Corticosteroids	-	-	100%	100%
Emergency Department				
Admittance Decision Time (minutes)[2]	700	68	125	98
Head CT Results Within 45 Min. of Arrival	36	89%	55%	57%
Patients Who Left ER Before Being Seen	34,170	5%	3%	2%
Time from ER Arrival to Admit. (minutes)[2]	701	270	323	274
Time from ER Arrival to Discharge (minutes)	402	177	168	134
Time in ER Before Being Evaluated (minutes)	472	50	29	26
Time to Pain Meds for Fractures (minutes)	58	96	62	57
Heart Attack Care				
Aspirin Given at Discharge	30	100%	99%	99%
Fibrinolytic Meds Within 30 Min. of Arrival[7]	-	-	73%	54%
PCI Within 90 Minutes of Arrival[1]	-	-	95%	96%
Statin Prescribed at Discharge	31	100%	98%	98%
Heart Failure Care				
ACE Inhibitor or ARB for LVSD	75	100%	97%	97%
Discharge Instructions Given	209	100%	94%	94%
Evaluation of LVS Function	248	100%	99%	99%
Medicare Spending				
Medicare Spending per Patient (ratio)	-	1.13	0.98	0.98
Pneumonia Care				
Appropriate Initial Antibiotic Given	106	100%	97%	95%
Blood Culture Timing	257	98%	98%	98%
Pregnancy and Delivery Care				
Newborn Deliveries Scheduled Early	88	0%	5%	6%
Preventive Care				
Immunization for Influenza[2]	512	91%	89%	90%
Immunization for Pneumonia[2]	658	93%	90%	92%
Stroke Care				
Anticoagulation Therapy for Atrial Fibrillation[1]	-	-	95%	95%
Antithrombotic Therapy Timing	44	89%	98%	98%
Assessed for Rehabilitation	53	79%	97%	97%
Discharged on Antithrombotic Therapy	44	93%	99%	99%
Discharged on Statin Medication	39	72%	94%	94%
Thrombolytic Therapy Timing[1]	-	-	72%	66%
Venous Thromboembolism Prophylaxis	51	63%	94%	94%
Written Stroke Educational Materials Given	26	58%	87%	88%
Surgical Care Improvement Project				
Appropriate Beta Blocker Usage	20	100%	97%	98%
Appropriate VTP Within 24 Hours	65	100%	98%	98%
Controlled Postoperative Blood Glucose[7]	-	-	96%	97%
Perioperative Temperature Management	71	100%	100%	100%
Prophylactic Antibiotic Selection	23	96%	99%	99%

NOTE: Hospital profiles are in alphabetical order by state, then city, then hospital within the city; Rankings exclude hospitals with less than 25 cases except for patient surveys which excludes hospitals with less than 100 cases; (a) 100-299 cases; (1) The number of cases/patients is too few to report; (2) Data submitted were based on a sample of cases/patients; (3) Results are based on a shorter time period than required; (4) Data suppressed by CMS for one or more quarters; (5) Results are not available for this reporting period; (6) Fewer than 100 patients completed the HCAHPS survey; (7) No cases met the criteria for this measure; (8) The lower limit of the confidence interval cannot be calculated if the number of observed infections equals zero; (9) No data are available from the state/territory for this reporting period; (10) The scores shown reflect fewer than 50 completed surveys; (11) There were discrepancies in the data collection process; (12) This measure does not apply to this hospital for this reporting period; (13) Results cannot be calculated for this reporting period; (14) The results for this state are combined with nearby states to protect confidentiality; Please refer to the User's Guide for a full explanation of data.

Measure	Cases	This Hosp.	State Avg.	U.S. Avg.
Prophylactic Antibiotic Selection (Outpatient)	57	95%	97%	98%
Prophylactic Antibiotic Stopped	17	100%	98%	98%
Prophylactic Antibiotic Timing	23	100%	99%	99%
Prophylactic Antibiotic Timing (Outpatient)	57	96%	97%	98%
Urinary Catheter Removal	27	100%	97%	97%
Survey of Patients' Hospital Experiences				
Area Around Room 'Always' Quiet at Night[11]	(a)	55%	51%	61%
Doctors 'Always' Communicated Well[11]	(a)	74%	78%	82%
Home Recovery Information Given[11]	(a)	82%	83%	85%
Hospital Given 9 or 10 on 10 Point Scale[11]	(a)	65%	68%	71%
Meds 'Always' Explained Before Given[11]	(a)	65%	61%	64%
Nurses 'Always' Communicated Well[11]	(a)	74%	74%	79%
Pain 'Always' Well Controlled[11]	(a)	62%	68%	71%
Room and Bathroom 'Always' Clean[11]	(a)	69%	70%	73%
Timely Help 'Always' Received[11]	(a)	60%	62%	68%
Would Definitely Recommend Hospital[11]	(a)	61%	70%	71%
Use of Medical Imaging				
Cardiac Imaging Stress Test before Surgery[1]	-	-	5.2%	5.3%
Combination Abdominal CT Scan	218	3.7%	13.4%	10.5%
Combination Brain/Sinus CT Scan	444	1.4%	2.2%	2.7%
Combination Chest CT Scan	210	0.0%	2.3%	2.7%
Follow-up Mammogram/Ultrasound[7]	-	-	8.2%	8.8%
Lumbar Spine MRI for Low Back Pain[1]	-	-	34.2%	37.2%

Colorado River Medical Center

1401 Bailey Ave
Needles, CA 92363
Phone: 760-326-4531
Fax: 760-326-4532
URL: www.prhc.net
Type: Critical Access Hospitals
Emergency Services: Yes
Ownership: Voluntary non-profit - Private
Beds: 49

Key Personnel:

Emergency Room . . . . John Alford
Chief of Medical Staff . . . . Kay Cunningham
CEO/President. . . . . Robert Mannix
Quality Assurance . . . . Rose Smith
Operating Room. . . . . Robyn Stein

Measure	Cases	This Hosp.	State Avg.	U.S. Avg.
Blood Clot Prevention and Treatment				
Anticoagulation Overlap Therapy[5]	-	-	92%	93%
ICU Venous Thromboembolism Prophylaxis[5]	-	-	92%	92%
Incidence of Potentially Preventable VTE[5]	-	-	11%	10%
UFH with Dosages/Platelet Monitoring[5]	-	-	96%	97%
Venous Thromboembolism Prophylaxis[5]	-	-	83%	85%
Warfarin Therapy Discharge Instructions[5]	-	-	75%	75%
Chest Pain/Possible Heart Attack Care				
Aspirin Given Within 24 Hours of Arrival	-	-	97%	96%
Fibrinolytic Meds Within 30 Min. of Arrival	-	-	62%	58%
Average Time to ECG (minutes)	-	-	9	7
Average Time to Transfer (minutes)	-	-	62	60
Children's Asthma Care				
Received Home Management Plan of Care	-	-	88%	88%
Received Reliever Medication	-	-	100%	100%
Received Systemic Corticosteroids	-	-	100%	100%
Emergency Department				
Admittance Decision Time (minutes)[5]	-	-	125	98
Head CT Results Within 45 Min. of Arrival	-	-	55%	57%
Patients Who Left ER Before Being Seen	-	-	3%	2%
Time from ER Arrival to Admit. (minutes)[5]	-	-	323	274
Time from ER Arrival to Discharge (minutes)	-	-	168	134
Time in ER Before Being Evaluated (minutes)	-	-	29	26
Time to Pain Meds for Fractures (minutes)	-	-	62	57
Heart Attack Care				
Aspirin Given at Discharge[5]	-	-	99%	99%
Fibrinolytic Meds Within 30 Min. of Arrival[5]	-	-	73%	54%
PCI Within 90 Minutes of Arrival[5]	-	-	95%	96%
Statin Prescribed at Discharge[5]	-	-	98%	98%
Heart Failure Care				
ACE Inhibitor or ARB for LVSD[2,3]	-	-	97%	97%
Discharge Instructions Given[1,2]	-	-	94%	94%
Evaluation of LVS Function[1,2]	-	-	99%	99%
Medicare Spending				
Medicare Spending per Patient (ratio)	-	-	0.98	0.98
Pneumonia Care				
Appropriate Initial Antibiotic Given[1,2]	-	-	97%	95%
Blood Culture Timing[1,2]	-	-	98%	98%
Pregnancy and Delivery Care				
Newborn Deliveries Scheduled Early[5]	-	-	5%	6%
Preventive Care				
Immunization for Influenza[5]	-	-	89%	90%
Immunization for Pneumonia[5]	-	-	90%	92%
Stroke Care				
Anticoagulation Therapy for Atrial Fibrillation[5]	-	-	95%	95%
Antithrombotic Therapy Timing[5]	-	-	98%	98%
Assessed for Rehabilitation[5]	-	-	97%	97%
Discharged on Antithrombotic Therapy[5]	-	-	99%	99%
Discharged on Statin Medication[5]	-	-	94%	94%
Thrombolytic Therapy Timing[5]	-	-	72%	66%
Venous Thromboembolism Prophylaxis[5]	-	-	94%	94%
Written Stroke Educational Materials Given[5]	-	-	87%	88%
Surgical Care Improvement Project				
Appropriate Beta Blocker Usage[5]	-	-	97%	98%
Appropriate VTP Within 24 Hours[5]	-	-	98%	98%
Controlled Postoperative Blood Glucose[5]	-	-	96%	97%
Perioperative Temperature Management[5]	-	-	100%	100%
Prophylactic Antibiotic Selection[5]	-	-	99%	99%
Prophylactic Antibiotic Selection (Outpatient)	-	-	97%	98%
Prophylactic Antibiotic Stopped[5]	-	-	98%	98%
Prophylactic Antibiotic Timing[5]	-	-	99%	99%
Prophylactic Antibiotic Timing (Outpatient)	-	-	97%	98%
Urinary Catheter Removal[5]	-	-	97%	97%
Survey of Patients' Hospital Experiences				
Area Around Room 'Always' Quiet at Night[5]	-	-	51%	61%
Doctors 'Always' Communicated Well[5]	-	-	78%	82%
Home Recovery Information Given[5]	-	-	83%	85%
Hospital Given 9 or 10 on 10 Point Scale[5]	-	-	68%	71%
Meds 'Always' Explained Before Given[5]	-	-	61%	64%
Nurses 'Always' Communicated Well[5]	-	-	74%	79%
Pain 'Always' Well Controlled[5]	-	-	68%	71%
Room and Bathroom 'Always' Clean[5]	-	-	70%	73%
Timely Help 'Always' Received[5]	-	-	62%	68%
Would Definitely Recommend Hospital[5]	-	-	70%	71%
Use of Medical Imaging				
Cardiac Imaging Stress Test before Surgery	-	-	5.2%	5.3%
Combination Abdominal CT Scan	-	-	13.4%	10.5%
Combination Brain/Sinus CT Scan	-	-	2.2%	2.7%
Combination Chest CT Scan	-	-	2.3%	2.7%
Follow-up Mammogram/Ultrasound	-	-	8.2%	8.8%
Lumbar Spine MRI for Low Back Pain	-	-	34.2%	37.2%

Hoag Memorial Hospital Presbyterian

One Hoag Drive
Newport Beach, CA 92663
Phone: 949-645-8600
Fax: 949-760-2138
URL: www.hoaghospital.org
Type: Acute Care Hospitals
Emergency Services: Yes
Ownership: Voluntary non-profit - Private

Key Personnel:

Emergency Room . . . . Eric Alcouloumre, MD
Chief of Medical Staff . . . . Neil M Barth, MD
Operating Room. . . . . Steven Beanes
Radiology. . . . . Frederick Bimberg, MD
Pediatric Ambulatory Care . . . . . . Andrew Blumberg, MD
CEO/President. . . . . Robert T. Braithwaite
Quality Assurance . . . . Jack L. Cox, M.D., M.M.M.
Infection Control. . . . . Rosalie DeSantis, RN

Measure	Cases	This Hosp.	State Avg.	U.S. Avg.
Blood Clot Prevention and Treatment				
Anticoagulation Overlap Therapy[2]	186	80%	92%	93%
ICU Venous Thromboembolism Prophylaxis[2]	146	89%	92%	92%
Incidence of Potentially Preventable VTE[2]	37	27%	11%	10%
UFH with Dosages/Platelet Monitoring[2]	177	2%	96%	97%
Venous Thromboembolism Prophylaxis[2]	416	77%	83%	85%
Warfarin Therapy Discharge Instructions[2]	128	9%	75%	75%
Chest Pain/Possible Heart Attack Care				
Aspirin Given Within 24 Hours of Arrival[1]	-	-	97%	96%
Fibrinolytic Meds Within 30 Min. of Arrival[3,7]	-	-	62%	58%
Average Time to ECG (minutes)[1]	-	-	9	7
Average Time to Transfer (minutes)[3,7]	-	-	62	60
Children's Asthma Care				
Received Home Management Plan of Care	-	-	88%	88%
Received Reliever Medication	-	-	100%	100%
Received Systemic Corticosteroids	-	-	100%	100%
Emergency Department				
Admittance Decision Time (minutes)[2]	906	75	125	98
Head CT Results Within 45 Min. of Arrival	21	14%	55%	57%
Patients Who Left ER Before Being Seen	68,348	2%	3%	2%
Time from ER Arrival to Admit. (minutes)[2]	917	276	323	274
Time from ER Arrival to Discharge (minutes)	646	164	168	134
Time in ER Before Being Evaluated (minutes)	340	34	29	26
Time to Pain Meds for Fractures (minutes)	607	50	62	57
Heart Attack Care				
Aspirin Given at Discharge	346	100%	99%	99%
Fibrinolytic Meds Within 30 Min. of Arrival[7]	-	-	73%	54%
PCI Within 90 Minutes of Arrival	101	97%	95%	96%
Statin Prescribed at Discharge	340	97%	98%	98%
Heart Failure Care				
ACE Inhibitor or ARB for LVSD	86	98%	97%	97%
Discharge Instructions Given	191	94%	94%	94%
Evaluation of LVS Function	236	100%	99%	99%
Medicare Spending				
Medicare Spending per Patient (ratio)	-	1.03	0.98	0.98
Pneumonia Care				
Appropriate Initial Antibiotic Given[2]	120	94%	97%	95%
Blood Culture Timing[2]	231	99%	98%	98%
Pregnancy and Delivery Care				
Newborn Deliveries Scheduled Early[2]	99	5%	5%	6%
Preventive Care				
Immunization for Influenza[2]	860	82%	89%	90%
Immunization for Pneumonia[2]	732	79%	90%	92%
Stroke Care				
Anticoagulation Therapy for Atrial Fibrillation	67	96%	95%	95%
Antithrombotic Therapy Timing	256	100%	98%	98%
Assessed for Rehabilitation	372	100%	97%	97%
Discharged on Antithrombotic Therapy	308	99%	99%	99%
Discharged on Statin Medication	253	99%	94%	94%
Thrombolytic Therapy Timing	27	93%	72%	66%
Venous Thromboembolism Prophylaxis	327	95%	94%	94%
Written Stroke Educational Materials Given	227	100%	87%	88%
Surgical Care Improvement Project				
Appropriate Beta Blocker Usage[2]	247	98%	97%	98%
Appropriate VTP Within 24 Hours[2]	477	96%	98%	98%
Controlled Postoperative Blood Glucose[2]	200	100%	96%	97%
Perioperative Temperature Management[2]	616	100%	100%	100%
Prophylactic Antibiotic Selection[2]	412	100%	99%	99%
Prophylactic Antibiotic Selection (Outpatient)	729	98%	97%	98%
Prophylactic Antibiotic Stopped[2]	401	99%	98%	98%
Prophylactic Antibiotic Timing[2]	415	99%	99%	99%
Prophylactic Antibiotic Timing (Outpatient)	730	99%	97%	98%
Urinary Catheter Removal[2]	434	95%	97%	97%
Survey of Patients' Hospital Experiences				
Area Around Room 'Always' Quiet at Night	300+	55%	51%	61%
Doctors 'Always' Communicated Well	300+	81%	78%	82%
Home Recovery Information Given	300+	85%	83%	85%
Hospital Given 9 or 10 on 10 Point Scale	300+	82%	68%	71%
Meds 'Always' Explained Before Given	300+	62%	61%	64%
Nurses 'Always' Communicated Well	300+	78%	74%	79%
Pain 'Always' Well Controlled	300+	72%	68%	71%
Room and Bathroom 'Always' Clean	300+	74%	70%	73%
Timely Help 'Always' Received	300+	61%	62%	68%
Would Definitely Recommend Hospital	300+	86%	70%	71%
Use of Medical Imaging				
Cardiac Imaging Stress Test before Surgery	494	8.3%	5.2%	5.3%
Combination Abdominal CT Scan	3,530	11.8%	13.4%	10.5%
Combination Brain/Sinus CT Scan	1,845	1.1%	2.2%	2.7%
Combination Chest CT Scan	2,596	6.2%	2.3%	2.7%
Follow-up Mammogram/Ultrasound	5,357	7.6%	8.2%	8.8%
Lumbar Spine MRI for Low Back Pain	259	35.5%	34.2%	37.2%

NOTE: Hospital profiles are in alphabetical order by state, then city, then hospital within the city; Rankings exclude hospitals with less than 25 cases except for patient surveys which excludes hospitals with less than 100 cases; (a) 100-299 cases; (1) The number of cases/patients is too few to report; (2) Data submitted were based on a sample of cases/patients; (3) Results are based on a shorter time period than required; (4) Data suppressed by CMS for one or more quarters; (5) Results are not available for this reporting period; (6) Fewer than 100 patients completed the HCAHPS survey; (7) No cases met the criteria for this measure; (8) The lower limit of the confidence interval cannot be calculated if the number of observed infections equals zero; (9) No data are available from the state/territory for this reporting period; (10) The scores shown reflect fewer than 50 completed surveys; (11) There were discrepancies in the data collection process; (12) This measure does not apply to this hospital for this reporting period; (13) Results cannot be calculated for this reporting period; (14) The results for this state are combined with nearby states to protect confidentiality; Please refer to the User's Guide for a full explanation of data.

Northridge Hospital Medical Center

18300 Roscoe Blvd Phone: 818-885-8500
Northridge, CA 91325 Fax: 818-885-5439
URL: www.northridgehospital.org
Type: Acute Care Hospitals Emergency Services: Yes
Ownership: Voluntary non-profit - Private Beds: 411

Key Personnel:
Pediatric In-Patient Care . . . . Kathy Alfe
Radiology. . . . . Nana Deeb
Chief of Medical Staff. . . . . Lamya Jarjour, MD
Infection Control. . . . . Vicki Kelley, RN
Operating Room. . . . . Martin Perez
CEO/President. . . . . Michael Wall
Quality Assurance . . . . Randi Young

Measure	Cases	This Hosp.	State Avg.	U.S. Avg.
Blood Clot Prevention and Treatment				
Anticoagulation Overlap Therapy[2]	73	97%	92%	93%
ICU Venous Thromboembolism Prophylaxis[2]	85	100%	92%	92%
Incidence of Potentially Preventable VTE[2]	19	0%	11%	10%
UFH with Dosages/Platelet Monitoring[2]	52	100%	96%	97%
Venous Thromboembolism Prophylaxis[2]	322	90%	83%	85%
Warfarin Therapy Discharge Instructions[2]	52	94%	75%	75%
Chest Pain/Possible Heart Attack Care				
Aspirin Given Within 24 Hours of Arrival	13	100%	97%	96%
Fibrinolytic Meds Within 30 Min. of Arrival[3,7]	-	-	62%	58%
Average Time to ECG (minutes)	15	8	9	7
Average Time to Transfer (minutes)[3,7]	-	-	62	60
Children's Asthma Care				
Received Home Management Plan of Care	-	-	88%	88%
Received Reliever Medication	-	-	100%	100%
Received Systemic Corticosteroids	-	-	100%	100%
Emergency Department				
Admittance Decision Time (minutes)[2]	783	115	125	98
Head CT Results Within 45 Min. of Arrival[1]	-	-	55%	57%
Patients Who Left ER Before Being Seen	58,288	1%	3%	2%
Time from ER Arrival to Admit. (minutes)[2]	783	329	323	274
Time from ER Arrival to Discharge (minutes)	397	168	168	134
Time in ER Before Being Evaluated (minutes)	428	23	29	26
Time to Pain Meds for Fractures (minutes)	198	62	62	57
Heart Attack Care				
Aspirin Given at Discharge	237	100%	99%	99%
Fibrinolytic Meds Within 30 Min. of Arrival[7]	-	-	73%	54%
PCI Within 90 Minutes of Arrival	31	90%	95%	96%
Statin Prescribed at Discharge	237	100%	98%	98%
Heart Failure Care				
ACE Inhibitor or ARB for LVSD	122	94%	97%	97%
Discharge Instructions Given	284	100%	94%	94%
Evaluation of LVS Function	347	100%	99%	99%
Medicare Spending				
Medicare Spending per Patient (ratio)	-	1.04	0.98	0.98
Pneumonia Care				
Appropriate Initial Antibiotic Given	161	99%	97%	95%
Blood Culture Timing	301	100%	98%	98%
Pregnancy and Delivery Care				
Newborn Deliveries Scheduled Early[2]	52	0%	5%	6%
Preventive Care				
Immunization for Influenza[2]	543	95%	89%	90%
Immunization for Pneumonia[2]	557	96%	90%	92%
Stroke Care				
Anticoagulation Therapy for Atrial Fibrillation	27	93%	95%	95%
Antithrombotic Therapy Timing	119	100%	98%	98%
Assessed for Rehabilitation	150	97%	97%	97%
Discharged on Antithrombotic Therapy	129	100%	99%	99%
Discharged on Statin Medication	102	98%	94%	94%
Thrombolytic Therapy Timing	16	88%	72%	66%
Venous Thromboembolism Prophylaxis	161	99%	94%	94%
Written Stroke Educational Materials Given	87	93%	87%	88%
Surgical Care Improvement Project				
Appropriate Beta Blocker Usage[2]	234	97%	97%	98%
Appropriate VTP Within 24 Hours[2]	728	97%	98%	98%
Controlled Postoperative Blood Glucose[2]	77	96%	96%	97%
Perioperative Temperature Management[2]	827	100%	100%	100%
Prophylactic Antibiotic Selection[2]	672	99%	99%	99%
Prophylactic Antibiotic Selection (Outpatient)	178	99%	97%	98%
Prophylactic Antibiotic Stopped[2]	642	98%	98%	98%
Prophylactic Antibiotic Timing[2]	671	98%	99%	99%
Prophylactic Antibiotic Timing (Outpatient)	172	97%	97%	98%
Urinary Catheter Removal[2]	634	99%	97%	97%
Survey of Patients' Hospital Experiences				
Area Around Room 'Always' Quiet at Night	300+	45%	51%	61%
Doctors 'Always' Communicated Well	300+	74%	78%	82%
Home Recovery Information Given	300+	82%	83%	85%
Hospital Given 9 or 10 on 10 Point Scale	300+	62%	68%	71%
Meds 'Always' Explained Before Given	300+	60%	61%	64%
Nurses 'Always' Communicated Well	300+	70%	74%	79%
Pain 'Always' Well Controlled	300+	65%	68%	71%
Room and Bathroom 'Always' Clean	300+	70%	70%	73%
Timely Help 'Always' Received	300+	51%	62%	68%
Would Definitely Recommend Hospital	300+	65%	70%	71%
Use of Medical Imaging				
Cardiac Imaging Stress Test before Surgery	293	7.5%	5.2%	5.3%
Combination Abdominal CT Scan	589	1.5%	13.4%	10.5%
Combination Brain/Sinus CT Scan	760	5.3%	2.2%	2.7%
Combination Chest CT Scan	272	2.2%	2.3%	2.7%
Follow-up Mammogram/Ultrasound	1,378	2.2%	8.2%	8.8%
Lumbar Spine MRI for Low Back Pain[1]	-	-	34.2%	37.2%

Coast Plaza Hospital

13100 Studerbaker Road Phone: 310-356-0550
Norwalk, CA 90650
Type: Acute Care Hospitals Emergency Services: Yes
Ownership: Proprietary

Measure	Cases	This Hosp.	State Avg.	U.S. Avg.
Blood Clot Prevention and Treatment				
Anticoagulation Overlap Therapy[1,2]	-	-	92%	93%
ICU Venous Thromboembolism Prophylaxis[2]	41	61%	92%	92%
Incidence of Potentially Preventable VTE[1,2]	-	-	11%	10%
UFH with Dosages/Platelet Monitoring[2,7]	-	-	96%	97%
Venous Thromboembolism Prophylaxis[2]	310	50%	83%	85%
Warfarin Therapy Discharge Instructions[2,7]	-	-	75%	75%
Chest Pain/Possible Heart Attack Care				
Aspirin Given Within 24 Hours of Arrival[3]	11	73%	97%	96%
Fibrinolytic Meds Within 30 Min. of Arrival[3,7]	-	-	62%	58%
Average Time to ECG (minutes)[3]	11	20	9	7
Average Time to Transfer (minutes)[1,3]	-	-	62	60
Children's Asthma Care				
Received Home Management Plan of Care	-	-	88%	88%
Received Reliever Medication	-	-	100%	100%
Received Systemic Corticosteroids	-	-	100%	100%
Emergency Department				
Admittance Decision Time (minutes)[2]	531	67	125	98
Head CT Results Within 45 Min. of Arrival[7]	-	-	55%	57%
Patients Who Left ER Before Being Seen	13,289	3%	3%	2%
Time from ER Arrival to Admit. (minutes)[2]	536	244	323	274
Time from ER Arrival to Discharge (minutes)	343	127	168	134
Time in ER Before Being Evaluated (minutes)	374	22	29	26
Time to Pain Meds for Fractures (minutes)	45	104	62	57
Heart Attack Care				
Aspirin Given at Discharge	18	78%	99%	99%
Fibrinolytic Meds Within 30 Min. of Arrival[7]	-	-	73%	54%
PCI Within 90 Minutes of Arrival[7]	-	-	95%	96%
Statin Prescribed at Discharge	15	73%	98%	98%
Heart Failure Care				
ACE Inhibitor or ARB for LVSD	17	76%	97%	97%
Discharge Instructions Given	61	92%	94%	94%
Evaluation of LVS Function	75	93%	99%	99%
Medicare Spending				
Medicare Spending per Patient (ratio)	-	1.19	0.98	0.98
Pneumonia Care				
Appropriate Initial Antibiotic Given	49	84%	97%	95%
Blood Culture Timing	139	97%	98%	98%
Pregnancy and Delivery Care				
Newborn Deliveries Scheduled Early[7]	-	-	5%	6%
Preventive Care				
Immunization for Influenza[2]	305	68%	89%	90%
Immunization for Pneumonia[2]	353	65%	90%	92%
Stroke Care				
Anticoagulation Therapy for Atrial Fibrillation[7]	-	-	95%	95%
Antithrombotic Therapy Timing	11	100%	98%	98%
Assessed for Rehabilitation	12	83%	97%	97%
Discharged on Antithrombotic Therapy[1]	-	-	99%	99%
Discharged on Statin Medication[1]	-	-	94%	94%
Thrombolytic Therapy Timing[1]	-	-	72%	66%
Venous Thromboembolism Prophylaxis	13	15%	94%	94%
Written Stroke Educational Materials Given[1]	-	-	87%	88%
Surgical Care Improvement Project				
Appropriate Beta Blocker Usage[1]	-	-	97%	98%
Appropriate VTP Within 24 Hours	27	81%	98%	98%
Controlled Postoperative Blood Glucose[7]	-	-	96%	97%
Perioperative Temperature Management	38	95%	100%	100%
Prophylactic Antibiotic Selection[1]	-	-	99%	99%
Prophylactic Antibiotic Selection (Outpatient)[1,3]	-	-	97%	98%
Prophylactic Antibiotic Stopped[1]	-	-	98%	98%
Prophylactic Antibiotic Timing[1]	-	-	99%	99%
Prophylactic Antibiotic Timing (Outpatient)[1,3]	-	-	97%	98%
Urinary Catheter Removal	18	61%	97%	97%
Survey of Patients' Hospital Experiences				
Area Around Room 'Always' Quiet at Night	300+	39%	51%	61%
Doctors 'Always' Communicated Well	300+	75%	78%	82%
Home Recovery Information Given	300+	77%	83%	85%
Hospital Given 9 or 10 on 10 Point Scale	300+	55%	68%	71%
Meds 'Always' Explained Before Given	300+	59%	61%	64%
Nurses 'Always' Communicated Well	300+	68%	74%	79%
Pain 'Always' Well Controlled	300+	63%	68%	71%
Room and Bathroom 'Always' Clean	300+	61%	70%	73%
Timely Help 'Always' Received	300+	60%	62%	68%
Would Definitely Recommend Hospital	300+	51%	70%	71%
Use of Medical Imaging				
Cardiac Imaging Stress Test before Surgery[7]	-	-	5.2%	5.3%
Combination Abdominal CT Scan	101	5.0%	13.4%	10.5%
Combination Brain/Sinus CT Scan[1]	-	-	2.2%	2.7%
Combination Chest CT Scan[1]	-	-	2.3%	2.7%
Follow-up Mammogram/Ultrasound[7]	-	-	8.2%	8.8%
Lumbar Spine MRI for Low Back Pain[1]	-	-	34.2%	37.2%

Novato Community Hospital

180 Rowland Way Phone: 415-209-1300
Novato, CA 94945 Fax: 415-492-4751
URL: www.novatocommunity.sutterhealth.org
Type: Acute Care Hospitals Emergency Services: Yes
Ownership: Voluntary non-profit - Other Beds: 47

Key Personnel:
CEO/President. . . . . David Bradley, RN
Quality Assurance . . . . Carole Cole
Chief of Medical Staff . . . . Timothy Murphy, MD
Emergency Room . . . . Peggy Parenti, RN
Operating Room. . . . . Jane Thom
Chair/CEO . . . . Robert M. Tomasello

Measure	Cases	This Hosp.	State Avg.	U.S. Avg.
Blood Clot Prevention and Treatment				
Anticoagulation Overlap Therapy[2]	15	100%	92%	93%
ICU Venous Thromboembolism Prophylaxis[2]	49	98%	92%	92%
Incidence of Potentially Preventable VTE[1,2]	-	-	11%	10%
UFH with Dosages/Platelet Monitoring[2]	11	100%	96%	97%
Venous Thromboembolism Prophylaxis[2]	135	91%	83%	85%
Warfarin Therapy Discharge Instructions[2]	12	100%	75%	75%
Chest Pain/Possible Heart Attack Care				
Aspirin Given Within 24 Hours of Arrival	29	90%	97%	96%
Fibrinolytic Meds Within 30 Min. of Arrival[7]	-	-	62%	58%
Average Time to ECG (minutes)	28	12	9	7
Average Time to Transfer (minutes)[1]	-	-	62	60
Children's Asthma Care				
Received Home Management Plan of Care	-	-	88%	88%
Received Reliever Medication	-	-	100%	100%
Received Systemic Corticosteroids	-	-	100%	100%
Emergency Department				
Admittance Decision Time (minutes)[2]	327	111	125	98
Head CT Results Within 45 Min. of Arrival[1,3]	-	-	55%	57%
Patients Who Left ER Before Being Seen	15,015	2%	3%	2%
Time from ER Arrival to Admit. (minutes)[2]	348	240	323	274

NOTE: Hospital profiles are in alphabetical order by state, then city, then hospital within the city; Rankings exclude hospitals with less than 25 cases except for patient surveys which excludes hospitals with less than 100 cases; (a) 100-299 cases; (1) The number of cases/patients is too few to report; (2) Data submitted were based on a sample of cases/patients; (3) Results are based on a shorter time period than required; (4) Data suppressed by CMS for one or more quarters; (5) Results are not available for this reporting period; (6) Fewer than 100 patients completed the HCAHPS survey; (7) No cases met the criteria for this measure; (8) The lower limit of the confidence interval cannot be calculated if the number of observed infections equals zero; (9) No data are available from the state/territory for this reporting period; (10) The scores shown reflect fewer than 50 completed surveys; (11) There were discrepancies in the data collection process; (12) This measure does not apply to this hospital for this reporting period; (13) Results cannot be calculated for this reporting period; (14) The results for this state are combined with nearby states to protect confidentiality; Please refer to the User's Guide for a full explanation of data.

Measure	Cases	This Hosp.	State Avg.	U.S. Avg.
Time from ER Arrival to Discharge (minutes)	359	90	168	134
Time in ER Before Being Evaluated (minutes)	358	17	29	26
Time to Pain Meds for Fractures (minutes)	83	34	62	57
Heart Attack Care				
Aspirin Given at Discharge[1,3]	-	-	99%	99%
Fibrinolytic Meds Within 30 Min. of Arrival[3,7]	-	-	73%	54%
PCI Within 90 Minutes of Arrival[3,7]	-	-	95%	96%
Statin Prescribed at Discharge[1,3]	-	-	98%	98%
Heart Failure Care				
ACE Inhibitor or ARB for LVSD	16	100%	97%	97%
Discharge Instructions Given	59	97%	94%	94%
Evaluation of LVS Function	72	100%	99%	99%
Medicare Spending				
Medicare Spending per Patient (ratio)	-	1.00	0.98	0.98
Pneumonia Care				
Appropriate Initial Antibiotic Given	38	97%	97%	95%
Blood Culture Timing	85	100%	98%	98%
Pregnancy and Delivery Care				
Newborn Deliveries Scheduled Early[7]	-	-	5%	6%
Preventive Care				
Immunization for Influenza[2]	299	98%	89%	90%
Immunization for Pneumonia[2]	463	98%	90%	92%
Stroke Care				
Anticoagulation Therapy for Atrial Fibrillation[1]	-	-	95%	95%
Antithrombotic Therapy Timing	16	100%	98%	98%
Assessed for Rehabilitation	22	95%	97%	97%
Discharged on Antithrombotic Therapy	19	100%	99%	99%
Discharged on Statin Medication	15	100%	94%	94%
Thrombolytic Therapy Timing[1]	-	-	72%	66%
Venous Thromboembolism Prophylaxis	22	100%	94%	94%
Written Stroke Educational Materials Given[1]	-	-	87%	88%
Surgical Care Improvement Project				
Appropriate Beta Blocker Usage	29	93%	97%	98%
Appropriate VTP Within 24 Hours	141	99%	98%	98%
Controlled Postoperative Blood Glucose[7]	-	-	96%	97%
Perioperative Temperature Management	156	100%	100%	100%
Prophylactic Antibiotic Selection	115	98%	99%	99%
Prophylactic Antibiotic Selection (Outpatient)	12	75%	97%	98%
Prophylactic Antibiotic Stopped	115	100%	98%	98%
Prophylactic Antibiotic Timing	115	100%	99%	99%
Prophylactic Antibiotic Timing (Outpatient)	12	100%	97%	98%
Urinary Catheter Removal	119	97%	97%	97%
Survey of Patients' Hospital Experiences				
Area Around Room 'Always' Quiet at Night	300+	64%	51%	61%
Doctors 'Always' Communicated Well	300+	83%	78%	82%
Home Recovery Information Given	300+	86%	83%	85%
Hospital Given 9 or 10 on 10 Point Scale	300+	84%	68%	71%
Meds 'Always' Explained Before Given	300+	64%	61%	64%
Nurses 'Always' Communicated Well	300+	82%	74%	79%
Pain 'Always' Well Controlled	300+	76%	68%	71%
Room and Bathroom 'Always' Clean	300+	77%	70%	73%
Timely Help 'Always' Received	300+	73%	62%	68%
Would Definitely Recommend Hospital	300+	88%	70%	71%
Use of Medical Imaging				
Cardiac Imaging Stress Test before Surgery[1]	-	-	5.2%	5.3%
Combination Abdominal CT Scan	364	4.7%	13.4%	10.5%
Combination Brain/Sinus CT Scan	313	1.3%	2.2%	2.7%
Combination Chest CT Scan	256	2.3%	2.3%	2.7%
Follow-up Mammogram/Ultrasound	1,134	6.1%	8.2%	8.8%
Lumbar Spine MRI for Low Back Pain	57	29.8%	34.2%	37.2%

Oak Valley District Hospital

350 S Oak Ave
Oakdale, CA 95361
Phone: 209-847-3011
Fax: 209-848-4110
URL: www.oakvalleycares.org
Type: Acute Care Hospitals
Emergency Services: Yes
Ownership: Govt - Hospital Dist/Auth
Beds: 141

Key Personnel:

Operating Room. . . . . Alan Abbott, RN
Chief of Medical Staff . . . . Krystyna Belski, MD
Pediatric Ambulatory Care . . . . . . Christina Belsky, MD
Pediatric In-Patient Care . . . . Christina Belsky, MD
Quality Assurance . . . . Charles P Francis
CEO/President. . . . . Wayne Mills
Emergency Room . . . . Vivian Thompson, RN

Measure	Cases	This Hosp.	State Avg.	U.S. Avg.
Blood Clot Prevention and Treatment				
Anticoagulation Overlap Therapy[1,2]	-	-	92%	93%
ICU Venous Thromboembolism Prophylaxis[2]	14	64%	92%	92%
Incidence of Potentially Preventable VTE[2,7]	-	-	11%	10%
UFH with Dosages/Platelet Monitoring[1,2]	-	-	96%	97%
Venous Thromboembolism Prophylaxis[2]	104	48%	83%	85%
Warfarin Therapy Discharge Instructions[1,2]	-	-	75%	75%
Chest Pain/Possible Heart Attack Care				
Aspirin Given Within 24 Hours of Arrival	40	95%	97%	96%
Fibrinolytic Meds Within 30 Min. of Arrival[7]	-	-	62%	58%
Average Time to ECG (minutes)	42	6	9	7
Average Time to Transfer (minutes)[1]	-	-	62	60
Children's Asthma Care				
Received Home Management Plan of Care	-	-	88%	88%
Received Reliever Medication	-	-	100%	100%
Received Systemic Corticosteroids	-	-	100%	100%
Emergency Department				
Admittance Decision Time (minutes)[2]	17	180	125	98
Head CT Results Within 45 Min. of Arrival[1]	-	-	55%	57%
Patients Who Left ER Before Being Seen	19,873	1%	3%	2%
Time from ER Arrival to Admit. (minutes)[2]	451	272	323	274
Time from ER Arrival to Discharge (minutes)	453	106	168	134
Time in ER Before Being Evaluated (minutes)	481	21	29	26
Time to Pain Meds for Fractures (minutes)	92	67	62	57
Heart Attack Care				
Aspirin Given at Discharge[1]	-	-	99%	99%
Fibrinolytic Meds Within 30 Min. of Arrival[7]	-	-	73%	54%
PCI Within 90 Minutes of Arrival[7]	-	-	95%	96%
Statin Prescribed at Discharge[1]	-	-	98%	98%
Heart Failure Care				
ACE Inhibitor or ARB for LVSD	15	93%	97%	97%
Discharge Instructions Given	32	97%	94%	94%
Evaluation of LVS Function	36	100%	99%	99%
Medicare Spending				
Medicare Spending per Patient (ratio)	-	0.93	0.98	0.98
Pneumonia Care				
Appropriate Initial Antibiotic Given	40	92%	97%	95%
Blood Culture Timing	43	93%	98%	98%
Pregnancy and Delivery Care				
Newborn Deliveries Scheduled Early[1,2]	-	-	5%	6%
Preventive Care				
Immunization for Influenza[2]	269	91%	89%	90%
Immunization for Pneumonia[2]	336	97%	90%	92%
Stroke Care				
Anticoagulation Therapy for Atrial Fibrillation[1]	-	-	95%	95%
Antithrombotic Therapy Timing[1]	-	-	98%	98%
Assessed for Rehabilitation[1]	-	-	97%	97%
Discharged on Antithrombotic Therapy[1]	-	-	99%	99%
Discharged on Statin Medication[1]	-	-	94%	94%
Thrombolytic Therapy Timing[7]	-	-	72%	66%
Venous Thromboembolism Prophylaxis[1]	-	-	94%	94%
Written Stroke Educational Materials Given[1]	-	-	87%	88%
Surgical Care Improvement Project				
Appropriate Beta Blocker Usage[1]	-	-	97%	98%
Appropriate VTP Within 24 Hours	34	100%	98%	98%
Controlled Postoperative Blood Glucose[7]	-	-	96%	97%
Perioperative Temperature Management	39	100%	100%	100%
Prophylactic Antibiotic Selection	24	100%	99%	99%
Prophylactic Antibiotic Selection (Outpatient)[1,3]	-	-	97%	98%
Prophylactic Antibiotic Stopped	22	100%	98%	98%
Prophylactic Antibiotic Timing	25	96%	99%	99%
Prophylactic Antibiotic Timing (Outpatient)[1,3]	-	-	97%	98%
Urinary Catheter Removal	11	82%	97%	97%
Survey of Patients' Hospital Experiences				
Area Around Room 'Always' Quiet at Night	(a)	42%	51%	61%
Doctors 'Always' Communicated Well	(a)	77%	78%	82%
Home Recovery Information Given	(a)	82%	83%	85%
Hospital Given 9 or 10 on 10 Point Scale	(a)	62%	68%	71%
Meds 'Always' Explained Before Given	(a)	52%	61%	64%
Nurses 'Always' Communicated Well	(a)	71%	74%	79%
Pain 'Always' Well Controlled	(a)	59%	68%	71%
Room and Bathroom 'Always' Clean	(a)	73%	70%	73%
Timely Help 'Always' Received	(a)	53%	62%	68%
Would Definitely Recommend Hospital	(a)	67%	70%	71%
Use of Medical Imaging				
Cardiac Imaging Stress Test before Surgery[7]	-	-	5.2%	5.3%
Combination Abdominal CT Scan	198	1.0%	13.4%	10.5%
Combination Brain/Sinus CT Scan[1]	-	-	2.2%	2.7%
Combination Chest CT Scan	95	0.0%	2.3%	2.7%
Follow-up Mammogram/Ultrasound	356	6.5%	8.2%	8.8%
Lumbar Spine MRI for Low Back Pain[1]	-	-	34.2%	37.2%

Alameda County Medical Center

1411 E 31st St
Oakland, CA 94602
Phone: 510-437-4800
Fax: 510-535-7759
E-mail: btate@acmedctr.org
URL: www.acmedctr.org
Type: Acute Care Hospitals
Emergency Services: Yes
Ownership: Govt - Hospital Dist/Auth
Beds: 308

Key Personnel:

CEO/President. . . . . Edwards A. Carladenise
Radiology. . . . . Ronald Eisenberg, MD
Quality Assurance . . . . Lea Henry, RN
Operating Room. . . . . Janet Johns
Pediatric Ambulatory Care . . . . . . Marian Johnson, MD
Pediatric In-Patient Care . . . . Marian Johnson, MD
Chief of Medical Staff . . . . Vallerie Ng, MD

Measure	Cases	This Hosp.	State Avg.	U.S. Avg.
Blood Clot Prevention and Treatment				
Anticoagulation Overlap Therapy[2]	47	96%	92%	93%
ICU Venous Thromboembolism Prophylaxis[2]	56	84%	92%	92%
Incidence of Potentially Preventable VTE[2]	11	36%	11%	10%
UFH with Dosages/Platelet Monitoring[2]	28	96%	96%	97%
Venous Thromboembolism Prophylaxis[2]	276	89%	83%	85%
Warfarin Therapy Discharge Instructions[2]	39	0%	75%	75%
Chest Pain/Possible Heart Attack Care				
Aspirin Given Within 24 Hours of Arrival[1,3]	-	-	97%	96%
Fibrinolytic Meds Within 30 Min. of Arrival[3,7]	-	-	62%	58%
Average Time to ECG (minutes)[1,3]	-	-	9	7
Average Time to Transfer (minutes)[3,7]	-	-	62	60
Children's Asthma Care				
Received Home Management Plan of Care	-	-	88%	88%
Received Reliever Medication	-	-	100%	100%
Received Systemic Corticosteroids	-	-	100%	100%
Emergency Department				
Admittance Decision Time (minutes)[2]	467	451	125	98
Head CT Results Within 45 Min. of Arrival[1]	-	-	55%	57%
Patients Who Left ER Before Being Seen	90,132	6%	3%	2%
Time from ER Arrival to Admit. (minutes)[2]	486	782	323	274
Time from ER Arrival to Discharge (minutes)	337	210	168	134
Time in ER Before Being Evaluated (minutes)	399	95	29	26
Time to Pain Meds for Fractures (minutes)	263	115	62	57
Heart Attack Care				
Aspirin Given at Discharge	99	100%	99%	99%
Fibrinolytic Meds Within 30 Min. of Arrival[7]	-	-	73%	54%
PCI Within 90 Minutes of Arrival	35	97%	95%	96%
Statin Prescribed at Discharge	99	100%	98%	98%
Heart Failure Care				
ACE Inhibitor or ARB for LVSD	207	100%	97%	97%
Discharge Instructions Given	331	39%	94%	94%
Evaluation of LVS Function	357	100%	99%	99%
Medicare Spending				
Medicare Spending per Patient (ratio)	-	1.02	0.98	0.98
Pneumonia Care				
Appropriate Initial Antibiotic Given	84	92%	97%	95%
Blood Culture Timing	162	86%	98%	98%
Pregnancy and Delivery Care				
Newborn Deliveries Scheduled Early[2]	18	6%	5%	6%
Preventive Care				
Immunization for Influenza[2]	548	69%	89%	90%
Immunization for Pneumonia[2]	408	72%	90%	92%
Stroke Care				
Anticoagulation Therapy for Atrial Fibrillation[1]	-	-	95%	95%
Antithrombotic Therapy Timing	69	99%	98%	98%
Assessed for Rehabilitation	92	87%	97%	97%

NOTE: Hospital profiles are in alphabetical order by state, then city, then hospital within the city; Rankings exclude hospitals with less than 25 cases except for patient surveys which excludes hospitals with less than 100 cases; (a) 100-299 cases; (1) The number of cases/patients is too few to report; (2) Data submitted were based on a sample of cases/patients; (3) Results are based on a shorter time period than required; (4) Data suppressed by CMS for one or more quarters; (5) Results are not available for this reporting period; (6) Fewer than 100 patients completed the HCAHPS survey; (7) No cases met the criteria for this measure; (8) The lower limit of the confidence interval cannot be calculated if the number of observed infections equals zero; (9) No data are available from the state/territory for this reporting period; (10) The scores shown reflect fewer than 50 completed surveys; (11) There were discrepancies in the data collection process; (12) This measure does not apply to this hospital for this reporting period; (13) Results cannot be calculated for this reporting period; (14) The results for this state are combined with nearby states to protect confidentiality; Please refer to the User's Guide for a full explanation of data.

Measure	Cases	This Hosp.	State Avg.	U.S. Avg.
Discharged on Antithrombotic Therapy	72	99%	99%	99%
Discharged on Statin Medication	65	100%	94%	94%
Thrombolytic Therapy Timing[1]	-	-	72%	66%
Venous Thromboembolism Prophylaxis	93	85%	94%	94%
Written Stroke Educational Materials Given	41	0%	87%	88%
Surgical Care Improvement Project				
Appropriate Beta Blocker Usage	38	87%	97%	98%
Appropriate VTP Within 24 Hours	363	98%	98%	98%
Controlled Postoperative Blood Glucose[1]	-	-	96%	97%
Perioperative Temperature Management	435	100%	100%	100%
Prophylactic Antibiotic Selection	178	94%	99%	99%
Prophylactic Antibiotic Selection (Outpatient)[3]	33	64%	97%	98%
Prophylactic Antibiotic Stopped	178	100%	98%	98%
Prophylactic Antibiotic Timing	179	93%	99%	99%
Prophylactic Antibiotic Timing (Outpatient)[3]	34	62%	97%	98%
Urinary Catheter Removal	170	95%	97%	97%
Survey of Patients' Hospital Experiences				
Area Around Room 'Always' Quiet at Night	300+	39%	51%	61%
Doctors 'Always' Communicated Well	300+	76%	78%	82%
Home Recovery Information Given	300+	80%	83%	85%
Hospital Given 9 or 10 on 10 Point Scale	300+	61%	68%	71%
Meds 'Always' Explained Before Given	300+	55%	61%	64%
Nurses 'Always' Communicated Well	300+	65%	74%	79%
Pain 'Always' Well Controlled	300+	64%	68%	71%
Room and Bathroom 'Always' Clean	300+	52%	70%	73%
Timely Help 'Always' Received	300+	52%	62%	68%
Would Definitely Recommend Hospital	300+	61%	70%	71%
Use of Medical Imaging				
Cardiac Imaging Stress Test before Surgery	62	0.0%	5.2%	5.3%
Combination Abdominal CT Scan	271	15.1%	13.4%	10.5%
Combination Brain/Sinus CT Scan[1]	-	-	2.2%	2.7%
Combination Chest CT Scan	192	8.9%	2.3%	2.7%
Follow-up Mammogram/Ultrasound	251	4.8%	8.2%	8.8%
Lumbar Spine MRI for Low Back Pain[1]	-	-	34.2%	37.2%

Alta Bates Summit Medical Center

350 Hawthorne Avenue
Oakland, CA 94609
Phone: 510-655-4000
Fax: 510-869-8980
URL: www.altabates.com
Type: Acute Care Hospitals
Emergency Services: Yes
Ownership: Voluntary non-profit - Private
Beds: 517

Key Personnel:

Chief of Medical Staff . . . . Samuel Dong, MD
Emergency Room . . . . Ellie Pecora
Quality Assurance . . . . Deanna Tarnow

Measure	Cases	This Hosp.	State Avg.	U.S. Avg.
Blood Clot Prevention and Treatment				
Anticoagulation Overlap Therapy[2]	51	84%	92%	93%
ICU Venous Thromboembolism Prophylaxis[2]	81	91%	92%	92%
Incidence of Potentially Preventable VTE[2]	18	22%	11%	10%
UFH with Dosages/Platelet Monitoring[2]	31	100%	96%	97%
Venous Thromboembolism Prophylaxis[2]	325	74%	83%	85%
Warfarin Therapy Discharge Instructions[2]	28	50%	75%	75%
Chest Pain/Possible Heart Attack Care				
Aspirin Given Within 24 Hours of Arrival[1,3]	-	-	97%	96%
Fibrinolytic Meds Within 30 Min. of Arrival[3,7]	-	-	62%	58%
Average Time to ECG (minutes)[1,3]	-	-	9	7
Average Time to Transfer (minutes)[3,7]	-	-	62	60
Children's Asthma Care				
Received Home Management Plan of Care	-	-	88%	88%
Received Reliever Medication	-	-	100%	100%
Received Systemic Corticosteroids	-	-	100%	100%
Emergency Department				
Admittance Decision Time (minutes)[2]	848	154	125	98
Head CT Results Within 45 Min. of Arrival	18	72%	55%	57%
Patients Who Left ER Before Being Seen	44,877	3%	3%	2%
Time from ER Arrival to Admit. (minutes)[2]	852	320	323	274
Time from ER Arrival to Discharge (minutes)	379	193	168	134
Time in ER Before Being Evaluated (minutes)	381	49	29	26
Time to Pain Meds for Fractures (minutes)	37	61	62	57
Heart Attack Care				
Aspirin Given at Discharge	377	100%	99%	99%
Fibrinolytic Meds Within 30 Min. of Arrival[7]	-	-	73%	54%
PCI Within 90 Minutes of Arrival	51	98%	95%	96%
Statin Prescribed at Discharge	376	99%	98%	98%
Heart Failure Care				
ACE Inhibitor or ARB for LVSD[2]	96	96%	97%	97%
Discharge Instructions Given[2]	241	69%	94%	94%
Evaluation of LVS Function[2]	300	99%	99%	99%
Medicare Spending				
Medicare Spending per Patient (ratio)	-	0.99	0.98	0.98
Pneumonia Care				
Appropriate Initial Antibiotic Given[2]	94	98%	97%	95%
Blood Culture Timing[2]	164	98%	98%	98%
Pregnancy and Delivery Care				
Newborn Deliveries Scheduled Early[7]	-	-	5%	6%
Preventive Care				
Immunization for Influenza[2]	616	90%	89%	90%
Immunization for Pneumonia[2]	952	72%	90%	92%
Stroke Care				
Anticoagulation Therapy for Atrial Fibrillation	16	100%	95%	95%
Antithrombotic Therapy Timing	164	98%	98%	98%
Assessed for Rehabilitation	177	99%	97%	97%
Discharged on Antithrombotic Therapy	161	99%	99%	99%
Discharged on Statin Medication	122	92%	94%	94%
Thrombolytic Therapy Timing	18	89%	72%	66%
Venous Thromboembolism Prophylaxis	198	92%	94%	94%
Written Stroke Educational Materials Given	75	83%	87%	88%
Surgical Care Improvement Project				
Appropriate Beta Blocker Usage[2]	236	98%	97%	98%
Appropriate VTP Within 24 Hours[2]	386	97%	98%	98%
Controlled Postoperative Blood Glucose[2]	186	97%	96%	97%
Perioperative Temperature Management[2]	447	100%	100%	100%
Prophylactic Antibiotic Selection[2]	454	100%	99%	99%
Prophylactic Antibiotic Selection (Outpatient)	301	98%	97%	98%
Prophylactic Antibiotic Stopped[2]	441	99%	98%	98%
Prophylactic Antibiotic Timing[2]	457	99%	99%	99%
Prophylactic Antibiotic Timing (Outpatient)	291	99%	97%	98%
Urinary Catheter Removal[2]	306	96%	97%	97%
Survey of Patients' Hospital Experiences				
Area Around Room 'Always' Quiet at Night	300+	43%	51%	61%
Doctors 'Always' Communicated Well	300+	76%	78%	82%
Home Recovery Information Given	300+	79%	83%	85%
Hospital Given 9 or 10 on 10 Point Scale	300+	55%	68%	71%
Meds 'Always' Explained Before Given	300+	52%	61%	64%
Nurses 'Always' Communicated Well	300+	69%	74%	79%
Pain 'Always' Well Controlled	300+	64%	68%	71%
Room and Bathroom 'Always' Clean	300+	53%	70%	73%
Timely Help 'Always' Received	300+	49%	62%	68%
Would Definitely Recommend Hospital	300+	63%	70%	71%
Use of Medical Imaging				
Cardiac Imaging Stress Test before Surgery	201	4.5%	5.2%	5.3%
Combination Abdominal CT Scan	678	10.2%	13.4%	10.5%
Combination Brain/Sinus CT Scan	730	2.3%	2.2%	2.7%
Combination Chest CT Scan	502	0.2%	2.3%	2.7%
Follow-up Mammogram/Ultrasound	2,650	5.7%	8.2%	8.8%
Lumbar Spine MRI for Low Back Pain[1]	-	-	34.2%	37.2%

Kaiser Foundation Hospital - Oakland/Richmond

280 W Macarthur Blvd
Oakland, CA 94611
Phone: 510-752-1000
Fax: 408-366-4182
E-mail: oakland-webmaster@kp.org
URL: www.oakland.kaiser.org
Type: Acute Care Hospitals
Emergency Services: Yes
Ownership: Voluntary non-profit - Private
Beds: 348

Key Personnel:

Quality Assurance . . . . Nancy Christman
Operating Room. . . . . Mary Diamond, RN
CEO/President. . . . . Mary Holland

Measure	Cases	This Hosp.	State Avg.	U.S. Avg.
Blood Clot Prevention and Treatment				
Anticoagulation Overlap Therapy[2]	82	100%	92%	93%
ICU Venous Thromboembolism Prophylaxis[2]	45	100%	92%	92%
Incidence of Potentially Preventable VTE[2]	15	0%	11%	10%
UFH with Dosages/Platelet Monitoring[2]	45	100%	96%	97%
Venous Thromboembolism Prophylaxis[2]	314	99%	83%	85%
Warfarin Therapy Discharge Instructions[2]	70	74%	75%	75%
Chest Pain/Possible Heart Attack Care				
Aspirin Given Within 24 Hours of Arrival	-	-	97%	96%
Fibrinolytic Meds Within 30 Min. of Arrival	-	-	62%	58%
Average Time to ECG (minutes)	-	-	9	7
Average Time to Transfer (minutes)	-	-	62	60
Children's Asthma Care				
Received Home Management Plan of Care	-	-	88%	88%
Received Reliever Medication	-	-	100%	100%
Received Systemic Corticosteroids	-	-	100%	100%
Emergency Department				
Admittance Decision Time (minutes)[2]	525	50	125	98
Head CT Results Within 45 Min. of Arrival	-	-	55%	57%
Patients Who Left ER Before Being Seen	-	-	3%	2%
Time from ER Arrival to Admit. (minutes)[2]	526	332	323	274
Time from ER Arrival to Discharge (minutes)	-	-	168	134
Time in ER Before Being Evaluated (minutes)	-	-	29	26
Time to Pain Meds for Fractures (minutes)	-	-	62	57
Heart Attack Care				
Aspirin Given at Discharge	80	99%	99%	99%
Fibrinolytic Meds Within 30 Min. of Arrival[1]	-	-	73%	54%
PCI Within 90 Minutes of Arrival[7]	-	-	95%	96%
Statin Prescribed at Discharge	83	100%	98%	98%
Heart Failure Care				
ACE Inhibitor or ARB for LVSD[2]	114	99%	97%	97%
Discharge Instructions Given[2]	381	100%	94%	94%
Evaluation of LVS Function[2]	416	100%	99%	99%
Medicare Spending				
Medicare Spending per Patient (ratio)	-	0.80	0.98	0.98
Pneumonia Care				
Appropriate Initial Antibiotic Given[2]	60	98%	97%	95%
Blood Culture Timing[2]	119	100%	98%	98%
Pregnancy and Delivery Care				
Newborn Deliveries Scheduled Early[2]	19	11%	5%	6%
Preventive Care				
Immunization for Influenza[2]	524	89%	89%	90%
Immunization for Pneumonia[2]	590	96%	90%	92%
Stroke Care				
Anticoagulation Therapy for Atrial Fibrillation[2]	18	100%	95%	95%
Antithrombotic Therapy Timing[2]	94	96%	98%	98%
Assessed for Rehabilitation[2]	128	97%	97%	97%
Discharged on Antithrombotic Therapy[2]	116	99%	99%	99%
Discharged on Statin Medication[2]	89	99%	94%	94%
Thrombolytic Therapy Timing[2]	14	79%	72%	66%
Venous Thromboembolism Prophylaxis[2]	118	97%	94%	94%
Written Stroke Educational Materials Given[2]	69	99%	87%	88%
Surgical Care Improvement Project				
Appropriate Beta Blocker Usage[2]	98	100%	97%	98%
Appropriate VTP Within 24 Hours[2]	389	98%	98%	98%
Controlled Postoperative Blood Glucose[2,7]	-	-	96%	97%
Perioperative Temperature Management[2]	494	100%	100%	100%
Prophylactic Antibiotic Selection[2]	329	100%	99%	99%
Prophylactic Antibiotic Selection (Outpatient)	-	-	97%	98%
Prophylactic Antibiotic Stopped[2]	322	100%	98%	98%
Prophylactic Antibiotic Timing[2]	329	100%	99%	99%
Prophylactic Antibiotic Timing (Outpatient)	-	-	97%	98%
Urinary Catheter Removal[2]	274	100%	97%	97%
Survey of Patients' Hospital Experiences				
Area Around Room 'Always' Quiet at Night	300+	40%	51%	61%
Doctors 'Always' Communicated Well	300+	78%	78%	82%
Home Recovery Information Given	300+	84%	83%	85%
Hospital Given 9 or 10 on 10 Point Scale	300+	60%	68%	71%
Meds 'Always' Explained Before Given	300+	56%	61%	64%
Nurses 'Always' Communicated Well	300+	68%	74%	79%
Pain 'Always' Well Controlled	300+	66%	68%	71%
Room and Bathroom 'Always' Clean	300+	62%	70%	73%
Timely Help 'Always' Received	300+	59%	62%	68%
Would Definitely Recommend Hospital	300+	65%	70%	71%
Use of Medical Imaging				
Cardiac Imaging Stress Test before Surgery	-	-	5.2%	5.3%
Combination Abdominal CT Scan	-	-	13.4%	10.5%
Combination Brain/Sinus CT Scan	-	-	2.2%	2.7%

NOTE: Hospital profiles are in alphabetical order by state, then city, then hospital within the city; Rankings exclude hospitals with less than 25 cases except for patient surveys which excludes hospitals with less than 100 cases; (a) 100-299 cases; (1) The number of cases/patients is too few to report; (2) Data submitted were based on a sample of cases/patients; (3) Results are based on a shorter time period than required; (4) Data suppressed by CMS for one or more quarters; (5) Results are not available for this reporting period; (6) Fewer than 100 patients completed the HCAHPS survey; (7) No cases met the criteria for this measure; (8) The lower limit of the confidence interval cannot be calculated if the number of observed infections equals zero; (9) No data are available from the state/territory for this reporting period; (10) The scores shown reflect fewer than 50 completed surveys; (11) There were discrepancies in the data collection process; (12) This measure does not apply to this hospital for this reporting period; (13) Results cannot be calculated for this reporting period; (14) The results for this state are combined with nearby states to protect confidentiality; Please refer to the User's Guide for a full explanation of data.

Combination Chest CT Scan	-	-	2.3%	2.7%
Follow-up Mammogram/Ultrasound	-	-	8.2%	8.8%
Lumbar Spine MRI for Low Back Pain	-	-	34.2%	37.2%

Tri - City Medical Center

4002 Vista Way
Oceanside, CA 92056
Phone: 760-724-8411
URL: www.tricitymed.org
Type: Acute Care Hospitals
Emergency Services: Yes
Ownership: Govt - Hospital Dist/Auth
Beds: 397

Key Personnel:
CEO .... Tim Moran

Measure	Cases	This Hosp.	State Avg.	U.S. Avg.
Blood Clot Prevention and Treatment				
Anticoagulation Overlap Therapy[2]	103	94%	92%	93%
ICU Venous Thromboembolism Prophylaxis[2]	68	99%	92%	92%
Incidence of Potentially Preventable VTE[1,2]	-	-	11%	10%
UFH with Dosages/Platelet Monitoring[2]	32	97%	96%	97%
Venous Thromboembolism Prophylaxis[2]	297	82%	83%	85%
Warfarin Therapy Discharge Instructions[2]	79	96%	75%	75%
Chest Pain/Possible Heart Attack Care				
Aspirin Given Within 24 Hours of Arrival	73	97%	97%	96%
Fibrinolytic Meds Within 30 Min. of Arrival[3,7]	-	-	62%	58%
Average Time to ECG (minutes)	78	0	9	7
Average Time to Transfer (minutes)[3,7]	-	-	62	60
Children's Asthma Care				
Received Home Management Plan of Care	-	-	88%	88%
Received Reliever Medication	-	-	100%	100%
Received Systemic Corticosteroids	-	-	100%	100%
Emergency Department				
Admittance Decision Time (minutes)[2]	563	92	125	98
Head CT Results Within 45 Min. of Arrival[1]	-	-	55%	57%
Patients Who Left ER Before Being Seen	69,898	5%	3%	2%
Time from ER Arrival to Admit. (minutes)[2]	568	364	323	274
Time from ER Arrival to Discharge (minutes)	19,168	221	168	134
Time in ER Before Being Evaluated (minutes)	21,797	43	29	26
Time to Pain Meds for Fractures (minutes)	204	74	62	57
Heart Attack Care				
Aspirin Given at Discharge[2]	271	100%	99%	99%
Fibrinolytic Meds Within 30 Min. of Arrival[2,7]	-	-	73%	54%
PCI Within 90 Minutes of Arrival[2]	62	98%	95%	96%
Statin Prescribed at Discharge[2]	261	100%	98%	98%
Heart Failure Care				
ACE Inhibitor or ARB for LVSD[2]	65	100%	97%	97%
Discharge Instructions Given[2]	205	100%	94%	94%
Evaluation of LVS Function[2]	259	100%	99%	99%
Medicare Spending				
Medicare Spending per Patient (ratio)	-	1.04	0.98	0.98
Pneumonia Care				
Appropriate Initial Antibiotic Given[2]	65	97%	97%	95%
Blood Culture Timing[2]	147	95%	98%	98%
Pregnancy and Delivery Care				
Newborn Deliveries Scheduled Early	178	4%	5%	6%
Preventive Care				
Immunization for Influenza[2]	505	82%	89%	90%
Immunization for Pneumonia[2]	545	85%	90%	92%
Stroke Care				
Anticoagulation Therapy for Atrial Fibrillation	38	100%	95%	95%
Antithrombotic Therapy Timing	108	99%	98%	98%
Assessed for Rehabilitation	209	100%	97%	97%
Discharged on Antithrombotic Therapy	167	99%	99%	99%
Discharged on Statin Medication	123	96%	94%	94%
Thrombolytic Therapy Timing	53	94%	72%	66%
Venous Thromboembolism Prophylaxis	207	99%	94%	94%
Written Stroke Educational Materials Given	103	100%	87%	88%
Surgical Care Improvement Project				
Appropriate Beta Blocker Usage[2]	154	99%	97%	98%
Appropriate VTP Within 24 Hours[2]	315	96%	98%	98%
Controlled Postoperative Blood Glucose[2]	94	96%	96%	97%
Perioperative Temperature Management[2]	390	100%	100%	100%
Prophylactic Antibiotic Selection[2]	351	99%	99%	99%
Prophylactic Antibiotic Selection (Outpatient)	342	98%	97%	98%
Prophylactic Antibiotic Stopped[2]	328	99%	98%	98%
Prophylactic Antibiotic Timing[2]	352	100%	99%	99%
Prophylactic Antibiotic Timing (Outpatient)	336	100%	97%	98%
Urinary Catheter Removal[2]	264	98%	97%	97%
Survey of Patients' Hospital Experiences				
Area Around Room 'Always' Quiet at Night	300+	43%	51%	61%
Doctors 'Always' Communicated Well	300+	77%	78%	82%
Home Recovery Information Given	300+	83%	83%	85%
Hospital Given 9 or 10 on 10 Point Scale	300+	59%	68%	71%
Meds 'Always' Explained Before Given	300+	62%	61%	64%
Nurses 'Always' Communicated Well	300+	75%	74%	79%
Pain 'Always' Well Controlled	300+	64%	68%	71%
Room and Bathroom 'Always' Clean	300+	66%	70%	73%
Timely Help 'Always' Received	300+	63%	62%	68%
Would Definitely Recommend Hospital	300+	65%	70%	71%
Use of Medical Imaging				
Cardiac Imaging Stress Test before Surgery	531	3.6%	5.2%	5.3%
Combination Abdominal CT Scan	894	5.1%	13.4%	10.5%
Combination Brain/Sinus CT Scan	966	1.0%	2.2%	2.7%
Combination Chest CT Scan	415	0.0%	2.3%	2.7%
Follow-up Mammogram/Ultrasound	1,716	6.2%	8.2%	8.8%
Lumbar Spine MRI for Low Back Pain	69	33.3%	34.2%	37.2%

Ojai Valley Community Hospital

1306 Maricopa Hwy
Ojai, CA 93023
Phone: 805-640-2280
Fax: 805-640-2204
URL: www.cmhshealth.org
Type: Acute Care Hospitals
Emergency Services: Yes
Ownership: Voluntary non-profit - Private
Beds: 103

Key Personnel:
Infection Control............. Anne Borchard, RN ICP
Emergency Room .... Kristi Cain, RN
Chief of Medical Staff.......... Stanley Frochtzwajg, MD
Intensive Care Unit............ Sunny Howard, RN
Operating Room............. Frederick Menninger III, MD
President/CEO.............. Gary K Wilde
Quality Assurance .... Sue Wood

Measure	Cases	This Hosp.	State Avg.	U.S. Avg.
Blood Clot Prevention and Treatment				
Anticoagulation Overlap Therapy[1,2]	-	-	92%	93%
ICU Venous Thromboembolism Prophylaxis[2]	15	87%	92%	92%
Incidence of Potentially Preventable VTE[1,2]	-	-	11%	10%
UFH with Dosages/Platelet Monitoring[1,2]	-	-	96%	97%
Venous Thromboembolism Prophylaxis[2]	77	83%	83%	85%
Warfarin Therapy Discharge Instructions[1,2]	-	-	75%	75%
Chest Pain/Possible Heart Attack Care				
Aspirin Given Within 24 Hours of Arrival[3]	16	100%	97%	96%
Fibrinolytic Meds Within 30 Min. of Arrival[3,7]	-	-	62%	58%
Average Time to ECG (minutes)[3]	17	4	9	7
Average Time to Transfer (minutes)[3,7]	-	-	62	60
Children's Asthma Care				
Received Home Management Plan of Care	-	-	88%	88%
Received Reliever Medication	-	-	100%	100%
Received Systemic Corticosteroids	-	-	100%	100%
Emergency Department				
Admittance Decision Time (minutes)[2]	410	74	125	98
Head CT Results Within 45 Min. of Arrival[1]	-	-	55%	57%
Patients Who Left ER Before Being Seen	8,106	1%	3%	2%
Time from ER Arrival to Admit. (minutes)[2]	474	231	323	274
Time from ER Arrival to Discharge (minutes)	334	107	168	134
Time in ER Before Being Evaluated (minutes)	380	19	29	26
Time to Pain Meds for Fractures (minutes)	22	32	62	57
Heart Attack Care				
Aspirin Given at Discharge[1]	-	-	99%	99%
Fibrinolytic Meds Within 30 Min. of Arrival[7]	-	-	73%	54%
PCI Within 90 Minutes of Arrival[7]	-	-	95%	96%
Statin Prescribed at Discharge[1]	-	-	98%	98%
Heart Failure Care				
ACE Inhibitor or ARB for LVSD[1]	-	-	97%	97%
Discharge Instructions Given	16	75%	94%	94%
Evaluation of LVS Function	20	100%	99%	99%
Medicare Spending				
Medicare Spending per Patient (ratio)	-	0.87	0.98	0.98
Pneumonia Care				
Appropriate Initial Antibiotic Given	26	88%	97%	95%
Blood Culture Timing	35	97%	98%	98%
Pregnancy and Delivery Care				
Newborn Deliveries Scheduled Early[7]	-	-	5%	6%
Preventive Care				
Immunization for Influenza[2]	264	89%	89%	90%
Immunization for Pneumonia[2]	403	86%	90%	92%
Stroke Care				
Anticoagulation Therapy for Atrial Fibrillation[7]	-	-	95%	95%
Antithrombotic Therapy Timing[1]	-	-	98%	98%
Assessed for Rehabilitation[1]	-	-	97%	97%
Discharged on Antithrombotic Therapy[1]	-	-	99%	99%
Discharged on Statin Medication[1]	-	-	94%	94%
Thrombolytic Therapy Timing[1]	-	-	72%	66%
Venous Thromboembolism Prophylaxis[1]	-	-	94%	94%
Written Stroke Educational Materials Given[1]	-	-	87%	88%
Surgical Care Improvement Project				
Appropriate Beta Blocker Usage[1]	-	-	97%	98%
Appropriate VTP Within 24 Hours	41	98%	98%	98%
Controlled Postoperative Blood Glucose[7]	-	-	96%	97%
Perioperative Temperature Management	45	100%	100%	100%
Prophylactic Antibiotic Selection	28	100%	99%	99%
Prophylactic Antibiotic Selection (Outpatient)[1,3]	-	-	97%	98%
Prophylactic Antibiotic Stopped	27	93%	98%	98%
Prophylactic Antibiotic Timing	29	97%	99%	99%
Prophylactic Antibiotic Timing (Outpatient)[1,3]	-	-	97%	98%
Urinary Catheter Removal	34	97%	97%	97%
Survey of Patients' Hospital Experiences				
Area Around Room 'Always' Quiet at Night	(a)	59%	51%	61%
Doctors 'Always' Communicated Well	(a)	84%	78%	82%
Home Recovery Information Given	(a)	86%	83%	85%
Hospital Given 9 or 10 on 10 Point Scale	(a)	70%	68%	71%
Meds 'Always' Explained Before Given	(a)	64%	61%	64%
Nurses 'Always' Communicated Well	(a)	87%	74%	79%
Pain 'Always' Well Controlled	(a)	75%	68%	71%
Room and Bathroom 'Always' Clean	(a)	80%	70%	73%
Timely Help 'Always' Received	(a)	75%	62%	68%
Would Definitely Recommend Hospital	(a)	74%	70%	71%
Use of Medical Imaging				
Cardiac Imaging Stress Test before Surgery[1]	-	-	5.2%	5.3%
Combination Abdominal CT Scan	161	16.1%	13.4%	10.5%
Combination Brain/Sinus CT Scan[1]	-	-	2.2%	2.7%
Combination Chest CT Scan	77	0.0%	2.3%	2.7%
Follow-up Mammogram/Ultrasound	304	8.6%	8.2%	8.8%
Lumbar Spine MRI for Low Back Pain[1]	-	-	34.2%	37.2%

Chapman Medical Center

2601 E Chapman Ave
Orange, CA 92869
Phone: 714-633-0011
Fax: 714-532-4345
URL: www.chapmanmedicalcenter.com
Type: Acute Care Hospitals
Emergency Services: Yes
Ownership: Proprietary
Beds: 114

Key Personnel:
Operating Room............. Alex Fernandez, RN
CEO .... Don Kreitz
Chief of Medical Staff.......... John Luster, MD
Intensive Care Unit............ Nancy McKinney, RN

Measure	Cases	This Hosp.	State Avg.	U.S. Avg.
Blood Clot Prevention and Treatment				
Anticoagulation Overlap Therapy[1,2]	-	-	92%	93%
ICU Venous Thromboembolism Prophylaxis[2]	60	92%	92%	92%
Incidence of Potentially Preventable VTE[1,2]	-	-	11%	10%
UFH with Dosages/Platelet Monitoring[1,2]	-	-	96%	97%
Venous Thromboembolism Prophylaxis[2]	111	87%	83%	85%
Warfarin Therapy Discharge Instructions[1,2]	-	-	75%	75%
Chest Pain/Possible Heart Attack Care				
Aspirin Given Within 24 Hours of Arrival[3]	13	100%	97%	96%
Fibrinolytic Meds Within 30 Min. of Arrival[3,7]	-	-	62%	58%
Average Time to ECG (minutes)[3]	13	11	9	7
Average Time to Transfer (minutes)[1,3]	-	-	62	60
Children's Asthma Care				
Received Home Management Plan of Care	-	-	88%	88%
Received Reliever Medication	-	-	100%	100%
Received Systemic Corticosteroids	-	-	100%	100%

NOTE: Hospital profiles are in alphabetical order by state, then city, then hospital within the city; Rankings exclude hospitals with less than 25 cases except for patient surveys which excludes hospitals with less than 100 cases; (a) 100-299 cases; (1) The number of cases/patients is too few to report; (2) Data submitted were based on a sample of cases/patients; (3) Results are based on a shorter time period than required; (4) Data suppressed by CMS for one or more quarters; (5) Results are not available for this reporting period; (6) Fewer than 100 patients completed the HCAHPS survey; (7) No cases met the criteria for this measure; (8) The lower limit of the confidence interval cannot be calculated if the number of observed infections equals zero; (9) No data are available from the state/territory for this reporting period; (10) The scores shown reflect fewer than 50 completed surveys; (11) There were discrepancies in the data collection process; (12) This measure does not apply to this hospital for this reporting period; (13) Results cannot be calculated for this reporting period; (14) The results for this state are combined with nearby states to protect confidentiality; Please refer to the User's Guide for a full explanation of data.

Measure	Cases	This Hosp.	State Avg.	U.S. Avg.
Emergency Department				
Admittance Decision Time (minutes)[2]	161	175	125	98
Head CT Results Within 45 Min. of Arrival[3,7]	-	-	55%	57%
Patients Who Left ER Before Being Seen	9,622	3%	3%	2%
Time from ER Arrival to Admit. (minutes)[2]	200	374	323	274
Time from ER Arrival to Discharge (minutes)	316	122	168	134
Time in ER Before Being Evaluated (minutes)	328	28	29	26
Time to Pain Meds for Fractures (minutes)	35	51	62	57
Heart Attack Care				
Aspirin Given at Discharge[1,3]	-	-	99%	99%
Fibrinolytic Meds Within 30 Min. of Arrival[3,7]	-	-	73%	54%
PCI Within 90 Minutes of Arrival[3,7]	-	-	95%	96%
Statin Prescribed at Discharge[1,3]	-	-	98%	98%
Heart Failure Care				
ACE Inhibitor or ARB for LVSD[1]	-	-	97%	97%
Discharge Instructions Given	17	88%	94%	94%
Evaluation of LVS Function	20	100%	99%	99%
Medicare Spending				
Medicare Spending per Patient (ratio)	-	1.09	0.98	0.98
Pneumonia Care				
Appropriate Initial Antibiotic Given	31	100%	97%	95%
Blood Culture Timing	59	98%	98%	98%
Pregnancy and Delivery Care				
Newborn Deliveries Scheduled Early[7]	-	-	5%	6%
Preventive Care				
Immunization for Influenza[2]	291	97%	89%	90%
Immunization for Pneumonia[2]	273	90%	90%	92%
Stroke Care				
Anticoagulation Therapy for Atrial Fibrillation[7]	-	-	95%	95%
Antithrombotic Therapy Timing[1]	-	-	98%	98%
Assessed for Rehabilitation[1]	-	-	97%	97%
Discharged on Antithrombotic Therapy[1]	-	-	99%	99%
Discharged on Statin Medication[1]	-	-	94%	94%
Thrombolytic Therapy Timing[7]	-	-	72%	66%
Venous Thromboembolism Prophylaxis	11	55%	94%	94%
Written Stroke Educational Materials Given[1]	-	-	87%	88%
Surgical Care Improvement Project				
Appropriate Beta Blocker Usage	39	95%	97%	98%
Appropriate VTP Within 24 Hours	116	98%	98%	98%
Controlled Postoperative Blood Glucose[7]	-	-	96%	97%
Perioperative Temperature Management	131	100%	100%	100%
Prophylactic Antibiotic Selection	85	99%	99%	99%
Prophylactic Antibiotic Selection (Outpatient)[1,3]	-	-	97%	98%
Prophylactic Antibiotic Stopped	84	99%	98%	98%
Prophylactic Antibiotic Timing	85	99%	99%	99%
Prophylactic Antibiotic Timing (Outpatient)[1,3]	-	-	97%	98%
Urinary Catheter Removal	89	97%	97%	97%
Survey of Patients' Hospital Experiences				
Area Around Room 'Always' Quiet at Night	300+	53%	51%	61%
Doctors 'Always' Communicated Well	300+	82%	78%	82%
Home Recovery Information Given	300+	83%	83%	85%
Hospital Given 9 or 10 on 10 Point Scale	300+	61%	68%	71%
Meds 'Always' Explained Before Given	300+	63%	61%	64%
Nurses 'Always' Communicated Well	300+	73%	74%	79%
Pain 'Always' Well Controlled	300+	72%	68%	71%
Room and Bathroom 'Always' Clean	300+	71%	70%	73%
Timely Help 'Always' Received	300+	55%	62%	68%
Would Definitely Recommend Hospital	300+	66%	70%	71%
Use of Medical Imaging				
Cardiac Imaging Stress Test before Surgery[1]	-	-	5.2%	5.3%
Combination Abdominal CT Scan	56	1.8%	13.4%	10.5%
Combination Brain/Sinus CT Scan[1]	-	-	2.2%	2.7%
Combination Chest CT Scan[1]	-	-	2.3%	2.7%
Follow-up Mammogram/Ultrasound[7]	-	-	8.2%	8.8%
Lumbar Spine MRI for Low Back Pain[1]	-	-	34.2%	37.2%

Saint Joseph Hospital

1100 West Stewart Dr
Orange, CA 92868
Phone: 714-633-9111
Fax: 714-744-8551
URL: www.sjo.org
Type: Acute Care Hospitals
Emergency Services: Yes
Ownership: Voluntary non-profit - Church
Beds: 412

Key Personnel:

Pediatric Ambulatory Care . . . . . . Allen Bobb, MD
Pediatric In-Patient Care . . . . Allen Bobb, MD
Chief of Medical Staff . . . . Raymond Casciari, MD
Coronary Care . . . . Carmen Farrell
CEO/President . . . . Steven C. Moreau
Infection Control . . . . Susan Parke
Radiology . . . . Wallace Peck, MD
Quality Assurance . . . . Diane Wynn

Measure	Cases	This Hosp.	State Avg.	U.S. Avg.
Blood Clot Prevention and Treatment				
Anticoagulation Overlap Therapy[2]	50	78%	92%	93%
ICU Venous Thromboembolism Prophylaxis[2]	74	93%	92%	92%
Incidence of Potentially Preventable VTE[1,2]	-	-	11%	10%
UFH with Dosages/Platelet Monitoring[2]	18	100%	96%	97%
Venous Thromboembolism Prophylaxis[2]	299	92%	83%	85%
Warfarin Therapy Discharge Instructions[2]	40	58%	75%	75%
Chest Pain/Possible Heart Attack Care				
Aspirin Given Within 24 Hours of Arrival	14	100%	97%	96%
Fibrinolytic Meds Within 30 Min. of Arrival[3,7]	-	-	62%	58%
Average Time to ECG (minutes)	15	6	9	7
Average Time to Transfer (minutes)[3,7]	-	-	62	60
Children's Asthma Care				
Received Home Management Plan of Care	-	-	88%	88%
Received Reliever Medication	-	-	100%	100%
Received Systemic Corticosteroids	-	-	100%	100%
Emergency Department				
Admittance Decision Time (minutes)[2]	79	151	125	98
Head CT Results Within 45 Min. of Arrival[1]	-	-	55%	57%
Patients Who Left ER Before Being Seen	>100k	3%	3%	2%
Time from ER Arrival to Admit. (minutes)[2]	88	326	323	274
Time from ER Arrival to Discharge (minutes)	220	180	168	134
Time in ER Before Being Evaluated (minutes)	382	61	29	26
Time to Pain Meds for Fractures (minutes)	302	75	62	57
Heart Attack Care				
Aspirin Given at Discharge	245	98%	99%	99%
Fibrinolytic Meds Within 30 Min. of Arrival[7]	-	-	73%	54%
PCI Within 90 Minutes of Arrival	38	95%	95%	96%
Statin Prescribed at Discharge	245	97%	98%	98%
Heart Failure Care				
ACE Inhibitor or ARB for LVSD	122	98%	97%	97%
Discharge Instructions Given	307	93%	94%	94%
Evaluation of LVS Function	368	100%	99%	99%
Medicare Spending				
Medicare Spending per Patient (ratio)	-	1.00	0.98	0.98
Pneumonia Care				
Appropriate Initial Antibiotic Given	168	99%	97%	95%
Blood Culture Timing	316	100%	98%	98%
Pregnancy and Delivery Care				
Newborn Deliveries Scheduled Early[2]	99	1%	5%	6%
Preventive Care				
Immunization for Influenza[2]	461	82%	89%	90%
Immunization for Pneumonia[2]	444	84%	90%	92%
Stroke Care				
Anticoagulation Therapy for Atrial Fibrillation	35	100%	95%	95%
Antithrombotic Therapy Timing	129	100%	98%	98%
Assessed for Rehabilitation	195	100%	97%	97%
Discharged on Antithrombotic Therapy	163	99%	99%	99%
Discharged on Statin Medication	123	98%	94%	94%
Thrombolytic Therapy Timing	13	85%	72%	66%
Venous Thromboembolism Prophylaxis	174	100%	94%	94%
Written Stroke Educational Materials Given	100	100%	87%	88%
Surgical Care Improvement Project				
Appropriate Beta Blocker Usage[2]	175	98%	97%	98%
Appropriate VTP Within 24 Hours[2]	304	97%	98%	98%
Controlled Postoperative Blood Glucose[2]	125	95%	96%	97%
Perioperative Temperature Management[2]	553	100%	100%	100%
Prophylactic Antibiotic Selection[2]	398	100%	99%	99%
Prophylactic Antibiotic Selection (Outpatient)	609	99%	97%	98%
Prophylactic Antibiotic Stopped[2]	377	98%	98%	98%
Prophylactic Antibiotic Timing[2]	398	99%	99%	99%
Prophylactic Antibiotic Timing (Outpatient)	612	97%	97%	98%
Urinary Catheter Removal[2]	332	99%	97%	97%
Survey of Patients' Hospital Experiences				
Area Around Room 'Always' Quiet at Night	300+	58%	51%	61%
Doctors 'Always' Communicated Well	300+	79%	78%	82%
Home Recovery Information Given	300+	85%	83%	85%
Hospital Given 9 or 10 on 10 Point Scale	300+	80%	68%	71%
Meds 'Always' Explained Before Given	300+	62%	61%	64%
Nurses 'Always' Communicated Well	300+	77%	74%	79%
Pain 'Always' Well Controlled	300+	70%	68%	71%
Room and Bathroom 'Always' Clean	300+	70%	70%	73%
Timely Help 'Always' Received	300+	62%	62%	68%
Would Definitely Recommend Hospital	300+	82%	70%	71%
Use of Medical Imaging				
Cardiac Imaging Stress Test before Surgery	300	6.7%	5.2%	5.3%
Combination Abdominal CT Scan	879	11.1%	13.4%	10.5%
Combination Brain/Sinus CT Scan	729	0.4%	2.2%	2.7%
Combination Chest CT Scan	696	0.0%	2.3%	2.7%
Follow-up Mammogram/Ultrasound	550	7.5%	8.2%	8.8%
Lumbar Spine MRI for Low Back Pain	59	30.5%	34.2%	37.2%

University of California Irvine Medical Center

101 City Drive South
Orange, CA 92868
Phone: 714-456-6112
Fax: 714-456-7927
E-mail: ucihealth@uci.edu
URL: www.ucihealth.com
Type: Acute Care Hospitals
Emergency Services: Yes
Ownership: Government - Local
Beds: 453

Key Personnel:

Operating Room. . . . . Amir Abolhoda, RN
Radiology. . . . . Michael A Arata
CEO/President. . . . . Ralph Cygan, MD
Infection Control. . . . . Linda Dickey, RN
Pediatric In-Patient Care . . . . Teri Donly, RN
Quality Assurance . . . . Nance Hove
Chief of Medical Staff . . . . Eugene Spiritus, MD

Measure	Cases	This Hosp.	State Avg.	U.S. Avg.
Blood Clot Prevention and Treatment				
Anticoagulation Overlap Therapy[2]	99	99%	92%	93%
ICU Venous Thromboembolism Prophylaxis[2]	104	100%	92%	92%
Incidence of Potentially Preventable VTE[2]	67	0%	11%	10%
UFH with Dosages/Platelet Monitoring[2]	71	100%	96%	97%
Venous Thromboembolism Prophylaxis[2]	247	95%	83%	85%
Warfarin Therapy Discharge Instructions[2]	75	97%	75%	75%
Chest Pain/Possible Heart Attack Care				
Aspirin Given Within 24 Hours of Arrival	36	83%	97%	96%
Fibrinolytic Meds Within 30 Min. of Arrival[5]	-	-	62%	58%
Average Time to ECG (minutes)	36	4	9	7
Average Time to Transfer (minutes)[5]	-	-	62	60
Children's Asthma Care				
Received Home Management Plan of Care	-	-	88%	88%
Received Reliever Medication	-	-	100%	100%
Received Systemic Corticosteroids	-	-	100%	100%
Emergency Department				
Admittance Decision Time (minutes)[2]	410	110	125	98
Head CT Results Within 45 Min. of Arrival[1,3]	-	-	55%	57%
Patients Who Left ER Before Being Seen	32,412	4%	3%	2%
Time from ER Arrival to Admit. (minutes)[2]	465	372	323	274
Time from ER Arrival to Discharge (minutes)	332	278	168	134
Time in ER Before Being Evaluated (minutes)	376	64	29	26
Time to Pain Meds for Fractures (minutes)	66	84	62	57
Heart Attack Care				
Aspirin Given at Discharge	123	98%	99%	99%
Fibrinolytic Meds Within 30 Min. of Arrival[7]	-	-	73%	54%
PCI Within 90 Minutes of Arrival	20	100%	95%	96%
Statin Prescribed at Discharge	122	100%	98%	98%
Heart Failure Care				
ACE Inhibitor or ARB for LVSD	110	100%	97%	97%
Discharge Instructions Given	228	98%	94%	94%
Evaluation of LVS Function	251	100%	99%	99%
Medicare Spending				
Medicare Spending per Patient (ratio)	-	1.02	0.98	0.98
Pneumonia Care				
Appropriate Initial Antibiotic Given	33	97%	97%	95%
Blood Culture Timing	122	98%	98%	98%
Pregnancy and Delivery Care				
Newborn Deliveries Scheduled Early[2]	23	4%	5%	6%
Preventive Care				

NOTE: Hospital profiles are in alphabetical order by state, then city, then hospital within the city; Rankings exclude hospitals with less than 25 cases except for patient surveys which excludes hospitals with less than 100 cases; (a) 100-299 cases; (1) The number of cases/patients is too few to report; (2) Data submitted were based on a sample of cases/patients; (3) Results are based on a shorter time period than required; (4) Data suppressed by CMS for one or more quarters; (5) Results are not available for this reporting period; (6) Fewer than 100 patients completed the HCAHPS survey; (7) No cases met the criteria for this measure; (8) The lower limit of the confidence interval cannot be calculated if the number of observed infections equals zero; (9) No data are available from the state/territory for this reporting period; (10) The scores shown reflect fewer than 50 completed surveys; (11) There were discrepancies in the data collection process; (12) This measure does not apply to this hospital for this reporting period; (13) Results cannot be calculated for this reporting period; (14) The results for this state are combined with nearby states to protect confidentiality; Please refer to the User's Guide for a full explanation of data.

Measure	Cases	This Hosp.	State Avg.	U.S. Avg.
Immunization for Influenza[2]	560	85%	89%	90%
Immunization for Pneumonia[2]	478	83%	90%	92%
Stroke Care				
Anticoagulation Therapy for Atrial Fibrillation	30	100%	95%	95%
Antithrombotic Therapy Timing	138	94%	98%	98%
Assessed for Rehabilitation	252	97%	97%	97%
Discharged on Antithrombotic Therapy	164	98%	99%	99%
Discharged on Statin Medication	131	98%	94%	94%
Thrombolytic Therapy Timing	18	89%	72%	66%
Venous Thromboembolism Prophylaxis	286	100%	94%	94%
Written Stroke Educational Materials Given	136	74%	87%	88%
Surgical Care Improvement Project				
Appropriate Beta Blocker Usage[2]	131	98%	97%	98%
Appropriate VTP Within 24 Hours[2]	335	98%	98%	98%
Controlled Postoperative Blood Glucose[2]	71	99%	96%	97%
Perioperative Temperature Management[2]	429	100%	100%	100%
Prophylactic Antibiotic Selection[2]	346	97%	99%	99%
Prophylactic Antibiotic Selection (Outpatient)	347	98%	97%	98%
Prophylactic Antibiotic Stopped[2]	329	99%	98%	98%
Prophylactic Antibiotic Timing[2]	346	100%	99%	99%
Prophylactic Antibiotic Timing (Outpatient)	266	97%	97%	98%
Urinary Catheter Removal[2]	243	97%	97%	97%
Survey of Patients' Hospital Experiences				
Area Around Room 'Always' Quiet at Night	300+	61%	51%	61%
Doctors 'Always' Communicated Well	300+	80%	78%	82%
Home Recovery Information Given	300+	86%	83%	85%
Hospital Given 9 or 10 on 10 Point Scale	300+	78%	68%	71%
Meds 'Always' Explained Before Given	300+	64%	61%	64%
Nurses 'Always' Communicated Well	300+	75%	74%	79%
Pain 'Always' Well Controlled	300+	69%	68%	71%
Room and Bathroom 'Always' Clean	300+	75%	70%	73%
Timely Help 'Always' Received	300+	65%	62%	68%
Would Definitely Recommend Hospital	300+	81%	70%	71%
Use of Medical Imaging				
Cardiac Imaging Stress Test before Surgery	381	6.3%	5.2%	5.3%
Combination Abdominal CT Scan	1,422	6.1%	13.4%	10.5%
Combination Brain/Sinus CT Scan	565	2.1%	2.2%	2.7%
Combination Chest CT Scan	1,176	2.0%	2.3%	2.7%
Follow-up Mammogram/Ultrasound	663	10.0%	8.2%	8.8%
Lumbar Spine MRI for Low Back Pain	79	34.2%	34.2%	37.2%

Oroville Hospital

2767 Olive Highway
Oroville, CA 95966
Phone: 530-533-8500
Fax: 530-532-8433
E-mail: info@orovillehospital.com
URL: www.orovillehospital.com
Type: Acute Care Hospitals
Emergency Services: Yes
Ownership: Voluntary non-profit - Private
Beds: 153

Key Personnel:
Coronary Care . . . . Rhonda Cheek, RN
Emergency Room . . . . Jodi Halligan, RN
Chief of Medical Staff . . . . Mark Heinrich
Radiology. . . . . William Moe
Infection Control. . . . . Kimberly Nixon, RN
Operating Room. . . . . Robyn North, RN
Anesthesiology. . . . . Osahon Oslfo, MD
CEO/President. . . . . Robert J Wentz

Measure	Cases	This Hosp.	State Avg.	U.S. Avg.
Blood Clot Prevention and Treatment				
Anticoagulation Overlap Therapy[2]	54	100%	92%	93%
ICU Venous Thromboembolism Prophylaxis[2]	26	88%	92%	92%
Incidence of Potentially Preventable VTE[2]	11	18%	11%	10%
UFH with Dosages/Platelet Monitoring[2]	21	100%	96%	97%
Venous Thromboembolism Prophylaxis[2]	417	85%	83%	85%
Warfarin Therapy Discharge Instructions[2]	39	97%	75%	75%
Chest Pain/Possible Heart Attack Care				
Aspirin Given Within 24 Hours of Arrival	40	95%	97%	96%
Fibrinolytic Meds Within 30 Min. of Arrival[7]	-	-	62%	58%
Average Time to ECG (minutes)	40	17	9	7
Average Time to Transfer (minutes)	14	60	62	60
Children's Asthma Care				
Received Home Management Plan of Care	-	-	88%	88%
Received Reliever Medication	-	-	100%	100%
Received Systemic Corticosteroids	-	-	100%	100%
Emergency Department				
Admittance Decision Time (minutes)[2]	996	168	125	98
Head CT Results Within 45 Min. of Arrival[1]	-	-	55%	57%
Patients Who Left ER Before Being Seen	34,910	6%	3%	2%
Time from ER Arrival to Admit. (minutes)[2]	996	300	323	274
Time from ER Arrival to Discharge (minutes)	390	146	168	134
Time in ER Before Being Evaluated (minutes)	397	49	29	26
Time to Pain Meds for Fractures (minutes)	91	101	62	57
Heart Attack Care				
Aspirin Given at Discharge	20	95%	99%	99%
Fibrinolytic Meds Within 30 Min. of Arrival[7]	-	-	73%	54%
PCI Within 90 Minutes of Arrival[7]	-	-	95%	96%
Statin Prescribed at Discharge	22	95%	98%	98%
Heart Failure Care				
ACE Inhibitor or ARB for LVSD	77	95%	97%	97%
Discharge Instructions Given	205	91%	94%	94%
Evaluation of LVS Function	241	100%	99%	99%
Medicare Spending				
Medicare Spending per Patient (ratio)	-	0.88	0.98	0.98
Pneumonia Care				
Appropriate Initial Antibiotic Given[2]	151	91%	97%	95%
Blood Culture Timing[2]	250	95%	98%	98%
Pregnancy and Delivery Care				
Newborn Deliveries Scheduled Early	38	29%	5%	6%
Preventive Care				
Immunization for Influenza[2]	509	86%	89%	90%
Immunization for Pneumonia[2]	978	83%	90%	92%
Stroke Care				
Anticoagulation Therapy for Atrial Fibrillation[1,2]	-	-	95%	95%
Antithrombotic Therapy Timing[2]	60	100%	98%	98%
Assessed for Rehabilitation[2]	61	100%	97%	97%
Discharged on Antithrombotic Therapy[2]	58	98%	99%	99%
Discharged on Statin Medication[2]	40	100%	94%	94%
Thrombolytic Therapy Timing[1,2]	-	-	72%	66%
Venous Thromboembolism Prophylaxis[2]	68	93%	94%	94%
Written Stroke Educational Materials Given[2]	40	100%	87%	88%
Surgical Care Improvement Project				
Appropriate Beta Blocker Usage[2]	79	92%	97%	98%
Appropriate VTP Within 24 Hours[2]	288	99%	98%	98%
Controlled Postoperative Blood Glucose[2,7]	-	-	96%	97%
Perioperative Temperature Management[2]	350	99%	100%	100%
Prophylactic Antibiotic Selection[2]	225	98%	99%	99%
Prophylactic Antibiotic Selection (Outpatient)	23	100%	97%	98%
Prophylactic Antibiotic Stopped[2]	223	98%	98%	98%
Prophylactic Antibiotic Timing[2]	225	92%	99%	99%
Prophylactic Antibiotic Timing (Outpatient)	30	70%	97%	98%
Urinary Catheter Removal[2]	177	86%	97%	97%
Survey of Patients' Hospital Experiences				
Area Around Room 'Always' Quiet at Night	300+	38%	51%	61%
Doctors 'Always' Communicated Well	300+	66%	78%	82%
Home Recovery Information Given	300+	76%	83%	85%
Hospital Given 9 or 10 on 10 Point Scale	300+	50%	68%	71%
Meds 'Always' Explained Before Given	300+	54%	61%	64%
Nurses 'Always' Communicated Well	300+	70%	74%	79%
Pain 'Always' Well Controlled	300+	68%	68%	71%
Room and Bathroom 'Always' Clean	300+	64%	70%	73%
Timely Help 'Always' Received	300+	55%	62%	68%
Would Definitely Recommend Hospital	300+	45%	70%	71%
Use of Medical Imaging				
Cardiac Imaging Stress Test before Surgery	291	6.2%	5.2%	5.3%
Combination Abdominal CT Scan	564	12.9%	13.4%	10.5%
Combination Brain/Sinus CT Scan	550	4.5%	2.2%	2.7%
Combination Chest CT Scan	425	0.9%	2.3%	2.7%
Follow-up Mammogram/Ultrasound	1,427	18.0%	8.2%	8.8%
Lumbar Spine MRI for Low Back Pain	112	26.8%	34.2%	37.2%

Saint Johns Regional Medical Center

1600 N Rose Ave
Oxnard, CA 93030
Phone: 805-988-2500
Fax: 805-981-4440
URL: www.stjohnshealth.org
Type: Acute Care Hospitals
Emergency Services: Yes
Ownership: Voluntary non-profit - Private
Beds: 230

Key Personnel:
Operating Room. . . . . Lisa L Babashoff, RN
Quality Assurance . . . . Pat Ballow, RN
Pediatric Ambulatory Care . . . . . . Jon D'Andrea, MD
Pediatric In-Patient Care . . . . Jon D'Andrea, MD
Emergency Room . . . . Eileen Hooper
CEO/President. . . . . Michael Merray
Radiology. . . . . Timothy O'Connor, MD
Chief of Medical Staff . . . . Zack Rotenderg

Measure	Cases	This Hosp.	State Avg.	U.S. Avg.
Blood Clot Prevention and Treatment				
Anticoagulation Overlap Therapy[2]	36	100%	92%	93%
ICU Venous Thromboembolism Prophylaxis[2]	99	99%	92%	92%
Incidence of Potentially Preventable VTE[1,2]	-	-	11%	10%
UFH with Dosages/Platelet Monitoring[2]	23	100%	96%	97%
Venous Thromboembolism Prophylaxis[2]	353	96%	83%	85%
Warfarin Therapy Discharge Instructions[2]	30	93%	75%	75%
Chest Pain/Possible Heart Attack Care				
Aspirin Given Within 24 Hours of Arrival	11	100%	97%	96%
Fibrinolytic Meds Within 30 Min. of Arrival[5]	-	-	62%	58%
Average Time to ECG (minutes)	11	15	9	7
Average Time to Transfer (minutes)[5]	-	-	62	60
Children's Asthma Care				
Received Home Management Plan of Care	-	-	88%	88%
Received Reliever Medication	-	-	100%	100%
Received Systemic Corticosteroids	-	-	100%	100%
Emergency Department				
Admittance Decision Time (minutes)[2]	463	178	125	98
Head CT Results Within 45 Min. of Arrival[1]	-	-	55%	57%
Patients Who Left ER Before Being Seen	49,229	1%	3%	2%
Time from ER Arrival to Admit. (minutes)[2]	471	356	323	274
Time from ER Arrival to Discharge (minutes)	414	140	168	134
Time in ER Before Being Evaluated (minutes)	430	19	29	26
Time to Pain Meds for Fractures (minutes)	212	53	62	57
Heart Attack Care				
Aspirin Given at Discharge	226	100%	99%	99%
Fibrinolytic Meds Within 30 Min. of Arrival[7]	-	-	73%	54%
PCI Within 90 Minutes of Arrival	31	97%	95%	96%
Statin Prescribed at Discharge	222	96%	98%	98%
Heart Failure Care				
ACE Inhibitor or ARB for LVSD	52	100%	97%	97%
Discharge Instructions Given	239	96%	94%	94%
Evaluation of LVS Function	272	100%	99%	99%
Medicare Spending				
Medicare Spending per Patient (ratio)	-	0.99	0.98	0.98
Pneumonia Care				
Appropriate Initial Antibiotic Given	134	99%	97%	95%
Blood Culture Timing	248	96%	98%	98%
Pregnancy and Delivery Care				
Newborn Deliveries Scheduled Early[2]	54	11%	5%	6%
Preventive Care				
Immunization for Influenza[2]	491	60%	89%	90%
Immunization for Pneumonia[2]	485	85%	90%	92%
Stroke Care				
Anticoagulation Therapy for Atrial Fibrillation	11	100%	95%	95%
Antithrombotic Therapy Timing	88	100%	98%	98%
Assessed for Rehabilitation	118	100%	97%	97%
Discharged on Antithrombotic Therapy	86	100%	99%	99%
Discharged on Statin Medication	67	90%	94%	94%
Thrombolytic Therapy Timing[1]	-	-	72%	66%
Venous Thromboembolism Prophylaxis	126	92%	94%	94%
Written Stroke Educational Materials Given	63	94%	87%	88%
Surgical Care Improvement Project				
Appropriate Beta Blocker Usage[2]	176	98%	97%	98%
Appropriate VTP Within 24 Hours[2]	381	98%	98%	98%
Controlled Postoperative Blood Glucose[2]	102	93%	96%	97%
Perioperative Temperature Management[2]	508	100%	100%	100%
Prophylactic Antibiotic Selection[2]	367	99%	99%	99%
Prophylactic Antibiotic Selection (Outpatient)	163	98%	97%	98%
Prophylactic Antibiotic Stopped[2]	339	100%	98%	98%
Prophylactic Antibiotic Timing[2]	367	99%	99%	99%
Prophylactic Antibiotic Timing (Outpatient)	165	93%	97%	98%
Urinary Catheter Removal[2]	312	98%	97%	97%
Survey of Patients' Hospital Experiences				
Area Around Room 'Always' Quiet at Night	300+	55%	51%	61%

NOTE: Hospital profiles are in alphabetical order by state, then city, then hospital within the city; Rankings exclude hospitals with less than 25 cases except for patient surveys which excludes hospitals with less than 100 cases; (a) 100-299 cases; (1) The number of cases/patients is too few to report; (2) Data submitted were based on a sample of cases/patients; (3) Results are based on a shorter time period than required; (4) Data suppressed by CMS for one or more quarters; (5) Results are not available for this reporting period; (6) Fewer than 100 patients completed the HCAHPS survey; (7) No cases met the criteria for this measure; (8) The lower limit of the confidence interval cannot be calculated if the number of observed infections equals zero; (9) No data are available from the state/territory for this reporting period; (10) The scores shown reflect fewer than 50 completed surveys; (11) There were discrepancies in the data collection process; (12) This measure does not apply to this hospital for this reporting period; (13) Results cannot be calculated for this reporting period; (14) The results for this state are combined with nearby states to protect confidentiality; Please refer to the User's Guide for a full explanation of data.

Measure	Cases	This Hosp.	State Avg.	U.S. Avg.
Doctors 'Always' Communicated Well	300+	75%	78%	82%
Home Recovery Information Given	300+	84%	83%	85%
Hospital Given 9 or 10 on 10 Point Scale	300+	69%	68%	71%
Meds 'Always' Explained Before Given	300+	61%	61%	64%
Nurses 'Always' Communicated Well	300+	72%	74%	79%
Pain 'Always' Well Controlled	300+	66%	68%	71%
Room and Bathroom 'Always' Clean	300+	70%	70%	73%
Timely Help 'Always' Received	300+	52%	62%	68%
Would Definitely Recommend Hospital	300+	70%	70%	71%
Use of Medical Imaging				
Cardiac Imaging Stress Test before Surgery	311	9.0%	5.2%	5.3%
Combination Abdominal CT Scan	596	0.5%	13.4%	10.5%
Combination Brain/Sinus CT Scan	824	1.9%	2.2%	2.7%
Combination Chest CT Scan	101	0.0%	2.3%	2.7%
Follow-up Mammogram/Ultrasound[7]	-	-	8.2%	8.8%
Lumbar Spine MRI for Low Back Pain[1]	-	-	34.2%	37.2%

Desert Regional Medical Center

1150 North Indian Canyon Drive
Palm Springs, CA 92262
Phone: 760-323-6511
Fax: 760-864-9577
URL: www.desertmedctr.com
Type: Acute Care Hospitals
Emergency Services: Yes
Ownership: Proprietary
Beds: 398

Key Personnel:
CEO/President. . . . . Carolyn Caldwell
Radiology. . . . . John Gilmore
Chair/CEO . . . . Jeanne Stanton, RN
Chief of Medical Staff . . . . Nancy Williams

Measure	Cases	This Hosp.	State Avg.	U.S. Avg.
Blood Clot Prevention and Treatment				
Anticoagulation Overlap Therapy[2]	93	88%	92%	93%
ICU Venous Thromboembolism Prophylaxis[2]	93	98%	92%	92%
Incidence of Potentially Preventable VTE[2]	22	0%	11%	10%
UFH with Dosages/Platelet Monitoring[2]	39	92%	96%	97%
Venous Thromboembolism Prophylaxis[2]	285	81%	83%	85%
Warfarin Therapy Discharge Instructions[2]	56	82%	75%	75%
Chest Pain/Possible Heart Attack Care				
Aspirin Given Within 24 Hours of Arrival[3,7]	-	-	97%	96%
Fibrinolytic Meds Within 30 Min. of Arrival[5]	-	-	62%	58%
Average Time to ECG (minutes)[1,3]	-	-	9	7
Average Time to Transfer (minutes)[5]	-	-	62	60
Children's Asthma Care				
Received Home Management Plan of Care	-	-	88%	88%
Received Reliever Medication	-	-	100%	100%
Received Systemic Corticosteroids	-	-	100%	100%
Emergency Department				
Admittance Decision Time (minutes)[2]	652	182	125	98
Head CT Results Within 45 Min. of Arrival[3,7]	-	-	55%	57%
Patients Who Left ER Before Being Seen	61,648	1%	3%	2%
Time from ER Arrival to Admit. (minutes)[2]	663	352	323	274
Time from ER Arrival to Discharge (minutes)	361	167	168	134
Time in ER Before Being Evaluated (minutes)	378	28	29	26
Time to Pain Meds for Fractures (minutes)	238	62	62	57
Heart Attack Care				
Aspirin Given at Discharge	363	99%	99%	99%
Fibrinolytic Meds Within 30 Min. of Arrival[7]	-	-	73%	54%
PCI Within 90 Minutes of Arrival	51	92%	95%	96%
Statin Prescribed at Discharge	354	99%	98%	98%
Heart Failure Care				
ACE Inhibitor or ARB for LVSD	162	98%	97%	97%
Discharge Instructions Given	273	98%	94%	94%
Evaluation of LVS Function	366	100%	99%	99%
Medicare Spending				
Medicare Spending per Patient (ratio)	-	0.99	0.98	0.98
Pneumonia Care				
Appropriate Initial Antibiotic Given[2]	126	99%	97%	95%
Blood Culture Timing[2]	167	98%	98%	98%
Pregnancy and Delivery Care				
Newborn Deliveries Scheduled Early[2]	60	5%	5%	6%
Preventive Care				
Immunization for Influenza[2]	545	94%	89%	90%
Immunization for Pneumonia[2]	559	96%	90%	92%
Stroke Care				
Anticoagulation Therapy for Atrial Fibrillation	37	97%	95%	95%
Antithrombotic Therapy Timing	168	98%	98%	98%
Assessed for Rehabilitation	310	97%	97%	97%
Discharged on Antithrombotic Therapy	230	100%	99%	99%
Discharged on Statin Medication	157	97%	94%	94%
Thrombolytic Therapy Timing	22	91%	72%	66%
Venous Thromboembolism Prophylaxis	294	99%	94%	94%
Written Stroke Educational Materials Given	164	95%	87%	88%
Surgical Care Improvement Project				
Appropriate Beta Blocker Usage[2]	160	98%	97%	98%
Appropriate VTP Within 24 Hours[2]	321	96%	98%	98%
Controlled Postoperative Blood Glucose[2]	130	97%	96%	97%
Perioperative Temperature Management[2]	508	100%	100%	100%
Prophylactic Antibiotic Selection[2]	444	99%	99%	99%
Prophylactic Antibiotic Selection (Outpatient)	189	98%	97%	98%
Prophylactic Antibiotic Stopped[2]	443	98%	98%	98%
Prophylactic Antibiotic Timing[2]	446	99%	99%	99%
Prophylactic Antibiotic Timing (Outpatient)	190	99%	97%	98%
Urinary Catheter Removal[2]	291	96%	97%	97%
Survey of Patients' Hospital Experiences				
Area Around Room 'Always' Quiet at Night	300+	49%	51%	61%
Doctors 'Always' Communicated Well	300+	78%	78%	82%
Home Recovery Information Given	300+	83%	83%	85%
Hospital Given 9 or 10 on 10 Point Scale	300+	75%	68%	71%
Meds 'Always' Explained Before Given	300+	64%	61%	64%
Nurses 'Always' Communicated Well	300+	77%	74%	79%
Pain 'Always' Well Controlled	300+	69%	68%	71%
Room and Bathroom 'Always' Clean	300+	69%	70%	73%
Timely Help 'Always' Received	300+	66%	62%	68%
Would Definitely Recommend Hospital	300+	76%	70%	71%
Use of Medical Imaging				
Cardiac Imaging Stress Test before Surgery	292	7.5%	5.2%	5.3%
Combination Abdominal CT Scan	822	7.2%	13.4%	10.5%
Combination Brain/Sinus CT Scan	609	2.0%	2.2%	2.7%
Combination Chest CT Scan	338	0.3%	2.3%	2.7%
Follow-up Mammogram/Ultrasound	1,373	13.5%	8.2%	8.8%
Lumbar Spine MRI for Low Back Pain	45	44.4%	34.2%	37.2%

Palmdale Regional Medical Center

38600 Medical Center Drive
Palmdale, CA 93552
Phone: 661-382-5000
URL: www.palmdaleregional.com
Type: Acute Care Hospitals
Emergency Services: Yes
Ownership: Proprietary
Beds: 121

Key Personnel:
CEO . . . . Richard Allen
Chief of Medical Staff. . . . . Bassel Hadaya, MD
Chairman/CEO . . . . Rick Norris

Measure	Cases	This Hosp.	State Avg.	U.S. Avg.
Blood Clot Prevention and Treatment				
Anticoagulation Overlap Therapy[2]	53	75%	92%	93%
ICU Venous Thromboembolism Prophylaxis[2]	84	85%	92%	92%
Incidence of Potentially Preventable VTE[1,2]	-	-	11%	10%
UFH with Dosages/Platelet Monitoring[2]	13	92%	96%	97%
Venous Thromboembolism Prophylaxis[2]	344	55%	83%	85%
Warfarin Therapy Discharge Instructions[2]	46	93%	75%	75%
Chest Pain/Possible Heart Attack Care				
Aspirin Given Within 24 Hours of Arrival[5]	-	-	97%	96%
Fibrinolytic Meds Within 30 Min. of Arrival[5]	-	-	62%	58%
Average Time to ECG (minutes)[5]	-	-	9	7
Average Time to Transfer (minutes)[5]	-	-	62	60
Children's Asthma Care				
Received Home Management Plan of Care	-	-	88%	88%
Received Reliever Medication	-	-	100%	100%
Received Systemic Corticosteroids	-	-	100%	100%
Emergency Department				
Admittance Decision Time (minutes)[2]	889	309	125	98
Head CT Results Within 45 Min. of Arrival[1,3]	-	-	55%	57%
Patients Who Left ER Before Being Seen	53,219	7%	3%	2%
Time from ER Arrival to Admit. (minutes)[2]	970	604	323	274
Time from ER Arrival to Discharge (minutes)	379	208	168	134
Time in ER Before Being Evaluated (minutes)	405	60	29	26
Time to Pain Meds for Fractures (minutes)	224	82	62	57
Heart Attack Care				
Aspirin Given at Discharge[2]	198	100%	99%	99%
Fibrinolytic Meds Within 30 Min. of Arrival[2,7]	-	-	73%	54%
PCI Within 90 Minutes of Arrival[2]	32	97%	95%	96%
Statin Prescribed at Discharge[2]	187	98%	98%	98%
Heart Failure Care				
ACE Inhibitor or ARB for LVSD[2]	110	97%	97%	97%
Discharge Instructions Given[2]	289	99%	94%	94%
Evaluation of LVS Function[2]	305	100%	99%	99%
Medicare Spending				
Medicare Spending per Patient (ratio)	-	0.99	0.98	0.98
Pneumonia Care				
Appropriate Initial Antibiotic Given[2]	110	95%	97%	95%
Blood Culture Timing[2]	95	94%	98%	98%
Pregnancy and Delivery Care				
Newborn Deliveries Scheduled Early[7]	-	-	5%	6%
Preventive Care				
Immunization for Influenza[2]	614	77%	89%	90%
Immunization for Pneumonia[2]	820	72%	90%	92%
Stroke Care				
Anticoagulation Therapy for Atrial Fibrillation[1]	-	-	95%	95%
Antithrombotic Therapy Timing	62	92%	98%	98%
Assessed for Rehabilitation	72	100%	97%	97%
Discharged on Antithrombotic Therapy	63	86%	99%	99%
Discharged on Statin Medication	52	85%	94%	94%
Thrombolytic Therapy Timing	43	2%	72%	66%
Venous Thromboembolism Prophylaxis	70	81%	94%	94%
Written Stroke Educational Materials Given	55	76%	87%	88%
Surgical Care Improvement Project				
Appropriate Beta Blocker Usage[2]	69	99%	97%	98%
Appropriate VTP Within 24 Hours[2]	364	97%	98%	98%
Controlled Postoperative Blood Glucose[1,2]	-	-	96%	97%
Perioperative Temperature Management[2]	402	100%	100%	100%
Prophylactic Antibiotic Selection[2]	255	98%	99%	99%
Prophylactic Antibiotic Selection (Outpatient)	68	97%	97%	98%
Prophylactic Antibiotic Stopped[2]	250	98%	98%	98%
Prophylactic Antibiotic Timing[2]	257	98%	99%	99%
Prophylactic Antibiotic Timing (Outpatient)	74	91%	97%	98%
Urinary Catheter Removal[2]	109	100%	97%	97%
Survey of Patients' Hospital Experiences				
Area Around Room 'Always' Quiet at Night	300+	70%	51%	61%
Doctors 'Always' Communicated Well	300+	77%	78%	82%
Home Recovery Information Given	300+	86%	83%	85%
Hospital Given 9 or 10 on 10 Point Scale	300+	75%	68%	71%
Meds 'Always' Explained Before Given	300+	65%	61%	64%
Nurses 'Always' Communicated Well	300+	76%	74%	79%
Pain 'Always' Well Controlled	300+	73%	68%	71%
Room and Bathroom 'Always' Clean	300+	77%	70%	73%
Timely Help 'Always' Received	300+	64%	62%	68%
Would Definitely Recommend Hospital	300+	76%	70%	71%
Use of Medical Imaging				
Cardiac Imaging Stress Test before Surgery[1]	-	-	5.2%	5.3%
Combination Abdominal CT Scan	461	1.7%	13.4%	10.5%
Combination Brain/Sinus CT Scan[1]	-	-	2.2%	2.7%
Combination Chest CT Scan	88	1.1%	2.3%	2.7%
Follow-up Mammogram/Ultrasound[7]	-	-	8.2%	8.8%
Lumbar Spine MRI for Low Back Pain[1]	-	-	34.2%	37.2%

Lucile Salter Packard Children's Hospital at Stanford

725 Welch Road
Palo Alto, CA 94304
Phone: 650-497-8000
Fax: 650-723-1225
URL: www.lpch.org
Type: Childrens
Emergency Services: No
Ownership: Voluntary non-profit - Private
Beds: 264

Key Personnel:
Quality Assurance . . . . David Bergman, MD
Chief of Medical Staff. . . . . Kenneth Cox, MD
CEO/President. . . . . Christopher G. Dawes
Intensive Care Unit. . . . . Lorry Frankel, MD
Infection Control. . . . . Jane Freeburn
Anesthesiology. . . . . Elliot Krane, MD
Surgery . . . . Thomas M. Krummel, MD
Radiology. . . . . William Northway, MD

NOTE: Hospital profiles are in alphabetical order by state, then city, then hospital within the city; Rankings exclude hospitals with less than 25 cases except for patient surveys which excludes hospitals with less than 100 cases; (a) 100-299 cases; (1) The number of cases/patients is too few to report; (2) Data submitted were based on a sample of cases/patients; (3) Results are based on a shorter time period than required; (4) Data suppressed by CMS for one or more quarters; (5) Results are not available for this reporting period; (6) Fewer than 100 patients completed the HCAHPS survey; (7) No cases met the criteria for this measure; (8) The lower limit of the confidence interval cannot be calculated if the number of observed infections equals zero; (9) No data are available from the state/territory for this reporting period; (10) The scores shown reflect fewer than 50 completed surveys; (11) There were discrepancies in the data collection process; (12) This measure does not apply to this hospital for this reporting period; (13) Results cannot be calculated for this reporting period; (14) The results for this state are combined with nearby states to protect confidentiality; Please refer to the User's Guide for a full explanation of data.

Measure	Cases	This Hosp.	State Avg.	U.S. Avg.
Blood Clot Prevention and Treatment				
Anticoagulation Overlap Therapy[5]	-	-	92%	93%
ICU Venous Thromboembolism Prophylaxis[5]	-	-	92%	92%
Incidence of Potentially Preventable VTE[5]	-	-	11%	10%
UFH with Dosages/Platelet Monitoring[5]	-	-	96%	97%
Venous Thromboembolism Prophylaxis[5]	-	-	83%	85%
Warfarin Therapy Discharge Instructions[5]	-	-	75%	75%
Chest Pain/Possible Heart Attack Care				
Aspirin Given Within 24 Hours of Arrival	-	-	97%	96%
Fibrinolytic Meds Within 30 Min. of Arrival	-	-	62%	58%
Average Time to ECG (minutes)	-	-	9	7
Average Time to Transfer (minutes)	-	-	62	60
Children's Asthma Care				
Received Home Management Plan of Care[2]	147	95%	88%	88%
Received Reliever Medication	147	100%	100%	100%
Received Systemic Corticosteroids	147	100%	100%	100%
Emergency Department				
Admittance Decision Time (minutes)[5]	-	-	125	98
Head CT Results Within 45 Min. of Arrival	-	-	55%	57%
Patients Who Left ER Before Being Seen	-	-	3%	2%
Time from ER Arrival to Admit. (minutes)[5]	-	-	323	274
Time from ER Arrival to Discharge (minutes)	-	-	168	134
Time in ER Before Being Evaluated (minutes)	-	-	29	26
Time to Pain Meds for Fractures (minutes)	-	-	62	57
Heart Attack Care				
Aspirin Given at Discharge[5]	-	-	99%	99%
Fibrinolytic Meds Within 30 Min. of Arrival[5]	-	-	73%	54%
PCI Within 90 Minutes of Arrival[5]	-	-	95%	96%
Statin Prescribed at Discharge[5]	-	-	98%	98%
Heart Failure Care				
ACE Inhibitor or ARB for LVSD[5]	-	-	97%	97%
Discharge Instructions Given[5]	-	-	94%	94%
Evaluation of LVS Function[5]	-	-	99%	99%
Medicare Spending				
Medicare Spending per Patient (ratio)	-	-	0.98	0.98
Pneumonia Care				
Appropriate Initial Antibiotic Given[5]	-	-	97%	95%
Blood Culture Timing[5]	-	-	98%	98%
Pregnancy and Delivery Care				
Newborn Deliveries Scheduled Early[5]	-	-	5%	6%
Preventive Care				
Immunization for Influenza[5]	-	-	89%	90%
Immunization for Pneumonia[5]	-	-	90%	92%
Stroke Care				
Anticoagulation Therapy for Atrial Fibrillation[5]	-	-	95%	95%
Antithrombotic Therapy Timing[5]	-	-	98%	98%
Assessed for Rehabilitation[5]	-	-	97%	97%
Discharged on Antithrombotic Therapy[5]	-	-	99%	99%
Discharged on Statin Medication[5]	-	-	94%	94%
Thrombolytic Therapy Timing[5]	-	-	72%	66%
Venous Thromboembolism Prophylaxis[5]	-	-	94%	94%
Written Stroke Educational Materials Given[5]	-	-	87%	88%
Surgical Care Improvement Project				
Appropriate Beta Blocker Usage[5]	-	-	97%	98%
Appropriate VTP Within 24 Hours[5]	-	-	98%	98%
Controlled Postoperative Blood Glucose[5]	-	-	96%	97%
Perioperative Temperature Management[5]	-	-	100%	100%
Prophylactic Antibiotic Selection[5]	-	-	99%	99%
Prophylactic Antibiotic Selection (Outpatient)	-	-	97%	98%
Prophylactic Antibiotic Stopped[5]	-	-	98%	98%
Prophylactic Antibiotic Timing[5]	-	-	99%	99%
Prophylactic Antibiotic Timing (Outpatient)	-	-	97%	98%
Urinary Catheter Removal[5]	-	-	97%	97%
Survey of Patients' Hospital Experiences				
Area Around Room 'Always' Quiet at Night[5]	-	-	51%	61%
Doctors 'Always' Communicated Well[5]	-	-	78%	82%
Home Recovery Information Given[5]	-	-	83%	85%
Hospital Given 9 or 10 on 10 Point Scale[5]	-	-	68%	71%
Meds 'Always' Explained Before Given[5]	-	-	61%	64%
Nurses 'Always' Communicated Well[5]	-	-	74%	79%
Pain 'Always' Well Controlled[5]	-	-	68%	71%
Room and Bathroom 'Always' Clean[5]	-	-	70%	73%
Timely Help 'Always' Received[5]	-	-	62%	68%
Would Definitely Recommend Hospital[5]	-	-	70%	71%
Use of Medical Imaging				
Cardiac Imaging Stress Test before Surgery	-	-	5.2%	5.3%
Combination Abdominal CT Scan	-	-	13.4%	10.5%
Combination Brain/Sinus CT Scan	-	-	2.2%	2.7%
Combination Chest CT Scan	-	-	2.3%	2.7%
Follow-up Mammogram/Ultrasound	-	-	8.2%	8.8%
Lumbar Spine MRI for Low Back Pain	-	-	34.2%	37.2%

Palo Alto VA Medical Center

3801 Miranda Avenue
Palo Alto, CA 94304
URL: www.palo-alto.med.va.gov
Type: Acute Care - VA
Ownership: Government Federal
Phone: 650-858-3939
Fax: 650-852-3228
Emergency Services: No
Beds: 900

Key Personnel:
Quality Assurance . . . . Patricia Allyn, RN
CEO/President. . . . . Lisa Freeman, FACHE
Chief of Medical Staff. . . . . Lawrence L. Leung, MD
Infection Control. . . . . Jeff Loutit
Intensive Care Unit. . . . . Shirley Paulson, RN
Emergency Room . . . . Don Schreiber, MD
Radiology. . . . . Paul Stark, MD
Operating Room. . . . . Cecilia Wu, RN

Measure	Cases	This Hosp.	State Avg.	U.S. Avg.
Blood Clot Prevention and Treatment				
Anticoagulation Overlap Therapy	-	-	92%	93%
ICU Venous Thromboembolism Prophylaxis	-	-	92%	92%
Incidence of Potentially Preventable VTE	-	-	11%	10%
UFH with Dosages/Platelet Monitoring	-	-	96%	97%
Venous Thromboembolism Prophylaxis	-	-	83%	85%
Warfarin Therapy Discharge Instructions	-	-	75%	75%
Chest Pain/Possible Heart Attack Care				
Aspirin Given Within 24 Hours of Arrival	-	-	97%	96%
Fibrinolytic Meds Within 30 Min. of Arrival	-	-	62%	58%
Average Time to ECG (minutes)	-	-	9	7
Average Time to Transfer (minutes)	-	-	62	60
Children's Asthma Care				
Received Home Management Plan of Care	-	-	88%	88%
Received Reliever Medication	-	-	100%	100%
Received Systemic Corticosteroids	-	-	100%	100%
Emergency Department				
Admittance Decision Time (minutes)	-	-	125	98
Head CT Results Within 45 Min. of Arrival	-	-	55%	57%
Patients Who Left ER Before Being Seen	-	-	3%	2%
Time from ER Arrival to Admit. (minutes)	-	-	323	274
Time from ER Arrival to Discharge (minutes)	-	-	168	134
Time in ER Before Being Evaluated (minutes)	-	-	29	26
Time to Pain Meds for Fractures (minutes)	-	-	62	57
Heart Attack Care				
Aspirin Given at Discharge	59	100%	99%	99%
Fibrinolytic Meds Within 30 Min. of Arrival[5]	-	-	73%	54%
PCI Within 90 Minutes of Arrival[1]	-	-	95%	96%
Statin Prescribed at Discharge	60	98%	98%	98%
Heart Failure Care				
ACE Inhibitor or ARB for LVSD	58	100%	97%	97%
Discharge Instructions Given	154	98%	94%	94%
Evaluation of LVS Function	175	100%	99%	99%
Medicare Spending				
Medicare Spending per Patient (ratio)	-	-	0.98	0.98
Pneumonia Care				
Appropriate Initial Antibiotic Given	57	88%	97%	95%
Blood Culture Timing	123	98%	98%	98%
Pregnancy and Delivery Care				
Newborn Deliveries Scheduled Early	-	-	5%	6%
Preventive Care				
Immunization for Influenza[5]	-	-	89%	90%
Immunization for Pneumonia[5]	-	-	90%	92%
Stroke Care				
Anticoagulation Therapy for Atrial Fibrillation	-	-	95%	95%
Antithrombotic Therapy Timing	-	-	98%	98%
Assessed for Rehabilitation	-	-	97%	97%
Discharged on Antithrombotic Therapy	-	-	99%	99%
Discharged on Statin Medication	-	-	94%	94%
Thrombolytic Therapy Timing	-	-	72%	66%
Venous Thromboembolism Prophylaxis	-	-	94%	94%
Written Stroke Educational Materials Given	-	-	87%	88%
Surgical Care Improvement Project				
Appropriate Beta Blocker Usage[2]	163	94%	97%	98%
Appropriate VTP Within 24 Hours[2]	395	99%	98%	98%
Controlled Postoperative Blood Glucose[2]	58	90%	96%	97%
Perioperative Temperature Management[2]	441	100%	100%	100%
Prophylactic Antibiotic Selection	396	100%	99%	99%
Prophylactic Antibiotic Selection (Outpatient)	-	-	97%	98%
Prophylactic Antibiotic Stopped	392	98%	98%	98%
Prophylactic Antibiotic Timing	396	98%	99%	99%
Prophylactic Antibiotic Timing (Outpatient)	-	-	97%	98%
Urinary Catheter Removal[2]	272	100%	97%	97%
Survey of Patients' Hospital Experiences				
Area Around Room 'Always' Quiet at Night	-	-	51%	61%
Doctors 'Always' Communicated Well	-	-	78%	82%
Home Recovery Information Given	-	-	83%	85%
Hospital Given 9 or 10 on 10 Point Scale	-	-	68%	71%
Meds 'Always' Explained Before Given	-	-	61%	64%
Nurses 'Always' Communicated Well	-	-	74%	79%
Pain 'Always' Well Controlled	-	-	68%	71%
Room and Bathroom 'Always' Clean	-	-	70%	73%
Timely Help 'Always' Received	-	-	62%	68%
Would Definitely Recommend Hospital	-	-	70%	71%
Use of Medical Imaging				
Cardiac Imaging Stress Test before Surgery	-	-	5.2%	5.3%
Combination Abdominal CT Scan	-	-	13.4%	10.5%
Combination Brain/Sinus CT Scan	-	-	2.2%	2.7%
Combination Chest CT Scan	-	-	2.3%	2.7%
Follow-up Mammogram/Ultrasound	-	-	8.2%	8.8%
Lumbar Spine MRI for Low Back Pain	-	-	34.2%	37.2%

Kaiser Foundation Hospital - Panorama City

13652 Cantara St
Panorama City, CA 91402
URL: www.kaiserpermanente.org
Type: Acute Care Hospitals
Ownership: Voluntary non-profit - Private
Phone: 818-375-3333
Fax: 818-375-2728
Emergency Services: Yes
Beds: 325

Key Personnel:
CEO/President. . . . . Dev Mahadevan
Quality Assurance . . . . Beverly Mosely
Operating Room. . . . . Anita Zermeno, RN

Measure	Cases	This Hosp.	State Avg.	U.S. Avg.
Blood Clot Prevention and Treatment				
Anticoagulation Overlap Therapy[2]	62	98%	92%	93%
ICU Venous Thromboembolism Prophylaxis[2]	40	95%	92%	92%
Incidence of Potentially Preventable VTE[1,2]	-	-	11%	10%
UFH with Dosages/Platelet Monitoring[1,2]	-	-	96%	97%
Venous Thromboembolism Prophylaxis[2]	295	84%	83%	85%
Warfarin Therapy Discharge Instructions[2]	51	78%	75%	75%
Chest Pain/Possible Heart Attack Care				
Aspirin Given Within 24 Hours of Arrival	-	-	97%	96%
Fibrinolytic Meds Within 30 Min. of Arrival	-	-	62%	58%
Average Time to ECG (minutes)	-	-	9	7
Average Time to Transfer (minutes)	-	-	62	60
Children's Asthma Care				
Received Home Management Plan of Care	-	-	88%	88%
Received Reliever Medication	-	-	100%	100%
Received Systemic Corticosteroids	-	-	100%	100%
Emergency Department				
Admittance Decision Time (minutes)[2]	505	92	125	98
Head CT Results Within 45 Min. of Arrival	-	-	55%	57%
Patients Who Left ER Before Being Seen	-	-	3%	2%
Time from ER Arrival to Admit. (minutes)[2]	512	302	323	274
Time from ER Arrival to Discharge (minutes)	-	-	168	134
Time in ER Before Being Evaluated (minutes)	-	-	29	26
Time to Pain Meds for Fractures (minutes)	-	-	62	57
Heart Attack Care				
Aspirin Given at Discharge	57	100%	99%	99%
Fibrinolytic Meds Within 30 Min. of Arrival[1]	-	-	73%	54%

NOTE: Hospital profiles are in alphabetical order by state, then city, then hospital within the city; Rankings exclude hospitals with less than 25 cases except for patient surveys which excludes hospitals with less than 100 cases; (a) 100-299 cases; (1) The number of cases/patients is too few to report; (2) Data submitted were based on a sample of cases/patients; (3) Results are based on a shorter time period than required; (4) Data suppressed by CMS for one or more quarters; (5) Results are not available for this reporting period; (6) Fewer than 100 patients completed the HCAHPS survey; (7) No cases met the criteria for this measure; (8) The lower limit of the confidence interval cannot be calculated if the number of observed infections equals zero; (9) No data are available from the state/territory for this reporting period; (10) The scores shown reflect fewer than 50 completed surveys; (11) There were discrepancies in the data collection process; (12) This measure does not apply to this hospital for this reporting period; (13) Results cannot be calculated for this reporting period; (14) The results for this state are combined with nearby states to protect confidentiality; Please refer to the User's Guide for a full explanation of data.

Measure	Cases	This Hosp.	State Avg.	U.S. Avg.
PCI Within 90 Minutes of Arrival[7]	-	-	95%	96%
Statin Prescribed at Discharge	63	100%	98%	98%
Heart Failure Care				
ACE Inhibitor or ARB for LVSD	49	96%	97%	97%
Discharge Instructions Given	213	100%	94%	94%
Evaluation of LVS Function	230	100%	99%	99%
Medicare Spending				
Medicare Spending per Patient (ratio)	-	0.80	0.98	0.98
Pneumonia Care				
Appropriate Initial Antibiotic Given[2]	69	99%	97%	95%
Blood Culture Timing[2]	156	99%	98%	98%
Pregnancy and Delivery Care				
Newborn Deliveries Scheduled Early[2]	132	0%	5%	6%
Preventive Care				
Immunization for Influenza[2]	506	97%	89%	90%
Immunization for Pneumonia[2]	602	97%	90%	92%
Stroke Care				
Anticoagulation Therapy for Atrial Fibrillation[2]	21	71%	95%	95%
Antithrombotic Therapy Timing[2]	84	99%	98%	98%
Assessed for Rehabilitation[2]	98	100%	97%	97%
Discharged on Antithrombotic Therapy[2]	90	100%	99%	99%
Discharged on Statin Medication[2]	77	99%	94%	94%
Thrombolytic Therapy Timing[1,2]	-	-	72%	66%
Venous Thromboembolism Prophylaxis[2]	94	100%	94%	94%
Written Stroke Educational Materials Given[2]	65	97%	87%	88%
Surgical Care Improvement Project				
Appropriate Beta Blocker Usage[2]	128	100%	97%	98%
Appropriate VTP Within 24 Hours[2]	378	100%	98%	98%
Controlled Postoperative Blood Glucose[2,7]	-	-	96%	97%
Perioperative Temperature Management[2]	461	100%	100%	100%
Prophylactic Antibiotic Selection[2]	310	100%	99%	99%
Prophylactic Antibiotic Selection (Outpatient)	-	-	97%	98%
Prophylactic Antibiotic Stopped[2]	307	99%	98%	98%
Prophylactic Antibiotic Timing[2]	310	100%	99%	99%
Prophylactic Antibiotic Timing (Outpatient)	-	-	97%	98%
Urinary Catheter Removal[2]	145	99%	97%	97%
Survey of Patients' Hospital Experiences				
Area Around Room 'Always' Quiet at Night	300+	61%	51%	61%
Doctors 'Always' Communicated Well	300+	81%	78%	82%
Home Recovery Information Given	300+	85%	83%	85%
Hospital Given 9 or 10 on 10 Point Scale	300+	78%	68%	71%
Meds 'Always' Explained Before Given	300+	62%	61%	64%
Nurses 'Always' Communicated Well	300+	74%	74%	79%
Pain 'Always' Well Controlled	300+	70%	68%	71%
Room and Bathroom 'Always' Clean	300+	79%	70%	73%
Timely Help 'Always' Received	300+	63%	62%	68%
Would Definitely Recommend Hospital	300+	79%	70%	71%
Use of Medical Imaging				
Cardiac Imaging Stress Test before Surgery	-	-	5.2%	5.3%
Combination Abdominal CT Scan	-	-	13.4%	10.5%
Combination Brain/Sinus CT Scan	-	-	2.2%	2.7%
Combination Chest CT Scan	-	-	2.3%	2.7%
Follow-up Mammogram/Ultrasound	-	-	8.2%	8.8%
Lumbar Spine MRI for Low Back Pain	-	-	34.2%	37.2%

Mission Community Hospital

14850 Roscoe Blvd
Panorama City, CA 91402
Phone: 818-904-3100
Fax: 818-904-3529
E-mail: info@mchonline.org
URL: www.mchonline.org
Type: Acute Care Hospitals
Emergency Services: Yes
Ownership: Voluntary non-profit - Private
Beds: 120

Key Personnel:

CEO/President. . . . . Heidi Lennartz
Quality Assurance . . . . Neil McAmiffe
Coronary Care . . . . Camila Mulrey
Intensive Care Unit. . . . . Camila Mulrey
Operating Room. . . . . Jeanette Nevarez
Patient Relations . . . . Ruby Pantoja
Chief of Medical Staff . . . . Robert E Thompson
Emergency Room . . . . James Webb

Measure	Cases	This Hosp.	State Avg.	U.S. Avg.
Blood Clot Prevention and Treatment				
Anticoagulation Overlap Therapy[1,2]	-	-	92%	93%
ICU Venous Thromboembolism Prophylaxis[2]	63	94%	92%	92%
Incidence of Potentially Preventable VTE[1,2]	-	-	11%	10%
UFH with Dosages/Platelet Monitoring[1,2]	-	-	96%	97%
Venous Thromboembolism Prophylaxis[2]	376	85%	83%	85%
Warfarin Therapy Discharge Instructions[1,2]	-	-	75%	75%
Chest Pain/Possible Heart Attack Care				
Aspirin Given Within 24 Hours of Arrival[1,3]	-	-	97%	96%
Fibrinolytic Meds Within 30 Min. of Arrival[3,7]	-	-	62%	58%
Average Time to ECG (minutes)[1,3]	-	-	9	7
Average Time to Transfer (minutes)[1,3]	-	-	62	60
Children's Asthma Care				
Received Home Management Plan of Care	-	-	88%	88%
Received Reliever Medication	-	-	100%	100%
Received Systemic Corticosteroids	-	-	100%	100%
Emergency Department				
Admittance Decision Time (minutes)[2]	316	71	125	98
Head CT Results Within 45 Min. of Arrival[5]	-	-	55%	57%
Patients Who Left ER Before Being Seen	19,964	3%	3%	2%
Time from ER Arrival to Admit. (minutes)[2]	472	238	323	274
Time from ER Arrival to Discharge (minutes)	328	121	168	134
Time in ER Before Being Evaluated (minutes)	328	23	29	26
Time to Pain Meds for Fractures (minutes)	38	57	62	57
Heart Attack Care				
Aspirin Given at Discharge	12	100%	99%	99%
Fibrinolytic Meds Within 30 Min. of Arrival[7]	-	-	73%	54%
PCI Within 90 Minutes of Arrival[7]	-	-	95%	96%
Statin Prescribed at Discharge[1]	-	-	98%	98%
Heart Failure Care				
ACE Inhibitor or ARB for LVSD	26	100%	97%	97%
Discharge Instructions Given	108	80%	94%	94%
Evaluation of LVS Function	154	100%	99%	99%
Medicare Spending				
Medicare Spending per Patient (ratio)	-	1.14	0.98	0.98
Pneumonia Care				
Appropriate Initial Antibiotic Given	59	97%	97%	95%
Blood Culture Timing	175	91%	98%	98%
Pregnancy and Delivery Care				
Newborn Deliveries Scheduled Early[7]	-	-	5%	6%
Preventive Care				
Immunization for Influenza[2]	439	80%	89%	90%
Immunization for Pneumonia[2]	689	78%	90%	92%
Stroke Care				
Anticoagulation Therapy for Atrial Fibrillation[1]	-	-	95%	95%
Antithrombotic Therapy Timing	27	96%	98%	98%
Assessed for Rehabilitation	29	83%	97%	97%
Discharged on Antithrombotic Therapy	26	92%	99%	99%
Discharged on Statin Medication	18	78%	94%	94%
Thrombolytic Therapy Timing[7]	-	-	72%	66%
Venous Thromboembolism Prophylaxis	32	94%	94%	94%
Written Stroke Educational Materials Given	12	50%	87%	88%
Surgical Care Improvement Project				
Appropriate Beta Blocker Usage	26	96%	97%	98%
Appropriate VTP Within 24 Hours	137	100%	98%	98%
Controlled Postoperative Blood Glucose[7]	-	-	96%	97%
Perioperative Temperature Management	190	100%	100%	100%
Prophylactic Antibiotic Selection	101	96%	99%	99%
Prophylactic Antibiotic Selection (Outpatient)	65	94%	97%	98%
Prophylactic Antibiotic Stopped	94	91%	98%	98%
Prophylactic Antibiotic Timing	101	93%	99%	99%
Prophylactic Antibiotic Timing (Outpatient)	66	95%	97%	98%
Urinary Catheter Removal	72	96%	97%	97%
Survey of Patients' Hospital Experiences				
Area Around Room 'Always' Quiet at Night	300+	45%	51%	61%
Doctors 'Always' Communicated Well	300+	70%	78%	82%
Home Recovery Information Given	300+	75%	83%	85%
Hospital Given 9 or 10 on 10 Point Scale	300+	54%	68%	71%
Meds 'Always' Explained Before Given	300+	48%	61%	64%
Nurses 'Always' Communicated Well	300+	62%	74%	79%
Pain 'Always' Well Controlled	300+	58%	68%	71%
Room and Bathroom 'Always' Clean	300+	71%	70%	73%
Timely Help 'Always' Received	300+	54%	62%	68%
Would Definitely Recommend Hospital	300+	52%	70%	71%
Use of Medical Imaging				
Cardiac Imaging Stress Test before Surgery	56	5.4%	5.2%	5.3%
Combination Abdominal CT Scan	202	5.9%	13.4%	10.5%
Combination Brain/Sinus CT Scan[1]	-	-	2.2%	2.7%
Combination Chest CT Scan[1]	-	-	2.3%	2.7%
Follow-up Mammogram/Ultrasound	140	2.1%	8.2%	8.8%
Lumbar Spine MRI for Low Back Pain[1]	-	-	34.2%	37.2%

Feather River Hospital

5974 Pentz Road
Paradise, CA 95969
Phone: 530-877-9361
Fax: 530-876-2157
E-mail: wisenemm@ah.org
URL: www.frhosp.org
Type: Acute Care Hospitals
Emergency Services: Yes
Ownership: Voluntary non-profit - Church
Beds: 101

Key Personnel:

Operating Room. . . . . Pat Bowen, RN
President/CEO. . . . . Kevin Erich
Infection Control. . . . . Carole Farmer
Quality Assurance . . . . Jean Higgins
Radiology. . . . . Margaret Murhpy
Chief of Medical Staff . . . . Anthony J Nasr, MD

Measure	Cases	This Hosp.	State Avg.	U.S. Avg.
Blood Clot Prevention and Treatment				
Anticoagulation Overlap Therapy[2]	38	97%	92%	93%
ICU Venous Thromboembolism Prophylaxis[2]	86	97%	92%	92%
Incidence of Potentially Preventable VTE[1,2]	-	-	11%	10%
UFH with Dosages/Platelet Monitoring[1,2]	-	-	96%	97%
Venous Thromboembolism Prophylaxis[2]	348	95%	83%	85%
Warfarin Therapy Discharge Instructions[2]	29	97%	75%	75%
Chest Pain/Possible Heart Attack Care				
Aspirin Given Within 24 Hours of Arrival	26	100%	97%	96%
Fibrinolytic Meds Within 30 Min. of Arrival[7]	-	-	62%	58%
Average Time to ECG (minutes)	26	14	9	7
Average Time to Transfer (minutes)[1]	-	-	62	60
Children's Asthma Care				
Received Home Management Plan of Care	-	-	88%	88%
Received Reliever Medication	-	-	100%	100%
Received Systemic Corticosteroids	-	-	100%	100%
Emergency Department				
Admittance Decision Time (minutes)[2]	614	108	125	98
Head CT Results Within 45 Min. of Arrival[7]	-	-	55%	57%
Patients Who Left ER Before Being Seen	23,224	2%	3%	2%
Time from ER Arrival to Admit. (minutes)[2]	717	297	323	274
Time from ER Arrival to Discharge (minutes)	355	163	168	134
Time in ER Before Being Evaluated (minutes)	363	29	29	26
Time to Pain Meds for Fractures (minutes)	46	74	62	57
Heart Attack Care				
Aspirin Given at Discharge	33	100%	99%	99%
Fibrinolytic Meds Within 30 Min. of Arrival[7]	-	-	73%	54%
PCI Within 90 Minutes of Arrival[7]	-	-	95%	96%
Statin Prescribed at Discharge	26	92%	98%	98%
Heart Failure Care				
ACE Inhibitor or ARB for LVSD	38	100%	97%	97%
Discharge Instructions Given	92	91%	94%	94%
Evaluation of LVS Function	111	99%	99%	99%
Medicare Spending				
Medicare Spending per Patient (ratio)	-	0.90	0.98	0.98
Pneumonia Care				
Appropriate Initial Antibiotic Given	146	95%	97%	95%
Blood Culture Timing	265	98%	98%	98%
Pregnancy and Delivery Care				
Newborn Deliveries Scheduled Early[2]	29	0%	5%	6%
Preventive Care				
Immunization for Influenza[2]	527	98%	89%	90%
Immunization for Pneumonia[2]	604	97%	90%	92%
Stroke Care				
Anticoagulation Therapy for Atrial Fibrillation[1]	-	-	95%	95%
Antithrombotic Therapy Timing	59	100%	98%	98%
Assessed for Rehabilitation	56	95%	97%	97%
Discharged on Antithrombotic Therapy	55	100%	99%	99%
Discharged on Statin Medication	34	100%	94%	94%
Thrombolytic Therapy Timing[1]	-	-	72%	66%
Venous Thromboembolism Prophylaxis	61	98%	94%	94%

NOTE: Hospital profiles are in alphabetical order by state, then city, then hospital within the city; Rankings exclude hospitals with less than 25 cases except for patient surveys which excludes hospitals with less than 100 cases; (a) 100-299 cases; (1) The number of cases/patients is too few to report; (2) Data submitted were based on a sample of cases/patients; (3) Results are based on a shorter time period than required; (4) Data suppressed by CMS for one or more quarters; (5) Results are not available for this reporting period; (6) Fewer than 100 patients completed the HCAHPS survey; (7) No cases met the criteria for this measure; (8) The lower limit of the confidence interval cannot be calculated if the number of observed infections equals zero; (9) No data are available from the state/territory for this reporting period; (10) The scores shown reflect fewer than 50 completed surveys; (11) There were discrepancies in the data collection process; (12) This measure does not apply to this hospital for this reporting period; (13) Results cannot be calculated for this reporting period; (14) The results for this state are combined with nearby states to protect confidentiality; Please refer to the User's Guide for a full explanation of data.

Measure	Cases	This Hosp.	State Avg.	U.S. Avg.
Written Stroke Educational Materials Given	34	79%	87%	88%
Surgical Care Improvement Project				
Appropriate Beta Blocker Usage[2]	92	98%	97%	98%
Appropriate VTP Within 24 Hours[2]	296	99%	98%	98%
Controlled Postoperative Blood Glucose[2,7]	-	-	96%	97%
Perioperative Temperature Management[2]	360	100%	100%	100%
Prophylactic Antibiotic Selection[2]	243	97%	99%	99%
Prophylactic Antibiotic Selection (Outpatient)	85	93%	97%	98%
Prophylactic Antibiotic Stopped[2]	237	98%	98%	98%
Prophylactic Antibiotic Timing[2]	243	99%	99%	99%
Prophylactic Antibiotic Timing (Outpatient)	85	92%	97%	98%
Urinary Catheter Removal[2]	214	99%	97%	97%
Survey of Patients' Hospital Experiences				
Area Around Room 'Always' Quiet at Night	300+	39%	51%	61%
Doctors 'Always' Communicated Well	300+	76%	78%	82%
Home Recovery Information Given	300+	87%	83%	85%
Hospital Given 9 or 10 on 10 Point Scale	300+	75%	68%	71%
Meds 'Always' Explained Before Given	300+	62%	61%	64%
Nurses 'Always' Communicated Well	300+	78%	74%	79%
Pain 'Always' Well Controlled	300+	68%	68%	71%
Room and Bathroom 'Always' Clean	300+	75%	70%	73%
Timely Help 'Always' Received	300+	63%	62%	68%
Would Definitely Recommend Hospital	300+	78%	70%	71%
Use of Medical Imaging				
Cardiac Imaging Stress Test before Surgery	424	5.0%	5.2%	5.3%
Combination Abdominal CT Scan	681	14.1%	13.4%	10.5%
Combination Brain/Sinus CT Scan	755	1.7%	2.2%	2.7%
Combination Chest CT Scan	471	4.5%	2.3%	2.7%
Follow-up Mammogram/Ultrasound	1,884	13.8%	8.2%	8.8%
Lumbar Spine MRI for Low Back Pain	159	30.8%	34.2%	37.2%

Huntington Memorial Hospital

100 W California Blvd — Phone: 626-397-5000
Pasadena, CA 91109 — Fax: 626-397-2903
URL: www.huntingtonhospital.com
Type: Acute Care Hospitals — Emergency Services: Yes
Ownership: Voluntary non-profit - Private — Beds: 606

Key Personnel:
Operating Room. . . . . Patricia Carter
Quality Assurance . . . . Sandra Davis
Cardiac Laboratory. . . . . Roth Fernando
Radiology. . . . . John Kassabian
CEO/President. . . . . Stephen Ralph
Chief of Medical Staff. . . . . Paula Verrette, MD
Pediatric Ambulatory Care . . . . . . William Vincent
Pediatric In-Patient Care . . . . William Vincent

Measure	Cases	This Hosp.	State Avg.	U.S. Avg.
Blood Clot Prevention and Treatment				
Anticoagulation Overlap Therapy[2]	119	87%	92%	93%
ICU Venous Thromboembolism Prophylaxis[2]	40	98%	92%	92%
Incidence of Potentially Preventable VTE[2]	61	31%	11%	10%
UFH with Dosages/Platelet Monitoring[2]	38	97%	96%	97%
Venous Thromboembolism Prophylaxis[2]	291	60%	83%	85%
Warfarin Therapy Discharge Instructions[2]	77	90%	75%	75%
Chest Pain/Possible Heart Attack Care				
Aspirin Given Within 24 Hours of Arrival[1,3]	-	-	97%	96%
Fibrinolytic Meds Within 30 Min. of Arrival[5]	-	-	62%	58%
Average Time to ECG (minutes)[1,3]	-	-	9	7
Average Time to Transfer (minutes)[5]	-	-	62	60
Children's Asthma Care				
Received Home Management Plan of Care	-	-	88%	88%
Received Reliever Medication	-	-	100%	100%
Received Systemic Corticosteroids	-	-	100%	100%
Emergency Department				
Admittance Decision Time (minutes)[2]	578	121	125	98
Head CT Results Within 45 Min. of Arrival[1]	-	-	55%	57%
Patients Who Left ER Before Being Seen	60,985	6%	3%	2%
Time from ER Arrival to Admit. (minutes)[2]	578	384	323	274
Time from ER Arrival to Discharge (minutes)	362	270	168	134
Time in ER Before Being Evaluated (minutes)	400	78	29	26
Time to Pain Meds for Fractures (minutes)	183	127	62	57
Heart Attack Care				
Aspirin Given at Discharge[2]	211	97%	99%	99%
Fibrinolytic Meds Within 30 Min. of Arrival[2,7]	-	-	73%	54%
PCI Within 90 Minutes of Arrival[2]	36	67%	95%	96%
Statin Prescribed at Discharge[2]	210	95%	98%	98%
Heart Failure Care				
ACE Inhibitor or ARB for LVSD[2]	111	83%	97%	97%
Discharge Instructions Given[2]	218	89%	94%	94%
Evaluation of LVS Function[2]	268	100%	99%	99%
Medicare Spending				
Medicare Spending per Patient (ratio)	-	0.98	0.98	0.98
Pneumonia Care				
Appropriate Initial Antibiotic Given[2]	89	80%	97%	95%
Blood Culture Timing[2]	133	95%	98%	98%
Pregnancy and Delivery Care				
Newborn Deliveries Scheduled Early[2]	65	12%	5%	6%
Preventive Care				
Immunization for Influenza[2]	512	87%	89%	90%
Immunization for Pneumonia[2]	541	82%	90%	92%
Stroke Care				
Anticoagulation Therapy for Atrial Fibrillation	33	94%	95%	95%
Antithrombotic Therapy Timing	189	94%	98%	98%
Assessed for Rehabilitation	239	99%	97%	97%
Discharged on Antithrombotic Therapy	196	98%	99%	99%
Discharged on Statin Medication	151	89%	94%	94%
Thrombolytic Therapy Timing	15	93%	72%	66%
Venous Thromboembolism Prophylaxis	258	90%	94%	94%
Written Stroke Educational Materials Given	131	85%	87%	88%
Surgical Care Improvement Project				
Appropriate Beta Blocker Usage[2]	152	97%	97%	98%
Appropriate VTP Within 24 Hours[2]	331	98%	98%	98%
Controlled Postoperative Blood Glucose[2]	123	94%	96%	97%
Perioperative Temperature Management[2]	421	100%	100%	100%
Prophylactic Antibiotic Selection[2]	373	98%	99%	99%
Prophylactic Antibiotic Selection (Outpatient)	230	96%	97%	98%
Prophylactic Antibiotic Stopped[2]	359	96%	98%	98%
Prophylactic Antibiotic Timing[2]	374	98%	99%	99%
Prophylactic Antibiotic Timing (Outpatient)	234	97%	97%	98%
Urinary Catheter Removal[2]	331	95%	97%	97%
Survey of Patients' Hospital Experiences				
Area Around Room 'Always' Quiet at Night	300+	58%	51%	61%
Doctors 'Always' Communicated Well	300+	82%	78%	82%
Home Recovery Information Given	300+	84%	83%	85%
Hospital Given 9 or 10 on 10 Point Scale	300+	82%	68%	71%
Meds 'Always' Explained Before Given	300+	66%	61%	64%
Nurses 'Always' Communicated Well	300+	81%	74%	79%
Pain 'Always' Well Controlled	300+	75%	68%	71%
Room and Bathroom 'Always' Clean	300+	70%	70%	73%
Timely Help 'Always' Received	300+	67%	62%	68%
Would Definitely Recommend Hospital	300+	87%	70%	71%
Use of Medical Imaging				
Cardiac Imaging Stress Test before Surgery	200	4.0%	5.2%	5.3%
Combination Abdominal CT Scan	437	0.9%	13.4%	10.5%
Combination Brain/Sinus CT Scan	729	2.2%	2.2%	2.7%
Combination Chest CT Scan	122	1.6%	2.3%	2.7%
Follow-up Mammogram/Ultrasound[7]	-	-	8.2%	8.8%
Lumbar Spine MRI for Low Back Pain[1]	-	-	34.2%	37.2%

Petaluma Valley Hospital

400 N Mcdowell Blvd — Phone: 707-778-1111
Petaluma, CA 94954 — Fax: 707-778-9117
URL: www.stjosephhealth.org
Type: Acute Care Hospitals — Emergency Services: Yes
Ownership: Voluntary non-profit - Other — Beds: 80

Key Personnel:
Coronary Care . . . . Nancy Corda, RN
Intensive Care Unit. . . . . Nancy Corda, RN
Infection Control. . . . . Leslie Fisher
Chief of Medical Staff. . . . . Gary Greenfweit
CEO/President. . . . . Kevin Kloekenga
Emergency Room . . . . Randeep Singh, MD

Measure	Cases	This Hosp.	State Avg.	U.S. Avg.
Blood Clot Prevention and Treatment				
Anticoagulation Overlap Therapy[2]	16	94%	92%	93%
ICU Venous Thromboembolism Prophylaxis[2]	32	81%	92%	92%
Incidence of Potentially Preventable VTE[1,2]	-	-	11%	10%
UFH with Dosages/Platelet Monitoring[1,2]	-	-	96%	97%
Venous Thromboembolism Prophylaxis[2]	161	83%	83%	85%
Warfarin Therapy Discharge Instructions[1,2]	-	-	75%	75%
Chest Pain/Possible Heart Attack Care				
Aspirin Given Within 24 Hours of Arrival	50	100%	97%	96%
Fibrinolytic Meds Within 30 Min. of Arrival[7]	-	-	62%	58%
Average Time to ECG (minutes)	53	10	9	7
Average Time to Transfer (minutes)[1]	-	-	62	60
Children's Asthma Care				
Received Home Management Plan of Care	-	-	88%	88%
Received Reliever Medication	-	-	100%	100%
Received Systemic Corticosteroids	-	-	100%	100%
Emergency Department				
Admittance Decision Time (minutes)[2]	339	147	125	98
Head CT Results Within 45 Min. of Arrival[1]	-	-	55%	57%
Patients Who Left ER Before Being Seen	17,267	1%	3%	2%
Time from ER Arrival to Admit. (minutes)[2]	341	354	323	274
Time from ER Arrival to Discharge (minutes)	342	160	168	134
Time in ER Before Being Evaluated (minutes)	317	24	29	26
Time to Pain Meds for Fractures (minutes)	87	65	62	57
Heart Attack Care				
Aspirin Given at Discharge	18	94%	99%	99%
Fibrinolytic Meds Within 30 Min. of Arrival[7]	-	-	73%	54%
PCI Within 90 Minutes of Arrival[7]	-	-	95%	96%
Statin Prescribed at Discharge	19	95%	98%	98%
Heart Failure Care				
ACE Inhibitor or ARB for LVSD	25	96%	97%	97%
Discharge Instructions Given	60	90%	94%	94%
Evaluation of LVS Function	74	99%	99%	99%
Medicare Spending				
Medicare Spending per Patient (ratio)	-	0.95	0.98	0.98
Pneumonia Care				
Appropriate Initial Antibiotic Given	58	95%	97%	95%
Blood Culture Timing	88	98%	98%	98%
Pregnancy and Delivery Care				
Newborn Deliveries Scheduled Early[2]	22	0%	5%	6%
Preventive Care				
Immunization for Influenza[2]	263	76%	89%	90%
Immunization for Pneumonia[2]	291	84%	90%	92%
Stroke Care				
Anticoagulation Therapy for Atrial Fibrillation[1]	-	-	95%	95%
Antithrombotic Therapy Timing	18	100%	98%	98%
Assessed for Rehabilitation	21	86%	97%	97%
Discharged on Antithrombotic Therapy	21	95%	99%	99%
Discharged on Statin Medication	17	82%	94%	94%
Thrombolytic Therapy Timing[1]	-	-	72%	66%
Venous Thromboembolism Prophylaxis	17	88%	94%	94%
Written Stroke Educational Materials Given	14	57%	87%	88%
Surgical Care Improvement Project				
Appropriate Beta Blocker Usage[2]	22	95%	97%	98%
Appropriate VTP Within 24 Hours[2]	124	94%	98%	98%
Controlled Postoperative Blood Glucose[2,7]	-	-	96%	97%
Perioperative Temperature Management[2]	141	99%	100%	100%
Prophylactic Antibiotic Selection[2]	96	99%	99%	99%
Prophylactic Antibiotic Selection (Outpatient)	40	100%	97%	98%
Prophylactic Antibiotic Stopped[2]	92	95%	98%	98%
Prophylactic Antibiotic Timing[2]	97	97%	99%	99%
Prophylactic Antibiotic Timing (Outpatient)	41	95%	97%	98%
Urinary Catheter Removal[2]	112	98%	97%	97%
Survey of Patients' Hospital Experiences				
Area Around Room 'Always' Quiet at Night	300+	54%	51%	61%
Doctors 'Always' Communicated Well	300+	77%	78%	82%
Home Recovery Information Given	300+	84%	83%	85%
Hospital Given 9 or 10 on 10 Point Scale	300+	68%	68%	71%
Meds 'Always' Explained Before Given	300+	64%	61%	64%
Nurses 'Always' Communicated Well	300+	77%	74%	79%
Pain 'Always' Well Controlled	300+	71%	68%	71%
Room and Bathroom 'Always' Clean	300+	81%	70%	73%
Timely Help 'Always' Received	300+	70%	62%	68%
Would Definitely Recommend Hospital	300+	71%	70%	71%
Use of Medical Imaging				
Cardiac Imaging Stress Test before Surgery[7]	-	-	5.2%	5.3%
Combination Abdominal CT Scan	319	1.9%	13.4%	10.5%

NOTE: Hospital profiles are in alphabetical order by state, then city, then hospital within the city; Rankings exclude hospitals with less than 25 cases except for patient surveys which excludes hospitals with less than 100 cases; (a) 100-299 cases; (1) The number of cases/patients is too few to report; (2) Data submitted were based on a sample of cases/patients; (3) Results are based on a shorter time period than required; (4) Data suppressed by CMS for one or more quarters; (5) Results are not available for this reporting period; (6) Fewer than 100 patients completed the HCAHPS survey; (7) No cases met the criteria for this measure; (8) The lower limit of the confidence interval cannot be calculated if the number of observed infections equals zero; (9) No data are available from the state/territory for this reporting period; (10) The scores shown reflect fewer than 50 completed surveys; (11) There were discrepancies in the data collection process; (12) This measure does not apply to this hospital for this reporting period; (13) Results cannot be calculated for this reporting period; (14) The results for this state are combined with nearby states to protect confidentiality; Please refer to the User's Guide for a full explanation of data.

Measure	Cases	This Hosp.	State Avg.	U.S. Avg.
Combination Brain/Sinus CT Scan[1]	-	-	2.2%	2.7%
Combination Chest CT Scan	193	0.0%	2.3%	2.7%
Follow-up Mammogram/Ultrasound	813	14.8%	8.2%	8.8%
Lumbar Spine MRI for Low Back Pain[1]	-	-	34.2%	37.2%

Placentia Linda Hospital

1301 N Rose Drive
Placentia, CA 92870
Phone: 714-993-2000
Fax: 714-961-8427
URL: www.placentialinda.com
Type: Acute Care Hospitals
Emergency Services: Yes
Ownership: Proprietary
Beds: 114

Key Personnel:
Cardiac Laboratory. . . . . Michael Babaeff, RPT
CEO/President. . . . . Kent Clayton
Chief of Medical Staff . . . . Paul Jordan, MD
Chair/CEO . . . . Scott Nelson, Mayor
Coronary Care . . . . Vicki Shrock, RN
Quality Assurance . . . . Earlene Tarr
Radiology. . . . . Harry Wolfe

Measure	Cases	This Hosp.	State Avg.	U.S. Avg.
Blood Clot Prevention and Treatment				
Anticoagulation Overlap Therapy[2]	22	86%	92%	93%
ICU Venous Thromboembolism Prophylaxis[2]	53	87%	92%	92%
Incidence of Potentially Preventable VTE[2,7]	-	-	11%	10%
UFH with Dosages/Platelet Monitoring[1,2]	-	-	96%	97%
Venous Thromboembolism Prophylaxis[2]	289	83%	83%	85%
Warfarin Therapy Discharge Instructions[2]	20	100%	75%	75%
Chest Pain/Possible Heart Attack Care				
Aspirin Given Within 24 Hours of Arrival	61	100%	97%	96%
Fibrinolytic Meds Within 30 Min. of Arrival[1]	-	-	62%	58%
Average Time to ECG (minutes)	65	3	9	7
Average Time to Transfer (minutes)	14	58	62	60
Children's Asthma Care				
Received Home Management Plan of Care	-	-	88%	88%
Received Reliever Medication	-	-	100%	100%
Received Systemic Corticosteroids	-	-	100%	100%
Emergency Department				
Admittance Decision Time (minutes)[2]	604	71	125	98
Head CT Results Within 45 Min. of Arrival[1]	-	-	55%	57%
Patients Who Left ER Before Being Seen	24,718	1%	3%	2%
Time from ER Arrival to Admit. (minutes)[2]	606	206	323	274
Time from ER Arrival to Discharge (minutes)	467	97	168	134
Time in ER Before Being Evaluated (minutes)	498	14	29	26
Time to Pain Meds for Fractures (minutes)	181	40	62	57
Heart Attack Care				
Aspirin Given at Discharge	15	100%	99%	99%
Fibrinolytic Meds Within 30 Min. of Arrival[7]	-	-	73%	54%
PCI Within 90 Minutes of Arrival[7]	-	-	95%	96%
Statin Prescribed at Discharge	19	100%	98%	98%
Heart Failure Care				
ACE Inhibitor or ARB for LVSD	24	88%	97%	97%
Discharge Instructions Given	89	92%	94%	94%
Evaluation of LVS Function	114	100%	99%	99%
Medicare Spending				
Medicare Spending per Patient (ratio)	-	1.07	0.98	0.98
Pneumonia Care				
Appropriate Initial Antibiotic Given[2]	83	96%	97%	95%
Blood Culture Timing[2]	132	100%	98%	98%
Pregnancy and Delivery Care				
Newborn Deliveries Scheduled Early[7]	-	-	5%	6%
Preventive Care				
Immunization for Influenza[2]	417	99%	89%	90%
Immunization for Pneumonia[2]	550	99%	90%	92%
Stroke Care				
Anticoagulation Therapy for Atrial Fibrillation[1]	-	-	95%	95%
Antithrombotic Therapy Timing	25	100%	98%	98%
Assessed for Rehabilitation	32	100%	97%	97%
Discharged on Antithrombotic Therapy	30	93%	99%	99%
Discharged on Statin Medication	27	96%	94%	94%
Thrombolytic Therapy Timing[1]	-	-	72%	66%
Venous Thromboembolism Prophylaxis	26	81%	94%	94%
Written Stroke Educational Materials Given	20	80%	87%	88%
Surgical Care Improvement Project				
Appropriate Beta Blocker Usage[2]	131	98%	97%	98%
Appropriate VTP Within 24 Hours[2]	475	100%	98%	98%
Controlled Postoperative Blood Glucose[2,7]	-	-	96%	97%
Perioperative Temperature Management[2]	509	100%	100%	100%
Prophylactic Antibiotic Selection[2]	407	100%	99%	99%
Prophylactic Antibiotic Selection (Outpatient)	76	96%	97%	98%
Prophylactic Antibiotic Stopped[2]	400	98%	98%	98%
Prophylactic Antibiotic Timing[2]	407	99%	99%	99%
Prophylactic Antibiotic Timing (Outpatient)	76	100%	97%	98%
Urinary Catheter Removal[2]	360	99%	97%	97%
Survey of Patients' Hospital Experiences				
Area Around Room 'Always' Quiet at Night	300+	52%	51%	61%
Doctors 'Always' Communicated Well	300+	83%	78%	82%
Home Recovery Information Given	300+	87%	83%	85%
Hospital Given 9 or 10 on 10 Point Scale	300+	75%	68%	71%
Meds 'Always' Explained Before Given	300+	71%	61%	64%
Nurses 'Always' Communicated Well	300+	81%	74%	79%
Pain 'Always' Well Controlled	300+	76%	68%	71%
Room and Bathroom 'Always' Clean	300+	75%	70%	73%
Timely Help 'Always' Received	300+	68%	62%	68%
Would Definitely Recommend Hospital	300+	76%	70%	71%
Use of Medical Imaging				
Cardiac Imaging Stress Test before Surgery[1]	-	-	5.2%	5.3%
Combination Abdominal CT Scan	380	9.2%	13.4%	10.5%
Combination Brain/Sinus CT Scan[1]	-	-	2.2%	2.7%
Combination Chest CT Scan	118	2.5%	2.3%	2.7%
Follow-up Mammogram/Ultrasound	309	13.9%	8.2%	8.8%
Lumbar Spine MRI for Low Back Pain	43	39.5%	34.2%	37.2%

Marshall Medical Center

1100 Marshall Way
Placerville, CA 95667
Phone: 530-622-1441
Fax: 530-622-7853
URL: www.marshallmedical.org
Type: Acute Care Hospitals
Emergency Services: Yes
Ownership: Voluntary non-profit - Other
Beds: 105

Key Personnel:
Radiology. . . . . Jerry Arnold
Infection Control. . . . . Sue Deal, RN
Quality Assurance . . . . Dibba Haymann
Cardiac Laboratory. . . . . Melinda Head, RN
Operating Room. . . . . Bonnie Line
Chief of Medical Staff. . . . . Rene Orona, MD
CEO . . . . James Whipple

Measure	Cases	This Hosp.	State Avg.	U.S. Avg.
Blood Clot Prevention and Treatment				
Anticoagulation Overlap Therapy[2]	49	100%	92%	93%
ICU Venous Thromboembolism Prophylaxis[2]	76	96%	92%	92%
Incidence of Potentially Preventable VTE[1,2]	-	-	11%	10%
UFH with Dosages/Platelet Monitoring[1,2]	-	-	96%	97%
Venous Thromboembolism Prophylaxis[2]	317	96%	83%	85%
Warfarin Therapy Discharge Instructions[2]	32	100%	75%	75%
Chest Pain/Possible Heart Attack Care				
Aspirin Given Within 24 Hours of Arrival	62	100%	97%	96%
Fibrinolytic Meds Within 30 Min. of Arrival	19	79%	62%	58%
Average Time to ECG (minutes)	67	9	9	7
Average Time to Transfer (minutes)[1]	-	-	62	60
Children's Asthma Care				
Received Home Management Plan of Care	-	-	88%	88%
Received Reliever Medication	-	-	100%	100%
Received Systemic Corticosteroids	-	-	100%	100%
Emergency Department				
Admittance Decision Time (minutes)[2]	666	98	125	98
Head CT Results Within 45 Min. of Arrival	11	64%	55%	57%
Patients Who Left ER Before Being Seen	27,700	2%	3%	2%
Time from ER Arrival to Admit. (minutes)[2]	692	328	323	274
Time from ER Arrival to Discharge (minutes)	371	170	168	134
Time in ER Before Being Evaluated (minutes)	404	23	29	26
Time to Pain Meds for Fractures (minutes)	123	49	62	57
Heart Attack Care				
Aspirin Given at Discharge	17	94%	99%	99%
Fibrinolytic Meds Within 30 Min. of Arrival[1]	-	-	73%	54%
PCI Within 90 Minutes of Arrival[7]	-	-	95%	96%
Statin Prescribed at Discharge	16	94%	98%	98%
Heart Failure Care				
ACE Inhibitor or ARB for LVSD	38	100%	97%	97%
Discharge Instructions Given	101	95%	94%	94%
Evaluation of LVS Function	134	100%	99%	99%
Medicare Spending				
Medicare Spending per Patient (ratio)	-	0.88	0.98	0.98
Pneumonia Care				
Appropriate Initial Antibiotic Given[2]	103	96%	97%	95%
Blood Culture Timing[2]	167	99%	98%	98%
Pregnancy and Delivery Care				
Newborn Deliveries Scheduled Early	77	3%	5%	6%
Preventive Care				
Immunization for Influenza[2]	523	97%	89%	90%
Immunization for Pneumonia[2]	673	96%	90%	92%
Stroke Care				
Anticoagulation Therapy for Atrial Fibrillation	12	100%	95%	95%
Antithrombotic Therapy Timing	64	100%	98%	98%
Assessed for Rehabilitation	72	100%	97%	97%
Discharged on Antithrombotic Therapy	69	100%	99%	99%
Discharged on Statin Medication	55	100%	94%	94%
Thrombolytic Therapy Timing[1]	-	-	72%	66%
Venous Thromboembolism Prophylaxis	64	100%	94%	94%
Written Stroke Educational Materials Given	42	98%	87%	88%
Surgical Care Improvement Project				
Appropriate Beta Blocker Usage[2]	87	100%	97%	98%
Appropriate VTP Within 24 Hours[2]	287	99%	98%	98%
Controlled Postoperative Blood Glucose[2,7]	-	-	96%	97%
Perioperative Temperature Management[2]	329	100%	100%	100%
Prophylactic Antibiotic Selection[2]	235	100%	99%	99%
Prophylactic Antibiotic Selection (Outpatient)	163	99%	97%	98%
Prophylactic Antibiotic Stopped[2]	225	99%	98%	98%
Prophylactic Antibiotic Timing[2]	235	100%	99%	99%
Prophylactic Antibiotic Timing (Outpatient)	163	100%	97%	98%
Urinary Catheter Removal[2]	226	96%	97%	97%
Survey of Patients' Hospital Experiences				
Area Around Room 'Always' Quiet at Night	300+	47%	51%	61%
Doctors 'Always' Communicated Well	300+	78%	78%	82%
Home Recovery Information Given	300+	86%	83%	85%
Hospital Given 9 or 10 on 10 Point Scale	300+	75%	68%	71%
Meds 'Always' Explained Before Given	300+	64%	61%	64%
Nurses 'Always' Communicated Well	300+	81%	74%	79%
Pain 'Always' Well Controlled	300+	74%	68%	71%
Room and Bathroom 'Always' Clean	300+	75%	70%	73%
Timely Help 'Always' Received	300+	68%	62%	68%
Would Definitely Recommend Hospital	300+	74%	70%	71%
Use of Medical Imaging				
Cardiac Imaging Stress Test before Surgery	604	5.6%	5.2%	5.3%
Combination Abdominal CT Scan	790	13.4%	13.4%	10.5%
Combination Brain/Sinus CT Scan	597	0.8%	2.2%	2.7%
Combination Chest CT Scan	370	1.1%	2.3%	2.7%
Follow-up Mammogram/Ultrasound	1,877	6.1%	8.2%	8.8%
Lumbar Spine MRI for Low Back Pain	132	38.6%	34.2%	37.2%

Valleycare Medical Center

5555 West Las Positas Boulevard
Pleasanton, CA 94588
Phone: 925-447-7000
URL: www.valleycare.com
Type: Acute Care Hospitals
Emergency Services: Yes
Ownership: Voluntary non-profit - Private

Key Personnel:
CEO . . . . Scott Gregerson

Measure	Cases	This Hosp.	State Avg.	U.S. Avg.
Blood Clot Prevention and Treatment				
Anticoagulation Overlap Therapy[2]	45	98%	92%	93%
ICU Venous Thromboembolism Prophylaxis[2]	186	88%	92%	92%
Incidence of Potentially Preventable VTE[1,2]	-	-	11%	10%
UFH with Dosages/Platelet Monitoring[2]	25	100%	96%	97%
Venous Thromboembolism Prophylaxis[2]	796	87%	83%	85%
Warfarin Therapy Discharge Instructions[2]	35	97%	75%	75%
Chest Pain/Possible Heart Attack Care				
Aspirin Given Within 24 Hours of Arrival[1,3]	-	-	97%	96%
Fibrinolytic Meds Within 30 Min. of Arrival[3,7]	-	-	62%	58%
Average Time to ECG (minutes)[1,3]	-	-	9	7
Average Time to Transfer (minutes)[3,7]	-	-	62	60
Children's Asthma Care				

NOTE: Hospital profiles are in alphabetical order by state, then city, then hospital within the city; Rankings exclude hospitals with less than 25 cases except for patient surveys which excludes hospitals with less than 100 cases; (a) 100-299 cases; (1) The number of cases/patients is too few to report; (2) Data submitted were based on a sample of cases/patients; (3) Results are based on a shorter time period than required; (4) Data suppressed by CMS for one or more quarters; (5) Results are not available for this reporting period; (6) Fewer than 100 patients completed the HCAHPS survey; (7) No cases met the criteria for this measure; (8) The lower limit of the confidence interval cannot be calculated if the number of observed infections equals zero; (9) No data are available from the state/territory for this reporting period; (10) The scores shown reflect fewer than 50 completed surveys; (11) There were discrepancies in the data collection process; (12) This measure does not apply to this hospital for this reporting period; (13) Results cannot be calculated for this reporting period; (14) The results for this state are combined with nearby states to protect confidentiality; Please refer to the User's Guide for a full explanation of data.

Measure	Cases	This Hosp.	State Avg.	U.S. Avg.
Received Home Management Plan of Care	-	-	88%	88%
Received Reliever Medication	-	-	100%	100%
Received Systemic Corticosteroids	-	-	100%	100%
Emergency Department				
Admittance Decision Time (minutes)[2]	597	113	125	98
Head CT Results Within 45 Min. of Arrival[1]	-	-	55%	57%
Patients Who Left ER Before Being Seen	30,229	1%	3%	2%
Time from ER Arrival to Admit. (minutes)[2]	600	264	323	274
Time from ER Arrival to Discharge (minutes)	339	128	168	134
Time in ER Before Being Evaluated (minutes)	398	19	29	26
Time to Pain Meds for Fractures (minutes)	217	48	62	57
Heart Attack Care				
Aspirin Given at Discharge	114	100%	99%	99%
Fibrinolytic Meds Within 30 Min. of Arrival[7]	-	-	73%	54%
PCI Within 90 Minutes of Arrival	45	98%	95%	96%
Statin Prescribed at Discharge	115	100%	98%	98%
Heart Failure Care				
ACE Inhibitor or ARB for LVSD	51	98%	97%	97%
Discharge Instructions Given	150	86%	94%	94%
Evaluation of LVS Function	197	100%	99%	99%
Medicare Spending				
Medicare Spending per Patient (ratio)	-	0.98	0.98	0.98
Pneumonia Care				
Appropriate Initial Antibiotic Given	157	93%	97%	95%
Blood Culture Timing	205	100%	98%	98%
Pregnancy and Delivery Care				
Newborn Deliveries Scheduled Early[2]	11	9%	5%	6%
Preventive Care				
Immunization for Influenza[2]	661	96%	89%	90%
Immunization for Pneumonia[2]	721	93%	90%	92%
Stroke Care				
Anticoagulation Therapy for Atrial Fibrillation[1]	-	-	95%	95%
Antithrombotic Therapy Timing	48	98%	98%	98%
Assessed for Rehabilitation	41	95%	97%	97%
Discharged on Antithrombotic Therapy	41	98%	99%	99%
Discharged on Statin Medication	28	86%	94%	94%
Thrombolytic Therapy Timing[7]	-	-	72%	66%
Venous Thromboembolism Prophylaxis	45	76%	94%	94%
Written Stroke Educational Materials Given	20	70%	87%	88%
Surgical Care Improvement Project				
Appropriate Beta Blocker Usage	206	100%	97%	98%
Appropriate VTP Within 24 Hours	537	98%	98%	98%
Controlled Postoperative Blood Glucose	38	92%	96%	97%
Perioperative Temperature Management	666	100%	100%	100%
Prophylactic Antibiotic Selection	562	99%	99%	99%
Prophylactic Antibiotic Selection (Outpatient)	166	98%	97%	98%
Prophylactic Antibiotic Stopped	552	99%	98%	98%
Prophylactic Antibiotic Timing	562	98%	99%	99%
Prophylactic Antibiotic Timing (Outpatient)	167	99%	97%	98%
Urinary Catheter Removal	452	98%	97%	97%
Survey of Patients' Hospital Experiences				
Area Around Room 'Always' Quiet at Night	300+	48%	51%	61%
Doctors 'Always' Communicated Well	300+	82%	78%	82%
Home Recovery Information Given	300+	87%	83%	85%
Hospital Given 9 or 10 on 10 Point Scale	300+	77%	68%	71%
Meds 'Always' Explained Before Given	300+	64%	61%	64%
Nurses 'Always' Communicated Well	300+	81%	74%	79%
Pain 'Always' Well Controlled	300+	73%	68%	71%
Room and Bathroom 'Always' Clean	300+	69%	70%	73%
Timely Help 'Always' Received	300+	72%	62%	68%
Would Definitely Recommend Hospital	300+	81%	70%	71%
Use of Medical Imaging				
Cardiac Imaging Stress Test before Surgery	353	5.1%	5.2%	5.3%
Combination Abdominal CT Scan	539	11.9%	13.4%	10.5%
Combination Brain/Sinus CT Scan	428	1.9%	2.2%	2.7%
Combination Chest CT Scan	290	0.0%	2.3%	2.7%
Follow-up Mammogram/Ultrasound	1,293	8.8%	8.2%	8.8%
Lumbar Spine MRI for Low Back Pain	66	34.8%	34.2%	37.2%

Pomona Valley Hospital Medical Center

1798 N Garey Ave — Phone: 909-865-9500
Pomona, CA 91767 — Fax: 909-865-9753
URL: www.pvhmc.com
Type: Acute Care Hospitals — Emergency Services: Yes
Ownership: Voluntary non-profit - Private — Beds: 453

Key Personnel:
Anesthesiology. . . . . Stephen Friedlander, MD
Operating Room. . . . . Karen Hughes, RN
Radiology. . . . . Johnson B Lightfoote, MD, MBA
Chief of Medical Staff. . . . . Kenneth Nakamoto, MD
Emergency Room . . . . Yvonne Nugent, RN
Quality Assurance . . . . Janie Ridgeway
Intensive Care Unit. . . . . Cyndy Tutt, RN
CEO/President. . . . . Rich Yochum

Measure	Cases	This Hosp.	State Avg.	U.S. Avg.
Blood Clot Prevention and Treatment				
Anticoagulation Overlap Therapy[2]	68	100%	92%	93%
ICU Venous Thromboembolism Prophylaxis[2]	114	98%	92%	92%
Incidence of Potentially Preventable VTE[2]	12	0%	11%	10%
UFH with Dosages/Platelet Monitoring[1,2]	-	-	96%	97%
Venous Thromboembolism Prophylaxis[2]	307	82%	83%	85%
Warfarin Therapy Discharge Instructions[2]	45	100%	75%	75%
Chest Pain/Possible Heart Attack Care				
Aspirin Given Within 24 Hours of Arrival	45	100%	97%	96%
Fibrinolytic Meds Within 30 Min. of Arrival[3,7]	-	-	62%	58%
Average Time to ECG (minutes)	47	0	9	7
Average Time to Transfer (minutes)[3,7]	-	-	62	60
Children's Asthma Care				
Received Home Management Plan of Care	-	-	88%	88%
Received Reliever Medication	-	-	100%	100%
Received Systemic Corticosteroids	-	-	100%	100%
Emergency Department				
Admittance Decision Time (minutes)[2]	337	233	125	98
Head CT Results Within 45 Min. of Arrival	20	80%	55%	57%
Patients Who Left ER Before Being Seen	81,925	0%	3%	2%
Time from ER Arrival to Admit. (minutes)[2]	356	446	323	274
Time from ER Arrival to Discharge (minutes)	347	181	168	134
Time in ER Before Being Evaluated (minutes)	351	28	29	26
Time to Pain Meds for Fractures (minutes)	348	64	62	57
Heart Attack Care				
Aspirin Given at Discharge[2]	243	98%	99%	99%
Fibrinolytic Meds Within 30 Min. of Arrival[2,7]	-	-	73%	54%
PCI Within 90 Minutes of Arrival[2]	53	100%	95%	96%
Statin Prescribed at Discharge[2]	250	96%	98%	98%
Heart Failure Care				
ACE Inhibitor or ARB for LVSD[2]	73	100%	97%	97%
Discharge Instructions Given[2]	239	95%	94%	94%
Evaluation of LVS Function[2]	307	100%	99%	99%
Medicare Spending				
Medicare Spending per Patient (ratio)	-	1.09	0.98	0.98
Pneumonia Care				
Appropriate Initial Antibiotic Given[2]	65	98%	97%	95%
Blood Culture Timing[2]	143	100%	98%	98%
Pregnancy and Delivery Care				
Newborn Deliveries Scheduled Early[2]	76	1%	5%	6%
Preventive Care				
Immunization for Influenza[2]	461	92%	89%	90%
Immunization for Pneumonia[2]	346	96%	90%	92%
Stroke Care				
Anticoagulation Therapy for Atrial Fibrillation[2]	24	92%	95%	95%
Antithrombotic Therapy Timing[2]	102	98%	98%	98%
Assessed for Rehabilitation[2]	146	100%	97%	97%
Discharged on Antithrombotic Therapy[2]	118	100%	99%	99%
Discharged on Statin Medication[2]	95	99%	94%	94%
Thrombolytic Therapy Timing[2]	16	100%	72%	66%
Venous Thromboembolism Prophylaxis[2]	144	94%	94%	94%
Written Stroke Educational Materials Given[2]	75	97%	87%	88%
Surgical Care Improvement Project				
Appropriate Beta Blocker Usage[2]	191	98%	97%	98%
Appropriate VTP Within 24 Hours[2]	355	99%	98%	98%
Controlled Postoperative Blood Glucose[2]	112	97%	96%	97%
Perioperative Temperature Management[2]	423	100%	100%	100%
Prophylactic Antibiotic Selection[2]	388	100%	99%	99%
Prophylactic Antibiotic Selection (Outpatient)	306	95%	97%	98%
Prophylactic Antibiotic Stopped[2]	371	98%	98%	98%
Prophylactic Antibiotic Timing[2]	388	100%	99%	99%
Prophylactic Antibiotic Timing (Outpatient)	309	96%	97%	98%
Urinary Catheter Removal[2]	327	100%	97%	97%
Survey of Patients' Hospital Experiences				
Area Around Room 'Always' Quiet at Night	300+	51%	51%	61%
Doctors 'Always' Communicated Well	300+	72%	78%	82%
Home Recovery Information Given	300+	81%	83%	85%
Hospital Given 9 or 10 on 10 Point Scale	300+	66%	68%	71%
Meds 'Always' Explained Before Given	300+	55%	61%	64%
Nurses 'Always' Communicated Well	300+	71%	74%	79%
Pain 'Always' Well Controlled	300+	62%	68%	71%
Room and Bathroom 'Always' Clean	300+	73%	70%	73%
Timely Help 'Always' Received	300+	55%	62%	68%
Would Definitely Recommend Hospital	300+	60%	70%	71%
Use of Medical Imaging				
Cardiac Imaging Stress Test before Surgery	111	7.2%	5.2%	5.3%
Combination Abdominal CT Scan	857	9.2%	13.4%	10.5%
Combination Brain/Sinus CT Scan	919	0.5%	2.2%	2.7%
Combination Chest CT Scan	332	0.0%	2.3%	2.7%
Follow-up Mammogram/Ultrasound	1,575	4.7%	8.2%	8.8%
Lumbar Spine MRI for Low Back Pain	112	27.7%	34.2%	37.2%

Sierra View District Hospital

465 W Putnam Ave — Phone: 559-784-1110
Porterville, CA 93257 — Fax: 559-788-6135
E-mail: webmaster@sierra-view.com
URL: www.sierra-view.com
Type: Acute Care Hospitals — Emergency Services: Yes
Ownership: Voluntary non-profit - Private — Beds: 163

Key Personnel:
CEO/President. . . . . Donna Hefner
Quality Assurance . . . . Donna Hefner
Infection Control. . . . . Betty Jones
Intensive Care Unit. . . . . Kris Reddell
Chief of Medical Staff. . . . . Harpreet Sandhu, MD
Operating Room. . . . . Pramod Srivastava
Radiology. . . . . Brenda Welling
Patient Relations . . . . Kathleen Widlund

Measure	Cases	This Hosp.	State Avg.	U.S. Avg.
Blood Clot Prevention and Treatment				
Anticoagulation Overlap Therapy[1,2]	-	-	92%	93%
ICU Venous Thromboembolism Prophylaxis[2]	82	80%	92%	92%
Incidence of Potentially Preventable VTE[1,2]	-	-	11%	10%
UFH with Dosages/Platelet Monitoring[1,2]	-	-	96%	97%
Venous Thromboembolism Prophylaxis[2]	435	76%	83%	85%
Warfarin Therapy Discharge Instructions[1,2]	-	-	75%	75%
Chest Pain/Possible Heart Attack Care				
Aspirin Given Within 24 Hours of Arrival	15	100%	97%	96%
Fibrinolytic Meds Within 30 Min. of Arrival[1]	-	-	62%	58%
Average Time to ECG (minutes)	17	10	9	7
Average Time to Transfer (minutes)[1]	-	-	62	60
Children's Asthma Care				
Received Home Management Plan of Care	-	-	88%	88%
Received Reliever Medication	-	-	100%	100%
Received Systemic Corticosteroids	-	-	100%	100%
Emergency Department				
Admittance Decision Time (minutes)[2]	668	105	125	98
Head CT Results Within 45 Min. of Arrival[1]	-	-	55%	57%
Patients Who Left ER Before Being Seen	43,805	3%	3%	2%
Time from ER Arrival to Admit. (minutes)[2]	680	389	323	274
Time from ER Arrival to Discharge (minutes)	464	176	168	134
Time in ER Before Being Evaluated (minutes)	441	44	29	26
Time to Pain Meds for Fractures (minutes)	86	93	62	57
Heart Attack Care				
Aspirin Given at Discharge	36	92%	99%	99%
Fibrinolytic Meds Within 30 Min. of Arrival[1]	-	-	73%	54%
PCI Within 90 Minutes of Arrival[7]	-	-	95%	96%
Statin Prescribed at Discharge	37	81%	98%	98%
Heart Failure Care				
ACE Inhibitor or ARB for LVSD	57	95%	97%	97%
Discharge Instructions Given	151	99%	94%	94%
Evaluation of LVS Function	170	95%	99%	99%

NOTE: Hospital profiles are in alphabetical order by state, then city, then hospital within the city; Rankings exclude hospitals with less than 25 cases except for patient surveys which excludes hospitals with less than 100 cases; (a) 100-299 cases; (1) The number of cases/patients is too few to report; (2) Data submitted were based on a sample of cases/patients; (3) Results are based on a shorter time period than required; (4) Data suppressed by CMS for one or more quarters; (5) Results are not available for this reporting period; (6) Fewer than 100 patients completed the HCAHPS survey; (7) No cases met the criteria for this measure; (8) The lower limit of the confidence interval cannot be calculated if the number of observed infections equals zero; (9) No data are available from the state/territory for this reporting period; (10) The scores shown reflect fewer than 50 completed surveys; (11) There were discrepancies in the data collection process; (12) This measure does not apply to this hospital for this reporting period; (13) Results cannot be calculated for this reporting period; (14) The results for this state are combined with nearby states to protect confidentiality; Please refer to the User's Guide for a full explanation of data.

Measure	Cases	This Hosp.	State Avg.	U.S. Avg.
Medicare Spending				
Medicare Spending per Patient (ratio)	-	0.93	0.98	0.98
Pneumonia Care				
Appropriate Initial Antibiotic Given	152	91%	97%	95%
Blood Culture Timing	200	97%	98%	98%
Pregnancy and Delivery Care				
Newborn Deliveries Scheduled Early[2]	51	14%	5%	6%
Preventive Care				
Immunization for Influenza[2]	553	94%	89%	90%
Immunization for Pneumonia[2]	528	93%	90%	92%
Stroke Care				
Anticoagulation Therapy for Atrial Fibrillation[1]	-	-	95%	95%
Antithrombotic Therapy Timing	57	98%	98%	98%
Assessed for Rehabilitation	54	83%	97%	97%
Discharged on Antithrombotic Therapy	50	96%	99%	99%
Discharged on Statin Medication	39	56%	94%	94%
Thrombolytic Therapy Timing	12	8%	72%	66%
Venous Thromboembolism Prophylaxis	58	84%	94%	94%
Written Stroke Educational Materials Given	30	77%	87%	88%
Surgical Care Improvement Project				
Appropriate Beta Blocker Usage	37	100%	97%	98%
Appropriate VTP Within 24 Hours	256	98%	98%	98%
Controlled Postoperative Blood Glucose[7]	-	-	96%	97%
Perioperative Temperature Management	271	100%	100%	100%
Prophylactic Antibiotic Selection	187	99%	99%	99%
Prophylactic Antibiotic Selection (Outpatient)	126	96%	97%	98%
Prophylactic Antibiotic Stopped	174	98%	98%	98%
Prophylactic Antibiotic Timing	187	100%	99%	99%
Prophylactic Antibiotic Timing (Outpatient)	128	98%	97%	98%
Urinary Catheter Removal	141	99%	97%	97%
Survey of Patients' Hospital Experiences				
Area Around Room 'Always' Quiet at Night	300+	53%	51%	61%
Doctors 'Always' Communicated Well	300+	79%	78%	82%
Home Recovery Information Given	300+	83%	83%	85%
Hospital Given 9 or 10 on 10 Point Scale	300+	63%	68%	71%
Meds 'Always' Explained Before Given	300+	66%	61%	64%
Nurses 'Always' Communicated Well	300+	76%	74%	79%
Pain 'Always' Well Controlled	300+	70%	68%	71%
Room and Bathroom 'Always' Clean	300+	70%	70%	73%
Timely Help 'Always' Received	300+	64%	62%	68%
Would Definitely Recommend Hospital	300+	56%	70%	71%
Use of Medical Imaging				
Cardiac Imaging Stress Test before Surgery[7]	-	-	5.2%	5.3%
Combination Abdominal CT Scan	642	24.0%	13.4%	10.5%
Combination Brain/Sinus CT Scan	732	2.2%	2.2%	2.7%
Combination Chest CT Scan	353	32.9%	2.3%	2.7%
Follow-up Mammogram/Ultrasound	1,463	9.0%	8.2%	8.8%
Lumbar Spine MRI for Low Back Pain	105	28.6%	34.2%	37.2%

Eastern Plumas Hospital - Portola Campus

500 First Avenue
Portola, CA 96122
Phone: 530-832-4277
Fax: 530-832-4494
E-mail: info@ephc.org
URL: www.ephc.org
Type: Critical Access Hospitals
Emergency Services: Yes
Ownership: Govt - Hospital Dist/Auth
Beds: 24

Key Personnel:
CEO . . . . Tom Hayes
Operating Room. . . . . Lisa Hogan, RN
Radiology. . . . . Robert Leckie, MD
Quality Assurance . . . . Leslie Solomon
Chief of Medical Staff . . . . Paul Swanson, M.D

Measure	Cases	This Hosp.	State Avg.	U.S. Avg.
Blood Clot Prevention and Treatment				
Anticoagulation Overlap Therapy[5]	-	-	92%	93%
ICU Venous Thromboembolism Prophylaxis[5]	-	-	92%	92%
Incidence of Potentially Preventable VTE[5]	-	-	11%	10%
UFH with Dosages/Platelet Monitoring[5]	-	-	96%	97%
Venous Thromboembolism Prophylaxis[5]	-	-	83%	85%
Warfarin Therapy Discharge Instructions[5]	-	-	75%	75%
Chest Pain/Possible Heart Attack Care				
Aspirin Given Within 24 Hours of Arrival[3]	16	100%	97%	96%
Fibrinolytic Meds Within 30 Min. of Arrival[1,3]	-	-	62%	58%
Average Time to ECG (minutes)[3]	18	12	9	7
Average Time to Transfer (minutes)[1,3]	-	-	62	60
Children's Asthma Care				
Received Home Management Plan of Care	-	-	88%	88%
Received Reliever Medication	-	-	100%	100%
Received Systemic Corticosteroids	-	-	100%	100%
Emergency Department				
Admittance Decision Time (minutes)[5]	-	-	125	98
Head CT Results Within 45 Min. of Arrival[1,3]	-	-	55%	57%
Patients Who Left ER Before Being Seen[5]	-	-	3%	2%
Time from ER Arrival to Admit. (minutes)[5]	-	-	323	274
Time from ER Arrival to Discharge (minutes)[5]	-	-	168	134
Time in ER Before Being Evaluated (minutes)[5]	-	-	29	26
Time to Pain Meds for Fractures (minutes)[5]	-	-	62	57
Heart Attack Care				
Aspirin Given at Discharge[5]	-	-	99%	99%
Fibrinolytic Meds Within 30 Min. of Arrival[5]	-	-	73%	54%
PCI Within 90 Minutes of Arrival[5]	-	-	95%	96%
Statin Prescribed at Discharge[5]	-	-	98%	98%
Heart Failure Care				
ACE Inhibitor or ARB for LVSD[1,3]	-	-	97%	97%
Discharge Instructions Given[1,3]	-	-	94%	94%
Evaluation of LVS Function[1,3]	-	-	99%	99%
Medicare Spending				
Medicare Spending per Patient (ratio)	-	-	0.98	0.98
Pneumonia Care				
Appropriate Initial Antibiotic Given[3]	14	79%	97%	95%
Blood Culture Timing[3]	17	88%	98%	98%
Pregnancy and Delivery Care				
Newborn Deliveries Scheduled Early[5]	-	-	5%	6%
Preventive Care				
Immunization for Influenza[5]	-	-	89%	90%
Immunization for Pneumonia[5]	-	-	90%	92%
Stroke Care				
Anticoagulation Therapy for Atrial Fibrillation[5]	-	-	95%	95%
Antithrombotic Therapy Timing[5]	-	-	98%	98%
Assessed for Rehabilitation[5]	-	-	97%	97%
Discharged on Antithrombotic Therapy[5]	-	-	99%	99%
Discharged on Statin Medication[5]	-	-	94%	94%
Thrombolytic Therapy Timing[5]	-	-	72%	66%
Venous Thromboembolism Prophylaxis[5]	-	-	94%	94%
Written Stroke Educational Materials Given[5]	-	-	87%	88%
Surgical Care Improvement Project				
Appropriate Beta Blocker Usage[5]	-	-	97%	98%
Appropriate VTP Within 24 Hours[5]	-	-	98%	98%
Controlled Postoperative Blood Glucose[5]	-	-	96%	97%
Perioperative Temperature Management[5]	-	-	100%	100%
Prophylactic Antibiotic Selection[5]	-	-	99%	99%
Prophylactic Antibiotic Selection (Outpatient)[5]	-	-	97%	98%
Prophylactic Antibiotic Stopped[5]	-	-	98%	98%
Prophylactic Antibiotic Timing[5]	-	-	99%	99%
Prophylactic Antibiotic Timing (Outpatient)[5]	-	-	97%	98%
Urinary Catheter Removal[5]	-	-	97%	97%
Survey of Patients' Hospital Experiences				
Area Around Room 'Always' Quiet at Night[5]	-	-	51%	61%
Doctors 'Always' Communicated Well[5]	-	-	78%	82%
Home Recovery Information Given[5]	-	-	83%	85%
Hospital Given 9 or 10 on 10 Point Scale[5]	-	-	68%	71%
Meds 'Always' Explained Before Given[5]	-	-	61%	64%
Nurses 'Always' Communicated Well[5]	-	-	74%	79%
Pain 'Always' Well Controlled[5]	-	-	68%	71%
Room and Bathroom 'Always' Clean[5]	-	-	70%	73%
Timely Help 'Always' Received[5]	-	-	62%	68%
Would Definitely Recommend Hospital[5]	-	-	70%	71%
Use of Medical Imaging				
Cardiac Imaging Stress Test before Surgery[7]	-	-	5.2%	5.3%
Combination Abdominal CT Scan	129	2.3%	13.4%	10.5%
Combination Brain/Sinus CT Scan[1]	-	-	2.2%	2.7%
Combination Chest CT Scan	47	0.0%	2.3%	2.7%
Follow-up Mammogram/Ultrasound	159	12.6%	8.2%	8.8%
Lumbar Spine MRI for Low Back Pain[1]	-	-	34.2%	37.2%

Pomerado Hospital

15615 Pomerado Road
Poway, CA 92064
Phone: 858-485-6511
Fax: 858-675-5077
URL: www.pph.org
Type: Acute Care Hospitals
Emergency Services: Yes
Ownership: Govt - Hospital Dist/Auth
Beds: 107

Key Personnel:
Administrator . . . . Sheila Brown
President/CEO. . . . . Michael H. Covert, FACHE
Quality Assurance . . . . Janie Fríncke, RN
Radiology. . . . . Thomas G Goergen, MD
Operating Room. . . . . Peggy Orr
Administrator . . . . David Tam, MD, FACHE
Infection Control. . . . . Val Tesoro, MD
Chief of Medical Staff . . . . Paul Tornambe

Measure	Cases	This Hosp.	State Avg.	U.S. Avg.
Blood Clot Prevention and Treatment				
Anticoagulation Overlap Therapy[2]	48	92%	92%	93%
ICU Venous Thromboembolism Prophylaxis[2]	71	87%	92%	92%
Incidence of Potentially Preventable VTE[1,2]	-	-	11%	10%
UFH with Dosages/Platelet Monitoring[2]	18	100%	96%	97%
Venous Thromboembolism Prophylaxis[2]	313	72%	83%	85%
Warfarin Therapy Discharge Instructions[2]	30	57%	75%	75%
Chest Pain/Possible Heart Attack Care				
Aspirin Given Within 24 Hours of Arrival	37	100%	97%	96%
Fibrinolytic Meds Within 30 Min. of Arrival[7]	-	-	62%	58%
Average Time to ECG (minutes)	37	14	9	7
Average Time to Transfer (minutes)	12	64	62	60
Children's Asthma Care				
Received Home Management Plan of Care	-	-	88%	88%
Received Reliever Medication	-	-	100%	100%
Received Systemic Corticosteroids	-	-	100%	100%
Emergency Department				
Admittance Decision Time (minutes)[2]	504	136	125	98
Head CT Results Within 45 Min. of Arrival	15	60%	55%	57%
Patients Who Left ER Before Being Seen	20,062	0%	3%	2%
Time from ER Arrival to Admit. (minutes)[2]	508	298	323	274
Time from ER Arrival to Discharge (minutes)	358	156	168	134
Time in ER Before Being Evaluated (minutes)	392	17	29	26
Time to Pain Meds for Fractures (minutes)	143	53	62	57
Heart Attack Care				
Aspirin Given at Discharge	33	97%	99%	99%
Fibrinolytic Meds Within 30 Min. of Arrival[7]	-	-	73%	54%
PCI Within 90 Minutes of Arrival[7]	-	-	95%	96%
Statin Prescribed at Discharge	28	86%	98%	98%
Heart Failure Care				
ACE Inhibitor or ARB for LVSD	41	95%	97%	97%
Discharge Instructions Given	134	100%	94%	94%
Evaluation of LVS Function	173	98%	99%	99%
Medicare Spending				
Medicare Spending per Patient (ratio)	-	0.95	0.98	0.98
Pneumonia Care				
Appropriate Initial Antibiotic Given	129	98%	97%	95%
Blood Culture Timing	169	96%	98%	98%
Pregnancy and Delivery Care				
Newborn Deliveries Scheduled Early[2]	28	0%	5%	6%
Preventive Care				
Immunization for Influenza[2]	484	77%	89%	90%
Immunization for Pneumonia[2]	530	81%	90%	92%
Stroke Care				
Anticoagulation Therapy for Atrial Fibrillation[1,2]	-	-	95%	95%
Antithrombotic Therapy Timing[2]	61	98%	98%	98%
Assessed for Rehabilitation[2]	59	100%	97%	97%
Discharged on Antithrombotic Therapy[2]	58	98%	99%	99%
Discharged on Statin Medication[2]	44	93%	94%	94%
Thrombolytic Therapy Timing[2]	12	42%	72%	66%
Venous Thromboembolism Prophylaxis[2]	62	87%	94%	94%
Written Stroke Educational Materials Given[2]	34	91%	87%	88%
Surgical Care Improvement Project				
Appropriate Beta Blocker Usage[2]	57	82%	97%	98%
Appropriate VTP Within 24 Hours[2]	279	98%	98%	98%
Controlled Postoperative Blood Glucose[2,7]	-	-	96%	97%
Perioperative Temperature Management[2]	338	100%	100%	100%
Prophylactic Antibiotic Selection[2]	219	100%	99%	99%

NOTE: Hospital profiles are in alphabetical order by state, then city, then hospital within the city; Rankings exclude hospitals with less than 25 cases except for patient surveys which excludes hospitals with less than 100 cases; (a) 100-299 cases; (1) The number of cases/patients is too few to report; (2) Data submitted were based on a sample of cases/patients; (3) Results are based on a shorter time period than required; (4) Data suppressed by CMS for one or more quarters; (5) Results are not available for this reporting period; (6) Fewer than 100 patients completed the HCAHPS survey; (7) No cases met the criteria for this measure; (8) The lower limit of the confidence interval cannot be calculated if the number of observed infections equals zero; (9) No data are available from the state/territory for this reporting period; (10) The scores shown reflect fewer than 50 completed surveys; (11) There were discrepancies in the data collection process; (12) This measure does not apply to this hospital for this reporting period; (13) Results cannot be calculated for this reporting period; (14) The results for this state are combined with nearby states to protect confidentiality; Please refer to the User's Guide for a full explanation of data.

Prophylactic Antibiotic Selection (Outpatient)	69	70%	97%	98%
Prophylactic Antibiotic Stopped[2]	217	99%	98%	98%
Prophylactic Antibiotic Timing[2]	219	99%	99%	99%
Prophylactic Antibiotic Timing (Outpatient)	69	84%	97%	98%
Urinary Catheter Removal[2]	172	93%	97%	97%
Survey of Patients' Hospital Experiences				
Area Around Room 'Always' Quiet at Night	300+	47%	51%	61%
Doctors 'Always' Communicated Well	300+	83%	78%	82%
Home Recovery Information Given	300+	81%	83%	85%
Hospital Given 9 or 10 on 10 Point Scale	300+	67%	68%	71%
Meds 'Always' Explained Before Given	300+	63%	61%	64%
Nurses 'Always' Communicated Well	300+	75%	74%	79%
Pain 'Always' Well Controlled	300+	71%	68%	71%
Room and Bathroom 'Always' Clean	300+	61%	70%	73%
Timely Help 'Always' Received	300+	70%	62%	68%
Would Definitely Recommend Hospital	300+	72%	70%	71%
Use of Medical Imaging				
Cardiac Imaging Stress Test before Surgery	130	3.1%	5.2%	5.3%
Combination Abdominal CT Scan	456	2.0%	13.4%	10.5%
Combination Brain/Sinus CT Scan	629	2.7%	2.2%	2.7%
Combination Chest CT Scan	126	0.0%	2.3%	2.7%
Follow-up Mammogram/Ultrasound	662	13.1%	8.2%	8.8%
Lumbar Spine MRI for Low Back Pain[1]	-	-	34.2%	37.2%

Plumas District Hospital

1065 Bucks Lake Road
Quincy, CA 95971
Phone: 530-283-2121
Fax: 530-283-7953
URL: www.pdh.org
Type: Critical Access Hospitals
Emergency Services: Yes
Ownership: Govt - Hospital Dist/Auth
Beds: 26

Key Personnel:
Infection Control. . . . . Linda Buddenbrock
CEO/President. . . . . Richard Hathaway
Quality Assurance . . . . Marilyn Johannson
Chief of Medical Staff. . . . . Jeffrey Kepple, MD
Emergency Room . . . . Mark Satterfield

Measure	Cases	This Hosp.	State Avg.	U.S. Avg.
Blood Clot Prevention and Treatment				
Anticoagulation Overlap Therapy[5]	-	-	92%	93%
ICU Venous Thromboembolism Prophylaxis[5]	-	-	92%	92%
Incidence of Potentially Preventable VTE[5]	-	-	11%	10%
UFH with Dosages/Platelet Monitoring[5]	-	-	96%	97%
Venous Thromboembolism Prophylaxis[5]	-	-	83%	85%
Warfarin Therapy Discharge Instructions[5]	-	-	75%	75%
Chest Pain/Possible Heart Attack Care				
Aspirin Given Within 24 Hours of Arrival	-	-	97%	96%
Fibrinolytic Meds Within 30 Min. of Arrival	-	-	62%	58%
Average Time to ECG (minutes)	-	-	9	7
Average Time to Transfer (minutes)	-	-	62	60
Children's Asthma Care				
Received Home Management Plan of Care	-	-	88%	88%
Received Reliever Medication	-	-	100%	100%
Received Systemic Corticosteroids	-	-	100%	100%
Emergency Department				
Admittance Decision Time (minutes)[5]	-	-	125	98
Head CT Results Within 45 Min. of Arrival	-	-	55%	57%
Patients Who Left ER Before Being Seen	-	-	3%	2%
Time from ER Arrival to Admit. (minutes)[5]	-	-	323	274
Time from ER Arrival to Discharge (minutes)	-	-	168	134
Time in ER Before Being Evaluated (minutes)	-	-	29	26
Time to Pain Meds for Fractures (minutes)	-	-	62	57
Heart Attack Care				
Aspirin Given at Discharge[5]	-	-	99%	99%
Fibrinolytic Meds Within 30 Min. of Arrival[6]	-	-	73%	54%
PCI Within 90 Minutes of Arrival[5]	-	-	95%	96%
Statin Prescribed at Discharge[5]	-	-	98%	98%
Heart Failure Care				
ACE Inhibitor or ARB for LVSD[5]	-	-	97%	97%
Discharge Instructions Given[5]	-	-	94%	94%
Evaluation of LVS Function[5]	-	-	99%	99%
Medicare Spending				
Medicare Spending per Patient (ratio)	-	-	0.98	0.98
Pneumonia Care				
Appropriate Initial Antibiotic Given[1,3]	-	-	97%	95%
Blood Culture Timing[1,3]	-	-	98%	98%
Pregnancy and Delivery Care				
Newborn Deliveries Scheduled Early[5]	-	-	5%	6%
Preventive Care				
Immunization for Influenza[5]	-	-	89%	90%
Immunization for Pneumonia[5]	-	-	90%	92%
Stroke Care				
Anticoagulation Therapy for Atrial Fibrillation[5]	-	-	95%	95%
Antithrombotic Therapy Timing[5]	-	-	98%	98%
Assessed for Rehabilitation[5]	-	-	97%	97%
Discharged on Antithrombotic Therapy[5]	-	-	99%	99%
Discharged on Statin Medication[5]	-	-	94%	94%
Thrombolytic Therapy Timing[5]	-	-	72%	66%
Venous Thromboembolism Prophylaxis[5]	-	-	94%	94%
Written Stroke Educational Materials Given[5]	-	-	87%	88%
Surgical Care Improvement Project				
Appropriate Beta Blocker Usage[5]	-	-	97%	98%
Appropriate VTP Within 24 Hours[5]	-	-	98%	98%
Controlled Postoperative Blood Glucose[5]	-	-	96%	97%
Perioperative Temperature Management[5]	-	-	100%	100%
Prophylactic Antibiotic Selection[5]	-	-	99%	99%
Prophylactic Antibiotic Selection (Outpatient)	-	-	97%	98%
Prophylactic Antibiotic Stopped[5]	-	-	98%	98%
Prophylactic Antibiotic Timing[5]	-	-	99%	99%
Prophylactic Antibiotic Timing (Outpatient)	-	-	97%	98%
Urinary Catheter Removal[5]	-	-	97%	97%
Survey of Patients' Hospital Experiences				
Area Around Room 'Always' Quiet at Night[5]	-	-	51%	61%
Doctors 'Always' Communicated Well[5]	-	-	78%	82%
Home Recovery Information Given[5]	-	-	83%	85%
Hospital Given 9 or 10 on 10 Point Scale[5]	-	-	68%	71%
Meds 'Always' Explained Before Given[5]	-	-	61%	64%
Nurses 'Always' Communicated Well[5]	-	-	74%	79%
Pain 'Always' Well Controlled[5]	-	-	68%	71%
Room and Bathroom 'Always' Clean[5]	-	-	70%	73%
Timely Help 'Always' Received[5]	-	-	62%	68%
Would Definitely Recommend Hospital[5]	-	-	70%	71%
Use of Medical Imaging				
Cardiac Imaging Stress Test before Surgery	-	-	5.2%	5.3%
Combination Abdominal CT Scan	-	-	13.4%	10.5%
Combination Brain/Sinus CT Scan	-	-	2.2%	2.7%
Combination Chest CT Scan	-	-	2.3%	2.7%
Follow-up Mammogram/Ultrasound	-	-	8.2%	8.8%
Lumbar Spine MRI for Low Back Pain	-	-	34.2%	37.2%

Eisenhower Medical Center

39-000 Bob Hope Drive
Rancho Mirage, CA 92270
Phone: 760-340-3911
Fax: 760-773-1421
URL: www.emc.org
Type: Acute Care Hospitals
Emergency Services: Yes
Ownership: Proprietary
Beds: 253

Key Personnel:
Quality Assurance . . . . Janice Campodallorto
Operating Room. . . . . Lynn Hart
Radiology. . . . . Brian Herman, MD
Pediatric Ambulatory Care . . . . . . Arturo Quintanilla, MD
Pediatric In-Patient Care . . . . Arturo Quintanilla, MD
Infection Control. . . . . Farzana Qureshi, MD
Chief of Medical Staff. . . . . Stephen Steele, DO
President. . . . . Shahriyar Tavakoli, MD

Measure	Cases	This Hosp.	State Avg.	U.S. Avg.
Blood Clot Prevention and Treatment				
Anticoagulation Overlap Therapy[2]	86	97%	92%	93%
ICU Venous Thromboembolism Prophylaxis[2]	44	98%	92%	92%
Incidence of Potentially Preventable VTE[2]	12	0%	11%	10%
UFH with Dosages/Platelet Monitoring[2]	69	100%	96%	97%
Venous Thromboembolism Prophylaxis[2]	332	75%	83%	85%
Warfarin Therapy Discharge Instructions[2]	65	88%	75%	75%
Chest Pain/Possible Heart Attack Care				
Aspirin Given Within 24 Hours of Arrival[1,3]	-	-	97%	96%
Fibrinolytic Meds Within 30 Min. of Arrival[5]	-	-	62%	58%
Average Time to ECG (minutes)[1,3]	-	-	9	7
Average Time to Transfer (minutes)[5]	-	-	62	60
Children's Asthma Care				
Received Home Management Plan of Care	-	-	88%	88%
Received Reliever Medication	-	-	100%	100%
Received Systemic Corticosteroids	-	-	100%	100%
Emergency Department				
Admittance Decision Time (minutes)[2]	1,240	114	125	98
Head CT Results Within 45 Min. of Arrival[1]	-	-	55%	57%
Patients Who Left ER Before Being Seen	68,057	1%	3%	2%
Time from ER Arrival to Admit. (minutes)[2]	1,246	320	323	274
Time from ER Arrival to Discharge (minutes)	387	205	168	134
Time in ER Before Being Evaluated (minutes)	397	43	29	26
Time to Pain Meds for Fractures (minutes)	319	79	62	57
Heart Attack Care				
Aspirin Given at Discharge	376	98%	99%	99%
Fibrinolytic Meds Within 30 Min. of Arrival[7]	-	-	73%	54%
PCI Within 90 Minutes of Arrival	56	89%	95%	96%
Statin Prescribed at Discharge	364	98%	98%	98%
Heart Failure Care				
ACE Inhibitor or ARB for LVSD	202	90%	97%	97%
Discharge Instructions Given	436	95%	94%	94%
Evaluation of LVS Function	543	100%	99%	99%
Medicare Spending				
Medicare Spending per Patient (ratio)	-	0.99	0.98	0.98
Pneumonia Care				
Appropriate Initial Antibiotic Given	328	99%	97%	95%
Blood Culture Timing	492	98%	98%	98%
Pregnancy and Delivery Care				
Newborn Deliveries Scheduled Early[7]	-	-	5%	6%
Preventive Care				
Immunization for Influenza[2]	932	82%	89%	90%
Immunization for Pneumonia[2]	1,308	81%	90%	92%
Stroke Care				
Anticoagulation Therapy for Atrial Fibrillation	46	100%	95%	95%
Antithrombotic Therapy Timing	295	99%	98%	98%
Assessed for Rehabilitation	408	97%	97%	97%
Discharged on Antithrombotic Therapy	369	100%	99%	99%
Discharged on Statin Medication	264	97%	94%	94%
Thrombolytic Therapy Timing	27	93%	72%	66%
Venous Thromboembolism Prophylaxis	369	95%	94%	94%
Written Stroke Educational Materials Given	221	97%	87%	88%
Surgical Care Improvement Project				
Appropriate Beta Blocker Usage	488	98%	97%	98%
Appropriate VTP Within 24 Hours	1,383	98%	98%	98%
Controlled Postoperative Blood Glucose	214	98%	96%	97%
Perioperative Temperature Management	1,634	100%	100%	100%
Prophylactic Antibiotic Selection	1,161	99%	99%	99%
Prophylactic Antibiotic Selection (Outpatient)	496	97%	97%	98%
Prophylactic Antibiotic Stopped	1,146	98%	98%	98%
Prophylactic Antibiotic Timing	1,163	99%	99%	99%
Prophylactic Antibiotic Timing (Outpatient)	499	96%	97%	98%
Urinary Catheter Removal	1,307	96%	97%	97%
Survey of Patients' Hospital Experiences				
Area Around Room 'Always' Quiet at Night	300+	58%	51%	61%
Doctors 'Always' Communicated Well	300+	79%	78%	82%
Home Recovery Information Given	300+	84%	83%	85%
Hospital Given 9 or 10 on 10 Point Scale	300+	77%	68%	71%
Meds 'Always' Explained Before Given	300+	63%	61%	64%
Nurses 'Always' Communicated Well	300+	77%	74%	79%
Pain 'Always' Well Controlled	300+	71%	68%	71%
Room and Bathroom 'Always' Clean	300+	73%	70%	73%
Timely Help 'Always' Received	300+	63%	62%	68%
Would Definitely Recommend Hospital	300+	83%	70%	71%
Use of Medical Imaging				
Cardiac Imaging Stress Test before Surgery	1,150	6.1%	5.2%	5.3%
Combination Abdominal CT Scan	1,272	49.7%	13.4%	10.5%
Combination Brain/Sinus CT Scan	1,210	2.4%	2.2%	2.7%
Combination Chest CT Scan	84	8.3%	2.3%	2.7%
Follow-up Mammogram/Ultrasound	6,860	8.9%	8.2%	8.8%
Lumbar Spine MRI for Low Back Pain[1]	-	-	34.2%	37.2%

NOTE: Hospital profiles are in alphabetical order by state, then city, then hospital within the city; Rankings exclude hospitals with less than 25 cases except for patient surveys which excludes hospitals with less than 100 cases; (a) 100-299 cases; (1) The number of cases/patients is too few to report; (2) Data submitted were based on a sample of cases/patients; (3) Results are based on a shorter time period than required; (4) Data suppressed by CMS for one or more quarters; (5) Results are not available for this reporting period; (6) Fewer than 100 patients completed the HCAHPS survey; (7) No cases met the criteria for this measure; (8) The lower limit of the confidence interval cannot be calculated if the number of observed infections equals zero; (9) No data are available from the state/territory for this reporting period; (10) The scores shown reflect fewer than 50 completed surveys; (11) There were discrepancies in the data collection process; (12) This measure does not apply to this hospital for this reporting period; (13) Results cannot be calculated for this reporting period; (14) The results for this state are combined with nearby states to protect confidentiality; Please refer to the User's Guide for a full explanation of data.

Saint Elizabeth Community Hospital

2550 Sister Mary Columba Drive Phone: 530-529-8012
Red Bluff, CA 96080 Fax: 530-529-8033
URL: www.redbluff.mercy.org
Type: Acute Care Hospitals Emergency Services: Yes
Ownership: Voluntary non-profit - Church Beds: 83

Key Personnel:
Chief of Medical Staff.......... George Bo-Linn, MD
Emergency Room .... Penny Costa, RN
Quality Assurance .... Charles P Francis
Pediatric Ambulatory Care ...... Joanne Heffner, RN
Pediatric In-Patient Care .... Joanne Heffner, RN
Radiology.................... Stephen L Hofkin, MD
CEO/President............... Tim Panks
Operating Room.............. Lauren P Strickland

Measure	Cases	This Hosp.	State Avg.	U.S. Avg.
Blood Clot Prevention and Treatment				
Anticoagulation Overlap Therapy[2]	11	73%	92%	93%
ICU Venous Thromboembolism Prophylaxis[1,2]	-	-	92%	92%
Incidence of Potentially Preventable VTE[1,2]	-	-	11%	10%
UFH with Dosages/Platelet Monitoring[1,2]	-	-	96%	97%
Venous Thromboembolism Prophylaxis[2]	194	84%	83%	85%
Warfarin Therapy Discharge Instructions[2]	12	58%	75%	75%
Chest Pain/Possible Heart Attack Care				
Aspirin Given Within 24 Hours of Arrival	77	96%	97%	96%
Fibrinolytic Meds Within 30 Min. of Arrival[7]	-	-	62%	58%
Average Time to ECG (minutes)	79	11	9	7
Average Time to Transfer (minutes)	21	108	62	60
Children's Asthma Care				
Received Home Management Plan of Care	-	-	88%	88%
Received Reliever Medication	-	-	100%	100%
Received Systemic Corticosteroids	-	-	100%	100%
Emergency Department				
Admittance Decision Time (minutes)[2]	330	106	125	98
Head CT Results Within 45 Min. of Arrival[1]	-	-	55%	57%
Patients Who Left ER Before Being Seen	30,472	1%	3%	2%
Time from ER Arrival to Admit. (minutes)[2]	364	270	323	274
Time from ER Arrival to Discharge (minutes)	382	146	168	134
Time in ER Before Being Evaluated (minutes)	396	17	29	26
Time to Pain Meds for Fractures (minutes)	164	50	62	57
Heart Attack Care				
Aspirin Given at Discharge[1]	-	-	99%	99%
Fibrinolytic Meds Within 30 Min. of Arrival[7]	-	-	73%	54%
PCI Within 90 Minutes of Arrival[7]	-	-	95%	96%
Statin Prescribed at Discharge[1]	-	-	98%	98%
Heart Failure Care				
ACE Inhibitor or ARB for LVSD	26	88%	97%	97%
Discharge Instructions Given	63	98%	94%	94%
Evaluation of LVS Function	77	97%	99%	99%
Medicare Spending				
Medicare Spending per Patient (ratio)	-	0.91	0.98	0.98
Pneumonia Care				
Appropriate Initial Antibiotic Given[2]	88	98%	97%	95%
Blood Culture Timing[2]	94	96%	98%	98%
Pregnancy and Delivery Care				
Newborn Deliveries Scheduled Early[2]	21	5%	5%	6%
Preventive Care				
Immunization for Influenza[2]	302	89%	89%	90%
Immunization for Pneumonia[2]	335	85%	90%	92%
Stroke Care				
Anticoagulation Therapy for Atrial Fibrillation[1]	-	-	95%	95%
Antithrombotic Therapy Timing	18	94%	98%	98%
Assessed for Rehabilitation	28	86%	97%	97%
Discharged on Antithrombotic Therapy	28	96%	99%	99%
Discharged on Statin Medication	27	44%	94%	94%
Thrombolytic Therapy Timing[1]	-	-	72%	66%
Venous Thromboembolism Prophylaxis	19	95%	94%	94%
Written Stroke Educational Materials Given	18	61%	87%	88%
Surgical Care Improvement Project				
Appropriate Beta Blocker Usage[2]	37	86%	97%	98%
Appropriate VTP Within 24 Hours[2]	146	97%	98%	98%
Controlled Postoperative Blood Glucose[2,7]	-	-	96%	97%
Perioperative Temperature Management[2]	237	100%	100%	100%
Prophylactic Antibiotic Selection[2]	149	99%	99%	99%
Prophylactic Antibiotic Selection (Outpatient)	79	100%	97%	98%
Prophylactic Antibiotic Stopped[2]	147	95%	98%	98%
Prophylactic Antibiotic Timing[2]	149	97%	99%	99%
Prophylactic Antibiotic Timing (Outpatient)	79	99%	97%	98%
Urinary Catheter Removal[2]	122	99%	97%	97%
Survey of Patients' Hospital Experiences				
Area Around Room 'Always' Quiet at Night	300+	47%	51%	61%
Doctors 'Always' Communicated Well	300+	81%	78%	82%
Home Recovery Information Given	300+	85%	83%	85%
Hospital Given 9 or 10 on 10 Point Scale	300+	67%	68%	71%
Meds 'Always' Explained Before Given	300+	63%	61%	64%
Nurses 'Always' Communicated Well	300+	75%	74%	79%
Pain 'Always' Well Controlled	300+	69%	68%	71%
Room and Bathroom 'Always' Clean	300+	72%	70%	73%
Timely Help 'Always' Received	300+	63%	62%	68%
Would Definitely Recommend Hospital	300+	69%	70%	71%
Use of Medical Imaging				
Cardiac Imaging Stress Test before Surgery	59	0.0%	5.2%	5.3%
Combination Abdominal CT Scan	755	5.2%	13.4%	10.5%
Combination Brain/Sinus CT Scan	606	3.8%	2.2%	2.7%
Combination Chest CT Scan	280	3.6%	2.3%	2.7%
Follow-up Mammogram/Ultrasound	568	5.1%	8.2%	8.8%
Lumbar Spine MRI for Low Back Pain	114	42.1%	34.2%	37.2%

Mercy Medical Center - Redding

2175 Rosaline Ave, Clairmont Hgts Phone: 530-225-6102
Redding, CA 96001 Fax: 530-225-6125
URL: www.redding.mercy.org
Type: Acute Care Hospitals Emergency Services: Yes
Ownership: Voluntary non-profit - Church Beds: 256

Key Personnel:
CEO/President............... Ray Barnet
Infection Control.............. Cathy Carl, RN
Operating Room.............. Lynn Heuer, RN
Intensive Care Unit............ Steven Struve, MD
Chief of Medical Staff.......... William de Vlaming, MD

Measure	Cases	This Hosp.	State Avg.	U.S. Avg.
Blood Clot Prevention and Treatment				
Anticoagulation Overlap Therapy[2]	61	93%	92%	93%
ICU Venous Thromboembolism Prophylaxis[2]	109	100%	92%	92%
Incidence of Potentially Preventable VTE[1,2]	-	-	11%	10%
UFH with Dosages/Platelet Monitoring[2]	25	100%	96%	97%
Venous Thromboembolism Prophylaxis[2]	273	91%	83%	85%
Warfarin Therapy Discharge Instructions[2]	40	100%	75%	75%
Chest Pain/Possible Heart Attack Care				
Aspirin Given Within 24 Hours of Arrival[1,3]	-	-	97%	96%
Fibrinolytic Meds Within 30 Min. of Arrival[5]	-	-	62%	58%
Average Time to ECG (minutes)[1,3]	-	-	9	7
Average Time to Transfer (minutes)[5]	-	-	62	60
Children's Asthma Care				
Received Home Management Plan of Care	-	-	88%	88%
Received Reliever Medication	-	-	100%	100%
Received Systemic Corticosteroids	-	-	100%	100%
Emergency Department				
Admittance Decision Time (minutes)[2]	508	173	125	98
Head CT Results Within 45 Min. of Arrival	14	36%	55%	57%
Patients Who Left ER Before Being Seen	48,804	2%	3%	2%
Time from ER Arrival to Admit. (minutes)[2]	537	355	323	274
Time from ER Arrival to Discharge (minutes)	364	166	168	134
Time in ER Before Being Evaluated (minutes)	405	21	29	26
Time to Pain Meds for Fractures (minutes)	207	62	62	57
Heart Attack Care				
Aspirin Given at Discharge[2]	234	100%	99%	99%
Fibrinolytic Meds Within 30 Min. of Arrival[2,7]	-	-	73%	54%
PCI Within 90 Minutes of Arrival[2]	29	90%	95%	96%
Statin Prescribed at Discharge[2]	232	100%	98%	98%
Heart Failure Care				
ACE Inhibitor or ARB for LVSD[2]	127	100%	97%	97%
Discharge Instructions Given[2]	229	97%	94%	94%
Evaluation of LVS Function[2]	307	100%	99%	99%
Medicare Spending				
Medicare Spending per Patient (ratio)	-	0.98	0.98	0.98
Pneumonia Care				
Appropriate Initial Antibiotic Given[2]	95	96%	97%	95%
Blood Culture Timing[2]	122	97%	98%	98%
Pregnancy and Delivery Care				
Newborn Deliveries Scheduled Early[2]	39	13%	5%	6%
Preventive Care				
Immunization for Influenza[2]	516	98%	89%	90%
Immunization for Pneumonia[2]	605	95%	90%	92%
Stroke Care				
Anticoagulation Therapy for Atrial Fibrillation	22	100%	95%	95%
Antithrombotic Therapy Timing	99	99%	98%	98%
Assessed for Rehabilitation	152	99%	97%	97%
Discharged on Antithrombotic Therapy	123	98%	99%	99%
Discharged on Statin Medication	91	93%	94%	94%
Thrombolytic Therapy Timing	14	100%	72%	66%
Venous Thromboembolism Prophylaxis	158	97%	94%	94%
Written Stroke Educational Materials Given	89	93%	87%	88%
Surgical Care Improvement Project				
Appropriate Beta Blocker Usage[2]	189	98%	97%	98%
Appropriate VTP Within 24 Hours[2]	399	98%	98%	98%
Controlled Postoperative Blood Glucose[2]	152	99%	96%	97%
Perioperative Temperature Management[2]	644	100%	100%	100%
Prophylactic Antibiotic Selection[2]	502	99%	99%	99%
Prophylactic Antibiotic Selection (Outpatient)	448	98%	97%	98%
Prophylactic Antibiotic Stopped[2]	495	97%	98%	98%
Prophylactic Antibiotic Timing[2]	506	99%	99%	99%
Prophylactic Antibiotic Timing (Outpatient)	448	99%	97%	98%
Urinary Catheter Removal[2]	458	97%	97%	97%
Survey of Patients' Hospital Experiences				
Area Around Room 'Always' Quiet at Night	300+	40%	51%	61%
Doctors 'Always' Communicated Well	300+	76%	78%	82%
Home Recovery Information Given	300+	85%	83%	85%
Hospital Given 9 or 10 on 10 Point Scale	300+	65%	68%	71%
Meds 'Always' Explained Before Given	300+	59%	61%	64%
Nurses 'Always' Communicated Well	300+	73%	74%	79%
Pain 'Always' Well Controlled	300+	65%	68%	71%
Room and Bathroom 'Always' Clean	300+	68%	70%	73%
Timely Help 'Always' Received	300+	56%	62%	68%
Would Definitely Recommend Hospital	300+	74%	70%	71%
Use of Medical Imaging				
Cardiac Imaging Stress Test before Surgery	134	3.7%	5.2%	5.3%
Combination Abdominal CT Scan	695	0.6%	13.4%	10.5%
Combination Brain/Sinus CT Scan	960	3.3%	2.2%	2.7%
Combination Chest CT Scan	148	0.7%	2.3%	2.7%
Follow-up Mammogram/Ultrasound[7]	-	-	8.2%	8.8%
Lumbar Spine MRI for Low Back Pain[1]	-	-	34.2%	37.2%

Patients' Hospital of Redding

2900 Eureka Way Phone: 530-225-8700
Redding, CA 96001
URL: www.patientshospital.com
Type: Acute Care Hospitals Emergency Services: No
Ownership: Proprietary

Measure	Cases	This Hosp.	State Avg.	U.S. Avg.
Blood Clot Prevention and Treatment				
Anticoagulation Overlap Therapy[7]	-	-	92%	93%
ICU Venous Thromboembolism Prophylaxis[7]	-	-	92%	92%
Incidence of Potentially Preventable VTE[7]	-	-	11%	10%
UFH with Dosages/Platelet Monitoring[7]	-	-	96%	97%
Venous Thromboembolism Prophylaxis	86	100%	83%	85%
Warfarin Therapy Discharge Instructions[7]	-	-	75%	75%
Chest Pain/Possible Heart Attack Care				
Aspirin Given Within 24 Hours of Arrival[5]	-	-	97%	96%
Fibrinolytic Meds Within 30 Min. of Arrival[5]	-	-	62%	58%
Average Time to ECG (minutes)[5]	-	-	9	7
Average Time to Transfer (minutes)[5]	-	-	62	60
Children's Asthma Care				
Received Home Management Plan of Care	-	-	88%	88%
Received Reliever Medication	-	-	100%	100%
Received Systemic Corticosteroids	-	-	100%	100%
Emergency Department				
Admittance Decision Time (minutes)[7]	-	-	125	98
Head CT Results Within 45 Min. of Arrival[5]	-	-	55%	57%

NOTE: Hospital profiles are in alphabetical order by state, then city, then hospital within the city; Rankings exclude hospitals with less than 25 cases except for patient surveys which excludes hospitals with less than 100 cases; (a) 100-299 cases; (1) The number of cases/patients is too few to report; (2) Data submitted were based on a sample of cases/patients; (3) Results are based on a shorter time period than required; (4) Data suppressed by CMS for one or more quarters; (5) Results are not available for this reporting period; (6) Fewer than 100 patients completed the HCAHPS survey; (7) No cases met the criteria for this measure; (8) The lower limit of the confidence interval cannot be calculated if the number of observed infections equals zero; (9) No data are available from the state/territory for this reporting period; (10) The scores shown reflect fewer than 50 completed surveys; (11) There were discrepancies in the data collection process; (12) This measure does not apply to this hospital for this reporting period; (13) Results cannot be calculated for this reporting period; (14) The results for this state are combined with nearby states to protect confidentiality; Please refer to the User's Guide for a full explanation of data.

Patients Who Left ER Before Being Seen[5]	-	-	3%	2%
Time from ER Arrival to Admit. (minutes)[7]	-	-	323	274
Time from ER Arrival to Discharge (minutes)[5]	-	-	168	134
Time in ER Before Being Evaluated (minutes)[5]	-	-	29	26
Time to Pain Meds for Fractures (minutes)[5]	-	-	62	57
Heart Attack Care				
Aspirin Given at Discharge[5]	-	-	99%	99%
Fibrinolytic Meds Within 30 Min. of Arrival[5]	-	-	73%	54%
PCI Within 90 Minutes of Arrival[5]	-	-	95%	96%
Statin Prescribed at Discharge[5]	-	-	98%	98%
Heart Failure Care				
ACE Inhibitor or ARB for LVSD[5]	-	-	97%	97%
Discharge Instructions Given[5]	-	-	94%	94%
Evaluation of LVS Function[5]	-	-	99%	99%
Medicare Spending				
Medicare Spending per Patient (ratio)	-	0.78	0.98	0.98
Pneumonia Care				
Appropriate Initial Antibiotic Given[5]	-	-	97%	95%
Blood Culture Timing[5]	-	-	98%	98%
Pregnancy and Delivery Care				
Newborn Deliveries Scheduled Early[7]	-	-	5%	6%
Preventive Care				
Immunization for Influenza	117	94%	89%	90%
Immunization for Pneumonia	96	91%	90%	92%
Stroke Care				
Anticoagulation Therapy for Atrial Fibrillation[5]	-	-	95%	95%
Antithrombotic Therapy Timing[5]	-	-	98%	98%
Assessed for Rehabilitation[5]	-	-	97%	97%
Discharged on Antithrombotic Therapy[5]	-	-	99%	99%
Discharged on Statin Medication[5]	-	-	94%	94%
Thrombolytic Therapy Timing[5]	-	-	72%	66%
Venous Thromboembolism Prophylaxis[5]	-	-	94%	94%
Written Stroke Educational Materials Given[5]	-	-	87%	88%
Surgical Care Improvement Project				
Appropriate Beta Blocker Usage[1]	-	-	97%	98%
Appropriate VTP Within 24 Hours	47	100%	98%	98%
Controlled Postoperative Blood Glucose[7]	-	-	96%	97%
Perioperative Temperature Management	51	100%	100%	100%
Prophylactic Antibiotic Selection	45	100%	99%	99%
Prophylactic Antibiotic Selection (Outpatient)	44	98%	97%	98%
Prophylactic Antibiotic Stopped	45	100%	98%	98%
Prophylactic Antibiotic Timing	45	100%	99%	99%
Prophylactic Antibiotic Timing (Outpatient)	44	100%	97%	98%
Urinary Catheter Removal	16	100%	97%	97%
Survey of Patients' Hospital Experiences				
Area Around Room 'Always' Quiet at Night	(a)	90%	51%	61%
Doctors 'Always' Communicated Well	(a)	89%	78%	82%
Home Recovery Information Given	(a)	93%	83%	85%
Hospital Given 9 or 10 on 10 Point Scale	(a)	95%	68%	71%
Meds 'Always' Explained Before Given	(a)	84%	61%	64%
Nurses 'Always' Communicated Well	(a)	94%	74%	79%
Pain 'Always' Well Controlled	(a)	82%	68%	71%
Room and Bathroom 'Always' Clean	(a)	90%	70%	73%
Timely Help 'Always' Received	(a)	93%	62%	68%
Would Definitely Recommend Hospital	(a)	96%	70%	71%
Use of Medical Imaging				
Cardiac Imaging Stress Test before Surgery[7]	-	-	5.2%	5.3%
Combination Abdominal CT Scan[7]	-	-	13.4%	10.5%
Combination Brain/Sinus CT Scan[7]	-	-	2.2%	2.7%
Combination Chest CT Scan[7]	-	-	2.3%	2.7%
Follow-up Mammogram/Ultrasound[7]	-	-	8.2%	8.8%
Lumbar Spine MRI for Low Back Pain[7]	-	-	34.2%	37.2%

Shasta Regional Medical Center

1100 Butte St
Redding, CA 96001
E-mail: info@shastaregional.com
URL: www.shastaregional.com
Type: Acute Care Hospitals
Ownership: Voluntary non-profit - Private

Phone: 530-244-5454
Fax: 530-244-5384
Emergency Services: Yes
Beds: 246

Key Personnel:
Cardiac Laboratory. . . . . Tamara Buadle
Quality Assurance . . . . Jan Chicoine
CEO . . . . Cyndy Gordon, RN, BSN, MBA
Emergency Room . . . . Marry House
Cardiac Laboratory. . . . . Mohamed Khan, MD
Chief of Medical Staff. . . . . Marcia McCampbell, MD
Infection Control. . . . . Matt Miles, MD
Anesthesiology. . . . . Rajnish Patel, MD

Measure	Cases	This Hosp.	State Avg.	U.S. Avg.
Blood Clot Prevention and Treatment				
Anticoagulation Overlap Therapy[2]	65	100%	92%	93%
ICU Venous Thromboembolism Prophylaxis[2]	72	96%	92%	92%
Incidence of Potentially Preventable VTE[1,2]	-	-	11%	10%
UFH with Dosages/Platelet Monitoring[2]	36	100%	96%	97%
Venous Thromboembolism Prophylaxis[2]	356	96%	83%	85%
Warfarin Therapy Discharge Instructions[2]	50	100%	75%	75%
Chest Pain/Possible Heart Attack Care				
Aspirin Given Within 24 Hours of Arrival[5]	-	-	97%	96%
Fibrinolytic Meds Within 30 Min. of Arrival[5]	-	-	62%	58%
Average Time to ECG (minutes)[5]	-	-	9	7
Average Time to Transfer (minutes)[5]	-	-	62	60
Children's Asthma Care				
Received Home Management Plan of Care	-	-	88%	88%
Received Reliever Medication	-	-	100%	100%
Received Systemic Corticosteroids	-	-	100%	100%
Emergency Department				
Admittance Decision Time (minutes)[2]	1,033	134	125	98
Head CT Results Within 45 Min. of Arrival[1]	-	-	55%	57%
Patients Who Left ER Before Being Seen	38,956	3%	3%	2%
Time from ER Arrival to Admit. (minutes)[2]	1,033	322	323	274
Time from ER Arrival to Discharge (minutes)	409	151	168	134
Time in ER Before Being Evaluated (minutes)	449	44	29	26
Time to Pain Meds for Fractures (minutes)	174	78	62	57
Heart Attack Care				
Aspirin Given at Discharge	160	99%	99%	99%
Fibrinolytic Meds Within 30 Min. of Arrival[7]	-	-	73%	54%
PCI Within 90 Minutes of Arrival	20	100%	95%	96%
Statin Prescribed at Discharge	144	99%	98%	98%
Heart Failure Care				
ACE Inhibitor or ARB for LVSD	95	100%	97%	97%
Discharge Instructions Given	245	100%	94%	94%
Evaluation of LVS Function	288	100%	99%	99%
Medicare Spending				
Medicare Spending per Patient (ratio)	-	0.92	0.98	0.98
Pneumonia Care				
Appropriate Initial Antibiotic Given	142	100%	97%	95%
Blood Culture Timing	212	100%	98%	98%
Pregnancy and Delivery Care				
Newborn Deliveries Scheduled Early[7]	-	-	5%	6%
Preventive Care				
Immunization for Influenza[2]	594	96%	89%	90%
Immunization for Pneumonia[2]	881	98%	90%	92%
Stroke Care				
Anticoagulation Therapy for Atrial Fibrillation	19	100%	95%	95%
Antithrombotic Therapy Timing	76	100%	98%	98%
Assessed for Rehabilitation	93	100%	97%	97%
Discharged on Antithrombotic Therapy	92	100%	99%	99%
Discharged on Statin Medication	63	100%	94%	94%
Thrombolytic Therapy Timing[1]	-	-	72%	66%
Venous Thromboembolism Prophylaxis	88	100%	94%	94%
Written Stroke Educational Materials Given	60	100%	87%	88%
Surgical Care Improvement Project				
Appropriate Beta Blocker Usage	144	99%	97%	98%
Appropriate VTP Within 24 Hours	453	99%	98%	98%
Controlled Postoperative Blood Glucose	83	100%	96%	97%
Perioperative Temperature Management	546	100%	100%	100%
Prophylactic Antibiotic Selection	418	100%	99%	99%
Prophylactic Antibiotic Selection (Outpatient)	218	99%	97%	98%
Prophylactic Antibiotic Stopped	410	99%	98%	98%
Prophylactic Antibiotic Timing	418	99%	99%	99%
Prophylactic Antibiotic Timing (Outpatient)	218	100%	97%	98%
Urinary Catheter Removal	412	98%	97%	97%
Survey of Patients' Hospital Experiences				
Area Around Room 'Always' Quiet at Night[11]	300+	50%	51%	61%
Doctors 'Always' Communicated Well[11]	300+	76%	78%	82%
Home Recovery Information Given[11]	300+	85%	83%	85%
Hospital Given 9 or 10 on 10 Point Scale[11]	300+	66%	68%	71%
Meds 'Always' Explained Before Given[11]	300+	60%	61%	64%
Nurses 'Always' Communicated Well[11]	300+	76%	74%	79%
Pain 'Always' Well Controlled[11]	300+	69%	68%	71%
Room and Bathroom 'Always' Clean[11]	300+	66%	70%	73%
Timely Help 'Always' Received[11]	300+	61%	62%	68%
Would Definitely Recommend Hospital[11]	300+	72%	70%	71%
Use of Medical Imaging				
Cardiac Imaging Stress Test before Surgery	65	3.1%	5.2%	5.3%
Combination Abdominal CT Scan	452	0.9%	13.4%	10.5%
Combination Brain/Sinus CT Scan	474	4.0%	2.2%	2.7%
Combination Chest CT Scan[1]	-	-	2.3%	2.7%
Follow-up Mammogram/Ultrasound[7]	-	-	8.2%	8.8%
Lumbar Spine MRI for Low Back Pain[1]	-	-	34.2%	37.2%

Redlands Community Hospital

350 Terracina Blvd
Redlands, CA 92373
URL: www.redlandshospital.com
Type: Acute Care Hospitals
Ownership: Government - Federal

Phone: 909-335-5500
Fax: 909-335-6497
Emergency Services: Yes
Beds: 172

Key Personnel:
Anesthesiology. . . . . Shelley Abdel-Sayed, MD
Surgery . . . . Bradley Basinger, MD
Quality Assurance . . . . Cathi Bell
CEO/President. . . . . James R Holmes
Chief of Medical Staff. . . . . Carolina Rosario

Measure	Cases	This Hosp.	State Avg.	U.S. Avg.
Blood Clot Prevention and Treatment				
Anticoagulation Overlap Therapy[2]	58	84%	92%	93%
ICU Venous Thromboembolism Prophylaxis[2]	49	82%	92%	92%
Incidence of Potentially Preventable VTE[1,2]	-	-	11%	10%
UFH with Dosages/Platelet Monitoring[2]	21	100%	96%	97%
Venous Thromboembolism Prophylaxis[2]	300	85%	83%	85%
Warfarin Therapy Discharge Instructions[2]	38	5%	75%	75%
Chest Pain/Possible Heart Attack Care				
Aspirin Given Within 24 Hours of Arrival	56	93%	97%	96%
Fibrinolytic Meds Within 30 Min. of Arrival[7]	-	-	62%	58%
Average Time to ECG (minutes)	58	10	9	7
Average Time to Transfer (minutes)	19	70	62	60
Children's Asthma Care				
Received Home Management Plan of Care	-	-	88%	88%
Received Reliever Medication	-	-	100%	100%
Received Systemic Corticosteroids	-	-	100%	100%
Emergency Department				
Admittance Decision Time (minutes)[2]	320	238	125	98
Head CT Results Within 45 Min. of Arrival	14	64%	55%	57%
Patients Who Left ER Before Being Seen	44,009	1%	3%	2%
Time from ER Arrival to Admit. (minutes)[2]	379	479	323	274
Time from ER Arrival to Discharge (minutes)	339	223	168	134
Time in ER Before Being Evaluated (minutes)	368	28	29	26
Time to Pain Meds for Fractures (minutes)	191	85	62	57
Heart Attack Care				
Aspirin Given at Discharge	60	97%	99%	99%
Fibrinolytic Meds Within 30 Min. of Arrival[7]	-	-	73%	54%
PCI Within 90 Minutes of Arrival[7]	-	-	95%	96%
Statin Prescribed at Discharge	58	97%	98%	98%
Heart Failure Care				
ACE Inhibitor or ARB for LVSD	74	92%	97%	97%
Discharge Instructions Given	162	93%	94%	94%
Evaluation of LVS Function	212	98%	99%	99%
Medicare Spending				
Medicare Spending per Patient (ratio)	-	0.96	0.98	0.98
Pneumonia Care				
Appropriate Initial Antibiotic Given[2]	75	99%	97%	95%
Blood Culture Timing[2]	132	98%	98%	98%
Pregnancy and Delivery Care				
Newborn Deliveries Scheduled Early	342	6%	5%	6%
Preventive Care				
Immunization for Influenza[2]	472	88%	89%	90%
Immunization for Pneumonia[2]	520	93%	90%	92%
Stroke Care				
Anticoagulation Therapy for Atrial Fibrillation	16	94%	95%	95%
Antithrombotic Therapy Timing	105	100%	98%	98%

NOTE: Hospital profiles are in alphabetical order by state, then city, then hospital within the city; Rankings exclude hospitals with less than 25 cases except for patient surveys which excludes hospitals with less than 100 cases; (a) 100-299 cases; (1) The number of cases/patients is too few to report; (2) Data submitted were based on a sample of cases/patients; (3) Results are based on a shorter time period than required; (4) Data suppressed by CMS for one or more quarters; (5) Results are not available for this reporting period; (6) Fewer than 100 patients completed the HCAHPS survey; (7) No cases met the criteria for this measure; (8) The lower limit of the confidence interval cannot be calculated if the number of observed infections equals zero; (9) No data are available from the state/territory for this reporting period; (10) The scores shown reflect fewer than 50 completed surveys; (11) There were discrepancies in the data collection process; (12) This measure does not apply to this hospital for this reporting period; (13) Results cannot be calculated for this reporting period; (14) The results for this state are combined with nearby states to protect confidentiality; Please refer to the User's Guide for a full explanation of data.

Assessed for Rehabilitation	119	99%	97%	97%
Discharged on Antithrombotic Therapy	110	98%	99%	99%
Discharged on Statin Medication	90	92%	94%	94%
Thrombolytic Therapy Timing[1]	-	-	72%	66%
Venous Thromboembolism Prophylaxis	121	82%	94%	94%
Written Stroke Educational Materials Given	58	90%	87%	88%
Surgical Care Improvement Project				
Appropriate Beta Blocker Usage[2]	280	99%	97%	98%
Appropriate VTP Within 24 Hours[2]	921	99%	98%	98%
Controlled Postoperative Blood Glucose[2,7]	-	-	96%	97%
Perioperative Temperature Management[2]	1,085	100%	100%	100%
Prophylactic Antibiotic Selection[2]	867	99%	99%	99%
Prophylactic Antibiotic Selection (Outpatient)	475	98%	97%	98%
Prophylactic Antibiotic Stopped[2]	852	97%	98%	98%
Prophylactic Antibiotic Timing[2]	868	99%	99%	99%
Prophylactic Antibiotic Timing (Outpatient)	475	99%	97%	98%
Urinary Catheter Removal[2]	621	99%	97%	97%
Survey of Patients' Hospital Experiences				
Area Around Room 'Always' Quiet at Night	300+	57%	51%	61%
Doctors 'Always' Communicated Well	300+	80%	78%	82%
Home Recovery Information Given	300+	86%	83%	85%
Hospital Given 9 or 10 on 10 Point Scale	300+	78%	68%	71%
Meds 'Always' Explained Before Given	300+	63%	61%	64%
Nurses 'Always' Communicated Well	300+	77%	74%	79%
Pain 'Always' Well Controlled	300+	71%	68%	71%
Room and Bathroom 'Always' Clean	300+	75%	70%	73%
Timely Help 'Always' Received	300+	65%	62%	68%
Would Definitely Recommend Hospital	300+	78%	70%	71%
Use of Medical Imaging				
Cardiac Imaging Stress Test before Surgery	103	2.9%	5.2%	5.3%
Combination Abdominal CT Scan	414	8.2%	13.4%	10.5%
Combination Brain/Sinus CT Scan	437	1.1%	2.2%	2.7%
Combination Chest CT Scan	214	0.0%	2.3%	2.7%
Follow-up Mammogram/Ultrasound	417	6.5%	8.2%	8.8%
Lumbar Spine MRI for Low Back Pain[1]	-	-	34.2%	37.2%

Kaiser Foundation Hospital - Redwood City

1150 Veterans Boulevard
Redwood City, CA 94063
Phone: 650-299-2000
Fax: 650-299-2421
URL: www.seiu-uhw.org/aboutuhw
Type: Acute Care Hospitals
Emergency Services: Yes
Ownership: Voluntary non-profit - Other
Beds: 171

Key Personnel:

Chief of Medical Staff.......... Henry Brodkin, MD
Operating Room.............. Joyce Delaney
Pediatric Ambulatory Care ...... Wayne Easter
Pediatric In-Patient Care .... Wayne Easter
CEO/President............... Sal Rosselli

Measure	Cases	This Hosp.	State Avg.	U.S. Avg.
Blood Clot Prevention and Treatment				
Anticoagulation Overlap Therapy[2]	56	100%	92%	93%
ICU Venous Thromboembolism Prophylaxis[2]	77	100%	92%	92%
Incidence of Potentially Preventable VTE[2]	15	0%	11%	10%
UFH with Dosages/Platelet Monitoring[2]	37	100%	96%	97%
Venous Thromboembolism Prophylaxis[2]	290	93%	83%	85%
Warfarin Therapy Discharge Instructions[2]	43	93%	75%	75%
Chest Pain/Possible Heart Attack Care				
Aspirin Given Within 24 Hours of Arrival	-	-	97%	96%
Fibrinolytic Meds Within 30 Min. of Arrival	-	-	62%	58%
Average Time to ECG (minutes)	-	-	9	7
Average Time to Transfer (minutes)	-	-	62	60
Children's Asthma Care				
Received Home Management Plan of Care	-	-	88%	88%
Received Reliever Medication	-	-	100%	100%
Received Systemic Corticosteroids	-	-	100%	100%
Emergency Department				
Admittance Decision Time (minutes)[2]	426	50	125	98
Head CT Results Within 45 Min. of Arrival	-	-	55%	57%
Patients Who Left ER Before Being Seen	-	-	3%	2%
Time from ER Arrival to Admit. (minutes)[2]	432	265	323	274
Time from ER Arrival to Discharge (minutes)	-	-	168	134
Time in ER Before Being Evaluated (minutes)	-	-	29	26
Time to Pain Meds for Fractures (minutes)	-	-	62	57
Heart Attack Care				
Aspirin Given at Discharge	57	100%	99%	99%
Fibrinolytic Meds Within 30 Min. of Arrival[7]	-	-	73%	54%
PCI Within 90 Minutes of Arrival	22	95%	95%	96%
Statin Prescribed at Discharge	55	100%	98%	98%
Heart Failure Care				
ACE Inhibitor or ARB for LVSD	27	100%	97%	97%
Discharge Instructions Given	91	100%	94%	94%
Evaluation of LVS Function	106	100%	99%	99%
Medicare Spending				
Medicare Spending per Patient (ratio)	-	0.81	0.98	0.98
Pneumonia Care				
Appropriate Initial Antibiotic Given[2]	67	97%	97%	95%
Blood Culture Timing[2]	133	99%	98%	98%
Pregnancy and Delivery Care				
Newborn Deliveries Scheduled Early[2]	27	0%	5%	6%
Preventive Care				
Immunization for Influenza[2]	500	94%	89%	90%
Immunization for Pneumonia[2]	570	97%	90%	92%
Stroke Care				
Anticoagulation Therapy for Atrial Fibrillation[2]	14	100%	95%	95%
Antithrombotic Therapy Timing[2]	43	100%	98%	98%
Assessed for Rehabilitation[2]	111	100%	97%	97%
Discharged on Antithrombotic Therapy[2]	50	100%	99%	99%
Discharged on Statin Medication[2]	36	100%	94%	94%
Thrombolytic Therapy Timing[1,2]	-	-	72%	66%
Venous Thromboembolism Prophylaxis[2]	128	99%	94%	94%
Written Stroke Educational Materials Given[2]	75	100%	87%	88%
Surgical Care Improvement Project				
Appropriate Beta Blocker Usage[2]	109	100%	97%	98%
Appropriate VTP Within 24 Hours[2]	350	100%	98%	98%
Controlled Postoperative Blood Glucose[2,7]	-	-	96%	97%
Perioperative Temperature Management[2]	381	100%	100%	100%
Prophylactic Antibiotic Selection[2]	233	100%	99%	99%
Prophylactic Antibiotic Selection (Outpatient)	-	-	97%	98%
Prophylactic Antibiotic Stopped[2]	230	100%	98%	98%
Prophylactic Antibiotic Timing[2]	233	100%	99%	99%
Prophylactic Antibiotic Timing (Outpatient)	-	-	97%	98%
Urinary Catheter Removal[2]	307	100%	97%	97%
Survey of Patients' Hospital Experiences				
Area Around Room 'Always' Quiet at Night	300+	46%	51%	61%
Doctors 'Always' Communicated Well	300+	82%	78%	82%
Home Recovery Information Given	300+	87%	83%	85%
Hospital Given 9 or 10 on 10 Point Scale	300+	68%	68%	71%
Meds 'Always' Explained Before Given	300+	62%	61%	64%
Nurses 'Always' Communicated Well	300+	75%	74%	79%
Pain 'Always' Well Controlled	300+	72%	68%	71%
Room and Bathroom 'Always' Clean	300+	72%	70%	73%
Timely Help 'Always' Received	300+	66%	62%	68%
Would Definitely Recommend Hospital	300+	73%	70%	71%
Use of Medical Imaging				
Cardiac Imaging Stress Test before Surgery	-	-	5.2%	5.3%
Combination Abdominal CT Scan	-	-	13.4%	10.5%
Combination Brain/Sinus CT Scan	-	-	2.2%	2.7%
Combination Chest CT Scan	-	-	2.3%	2.7%
Follow-up Mammogram/Ultrasound	-	-	8.2%	8.8%
Lumbar Spine MRI for Low Back Pain	-	-	34.2%	37.2%

Sequoia Hospital

170 Alameda De Las Pulgas
Redwood City, CA 94062
Phone: 650-367-5551
Fax: 650-367-5100
URL: www.sequoiahospital.org
Type: Acute Care Hospitals
Emergency Services: Yes
Ownership: Voluntary non-profit - Private

Key Personnel:

CEO/President................ Glenna Vaskelis
Radiology.................... Richard L Wheat
Chief of Medical Staff.......... Rachel Young

Measure	Cases	This Hosp.	State Avg.	U.S. Avg.
Blood Clot Prevention and Treatment				
Anticoagulation Overlap Therapy[2]	15	80%	92%	93%
ICU Venous Thromboembolism Prophylaxis[2]	69	96%	92%	92%
Incidence of Potentially Preventable VTE[1,2]	-	-	11%	10%
UFH with Dosages/Platelet Monitoring[2]	16	69%	96%	97%
Venous Thromboembolism Prophylaxis[2]	309	92%	83%	85%
Warfarin Therapy Discharge Instructions[2]	11	82%	75%	75%
Chest Pain/Possible Heart Attack Care				
Aspirin Given Within 24 Hours of Arrival[3,7]	-	-	97%	96%
Fibrinolytic Meds Within 30 Min. of Arrival[5]	-	-	62%	58%
Average Time to ECG (minutes)[3,7]	-	-	9	7
Average Time to Transfer (minutes)[5]	-	-	62	60
Children's Asthma Care				
Received Home Management Plan of Care	-	-	88%	88%
Received Reliever Medication	-	-	100%	100%
Received Systemic Corticosteroids	-	-	100%	100%
Emergency Department				
Admittance Decision Time (minutes)[2]	452	96	125	98
Head CT Results Within 45 Min. of Arrival[1]	-	-	55%	57%
Patients Who Left ER Before Being Seen	21,019	1%	3%	2%
Time from ER Arrival to Admit. (minutes)[2]	458	232	323	274
Time from ER Arrival to Discharge (minutes)	390	115	168	134
Time in ER Before Being Evaluated (minutes)	401	16	29	26
Time to Pain Meds for Fractures (minutes)	113	44	62	57
Heart Attack Care				
Aspirin Given at Discharge	76	100%	99%	99%
Fibrinolytic Meds Within 30 Min. of Arrival[7]	-	-	73%	54%
PCI Within 90 Minutes of Arrival	21	100%	95%	96%
Statin Prescribed at Discharge	74	100%	98%	98%
Heart Failure Care				
ACE Inhibitor or ARB for LVSD	30	100%	97%	97%
Discharge Instructions Given	150	93%	94%	94%
Evaluation of LVS Function	179	100%	99%	99%
Medicare Spending				
Medicare Spending per Patient (ratio)	-	0.96	0.98	0.98
Pneumonia Care				
Appropriate Initial Antibiotic Given[2]	81	94%	97%	95%
Blood Culture Timing[2]	114	99%	98%	98%
Pregnancy and Delivery Care				
Newborn Deliveries Scheduled Early[2]	29	3%	5%	6%
Preventive Care				
Immunization for Influenza[2]	486	97%	89%	90%
Immunization for Pneumonia[2]	536	95%	90%	92%
Stroke Care				
Anticoagulation Therapy for Atrial Fibrillation	17	76%	95%	95%
Antithrombotic Therapy Timing	45	100%	98%	98%
Assessed for Rehabilitation	65	98%	97%	97%
Discharged on Antithrombotic Therapy	62	98%	99%	99%
Discharged on Statin Medication	56	96%	94%	94%
Thrombolytic Therapy Timing[1]	-	-	72%	66%
Venous Thromboembolism Prophylaxis	57	95%	94%	94%
Written Stroke Educational Materials Given	37	84%	87%	88%
Surgical Care Improvement Project				
Appropriate Beta Blocker Usage[2]	155	98%	97%	98%
Appropriate VTP Within 24 Hours[2]	339	99%	98%	98%
Controlled Postoperative Blood Glucose[2]	136	97%	96%	97%
Perioperative Temperature Management[2]	437	100%	100%	100%
Prophylactic Antibiotic Selection[2]	408	100%	99%	99%
Prophylactic Antibiotic Selection (Outpatient)	274	99%	97%	98%
Prophylactic Antibiotic Stopped[2]	393	98%	98%	98%
Prophylactic Antibiotic Timing[2]	408	98%	99%	99%
Prophylactic Antibiotic Timing (Outpatient)	274	100%	97%	98%
Urinary Catheter Removal[2]	407	98%	97%	97%
Survey of Patients' Hospital Experiences				
Area Around Room 'Always' Quiet at Night	300+	43%	51%	61%
Doctors 'Always' Communicated Well	300+	82%	78%	82%
Home Recovery Information Given	300+	82%	83%	85%
Hospital Given 9 or 10 on 10 Point Scale	300+	65%	68%	71%
Meds 'Always' Explained Before Given	300+	56%	61%	64%
Nurses 'Always' Communicated Well	300+	70%	74%	79%
Pain 'Always' Well Controlled	300+	65%	68%	71%
Room and Bathroom 'Always' Clean	300+	68%	70%	73%
Timely Help 'Always' Received	300+	48%	62%	68%
Would Definitely Recommend Hospital	300+	71%	70%	71%
Use of Medical Imaging				
Cardiac Imaging Stress Test before Surgery[1]	-	-	5.2%	5.3%

NOTE: Hospital profiles are in alphabetical order by state, then city, then hospital within the city; Rankings exclude hospitals with less than 25 cases except for patient surveys which excludes hospitals with less than 100 cases; (a) 100-299 cases; (1) The number of cases/patients is too few to report; (2) Data submitted were based on a sample of cases/patients; (3) Results are based on a shorter time period than required; (4) Data suppressed by CMS for one or more quarters; (5) Results are not available for this reporting period; (6) Fewer than 100 patients completed the HCAHPS survey; (7) No cases met the criteria for this measure; (8) The lower limit of the confidence interval cannot be calculated if the number of observed infections equals zero; (9) No data are available from the state/territory for this reporting period; (10) The scores shown reflect fewer than 50 completed surveys; (11) There were discrepancies in the data collection process; (12) This measure does not apply to this hospital for this reporting period; (13) Results cannot be calculated for this reporting period; (14) The results for this state are combined with nearby states to protect confidentiality; Please refer to the User's Guide for a full explanation of data.

Measure	Cases	This Hosp.	State Avg.	U.S. Avg.
Combination Abdominal CT Scan	432	6.9%	13.4%	10.5%
Combination Brain/Sinus CT Scan	440	1.4%	2.2%	2.7%
Combination Chest CT Scan	431	1.4%	2.3%	2.7%
Follow-up Mammogram/Ultrasound	943	5.9%	8.2%	8.8%
Lumbar Spine MRI for Low Back Pain[1]	-	-	34.2%	37.2%

Adventist Medical Center - Reedley

372 W Cypress Ave Phone: 559-638-8155
Reedley, CA 93654 Fax: 559-637-7553
URL: www.skdh.org
Type: Acute Care Hospitals Emergency Services: Yes
Ownership: Govt - Hospital Dist/Auth Beds: 44
Key Personnel:
Infection Control. . . . . Lori Bray, RN
CEO/President. . . . . Wayne Ferch
Radiology. . . . . Don Helland, Jr
Operating Room. . . . . Calvin Schuster
Chief of Medical Staff. . . . . Todd Spencer, MD
Chairman/CEO . . . . Bill Wing
Emergency Room . . . . Oleh Wolowodiuk, MD

Measure	Cases	This Hosp.	State Avg.	U.S. Avg.
Blood Clot Prevention and Treatment				
Anticoagulation Overlap Therapy[1,2]	-	-	92%	93%
ICU Venous Thromboembolism Prophylaxis[2,7]	-	-	92%	92%
Incidence of Potentially Preventable VTE[1,2]	-	-	11%	10%
UFH with Dosages/Platelet Monitoring[2,7]	-	-	96%	97%
Venous Thromboembolism Prophylaxis[2]	154	71%	83%	85%
Warfarin Therapy Discharge Instructions[1,2]	-	-	75%	75%
Chest Pain/Possible Heart Attack Care				
Aspirin Given Within 24 Hours of Arrival	14	93%	97%	96%
Fibrinolytic Meds Within 30 Min. of Arrival[7]	-	-	62%	58%
Average Time to ECG (minutes)	14	24	9	7
Average Time to Transfer (minutes)[1]	-	-	62	60
Children's Asthma Care				
Received Home Management Plan of Care	-	-	88%	88%
Received Reliever Medication	-	-	100%	100%
Received Systemic Corticosteroids	-	-	100%	100%
Emergency Department				
Admittance Decision Time (minutes)[2]	69	105	125	98
Head CT Results Within 45 Min. of Arrival[1]	-	-	55%	57%
Patients Who Left ER Before Being Seen	48,835	0%	3%	2%
Time from ER Arrival to Admit. (minutes)[2]	139	336	323	274
Time from ER Arrival to Discharge (minutes)	366	137	168	134
Time in ER Before Being Evaluated (minutes)	372	30	29	26
Time to Pain Meds for Fractures (minutes)	74	68	62	57
Heart Attack Care				
Aspirin Given at Discharge[1,3]	-	-	99%	99%
Fibrinolytic Meds Within 30 Min. of Arrival[3,7]	-	-	73%	54%
PCI Within 90 Minutes of Arrival[3,7]	-	-	95%	96%
Statin Prescribed at Discharge[1,3]	-	-	98%	98%
Heart Failure Care				
ACE Inhibitor or ARB for LVSD[1]	-	-	97%	97%
Discharge Instructions Given	15	80%	94%	94%
Evaluation of LVS Function	20	80%	99%	99%
Medicare Spending				
Medicare Spending per Patient (ratio)	-	0.99	0.98	0.98
Pneumonia Care				
Appropriate Initial Antibiotic Given	34	94%	97%	95%
Blood Culture Timing	43	93%	98%	98%
Pregnancy and Delivery Care				
Newborn Deliveries Scheduled Early[2]	40	18%	5%	6%
Preventive Care				
Immunization for Influenza[2]	235	81%	89%	90%
Immunization for Pneumonia[2]	130	72%	90%	92%
Stroke Care				
Anticoagulation Therapy for Atrial Fibrillation[5]	-	-	95%	95%
Antithrombotic Therapy Timing[5]	-	-	98%	98%
Assessed for Rehabilitation[5]	-	-	97%	97%
Discharged on Antithrombotic Therapy[5]	-	-	99%	99%
Discharged on Statin Medication[5]	-	-	94%	94%
Thrombolytic Therapy Timing[5]	-	-	72%	66%
Venous Thromboembolism Prophylaxis[5]	-	-	94%	94%
Written Stroke Educational Materials Given[5]	-	-	87%	88%
Surgical Care Improvement Project				
Appropriate Beta Blocker Usage[1]	-	-	97%	98%
Appropriate VTP Within 24 Hours	17	88%	98%	98%
Controlled Postoperative Blood Glucose[7]	-	-	96%	97%
Perioperative Temperature Management	22	91%	100%	100%
Prophylactic Antibiotic Selection[1]	-	-	99%	99%
Prophylactic Antibiotic Selection (Outpatient)[3,7]	-	-	97%	98%
Prophylactic Antibiotic Stopped[1]	-	-	98%	98%
Prophylactic Antibiotic Timing[1]	-	-	99%	99%
Prophylactic Antibiotic Timing (Outpatient)[1,3]	-	-	97%	98%
Urinary Catheter Removal[1]	-	-	97%	97%
Survey of Patients' Hospital Experiences				
Area Around Room 'Always' Quiet at Night	(a)	51%	51%	61%
Doctors 'Always' Communicated Well	(a)	78%	78%	82%
Home Recovery Information Given	(a)	79%	83%	85%
Hospital Given 9 or 10 on 10 Point Scale	(a)	60%	68%	71%
Meds 'Always' Explained Before Given	(a)	61%	61%	64%
Nurses 'Always' Communicated Well	(a)	72%	74%	79%
Pain 'Always' Well Controlled	(a)	67%	68%	71%
Room and Bathroom 'Always' Clean	(a)	65%	70%	73%
Timely Help 'Always' Received	(a)	59%	62%	68%
Would Definitely Recommend Hospital	(a)	60%	70%	71%
Use of Medical Imaging				
Cardiac Imaging Stress Test before Surgery[7]	-	-	5.2%	5.3%
Combination Abdominal CT Scan	177	23.2%	13.4%	10.5%
Combination Brain/Sinus CT Scan[1]	-	-	2.2%	2.7%
Combination Chest CT Scan[1]	-	-	2.3%	2.7%
Follow-up Mammogram/Ultrasound	393	7.6%	8.2%	8.8%
Lumbar Spine MRI for Low Back Pain[1]	-	-	34.2%	37.2%

Kaiser Foundation Hospital - Riverside

10800 Magnolia Avenue Phone: 951-353-2000
Riverside, CA 92505
Type: Acute Care Hospitals Emergency Services: Yes
Ownership: Govt - Hospital Dist/Auth Beds: 215

Measure	Cases	This Hosp.	State Avg.	U.S. Avg.
Blood Clot Prevention and Treatment				
Anticoagulation Overlap Therapy[2]	82	91%	92%	93%
ICU Venous Thromboembolism Prophylaxis[2]	51	90%	92%	92%
Incidence of Potentially Preventable VTE[1,2]	-	-	11%	10%
UFH with Dosages/Platelet Monitoring[2]	73	99%	96%	97%
Venous Thromboembolism Prophylaxis[2]	295	85%	83%	85%
Warfarin Therapy Discharge Instructions[2]	76	96%	75%	75%
Chest Pain/Possible Heart Attack Care				
Aspirin Given Within 24 Hours of Arrival	-	-	97%	96%
Fibrinolytic Meds Within 30 Min. of Arrival	-	-	62%	58%
Average Time to ECG (minutes)	-	-	9	7
Average Time to Transfer (minutes)	-	-	62	60
Children's Asthma Care				
Received Home Management Plan of Care	-	-	88%	88%
Received Reliever Medication	-	-	100%	100%
Received Systemic Corticosteroids	-	-	100%	100%
Emergency Department				
Admittance Decision Time (minutes)[2]	298	97	125	98
Head CT Results Within 45 Min. of Arrival	-	-	55%	57%
Patients Who Left ER Before Being Seen	-	-	3%	2%
Time from ER Arrival to Admit. (minutes)[2]	335	315	323	274
Time from ER Arrival to Discharge (minutes)	-	-	168	134
Time in ER Before Being Evaluated (minutes)	-	-	29	26
Time to Pain Meds for Fractures (minutes)	-	-	62	57
Heart Attack Care				
Aspirin Given at Discharge	86	99%	99%	99%
Fibrinolytic Meds Within 30 Min. of Arrival[1]	-	-	73%	54%
PCI Within 90 Minutes of Arrival[7]	-	-	95%	96%
Statin Prescribed at Discharge	87	100%	98%	98%
Heart Failure Care				
ACE Inhibitor or ARB for LVSD	92	100%	97%	97%
Discharge Instructions Given	251	100%	94%	94%
Evaluation of LVS Function	268	100%	99%	99%
Medicare Spending				
Medicare Spending per Patient (ratio)	-	0.81	0.98	0.98
Pneumonia Care				
Appropriate Initial Antibiotic Given[2]	85	100%	97%	95%
Blood Culture Timing[2]	111	98%	98%	98%
Pregnancy and Delivery Care				
Newborn Deliveries Scheduled Early	237	0%	5%	6%
Preventive Care				
Immunization for Influenza[2]	497	95%	89%	90%
Immunization for Pneumonia[2]	516	95%	90%	92%
Stroke Care				
Anticoagulation Therapy for Atrial Fibrillation[2]	13	92%	95%	95%
Antithrombotic Therapy Timing[2]	69	99%	98%	98%
Assessed for Rehabilitation[2]	91	95%	97%	97%
Discharged on Antithrombotic Therapy[2]	83	100%	99%	99%
Discharged on Statin Medication[2]	66	95%	94%	94%
Thrombolytic Therapy Timing[1,2]	-	-	72%	66%
Venous Thromboembolism Prophylaxis[2]	69	99%	94%	94%
Written Stroke Educational Materials Given[2]	62	97%	87%	88%
Surgical Care Improvement Project				
Appropriate Beta Blocker Usage[2]	106	97%	97%	98%
Appropriate VTP Within 24 Hours[2]	398	99%	98%	98%
Controlled Postoperative Blood Glucose[2,7]	-	-	96%	97%
Perioperative Temperature Management[2]	448	100%	100%	100%
Prophylactic Antibiotic Selection[2]	264	99%	99%	99%
Prophylactic Antibiotic Selection (Outpatient)	-	-	97%	98%
Prophylactic Antibiotic Stopped[2]	251	98%	98%	98%
Prophylactic Antibiotic Timing[2]	264	100%	99%	99%
Prophylactic Antibiotic Timing (Outpatient)	-	-	97%	98%
Urinary Catheter Removal[2]	265	99%	97%	97%
Survey of Patients' Hospital Experiences				
Area Around Room 'Always' Quiet at Night	300+	44%	51%	61%
Doctors 'Always' Communicated Well	300+	81%	78%	82%
Home Recovery Information Given	300+	85%	83%	85%
Hospital Given 9 or 10 on 10 Point Scale	300+	74%	68%	71%
Meds 'Always' Explained Before Given	300+	64%	61%	64%
Nurses 'Always' Communicated Well	300+	74%	74%	79%
Pain 'Always' Well Controlled	300+	71%	68%	71%
Room and Bathroom 'Always' Clean	300+	75%	70%	73%
Timely Help 'Always' Received	300+	64%	62%	68%
Would Definitely Recommend Hospital	300+	75%	70%	71%
Use of Medical Imaging				
Cardiac Imaging Stress Test before Surgery	-	-	5.2%	5.3%
Combination Abdominal CT Scan	-	-	13.4%	10.5%
Combination Brain/Sinus CT Scan	-	-	2.2%	2.7%
Combination Chest CT Scan	-	-	2.3%	2.7%
Follow-up Mammogram/Ultrasound	-	-	8.2%	8.8%
Lumbar Spine MRI for Low Back Pain	-	-	34.2%	37.2%

Parkview Community Hospital Medical Center

3865 Jackson Street Phone: 951-688-2211
Riverside, CA 92503 Fax: 951-352-5394
URL: www.pchmc.org
Type: Acute Care Hospitals Emergency Services: Yes
Ownership: Proprietary Beds: 193
Key Personnel:
CEO/President. . . . . Douglas Drumwright
Radiology. . . . . Bienvenido Jr, Jr

Measure	Cases	This Hosp.	State Avg.	U.S. Avg.
Blood Clot Prevention and Treatment				
Anticoagulation Overlap Therapy[2]	20	70%	92%	93%
ICU Venous Thromboembolism Prophylaxis[2]	38	76%	92%	92%
Incidence of Potentially Preventable VTE[2]	14	14%	11%	10%
UFH with Dosages/Platelet Monitoring[1,2]	-	-	96%	97%
Venous Thromboembolism Prophylaxis[2]	336	59%	83%	85%
Warfarin Therapy Discharge Instructions[2]	11	27%	75%	75%
Chest Pain/Possible Heart Attack Care				
Aspirin Given Within 24 Hours of Arrival[3]	31	97%	97%	96%
Fibrinolytic Meds Within 30 Min. of Arrival[3,7]	-	-	62%	58%
Average Time to ECG (minutes)[3]	33	25	9	7
Average Time to Transfer (minutes)[3,7]	-	-	62	60
Children's Asthma Care				
Received Home Management Plan of Care	-	-	88%	88%
Received Reliever Medication	-	-	100%	100%
Received Systemic Corticosteroids	-	-	100%	100%
Emergency Department				
Admittance Decision Time (minutes)[2]	218	102	125	98

NOTE: Hospital profiles are in alphabetical order by state, then city, then hospital within the city; Rankings exclude hospitals with less than 25 cases except for patient surveys which excludes hospitals with less than 100 cases; (a) 100-299 cases; (1) The number of cases/patients is too few to report; (2) Data submitted were based on a sample of cases/patients; (3) Results are based on a shorter time period than required; (4) Data suppressed by CMS for one or more quarters; (5) Results are not available for this reporting period; (6) Fewer than 100 patients completed the HCAHPS survey; (7) No cases met the criteria for this measure; (8) The lower limit of the confidence interval cannot be calculated if the number of observed infections equals zero; (9) No data are available from the state/territory for this reporting period; (10) The scores shown reflect fewer than 50 completed surveys; (11) There were discrepancies in the data collection process; (12) This measure does not apply to this hospital for this reporting period; (13) Results cannot be calculated for this reporting period; (14) The results for this state are combined with nearby states to protect confidentiality; Please refer to the User's Guide for a full explanation of data.

Head CT Results Within 45 Min. of Arrival[3,7]	-	-	55%	57%
Patients Who Left ER Before Being Seen	43,901	3%	3%	2%
Time from ER Arrival to Admit. (minutes)[2]	219	296	323	274
Time from ER Arrival to Discharge (minutes)	938	125	168	134
Time in ER Before Being Evaluated (minutes)	1,293	37	29	26
Time to Pain Meds for Fractures (minutes)	19	85	62	57
Heart Attack Care				
Aspirin Given at Discharge	12	100%	99%	99%
Fibrinolytic Meds Within 30 Min. of Arrival[7]	-	-	73%	54%
PCI Within 90 Minutes of Arrival[7]	-	-	95%	96%
Statin Prescribed at Discharge	11	64%	98%	98%
Heart Failure Care				
ACE Inhibitor or ARB for LVSD[2]	48	92%	97%	97%
Discharge Instructions Given[2]	157	71%	94%	94%
Evaluation of LVS Function[2]	214	95%	99%	99%
Medicare Spending				
Medicare Spending per Patient (ratio)	-	1.13	0.98	0.98
Pneumonia Care				
Appropriate Initial Antibiotic Given[2]	150	93%	97%	95%
Blood Culture Timing[2]	317	94%	98%	98%
Pregnancy and Delivery Care				
Newborn Deliveries Scheduled Early	179	8%	5%	6%
Preventive Care				
Immunization for Influenza[2]	462	86%	89%	90%
Immunization for Pneumonia[2]	461	75%	90%	92%
Stroke Care				
Anticoagulation Therapy for Atrial Fibrillation[1]	-	-	95%	95%
Antithrombotic Therapy Timing	71	100%	98%	98%
Assessed for Rehabilitation	75	84%	97%	97%
Discharged on Antithrombotic Therapy	72	92%	99%	99%
Discharged on Statin Medication	60	78%	94%	94%
Thrombolytic Therapy Timing	12	33%	72%	66%
Venous Thromboembolism Prophylaxis	75	71%	94%	94%
Written Stroke Educational Materials Given	39	26%	87%	88%
Surgical Care Improvement Project				
Appropriate Beta Blocker Usage[2]	110	91%	97%	98%
Appropriate VTP Within 24 Hours[2]	493	90%	98%	98%
Controlled Postoperative Blood Glucose[2,7]	-	-	96%	97%
Perioperative Temperature Management[2]	530	99%	100%	100%
Prophylactic Antibiotic Selection[2]	420	97%	99%	99%
Prophylactic Antibiotic Selection (Outpatient)	30	93%	97%	98%
Prophylactic Antibiotic Stopped[2]	419	94%	98%	98%
Prophylactic Antibiotic Timing[2]	423	96%	99%	99%
Prophylactic Antibiotic Timing (Outpatient)	33	82%	97%	98%
Urinary Catheter Removal[2]	387	94%	97%	97%
Survey of Patients' Hospital Experiences				
Area Around Room 'Always' Quiet at Night	300+	35%	51%	61%
Doctors 'Always' Communicated Well	300+	70%	78%	82%
Home Recovery Information Given	300+	81%	83%	85%
Hospital Given 9 or 10 on 10 Point Scale	300+	49%	68%	71%
Meds 'Always' Explained Before Given	300+	51%	61%	64%
Nurses 'Always' Communicated Well	300+	66%	74%	79%
Pain 'Always' Well Controlled	300+	64%	68%	71%
Room and Bathroom 'Always' Clean	300+	64%	70%	73%
Timely Help 'Always' Received	300+	55%	62%	68%
Would Definitely Recommend Hospital	300+	50%	70%	71%
Use of Medical Imaging				
Cardiac Imaging Stress Test before Surgery[1]	-	-	5.2%	5.3%
Combination Abdominal CT Scan	310	14.8%	13.4%	10.5%
Combination Brain/Sinus CT Scan[1]	-	-	2.2%	2.7%
Combination Chest CT Scan	101	15.8%	2.3%	2.7%
Follow-up Mammogram/Ultrasound	230	6.5%	8.2%	8.8%
Lumbar Spine MRI for Low Back Pain[1]	-	-	34.2%	37.2%

Riverside Community Hospital

4445 Magnolia Avenue Phone: 951-788-3000
Riverside, CA 92501
URL: www.rchc.org
Type: Acute Care Hospitals Emergency Services: Yes
Ownership: Government - State
Key Personnel:
CEO . . . . Patrick Brilliant

Measure	Cases	This Hosp.	State Avg.	U.S. Avg.
Blood Clot Prevention and Treatment				
Anticoagulation Overlap Therapy[2]	112	83%	92%	93%
ICU Venous Thromboembolism Prophylaxis[2]	80	90%	92%	92%
Incidence of Potentially Preventable VTE[2]	25	24%	11%	10%
UFH with Dosages/Platelet Monitoring[2]	40	100%	96%	97%
Venous Thromboembolism Prophylaxis[2]	353	82%	83%	85%
Warfarin Therapy Discharge Instructions[2]	67	85%	75%	75%
Chest Pain/Possible Heart Attack Care				
Aspirin Given Within 24 Hours of Arrival[1,3]	-	-	97%	96%
Fibrinolytic Meds Within 30 Min. of Arrival[3,7]	-	-	62%	58%
Average Time to ECG (minutes)[1,3]	-	-	9	7
Average Time to Transfer (minutes)[3,7]	-	-	62	60
Children's Asthma Care				
Received Home Management Plan of Care	-	-	88%	88%
Received Reliever Medication	-	-	100%	100%
Received Systemic Corticosteroids	-	-	100%	100%
Emergency Department				
Admittance Decision Time (minutes)[2]	644	260	125	98
Head CT Results Within 45 Min. of Arrival	17	65%	55%	57%
Patients Who Left ER Before Being Seen	81,747	1%	3%	2%
Time from ER Arrival to Admit. (minutes)[2]	644	453	323	274
Time from ER Arrival to Discharge (minutes)	412	142	168	134
Time in ER Before Being Evaluated (minutes)	437	10	29	26
Time to Pain Meds for Fractures (minutes)	247	59	62	57
Heart Attack Care				
Aspirin Given at Discharge[2]	278	100%	99%	99%
Fibrinolytic Meds Within 30 Min. of Arrival[2,7]	-	-	73%	54%
PCI Within 90 Minutes of Arrival[2]	57	100%	95%	96%
Statin Prescribed at Discharge[2]	269	100%	98%	98%
Heart Failure Care				
ACE Inhibitor or ARB for LVSD[2]	113	100%	97%	97%
Discharge Instructions Given[2]	235	100%	94%	94%
Evaluation of LVS Function[2]	290	100%	99%	99%
Medicare Spending				
Medicare Spending per Patient (ratio)	-	1.05	0.98	0.98
Pneumonia Care				
Appropriate Initial Antibiotic Given[2]	81	99%	97%	95%
Blood Culture Timing[2]	137	100%	98%	98%
Pregnancy and Delivery Care				
Newborn Deliveries Scheduled Early[2]	73	0%	5%	6%
Preventive Care				
Immunization for Influenza[2]	551	95%	89%	90%
Immunization for Pneumonia[2]	600	97%	90%	92%
Stroke Care				
Anticoagulation Therapy for Atrial Fibrillation[2]	12	92%	95%	95%
Antithrombotic Therapy Timing[2]	84	95%	98%	98%
Assessed for Rehabilitation[2]	106	95%	97%	97%
Discharged on Antithrombotic Therapy[2]	87	97%	99%	99%
Discharged on Statin Medication[2]	72	94%	94%	94%
Thrombolytic Therapy Timing[1,2]	-	-	72%	66%
Venous Thromboembolism Prophylaxis[2]	114	84%	94%	94%
Written Stroke Educational Materials Given[2]	45	100%	87%	88%
Surgical Care Improvement Project				
Appropriate Beta Blocker Usage[2]	225	99%	97%	98%
Appropriate VTP Within 24 Hours[2]	460	100%	98%	98%
Controlled Postoperative Blood Glucose[2]	152	97%	96%	97%
Perioperative Temperature Management[2]	568	100%	100%	100%
Prophylactic Antibiotic Selection[2]	502	100%	99%	99%
Prophylactic Antibiotic Selection (Outpatient)	455	96%	97%	98%
Prophylactic Antibiotic Stopped[2]	470	99%	98%	98%
Prophylactic Antibiotic Timing[2]	503	100%	99%	99%
Prophylactic Antibiotic Timing (Outpatient)	459	98%	97%	98%
Urinary Catheter Removal[2]	337	99%	97%	97%
Survey of Patients' Hospital Experiences				
Area Around Room 'Always' Quiet at Night	300+	38%	51%	61%
Doctors 'Always' Communicated Well	300+	74%	78%	82%
Home Recovery Information Given	300+	83%	83%	85%
Hospital Given 9 or 10 on 10 Point Scale	300+	57%	68%	71%
Meds 'Always' Explained Before Given	300+	54%	61%	64%
Nurses 'Always' Communicated Well	300+	69%	74%	79%
Pain 'Always' Well Controlled	300+	66%	68%	71%
Room and Bathroom 'Always' Clean	300+	61%	70%	73%
Timely Help 'Always' Received	300+	50%	62%	68%
Would Definitely Recommend Hospital	300+	60%	70%	71%
Use of Medical Imaging				
Cardiac Imaging Stress Test before Surgery	165	9.7%	5.2%	5.3%
Combination Abdominal CT Scan	702	15.0%	13.4%	10.5%
Combination Brain/Sinus CT Scan	650	2.3%	2.2%	2.7%
Combination Chest CT Scan	299	13.4%	2.3%	2.7%
Follow-up Mammogram/Ultrasound	637	13.0%	8.2%	8.8%
Lumbar Spine MRI for Low Back Pain[1]	-	-	34.2%	37.2%

Kaiser Foundation Hospital - Roseville

1600 Eureka Road Phone: 916-784-4000
Roseville, CA 95661
URL: www.kaiserpermanente.org/roseville
Type: Acute Care Hospitals Emergency Services: Yes
Ownership: Voluntary non-profit - Private

Measure	Cases	This Hosp.	State Avg.	U.S. Avg.
Blood Clot Prevention and Treatment				
Anticoagulation Overlap Therapy[2]	93	100%	92%	93%
ICU Venous Thromboembolism Prophylaxis[2]	86	100%	92%	92%
Incidence of Potentially Preventable VTE[1,2]	-	-	11%	10%
UFH with Dosages/Platelet Monitoring[2]	62	100%	96%	97%
Venous Thromboembolism Prophylaxis[2]	232	99%	83%	85%
Warfarin Therapy Discharge Instructions[2]	86	97%	75%	75%
Chest Pain/Possible Heart Attack Care				
Aspirin Given Within 24 Hours of Arrival	-	-	97%	96%
Fibrinolytic Meds Within 30 Min. of Arrival	-	-	62%	58%
Average Time to ECG (minutes)	-	-	9	7
Average Time to Transfer (minutes)	-	-	62	60
Children's Asthma Care				
Received Home Management Plan of Care	-	-	88%	88%
Received Reliever Medication	-	-	100%	100%
Received Systemic Corticosteroids	-	-	100%	100%
Emergency Department				
Admittance Decision Time (minutes)[2]	418	48	125	98
Head CT Results Within 45 Min. of Arrival	-	-	55%	57%
Patients Who Left ER Before Being Seen	-	-	3%	2%
Time from ER Arrival to Admit. (minutes)[2]	420	292	323	274
Time from ER Arrival to Discharge (minutes)	-	-	168	134
Time in ER Before Being Evaluated (minutes)	-	-	29	26
Time to Pain Meds for Fractures (minutes)	-	-	62	57
Heart Attack Care				
Aspirin Given at Discharge[2]	216	98%	99%	99%
Fibrinolytic Meds Within 30 Min. of Arrival[1,2]	-	-	73%	54%
PCI Within 90 Minutes of Arrival[2]	73	99%	95%	96%
Statin Prescribed at Discharge[2]	217	99%	98%	98%
Heart Failure Care				
ACE Inhibitor or ARB for LVSD[2]	58	100%	97%	97%
Discharge Instructions Given[2]	254	100%	94%	94%
Evaluation of LVS Function[2]	284	100%	99%	99%
Medicare Spending				
Medicare Spending per Patient (ratio)	-	0.88	0.98	0.98
Pneumonia Care				
Appropriate Initial Antibiotic Given[2]	87	100%	97%	95%
Blood Culture Timing[2]	127	99%	98%	98%
Pregnancy and Delivery Care				
Newborn Deliveries Scheduled Early[2]	54	2%	5%	6%
Preventive Care				
Immunization for Influenza[2]	469	94%	89%	90%
Immunization for Pneumonia[2]	445	98%	90%	92%
Stroke Care				
Anticoagulation Therapy for Atrial Fibrillation[2]	20	95%	95%	95%
Antithrombotic Therapy Timing[2]	75	97%	98%	98%
Assessed for Rehabilitation[2]	124	99%	97%	97%
Discharged on Antithrombotic Therapy[2]	117	100%	99%	99%
Discharged on Statin Medication[2]	97	100%	94%	94%
Thrombolytic Therapy Timing[2]	18	94%	72%	66%
Venous Thromboembolism Prophylaxis[2]	87	100%	94%	94%
Written Stroke Educational Materials Given[2]	73	97%	87%	88%
Surgical Care Improvement Project				
Appropriate Beta Blocker Usage[2]	124	99%	97%	98%
Appropriate VTP Within 24 Hours[2]	373	100%	98%	98%

NOTE: Hospital profiles are in alphabetical order by state, then city, then hospital within the city; Rankings exclude hospitals with less than 25 cases except for patient surveys which excludes hospitals with less than 100 cases; (a) 100-299 cases; (1) The number of cases/patients is too few to report; (2) Data submitted were based on a sample of cases/patients; (3) Results are based on a shorter time period than required; (4) Data suppressed by CMS for one or more quarters; (5) Results are not available for this reporting period; (6) Fewer than 100 patients completed the HCAHPS survey; (7) No cases met the criteria for this measure; (8) The lower limit of the confidence interval cannot be calculated if the number of observed infections equals zero; (9) No data are available from the state/territory for this reporting period; (10) The scores shown reflect fewer than 50 completed surveys; (11) There were discrepancies in the data collection process; (12) This measure does not apply to this hospital for this reporting period; (13) Results cannot be calculated for this reporting period; (14) The results for this state are combined with nearby states to protect confidentiality; Please refer to the User's Guide for a full explanation of data.

Controlled Postoperative Blood Glucose[2,7]	-	-	96%	97%
Perioperative Temperature Management[2]	477	100%	100%	100%
Prophylactic Antibiotic Selection[2]	316	100%	99%	99%
Prophylactic Antibiotic Selection (Outpatient)	-	-	97%	98%
Prophylactic Antibiotic Stopped[2]	316	100%	98%	98%
Prophylactic Antibiotic Timing[2]	317	99%	99%	99%
Prophylactic Antibiotic Timing (Outpatient)	-	-	97%	98%
Urinary Catheter Removal[2]	323	100%	97%	97%
Survey of Patients' Hospital Experiences				
Area Around Room 'Always' Quiet at Night	300+	52%	51%	61%
Doctors 'Always' Communicated Well	300+	81%	78%	82%
Home Recovery Information Given	300+	86%	83%	85%
Hospital Given 9 or 10 on 10 Point Scale	300+	78%	68%	71%
Meds 'Always' Explained Before Given	300+	63%	61%	64%
Nurses 'Always' Communicated Well	300+	76%	74%	79%
Pain 'Always' Well Controlled	300+	73%	68%	71%
Room and Bathroom 'Always' Clean	300+	73%	70%	73%
Timely Help 'Always' Received	300+	63%	62%	68%
Would Definitely Recommend Hospital	300+	81%	70%	71%
Use of Medical Imaging				
Cardiac Imaging Stress Test before Surgery	-	-	5.2%	5.3%
Combination Abdominal CT Scan	-	-	13.4%	10.5%
Combination Brain/Sinus CT Scan	-	-	2.2%	2.7%
Combination Chest CT Scan	-	-	2.3%	2.7%
Follow-up Mammogram/Ultrasound	-	-	8.2%	8.8%
Lumbar Spine MRI for Low Back Pain	-	-	34.2%	37.2%

Sutter Roseville Medical Center

One Medical Plaza
Roseville, CA 95661
URL: www.sutterroseville.org
Type: Acute Care Hospitals
Ownership: Voluntary non-profit - Other
Phone: 916-781-1000
Fax: 916-781-1605
Emergency Services: Yes
Beds: 172

Key Personnel:
Radiology. . . . . Jerry P Arnold
Chief of Medical Staff . . . . Stuart G Brostrom
CEO/President. . . . . Sarah Krevans

Measure	Cases	This Hosp.	State Avg.	U.S. Avg.
Blood Clot Prevention and Treatment				
Anticoagulation Overlap Therapy[2]	164	97%	92%	93%
ICU Venous Thromboembolism Prophylaxis[2]	90	96%	92%	92%
Incidence of Potentially Preventable VTE[2]	20	10%	11%	10%
UFH with Dosages/Platelet Monitoring[2]	28	96%	96%	97%
Venous Thromboembolism Prophylaxis[2]	310	88%	83%	85%
Warfarin Therapy Discharge Instructions[2]	117	88%	75%	75%
Chest Pain/Possible Heart Attack Care				
Aspirin Given Within 24 Hours of Arrival	16	94%	97%	96%
Fibrinolytic Meds Within 30 Min. of Arrival[1]	-	-	62%	58%
Average Time to ECG (minutes)	16	8	9	7
Average Time to Transfer (minutes)[7]	-	-	62	60
Children's Asthma Care				
Received Home Management Plan of Care	-	-	88%	88%
Received Reliever Medication	-	-	100%	100%
Received Systemic Corticosteroids	-	-	100%	100%
Emergency Department				
Admittance Decision Time (minutes)[2]	705	150	125	98
Head CT Results Within 45 Min. of Arrival[1]	-	-	55%	57%
Patients Who Left ER Before Being Seen	74,081	2%	3%	2%
Time from ER Arrival to Admit. (minutes)[2]	710	362	323	274
Time from ER Arrival to Discharge (minutes)	379	188	168	134
Time in ER Before Being Evaluated (minutes)	385	31	29	26
Time to Pain Meds for Fractures (minutes)	334	79	62	57
Heart Attack Care				
Aspirin Given at Discharge	234	99%	99%	99%
Fibrinolytic Meds Within 30 Min. of Arrival[7]	-	-	73%	54%
PCI Within 90 Minutes of Arrival	63	95%	95%	96%
Statin Prescribed at Discharge	231	100%	98%	98%
Heart Failure Care				
ACE Inhibitor or ARB for LVSD[2]	84	100%	97%	97%
Discharge Instructions Given[2]	225	98%	94%	94%
Evaluation of LVS Function[2]	250	100%	99%	99%
Medicare Spending				
Medicare Spending per Patient (ratio)	-	0.94	0.98	0.98
Pneumonia Care				
Appropriate Initial Antibiotic Given[2]	90	97%	97%	95%
Blood Culture Timing[2]	157	97%	98%	98%
Pregnancy and Delivery Care				
Newborn Deliveries Scheduled Early	240	1%	5%	6%
Preventive Care				
Immunization for Influenza[2]	524	96%	89%	90%
Immunization for Pneumonia[2]	539	98%	90%	92%
Stroke Care				
Anticoagulation Therapy for Atrial Fibrillation	27	93%	95%	95%
Antithrombotic Therapy Timing	172	97%	98%	98%
Assessed for Rehabilitation	198	99%	97%	97%
Discharged on Antithrombotic Therapy	172	100%	99%	99%
Discharged on Statin Medication	141	99%	94%	94%
Thrombolytic Therapy Timing	12	100%	72%	66%
Venous Thromboembolism Prophylaxis	223	99%	94%	94%
Written Stroke Educational Materials Given	104	93%	87%	88%
Surgical Care Improvement Project				
Appropriate Beta Blocker Usage[2]	117	94%	97%	98%
Appropriate VTP Within 24 Hours[2]	404	98%	98%	98%
Controlled Postoperative Blood Glucose[2,7]	-	-	96%	97%
Perioperative Temperature Management[2]	525	100%	100%	100%
Prophylactic Antibiotic Selection[2]	353	100%	99%	99%
Prophylactic Antibiotic Selection (Outpatient)	241	98%	97%	98%
Prophylactic Antibiotic Stopped[2]	347	98%	98%	98%
Prophylactic Antibiotic Timing[2]	353	99%	99%	99%
Prophylactic Antibiotic Timing (Outpatient)	242	99%	97%	98%
Urinary Catheter Removal[2]	304	95%	97%	97%
Survey of Patients' Hospital Experiences				
Area Around Room 'Always' Quiet at Night	300+	55%	51%	61%
Doctors 'Always' Communicated Well	300+	78%	78%	82%
Home Recovery Information Given	300+	85%	83%	85%
Hospital Given 9 or 10 on 10 Point Scale	300+	75%	68%	71%
Meds 'Always' Explained Before Given	300+	61%	61%	64%
Nurses 'Always' Communicated Well	300+	76%	74%	79%
Pain 'Always' Well Controlled	300+	70%	68%	71%
Room and Bathroom 'Always' Clean	300+	70%	70%	73%
Timely Help 'Always' Received	300+	68%	62%	68%
Would Definitely Recommend Hospital	300+	79%	70%	71%
Use of Medical Imaging				
Cardiac Imaging Stress Test before Surgery	269	4.1%	5.2%	5.3%
Combination Abdominal CT Scan	721	0.0%	13.4%	10.5%
Combination Brain/Sinus CT Scan	981	2.3%	2.2%	2.7%
Combination Chest CT Scan	279	0.0%	2.3%	2.7%
Follow-up Mammogram/Ultrasound[7]	-	-	8.2%	8.8%
Lumbar Spine MRI for Low Back Pain[1]	-	-	34.2%	37.2%

Kaiser Foundation Hospital - Sacramento

2025 Morse Avenue
Sacramento, CA 95825
URL: www.kaiserpermanente.org
Type: Acute Care Hospitals
Ownership: Voluntary non-profit - Private
Phone: 916-973-5000
Fax: 916-973-6222
Emergency Services: No
Beds: 340

Key Personnel:
Radiology. . . . . William Brown, MD
Quality Assurance . . . . Barbara Crawford
CEO/President. . . . . Edd Glavis
Operating Room. . . . . Theresa Lee
Pediatric Ambulatory Care . . . . . . Paul Phinney, MD
Pediatric In-Patient Care . . . . Paul Phinney, MD

Measure	Cases	This Hosp.	State Avg.	U.S. Avg.
Blood Clot Prevention and Treatment				
Anticoagulation Overlap Therapy[2]	59	98%	92%	93%
ICU Venous Thromboembolism Prophylaxis[2]	112	98%	92%	92%
Incidence of Potentially Preventable VTE[2]	21	5%	11%	10%
UFH with Dosages/Platelet Monitoring[2]	33	100%	96%	97%
Venous Thromboembolism Prophylaxis[2]	272	97%	83%	85%
Warfarin Therapy Discharge Instructions[2]	47	94%	75%	75%
Chest Pain/Possible Heart Attack Care				
Aspirin Given Within 24 Hours of Arrival	-	-	97%	96%
Fibrinolytic Meds Within 30 Min. of Arrival	-	-	62%	58%
Average Time to ECG (minutes)	-	-	9	7
Average Time to Transfer (minutes)	-	-	62	60
Children's Asthma Care				
Received Home Management Plan of Care	-	-	88%	88%
Received Reliever Medication	-	-	100%	100%
Received Systemic Corticosteroids	-	-	100%	100%
Emergency Department				
Admittance Decision Time (minutes)[2]	667	47	125	98
Head CT Results Within 45 Min. of Arrival	-	-	55%	57%
Patients Who Left ER Before Being Seen	-	-	3%	2%
Time from ER Arrival to Admit. (minutes)[2]	670	306	323	274
Time from ER Arrival to Discharge (minutes)	-	-	168	134
Time in ER Before Being Evaluated (minutes)	-	-	29	26
Time to Pain Meds for Fractures (minutes)	-	-	62	57
Heart Attack Care				
Aspirin Given at Discharge	79	100%	99%	99%
Fibrinolytic Meds Within 30 Min. of Arrival[7]	-	-	73%	54%
PCI Within 90 Minutes of Arrival[7]	-	-	95%	96%
Statin Prescribed at Discharge	84	100%	98%	98%
Heart Failure Care				
ACE Inhibitor or ARB for LVSD	57	100%	97%	97%
Discharge Instructions Given	156	100%	94%	94%
Evaluation of LVS Function	180	100%	99%	99%
Medicare Spending				
Medicare Spending per Patient (ratio)	-	0.87	0.98	0.98
Pneumonia Care				
Appropriate Initial Antibiotic Given[2]	62	97%	97%	95%
Blood Culture Timing[2]	132	98%	98%	98%
Pregnancy and Delivery Care				
Newborn Deliveries Scheduled Early[7]	-	-	5%	6%
Preventive Care				
Immunization for Influenza[2]	616	92%	89%	90%
Immunization for Pneumonia[2]	844	96%	90%	92%
Stroke Care				
Anticoagulation Therapy for Atrial Fibrillation[2]	12	92%	95%	95%
Antithrombotic Therapy Timing[2]	44	100%	98%	98%
Assessed for Rehabilitation[2]	122	98%	97%	97%
Discharged on Antithrombotic Therapy[2]	61	98%	99%	99%
Discharged on Statin Medication[2]	50	96%	94%	94%
Thrombolytic Therapy Timing[1,2]	-	-	72%	66%
Venous Thromboembolism Prophylaxis[2]	117	100%	94%	94%
Written Stroke Educational Materials Given[2]	81	95%	87%	88%
Surgical Care Improvement Project				
Appropriate Beta Blocker Usage[2]	122	98%	97%	98%
Appropriate VTP Within 24 Hours[2]	423	100%	98%	98%
Controlled Postoperative Blood Glucose[2,7]	-	-	96%	97%
Perioperative Temperature Management[2]	487	100%	100%	100%
Prophylactic Antibiotic Selection[2]	324	99%	99%	99%
Prophylactic Antibiotic Selection (Outpatient)	-	-	97%	98%
Prophylactic Antibiotic Stopped[2]	322	100%	98%	98%
Prophylactic Antibiotic Timing[2]	324	100%	99%	99%
Prophylactic Antibiotic Timing (Outpatient)	-	-	97%	98%
Urinary Catheter Removal[2]	284	100%	97%	97%
Survey of Patients' Hospital Experiences				
Area Around Room 'Always' Quiet at Night	300+	41%	51%	61%
Doctors 'Always' Communicated Well	300+	83%	78%	82%
Home Recovery Information Given	300+	88%	83%	85%
Hospital Given 9 or 10 on 10 Point Scale	300+	69%	68%	71%
Meds 'Always' Explained Before Given	300+	62%	61%	64%
Nurses 'Always' Communicated Well	300+	76%	74%	79%
Pain 'Always' Well Controlled	300+	73%	68%	71%
Room and Bathroom 'Always' Clean	300+	71%	70%	73%
Timely Help 'Always' Received	300+	68%	62%	68%
Would Definitely Recommend Hospital	300+	72%	70%	71%
Use of Medical Imaging				
Cardiac Imaging Stress Test before Surgery	-	-	5.2%	5.3%
Combination Abdominal CT Scan	-	-	13.4%	10.5%
Combination Brain/Sinus CT Scan	-	-	2.2%	2.7%
Combination Chest CT Scan	-	-	2.3%	2.7%
Follow-up Mammogram/Ultrasound	-	-	8.2%	8.8%
Lumbar Spine MRI for Low Back Pain	-	-	34.2%	37.2%

NOTE: Hospital profiles are in alphabetical order by state, then city, then hospital within the city; Rankings exclude hospitals with less than 25 cases except for patient surveys which excludes hospitals with less than 100 cases; (a) 100-299 cases; (1) The number of cases/patients is too few to report; (2) Data submitted were based on a sample of cases/patients; (3) Results are based on a shorter time period than required; (4) Data suppressed by CMS for one or more quarters; (5) Results are not available for this reporting period; (6) Fewer than 100 patients completed the HCAHPS survey; (7) No cases met the criteria for this measure; (8) The lower limit of the confidence interval cannot be calculated if the number of observed infections equals zero; (9) No data are available from the state/territory for this reporting period; (10) The scores shown reflect fewer than 50 completed surveys; (11) There were discrepancies in the data collection process; (12) This measure does not apply to this hospital for this reporting period; (13) Results cannot be calculated for this reporting period; (14) The results for this state are combined with nearby states to protect confidentiality; Please refer to the User's Guide for a full explanation of data.

Kaiser Foundation Hospital South Sacramento

6600 Bruceville Road | Phone: 916-688-2000
Sacramento, CA 95823
URL: www.mydoctor.kaiserpermanente.org
Type: Acute Care Hospitals | Emergency Services: Yes
Ownership: Voluntary non-profit - Other | Beds: 161

Measure	Cases	This Hosp.	State Avg.	U.S. Avg.
Blood Clot Prevention and Treatment				
Anticoagulation Overlap Therapy[2]	89	99%	92%	93%
ICU Venous Thromboembolism Prophylaxis[2]	76	99%	92%	92%
Incidence of Potentially Preventable VTE[2]	14	0%	11%	10%
UFH with Dosages/Platelet Monitoring[2]	52	100%	96%	97%
Venous Thromboembolism Prophylaxis[2]	269	95%	83%	85%
Warfarin Therapy Discharge Instructions[2]	74	97%	75%	75%
Chest Pain/Possible Heart Attack Care				
Aspirin Given Within 24 Hours of Arrival	-	-	97%	96%
Fibrinolytic Meds Within 30 Min. of Arrival	-	-	62%	58%
Average Time to ECG (minutes)	-	-	9	7
Average Time to Transfer (minutes)	-	-	62	60
Children's Asthma Care				
Received Home Management Plan of Care	-	-	88%	88%
Received Reliever Medication	-	-	100%	100%
Received Systemic Corticosteroids	-	-	100%	100%
Emergency Department				
Admittance Decision Time (minutes)[2]	565	53	125	98
Head CT Results Within 45 Min. of Arrival	-	-	55%	57%
Patients Who Left ER Before Being Seen	-	-	3%	2%
Time from ER Arrival to Admit. (minutes)[2]	584	310	323	274
Time from ER Arrival to Discharge (minutes)	-	-	168	134
Time in ER Before Being Evaluated (minutes)	-	-	29	26
Time to Pain Meds for Fractures (minutes)	-	-	62	57
Heart Attack Care				
Aspirin Given at Discharge	107	100%	99%	99%
Fibrinolytic Meds Within 30 Min. of Arrival[7]	-	-	73%	54%
PCI Within 90 Minutes of Arrival[1]	-	-	95%	96%
Statin Prescribed at Discharge	114	100%	98%	98%
Heart Failure Care				
ACE Inhibitor or ARB for LVSD[2]	74	100%	97%	97%
Discharge Instructions Given[2]	283	100%	94%	94%
Evaluation of LVS Function[2]	308	100%	99%	99%
Medicare Spending				
Medicare Spending per Patient (ratio)	-	0.84	0.98	0.98
Pneumonia Care				
Appropriate Initial Antibiotic Given[2]	84	100%	97%	95%
Blood Culture Timing[2]	132	95%	98%	98%
Pregnancy and Delivery Care				
Newborn Deliveries Scheduled Early[2]	30	0%	5%	6%
Preventive Care				
Immunization for Influenza[2]	490	92%	89%	90%
Immunization for Pneumonia[2]	588	94%	90%	92%
Stroke Care				
Anticoagulation Therapy for Atrial Fibrillation[2]	12	100%	95%	95%
Antithrombotic Therapy Timing[2]	72	100%	98%	98%
Assessed for Rehabilitation[2]	124	100%	97%	97%
Discharged on Antithrombotic Therapy[2]	111	99%	99%	99%
Discharged on Statin Medication[2]	82	99%	94%	94%
Thrombolytic Therapy Timing[2]	12	100%	72%	66%
Venous Thromboembolism Prophylaxis[2]	86	100%	94%	94%
Written Stroke Educational Materials Given[2]	78	99%	87%	88%
Surgical Care Improvement Project				
Appropriate Beta Blocker Usage[2]	110	99%	97%	98%
Appropriate VTP Within 24 Hours[2]	322	98%	98%	98%
Controlled Postoperative Blood Glucose[2,7]	-	-	96%	97%
Perioperative Temperature Management[2]	467	99%	100%	100%
Prophylactic Antibiotic Selection[2]	313	99%	99%	99%
Prophylactic Antibiotic Selection (Outpatient)	-	-	97%	98%
Prophylactic Antibiotic Stopped[2]	310	100%	98%	98%
Prophylactic Antibiotic Timing[2]	313	98%	99%	99%
Prophylactic Antibiotic Timing (Outpatient)	-	-	97%	98%
Urinary Catheter Removal[2]	241	98%	97%	97%
Survey of Patients' Hospital Experiences				
Area Around Room 'Always' Quiet at Night	300+	49%	51%	61%
Doctors 'Always' Communicated Well	300+	83%	78%	82%
Home Recovery Information Given	300+	87%	83%	85%
Hospital Given 9 or 10 on 10 Point Scale	300+	73%	68%	71%
Meds 'Always' Explained Before Given	300+	64%	61%	64%
Nurses 'Always' Communicated Well	300+	75%	74%	79%
Pain 'Always' Well Controlled	300+	71%	68%	71%
Room and Bathroom 'Always' Clean	300+	70%	70%	73%
Timely Help 'Always' Received	300+	63%	62%	68%
Would Definitely Recommend Hospital	300+	75%	70%	71%
Use of Medical Imaging				
Cardiac Imaging Stress Test before Surgery	-	-	5.2%	5.3%
Combination Abdominal CT Scan	-	-	13.4%	10.5%
Combination Brain/Sinus CT Scan	-	-	2.2%	2.7%
Combination Chest CT Scan	-	-	2.3%	2.7%
Follow-up Mammogram/Ultrasound	-	-	8.2%	8.8%
Lumbar Spine MRI for Low Back Pain	-	-	34.2%	37.2%

Mercy General Hospital

4001 J St | Phone: 916-453-4545
Sacramento, CA 95819 | Fax: 916-453-4587
URL: www.mercygeneral.org
Type: Acute Care Hospitals | Emergency Services: Yes
Ownership: Voluntary non-profit - Church | Beds: 399

Key Personnel:
Chief of Medical Staff.......... Richard Atkinson, MD
Operating Room.............. Sherry Franceschi
Hemotology Center .... Allison Jones
Cardiac Laboratory............ Jim Roxburgh
Radiology.................... Parrish Scarboro
Emergency Room .... Mark Smedley, MD
Infection Control............ Roberta Stultz
Quality Assurance .... Linda Ubaldi

Measure	Cases	This Hosp.	State Avg.	U.S. Avg.
Blood Clot Prevention and Treatment				
Anticoagulation Overlap Therapy[2]	91	100%	92%	93%
ICU Venous Thromboembolism Prophylaxis[2]	130	100%	92%	92%
Incidence of Potentially Preventable VTE[1,2]	-	-	11%	10%
UFH with Dosages/Platelet Monitoring[2]	90	100%	96%	97%
Venous Thromboembolism Prophylaxis[2]	266	96%	83%	85%
Warfarin Therapy Discharge Instructions[2]	70	97%	75%	75%
Chest Pain/Possible Heart Attack Care				
Aspirin Given Within 24 Hours of Arrival[1]	-	-	97%	96%
Fibrinolytic Meds Within 30 Min. of Arrival[3,7]	-	-	62%	58%
Average Time to ECG (minutes)[1]	-	-	9	7
Average Time to Transfer (minutes)[3,7]	-	-	62	60
Children's Asthma Care				
Received Home Management Plan of Care	-	-	88%	88%
Received Reliever Medication	-	-	100%	100%
Received Systemic Corticosteroids	-	-	100%	100%
Emergency Department				
Admittance Decision Time (minutes)[2]	422	85	125	98
Head CT Results Within 45 Min. of Arrival[1]	-	-	55%	57%
Patients Who Left ER Before Being Seen	41,070	1%	3%	2%
Time from ER Arrival to Admit. (minutes)[2]	434	307	323	274
Time from ER Arrival to Discharge (minutes)	358	159	168	134
Time in ER Before Being Evaluated (minutes)	408	15	29	26
Time to Pain Meds for Fractures (minutes)	79	63	62	57
Heart Attack Care				
Aspirin Given at Discharge	1,112	100%	99%	99%
Fibrinolytic Meds Within 30 Min. of Arrival[1]	-	-	73%	54%
PCI Within 90 Minutes of Arrival	88	91%	95%	96%
Statin Prescribed at Discharge	1,099	100%	98%	98%
Heart Failure Care				
ACE Inhibitor or ARB for LVSD	164	99%	97%	97%
Discharge Instructions Given	383	99%	94%	94%
Evaluation of LVS Function	444	100%	99%	99%
Medicare Spending				
Medicare Spending per Patient (ratio)	-	0.94	0.98	0.98
Pneumonia Care				
Appropriate Initial Antibiotic Given	141	100%	97%	95%
Blood Culture Timing	228	100%	98%	98%
Pregnancy and Delivery Care				
Newborn Deliveries Scheduled Early[2]	39	5%	5%	6%
Preventive Care				
Immunization for Influenza[2]	547	99%	89%	90%
Immunization for Pneumonia[2]	706	98%	90%	92%
Stroke Care				
Anticoagulation Therapy for Atrial Fibrillation	19	100%	95%	95%
Antithrombotic Therapy Timing	149	99%	98%	98%
Assessed for Rehabilitation	240	98%	97%	97%
Discharged on Antithrombotic Therapy	194	98%	99%	99%
Discharged on Statin Medication	151	96%	94%	94%
Thrombolytic Therapy Timing	30	60%	72%	66%
Venous Thromboembolism Prophylaxis	232	97%	94%	94%
Written Stroke Educational Materials Given	125	92%	87%	88%
Surgical Care Improvement Project				
Appropriate Beta Blocker Usage[2]	242	97%	97%	98%
Appropriate VTP Within 24 Hours[2]	390	99%	98%	98%
Controlled Postoperative Blood Glucose[2]	228	98%	96%	97%
Perioperative Temperature Management[2]	531	100%	100%	100%
Prophylactic Antibiotic Selection[2]	585	99%	99%	99%
Prophylactic Antibiotic Selection (Outpatient)	394	99%	97%	98%
Prophylactic Antibiotic Stopped[2]	566	100%	98%	98%
Prophylactic Antibiotic Timing[2]	585	100%	99%	99%
Prophylactic Antibiotic Timing (Outpatient)	395	99%	97%	98%
Urinary Catheter Removal[2]	350	100%	97%	97%
Survey of Patients' Hospital Experiences				
Area Around Room 'Always' Quiet at Night	300+	49%	51%	61%
Doctors 'Always' Communicated Well	300+	80%	78%	82%
Home Recovery Information Given	300+	86%	83%	85%
Hospital Given 9 or 10 on 10 Point Scale	300+	68%	68%	71%
Meds 'Always' Explained Before Given	300+	63%	61%	64%
Nurses 'Always' Communicated Well	300+	77%	74%	79%
Pain 'Always' Well Controlled	300+	69%	68%	71%
Room and Bathroom 'Always' Clean	300+	68%	70%	73%
Timely Help 'Always' Received	300+	63%	62%	68%
Would Definitely Recommend Hospital	300+	70%	70%	71%
Use of Medical Imaging				
Cardiac Imaging Stress Test before Surgery	342	5.3%	5.2%	5.3%
Combination Abdominal CT Scan	542	1.1%	13.4%	10.5%
Combination Brain/Sinus CT Scan	716	1.3%	2.2%	2.7%
Combination Chest CT Scan	95	0.0%	2.3%	2.7%
Follow-up Mammogram/Ultrasound[7]	-	-	8.2%	8.8%
Lumbar Spine MRI for Low Back Pain[1]	-	-	34.2%	37.2%

Methodist Hospital of Sacramento

7500 Hospital Drive | Phone: 916-423-6010
Sacramento, CA 95823 | Fax: 916-689-7833
URL: www.methodistsacramento.org
Type: Acute Care Hospitals | Emergency Services: Yes
Ownership: Voluntary non-profit - Other | Beds: 355

Key Personnel:
Chief of Medical Staff.......... George Bo-Linn, MD
Operating Room.............. Rondi Crowley
Quality Assurance .... Charles P Francis
Pediatric Ambulatory Care ..... Maureen McGinley
CEO/President............... Timothy Moran
Emergency Room .... Sindy Myas
Radiology................... Stan Wardlaw

Measure	Cases	This Hosp.	State Avg.	U.S. Avg.
Blood Clot Prevention and Treatment				
Anticoagulation Overlap Therapy[2]	41	90%	92%	93%
ICU Venous Thromboembolism Prophylaxis[2]	76	99%	92%	92%
Incidence of Potentially Preventable VTE[1,2]	-	-	11%	10%
UFH with Dosages/Platelet Monitoring[2]	16	100%	96%	97%
Venous Thromboembolism Prophylaxis[2]	329	97%	83%	85%
Warfarin Therapy Discharge Instructions[2]	28	100%	75%	75%
Chest Pain/Possible Heart Attack Care				
Aspirin Given Within 24 Hours of Arrival	91	98%	97%	96%
Fibrinolytic Meds Within 30 Min. of Arrival	13	38%	62%	58%
Average Time to ECG (minutes)	94	10	9	7
Average Time to Transfer (minutes)[1]	-	-	62	60
Children's Asthma Care				
Received Home Management Plan of Care	-	-	88%	88%
Received Reliever Medication	-	-	100%	100%
Received Systemic Corticosteroids	-	-	100%	100%
Emergency Department				
Admittance Decision Time (minutes)[2]	660	194	125	98

NOTE: Hospital profiles are in alphabetical order by state, then city, then hospital within the city; Rankings exclude hospitals with less than 25 cases except for patient surveys which excludes hospitals with less than 100 cases; (a) 100-299 cases; (1) The number of cases/patients is too few to report; (2) Data submitted were based on a sample of cases/patients; (3) Results are based on a shorter time period than required; (4) Data suppressed by CMS for one or more quarters; (5) Results are not available for this reporting period; (6) Fewer than 100 patients completed the HCAHPS survey; (7) No cases met the criteria for this measure; (8) The lower limit of the confidence interval cannot be calculated if the number of observed infections equals zero; (9) No data are available from the state/territory for this reporting period; (10) The scores shown reflect fewer than 50 completed surveys; (11) There were discrepancies in the data collection process; (12) This measure does not apply to this hospital for this reporting period; (13) Results cannot be calculated for this reporting period; (14) The results for this state are combined with nearby states to protect confidentiality; Please refer to the User's Guide for a full explanation of data.

Measure	Cases	This Hosp.	State Avg.	U.S. Avg.
Head CT Results Within 45 Min. of Arrival	30	87%	55%	57%
Patients Who Left ER Before Being Seen	56,353	1%	3%	2%
Time from ER Arrival to Admit. (minutes)[2]	661	444	323	274
Time from ER Arrival to Discharge (minutes)	377	159	168	134
Time in ER Before Being Evaluated (minutes)	425	19	29	26
Time to Pain Meds for Fractures (minutes)	220	54	62	57
Heart Attack Care				
Aspirin Given at Discharge	19	95%	99%	99%
Fibrinolytic Meds Within 30 Min. of Arrival[7]	-	-	73%	54%
PCI Within 90 Minutes of Arrival[7]	-	-	95%	96%
Statin Prescribed at Discharge	19	100%	98%	98%
Heart Failure Care				
ACE Inhibitor or ARB for LVSD[2]	84	99%	97%	97%
Discharge Instructions Given[2]	245	100%	94%	94%
Evaluation of LVS Function[2]	274	100%	99%	99%
Medicare Spending				
Medicare Spending per Patient (ratio)	-	0.88	0.98	0.98
Pneumonia Care				
Appropriate Initial Antibiotic Given[2]	87	99%	97%	95%
Blood Culture Timing[2]	138	96%	98%	98%
Pregnancy and Delivery Care				
Newborn Deliveries Scheduled Early[2]	35	9%	5%	6%
Preventive Care				
Immunization for Influenza[2]	511	99%	89%	90%
Immunization for Pneumonia[2]	596	96%	90%	92%
Stroke Care				
Anticoagulation Therapy for Atrial Fibrillation	16	100%	95%	95%
Antithrombotic Therapy Timing	136	100%	98%	98%
Assessed for Rehabilitation	144	99%	97%	97%
Discharged on Antithrombotic Therapy	132	100%	99%	99%
Discharged on Statin Medication	107	99%	94%	94%
Thrombolytic Therapy Timing[1]	-	-	72%	66%
Venous Thromboembolism Prophylaxis	148	99%	94%	94%
Written Stroke Educational Materials Given	106	100%	87%	88%
Surgical Care Improvement Project				
Appropriate Beta Blocker Usage[2]	63	98%	97%	98%
Appropriate VTP Within 24 Hours[2]	323	97%	98%	98%
Controlled Postoperative Blood Glucose[2,7]	-	-	96%	97%
Perioperative Temperature Management[2]	444	100%	100%	100%
Prophylactic Antibiotic Selection[2]	304	96%	99%	99%
Prophylactic Antibiotic Selection (Outpatient)	16	100%	97%	98%
Prophylactic Antibiotic Stopped[2]	304	100%	98%	98%
Prophylactic Antibiotic Timing[2]	304	100%	99%	99%
Prophylactic Antibiotic Timing (Outpatient)	16	88%	97%	98%
Urinary Catheter Removal[2]	56	100%	97%	97%
Survey of Patients' Hospital Experiences				
Area Around Room 'Always' Quiet at Night	300+	49%	51%	61%
Doctors 'Always' Communicated Well	300+	75%	78%	82%
Home Recovery Information Given	300+	88%	83%	85%
Hospital Given 9 or 10 on 10 Point Scale	300+	65%	68%	71%
Meds 'Always' Explained Before Given	300+	63%	61%	64%
Nurses 'Always' Communicated Well	300+	73%	74%	79%
Pain 'Always' Well Controlled	300+	65%	68%	71%
Room and Bathroom 'Always' Clean	300+	67%	70%	73%
Timely Help 'Always' Received	300+	60%	62%	68%
Would Definitely Recommend Hospital	300+	65%	70%	71%
Use of Medical Imaging				
Cardiac Imaging Stress Test before Surgery	240	4.6%	5.2%	5.3%
Combination Abdominal CT Scan	656	1.5%	13.4%	10.5%
Combination Brain/Sinus CT Scan	800	2.3%	2.2%	2.7%
Combination Chest CT Scan	115	0.0%	2.3%	2.7%
Follow-up Mammogram/Ultrasound[7]	-	-	8.2%	8.8%
Lumbar Spine MRI for Low Back Pain[1]	-	-	34.2%	37.2%

Sutter General Hospital

2801 L Street
Sacramento, CA 95816
Phone: 916-733-8999
Fax: 916-733-8388
URL: www.suttermedicalcenter.org
Type: Acute Care Hospitals
Emergency Services: Yes
Ownership: Voluntary non-profit - Private
Beds: 306

Key Personnel:

Chief of Medical Staff. . . . . Stuart G Bostrom, MD
CEO/President. . . . . Sarah Krevans

Measure	Cases	This Hosp.	State Avg.	U.S. Avg.
Blood Clot Prevention and Treatment				
Anticoagulation Overlap Therapy[2]	132	97%	92%	93%
ICU Venous Thromboembolism Prophylaxis[2]	111	94%	92%	92%
Incidence of Potentially Preventable VTE[2]	20	5%	11%	10%
UFH with Dosages/Platelet Monitoring[2]	46	98%	96%	97%
Venous Thromboembolism Prophylaxis[2]	276	86%	83%	85%
Warfarin Therapy Discharge Instructions[2]	105	93%	75%	75%
Chest Pain/Possible Heart Attack Care				
Aspirin Given Within 24 Hours of Arrival	61	98%	97%	96%
Fibrinolytic Meds Within 30 Min. of Arrival[1]	-	-	62%	58%
Average Time to ECG (minutes)	64	6	9	7
Average Time to Transfer (minutes)[7]	-	-	62	60
Children's Asthma Care				
Received Home Management Plan of Care	-	-	88%	88%
Received Reliever Medication	-	-	100%	100%
Received Systemic Corticosteroids	-	-	100%	100%
Emergency Department				
Admittance Decision Time (minutes)[2]	362	191	125	98
Head CT Results Within 45 Min. of Arrival[1]	-	-	55%	57%
Patients Who Left ER Before Being Seen	88,048	3%	3%	2%
Time from ER Arrival to Admit. (minutes)[2]	382	430	323	274
Time from ER Arrival to Discharge (minutes)	359	177	168	134
Time in ER Before Being Evaluated (minutes)	403	42	29	26
Time to Pain Meds for Fractures (minutes)	238	67	62	57
Heart Attack Care				
Aspirin Given at Discharge	436	100%	99%	99%
Fibrinolytic Meds Within 30 Min. of Arrival[7]	-	-	73%	54%
PCI Within 90 Minutes of Arrival	18	100%	95%	96%
Statin Prescribed at Discharge	416	100%	98%	98%
Heart Failure Care				
ACE Inhibitor or ARB for LVSD[2]	108	100%	97%	97%
Discharge Instructions Given[2]	280	98%	94%	94%
Evaluation of LVS Function[2]	317	100%	99%	99%
Medicare Spending				
Medicare Spending per Patient (ratio)	-	0.93	0.98	0.98
Pneumonia Care				
Appropriate Initial Antibiotic Given[2]	79	99%	97%	95%
Blood Culture Timing[2]	163	98%	98%	98%
Pregnancy and Delivery Care				
Newborn Deliveries Scheduled Early	398	1%	5%	6%
Preventive Care				
Immunization for Influenza[2]	502	92%	89%	90%
Immunization for Pneumonia[2]	473	94%	90%	92%
Stroke Care				
Anticoagulation Therapy for Atrial Fibrillation	20	100%	95%	95%
Antithrombotic Therapy Timing	207	100%	98%	98%
Assessed for Rehabilitation	273	97%	97%	97%
Discharged on Antithrombotic Therapy	223	100%	99%	99%
Discharged on Statin Medication	170	96%	94%	94%
Thrombolytic Therapy Timing	15	53%	72%	66%
Venous Thromboembolism Prophylaxis	270	94%	94%	94%
Written Stroke Educational Materials Given	174	90%	87%	88%
Surgical Care Improvement Project				
Appropriate Beta Blocker Usage[2]	299	100%	97%	98%
Appropriate VTP Within 24 Hours[2]	429	98%	98%	98%
Controlled Postoperative Blood Glucose[2]	191	99%	96%	97%
Perioperative Temperature Management[2]	632	100%	100%	100%
Prophylactic Antibiotic Selection[2]	592	99%	99%	99%
Prophylactic Antibiotic Selection (Outpatient)	467	99%	97%	98%
Prophylactic Antibiotic Stopped[2]	581	100%	98%	98%
Prophylactic Antibiotic Timing[2]	593	99%	99%	99%
Prophylactic Antibiotic Timing (Outpatient)	469	100%	97%	98%
Urinary Catheter Removal[2]	544	100%	97%	97%
Survey of Patients' Hospital Experiences				
Area Around Room 'Always' Quiet at Night	300+	49%	51%	61%
Doctors 'Always' Communicated Well	300+	81%	78%	82%
Home Recovery Information Given	300+	87%	83%	85%
Hospital Given 9 or 10 on 10 Point Scale	300+	68%	68%	71%
Meds 'Always' Explained Before Given	300+	62%	61%	64%
Nurses 'Always' Communicated Well	300+	78%	74%	79%
Pain 'Always' Well Controlled	300+	70%	68%	71%
Room and Bathroom 'Always' Clean	300+	71%	70%	73%
Timely Help 'Always' Received	300+	59%	62%	68%
Would Definitely Recommend Hospital	300+	72%	70%	71%
Use of Medical Imaging				
Cardiac Imaging Stress Test before Surgery	177	4.5%	5.2%	5.3%
Combination Abdominal CT Scan	585	0.3%	13.4%	10.5%
Combination Brain/Sinus CT Scan	703	2.0%	2.2%	2.7%
Combination Chest CT Scan	250	1.2%	2.3%	2.7%
Follow-up Mammogram/Ultrasound[7]	-	-	8.2%	8.8%
Lumbar Spine MRI for Low Back Pain[1]	-	-	34.2%	37.2%

University of California Davis Medical Center

2315 Stockton Boulevard
Sacramento, CA 95817
Phone: 916-734-2011
Fax: 916-734-8080
URL: www.ucdmc.ucdavis.edu
Type: Acute Care Hospitals
Emergency Services: Yes
Ownership: Voluntary non-profit - Other
Beds: 528

Key Personnel:

Radiology. . . . . James Brunberg
Quality Assurance . . . . Joanne Castello
CEO/President. . . . . Robert Chason
Infection Control. . . . . Marsha Koopman
Pediatric Ambulatory Care . . . . . . Morgan Moncada
Chief of Medical Staff. . . . . Gibbe Parsons, MD
Pediatric In-Patient Care . . . . Lisa Trask
Coronary Care. . . . . Rob Underwood

Measure	Cases	This Hosp.	State Avg.	U.S. Avg.
Blood Clot Prevention and Treatment				
Anticoagulation Overlap Therapy[2]	163	100%	92%	93%
ICU Venous Thromboembolism Prophylaxis[2]	86	94%	92%	92%
Incidence of Potentially Preventable VTE[2]	55	4%	11%	10%
UFH with Dosages/Platelet Monitoring[2]	134	100%	96%	97%
Venous Thromboembolism Prophylaxis[2]	292	85%	83%	85%
Warfarin Therapy Discharge Instructions[2]	118	84%	75%	75%
Chest Pain/Possible Heart Attack Care				
Aspirin Given Within 24 Hours of Arrival[5]	-	-	97%	96%
Fibrinolytic Meds Within 30 Min. of Arrival[5]	-	-	62%	58%
Average Time to ECG (minutes)[5]	-	-	9	7
Average Time to Transfer (minutes)[5]	-	-	62	60
Children's Asthma Care				
Received Home Management Plan of Care[2]	132	54%	88%	88%
Received Reliever Medication	132	98%	100%	100%
Received Systemic Corticosteroids	131	100%	100%	100%
Emergency Department				
Admittance Decision Time (minutes)[2]	597	262	125	98
Head CT Results Within 45 Min. of Arrival[1]	-	-	55%	57%
Patients Who Left ER Before Being Seen	69,293	10%	3%	2%
Time from ER Arrival to Admit. (minutes)[2]	597	555	323	274
Time from ER Arrival to Discharge (minutes)	345	267	168	134
Time in ER Before Being Evaluated (minutes)	372	38	29	26
Time to Pain Meds for Fractures (minutes)	231	85	62	57
Heart Attack Care				
Aspirin Given at Discharge[2]	251	98%	99%	99%
Fibrinolytic Meds Within 30 Min. of Arrival[2,7]	-	-	73%	54%
PCI Within 90 Minutes of Arrival[2]	42	86%	95%	96%
Statin Prescribed at Discharge[2]	251	97%	98%	98%
Heart Failure Care				
ACE Inhibitor or ARB for LVSD[2]	115	89%	97%	97%
Discharge Instructions Given[2]	274	92%	94%	94%
Evaluation of LVS Function[2]	289	100%	99%	99%
Medicare Spending				
Medicare Spending per Patient (ratio)	-	0.90	0.98	0.98
Pneumonia Care				
Appropriate Initial Antibiotic Given[2]	55	100%	97%	95%
Blood Culture Timing[2]	134	99%	98%	98%
Pregnancy and Delivery Care				
Newborn Deliveries Scheduled Early[2]	17	0%	5%	6%
Preventive Care				
Immunization for Influenza[2]	529	84%	89%	90%
Immunization for Pneumonia[2]	507	92%	90%	92%
Stroke Care				
Anticoagulation Therapy for Atrial Fibrillation[2]	12	100%	95%	95%
Antithrombotic Therapy Timing[2]	64	95%	98%	98%
Assessed for Rehabilitation[2]	96	100%	97%	97%

NOTE: Hospital profiles are in alphabetical order by state, then city, then hospital within the city; Rankings exclude hospitals with less than 25 cases except for patient surveys which excludes hospitals with less than 100 cases; (a) 100-299 cases; (1) The number of cases/patients is too few to report; (2) Data submitted were based on a sample of cases/patients; (3) Results are based on a shorter time period than required; (4) Data suppressed by CMS for one or more quarters; (5) Results are not available for this reporting period; (6) Fewer than 100 patients completed the HCAHPS survey; (7) No cases met the criteria for this measure; (8) The lower limit of the confidence interval cannot be calculated if the number of observed infections equals zero; (9) No data are available from the state/territory for this reporting period; (10) The scores shown reflect fewer than 50 completed surveys; (11) There were discrepancies in the data collection process; (12) This measure does not apply to this hospital for this reporting period; (13) Results cannot be calculated for this reporting period; (14) The results for this state are combined with nearby states to protect confidentiality; Please refer to the User's Guide for a full explanation of data.

Measure	Cases	This Hosp.	State Avg.	U.S. Avg.
Discharged on Antithrombotic Therapy[2]	76	100%	99%	99%
Discharged on Statin Medication[2]	57	100%	94%	94%
Thrombolytic Therapy Timing[1,2]	-	-	72%	66%
Venous Thromboembolism Prophylaxis[2]	92	95%	94%	94%
Written Stroke Educational Materials Given[2]	65	63%	87%	88%
Surgical Care Improvement Project				
Appropriate Beta Blocker Usage[2]	153	99%	97%	98%
Appropriate VTP Within 24 Hours[2]	337	97%	98%	98%
Controlled Postoperative Blood Glucose[2]	98	93%	96%	97%
Perioperative Temperature Management[2]	466	100%	100%	100%
Prophylactic Antibiotic Selection[2]	350	99%	99%	99%
Prophylactic Antibiotic Selection (Outpatient)	470	98%	97%	98%
Prophylactic Antibiotic Stopped[2]	334	98%	98%	98%
Prophylactic Antibiotic Timing[2]	351	98%	99%	99%
Prophylactic Antibiotic Timing (Outpatient)	235	100%	97%	98%
Urinary Catheter Removal[2]	250	98%	97%	97%
Survey of Patients' Hospital Experiences				
Area Around Room 'Always' Quiet at Night	300+	46%	51%	61%
Doctors 'Always' Communicated Well	300+	79%	78%	82%
Home Recovery Information Given	300+	87%	83%	85%
Hospital Given 9 or 10 on 10 Point Scale	300+	70%	68%	71%
Meds 'Always' Explained Before Given	300+	63%	61%	64%
Nurses 'Always' Communicated Well	300+	75%	74%	79%
Pain 'Always' Well Controlled	300+	69%	68%	71%
Room and Bathroom 'Always' Clean	300+	59%	70%	73%
Timely Help 'Always' Received	300+	61%	62%	68%
Would Definitely Recommend Hospital	300+	75%	70%	71%
Use of Medical Imaging				
Cardiac Imaging Stress Test before Surgery	680	7.8%	5.2%	5.3%
Combination Abdominal CT Scan	2,010	13.9%	13.4%	10.5%
Combination Brain/Sinus CT Scan	1,049	2.9%	2.2%	2.7%
Combination Chest CT Scan	2,093	0.2%	2.3%	2.7%
Follow-up Mammogram/Ultrasound	3,031	7.5%	8.2%	8.8%
Lumbar Spine MRI for Low Back Pain	331	30.2%	34.2%	37.2%

Saint Helena Hospital

10 Woodland Road
Saint Helena, CA 94574
URL: www.sthelenahospital.org
Type: Acute Care Hospitals
Ownership: Voluntary non-profit - Private
Phone: 707-963-3611
Fax: 707-963-6461
Emergency Services: No
Beds: 181

Key Personnel:
Radiology. . . . . William Duqe
Emergency Room . . . . Tami Gash-Kim
CEO/President. . . . . Steven Herber, MD, FACS
Chief of Medical Staff. . . . . Pam Lomar
Cardiac Laboratory. . . . . Dave Tilton

Measure	Cases	This Hosp.	State Avg.	U.S. Avg.
Blood Clot Prevention and Treatment				
Anticoagulation Overlap Therapy[2]	12	92%	92%	93%
ICU Venous Thromboembolism Prophylaxis[2]	74	73%	92%	92%
Incidence of Potentially Preventable VTE[1,2]	-	-	11%	10%
UFH with Dosages/Platelet Monitoring[1,2]	-	-	96%	97%
Venous Thromboembolism Prophylaxis[2]	178	63%	83%	85%
Warfarin Therapy Discharge Instructions[1,2]	-	-	75%	75%
Chest Pain/Possible Heart Attack Care				
Aspirin Given Within 24 Hours of Arrival[1,3]	-	-	97%	96%
Fibrinolytic Meds Within 30 Min. of Arrival[5]	-	-	62%	58%
Average Time to ECG (minutes)[1,3]	-	-	9	7
Average Time to Transfer (minutes)[5]	-	-	62	60
Children's Asthma Care				
Received Home Management Plan of Care	-	-	88%	88%
Received Reliever Medication	-	-	100%	100%
Received Systemic Corticosteroids	-	-	100%	100%
Emergency Department				
Admittance Decision Time (minutes)[2]	135	88	125	98
Head CT Results Within 45 Min. of Arrival[1]	-	-	55%	57%
Patients Who Left ER Before Being Seen	7,446	0%	3%	2%
Time from ER Arrival to Admit. (minutes)[2]	220	210	323	274
Time from ER Arrival to Discharge (minutes)	360	113	168	134
Time in ER Before Being Evaluated (minutes)	381	3	29	26
Time to Pain Meds for Fractures (minutes)	45	46	62	57
Heart Attack Care				
Aspirin Given at Discharge	118	95%	99%	99%
Fibrinolytic Meds Within 30 Min. of Arrival[7]	-	-	73%	54%
PCI Within 90 Minutes of Arrival[1]	-	-	95%	96%
Statin Prescribed at Discharge	115	95%	98%	98%
Heart Failure Care				
ACE Inhibitor or ARB for LVSD	38	92%	97%	97%
Discharge Instructions Given	100	95%	94%	94%
Evaluation of LVS Function	119	100%	99%	99%
Medicare Spending				
Medicare Spending per Patient (ratio)	-	0.84	0.98	0.98
Pneumonia Care				
Appropriate Initial Antibiotic Given	18	89%	97%	95%
Blood Culture Timing	26	100%	98%	98%
Pregnancy and Delivery Care				
Newborn Deliveries Scheduled Early[2]	21	24%	5%	6%
Preventive Care				
Immunization for Influenza[2]	524	55%	89%	90%
Immunization for Pneumonia[2]	604	59%	90%	92%
Stroke Care				
Anticoagulation Therapy for Atrial Fibrillation[1]	-	-	95%	95%
Antithrombotic Therapy Timing	18	100%	98%	98%
Assessed for Rehabilitation	19	95%	97%	97%
Discharged on Antithrombotic Therapy	19	100%	99%	99%
Discharged on Statin Medication	12	100%	94%	94%
Thrombolytic Therapy Timing[7]	-	-	72%	66%
Venous Thromboembolism Prophylaxis	21	95%	94%	94%
Written Stroke Educational Materials Given	13	100%	87%	88%
Surgical Care Improvement Project				
Appropriate Beta Blocker Usage	298	99%	97%	98%
Appropriate VTP Within 24 Hours	159	91%	98%	98%
Controlled Postoperative Blood Glucose	105	93%	96%	97%
Perioperative Temperature Management	1,096	100%	100%	100%
Prophylactic Antibiotic Selection	1,000	99%	99%	99%
Prophylactic Antibiotic Selection (Outpatient)	184	80%	97%	98%
Prophylactic Antibiotic Stopped	993	99%	98%	98%
Prophylactic Antibiotic Timing	1,000	100%	99%	99%
Prophylactic Antibiotic Timing (Outpatient)	155	92%	97%	98%
Urinary Catheter Removal	193	95%	97%	97%
Survey of Patients' Hospital Experiences				
Area Around Room 'Always' Quiet at Night	300+	58%	51%	61%
Doctors 'Always' Communicated Well	300+	80%	78%	82%
Home Recovery Information Given	300+	89%	83%	85%
Hospital Given 9 or 10 on 10 Point Scale	300+	79%	68%	71%
Meds 'Always' Explained Before Given	300+	69%	61%	64%
Nurses 'Always' Communicated Well	300+	83%	74%	79%
Pain 'Always' Well Controlled	300+	76%	68%	71%
Room and Bathroom 'Always' Clean	300+	79%	70%	73%
Timely Help 'Always' Received	300+	70%	62%	68%
Would Definitely Recommend Hospital	300+	83%	70%	71%
Use of Medical Imaging				
Cardiac Imaging Stress Test before Surgery	227	3.1%	5.2%	5.3%
Combination Abdominal CT Scan	265	5.7%	13.4%	10.5%
Combination Brain/Sinus CT Scan[1]	-	-	2.2%	2.7%
Combination Chest CT Scan	235	0.4%	2.3%	2.7%
Follow-up Mammogram/Ultrasound	413	8.0%	8.2%	8.8%
Lumbar Spine MRI for Low Back Pain[1]	-	-	34.2%	37.2%

Natividad Medical Center

1441 Constitution Boulevard
Salinas, CA 93906
URL: www.natividad.com
Type: Acute Care Hospitals
Ownership: Govt - Hospital Dist/Auth
Phone: 831-755-4195
Fax: 831-755-6254
Emergency Services: Yes
Beds: 172

Key Personnel:
Pediatric Ambulatory Care . . . . . . Valerie Barnes, MD
Pediatric In-Patient Care . . . . Valerie Barnes, MD
Radiology. . . . . Michael Basse
CEO/President. . . . . Fernando R. Elizondo
Quality Assurance . . . . Jane Finney
Chief of Medical Staff. . . . . Gary Gary, MD
Emergency Room . . . . Judy Jackson, RN
Operating Room. . . . . Alexander Di Stante, RN

Measure	Cases	This Hosp.	State Avg.	U.S. Avg.
Blood Clot Prevention and Treatment				
Anticoagulation Overlap Therapy[1,2]	-	-	92%	93%
ICU Venous Thromboembolism Prophylaxis[2]	45	98%	92%	92%
Incidence of Potentially Preventable VTE[1,2]	-	-	11%	10%
UFH with Dosages/Platelet Monitoring[1,2]	-	-	96%	97%
Venous Thromboembolism Prophylaxis[2]	272	99%	83%	85%
Warfarin Therapy Discharge Instructions[1,2]	-	-	75%	75%
Chest Pain/Possible Heart Attack Care				
Aspirin Given Within 24 Hours of Arrival	15	100%	97%	96%
Fibrinolytic Meds Within 30 Min. of Arrival[7]	-	-	62%	58%
Average Time to ECG (minutes)	15	32	9	7
Average Time to Transfer (minutes)[1]	-	-	62	60
Children's Asthma Care				
Received Home Management Plan of Care	-	-	88%	88%
Received Reliever Medication	-	-	100%	100%
Received Systemic Corticosteroids	-	-	100%	100%
Emergency Department				
Admittance Decision Time (minutes)[2]	362	146	125	98
Head CT Results Within 45 Min. of Arrival	24	25%	55%	57%
Patients Who Left ER Before Being Seen	46,413	1%	3%	2%
Time from ER Arrival to Admit. (minutes)[2]	363	394	323	274
Time from ER Arrival to Discharge (minutes)	589	115	168	134
Time in ER Before Being Evaluated (minutes)	637	26	29	26
Time to Pain Meds for Fractures (minutes)	147	46	62	57
Heart Attack Care				
Aspirin Given at Discharge[1]	-	-	99%	99%
Fibrinolytic Meds Within 30 Min. of Arrival[7]	-	-	73%	54%
PCI Within 90 Minutes of Arrival[7]	-	-	95%	96%
Statin Prescribed at Discharge[1]	-	-	98%	98%
Heart Failure Care				
ACE Inhibitor or ARB for LVSD	38	95%	97%	97%
Discharge Instructions Given	83	77%	94%	94%
Evaluation of LVS Function	91	99%	99%	99%
Medicare Spending				
Medicare Spending per Patient (ratio)	-	0.94	0.98	0.98
Pneumonia Care				
Appropriate Initial Antibiotic Given	40	90%	97%	95%
Blood Culture Timing	64	91%	98%	98%
Pregnancy and Delivery Care				
Newborn Deliveries Scheduled Early[2]	35	3%	5%	6%
Preventive Care				
Immunization for Influenza[2]	438	60%	89%	90%
Immunization for Pneumonia[2]	262	84%	90%	92%
Stroke Care				
Anticoagulation Therapy for Atrial Fibrillation[1]	-	-	95%	95%
Antithrombotic Therapy Timing	20	100%	98%	98%
Assessed for Rehabilitation	21	95%	97%	97%
Discharged on Antithrombotic Therapy	19	95%	99%	99%
Discharged on Statin Medication	11	82%	94%	94%
Thrombolytic Therapy Timing[1]	-	-	72%	66%
Venous Thromboembolism Prophylaxis	21	95%	94%	94%
Written Stroke Educational Materials Given	18	50%	87%	88%
Surgical Care Improvement Project				
Appropriate Beta Blocker Usage	20	85%	97%	98%
Appropriate VTP Within 24 Hours	134	91%	98%	98%
Controlled Postoperative Blood Glucose[7]	-	-	96%	97%
Perioperative Temperature Management	163	98%	100%	100%
Prophylactic Antibiotic Selection	76	96%	99%	99%
Prophylactic Antibiotic Selection (Outpatient)[5]	-	-	97%	98%
Prophylactic Antibiotic Stopped	75	95%	98%	98%
Prophylactic Antibiotic Timing	78	94%	99%	99%
Prophylactic Antibiotic Timing (Outpatient)[5]	-	-	97%	98%
Urinary Catheter Removal	68	91%	97%	97%
Survey of Patients' Hospital Experiences				
Area Around Room 'Always' Quiet at Night	300+	46%	51%	61%
Doctors 'Always' Communicated Well	300+	79%	78%	82%
Home Recovery Information Given	300+	86%	83%	85%
Hospital Given 9 or 10 on 10 Point Scale	300+	73%	68%	71%
Meds 'Always' Explained Before Given	300+	66%	61%	64%
Nurses 'Always' Communicated Well	300+	74%	74%	79%
Pain 'Always' Well Controlled	300+	67%	68%	71%
Room and Bathroom 'Always' Clean	300+	68%	70%	73%
Timely Help 'Always' Received	300+	59%	62%	68%

NOTE: Hospital profiles are in alphabetical order by state, then city, then hospital within the city; Rankings exclude hospitals with less than 25 cases except for patient surveys which excludes hospitals with less than 100 cases; (a) 100-299 cases; (1) The number of cases/patients is too few to report; (2) Data submitted were based on a sample of cases/patients; (3) Results are based on a shorter time period than required; (4) Data suppressed by CMS for one or more quarters; (5) Results are not available for this reporting period; (6) Fewer than 100 patients completed the HCAHPS survey; (7) No cases met the criteria for this measure; (8) The lower limit of the confidence interval cannot be calculated if the number of observed infections equals zero; (9) No data are available from the state/territory for this reporting period; (10) The scores shown reflect fewer than 50 completed surveys; (11) There were discrepancies in the data collection process; (12) This measure does not apply to this hospital for this reporting period; (13) Results cannot be calculated for this reporting period; (14) The results for this state are combined with nearby states to protect confidentiality; Please refer to the User's Guide for a full explanation of data.

Measure	Cases	This Hosp.	State Avg.	U.S. Avg.
Would Definitely Recommend Hospital	300+	71%	70%	71%
Use of Medical Imaging				
Cardiac Imaging Stress Test before Surgery	99	3.0%	5.2%	5.3%
Combination Abdominal CT Scan	147	8.8%	13.4%	10.5%
Combination Brain/Sinus CT Scan[1]	-	-	2.2%	2.7%
Combination Chest CT Scan[1]	-	-	2.3%	2.7%
Follow-up Mammogram/Ultrasound	213	11.3%	8.2%	8.8%
Lumbar Spine MRI for Low Back Pain[1]	-	-	34.2%	37.2%

Salinas Valley Memorial Hospital

450 East Romie Lane
Salinas, CA 93901
URL: www.svmh.com
Phone: 831-757-4333
Fax: 831-753-6297
Type: Acute Care Hospitals
Emergency Services: Yes
Ownership: Voluntary non-profit - Other
Beds: 266

Key Personnel:

CEO/President.............. Pete Delgado
Operating Room............. Steven M Denmark
Infection Control.......... Wendy Oliva
Radiology.................. F Scott Pereles
Chief of Medical Staff..... Allen Radner, MD
Quality Assurance.......... Anne Robinson
Coronary Care.............. Annette Schuessler
Cardiac Laboratory......... Lesley Turpin

Measure	Cases	This Hosp.	State Avg.	U.S. Avg.
Blood Clot Prevention and Treatment				
Anticoagulation Overlap Therapy[2]	52	92%	92%	93%
ICU Venous Thromboembolism Prophylaxis[2]	51	98%	92%	92%
Incidence of Potentially Preventable VTE[2]	13	0%	11%	10%
UFH with Dosages/Platelet Monitoring[2]	42	100%	96%	97%
Venous Thromboembolism Prophylaxis[2]	352	95%	83%	85%
Warfarin Therapy Discharge Instructions[2]	31	90%	75%	75%
Chest Pain/Possible Heart Attack Care				
Aspirin Given Within 24 Hours of Arrival[5]	-	-	97%	96%
Fibrinolytic Meds Within 30 Min. of Arrival[5]	-	-	62%	58%
Average Time to ECG (minutes)[5]	-	-	9	7
Average Time to Transfer (minutes)[5]	-	-	62	60
Children's Asthma Care				
Received Home Management Plan of Care	-	-	88%	88%
Received Reliever Medication	-	-	100%	100%
Received Systemic Corticosteroids	-	-	100%	100%
Emergency Department				
Admittance Decision Time (minutes)[2]	555	119	125	98
Head CT Results Within 45 Min. of Arrival[1]	-	-	55%	57%
Patients Who Left ER Before Being Seen	43,272	1%	3%	2%
Time from ER Arrival to Admit. (minutes)[2]	570	271	323	274
Time from ER Arrival to Discharge (minutes)	384	155	168	134
Time in ER Before Being Evaluated (minutes)	410	38	29	26
Time to Pain Meds for Fractures (minutes)	168	74	62	57
Heart Attack Care				
Aspirin Given at Discharge	202	100%	99%	99%
Fibrinolytic Meds Within 30 Min. of Arrival[7]	-	-	73%	54%
PCI Within 90 Minutes of Arrival	31	100%	95%	96%
Statin Prescribed at Discharge	192	99%	98%	98%
Heart Failure Care				
ACE Inhibitor or ARB for LVSD[2]	77	100%	97%	97%
Discharge Instructions Given[2]	213	99%	94%	94%
Evaluation of LVS Function[2]	271	100%	99%	99%
Medicare Spending				
Medicare Spending per Patient (ratio)	-	0.98	0.98	0.98
Pneumonia Care				
Appropriate Initial Antibiotic Given[2]	76	93%	97%	95%
Blood Culture Timing[2]	131	98%	98%	98%
Pregnancy and Delivery Care				
Newborn Deliveries Scheduled Early[2]	304	2%	5%	6%
Preventive Care				
Immunization for Influenza[2]	513	89%	89%	90%
Immunization for Pneumonia[2]	555	97%	90%	92%
Stroke Care				
Anticoagulation Therapy for Atrial Fibrillation[2]	21	100%	95%	95%
Antithrombotic Therapy Timing[2]	112	100%	98%	98%
Assessed for Rehabilitation[2]	120	100%	97%	97%
Discharged on Antithrombotic Therapy[2]	112	100%	99%	99%
Discharged on Statin Medication[2]	81	100%	94%	94%
Thrombolytic Therapy Timing[1,2]	-	-	72%	66%
Venous Thromboembolism Prophylaxis[2]	126	100%	94%	94%
Written Stroke Educational Materials Given[2]	54	100%	87%	88%
Surgical Care Improvement Project				
Appropriate Beta Blocker Usage[2]	137	100%	97%	98%
Appropriate VTP Within 24 Hours[2]	322	100%	98%	98%
Controlled Postoperative Blood Glucose[2]	104	98%	96%	97%
Perioperative Temperature Management[2]	400	100%	100%	100%
Prophylactic Antibiotic Selection[2]	380	100%	99%	99%
Prophylactic Antibiotic Selection (Outpatient)	183	100%	97%	98%
Prophylactic Antibiotic Stopped[2]	376	99%	98%	98%
Prophylactic Antibiotic Timing[2]	380	100%	99%	99%
Prophylactic Antibiotic Timing (Outpatient)	184	99%	97%	98%
Urinary Catheter Removal[2]	284	100%	97%	97%
Survey of Patients' Hospital Experiences				
Area Around Room 'Always' Quiet at Night	300+	41%	51%	61%
Doctors 'Always' Communicated Well	300+	79%	78%	82%
Home Recovery Information Given	300+	85%	83%	85%
Hospital Given 9 or 10 on 10 Point Scale	300+	67%	68%	71%
Meds 'Always' Explained Before Given	300+	61%	61%	64%
Nurses 'Always' Communicated Well	300+	73%	74%	79%
Pain 'Always' Well Controlled	300+	70%	68%	71%
Room and Bathroom 'Always' Clean	300+	67%	70%	73%
Timely Help 'Always' Received	300+	56%	62%	68%
Would Definitely Recommend Hospital	300+	71%	70%	71%
Use of Medical Imaging				
Cardiac Imaging Stress Test before Surgery	389	2.3%	5.2%	5.3%
Combination Abdominal CT Scan	478	0.4%	13.4%	10.5%
Combination Brain/Sinus CT Scan	665	2.3%	2.2%	2.7%
Combination Chest CT Scan	96	0.0%	2.3%	2.7%
Follow-up Mammogram/Ultrasound	3,007	11.2%	8.2%	8.8%
Lumbar Spine MRI for Low Back Pain[1]	-	-	34.2%	37.2%

Mark Twain Medical Center

768 Mountain Ranch Rd
San Andreas, CA 95249
Phone: 209-754-2515
Type: Critical Access Hospitals
Emergency Services: Yes
Ownership: Voluntary non-profit - Other

Measure	Cases	This Hosp.	State Avg.	U.S. Avg.
Blood Clot Prevention and Treatment				
Anticoagulation Overlap Therapy[1,2]	-	-	92%	93%
ICU Venous Thromboembolism Prophylaxis[2]	37	97%	92%	92%
Incidence of Potentially Preventable VTE[2,7]	-	-	11%	10%
UFH with Dosages/Platelet Monitoring[1,2]	-	-	96%	97%
Venous Thromboembolism Prophylaxis[2]	119	90%	83%	85%
Warfarin Therapy Discharge Instructions[1,2]	-	-	75%	75%
Chest Pain/Possible Heart Attack Care				
Aspirin Given Within 24 Hours of Arrival[5]	-	-	97%	96%
Fibrinolytic Meds Within 30 Min. of Arrival[5]	-	-	62%	58%
Average Time to ECG (minutes)[5]	-	-	9	7
Average Time to Transfer (minutes)[5]	-	-	62	60
Children's Asthma Care				
Received Home Management Plan of Care	-	-	88%	88%
Received Reliever Medication	-	-	100%	100%
Received Systemic Corticosteroids	-	-	100%	100%
Emergency Department				
Admittance Decision Time (minutes)[2]	534	80	125	98
Head CT Results Within 45 Min. of Arrival[5]	-	-	55%	57%
Patients Who Left ER Before Being Seen	9,398	0%	3%	2%
Time from ER Arrival to Admit. (minutes)[2]	552	246	323	274
Time from ER Arrival to Discharge (minutes)[5]	-	-	168	134
Time in ER Before Being Evaluated (minutes)[5]	-	-	29	26
Time to Pain Meds for Fractures (minutes)[5]	-	-	62	57
Heart Attack Care				
Aspirin Given at Discharge[1,3]	-	-	99%	99%
Fibrinolytic Meds Within 30 Min. of Arrival[3,7]	-	-	73%	54%
PCI Within 90 Minutes of Arrival[3,7]	-	-	95%	96%
Statin Prescribed at Discharge[1,3]	-	-	98%	98%
Heart Failure Care				
ACE Inhibitor or ARB for LVSD	25	96%	97%	97%
Discharge Instructions Given	48	96%	94%	94%
Evaluation of LVS Function	55	100%	99%	99%
Medicare Spending				
Medicare Spending per Patient (ratio)	-	-	0.98	0.98
Pneumonia Care				
Appropriate Initial Antibiotic Given	39	92%	97%	95%
Blood Culture Timing	69	97%	98%	98%
Pregnancy and Delivery Care				
Newborn Deliveries Scheduled Early[7]	-	-	5%	6%
Preventive Care				
Immunization for Influenza[2]	298	90%	89%	90%
Immunization for Pneumonia[2]	482	88%	90%	92%
Stroke Care				
Anticoagulation Therapy for Atrial Fibrillation[1]	-	-	95%	95%
Antithrombotic Therapy Timing[1]	-	-	98%	98%
Assessed for Rehabilitation	11	91%	97%	97%
Discharged on Antithrombotic Therapy[1]	-	-	99%	99%
Discharged on Statin Medication[1]	-	-	94%	94%
Thrombolytic Therapy Timing[7]	-	-	72%	66%
Venous Thromboembolism Prophylaxis	12	92%	94%	94%
Written Stroke Educational Materials Given[1]	-	-	87%	88%
Surgical Care Improvement Project				
Appropriate Beta Blocker Usage[2]	27	100%	97%	98%
Appropriate VTP Within 24 Hours[2]	79	99%	98%	98%
Controlled Postoperative Blood Glucose[2,3]	-	-	96%	97%
Perioperative Temperature Management[2]	88	100%	100%	100%
Prophylactic Antibiotic Selection[2]	52	100%	99%	99%
Prophylactic Antibiotic Selection (Outpatient)[5]	-	-	97%	98%
Prophylactic Antibiotic Stopped[2]	51	100%	98%	98%
Prophylactic Antibiotic Timing[2]	52	100%	99%	99%
Prophylactic Antibiotic Timing (Outpatient)[5]	-	-	97%	98%
Urinary Catheter Removal[2]	32	94%	97%	97%
Survey of Patients' Hospital Experiences				
Area Around Room 'Always' Quiet at Night	(a)	58%	51%	61%
Doctors 'Always' Communicated Well	(a)	77%	78%	82%
Home Recovery Information Given	(a)	83%	83%	85%
Hospital Given 9 or 10 on 10 Point Scale	(a)	64%	68%	71%
Meds 'Always' Explained Before Given	(a)	60%	61%	64%
Nurses 'Always' Communicated Well	(a)	73%	74%	79%
Pain 'Always' Well Controlled	(a)	70%	68%	71%
Room and Bathroom 'Always' Clean	(a)	72%	70%	73%
Timely Help 'Always' Received	(a)	64%	62%	68%
Would Definitely Recommend Hospital	(a)	60%	70%	71%
Use of Medical Imaging				
Cardiac Imaging Stress Test before Surgery	117	6.0%	5.2%	5.3%
Combination Abdominal CT Scan	274	3.6%	13.4%	10.5%
Combination Brain/Sinus CT Scan[1]	-	-	2.2%	2.7%
Combination Chest CT Scan	112	2.7%	2.3%	2.7%
Follow-up Mammogram/Ultrasound	688	7.4%	8.2%	8.8%
Lumbar Spine MRI for Low Back Pain	54	40.7%	34.2%	37.2%

Community Hospital of San Bernardino

1805 Medical Center Drive
San Bernardino, CA 92411
URL: www.chw.edu
Phone: 909-887-6333
Fax: 909-887-6468
Type: Acute Care Hospitals
Emergency Services: Yes
Ownership: Voluntary non-profit - Private
Beds: 374

Key Personnel:

CEO/President.............. June Collison
Operating Room............. Pauline Fernandez, RN
Radiology.................. Phil Liang, MD
Chief of Medical Staff..... Edward Puttre
Quality Assurance.......... Carolyn Swinton

Measure	Cases	This Hosp.	State Avg.	U.S. Avg.
Blood Clot Prevention and Treatment				
Anticoagulation Overlap Therapy[1,2]	-	-	92%	93%
ICU Venous Thromboembolism Prophylaxis[2]	100	91%	92%	92%
Incidence of Potentially Preventable VTE[1,2]	-	-	11%	10%
UFH with Dosages/Platelet Monitoring[1,2]	-	-	96%	97%
Venous Thromboembolism Prophylaxis[2]	333	87%	83%	85%
Warfarin Therapy Discharge Instructions[1,2]	-	-	75%	75%
Chest Pain/Possible Heart Attack Care				
Aspirin Given Within 24 Hours of Arrival	39	100%	97%	96%
Fibrinolytic Meds Within 30 Min. of Arrival[7]	-	-	62%	58%
Average Time to ECG (minutes)	42	6	9	7

NOTE: Hospital profiles are in alphabetical order by state, then city, then hospital within the city; Rankings exclude hospitals with less than 25 cases except for patient surveys which excludes hospitals with less than 100 cases; (a) 100-299 cases; (1) The number of cases/patients is too few to report; (2) Data submitted were based on a sample of cases/patients; (3) Results are based on a shorter time period than required; (4) Data suppressed by CMS for one or more quarters; (5) Results are not available for this reporting period; (6) Fewer than 100 patients completed the HCAHPS survey; (7) No cases met the criteria for this measure; (8) The lower limit of the confidence interval cannot be calculated if the number of observed infections equals zero; (9) No data are available from the state/territory for this reporting period; (10) The scores shown reflect fewer than 50 completed surveys; (11) There were discrepancies in the data collection process; (12) This measure does not apply to this hospital for this reporting period; (13) Results cannot be calculated for this reporting period; (14) The results for this state are combined with nearby states to protect confidentiality; Please refer to the User's Guide for a full explanation of data.

Measure	Cases	This Hosp.	State Avg.	U.S. Avg.
Average Time to Transfer (minutes)	11	30	62	60
Children's Asthma Care				
Received Home Management Plan of Care	-	-	88%	88%
Received Reliever Medication	-	-	100%	100%
Received Systemic Corticosteroids	-	-	100%	100%
Emergency Department				
Admittance Decision Time (minutes)[2]	226	170	125	98
Head CT Results Within 45 Min. of Arrival[1]	-	-	55%	57%
Patients Who Left ER Before Being Seen	51,113	1%	3%	2%
Time from ER Arrival to Admit. (minutes)[2]	237	349	323	274
Time from ER Arrival to Discharge (minutes)	325	138	168	134
Time in ER Before Being Evaluated (minutes)	382	8	29	26
Time to Pain Meds for Fractures (minutes)	219	42	62	57
Heart Attack Care				
Aspirin Given at Discharge	24	83%	99%	99%
Fibrinolytic Meds Within 30 Min. of Arrival[7]	-	-	73%	54%
PCI Within 90 Minutes of Arrival[7]	-	-	95%	96%
Statin Prescribed at Discharge	25	88%	98%	98%
Heart Failure Care				
ACE Inhibitor or ARB for LVSD	32	100%	97%	97%
Discharge Instructions Given	94	100%	94%	94%
Evaluation of LVS Function	95	99%	99%	99%
Medicare Spending				
Medicare Spending per Patient (ratio)	-	1.02	0.98	0.98
Pneumonia Care				
Appropriate Initial Antibiotic Given[2]	52	94%	97%	95%
Blood Culture Timing[2]	119	97%	98%	98%
Pregnancy and Delivery Care				
Newborn Deliveries Scheduled Early[2]	44	2%	5%	6%
Preventive Care				
Immunization for Influenza[2]	467	97%	89%	90%
Immunization for Pneumonia[2]	387	97%	90%	92%
Stroke Care				
Anticoagulation Therapy for Atrial Fibrillation[1]	-	-	95%	95%
Antithrombotic Therapy Timing	14	100%	98%	98%
Assessed for Rehabilitation	15	100%	97%	97%
Discharged on Antithrombotic Therapy	12	83%	99%	99%
Discharged on Statin Medication	11	73%	94%	94%
Thrombolytic Therapy Timing[7]	-	-	72%	66%
Venous Thromboembolism Prophylaxis	17	94%	94%	94%
Written Stroke Educational Materials Given[1]	-	-	87%	88%
Surgical Care Improvement Project				
Appropriate Beta Blocker Usage[2]	18	89%	97%	98%
Appropriate VTP Within 24 Hours[2]	107	99%	98%	98%
Controlled Postoperative Blood Glucose[2,7]	-	-	96%	97%
Perioperative Temperature Management[2]	132	99%	100%	100%
Prophylactic Antibiotic Selection[2]	56	96%	99%	99%
Prophylactic Antibiotic Selection (Outpatient)	29	97%	97%	98%
Prophylactic Antibiotic Stopped[2]	55	100%	98%	98%
Prophylactic Antibiotic Timing[2]	57	98%	99%	99%
Prophylactic Antibiotic Timing (Outpatient)	31	84%	97%	98%
Urinary Catheter Removal[2]	29	97%	97%	97%
Survey of Patients' Hospital Experiences				
Area Around Room 'Always' Quiet at Night	300+	56%	51%	61%
Doctors 'Always' Communicated Well	300+	66%	78%	82%
Home Recovery Information Given	300+	80%	83%	85%
Hospital Given 9 or 10 on 10 Point Scale	300+	64%	68%	71%
Meds 'Always' Explained Before Given	300+	66%	61%	64%
Nurses 'Always' Communicated Well	300+	70%	74%	79%
Pain 'Always' Well Controlled	300+	64%	68%	71%
Room and Bathroom 'Always' Clean	300+	67%	70%	73%
Timely Help 'Always' Received	300+	52%	62%	68%
Would Definitely Recommend Hospital	300+	62%	70%	71%
Use of Medical Imaging				
Cardiac Imaging Stress Test before Surgery[1]	-	-	5.2%	5.3%
Combination Abdominal CT Scan	213	12.2%	13.4%	10.5%
Combination Brain/Sinus CT Scan[1]	-	-	2.2%	2.7%
Combination Chest CT Scan[1]	-	-	2.3%	2.7%
Follow-up Mammogram/Ultrasound	104	4.8%	8.2%	8.8%
Lumbar Spine MRI for Low Back Pain[1]	-	-	34.2%	37.2%

Saint Bernardine Medical Center

2101 N Waterman Ave — Phone: 909-881-4440
San Bernardino, CA 92404 — Fax: 909-881-4481
URL: www.stbernardinemedicalcenter.com
Type: Acute Care Hospitals — Emergency Services: Yes
Ownership: Voluntary non-profit - Private — Beds: 463

Key Personnel:
CEO/President. . . . . Steven R Barron
Radiology. . . . . Joel H Block
Infection Control. . . . . Bridget Connell
Pediatric Ambulatory Care . . . . . . Ernesto Cruz
Pediatric In-Patient Care . . . . Ernesto Cruz
Operating Room. . . . . Paul Godfrey
Coronary Care . . . . Aaron Jordan
Chief of Medical Staff . . . . John Udeh

Measure	Cases	This Hosp.	State Avg.	U.S. Avg.
Blood Clot Prevention and Treatment				
Anticoagulation Overlap Therapy[2]	67	88%	92%	93%
ICU Venous Thromboembolism Prophylaxis[2]	113	100%	92%	92%
Incidence of Potentially Preventable VTE[2]	29	0%	11%	10%
UFH with Dosages/Platelet Monitoring[2]	83	100%	96%	97%
Venous Thromboembolism Prophylaxis[2]	276	89%	83%	85%
Warfarin Therapy Discharge Instructions[2]	45	100%	75%	75%
Chest Pain/Possible Heart Attack Care				
Aspirin Given Within 24 Hours of Arrival	18	94%	97%	96%
Fibrinolytic Meds Within 30 Min. of Arrival[3,7]	-	-	62%	58%
Average Time to ECG (minutes)	18	0	9	7
Average Time to Transfer (minutes)[3,7]	-	-	62	60
Children's Asthma Care				
Received Home Management Plan of Care	-	-	88%	88%
Received Reliever Medication	-	-	100%	100%
Received Systemic Corticosteroids	-	-	100%	100%
Emergency Department				
Admittance Decision Time (minutes)[2]	445	300	125	98
Head CT Results Within 45 Min. of Arrival[1]	-	-	55%	57%
Patients Who Left ER Before Being Seen	73,545	0%	3%	2%
Time from ER Arrival to Admit. (minutes)[2]	465	520	323	274
Time from ER Arrival to Discharge (minutes)	391	93	168	134
Time in ER Before Being Evaluated (minutes)	422	0	29	26
Time to Pain Meds for Fractures (minutes)	208	44	62	57
Heart Attack Care				
Aspirin Given at Discharge[2]	296	100%	99%	99%
Fibrinolytic Meds Within 30 Min. of Arrival[2,7]	-	-	73%	54%
PCI Within 90 Minutes of Arrival[2]	24	83%	95%	96%
Statin Prescribed at Discharge[2]	290	99%	98%	98%
Heart Failure Care				
ACE Inhibitor or ARB for LVSD[2]	119	99%	97%	97%
Discharge Instructions Given[2]	254	96%	94%	94%
Evaluation of LVS Function[2]	288	99%	99%	99%
Medicare Spending				
Medicare Spending per Patient (ratio)	-	1.05	0.98	0.98
Pneumonia Care				
Appropriate Initial Antibiotic Given[2]	59	95%	97%	95%
Blood Culture Timing[2]	125	99%	98%	98%
Pregnancy and Delivery Care				
Newborn Deliveries Scheduled Early[2]	47	2%	5%	6%
Preventive Care				
Immunization for Influenza[2]	553	95%	89%	90%
Immunization for Pneumonia[2]	705	93%	90%	92%
Stroke Care				
Anticoagulation Therapy for Atrial Fibrillation[1]	-	-	95%	95%
Antithrombotic Therapy Timing	82	99%	98%	98%
Assessed for Rehabilitation	100	91%	97%	97%
Discharged on Antithrombotic Therapy	81	99%	99%	99%
Discharged on Statin Medication	66	85%	94%	94%
Thrombolytic Therapy Timing[1]	-	-	72%	66%
Venous Thromboembolism Prophylaxis	102	90%	94%	94%
Written Stroke Educational Materials Given	63	22%	87%	88%
Surgical Care Improvement Project				
Appropriate Beta Blocker Usage[2]	210	92%	97%	98%
Appropriate VTP Within 24 Hours[2]	409	96%	98%	98%
Controlled Postoperative Blood Glucose[2]	192	98%	96%	97%
Perioperative Temperature Management[2]	451	100%	100%	100%
Prophylactic Antibiotic Selection[2]	477	99%	99%	99%
Prophylactic Antibiotic Selection (Outpatient)	152	99%	97%	98%
Prophylactic Antibiotic Stopped[2]	466	96%	98%	98%
Prophylactic Antibiotic Timing[2]	478	99%	99%	99%
Prophylactic Antibiotic Timing (Outpatient)	155	97%	97%	98%
Urinary Catheter Removal[2]	314	94%	97%	97%
Survey of Patients' Hospital Experiences				
Area Around Room 'Always' Quiet at Night	300+	57%	51%	61%
Doctors 'Always' Communicated Well	300+	76%	78%	82%
Home Recovery Information Given	300+	81%	83%	85%
Hospital Given 9 or 10 on 10 Point Scale	300+	70%	68%	71%
Meds 'Always' Explained Before Given	300+	61%	61%	64%
Nurses 'Always' Communicated Well	300+	74%	74%	79%
Pain 'Always' Well Controlled	300+	69%	68%	71%
Room and Bathroom 'Always' Clean	300+	65%	70%	73%
Timely Help 'Always' Received	300+	58%	62%	68%
Would Definitely Recommend Hospital	300+	71%	70%	71%
Use of Medical Imaging				
Cardiac Imaging Stress Test before Surgery	251	6.4%	5.2%	5.3%
Combination Abdominal CT Scan	602	16.1%	13.4%	10.5%
Combination Brain/Sinus CT Scan	607	1.8%	2.2%	2.7%
Combination Chest CT Scan	170	22.4%	2.3%	2.7%
Follow-up Mammogram/Ultrasound	247	11.3%	8.2%	8.8%
Lumbar Spine MRI for Low Back Pain[1]	-	-	34.2%	37.2%

Alvarado Hospital Medical Center

6655 Alvarado Road — Phone: 619-229-3172
San Diego, CA 92120 — Fax: 619-229-7020
URL: www.alvaradohospital.com
Type: Acute Care Hospitals — Emergency Services: Yes
Ownership: Government - Federal — Beds: 231

Key Personnel:
Quality Assurance . . . . Wendy Campbell
Operating Room. . . . . Paul Goldfarb
Administrator . . . . Robin Gomez, RN
President/CEO. . . . . Prem Reddy, MD
Chief of Medical Staff . . . . Lauren Stephen-Porte

Measure	Cases	This Hosp.	State Avg.	U.S. Avg.
Blood Clot Prevention and Treatment				
Anticoagulation Overlap Therapy[2]	40	95%	92%	93%
ICU Venous Thromboembolism Prophylaxis[2]	72	90%	92%	92%
Incidence of Potentially Preventable VTE[1,2]	-	-	11%	10%
UFH with Dosages/Platelet Monitoring[2]	20	100%	96%	97%
Venous Thromboembolism Prophylaxis[2]	339	77%	83%	85%
Warfarin Therapy Discharge Instructions[2]	24	96%	75%	75%
Chest Pain/Possible Heart Attack Care				
Aspirin Given Within 24 Hours of Arrival[3,7]	-	-	97%	96%
Fibrinolytic Meds Within 30 Min. of Arrival[5]	-	-	62%	58%
Average Time to ECG (minutes)[3,7]	-	-	9	7
Average Time to Transfer (minutes)[5]	-	-	62	60
Children's Asthma Care				
Received Home Management Plan of Care	-	-	88%	88%
Received Reliever Medication	-	-	100%	100%
Received Systemic Corticosteroids	-	-	100%	100%
Emergency Department				
Admittance Decision Time (minutes)[2]	423	97	125	98
Head CT Results Within 45 Min. of Arrival[3,7]	-	-	55%	57%
Patients Who Left ER Before Being Seen	25,779	5%	3%	2%
Time from ER Arrival to Admit. (minutes)[2]	434	275	323	274
Time from ER Arrival to Discharge (minutes)	329	170	168	134
Time in ER Before Being Evaluated (minutes)	198	50	29	26
Time to Pain Meds for Fractures (minutes)	22	88	62	57
Heart Attack Care				
Aspirin Given at Discharge	87	100%	99%	99%
Fibrinolytic Meds Within 30 Min. of Arrival[7]	-	-	73%	54%
PCI Within 90 Minutes of Arrival	14	79%	95%	96%
Statin Prescribed at Discharge	79	96%	98%	98%
Heart Failure Care				
ACE Inhibitor or ARB for LVSD	79	92%	97%	97%
Discharge Instructions Given	118	81%	94%	94%
Evaluation of LVS Function	176	100%	99%	99%
Medicare Spending				
Medicare Spending per Patient (ratio)	-	1.07	0.98	0.98
Pneumonia Care				

NOTE: Hospital profiles are in alphabetical order by state, then city, then hospital within the city; Rankings exclude hospitals with less than 25 cases except for patient surveys which excludes hospitals with less than 100 cases; (a) 100-299 cases; (1) The number of cases/patients is too few to report; (2) Data submitted were based on a sample of cases/patients; (3) Results are based on a shorter time period than required; (4) Data suppressed by CMS for one or more quarters; (5) Results are not available for this reporting period; (6) Fewer than 100 patients completed the HCAHPS survey; (7) No cases met the criteria for this measure; (8) The lower limit of the confidence interval cannot be calculated if the number of observed infections equals zero; (9) No data are available from the state/territory for this reporting period; (10) The scores shown reflect fewer than 50 completed surveys; (11) There were discrepancies in the data collection process; (12) This measure does not apply to this hospital for this reporting period; (13) Results cannot be calculated for this reporting period; (14) The results for this state are combined with nearby states to protect confidentiality; Please refer to the User's Guide for a full explanation of data.

Measure	Cases	This Hosp.	State Avg.	U.S. Avg.
Appropriate Initial Antibiotic Given[2]	73	99%	97%	95%
Blood Culture Timing[2]	136	99%	98%	98%
Pregnancy and Delivery Care				
Newborn Deliveries Scheduled Early[7]	-	-	5%	6%
Preventive Care				
Immunization for Influenza[2]	631	95%	89%	90%
Immunization for Pneumonia[2]	902	97%	90%	92%
Stroke Care				
Anticoagulation Therapy for Atrial Fibrillation[1]	-	-	95%	95%
Antithrombotic Therapy Timing	51	92%	98%	98%
Assessed for Rehabilitation	63	98%	97%	97%
Discharged on Antithrombotic Therapy	56	95%	99%	99%
Discharged on Statin Medication	42	88%	94%	94%
Thrombolytic Therapy Timing[1]	-	-	72%	66%
Venous Thromboembolism Prophylaxis	66	79%	94%	94%
Written Stroke Educational Materials Given	38	74%	87%	88%
Surgical Care Improvement Project				
Appropriate Beta Blocker Usage	145	93%	97%	98%
Appropriate VTP Within 24 Hours	237	93%	98%	98%
Controlled Postoperative Blood Glucose	50	80%	96%	97%
Perioperative Temperature Management	301	99%	100%	100%
Prophylactic Antibiotic Selection	209	98%	99%	99%
Prophylactic Antibiotic Selection (Outpatient)	101	98%	97%	98%
Prophylactic Antibiotic Stopped	202	96%	98%	98%
Prophylactic Antibiotic Timing	209	99%	99%	99%
Prophylactic Antibiotic Timing (Outpatient)	102	97%	97%	98%
Urinary Catheter Removal	232	94%	97%	97%
Survey of Patients' Hospital Experiences				
Area Around Room 'Always' Quiet at Night	300+	54%	51%	61%
Doctors 'Always' Communicated Well	300+	76%	78%	82%
Home Recovery Information Given	300+	84%	83%	85%
Hospital Given 9 or 10 on 10 Point Scale	300+	61%	68%	71%
Meds 'Always' Explained Before Given	300+	54%	61%	64%
Nurses 'Always' Communicated Well	300+	69%	74%	79%
Pain 'Always' Well Controlled	300+	62%	68%	71%
Room and Bathroom 'Always' Clean	300+	65%	70%	73%
Timely Help 'Always' Received	300+	57%	62%	68%
Would Definitely Recommend Hospital	300+	62%	70%	71%
Use of Medical Imaging				
Cardiac Imaging Stress Test before Surgery	159	8.2%	5.2%	5.3%
Combination Abdominal CT Scan	291	5.5%	13.4%	10.5%
Combination Brain/Sinus CT Scan	418	2.2%	2.2%	2.7%
Combination Chest CT Scan	96	0.0%	2.3%	2.7%
Follow-up Mammogram/Ultrasound[1]	-	-	8.2%	8.8%
Lumbar Spine MRI for Low Back Pain[1]	-	-	34.2%	37.2%

Kaiser Foundation Hospital - San Diego

4647 Zion Ave
San Diego, CA 92120
Phone: 619-528-5000
Fax: 626-405-3176
URL: www.members.kaiserpermanente.org
Type: Acute Care Hospitals
Emergency Services: Yes
Ownership: Voluntary non-profit - Other
Beds: 392

Key Personnel:
Chief of Medical Staff.......... Daniel Anderson, MD
Infection Control.............. Roger Bitar, MD
Pediatric In-Patient Care .... Charles Freedman, MD
Quality Assurance .... Louise L Lang
Emergency Room .... Raymond Poliakoff, MD
Anesthesiology................ Diane Rand, MD
CEO/President............... Mary Ann Thode

Measure	Cases	This Hosp.	State Avg.	U.S. Avg.
Blood Clot Prevention and Treatment				
Anticoagulation Overlap Therapy[2]	135	98%	92%	93%
ICU Venous Thromboembolism Prophylaxis[2]	22	95%	92%	92%
Incidence of Potentially Preventable VTE[2]	27	4%	11%	10%
UFH with Dosages/Platelet Monitoring[2]	96	100%	96%	97%
Venous Thromboembolism Prophylaxis[2]	361	88%	83%	85%
Warfarin Therapy Discharge Instructions[2]	107	97%	75%	75%
Chest Pain/Possible Heart Attack Care				
Aspirin Given Within 24 Hours of Arrival	-	-	97%	96%
Fibrinolytic Meds Within 30 Min. of Arrival	-	-	62%	58%
Average Time to ECG (minutes)	-	-	9	7
Average Time to Transfer (minutes)	-	-	62	60
Children's Asthma Care				
Received Home Management Plan of Care	-	-	88%	88%
Received Reliever Medication	-	-	100%	100%
Received Systemic Corticosteroids	-	-	100%	100%
Emergency Department				
Admittance Decision Time (minutes)[2]	411	96	125	98
Head CT Results Within 45 Min. of Arrival	-	-	55%	57%
Patients Who Left ER Before Being Seen	-	-	3%	2%
Time from ER Arrival to Admit. (minutes)[2]	505	418	323	274
Time from ER Arrival to Discharge (minutes)	-	-	168	134
Time in ER Before Being Evaluated (minutes)	-	-	29	26
Time to Pain Meds for Fractures (minutes)	-	-	62	57
Heart Attack Care				
Aspirin Given at Discharge	105	100%	99%	99%
Fibrinolytic Meds Within 30 Min. of Arrival[7]	-	-	73%	54%
PCI Within 90 Minutes of Arrival[7]	-	-	95%	96%
Statin Prescribed at Discharge	108	100%	98%	98%
Heart Failure Care				
ACE Inhibitor or ARB for LVSD	168	99%	97%	97%
Discharge Instructions Given	630	100%	94%	94%
Evaluation of LVS Function	683	100%	99%	99%
Medicare Spending				
Medicare Spending per Patient (ratio)	-	0.73	0.98	0.98
Pneumonia Care				
Appropriate Initial Antibiotic Given[2]	47	98%	97%	95%
Blood Culture Timing[2]	152	99%	98%	98%
Pregnancy and Delivery Care				
Newborn Deliveries Scheduled Early	345	3%	5%	6%
Preventive Care				
Immunization for Influenza[2]	493	92%	89%	90%
Immunization for Pneumonia[2]	533	95%	90%	92%
Stroke Care				
Anticoagulation Therapy for Atrial Fibrillation[2]	18	100%	95%	95%
Antithrombotic Therapy Timing[2]	66	100%	98%	98%
Assessed for Rehabilitation[2]	120	99%	97%	97%
Discharged on Antithrombotic Therapy[2]	96	100%	99%	99%
Discharged on Statin Medication[2]	79	100%	94%	94%
Thrombolytic Therapy Timing[1,2]	-	-	72%	66%
Venous Thromboembolism Prophylaxis[2]	86	99%	94%	94%
Written Stroke Educational Materials Given[2]	78	100%	87%	88%
Surgical Care Improvement Project				
Appropriate Beta Blocker Usage[2]	134	99%	97%	98%
Appropriate VTP Within 24 Hours[2]	358	100%	98%	98%
Controlled Postoperative Blood Glucose[2,7]	-	-	96%	97%
Perioperative Temperature Management[2]	469	100%	100%	100%
Prophylactic Antibiotic Selection[2]	271	100%	99%	99%
Prophylactic Antibiotic Selection (Outpatient)	-	-	97%	98%
Prophylactic Antibiotic Stopped[2]	257	100%	98%	98%
Prophylactic Antibiotic Timing[2]	271	99%	99%	99%
Prophylactic Antibiotic Timing (Outpatient)	-	-	97%	98%
Urinary Catheter Removal[2]	311	100%	97%	97%
Survey of Patients' Hospital Experiences				
Area Around Room 'Always' Quiet at Night	300+	45%	51%	61%
Doctors 'Always' Communicated Well	300+	81%	78%	82%
Home Recovery Information Given	300+	87%	83%	85%
Hospital Given 9 or 10 on 10 Point Scale	300+	71%	68%	71%
Meds 'Always' Explained Before Given	300+	64%	61%	64%
Nurses 'Always' Communicated Well	300+	77%	74%	79%
Pain 'Always' Well Controlled	300+	72%	68%	71%
Room and Bathroom 'Always' Clean	300+	72%	70%	73%
Timely Help 'Always' Received	300+	66%	62%	68%
Would Definitely Recommend Hospital	300+	73%	70%	71%
Use of Medical Imaging				
Cardiac Imaging Stress Test before Surgery	-	-	5.2%	5.3%
Combination Abdominal CT Scan	-	-	13.4%	10.5%
Combination Brain/Sinus CT Scan	-	-	2.2%	2.7%
Combination Chest CT Scan	-	-	2.3%	2.7%
Follow-up Mammogram/Ultrasound	-	-	8.2%	8.8%
Lumbar Spine MRI for Low Back Pain	-	-	34.2%	37.2%

Scripps Mercy Hospital

4077 5th Ave
San Diego, CA 92103
Phone: 619-294-8111
Fax: 619-686-3530
URL: www.scrippshealth.org
Type: Acute Care Hospitals
Emergency Services: Yes
Ownership: Voluntary non-profit - Private
Beds: 700

Key Personnel:
Pediatric Ambulatory Care .... William Fischer, MD
Pediatric In-Patient Care .... William Fischer, MD
Quality Assurance .... Ellen Kealy-Pels
CEO/President............... Chris Van Gorder, FACHE

Measure	Cases	This Hosp.	State Avg.	U.S. Avg.
Blood Clot Prevention and Treatment				
Anticoagulation Overlap Therapy[2]	203	93%	92%	93%
ICU Venous Thromboembolism Prophylaxis[2]	65	95%	92%	92%
Incidence of Potentially Preventable VTE[2]	28	4%	11%	10%
UFH with Dosages/Platelet Monitoring[2]	168	98%	96%	97%
Venous Thromboembolism Prophylaxis[2]	361	86%	83%	85%
Warfarin Therapy Discharge Instructions[2]	137	10%	75%	75%
Chest Pain/Possible Heart Attack Care				
Aspirin Given Within 24 Hours of Arrival	37	97%	97%	96%
Fibrinolytic Meds Within 30 Min. of Arrival[7]	-	-	62%	58%
Average Time to ECG (minutes)	34	11	9	7
Average Time to Transfer (minutes)[1]	-	-	62	60
Children's Asthma Care				
Received Home Management Plan of Care	-	-	88%	88%
Received Reliever Medication	-	-	100%	100%
Received Systemic Corticosteroids	-	-	100%	100%
Emergency Department				
Admittance Decision Time (minutes)[2]	581	146	125	98
Head CT Results Within 45 Min. of Arrival	38	79%	55%	57%
Patients Who Left ER Before Being Seen	>100k	2%	3%	2%
Time from ER Arrival to Admit. (minutes)[2]	601	344	323	274
Time from ER Arrival to Discharge (minutes)	363	197	168	134
Time in ER Before Being Evaluated (minutes)	400	21	29	26
Time to Pain Meds for Fractures (minutes)	186	44	62	57
Heart Attack Care				
Aspirin Given at Discharge	353	99%	99%	99%
Fibrinolytic Meds Within 30 Min. of Arrival[1]	-	-	73%	54%
PCI Within 90 Minutes of Arrival	69	94%	95%	96%
Statin Prescribed at Discharge	359	99%	98%	98%
Heart Failure Care				
ACE Inhibitor or ARB for LVSD[2]	197	98%	97%	97%
Discharge Instructions Given[2]	444	96%	94%	94%
Evaluation of LVS Function[2]	551	100%	99%	99%
Medicare Spending				
Medicare Spending per Patient (ratio)	-	1.04	0.98	0.98
Pneumonia Care				
Appropriate Initial Antibiotic Given[2]	68	100%	97%	95%
Blood Culture Timing[2]	136	100%	98%	98%
Pregnancy and Delivery Care				
Newborn Deliveries Scheduled Early[2]	81	0%	5%	6%
Preventive Care				
Immunization for Influenza[2]	537	94%	89%	90%
Immunization for Pneumonia[2]	615	94%	90%	92%
Stroke Care				
Anticoagulation Therapy for Atrial Fibrillation	50	100%	95%	95%
Antithrombotic Therapy Timing	265	99%	98%	98%
Assessed for Rehabilitation	325	100%	97%	97%
Discharged on Antithrombotic Therapy	288	100%	99%	99%
Discharged on Statin Medication	227	97%	94%	94%
Thrombolytic Therapy Timing	27	96%	72%	66%
Venous Thromboembolism Prophylaxis	333	94%	94%	94%
Written Stroke Educational Materials Given	173	100%	87%	88%
Surgical Care Improvement Project				
Appropriate Beta Blocker Usage[2]	249	100%	97%	98%
Appropriate VTP Within 24 Hours[2]	420	98%	98%	98%
Controlled Postoperative Blood Glucose[2]	144	100%	96%	97%
Perioperative Temperature Management[2]	529	100%	100%	100%
Prophylactic Antibiotic Selection[2]	466	99%	99%	99%
Prophylactic Antibiotic Selection (Outpatient)	485	95%	97%	98%
Prophylactic Antibiotic Stopped[2]	453	99%	98%	98%
Prophylactic Antibiotic Timing[2]	466	99%	99%	99%

NOTE: Hospital profiles are in alphabetical order by state, then city, then hospital within the city; Rankings exclude hospitals with less than 25 cases except for patient surveys which excludes hospitals with less than 100 cases; (a) 100-299 cases; (1) The number of cases/patients is too few to report; (2) Data submitted were based on a sample of cases/patients; (3) Results are based on a shorter time period than required; (4) Data suppressed by CMS for one or more quarters; (5) Results are not available for this reporting period; (6) Fewer than 100 patients completed the HCAHPS survey; (7) No cases met the criteria for this measure; (8) The lower limit of the confidence interval cannot be calculated if the number of observed infections equals zero; (9) No data are available from the state/territory for this reporting period; (10) The scores shown reflect fewer than 50 completed surveys; (11) There were discrepancies in the data collection process; (12) This measure does not apply to this hospital for this reporting period; (13) Results cannot be calculated for this reporting period; (14) The results for this state are combined with nearby states to protect confidentiality; Please refer to the User's Guide for a full explanation of data.

Measure	Cases	This Hosp.	State Avg.	U.S. Avg.
Prophylactic Antibiotic Timing (Outpatient)	501	94%	97%	98%
Urinary Catheter Removal[2]	422	99%	97%	97%
Survey of Patients' Hospital Experiences				
Area Around Room 'Always' Quiet at Night	300+	48%	51%	61%
Doctors 'Always' Communicated Well	300+	79%	78%	82%
Home Recovery Information Given	300+	83%	83%	85%
Hospital Given 9 or 10 on 10 Point Scale	300+	66%	68%	71%
Meds 'Always' Explained Before Given	300+	63%	61%	64%
Nurses 'Always' Communicated Well	300+	74%	74%	79%
Pain 'Always' Well Controlled	300+	69%	68%	71%
Room and Bathroom 'Always' Clean	300+	66%	70%	73%
Timely Help 'Always' Received	300+	58%	62%	68%
Would Definitely Recommend Hospital	300+	69%	70%	71%
Use of Medical Imaging				
Cardiac Imaging Stress Test before Surgery	221	5.9%	5.2%	5.3%
Combination Abdominal CT Scan	1,453	4.4%	13.4%	10.5%
Combination Brain/Sinus CT Scan	1,717	4.2%	2.2%	2.7%
Combination Chest CT Scan	726	1.2%	2.3%	2.7%
Follow-up Mammogram/Ultrasound	1,642	6.1%	8.2%	8.8%
Lumbar Spine MRI for Low Back Pain	175	27.4%	34.2%	37.2%

Sharp Memorial Hospital

7901 Frost St
San Diego, CA 92123
Phone: 858-939-3400
Fax: 858-939-3514
URL: www.sharp.com/memorial
Type: Acute Care Hospitals
Emergency Services: Yes
Ownership: Voluntary non-profit - Other
Beds: 464

Key Personnel:
Operating Room. . . . . Mary Diamond
Emergency Room . . . . Denise Foster
Chief of Medical Staff. . . . . Peter M Hoagland, MD
Patient Relations . . . . Cindy Murphy
Infection Control. . . . . Shannon Oriola
Cardiac Laboratory. . . . . Tim Smith
Radiology. . . . . Sharon Stromme
Ambulatory Care . . . . Lori Wells

Measure	Cases	This Hosp.	State Avg.	U.S. Avg.
Blood Clot Prevention and Treatment				
Anticoagulation Overlap Therapy[2]	140	95%	92%	93%
ICU Venous Thromboembolism Prophylaxis[2]	66	92%	92%	92%
Incidence of Potentially Preventable VTE[2]	32	9%	11%	10%
UFH with Dosages/Platelet Monitoring[2]	33	100%	96%	97%
Venous Thromboembolism Prophylaxis[2]	332	81%	83%	85%
Warfarin Therapy Discharge Instructions[2]	110	83%	75%	75%
Chest Pain/Possible Heart Attack Care				
Aspirin Given Within 24 Hours of Arrival[1,3]	-	-	97%	96%
Fibrinolytic Meds Within 30 Min. of Arrival[3,7]	-	-	62%	58%
Average Time to ECG (minutes)[1,3]	-	-	9	7
Average Time to Transfer (minutes)[1,3]	-	-	62	60
Children's Asthma Care				
Received Home Management Plan of Care	-	-	88%	88%
Received Reliever Medication	-	-	100%	100%
Received Systemic Corticosteroids	-	-	100%	100%
Emergency Department				
Admittance Decision Time (minutes)[2]	443	75	125	98
Head CT Results Within 45 Min. of Arrival[1]	-	-	55%	57%
Patients Who Left ER Before Being Seen	70,523	1%	3%	2%
Time from ER Arrival to Admit. (minutes)[2]	459	232	323	274
Time from ER Arrival to Discharge (minutes)	406	180	168	134
Time in ER Before Being Evaluated (minutes)	385	26	29	26
Time to Pain Meds for Fractures (minutes)	163	50	62	57
Heart Attack Care				
Aspirin Given at Discharge	236	100%	99%	99%
Fibrinolytic Meds Within 30 Min. of Arrival[7]	-	-	73%	54%
PCI Within 90 Minutes of Arrival	50	96%	95%	96%
Statin Prescribed at Discharge	236	100%	98%	98%
Heart Failure Care				
ACE Inhibitor or ARB for LVSD	148	100%	97%	97%
Discharge Instructions Given	448	96%	94%	94%
Evaluation of LVS Function	534	100%	99%	99%
Medicare Spending				
Medicare Spending per Patient (ratio)	-	1.00	0.98	0.98
Pneumonia Care				
Appropriate Initial Antibiotic Given	274	99%	97%	95%
Blood Culture Timing	401	100%	98%	98%
Pregnancy and Delivery Care				
Newborn Deliveries Scheduled Early	876	2%	5%	6%
Preventive Care				
Immunization for Influenza[2]	532	97%	89%	90%
Immunization for Pneumonia[2]	417	95%	90%	92%
Stroke Care				
Anticoagulation Therapy for Atrial Fibrillation	35	97%	95%	95%
Antithrombotic Therapy Timing	191	98%	98%	98%
Assessed for Rehabilitation	296	99%	97%	97%
Discharged on Antithrombotic Therapy	234	99%	99%	99%
Discharged on Statin Medication	161	94%	94%	94%
Thrombolytic Therapy Timing	27	78%	72%	66%
Venous Thromboembolism Prophylaxis	280	98%	94%	94%
Written Stroke Educational Materials Given	159	96%	87%	88%
Surgical Care Improvement Project				
Appropriate Beta Blocker Usage[2]	476	99%	97%	98%
Appropriate VTP Within 24 Hours[2]	1,341	99%	98%	98%
Controlled Postoperative Blood Glucose[2]	253	99%	96%	97%
Perioperative Temperature Management[2]	1,500	100%	100%	100%
Prophylactic Antibiotic Selection[2]	1,418	100%	99%	99%
Prophylactic Antibiotic Selection (Outpatient)	577	99%	97%	98%
Prophylactic Antibiotic Stopped[2]	1,371	99%	98%	98%
Prophylactic Antibiotic Timing[2]	1,417	100%	99%	99%
Prophylactic Antibiotic Timing (Outpatient)	577	100%	97%	98%
Urinary Catheter Removal[2]	1,245	99%	97%	97%
Survey of Patients' Hospital Experiences				
Area Around Room 'Always' Quiet at Night	300+	66%	51%	61%
Doctors 'Always' Communicated Well	300+	82%	78%	82%
Home Recovery Information Given	300+	87%	83%	85%
Hospital Given 9 or 10 on 10 Point Scale	300+	85%	68%	71%
Meds 'Always' Explained Before Given	300+	67%	61%	64%
Nurses 'Always' Communicated Well	300+	83%	74%	79%
Pain 'Always' Well Controlled	300+	76%	68%	71%
Room and Bathroom 'Always' Clean	300+	77%	70%	73%
Timely Help 'Always' Received	300+	71%	62%	68%
Would Definitely Recommend Hospital	300+	86%	70%	71%
Use of Medical Imaging				
Cardiac Imaging Stress Test before Surgery	267	4.9%	5.2%	5.3%
Combination Abdominal CT Scan	1,075	1.1%	13.4%	10.5%
Combination Brain/Sinus CT Scan	1,309	3.5%	2.2%	2.7%
Combination Chest CT Scan	435	4.8%	2.3%	2.7%
Follow-up Mammogram/Ultrasound	1,636	7.8%	8.2%	8.8%
Lumbar Spine MRI for Low Back Pain[1]	-	-	34.2%	37.2%

University of California San Diego Medical Center

200 West Arbor Drive
San Diego, CA 92103
Phone: 619-543-6222
Fax: 619-543-5423
URL: www.health.ucsd.edu
Type: Acute Care Hospitals
Emergency Services: Yes
Ownership: Voluntary non-profit - Other
Beds: 558

Key Personnel:
Intensive Care Unit. . . . . David Hoyt, MD
Emergency Room . . . . Kevin Jones
Radiology. . . . . George Leopold, MD
CEO/President. . . . . Richard Liekweg
Pediatric Ambulatory Care . . . . . . Stanley Mendoza, MD
Pediatric In-Patient Care . . . . Stanley Mendoza, MD
Infection Control. . . . . S Spencer, MD
Chief of Medical Staff. . . . . Stephen I Wasserman

Measure	Cases	This Hosp.	State Avg.	U.S. Avg.
Blood Clot Prevention and Treatment				
Anticoagulation Overlap Therapy[2]	122	93%	92%	93%
ICU Venous Thromboembolism Prophylaxis[2]	75	100%	92%	92%
Incidence of Potentially Preventable VTE[2]	82	6%	11%	10%
UFH with Dosages/Platelet Monitoring[2]	86	100%	96%	97%
Venous Thromboembolism Prophylaxis[2]	311	93%	83%	85%
Warfarin Therapy Discharge Instructions[2]	99	4%	75%	75%
Chest Pain/Possible Heart Attack Care				
Aspirin Given Within 24 Hours of Arrival[1]	-	-	97%	96%
Fibrinolytic Meds Within 30 Min. of Arrival[5]	-	-	62%	58%
Average Time to ECG (minutes)[1]	-	-	9	7
Average Time to Transfer (minutes)[5]	-	-	62	60
Children's Asthma Care				
Received Home Management Plan of Care	-	-	88%	88%
Received Reliever Medication	-	-	100%	100%
Received Systemic Corticosteroids	-	-	100%	100%
Emergency Department				
Admittance Decision Time (minutes)[2]	494	287	125	98
Head CT Results Within 45 Min. of Arrival[3,7]	-	-	55%	57%
Patients Who Left ER Before Being Seen	66,694	2%	3%	2%
Time from ER Arrival to Admit. (minutes)[2]	494	427	323	274
Time from ER Arrival to Discharge (minutes)	342	244	168	134
Time in ER Before Being Evaluated (minutes)	383	20	29	26
Time to Pain Meds for Fractures (minutes)	94	66	62	57
Heart Attack Care				
Aspirin Given at Discharge	266	100%	99%	99%
Fibrinolytic Meds Within 30 Min. of Arrival[7]	-	-	73%	54%
PCI Within 90 Minutes of Arrival	40	98%	95%	96%
Statin Prescribed at Discharge	263	100%	98%	98%
Heart Failure Care				
ACE Inhibitor or ARB for LVSD[2]	101	96%	97%	97%
Discharge Instructions Given[2]	242	92%	94%	94%
Evaluation of LVS Function[2]	270	100%	99%	99%
Medicare Spending				
Medicare Spending per Patient (ratio)	-	0.97	0.98	0.98
Pneumonia Care				
Appropriate Initial Antibiotic Given[2]	40	90%	97%	95%
Blood Culture Timing[2]	136	96%	98%	98%
Pregnancy and Delivery Care				
Newborn Deliveries Scheduled Early[2]	16	0%	5%	6%
Preventive Care				
Immunization for Influenza[2]	527	90%	89%	90%
Immunization for Pneumonia[2]	535	82%	90%	92%
Stroke Care				
Anticoagulation Therapy for Atrial Fibrillation	26	100%	95%	95%
Antithrombotic Therapy Timing	129	100%	98%	98%
Assessed for Rehabilitation	188	99%	97%	97%
Discharged on Antithrombotic Therapy	148	100%	99%	99%
Discharged on Statin Medication	101	98%	94%	94%
Thrombolytic Therapy Timing	15	93%	72%	66%
Venous Thromboembolism Prophylaxis	179	99%	94%	94%
Written Stroke Educational Materials Given	121	93%	87%	88%
Surgical Care Improvement Project				
Appropriate Beta Blocker Usage[2]	168	98%	97%	98%
Appropriate VTP Within 24 Hours[2]	324	98%	98%	98%
Controlled Postoperative Blood Glucose[2]	138	99%	96%	97%
Perioperative Temperature Management[2]	470	99%	100%	100%
Prophylactic Antibiotic Selection[2]	372	99%	99%	99%
Prophylactic Antibiotic Selection (Outpatient)	349	99%	97%	98%
Prophylactic Antibiotic Stopped[2]	348	96%	98%	98%
Prophylactic Antibiotic Timing[2]	371	98%	99%	99%
Prophylactic Antibiotic Timing (Outpatient)	241	97%	97%	98%
Urinary Catheter Removal[2]	316	98%	97%	97%
Survey of Patients' Hospital Experiences				
Area Around Room 'Always' Quiet at Night	300+	56%	51%	61%
Doctors 'Always' Communicated Well	300+	80%	78%	82%
Home Recovery Information Given	300+	86%	83%	85%
Hospital Given 9 or 10 on 10 Point Scale	300+	70%	68%	71%
Meds 'Always' Explained Before Given	300+	66%	61%	64%
Nurses 'Always' Communicated Well	300+	76%	74%	79%
Pain 'Always' Well Controlled	300+	70%	68%	71%
Room and Bathroom 'Always' Clean	300+	72%	70%	73%
Timely Help 'Always' Received	300+	64%	62%	68%
Would Definitely Recommend Hospital	300+	78%	70%	71%
Use of Medical Imaging				
Cardiac Imaging Stress Test before Surgery	898	5.7%	5.2%	5.3%
Combination Abdominal CT Scan	2,173	9.7%	13.4%	10.5%
Combination Brain/Sinus CT Scan	823	3.3%	2.2%	2.7%
Combination Chest CT Scan	2,241	0.2%	2.3%	2.7%
Follow-up Mammogram/Ultrasound	1,370	9.3%	8.2%	8.8%
Lumbar Spine MRI for Low Back Pain	146	36.3%	34.2%	37.2%

NOTE: Hospital profiles are in alphabetical order by state, then city, then hospital within the city; Rankings exclude hospitals with less than 25 cases except for patient surveys which excludes hospitals with less than 100 cases; (a) 100-299 cases; (1) The number of cases/patients is too few to report; (2) Data submitted were based on a sample of cases/patients; (3) Results are based on a shorter time period than required; (4) Data suppressed by CMS for one or more quarters; (5) Results are not available for this reporting period; (6) Fewer than 100 patients completed the HCAHPS survey; (7) No cases met the criteria for this measure; (8) The lower limit of the confidence interval cannot be calculated if the number of observed infections equals zero; (9) No data are available from the state/territory for this reporting period; (10) The scores shown reflect fewer than 50 completed surveys; (11) There were discrepancies in the data collection process; (12) This measure does not apply to this hospital for this reporting period; (13) Results cannot be calculated for this reporting period; (14) The results for this state are combined with nearby states to protect confidentiality; Please refer to the User's Guide for a full explanation of data.

VA San Diego Healthcare System

3350 La Jolla Village Drive Phone: 858-552-8585
San Diego, CA 92161 Fax: 858-552-7509
URL: www.san-diego.med.va.gov
Type: Acute Care - VA Emergency Services: No
Ownership: Government Federal Beds: 238

Key Personnel:
Patient Relations . . . . Marilyn Dennis
Infection Control. . . . . Grace Hamilton, RN
Emergency Room . . . . Pat Hlavin, MD
Anesthesiology. . . . . Mark Mitchel, MD
CEO/President. . . . . Gary J Rossio
Intensive Care Unit. . . . . Robert Smith
Operating Room. . . . . Pam Stevens, RN
Quality Assurance . . . . Janet Tremblay

Measure	Cases	This Hosp.	State Avg.	U.S. Avg.
Blood Clot Prevention and Treatment				
Anticoagulation Overlap Therapy	-	-	92%	93%
ICU Venous Thromboembolism Prophylaxis	-	-	92%	92%
Incidence of Potentially Preventable VTE	-	-	11%	10%
UFH with Dosages/Platelet Monitoring	-	-	96%	97%
Venous Thromboembolism Prophylaxis	-	-	83%	85%
Warfarin Therapy Discharge Instructions	-	-	75%	75%
Chest Pain/Possible Heart Attack Care				
Aspirin Given Within 24 Hours of Arrival	-	-	97%	96%
Fibrinolytic Meds Within 30 Min. of Arrival	-	-	62%	58%
Average Time to ECG (minutes)	-	-	9	7
Average Time to Transfer (minutes)	-	-	62	60
Children's Asthma Care				
Received Home Management Plan of Care	-	-	88%	88%
Received Reliever Medication	-	-	100%	100%
Received Systemic Corticosteroids	-	-	100%	100%
Emergency Department				
Admittance Decision Time (minutes)	-	-	125	98
Head CT Results Within 45 Min. of Arrival	-	-	55%	57%
Patients Who Left ER Before Being Seen	-	-	3%	2%
Time from ER Arrival to Admit. (minutes)	-	-	323	274
Time from ER Arrival to Discharge (minutes)	-	-	168	134
Time in ER Before Being Evaluated (minutes)	-	-	29	26
Time to Pain Meds for Fractures (minutes)	-	-	62	57
Heart Attack Care				
Aspirin Given at Discharge	79	100%	99%	99%
Fibrinolytic Meds Within 30 Min. of Arrival[5]	-	-	73%	54%
PCI Within 90 Minutes of Arrival[1]	-	-	95%	96%
Statin Prescribed at Discharge	77	99%	98%	98%
Heart Failure Care				
ACE Inhibitor or ARB for LVSD	87	100%	97%	97%
Discharge Instructions Given	282	99%	94%	94%
Evaluation of LVS Function	293	100%	99%	99%
Medicare Spending				
Medicare Spending per Patient (ratio)	-	-	0.98	0.98
Pneumonia Care				
Appropriate Initial Antibiotic Given	59	100%	97%	95%
Blood Culture Timing	150	99%	98%	98%
Pregnancy and Delivery Care				
Newborn Deliveries Scheduled Early	-	-	5%	6%
Preventive Care				
Immunization for Influenza[5]	-	-	89%	90%
Immunization for Pneumonia[5]	-	-	90%	92%
Stroke Care				
Anticoagulation Therapy for Atrial Fibrillation	-	-	95%	95%
Antithrombotic Therapy Timing	-	-	98%	98%
Assessed for Rehabilitation	-	-	97%	97%
Discharged on Antithrombotic Therapy	-	-	99%	99%
Discharged on Statin Medication	-	-	94%	94%
Thrombolytic Therapy Timing	-	-	72%	66%
Venous Thromboembolism Prophylaxis	-	-	94%	94%
Written Stroke Educational Materials Given	-	-	87%	88%
Surgical Care Improvement Project				
Appropriate Beta Blocker Usage[2]	182	100%	97%	98%
Appropriate VTP Within 24 Hours[2]	260	100%	98%	98%
Controlled Postoperative Blood Glucose[2]	85	99%	96%	97%
Perioperative Temperature Management[2]	419	100%	100%	100%
Prophylactic Antibiotic Selection	259	100%	99%	99%
Prophylactic Antibiotic Selection (Outpatient)	-	-	97%	98%
Prophylactic Antibiotic Stopped	256	99%	98%	98%
Prophylactic Antibiotic Timing	259	100%	99%	99%
Prophylactic Antibiotic Timing (Outpatient)	-	-	97%	98%
Urinary Catheter Removal[2]	288	100%	97%	97%
Survey of Patients' Hospital Experiences				
Area Around Room 'Always' Quiet at Night	-	-	51%	61%
Doctors 'Always' Communicated Well	-	-	78%	82%
Home Recovery Information Given	-	-	83%	85%
Hospital Given 9 or 10 on 10 Point Scale	-	-	68%	71%
Meds 'Always' Explained Before Given	-	-	61%	64%
Nurses 'Always' Communicated Well	-	-	74%	79%
Pain 'Always' Well Controlled	-	-	68%	71%
Room and Bathroom 'Always' Clean	-	-	70%	73%
Timely Help 'Always' Received	-	-	62%	68%
Would Definitely Recommend Hospital	-	-	70%	71%
Use of Medical Imaging				
Cardiac Imaging Stress Test before Surgery	-	-	5.2%	5.3%
Combination Abdominal CT Scan	-	-	13.4%	10.5%
Combination Brain/Sinus CT Scan	-	-	2.2%	2.7%
Combination Chest CT Scan	-	-	2.3%	2.7%
Follow-up Mammogram/Ultrasound	-	-	8.2%	8.8%
Lumbar Spine MRI for Low Back Pain	-	-	34.2%	37.2%

San Dimas Community Hospital

1350 W Covina Blvd Phone: 909-599-6811
San Dimas, CA 91773 Fax: 909-305-5677
E-mail: ketsana.nobouphasavanh@tenethealth.com
URL: www.sandimashospital.com
Type: Acute Care Hospitals Emergency Services: Yes
Ownership: Proprietary Beds: 93

Key Personnel:
Hemotology Center . . . . Hany Boutros
Emergency Room . . . . Mary Dahl
Intensive Care Unit. . . . . Mary Dahl
CEO/President. . . . . Kevin Metcalfa
Infection Control. . . . . Jean Rathod
Operating Room. . . . . Regina Rico
Quality Assurance . . . . Joann Roset
Chair/CEO . . . . Zuhair Yahya

Measure	Cases	This Hosp.	State Avg.	U.S. Avg.
Blood Clot Prevention and Treatment				
Anticoagulation Overlap Therapy[2]	16	88%	92%	93%
ICU Venous Thromboembolism Prophylaxis[2]	45	69%	92%	92%
Incidence of Potentially Preventable VTE[1,2]	-	-	11%	10%
UFH with Dosages/Platelet Monitoring[1,2]	-	-	96%	97%
Venous Thromboembolism Prophylaxis[2]	249	75%	83%	85%
Warfarin Therapy Discharge Instructions[1,2]	-	-	75%	75%
Chest Pain/Possible Heart Attack Care				
Aspirin Given Within 24 Hours of Arrival	13	100%	97%	96%
Fibrinolytic Meds Within 30 Min. of Arrival[7]	-	-	62%	58%
Average Time to ECG (minutes)	13	8	9	7
Average Time to Transfer (minutes)[1]	-	-	62	60
Children's Asthma Care				
Received Home Management Plan of Care	-	-	88%	88%
Received Reliever Medication	-	-	100%	100%
Received Systemic Corticosteroids	-	-	100%	100%
Emergency Department				
Admittance Decision Time (minutes)[2]	593	67	125	98
Head CT Results Within 45 Min. of Arrival[1]	-	-	55%	57%
Patients Who Left ER Before Being Seen	15,307	2%	3%	2%
Time from ER Arrival to Admit. (minutes)[2]	617	209	323	274
Time from ER Arrival to Discharge (minutes)	377	135	168	134
Time in ER Before Being Evaluated (minutes)	395	14	29	26
Time to Pain Meds for Fractures (minutes)	83	54	62	57
Heart Attack Care				
Aspirin Given at Discharge[1]	-	-	99%	99%
Fibrinolytic Meds Within 30 Min. of Arrival[7]	-	-	73%	54%
PCI Within 90 Minutes of Arrival[7]	-	-	95%	96%
Statin Prescribed at Discharge[1]	-	-	98%	98%
Heart Failure Care				
ACE Inhibitor or ARB for LVSD	22	100%	97%	97%
Discharge Instructions Given	49	96%	94%	94%
Evaluation of LVS Function	80	99%	99%	99%
Medicare Spending				
Medicare Spending per Patient (ratio)	-	1.15	0.98	0.98
Pneumonia Care				
Appropriate Initial Antibiotic Given[2]	45	93%	97%	95%
Blood Culture Timing[2]	120	97%	98%	98%
Pregnancy and Delivery Care				
Newborn Deliveries Scheduled Early[2]	35	0%	5%	6%
Preventive Care				
Immunization for Influenza[2]	388	95%	89%	90%
Immunization for Pneumonia[2]	440	97%	90%	92%
Stroke Care				
Anticoagulation Therapy for Atrial Fibrillation[1]	-	-	95%	95%
Antithrombotic Therapy Timing	24	96%	98%	98%
Assessed for Rehabilitation	25	96%	97%	97%
Discharged on Antithrombotic Therapy	22	95%	99%	99%
Discharged on Statin Medication	13	77%	94%	94%
Thrombolytic Therapy Timing[7]	-	-	72%	66%
Venous Thromboembolism Prophylaxis	26	54%	94%	94%
Written Stroke Educational Materials Given	13	92%	87%	88%
Surgical Care Improvement Project				
Appropriate Beta Blocker Usage[2]	59	97%	97%	98%
Appropriate VTP Within 24 Hours[2]	194	95%	98%	98%
Controlled Postoperative Blood Glucose[2,7]	-	-	96%	97%
Perioperative Temperature Management[2]	223	100%	100%	100%
Prophylactic Antibiotic Selection[2]	172	99%	99%	99%
Prophylactic Antibiotic Selection (Outpatient)	20	90%	97%	98%
Prophylactic Antibiotic Stopped[2]	167	98%	98%	98%
Prophylactic Antibiotic Timing[2]	172	97%	99%	99%
Prophylactic Antibiotic Timing (Outpatient)	20	95%	97%	98%
Urinary Catheter Removal[2]	157	99%	97%	97%
Survey of Patients' Hospital Experiences				
Area Around Room 'Always' Quiet at Night[11]	300+	53%	51%	61%
Doctors 'Always' Communicated Well[11]	300+	75%	78%	82%
Home Recovery Information Given[11]	300+	82%	83%	85%
Hospital Given 9 or 10 on 10 Point Scale[11]	300+	65%	68%	71%
Meds 'Always' Explained Before Given[11]	300+	53%	61%	64%
Nurses 'Always' Communicated Well[11]	300+	74%	74%	79%
Pain 'Always' Well Controlled[11]	300+	66%	68%	71%
Room and Bathroom 'Always' Clean[11]	300+	70%	70%	73%
Timely Help 'Always' Received[11]	300+	58%	62%	68%
Would Definitely Recommend Hospital[11]	300+	66%	70%	71%
Use of Medical Imaging				
Cardiac Imaging Stress Test before Surgery[1]	-	-	5.2%	5.3%
Combination Abdominal CT Scan	101	1.0%	13.4%	10.5%
Combination Brain/Sinus CT Scan[1]	-	-	2.2%	2.7%
Combination Chest CT Scan[1]	-	-	2.3%	2.7%
Follow-up Mammogram/Ultrasound	77	2.6%	8.2%	8.8%
Lumbar Spine MRI for Low Back Pain[1]	-	-	34.2%	37.2%

California Pacific Medical Center - Davies Campus Hospital

601 Duboce Ave Phone: 415-600-6000
San Francisco, CA 94117
URL: www.daviesmed.org
Type: Acute Care Hospitals Emergency Services: Yes
Ownership: Voluntary non-profit - Other Beds: 341

Measure	Cases	This Hosp.	State Avg.	U.S. Avg.
Blood Clot Prevention and Treatment				
Anticoagulation Overlap Therapy[2]	18	100%	92%	93%
ICU Venous Thromboembolism Prophylaxis[2]	79	100%	92%	92%
Incidence of Potentially Preventable VTE[1,2]	-	-	11%	10%
UFH with Dosages/Platelet Monitoring[1,2]	-	-	96%	97%
Venous Thromboembolism Prophylaxis[2]	247	84%	83%	85%
Warfarin Therapy Discharge Instructions[2]	12	8%	75%	75%
Chest Pain/Possible Heart Attack Care				
Aspirin Given Within 24 Hours of Arrival[1]	-	-	97%	96%
Fibrinolytic Meds Within 30 Min. of Arrival[3,7]	-	-	62%	58%
Average Time to ECG (minutes)[1]	-	-	9	7
Average Time to Transfer (minutes)[1,3]	-	-	62	60
Children's Asthma Care				
Received Home Management Plan of Care	-	-	88%	88%
Received Reliever Medication	-	-	100%	100%

NOTE: Hospital profiles are in alphabetical order by state, then city, then hospital within the city; Rankings exclude hospitals with less than 25 cases except for patient surveys which excludes hospitals with less than 100 cases; (a) 100-299 cases; (1) The number of cases/patients is too few to report; (2) Data submitted were based on a sample of cases/patients; (3) Results are based on a shorter time period than required; (4) Data suppressed by CMS for one or more quarters; (5) Results are not available for this reporting period; (6) Fewer than 100 patients completed the HCAHPS survey; (7) No cases met the criteria for this measure; (8) The lower limit of the confidence interval cannot be calculated if the number of observed infections equals zero; (9) No data are available from the state/territory for this reporting period; (10) The scores shown reflect fewer than 50 completed surveys; (11) There were discrepancies in the data collection process; (12) This measure does not apply to this hospital for this reporting period; (13) Results cannot be calculated for this reporting period; (14) The results for this state are combined with nearby states to protect confidentiality; Please refer to the User's Guide for a full explanation of data.

Measure	Cases	This Hosp.	State Avg.	U.S. Avg.
Received Systemic Corticosteroids	-	-	100%	100%
Emergency Department				
Admittance Decision Time (minutes)[2]	254	115	125	98
Head CT Results Within 45 Min. of Arrival[7]	-	-	55%	57%
Patients Who Left ER Before Being Seen	14,323	1%	3%	2%
Time from ER Arrival to Admit. (minutes)[2]	254	239	323	274
Time from ER Arrival to Discharge (minutes)	371	120	168	134
Time in ER Before Being Evaluated (minutes)	409	20	29	26
Time to Pain Meds for Fractures (minutes)	36	38	62	57
Heart Attack Care				
Aspirin Given at Discharge[1]	-	-	99%	99%
Fibrinolytic Meds Within 30 Min. of Arrival[7]	-	-	73%	54%
PCI Within 90 Minutes of Arrival[7]	-	-	95%	96%
Statin Prescribed at Discharge[1]	-	-	98%	98%
Heart Failure Care				
ACE Inhibitor or ARB for LVSD[1]	-	-	97%	97%
Discharge Instructions Given	21	100%	94%	94%
Evaluation of LVS Function	28	100%	99%	99%
Medicare Spending				
Medicare Spending per Patient (ratio)	-	0.99	0.98	0.98
Pneumonia Care				
Appropriate Initial Antibiotic Given	27	100%	97%	95%
Blood Culture Timing	52	98%	98%	98%
Pregnancy and Delivery Care				
Newborn Deliveries Scheduled Early[7]	-	-	5%	6%
Preventive Care				
Immunization for Influenza[2]	327	95%	89%	90%
Immunization for Pneumonia[2]	328	89%	90%	92%
Stroke Care				
Anticoagulation Therapy for Atrial Fibrillation	47	100%	95%	95%
Antithrombotic Therapy Timing	71	100%	98%	98%
Assessed for Rehabilitation	213	100%	97%	97%
Discharged on Antithrombotic Therapy	147	100%	99%	99%
Discharged on Statin Medication	113	100%	94%	94%
Thrombolytic Therapy Timing[1]	-	-	72%	66%
Venous Thromboembolism Prophylaxis	246	100%	94%	94%
Written Stroke Educational Materials Given	91	97%	87%	88%
Surgical Care Improvement Project				
Appropriate Beta Blocker Usage[2]	24	96%	97%	98%
Appropriate VTP Within 24 Hours[2]	94	96%	98%	98%
Controlled Postoperative Blood Glucose[2,7]	-	-	96%	97%
Perioperative Temperature Management[2]	108	100%	100%	100%
Prophylactic Antibiotic Selection[1,2]	-	-	99%	99%
Prophylactic Antibiotic Selection (Outpatient)	148	99%	97%	98%
Prophylactic Antibiotic Stopped[1,2]	-	-	98%	98%
Prophylactic Antibiotic Timing[1,2]	-	-	99%	99%
Prophylactic Antibiotic Timing (Outpatient)	153	93%	97%	98%
Urinary Catheter Removal[2]	63	94%	97%	97%
Survey of Patients' Hospital Experiences				
Area Around Room 'Always' Quiet at Night	300+	42%	51%	61%
Doctors 'Always' Communicated Well	300+	80%	78%	82%
Home Recovery Information Given	300+	80%	83%	85%
Hospital Given 9 or 10 on 10 Point Scale	300+	65%	68%	71%
Meds 'Always' Explained Before Given	300+	61%	61%	64%
Nurses 'Always' Communicated Well	300+	72%	74%	79%
Pain 'Always' Well Controlled	300+	65%	68%	71%
Room and Bathroom 'Always' Clean	300+	67%	70%	73%
Timely Help 'Always' Received	300+	48%	62%	68%
Would Definitely Recommend Hospital	300+	69%	70%	71%
Use of Medical Imaging				
Cardiac Imaging Stress Test before Surgery[1]	-	-	5.2%	5.3%
Combination Abdominal CT Scan	310	16.5%	13.4%	10.5%
Combination Brain/Sinus CT Scan[1]	-	-	2.2%	2.7%
Combination Chest CT Scan	185	0.0%	2.3%	2.7%
Follow-up Mammogram/Ultrasound[7]	-	-	8.2%	8.8%
Lumbar Spine MRI for Low Back Pain	42	40.5%	34.2%	37.2%

California Pacific Medical Center - Pacific Campus Hospital

2333 Buchanan Street
San Francisco, CA 94115
Phone: 415-600-6000
Fax: 415-600-2985
E-mail: cpmcadmin@sutterhealth.org
URL: www.cpmc.org
Type: Acute Care Hospitals
Emergency Services: Yes
Ownership: Voluntary non-profit - Private
Beds: 341

Key Personnel:
CEO/President. . . . . Warren Browner, MD, MPH
Anesthesiology. . . . . Edward A Eisler, MD
Quality Assurance . . . . Thomas Knight, MD
Operating Room. . . . . Stephen Lockhart, MD
Radiology. . . . . Kirk L Moon, MD
Cardiac Laboratory. . . . . Soon J Park, MD
Emergency Room . . . . Michael H Rokeach, MD
Pediatric In-Patient Care . . . . David Tejeda, MD

Measure	Cases	This Hosp.	State Avg.	U.S. Avg.
Blood Clot Prevention and Treatment				
Anticoagulation Overlap Therapy[2]	80	100%	92%	93%
ICU Venous Thromboembolism Prophylaxis[2]	104	97%	92%	92%
Incidence of Potentially Preventable VTE[2]	15	20%	11%	10%
UFH with Dosages/Platelet Monitoring[2]	37	100%	96%	97%
Venous Thromboembolism Prophylaxis[2]	245	79%	83%	85%
Warfarin Therapy Discharge Instructions[2]	65	2%	75%	75%
Chest Pain/Possible Heart Attack Care				
Aspirin Given Within 24 Hours of Arrival[1]	-	-	97%	96%
Fibrinolytic Meds Within 30 Min. of Arrival[3,7]	-	-	62%	58%
Average Time to ECG (minutes)[1]	-	-	9	7
Average Time to Transfer (minutes)[3,7]	-	-	62	60
Children's Asthma Care				
Received Home Management Plan of Care	73	79%	88%	88%
Received Reliever Medication	74	100%	100%	100%
Received Systemic Corticosteroids	74	100%	100%	100%
Emergency Department				
Admittance Decision Time (minutes)[2]	296	95	125	98
Head CT Results Within 45 Min. of Arrival[7]	-	-	55%	57%
Patients Who Left ER Before Being Seen	49,007	1%	3%	2%
Time from ER Arrival to Admit. (minutes)[2]	297	246	323	274
Time from ER Arrival to Discharge (minutes)	378	148	168	134
Time in ER Before Being Evaluated (minutes)	413	20	29	26
Time to Pain Meds for Fractures (minutes)	172	28	62	57
Heart Attack Care				
Aspirin Given at Discharge	199	100%	99%	99%
Fibrinolytic Meds Within 30 Min. of Arrival[7]	-	-	73%	54%
PCI Within 90 Minutes of Arrival	30	100%	95%	96%
Statin Prescribed at Discharge	200	100%	98%	98%
Heart Failure Care				
ACE Inhibitor or ARB for LVSD[2]	65	98%	97%	97%
Discharge Instructions Given[2]	264	97%	94%	94%
Evaluation of LVS Function[2]	296	100%	99%	99%
Medicare Spending				
Medicare Spending per Patient (ratio)	-	0.90	0.98	0.98
Pneumonia Care				
Appropriate Initial Antibiotic Given[2]	77	100%	97%	95%
Blood Culture Timing[2]	161	100%	98%	98%
Pregnancy and Delivery Care				
Newborn Deliveries Scheduled Early	222	0%	5%	6%
Preventive Care				
Immunization for Influenza[2]	481	93%	89%	90%
Immunization for Pneumonia[2]	440	88%	90%	92%
Stroke Care				
Anticoagulation Therapy for Atrial Fibrillation	30	100%	95%	95%
Antithrombotic Therapy Timing	98	100%	98%	98%
Assessed for Rehabilitation	169	100%	97%	97%
Discharged on Antithrombotic Therapy	131	100%	99%	99%
Discharged on Statin Medication	100	100%	94%	94%
Thrombolytic Therapy Timing	13	69%	72%	66%
Venous Thromboembolism Prophylaxis	158	100%	94%	94%
Written Stroke Educational Materials Given	93	95%	87%	88%
Surgical Care Improvement Project				
Appropriate Beta Blocker Usage[2]	200	98%	97%	98%
Appropriate VTP Within 24 Hours[2]	452	98%	98%	98%
Controlled Postoperative Blood Glucose[2]	145	98%	96%	97%
Perioperative Temperature Management[2]	551	100%	100%	100%
Prophylactic Antibiotic Selection[2]	496	100%	99%	99%
Prophylactic Antibiotic Selection (Outpatient)	359	99%	97%	98%
Prophylactic Antibiotic Stopped[2]	477	100%	98%	98%
Prophylactic Antibiotic Timing[2]	497	100%	99%	99%
Prophylactic Antibiotic Timing (Outpatient)	363	97%	97%	98%
Urinary Catheter Removal[2]	454	98%	97%	97%
Survey of Patients' Hospital Experiences				
Area Around Room 'Always' Quiet at Night	300+	37%	51%	61%
Doctors 'Always' Communicated Well	300+	76%	78%	82%
Home Recovery Information Given	300+	81%	83%	85%
Hospital Given 9 or 10 on 10 Point Scale	300+	66%	68%	71%
Meds 'Always' Explained Before Given	300+	57%	61%	64%
Nurses 'Always' Communicated Well	300+	73%	74%	79%
Pain 'Always' Well Controlled	300+	68%	68%	71%
Room and Bathroom 'Always' Clean	300+	68%	70%	73%
Timely Help 'Always' Received	300+	64%	62%	68%
Would Definitely Recommend Hospital	300+	74%	70%	71%
Use of Medical Imaging				
Cardiac Imaging Stress Test before Surgery	609	5.3%	5.2%	5.3%
Combination Abdominal CT Scan	1,362	16.9%	13.4%	10.5%
Combination Brain/Sinus CT Scan	541	0.2%	2.2%	2.7%
Combination Chest CT Scan	1,175	0.3%	2.3%	2.7%
Follow-up Mammogram/Ultrasound	3,984	4.6%	8.2%	8.8%
Lumbar Spine MRI for Low Back Pain[1]	-	-	34.2%	37.2%

California Pacific Medical Center - Saint Luke's Campus

3555 Cesar Chavez Street
San Francisco, CA 94110
Phone: 415-641-6562
E-mail: seidera@suuterhealth.org
URL: www.stlukes.sf.org
Type: Acute Care Hospitals
Emergency Services: Yes
Ownership: Voluntary non-profit - Church
Beds: 260

Key Personnel:
CEO/President. . . . . Warren Browner, MD, MPH
Quality Assurance . . . . Emmett Ervin
Coronary Care . . . . Tommye Farley, RN
Chief of Medical Staff. . . . . Vernon L. Giang, MD
Radiology. . . . . Mitch Matcovsky
Pediatric Ambulatory Care . . . . . Robert Roth, MD
Pediatric In-Patient Care . . . . Louise Todd, RN

Measure	Cases	This Hosp.	State Avg.	U.S. Avg.
Blood Clot Prevention and Treatment				
Anticoagulation Overlap Therapy[1,2]	-	-	92%	93%
ICU Venous Thromboembolism Prophylaxis[2]	56	96%	92%	92%
Incidence of Potentially Preventable VTE[1,2]	-	-	11%	10%
UFH with Dosages/Platelet Monitoring[1,2]	-	-	96%	97%
Venous Thromboembolism Prophylaxis[2]	218	85%	83%	85%
Warfarin Therapy Discharge Instructions[1,2]	-	-	75%	75%
Chest Pain/Possible Heart Attack Care				
Aspirin Given Within 24 Hours of Arrival	17	100%	97%	96%
Fibrinolytic Meds Within 30 Min. of Arrival[7]	-	-	62%	58%
Average Time to ECG (minutes)	16	0	9	7
Average Time to Transfer (minutes)[1]	-	-	62	60
Children's Asthma Care				
Received Home Management Plan of Care[1]	-	-	88%	88%
Received Reliever Medication[1]	-	-	100%	100%
Received Systemic Corticosteroids[1]	-	-	100%	100%
Emergency Department				
Admittance Decision Time (minutes)[2]	342	123	125	98
Head CT Results Within 45 Min. of Arrival[1]	-	-	55%	57%
Patients Who Left ER Before Being Seen	27,639	4%	3%	2%
Time from ER Arrival to Admit. (minutes)[2]	342	268	323	274
Time from ER Arrival to Discharge (minutes)	355	144	168	134
Time in ER Before Being Evaluated (minutes)	411	36	29	26
Time to Pain Meds for Fractures (minutes)	68	63	62	57
Heart Attack Care				
Aspirin Given at Discharge	12	100%	99%	99%
Fibrinolytic Meds Within 30 Min. of Arrival[7]	-	-	73%	54%
PCI Within 90 Minutes of Arrival[7]	-	-	95%	96%
Statin Prescribed at Discharge	13	100%	98%	98%
Heart Failure Care				
ACE Inhibitor or ARB for LVSD	24	100%	97%	97%

NOTE: Hospital profiles are in alphabetical order by state, then city, then hospital within the city; Rankings exclude hospitals with less than 25 cases except for patient surveys which excludes hospitals with less than 100 cases; (a) 100-299 cases; (1) The number of cases/patients is too few to report; (2) Data submitted were based on a sample of cases/patients; (3) Results are based on a shorter time period than required; (4) Data suppressed by CMS for one or more quarters; (5) Results are not available for this reporting period; (6) Fewer than 100 patients completed the HCAHPS survey; (7) No cases met the criteria for this measure; (8) The lower limit of the confidence interval cannot be calculated if the number of observed infections equals zero; (9) No data are available from the state/territory for this reporting period; (10) The scores shown reflect fewer than 50 completed surveys; (11) There were discrepancies in the data collection process; (12) This measure does not apply to this hospital for this reporting period; (13) Results cannot be calculated for this reporting period; (14) The results for this state are combined with nearby states to protect confidentiality; Please refer to the User's Guide for a full explanation of data.

Measure	Cases	This Hosp.	State Avg.	U.S. Avg.
Discharge Instructions Given	97	99%	94%	94%
Evaluation of LVS Function	105	100%	99%	99%
Medicare Spending				
Medicare Spending per Patient (ratio)	-	0.90	0.98	0.98
Pneumonia Care				
Appropriate Initial Antibiotic Given[2]	57	100%	97%	95%
Blood Culture Timing[2]	87	100%	98%	98%
Pregnancy and Delivery Care				
Newborn Deliveries Scheduled Early	60	0%	5%	6%
Preventive Care				
Immunization for Influenza[2]	378	85%	89%	90%
Immunization for Pneumonia[2]	360	93%	90%	92%
Stroke Care				
Anticoagulation Therapy for Atrial Fibrillation[1]	-	-	95%	95%
Antithrombotic Therapy Timing	12	100%	98%	98%
Assessed for Rehabilitation	15	100%	97%	97%
Discharged on Antithrombotic Therapy	13	92%	99%	99%
Discharged on Statin Medication	13	100%	94%	94%
Thrombolytic Therapy Timing[7]	-	-	72%	66%
Venous Thromboembolism Prophylaxis	19	100%	94%	94%
Written Stroke Educational Materials Given[1]	-	-	87%	88%
Surgical Care Improvement Project				
Appropriate Beta Blocker Usage[2]	34	94%	97%	98%
Appropriate VTP Within 24 Hours[2]	152	95%	98%	98%
Controlled Postoperative Blood Glucose[2,7]	-	-	96%	97%
Perioperative Temperature Management[2]	178	100%	100%	100%
Prophylactic Antibiotic Selection[2]	98	99%	99%	99%
Prophylactic Antibiotic Selection (Outpatient)	31	97%	97%	98%
Prophylactic Antibiotic Stopped[2]	91	97%	98%	98%
Prophylactic Antibiotic Timing[2]	98	99%	99%	99%
Prophylactic Antibiotic Timing (Outpatient)	33	88%	97%	98%
Urinary Catheter Removal[2]	89	96%	97%	97%
Survey of Patients' Hospital Experiences				
Area Around Room 'Always' Quiet at Night	300+	49%	51%	61%
Doctors 'Always' Communicated Well	300+	76%	78%	82%
Home Recovery Information Given	300+	81%	83%	85%
Hospital Given 9 or 10 on 10 Point Scale	300+	58%	68%	71%
Meds 'Always' Explained Before Given	300+	58%	61%	64%
Nurses 'Always' Communicated Well	300+	70%	74%	79%
Pain 'Always' Well Controlled	300+	69%	68%	71%
Room and Bathroom 'Always' Clean	300+	67%	70%	73%
Timely Help 'Always' Received	300+	59%	62%	68%
Would Definitely Recommend Hospital	300+	67%	70%	71%
Use of Medical Imaging				
Cardiac Imaging Stress Test before Surgery	211	4.3%	5.2%	5.3%
Combination Abdominal CT Scan	301	3.0%	13.4%	10.5%
Combination Brain/Sinus CT Scan[1]	-	-	2.2%	2.7%
Combination Chest CT Scan	115	0.0%	2.3%	2.7%
Follow-up Mammogram/Ultrasound	896	3.2%	8.2%	8.8%
Lumbar Spine MRI for Low Back Pain[1]	-	-	34.2%	37.2%

Chinese Hospital

845 Jackson St
San Francisco, CA 94133
Phone: 415-982-2400
Fax: 415-217-4188
URL: www.chinesehospital-sf.org
Type: Acute Care Hospitals
Emergency Services: Yes
Ownership: Voluntary non-profit - Private
Beds: 54

Key Personnel:

Anesthesiology. . . . . Irwin Chow, MD
Patient Relations . . . . Sandra Chow
Quality Assurance . . . . Patricia Chung
Chief of Medical Staff. . . . . William S. Chung, MD
Infection Control. . . . . Stuart Fong
Operating Room. . . . . Dolores Ong
Emergency Room . . . . Michael L Shafer, MD
CEO/President. . . . . Brenda Yee, RN, MSN

Measure	Cases	This Hosp.	State Avg.	U.S. Avg.
Blood Clot Prevention and Treatment				
Anticoagulation Overlap Therapy[1,2]	-	-	92%	93%
ICU Venous Thromboembolism Prophylaxis[2]	23	61%	92%	92%
Incidence of Potentially Preventable VTE[2,7]	-	-	11%	10%
UFH with Dosages/Platelet Monitoring[2,7]	-	-	96%	97%
Venous Thromboembolism Prophylaxis[2]	219	42%	83%	85%
Warfarin Therapy Discharge Instructions[1,2]	-	-	75%	75%
Chest Pain/Possible Heart Attack Care				
Aspirin Given Within 24 Hours of Arrival[1]	-	-	97%	96%
Fibrinolytic Meds Within 30 Min. of Arrival[3,7]	-	-	62%	58%
Average Time to ECG (minutes)[1]	-	-	9	7
Average Time to Transfer (minutes)[1,3]	-	-	62	60
Children's Asthma Care				
Received Home Management Plan of Care	-	-	88%	88%
Received Reliever Medication	-	-	100%	100%
Received Systemic Corticosteroids	-	-	100%	100%
Emergency Department				
Admittance Decision Time (minutes)[2]	454	75	125	98
Head CT Results Within 45 Min. of Arrival[1]	-	-	55%	57%
Patients Who Left ER Before Being Seen	6,187	1%	3%	2%
Time from ER Arrival to Admit. (minutes)[2]	465	227	323	274
Time from ER Arrival to Discharge (minutes)	973	140	168	134
Time in ER Before Being Evaluated (minutes)	1,043	26	29	26
Time to Pain Meds for Fractures (minutes)[1]	-	-	62	57
Heart Attack Care				
Aspirin Given at Discharge[1]	-	-	99%	99%
Fibrinolytic Meds Within 30 Min. of Arrival[7]	-	-	73%	54%
PCI Within 90 Minutes of Arrival[7]	-	-	95%	96%
Statin Prescribed at Discharge	11	91%	98%	98%
Heart Failure Care				
ACE Inhibitor or ARB for LVSD	30	93%	97%	97%
Discharge Instructions Given	109	94%	94%	94%
Evaluation of LVS Function	116	99%	99%	99%
Medicare Spending				
Medicare Spending per Patient (ratio)	-	0.94	0.98	0.98
Pneumonia Care				
Appropriate Initial Antibiotic Given	78	97%	97%	95%
Blood Culture Timing	108	95%	98%	98%
Pregnancy and Delivery Care				
Newborn Deliveries Scheduled Early[7]	-	-	5%	6%
Preventive Care				
Immunization for Influenza[2]	281	77%	89%	90%
Immunization for Pneumonia[2]	519	93%	90%	92%
Stroke Care				
Anticoagulation Therapy for Atrial Fibrillation[1]	-	-	95%	95%
Antithrombotic Therapy Timing	36	94%	98%	98%
Assessed for Rehabilitation	36	97%	97%	97%
Discharged on Antithrombotic Therapy	34	94%	99%	99%
Discharged on Statin Medication	32	81%	94%	94%
Thrombolytic Therapy Timing[7]	-	-	72%	66%
Venous Thromboembolism Prophylaxis	39	44%	94%	94%
Written Stroke Educational Materials Given	11	0%	87%	88%
Surgical Care Improvement Project				
Appropriate Beta Blocker Usage	42	60%	97%	98%
Appropriate VTP Within 24 Hours	115	92%	98%	98%
Controlled Postoperative Blood Glucose[7]	-	-	96%	97%
Perioperative Temperature Management	127	100%	100%	100%
Prophylactic Antibiotic Selection	87	99%	99%	99%
Prophylactic Antibiotic Selection (Outpatient)	18	89%	97%	98%
Prophylactic Antibiotic Stopped	81	99%	98%	98%
Prophylactic Antibiotic Timing	87	98%	99%	99%
Prophylactic Antibiotic Timing (Outpatient)	18	78%	97%	98%
Urinary Catheter Removal	78	82%	97%	97%
Survey of Patients' Hospital Experiences				
Area Around Room 'Always' Quiet at Night	300+	40%	51%	61%
Doctors 'Always' Communicated Well	300+	69%	78%	82%
Home Recovery Information Given	300+	83%	83%	85%
Hospital Given 9 or 10 on 10 Point Scale	300+	44%	68%	71%
Meds 'Always' Explained Before Given	300+	56%	61%	64%
Nurses 'Always' Communicated Well	300+	63%	74%	79%
Pain 'Always' Well Controlled	300+	50%	68%	71%
Room and Bathroom 'Always' Clean	300+	62%	70%	73%
Timely Help 'Always' Received	300+	64%	62%	68%
Would Definitely Recommend Hospital	300+	47%	70%	71%
Use of Medical Imaging				
Cardiac Imaging Stress Test before Surgery	293	4.8%	5.2%	5.3%
Combination Abdominal CT Scan	353	4.0%	13.4%	10.5%
Combination Brain/Sinus CT Scan	361	0.6%	2.2%	2.7%
Combination Chest CT Scan	239	0.0%	2.3%	2.7%
Follow-up Mammogram/Ultrasound	735	1.8%	8.2%	8.8%
Lumbar Spine MRI for Low Back Pain[7]	-	-	34.2%	37.2%

Kaiser Foundation Hospital - San Francisco

2425 Geary Blvd
San Francisco, CA 94115
Phone: 415-833-2646
Fax: 415-833-4567
URL: www.permanente.net
Type: Acute Care Hospitals
Emergency Services: Yes
Ownership: Voluntary non-profit - Other
Beds: 620

Key Personnel:

Radiology. . . . . Stefan Arnon, MD
Chief of Medical Staff . . . . Paul Feigenbaum, MD
Quality Assurance . . . . Lynn Forsee
Infection Control. . . . . Barbara Lamberto
Emergency Room . . . . Steve Lauterbach, MD
CEO/President. . . . . Mary Ann Theodore
Pediatric Ambulatory Care . . . . . . Marie Waters, RN
Pediatric In-Patient Care . . . . Marie Waters, RN

Measure	Cases	This Hosp.	State Avg.	U.S. Avg.
Blood Clot Prevention and Treatment				
Anticoagulation Overlap Therapy[2]	54	100%	92%	93%
ICU Venous Thromboembolism Prophylaxis[2]	119	98%	92%	92%
Incidence of Potentially Preventable VTE[1,2]	-	-	11%	10%
UFH with Dosages/Platelet Monitoring[2]	43	100%	96%	97%
Venous Thromboembolism Prophylaxis[2]	267	96%	83%	85%
Warfarin Therapy Discharge Instructions[2]	49	80%	75%	75%
Chest Pain/Possible Heart Attack Care				
Aspirin Given Within 24 Hours of Arrival	-	-	97%	96%
Fibrinolytic Meds Within 30 Min. of Arrival	-	-	62%	58%
Average Time to ECG (minutes)	-	-	9	7
Average Time to Transfer (minutes)	-	-	62	60
Children's Asthma Care				
Received Home Management Plan of Care	-	-	88%	88%
Received Reliever Medication	-	-	100%	100%
Received Systemic Corticosteroids	-	-	100%	100%
Emergency Department				
Admittance Decision Time (minutes)[2]	332	41	125	98
Head CT Results Within 45 Min. of Arrival	-	-	55%	57%
Patients Who Left ER Before Being Seen	-	-	3%	2%
Time from ER Arrival to Admit. (minutes)[2]	332	276	323	274
Time from ER Arrival to Discharge (minutes)	-	-	168	134
Time in ER Before Being Evaluated (minutes)	-	-	29	26
Time to Pain Meds for Fractures (minutes)	-	-	62	57
Heart Attack Care				
Aspirin Given at Discharge[2]	286	99%	99%	99%
Fibrinolytic Meds Within 30 Min. of Arrival[2,7]	-	-	73%	54%
PCI Within 90 Minutes of Arrival[2]	20	100%	95%	96%
Statin Prescribed at Discharge[2]	281	100%	98%	98%
Heart Failure Care				
ACE Inhibitor or ARB for LVSD	63	100%	97%	97%
Discharge Instructions Given	245	100%	94%	94%
Evaluation of LVS Function	265	100%	99%	99%
Medicare Spending				
Medicare Spending per Patient (ratio)	-	0.73	0.98	0.98
Pneumonia Care				
Appropriate Initial Antibiotic Given[2]	107	99%	97%	95%
Blood Culture Timing[2]	161	98%	98%	98%
Pregnancy and Delivery Care				
Newborn Deliveries Scheduled Early[2]	26	0%	5%	6%
Preventive Care				
Immunization for Influenza[2]	505	97%	89%	90%
Immunization for Pneumonia[2]	536	98%	90%	92%
Stroke Care				
Anticoagulation Therapy for Atrial Fibrillation[2]	17	100%	95%	95%
Antithrombotic Therapy Timing[2]	77	97%	98%	98%
Assessed for Rehabilitation[2]	109	99%	97%	97%
Discharged on Antithrombotic Therapy[2]	94	96%	99%	99%
Discharged on Statin Medication[2]	82	94%	94%	94%
Thrombolytic Therapy Timing[1,2]	-	-	72%	66%
Venous Thromboembolism Prophylaxis[2]	96	100%	94%	94%
Written Stroke Educational Materials Given[2]	71	96%	87%	88%
Surgical Care Improvement Project				
Appropriate Beta Blocker Usage[2]	283	99%	97%	98%
Appropriate VTP Within 24 Hours[2]	379	99%	98%	98%

NOTE: Hospital profiles are in alphabetical order by state, then city, then hospital within the city; Rankings exclude hospitals with less than 25 cases except for patient surveys which excludes hospitals with less than 100 cases; (a) 100-299 cases; (1) The number of cases/patients is too few to report; (2) Data submitted were based on a sample of cases/patients; (3) Results are based on a shorter time period than required; (4) Data suppressed by CMS for one or more quarters; (5) Results are not available for this reporting period; (6) Fewer than 100 patients completed the HCAHPS survey; (7) No cases met the criteria for this measure; (8) The lower limit of the confidence interval cannot be calculated if the number of observed infections equals zero; (9) No data are available from the state/territory for this reporting period; (10) The scores shown reflect fewer than 50 completed surveys; (11) There were discrepancies in the data collection process; (12) This measure does not apply to this hospital for this reporting period; (13) Results cannot be calculated for this reporting period; (14) The results for this state are combined with nearby states to protect confidentiality; Please refer to the User's Guide for a full explanation of data.

Measure	Cases	This Hosp.	State Avg.	U.S. Avg.
Controlled Postoperative Blood Glucose[2]	173	98%	96%	97%
Perioperative Temperature Management[2]	487	100%	100%	100%
Prophylactic Antibiotic Selection[2]	488	99%	99%	99%
Prophylactic Antibiotic Selection (Outpatient)	-	-	97%	98%
Prophylactic Antibiotic Stopped[2]	471	97%	98%	98%
Prophylactic Antibiotic Timing[2]	488	99%	99%	99%
Prophylactic Antibiotic Timing (Outpatient)	-	-	97%	98%
Urinary Catheter Removal[2]	445	100%	97%	97%
Survey of Patients' Hospital Experiences				
Area Around Room 'Always' Quiet at Night	300+	52%	51%	61%
Doctors 'Always' Communicated Well	300+	81%	78%	82%
Home Recovery Information Given	300+	86%	83%	85%
Hospital Given 9 or 10 on 10 Point Scale	300+	74%	68%	71%
Meds 'Always' Explained Before Given	300+	64%	61%	64%
Nurses 'Always' Communicated Well	300+	77%	74%	79%
Pain 'Always' Well Controlled	300+	73%	68%	71%
Room and Bathroom 'Always' Clean	300+	68%	70%	73%
Timely Help 'Always' Received	300+	67%	62%	68%
Would Definitely Recommend Hospital	300+	77%	70%	71%
Use of Medical Imaging				
Cardiac Imaging Stress Test before Surgery	-	-	5.2%	5.3%
Combination Abdominal CT Scan	-	-	13.4%	10.5%
Combination Brain/Sinus CT Scan	-	-	2.2%	2.7%
Combination Chest CT Scan	-	-	2.3%	2.7%
Follow-up Mammogram/Ultrasound	-	-	8.2%	8.8%
Lumbar Spine MRI for Low Back Pain	-	-	34.2%	37.2%

Laguna Honda Hospital & Rehabilitation Center

375 Laguna Honda Blvd
San Francisco, CA 94116
Phone: 415-759-2300
Fax: 415-759-2374
URL: www.dph.sf.ca.us/chn/lagunahondahosp
Type: Acute Care Hospitals
Emergency Services: No
Ownership: Voluntary non-profit - Other
Beds: 1,147

Measure	Cases	This Hosp.	State Avg.	U.S. Avg.
Blood Clot Prevention and Treatment				
Anticoagulation Overlap Therapy[7]	-	-	92%	93%
ICU Venous Thromboembolism Prophylaxis[7]	-	-	92%	92%
Incidence of Potentially Preventable VTE[7]	-	-	11%	10%
UFH with Dosages/Platelet Monitoring[7]	-	-	96%	97%
Venous Thromboembolism Prophylaxis	64	16%	83%	85%
Warfarin Therapy Discharge Instructions[7]	-	-	75%	75%
Chest Pain/Possible Heart Attack Care				
Aspirin Given Within 24 Hours of Arrival[5]	-	-	97%	96%
Fibrinolytic Meds Within 30 Min. of Arrival[5]	-	-	62%	58%
Average Time to ECG (minutes)[5]	-	-	9	7
Average Time to Transfer (minutes)[5]	-	-	62	60
Children's Asthma Care				
Received Home Management Plan of Care	-	-	88%	88%
Received Reliever Medication	-	-	100%	100%
Received Systemic Corticosteroids	-	-	100%	100%
Emergency Department				
Admittance Decision Time (minutes)[7]	-	-	125	98
Head CT Results Within 45 Min. of Arrival[5]	-	-	55%	57%
Patients Who Left ER Before Being Seen[5]	-	-	3%	2%
Time from ER Arrival to Admit. (minutes)[7]	-	-	323	274
Time from ER Arrival to Discharge (minutes)[5]	-	-	168	134
Time in ER Before Being Evaluated (minutes)[5]	-	-	29	26
Time to Pain Meds for Fractures (minutes)[5]	-	-	62	57
Heart Attack Care				
Aspirin Given at Discharge[5]	-	-	99%	99%
Fibrinolytic Meds Within 30 Min. of Arrival[5]	-	-	73%	54%
PCI Within 90 Minutes of Arrival[5]	-	-	95%	96%
Statin Prescribed at Discharge[5]	-	-	98%	98%
Heart Failure Care				
ACE Inhibitor or ARB for LVSD[5]	-	-	97%	97%
Discharge Instructions Given[5]	-	-	94%	94%
Evaluation of LVS Function[5]	-	-	99%	99%
Medicare Spending				
Medicare Spending per Patient (ratio)	-	0.62	0.98	0.98
Pneumonia Care				
Appropriate Initial Antibiotic Given[3,7]	-	-	97%	95%
Blood Culture Timing[3,7]	-	-	98%	98%
Pregnancy and Delivery Care				
Newborn Deliveries Scheduled Early[7]	-	-	5%	6%
Preventive Care				
Immunization for Influenza	47	83%	89%	90%
Immunization for Pneumonia	61	92%	90%	92%
Stroke Care				
Anticoagulation Therapy for Atrial Fibrillation[5]	-	-	95%	95%
Antithrombotic Therapy Timing[5]	-	-	98%	98%
Assessed for Rehabilitation[5]	-	-	97%	97%
Discharged on Antithrombotic Therapy[5]	-	-	99%	99%
Discharged on Statin Medication[5]	-	-	94%	94%
Thrombolytic Therapy Timing[5]	-	-	72%	66%
Venous Thromboembolism Prophylaxis[5]	-	-	94%	94%
Written Stroke Educational Materials Given[5]	-	-	87%	88%
Surgical Care Improvement Project				
Appropriate Beta Blocker Usage[5]	-	-	97%	98%
Appropriate VTP Within 24 Hours[5]	-	-	98%	98%
Controlled Postoperative Blood Glucose[5]	-	-	96%	97%
Perioperative Temperature Management[5]	-	-	100%	100%
Prophylactic Antibiotic Selection[5]	-	-	99%	99%
Prophylactic Antibiotic Selection (Outpatient)[5]	-	-	97%	98%
Prophylactic Antibiotic Stopped[5]	-	-	98%	98%
Prophylactic Antibiotic Timing[5]	-	-	99%	99%
Prophylactic Antibiotic Timing (Outpatient)[5]	-	-	97%	98%
Urinary Catheter Removal[5]	-	-	97%	97%
Survey of Patients' Hospital Experiences				
Area Around Room 'Always' Quiet at Night[1]	-	-	51%	61%
Doctors 'Always' Communicated Well[1]	-	-	78%	82%
Home Recovery Information Given[1]	-	-	83%	85%
Hospital Given 9 or 10 on 10 Point Scale[1]	-	-	68%	71%
Meds 'Always' Explained Before Given[1]	-	-	61%	64%
Nurses 'Always' Communicated Well[1]	-	-	74%	79%
Pain 'Always' Well Controlled[1]	-	-	68%	71%
Room and Bathroom 'Always' Clean[1]	-	-	70%	73%
Timely Help 'Always' Received[1]	-	-	62%	68%
Would Definitely Recommend Hospital[1]	-	-	70%	71%
Use of Medical Imaging				
Cardiac Imaging Stress Test before Surgery[7]	-	-	5.2%	5.3%
Combination Abdominal CT Scan[7]	-	-	13.4%	10.5%
Combination Brain/Sinus CT Scan[7]	-	-	2.2%	2.7%
Combination Chest CT Scan[7]	-	-	2.3%	2.7%
Follow-up Mammogram/Ultrasound[7]	-	-	8.2%	8.8%
Lumbar Spine MRI for Low Back Pain[7]	-	-	34.2%	37.2%

Saint Francis Memorial Hospital

900 Hyde St
San Francisco, CA 94109
Phone: 415-353-6000
Fax: 415-353-6912
URL: www.saintfrancismemorial.org
Type: Acute Care Hospitals
Emergency Services: Yes
Ownership: Voluntary non-profit - Private
Beds: 356

Key Personnel:
Anesthesiology. . . . . Thomas Alberg, MD
Intensive Care Unit. . . . . Nancy Carewe
Infection Control. . . . . Fred Deneau
CEO/President. . . . . Robert Dureault
Radiology. . . . . John L Meyer, MD
Emergency Room . . . . Richard Naidus, MD
Chief of Medical Staff. . . . . Roger R Smith, MD

Measure	Cases	This Hosp.	State Avg.	U.S. Avg.
Blood Clot Prevention and Treatment				
Anticoagulation Overlap Therapy[2]	15	93%	92%	93%
ICU Venous Thromboembolism Prophylaxis[2]	177	99%	92%	92%
Incidence of Potentially Preventable VTE[1,2]	-	-	11%	10%
UFH with Dosages/Platelet Monitoring[1,2]	-	-	96%	97%
Venous Thromboembolism Prophylaxis[2]	236	97%	83%	85%
Warfarin Therapy Discharge Instructions[2]	11	100%	75%	75%
Chest Pain/Possible Heart Attack Care				
Aspirin Given Within 24 Hours of Arrival	28	100%	97%	96%
Fibrinolytic Meds Within 30 Min. of Arrival[7]	-	-	62%	58%
Average Time to ECG (minutes)	28	22	9	7
Average Time to Transfer (minutes)[1]	-	-	62	60
Children's Asthma Care				
Received Home Management Plan of Care	-	-	88%	88%
Received Reliever Medication	-	-	100%	100%
Received Systemic Corticosteroids	-	-	100%	100%
Emergency Department				
Admittance Decision Time (minutes)[2]	643	148	125	98
Head CT Results Within 45 Min. of Arrival[1]	-	-	55%	57%
Patients Who Left ER Before Being Seen	33,052	1%	3%	2%
Time from ER Arrival to Admit. (minutes)[2]	649	314	323	274
Time from ER Arrival to Discharge (minutes)	341	125	168	134
Time in ER Before Being Evaluated (minutes)	402	12	29	26
Time to Pain Meds for Fractures (minutes)	50	47	62	57
Heart Attack Care				
Aspirin Given at Discharge[1]	-	-	99%	99%
Fibrinolytic Meds Within 30 Min. of Arrival[7]	-	-	73%	54%
PCI Within 90 Minutes of Arrival[7]	-	-	95%	96%
Statin Prescribed at Discharge	11	82%	98%	98%
Heart Failure Care				
ACE Inhibitor or ARB for LVSD	36	100%	97%	97%
Discharge Instructions Given	108	98%	94%	94%
Evaluation of LVS Function	123	99%	99%	99%
Medicare Spending				
Medicare Spending per Patient (ratio)	-	1.08	0.98	0.98
Pneumonia Care				
Appropriate Initial Antibiotic Given[2]	80	98%	97%	95%
Blood Culture Timing[2]	165	99%	98%	98%
Pregnancy and Delivery Care				
Newborn Deliveries Scheduled Early[7]	-	-	5%	6%
Preventive Care				
Immunization for Influenza[2]	432	98%	89%	90%
Immunization for Pneumonia[2]	495	96%	90%	92%
Stroke Care				
Anticoagulation Therapy for Atrial Fibrillation	12	100%	95%	95%
Antithrombotic Therapy Timing	56	100%	98%	98%
Assessed for Rehabilitation	60	97%	97%	97%
Discharged on Antithrombotic Therapy	52	96%	99%	99%
Discharged on Statin Medication	39	92%	94%	94%
Thrombolytic Therapy Timing[1]	-	-	72%	66%
Venous Thromboembolism Prophylaxis	76	99%	94%	94%
Written Stroke Educational Materials Given	25	96%	87%	88%
Surgical Care Improvement Project				
Appropriate Beta Blocker Usage[2]	54	100%	97%	98%
Appropriate VTP Within 24 Hours[2]	255	99%	98%	98%
Controlled Postoperative Blood Glucose[2,7]	-	-	96%	97%
Perioperative Temperature Management[2]	299	100%	100%	100%
Prophylactic Antibiotic Selection[2]	211	100%	99%	99%
Prophylactic Antibiotic Selection (Outpatient)	24	100%	97%	98%
Prophylactic Antibiotic Stopped[2]	207	100%	98%	98%
Prophylactic Antibiotic Timing[2]	211	100%	99%	99%
Prophylactic Antibiotic Timing (Outpatient)	23	87%	97%	98%
Urinary Catheter Removal[2]	222	100%	97%	97%
Survey of Patients' Hospital Experiences				
Area Around Room 'Always' Quiet at Night	300+	44%	51%	61%
Doctors 'Always' Communicated Well	300+	74%	78%	82%
Home Recovery Information Given	300+	83%	83%	85%
Hospital Given 9 or 10 on 10 Point Scale	300+	66%	68%	71%
Meds 'Always' Explained Before Given	300+	57%	61%	64%
Nurses 'Always' Communicated Well	300+	66%	74%	79%
Pain 'Always' Well Controlled	300+	62%	68%	71%
Room and Bathroom 'Always' Clean	300+	64%	70%	73%
Timely Help 'Always' Received	300+	53%	62%	68%
Would Definitely Recommend Hospital	300+	68%	70%	71%
Use of Medical Imaging				
Cardiac Imaging Stress Test before Surgery	84	3.6%	5.2%	5.3%
Combination Abdominal CT Scan	259	3.9%	13.4%	10.5%
Combination Brain/Sinus CT Scan[1]	-	-	2.2%	2.7%
Combination Chest CT Scan	102	1.0%	2.3%	2.7%
Follow-up Mammogram/Ultrasound	269	9.7%	8.2%	8.8%
Lumbar Spine MRI for Low Back Pain[1]	-	-	34.2%	37.2%

NOTE: Hospital profiles are in alphabetical order by state, then city, then hospital within the city; Rankings exclude hospitals with less than 25 cases except for patient surveys which excludes hospitals with less than 100 cases; (a) 100-299 cases; (1) The number of cases/patients is too few to report; (2) Data submitted were based on a sample of cases/patients; (3) Results are based on a shorter time period than required; (4) Data suppressed by CMS for one or more quarters; (5) Results are not available for this reporting period; (6) Fewer than 100 patients completed the HCAHPS survey; (7) No cases met the criteria for this measure; (8) The lower limit of the confidence interval cannot be calculated if the number of observed infections equals zero; (9) No data are available from the state/territory for this reporting period; (10) The scores shown reflect fewer than 50 completed surveys; (11) There were discrepancies in the data collection process; (12) This measure does not apply to this hospital for this reporting period; (13) Results cannot be calculated for this reporting period; (14) The results for this state are combined with nearby states to protect confidentiality; Please refer to the User's Guide for a full explanation of data.

Saint Mary's Medical Center

450 Stanyan St
San Francisco, CA 94117
Phone: 415-668-1000
Fax: 415-668-4531
URL: www.stmarysmedicalcenter.org
Type: Acute Care Hospitals
Emergency Services: Yes
Ownership: Voluntary non-profit - Private
Beds: 531

Key Personnel:
Operating Room. . . . . Rose Calhan
CEO/President. . . . . Lloyd H Dean
Quality Assurance . . . . Charles P Francis
Radiology. . . . . James Gorder, MD
Emergency Room . . . . Robert Mueller
Cardiac Laboratory. . . . . James Seene

Measure	Cases	This Hosp.	State Avg.	U.S. Avg.
Blood Clot Prevention and Treatment				
Anticoagulation Overlap Therapy[2]	23	100%	92%	93%
ICU Venous Thromboembolism Prophylaxis[2]	123	99%	92%	92%
Incidence of Potentially Preventable VTE[1,2]	-	-	11%	10%
UFH with Dosages/Platelet Monitoring[2]	11	100%	96%	97%
Venous Thromboembolism Prophylaxis[2]	321	98%	83%	85%
Warfarin Therapy Discharge Instructions[2]	15	87%	75%	75%
Chest Pain/Possible Heart Attack Care				
Aspirin Given Within 24 Hours of Arrival[5]	-	-	97%	96%
Fibrinolytic Meds Within 30 Min. of Arrival[5]	-	-	62%	58%
Average Time to ECG (minutes)[5]	-	-	9	7
Average Time to Transfer (minutes)[5]	-	-	62	60
Children's Asthma Care				
Received Home Management Plan of Care	-	-	88%	88%
Received Reliever Medication	-	-	100%	100%
Received Systemic Corticosteroids	-	-	100%	100%
Emergency Department				
Admittance Decision Time (minutes)[2]	459	57	125	98
Head CT Results Within 45 Min. of Arrival[3,7]	-	-	55%	57%
Patients Who Left ER Before Being Seen	17,503	0%	3%	2%
Time from ER Arrival to Admit. (minutes)[2]	674	285	323	274
Time from ER Arrival to Discharge (minutes)	365	153	168	134
Time in ER Before Being Evaluated (minutes)	404	14	29	26
Time to Pain Meds for Fractures (minutes)	80	52	62	57
Heart Attack Care				
Aspirin Given at Discharge	95	99%	99%	99%
Fibrinolytic Meds Within 30 Min. of Arrival[7]	-	-	73%	54%
PCI Within 90 Minutes of Arrival	21	95%	95%	96%
Statin Prescribed at Discharge	97	100%	98%	98%
Heart Failure Care				
ACE Inhibitor or ARB for LVSD	69	99%	97%	97%
Discharge Instructions Given	141	100%	94%	94%
Evaluation of LVS Function	185	98%	99%	99%
Medicare Spending				
Medicare Spending per Patient (ratio)	-	0.95	0.98	0.98
Pneumonia Care				
Appropriate Initial Antibiotic Given	120	99%	97%	95%
Blood Culture Timing	232	100%	98%	98%
Pregnancy and Delivery Care				
Newborn Deliveries Scheduled Early[7]	-	-	5%	6%
Preventive Care				
Immunization for Influenza[2]	474	96%	89%	90%
Immunization for Pneumonia[2]	692	97%	90%	92%
Stroke Care				
Anticoagulation Therapy for Atrial Fibrillation	20	100%	95%	95%
Antithrombotic Therapy Timing	53	100%	98%	98%
Assessed for Rehabilitation	59	100%	97%	97%
Discharged on Antithrombotic Therapy	56	100%	99%	99%
Discharged on Statin Medication	51	100%	94%	94%
Thrombolytic Therapy Timing[1]	-	-	72%	66%
Venous Thromboembolism Prophylaxis	57	100%	94%	94%
Written Stroke Educational Materials Given	30	100%	87%	88%
Surgical Care Improvement Project				
Appropriate Beta Blocker Usage[2]	81	98%	97%	98%
Appropriate VTP Within 24 Hours[2]	304	98%	98%	98%
Controlled Postoperative Blood Glucose[2]	25	92%	96%	97%
Perioperative Temperature Management[2]	351	100%	100%	100%
Prophylactic Antibiotic Selection[2]	249	98%	99%	99%
Prophylactic Antibiotic Selection (Outpatient)	99	97%	97%	98%
Prophylactic Antibiotic Stopped[2]	247	99%	98%	98%
Prophylactic Antibiotic Timing[2]	249	99%	99%	99%
Prophylactic Antibiotic Timing (Outpatient)	100	97%	97%	98%
Urinary Catheter Removal[2]	109	99%	97%	97%
Survey of Patients' Hospital Experiences				
Area Around Room 'Always' Quiet at Night	300+	38%	51%	61%
Doctors 'Always' Communicated Well	300+	76%	78%	82%
Home Recovery Information Given	300+	85%	83%	85%
Hospital Given 9 or 10 on 10 Point Scale	300+	67%	68%	71%
Meds 'Always' Explained Before Given	300+	63%	61%	64%
Nurses 'Always' Communicated Well	300+	72%	74%	79%
Pain 'Always' Well Controlled	300+	67%	68%	71%
Room and Bathroom 'Always' Clean	300+	71%	70%	73%
Timely Help 'Always' Received	300+	59%	62%	68%
Would Definitely Recommend Hospital	300+	69%	70%	71%
Use of Medical Imaging				
Cardiac Imaging Stress Test before Surgery	147	7.5%	5.2%	5.3%
Combination Abdominal CT Scan	360	6.7%	13.4%	10.5%
Combination Brain/Sinus CT Scan[1]	-	-	2.2%	2.7%
Combination Chest CT Scan	192	0.0%	2.3%	2.7%
Follow-up Mammogram/Ultrasound	628	7.3%	8.2%	8.8%
Lumbar Spine MRI for Low Back Pain	172	28.5%	34.2%	37.2%

San Francisco General Hospital

1001 Potrero Avenue
San Francisco, CA 94110
Phone: 415-206-8000
Fax: 415-206-3434
URL: www.dph.sf.ca.us/chn/sfgh/default.asp
Type: Acute Care Hospitals
Emergency Services: Yes
Ownership: Government - Local
Beds: 639

Key Personnel:
Emergency Room . . . . Chris Barton, MD
Chief of Medical Staff. . . . . Jeff Critchfield, MD
CEO/President. . . . . Susan A Currin, RN, MS
Pediatric Ambulatory Care . . . . . . Elena Fuestes Afflick, MD
Pediatric In-Patient Care . . . . Elena Fuestes Afflick, MD
Infection Control. . . . . John Luce, MD
Quality Assurance . . . . John Luce, MD
Radiology. . . . . Mark Wilson, MD

Measure	Cases	This Hosp.	State Avg.	U.S. Avg.
Blood Clot Prevention and Treatment				
Anticoagulation Overlap Therapy[2]	65	100%	92%	93%
ICU Venous Thromboembolism Prophylaxis[2]	49	86%	92%	92%
Incidence of Potentially Preventable VTE[2]	32	12%	11%	10%
UFH with Dosages/Platelet Monitoring[2]	47	100%	96%	97%
Venous Thromboembolism Prophylaxis[2]	328	79%	83%	85%
Warfarin Therapy Discharge Instructions[2]	42	69%	75%	75%
Chest Pain/Possible Heart Attack Care				
Aspirin Given Within 24 Hours of Arrival[1,3]	-	-	97%	96%
Fibrinolytic Meds Within 30 Min. of Arrival[3,7]	-	-	62%	58%
Average Time to ECG (minutes)[1,3]	-	-	9	7
Average Time to Transfer (minutes)[3,7]	-	-	62	60
Children's Asthma Care				
Received Home Management Plan of Care	-	-	88%	88%
Received Reliever Medication	-	-	100%	100%
Received Systemic Corticosteroids	-	-	100%	100%
Emergency Department				
Admittance Decision Time (minutes)[2]	730	242	125	98
Head CT Results Within 45 Min. of Arrival[3,7]	-	-	55%	57%
Patients Who Left ER Before Being Seen	63,335	9%	3%	2%
Time from ER Arrival to Admit. (minutes)[2]	730	456	323	274
Time from ER Arrival to Discharge (minutes)	281	263	168	134
Time in ER Before Being Evaluated (minutes)	358	40	29	26
Time to Pain Meds for Fractures (minutes)	226	72	62	57
Heart Attack Care				
Aspirin Given at Discharge	144	98%	99%	99%
Fibrinolytic Meds Within 30 Min. of Arrival[7]	-	-	73%	54%
PCI Within 90 Minutes of Arrival	31	94%	95%	96%
Statin Prescribed at Discharge	145	97%	98%	98%
Heart Failure Care				
ACE Inhibitor or ARB for LVSD[2]	162	96%	97%	97%
Discharge Instructions Given[2]	254	90%	94%	94%
Evaluation of LVS Function[2]	266	100%	99%	99%
Medicare Spending				
Medicare Spending per Patient (ratio)	-	0.92	0.98	0.98
Pneumonia Care				
Appropriate Initial Antibiotic Given[2]	74	99%	97%	95%
Blood Culture Timing[2]	143	84%	98%	98%
Pregnancy and Delivery Care				
Newborn Deliveries Scheduled Early[2]	17	0%	5%	6%
Preventive Care				
Immunization for Influenza[2]	524	75%	89%	90%
Immunization for Pneumonia[2]	476	79%	90%	92%
Stroke Care				
Anticoagulation Therapy for Atrial Fibrillation[1,2]	-	-	95%	95%
Antithrombotic Therapy Timing[2]	56	100%	98%	98%
Assessed for Rehabilitation[2]	86	98%	97%	97%
Discharged on Antithrombotic Therapy[2]	61	98%	99%	99%
Discharged on Statin Medication[2]	47	96%	94%	94%
Thrombolytic Therapy Timing[2]	15	87%	72%	66%
Venous Thromboembolism Prophylaxis[2]	103	92%	94%	94%
Written Stroke Educational Materials Given[2]	45	89%	87%	88%
Surgical Care Improvement Project				
Appropriate Beta Blocker Usage[2]	56	100%	97%	98%
Appropriate VTP Within 24 Hours[2]	244	99%	98%	98%
Controlled Postoperative Blood Glucose[2,7]	-	-	96%	97%
Perioperative Temperature Management[2]	292	100%	100%	100%
Prophylactic Antibiotic Selection[2]	190	99%	99%	99%
Prophylactic Antibiotic Selection (Outpatient)	50	100%	97%	98%
Prophylactic Antibiotic Stopped[2]	190	96%	98%	98%
Prophylactic Antibiotic Timing[2]	190	99%	99%	99%
Prophylactic Antibiotic Timing (Outpatient)	14	100%	97%	98%
Urinary Catheter Removal[2]	150	99%	97%	97%
Survey of Patients' Hospital Experiences				
Area Around Room 'Always' Quiet at Night	(a)	35%	51%	61%
Doctors 'Always' Communicated Well	(a)	65%	78%	82%
Home Recovery Information Given	(a)	86%	83%	85%
Hospital Given 9 or 10 on 10 Point Scale	(a)	58%	68%	71%
Meds 'Always' Explained Before Given	(a)	49%	61%	64%
Nurses 'Always' Communicated Well	(a)	62%	74%	79%
Pain 'Always' Well Controlled	(a)	57%	68%	71%
Room and Bathroom 'Always' Clean	(a)	55%	70%	73%
Timely Help 'Always' Received	(a)	48%	62%	68%
Would Definitely Recommend Hospital	(a)	58%	70%	71%
Use of Medical Imaging				
Cardiac Imaging Stress Test before Surgery[7]	-	-	5.2%	5.3%
Combination Abdominal CT Scan	628	10.2%	13.4%	10.5%
Combination Brain/Sinus CT Scan	424	5.9%	2.2%	2.7%
Combination Chest CT Scan	455	0.2%	2.3%	2.7%
Follow-up Mammogram/Ultrasound	950	4.7%	8.2%	8.8%
Lumbar Spine MRI for Low Back Pain[1]	-	-	34.2%	37.2%

San Francisco VA Medical Center

4150 Clement Street
San Francisco, CA 94121
Phone: 415-221-4810
Fax: 415-750-2177
URL: www.sanfrancisco.va.gov
Type: Acute Care - VA
Emergency Services: No
Ownership: Government Federal
Beds: 244

Key Personnel:
Hemotology Center . . . . Patricia Cornett, MD
Emergency Room . . . . Jody Garber, MD
Infection Control. . . . . Peter Jensen, MD
Chief of Medical Staff. . . . . C Diana Nicoll, MD, PhD
Coronary Care . . . . Mark Ratcliff, MD
Operating Room. . . . . Mark Ratcliff, RN
Intensive Care Unit. . . . . Leslie Zimmerman, MD

Measure	Cases	This Hosp.	State Avg.	U.S. Avg.
Blood Clot Prevention and Treatment				
Anticoagulation Overlap Therapy	-	-	92%	93%
ICU Venous Thromboembolism Prophylaxis	-	-	92%	92%
Incidence of Potentially Preventable VTE	-	-	11%	10%
UFH with Dosages/Platelet Monitoring	-	-	96%	97%
Venous Thromboembolism Prophylaxis	-	-	83%	85%
Warfarin Therapy Discharge Instructions	-	-	75%	75%
Chest Pain/Possible Heart Attack Care				
Aspirin Given Within 24 Hours of Arrival	-	-	97%	96%
Fibrinolytic Meds Within 30 Min. of Arrival	-	-	62%	58%
Average Time to ECG (minutes)	-	-	9	7
Average Time to Transfer (minutes)	-	-	62	60
Children's Asthma Care				

NOTE: *Hospital profiles are in alphabetical order by state, then city, then hospital within the city; Rankings exclude hospitals with less than 25 cases except for patient surveys which excludes hospitals with less than 100 cases; (a) 100-299 cases; (1) The number of cases/patients is too few to report; (2) Data submitted were based on a sample of cases/patients; (3) Results are based on a shorter time period than required; (4) Data suppressed by CMS for one or more quarters; (5) Results are not available for this reporting period; (6) Fewer than 100 patients completed the HCAHPS survey; (7) No cases met the criteria for this measure; (8) The lower limit of the confidence interval cannot be calculated if the number of observed infections equals zero; (9) No data are available from the state/territory for this reporting period; (10) The scores shown reflect fewer than 50 completed surveys; (11) There were discrepancies in the data collection process; (12) This measure does not apply to this hospital for this reporting period; (13) Results cannot be calculated for this reporting period; (14) The results for this state are combined with nearby states to protect confidentiality; Please refer to the User's Guide for a full explanation of data.*

Measure	Cases	This Hosp.	State Avg.	U.S. Avg.
Received Home Management Plan of Care	-	-	88%	88%
Received Reliever Medication	-	-	100%	100%
Received Systemic Corticosteroids	-	-	100%	100%
Emergency Department				
Admittance Decision Time (minutes)	-	-	125	98
Head CT Results Within 45 Min. of Arrival	-	-	55%	57%
Patients Who Left ER Before Being Seen	-	-	3%	2%
Time from ER Arrival to Admit. (minutes)	-	-	323	274
Time from ER Arrival to Discharge (minutes)	-	-	168	134
Time in ER Before Being Evaluated (minutes)	-	-	29	26
Time to Pain Meds for Fractures (minutes)	-	-	62	57
Heart Attack Care				
Aspirin Given at Discharge	39	100%	99%	99%
Fibrinolytic Meds Within 30 Min. of Arrival[5]	-	-	73%	54%
PCI Within 90 Minutes of Arrival[5]	-	-	95%	96%
Statin Prescribed at Discharge	39	100%	98%	98%
Heart Failure Care				
ACE Inhibitor or ARB for LVSD	45	96%	97%	97%
Discharge Instructions Given	147	97%	94%	94%
Evaluation of LVS Function	157	99%	99%	99%
Medicare Spending				
Medicare Spending per Patient (ratio)	-	-	0.98	0.98
Pneumonia Care				
Appropriate Initial Antibiotic Given	41	98%	97%	95%
Blood Culture Timing	90	98%	98%	98%
Pregnancy and Delivery Care				
Newborn Deliveries Scheduled Early	-	-	5%	6%
Preventive Care				
Immunization for Influenza[5]	-	-	89%	90%
Immunization for Pneumonia[5]	-	-	90%	92%
Stroke Care				
Anticoagulation Therapy for Atrial Fibrillation	-	-	95%	95%
Antithrombotic Therapy Timing	-	-	98%	98%
Assessed for Rehabilitation	-	-	97%	97%
Discharged on Antithrombotic Therapy	-	-	99%	99%
Discharged on Statin Medication	-	-	94%	94%
Thrombolytic Therapy Timing	-	-	72%	66%
Venous Thromboembolism Prophylaxis	-	-	94%	94%
Written Stroke Educational Materials Given	-	-	87%	88%
Surgical Care Improvement Project				
Appropriate Beta Blocker Usage[2]	216	98%	97%	98%
Appropriate VTP Within 24 Hours[2]	339	99%	98%	98%
Controlled Postoperative Blood Glucose[2]	71	99%	96%	97%
Perioperative Temperature Management[2]	388	100%	100%	100%
Prophylactic Antibiotic Selection	315	100%	99%	99%
Prophylactic Antibiotic Selection (Outpatient)	-	-	97%	98%
Prophylactic Antibiotic Stopped	309	97%	98%	98%
Prophylactic Antibiotic Timing	315	100%	99%	99%
Prophylactic Antibiotic Timing (Outpatient)	-	-	97%	98%
Urinary Catheter Removal[2]	338	97%	97%	97%
Survey of Patients' Hospital Experiences				
Area Around Room 'Always' Quiet at Night	-	-	51%	61%
Doctors 'Always' Communicated Well	-	-	78%	82%
Home Recovery Information Given	-	-	83%	85%
Hospital Given 9 or 10 on 10 Point Scale	-	-	68%	71%
Meds 'Always' Explained Before Given	-	-	61%	64%
Nurses 'Always' Communicated Well	-	-	74%	79%
Pain 'Always' Well Controlled	-	-	68%	71%
Room and Bathroom 'Always' Clean	-	-	70%	73%
Timely Help 'Always' Received	-	-	62%	68%
Would Definitely Recommend Hospital	-	-	70%	71%
Use of Medical Imaging				
Cardiac Imaging Stress Test before Surgery	-	-	5.2%	5.3%
Combination Abdominal CT Scan	-	-	13.4%	10.5%
Combination Brain/Sinus CT Scan	-	-	2.2%	2.7%
Combination Chest CT Scan	-	-	2.3%	2.7%
Follow-up Mammogram/Ultrasound	-	-	8.2%	8.8%
Lumbar Spine MRI for Low Back Pain	-	-	34.2%	37.2%

UCSF Medical Center

505 Parnassus Ave, Box 0296 Phone: 415-353-2733
San Francisco, CA 94143
E-mail: referral.center@ucsfmedicalcenter.org
URL: www.ucsfhealth.org
Type: Acute Care Hospitals Emergency Services: Yes
Ownership: Voluntary non-profit - Other Beds: 688

Key Personnel:
Radiology. . . . . David Edward Avrin, MD
Operating Room. . . . . Guilherme MR Campos, RN
Pediatric In-Patient Care . . . . Roxanne Fernandes, RN
Quality Assurance . . . . Virginia Fleming
Cardiac Laboratory. . . . . William Grossman
CEO/President. . . . . Mark R. Laret
Infection Control. . . . . Amy Nichols, MD
Chief of Medical Staff . . . . Ernest Ring, MD

Measure	Cases	This Hosp.	State Avg.	U.S. Avg.
Blood Clot Prevention and Treatment				
Anticoagulation Overlap Therapy[2]	71	99%	92%	93%
ICU Venous Thromboembolism Prophylaxis[2]	87	84%	92%	92%
Incidence of Potentially Preventable VTE[2]	82	20%	11%	10%
UFH with Dosages/Platelet Monitoring[2]	88	100%	96%	97%
Venous Thromboembolism Prophylaxis[2]	296	71%	83%	85%
Warfarin Therapy Discharge Instructions[2]	63	0%	75%	75%
Chest Pain/Possible Heart Attack Care				
Aspirin Given Within 24 Hours of Arrival[1,3]	-	-	97%	96%
Fibrinolytic Meds Within 30 Min. of Arrival[5]	-	-	62%	58%
Average Time to ECG (minutes)[1,3]	-	-	9	7
Average Time to Transfer (minutes)[5]	-	-	62	60
Children's Asthma Care				
Received Home Management Plan of Care	32	97%	88%	88%
Received Reliever Medication	32	100%	100%	100%
Received Systemic Corticosteroids	32	100%	100%	100%
Emergency Department				
Admittance Decision Time (minutes)[2]	233	218	125	98
Head CT Results Within 45 Min. of Arrival[1]	-	-	55%	57%
Patients Who Left ER Before Being Seen	38,764	4%	3%	2%
Time from ER Arrival to Admit. (minutes)[2]	233	417	323	274
Time from ER Arrival to Discharge (minutes)	351	229	168	134
Time in ER Before Being Evaluated (minutes)	383	34	29	26
Time to Pain Meds for Fractures (minutes)	71	58	62	57
Heart Attack Care				
Aspirin Given at Discharge	136	100%	99%	99%
Fibrinolytic Meds Within 30 Min. of Arrival[7]	-	-	73%	54%
PCI Within 90 Minutes of Arrival	26	100%	95%	96%
Statin Prescribed at Discharge	135	100%	98%	98%
Heart Failure Care				
ACE Inhibitor or ARB for LVSD[2]	65	100%	97%	97%
Discharge Instructions Given[2]	219	93%	94%	94%
Evaluation of LVS Function[2]	238	100%	99%	99%
Medicare Spending				
Medicare Spending per Patient (ratio)	-	0.97	0.98	0.98
Pneumonia Care				
Appropriate Initial Antibiotic Given[2]	53	98%	97%	95%
Blood Culture Timing[2]	121	94%	98%	98%
Pregnancy and Delivery Care				
Newborn Deliveries Scheduled Early	69	4%	5%	6%
Preventive Care				
Immunization for Influenza[2]	529	74%	89%	90%
Immunization for Pneumonia[2]	408	77%	90%	92%
Stroke Care				
Anticoagulation Therapy for Atrial Fibrillation[2]	15	100%	95%	95%
Antithrombotic Therapy Timing[2]	46	98%	98%	98%
Assessed for Rehabilitation[2]	128	98%	97%	97%
Discharged on Antithrombotic Therapy[2]	62	100%	99%	99%
Discharged on Statin Medication[2]	50	98%	94%	94%
Thrombolytic Therapy Timing[1,2]	-	-	72%	66%
Venous Thromboembolism Prophylaxis[2]	149	95%	94%	94%
Written Stroke Educational Materials Given[2]	61	77%	87%	88%
Surgical Care Improvement Project				
Appropriate Beta Blocker Usage[2]	139	99%	97%	98%
Appropriate VTP Within 24 Hours[2]	403	100%	98%	98%
Controlled Postoperative Blood Glucose[2]	91	96%	96%	97%
Perioperative Temperature Management[2]	533	98%	100%	100%
Prophylactic Antibiotic Selection[2]	354	99%	99%	99%
Prophylactic Antibiotic Selection (Outpatient)	802	99%	97%	98%
Prophylactic Antibiotic Stopped[2]	343	97%	98%	98%
Prophylactic Antibiotic Timing[2]	355	97%	99%	99%
Prophylactic Antibiotic Timing (Outpatient)	479	97%	97%	98%
Urinary Catheter Removal[2]	368	92%	97%	97%
Survey of Patients' Hospital Experiences				
Area Around Room 'Always' Quiet at Night	300+	55%	51%	61%
Doctors 'Always' Communicated Well	300+	81%	78%	82%
Home Recovery Information Given	300+	88%	83%	85%
Hospital Given 9 or 10 on 10 Point Scale	300+	78%	68%	71%
Meds 'Always' Explained Before Given	300+	67%	61%	64%
Nurses 'Always' Communicated Well	300+	80%	74%	79%
Pain 'Always' Well Controlled	300+	66%	68%	71%
Room and Bathroom 'Always' Clean	300+	72%	70%	73%
Timely Help 'Always' Received	300+	63%	62%	68%
Would Definitely Recommend Hospital	300+	82%	70%	71%
Use of Medical Imaging				
Cardiac Imaging Stress Test before Surgery	697	4.6%	5.2%	5.3%
Combination Abdominal CT Scan	2,186	19.8%	13.4%	10.5%
Combination Brain/Sinus CT Scan	560	1.1%	2.2%	2.7%
Combination Chest CT Scan	2,875	0.4%	2.3%	2.7%
Follow-up Mammogram/Ultrasound	2,361	6.3%	8.2%	8.8%
Lumbar Spine MRI for Low Back Pain	238	30.3%	34.2%	37.2%

San Gabriel Valley Medical Center

438 W Las Tunas Drive Phone: 626-289-5454
San Gabriel, CA 91776 Fax: 626-570-6555
URL: www.sangabrielvalleymedctr.org
Type: Acute Care Hospitals Emergency Services: Yes
Ownership: Physician Beds: 274

Key Personnel:
Chief of Medical Staff . . . . Sergio Blesa, MD
Cardiac Laboratory. . . . . Delia DelAngel
Infection Control. . . . . Susan Feliciano
CEO/President. . . . . Makato Nakayama
Operating Room. . . . . Mike Nassman
Quality Assurance . . . . Debra Starr-Knecht
Radiology. . . . . A Franklin Turner, MD
Emergency Room . . . . Geri Woessner, RN

Measure	Cases	This Hosp.	State Avg.	U.S. Avg.
Blood Clot Prevention and Treatment				
Anticoagulation Overlap Therapy[2]	17	71%	92%	93%
ICU Venous Thromboembolism Prophylaxis[2]	58	97%	92%	92%
Incidence of Potentially Preventable VTE[2,7]	-	-	11%	10%
UFH with Dosages/Platelet Monitoring[1,2]	-	-	96%	97%
Venous Thromboembolism Prophylaxis[2]	301	94%	83%	85%
Warfarin Therapy Discharge Instructions[1,2]	-	-	75%	75%
Chest Pain/Possible Heart Attack Care				
Aspirin Given Within 24 Hours of Arrival	15	93%	97%	96%
Fibrinolytic Meds Within 30 Min. of Arrival[7]	-	-	62%	58%
Average Time to ECG (minutes)	15	19	9	7
Average Time to Transfer (minutes)[1]	-	-	62	60
Children's Asthma Care				
Received Home Management Plan of Care	-	-	88%	88%
Received Reliever Medication	-	-	100%	100%
Received Systemic Corticosteroids	-	-	100%	100%
Emergency Department				
Admittance Decision Time (minutes)[2]	472	84	125	98
Head CT Results Within 45 Min. of Arrival[1]	-	-	55%	57%
Patients Who Left ER Before Being Seen	25,408	1%	3%	2%
Time from ER Arrival to Admit. (minutes)[2]	472	255	323	274
Time from ER Arrival to Discharge (minutes)	369	144	168	134
Time in ER Before Being Evaluated (minutes)	413	25	29	26
Time to Pain Meds for Fractures (minutes)	114	66	62	57
Heart Attack Care				
Aspirin Given at Discharge	32	100%	99%	99%
Fibrinolytic Meds Within 30 Min. of Arrival[7]	-	-	73%	54%
PCI Within 90 Minutes of Arrival[7]	-	-	95%	96%
Statin Prescribed at Discharge	34	100%	98%	98%
Heart Failure Care				
ACE Inhibitor or ARB for LVSD	46	100%	97%	97%
Discharge Instructions Given	155	99%	94%	94%
Evaluation of LVS Function	234	99%	99%	99%

NOTE: Hospital profiles are in alphabetical order by state, then city, then hospital within the city; Rankings exclude hospitals with less than 25 cases except for patient surveys which excludes hospitals with less than 100 cases; (a) 100-299 cases; (1) The number of cases/patients is too few to report; (2) Data submitted were based on a sample of cases/patients; (3) Results are based on a shorter time period than required; (4) Data suppressed by CMS for one or more quarters; (5) Results are not available for this reporting period; (6) Fewer than 100 patients completed the HCAHPS survey; (7) No cases met the criteria for this measure; (8) The lower limit of the confidence interval cannot be calculated if the number of observed infections equals zero; (9) No data are available from the state/territory for this reporting period; (10) The scores shown reflect fewer than 50 completed surveys; (11) There were discrepancies in the data collection process; (12) This measure does not apply to this hospital for this reporting period; (13) Results cannot be calculated for this reporting period; (14) The results for this state are combined with nearby states to protect confidentiality; Please refer to the User's Guide for a full explanation of data.

Measure	Cases	This Hosp.	State Avg.	U.S. Avg.
Medicare Spending				
Medicare Spending per Patient (ratio)	-	1.14	0.98	0.98
Pneumonia Care				
Appropriate Initial Antibiotic Given[2]	49	96%	97%	95%
Blood Culture Timing[2]	162	99%	98%	98%
Pregnancy and Delivery Care				
Newborn Deliveries Scheduled Early[2]	452	17%	5%	6%
Preventive Care				
Immunization for Influenza[2]	454	62%	89%	90%
Immunization for Pneumonia[2]	462	90%	90%	92%
Stroke Care				
Anticoagulation Therapy for Atrial Fibrillation[1]	-	-	95%	95%
Antithrombotic Therapy Timing	38	100%	98%	98%
Assessed for Rehabilitation	49	100%	97%	97%
Discharged on Antithrombotic Therapy	40	100%	99%	99%
Discharged on Statin Medication	26	100%	94%	94%
Thrombolytic Therapy Timing[1]	-	-	72%	66%
Venous Thromboembolism Prophylaxis	48	100%	94%	94%
Written Stroke Educational Materials Given	26	100%	87%	88%
Surgical Care Improvement Project				
Appropriate Beta Blocker Usage[2]	52	98%	97%	98%
Appropriate VTP Within 24 Hours[2]	277	100%	98%	98%
Controlled Postoperative Blood Glucose[2,7]	-	-	96%	97%
Perioperative Temperature Management[2]	308	100%	100%	100%
Prophylactic Antibiotic Selection[2]	184	97%	99%	99%
Prophylactic Antibiotic Selection (Outpatient)	52	90%	97%	98%
Prophylactic Antibiotic Stopped[2]	170	97%	98%	98%
Prophylactic Antibiotic Timing[2]	184	99%	99%	99%
Prophylactic Antibiotic Timing (Outpatient)	52	100%	97%	98%
Urinary Catheter Removal[2]	154	100%	97%	97%
Survey of Patients' Hospital Experiences				
Area Around Room 'Always' Quiet at Night	300+	44%	51%	61%
Doctors 'Always' Communicated Well	300+	70%	78%	82%
Home Recovery Information Given	300+	78%	83%	85%
Hospital Given 9 or 10 on 10 Point Scale	300+	53%	68%	71%
Meds 'Always' Explained Before Given	300+	53%	61%	64%
Nurses 'Always' Communicated Well	300+	64%	74%	79%
Pain 'Always' Well Controlled	300+	59%	68%	71%
Room and Bathroom 'Always' Clean	300+	63%	70%	73%
Timely Help 'Always' Received	300+	52%	62%	68%
Would Definitely Recommend Hospital	300+	55%	70%	71%
Use of Medical Imaging				
Cardiac Imaging Stress Test before Surgery[7]	-	-	5.2%	5.3%
Combination Abdominal CT Scan	235	5.5%	13.4%	10.5%
Combination Brain/Sinus CT Scan[1]	-	-	2.2%	2.7%
Combination Chest CT Scan	89	1.1%	2.3%	2.7%
Follow-up Mammogram/Ultrasound	132	11.4%	8.2%	8.8%
Lumbar Spine MRI for Low Back Pain[1]	-	-	34.2%	37.2%

Good Samaritan Hospital

2425 Samaritan Drive
San Jose, CA 95124
Phone: 408-559-2011
Fax: 408-559-2662
URL: www.goodsamsj.org
Type: Acute Care Hospitals
Emergency Services: Yes
Ownership: Proprietary
Beds: 474
Key Personnel:
CEO/President. . . . . Paul Beaupre, MD

Measure	Cases	This Hosp.	State Avg.	U.S. Avg.
Blood Clot Prevention and Treatment				
Anticoagulation Overlap Therapy[2]	93	95%	92%	93%
ICU Venous Thromboembolism Prophylaxis[2]	87	97%	92%	92%
Incidence of Potentially Preventable VTE[2]	13	0%	11%	10%
UFH with Dosages/Platelet Monitoring[2]	66	100%	96%	97%
Venous Thromboembolism Prophylaxis[2]	325	72%	83%	85%
Warfarin Therapy Discharge Instructions[2]	67	85%	75%	75%
Chest Pain/Possible Heart Attack Care				
Aspirin Given Within 24 Hours of Arrival[1]	-	-	97%	96%
Fibrinolytic Meds Within 30 Min. of Arrival[5]	-	-	62%	58%
Average Time to ECG (minutes)[1]	-	-	9	7
Average Time to Transfer (minutes)[5]	-	-	62	60
Children's Asthma Care				
Received Home Management Plan of Care	-	-	88%	88%
Received Reliever Medication	-	-	100%	100%
Received Systemic Corticosteroids	-	-	100%	100%
Emergency Department				
Admittance Decision Time (minutes)[2]	555	175	125	98
Head CT Results Within 45 Min. of Arrival[1]	-	-	55%	57%
Patients Who Left ER Before Being Seen	44,761	1%	3%	2%
Time from ER Arrival to Admit. (minutes)[2]	560	301	323	274
Time from ER Arrival to Discharge (minutes)	429	140	168	134
Time in ER Before Being Evaluated (minutes)	455	7	29	26
Time to Pain Meds for Fractures (minutes)	187	38	62	57
Heart Attack Care				
Aspirin Given at Discharge	198	100%	99%	99%
Fibrinolytic Meds Within 30 Min. of Arrival[7]	-	-	73%	54%
PCI Within 90 Minutes of Arrival	51	100%	95%	96%
Statin Prescribed at Discharge	192	100%	98%	98%
Heart Failure Care				
ACE Inhibitor or ARB for LVSD	51	100%	97%	97%
Discharge Instructions Given	195	98%	94%	94%
Evaluation of LVS Function	249	100%	99%	99%
Medicare Spending				
Medicare Spending per Patient (ratio)	-	1.02	0.98	0.98
Pneumonia Care				
Appropriate Initial Antibiotic Given[2]	118	97%	97%	95%
Blood Culture Timing[2]	179	100%	98%	98%
Pregnancy and Delivery Care				
Newborn Deliveries Scheduled Early[2]	49	0%	5%	6%
Preventive Care				
Immunization for Influenza[2]	513	97%	89%	90%
Immunization for Pneumonia[2]	488	96%	90%	92%
Stroke Care				
Anticoagulation Therapy for Atrial Fibrillation[2]	20	100%	95%	95%
Antithrombotic Therapy Timing[2]	78	100%	98%	98%
Assessed for Rehabilitation[2]	120	100%	97%	97%
Discharged on Antithrombotic Therapy[2]	95	100%	99%	99%
Discharged on Statin Medication[2]	76	100%	94%	94%
Thrombolytic Therapy Timing[1,2]	-	-	72%	66%
Venous Thromboembolism Prophylaxis[2]	121	98%	94%	94%
Written Stroke Educational Materials Given[2]	70	99%	87%	88%
Surgical Care Improvement Project				
Appropriate Beta Blocker Usage[2]	212	98%	97%	98%
Appropriate VTP Within 24 Hours[2]	470	99%	98%	98%
Controlled Postoperative Blood Glucose[2]	131	99%	96%	97%
Perioperative Temperature Management[2]	557	100%	100%	100%
Prophylactic Antibiotic Selection[2]	470	100%	99%	99%
Prophylactic Antibiotic Selection (Outpatient)	439	95%	97%	98%
Prophylactic Antibiotic Stopped[2]	459	99%	98%	98%
Prophylactic Antibiotic Timing[2]	470	99%	99%	99%
Prophylactic Antibiotic Timing (Outpatient)	440	95%	97%	98%
Urinary Catheter Removal[2]	347	99%	97%	97%
Survey of Patients' Hospital Experiences				
Area Around Room 'Always' Quiet at Night	300+	49%	51%	61%
Doctors 'Always' Communicated Well	300+	78%	78%	82%
Home Recovery Information Given	300+	81%	83%	85%
Hospital Given 9 or 10 on 10 Point Scale	300+	64%	68%	71%
Meds 'Always' Explained Before Given	300+	51%	61%	64%
Nurses 'Always' Communicated Well	300+	71%	74%	79%
Pain 'Always' Well Controlled	300+	67%	68%	71%
Room and Bathroom 'Always' Clean	300+	63%	70%	73%
Timely Help 'Always' Received	300+	52%	62%	68%
Would Definitely Recommend Hospital	300+	70%	70%	71%
Use of Medical Imaging				
Cardiac Imaging Stress Test before Surgery	55	5.5%	5.2%	5.3%
Combination Abdominal CT Scan	762	4.1%	13.4%	10.5%
Combination Brain/Sinus CT Scan	701	0.9%	2.2%	2.7%
Combination Chest CT Scan	387	0.0%	2.3%	2.7%
Follow-up Mammogram/Ultrasound	2,867	14.1%	8.2%	8.8%
Lumbar Spine MRI for Low Back Pain[1]	-	-	34.2%	37.2%

Kaiser Foundation Hospital - San Jose

250 Hospital Parkway
San Jose, CA 95119
Phone: 408-972-7000
Fax: 888-805-7562
URL: www.mydoctor.kaiserpermanente.org
Type: Acute Care Hospitals
Emergency Services: Yes
Ownership: Voluntary non-profit - Other
Beds: 228
Key Personnel:
CEO/President. . . . . George Ajlverson
Radiology. . . . . Andrea L Baron
Chief of Medical Staff . . . . Raj Bhandari, MD
Emergency Room . . . . Robin Parsons, RN
Coronary Care. . . . . Kwaiben Valley

Measure	Cases	This Hosp.	State Avg.	U.S. Avg.
Blood Clot Prevention and Treatment				
Anticoagulation Overlap Therapy[2]	68	100%	92%	93%
ICU Venous Thromboembolism Prophylaxis[2]	67	94%	92%	92%
Incidence of Potentially Preventable VTE[1,2]	-	-	11%	10%
UFH with Dosages/Platelet Monitoring[2]	47	100%	96%	97%
Venous Thromboembolism Prophylaxis[2]	309	93%	83%	85%
Warfarin Therapy Discharge Instructions[2]	59	68%	75%	75%
Chest Pain/Possible Heart Attack Care				
Aspirin Given Within 24 Hours of Arrival	-	-	97%	96%
Fibrinolytic Meds Within 30 Min. of Arrival	-	-	62%	58%
Average Time to ECG (minutes)	-	-	9	7
Average Time to Transfer (minutes)	-	-	62	60
Children's Asthma Care				
Received Home Management Plan of Care	-	-	88%	88%
Received Reliever Medication	-	-	100%	100%
Received Systemic Corticosteroids	-	-	100%	100%
Emergency Department				
Admittance Decision Time (minutes)[2]	507	57	125	98
Head CT Results Within 45 Min. of Arrival	-	-	55%	57%
Patients Who Left ER Before Being Seen	-	-	3%	2%
Time from ER Arrival to Admit. (minutes)[2]	512	301	323	274
Time from ER Arrival to Discharge (minutes)	-	-	168	134
Time in ER Before Being Evaluated (minutes)	-	-	29	26
Time to Pain Meds for Fractures (minutes)	-	-	62	57
Heart Attack Care				
Aspirin Given at Discharge	116	99%	99%	99%
Fibrinolytic Meds Within 30 Min. of Arrival[7]	-	-	73%	54%
PCI Within 90 Minutes of Arrival	55	100%	95%	96%
Statin Prescribed at Discharge	117	99%	98%	98%
Heart Failure Care				
ACE Inhibitor or ARB for LVSD	49	100%	97%	97%
Discharge Instructions Given	239	100%	94%	94%
Evaluation of LVS Function	260	100%	99%	99%
Medicare Spending				
Medicare Spending per Patient (ratio)	-	0.87	0.98	0.98
Pneumonia Care				
Appropriate Initial Antibiotic Given[2]	80	100%	97%	95%
Blood Culture Timing[2]	135	100%	98%	98%
Pregnancy and Delivery Care				
Newborn Deliveries Scheduled Early[2]	25	0%	5%	6%
Preventive Care				
Immunization for Influenza[2]	497	86%	89%	90%
Immunization for Pneumonia[2]	597	93%	90%	92%
Stroke Care				
Anticoagulation Therapy for Atrial Fibrillation[2]	17	100%	95%	95%
Antithrombotic Therapy Timing[2]	77	100%	98%	98%
Assessed for Rehabilitation[2]	121	99%	97%	97%
Discharged on Antithrombotic Therapy[2]	102	99%	99%	99%
Discharged on Statin Medication[2]	85	99%	94%	94%
Thrombolytic Therapy Timing[2]	12	92%	72%	66%
Venous Thromboembolism Prophylaxis[2]	94	94%	94%	94%
Written Stroke Educational Materials Given[2]	81	99%	87%	88%
Surgical Care Improvement Project				
Appropriate Beta Blocker Usage[2]	126	99%	97%	98%
Appropriate VTP Within 24 Hours[2]	374	100%	98%	98%
Controlled Postoperative Blood Glucose[2,7]	-	-	96%	97%
Perioperative Temperature Management[2]	459	100%	100%	100%
Prophylactic Antibiotic Selection[2]	314	100%	99%	99%
Prophylactic Antibiotic Selection (Outpatient)	-	-	97%	98%
Prophylactic Antibiotic Stopped[2]	314	100%	98%	98%

NOTE: Hospital profiles are in alphabetical order by state, then city, then hospital within the city; Rankings exclude hospitals with less than 25 cases except for patient surveys which excludes hospitals with less than 100 cases; (a) 100-299 cases; (1) The number of cases/patients is too few to report; (2) Data submitted were based on a sample of cases/patients; (3) Results are based on a shorter time period than required; (4) Data suppressed by CMS for one or more quarters; (5) Results are not available for this reporting period; (6) Fewer than 100 patients completed the HCAHPS survey; (7) No cases met the criteria for this measure; (8) The lower limit of the confidence interval cannot be calculated if the number of observed infections equals zero; (9) No data are available from the state/territory for this reporting period; (10) The scores shown reflect fewer than 50 completed surveys; (11) There were discrepancies in the data collection process; (12) This measure does not apply to this hospital for this reporting period; (13) Results cannot be calculated for this reporting period; (14) The results for this state are combined with nearby states to protect confidentiality; Please refer to the User's Guide for a full explanation of data.

Measure	Cases	This Hosp.	State Avg.	U.S. Avg.
Prophylactic Antibiotic Timing[2]	314	100%	99%	99%
Prophylactic Antibiotic Timing (Outpatient)	-	-	97%	98%
Urinary Catheter Removal[2]	290	100%	97%	97%
Survey of Patients' Hospital Experiences				
Area Around Room 'Always' Quiet at Night	300+	47%	51%	61%
Doctors 'Always' Communicated Well	300+	81%	78%	82%
Home Recovery Information Given	300+	87%	83%	85%
Hospital Given 9 or 10 on 10 Point Scale	300+	68%	68%	71%
Meds 'Always' Explained Before Given	300+	61%	61%	64%
Nurses 'Always' Communicated Well	300+	73%	74%	79%
Pain 'Always' Well Controlled	300+	71%	68%	71%
Room and Bathroom 'Always' Clean	300+	69%	70%	73%
Timely Help 'Always' Received	300+	60%	62%	68%
Would Definitely Recommend Hospital	300+	71%	70%	71%
Use of Medical Imaging				
Cardiac Imaging Stress Test before Surgery	-	-	5.2%	5.3%
Combination Abdominal CT Scan	-	-	13.4%	10.5%
Combination Brain/Sinus CT Scan	-	-	2.2%	2.7%
Combination Chest CT Scan	-	-	2.3%	2.7%
Follow-up Mammogram/Ultrasound	-	-	8.2%	8.8%
Lumbar Spine MRI for Low Back Pain	-	-	34.2%	37.2%

O'Connor Hospital

2105 Forest Avenue Phone: 408-947-2500
San Jose, CA 95128 Fax: 408-283-7778
URL: www.oconnorhospital.org
Type: Acute Care Hospitals Emergency Services: Yes
Ownership: Voluntary non-profit - Church Beds: 358
Key Personnel:
Chief of Medical Staff.......... George Block, MD
CEO/President.............. James F. Dover, FACHE
Cardiac Laboratory............ Claudia Rod
Emergency Room .... Brian Saavedra
Patient Relations .... Pamela Sedano, MD, RN
Infection Control.............. Rosalie Sheveland

Measure	Cases	This Hosp.	State Avg.	U.S. Avg.
Blood Clot Prevention and Treatment				
Anticoagulation Overlap Therapy[2]	45	98%	92%	93%
ICU Venous Thromboembolism Prophylaxis[2]	82	93%	92%	92%
Incidence of Potentially Preventable VTE[1,2]	-	-	11%	10%
UFH with Dosages/Platelet Monitoring[2]	24	88%	96%	97%
Venous Thromboembolism Prophylaxis[2]	321	96%	83%	85%
Warfarin Therapy Discharge Instructions[2]	29	38%	75%	75%
Chest Pain/Possible Heart Attack Care				
Aspirin Given Within 24 Hours of Arrival[5]	-	-	97%	96%
Fibrinolytic Meds Within 30 Min. of Arrival[5]	-	-	62%	58%
Average Time to ECG (minutes)[5]	-	-	9	7
Average Time to Transfer (minutes)[5]	-	-	62	60
Children's Asthma Care				
Received Home Management Plan of Care	-	-	88%	88%
Received Reliever Medication	-	-	100%	100%
Received Systemic Corticosteroids	-	-	100%	100%
Emergency Department				
Admittance Decision Time (minutes)[2]	455	175	125	98
Head CT Results Within 45 Min. of Arrival[1]	-	-	55%	57%
Patients Who Left ER Before Being Seen	54,195	2%	3%	2%
Time from ER Arrival to Admit. (minutes)[2]	467	321	323	274
Time from ER Arrival to Discharge (minutes)	378	137	168	134
Time in ER Before Being Evaluated (minutes)	396	23	29	26
Time to Pain Meds for Fractures (minutes)	112	64	62	57
Heart Attack Care				
Aspirin Given at Discharge	170	99%	99%	99%
Fibrinolytic Meds Within 30 Min. of Arrival[7]	-	-	73%	54%
PCI Within 90 Minutes of Arrival	34	85%	95%	96%
Statin Prescribed at Discharge	166	99%	98%	98%
Heart Failure Care				
ACE Inhibitor or ARB for LVSD	66	98%	97%	97%
Discharge Instructions Given	234	98%	94%	94%
Evaluation of LVS Function	300	100%	99%	99%
Medicare Spending				
Medicare Spending per Patient (ratio)	-	0.98	0.98	0.98
Pneumonia Care				
Appropriate Initial Antibiotic Given	153	97%	97%	95%
Blood Culture Timing	247	99%	98%	98%
Pregnancy and Delivery Care				
Newborn Deliveries Scheduled Early[2]	67	9%	5%	6%
Preventive Care				
Immunization for Influenza[2]	457	93%	89%	90%
Immunization for Pneumonia[2]	433	95%	90%	92%
Stroke Care				
Anticoagulation Therapy for Atrial Fibrillation[2]	12	100%	95%	95%
Antithrombotic Therapy Timing[2]	67	99%	98%	98%
Assessed for Rehabilitation[2]	83	100%	97%	97%
Discharged on Antithrombotic Therapy[2]	65	98%	99%	99%
Discharged on Statin Medication[2]	52	98%	94%	94%
Thrombolytic Therapy Timing[1,2]	-	-	72%	66%
Venous Thromboembolism Prophylaxis[2]	85	99%	94%	94%
Written Stroke Educational Materials Given[2]	47	100%	87%	88%
Surgical Care Improvement Project				
Appropriate Beta Blocker Usage[2]	174	98%	97%	98%
Appropriate VTP Within 24 Hours[2]	495	98%	98%	98%
Controlled Postoperative Blood Glucose[2]	46	98%	96%	97%
Perioperative Temperature Management[2]	614	100%	100%	100%
Prophylactic Antibiotic Selection[2]	478	99%	99%	99%
Prophylactic Antibiotic Selection (Outpatient)	150	81%	97%	98%
Prophylactic Antibiotic Stopped[2]	454	99%	98%	98%
Prophylactic Antibiotic Timing[2]	479	100%	99%	99%
Prophylactic Antibiotic Timing (Outpatient)	151	94%	97%	98%
Urinary Catheter Removal[2]	119	92%	97%	97%
Survey of Patients' Hospital Experiences				
Area Around Room 'Always' Quiet at Night	300+	54%	51%	61%
Doctors 'Always' Communicated Well	300+	79%	78%	82%
Home Recovery Information Given	300+	83%	83%	85%
Hospital Given 9 or 10 on 10 Point Scale	300+	67%	68%	71%
Meds 'Always' Explained Before Given	300+	56%	61%	64%
Nurses 'Always' Communicated Well	300+	73%	74%	79%
Pain 'Always' Well Controlled	300+	66%	68%	71%
Room and Bathroom 'Always' Clean	300+	66%	70%	73%
Timely Help 'Always' Received	300+	59%	62%	68%
Would Definitely Recommend Hospital	300+	72%	70%	71%
Use of Medical Imaging				
Cardiac Imaging Stress Test before Surgery	156	4.5%	5.2%	5.3%
Combination Abdominal CT Scan	870	1.8%	13.4%	10.5%
Combination Brain/Sinus CT Scan	764	1.8%	2.2%	2.7%
Combination Chest CT Scan	304	0.0%	2.3%	2.7%
Follow-up Mammogram/Ultrasound	590	6.4%	8.2%	8.8%
Lumbar Spine MRI for Low Back Pain	87	33.3%	34.2%	37.2%

Regional Medical Center of San Jose

225 N Jackson Avenue Phone: 408-259-5000
San Jose, CA 95116 Fax: 408-729-2884
URL: www.regionalmedicalsanjose.com
Type: Acute Care Hospitals Emergency Services: Yes
Ownership: Voluntary non-profit - Church Beds: 204
Key Personnel:
CEO/President.............. William L Gilbert
Radiology.................. Reza Malek
Chief of Medical Staff.......... Elaine Nelson

Measure	Cases	This Hosp.	State Avg.	U.S. Avg.
Blood Clot Prevention and Treatment				
Anticoagulation Overlap Therapy[2]	52	81%	92%	93%
ICU Venous Thromboembolism Prophylaxis[2]	97	100%	92%	92%
Incidence of Potentially Preventable VTE[2]	19	0%	11%	10%
UFH with Dosages/Platelet Monitoring[2]	47	98%	96%	97%
Venous Thromboembolism Prophylaxis[2]	381	90%	83%	85%
Warfarin Therapy Discharge Instructions[2]	39	100%	75%	75%
Chest Pain/Possible Heart Attack Care				
Aspirin Given Within 24 Hours of Arrival	11	100%	97%	96%
Fibrinolytic Meds Within 30 Min. of Arrival[3,7]	-	-	62%	58%
Average Time to ECG (minutes)	15	16	9	7
Average Time to Transfer (minutes)[3,7]	-	-	62	60
Children's Asthma Care				
Received Home Management Plan of Care	-	-	88%	88%
Received Reliever Medication	-	-	100%	100%
Received Systemic Corticosteroids	-	-	100%	100%
Emergency Department				
Admittance Decision Time (minutes)[2]	1,138	258	125	98
Head CT Results Within 45 Min. of Arrival[1]	-	-	55%	57%
Patients Who Left ER Before Being Seen	61,126	2%	3%	2%
Time from ER Arrival to Admit. (minutes)[2]	1,138	373	323	274
Time from ER Arrival to Discharge (minutes)	450	164	168	134
Time in ER Before Being Evaluated (minutes)	496	8	29	26
Time to Pain Meds for Fractures (minutes)	191	77	62	57
Heart Attack Care				
Aspirin Given at Discharge	235	98%	99%	99%
Fibrinolytic Meds Within 30 Min. of Arrival[1]	-	-	73%	54%
PCI Within 90 Minutes of Arrival	43	98%	95%	96%
Statin Prescribed at Discharge	235	98%	98%	98%
Heart Failure Care				
ACE Inhibitor or ARB for LVSD	137	89%	97%	97%
Discharge Instructions Given	407	98%	94%	94%
Evaluation of LVS Function	501	98%	99%	99%
Medicare Spending				
Medicare Spending per Patient (ratio)	-	0.98	0.98	0.98
Pneumonia Care				
Appropriate Initial Antibiotic Given[2]	98	100%	97%	95%
Blood Culture Timing[2]	136	100%	98%	98%
Pregnancy and Delivery Care				
Newborn Deliveries Scheduled Early[2]	50	0%	5%	6%
Preventive Care				
Immunization for Influenza[2]	574	93%	89%	90%
Immunization for Pneumonia[2]	875	95%	90%	92%
Stroke Care				
Anticoagulation Therapy for Atrial Fibrillation[2]	12	92%	95%	95%
Antithrombotic Therapy Timing[2]	88	100%	98%	98%
Assessed for Rehabilitation[2]	118	99%	97%	97%
Discharged on Antithrombotic Therapy[2]	91	99%	99%	99%
Discharged on Statin Medication[2]	69	99%	94%	94%
Thrombolytic Therapy Timing[1,2]	-	-	72%	66%
Venous Thromboembolism Prophylaxis[2]	128	99%	94%	94%
Written Stroke Educational Materials Given[2]	52	98%	87%	88%
Surgical Care Improvement Project				
Appropriate Beta Blocker Usage[2]	118	94%	97%	98%
Appropriate VTP Within 24 Hours[2]	259	89%	98%	98%
Controlled Postoperative Blood Glucose[2]	76	99%	96%	97%
Perioperative Temperature Management[2]	297	100%	100%	100%
Prophylactic Antibiotic Selection[2]	209	98%	99%	99%
Prophylactic Antibiotic Selection (Outpatient)	133	98%	97%	98%
Prophylactic Antibiotic Stopped[2]	197	92%	98%	98%
Prophylactic Antibiotic Timing[2]	209	99%	99%	99%
Prophylactic Antibiotic Timing (Outpatient)	135	99%	97%	98%
Urinary Catheter Removal[2]	194	91%	97%	97%
Survey of Patients' Hospital Experiences				
Area Around Room 'Always' Quiet at Night	300+	49%	51%	61%
Doctors 'Always' Communicated Well	300+	71%	78%	82%
Home Recovery Information Given	300+	79%	83%	85%
Hospital Given 9 or 10 on 10 Point Scale	300+	57%	68%	71%
Meds 'Always' Explained Before Given	300+	54%	61%	64%
Nurses 'Always' Communicated Well	300+	65%	74%	79%
Pain 'Always' Well Controlled	300+	62%	68%	71%
Room and Bathroom 'Always' Clean	300+	62%	70%	73%
Timely Help 'Always' Received	300+	54%	62%	68%
Would Definitely Recommend Hospital	300+	56%	70%	71%
Use of Medical Imaging				
Cardiac Imaging Stress Test before Surgery	253	4.0%	5.2%	5.3%
Combination Abdominal CT Scan	752	1.7%	13.4%	10.5%
Combination Brain/Sinus CT Scan	916	0.8%	2.2%	2.7%
Combination Chest CT Scan	259	0.0%	2.3%	2.7%
Follow-up Mammogram/Ultrasound	504	3.8%	8.2%	8.8%
Lumbar Spine MRI for Low Back Pain[1]	-	-	34.2%	37.2%

Santa Clara Valley Medical Center

751 South Bascom Avenue Phone: 408-885-5000
San Jose, CA 95128 Fax: 408-885-6459
URL: www.sccgov.org
Type: Acute Care Hospitals Emergency Services: Yes
Ownership: Government - Local Beds: 524
Key Personnel:
Chief of Medical Staff.......... Jeffrey Arnold, MD
Radiology.................. Young S Kang, MD PhD
CEO .... Paul E. Lorenz

NOTE: Hospital profiles are in alphabetical order by state, then city, then hospital within the city; Rankings exclude hospitals with less than 25 cases except for patient surveys which excludes hospitals with less than 100 cases; (a) 100-299 cases; (1) The number of cases/patients is too few to report; (2) Data submitted were based on a sample of cases/patients; (3) Results are based on a shorter time period than required; (4) Data suppressed by CMS for one or more quarters; (5) Results are not available for this reporting period; (6) Fewer than 100 patients completed the HCAHPS survey; (7) No cases met the criteria for this measure; (8) The lower limit of the confidence interval cannot be calculated if the number of observed infections equals zero; (9) No data are available from the state/territory for this reporting period; (10) The scores shown reflect fewer than 50 completed surveys; (11) There were discrepancies in the data collection process; (12) This measure does not apply to this hospital for this reporting period; (13) Results cannot be calculated for this reporting period; (14) The results for this state are combined with nearby states to protect confidentiality; Please refer to the User's Guide for a full explanation of data.

Ambulatory Care . . . . Sonia Menzies, RN
Anesthesiology. . . . . Tim Park, MD

Measure	Cases	This Hosp.	State Avg.	U.S. Avg.
Blood Clot Prevention and Treatment				
Anticoagulation Overlap Therapy[2]	57	98%	92%	93%
ICU Venous Thromboembolism Prophylaxis[2]	55	93%	92%	92%
Incidence of Potentially Preventable VTE[2]	15	13%	11%	10%
UFH with Dosages/Platelet Monitoring[2]	39	100%	96%	97%
Venous Thromboembolism Prophylaxis[2]	307	84%	83%	85%
Warfarin Therapy Discharge Instructions[2]	50	72%	75%	75%
Chest Pain/Possible Heart Attack Care				
Aspirin Given Within 24 Hours of Arrival[1]	-	-	97%	96%
Fibrinolytic Meds Within 30 Min. of Arrival[5]	-	-	62%	58%
Average Time to ECG (minutes)[1]	-	-	9	7
Average Time to Transfer (minutes)[5]	-	-	62	60
Children's Asthma Care				
Received Home Management Plan of Care	-	-	88%	88%
Received Reliever Medication	-	-	100%	100%
Received Systemic Corticosteroids	-	-	100%	100%
Emergency Department				
Admittance Decision Time (minutes)[2]	545	227	125	98
Head CT Results Within 45 Min. of Arrival[1]	-	-	55%	57%
Patients Who Left ER Before Being Seen	71,611	4%	3%	2%
Time from ER Arrival to Admit. (minutes)[2]	545	491	323	274
Time from ER Arrival to Discharge (minutes)	340	199	168	134
Time in ER Before Being Evaluated (minutes)	382	33	29	26
Time to Pain Meds for Fractures (minutes)	134	106	62	57
Heart Attack Care				
Aspirin Given at Discharge	177	100%	99%	99%
Fibrinolytic Meds Within 30 Min. of Arrival[7]	-	-	73%	54%
PCI Within 90 Minutes of Arrival	24	100%	95%	96%
Statin Prescribed at Discharge	178	98%	98%	98%
Heart Failure Care				
ACE Inhibitor or ARB for LVSD[2]	119	100%	97%	97%
Discharge Instructions Given[2]	266	94%	94%	94%
Evaluation of LVS Function[2]	284	100%	99%	99%
Medicare Spending				
Medicare Spending per Patient (ratio)	-	0.97	0.98	0.98
Pneumonia Care				
Appropriate Initial Antibiotic Given[2]	52	100%	97%	95%
Blood Culture Timing[2]	124	98%	98%	98%
Pregnancy and Delivery Care				
Newborn Deliveries Scheduled Early[2]	54	2%	5%	6%
Preventive Care				
Immunization for Influenza[2]	470	86%	89%	90%
Immunization for Pneumonia[2]	411	70%	90%	92%
Stroke Care				
Anticoagulation Therapy for Atrial Fibrillation[2]	12	83%	95%	95%
Antithrombotic Therapy Timing[2]	77	92%	98%	98%
Assessed for Rehabilitation[2]	109	95%	97%	97%
Discharged on Antithrombotic Therapy[2]	89	97%	99%	99%
Discharged on Statin Medication[2]	77	95%	94%	94%
Thrombolytic Therapy Timing[1,2]	-	-	72%	66%
Venous Thromboembolism Prophylaxis[2]	99	83%	94%	94%
Written Stroke Educational Materials Given[2]	86	77%	87%	88%
Surgical Care Improvement Project				
Appropriate Beta Blocker Usage[2]	154	95%	97%	98%
Appropriate VTP Within 24 Hours[2]	282	98%	98%	98%
Controlled Postoperative Blood Glucose[2]	102	93%	96%	97%
Perioperative Temperature Management[2]	328	100%	100%	100%
Prophylactic Antibiotic Selection[2]	309	98%	99%	99%
Prophylactic Antibiotic Selection (Outpatient)	288	95%	97%	98%
Prophylactic Antibiotic Stopped[2]	292	92%	98%	98%
Prophylactic Antibiotic Timing[2]	310	99%	99%	99%
Prophylactic Antibiotic Timing (Outpatient)	121	98%	97%	98%
Urinary Catheter Removal[2]	218	96%	97%	97%
Survey of Patients' Hospital Experiences				
Area Around Room 'Always' Quiet at Night	300+	38%	51%	61%
Doctors 'Always' Communicated Well	300+	76%	78%	82%
Home Recovery Information Given	300+	77%	83%	85%
Hospital Given 9 or 10 on 10 Point Scale	300+	59%	68%	71%
Meds 'Always' Explained Before Given	300+	57%	61%	64%
Nurses 'Always' Communicated Well	300+	68%	74%	79%
Pain 'Always' Well Controlled	300+	65%	68%	71%
Room and Bathroom 'Always' Clean	300+	59%	70%	73%
Timely Help 'Always' Received	300+	49%	62%	68%
Would Definitely Recommend Hospital	300+	53%	70%	71%
Use of Medical Imaging				
Cardiac Imaging Stress Test before Surgery	573	1.7%	5.2%	5.3%
Combination Abdominal CT Scan	1,024	21.4%	13.4%	10.5%
Combination Brain/Sinus CT Scan	967	2.5%	2.2%	2.7%
Combination Chest CT Scan	609	2.6%	2.3%	2.7%
Follow-up Mammogram/Ultrasound	673	5.1%	8.2%	8.8%
Lumbar Spine MRI for Low Back Pain	65	36.9%	34.2%	37.2%

San Leandro Hospital

13855 E 14th Street Phone: 510-357-6500
San Leandro, CA 94578
Type: Acute Care Hospitals Emergency Services: Yes
Ownership: Voluntary non-profit - Other

Measure	Cases	This Hosp.	State Avg.	U.S. Avg.
Blood Clot Prevention and Treatment				
Anticoagulation Overlap Therapy[2,3]	26	100%	92%	93%
ICU Venous Thromboembolism Prophylaxis[2,3]	51	80%	92%	92%
Incidence of Potentially Preventable VTE[1,2]	-	-	11%	10%
UFH with Dosages/Platelet Monitoring[2,3]	19	100%	96%	97%
Venous Thromboembolism Prophylaxis[2,3]	166	60%	83%	85%
Warfarin Therapy Discharge Instructions[2,3]	20	90%	75%	75%
Chest Pain/Possible Heart Attack Care				
Aspirin Given Within 24 Hours of Arrival[3]	11	100%	97%	96%
Fibrinolytic Meds Within 30 Min. of Arrival[3,7]	-	-	62%	58%
Average Time to ECG (minutes)[3]	11	14	9	7
Average Time to Transfer (minutes)[1,3]	-	-	62	60
Children's Asthma Care				
Received Home Management Plan of Care	-	-	88%	88%
Received Reliever Medication	-	-	100%	100%
Received Systemic Corticosteroids	-	-	100%	100%
Emergency Department				
Admittance Decision Time (minutes)[2,3]	224	145	125	98
Head CT Results Within 45 Min. of Arrival[3,7]	-	-	55%	57%
Patients Who Left ER Before Being Seen	9,305	5%	3%	2%
Time from ER Arrival to Admit. (minutes)[2,3]	237	350	323	274
Time from ER Arrival to Discharge (minutes)[3]	187	180	168	134
Time in ER Before Being Evaluated (minutes)[3]	200	53	29	26
Time to Pain Meds for Fractures (minutes)[3]	18	92	62	57
Heart Attack Care				
Aspirin Given at Discharge[1,3]	-	-	99%	99%
Fibrinolytic Meds Within 30 Min. of Arrival[3,7]	-	-	73%	54%
PCI Within 90 Minutes of Arrival[3,7]	-	-	95%	96%
Statin Prescribed at Discharge[1,3]	-	-	98%	98%
Heart Failure Care				
ACE Inhibitor or ARB for LVSD[3]	25	100%	97%	97%
Discharge Instructions Given[3]	74	91%	94%	94%
Evaluation of LVS Function[3]	80	100%	99%	99%
Medicare Spending				
Medicare Spending per Patient (ratio)[1]	-	-	0.98	0.98
Pneumonia Care				
Appropriate Initial Antibiotic Given[3]	11	100%	97%	95%
Blood Culture Timing[3]	21	100%	98%	98%
Pregnancy and Delivery Care				
Newborn Deliveries Scheduled Early[3,7]	-	-	5%	6%
Preventive Care				
Immunization for Influenza[5]	-	-	89%	90%
Immunization for Pneumonia[2,3]	242	83%	90%	92%
Stroke Care				
Anticoagulation Therapy for Atrial Fibrillation[1,3]	-	-	95%	95%
Antithrombotic Therapy Timing[3]	18	100%	98%	98%
Assessed for Rehabilitation[3]	16	94%	97%	97%
Discharged on Antithrombotic Therapy[3]	16	100%	99%	99%
Discharged on Statin Medication[3]	15	80%	94%	94%
Thrombolytic Therapy Timing[3,7]	-	-	72%	66%
Venous Thromboembolism Prophylaxis[3]	19	58%	94%	94%
Written Stroke Educational Materials Given[1,3]	-	-	87%	88%
Surgical Care Improvement Project				
Appropriate Beta Blocker Usage[3]	15	87%	97%	98%
Appropriate VTP Within 24 Hours[3]	13	92%	98%	98%
Controlled Postoperative Blood Glucose[3,7]	-	-	96%	97%
Perioperative Temperature Management[3]	28	100%	100%	100%
Prophylactic Antibiotic Selection[1,3]	-	-	99%	99%
Prophylactic Antibiotic Selection (Outpatient)[3]	35	100%	97%	98%
Prophylactic Antibiotic Stopped[1,3]	-	-	98%	98%
Prophylactic Antibiotic Timing[1,3]	-	-	99%	99%
Prophylactic Antibiotic Timing (Outpatient)[3]	35	100%	97%	98%
Urinary Catheter Removal[3]	14	86%	97%	97%
Survey of Patients' Hospital Experiences				
Area Around Room 'Always' Quiet at Night	(a)	53%	51%	61%
Doctors 'Always' Communicated Well	(a)	79%	78%	82%
Home Recovery Information Given	(a)	80%	83%	85%
Hospital Given 9 or 10 on 10 Point Scale	(a)	58%	68%	71%
Meds 'Always' Explained Before Given	(a)	63%	61%	64%
Nurses 'Always' Communicated Well	(a)	71%	74%	79%
Pain 'Always' Well Controlled	(a)	69%	68%	71%
Room and Bathroom 'Always' Clean	(a)	58%	70%	73%
Timely Help 'Always' Received	(a)	55%	62%	68%
Would Definitely Recommend Hospital	(a)	65%	70%	71%
Use of Medical Imaging				
Cardiac Imaging Stress Test before Surgery[1]	-	-	5.2%	5.3%
Combination Abdominal CT Scan	93	1.1%	13.4%	10.5%
Combination Brain/Sinus CT Scan[1]	-	-	2.2%	2.7%
Combination Chest CT Scan[1]	-	-	2.3%	2.7%
Follow-up Mammogram/Ultrasound[7]	-	-	8.2%	8.8%
Lumbar Spine MRI for Low Back Pain[7]	-	-	34.2%	37.2%

French Hospital Medical Center

1911 Johnson Ave Phone: 805-543-5353
San Luis Obispo, CA 93401
URL: www.frenchmedicalcenter.org
Type: Acute Care Hospitals Emergency Services: Yes
Ownership: Voluntary non-profit - Other Beds: 112

Key Personnel:
CEO/President. . . . . Alan E Atiniuk
Radiology. . . . . Ken Hritz
Chief of Medical Staff . . . . Jim Malone, MD
Operating Room. . . . . Jim ton L Paulsen
Cardiac Laboratory. . . . . Charlie Tagawa
Quality Assurance . . . . Karen Trask, RN
Infection Control. . . . . Vicki Warnock

Measure	Cases	This Hosp.	State Avg.	U.S. Avg.
Blood Clot Prevention and Treatment				
Anticoagulation Overlap Therapy[2]	33	91%	92%	93%
ICU Venous Thromboembolism Prophylaxis[2]	90	100%	92%	92%
Incidence of Potentially Preventable VTE[1,2]	-	-	11%	10%
UFH with Dosages/Platelet Monitoring[2]	21	100%	96%	97%
Venous Thromboembolism Prophylaxis[2]	247	100%	83%	85%
Warfarin Therapy Discharge Instructions[2]	24	100%	75%	75%
Chest Pain/Possible Heart Attack Care				
Aspirin Given Within 24 Hours of Arrival[3,7]	-	-	97%	96%
Fibrinolytic Meds Within 30 Min. of Arrival[5]	-	-	62%	58%
Average Time to ECG (minutes)[3,7]	-	-	9	7
Average Time to Transfer (minutes)[5]	-	-	62	60
Children's Asthma Care				
Received Home Management Plan of Care	-	-	88%	88%
Received Reliever Medication	-	-	100%	100%
Received Systemic Corticosteroids	-	-	100%	100%
Emergency Department				
Admittance Decision Time (minutes)[2]	440	78	125	98
Head CT Results Within 45 Min. of Arrival[1]	-	-	55%	57%
Patients Who Left ER Before Being Seen	16,875	0%	3%	2%
Time from ER Arrival to Admit. (minutes)[2]	461	218	323	274
Time from ER Arrival to Discharge (minutes)	382	116	168	134
Time in ER Before Being Evaluated (minutes)	405	10	29	26
Time to Pain Meds for Fractures (minutes)	66	42	62	57
Heart Attack Care				
Aspirin Given at Discharge[2]	268	100%	99%	99%
Fibrinolytic Meds Within 30 Min. of Arrival[2,7]	-	-	73%	54%
PCI Within 90 Minutes of Arrival[2]	36	100%	95%	96%
Statin Prescribed at Discharge[2]	253	98%	98%	98%
Heart Failure Care				

NOTE: Hospital profiles are in alphabetical order by state, then city, then hospital within the city; Rankings exclude hospitals with less than 25 cases except for patient surveys which excludes hospitals with less than 100 cases; (a) 100-299 cases; (1) The number of cases/patients is too few to report; (2) Data submitted were based on a sample of cases/patients; (3) Results are based on a shorter time period than required; (4) Data suppressed by CMS for one or more quarters; (5) Results are not available for this reporting period; (6) Fewer than 100 patients completed the HCAHPS survey; (7) No cases met the criteria for this measure; (8) The lower limit of the confidence interval cannot be calculated if the number of observed infections equals zero; (9) No data are available from the state/territory for this reporting period; (10) The scores shown reflect fewer than 50 completed surveys; (11) There were discrepancies in the data collection process; (12) This measure does not apply to this hospital for this reporting period; (13) Results cannot be calculated for this reporting period; (14) The results for this state are combined with nearby states to protect confidentiality; Please refer to the User's Guide for a full explanation of data.

ACE Inhibitor or ARB for LVSD	53	100%	97%	97%
Discharge Instructions Given	95	97%	94%	94%
Evaluation of LVS Function	118	99%	99%	99%
Medicare Spending				
Medicare Spending per Patient (ratio)	-	0.96	0.98	0.98
Pneumonia Care				
Appropriate Initial Antibiotic Given[2]	64	98%	97%	95%
Blood Culture Timing[2]	104	99%	98%	98%
Pregnancy and Delivery Care				
Newborn Deliveries Scheduled Early	30	0%	5%	6%
Preventive Care				
Immunization for Influenza[2]	455	98%	89%	90%
Immunization for Pneumonia[2]	551	99%	90%	92%
Stroke Care				
Anticoagulation Therapy for Atrial Fibrillation[1]	-	-	95%	95%
Antithrombotic Therapy Timing	35	100%	98%	98%
Assessed for Rehabilitation	36	100%	97%	97%
Discharged on Antithrombotic Therapy	36	100%	99%	99%
Discharged on Statin Medication	26	100%	94%	94%
Thrombolytic Therapy Timing[1]	-	-	72%	66%
Venous Thromboembolism Prophylaxis	34	100%	94%	94%
Written Stroke Educational Materials Given	17	100%	87%	88%
Surgical Care Improvement Project				
Appropriate Beta Blocker Usage[2]	156	98%	97%	98%
Appropriate VTP Within 24 Hours[2]	297	99%	98%	98%
Controlled Postoperative Blood Glucose[2]	143	97%	96%	97%
Perioperative Temperature Management[2]	390	100%	100%	100%
Prophylactic Antibiotic Selection[2]	407	99%	99%	99%
Prophylactic Antibiotic Selection (Outpatient)	169	96%	97%	98%
Prophylactic Antibiotic Stopped[2]	401	100%	98%	98%
Prophylactic Antibiotic Timing[2]	407	100%	99%	99%
Prophylactic Antibiotic Timing (Outpatient)	169	100%	97%	98%
Urinary Catheter Removal[2]	350	99%	97%	97%
Survey of Patients' Hospital Experiences				
Area Around Room 'Always' Quiet at Night	300+	45%	51%	61%
Doctors 'Always' Communicated Well	300+	81%	78%	82%
Home Recovery Information Given	300+	85%	83%	85%
Hospital Given 9 or 10 on 10 Point Scale	300+	75%	68%	71%
Meds 'Always' Explained Before Given	300+	66%	61%	64%
Nurses 'Always' Communicated Well	300+	80%	74%	79%
Pain 'Always' Well Controlled	300+	74%	68%	71%
Room and Bathroom 'Always' Clean	300+	69%	70%	73%
Timely Help 'Always' Received	300+	70%	62%	68%
Would Definitely Recommend Hospital	300+	82%	70%	71%
Use of Medical Imaging				
Cardiac Imaging Stress Test before Surgery[1]	-	-	5.2%	5.3%
Combination Abdominal CT Scan	419	22.4%	13.4%	10.5%
Combination Brain/Sinus CT Scan	487	1.8%	2.2%	2.7%
Combination Chest CT Scan	205	10.2%	2.3%	2.7%
Follow-up Mammogram/Ultrasound	474	7.8%	8.2%	8.8%
Lumbar Spine MRI for Low Back Pain[1]	-	-	34.2%	37.2%

Sierra Vista Regional Medical Center

1010 Murray St
San Luis Obispo, CA 93405
URL: www.sierravistaregional.com
Type: Acute Care Hospitals
Ownership: Proprietary
Phone: 850-546-7600
Fax: 805-546-7892
Emergency Services: Yes
Beds: 201

Key Personnel:

CEO . . . . Joseph DeSchryver
Quality Assurance . . . . Stephanie Gigsby
Emergency Room . . . . George Hansen
Operating Room. . . . . Howard Hayashi
Cardiac Laboratory. . . . . Marirose Rhee
Chief of Medical Staff . . . . Patrick Vaughn, MD

Measure	Cases	This Hosp.	State Avg.	U.S. Avg.
Blood Clot Prevention and Treatment				
Anticoagulation Overlap Therapy[2]	18	100%	92%	93%
ICU Venous Thromboembolism Prophylaxis[2]	74	97%	92%	92%
Incidence of Potentially Preventable VTE[2,7]	-	-	11%	10%
UFH with Dosages/Platelet Monitoring[1,2]	-	-	96%	97%
Venous Thromboembolism Prophylaxis[2]	279	92%	83%	85%
Warfarin Therapy Discharge Instructions[2]	15	100%	75%	75%
Chest Pain/Possible Heart Attack Care				
Aspirin Given Within 24 Hours of Arrival	29	97%	97%	96%
Fibrinolytic Meds Within 30 Min. of Arrival[7]	-	-	62%	58%
Average Time to ECG (minutes)	29	15	9	7
Average Time to Transfer (minutes)[1]	-	-	62	60
Children's Asthma Care				
Received Home Management Plan of Care	-	-	88%	88%
Received Reliever Medication	-	-	100%	100%
Received Systemic Corticosteroids	-	-	100%	100%
Emergency Department				
Admittance Decision Time (minutes)[2]	475	86	125	98
Head CT Results Within 45 Min. of Arrival[1]	-	-	55%	57%
Patients Who Left ER Before Being Seen	21,387	0%	3%	2%
Time from ER Arrival to Admit. (minutes)[2]	475	248	323	274
Time from ER Arrival to Discharge (minutes)	449	133	168	134
Time in ER Before Being Evaluated (minutes)	487	26	29	26
Time to Pain Meds for Fractures (minutes)	151	56	62	57
Heart Attack Care				
Aspirin Given at Discharge[1]	-	-	99%	99%
Fibrinolytic Meds Within 30 Min. of Arrival[7]	-	-	73%	54%
PCI Within 90 Minutes of Arrival[7]	-	-	95%	96%
Statin Prescribed at Discharge[1]	-	-	98%	98%
Heart Failure Care				
ACE Inhibitor or ARB for LVSD[1]	-	-	97%	97%
Discharge Instructions Given	33	97%	94%	94%
Evaluation of LVS Function	45	100%	99%	99%
Medicare Spending				
Medicare Spending per Patient (ratio)	-	1.00	0.98	0.98
Pneumonia Care				
Appropriate Initial Antibiotic Given	43	98%	97%	95%
Blood Culture Timing	46	98%	98%	98%
Pregnancy and Delivery Care				
Newborn Deliveries Scheduled Early[2]	24	0%	5%	6%
Preventive Care				
Immunization for Influenza[2]	490	96%	89%	90%
Immunization for Pneumonia[2]	402	98%	90%	92%
Stroke Care				
Anticoagulation Therapy for Atrial Fibrillation[1]	-	-	95%	95%
Antithrombotic Therapy Timing	30	97%	98%	98%
Assessed for Rehabilitation	69	96%	97%	97%
Discharged on Antithrombotic Therapy	44	98%	99%	99%
Discharged on Statin Medication	38	87%	94%	94%
Thrombolytic Therapy Timing[1]	-	-	72%	66%
Venous Thromboembolism Prophylaxis	74	99%	94%	94%
Written Stroke Educational Materials Given	32	94%	87%	88%
Surgical Care Improvement Project				
Appropriate Beta Blocker Usage	96	100%	97%	98%
Appropriate VTP Within 24 Hours	388	98%	98%	98%
Controlled Postoperative Blood Glucose[7]	-	-	96%	97%
Perioperative Temperature Management	460	100%	100%	100%
Prophylactic Antibiotic Selection	240	100%	99%	99%
Prophylactic Antibiotic Selection (Outpatient)	28	96%	97%	98%
Prophylactic Antibiotic Stopped	240	100%	98%	98%
Prophylactic Antibiotic Timing	240	99%	99%	99%
Prophylactic Antibiotic Timing (Outpatient)	29	97%	97%	98%
Urinary Catheter Removal	284	97%	97%	97%
Survey of Patients' Hospital Experiences				
Area Around Room 'Always' Quiet at Night	300+	48%	51%	61%
Doctors 'Always' Communicated Well	300+	83%	78%	82%
Home Recovery Information Given	300+	88%	83%	85%
Hospital Given 9 or 10 on 10 Point Scale	300+	73%	68%	71%
Meds 'Always' Explained Before Given	300+	68%	61%	64%
Nurses 'Always' Communicated Well	300+	81%	74%	79%
Pain 'Always' Well Controlled	300+	73%	68%	71%
Room and Bathroom 'Always' Clean	300+	62%	70%	73%
Timely Help 'Always' Received	300+	70%	62%	68%
Would Definitely Recommend Hospital	300+	80%	70%	71%
Use of Medical Imaging				
Cardiac Imaging Stress Test before Surgery[1]	-	-	5.2%	5.3%
Combination Abdominal CT Scan	275	12.0%	13.4%	10.5%
Combination Brain/Sinus CT Scan	304	1.0%	2.2%	2.7%
Combination Chest CT Scan	133	6.0%	2.3%	2.7%
Follow-up Mammogram/Ultrasound	371	7.5%	8.2%	8.8%
Lumbar Spine MRI for Low Back Pain[1]	-	-	34.2%	37.2%

San Mateo Medical Center

222 W 39th Ave
San Mateo, CA 94403
URL: www.sanmateomedicalcenter.org
Type: Acute Care Hospitals
Ownership: Government - Local
Phone: 650-573-2222
Fax: 650-573-2950
Emergency Services: Yes
Beds: 509

Key Personnel:

CEO/President. . . . . Susan P. Ehrlich, MD, MPP
Chief of Medical Staff . . . . Chester Kunnappilly, MD
Emergency Room . . . . Serena Lee, MD
Intensive Care Unit. . . . . Jim Lonergan
Radiology. . . . . David Marcus
Quality Assurance . . . . Edgar Pierluissi, MD
Operating Room. . . . . Barry Sanchez
Infection Control . . . . Mary Webb

Measure	Cases	This Hosp.	State Avg.	U.S. Avg.
Blood Clot Prevention and Treatment				
Anticoagulation Overlap Therapy[1,2]	-	-	92%	93%
ICU Venous Thromboembolism Prophylaxis[2]	43	95%	92%	92%
Incidence of Potentially Preventable VTE[2,7]	-	-	11%	10%
UFH with Dosages/Platelet Monitoring[1,2]	-	-	96%	97%
Venous Thromboembolism Prophylaxis[2]	237	74%	83%	85%
Warfarin Therapy Discharge Instructions[1,2]	-	-	75%	75%
Chest Pain/Possible Heart Attack Care				
Aspirin Given Within 24 Hours of Arrival	40	95%	97%	96%
Fibrinolytic Meds Within 30 Min. of Arrival[7]	-	-	62%	58%
Average Time to ECG (minutes)	43	15	9	7
Average Time to Transfer (minutes)	11	94	62	60
Children's Asthma Care				
Received Home Management Plan of Care	-	-	88%	88%
Received Reliever Medication	-	-	100%	100%
Received Systemic Corticosteroids	-	-	100%	100%
Emergency Department				
Admittance Decision Time (minutes)[2]	418	173	125	98
Head CT Results Within 45 Min. of Arrival[7]	-	-	55%	57%
Patients Who Left ER Before Being Seen	42,570	4%	3%	2%
Time from ER Arrival to Admit. (minutes)[2]	419	381	323	274
Time from ER Arrival to Discharge (minutes)	347	193	168	134
Time in ER Before Being Evaluated (minutes)	379	54	29	26
Time to Pain Meds for Fractures (minutes)	81	91	62	57
Heart Attack Care				
Aspirin Given at Discharge	14	100%	99%	99%
Fibrinolytic Meds Within 30 Min. of Arrival[7]	-	-	73%	54%
PCI Within 90 Minutes of Arrival[7]	-	-	95%	96%
Statin Prescribed at Discharge	12	100%	98%	98%
Heart Failure Care				
ACE Inhibitor or ARB for LVSD	44	100%	97%	97%
Discharge Instructions Given	83	92%	94%	94%
Evaluation of LVS Function	92	100%	99%	99%
Medicare Spending				
Medicare Spending per Patient (ratio)	-	0.90	0.98	0.98
Pneumonia Care				
Appropriate Initial Antibiotic Given	53	96%	97%	95%
Blood Culture Timing	66	95%	98%	98%
Pregnancy and Delivery Care				
Newborn Deliveries Scheduled Early[7]	-	-	5%	6%
Preventive Care				
Immunization for Influenza[2]	332	70%	89%	90%
Immunization for Pneumonia[2]	290	73%	90%	92%
Stroke Care				
Anticoagulation Therapy for Atrial Fibrillation[1]	-	-	95%	95%
Antithrombotic Therapy Timing	15	100%	98%	98%
Assessed for Rehabilitation	20	100%	97%	97%
Discharged on Antithrombotic Therapy	18	100%	99%	99%
Discharged on Statin Medication	16	81%	94%	94%
Thrombolytic Therapy Timing[7]	-	-	72%	66%
Venous Thromboembolism Prophylaxis	15	80%	94%	94%
Written Stroke Educational Materials Given[1]	-	-	87%	88%
Surgical Care Improvement Project				
Appropriate Beta Blocker Usage	36	94%	97%	98%
Appropriate VTP Within 24 Hours	152	99%	98%	98%
Controlled Postoperative Blood Glucose[7]	-	-	96%	97%

NOTE: Hospital profiles are in alphabetical order by state, then city, then hospital within the city; Rankings exclude hospitals with less than 25 cases except for patient surveys which excludes hospitals with less than 100 cases; (a) 100-299 cases; (1) The number of cases/patients is too few to report; (2) Data submitted were based on a sample of cases/patients; (3) Results are based on a shorter time period than required; (4) Data suppressed by CMS for one or more quarters; (5) Results are not available for this reporting period; (6) Fewer than 100 patients completed the HCAHPS survey; (7) No cases met the criteria for this measure; (8) The lower limit of the confidence interval cannot be calculated if the number of observed infections equals zero; (9) No data are available from the state/territory for this reporting period; (10) The scores shown reflect fewer than 50 completed surveys; (11) There were discrepancies in the data collection process; (12) This measure does not apply to this hospital for this reporting period; (13) Results cannot be calculated for this reporting period; (14) The results for this state are combined with nearby states to protect confidentiality; Please refer to the User's Guide for a full explanation of data.

Perioperative Temperature Management	165	100%	100%	100%
Prophylactic Antibiotic Selection	100	99%	99%	99%
Prophylactic Antibiotic Selection (Outpatient)	97	100%	97%	98%
Prophylactic Antibiotic Stopped	98	99%	98%	98%
Prophylactic Antibiotic Timing	100	99%	99%	99%
Prophylactic Antibiotic Timing (Outpatient)	66	92%	97%	98%
Urinary Catheter Removal	92	99%	97%	97%
Survey of Patients' Hospital Experiences				
Area Around Room 'Always' Quiet at Night	300+	44%	51%	61%
Doctors 'Always' Communicated Well	300+	75%	78%	82%
Home Recovery Information Given	300+	78%	83%	85%
Hospital Given 9 or 10 on 10 Point Scale	300+	61%	68%	71%
Meds 'Always' Explained Before Given	300+	57%	61%	64%
Nurses 'Always' Communicated Well	300+	69%	74%	79%
Pain 'Always' Well Controlled	300+	64%	68%	71%
Room and Bathroom 'Always' Clean	300+	65%	70%	73%
Timely Help 'Always' Received	300+	52%	62%	68%
Would Definitely Recommend Hospital	300+	64%	70%	71%
Use of Medical Imaging				
Cardiac Imaging Stress Test before Surgery	60	1.7%	5.2%	5.3%
Combination Abdominal CT Scan	123	5.7%	13.4%	10.5%
Combination Brain/Sinus CT Scan	102	0.0%	2.2%	2.7%
Combination Chest CT Scan	73	6.8%	2.3%	2.7%
Follow-up Mammogram/Ultrasound	263	9.1%	8.2%	8.8%
Lumbar Spine MRI for Low Back Pain[1]	-	-	34.2%	37.2%

Doctors Medical Center - San Pablo

2000 Vale Rd
San Pablo, CA 94806
Phone: 510-970-5000
Fax: 510-970-5730
URL: www.doctorsmedicalcenter.org
Type: Acute Care Hospitals
Emergency Services: Yes
Ownership: Govt - Hospital Dist/Auth
Beds: 247

Key Personnel:

Patient Relations . . . . Toni Alcott
Emergency Room . . . . Susan Ancell, RN
CEO/President. . . . . Irwin Hansen
Infection Control. . . . . Nayda Ramiro
Chief of Medical Staff . . . . Paul Ryan, MD
Intensive Care Unit. . . . . Ronica Shelton
Radiology. . . . . Carol Towarnick

Measure	Cases	This Hosp.	State Avg.	U.S. Avg.
Blood Clot Prevention and Treatment				
Anticoagulation Overlap Therapy[2]	29	93%	92%	93%
ICU Venous Thromboembolism Prophylaxis[2]	96	95%	92%	92%
Incidence of Potentially Preventable VTE[1,2]	-	-	11%	10%
UFH with Dosages/Platelet Monitoring[2]	26	100%	96%	97%
Venous Thromboembolism Prophylaxis[2]	345	81%	83%	85%
Warfarin Therapy Discharge Instructions[2]	24	71%	75%	75%
Chest Pain/Possible Heart Attack Care				
Aspirin Given Within 24 Hours of Arrival[1]	-	-	97%	96%
Fibrinolytic Meds Within 30 Min. of Arrival[3,7]	-	-	62%	58%
Average Time to ECG (minutes)[1]	-	-	9	7
Average Time to Transfer (minutes)[3,7]	-	-	62	60
Children's Asthma Care				
Received Home Management Plan of Care	-	-	88%	88%
Received Reliever Medication	-	-	100%	100%
Received Systemic Corticosteroids	-	-	100%	100%
Emergency Department				
Admittance Decision Time (minutes)[2]	490	80	125	98
Head CT Results Within 45 Min. of Arrival	12	100%	55%	57%
Patients Who Left ER Before Being Seen	90,506	1%	3%	2%
Time from ER Arrival to Admit. (minutes)[2]	500	334	323	274
Time from ER Arrival to Discharge (minutes)	265	130	168	134
Time in ER Before Being Evaluated (minutes)	355	31	29	26
Time to Pain Meds for Fractures (minutes)	159	53	62	57
Heart Attack Care				
Aspirin Given at Discharge	136	100%	99%	99%
Fibrinolytic Meds Within 30 Min. of Arrival[7]	-	-	73%	54%
PCI Within 90 Minutes of Arrival	19	89%	95%	96%
Statin Prescribed at Discharge	125	100%	98%	98%
Heart Failure Care				
ACE Inhibitor or ARB for LVSD[2]	119	98%	97%	97%
Discharge Instructions Given[2]	274	87%	94%	94%
Evaluation of LVS Function[2]	325	99%	99%	99%
Medicare Spending				
Medicare Spending per Patient (ratio)	-	0.95	0.98	0.98
Pneumonia Care				
Appropriate Initial Antibiotic Given[2]	70	97%	97%	95%
Blood Culture Timing[2]	151	97%	98%	98%
Pregnancy and Delivery Care				
Newborn Deliveries Scheduled Early[7]	-	-	5%	6%
Preventive Care				
Immunization for Influenza[2]	592	87%	89%	90%
Immunization for Pneumonia[2]	905	88%	90%	92%
Stroke Care				
Anticoagulation Therapy for Atrial Fibrillation	12	100%	95%	95%
Antithrombotic Therapy Timing	99	98%	98%	98%
Assessed for Rehabilitation	105	99%	97%	97%
Discharged on Antithrombotic Therapy	101	100%	99%	99%
Discharged on Statin Medication	76	99%	94%	94%
Thrombolytic Therapy Timing	14	100%	72%	66%
Venous Thromboembolism Prophylaxis	103	92%	94%	94%
Written Stroke Educational Materials Given	59	97%	87%	88%
Surgical Care Improvement Project				
Appropriate Beta Blocker Usage[2]	65	98%	97%	98%
Appropriate VTP Within 24 Hours[2]	186	92%	98%	98%
Controlled Postoperative Blood Glucose[2,7]	-	-	96%	97%
Perioperative Temperature Management[2]	206	100%	100%	100%
Prophylactic Antibiotic Selection[2]	117	97%	99%	99%
Prophylactic Antibiotic Selection (Outpatient)	107	74%	97%	98%
Prophylactic Antibiotic Stopped[2]	113	95%	98%	98%
Prophylactic Antibiotic Timing[2]	117	97%	99%	99%
Prophylactic Antibiotic Timing (Outpatient)	106	95%	97%	98%
Urinary Catheter Removal[2]	155	95%	97%	97%
Survey of Patients' Hospital Experiences				
Area Around Room 'Always' Quiet at Night	300+	38%	51%	61%
Doctors 'Always' Communicated Well	300+	72%	78%	82%
Home Recovery Information Given	300+	74%	83%	85%
Hospital Given 9 or 10 on 10 Point Scale	300+	48%	68%	71%
Meds 'Always' Explained Before Given	300+	54%	61%	64%
Nurses 'Always' Communicated Well	300+	66%	74%	79%
Pain 'Always' Well Controlled	300+	61%	68%	71%
Room and Bathroom 'Always' Clean	300+	61%	70%	73%
Timely Help 'Always' Received	300+	50%	62%	68%
Would Definitely Recommend Hospital	300+	49%	70%	71%
Use of Medical Imaging				
Cardiac Imaging Stress Test before Surgery	61	1.6%	5.2%	5.3%
Combination Abdominal CT Scan	369	4.6%	13.4%	10.5%
Combination Brain/Sinus CT Scan	475	1.5%	2.2%	2.7%
Combination Chest CT Scan	191	0.0%	2.3%	2.7%
Follow-up Mammogram/Ultrasound	911	6.0%	8.2%	8.8%
Lumbar Spine MRI for Low Back Pain[1]	-	-	34.2%	37.2%

Providence Little Co of Mary Medical Center San Pedro

1300 W 7th St
San Pedro, CA 90732
Phone: 310-832-3311
Fax: 310-514-5314
URL: www.lcmweb.org
Type: Acute Care Hospitals
Emergency Services: Yes
Ownership: Voluntary non-profit - Private
Beds: 387

Key Personnel:

Anesthesiology. . . . . Paramjit Bhalla, MD
Pediatric Ambulatory Care . . . . . . Frank Brow, MD
Pediatric In-Patient Care . . . . Frank Brow, MD
Radiology. . . . . Neil Chafetz, MD
Chief of Medical Staff. . . . . Laurence Eason, MD
Quality Assurance . . . . Vicky Ryan
Emergency Room . . . . Miles Shaw, MD

Measure	Cases	This Hosp.	State Avg.	U.S. Avg.
Blood Clot Prevention and Treatment				
Anticoagulation Overlap Therapy[2]	20	65%	92%	93%
ICU Venous Thromboembolism Prophylaxis[2]	59	95%	92%	92%
Incidence of Potentially Preventable VTE[1,2]	-	-	11%	10%
UFH with Dosages/Platelet Monitoring[1,2]	-	-	96%	97%
Venous Thromboembolism Prophylaxis[2]	282	96%	83%	85%
Warfarin Therapy Discharge Instructions[2]	16	94%	75%	75%
Chest Pain/Possible Heart Attack Care				
Aspirin Given Within 24 Hours of Arrival[3]	23	100%	97%	96%
Fibrinolytic Meds Within 30 Min. of Arrival[3,7]	-	-	62%	58%
Average Time to ECG (minutes)[3]	25	10	9	7
Average Time to Transfer (minutes)[3,7]	-	-	62	60
Children's Asthma Care				
Received Home Management Plan of Care	-	-	88%	88%
Received Reliever Medication	-	-	100%	100%
Received Systemic Corticosteroids	-	-	100%	100%
Emergency Department				
Admittance Decision Time (minutes)[2]	703	126	125	98
Head CT Results Within 45 Min. of Arrival[5]	-	-	55%	57%
Patients Who Left ER Before Being Seen	37,199	1%	3%	2%
Time from ER Arrival to Admit. (minutes)[2]	705	277	323	274
Time from ER Arrival to Discharge (minutes)	383	134	168	134
Time in ER Before Being Evaluated (minutes)	408	21	29	26
Time to Pain Meds for Fractures (minutes)	150	40	62	57
Heart Attack Care				
Aspirin Given at Discharge	16	100%	99%	99%
Fibrinolytic Meds Within 30 Min. of Arrival[7]	-	-	73%	54%
PCI Within 90 Minutes of Arrival[7]	-	-	95%	96%
Statin Prescribed at Discharge	18	100%	98%	98%
Heart Failure Care				
ACE Inhibitor or ARB for LVSD	56	96%	97%	97%
Discharge Instructions Given	116	97%	94%	94%
Evaluation of LVS Function	136	100%	99%	99%
Medicare Spending				
Medicare Spending per Patient (ratio)	-	1.00	0.98	0.98
Pneumonia Care				
Appropriate Initial Antibiotic Given	106	95%	97%	95%
Blood Culture Timing	198	97%	98%	98%
Pregnancy and Delivery Care				
Newborn Deliveries Scheduled Early[2]	162	3%	5%	6%
Preventive Care				
Immunization for Influenza[2]	507	90%	89%	90%
Immunization for Pneumonia[2]	562	94%	90%	92%
Stroke Care				
Anticoagulation Therapy for Atrial Fibrillation[1]	-	-	95%	95%
Antithrombotic Therapy Timing	47	98%	98%	98%
Assessed for Rehabilitation	62	97%	97%	97%
Discharged on Antithrombotic Therapy	56	100%	99%	99%
Discharged on Statin Medication	45	96%	94%	94%
Thrombolytic Therapy Timing[1]	-	-	72%	66%
Venous Thromboembolism Prophylaxis	53	96%	94%	94%
Written Stroke Educational Materials Given	24	96%	87%	88%
Surgical Care Improvement Project				
Appropriate Beta Blocker Usage[2]	42	98%	97%	98%
Appropriate VTP Within 24 Hours[2]	200	94%	98%	98%
Controlled Postoperative Blood Glucose[2,7]	-	-	96%	97%
Perioperative Temperature Management[2]	246	100%	100%	100%
Prophylactic Antibiotic Selection[2]	134	99%	99%	99%
Prophylactic Antibiotic Selection (Outpatient)	44	86%	97%	98%
Prophylactic Antibiotic Stopped[2]	131	94%	98%	98%
Prophylactic Antibiotic Timing[2]	134	98%	99%	99%
Prophylactic Antibiotic Timing (Outpatient)	47	94%	97%	98%
Urinary Catheter Removal[2]	126	99%	97%	97%
Survey of Patients' Hospital Experiences				
Area Around Room 'Always' Quiet at Night	300+	49%	51%	61%
Doctors 'Always' Communicated Well	300+	80%	78%	82%
Home Recovery Information Given	300+	81%	83%	85%
Hospital Given 9 or 10 on 10 Point Scale	300+	72%	68%	71%
Meds 'Always' Explained Before Given	300+	63%	61%	64%
Nurses 'Always' Communicated Well	300+	78%	74%	79%
Pain 'Always' Well Controlled	300+	74%	68%	71%
Room and Bathroom 'Always' Clean	300+	79%	70%	73%
Timely Help 'Always' Received	300+	66%	62%	68%
Would Definitely Recommend Hospital	300+	75%	70%	71%
Use of Medical Imaging				
Cardiac Imaging Stress Test before Surgery	122	7.4%	5.2%	5.3%
Combination Abdominal CT Scan	400	5.5%	13.4%	10.5%
Combination Brain/Sinus CT Scan	409	1.5%	2.2%	2.7%
Combination Chest CT Scan	125	1.6%	2.3%	2.7%
Follow-up Mammogram/Ultrasound	669	12.0%	8.2%	8.8%
Lumbar Spine MRI for Low Back Pain	63	42.9%	34.2%	37.2%

NOTE: Hospital profiles are in alphabetical order by state, then city, then hospital within the city; Rankings exclude hospitals with less than 25 cases except for patient surveys which excludes hospitals with less than 100 cases; (a) 100-299 cases; (1) The number of cases/patients is too few to report; (2) Data submitted were based on a sample of cases/patients; (3) Results are based on a shorter time period than required; (4) Data suppressed by CMS for one or more quarters; (5) Results are not available for this reporting period; (6) Fewer than 100 patients completed the HCAHPS survey; (7) No cases met the criteria for this measure; (8) The lower limit of the confidence interval cannot be calculated if the number of observed infections equals zero; (9) No data are available from the state/territory for this reporting period; (10) The scores shown reflect fewer than 50 completed surveys; (11) There were discrepancies in the data collection process; (12) This measure does not apply to this hospital for this reporting period; (13) Results cannot be calculated for this reporting period; (14) The results for this state are combined with nearby states to protect confidentiality; Please refer to the User's Guide for a full explanation of data.

Kaiser Foundation Hospital

99 Montecillo Rd
San Rafael, CA 94903
Phone: 415-444-2000
Fax: 415-444-2492
URL: www.kaisersanrafael.org
Type: Acute Care Hospitals
Emergency Services: Yes
Ownership: Voluntary non-profit - Other
Beds: 120

Key Personnel:
Cardiac Laboratory. . . . . Scott Adelman
Radiology. . . . . Diane Michelle Barnes, MD
Operating Room. . . . . Ada Fernandez
CEO/President. . . . . Dan Leetz
Chief of Medical Staff. . . . . James Martin
Quality Assurance . . . . Sandy McCreary
Pediatric Ambulatory Care . . . . . . Aimy Taniguchi
Pediatric In-Patient Care . . . . Aimy Taniguchi

Measure	Cases	This Hosp.	State Avg.	U.S. Avg.
Blood Clot Prevention and Treatment				
Anticoagulation Overlap Therapy[2]	34	100%	92%	93%
ICU Venous Thromboembolism Prophylaxis[2]	63	94%	92%	92%
Incidence of Potentially Preventable VTE[1,2]	-	-	11%	10%
UFH with Dosages/Platelet Monitoring[2]	12	100%	96%	97%
Venous Thromboembolism Prophylaxis[2]	251	92%	83%	85%
Warfarin Therapy Discharge Instructions[2]	33	39%	75%	75%
Chest Pain/Possible Heart Attack Care				
Aspirin Given Within 24 Hours of Arrival	-	-	97%	96%
Fibrinolytic Meds Within 30 Min. of Arrival	-	-	62%	58%
Average Time to ECG (minutes)	-	-	9	7
Average Time to Transfer (minutes)	-	-	62	60
Children's Asthma Care				
Received Home Management Plan of Care	-	-	88%	88%
Received Reliever Medication	-	-	100%	100%
Received Systemic Corticosteroids	-	-	100%	100%
Emergency Department				
Admittance Decision Time (minutes)[2]	665	47	125	98
Head CT Results Within 45 Min. of Arrival	-	-	55%	57%
Patients Who Left ER Before Being Seen	-	-	3%	2%
Time from ER Arrival to Admit. (minutes)[2]	666	269	323	274
Time from ER Arrival to Discharge (minutes)	-	-	168	134
Time in ER Before Being Evaluated (minutes)	-	-	29	26
Time to Pain Meds for Fractures (minutes)	-	-	62	57
Heart Attack Care				
Aspirin Given at Discharge	43	100%	99%	99%
Fibrinolytic Meds Within 30 Min. of Arrival[7]	-	-	73%	54%
PCI Within 90 Minutes of Arrival	14	93%	95%	96%
Statin Prescribed at Discharge	51	98%	98%	98%
Heart Failure Care				
ACE Inhibitor or ARB for LVSD	22	100%	97%	97%
Discharge Instructions Given	104	97%	94%	94%
Evaluation of LVS Function	107	100%	99%	99%
Medicare Spending				
Medicare Spending per Patient (ratio)	-	1.01	0.98	0.98
Pneumonia Care				
Appropriate Initial Antibiotic Given[2]	60	100%	97%	95%
Blood Culture Timing[2]	110	95%	98%	98%
Pregnancy and Delivery Care				
Newborn Deliveries Scheduled Early[7]	-	-	5%	6%
Preventive Care				
Immunization for Influenza[2]	442	91%	89%	90%
Immunization for Pneumonia[2]	691	96%	90%	92%
Stroke Care				
Anticoagulation Therapy for Atrial Fibrillation[2]	26	100%	95%	95%
Antithrombotic Therapy Timing[2]	77	99%	98%	98%
Assessed for Rehabilitation[2]	105	100%	97%	97%
Discharged on Antithrombotic Therapy[2]	96	99%	99%	99%
Discharged on Statin Medication[2]	78	99%	94%	94%
Thrombolytic Therapy Timing[1,2]	-	-	72%	66%
Venous Thromboembolism Prophylaxis[2]	93	94%	94%	94%
Written Stroke Educational Materials Given[2]	70	99%	87%	88%
Surgical Care Improvement Project				
Appropriate Beta Blocker Usage[2]	96	100%	97%	98%
Appropriate VTP Within 24 Hours[2]	343	100%	98%	98%
Controlled Postoperative Blood Glucose[2,7]	-	-	96%	97%
Perioperative Temperature Management[2]	396	100%	100%	100%
Prophylactic Antibiotic Selection[2]	264	100%	99%	99%
Prophylactic Antibiotic Selection (Outpatient)	-	-	97%	98%
Prophylactic Antibiotic Stopped[2]	259	99%	98%	98%
Prophylactic Antibiotic Timing[2]	264	100%	99%	99%
Prophylactic Antibiotic Timing (Outpatient)	-	-	97%	98%
Urinary Catheter Removal[2]	325	100%	97%	97%
Survey of Patients' Hospital Experiences				
Area Around Room 'Always' Quiet at Night	300+	39%	51%	61%
Doctors 'Always' Communicated Well	300+	83%	78%	82%
Home Recovery Information Given	300+	88%	83%	85%
Hospital Given 9 or 10 on 10 Point Scale	300+	73%	68%	71%
Meds 'Always' Explained Before Given	300+	63%	61%	64%
Nurses 'Always' Communicated Well	300+	75%	74%	79%
Pain 'Always' Well Controlled	300+	72%	68%	71%
Room and Bathroom 'Always' Clean	300+	69%	70%	73%
Timely Help 'Always' Received	300+	68%	62%	68%
Would Definitely Recommend Hospital	300+	77%	70%	71%
Use of Medical Imaging				
Cardiac Imaging Stress Test before Surgery	-	-	5.2%	5.3%
Combination Abdominal CT Scan	-	-	13.4%	10.5%
Combination Brain/Sinus CT Scan	-	-	2.2%	2.7%
Combination Chest CT Scan	-	-	2.3%	2.7%
Follow-up Mammogram/Ultrasound	-	-	8.2%	8.8%
Lumbar Spine MRI for Low Back Pain	-	-	34.2%	37.2%

San Ramon Regional Medical Center

6001 Norris Canyon Road
San Ramon, CA 94583
Phone: 925-275-9200
Fax: 925-275-0107
URL: www.sanramonmedctr.com
Type: Acute Care Hospitals
Emergency Services: Yes
Ownership: Proprietary
Beds: 123

Key Personnel:
Chief of Medical Staff. . . . . Carl Critc
CEO/President. . . . . Trevor Fetter
Cardiac Laboratory. . . . . Candy Hogan
Emergency Room . . . . Michael Kazemi
Radiology. . . . . Yuriria Lobato
CEO . . . . Gary Sloan

Measure	Cases	This Hosp.	State Avg.	U.S. Avg.
Blood Clot Prevention and Treatment				
Anticoagulation Overlap Therapy[2]	27	81%	92%	93%
ICU Venous Thromboembolism Prophylaxis[2]	69	84%	92%	92%
Incidence of Potentially Preventable VTE[2,7]	-	-	11%	10%
UFH with Dosages/Platelet Monitoring[2]	13	100%	96%	97%
Venous Thromboembolism Prophylaxis[2]	279	64%	83%	85%
Warfarin Therapy Discharge Instructions[2]	23	83%	75%	75%
Chest Pain/Possible Heart Attack Care				
Aspirin Given Within 24 Hours of Arrival[1]	-	-	97%	96%
Fibrinolytic Meds Within 30 Min. of Arrival[5]	-	-	62%	58%
Average Time to ECG (minutes)[1]	-	-	9	7
Average Time to Transfer (minutes)[5]	-	-	62	60
Children's Asthma Care				
Received Home Management Plan of Care	-	-	88%	88%
Received Reliever Medication	-	-	100%	100%
Received Systemic Corticosteroids	-	-	100%	100%
Emergency Department				
Admittance Decision Time (minutes)[2]	491	89	125	98
Head CT Results Within 45 Min. of Arrival	19	95%	55%	57%
Patients Who Left ER Before Being Seen	16,969	1%	3%	2%
Time from ER Arrival to Admit. (minutes)[2]	491	265	323	274
Time from ER Arrival to Discharge (minutes)	394	158	168	134
Time in ER Before Being Evaluated (minutes)	413	32	29	26
Time to Pain Meds for Fractures (minutes)	148	68	62	57
Heart Attack Care				
Aspirin Given at Discharge	56	100%	99%	99%
Fibrinolytic Meds Within 30 Min. of Arrival[7]	-	-	73%	54%
PCI Within 90 Minutes of Arrival[1]	-	-	95%	96%
Statin Prescribed at Discharge	54	100%	98%	98%
Heart Failure Care				
ACE Inhibitor or ARB for LVSD	19	100%	97%	97%
Discharge Instructions Given	50	100%	94%	94%
Evaluation of LVS Function	64	100%	99%	99%
Medicare Spending				
Medicare Spending per Patient (ratio)	-	1.01	0.98	0.98
Pneumonia Care				
Appropriate Initial Antibiotic Given	70	99%	97%	95%
Blood Culture Timing	108	100%	98%	98%
Pregnancy and Delivery Care				
Newborn Deliveries Scheduled Early[2]	18	0%	5%	6%
Preventive Care				
Immunization for Influenza[2]	482	69%	89%	90%
Immunization for Pneumonia[2]	451	79%	90%	92%
Stroke Care				
Anticoagulation Therapy for Atrial Fibrillation	17	100%	95%	95%
Antithrombotic Therapy Timing	42	100%	98%	98%
Assessed for Rehabilitation	67	100%	97%	97%
Discharged on Antithrombotic Therapy	61	100%	99%	99%
Discharged on Statin Medication	49	100%	94%	94%
Thrombolytic Therapy Timing	18	100%	72%	66%
Venous Thromboembolism Prophylaxis	67	100%	94%	94%
Written Stroke Educational Materials Given	39	100%	87%	88%
Surgical Care Improvement Project				
Appropriate Beta Blocker Usage[2]	64	97%	97%	98%
Appropriate VTP Within 24 Hours[2]	213	96%	98%	98%
Controlled Postoperative Blood Glucose[2]	31	100%	96%	97%
Perioperative Temperature Management[2]	240	100%	100%	100%
Prophylactic Antibiotic Selection[2]	168	99%	99%	99%
Prophylactic Antibiotic Selection (Outpatient)	194	99%	97%	98%
Prophylactic Antibiotic Stopped[2]	162	98%	98%	98%
Prophylactic Antibiotic Timing[2]	168	99%	99%	99%
Prophylactic Antibiotic Timing (Outpatient)	195	99%	97%	98%
Urinary Catheter Removal[2]	154	99%	97%	97%
Survey of Patients' Hospital Experiences				
Area Around Room 'Always' Quiet at Night	300+	52%	51%	61%
Doctors 'Always' Communicated Well	300+	81%	78%	82%
Home Recovery Information Given	300+	83%	83%	85%
Hospital Given 9 or 10 on 10 Point Scale	300+	74%	68%	71%
Meds 'Always' Explained Before Given	300+	65%	61%	64%
Nurses 'Always' Communicated Well	300+	78%	74%	79%
Pain 'Always' Well Controlled	300+	69%	68%	71%
Room and Bathroom 'Always' Clean	300+	70%	70%	73%
Timely Help 'Always' Received	300+	67%	62%	68%
Would Definitely Recommend Hospital	300+	78%	70%	71%
Use of Medical Imaging				
Cardiac Imaging Stress Test before Surgery	133	11.3%	5.2%	5.3%
Combination Abdominal CT Scan	327	10.4%	13.4%	10.5%
Combination Brain/Sinus CT Scan[1]	-	-	2.2%	2.7%
Combination Chest CT Scan	148	0.0%	2.3%	2.7%
Follow-up Mammogram/Ultrasound	815	4.7%	8.2%	8.8%
Lumbar Spine MRI for Low Back Pain[7]	-	-	34.2%	37.2%

Coastal Communities Hospital

2701 S Bristol St
Santa Ana, CA 92704
Phone: 714-754-5454
URL: www.coastalcommhospital.com
Type: Acute Care Hospitals
Emergency Services: Yes
Ownership: Proprietary
Beds: 178

Key Personnel:
Infection Control. . . . . Jennifer Cox
Radiology. . . . . Jennifer Douglas
Coronary Care . . . . Carol Frank, RN
Emergency Room . . . . Carol Frank, RN
Operating Room. . . . . Lisa Molina
CEO/President. . . . . Craig Myers
Chief of Medical Staff . . . . Shahin Samim, MD

Measure	Cases	This Hosp.	State Avg.	U.S. Avg.
Blood Clot Prevention and Treatment				
Anticoagulation Overlap Therapy[1,2]	-	-	92%	93%
ICU Venous Thromboembolism Prophylaxis[2]	50	62%	92%	92%
Incidence of Potentially Preventable VTE[1,2]	-	-	11%	10%
UFH with Dosages/Platelet Monitoring[2,7]	-	-	96%	97%
Venous Thromboembolism Prophylaxis[2]	199	51%	83%	85%
Warfarin Therapy Discharge Instructions[1,2]	-	-	75%	75%
Chest Pain/Possible Heart Attack Care				
Aspirin Given Within 24 Hours of Arrival[1,3]	-	-	97%	96%
Fibrinolytic Meds Within 30 Min. of Arrival[3,7]	-	-	62%	58%
Average Time to ECG (minutes)[1,3]	-	-	9	7
Average Time to Transfer (minutes)[3,7]	-	-	62	60
Children's Asthma Care				

NOTE: Hospital profiles are in alphabetical order by state, then city, then hospital within the city; Rankings exclude hospitals with less than 25 cases except for patient surveys which excludes hospitals with less than 100 cases; (a) 100-299 cases; (1) The number of cases/patients is too few to report; (2) Data submitted were based on a sample of cases/patients; (3) Results are based on a shorter time period than required; (4) Data suppressed by CMS for one or more quarters; (5) Results are not available for this reporting period; (6) Fewer than 100 patients completed the HCAHPS survey; (7) No cases met the criteria for this measure; (8) The lower limit of the confidence interval cannot be calculated if the number of observed infections equals zero; (9) No data are available from the state/territory for this reporting period; (10) The scores shown reflect fewer than 50 completed surveys; (11) There were discrepancies in the data collection process; (12) This measure does not apply to this hospital for this reporting period; (13) Results cannot be calculated for this reporting period; (14) The results for this state are combined with nearby states to protect confidentiality; Please refer to the User's Guide for a full explanation of data.

Measure	Cases	This Hosp.	State Avg.	U.S. Avg.
Received Home Management Plan of Care	-	-	88%	88%
Received Reliever Medication	-	-	100%	100%
Received Systemic Corticosteroids	-	-	100%	100%
Emergency Department				
Admittance Decision Time (minutes)[2]	274	75	125	98
Head CT Results Within 45 Min. of Arrival[1,3]	-	-	55%	57%
Patients Who Left ER Before Being Seen	21,305	1%	3%	2%
Time from ER Arrival to Admit. (minutes)[2]	278	249	323	274
Time from ER Arrival to Discharge (minutes)	345	105	168	134
Time in ER Before Being Evaluated (minutes)	366	28	29	26
Time to Pain Meds for Fractures (minutes)	76	38	62	57
Heart Attack Care				
Aspirin Given at Discharge[1]	-	-	99%	99%
Fibrinolytic Meds Within 30 Min. of Arrival[7]	-	-	73%	54%
PCI Within 90 Minutes of Arrival[7]	-	-	95%	96%
Statin Prescribed at Discharge[1]	-	-	98%	98%
Heart Failure Care				
ACE Inhibitor or ARB for LVSD	16	100%	97%	97%
Discharge Instructions Given	50	94%	94%	94%
Evaluation of LVS Function	61	97%	99%	99%
Medicare Spending				
Medicare Spending per Patient (ratio)	-	1.28	0.98	0.98
Pneumonia Care				
Appropriate Initial Antibiotic Given	46	100%	97%	95%
Blood Culture Timing	93	99%	98%	98%
Pregnancy and Delivery Care				
Newborn Deliveries Scheduled Early[2]	25	0%	5%	6%
Preventive Care				
Immunization for Influenza[2]	375	97%	89%	90%
Immunization for Pneumonia[2]	284	90%	90%	92%
Stroke Care				
Anticoagulation Therapy for Atrial Fibrillation[7]	-	-	95%	95%
Antithrombotic Therapy Timing	12	92%	98%	98%
Assessed for Rehabilitation[1]	-	-	97%	97%
Discharged on Antithrombotic Therapy[1]	-	-	99%	99%
Discharged on Statin Medication[1]	-	-	94%	94%
Thrombolytic Therapy Timing[7]	-	-	72%	66%
Venous Thromboembolism Prophylaxis	12	50%	94%	94%
Written Stroke Educational Materials Given[1]	-	-	87%	88%
Surgical Care Improvement Project				
Appropriate Beta Blocker Usage	14	93%	97%	98%
Appropriate VTP Within 24 Hours	148	97%	98%	98%
Controlled Postoperative Blood Glucose[7]	-	-	96%	97%
Perioperative Temperature Management	164	99%	100%	100%
Prophylactic Antibiotic Selection	90	98%	99%	99%
Prophylactic Antibiotic Selection (Outpatient)	26	92%	97%	98%
Prophylactic Antibiotic Stopped	88	98%	98%	98%
Prophylactic Antibiotic Timing	90	98%	99%	99%
Prophylactic Antibiotic Timing (Outpatient)	29	83%	97%	98%
Urinary Catheter Removal	20	80%	97%	97%
Survey of Patients' Hospital Experiences				
Area Around Room 'Always' Quiet at Night	300+	39%	51%	61%
Doctors 'Always' Communicated Well	300+	82%	78%	82%
Home Recovery Information Given	300+	78%	83%	85%
Hospital Given 9 or 10 on 10 Point Scale	300+	68%	68%	71%
Meds 'Always' Explained Before Given	300+	64%	61%	64%
Nurses 'Always' Communicated Well	300+	74%	74%	79%
Pain 'Always' Well Controlled	300+	69%	68%	71%
Room and Bathroom 'Always' Clean	300+	73%	70%	73%
Timely Help 'Always' Received	300+	60%	62%	68%
Would Definitely Recommend Hospital	300+	64%	70%	71%
Use of Medical Imaging				
Cardiac Imaging Stress Test before Surgery[1]	-	-	5.2%	5.3%
Combination Abdominal CT Scan[1]	-	-	13.4%	10.5%
Combination Brain/Sinus CT Scan	93	0.0%	2.2%	2.7%
Combination Chest CT Scan[1]	-	-	2.3%	2.7%
Follow-up Mammogram/Ultrasound	77	7.8%	8.2%	8.8%
Lumbar Spine MRI for Low Back Pain[7]	-	-	34.2%	37.2%

Western Medical Center Santa Ana

1001 North Tustin Avenue
Santa Ana, CA 92705
Phone: 714-953-3331
Fax: 714-953-3613
URL: www.westernmedicalcenter.com
Type: Acute Care Hospitals
Emergency Services: Yes
Ownership: Proprietary
Beds: 282

Key Personnel:

Radiology. . . . . Joseph Brogman, MD
Quality Assurance . . . . Lee Dawson
Operating Room. . . . . Helen Evans, RN
Emergency Room . . . . S Jones, RN
Pediatric Ambulatory Care . . . . . . Araceli Quimbo, MD
Pediatric In-Patient Care . . . . Araceli Quimbo, MD
CEO/President. . . . . Suzanne Richards
Chief of Medical Staff. . . . . David Stanton, MD

Measure	Cases	This Hosp.	State Avg.	U.S. Avg.
Blood Clot Prevention and Treatment				
Anticoagulation Overlap Therapy[2]	16	88%	92%	93%
ICU Venous Thromboembolism Prophylaxis[2]	145	99%	92%	92%
Incidence of Potentially Preventable VTE[1,2]	-	-	11%	10%
UFH with Dosages/Platelet Monitoring[1,2]	-	-	96%	97%
Venous Thromboembolism Prophylaxis[2]	267	87%	83%	85%
Warfarin Therapy Discharge Instructions[1,2]	-	-	75%	75%
Chest Pain/Possible Heart Attack Care				
Aspirin Given Within 24 Hours of Arrival[1]	-	-	97%	96%
Fibrinolytic Meds Within 30 Min. of Arrival[5]	-	-	62%	58%
Average Time to ECG (minutes)[1]	-	-	9	7
Average Time to Transfer (minutes)[5]	-	-	62	60
Children's Asthma Care				
Received Home Management Plan of Care	-	-	88%	88%
Received Reliever Medication	-	-	100%	100%
Received Systemic Corticosteroids	-	-	100%	100%
Emergency Department				
Admittance Decision Time (minutes)[2]	113	58	125	98
Head CT Results Within 45 Min. of Arrival[1]	-	-	55%	57%
Patients Who Left ER Before Being Seen	25,160	3%	3%	2%
Time from ER Arrival to Admit. (minutes)[2]	990	216	323	274
Time from ER Arrival to Discharge (minutes)	310	176	168	134
Time in ER Before Being Evaluated (minutes)	84	30	29	26
Time to Pain Meds for Fractures (minutes)	65	43	62	57
Heart Attack Care				
Aspirin Given at Discharge	184	99%	99%	99%
Fibrinolytic Meds Within 30 Min. of Arrival[7]	-	-	73%	54%
PCI Within 90 Minutes of Arrival	22	91%	95%	96%
Statin Prescribed at Discharge	193	96%	98%	98%
Heart Failure Care				
ACE Inhibitor or ARB for LVSD	41	93%	97%	97%
Discharge Instructions Given	76	95%	94%	94%
Evaluation of LVS Function	84	98%	99%	99%
Medicare Spending				
Medicare Spending per Patient (ratio)	-	1.08	0.98	0.98
Pneumonia Care				
Appropriate Initial Antibiotic Given	53	96%	97%	95%
Blood Culture Timing	119	97%	98%	98%
Pregnancy and Delivery Care				
Newborn Deliveries Scheduled Early[2]	247	2%	5%	6%
Preventive Care				
Immunization for Influenza[2]	1,101	91%	89%	90%
Immunization for Pneumonia[2]	832	87%	90%	92%
Stroke Care				
Anticoagulation Therapy for Atrial Fibrillation	11	91%	95%	95%
Antithrombotic Therapy Timing	77	92%	98%	98%
Assessed for Rehabilitation	115	95%	97%	97%
Discharged on Antithrombotic Therapy	75	100%	99%	99%
Discharged on Statin Medication	59	92%	94%	94%
Thrombolytic Therapy Timing	12	100%	72%	66%
Venous Thromboembolism Prophylaxis	143	99%	94%	94%
Written Stroke Educational Materials Given	55	87%	87%	88%
Surgical Care Improvement Project				
Appropriate Beta Blocker Usage	82	90%	97%	98%
Appropriate VTP Within 24 Hours	303	92%	98%	98%
Controlled Postoperative Blood Glucose	79	81%	96%	97%
Perioperative Temperature Management	346	99%	100%	100%
Prophylactic Antibiotic Selection	207	95%	99%	99%
Prophylactic Antibiotic Selection (Outpatient)	79	97%	97%	98%
Prophylactic Antibiotic Stopped	204	88%	98%	98%
Prophylactic Antibiotic Timing	208	96%	99%	99%
Prophylactic Antibiotic Timing (Outpatient)	81	94%	97%	98%
Urinary Catheter Removal	136	76%	97%	97%
Survey of Patients' Hospital Experiences				
Area Around Room 'Always' Quiet at Night	300+	42%	51%	61%
Doctors 'Always' Communicated Well	300+	81%	78%	82%
Home Recovery Information Given	300+	81%	83%	85%
Hospital Given 9 or 10 on 10 Point Scale	300+	68%	68%	71%
Meds 'Always' Explained Before Given	300+	63%	61%	64%
Nurses 'Always' Communicated Well	300+	76%	74%	79%
Pain 'Always' Well Controlled	300+	73%	68%	71%
Room and Bathroom 'Always' Clean	300+	70%	70%	73%
Timely Help 'Always' Received	300+	61%	62%	68%
Would Definitely Recommend Hospital	300+	65%	70%	71%
Use of Medical Imaging				
Cardiac Imaging Stress Test before Surgery[1]	-	-	5.2%	5.3%
Combination Abdominal CT Scan	130	3.1%	13.4%	10.5%
Combination Brain/Sinus CT Scan	301	5.0%	2.2%	2.7%
Combination Chest CT Scan	45	0.0%	2.3%	2.7%
Follow-up Mammogram/Ultrasound[7]	-	-	8.2%	8.8%
Lumbar Spine MRI for Low Back Pain[7]	-	-	34.2%	37.2%

Goleta Valley Cottage Hospital

351 S Patterson Ave
Santa Barbara, CA 93111
Phone: 805-681-6446
Fax: 805-681-6437
URL: www.sbch.org
Type: Acute Care Hospitals
Emergency Services: Yes
Ownership: Voluntary non-profit - Other
Beds: 122

Key Personnel:

Operating Room. . . . . Steffanie Carty
Chief of Medical Staff. . . . . Christopher Flynn, MD
Emergency Room . . . . Leslie Houston
Quality Assurance . . . . Sharon Lutz
Radiology. . . . . Carol Mathys
Chair/CEO . . . . Robert E Nourse
CEO/President. . . . . Ron Werft

Measure	Cases	This Hosp.	State Avg.	U.S. Avg.
Blood Clot Prevention and Treatment				
Anticoagulation Overlap Therapy[1,2]	-	-	92%	93%
ICU Venous Thromboembolism Prophylaxis[2]	14	71%	92%	92%
Incidence of Potentially Preventable VTE[2,7]	-	-	11%	10%
UFH with Dosages/Platelet Monitoring[2,7]	-	-	96%	97%
Venous Thromboembolism Prophylaxis[2]	46	74%	83%	85%
Warfarin Therapy Discharge Instructions[1,2]	-	-	75%	75%
Chest Pain/Possible Heart Attack Care				
Aspirin Given Within 24 Hours of Arrival	37	86%	97%	96%
Fibrinolytic Meds Within 30 Min. of Arrival[7]	-	-	62%	58%
Average Time to ECG (minutes)	38	12	9	7
Average Time to Transfer (minutes)[1]	-	-	62	60
Children's Asthma Care				
Received Home Management Plan of Care	-	-	88%	88%
Received Reliever Medication	-	-	100%	100%
Received Systemic Corticosteroids	-	-	100%	100%
Emergency Department				
Admittance Decision Time (minutes)[2]	249	85	125	98
Head CT Results Within 45 Min. of Arrival[1]	-	-	55%	57%
Patients Who Left ER Before Being Seen	18,694	1%	3%	2%
Time from ER Arrival to Admit. (minutes)[2]	249	230	323	274
Time from ER Arrival to Discharge (minutes)	348	110	168	134
Time in ER Before Being Evaluated (minutes)	392	25	29	26
Time to Pain Meds for Fractures (minutes)	97	34	62	57
Heart Attack Care				
Aspirin Given at Discharge[5]	-	-	99%	99%
Fibrinolytic Meds Within 30 Min. of Arrival[5]	-	-	73%	54%
PCI Within 90 Minutes of Arrival[5]	-	-	95%	96%
Statin Prescribed at Discharge[5]	-	-	98%	98%
Heart Failure Care				
ACE Inhibitor or ARB for LVSD[1]	-	-	97%	97%
Discharge Instructions Given[1]	-	-	94%	94%
Evaluation of LVS Function[1]	-	-	99%	99%
Medicare Spending				
Medicare Spending per Patient (ratio)	-	0.94	0.98	0.98

NOTE: Hospital profiles are in alphabetical order by state, then city, then hospital within the city; Rankings exclude hospitals with less than 25 cases except for patient surveys which excludes hospitals with less than 100 cases; (a) 100-299 cases; (1) The number of cases/patients is too few to report; (2) Data submitted were based on a sample of cases/patients; (3) Results are based on a shorter time period than required; (4) Data suppressed by CMS for one or more quarters; (5) Results are not available for this reporting period; (6) Fewer than 100 patients completed the HCAHPS survey; (7) No cases met the criteria for this measure; (8) The lower limit of the confidence interval cannot be calculated if the number of observed infections equals zero; (9) No data are available from the state/territory for this reporting period; (10) The scores shown reflect fewer than 50 completed surveys; (11) There were discrepancies in the data collection process; (12) This measure does not apply to this hospital for this reporting period; (13) Results cannot be calculated for this reporting period; (14) The results for this state are combined with nearby states to protect confidentiality; Please refer to the User's Guide for a full explanation of data.

Measure	Cases	This Hosp.	State Avg.	U.S. Avg.
Pneumonia Care				
Appropriate Initial Antibiotic Given	16	88%	97%	95%
Blood Culture Timing	29	93%	98%	98%
Pregnancy and Delivery Care				
Newborn Deliveries Scheduled Early[7]	-	-	5%	6%
Preventive Care				
Immunization for Influenza[2]	321	89%	89%	90%
Immunization for Pneumonia[2]	382	94%	90%	92%
Stroke Care				
Anticoagulation Therapy for Atrial Fibrillation[1,3]	-	-	95%	95%
Antithrombotic Therapy Timing[1,3]	-	-	98%	98%
Assessed for Rehabilitation[1,3]	-	-	97%	97%
Discharged on Antithrombotic Therapy[1,3]	-	-	99%	99%
Discharged on Statin Medication[1,3]	-	-	94%	94%
Thrombolytic Therapy Timing[3,7]	-	-	72%	66%
Venous Thromboembolism Prophylaxis[1,3]	-	-	94%	94%
Written Stroke Educational Materials Given[3,7]	-	-	87%	88%
Surgical Care Improvement Project				
Appropriate Beta Blocker Usage[2]	56	93%	97%	98%
Appropriate VTP Within 24 Hours[2]	297	98%	98%	98%
Controlled Postoperative Blood Glucose[2,7]	-	-	96%	97%
Perioperative Temperature Management[2]	317	100%	100%	100%
Prophylactic Antibiotic Selection[2]	237	100%	99%	99%
Prophylactic Antibiotic Selection (Outpatient)	33	85%	97%	98%
Prophylactic Antibiotic Stopped[2]	230	98%	98%	98%
Prophylactic Antibiotic Timing[2]	237	97%	99%	99%
Prophylactic Antibiotic Timing (Outpatient)	28	89%	97%	98%
Urinary Catheter Removal[2]	295	99%	97%	97%
Survey of Patients' Hospital Experiences				
Area Around Room 'Always' Quiet at Night	300+	52%	51%	61%
Doctors 'Always' Communicated Well	300+	84%	78%	82%
Home Recovery Information Given	300+	89%	83%	85%
Hospital Given 9 or 10 on 10 Point Scale	300+	78%	68%	71%
Meds 'Always' Explained Before Given	300+	65%	61%	64%
Nurses 'Always' Communicated Well	300+	83%	74%	79%
Pain 'Always' Well Controlled	300+	74%	68%	71%
Room and Bathroom 'Always' Clean	300+	79%	70%	73%
Timely Help 'Always' Received	300+	77%	62%	68%
Would Definitely Recommend Hospital	300+	84%	70%	71%
Use of Medical Imaging				
Cardiac Imaging Stress Test before Surgery[1]	-	-	5.2%	5.3%
Combination Abdominal CT Scan	219	4.1%	13.4%	10.5%
Combination Brain/Sinus CT Scan[1]	-	-	2.2%	2.7%
Combination Chest CT Scan	111	0.9%	2.3%	2.7%
Follow-up Mammogram/Ultrasound	631	5.1%	8.2%	8.8%
Lumbar Spine MRI for Low Back Pain[1]	-	-	34.2%	37.2%

Santa Barbara Cottage Hospital

400 West Pueblo — Phone: 805-682-7111
Santa Barbara, CA 93102 — Fax: 805-569-8368
E-mail: joneill@cottagehealthsystem.org
URL: www.cottagehealthsystem.org
Type: Acute Care Hospitals — Emergency Services: Yes
Ownership: Voluntary non-profit - Private — Beds: 404

Key Personnel:
Chief of Medical Staff.......... Jason Boyatt, MD
Radiology.................... Bernard Chow
Cardiac Laboratory............ Rick Donovan
Surgery...................... Deborah Fanning
Emergency Room .... Denise McDonald
Cardiology................... Kit Robbins
Infection Control............. Leslie Stanfield
CEO/President............... Ronald C. Werft

Measure	Cases	This Hosp.	State Avg.	U.S. Avg.
Blood Clot Prevention and Treatment				
Anticoagulation Overlap Therapy[2]	56	95%	92%	93%
ICU Venous Thromboembolism Prophylaxis[2]	103	96%	92%	92%
Incidence of Potentially Preventable VTE[2]	22	9%	11%	10%
UFH with Dosages/Platelet Monitoring[2]	25	96%	96%	97%
Venous Thromboembolism Prophylaxis[2]	311	79%	83%	85%
Warfarin Therapy Discharge Instructions[2]	39	92%	75%	75%
Chest Pain/Possible Heart Attack Care				
Aspirin Given Within 24 Hours of Arrival[5]	-	-	97%	96%
Fibrinolytic Meds Within 30 Min. of Arrival[5]	-	-	62%	58%
Average Time to ECG (minutes)[5]	-	-	9	7
Average Time to Transfer (minutes)[5]	-	-	62	60
Children's Asthma Care				
Received Home Management Plan of Care	-	-	88%	88%
Received Reliever Medication	-	-	100%	100%
Received Systemic Corticosteroids	-	-	100%	100%
Emergency Department				
Admittance Decision Time (minutes)[2]	525	99	125	98
Head CT Results Within 45 Min. of Arrival[1,3]	-	-	55%	57%
Patients Who Left ER Before Being Seen	44,200	1%	3%	2%
Time from ER Arrival to Admit. (minutes)[2]	525	266	323	274
Time from ER Arrival to Discharge (minutes)	357	158	168	134
Time in ER Before Being Evaluated (minutes)	402	38	29	26
Time to Pain Meds for Fractures (minutes)	181	54	62	57
Heart Attack Care				
Aspirin Given at Discharge	230	100%	99%	99%
Fibrinolytic Meds Within 30 Min. of Arrival[7]	-	-	73%	54%
PCI Within 90 Minutes of Arrival	39	95%	95%	96%
Statin Prescribed at Discharge	225	99%	98%	98%
Heart Failure Care				
ACE Inhibitor or ARB for LVSD	85	95%	97%	97%
Discharge Instructions Given	232	86%	94%	94%
Evaluation of LVS Function	298	100%	99%	99%
Medicare Spending				
Medicare Spending per Patient (ratio)	-	0.94	0.98	0.98
Pneumonia Care				
Appropriate Initial Antibiotic Given	144	92%	97%	95%
Blood Culture Timing	252	98%	98%	98%
Pregnancy and Delivery Care				
Newborn Deliveries Scheduled Early	155	6%	5%	6%
Preventive Care				
Immunization for Influenza[2]	542	73%	89%	90%
Immunization for Pneumonia[2]	535	78%	90%	92%
Stroke Care				
Anticoagulation Therapy for Atrial Fibrillation	50	96%	95%	95%
Antithrombotic Therapy Timing	197	96%	98%	98%
Assessed for Rehabilitation	335	96%	97%	97%
Discharged on Antithrombotic Therapy	239	100%	99%	99%
Discharged on Statin Medication	171	91%	94%	94%
Thrombolytic Therapy Timing	21	76%	72%	66%
Venous Thromboembolism Prophylaxis	364	96%	94%	94%
Written Stroke Educational Materials Given	168	93%	87%	88%
Surgical Care Improvement Project				
Appropriate Beta Blocker Usage[2]	110	96%	97%	98%
Appropriate VTP Within 24 Hours[2]	400	97%	98%	98%
Controlled Postoperative Blood Glucose[2]	159	95%	96%	97%
Perioperative Temperature Management[2]	548	99%	100%	100%
Prophylactic Antibiotic Selection[2]	534	98%	99%	99%
Prophylactic Antibiotic Selection (Outpatient)	632	99%	97%	98%
Prophylactic Antibiotic Stopped[2]	524	96%	98%	98%
Prophylactic Antibiotic Timing[2]	535	99%	99%	99%
Prophylactic Antibiotic Timing (Outpatient)	634	98%	97%	98%
Urinary Catheter Removal[2]	406	96%	97%	97%
Survey of Patients' Hospital Experiences				
Area Around Room 'Always' Quiet at Night	300+	60%	51%	61%
Doctors 'Always' Communicated Well	300+	80%	78%	82%
Home Recovery Information Given	300+	83%	83%	85%
Hospital Given 9 or 10 on 10 Point Scale	300+	82%	68%	71%
Meds 'Always' Explained Before Given	300+	65%	61%	64%
Nurses 'Always' Communicated Well	300+	80%	74%	79%
Pain 'Always' Well Controlled	300+	74%	68%	71%
Room and Bathroom 'Always' Clean	300+	76%	70%	73%
Timely Help 'Always' Received	300+	63%	62%	68%
Would Definitely Recommend Hospital	300+	87%	70%	71%
Use of Medical Imaging				
Cardiac Imaging Stress Test before Surgery	192	4.2%	5.2%	5.3%
Combination Abdominal CT Scan	670	3.1%	13.4%	10.5%
Combination Brain/Sinus CT Scan[1]	-	-	2.2%	2.7%
Combination Chest CT Scan	905	0.1%	2.3%	2.7%
Follow-up Mammogram/Ultrasound	184	5.4%	8.2%	8.8%
Lumbar Spine MRI for Low Back Pain	108	30.6%	34.2%	37.2%

Kaiser Foundation Hospital - Santa Clara

700 Lawrence Expressway — Phone: 408-236-6400
Santa Clara, CA 95051 — Fax: 888-805-7562
URL: www.members.kaiserpermanente.org
Type: Acute Care Hospitals — Emergency Services: Yes
Ownership: Government - Federal — Beds: 286

Key Personnel:
Emergency Room .... Eric Koscove, MD
Infection Control............. Mark Lillo, MD
Chief of Medical Staff.......... Bernadette Loftus, MD
Pediatric Ambulatory Care ...... Robert Maddox, MD
Anesthesiology............... Thomas Schares, MD

Measure	Cases	This Hosp.	State Avg.	U.S. Avg.
Blood Clot Prevention and Treatment				
Anticoagulation Overlap Therapy[2]	61	100%	92%	93%
ICU Venous Thromboembolism Prophylaxis[2]	64	98%	92%	92%
Incidence of Potentially Preventable VTE[2]	23	0%	11%	10%
UFH with Dosages/Platelet Monitoring[2]	47	100%	96%	97%
Venous Thromboembolism Prophylaxis[2]	270	90%	83%	85%
Warfarin Therapy Discharge Instructions[2]	58	72%	75%	75%
Chest Pain/Possible Heart Attack Care				
Aspirin Given Within 24 Hours of Arrival	-	-	97%	96%
Fibrinolytic Meds Within 30 Min. of Arrival	-	-	62%	58%
Average Time to ECG (minutes)	-	-	9	7
Average Time to Transfer (minutes)	-	-	62	60
Children's Asthma Care				
Received Home Management Plan of Care	-	-	88%	88%
Received Reliever Medication	-	-	100%	100%
Received Systemic Corticosteroids	-	-	100%	100%
Emergency Department				
Admittance Decision Time (minutes)[2]	428	51	125	98
Head CT Results Within 45 Min. of Arrival	-	-	55%	57%
Patients Who Left ER Before Being Seen	-	-	3%	2%
Time from ER Arrival to Admit. (minutes)[2]	431	335	323	274
Time from ER Arrival to Discharge (minutes)	-	-	168	134
Time in ER Before Being Evaluated (minutes)	-	-	29	26
Time to Pain Meds for Fractures (minutes)	-	-	62	57
Heart Attack Care				
Aspirin Given at Discharge[2]	291	100%	99%	99%
Fibrinolytic Meds Within 30 Min. of Arrival[2,7]	-	-	73%	54%
PCI Within 90 Minutes of Arrival[2]	16	100%	95%	96%
Statin Prescribed at Discharge[2]	287	100%	98%	98%
Heart Failure Care				
ACE Inhibitor or ARB for LVSD[2]	76	100%	97%	97%
Discharge Instructions Given[2]	264	100%	94%	94%
Evaluation of LVS Function[2]	282	100%	99%	99%
Medicare Spending				
Medicare Spending per Patient (ratio)	-	0.81	0.98	0.98
Pneumonia Care				
Appropriate Initial Antibiotic Given[2]	64	100%	97%	95%
Blood Culture Timing[2]	128	100%	98%	98%
Pregnancy and Delivery Care				
Newborn Deliveries Scheduled Early[2]	35	3%	5%	6%
Preventive Care				
Immunization for Influenza[2]	504	94%	89%	90%
Immunization for Pneumonia[2]	562	94%	90%	92%
Stroke Care				
Anticoagulation Therapy for Atrial Fibrillation[2]	24	96%	95%	95%
Antithrombotic Therapy Timing[2]	75	100%	98%	98%
Assessed for Rehabilitation[2]	134	99%	97%	97%
Discharged on Antithrombotic Therapy[2]	115	98%	99%	99%
Discharged on Statin Medication[2]	91	100%	94%	94%
Thrombolytic Therapy Timing[1,2]	-	-	72%	66%
Venous Thromboembolism Prophylaxis[2]	104	99%	94%	94%
Written Stroke Educational Materials Given[2]	92	100%	87%	88%
Surgical Care Improvement Project				
Appropriate Beta Blocker Usage[2]	260	100%	97%	98%
Appropriate VTP Within 24 Hours[2]	350	100%	98%	98%
Controlled Postoperative Blood Glucose[2]	174	96%	96%	97%
Perioperative Temperature Management[2]	519	100%	100%	100%
Prophylactic Antibiotic Selection[2]	487	100%	99%	99%
Prophylactic Antibiotic Selection (Outpatient)	-	-	97%	98%
Prophylactic Antibiotic Stopped[2]	486	100%	98%	98%

NOTE: Hospital profiles are in alphabetical order by state, then city, then hospital within the city; Rankings exclude hospitals with less than 25 cases except for patient surveys which excludes hospitals with less than 100 cases; (a) 100-299 cases; (1) The number of cases/patients is too few to report; (2) Data submitted were based on a sample of cases/patients; (3) Results are based on a shorter time period than required; (4) Data suppressed by CMS for one or more quarters; (5) Results are not available for this reporting period; (6) Fewer than 100 patients completed the HCAHPS survey; (7) No cases met the criteria for this measure; (8) The lower limit of the confidence interval cannot be calculated if the number of observed infections equals zero; (9) No data are available from the state/territory for this reporting period; (10) The scores shown reflect fewer than 50 completed surveys; (11) There were discrepancies in the data collection process; (12) This measure does not apply to this hospital for this reporting period; (13) Results cannot be calculated for this reporting period; (14) The results for this state are combined with nearby states to protect confidentiality; Please refer to the User's Guide for a full explanation of data.

Measure	Cases	This Hosp.	State Avg.	U.S. Avg.
Prophylactic Antibiotic Timing[2]	487	100%	99%	99%
Prophylactic Antibiotic Timing (Outpatient)	-	-	97%	98%
Urinary Catheter Removal[2]	346	100%	97%	97%
Survey of Patients' Hospital Experiences				
Area Around Room 'Always' Quiet at Night	300+	55%	51%	61%
Doctors 'Always' Communicated Well	300+	82%	78%	82%
Home Recovery Information Given	300+	87%	83%	85%
Hospital Given 9 or 10 on 10 Point Scale	300+	79%	68%	71%
Meds 'Always' Explained Before Given	300+	65%	61%	64%
Nurses 'Always' Communicated Well	300+	79%	74%	79%
Pain 'Always' Well Controlled	300+	73%	68%	71%
Room and Bathroom 'Always' Clean	300+	73%	70%	73%
Timely Help 'Always' Received	300+	67%	62%	68%
Would Definitely Recommend Hospital	300+	81%	70%	71%
Use of Medical Imaging				
Cardiac Imaging Stress Test before Surgery	-	-	5.2%	5.3%
Combination Abdominal CT Scan	-	-	13.4%	10.5%
Combination Brain/Sinus CT Scan	-	-	2.2%	2.7%
Combination Chest CT Scan	-	-	2.3%	2.7%
Follow-up Mammogram/Ultrasound	-	-	8.2%	8.8%
Lumbar Spine MRI for Low Back Pain	-	-	34.2%	37.2%

Dominican Hospital

1555 Soquel Drive
Santa Cruz, CA 95065
URL: www.dominicanhospital.org
Type: Acute Care Hospitals
Ownership: Voluntary non-profit - Church
Phone: 831-462-7700
Fax: 831-464-8813
Emergency Services: Yes
Beds: 379

Key Personnel:
Radiology. . . . . Richard Crescini
Quality Assurance . . . . Kathy Dean, RN
Operating Room. . . . . Mary Ann Dunlap, RN
CEO/President. . . . . Julie Hyer
Chief of Medical Staff . . . . Dean Kashino, MD
Pediatric In-Patient Care . . . . Salem Magarian, MD
Infection Control. . . . . Nanette Mickiewicz, MD

Measure	Cases	This Hosp.	State Avg.	U.S. Avg.
Blood Clot Prevention and Treatment				
Anticoagulation Overlap Therapy[2]	59	100%	92%	93%
ICU Venous Thromboembolism Prophylaxis[2]	85	95%	92%	92%
Incidence of Potentially Preventable VTE[1,2]	-	-	11%	10%
UFH with Dosages/Platelet Monitoring[2]	31	94%	96%	97%
Venous Thromboembolism Prophylaxis[2]	317	94%	83%	85%
Warfarin Therapy Discharge Instructions[2]	40	100%	75%	75%
Chest Pain/Possible Heart Attack Care				
Aspirin Given Within 24 Hours of Arrival[1]	-	-	97%	96%
Fibrinolytic Meds Within 30 Min. of Arrival[5]	-	-	62%	58%
Average Time to ECG (minutes)[1]	-	-	9	7
Average Time to Transfer (minutes)[5]	-	-	62	60
Children's Asthma Care				
Received Home Management Plan of Care	-	-	88%	88%
Received Reliever Medication	-	-	100%	100%
Received Systemic Corticosteroids	-	-	100%	100%
Emergency Department				
Admittance Decision Time (minutes)[2]	725	117	125	98
Head CT Results Within 45 Min. of Arrival[1]	-	-	55%	57%
Patients Who Left ER Before Being Seen	42,944	2%	3%	2%
Time from ER Arrival to Admit. (minutes)[2]	742	306	323	274
Time from ER Arrival to Discharge (minutes)	375	166	168	134
Time in ER Before Being Evaluated (minutes)	417	18	29	26
Time to Pain Meds for Fractures (minutes)	207	75	62	57
Heart Attack Care				
Aspirin Given at Discharge[2]	220	99%	99%	99%
Fibrinolytic Meds Within 30 Min. of Arrival[2,7]	-	-	73%	54%
PCI Within 90 Minutes of Arrival[2]	72	99%	95%	96%
Statin Prescribed at Discharge[2]	209	99%	98%	98%
Heart Failure Care				
ACE Inhibitor or ARB for LVSD[2]	84	100%	97%	97%
Discharge Instructions Given[2]	216	100%	94%	94%
Evaluation of LVS Function[2]	225	100%	99%	99%
Medicare Spending				
Medicare Spending per Patient (ratio)	-	0.99	0.98	0.98
Pneumonia Care				
Appropriate Initial Antibiotic Given[2]	107	100%	97%	95%
Blood Culture Timing[2]	170	100%	98%	98%
Pregnancy and Delivery Care				
Newborn Deliveries Scheduled Early[2]	18	6%	5%	6%
Preventive Care				
Immunization for Influenza[2]	528	84%	89%	90%
Immunization for Pneumonia[2]	628	78%	90%	92%
Stroke Care				
Anticoagulation Therapy for Atrial Fibrillation	18	100%	95%	95%
Antithrombotic Therapy Timing	75	99%	98%	98%
Assessed for Rehabilitation	112	100%	97%	97%
Discharged on Antithrombotic Therapy	94	100%	99%	99%
Discharged on Statin Medication	71	99%	94%	94%
Thrombolytic Therapy Timing	11	100%	72%	66%
Venous Thromboembolism Prophylaxis	104	98%	94%	94%
Written Stroke Educational Materials Given	41	95%	87%	88%
Surgical Care Improvement Project				
Appropriate Beta Blocker Usage[2]	121	99%	97%	98%
Appropriate VTP Within 24 Hours[2]	382	99%	98%	98%
Controlled Postoperative Blood Glucose[2]	93	96%	96%	97%
Perioperative Temperature Management[2]	505	100%	100%	100%
Prophylactic Antibiotic Selection[2]	394	99%	99%	99%
Prophylactic Antibiotic Selection (Outpatient)	126	99%	97%	98%
Prophylactic Antibiotic Stopped[2]	392	98%	98%	98%
Prophylactic Antibiotic Timing[2]	394	100%	99%	99%
Prophylactic Antibiotic Timing (Outpatient)	126	100%	97%	98%
Urinary Catheter Removal[2]	288	100%	97%	97%
Survey of Patients' Hospital Experiences				
Area Around Room 'Always' Quiet at Night	300+	34%	51%	61%
Doctors 'Always' Communicated Well	300+	77%	78%	82%
Home Recovery Information Given	300+	84%	83%	85%
Hospital Given 9 or 10 on 10 Point Scale	300+	60%	68%	71%
Meds 'Always' Explained Before Given	300+	57%	61%	64%
Nurses 'Always' Communicated Well	300+	71%	74%	79%
Pain 'Always' Well Controlled	300+	66%	68%	71%
Room and Bathroom 'Always' Clean	300+	62%	70%	73%
Timely Help 'Always' Received	300+	55%	62%	68%
Would Definitely Recommend Hospital	300+	64%	70%	71%
Use of Medical Imaging				
Cardiac Imaging Stress Test before Surgery	162	5.6%	5.2%	5.3%
Combination Abdominal CT Scan	542	2.2%	13.4%	10.5%
Combination Brain/Sinus CT Scan	795	1.0%	2.2%	2.7%
Combination Chest CT Scan	255	0.0%	2.3%	2.7%
Follow-up Mammogram/Ultrasound[7]	-	-	8.2%	8.8%
Lumbar Spine MRI for Low Back Pain[7]	-	-	34.2%	37.2%

Sutter Maternity & Surgery Center of Santa Cruz

2900 Chanticleer Avenue
Santa Cruz, CA 95065
URL: www.suttermatsurg.org
Type: Acute Care Hospitals
Ownership: Voluntary non-profit - Private
Phone: 831-477-2200
Emergency Services: No
Beds: 30

Measure	Cases	This Hosp.	State Avg.	U.S. Avg.
Blood Clot Prevention and Treatment				
Anticoagulation Overlap Therapy[7]	-	-	92%	93%
ICU Venous Thromboembolism Prophylaxis[7]	-	-	92%	92%
Incidence of Potentially Preventable VTE[7]	-	-	11%	10%
UFH with Dosages/Platelet Monitoring[7]	-	-	96%	97%
Venous Thromboembolism Prophylaxis	72	93%	83%	85%
Warfarin Therapy Discharge Instructions[7]	-	-	75%	75%
Chest Pain/Possible Heart Attack Care				
Aspirin Given Within 24 Hours of Arrival[5]	-	-	97%	96%
Fibrinolytic Meds Within 30 Min. of Arrival[5]	-	-	62%	58%
Average Time to ECG (minutes)[5]	-	-	9	7
Average Time to Transfer (minutes)[5]	-	-	62	60
Children's Asthma Care				
Received Home Management Plan of Care	-	-	88%	88%
Received Reliever Medication	-	-	100%	100%
Received Systemic Corticosteroids	-	-	100%	100%
Emergency Department				
Admittance Decision Time (minutes)[2,7]	-	-	125	98
Head CT Results Within 45 Min. of Arrival[5]	-	-	55%	57%
Patients Who Left ER Before Being Seen[5]	-	-	3%	2%
Time from ER Arrival to Admit. (minutes)[2,7]	-	-	323	274
Time from ER Arrival to Discharge (minutes)[5]	-	-	168	134
Time in ER Before Being Evaluated (minutes)[5]	-	-	29	26
Time to Pain Meds for Fractures (minutes)[5]	-	-	62	57
Heart Attack Care				
Aspirin Given at Discharge[5]	-	-	99%	99%
Fibrinolytic Meds Within 30 Min. of Arrival[5]	-	-	73%	54%
PCI Within 90 Minutes of Arrival[5]	-	-	95%	96%
Statin Prescribed at Discharge[5]	-	-	98%	98%
Heart Failure Care				
ACE Inhibitor or ARB for LVSD[5]	-	-	97%	97%
Discharge Instructions Given[5]	-	-	94%	94%
Evaluation of LVS Function[5]	-	-	99%	99%
Medicare Spending				
Medicare Spending per Patient (ratio)	-	0.91	0.98	0.98
Pneumonia Care				
Appropriate Initial Antibiotic Given[3,7]	-	-	97%	95%
Blood Culture Timing[3,7]	-	-	98%	98%
Pregnancy and Delivery Care				
Newborn Deliveries Scheduled Early	43	2%	5%	6%
Preventive Care				
Immunization for Influenza[2]	190	87%	89%	90%
Immunization for Pneumonia[2]	78	88%	90%	92%
Stroke Care				
Anticoagulation Therapy for Atrial Fibrillation[5]	-	-	95%	95%
Antithrombotic Therapy Timing[5]	-	-	98%	98%
Assessed for Rehabilitation[5]	-	-	97%	97%
Discharged on Antithrombotic Therapy[5]	-	-	99%	99%
Discharged on Statin Medication[5]	-	-	94%	94%
Thrombolytic Therapy Timing[5]	-	-	72%	66%
Venous Thromboembolism Prophylaxis[5]	-	-	94%	94%
Written Stroke Educational Materials Given[5]	-	-	87%	88%
Surgical Care Improvement Project				
Appropriate Beta Blocker Usage	44	100%	97%	98%
Appropriate VTP Within 24 Hours	224	100%	98%	98%
Controlled Postoperative Blood Glucose[7]	-	-	96%	97%
Perioperative Temperature Management	261	100%	100%	100%
Prophylactic Antibiotic Selection	190	98%	99%	99%
Prophylactic Antibiotic Selection (Outpatient)	117	97%	97%	98%
Prophylactic Antibiotic Stopped	188	99%	98%	98%
Prophylactic Antibiotic Timing	190	99%	99%	99%
Prophylactic Antibiotic Timing (Outpatient)	118	98%	97%	98%
Urinary Catheter Removal	163	100%	97%	97%
Survey of Patients' Hospital Experiences				
Area Around Room 'Always' Quiet at Night	300+	73%	51%	61%
Doctors 'Always' Communicated Well	300+	79%	78%	82%
Home Recovery Information Given	300+	87%	83%	85%
Hospital Given 9 or 10 on 10 Point Scale	300+	88%	68%	71%
Meds 'Always' Explained Before Given	300+	68%	61%	64%
Nurses 'Always' Communicated Well	300+	83%	74%	79%
Pain 'Always' Well Controlled	300+	74%	68%	71%
Room and Bathroom 'Always' Clean	300+	80%	70%	73%
Timely Help 'Always' Received	300+	75%	62%	68%
Would Definitely Recommend Hospital	300+	91%	70%	71%
Use of Medical Imaging				
Cardiac Imaging Stress Test before Surgery[7]	-	-	5.2%	5.3%
Combination Abdominal CT Scan[7]	-	-	13.4%	10.5%
Combination Brain/Sinus CT Scan[7]	-	-	2.2%	2.7%
Combination Chest CT Scan[7]	-	-	2.3%	2.7%
Follow-up Mammogram/Ultrasound[7]	-	-	8.2%	8.8%
Lumbar Spine MRI for Low Back Pain[7]	-	-	34.2%	37.2%

Marian Regional Medical Center

1400 E Church St
Santa Maria, CA 93454
URL: www.marianmedicalcenter.org
Type: Acute Care Hospitals
Ownership: Voluntary non-profit - Church
Phone: 805-739-3000
Fax: 805-739-3060
Emergency Services: Yes
Beds: 227

Key Personnel:
Infection Control. . . . . Leslie Anderson
Chief of Medical Staff . . . . Todd Bailey
CEO/President. . . . . Charles Cova
Quality Assurance . . . . Julie Orr
Operating Room. . . . . William Pierce
Pediatric Ambulatory Care . . . . . . Himat Tank, MD

NOTE: Hospital profiles are in alphabetical order by state, then city, then hospital within the city; Rankings exclude hospitals with less than 25 cases except for patient surveys which excludes hospitals with less than 100 cases; (a) 100-299 cases; (1) The number of cases/patients is too few to report; (2) Data submitted were based on a sample of cases/patients; (3) Results are based on a shorter time period than required; (4) Data suppressed by CMS for one or more quarters; (5) Results are not available for this reporting period; (6) Fewer than 100 patients completed the HCAHPS survey; (7) No cases met the criteria for this measure; (8) The lower limit of the confidence interval cannot be calculated if the number of observed infections equals zero; (9) No data are available from the state/territory for this reporting period; (10) The scores shown reflect fewer than 50 completed surveys; (11) There were discrepancies in the data collection process; (12) This measure does not apply to this hospital for this reporting period; (13) Results cannot be calculated for this reporting period; (14) The results for this state are combined with nearby states to protect confidentiality; Please refer to the User's Guide for a full explanation of data.

Pediatric In-Patient Care .... Himat Tank, MD
Radiology................... Mark A Ziemba

Measure	Cases	This Hosp.	State Avg.	U.S. Avg.
Blood Clot Prevention and Treatment				
Anticoagulation Overlap Therapy[2]	43	98%	92%	93%
ICU Venous Thromboembolism Prophylaxis[2]	112	94%	92%	92%
Incidence of Potentially Preventable VTE[1,2]	-	-	11%	10%
UFH with Dosages/Platelet Monitoring[2]	17	100%	96%	97%
Venous Thromboembolism Prophylaxis[2]	419	94%	83%	85%
Warfarin Therapy Discharge Instructions[2]	34	91%	75%	75%
Chest Pain/Possible Heart Attack Care				
Aspirin Given Within 24 Hours of Arrival[3]	24	96%	97%	96%
Fibrinolytic Meds Within 30 Min. of Arrival[3,7]	-	-	62%	58%
Average Time to ECG (minutes)[3]	26	12	9	7
Average Time to Transfer (minutes)[1,3]	-	-	62	60
Children's Asthma Care				
Received Home Management Plan of Care	-	-	88%	88%
Received Reliever Medication	-	-	100%	100%
Received Systemic Corticosteroids	-	-	100%	100%
Emergency Department				
Admittance Decision Time (minutes)[2]	765	118	125	98
Head CT Results Within 45 Min. of Arrival	19	68%	55%	57%
Patients Who Left ER Before Being Seen	61,779	1%	3%	2%
Time from ER Arrival to Admit. (minutes)[2]	789	275	323	274
Time from ER Arrival to Discharge (minutes)	591	110	168	134
Time in ER Before Being Evaluated (minutes)	620	16	29	26
Time to Pain Meds for Fractures (minutes)	260	45	62	57
Heart Attack Care				
Aspirin Given at Discharge	146	97%	99%	99%
Fibrinolytic Meds Within 30 Min. of Arrival[7]	-	-	73%	54%
PCI Within 90 Minutes of Arrival	42	93%	95%	96%
Statin Prescribed at Discharge	135	99%	98%	98%
Heart Failure Care				
ACE Inhibitor or ARB for LVSD	87	97%	97%	97%
Discharge Instructions Given	202	99%	94%	94%
Evaluation of LVS Function	253	100%	99%	99%
Medicare Spending				
Medicare Spending per Patient (ratio)	-	0.94	0.98	0.98
Pneumonia Care				
Appropriate Initial Antibiotic Given	186	99%	97%	95%
Blood Culture Timing	280	99%	98%	98%
Pregnancy and Delivery Care				
Newborn Deliveries Scheduled Early[2]	53	0%	5%	6%
Preventive Care				
Immunization for Influenza[2]	488	93%	89%	90%
Immunization for Pneumonia[2]	665	92%	90%	92%
Stroke Care				
Anticoagulation Therapy for Atrial Fibrillation[1]	-	-	95%	95%
Antithrombotic Therapy Timing	91	98%	98%	98%
Assessed for Rehabilitation	119	97%	97%	97%
Discharged on Antithrombotic Therapy	107	99%	99%	99%
Discharged on Statin Medication	91	90%	94%	94%
Thrombolytic Therapy Timing[1]	-	-	72%	66%
Venous Thromboembolism Prophylaxis	109	96%	94%	94%
Written Stroke Educational Materials Given	62	60%	87%	88%
Surgical Care Improvement Project				
Appropriate Beta Blocker Usage[2]	179	97%	97%	98%
Appropriate VTP Within 24 Hours[2]	453	96%	98%	98%
Controlled Postoperative Blood Glucose[2]	84	89%	96%	97%
Perioperative Temperature Management[2]	558	100%	100%	100%
Prophylactic Antibiotic Selection[2]	445	100%	99%	99%
Prophylactic Antibiotic Selection (Outpatient)	316	99%	97%	98%
Prophylactic Antibiotic Stopped[2]	441	99%	98%	98%
Prophylactic Antibiotic Timing[2]	445	99%	99%	99%
Prophylactic Antibiotic Timing (Outpatient)	317	98%	97%	98%
Urinary Catheter Removal[2]	391	98%	97%	97%
Survey of Patients' Hospital Experiences				
Area Around Room 'Always' Quiet at Night	300+	62%	51%	61%
Doctors 'Always' Communicated Well	300+	76%	78%	82%
Home Recovery Information Given	300+	85%	83%	85%
Hospital Given 9 or 10 on 10 Point Scale	300+	74%	68%	71%
Meds 'Always' Explained Before Given	300+	67%	61%	64%
Nurses 'Always' Communicated Well	300+	75%	74%	79%
Pain 'Always' Well Controlled	300+	67%	68%	71%
Room and Bathroom 'Always' Clean	300+	78%	70%	73%
Timely Help 'Always' Received	300+	59%	62%	68%
Would Definitely Recommend Hospital	300+	75%	70%	71%
Use of Medical Imaging				
Cardiac Imaging Stress Test before Surgery	334	6.6%	5.2%	5.3%
Combination Abdominal CT Scan	1,390	8.9%	13.4%	10.5%
Combination Brain/Sinus CT Scan	1,498	0.9%	2.2%	2.7%
Combination Chest CT Scan	594	1.2%	2.3%	2.7%
Follow-up Mammogram/Ultrasound	2,985	7.8%	8.2%	8.8%
Lumbar Spine MRI for Low Back Pain	141	31.9%	34.2%	37.2%

Providence Saint John's Health Center

2121 Santa Monica Blvd — Phone: 310-829-5511
Santa Monica, CA 90404 — Fax: 310-829-8005
URL: www.stjohns.org
Type: Acute Care Hospitals — Emergency Services: Yes
Ownership: Voluntary non-profit - Private — Beds: 237
Key Personnel:
Radiology..................... Richard Goldstein, MD
Cardiac Laboratory............ Donna Hendel
CEO/President.............. Lourdes Lazatin
Pediatric Ambulatory Care ...... Edward Malphus, MD
Pediatric In-Patient Care .... Edward Malphus, MD
Quality Assurance .... Janet McLaughlin
Chief of Medical Staff.......... Charles Pietrasesa
Operating Room............. Decio Rangel

Measure	Cases	This Hosp.	State Avg.	U.S. Avg.
Blood Clot Prevention and Treatment				
Anticoagulation Overlap Therapy[2]	34	91%	92%	93%
ICU Venous Thromboembolism Prophylaxis[2]	74	80%	92%	92%
Incidence of Potentially Preventable VTE[2]	14	14%	11%	10%
UFH with Dosages/Platelet Monitoring[2]	39	90%	96%	97%
Venous Thromboembolism Prophylaxis[2]	241	73%	83%	85%
Warfarin Therapy Discharge Instructions[2]	30	97%	75%	75%
Chest Pain/Possible Heart Attack Care				
Aspirin Given Within 24 Hours of Arrival[5]	-	-	97%	96%
Fibrinolytic Meds Within 30 Min. of Arrival[5]	-	-	62%	58%
Average Time to ECG (minutes)[5]	-	-	9	7
Average Time to Transfer (minutes)[5]	-	-	62	60
Children's Asthma Care				
Received Home Management Plan of Care	-	-	88%	88%
Received Reliever Medication	-	-	100%	100%
Received Systemic Corticosteroids	-	-	100%	100%
Emergency Department				
Admittance Decision Time (minutes)[2]	233	170	125	98
Head CT Results Within 45 Min. of Arrival[1]	-	-	55%	57%
Patients Who Left ER Before Being Seen	30,372	2%	3%	2%
Time from ER Arrival to Admit. (minutes)[2]	237	318	323	274
Time from ER Arrival to Discharge (minutes)	486	142	168	134
Time in ER Before Being Evaluated (minutes)	458	22	29	26
Time to Pain Meds for Fractures (minutes)	140	59	62	57
Heart Attack Care				
Aspirin Given at Discharge	124	100%	99%	99%
Fibrinolytic Meds Within 30 Min. of Arrival[7]	-	-	73%	54%
PCI Within 90 Minutes of Arrival	34	94%	95%	96%
Statin Prescribed at Discharge	122	100%	98%	98%
Heart Failure Care				
ACE Inhibitor or ARB for LVSD	64	100%	97%	97%
Discharge Instructions Given	145	99%	94%	94%
Evaluation of LVS Function	186	100%	99%	99%
Medicare Spending				
Medicare Spending per Patient (ratio)	-	0.97	0.98	0.98
Pneumonia Care				
Appropriate Initial Antibiotic Given	108	98%	97%	95%
Blood Culture Timing	193	100%	98%	98%
Pregnancy and Delivery Care				
Newborn Deliveries Scheduled Early[2]	19	0%	5%	6%
Preventive Care				
Immunization for Influenza[2]	515	73%	89%	90%
Immunization for Pneumonia[2]	608	73%	90%	92%
Stroke Care				
Anticoagulation Therapy for Atrial Fibrillation[1]	-	-	95%	95%
Antithrombotic Therapy Timing	54	98%	98%	98%
Assessed for Rehabilitation	60	87%	97%	97%
Discharged on Antithrombotic Therapy	43	98%	99%	99%
Discharged on Statin Medication	39	85%	94%	94%
Thrombolytic Therapy Timing	14	0%	72%	66%
Venous Thromboembolism Prophylaxis	71	79%	94%	94%
Written Stroke Educational Materials Given	36	92%	87%	88%
Surgical Care Improvement Project				
Appropriate Beta Blocker Usage[2]	113	100%	97%	98%
Appropriate VTP Within 24 Hours[2]	347	100%	98%	98%
Controlled Postoperative Blood Glucose[2]	83	100%	96%	97%
Perioperative Temperature Management[2]	408	100%	100%	100%
Prophylactic Antibiotic Selection[2]	367	99%	99%	99%
Prophylactic Antibiotic Selection (Outpatient)	311	92%	97%	98%
Prophylactic Antibiotic Stopped[2]	334	99%	98%	98%
Prophylactic Antibiotic Timing[2]	372	99%	99%	99%
Prophylactic Antibiotic Timing (Outpatient)	299	95%	97%	98%
Urinary Catheter Removal[2]	269	100%	97%	97%
Survey of Patients' Hospital Experiences				
Area Around Room 'Always' Quiet at Night	300+	58%	51%	61%
Doctors 'Always' Communicated Well	300+	78%	78%	82%
Home Recovery Information Given	300+	83%	83%	85%
Hospital Given 9 or 10 on 10 Point Scale	300+	70%	68%	71%
Meds 'Always' Explained Before Given	300+	55%	61%	64%
Nurses 'Always' Communicated Well	300+	69%	74%	79%
Pain 'Always' Well Controlled	300+	65%	68%	71%
Room and Bathroom 'Always' Clean	300+	67%	70%	73%
Timely Help 'Always' Received	300+	50%	62%	68%
Would Definitely Recommend Hospital	300+	77%	70%	71%
Use of Medical Imaging				
Cardiac Imaging Stress Test before Surgery	176	8.0%	5.2%	5.3%
Combination Abdominal CT Scan	568	4.2%	13.4%	10.5%
Combination Brain/Sinus CT Scan[1]	-	-	2.2%	2.7%
Combination Chest CT Scan	222	2.3%	2.3%	2.7%
Follow-up Mammogram/Ultrasound	689	7.3%	8.2%	8.8%
Lumbar Spine MRI for Low Back Pain	68	29.4%	34.2%	37.2%

Santa Monica - UCLA Medical Center & Orthopaedic Hospital

1250 16th Street — Phone: 310-319-4000
Santa Monica, CA 90404 — Fax: 310-319-4821
URL: www.healthcare.ucla.edu
Type: Acute Care Hospitals — Emergency Services: Yes
Ownership: Government - State — Beds: 600
Key Personnel:
CEO/President............... Posie Carpenter, RN
Quality Assurance .... Pamela Christensen
Infection Control............. Laverne Kroemer
Pediatric Ambulatory Care ...... Richard Levy, MD
Pediatric In-Patient Care .... Richard Levy, MD
Chief of Medical Staff.......... Stephen Ross, MD
Radiology................... Vino Salazan

Measure	Cases	This Hosp.	State Avg.	U.S. Avg.
Blood Clot Prevention and Treatment				
Anticoagulation Overlap Therapy[2]	60	100%	92%	93%
ICU Venous Thromboembolism Prophylaxis[2]	50	96%	92%	92%
Incidence of Potentially Preventable VTE[2]	14	0%	11%	10%
UFH with Dosages/Platelet Monitoring[2]	58	93%	96%	97%
Venous Thromboembolism Prophylaxis[2]	351	89%	83%	85%
Warfarin Therapy Discharge Instructions[2]	47	64%	75%	75%
Chest Pain/Possible Heart Attack Care				
Aspirin Given Within 24 Hours of Arrival[5]	-	-	97%	96%
Fibrinolytic Meds Within 30 Min. of Arrival[5]	-	-	62%	58%
Average Time to ECG (minutes)[5]	-	-	9	7
Average Time to Transfer (minutes)[5]	-	-	62	60
Children's Asthma Care				
Received Home Management Plan of Care	-	-	88%	88%
Received Reliever Medication	-	-	100%	100%
Received Systemic Corticosteroids	-	-	100%	100%
Emergency Department				
Admittance Decision Time (minutes)[2]	547	291	125	98
Head CT Results Within 45 Min. of Arrival[1,3]	-	-	55%	57%
Patients Who Left ER Before Being Seen	41,070	1%	3%	2%
Time from ER Arrival to Admit. (minutes)[2]	547	409	323	274

NOTE: Hospital profiles are in alphabetical order by state, then city, then hospital within the city; Rankings exclude hospitals with less than 25 cases except for patient surveys which excludes hospitals with less than 100 cases; (a) 100-299 cases; (1) The number of cases/patients is too few to report; (2) Data submitted were based on a sample of cases/patients; (3) Results are based on a shorter time period than required; (4) Data suppressed by CMS for one or more quarters; (5) Results are not available for this reporting period; (6) Fewer than 100 patients completed the HCAHPS survey; (7) No cases met the criteria for this measure; (8) The lower limit of the confidence interval cannot be calculated if the number of observed infections equals zero; (9) No data are available from the state/territory for this reporting period; (10) The scores shown reflect fewer than 50 completed surveys; (11) There were discrepancies in the data collection process; (12) This measure does not apply to this hospital for this reporting period; (13) Results cannot be calculated for this reporting period; (14) The results for this state are combined with nearby states to protect confidentiality; Please refer to the User's Guide for a full explanation of data.

Time from ER Arrival to Discharge (minutes)	410	148	168	134
Time in ER Before Being Evaluated (minutes)	430	24	29	26
Time to Pain Meds for Fractures (minutes)	141	56	62	57
Heart Attack Care				
Aspirin Given at Discharge	150	100%	99%	99%
Fibrinolytic Meds Within 30 Min. of Arrival[7]	-	-	73%	54%
PCI Within 90 Minutes of Arrival	20	100%	95%	96%
Statin Prescribed at Discharge	147	99%	98%	98%
Heart Failure Care				
ACE Inhibitor or ARB for LVSD[2]	54	100%	97%	97%
Discharge Instructions Given[2]	215	81%	94%	94%
Evaluation of LVS Function[2]	272	100%	99%	99%
Medicare Spending				
Medicare Spending per Patient (ratio)	-	1.01	0.98	0.98
Pneumonia Care				
Appropriate Initial Antibiotic Given[2]	58	97%	97%	95%
Blood Culture Timing[2]	100	100%	98%	98%
Pregnancy and Delivery Care				
Newborn Deliveries Scheduled Early[2]	23	13%	5%	6%
Preventive Care				
Immunization for Influenza[2]	539	81%	89%	90%
Immunization for Pneumonia[2]	604	87%	90%	92%
Stroke Care				
Anticoagulation Therapy for Atrial Fibrillation[1]	-	-	95%	95%
Antithrombotic Therapy Timing	62	100%	98%	98%
Assessed for Rehabilitation	70	99%	97%	97%
Discharged on Antithrombotic Therapy	69	100%	99%	99%
Discharged on Statin Medication	50	100%	94%	94%
Thrombolytic Therapy Timing[1]	-	-	72%	66%
Venous Thromboembolism Prophylaxis	66	92%	94%	94%
Written Stroke Educational Materials Given	35	66%	87%	88%
Surgical Care Improvement Project				
Appropriate Beta Blocker Usage[2]	80	100%	97%	98%
Appropriate VTP Within 24 Hours[2]	279	100%	98%	98%
Controlled Postoperative Blood Glucose[2,7]	-	-	96%	97%
Perioperative Temperature Management[2]	350	100%	100%	100%
Prophylactic Antibiotic Selection[2]	221	98%	99%	99%
Prophylactic Antibiotic Selection (Outpatient)	208	99%	97%	98%
Prophylactic Antibiotic Stopped[2]	211	99%	98%	98%
Prophylactic Antibiotic Timing[2]	222	100%	99%	99%
Prophylactic Antibiotic Timing (Outpatient)	211	96%	97%	98%
Urinary Catheter Removal[2]	211	100%	97%	97%
Survey of Patients' Hospital Experiences				
Area Around Room 'Always' Quiet at Night	300+	57%	51%	61%
Doctors 'Always' Communicated Well	300+	77%	78%	82%
Home Recovery Information Given	300+	79%	83%	85%
Hospital Given 9 or 10 on 10 Point Scale	300+	73%	68%	71%
Meds 'Always' Explained Before Given	300+	60%	61%	64%
Nurses 'Always' Communicated Well	300+	71%	74%	79%
Pain 'Always' Well Controlled	300+	66%	68%	71%
Room and Bathroom 'Always' Clean	300+	70%	70%	73%
Timely Help 'Always' Received	300+	60%	62%	68%
Would Definitely Recommend Hospital	300+	77%	70%	71%
Use of Medical Imaging				
Cardiac Imaging Stress Test before Surgery[1]	-	-	5.2%	5.3%
Combination Abdominal CT Scan	424	39.9%	13.4%	10.5%
Combination Brain/Sinus CT Scan[1]	-	-	2.2%	2.7%
Combination Chest CT Scan	247	13.0%	2.3%	2.7%
Follow-up Mammogram/Ultrasound[7]	-	-	8.2%	8.8%
Lumbar Spine MRI for Low Back Pain	103	33.0%	34.2%	37.2%

Kaiser Foundation Hospital - Santa Rosa

401 Bicentennial Way
Santa Rosa, CA 95403
Phone: 707-571-4000
URL: www.kaisersantarosa.org
Type: Acute Care Hospitals
Emergency Services: Yes
Ownership: Voluntary non-profit - Other
Beds: 117

Measure	Cases	This Hosp.	State Avg.	U.S. Avg.
Blood Clot Prevention and Treatment				
Anticoagulation Overlap Therapy[2]	44	100%	92%	93%
ICU Venous Thromboembolism Prophylaxis[2]	51	98%	92%	92%
Incidence of Potentially Preventable VTE[1,2]	-	-	11%	10%
UFH with Dosages/Platelet Monitoring[2]	21	100%	96%	97%
Venous Thromboembolism Prophylaxis[2]	306	92%	83%	85%
Warfarin Therapy Discharge Instructions[2]	38	63%	75%	75%
Chest Pain/Possible Heart Attack Care				
Aspirin Given Within 24 Hours of Arrival	-	-	97%	96%
Fibrinolytic Meds Within 30 Min. of Arrival	-	-	62%	58%
Average Time to ECG (minutes)	-	-	9	7
Average Time to Transfer (minutes)	-	-	62	60
Children's Asthma Care				
Received Home Management Plan of Care	-	-	88%	88%
Received Reliever Medication	-	-	100%	100%
Received Systemic Corticosteroids	-	-	100%	100%
Emergency Department				
Admittance Decision Time (minutes)[2]	509	45	125	98
Head CT Results Within 45 Min. of Arrival	-	-	55%	57%
Patients Who Left ER Before Being Seen	-	-	3%	2%
Time from ER Arrival to Admit. (minutes)[2]	518	280	323	274
Time from ER Arrival to Discharge (minutes)	-	-	168	134
Time in ER Before Being Evaluated (minutes)	-	-	29	26
Time to Pain Meds for Fractures (minutes)	-	-	62	57
Heart Attack Care				
Aspirin Given at Discharge	51	100%	99%	99%
Fibrinolytic Meds Within 30 Min. of Arrival[7]	-	-	73%	54%
PCI Within 90 Minutes of Arrival[7]	-	-	95%	96%
Statin Prescribed at Discharge	57	100%	98%	98%
Heart Failure Care				
ACE Inhibitor or ARB for LVSD	30	100%	97%	97%
Discharge Instructions Given	98	98%	94%	94%
Evaluation of LVS Function	112	99%	99%	99%
Medicare Spending				
Medicare Spending per Patient (ratio)	-	0.86	0.98	0.98
Pneumonia Care				
Appropriate Initial Antibiotic Given[2]	90	99%	97%	95%
Blood Culture Timing[2]	139	96%	98%	98%
Pregnancy and Delivery Care				
Newborn Deliveries Scheduled Early[2]	19	0%	5%	6%
Preventive Care				
Immunization for Influenza[2]	466	90%	89%	90%
Immunization for Pneumonia[2]	530	93%	90%	92%
Stroke Care				
Anticoagulation Therapy for Atrial Fibrillation[2]	16	100%	95%	95%
Antithrombotic Therapy Timing[2]	53	92%	98%	98%
Assessed for Rehabilitation[2]	85	99%	97%	97%
Discharged on Antithrombotic Therapy[2]	69	100%	99%	99%
Discharged on Statin Medication[2]	67	100%	94%	94%
Thrombolytic Therapy Timing[2]	17	94%	72%	66%
Venous Thromboembolism Prophylaxis[2]	81	94%	94%	94%
Written Stroke Educational Materials Given[2]	41	90%	87%	88%
Surgical Care Improvement Project				
Appropriate Beta Blocker Usage[2]	131	98%	97%	98%
Appropriate VTP Within 24 Hours[2]	368	100%	98%	98%
Controlled Postoperative Blood Glucose[2,7]	-	-	96%	97%
Perioperative Temperature Management[2]	437	100%	100%	100%
Prophylactic Antibiotic Selection[2]	283	100%	99%	99%
Prophylactic Antibiotic Selection (Outpatient)	-	-	97%	98%
Prophylactic Antibiotic Stopped[2]	275	98%	98%	98%
Prophylactic Antibiotic Timing[2]	283	99%	99%	99%
Prophylactic Antibiotic Timing (Outpatient)	-	-	97%	98%
Urinary Catheter Removal[2]	368	100%	97%	97%
Survey of Patients' Hospital Experiences				
Area Around Room 'Always' Quiet at Night	300+	55%	51%	61%
Doctors 'Always' Communicated Well	300+	80%	78%	82%
Home Recovery Information Given	300+	87%	83%	85%
Hospital Given 9 or 10 on 10 Point Scale	300+	78%	68%	71%
Meds 'Always' Explained Before Given	300+	65%	61%	64%
Nurses 'Always' Communicated Well	300+	77%	74%	79%
Pain 'Always' Well Controlled	300+	74%	68%	71%
Room and Bathroom 'Always' Clean	300+	75%	70%	73%
Timely Help 'Always' Received	300+	64%	62%	68%
Would Definitely Recommend Hospital	300+	81%	70%	71%
Use of Medical Imaging				
Cardiac Imaging Stress Test before Surgery	-	-	5.2%	5.3%
Combination Abdominal CT Scan	-	-	13.4%	10.5%
Combination Brain/Sinus CT Scan	-	-	2.2%	2.7%
Combination Chest CT Scan	-	-	2.3%	2.7%
Follow-up Mammogram/Ultrasound	-	-	8.2%	8.8%
Lumbar Spine MRI for Low Back Pain	-	-	34.2%	37.2%

Santa Rosa Memorial Hospital

1165 Montgomery Dr
Santa Rosa, CA 95405
Phone: 707-525-5300
Fax: 707-522-1522
URL: www.stjosephhealth.org
Type: Acute Care Hospitals
Emergency Services: Yes
Ownership: Voluntary non-profit - Private
Beds: 209

Key Personnel:
Quality Assurance . . . . Nancy Boostrom
Pediatric Ambulatory Care . . . . . . Dorthy Coleman-Riese, MD
Pediatric In-Patient Care . . . . Dorthy Coleman-Riese, MD
Chief of Medical Staff . . . . Jan Fonander, MD
Emergency Room . . . . Kristy Gaub, Dir
Radiology. . . . . Ralph Hanahan, MD
President/CEO. . . . . Kevin Klockenga
Operating Room. . . . . Gail Sarlatte

Measure	Cases	This Hosp.	State Avg.	U.S. Avg.
Blood Clot Prevention and Treatment				
Anticoagulation Overlap Therapy[2]	54	96%	92%	93%
ICU Venous Thromboembolism Prophylaxis[2]	54	96%	92%	92%
Incidence of Potentially Preventable VTE[2]	20	10%	11%	10%
UFH with Dosages/Platelet Monitoring[2]	24	96%	96%	97%
Venous Thromboembolism Prophylaxis[2]	330	90%	83%	85%
Warfarin Therapy Discharge Instructions[2]	42	43%	75%	75%
Chest Pain/Possible Heart Attack Care				
Aspirin Given Within 24 Hours of Arrival	18	94%	97%	96%
Fibrinolytic Meds Within 30 Min. of Arrival[7]	-	-	62%	58%
Average Time to ECG (minutes)	18	8	9	7
Average Time to Transfer (minutes)[7]	-	-	62	60
Children's Asthma Care				
Received Home Management Plan of Care	-	-	88%	88%
Received Reliever Medication	-	-	100%	100%
Received Systemic Corticosteroids	-	-	100%	100%
Emergency Department				
Admittance Decision Time (minutes)[2]	679	146	125	98
Head CT Results Within 45 Min. of Arrival[1]	-	-	55%	57%
Patients Who Left ER Before Being Seen	36,961	4%	3%	2%
Time from ER Arrival to Admit. (minutes)[2]	682	329	323	274
Time from ER Arrival to Discharge (minutes)	333	176	168	134
Time in ER Before Being Evaluated (minutes)	314	34	29	26
Time to Pain Meds for Fractures (minutes)	125	85	62	57
Heart Attack Care				
Aspirin Given at Discharge	219	99%	99%	99%
Fibrinolytic Meds Within 30 Min. of Arrival[7]	-	-	73%	54%
PCI Within 90 Minutes of Arrival	48	92%	95%	96%
Statin Prescribed at Discharge	210	97%	98%	98%
Heart Failure Care				
ACE Inhibitor or ARB for LVSD	83	95%	97%	97%
Discharge Instructions Given	160	94%	94%	94%
Evaluation of LVS Function	223	98%	99%	99%
Medicare Spending				
Medicare Spending per Patient (ratio)	-	0.97	0.98	0.98
Pneumonia Care				
Appropriate Initial Antibiotic Given	111	97%	97%	95%
Blood Culture Timing	169	97%	98%	98%
Pregnancy and Delivery Care				
Newborn Deliveries Scheduled Early[2]	23	13%	5%	6%
Preventive Care				
Immunization for Influenza[2]	527	75%	89%	90%
Immunization for Pneumonia[2]	605	82%	90%	92%
Stroke Care				
Anticoagulation Therapy for Atrial Fibrillation[2]	24	88%	95%	95%
Antithrombotic Therapy Timing[2]	87	95%	98%	98%
Assessed for Rehabilitation[2]	130	95%	97%	97%
Discharged on Antithrombotic Therapy[2]	108	98%	99%	99%
Discharged on Statin Medication[2]	77	88%	94%	94%
Thrombolytic Therapy Timing[2]	14	93%	72%	66%
Venous Thromboembolism Prophylaxis[2]	141	99%	94%	94%
Written Stroke Educational Materials Given[2]	70	91%	87%	88%

NOTE: Hospital profiles are in alphabetical order by state, then city, then hospital within the city; Rankings exclude hospitals with less than 25 cases except for patient surveys which excludes hospitals with less than 100 cases; (a) 100-299 cases; (1) The number of cases/patients is too few to report; (2) Data submitted were based on a sample of cases/patients; (3) Results are based on a shorter time period than required; (4) Data suppressed by CMS for one or more quarters; (5) Results are not available for this reporting period; (6) Fewer than 100 patients completed the HCAHPS survey; (7) No cases met the criteria for this measure; (8) The lower limit of the confidence interval cannot be calculated if the number of observed infections equals zero; (9) No data are available from the state/territory for this reporting period; (10) The scores shown reflect fewer than 50 completed surveys; (11) There were discrepancies in the data collection process; (12) This measure does not apply to this hospital for this reporting period; (13) Results cannot be calculated for this reporting period; (14) The results for this state are combined with nearby states to protect confidentiality; Please refer to the User's Guide for a full explanation of data.

Measure	Cases	This Hosp.	State Avg.	U.S. Avg.
Surgical Care Improvement Project				
Appropriate Beta Blocker Usage[2]	87	98%	97%	98%
Appropriate VTP Within 24 Hours[2]	263	93%	98%	98%
Controlled Postoperative Blood Glucose[2]	89	92%	96%	97%
Perioperative Temperature Management[2]	336	100%	100%	100%
Prophylactic Antibiotic Selection[2]	265	97%	99%	99%
Prophylactic Antibiotic Selection (Outpatient)	363	96%	97%	98%
Prophylactic Antibiotic Stopped[2]	261	98%	98%	98%
Prophylactic Antibiotic Timing[2]	265	98%	99%	99%
Prophylactic Antibiotic Timing (Outpatient)	361	99%	97%	98%
Urinary Catheter Removal[2]	272	95%	97%	97%
Survey of Patients' Hospital Experiences				
Area Around Room 'Always' Quiet at Night	300+	43%	51%	61%
Doctors 'Always' Communicated Well	300+	74%	78%	82%
Home Recovery Information Given	300+	83%	83%	85%
Hospital Given 9 or 10 on 10 Point Scale	300+	63%	68%	71%
Meds 'Always' Explained Before Given	300+	57%	61%	64%
Nurses 'Always' Communicated Well	300+	72%	74%	79%
Pain 'Always' Well Controlled	300+	68%	68%	71%
Room and Bathroom 'Always' Clean	300+	70%	70%	73%
Timely Help 'Always' Received	300+	61%	62%	68%
Would Definitely Recommend Hospital	300+	70%	70%	71%
Use of Medical Imaging				
Cardiac Imaging Stress Test before Surgery	229	3.1%	5.2%	5.3%
Combination Abdominal CT Scan	651	2.6%	13.4%	10.5%
Combination Brain/Sinus CT Scan	768	1.8%	2.2%	2.7%
Combination Chest CT Scan	189	2.1%	2.3%	2.7%
Follow-up Mammogram/Ultrasound[7]	-	-	8.2%	8.8%
Lumbar Spine MRI for Low Back Pain[1]	-	-	34.2%	37.2%

Sutter Medical Center of Santa Rosa

3325 Chanate Rd Phone: 707-576-4000
Santa Rosa, CA 95404 Fax: 707-576-4318
E-mail: srsutter@sutterhealth.org
URL: www.suttersantarosa.org
Type: Acute Care Hospitals Emergency Services: Yes
Ownership: Government - Local Beds: 175

Key Personnel:
Radiology.................. Brendan Bottari
Pediatric Ambulatory Care...... Fred Brewer, MD
Pediatric In-Patient Care....... Fred Brewer, MD
CEO/President............... Michael J Cohill
Chief of Medical Staff.......... Robert P Heckey, MD
Quality Assurance............ Marsha Lose, RN
Infection Control............. Marion McDonald, RN
Patient Relations............. Sandra Stewart

Measure	Cases	This Hosp.	State Avg.	U.S. Avg.
Blood Clot Prevention and Treatment				
Anticoagulation Overlap Therapy[2]	27	96%	92%	93%
ICU Venous Thromboembolism Prophylaxis[2]	112	98%	92%	92%
Incidence of Potentially Preventable VTE[1,2]	-	-	11%	10%
UFH with Dosages/Platelet Monitoring[1,2]	-	-	96%	97%
Venous Thromboembolism Prophylaxis[2]	431	90%	83%	85%
Warfarin Therapy Discharge Instructions[2]	24	88%	75%	75%
Chest Pain/Possible Heart Attack Care				
Aspirin Given Within 24 Hours of Arrival[1,3]	-	-	97%	96%
Fibrinolytic Meds Within 30 Min. of Arrival[3,7]	-	-	62%	58%
Average Time to ECG (minutes)[1,3]	-	-	9	7
Average Time to Transfer (minutes)[3,7]	-	-	62	60
Children's Asthma Care				
Received Home Management Plan of Care	-	-	88%	88%
Received Reliever Medication	-	-	100%	100%
Received Systemic Corticosteroids	-	-	100%	100%
Emergency Department				
Admittance Decision Time (minutes)[2]	337	150	125	98
Head CT Results Within 45 Min. of Arrival[1]	-	-	55%	57%
Patients Who Left ER Before Being Seen	26,618	3%	3%	2%
Time from ER Arrival to Admit. (minutes)[2]	349	346	323	274
Time from ER Arrival to Discharge (minutes)	377	165	168	134
Time in ER Before Being Evaluated (minutes)	359	35	29	26
Time to Pain Meds for Fractures (minutes)	60	55	62	57
Heart Attack Care				
Aspirin Given at Discharge	147	100%	99%	99%
Fibrinolytic Meds Within 30 Min. of Arrival[7]	-	-	73%	54%
PCI Within 90 Minutes of Arrival	19	100%	95%	96%
Statin Prescribed at Discharge	149	100%	98%	98%
Heart Failure Care				
ACE Inhibitor or ARB for LVSD	51	100%	97%	97%
Discharge Instructions Given	125	100%	94%	94%
Evaluation of LVS Function	137	100%	99%	99%
Medicare Spending				
Medicare Spending per Patient (ratio)	-	0.99	0.98	0.98
Pneumonia Care				
Appropriate Initial Antibiotic Given[2]	44	100%	97%	95%
Blood Culture Timing[2]	98	100%	98%	98%
Pregnancy and Delivery Care				
Newborn Deliveries Scheduled Early	61	0%	5%	6%
Preventive Care				
Immunization for Influenza[2]	499	90%	89%	90%
Immunization for Pneumonia[2]	474	88%	90%	92%
Stroke Care				
Anticoagulation Therapy for Atrial Fibrillation[1]	-	-	95%	95%
Antithrombotic Therapy Timing	36	100%	98%	98%
Assessed for Rehabilitation	43	100%	97%	97%
Discharged on Antithrombotic Therapy	41	100%	99%	99%
Discharged on Statin Medication	31	97%	94%	94%
Thrombolytic Therapy Timing[1]	-	-	72%	66%
Venous Thromboembolism Prophylaxis	40	100%	94%	94%
Written Stroke Educational Materials Given	32	97%	87%	88%
Surgical Care Improvement Project				
Appropriate Beta Blocker Usage[2]	131	99%	97%	98%
Appropriate VTP Within 24 Hours[2]	327	99%	98%	98%
Controlled Postoperative Blood Glucose[2]	111	96%	96%	97%
Perioperative Temperature Management[2]	497	100%	100%	100%
Prophylactic Antibiotic Selection[2]	340	100%	99%	99%
Prophylactic Antibiotic Selection (Outpatient)	144	99%	97%	98%
Prophylactic Antibiotic Stopped[2]	331	99%	98%	98%
Prophylactic Antibiotic Timing[2]	340	100%	99%	99%
Prophylactic Antibiotic Timing (Outpatient)	122	99%	97%	98%
Urinary Catheter Removal[2]	343	99%	97%	97%
Survey of Patients' Hospital Experiences				
Area Around Room 'Always' Quiet at Night	300+	41%	51%	61%
Doctors 'Always' Communicated Well	300+	82%	78%	82%
Home Recovery Information Given	300+	85%	83%	85%
Hospital Given 9 or 10 on 10 Point Scale	300+	69%	68%	71%
Meds 'Always' Explained Before Given	300+	65%	61%	64%
Nurses 'Always' Communicated Well	300+	81%	74%	79%
Pain 'Always' Well Controlled	300+	75%	68%	71%
Room and Bathroom 'Always' Clean	300+	70%	70%	73%
Timely Help 'Always' Received	300+	65%	62%	68%
Would Definitely Recommend Hospital	300+	71%	70%	71%
Use of Medical Imaging				
Cardiac Imaging Stress Test before Surgery[1]	-	-	5.2%	5.3%
Combination Abdominal CT Scan	209	2.9%	13.4%	10.5%
Combination Brain/Sinus CT Scan[1]	-	-	2.2%	2.7%
Combination Chest CT Scan	108	1.9%	2.3%	2.7%
Follow-up Mammogram/Ultrasound[7]	-	-	8.2%	8.8%
Lumbar Spine MRI for Low Back Pain[1]	-	-	34.2%	37.2%

Palm Drive Hospital

501 Petaluma Ave Phone: 707-823-8511
Sebastopol, CA 95472 Fax: 707-829-4178
URL: www.palmdrivehospital.com
Type: Acute Care Hospitals Emergency Services: Yes
Ownership: Voluntary non-profit - Other Beds: 37

Key Personnel:
Quality Assurance............ Alison Juric, RN
Chief of Medical Staff.......... Sue Platts
Emergency Room............ Malissa Reinders, RN
CEO/President............... Neil Todhunter

Measure	Cases	This Hosp.	State Avg.	U.S. Avg.
Blood Clot Prevention and Treatment				
Anticoagulation Overlap Therapy[1,2]	-	-	92%	93%
ICU Venous Thromboembolism Prophylaxis[2]	30	97%	92%	92%
Incidence of Potentially Preventable VTE[1,2]	-	-	11%	10%
UFH with Dosages/Platelet Monitoring[2,7]	-	-	96%	97%
Venous Thromboembolism Prophylaxis[2]	75	95%	83%	85%
Warfarin Therapy Discharge Instructions[1,2]	-	-	75%	75%
Chest Pain/Possible Heart Attack Care				
Aspirin Given Within 24 Hours of Arrival[3]	11	100%	97%	96%
Fibrinolytic Meds Within 30 Min. of Arrival[3,7]	-	-	62%	58%
Average Time to ECG (minutes)[3]	11	10	9	7
Average Time to Transfer (minutes)[1,3]	-	-	62	60
Children's Asthma Care				
Received Home Management Plan of Care	-	-	88%	88%
Received Reliever Medication	-	-	100%	100%
Received Systemic Corticosteroids	-	-	100%	100%
Emergency Department				
Admittance Decision Time (minutes)[2]	387	130	125	98
Head CT Results Within 45 Min. of Arrival[1,3]	-	-	55%	57%
Patients Who Left ER Before Being Seen	7,801	3%	3%	2%
Time from ER Arrival to Admit. (minutes)[2]	403	312	323	274
Time from ER Arrival to Discharge (minutes)	401	130	168	134
Time in ER Before Being Evaluated (minutes)	395	33	29	26
Time to Pain Meds for Fractures (minutes)	47	61	62	57
Heart Attack Care				
Aspirin Given at Discharge[5]	-	-	99%	99%
Fibrinolytic Meds Within 30 Min. of Arrival[5]	-	-	73%	54%
PCI Within 90 Minutes of Arrival[5]	-	-	95%	96%
Statin Prescribed at Discharge[5]	-	-	98%	98%
Heart Failure Care				
ACE Inhibitor or ARB for LVSD[1,3]	-	-	97%	97%
Discharge Instructions Given[3]	20	100%	94%	94%
Evaluation of LVS Function[3]	23	96%	99%	99%
Medicare Spending				
Medicare Spending per Patient (ratio)	-	0.94	0.98	0.98
Pneumonia Care				
Appropriate Initial Antibiotic Given	39	95%	97%	95%
Blood Culture Timing	47	96%	98%	98%
Pregnancy and Delivery Care				
Newborn Deliveries Scheduled Early[7]	-	-	5%	6%
Preventive Care				
Immunization for Influenza[2]	327	99%	89%	90%
Immunization for Pneumonia[2]	473	95%	90%	92%
Stroke Care				
Anticoagulation Therapy for Atrial Fibrillation[1]	-	-	95%	95%
Antithrombotic Therapy Timing[1]	-	-	98%	98%
Assessed for Rehabilitation	20	95%	97%	97%
Discharged on Antithrombotic Therapy	20	100%	99%	99%
Discharged on Statin Medication	16	100%	94%	94%
Thrombolytic Therapy Timing[1]	-	-	72%	66%
Venous Thromboembolism Prophylaxis	18	89%	94%	94%
Written Stroke Educational Materials Given	12	83%	87%	88%
Surgical Care Improvement Project				
Appropriate Beta Blocker Usage[2]	26	88%	97%	98%
Appropriate VTP Within 24 Hours[2]	129	95%	98%	98%
Controlled Postoperative Blood Glucose[2,7]	-	-	96%	97%
Perioperative Temperature Management[2]	138	100%	100%	100%
Prophylactic Antibiotic Selection[2]	116	100%	99%	99%
Prophylactic Antibiotic Selection (Outpatient)[5]	-	-	97%	98%
Prophylactic Antibiotic Stopped[2]	115	99%	98%	98%
Prophylactic Antibiotic Timing[2]	116	94%	99%	99%
Prophylactic Antibiotic Timing (Outpatient)[5]	-	-	97%	98%
Urinary Catheter Removal[2]	44	95%	97%	97%
Survey of Patients' Hospital Experiences				
Area Around Room 'Always' Quiet at Night	(a)	51%	51%	61%
Doctors 'Always' Communicated Well	(a)	81%	78%	82%
Home Recovery Information Given	(a)	85%	83%	85%
Hospital Given 9 or 10 on 10 Point Scale	(a)	70%	68%	71%
Meds 'Always' Explained Before Given	(a)	66%	61%	64%
Nurses 'Always' Communicated Well	(a)	79%	74%	79%
Pain 'Always' Well Controlled	(a)	70%	68%	71%
Room and Bathroom 'Always' Clean	(a)	75%	70%	73%
Timely Help 'Always' Received	(a)	69%	62%	68%
Would Definitely Recommend Hospital	(a)	79%	70%	71%
Use of Medical Imaging				
Cardiac Imaging Stress Test before Surgery[7]	-	-	5.2%	5.3%
Combination Abdominal CT Scan	187	2.7%	13.4%	10.5%
Combination Brain/Sinus CT Scan[1]	-	-	2.2%	2.7%

NOTE: Hospital profiles are in alphabetical order by state, then city, then hospital within the city; Rankings exclude hospitals with less than 25 cases except for patient surveys which excludes hospitals with less than 100 cases; (a) 100-299 cases; (1) The number of cases/patients is too few to report; (2) Data submitted were based on a sample of cases/patients; (3) Results are based on a shorter time period than required; (4) Data suppressed by CMS for one or more quarters; (5) Results are not available for this reporting period; (6) Fewer than 100 patients completed the HCAHPS survey; (7) No cases met the criteria for this measure; (8) The lower limit of the confidence interval cannot be calculated if the number of observed infections equals zero; (9) No data are available from the state/territory for this reporting period; (10) The scores shown reflect fewer than 50 completed surveys; (11) There were discrepancies in the data collection process; (12) This measure does not apply to this hospital for this reporting period; (13) Results cannot be calculated for this reporting period; (14) The results for this state are combined with nearby states to protect confidentiality; Please refer to the User's Guide for a full explanation of data.

Measure	Cases	This Hosp.	State Avg.	U.S. Avg.
Combination Chest CT Scan	75	1.3%	2.3%	2.7%
Follow-up Mammogram/Ultrasound	299	10.7%	8.2%	8.8%
Lumbar Spine MRI for Low Back Pain[1]	-	-	34.2%	37.2%

Sherman Oaks Hospital

4929 Van Nuys Blvd
Sherman Oaks, CA 91403
Phone: 818-981-7111
Fax: 818-907-4539
E-mail: info@shermanoakshospital.com
URL: www.shermanoakshospital.com
Type: Acute Care Hospitals
Emergency Services: Yes
Ownership: Voluntary non-profit - Private
Beds: 153

Key Personnel:
Chair/CEO . . . . Sandeep Bhatia, MD
CEO/President. . . . . Dr. Prem Reddy, MBA, MHA
Chief of Medical Staff . . . . J. Nathan Rubin, MD

Measure	Cases	This Hosp.	State Avg.	U.S. Avg.
Blood Clot Prevention and Treatment				
Anticoagulation Overlap Therapy[2]	11	91%	92%	93%
ICU Venous Thromboembolism Prophylaxis[2]	65	91%	92%	92%
Incidence of Potentially Preventable VTE[1,2]	-	-	11%	10%
UFH with Dosages/Platelet Monitoring[1,2]	-	-	96%	97%
Venous Thromboembolism Prophylaxis[2]	306	63%	83%	85%
Warfarin Therapy Discharge Instructions[1,2]	-	-	75%	75%
Chest Pain/Possible Heart Attack Care				
Aspirin Given Within 24 Hours of Arrival	29	100%	97%	96%
Fibrinolytic Meds Within 30 Min. of Arrival[7]	-	-	62%	58%
Average Time to ECG (minutes)	29	9	9	7
Average Time to Transfer (minutes)	12	73	62	60
Children's Asthma Care				
Received Home Management Plan of Care	-	-	88%	88%
Received Reliever Medication	-	-	100%	100%
Received Systemic Corticosteroids	-	-	100%	100%
Emergency Department				
Admittance Decision Time (minutes)[2]	654	110	125	98
Head CT Results Within 45 Min. of Arrival[7]	-	-	55%	57%
Patients Who Left ER Before Being Seen	20,962	1%	3%	2%
Time from ER Arrival to Admit. (minutes)[2]	655	211	323	274
Time from ER Arrival to Discharge (minutes)	320	107	168	134
Time in ER Before Being Evaluated (minutes)	380	14	29	26
Time to Pain Meds for Fractures (minutes)	117	40	62	57
Heart Attack Care				
Aspirin Given at Discharge	65	100%	99%	99%
Fibrinolytic Meds Within 30 Min. of Arrival[7]	-	-	73%	54%
PCI Within 90 Minutes of Arrival[7]	-	-	95%	96%
Statin Prescribed at Discharge	55	100%	98%	98%
Heart Failure Care				
ACE Inhibitor or ARB for LVSD	13	92%	97%	97%
Discharge Instructions Given	76	100%	94%	94%
Evaluation of LVS Function	104	98%	99%	99%
Medicare Spending				
Medicare Spending per Patient (ratio)	-	1.08	0.98	0.98
Pneumonia Care				
Appropriate Initial Antibiotic Given	65	94%	97%	95%
Blood Culture Timing	147	99%	98%	98%
Pregnancy and Delivery Care				
Newborn Deliveries Scheduled Early[7]	-	-	5%	6%
Preventive Care				
Immunization for Influenza[2]	365	100%	89%	90%
Immunization for Pneumonia[2]	499	100%	90%	92%
Stroke Care				
Anticoagulation Therapy for Atrial Fibrillation[1]	-	-	95%	95%
Antithrombotic Therapy Timing	11	100%	98%	98%
Assessed for Rehabilitation	11	82%	97%	97%
Discharged on Antithrombotic Therapy	11	100%	99%	99%
Discharged on Statin Medication[1]	-	-	94%	94%
Thrombolytic Therapy Timing[7]	-	-	72%	66%
Venous Thromboembolism Prophylaxis	11	100%	94%	94%
Written Stroke Educational Materials Given[1]	-	-	87%	88%
Surgical Care Improvement Project				
Appropriate Beta Blocker Usage	22	91%	97%	98%
Appropriate VTP Within 24 Hours	107	100%	98%	98%
Controlled Postoperative Blood Glucose[7]	-	-	96%	97%
Perioperative Temperature Management	114	100%	100%	100%
Prophylactic Antibiotic Selection	76	99%	99%	99%
Prophylactic Antibiotic Selection (Outpatient)[1]	-	-	97%	98%
Prophylactic Antibiotic Stopped	76	100%	98%	98%
Prophylactic Antibiotic Timing	76	100%	99%	99%
Prophylactic Antibiotic Timing (Outpatient)[1]	-	-	97%	98%
Urinary Catheter Removal	54	98%	97%	97%
Survey of Patients' Hospital Experiences				
Area Around Room 'Always' Quiet at Night[11]	(a)	49%	51%	61%
Doctors 'Always' Communicated Well[11]	(a)	69%	78%	82%
Home Recovery Information Given[11]	(a)	79%	83%	85%
Hospital Given 9 or 10 on 10 Point Scale[11]	(a)	54%	68%	71%
Meds 'Always' Explained Before Given[11]	(a)	56%	61%	64%
Nurses 'Always' Communicated Well[11]	(a)	64%	74%	79%
Pain 'Always' Well Controlled[11]	(a)	57%	68%	71%
Room and Bathroom 'Always' Clean[11]	(a)	67%	70%	73%
Timely Help 'Always' Received[11]	(a)	46%	62%	68%
Would Definitely Recommend Hospital[11]	(a)	45%	70%	71%
Use of Medical Imaging				
Cardiac Imaging Stress Test before Surgery	66	6.1%	5.2%	5.3%
Combination Abdominal CT Scan	174	1.1%	13.4%	10.5%
Combination Brain/Sinus CT Scan[1]	-	-	2.2%	2.7%
Combination Chest CT Scan[1]	-	-	2.3%	2.7%
Follow-up Mammogram/Ultrasound[7]	-	-	8.2%	8.8%
Lumbar Spine MRI for Low Back Pain[7]	-	-	34.2%	37.2%

Simi Valley Hospital & Health Care Services

2975 N Sycamore Dr
Simi Valley, CA 93065
Phone: 805-955-6000
Fax: 805-526-0837
URL: www.simivalleyhospital.com
Type: Acute Care Hospitals
Emergency Services: Yes
Ownership: Voluntary non-profit - Church
Beds: 185

Key Personnel:
Radiology. . . . . Robert Acquarelli, MD
Infection Control. . . . . Ken Archulet
Emergency Room . . . . Peter Cho, MD
Operating Room. . . . . KwanHo Chong
Chief of Medical Staff. . . . . Jonathan Kurohara
Patient Relations . . . . Susan Myers
CEO/President. . . . . Darwin Remboldt
Quality Assurance . . . . Vicki Vander Toorn

Measure	Cases	This Hosp.	State Avg.	U.S. Avg.
Blood Clot Prevention and Treatment				
Anticoagulation Overlap Therapy[2]	42	98%	92%	93%
ICU Venous Thromboembolism Prophylaxis[2]	64	84%	92%	92%
Incidence of Potentially Preventable VTE[1,2]	-	-	11%	10%
UFH with Dosages/Platelet Monitoring[1,2]	-	-	96%	97%
Venous Thromboembolism Prophylaxis[2]	312	77%	83%	85%
Warfarin Therapy Discharge Instructions[2]	30	83%	75%	75%
Chest Pain/Possible Heart Attack Care				
Aspirin Given Within 24 Hours of Arrival	78	100%	97%	96%
Fibrinolytic Meds Within 30 Min. of Arrival[7]	-	-	62%	58%
Average Time to ECG (minutes)	83	6	9	7
Average Time to Transfer (minutes)	14	30	62	60
Children's Asthma Care				
Received Home Management Plan of Care	-	-	88%	88%
Received Reliever Medication	-	-	100%	100%
Received Systemic Corticosteroids	-	-	100%	100%
Emergency Department				
Admittance Decision Time (minutes)[2]	771	116	125	98
Head CT Results Within 45 Min. of Arrival	12	67%	55%	57%
Patients Who Left ER Before Being Seen	30,155	0%	3%	2%
Time from ER Arrival to Admit. (minutes)[2]	772	259	323	274
Time from ER Arrival to Discharge (minutes)	368	151	168	134
Time in ER Before Being Evaluated (minutes)	408	12	29	26
Time to Pain Meds for Fractures (minutes)	90	41	62	57
Heart Attack Care				
Aspirin Given at Discharge	13	100%	99%	99%
Fibrinolytic Meds Within 30 Min. of Arrival[7]	-	-	73%	54%
PCI Within 90 Minutes of Arrival[7]	-	-	95%	96%
Statin Prescribed at Discharge	15	100%	98%	98%
Heart Failure Care				
ACE Inhibitor or ARB for LVSD	17	100%	97%	97%
Discharge Instructions Given	76	97%	94%	94%
Evaluation of LVS Function	88	100%	99%	99%
Medicare Spending				
Medicare Spending per Patient (ratio)	-	1.02	0.98	0.98
Pneumonia Care				
Appropriate Initial Antibiotic Given	76	95%	97%	95%
Blood Culture Timing	125	99%	98%	98%
Pregnancy and Delivery Care				
Newborn Deliveries Scheduled Early[2]	26	4%	5%	6%
Preventive Care				
Immunization for Influenza[2]	504	96%	89%	90%
Immunization for Pneumonia[2]	555	95%	90%	92%
Stroke Care				
Anticoagulation Therapy for Atrial Fibrillation	12	92%	95%	95%
Antithrombotic Therapy Timing	48	98%	98%	98%
Assessed for Rehabilitation	60	97%	97%	97%
Discharged on Antithrombotic Therapy	52	96%	99%	99%
Discharged on Statin Medication	44	91%	94%	94%
Thrombolytic Therapy Timing[1]	-	-	72%	66%
Venous Thromboembolism Prophylaxis	63	94%	94%	94%
Written Stroke Educational Materials Given	38	82%	87%	88%
Surgical Care Improvement Project				
Appropriate Beta Blocker Usage[2]	67	87%	97%	98%
Appropriate VTP Within 24 Hours[2]	266	94%	98%	98%
Controlled Postoperative Blood Glucose[2,7]	-	-	96%	97%
Perioperative Temperature Management[2]	322	99%	100%	100%
Prophylactic Antibiotic Selection[2]	193	96%	99%	99%
Prophylactic Antibiotic Selection (Outpatient)	50	96%	97%	98%
Prophylactic Antibiotic Stopped[2]	187	94%	98%	98%
Prophylactic Antibiotic Timing[2]	193	99%	99%	99%
Prophylactic Antibiotic Timing (Outpatient)	50	96%	97%	98%
Urinary Catheter Removal[2]	169	86%	97%	97%
Survey of Patients' Hospital Experiences				
Area Around Room 'Always' Quiet at Night	300+	56%	51%	61%
Doctors 'Always' Communicated Well	300+	76%	78%	82%
Home Recovery Information Given	300+	83%	83%	85%
Hospital Given 9 or 10 on 10 Point Scale	300+	70%	68%	71%
Meds 'Always' Explained Before Given	300+	61%	61%	64%
Nurses 'Always' Communicated Well	300+	71%	74%	79%
Pain 'Always' Well Controlled	300+	66%	68%	71%
Room and Bathroom 'Always' Clean	300+	75%	70%	73%
Timely Help 'Always' Received	300+	62%	62%	68%
Would Definitely Recommend Hospital	300+	69%	70%	71%
Use of Medical Imaging				
Cardiac Imaging Stress Test before Surgery[1]	-	-	5.2%	5.3%
Combination Abdominal CT Scan	566	14.7%	13.4%	10.5%
Combination Brain/Sinus CT Scan	426	0.5%	2.2%	2.7%
Combination Chest CT Scan	210	0.0%	2.3%	2.7%
Follow-up Mammogram/Ultrasound	1,025	11.2%	8.2%	8.8%
Lumbar Spine MRI for Low Back Pain	53	30.2%	34.2%	37.2%

Santa Ynez Valley Cottage Hospital

2050 Viborg Rd
Solvang, CA 93463
Phone: 805-688-6431
Fax: 805-686-5561
E-mail: bkline@sbch.org
URL: www.cottagehealthsystem.org
Type: Critical Access Hospitals
Emergency Services: Yes
Ownership: Voluntary non-profit - Private
Beds: 20

Key Personnel:
Radiology. . . . . James M Benzian
Patient Relations . . . . Herb Geary
Chief of Medical Staff . . . . Laurel Hansch
Pediatric Ambulatory Care . . . . . . Gina Randal
Pediatric In-Patient Care . . . . Gina Randall
Infection Control. . . . . Leslie Stanfield
Anesthesiology. . . . . Kathryn Von Dollen
CEO/President. . . . . Ronald C Werft

Measure	Cases	This Hosp.	State Avg.	U.S. Avg.
Blood Clot Prevention and Treatment				
Anticoagulation Overlap Therapy[1,2]	-	-	92%	93%
ICU Venous Thromboembolism Prophylaxis[2,7]	-	-	92%	92%
Incidence of Potentially Preventable VTE[1,2]	-	-	11%	10%
UFH with Dosages/Platelet Monitoring[2,7]	-	-	96%	97%
Venous Thromboembolism Prophylaxis[2]	112	85%	83%	85%
Warfarin Therapy Discharge Instructions[1,2]	-	-	75%	75%
Chest Pain/Possible Heart Attack Care				

NOTE: Hospital profiles are in alphabetical order by state, then city, then hospital within the city; Rankings exclude hospitals with less than 25 cases except for patient surveys which excludes hospitals with less than 100 cases; (a) 100-299 cases; (1) The number of cases/patients is too few to report; (2) Data submitted were based on a sample of cases/patients; (3) Results are based on a shorter time period than required; (4) Data suppressed by CMS for one or more quarters; (5) Results are not available for this reporting period; (6) Fewer than 100 patients completed the HCAHPS survey; (7) No cases met the criteria for this measure; (8) The lower limit of the confidence interval cannot be calculated if the number of observed infections equals zero; (9) No data are available from the state/territory for this reporting period; (10) The scores shown reflect fewer than 50 completed surveys; (11) There were discrepancies in the data collection process; (12) This measure does not apply to this hospital for this reporting period; (13) Results cannot be calculated for this reporting period; (14) The results for this state are combined with nearby states to protect confidentiality; Please refer to the User's Guide for a full explanation of data.

Measure	Cases	This Hosp.	State Avg.	U.S. Avg.
Aspirin Given Within 24 Hours of Arrival	34	97%	97%	96%
Fibrinolytic Meds Within 30 Min. of Arrival[7]	-	-	62%	58%
Average Time to ECG (minutes)	35	5	9	7
Average Time to Transfer (minutes)[1]	-	-	62	60
Children's Asthma Care				
Received Home Management Plan of Care	-	-	88%	88%
Received Reliever Medication	-	-	100%	100%
Received Systemic Corticosteroids	-	-	100%	100%
Emergency Department				
Admittance Decision Time (minutes)	175	77	125	98
Head CT Results Within 45 Min. of Arrival[1]	-	-	55%	57%
Patients Who Left ER Before Being Seen	6,696	0%	3%	2%
Time from ER Arrival to Admit. (minutes)	175	252	323	274
Time from ER Arrival to Discharge (minutes)	364	113	168	134
Time in ER Before Being Evaluated (minutes)	384	16	29	26
Time to Pain Meds for Fractures (minutes)	33	19	62	57
Heart Attack Care				
Aspirin Given at Discharge[3,7]	-	-	99%	99%
Fibrinolytic Meds Within 30 Min. of Arrival[3,7]	-	-	73%	54%
PCI Within 90 Minutes of Arrival[3,7]	-	-	95%	96%
Statin Prescribed at Discharge[3,7]	-	-	98%	98%
Heart Failure Care				
ACE Inhibitor or ARB for LVSD[1]	-	-	97%	97%
Discharge Instructions Given	12	100%	94%	94%
Evaluation of LVS Function	14	100%	99%	99%
Medicare Spending				
Medicare Spending per Patient (ratio)	-	-	0.98	0.98
Pneumonia Care				
Appropriate Initial Antibiotic Given[1]	-	-	97%	95%
Blood Culture Timing	22	100%	98%	98%
Pregnancy and Delivery Care				
Newborn Deliveries Scheduled Early[3,7]	-	-	5%	6%
Preventive Care				
Immunization for Influenza	112	94%	89%	90%
Immunization for Pneumonia	169	95%	90%	92%
Stroke Care				
Anticoagulation Therapy for Atrial Fibrillation[1,3]	-	-	95%	95%
Antithrombotic Therapy Timing[1,3]	-	-	98%	98%
Assessed for Rehabilitation[1,3]	-	-	97%	97%
Discharged on Antithrombotic Therapy[1,3]	-	-	99%	99%
Discharged on Statin Medication[1,3]	-	-	94%	94%
Thrombolytic Therapy Timing[1,3]	-	-	72%	66%
Venous Thromboembolism Prophylaxis[1,3]	-	-	94%	94%
Written Stroke Educational Materials Given[1,3]	-	-	87%	88%
Surgical Care Improvement Project				
Appropriate Beta Blocker Usage[5]	-	-	97%	98%
Appropriate VTP Within 24 Hours[5]	-	-	98%	98%
Controlled Postoperative Blood Glucose[5]	-	-	96%	97%
Perioperative Temperature Management[5]	-	-	100%	100%
Prophylactic Antibiotic Selection[5]	-	-	99%	99%
Prophylactic Antibiotic Selection (Outpatient)[1]	-	-	97%	98%
Prophylactic Antibiotic Stopped[5]	-	-	98%	98%
Prophylactic Antibiotic Timing[5]	-	-	99%	99%
Prophylactic Antibiotic Timing (Outpatient)[1]	-	-	97%	98%
Urinary Catheter Removal[5]	-	-	97%	97%
Survey of Patients' Hospital Experiences				
Area Around Room 'Always' Quiet at Night[6]	<100	94%	51%	61%
Doctors 'Always' Communicated Well[6]	<100	98%	78%	82%
Home Recovery Information Given[6]	<100	91%	83%	85%
Hospital Given 9 or 10 on 10 Point Scale[6]	<100	97%	68%	71%
Meds 'Always' Explained Before Given[6]	<100	84%	61%	64%
Nurses 'Always' Communicated Well[6]	<100	95%	74%	79%
Pain 'Always' Well Controlled[6]	<100	94%	68%	71%
Room and Bathroom 'Always' Clean[6]	<100	94%	70%	73%
Timely Help 'Always' Received[6]	<100	98%	62%	68%
Would Definitely Recommend Hospital[6]	<100	97%	70%	71%
Use of Medical Imaging				
Cardiac Imaging Stress Test before Surgery[7]	-	-	5.2%	5.3%
Combination Abdominal CT Scan	349	14.3%	13.4%	10.5%
Combination Brain/Sinus CT Scan[1]	-	-	2.2%	2.7%
Combination Chest CT Scan	272	0.7%	2.3%	2.7%
Follow-up Mammogram/Ultrasound	454	4.8%	8.2%	8.8%
Lumbar Spine MRI for Low Back Pain	39	41.0%	34.2%	37.2%

Sonoma Valley Hospital

347 Andrieux St
Sonoma, CA 95476
Phone: 707-935-5000
Fax: 707-938-0166
E-mail: administration@svh.com.
URL: www.svh.com
Type: Acute Care Hospitals
Emergency Services: Yes
Ownership: Govt - Hospital Dist/Auth
Beds: 49

Key Personnel:

Radiology. . . . . Tom Atkin
Anesthesiology. . . . . Phyllis Carter
Patient Relations . . . . Mary Kelly, RN
CEO/President. . . . . Jim McSweeney
Chair/CEO . . . . Sharon Nevins

Measure	Cases	This Hosp.	State Avg.	U.S. Avg.
Blood Clot Prevention and Treatment				
Anticoagulation Overlap Therapy[1,2]	-	-	92%	93%
ICU Venous Thromboembolism Prophylaxis[2]	44	91%	92%	92%
Incidence of Potentially Preventable VTE[2,7]	-	-	11%	10%
UFH with Dosages/Platelet Monitoring[2,7]	-	-	96%	97%
Venous Thromboembolism Prophylaxis[2]	85	94%	83%	85%
Warfarin Therapy Discharge Instructions[1,2]	-	-	75%	75%
Chest Pain/Possible Heart Attack Care				
Aspirin Given Within 24 Hours of Arrival	21	95%	97%	96%
Fibrinolytic Meds Within 30 Min. of Arrival[7]	-	-	62%	58%
Average Time to ECG (minutes)	20	13	9	7
Average Time to Transfer (minutes)[1]	-	-	62	60
Children's Asthma Care				
Received Home Management Plan of Care	-	-	88%	88%
Received Reliever Medication	-	-	100%	100%
Received Systemic Corticosteroids	-	-	100%	100%
Emergency Department				
Admittance Decision Time (minutes)[2]	168	45	125	98
Head CT Results Within 45 Min. of Arrival[1]	-	-	55%	57%
Patients Who Left ER Before Being Seen	9,492	2%	3%	2%
Time from ER Arrival to Admit. (minutes)[2]	269	257	323	274
Time from ER Arrival to Discharge (minutes)	360	124	168	134
Time in ER Before Being Evaluated (minutes)	44	14	29	26
Time to Pain Meds for Fractures (minutes)	61	63	62	57
Heart Attack Care				
Aspirin Given at Discharge[1,3]	-	-	99%	99%
Fibrinolytic Meds Within 30 Min. of Arrival[3,7]	-	-	73%	54%
PCI Within 90 Minutes of Arrival[3,7]	-	-	95%	96%
Statin Prescribed at Discharge[1,3]	-	-	98%	98%
Heart Failure Care				
ACE Inhibitor or ARB for LVSD[1]	-	-	97%	97%
Discharge Instructions Given	18	89%	94%	94%
Evaluation of LVS Function	31	100%	99%	99%
Medicare Spending				
Medicare Spending per Patient (ratio)	-	0.87	0.98	0.98
Pneumonia Care				
Appropriate Initial Antibiotic Given	29	93%	97%	95%
Blood Culture Timing	47	98%	98%	98%
Pregnancy and Delivery Care				
Newborn Deliveries Scheduled Early[1]	-	-	5%	6%
Preventive Care				
Immunization for Influenza[2]	286	92%	89%	90%
Immunization for Pneumonia[2]	348	88%	90%	92%
Stroke Care				
Anticoagulation Therapy for Atrial Fibrillation[1]	-	-	95%	95%
Antithrombotic Therapy Timing	21	95%	98%	98%
Assessed for Rehabilitation	22	100%	97%	97%
Discharged on Antithrombotic Therapy	21	100%	99%	99%
Discharged on Statin Medication	19	100%	94%	94%
Thrombolytic Therapy Timing[1]	-	-	72%	66%
Venous Thromboembolism Prophylaxis	26	96%	94%	94%
Written Stroke Educational Materials Given[1]	-	-	87%	88%
Surgical Care Improvement Project				
Appropriate Beta Blocker Usage	23	100%	97%	98%
Appropriate VTP Within 24 Hours	124	99%	98%	98%
Controlled Postoperative Blood Glucose[7]	-	-	96%	97%
Perioperative Temperature Management	139	100%	100%	100%
Prophylactic Antibiotic Selection	96	99%	99%	99%
Prophylactic Antibiotic Selection (Outpatient)	30	100%	97%	98%
Prophylactic Antibiotic Stopped	93	99%	98%	98%
Prophylactic Antibiotic Timing	96	99%	99%	99%
Prophylactic Antibiotic Timing (Outpatient)	30	93%	97%	98%
Urinary Catheter Removal	108	98%	97%	97%
Survey of Patients' Hospital Experiences				
Area Around Room 'Always' Quiet at Night	(a)	50%	51%	61%
Doctors 'Always' Communicated Well	(a)	79%	78%	82%
Home Recovery Information Given	(a)	86%	83%	85%
Hospital Given 9 or 10 on 10 Point Scale	(a)	63%	68%	71%
Meds 'Always' Explained Before Given	(a)	63%	61%	64%
Nurses 'Always' Communicated Well	(a)	76%	74%	79%
Pain 'Always' Well Controlled	(a)	72%	68%	71%
Room and Bathroom 'Always' Clean	(a)	69%	70%	73%
Timely Help 'Always' Received	(a)	67%	62%	68%
Would Definitely Recommend Hospital	(a)	67%	70%	71%
Use of Medical Imaging				
Cardiac Imaging Stress Test before Surgery	139	2.2%	5.2%	5.3%
Combination Abdominal CT Scan	265	8.3%	13.4%	10.5%
Combination Brain/Sinus CT Scan[1]	-	-	2.2%	2.7%
Combination Chest CT Scan	145	0.0%	2.3%	2.7%
Follow-up Mammogram/Ultrasound	800	5.3%	8.2%	8.8%
Lumbar Spine MRI for Low Back Pain	58	39.7%	34.2%	37.2%

Sonora Regional Medical Center

1000 Greenley Road
Sonora, CA 95370
Phone: 209-532-3161
Fax: 209-536-3500
URL: www.sonorahospital.org
Type: Acute Care Hospitals
Emergency Services: Yes
Ownership: Voluntary non-profit - Church
Beds: 152

Key Personnel:

Emergency Room . . . . Penny H Ablin, RN
Infection Control. . . . . Marti Carter, RN
Chief of Medical Staff . . . . Edward Clinite, DO
Quality Assurance . . . . Dixie Hukari
CEO/President. . . . . Andrew Jahn
Patient Relations . . . . Julie Kline, RN
Operating Room. . . . . Marylou Meersman
Radiology. . . . . Matthew J Nesper

Measure	Cases	This Hosp.	State Avg.	U.S. Avg.
Blood Clot Prevention and Treatment				
Anticoagulation Overlap Therapy[2]	53	100%	92%	93%
ICU Venous Thromboembolism Prophylaxis[2]	52	96%	92%	92%
Incidence of Potentially Preventable VTE[1,2]	-	-	11%	10%
UFH with Dosages/Platelet Monitoring[1,2]	-	-	96%	97%
Venous Thromboembolism Prophylaxis[2]	331	91%	83%	85%
Warfarin Therapy Discharge Instructions[2]	43	100%	75%	75%
Chest Pain/Possible Heart Attack Care				
Aspirin Given Within 24 Hours of Arrival	86	100%	97%	96%
Fibrinolytic Meds Within 30 Min. of Arrival	11	91%	62%	58%
Average Time to ECG (minutes)	86	11	9	7
Average Time to Transfer (minutes)[7]	-	-	62	60
Children's Asthma Care				
Received Home Management Plan of Care	-	-	88%	88%
Received Reliever Medication	-	-	100%	100%
Received Systemic Corticosteroids	-	-	100%	100%
Emergency Department				
Admittance Decision Time (minutes)[2]	446	129	125	98
Head CT Results Within 45 Min. of Arrival[1]	-	-	55%	57%
Patients Who Left ER Before Being Seen	26,725	1%	3%	2%
Time from ER Arrival to Admit. (minutes)[2]	635	297	323	274
Time from ER Arrival to Discharge (minutes)	289	159	168	134
Time in ER Before Being Evaluated (minutes)	372	18	29	26
Time to Pain Meds for Fractures (minutes)	145	75	62	57
Heart Attack Care				
Aspirin Given at Discharge	20	100%	99%	99%
Fibrinolytic Meds Within 30 Min. of Arrival[1]	-	-	73%	54%
PCI Within 90 Minutes of Arrival[7]	-	-	95%	96%
Statin Prescribed at Discharge	20	100%	98%	98%
Heart Failure Care				
ACE Inhibitor or ARB for LVSD	22	95%	97%	97%
Discharge Instructions Given	87	100%	94%	94%
Evaluation of LVS Function	97	99%	99%	99%
Medicare Spending				

NOTE: Hospital profiles are in alphabetical order by state, then city, then hospital within the city; Rankings exclude hospitals with less than 25 cases except for patient surveys which excludes hospitals with less than 100 cases; (a) 100-299 cases; (1) The number of cases/patients is too few to report; (2) Data submitted were based on a sample of cases/patients; (3) Results are based on a shorter time period than required; (4) Data suppressed by CMS for one or more quarters; (5) Results are not available for this reporting period; (6) Fewer than 100 patients completed the HCAHPS survey; (7) No cases met the criteria for this measure; (8) The lower limit of the confidence interval cannot be calculated if the number of observed infections equals zero; (9) No data are available from the state/territory for this reporting period; (10) The scores shown reflect fewer than 50 completed surveys; (11) There were discrepancies in the data collection process; (12) This measure does not apply to this hospital for this reporting period; (13) Results cannot be calculated for this reporting period; (14) The results for this state are combined with nearby states to protect confidentiality; Please refer to the User's Guide for a full explanation of data.

Measure	Cases	This Hosp.	State Avg.	U.S. Avg.
Medicare Spending per Patient (ratio)	-	0.85	0.98	0.98
Pneumonia Care				
Appropriate Initial Antibiotic Given	136	99%	97%	95%
Blood Culture Timing	197	99%	98%	98%
Pregnancy and Delivery Care				
Newborn Deliveries Scheduled Early[2]	21	0%	5%	6%
Preventive Care				
Immunization for Influenza[2]	450	97%	89%	90%
Immunization for Pneumonia[2]	552	97%	90%	92%
Stroke Care				
Anticoagulation Therapy for Atrial Fibrillation[1]	-	-	95%	95%
Antithrombotic Therapy Timing	55	100%	98%	98%
Assessed for Rehabilitation	59	100%	97%	97%
Discharged on Antithrombotic Therapy	56	100%	99%	99%
Discharged on Statin Medication	47	96%	94%	94%
Thrombolytic Therapy Timing[7]	-	-	72%	66%
Venous Thromboembolism Prophylaxis	58	98%	94%	94%
Written Stroke Educational Materials Given	35	100%	87%	88%
Surgical Care Improvement Project				
Appropriate Beta Blocker Usage	100	100%	97%	98%
Appropriate VTP Within 24 Hours	359	99%	98%	98%
Controlled Postoperative Blood Glucose[7]	-	-	96%	97%
Perioperative Temperature Management	471	100%	100%	100%
Prophylactic Antibiotic Selection	361	99%	99%	99%
Prophylactic Antibiotic Selection (Outpatient)	133	95%	97%	98%
Prophylactic Antibiotic Stopped	350	99%	98%	98%
Prophylactic Antibiotic Timing	363	99%	99%	99%
Prophylactic Antibiotic Timing (Outpatient)	134	98%	97%	98%
Urinary Catheter Removal	320	99%	97%	97%
Survey of Patients' Hospital Experiences				
Area Around Room 'Always' Quiet at Night	300+	46%	51%	61%
Doctors 'Always' Communicated Well	300+	77%	78%	82%
Home Recovery Information Given	300+	87%	83%	85%
Hospital Given 9 or 10 on 10 Point Scale	300+	66%	68%	71%
Meds 'Always' Explained Before Given	300+	62%	61%	64%
Nurses 'Always' Communicated Well	300+	77%	74%	79%
Pain 'Always' Well Controlled	300+	68%	68%	71%
Room and Bathroom 'Always' Clean	300+	76%	70%	73%
Timely Help 'Always' Received	300+	67%	62%	68%
Would Definitely Recommend Hospital	300+	67%	70%	71%
Use of Medical Imaging				
Cardiac Imaging Stress Test before Surgery	533	4.1%	5.2%	5.3%
Combination Abdominal CT Scan	859	6.9%	13.4%	10.5%
Combination Brain/Sinus CT Scan	729	1.5%	2.2%	2.7%
Combination Chest CT Scan	406	0.2%	2.3%	2.7%
Follow-up Mammogram/Ultrasound	2,401	9.5%	8.2%	8.8%
Lumbar Spine MRI for Low Back Pain	277	28.5%	34.2%	37.2%

Greater El Monte Community Hospital

1701 Santa Anita Ave
South El Monte, CA 91733
Phone: 626-350-7975
Fax: 626-350-0368
URL: www.greaterelmonte.com
Type: Acute Care Hospitals
Emergency Services: No
Ownership: Voluntary non-profit - Private
Beds: 117

Key Personnel:
CEO/President. . . . . Philip A Cohen

Measure	Cases	This Hosp.	State Avg.	U.S. Avg.
Blood Clot Prevention and Treatment				
Anticoagulation Overlap Therapy[1,2]	-	-	92%	93%
ICU Venous Thromboembolism Prophylaxis[2]	47	74%	92%	92%
Incidence of Potentially Preventable VTE[1,2]	-	-	11%	10%
UFH with Dosages/Platelet Monitoring[1,2]	-	-	96%	97%
Venous Thromboembolism Prophylaxis[2]	176	78%	83%	85%
Warfarin Therapy Discharge Instructions[2,7]	-	-	75%	75%
Chest Pain/Possible Heart Attack Care				
Aspirin Given Within 24 Hours of Arrival[1,3]	-	-	97%	96%
Fibrinolytic Meds Within 30 Min. of Arrival[3,7]	-	-	62%	58%
Average Time to ECG (minutes)[1,3]	-	-	9	7
Average Time to Transfer (minutes)[3,7]	-	-	62	60
Children's Asthma Care				
Received Home Management Plan of Care	-	-	88%	88%
Received Reliever Medication	-	-	100%	100%
Received Systemic Corticosteroids	-	-	100%	100%
Emergency Department				
Admittance Decision Time (minutes)[2]	417	85	125	98
Head CT Results Within 45 Min. of Arrival[3,7]	-	-	55%	57%
Patients Who Left ER Before Being Seen	18,927	4%	3%	2%
Time from ER Arrival to Admit. (minutes)[2]	420	326	323	274
Time from ER Arrival to Discharge (minutes)	320	177	168	134
Time in ER Before Being Evaluated (minutes)	356	40	29	26
Time to Pain Meds for Fractures (minutes)	79	77	62	57
Heart Attack Care				
Aspirin Given at Discharge[1]	-	-	99%	99%
Fibrinolytic Meds Within 30 Min. of Arrival[7]	-	-	73%	54%
PCI Within 90 Minutes of Arrival[7]	-	-	95%	96%
Statin Prescribed at Discharge[1]	-	-	98%	98%
Heart Failure Care				
ACE Inhibitor or ARB for LVSD	23	96%	97%	97%
Discharge Instructions Given	63	83%	94%	94%
Evaluation of LVS Function	76	99%	99%	99%
Medicare Spending				
Medicare Spending per Patient (ratio)	-	1.23	0.98	0.98
Pneumonia Care				
Appropriate Initial Antibiotic Given[2]	31	100%	97%	95%
Blood Culture Timing[2]	110	98%	98%	98%
Pregnancy and Delivery Care				
Newborn Deliveries Scheduled Early[2]	43	5%	5%	6%
Preventive Care				
Immunization for Influenza[2]	375	67%	89%	90%
Immunization for Pneumonia[2]	259	96%	90%	92%
Stroke Care				
Anticoagulation Therapy for Atrial Fibrillation[1]	-	-	95%	95%
Antithrombotic Therapy Timing	13	92%	98%	98%
Assessed for Rehabilitation	13	92%	97%	97%
Discharged on Antithrombotic Therapy	13	85%	99%	99%
Discharged on Statin Medication	11	64%	94%	94%
Thrombolytic Therapy Timing[7]	-	-	72%	66%
Venous Thromboembolism Prophylaxis	12	67%	94%	94%
Written Stroke Educational Materials Given[1]	-	-	87%	88%
Surgical Care Improvement Project				
Appropriate Beta Blocker Usage[1]	-	-	97%	98%
Appropriate VTP Within 24 Hours	42	81%	98%	98%
Controlled Postoperative Blood Glucose[7]	-	-	96%	97%
Perioperative Temperature Management	52	98%	100%	100%
Prophylactic Antibiotic Selection	18	100%	99%	99%
Prophylactic Antibiotic Selection (Outpatient)[1]	-	-	97%	98%
Prophylactic Antibiotic Stopped	18	100%	98%	98%
Prophylactic Antibiotic Timing	18	100%	99%	99%
Prophylactic Antibiotic Timing (Outpatient)[1]	-	-	97%	98%
Urinary Catheter Removal	13	92%	97%	97%
Survey of Patients' Hospital Experiences				
Area Around Room 'Always' Quiet at Night	300+	50%	51%	61%
Doctors 'Always' Communicated Well	300+	70%	78%	82%
Home Recovery Information Given	300+	79%	83%	85%
Hospital Given 9 or 10 on 10 Point Scale	300+	51%	68%	71%
Meds 'Always' Explained Before Given	300+	50%	61%	64%
Nurses 'Always' Communicated Well	300+	61%	74%	79%
Pain 'Always' Well Controlled	300+	57%	68%	71%
Room and Bathroom 'Always' Clean	300+	62%	70%	73%
Timely Help 'Always' Received	300+	51%	62%	68%
Would Definitely Recommend Hospital	300+	49%	70%	71%
Use of Medical Imaging				
Cardiac Imaging Stress Test before Surgery[1]	-	-	5.2%	5.3%
Combination Abdominal CT Scan[1]	-	-	13.4%	10.5%
Combination Brain/Sinus CT Scan[1]	-	-	2.2%	2.7%
Combination Chest CT Scan[1]	-	-	2.3%	2.7%
Follow-up Mammogram/Ultrasound[7]	-	-	8.2%	8.8%
Lumbar Spine MRI for Low Back Pain[7]	-	-	34.2%	37.2%

Barton Memorial Hospital

2170 South Avenue
South Lake Tahoe, CA 96150
Phone: 530-541-3420
Fax: 530-542-3740
E-mail: publicrelations@bartonhealth.org
URL: www.bartonhealth.org
Type: Acute Care Hospitals
Emergency Services: Yes
Ownership: Voluntary non-profit - Private
Beds: 75

Key Personnel:
Radiology. Jeffrey V Behar
Quality Assurance . . . . Katherine Biasotti
Emergency Room . . . . Peter Chau, MD
Operating Room. . . . . Gregory Eyre
Intensive Care Unit. . . . . Kenneth Harvey
Chief of Medical Staff . . . . Dr. Clint Purvance
Infection Control. . . . . Dawn Spicer
CEO/President. . . . . John G Williams

Measure	Cases	This Hosp.	State Avg.	U.S. Avg.
Blood Clot Prevention and Treatment				
Anticoagulation Overlap Therapy[2]	19	100%	92%	93%
ICU Venous Thromboembolism Prophylaxis[2]	45	98%	92%	92%
Incidence of Potentially Preventable VTE[1,2]	-	-	11%	10%
UFH with Dosages/Platelet Monitoring[1,2]	-	-	96%	97%
Venous Thromboembolism Prophylaxis[2]	148	97%	83%	85%
Warfarin Therapy Discharge Instructions[2]	16	94%	75%	75%
Chest Pain/Possible Heart Attack Care				
Aspirin Given Within 24 Hours of Arrival	34	94%	97%	96%
Fibrinolytic Meds Within 30 Min. of Arrival[7]	-	-	62%	58%
Average Time to ECG (minutes)	39	6	9	7
Average Time to Transfer (minutes)[1]	-	-	62	60
Children's Asthma Care				
Received Home Management Plan of Care	-	-	88%	88%
Received Reliever Medication	-	-	100%	100%
Received Systemic Corticosteroids	-	-	100%	100%
Emergency Department				
Admittance Decision Time (minutes)[2]	270	134	125	98
Head CT Results Within 45 Min. of Arrival[1]	-	-	55%	57%
Patients Who Left ER Before Being Seen	19,024	2%	3%	2%
Time from ER Arrival to Admit. (minutes)[2]	272	284	323	274
Time from ER Arrival to Discharge (minutes)	349	131	168	134
Time in ER Before Being Evaluated (minutes)	376	24	29	26
Time to Pain Meds for Fractures (minutes)	133	54	62	57
Heart Attack Care				
Aspirin Given at Discharge[1]	-	-	99%	99%
Fibrinolytic Meds Within 30 Min. of Arrival[7]	-	-	73%	54%
PCI Within 90 Minutes of Arrival[7]	-	-	95%	96%
Statin Prescribed at Discharge[1]	-	-	98%	98%
Heart Failure Care				
ACE Inhibitor or ARB for LVSD	13	100%	97%	97%
Discharge Instructions Given	43	77%	94%	94%
Evaluation of LVS Function	45	98%	99%	99%
Medicare Spending				
Medicare Spending per Patient (ratio)	-	0.87	0.98	0.98
Pneumonia Care				
Appropriate Initial Antibiotic Given	48	92%	97%	95%
Blood Culture Timing	83	99%	98%	98%
Pregnancy and Delivery Care				
Newborn Deliveries Scheduled Early[2]	27	0%	5%	6%
Preventive Care				
Immunization for Influenza[2]	256	96%	89%	90%
Immunization for Pneumonia[2]	236	95%	90%	92%
Stroke Care				
Anticoagulation Therapy for Atrial Fibrillation[1,2]	-	-	95%	95%
Antithrombotic Therapy Timing[1,2]	-	-	98%	98%
Assessed for Rehabilitation[1,2]	-	-	97%	97%
Discharged on Antithrombotic Therapy[1,2]	-	-	99%	99%
Discharged on Statin Medication[1,2]	-	-	94%	94%
Thrombolytic Therapy Timing[1,2]	-	-	72%	66%
Venous Thromboembolism Prophylaxis[1,2]	-	-	94%	94%
Written Stroke Educational Materials Given[1,2]	-	-	87%	88%
Surgical Care Improvement Project				
Appropriate Beta Blocker Usage	40	95%	97%	98%
Appropriate VTP Within 24 Hours	225	99%	98%	98%
Controlled Postoperative Blood Glucose[7]	-	-	96%	97%
Perioperative Temperature Management	245	100%	100%	100%

NOTE: Hospital profiles are in alphabetical order by state, then city, then hospital within the city; Rankings exclude hospitals with less than 25 cases except for patient surveys which excludes hospitals with less than 100 cases; (a) 100-299 cases; (1) The number of cases/patients is too few to report; (2) Data submitted were based on a sample of cases/patients; (3) Results are based on a shorter time period than required; (4) Data suppressed by CMS for one or more quarters; (5) Results are not available for this reporting period; (6) Fewer than 100 patients completed the HCAHPS survey; (7) No cases met the criteria for this measure; (8) The lower limit of the confidence interval cannot be calculated if the number of observed infections equals zero; (9) No data are available from the state/territory for this reporting period; (10) The scores shown reflect fewer than 50 completed surveys; (11) There were discrepancies in the data collection process; (12) This measure does not apply to this hospital for this reporting period; (13) Results cannot be calculated for this reporting period; (14) The results for this state are combined with nearby states to protect confidentiality; Please refer to the User's Guide for a full explanation of data.

Measure	Cases	This Hosp.	State Avg.	U.S. Avg.
Prophylactic Antibiotic Selection	183	100%	99%	99%
Prophylactic Antibiotic Selection (Outpatient)	87	99%	97%	98%
Prophylactic Antibiotic Stopped	180	99%	98%	98%
Prophylactic Antibiotic Timing	183	100%	99%	99%
Prophylactic Antibiotic Timing (Outpatient)	89	96%	97%	98%
Urinary Catheter Removal	207	100%	97%	97%
Survey of Patients' Hospital Experiences				
Area Around Room 'Always' Quiet at Night	300+	53%	51%	61%
Doctors 'Always' Communicated Well	300+	79%	78%	82%
Home Recovery Information Given	300+	91%	83%	85%
Hospital Given 9 or 10 on 10 Point Scale	300+	71%	68%	71%
Meds 'Always' Explained Before Given	300+	64%	61%	64%
Nurses 'Always' Communicated Well	300+	76%	74%	79%
Pain 'Always' Well Controlled	300+	71%	68%	71%
Room and Bathroom 'Always' Clean	300+	80%	70%	73%
Timely Help 'Always' Received	300+	69%	62%	68%
Would Definitely Recommend Hospital	300+	71%	70%	71%
Use of Medical Imaging				
Cardiac Imaging Stress Test before Surgery	210	5.2%	5.2%	5.3%
Combination Abdominal CT Scan	300	8.7%	13.4%	10.5%
Combination Brain/Sinus CT Scan[1]	-	-	2.2%	2.7%
Combination Chest CT Scan	230	3.0%	2.3%	2.7%
Follow-up Mammogram/Ultrasound	533	8.1%	8.2%	8.8%
Lumbar Spine MRI for Low Back Pain	60	41.7%	34.2%	37.2%

Kaiser Foundation Hospital - South San Francisco

1200 El Camino Real
South San Francisco, CA 94080
Phone: 650-742-3200
Fax: 888-805-7562
URL: www.healthy.kaiserpermanente.org
Type: Acute Care Hospitals
Emergency Services: Yes
Ownership: Voluntary non-profit - Private
Beds: 127

Key Personnel:

Operating Room. . . . . Ramzi Alami
Radiology. . . . . Amita Bhandari, MD
Quality Assurance . . . . Michelle Caughey, MD
Intensive Care Unit. . . . . Tommy Farley
Anesthesiology. . . . . Hamid Motamed
Infection Control. . . . . Ronald Tempesta, MD
Chief of Medical Staff . . . . Laurie Weisberg, MD

Measure	Cases	This Hosp.	State Avg.	U.S. Avg.
Blood Clot Prevention and Treatment				
Anticoagulation Overlap Therapy[2]	37	100%	92%	93%
ICU Venous Thromboembolism Prophylaxis[2]	69	100%	92%	92%
Incidence of Potentially Preventable VTE[1,2]	-	-	11%	10%
UFH with Dosages/Platelet Monitoring[2]	21	100%	96%	97%
Venous Thromboembolism Prophylaxis[2]	272	98%	83%	85%
Warfarin Therapy Discharge Instructions[2]	34	82%	75%	75%
Chest Pain/Possible Heart Attack Care				
Aspirin Given Within 24 Hours of Arrival	-	-	97%	96%
Fibrinolytic Meds Within 30 Min. of Arrival	-	-	62%	58%
Average Time to ECG (minutes)	-	-	9	7
Average Time to Transfer (minutes)	-	-	62	60
Children's Asthma Care				
Received Home Management Plan of Care	-	-	88%	88%
Received Reliever Medication	-	-	100%	100%
Received Systemic Corticosteroids	-	-	100%	100%
Emergency Department				
Admittance Decision Time (minutes)[2]	624	44	125	98
Head CT Results Within 45 Min. of Arrival	-	-	55%	57%
Patients Who Left ER Before Being Seen	-	-	3%	2%
Time from ER Arrival to Admit. (minutes)[2]	624	247	323	274
Time from ER Arrival to Discharge (minutes)	-	-	168	134
Time in ER Before Being Evaluated (minutes)	-	-	29	26
Time to Pain Meds for Fractures (minutes)	-	-	62	57
Heart Attack Care				
Aspirin Given at Discharge	25	100%	99%	99%
Fibrinolytic Meds Within 30 Min. of Arrival[7]	-	-	73%	54%
PCI Within 90 Minutes of Arrival[7]	-	-	95%	96%
Statin Prescribed at Discharge	26	100%	98%	98%
Heart Failure Care				
ACE Inhibitor or ARB for LVSD	38	100%	97%	97%
Discharge Instructions Given	187	100%	94%	94%
Evaluation of LVS Function	198	100%	99%	99%
Medicare Spending				
Medicare Spending per Patient (ratio)	-	0.73	0.98	0.98
Pneumonia Care				
Appropriate Initial Antibiotic Given[2]	88	100%	97%	95%
Blood Culture Timing[2]	127	98%	98%	98%
Pregnancy and Delivery Care				
Newborn Deliveries Scheduled Early[7]	-	-	5%	6%
Preventive Care				
Immunization for Influenza[2]	547	97%	89%	90%
Immunization for Pneumonia[2]	793	99%	90%	92%
Stroke Care				
Anticoagulation Therapy for Atrial Fibrillation[2]	12	100%	95%	95%
Antithrombotic Therapy Timing[2]	76	100%	98%	98%
Assessed for Rehabilitation[2]	83	100%	97%	97%
Discharged on Antithrombotic Therapy[2]	68	100%	99%	99%
Discharged on Statin Medication[2]	56	100%	94%	94%
Thrombolytic Therapy Timing[1,2]	-	-	72%	66%
Venous Thromboembolism Prophylaxis[2]	96	100%	94%	94%
Written Stroke Educational Materials Given[2]	46	100%	87%	88%
Surgical Care Improvement Project				
Appropriate Beta Blocker Usage[2]	156	97%	97%	98%
Appropriate VTP Within 24 Hours[2]	351	99%	98%	98%
Controlled Postoperative Blood Glucose[2,7]	-	-	96%	97%
Perioperative Temperature Management[2]	382	100%	100%	100%
Prophylactic Antibiotic Selection[2]	250	100%	99%	99%
Prophylactic Antibiotic Selection (Outpatient)	-	-	97%	98%
Prophylactic Antibiotic Stopped[2]	247	100%	98%	98%
Prophylactic Antibiotic Timing[2]	250	100%	99%	99%
Prophylactic Antibiotic Timing (Outpatient)	-	-	97%	98%
Urinary Catheter Removal[2]	284	100%	97%	97%
Survey of Patients' Hospital Experiences				
Area Around Room 'Always' Quiet at Night	300+	45%	51%	61%
Doctors 'Always' Communicated Well	300+	82%	78%	82%
Home Recovery Information Given	300+	86%	83%	85%
Hospital Given 9 or 10 on 10 Point Scale	300+	73%	68%	71%
Meds 'Always' Explained Before Given	300+	65%	61%	64%
Nurses 'Always' Communicated Well	300+	78%	74%	79%
Pain 'Always' Well Controlled	300+	73%	68%	71%
Room and Bathroom 'Always' Clean	300+	72%	70%	73%
Timely Help 'Always' Received	300+	67%	62%	68%
Would Definitely Recommend Hospital	300+	76%	70%	71%
Use of Medical Imaging				
Cardiac Imaging Stress Test before Surgery	-	-	5.2%	5.3%
Combination Abdominal CT Scan	-	-	13.4%	10.5%
Combination Brain/Sinus CT Scan	-	-	2.2%	2.7%
Combination Chest CT Scan	-	-	2.3%	2.7%
Follow-up Mammogram/Ultrasound	-	-	8.2%	8.8%
Lumbar Spine MRI for Low Back Pain	-	-	34.2%	37.2%

Stanford Hospital

300 Pasteur Drive
Stanford, CA 94305
Phone: 650-723-5708
Fax: 650-723-0074
URL: www.stanfordhospital.com
Type: Acute Care Hospitals
Emergency Services: Yes
Ownership: Voluntary non-profit - Private
Beds: 613

Key Personnel:

Radiology. . . . . Scott Alan Alexander
Chief of Medical Staff . . . . Bryan D Bohman, MD
Operating Room. . . . . Jay Brodsky, MD
Patient Relations . . . . Cindy Day
CEO/President. . . . . Martha Marsh
Ambulatory Care . . . . Gerald Shefren, MD
Quality Assurance . . . . Kevin Tabb, MD

Measure	Cases	This Hosp.	State Avg.	U.S. Avg.
Blood Clot Prevention and Treatment				
Anticoagulation Overlap Therapy[2]	116	96%	92%	93%
ICU Venous Thromboembolism Prophylaxis[2]	63	95%	92%	92%
Incidence of Potentially Preventable VTE[2]	76	5%	11%	10%
UFH with Dosages/Platelet Monitoring[2]	103	98%	96%	97%
Venous Thromboembolism Prophylaxis[2]	314	75%	83%	85%
Warfarin Therapy Discharge Instructions[2]	98	48%	75%	75%
Chest Pain/Possible Heart Attack Care				
Aspirin Given Within 24 Hours of Arrival[1]	-	-	97%	96%
Fibrinolytic Meds Within 30 Min. of Arrival[5]	-	-	62%	58%
Average Time to ECG (minutes)[1]	-	-	9	7
Average Time to Transfer (minutes)[5]	-	-	62	60
Children's Asthma Care				
Received Home Management Plan of Care	-	-	88%	88%
Received Reliever Medication	-	-	100%	100%
Received Systemic Corticosteroids	-	-	100%	100%
Emergency Department				
Admittance Decision Time (minutes)[2]	409	152	125	98
Head CT Results Within 45 Min. of Arrival[1]	-	-	55%	57%
Patients Who Left ER Before Being Seen	54,101	0%	3%	2%
Time from ER Arrival to Admit. (minutes)[2]	414	348	323	274
Time from ER Arrival to Discharge (minutes)	363	210	168	134
Time in ER Before Being Evaluated (minutes)	400	27	29	26
Time to Pain Meds for Fractures (minutes)	326	59	62	57
Heart Attack Care				
Aspirin Given at Discharge	184	100%	99%	99%
Fibrinolytic Meds Within 30 Min. of Arrival[7]	-	-	73%	54%
PCI Within 90 Minutes of Arrival	27	89%	95%	96%
Statin Prescribed at Discharge	179	99%	98%	98%
Heart Failure Care				
ACE Inhibitor or ARB for LVSD	127	99%	97%	97%
Discharge Instructions Given	292	99%	94%	94%
Evaluation of LVS Function	326	100%	99%	99%
Medicare Spending				
Medicare Spending per Patient (ratio)	-	0.99	0.98	0.98
Pneumonia Care				
Appropriate Initial Antibiotic Given	126	98%	97%	95%
Blood Culture Timing	319	100%	98%	98%
Pregnancy and Delivery Care				
Newborn Deliveries Scheduled Early[1]	-	-	5%	6%
Preventive Care				
Immunization for Influenza[2]	613	98%	89%	90%
Immunization for Pneumonia[2]	722	99%	90%	92%
Stroke Care				
Anticoagulation Therapy for Atrial Fibrillation	46	98%	95%	95%
Antithrombotic Therapy Timing	119	96%	98%	98%
Assessed for Rehabilitation	289	98%	97%	97%
Discharged on Antithrombotic Therapy	180	100%	99%	99%
Discharged on Statin Medication	150	97%	94%	94%
Thrombolytic Therapy Timing	20	100%	72%	66%
Venous Thromboembolism Prophylaxis	287	99%	94%	94%
Written Stroke Educational Materials Given	163	94%	87%	88%
Surgical Care Improvement Project				
Appropriate Beta Blocker Usage[2]	220	100%	97%	98%
Appropriate VTP Within 24 Hours[2]	590	99%	98%	98%
Controlled Postoperative Blood Glucose[2]	175	95%	96%	97%
Perioperative Temperature Management[2]	705	100%	100%	100%
Prophylactic Antibiotic Selection[2]	588	99%	99%	99%
Prophylactic Antibiotic Selection (Outpatient)	691	98%	97%	98%
Prophylactic Antibiotic Stopped[2]	564	99%	98%	98%
Prophylactic Antibiotic Timing[2]	588	99%	99%	99%
Prophylactic Antibiotic Timing (Outpatient)	637	97%	97%	98%
Urinary Catheter Removal[2]	458	100%	97%	97%
Survey of Patients' Hospital Experiences				
Area Around Room 'Always' Quiet at Night	300+	39%	51%	61%
Doctors 'Always' Communicated Well	300+	85%	78%	82%
Home Recovery Information Given	300+	87%	83%	85%
Hospital Given 9 or 10 on 10 Point Scale	300+	79%	68%	71%
Meds 'Always' Explained Before Given	300+	64%	61%	64%
Nurses 'Always' Communicated Well	300+	82%	74%	79%
Pain 'Always' Well Controlled	300+	70%	68%	71%
Room and Bathroom 'Always' Clean	300+	72%	70%	73%
Timely Help 'Always' Received	300+	68%	62%	68%
Would Definitely Recommend Hospital	300+	85%	70%	71%
Use of Medical Imaging				
Cardiac Imaging Stress Test before Surgery	1,107	6.9%	5.2%	5.3%
Combination Abdominal CT Scan	2,654	7.6%	13.4%	10.5%
Combination Brain/Sinus CT Scan	972	3.5%	2.2%	2.7%
Combination Chest CT Scan	3,376	0.2%	2.3%	2.7%
Follow-up Mammogram/Ultrasound	1,127	7.0%	8.2%	8.8%
Lumbar Spine MRI for Low Back Pain	317	35.3%	34.2%	37.2%

NOTE: Hospital profiles are in alphabetical order by state, then city, then hospital within the city; Rankings exclude hospitals with less than 25 cases except for patient surveys which excludes hospitals with less than 100 cases; (a) 100-299 cases; (1) The number of cases/patients is too few to report; (2) Data submitted were based on a sample of cases/patients; (3) Results are based on a shorter time period than required; (4) Data suppressed by CMS for one or more quarters; (5) Results are not available for this reporting period; (6) Fewer than 100 patients completed the HCAHPS survey; (7) No cases met the criteria for this measure; (8) The lower limit of the confidence interval cannot be calculated if the number of observed infections equals zero; (9) No data are available from the state/territory for this reporting period; (10) The scores shown reflect fewer than 50 completed surveys; (11) There were discrepancies in the data collection process; (12) This measure does not apply to this hospital for this reporting period; (13) Results cannot be calculated for this reporting period; (14) The results for this state are combined with nearby states to protect confidentiality; Please refer to the User's Guide for a full explanation of data.

Dameron Hospital

525 West Acacia Street
Stockton, CA 95203
E-mail: info@dameronhospital.org
URL: www.dameronhospital.org
Type: Acute Care Hospitals
Ownership: Voluntary non-profit - Other
Phone: 209-944-5550
Fax: 209-461-7578
Emergency Services: Yes
Beds: 188

Key Personnel:
CEO/President. . . . . Christopher Arismendi, MD
Infection Control. . . . . Linda Knowles, RN
Quality Assurance . . . . Mark Koenig
Chief of Medical Staff. . . . . Robert Lawrence, MD
Operating Room. . . . . Sandra Mayer, RN
Pediatric Ambulatory Care . . . . . . Carolyn Sanders, RN
Pediatric In-Patient Care . . . . Carolyn Sanders
Patient Relations . . . . Marla Scott, RN

Measure	Cases	This Hosp.	State Avg.	U.S. Avg.
Blood Clot Prevention and Treatment				
Anticoagulation Overlap Therapy[2]	47	100%	92%	93%
ICU Venous Thromboembolism Prophylaxis[2]	106	94%	92%	92%
Incidence of Potentially Preventable VTE[1,2]	-	-	11%	10%
UFH with Dosages/Platelet Monitoring[2]	34	100%	96%	97%
Venous Thromboembolism Prophylaxis[2]	277	90%	83%	85%
Warfarin Therapy Discharge Instructions[2]	36	100%	75%	75%
Chest Pain/Possible Heart Attack Care				
Aspirin Given Within 24 Hours of Arrival[1,3]	-	-	97%	96%
Fibrinolytic Meds Within 30 Min. of Arrival[3,7]	-	-	62%	58%
Average Time to ECG (minutes)[1,3]	-	-	9	7
Average Time to Transfer (minutes)[3,7]	-	-	62	60
Children's Asthma Care				
Received Home Management Plan of Care	-	-	88%	88%
Received Reliever Medication	-	-	100%	100%
Received Systemic Corticosteroids	-	-	100%	100%
Emergency Department				
Admittance Decision Time (minutes)[2]	531	152	125	98
Head CT Results Within 45 Min. of Arrival[1]	-	-	55%	57%
Patients Who Left ER Before Being Seen	43,601	0%	3%	2%
Time from ER Arrival to Admit. (minutes)[2]	531	333	323	274
Time from ER Arrival to Discharge (minutes)	336	154	168	134
Time in ER Before Being Evaluated (minutes)	384	10	29	26
Time to Pain Meds for Fractures (minutes)	121	64	62	57
Heart Attack Care				
Aspirin Given at Discharge	261	99%	99%	99%
Fibrinolytic Meds Within 30 Min. of Arrival[1]	-	-	73%	54%
PCI Within 90 Minutes of Arrival	26	88%	95%	96%
Statin Prescribed at Discharge	266	97%	98%	98%
Heart Failure Care				
ACE Inhibitor or ARB for LVSD	60	95%	97%	97%
Discharge Instructions Given	149	100%	94%	94%
Evaluation of LVS Function	187	100%	99%	99%
Medicare Spending				
Medicare Spending per Patient (ratio)	-	1.02	0.98	0.98
Pneumonia Care				
Appropriate Initial Antibiotic Given	96	98%	97%	95%
Blood Culture Timing	179	100%	98%	98%
Pregnancy and Delivery Care				
Newborn Deliveries Scheduled Early	90	1%	5%	6%
Preventive Care				
Immunization for Influenza[2]	480	96%	89%	90%
Immunization for Pneumonia[2]	542	99%	90%	92%
Stroke Care				
Anticoagulation Therapy for Atrial Fibrillation[1]	-	-	95%	95%
Antithrombotic Therapy Timing	57	100%	98%	98%
Assessed for Rehabilitation	61	100%	97%	97%
Discharged on Antithrombotic Therapy	58	100%	99%	99%
Discharged on Statin Medication	47	91%	94%	94%
Thrombolytic Therapy Timing[7]	-	-	72%	66%
Venous Thromboembolism Prophylaxis	62	92%	94%	94%
Written Stroke Educational Materials Given	32	100%	87%	88%
Surgical Care Improvement Project				
Appropriate Beta Blocker Usage	190	99%	97%	98%
Appropriate VTP Within 24 Hours	610	100%	98%	98%
Controlled Postoperative Blood Glucose	11	82%	96%	97%
Perioperative Temperature Management	658	100%	100%	100%
Prophylactic Antibiotic Selection	522	100%	99%	99%
Prophylactic Antibiotic Selection (Outpatient)	116	99%	97%	98%
Prophylactic Antibiotic Stopped	522	100%	98%	98%
Prophylactic Antibiotic Timing	522	99%	99%	99%
Prophylactic Antibiotic Timing (Outpatient)	116	99%	97%	98%
Urinary Catheter Removal	544	100%	97%	97%
Survey of Patients' Hospital Experiences				
Area Around Room 'Always' Quiet at Night	300+	48%	51%	61%
Doctors 'Always' Communicated Well	300+	78%	78%	82%
Home Recovery Information Given	300+	84%	83%	85%
Hospital Given 9 or 10 on 10 Point Scale	300+	67%	68%	71%
Meds 'Always' Explained Before Given	300+	63%	61%	64%
Nurses 'Always' Communicated Well	300+	75%	74%	79%
Pain 'Always' Well Controlled	300+	70%	68%	71%
Room and Bathroom 'Always' Clean	300+	73%	70%	73%
Timely Help 'Always' Received	300+	63%	62%	68%
Would Definitely Recommend Hospital	300+	67%	70%	71%
Use of Medical Imaging				
Cardiac Imaging Stress Test before Surgery	127	3.1%	5.2%	5.3%
Combination Abdominal CT Scan	309	0.0%	13.4%	10.5%
Combination Brain/Sinus CT Scan[1]	-	-	2.2%	2.7%
Combination Chest CT Scan	101	0.0%	2.3%	2.7%
Follow-up Mammogram/Ultrasound[7]	-	-	8.2%	8.8%
Lumbar Spine MRI for Low Back Pain[7]	-	-	34.2%	37.2%

Saint Joseph's Medical Center of Stockton

1800 N California St
Stockton, CA 95204
URL: www.stjospehscares.org
Type: Acute Care Hospitals
Ownership: Voluntary non-profit - Church
Phone: 209-943-2000
Fax: 209-461-3299
Emergency Services: Yes
Beds: 294

Key Personnel:
Operating Room. . . . . Barbara Chalmers, RN
Pediatric Ambulatory Care . . . . . . Norma Espiritu, MD
Pediatric In-Patient Care . . . . Norma Espiritu, MD
Radiology. . . . . Jack Funamura, MD
Chief of Medical Staff. . . . . Masanobu Kamigaki, MD
Quality Assurance . . . . Liz Mitchell
CEO/President. . . . . Donald Wiley

Measure	Cases	This Hosp.	State Avg.	U.S. Avg.
Blood Clot Prevention and Treatment				
Anticoagulation Overlap Therapy[2]	69	91%	92%	93%
ICU Venous Thromboembolism Prophylaxis[2]	118	100%	92%	92%
Incidence of Potentially Preventable VTE[1,2]	-	-	11%	10%
UFH with Dosages/Platelet Monitoring[2]	81	100%	96%	97%
Venous Thromboembolism Prophylaxis[2]	368	98%	83%	85%
Warfarin Therapy Discharge Instructions[2]	43	100%	75%	75%
Chest Pain/Possible Heart Attack Care				
Aspirin Given Within 24 Hours of Arrival[1,3]	-	-	97%	96%
Fibrinolytic Meds Within 30 Min. of Arrival[5]	-	-	62%	58%
Average Time to ECG (minutes)[1,3]	-	-	9	7
Average Time to Transfer (minutes)[5]	-	-	62	60
Children's Asthma Care				
Received Home Management Plan of Care	-	-	88%	88%
Received Reliever Medication	-	-	100%	100%
Received Systemic Corticosteroids	-	-	100%	100%
Emergency Department				
Admittance Decision Time (minutes)[2]	730	180	125	98
Head CT Results Within 45 Min. of Arrival	17	82%	55%	57%
Patients Who Left ER Before Being Seen	54,159	1%	3%	2%
Time from ER Arrival to Admit. (minutes)[2]	734	390	323	274
Time from ER Arrival to Discharge (minutes)	385	163	168	134
Time in ER Before Being Evaluated (minutes)	422	19	29	26
Time to Pain Meds for Fractures (minutes)	151	61	62	57
Heart Attack Care				
Aspirin Given at Discharge	326	100%	99%	99%
Fibrinolytic Meds Within 30 Min. of Arrival[1]	-	-	73%	54%
PCI Within 90 Minutes of Arrival	40	100%	95%	96%
Statin Prescribed at Discharge	323	100%	98%	98%
Heart Failure Care				
ACE Inhibitor or ARB for LVSD[2]	145	99%	97%	97%
Discharge Instructions Given[2]	231	96%	94%	94%
Evaluation of LVS Function[2]	314	100%	99%	99%
Medicare Spending				
Medicare Spending per Patient (ratio)	-	1.01	0.98	0.98
Pneumonia Care				
Appropriate Initial Antibiotic Given[2]	85	96%	97%	95%
Blood Culture Timing[2]	158	98%	98%	98%
Pregnancy and Delivery Care				
Newborn Deliveries Scheduled Early[2]	72	0%	5%	6%
Preventive Care				
Immunization for Influenza[2]	515	91%	89%	90%
Immunization for Pneumonia[2]	641	95%	90%	92%
Stroke Care				
Anticoagulation Therapy for Atrial Fibrillation[2]	11	100%	95%	95%
Antithrombotic Therapy Timing[2]	94	95%	98%	98%
Assessed for Rehabilitation[2]	100	97%	97%	97%
Discharged on Antithrombotic Therapy[2]	88	98%	99%	99%
Discharged on Statin Medication[2]	72	96%	94%	94%
Thrombolytic Therapy Timing[1,2]	-	-	72%	66%
Venous Thromboembolism Prophylaxis[2]	112	95%	94%	94%
Written Stroke Educational Materials Given[2]	45	93%	87%	88%
Surgical Care Improvement Project				
Appropriate Beta Blocker Usage[2]	218	100%	97%	98%
Appropriate VTP Within 24 Hours[2]	338	98%	98%	98%
Controlled Postoperative Blood Glucose[2]	181	98%	96%	97%
Perioperative Temperature Management[2]	565	100%	100%	100%
Prophylactic Antibiotic Selection[2]	460	99%	99%	99%
Prophylactic Antibiotic Selection (Outpatient)	248	98%	97%	98%
Prophylactic Antibiotic Stopped[2]	448	98%	98%	98%
Prophylactic Antibiotic Timing[2]	461	100%	99%	99%
Prophylactic Antibiotic Timing (Outpatient)	249	99%	97%	98%
Urinary Catheter Removal[2]	263	98%	97%	97%
Survey of Patients' Hospital Experiences				
Area Around Room 'Always' Quiet at Night	300+	48%	51%	61%
Doctors 'Always' Communicated Well	300+	75%	78%	82%
Home Recovery Information Given	300+	81%	83%	85%
Hospital Given 9 or 10 on 10 Point Scale	300+	64%	68%	71%
Meds 'Always' Explained Before Given	300+	58%	61%	64%
Nurses 'Always' Communicated Well	300+	71%	74%	79%
Pain 'Always' Well Controlled	300+	67%	68%	71%
Room and Bathroom 'Always' Clean	300+	64%	70%	73%
Timely Help 'Always' Received	300+	56%	62%	68%
Would Definitely Recommend Hospital	300+	68%	70%	71%
Use of Medical Imaging				
Cardiac Imaging Stress Test before Surgery	50	2.0%	5.2%	5.3%
Combination Abdominal CT Scan	873	2.6%	13.4%	10.5%
Combination Brain/Sinus CT Scan	994	2.5%	2.2%	2.7%
Combination Chest CT Scan	349	2.0%	2.3%	2.7%
Follow-up Mammogram/Ultrasound	1,722	6.5%	8.2%	8.8%
Lumbar Spine MRI for Low Back Pain	55	38.2%	34.2%	37.2%

Menifee Valley Medical Center

28400 Mccall B0ulevard
Sun City, CA 92585
URL: www.valleyhealthsystem.com
Type: Acute Care Hospitals
Ownership: Govt - Hospital Dist/Auth
Phone: 951-679-8888
Fax: 951-672-7050
Emergency Services: Yes
Beds: 84

Key Personnel:
CEO/President. . . . . Fred Harper
Chief of Medical Staff. . . . . Surendra Sharma, MD
Quality Assurance . . . . Lynda Wills, RN
Operating Room. . . . . Denise Wilson-Allen, RN
Radiology. . . . . Thavinsak di Vir, MD

Measure	Cases	This Hosp.	State Avg.	U.S. Avg.
Blood Clot Prevention and Treatment				
Anticoagulation Overlap Therapy[2]	22	55%	92%	93%
ICU Venous Thromboembolism Prophylaxis[2]	61	61%	92%	92%
Incidence of Potentially Preventable VTE[1,2]	-	-	11%	10%
UFH with Dosages/Platelet Monitoring[1,2]	-	-	96%	97%
Venous Thromboembolism Prophylaxis[2]	293	52%	83%	85%
Warfarin Therapy Discharge Instructions[2]	12	50%	75%	75%
Chest Pain/Possible Heart Attack Care				
Aspirin Given Within 24 Hours of Arrival	27	96%	97%	96%
Fibrinolytic Meds Within 30 Min. of Arrival[7]	-	-	62%	58%
Average Time to ECG (minutes)	27	0	9	7
Average Time to Transfer (minutes)[1]	-	-	62	60

NOTE: Hospital profiles are in alphabetical order by state, then city, then hospital within the city; Rankings exclude hospitals with less than 25 cases except for patient surveys which excludes hospitals with less than 100 cases; (a) 100-299 cases; (1) The number of cases/patients is too few to report; (2) Data submitted were based on a sample of cases/patients; (3) Results are based on a shorter time period than required; (4) Data suppressed by CMS for one or more quarters; (5) Results are not available for this reporting period; (6) Fewer than 100 patients completed the HCAHPS survey; (7) No cases met the criteria for this measure; (8) The lower limit of the confidence interval cannot be calculated if the number of observed infections equals zero; (9) No data are available from the state/territory for this reporting period; (10) The scores shown reflect fewer than 50 completed surveys; (11) There were discrepancies in the data collection process; (12) This measure does not apply to this hospital for this reporting period; (13) Results cannot be calculated for this reporting period; (14) The results for this state are combined with nearby states to protect confidentiality; Please refer to the User's Guide for a full explanation of data.

Measure	Cases	This Hosp.	State Avg.	U.S. Avg.
Children's Asthma Care				
Received Home Management Plan of Care	-	-	88%	88%
Received Reliever Medication	-	-	100%	100%
Received Systemic Corticosteroids	-	-	100%	100%
Emergency Department				
Admittance Decision Time (minutes)[2]	275	150	125	98
Head CT Results Within 45 Min. of Arrival[1,3]	-	-	55%	57%
Patients Who Left ER Before Being Seen	16,930	3%	3%	2%
Time from ER Arrival to Admit. (minutes)[2]	276	401	323	274
Time from ER Arrival to Discharge (minutes)	319	218	168	134
Time in ER Before Being Evaluated (minutes)	201	55	29	26
Time to Pain Meds for Fractures (minutes)	23	65	62	57
Heart Attack Care				
Aspirin Given at Discharge	37	95%	99%	99%
Fibrinolytic Meds Within 30 Min. of Arrival[7]	-	-	73%	54%
PCI Within 90 Minutes of Arrival[7]	-	-	95%	96%
Statin Prescribed at Discharge	36	92%	98%	98%
Heart Failure Care				
ACE Inhibitor or ARB for LVSD	45	87%	97%	97%
Discharge Instructions Given	107	89%	94%	94%
Evaluation of LVS Function	131	93%	99%	99%
Medicare Spending				
Medicare Spending per Patient (ratio)	-	0.98	0.98	0.98
Pneumonia Care				
Appropriate Initial Antibiotic Given[2]	66	95%	97%	95%
Blood Culture Timing[2]	93	99%	98%	98%
Pregnancy and Delivery Care				
Newborn Deliveries Scheduled Early[7]	-	-	5%	6%
Preventive Care				
Immunization for Influenza[2]	315	95%	89%	90%
Immunization for Pneumonia[2]	494	89%	90%	92%
Stroke Care				
Anticoagulation Therapy for Atrial Fibrillation[1]	-	-	95%	95%
Antithrombotic Therapy Timing	52	96%	98%	98%
Assessed for Rehabilitation	50	88%	97%	97%
Discharged on Antithrombotic Therapy	48	98%	99%	99%
Discharged on Statin Medication	46	74%	94%	94%
Thrombolytic Therapy Timing[1]	-	-	72%	66%
Venous Thromboembolism Prophylaxis	53	57%	94%	94%
Written Stroke Educational Materials Given	22	23%	87%	88%
Surgical Care Improvement Project				
Appropriate Beta Blocker Usage[2]	70	90%	97%	98%
Appropriate VTP Within 24 Hours[2]	167	95%	98%	98%
Controlled Postoperative Blood Glucose[2,7]	-	-	96%	97%
Perioperative Temperature Management[2]	189	98%	100%	100%
Prophylactic Antibiotic Selection[2]	131	96%	99%	99%
Prophylactic Antibiotic Selection (Outpatient)	30	100%	97%	98%
Prophylactic Antibiotic Stopped[2]	121	83%	98%	98%
Prophylactic Antibiotic Timing[2]	133	91%	99%	99%
Prophylactic Antibiotic Timing (Outpatient)	31	97%	97%	98%
Urinary Catheter Removal[2]	106	94%	97%	97%
Survey of Patients' Hospital Experiences				
Area Around Room 'Always' Quiet at Night	300+	50%	51%	61%
Doctors 'Always' Communicated Well	300+	73%	78%	82%
Home Recovery Information Given	300+	79%	83%	85%
Hospital Given 9 or 10 on 10 Point Scale	300+	59%	68%	71%
Meds 'Always' Explained Before Given	300+	55%	61%	64%
Nurses 'Always' Communicated Well	300+	71%	74%	79%
Pain 'Always' Well Controlled	300+	62%	68%	71%
Room and Bathroom 'Always' Clean	300+	69%	70%	73%
Timely Help 'Always' Received	300+	59%	62%	68%
Would Definitely Recommend Hospital	300+	60%	70%	71%
Use of Medical Imaging				
Cardiac Imaging Stress Test before Surgery[1]	-	-	5.2%	5.3%
Combination Abdominal CT Scan	105	36.2%	13.4%	10.5%
Combination Brain/Sinus CT Scan[1]	-	-	2.2%	2.7%
Combination Chest CT Scan	51	0.0%	2.3%	2.7%
Follow-up Mammogram/Ultrasound	126	15.9%	8.2%	8.8%
Lumbar Spine MRI for Low Back Pain[7]	-	-	34.2%	37.2%

Pacifica Hospital of the Valley

9449 San Fernando Rd
Sun Valley, CA 91352
Phone: 818-767-3310
Fax: 818-252-2439
URL: www.pacificahospital.com
Type: Acute Care Hospitals
Emergency Services: Yes
Ownership: Proprietary
Beds: 248
Key Personnel:
Chief of Medical Staff. . . . . Allison Cunning
CEO/President. . . . . SK Durairaj
Emergency Room . . . . Jannet Latto

Measure	Cases	This Hosp.	State Avg.	U.S. Avg.
Blood Clot Prevention and Treatment				
Anticoagulation Overlap Therapy[1,2]	-	-	92%	93%
ICU Venous Thromboembolism Prophylaxis[2]	21	71%	92%	92%
Incidence of Potentially Preventable VTE[2,7]	-	-	11%	10%
UFH with Dosages/Platelet Monitoring[1,2]	-	-	96%	97%
Venous Thromboembolism Prophylaxis[2]	220	38%	83%	85%
Warfarin Therapy Discharge Instructions[1,2]	-	-	75%	75%
Chest Pain/Possible Heart Attack Care				
Aspirin Given Within 24 Hours of Arrival[1,3]	-	-	97%	96%
Fibrinolytic Meds Within 30 Min. of Arrival[3,7]	-	-	62%	58%
Average Time to ECG (minutes)[1,3]	-	-	9	7
Average Time to Transfer (minutes)[3,7]	-	-	62	60
Children's Asthma Care				
Received Home Management Plan of Care	-	-	88%	88%
Received Reliever Medication	-	-	100%	100%
Received Systemic Corticosteroids	-	-	100%	100%
Emergency Department				
Admittance Decision Time (minutes)[2]	435	97	125	98
Head CT Results Within 45 Min. of Arrival[1]	-	-	55%	57%
Patients Who Left ER Before Being Seen	12,756	4%	3%	2%
Time from ER Arrival to Admit. (minutes)[2]	445	103	323	274
Time from ER Arrival to Discharge (minutes)[3]	102	134	168	134
Time in ER Before Being Evaluated (minutes)	116	55	29	26
Time to Pain Meds for Fractures (minutes)	42	55	62	57
Heart Attack Care				
Aspirin Given at Discharge[1]	-	-	99%	99%
Fibrinolytic Meds Within 30 Min. of Arrival[1]	-	-	73%	54%
PCI Within 90 Minutes of Arrival[7]	-	-	95%	96%
Statin Prescribed at Discharge[1]	-	-	98%	98%
Heart Failure Care				
ACE Inhibitor or ARB for LVSD	18	94%	97%	97%
Discharge Instructions Given	54	56%	94%	94%
Evaluation of LVS Function	73	71%	99%	99%
Medicare Spending				
Medicare Spending per Patient (ratio)	-	1.11	0.98	0.98
Pneumonia Care				
Appropriate Initial Antibiotic Given	24	88%	97%	95%
Blood Culture Timing	53	91%	98%	98%
Pregnancy and Delivery Care				
Newborn Deliveries Scheduled Early[2]	139	15%	5%	6%
Preventive Care				
Immunization for Influenza[2]	496	16%	89%	90%
Immunization for Pneumonia[2]	419	13%	90%	92%
Stroke Care				
Anticoagulation Therapy for Atrial Fibrillation[1]	-	-	95%	95%
Antithrombotic Therapy Timing[1]	-	-	98%	98%
Assessed for Rehabilitation	20	75%	97%	97%
Discharged on Antithrombotic Therapy	17	94%	99%	99%
Discharged on Statin Medication	16	88%	94%	94%
Thrombolytic Therapy Timing[1]	-	-	72%	66%
Venous Thromboembolism Prophylaxis	21	71%	94%	94%
Written Stroke Educational Materials Given	12	92%	87%	88%
Surgical Care Improvement Project				
Appropriate Beta Blocker Usage[1]	-	-	97%	98%
Appropriate VTP Within 24 Hours	52	73%	98%	98%
Controlled Postoperative Blood Glucose[7]	-	-	96%	97%
Perioperative Temperature Management	62	85%	100%	100%
Prophylactic Antibiotic Selection	30	97%	99%	99%
Prophylactic Antibiotic Selection (Outpatient)[1]	-	-	97%	98%
Prophylactic Antibiotic Stopped	29	62%	98%	98%
Prophylactic Antibiotic Timing	30	83%	99%	99%
Prophylactic Antibiotic Timing (Outpatient)[1]	-	-	97%	98%
Urinary Catheter Removal	20	75%	97%	97%
Survey of Patients' Hospital Experiences				
Area Around Room 'Always' Quiet at Night	(a)	51%	51%	61%
Doctors 'Always' Communicated Well	(a)	76%	78%	82%
Home Recovery Information Given	(a)	73%	83%	85%
Hospital Given 9 or 10 on 10 Point Scale	(a)	60%	68%	71%
Meds 'Always' Explained Before Given	(a)	55%	61%	64%
Nurses 'Always' Communicated Well	(a)	72%	74%	79%
Pain 'Always' Well Controlled	(a)	71%	68%	71%
Room and Bathroom 'Always' Clean	(a)	73%	70%	73%
Timely Help 'Always' Received	(a)	59%	62%	68%
Would Definitely Recommend Hospital	(a)	57%	70%	71%
Use of Medical Imaging				
Cardiac Imaging Stress Test before Surgery[7]	-	-	5.2%	5.3%
Combination Abdominal CT Scan[1]	-	-	13.4%	10.5%
Combination Brain/Sinus CT Scan[1]	-	-	2.2%	2.7%
Combination Chest CT Scan[1]	-	-	2.3%	2.7%
Follow-up Mammogram/Ultrasound[7]	-	-	8.2%	8.8%
Lumbar Spine MRI for Low Back Pain[1]	-	-	34.2%	37.2%

Banner Lassen Medical Center

1800 Spring Ridge Drive
Susanville, CA 96130
Phone: 530-252-2000
Type: Critical Access Hospitals
Emergency Services: Yes
Ownership: Voluntary non-profit - Private
Key Personnel:
Infection Control. . . . . Brenda Bassett
Radiology. . . . . William Dockery, MD
Administrator . . . . Amanda Gonzalez
Anesthesiology. . . . . Richard Hrezo
Chief of Medical Staff . . . . Kevin Wheelan, MD
CEO/President. . . . . Elizabeth Woodyard

Measure	Cases	This Hosp.	State Avg.	U.S. Avg.
Blood Clot Prevention and Treatment				
Anticoagulation Overlap Therapy[5]	-	-	92%	93%
ICU Venous Thromboembolism Prophylaxis[5]	-	-	92%	92%
Incidence of Potentially Preventable VTE[5]	-	-	11%	10%
UFH with Dosages/Platelet Monitoring[5]	-	-	96%	97%
Venous Thromboembolism Prophylaxis[5]	-	-	83%	85%
Warfarin Therapy Discharge Instructions[5]	-	-	75%	75%
Chest Pain/Possible Heart Attack Care				
Aspirin Given Within 24 Hours of Arrival	32	97%	97%	96%
Fibrinolytic Meds Within 30 Min. of Arrival[1,3]	-	-	62%	58%
Average Time to ECG (minutes)	36	12	9	7
Average Time to Transfer (minutes)[3,7]	-	-	62	60
Children's Asthma Care				
Received Home Management Plan of Care	-	-	88%	88%
Received Reliever Medication	-	-	100%	100%
Received Systemic Corticosteroids	-	-	100%	100%
Emergency Department				
Admittance Decision Time (minutes)[5]	-	-	125	98
Head CT Results Within 45 Min. of Arrival[5]	-	-	55%	57%
Patients Who Left ER Before Being Seen	10,637	2%	3%	2%
Time from ER Arrival to Admit. (minutes)[5]	-	-	323	274
Time from ER Arrival to Discharge (minutes)[5]	-	-	168	134
Time in ER Before Being Evaluated (minutes)[5]	-	-	29	26
Time to Pain Meds for Fractures (minutes)[5]	-	-	62	57
Heart Attack Care				
Aspirin Given at Discharge[1,3]	-	-	99%	99%
Fibrinolytic Meds Within 30 Min. of Arrival[3,7]	-	-	73%	54%
PCI Within 90 Minutes of Arrival[3,7]	-	-	95%	96%
Statin Prescribed at Discharge[1,3]	-	-	98%	98%
Heart Failure Care				
ACE Inhibitor or ARB for LVSD[1]	-	-	97%	97%
Discharge Instructions Given	11	91%	94%	94%
Evaluation of LVS Function	12	100%	99%	99%
Medicare Spending				
Medicare Spending per Patient (ratio)	-	-	0.98	0.98
Pneumonia Care				
Appropriate Initial Antibiotic Given[2]	33	88%	97%	95%
Blood Culture Timing[2]	33	94%	98%	98%
Pregnancy and Delivery Care				
Newborn Deliveries Scheduled Early[3,7]	-	-	5%	6%
Preventive Care				

NOTE: Hospital profiles are in alphabetical order by state, then city, then hospital within the city; Rankings exclude hospitals with less than 25 cases except for patient surveys which excludes hospitals with less than 100 cases; (a) 100-299 cases; (1) The number of cases/patients is too few to report; (2) Data submitted were based on a sample of cases/patients; (3) Results are based on a shorter time period than required; (4) Data suppressed by CMS for one or more quarters; (5) Results are not available for this reporting period; (6) Fewer than 100 patients completed the HCAHPS survey; (7) No cases met the criteria for this measure; (8) The lower limit of the confidence interval cannot be calculated if the number of observed infections equals zero; (9) No data are available from the state/territory for this reporting period; (10) The scores shown reflect fewer than 50 completed surveys; (11) There were discrepancies in the data collection process; (12) This measure does not apply to this hospital for this reporting period; (13) Results cannot be calculated for this reporting period; (14) The results for this state are combined with nearby states to protect confidentiality; Please refer to the User's Guide for a full explanation of data.

Immunization for Influenza[5]	-	-	89%	90%
Immunization for Pneumonia[5]	-	-	90%	92%
Stroke Care				
Anticoagulation Therapy for Atrial Fibrillation[5]	-	-	95%	95%
Antithrombotic Therapy Timing[5]	-	-	98%	98%
Assessed for Rehabilitation[5]	-	-	97%	97%
Discharged on Antithrombotic Therapy[5]	-	-	99%	99%
Discharged on Statin Medication[5]	-	-	94%	94%
Thrombolytic Therapy Timing[5]	-	-	72%	66%
Venous Thromboembolism Prophylaxis[5]	-	-	94%	94%
Written Stroke Educational Materials Given[5]	-	-	87%	88%
Surgical Care Improvement Project				
Appropriate Beta Blocker Usage[1]	-	-	97%	98%
Appropriate VTP Within 24 Hours	18	89%	98%	98%
Controlled Postoperative Blood Glucose[7]	-	-	96%	97%
Perioperative Temperature Management	20	100%	100%	100%
Prophylactic Antibiotic Selection[1]	-	-	99%	99%
Prophylactic Antibiotic Selection (Outpatient)	16	94%	97%	98%
Prophylactic Antibiotic Stopped[1]	-	-	98%	98%
Prophylactic Antibiotic Timing[1]	-	-	99%	99%
Prophylactic Antibiotic Timing (Outpatient)	16	100%	97%	98%
Urinary Catheter Removal[1]	-	-	97%	97%
Survey of Patients' Hospital Experiences				
Area Around Room 'Always' Quiet at Night[11]	(a)	65%	51%	61%
Doctors 'Always' Communicated Well[11]	(a)	84%	78%	82%
Home Recovery Information Given[11]	(a)	91%	83%	85%
Hospital Given 9 or 10 on 10 Point Scale[11]	(a)	78%	68%	71%
Meds 'Always' Explained Before Given[11]	(a)	72%	61%	64%
Nurses 'Always' Communicated Well[11]	(a)	83%	74%	79%
Pain 'Always' Well Controlled[11]	(a)	76%	68%	71%
Room and Bathroom 'Always' Clean[11]	(a)	71%	70%	73%
Timely Help 'Always' Received[11]	(a)	74%	62%	68%
Would Definitely Recommend Hospital[11]	(a)	74%	70%	71%
Use of Medical Imaging				
Cardiac Imaging Stress Test before Surgery[1]	-	-	5.2%	5.3%
Combination Abdominal CT Scan	193	5.7%	13.4%	10.5%
Combination Brain/Sinus CT Scan	228	5.3%	2.2%	2.7%
Combination Chest CT Scan	91	0.0%	2.3%	2.7%
Follow-up Mammogram/Ultrasound	367	7.1%	8.2%	8.8%
Lumbar Spine MRI for Low Back Pain	42	47.6%	34.2%	37.2%

LAC/Olive View - UCLA Medical Center

14445 Olive View Drive
Sylmar, CA 91342
URL: www.ladhs.org
Type: Acute Care Hospitals
Ownership: Voluntary non-profit - Other
Phone: 818-364-1555
Fax: 818-364-4206
Emergency Services: Yes
Beds: 377

Key Personnel:
Operating Room. . . . . Zan Barney, RN
Anesthesiology. . . . . Selma H Calmes, MD
Quality Assurance . . . . Stephanie Johnson
Infection Control. . . . . Glenn Mathison, MD
CEO/President. . . . . Gretchen McGinley
Emergency Room . . . . David Talan, MD
Radiology. . . . . Ramesh Verma, MD
Chief of Medical Staff. . . . . Irwin Ziment, MD

Measure	Cases	This Hosp.	State Avg.	U.S. Avg.
Blood Clot Prevention and Treatment				
Anticoagulation Overlap Therapy[2]	53	96%	92%	93%
ICU Venous Thromboembolism Prophylaxis[2]	43	95%	92%	92%
Incidence of Potentially Preventable VTE[1,2]	-	-	11%	10%
UFH with Dosages/Platelet Monitoring[2]	60	95%	96%	97%
Venous Thromboembolism Prophylaxis[2]	304	87%	83%	85%
Warfarin Therapy Discharge Instructions[2]	42	74%	75%	75%
Chest Pain/Possible Heart Attack Care				
Aspirin Given Within 24 Hours of Arrival	28	96%	97%	96%
Fibrinolytic Meds Within 30 Min. of Arrival[7]	-	-	62%	58%
Average Time to ECG (minutes)	30	10	9	7
Average Time to Transfer (minutes)	11	50	62	60
Children's Asthma Care				
Received Home Management Plan of Care	-	-	88%	88%
Received Reliever Medication	-	-	100%	100%
Received Systemic Corticosteroids	-	-	100%	100%
Emergency Department				
Admittance Decision Time (minutes)[2]	833	291	125	98
Head CT Results Within 45 Min. of Arrival[7]	-	-	55%	57%
Patients Who Left ER Before Being Seen	64,917	9%	3%	2%
Time from ER Arrival to Admit. (minutes)[2]	833	678	323	274
Time from ER Arrival to Discharge (minutes)	319	448	168	134
Time in ER Before Being Evaluated (minutes)	371	101	29	26
Time to Pain Meds for Fractures (minutes)	78	85	62	57
Heart Attack Care				
Aspirin Given at Discharge	92	100%	99%	99%
Fibrinolytic Meds Within 30 Min. of Arrival[7]	-	-	73%	54%
PCI Within 90 Minutes of Arrival[1]	-	-	95%	96%
Statin Prescribed at Discharge	92	100%	98%	98%
Heart Failure Care				
ACE Inhibitor or ARB for LVSD[2]	130	98%	97%	97%
Discharge Instructions Given[2]	257	87%	94%	94%
Evaluation of LVS Function[2]	260	100%	99%	99%
Medicare Spending				
Medicare Spending per Patient (ratio)	-	0.86	0.98	0.98
Pneumonia Care				
Appropriate Initial Antibiotic Given[2]	39	97%	97%	95%
Blood Culture Timing[2]	73	93%	98%	98%
Pregnancy and Delivery Care				
Newborn Deliveries Scheduled Early[2]	20	0%	5%	6%
Preventive Care				
Immunization for Influenza[2]	565	89%	89%	90%
Immunization for Pneumonia[2]	501	83%	90%	92%
Stroke Care				
Anticoagulation Therapy for Atrial Fibrillation[1]	-	-	95%	95%
Antithrombotic Therapy Timing	64	98%	98%	98%
Assessed for Rehabilitation	73	86%	97%	97%
Discharged on Antithrombotic Therapy	66	100%	99%	99%
Discharged on Statin Medication	61	100%	94%	94%
Thrombolytic Therapy Timing[1]	-	-	72%	66%
Venous Thromboembolism Prophylaxis	75	80%	94%	94%
Written Stroke Educational Materials Given	65	20%	87%	88%
Surgical Care Improvement Project				
Appropriate Beta Blocker Usage[2]	17	100%	97%	98%
Appropriate VTP Within 24 Hours[2]	192	99%	98%	98%
Controlled Postoperative Blood Glucose[2,7]	-	-	96%	97%
Perioperative Temperature Management[2]	218	100%	100%	100%
Prophylactic Antibiotic Selection[2]	116	98%	99%	99%
Prophylactic Antibiotic Selection (Outpatient)	204	99%	97%	98%
Prophylactic Antibiotic Stopped[2]	116	100%	98%	98%
Prophylactic Antibiotic Timing[2]	116	99%	99%	99%
Prophylactic Antibiotic Timing (Outpatient)	46	98%	97%	98%
Urinary Catheter Removal[2]	57	98%	97%	97%
Survey of Patients' Hospital Experiences				
Area Around Room 'Always' Quiet at Night	300+	37%	51%	61%
Doctors 'Always' Communicated Well	300+	80%	78%	82%
Home Recovery Information Given	300+	81%	83%	85%
Hospital Given 9 or 10 on 10 Point Scale	300+	67%	68%	71%
Meds 'Always' Explained Before Given	300+	61%	61%	64%
Nurses 'Always' Communicated Well	300+	71%	74%	79%
Pain 'Always' Well Controlled	300+	68%	68%	71%
Room and Bathroom 'Always' Clean	300+	65%	70%	73%
Timely Help 'Always' Received	300+	56%	62%	68%
Would Definitely Recommend Hospital	300+	73%	70%	71%
Use of Medical Imaging				
Cardiac Imaging Stress Test before Surgery[1]	-	-	5.2%	5.3%
Combination Abdominal CT Scan	84	2.4%	13.4%	10.5%
Combination Brain/Sinus CT Scan[1]	-	-	2.2%	2.7%
Combination Chest CT Scan	63	1.6%	2.3%	2.7%
Follow-up Mammogram/Ultrasound[7]	-	-	8.2%	8.8%
Lumbar Spine MRI for Low Back Pain[7]	-	-	34.2%	37.2%

Providence Tarzana Medical Center

18321 Clark Street
Tarzana, CA 91356
E-mail: etrmcpublicrelations@tenethealth.com
URL: www.encino-tarzana.com
Type: Acute Care Hospitals
Ownership: Voluntary non-profit - Private
Phone: 818-881-0800
Fax: 818-708-5565
Emergency Services: Yes
Beds: 396

Key Personnel:
Pediatric Ambulatory Care . . . . . . Robert Barnhard, MD
Pediatric In-Patient Care . . . . Robert Barnhard, MD
Radiology. . . . . Leroy Clark, MD
Chief of Medical Staff . . . . Dr Jennifer Daly
Quality Assurance . . . . Sharon Gross
Chair/CEO . . . . Lee Kanon Alpert, Esq.
CEO/President. . . . . Dale Surowitz
Operating Room. . . . . Katie Walter, RN

Measure	Cases	This Hosp.	State Avg.	U.S. Avg.
Blood Clot Prevention and Treatment				
Anticoagulation Overlap Therapy[2]	68	82%	92%	93%
ICU Venous Thromboembolism Prophylaxis[2]	67	96%	92%	92%
Incidence of Potentially Preventable VTE[2]	18	6%	11%	10%
UFH with Dosages/Platelet Monitoring[2]	25	92%	96%	97%
Venous Thromboembolism Prophylaxis[2]	350	94%	83%	85%
Warfarin Therapy Discharge Instructions[2]	46	67%	75%	75%
Chest Pain/Possible Heart Attack Care				
Aspirin Given Within 24 Hours of Arrival[5]	-	-	97%	96%
Fibrinolytic Meds Within 30 Min. of Arrival[5]	-	-	62%	58%
Average Time to ECG (minutes)[5]	-	-	9	7
Average Time to Transfer (minutes)[5]	-	-	62	60
Children's Asthma Care				
Received Home Management Plan of Care	-	-	88%	88%
Received Reliever Medication	-	-	100%	100%
Received Systemic Corticosteroids	-	-	100%	100%
Emergency Department				
Admittance Decision Time (minutes)[2]	609	166	125	98
Head CT Results Within 45 Min. of Arrival[1]	-	-	55%	57%
Patients Who Left ER Before Being Seen	34,829	2%	3%	2%
Time from ER Arrival to Admit. (minutes)[2]	613	291	323	274
Time from ER Arrival to Discharge (minutes)	371	125	168	134
Time in ER Before Being Evaluated (minutes)	383	21	29	26
Time to Pain Meds for Fractures (minutes)	137	46	62	57
Heart Attack Care				
Aspirin Given at Discharge	122	99%	99%	99%
Fibrinolytic Meds Within 30 Min. of Arrival[7]	-	-	73%	54%
PCI Within 90 Minutes of Arrival	14	86%	95%	96%
Statin Prescribed at Discharge	124	100%	98%	98%
Heart Failure Care				
ACE Inhibitor or ARB for LVSD	86	95%	97%	97%
Discharge Instructions Given	233	91%	94%	94%
Evaluation of LVS Function	304	100%	99%	99%
Medicare Spending				
Medicare Spending per Patient (ratio)	-	1.02	0.98	0.98
Pneumonia Care				
Appropriate Initial Antibiotic Given	130	98%	97%	95%
Blood Culture Timing	370	99%	98%	98%
Pregnancy and Delivery Care				
Newborn Deliveries Scheduled Early[2]	69	9%	5%	6%
Preventive Care				
Immunization for Influenza[2]	479	92%	89%	90%
Immunization for Pneumonia[2]	558	96%	90%	92%
Stroke Care				
Anticoagulation Therapy for Atrial Fibrillation	15	93%	95%	95%
Antithrombotic Therapy Timing	81	94%	98%	98%
Assessed for Rehabilitation	93	95%	97%	97%
Discharged on Antithrombotic Therapy	84	100%	99%	99%
Discharged on Statin Medication	73	95%	94%	94%
Thrombolytic Therapy Timing[1]	-	-	72%	66%
Venous Thromboembolism Prophylaxis	93	92%	94%	94%
Written Stroke Educational Materials Given	53	77%	87%	88%
Surgical Care Improvement Project				
Appropriate Beta Blocker Usage[2]	143	99%	97%	98%
Appropriate VTP Within 24 Hours[2]	281	99%	98%	98%
Controlled Postoperative Blood Glucose[2]	69	97%	96%	97%
Perioperative Temperature Management[2]	384	100%	100%	100%
Prophylactic Antibiotic Selection[2]	270	98%	99%	99%
Prophylactic Antibiotic Selection (Outpatient)	292	90%	97%	98%
Prophylactic Antibiotic Stopped[2]	253	98%	98%	98%
Prophylactic Antibiotic Timing[2]	270	99%	99%	99%
Prophylactic Antibiotic Timing (Outpatient)	292	99%	97%	98%
Urinary Catheter Removal[2]	205	99%	97%	97%
Survey of Patients' Hospital Experiences				
Area Around Room 'Always' Quiet at Night	300+	39%	51%	61%

NOTE: Hospital profiles are in alphabetical order by state, then city, then hospital within the city; Rankings exclude hospitals with less than 25 cases except for patient surveys which excludes hospitals with less than 100 cases; (a) 100-299 cases; (1) The number of cases/patients is too few to report; (2) Data submitted were based on a sample of cases/patients; (3) Results are based on a shorter time period than required; (4) Data suppressed by CMS for one or more quarters; (5) Results are not available for this reporting period; (6) Fewer than 100 patients completed the HCAHPS survey; (7) No cases met the criteria for this measure; (8) The lower limit of the confidence interval cannot be calculated if the number of observed infections equals zero; (9) No data are available from the state/territory for this reporting period; (10) The scores shown reflect fewer than 50 completed surveys; (11) There were discrepancies in the data collection process; (12) This measure does not apply to this hospital for this reporting period; (13) Results cannot be calculated for this reporting period; (14) The results for this state are combined with nearby states to protect confidentiality; Please refer to the User's Guide for a full explanation of data.

Measure	Cases	This Hosp.	State Avg.	U.S. Avg.
Doctors 'Always' Communicated Well	300+	80%	78%	82%
Home Recovery Information Given	300+	79%	83%	85%
Hospital Given 9 or 10 on 10 Point Scale	300+	57%	68%	71%
Meds 'Always' Explained Before Given	300+	54%	61%	64%
Nurses 'Always' Communicated Well	300+	68%	74%	79%
Pain 'Always' Well Controlled	300+	62%	68%	71%
Room and Bathroom 'Always' Clean	300+	62%	70%	73%
Timely Help 'Always' Received	300+	52%	62%	68%
Would Definitely Recommend Hospital	300+	61%	70%	71%
Use of Medical Imaging				
Cardiac Imaging Stress Test before Surgery	310	5.2%	5.2%	5.3%
Combination Abdominal CT Scan	445	6.5%	13.4%	10.5%
Combination Brain/Sinus CT Scan	651	3.2%	2.2%	2.7%
Combination Chest CT Scan	169	1.2%	2.3%	2.7%
Follow-up Mammogram/Ultrasound	3,123	4.7%	8.2%	8.8%
Lumbar Spine MRI for Low Back Pain[1]	-	-	34.2%	37.2%

Tehachapi Hospital

115 West E Street
Tehachapi, CA 93561
Phone: 661-822-3241
Fax: 661-823-3081
E-mail: lmizumoto@tvhd.org
URL: www.tvhd.org
Type: Critical Access Hospitals
Emergency Services: Yes
Ownership: Govt - Hospital Dist/Auth
Beds: 28

Key Personnel:
Emergency Room . . . . Regina Clark
President . . . . Sam Conklin, MD
Radiology. . . . . Ramesh Gopi, MD
Operating Room. . . . . Gary Olsen, RN
Chief of Medical Staff . . . . Susan J P Hall, MD
Quality Assurance . . . . Christine Sherrill

Measure	Cases	This Hosp.	State Avg.	U.S. Avg.
Blood Clot Prevention and Treatment				
Anticoagulation Overlap Therapy[5]	-	-	92%	93%
ICU Venous Thromboembolism Prophylaxis[5]	-	-	92%	92%
Incidence of Potentially Preventable VTE[5]	-	-	11%	10%
UFH with Dosages/Platelet Monitoring[5]	-	-	96%	97%
Venous Thromboembolism Prophylaxis[5]	-	-	83%	85%
Warfarin Therapy Discharge Instructions[5]	-	-	75%	75%
Chest Pain/Possible Heart Attack Care				
Aspirin Given Within 24 Hours of Arrival	-	-	97%	96%
Fibrinolytic Meds Within 30 Min. of Arrival	-	-	62%	58%
Average Time to ECG (minutes)	-	-	9	7
Average Time to Transfer (minutes)	-	-	62	60
Children's Asthma Care				
Received Home Management Plan of Care	-	-	88%	88%
Received Reliever Medication	-	-	100%	100%
Received Systemic Corticosteroids	-	-	100%	100%
Emergency Department				
Admittance Decision Time (minutes)[5]	-	-	125	98
Head CT Results Within 45 Min. of Arrival	-	-	55%	57%
Patients Who Left ER Before Being Seen	-	-	3%	2%
Time from ER Arrival to Admit. (minutes)[5]	-	-	323	274
Time from ER Arrival to Discharge (minutes)	-	-	168	134
Time in ER Before Being Evaluated (minutes)	-	-	29	26
Time to Pain Meds for Fractures (minutes)	-	-	62	57
Heart Attack Care				
Aspirin Given at Discharge[5]	-	-	99%	99%
Fibrinolytic Meds Within 30 Min. of Arrival[5]	-	-	73%	54%
PCI Within 90 Minutes of Arrival[5]	-	-	95%	96%
Statin Prescribed at Discharge[5]	-	-	98%	98%
Heart Failure Care				
ACE Inhibitor or ARB for LVSD[3,7]	-	-	97%	97%
Discharge Instructions Given[1,3]	-	-	94%	94%
Evaluation of LVS Function[1,3]	-	-	99%	99%
Medicare Spending				
Medicare Spending per Patient (ratio)	-	-	0.98	0.98
Pneumonia Care				
Appropriate Initial Antibiotic Given[1]	-	-	97%	95%
Blood Culture Timing[1]	-	-	98%	98%
Pregnancy and Delivery Care				
Newborn Deliveries Scheduled Early[5]	-	-	5%	6%
Preventive Care				
Immunization for Influenza[5]	-	-	89%	90%
Immunization for Pneumonia[5]	-	-	90%	92%
Stroke Care				
Anticoagulation Therapy for Atrial Fibrillation[5]	-	-	95%	95%
Antithrombotic Therapy Timing[5]	-	-	98%	98%
Assessed for Rehabilitation[5]	-	-	97%	97%
Discharged on Antithrombotic Therapy[5]	-	-	99%	99%
Discharged on Statin Medication[5]	-	-	94%	94%
Thrombolytic Therapy Timing[5]	-	-	72%	66%
Venous Thromboembolism Prophylaxis[5]	-	-	94%	94%
Written Stroke Educational Materials Given[5]	-	-	87%	88%
Surgical Care Improvement Project				
Appropriate Beta Blocker Usage[5]	-	-	97%	98%
Appropriate VTP Within 24 Hours[5]	-	-	98%	98%
Controlled Postoperative Blood Glucose[5]	-	-	96%	97%
Perioperative Temperature Management[5]	-	-	100%	100%
Prophylactic Antibiotic Selection[5]	-	-	99%	99%
Prophylactic Antibiotic Selection (Outpatient)	-	-	97%	98%
Prophylactic Antibiotic Stopped[5]	-	-	98%	98%
Prophylactic Antibiotic Timing[5]	-	-	99%	99%
Prophylactic Antibiotic Timing (Outpatient)	-	-	97%	98%
Urinary Catheter Removal[5]	-	-	97%	97%
Survey of Patients' Hospital Experiences				
Area Around Room 'Always' Quiet at Night[10]	<100	41%	51%	61%
Doctors 'Always' Communicated Well[10]	<100	75%	78%	82%
Home Recovery Information Given[10]	<100	81%	83%	85%
Hospital Given 9 or 10 on 10 Point Scale[10]	<100	40%	68%	71%
Meds 'Always' Explained Before Given[10]	<100	52%	61%	64%
Nurses 'Always' Communicated Well[10]	<100	73%	74%	79%
Pain 'Always' Well Controlled[10]	<100	30%	68%	71%
Room and Bathroom 'Always' Clean[10]	<100	63%	70%	73%
Timely Help 'Always' Received[10]	<100	58%	62%	68%
Would Definitely Recommend Hospital[10]	<100	51%	70%	71%
Use of Medical Imaging				
Cardiac Imaging Stress Test before Surgery	-	-	5.2%	5.3%
Combination Abdominal CT Scan	-	-	13.4%	10.5%
Combination Brain/Sinus CT Scan	-	-	2.2%	2.7%
Combination Chest CT Scan	-	-	2.3%	2.7%
Follow-up Mammogram/Ultrasound	-	-	8.2%	8.8%
Lumbar Spine MRI for Low Back Pain	-	-	34.2%	37.2%

Twin Cities Community Hospital

1100 Las Tablas Rd
Templeton, CA 93465
Phone: 805-434-3500
Fax: 805-434-2913
URL: www.twincitieshospital.com
Type: Acute Care Hospitals
Emergency Services: Yes
Ownership: Proprietary
Beds: 84

Key Personnel:
Chief of Medical Staff. . . . . Keven Colton
Radiology. . . . . Blake Evernden
Operating Room. . . . . John Henry, RN
CEO/President. . . . . Richard D Lyons
Pediatric Ambulatory Care . . . . . . Mary Nave, MD
Infection Control. . . . . Jeanette Tosh
Quality Assurance . . . . Ellen Walsh, RN
Intensive Care Unit. . . . . Doris Warren, RN

Measure	Cases	This Hosp.	State Avg.	U.S. Avg.
Blood Clot Prevention and Treatment				
Anticoagulation Overlap Therapy[2]	49	88%	92%	93%
ICU Venous Thromboembolism Prophylaxis[2]	49	98%	92%	92%
Incidence of Potentially Preventable VTE[1,2]	-	-	11%	10%
UFH with Dosages/Platelet Monitoring[2]	16	94%	96%	97%
Venous Thromboembolism Prophylaxis[2]	358	85%	83%	85%
Warfarin Therapy Discharge Instructions[2]	39	92%	75%	75%
Chest Pain/Possible Heart Attack Care				
Aspirin Given Within 24 Hours of Arrival	66	98%	97%	96%
Fibrinolytic Meds Within 30 Min. of Arrival[7]	-	-	62%	58%
Average Time to ECG (minutes)	72	6	9	7
Average Time to Transfer (minutes)	11	38	62	60
Children's Asthma Care				
Received Home Management Plan of Care	-	-	88%	88%
Received Reliever Medication	-	-	100%	100%
Received Systemic Corticosteroids	-	-	100%	100%
Emergency Department				
Admittance Decision Time (minutes)[2]	787	144	125	98
Head CT Results Within 45 Min. of Arrival	16	81%	55%	57%
Patients Who Left ER Before Being Seen	27,524	1%	3%	2%
Time from ER Arrival to Admit. (minutes)[2]	787	277	323	274
Time from ER Arrival to Discharge (minutes)	481	115	168	134
Time in ER Before Being Evaluated (minutes)	502	27	29	26
Time to Pain Meds for Fractures (minutes)	152	53	62	57
Heart Attack Care				
Aspirin Given at Discharge[1]	-	-	99%	99%
Fibrinolytic Meds Within 30 Min. of Arrival[7]	-	-	73%	54%
PCI Within 90 Minutes of Arrival[7]	-	-	95%	96%
Statin Prescribed at Discharge[1]	-	-	98%	98%
Heart Failure Care				
ACE Inhibitor or ARB for LVSD	30	100%	97%	97%
Discharge Instructions Given	93	100%	94%	94%
Evaluation of LVS Function	110	100%	99%	99%
Medicare Spending				
Medicare Spending per Patient (ratio)	-	0.98	0.98	0.98
Pneumonia Care				
Appropriate Initial Antibiotic Given	122	99%	97%	95%
Blood Culture Timing	131	100%	98%	98%
Pregnancy and Delivery Care				
Newborn Deliveries Scheduled Early[2]	31	6%	5%	6%
Preventive Care				
Immunization for Influenza[2]	542	99%	89%	90%
Immunization for Pneumonia[2]	611	98%	90%	92%
Stroke Care				
Anticoagulation Therapy for Atrial Fibrillation[1]	-	-	95%	95%
Antithrombotic Therapy Timing	54	100%	98%	98%
Assessed for Rehabilitation	64	92%	97%	97%
Discharged on Antithrombotic Therapy	59	93%	99%	99%
Discharged on Statin Medication	48	90%	94%	94%
Thrombolytic Therapy Timing[1]	-	-	72%	66%
Venous Thromboembolism Prophylaxis	58	95%	94%	94%
Written Stroke Educational Materials Given	39	79%	87%	88%
Surgical Care Improvement Project				
Appropriate Beta Blocker Usage	109	98%	97%	98%
Appropriate VTP Within 24 Hours	484	99%	98%	98%
Controlled Postoperative Blood Glucose[7]	-	-	96%	97%
Perioperative Temperature Management	539	100%	100%	100%
Prophylactic Antibiotic Selection	393	99%	99%	99%
Prophylactic Antibiotic Selection (Outpatient)	68	97%	97%	98%
Prophylactic Antibiotic Stopped	384	99%	98%	98%
Prophylactic Antibiotic Timing	393	100%	99%	99%
Prophylactic Antibiotic Timing (Outpatient)	70	96%	97%	98%
Urinary Catheter Removal	327	97%	97%	97%
Survey of Patients' Hospital Experiences				
Area Around Room 'Always' Quiet at Night	300+	50%	51%	61%
Doctors 'Always' Communicated Well	300+	82%	78%	82%
Home Recovery Information Given	300+	87%	83%	85%
Hospital Given 9 or 10 on 10 Point Scale	300+	69%	68%	71%
Meds 'Always' Explained Before Given	300+	67%	61%	64%
Nurses 'Always' Communicated Well	300+	80%	74%	79%
Pain 'Always' Well Controlled	300+	71%	68%	71%
Room and Bathroom 'Always' Clean	300+	71%	70%	73%
Timely Help 'Always' Received	300+	70%	62%	68%
Would Definitely Recommend Hospital	300+	71%	70%	71%
Use of Medical Imaging				
Cardiac Imaging Stress Test before Surgery[1]	-	-	5.2%	5.3%
Combination Abdominal CT Scan	405	5.4%	13.4%	10.5%
Combination Brain/Sinus CT Scan	513	0.8%	2.2%	2.7%
Combination Chest CT Scan[1]	-	-	2.3%	2.7%
Follow-up Mammogram/Ultrasound[7]	-	-	8.2%	8.8%
Lumbar Spine MRI for Low Back Pain[1]	-	-	34.2%	37.2%

Los Robles Hospital & Medical Center

215 W Janss Rd
Thousand Oaks, CA 91360
Phone: 805-497-2727
Fax: 805-446-7701
URL: www.losrobleshospital.com
Type: Acute Care Hospitals
Emergency Services: Yes
Ownership: Proprietary
Beds: 395

Key Personnel:
Pediatric In-Patient Care . . . . Simon Boostanfar
Infection Control. . . . . Diane Duff, RN
Quality Assurance . . . . Donna Hartman, RN

NOTE: Hospital profiles are in alphabetical order by state, then city, then hospital within the city; Rankings exclude hospitals with less than 25 cases except for patient surveys which excludes hospitals with less than 100 cases; (a) 100-299 cases; (1) The number of cases/patients is too few to report; (2) Data submitted were based on a sample of cases/patients; (3) Results are based on a shorter time period than required; (4) Data suppressed by CMS for one or more quarters; (5) Results are not available for this reporting period; (6) Fewer than 100 patients completed the HCAHPS survey; (7) No cases met the criteria for this measure; (8) The lower limit of the confidence interval cannot be calculated if the number of observed infections equals zero; (9) No data are available from the state/territory for this reporting period; (10) The scores shown reflect fewer than 50 completed surveys; (11) There were discrepancies in the data collection process; (12) This measure does not apply to this hospital for this reporting period; (13) Results cannot be calculated for this reporting period; (14) The results for this state are combined with nearby states to protect confidentiality; Please refer to the User's Guide for a full explanation of data.

CEO/President . . . . Natalie Mussi
Chief of Medical Staff . . . . David Newman, MD
Pediatric Ambulatory Care . . . . . . Kenneth Saul, MD
Coronary Care . . . . Lisa Shaper, RN
Radiology . . . . TJ Turkat, MD

Measure	Cases	This Hosp.	State Avg.	U.S. Avg.
Blood Clot Prevention and Treatment				
Anticoagulation Overlap Therapy[2]	68	78%	92%	93%
ICU Venous Thromboembolism Prophylaxis[2]	87	92%	92%	92%
Incidence of Potentially Preventable VTE[2]	14	21%	11%	10%
UFH with Dosages/Platelet Monitoring[1,2]	-	-	96%	97%
Venous Thromboembolism Prophylaxis[2]	336	84%	83%	85%
Warfarin Therapy Discharge Instructions[2]	47	100%	75%	75%
Chest Pain/Possible Heart Attack Care				
Aspirin Given Within 24 Hours of Arrival	29	100%	97%	96%
Fibrinolytic Meds Within 30 Min. of Arrival[3,7]	-	-	62%	58%
Average Time to ECG (minutes)	32	8	9	7
Average Time to Transfer (minutes)[3,7]	-	-	62	60
Children's Asthma Care				
Received Home Management Plan of Care	-	-	88%	88%
Received Reliever Medication	-	-	100%	100%
Received Systemic Corticosteroids	-	-	100%	100%
Emergency Department				
Admittance Decision Time (minutes)[2]	695	165	125	98
Head CT Results Within 45 Min. of Arrival[1]	-	-	55%	57%
Patients Who Left ER Before Being Seen	40,563	0%	3%	2%
Time from ER Arrival to Admit. (minutes)[2]	696	322	323	274
Time from ER Arrival to Discharge (minutes)	421	176	168	134
Time in ER Before Being Evaluated (minutes)	452	6	29	26
Time to Pain Meds for Fractures (minutes)	219	75	62	57
Heart Attack Care				
Aspirin Given at Discharge	296	100%	99%	99%
Fibrinolytic Meds Within 30 Min. of Arrival[7]	-	-	73%	54%
PCI Within 90 Minutes of Arrival	64	100%	95%	96%
Statin Prescribed at Discharge	276	100%	98%	98%
Heart Failure Care				
ACE Inhibitor or ARB for LVSD	80	100%	97%	97%
Discharge Instructions Given	228	100%	94%	94%
Evaluation of LVS Function	287	100%	99%	99%
Medicare Spending				
Medicare Spending per Patient (ratio)	-	0.99	0.98	0.98
Pneumonia Care				
Appropriate Initial Antibiotic Given	125	99%	97%	95%
Blood Culture Timing	228	99%	98%	98%
Pregnancy and Delivery Care				
Newborn Deliveries Scheduled Early[2]	45	0%	5%	6%
Preventive Care				
Immunization for Influenza[2]	591	94%	89%	90%
Immunization for Pneumonia[2]	686	94%	90%	92%
Stroke Care				
Anticoagulation Therapy for Atrial Fibrillation[2]	19	100%	95%	95%
Antithrombotic Therapy Timing[2]	70	99%	98%	98%
Assessed for Rehabilitation[2]	86	99%	97%	97%
Discharged on Antithrombotic Therapy[2]	78	100%	99%	99%
Discharged on Statin Medication[2]	61	98%	94%	94%
Thrombolytic Therapy Timing[2]	12	100%	72%	66%
Venous Thromboembolism Prophylaxis[2]	88	95%	94%	94%
Written Stroke Educational Materials Given[2]	45	100%	87%	88%
Surgical Care Improvement Project				
Appropriate Beta Blocker Usage[2]	187	98%	97%	98%
Appropriate VTP Within 24 Hours[2]	451	99%	98%	98%
Controlled Postoperative Blood Glucose[2]	118	97%	96%	97%
Perioperative Temperature Management[2]	587	100%	100%	100%
Prophylactic Antibiotic Selection[2]	460	100%	99%	99%
Prophylactic Antibiotic Selection (Outpatient)	243	98%	97%	98%
Prophylactic Antibiotic Stopped[2]	446	99%	98%	98%
Prophylactic Antibiotic Timing[2]	461	100%	99%	99%
Prophylactic Antibiotic Timing (Outpatient)	245	99%	97%	98%
Urinary Catheter Removal[2]	425	98%	97%	97%
Survey of Patients' Hospital Experiences				
Area Around Room 'Always' Quiet at Night	300+	52%	51%	61%
Doctors 'Always' Communicated Well	300+	75%	78%	82%
Home Recovery Information Given	300+	83%	83%	85%
Hospital Given 9 or 10 on 10 Point Scale	300+	69%	68%	71%
Meds 'Always' Explained Before Given	300+	54%	61%	64%
Nurses 'Always' Communicated Well	300+	72%	74%	79%
Pain 'Always' Well Controlled	300+	66%	68%	71%
Room and Bathroom 'Always' Clean	300+	68%	70%	73%
Timely Help 'Always' Received	300+	53%	62%	68%
Would Definitely Recommend Hospital	300+	71%	70%	71%
Use of Medical Imaging				
Cardiac Imaging Stress Test before Surgery	111	3.6%	5.2%	5.3%
Combination Abdominal CT Scan	784	37.0%	13.4%	10.5%
Combination Brain/Sinus CT Scan	751	3.1%	2.2%	2.7%
Combination Chest CT Scan	238	0.0%	2.3%	2.7%
Follow-up Mammogram/Ultrasound	79	11.4%	8.2%	8.8%
Lumbar Spine MRI for Low Back Pain[1]	-	-	34.2%	37.2%

LAC/Harbor - UCLA Medical Center

1000 W Carson St
Torrance, CA 90509
URL: www.harbor-ucla.org
Type: Acute Care Hospitals
Ownership: Government - Local
Phone: 310-222-2101
Fax: 310-328-8450
Emergency Services: Yes
Beds: 553

Key Personnel:
Radiology . . . . Michael Diament, MD
CEO . . . . Delvecchio Finley, MPP, FACHE
Quality Assurance . . . . Tony Greenberg, MD
CEO/President . . . . Darrell W Harrington
Emergency Room . . . . Robert Hockberger, MD
Pediatric Ambulatory Care . . . . . . Adam Jonas, MD
Anesthesiology . . . . John McDonald, MD
Infection Control . . . . Joel Ward, MD

Measure	Cases	This Hosp.	State Avg.	U.S. Avg.
Blood Clot Prevention and Treatment				
Anticoagulation Overlap Therapy[2]	56	98%	92%	93%
ICU Venous Thromboembolism Prophylaxis[2]	75	99%	92%	92%
Incidence of Potentially Preventable VTE[2]	15	0%	11%	10%
UFH with Dosages/Platelet Monitoring[2]	60	100%	96%	97%
Venous Thromboembolism Prophylaxis[2]	308	91%	83%	85%
Warfarin Therapy Discharge Instructions[2]	54	94%	75%	75%
Chest Pain/Possible Heart Attack Care				
Aspirin Given Within 24 Hours of Arrival	15	93%	97%	96%
Fibrinolytic Meds Within 30 Min. of Arrival[3,7]	-	-	62%	58%
Average Time to ECG (minutes)	15	19	9	7
Average Time to Transfer (minutes)[3,7]	-	-	62	60
Children's Asthma Care				
Received Home Management Plan of Care	-	-	88%	88%
Received Reliever Medication	-	-	100%	100%
Received Systemic Corticosteroids	-	-	100%	100%
Emergency Department				
Admittance Decision Time (minutes)[2]	731	230	125	98
Head CT Results Within 45 Min. of Arrival[1,3]	-	-	55%	57%
Patients Who Left ER Before Being Seen	>100k	10%	3%	2%
Time from ER Arrival to Admit. (minutes)[2]	799	637	323	274
Time from ER Arrival to Discharge (minutes)	288	316	168	134
Time in ER Before Being Evaluated (minutes)	373	59	29	26
Time to Pain Meds for Fractures (minutes)	204	65	62	57
Heart Attack Care				
Aspirin Given at Discharge[2]	237	99%	99%	99%
Fibrinolytic Meds Within 30 Min. of Arrival[2,7]	-	-	73%	54%
PCI Within 90 Minutes of Arrival[2]	37	86%	95%	96%
Statin Prescribed at Discharge[2]	237	99%	98%	98%
Heart Failure Care				
ACE Inhibitor or ARB for LVSD[2]	144	96%	97%	97%
Discharge Instructions Given[2]	280	94%	94%	94%
Evaluation of LVS Function[2]	283	100%	99%	99%
Medicare Spending				
Medicare Spending per Patient (ratio)	-	0.89	0.98	0.98
Pneumonia Care				
Appropriate Initial Antibiotic Given[2]	74	88%	97%	95%
Blood Culture Timing[2]	96	93%	98%	98%
Pregnancy and Delivery Care				
Newborn Deliveries Scheduled Early[2]	33	39%	5%	6%
Preventive Care				
Immunization for Influenza[2]	558	88%	89%	90%
Immunization for Pneumonia[2]	428	86%	90%	92%
Stroke Care				
Anticoagulation Therapy for Atrial Fibrillation[1,2]	-	-	95%	95%
Antithrombotic Therapy Timing[2]	97	100%	98%	98%
Assessed for Rehabilitation[2]	115	77%	97%	97%
Discharged on Antithrombotic Therapy[2]	96	99%	99%	99%
Discharged on Statin Medication[2]	82	96%	94%	94%
Thrombolytic Therapy Timing[1,2]	-	-	72%	66%
Venous Thromboembolism Prophylaxis[2]	128	80%	94%	94%
Written Stroke Educational Materials Given[2]	85	48%	87%	88%
Surgical Care Improvement Project				
Appropriate Beta Blocker Usage[2]	133	99%	97%	98%
Appropriate VTP Within 24 Hours[2]	285	98%	98%	98%
Controlled Postoperative Blood Glucose[2]	102	100%	96%	97%
Perioperative Temperature Management[2]	354	100%	100%	100%
Prophylactic Antibiotic Selection[2]	309	99%	99%	99%
Prophylactic Antibiotic Selection (Outpatient)	69	97%	97%	98%
Prophylactic Antibiotic Stopped[2]	294	97%	98%	98%
Prophylactic Antibiotic Timing[2]	312	99%	99%	99%
Prophylactic Antibiotic Timing (Outpatient)	71	97%	97%	98%
Urinary Catheter Removal[2]	181	98%	97%	97%
Survey of Patients' Hospital Experiences				
Area Around Room 'Always' Quiet at Night	300+	40%	51%	61%
Doctors 'Always' Communicated Well	300+	81%	78%	82%
Home Recovery Information Given	300+	80%	83%	85%
Hospital Given 9 or 10 on 10 Point Scale	300+	59%	68%	71%
Meds 'Always' Explained Before Given	300+	56%	61%	64%
Nurses 'Always' Communicated Well	300+	71%	74%	79%
Pain 'Always' Well Controlled	300+	66%	68%	71%
Room and Bathroom 'Always' Clean	300+	59%	70%	73%
Timely Help 'Always' Received	300+	54%	62%	68%
Would Definitely Recommend Hospital	300+	64%	70%	71%
Use of Medical Imaging				
Cardiac Imaging Stress Test before Surgery[1]	-	-	5.2%	5.3%
Combination Abdominal CT Scan	133	21.1%	13.4%	10.5%
Combination Brain/Sinus CT Scan[1]	-	-	2.2%	2.7%
Combination Chest CT Scan	90	6.7%	2.3%	2.7%
Follow-up Mammogram/Ultrasound[1]	-	-	8.2%	8.8%
Lumbar Spine MRI for Low Back Pain[7]	-	-	34.2%	37.2%

Providence Little Co of Mary Medical Center Torrance

4101 Torrance Blvd
Torrance, CA 90503
URL: www.lcmhs.org
Type: Acute Care Hospitals
Ownership: Voluntary non-profit - Church
Phone: 310-540-7676
Fax: 310-540-8408
Emergency Services: Yes
Beds: 317

Key Personnel:
Operating Room . . . . Doreen Barry
Pediatric Ambulatory Care . . . . . . Reeta Demonteverdo, MD
Pediatric In-Patient Care . . . . Reeta Demonteverdo, MD
CEO/President . . . . Liz Dunne
Chief of Medical Staff . . . . Richard Glimp, MD
Radiology . . . . Lee Secrist
Quality Assurance . . . . Pam Stahl

Measure	Cases	This Hosp.	State Avg.	U.S. Avg.
Blood Clot Prevention and Treatment				
Anticoagulation Overlap Therapy[2]	96	100%	92%	93%
ICU Venous Thromboembolism Prophylaxis[2]	70	96%	92%	92%
Incidence of Potentially Preventable VTE[2]	23	0%	11%	10%
UFH with Dosages/Platelet Monitoring[2]	18	100%	96%	97%
Venous Thromboembolism Prophylaxis[2]	328	92%	83%	85%
Warfarin Therapy Discharge Instructions[2]	74	100%	75%	75%
Chest Pain/Possible Heart Attack Care				
Aspirin Given Within 24 Hours of Arrival	70	100%	97%	96%
Fibrinolytic Meds Within 30 Min. of Arrival[3,7]	-	-	62%	58%
Average Time to ECG (minutes)	77	2	9	7
Average Time to Transfer (minutes)[3,7]	-	-	62	60
Children's Asthma Care				
Received Home Management Plan of Care	-	-	88%	88%
Received Reliever Medication	-	-	100%	100%
Received Systemic Corticosteroids	-	-	100%	100%
Emergency Department				
Admittance Decision Time (minutes)[2]	727	247	125	98

NOTE: Hospital profiles are in alphabetical order by state, then city, then hospital within the city; Rankings exclude hospitals with less than 25 cases except for patient surveys which excludes hospitals with less than 100 cases; (a) 100-299 cases; (1) The number of cases/patients is too few to report; (2) Data submitted were based on a sample of cases/patients; (3) Results are based on a shorter time period than required; (4) Data suppressed by CMS for one or more quarters; (5) Results are not available for this reporting period; (6) Fewer than 100 patients completed the HCAHPS survey; (7) No cases met the criteria for this measure; (8) The lower limit of the confidence interval cannot be calculated if the number of observed infections equals zero; (9) No data are available from the state/territory for this reporting period; (10) The scores shown reflect fewer than 50 completed surveys; (11) There were discrepancies in the data collection process; (12) This measure does not apply to this hospital for this reporting period; (13) Results cannot be calculated for this reporting period; (14) The results for this state are combined with nearby states to protect confidentiality; Please refer to the User's Guide for a full explanation of data.

Measure	Cases	This Hosp.	State Avg.	U.S. Avg.
Head CT Results Within 45 Min. of Arrival	13	38%	55%	57%
Patients Who Left ER Before Being Seen	66,748	3%	3%	2%
Time from ER Arrival to Admit. (minutes)[2]	739	476	323	274
Time from ER Arrival to Discharge (minutes)	389	222	168	134
Time in ER Before Being Evaluated (minutes)	430	37	29	26
Time to Pain Meds for Fractures (minutes)	206	82	62	57
Heart Attack Care				
Aspirin Given at Discharge	307	100%	99%	99%
Fibrinolytic Meds Within 30 Min. of Arrival[7]	-	-	73%	54%
PCI Within 90 Minutes of Arrival	28	100%	95%	96%
Statin Prescribed at Discharge	295	100%	98%	98%
Heart Failure Care				
ACE Inhibitor or ARB for LVSD[2]	113	100%	97%	97%
Discharge Instructions Given[2]	257	100%	94%	94%
Evaluation of LVS Function[2]	331	100%	99%	99%
Medicare Spending				
Medicare Spending per Patient (ratio)	-	1.01	0.98	0.98
Pneumonia Care				
Appropriate Initial Antibiotic Given[2]	89	93%	97%	95%
Blood Culture Timing[2]	191	98%	98%	98%
Pregnancy and Delivery Care				
Newborn Deliveries Scheduled Early[2]	84	2%	5%	6%
Preventive Care				
Immunization for Influenza[2]	543	98%	89%	90%
Immunization for Pneumonia[2]	595	98%	90%	92%
Stroke Care				
Anticoagulation Therapy for Atrial Fibrillation	25	80%	95%	95%
Antithrombotic Therapy Timing	162	98%	98%	98%
Assessed for Rehabilitation	241	98%	97%	97%
Discharged on Antithrombotic Therapy	203	99%	99%	99%
Discharged on Statin Medication	166	92%	94%	94%
Thrombolytic Therapy Timing[1]	-	-	72%	66%
Venous Thromboembolism Prophylaxis	224	94%	94%	94%
Written Stroke Educational Materials Given	106	90%	87%	88%
Surgical Care Improvement Project				
Appropriate Beta Blocker Usage[2]	148	99%	97%	98%
Appropriate VTP Within 24 Hours[2]	447	100%	98%	98%
Controlled Postoperative Blood Glucose[2]	102	96%	96%	97%
Perioperative Temperature Management[2]	551	100%	100%	100%
Prophylactic Antibiotic Selection[2]	411	100%	99%	99%
Prophylactic Antibiotic Selection (Outpatient)	289	99%	97%	98%
Prophylactic Antibiotic Stopped[2]	390	99%	98%	98%
Prophylactic Antibiotic Timing[2]	411	100%	99%	99%
Prophylactic Antibiotic Timing (Outpatient)	289	100%	97%	98%
Urinary Catheter Removal[2]	351	100%	97%	97%
Survey of Patients' Hospital Experiences				
Area Around Room 'Always' Quiet at Night	300+	53%	51%	61%
Doctors 'Always' Communicated Well	300+	80%	78%	82%
Home Recovery Information Given	300+	83%	83%	85%
Hospital Given 9 or 10 on 10 Point Scale	300+	76%	68%	71%
Meds 'Always' Explained Before Given	300+	63%	61%	64%
Nurses 'Always' Communicated Well	300+	77%	74%	79%
Pain 'Always' Well Controlled	300+	72%	68%	71%
Room and Bathroom 'Always' Clean	300+	71%	70%	73%
Timely Help 'Always' Received	300+	59%	62%	68%
Would Definitely Recommend Hospital	300+	80%	70%	71%
Use of Medical Imaging				
Cardiac Imaging Stress Test before Surgery	672	4.9%	5.2%	5.3%
Combination Abdominal CT Scan	1,108	3.0%	13.4%	10.5%
Combination Brain/Sinus CT Scan	1,127	2.2%	2.2%	2.7%
Combination Chest CT Scan	304	1.0%	2.3%	2.7%
Follow-up Mammogram/Ultrasound	2,231	6.1%	8.2%	8.8%
Lumbar Spine MRI for Low Back Pain	68	33.8%	34.2%	37.2%

Torrance Memorial Medical Center

3330 Lomita Blvd
Torrance, CA 90509
Phone: 310-325-9110
Fax: 310-784-4801
URL: www.torrancememorial.org
Type: Acute Care Hospitals
Emergency Services: Yes
Ownership: Voluntary non-profit - Other
Beds: 335

Key Personnel:

Operating Room. . . . . Riad Adoumie, RN
Radiology. . . . . Donny Baek, MD
Quality Assurance . . . . Linda Dobie, RN
Cardiac Laboratory. . . . . Peggy Gould
CEO/President. . . . . Craig Leach
Chief of Medical Staff . . . . John McNamara, MD
Pediatric Ambulatory Care . . . . . . William Pazdral, MD
Pediatric In-Patient Care . . . . William Pazdral, MD

Measure	Cases	This Hosp.	State Avg.	U.S. Avg.
Blood Clot Prevention and Treatment				
Anticoagulation Overlap Therapy[2]	85	100%	92%	93%
ICU Venous Thromboembolism Prophylaxis[2]	69	100%	92%	92%
Incidence of Potentially Preventable VTE[2]	11	9%	11%	10%
UFH with Dosages/Platelet Monitoring[2]	22	100%	96%	97%
Venous Thromboembolism Prophylaxis[2]	408	86%	83%	85%
Warfarin Therapy Discharge Instructions[2]	67	88%	75%	75%
Chest Pain/Possible Heart Attack Care				
Aspirin Given Within 24 Hours of Arrival	16	100%	97%	96%
Fibrinolytic Meds Within 30 Min. of Arrival[5]	-	-	62%	58%
Average Time to ECG (minutes)	17	2	9	7
Average Time to Transfer (minutes)[5]	-	-	62	60
Children's Asthma Care				
Received Home Management Plan of Care	-	-	88%	88%
Received Reliever Medication	-	-	100%	100%
Received Systemic Corticosteroids	-	-	100%	100%
Emergency Department				
Admittance Decision Time (minutes)[2]	828	112	125	98
Head CT Results Within 45 Min. of Arrival	13	92%	55%	57%
Patients Who Left ER Before Being Seen	16,718	4%	3%	2%
Time from ER Arrival to Admit. (minutes)[2]	829	331	323	274
Time from ER Arrival to Discharge (minutes)	1,475	223	168	134
Time in ER Before Being Evaluated (minutes)	1,552	77	29	26
Time to Pain Meds for Fractures (minutes)	276	72	62	57
Heart Attack Care				
Aspirin Given at Discharge	341	99%	99%	99%
Fibrinolytic Meds Within 30 Min. of Arrival[7]	-	-	73%	54%
PCI Within 90 Minutes of Arrival	71	99%	95%	96%
Statin Prescribed at Discharge	323	98%	98%	98%
Heart Failure Care				
ACE Inhibitor or ARB for LVSD	167	99%	97%	97%
Discharge Instructions Given	405	99%	94%	94%
Evaluation of LVS Function	536	100%	99%	99%
Medicare Spending				
Medicare Spending per Patient (ratio)	-	0.98	0.98	0.98
Pneumonia Care				
Appropriate Initial Antibiotic Given[2]	77	94%	97%	95%
Blood Culture Timing[2]	140	96%	98%	98%
Pregnancy and Delivery Care				
Newborn Deliveries Scheduled Early[2]	54	0%	5%	6%
Preventive Care				
Immunization for Influenza[2]	697	95%	89%	90%
Immunization for Pneumonia[2]	829	94%	90%	92%
Stroke Care				
Anticoagulation Therapy for Atrial Fibrillation	36	100%	95%	95%
Antithrombotic Therapy Timing	183	99%	98%	98%
Assessed for Rehabilitation	265	99%	97%	97%
Discharged on Antithrombotic Therapy	230	100%	99%	99%
Discharged on Statin Medication	189	98%	94%	94%
Thrombolytic Therapy Timing	17	100%	72%	66%
Venous Thromboembolism Prophylaxis	241	99%	94%	94%
Written Stroke Educational Materials Given	141	97%	87%	88%
Surgical Care Improvement Project				
Appropriate Beta Blocker Usage[2]	237	99%	97%	98%
Appropriate VTP Within 24 Hours[2]	775	99%	98%	98%
Controlled Postoperative Blood Glucose[2]	89	99%	96%	97%
Perioperative Temperature Management[2]	915	100%	100%	100%
Prophylactic Antibiotic Selection[2]	617	100%	99%	99%
Prophylactic Antibiotic Selection (Outpatient)	380	99%	97%	98%
Prophylactic Antibiotic Stopped[2]	585	99%	98%	98%
Prophylactic Antibiotic Timing[2]	617	100%	99%	99%
Prophylactic Antibiotic Timing (Outpatient)	386	97%	97%	98%
Urinary Catheter Removal[2]	551	99%	97%	97%
Survey of Patients' Hospital Experiences				
Area Around Room 'Always' Quiet at Night	300+	50%	51%	61%
Doctors 'Always' Communicated Well	300+	78%	78%	82%
Home Recovery Information Given	300+	84%	83%	85%
Hospital Given 9 or 10 on 10 Point Scale	300+	75%	68%	71%
Meds 'Always' Explained Before Given	300+	62%	61%	64%
Nurses 'Always' Communicated Well	300+	77%	74%	79%
Pain 'Always' Well Controlled	300+	70%	68%	71%
Room and Bathroom 'Always' Clean	300+	72%	70%	73%
Timely Help 'Always' Received	300+	60%	62%	68%
Would Definitely Recommend Hospital	300+	79%	70%	71%
Use of Medical Imaging				
Cardiac Imaging Stress Test before Surgery	682	5.6%	5.2%	5.3%
Combination Abdominal CT Scan	1,462	12.7%	13.4%	10.5%
Combination Brain/Sinus CT Scan	873	0.8%	2.2%	2.7%
Combination Chest CT Scan	966	0.1%	2.3%	2.7%
Follow-up Mammogram/Ultrasound	5,028	8.9%	8.2%	8.8%
Lumbar Spine MRI for Low Back Pain	190	35.3%	34.2%	37.2%

Sutter Tracy Community Hospital

1420 N Tracy Blvd
Tracy, CA 95376
Phone: 209-835-1500
Fax: 209-832-6091
E-mail: alonzot@sutterhealth.org
URL: www.suttertracy.org
Type: Acute Care Hospitals
Emergency Services: Yes
Ownership: Voluntary non-profit - Private
Beds: 79

Key Personnel:

Cardiology . . . . Jonthan Bridges
Cardiology . . . . Lance Briggs, MD
Cardiology . . . . James Clayburg
Emergency Room . . . . Denise Drewry, RN
Radiology. . . . . Sam Kokoris, MD
CEO/President. . . . . Robert Reed
Quality Assurance . . . . Sandy Williams

Measure	Cases	This Hosp.	State Avg.	U.S. Avg.
Blood Clot Prevention and Treatment				
Anticoagulation Overlap Therapy[2]	27	85%	92%	93%
ICU Venous Thromboembolism Prophylaxis[2]	73	97%	92%	92%
Incidence of Potentially Preventable VTE[1,2]	-	-	11%	10%
UFH with Dosages/Platelet Monitoring[2]	23	100%	96%	97%
Venous Thromboembolism Prophylaxis[2]	238	96%	83%	85%
Warfarin Therapy Discharge Instructions[2]	18	100%	75%	75%
Chest Pain/Possible Heart Attack Care				
Aspirin Given Within 24 Hours of Arrival[1]	-	-	97%	96%
Fibrinolytic Meds Within 30 Min. of Arrival[1,3]	-	-	62%	58%
Average Time to ECG (minutes)[1]	-	-	9	7
Average Time to Transfer (minutes)[1,3]	-	-	62	60
Children's Asthma Care				
Received Home Management Plan of Care	-	-	88%	88%
Received Reliever Medication	-	-	100%	100%
Received Systemic Corticosteroids	-	-	100%	100%
Emergency Department				
Admittance Decision Time (minutes)[2]	468	95	125	98
Head CT Results Within 45 Min. of Arrival	15	33%	55%	57%
Patients Who Left ER Before Being Seen	32,559	3%	3%	2%
Time from ER Arrival to Admit. (minutes)[2]	469	281	323	274
Time from ER Arrival to Discharge (minutes)	402	158	168	134
Time in ER Before Being Evaluated (minutes)	422	32	29	26
Time to Pain Meds for Fractures (minutes)	173	66	62	57
Heart Attack Care				
Aspirin Given at Discharge	30	100%	99%	99%
Fibrinolytic Meds Within 30 Min. of Arrival[1]	-	-	73%	54%
PCI Within 90 Minutes of Arrival[7]	-	-	95%	96%
Statin Prescribed at Discharge	28	100%	98%	98%
Heart Failure Care				
ACE Inhibitor or ARB for LVSD	30	100%	97%	97%
Discharge Instructions Given	76	97%	94%	94%
Evaluation of LVS Function	95	99%	99%	99%
Medicare Spending				
Medicare Spending per Patient (ratio)	-	0.97	0.98	0.98
Pneumonia Care				
Appropriate Initial Antibiotic Given	54	100%	97%	95%
Blood Culture Timing	99	99%	98%	98%
Pregnancy and Delivery Care				
Newborn Deliveries Scheduled Early	39	0%	5%	6%
Preventive Care				
Immunization for Influenza[2]	361	99%	89%	90%

NOTE: Hospital profiles are in alphabetical order by state, then city, then hospital within the city; Rankings exclude hospitals with less than 25 cases except for patient surveys which excludes hospitals with less than 100 cases; (a) 100-299 cases; (1) The number of cases/patients is too few to report; (2) Data submitted were based on a sample of cases/patients; (3) Results are based on a shorter time period than required; (4) Data suppressed by CMS for one or more quarters; (5) Results are not available for this reporting period; (6) Fewer than 100 patients completed the HCAHPS survey; (7) No cases met the criteria for this measure; (8) The lower limit of the confidence interval cannot be calculated if the number of observed infections equals zero; (9) No data are available from the state/territory for this reporting period; (10) The scores shown reflect fewer than 50 completed surveys; (11) There were discrepancies in the data collection process; (12) This measure does not apply to this hospital for this reporting period; (13) Results cannot be calculated for this reporting period; (14) The results for this state are combined with nearby states to protect confidentiality; Please refer to the User's Guide for a full explanation of data.

Measure	Cases	This Hosp.	State Avg.	U.S. Avg.
Immunization for Pneumonia[2]	398	98%	90%	92%
Stroke Care				
Anticoagulation Therapy for Atrial Fibrillation[1]	-	-	95%	95%
Antithrombotic Therapy Timing	14	93%	98%	98%
Assessed for Rehabilitation	22	95%	97%	97%
Discharged on Antithrombotic Therapy	21	90%	99%	99%
Discharged on Statin Medication	20	90%	94%	94%
Thrombolytic Therapy Timing[1]	-	-	72%	66%
Venous Thromboembolism Prophylaxis	19	89%	94%	94%
Written Stroke Educational Materials Given	16	81%	87%	88%
Surgical Care Improvement Project				
Appropriate Beta Blocker Usage	45	98%	97%	98%
Appropriate VTP Within 24 Hours	147	100%	98%	98%
Controlled Postoperative Blood Glucose[7]	-	-	96%	97%
Perioperative Temperature Management	194	100%	100%	100%
Prophylactic Antibiotic Selection	150	100%	99%	99%
Prophylactic Antibiotic Selection (Outpatient)	91	100%	97%	98%
Prophylactic Antibiotic Stopped	144	99%	98%	98%
Prophylactic Antibiotic Timing	150	100%	99%	99%
Prophylactic Antibiotic Timing (Outpatient)	91	100%	97%	98%
Urinary Catheter Removal	126	100%	97%	97%
Survey of Patients' Hospital Experiences				
Area Around Room 'Always' Quiet at Night	300+	57%	51%	61%
Doctors 'Always' Communicated Well	300+	81%	78%	82%
Home Recovery Information Given	300+	84%	83%	85%
Hospital Given 9 or 10 on 10 Point Scale	300+	77%	68%	71%
Meds 'Always' Explained Before Given	300+	65%	61%	64%
Nurses 'Always' Communicated Well	300+	80%	74%	79%
Pain 'Always' Well Controlled	300+	73%	68%	71%
Room and Bathroom 'Always' Clean	300+	76%	70%	73%
Timely Help 'Always' Received	300+	65%	62%	68%
Would Definitely Recommend Hospital	300+	79%	70%	71%
Use of Medical Imaging				
Cardiac Imaging Stress Test before Surgery[1]	-	-	5.2%	5.3%
Combination Abdominal CT Scan	474	4.6%	13.4%	10.5%
Combination Brain/Sinus CT Scan[1]	-	-	2.2%	2.7%
Combination Chest CT Scan	181	2.8%	2.3%	2.7%
Follow-up Mammogram/Ultrasound	858	5.4%	8.2%	8.8%
Lumbar Spine MRI for Low Back Pain[1]	-	-	34.2%	37.2%

Tahoe Forest Hospital

10121 Pine Ave
Truckee, CA 96161
E-mail: information@tfhd.com
URL: www.tfhd.com
Type: Critical Access Hospitals
Ownership: Govt - Hospital Dist/Auth

Phone: 530-587-6011
Fax: 530-587-2532
Emergency Services: Yes
Beds: 25

Key Personnel:

Operating Room. . . . . Helmuth Billy
Emergency Room . . . . Charles Clemons
Infection Control. . . . . Laurel Holmer, RN
Radiology. . . . . Myron Kamenetsky
Quality Assurance . . . . Judy Newland
CEO . . . . Robert A Schapper
Chief of Medical Staff . . . . Terri Schnieder, MD
Intensive Care Unit. . . . . Carolyn Willette

Measure	Cases	This Hosp.	State Avg.	U.S. Avg.
Blood Clot Prevention and Treatment				
Anticoagulation Overlap Therapy[2]	11	91%	92%	93%
ICU Venous Thromboembolism Prophylaxis[2]	27	74%	92%	92%
Incidence of Potentially Preventable VTE[2,7]	-	-	11%	10%
UFH with Dosages/Platelet Monitoring[1,2]	-	-	96%	97%
Venous Thromboembolism Prophylaxis[2]	74	69%	83%	85%
Warfarin Therapy Discharge Instructions[1,2]	-	-	75%	75%
Chest Pain/Possible Heart Attack Care				
Aspirin Given Within 24 Hours of Arrival	-	-	97%	96%
Fibrinolytic Meds Within 30 Min. of Arrival	-	-	62%	58%
Average Time to ECG (minutes)	-	-	9	7
Average Time to Transfer (minutes)	-	-	62	60
Children's Asthma Care				
Received Home Management Plan of Care	-	-	88%	88%
Received Reliever Medication	-	-	100%	100%
Received Systemic Corticosteroids	-	-	100%	100%
Emergency Department				
Admittance Decision Time (minutes)[2]	275	99	125	98
Head CT Results Within 45 Min. of Arrival	-	-	55%	57%
Patients Who Left ER Before Being Seen	-	-	3%	2%
Time from ER Arrival to Admit. (minutes)[2]	280	242	323	274
Time from ER Arrival to Discharge (minutes)	-	-	168	134
Time in ER Before Being Evaluated (minutes)	-	-	29	26
Time to Pain Meds for Fractures (minutes)	-	-	62	57
Heart Attack Care				
Aspirin Given at Discharge[1,3]	-	-	99%	99%
Fibrinolytic Meds Within 30 Min. of Arrival[3,7]	-	-	73%	54%
PCI Within 90 Minutes of Arrival[3,7]	-	-	95%	96%
Statin Prescribed at Discharge[1,3]	-	-	98%	98%
Heart Failure Care				
ACE Inhibitor or ARB for LVSD[1]	-	-	97%	97%
Discharge Instructions Given	12	100%	94%	94%
Evaluation of LVS Function	13	100%	99%	99%
Medicare Spending				
Medicare Spending per Patient (ratio)	-	-	0.98	0.98
Pneumonia Care				
Appropriate Initial Antibiotic Given[1]	-	-	97%	95%
Blood Culture Timing[1]	-	-	98%	98%
Pregnancy and Delivery Care				
Newborn Deliveries Scheduled Early[5]	-	-	5%	6%
Preventive Care				
Immunization for Influenza[2]	290	87%	89%	90%
Immunization for Pneumonia[2]	225	85%	90%	92%
Stroke Care				
Anticoagulation Therapy for Atrial Fibrillation[1,3]	-	-	95%	95%
Antithrombotic Therapy Timing[1,3]	-	-	98%	98%
Assessed for Rehabilitation[1,3]	-	-	97%	97%
Discharged on Antithrombotic Therapy[1,3]	-	-	99%	99%
Discharged on Statin Medication[1,3]	-	-	94%	94%
Thrombolytic Therapy Timing[1,3]	-	-	72%	66%
Venous Thromboembolism Prophylaxis[1,3]	-	-	94%	94%
Written Stroke Educational Materials Given[1,3]	-	-	87%	88%
Surgical Care Improvement Project				
Appropriate Beta Blocker Usage	33	85%	97%	98%
Appropriate VTP Within 24 Hours	177	95%	98%	98%
Controlled Postoperative Blood Glucose[7]	-	-	96%	97%
Perioperative Temperature Management	218	100%	100%	100%
Prophylactic Antibiotic Selection	170	99%	99%	99%
Prophylactic Antibiotic Selection (Outpatient)	-	-	97%	98%
Prophylactic Antibiotic Stopped	167	94%	98%	98%
Prophylactic Antibiotic Timing	170	98%	99%	99%
Prophylactic Antibiotic Timing (Outpatient)	-	-	97%	98%
Urinary Catheter Removal	158	94%	97%	97%
Survey of Patients' Hospital Experiences				
Area Around Room 'Always' Quiet at Night	(a)	62%	51%	61%
Doctors 'Always' Communicated Well	(a)	81%	78%	82%
Home Recovery Information Given	(a)	86%	83%	85%
Hospital Given 9 or 10 on 10 Point Scale	(a)	83%	68%	71%
Meds 'Always' Explained Before Given	(a)	66%	61%	64%
Nurses 'Always' Communicated Well	(a)	85%	74%	79%
Pain 'Always' Well Controlled	(a)	72%	68%	71%
Room and Bathroom 'Always' Clean	(a)	86%	70%	73%
Timely Help 'Always' Received	(a)	73%	62%	68%
Would Definitely Recommend Hospital	(a)	86%	70%	71%
Use of Medical Imaging				
Cardiac Imaging Stress Test before Surgery	-	-	5.2%	5.3%
Combination Abdominal CT Scan	-	-	13.4%	10.5%
Combination Brain/Sinus CT Scan	-	-	2.2%	2.7%
Combination Chest CT Scan	-	-	2.3%	2.7%
Follow-up Mammogram/Ultrasound	-	-	8.2%	8.8%
Lumbar Spine MRI for Low Back Pain	-	-	34.2%	37.2%

Tulare Regional Medical Center

869 Cherry Avenue
Tulare, CA 93274
E-mail: info@tdhs.org
URL: www.tdhs.org
Type: Acute Care Hospitals
Ownership: Govt - Hospital Dist/Auth

Phone: 559-688-0821
Fax: 559-685-3875
Emergency Services: Yes
Beds: 112

Key Personnel:

Chief of Medical Staff. . . . . Denise Cerry
Quality Assurance . . . . Melissa Janes
CEO/President. . . . . Robert Montain

Measure	Cases	This Hosp.	State Avg.	U.S. Avg.
Blood Clot Prevention and Treatment				
Anticoagulation Overlap Therapy[2]	21	52%	92%	93%
ICU Venous Thromboembolism Prophylaxis[2]	67	91%	92%	92%
Incidence of Potentially Preventable VTE[1,2]	-	-	11%	10%
UFH with Dosages/Platelet Monitoring[1,2]	-	-	96%	97%
Venous Thromboembolism Prophylaxis[2]	288	83%	83%	85%
Warfarin Therapy Discharge Instructions[2]	15	47%	75%	75%
Chest Pain/Possible Heart Attack Care				
Aspirin Given Within 24 Hours of Arrival[1,3]	-	-	97%	96%
Fibrinolytic Meds Within 30 Min. of Arrival[3,7]	-	-	62%	58%
Average Time to ECG (minutes)[1,3]	-	-	9	7
Average Time to Transfer (minutes)[1,3]	-	-	62	60
Children's Asthma Care				
Received Home Management Plan of Care	-	-	88%	88%
Received Reliever Medication	-	-	100%	100%
Received Systemic Corticosteroids	-	-	100%	100%
Emergency Department				
Admittance Decision Time (minutes)[2]	360	104	125	98
Head CT Results Within 45 Min. of Arrival	12	42%	55%	57%
Patients Who Left ER Before Being Seen	31,590	7%	3%	2%
Time from ER Arrival to Admit. (minutes)[2]	372	306	323	274
Time from ER Arrival to Discharge (minutes)	406	168	168	134
Time in ER Before Being Evaluated (minutes)	398	70	29	26
Time to Pain Meds for Fractures (minutes)	124	72	62	57
Heart Attack Care				
Aspirin Given at Discharge	26	100%	99%	99%
Fibrinolytic Meds Within 30 Min. of Arrival[1]	-	-	73%	54%
PCI Within 90 Minutes of Arrival[7]	-	-	95%	96%
Statin Prescribed at Discharge	21	100%	98%	98%
Heart Failure Care				
ACE Inhibitor or ARB for LVSD	26	100%	97%	97%
Discharge Instructions Given	87	100%	94%	94%
Evaluation of LVS Function	105	100%	99%	99%
Medicare Spending				
Medicare Spending per Patient (ratio)	-	0.96	0.98	0.98
Pneumonia Care				
Appropriate Initial Antibiotic Given	107	99%	97%	95%
Blood Culture Timing	148	97%	98%	98%
Pregnancy and Delivery Care				
Newborn Deliveries Scheduled Early[2]	56	9%	5%	6%
Preventive Care				
Immunization for Influenza[2]	392	69%	89%	90%
Immunization for Pneumonia[2]	316	82%	90%	92%
Stroke Care				
Anticoagulation Therapy for Atrial Fibrillation[1]	-	-	95%	95%
Antithrombotic Therapy Timing	25	80%	98%	98%
Assessed for Rehabilitation	25	76%	97%	97%
Discharged on Antithrombotic Therapy	23	83%	99%	99%
Discharged on Statin Medication	23	52%	94%	94%
Thrombolytic Therapy Timing[7]	-	-	72%	66%
Venous Thromboembolism Prophylaxis	24	83%	94%	94%
Written Stroke Educational Materials Given	14	43%	87%	88%
Surgical Care Improvement Project				
Appropriate Beta Blocker Usage	20	100%	97%	98%
Appropriate VTP Within 24 Hours	109	96%	98%	98%
Controlled Postoperative Blood Glucose[7]	-	-	96%	97%
Perioperative Temperature Management	129	99%	100%	100%
Prophylactic Antibiotic Selection	52	94%	99%	99%
Prophylactic Antibiotic Selection (Outpatient)	112	98%	97%	98%
Prophylactic Antibiotic Stopped	49	96%	98%	98%
Prophylactic Antibiotic Timing	52	92%	99%	99%
Prophylactic Antibiotic Timing (Outpatient)	114	98%	97%	98%
Urinary Catheter Removal	43	98%	97%	97%
Survey of Patients' Hospital Experiences				
Area Around Room 'Always' Quiet at Night	300+	45%	51%	61%
Doctors 'Always' Communicated Well	300+	75%	78%	82%
Home Recovery Information Given	300+	76%	83%	85%
Hospital Given 9 or 10 on 10 Point Scale	300+	55%	68%	71%
Meds 'Always' Explained Before Given	300+	63%	61%	64%

NOTE: Hospital profiles are in alphabetical order by state, then city, then hospital within the city; Rankings exclude hospitals with less than 25 cases except for patient surveys which excludes hospitals with less than 100 cases; (a) 100-299 cases; (1) The number of cases/patients is too few to report; (2) Data submitted were based on a sample of cases/patients; (3) Results are based on a shorter time period than required; (4) Data suppressed by CMS for one or more quarters; (5) Results are not available for this reporting period; (6) Fewer than 100 patients completed the HCAHPS survey; (7) No cases met the criteria for this measure; (8) The lower limit of the confidence interval cannot be calculated if the number of observed infections equals zero; (9) No data are available from the state/territory for this reporting period; (10) The scores shown reflect fewer than 50 completed surveys; (11) There were discrepancies in the data collection process; (12) This measure does not apply to this hospital for this reporting period; (13) Results cannot be calculated for this reporting period; (14) The results for this state are combined with nearby states to protect confidentiality; Please refer to the User's Guide for a full explanation of data.

Measure	Cases	This Hosp.	State Avg.	U.S. Avg.
Nurses 'Always' Communicated Well	300+	70%	74%	79%
Pain 'Always' Well Controlled	300+	64%	68%	71%
Room and Bathroom 'Always' Clean	300+	61%	70%	73%
Timely Help 'Always' Received	300+	51%	62%	68%
Would Definitely Recommend Hospital	300+	53%	70%	71%
Use of Medical Imaging				
Cardiac Imaging Stress Test before Surgery[1]	-	-	5.2%	5.3%
Combination Abdominal CT Scan	482	2.3%	13.4%	10.5%
Combination Brain/Sinus CT Scan[1]	-	-	2.2%	2.7%
Combination Chest CT Scan	158	4.4%	2.3%	2.7%
Follow-up Mammogram/Ultrasound	726	7.7%	8.2%	8.8%
Lumbar Spine MRI for Low Back Pain	47	40.4%	34.2%	37.2%

Emanuel Medical Center

825 Delbon Ave
Turlock, CA 95382
Phone: 209-667-4200
Fax: 209-669-2372
URL: www.emanuelmedicalcenter.org
Type: Acute Care Hospitals
Emergency Services: Yes
Ownership: Voluntary non-profit - Church
Beds: 150

Key Personnel:

Radiology. . . . . Dennis J Alsofrom
Chief of Medical Staff. . . . . Ronald Arakelian, MD
Patient Relations . . . . Connie Fairchilds
CEO . . . . Sue Micheletti
Quality Assurance . . . . Julie Riddick
CEO/President. . . . . John Sigsbury

Measure	Cases	This Hosp.	State Avg.	U.S. Avg.
Blood Clot Prevention and Treatment				
Anticoagulation Overlap Therapy[2]	43	86%	92%	93%
ICU Venous Thromboembolism Prophylaxis[2]	19	100%	92%	92%
Incidence of Potentially Preventable VTE[2]	12	25%	11%	10%
UFH with Dosages/Platelet Monitoring[2]	24	100%	96%	97%
Venous Thromboembolism Prophylaxis[2]	478	89%	83%	85%
Warfarin Therapy Discharge Instructions[2]	30	40%	75%	75%
Chest Pain/Possible Heart Attack Care				
Aspirin Given Within 24 Hours of Arrival[3]	12	100%	97%	96%
Fibrinolytic Meds Within 30 Min. of Arrival[3,7]	-	-	62%	58%
Average Time to ECG (minutes)[3]	13	11	9	7
Average Time to Transfer (minutes)[3,7]	-	-	62	60
Children's Asthma Care				
Received Home Management Plan of Care	-	-	88%	88%
Received Reliever Medication	-	-	100%	100%
Received Systemic Corticosteroids	-	-	100%	100%
Emergency Department				
Admittance Decision Time (minutes)[2]	883	141	125	98
Head CT Results Within 45 Min. of Arrival	29	24%	55%	57%
Patients Who Left ER Before Being Seen	61,364	1%	3%	2%
Time from ER Arrival to Admit. (minutes)[2]	941	372	323	274
Time from ER Arrival to Discharge (minutes)	457	121	168	134
Time in ER Before Being Evaluated (minutes)	424	28	29	26
Time to Pain Meds for Fractures (minutes)	204	44	62	57
Heart Attack Care				
Aspirin Given at Discharge	245	100%	99%	99%
Fibrinolytic Meds Within 30 Min. of Arrival[7]	-	-	73%	54%
PCI Within 90 Minutes of Arrival	52	92%	95%	96%
Statin Prescribed at Discharge	237	98%	98%	98%
Heart Failure Care				
ACE Inhibitor or ARB for LVSD	90	100%	97%	97%
Discharge Instructions Given	221	90%	94%	94%
Evaluation of LVS Function	288	100%	99%	99%
Medicare Spending				
Medicare Spending per Patient (ratio)	-	0.95	0.98	0.98
Pneumonia Care				
Appropriate Initial Antibiotic Given	259	95%	97%	95%
Blood Culture Timing	332	99%	98%	98%
Pregnancy and Delivery Care				
Newborn Deliveries Scheduled Early[2]	36	3%	5%	6%
Preventive Care				
Immunization for Influenza[2]	599	97%	89%	90%
Immunization for Pneumonia[2]	693	96%	90%	92%
Stroke Care				
Anticoagulation Therapy for Atrial Fibrillation	11	100%	95%	95%
Antithrombotic Therapy Timing	49	100%	98%	98%
Assessed for Rehabilitation	52	90%	97%	97%
Discharged on Antithrombotic Therapy	48	100%	99%	99%
Discharged on Statin Medication	42	95%	94%	94%
Thrombolytic Therapy Timing	12	0%	72%	66%
Venous Thromboembolism Prophylaxis	56	89%	94%	94%
Written Stroke Educational Materials Given	33	70%	87%	88%
Surgical Care Improvement Project				
Appropriate Beta Blocker Usage	105	100%	97%	98%
Appropriate VTP Within 24 Hours	304	95%	98%	98%
Controlled Postoperative Blood Glucose	39	100%	96%	97%
Perioperative Temperature Management	424	100%	100%	100%
Prophylactic Antibiotic Selection	323	98%	99%	99%
Prophylactic Antibiotic Selection (Outpatient)	84	93%	97%	98%
Prophylactic Antibiotic Stopped	317	98%	98%	98%
Prophylactic Antibiotic Timing	323	98%	99%	99%
Prophylactic Antibiotic Timing (Outpatient)	88	86%	97%	98%
Urinary Catheter Removal	184	99%	97%	97%
Survey of Patients' Hospital Experiences				
Area Around Room 'Always' Quiet at Night	300+	40%	51%	61%
Doctors 'Always' Communicated Well	300+	68%	78%	82%
Home Recovery Information Given	300+	79%	83%	85%
Hospital Given 9 or 10 on 10 Point Scale	300+	57%	68%	71%
Meds 'Always' Explained Before Given	300+	57%	61%	64%
Nurses 'Always' Communicated Well	300+	69%	74%	79%
Pain 'Always' Well Controlled	300+	62%	68%	71%
Room and Bathroom 'Always' Clean	300+	66%	70%	73%
Timely Help 'Always' Received	300+	52%	62%	68%
Would Definitely Recommend Hospital	300+	58%	70%	71%
Use of Medical Imaging				
Cardiac Imaging Stress Test before Surgery	245	2.0%	5.2%	5.3%
Combination Abdominal CT Scan	375	1.3%	13.4%	10.5%
Combination Brain/Sinus CT Scan	572	2.3%	2.2%	2.7%
Combination Chest CT Scan	103	0.0%	2.3%	2.7%
Follow-up Mammogram/Ultrasound	1,324	5.5%	8.2%	8.8%
Lumbar Spine MRI for Low Back Pain[1]	-	-	34.2%	37.2%

Ukiah Valley Medical Center

275 Hospital Drive
Ukiah, CA 95482
Phone: 707-462-3111
Fax: 707-463-7384
URL: www.uvmc.org
Type: Acute Care Hospitals
Emergency Services: Yes
Ownership: Voluntary non-profit - Church
Beds: 101

Key Personnel:

Cardiac Laboratory. . . . . Jill Bartolomie, RN
Coronary Care . . . . Jill Bartolomie, RN
Pediatric Ambulatory Care . . . . . . Jill Bartolomie, RN
Radiology. . . . . Randall L Bivens
Operating Room. . . . . Fredrick A Burris, RN
Chief of Medical Staff. . . . . Geoffrey Esselman, MD
Infection Control. . . . . Sue Mason, RN

Measure	Cases	This Hosp.	State Avg.	U.S. Avg.
Blood Clot Prevention and Treatment				
Anticoagulation Overlap Therapy[2]	15	80%	92%	93%
ICU Venous Thromboembolism Prophylaxis[2]	47	77%	92%	92%
Incidence of Potentially Preventable VTE[1,2]	-	-	11%	10%
UFH with Dosages/Platelet Monitoring[1,2]	-	-	96%	97%
Venous Thromboembolism Prophylaxis[2]	221	83%	83%	85%
Warfarin Therapy Discharge Instructions[2]	13	62%	75%	75%
Chest Pain/Possible Heart Attack Care				
Aspirin Given Within 24 Hours of Arrival	37	100%	97%	96%
Fibrinolytic Meds Within 30 Min. of Arrival[1]	-	-	62%	58%
Average Time to ECG (minutes)	40	14	9	7
Average Time to Transfer (minutes)[1]	-	-	62	60
Children's Asthma Care				
Received Home Management Plan of Care	-	-	88%	88%
Received Reliever Medication	-	-	100%	100%
Received Systemic Corticosteroids	-	-	100%	100%
Emergency Department				
Admittance Decision Time (minutes)[2]	456	85	125	98
Head CT Results Within 45 Min. of Arrival[1]	-	-	55%	57%
Patients Who Left ER Before Being Seen	22,200	1%	3%	2%
Time from ER Arrival to Admit. (minutes)[2]	463	236	323	274
Time from ER Arrival to Discharge (minutes)	346	136	168	134
Time in ER Before Being Evaluated (minutes)	143	21	29	26
Time to Pain Meds for Fractures (minutes)	36	46	62	57
Heart Attack Care				
Aspirin Given at Discharge[1]	-	-	99%	99%
Fibrinolytic Meds Within 30 Min. of Arrival[7]	-	-	73%	54%
PCI Within 90 Minutes of Arrival[7]	-	-	95%	96%
Statin Prescribed at Discharge[1]	-	-	98%	98%
Heart Failure Care				
ACE Inhibitor or ARB for LVSD	24	92%	97%	97%
Discharge Instructions Given	81	86%	94%	94%
Evaluation of LVS Function	90	99%	99%	99%
Medicare Spending				
Medicare Spending per Patient (ratio)	-	0.88	0.98	0.98
Pneumonia Care				
Appropriate Initial Antibiotic Given	89	97%	97%	95%
Blood Culture Timing	120	100%	98%	98%
Pregnancy and Delivery Care				
Newborn Deliveries Scheduled Early[2]	26	4%	5%	6%
Preventive Care				
Immunization for Influenza[2]	361	70%	89%	90%
Immunization for Pneumonia[2]	402	76%	90%	92%
Stroke Care				
Anticoagulation Therapy for Atrial Fibrillation[1]	-	-	95%	95%
Antithrombotic Therapy Timing	38	95%	98%	98%
Assessed for Rehabilitation	43	91%	97%	97%
Discharged on Antithrombotic Therapy	40	95%	99%	99%
Discharged on Statin Medication	35	80%	94%	94%
Thrombolytic Therapy Timing[1]	-	-	72%	66%
Venous Thromboembolism Prophylaxis	46	80%	94%	94%
Written Stroke Educational Materials Given	22	55%	87%	88%
Surgical Care Improvement Project				
Appropriate Beta Blocker Usage	26	92%	97%	98%
Appropriate VTP Within 24 Hours	162	91%	98%	98%
Controlled Postoperative Blood Glucose[7]	-	-	96%	97%
Perioperative Temperature Management	190	100%	100%	100%
Prophylactic Antibiotic Selection	114	98%	99%	99%
Prophylactic Antibiotic Selection (Outpatient)	46	93%	97%	98%
Prophylactic Antibiotic Stopped	113	91%	98%	98%
Prophylactic Antibiotic Timing	115	94%	99%	99%
Prophylactic Antibiotic Timing (Outpatient)	46	100%	97%	98%
Urinary Catheter Removal	109	94%	97%	97%
Survey of Patients' Hospital Experiences				
Area Around Room 'Always' Quiet at Night	300+	39%	51%	61%
Doctors 'Always' Communicated Well	300+	80%	78%	82%
Home Recovery Information Given	300+	88%	83%	85%
Hospital Given 9 or 10 on 10 Point Scale	300+	68%	68%	71%
Meds 'Always' Explained Before Given	300+	64%	61%	64%
Nurses 'Always' Communicated Well	300+	78%	74%	79%
Pain 'Always' Well Controlled	300+	71%	68%	71%
Room and Bathroom 'Always' Clean	300+	70%	70%	73%
Timely Help 'Always' Received	300+	64%	62%	68%
Would Definitely Recommend Hospital	300+	70%	70%	71%
Use of Medical Imaging				
Cardiac Imaging Stress Test before Surgery	346	2.9%	5.2%	5.3%
Combination Abdominal CT Scan	488	8.2%	13.4%	10.5%
Combination Brain/Sinus CT Scan	338	8.0%	2.2%	2.7%
Combination Chest CT Scan	217	3.2%	2.3%	2.7%
Follow-up Mammogram/Ultrasound	1,338	5.6%	8.2%	8.8%
Lumbar Spine MRI for Low Back Pain	98	30.6%	34.2%	37.2%

San Antonio Community Hospital

999 San Bernardino Rd
Upland, CA 91786
Phone: 714-985-2811
Fax: 909-920-6357
URL: www.sach.org
Type: Acute Care Hospitals
Emergency Services: Yes
Ownership: Voluntary non-profit - Other
Beds: 329

Key Personnel:

CEO/President. . . . . Harvey Cohen, MD
Infection Control. . . . . Karen Drinkwine
Operating Room. . . . . Regina Millard, RN
Quality Assurance . . . . Debbie Nicol
Emergency Room . . . . Matthew Potts, MD
Patient Relations . . . . Meri Ravenkamp
Anesthesiology. . . . . Thuan Tu, MD
Radiology. . . . . Peter Yoo, MD

Measure	Cases	This Hosp.	State Avg.	U.S. Avg.

NOTE: Hospital profiles are in alphabetical order by state, then city, then hospital within the city; Rankings exclude hospitals with less than 25 cases except for patient surveys which excludes hospitals with less than 100 cases; (a) 100-299 cases; (1) The number of cases/patients is too few to report; (2) Data submitted were based on a sample of cases/patients; (3) Results are based on a shorter time period than required; (4) Data suppressed by CMS for one or more quarters; (5) Results are not available for this reporting period; (6) Fewer than 100 patients completed the HCAHPS survey; (7) No cases met the criteria for this measure; (8) The lower limit of the confidence interval cannot be calculated if the number of observed infections equals zero; (9) No data are available from the state/territory for this reporting period; (10) The scores shown reflect fewer than 50 completed surveys; (11) There were discrepancies in the data collection process; (12) This measure does not apply to this hospital for this reporting period; (13) Results cannot be calculated for this reporting period; (14) The results for this state are combined with nearby states to protect confidentiality; Please refer to the User's Guide for a full explanation of data.

Measure	Cases	This Hosp.	State Avg.	U.S. Avg.
Blood Clot Prevention and Treatment				
Anticoagulation Overlap Therapy[2]	65	92%	92%	93%
ICU Venous Thromboembolism Prophylaxis[2]	36	94%	92%	92%
Incidence of Potentially Preventable VTE[2]	19	11%	11%	10%
UFH with Dosages/Platelet Monitoring[2]	26	100%	96%	97%
Venous Thromboembolism Prophylaxis[2]	303	79%	83%	85%
Warfarin Therapy Discharge Instructions[2]	44	86%	75%	75%
Chest Pain/Possible Heart Attack Care				
Aspirin Given Within 24 Hours of Arrival[1,3]	-	-	97%	96%
Fibrinolytic Meds Within 30 Min. of Arrival[3,7]	-	-	62%	58%
Average Time to ECG (minutes)[1,3]	-	-	9	7
Average Time to Transfer (minutes)[3,7]	-	-	62	60
Children's Asthma Care				
Received Home Management Plan of Care	-	-	88%	88%
Received Reliever Medication	-	-	100%	100%
Received Systemic Corticosteroids	-	-	100%	100%
Emergency Department				
Admittance Decision Time (minutes)[2]	656	167	125	98
Head CT Results Within 45 Min. of Arrival[1]	-	-	55%	57%
Patients Who Left ER Before Being Seen	74,197	2%	3%	2%
Time from ER Arrival to Admit. (minutes)[2]	656	334	323	274
Time from ER Arrival to Discharge (minutes)	343	221	168	134
Time in ER Before Being Evaluated (minutes)	389	51	29	26
Time to Pain Meds for Fractures (minutes)	64	76	62	57
Heart Attack Care				
Aspirin Given at Discharge	325	99%	99%	99%
Fibrinolytic Meds Within 30 Min. of Arrival[1]	-	-	73%	54%
PCI Within 90 Minutes of Arrival	53	91%	95%	96%
Statin Prescribed at Discharge	359	97%	98%	98%
Heart Failure Care				
ACE Inhibitor or ARB for LVSD	133	96%	97%	97%
Discharge Instructions Given	333	100%	94%	94%
Evaluation of LVS Function	397	98%	99%	99%
Medicare Spending				
Medicare Spending per Patient (ratio)	-	1.04	0.98	0.98
Pneumonia Care				
Appropriate Initial Antibiotic Given[2]	77	99%	97%	95%
Blood Culture Timing[2]	161	95%	98%	98%
Pregnancy and Delivery Care				
Newborn Deliveries Scheduled Early[2]	46	2%	5%	6%
Preventive Care				
Immunization for Influenza[2]	545	85%	89%	90%
Immunization for Pneumonia[2]	589	91%	90%	92%
Stroke Care				
Anticoagulation Therapy for Atrial Fibrillation	26	100%	95%	95%
Antithrombotic Therapy Timing	123	98%	98%	98%
Assessed for Rehabilitation	199	99%	97%	97%
Discharged on Antithrombotic Therapy	149	98%	99%	99%
Discharged on Statin Medication	121	94%	94%	94%
Thrombolytic Therapy Timing	26	96%	72%	66%
Venous Thromboembolism Prophylaxis	190	99%	94%	94%
Written Stroke Educational Materials Given	88	99%	87%	88%
Surgical Care Improvement Project				
Appropriate Beta Blocker Usage[2]	229	100%	97%	98%
Appropriate VTP Within 24 Hours[2]	352	95%	98%	98%
Controlled Postoperative Blood Glucose[2]	117	97%	96%	97%
Perioperative Temperature Management[2]	422	100%	100%	100%
Prophylactic Antibiotic Selection[2]	387	100%	99%	99%
Prophylactic Antibiotic Selection (Outpatient)	369	96%	97%	98%
Prophylactic Antibiotic Stopped[2]	368	96%	98%	98%
Prophylactic Antibiotic Timing[2]	388	98%	99%	99%
Prophylactic Antibiotic Timing (Outpatient)	370	97%	97%	98%
Urinary Catheter Removal[2]	300	96%	97%	97%
Survey of Patients' Hospital Experiences				
Area Around Room 'Always' Quiet at Night	300+	43%	51%	61%
Doctors 'Always' Communicated Well	300+	78%	78%	82%
Home Recovery Information Given	300+	85%	83%	85%
Hospital Given 9 or 10 on 10 Point Scale	300+	71%	68%	71%
Meds 'Always' Explained Before Given	300+	62%	61%	64%
Nurses 'Always' Communicated Well	300+	77%	74%	79%
Pain 'Always' Well Controlled	300+	70%	68%	71%
Room and Bathroom 'Always' Clean	300+	66%	70%	73%
Timely Help 'Always' Received	300+	58%	62%	68%
Would Definitely Recommend Hospital	300+	76%	70%	71%
Use of Medical Imaging				
Cardiac Imaging Stress Test before Surgery	144	9.0%	5.2%	5.3%
Combination Abdominal CT Scan	1,016	14.3%	13.4%	10.5%
Combination Brain/Sinus CT Scan	924	1.6%	2.2%	2.7%
Combination Chest CT Scan	624	1.1%	2.3%	2.7%
Follow-up Mammogram/Ultrasound	1,645	12.1%	8.2%	8.8%
Lumbar Spine MRI for Low Back Pain	70	34.3%	34.2%	37.2%

Kaiser Foundation Hospital - Vacaville

1 Quality Drive
Vacaville, CA 95688
Phone: 707-624-4000
URL: www.kaiserpermanente.org
Type: Acute Care Hospitals
Emergency Services: Yes
Ownership: Proprietary

Measure	Cases	This Hosp.	State Avg.	U.S. Avg.
Blood Clot Prevention and Treatment				
Anticoagulation Overlap Therapy[2]	36	94%	92%	93%
ICU Venous Thromboembolism Prophylaxis[2]	80	98%	92%	92%
Incidence of Potentially Preventable VTE[1,2]	-	-	11%	10%
UFH with Dosages/Platelet Monitoring[2]	20	100%	96%	97%
Venous Thromboembolism Prophylaxis[2]	321	92%	83%	85%
Warfarin Therapy Discharge Instructions[2]	25	60%	75%	75%
Chest Pain/Possible Heart Attack Care				
Aspirin Given Within 24 Hours of Arrival	-	-	97%	96%
Fibrinolytic Meds Within 30 Min. of Arrival	-	-	62%	58%
Average Time to ECG (minutes)	-	-	9	7
Average Time to Transfer (minutes)	-	-	62	60
Children's Asthma Care				
Received Home Management Plan of Care	-	-	88%	88%
Received Reliever Medication	-	-	100%	100%
Received Systemic Corticosteroids	-	-	100%	100%
Emergency Department				
Admittance Decision Time (minutes)[2]	627	41	125	98
Head CT Results Within 45 Min. of Arrival	-	-	55%	57%
Patients Who Left ER Before Being Seen	-	-	3%	2%
Time from ER Arrival to Admit. (minutes)[2]	630	318	323	274
Time from ER Arrival to Discharge (minutes)	-	-	168	134
Time in ER Before Being Evaluated (minutes)	-	-	29	26
Time to Pain Meds for Fractures (minutes)	-	-	62	57
Heart Attack Care				
Aspirin Given at Discharge	65	100%	99%	99%
Fibrinolytic Meds Within 30 Min. of Arrival[7]	-	-	73%	54%
PCI Within 90 Minutes of Arrival[7]	-	-	95%	96%
Statin Prescribed at Discharge	69	100%	98%	98%
Heart Failure Care				
ACE Inhibitor or ARB for LVSD	21	100%	97%	97%
Discharge Instructions Given	104	100%	94%	94%
Evaluation of LVS Function	120	100%	99%	99%
Medicare Spending				
Medicare Spending per Patient (ratio)	-	0.74	0.98	0.98
Pneumonia Care				
Appropriate Initial Antibiotic Given[2]	113	98%	97%	95%
Blood Culture Timing[2]	146	99%	98%	98%
Pregnancy and Delivery Care				
Newborn Deliveries Scheduled Early[7]	-	-	5%	6%
Preventive Care				
Immunization for Influenza[2]	383	93%	89%	90%
Immunization for Pneumonia[2]	572	96%	90%	92%
Stroke Care				
Anticoagulation Therapy for Atrial Fibrillation[1]	-	-	95%	95%
Antithrombotic Therapy Timing	54	100%	98%	98%
Assessed for Rehabilitation	65	100%	97%	97%
Discharged on Antithrombotic Therapy	62	94%	99%	99%
Discharged on Statin Medication	42	88%	94%	94%
Thrombolytic Therapy Timing[1]	-	-	72%	66%
Venous Thromboembolism Prophylaxis	56	100%	94%	94%
Written Stroke Educational Materials Given	45	93%	87%	88%
Surgical Care Improvement Project				
Appropriate Beta Blocker Usage[2]	107	100%	97%	98%
Appropriate VTP Within 24 Hours[2]	289	100%	98%	98%
Controlled Postoperative Blood Glucose[2,7]	-	-	96%	97%
Perioperative Temperature Management[2]	325	100%	100%	100%
Prophylactic Antibiotic Selection[2]	195	99%	99%	99%
Prophylactic Antibiotic Selection (Outpatient)	-	-	97%	98%
Prophylactic Antibiotic Stopped[2]	195	100%	98%	98%
Prophylactic Antibiotic Timing[2]	195	97%	99%	99%
Prophylactic Antibiotic Timing (Outpatient)	-	-	97%	98%
Urinary Catheter Removal[2]	267	100%	97%	97%
Survey of Patients' Hospital Experiences				
Area Around Room 'Always' Quiet at Night	300+	55%	51%	61%
Doctors 'Always' Communicated Well	300+	80%	78%	82%
Home Recovery Information Given	300+	86%	83%	85%
Hospital Given 9 or 10 on 10 Point Scale	300+	81%	68%	71%
Meds 'Always' Explained Before Given	300+	66%	61%	64%
Nurses 'Always' Communicated Well	300+	78%	74%	79%
Pain 'Always' Well Controlled	300+	72%	68%	71%
Room and Bathroom 'Always' Clean	300+	77%	70%	73%
Timely Help 'Always' Received	300+	66%	62%	68%
Would Definitely Recommend Hospital	300+	82%	70%	71%
Use of Medical Imaging				
Cardiac Imaging Stress Test before Surgery	-	-	5.2%	5.3%
Combination Abdominal CT Scan	-	-	13.4%	10.5%
Combination Brain/Sinus CT Scan	-	-	2.2%	2.7%
Combination Chest CT Scan	-	-	2.3%	2.7%
Follow-up Mammogram/Ultrasound	-	-	8.2%	8.8%
Lumbar Spine MRI for Low Back Pain	-	-	34.2%	37.2%

Henry Mayo Newhall Memorial Hospital

23845 Mcbean Pkwy
Valencia, CA 91355
Phone: 661-253-8000
Fax: 661-253-8142
URL: www.henrymayo.com
Type: Acute Care Hospitals
Emergency Services: Yes
Ownership: Voluntary non-profit - Private
Beds: 217

Key Personnel:
Operating Room. . . . . Larry M Isaacs, RN
Chief of Medical Staff . . . . Chand Khanna, MD
Quality Assurance . . . . Kathy Menard
CEO/President. . . . . James Yoshikora

Measure	Cases	This Hosp.	State Avg.	U.S. Avg.
Blood Clot Prevention and Treatment				
Anticoagulation Overlap Therapy[2]	54	74%	92%	93%
ICU Venous Thromboembolism Prophylaxis[2]	75	97%	92%	92%
Incidence of Potentially Preventable VTE[2]	11	0%	11%	10%
UFH with Dosages/Platelet Monitoring[2]	12	100%	96%	97%
Venous Thromboembolism Prophylaxis[2]	292	87%	83%	85%
Warfarin Therapy Discharge Instructions[2]	35	69%	75%	75%
Chest Pain/Possible Heart Attack Care				
Aspirin Given Within 24 Hours of Arrival	145	100%	97%	96%
Fibrinolytic Meds Within 30 Min. of Arrival[7]	-	-	62%	58%
Average Time to ECG (minutes)	147	0	9	7
Average Time to Transfer (minutes)	14	34	62	60
Children's Asthma Care				
Received Home Management Plan of Care	-	-	88%	88%
Received Reliever Medication	-	-	100%	100%
Received Systemic Corticosteroids	-	-	100%	100%
Emergency Department				
Admittance Decision Time (minutes)[2]	770	158	125	98
Head CT Results Within 45 Min. of Arrival[1]	-	-	55%	57%
Patients Who Left ER Before Being Seen	49,684	3%	3%	2%
Time from ER Arrival to Admit. (minutes)[2]	809	349	323	274
Time from ER Arrival to Discharge (minutes)	364	146	168	134
Time in ER Before Being Evaluated (minutes)	407	16	29	26
Time to Pain Meds for Fractures (minutes)	243	43	62	57
Heart Attack Care				
Aspirin Given at Discharge	160	100%	99%	99%
Fibrinolytic Meds Within 30 Min. of Arrival[7]	-	-	73%	54%
PCI Within 90 Minutes of Arrival[1]	-	-	95%	96%
Statin Prescribed at Discharge	157	99%	98%	98%
Heart Failure Care				
ACE Inhibitor or ARB for LVSD[2]	64	100%	97%	97%
Discharge Instructions Given[2]	254	99%	94%	94%
Evaluation of LVS Function[2]	299	100%	99%	99%
Medicare Spending				

NOTE: Hospital profiles are in alphabetical order by state, then city, then hospital within the city; Rankings exclude hospitals with less than 25 cases except for patient surveys which excludes hospitals with less than 100 cases; (a) 100-299 cases; (1) The number of cases/patients is too few to report; (2) Data submitted were based on a sample of cases/patients; (3) Results are based on a shorter time period than required; (4) Data suppressed by CMS for one or more quarters; (5) Results are not available for this reporting period; (6) Fewer than 100 patients completed the HCAHPS survey; (7) No cases met the criteria for this measure; (8) The lower limit of the confidence interval cannot be calculated if the number of observed infections equals zero; (9) No data are available from the state/territory for this reporting period; (10) The scores shown reflect fewer than 50 completed surveys; (11) There were discrepancies in the data collection process; (12) This measure does not apply to this hospital for this reporting period; (13) Results cannot be calculated for this reporting period; (14) The results for this state are combined with nearby states to protect confidentiality; Please refer to the User's Guide for a full explanation of data.

Measure	Cases	This Hosp.	State Avg.	U.S. Avg.
Medicare Spending per Patient (ratio)	-	1.03	0.98	0.98
Pneumonia Care				
Appropriate Initial Antibiotic Given[2]	96	100%	97%	95%
Blood Culture Timing[2]	169	99%	98%	98%
Pregnancy and Delivery Care				
Newborn Deliveries Scheduled Early	268	0%	5%	6%
Preventive Care				
Immunization for Influenza[2]	557	98%	89%	90%
Immunization for Pneumonia[2]	628	100%	90%	92%
Stroke Care				
Anticoagulation Therapy for Atrial Fibrillation	13	85%	95%	95%
Antithrombotic Therapy Timing	112	97%	98%	98%
Assessed for Rehabilitation	136	96%	97%	97%
Discharged on Antithrombotic Therapy	122	100%	99%	99%
Discharged on Statin Medication	103	94%	94%	94%
Thrombolytic Therapy Timing	15	93%	72%	66%
Venous Thromboembolism Prophylaxis	146	100%	94%	94%
Written Stroke Educational Materials Given	81	94%	87%	88%
Surgical Care Improvement Project				
Appropriate Beta Blocker Usage[2]	107	96%	97%	98%
Appropriate VTP Within 24 Hours[2]	314	98%	98%	98%
Controlled Postoperative Blood Glucose[2]	17	94%	96%	97%
Perioperative Temperature Management[2]	460	100%	100%	100%
Prophylactic Antibiotic Selection[2]	294	95%	99%	99%
Prophylactic Antibiotic Selection (Outpatient)	63	95%	97%	98%
Prophylactic Antibiotic Stopped[2]	282	99%	98%	98%
Prophylactic Antibiotic Timing[2]	297	99%	99%	99%
Prophylactic Antibiotic Timing (Outpatient)	64	97%	97%	98%
Urinary Catheter Removal[2]	209	97%	97%	97%
Survey of Patients' Hospital Experiences				
Area Around Room 'Always' Quiet at Night	300+	44%	51%	61%
Doctors 'Always' Communicated Well	300+	75%	78%	82%
Home Recovery Information Given	300+	82%	83%	85%
Hospital Given 9 or 10 on 10 Point Scale	300+	66%	68%	71%
Meds 'Always' Explained Before Given	300+	60%	61%	64%
Nurses 'Always' Communicated Well	300+	75%	74%	79%
Pain 'Always' Well Controlled	300+	69%	68%	71%
Room and Bathroom 'Always' Clean	300+	66%	70%	73%
Timely Help 'Always' Received	300+	62%	62%	68%
Would Definitely Recommend Hospital	300+	65%	70%	71%
Use of Medical Imaging				
Cardiac Imaging Stress Test before Surgery	226	8.4%	5.2%	5.3%
Combination Abdominal CT Scan	407	0.2%	13.4%	10.5%
Combination Brain/Sinus CT Scan	458	4.4%	2.2%	2.7%
Combination Chest CT Scan	78	1.3%	2.3%	2.7%
Follow-up Mammogram/Ultrasound	1,336	5.8%	8.2%	8.8%
Lumbar Spine MRI for Low Back Pain[1]	-	-	34.2%	37.2%

Kaiser Foundation Hospital & Rehab Center

975 Sereno Dr
Vallejo, CA 94589
Phone: 707-651-1000
Type: Acute Care Hospitals
Emergency Services: Yes
Ownership: Voluntary non-profit - Other
Beds: 267
Key Personnel:
Radiology. . . . . Michael Hines

Measure	Cases	This Hosp.	State Avg.	U.S. Avg.
Blood Clot Prevention and Treatment				
Anticoagulation Overlap Therapy[2]	50	96%	92%	93%
ICU Venous Thromboembolism Prophylaxis[2]	83	100%	92%	92%
Incidence of Potentially Preventable VTE[2]	12	25%	11%	10%
UFH with Dosages/Platelet Monitoring[2]	40	100%	96%	97%
Venous Thromboembolism Prophylaxis[2]	320	88%	83%	85%
Warfarin Therapy Discharge Instructions[2]	53	64%	75%	75%
Chest Pain/Possible Heart Attack Care				
Aspirin Given Within 24 Hours of Arrival	-	-	97%	96%
Fibrinolytic Meds Within 30 Min. of Arrival	-	-	62%	58%
Average Time to ECG (minutes)	-	-	9	7
Average Time to Transfer (minutes)	-	-	62	60
Children's Asthma Care				
Received Home Management Plan of Care	-	-	88%	88%
Received Reliever Medication	-	-	100%	100%
Received Systemic Corticosteroids	-	-	100%	100%
Emergency Department				
Admittance Decision Time (minutes)[2]	494	52	125	98
Head CT Results Within 45 Min. of Arrival	-	-	55%	57%
Patients Who Left ER Before Being Seen	-	-	3%	2%
Time from ER Arrival to Admit. (minutes)[2]	502	340	323	274
Time from ER Arrival to Discharge (minutes)	-	-	168	134
Time in ER Before Being Evaluated (minutes)	-	-	29	26
Time to Pain Meds for Fractures (minutes)	-	-	62	57
Heart Attack Care				
Aspirin Given at Discharge	146	100%	99%	99%
Fibrinolytic Meds Within 30 Min. of Arrival[7]	-	-	73%	54%
PCI Within 90 Minutes of Arrival	41	100%	95%	96%
Statin Prescribed at Discharge	142	99%	98%	98%
Heart Failure Care				
ACE Inhibitor or ARB for LVSD	49	100%	97%	97%
Discharge Instructions Given	247	100%	94%	94%
Evaluation of LVS Function	270	100%	99%	99%
Medicare Spending				
Medicare Spending per Patient (ratio)	-	0.79	0.98	0.98
Pneumonia Care				
Appropriate Initial Antibiotic Given[2]	93	98%	97%	95%
Blood Culture Timing[2]	152	95%	98%	98%
Pregnancy and Delivery Care				
Newborn Deliveries Scheduled Early[2]	32	0%	5%	6%
Preventive Care				
Immunization for Influenza[2]	481	93%	89%	90%
Immunization for Pneumonia[2]	592	93%	90%	92%
Stroke Care				
Anticoagulation Therapy for Atrial Fibrillation[2]	14	86%	95%	95%
Antithrombotic Therapy Timing[2]	96	98%	98%	98%
Assessed for Rehabilitation[2]	120	100%	97%	97%
Discharged on Antithrombotic Therapy[2]	106	92%	99%	99%
Discharged on Statin Medication[2]	88	92%	94%	94%
Thrombolytic Therapy Timing[1,2]	-	-	72%	66%
Venous Thromboembolism Prophylaxis[2]	96	98%	94%	94%
Written Stroke Educational Materials Given[2]	80	96%	87%	88%
Surgical Care Improvement Project				
Appropriate Beta Blocker Usage[2]	144	99%	97%	98%
Appropriate VTP Within 24 Hours[2]	342	99%	98%	98%
Controlled Postoperative Blood Glucose[2,7]	-	-	96%	97%
Perioperative Temperature Management[2]	427	100%	100%	100%
Prophylactic Antibiotic Selection[2]	283	99%	99%	99%
Prophylactic Antibiotic Selection (Outpatient)	-	-	97%	98%
Prophylactic Antibiotic Stopped[2]	283	100%	98%	98%
Prophylactic Antibiotic Timing[2]	283	99%	99%	99%
Prophylactic Antibiotic Timing (Outpatient)	-	-	97%	98%
Urinary Catheter Removal[2]	304	99%	97%	97%
Survey of Patients' Hospital Experiences				
Area Around Room 'Always' Quiet at Night	300+	54%	51%	61%
Doctors 'Always' Communicated Well	300+	80%	78%	82%
Home Recovery Information Given	300+	86%	83%	85%
Hospital Given 9 or 10 on 10 Point Scale	300+	72%	68%	71%
Meds 'Always' Explained Before Given	300+	62%	61%	64%
Nurses 'Always' Communicated Well	300+	74%	74%	79%
Pain 'Always' Well Controlled	300+	69%	68%	71%
Room and Bathroom 'Always' Clean	300+	68%	70%	73%
Timely Help 'Always' Received	300+	63%	62%	68%
Would Definitely Recommend Hospital	300+	75%	70%	71%
Use of Medical Imaging				
Cardiac Imaging Stress Test before Surgery	-	-	5.2%	5.3%
Combination Abdominal CT Scan	-	-	13.4%	10.5%
Combination Brain/Sinus CT Scan	-	-	2.2%	2.7%
Combination Chest CT Scan	-	-	2.3%	2.7%
Follow-up Mammogram/Ultrasound	-	-	8.2%	8.8%
Lumbar Spine MRI for Low Back Pain	-	-	34.2%	37.2%

Sutter Solano Medical Center

300 Hospital Dr
Vallejo, CA 94589
Phone: 707-554-5280
Fax: 707-648-3227
URL: www.suttersolano.org
Type: Acute Care Hospitals
Emergency Services: Yes
Ownership: Voluntary non-profit - Private
Beds: 111
Key Personnel:
Radiology. . . . . Christian B Anderson
Chief of Medical Staff . . . . Gregory Coe
President/CEO. . . . . Patricia Fong Kushida
CEO . . . . Christopher Johnson
President . . . . Dick Kramer
Quality Assurance . . . . Leslie Morrison

Measure	Cases	This Hosp.	State Avg.	U.S. Avg.
Blood Clot Prevention and Treatment				
Anticoagulation Overlap Therapy[2]	18	100%	92%	93%
ICU Venous Thromboembolism Prophylaxis[2]	129	95%	92%	92%
Incidence of Potentially Preventable VTE[1,2]	-	-	11%	10%
UFH with Dosages/Platelet Monitoring[1,2]	-	-	96%	97%
Venous Thromboembolism Prophylaxis[2]	277	92%	83%	85%
Warfarin Therapy Discharge Instructions[2]	13	100%	75%	75%
Chest Pain/Possible Heart Attack Care				
Aspirin Given Within 24 Hours of Arrival	32	100%	97%	96%
Fibrinolytic Meds Within 30 Min. of Arrival[1]	-	-	62%	58%
Average Time to ECG (minutes)	33	10	9	7
Average Time to Transfer (minutes)[1]	-	-	62	60
Children's Asthma Care				
Received Home Management Plan of Care	-	-	88%	88%
Received Reliever Medication	-	-	100%	100%
Received Systemic Corticosteroids	-	-	100%	100%
Emergency Department				
Admittance Decision Time (minutes)[2]	646	236	125	98
Head CT Results Within 45 Min. of Arrival	21	86%	55%	57%
Patients Who Left ER Before Being Seen	39,175	2%	3%	2%
Time from ER Arrival to Admit. (minutes)[2]	649	423	323	274
Time from ER Arrival to Discharge (minutes)	375	134	168	134
Time in ER Before Being Evaluated (minutes)	408	39	29	26
Time to Pain Meds for Fractures (minutes)	85	59	62	57
Heart Attack Care				
Aspirin Given at Discharge[1]	-	-	99%	99%
Fibrinolytic Meds Within 30 Min. of Arrival[7]	-	-	73%	54%
PCI Within 90 Minutes of Arrival[7]	-	-	95%	96%
Statin Prescribed at Discharge[1]	-	-	98%	98%
Heart Failure Care				
ACE Inhibitor or ARB for LVSD	55	100%	97%	97%
Discharge Instructions Given	110	100%	94%	94%
Evaluation of LVS Function	129	100%	99%	99%
Medicare Spending				
Medicare Spending per Patient (ratio)	-	1.02	0.98	0.98
Pneumonia Care				
Appropriate Initial Antibiotic Given[2]	76	97%	97%	95%
Blood Culture Timing[2]	130	96%	98%	98%
Pregnancy and Delivery Care				
Newborn Deliveries Scheduled Early	82	0%	5%	6%
Preventive Care				
Immunization for Influenza[2]	493	98%	89%	90%
Immunization for Pneumonia[2]	574	99%	90%	92%
Stroke Care				
Anticoagulation Therapy for Atrial Fibrillation[1]	-	-	95%	95%
Antithrombotic Therapy Timing	62	98%	98%	98%
Assessed for Rehabilitation	57	100%	97%	97%
Discharged on Antithrombotic Therapy	53	100%	99%	99%
Discharged on Statin Medication	46	96%	94%	94%
Thrombolytic Therapy Timing[7]	-	-	72%	66%
Venous Thromboembolism Prophylaxis	64	98%	94%	94%
Written Stroke Educational Materials Given	29	93%	87%	88%
Surgical Care Improvement Project				
Appropriate Beta Blocker Usage[2]	110	98%	97%	98%
Appropriate VTP Within 24 Hours[2]	340	99%	98%	98%
Controlled Postoperative Blood Glucose[2,7]	-	-	96%	97%
Perioperative Temperature Management[2]	364	100%	100%	100%
Prophylactic Antibiotic Selection[2]	212	100%	99%	99%
Prophylactic Antibiotic Selection (Outpatient)	92	97%	97%	98%
Prophylactic Antibiotic Stopped[2]	202	99%	98%	98%
Prophylactic Antibiotic Timing[2]	212	100%	99%	99%
Prophylactic Antibiotic Timing (Outpatient)	93	99%	97%	98%
Urinary Catheter Removal[2]	249	100%	97%	97%
Survey of Patients' Hospital Experiences				
Area Around Room 'Always' Quiet at Night	300+	59%	51%	61%
Doctors 'Always' Communicated Well	300+	78%	78%	82%

NOTE: Hospital profiles are in alphabetical order by state, then city, then hospital within the city; Rankings exclude hospitals with less than 25 cases except for patient surveys which excludes hospitals with less than 100 cases; (a) 100-299 cases; (1) The number of cases/patients is too few to report; (2) Data submitted were based on a sample of cases/patients; (3) Results are based on a shorter time period than required; (4) Data suppressed by CMS for one or more quarters; (5) Results are not available for this reporting period; (6) Fewer than 100 patients completed the HCAHPS survey; (7) No cases met the criteria for this measure; (8) The lower limit of the confidence interval cannot be calculated if the number of observed infections equals zero; (9) No data are available from the state/territory for this reporting period; (10) The scores shown reflect fewer than 50 completed surveys; (11) There were discrepancies in the data collection process; (12) This measure does not apply to this hospital for this reporting period; (13) Results cannot be calculated for this reporting period; (14) The results for this state are combined with nearby states to protect confidentiality; Please refer to the User's Guide for a full explanation of data.

Home Recovery Information Given	300+	83%	83%	85%
Hospital Given 9 or 10 on 10 Point Scale	300+	65%	68%	71%
Meds 'Always' Explained Before Given	300+	61%	61%	64%
Nurses 'Always' Communicated Well	300+	76%	74%	79%
Pain 'Always' Well Controlled	300+	69%	68%	71%
Room and Bathroom 'Always' Clean	300+	72%	70%	73%
Timely Help 'Always' Received	300+	61%	62%	68%
Would Definitely Recommend Hospital	300+	68%	70%	71%
Use of Medical Imaging				
Cardiac Imaging Stress Test before Surgery	152	3.9%	5.2%	5.3%
Combination Abdominal CT Scan	301	6.6%	13.4%	10.5%
Combination Brain/Sinus CT Scan	268	5.2%	2.2%	2.7%
Combination Chest CT Scan	134	0.7%	2.3%	2.7%
Follow-up Mammogram/Ultrasound	461	5.9%	8.2%	8.8%
Lumbar Spine MRI for Low Back Pain[1]	-	-	34.2%	37.2%

Valley Presbyterian Hospital

15107 Vanowen St
Van Nuys, CA 91406
Phone: 818-902-3906
Fax: 818-902-3949
URL: www.valleypres.org
Type: Acute Care Hospitals
Emergency Services: Yes
Ownership: Voluntary non-profit - Other
Beds: 350

Key Personnel:
Chairman/CEO . . . . Greg Kay, MD
CEO/President. . . . . Gustavo Valdespino

Measure	Cases	This Hosp.	State Avg.	U.S. Avg.
Blood Clot Prevention and Treatment				
Anticoagulation Overlap Therapy[2]	46	78%	92%	93%
ICU Venous Thromboembolism Prophylaxis[2]	68	71%	92%	92%
Incidence of Potentially Preventable VTE[2]	19	16%	11%	10%
UFH with Dosages/Platelet Monitoring[1,2]	-	-	96%	97%
Venous Thromboembolism Prophylaxis[2]	329	66%	83%	85%
Warfarin Therapy Discharge Instructions[2]	33	27%	75%	75%
Chest Pain/Possible Heart Attack Care				
Aspirin Given Within 24 Hours of Arrival[1,3]	-	-	97%	96%
Fibrinolytic Meds Within 30 Min. of Arrival[5]	-	-	62%	58%
Average Time to ECG (minutes)[1,3]	-	-	9	7
Average Time to Transfer (minutes)[5]	-	-	62	60
Children's Asthma Care				
Received Home Management Plan of Care	-	-	88%	88%
Received Reliever Medication	-	-	100%	100%
Received Systemic Corticosteroids	-	-	100%	100%
Emergency Department				
Admittance Decision Time (minutes)[2]	160	151	125	98
Head CT Results Within 45 Min. of Arrival[1]	-	-	55%	57%
Patients Who Left ER Before Being Seen	60,812	4%	3%	2%
Time from ER Arrival to Admit. (minutes)[2]	176	320	323	274
Time from ER Arrival to Discharge (minutes)	355	191	168	134
Time in ER Before Being Evaluated (minutes)	279	60	29	26
Time to Pain Meds for Fractures (minutes)	112	76	62	57
Heart Attack Care				
Aspirin Given at Discharge	201	98%	99%	99%
Fibrinolytic Meds Within 30 Min. of Arrival[7]	-	-	73%	54%
PCI Within 90 Minutes of Arrival	43	86%	95%	96%
Statin Prescribed at Discharge	192	95%	98%	98%
Heart Failure Care				
ACE Inhibitor or ARB for LVSD	107	91%	97%	97%
Discharge Instructions Given	280	95%	94%	94%
Evaluation of LVS Function	349	97%	99%	99%
Medicare Spending				
Medicare Spending per Patient (ratio)	-	1.10	0.98	0.98
Pneumonia Care				
Appropriate Initial Antibiotic Given[2]	81	93%	97%	95%
Blood Culture Timing[2]	189	94%	98%	98%
Pregnancy and Delivery Care				
Newborn Deliveries Scheduled Early[2]	116	2%	5%	6%
Preventive Care				
Immunization for Influenza[2]	596	63%	89%	90%
Immunization for Pneumonia[2]	457	75%	90%	92%
Stroke Care				
Anticoagulation Therapy for Atrial Fibrillation	14	79%	95%	95%
Antithrombotic Therapy Timing	86	97%	98%	98%
Assessed for Rehabilitation	110	90%	97%	97%
Discharged on Antithrombotic Therapy	94	98%	99%	99%
Discharged on Statin Medication	66	83%	94%	94%
Thrombolytic Therapy Timing	14	100%	72%	66%
Venous Thromboembolism Prophylaxis	117	86%	94%	94%
Written Stroke Educational Materials Given	60	88%	87%	88%
Surgical Care Improvement Project				
Appropriate Beta Blocker Usage[2]	154	90%	97%	98%
Appropriate VTP Within 24 Hours[2]	560	98%	98%	98%
Controlled Postoperative Blood Glucose[2]	47	94%	96%	97%
Perioperative Temperature Management[2]	622	100%	100%	100%
Prophylactic Antibiotic Selection[2]	466	99%	99%	99%
Prophylactic Antibiotic Selection (Outpatient)	89	100%	97%	98%
Prophylactic Antibiotic Stopped[2]	454	90%	98%	98%
Prophylactic Antibiotic Timing[2]	467	93%	99%	99%
Prophylactic Antibiotic Timing (Outpatient)	98	90%	97%	98%
Urinary Catheter Removal[2]	434	91%	97%	97%
Survey of Patients' Hospital Experiences				
Area Around Room 'Always' Quiet at Night	300+	47%	51%	61%
Doctors 'Always' Communicated Well	300+	74%	78%	82%
Home Recovery Information Given	300+	79%	83%	85%
Hospital Given 9 or 10 on 10 Point Scale	300+	62%	68%	71%
Meds 'Always' Explained Before Given	300+	56%	61%	64%
Nurses 'Always' Communicated Well	300+	69%	74%	79%
Pain 'Always' Well Controlled	300+	69%	68%	71%
Room and Bathroom 'Always' Clean	300+	64%	70%	73%
Timely Help 'Always' Received	300+	53%	62%	68%
Would Definitely Recommend Hospital	300+	64%	70%	71%
Use of Medical Imaging				
Cardiac Imaging Stress Test before Surgery	123	4.1%	5.2%	5.3%
Combination Abdominal CT Scan	444	5.9%	13.4%	10.5%
Combination Brain/Sinus CT Scan	561	2.1%	2.2%	2.7%
Combination Chest CT Scan	91	0.0%	2.3%	2.7%
Follow-up Mammogram/Ultrasound[7]	-	-	8.2%	8.8%
Lumbar Spine MRI for Low Back Pain[1]	-	-	34.2%	37.2%

Community Memorial Hospital San Buenaventura

147 N Brent St
Ventura, CA 93003
Phone: 805-652-5011
Fax: 805-643-7554
E-mail: jmasterson@cmhhospital.org
URL: www.cmhhospital.org
Type: Acute Care Hospitals
Emergency Services: Yes
Ownership: Government - Federal
Beds: 240

Key Personnel:
Quality Assurance . . . . Idolia Barbee
Pediatric Ambulatory Care . . . . . . Vicki Beaver
Cardiac Laboratory. . . . . Carolyn Estrada
Chief of Medical Staff. . . . . Peter Gaal
Infection Control. . . . . Chris Ouellette
Radiology. . . . . Kirk Pieper
Operating Room. . . . . Peggy Strople, RN
CEO/President. . . . . Gary Wilde

Measure	Cases	This Hosp.	State Avg.	U.S. Avg.
Blood Clot Prevention and Treatment				
Anticoagulation Overlap Therapy[2]	73	84%	92%	93%
ICU Venous Thromboembolism Prophylaxis[2]	73	86%	92%	92%
Incidence of Potentially Preventable VTE[2]	14	14%	11%	10%
UFH with Dosages/Platelet Monitoring[2]	29	97%	96%	97%
Venous Thromboembolism Prophylaxis[2]	293	81%	83%	85%
Warfarin Therapy Discharge Instructions[2]	53	53%	75%	75%
Chest Pain/Possible Heart Attack Care				
Aspirin Given Within 24 Hours of Arrival[5]	-	-	97%	96%
Fibrinolytic Meds Within 30 Min. of Arrival[5]	-	-	62%	58%
Average Time to ECG (minutes)[5]	-	-	9	7
Average Time to Transfer (minutes)[5]	-	-	62	60
Children's Asthma Care				
Received Home Management Plan of Care	-	-	88%	88%
Received Reliever Medication	-	-	100%	100%
Received Systemic Corticosteroids	-	-	100%	100%
Emergency Department				
Admittance Decision Time (minutes)[2]	445	151	125	98
Head CT Results Within 45 Min. of Arrival[1]	-	-	55%	57%
Patients Who Left ER Before Being Seen	40,782	1%	3%	2%
Time from ER Arrival to Admit. (minutes)[2]	461	319	323	274
Time from ER Arrival to Discharge (minutes)	366	164	168	134
Time in ER Before Being Evaluated (minutes)	358	47	29	26
Time to Pain Meds for Fractures (minutes)	37	91	62	57
Heart Attack Care				
Aspirin Given at Discharge	219	100%	99%	99%
Fibrinolytic Meds Within 30 Min. of Arrival[7]	-	-	73%	54%
PCI Within 90 Minutes of Arrival	38	95%	95%	96%
Statin Prescribed at Discharge	214	99%	98%	98%
Heart Failure Care				
ACE Inhibitor or ARB for LVSD	81	100%	97%	97%
Discharge Instructions Given	223	92%	94%	94%
Evaluation of LVS Function	265	100%	99%	99%
Medicare Spending				
Medicare Spending per Patient (ratio)	-	0.94	0.98	0.98
Pneumonia Care				
Appropriate Initial Antibiotic Given	177	97%	97%	95%
Blood Culture Timing	242	95%	98%	98%
Pregnancy and Delivery Care				
Newborn Deliveries Scheduled Early	209	9%	5%	6%
Preventive Care				
Immunization for Influenza[2]	485	81%	89%	90%
Immunization for Pneumonia[2]	532	82%	90%	92%
Stroke Care				
Anticoagulation Therapy for Atrial Fibrillation	38	82%	95%	95%
Antithrombotic Therapy Timing	92	92%	98%	98%
Assessed for Rehabilitation	131	97%	97%	97%
Discharged on Antithrombotic Therapy	109	97%	99%	99%
Discharged on Statin Medication	86	97%	94%	94%
Thrombolytic Therapy Timing	17	65%	72%	66%
Venous Thromboembolism Prophylaxis	119	78%	94%	94%
Written Stroke Educational Materials Given	88	57%	87%	88%
Surgical Care Improvement Project				
Appropriate Beta Blocker Usage[2]	152	93%	97%	98%
Appropriate VTP Within 24 Hours[2]	300	97%	98%	98%
Controlled Postoperative Blood Glucose[2]	101	100%	96%	97%
Perioperative Temperature Management[2]	385	100%	100%	100%
Prophylactic Antibiotic Selection[2]	356	97%	99%	99%
Prophylactic Antibiotic Selection (Outpatient)	406	93%	97%	98%
Prophylactic Antibiotic Stopped[2]	347	98%	98%	98%
Prophylactic Antibiotic Timing[2]	357	98%	99%	99%
Prophylactic Antibiotic Timing (Outpatient)	397	97%	97%	98%
Urinary Catheter Removal[2]	297	97%	97%	97%
Survey of Patients' Hospital Experiences				
Area Around Room 'Always' Quiet at Night	300+	46%	51%	61%
Doctors 'Always' Communicated Well	300+	81%	78%	82%
Home Recovery Information Given	300+	82%	83%	85%
Hospital Given 9 or 10 on 10 Point Scale	300+	66%	68%	71%
Meds 'Always' Explained Before Given	300+	61%	61%	64%
Nurses 'Always' Communicated Well	300+	78%	74%	79%
Pain 'Always' Well Controlled	300+	72%	68%	71%
Room and Bathroom 'Always' Clean	300+	68%	70%	73%
Timely Help 'Always' Received	300+	64%	62%	68%
Would Definitely Recommend Hospital	300+	72%	70%	71%
Use of Medical Imaging				
Cardiac Imaging Stress Test before Surgery	254	5.1%	5.2%	5.3%
Combination Abdominal CT Scan	582	14.9%	13.4%	10.5%
Combination Brain/Sinus CT Scan	613	1.0%	2.2%	2.7%
Combination Chest CT Scan	188	21.8%	2.3%	2.7%
Follow-up Mammogram/Ultrasound[7]	-	-	8.2%	8.8%
Lumbar Spine MRI for Low Back Pain	50	36.0%	34.2%	37.2%

Ventura County Medical Center

3291 Loma Vista Rd
Ventura, CA 93003
Phone: 805-652-6075
Fax: 805-652-6188
URL: www.vchca.org
Type: Acute Care Hospitals
Emergency Services: Yes
Ownership: Government - Local
Beds: 208

Key Personnel:
Coronary Care . . . . Daniel Clark, MD
Chief of Medical Staff . . . . Joseph Esherick, MD
Pediatric In-Patient Care . . . . Todd Flosi, MD
Pediatric Ambulatory Care . . . . . . Chris Landon, MD
CEO/President. . . . . Paul E Lorentz
Quality Assurance . . . . Paul Lorenz
Infection Control. . . . . Elise McKee
Operating Room. . . . . Rosario Oropesa

NOTE: Hospital profiles are in alphabetical order by state, then city, then hospital within the city; Rankings exclude hospitals with less than 25 cases except for patient surveys which excludes hospitals with less than 100 cases; (a) 100-299 cases; (1) The number of cases/patients is too few to report; (2) Data submitted were based on a sample of cases/patients; (3) Results are based on a shorter time period than required; (4) Data suppressed by CMS for one or more quarters; (5) Results are not available for this reporting period; (6) Fewer than 100 patients completed the HCAHPS survey; (7) No cases met the criteria for this measure; (8) The lower limit of the confidence interval cannot be calculated if the number of observed infections equals zero; (9) No data are available from the state/territory for this reporting period; (10) The scores shown reflect fewer than 50 completed surveys; (11) There were discrepancies in the data collection process; (12) This measure does not apply to this hospital for this reporting period; (13) Results cannot be calculated for this reporting period; (14) The results for this state are combined with nearby states to protect confidentiality; Please refer to the User's Guide for a full explanation of data.

Measure	Cases	This Hosp.	State Avg.	U.S. Avg.
Blood Clot Prevention and Treatment				
Anticoagulation Overlap Therapy[2]	14	93%	92%	93%
ICU Venous Thromboembolism Prophylaxis[2]	55	95%	92%	92%
Incidence of Potentially Preventable VTE[1,2]	-	-	11%	10%
UFH with Dosages/Platelet Monitoring[1,2]	-	-	96%	97%
Venous Thromboembolism Prophylaxis[2]	301	82%	83%	85%
Warfarin Therapy Discharge Instructions[2]	13	46%	75%	75%
Chest Pain/Possible Heart Attack Care				
Aspirin Given Within 24 Hours of Arrival[5]	-	-	97%	96%
Fibrinolytic Meds Within 30 Min. of Arrival[5]	-	-	62%	58%
Average Time to ECG (minutes)[5]	-	-	9	7
Average Time to Transfer (minutes)[5]	-	-	62	60
Children's Asthma Care				
Received Home Management Plan of Care	-	-	88%	88%
Received Reliever Medication	-	-	100%	100%
Received Systemic Corticosteroids	-	-	100%	100%
Emergency Department				
Admittance Decision Time (minutes)[2]	526	260	125	98
Head CT Results Within 45 Min. of Arrival[1,3]	-	-	55%	57%
Patients Who Left ER Before Being Seen	52,387	4%	3%	2%
Time from ER Arrival to Admit. (minutes)[2]	529	390	323	274
Time from ER Arrival to Discharge (minutes)[3]	282	174	168	134
Time in ER Before Being Evaluated (minutes)[3]	298	57	29	26
Time to Pain Meds for Fractures (minutes)[3]	183	83	62	57
Heart Attack Care				
Aspirin Given at Discharge	34	94%	99%	99%
Fibrinolytic Meds Within 30 Min. of Arrival[7]	-	-	73%	54%
PCI Within 90 Minutes of Arrival[7]	-	-	95%	96%
Statin Prescribed at Discharge	34	97%	98%	98%
Heart Failure Care				
ACE Inhibitor or ARB for LVSD[2]	41	85%	97%	97%
Discharge Instructions Given[2]	119	80%	94%	94%
Evaluation of LVS Function[2]	138	98%	99%	99%
Medicare Spending				
Medicare Spending per Patient (ratio)	-	0.92	0.98	0.98
Pneumonia Care				
Appropriate Initial Antibiotic Given[2]	99	91%	97%	95%
Blood Culture Timing[2]	167	95%	98%	98%
Pregnancy and Delivery Care				
Newborn Deliveries Scheduled Early[2]	11	0%	5%	6%
Preventive Care				
Immunization for Influenza[2]	461	92%	89%	90%
Immunization for Pneumonia[2]	384	69%	90%	92%
Stroke Care				
Anticoagulation Therapy for Atrial Fibrillation[1]	-	-	95%	95%
Antithrombotic Therapy Timing	35	100%	98%	98%
Assessed for Rehabilitation	49	100%	97%	97%
Discharged on Antithrombotic Therapy	39	100%	99%	99%
Discharged on Statin Medication	21	95%	94%	94%
Thrombolytic Therapy Timing	12	17%	72%	66%
Venous Thromboembolism Prophylaxis	48	98%	94%	94%
Written Stroke Educational Materials Given	43	100%	87%	88%
Surgical Care Improvement Project				
Appropriate Beta Blocker Usage[2]	53	92%	97%	98%
Appropriate VTP Within 24 Hours[2]	404	95%	98%	98%
Controlled Postoperative Blood Glucose[1,2]	-	-	96%	97%
Perioperative Temperature Management[2]	497	98%	100%	100%
Prophylactic Antibiotic Selection[2]	258	99%	99%	99%
Prophylactic Antibiotic Selection (Outpatient)[5]	-	-	97%	98%
Prophylactic Antibiotic Stopped[2]	250	100%	98%	98%
Prophylactic Antibiotic Timing[2]	260	96%	99%	99%
Prophylactic Antibiotic Timing (Outpatient)[5]	-	-	97%	98%
Urinary Catheter Removal[2]	245	95%	97%	97%
Survey of Patients' Hospital Experiences				
Area Around Room 'Always' Quiet at Night	300+	42%	51%	61%
Doctors 'Always' Communicated Well	300+	79%	78%	82%
Home Recovery Information Given	300+	77%	83%	85%
Hospital Given 9 or 10 on 10 Point Scale	300+	64%	68%	71%
Meds 'Always' Explained Before Given	300+	57%	61%	64%
Nurses 'Always' Communicated Well	300+	71%	74%	79%
Pain 'Always' Well Controlled	300+	64%	68%	71%
Room and Bathroom 'Always' Clean	300+	69%	70%	73%
Timely Help 'Always' Received	300+	54%	62%	68%
Would Definitely Recommend Hospital	300+	66%	70%	71%
Use of Medical Imaging				
Cardiac Imaging Stress Test before Surgery	190	6.8%	5.2%	5.3%
Combination Abdominal CT Scan	245	16.7%	13.4%	10.5%
Combination Brain/Sinus CT Scan[1]	-	-	2.2%	2.7%
Combination Chest CT Scan	108	2.8%	2.3%	2.7%
Follow-up Mammogram/Ultrasound	305	5.6%	8.2%	8.8%
Lumbar Spine MRI for Low Back Pain[1]	-	-	34.2%	37.2%

Desert Valley Hospital

16850 Bear Valley Rd
Victorville, CA 92395
Phone: 760-241-8000
Fax: 760-245-0156
E-mail: patientrelations@dvmc.com
URL: www.dvmc.com
Type: Acute Care Hospitals
Emergency Services: Yes
Ownership: Proprietary
Beds: 83
Key Personnel:
Chief of Medical Staff. . . . . R Bearman, MD
CEO/President. . . . . Lex Reddy, MBA MHA

Measure	Cases	This Hosp.	State Avg.	U.S. Avg.
Blood Clot Prevention and Treatment				
Anticoagulation Overlap Therapy[2]	59	100%	92%	93%
ICU Venous Thromboembolism Prophylaxis[2]	41	98%	92%	92%
Incidence of Potentially Preventable VTE[1,2]	-	-	11%	10%
UFH with Dosages/Platelet Monitoring[1,2]	-	-	96%	97%
Venous Thromboembolism Prophylaxis[2]	377	98%	83%	85%
Warfarin Therapy Discharge Instructions[2]	55	100%	75%	75%
Chest Pain/Possible Heart Attack Care				
Aspirin Given Within 24 Hours of Arrival[1]	-	-	97%	96%
Fibrinolytic Meds Within 30 Min. of Arrival[3,7]	-	-	62%	58%
Average Time to ECG (minutes)[1]	-	-	9	7
Average Time to Transfer (minutes)[3,7]	-	-	62	60
Children's Asthma Care				
Received Home Management Plan of Care	-	-	88%	88%
Received Reliever Medication	-	-	100%	100%
Received Systemic Corticosteroids	-	-	100%	100%
Emergency Department				
Admittance Decision Time (minutes)[2]	877	246	125	98
Head CT Results Within 45 Min. of Arrival[1]	-	-	55%	57%
Patients Who Left ER Before Being Seen	36,887	7%	3%	2%
Time from ER Arrival to Admit. (minutes)[2]	878	483	323	274
Time from ER Arrival to Discharge (minutes)	350	212	168	134
Time in ER Before Being Evaluated (minutes)	382	58	29	26
Time to Pain Meds for Fractures (minutes)	181	98	62	57
Heart Attack Care				
Aspirin Given at Discharge	152	100%	99%	99%
Fibrinolytic Meds Within 30 Min. of Arrival[7]	-	-	73%	54%
PCI Within 90 Minutes of Arrival	37	65%	95%	96%
Statin Prescribed at Discharge	150	100%	98%	98%
Heart Failure Care				
ACE Inhibitor or ARB for LVSD[2]	114	100%	97%	97%
Discharge Instructions Given[2]	276	100%	94%	94%
Evaluation of LVS Function[2]	288	100%	99%	99%
Medicare Spending				
Medicare Spending per Patient (ratio)	-	0.89	0.98	0.98
Pneumonia Care				
Appropriate Initial Antibiotic Given[2]	76	99%	97%	95%
Blood Culture Timing[2]	114	96%	98%	98%
Pregnancy and Delivery Care				
Newborn Deliveries Scheduled Early[2]	49	4%	5%	6%
Preventive Care				
Immunization for Influenza[2]	543	97%	89%	90%
Immunization for Pneumonia[2]	735	99%	90%	92%
Stroke Care				
Anticoagulation Therapy for Atrial Fibrillation[1]	-	-	95%	95%
Antithrombotic Therapy Timing	85	100%	98%	98%
Assessed for Rehabilitation	94	100%	97%	97%
Discharged on Antithrombotic Therapy	84	100%	99%	99%
Discharged on Statin Medication	59	100%	94%	94%
Thrombolytic Therapy Timing[7]	-	-	72%	66%
Venous Thromboembolism Prophylaxis	93	98%	94%	94%
Written Stroke Educational Materials Given	85	61%	87%	88%
Surgical Care Improvement Project				
Appropriate Beta Blocker Usage[2]	39	100%	97%	98%
Appropriate VTP Within 24 Hours[2]	153	100%	98%	98%
Controlled Postoperative Blood Glucose[2]	22	95%	96%	97%
Perioperative Temperature Management[2]	198	100%	100%	100%
Prophylactic Antibiotic Selection[2]	98	96%	99%	99%
Prophylactic Antibiotic Selection (Outpatient)	23	100%	97%	98%
Prophylactic Antibiotic Stopped[2]	67	100%	98%	98%
Prophylactic Antibiotic Timing[2]	98	100%	99%	99%
Prophylactic Antibiotic Timing (Outpatient)	23	100%	97%	98%
Urinary Catheter Removal[2]	94	99%	97%	97%
Survey of Patients' Hospital Experiences				
Area Around Room 'Always' Quiet at Night	300+	55%	51%	61%
Doctors 'Always' Communicated Well	300+	74%	78%	82%
Home Recovery Information Given	300+	78%	83%	85%
Hospital Given 9 or 10 on 10 Point Scale	300+	63%	68%	71%
Meds 'Always' Explained Before Given	300+	53%	61%	64%
Nurses 'Always' Communicated Well	300+	72%	74%	79%
Pain 'Always' Well Controlled	300+	66%	68%	71%
Room and Bathroom 'Always' Clean	300+	66%	70%	73%
Timely Help 'Always' Received	300+	61%	62%	68%
Would Definitely Recommend Hospital	300+	64%	70%	71%
Use of Medical Imaging				
Cardiac Imaging Stress Test before Surgery	50	4.0%	5.2%	5.3%
Combination Abdominal CT Scan	216	7.4%	13.4%	10.5%
Combination Brain/Sinus CT Scan[1]	-	-	2.2%	2.7%
Combination Chest CT Scan	85	0.0%	2.3%	2.7%
Follow-up Mammogram/Ultrasound[7]	-	-	8.2%	8.8%
Lumbar Spine MRI for Low Back Pain[1]	-	-	34.2%	37.2%

Victor Valley Global Medical Center

15248 11th St
Victorville, CA 92392
Phone: 760-245-8691
Fax: 760-952-1461
E-mail: hr@vvch.org
URL: www.vvch.org
Type: Acute Care Hospitals
Emergency Services: Yes
Ownership: Voluntary non-profit - Private
Beds: 119
Key Personnel:
Radiology. . . . . Mohinder Ahlwalia
Operating Room. . . . . Vincente E Ajanwachuku
Infection Control. . . . . Darcel Black, RN
Quality Assurance . . . . Patrick Chambers
CEO/President. . . . . Dexter Degoma
Ambulatory Care . . . . Flor Gamurot
Emergency Room . . . . N Johnson
Pediatric Ambulatory Care . . . . . . Celestine de La Cruz, MD

Measure	Cases	This Hosp.	State Avg.	U.S. Avg.
Blood Clot Prevention and Treatment				
Anticoagulation Overlap Therapy[2]	34	74%	92%	93%
ICU Venous Thromboembolism Prophylaxis[2]	65	63%	92%	92%
Incidence of Potentially Preventable VTE[1,2]	-	-	11%	10%
UFH with Dosages/Platelet Monitoring[1,2]	-	-	96%	97%
Venous Thromboembolism Prophylaxis[2]	345	30%	83%	85%
Warfarin Therapy Discharge Instructions[2]	31	19%	75%	75%
Chest Pain/Possible Heart Attack Care				
Aspirin Given Within 24 Hours of Arrival[1,3]	-	-	97%	96%
Fibrinolytic Meds Within 30 Min. of Arrival[3,7]	-	-	62%	58%
Average Time to ECG (minutes)[1,3]	-	-	9	7
Average Time to Transfer (minutes)[3,7]	-	-	62	60
Children's Asthma Care				
Received Home Management Plan of Care	-	-	88%	88%
Received Reliever Medication	-	-	100%	100%
Received Systemic Corticosteroids	-	-	100%	100%
Emergency Department				
Admittance Decision Time (minutes)[2]	415	182	125	98
Head CT Results Within 45 Min. of Arrival[1]	-	-	55%	57%
Patients Who Left ER Before Being Seen	35,482	7%	3%	2%
Time from ER Arrival to Admit. (minutes)[2]	461	505	323	274
Time from ER Arrival to Discharge (minutes)	342	170	168	134
Time in ER Before Being Evaluated (minutes)	366	36	29	26
Time to Pain Meds for Fractures (minutes)	36	69	62	57
Heart Attack Care				
Aspirin Given at Discharge	19	79%	99%	99%

NOTE: Hospital profiles are in alphabetical order by state, then city, then hospital within the city; Rankings exclude hospitals with less than 25 cases except for patient surveys which excludes hospitals with less than 100 cases; (a) 100-299 cases; (1) The number of cases/patients is too few to report; (2) Data submitted were based on a sample of cases/patients; (3) Results are based on a shorter time period than required; (4) Data suppressed by CMS for one or more quarters; (5) Results are not available for this reporting period; (6) Fewer than 100 patients completed the HCAHPS survey; (7) No cases met the criteria for this measure; (8) The lower limit of the confidence interval cannot be calculated if the number of observed infections equals zero; (9) No data are available from the state/territory for this reporting period; (10) The scores shown reflect fewer than 50 completed surveys; (11) There were discrepancies in the data collection process; (12) This measure does not apply to this hospital for this reporting period; (13) Results cannot be calculated for this reporting period; (14) The results for this state are combined with nearby states to protect confidentiality; Please refer to the User's Guide for a full explanation of data.

Fibrinolytic Meds Within 30 Min. of Arrival[7]	-	-	73%	54%
PCI Within 90 Minutes of Arrival[7]	-	-	95%	96%
Statin Prescribed at Discharge	19	74%	98%	98%
Heart Failure Care				
ACE Inhibitor or ARB for LVSD	58	97%	97%	97%
Discharge Instructions Given	151	79%	94%	94%
Evaluation of LVS Function	154	92%	99%	99%
Medicare Spending				
Medicare Spending per Patient (ratio)	-	0.98	0.98	0.98
Pneumonia Care				
Appropriate Initial Antibiotic Given[2]	56	96%	97%	95%
Blood Culture Timing[2]	103	92%	98%	98%
Pregnancy and Delivery Care				
Newborn Deliveries Scheduled Early[2]	48	21%	5%	6%
Preventive Care				
Immunization for Influenza[2]	524	86%	89%	90%
Immunization for Pneumonia[2]	423	94%	90%	92%
Stroke Care				
Anticoagulation Therapy for Atrial Fibrillation[1]	-	-	95%	95%
Antithrombotic Therapy Timing	46	80%	98%	98%
Assessed for Rehabilitation	47	77%	97%	97%
Discharged on Antithrombotic Therapy	46	96%	99%	99%
Discharged on Statin Medication	36	81%	94%	94%
Thrombolytic Therapy Timing[1]	-	-	72%	66%
Venous Thromboembolism Prophylaxis	51	49%	94%	94%
Written Stroke Educational Materials Given	40	52%	87%	88%
Surgical Care Improvement Project				
Appropriate Beta Blocker Usage[2]	67	91%	97%	98%
Appropriate VTP Within 24 Hours[2]	265	91%	98%	98%
Controlled Postoperative Blood Glucose[2,7]	-	-	96%	97%
Perioperative Temperature Management[2]	340	100%	100%	100%
Prophylactic Antibiotic Selection[2]	220	99%	99%	99%
Prophylactic Antibiotic Selection (Outpatient)	20	95%	97%	98%
Prophylactic Antibiotic Stopped[2]	215	90%	98%	98%
Prophylactic Antibiotic Timing[2]	222	99%	99%	99%
Prophylactic Antibiotic Timing (Outpatient)	22	86%	97%	98%
Urinary Catheter Removal[2]	165	88%	97%	97%
Survey of Patients' Hospital Experiences				
Area Around Room 'Always' Quiet at Night	300+	50%	51%	61%
Doctors 'Always' Communicated Well	300+	74%	78%	82%
Home Recovery Information Given	300+	81%	83%	85%
Hospital Given 9 or 10 on 10 Point Scale	300+	56%	68%	71%
Meds 'Always' Explained Before Given	300+	61%	61%	64%
Nurses 'Always' Communicated Well	300+	71%	74%	79%
Pain 'Always' Well Controlled	300+	61%	68%	71%
Room and Bathroom 'Always' Clean	300+	67%	70%	73%
Timely Help 'Always' Received	300+	52%	62%	68%
Would Definitely Recommend Hospital	300+	54%	70%	71%
Use of Medical Imaging				
Cardiac Imaging Stress Test before Surgery[1]	-	-	5.2%	5.3%
Combination Abdominal CT Scan	155	3.9%	13.4%	10.5%
Combination Brain/Sinus CT Scan[1]	-	-	2.2%	2.7%
Combination Chest CT Scan[1]	-	-	2.3%	2.7%
Follow-up Mammogram/Ultrasound	156	7.7%	8.2%	8.8%
Lumbar Spine MRI for Low Back Pain[1]	-	-	34.2%	37.2%

Kaweah Delta Medical Center

400 W Mineral King Ave Phone: 559-624-2000
Visalia, CA 93291 Fax: 559-635-4021
E-mail: cjohnson@kdhcd.org
URL: www.kaweahdelta.org
Type: Acute Care Hospitals Emergency Services: Yes
Ownership: Govt - Hospital Dist/Auth Beds: 495
Key Personnel:
Infection Control. . . . . Daniel Boken, MD
Radiology. . . . . Richard Clutson, MD
Anesthesiology. . . . . Adam Dorin, MD
Emergency Room . . . . Jerry I Jacobson, MD
CEO . . . . Lindsay K. Mann
Pediatric In-Patient Care . . . . Christine Nelson, MD
Quality Assurance . . . . Barbara Porter
Chief of Medical Staff. . . . . William Roach, MD

Measure	Cases	This Hosp.	State Avg.	U.S. Avg.
Blood Clot Prevention and Treatment				
Anticoagulation Overlap Therapy[2]	90	81%	92%	93%
ICU Venous Thromboembolism Prophylaxis[2]	57	98%	92%	92%
Incidence of Potentially Preventable VTE[1,2]	-	-	11%	10%
UFH with Dosages/Platelet Monitoring[2]	27	100%	96%	97%
Venous Thromboembolism Prophylaxis[2]	363	92%	83%	85%
Warfarin Therapy Discharge Instructions[2]	72	56%	75%	75%
Chest Pain/Possible Heart Attack Care				
Aspirin Given Within 24 Hours of Arrival[1,3]	-	-	97%	96%
Fibrinolytic Meds Within 30 Min. of Arrival[5]	-	-	62%	58%
Average Time to ECG (minutes)[1,3]	-	-	9	7
Average Time to Transfer (minutes)[5]	-	-	62	60
Children's Asthma Care				
Received Home Management Plan of Care	-	-	88%	88%
Received Reliever Medication	-	-	100%	100%
Received Systemic Corticosteroids	-	-	100%	100%
Emergency Department				
Admittance Decision Time (minutes)[2]	612	105	125	98
Head CT Results Within 45 Min. of Arrival	21	86%	55%	57%
Patients Who Left ER Before Being Seen	85,222	1%	3%	2%
Time from ER Arrival to Admit. (minutes)[2]	614	305	323	274
Time from ER Arrival to Discharge (minutes)	362	186	168	134
Time in ER Before Being Evaluated (minutes)	405	13	29	26
Time to Pain Meds for Fractures (minutes)	330	62	62	57
Heart Attack Care				
Aspirin Given at Discharge[2]	314	98%	99%	99%
Fibrinolytic Meds Within 30 Min. of Arrival[1,2]	-	-	73%	54%
PCI Within 90 Minutes of Arrival[2]	73	92%	95%	96%
Statin Prescribed at Discharge[2]	310	95%	98%	98%
Heart Failure Care				
ACE Inhibitor or ARB for LVSD[2]	110	97%	97%	97%
Discharge Instructions Given[2]	261	94%	94%	94%
Evaluation of LVS Function[2]	295	100%	99%	99%
Medicare Spending				
Medicare Spending per Patient (ratio)	-	0.96	0.98	0.98
Pneumonia Care				
Appropriate Initial Antibiotic Given[2]	78	95%	97%	95%
Blood Culture Timing[2]	161	98%	98%	98%
Pregnancy and Delivery Care				
Newborn Deliveries Scheduled Early	448	21%	5%	6%
Preventive Care				
Immunization for Influenza[2]	513	94%	89%	90%
Immunization for Pneumonia[2]	529	97%	90%	92%
Stroke Care				
Anticoagulation Therapy for Atrial Fibrillation[2]	14	86%	95%	95%
Antithrombotic Therapy Timing[2]	74	99%	98%	98%
Assessed for Rehabilitation[2]	87	86%	97%	97%
Discharged on Antithrombotic Therapy[2]	83	99%	99%	99%
Discharged on Statin Medication[2]	64	78%	94%	94%
Thrombolytic Therapy Timing[2]	13	62%	72%	66%
Venous Thromboembolism Prophylaxis[2]	83	96%	94%	94%
Written Stroke Educational Materials Given[2]	47	81%	87%	88%
Surgical Care Improvement Project				
Appropriate Beta Blocker Usage[2]	200	96%	97%	98%
Appropriate VTP Within 24 Hours[2]	425	96%	98%	98%
Controlled Postoperative Blood Glucose[2]	124	97%	96%	97%
Perioperative Temperature Management[2]	526	100%	100%	100%
Prophylactic Antibiotic Selection[2]	487	99%	99%	99%
Prophylactic Antibiotic Selection (Outpatient)	320	97%	97%	98%
Prophylactic Antibiotic Stopped[2]	468	92%	98%	98%
Prophylactic Antibiotic Timing[2]	491	98%	99%	99%
Prophylactic Antibiotic Timing (Outpatient)	322	96%	97%	98%
Urinary Catheter Removal[2]	281	92%	97%	97%
Survey of Patients' Hospital Experiences				
Area Around Room 'Always' Quiet at Night	300+	53%	51%	61%
Doctors 'Always' Communicated Well	300+	75%	78%	82%
Home Recovery Information Given	300+	81%	83%	85%
Hospital Given 9 or 10 on 10 Point Scale	300+	64%	68%	71%
Meds 'Always' Explained Before Given	300+	58%	61%	64%
Nurses 'Always' Communicated Well	300+	77%	74%	79%
Pain 'Always' Well Controlled	300+	68%	68%	71%
Room and Bathroom 'Always' Clean	300+	66%	70%	73%
Timely Help 'Always' Received	300+	61%	62%	68%
Would Definitely Recommend Hospital	300+	69%	70%	71%
Use of Medical Imaging				
Cardiac Imaging Stress Test before Surgery	469	1.9%	5.2%	5.3%
Combination Abdominal CT Scan	1,336	25.9%	13.4%	10.5%
Combination Brain/Sinus CT Scan	1,349	1.6%	2.2%	2.7%
Combination Chest CT Scan	618	1.5%	2.3%	2.7%
Follow-up Mammogram/Ultrasound	1,260	7.7%	8.2%	8.8%
Lumbar Spine MRI for Low Back Pain	171	36.3%	34.2%	37.2%

John Muir Medical Center - Walnut Creek Campus

1601 Ygnacio Valley Rd Phone: 925-939-3000
Walnut Creek, CA 94598 Fax: 925-947-4497
URL: www.jmmdhs.com
Type: Acute Care Hospitals Emergency Services: Yes
Ownership: Voluntary non-profit - Other Beds: 321
Key Personnel:
Operating Room. . . . . Nancy Cotton, RN
Chief of Medical Staff . . . . Sally Davis
CEO/President. . . . . Jane A. Willemsen

Measure	Cases	This Hosp.	State Avg.	U.S. Avg.
Blood Clot Prevention and Treatment				
Anticoagulation Overlap Therapy[2]	82	99%	92%	93%
ICU Venous Thromboembolism Prophylaxis[2]	83	99%	92%	92%
Incidence of Potentially Preventable VTE[2]	16	0%	11%	10%
UFH with Dosages/Platelet Monitoring[2]	24	100%	96%	97%
Venous Thromboembolism Prophylaxis[2]	311	95%	83%	85%
Warfarin Therapy Discharge Instructions[2]	54	98%	75%	75%
Chest Pain/Possible Heart Attack Care				
Aspirin Given Within 24 Hours of Arrival	46	100%	97%	96%
Fibrinolytic Meds Within 30 Min. of Arrival[7]	-	-	62%	58%
Average Time to ECG (minutes)	46	8	9	7
Average Time to Transfer (minutes)[7]	-	-	62	60
Children's Asthma Care				
Received Home Management Plan of Care	-	-	88%	88%
Received Reliever Medication	-	-	100%	100%
Received Systemic Corticosteroids	-	-	100%	100%
Emergency Department				
Admittance Decision Time (minutes)[2]	591	161	125	98
Head CT Results Within 45 Min. of Arrival[1]	-	-	55%	57%
Patients Who Left ER Before Being Seen	47,283	0%	3%	2%
Time from ER Arrival to Admit. (minutes)[2]	607	305	323	274
Time from ER Arrival to Discharge (minutes)	384	142	168	134
Time in ER Before Being Evaluated (minutes)	432	16	29	26
Time to Pain Meds for Fractures (minutes)	192	58	62	57
Heart Attack Care				
Aspirin Given at Discharge	81	100%	99%	99%
Fibrinolytic Meds Within 30 Min. of Arrival[7]	-	-	73%	54%
PCI Within 90 Minutes of Arrival	22	100%	95%	96%
Statin Prescribed at Discharge	76	97%	98%	98%
Heart Failure Care				
ACE Inhibitor or ARB for LVSD	61	98%	97%	97%
Discharge Instructions Given	234	99%	94%	94%
Evaluation of LVS Function	307	100%	99%	99%
Medicare Spending				
Medicare Spending per Patient (ratio)	-	1.05	0.98	0.98
Pneumonia Care				
Appropriate Initial Antibiotic Given[2]	108	97%	97%	95%
Blood Culture Timing[2]	124	98%	98%	98%
Pregnancy and Delivery Care				
Newborn Deliveries Scheduled Early[2]	53	15%	5%	6%
Preventive Care				
Immunization for Influenza[2]	528	90%	89%	90%
Immunization for Pneumonia[2]	568	88%	90%	92%
Stroke Care				
Anticoagulation Therapy for Atrial Fibrillation	43	98%	95%	95%
Antithrombotic Therapy Timing	128	98%	98%	98%
Assessed for Rehabilitation	253	99%	97%	97%
Discharged on Antithrombotic Therapy	167	99%	99%	99%
Discharged on Statin Medication	120	95%	94%	94%
Thrombolytic Therapy Timing	12	100%	72%	66%
Venous Thromboembolism Prophylaxis	291	97%	94%	94%
Written Stroke Educational Materials Given	119	83%	87%	88%
Surgical Care Improvement Project				

NOTE: Hospital profiles are in alphabetical order by state, then city, then hospital within the city; Rankings exclude hospitals with less than 25 cases except for patient surveys which excludes hospitals with less than 100 cases; (a) 100-299 cases; (1) The number of cases/patients is too few to report; (2) Data submitted were based on a sample of cases/patients; (3) Results are based on a shorter time period than required; (4) Data suppressed by CMS for one or more quarters; (5) Results are not available for this reporting period; (6) Fewer than 100 patients completed the HCAHPS survey; (7) No cases met the criteria for this measure; (8) The lower limit of the confidence interval cannot be calculated if the number of observed infections equals zero; (9) No data are available from the state/territory for this reporting period; (10) The scores shown reflect fewer than 50 completed surveys; (11) There were discrepancies in the data collection process; (12) This measure does not apply to this hospital for this reporting period; (13) Results cannot be calculated for this reporting period; (14) The results for this state are combined with nearby states to protect confidentiality; Please refer to the User's Guide for a full explanation of data.

Measure	Cases	This Hosp.	State Avg.	U.S. Avg.
Appropriate Beta Blocker Usage[2]	100	100%	97%	98%
Appropriate VTP Within 24 Hours[2]	437	97%	98%	98%
Controlled Postoperative Blood Glucose[2,7]	-	-	96%	97%
Perioperative Temperature Management[2]	483	100%	100%	100%
Prophylactic Antibiotic Selection[2]	329	99%	99%	99%
Prophylactic Antibiotic Selection (Outpatient)	260	96%	97%	98%
Prophylactic Antibiotic Stopped[2]	314	98%	98%	98%
Prophylactic Antibiotic Timing[2]	329	100%	99%	99%
Prophylactic Antibiotic Timing (Outpatient)	261	100%	97%	98%
Urinary Catheter Removal[2]	297	98%	97%	97%
Survey of Patients' Hospital Experiences				
Area Around Room 'Always' Quiet at Night	300+	59%	51%	61%
Doctors 'Always' Communicated Well	300+	78%	78%	82%
Home Recovery Information Given	300+	81%	83%	85%
Hospital Given 9 or 10 on 10 Point Scale	300+	80%	68%	71%
Meds 'Always' Explained Before Given	300+	61%	61%	64%
Nurses 'Always' Communicated Well	300+	77%	74%	79%
Pain 'Always' Well Controlled	300+	72%	68%	71%
Room and Bathroom 'Always' Clean	300+	76%	70%	73%
Timely Help 'Always' Received	300+	61%	62%	68%
Would Definitely Recommend Hospital	300+	84%	70%	71%
Use of Medical Imaging				
Cardiac Imaging Stress Test before Surgery	305	6.6%	5.2%	5.3%
Combination Abdominal CT Scan	570	5.8%	13.4%	10.5%
Combination Brain/Sinus CT Scan	836	2.9%	2.2%	2.7%
Combination Chest CT Scan	134	0.0%	2.3%	2.7%
Follow-up Mammogram/Ultrasound	4,759	6.8%	8.2%	8.8%
Lumbar Spine MRI for Low Back Pain	54	40.7%	34.2%	37.2%

Kaiser Foundation Hospital - Walnut Creek

1425 S Main St Phone: 925-295-4000
Walnut Creek, CA 94596
Type: Acute Care Hospitals Emergency Services: Yes
Ownership: Voluntary non-profit - Other Beds: 362

Measure	Cases	This Hosp.	State Avg.	U.S. Avg.
Blood Clot Prevention and Treatment				
Anticoagulation Overlap Therapy[2]	103	100%	92%	93%
ICU Venous Thromboembolism Prophylaxis[2]	76	97%	92%	92%
Incidence of Potentially Preventable VTE[1,2]	-	-	11%	10%
UFH with Dosages/Platelet Monitoring[2]	37	100%	96%	97%
Venous Thromboembolism Prophylaxis[2]	307	95%	83%	85%
Warfarin Therapy Discharge Instructions[2]	93	75%	75%	75%
Chest Pain/Possible Heart Attack Care				
Aspirin Given Within 24 Hours of Arrival	-	-	97%	96%
Fibrinolytic Meds Within 30 Min. of Arrival	-	-	62%	58%
Average Time to ECG (minutes)	-	-	9	7
Average Time to Transfer (minutes)	-	-	62	60
Children's Asthma Care				
Received Home Management Plan of Care	-	-	88%	88%
Received Reliever Medication	-	-	100%	100%
Received Systemic Corticosteroids	-	-	100%	100%
Emergency Department				
Admittance Decision Time (minutes)[2]	557	59	125	98
Head CT Results Within 45 Min. of Arrival	-	-	55%	57%
Patients Who Left ER Before Being Seen	-	-	3%	2%
Time from ER Arrival to Admit. (minutes)[2]	560	360	323	274
Time from ER Arrival to Discharge (minutes)	-	-	168	134
Time in ER Before Being Evaluated (minutes)	-	-	29	26
Time to Pain Meds for Fractures (minutes)	-	-	62	57
Heart Attack Care				
Aspirin Given at Discharge	204	100%	99%	99%
Fibrinolytic Meds Within 30 Min. of Arrival[7]	-	-	73%	54%
PCI Within 90 Minutes of Arrival	44	98%	95%	96%
Statin Prescribed at Discharge	200	100%	98%	98%
Heart Failure Care				
ACE Inhibitor or ARB for LVSD	40	100%	97%	97%
Discharge Instructions Given	232	100%	94%	94%
Evaluation of LVS Function	263	100%	99%	99%
Medicare Spending				
Medicare Spending per Patient (ratio)	-	0.80	0.98	0.98
Pneumonia Care				
Appropriate Initial Antibiotic Given[2]	73	100%	97%	95%
Blood Culture Timing[2]	150	98%	98%	98%
Pregnancy and Delivery Care				
Newborn Deliveries Scheduled Early[2]	41	0%	5%	6%
Preventive Care				
Immunization for Influenza[2]	477	95%	89%	90%
Immunization for Pneumonia[2]	534	96%	90%	92%
Stroke Care				
Anticoagulation Therapy for Atrial Fibrillation[2]	28	96%	95%	95%
Antithrombotic Therapy Timing[2]	87	100%	98%	98%
Assessed for Rehabilitation[2]	118	98%	97%	97%
Discharged on Antithrombotic Therapy[2]	102	99%	99%	99%
Discharged on Statin Medication[2]	85	99%	94%	94%
Thrombolytic Therapy Timing[1,2]	-	-	72%	66%
Venous Thromboembolism Prophylaxis[2]	99	95%	94%	94%
Written Stroke Educational Materials Given[2]	61	97%	87%	88%
Surgical Care Improvement Project				
Appropriate Beta Blocker Usage[2]	152	100%	97%	98%
Appropriate VTP Within 24 Hours[2]	391	99%	98%	98%
Controlled Postoperative Blood Glucose[2,7]	-	-	96%	97%
Perioperative Temperature Management[2]	456	100%	100%	100%
Prophylactic Antibiotic Selection[2]	294	99%	99%	99%
Prophylactic Antibiotic Selection (Outpatient)	-	-	97%	98%
Prophylactic Antibiotic Stopped[2]	288	98%	98%	98%
Prophylactic Antibiotic Timing[2]	294	99%	99%	99%
Prophylactic Antibiotic Timing (Outpatient)	-	-	97%	98%
Urinary Catheter Removal[2]	291	99%	97%	97%
Survey of Patients' Hospital Experiences				
Area Around Room 'Always' Quiet at Night	300+	40%	51%	61%
Doctors 'Always' Communicated Well	300+	79%	78%	82%
Home Recovery Information Given	300+	85%	83%	85%
Hospital Given 9 or 10 on 10 Point Scale	300+	66%	68%	71%
Meds 'Always' Explained Before Given	300+	57%	61%	64%
Nurses 'Always' Communicated Well	300+	71%	74%	79%
Pain 'Always' Well Controlled	300+	69%	68%	71%
Room and Bathroom 'Always' Clean	300+	67%	70%	73%
Timely Help 'Always' Received	300+	58%	62%	68%
Would Definitely Recommend Hospital	300+	71%	70%	71%
Use of Medical Imaging				
Cardiac Imaging Stress Test before Surgery	-	-	5.2%	5.3%
Combination Abdominal CT Scan	-	-	13.4%	10.5%
Combination Brain/Sinus CT Scan	-	-	2.2%	2.7%
Combination Chest CT Scan	-	-	2.3%	2.7%
Follow-up Mammogram/Ultrasound	-	-	8.2%	8.8%
Lumbar Spine MRI for Low Back Pain	-	-	34.2%	37.2%

Watsonville Community Hospital

75 Nielson Street Phone: 831-724-4741
Watsonville, CA 95076 Fax: 831-728-4758
URL: www.watsonvillehospital.com
Type: Acute Care Hospitals Emergency Services: Yes
Ownership: Proprietary Beds: 106
Key Personnel:
CEO/President. . . . . Joe Dale
Quality Assurance . . . . Diane Howery
Chief of Medical Staff. . . . . Gordon M Kaplan, MD

Measure	Cases	This Hosp.	State Avg.	U.S. Avg.
Blood Clot Prevention and Treatment				
Anticoagulation Overlap Therapy[2]	16	100%	92%	93%
ICU Venous Thromboembolism Prophylaxis[2]	47	96%	92%	92%
Incidence of Potentially Preventable VTE[1,2]	-	-	11%	10%
UFH with Dosages/Platelet Monitoring[1,2]	-	-	96%	97%
Venous Thromboembolism Prophylaxis[2]	236	95%	83%	85%
Warfarin Therapy Discharge Instructions[1,2]	-	-	75%	75%
Chest Pain/Possible Heart Attack Care				
Aspirin Given Within 24 Hours of Arrival[1]	-	-	97%	96%
Fibrinolytic Meds Within 30 Min. of Arrival[7]	-	-	62%	58%
Average Time to ECG (minutes)[1]	-	-	9	7
Average Time to Transfer (minutes)[1]	-	-	62	60
Children's Asthma Care				
Received Home Management Plan of Care	-	-	88%	88%
Received Reliever Medication	-	-	100%	100%
Received Systemic Corticosteroids	-	-	100%	100%
Emergency Department				
Admittance Decision Time (minutes)[2]	444	57	125	98
Head CT Results Within 45 Min. of Arrival[1]	-	-	55%	57%
Patients Who Left ER Before Being Seen	27,535	2%	3%	2%
Time from ER Arrival to Admit. (minutes)[2]	501	247	323	274
Time from ER Arrival to Discharge (minutes)	355	157	168	134
Time in ER Before Being Evaluated (minutes)	381	12	29	26
Time to Pain Meds for Fractures (minutes)	48	45	62	57
Heart Attack Care				
Aspirin Given at Discharge[1]	-	-	99%	99%
Fibrinolytic Meds Within 30 Min. of Arrival[7]	-	-	73%	54%
PCI Within 90 Minutes of Arrival[7]	-	-	95%	96%
Statin Prescribed at Discharge[1]	-	-	98%	98%
Heart Failure Care				
ACE Inhibitor or ARB for LVSD	19	100%	97%	97%
Discharge Instructions Given	71	99%	94%	94%
Evaluation of LVS Function	93	100%	99%	99%
Medicare Spending				
Medicare Spending per Patient (ratio)	-	0.92	0.98	0.98
Pneumonia Care				
Appropriate Initial Antibiotic Given	87	97%	97%	95%
Blood Culture Timing	120	98%	98%	98%
Pregnancy and Delivery Care				
Newborn Deliveries Scheduled Early[2]	32	0%	5%	6%
Preventive Care				
Immunization for Influenza[2]	505	99%	89%	90%
Immunization for Pneumonia[2]	433	99%	90%	92%
Stroke Care				
Anticoagulation Therapy for Atrial Fibrillation[1]	-	-	95%	95%
Antithrombotic Therapy Timing	45	100%	98%	98%
Assessed for Rehabilitation	48	98%	97%	97%
Discharged on Antithrombotic Therapy	45	100%	99%	99%
Discharged on Statin Medication	39	97%	94%	94%
Thrombolytic Therapy Timing[7]	-	-	72%	66%
Venous Thromboembolism Prophylaxis	47	96%	94%	94%
Written Stroke Educational Materials Given	27	96%	87%	88%
Surgical Care Improvement Project				
Appropriate Beta Blocker Usage	45	100%	97%	98%
Appropriate VTP Within 24 Hours	198	99%	98%	98%
Controlled Postoperative Blood Glucose[7]	-	-	96%	97%
Perioperative Temperature Management	249	100%	100%	100%
Prophylactic Antibiotic Selection	102	100%	99%	99%
Prophylactic Antibiotic Selection (Outpatient)	53	98%	97%	98%
Prophylactic Antibiotic Stopped	101	100%	98%	98%
Prophylactic Antibiotic Timing	102	100%	99%	99%
Prophylactic Antibiotic Timing (Outpatient)	55	95%	97%	98%
Urinary Catheter Removal	61	100%	97%	97%
Survey of Patients' Hospital Experiences				
Area Around Room 'Always' Quiet at Night	300+	52%	51%	61%
Doctors 'Always' Communicated Well	300+	79%	78%	82%
Home Recovery Information Given	300+	82%	83%	85%
Hospital Given 9 or 10 on 10 Point Scale	300+	72%	68%	71%
Meds 'Always' Explained Before Given	300+	61%	61%	64%
Nurses 'Always' Communicated Well	300+	75%	74%	79%
Pain 'Always' Well Controlled	300+	72%	68%	71%
Room and Bathroom 'Always' Clean	300+	67%	70%	73%
Timely Help 'Always' Received	300+	61%	62%	68%
Would Definitely Recommend Hospital	300+	62%	70%	71%
Use of Medical Imaging				
Cardiac Imaging Stress Test before Surgery	51	0.0%	5.2%	5.3%
Combination Abdominal CT Scan	283	4.2%	13.4%	10.5%
Combination Brain/Sinus CT Scan	371	0.3%	2.2%	2.7%
Combination Chest CT Scan	110	1.8%	2.3%	2.7%
Follow-up Mammogram/Ultrasound	1,032	3.6%	8.2%	8.8%
Lumbar Spine MRI for Low Back Pain[1]	-	-	34.2%	37.2%

Trinity Hospital

60 Easter Avenue Phone: 530-623-5541
Weaverville, CA 96093
Type: Critical Access Hospitals Emergency Services: Yes
Ownership: Govt - Hospital Dist/Auth

Measure	Cases	This Hosp.	State Avg.	U.S. Avg.
Blood Clot Prevention and Treatment				

NOTE: Hospital profiles are in alphabetical order by state, then city, then hospital within the city; Rankings exclude hospitals with less than 25 cases except for patient surveys which excludes hospitals with less than 100 cases; (a) 100-299 cases; (1) The number of cases/patients is too few to report; (2) Data submitted were based on a sample of cases/patients; (3) Results are based on a shorter time period than required; (4) Data suppressed by CMS for one or more quarters; (5) Results are not available for this reporting period; (6) Fewer than 100 patients completed the HCAHPS survey; (7) No cases met the criteria for this measure; (8) The lower limit of the confidence interval cannot be calculated if the number of observed infections equals zero; (9) No data are available from the state/territory for this reporting period; (10) The scores shown reflect fewer than 50 completed surveys; (11) There were discrepancies in the data collection process; (12) This measure does not apply to this hospital for this reporting period; (13) Results cannot be calculated for this reporting period; (14) The results for this state are combined with nearby states to protect confidentiality; Please refer to the User's Guide for a full explanation of data.

Anticoagulation Overlap Therapy[5]	-	-	92%	93%
ICU Venous Thromboembolism Prophylaxis[5]	-	-	92%	92%
Incidence of Potentially Preventable VTE[5]	-	-	11%	10%
UFH with Dosages/Platelet Monitoring[5]	-	-	96%	97%
Venous Thromboembolism Prophylaxis[5]	-	-	83%	85%
Warfarin Therapy Discharge Instructions[5]	-	-	75%	75%
Chest Pain/Possible Heart Attack Care				
Aspirin Given Within 24 Hours of Arrival[5]	-	-	97%	96%
Fibrinolytic Meds Within 30 Min. of Arrival[5]	-	-	62%	58%
Average Time to ECG (minutes)[5]	-	-	9	7
Average Time to Transfer (minutes)[5]	-	-	62	60
Children's Asthma Care				
Received Home Management Plan of Care	-	-	88%	88%
Received Reliever Medication	-	-	100%	100%
Received Systemic Corticosteroids	-	-	100%	100%
Emergency Department				
Admittance Decision Time (minutes)[5]	-	-	125	98
Head CT Results Within 45 Min. of Arrival[5]	-	-	55%	57%
Patients Who Left ER Before Being Seen[5]	-	-	3%	2%
Time from ER Arrival to Admit. (minutes)[5]	-	-	323	274
Time from ER Arrival to Discharge (minutes)[5]	-	-	168	134
Time in ER Before Being Evaluated (minutes)[5]	-	-	29	26
Time to Pain Meds for Fractures (minutes)[5]	-	-	62	57
Heart Attack Care				
Aspirin Given at Discharge[5]	-	-	99%	99%
Fibrinolytic Meds Within 30 Min. of Arrival[5]	-	-	73%	54%
PCI Within 90 Minutes of Arrival[5]	-	-	95%	96%
Statin Prescribed at Discharge[5]	-	-	98%	98%
Heart Failure Care				
ACE Inhibitor or ARB for LVSD[5]	-	-	97%	97%
Discharge Instructions Given[5]	-	-	94%	94%
Evaluation of LVS Function[5]	-	-	99%	99%
Medicare Spending				
Medicare Spending per Patient (ratio)	-	-	0.98	0.98
Pneumonia Care				
Appropriate Initial Antibiotic Given[5]	-	-	97%	95%
Blood Culture Timing[5]	-	-	98%	98%
Pregnancy and Delivery Care				
Newborn Deliveries Scheduled Early[5]	-	-	5%	6%
Preventive Care				
Immunization for Influenza[5]	-	-	89%	90%
Immunization for Pneumonia[5]	-	-	90%	92%
Stroke Care				
Anticoagulation Therapy for Atrial Fibrillation[5]	-	-	95%	95%
Antithrombotic Therapy Timing[5]	-	-	98%	98%
Assessed for Rehabilitation[5]	-	-	97%	97%
Discharged on Antithrombotic Therapy[5]	-	-	99%	99%
Discharged on Statin Medication[5]	-	-	94%	94%
Thrombolytic Therapy Timing[5]	-	-	72%	66%
Venous Thromboembolism Prophylaxis[5]	-	-	94%	94%
Written Stroke Educational Materials Given[5]	-	-	87%	88%
Surgical Care Improvement Project				
Appropriate Beta Blocker Usage[5]	-	-	97%	98%
Appropriate VTP Within 24 Hours[5]	-	-	98%	98%
Controlled Postoperative Blood Glucose[5]	-	-	96%	97%
Perioperative Temperature Management[5]	-	-	100%	100%
Prophylactic Antibiotic Selection[5]	-	-	99%	99%
Prophylactic Antibiotic Selection (Outpatient)[5]	-	-	97%	98%
Prophylactic Antibiotic Stopped[5]	-	-	98%	98%
Prophylactic Antibiotic Timing[5]	-	-	99%	99%
Prophylactic Antibiotic Timing (Outpatient)[5]	-	-	97%	98%
Urinary Catheter Removal[5]	-	-	97%	97%
Survey of Patients' Hospital Experiences				
Area Around Room 'Always' Quiet at Night[5]	-	-	51%	61%
Doctors 'Always' Communicated Well[5]	-	-	78%	82%
Home Recovery Information Given[5]	-	-	83%	85%
Hospital Given 9 or 10 on 10 Point Scale[5]	-	-	68%	71%
Meds 'Always' Explained Before Given[5]	-	-	61%	64%
Nurses 'Always' Communicated Well[5]	-	-	74%	79%
Pain 'Always' Well Controlled[5]	-	-	68%	71%
Room and Bathroom 'Always' Clean[5]	-	-	70%	73%
Timely Help 'Always' Received[5]	-	-	62%	68%
Would Definitely Recommend Hospital[5]	-	-	70%	71%
Use of Medical Imaging				
Cardiac Imaging Stress Test before Surgery[7]	-	-	5.2%	5.3%
Combination Abdominal CT Scan	137	11.7%	13.4%	10.5%
Combination Brain/Sinus CT Scan[1]	-	-	2.2%	2.7%
Combination Chest CT Scan	73	11.0%	2.3%	2.7%
Follow-up Mammogram/Ultrasound[7]	-	-	8.2%	8.8%
Lumbar Spine MRI for Low Back Pain[7]	-	-	34.2%	37.2%

Doctors Hospital of West Covina

725 S Orange Ave
West Covina, CA 91790
Phone: 626-338-8481
Fax: 626-960-9178
Type: Acute Care Hospitals
Emergency Services: No
Ownership: Proprietary
Beds: 51

Key Personnel:
Chief of Medical Staff. . . . . Nashat Ateia, MD
Anesthesiology. . . . . Erich Pollak, MD
Infection Control. . . . . Milad Shokair
Operating Room. . . . . Lisa Torres
Quality Assurance . . . . Gerald Wallman

Measure	Cases	This Hosp.	State Avg.	U.S. Avg.
Blood Clot Prevention and Treatment				
Anticoagulation Overlap Therapy[7]	-	-	92%	93%
ICU Venous Thromboembolism Prophylaxis[7]	-	-	92%	92%
Incidence of Potentially Preventable VTE[7]	-	-	11%	10%
UFH with Dosages/Platelet Monitoring[7]	-	-	96%	97%
Venous Thromboembolism Prophylaxis	30	27%	83%	85%
Warfarin Therapy Discharge Instructions[7]	-	-	75%	75%
Chest Pain/Possible Heart Attack Care				
Aspirin Given Within 24 Hours of Arrival[5]	-	-	97%	96%
Fibrinolytic Meds Within 30 Min. of Arrival[5]	-	-	62%	58%
Average Time to ECG (minutes)[5]	-	-	9	7
Average Time to Transfer (minutes)[5]	-	-	62	60
Children's Asthma Care				
Received Home Management Plan of Care	-	-	88%	88%
Received Reliever Medication	-	-	100%	100%
Received Systemic Corticosteroids	-	-	100%	100%
Emergency Department				
Admittance Decision Time (minutes)[7]	-	-	125	98
Head CT Results Within 45 Min. of Arrival[5]	-	-	55%	57%
Patients Who Left ER Before Being Seen[5]	-	-	3%	2%
Time from ER Arrival to Admit. (minutes)[7]	-	-	323	274
Time from ER Arrival to Discharge (minutes)[5]	-	-	168	134
Time in ER Before Being Evaluated (minutes)[5]	-	-	29	26
Time to Pain Meds for Fractures (minutes)[5]	-	-	62	57
Heart Attack Care				
Aspirin Given at Discharge[5]	-	-	99%	99%
Fibrinolytic Meds Within 30 Min. of Arrival[5]	-	-	73%	54%
PCI Within 90 Minutes of Arrival[5]	-	-	95%	96%
Statin Prescribed at Discharge[5]	-	-	98%	98%
Heart Failure Care				
ACE Inhibitor or ARB for LVSD[5]	-	-	97%	97%
Discharge Instructions Given[5]	-	-	94%	94%
Evaluation of LVS Function[5]	-	-	99%	99%
Medicare Spending				
Medicare Spending per Patient (ratio)	-	0.89	0.98	0.98
Pneumonia Care				
Appropriate Initial Antibiotic Given[1,3]	-	-	97%	95%
Blood Culture Timing[3,7]	-	-	98%	98%
Pregnancy and Delivery Care				
Newborn Deliveries Scheduled Early[7]	-	-	5%	6%
Preventive Care				
Immunization for Influenza	58	76%	89%	90%
Immunization for Pneumonia	49	88%	90%	92%
Stroke Care				
Anticoagulation Therapy for Atrial Fibrillation[5]	-	-	95%	95%
Antithrombotic Therapy Timing[5]	-	-	98%	98%
Assessed for Rehabilitation[5]	-	-	97%	97%
Discharged on Antithrombotic Therapy[5]	-	-	99%	99%
Discharged on Statin Medication[5]	-	-	94%	94%
Thrombolytic Therapy Timing[5]	-	-	72%	66%
Venous Thromboembolism Prophylaxis[5]	-	-	94%	94%
Written Stroke Educational Materials Given[5]	-	-	87%	88%
Surgical Care Improvement Project				
Appropriate Beta Blocker Usage[1]	-	-	97%	98%
Appropriate VTP Within 24 Hours	54	98%	98%	98%
Controlled Postoperative Blood Glucose[7]	-	-	96%	97%
Perioperative Temperature Management	54	100%	100%	100%
Prophylactic Antibiotic Selection	44	98%	99%	99%
Prophylactic Antibiotic Selection (Outpatient)[5]	-	-	97%	98%
Prophylactic Antibiotic Stopped	45	84%	98%	98%
Prophylactic Antibiotic Timing	45	89%	99%	99%
Prophylactic Antibiotic Timing (Outpatient)[5]	-	-	97%	98%
Urinary Catheter Removal[1]	-	-	97%	97%
Survey of Patients' Hospital Experiences				
Area Around Room 'Always' Quiet at Night[10]	<100	100%	51%	61%
Doctors 'Always' Communicated Well[10]	<100	100%	78%	82%
Home Recovery Information Given[10]	<100	99%	83%	85%
Hospital Given 9 or 10 on 10 Point Scale[10]	<100	89%	68%	71%
Meds 'Always' Explained Before Given[10]	<100	79%	61%	64%
Nurses 'Always' Communicated Well[10]	<100	92%	74%	79%
Pain 'Always' Well Controlled[10]	<100	94%	68%	71%
Room and Bathroom 'Always' Clean[10]	<100	88%	70%	73%
Timely Help 'Always' Received[10]	<100	93%	62%	68%
Would Definitely Recommend Hospital[10]	<100	89%	70%	71%
Use of Medical Imaging				
Cardiac Imaging Stress Test before Surgery[7]	-	-	5.2%	5.3%
Combination Abdominal CT Scan[7]	-	-	13.4%	10.5%
Combination Brain/Sinus CT Scan[7]	-	-	2.2%	2.7%
Combination Chest CT Scan[7]	-	-	2.3%	2.7%
Follow-up Mammogram/Ultrasound[7]	-	-	8.2%	8.8%
Lumbar Spine MRI for Low Back Pain[7]	-	-	34.2%	37.2%

West Hills Hospital & Medical Center

7300 Medical Center Dr
West Hills, CA 91307
Phone: 818-676-4100
Fax: 818-347-4519
URL: www.westhillshospital.com
Type: Acute Care Hospitals
Emergency Services: Yes
Ownership: Proprietary
Beds: 220

Key Personnel:
Chief of Medical Staff. . . . . Frank C Candela, MD
President/CEO. . . . . Douglas Long

Measure	Cases	This Hosp.	State Avg.	U.S. Avg.
Blood Clot Prevention and Treatment				
Anticoagulation Overlap Therapy[2]	48	94%	92%	93%
ICU Venous Thromboembolism Prophylaxis[2]	92	95%	92%	92%
Incidence of Potentially Preventable VTE[2]	12	17%	11%	10%
UFH with Dosages/Platelet Monitoring[2]	22	100%	96%	97%
Venous Thromboembolism Prophylaxis[2]	318	93%	83%	85%
Warfarin Therapy Discharge Instructions[2]	32	84%	75%	75%
Chest Pain/Possible Heart Attack Care				
Aspirin Given Within 24 Hours of Arrival[1,3]	-	-	97%	96%
Fibrinolytic Meds Within 30 Min. of Arrival[5]	-	-	62%	58%
Average Time to ECG (minutes)[1,3]	-	-	9	7
Average Time to Transfer (minutes)[5]	-	-	62	60
Children's Asthma Care				
Received Home Management Plan of Care	-	-	88%	88%
Received Reliever Medication	-	-	100%	100%
Received Systemic Corticosteroids	-	-	100%	100%
Emergency Department				
Admittance Decision Time (minutes)[2]	759	265	125	98
Head CT Results Within 45 Min. of Arrival	15	73%	55%	57%
Patients Who Left ER Before Being Seen	39,178	0%	3%	2%
Time from ER Arrival to Admit. (minutes)[2]	759	362	323	274
Time from ER Arrival to Discharge (minutes)	468	141	168	134
Time in ER Before Being Evaluated (minutes)	536	6	29	26
Time to Pain Meds for Fractures (minutes)	171	45	62	57
Heart Attack Care				
Aspirin Given at Discharge	152	99%	99%	99%
Fibrinolytic Meds Within 30 Min. of Arrival[7]	-	-	73%	54%
PCI Within 90 Minutes of Arrival	42	90%	95%	96%
Statin Prescribed at Discharge	156	98%	98%	98%
Heart Failure Care				
ACE Inhibitor or ARB for LVSD	68	99%	97%	97%
Discharge Instructions Given	147	98%	94%	94%
Evaluation of LVS Function	196	99%	99%	99%

NOTE: Hospital profiles are in alphabetical order by state, then city, then hospital within the city; Rankings exclude hospitals with less than 25 cases except for patient surveys which excludes hospitals with less than 100 cases; (a) 100-299 cases; (1) The number of cases/patients is too few to report; (2) Data submitted were based on a sample of cases/patients; (3) Results are based on a shorter time period than required; (4) Data suppressed by CMS for one or more quarters; (5) Results are not available for this reporting period; (6) Fewer than 100 patients completed the HCAHPS survey; (7) No cases met the criteria for this measure; (8) The lower limit of the confidence interval cannot be calculated if the number of observed infections equals zero; (9) No data are available from the state/territory for this reporting period; (10) The scores shown reflect fewer than 50 completed surveys; (11) There were discrepancies in the data collection process; (12) This measure does not apply to this hospital for this reporting period; (13) Results cannot be calculated for this reporting period; (14) The results for this state are combined with nearby states to protect confidentiality; Please refer to the User's Guide for a full explanation of data.

Measure	Cases	This Hosp.	State Avg.	U.S. Avg.
Medicare Spending				
Medicare Spending per Patient (ratio)	-	1.10	0.98	0.98
Pneumonia Care				
Appropriate Initial Antibiotic Given[2]	61	98%	97%	95%
Blood Culture Timing[2]	155	100%	98%	98%
Pregnancy and Delivery Care				
Newborn Deliveries Scheduled Early[2]	23	0%	5%	6%
Preventive Care				
Immunization for Influenza[2]	540	99%	89%	90%
Immunization for Pneumonia[2]	679	98%	90%	92%
Stroke Care				
Anticoagulation Therapy for Atrial Fibrillation[2]	18	94%	95%	95%
Antithrombotic Therapy Timing[2]	73	99%	98%	98%
Assessed for Rehabilitation[2]	89	93%	97%	97%
Discharged on Antithrombotic Therapy[2]	73	100%	99%	99%
Discharged on Statin Medication[2]	58	97%	94%	94%
Thrombolytic Therapy Timing[1,2]	-	-	72%	66%
Venous Thromboembolism Prophylaxis[2]	92	95%	94%	94%
Written Stroke Educational Materials Given[2]	52	100%	87%	88%
Surgical Care Improvement Project				
Appropriate Beta Blocker Usage[2]	114	99%	97%	98%
Appropriate VTP Within 24 Hours[2]	343	99%	98%	98%
Controlled Postoperative Blood Glucose[2]	56	96%	96%	97%
Perioperative Temperature Management[2]	401	100%	100%	100%
Prophylactic Antibiotic Selection[2]	305	99%	99%	99%
Prophylactic Antibiotic Selection (Outpatient)	136	96%	97%	98%
Prophylactic Antibiotic Stopped[2]	300	99%	98%	98%
Prophylactic Antibiotic Timing[2]	305	100%	99%	99%
Prophylactic Antibiotic Timing (Outpatient)	138	98%	97%	98%
Urinary Catheter Removal[2]	274	100%	97%	97%
Survey of Patients' Hospital Experiences				
Area Around Room 'Always' Quiet at Night	300+	44%	51%	61%
Doctors 'Always' Communicated Well	300+	75%	78%	82%
Home Recovery Information Given	300+	82%	83%	85%
Hospital Given 9 or 10 on 10 Point Scale	300+	56%	68%	71%
Meds 'Always' Explained Before Given	300+	53%	61%	64%
Nurses 'Always' Communicated Well	300+	64%	74%	79%
Pain 'Always' Well Controlled	300+	64%	68%	71%
Room and Bathroom 'Always' Clean	300+	56%	70%	73%
Timely Help 'Always' Received	300+	47%	62%	68%
Would Definitely Recommend Hospital	300+	61%	70%	71%
Use of Medical Imaging				
Cardiac Imaging Stress Test before Surgery	222	6.8%	5.2%	5.3%
Combination Abdominal CT Scan	347	0.6%	13.4%	10.5%
Combination Brain/Sinus CT Scan	594	1.7%	2.2%	2.7%
Combination Chest CT Scan	80	0.0%	2.3%	2.7%
Follow-up Mammogram/Ultrasound	1,465	9.1%	8.2%	8.8%
Lumbar Spine MRI for Low Back Pain[1]	-	-	34.2%	37.2%

VA Greater Los Angeles Healthcare System

11301 Wilshire Blvd. — Phone: 310-478-3711
West Los Angeles, CA 90073 — Fax: 310-268-4642
URL: www1.va.gov
Type: Acute Care - VA — Emergency Services: No
Ownership: Government Federal — Beds: 945

Key Personnel:
Cardiac Laboratory. . . . . Abbas Ardihali
CEO/President. . . . . Donna M Breiter, RN, MSN
Infection Control. . . . . Matthew Goetz, MD
Radiology. . . . . Edward Grant, MD
Quality Assurance . . . . Lester Jones, MD
Chief of Medical Staff . . . . Dean C Norman, MD
Operating Room. . . . . Mark Sawicki, RN

Measure	Cases	This Hosp.	State Avg.	U.S. Avg.
Blood Clot Prevention and Treatment				
Anticoagulation Overlap Therapy	-	-	92%	93%
ICU Venous Thromboembolism Prophylaxis	-	-	92%	92%
Incidence of Potentially Preventable VTE	-	-	11%	10%
UFH with Dosages/Platelet Monitoring	-	-	96%	97%
Venous Thromboembolism Prophylaxis	-	-	83%	85%
Warfarin Therapy Discharge Instructions	-	-	75%	75%
Chest Pain/Possible Heart Attack Care				
Aspirin Given Within 24 Hours of Arrival	-	-	97%	96%
Fibrinolytic Meds Within 30 Min. of Arrival	-	-	62%	58%
Average Time to ECG (minutes)	-	-	9	7
Average Time to Transfer (minutes)	-	-	62	60
Children's Asthma Care				
Received Home Management Plan of Care	-	-	88%	88%
Received Reliever Medication	-	-	100%	100%
Received Systemic Corticosteroids	-	-	100%	100%
Emergency Department				
Admittance Decision Time (minutes)	-	-	125	98
Head CT Results Within 45 Min. of Arrival	-	-	55%	57%
Patients Who Left ER Before Being Seen	-	-	3%	2%
Time from ER Arrival to Admit. (minutes)	-	-	323	274
Time from ER Arrival to Discharge (minutes)	-	-	168	134
Time in ER Before Being Evaluated (minutes)	-	-	29	26
Time to Pain Meds for Fractures (minutes)	-	-	62	57
Heart Attack Care				
Aspirin Given at Discharge	103	98%	99%	99%
Fibrinolytic Meds Within 30 Min. of Arrival[5]	-	-	73%	54%
PCI Within 90 Minutes of Arrival[5]	-	-	95%	96%
Statin Prescribed at Discharge	101	97%	98%	98%
Heart Failure Care				
ACE Inhibitor or ARB for LVSD	116	97%	97%	97%
Discharge Instructions Given	289	99%	94%	94%
Evaluation of LVS Function	320	100%	99%	99%
Medicare Spending				
Medicare Spending per Patient (ratio)	-	-	0.98	0.98
Pneumonia Care				
Appropriate Initial Antibiotic Given	50	96%	97%	95%
Blood Culture Timing	101	98%	98%	98%
Pregnancy and Delivery Care				
Newborn Deliveries Scheduled Early	-	-	5%	6%
Preventive Care				
Immunization for Influenza[5]	-	-	89%	90%
Immunization for Pneumonia[5]	-	-	90%	92%
Stroke Care				
Anticoagulation Therapy for Atrial Fibrillation	-	-	95%	95%
Antithrombotic Therapy Timing	-	-	98%	98%
Assessed for Rehabilitation	-	-	97%	97%
Discharged on Antithrombotic Therapy	-	-	99%	99%
Discharged on Statin Medication	-	-	94%	94%
Thrombolytic Therapy Timing	-	-	72%	66%
Venous Thromboembolism Prophylaxis	-	-	94%	94%
Written Stroke Educational Materials Given	-	-	87%	88%
Surgical Care Improvement Project				
Appropriate Beta Blocker Usage[2]	172	95%	97%	98%
Appropriate VTP Within 24 Hours[2]	257	99%	98%	98%
Controlled Postoperative Blood Glucose[2]	106	94%	96%	97%
Perioperative Temperature Management[2]	316	100%	100%	100%
Prophylactic Antibiotic Selection	279	100%	99%	99%
Prophylactic Antibiotic Selection (Outpatient)	-	-	97%	98%
Prophylactic Antibiotic Stopped	262	95%	98%	98%
Prophylactic Antibiotic Timing	279	97%	99%	99%
Prophylactic Antibiotic Timing (Outpatient)	-	-	97%	98%
Urinary Catheter Removal[2]	255	99%	97%	97%
Survey of Patients' Hospital Experiences				
Area Around Room 'Always' Quiet at Night	-	-	51%	61%
Doctors 'Always' Communicated Well	-	-	78%	82%
Home Recovery Information Given	-	-	83%	85%
Hospital Given 9 or 10 on 10 Point Scale	-	-	68%	71%
Meds 'Always' Explained Before Given	-	-	61%	64%
Nurses 'Always' Communicated Well	-	-	74%	79%
Pain 'Always' Well Controlled	-	-	68%	71%
Room and Bathroom 'Always' Clean	-	-	70%	73%
Timely Help 'Always' Received	-	-	62%	68%
Would Definitely Recommend Hospital	-	-	70%	71%
Use of Medical Imaging				
Cardiac Imaging Stress Test before Surgery	-	-	5.2%	5.3%
Combination Abdominal CT Scan	-	-	13.4%	10.5%
Combination Brain/Sinus CT Scan	-	-	2.2%	2.7%
Combination Chest CT Scan	-	-	2.3%	2.7%
Follow-up Mammogram/Ultrasound	-	-	8.2%	8.8%
Lumbar Spine MRI for Low Back Pain	-	-	34.2%	37.2%

Presbyterian Intercommunity Hospital

12401 E Washington Blvd — Phone: 526-698-0811
Whittier, CA 90602 — Fax: 562-945-6854
URL: www.whittierpres.com
Type: Acute Care Hospitals — Emergency Services: Yes
Ownership: Voluntary non-profit - Private — Beds: 444

Key Personnel:
Patient Relations . . . . Nanette Herrera
Radiology. . . . . Stacy Johnson
Pediatric In-Patient Care . . . . Juliet Lener, MD
Chief of Medical Staff . . . . Rosalio Lopez, MD
Quality Assurance . . . . Judy Pugach
Emergency Room . . . . Joan Rolland, RN
Operating Room. . . . . Todd Salnas
CEO/President. . . . . Jim West

Measure	Cases	This Hosp.	State Avg.	U.S. Avg.
Blood Clot Prevention and Treatment				
Anticoagulation Overlap Therapy[2]	106	92%	92%	93%
ICU Venous Thromboembolism Prophylaxis[2]	77	99%	92%	92%
Incidence of Potentially Preventable VTE[2]	22	9%	11%	10%
UFH with Dosages/Platelet Monitoring[2]	100	100%	96%	97%
Venous Thromboembolism Prophylaxis[2]	329	92%	83%	85%
Warfarin Therapy Discharge Instructions[2]	82	57%	75%	75%
Chest Pain/Possible Heart Attack Care				
Aspirin Given Within 24 Hours of Arrival	42	100%	97%	96%
Fibrinolytic Meds Within 30 Min. of Arrival[3,7]	-	-	62%	58%
Average Time to ECG (minutes)	42	2	9	7
Average Time to Transfer (minutes)[3,7]	-	-	62	60
Children's Asthma Care				
Received Home Management Plan of Care	-	-	88%	88%
Received Reliever Medication	-	-	100%	100%
Received Systemic Corticosteroids	-	-	100%	100%
Emergency Department				
Admittance Decision Time (minutes)[2]	587	115	125	98
Head CT Results Within 45 Min. of Arrival	30	70%	55%	57%
Patients Who Left ER Before Being Seen	70,349	3%	3%	2%
Time from ER Arrival to Admit. (minutes)[2]	606	320	323	274
Time from ER Arrival to Discharge (minutes)	385	220	168	134
Time in ER Before Being Evaluated (minutes)	421	14	29	26
Time to Pain Meds for Fractures (minutes)	166	62	62	57
Heart Attack Care				
Aspirin Given at Discharge[2]	252	100%	99%	99%
Fibrinolytic Meds Within 30 Min. of Arrival[1,2]	-	-	73%	54%
PCI Within 90 Minutes of Arrival[2]	18	100%	95%	96%
Statin Prescribed at Discharge[2]	259	99%	98%	98%
Heart Failure Care				
ACE Inhibitor or ARB for LVSD[2]	84	95%	97%	97%
Discharge Instructions Given[2]	247	99%	94%	94%
Evaluation of LVS Function[2]	305	100%	99%	99%
Medicare Spending				
Medicare Spending per Patient (ratio)	-	1.01	0.98	0.98
Pneumonia Care				
Appropriate Initial Antibiotic Given[2]	79	99%	97%	95%
Blood Culture Timing[2]	169	98%	98%	98%
Pregnancy and Delivery Care				
Newborn Deliveries Scheduled Early[2]	101	0%	5%	6%
Preventive Care				
Immunization for Influenza[2]	661	97%	89%	90%
Immunization for Pneumonia[2]	725	97%	90%	92%
Stroke Care				
Anticoagulation Therapy for Atrial Fibrillation[2]	28	100%	95%	95%
Antithrombotic Therapy Timing[2]	140	99%	98%	98%
Assessed for Rehabilitation[2]	197	99%	97%	97%
Discharged on Antithrombotic Therapy[2]	164	98%	99%	99%
Discharged on Statin Medication[2]	130	98%	94%	94%
Thrombolytic Therapy Timing[2]	17	100%	72%	66%
Venous Thromboembolism Prophylaxis[2]	190	94%	94%	94%
Written Stroke Educational Materials Given[2]	103	97%	87%	88%
Surgical Care Improvement Project				
Appropriate Beta Blocker Usage[2]	134	98%	97%	98%
Appropriate VTP Within 24 Hours[2]	362	99%	98%	98%
Controlled Postoperative Blood Glucose[2]	109	96%	96%	97%
Perioperative Temperature Management[2]	408	100%	100%	100%
Prophylactic Antibiotic Selection[2]	356	98%	99%	99%

NOTE: Hospital profiles are in alphabetical order by state, then city, then hospital within the city; Rankings exclude hospitals with less than 25 cases except for patient surveys which excludes hospitals with less than 100 cases; (a) 100-299 cases; (1) The number of cases/patients is too few to report; (2) Data submitted were based on a sample of cases/patients; (3) Results are based on a shorter time period than required; (4) Data suppressed by CMS for one or more quarters; (5) Results are not available for this reporting period; (6) Fewer than 100 patients completed the HCAHPS survey; (7) No cases met the criteria for this measure; (8) The lower limit of the confidence interval cannot be calculated if the number of observed infections equals zero; (9) No data are available from the state/territory for this reporting period; (10) The scores shown reflect fewer than 50 completed surveys; (11) There were discrepancies in the data collection process; (12) This measure does not apply to this hospital for this reporting period; (13) Results cannot be calculated for this reporting period; (14) The results for this state are combined with nearby states to protect confidentiality; Please refer to the User's Guide for a full explanation of data.

Measure	Cases	This Hosp.	State Avg.	U.S. Avg.
Prophylactic Antibiotic Selection (Outpatient)	234	98%	97%	98%
Prophylactic Antibiotic Stopped[2]	339	98%	98%	98%
Prophylactic Antibiotic Timing[2]	357	100%	99%	99%
Prophylactic Antibiotic Timing (Outpatient)	241	95%	97%	98%
Urinary Catheter Removal[2]	327	98%	97%	97%
Survey of Patients' Hospital Experiences				
Area Around Room 'Always' Quiet at Night	300+	58%	51%	61%
Doctors 'Always' Communicated Well	300+	80%	78%	82%
Home Recovery Information Given	300+	83%	83%	85%
Hospital Given 9 or 10 on 10 Point Scale	300+	81%	68%	71%
Meds 'Always' Explained Before Given	300+	63%	61%	64%
Nurses 'Always' Communicated Well	300+	78%	74%	79%
Pain 'Always' Well Controlled	300+	74%	68%	71%
Room and Bathroom 'Always' Clean	300+	73%	70%	73%
Timely Help 'Always' Received	300+	63%	62%	68%
Would Definitely Recommend Hospital	300+	82%	70%	71%
Use of Medical Imaging				
Cardiac Imaging Stress Test before Surgery	386	4.4%	5.2%	5.3%
Combination Abdominal CT Scan	880	36.9%	13.4%	10.5%
Combination Brain/Sinus CT Scan	794	0.9%	2.2%	2.7%
Combination Chest CT Scan	623	1.1%	2.3%	2.7%
Follow-up Mammogram/Ultrasound	1,576	10.7%	8.2%	8.8%
Lumbar Spine MRI for Low Back Pain	155	37.4%	34.2%	37.2%

Whittier Hospital Medical Center

9080 Colima Rd — Phone: 562-945-3561
Whittier, CA 90605 — Fax: 562-693-6811
URL: www.whittierhospital.com
Type: Acute Care Hospitals — Emergency Services: Yes
Ownership: Proprietary — Beds: 181

Key Personnel:
Intensive Care Unit. . . . . Sandra Alderman
Quality Assurance . . . . Sharon Alex
Pediatric In-Patient Care . . . . Nanette Buenavidez
CEO . . . . Richard Castro
Pediatric Ambulatory Care . . . . . . Dinesh Ghiya, MD
Infection Control. . . . . Kym Lengyel
Cardiac Laboratory. . . . . Ernie Matsuo
Operating Room. . . . . Lunice Siiter

Measure	Cases	This Hosp.	State Avg.	U.S. Avg.
Blood Clot Prevention and Treatment				
Anticoagulation Overlap Therapy[2]	19	100%	92%	93%
ICU Venous Thromboembolism Prophylaxis[2]	99	94%	92%	92%
Incidence of Potentially Preventable VTE[1,2]	-	-	11%	10%
UFH with Dosages/Platelet Monitoring[1,2]	-	-	96%	97%
Venous Thromboembolism Prophylaxis[2]	321	96%	83%	85%
Warfarin Therapy Discharge Instructions[2]	12	92%	75%	75%
Chest Pain/Possible Heart Attack Care				
Aspirin Given Within 24 Hours of Arrival	36	100%	97%	96%
Fibrinolytic Meds Within 30 Min. of Arrival[3,7]	-	-	62%	58%
Average Time to ECG (minutes)	33	10	9	7
Average Time to Transfer (minutes)[1,3]	-	-	62	60
Children's Asthma Care				
Received Home Management Plan of Care	-	-	88%	88%
Received Reliever Medication	-	-	100%	100%
Received Systemic Corticosteroids	-	-	100%	100%
Emergency Department				
Admittance Decision Time (minutes)[2]	372	84	125	98
Head CT Results Within 45 Min. of Arrival[1]	-	-	55%	57%
Patients Who Left ER Before Being Seen	26,843	1%	3%	2%
Time from ER Arrival to Admit. (minutes)[2]	386	295	323	274
Time from ER Arrival to Discharge (minutes)	342	171	168	134
Time in ER Before Being Evaluated (minutes)	367	21	29	26
Time to Pain Meds for Fractures (minutes)	136	62	62	57
Heart Attack Care				
Aspirin Given at Discharge	23	96%	99%	99%
Fibrinolytic Meds Within 30 Min. of Arrival[7]	-	-	73%	54%
PCI Within 90 Minutes of Arrival[7]	-	-	95%	96%
Statin Prescribed at Discharge	25	96%	98%	98%
Heart Failure Care				
ACE Inhibitor or ARB for LVSD	58	100%	97%	97%
Discharge Instructions Given	141	99%	94%	94%
Evaluation of LVS Function	187	100%	99%	99%
Medicare Spending				
Medicare Spending per Patient (ratio)	-	1.30	0.98	0.98
Pneumonia Care				
Appropriate Initial Antibiotic Given	92	98%	97%	95%
Blood Culture Timing	204	98%	98%	98%
Pregnancy and Delivery Care				
Newborn Deliveries Scheduled Early[2]	33	0%	5%	6%
Preventive Care				
Immunization for Influenza[2]	448	94%	89%	90%
Immunization for Pneumonia[2]	376	97%	90%	92%
Stroke Care				
Anticoagulation Therapy for Atrial Fibrillation[1]	-	-	95%	95%
Antithrombotic Therapy Timing	34	97%	98%	98%
Assessed for Rehabilitation	42	95%	97%	97%
Discharged on Antithrombotic Therapy	33	100%	99%	99%
Discharged on Statin Medication	31	97%	94%	94%
Thrombolytic Therapy Timing[1]	-	-	72%	66%
Venous Thromboembolism Prophylaxis	44	95%	94%	94%
Written Stroke Educational Materials Given	29	90%	87%	88%
Surgical Care Improvement Project				
Appropriate Beta Blocker Usage	40	88%	97%	98%
Appropriate VTP Within 24 Hours	179	98%	98%	98%
Controlled Postoperative Blood Glucose[7]	-	-	96%	97%
Perioperative Temperature Management	197	100%	100%	100%
Prophylactic Antibiotic Selection	103	96%	99%	99%
Prophylactic Antibiotic Selection (Outpatient)	42	95%	97%	98%
Prophylactic Antibiotic Stopped	100	92%	98%	98%
Prophylactic Antibiotic Timing	103	99%	99%	99%
Prophylactic Antibiotic Timing (Outpatient)	43	93%	97%	98%
Urinary Catheter Removal	59	98%	97%	97%
Survey of Patients' Hospital Experiences				
Area Around Room 'Always' Quiet at Night	300+	46%	51%	61%
Doctors 'Always' Communicated Well	300+	74%	78%	82%
Home Recovery Information Given	300+	81%	83%	85%
Hospital Given 9 or 10 on 10 Point Scale	300+	59%	68%	71%
Meds 'Always' Explained Before Given	300+	59%	61%	64%
Nurses 'Always' Communicated Well	300+	70%	74%	79%
Pain 'Always' Well Controlled	300+	67%	68%	71%
Room and Bathroom 'Always' Clean	300+	75%	70%	73%
Timely Help 'Always' Received	300+	58%	62%	68%
Would Definitely Recommend Hospital	300+	58%	70%	71%
Use of Medical Imaging				
Cardiac Imaging Stress Test before Surgery[1]	-	-	5.2%	5.3%
Combination Abdominal CT Scan	159	18.9%	13.4%	10.5%
Combination Brain/Sinus CT Scan[1]	-	-	2.2%	2.7%
Combination Chest CT Scan	52	3.8%	2.3%	2.7%
Follow-up Mammogram/Ultrasound	130	4.6%	8.2%	8.8%
Lumbar Spine MRI for Low Back Pain[1]	-	-	34.2%	37.2%

Frank R Howard Memorial Hospital

1 Madrone Street — Phone: 707-459-6801
Willits, CA 95490 — Fax: 707-459-9486
URL: www.howardhospital.com
Type: Critical Access Hospitals — Emergency Services: Yes
Ownership: Voluntary non-profit - Church — Beds: 38

Key Personnel:
Operating Room. . . . . Tedd Dawson
Emergency Room . . . . Marilyn Depew
CEO/President. . . . . Kevin Erich
Chief of Medical Staff. . . . . Carla Longthamp
Quality Assurance . . . . Diane Moratti

Measure	Cases	This Hosp.	State Avg.	U.S. Avg.
Blood Clot Prevention and Treatment				
Anticoagulation Overlap Therapy[1,2]	-	-	92%	93%
ICU Venous Thromboembolism Prophylaxis[2]	28	79%	92%	92%
Incidence of Potentially Preventable VTE[1,2]	-	-	11%	10%
UFH with Dosages/Platelet Monitoring[2,7]	-	-	96%	97%
Venous Thromboembolism Prophylaxis[2]	94	80%	83%	85%
Warfarin Therapy Discharge Instructions[1,2]	-	-	75%	75%
Chest Pain/Possible Heart Attack Care				
Aspirin Given Within 24 Hours of Arrival	-	-	97%	96%
Fibrinolytic Meds Within 30 Min. of Arrival	-	-	62%	58%
Average Time to ECG (minutes)	-	-	9	7
Average Time to Transfer (minutes)	-	-	62	60
Children's Asthma Care				
Received Home Management Plan of Care	-	-	88%	88%
Received Reliever Medication	-	-	100%	100%
Received Systemic Corticosteroids	-	-	100%	100%
Emergency Department				
Admittance Decision Time (minutes)[5]	-	-	125	98
Head CT Results Within 45 Min. of Arrival	-	-	55%	57%
Patients Who Left ER Before Being Seen	-	-	3%	2%
Time from ER Arrival to Admit. (minutes)[5]	-	-	323	274
Time from ER Arrival to Discharge (minutes)	-	-	168	134
Time in ER Before Being Evaluated (minutes)	-	-	29	26
Time to Pain Meds for Fractures (minutes)	-	-	62	57
Heart Attack Care				
Aspirin Given at Discharge[3,7]	-	-	99%	99%
Fibrinolytic Meds Within 30 Min. of Arrival[3,7]	-	-	73%	54%
PCI Within 90 Minutes of Arrival[3,7]	-	-	95%	96%
Statin Prescribed at Discharge[3,7]	-	-	98%	98%
Heart Failure Care				
ACE Inhibitor or ARB for LVSD	14	93%	97%	97%
Discharge Instructions Given	35	94%	94%	94%
Evaluation of LVS Function	39	100%	99%	99%
Medicare Spending				
Medicare Spending per Patient (ratio)	-	-	0.98	0.98
Pneumonia Care				
Appropriate Initial Antibiotic Given	16	94%	97%	95%
Blood Culture Timing	29	100%	98%	98%
Pregnancy and Delivery Care				
Newborn Deliveries Scheduled Early[5]	-	-	5%	6%
Preventive Care				
Immunization for Influenza[5]	-	-	89%	90%
Immunization for Pneumonia[5]	-	-	90%	92%
Stroke Care				
Anticoagulation Therapy for Atrial Fibrillation[1]	-	-	95%	95%
Antithrombotic Therapy Timing[1]	-	-	98%	98%
Assessed for Rehabilitation	17	88%	97%	97%
Discharged on Antithrombotic Therapy	15	93%	99%	99%
Discharged on Statin Medication	16	88%	94%	94%
Thrombolytic Therapy Timing[1]	-	-	72%	66%
Venous Thromboembolism Prophylaxis	12	50%	94%	94%
Written Stroke Educational Materials Given[1]	-	-	87%	88%
Surgical Care Improvement Project				
Appropriate Beta Blocker Usage	45	100%	97%	98%
Appropriate VTP Within 24 Hours	246	96%	98%	98%
Controlled Postoperative Blood Glucose[7]	-	-	96%	97%
Perioperative Temperature Management	266	100%	100%	100%
Prophylactic Antibiotic Selection	211	99%	99%	99%
Prophylactic Antibiotic Selection (Outpatient)	-	-	97%	98%
Prophylactic Antibiotic Stopped	208	98%	98%	98%
Prophylactic Antibiotic Timing	211	99%	99%	99%
Prophylactic Antibiotic Timing (Outpatient)	-	-	97%	98%
Urinary Catheter Removal	36	94%	97%	97%
Survey of Patients' Hospital Experiences				
Area Around Room 'Always' Quiet at Night	300+	41%	51%	61%
Doctors 'Always' Communicated Well	300+	85%	78%	82%
Home Recovery Information Given	300+	89%	83%	85%
Hospital Given 9 or 10 on 10 Point Scale	300+	78%	68%	71%
Meds 'Always' Explained Before Given	300+	69%	61%	64%
Nurses 'Always' Communicated Well	300+	83%	74%	79%
Pain 'Always' Well Controlled	300+	73%	68%	71%
Room and Bathroom 'Always' Clean	300+	81%	70%	73%
Timely Help 'Always' Received	300+	74%	62%	68%
Would Definitely Recommend Hospital	300+	80%	70%	71%
Use of Medical Imaging				
Cardiac Imaging Stress Test before Surgery	-	-	5.2%	5.3%
Combination Abdominal CT Scan	-	-	13.4%	10.5%
Combination Brain/Sinus CT Scan	-	-	2.2%	2.7%
Combination Chest CT Scan	-	-	2.3%	2.7%
Follow-up Mammogram/Ultrasound	-	-	8.2%	8.8%
Lumbar Spine MRI for Low Back Pain	-	-	34.2%	37.2%

NOTE: Hospital profiles are in alphabetical order by state, then city, then hospital within the city; Rankings exclude hospitals with less than 25 cases except for patient surveys which excludes hospitals with less than 100 cases; (a) 100-299 cases; (1) The number of cases/patients is too few to report; (2) Data submitted were based on a sample of cases/patients; (3) Results are based on a shorter time period than required; (4) Data suppressed by CMS for one or more quarters; (5) Results are not available for this reporting period; (6) Fewer than 100 patients completed the HCAHPS survey; (7) No cases met the criteria for this measure; (8) The lower limit of the confidence interval cannot be calculated if the number of observed infections equals zero; (9) No data are available from the state/territory for this reporting period; (10) The scores shown reflect fewer than 50 completed surveys; (11) There were discrepancies in the data collection process; (12) This measure does not apply to this hospital for this reporting period; (13) Results cannot be calculated for this reporting period; (14) The results for this state are combined with nearby states to protect confidentiality; Please refer to the User's Guide for a full explanation of data.

Glenn Medical Center

1133 W Sycamore St Phone: 530-934-1818
Willows, CA 95988
URL: www.glennmed.org
Type: Critical Access Hospitals Emergency Services: Yes
Ownership: Voluntary non-profit - Private
Key Personnel:
Pediatrics. . . . . Irmeen Ashraf, FAAP
Radiology. . . . . Dawna Keolanui
CEO/President. . . . . Woody Laughnan Jr
Cardiology . . . . Peter J. Wolk, M.D.

Measure	Cases	This Hosp.	State Avg.	U.S. Avg.
Blood Clot Prevention and Treatment				
Anticoagulation Overlap Therapy[5]	-	-	92%	93%
ICU Venous Thromboembolism Prophylaxis[5]	-	-	92%	92%
Incidence of Potentially Preventable VTE[5]	-	-	11%	10%
UFH with Dosages/Platelet Monitoring[5]	-	-	96%	97%
Venous Thromboembolism Prophylaxis[5]	-	-	83%	85%
Warfarin Therapy Discharge Instructions[5]	-	-	75%	75%
Chest Pain/Possible Heart Attack Care				
Aspirin Given Within 24 Hours of Arrival	-	-	97%	96%
Fibrinolytic Meds Within 30 Min. of Arrival	-	-	62%	58%
Average Time to ECG (minutes)	-	-	9	7
Average Time to Transfer (minutes)	-	-	62	60
Children's Asthma Care				
Received Home Management Plan of Care	-	-	88%	88%
Received Reliever Medication	-	-	100%	100%
Received Systemic Corticosteroids	-	-	100%	100%
Emergency Department				
Admittance Decision Time (minutes)[5]	-	-	125	98
Head CT Results Within 45 Min. of Arrival	-	-	55%	57%
Patients Who Left ER Before Being Seen	-	-	3%	2%
Time from ER Arrival to Admit. (minutes)[5]	-	-	323	274
Time from ER Arrival to Discharge (minutes)	-	-	168	134
Time in ER Before Being Evaluated (minutes)	-	-	29	26
Time to Pain Meds for Fractures (minutes)	-	-	62	57
Heart Attack Care				
Aspirin Given at Discharge[5]	-	-	99%	99%
Fibrinolytic Meds Within 30 Min. of Arrival[5]	-	-	73%	54%
PCI Within 90 Minutes of Arrival[5]	-	-	95%	96%
Statin Prescribed at Discharge[5]	-	-	98%	98%
Heart Failure Care				
ACE Inhibitor or ARB for LVSD[1,3]	-	-	97%	97%
Discharge Instructions Given[1,3]	-	-	94%	94%
Evaluation of LVS Function[1,3]	-	-	99%	99%
Medicare Spending				
Medicare Spending per Patient (ratio)	-	-	0.98	0.98
Pneumonia Care				
Appropriate Initial Antibiotic Given[1,2]	-	-	97%	95%
Blood Culture Timing[2]	23	100%	98%	98%
Pregnancy and Delivery Care				
Newborn Deliveries Scheduled Early[5]	-	-	5%	6%
Preventive Care				
Immunization for Influenza[5]	-	-	89%	90%
Immunization for Pneumonia[5]	-	-	90%	92%
Stroke Care				
Anticoagulation Therapy for Atrial Fibrillation[5]	-	-	95%	95%
Antithrombotic Therapy Timing[5]	-	-	98%	98%
Assessed for Rehabilitation[5]	-	-	97%	97%
Discharged on Antithrombotic Therapy[5]	-	-	99%	99%
Discharged on Statin Medication[5]	-	-	94%	94%
Thrombolytic Therapy Timing[5]	-	-	72%	66%
Venous Thromboembolism Prophylaxis[5]	-	-	94%	94%
Written Stroke Educational Materials Given[5]	-	-	87%	88%
Surgical Care Improvement Project				
Appropriate Beta Blocker Usage[5]	-	-	97%	98%
Appropriate VTP Within 24 Hours[5]	-	-	98%	98%
Controlled Postoperative Blood Glucose[5]	-	-	96%	97%
Perioperative Temperature Management[5]	-	-	100%	100%
Prophylactic Antibiotic Selection[5]	-	-	99%	99%
Prophylactic Antibiotic Selection (Outpatient)	-	-	97%	98%
Prophylactic Antibiotic Stopped[5]	-	-	98%	98%
Prophylactic Antibiotic Timing[5]	-	-	99%	99%
Prophylactic Antibiotic Timing (Outpatient)	-	-	97%	98%
Urinary Catheter Removal[5]	-	-	97%	97%
Survey of Patients' Hospital Experiences				
Area Around Room 'Always' Quiet at Night[5]	-	-	51%	61%
Doctors 'Always' Communicated Well[5]	-	-	78%	82%
Home Recovery Information Given[5]	-	-	83%	85%
Hospital Given 9 or 10 on 10 Point Scale[5]	-	-	68%	71%
Meds 'Always' Explained Before Given[5]	-	-	61%	64%
Nurses 'Always' Communicated Well[5]	-	-	74%	79%
Pain 'Always' Well Controlled[5]	-	-	68%	71%
Room and Bathroom 'Always' Clean[5]	-	-	70%	73%
Timely Help 'Always' Received[5]	-	-	62%	68%
Would Definitely Recommend Hospital[5]	-	-	70%	71%
Use of Medical Imaging				
Cardiac Imaging Stress Test before Surgery	-	-	5.2%	5.3%
Combination Abdominal CT Scan	-	-	13.4%	10.5%
Combination Brain/Sinus CT Scan	-	-	2.2%	2.7%
Combination Chest CT Scan	-	-	2.3%	2.7%
Follow-up Mammogram/Ultrasound	-	-	8.2%	8.8%
Lumbar Spine MRI for Low Back Pain	-	-	34.2%	37.2%

Woodland Memorial Hospital

1325 Cottonwood Street Phone: 530-662-3961
Woodland, CA 95695 Fax: 530-666-7948
URL: www.woodlandhealthcare.org
Type: Acute Care Hospitals Emergency Services: Yes
Ownership: Voluntary non-profit - Other Beds: 103
Key Personnel:
Pediatric Ambulatory Care . . . . . . Tom March, MD
Pediatric In-Patient Care . . . . Tom March, MD
Chief of Medical Staff. . . . . Liana Turkot, MD
CEO/President. . . . . Kevin Vaziri
Radiology. . . . . Virgil Williams, MD

Measure	Cases	This Hosp.	State Avg.	U.S. Avg.
Blood Clot Prevention and Treatment				
Anticoagulation Overlap Therapy[2]	22	100%	92%	93%
ICU Venous Thromboembolism Prophylaxis[2]	71	100%	92%	92%
Incidence of Potentially Preventable VTE[2,7]	-	-	11%	10%
UFH with Dosages/Platelet Monitoring[1,2]	-	-	96%	97%
Venous Thromboembolism Prophylaxis[2]	144	100%	83%	85%
Warfarin Therapy Discharge Instructions[2]	17	100%	75%	75%
Chest Pain/Possible Heart Attack Care				
Aspirin Given Within 24 Hours of Arrival	47	100%	97%	96%
Fibrinolytic Meds Within 30 Min. of Arrival	13	85%	62%	58%
Average Time to ECG (minutes)	48	12	9	7
Average Time to Transfer (minutes)[7]	-	-	62	60
Children's Asthma Care				
Received Home Management Plan of Care	-	-	88%	88%
Received Reliever Medication	-	-	100%	100%
Received Systemic Corticosteroids	-	-	100%	100%
Emergency Department				
Admittance Decision Time (minutes)[2]	345	71	125	98
Head CT Results Within 45 Min. of Arrival	21	71%	55%	57%
Patients Who Left ER Before Being Seen	21,134	1%	3%	2%
Time from ER Arrival to Admit. (minutes)[2]	345	290	323	274
Time from ER Arrival to Discharge (minutes)	401	117	168	134
Time in ER Before Being Evaluated (minutes)	409	19	29	26
Time to Pain Meds for Fractures (minutes)	114	50	62	57
Heart Attack Care				
Aspirin Given at Discharge	12	100%	99%	99%
Fibrinolytic Meds Within 30 Min. of Arrival[7]	-	-	73%	54%
PCI Within 90 Minutes of Arrival[7]	-	-	95%	96%
Statin Prescribed at Discharge[1]	-	-	98%	98%
Heart Failure Care				
ACE Inhibitor or ARB for LVSD	17	100%	97%	97%
Discharge Instructions Given	36	100%	94%	94%
Evaluation of LVS Function	50	100%	99%	99%
Medicare Spending				
Medicare Spending per Patient (ratio)	-	0.93	0.98	0.98
Pneumonia Care				
Appropriate Initial Antibiotic Given[2]	57	95%	97%	95%
Blood Culture Timing[2]	114	100%	98%	98%
Pregnancy and Delivery Care				
Newborn Deliveries Scheduled Early[2]	22	5%	5%	6%
Preventive Care				
Immunization for Influenza[2]	323	96%	89%	90%
Immunization for Pneumonia[2]	301	96%	90%	92%
Stroke Care				
Anticoagulation Therapy for Atrial Fibrillation[1]	-	-	95%	95%
Antithrombotic Therapy Timing	19	100%	98%	98%
Assessed for Rehabilitation	32	94%	97%	97%
Discharged on Antithrombotic Therapy	29	100%	99%	99%
Discharged on Statin Medication	17	88%	94%	94%
Thrombolytic Therapy Timing[1]	-	-	72%	66%
Venous Thromboembolism Prophylaxis	21	100%	94%	94%
Written Stroke Educational Materials Given	21	100%	87%	88%
Surgical Care Improvement Project				
Appropriate Beta Blocker Usage[2]	54	100%	97%	98%
Appropriate VTP Within 24 Hours[2]	219	100%	98%	98%
Controlled Postoperative Blood Glucose[2,7]	-	-	96%	97%
Perioperative Temperature Management[2]	257	100%	100%	100%
Prophylactic Antibiotic Selection[2]	178	97%	99%	99%
Prophylactic Antibiotic Selection (Outpatient)	67	100%	97%	98%
Prophylactic Antibiotic Stopped[2]	177	100%	98%	98%
Prophylactic Antibiotic Timing[2]	178	100%	99%	99%
Prophylactic Antibiotic Timing (Outpatient)	72	93%	97%	98%
Urinary Catheter Removal[2]	128	100%	97%	97%
Survey of Patients' Hospital Experiences				
Area Around Room 'Always' Quiet at Night	(a)	49%	51%	61%
Doctors 'Always' Communicated Well	(a)	82%	78%	82%
Home Recovery Information Given	(a)	86%	83%	85%
Hospital Given 9 or 10 on 10 Point Scale	(a)	69%	68%	71%
Meds 'Always' Explained Before Given	(a)	68%	61%	64%
Nurses 'Always' Communicated Well	(a)	76%	74%	79%
Pain 'Always' Well Controlled	(a)	74%	68%	71%
Room and Bathroom 'Always' Clean	(a)	73%	70%	73%
Timely Help 'Always' Received	(a)	65%	62%	68%
Would Definitely Recommend Hospital	(a)	75%	70%	71%
Use of Medical Imaging				
Cardiac Imaging Stress Test before Surgery	63	6.3%	5.2%	5.3%
Combination Abdominal CT Scan	272	6.3%	13.4%	10.5%
Combination Brain/Sinus CT Scan[1]	-	-	2.2%	2.7%
Combination Chest CT Scan	158	0.0%	2.3%	2.7%
Follow-up Mammogram/Ultrasound[7]	-	-	8.2%	8.8%
Lumbar Spine MRI for Low Back Pain[1]	-	-	34.2%	37.2%

Kaiser Foundation Hospital - Woodland Hills

5601 De Soto Phone: 818-719-3800
Woodland Hills, CA 91367
Type: Acute Care Hospitals Emergency Services: Yes
Ownership: Voluntary non-profit - Private Beds: 218
Key Personnel:
President. . . . . Richard Tofel

Measure	Cases	This Hosp.	State Avg.	U.S. Avg.
Blood Clot Prevention and Treatment				
Anticoagulation Overlap Therapy[2]	72	94%	92%	93%
ICU Venous Thromboembolism Prophylaxis[2]	36	97%	92%	92%
Incidence of Potentially Preventable VTE[2]	11	0%	11%	10%
UFH with Dosages/Platelet Monitoring[2]	21	100%	96%	97%
Venous Thromboembolism Prophylaxis[2]	309	95%	83%	85%
Warfarin Therapy Discharge Instructions[2]	65	95%	75%	75%
Chest Pain/Possible Heart Attack Care				
Aspirin Given Within 24 Hours of Arrival	-	-	97%	96%
Fibrinolytic Meds Within 30 Min. of Arrival	-	-	62%	58%
Average Time to ECG (minutes)	-	-	9	7
Average Time to Transfer (minutes)	-	-	62	60
Children's Asthma Care				
Received Home Management Plan of Care	-	-	88%	88%
Received Reliever Medication	-	-	100%	100%
Received Systemic Corticosteroids	-	-	100%	100%
Emergency Department				
Admittance Decision Time (minutes)[2]	369	87	125	98
Head CT Results Within 45 Min. of Arrival	-	-	55%	57%
Patients Who Left ER Before Being Seen	-	-	3%	2%
Time from ER Arrival to Admit. (minutes)[2]	374	336	323	274
Time from ER Arrival to Discharge (minutes)	-	-	168	134

NOTE: Hospital profiles are in alphabetical order by state, then city, then hospital within the city; Rankings exclude hospitals with less than 25 cases except for patient surveys which excludes hospitals with less than 100 cases; (a) 100-299 cases; (1) The number of cases/patients is too few to report; (2) Data submitted were based on a sample of cases/patients; (3) Results are based on a shorter time period than required; (4) Data suppressed by CMS for one or more quarters; (5) Results are not available for this reporting period; (6) Fewer than 100 patients completed the HCAHPS survey; (7) No cases met the criteria for this measure; (8) The lower limit of the confidence interval cannot be calculated if the number of observed infections equals zero; (9) No data are available from the state/territory for this reporting period; (10) The scores shown reflect fewer than 50 completed surveys; (11) There were discrepancies in the data collection process; (12) This measure does not apply to this hospital for this reporting period; (13) Results cannot be calculated for this reporting period; (14) The results for this state are combined with nearby states to protect confidentiality; Please refer to the User's Guide for a full explanation of data.

Measure	Cases	This Hosp.	State Avg.	U.S. Avg.
Time in ER Before Being Evaluated (minutes)	-	-	29	26
Time to Pain Meds for Fractures (minutes)	-	-	62	57
Heart Attack Care				
Aspirin Given at Discharge	93	100%	99%	99%
Fibrinolytic Meds Within 30 Min. of Arrival[1]	-	-	73%	54%
PCI Within 90 Minutes of Arrival[7]	-	-	95%	96%
Statin Prescribed at Discharge	93	100%	98%	98%
Heart Failure Care				
ACE Inhibitor or ARB for LVSD	42	100%	97%	97%
Discharge Instructions Given	247	98%	94%	94%
Evaluation of LVS Function	264	100%	99%	99%
Medicare Spending				
Medicare Spending per Patient (ratio)	-	0.82	0.98	0.98
Pneumonia Care				
Appropriate Initial Antibiotic Given[2]	80	99%	97%	95%
Blood Culture Timing[2]	128	98%	98%	98%
Pregnancy and Delivery Care				
Newborn Deliveries Scheduled Early[2]	143	1%	5%	6%
Preventive Care				
Immunization for Influenza[2]	514	96%	89%	90%
Immunization for Pneumonia[2]	639	98%	90%	92%
Stroke Care				
Anticoagulation Therapy for Atrial Fibrillation[2]	18	100%	95%	95%
Antithrombotic Therapy Timing[2]	73	99%	98%	98%
Assessed for Rehabilitation[2]	90	100%	97%	97%
Discharged on Antithrombotic Therapy[2]	85	100%	99%	99%
Discharged on Statin Medication[2]	74	97%	94%	94%
Thrombolytic Therapy Timing[1,2]	-	-	72%	66%
Venous Thromboembolism Prophylaxis[2]	83	100%	94%	94%
Written Stroke Educational Materials Given[2]	66	100%	87%	88%
Surgical Care Improvement Project				
Appropriate Beta Blocker Usage[2]	117	99%	97%	98%
Appropriate VTP Within 24 Hours[2]	318	100%	98%	98%
Controlled Postoperative Blood Glucose[2,7]	-	-	96%	97%
Perioperative Temperature Management[2]	443	100%	100%	100%
Prophylactic Antibiotic Selection[2]	290	100%	99%	99%
Prophylactic Antibiotic Selection (Outpatient)	-	-	97%	98%
Prophylactic Antibiotic Stopped[2]	283	100%	98%	98%
Prophylactic Antibiotic Timing[2]	290	99%	99%	99%
Prophylactic Antibiotic Timing (Outpatient)	-	-	97%	98%
Urinary Catheter Removal[2]	255	100%	97%	97%
Survey of Patients' Hospital Experiences				
Area Around Room 'Always' Quiet at Night	300+	51%	51%	61%
Doctors 'Always' Communicated Well	300+	82%	78%	82%
Home Recovery Information Given	300+	85%	83%	85%
Hospital Given 9 or 10 on 10 Point Scale	300+	79%	68%	71%
Meds 'Always' Explained Before Given	300+	65%	61%	64%
Nurses 'Always' Communicated Well	300+	79%	74%	79%
Pain 'Always' Well Controlled	300+	74%	68%	71%
Room and Bathroom 'Always' Clean	300+	76%	70%	73%
Timely Help 'Always' Received	300+	71%	62%	68%
Would Definitely Recommend Hospital	300+	79%	70%	71%
Use of Medical Imaging				
Cardiac Imaging Stress Test before Surgery	-	-	5.2%	5.3%
Combination Abdominal CT Scan	-	-	13.4%	10.5%
Combination Brain/Sinus CT Scan	-	-	2.2%	2.7%
Combination Chest CT Scan	-	-	2.3%	2.7%
Follow-up Mammogram/Ultrasound	-	-	8.2%	8.8%
Lumbar Spine MRI for Low Back Pain	-	-	34.2%	37.2%

Motion Picture & Television Hospital

23388 Mulholland Drive
Woodland Hills, CA 91364
URL: www.mptvfund.org
Phone: 818-876-1888
Fax: 818-876-1079
Type: Acute Care Hospitals
Ownership: Voluntary non-profit - Other
Emergency Services: No
Beds: 256

Key Personnel:
Operating Room. . . . . Sarah DeLaughter, RN
Chief of Medical Staff. . . . . Saeed Humaun
Quality Assurance . . . . Terry Sepulveda
Radiology. . . . . Bruce Shragg, MD
CEO/President. . . . . David Tillman, MD

Measure	Cases	This Hosp.	State Avg.	U.S. Avg.
Blood Clot Prevention and Treatment				
Anticoagulation Overlap Therapy[1]	-	-	92%	93%
ICU Venous Thromboembolism Prophylaxis[7]	-	-	92%	92%
Incidence of Potentially Preventable VTE[7]	-	-	11%	10%
UFH with Dosages/Platelet Monitoring[7]	-	-	96%	97%
Venous Thromboembolism Prophylaxis	33	12%	83%	85%
Warfarin Therapy Discharge Instructions[7]	-	-	75%	75%
Chest Pain/Possible Heart Attack Care				
Aspirin Given Within 24 Hours of Arrival[5]	-	-	97%	96%
Fibrinolytic Meds Within 30 Min. of Arrival[5]	-	-	62%	58%
Average Time to ECG (minutes)[5]	-	-	9	7
Average Time to Transfer (minutes)[5]	-	-	62	60
Children's Asthma Care				
Received Home Management Plan of Care	-	-	88%	88%
Received Reliever Medication	-	-	100%	100%
Received Systemic Corticosteroids	-	-	100%	100%
Emergency Department				
Admittance Decision Time (minutes)[7]	-	-	125	98
Head CT Results Within 45 Min. of Arrival[5]	-	-	55%	57%
Patients Who Left ER Before Being Seen[5]	-	-	3%	2%
Time from ER Arrival to Admit. (minutes)[7]	-	-	323	274
Time from ER Arrival to Discharge (minutes)[5]	-	-	168	134
Time in ER Before Being Evaluated (minutes)[5]	-	-	29	26
Time to Pain Meds for Fractures (minutes)[5]	-	-	62	57
Heart Attack Care				
Aspirin Given at Discharge[3,7]	-	-	99%	99%
Fibrinolytic Meds Within 30 Min. of Arrival[3,7]	-	-	73%	54%
PCI Within 90 Minutes of Arrival[3,7]	-	-	95%	96%
Statin Prescribed at Discharge[3,7]	-	-	98%	98%
Heart Failure Care				
ACE Inhibitor or ARB for LVSD[3,7]	-	-	97%	97%
Discharge Instructions Given[3,7]	-	-	94%	94%
Evaluation of LVS Function[3,7]	-	-	99%	99%
Medicare Spending				
Medicare Spending per Patient (ratio)	-	0.81	0.98	0.98
Pneumonia Care				
Appropriate Initial Antibiotic Given[1]	-	-	97%	95%
Blood Culture Timing[7]	-	-	98%	98%
Pregnancy and Delivery Care				
Newborn Deliveries Scheduled Early[7]	-	-	5%	6%
Preventive Care				
Immunization for Influenza	94	43%	89%	90%
Immunization for Pneumonia	116	54%	90%	92%
Stroke Care				
Anticoagulation Therapy for Atrial Fibrillation[5]	-	-	95%	95%
Antithrombotic Therapy Timing[5]	-	-	98%	98%
Assessed for Rehabilitation[5]	-	-	97%	97%
Discharged on Antithrombotic Therapy[5]	-	-	99%	99%
Discharged on Statin Medication[5]	-	-	94%	94%
Thrombolytic Therapy Timing[5]	-	-	72%	66%
Venous Thromboembolism Prophylaxis[5]	-	-	94%	94%
Written Stroke Educational Materials Given[5]	-	-	87%	88%
Surgical Care Improvement Project				
Appropriate Beta Blocker Usage[5]	-	-	97%	98%
Appropriate VTP Within 24 Hours[5]	-	-	98%	98%
Controlled Postoperative Blood Glucose[5]	-	-	96%	97%
Perioperative Temperature Management[5]	-	-	100%	100%
Prophylactic Antibiotic Selection[5]	-	-	99%	99%
Prophylactic Antibiotic Selection (Outpatient)[1,3]	-	-	97%	98%
Prophylactic Antibiotic Stopped[5]	-	-	98%	98%
Prophylactic Antibiotic Timing[5]	-	-	99%	99%
Prophylactic Antibiotic Timing (Outpatient)[1,3]	-	-	97%	98%
Urinary Catheter Removal[5]	-	-	97%	97%
Survey of Patients' Hospital Experiences				
Area Around Room 'Always' Quiet at Night[5]	-	-	51%	61%
Doctors 'Always' Communicated Well[5]	-	-	78%	82%
Home Recovery Information Given[5]	-	-	83%	85%
Hospital Given 9 or 10 on 10 Point Scale[5]	-	-	68%	71%
Meds 'Always' Explained Before Given[5]	-	-	61%	64%
Nurses 'Always' Communicated Well[5]	-	-	74%	79%
Pain 'Always' Well Controlled[5]	-	-	68%	71%
Room and Bathroom 'Always' Clean[5]	-	-	70%	73%
Timely Help 'Always' Received[5]	-	-	62%	68%
Would Definitely Recommend Hospital[5]	-	-	70%	71%
Use of Medical Imaging				
Cardiac Imaging Stress Test before Surgery[7]	-	-	5.2%	5.3%
Combination Abdominal CT Scan	81	22.2%	13.4%	10.5%
Combination Brain/Sinus CT Scan[1]	-	-	2.2%	2.7%
Combination Chest CT Scan[1]	-	-	2.3%	2.7%
Follow-up Mammogram/Ultrasound	627	6.7%	8.2%	8.8%
Lumbar Spine MRI for Low Back Pain[7]	-	-	34.2%	37.2%

Fairchild Medical Center

444 Bruce Street
Yreka, CA 96097
E-mail: inquiries@fairchildmed.org
URL: www.fairchildmed.org
Phone: 530-842-4121
Fax: 530-841-0913
Type: Critical Access Hospitals
Ownership: Voluntary non-profit - Other
Emergency Services: Yes
Beds: 25

Key Personnel:
CEO . . . . Jonathon Andrus
Chief of Medical Staff. . . . . Judi Rowland

Measure	Cases	This Hosp.	State Avg.	U.S. Avg.
Blood Clot Prevention and Treatment				
Anticoagulation Overlap Therapy[1,2]	-	-	92%	93%
ICU Venous Thromboembolism Prophylaxis[2]	117	96%	92%	92%
Incidence of Potentially Preventable VTE[1,2]	-	-	11%	10%
UFH with Dosages/Platelet Monitoring[1,2]	-	-	96%	97%
Venous Thromboembolism Prophylaxis[2]	502	91%	83%	85%
Warfarin Therapy Discharge Instructions[2]	11	100%	75%	75%
Chest Pain/Possible Heart Attack Care				
Aspirin Given Within 24 Hours of Arrival	-	-	97%	96%
Fibrinolytic Meds Within 30 Min. of Arrival	-	-	62%	58%
Average Time to ECG (minutes)	-	-	9	7
Average Time to Transfer (minutes)	-	-	62	60
Children's Asthma Care				
Received Home Management Plan of Care	-	-	88%	88%
Received Reliever Medication	-	-	100%	100%
Received Systemic Corticosteroids	-	-	100%	100%
Emergency Department				
Admittance Decision Time (minutes)[2,3]	216	60	125	98
Head CT Results Within 45 Min. of Arrival	-	-	55%	57%
Patients Who Left ER Before Being Seen	-	-	3%	2%
Time from ER Arrival to Admit. (minutes)[2,3]	260	221	323	274
Time from ER Arrival to Discharge (minutes)	-	-	168	134
Time in ER Before Being Evaluated (minutes)	-	-	29	26
Time to Pain Meds for Fractures (minutes)	-	-	62	57
Heart Attack Care				
Aspirin Given at Discharge[1]	-	-	99%	99%
Fibrinolytic Meds Within 30 Min. of Arrival[7]	-	-	73%	54%
PCI Within 90 Minutes of Arrival[7]	-	-	95%	96%
Statin Prescribed at Discharge[1]	-	-	98%	98%
Heart Failure Care				
ACE Inhibitor or ARB for LVSD	11	100%	97%	97%
Discharge Instructions Given	32	94%	94%	94%
Evaluation of LVS Function	27	93%	99%	99%
Medicare Spending				
Medicare Spending per Patient (ratio)	-	-	0.98	0.98
Pneumonia Care				
Appropriate Initial Antibiotic Given	69	96%	97%	95%
Blood Culture Timing	75	95%	98%	98%
Pregnancy and Delivery Care				
Newborn Deliveries Scheduled Early[1,3]	-	-	5%	6%
Preventive Care				
Immunization for Influenza[5]	-	-	89%	90%
Immunization for Pneumonia[2,3]	230	97%	90%	92%
Stroke Care				
Anticoagulation Therapy for Atrial Fibrillation[1]	-	-	95%	95%
Antithrombotic Therapy Timing	14	100%	98%	98%
Assessed for Rehabilitation	19	100%	97%	97%
Discharged on Antithrombotic Therapy	17	94%	99%	99%
Discharged on Statin Medication	13	77%	94%	94%
Thrombolytic Therapy Timing[7]	-	-	72%	66%
Venous Thromboembolism Prophylaxis	16	94%	94%	94%
Written Stroke Educational Materials Given	14	64%	87%	88%
Surgical Care Improvement Project				

NOTE: Hospital profiles are in alphabetical order by state, then city, then hospital within the city; Rankings exclude hospitals with less than 25 cases except for patient surveys which excludes hospitals with less than 100 cases; (a) 100-299 cases; (1) The number of cases/patients is too few to report; (2) Data submitted were based on a sample of cases/patients; (3) Results are based on a shorter time period than required; (4) Data suppressed by CMS for one or more quarters; (5) Results are not available for this reporting period; (6) Fewer than 100 patients completed the HCAHPS survey; (7) No cases met the criteria for this measure; (8) The lower limit of the confidence interval cannot be calculated if the number of observed infections equals zero; (9) No data are available from the state/territory for this reporting period; (10) The scores shown reflect fewer than 50 completed surveys; (11) There were discrepancies in the data collection process; (12) This measure does not apply to this hospital for this reporting period; (13) Results cannot be calculated for this reporting period; (14) The results for this state are combined with nearby states to protect confidentiality; Please refer to the User's Guide for a full explanation of data.

Measure	Cases	This Hosp.	State Avg.	U.S. Avg.
Appropriate Beta Blocker Usage	18	94%	97%	98%
Appropriate VTP Within 24 Hours	134	94%	98%	98%
Controlled Postoperative Blood Glucose[7]	-	-	96%	97%
Perioperative Temperature Management	164	100%	100%	100%
Prophylactic Antibiotic Selection	129	97%	99%	99%
Prophylactic Antibiotic Selection (Outpatient)	-	-	97%	98%
Prophylactic Antibiotic Stopped	129	100%	98%	98%
Prophylactic Antibiotic Timing	129	97%	99%	99%
Prophylactic Antibiotic Timing (Outpatient)	-	-	97%	98%
Urinary Catheter Removal	93	98%	97%	97%
Survey of Patients' Hospital Experiences				
Area Around Room 'Always' Quiet at Night	300+	53%	51%	61%
Doctors 'Always' Communicated Well	300+	77%	78%	82%
Home Recovery Information Given	300+	85%	83%	85%
Hospital Given 9 or 10 on 10 Point Scale	300+	58%	68%	71%
Meds 'Always' Explained Before Given	300+	63%	61%	64%
Nurses 'Always' Communicated Well	300+	74%	74%	79%
Pain 'Always' Well Controlled	300+	65%	68%	71%
Room and Bathroom 'Always' Clean	300+	75%	70%	73%
Timely Help 'Always' Received	300+	61%	62%	68%
Would Definitely Recommend Hospital	300+	58%	70%	71%
Use of Medical Imaging				
Cardiac Imaging Stress Test before Surgery	-	-	5.2%	5.3%
Combination Abdominal CT Scan	-	-	13.4%	10.5%
Combination Brain/Sinus CT Scan	-	-	2.2%	2.7%
Combination Chest CT Scan	-	-	2.3%	2.7%
Follow-up Mammogram/Ultrasound	-	-	8.2%	8.8%
Lumbar Spine MRI for Low Back Pain	-	-	34.2%	37.2%

Sutter Surgical Hospital - North Valley

455 Plumas Blvd
Yuba City, CA 95991
Phone: 530-749-5700
URL: www.suttersurgicalhospitalnorthvalley.org
Type: Acute Care Hospitals
Emergency Services: Yes
Ownership: Proprietary
Key Personnel:
CEO . . . . Toni Morris

Measure	Cases	This Hosp.	State Avg.	U.S. Avg.
Blood Clot Prevention and Treatment				
Anticoagulation Overlap Therapy[2,7]	-	-	92%	93%
ICU Venous Thromboembolism Prophylaxis[2,7]	-	-	92%	92%
Incidence of Potentially Preventable VTE[2,7]	-	-	11%	10%
UFH with Dosages/Platelet Monitoring[2,7]	-	-	96%	97%
Venous Thromboembolism Prophylaxis[2]	111	99%	83%	85%
Warfarin Therapy Discharge Instructions[2,7]	-	-	75%	75%
Chest Pain/Possible Heart Attack Care				
Aspirin Given Within 24 Hours of Arrival[5]	-	-	97%	96%
Fibrinolytic Meds Within 30 Min. of Arrival[5]	-	-	62%	58%
Average Time to ECG (minutes)[5]	-	-	9	7
Average Time to Transfer (minutes)[5]	-	-	62	60
Children's Asthma Care				
Received Home Management Plan of Care	-	-	88%	88%
Received Reliever Medication	-	-	100%	100%
Received Systemic Corticosteroids	-	-	100%	100%
Emergency Department				
Admittance Decision Time (minutes)[7]	-	-	125	98
Head CT Results Within 45 Min. of Arrival[5]	-	-	55%	57%
Patients Who Left ER Before Being Seen[5]	-	-	3%	2%
Time from ER Arrival to Admit. (minutes)[7]	-	-	323	274
Time from ER Arrival to Discharge (minutes)[5]	-	-	168	134
Time in ER Before Being Evaluated (minutes)[5]	-	-	29	26
Time to Pain Meds for Fractures (minutes)[5]	-	-	62	57
Heart Attack Care				
Aspirin Given at Discharge[5]	-	-	99%	99%
Fibrinolytic Meds Within 30 Min. of Arrival[5]	-	-	73%	54%
PCI Within 90 Minutes of Arrival[5]	-	-	95%	96%
Statin Prescribed at Discharge[5]	-	-	98%	98%
Heart Failure Care				
ACE Inhibitor or ARB for LVSD[5]	-	-	97%	97%
Discharge Instructions Given[5]	-	-	94%	94%
Evaluation of LVS Function[5]	-	-	99%	99%
Medicare Spending				
Medicare Spending per Patient (ratio)	-	0.92	0.98	0.98
Pneumonia Care				
Appropriate Initial Antibiotic Given[5]	-	-	97%	95%
Blood Culture Timing[5]	-	-	98%	98%
Pregnancy and Delivery Care				
Newborn Deliveries Scheduled Early[7]	-	-	5%	6%
Preventive Care				
Immunization for Influenza	253	92%	89%	90%
Immunization for Pneumonia	316	91%	90%	92%
Stroke Care				
Anticoagulation Therapy for Atrial Fibrillation[5]	-	-	95%	95%
Antithrombotic Therapy Timing[5]	-	-	98%	98%
Assessed for Rehabilitation[5]	-	-	97%	97%
Discharged on Antithrombotic Therapy[5]	-	-	99%	99%
Discharged on Statin Medication[5]	-	-	94%	94%
Thrombolytic Therapy Timing[5]	-	-	72%	66%
Venous Thromboembolism Prophylaxis[5]	-	-	94%	94%
Written Stroke Educational Materials Given[5]	-	-	87%	88%
Surgical Care Improvement Project				
Appropriate Beta Blocker Usage	57	100%	97%	98%
Appropriate VTP Within 24 Hours	280	98%	98%	98%
Controlled Postoperative Blood Glucose[7]	-	-	96%	97%
Perioperative Temperature Management	320	100%	100%	100%
Prophylactic Antibiotic Selection	271	99%	99%	99%
Prophylactic Antibiotic Selection (Outpatient)	47	98%	97%	98%
Prophylactic Antibiotic Stopped	269	100%	98%	98%
Prophylactic Antibiotic Timing	271	100%	99%	99%
Prophylactic Antibiotic Timing (Outpatient)	47	98%	97%	98%
Urinary Catheter Removal	236	98%	97%	97%
Survey of Patients' Hospital Experiences				
Area Around Room 'Always' Quiet at Night	(a)	77%	51%	61%
Doctors 'Always' Communicated Well	(a)	85%	78%	82%
Home Recovery Information Given	(a)	88%	83%	85%
Hospital Given 9 or 10 on 10 Point Scale	(a)	88%	68%	71%
Meds 'Always' Explained Before Given	(a)	75%	61%	64%
Nurses 'Always' Communicated Well	(a)	87%	74%	79%
Pain 'Always' Well Controlled	(a)	77%	68%	71%
Room and Bathroom 'Always' Clean	(a)	87%	70%	73%
Timely Help 'Always' Received	(a)	85%	62%	68%
Would Definitely Recommend Hospital	(a)	93%	70%	71%
Use of Medical Imaging				
Cardiac Imaging Stress Test before Surgery[7]	-	-	5.2%	5.3%
Combination Abdominal CT Scan[7]	-	-	13.4%	10.5%
Combination Brain/Sinus CT Scan[7]	-	-	2.2%	2.7%
Combination Chest CT Scan[7]	-	-	2.3%	2.7%
Follow-up Mammogram/Ultrasound[7]	-	-	8.2%	8.8%
Lumbar Spine MRI for Low Back Pain[1]	-	-	34.2%	37.2%

NOTE: Hospital profiles are in alphabetical order by state, then city, then hospital within the city; Rankings exclude hospitals with less than 25 cases except for patient surveys which excludes hospitals with less than 100 cases; (a) 100-299 cases; (1) The number of cases/patients is too few to report; (2) Data submitted were based on a sample of cases/patients; (3) Results are based on a shorter time period than required; (4) Data suppressed by CMS for one or more quarters; (5) Results are not available for this reporting period; (6) Fewer than 100 patients completed the HCAHPS survey; (7) No cases met the criteria for this measure; (8) The lower limit of the confidence interval cannot be calculated if the number of observed infections equals zero; (9) No data are available from the state/territory for this reporting period; (10) The scores shown reflect fewer than 50 completed surveys; (11) There were discrepancies in the data collection process; (12) This measure does not apply to this hospital for this reporting period; (13) Results cannot be calculated for this reporting period; (14) The results for this state are combined with nearby states to protect confidentiality; Please refer to the User's Guide for a full explanation of data.

Blood Clot Prevention and Treatment

Anticoagulation Overlap Therapy

Hospital Name	City	Rate	Cases
Boulder Community Hospital[2]	Boulder	100%	97
Centura Health-St Mary Corwin Med Ctr[2]	Pueblo	100%	63
McKee Medical Center[2]	Loveland	100%	31
The Medical Center of Aurora[2]	Aurora	100%	160
Montrose Memorial Hospital[2]	Montrose	100%	33
North Suburban Medical Center[2]	Thornton	100%	49
Rose Medical Center[2]	Denver	100%	119
Centura Health-Littleton Adventist Hosp[2]	Littleton	99%	113
Centura Health - Saint Anthony Hospital[2]	Lakewood	99%	136
Exempla Good Samaritan Medical Center[2]	Lafayette	99%	119
Longmont United Hospital[2]	Longmont	99%	81
Presbyterian Saint Lukes Medical Center[2]	Denver	99%	69
Saint Marys Hospital & Medical Center	Grand Junction	99%	94
Sky Ridge Medical Center[2]	Lone Tree	99%	114
University of Colorado Hospital[2]	Aurora	99%	163
Denver Health Medical Center[2]	Denver	98%	98
Exempla Lutheran Medical Center[2]	Wheat Ridge	98%	110
Exempla Saint Joseph Hospital[2]	Denver	98%	134
Centura Health-Penrose St Francis[2]	Colorado Spgs	97%	216
Centura Health-Porter Adventist Hosp[2]	Denver	97%	64
North Colorado Medical Center[2]	Greeley	97%	112
Centura Health-Avista Adventist Hosp[2]	Louisville	95%	39
Parker Adventist Hospital[2]	Parker	95%	60
Univ of CO Health Mem Hosp[2]	Colorado Spgs	95%	188
Parkview Medical Center[2]	Pueblo	94%	167
Delta County Memorial Hospital[2]	Delta	93%	28
Mercy Regional Medical Center[2]	Durango	93%	46
Poudre Valley Hospital[2]	Fort Collins	93%	119
Swedish Medical Center[2]	Englewood	93%	189
Centura Health-St Anthony North Hosp[2]	Westminster	86%	51
Medical Center of the Rockies[2]	Loveland	81%	93

ICU Venous Thromboembolism Prophylaxis

Hospital Name	City	Rate	Cases
Centura Health - Saint Anthony Hospital[2]	Lakewood	100%	179
Community Hospital[2]	Grand Junction	100%	26
The Medical Center of Aurora[2]	Aurora	100%	97
North Suburban Medical Center[2]	Thornton	100%	110
Platte Valley Medical Center[2]	Brighton	100%	34
Rose Medical Center[2]	Denver	100%	67
San Luis Valley Regional Medical Center[2]	Alamosa	100%	36
Valley View Hospital Association[2]	Glenwood Spgs	100%	51
Sky Ridge Medical Center[2]	Lone Tree	99%	75
Univ of CO Health Mem Hosp[2]	Colorado Spgs	99%	90
University of Colorado Hospital[2]	Aurora	99%	102
Centura Health-Littleton Adventist Hosp[2]	Littleton	98%	81
Centura Health-St Anthony North Hosp[2]	Westminster	98%	54
Parker Adventist Hospital[2]	Parker	98%	96
Presbyterian Saint Lukes Medical Center[2]	Denver	98%	82
Swedish Medical Center[2]	Englewood	98%	95
Vail Valley Medical Center[2]	Vail	98%	41
Exempla Good Samaritan Medical Center[2]	Lafayette	97%	61
McKee Medical Center[2]	Loveland	97%	30
Medical Center of the Rockies[2]	Loveland	97%	93
North Colorado Medical Center[2]	Greeley	97%	58
Boulder Community Hospital[2]	Boulder	96%	75
Centura Health-St Mary Corwin Med Ctr[2]	Pueblo	96%	84
Exempla Saint Joseph Hospital[2]	Denver	95%	83
Montrose Memorial Hospital[2]	Montrose	95%	43
Poudre Valley Hospital[2]	Fort Collins	94%	34
Saint Marys Hospital & Medical Center	Grand Junction	94%	1060
Exempla Lutheran Medical Center[2]	Wheat Ridge	93%	83
Parkview Medical Center[2]	Pueblo	93%	88
Centura Health-Penrose St Francis[2]	Colorado Spgs	91%	70
Delta County Memorial Hospital[2]	Delta	91%	44
Centura Health-St Thomas More Hosp[2]	Canon City	90%	39
Centura Health-Porter Adventist Hosp[2]	Denver	89%	92
Arkansas Valley Regional Medical Center[2]	La Junta	88%	56
Denver Health Medical Center[2]	Denver	87%	113
Mercy Regional Medical Center[2]	Durango	87%	47
Centura Health-Avista Adventist Hosp[2]	Louisville	85%	46
Longmont United Hospital[2]	Longmont	79%	89

Incidence of Potentially Preventable VTE

Hospital Name	City	Rate	Cases
The Medical Center of Aurora[2]	Aurora	0%	25
Rose Medical Center[2]	Denver	4%	27
University of Colorado Hospital[2]	Aurora	6%	54
Denver Health Medical Center[2]	Denver	11%	47
Swedish Medical Center[2]	Englewood	11%	55
Centura Health-Littleton Adventist Hosp[2]	Littleton	12%	26
Centura Health - Saint Anthony Hospital[2]	Lakewood	25%	28

UFH with Dosages/Platelet Count Monitoring

Hospital Name	City	Rate	Cases
Boulder Community Hospital[2]	Boulder	100%	72
Centura Health-Penrose St Francis[2]	Colorado Spgs	100%	64
Centura Health-Porter Adventist Hosp[2]	Denver	100%	53
Longmont United Hospital[2]	Longmont	100%	79
The Medical Center of Aurora[2]	Aurora	100%	110
North Suburban Medical Center[2]	Thornton	100%	27
Parkview Medical Center[2]	Pueblo	100%	47
Presbyterian Saint Lukes Medical Center[2]	Denver	100%	50
Rose Medical Center[2]	Denver	100%	93
Saint Marys Hospital & Medical Center	Grand Junction	100%	54
Sky Ridge Medical Center[2]	Lone Tree	100%	82
Exempla Good Samaritan Medical Center[2]	Lafayette	99%	82
Exempla Lutheran Medical Center[2]	Wheat Ridge	99%	71
Univ of CO Health Mem Hosp[2]	Colorado Spgs	99%	85
Exempla Saint Joseph Hospital[2]	Denver	98%	127
North Colorado Medical Center[2]	Greeley	98%	50
Centura Health-St Anthony North Hosp[2]	Westminster	97%	35
Centura Health-Littleton Adventist Hosp[2]	Littleton	96%	120
Centura Health - Saint Anthony Hospital[2]	Lakewood	96%	96
Denver Health Medical Center[2]	Denver	96%	80
Parker Adventist Hospital[2]	Parker	96%	56
University of Colorado Hospital[2]	Aurora	95%	182
Poudre Valley Hospital[2]	Fort Collins	94%	48
Medical Center of the Rockies[2]	Loveland	90%	48
Swedish Medical Center[2]	Englewood	88%	110

Venous Thromboembolism Prophylaxis

Hospital Name	City	Rate	Cases
Orthocolorado Hosp-St Anthony Med Camp[2]	Lakewood	100%	64
Colorado Plains Medical Center[2]	Fort Morgan	99%	71
Rose Medical Center[2]	Denver	99%	321
Sky Ridge Medical Center[2]	Lone Tree	99%	349
Community Hospital[2]	Grand Junction	98%	116
North Suburban Medical Center[2]	Thornton	98%	307
Platte Valley Medical Center[2]	Brighton	98%	206
Vail Valley Medical Center[2]	Vail	98%	105
McKee Medical Center[2]	Loveland	96%	268
Saint Anthony Summit Medical Center[2]	Frisco	96%	105
Yampa Valley Medical Center[2]	Steamboat Spgs	96%	83
Montrose Memorial Hospital[2]	Montrose	95%	147
Parker Adventist Hospital[2]	Parker	95%	313
Valley View Hospital Association[2]	Glenwood Spgs	95%	121
Boulder Community Hospital[2]	Boulder	94%	304
Centura Health-St Anthony North Hosp[2]	Westminster	94%	348
Exempla Good Samaritan Medical Center[2]	Lafayette	94%	319
The Medical Center of Aurora[2]	Aurora	94%	352
North Colorado Medical Center[2]	Greeley	93%	296
Exempla Saint Joseph Hospital[2]	Denver	92%	304
Presbyterian Saint Lukes Medical Center[2]	Denver	92%	322
Saint Marys Hospital & Medical Center	Grand Junction	92%	3546
University of Colorado Hospital[2]	Aurora	92%	268
Centura Health - Saint Anthony Hospital[2]	Lakewood	91%	274
Southwest Memorial Hospital[2]	Cortez	91%	109
Sterling Regional Medcenter[2]	Sterling	91%	93
San Luis Valley Regional Medical Center[2]	Alamosa	90%	99
Delta County Memorial Hospital[2]	Delta	89%	209
Mercy Regional Medical Center[2]	Durango	89%	282
Centura Health-Littleton Adventist Hosp[2]	Littleton	88%	336
Centura Health-St Mary Corwin Med Ctr[2]	Pueblo	88%	347
Exempla Lutheran Medical Center[2]	Wheat Ridge	88%	365
Poudre Valley Hospital[2]	Fort Collins	88%	256
Parkview Medical Center[2]	Pueblo	87%	322
Centura Health-St Thomas More Hosp[2]	Canon City	86%	105
Pikes Peak Regional Hospital[2]	Woodland Park	86%	94
Medical Center of the Rockies[2]	Loveland	85%	294
Swedish Medical Center[2]	Englewood	84%	327
Univ of CO Health Mem Hosp[2]	Colorado Spgs	83%	493
Centura Health-Porter Adventist Hosp[2]	Denver	82%	247
Centura Health-Avista Adventist Hosp[2]	Louisville	81%	140
Arkansas Valley Regional Medical Center[2]	La Junta	80%	193
Animas Surgical Hospital[2]	Durango	77%	26
Grand River Medical Center[2]	Rifle	77%	83
Longmont United Hospital[2]	Longmont	77%	297
Denver Health Medical Center[2]	Denver	74%	309
Centura Health-Penrose St Francis[2]	Colorado Spgs	70%	299
Keefe Memorial Hospital[2]	Cheyenne Wells	0%	40

Warfarin Therapy Discharge Instructions

Hospital Name	City	Rate	Cases
The Medical Center of Aurora[2]	Aurora	100%	123
Rose Medical Center[2]	Denver	100%	82
Parkview Medical Center[2]	Pueblo	97%	134
Boulder Community Hospital[2]	Boulder	96%	77
Centura Health-St Mary Corwin Med Ctr[2]	Pueblo	96%	52
Saint Marys Hospital & Medical Center	Grand Junction	96%	79
Sky Ridge Medical Center[2]	Lone Tree	96%	92
North Suburban Medical Center[2]	Thornton	91%	45
Exempla Good Samaritan Medical Center[2]	Lafayette	86%	100
Denver Health Medical Center[2]	Denver	85%	78
Exempla Saint Joseph Hospital[2]	Denver	84%	99
Montrose Memorial Hospital[2]	Montrose	83%	35
Exempla Lutheran Medical Center[2]	Wheat Ridge	74%	90
Univ of CO Health Mem Hosp[2]	Colorado Spgs	74%	148
Swedish Medical Center[2]	Englewood	70%	132
Presbyterian Saint Lukes Medical Center[2]	Denver	69%	61
Poudre Valley Hospital[2]	Fort Collins	68%	101
Centura Health - Saint Anthony Hospital[2]	Lakewood	67%	94
McKee Medical Center[2]	Loveland	63%	27
University of Colorado Hospital[2]	Aurora	62%	139
Parker Adventist Hospital[2]	Parker	58%	45
North Colorado Medical Center[2]	Greeley	57%	84
Medical Center of the Rockies[2]	Loveland	56%	77
Longmont United Hospital[2]	Longmont	44%	70
Mercy Regional Medical Center[2]	Durango	36%	39
Centura Health-Littleton Adventist Hosp[2]	Littleton	30%	92
Centura Health-Avista Adventist Hosp[2]	Louisville	28%	32
Centura Health-Penrose St Francis[2]	Colorado Spgs	17%	173
Centura Health-St Anthony North Hosp[2]	Westminster	15%	41
Centura Health-Porter Adventist Hosp[2]	Denver	13%	52

Chest Pain/Possible Heart Attack Care

Aspirin Given Within 24 Hours of Arrival

Hospital Name	City	Rate	Cases
Colorado Plains Medical Center	Fort Morgan	100%	33
Sterling Regional Medcenter	Sterling	100%	29
Vail Valley Medical Center	Vail	100%	76
Centura Health-Littleton Adventist Hosp	Littleton	99%	99
Centura Health-St Thomas More Hosp	Canon City	99%	93
Arkansas Valley Regional Medical Center	La Junta	98%	61
The Medical Center of Aurora	Aurora	98%	42
San Luis Valley Regional Medical Center	Alamosa	98%	41
Delta County Memorial Hospital	Delta	96%	51
Saint Anthony Summit Medical Center	Frisco	96%	54

Average Time to ECG (minutes)

Hospital Name	City	Min.	Cases
Colorado Plains Medical Center	Fort Morgan	5	35
Centura Health-Littleton Adventist Hosp	Littleton	6	100
The Medical Center of Aurora	Aurora	6	44
Sterling Regional Medcenter	Sterling	6	29
Delta County Memorial Hospital	Delta	7	50
Saint Anthony Summit Medical Center	Frisco	7	54
San Luis Valley Regional Medical Center	Alamosa	7	42
Centura Health-St Thomas More Hosp	Canon City	8	92
Vail Valley Medical Center	Vail	12	76
Arkansas Valley Regional Medical Center	La Junta	18	63
Southwest Memorial Hospital	Cortez	19	28

Children's Asthma Care

Received Home Management Plan of Care

Hospital Name	City	Rate	Cases
Childrens Hospital Colorado	Aurora	94%	813

Received Reliever Medication

Hospital Name	City	Rate	Cases
Childrens Hospital Colorado	Aurora	100%	814

Received Systemic Corticosteroids

Hospital Name	City	Rate	Cases
Childrens Hospital Colorado	Aurora	100%	814

Emergency Department

Admittance Decision Time (minutes)

Hospital Name	City	Min.	Cases
Keefe Memorial Hospital[2]	Cheyenne Wells	13	31
Sterling Regional Medcenter[2]	Sterling	38	247
Rio Grande Hospital[2,3]	Del Norte	40	119
Southwest Memorial Hospital[2,3]	Cortez	48	252
Platte Valley Medical Center[2]	Brighton	52	328
Colorado Plains Medical Center[2]	Fort Morgan	56	182
Arkansas Valley Regional Medical Center[2]	La Junta	57	304
Centura Health-St Thomas More Hosp[2]	Canon City	64	348
McKee Medical Center[2]	Loveland	64	559
North Colorado Medical Center[2]	Greeley	64	451
Saint Anthony Summit Medical Center[2]	Frisco	65	152
Community Hospital[2]	Grand Junction	68	324
Delta County Memorial Hospital[2]	Delta	70	264
Vail Valley Medical Center[2]	Vail	70	99
Boulder Community Hospital[2]	Boulder	71	423
Univ of CO Health Mem Hosp[2]	Colorado Spgs	71	462
Yampa Valley Medical Center[2]	Steamboat Spgs	71	191
Exempla Lutheran Medical Center[2]	Wheat Ridge	75	623

NOTE: Hospital profiles are in alphabetical order by state, then city, then hospital within the city; Rankings exclude hospitals with less than 25 cases except for patient surveys which excludes hospitals with less than 100 cases; (a) 100-299 cases; (1) The number of cases/patients is too few to report; (2) Data submitted were based on a sample of cases/patients; (3) Results are based on a shorter time period than required; (4) Data suppressed by CMS for one or more quarters; (5) Results are not available for this reporting period; (6) Fewer than 100 patients completed the HCAHPS survey; (7) No cases met the criteria for this measure; (8) The lower limit of the confidence interval cannot be calculated if the number of observed infections equals zero; (9) No data are available from the state/territory for this reporting period; (10) The scores shown reflect fewer than 50 completed surveys; (11) There were discrepancies in the data collection process; (12) This measure does not apply to this hospital for this reporting period; (13) Results cannot be calculated for this reporting period; (14) The results for this state are combined with nearby states to protect confidentiality; Please refer to the User's Guide for a full explanation of data.

Longmont United Hospital[2]	Longmont	75	701
Poudre Valley Hospital[2]	Fort Collins	75	320
Presbyterian Saint Lukes Medical Center[2]	Denver	79	440
Rose Medical Center[2]	Denver	80	435
Exempla Good Samaritan Medical Center[2]	Lafayette	81	579
Centura Health - Saint Anthony Hospital[2]	Lakewood	82	783
North Suburban Medical Center[2]	Thornton	85	508
Centura Health-Avista Adventist Hosp[2]	Louisville	92	194
Centura Health-Penrose St Francis[2]	Colorado Spgs	93	659
Mercy Regional Medical Center[2]	Durango	96	242
Valley View Hospital Association[2]	Glenwood Spgs	98	166
Exempla Saint Joseph Hospital[2]	Denver	100	400
Swedish Medical Center[2]	Englewood	107	695
San Luis Valley Regional Medical Center[2]	Alamosa	108	156
Medical Center of the Rockies[2]	Loveland	113	392
Parker Adventist Hospital[2]	Parker	113	448
Montrose Memorial Hospital[2]	Montrose	116	304
Saint Marys Hospital & Medical Center	Grand Junction	116	4618
Parkview Medical Center[2]	Pueblo	118	464
Sky Ridge Medical Center[2]	Lone Tree	119	379
The Medical Center of Aurora[2]	Aurora	120	789
University of Colorado Hospital[2]	Aurora	126	344
Denver Health Medical Center[2]	Denver	134	436
Centura Health-Littleton Adventist Hosp[2]	Littleton	135	653
Centura Health-St Anthony North Hosp[2]	Westminster	138	691
Centura Health-St Mary Corwin Med Ctr[2]	Pueblo	146	486
Centura Health-Porter Adventist Hosp[2]	Denver	157	531

Head CT Results Within 45 Minutes of Arrival

Hospital Name	City	Rate	Cases
North Suburban Medical Center	Thornton	88%	33
Centura Health-St Anthony North Hosp	Westminster	76%	45
Centura Health-Penrose St Francis	Colorado Spgs	74%	27

Patients Who Left ER Before Being Seen

Hospital Name	City	Rate	Cases
Animas Surgical Hospital	Durango	0%	5980
Centura Health-Avista Adventist Hosp	Louisville	0%	11999
Centura Health-Porter Adventist Hosp	Denver	0%	25575
Centura Health - Saint Anthony Hospital	Lakewood	0%	46501
Colorado Plains Medical Center	Fort Morgan	0%	7092
Community Hospital	Grand Junction	0%	15624
Delta County Memorial Hospital	Delta	0%	13846
East Morgan County Hospital	Brush	0%	4506
Exempla Good Samaritan Medical Center	Lafayette	0%	40863
Exempla Lutheran Medical Center	Wheat Ridge	0%	72155
Keefe Memorial Hospital	Cheyenne Wells	0%	651
The Memorial Hospital	Craig	0%	5036
Mercy Regional Medical Center	Durango	0%	15216
Platte Valley Medical Center	Brighton	0%	21226
Presbyterian Saint Lukes Medical Center	Denver	0%	25863
Rose Medical Center	Denver	0%	35920
Saint Anthony Summit Medical Center	Frisco	0%	11760
Sky Ridge Medical Center	Lone Tree	0%	36596
Swedish Medical Center	Englewood	0%	77386
Arkansas Valley Regional Medical Center	La Junta	1%	6178
Boulder Community Hospital	Boulder	1%	32571
Centura Health-Littleton Adventist Hosp	Littleton	1%	35786
Centura Health-Penrose St Francis	Colorado Spgs	1%	91199
Centura Health-St Mary Corwin Med Ctr	Pueblo	1%	35223
Centura Health-St Thomas More Hosp	Canon City	1%	18802
Exempla Saint Joseph Hospital	Denver	1%	51961
Kit Carson County Memorial Hospital	Burlington	1%	2207
Longmont United Hospital	Longmont	1%	16486
McKee Medical Center	Loveland	1%	27515
The Medical Center of Aurora	Aurora	1%	76851
Montrose Memorial Hospital	Montrose	1%	16650
North Colorado Medical Center	Greeley	1%	58575
North Suburban Medical Center	Thornton	1%	56259
Parker Adventist Hospital	Parker	1%	25556
Poudre Valley Hospital	Fort Collins	1%	44576
Southwest Memorial Hospital	Cortez	1%	12030
Sterling Regional Medcenter	Sterling	1%	7850
Vail Valley Medical Center	Vail	1%	11610
Valley View Hospital Association	Glenwood Spgs	1%	10755
Yampa Valley Medical Center	Steamboat Spgs	1%	8028
Medical Center of the Rockies	Loveland	2%	4365
Saint Marys Hospital & Medical Center	Grand Junction	2%	39725
San Luis Valley Regional Medical Center	Alamosa	2%	12705
Centura Health-St Anthony North Hosp	Westminster	3%	36801
Parkview Medical Center	Pueblo	3%	60705
Univ of CO Health Mem Hosp	Colorado Spgs	3%	140015
University of Colorado Hospital	Aurora	5%	70430
Denver Health Medical Center	Denver	6%	87569

Time from ER Arrival to Being Admitted (minutes)

Hospital Name	City	Min.	Cases
Keefe Memorial Hospital[2]	Cheyenne Wells	106	35
Yuma District Hospital	Yuma	120	98
Southeast Colorado Hospital	Springfield	122	86
Southwest Memorial Hospital[2,3]	Cortez	171	252
Colorado Plains Medical Center[2]	Fort Morgan	178	182
Presbyterian Saint Lukes Medical Center[2]	Denver	178	440
Sterling Regional Medcenter[2]	Sterling	178	285
Yampa Valley Medical Center[2]	Steamboat Spgs	181	208
Boulder Community Hospital[2]	Boulder	188	438
Longmont United Hospital[2]	Longmont	194	701
Rose Medical Center[2]	Denver	195	435
Poudre Valley Hospital[2]	Fort Collins	196	423
Centura Health - Saint Anthony Hospital[2]	Lakewood	202	810
Saint Anthony Summit Medical Center[2]	Frisco	203	229
Delta County Memorial Hospital[2]	Delta	209	293
Centura Health-St Thomas More Hosp[2]	Canon City	212	364
Platte Valley Medical Center[2]	Brighton	214	340
Rio Grande Hospital[2,3]	Del Norte	215	145
Medical Center of the Rockies[2]	Loveland	216	449
Sky Ridge Medical Center[2]	Lone Tree	219	379
North Colorado Medical Center[2]	Greeley	220	464
Centura Health-Avista Adventist Hosp[2]	Louisville	222	196
Swedish Medical Center[2]	Englewood	222	698
Montrose Memorial Hospital[2]	Montrose	223	304
Vail Valley Medical Center[2]	Vail	223	116
McKee Medical Center[2]	Loveland	226	578
North Suburban Medical Center[2]	Thornton	228	508
Community Hospital[2]	Grand Junction	231	380
Arkansas Valley Regional Medical Center[2]	La Junta	243	317
Parkview Medical Center[2]	Pueblo	250	468
Valley View Hospital Association[2]	Glenwood Spgs	256	191
The Medical Center of Aurora[2]	Aurora	257	789
Exempla Good Samaritan Medical Center[2]	Lafayette	258	581
Centura Health-Penrose St Francis[2]	Colorado Spgs	267	677
Exempla Lutheran Medical Center[2]	Wheat Ridge	271	624
Centura Health-St Mary Corwin Med Ctr[2]	Pueblo	272	499
Parker Adventist Hospital[2]	Parker	274	453
Mercy Regional Medical Center[2]	Durango	276	258
Saint Marys Hospital & Medical Center	Grand Junction	277	4745
San Luis Valley Regional Medical Center[2]	Alamosa	278	263
Centura Health-St Anthony North Hosp[2]	Westminster	280	738
Univ of CO Health Mem Hosp[2]	Colorado Spgs	287	565
Centura Health-Littleton Adventist Hosp[2]	Littleton	294	701
Exempla Saint Joseph Hospital[2]	Denver	299	403
Centura Health-Porter Adventist Hosp[2]	Denver	319	542
Denver Health Medical Center[2]	Denver	319	445
University of Colorado Hospital[2]	Aurora	353	345

Time from ER Arrival to Discharge (minutes)

Hospital Name	City	Min.	Cases
Animas Surgical Hospital	Durango	74	359
The Memorial Hospital[3]	Craig	85	387
Yampa Valley Medical Center	Steamboat Spgs	94	361
Colorado Plains Medical Center	Fort Morgan	96	360
Vail Valley Medical Center	Vail	101	574
Montrose Memorial Hospital	Montrose	102	428
Keefe Memorial Hospital	Cheyenne Wells	106	240
Saint Anthony Summit Medical Center	Frisco	107	423
Arkansas Valley Regional Medical Center	La Junta	114	340
Sterling Regional Medcenter	Sterling	114	346
Centura Health-St Mary Corwin Med Ctr	Pueblo	116	466
North Colorado Medical Center	Greeley	119	317
Boulder Community Hospital	Boulder	120	316
Centura Health - Saint Anthony Hospital	Lakewood	126	424
Delta County Memorial Hospital	Delta	127	455
Centura Health-St Thomas More Hosp	Canon City	128	469
McKee Medical Center	Loveland	128	337
Centura Health-St Anthony North Hosp	Westminster	129	441
North Suburban Medical Center	Thornton	129	477
Swedish Medical Center	Englewood	130	460
Community Hospital	Grand Junction	133	396
Medical Center of the Rockies	Loveland	133	443
Centura Health-Avista Adventist Hosp	Louisville	136	420
Longmont United Hospital	Longmont	138	363
Presbyterian Saint Lukes Medical Center	Denver	138	457
Rose Medical Center	Denver	139	488
The Medical Center of Aurora	Aurora	140	458
San Luis Valley Regional Medical Center	Alamosa	140	355
Poudre Valley Hospital	Fort Collins	146	380
Parkview Medical Center	Pueblo	147	349
Sky Ridge Medical Center	Lone Tree	149	445
Valley View Hospital Association	Glenwood Spgs	152	353
Platte Valley Medical Center	Brighton	158	489
Saint Marys Hospital & Medical Center	Grand Junction	158	4027
Centura Health-Littleton Adventist Hosp	Littleton	161	435
Mercy Regional Medical Center	Durango	165	450
Centura Health-Penrose St Francis	Colorado Spgs	166	465
Centura Health-Porter Adventist Hosp	Denver	169	420
Univ of CO Health Mem Hosp	Colorado Spgs	170	495
Exempla Lutheran Medical Center	Wheat Ridge	172	315
Exempla Saint Joseph Hospital	Denver	172	296
Exempla Good Samaritan Medical Center	Lafayette	181	323
University of Colorado Hospital	Aurora	185	333
Parker Adventist Hospital	Parker	198	434
Denver Health Medical Center	Denver	268	296

Time in ER Before Being Evaluated (minutes)

Hospital Name	City	Min.	Cases
Colorado Plains Medical Center	Fort Morgan	7	404
Community Hospital	Grand Junction	7	415
Presbyterian Saint Lukes Medical Center	Denver	7	503
Centura Health - Saint Anthony Hospital	Lakewood	8	243
Rose Medical Center	Denver	8	523
Centura Health-St Anthony North Hosp	Westminster	10	364
Keefe Memorial Hospital	Cheyenne Wells	11	249
Saint Anthony Summit Medical Center	Frisco	11	438
Centura Health-Avista Adventist Hosp	Louisville	12	499
The Medical Center of Aurora	Aurora	12	525
North Colorado Medical Center	Greeley	13	382
Centura Health-Littleton Adventist Hosp	Littleton	14	447
Yampa Valley Medical Center	Steamboat Spgs	14	392
Centura Health-Porter Adventist Hosp	Denver	15	445
The Memorial Hospital[3]	Craig	15	311
Montrose Memorial Hospital	Montrose	15	472
North Suburban Medical Center	Thornton	15	529
Sky Ridge Medical Center	Lone Tree	15	523
Swedish Medical Center	Englewood	15	520
Exempla Good Samaritan Medical Center	Lafayette	16	382
Parker Adventist Hospital	Parker	17	462
Exempla Saint Joseph Hospital	Denver	18	382
McKee Medical Center	Loveland	18	349
Medical Center of the Rockies	Loveland	18	461
Denver Health Medical Center	Denver	19	389
Animas Surgical Hospital	Durango	20	360
San Luis Valley Regional Medical Center	Alamosa	20	370
Sterling Regional Medcenter	Sterling	20	339
Boulder Community Hospital	Boulder	21	376
University of Colorado Hospital	Aurora	21	378
Centura Health-St Thomas More Hosp	Canon City	22	362
Arkansas Valley Regional Medical Center	La Junta	24	372
Vail Valley Medical Center	Vail	25	592
Univ of CO Health Mem Hosp	Colorado Spgs	27	559
Platte Valley Medical Center	Brighton	28	215
Poudre Valley Hospital	Fort Collins	29	383
Valley View Hospital Association	Glenwood Spgs	29	193
Delta County Memorial Hospital	Delta	32	430
Exempla Lutheran Medical Center	Wheat Ridge	32	383
Longmont United Hospital	Longmont	32	368
Mercy Regional Medical Center	Durango	32	471
Centura Health-Penrose St Francis	Colorado Spgs	35	357
Centura Health-St Mary Corwin Med Ctr	Pueblo	36	496
Parkview Medical Center	Pueblo	37	392
Saint Marys Hospital & Medical Center	Grand Junction	37	3746

Time to Pain Meds for Bone Fractures (minutes)

Hospital Name	City	Min.	Cases
Colorado Plains Medical Center	Fort Morgan	25	38
Denver Health Medical Center	Denver	25	335
Presbyterian Saint Lukes Medical Center	Denver	30	78
Longmont United Hospital	Longmont	32	118
North Suburban Medical Center	Thornton	33	212
Boulder Community Hospital	Boulder	34	160
The Medical Center of Aurora	Aurora	34	197
Sky Ridge Medical Center	Lone Tree	35	184
Centura Health - Saint Anthony Hospital	Lakewood	36	232
Univ of CO Health Mem Hosp	Colorado Spgs	37	390
Montrose Memorial Hospital	Montrose	38	36
Swedish Medical Center	Englewood	38	311
Yampa Valley Medical Center	Steamboat Spgs	39	103
Platte Valley Medical Center	Brighton	40	101
North Colorado Medical Center	Greeley	41	167
Southwest Memorial Hospital[3]	Cortez	41	69
Delta County Memorial Hospital	Delta	42	72
Rose Medical Center	Denver	43	107
Centura Health-Littleton Adventist Hosp	Littleton	44	196
Centura Health-St Thomas More Hosp	Canon City	45	62
Parkview Medical Center	Pueblo	47	217
McKee Medical Center	Loveland	48	106
Sterling Regional Medcenter	Sterling	48	31
Vail Valley Medical Center	Vail	48	102
Centura Health-St Anthony North Hosp	Westminster	50	180
University of Colorado Hospital	Aurora	51	72
Exempla Lutheran Medical Center	Wheat Ridge	52	196
San Luis Valley Regional Medical Center	Alamosa	52	73
Community Hospital	Grand Junction	53	77
Saint Anthony Summit Medical Center	Frisco	53	99
Exempla Good Samaritan Medical Center	Lafayette	54	197
Centura Health-Porter Adventist Hosp	Denver	56	47
Parker Adventist Hospital	Parker	56	138
Centura Health-Avista Adventist Hosp	Louisville	57	51
Centura Health-St Mary Corwin Med Ctr	Pueblo	58	100
Valley View Hospital Association	Glenwood Spgs	58	63
Saint Marys Hospital & Medical Center	Grand Junction	60	163
Centura Health-Penrose St Francis	Colorado Spgs	64	249

NOTE: Hospital profiles are in alphabetical order by state, then city, then hospital within the city; Rankings exclude hospitals with less than 25 cases except for patient surveys which excludes hospitals with less than 100 cases; (a) 100-299 cases; (1) The number of cases/patients is too few to report; (2) Data submitted were based on a sample of cases/patients; (3) Results are based on a shorter time period than required; (4) Data suppressed by CMS for one or more quarters; (5) Results are not available for this reporting period; (6) Fewer than 100 patients completed the HCAHPS survey; (7) No cases met the criteria for this measure; (8) The lower limit of the confidence interval cannot be calculated if the number of observed infections equals zero; (9) No data are available from the state/territory for this reporting period; (10) The scores shown reflect fewer than 50 completed surveys; (11) There were discrepancies in the data collection process; (12) This measure does not apply to this hospital for this reporting period; (13) Results cannot be calculated for this reporting period; (14) The results for this state are combined with nearby states to protect confidentiality; Please refer to the User's Guide for a full explanation of data.

Hospital Name	City	Rate	Cases
Mercy Regional Medical Center	Durango	65	77
Medical Center of the Rockies	Loveland	66	168
Poudre Valley Hospital	Fort Collins	70	266
Exempla Saint Joseph Hospital	Denver	71	78

Heart Attack Care

Aspirin Given at Discharge

Hospital Name	City	Rate	Cases
Centura Health-Littleton Adventist Hosp	Littleton	100%	115
Centura Health-Penrose St Francis	Colorado Spgs	100%	426
Centura Health-Porter Adventist Hosp	Denver	100%	92
Centura Health - Saint Anthony Hospital	Lakewood	100%	288
Centura Health-St Mary Corwin Med Ctr	Pueblo	100%	161
Exempla Good Samaritan Medical Center	Lafayette	100%	147
Exempla Lutheran Medical Center	Wheat Ridge	100%	257
Longmont United Hospital	Longmont	100%	107
McKee Medical Center	Loveland	100%	91
The Medical Center of Aurora[2]	Aurora	100%	260
Medical Center of the Rockies[2]	Loveland	100%	356
Mercy Regional Medical Center	Durango	100%	69
Montrose Memorial Hospital	Montrose	100%	45
North Colorado Medical Center[2]	Greeley	100%	275
North Suburban Medical Center[2]	Thornton	100%	115
Parker Adventist Hospital	Parker	100%	63
Poudre Valley Hospital	Fort Collins	100%	122
Presbyterian Saint Lukes Medical Center	Denver	100%	78
Rose Medical Center	Denver	100%	104
Saint Marys Hospital & Medical Center	Grand Junction	100%	320
Sky Ridge Medical Center	Lone Tree	100%	118
Swedish Medical Center[2]	Englewood	100%	183
Univ of CO Health Mem Hosp	Colorado Spgs	100%	371
University of Colorado Hospital	Aurora	100%	227
Valley View Hospital Association	Glenwood Spgs	100%	37
Boulder Community Hospital	Boulder	99%	68
Centura Health-St Anthony North Hosp	Westminster	99%	163
Denver Health Medical Center	Denver	99%	156
Exempla Saint Joseph Hospital[2]	Denver	99%	153
Parkview Medical Center	Pueblo	98%	255
Platte Valley Medical Center	Brighton	98%	53
VA Eastern Colorado Healthcare System	Denver	98%	52

PCI Within 90 Minutes of Arrival

Hospital Name	City	Rate	Cases
Centura Health-Littleton Adventist Hosp	Littleton	100%	59
Centura Health-St Mary Corwin Med Ctr	Pueblo	100%	33
Exempla Good Samaritan Medical Center	Lafayette	100%	35
Exempla Lutheran Medical Center	Wheat Ridge	100%	61
Longmont United Hospital	Longmont	100%	44
Medical Center of the Rockies[2]	Loveland	100%	58
North Suburban Medical Center[2]	Thornton	100%	34
Rose Medical Center	Denver	100%	27
Saint Marys Hospital & Medical Center	Grand Junction	100%	44
Sky Ridge Medical Center	Lone Tree	100%	38
Univ of CO Health Mem Hosp	Colorado Spgs	99%	81
Centura Health-Penrose St Francis	Colorado Spgs	98%	92
Parkview Medical Center	Pueblo	98%	50
Swedish Medical Center[2]	Englewood	98%	64
Centura Health - Saint Anthony Hospital	Lakewood	97%	106
The Medical Center of Aurora[2]	Aurora	97%	61
Poudre Valley Hospital	Fort Collins	96%	27
North Colorado Medical Center[2]	Greeley	95%	38
Centura Health-St Anthony North Hosp	Westminster	94%	48
University of Colorado Hospital	Aurora	93%	42
Mercy Regional Medical Center	Durango	84%	25
Denver Health Medical Center	Denver	79%	38

Statin Prescribed at Discharge

Hospital Name	City	Rate	Cases
Centura Health-Littleton Adventist Hosp	Littleton	100%	119
Centura Health-Porter Adventist Hosp	Denver	100%	91
Centura Health - Saint Anthony Hospital	Lakewood	100%	290
Exempla Good Samaritan Medical Center	Lafayette	100%	140
Exempla Saint Joseph Hospital[2]	Denver	100%	144
McKee Medical Center	Loveland	100%	79
The Medical Center of Aurora[2]	Aurora	100%	255
Mercy Regional Medical Center	Durango	100%	67
North Colorado Medical Center[2]	Greeley	100%	269
North Suburban Medical Center[2]	Thornton	100%	110
Parker Adventist Hospital	Parker	100%	59
Platte Valley Medical Center	Brighton	100%	49
Presbyterian Saint Lukes Medical Center	Denver	100%	77
Rose Medical Center	Denver	100%	104
Sky Ridge Medical Center	Lone Tree	100%	116
Swedish Medical Center[2]	Englewood	100%	178
VA Eastern Colorado Healthcare System	Denver	100%	53
Valley View Hospital Association	Glenwood Spgs	100%	37
Centura Health-Penrose St Francis	Colorado Spgs	99%	441
Centura Health-St Anthony North Hosp	Westminster	99%	159
Centura Health-St Mary Corwin Med Ctr	Pueblo	99%	164
Denver Health Medical Center	Denver	99%	158
Exempla Lutheran Medical Center	Wheat Ridge	99%	248
Medical Center of the Rockies[2]	Loveland	99%	330
Parkview Medical Center	Pueblo	99%	257
Poudre Valley Hospital	Fort Collins	99%	112
Saint Marys Hospital & Medical Center	Grand Junction	99%	303
Univ of CO Health Mem Hosp	Colorado Spgs	99%	362
University of Colorado Hospital	Aurora	99%	220
Montrose Memorial Hospital	Montrose	98%	40
Boulder Community Hospital	Boulder	97%	68
Longmont United Hospital	Longmont	97%	103

Heart Failure Care

ACE Inhibitor or ARB for LVSD

Hospital Name	City	Rate	Cases
Centura Health-Littleton Adventist Hosp	Littleton	100%	32
Centura Health - Saint Anthony Hospital	Lakewood	100%	56
Centura Health-St Anthony North Hosp	Westminster	100%	43
Centura Health-St Mary Corwin Med Ctr	Pueblo	100%	38
Exempla Lutheran Medical Center[2]	Wheat Ridge	100%	50
North Colorado Medical Center[2]	Greeley	100%	53
Poudre Valley Hospital	Fort Collins	100%	41
Presbyterian Saint Lukes Medical Center	Denver	100%	27
Rose Medical Center	Denver	100%	40
Sky Ridge Medical Center	Lone Tree	100%	29
Swedish Medical Center[2]	Englewood	100%	62
Denver Health Medical Center	Denver	99%	145
Exempla Saint Joseph Hospital[2]	Denver	99%	82
University of Colorado Hospital[2]	Aurora	99%	110
Saint Marys Hospital & Medical Center	Grand Junction	98%	42
The Medical Center of Aurora[2]	Aurora	97%	91
Parkview Medical Center	Pueblo	97%	63
VA Eastern Colorado Healthcare System	Denver	97%	62
Exempla Good Samaritan Medical Center	Lafayette	96%	73
Medical Center of the Rockies	Loveland	96%	49
Univ of CO Health Mem Hosp	Colorado Spgs	96%	120
Centura Health-Penrose St Francis	Colorado Spgs	95%	129
Centura Health-Porter Adventist Hosp	Denver	95%	39
Boulder Community Hospital	Boulder	94%	34

Discharge Instructions Given

Hospital Name	City	Rate	Cases
Delta County Memorial Hospital	Delta	100%	27
Exempla Good Samaritan Medical Center	Lafayette	100%	251
Grand Junction VA Medical Center	Grand Junction	100%	27
North Suburban Medical Center[2]	Thornton	100%	56
Rose Medical Center	Denver	100%	124
Sterling Regional Medcenter	Sterling	100%	26
Centura Health-Porter Adventist Hosp	Denver	99%	105
Exempla Lutheran Medical Center[2]	Wheat Ridge	99%	154
McKee Medical Center[2]	Loveland	99%	69
Sky Ridge Medical Center	Lone Tree	99%	104
Exempla Saint Joseph Hospital[2]	Denver	98%	284
Mercy Regional Medical Center	Durango	98%	53
Platte Valley Medical Center	Brighton	98%	64
Presbyterian Saint Lukes Medical Center	Denver	98%	65
Swedish Medical Center[2]	Englewood	98%	163
Community Hospital	Grand Junction	97%	29
The Medical Center of Aurora[2]	Aurora	97%	204
North Colorado Medical Center[2]	Greeley	97%	189
Poudre Valley Hospital	Fort Collins	97%	130
Univ of CO Health Mem Hosp	Colorado Spgs	97%	246
VA Eastern Colorado Healthcare System	Denver	97%	172
Arkansas Valley Regional Medical Center[2]	La Junta	96%	25
Centura Health - Saint Anthony Hospital	Lakewood	96%	148
Centura Health-St Mary Corwin Med Ctr	Pueblo	96%	93
Centura Health-Littleton Adventist Hosp	Littleton	95%	105
Centura Health-St Anthony North Hosp	Westminster	95%	141
Medical Center of the Rockies	Loveland	95%	129
Parkview Medical Center	Pueblo	95%	182
Longmont United Hospital	Longmont	94%	106
Montrose Memorial Hospital	Montrose	94%	47
Parker Adventist Hospital	Parker	92%	72
Denver Health Medical Center	Denver	91%	330
University of Colorado Hospital[2]	Aurora	91%	262
Saint Marys Hospital & Medical Center	Grand Junction	87%	117
Centura Health-Penrose St Francis	Colorado Spgs	83%	321
Boulder Community Hospital	Boulder	66%	111

Evaluation of LVS Function

Hospital Name	City	Rate	Cases
Boulder Community Hospital	Boulder	100%	150
Centura Health-Littleton Adventist Hosp	Littleton	100%	133
Centura Health-Porter Adventist Hosp	Denver	100%	139
Centura Health - Saint Anthony Hospital	Lakewood	100%	201
Centura Health-St Anthony North Hosp	Westminster	100%	166
Centura Health-St Mary Corwin Med Ctr	Pueblo	100%	116
Centura Health-St Thomas More Hosp	Canon City	100%	30
Colorado Plains Medical Center	Fort Morgan	100%	29
Community Hospital	Grand Junction	100%	42
Denver Health Medical Center	Denver	100%	348
Exempla Good Samaritan Medical Center	Lafayette	100%	285
Exempla Saint Joseph Hospital[2]	Denver	100%	334
Grand Junction VA Medical Center	Grand Junction	100%	31
McKee Medical Center[2]	Loveland	100%	84
Medical Center of the Rockies	Loveland	100%	148
Montrose Memorial Hospital	Montrose	100%	54
North Colorado Medical Center[2]	Greeley	100%	234
North Suburban Medical Center[2]	Thornton	100%	69
Parkview Medical Center	Pueblo	100%	219
Platte Valley Medical Center	Brighton	100%	69
Poudre Valley Hospital	Fort Collins	100%	171
Presbyterian Saint Lukes Medical Center	Denver	100%	82
Rose Medical Center	Denver	100%	153
Saint Marys Hospital & Medical Center	Grand Junction	100%	138
San Luis Valley Regional Medical Center	Alamosa	100%	34
Sky Ridge Medical Center	Lone Tree	100%	129
Southwest Memorial Hospital	Cortez	100%	25
Sterling Regional Medcenter	Sterling	100%	28
Swedish Medical Center[2]	Englewood	100%	235
Univ of CO Health Mem Hosp	Colorado Spgs	100%	314
University of Colorado Hospital[2]	Aurora	100%	296
VA Eastern Colorado Healthcare System	Denver	100%	183
Centura Health-Penrose St Francis	Colorado Spgs	99%	409
Exempla Lutheran Medical Center[2]	Wheat Ridge	99%	189
Longmont United Hospital	Longmont	99%	141
The Medical Center of Aurora[2]	Aurora	99%	269
Parker Adventist Hospital	Parker	99%	88
Delta County Memorial Hospital	Delta	98%	44
Mercy Regional Medical Center	Durango	98%	57
Arkansas Valley Regional Medical Center[2]	La Junta	95%	40
Heart of the Rockies Reg Med Ctr	Salida	84%	25

Medicare Spending

Medicare Spending per Patient (ratio)

Hospital Name	City	Ratio	Cases
Keefe Memorial Hospital	Cheyenne Wells	0.67	-
Saint Anthony Summit Medical Center	Frisco	0.84	-
Animas Surgical Hospital	Durango	0.89	-
Arkansas Valley Regional Medical Center	La Junta	0.89	-
Montrose Memorial Hospital	Montrose	0.90	-
Orthocolorado Hosp-St Anthony Med Camp	Lakewood	0.90	-
Yampa Valley Medical Center	Steamboat Spgs	0.90	-
Centura Health-St Thomas More Hosp	Canon City	0.91	-
Delta County Memorial Hospital	Delta	0.91	-
Sterling Regional Medcenter	Sterling	0.92	-
McKee Medical Center	Loveland	0.93	-
Valley View Hospital Association	Glenwood Spgs	0.93	-
Colorado Plains Medical Center	Fort Morgan	0.94	-
Denver Health Medical Center	Denver	0.94	-
Parkview Medical Center	Pueblo	0.94	-
Community Hospital	Grand Junction	0.95	-
Poudre Valley Hospital	Fort Collins	0.95	-
Saint Marys Hospital & Medical Center	Grand Junction	0.95	-
University of Colorado Hospital	Aurora	0.95	-
Parker Adventist Hospital	Parker	0.96	-
Vail Valley Medical Center	Vail	0.96	-
Exempla Saint Joseph Hospital	Denver	0.97	-
Longmont United Hospital	Longmont	0.97	-
Mercy Regional Medical Center	Durango	0.97	-
Rose Medical Center	Denver	0.97	-
Boulder Community Hospital	Boulder	0.98	-
Platte Valley Medical Center	Brighton	0.98	-
Centura Health-Avista Adventist Hosp	Louisville	0.99	-
Centura Health-Penrose St Francis	Colorado Spgs	0.99	-
Centura Health-Porter Adventist Hosp	Denver	0.99	-
Centura Health-St Anthony North Hosp	Westminster	0.99	-
North Colorado Medical Center	Greeley	0.99	-
Sky Ridge Medical Center	Lone Tree	0.99	-
Centura Health-St Mary Corwin Med Ctr	Pueblo	1.00	-
Exempla Good Samaritan Medical Center	Lafayette	1.00	-
Exempla Lutheran Medical Center	Wheat Ridge	1.00	-
Centura Health-Littleton Adventist Hosp	Littleton	1.01	-
Swedish Medical Center	Englewood	1.01	-
Centura Health - Saint Anthony Hospital	Lakewood	1.02	-
Medical Center of the Rockies	Loveland	1.02	-
Univ of CO Health Mem Hosp	Colorado Spgs	1.02	-
North Suburban Medical Center	Thornton	1.03	-
Presbyterian Saint Lukes Medical Center	Denver	1.03	-
The Medical Center of Aurora	Aurora	1.04	-
San Luis Valley Regional Medical Center	Alamosa	1.04	-

NOTE: Hospital profiles are in alphabetical order by state, then city, then hospital within the city; Rankings exclude hospitals with less than 25 cases except for patient surveys which excludes hospitals with less than 100 cases; (a) 100-299 cases; (1) The number of cases/patients is too few to report; (2) Data submitted were based on a sample of cases/patients; (3) Results are based on a shorter time period than required; (4) Data suppressed by CMS for one or more quarters; (5) Results are not available for this reporting period; (6) Fewer than 100 patients completed the HCAHPS survey; (7) No cases met the criteria for this measure; (8) The lower limit of the confidence interval cannot be calculated if the number of observed infections equals zero; (9) No data are available from the state/territory for this reporting period; (10) The scores shown reflect fewer than 50 completed surveys; (11) There were discrepancies in the data collection process; (12) This measure does not apply to this hospital for this reporting period; (13) Results cannot be calculated for this reporting period; (14) The results for this state are combined with nearby states to protect confidentiality; Please refer to the User's Guide for a full explanation of data.

Pneumonia Care

Appropriate Initial Antibiotic Given

Hospital Name	City	Rate	Cases
Centura Health - Saint Anthony Hospital[2]	Lakewood	100%	93
Exempla Lutheran Medical Center	Wheat Ridge	100%	192
North Suburban Medical Center[2]	Thornton	100%	72
Parker Adventist Hospital	Parker	100%	106
Platte Valley Medical Center	Brighton	100%	70
Rose Medical Center	Denver	100%	113
Centura Health-St Mary Corwin Med Ctr	Pueblo	99%	76
Exempla Good Samaritan Medical Center	Lafayette	99%	155
McKee Medical Center[2]	Loveland	99%	73
University of Colorado Hospital[2]	Aurora	99%	86
Community Hospital	Grand Junction	98%	63
The Medical Center of Aurora[2]	Aurora	98%	106
Poudre Valley Hospital[2]	Fort Collins	98%	120
Sky Ridge Medical Center[2]	Lone Tree	98%	88
Centura Health-Littleton Adventist Hosp	Littleton	97%	124
Centura Health-Penrose St Francis[2]	Colorado Spgs	97%	230
Centura Health-St Anthony North Hosp	Westminster	97%	149
Grand Junction VA Medical Center	Grand Junction	97%	29
Parkview Medical Center[2]	Pueblo	97%	70
Presbyterian Saint Lukes Medical Center	Denver	97%	37
Centura Health-Avista Adventist Hosp	Louisville	96%	57
Centura Health-Porter Adventist Hosp	Denver	96%	105
Montrose Memorial Hospital	Montrose	96%	54
Exempla Saint Joseph Hospital	Denver	95%	201
Saint Marys Hospital & Medical Center	Grand Junction	95%	132
Denver Health Medical Center[2]	Denver	94%	65
Longmont United Hospital	Longmont	94%	83
North Colorado Medical Center[2]	Greeley	94%	67
Swedish Medical Center[2]	Englewood	94%	65
Univ of CO Health Mem Hosp	Colorado Spgs	94%	265
Boulder Community Hospital	Boulder	92%	86
Medical Center of the Rockies[2]	Loveland	91%	76
Mercy Regional Medical Center	Durango	91%	45
San Luis Valley Regional Medical Center	Alamosa	89%	37
Delta County Memorial Hospital	Delta	88%	50
Centura Health-St Thomas More Hosp	Canon City	86%	43
VA Eastern Colorado Healthcare System	Denver	82%	33
Arkansas Valley Regional Medical Center[2]	La Junta	74%	105

Blood Culture Timing

Hospital Name	City	Rate	Cases
Centura Health-St Anthony North Hosp	Westminster	100%	114
Centura Health-St Mary Corwin Med Ctr	Pueblo	100%	114
East Morgan County Hospital	Brush	100%	25
Exempla Good Samaritan Medical Center	Lafayette	100%	291
Grand Junction VA Medical Center	Grand Junction	100%	38
McKee Medical Center[2]	Loveland	100%	131
The Medical Center of Aurora[2]	Aurora	100%	156
North Colorado Medical Center[2]	Greeley	100%	114
North Suburban Medical Center[2]	Thornton	100%	156
Presbyterian Saint Lukes Medical Center	Denver	100%	109
Rose Medical Center	Denver	100%	252
Swedish Medical Center[2]	Englewood	100%	103
VA Eastern Colorado Healthcare System	Denver	100%	54
Valley View Hospital Association	Glenwood Spgs	100%	41
Exempla Lutheran Medical Center	Wheat Ridge	99%	391
Longmont United Hospital	Longmont	99%	90
Medical Center of the Rockies[2]	Loveland	99%	158
Platte Valley Medical Center	Brighton	99%	109
Poudre Valley Hospital[2]	Fort Collins	99%	214
Sky Ridge Medical Center[2]	Lone Tree	99%	120
Centura Health-Penrose St Francis[2]	Colorado Spgs	98%	287
Centura Health-Porter Adventist Hosp	Denver	98%	175
Centura Health-St Thomas More Hosp	Canon City	98%	62
Exempla Saint Joseph Hospital	Denver	98%	369
Parker Adventist Hospital	Parker	98%	117
San Luis Valley Regional Medical Center	Alamosa	98%	47
Centura Health-Littleton Adventist Hosp	Littleton	97%	166
Colorado Plains Medical Center	Fort Morgan	97%	33
Grand River Medical Center	Rifle	97%	32
Parkview Medical Center[2]	Pueblo	97%	119
Southwest Memorial Hospital	Cortez	97%	39
Sterling Regional Medcenter	Sterling	97%	31
Univ of CO Health Mem Hosp	Colorado Spgs	97%	398
Centura Health - Saint Anthony Hospital[2]	Lakewood	96%	137
Mercy Regional Medical Center	Durango	96%	78
Saint Marys Hospital & Medical Center	Grand Junction	96%	224
Boulder Community Hospital	Boulder	95%	140
Community Hospital	Grand Junction	95%	81
Centura Health-Avista Adventist Hosp	Louisville	94%	63
Arkansas Valley Regional Medical Center[2]	La Junta	93%	107
Spanish Peaks Regional Health Center	Walsenburg	93%	29
Delta County Memorial Hospital	Delta	92%	65
University of Colorado Hospital[2]	Aurora	92%	145
Montrose Memorial Hospital	Montrose	89%	66
Denver Health Medical Center[2]	Denver	87%	39

Pregnancy and Delivery Care

Newborns whose Deliveries were Scheduled Early

Hospital Name	City	Rate	Cases
Arkansas Valley Regional Medical Center[2]	La Junta	0%	27
Denver Health Medical Center[2]	Denver	0%	50
Exempla Lutheran Medical Center	Wheat Ridge	0%	208
The Medical Center of Aurora[2]	Aurora	0%	49
Medical Center of the Rockies[2]	Loveland	0%	31
North Suburban Medical Center[2]	Thornton	0%	35
Sky Ridge Medical Center[2]	Lone Tree	0%	78
University of Colorado Hospital[2]	Aurora	0%	39
Valley View Hospital Association	Glenwood Spgs	0%	78
Exempla Saint Joseph Hospital	Denver	1%	265
Longmont United Hospital	Longmont	1%	106
Centura Health-Penrose St Francis[2]	Colorado Spgs	2%	43
Centura Health-St Mary Corwin Med Ctr	Pueblo	2%	58
Parkview Medical Center	Pueblo	2%	173
Platte Valley Medical Center	Brighton	2%	122
Rose Medical Center[2]	Denver	2%	43
Saint Marys Hospital & Medical Center	Grand Junction	2%	181
Swedish Medical Center[2]	Englewood	2%	53
Exempla Good Samaritan Medical Center	Lafayette	3%	157
North Colorado Medical Center[2]	Greeley	3%	32
Parker Adventist Hospital[2]	Parker	3%	32
Presbyterian Saint Lukes Medical Center[2]	Denver	3%	67
Univ of CO Health Mem Hosp[2]	Colorado Spgs	3%	154
Saint Anthony Summit Medical Center[2]	Frisco	4%	27
Vail Valley Medical Center	Vail	4%	48
Centura Health-Avista Adventist Hosp[2]	Louisville	5%	38
Boulder Community Hospital[2]	Boulder	6%	31
Mercy Regional Medical Center[2]	Durango	6%	33
Poudre Valley Hospital[2]	Fort Collins	6%	35
Montrose Memorial Hospital	Montrose	8%	37
San Luis Valley Regional Medical Center[2]	Alamosa	9%	45
Centura Health-Littleton Adventist Hosp[2]	Littleton	10%	42
McKee Medical Center[2]	Loveland	16%	32

Preventive Care

Immunization for Influenza

Hospital Name	City	Rate	Cases
Centura Health-Avista Adventist Hosp[2]	Louisville	99%	427
The Medical Center of Aurora[2]	Aurora	99%	590
North Suburban Medical Center[2]	Thornton	99%	499
Rose Medical Center[2]	Denver	99%	535
McKee Medical Center[2]	Loveland	98%	519
Valley View Hospital Association[2]	Glenwood Spgs	98%	243
Centura Health-St Mary Corwin Med Ctr[2]	Pueblo	97%	588
Colorado Plains Medical Center[2]	Fort Morgan	97%	210
North Colorado Medical Center[2]	Greeley	97%	497
Sky Ridge Medical Center[2]	Lone Tree	97%	574
Swedish Medical Center[2]	Englewood	97%	638
Centura Health-St Anthony North Hosp[2]	Westminster	96%	542
Montrose Memorial Hospital[2]	Montrose	96%	279
Sterling Regional Medcenter[2]	Sterling	96%	229
Vail Valley Medical Center[2]	Vail	96%	249
Centura Health-Littleton Adventist Hosp[2]	Littleton	95%	550
Centura Health-St Thomas More Hosp[2]	Canon City	95%	308
Presbyterian Saint Lukes Medical Center[2]	Denver	95%	528
Saint Marys Hospital & Medical Center	Grand Junction	95%	5869
Centura Health - Saint Anthony Hospital[2]	Lakewood	94%	644
Longmont United Hospital[2]	Longmont	94%	544
Univ of CO Health Mem Hosp[2]	Colorado Spgs	94%	764
Centura Health-Porter Adventist Hosp[2]	Denver	93%	632
Exempla Good Samaritan Medical Center[2]	Lafayette	93%	521
Saint Anthony Summit Medical Center[2]	Frisco	93%	283
Yampa Valley Medical Center[2]	Steamboat Spgs	93%	251
Parkview Medical Center[2]	Pueblo	92%	524
Platte Valley Medical Center[2]	Brighton	92%	312
Centura Health-Penrose St Francis[2]	Colorado Spgs	91%	590
Exempla Lutheran Medical Center[2]	Wheat Ridge	91%	487
Arkansas Valley Regional Medical Center[2]	La Junta	90%	252
Community Hospital[2]	Grand Junction	90%	329
Mercy Regional Medical Center[2]	Durango	90%	434
Exempla Saint Joseph Hospital[2]	Denver	89%	502
Parker Adventist Hospital[2]	Parker	88%	524
Boulder Community Hospital[2]	Boulder	87%	533
Poudre Valley Hospital[2]	Fort Collins	85%	529
Denver Health Medical Center[2]	Denver	84%	487
Keefe Memorial Hospital[2]	Cheyenne Wells	83%	30
Rio Grande Hospital[3]	Del Norte	83%	59
Medical Center of the Rockies[2]	Loveland	78%	579
Orthocolorado Hosp-St Anthony Med Camp[2]	Lakewood	78%	358
Yuma District Hospital	Yuma	71%	83
Delta County Memorial Hospital[2]	Delta	70%	328
San Luis Valley Regional Medical Center[2]	Alamosa	69%	261
University of Colorado Hospital[2]	Aurora	69%	513
Southwest Memorial Hospital[2,3]	Cortez	67%	132
Southeast Colorado Hospital[2]	Springfield	32%	34
Animas Surgical Hospital[2,3]	Durango	7%	82

Immunization for Pneumonia

Hospital Name	City	Rate	Cases
Centura Health-St Anthony North Hosp[2]	Westminster	99%	719
Rose Medical Center[2]	Denver	99%	497
The Medical Center of Aurora[2]	Aurora	98%	739
North Suburban Medical Center[2]	Thornton	98%	495
Centura Health-Littleton Adventist Hosp[2]	Littleton	97%	565
Centura Health-St Mary Corwin Med Ctr[2]	Pueblo	97%	748
Swedish Medical Center[2]	Englewood	97%	698
Yampa Valley Medical Center[2]	Steamboat Spgs	97%	184
Centura Health-Avista Adventist Hosp[2]	Louisville	96%	262
Centura Health-St Thomas More Hosp[2]	Canon City	96%	377
Sky Ridge Medical Center[2]	Lone Tree	96%	504
Colorado Plains Medical Center[2]	Fort Morgan	95%	154
Exempla Good Samaritan Medical Center[2]	Lafayette	95%	610
Montrose Memorial Hospital[2]	Montrose	95%	310
Platte Valley Medical Center[2]	Brighton	95%	283
Presbyterian Saint Lukes Medical Center[2]	Denver	95%	413
Saint Marys Hospital & Medical Center	Grand Junction	95%	5956
Sterling Regional Medcenter[2]	Sterling	95%	306
Valley View Hospital Association[2]	Glenwood Spgs	95%	198
Arkansas Valley Regional Medical Center[2]	La Junta	94%	316
McKee Medical Center[2]	Loveland	94%	619
North Colorado Medical Center[2]	Greeley	94%	582
Centura Health - Saint Anthony Hospital[2]	Lakewood	93%	805
Centura Health-Porter Adventist Hosp[2]	Denver	92%	822
Exempla Lutheran Medical Center[2]	Wheat Ridge	92%	534
Exempla Saint Joseph Hospital[2]	Denver	92%	560
Longmont United Hospital[2]	Longmont	92%	624
Univ of CO Health Mem Hosp[2]	Colorado Spgs	92%	704
Centura Health-Penrose St Francis[2]	Colorado Spgs	91%	699
Vail Valley Medical Center[2]	Vail	91%	153
Boulder Community Hospital[2]	Boulder	89%	534
Community Hospital[2]	Grand Junction	89%	445
Mercy Regional Medical Center[2]	Durango	88%	421
Poudre Valley Hospital[2]	Fort Collins	87%	549
Aspen Valley Hospital[2,3]	Aspen	86%	74
Denver Health Medical Center[2]	Denver	86%	436
Parker Adventist Hospital[2]	Parker	86%	475
Parkview Medical Center[2]	Pueblo	85%	594
Orthocolorado Hosp-St Anthony Med Camp[2]	Lakewood	84%	456
Medical Center of the Rockies[2]	Loveland	79%	707
Yuma District Hospital	Yuma	77%	159
Rio Grande Hospital[3]	Del Norte	76%	123
Southeast Colorado Hospital[2]	Springfield	76%	62
Saint Anthony Summit Medical Center[2]	Frisco	75%	131
Southwest Memorial Hospital[2,3]	Cortez	74%	232
University of Colorado Hospital[2]	Aurora	74%	494
Delta County Memorial Hospital[2]	Delta	73%	452
Keefe Memorial Hospital[2]	Cheyenne Wells	73%	44
San Luis Valley Regional Medical Center[2]	Alamosa	70%	196
Animas Surgical Hospital[2,3]	Durango	55%	202

Stroke Care

Anticoagulation Therapy for Atrial Fibrillation

Hospital Name	City	Rate	Cases
Centura Health - Saint Anthony Hospital	Lakewood	100%	35
Exempla Lutheran Medical Center	Wheat Ridge	100%	33
Swedish Medical Center[2]	Englewood	97%	31
Saint Marys Hospital & Medical Center	Grand Junction	96%	25

Antithrombotic Therapy Timing

Hospital Name	City	Rate	Cases
Boulder Community Hospital	Boulder	100%	65
Centura Health-Littleton Adventist Hosp	Littleton	100%	84
Centura Health-Porter Adventist Hosp	Denver	100%	35
Centura Health-St Mary Corwin Med Ctr	Pueblo	100%	59
Mercy Regional Medical Center	Durango	100%	25
North Suburban Medical Center[2]	Thornton	100%	38
Parker Adventist Hospital	Parker	100%	43
Parkview Medical Center	Pueblo	100%	115
Platte Valley Medical Center	Brighton	100%	25
Poudre Valley Hospital	Fort Collins	100%	47
Presbyterian Saint Lukes Medical Center[2]	Denver	100%	25
Saint Marys Hospital & Medical Center	Grand Junction	100%	89
Sky Ridge Medical Center[2]	Lone Tree	100%	46
University of Colorado Hospital[2]	Aurora	100%	50
Exempla Good Samaritan Medical Center	Lafayette	99%	91
Exempla Saint Joseph Hospital	Denver	99%	89
The Medical Center of Aurora[2]	Aurora	99%	73
North Colorado Medical Center	Greeley	99%	75
Centura Health - Saint Anthony Hospital	Lakewood	98%	132
Centura Health-St Anthony North Hosp	Westminster	98%	41
McKee Medical Center	Loveland	98%	44
Medical Center of the Rockies	Loveland	98%	47
Rose Medical Center[2]	Denver	98%	58

NOTE: Hospital profiles are in alphabetical order by state, then city, then hospital within the city; Rankings exclude hospitals with less than 25 cases except for patient surveys which excludes hospitals with less than 100 cases; (a) 100-299 cases; (1) The number of cases/patients is too few to report; (2) Data submitted were based on a sample of cases/patients; (3) Results are based on a shorter time period than required; (4) Data suppressed by CMS for one or more quarters; (5) Results are not available for this reporting period; (6) Fewer than 100 patients completed the HCAHPS survey; (7) No cases met the criteria for this measure; (8) The lower limit of the confidence interval cannot be calculated if the number of observed infections equals zero; (9) No data are available from the state/territory for this reporting period; (10) The scores shown reflect fewer than 50 completed surveys; (11) There were discrepancies in the data collection process; (12) This measure does not apply to this hospital for this reporting period; (13) Results cannot be calculated for this reporting period; (14) The results for this state are combined with nearby states to protect confidentiality; Please refer to the User's Guide for a full explanation of data.

Swedish Medical Center[2]	Englewood	98%	88
Univ of CO Health Mem Hosp	Colorado Spgs	97%	157
Centura Health-Penrose St Francis[2]	Colorado Spgs	96%	78
Exempla Lutheran Medical Center	Wheat Ridge	96%	104
Denver Health Medical Center	Denver	95%	65
Longmont United Hospital	Longmont	95%	59

Assessed for Rehabilitation

Hospital Name	City	Rate	Cases
Centura Health-St Anthony North Hosp	Westminster	100%	42
Centura Health-St Mary Corwin Med Ctr	Pueblo	100%	83
McKee Medical Center	Loveland	100%	60
The Medical Center of Aurora[2]	Aurora	100%	97
Medical Center of the Rockies	Loveland	100%	66
Mercy Regional Medical Center	Durango	100%	26
Montrose Memorial Hospital	Montrose	100%	28
North Suburban Medical Center[2]	Thornton	100%	38
Platte Valley Medical Center	Brighton	100%	33
Presbyterian Saint Lukes Medical Center[2]	Denver	100%	28
Saint Marys Hospital & Medical Center	Grand Junction	100%	133
Sky Ridge Medical Center[2]	Lone Tree	100%	59
Centura Health - Saint Anthony Hospital	Lakewood	99%	268
Exempla Good Samaritan Medical Center	Lafayette	99%	146
Exempla Lutheran Medical Center	Wheat Ridge	99%	158
Poudre Valley Hospital	Fort Collins	99%	84
Rose Medical Center[2]	Denver	99%	82
Swedish Medical Center[2]	Englewood	99%	146
Univ of CO Health Mem Hosp	Colorado Spgs	99%	203
University of Colorado Hospital[2]	Aurora	99%	131
Centura Health-Littleton Adventist Hosp	Littleton	98%	142
Centura Health-Porter Adventist Hosp	Denver	98%	40
Parker Adventist Hospital	Parker	98%	65
Boulder Community Hospital	Boulder	97%	91
Exempla Saint Joseph Hospital	Denver	97%	118
Longmont United Hospital	Longmont	97%	65
Parkview Medical Center	Pueblo	97%	134
Centura Health-Penrose St Francis[2]	Colorado Spgs	96%	105
North Colorado Medical Center	Greeley	92%	87
Denver Health Medical Center	Denver	90%	86

Discharged on Antithrombotic Therapy

Hospital Name	City	Rate	Cases
Boulder Community Hospital	Boulder	100%	78
Centura Health-Penrose St Francis[2]	Colorado Spgs	100%	85
Centura Health-Porter Adventist Hosp	Denver	100%	40
Centura Health-St Anthony North Hosp	Westminster	100%	41
Denver Health Medical Center	Denver	100%	78
Exempla Good Samaritan Medical Center	Lafayette	100%	131
Exempla Lutheran Medical Center	Wheat Ridge	100%	134
Exempla Saint Joseph Hospital	Denver	100%	108
The Medical Center of Aurora[2]	Aurora	100%	87
Medical Center of the Rockies	Loveland	100%	54
Mercy Regional Medical Center	Durango	100%	25
Montrose Memorial Hospital	Montrose	100%	27
North Colorado Medical Center	Greeley	100%	77
North Suburban Medical Center[2]	Thornton	100%	36
Parker Adventist Hospital	Parker	100%	59
Platte Valley Medical Center	Brighton	100%	33
Poudre Valley Hospital	Fort Collins	100%	69
Presbyterian Saint Lukes Medical Center[2]	Denver	100%	26
Rose Medical Center[2]	Denver	100%	73
Saint Marys Hospital & Medical Center	Grand Junction	100%	117
Sky Ridge Medical Center[2]	Lone Tree	100%	52
University of Colorado Hospital[2]	Aurora	100%	80
Centura Health-Littleton Adventist Hosp	Littleton	99%	110
Centura Health - Saint Anthony Hospital	Lakewood	99%	197
Centura Health-St Mary Corwin Med Ctr	Pueblo	99%	70
Swedish Medical Center[2]	Englewood	99%	124
Univ of CO Health Mem Hosp	Colorado Spgs	99%	176
Longmont United Hospital	Longmont	98%	60
McKee Medical Center	Loveland	98%	58
Parkview Medical Center	Pueblo	98%	125

Discharged on Statin Medication

Hospital Name	City	Rate	Cases
Centura Health-Porter Adventist Hosp	Denver	100%	25
The Medical Center of Aurora[2]	Aurora	100%	60
North Suburban Medical Center[2]	Thornton	100%	25
Platte Valley Medical Center	Brighton	100%	26
Sky Ridge Medical Center[2]	Lone Tree	100%	41
University of Colorado Hospital[2]	Aurora	100%	45
Centura Health-Littleton Adventist Hosp	Littleton	99%	83
Exempla Good Samaritan Medical Center	Lafayette	99%	98
Saint Marys Hospital & Medical Center	Grand Junction	99%	83
Rose Medical Center[2]	Denver	98%	53
Exempla Lutheran Medical Center	Wheat Ridge	97%	103
Boulder Community Hospital	Boulder	96%	47
Poudre Valley Hospital	Fort Collins	96%	48
Univ of CO Health Mem Hosp	Colorado Spgs	96%	124
Exempla Saint Joseph Hospital	Denver	95%	91
Medical Center of the Rockies	Loveland	95%	40
North Colorado Medical Center	Greeley	95%	59
Parker Adventist Hospital	Parker	95%	42
Centura Health - Saint Anthony Hospital	Lakewood	93%	123
Centura Health-St Anthony North Hosp	Westminster	93%	29
Centura Health-St Mary Corwin Med Ctr	Pueblo	93%	43
Parkview Medical Center	Pueblo	93%	86
Swedish Medical Center[2]	Englewood	93%	95
Centura Health-Penrose St Francis[2]	Colorado Spgs	92%	65
Denver Health Medical Center	Denver	90%	59
McKee Medical Center	Loveland	90%	48
Longmont United Hospital	Longmont	72%	47

Thrombolytic Therapy Timing

Hospital Name	City	Rate	Cases
Centura Health - Saint Anthony Hospital	Lakewood	40%	50

Venous Thromboembolism (VTE) Prophylaxis

Hospital Name	City	Rate	Cases
Centura Health-Littleton Adventist Hosp	Littleton	100%	141
The Medical Center of Aurora[2]	Aurora	100%	98
North Suburban Medical Center[2]	Thornton	100%	34
Parker Adventist Hospital	Parker	100%	56
Presbyterian Saint Lukes Medical Center[2]	Denver	100%	25
Rose Medical Center[2]	Denver	100%	75
Saint Marys Hospital & Medical Center	Grand Junction	100%	138
Sky Ridge Medical Center[2]	Lone Tree	100%	59
Exempla Good Samaritan Medical Center	Lafayette	99%	119
Swedish Medical Center[2]	Englewood	99%	142
Univ of CO Health Mem Hosp	Colorado Spgs	99%	224
Centura Health - Saint Anthony Hospital	Lakewood	98%	274
McKee Medical Center	Loveland	98%	46
Centura Health-St Anthony North Hosp	Westminster	97%	39
Centura Health-St Mary Corwin Med Ctr	Pueblo	97%	90
Exempla Lutheran Medical Center	Wheat Ridge	97%	156
Platte Valley Medical Center	Brighton	97%	30
University of Colorado Hospital[2]	Aurora	97%	135
Centura Health-Penrose St Francis[2]	Colorado Spgs	96%	105
Mercy Regional Medical Center	Durango	96%	26
Boulder Community Hospital	Boulder	95%	87
Centura Health-Porter Adventist Hosp	Denver	95%	42
Parkview Medical Center	Pueblo	94%	139
Exempla Saint Joseph Hospital	Denver	92%	101
Medical Center of the Rockies	Loveland	92%	65
North Colorado Medical Center	Greeley	90%	93
Poudre Valley Hospital	Fort Collins	89%	74
Denver Health Medical Center	Denver	87%	86
Longmont United Hospital	Longmont	77%	78

Written Stroke Educational Materials Given

Hospital Name	City	Rate	Cases
Parkview Medical Center	Pueblo	99%	85
Centura Health - Saint Anthony Hospital	Lakewood	97%	141
Centura Health-St Mary Corwin Med Ctr	Pueblo	97%	37
Exempla Good Samaritan Medical Center	Lafayette	96%	85
Poudre Valley Hospital	Fort Collins	96%	55
Rose Medical Center[2]	Denver	96%	47
Saint Marys Hospital & Medical Center	Grand Junction	96%	76
Univ of CO Health Mem Hosp	Colorado Spgs	96%	107
University of Colorado Hospital[2]	Aurora	96%	80
Exempla Lutheran Medical Center	Wheat Ridge	93%	81
The Medical Center of Aurora[2]	Aurora	93%	59
Sky Ridge Medical Center[2]	Lone Tree	93%	30
Centura Health-Penrose St Francis[2]	Colorado Spgs	89%	62
North Colorado Medical Center	Greeley	89%	46
Swedish Medical Center[2]	Englewood	89%	87
Exempla Saint Joseph Hospital	Denver	81%	75
Medical Center of the Rockies	Loveland	81%	32
Denver Health Medical Center	Denver	80%	51
Longmont United Hospital	Longmont	76%	37
Boulder Community Hospital	Boulder	73%	45
McKee Medical Center	Loveland	70%	33
Parker Adventist Hospital	Parker	67%	39
Centura Health-Littleton Adventist Hosp	Littleton	62%	58

Surgical Care Improvement Project

Appropriate Beta Blocker Usage

Hospital Name	City	Rate	Cases
Centura Health-Avista Adventist Hosp	Louisville	100%	67
Centura Health-St Anthony North Hosp	Westminster	100%	74
Denver Health Medical Center[2]	Denver	100%	48
Exempla Good Samaritan Medical Center[2]	Lafayette	100%	197
Exempla Lutheran Medical Center[2]	Wheat Ridge	100%	138
Medical Center of the Rockies[2]	Loveland	100%	209
North Suburban Medical Center[2]	Thornton	100%	53
Platte Valley Medical Center	Brighton	100%	39
Poudre Valley Hospital[2]	Fort Collins	100%	93
Presbyterian Saint Lukes Medical Center[2]	Denver	100%	127
Rose Medical Center[2]	Denver	100%	130
Sky Ridge Medical Center[2]	Lone Tree	100%	119
Swedish Medical Center[2]	Englewood	100%	165
Exempla Saint Joseph Hospital[2]	Denver	99%	265
The Medical Center of Aurora[2]	Aurora	99%	158
Saint Marys Hospital & Medical Center	Grand Junction	99%	387
Univ of CO Health Mem Hosp[2]	Colorado Spgs	99%	297
Centura Health-Littleton Adventist Hosp[2]	Littleton	98%	113
Centura Health-Penrose St Francis[2]	Colorado Spgs	98%	272
Centura Health-Porter Adventist Hosp[2]	Denver	98%	187
Centura Health-St Mary Corwin Med Ctr	Pueblo	98%	113
Community Hospital	Grand Junction	98%	48
Delta County Memorial Hospital	Delta	98%	43
McKee Medical Center[2]	Loveland	98%	82
Parker Adventist Hospital	Parker	98%	126
Centura Health - Saint Anthony Hospital[2]	Lakewood	97%	170
Mercy Regional Medical Center	Durango	97%	70
Montrose Memorial Hospital[2]	Montrose	97%	67
North Colorado Medical Center[2]	Greeley	97%	154
Parkview Medical Center[2]	Pueblo	97%	146
University of Colorado Hospital[2]	Aurora	97%	152
Vail Valley Medical Center	Vail	97%	29
Longmont United Hospital	Longmont	96%	121
Orthocolorado Hosp-St Anthony Med Camp[2]	Lakewood	96%	82
Boulder Community Hospital[2]	Boulder	95%	115
Centura Health-St Thomas More Hosp	Canon City	95%	39
Valley View Hospital Association	Glenwood Spgs	95%	37
VA Eastern Colorado Healthcare System[2]	Denver	94%	108
Colorado Plains Medical Center	Fort Morgan	93%	27
Animas Surgical Hospital[2]	Durango	90%	42

Appropriate VTP Within 24 Hours

Hospital Name	City	Rate	Cases
Animas Surgical Hospital[2]	Durango	100%	235
Arkansas Valley Regional Medical Center[2]	La Junta	100%	44
Aspen Valley Hospital[3]	Aspen	100%	100
Exempla Good Samaritan Medical Center[2]	Lafayette	100%	577
Exempla Lutheran Medical Center[2]	Wheat Ridge	100%	257
Exempla Saint Joseph Hospital[2]	Denver	100%	372
Grand Junction VA Medical Center[2]	Grand Junction	100%	56
North Suburban Medical Center[2]	Thornton	100%	280
Orthocolorado Hosp-St Anthony Med Camp[2]	Lakewood	100%	308
Pikes Peak Regional Hospital	Woodland Park	100%	44
Rose Medical Center[2]	Denver	100%	441
Sky Ridge Medical Center[2]	Lone Tree	100%	443
University of Colorado Hospital[2]	Aurora	100%	338
Centura Health-Littleton Adventist Hosp[2]	Littleton	99%	418
Centura Health-Penrose St Francis[2]	Colorado Spgs	99%	683
Centura Health-St Thomas More Hosp	Canon City	99%	195
Colorado Plains Medical Center	Fort Morgan	99%	124
Community Hospital	Grand Junction	99%	228
The Medical Center of Aurora[2]	Aurora	99%	434
North Colorado Medical Center[2]	Greeley	99%	348
Parker Adventist Hospital	Parker	99%	449
Presbyterian Saint Lukes Medical Center[2]	Denver	99%	361
Saint Marys Hospital & Medical Center	Grand Junction	99%	1089
San Luis Valley Regional Medical Center	Alamosa	99%	103
Southwest Memorial Hospital	Cortez	99%	72
Swedish Medical Center[2]	Englewood	99%	516
Centura Health - Saint Anthony Hospital[2]	Lakewood	98%	337
Centura Health-St Mary Corwin Med Ctr	Pueblo	98%	454
Denver Health Medical Center[2]	Denver	98%	276
Longmont United Hospital	Longmont	98%	538
Mercy Regional Medical Center	Durango	98%	325
Montrose Memorial Hospital[2]	Montrose	98%	274
Univ of CO Health Mem Hosp[2]	Colorado Spgs	98%	970
Centura Health-Avista Adventist Hosp	Louisville	97%	227
McKee Medical Center[2]	Loveland	97%	287
Medical Center of the Rockies[2]	Loveland	97%	345
Vail Valley Medical Center	Vail	97%	178
Valley View Hospital Association	Glenwood Spgs	97%	178
Yampa Valley Medical Center[2]	Steamboat Spgs	97%	140
Centura Health-Porter Adventist Hosp[2]	Denver	96%	353
Centura Health-St Anthony North Hosp	Westminster	96%	297
Delta County Memorial Hospital	Delta	96%	188
Platte Valley Medical Center	Brighton	96%	157
VA Eastern Colorado Healthcare System[2]	Denver	96%	215
The Memorial Hospital	Craig	95%	38
Parkview Medical Center[2]	Pueblo	95%	397
Boulder Community Hospital[2]	Boulder	94%	284
Poudre Valley Hospital[2]	Fort Collins	94%	420
Saint Anthony Summit Medical Center	Frisco	92%	48
Sterling Regional Medcenter	Sterling	92%	78

Controlled Postoperative Blood Glucose

Hospital Name	City	Rate	Cases
Presbyterian Saint Lukes Medical Center[2]	Denver	100%	37
Exempla Saint Joseph Hospital[2]	Denver	99%	137
The Medical Center of Aurora[2]	Aurora	99%	75
North Colorado Medical Center[2]	Greeley	99%	92

NOTE: Hospital profiles are in alphabetical order by state, then city, then hospital within the city; Rankings exclude hospitals with less than 25 cases except for patient surveys which excludes hospitals with less than 100 cases; (a) 100-299 cases; (1) The number of cases/patients is too few to report; (2) Data submitted were based on a sample of cases/patients; (3) Results are based on a shorter time period than required; (4) Data suppressed by CMS for one or more quarters; (5) Results are not available for this reporting period; (6) Fewer than 100 patients completed the HCAHPS survey; (7) No cases met the criteria for this measure; (8) The lower limit of the confidence interval cannot be calculated if the number of observed infections equals zero; (9) No data are available from the state/territory for this reporting period; (10) The scores shown reflect fewer than 50 completed surveys; (11) There were discrepancies in the data collection process; (12) This measure does not apply to this hospital for this reporting period; (13) Results cannot be calculated for this reporting period; (14) The results for this state are combined with nearby states to protect confidentiality; Please refer to the User's Guide for a full explanation of data.

Hospital Name	City	Rate	Cases
Saint Marys Hospital & Medical Center	Grand Junction	99%	141
Univ of CO Health Mem Hosp[2]	Colorado Spgs	99%	199
Exempla Lutheran Medical Center[2]	Wheat Ridge	98%	106
VA Eastern Colorado Healthcare System[2]	Denver	98%	61
Medical Center of the Rockies[2]	Loveland	97%	211
Centura Health-Porter Adventist Hosp[2]	Denver	95%	182
Centura Health - Saint Anthony Hospital[2]	Lakewood	95%	104
Swedish Medical Center[2]	Englewood	94%	69
Centura Health-Penrose St Francis[2]	Colorado Spgs	93%	250
Boulder Community Hospital[2]	Boulder	92%	106
Sky Ridge Medical Center[2]	Lone Tree	91%	33
Parkview Medical Center[2]	Pueblo	90%	51
University of Colorado Hospital[2]	Aurora	90%	136

Perioperative Temperature Management

Hospital Name	City	Rate	Cases
Arkansas Valley Regional Medical Center[2]	La Junta	100%	45
Aspen Valley Hospital[3]	Aspen	100%	123
Boulder Community Hospital[2]	Boulder	100%	366
Centura Health-Littleton Adventist Hosp[2]	Littleton	100%	470
Centura Health-Penrose St Francis[2]	Colorado Spgs	100%	818
Centura Health-Porter Adventist Hosp[2]	Denver	100%	435
Centura Health - Saint Anthony Hospital[2]	Lakewood	100%	420
Centura Health-St Anthony North Hosp	Westminster	100%	327
Centura Health-St Mary Corwin Med Ctr	Pueblo	100%	493
Centura Health-St Thomas More Hosp	Canon City	100%	213
Colorado Plains Medical Center	Fort Morgan	100%	142
Community Hospital	Grand Junction	100%	240
Delta County Memorial Hospital	Delta	100%	234
Exempla Good Samaritan Medical Center[2]	Lafayette	100%	628
Exempla Lutheran Medical Center[2]	Wheat Ridge	100%	330
Exempla Saint Joseph Hospital[2]	Denver	100%	455
Grand Junction VA Medical Center[2]	Grand Junction	100%	60
Grand River Medical Center[3]	Rifle	100%	31
Longmont United Hospital	Longmont	100%	612
McKee Medical Center[2]	Loveland	100%	332
The Medical Center of Aurora[2]	Aurora	100%	487
Medical Center of the Rockies[2]	Loveland	100%	454
Mercy Regional Medical Center	Durango	100%	358
North Colorado Medical Center[2]	Greeley	100%	401
North Suburban Medical Center[2]	Thornton	100%	310
Orthocolorado Hosp-St Anthony Med Camp[2]	Lakewood	100%	352
Parker Adventist Hospital	Parker	100%	656
Parkview Medical Center[2]	Pueblo	100%	437
Pikes Peak Regional Hospital	Woodland Park	100%	48
Platte Valley Medical Center	Brighton	100%	169
Poudre Valley Hospital[2]	Fort Collins	100%	464
Presbyterian Saint Lukes Medical Center[2]	Denver	100%	500
Rose Medical Center[2]	Denver	100%	556
Saint Anthony Summit Medical Center	Frisco	100%	54
Saint Marys Hospital & Medical Center	Grand Junction	100%	1306
San Luis Valley Regional Medical Center	Alamosa	100%	128
Sky Ridge Medical Center[2]	Lone Tree	100%	568
Southwest Memorial Hospital	Cortez	100%	91
Sterling Regional Medcenter	Sterling	100%	85
Swedish Medical Center[2]	Englewood	100%	627
Univ of CO Health Mem Hosp[2]	Colorado Spgs	100%	1153
University of Colorado Hospital[2]	Aurora	100%	458
VA Eastern Colorado Healthcare System[2]	Denver	100%	253
Valley View Hospital Association	Glenwood Spgs	100%	198
Wray Community District Hospital	Wray	100%	26
Yampa Valley Medical Center[2]	Steamboat Spgs	100%	155
Centura Health-Avista Adventist Hosp	Louisville	99%	341
Montrose Memorial Hospital[2]	Montrose	99%	300
Vail Valley Medical Center	Vail	99%	183
The Memorial Hospital	Craig	98%	47
Denver Health Medical Center[2]	Denver	97%	341
Animas Surgical Hospital[2]	Durango	25%	281

Prophylactic Antibiotic Selection

Hospital Name	City	Rate	Cases
Centura Health-Avista Adventist Hosp	Louisville	100%	247
Centura Health-Penrose St Francis[2]	Colorado Spgs	100%	764
Centura Health-St Mary Corwin Med Ctr	Pueblo	100%	312
Denver Health Medical Center[2]	Denver	100%	220
Exempla Good Samaritan Medical Center[2]	Lafayette	100%	457
Exempla Lutheran Medical Center[2]	Wheat Ridge	100%	296
Exempla Saint Joseph Hospital[2]	Denver	100%	446
Grand Junction VA Medical Center	Grand Junction	100%	54
McKee Medical Center[2]	Loveland	100%	216
The Medical Center of Aurora[2]	Aurora	100%	335
Montrose Memorial Hospital[2]	Montrose	100%	213
North Suburban Medical Center[2]	Thornton	100%	180
Orthocolorado Hosp-St Anthony Med Camp[2]	Lakewood	100%	267
Poudre Valley Hospital[2]	Fort Collins	100%	284
Presbyterian Saint Lukes Medical Center[2]	Denver	100%	326
Rose Medical Center[2]	Denver	100%	415
Saint Marys Hospital & Medical Center	Grand Junction	100%	852
Sky Ridge Medical Center[2]	Lone Tree	100%	386
Swedish Medical Center[2]	Englewood	100%	414
Animas Surgical Hospital[2]	Durango	99%	254
Centura Health-Littleton Adventist Hosp[2]	Littleton	99%	301
Centura Health-Porter Adventist Hosp[2]	Denver	99%	441
Centura Health - Saint Anthony Hospital[2]	Lakewood	99%	349
Colorado Plains Medical Center	Fort Morgan	99%	113
Medical Center of the Rockies[2]	Loveland	99%	434
Mercy Regional Medical Center	Durango	99%	272
North Colorado Medical Center[2]	Greeley	99%	318
Parker Adventist Hospital	Parker	99%	349
Parkview Medical Center[2]	Pueblo	99%	326
Univ of CO Health Mem Hosp[2]	Colorado Spgs	99%	901
University of Colorado Hospital[2]	Aurora	99%	397
VA Eastern Colorado Healthcare System	Denver	99%	188
Vail Valley Medical Center	Vail	99%	150
Valley View Hospital Association	Glenwood Spgs	99%	128
Yampa Valley Medical Center[2]	Steamboat Spgs	99%	111
Aspen Valley Hospital[3]	Aspen	98%	108
Centura Health-St Thomas More Hosp	Canon City	98%	138
Longmont United Hospital	Longmont	98%	375
Pikes Peak Regional Hospital	Woodland Park	98%	40
Platte Valley Medical Center	Brighton	98%	116
Saint Anthony Summit Medical Center	Frisco	98%	40
San Luis Valley Regional Medical Center	Alamosa	98%	98
Sterling Regional Medcenter	Sterling	98%	57
Centura Health-St Anthony North Hosp	Westminster	97%	177
Community Hospital	Grand Junction	97%	186
The Memorial Hospital	Craig	97%	38
Southwest Memorial Hospital	Cortez	97%	67
Boulder Community Hospital[2]	Boulder	96%	311
Delta County Memorial Hospital	Delta	96%	158
Arkansas Valley Regional Medical Center[2]	La Junta	87%	30

Prophylactic Antibiotic Selection (Outpatient)

Hospital Name	City	Rate	Cases
Animas Surgical Hospital	Durango	100%	29
Centura Health-Avista Adventist Hosp	Louisville	100%	129
Centura Health - Saint Anthony Hospital	Lakewood	100%	264
The Medical Center of Aurora	Aurora	100%	308
North Suburban Medical Center	Thornton	100%	178
Orthocolorado Hosp-St Anthony Med Camp	Lakewood	100%	174
Platte Valley Medical Center	Brighton	100%	82
Saint Anthony Summit Medical Center	Frisco	100%	48
Swedish Medical Center	Englewood	100%	440
Exempla Good Samaritan Medical Center	Lafayette	99%	365
Exempla Lutheran Medical Center	Wheat Ridge	99%	533
Exempla Saint Joseph Hospital	Denver	99%	680
Medical Center of the Rockies	Loveland	99%	367
Mercy Regional Medical Center	Durango	99%	182
North Colorado Medical Center	Greeley	99%	428
Rose Medical Center	Denver	99%	609
Sky Ridge Medical Center	Lone Tree	99%	561
Valley View Hospital Association	Glenwood Spgs	99%	150
Boulder Community Hospital	Boulder	98%	274
Centura Health-Porter Adventist Hosp	Denver	98%	434
Centura Health-St Anthony North Hosp	Westminster	98%	84
Longmont United Hospital	Longmont	98%	224
McKee Medical Center	Loveland	98%	110
Parkview Medical Center	Pueblo	98%	483
Poudre Valley Hospital	Fort Collins	98%	444
Presbyterian Saint Lukes Medical Center	Denver	98%	265
University of Colorado Hospital	Aurora	98%	288
Vail Valley Medical Center	Vail	98%	132
Yampa Valley Medical Center	Steamboat Spgs	98%	113
Centura Health-Penrose St Francis	Colorado Spgs	97%	814
Centura Health-St Mary Corwin Med Ctr	Pueblo	97%	224
Centura Health-St Thomas More Hosp	Canon City	97%	39
Denver Health Medical Center	Denver	97%	339
Parker Adventist Hospital	Parker	97%	337
Saint Marys Hospital & Medical Center	Grand Junction	97%	548
Centura Health-Littleton Adventist Hosp	Littleton	96%	368
Delta County Memorial Hospital	Delta	96%	28
Montrose Memorial Hospital	Montrose	95%	153
Univ of CO Health Mem Hosp	Colorado Spgs	95%	1180
Community Hospital	Grand Junction	93%	117

Prophylactic Antibiotic Stopped

Hospital Name	City	Rate	Cases
Animas Surgical Hospital[2]	Durango	100%	254
Arkansas Valley Regional Medical Center[2]	La Junta	100%	28
Centura Health-Avista Adventist Hosp	Louisville	100%	243
Centura Health-St Mary Corwin Med Ctr	Pueblo	100%	305
Exempla Good Samaritan Medical Center[2]	Lafayette	100%	452
Grand Junction VA Medical Center	Grand Junction	100%	54
North Suburban Medical Center[2]	Thornton	100%	171
Orthocolorado Hosp-St Anthony Med Camp[2]	Lakewood	100%	266
Platte Valley Medical Center	Brighton	100%	116
Presbyterian Saint Lukes Medical Center[2]	Denver	100%	315
Rose Medical Center[2]	Denver	100%	398
Saint Anthony Summit Medical Center	Frisco	100%	40
San Luis Valley Regional Medical Center	Alamosa	100%	98
Sky Ridge Medical Center[2]	Lone Tree	100%	375
Southwest Memorial Hospital	Cortez	100%	66
Yampa Valley Medical Center[2]	Steamboat Spgs	100%	111
Exempla Saint Joseph Hospital[2]	Denver	99%	440
Mercy Regional Medical Center	Durango	99%	271
Montrose Memorial Hospital[2]	Montrose	99%	212
North Colorado Medical Center[2]	Greeley	99%	309
Parker Adventist Hospital	Parker	99%	341
Poudre Valley Hospital[2]	Fort Collins	99%	282
Swedish Medical Center[2]	Englewood	99%	398
Univ of CO Health Mem Hosp[2]	Colorado Spgs	99%	894
Centura Health-Littleton Adventist Hosp[2]	Littleton	98%	291
Exempla Lutheran Medical Center[2]	Wheat Ridge	98%	285
Longmont United Hospital	Longmont	98%	370
McKee Medical Center[2]	Loveland	98%	212
Saint Marys Hospital & Medical Center	Grand Junction	98%	827
Centura Health-Penrose St Francis[2]	Colorado Spgs	97%	743
Centura Health-Porter Adventist Hosp[2]	Denver	97%	437
Centura Health - Saint Anthony Hospital[2]	Lakewood	97%	336
Centura Health-St Anthony North Hosp	Westminster	97%	169
Colorado Plains Medical Center	Fort Morgan	97%	109
Delta County Memorial Hospital	Delta	97%	153
The Medical Center of Aurora[2]	Aurora	97%	313
VA Eastern Colorado Healthcare System	Denver	97%	187
Vail Valley Medical Center	Vail	97%	149
Valley View Hospital Association	Glenwood Spgs	97%	126
Aspen Valley Hospital[3]	Aspen	96%	107
Boulder Community Hospital[2]	Boulder	96%	305
Medical Center of the Rockies[2]	Loveland	96%	426
Sterling Regional Medcenter	Sterling	96%	55
University of Colorado Hospital[2]	Aurora	96%	381
Centura Health-St Thomas More Hosp	Canon City	95%	135
Parkview Medical Center[2]	Pueblo	95%	311
Pikes Peak Regional Hospital	Woodland Park	95%	38
Community Hospital	Grand Junction	94%	181
Denver Health Medical Center[2]	Denver	94%	212
The Memorial Hospital	Craig	92%	37

Prophylactic Antibiotic Timing

Hospital Name	City	Rate	Cases
Centura Health-Porter Adventist Hosp[2]	Denver	100%	441
Centura Health-St Mary Corwin Med Ctr	Pueblo	100%	312
Centura Health-St Thomas More Hosp	Canon City	100%	138
Colorado Plains Medical Center	Fort Morgan	100%	113
Exempla Good Samaritan Medical Center[2]	Lafayette	100%	457
Grand Junction VA Medical Center	Grand Junction	100%	54
McKee Medical Center[2]	Loveland	100%	216
The Medical Center of Aurora[2]	Aurora	100%	336
Mercy Regional Medical Center	Durango	100%	272
North Suburban Medical Center[2]	Thornton	100%	180
Platte Valley Medical Center	Brighton	100%	116
Presbyterian Saint Lukes Medical Center[2]	Denver	100%	326
Rose Medical Center[2]	Denver	100%	415
Sky Ridge Medical Center[2]	Lone Tree	100%	387
Sterling Regional Medcenter	Sterling	100%	57
Swedish Medical Center[2]	Englewood	100%	415
Valley View Hospital Association	Glenwood Spgs	100%	128
Centura Health - Saint Anthony Hospital[2]	Lakewood	99%	349
Centura Health-St Anthony North Hosp	Westminster	99%	177
Exempla Lutheran Medical Center[2]	Wheat Ridge	99%	295
Longmont United Hospital	Longmont	99%	375
North Colorado Medical Center[2]	Greeley	99%	319
Orthocolorado Hosp-St Anthony Med Camp[2]	Lakewood	99%	267
Parker Adventist Hospital	Parker	99%	350
Poudre Valley Hospital[2]	Fort Collins	99%	285
Saint Marys Hospital & Medical Center	Grand Junction	99%	857
VA Eastern Colorado Healthcare System	Denver	99%	188
Aspen Valley Hospital[3]	Aspen	98%	108
Centura Health-Avista Adventist Hosp	Louisville	98%	247
Centura Health-Penrose St Francis[2]	Colorado Spgs	98%	764
Exempla Saint Joseph Hospital[2]	Denver	98%	446
Medical Center of the Rockies[2]	Loveland	98%	436
Parkview Medical Center[2]	Pueblo	98%	326
Pikes Peak Regional Hospital	Woodland Park	98%	40
Saint Anthony Summit Medical Center	Frisco	98%	40
Univ of CO Health Mem Hosp[2]	Colorado Spgs	98%	905
University of Colorado Hospital[2]	Aurora	98%	396
Boulder Community Hospital[2]	Boulder	97%	312
Centura Health-Littleton Adventist Hosp[2]	Littleton	97%	300
Denver Health Medical Center[2]	Denver	97%	221
Yampa Valley Medical Center[2]	Steamboat Spgs	97%	112
Community Hospital	Grand Junction	96%	186
Delta County Memorial Hospital	Delta	95%	159
Montrose Memorial Hospital[2]	Montrose	95%	214
Vail Valley Medical Center	Vail	95%	150
Southwest Memorial Hospital	Cortez	94%	68
Animas Surgical Hospital[2]	Durango	92%	254
Arkansas Valley Regional Medical Center[2]	La Junta	90%	30
The Memorial Hospital	Craig	87%	38
San Luis Valley Regional Medical Center	Alamosa	80%	100

NOTE: Hospital profiles are in alphabetical order by state, then city, then hospital within the city; Rankings exclude hospitals with less than 25 cases except for patient surveys which excludes hospitals with less than 100 cases; (a) 100-299 cases; (1) The number of cases/patients is too few to report; (2) Data submitted were based on a sample of cases/patients; (3) Results are based on a shorter time period than required; (4) Data suppressed by CMS for one or more quarters; (5) Results are not available for this reporting period; (6) Fewer than 100 patients completed the HCAHPS survey; (7) No cases met the criteria for this measure; (8) The lower limit of the confidence interval cannot be calculated if the number of observed infections equals zero; (9) No data are available from the state/territory for this reporting period; (10) The scores shown reflect fewer than 50 completed surveys; (11) There were discrepancies in the data collection process; (12) This measure does not apply to this hospital for this reporting period; (13) Results cannot be calculated for this reporting period; (14) The results for this state are combined with nearby states to protect confidentiality; Please refer to the User's Guide for a full explanation of data.

Prophylactic Antibiotic Timing (Outpatient)

Hospital Name	City	Rate	Cases
Centura Health-Porter Adventist Hosp	Denver	100%	434
Centura Health-St Mary Corwin Med Ctr	Pueblo	100%	224
Centura Health-St Thomas More Hosp	Canon City	100%	39
Delta County Memorial Hospital	Delta	100%	28
North Colorado Medical Center	Greeley	100%	429
North Suburban Medical Center	Thornton	100%	178
Rose Medical Center	Denver	100%	609
Sky Ridge Medical Center	Lone Tree	100%	561
University of Colorado Hospital	Aurora	100%	47
Centura Health-Littleton Adventist Hosp	Littleton	99%	370
Centura Health-St Anthony North Hosp	Westminster	99%	84
Community Hospital	Grand Junction	99%	117
Exempla Good Samaritan Medical Center	Lafayette	99%	366
Exempla Lutheran Medical Center	Wheat Ridge	99%	534
Longmont United Hospital	Longmont	99%	225
The Medical Center of Aurora	Aurora	99%	309
Medical Center of the Rockies	Loveland	99%	368
Orthocolorado Hosp-St Anthony Med Camp	Lakewood	99%	174
Parker Adventist Hospital	Parker	99%	338
Presbyterian Saint Lukes Medical Center	Denver	99%	268
Swedish Medical Center	Englewood	99%	440
Centura Health-Avista Adventist Hosp	Louisville	98%	129
Mercy Regional Medical Center	Durango	98%	183
Platte Valley Medical Center	Brighton	98%	82
Poudre Valley Hospital	Fort Collins	98%	449
Saint Anthony Summit Medical Center	Frisco	98%	48
Valley View Hospital Association	Glenwood Spgs	98%	145
Exempla Saint Joseph Hospital	Denver	97%	684
McKee Medical Center	Loveland	97%	112
Saint Marys Hospital & Medical Center	Grand Junction	97%	551
Centura Health-Penrose St Francis	Colorado Spgs	96%	810
Centura Health - Saint Anthony Hospital	Lakewood	96%	266
Yampa Valley Medical Center	Steamboat Spgs	96%	114
Boulder Community Hospital	Boulder	95%	279
Montrose Memorial Hospital	Montrose	95%	156
Parkview Medical Center	Pueblo	95%	485
Univ of CO Health Mem Hosp	Colorado Spgs	95%	1189
Vail Valley Medical Center	Vail	95%	132
Denver Health Medical Center	Denver	94%	200
Animas Surgical Hospital	Durango	93%	29

Urinary Catheter Removal

Hospital Name	City	Rate	Cases
Exempla Good Samaritan Medical Center[2]	Lafayette	100%	423
North Suburban Medical Center[2]	Thornton	100%	180
Orthocolorado Hosp-St Anthony Med Camp[2]	Lakewood	100%	325
Rose Medical Center[2]	Denver	100%	325
Sterling Regional Medcenter	Sterling	100%	50
Univ of CO Health Mem Hosp[2]	Colorado Spgs	100%	786
Animas Surgical Hospital[2]	Durango	99%	140
Aspen Valley Hospital[3]	Aspen	99%	71
Centura Health-Avista Adventist Hosp	Louisville	99%	179
Centura Health-Littleton Adventist Hosp[2]	Littleton	99%	309
Centura Health-St Anthony North Hosp	Westminster	99%	242
Centura Health-St Thomas More Hosp	Canon City	99%	138
Colorado Plains Medical Center	Fort Morgan	99%	74
Exempla Saint Joseph Hospital[2]	Denver	99%	296
The Medical Center of Aurora[2]	Aurora	99%	360
North Colorado Medical Center[2]	Greeley	99%	250
Poudre Valley Hospital[2]	Fort Collins	99%	326
Sky Ridge Medical Center[2]	Lone Tree	99%	175
Yampa Valley Medical Center[2]	Steamboat Spgs	99%	108
Arkansas Valley Regional Medical Center[2]	La Junta	98%	41
Boulder Community Hospital[2]	Boulder	98%	311
Pikes Peak Regional Hospital	Woodland Park	98%	44
Presbyterian Saint Lukes Medical Center[2]	Denver	98%	235
Southwest Memorial Hospital	Cortez	98%	55
Swedish Medical Center[2]	Englewood	98%	277
VA Eastern Colorado Healthcare System[2]	Denver	98%	192
Centura Health-Porter Adventist Hosp[2]	Denver	97%	473
Community Hospital	Grand Junction	97%	118
Denver Health Medical Center[2]	Denver	97%	167
Exempla Lutheran Medical Center[2]	Wheat Ridge	97%	197
Mercy Regional Medical Center	Durango	97%	260
Platte Valley Medical Center	Brighton	97%	117
Saint Anthony Summit Medical Center	Frisco	97%	39
Saint Marys Hospital & Medical Center	Grand Junction	97%	874
Vail Valley Medical Center	Vail	97%	148
Valley View Hospital Association	Glenwood Spgs	97%	113
Centura Health - Saint Anthony Hospital[2]	Lakewood	96%	307
McKee Medical Center[2]	Loveland	96%	117
Medical Center of the Rockies[2]	Loveland	96%	411
Montrose Memorial Hospital[2]	Montrose	96%	238
San Luis Valley Regional Medical Center	Alamosa	96%	78
Longmont United Hospital	Longmont	94%	368
Parkview Medical Center[2]	Pueblo	94%	307
University of Colorado Hospital[2]	Aurora	94%	349
Delta County Memorial Hospital	Delta	93%	61
Centura Health-Penrose St Francis[2]	Colorado Spgs	92%	691
Parker Adventist Hospital	Parker	92%	256
Centura Health-St Mary Corwin Med Ctr	Pueblo	90%	103

Survey of Patients' Hospital Experiences

Area Around Room 'Always' Quiet at Night

Hospital Name	City	Rate	Cases
Animas Surgical Hospital	Durango	81%	300+
Gunnison Valley Hospital	Gunnison	78%	(a)
Pikes Peak Regional Hospital	Woodland Park	76%	(a)
Orthocolorado Hosp-St Anthony Med Camp	Lakewood	75%	300+
Aspen Valley Hospital	Aspen	74%	(a)
Saint Anthony Summit Medical Center	Frisco	72%	300+
Yampa Valley Medical Center	Steamboat Spgs	70%	300+
Heart of the Rockies Reg Med Ctr	Salida	69%	(a)
Longmont United Hospital	Longmont	68%	300+
Medical Center of the Rockies	Loveland	67%	300+
Sterling Regional Medcenter[11]	Sterling	67%	(a)
Vail Valley Medical Center	Vail	67%	300+
Centura Health-Avista Adventist Hosp	Louisville	65%	300+
Rose Medical Center	Denver	65%	300+
Colorado Plains Medical Center	Fort Morgan	64%	300+
Exempla Good Samaritan Medical Center	Lafayette	64%	300+
McKee Medical Center[11]	Loveland	64%	300+
Parker Adventist Hospital	Parker	64%	300+
Platte Valley Medical Center	Brighton	64%	300+
Sky Ridge Medical Center	Lone Tree	64%	300+
Valley View Hospital Association	Glenwood Spgs	64%	300+
Centura Health-Penrose St Francis	Colorado Spgs	63%	300+
Southwest Memorial Hospital	Cortez	63%	(a)
University of Colorado Hospital	Aurora	63%	300+
The Medical Center of Aurora	Aurora	62%	300+
Montrose Memorial Hospital	Montrose	62%	300+
Presbyterian Saint Lukes Medical Center	Denver	62%	300+
Denver Health Medical Center	Denver	61%	300+
The Memorial Hospital	Craig	61%	(a)
Boulder Community Hospital	Boulder	60%	300+
Centura Health-Porter Adventist Hosp	Denver	60%	300+
Centura Health - Saint Anthony Hospital	Lakewood	60%	300+
Exempla Lutheran Medical Center	Wheat Ridge	60%	300+
North Colorado Medical Center[11]	Greeley	60%	300+
Mercy Regional Medical Center	Durango	58%	300+
Parkview Medical Center	Pueblo	58%	300+
Poudre Valley Hospital	Fort Collins	58%	300+
Centura Health-St Thomas More Hosp	Canon City	57%	300+
Exempla Saint Joseph Hospital	Denver	57%	300+
Swedish Medical Center	Englewood	57%	300+
Arkansas Valley Regional Medical Center	La Junta	56%	300+
Centura Health-St Mary Corwin Med Ctr	Pueblo	56%	300+
Delta County Memorial Hospital	Delta	56%	(a)
Mount San Rafael Hospital	Trinidad	56%	(a)
North Suburban Medical Center	Thornton	56%	300+
Saint Marys Hospital & Medical Center	Grand Junction	56%	300+
Estes Park Medical Center	Estes Park	55%	(a)
Centura Health-Littleton Adventist Hosp	Littleton	54%	300+
Centura Health-St Anthony North Hosp	Westminster	54%	300+
Community Hospital[11]	Grand Junction	52%	300+
Univ of CO Health Mem Hosp	Colorado Spgs	52%	300+
San Luis Valley Regional Medical Center	Alamosa	48%	300+

Doctors 'Always' Communicated Well

Hospital Name	City	Rate	Cases
Animas Surgical Hospital	Durango	90%	300+
Southwest Memorial Hospital	Cortez	86%	(a)
Estes Park Medical Center	Estes Park	85%	(a)
Heart of the Rockies Reg Med Ctr	Salida	85%	(a)
Mercy Regional Medical Center	Durango	85%	300+
Orthocolorado Hosp-St Anthony Med Camp	Lakewood	85%	300+
Yampa Valley Medical Center	Steamboat Spgs	85%	300+
Aspen Valley Hospital	Aspen	84%	(a)
Gunnison Valley Hospital	Gunnison	84%	(a)
Sterling Regional Medcenter[11]	Sterling	84%	(a)
McKee Medical Center[11]	Loveland	83%	300+
Mount San Rafael Hospital	Trinidad	83%	(a)
Pikes Peak Regional Hospital	Woodland Park	83%	(a)
Vail Valley Medical Center	Vail	83%	300+
Centura Health-Avista Adventist Hosp	Louisville	82%	300+
Colorado Plains Medical Center	Fort Morgan	82%	300+
Platte Valley Medical Center	Brighton	82%	300+
Valley View Hospital Association	Glenwood Spgs	82%	300+
Boulder Community Hospital	Boulder	81%	300+
Centura Health-Penrose St Francis	Colorado Spgs	81%	300+
Centura Health-St Thomas More Hosp	Canon City	81%	300+
Community Hospital[11]	Grand Junction	81%	300+
Exempla Good Samaritan Medical Center	Lafayette	81%	300+
The Memorial Hospital	Craig	81%	(a)
Montrose Memorial Hospital	Montrose	81%	300+
North Colorado Medical Center[11]	Greeley	81%	300+
Saint Marys Hospital & Medical Center	Grand Junction	81%	300+
Arkansas Valley Regional Medical Center	La Junta	80%	300+
Centura Health-Porter Adventist Hosp	Denver	80%	300+
Centura Health-St Mary Corwin Med Ctr	Pueblo	80%	300+
Exempla Saint Joseph Hospital	Denver	80%	300+
Parker Adventist Hospital	Parker	80%	300+
Centura Health-Littleton Adventist Hosp	Littleton	79%	300+
Delta County Memorial Hospital	Delta	79%	(a)
Medical Center of the Rockies	Loveland	79%	300+
Presbyterian Saint Lukes Medical Center	Denver	79%	300+
Rose Medical Center	Denver	79%	300+
University of Colorado Hospital	Aurora	79%	300+
Centura Health - Saint Anthony Hospital	Lakewood	78%	300+
Denver Health Medical Center	Denver	78%	300+
Exempla Lutheran Medical Center	Wheat Ridge	78%	300+
Longmont United Hospital	Longmont	78%	300+
Poudre Valley Hospital	Fort Collins	78%	300+
Saint Anthony Summit Medical Center	Frisco	78%	300+
Centura Health-St Anthony North Hosp	Westminster	77%	300+
San Luis Valley Regional Medical Center	Alamosa	77%	300+
North Suburban Medical Center	Thornton	76%	300+
Parkview Medical Center	Pueblo	76%	300+
Sky Ridge Medical Center	Lone Tree	76%	300+
Swedish Medical Center	Englewood	76%	300+
Univ of CO Health Mem Hosp	Colorado Spgs	76%	300+
The Medical Center of Aurora	Aurora	74%	300+

Home Recovery Information Given

Hospital Name	City	Rate	Cases
McKee Medical Center[11]	Loveland	92%	300+
Sterling Regional Medcenter[11]	Sterling	92%	(a)
North Colorado Medical Center[11]	Greeley	91%	300+
Orthocolorado Hosp-St Anthony Med Camp	Lakewood	91%	300+
Parker Adventist Hospital	Parker	91%	300+
Pikes Peak Regional Hospital	Woodland Park	91%	(a)
Southwest Memorial Hospital	Cortez	91%	(a)
Animas Surgical Hospital	Durango	90%	300+
Centura Health-Avista Adventist Hosp	Louisville	90%	300+
Exempla Good Samaritan Medical Center	Lafayette	90%	300+
Exempla Saint Joseph Hospital	Denver	90%	300+
Saint Anthony Summit Medical Center	Frisco	90%	300+
Vail Valley Medical Center	Vail	90%	300+
Centura Health-Porter Adventist Hosp	Denver	89%	300+
Estes Park Medical Center	Estes Park	89%	(a)
Heart of the Rockies Reg Med Ctr	Salida	89%	(a)
Mercy Regional Medical Center	Durango	89%	300+
Platte Valley Medical Center	Brighton	89%	300+
Rose Medical Center	Denver	89%	300+
Yampa Valley Medical Center	Steamboat Spgs	89%	300+
Boulder Community Hospital	Boulder	88%	300+
Centura Health - Saint Anthony Hospital	Lakewood	88%	300+
Centura Health-St Mary Corwin Med Ctr	Pueblo	88%	300+
Colorado Plains Medical Center	Fort Morgan	88%	300+
Exempla Lutheran Medical Center	Wheat Ridge	88%	300+
Longmont United Hospital	Longmont	88%	300+
Medical Center of the Rockies	Loveland	88%	300+
The Memorial Hospital	Craig	88%	(a)
Poudre Valley Hospital	Fort Collins	88%	300+
Presbyterian Saint Lukes Medical Center	Denver	88%	300+
Sky Ridge Medical Center	Lone Tree	88%	300+
Centura Health-Littleton Adventist Hosp	Littleton	87%	300+
Centura Health-Penrose St Francis	Colorado Spgs	87%	300+
Gunnison Valley Hospital	Gunnison	87%	(a)
Saint Marys Hospital & Medical Center	Grand Junction	87%	300+
Valley View Hospital Association	Glenwood Spgs	87%	300+
Aspen Valley Hospital	Aspen	86%	(a)
Centura Health-St Anthony North Hosp	Westminster	86%	300+
Delta County Memorial Hospital	Delta	86%	(a)
North Suburban Medical Center	Thornton	86%	300+
Centura Health-St Thomas More Hosp	Canon City	85%	300+
Community Hospital[11]	Grand Junction	85%	300+
Denver Health Medical Center	Denver	85%	300+
The Medical Center of Aurora	Aurora	85%	300+
Swedish Medical Center	Englewood	85%	300+
University of Colorado Hospital	Aurora	85%	300+
Montrose Memorial Hospital	Montrose	84%	300+
Mount San Rafael Hospital	Trinidad	84%	(a)
Parkview Medical Center	Pueblo	84%	300+
Univ of CO Health Mem Hosp	Colorado Spgs	84%	300+
San Luis Valley Regional Medical Center	Alamosa	81%	300+
Arkansas Valley Regional Medical Center	La Junta	78%	300+

Hospital Given 9 or 10 on 10 Point Scale

Hospital Name	City	Rate	Cases
Animas Surgical Hospital	Durango	90%	300+
Saint Anthony Summit Medical Center	Frisco	84%	300+
Yampa Valley Medical Center	Steamboat Spgs	83%	300+
Heart of the Rockies Reg Med Ctr	Salida	82%	(a)
Medical Center of the Rockies	Loveland	82%	300+
Aspen Valley Hospital	Aspen	81%	(a)
Orthocolorado Hosp-St Anthony Med Camp	Lakewood	81%	300+

NOTE: Hospital profiles are in alphabetical order by state, then city, then hospital within the city; Rankings exclude hospitals with less than 25 cases except for patient surveys which excludes hospitals with less than 100 cases; (a) 100-299 cases; (1) The number of cases/patients is too few to report; (2) Data submitted were based on a sample of cases/patients; (3) Results are based on a shorter time period than required; (4) Data suppressed by CMS for one or more quarters; (5) Results are not available for this reporting period; (6) Fewer than 100 patients completed the HCAHPS survey; (7) No cases met the criteria for this measure; (8) The lower limit of the confidence interval cannot be calculated if the number of observed infections equals zero; (9) No data are available from the state/territory for this reporting period; (10) The scores shown reflect fewer than 50 completed surveys; (11) There were discrepancies in the data collection process; (12) This measure does not apply to this hospital for this reporting period; (13) Results cannot be calculated for this reporting period; (14) The results for this state are combined with nearby states to protect confidentiality; Please refer to the User's Guide for a full explanation of data.

Centura Health-Avista Adventist Hosp	Louisville	80%	300+
Valley View Hospital Association	Glenwood Spgs	80%	300+
Pikes Peak Regional Hospital	Woodland Park	79%	(a)
Vail Valley Medical Center	Vail	79%	300+
Gunnison Valley Hospital	Gunnison	78%	(a)
Mercy Regional Medical Center	Durango	78%	300+
Rose Medical Center	Denver	78%	300+
Exempla Good Samaritan Medical Center	Lafayette	77%	300+
Platte Valley Medical Center	Brighton	77%	300+
Poudre Valley Hospital	Fort Collins	77%	300+
Sterling Regional Medcenter[11]	Sterling	77%	(a)
University of Colorado Hospital	Aurora	77%	300+
Centura Health - Saint Anthony Hospital	Lakewood	76%	300+
Longmont United Hospital	Longmont	76%	300+
Parker Adventist Hospital	Parker	76%	300+
Parkview Medical Center	Pueblo	76%	300+
Exempla Lutheran Medical Center	Wheat Ridge	75%	300+
McKee Medical Center[11]	Loveland	75%	300+
Sky Ridge Medical Center	Lone Tree	75%	300+
Community Hospital[11]	Grand Junction	74%	300+
Exempla Saint Joseph Hospital	Denver	74%	300+
Montrose Memorial Hospital	Montrose	74%	300+
North Colorado Medical Center[11]	Greeley	74%	300+
Saint Marys Hospital & Medical Center	Grand Junction	74%	300+
Centura Health-Littleton Adventist Hosp	Littleton	73%	300+
Centura Health-Penrose St Francis	Colorado Spgs	73%	300+
Centura Health-Porter Adventist Hosp	Denver	73%	300+
Delta County Memorial Hospital	Delta	73%	(a)
Estes Park Medical Center	Estes Park	73%	(a)
Boulder Community Hospital	Boulder	72%	300+
Colorado Plains Medical Center	Fort Morgan	72%	300+
Centura Health-St Mary Corwin Med Ctr	Pueblo	71%	300+
Presbyterian Saint Lukes Medical Center	Denver	71%	300+
The Medical Center of Aurora	Aurora	70%	300+
Swedish Medical Center	Englewood	69%	300+
Centura Health-St Anthony North Hosp	Westminster	68%	300+
Denver Health Medical Center	Denver	68%	300+
Centura Health-St Thomas More Hosp	Canon City	67%	300+
Southwest Memorial Hospital	Cortez	67%	(a)
Mount San Rafael Hospital	Trinidad	66%	(a)
North Suburban Medical Center	Thornton	66%	300+
Univ of CO Health Mem Hosp	Colorado Spgs	64%	300+
The Memorial Hospital	Craig	61%	(a)
Arkansas Valley Regional Medical Center	La Junta	51%	300+
San Luis Valley Regional Medical Center	Alamosa	49%	300+

Meds 'Always' Explained Before Given

Hospital Name	City	Rate	Cases
Heart of the Rockies Reg Med Ctr	Salida	78%	(a)
Animas Surgical Hospital	Durango	76%	300+
Gunnison Valley Hospital	Gunnison	71%	(a)
Estes Park Medical Center	Estes Park	70%	(a)
McKee Medical Center[11]	Loveland	70%	300+
Platte Valley Medical Center	Brighton	70%	300+
Community Hospital[11]	Grand Junction	69%	300+
Orthocolorado Hosp-St Anthony Med Camp	Lakewood	69%	300+
Pikes Peak Regional Hospital	Woodland Park	69%	(a)
Southwest Memorial Hospital	Cortez	69%	(a)
Sterling Regional Medcenter[11]	Sterling	69%	(a)
Yampa Valley Medical Center	Steamboat Spgs	69%	300+
Centura Health-St Mary Corwin Med Ctr	Pueblo	68%	300+
The Memorial Hospital	Craig	68%	(a)
North Colorado Medical Center[11]	Greeley	68%	300+
Colorado Plains Medical Center	Fort Morgan	67%	300+
Mercy Regional Medical Center	Durango	67%	300+
Saint Anthony Summit Medical Center	Frisco	67%	300+
Aspen Valley Hospital	Aspen	66%	(a)
Centura Health-Avista Adventist Hosp	Louisville	66%	300+
Exempla Saint Joseph Hospital	Denver	66%	300+
Medical Center of the Rockies	Loveland	66%	300+
Montrose Memorial Hospital	Montrose	66%	300+
Mount San Rafael Hospital	Trinidad	66%	(a)
Rose Medical Center	Denver	66%	300+
Vail Valley Medical Center	Vail	66%	300+
Exempla Good Samaritan Medical Center	Lafayette	65%	300+
Presbyterian Saint Lukes Medical Center	Denver	65%	300+
University of Colorado Hospital	Aurora	65%	300+
Valley View Hospital Association	Glenwood Spgs	65%	300+
Boulder Community Hospital	Boulder	64%	300+
Centura Health-St Anthony North Hosp	Westminster	64%	300+
Centura Health-St Thomas More Hosp	Canon City	64%	300+
The Medical Center of Aurora	Aurora	64%	300+
Parker Adventist Hospital	Parker	64%	300+
Poudre Valley Hospital	Fort Collins	64%	300+
Denver Health Medical Center	Denver	63%	300+
North Suburban Medical Center	Thornton	63%	300+
Saint Marys Hospital & Medical Center	Grand Junction	63%	300+
Sky Ridge Medical Center	Lone Tree	63%	300+
Centura Health-Penrose St Francis	Colorado Spgs	62%	300+
Centura Health-Porter Adventist Hosp	Denver	62%	300+
Centura Health - Saint Anthony Hospital	Lakewood	62%	300+
Exempla Lutheran Medical Center	Wheat Ridge	62%	300+
Longmont United Hospital	Longmont	62%	300+
Parkview Medical Center	Pueblo	62%	300+
Centura Health-Littleton Adventist Hosp	Littleton	61%	300+
Delta County Memorial Hospital	Delta	61%	(a)
Univ of CO Health Mem Hosp	Colorado Spgs	61%	300+
San Luis Valley Regional Medical Center	Alamosa	59%	300+
Swedish Medical Center	Englewood	59%	300+
Arkansas Valley Regional Medical Center	La Junta	57%	300+

Nurses 'Always' Communicated Well

Hospital Name	City	Rate	Cases
Animas Surgical Hospital	Durango	86%	300+
Heart of the Rockies Reg Med Ctr	Salida	85%	(a)
Sterling Regional Medcenter[11]	Sterling	84%	(a)
Pikes Peak Regional Hospital	Woodland Park	83%	(a)
Saint Anthony Summit Medical Center	Frisco	83%	300+
Colorado Plains Medical Center	Fort Morgan	82%	300+
Community Hospital[11]	Grand Junction	82%	300+
Gunnison Valley Hospital	Gunnison	82%	(a)
McKee Medical Center[11]	Loveland	82%	300+
Vail Valley Medical Center	Vail	82%	300+
Aspen Valley Hospital	Aspen	81%	(a)
The Memorial Hospital	Craig	81%	(a)
Mercy Regional Medical Center	Durango	81%	300+
North Colorado Medical Center[11]	Greeley	81%	300+
Orthocolorado Hosp-St Anthony Med Camp	Lakewood	81%	300+
Yampa Valley Medical Center	Steamboat Spgs	81%	300+
Centura Health-Avista Adventist Hosp	Louisville	79%	300+
Estes Park Medical Center	Estes Park	79%	(a)
Longmont United Hospital	Longmont	79%	300+
Medical Center of the Rockies	Loveland	79%	300+
Parker Adventist Hospital	Parker	79%	300+
Poudre Valley Hospital	Fort Collins	79%	300+
Southwest Memorial Hospital	Cortez	79%	(a)
University of Colorado Hospital	Aurora	79%	300+
Valley View Hospital Association	Glenwood Spgs	79%	300+
Boulder Community Hospital	Boulder	78%	300+
Centura Health-St Thomas More Hosp	Canon City	78%	300+
Exempla Lutheran Medical Center	Wheat Ridge	78%	300+
Exempla Saint Joseph Hospital	Denver	78%	300+
Montrose Memorial Hospital	Montrose	78%	300+
Parkview Medical Center	Pueblo	78%	300+
Platte Valley Medical Center	Brighton	78%	300+
Centura Health-Littleton Adventist Hosp	Littleton	77%	300+
Centura Health-Penrose St Francis	Colorado Spgs	77%	300+
Centura Health-Porter Adventist Hosp	Denver	77%	300+
Centura Health - Saint Anthony Hospital	Lakewood	77%	300+
Centura Health-St Mary Corwin Med Ctr	Pueblo	77%	300+
Exempla Good Samaritan Medical Center	Lafayette	77%	300+
The Medical Center of Aurora	Aurora	77%	300+
Rose Medical Center	Denver	77%	300+
Saint Marys Hospital & Medical Center	Grand Junction	77%	300+
Centura Health-St Anthony North Hosp	Westminster	76%	300+
Sky Ridge Medical Center	Lone Tree	76%	300+
Delta County Memorial Hospital	Delta	75%	(a)
North Suburban Medical Center	Thornton	75%	300+
Presbyterian Saint Lukes Medical Center	Denver	75%	300+
Denver Health Medical Center	Denver	74%	300+
Swedish Medical Center	Englewood	74%	300+
Arkansas Valley Regional Medical Center	La Junta	73%	300+
Univ of CO Health Mem Hosp	Colorado Spgs	73%	300+
Mount San Rafael Hospital	Trinidad	72%	(a)
San Luis Valley Regional Medical Center	Alamosa	71%	300+

Pain 'Always' Well Controlled

Hospital Name	City	Rate	Cases
Gunnison Valley Hospital	Gunnison	85%	(a)
Animas Surgical Hospital	Durango	83%	300+
Heart of the Rockies Reg Med Ctr	Salida	79%	(a)
The Memorial Hospital	Craig	76%	(a)
McKee Medical Center[11]	Loveland	75%	300+
Pikes Peak Regional Hospital	Woodland Park	74%	(a)
Vail Valley Medical Center	Vail	74%	300+
Aspen Valley Hospital	Aspen	73%	(a)
Colorado Plains Medical Center	Fort Morgan	73%	300+
Medical Center of the Rockies	Loveland	73%	300+
Mercy Regional Medical Center	Durango	73%	300+
Orthocolorado Hosp-St Anthony Med Camp	Lakewood	73%	300+
Saint Anthony Summit Medical Center	Frisco	73%	300+
Southwest Memorial Hospital	Cortez	73%	(a)
Sterling Regional Medcenter[11]	Sterling	73%	(a)
Boulder Community Hospital	Boulder	72%	300+
Centura Health-Avista Adventist Hosp	Louisville	72%	300+
Centura Health-St Thomas More Hosp	Canon City	72%	300+
Delta County Memorial Hospital	Delta	72%	(a)
Rose Medical Center	Denver	72%	300+
Yampa Valley Medical Center	Steamboat Spgs	72%	300+
Estes Park Medical Center	Estes Park	71%	(a)
Exempla Lutheran Medical Center	Wheat Ridge	71%	300+
Poudre Valley Hospital	Fort Collins	71%	300+
Centura Health-Littleton Adventist Hosp	Littleton	70%	300+
Centura Health - Saint Anthony Hospital	Lakewood	70%	300+
Exempla Saint Joseph Hospital	Denver	70%	300+
The Medical Center of Aurora	Aurora	70%	300+
North Colorado Medical Center[11]	Greeley	70%	300+
North Suburban Medical Center	Thornton	70%	300+
Parkview Medical Center	Pueblo	70%	300+
Saint Marys Hospital & Medical Center	Grand Junction	70%	300+
University of Colorado Hospital	Aurora	70%	300+
Centura Health-St Mary Corwin Med Ctr	Pueblo	69%	300+
Community Hospital[11]	Grand Junction	69%	300+
Exempla Good Samaritan Medical Center	Lafayette	69%	300+
Longmont United Hospital	Longmont	69%	300+
Montrose Memorial Hospital	Montrose	69%	300+
Parker Adventist Hospital	Parker	69%	300+
Platte Valley Medical Center	Brighton	69%	300+
San Luis Valley Regional Medical Center	Alamosa	69%	300+
Valley View Hospital Association	Glenwood Spgs	69%	300+
Centura Health-Penrose St Francis	Colorado Spgs	68%	300+
Centura Health-Porter Adventist Hosp	Denver	68%	300+
Presbyterian Saint Lukes Medical Center	Denver	68%	300+
Sky Ridge Medical Center	Lone Tree	68%	300+
Arkansas Valley Regional Medical Center	La Junta	67%	300+
Swedish Medical Center	Englewood	67%	300+
Univ of CO Health Mem Hosp	Colorado Spgs	66%	300+
Centura Health-St Anthony North Hosp	Westminster	65%	300+
Denver Health Medical Center	Denver	65%	300+
Mount San Rafael Hospital	Trinidad	62%	(a)

Room and Bathroom 'Always' Clean

Hospital Name	City	Rate	Cases
Animas Surgical Hospital	Durango	87%	300+
Montrose Memorial Hospital	Montrose	86%	300+
Aspen Valley Hospital	Aspen	85%	(a)
Vail Valley Medical Center	Vail	85%	300+
Mount San Rafael Hospital	Trinidad	84%	(a)
Orthocolorado Hosp-St Anthony Med Camp	Lakewood	84%	300+
Gunnison Valley Hospital	Gunnison	82%	(a)
Parkview Medical Center	Pueblo	81%	300+
Delta County Memorial Hospital	Delta	80%	(a)
Medical Center of the Rockies	Loveland	80%	300+
Yampa Valley Medical Center	Steamboat Spgs	79%	300+
Heart of the Rockies Reg Med Ctr	Salida	78%	(a)
McKee Medical Center[11]	Loveland	78%	300+
The Memorial Hospital	Craig	78%	(a)
Platte Valley Medical Center	Brighton	78%	300+
Valley View Hospital Association	Glenwood Spgs	78%	300+
Pikes Peak Regional Hospital	Woodland Park	77%	(a)
Poudre Valley Hospital	Fort Collins	77%	300+
Colorado Plains Medical Center	Fort Morgan	76%	300+
Mercy Regional Medical Center	Durango	76%	300+
Saint Anthony Summit Medical Center	Frisco	76%	300+
Sterling Regional Medcenter[11]	Sterling	76%	(a)
Arkansas Valley Regional Medical Center	La Junta	75%	300+
Estes Park Medical Center	Estes Park	74%	(a)
Centura Health-Avista Adventist Hosp	Louisville	73%	300+
Centura Health - Saint Anthony Hospital	Lakewood	73%	300+
Community Hospital[11]	Grand Junction	73%	300+
North Colorado Medical Center[11]	Greeley	73%	300+
Rose Medical Center	Denver	73%	300+
San Luis Valley Regional Medical Center	Alamosa	73%	300+
Sky Ridge Medical Center	Lone Tree	73%	300+
Centura Health-Porter Adventist Hosp	Denver	72%	300+
Longmont United Hospital	Longmont	72%	300+
North Suburban Medical Center	Thornton	72%	300+
Parker Adventist Hospital	Parker	72%	300+
Boulder Community Hospital	Boulder	71%	300+
Centura Health-St Mary Corwin Med Ctr	Pueblo	71%	300+
Presbyterian Saint Lukes Medical Center	Denver	71%	300+
Saint Marys Hospital & Medical Center	Grand Junction	71%	300+
Swedish Medical Center	Englewood	71%	300+
Exempla Lutheran Medical Center	Wheat Ridge	70%	300+
The Medical Center of Aurora	Aurora	70%	300+
University of Colorado Hospital	Aurora	70%	300+
Centura Health-Littleton Adventist Hosp	Littleton	69%	300+
Exempla Good Samaritan Medical Center	Lafayette	69%	300+
Centura Health-St Thomas More Hosp	Canon City	68%	300+
Exempla Saint Joseph Hospital	Denver	67%	300+
Centura Health-Penrose St Francis	Colorado Spgs	66%	300+
Centura Health-St Anthony North Hosp	Westminster	66%	300+
Univ of CO Health Mem Hosp	Colorado Spgs	65%	300+
Southwest Memorial Hospital	Cortez	61%	(a)
Denver Health Medical Center	Denver	60%	300+

Timely Help 'Always' Received

Hospital Name	City	Rate	Cases
Animas Surgical Hospital	Durango	87%	300+
Heart of the Rockies Reg Med Ctr	Salida	82%	(a)
Gunnison Valley Hospital	Gunnison	81%	(a)

NOTE: Hospital profiles are in alphabetical order by state, then city, then hospital within the city; Rankings exclude hospitals with less than 25 cases except for patient surveys which excludes hospitals with less than 100 cases; (a) 100-299 cases; (1) The number of cases/patients is too few to report; (2) Data submitted were based on a sample of cases/patients; (3) Results are based on a shorter time period than required; (4) Data suppressed by CMS for one or more quarters; (5) Results are not available for this reporting period; (6) Fewer than 100 patients completed the HCAHPS survey; (7) No cases met the criteria for this measure; (8) The lower limit of the confidence interval cannot be calculated if the number of observed infections equals zero; (9) No data are available from the state/territory for this reporting period; (10) The scores shown reflect fewer than 50 completed surveys; (11) There were discrepancies in the data collection process; (12) This measure does not apply to this hospital for this reporting period; (13) Results cannot be calculated for this reporting period; (14) The results for this state are combined with nearby states to protect confidentiality; Please refer to the User's Guide for a full explanation of data.

The Memorial Hospital	Craig	81%	(a)
Yampa Valley Medical Center	Steamboat Spgs	79%	300+
Pikes Peak Regional Hospital	Woodland Park	77%	(a)
Saint Anthony Summit Medical Center	Frisco	77%	300+
Aspen Valley Hospital	Aspen	75%	(a)
Southwest Memorial Hospital	Cortez	75%	(a)
Sterling Regional Medcenter[11]	Sterling	75%	(a)
Vail Valley Medical Center	Vail	74%	300+
Estes Park Medical Center	Estes Park	73%	(a)
Montrose Memorial Hospital	Montrose	73%	300+
Centura Health-Avista Adventist Hosp	Louisville	71%	300+
Colorado Plains Medical Center	Fort Morgan	71%	300+
Community Hospital[11]	Grand Junction	71%	300+
Valley View Hospital Association	Glenwood Spgs	71%	300+
McKee Medical Center[11]	Loveland	70%	300+
Mercy Regional Medical Center	Durango	70%	300+
Platte Valley Medical Center	Brighton	70%	300+
Boulder Community Hospital	Boulder	69%	300+
Exempla Saint Joseph Hospital	Denver	69%	300+
Longmont United Hospital	Longmont	68%	300+
Mount San Rafael Hospital	Trinidad	68%	(a)
Poudre Valley Hospital	Fort Collins	68%	300+
Delta County Memorial Hospital	Delta	67%	(a)
North Colorado Medical Center[11]	Greeley	67%	300+
Centura Health-Porter Adventist Hosp	Denver	66%	300+
Centura Health-St Thomas More Hosp	Canon City	66%	300+
Orthocolorado Hosp-St Anthony Med Camp	Lakewood	66%	300+
Rose Medical Center	Denver	66%	300+
Arkansas Valley Regional Medical Center	La Junta	65%	300+
The Medical Center of Aurora	Aurora	65%	300+
Medical Center of the Rockies	Loveland	65%	300+
University of Colorado Hospital	Aurora	65%	300+
Centura Health - Saint Anthony Hospital	Lakewood	64%	300+
Centura Health-St Mary Corwin Med Ctr	Pueblo	64%	300+
Parkview Medical Center	Pueblo	64%	300+
Saint Marys Hospital & Medical Center	Grand Junction	64%	300+
Sky Ridge Medical Center	Lone Tree	64%	300+
Centura Health-Littleton Adventist Hosp	Littleton	63%	300+
Centura Health-Penrose St Francis	Colorado Spgs	63%	300+
Exempla Good Samaritan Medical Center	Lafayette	63%	300+
Exempla Lutheran Medical Center	Wheat Ridge	63%	300+
North Suburban Medical Center	Thornton	63%	300+
Parker Adventist Hospital	Parker	63%	300+
Presbyterian Saint Lukes Medical Center	Denver	62%	300+
Univ of CO Health Mem Hosp	Colorado Spgs	62%	300+
San Luis Valley Regional Medical Center	Alamosa	60%	300+
Swedish Medical Center	Englewood	60%	300+
Denver Health Medical Center	Denver	59%	300+
Centura Health-St Anthony North Hosp	Westminster	58%	300+

Would Definitely Recommend Hospital

Hospital Name	City	Rate	Cases
Animas Surgical Hospital	Durango	91%	300+
Yampa Valley Medical Center	Steamboat Spgs	85%	300+
Medical Center of the Rockies	Loveland	83%	300+
Orthocolorado Hosp-St Anthony Med Camp	Lakewood	83%	300+
Community Hospital[11]	Grand Junction	82%	300+
Mercy Regional Medical Center	Durango	82%	300+
Saint Anthony Summit Medical Center	Frisco	82%	300+
Vail Valley Medical Center	Vail	82%	300+
Centura Health-Avista Adventist Hosp	Louisville	81%	300+
Exempla Good Samaritan Medical Center	Lafayette	81%	300+
Heart of the Rockies Reg Med Ctr	Salida	81%	(a)
Valley View Hospital Association	Glenwood Spgs	81%	300+
Gunnison Valley Hospital	Gunnison	80%	(a)
Parkview Medical Center	Pueblo	80%	300+
Poudre Valley Hospital	Fort Collins	80%	300+
Rose Medical Center	Denver	80%	300+
University of Colorado Hospital	Aurora	80%	300+
Centura Health - Saint Anthony Hospital	Lakewood	79%	300+
Parker Adventist Hospital	Parker	79%	300+
Aspen Valley Hospital	Aspen	78%	(a)
Pikes Peak Regional Hospital	Woodland Park	78%	(a)
Centura Health-Littleton Adventist Hosp	Littleton	77%	300+
Centura Health-Penrose St Francis	Colorado Spgs	77%	300+
McKee Medical Center[11]	Loveland	77%	300+
Saint Marys Hospital & Medical Center	Grand Junction	77%	300+
Sky Ridge Medical Center	Lone Tree	77%	300+
Estes Park Medical Center	Estes Park	76%	(a)
Exempla Lutheran Medical Center	Wheat Ridge	76%	300+
Exempla Saint Joseph Hospital	Denver	76%	300+
Platte Valley Medical Center	Brighton	76%	300+
Boulder Community Hospital	Boulder	75%	300+
Centura Health-Porter Adventist Hosp	Denver	75%	300+
Centura Health-St Mary Corwin Med Ctr	Pueblo	74%	300+
Longmont United Hospital	Longmont	74%	300+
Presbyterian Saint Lukes Medical Center	Denver	74%	300+
Delta County Memorial Hospital	Delta	73%	(a)
Montrose Memorial Hospital	Montrose	73%	300+
North Colorado Medical Center[11]	Greeley	72%	300+
Swedish Medical Center	Englewood	72%	300+
The Medical Center of Aurora	Aurora	71%	300+
Colorado Plains Medical Center	Fort Morgan	70%	300+
Sterling Regional Medcenter[11]	Sterling	69%	(a)
Centura Health-St Anthony North Hosp	Westminster	68%	300+
Univ of CO Health Mem Hosp	Colorado Spgs	68%	300+
Denver Health Medical Center	Denver	67%	300+
Southwest Memorial Hospital	Cortez	66%	(a)
North Suburban Medical Center	Thornton	65%	300+
The Memorial Hospital	Craig	64%	(a)
Centura Health-St Thomas More Hosp	Canon City	63%	300+
Mount San Rafael Hospital	Trinidad	60%	(a)
Arkansas Valley Regional Medical Center	La Junta	47%	300+
San Luis Valley Regional Medical Center	Alamosa	45%	300+

Use of Medical Imaging

Cardiac Imaging Stress Test before OP Surgery

Hospital Name	City	Rate	Cases
Denver Health Medical Center	Denver	0.7%	137
Arkansas Valley Regional Medical Center	La Junta	1.9%	54
Swedish Medical Center	Englewood	2.2%	92
Longmont United Hospital	Longmont	2.4%	82
Exempla Saint Joseph Hospital	Denver	2.5%	79
North Colorado Medical Center	Greeley	3.1%	413
Parker Adventist Hospital	Parker	3.1%	161
North Suburban Medical Center	Thornton	3.2%	124
Colorado Plains Medical Center	Fort Morgan	3.6%	56
Mercy Regional Medical Center	Durango	3.6%	646
Poudre Valley Hospital	Fort Collins	3.6%	964
Centura Health-St Anthony North Hosp	Westminster	3.7%	107
San Luis Valley Regional Medical Center	Alamosa	3.7%	107
Univ of CO Health Mem Hosp	Colorado Spgs	4.0%	1159
Medical Center of the Rockies	Loveland	4.1%	511
Sky Ridge Medical Center	Lone Tree	4.2%	237
Southwest Memorial Hospital	Cortez	4.4%	91
Delta County Memorial Hospital	Delta	4.5%	110
Sterling Regional Medcenter	Sterling	4.6%	108
Centura Health-Littleton Adventist Hosp	Littleton	4.8%	1180
Centura Health-St Mary Corwin Med Ctr	Pueblo	4.8%	165
Boulder Community Hospital	Boulder	5.1%	530
Montrose Memorial Hospital	Montrose	5.2%	267
Yampa Valley Medical Center	Steamboat Spgs	5.2%	77
Centura Health-St Thomas More Hosp	Canon City	5.4%	74
McKee Medical Center	Loveland	5.4%	185
Centura Health-Penrose St Francis	Colorado Spgs	5.6%	1076
Presbyterian Saint Lukes Medical Center	Denver	5.6%	108
Aspen Valley Hospital	Aspen	5.7%	174
The Medical Center of Aurora	Aurora	5.7%	263
Platte Valley Medical Center	Brighton	5.9%	119
Exempla Lutheran Medical Center	Wheat Ridge	6.1%	181
Parkview Medical Center	Pueblo	6.1%	870
Rose Medical Center	Denver	6.1%	99
Saint Anthony Summit Medical Center	Frisco	6.3%	64
Exempla Good Samaritan Medical Center	Lafayette	6.5%	93
Centura Health-Porter Adventist Hosp	Denver	6.7%	179
Valley View Hospital Association	Glenwood Spgs	7.0%	186
University of Colorado Hospital	Aurora	7.1%	420
Vail Valley Medical Center	Vail	7.1%	127
Estes Park Medical Center	Estes Park	7.2%	97
Saint Marys Hospital & Medical Center	Grand Junction	7.9%	101
Centura Health-Avista Adventist Hosp	Louisville	8.4%	83
Centura Health - Saint Anthony Hospital	Lakewood	9.6%	136
National Jewish Health	Denver	9.6%	345

Combination Abdominal CT Scan

Hospital Name	City	Rate	Cases
Denver Health Medical Center	Denver	0.2%	532
Arkansas Valley Regional Medical Center	La Junta	1.0%	198
Kit Carson County Memorial Hospital	Burlington	1.5%	67
The Memorial Hospital	Craig	2.9%	104
Southwest Memorial Hospital	Cortez	3.0%	338
Centura Health - Saint Anthony Hospital	Lakewood	3.4%	507
Exempla Lutheran Medical Center	Wheat Ridge	3.4%	901
North Suburban Medical Center	Thornton	3.5%	371
Centura Health-St Anthony North Hosp	Westminster	3.6%	413
The Medical Center of Aurora	Aurora	3.9%	684
Rose Medical Center	Denver	3.9%	741
Exempla Saint Joseph Hospital	Denver	4.3%	231
Mercy Regional Medical Center	Durango	4.4%	410
Centura Health-Penrose St Francis	Colorado Spgs	4.7%	965
North Colorado Medical Center	Greeley	4.7%	738
Presbyterian Saint Lukes Medical Center	Denver	4.9%	390
Yuma District Hospital	Yuma	5.1%	98
Parkview Medical Center	Pueblo	5.6%	1526
National Jewish Health	Denver	5.8%	86
Platte Valley Medical Center	Brighton	5.8%	224
Colorado Plains Medical Center	Fort Morgan	5.9%	187
Saint Anthony Summit Medical Center	Frisco	6.4%	110
University of Colorado Hospital	Aurora	6.8%	2535
Yampa Valley Medical Center	Steamboat Spgs	7.7%	156
Poudre Valley Hospital	Fort Collins	8.1%	887
Exempla Good Samaritan Medical Center	Lafayette	8.3%	217
Swedish Medical Center	Englewood	8.7%	759
Boulder Community Hospital	Boulder	9.1%	561
Medical Center of the Rockies	Loveland	9.1%	877
Centura Health-Avista Adventist Hosp	Louisville	9.6%	187
Valley View Hospital Association	Glenwood Spgs	9.8%	235
Sky Ridge Medical Center	Lone Tree	10.0%	519
Spanish Peaks Regional Health Center	Walsenburg	10.3%	116
Vail Valley Medical Center	Vail	11.0%	173
Delta County Memorial Hospital	Delta	11.2%	383
Estes Park Medical Center	Estes Park	11.5%	122
Longmont United Hospital	Longmont	11.6%	336
Centura Health-St Mary Corwin Med Ctr	Pueblo	11.7%	652
Aspen Valley Hospital	Aspen	11.8%	144
Centura Health-St Thomas More Hosp	Canon City	11.9%	506
McKee Medical Center	Loveland	12.0%	592
Parker Adventist Hospital	Parker	12.2%	458
Rio Grande Hospital	Del Norte	12.2%	115
Gunnison Valley Hospital	Gunnison	12.6%	95
Saint Marys Hospital & Medical Center	Grand Junction	13.7%	739
Centura Health-Littleton Adventist Hosp	Littleton	15.5%	582
Community Hospital	Grand Junction	18.7%	283
Montrose Memorial Hospital	Montrose	20.6%	462
Sterling Regional Medcenter	Sterling	20.6%	253
San Luis Valley Regional Medical Center	Alamosa	22.8%	237
Animas Surgical Hospital	Durango	25.3%	79
Univ of CO Health Mem Hosp	Colorado Spgs	25.9%	1763
Centura Health-Porter Adventist Hosp	Denver	26.5%	468
East Morgan County Hospital	Brush	33.3%	159

Combination Brain/Sinus CT Scan

Hospital Name	City	Rate	Cases
Arkansas Valley Regional Medical Center	La Junta	0.0%	168
Exempla Saint Joseph Hospital	Denver	0.0%	134
Melissa Memorial Hospital	Holyoke	0.0%	37
Rio Grande Hospital	Del Norte	0.0%	87
Sedgwick County Memorial Hospital	Julesburg	0.0%	33
Denver Health Medical Center	Denver	0.5%	416
Presbyterian Saint Lukes Medical Center	Denver	0.9%	223
Centura Health-St Thomas More Hosp	Canon City	1.0%	388
Platte Valley Medical Center	Brighton	1.0%	210
Centura Health-Porter Adventist Hosp	Denver	1.1%	348
Montrose Memorial Hospital	Montrose	1.1%	265
Medical Center of the Rockies	Loveland	1.2%	492
San Luis Valley Regional Medical Center	Alamosa	1.2%	171
Boulder Community Hospital	Boulder	1.4%	418
Exempla Lutheran Medical Center	Wheat Ridge	1.6%	810
Longmont United Hospital	Longmont	1.6%	425
Mercy Regional Medical Center	Durango	1.7%	350
Poudre Valley Hospital	Fort Collins	1.8%	781
University of Colorado Hospital	Aurora	1.8%	613
Centura Health-Penrose St Francis	Colorado Spgs	2.0%	1221
The Medical Center of Aurora	Aurora	2.0%	615
Parkview Medical Center	Pueblo	2.2%	1156
Swedish Medical Center	Englewood	2.3%	525
Centura Health-Littleton Adventist Hosp	Littleton	2.4%	542
Univ of CO Health Mem Hosp	Colorado Spgs	2.5%	1708
North Colorado Medical Center	Greeley	3.4%	738
Colorado Plains Medical Center	Fort Morgan	5.4%	149
Saint Anthony Summit Medical Center	Frisco	5.9%	118
Yuma District Hospital	Yuma	8.7%	69

Combination Chest CT Scan

Hospital Name	City	Rate	Cases
Boulder Community Hospital	Boulder	0.0%	345
The Memorial Hospital	Craig	0.0%	53
National Jewish Health	Denver	0.0%	2829
North Suburban Medical Center	Thornton	0.0%	60
Rio Grande Hospital	Del Norte	0.0%	97
Vail Valley Medical Center	Vail	0.0%	99
Yampa Valley Medical Center	Steamboat Spgs	0.0%	133
Parkview Medical Center	Pueblo	0.2%	520
Saint Marys Hospital & Medical Center	Grand Junction	0.2%	544
University of Colorado Hospital	Aurora	0.2%	2935
Presbyterian Saint Lukes Medical Center	Denver	0.3%	368
Exempla Good Samaritan Medical Center	Lafayette	0.5%	185
Exempla Lutheran Medical Center	Wheat Ridge	0.5%	548
Sky Ridge Medical Center	Lone Tree	0.5%	380
Southwest Memorial Hospital	Cortez	0.5%	184
Rose Medical Center	Denver	0.6%	362
Swedish Medical Center	Englewood	0.6%	355
Platte Valley Medical Center	Brighton	0.8%	131
Exempla Saint Joseph Hospital	Denver	0.9%	117
The Medical Center of Aurora	Aurora	0.9%	216
Valley View Hospital Association	Glenwood Spgs	1.1%	175
Centura Health - Saint Anthony Hospital	Lakewood	1.2%	255
Arkansas Valley Regional Medical Center	La Junta	1.3%	78
Centura Health-Penrose St Francis	Colorado Spgs	1.3%	388
Medical Center of the Rockies	Loveland	1.5%	467

NOTE: Hospital profiles are in alphabetical order by state, then city, then hospital within the city; Rankings exclude hospitals with less than 25 cases except for patient surveys which excludes hospitals with less than 100 cases; (a) 100-299 cases; (1) The number of cases/patients is too few to report; (2) Data submitted were based on a sample of cases/patients; (3) Results are based on a shorter time period than required; (4) Data suppressed by CMS for one or more quarters; (5) Results are not available for this reporting period; (6) Fewer than 100 patients completed the HCAHPS survey; (7) No cases met the criteria for this measure; (8) The lower limit of the confidence interval cannot be calculated if the number of observed infections equals zero; (9) No data are available from the state/territory for this reporting period; (10) The scores shown reflect fewer than 50 completed surveys; (11) There were discrepancies in the data collection process; (12) This measure does not apply to this hospital for this reporting period; (13) Results cannot be calculated for this reporting period; (14) The results for this state are combined with nearby states to protect confidentiality; Please refer to the User's Guide for a full explanation of data.

Delta County Memorial Hospital	Delta	1.7%	302
Mercy Regional Medical Center	Durango	1.7%	239
Centura Health-Avista Adventist Hosp	Louisville	1.8%	56
Yuma District Hospital	Yuma	1.8%	57
North Colorado Medical Center	Greeley	2.3%	436
Community Hospital	Grand Junction	2.4%	84
Aspen Valley Hospital	Aspen	2.7%	225
Poudre Valley Hospital	Fort Collins	2.8%	435
Colorado Plains Medical Center	Fort Morgan	2.9%	69
Longmont United Hospital	Longmont	2.9%	103
Saint Anthony Summit Medical Center	Frisco	2.9%	69
Centura Health-St Anthony North Hosp	Westminster	3.7%	189
Denver Health Medical Center	Denver	4.0%	379
Spanish Peaks Regional Health Center	Walsenburg	4.0%	75
Centura Health-St Thomas More Hosp	Canon City	5.0%	221
Centura Health-Littleton Adventist Hosp	Littleton	5.9%	289
McKee Medical Center	Loveland	6.4%	235
Centura Health-Porter Adventist Hosp	Denver	6.9%	262
Centura Health-St Mary Corwin Med Ctr	Pueblo	8.3%	363
Sterling Regional Medcenter	Sterling	9.5%	148
Parker Adventist Hospital	Parker	9.9%	233
Montrose Memorial Hospital	Montrose	11.9%	226
San Luis Valley Regional Medical Center	Alamosa	17.9%	117
Univ of CO Health Mem Hosp	Colorado Spgs	20.3%	988
East Morgan County Hospital	Brush	20.6%	63

Follow-up Mammogram/Ultrasound

A follow-up rate near zero may indicate missed cancer; a rate higher than 14% may mean there is unnecessary follow up.

Hospital Name	City	Rate	Cases
Arkansas Valley Regional Medical Center	La Junta	1.2%	508
Gunnison Valley Hospital	Gunnison	3.7%	219
Kit Carson County Memorial Hospital	Burlington	4.1%	74
Longmont United Hospital	Longmont	4.6%	1035
Rose Medical Center	Denver	5.0%	2005
Exempla Saint Joseph Hospital	Denver	5.4%	441
Aspen Valley Hospital	Aspen	5.5%	220
Medical Center of the Rockies	Loveland	5.7%	1065
Community Hospital	Grand Junction	6.2%	679
Pioneers Medical Center	Meeker	6.3%	64
Poudre Valley Hospital	Fort Collins	6.3%	2840
McKee Medical Center	Loveland	6.5%	1560
North Colorado Medical Center	Greeley	6.6%	1895
Univ of CO Health Mem Hosp	Colorado Spgs	6.6%	3043
Centura Health-Avista Adventist Hosp	Louisville	6.7%	511
Estes Park Medical Center	Estes Park	6.7%	298
Yampa Valley Medical Center	Steamboat Spgs	7.2%	332
Vail Valley Medical Center	Vail	7.3%	509
Sedgwick County Memorial Hospital	Julesburg	7.5%	67
Colorado Plains Medical Center	Fort Morgan	7.6%	237
The Medical Center of Aurora	Aurora	7.9%	2103
East Morgan County Hospital	Brush	8.0%	275
Centura Health - Saint Anthony Hospital	Lakewood	8.1%	297
Mercy Regional Medical Center	Durango	8.1%	1267
The Memorial Hospital	Craig	8.2%	195
Centura Health-St Anthony North Hosp	Westminster	8.3%	641
Centura Health-St Thomas More Hosp	Canon City	8.3%	785
Southwest Memorial Hospital	Cortez	8.4%	454
Yuma District Hospital	Yuma	8.5%	165
Presbyterian Saint Lukes Medical Center	Denver	8.6%	567
University of Colorado Hospital	Aurora	8.6%	2348
Valley View Hospital Association	Glenwood Spgs	8.7%	584
Denver Health Medical Center	Denver	8.9%	700
Centura Health-St Mary Corwin Med Ctr	Pueblo	9.2%	1836
Centura Health-Littleton Adventist Hosp	Littleton	9.8%	633
Montrose Memorial Hospital	Montrose	10.0%	956
North Suburban Medical Center	Thornton	10.4%	412
Saint Marys Hospital & Medical Center	Grand Junction	10.9%	1316
Boulder Community Hospital	Boulder	11.4%	2932
Platte Valley Medical Center	Brighton	11.4%	482
Exempla Lutheran Medical Center	Wheat Ridge	11.6%	2197
Parker Adventist Hospital	Parker	11.6%	422
Saint Anthony Summit Medical Center	Frisco	12.0%	250
San Luis Valley Regional Medical Center	Alamosa	12.0%	326
Parkview Medical Center	Pueblo	12.2%	605
Centura Health-Porter Adventist Hosp	Denver	13.4%	582
Exempla Good Samaritan Medical Center	Lafayette	14.5%	186
Centura Health-Penrose St Francis	Colorado Spgs	15.1%	781
Sterling Regional Medcenter	Sterling	15.4%	649
Delta County Memorial Hospital	Delta	18.1%	735

Lumbar Spine MRI for Low Back Pain

Hospital Name	City	Rate	Cases
Exempla Lutheran Medical Center	Wheat Ridge	34.2%	117
The Medical Center of Aurora	Aurora	35.0%	60
Montrose Memorial Hospital	Montrose	35.1%	114
Parker Adventist Hospital	Parker	35.6%	73
Univ of CO Health Mem Hosp	Colorado Spgs	35.8%	293
Poudre Valley Hospital	Fort Collins	36.3%	179
Saint Marys Hospital & Medical Center	Grand Junction	36.4%	99
University of Colorado Hospital	Aurora	36.9%	179
Medical Center of the Rockies	Loveland	38.0%	192
Rose Medical Center	Denver	38.1%	160
Swedish Medical Center	Englewood	38.1%	42
Boulder Community Hospital	Boulder	38.4%	185
McKee Medical Center	Loveland	38.8%	116
Parkview Medical Center	Pueblo	39.2%	143
North Colorado Medical Center	Greeley	40.1%	157
Animas Surgical Hospital	Durango	41.0%	61
Centura Health-St Mary Corwin Med Ctr	Pueblo	41.9%	74
Centura Health - Saint Anthony Hospital	Lakewood	42.4%	59
Delta County Memorial Hospital	Delta	42.4%	59
Presbyterian Saint Lukes Medical Center	Denver	42.5%	40
San Luis Valley Regional Medical Center	Alamosa	42.5%	40
Community Hospital	Grand Junction	42.6%	54
Centura Health-Littleton Adventist Hosp	Littleton	42.9%	49
Sterling Regional Medcenter	Sterling	42.9%	63
Longmont United Hospital	Longmont	43.9%	57
Valley View Hospital Association	Glenwood Spgs	44.1%	59
Exempla Good Samaritan Medical Center	Lafayette	47.4%	38
Centura Health-St Thomas More Hosp	Canon City	47.7%	88
Platte Valley Medical Center	Brighton	47.7%	65
Arkansas Valley Regional Medical Center	La Junta	48.8%	41
Yampa Valley Medical Center	Steamboat Spgs	49.0%	51
Sky Ridge Medical Center	Lone Tree	54.8%	104
Denver Health Medical Center	Denver	55.8%	52

NOTE: Hospital profiles are in alphabetical order by state, then hospital within the city; Rankings exclude hospitals with less than 25 cases except for patient surveys which excludes hospitals with less than 100 cases; (a) 100-299 cases; (1) The number of cases/patients is too few to report; (2) Data submitted were based on a sample of cases/patients; (3) Results are based on a shorter time period than required; (4) Data suppressed by CMS for one or more quarters; (5) Results are not available for this reporting period; (6) Fewer than 100 patients completed the HCAHPS survey; (7) No cases met the criteria for this measure; (8) The lower limit of the confidence interval cannot be calculated if the number of observed infections equals zero; (9) No data are available from the state/territory for this reporting period; (10) The scores shown reflect fewer than 50 completed surveys; (11) There were discrepancies in the data collection process; (12) This measure does not apply to this hospital for this reporting period; (13) Results cannot be calculated for this reporting period; (14) The results for this state are combined with nearby states to protect confidentiality; Please refer to the User's Guide for a full explanation of data.

San Luis Valley Regional Medical Center

106 Blanca Ave Phone: 719-589-2511
Alamosa, CO 81101 Fax: 719-587-1372
URL: www.slvrmc.org
Type: Acute Care Hospitals Emergency Services: Yes
Ownership: Voluntary non-profit - Private Beds: 85

Key Personnel:
Radiology. . . . . Samuel Andelman
CEO/President. . . . . Larry Pochardt
Infection Control. . . . . Leonard Snow
Quality Assurance . . . . Leonard Snow

Measure	Cases	This Hosp.	State Avg.	U.S. Avg.
Blood Clot Prevention and Treatment				
Anticoagulation Overlap Therapy[2]	15	87%	97%	93%
ICU Venous Thromboembolism Prophylaxis[2]	36	100%	95%	92%
Incidence of Potentially Preventable VTE[1,2]	-	-	8%	10%
UFH with Dosages/Platelet Monitoring[2,7]	-	-	97%	97%
Venous Thromboembolism Prophylaxis[2]	99	90%	90%	85%
Warfarin Therapy Discharge Instructions[1,2]	-	-	69%	75%
Chest Pain/Possible Heart Attack Care				
Aspirin Given Within 24 Hours of Arrival	41	98%	97%	96%
Fibrinolytic Meds Within 30 Min. of Arrival[1]	-	-	55%	58%
Average Time to ECG (minutes)	42	7	8	7
Average Time to Transfer (minutes)[7]	-	-	74	60
Children's Asthma Care				
Received Home Management Plan of Care	-	-	-	88%
Received Reliever Medication	-	-	-	100%
Received Systemic Corticosteroids	-	-	-	100%
Emergency Department				
Admittance Decision Time (minutes)[2]	156	108	96	98
Head CT Results Within 45 Min. of Arrival[1]	-	-	67%	57%
Patients Who Left ER Before Being Seen	12,705	2%	2%	2%
Time from ER Arrival to Admit. (minutes)[2]	263	278	244	274
Time from ER Arrival to Discharge (minutes)	355	140	139	134
Time in ER Before Being Evaluated (minutes)	370	20	20	26
Time to Pain Meds for Fractures (minutes)	73	52	45	57
Heart Attack Care				
Aspirin Given at Discharge[1]	-	-	100%	99%
Fibrinolytic Meds Within 30 Min. of Arrival[7]	-	-	20%	54%
PCI Within 90 Minutes of Arrival[7]	-	-	97%	96%
Statin Prescribed at Discharge[1]	-	-	99%	98%
Heart Failure Care				
ACE Inhibitor or ARB for LVSD[1]	-	-	97%	97%
Discharge Instructions Given	23	74%	93%	94%
Evaluation of LVS Function	34	100%	99%	99%
Medicare Spending				
Medicare Spending per Patient (ratio)	-	1.04	0.95	0.98
Pneumonia Care				
Appropriate Initial Antibiotic Given	37	89%	95%	95%
Blood Culture Timing	47	98%	98%	98%
Pregnancy and Delivery Care				
Newborn Deliveries Scheduled Early[2]	45	9%	2%	6%
Preventive Care				
Immunization for Influenza[2]	261	69%	92%	90%
Immunization for Pneumonia[2]	196	70%	92%	92%
Stroke Care				
Anticoagulation Therapy for Atrial Fibrillation[7]	-	-	97%	95%
Antithrombotic Therapy Timing	12	92%	98%	98%
Assessed for Rehabilitation[1]	-	-	98%	97%
Discharged on Antithrombotic Therapy[1]	-	-	100%	99%
Discharged on Statin Medication[1]	-	-	94%	94%
Thrombolytic Therapy Timing[7]	-	-	78%	66%
Venous Thromboembolism Prophylaxis[1]	-	-	96%	94%
Written Stroke Educational Materials Given[1]	-	-	87%	88%
Surgical Care Improvement Project				
Appropriate Beta Blocker Usage	20	90%	98%	98%
Appropriate VTP Within 24 Hours	103	99%	98%	98%
Controlled Postoperative Blood Glucose[7]	-	-	96%	97%
Perioperative Temperature Management	128	100%	99%	100%
Prophylactic Antibiotic Selection	98	98%	99%	99%
Prophylactic Antibiotic Selection (Outpatient)[3,7]	-	-	98%	98%
Prophylactic Antibiotic Stopped	98	100%	98%	98%
Prophylactic Antibiotic Timing	100	80%	98%	99%
Prophylactic Antibiotic Timing (Outpatient)[1,3]	-	-	98%	98%
Urinary Catheter Removal	78	96%	97%	97%
Survey of Patients' Hospital Experiences				
Area Around Room 'Always' Quiet at Night	300+	48%	64%	61%
Doctors 'Always' Communicated Well	300+	77%	81%	82%
Home Recovery Information Given	300+	81%	87%	85%
Hospital Given 9 or 10 on 10 Point Scale	300+	49%	75%	71%
Meds 'Always' Explained Before Given	300+	59%	67%	64%
Nurses 'Always' Communicated Well	300+	71%	79%	79%
Pain 'Always' Well Controlled	300+	69%	72%	71%
Room and Bathroom 'Always' Clean	300+	73%	74%	73%
Timely Help 'Always' Received	300+	60%	70%	68%
Would Definitely Recommend Hospital	300+	45%	76%	71%
Use of Medical Imaging				
Cardiac Imaging Stress Test before Surgery	107	3.7%	5%	5.3%
Combination Abdominal CT Scan	237	22.8%	10%	10.5%
Combination Brain/Sinus CT Scan	171	1.2%	2.1%	2.7%
Combination Chest CT Scan	117	17.9%	3.1%	2.7%
Follow-up Mammogram/Ultrasound	326	12.0%	8.7%	8.8%
Lumbar Spine MRI for Low Back Pain	40	42.5%	39.7%	37.2%

Aspen Valley Hospital

0401 Castle Creek Road Phone: 970-544-1261
Aspen, CO 81611 Fax: 970-544-1585
URL: www.avhaspen.org
Type: Critical Access Hospitals Emergency Services: Yes
Ownership: Govt - Hospital Dist/Auth Beds: 25

Key Personnel:
Operating Room. . . . . Todd Bartlett, RN
Chief of Medical Staff. . . . . Chris Beck, MD
Coronary Care . . . . Joseph Dunn, RN
Pediatric In-Patient Care . . . . . . Joseph Dunn, RN
Radiology. . . . . Bart Dutzen, RT
Infection Control. . . . . Kathy Gibbard, RN
Quality Assurance . . . . Annette Kremer
CEO/President. . . . . Dave Ressler

Measure	Cases	This Hosp.	State Avg.	U.S. Avg.
Blood Clot Prevention and Treatment				
Anticoagulation Overlap Therapy[5]	-	-	97%	93%
ICU Venous Thromboembolism Prophylaxis[5]	-	-	95%	92%
Incidence of Potentially Preventable VTE[5]	-	-	8%	10%
UFH with Dosages/Platelet Monitoring[5]	-	-	97%	97%
Venous Thromboembolism Prophylaxis[5]	-	-	90%	85%
Warfarin Therapy Discharge Instructions[5]	-	-	69%	75%
Chest Pain/Possible Heart Attack Care				
Aspirin Given Within 24 Hours of Arrival[1]	-	-	97%	96%
Fibrinolytic Meds Within 30 Min. of Arrival[1]	-	-	55%	58%
Average Time to ECG (minutes)	11	11	8	7
Average Time to Transfer (minutes)[1]	-	-	74	60
Children's Asthma Care				
Received Home Management Plan of Care	-	-	-	88%
Received Reliever Medication	-	-	-	100%
Received Systemic Corticosteroids	-	-	-	100%
Emergency Department				
Admittance Decision Time (minutes)[5]	-	-	96	98
Head CT Results Within 45 Min. of Arrival[5]	-	-	67%	57%
Patients Who Left ER Before Being Seen[5]	-	-	2%	2%
Time from ER Arrival to Admit. (minutes)[5]	-	-	244	274
Time from ER Arrival to Discharge (minutes)[5]	-	-	139	134
Time in ER Before Being Evaluated (minutes)[5]	-	-	20	26
Time to Pain Meds for Fractures (minutes)[5]	-	-	45	57
Heart Attack Care				
Aspirin Given at Discharge[3,7]	-	-	100%	99%
Fibrinolytic Meds Within 30 Min. of Arrival[3,7]	-	-	20%	54%
PCI Within 90 Minutes of Arrival[3,7]	-	-	97%	96%
Statin Prescribed at Discharge[3,7]	-	-	99%	98%
Heart Failure Care				
ACE Inhibitor or ARB for LVSD[1]	-	-	97%	97%
Discharge Instructions Given	11	100%	93%	94%
Evaluation of LVS Function	11	100%	99%	99%
Medicare Spending				
Medicare Spending per Patient (ratio)	-	-	0.95	0.98
Pneumonia Care				
Appropriate Initial Antibiotic Given[1]	-	-	95%	95%
Blood Culture Timing[1]	-	-	98%	98%
Pregnancy and Delivery Care				
Newborn Deliveries Scheduled Early[5]	-	-	2%	6%
Preventive Care				
Immunization for Influenza[5]	-	-	92%	90%
Immunization for Pneumonia[2,3]	74	86%	92%	92%
Stroke Care				
Anticoagulation Therapy for Atrial Fibrillation[5]	-	-	97%	95%
Antithrombotic Therapy Timing[5]	-	-	98%	98%
Assessed for Rehabilitation[5]	-	-	98%	97%
Discharged on Antithrombotic Therapy[5]	-	-	100%	99%
Discharged on Statin Medication[5]	-	-	94%	94%
Thrombolytic Therapy Timing[5]	-	-	78%	66%
Venous Thromboembolism Prophylaxis[5]	-	-	96%	94%
Written Stroke Educational Materials Given[5]	-	-	87%	88%
Surgical Care Improvement Project				
Appropriate Beta Blocker Usage[3]	19	100%	98%	98%
Appropriate VTP Within 24 Hours[3]	100	100%	98%	98%
Controlled Postoperative Blood Glucose[3,7]	-	-	96%	97%
Perioperative Temperature Management[3]	123	100%	99%	100%
Prophylactic Antibiotic Selection[3]	108	98%	99%	99%
Prophylactic Antibiotic Selection (Outpatient)[5]	-	-	98%	98%
Prophylactic Antibiotic Stopped[3]	107	96%	98%	98%
Prophylactic Antibiotic Timing[3]	108	98%	98%	99%
Prophylactic Antibiotic Timing (Outpatient)[5]	-	-	98%	98%
Urinary Catheter Removal[3]	71	99%	97%	97%
Survey of Patients' Hospital Experiences				
Area Around Room 'Always' Quiet at Night	(a)	74%	64%	61%
Doctors 'Always' Communicated Well	(a)	84%	81%	82%
Home Recovery Information Given	(a)	86%	87%	85%
Hospital Given 9 or 10 on 10 Point Scale	(a)	81%	75%	71%
Meds 'Always' Explained Before Given	(a)	66%	67%	64%
Nurses 'Always' Communicated Well	(a)	81%	79%	79%
Pain 'Always' Well Controlled	(a)	73%	72%	71%
Room and Bathroom 'Always' Clean	(a)	85%	74%	73%
Timely Help 'Always' Received	(a)	75%	70%	68%
Would Definitely Recommend Hospital	(a)	78%	76%	71%
Use of Medical Imaging				
Cardiac Imaging Stress Test before Surgery	174	5.7%	5%	5.3%
Combination Abdominal CT Scan	144	11.8%	10%	10.5%
Combination Brain/Sinus CT Scan[1]	-	-	2.1%	2.7%
Combination Chest CT Scan	225	2.7%	3.1%	2.7%
Follow-up Mammogram/Ultrasound	220	5.5%	8.7%	8.8%
Lumbar Spine MRI for Low Back Pain[1]	-	-	39.7%	37.2%

Childrens Hospital Colorado

13123 East 16th Avenue Phone: 720-777-1234
Aurora, CO 80045
URL: www.childrenscolorado.org
Type: Childrens Emergency Services: No
Ownership: Voluntary non-profit - Private Beds: 318

Key Personnel:
President/CEO. . . . . Jim Shmerling, DHA, FACHE

Measure	Cases	This Hosp.	State Avg.	U.S. Avg.
Blood Clot Prevention and Treatment				
Anticoagulation Overlap Therapy[5]	-	-	97%	93%
ICU Venous Thromboembolism Prophylaxis[5]	-	-	95%	92%
Incidence of Potentially Preventable VTE[5]	-	-	8%	10%
UFH with Dosages/Platelet Monitoring[5]	-	-	97%	97%
Venous Thromboembolism Prophylaxis[5]	-	-	90%	85%
Warfarin Therapy Discharge Instructions[5]	-	-	69%	75%
Chest Pain/Possible Heart Attack Care				
Aspirin Given Within 24 Hours of Arrival	-	-	97%	96%
Fibrinolytic Meds Within 30 Min. of Arrival	-	-	55%	58%
Average Time to ECG (minutes)	-	-	8	7
Average Time to Transfer (minutes)	-	-	74	60
Children's Asthma Care				
Received Home Management Plan of Care	813	94%	-	88%
Received Reliever Medication	814	100%	-	100%
Received Systemic Corticosteroids	814	100%	-	100%
Emergency Department				
Admittance Decision Time (minutes)[5]	-	-	96	98
Head CT Results Within 45 Min. of Arrival	-	-	67%	57%

NOTE: Hospital profiles are in alphabetical order by state, then city, then hospital within the city; Rankings exclude hospitals with less than 25 cases except for patient surveys which excludes hospitals with less than 100 cases; (a) 100-299 cases; (1) The number of cases/patients is too few to report; (2) Data submitted were based on a sample of cases/patients; (3) Results are based on a shorter time period than required; (4) Data suppressed by CMS for one or more quarters; (5) Results are not available for this reporting period; (6) Fewer than 100 patients completed the HCAHPS survey; (7) No cases met the criteria for this measure; (8) The lower limit of the confidence interval cannot be calculated if the number of observed infections equals zero; (9) No data are available from the state/territory for this reporting period; (10) The scores shown reflect fewer than 50 completed surveys; (11) There were discrepancies in the data collection process; (12) This measure does not apply to this hospital for this reporting period; (13) Results cannot be calculated for this reporting period; (14) The results for this state are combined with nearby states to protect confidentiality; Please refer to the User's Guide for a full explanation of data.

Measure	Cases	This Hosp.	State Avg.	U.S. Avg.
Patients Who Left ER Before Being Seen	-	-	2%	2%
Time from ER Arrival to Admit. (minutes)[5]	-	-	244	274
Time from ER Arrival to Discharge (minutes)	-	-	139	134
Time in ER Before Being Evaluated (minutes)	-	-	20	26
Time to Pain Meds for Fractures (minutes)	-	-	45	57
Heart Attack Care				
Aspirin Given at Discharge[5]	-	-	100%	99%
Fibrinolytic Meds Within 30 Min. of Arrival[5]	-	-	20%	54%
PCI Within 90 Minutes of Arrival[5]	-	-	97%	96%
Statin Prescribed at Discharge[5]	-	-	99%	98%
Heart Failure Care				
ACE Inhibitor or ARB for LVSD[5]	-	-	97%	97%
Discharge Instructions Given[5]	-	-	93%	94%
Evaluation of LVS Function[5]	-	-	99%	99%
Medicare Spending				
Medicare Spending per Patient (ratio)	-	-	0.95	0.98
Pneumonia Care				
Appropriate Initial Antibiotic Given[5]	-	-	95%	95%
Blood Culture Timing[5]	-	-	98%	98%
Pregnancy and Delivery Care				
Newborn Deliveries Scheduled Early[5]	-	-	2%	6%
Preventive Care				
Immunization for Influenza[5]	-	-	92%	90%
Immunization for Pneumonia[5]	-	-	92%	92%
Stroke Care				
Anticoagulation Therapy for Atrial Fibrillation[5]	-	-	97%	95%
Antithrombotic Therapy Timing[5]	-	-	98%	98%
Assessed for Rehabilitation[5]	-	-	98%	97%
Discharged on Antithrombotic Therapy[5]	-	-	100%	99%
Discharged on Statin Medication[5]	-	-	94%	94%
Thrombolytic Therapy Timing[5]	-	-	78%	66%
Venous Thromboembolism Prophylaxis[5]	-	-	96%	94%
Written Stroke Educational Materials Given[5]	-	-	87%	88%
Surgical Care Improvement Project				
Appropriate Beta Blocker Usage[5]	-	-	98%	98%
Appropriate VTP Within 24 Hours[5]	-	-	98%	98%
Controlled Postoperative Blood Glucose[5]	-	-	96%	97%
Perioperative Temperature Management[5]	-	-	99%	100%
Prophylactic Antibiotic Selection[5]	-	-	99%	99%
Prophylactic Antibiotic Selection (Outpatient)	-	-	98%	98%
Prophylactic Antibiotic Stopped[5]	-	-	98%	98%
Prophylactic Antibiotic Timing[5]	-	-	98%	99%
Prophylactic Antibiotic Timing (Outpatient)	-	-	98%	98%
Urinary Catheter Removal[5]	-	-	97%	97%
Survey of Patients' Hospital Experiences				
Area Around Room 'Always' Quiet at Night[5]	-	-	64%	61%
Doctors 'Always' Communicated Well[5]	-	-	81%	82%
Home Recovery Information Given[5]	-	-	87%	85%
Hospital Given 9 or 10 on 10 Point Scale[5]	-	-	75%	71%
Meds 'Always' Explained Before Given[5]	-	-	67%	64%
Nurses 'Always' Communicated Well[5]	-	-	79%	79%
Pain 'Always' Well Controlled[5]	-	-	72%	71%
Room and Bathroom 'Always' Clean[5]	-	-	74%	73%
Timely Help 'Always' Received[5]	-	-	70%	68%
Would Definitely Recommend Hospital[5]	-	-	76%	71%
Use of Medical Imaging				
Cardiac Imaging Stress Test before Surgery	-	-	5%	5.3%
Combination Abdominal CT Scan	-	-	10%	10.5%
Combination Brain/Sinus CT Scan	-	-	2.1%	2.7%
Combination Chest CT Scan	-	-	3.1%	2.7%
Follow-up Mammogram/Ultrasound	-	-	8.7%	8.8%
Lumbar Spine MRI for Low Back Pain	-	-	39.7%	37.2%

The Medical Center of Aurora

1501 S Potomac St — Phone: 303-695-2600
Aurora, CO 80012 — Fax: 303-873-5682
URL: www.auroramed.com
Type: Acute Care Hospitals — Emergency Services: Yes
Ownership: Proprietary — Beds: 372
Key Personnel:
CEO/President. . . . . Richard Hammett
Quality Assurance . . . . Donna Kusuda
Chief of Medical Staff. . . . . Dr. Dianne McCallister
Operating Room. . . . . Linda Young

Measure	Cases	This Hosp.	State Avg.	U.S. Avg.
Blood Clot Prevention and Treatment				
Anticoagulation Overlap Therapy[2]	160	100%	97%	93%
ICU Venous Thromboembolism Prophylaxis[2]	97	100%	95%	92%
Incidence of Potentially Preventable VTE[2]	25	0%	8%	10%
UFH with Dosages/Platelet Monitoring[2]	110	100%	97%	97%
Venous Thromboembolism Prophylaxis[2]	352	94%	90%	85%
Warfarin Therapy Discharge Instructions[2]	123	100%	69%	75%
Chest Pain/Possible Heart Attack Care				
Aspirin Given Within 24 Hours of Arrival	42	98%	97%	96%
Fibrinolytic Meds Within 30 Min. of Arrival[3,7]	-	-	55%	58%
Average Time to ECG (minutes)	44	6	8	7
Average Time to Transfer (minutes)[1,3]	-	-	74	60
Children's Asthma Care				
Received Home Management Plan of Care	-	-	-	88%
Received Reliever Medication	-	-	-	100%
Received Systemic Corticosteroids	-	-	-	100%
Emergency Department				
Admittance Decision Time (minutes)[2]	789	120	96	98
Head CT Results Within 45 Min. of Arrival	15	60%	67%	57%
Patients Who Left ER Before Being Seen	76,851	1%	2%	2%
Time from ER Arrival to Admit. (minutes)[2]	789	257	244	274
Time from ER Arrival to Discharge (minutes)	458	140	139	134
Time in ER Before Being Evaluated (minutes)	525	12	20	26
Time to Pain Meds for Fractures (minutes)	197	34	45	57
Heart Attack Care				
Aspirin Given at Discharge[2]	260	100%	100%	99%
Fibrinolytic Meds Within 30 Min. of Arrival[2,7]	-	-	20%	54%
PCI Within 90 Minutes of Arrival[2]	61	97%	97%	96%
Statin Prescribed at Discharge[2]	255	100%	99%	98%
Heart Failure Care				
ACE Inhibitor or ARB for LVSD[2]	91	97%	97%	97%
Discharge Instructions Given[2]	204	97%	93%	94%
Evaluation of LVS Function[2]	269	99%	99%	99%
Medicare Spending				
Medicare Spending per Patient (ratio)	-	1.04	0.95	0.98
Pneumonia Care				
Appropriate Initial Antibiotic Given[2]	106	98%	95%	95%
Blood Culture Timing[2]	156	100%	98%	98%
Pregnancy and Delivery Care				
Newborn Deliveries Scheduled Early[2]	49	0%	2%	6%
Preventive Care				
Immunization for Influenza[2]	590	99%	92%	90%
Immunization for Pneumonia[2]	739	98%	92%	92%
Stroke Care				
Anticoagulation Therapy for Atrial Fibrillation[2]	13	92%	97%	95%
Antithrombotic Therapy Timing[2]	73	99%	98%	98%
Assessed for Rehabilitation[2]	97	100%	98%	97%
Discharged on Antithrombotic Therapy[2]	87	100%	100%	99%
Discharged on Statin Medication[2]	60	100%	94%	94%
Thrombolytic Therapy Timing[2]	14	93%	78%	66%
Venous Thromboembolism Prophylaxis[2]	98	100%	96%	94%
Written Stroke Educational Materials Given[2]	59	93%	87%	88%
Surgical Care Improvement Project				
Appropriate Beta Blocker Usage[2]	158	99%	98%	98%
Appropriate VTP Within 24 Hours[2]	434	99%	98%	98%
Controlled Postoperative Blood Glucose[2]	75	99%	96%	97%
Perioperative Temperature Management[2]	487	100%	99%	100%
Prophylactic Antibiotic Selection[2]	335	100%	99%	99%
Prophylactic Antibiotic Selection (Outpatient)	308	100%	98%	98%
Prophylactic Antibiotic Stopped[2]	313	97%	98%	98%
Prophylactic Antibiotic Timing[2]	336	100%	98%	99%
Prophylactic Antibiotic Timing (Outpatient)	309	99%	98%	98%
Urinary Catheter Removal[2]	360	99%	97%	97%
Survey of Patients' Hospital Experiences				
Area Around Room 'Always' Quiet at Night	300+	62%	64%	61%
Doctors 'Always' Communicated Well	300+	74%	81%	82%
Home Recovery Information Given	300+	85%	87%	85%
Hospital Given 9 or 10 on 10 Point Scale	300+	70%	75%	71%
Meds 'Always' Explained Before Given	300+	64%	67%	64%
Nurses 'Always' Communicated Well	300+	77%	79%	79%
Pain 'Always' Well Controlled	300+	70%	72%	71%
Room and Bathroom 'Always' Clean	300+	70%	74%	73%
Timely Help 'Always' Received	300+	65%	70%	68%
Would Definitely Recommend Hospital	300+	71%	76%	71%
Use of Medical Imaging				
Cardiac Imaging Stress Test before Surgery	263	5.7%	5%	5.3%
Combination Abdominal CT Scan	684	3.9%	10%	10.5%
Combination Brain/Sinus CT Scan	615	2.0%	2.1%	2.7%
Combination Chest CT Scan	216	0.9%	3.1%	2.7%
Follow-up Mammogram/Ultrasound	2,103	7.9%	8.7%	8.8%
Lumbar Spine MRI for Low Back Pain	60	35.0%	39.7%	37.2%

University of Colorado Hospital

12605 East 16th Avenue — Phone: 720-848-0000
Aurora, CO 80045
URL: www.uch.edu
Type: Acute Care Hospitals — Emergency Services: Yes
Ownership: Govt - Hospital Dist/Auth
Key Personnel:
President/CEO. . . . . John P. Harney

Measure	Cases	This Hosp.	State Avg.	U.S. Avg.
Blood Clot Prevention and Treatment				
Anticoagulation Overlap Therapy[2]	163	99%	97%	93%
ICU Venous Thromboembolism Prophylaxis[2]	102	99%	95%	92%
Incidence of Potentially Preventable VTE[2]	54	6%	8%	10%
UFH with Dosages/Platelet Monitoring[2]	182	95%	97%	97%
Venous Thromboembolism Prophylaxis[2]	268	92%	90%	85%
Warfarin Therapy Discharge Instructions[2]	139	62%	69%	75%
Chest Pain/Possible Heart Attack Care				
Aspirin Given Within 24 Hours of Arrival[3,7]	-	-	97%	96%
Fibrinolytic Meds Within 30 Min. of Arrival[5]	-	-	55%	58%
Average Time to ECG (minutes)[3,7]	-	-	8	7
Average Time to Transfer (minutes)[5]	-	-	74	60
Children's Asthma Care				
Received Home Management Plan of Care	-	-	-	88%
Received Reliever Medication	-	-	-	100%
Received Systemic Corticosteroids	-	-	-	100%
Emergency Department				
Admittance Decision Time (minutes)[2]	344	126	96	98
Head CT Results Within 45 Min. of Arrival[1]	-	-	67%	57%
Patients Who Left ER Before Being Seen	70,430	5%	2%	2%
Time from ER Arrival to Admit. (minutes)[2]	345	353	244	274
Time from ER Arrival to Discharge (minutes)	333	185	139	134
Time in ER Before Being Evaluated (minutes)	378	21	20	26
Time to Pain Meds for Fractures (minutes)	72	51	45	57
Heart Attack Care				
Aspirin Given at Discharge	227	100%	100%	99%
Fibrinolytic Meds Within 30 Min. of Arrival[7]	-	-	20%	54%
PCI Within 90 Minutes of Arrival	42	93%	97%	96%
Statin Prescribed at Discharge	220	99%	99%	98%
Heart Failure Care				
ACE Inhibitor or ARB for LVSD[2]	110	99%	97%	97%
Discharge Instructions Given[2]	262	91%	93%	94%
Evaluation of LVS Function[2]	296	100%	99%	99%
Medicare Spending				
Medicare Spending per Patient (ratio)	-	0.95	0.95	0.98
Pneumonia Care				
Appropriate Initial Antibiotic Given[2]	86	99%	95%	95%
Blood Culture Timing[2]	145	92%	98%	98%
Pregnancy and Delivery Care				
Newborn Deliveries Scheduled Early[2]	39	0%	2%	6%
Preventive Care				
Immunization for Influenza[2]	513	69%	92%	90%
Immunization for Pneumonia[2]	494	74%	92%	92%
Stroke Care				
Anticoagulation Therapy for Atrial Fibrillation[2]	13	100%	97%	95%
Antithrombotic Therapy Timing[2]	50	100%	98%	98%
Assessed for Rehabilitation[2]	131	99%	98%	97%
Discharged on Antithrombotic Therapy[2]	80	100%	100%	99%
Discharged on Statin Medication[2]	45	100%	94%	94%
Thrombolytic Therapy Timing[2]	17	88%	78%	66%
Venous Thromboembolism Prophylaxis[2]	135	97%	96%	94%
Written Stroke Educational Materials Given[2]	80	96%	87%	88%
Surgical Care Improvement Project				

NOTE: Hospital profiles are in alphabetical order by state, then city, then hospital within the city; Rankings exclude hospitals with less than 25 cases except for patient surveys which excludes hospitals with less than 100 cases; (a) 100-299 cases; (1) The number of cases/patients is too few to report; (2) Data submitted were based on a sample of cases/patients; (3) Results are based on a shorter time period than required; (4) Data suppressed by CMS for one or more quarters; (5) Results are not available for this reporting period; (6) Fewer than 100 patients completed the HCAHPS survey; (7) No cases met the criteria for this measure; (8) The lower limit of the confidence interval cannot be calculated if the number of observed infections equals zero; (9) No data are available from the state/territory for this reporting period; (10) The scores shown reflect fewer than 50 completed surveys; (11) There were discrepancies in the data collection process; (12) This measure does not apply to this hospital for this reporting period; (13) Results cannot be calculated for this reporting period; (14) The results for this state are combined with nearby states to protect confidentiality; Please refer to the User's Guide for a full explanation of data.

Appropriate Beta Blocker Usage[2]	152	97%	98%	98%
Appropriate VTP Within 24 Hours[2]	338	100%	98%	98%
Controlled Postoperative Blood Glucose[2]	136	90%	96%	97%
Perioperative Temperature Management[2]	458	100%	99%	100%
Prophylactic Antibiotic Selection[2]	397	99%	99%	99%
Prophylactic Antibiotic Selection (Outpatient)	288	98%	98%	98%
Prophylactic Antibiotic Stopped[2]	381	96%	98%	98%
Prophylactic Antibiotic Timing[2]	396	98%	98%	99%
Prophylactic Antibiotic Timing (Outpatient)	47	100%	98%	98%
Urinary Catheter Removal[2]	349	94%	97%	97%
Survey of Patients' Hospital Experiences				
Area Around Room 'Always' Quiet at Night	300+	63%	64%	61%
Doctors 'Always' Communicated Well	300+	79%	81%	82%
Home Recovery Information Given	300+	85%	87%	85%
Hospital Given 9 or 10 on 10 Point Scale	300+	77%	75%	71%
Meds 'Always' Explained Before Given	300+	65%	67%	64%
Nurses 'Always' Communicated Well	300+	79%	79%	79%
Pain 'Always' Well Controlled	300+	70%	72%	71%
Room and Bathroom 'Always' Clean	300+	70%	74%	73%
Timely Help 'Always' Received	300+	65%	70%	68%
Would Definitely Recommend Hospital	300+	80%	76%	71%
Use of Medical Imaging				
Cardiac Imaging Stress Test before Surgery	420	7.1%	5%	5.3%
Combination Abdominal CT Scan	2,535	6.8%	10%	10.5%
Combination Brain/Sinus CT Scan	613	1.8%	2.1%	2.7%
Combination Chest CT Scan	2,935	0.2%	3.1%	2.7%
Follow-up Mammogram/Ultrasound	2,348	8.6%	8.7%	8.8%
Lumbar Spine MRI for Low Back Pain	179	36.9%	39.7%	37.2%

Boulder Community Hospital

1100 Balsam Avenue
Boulder, CO 80304
Phone: 303-440-2273
Fax: 303-441-0478
E-mail: pr@bch.org
URL: www.bch.org
Type: Acute Care Hospitals
Emergency Services: Yes
Ownership: Voluntary non-profit - Private
Beds: 265

Key Personnel:
Hemotology Center . . . . Connie Holden
CEO/President. . . . . Mark King, MD
Surgery . . . . Robert Koch, MD
Chief of Medical Staff . . . . Paul Lewis, MD
Radiology. . . . . Joe Mikoni

Measure	Cases	This Hosp.	State Avg.	U.S. Avg.
Blood Clot Prevention and Treatment				
Anticoagulation Overlap Therapy[2]	97	100%	97%	93%
ICU Venous Thromboembolism Prophylaxis[2]	75	96%	95%	92%
Incidence of Potentially Preventable VTE[2]	16	0%	8%	10%
UFH with Dosages/Platelet Monitoring[2]	72	100%	97%	97%
Venous Thromboembolism Prophylaxis[2]	304	94%	90%	85%
Warfarin Therapy Discharge Instructions[2]	77	96%	69%	75%
Chest Pain/Possible Heart Attack Care				
Aspirin Given Within 24 Hours of Arrival[1,3]	-	-	97%	96%
Fibrinolytic Meds Within 30 Min. of Arrival[5]	-	-	55%	58%
Average Time to ECG (minutes)[1,3]	-	-	8	7
Average Time to Transfer (minutes)[5]	-	-	74	60
Children's Asthma Care				
Received Home Management Plan of Care	-	-	-	88%
Received Reliever Medication	-	-	-	100%
Received Systemic Corticosteroids	-	-	-	100%
Emergency Department				
Admittance Decision Time (minutes)[2]	423	71	96	98
Head CT Results Within 45 Min. of Arrival[1]	-	-	67%	57%
Patients Who Left ER Before Being Seen	32,571	1%	2%	2%
Time from ER Arrival to Admit. (minutes)[2]	438	188	244	274
Time from ER Arrival to Discharge (minutes)	316	120	139	134
Time in ER Before Being Evaluated (minutes)	376	21	20	26
Time to Pain Meds for Fractures (minutes)	160	34	45	57
Heart Attack Care				
Aspirin Given at Discharge	68	99%	100%	99%
Fibrinolytic Meds Within 30 Min. of Arrival[7]	-	-	20%	54%
PCI Within 90 Minutes of Arrival	16	94%	97%	96%
Statin Prescribed at Discharge	68	97%	99%	98%
Heart Failure Care				
ACE Inhibitor or ARB for LVSD	34	94%	97%	97%
Discharge Instructions Given	111	66%	93%	94%
Evaluation of LVS Function	150	100%	99%	99%
Medicare Spending				
Medicare Spending per Patient (ratio)	-	0.98	0.95	0.98
Pneumonia Care				
Appropriate Initial Antibiotic Given	86	92%	95%	95%
Blood Culture Timing	140	95%	98%	98%
Pregnancy and Delivery Care				
Newborn Deliveries Scheduled Early[2]	31	6%	2%	6%
Preventive Care				
Immunization for Influenza[2]	533	87%	92%	90%
Immunization for Pneumonia[2]	534	89%	92%	92%
Stroke Care				
Anticoagulation Therapy for Atrial Fibrillation	16	100%	97%	95%
Antithrombotic Therapy Timing	65	100%	98%	98%
Assessed for Rehabilitation	91	97%	98%	97%
Discharged on Antithrombotic Therapy	78	100%	100%	99%
Discharged on Statin Medication	47	96%	94%	94%
Thrombolytic Therapy Timing	12	100%	78%	66%
Venous Thromboembolism Prophylaxis	87	95%	96%	94%
Written Stroke Educational Materials Given	45	73%	87%	88%
Surgical Care Improvement Project				
Appropriate Beta Blocker Usage[2]	115	95%	98%	98%
Appropriate VTP Within 24 Hours[2]	284	94%	98%	98%
Controlled Postoperative Blood Glucose[2]	106	92%	96%	97%
Perioperative Temperature Management[2]	366	100%	99%	100%
Prophylactic Antibiotic Selection[2]	311	96%	99%	99%
Prophylactic Antibiotic Selection (Outpatient)	274	98%	98%	98%
Prophylactic Antibiotic Stopped[2]	305	96%	98%	98%
Prophylactic Antibiotic Timing[2]	312	97%	98%	99%
Prophylactic Antibiotic Timing (Outpatient)	279	95%	98%	98%
Urinary Catheter Removal[2]	311	98%	97%	97%
Survey of Patients' Hospital Experiences				
Area Around Room 'Always' Quiet at Night	300+	60%	64%	61%
Doctors 'Always' Communicated Well	300+	81%	81%	82%
Home Recovery Information Given	300+	88%	87%	85%
Hospital Given 9 or 10 on 10 Point Scale	300+	72%	75%	71%
Meds 'Always' Explained Before Given	300+	64%	67%	64%
Nurses 'Always' Communicated Well	300+	78%	79%	79%
Pain 'Always' Well Controlled	300+	72%	72%	71%
Room and Bathroom 'Always' Clean	300+	71%	74%	73%
Timely Help 'Always' Received	300+	69%	70%	68%
Would Definitely Recommend Hospital	300+	75%	76%	71%
Use of Medical Imaging				
Cardiac Imaging Stress Test before Surgery	530	5.1%	5%	5.3%
Combination Abdominal CT Scan	561	9.1%	10%	10.5%
Combination Brain/Sinus CT Scan	418	1.4%	2.1%	2.7%
Combination Chest CT Scan	345	0.0%	3.1%	2.7%
Follow-up Mammogram/Ultrasound	2,932	11.4%	8.7%	8.8%
Lumbar Spine MRI for Low Back Pain	185	38.4%	39.7%	37.2%

Platte Valley Medical Center

1600 Prairie Center Parkway
Brighton, CO 80601
Phone: 303-498-1601
URL: www.pvmc.org
Type: Acute Care Hospitals
Emergency Services: Yes
Ownership: Voluntary non-profit - Private
Beds: 98

Key Personnel:
Infection Control. . . . . Colleen Casaceli, RN
Anesthesiology. . . . . Matthew Flaherty
CEO/President. . . . . John Hicks
Quality Assurance . . . . Elaine Massie
Radiology. . . . . Eric Robbins
Intensive Care Unit. . . . . Michele Slem
Operating Room. . . . . Karen Welz, RN
Emergency Room . . . . Fred O Williams

Measure	Cases	This Hosp.	State Avg.	U.S. Avg.
Blood Clot Prevention and Treatment				
Anticoagulation Overlap Therapy[2]	18	94%	97%	93%
ICU Venous Thromboembolism Prophylaxis[2]	34	100%	95%	92%
Incidence of Potentially Preventable VTE[1,2]	-	-	8%	10%
UFH with Dosages/Platelet Monitoring[2]	11	100%	97%	97%
Venous Thromboembolism Prophylaxis[2]	206	98%	90%	85%
Warfarin Therapy Discharge Instructions[2]	15	87%	69%	75%
Chest Pain/Possible Heart Attack Care				
Aspirin Given Within 24 Hours of Arrival	17	100%	97%	96%
Fibrinolytic Meds Within 30 Min. of Arrival[7]	-	-	55%	58%
Average Time to ECG (minutes)	17	4	8	7
Average Time to Transfer (minutes)[1]	-	-	74	60
Children's Asthma Care				
Received Home Management Plan of Care	-	-	-	88%
Received Reliever Medication	-	-	-	100%
Received Systemic Corticosteroids	-	-	-	100%
Emergency Department				
Admittance Decision Time (minutes)[2]	328	52	96	98
Head CT Results Within 45 Min. of Arrival[1]	-	-	67%	57%
Patients Who Left ER Before Being Seen	21,226	0%	2%	2%
Time from ER Arrival to Admit. (minutes)[2]	340	214	244	274
Time from ER Arrival to Discharge (minutes)	489	158	139	134
Time in ER Before Being Evaluated (minutes)	215	28	20	26
Time to Pain Meds for Fractures (minutes)	101	40	45	57
Heart Attack Care				
Aspirin Given at Discharge	53	98%	100%	99%
Fibrinolytic Meds Within 30 Min. of Arrival[7]	-	-	20%	54%
PCI Within 90 Minutes of Arrival[1]	-	-	97%	96%
Statin Prescribed at Discharge	49	100%	99%	98%
Heart Failure Care				
ACE Inhibitor or ARB for LVSD	24	100%	97%	97%
Discharge Instructions Given	64	98%	93%	94%
Evaluation of LVS Function	69	100%	99%	99%
Medicare Spending				
Medicare Spending per Patient (ratio)	-	0.98	0.95	0.98
Pneumonia Care				
Appropriate Initial Antibiotic Given	70	100%	95%	95%
Blood Culture Timing	109	99%	98%	98%
Pregnancy and Delivery Care				
Newborn Deliveries Scheduled Early	122	2%	2%	6%
Preventive Care				
Immunization for Influenza[2]	312	92%	92%	90%
Immunization for Pneumonia[2]	283	95%	92%	92%
Stroke Care				
Anticoagulation Therapy for Atrial Fibrillation[1]	-	-	97%	95%
Antithrombotic Therapy Timing	25	100%	98%	98%
Assessed for Rehabilitation	33	100%	98%	97%
Discharged on Antithrombotic Therapy	33	100%	100%	99%
Discharged on Statin Medication	26	100%	94%	94%
Thrombolytic Therapy Timing[1]	-	-	78%	66%
Venous Thromboembolism Prophylaxis	30	97%	96%	94%
Written Stroke Educational Materials Given	22	100%	87%	88%
Surgical Care Improvement Project				
Appropriate Beta Blocker Usage	39	100%	98%	98%
Appropriate VTP Within 24 Hours	157	96%	98%	98%
Controlled Postoperative Blood Glucose[7]	-	-	96%	97%
Perioperative Temperature Management	169	100%	99%	100%
Prophylactic Antibiotic Selection	116	98%	99%	99%
Prophylactic Antibiotic Selection (Outpatient)	82	100%	98%	98%
Prophylactic Antibiotic Stopped	116	100%	98%	98%
Prophylactic Antibiotic Timing	116	100%	98%	99%
Prophylactic Antibiotic Timing (Outpatient)	82	98%	98%	98%
Urinary Catheter Removal	117	97%	97%	97%
Survey of Patients' Hospital Experiences				
Area Around Room 'Always' Quiet at Night	300+	64%	64%	61%
Doctors 'Always' Communicated Well	300+	82%	81%	82%
Home Recovery Information Given	300+	89%	87%	85%
Hospital Given 9 or 10 on 10 Point Scale	300+	77%	75%	71%
Meds 'Always' Explained Before Given	300+	70%	67%	64%
Nurses 'Always' Communicated Well	300+	78%	79%	79%
Pain 'Always' Well Controlled	300+	69%	72%	71%
Room and Bathroom 'Always' Clean	300+	78%	74%	73%
Timely Help 'Always' Received	300+	70%	70%	68%
Would Definitely Recommend Hospital	300+	76%	76%	71%
Use of Medical Imaging				
Cardiac Imaging Stress Test before Surgery	119	5.9%	5%	5.3%
Combination Abdominal CT Scan	224	5.8%	10%	10.5%
Combination Brain/Sinus CT Scan	210	1.0%	2.1%	2.7%
Combination Chest CT Scan	131	0.8%	3.1%	2.7%

NOTE: Hospital profiles are in alphabetical order by state, then city, then hospital within the city; Rankings exclude hospitals with less than 25 cases except for patient surveys which excludes hospitals with less than 100 cases; (a) 100-299 cases; (1) The number of cases/patients is too few to report; (2) Data submitted were based on a sample of cases/patients; (3) Results are based on a shorter time period than required; (4) Data suppressed by CMS for one or more quarters; (5) Results are not available for this reporting period; (6) Fewer than 100 patients completed the HCAHPS survey; (7) No cases met the criteria for this measure; (8) The lower limit of the confidence interval cannot be calculated if the number of observed infections equals zero; (9) No data are available from the state/territory for this reporting period; (10) The scores shown reflect fewer than 50 completed surveys; (11) There were discrepancies in the data collection process; (12) This measure does not apply to this hospital for this reporting period; (13) Results cannot be calculated for this reporting period; (14) The results for this state are combined with nearby states to protect confidentiality; Please refer to the User's Guide for a full explanation of data.

Measure	Cases	This Hosp.	State Avg.	U.S. Avg.
Follow-up Mammogram/Ultrasound	482	11.4%	8.7%	8.8%
Lumbar Spine MRI for Low Back Pain	65	47.7%	39.7%	37.2%

East Morgan County Hospital

2400 W Edison St
Brush, CO 80723
Phone: 970-842-6200
Fax: 970-842-4827
URL: www.emchbrush.comorwww.bannerhealth.com
Type: Critical Access Hospitals
Emergency Services: Yes
Ownership: Govt - Hospital Dist/Auth
Beds: 25

Key Personnel:
Patient Relations . . . . Kathy Batrez
Emergency Room . . . . Ralph Mc Clure
Chief of Medical Staff . . . . Paula Pattee
Infection Control . . . . Kelly Plessman
CEO . . . . Linda Thorpe

Measure	Cases	This Hosp.	State Avg.	U.S. Avg.
Blood Clot Prevention and Treatment				
Anticoagulation Overlap Therapy[5]	-	-	97%	93%
ICU Venous Thromboembolism Prophylaxis[5]	-	-	95%	92%
Incidence of Potentially Preventable VTE[5]	-	-	8%	10%
UFH with Dosages/Platelet Monitoring[5]	-	-	97%	97%
Venous Thromboembolism Prophylaxis[5]	-	-	90%	85%
Warfarin Therapy Discharge Instructions[5]	-	-	69%	75%
Chest Pain/Possible Heart Attack Care				
Aspirin Given Within 24 Hours of Arrival	19	89%	97%	96%
Fibrinolytic Meds Within 30 Min. of Arrival[1]	-	-	55%	58%
Average Time to ECG (minutes)	19	4	8	7
Average Time to Transfer (minutes)[7]	-	-	74	60
Children's Asthma Care				
Received Home Management Plan of Care	-	-	-	88%
Received Reliever Medication	-	-	-	100%
Received Systemic Corticosteroids	-	-	-	100%
Emergency Department				
Admittance Decision Time (minutes)[5]	-	-	96	98
Head CT Results Within 45 Min. of Arrival[5]	-	-	67%	57%
Patients Who Left ER Before Being Seen	4,506	0%	2%	2%
Time from ER Arrival to Admit. (minutes)[5]	-	-	244	274
Time from ER Arrival to Discharge (minutes)[5]	-	-	139	134
Time in ER Before Being Evaluated (minutes)[5]	-	-	20	26
Time to Pain Meds for Fractures (minutes)[5]	-	-	45	57
Heart Attack Care				
Aspirin Given at Discharge[1]	-	-	100%	99%
Fibrinolytic Meds Within 30 Min. of Arrival[7]	-	-	20%	54%
PCI Within 90 Minutes of Arrival[7]	-	-	97%	96%
Statin Prescribed at Discharge[7]	-	-	99%	98%
Heart Failure Care				
ACE Inhibitor or ARB for LVSD[1]	-	-	97%	97%
Discharge Instructions Given	11	91%	93%	94%
Evaluation of LVS Function	14	100%	99%	99%
Medicare Spending				
Medicare Spending per Patient (ratio)	-	-	0.95	0.98
Pneumonia Care				
Appropriate Initial Antibiotic Given	19	84%	95%	95%
Blood Culture Timing	25	100%	98%	98%
Pregnancy and Delivery Care				
Newborn Deliveries Scheduled Early[3,7]	-	-	2%	6%
Preventive Care				
Immunization for Influenza[5]	-	-	92%	90%
Immunization for Pneumonia[5]	-	-	92%	92%
Stroke Care				
Anticoagulation Therapy for Atrial Fibrillation[5]	-	-	97%	95%
Antithrombotic Therapy Timing[5]	-	-	98%	98%
Assessed for Rehabilitation[5]	-	-	98%	97%
Discharged on Antithrombotic Therapy[5]	-	-	100%	99%
Discharged on Statin Medication[5]	-	-	94%	94%
Thrombolytic Therapy Timing[5]	-	-	78%	66%
Venous Thromboembolism Prophylaxis[5]	-	-	96%	94%
Written Stroke Educational Materials Given[5]	-	-	87%	88%
Surgical Care Improvement Project				
Appropriate Beta Blocker Usage[1,3]	-	-	98%	98%
Appropriate VTP Within 24 Hours[1,3]	-	-	98%	98%
Controlled Postoperative Blood Glucose[3,7]	-	-	96%	97%
Perioperative Temperature Management[1,3]	-	-	99%	100%
Prophylactic Antibiotic Selection[1,3]	-	-	99%	99%
Prophylactic Antibiotic Selection (Outpatient)[1,3]	-	-	98%	98%
Prophylactic Antibiotic Stopped[1,3]	-	-	98%	98%
Prophylactic Antibiotic Timing[1,3]	-	-	98%	99%
Prophylactic Antibiotic Timing (Outpatient)[1,3]	-	-	98%	98%
Urinary Catheter Removal[1,3]	-	-	97%	97%
Survey of Patients' Hospital Experiences				
Area Around Room 'Always' Quiet at Night[6,11]	<100	62%	64%	61%
Doctors 'Always' Communicated Well[6,11]	<100	82%	81%	82%
Home Recovery Information Given[6,11]	<100	88%	87%	85%
Hospital Given 9 or 10 on 10 Point Scale[6,11]	<100	80%	75%	71%
Meds 'Always' Explained Before Given[6,11]	<100	72%	67%	64%
Nurses 'Always' Communicated Well[6,11]	<100	87%	79%	79%
Pain 'Always' Well Controlled[6,11]	<100	73%	72%	71%
Room and Bathroom 'Always' Clean[6,11]	<100	84%	74%	73%
Timely Help 'Always' Received[6,11]	<100	75%	70%	68%
Would Definitely Recommend Hospital[6,11]	<100	79%	76%	71%
Use of Medical Imaging				
Cardiac Imaging Stress Test before Surgery[1]	-	-	5%	5.3%
Combination Abdominal CT Scan	159	33.3%	10%	10.5%
Combination Brain/Sinus CT Scan[1]	-	-	2.1%	2.7%
Combination Chest CT Scan	63	20.6%	3.1%	2.7%
Follow-up Mammogram/Ultrasound	275	8.0%	8.7%	8.8%
Lumbar Spine MRI for Low Back Pain[1]	-	-	39.7%	37.2%

Kit Carson County Memorial Hospital

286 16th Street
Burlington, CO 80807
Phone: 719-346-5311
Fax: 719-346-5252
URL: www.kccmh.org
Type: Critical Access Hospitals
Emergency Services: Yes
Ownership: Govt - Hospital Dist/Auth
Beds: 25

Key Personnel:
Radiology. . . . . Carl Fieser
Operating Room. . . . . Charles Frankum
Quality Assurance . . . . Regina Korsvold, RN
Pediatric In-Patient Care . . . . Diane Mettling
Chief of Medical Staff. . . . . Zach Pimentel, MD
Cardiac Laboratory. . . . . Tonda Scott, RN
CEO . . . . Donald Wade
Infection Control. . . . . Linda Wardlaw

Measure	Cases	This Hosp.	State Avg.	U.S. Avg.
Blood Clot Prevention and Treatment				
Anticoagulation Overlap Therapy[5]	-	-	97%	93%
ICU Venous Thromboembolism Prophylaxis[5]	-	-	95%	92%
Incidence of Potentially Preventable VTE[5]	-	-	8%	10%
UFH with Dosages/Platelet Monitoring[5]	-	-	97%	97%
Venous Thromboembolism Prophylaxis[5]	-	-	90%	85%
Warfarin Therapy Discharge Instructions[5]	-	-	69%	75%
Chest Pain/Possible Heart Attack Care				
Aspirin Given Within 24 Hours of Arrival[5]	-	-	97%	96%
Fibrinolytic Meds Within 30 Min. of Arrival[5]	-	-	55%	58%
Average Time to ECG (minutes)[5]	-	-	8	7
Average Time to Transfer (minutes)[5]	-	-	74	60
Children's Asthma Care				
Received Home Management Plan of Care	-	-	-	88%
Received Reliever Medication	-	-	-	100%
Received Systemic Corticosteroids	-	-	-	100%
Emergency Department				
Admittance Decision Time (minutes)[5]	-	-	96	98
Head CT Results Within 45 Min. of Arrival[5]	-	-	67%	57%
Patients Who Left ER Before Being Seen	2,207	1%	2%	2%
Time from ER Arrival to Admit. (minutes)[5]	-	-	244	274
Time from ER Arrival to Discharge (minutes)[5]	-	-	139	134
Time in ER Before Being Evaluated (minutes)[5]	-	-	20	26
Time to Pain Meds for Fractures (minutes)[5]	-	-	45	57
Heart Attack Care				
Aspirin Given at Discharge[5]	-	-	100%	99%
Fibrinolytic Meds Within 30 Min. of Arrival[5]	-	-	20%	54%
PCI Within 90 Minutes of Arrival[5]	-	-	97%	96%
Statin Prescribed at Discharge[5]	-	-	99%	98%
Heart Failure Care				
ACE Inhibitor or ARB for LVSD[1,2]	-	-	97%	97%
Discharge Instructions Given[1,2]	-	-	93%	94%
Evaluation of LVS Function[1,2]	-	-	99%	99%
Medicare Spending				
Medicare Spending per Patient (ratio)	-	-	0.95	0.98
Pneumonia Care				
Appropriate Initial Antibiotic Given[1,2]	-	-	95%	95%
Blood Culture Timing[1,2]	-	-	98%	98%
Pregnancy and Delivery Care				
Newborn Deliveries Scheduled Early[5]	-	-	2%	6%
Preventive Care				
Immunization for Influenza[5]	-	-	92%	90%
Immunization for Pneumonia[5]	-	-	92%	92%
Stroke Care				
Anticoagulation Therapy for Atrial Fibrillation[5]	-	-	97%	95%
Antithrombotic Therapy Timing[5]	-	-	98%	98%
Assessed for Rehabilitation[5]	-	-	98%	97%
Discharged on Antithrombotic Therapy[5]	-	-	100%	99%
Discharged on Statin Medication[5]	-	-	94%	94%
Thrombolytic Therapy Timing[5]	-	-	78%	66%
Venous Thromboembolism Prophylaxis[5]	-	-	96%	94%
Written Stroke Educational Materials Given[5]	-	-	87%	88%
Surgical Care Improvement Project				
Appropriate Beta Blocker Usage[5]	-	-	98%	98%
Appropriate VTP Within 24 Hours[5]	-	-	98%	98%
Controlled Postoperative Blood Glucose[5]	-	-	96%	97%
Perioperative Temperature Management[5]	-	-	99%	100%
Prophylactic Antibiotic Selection[5]	-	-	99%	99%
Prophylactic Antibiotic Selection (Outpatient)[5]	-	-	98%	98%
Prophylactic Antibiotic Stopped[5]	-	-	98%	98%
Prophylactic Antibiotic Timing[5]	-	-	98%	99%
Prophylactic Antibiotic Timing (Outpatient)[5]	-	-	98%	98%
Urinary Catheter Removal[5]	-	-	97%	97%
Survey of Patients' Hospital Experiences				
Area Around Room 'Always' Quiet at Night[10]	<100	83%	64%	61%
Doctors 'Always' Communicated Well[10]	<100	88%	81%	82%
Home Recovery Information Given[10]	<100	90%	87%	85%
Hospital Given 9 or 10 on 10 Point Scale[10]	<100	82%	75%	71%
Meds 'Always' Explained Before Given[10]	<100	79%	67%	64%
Nurses 'Always' Communicated Well[10]	<100	89%	79%	79%
Pain 'Always' Well Controlled[10]	<100	75%	72%	71%
Room and Bathroom 'Always' Clean[10]	<100	85%	74%	73%
Timely Help 'Always' Received[10]	<100	78%	70%	68%
Would Definitely Recommend Hospital[10]	<100	74%	76%	71%
Use of Medical Imaging				
Cardiac Imaging Stress Test before Surgery[1]	-	-	5%	5.3%
Combination Abdominal CT Scan	67	1.5%	10%	10.5%
Combination Brain/Sinus CT Scan[1]	-	-	2.1%	2.7%
Combination Chest CT Scan[1]	-	-	3.1%	2.7%
Follow-up Mammogram/Ultrasound	74	4.1%	8.7%	8.8%
Lumbar Spine MRI for Low Back Pain[1]	-	-	39.7%	37.2%

Centura Health - Saint Thomas More Hospital

1338 Phay Ave
Canon City, CO 81212
Phone: 719-285-2000
Fax: 719-285-2016
URL: www.stthomasmorehosp.org
Type: Acute Care Hospitals
Emergency Services: Yes
Ownership: Voluntary non-profit - Church
Beds: 55

Key Personnel:
Emergency Room . . . . Paul Bleim, RN
Operating Room. . . . . Tom Cravens, CRNA
Infection Control. . . . . Pam Galkowski
Quality Assurance . . . . Pam Galkowski
Intensive Care Unit. . . . . Barb Sherriff
Patient Relations . . . . Millie Stacey-Langley, RN
CEO/President. . . . . Diane Swagger
Chief of Medical Staff . . . . Victoria Tori King, MD

Measure	Cases	This Hosp.	State Avg.	U.S. Avg.
Blood Clot Prevention and Treatment				
Anticoagulation Overlap Therapy[2]	21	90%	97%	93%
ICU Venous Thromboembolism Prophylaxis[2]	39	90%	95%	92%
Incidence of Potentially Preventable VTE[1,2]	-	-	8%	10%
UFH with Dosages/Platelet Monitoring[2,7]	-	-	97%	97%
Venous Thromboembolism Prophylaxis[2]	105	86%	90%	85%
Warfarin Therapy Discharge Instructions[2]	17	94%	69%	75%
Chest Pain/Possible Heart Attack Care				
Aspirin Given Within 24 Hours of Arrival	93	99%	97%	96%
Fibrinolytic Meds Within 30 Min. of Arrival[1]	-	-	55%	58%

NOTE: Hospital profiles are in alphabetical order by state, then city, then hospital within the city; Rankings exclude hospitals with less than 25 cases except for patient surveys which excludes hospitals with less than 100 cases; (a) 100-299 cases; (1) The number of cases/patients is too few to report; (2) Data submitted were based on a sample of cases/patients; (3) Results are based on a shorter time period than required; (4) Data suppressed by CMS for one or more quarters; (5) Results are not available for this reporting period; (6) Fewer than 100 patients completed the HCAHPS survey; (7) No cases met the criteria for this measure; (8) The lower limit of the confidence interval cannot be calculated if the number of observed infections equals zero; (9) No data are available from the state/territory for this reporting period; (10) The scores shown reflect fewer than 50 completed surveys; (11) There were discrepancies in the data collection process; (12) This measure does not apply to this hospital for this reporting period; (13) Results cannot be calculated for this reporting period; (14) The results for this state are combined with nearby states to protect confidentiality; Please refer to the User's Guide for a full explanation of data.

Measure	Cases	This Hosp.	State Avg.	U.S. Avg.
Average Time to ECG (minutes)	92	8	8	7
Average Time to Transfer (minutes)[1]	-	-	74	60
Children's Asthma Care				
Received Home Management Plan of Care	-	-	-	88%
Received Reliever Medication	-	-	-	100%
Received Systemic Corticosteroids	-	-	-	100%
Emergency Department				
Admittance Decision Time (minutes)[2]	348	64	96	98
Head CT Results Within 45 Min. of Arrival	15	80%	67%	57%
Patients Who Left ER Before Being Seen	18,802	1%	2%	2%
Time from ER Arrival to Admit. (minutes)[2]	364	212	244	274
Time from ER Arrival to Discharge (minutes)	469	128	139	134
Time in ER Before Being Evaluated (minutes)	362	22	20	26
Time to Pain Meds for Fractures (minutes)	62	45	45	57
Heart Attack Care				
Aspirin Given at Discharge[1,3]	-	-	100%	99%
Fibrinolytic Meds Within 30 Min. of Arrival[3,7]	-	-	20%	54%
PCI Within 90 Minutes of Arrival[3,7]	-	-	97%	96%
Statin Prescribed at Discharge[1,3]	-	-	99%	98%
Heart Failure Care				
ACE Inhibitor or ARB for LVSD[1]	-	-	97%	97%
Discharge Instructions Given	21	81%	93%	94%
Evaluation of LVS Function	30	100%	99%	99%
Medicare Spending				
Medicare Spending per Patient (ratio)	-	0.91	0.95	0.98
Pneumonia Care				
Appropriate Initial Antibiotic Given	43	86%	95%	95%
Blood Culture Timing	62	98%	98%	98%
Pregnancy and Delivery Care				
Newborn Deliveries Scheduled Early[2]	18	0%	2%	6%
Preventive Care				
Immunization for Influenza[2]	308	95%	92%	90%
Immunization for Pneumonia[2]	377	96%	92%	92%
Stroke Care				
Anticoagulation Therapy for Atrial Fibrillation[1]	-	-	97%	95%
Antithrombotic Therapy Timing	13	100%	98%	98%
Assessed for Rehabilitation	14	100%	98%	97%
Discharged on Antithrombotic Therapy	14	100%	100%	99%
Discharged on Statin Medication	12	67%	94%	94%
Thrombolytic Therapy Timing[1]	-	-	78%	66%
Venous Thromboembolism Prophylaxis	15	93%	96%	94%
Written Stroke Educational Materials Given[1]	-	-	87%	88%
Surgical Care Improvement Project				
Appropriate Beta Blocker Usage	39	95%	98%	98%
Appropriate VTP Within 24 Hours	195	99%	98%	98%
Controlled Postoperative Blood Glucose[7]	-	-	96%	97%
Perioperative Temperature Management	213	100%	99%	100%
Prophylactic Antibiotic Selection	138	98%	99%	99%
Prophylactic Antibiotic Selection (Outpatient)	39	97%	98%	98%
Prophylactic Antibiotic Stopped	135	95%	98%	98%
Prophylactic Antibiotic Timing	138	100%	98%	99%
Prophylactic Antibiotic Timing (Outpatient)	39	100%	98%	98%
Urinary Catheter Removal	138	99%	97%	97%
Survey of Patients' Hospital Experiences				
Area Around Room 'Always' Quiet at Night	300+	57%	64%	61%
Doctors 'Always' Communicated Well	300+	81%	81%	82%
Home Recovery Information Given	300+	85%	87%	85%
Hospital Given 9 or 10 on 10 Point Scale	300+	67%	75%	71%
Meds 'Always' Explained Before Given	300+	64%	67%	64%
Nurses 'Always' Communicated Well	300+	78%	79%	79%
Pain 'Always' Well Controlled	300+	72%	72%	71%
Room and Bathroom 'Always' Clean	300+	68%	74%	73%
Timely Help 'Always' Received	300+	66%	70%	68%
Would Definitely Recommend Hospital	300+	63%	76%	71%
Use of Medical Imaging				
Cardiac Imaging Stress Test before Surgery	74	5.4%	5%	5.3%
Combination Abdominal CT Scan	506	11.9%	10%	10.5%
Combination Brain/Sinus CT Scan	388	1.0%	2.1%	2.7%
Combination Chest CT Scan	221	5.0%	3.1%	2.7%
Follow-up Mammogram/Ultrasound	785	8.3%	8.7%	8.8%
Lumbar Spine MRI for Low Back Pain	88	47.7%	39.7%	37.2%

Castle Rock Adventist Hospital

2350 Meadows Blvd
Phone: 720-455-2500
Castle Rock, CO 80109
Type: Acute Care Hospitals
Emergency Services: Yes
Ownership: Voluntary non-profit - Private

Measure	Cases	This Hosp.	State Avg.	U.S. Avg.
Blood Clot Prevention and Treatment				
Anticoagulation Overlap Therapy[5]	-	-	97%	93%
ICU Venous Thromboembolism Prophylaxis[5]	-	-	95%	92%
Incidence of Potentially Preventable VTE[5]	-	-	8%	10%
UFH with Dosages/Platelet Monitoring[5]	-	-	97%	97%
Venous Thromboembolism Prophylaxis[5]	-	-	90%	85%
Warfarin Therapy Discharge Instructions[5]	-	-	69%	75%
Chest Pain/Possible Heart Attack Care				
Aspirin Given Within 24 Hours of Arrival[5]	-	-	97%	96%
Fibrinolytic Meds Within 30 Min. of Arrival[5]	-	-	55%	58%
Average Time to ECG (minutes)[5]	-	-	8	7
Average Time to Transfer (minutes)[5]	-	-	74	60
Children's Asthma Care				
Received Home Management Plan of Care	-	-	-	88%
Received Reliever Medication	-	-	-	100%
Received Systemic Corticosteroids	-	-	-	100%
Emergency Department				
Admittance Decision Time (minutes)[5]	-	-	96	98
Head CT Results Within 45 Min. of Arrival[5]	-	-	67%	57%
Patients Who Left ER Before Being Seen[5]	-	-	2%	2%
Time from ER Arrival to Admit. (minutes)[5]	-	-	244	274
Time from ER Arrival to Discharge (minutes)[5]	-	-	139	134
Time in ER Before Being Evaluated (minutes)[5]	-	-	20	26
Time to Pain Meds for Fractures (minutes)[5]	-	-	45	57
Heart Attack Care				
Aspirin Given at Discharge[5]	-	-	100%	99%
Fibrinolytic Meds Within 30 Min. of Arrival[5]	-	-	20%	54%
PCI Within 90 Minutes of Arrival[5]	-	-	97%	96%
Statin Prescribed at Discharge[5]	-	-	99%	98%
Heart Failure Care				
ACE Inhibitor or ARB for LVSD[5]	-	-	97%	97%
Discharge Instructions Given[5]	-	-	93%	94%
Evaluation of LVS Function[5]	-	-	99%	99%
Medicare Spending				
Medicare Spending per Patient (ratio)	-	-	0.95	0.98
Pneumonia Care				
Appropriate Initial Antibiotic Given[5]	-	-	95%	95%
Blood Culture Timing[5]	-	-	98%	98%
Pregnancy and Delivery Care				
Newborn Deliveries Scheduled Early[5]	-	-	2%	6%
Preventive Care				
Immunization for Influenza[5]	-	-	92%	90%
Immunization for Pneumonia[5]	-	-	92%	92%
Stroke Care				
Anticoagulation Therapy for Atrial Fibrillation[5]	-	-	97%	95%
Antithrombotic Therapy Timing[5]	-	-	98%	98%
Assessed for Rehabilitation[5]	-	-	98%	97%
Discharged on Antithrombotic Therapy[5]	-	-	100%	99%
Discharged on Statin Medication[5]	-	-	94%	94%
Thrombolytic Therapy Timing[5]	-	-	78%	66%
Venous Thromboembolism Prophylaxis[5]	-	-	96%	94%
Written Stroke Educational Materials Given[5]	-	-	87%	88%
Surgical Care Improvement Project				
Appropriate Beta Blocker Usage[5]	-	-	98%	98%
Appropriate VTP Within 24 Hours[5]	-	-	98%	98%
Controlled Postoperative Blood Glucose[5]	-	-	96%	97%
Perioperative Temperature Management[5]	-	-	99%	100%
Prophylactic Antibiotic Selection[5]	-	-	99%	99%
Prophylactic Antibiotic Selection (Outpatient)[5]	-	-	98%	98%
Prophylactic Antibiotic Stopped[5]	-	-	98%	98%
Prophylactic Antibiotic Timing[5]	-	-	98%	99%
Prophylactic Antibiotic Timing (Outpatient)[5]	-	-	98%	98%
Urinary Catheter Removal[5]	-	-	97%	97%
Survey of Patients' Hospital Experiences				
Area Around Room 'Always' Quiet at Night[5]	-	-	64%	61%
Doctors 'Always' Communicated Well[5]	-	-	81%	82%
Home Recovery Information Given[5]	-	-	87%	85%
Hospital Given 9 or 10 on 10 Point Scale[5]	-	-	75%	71%
Meds 'Always' Explained Before Given[5]	-	-	67%	64%
Nurses 'Always' Communicated Well[5]	-	-	79%	79%
Pain 'Always' Well Controlled[5]	-	-	72%	71%
Room and Bathroom 'Always' Clean[5]	-	-	74%	73%
Timely Help 'Always' Received[5]	-	-	70%	68%
Would Definitely Recommend Hospital[5]	-	-	76%	71%
Use of Medical Imaging				
Cardiac Imaging Stress Test before Surgery[5]	-	-	5%	5.3%
Combination Abdominal CT Scan[5]	-	-	10%	10.5%
Combination Brain/Sinus CT Scan[5]	-	-	2.1%	2.7%
Combination Chest CT Scan[5]	-	-	3.1%	2.7%
Follow-up Mammogram/Ultrasound[5]	-	-	8.7%	8.8%
Lumbar Spine MRI for Low Back Pain[5]	-	-	39.7%	37.2%

Keefe Memorial Hospital

602 N 6th W St
Phone: 719-767-5661
Cheyenne Wells, CO 80810
Fax: 719-767-8042
Type: Acute Care Hospitals
Emergency Services: Yes
Ownership: Government - Local
Beds: 32

Key Personnel:

Chief of Medical Staff . . . . Saied Ahmad Pour
Imaging . . . . Kathy Dwyer-keefe
Quality Assurance . . . . Rose Galli
CEO . . . . Ginny Hallagin
Operating Room. . . . . Sue Kern, RN

Measure	Cases	This Hosp.	State Avg.	U.S. Avg.
Blood Clot Prevention and Treatment				
Anticoagulation Overlap Therapy[2,7]	-	-	97%	93%
ICU Venous Thromboembolism Prophylaxis[2,7]	-	-	95%	92%
Incidence of Potentially Preventable VTE[2,7]	-	-	8%	10%
UFH with Dosages/Platelet Monitoring[2,7]	-	-	97%	97%
Venous Thromboembolism Prophylaxis[2]	40	0%	90%	85%
Warfarin Therapy Discharge Instructions[2,7]	-	-	69%	75%
Chest Pain/Possible Heart Attack Care				
Aspirin Given Within 24 Hours of Arrival[5]	-	-	97%	96%
Fibrinolytic Meds Within 30 Min. of Arrival[5]	-	-	55%	58%
Average Time to ECG (minutes)[5]	-	-	8	7
Average Time to Transfer (minutes)[5]	-	-	74	60
Children's Asthma Care				
Received Home Management Plan of Care	-	-	-	88%
Received Reliever Medication	-	-	-	100%
Received Systemic Corticosteroids	-	-	-	100%
Emergency Department				
Admittance Decision Time (minutes)[2]	31	13	96	98
Head CT Results Within 45 Min. of Arrival[5]	-	-	67%	57%
Patients Who Left ER Before Being Seen	651	0%	2%	2%
Time from ER Arrival to Admit. (minutes)[2]	35	106	244	274
Time from ER Arrival to Discharge (minutes)	240	106	139	134
Time in ER Before Being Evaluated (minutes)	249	11	20	26
Time to Pain Meds for Fractures (minutes)[5]	-	-	45	57
Heart Attack Care				
Aspirin Given at Discharge[5]	-	-	100%	99%
Fibrinolytic Meds Within 30 Min. of Arrival[5]	-	-	20%	54%
PCI Within 90 Minutes of Arrival[5]	-	-	97%	96%
Statin Prescribed at Discharge[5]	-	-	99%	98%
Heart Failure Care				
ACE Inhibitor or ARB for LVSD[2,7]	-	-	97%	97%
Discharge Instructions Given[1,2]	-	-	93%	94%
Evaluation of LVS Function[1,2]	-	-	99%	99%
Medicare Spending				
Medicare Spending per Patient (ratio)	-	0.67	0.95	0.98
Pneumonia Care				
Appropriate Initial Antibiotic Given[2]	16	69%	95%	95%
Blood Culture Timing[1,2]	-	-	98%	98%
Pregnancy and Delivery Care				
Newborn Deliveries Scheduled Early[2,7]	-	-	2%	6%
Preventive Care				
Immunization for Influenza[2]	30	83%	92%	90%
Immunization for Pneumonia[2]	44	73%	92%	92%
Stroke Care				
Anticoagulation Therapy for Atrial Fibrillation[5]	-	-	97%	95%

NOTE: Hospital profiles are in alphabetical order by state, then city, then hospital within the city; Rankings exclude hospitals with less than 25 cases except for patient surveys which excludes hospitals with less than 100 cases; (a) 100-299 cases; (1) The number of cases/patients is too few to report; (2) Data submitted were based on a sample of cases/patients; (3) Results are based on a shorter time period than required; (4) Data suppressed by CMS for one or more quarters; (5) Results are not available for this reporting period; (6) Fewer than 100 patients completed the HCAHPS survey; (7) No cases met the criteria for this measure; (8) The lower limit of the confidence interval cannot be calculated if the number of observed infections equals zero; (9) No data are available from the state/territory for this reporting period; (10) The scores shown reflect fewer than 50 completed surveys; (11) There were discrepancies in the data collection process; (12) This measure does not apply to this hospital for this reporting period; (13) Results cannot be calculated for this reporting period; (14) The results for this state are combined with nearby states to protect confidentiality; Please refer to the User's Guide for a full explanation of data.

Antithrombotic Therapy Timing[5]	-	-	98%	98%
Assessed for Rehabilitation[5]	-	-	98%	97%
Discharged on Antithrombotic Therapy[5]	-	-	100%	99%
Discharged on Statin Medication[5]	-	-	94%	94%
Thrombolytic Therapy Timing[5]	-	-	78%	66%
Venous Thromboembolism Prophylaxis[5]	-	-	96%	94%
Written Stroke Educational Materials Given[5]	-	-	87%	88%
Surgical Care Improvement Project				
Appropriate Beta Blocker Usage[5]	-	-	98%	98%
Appropriate VTP Within 24 Hours[5]	-	-	98%	98%
Controlled Postoperative Blood Glucose[5]	-	-	96%	97%
Perioperative Temperature Management[5]	-	-	99%	100%
Prophylactic Antibiotic Selection[5]	-	-	99%	99%
Prophylactic Antibiotic Selection (Outpatient)[5]	-	-	98%	98%
Prophylactic Antibiotic Stopped[5]	-	-	98%	98%
Prophylactic Antibiotic Timing[5]	-	-	98%	99%
Prophylactic Antibiotic Timing (Outpatient)[5]	-	-	98%	98%
Urinary Catheter Removal[5]	-	-	97%	97%
Survey of Patients' Hospital Experiences				
Area Around Room 'Always' Quiet at Night[10]	<100	72%	64%	61%
Doctors 'Always' Communicated Well[10]	<100	95%	81%	82%
Home Recovery Information Given[10]	<100	92%	87%	85%
Hospital Given 9 or 10 on 10 Point Scale[10]	<100	97%	75%	71%
Meds 'Always' Explained Before Given[10]	<100	-	67%	64%
Nurses 'Always' Communicated Well[10]	<100	99%	79%	79%
Pain 'Always' Well Controlled[10]	<100	95%	72%	71%
Room and Bathroom 'Always' Clean[10]	<100	90%	74%	73%
Timely Help 'Always' Received[10]	<100	79%	70%	68%
Would Definitely Recommend Hospital[10]	<100	98%	76%	71%
Use of Medical Imaging				
Cardiac Imaging Stress Test before Surgery[1]	-	-	5%	5.3%
Combination Abdominal CT Scan[1]	-	-	10%	10.5%
Combination Brain/Sinus CT Scan[1]	-	-	2.1%	2.7%
Combination Chest CT Scan[1]	-	-	3.1%	2.7%
Follow-up Mammogram/Ultrasound[1]	-	-	8.7%	8.8%
Lumbar Spine MRI for Low Back Pain[1]	-	-	39.7%	37.2%

Centura Health - Penrose Saint Francis Health Services

2222 N Nevada Ave Phone: 719-776-5000
Colorado Springs, CO 80907 Fax: 719-776-2770
URL: www.centurahealth.com
Type: Acute Care Hospitals Emergency Services: Yes
Ownership: Voluntary non-profit - Private Beds: 522

Key Personnel:
Operating Room. . . . . Steve Butler
Radiology. . . . . Jeanne Giustra
Cardiac Laboratory. . . . . Keathe Hanley
Infection Control. . . . . Marie Lucero
Coronary Care . . . . Kate McCord
CEO/President. . . . . Margaret Sabin
Chief of Medical Staff . . . . Peter Walsh, MD

Measure	Cases	This Hosp.	State Avg.	U.S. Avg.
Blood Clot Prevention and Treatment				
Anticoagulation Overlap Therapy[2]	216	97%	97%	93%
ICU Venous Thromboembolism Prophylaxis[2]	70	91%	95%	92%
Incidence of Potentially Preventable VTE[2]	21	14%	8%	10%
UFH with Dosages/Platelet Monitoring[2]	64	100%	97%	97%
Venous Thromboembolism Prophylaxis[2]	299	70%	90%	85%
Warfarin Therapy Discharge Instructions[2]	173	17%	69%	75%
Chest Pain/Possible Heart Attack Care				
Aspirin Given Within 24 Hours of Arrival[1,3]	-	-	97%	96%
Fibrinolytic Meds Within 30 Min. of Arrival[5]	-	-	55%	58%
Average Time to ECG (minutes)[1,3]	-	-	8	7
Average Time to Transfer (minutes)[5]	-	-	74	60
Children's Asthma Care				
Received Home Management Plan of Care	-	-	-	88%
Received Reliever Medication	-	-	-	100%
Received Systemic Corticosteroids	-	-	-	100%
Emergency Department				
Admittance Decision Time (minutes)[2]	659	93	96	98
Head CT Results Within 45 Min. of Arrival	27	74%	67%	57%
Patients Who Left ER Before Being Seen	91,199	1%	2%	2%
Time from ER Arrival to Admit. (minutes)[2]	677	267	244	274
Time from ER Arrival to Discharge (minutes)	465	166	139	134
Time in ER Before Being Evaluated (minutes)	357	35	20	26
Time to Pain Meds for Fractures (minutes)	249	64	45	57
Heart Attack Care				
Aspirin Given at Discharge	426	100%	100%	99%
Fibrinolytic Meds Within 30 Min. of Arrival[7]	-	-	20%	54%
PCI Within 90 Minutes of Arrival	92	98%	97%	96%
Statin Prescribed at Discharge	441	99%	99%	98%
Heart Failure Care				
ACE Inhibitor or ARB for LVSD	129	95%	97%	97%
Discharge Instructions Given	321	83%	93%	94%
Evaluation of LVS Function	409	99%	99%	99%
Medicare Spending				
Medicare Spending per Patient (ratio)	-	0.99	0.95	0.98
Pneumonia Care				
Appropriate Initial Antibiotic Given[2]	230	97%	95%	95%
Blood Culture Timing[2]	287	98%	98%	98%
Pregnancy and Delivery Care				
Newborn Deliveries Scheduled Early[2]	43	2%	2%	6%
Preventive Care				
Immunization for Influenza[2]	590	91%	92%	90%
Immunization for Pneumonia[2]	699	91%	92%	92%
Stroke Care				
Anticoagulation Therapy for Atrial Fibrillation[1,2]	-	-	97%	95%
Antithrombotic Therapy Timing[2]	78	96%	98%	98%
Assessed for Rehabilitation[2]	105	96%	98%	97%
Discharged on Antithrombotic Therapy[2]	85	100%	100%	99%
Discharged on Statin Medication[2]	65	92%	94%	94%
Thrombolytic Therapy Timing[1,2]	-	-	78%	66%
Venous Thromboembolism Prophylaxis[2]	105	96%	96%	94%
Written Stroke Educational Materials Given[2]	62	89%	87%	88%
Surgical Care Improvement Project				
Appropriate Beta Blocker Usage[2]	272	98%	98%	98%
Appropriate VTP Within 24 Hours[2]	683	99%	98%	98%
Controlled Postoperative Blood Glucose[2]	250	93%	96%	97%
Perioperative Temperature Management[2]	818	100%	99%	100%
Prophylactic Antibiotic Selection[2]	764	100%	99%	99%
Prophylactic Antibiotic Selection (Outpatient)	814	97%	98%	98%
Prophylactic Antibiotic Stopped[2]	743	97%	98%	98%
Prophylactic Antibiotic Timing[2]	764	98%	98%	99%
Prophylactic Antibiotic Timing (Outpatient)	810	96%	98%	98%
Urinary Catheter Removal[2]	691	92%	97%	97%
Survey of Patients' Hospital Experiences				
Area Around Room 'Always' Quiet at Night	300+	63%	64%	61%
Doctors 'Always' Communicated Well	300+	81%	81%	82%
Home Recovery Information Given	300+	87%	87%	85%
Hospital Given 9 or 10 on 10 Point Scale	300+	73%	75%	71%
Meds 'Always' Explained Before Given	300+	62%	67%	64%
Nurses 'Always' Communicated Well	300+	77%	79%	79%
Pain 'Always' Well Controlled	300+	68%	72%	71%
Room and Bathroom 'Always' Clean	300+	66%	74%	73%
Timely Help 'Always' Received	300+	63%	70%	68%
Would Definitely Recommend Hospital	300+	77%	76%	71%
Use of Medical Imaging				
Cardiac Imaging Stress Test before Surgery	1,076	5.6%	5%	5.3%
Combination Abdominal CT Scan	965	4.7%	10%	10.5%
Combination Brain/Sinus CT Scan	1,221	2.0%	2.1%	2.7%
Combination Chest CT Scan	388	1.3%	3.1%	2.7%
Follow-up Mammogram/Ultrasound	781	15.1%	8.7%	8.8%
Lumbar Spine MRI for Low Back Pain[1]	-	-	39.7%	37.2%

University Colo Health Memorial Hospital Central

1400 E Boulder St Phone: 719-365-5000
Colorado Springs, CO 80909 Fax: 719-365-2472
E-mail: info@memorialhealthsystem.com
URL: www.memorialhospital.com
Type: Acute Care Hospitals Emergency Services: Yes
Ownership: Government - Local Beds: 386

Key Personnel:
Radiology. . . . . Maxwell B Abbott, MD
Quality Assurance . . . . Ron Burnside
Chief of Medical Staff . . . . Patrick Faricy, MD
Pediatric Ambulatory Care . . . . . . Kenneth M Gheen, MD
Pediatric In-Patient Care . . . . Kenneth M Gheen, MD
CEO/President. . . . . George Hayes
Infection Control. . . . . Joan Walker, RN

Measure	Cases	This Hosp.	State Avg.	U.S. Avg.
Blood Clot Prevention and Treatment				
Anticoagulation Overlap Therapy[2]	188	95%	97%	93%
ICU Venous Thromboembolism Prophylaxis[2]	90	99%	95%	92%
Incidence of Potentially Preventable VTE[2]	24	4%	8%	10%
UFH with Dosages/Platelet Monitoring[2]	85	99%	97%	97%
Venous Thromboembolism Prophylaxis[2]	493	83%	90%	85%
Warfarin Therapy Discharge Instructions[2]	148	74%	69%	75%
Chest Pain/Possible Heart Attack Care				
Aspirin Given Within 24 Hours of Arrival[1,3]	-	-	97%	96%
Fibrinolytic Meds Within 30 Min. of Arrival[5]	-	-	55%	58%
Average Time to ECG (minutes)[1,3]	-	-	8	7
Average Time to Transfer (minutes)[5]	-	-	74	60
Children's Asthma Care				
Received Home Management Plan of Care	-	-	-	88%
Received Reliever Medication	-	-	-	100%
Received Systemic Corticosteroids	-	-	-	100%
Emergency Department				
Admittance Decision Time (minutes)[2]	462	71	96	98
Head CT Results Within 45 Min. of Arrival	19	63%	67%	57%
Patients Who Left ER Before Being Seen	>100k	3%	2%	2%
Time from ER Arrival to Admit. (minutes)[2]	565	287	244	274
Time from ER Arrival to Discharge (minutes)	495	170	139	134
Time in ER Before Being Evaluated (minutes)	559	27	20	26
Time to Pain Meds for Fractures (minutes)	390	37	45	57
Heart Attack Care				
Aspirin Given at Discharge	371	100%	100%	99%
Fibrinolytic Meds Within 30 Min. of Arrival[7]	-	-	20%	54%
PCI Within 90 Minutes of Arrival	81	99%	97%	96%
Statin Prescribed at Discharge	362	99%	99%	98%
Heart Failure Care				
ACE Inhibitor or ARB for LVSD	120	96%	97%	97%
Discharge Instructions Given	246	97%	93%	94%
Evaluation of LVS Function	314	100%	99%	99%
Medicare Spending				
Medicare Spending per Patient (ratio)	-	1.02	0.95	0.98
Pneumonia Care				
Appropriate Initial Antibiotic Given	265	94%	95%	95%
Blood Culture Timing	398	97%	98%	98%
Pregnancy and Delivery Care				
Newborn Deliveries Scheduled Early[2]	154	3%	2%	6%
Preventive Care				
Immunization for Influenza[2]	764	94%	92%	90%
Immunization for Pneumonia[2]	704	92%	92%	92%
Stroke Care				
Anticoagulation Therapy for Atrial Fibrillation	23	100%	97%	95%
Antithrombotic Therapy Timing	157	97%	98%	98%
Assessed for Rehabilitation	203	99%	98%	97%
Discharged on Antithrombotic Therapy	176	99%	100%	99%
Discharged on Statin Medication	124	96%	94%	94%
Thrombolytic Therapy Timing	24	92%	78%	66%
Venous Thromboembolism Prophylaxis	224	99%	96%	94%
Written Stroke Educational Materials Given	107	96%	87%	88%
Surgical Care Improvement Project				
Appropriate Beta Blocker Usage[2]	297	99%	98%	98%
Appropriate VTP Within 24 Hours[2]	970	98%	98%	98%
Controlled Postoperative Blood Glucose[2]	199	99%	96%	97%
Perioperative Temperature Management[2]	1,153	100%	99%	100%
Prophylactic Antibiotic Selection[2]	901	99%	99%	99%
Prophylactic Antibiotic Selection (Outpatient)	1,180	95%	98%	98%
Prophylactic Antibiotic Stopped[2]	894	99%	98%	98%
Prophylactic Antibiotic Timing[2]	905	98%	98%	99%
Prophylactic Antibiotic Timing (Outpatient)	1,189	95%	98%	98%
Urinary Catheter Removal[2]	786	100%	97%	97%
Survey of Patients' Hospital Experiences				
Area Around Room 'Always' Quiet at Night	300+	52%	64%	61%
Doctors 'Always' Communicated Well	300+	76%	81%	82%
Home Recovery Information Given	300+	84%	87%	85%
Hospital Given 9 or 10 on 10 Point Scale	300+	64%	75%	71%
Meds 'Always' Explained Before Given	300+	61%	67%	64%

NOTE: Hospital profiles are in alphabetical order by state, then city, then hospital within the city; Rankings exclude hospitals with less than 25 cases except for patient surveys which excludes hospitals with less than 100 cases; (a) 100-299 cases; (1) The number of cases/patients is too few to report; (2) Data submitted were based on a sample of cases/patients; (3) Results are based on a shorter time period than required; (4) Data suppressed by CMS for one or more quarters; (5) Results are not available for this reporting period; (6) Fewer than 100 patients completed the HCAHPS survey; (7) No cases met the criteria for this measure; (8) The lower limit of the confidence interval cannot be calculated if the number of observed infections equals zero; (9) No data are available from the state/territory for this reporting period; (10) The scores shown reflect fewer than 50 completed surveys; (11) There were discrepancies in the data collection process; (12) This measure does not apply to this hospital for this reporting period; (13) Results cannot be calculated for this reporting period; (14) The results for this state are combined with nearby states to protect confidentiality; Please refer to the User's Guide for a full explanation of data.

Measure	Cases	This Hosp.	State Avg.	U.S. Avg.
Nurses 'Always' Communicated Well	300+	73%	79%	79%
Pain 'Always' Well Controlled	300+	66%	72%	71%
Room and Bathroom 'Always' Clean	300+	65%	74%	73%
Timely Help 'Always' Received	300+	62%	70%	68%
Would Definitely Recommend Hospital	300+	68%	76%	71%
Use of Medical Imaging				
Cardiac Imaging Stress Test before Surgery	1,159	4.0%	5%	5.3%
Combination Abdominal CT Scan	1,763	25.9%	10%	10.5%
Combination Brain/Sinus CT Scan	1,708	2.5%	2.1%	2.7%
Combination Chest CT Scan	988	20.3%	3.1%	2.7%
Follow-up Mammogram/Ultrasound	3,043	6.6%	8.7%	8.8%
Lumbar Spine MRI for Low Back Pain	293	35.8%	39.7%	37.2%

Southwest Memorial Hospital

1311 N Mildred Rd
Cortez, CO 81321
Phone: 970-565-6666
Fax: 970-564-2403
URL: www.swhealth.org
Type: Critical Access Hospitals
Emergency Services: Yes
Ownership: Voluntary non-profit - Private
Beds: 61

Key Personnel:

Operating Room. . . . . Kyle Cruzan
Imaging . . . . Wendell Heck, RT(R)MR
Emergency Room . . . . Dennis Keown, RN
Surgery . . . . Heather Nowlin, MSN, RN, CNOR
Chair/CEO . . . . Judy Schuenemeyer
CEO/President. . . . . Liz Sellers, MSN, MHA
Chief of Medical Staff . . . . Kameo L. Smith, DO

Measure	Cases	This Hosp.	State Avg.	U.S. Avg.
Blood Clot Prevention and Treatment				
Anticoagulation Overlap Therapy[2]	11	100%	97%	93%
ICU Venous Thromboembolism Prophylaxis[2]	15	93%	95%	92%
Incidence of Potentially Preventable VTE[2,7]	-	-	8%	10%
UFH with Dosages/Platelet Monitoring[1,2]	-	-	97%	97%
Venous Thromboembolism Prophylaxis[2]	109	91%	90%	85%
Warfarin Therapy Discharge Instructions[1,2]	-	-	69%	75%
Chest Pain/Possible Heart Attack Care				
Aspirin Given Within 24 Hours of Arrival	21	100%	97%	96%
Fibrinolytic Meds Within 30 Min. of Arrival[1]	-	-	55%	58%
Average Time to ECG (minutes)	28	19	8	7
Average Time to Transfer (minutes)[1]	-	-	74	60
Children's Asthma Care				
Received Home Management Plan of Care	-	-	-	88%
Received Reliever Medication	-	-	-	100%
Received Systemic Corticosteroids	-	-	-	100%
Emergency Department				
Admittance Decision Time (minutes)[2,3]	252	48	96	98
Head CT Results Within 45 Min. of Arrival[1]	-	-	67%	57%
Patients Who Left ER Before Being Seen	12,030	1%	2%	2%
Time from ER Arrival to Admit. (minutes)[2,3]	252	171	244	274
Time from ER Arrival to Discharge (minutes)[5]	-	-	139	134
Time in ER Before Being Evaluated (minutes)[5]	-	-	20	26
Time to Pain Meds for Fractures (minutes)[3]	69	41	45	57
Heart Attack Care				
Aspirin Given at Discharge[1]	-	-	100%	99%
Fibrinolytic Meds Within 30 Min. of Arrival[7]	-	-	20%	54%
PCI Within 90 Minutes of Arrival[7]	-	-	97%	96%
Statin Prescribed at Discharge[1]	-	-	99%	98%
Heart Failure Care				
ACE Inhibitor or ARB for LVSD	12	92%	97%	97%
Discharge Instructions Given	23	100%	93%	94%
Evaluation of LVS Function	25	100%	99%	99%
Medicare Spending				
Medicare Spending per Patient (ratio)	-	-	0.95	0.98
Pneumonia Care				
Appropriate Initial Antibiotic Given	22	100%	95%	95%
Blood Culture Timing	39	97%	98%	98%
Pregnancy and Delivery Care				
Newborn Deliveries Scheduled Early[5]	-	-	2%	6%
Preventive Care				
Immunization for Influenza[2,3]	132	67%	92%	90%
Immunization for Pneumonia[2,3]	232	74%	92%	92%
Stroke Care				
Anticoagulation Therapy for Atrial Fibrillation[1]	-	-	97%	95%
Antithrombotic Therapy Timing[1]	-	-	98%	98%
Assessed for Rehabilitation[1]	-	-	98%	97%
Discharged on Antithrombotic Therapy[1]	-	-	100%	99%
Discharged on Statin Medication[1]	-	-	94%	94%
Thrombolytic Therapy Timing[7]	-	-	78%	66%
Venous Thromboembolism Prophylaxis[1]	-	-	96%	94%
Written Stroke Educational Materials Given[1]	-	-	87%	88%
Surgical Care Improvement Project				
Appropriate Beta Blocker Usage	11	100%	98%	98%
Appropriate VTP Within 24 Hours	72	99%	98%	98%
Controlled Postoperative Blood Glucose[7]	-	-	96%	97%
Perioperative Temperature Management	91	100%	99%	100%
Prophylactic Antibiotic Selection	67	97%	99%	99%
Prophylactic Antibiotic Selection (Outpatient)[1]	-	-	98%	98%
Prophylactic Antibiotic Stopped	66	100%	98%	98%
Prophylactic Antibiotic Timing	68	94%	98%	99%
Prophylactic Antibiotic Timing (Outpatient)[1]	-	-	98%	98%
Urinary Catheter Removal	55	98%	97%	97%
Survey of Patients' Hospital Experiences				
Area Around Room 'Always' Quiet at Night	(a)	63%	64%	61%
Doctors 'Always' Communicated Well	(a)	86%	81%	82%
Home Recovery Information Given	(a)	91%	87%	85%
Hospital Given 9 or 10 on 10 Point Scale	(a)	67%	75%	71%
Meds 'Always' Explained Before Given	(a)	69%	67%	64%
Nurses 'Always' Communicated Well	(a)	79%	79%	79%
Pain 'Always' Well Controlled	(a)	73%	72%	71%
Room and Bathroom 'Always' Clean	(a)	61%	74%	73%
Timely Help 'Always' Received	(a)	75%	70%	68%
Would Definitely Recommend Hospital	(a)	66%	76%	71%
Use of Medical Imaging				
Cardiac Imaging Stress Test before Surgery	91	4.4%	5%	5.3%
Combination Abdominal CT Scan	338	3.0%	10%	10.5%
Combination Brain/Sinus CT Scan[1]	-	-	2.1%	2.7%
Combination Chest CT Scan	184	0.5%	3.1%	2.7%
Follow-up Mammogram/Ultrasound	454	8.4%	8.7%	8.8%
Lumbar Spine MRI for Low Back Pain[1]	-	-	39.7%	37.2%

The Memorial Hospital

750 Hospital Loop
Craig, CO 81625
Phone: 970-824-9411
Fax: 970-824-2235
URL: www.thememorialhospital.com
Type: Critical Access Hospitals
Emergency Services: Yes
Ownership: Government - Local
Beds: 29

Key Personnel:

Quality Assurance . . . . Betsy Bair
Operating Room. . . . . William Bertram
Cardiac Laboratory. . . . . Chris Evans
Hemotology Center . . . . Marle Kettle
Emergency Room . . . . Tom Soos
Radiology. . . . . Malaika C. Thompson
Chief of Medical Staff. . . . . Amy Updike
Infection Control. . . . . Beka Warren

Measure	Cases	This Hosp.	State Avg.	U.S. Avg.
Blood Clot Prevention and Treatment				
Anticoagulation Overlap Therapy[5]	-	-	97%	93%
ICU Venous Thromboembolism Prophylaxis[5]	-	-	95%	92%
Incidence of Potentially Preventable VTE[5]	-	-	8%	10%
UFH with Dosages/Platelet Monitoring[5]	-	-	97%	97%
Venous Thromboembolism Prophylaxis[5]	-	-	90%	85%
Warfarin Therapy Discharge Instructions[5]	-	-	69%	75%
Chest Pain/Possible Heart Attack Care				
Aspirin Given Within 24 Hours of Arrival[5]	-	-	97%	96%
Fibrinolytic Meds Within 30 Min. of Arrival[5]	-	-	55%	58%
Average Time to ECG (minutes)[5]	-	-	8	7
Average Time to Transfer (minutes)[5]	-	-	74	60
Children's Asthma Care				
Received Home Management Plan of Care	-	-	-	88%
Received Reliever Medication	-	-	-	100%
Received Systemic Corticosteroids	-	-	-	100%
Emergency Department				
Admittance Decision Time (minutes)[5]	-	-	96	98
Head CT Results Within 45 Min. of Arrival[5]	-	-	67%	57%
Patients Who Left ER Before Being Seen	5,036	0%	2%	2%
Time from ER Arrival to Admit. (minutes)[5]	-	-	244	274
Time from ER Arrival to Discharge (minutes)[3]	387	85	139	134
Time in ER Before Being Evaluated (minutes)[3]	311	15	20	26
Time to Pain Meds for Fractures (minutes)[5]	-	-	45	57
Heart Attack Care				
Aspirin Given at Discharge[1]	-	-	100%	99%
Fibrinolytic Meds Within 30 Min. of Arrival[7]	-	-	20%	54%
PCI Within 90 Minutes of Arrival[3,7]	-	-	97%	96%
Statin Prescribed at Discharge[7]	-	-	99%	98%
Heart Failure Care				
ACE Inhibitor or ARB for LVSD[1]	-	-	97%	97%
Discharge Instructions Given[1]	-	-	93%	94%
Evaluation of LVS Function[1]	-	-	99%	99%
Medicare Spending				
Medicare Spending per Patient (ratio)	-	-	0.95	0.98
Pneumonia Care				
Appropriate Initial Antibiotic Given	20	90%	95%	95%
Blood Culture Timing	20	90%	98%	98%
Pregnancy and Delivery Care				
Newborn Deliveries Scheduled Early[5]	-	-	2%	6%
Preventive Care				
Immunization for Influenza[5]	-	-	92%	90%
Immunization for Pneumonia[5]	-	-	92%	92%
Stroke Care				
Anticoagulation Therapy for Atrial Fibrillation[1]	-	-	97%	95%
Antithrombotic Therapy Timing[1]	-	-	98%	98%
Assessed for Rehabilitation[1]	-	-	98%	97%
Discharged on Antithrombotic Therapy[1]	-	-	100%	99%
Discharged on Statin Medication[1]	-	-	94%	94%
Thrombolytic Therapy Timing[1]	-	-	78%	66%
Venous Thromboembolism Prophylaxis[1]	-	-	96%	94%
Written Stroke Educational Materials Given[1]	-	-	87%	88%
Surgical Care Improvement Project				
Appropriate Beta Blocker Usage	17	41%	98%	98%
Appropriate VTP Within 24 Hours	38	95%	98%	98%
Controlled Postoperative Blood Glucose[7]	-	-	96%	97%
Perioperative Temperature Management	47	98%	99%	100%
Prophylactic Antibiotic Selection	38	97%	99%	99%
Prophylactic Antibiotic Selection (Outpatient)[5]	-	-	98%	98%
Prophylactic Antibiotic Stopped	37	92%	98%	98%
Prophylactic Antibiotic Timing	38	87%	98%	99%
Prophylactic Antibiotic Timing (Outpatient)[5]	-	-	98%	98%
Urinary Catheter Removal	19	95%	97%	97%
Survey of Patients' Hospital Experiences				
Area Around Room 'Always' Quiet at Night	(a)	61%	64%	61%
Doctors 'Always' Communicated Well	(a)	81%	81%	82%
Home Recovery Information Given	(a)	88%	87%	85%
Hospital Given 9 or 10 on 10 Point Scale	(a)	61%	75%	71%
Meds 'Always' Explained Before Given	(a)	68%	67%	64%
Nurses 'Always' Communicated Well	(a)	81%	79%	79%
Pain 'Always' Well Controlled	(a)	76%	72%	71%
Room and Bathroom 'Always' Clean	(a)	78%	74%	73%
Timely Help 'Always' Received	(a)	81%	70%	68%
Would Definitely Recommend Hospital	(a)	64%	76%	71%
Use of Medical Imaging				
Cardiac Imaging Stress Test before Surgery[1]	-	-	5%	5.3%
Combination Abdominal CT Scan	104	2.9%	10%	10.5%
Combination Brain/Sinus CT Scan[1]	-	-	2.1%	2.7%
Combination Chest CT Scan	53	0.0%	3.1%	2.7%
Follow-up Mammogram/Ultrasound	195	8.2%	8.7%	8.8%
Lumbar Spine MRI for Low Back Pain[1]	-	-	39.7%	37.2%

Rio Grande Hospital

310 County Rd 14
Del Norte, CO 81132
Phone: 719-657-2510
URL: www.rio-grande-hospital.org
Type: Critical Access Hospitals
Emergency Services: Yes
Ownership: Voluntary non-profit - Private

Key Personnel:

CEO . . . . Arlene Helms
Radiology. . . . . Chris Lefavre

Measure	Cases	This Hosp.	State Avg.	U.S. Avg.
Blood Clot Prevention and Treatment				
Anticoagulation Overlap Therapy[1,3]	-	-	97%	93%
ICU Venous Thromboembolism Prophylaxis[3,7]	-	-	95%	92%

NOTE: Hospital profiles are in alphabetical order by state, then city, then hospital within the city; Rankings exclude hospitals with less than 25 cases except for patient surveys which excludes hospitals with less than 100 cases; (a) 100-299 cases; (1) The number of cases/patients is too few to report; (2) Data submitted were based on a sample of cases/patients; (3) Results are based on a shorter time period than required; (4) Data suppressed by CMS for one or more quarters; (5) Results are not available for this reporting period; (6) Fewer than 100 patients completed the HCAHPS survey; (7) No cases met the criteria for this measure; (8) The lower limit of the confidence interval cannot be calculated if the number of observed infections equals zero; (9) No data are available from the state/territory for this reporting period; (10) The scores shown reflect fewer than 50 completed surveys; (11) There were discrepancies in the data collection process; (12) This measure does not apply to this hospital for this reporting period; (13) Results cannot be calculated for this reporting period; (14) The results for this state are combined with nearby states to protect confidentiality; Please refer to the User's Guide for a full explanation of data.

Measure	Cases	This Hosp.	State Avg.	U.S. Avg.
Incidence of Potentially Preventable VTE[3,7]	-	-	8%	10%
UFH with Dosages/Platelet Monitoring[1,3]	-	-	97%	97%
Venous Thromboembolism Prophylaxis[1,3]	-	-	90%	85%
Warfarin Therapy Discharge Instructions[1,3]	-	-	69%	75%
Chest Pain/Possible Heart Attack Care				
Aspirin Given Within 24 Hours of Arrival[3]	11	91%	97%	96%
Fibrinolytic Meds Within 30 Min. of Arrival[1,3]	-	-	55%	58%
Average Time to ECG (minutes)[3]	11	4	8	7
Average Time to Transfer (minutes)[1,3]	-	-	74	60
Children's Asthma Care				
Received Home Management Plan of Care	-	-	-	88%
Received Reliever Medication	-	-	-	100%
Received Systemic Corticosteroids	-	-	-	100%
Emergency Department				
Admittance Decision Time (minutes)[2,3]	119	40	96	98
Head CT Results Within 45 Min. of Arrival[1,3]	-	-	67%	57%
Patients Who Left ER Before Being Seen[5]	-	-	2%	2%
Time from ER Arrival to Admit. (minutes)[2,3]	145	215	244	274
Time from ER Arrival to Discharge (minutes)[3,7]	-	-	139	134
Time in ER Before Being Evaluated (minutes)[3]	18	0	20	26
Time to Pain Meds for Fractures (minutes)[1,3]	-	-	45	57
Heart Attack Care				
Aspirin Given at Discharge[1,3]	-	-	100%	99%
Fibrinolytic Meds Within 30 Min. of Arrival[3,7]	-	-	20%	54%
PCI Within 90 Minutes of Arrival[3,7]	-	-	97%	96%
Statin Prescribed at Discharge[1,3]	-	-	99%	98%
Heart Failure Care				
ACE Inhibitor or ARB for LVSD[1,3]	-	-	97%	97%
Discharge Instructions Given[1,3]	-	-	93%	94%
Evaluation of LVS Function[1,3]	-	-	99%	99%
Medicare Spending				
Medicare Spending per Patient (ratio)	-	-	0.95	0.98
Pneumonia Care				
Appropriate Initial Antibiotic Given[1,3]	-	-	95%	95%
Blood Culture Timing[3]	15	87%	98%	98%
Pregnancy and Delivery Care				
Newborn Deliveries Scheduled Early[5]	-	-	2%	6%
Preventive Care				
Immunization for Influenza[3]	59	83%	92%	90%
Immunization for Pneumonia[3]	123	76%	92%	92%
Stroke Care				
Anticoagulation Therapy for Atrial Fibrillation[3,7]	-	-	97%	95%
Antithrombotic Therapy Timing[1,3]	-	-	98%	98%
Assessed for Rehabilitation[1,3]	-	-	98%	97%
Discharged on Antithrombotic Therapy[3,7]	-	-	100%	99%
Discharged on Statin Medication[1,3]	-	-	94%	94%
Thrombolytic Therapy Timing[3,7]	-	-	78%	66%
Venous Thromboembolism Prophylaxis[1,3]	-	-	96%	94%
Written Stroke Educational Materials Given[3,7]	-	-	87%	88%
Surgical Care Improvement Project				
Appropriate Beta Blocker Usage[5]	-	-	98%	98%
Appropriate VTP Within 24 Hours[5]	-	-	98%	98%
Controlled Postoperative Blood Glucose[5]	-	-	96%	97%
Perioperative Temperature Management[5]	-	-	99%	100%
Prophylactic Antibiotic Selection[5]	-	-	99%	99%
Prophylactic Antibiotic Selection (Outpatient)[5]	-	-	98%	98%
Prophylactic Antibiotic Stopped[5]	-	-	98%	98%
Prophylactic Antibiotic Timing[5]	-	-	98%	99%
Prophylactic Antibiotic Timing (Outpatient)[5]	-	-	98%	98%
Urinary Catheter Removal[5]	-	-	97%	97%
Survey of Patients' Hospital Experiences				
Area Around Room 'Always' Quiet at Night[6]	<100	73%	64%	61%
Doctors 'Always' Communicated Well[6]	<100	77%	81%	82%
Home Recovery Information Given[6]	<100	84%	87%	85%
Hospital Given 9 or 10 on 10 Point Scale[6]	<100	81%	75%	71%
Meds 'Always' Explained Before Given[6]	<100	75%	67%	64%
Nurses 'Always' Communicated Well[6]	<100	76%	79%	79%
Pain 'Always' Well Controlled[6]	<100	70%	72%	71%
Room and Bathroom 'Always' Clean[6]	<100	79%	74%	73%
Timely Help 'Always' Received[6]	<100	71%	70%	68%
Would Definitely Recommend Hospital[6]	<100	73%	76%	71%
Use of Medical Imaging				
Cardiac Imaging Stress Test before Surgery[1]	-	-	5%	5.3%
Combination Abdominal CT Scan	115	12.2%	10%	10.5%
Combination Brain/Sinus CT Scan	87	0.0%	2.1%	2.7%
Combination Chest CT Scan	97	0.0%	3.1%	2.7%
Follow-up Mammogram/Ultrasound[7]	-	-	8.7%	8.8%
Lumbar Spine MRI for Low Back Pain[1]	-	-	39.7%	37.2%

Delta County Memorial Hospital

1501 E 3rd Street
Delta, CO 81416
Phone: 970-874-7681
Fax: 970-874-2204
E-mail: info@deltahospital.org
URL: www.deltahospital.org
Type: Acute Care Hospitals
Emergency Services: Yes
Ownership: Government - Local
Key Personnel:
Radiology . . . . Steven Bernstein
Emergency Room . . . . Charles Bibby
CEO/President . . . . Tom Mingen

Measure	Cases	This Hosp.	State Avg.	U.S. Avg.
Blood Clot Prevention and Treatment				
Anticoagulation Overlap Therapy[2]	28	93%	97%	93%
ICU Venous Thromboembolism Prophylaxis[2]	44	91%	95%	92%
Incidence of Potentially Preventable VTE[1,2]	-	-	8%	10%
UFH with Dosages/Platelet Monitoring[1,2]	-	-	97%	97%
Venous Thromboembolism Prophylaxis[2]	209	89%	90%	85%
Warfarin Therapy Discharge Instructions[2]	21	76%	69%	75%
Chest Pain/Possible Heart Attack Care				
Aspirin Given Within 24 Hours of Arrival	51	96%	97%	96%
Fibrinolytic Meds Within 30 Min. of Arrival	11	73%	55%	58%
Average Time to ECG (minutes)	50	7	8	7
Average Time to Transfer (minutes)[7]	-	-	74	60
Children's Asthma Care				
Received Home Management Plan of Care	-	-	-	88%
Received Reliever Medication	-	-	-	100%
Received Systemic Corticosteroids	-	-	-	100%
Emergency Department				
Admittance Decision Time (minutes)[2]	264	70	96	98
Head CT Results Within 45 Min. of Arrival[1]	-	-	67%	57%
Patients Who Left ER Before Being Seen	13,846	0%	2%	2%
Time from ER Arrival to Admit. (minutes)[2]	293	209	244	274
Time from ER Arrival to Discharge (minutes)	455	127	139	134
Time in ER Before Being Evaluated (minutes)	430	32	20	26
Time to Pain Meds for Fractures (minutes)	72	42	45	57
Heart Attack Care				
Aspirin Given at Discharge	11	100%	100%	99%
Fibrinolytic Meds Within 30 Min. of Arrival[1]	-	-	20%	54%
PCI Within 90 Minutes of Arrival[7]	-	-	97%	96%
Statin Prescribed at Discharge[1]	-	-	99%	98%
Heart Failure Care				
ACE Inhibitor or ARB for LVSD	16	94%	97%	97%
Discharge Instructions Given	27	100%	93%	94%
Evaluation of LVS Function	44	98%	99%	99%
Medicare Spending				
Medicare Spending per Patient (ratio)	-	0.91	0.95	0.98
Pneumonia Care				
Appropriate Initial Antibiotic Given	50	88%	95%	95%
Blood Culture Timing	65	92%	98%	98%
Pregnancy and Delivery Care				
Newborn Deliveries Scheduled Early	19	0%	2%	6%
Preventive Care				
Immunization for Influenza[2]	328	70%	92%	90%
Immunization for Pneumonia[2]	452	73%	92%	92%
Stroke Care				
Anticoagulation Therapy for Atrial Fibrillation[1]	-	-	97%	95%
Antithrombotic Therapy Timing	16	100%	98%	98%
Assessed for Rehabilitation	20	100%	98%	97%
Discharged on Antithrombotic Therapy	17	100%	100%	99%
Discharged on Statin Medication	13	85%	94%	94%
Thrombolytic Therapy Timing[7]	-	-	78%	66%
Venous Thromboembolism Prophylaxis	19	100%	96%	94%
Written Stroke Educational Materials Given[1]	-	-	87%	88%
Surgical Care Improvement Project				
Appropriate Beta Blocker Usage	43	98%	98%	98%
Appropriate VTP Within 24 Hours	188	96%	98%	98%
Controlled Postoperative Blood Glucose[7]	-	-	96%	97%
Perioperative Temperature Management	234	100%	99%	100%
Prophylactic Antibiotic Selection	158	96%	99%	99%
Prophylactic Antibiotic Selection (Outpatient)	28	96%	98%	98%
Prophylactic Antibiotic Stopped	153	97%	98%	98%
Prophylactic Antibiotic Timing	159	95%	98%	99%
Prophylactic Antibiotic Timing (Outpatient)	28	100%	98%	98%
Urinary Catheter Removal	61	93%	97%	97%
Survey of Patients' Hospital Experiences				
Area Around Room 'Always' Quiet at Night	(a)	56%	64%	61%
Doctors 'Always' Communicated Well	(a)	79%	81%	82%
Home Recovery Information Given	(a)	86%	87%	85%
Hospital Given 9 or 10 on 10 Point Scale	(a)	73%	75%	71%
Meds 'Always' Explained Before Given	(a)	61%	67%	64%
Nurses 'Always' Communicated Well	(a)	75%	79%	79%
Pain 'Always' Well Controlled	(a)	72%	72%	71%
Room and Bathroom 'Always' Clean	(a)	80%	74%	73%
Timely Help 'Always' Received	(a)	67%	70%	68%
Would Definitely Recommend Hospital	(a)	73%	76%	71%
Use of Medical Imaging				
Cardiac Imaging Stress Test before Surgery	110	4.5%	5%	5.3%
Combination Abdominal CT Scan	383	11.2%	10%	10.5%
Combination Brain/Sinus CT Scan[1]	-	-	2.1%	2.7%
Combination Chest CT Scan	302	1.7%	3.1%	2.7%
Follow-up Mammogram/Ultrasound	735	18.1%	8.7%	8.8%
Lumbar Spine MRI for Low Back Pain	59	42.4%	39.7%	37.2%

Centura Health - Porter Adventist Hospital

2525 S Downing St
Denver, CO 80210
Phone: 303-778-1955
Fax: 303-778-5252
URL: www.centura.org
Type: Acute Care Hospitals
Emergency Services: Yes
Ownership: Voluntary non-profit - Church
Beds: 368
Key Personnel:
Radiology . . . . Simeon David Abramson
Pediatric In-Patient Care . . . . Janell Dillard
Chief of Medical Staff . . . . Thomas Drake, MD
Pediatric Ambulatory Care . . . . . . Marlene Ellstrom
CEO/President . . . . Randy Haffner, PhD
Quality Assurance . . . . Richard Osborn
Coronary Care . . . . Karolyn Scheneman
Infection Control . . . . Cindy Thistel

Measure	Cases	This Hosp.	State Avg.	U.S. Avg.
Blood Clot Prevention and Treatment				
Anticoagulation Overlap Therapy[2]	64	97%	97%	93%
ICU Venous Thromboembolism Prophylaxis[2]	92	89%	95%	92%
Incidence of Potentially Preventable VTE[2]	12	0%	8%	10%
UFH with Dosages/Platelet Monitoring[2]	53	100%	97%	97%
Venous Thromboembolism Prophylaxis[2]	247	82%	90%	85%
Warfarin Therapy Discharge Instructions[2]	52	13%	69%	75%
Chest Pain/Possible Heart Attack Care				
Aspirin Given Within 24 Hours of Arrival[1,3]	-	-	97%	96%
Fibrinolytic Meds Within 30 Min. of Arrival[3,7]	-	-	55%	58%
Average Time to ECG (minutes)[1,3]	-	-	8	7
Average Time to Transfer (minutes)[3,7]	-	-	74	60
Children's Asthma Care				
Received Home Management Plan of Care	-	-	-	88%
Received Reliever Medication	-	-	-	100%
Received Systemic Corticosteroids	-	-	-	100%
Emergency Department				
Admittance Decision Time (minutes)[2]	531	157	96	98
Head CT Results Within 45 Min. of Arrival[1]	-	-	67%	57%
Patients Who Left ER Before Being Seen	25,575	0%	2%	2%
Time from ER Arrival to Admit. (minutes)[2]	542	319	244	274
Time from ER Arrival to Discharge (minutes)	420	169	139	134
Time in ER Before Being Evaluated (minutes)	445	15	20	26
Time to Pain Meds for Fractures (minutes)	47	56	45	57
Heart Attack Care				
Aspirin Given at Discharge	92	100%	100%	99%
Fibrinolytic Meds Within 30 Min. of Arrival[7]	-	-	20%	54%
PCI Within 90 Minutes of Arrival	20	95%	97%	96%
Statin Prescribed at Discharge	91	100%	99%	98%
Heart Failure Care				

NOTE: Hospital profiles are in alphabetical order by state, then city, then hospital within the city; Rankings exclude hospitals with less than 25 cases except for patient surveys which excludes hospitals with less than 100 cases; (a) 100-299 cases; (1) The number of cases/patients is too few to report; (2) Data submitted were based on a sample of cases/patients; (3) Results are based on a shorter time period than required; (4) Data suppressed by CMS for one or more quarters; (5) Results are not available for this reporting period; (6) Fewer than 100 patients completed the HCAHPS survey; (7) No cases met the criteria for this measure; (8) The lower limit of the confidence interval cannot be calculated if the number of observed infections equals zero; (9) No data are available from the state/territory for this reporting period; (10) The scores shown reflect fewer than 50 completed surveys; (11) There were discrepancies in the data collection process; (12) This measure does not apply to this hospital for this reporting period; (13) Results cannot be calculated for this reporting period; (14) The results for this state are combined with nearby states to protect confidentiality; Please refer to the User's Guide for a full explanation of data.

Measure	Cases	This Hosp.	State Avg.	U.S. Avg.
ACE Inhibitor or ARB for LVSD	39	95%	97%	97%
Discharge Instructions Given	105	99%	93%	94%
Evaluation of LVS Function	139	100%	99%	99%
Medicare Spending				
Medicare Spending per Patient (ratio)	-	0.99	0.95	0.98
Pneumonia Care				
Appropriate Initial Antibiotic Given	105	96%	95%	95%
Blood Culture Timing	175	98%	98%	98%
Pregnancy and Delivery Care				
Newborn Deliveries Scheduled Early[7]	-	-	2%	6%
Preventive Care				
Immunization for Influenza[2]	632	93%	92%	90%
Immunization for Pneumonia[2]	822	92%	92%	92%
Stroke Care				
Anticoagulation Therapy for Atrial Fibrillation[1]	-	-	97%	95%
Antithrombotic Therapy Timing	35	100%	98%	98%
Assessed for Rehabilitation	40	98%	98%	97%
Discharged on Antithrombotic Therapy	40	100%	100%	99%
Discharged on Statin Medication	25	100%	94%	94%
Thrombolytic Therapy Timing[1]	-	-	78%	66%
Venous Thromboembolism Prophylaxis	42	95%	96%	94%
Written Stroke Educational Materials Given	15	33%	87%	88%
Surgical Care Improvement Project				
Appropriate Beta Blocker Usage[2]	187	98%	98%	98%
Appropriate VTP Within 24 Hours[2]	353	96%	98%	98%
Controlled Postoperative Blood Glucose[2]	182	95%	96%	97%
Perioperative Temperature Management[2]	435	100%	99%	100%
Prophylactic Antibiotic Selection[2]	441	99%	99%	99%
Prophylactic Antibiotic Selection (Outpatient)	434	98%	98%	98%
Prophylactic Antibiotic Stopped[2]	437	97%	98%	98%
Prophylactic Antibiotic Timing[2]	441	100%	98%	99%
Prophylactic Antibiotic Timing (Outpatient)	434	100%	98%	98%
Urinary Catheter Removal[2]	473	97%	97%	97%
Survey of Patients' Hospital Experiences				
Area Around Room 'Always' Quiet at Night	300+	60%	64%	61%
Doctors 'Always' Communicated Well	300+	80%	81%	82%
Home Recovery Information Given	300+	89%	87%	85%
Hospital Given 9 or 10 on 10 Point Scale	300+	73%	75%	71%
Meds 'Always' Explained Before Given	300+	62%	67%	64%
Nurses 'Always' Communicated Well	300+	77%	79%	79%
Pain 'Always' Well Controlled	300+	68%	72%	71%
Room and Bathroom 'Always' Clean	300+	72%	74%	73%
Timely Help 'Always' Received	300+	66%	70%	68%
Would Definitely Recommend Hospital	300+	75%	76%	71%
Use of Medical Imaging				
Cardiac Imaging Stress Test before Surgery	179	6.7%	5%	5.3%
Combination Abdominal CT Scan	468	26.5%	10%	10.5%
Combination Brain/Sinus CT Scan	348	1.1%	2.1%	2.7%
Combination Chest CT Scan	262	6.9%	3.1%	2.7%
Follow-up Mammogram/Ultrasound	582	13.4%	8.7%	8.8%
Lumbar Spine MRI for Low Back Pain[1]	-	-	39.7%	37.2%

Denver Health Medical Center

777 Bannock St
Denver, CO 80204
Phone: 303-436-6000
Fax: 303-436-7159
URL: www.denverhealth.org
Type: Acute Care Hospitals
Emergency Services: Yes
Ownership: Government - State
Beds: 477

Key Personnel:

CEO/President. . . . . Arthur Gonzalez, P.H., FACHE
Pediatric Ambulatory Care . . . . . . Simon Hambrdge, MD
Quality Assurance . . . . Dave Krapil
Coronary Care. . . . . Caroline Long, MD
Chief of Medical Staff. . . . . Philip Mehler, MD
Pediatric In-Patient Care . . . . John O, MD
Infection Control. . . . . Connie Price, MD
Radiology. . . . . Ron Townsend, MD

Measure	Cases	This Hosp.	State Avg.	U.S. Avg.
Blood Clot Prevention and Treatment				
Anticoagulation Overlap Therapy[2]	98	98%	97%	93%
ICU Venous Thromboembolism Prophylaxis[2]	113	87%	95%	92%
Incidence of Potentially Preventable VTE[2]	47	11%	8%	10%
UFH with Dosages/Platelet Monitoring[2]	80	96%	97%	97%
Venous Thromboembolism Prophylaxis[2]	309	74%	90%	85%
Warfarin Therapy Discharge Instructions[2]	78	85%	69%	75%
Chest Pain/Possible Heart Attack Care				
Aspirin Given Within 24 Hours of Arrival[3,7]	-	-	97%	96%
Fibrinolytic Meds Within 30 Min. of Arrival[5]	-	-	55%	58%
Average Time to ECG (minutes)[1,3]	-	-	8	7
Average Time to Transfer (minutes)[5]	-	-	74	60
Children's Asthma Care				
Received Home Management Plan of Care	-	-	-	88%
Received Reliever Medication	-	-	-	100%
Received Systemic Corticosteroids	-	-	-	100%
Emergency Department				
Admittance Decision Time (minutes)[2]	436	134	96	98
Head CT Results Within 45 Min. of Arrival[1]	-	-	67%	57%
Patients Who Left ER Before Being Seen	87,569	6%	2%	2%
Time from ER Arrival to Admit. (minutes)[2]	445	319	244	274
Time from ER Arrival to Discharge (minutes)	296	268	139	134
Time in ER Before Being Evaluated (minutes)	389	19	20	26
Time to Pain Meds for Fractures (minutes)	335	25	45	57
Heart Attack Care				
Aspirin Given at Discharge	156	99%	100%	99%
Fibrinolytic Meds Within 30 Min. of Arrival[7]	-	-	20%	54%
PCI Within 90 Minutes of Arrival	38	79%	97%	96%
Statin Prescribed at Discharge	158	99%	99%	98%
Heart Failure Care				
ACE Inhibitor or ARB for LVSD	145	99%	97%	97%
Discharge Instructions Given	330	91%	93%	94%
Evaluation of LVS Function	348	100%	99%	99%
Medicare Spending				
Medicare Spending per Patient (ratio)	-	0.94	0.95	0.98
Pneumonia Care				
Appropriate Initial Antibiotic Given[2]	65	94%	95%	95%
Blood Culture Timing[2]	39	87%	98%	98%
Pregnancy and Delivery Care				
Newborn Deliveries Scheduled Early[2]	50	0%	2%	6%
Preventive Care				
Immunization for Influenza[2]	487	84%	92%	90%
Immunization for Pneumonia[2]	436	86%	92%	92%
Stroke Care				
Anticoagulation Therapy for Atrial Fibrillation	11	100%	97%	95%
Antithrombotic Therapy Timing	65	95%	98%	98%
Assessed for Rehabilitation	86	90%	98%	97%
Discharged on Antithrombotic Therapy	78	100%	100%	99%
Discharged on Statin Medication	59	90%	94%	94%
Thrombolytic Therapy Timing[1]	-	-	78%	66%
Venous Thromboembolism Prophylaxis	86	87%	96%	94%
Written Stroke Educational Materials Given	51	80%	87%	88%
Surgical Care Improvement Project				
Appropriate Beta Blocker Usage[2]	48	100%	98%	98%
Appropriate VTP Within 24 Hours[2]	276	98%	98%	98%
Controlled Postoperative Blood Glucose[2,7]	-	-	96%	97%
Perioperative Temperature Management[2]	341	97%	99%	100%
Prophylactic Antibiotic Selection[2]	220	100%	99%	99%
Prophylactic Antibiotic Selection (Outpatient)	339	97%	98%	98%
Prophylactic Antibiotic Stopped[2]	212	94%	98%	98%
Prophylactic Antibiotic Timing[2]	221	97%	98%	99%
Prophylactic Antibiotic Timing (Outpatient)	200	94%	98%	98%
Urinary Catheter Removal[2]	167	97%	97%	97%
Survey of Patients' Hospital Experiences				
Area Around Room 'Always' Quiet at Night	300+	61%	64%	61%
Doctors 'Always' Communicated Well	300+	78%	81%	82%
Home Recovery Information Given	300+	85%	87%	85%
Hospital Given 9 or 10 on 10 Point Scale	300+	68%	75%	71%
Meds 'Always' Explained Before Given	300+	63%	67%	64%
Nurses 'Always' Communicated Well	300+	74%	79%	79%
Pain 'Always' Well Controlled	300+	65%	72%	71%
Room and Bathroom 'Always' Clean	300+	60%	74%	73%
Timely Help 'Always' Received	300+	59%	70%	68%
Would Definitely Recommend Hospital	300+	67%	76%	71%
Use of Medical Imaging				
Cardiac Imaging Stress Test before Surgery	137	0.7%	5%	5.3%
Combination Abdominal CT Scan	532	0.2%	10%	10.5%
Combination Brain/Sinus CT Scan	416	0.5%	2.1%	2.7%
Combination Chest CT Scan	379	4.0%	3.1%	2.7%
Follow-up Mammogram/Ultrasound	700	8.9%	8.7%	8.8%
Lumbar Spine MRI for Low Back Pain	52	55.8%	39.7%	37.2%

Exempla Saint Joseph Hospital

1835 Franklin St
Denver, CO 80218
Phone: 303-837-7111
Fax: 303-318-2115
URL: www.exempla.org
Type: Acute Care Hospitals
Emergency Services: Yes
Ownership: Voluntary non-profit - Private
Beds: 565

Key Personnel:

Chief of Medical Staff . . . . Shawn Dufford, MD, MBA
CEO/President. . . . . Bain J. Farris

Measure	Cases	This Hosp.	State Avg.	U.S. Avg.
Blood Clot Prevention and Treatment				
Anticoagulation Overlap Therapy[2]	134	98%	97%	93%
ICU Venous Thromboembolism Prophylaxis[2]	83	95%	95%	92%
Incidence of Potentially Preventable VTE[2]	17	0%	8%	10%
UFH with Dosages/Platelet Monitoring[2]	127	98%	97%	97%
Venous Thromboembolism Prophylaxis[2]	304	92%	90%	85%
Warfarin Therapy Discharge Instructions[2]	99	84%	69%	75%
Chest Pain/Possible Heart Attack Care				
Aspirin Given Within 24 Hours of Arrival[1,3]	-	-	97%	96%
Fibrinolytic Meds Within 30 Min. of Arrival[5]	-	-	55%	58%
Average Time to ECG (minutes)[1,3]	-	-	8	7
Average Time to Transfer (minutes)[5]	-	-	74	60
Children's Asthma Care				
Received Home Management Plan of Care	-	-	-	88%
Received Reliever Medication	-	-	-	100%
Received Systemic Corticosteroids	-	-	-	100%
Emergency Department				
Admittance Decision Time (minutes)[2]	400	100	96	98
Head CT Results Within 45 Min. of Arrival[1]	-	-	67%	57%
Patients Who Left ER Before Being Seen	51,961	1%	2%	2%
Time from ER Arrival to Admit. (minutes)[2]	403	299	244	274
Time from ER Arrival to Discharge (minutes)	296	172	139	134
Time in ER Before Being Evaluated (minutes)	382	18	20	26
Time to Pain Meds for Fractures (minutes)	78	71	45	57
Heart Attack Care				
Aspirin Given at Discharge[2]	153	99%	100%	99%
Fibrinolytic Meds Within 30 Min. of Arrival[2,7]	-	-	20%	54%
PCI Within 90 Minutes of Arrival[2]	13	85%	97%	96%
Statin Prescribed at Discharge[2]	144	100%	99%	98%
Heart Failure Care				
ACE Inhibitor or ARB for LVSD[2]	82	99%	97%	97%
Discharge Instructions Given[2]	284	98%	93%	94%
Evaluation of LVS Function[2]	334	100%	99%	99%
Medicare Spending				
Medicare Spending per Patient (ratio)	-	0.97	0.95	0.98
Pneumonia Care				
Appropriate Initial Antibiotic Given	201	95%	95%	95%
Blood Culture Timing	369	98%	98%	98%
Pregnancy and Delivery Care				
Newborn Deliveries Scheduled Early	265	1%	2%	6%
Preventive Care				
Immunization for Influenza[2]	502	89%	92%	90%
Immunization for Pneumonia[2]	560	92%	92%	92%
Stroke Care				
Anticoagulation Therapy for Atrial Fibrillation	13	100%	97%	95%
Antithrombotic Therapy Timing	89	99%	98%	98%
Assessed for Rehabilitation	118	97%	98%	97%
Discharged on Antithrombotic Therapy	108	100%	100%	99%
Discharged on Statin Medication	91	95%	94%	94%
Thrombolytic Therapy Timing[1]	-	-	78%	66%
Venous Thromboembolism Prophylaxis	101	92%	96%	94%
Written Stroke Educational Materials Given	75	81%	87%	88%
Surgical Care Improvement Project				
Appropriate Beta Blocker Usage[2]	265	99%	98%	98%
Appropriate VTP Within 24 Hours[2]	372	100%	98%	98%
Controlled Postoperative Blood Glucose[2]	137	99%	96%	97%
Perioperative Temperature Management[2]	455	100%	99%	100%
Prophylactic Antibiotic Selection[2]	446	100%	99%	99%
Prophylactic Antibiotic Selection (Outpatient)	680	99%	98%	98%

NOTE: Hospital profiles are in alphabetical order by state, then city, then hospital within the city; Rankings exclude hospitals with less than 25 cases except for patient surveys which excludes hospitals with less than 100 cases; (a) 100-299 cases; (1) The number of cases/patients is too few to report; (2) Data submitted were based on a sample of cases/patients; (3) Results are based on a shorter time period than required; (4) Data suppressed by CMS for one or more quarters; (5) Results are not available for this reporting period; (6) Fewer than 100 patients completed the HCAHPS survey; (7) No cases met the criteria for this measure; (8) The lower limit of the confidence interval cannot be calculated if the number of observed infections equals zero; (9) No data are available from the state/territory for this reporting period; (10) The scores shown reflect fewer than 50 completed surveys; (11) There were discrepancies in the data collection process; (12) This measure does not apply to this hospital for this reporting period; (13) Results cannot be calculated for this reporting period; (14) The results for this state are combined with nearby states to protect confidentiality; Please refer to the User's Guide for a full explanation of data.

Measure	Cases	This Hosp.	State Avg.	U.S. Avg.
Prophylactic Antibiotic Stopped[2]	440	99%	98%	98%
Prophylactic Antibiotic Timing[2]	446	98%	98%	99%
Prophylactic Antibiotic Timing (Outpatient)	684	97%	98%	98%
Urinary Catheter Removal[2]	296	99%	97%	97%
Survey of Patients' Hospital Experiences				
Area Around Room 'Always' Quiet at Night	300+	57%	64%	61%
Doctors 'Always' Communicated Well	300+	80%	81%	82%
Home Recovery Information Given	300+	90%	87%	85%
Hospital Given 9 or 10 on 10 Point Scale	300+	74%	75%	71%
Meds 'Always' Explained Before Given	300+	66%	67%	64%
Nurses 'Always' Communicated Well	300+	78%	79%	79%
Pain 'Always' Well Controlled	300+	70%	72%	71%
Room and Bathroom 'Always' Clean	300+	67%	74%	73%
Timely Help 'Always' Received	300+	69%	70%	68%
Would Definitely Recommend Hospital	300+	76%	76%	71%
Use of Medical Imaging				
Cardiac Imaging Stress Test before Surgery	79	2.5%	5%	5.3%
Combination Abdominal CT Scan	231	4.3%	10%	10.5%
Combination Brain/Sinus CT Scan	134	0.0%	2.1%	2.7%
Combination Chest CT Scan	117	0.9%	3.1%	2.7%
Follow-up Mammogram/Ultrasound	441	5.4%	8.7%	8.8%
Lumbar Spine MRI for Low Back Pain[1]	-	-	39.7%	37.2%

National Jewish Health

1400 Jackson St
Denver, CO 80206
Phone: 303-388-4461
Fax: 303-270-2165
E-mail: lungline@njc.org
URL: www.njc.org
Type: Acute Care Hospitals
Emergency Services: No
Ownership: Voluntary non-profit - Private
Beds: 46

Key Personnel:

Pediatrics. . . . . Erwin W. Gelfand, MD
Radiology. . . . . John D Newell, MD
CEO/President. . . . . Michael Salem, MD
Chair/CEO . . . . Richard A. Schierburg

Measure	Cases	This Hosp.	State Avg.	U.S. Avg.
Blood Clot Prevention and Treatment				
Anticoagulation Overlap Therapy[7]	-	-	97%	93%
ICU Venous Thromboembolism Prophylaxis[7]	-	-	95%	92%
Incidence of Potentially Preventable VTE[7]	-	-	8%	10%
UFH with Dosages/Platelet Monitoring[7]	-	-	97%	97%
Venous Thromboembolism Prophylaxis[1]	-	-	90%	85%
Warfarin Therapy Discharge Instructions[7]	-	-	69%	75%
Chest Pain/Possible Heart Attack Care				
Aspirin Given Within 24 Hours of Arrival[5]	-	-	97%	96%
Fibrinolytic Meds Within 30 Min. of Arrival[5]	-	-	55%	58%
Average Time to ECG (minutes)[5]	-	-	8	7
Average Time to Transfer (minutes)[5]	-	-	74	60
Children's Asthma Care				
Received Home Management Plan of Care	-	-	-	88%
Received Reliever Medication	-	-	-	100%
Received Systemic Corticosteroids	-	-	-	100%
Emergency Department				
Admittance Decision Time (minutes)[7]	-	-	96	98
Head CT Results Within 45 Min. of Arrival[5]	-	-	67%	57%
Patients Who Left ER Before Being Seen[5]	-	-	2%	2%
Time from ER Arrival to Admit. (minutes)[7]	-	-	244	274
Time from ER Arrival to Discharge (minutes)[5]	-	-	139	134
Time in ER Before Being Evaluated (minutes)[5]	-	-	20	26
Time to Pain Meds for Fractures (minutes)[5]	-	-	45	57
Heart Attack Care				
Aspirin Given at Discharge[5]	-	-	100%	99%
Fibrinolytic Meds Within 30 Min. of Arrival[5]	-	-	20%	54%
PCI Within 90 Minutes of Arrival[5]	-	-	97%	96%
Statin Prescribed at Discharge[5]	-	-	99%	98%
Heart Failure Care				
ACE Inhibitor or ARB for LVSD[5]	-	-	97%	97%
Discharge Instructions Given[5]	-	-	93%	94%
Evaluation of LVS Function[5]	-	-	99%	99%
Medicare Spending				
Medicare Spending per Patient (ratio)[1]	-	-	0.95	0.98
Pneumonia Care				
Appropriate Initial Antibiotic Given[3,7]	-	-	95%	95%
Blood Culture Timing[3,7]	-	-	98%	98%
Pregnancy and Delivery Care				
Newborn Deliveries Scheduled Early[7]	-	-	2%	6%
Preventive Care				
Immunization for Influenza[2]	23	61%	92%	90%
Immunization for Pneumonia[1,2]	-	-	92%	92%
Stroke Care				
Anticoagulation Therapy for Atrial Fibrillation[5]	-	-	97%	95%
Antithrombotic Therapy Timing[5]	-	-	98%	98%
Assessed for Rehabilitation[5]	-	-	98%	97%
Discharged on Antithrombotic Therapy[5]	-	-	100%	99%
Discharged on Statin Medication[5]	-	-	94%	94%
Thrombolytic Therapy Timing[5]	-	-	78%	66%
Venous Thromboembolism Prophylaxis[5]	-	-	96%	94%
Written Stroke Educational Materials Given[5]	-	-	87%	88%
Surgical Care Improvement Project				
Appropriate Beta Blocker Usage[5]	-	-	98%	98%
Appropriate VTP Within 24 Hours[5]	-	-	98%	98%
Controlled Postoperative Blood Glucose[5]	-	-	96%	97%
Perioperative Temperature Management[5]	-	-	99%	100%
Prophylactic Antibiotic Selection[5]	-	-	99%	99%
Prophylactic Antibiotic Selection (Outpatient)[5]	-	-	98%	98%
Prophylactic Antibiotic Stopped[5]	-	-	98%	98%
Prophylactic Antibiotic Timing[5]	-	-	98%	99%
Prophylactic Antibiotic Timing (Outpatient)[5]	-	-	98%	98%
Urinary Catheter Removal[5]	-	-	97%	97%
Survey of Patients' Hospital Experiences				
Area Around Room 'Always' Quiet at Night[10]	<100	100%	64%	61%
Doctors 'Always' Communicated Well[10]	<100	82%	81%	82%
Home Recovery Information Given[10]	<100	100%	87%	85%
Hospital Given 9 or 10 on 10 Point Scale[10]	<100	100%	75%	71%
Meds 'Always' Explained Before Given[10]	<100	100%	67%	64%
Nurses 'Always' Communicated Well[10]	<100	98%	79%	79%
Pain 'Always' Well Controlled[10]	<100	-	72%	71%
Room and Bathroom 'Always' Clean[10]	<100	8%	74%	73%
Timely Help 'Always' Received[10]	<100	71%	70%	68%
Would Definitely Recommend Hospital[10]	<100	100%	76%	71%
Use of Medical Imaging				
Cardiac Imaging Stress Test before Surgery	345	9.6%	5%	5.3%
Combination Abdominal CT Scan	86	5.8%	10%	10.5%
Combination Brain/Sinus CT Scan[1]	-	-	2.1%	2.7%
Combination Chest CT Scan	2,829	0.0%	3.1%	2.7%
Follow-up Mammogram/Ultrasound[7]	-	-	8.7%	8.8%
Lumbar Spine MRI for Low Back Pain[1]	-	-	39.7%	37.2%

Presbyterian Saint Lukes Medical Center

1719 E 19th Ave
Denver, CO 80218
Phone: 303-839-6000
Fax: 303-839-7294
E-mail: paula.cooper@healthonecares.com
URL: www.pslmc.com
Type: Acute Care Hospitals
Emergency Services: Yes
Ownership: Government - State
Beds: 680

Key Personnel:

Quality Assurance . . . . Jeanine Legg
Radiology. . . . . Jane O'Connor
Chief of Medical Staff. . . . . Steve Quach, MD
CEO/President. . . . . Maureen Tarrant
Pediatric In-Patient Care . . . . Mary Wintz
Cardiac Laboratory. . . . . Tammy Woolley

Measure	Cases	This Hosp.	State Avg.	U.S. Avg.
Blood Clot Prevention and Treatment				
Anticoagulation Overlap Therapy[2]	69	99%	97%	93%
ICU Venous Thromboembolism Prophylaxis[2]	82	98%	95%	92%
Incidence of Potentially Preventable VTE[2]	15	7%	8%	10%
UFH with Dosages/Platelet Monitoring[2]	50	100%	97%	97%
Venous Thromboembolism Prophylaxis[2]	322	92%	90%	85%
Warfarin Therapy Discharge Instructions[2]	61	69%	69%	75%
Chest Pain/Possible Heart Attack Care				
Aspirin Given Within 24 Hours of Arrival[3,7]	-	-	97%	96%
Fibrinolytic Meds Within 30 Min. of Arrival[5]	-	-	55%	58%
Average Time to ECG (minutes)[1,3]	-	-	8	7
Average Time to Transfer (minutes)[5]	-	-	74	60
Children's Asthma Care				
Received Home Management Plan of Care	-	-	-	88%
Received Reliever Medication	-	-	-	100%
Received Systemic Corticosteroids	-	-	-	100%
Emergency Department				
Admittance Decision Time (minutes)[2]	440	79	96	98
Head CT Results Within 45 Min. of Arrival[1,3]	-	-	67%	57%
Patients Who Left ER Before Being Seen	25,863	0%	2%	2%
Time from ER Arrival to Admit. (minutes)[2]	440	178	244	274
Time from ER Arrival to Discharge (minutes)	457	138	139	134
Time in ER Before Being Evaluated (minutes)	503	7	20	26
Time to Pain Meds for Fractures (minutes)	78	30	45	57
Heart Attack Care				
Aspirin Given at Discharge	78	100%	100%	99%
Fibrinolytic Meds Within 30 Min. of Arrival[7]	-	-	20%	54%
PCI Within 90 Minutes of Arrival	12	100%	97%	96%
Statin Prescribed at Discharge	77	100%	99%	98%
Heart Failure Care				
ACE Inhibitor or ARB for LVSD	27	100%	97%	97%
Discharge Instructions Given	65	98%	93%	94%
Evaluation of LVS Function	82	100%	99%	99%
Medicare Spending				
Medicare Spending per Patient (ratio)	-	1.03	0.95	0.98
Pneumonia Care				
Appropriate Initial Antibiotic Given	37	97%	95%	95%
Blood Culture Timing	109	100%	98%	98%
Pregnancy and Delivery Care				
Newborn Deliveries Scheduled Early[2]	67	3%	2%	6%
Preventive Care				
Immunization for Influenza[2]	528	95%	92%	90%
Immunization for Pneumonia[2]	413	95%	92%	92%
Stroke Care				
Anticoagulation Therapy for Atrial Fibrillation[1,2]	-	-	97%	95%
Antithrombotic Therapy Timing[2]	25	100%	98%	98%
Assessed for Rehabilitation[2]	28	100%	98%	97%
Discharged on Antithrombotic Therapy[2]	26	100%	100%	99%
Discharged on Statin Medication[2]	16	94%	94%	94%
Thrombolytic Therapy Timing[2,7]	-	-	78%	66%
Venous Thromboembolism Prophylaxis[2]	25	100%	96%	94%
Written Stroke Educational Materials Given[2]	20	90%	87%	88%
Surgical Care Improvement Project				
Appropriate Beta Blocker Usage[2]	127	100%	98%	98%
Appropriate VTP Within 24 Hours[2]	361	99%	98%	98%
Controlled Postoperative Blood Glucose[2]	37	100%	96%	97%
Perioperative Temperature Management[2]	500	100%	99%	100%
Prophylactic Antibiotic Selection[2]	326	100%	99%	99%
Prophylactic Antibiotic Selection (Outpatient)	265	98%	98%	98%
Prophylactic Antibiotic Stopped[2]	315	100%	98%	98%
Prophylactic Antibiotic Timing[2]	326	100%	98%	99%
Prophylactic Antibiotic Timing (Outpatient)	268	99%	98%	98%
Urinary Catheter Removal[2]	235	98%	97%	97%
Survey of Patients' Hospital Experiences				
Area Around Room 'Always' Quiet at Night	300+	62%	64%	61%
Doctors 'Always' Communicated Well	300+	79%	81%	82%
Home Recovery Information Given	300+	88%	87%	85%
Hospital Given 9 or 10 on 10 Point Scale	300+	71%	75%	71%
Meds 'Always' Explained Before Given	300+	65%	67%	64%
Nurses 'Always' Communicated Well	300+	75%	79%	79%
Pain 'Always' Well Controlled	300+	68%	72%	71%
Room and Bathroom 'Always' Clean	300+	71%	74%	73%
Timely Help 'Always' Received	300+	62%	70%	68%
Would Definitely Recommend Hospital	300+	74%	76%	71%
Use of Medical Imaging				
Cardiac Imaging Stress Test before Surgery	108	5.6%	5%	5.3%
Combination Abdominal CT Scan	390	4.9%	10%	10.5%
Combination Brain/Sinus CT Scan	223	0.9%	2.1%	2.7%
Combination Chest CT Scan	368	0.3%	3.1%	2.7%
Follow-up Mammogram/Ultrasound	567	8.6%	8.7%	8.8%
Lumbar Spine MRI for Low Back Pain	40	42.5%	39.7%	37.2%

NOTE: Hospital profiles are in alphabetical order by state, then city, then hospital within the city; Rankings exclude hospitals with less than 25 cases except for patient surveys which excludes hospitals with less than 100 cases; (a) 100-299 cases; (1) The number of cases/patients is too few to report; (2) Data submitted were based on a sample of cases/patients; (3) Results are based on a shorter time period than required; (4) Data suppressed by CMS for one or more quarters; (5) Results are not available for this reporting period; (6) Fewer than 100 patients completed the HCAHPS survey; (7) No cases met the criteria for this measure; (8) The lower limit of the confidence interval cannot be calculated if the number of observed infections equals zero; (9) No data are available from the state/territory for this reporting period; (10) The scores shown reflect fewer than 50 completed surveys; (11) There were discrepancies in the data collection process; (12) This measure does not apply to this hospital for this reporting period; (13) Results cannot be calculated for this reporting period; (14) The results for this state are combined with nearby states to protect confidentiality; Please refer to the User's Guide for a full explanation of data.

Rose Medical Center

4567 E 9th Avenue Phone: 303-320-2121
Denver, CO 80220 Fax: 303-320-2200
URL: www.rosemed.com
Type: Acute Care Hospitals Emergency Services: Yes
Ownership: Proprietary Beds: 420

Key Personnel:
Pediatric In-Patient Care . . . . James Banks, MD
CEO/President. . . . . Kenneth H Feiler
Operating Room. . . . . Nancy Gundersen
Radiology. . . . . Jennifer Kemp, MD
Pediatric Ambulatory Care . . . . . . Susan Larson, MD
Chief of Medical Staff . . . . Hal Levy, MD
Quality Assurance . . . . Lynette Shannon
Emergency Room . . . . Andy Ziller, MD

Measure	Cases	This Hosp.	State Avg.	U.S. Avg.
Blood Clot Prevention and Treatment				
Anticoagulation Overlap Therapy[2]	119	100%	97%	93%
ICU Venous Thromboembolism Prophylaxis[2]	67	100%	95%	92%
Incidence of Potentially Preventable VTE[2]	27	4%	8%	10%
UFH with Dosages/Platelet Monitoring[2]	93	100%	97%	97%
Venous Thromboembolism Prophylaxis[2]	321	99%	90%	85%
Warfarin Therapy Discharge Instructions[2]	82	100%	69%	75%
Chest Pain/Possible Heart Attack Care				
Aspirin Given Within 24 Hours of Arrival[1,3]	-	-	97%	96%
Fibrinolytic Meds Within 30 Min. of Arrival[3,7]	-	-	55%	58%
Average Time to ECG (minutes)[1,3]	-	-	8	7
Average Time to Transfer (minutes)[3,7]	-	-	74	60
Children's Asthma Care				
Received Home Management Plan of Care	-	-	-	88%
Received Reliever Medication	-	-	-	100%
Received Systemic Corticosteroids	-	-	-	100%
Emergency Department				
Admittance Decision Time (minutes)[2]	435	80	96	98
Head CT Results Within 45 Min. of Arrival[1]	-	-	67%	57%
Patients Who Left ER Before Being Seen	35,920	0%	2%	2%
Time from ER Arrival to Admit. (minutes)[2]	435	195	244	274
Time from ER Arrival to Discharge (minutes)	488	139	139	134
Time in ER Before Being Evaluated (minutes)	523	8	20	26
Time to Pain Meds for Fractures (minutes)	107	43	45	57
Heart Attack Care				
Aspirin Given at Discharge	104	100%	100%	99%
Fibrinolytic Meds Within 30 Min. of Arrival[7]	-	-	20%	54%
PCI Within 90 Minutes of Arrival	27	100%	97%	96%
Statin Prescribed at Discharge	104	100%	99%	98%
Heart Failure Care				
ACE Inhibitor or ARB for LVSD	40	100%	97%	97%
Discharge Instructions Given	124	100%	93%	94%
Evaluation of LVS Function	153	100%	99%	99%
Medicare Spending				
Medicare Spending per Patient (ratio)	-	0.97	0.95	0.98
Pneumonia Care				
Appropriate Initial Antibiotic Given	113	100%	95%	95%
Blood Culture Timing	252	100%	98%	98%
Pregnancy and Delivery Care				
Newborn Deliveries Scheduled Early[2]	43	2%	2%	6%
Preventive Care				
Immunization for Influenza[2]	535	99%	92%	90%
Immunization for Pneumonia[2]	497	99%	92%	92%
Stroke Care				
Anticoagulation Therapy for Atrial Fibrillation[2]	13	100%	97%	95%
Antithrombotic Therapy Timing[2]	58	98%	98%	98%
Assessed for Rehabilitation[2]	82	99%	98%	97%
Discharged on Antithrombotic Therapy[2]	73	100%	100%	99%
Discharged on Statin Medication[2]	53	98%	94%	94%
Thrombolytic Therapy Timing[1,2]	-	-	78%	66%
Venous Thromboembolism Prophylaxis[2]	75	100%	96%	94%
Written Stroke Educational Materials Given[2]	47	96%	87%	88%
Surgical Care Improvement Project				
Appropriate Beta Blocker Usage[2]	130	100%	98%	98%
Appropriate VTP Within 24 Hours[2]	441	100%	98%	98%
Controlled Postoperative Blood Glucose[2]	22	100%	96%	97%
Perioperative Temperature Management[2]	556	100%	99%	100%
Prophylactic Antibiotic Selection[2]	415	100%	99%	99%
Prophylactic Antibiotic Selection (Outpatient)	609	99%	98%	98%
Prophylactic Antibiotic Stopped[2]	398	100%	98%	98%
Prophylactic Antibiotic Timing[2]	415	100%	98%	99%
Prophylactic Antibiotic Timing (Outpatient)	609	100%	98%	98%
Urinary Catheter Removal[2]	325	100%	97%	97%
Survey of Patients' Hospital Experiences				
Area Around Room 'Always' Quiet at Night	300+	65%	64%	61%
Doctors 'Always' Communicated Well	300+	79%	81%	82%
Home Recovery Information Given	300+	89%	87%	85%
Hospital Given 9 or 10 on 10 Point Scale	300+	78%	75%	71%
Meds 'Always' Explained Before Given	300+	66%	67%	64%
Nurses 'Always' Communicated Well	300+	77%	79%	79%
Pain 'Always' Well Controlled	300+	72%	72%	71%
Room and Bathroom 'Always' Clean	300+	73%	74%	73%
Timely Help 'Always' Received	300+	66%	70%	68%
Would Definitely Recommend Hospital	300+	80%	76%	71%
Use of Medical Imaging				
Cardiac Imaging Stress Test before Surgery	99	6.1%	5%	5.3%
Combination Abdominal CT Scan	741	3.9%	10%	10.5%
Combination Brain/Sinus CT Scan[1]	-	-	2.1%	2.7%
Combination Chest CT Scan	362	0.6%	3.1%	2.7%
Follow-up Mammogram/Ultrasound	2,005	5.0%	8.7%	8.8%
Lumbar Spine MRI for Low Back Pain	160	38.1%	39.7%	37.2%

VA Eastern Colorado Healthcare System

1055 Clermont Street Phone: 303-393-2800
Denver, CO 80220 Fax: 303-393-2861
URL: www.va.gov/visn19
Type: Acute Care - VA Emergency Services: No
Ownership: Government Federal Beds: 128

Key Personnel:
Infection Control. . . . . Mary Bessesen
Emergency Room . . . . Michael Bleiden, MD
Operating Room. . . . . Nancy Detweiler, RN
Hemotology Center . . . . Madeleine Kane, MD
Chief of Medical Staff . . . . Ellen J Mangione, MD
Quality Assurance . . . . Rebecca Pedot, RN
Patient Relations . . . . Sara Tribble
Intensive Care Unit. . . . . Carol Welch, MD

Measure	Cases	This Hosp.	State Avg.	U.S. Avg.
Blood Clot Prevention and Treatment				
Anticoagulation Overlap Therapy	-	-	97%	93%
ICU Venous Thromboembolism Prophylaxis	-	-	95%	92%
Incidence of Potentially Preventable VTE	-	-	8%	10%
UFH with Dosages/Platelet Monitoring	-	-	97%	97%
Venous Thromboembolism Prophylaxis	-	-	90%	85%
Warfarin Therapy Discharge Instructions	-	-	69%	75%
Chest Pain/Possible Heart Attack Care				
Aspirin Given Within 24 Hours of Arrival	-	-	97%	96%
Fibrinolytic Meds Within 30 Min. of Arrival	-	-	55%	58%
Average Time to ECG (minutes)	-	-	8	7
Average Time to Transfer (minutes)	-	-	74	60
Children's Asthma Care				
Received Home Management Plan of Care	-	-	-	88%
Received Reliever Medication	-	-	-	100%
Received Systemic Corticosteroids	-	-	-	100%
Emergency Department				
Admittance Decision Time (minutes)	-	-	96	98
Head CT Results Within 45 Min. of Arrival	-	-	67%	57%
Patients Who Left ER Before Being Seen	-	-	2%	2%
Time from ER Arrival to Admit. (minutes)	-	-	244	274
Time from ER Arrival to Discharge (minutes)	-	-	139	134
Time in ER Before Being Evaluated (minutes)	-	-	20	26
Time to Pain Meds for Fractures (minutes)	-	-	45	57
Heart Attack Care				
Aspirin Given at Discharge	52	98%	100%	99%
Fibrinolytic Meds Within 30 Min. of Arrival[1]	-	-	20%	54%
PCI Within 90 Minutes of Arrival[1]	-	-	97%	96%
Statin Prescribed at Discharge	53	100%	99%	98%
Heart Failure Care				
ACE Inhibitor or ARB for LVSD	62	97%	97%	97%
Discharge Instructions Given	172	97%	93%	94%
Evaluation of LVS Function	183	100%	99%	99%
Medicare Spending				
Medicare Spending per Patient (ratio)	-	-	0.95	0.98
Pneumonia Care				
Appropriate Initial Antibiotic Given	33	82%	95%	95%
Blood Culture Timing	54	100%	98%	98%
Pregnancy and Delivery Care				
Newborn Deliveries Scheduled Early	-	-	2%	6%
Preventive Care				
Immunization for Influenza[5]	-	-	92%	90%
Immunization for Pneumonia[5]	-	-	92%	92%
Stroke Care				
Anticoagulation Therapy for Atrial Fibrillation	-	-	97%	95%
Antithrombotic Therapy Timing	-	-	98%	98%
Assessed for Rehabilitation	-	-	98%	97%
Discharged on Antithrombotic Therapy	-	-	100%	99%
Discharged on Statin Medication	-	-	94%	94%
Thrombolytic Therapy Timing	-	-	78%	66%
Venous Thromboembolism Prophylaxis	-	-	96%	94%
Written Stroke Educational Materials Given	-	-	87%	88%
Surgical Care Improvement Project				
Appropriate Beta Blocker Usage[2]	108	94%	98%	98%
Appropriate VTP Within 24 Hours[2]	215	96%	98%	98%
Controlled Postoperative Blood Glucose[2]	61	98%	96%	97%
Perioperative Temperature Management[2]	253	100%	99%	100%
Prophylactic Antibiotic Selection	188	99%	99%	99%
Prophylactic Antibiotic Selection (Outpatient)	-	-	98%	98%
Prophylactic Antibiotic Stopped	187	97%	98%	98%
Prophylactic Antibiotic Timing	188	99%	98%	99%
Prophylactic Antibiotic Timing (Outpatient)	-	-	98%	98%
Urinary Catheter Removal[2]	192	98%	97%	97%
Survey of Patients' Hospital Experiences				
Area Around Room 'Always' Quiet at Night	-	-	64%	61%
Doctors 'Always' Communicated Well	-	-	81%	82%
Home Recovery Information Given	-	-	87%	85%
Hospital Given 9 or 10 on 10 Point Scale	-	-	75%	71%
Meds 'Always' Explained Before Given	-	-	67%	64%
Nurses 'Always' Communicated Well	-	-	79%	79%
Pain 'Always' Well Controlled	-	-	72%	71%
Room and Bathroom 'Always' Clean	-	-	74%	73%
Timely Help 'Always' Received	-	-	70%	68%
Would Definitely Recommend Hospital	-	-	76%	71%
Use of Medical Imaging				
Cardiac Imaging Stress Test before Surgery	-	-	5%	5.3%
Combination Abdominal CT Scan	-	-	10%	10.5%
Combination Brain/Sinus CT Scan	-	-	2.1%	2.7%
Combination Chest CT Scan	-	-	3.1%	2.7%
Follow-up Mammogram/Ultrasound	-	-	8.7%	8.8%
Lumbar Spine MRI for Low Back Pain	-	-	39.7%	37.2%

Animas Surgical Hospital

575 Rivergate Lane Phone: 970-247-3537
Durango, CO 81301
URL: www.animassurgical.com
Type: Acute Care Hospitals Emergency Services: Yes
Ownership: Proprietary Beds: 12

Key Personnel:
Cardiology. . . . . Bruce Andrea, MD
Emergency Room . . . . Daniel Caplin
Pediatrics. . . . . Kimberly Caruso, MD
Radiology. . . . . Jonathan DeLacey, MD

Measure	Cases	This Hosp.	State Avg.	U.S. Avg.
Blood Clot Prevention and Treatment				
Anticoagulation Overlap Therapy[2,7]	-	-	97%	93%
ICU Venous Thromboembolism Prophylaxis[2,7]	-	-	95%	92%
Incidence of Potentially Preventable VTE[2,7]	-	-	8%	10%
UFH with Dosages/Platelet Monitoring[2,7]	-	-	97%	97%
Venous Thromboembolism Prophylaxis[2]	26	77%	90%	85%
Warfarin Therapy Discharge Instructions[2,7]	-	-	69%	75%
Chest Pain/Possible Heart Attack Care				
Aspirin Given Within 24 Hours of Arrival[1,3]	-	-	97%	96%
Fibrinolytic Meds Within 30 Min. of Arrival[3,7]	-	-	55%	58%
Average Time to ECG (minutes)[1,3]	-	-	8	7
Average Time to Transfer (minutes)[3,7]	-	-	74	60
Children's Asthma Care				

NOTE: Hospital profiles are in alphabetical order by state, then city, then hospital within the city; Rankings exclude hospitals with less than 25 cases except for patient surveys which excludes hospitals with less than 100 cases; (a) 100-299 cases; (1) The number of cases/patients is too few to report; (2) Data submitted were based on a sample of cases/patients; (3) Results are based on a shorter time period than required; (4) Data suppressed by CMS for one or more quarters; (5) Results are not available for this reporting period; (6) Fewer than 100 patients completed the HCAHPS survey; (7) No cases met the criteria for this measure; (8) The lower limit of the confidence interval cannot be calculated if the number of observed infections equals zero; (9) No data are available from the state/territory for this reporting period; (10) The scores shown reflect fewer than 50 completed surveys; (11) There were discrepancies in the data collection process; (12) This measure does not apply to this hospital for this reporting period; (13) Results cannot be calculated for this reporting period; (14) The results for this state are combined with nearby states to protect confidentiality; Please refer to the User's Guide for a full explanation of data.

Measure	Cases	This Hosp.	State Avg.	U.S. Avg.
Received Home Management Plan of Care	-	-	-	88%
Received Reliever Medication	-	-	-	100%
Received Systemic Corticosteroids	-	-	-	100%
Emergency Department				
Admittance Decision Time (minutes)[2,3]	12	69	96	98
Head CT Results Within 45 Min. of Arrival[3,7]	-	-	67%	57%
Patients Who Left ER Before Being Seen	5,980	0%	2%	2%
Time from ER Arrival to Admit. (minutes)[2,3]	23	145	244	274
Time from ER Arrival to Discharge (minutes)	359	74	139	134
Time in ER Before Being Evaluated (minutes)	360	20	20	26
Time to Pain Meds for Fractures (minutes)[3]	19	38	45	57
Heart Attack Care				
Aspirin Given at Discharge[5]	-	-	100%	99%
Fibrinolytic Meds Within 30 Min. of Arrival[5]	-	-	20%	54%
PCI Within 90 Minutes of Arrival[5]	-	-	97%	96%
Statin Prescribed at Discharge[5]	-	-	99%	98%
Heart Failure Care				
ACE Inhibitor or ARB for LVSD[5]	-	-	97%	97%
Discharge Instructions Given[5]	-	-	93%	94%
Evaluation of LVS Function[5]	-	-	99%	99%
Medicare Spending				
Medicare Spending per Patient (ratio)	-	0.89	0.95	0.98
Pneumonia Care				
Appropriate Initial Antibiotic Given[5]	-	-	95%	95%
Blood Culture Timing[5]	-	-	98%	98%
Pregnancy and Delivery Care				
Newborn Deliveries Scheduled Early[7]	-	-	2%	6%
Preventive Care				
Immunization for Influenza[2,3]	82	7%	92%	90%
Immunization for Pneumonia[2,3]	202	55%	92%	92%
Stroke Care				
Anticoagulation Therapy for Atrial Fibrillation[5]	-	-	97%	95%
Antithrombotic Therapy Timing[5]	-	-	98%	98%
Assessed for Rehabilitation[5]	-	-	98%	97%
Discharged on Antithrombotic Therapy[5]	-	-	100%	99%
Discharged on Statin Medication[5]	-	-	94%	94%
Thrombolytic Therapy Timing[5]	-	-	78%	66%
Venous Thromboembolism Prophylaxis[5]	-	-	96%	94%
Written Stroke Educational Materials Given[5]	-	-	87%	88%
Surgical Care Improvement Project				
Appropriate Beta Blocker Usage[2]	42	90%	98%	98%
Appropriate VTP Within 24 Hours[2]	235	100%	98%	98%
Controlled Postoperative Blood Glucose[2,7]	-	-	96%	97%
Perioperative Temperature Management[2]	281	25%	99%	100%
Prophylactic Antibiotic Selection[2]	254	99%	99%	99%
Prophylactic Antibiotic Selection (Outpatient)	29	100%	98%	98%
Prophylactic Antibiotic Stopped[2]	254	100%	98%	98%
Prophylactic Antibiotic Timing[2]	254	92%	98%	99%
Prophylactic Antibiotic Timing (Outpatient)	29	93%	98%	98%
Urinary Catheter Removal[2]	140	99%	97%	97%
Survey of Patients' Hospital Experiences				
Area Around Room 'Always' Quiet at Night	300+	81%	64%	61%
Doctors 'Always' Communicated Well	300+	90%	81%	82%
Home Recovery Information Given	300+	90%	87%	85%
Hospital Given 9 or 10 on 10 Point Scale	300+	90%	75%	71%
Meds 'Always' Explained Before Given	300+	76%	67%	64%
Nurses 'Always' Communicated Well	300+	86%	79%	79%
Pain 'Always' Well Controlled	300+	83%	72%	71%
Room and Bathroom 'Always' Clean	300+	87%	74%	73%
Timely Help 'Always' Received	300+	87%	70%	68%
Would Definitely Recommend Hospital	300+	91%	76%	71%
Use of Medical Imaging				
Cardiac Imaging Stress Test before Surgery[7]	-	-	5%	5.3%
Combination Abdominal CT Scan	79	25.3%	10%	10.5%
Combination Brain/Sinus CT Scan[1]	-	-	2.1%	2.7%
Combination Chest CT Scan[1]	-	-	3.1%	2.7%
Follow-up Mammogram/Ultrasound[7]	-	-	8.7%	8.8%
Lumbar Spine MRI for Low Back Pain	61	41.0%	39.7%	37.2%

Mercy Regional Medical Center

1010 Three Springs Blvd
Durango, CO 81301
URL: www.mercydurango.org
Phone: 970-247-4311
Fax: 970-764-3759
Type: Acute Care Hospitals
Emergency Services: Yes
Ownership: Voluntary non-profit - Church
Beds: 110

Key Personnel:
Emergency Room . . . . Donald Bader
Operating Room. . . . . Kathleen Bradshaw
Radiology. . . . . Jonathan DeLacey
Cardiac Laboratory. . . . . Amry Elliott
President/CEO. . . . . Thomas D. Gessel, FACHE
Chief of Medical Staff . . . . Karen Otterstein
Intensive Care Unit. . . . . Linda Riggle
Quality Assurance . . . . Jane Schrier

Measure	Cases	This Hosp.	State Avg.	U.S. Avg.
Blood Clot Prevention and Treatment				
Anticoagulation Overlap Therapy[2]	46	93%	97%	93%
ICU Venous Thromboembolism Prophylaxis[2]	47	87%	95%	92%
Incidence of Potentially Preventable VTE[1,2]	-	-	8%	10%
UFH with Dosages/Platelet Monitoring[2]	16	81%	97%	97%
Venous Thromboembolism Prophylaxis[2]	282	89%	90%	85%
Warfarin Therapy Discharge Instructions[2]	39	36%	69%	75%
Chest Pain/Possible Heart Attack Care				
Aspirin Given Within 24 Hours of Arrival[1,3]	-	-	97%	96%
Fibrinolytic Meds Within 30 Min. of Arrival[3,7]	-	-	55%	58%
Average Time to ECG (minutes)[1,3]	-	-	8	7
Average Time to Transfer (minutes)[3,7]	-	-	74	60
Children's Asthma Care				
Received Home Management Plan of Care	-	-	-	88%
Received Reliever Medication	-	-	-	100%
Received Systemic Corticosteroids	-	-	-	100%
Emergency Department				
Admittance Decision Time (minutes)[2]	242	96	96	98
Head CT Results Within 45 Min. of Arrival	11	36%	67%	57%
Patients Who Left ER Before Being Seen	15,216	0%	2%	2%
Time from ER Arrival to Admit. (minutes)[2]	258	276	244	274
Time from ER Arrival to Discharge (minutes)	450	165	139	134
Time in ER Before Being Evaluated (minutes)	471	32	20	26
Time to Pain Meds for Fractures (minutes)	77	65	45	57
Heart Attack Care				
Aspirin Given at Discharge	69	100%	100%	99%
Fibrinolytic Meds Within 30 Min. of Arrival[7]	-	-	20%	54%
PCI Within 90 Minutes of Arrival	25	84%	97%	96%
Statin Prescribed at Discharge	67	100%	99%	98%
Heart Failure Care				
ACE Inhibitor or ARB for LVSD	20	100%	97%	97%
Discharge Instructions Given	53	98%	93%	94%
Evaluation of LVS Function	57	98%	99%	99%
Medicare Spending				
Medicare Spending per Patient (ratio)	-	0.97	0.95	0.98
Pneumonia Care				
Appropriate Initial Antibiotic Given	45	91%	95%	95%
Blood Culture Timing	78	96%	98%	98%
Pregnancy and Delivery Care				
Newborn Deliveries Scheduled Early[2]	33	6%	2%	6%
Preventive Care				
Immunization for Influenza[2]	434	90%	92%	90%
Immunization for Pneumonia[2]	421	88%	92%	92%
Stroke Care				
Anticoagulation Therapy for Atrial Fibrillation[1]	-	-	97%	95%
Antithrombotic Therapy Timing	25	100%	98%	98%
Assessed for Rehabilitation	26	100%	98%	97%
Discharged on Antithrombotic Therapy	25	100%	100%	99%
Discharged on Statin Medication	17	88%	94%	94%
Thrombolytic Therapy Timing[7]	-	-	78%	66%
Venous Thromboembolism Prophylaxis	26	96%	96%	94%
Written Stroke Educational Materials Given	13	54%	87%	88%
Surgical Care Improvement Project				
Appropriate Beta Blocker Usage	70	97%	98%	98%
Appropriate VTP Within 24 Hours	325	98%	98%	98%
Controlled Postoperative Blood Glucose[7]	-	-	96%	97%
Perioperative Temperature Management	358	100%	99%	100%
Prophylactic Antibiotic Selection	272	99%	99%	99%
Prophylactic Antibiotic Selection (Outpatient)	182	99%	98%	98%
Prophylactic Antibiotic Stopped	271	99%	98%	98%
Prophylactic Antibiotic Timing	272	100%	98%	99%
Prophylactic Antibiotic Timing (Outpatient)	183	98%	98%	98%
Urinary Catheter Removal	260	97%	97%	97%
Survey of Patients' Hospital Experiences				
Area Around Room 'Always' Quiet at Night	300+	58%	64%	61%
Doctors 'Always' Communicated Well	300+	85%	81%	82%
Home Recovery Information Given	300+	89%	87%	85%
Hospital Given 9 or 10 on 10 Point Scale	300+	78%	75%	71%
Meds 'Always' Explained Before Given	300+	67%	67%	64%
Nurses 'Always' Communicated Well	300+	81%	79%	79%
Pain 'Always' Well Controlled	300+	73%	72%	71%
Room and Bathroom 'Always' Clean	300+	76%	74%	73%
Timely Help 'Always' Received	300+	70%	70%	68%
Would Definitely Recommend Hospital	300+	82%	76%	71%
Use of Medical Imaging				
Cardiac Imaging Stress Test before Surgery	646	3.6%	5%	5.3%
Combination Abdominal CT Scan	410	4.4%	10%	10.5%
Combination Brain/Sinus CT Scan	350	1.7%	2.1%	2.7%
Combination Chest CT Scan	239	1.7%	3.1%	2.7%
Follow-up Mammogram/Ultrasound	1,267	8.1%	8.7%	8.8%
Lumbar Spine MRI for Low Back Pain[1]	-	-	39.7%	37.2%

Weisbrod Memorial County Hospital

1208 Luther Street
Eads, CO 81036
Phone: 719-438-5401
Type: Critical Access Hospitals
Emergency Services: Yes
Ownership: Govt - Hospital Dist/Auth

Measure	Cases	This Hosp.	State Avg.	U.S. Avg.
Blood Clot Prevention and Treatment				
Anticoagulation Overlap Therapy[3,7]	-	-	97%	93%
ICU Venous Thromboembolism Prophylaxis[3,7]	-	-	95%	92%
Incidence of Potentially Preventable VTE[3,7]	-	-	8%	10%
UFH with Dosages/Platelet Monitoring[3,7]	-	-	97%	97%
Venous Thromboembolism Prophylaxis[1,3]	-	-	90%	85%
Warfarin Therapy Discharge Instructions[3,7]	-	-	69%	75%
Chest Pain/Possible Heart Attack Care				
Aspirin Given Within 24 Hours of Arrival	-	-	97%	96%
Fibrinolytic Meds Within 30 Min. of Arrival	-	-	55%	58%
Average Time to ECG (minutes)	-	-	8	7
Average Time to Transfer (minutes)	-	-	74	60
Children's Asthma Care				
Received Home Management Plan of Care	-	-	-	88%
Received Reliever Medication	-	-	-	100%
Received Systemic Corticosteroids	-	-	-	100%
Emergency Department				
Admittance Decision Time (minutes)[5]	-	-	96	98
Head CT Results Within 45 Min. of Arrival	-	-	67%	57%
Patients Who Left ER Before Being Seen	-	-	2%	2%
Time from ER Arrival to Admit. (minutes)[5]	-	-	244	274
Time from ER Arrival to Discharge (minutes)	-	-	139	134
Time in ER Before Being Evaluated (minutes)	-	-	20	26
Time to Pain Meds for Fractures (minutes)	-	-	45	57
Heart Attack Care				
Aspirin Given at Discharge[5]	-	-	100%	99%
Fibrinolytic Meds Within 30 Min. of Arrival[5]	-	-	20%	54%
PCI Within 90 Minutes of Arrival[5]	-	-	97%	96%
Statin Prescribed at Discharge[5]	-	-	99%	98%
Heart Failure Care				
ACE Inhibitor or ARB for LVSD[5]	-	-	97%	97%
Discharge Instructions Given[5]	-	-	93%	94%
Evaluation of LVS Function[5]	-	-	99%	99%
Medicare Spending				
Medicare Spending per Patient (ratio)	-	-	0.95	0.98
Pneumonia Care				
Appropriate Initial Antibiotic Given[1,3]	-	-	95%	95%
Blood Culture Timing[3,7]	-	-	98%	98%
Pregnancy and Delivery Care				
Newborn Deliveries Scheduled Early[5]	-	-	2%	6%
Preventive Care				
Immunization for Influenza[5]	-	-	92%	90%

NOTE: Hospital profiles are in alphabetical order by state, then city, then hospital within the city; Rankings exclude hospitals with less than 25 cases except for patient surveys which excludes hospitals with less than 100 cases; (a) 100-299 cases; (1) The number of cases/patients is too few to report; (2) Data submitted were based on a sample of cases/patients; (3) Results are based on a shorter time period than required; (4) Data suppressed by CMS for one or more quarters; (5) Results are not available for this reporting period; (6) Fewer than 100 patients completed the HCAHPS survey; (7) No cases met the criteria for this measure; (8) The lower limit of the confidence interval cannot be calculated if the number of observed infections equals zero; (9) No data are available from the state/territory for this reporting period; (10) The scores shown reflect fewer than 50 completed surveys; (11) There were discrepancies in the data collection process; (12) This measure does not apply to this hospital for this reporting period; (13) Results cannot be calculated for this reporting period; (14) The results for this state are combined with nearby states to protect confidentiality; Please refer to the User's Guide for a full explanation of data.

Measure	Cases	This Hosp.	State Avg.	U.S. Avg.
Immunization for Pneumonia[1,3]	-	-	92%	92%
Stroke Care				
Anticoagulation Therapy for Atrial Fibrillation[5]	-	-	97%	95%
Antithrombotic Therapy Timing[5]	-	-	98%	98%
Assessed for Rehabilitation[5]	-	-	98%	97%
Discharged on Antithrombotic Therapy[5]	-	-	100%	99%
Discharged on Statin Medication[5]	-	-	94%	94%
Thrombolytic Therapy Timing[5]	-	-	78%	66%
Venous Thromboembolism Prophylaxis[5]	-	-	96%	94%
Written Stroke Educational Materials Given[5]	-	-	87%	88%
Surgical Care Improvement Project				
Appropriate Beta Blocker Usage[5]	-	-	98%	98%
Appropriate VTP Within 24 Hours[5]	-	-	98%	98%
Controlled Postoperative Blood Glucose[5]	-	-	96%	97%
Perioperative Temperature Management[5]	-	-	99%	100%
Prophylactic Antibiotic Selection[5]	-	-	99%	99%
Prophylactic Antibiotic Selection (Outpatient)	-	-	98%	98%
Prophylactic Antibiotic Stopped[5]	-	-	98%	98%
Prophylactic Antibiotic Timing[5]	-	-	98%	99%
Prophylactic Antibiotic Timing (Outpatient)	-	-	98%	98%
Urinary Catheter Removal[5]	-	-	97%	97%
Survey of Patients' Hospital Experiences				
Area Around Room 'Always' Quiet at Night[5]	-	-	64%	61%
Doctors 'Always' Communicated Well[5]	-	-	81%	82%
Home Recovery Information Given[5]	-	-	87%	85%
Hospital Given 9 or 10 on 10 Point Scale[5]	-	-	75%	71%
Meds 'Always' Explained Before Given[5]	-	-	67%	64%
Nurses 'Always' Communicated Well[5]	-	-	79%	79%
Pain 'Always' Well Controlled[5]	-	-	72%	71%
Room and Bathroom 'Always' Clean[5]	-	-	74%	73%
Timely Help 'Always' Received[5]	-	-	70%	68%
Would Definitely Recommend Hospital[5]	-	-	76%	71%
Use of Medical Imaging				
Cardiac Imaging Stress Test before Surgery	-	-	5%	5.3%
Combination Abdominal CT Scan	-	-	10%	10.5%
Combination Brain/Sinus CT Scan	-	-	2.1%	2.7%
Combination Chest CT Scan	-	-	3.1%	2.7%
Follow-up Mammogram/Ultrasound	-	-	8.7%	8.8%
Lumbar Spine MRI for Low Back Pain	-	-	39.7%	37.2%

Swedish Medical Center

501 E Hampden Avenue
Englewood, CO 80113
Phone: 303-788-5000
Fax: 303-788-6029
URL: www.swedishhospital.com/default.asp
Type: Acute Care Hospitals
Emergency Services: Yes
Ownership: Proprietary
Beds: 368

Key Personnel:

Pediatric In-Patient Care .... Martin Alswanger, CHRM
Anesthesiology.............. Ron Ellis, CHRM
Chief of Medical Staff.......... Paul Hancock, MD
Emergency Room .... Mark Kozlowski
Operating Room.............. Mary Reno
Quality Assurance .... Dawn Shafferman
President/CEO.............. Mary M. White
Radiology.................. Wayne F Yakes, MD

Measure	Cases	This Hosp.	State Avg.	U.S. Avg.
Blood Clot Prevention and Treatment				
Anticoagulation Overlap Therapy[2]	189	93%	97%	93%
ICU Venous Thromboembolism Prophylaxis[2]	95	98%	95%	92%
Incidence of Potentially Preventable VTE[2]	55	11%	8%	10%
UFH with Dosages/Platelet Monitoring[2]	110	88%	97%	97%
Venous Thromboembolism Prophylaxis[2]	327	84%	90%	85%
Warfarin Therapy Discharge Instructions[2]	132	70%	69%	75%
Chest Pain/Possible Heart Attack Care				
Aspirin Given Within 24 Hours of Arrival[1,3]	-	-	97%	96%
Fibrinolytic Meds Within 30 Min. of Arrival[3,7]	-	-	55%	58%
Average Time to ECG (minutes)[1,3]	-	-	8	7
Average Time to Transfer (minutes)[3,7]	-	-	74	60
Children's Asthma Care				
Received Home Management Plan of Care	-	-	-	88%
Received Reliever Medication	-	-	-	100%
Received Systemic Corticosteroids	-	-	-	100%
Emergency Department				
Admittance Decision Time (minutes)[2]	695	107	96	98
Head CT Results Within 45 Min. of Arrival[1]	-	-	67%	57%
Patients Who Left ER Before Being Seen	77,386	0%	2%	2%
Time from ER Arrival to Admit. (minutes)[2]	698	222	244	274
Time from ER Arrival to Discharge (minutes)	460	130	139	134
Time in ER Before Being Evaluated (minutes)	520	15	20	26
Time to Pain Meds for Fractures (minutes)	311	38	45	57
Heart Attack Care				
Aspirin Given at Discharge[2]	183	100%	100%	99%
Fibrinolytic Meds Within 30 Min. of Arrival[2,7]	-	-	20%	54%
PCI Within 90 Minutes of Arrival[2]	64	98%	97%	96%
Statin Prescribed at Discharge[2]	178	100%	99%	98%
Heart Failure Care				
ACE Inhibitor or ARB for LVSD[2]	62	100%	97%	97%
Discharge Instructions Given[2]	163	98%	93%	94%
Evaluation of LVS Function[2]	235	100%	99%	99%
Medicare Spending				
Medicare Spending per Patient (ratio)	-	1.01	0.95	0.98
Pneumonia Care				
Appropriate Initial Antibiotic Given[2]	65	94%	95%	95%
Blood Culture Timing[2]	103	100%	98%	98%
Pregnancy and Delivery Care				
Newborn Deliveries Scheduled Early[2]	53	2%	2%	6%
Preventive Care				
Immunization for Influenza[2]	638	97%	92%	90%
Immunization for Pneumonia[2]	698	97%	92%	92%
Stroke Care				
Anticoagulation Therapy for Atrial Fibrillation[2]	31	97%	97%	95%
Antithrombotic Therapy Timing[2]	88	98%	98%	98%
Assessed for Rehabilitation[2]	146	99%	98%	97%
Discharged on Antithrombotic Therapy[2]	124	99%	100%	99%
Discharged on Statin Medication[2]	95	93%	94%	94%
Thrombolytic Therapy Timing[1,2]	-	-	78%	66%
Venous Thromboembolism Prophylaxis[2]	142	99%	96%	94%
Written Stroke Educational Materials Given[2]	87	89%	87%	88%
Surgical Care Improvement Project				
Appropriate Beta Blocker Usage[2]	165	100%	98%	98%
Appropriate VTP Within 24 Hours[2]	516	99%	98%	98%
Controlled Postoperative Blood Glucose[2]	69	94%	96%	97%
Perioperative Temperature Management[2]	627	100%	99%	100%
Prophylactic Antibiotic Selection[2]	414	100%	99%	99%
Prophylactic Antibiotic Selection (Outpatient)	440	100%	98%	98%
Prophylactic Antibiotic Stopped[2]	398	99%	98%	98%
Prophylactic Antibiotic Timing[2]	415	100%	98%	99%
Prophylactic Antibiotic Timing (Outpatient)	440	99%	98%	98%
Urinary Catheter Removal[2]	277	98%	97%	97%
Survey of Patients' Hospital Experiences				
Area Around Room 'Always' Quiet at Night	300+	57%	64%	61%
Doctors 'Always' Communicated Well	300+	76%	81%	82%
Home Recovery Information Given	300+	85%	87%	85%
Hospital Given 9 or 10 on 10 Point Scale	300+	69%	75%	71%
Meds 'Always' Explained Before Given	300+	59%	67%	64%
Nurses 'Always' Communicated Well	300+	74%	79%	79%
Pain 'Always' Well Controlled	300+	67%	72%	71%
Room and Bathroom 'Always' Clean	300+	71%	74%	73%
Timely Help 'Always' Received	300+	60%	70%	68%
Would Definitely Recommend Hospital	300+	72%	76%	71%
Use of Medical Imaging				
Cardiac Imaging Stress Test before Surgery	92	2.2%	5%	5.3%
Combination Abdominal CT Scan	759	8.7%	10%	10.5%
Combination Brain/Sinus CT Scan	525	2.3%	2.1%	2.7%
Combination Chest CT Scan	355	0.6%	3.1%	2.7%
Follow-up Mammogram/Ultrasound[7]	-	-	8.7%	8.8%
Lumbar Spine MRI for Low Back Pain	42	38.1%	39.7%	37.2%

Estes Park Medical Center

555 Prospect Avenue
Estes Park, CO 80517
Phone: 970-586-2317
Fax: 970-586-0109
E-mail: info@epmedcenter.com
URL: www.epmedcenter.com
Type: Critical Access Hospitals
Emergency Services: Yes
Ownership: Govt - Hospital Dist/Auth
Beds: 15

Key Personnel:

Emergency Room .... Cindy Bauinghatt, RN
Anesthesiology............ David Brunner, CRNA
Radiology.................. Mark J Hansen
Chief of Medical Staff.......... Martin Koschnitzke, MD
Pediatrics.................. Mark Wiesner, DO
CEO/President............... Andrew Wills

Measure	Cases	This Hosp.	State Avg.	U.S. Avg.
Blood Clot Prevention and Treatment				
Anticoagulation Overlap Therapy[5]	-	-	97%	93%
ICU Venous Thromboembolism Prophylaxis[5]	-	-	95%	92%
Incidence of Potentially Preventable VTE[5]	-	-	8%	10%
UFH with Dosages/Platelet Monitoring[5]	-	-	97%	97%
Venous Thromboembolism Prophylaxis[5]	-	-	90%	85%
Warfarin Therapy Discharge Instructions[5]	-	-	69%	75%
Chest Pain/Possible Heart Attack Care				
Aspirin Given Within 24 Hours of Arrival[1]	-	-	97%	96%
Fibrinolytic Meds Within 30 Min. of Arrival[5]	-	-	55%	58%
Average Time to ECG (minutes)[1]	-	-	8	7
Average Time to Transfer (minutes)[5]	-	-	74	60
Children's Asthma Care				
Received Home Management Plan of Care	-	-	-	88%
Received Reliever Medication	-	-	-	100%
Received Systemic Corticosteroids	-	-	-	100%
Emergency Department				
Admittance Decision Time (minutes)[5]	-	-	96	98
Head CT Results Within 45 Min. of Arrival[5]	-	-	67%	57%
Patients Who Left ER Before Being Seen[5]	-	-	2%	2%
Time from ER Arrival to Admit. (minutes)[5]	-	-	244	274
Time from ER Arrival to Discharge (minutes)[5]	-	-	139	134
Time in ER Before Being Evaluated (minutes)[5]	-	-	20	26
Time to Pain Meds for Fractures (minutes)[5]	-	-	45	57
Heart Attack Care				
Aspirin Given at Discharge[5]	-	-	100%	99%
Fibrinolytic Meds Within 30 Min. of Arrival[5]	-	-	20%	54%
PCI Within 90 Minutes of Arrival[5]	-	-	97%	96%
Statin Prescribed at Discharge[5]	-	-	99%	98%
Heart Failure Care				
ACE Inhibitor or ARB for LVSD[5]	-	-	97%	97%
Discharge Instructions Given[5]	-	-	93%	94%
Evaluation of LVS Function[5]	-	-	99%	99%
Medicare Spending				
Medicare Spending per Patient (ratio)	-	-	0.95	0.98
Pneumonia Care				
Appropriate Initial Antibiotic Given[5]	-	-	95%	95%
Blood Culture Timing[5]	-	-	98%	98%
Pregnancy and Delivery Care				
Newborn Deliveries Scheduled Early[5]	-	-	2%	6%
Preventive Care				
Immunization for Influenza[5]	-	-	92%	90%
Immunization for Pneumonia[5]	-	-	92%	92%
Stroke Care				
Anticoagulation Therapy for Atrial Fibrillation[5]	-	-	97%	95%
Antithrombotic Therapy Timing[5]	-	-	98%	98%
Assessed for Rehabilitation[5]	-	-	98%	97%
Discharged on Antithrombotic Therapy[5]	-	-	100%	99%
Discharged on Statin Medication[5]	-	-	94%	94%
Thrombolytic Therapy Timing[5]	-	-	78%	66%
Venous Thromboembolism Prophylaxis[5]	-	-	96%	94%
Written Stroke Educational Materials Given[5]	-	-	87%	88%
Surgical Care Improvement Project				
Appropriate Beta Blocker Usage[3,7]	-	-	98%	98%
Appropriate VTP Within 24 Hours[1,3]	-	-	98%	98%
Controlled Postoperative Blood Glucose[3,7]	-	-	96%	97%
Perioperative Temperature Management[1,3]	-	-	99%	100%
Prophylactic Antibiotic Selection[1,3]	-	-	99%	99%
Prophylactic Antibiotic Selection (Outpatient)[5]	-	-	98%	98%
Prophylactic Antibiotic Stopped[1,3]	-	-	98%	98%
Prophylactic Antibiotic Timing[1,3]	-	-	98%	99%
Prophylactic Antibiotic Timing (Outpatient)[5]	-	-	98%	98%
Urinary Catheter Removal	15	100%	97%	97%
Survey of Patients' Hospital Experiences				
Area Around Room 'Always' Quiet at Night	(a)	55%	64%	61%
Doctors 'Always' Communicated Well	(a)	85%	81%	82%
Home Recovery Information Given	(a)	89%	87%	85%

NOTE: Hospital profiles are in alphabetical order by state, then city, then hospital within the city; Rankings exclude hospitals with less than 25 cases except for patient surveys which excludes hospitals with less than 100 cases; (a) 100-299 cases; (1) The number of cases/patients is too few to report; (2) Data submitted were based on a sample of cases/patients; (3) Results are based on a shorter time period than required; (4) Data suppressed by CMS for one or more quarters; (5) Results are not available for this reporting period; (6) Fewer than 100 patients completed the HCAHPS survey; (7) No cases met the criteria for this measure; (8) The lower limit of the confidence interval cannot be calculated if the number of observed infections equals zero; (9) No data are available from the state/territory for this reporting period; (10) The scores shown reflect fewer than 50 completed surveys; (11) There were discrepancies in the data collection process; (12) This measure does not apply to this hospital for this reporting period; (13) Results cannot be calculated for this reporting period; (14) The results for this state are combined with nearby states to protect confidentiality; Please refer to the User's Guide for a full explanation of data.

Hospital Given 9 or 10 on 10 Point Scale	(a)	73%	75%	71%
Meds 'Always' Explained Before Given	(a)	70%	67%	64%
Nurses 'Always' Communicated Well	(a)	79%	79%	79%
Pain 'Always' Well Controlled	(a)	71%	72%	71%
Room and Bathroom 'Always' Clean	(a)	74%	74%	73%
Timely Help 'Always' Received	(a)	73%	70%	68%
Would Definitely Recommend Hospital	(a)	76%	76%	71%
Use of Medical Imaging				
Cardiac Imaging Stress Test before Surgery	97	7.2%	5%	5.3%
Combination Abdominal CT Scan	122	11.5%	10%	10.5%
Combination Brain/Sinus CT Scan[1]	-	-	2.1%	2.7%
Combination Chest CT Scan[1]	-	-	3.1%	2.7%
Follow-up Mammogram/Ultrasound	298	6.7%	8.7%	8.8%
Lumbar Spine MRI for Low Back Pain[1]	-	-	39.7%	37.2%

Poudre Valley Hospital

1024 S Lemay Ave | Phone: 970-495-7000
Fort Collins, CO 80524 | Fax: 970-495-7600
E-mail: pvhs@pvh.org
URL: www.pvhs.org
Type: Acute Care Hospitals | Emergency Services: Yes
Ownership: Voluntary non-profit - Private | Beds: 235

Key Personnel:
Radiology.................. Bruce A Berkowitz
Patient Relations .... Craig Luzinski
Chief of Medical Staff.......... William Miller, MD
Pediatric Ambulatory Care .... Jan Paisley, MD
Pediatric In-Patient Care .... Jan Paisley, MD
Quality Assurance .... Judy Robinson
CEO/President............... Kevin Unger

Measure	Cases	This Hosp.	State Avg.	U.S. Avg.
Blood Clot Prevention and Treatment				
Anticoagulation Overlap Therapy[2]	119	93%	97%	93%
ICU Venous Thromboembolism Prophylaxis[2]	34	94%	95%	92%
Incidence of Potentially Preventable VTE[1,2]	-	-	8%	10%
UFH with Dosages/Platelet Monitoring[2]	48	94%	97%	97%
Venous Thromboembolism Prophylaxis[2]	256	88%	90%	85%
Warfarin Therapy Discharge Instructions[2]	101	68%	69%	75%
Chest Pain/Possible Heart Attack Care				
Aspirin Given Within 24 Hours of Arrival[3,7]	-	-	97%	96%
Fibrinolytic Meds Within 30 Min. of Arrival[5]	-	-	55%	58%
Average Time to ECG (minutes)[3,7]	-	-	8	7
Average Time to Transfer (minutes)[5]	-	-	74	60
Children's Asthma Care				
Received Home Management Plan of Care	-	-	-	88%
Received Reliever Medication	-	-	-	100%
Received Systemic Corticosteroids	-	-	-	100%
Emergency Department				
Admittance Decision Time (minutes)[2]	320	75	96	98
Head CT Results Within 45 Min. of Arrival[1]	-	-	67%	57%
Patients Who Left ER Before Being Seen	44,576	1%	2%	2%
Time from ER Arrival to Admit. (minutes)[2]	423	196	244	274
Time from ER Arrival to Discharge (minutes)	380	146	139	134
Time in ER Before Being Evaluated (minutes)	383	29	20	26
Time to Pain Meds for Fractures (minutes)	266	70	45	57
Heart Attack Care				
Aspirin Given at Discharge	122	100%	100%	99%
Fibrinolytic Meds Within 30 Min. of Arrival[7]	-	-	20%	54%
PCI Within 90 Minutes of Arrival	27	96%	97%	96%
Statin Prescribed at Discharge	112	99%	99%	98%
Heart Failure Care				
ACE Inhibitor or ARB for LVSD	41	100%	97%	97%
Discharge Instructions Given	130	97%	93%	94%
Evaluation of LVS Function	171	100%	99%	99%
Medicare Spending				
Medicare Spending per Patient (ratio)	-	0.95	0.95	0.98
Pneumonia Care				
Appropriate Initial Antibiotic Given[2]	120	98%	95%	95%
Blood Culture Timing[2]	214	99%	98%	98%
Pregnancy and Delivery Care				
Newborn Deliveries Scheduled Early[2]	35	6%	2%	6%
Preventive Care				
Immunization for Influenza[2]	529	85%	92%	90%
Immunization for Pneumonia[2]	549	87%	92%	92%
Stroke Care				
Anticoagulation Therapy for Atrial Fibrillation	19	89%	97%	95%
Antithrombotic Therapy Timing	47	100%	98%	98%
Assessed for Rehabilitation	84	99%	98%	97%
Discharged on Antithrombotic Therapy	69	100%	100%	99%
Discharged on Statin Medication	48	96%	94%	94%
Thrombolytic Therapy Timing	14	93%	78%	66%
Venous Thromboembolism Prophylaxis	74	89%	96%	94%
Written Stroke Educational Materials Given	55	96%	87%	88%
Surgical Care Improvement Project				
Appropriate Beta Blocker Usage[2]	93	100%	98%	98%
Appropriate VTP Within 24 Hours[2]	420	94%	98%	98%
Controlled Postoperative Blood Glucose[2,7]	-	-	96%	97%
Perioperative Temperature Management[2]	464	100%	99%	100%
Prophylactic Antibiotic Selection[2]	284	100%	99%	99%
Prophylactic Antibiotic Selection (Outpatient)	444	98%	98%	98%
Prophylactic Antibiotic Stopped[2]	282	99%	98%	98%
Prophylactic Antibiotic Timing[2]	285	99%	98%	99%
Prophylactic Antibiotic Timing (Outpatient)	449	98%	98%	98%
Urinary Catheter Removal[2]	326	99%	97%	97%
Survey of Patients' Hospital Experiences				
Area Around Room 'Always' Quiet at Night	300+	58%	64%	61%
Doctors 'Always' Communicated Well	300+	78%	81%	82%
Home Recovery Information Given	300+	88%	87%	85%
Hospital Given 9 or 10 on 10 Point Scale	300+	77%	75%	71%
Meds 'Always' Explained Before Given	300+	64%	67%	64%
Nurses 'Always' Communicated Well	300+	79%	79%	79%
Pain 'Always' Well Controlled	300+	71%	72%	71%
Room and Bathroom 'Always' Clean	300+	77%	74%	73%
Timely Help 'Always' Received	300+	68%	70%	68%
Would Definitely Recommend Hospital	300+	80%	76%	71%
Use of Medical Imaging				
Cardiac Imaging Stress Test before Surgery	964	3.6%	5%	5.3%
Combination Abdominal CT Scan	887	8.1%	10%	10.5%
Combination Brain/Sinus CT Scan	781	1.8%	2.1%	2.7%
Combination Chest CT Scan	435	2.8%	3.1%	2.7%
Follow-up Mammogram/Ultrasound	2,840	6.3%	8.7%	8.8%
Lumbar Spine MRI for Low Back Pain	179	36.3%	39.7%	37.2%

Colorado Plains Medical Center

1000 Lincoln St | Phone: 970-867-3391
Fort Morgan, CO 80701 | Fax: 970-542-4352
URL: www.coloradoplainsmedicalcenter.com
Type: Acute Care Hospitals | Emergency Services: Yes
Ownership: Voluntary non-profit - Other | Beds: 50

Key Personnel:
CEO/President............... Michael A Anaya Sr, FACHE
Chief of Medical Staff.......... Lois Elliot
CEO .... Mike Patterson

Measure	Cases	This Hosp.	State Avg.	U.S. Avg.
Blood Clot Prevention and Treatment				
Anticoagulation Overlap Therapy[1,2]	-	-	97%	93%
ICU Venous Thromboembolism Prophylaxis[1,2]	-	-	95%	92%
Incidence of Potentially Preventable VTE[2,7]	-	-	8%	10%
UFH with Dosages/Platelet Monitoring[1,2]	-	-	97%	97%
Venous Thromboembolism Prophylaxis[2]	71	99%	90%	85%
Warfarin Therapy Discharge Instructions[1,2]	-	-	69%	75%
Chest Pain/Possible Heart Attack Care				
Aspirin Given Within 24 Hours of Arrival	33	100%	97%	96%
Fibrinolytic Meds Within 30 Min. of Arrival[1]	-	-	55%	58%
Average Time to ECG (minutes)	35	5	8	7
Average Time to Transfer (minutes)[7]	-	-	74	60
Children's Asthma Care				
Received Home Management Plan of Care	-	-	-	88%
Received Reliever Medication	-	-	-	100%
Received Systemic Corticosteroids	-	-	-	100%
Emergency Department				
Admittance Decision Time (minutes)[2]	182	56	96	98
Head CT Results Within 45 Min. of Arrival[1]	-	-	67%	57%
Patients Who Left ER Before Being Seen	7,092	0%	2%	2%
Time from ER Arrival to Admit. (minutes)[2]	182	178	244	274
Time from ER Arrival to Discharge (minutes)	360	96	139	134
Time in ER Before Being Evaluated (minutes)	404	7	20	26
Time to Pain Meds for Fractures (minutes)	38	25	45	57
Heart Attack Care				
Aspirin Given at Discharge[1]	-	-	100%	99%
Fibrinolytic Meds Within 30 Min. of Arrival[7]	-	-	20%	54%
PCI Within 90 Minutes of Arrival[7]	-	-	97%	96%
Statin Prescribed at Discharge[1]	-	-	99%	98%
Heart Failure Care				
ACE Inhibitor or ARB for LVSD[1]	-	-	97%	97%
Discharge Instructions Given	18	89%	93%	94%
Evaluation of LVS Function	29	100%	99%	99%
Medicare Spending				
Medicare Spending per Patient (ratio)	-	0.94	0.95	0.98
Pneumonia Care				
Appropriate Initial Antibiotic Given	20	100%	95%	95%
Blood Culture Timing	33	97%	98%	98%
Pregnancy and Delivery Care				
Newborn Deliveries Scheduled Early[2]	19	11%	2%	6%
Preventive Care				
Immunization for Influenza[2]	210	97%	92%	90%
Immunization for Pneumonia[2]	154	95%	92%	92%
Stroke Care				
Anticoagulation Therapy for Atrial Fibrillation[7]	-	-	97%	95%
Antithrombotic Therapy Timing[1]	-	-	98%	98%
Assessed for Rehabilitation[1]	-	-	98%	97%
Discharged on Antithrombotic Therapy[1]	-	-	100%	99%
Discharged on Statin Medication[1]	-	-	94%	94%
Thrombolytic Therapy Timing[1]	-	-	78%	66%
Venous Thromboembolism Prophylaxis[1]	-	-	96%	94%
Written Stroke Educational Materials Given[1]	-	-	87%	88%
Surgical Care Improvement Project				
Appropriate Beta Blocker Usage	27	93%	98%	98%
Appropriate VTP Within 24 Hours	124	99%	98%	98%
Controlled Postoperative Blood Glucose[7]	-	-	96%	97%
Perioperative Temperature Management	142	100%	99%	100%
Prophylactic Antibiotic Selection	113	99%	99%	99%
Prophylactic Antibiotic Selection (Outpatient)	12	92%	98%	98%
Prophylactic Antibiotic Stopped	109	97%	98%	98%
Prophylactic Antibiotic Timing	113	100%	98%	99%
Prophylactic Antibiotic Timing (Outpatient)	13	92%	98%	98%
Urinary Catheter Removal	74	99%	97%	97%
Survey of Patients' Hospital Experiences				
Area Around Room 'Always' Quiet at Night	300+	64%	64%	61%
Doctors 'Always' Communicated Well	300+	82%	81%	82%
Home Recovery Information Given	300+	88%	87%	85%
Hospital Given 9 or 10 on 10 Point Scale	300+	72%	75%	71%
Meds 'Always' Explained Before Given	300+	67%	67%	64%
Nurses 'Always' Communicated Well	300+	82%	79%	79%
Pain 'Always' Well Controlled	300+	73%	72%	71%
Room and Bathroom 'Always' Clean	300+	76%	74%	73%
Timely Help 'Always' Received	300+	71%	70%	68%
Would Definitely Recommend Hospital	300+	70%	76%	71%
Use of Medical Imaging				
Cardiac Imaging Stress Test before Surgery	56	3.6%	5%	5.3%
Combination Abdominal CT Scan	187	5.9%	10%	10.5%
Combination Brain/Sinus CT Scan	149	5.4%	2.1%	2.7%
Combination Chest CT Scan	69	2.9%	3.1%	2.7%
Follow-up Mammogram/Ultrasound	237	7.6%	8.7%	8.8%
Lumbar Spine MRI for Low Back Pain[1]	-	-	39.7%	37.2%

Saint Anthony Summit Medical Center

340 Peak One Drive | Phone: 970-668-3300
Frisco, CO 80443 | Fax: 970-668-1517
Type: Acute Care Hospitals | Emergency Services: No
Ownership: Voluntary non-profit - Church | Beds: 9

Key Personnel:
CEO .... Paul Chodkowski
Chief of Medical Staff.......... Alan Dulit
Quality Assurance .... Wes Hunter, RN
Operating Room.............. Trilok Khanna, RN
Emergency Room .... Lory Profota, RN

Measure	Cases	This Hosp.	State Avg.	U.S. Avg.
Blood Clot Prevention and Treatment				
Anticoagulation Overlap Therapy[1,2]	-	-	97%	93%

NOTE: Hospital profiles are in alphabetical order by state, then city, then hospital within the city; Rankings exclude hospitals with less than 25 cases except for patient surveys which excludes hospitals with less than 100 cases; (a) 100-299 cases; (1) The number of cases/patients is too few to report; (2) Data submitted were based on a sample of cases/patients; (3) Results are based on a shorter time period than required; (4) Data suppressed by CMS for one or more quarters; (5) Results are not available for this reporting period; (6) Fewer than 100 patients completed the HCAHPS survey; (7) No cases met the criteria for this measure; (8) The lower limit of the confidence interval cannot be calculated if the number of observed infections equals zero; (9) No data are available from the state/territory for this reporting period; (10) The scores shown reflect fewer than 50 completed surveys; (11) There were discrepancies in the data collection process; (12) This measure does not apply to this hospital for this reporting period; (13) Results cannot be calculated for this reporting period; (14) The results for this state are combined with nearby states to protect confidentiality; Please refer to the User's Guide for a full explanation of data.

Measure	Cases	This Hosp.	State Avg.	U.S. Avg.
ICU Venous Thromboembolism Prophylaxis[2]	14	86%	95%	92%
Incidence of Potentially Preventable VTE[2,7]	-	-	8%	10%
UFH with Dosages/Platelet Monitoring[1,2]	-	-	97%	97%
Venous Thromboembolism Prophylaxis[2]	105	96%	90%	85%
Warfarin Therapy Discharge Instructions[1,2]	-	-	69%	75%
Chest Pain/Possible Heart Attack Care				
Aspirin Given Within 24 Hours of Arrival	54	96%	97%	96%
Fibrinolytic Meds Within 30 Min. of Arrival[1]	-	-	55%	58%
Average Time to ECG (minutes)	54	7	8	7
Average Time to Transfer (minutes)[1]	-	-	74	60
Children's Asthma Care				
Received Home Management Plan of Care	-	-	-	88%
Received Reliever Medication	-	-	-	100%
Received Systemic Corticosteroids	-	-	-	100%
Emergency Department				
Admittance Decision Time (minutes)[2]	152	65	96	98
Head CT Results Within 45 Min. of Arrival[1]	-	-	67%	57%
Patients Who Left ER Before Being Seen	11,760	0%	2%	2%
Time from ER Arrival to Admit. (minutes)[2]	229	203	244	274
Time from ER Arrival to Discharge (minutes)	423	107	139	134
Time in ER Before Being Evaluated (minutes)	438	11	20	26
Time to Pain Meds for Fractures (minutes)	99	53	45	57
Heart Attack Care				
Aspirin Given at Discharge[5]	-	-	100%	99%
Fibrinolytic Meds Within 30 Min. of Arrival[5]	-	-	20%	54%
PCI Within 90 Minutes of Arrival[5]	-	-	97%	96%
Statin Prescribed at Discharge[5]	-	-	99%	98%
Heart Failure Care				
ACE Inhibitor or ARB for LVSD[1]	-	-	97%	97%
Discharge Instructions Given[1]	-	-	93%	94%
Evaluation of LVS Function[1]	-	-	99%	99%
Medicare Spending				
Medicare Spending per Patient (ratio)	-	0.84	0.95	0.98
Pneumonia Care				
Appropriate Initial Antibiotic Given	19	100%	95%	95%
Blood Culture Timing	20	100%	98%	98%
Pregnancy and Delivery Care				
Newborn Deliveries Scheduled Early[2]	27	4%	2%	6%
Preventive Care				
Immunization for Influenza[2]	283	93%	92%	90%
Immunization for Pneumonia[2]	131	75%	92%	92%
Stroke Care				
Anticoagulation Therapy for Atrial Fibrillation[3,7]	-	-	97%	95%
Antithrombotic Therapy Timing[3,7]	-	-	98%	98%
Assessed for Rehabilitation[1,3]	-	-	98%	97%
Discharged on Antithrombotic Therapy[1,3]	-	-	100%	99%
Discharged on Statin Medication[1,3]	-	-	94%	94%
Thrombolytic Therapy Timing[3,7]	-	-	78%	66%
Venous Thromboembolism Prophylaxis[3,7]	-	-	96%	94%
Written Stroke Educational Materials Given[1,3]	-	-	87%	88%
Surgical Care Improvement Project				
Appropriate Beta Blocker Usage[1]	-	-	98%	98%
Appropriate VTP Within 24 Hours	48	92%	98%	98%
Controlled Postoperative Blood Glucose[7]	-	-	96%	97%
Perioperative Temperature Management	54	100%	99%	100%
Prophylactic Antibiotic Selection	40	98%	99%	99%
Prophylactic Antibiotic Selection (Outpatient)	48	100%	98%	98%
Prophylactic Antibiotic Stopped	40	100%	98%	98%
Prophylactic Antibiotic Timing	40	98%	98%	99%
Prophylactic Antibiotic Timing (Outpatient)	48	98%	98%	98%
Urinary Catheter Removal	39	97%	97%	97%
Survey of Patients' Hospital Experiences				
Area Around Room 'Always' Quiet at Night	300+	72%	64%	61%
Doctors 'Always' Communicated Well	300+	78%	81%	82%
Home Recovery Information Given	300+	90%	87%	85%
Hospital Given 9 or 10 on 10 Point Scale	300+	84%	75%	71%
Meds 'Always' Explained Before Given	300+	67%	67%	64%
Nurses 'Always' Communicated Well	300+	83%	79%	79%
Pain 'Always' Well Controlled	300+	73%	72%	71%
Room and Bathroom 'Always' Clean	300+	76%	74%	73%
Timely Help 'Always' Received	300+	77%	70%	68%
Would Definitely Recommend Hospital	300+	82%	76%	71%
Use of Medical Imaging				
Cardiac Imaging Stress Test before Surgery	64	6.3%	5%	5.3%
Combination Abdominal CT Scan	110	6.4%	10%	10.5%
Combination Brain/Sinus CT Scan	118	5.9%	2.1%	2.7%
Combination Chest CT Scan	69	2.9%	3.1%	2.7%
Follow-up Mammogram/Ultrasound	250	12.0%	8.7%	8.8%
Lumbar Spine MRI for Low Back Pain[1]	-	-	39.7%	37.2%

Family Health West Hospital

300 West Ottley Avenue
Fruita, CO 81521
Phone: 970-858-9871
Type: Critical Access Hospitals
Emergency Services: Yes
Ownership: Voluntary non-profit - Private

Measure	Cases	This Hosp.	State Avg.	U.S. Avg.
Blood Clot Prevention and Treatment				
Anticoagulation Overlap Therapy[5]	-	-	97%	93%
ICU Venous Thromboembolism Prophylaxis[5]	-	-	95%	92%
Incidence of Potentially Preventable VTE[5]	-	-	8%	10%
UFH with Dosages/Platelet Monitoring[5]	-	-	97%	97%
Venous Thromboembolism Prophylaxis[5]	-	-	90%	85%
Warfarin Therapy Discharge Instructions[5]	-	-	69%	75%
Chest Pain/Possible Heart Attack Care				
Aspirin Given Within 24 Hours of Arrival	-	-	97%	96%
Fibrinolytic Meds Within 30 Min. of Arrival	-	-	55%	58%
Average Time to ECG (minutes)	-	-	8	7
Average Time to Transfer (minutes)	-	-	74	60
Children's Asthma Care				
Received Home Management Plan of Care	-	-	-	88%
Received Reliever Medication	-	-	-	100%
Received Systemic Corticosteroids	-	-	-	100%
Emergency Department				
Admittance Decision Time (minutes)[5]	-	-	96	98
Head CT Results Within 45 Min. of Arrival	-	-	67%	57%
Patients Who Left ER Before Being Seen	-	-	2%	2%
Time from ER Arrival to Admit. (minutes)[5]	-	-	244	274
Time from ER Arrival to Discharge (minutes)	-	-	139	134
Time in ER Before Being Evaluated (minutes)	-	-	20	26
Time to Pain Meds for Fractures (minutes)	-	-	45	57
Heart Attack Care				
Aspirin Given at Discharge[5]	-	-	100%	99%
Fibrinolytic Meds Within 30 Min. of Arrival[5]	-	-	20%	54%
PCI Within 90 Minutes of Arrival[5]	-	-	97%	96%
Statin Prescribed at Discharge[5]	-	-	99%	98%
Heart Failure Care				
ACE Inhibitor or ARB for LVSD[5]	-	-	97%	97%
Discharge Instructions Given[5]	-	-	93%	94%
Evaluation of LVS Function[5]	-	-	99%	99%
Medicare Spending				
Medicare Spending per Patient (ratio)	-	-	0.95	0.98
Pneumonia Care				
Appropriate Initial Antibiotic Given[5]	-	-	95%	95%
Blood Culture Timing[5]	-	-	98%	98%
Pregnancy and Delivery Care				
Newborn Deliveries Scheduled Early[5]	-	-	2%	6%
Preventive Care				
Immunization for Influenza[5]	-	-	92%	90%
Immunization for Pneumonia[5]	-	-	92%	92%
Stroke Care				
Anticoagulation Therapy for Atrial Fibrillation[5]	-	-	97%	95%
Antithrombotic Therapy Timing[5]	-	-	98%	98%
Assessed for Rehabilitation[5]	-	-	98%	97%
Discharged on Antithrombotic Therapy[5]	-	-	100%	99%
Discharged on Statin Medication[5]	-	-	94%	94%
Thrombolytic Therapy Timing[5]	-	-	78%	66%
Venous Thromboembolism Prophylaxis[5]	-	-	96%	94%
Written Stroke Educational Materials Given[5]	-	-	87%	88%
Surgical Care Improvement Project				
Appropriate Beta Blocker Usage[5]	-	-	98%	98%
Appropriate VTP Within 24 Hours[5]	-	-	98%	98%
Controlled Postoperative Blood Glucose[5]	-	-	96%	97%
Perioperative Temperature Management[5]	-	-	99%	100%
Prophylactic Antibiotic Selection[5]	-	-	99%	99%
Prophylactic Antibiotic Selection (Outpatient)	-	-	98%	98%
Prophylactic Antibiotic Stopped[5]	-	-	98%	98%
Prophylactic Antibiotic Timing[5]	-	-	98%	99%
Prophylactic Antibiotic Timing (Outpatient)	-	-	98%	98%
Urinary Catheter Removal[5]	-	-	97%	97%
Survey of Patients' Hospital Experiences				
Area Around Room 'Always' Quiet at Night[6]	<100	70%	64%	61%
Doctors 'Always' Communicated Well[6]	<100	92%	81%	82%
Home Recovery Information Given[6]	<100	85%	87%	85%
Hospital Given 9 or 10 on 10 Point Scale[6]	<100	88%	75%	71%
Meds 'Always' Explained Before Given[6]	<100	81%	67%	64%
Nurses 'Always' Communicated Well[6]	<100	85%	79%	79%
Pain 'Always' Well Controlled[6]	<100	76%	72%	71%
Room and Bathroom 'Always' Clean[6]	<100	84%	74%	73%
Timely Help 'Always' Received[6]	<100	74%	70%	68%
Would Definitely Recommend Hospital[6]	<100	80%	76%	71%
Use of Medical Imaging				
Cardiac Imaging Stress Test before Surgery	-	-	5%	5.3%
Combination Abdominal CT Scan	-	-	10%	10.5%
Combination Brain/Sinus CT Scan	-	-	2.1%	2.7%
Combination Chest CT Scan	-	-	3.1%	2.7%
Follow-up Mammogram/Ultrasound	-	-	8.7%	8.8%
Lumbar Spine MRI for Low Back Pain	-	-	39.7%	37.2%

Valley View Hospital Association

1906 Blake Ave
Glenwood Springs, CO 81601
Phone: 970-945-6535
Fax: 970-945-2073
E-mail: vvhadmin@ruralhealth.org
Type: Acute Care Hospitals
Emergency Services: Yes
Ownership: Voluntary non-profit - Private
Beds: 80

Key Personnel:

CEO/President. . . . . Gary Brewer
Pediatric Ambulatory Care . . . . . . David & Ellen Brooks, MD
Infection Control. . . . . Trish Cerise
Quality Assurance . . . . Cathy Desantels
Radiology. . . . . Charles Fowler, MD
Operating Room. . . . . Jean-Marie Heagerty
Chief of Medical Staff . . . . Rob Macaulay

Measure	Cases	This Hosp.	State Avg.	U.S. Avg.
Blood Clot Prevention and Treatment				
Anticoagulation Overlap Therapy[2]	23	100%	97%	93%
ICU Venous Thromboembolism Prophylaxis[2]	51	100%	95%	92%
Incidence of Potentially Preventable VTE[1,2]	-	-	8%	10%
UFH with Dosages/Platelet Monitoring[2]	12	100%	97%	97%
Venous Thromboembolism Prophylaxis[2]	121	95%	90%	85%
Warfarin Therapy Discharge Instructions[2]	18	100%	69%	75%
Chest Pain/Possible Heart Attack Care				
Aspirin Given Within 24 Hours of Arrival[1,3]	-	-	97%	96%
Fibrinolytic Meds Within 30 Min. of Arrival[3,7]	-	-	55%	58%
Average Time to ECG (minutes)[1,3]	-	-	8	7
Average Time to Transfer (minutes)[3,7]	-	-	74	60
Children's Asthma Care				
Received Home Management Plan of Care	-	-	-	88%
Received Reliever Medication	-	-	-	100%
Received Systemic Corticosteroids	-	-	-	100%
Emergency Department				
Admittance Decision Time (minutes)[2]	166	98	96	98
Head CT Results Within 45 Min. of Arrival[1]	-	-	67%	57%
Patients Who Left ER Before Being Seen	10,755	1%	2%	2%
Time from ER Arrival to Admit. (minutes)[2]	191	256	244	274
Time from ER Arrival to Discharge (minutes)	353	152	139	134
Time in ER Before Being Evaluated (minutes)	193	29	20	26
Time to Pain Meds for Fractures (minutes)	63	58	45	57
Heart Attack Care				
Aspirin Given at Discharge	37	100%	100%	99%
Fibrinolytic Meds Within 30 Min. of Arrival[7]	-	-	20%	54%
PCI Within 90 Minutes of Arrival[1]	-	-	97%	96%
Statin Prescribed at Discharge	37	100%	99%	98%
Heart Failure Care				
ACE Inhibitor or ARB for LVSD[1]	-	-	97%	97%
Discharge Instructions Given	18	89%	93%	94%
Evaluation of LVS Function	21	100%	99%	99%
Medicare Spending				
Medicare Spending per Patient (ratio)	-	0.93	0.95	0.98

NOTE: Hospital profiles are in alphabetical order by state, then city, then hospital within the city; Rankings exclude hospitals with less than 25 cases except for patient surveys which excludes hospitals with less than 100 cases; (a) 100-299 cases; (1) The number of cases/patients is too few to report; (2) Data submitted were based on a sample of cases/patients; (3) Results are based on a shorter time period than required; (4) Data suppressed by CMS for one or more quarters; (5) Results are not available for this reporting period; (6) Fewer than 100 patients completed the HCAHPS survey; (7) No cases met the criteria for this measure; (8) The lower limit of the confidence interval cannot be calculated if the number of observed infections equals zero; (9) No data are available from the state/territory for this reporting period; (10) The scores shown reflect fewer than 50 completed surveys; (11) There were discrepancies in the data collection process; (12) This measure does not apply to this hospital for this reporting period; (13) Results cannot be calculated for this reporting period; (14) The results for this state are combined with nearby states to protect confidentiality; Please refer to the User's Guide for a full explanation of data.

Measure	Cases	This Hosp.	State Avg.	U.S. Avg.
Pneumonia Care				
Appropriate Initial Antibiotic Given	22	100%	95%	95%
Blood Culture Timing	41	100%	98%	98%
Pregnancy and Delivery Care				
Newborn Deliveries Scheduled Early	78	0%	2%	6%
Preventive Care				
Immunization for Influenza[2]	243	98%	92%	90%
Immunization for Pneumonia[2]	198	95%	92%	92%
Stroke Care				
Anticoagulation Therapy for Atrial Fibrillation[1]	-	-	97%	95%
Antithrombotic Therapy Timing	11	100%	98%	98%
Assessed for Rehabilitation	12	92%	98%	97%
Discharged on Antithrombotic Therapy	12	100%	100%	99%
Discharged on Statin Medication[1]	-	-	94%	94%
Thrombolytic Therapy Timing[7]	-	-	78%	66%
Venous Thromboembolism Prophylaxis[1]	-	-	96%	94%
Written Stroke Educational Materials Given[1]	-	-	87%	88%
Surgical Care Improvement Project				
Appropriate Beta Blocker Usage	37	95%	98%	98%
Appropriate VTP Within 24 Hours	178	97%	98%	98%
Controlled Postoperative Blood Glucose[7]	-	-	96%	97%
Perioperative Temperature Management	198	100%	99%	100%
Prophylactic Antibiotic Selection	128	99%	99%	99%
Prophylactic Antibiotic Selection (Outpatient)	150	99%	98%	98%
Prophylactic Antibiotic Stopped	126	97%	98%	98%
Prophylactic Antibiotic Timing	128	100%	98%	99%
Prophylactic Antibiotic Timing (Outpatient)	145	98%	98%	98%
Urinary Catheter Removal	113	97%	97%	97%
Survey of Patients' Hospital Experiences				
Area Around Room 'Always' Quiet at Night	300+	64%	64%	61%
Doctors 'Always' Communicated Well	300+	82%	81%	82%
Home Recovery Information Given	300+	87%	87%	85%
Hospital Given 9 or 10 on 10 Point Scale	300+	80%	75%	71%
Meds 'Always' Explained Before Given	300+	65%	67%	64%
Nurses 'Always' Communicated Well	300+	79%	79%	79%
Pain 'Always' Well Controlled	300+	69%	72%	71%
Room and Bathroom 'Always' Clean	300+	78%	74%	73%
Timely Help 'Always' Received	300+	71%	70%	68%
Would Definitely Recommend Hospital	300+	81%	76%	71%
Use of Medical Imaging				
Cardiac Imaging Stress Test before Surgery	186	7.0%	5%	5.3%
Combination Abdominal CT Scan	235	9.8%	10%	10.5%
Combination Brain/Sinus CT Scan[1]	-	-	2.1%	2.7%
Combination Chest CT Scan	175	1.1%	3.1%	2.7%
Follow-up Mammogram/Ultrasound	584	8.7%	8.7%	8.8%
Lumbar Spine MRI for Low Back Pain	59	44.1%	39.7%	37.2%

Community Hospital

2021 N 12th St
Grand Junction, CO 81501
Phone: 970-256-6201
Fax: 970-256-6510
E-mail: bjessen@gjhosp.org
URL: www.gjhosp.org
Type: Acute Care Hospitals
Emergency Services: Yes
Ownership: Voluntary non-profit - Private
Beds: 78

Key Personnel:
Operating Room. . . . . Stuart H Ackley
Radiology. . . . . Jeff Amans
CEO/President. . . . . Mark Francis
Chief of Medical Staff. . . . . Mann Mariekjosa
Cardiac Laboratory. . . . . Shary Shafer

Measure	Cases	This Hosp.	State Avg.	U.S. Avg.
Blood Clot Prevention and Treatment				
Anticoagulation Overlap Therapy[2]	15	93%	97%	93%
ICU Venous Thromboembolism Prophylaxis[2]	26	100%	95%	92%
Incidence of Potentially Preventable VTE[1,2]	-	-	8%	10%
UFH with Dosages/Platelet Monitoring[1,2]	-	-	97%	97%
Venous Thromboembolism Prophylaxis[2]	116	98%	90%	85%
Warfarin Therapy Discharge Instructions[1,2]	-	-	69%	75%
Chest Pain/Possible Heart Attack Care				
Aspirin Given Within 24 Hours of Arrival[3]	12	100%	97%	96%
Fibrinolytic Meds Within 30 Min. of Arrival[1,3]	-	-	55%	58%
Average Time to ECG (minutes)[3]	12	12	8	7
Average Time to Transfer (minutes)[3,7]	-	-	74	60
Children's Asthma Care				
Received Home Management Plan of Care	-	-	-	88%
Received Reliever Medication	-	-	-	100%
Received Systemic Corticosteroids	-	-	-	100%
Emergency Department				
Admittance Decision Time (minutes)[2]	324	68	96	98
Head CT Results Within 45 Min. of Arrival[3,7]	-	-	67%	57%
Patients Who Left ER Before Being Seen	15,624	0%	2%	2%
Time from ER Arrival to Admit. (minutes)[2]	380	231	244	274
Time from ER Arrival to Discharge (minutes)	396	133	139	134
Time in ER Before Being Evaluated (minutes)	415	7	20	26
Time to Pain Meds for Fractures (minutes)	77	53	45	57
Heart Attack Care				
Aspirin Given at Discharge[1]	-	-	100%	99%
Fibrinolytic Meds Within 30 Min. of Arrival[7]	-	-	20%	54%
PCI Within 90 Minutes of Arrival[7]	-	-	97%	96%
Statin Prescribed at Discharge[1]	-	-	99%	98%
Heart Failure Care				
ACE Inhibitor or ARB for LVSD	16	94%	97%	97%
Discharge Instructions Given	29	97%	93%	94%
Evaluation of LVS Function	42	100%	99%	99%
Medicare Spending				
Medicare Spending per Patient (ratio)	-	0.95	0.95	0.98
Pneumonia Care				
Appropriate Initial Antibiotic Given	63	98%	95%	95%
Blood Culture Timing	81	95%	98%	98%
Pregnancy and Delivery Care				
Newborn Deliveries Scheduled Early[7]	-	-	2%	6%
Preventive Care				
Immunization for Influenza[2]	329	90%	92%	90%
Immunization for Pneumonia[2]	445	89%	92%	92%
Stroke Care				
Anticoagulation Therapy for Atrial Fibrillation[1]	-	-	97%	95%
Antithrombotic Therapy Timing[1]	-	-	98%	98%
Assessed for Rehabilitation[1]	-	-	98%	97%
Discharged on Antithrombotic Therapy[1]	-	-	100%	99%
Discharged on Statin Medication[1]	-	-	94%	94%
Thrombolytic Therapy Timing[1]	-	-	78%	66%
Venous Thromboembolism Prophylaxis	11	100%	96%	94%
Written Stroke Educational Materials Given[1]	-	-	87%	88%
Surgical Care Improvement Project				
Appropriate Beta Blocker Usage	48	98%	98%	98%
Appropriate VTP Within 24 Hours	228	99%	98%	98%
Controlled Postoperative Blood Glucose[7]	-	-	96%	97%
Perioperative Temperature Management	240	100%	99%	100%
Prophylactic Antibiotic Selection	186	97%	99%	99%
Prophylactic Antibiotic Selection (Outpatient)	117	93%	98%	98%
Prophylactic Antibiotic Stopped	181	94%	98%	98%
Prophylactic Antibiotic Timing	186	96%	98%	99%
Prophylactic Antibiotic Timing (Outpatient)	117	99%	98%	98%
Urinary Catheter Removal	118	97%	97%	97%
Survey of Patients' Hospital Experiences				
Area Around Room 'Always' Quiet at Night[11]	300+	52%	64%	61%
Doctors 'Always' Communicated Well[11]	300+	81%	81%	82%
Home Recovery Information Given[11]	300+	85%	87%	85%
Hospital Given 9 or 10 on 10 Point Scale[11]	300+	74%	75%	71%
Meds 'Always' Explained Before Given[11]	300+	69%	67%	64%
Nurses 'Always' Communicated Well[11]	300+	82%	79%	79%
Pain 'Always' Well Controlled[11]	300+	69%	72%	71%
Room and Bathroom 'Always' Clean[11]	300+	73%	74%	73%
Timely Help 'Always' Received[11]	300+	71%	70%	68%
Would Definitely Recommend Hospital[11]	300+	82%	76%	71%
Use of Medical Imaging				
Cardiac Imaging Stress Test before Surgery[1]	-	-	5%	5.3%
Combination Abdominal CT Scan	283	18.7%	10%	10.5%
Combination Brain/Sinus CT Scan[1]	-	-	2.1%	2.7%
Combination Chest CT Scan	84	2.4%	3.1%	2.7%
Follow-up Mammogram/Ultrasound	679	6.2%	8.7%	8.8%
Lumbar Spine MRI for Low Back Pain	54	42.6%	39.7%	37.2%

Grand Junction VA Medical Center

2121 N. Avenue
Grand Junction, CO 81501
Phone: 970-244-1329
Fax: 970-244-1303
Type: Acute Care - VA
Emergency Services: No
Ownership: Government Federal
Beds: 53

Key Personnel:
Patient Relations . . . . Karl Coleman
Quality Assurance . . . . Charles Hensel
Infection Control. . . . . Sharon Kautzsch
Ambulatory Care . . . . Karen Nelson
Operating Room. . . . . Douglas Rosendale, MD
Chief of Medical Staff. . . . . Jerold L Saef, MD
CEO/President. . . . . Kurt W Schlegelmilch, MD

Measure	Cases	This Hosp.	State Avg.	U.S. Avg.
Blood Clot Prevention and Treatment				
Anticoagulation Overlap Therapy	-	-	97%	93%
ICU Venous Thromboembolism Prophylaxis	-	-	95%	92%
Incidence of Potentially Preventable VTE	-	-	8%	10%
UFH with Dosages/Platelet Monitoring	-	-	97%	97%
Venous Thromboembolism Prophylaxis	-	-	90%	85%
Warfarin Therapy Discharge Instructions	-	-	69%	75%
Chest Pain/Possible Heart Attack Care				
Aspirin Given Within 24 Hours of Arrival	-	-	97%	96%
Fibrinolytic Meds Within 30 Min. of Arrival	-	-	55%	58%
Average Time to ECG (minutes)	-	-	8	7
Average Time to Transfer (minutes)	-	-	74	60
Children's Asthma Care				
Received Home Management Plan of Care	-	-	-	88%
Received Reliever Medication	-	-	-	100%
Received Systemic Corticosteroids	-	-	-	100%
Emergency Department				
Admittance Decision Time (minutes)	-	-	96	98
Head CT Results Within 45 Min. of Arrival	-	-	67%	57%
Patients Who Left ER Before Being Seen	-	-	2%	2%
Time from ER Arrival to Admit. (minutes)	-	-	244	274
Time from ER Arrival to Discharge (minutes)	-	-	139	134
Time in ER Before Being Evaluated (minutes)	-	-	20	26
Time to Pain Meds for Fractures (minutes)	-	-	45	57
Heart Attack Care				
Aspirin Given at Discharge[5]	-	-	100%	99%
Fibrinolytic Meds Within 30 Min. of Arrival[5]	-	-	20%	54%
PCI Within 90 Minutes of Arrival[5]	-	-	97%	96%
Statin Prescribed at Discharge[5]	-	-	99%	98%
Heart Failure Care				
ACE Inhibitor or ARB for LVSD[1]	15	100%	97%	97%
Discharge Instructions Given	27	100%	93%	94%
Evaluation of LVS Function	31	100%	99%	99%
Medicare Spending				
Medicare Spending per Patient (ratio)	-	-	0.95	0.98
Pneumonia Care				
Appropriate Initial Antibiotic Given	29	97%	95%	95%
Blood Culture Timing	38	100%	98%	98%
Pregnancy and Delivery Care				
Newborn Deliveries Scheduled Early	-	-	2%	6%
Preventive Care				
Immunization for Influenza[5]	-	-	92%	90%
Immunization for Pneumonia[5]	-	-	92%	92%
Stroke Care				
Anticoagulation Therapy for Atrial Fibrillation	-	-	97%	95%
Antithrombotic Therapy Timing	-	-	98%	98%
Assessed for Rehabilitation	-	-	98%	97%
Discharged on Antithrombotic Therapy	-	-	100%	99%
Discharged on Statin Medication	-	-	94%	94%
Thrombolytic Therapy Timing	-	-	78%	66%
Venous Thromboembolism Prophylaxis	-	-	96%	94%
Written Stroke Educational Materials Given	-	-	87%	88%
Surgical Care Improvement Project				
Appropriate Beta Blocker Usage[1,2]	-	-	98%	98%
Appropriate VTP Within 24 Hours[2]	56	100%	98%	98%
Controlled Postoperative Blood Glucose[5]	-	-	96%	97%
Perioperative Temperature Management[2]	60	100%	99%	100%
Prophylactic Antibiotic Selection	54	100%	99%	99%
Prophylactic Antibiotic Selection (Outpatient)	-	-	98%	98%
Prophylactic Antibiotic Stopped	54	100%	98%	98%

NOTE: Hospital profiles are in alphabetical order by state, then city, then hospital within the city; Rankings exclude hospitals with less than 25 cases except for patient surveys which excludes hospitals with less than 100 cases; (a) 100-299 cases; (1) The number of cases/patients is too few to report; (2) Data submitted were based on a sample of cases/patients; (3) Results are based on a shorter time period than required; (4) Data suppressed by CMS for one or more quarters; (5) Results are not available for this reporting period; (6) Fewer than 100 patients completed the HCAHPS survey; (7) No cases met the criteria for this measure; (8) The lower limit of the confidence interval cannot be calculated if the number of observed infections equals zero; (9) No data are available from the state/territory for this reporting period; (10) The scores shown reflect fewer than 50 completed surveys; (11) There were discrepancies in the data collection process; (12) This measure does not apply to this hospital for this reporting period; (13) Results cannot be calculated for this reporting period; (14) The results for this state are combined with nearby states to protect confidentiality; Please refer to the User's Guide for a full explanation of data.

Measure	Cases	This Hosp.	State Avg.	U.S. Avg.
Prophylactic Antibiotic Timing	54	100%	98%	99%
Prophylactic Antibiotic Timing (Outpatient)	-	-	98%	98%
Urinary Catheter Removal[1,2]	20	100%	97%	97%
Survey of Patients' Hospital Experiences				
Area Around Room 'Always' Quiet at Night	-	-	64%	61%
Doctors 'Always' Communicated Well	-	-	81%	82%
Home Recovery Information Given	-	-	87%	85%
Hospital Given 9 or 10 on 10 Point Scale	-	-	75%	71%
Meds 'Always' Explained Before Given	-	-	67%	64%
Nurses 'Always' Communicated Well	-	-	79%	79%
Pain 'Always' Well Controlled	-	-	72%	71%
Room and Bathroom 'Always' Clean	-	-	74%	73%
Timely Help 'Always' Received	-	-	70%	68%
Would Definitely Recommend Hospital	-	-	76%	71%
Use of Medical Imaging				
Cardiac Imaging Stress Test before Surgery	-	-	5%	5.3%
Combination Abdominal CT Scan	-	-	10%	10.5%
Combination Brain/Sinus CT Scan	-	-	2.1%	2.7%
Combination Chest CT Scan	-	-	3.1%	2.7%
Follow-up Mammogram/Ultrasound	-	-	8.7%	8.8%
Lumbar Spine MRI for Low Back Pain	-	-	39.7%	37.2%

Saint Marys Hospital & Medical Center

2635 N 7th Street
Grand Junction, CO 81502
URL: www.stmarygj.org
Type: Acute Care Hospitals
Ownership: Voluntary non-profit - Church
Phone: 970-298-1950
Fax: 970-244-7510
Emergency Services: Yes
Beds: 277

Key Personnel:
Infection Control. . . . . William Cobb, MD
Emergency Room . . . . Roy Cromer, MD
Radiology. . . . . Richard Fulton, MD
Anesthesiology. . . . . Steven Gardner, MD
Chief of Medical Staff . . . . Robert Halpenny, MD
CEO/President. . . . . Michael McBride
Hemotology Center . . . . Cindy Thomas, RN
Pediatric In-Patient Care . . . . Michael Whistler, MD

Measure	Cases	This Hosp.	State Avg.	U.S. Avg.
Blood Clot Prevention and Treatment				
Anticoagulation Overlap Therapy	94	99%	97%	93%
ICU Venous Thromboembolism Prophylaxis	1,060	94%	95%	92%
Incidence of Potentially Preventable VTE	15	7%	8%	10%
UFH with Dosages/Platelet Monitoring	54	100%	97%	97%
Venous Thromboembolism Prophylaxis	3,546	92%	90%	85%
Warfarin Therapy Discharge Instructions	79	96%	69%	75%
Chest Pain/Possible Heart Attack Care				
Aspirin Given Within 24 Hours of Arrival[1,3]	-	-	97%	96%
Fibrinolytic Meds Within 30 Min. of Arrival[3,7]	-	-	55%	58%
Average Time to ECG (minutes)[1,3]	-	-	8	7
Average Time to Transfer (minutes)[3,7]	-	-	74	60
Children's Asthma Care				
Received Home Management Plan of Care	-	-	-	88%
Received Reliever Medication	-	-	-	100%
Received Systemic Corticosteroids	-	-	-	100%
Emergency Department				
Admittance Decision Time (minutes)	4,618	116	96	98
Head CT Results Within 45 Min. of Arrival[1]	-	-	67%	57%
Patients Who Left ER Before Being Seen	39,725	2%	2%	2%
Time from ER Arrival to Admit. (minutes)	4,745	277	244	274
Time from ER Arrival to Discharge (minutes)	4,027	158	139	134
Time in ER Before Being Evaluated (minutes)	3,746	37	20	26
Time to Pain Meds for Fractures (minutes)	163	60	45	57
Heart Attack Care				
Aspirin Given at Discharge	320	100%	100%	99%
Fibrinolytic Meds Within 30 Min. of Arrival[7]	-	-	20%	54%
PCI Within 90 Minutes of Arrival	44	100%	97%	96%
Statin Prescribed at Discharge	303	99%	99%	98%
Heart Failure Care				
ACE Inhibitor or ARB for LVSD	42	98%	97%	97%
Discharge Instructions Given	117	87%	93%	94%
Evaluation of LVS Function	138	100%	99%	99%
Medicare Spending				
Medicare Spending per Patient (ratio)	-	0.95	0.95	0.98
Pneumonia Care				
Appropriate Initial Antibiotic Given	132	95%	95%	95%
Blood Culture Timing	224	96%	98%	98%
Pregnancy and Delivery Care				
Newborn Deliveries Scheduled Early	181	2%	2%	6%
Preventive Care				
Immunization for Influenza	5,869	95%	92%	90%
Immunization for Pneumonia	5,956	95%	92%	92%
Stroke Care				
Anticoagulation Therapy for Atrial Fibrillation	25	96%	97%	95%
Antithrombotic Therapy Timing	89	100%	98%	98%
Assessed for Rehabilitation	133	100%	98%	97%
Discharged on Antithrombotic Therapy	117	100%	100%	99%
Discharged on Statin Medication	83	99%	94%	94%
Thrombolytic Therapy Timing	18	94%	78%	66%
Venous Thromboembolism Prophylaxis	138	100%	96%	94%
Written Stroke Educational Materials Given	76	96%	87%	88%
Surgical Care Improvement Project				
Appropriate Beta Blocker Usage	387	99%	98%	98%
Appropriate VTP Within 24 Hours	1,089	99%	98%	98%
Controlled Postoperative Blood Glucose	141	99%	96%	97%
Perioperative Temperature Management	1,306	100%	99%	100%
Prophylactic Antibiotic Selection	852	100%	99%	99%
Prophylactic Antibiotic Selection (Outpatient)	548	97%	98%	98%
Prophylactic Antibiotic Stopped	827	98%	98%	98%
Prophylactic Antibiotic Timing	857	99%	98%	99%
Prophylactic Antibiotic Timing (Outpatient)	551	97%	98%	98%
Urinary Catheter Removal	874	97%	97%	97%
Survey of Patients' Hospital Experiences				
Area Around Room 'Always' Quiet at Night	300+	56%	64%	61%
Doctors 'Always' Communicated Well	300+	81%	81%	82%
Home Recovery Information Given	300+	87%	87%	85%
Hospital Given 9 or 10 on 10 Point Scale	300+	74%	75%	71%
Meds 'Always' Explained Before Given	300+	63%	67%	64%
Nurses 'Always' Communicated Well	300+	77%	79%	79%
Pain 'Always' Well Controlled	300+	70%	72%	71%
Room and Bathroom 'Always' Clean	300+	71%	74%	73%
Timely Help 'Always' Received	300+	64%	70%	68%
Would Definitely Recommend Hospital	300+	77%	76%	71%
Use of Medical Imaging				
Cardiac Imaging Stress Test before Surgery	101	7.9%	5%	5.3%
Combination Abdominal CT Scan	739	13.7%	10%	10.5%
Combination Brain/Sinus CT Scan[1]	-	-	2.1%	2.7%
Combination Chest CT Scan	544	0.2%	3.1%	2.7%
Follow-up Mammogram/Ultrasound	1,316	10.9%	8.7%	8.8%
Lumbar Spine MRI for Low Back Pain	99	36.4%	39.7%	37.2%

North Colorado Medical Center

1801 16th Street
Greeley, CO 80631
URL: www.bannerhealth.com
Type: Acute Care Hospitals
Ownership: Voluntary non-profit - Private
Phone: 970-352-4121
Fax: 970-350-6114
Emergency Services: Yes
Beds: 326

Key Personnel:
Emergency Room . . . . April Asdury
Cardiac Laboratory. . . . . Dayle Hosek
CEO/President. . . . . Richard O'Sutton
Quality Assurance . . . . Lynn Runyon

Measure	Cases	This Hosp.	State Avg.	U.S. Avg.
Blood Clot Prevention and Treatment				
Anticoagulation Overlap Therapy[2]	112	97%	97%	93%
ICU Venous Thromboembolism Prophylaxis[2]	58	97%	95%	92%
Incidence of Potentially Preventable VTE[2]	17	0%	8%	10%
UFH with Dosages/Platelet Monitoring[2]	50	98%	97%	97%
Venous Thromboembolism Prophylaxis[2]	296	93%	90%	85%
Warfarin Therapy Discharge Instructions[2]	84	57%	69%	75%
Chest Pain/Possible Heart Attack Care				
Aspirin Given Within 24 Hours of Arrival[3,7]	-	-	97%	96%
Fibrinolytic Meds Within 30 Min. of Arrival[5]	-	-	55%	58%
Average Time to ECG (minutes)[3,7]	-	-	8	7
Average Time to Transfer (minutes)[5]	-	-	74	60
Children's Asthma Care				
Received Home Management Plan of Care	-	-	-	88%
Received Reliever Medication	-	-	-	100%
Received Systemic Corticosteroids	-	-	-	100%
Emergency Department				
Admittance Decision Time (minutes)[2]	451	64	96	98
Head CT Results Within 45 Min. of Arrival	16	75%	67%	57%
Patients Who Left ER Before Being Seen	58,575	1%	2%	2%
Time from ER Arrival to Admit. (minutes)[2]	464	220	244	274
Time from ER Arrival to Discharge (minutes)	317	119	139	134
Time in ER Before Being Evaluated (minutes)	382	13	20	26
Time to Pain Meds for Fractures (minutes)	167	41	45	57
Heart Attack Care				
Aspirin Given at Discharge[2]	275	100%	100%	99%
Fibrinolytic Meds Within 30 Min. of Arrival[2,7]	-	-	20%	54%
PCI Within 90 Minutes of Arrival[2]	38	95%	97%	96%
Statin Prescribed at Discharge[2]	269	100%	99%	98%
Heart Failure Care				
ACE Inhibitor or ARB for LVSD[2]	53	100%	97%	97%
Discharge Instructions Given[2]	189	97%	93%	94%
Evaluation of LVS Function[2]	234	100%	99%	99%
Medicare Spending				
Medicare Spending per Patient (ratio)	-	0.99	0.95	0.98
Pneumonia Care				
Appropriate Initial Antibiotic Given[2]	67	94%	95%	95%
Blood Culture Timing[2]	114	100%	98%	98%
Pregnancy and Delivery Care				
Newborn Deliveries Scheduled Early[2]	32	3%	2%	6%
Preventive Care				
Immunization for Influenza[2]	497	97%	92%	90%
Immunization for Pneumonia[2]	582	94%	92%	92%
Stroke Care				
Anticoagulation Therapy for Atrial Fibrillation	11	91%	97%	95%
Antithrombotic Therapy Timing	75	99%	98%	98%
Assessed for Rehabilitation	87	92%	98%	97%
Discharged on Antithrombotic Therapy	77	100%	100%	99%
Discharged on Statin Medication	59	95%	94%	94%
Thrombolytic Therapy Timing	11	73%	78%	66%
Venous Thromboembolism Prophylaxis	93	90%	96%	94%
Written Stroke Educational Materials Given	46	89%	87%	88%
Surgical Care Improvement Project				
Appropriate Beta Blocker Usage[2]	154	97%	98%	98%
Appropriate VTP Within 24 Hours[2]	348	99%	98%	98%
Controlled Postoperative Blood Glucose[2]	92	99%	96%	97%
Perioperative Temperature Management[2]	401	100%	99%	100%
Prophylactic Antibiotic Selection[2]	318	99%	99%	99%
Prophylactic Antibiotic Selection (Outpatient)	428	99%	98%	98%
Prophylactic Antibiotic Stopped[2]	309	99%	98%	98%
Prophylactic Antibiotic Timing[2]	319	99%	98%	99%
Prophylactic Antibiotic Timing (Outpatient)	429	100%	98%	98%
Urinary Catheter Removal[2]	250	99%	97%	97%
Survey of Patients' Hospital Experiences				
Area Around Room 'Always' Quiet at Night[11]	300+	60%	64%	61%
Doctors 'Always' Communicated Well[11]	300+	81%	81%	82%
Home Recovery Information Given[11]	300+	91%	87%	85%
Hospital Given 9 or 10 on 10 Point Scale[11]	300+	74%	75%	71%
Meds 'Always' Explained Before Given[11]	300+	68%	67%	64%
Nurses 'Always' Communicated Well[11]	300+	81%	79%	79%
Pain 'Always' Well Controlled[11]	300+	70%	72%	71%
Room and Bathroom 'Always' Clean[11]	300+	73%	74%	73%
Timely Help 'Always' Received[11]	300+	67%	70%	68%
Would Definitely Recommend Hospital[11]	300+	72%	76%	71%
Use of Medical Imaging				
Cardiac Imaging Stress Test before Surgery	413	3.1%	5%	5.3%
Combination Abdominal CT Scan	738	4.7%	10%	10.5%
Combination Brain/Sinus CT Scan	738	3.4%	2.1%	2.7%
Combination Chest CT Scan	436	2.3%	3.1%	2.7%
Follow-up Mammogram/Ultrasound	1,895	6.6%	8.7%	8.8%
Lumbar Spine MRI for Low Back Pain	157	40.1%	39.7%	37.2%

NOTE: Hospital profiles are in alphabetical order by state, then city, then hospital within the city; Rankings exclude hospitals with less than 25 cases except for patient surveys which excludes hospitals with less than 100 cases; (a) 100-299 cases; (1) The number of cases/patients is too few to report; (2) Data submitted were based on a sample of cases/patients; (3) Results are based on a shorter time period than required; (4) Data suppressed by CMS for one or more quarters; (5) Results are not available for this reporting period; (6) Fewer than 100 patients completed the HCAHPS survey; (7) No cases met the criteria for this measure; (8) The lower limit of the confidence interval cannot be calculated if the number of observed infections equals zero; (9) No data are available from the state/territory for this reporting period; (10) The scores shown reflect fewer than 50 completed surveys; (11) There were discrepancies in the data collection process; (12) This measure does not apply to this hospital for this reporting period; (13) Results cannot be calculated for this reporting period; (14) The results for this state are combined with nearby states to protect confidentiality; Please refer to the User's Guide for a full explanation of data.

Gunnison Valley Hospital

711 N Taylor Street Phone: 970-641-1456
Gunnison, CO 81230 Fax: 970-641-4461
URL: www.gvh-colorado.org
Type: Critical Access Hospitals Emergency Services: Yes
Ownership: Government - Local Beds: 21
Key Personnel:
Operating Room. . . . . John Bishop, RN
Chief of Medical Staff . . . . Lauretta F Garren, MD
Cardiology . . . . Bradley D. Huhta, MD, FACC
Emergency Room . . . . Leandra Lynch, RN
Quality Assurance . . . . Donna Neilsen
CEO/President. . . . . Randy Phelps
Radiology. . . . . Gareth Roberts, MD
Anesthesiology. . . . . Jim Woelk

Measure	Cases	This Hosp.	State Avg.	U.S. Avg.
Blood Clot Prevention and Treatment				
Anticoagulation Overlap Therapy[5]	-	-	97%	93%
ICU Venous Thromboembolism Prophylaxis[5]	-	-	95%	92%
Incidence of Potentially Preventable VTE[5]	-	-	8%	10%
UFH with Dosages/Platelet Monitoring[5]	-	-	97%	97%
Venous Thromboembolism Prophylaxis[5]	-	-	90%	85%
Warfarin Therapy Discharge Instructions[5]	-	-	69%	75%
Chest Pain/Possible Heart Attack Care				
Aspirin Given Within 24 Hours of Arrival	12	100%	97%	96%
Fibrinolytic Meds Within 30 Min. of Arrival[1]	-	-	55%	58%
Average Time to ECG (minutes)	12	13	8	7
Average Time to Transfer (minutes)[7]	-	-	74	60
Children's Asthma Care				
Received Home Management Plan of Care	-	-	-	88%
Received Reliever Medication	-	-	-	100%
Received Systemic Corticosteroids	-	-	-	100%
Emergency Department				
Admittance Decision Time (minutes)[5]	-	-	96	98
Head CT Results Within 45 Min. of Arrival[5]	-	-	67%	57%
Patients Who Left ER Before Being Seen[5]	-	-	2%	2%
Time from ER Arrival to Admit. (minutes)[5]	-	-	244	274
Time from ER Arrival to Discharge (minutes)[5]	-	-	139	134
Time in ER Before Being Evaluated (minutes)[5]	-	-	20	26
Time to Pain Meds for Fractures (minutes)[5]	-	-	45	57
Heart Attack Care				
Aspirin Given at Discharge[5]	-	-	100%	99%
Fibrinolytic Meds Within 30 Min. of Arrival[5]	-	-	20%	54%
PCI Within 90 Minutes of Arrival[5]	-	-	97%	96%
Statin Prescribed at Discharge[5]	-	-	99%	98%
Heart Failure Care				
ACE Inhibitor or ARB for LVSD[1,2]	-	-	97%	97%
Discharge Instructions Given[2]	12	92%	93%	94%
Evaluation of LVS Function[2]	16	62%	99%	99%
Medicare Spending				
Medicare Spending per Patient (ratio)	-	-	0.95	0.98
Pneumonia Care				
Appropriate Initial Antibiotic Given[1]	-	-	95%	95%
Blood Culture Timing[1]	-	-	98%	98%
Pregnancy and Delivery Care				
Newborn Deliveries Scheduled Early[5]	-	-	2%	6%
Preventive Care				
Immunization for Influenza[5]	-	-	92%	90%
Immunization for Pneumonia[5]	-	-	92%	92%
Stroke Care				
Anticoagulation Therapy for Atrial Fibrillation[5]	-	-	97%	95%
Antithrombotic Therapy Timing[5]	-	-	98%	98%
Assessed for Rehabilitation[5]	-	-	98%	97%
Discharged on Antithrombotic Therapy[5]	-	-	100%	99%
Discharged on Statin Medication[5]	-	-	94%	94%
Thrombolytic Therapy Timing[5]	-	-	78%	66%
Venous Thromboembolism Prophylaxis[5]	-	-	96%	94%
Written Stroke Educational Materials Given[5]	-	-	87%	88%
Surgical Care Improvement Project				
Appropriate Beta Blocker Usage[1,3]	-	-	98%	98%
Appropriate VTP Within 24 Hours[3]	12	75%	98%	98%
Controlled Postoperative Blood Glucose[3,7]	-	-	96%	97%
Perioperative Temperature Management[3]	16	100%	99%	100%
Prophylactic Antibiotic Selection[1,3]	-	-	99%	99%
Prophylactic Antibiotic Selection (Outpatient)[1,3]	-	-	98%	98%
Prophylactic Antibiotic Stopped[1,3]	-	-	98%	98%
Prophylactic Antibiotic Timing[1,3]	-	-	98%	99%
Prophylactic Antibiotic Timing (Outpatient)[1,3]	-	-	98%	98%
Urinary Catheter Removal[1,3]	-	-	97%	97%
Survey of Patients' Hospital Experiences				
Area Around Room 'Always' Quiet at Night	(a)	78%	64%	61%
Doctors 'Always' Communicated Well	(a)	84%	81%	82%
Home Recovery Information Given	(a)	87%	87%	85%
Hospital Given 9 or 10 on 10 Point Scale	(a)	78%	75%	71%
Meds 'Always' Explained Before Given	(a)	71%	67%	64%
Nurses 'Always' Communicated Well	(a)	82%	79%	79%
Pain 'Always' Well Controlled	(a)	85%	72%	71%
Room and Bathroom 'Always' Clean	(a)	82%	74%	73%
Timely Help 'Always' Received	(a)	81%	70%	68%
Would Definitely Recommend Hospital	(a)	80%	76%	71%
Use of Medical Imaging				
Cardiac Imaging Stress Test before Surgery[7]	-	-	5%	5.3%
Combination Abdominal CT Scan	95	12.6%	10%	10.5%
Combination Brain/Sinus CT Scan[1]	-	-	2.1%	2.7%
Combination Chest CT Scan[1]	-	-	3.1%	2.7%
Follow-up Mammogram/Ultrasound	219	3.7%	8.7%	8.8%
Lumbar Spine MRI for Low Back Pain[1]	-	-	39.7%	37.2%

Haxtun Hospital District

235 W Fletcher Street Phone: 970-774-6123
Haxtun, CO 80731
Type: Critical Access Hospitals Emergency Services: Yes
Ownership: Govt - Hospital Dist/Auth

Measure	Cases	This Hosp.	State Avg.	U.S. Avg.
Blood Clot Prevention and Treatment				
Anticoagulation Overlap Therapy[5]	-	-	97%	93%
ICU Venous Thromboembolism Prophylaxis[5]	-	-	95%	92%
Incidence of Potentially Preventable VTE[5]	-	-	8%	10%
UFH with Dosages/Platelet Monitoring[5]	-	-	97%	97%
Venous Thromboembolism Prophylaxis[5]	-	-	90%	85%
Warfarin Therapy Discharge Instructions[5]	-	-	69%	75%
Chest Pain/Possible Heart Attack Care				
Aspirin Given Within 24 Hours of Arrival	-	-	97%	96%
Fibrinolytic Meds Within 30 Min. of Arrival	-	-	55%	58%
Average Time to ECG (minutes)	-	-	8	7
Average Time to Transfer (minutes)	-	-	74	60
Children's Asthma Care				
Received Home Management Plan of Care	-	-	-	88%
Received Reliever Medication	-	-	-	100%
Received Systemic Corticosteroids	-	-	-	100%
Emergency Department				
Admittance Decision Time (minutes)[5]	-	-	96	98
Head CT Results Within 45 Min. of Arrival	-	-	67%	57%
Patients Who Left ER Before Being Seen	-	-	2%	2%
Time from ER Arrival to Admit. (minutes)[5]	-	-	244	274
Time from ER Arrival to Discharge (minutes)	-	-	139	134
Time in ER Before Being Evaluated (minutes)	-	-	20	26
Time to Pain Meds for Fractures (minutes)	-	-	45	57
Heart Attack Care				
Aspirin Given at Discharge[5]	-	-	100%	99%
Fibrinolytic Meds Within 30 Min. of Arrival[5]	-	-	20%	54%
PCI Within 90 Minutes of Arrival[5]	-	-	97%	96%
Statin Prescribed at Discharge[5]	-	-	99%	98%
Heart Failure Care				
ACE Inhibitor or ARB for LVSD[5]	-	-	97%	97%
Discharge Instructions Given[5]	-	-	93%	94%
Evaluation of LVS Function[5]	-	-	99%	99%
Medicare Spending				
Medicare Spending per Patient (ratio)	-	-	0.95	0.98
Pneumonia Care				
Appropriate Initial Antibiotic Given[5]	-	-	95%	95%
Blood Culture Timing[5]	-	-	98%	98%
Pregnancy and Delivery Care				
Newborn Deliveries Scheduled Early[5]	-	-	2%	6%
Preventive Care				
Immunization for Influenza[5]	-	-	92%	90%
Immunization for Pneumonia[5]	-	-	92%	92%
Stroke Care				
Anticoagulation Therapy for Atrial Fibrillation[5]	-	-	97%	95%
Antithrombotic Therapy Timing[5]	-	-	98%	98%
Assessed for Rehabilitation[5]	-	-	98%	97%
Discharged on Antithrombotic Therapy[5]	-	-	100%	99%
Discharged on Statin Medication[5]	-	-	94%	94%
Thrombolytic Therapy Timing[5]	-	-	78%	66%
Venous Thromboembolism Prophylaxis[5]	-	-	96%	94%
Written Stroke Educational Materials Given[5]	-	-	87%	88%
Surgical Care Improvement Project				
Appropriate Beta Blocker Usage[5]	-	-	98%	98%
Appropriate VTP Within 24 Hours[5]	-	-	98%	98%
Controlled Postoperative Blood Glucose[5]	-	-	96%	97%
Perioperative Temperature Management[5]	-	-	99%	100%
Prophylactic Antibiotic Selection[5]	-	-	99%	99%
Prophylactic Antibiotic Selection (Outpatient)	-	-	98%	98%
Prophylactic Antibiotic Stopped[5]	-	-	98%	98%
Prophylactic Antibiotic Timing[5]	-	-	98%	99%
Prophylactic Antibiotic Timing (Outpatient)	-	-	98%	98%
Urinary Catheter Removal[5]	-	-	97%	97%
Survey of Patients' Hospital Experiences				
Area Around Room 'Always' Quiet at Night[10]	<100	72%	64%	61%
Doctors 'Always' Communicated Well[10]	<100	77%	81%	82%
Home Recovery Information Given[10]	<100	63%	87%	85%
Hospital Given 9 or 10 on 10 Point Scale[10]	<100	70%	75%	71%
Meds 'Always' Explained Before Given[10]	<100	51%	67%	64%
Nurses 'Always' Communicated Well[10]	<100	59%	79%	79%
Pain 'Always' Well Controlled[10]	<100	60%	72%	71%
Room and Bathroom 'Always' Clean[10]	<100	76%	74%	73%
Timely Help 'Always' Received[10]	<100	73%	70%	68%
Would Definitely Recommend Hospital[10]	<100	86%	76%	71%
Use of Medical Imaging				
Cardiac Imaging Stress Test before Surgery	-	-	5%	5.3%
Combination Abdominal CT Scan	-	-	10%	10.5%
Combination Brain/Sinus CT Scan	-	-	2.1%	2.7%
Combination Chest CT Scan	-	-	3.1%	2.7%
Follow-up Mammogram/Ultrasound	-	-	8.7%	8.8%
Lumbar Spine MRI for Low Back Pain	-	-	39.7%	37.2%

Melissa Memorial Hospital

1001 E Johnson Street Phone: 970-854-2241
Holyoke, CO 80734 Fax: 970-854-3821
E-mail: john.ayoub@bannerhealth.com
URL: www.melissamemorial.org
Type: Critical Access Hospitals Emergency Services: Yes
Ownership: Govt - Hospital Dist/Auth Beds: 15
Key Personnel:
Quality Assurance . . . . John Ayoub
Anesthesiology. . . . . Carol Deslauriers
Chief of Medical Staff . . . . Dennis Jelden
Operating Room. . . . . Cindy Lock
Infection Control. . . . . Claudia Powell, RN
President . . . . Steve Young

Measure	Cases	This Hosp.	State Avg.	U.S. Avg.
Blood Clot Prevention and Treatment				
Anticoagulation Overlap Therapy[5]	-	-	97%	93%
ICU Venous Thromboembolism Prophylaxis[5]	-	-	95%	92%
Incidence of Potentially Preventable VTE[5]	-	-	8%	10%
UFH with Dosages/Platelet Monitoring[5]	-	-	97%	97%
Venous Thromboembolism Prophylaxis[5]	-	-	90%	85%
Warfarin Therapy Discharge Instructions[5]	-	-	69%	75%
Chest Pain/Possible Heart Attack Care				
Aspirin Given Within 24 Hours of Arrival[5]	-	-	97%	96%
Fibrinolytic Meds Within 30 Min. of Arrival[5]	-	-	55%	58%
Average Time to ECG (minutes)[5]	-	-	8	7
Average Time to Transfer (minutes)[5]	-	-	74	60
Children's Asthma Care				
Received Home Management Plan of Care	-	-	-	88%
Received Reliever Medication	-	-	-	100%
Received Systemic Corticosteroids	-	-	-	100%
Emergency Department				
Admittance Decision Time (minutes)[5]	-	-	96	98
Head CT Results Within 45 Min. of Arrival[5]	-	-	67%	57%

NOTE: Hospital profiles are in alphabetical order by state, then city, then hospital within the city; Rankings exclude hospitals with less than 25 cases except for patient surveys which excludes hospitals with less than 100 cases; (a) 100-299 cases; (1) The number of cases/patients is too few to report; (2) Data submitted were based on a sample of cases/patients; (3) Results are based on a shorter time period than required; (4) Data suppressed by CMS for one or more quarters; (5) Results are not available for this reporting period; (6) Fewer than 100 patients completed the HCAHPS survey; (7) No cases met the criteria for this measure; (8) The lower limit of the confidence interval cannot be calculated if the number of observed infections equals zero; (9) No data are available from the state/territory for this reporting period; (10) The scores shown reflect fewer than 50 completed surveys; (11) There were discrepancies in the data collection process; (12) This measure does not apply to this hospital for this reporting period; (13) Results cannot be calculated for this reporting period; (14) The results for this state are combined with nearby states to protect confidentiality; Please refer to the User's Guide for a full explanation of data.

Patients Who Left ER Before Being Seen[5]	-	-	2%	2%
Time from ER Arrival to Admit. (minutes)[5]	-	-	244	274
Time from ER Arrival to Discharge (minutes)[5]	-	-	139	134
Time in ER Before Being Evaluated (minutes)[5]	-	-	20	26
Time to Pain Meds for Fractures (minutes)[5]	-	-	45	57
Heart Attack Care				
Aspirin Given at Discharge[3,7]	-	-	100%	99%
Fibrinolytic Meds Within 30 Min. of Arrival[3,7]	-	-	20%	54%
PCI Within 90 Minutes of Arrival[3,7]	-	-	97%	96%
Statin Prescribed at Discharge[3,7]	-	-	99%	98%
Heart Failure Care				
ACE Inhibitor or ARB for LVSD[1,3]	-	-	97%	97%
Discharge Instructions Given[1,3]	-	-	93%	94%
Evaluation of LVS Function[1,3]	-	-	99%	99%
Medicare Spending				
Medicare Spending per Patient (ratio)	-	-	0.95	0.98
Pneumonia Care				
Appropriate Initial Antibiotic Given[3,7]	-	-	95%	95%
Blood Culture Timing[1,3]	-	-	98%	98%
Pregnancy and Delivery Care				
Newborn Deliveries Scheduled Early[5]	-	-	2%	6%
Preventive Care				
Immunization for Influenza[5]	-	-	92%	90%
Immunization for Pneumonia[5]	-	-	92%	92%
Stroke Care				
Anticoagulation Therapy for Atrial Fibrillation[5]	-	-	97%	95%
Antithrombotic Therapy Timing[5]	-	-	98%	98%
Assessed for Rehabilitation[5]	-	-	98%	97%
Discharged on Antithrombotic Therapy[5]	-	-	100%	99%
Discharged on Statin Medication[5]	-	-	94%	94%
Thrombolytic Therapy Timing[5]	-	-	78%	66%
Venous Thromboembolism Prophylaxis[5]	-	-	96%	94%
Written Stroke Educational Materials Given[5]	-	-	87%	88%
Surgical Care Improvement Project				
Appropriate Beta Blocker Usage[5]	-	-	98%	98%
Appropriate VTP Within 24 Hours[5]	-	-	98%	98%
Controlled Postoperative Blood Glucose[5]	-	-	96%	97%
Perioperative Temperature Management[5]	-	-	99%	100%
Prophylactic Antibiotic Selection[5]	-	-	99%	99%
Prophylactic Antibiotic Selection (Outpatient)[5]	-	-	98%	98%
Prophylactic Antibiotic Stopped[5]	-	-	98%	98%
Prophylactic Antibiotic Timing[5]	-	-	98%	99%
Prophylactic Antibiotic Timing (Outpatient)[5]	-	-	98%	98%
Urinary Catheter Removal[5]	-	-	97%	97%
Survey of Patients' Hospital Experiences				
Area Around Room 'Always' Quiet at Night[5]	-	-	64%	61%
Doctors 'Always' Communicated Well[5]	-	-	81%	82%
Home Recovery Information Given[5]	-	-	87%	85%
Hospital Given 9 or 10 on 10 Point Scale[5]	-	-	75%	71%
Meds 'Always' Explained Before Given[5]	-	-	67%	64%
Nurses 'Always' Communicated Well[5]	-	-	79%	79%
Pain 'Always' Well Controlled[5]	-	-	72%	71%
Room and Bathroom 'Always' Clean[5]	-	-	74%	73%
Timely Help 'Always' Received[5]	-	-	70%	68%
Would Definitely Recommend Hospital[5]	-	-	76%	71%
Use of Medical Imaging				
Cardiac Imaging Stress Test before Surgery[1]	-	-	5%	5.3%
Combination Abdominal CT Scan[1]	-	-	10%	10.5%
Combination Brain/Sinus CT Scan	37	0.0%	2.1%	2.7%
Combination Chest CT Scan[1]	-	-	3.1%	2.7%
Follow-up Mammogram/Ultrasound[1]	-	-	8.7%	8.8%
Lumbar Spine MRI for Low Back Pain[1]	-	-	39.7%	37.2%

Lincoln Community Hospital

111 6th St
Hugo, CO 80821
Phone: 719-743-2421
Type: Critical Access Hospitals
Emergency Services: Yes
Ownership: Voluntary non-profit - Other

Measure	Cases	This Hosp.	State Avg.	U.S. Avg.
Blood Clot Prevention and Treatment				
Anticoagulation Overlap Therapy[5]	-	-	97%	93%
ICU Venous Thromboembolism Prophylaxis[5]	-	-	95%	92%
Incidence of Potentially Preventable VTE[5]	-	-	8%	10%
UFH with Dosages/Platelet Monitoring[5]	-	-	97%	97%
Venous Thromboembolism Prophylaxis[5]	-	-	90%	85%
Warfarin Therapy Discharge Instructions[5]	-	-	69%	75%
Chest Pain/Possible Heart Attack Care				
Aspirin Given Within 24 Hours of Arrival	-	-	97%	96%
Fibrinolytic Meds Within 30 Min. of Arrival	-	-	55%	58%
Average Time to ECG (minutes)	-	-	8	7
Average Time to Transfer (minutes)	-	-	74	60
Children's Asthma Care				
Received Home Management Plan of Care	-	-	-	88%
Received Reliever Medication	-	-	-	100%
Received Systemic Corticosteroids	-	-	-	100%
Emergency Department				
Admittance Decision Time (minutes)[5]	-	-	96	98
Head CT Results Within 45 Min. of Arrival	-	-	67%	57%
Patients Who Left ER Before Being Seen	-	-	2%	2%
Time from ER Arrival to Admit. (minutes)[5]	-	-	244	274
Time from ER Arrival to Discharge (minutes)	-	-	139	134
Time in ER Before Being Evaluated (minutes)	-	-	20	26
Time to Pain Meds for Fractures (minutes)	-	-	45	57
Heart Attack Care				
Aspirin Given at Discharge[5]	-	-	100%	99%
Fibrinolytic Meds Within 30 Min. of Arrival[5]	-	-	20%	54%
PCI Within 90 Minutes of Arrival[5]	-	-	97%	96%
Statin Prescribed at Discharge[5]	-	-	99%	98%
Heart Failure Care				
ACE Inhibitor or ARB for LVSD[1,3]	-	-	97%	97%
Discharge Instructions Given[1,3]	-	-	93%	94%
Evaluation of LVS Function[1,3]	-	-	99%	99%
Medicare Spending				
Medicare Spending per Patient (ratio)	-	-	0.95	0.98
Pneumonia Care				
Appropriate Initial Antibiotic Given[3]	11	91%	95%	95%
Blood Culture Timing[3]	12	83%	98%	98%
Pregnancy and Delivery Care				
Newborn Deliveries Scheduled Early[5]	-	-	2%	6%
Preventive Care				
Immunization for Influenza[5]	-	-	92%	90%
Immunization for Pneumonia[5]	-	-	92%	92%
Stroke Care				
Anticoagulation Therapy for Atrial Fibrillation[5]	-	-	97%	95%
Antithrombotic Therapy Timing[5]	-	-	98%	98%
Assessed for Rehabilitation[5]	-	-	98%	97%
Discharged on Antithrombotic Therapy[5]	-	-	100%	99%
Discharged on Statin Medication[5]	-	-	94%	94%
Thrombolytic Therapy Timing[5]	-	-	78%	66%
Venous Thromboembolism Prophylaxis[5]	-	-	96%	94%
Written Stroke Educational Materials Given[5]	-	-	87%	88%
Surgical Care Improvement Project				
Appropriate Beta Blocker Usage[5]	-	-	98%	98%
Appropriate VTP Within 24 Hours[5]	-	-	98%	98%
Controlled Postoperative Blood Glucose[5]	-	-	96%	97%
Perioperative Temperature Management[5]	-	-	99%	100%
Prophylactic Antibiotic Selection[5]	-	-	99%	99%
Prophylactic Antibiotic Selection (Outpatient)	-	-	98%	98%
Prophylactic Antibiotic Stopped[5]	-	-	98%	98%
Prophylactic Antibiotic Timing[5]	-	-	98%	99%
Prophylactic Antibiotic Timing (Outpatient)	-	-	98%	98%
Urinary Catheter Removal[5]	-	-	97%	97%
Survey of Patients' Hospital Experiences				
Area Around Room 'Always' Quiet at Night[5]	-	-	64%	61%
Doctors 'Always' Communicated Well[5]	-	-	81%	82%
Home Recovery Information Given[5]	-	-	87%	85%
Hospital Given 9 or 10 on 10 Point Scale[5]	-	-	75%	71%
Meds 'Always' Explained Before Given[5]	-	-	67%	64%
Nurses 'Always' Communicated Well[5]	-	-	79%	79%
Pain 'Always' Well Controlled[5]	-	-	72%	71%
Room and Bathroom 'Always' Clean[5]	-	-	74%	73%
Timely Help 'Always' Received[5]	-	-	70%	68%
Would Definitely Recommend Hospital[5]	-	-	76%	71%
Use of Medical Imaging				
Cardiac Imaging Stress Test before Surgery	-	-	5%	5.3%
Combination Abdominal CT Scan	-	-	10%	10.5%
Combination Brain/Sinus CT Scan	-	-	2.1%	2.7%
Combination Chest CT Scan	-	-	3.1%	2.7%
Follow-up Mammogram/Ultrasound	-	-	8.7%	8.8%
Lumbar Spine MRI for Low Back Pain	-	-	39.7%	37.2%

Sedgwick County Memorial Hospital

900 Cedar Street
Julesburg, CO 80737
Phone: 970-474-3323
Type: Critical Access Hospitals
Emergency Services: No
Ownership: Government - Local

Measure	Cases	This Hosp.	State Avg.	U.S. Avg.
Blood Clot Prevention and Treatment				
Anticoagulation Overlap Therapy[5]	-	-	97%	93%
ICU Venous Thromboembolism Prophylaxis[5]	-	-	95%	92%
Incidence of Potentially Preventable VTE[5]	-	-	8%	10%
UFH with Dosages/Platelet Monitoring[5]	-	-	97%	97%
Venous Thromboembolism Prophylaxis[5]	-	-	90%	85%
Warfarin Therapy Discharge Instructions[5]	-	-	69%	75%
Chest Pain/Possible Heart Attack Care				
Aspirin Given Within 24 Hours of Arrival[5]	-	-	97%	96%
Fibrinolytic Meds Within 30 Min. of Arrival[5]	-	-	55%	58%
Average Time to ECG (minutes)[5]	-	-	8	7
Average Time to Transfer (minutes)[5]	-	-	74	60
Children's Asthma Care				
Received Home Management Plan of Care	-	-	-	88%
Received Reliever Medication	-	-	-	100%
Received Systemic Corticosteroids	-	-	-	100%
Emergency Department				
Admittance Decision Time (minutes)[5]	-	-	96	98
Head CT Results Within 45 Min. of Arrival[5]	-	-	67%	57%
Patients Who Left ER Before Being Seen[5]	-	-	2%	2%
Time from ER Arrival to Admit. (minutes)[5]	-	-	244	274
Time from ER Arrival to Discharge (minutes)[5]	-	-	139	134
Time in ER Before Being Evaluated (minutes)[5]	-	-	20	26
Time to Pain Meds for Fractures (minutes)[5]	-	-	45	57
Heart Attack Care				
Aspirin Given at Discharge[5]	-	-	100%	99%
Fibrinolytic Meds Within 30 Min. of Arrival[5]	-	-	20%	54%
PCI Within 90 Minutes of Arrival[5]	-	-	97%	96%
Statin Prescribed at Discharge[5]	-	-	99%	98%
Heart Failure Care				
ACE Inhibitor or ARB for LVSD[5]	-	-	97%	97%
Discharge Instructions Given[5]	-	-	93%	94%
Evaluation of LVS Function[5]	-	-	99%	99%
Medicare Spending				
Medicare Spending per Patient (ratio)	-	-	0.95	0.98
Pneumonia Care				
Appropriate Initial Antibiotic Given[5]	-	-	95%	95%
Blood Culture Timing[5]	-	-	98%	98%
Pregnancy and Delivery Care				
Newborn Deliveries Scheduled Early[5]	-	-	2%	6%
Preventive Care				
Immunization for Influenza[5]	-	-	92%	90%
Immunization for Pneumonia[5]	-	-	92%	92%
Stroke Care				
Anticoagulation Therapy for Atrial Fibrillation[5]	-	-	97%	95%
Antithrombotic Therapy Timing[5]	-	-	98%	98%
Assessed for Rehabilitation[5]	-	-	98%	97%
Discharged on Antithrombotic Therapy[5]	-	-	100%	99%
Discharged on Statin Medication[5]	-	-	94%	94%
Thrombolytic Therapy Timing[5]	-	-	78%	66%
Venous Thromboembolism Prophylaxis[5]	-	-	96%	94%
Written Stroke Educational Materials Given[5]	-	-	87%	88%
Surgical Care Improvement Project				
Appropriate Beta Blocker Usage[5]	-	-	98%	98%
Appropriate VTP Within 24 Hours[5]	-	-	98%	98%
Controlled Postoperative Blood Glucose[5]	-	-	96%	97%
Perioperative Temperature Management[5]	-	-	99%	100%
Prophylactic Antibiotic Selection[5]	-	-	99%	99%
Prophylactic Antibiotic Selection (Outpatient)[5]	-	-	98%	98%

NOTE: Hospital profiles are in alphabetical order by state, then city, then hospital within the city; Rankings exclude hospitals with less than 25 cases except for patient surveys which excludes hospitals with less than 100 cases; (a) 100-299 cases; (1) The number of cases/patients is too few to report; (2) Data submitted were based on a sample of cases/patients; (3) Results are based on a shorter time period than required; (4) Data suppressed by CMS for one or more quarters; (5) Results are not available for this reporting period; (6) Fewer than 100 patients completed the HCAHPS survey; (7) No cases met the criteria for this measure; (8) The lower limit of the confidence interval cannot be calculated if the number of observed infections equals zero; (9) No data are available from the state/territory for this reporting period; (10) The scores shown reflect fewer than 50 completed surveys; (11) There were discrepancies in the data collection process; (12) This measure does not apply to this hospital for this reporting period; (13) Results cannot be calculated for this reporting period; (14) The results for this state are combined with nearby states to protect confidentiality; Please refer to the User's Guide for a full explanation of data.

Measure	Cases	This Hosp.	State Avg.	U.S. Avg.
Prophylactic Antibiotic Stopped[5]	-	-	98%	98%
Prophylactic Antibiotic Timing[5]	-	-	98%	99%
Prophylactic Antibiotic Timing (Outpatient)[5]	-	-	98%	98%
Urinary Catheter Removal[5]	-	-	97%	97%
Survey of Patients' Hospital Experiences				
Area Around Room 'Always' Quiet at Night[5]	-	-	64%	61%
Doctors 'Always' Communicated Well[5]	-	-	81%	82%
Home Recovery Information Given[5]	-	-	87%	85%
Hospital Given 9 or 10 on 10 Point Scale[5]	-	-	75%	71%
Meds 'Always' Explained Before Given[5]	-	-	67%	64%
Nurses 'Always' Communicated Well[5]	-	-	79%	79%
Pain 'Always' Well Controlled[5]	-	-	72%	71%
Room and Bathroom 'Always' Clean[5]	-	-	74%	73%
Timely Help 'Always' Received[5]	-	-	70%	68%
Would Definitely Recommend Hospital[5]	-	-	76%	71%
Use of Medical Imaging				
Cardiac Imaging Stress Test before Surgery[1]	-	-	5%	5.3%
Combination Abdominal CT Scan[1]	-	-	10%	10.5%
Combination Brain/Sinus CT Scan	33	0.0%	2.1%	2.7%
Combination Chest CT Scan[1]	-	-	3.1%	2.7%
Follow-up Mammogram/Ultrasound	67	7.5%	8.7%	8.8%
Lumbar Spine MRI for Low Back Pain[1]	-	-	39.7%	37.2%

Middle Park Medical Center

214 S 4th Street Phone: 970-724-3442
Kremmling, CO 80459
Type: Critical Access Hospitals Emergency Services: Yes
Ownership: Govt - Hospital Dist/Auth

Measure	Cases	This Hosp.	State Avg.	U.S. Avg.
Blood Clot Prevention and Treatment				
Anticoagulation Overlap Therapy[5]	-	-	97%	93%
ICU Venous Thromboembolism Prophylaxis[5]	-	-	95%	92%
Incidence of Potentially Preventable VTE[5]	-	-	8%	10%
UFH with Dosages/Platelet Monitoring[5]	-	-	97%	97%
Venous Thromboembolism Prophylaxis[5]	-	-	90%	85%
Warfarin Therapy Discharge Instructions[5]	-	-	69%	75%
Chest Pain/Possible Heart Attack Care				
Aspirin Given Within 24 Hours of Arrival	-	-	97%	96%
Fibrinolytic Meds Within 30 Min. of Arrival	-	-	55%	58%
Average Time to ECG (minutes)	-	-	8	7
Average Time to Transfer (minutes)	-	-	74	60
Children's Asthma Care				
Received Home Management Plan of Care	-	-	-	88%
Received Reliever Medication	-	-	-	100%
Received Systemic Corticosteroids	-	-	-	100%
Emergency Department				
Admittance Decision Time (minutes)[5]	-	-	96	98
Head CT Results Within 45 Min. of Arrival	-	-	67%	57%
Patients Who Left ER Before Being Seen	-	-	2%	2%
Time from ER Arrival to Admit. (minutes)[5]	-	-	244	274
Time from ER Arrival to Discharge (minutes)	-	-	139	134
Time in ER Before Being Evaluated (minutes)	-	-	20	26
Time to Pain Meds for Fractures (minutes)	-	-	45	57
Heart Attack Care				
Aspirin Given at Discharge[5]	-	-	100%	99%
Fibrinolytic Meds Within 30 Min. of Arrival[5]	-	-	20%	54%
PCI Within 90 Minutes of Arrival[5]	-	-	97%	96%
Statin Prescribed at Discharge[5]	-	-	99%	98%
Heart Failure Care				
ACE Inhibitor or ARB for LVSD[3,7]	-	-	97%	97%
Discharge Instructions Given[1,3]	-	-	93%	94%
Evaluation of LVS Function[1,3]	-	-	99%	99%
Medicare Spending				
Medicare Spending per Patient (ratio)	-	-	0.95	0.98
Pneumonia Care				
Appropriate Initial Antibiotic Given[1,2]	-	-	95%	95%
Blood Culture Timing[1,2]	-	-	98%	98%
Pregnancy and Delivery Care				
Newborn Deliveries Scheduled Early[5]	-	-	2%	6%
Preventive Care				
Immunization for Influenza[5]	-	-	92%	90%
Immunization for Pneumonia[5]	-	-	92%	92%
Stroke Care				
Anticoagulation Therapy for Atrial Fibrillation[5]	-	-	97%	95%
Antithrombotic Therapy Timing[5]	-	-	98%	98%
Assessed for Rehabilitation[5]	-	-	98%	97%
Discharged on Antithrombotic Therapy[5]	-	-	100%	99%
Discharged on Statin Medication[5]	-	-	94%	94%
Thrombolytic Therapy Timing[5]	-	-	78%	66%
Venous Thromboembolism Prophylaxis[5]	-	-	96%	94%
Written Stroke Educational Materials Given[5]	-	-	87%	88%
Surgical Care Improvement Project				
Appropriate Beta Blocker Usage[5]	-	-	98%	98%
Appropriate VTP Within 24 Hours[5]	-	-	98%	98%
Controlled Postoperative Blood Glucose[5]	-	-	96%	97%
Perioperative Temperature Management[5]	-	-	99%	100%
Prophylactic Antibiotic Selection[5]	-	-	99%	99%
Prophylactic Antibiotic Selection (Outpatient)	-	-	98%	98%
Prophylactic Antibiotic Stopped[5]	-	-	98%	98%
Prophylactic Antibiotic Timing[5]	-	-	98%	99%
Prophylactic Antibiotic Timing (Outpatient)	-	-	98%	98%
Urinary Catheter Removal[5]	-	-	97%	97%
Survey of Patients' Hospital Experiences				
Area Around Room 'Always' Quiet at Night[5]	-	-	64%	61%
Doctors 'Always' Communicated Well[5]	-	-	81%	82%
Home Recovery Information Given[5]	-	-	87%	85%
Hospital Given 9 or 10 on 10 Point Scale[5]	-	-	75%	71%
Meds 'Always' Explained Before Given[5]	-	-	67%	64%
Nurses 'Always' Communicated Well[5]	-	-	79%	79%
Pain 'Always' Well Controlled[5]	-	-	72%	71%
Room and Bathroom 'Always' Clean[5]	-	-	74%	73%
Timely Help 'Always' Received[5]	-	-	70%	68%
Would Definitely Recommend Hospital[5]	-	-	76%	71%
Use of Medical Imaging				
Cardiac Imaging Stress Test before Surgery	-	-	5%	5.3%
Combination Abdominal CT Scan	-	-	10%	10.5%
Combination Brain/Sinus CT Scan	-	-	2.1%	2.7%
Combination Chest CT Scan	-	-	3.1%	2.7%
Follow-up Mammogram/Ultrasound	-	-	8.7%	8.8%
Lumbar Spine MRI for Low Back Pain	-	-	39.7%	37.2%

San Luis Valley Health Conejos County Hospital

19021 Us Hwy 285 Phone: 719-274-5121
La Jara, CO 81140
Type: Critical Access Hospitals Emergency Services: Yes
Ownership: Voluntary non-profit - Private

Measure	Cases	This Hosp.	State Avg.	U.S. Avg.
Blood Clot Prevention and Treatment				
Anticoagulation Overlap Therapy[5]	-	-	97%	93%
ICU Venous Thromboembolism Prophylaxis[5]	-	-	95%	92%
Incidence of Potentially Preventable VTE[5]	-	-	8%	10%
UFH with Dosages/Platelet Monitoring[5]	-	-	97%	97%
Venous Thromboembolism Prophylaxis[5]	-	-	90%	85%
Warfarin Therapy Discharge Instructions[5]	-	-	69%	75%
Chest Pain/Possible Heart Attack Care				
Aspirin Given Within 24 Hours of Arrival	-	-	97%	96%
Fibrinolytic Meds Within 30 Min. of Arrival	-	-	55%	58%
Average Time to ECG (minutes)	-	-	8	7
Average Time to Transfer (minutes)	-	-	74	60
Children's Asthma Care				
Received Home Management Plan of Care	-	-	-	88%
Received Reliever Medication	-	-	-	100%
Received Systemic Corticosteroids	-	-	-	100%
Emergency Department				
Admittance Decision Time (minutes)[5]	-	-	96	98
Head CT Results Within 45 Min. of Arrival	-	-	67%	57%
Patients Who Left ER Before Being Seen	-	-	2%	2%
Time from ER Arrival to Admit. (minutes)[5]	-	-	244	274
Time from ER Arrival to Discharge (minutes)	-	-	139	134
Time in ER Before Being Evaluated (minutes)	-	-	20	26
Time to Pain Meds for Fractures (minutes)	-	-	45	57
Heart Attack Care				
Aspirin Given at Discharge[5]	-	-	100%	99%
Fibrinolytic Meds Within 30 Min. of Arrival[5]	-	-	20%	54%
PCI Within 90 Minutes of Arrival[5]	-	-	97%	96%
Statin Prescribed at Discharge[5]	-	-	99%	98%
Heart Failure Care				
ACE Inhibitor or ARB for LVSD[3,7]	-	-	97%	97%
Discharge Instructions Given[1,3]	-	-	93%	94%
Evaluation of LVS Function[1,3]	-	-	99%	99%
Medicare Spending				
Medicare Spending per Patient (ratio)	-	-	0.95	0.98
Pneumonia Care				
Appropriate Initial Antibiotic Given[1,3]	-	-	95%	95%
Blood Culture Timing[3,7]	-	-	98%	98%
Pregnancy and Delivery Care				
Newborn Deliveries Scheduled Early[5]	-	-	2%	6%
Preventive Care				
Immunization for Influenza[5]	-	-	92%	90%
Immunization for Pneumonia[5]	-	-	92%	92%
Stroke Care				
Anticoagulation Therapy for Atrial Fibrillation[5]	-	-	97%	95%
Antithrombotic Therapy Timing[5]	-	-	98%	98%
Assessed for Rehabilitation[5]	-	-	98%	97%
Discharged on Antithrombotic Therapy[5]	-	-	100%	99%
Discharged on Statin Medication[5]	-	-	94%	94%
Thrombolytic Therapy Timing[5]	-	-	78%	66%
Venous Thromboembolism Prophylaxis[5]	-	-	96%	94%
Written Stroke Educational Materials Given[5]	-	-	87%	88%
Surgical Care Improvement Project				
Appropriate Beta Blocker Usage[5]	-	-	98%	98%
Appropriate VTP Within 24 Hours[5]	-	-	98%	98%
Controlled Postoperative Blood Glucose[5]	-	-	96%	97%
Perioperative Temperature Management[5]	-	-	99%	100%
Prophylactic Antibiotic Selection[5]	-	-	99%	99%
Prophylactic Antibiotic Selection (Outpatient)	-	-	98%	98%
Prophylactic Antibiotic Stopped[5]	-	-	98%	98%
Prophylactic Antibiotic Timing[5]	-	-	98%	99%
Prophylactic Antibiotic Timing (Outpatient)	-	-	98%	98%
Urinary Catheter Removal[5]	-	-	97%	97%
Survey of Patients' Hospital Experiences				
Area Around Room 'Always' Quiet at Night[5]	-	-	64%	61%
Doctors 'Always' Communicated Well[5]	-	-	81%	82%
Home Recovery Information Given[5]	-	-	87%	85%
Hospital Given 9 or 10 on 10 Point Scale[5]	-	-	75%	71%
Meds 'Always' Explained Before Given[5]	-	-	67%	64%
Nurses 'Always' Communicated Well[5]	-	-	79%	79%
Pain 'Always' Well Controlled[5]	-	-	72%	71%
Room and Bathroom 'Always' Clean[5]	-	-	74%	73%
Timely Help 'Always' Received[5]	-	-	70%	68%
Would Definitely Recommend Hospital[5]	-	-	76%	71%
Use of Medical Imaging				
Cardiac Imaging Stress Test before Surgery	-	-	5%	5.3%
Combination Abdominal CT Scan	-	-	10%	10.5%
Combination Brain/Sinus CT Scan	-	-	2.1%	2.7%
Combination Chest CT Scan	-	-	3.1%	2.7%
Follow-up Mammogram/Ultrasound	-	-	8.7%	8.8%
Lumbar Spine MRI for Low Back Pain	-	-	39.7%	37.2%

Arkansas Valley Regional Medical Center

1100 Carson Avenue Phone: 719-383-6000
La Junta, CO 81050 Fax: 719-383-6005
URL: www.avrmc.org
Type: Acute Care Hospitals Emergency Services: Yes
Ownership: Voluntary non-profit - Private Beds: 203

Key Personnel:

Emergency Room . . . . Mike Archulefer
Radiology. . . . . Joseph L Collins
CEO/President. . . . . Lynn Crowell
Infection Control. . . . . Norman Finkner
Quality Assurance . . . . Cathy Hammons
Operating Room. . . . . Tonya Kersey
Intensive Care Unit. . . . . Amy Piquette
Chief of Medical Staff . . . . Jason Sims DO

Measure	Cases	This Hosp.	State Avg.	U.S. Avg.
Blood Clot Prevention and Treatment				
Anticoagulation Overlap Therapy[2]	12	92%	97%	93%
ICU Venous Thromboembolism Prophylaxis[2]	56	88%	95%	92%

NOTE: Hospital profiles are in alphabetical order by state, then city, then hospital within the city; Rankings exclude hospitals with less than 25 cases except for patient surveys which excludes hospitals with less than 100 cases; (a) 100-299 cases; (1) The number of cases/patients is too few to report; (2) Data submitted were based on a sample of cases/patients; (3) Results are based on a shorter time period than required; (4) Data suppressed by CMS for one or more quarters; (5) Results are not available for this reporting period; (6) Fewer than 100 patients completed the HCAHPS survey; (7) No cases met the criteria for this measure; (8) The lower limit of the confidence interval cannot be calculated if the number of observed infections equals zero; (9) No data are available from the state/territory for this reporting period; (10) The scores shown reflect fewer than 50 completed surveys; (11) There were discrepancies in the data collection process; (12) This measure does not apply to this hospital for this reporting period; (13) Results cannot be calculated for this reporting period; (14) The results for this state are combined with nearby states to protect confidentiality; Please refer to the User's Guide for a full explanation of data.

Incidence of Potentially Preventable VTE[2,7]	-	-	8%	10%
UFH with Dosages/Platelet Monitoring[1,2]	-	-	97%	97%
Venous Thromboembolism Prophylaxis[2]	193	80%	90%	85%
Warfarin Therapy Discharge Instructions[2]	12	100%	69%	75%
Chest Pain/Possible Heart Attack Care				
Aspirin Given Within 24 Hours of Arrival	61	98%	97%	96%
Fibrinolytic Meds Within 30 Min. of Arrival[1]	-	-	55%	58%
Average Time to ECG (minutes)	63	18	8	7
Average Time to Transfer (minutes)[1]	-	-	74	60
Children's Asthma Care				
Received Home Management Plan of Care	-	-	-	88%
Received Reliever Medication	-	-	-	100%
Received Systemic Corticosteroids	-	-	-	100%
Emergency Department				
Admittance Decision Time (minutes)[2]	304	57	96	98
Head CT Results Within 45 Min. of Arrival[1]	-	-	67%	57%
Patients Who Left ER Before Being Seen	6,178	1%	2%	2%
Time from ER Arrival to Admit. (minutes)[2]	317	243	244	274
Time from ER Arrival to Discharge (minutes)	340	114	139	134
Time in ER Before Being Evaluated (minutes)	372	24	20	26
Time to Pain Meds for Fractures (minutes)	20	54	45	57
Heart Attack Care				
Aspirin Given at Discharge[1,2]	-	-	100%	99%
Fibrinolytic Meds Within 30 Min. of Arrival[2,7]	-	-	20%	54%
PCI Within 90 Minutes of Arrival[2,7]	-	-	97%	96%
Statin Prescribed at Discharge[1,2]	-	-	99%	98%
Heart Failure Care				
ACE Inhibitor or ARB for LVSD[2]	14	93%	97%	97%
Discharge Instructions Given[2]	25	96%	93%	94%
Evaluation of LVS Function[2]	40	95%	99%	99%
Medicare Spending				
Medicare Spending per Patient (ratio)	-	0.89	0.95	0.98
Pneumonia Care				
Appropriate Initial Antibiotic Given[2]	105	74%	95%	95%
Blood Culture Timing[2]	107	93%	98%	98%
Pregnancy and Delivery Care				
Newborn Deliveries Scheduled Early[2]	27	0%	2%	6%
Preventive Care				
Immunization for Influenza[2]	252	90%	92%	90%
Immunization for Pneumonia[2]	316	94%	92%	92%
Stroke Care				
Anticoagulation Therapy for Atrial Fibrillation[1,2]	-	-	97%	95%
Antithrombotic Therapy Timing[1,2]	-	-	98%	98%
Assessed for Rehabilitation[2]	14	100%	98%	97%
Discharged on Antithrombotic Therapy[2]	11	100%	100%	99%
Discharged on Statin Medication[1,2]	-	-	94%	94%
Thrombolytic Therapy Timing[1,2]	-	-	78%	66%
Venous Thromboembolism Prophylaxis[2]	15	93%	96%	94%
Written Stroke Educational Materials Given[1,2]	-	-	87%	88%
Surgical Care Improvement Project				
Appropriate Beta Blocker Usage[2]	12	83%	98%	98%
Appropriate VTP Within 24 Hours[2]	44	100%	98%	98%
Controlled Postoperative Blood Glucose[2,7]	-	-	96%	97%
Perioperative Temperature Management[2]	45	100%	99%	100%
Prophylactic Antibiotic Selection[2]	30	87%	99%	99%
Prophylactic Antibiotic Selection (Outpatient)[3,7]	-	-	98%	98%
Prophylactic Antibiotic Stopped[2]	28	100%	98%	98%
Prophylactic Antibiotic Timing[2]	30	90%	98%	99%
Prophylactic Antibiotic Timing (Outpatient)[1,3]	-	-	98%	98%
Urinary Catheter Removal[2]	41	98%	97%	97%
Survey of Patients' Hospital Experiences				
Area Around Room 'Always' Quiet at Night	300+	56%	64%	61%
Doctors 'Always' Communicated Well	300+	80%	81%	82%
Home Recovery Information Given	300+	78%	87%	85%
Hospital Given 9 or 10 on 10 Point Scale	300+	51%	75%	71%
Meds 'Always' Explained Before Given	300+	57%	67%	64%
Nurses 'Always' Communicated Well	300+	73%	79%	79%
Pain 'Always' Well Controlled	300+	67%	72%	71%
Room and Bathroom 'Always' Clean	300+	75%	74%	73%
Timely Help 'Always' Received	300+	65%	70%	68%
Would Definitely Recommend Hospital	300+	47%	76%	71%
Use of Medical Imaging				
Cardiac Imaging Stress Test before Surgery	54	1.9%	5%	5.3%
Combination Abdominal CT Scan	198	1.0%	10%	10.5%
Combination Brain/Sinus CT Scan	168	0.0%	2.1%	2.7%
Combination Chest CT Scan	78	1.3%	3.1%	2.7%
Follow-up Mammogram/Ultrasound	508	1.2%	8.7%	8.8%
Lumbar Spine MRI for Low Back Pain	41	48.8%	39.7%	37.2%

Exempla Good Samaritan Medical Center

200 Exempla Circle Phone: 303-689-4000
Lafayette, CO 80026
URL: www.exempla.org
Type: Acute Care Hospitals Emergency Services: Yes
Ownership: Voluntary non-profit - Private Beds: 202
Key Personnel:
Quality Assurance . . . . Barbara Davis
President/CEO. . . . . David Hamm
Chief of Medical Staff. . . . . Todd Mydler, MD

Measure	Cases	This Hosp.	State Avg.	U.S. Avg.
Blood Clot Prevention and Treatment				
Anticoagulation Overlap Therapy[2]	119	99%	97%	93%
ICU Venous Thromboembolism Prophylaxis[2]	61	97%	95%	92%
Incidence of Potentially Preventable VTE[1,2]	-	-	8%	10%
UFH with Dosages/Platelet Monitoring[2]	82	99%	97%	97%
Venous Thromboembolism Prophylaxis[2]	319	94%	90%	85%
Warfarin Therapy Discharge Instructions[2]	100	86%	69%	75%
Chest Pain/Possible Heart Attack Care				
Aspirin Given Within 24 Hours of Arrival[1,3]	-	-	97%	96%
Fibrinolytic Meds Within 30 Min. of Arrival[5]	-	-	55%	58%
Average Time to ECG (minutes)[1,3]	-	-	8	7
Average Time to Transfer (minutes)[5]	-	-	74	60
Children's Asthma Care				
Received Home Management Plan of Care	-	-	-	88%
Received Reliever Medication	-	-	-	100%
Received Systemic Corticosteroids	-	-	-	100%
Emergency Department				
Admittance Decision Time (minutes)[2]	579	81	96	98
Head CT Results Within 45 Min. of Arrival[1]	-	-	67%	57%
Patients Who Left ER Before Being Seen	40,863	0%	2%	2%
Time from ER Arrival to Admit. (minutes)[2]	581	258	244	274
Time from ER Arrival to Discharge (minutes)	323	181	139	134
Time in ER Before Being Evaluated (minutes)	382	16	20	26
Time to Pain Meds for Fractures (minutes)	197	54	45	57
Heart Attack Care				
Aspirin Given at Discharge	147	100%	100%	99%
Fibrinolytic Meds Within 30 Min. of Arrival[7]	-	-	20%	54%
PCI Within 90 Minutes of Arrival	35	100%	97%	96%
Statin Prescribed at Discharge	140	100%	99%	98%
Heart Failure Care				
ACE Inhibitor or ARB for LVSD	73	96%	97%	97%
Discharge Instructions Given	251	100%	93%	94%
Evaluation of LVS Function	285	100%	99%	99%
Medicare Spending				
Medicare Spending per Patient (ratio)	-	1.00	0.95	0.98
Pneumonia Care				
Appropriate Initial Antibiotic Given	155	99%	95%	95%
Blood Culture Timing	291	100%	98%	98%
Pregnancy and Delivery Care				
Newborn Deliveries Scheduled Early	157	3%	2%	6%
Preventive Care				
Immunization for Influenza[2]	521	93%	92%	90%
Immunization for Pneumonia[2]	610	95%	92%	92%
Stroke Care				
Anticoagulation Therapy for Atrial Fibrillation	15	100%	97%	95%
Antithrombotic Therapy Timing	91	99%	98%	98%
Assessed for Rehabilitation	146	99%	98%	97%
Discharged on Antithrombotic Therapy	131	100%	100%	99%
Discharged on Statin Medication	98	99%	94%	94%
Thrombolytic Therapy Timing	11	100%	78%	66%
Venous Thromboembolism Prophylaxis	119	99%	96%	94%
Written Stroke Educational Materials Given	85	96%	87%	88%
Surgical Care Improvement Project				
Appropriate Beta Blocker Usage[2]	197	100%	98%	98%
Appropriate VTP Within 24 Hours[2]	577	100%	98%	98%
Controlled Postoperative Blood Glucose[2,7]	-	-	96%	97%
Perioperative Temperature Management[2]	628	100%	99%	100%
Prophylactic Antibiotic Selection[2]	457	100%	99%	99%
Prophylactic Antibiotic Selection (Outpatient)	365	99%	98%	98%
Prophylactic Antibiotic Stopped[2]	452	100%	98%	98%
Prophylactic Antibiotic Timing[2]	457	100%	98%	99%
Prophylactic Antibiotic Timing (Outpatient)	366	99%	98%	98%
Urinary Catheter Removal[2]	423	100%	97%	97%
Survey of Patients' Hospital Experiences				
Area Around Room 'Always' Quiet at Night	300+	64%	64%	61%
Doctors 'Always' Communicated Well	300+	81%	81%	82%
Home Recovery Information Given	300+	90%	87%	85%
Hospital Given 9 or 10 on 10 Point Scale	300+	77%	75%	71%
Meds 'Always' Explained Before Given	300+	65%	67%	64%
Nurses 'Always' Communicated Well	300+	77%	79%	79%
Pain 'Always' Well Controlled	300+	69%	72%	71%
Room and Bathroom 'Always' Clean	300+	69%	74%	73%
Timely Help 'Always' Received	300+	63%	70%	68%
Would Definitely Recommend Hospital	300+	81%	76%	71%
Use of Medical Imaging				
Cardiac Imaging Stress Test before Surgery	93	6.5%	5%	5.3%
Combination Abdominal CT Scan	217	8.3%	10%	10.5%
Combination Brain/Sinus CT Scan[1]	-	-	2.1%	2.7%
Combination Chest CT Scan	185	0.5%	3.1%	2.7%
Follow-up Mammogram/Ultrasound	186	14.5%	8.7%	8.8%
Lumbar Spine MRI for Low Back Pain	38	47.4%	39.7%	37.2%

Centura Health - Saint Anthony Hospital

11600 West 2nd Place Phone: 720-321-0000
Lakewood, CO 80228 Fax: 303-629-2318
URL: www.stanthonyhosp.org
Type: Acute Care Hospitals Emergency Services: Yes
Ownership: Voluntary non-profit - Church Beds: 498
Key Personnel:
Radiology. . . . . Clinton Mark Anderson
Chief of Medical Staff . . . . Christopher J. Ott, MD, FACEP
CEO/President. . . . . George A Zara

Measure	Cases	This Hosp.	State Avg.	U.S. Avg.
Blood Clot Prevention and Treatment				
Anticoagulation Overlap Therapy[2]	136	99%	97%	93%
ICU Venous Thromboembolism Prophylaxis[2]	179	100%	95%	92%
Incidence of Potentially Preventable VTE[2]	28	25%	8%	10%
UFH with Dosages/Platelet Monitoring[2]	96	96%	97%	97%
Venous Thromboembolism Prophylaxis[2]	274	91%	90%	85%
Warfarin Therapy Discharge Instructions[2]	94	67%	69%	75%
Chest Pain/Possible Heart Attack Care				
Aspirin Given Within 24 Hours of Arrival[1,3]	-	-	97%	96%
Fibrinolytic Meds Within 30 Min. of Arrival[5]	-	-	55%	58%
Average Time to ECG (minutes)[1,3]	-	-	8	7
Average Time to Transfer (minutes)[5]	-	-	74	60
Children's Asthma Care				
Received Home Management Plan of Care	-	-	-	88%
Received Reliever Medication	-	-	-	100%
Received Systemic Corticosteroids	-	-	-	100%
Emergency Department				
Admittance Decision Time (minutes)[2]	783	82	96	98
Head CT Results Within 45 Min. of Arrival[1]	-	-	67%	57%
Patients Who Left ER Before Being Seen	46,501	0%	2%	2%
Time from ER Arrival to Admit. (minutes)[2]	810	202	244	274
Time from ER Arrival to Discharge (minutes)	424	126	139	134
Time in ER Before Being Evaluated (minutes)	243	8	20	26
Time to Pain Meds for Fractures (minutes)	232	36	45	57
Heart Attack Care				
Aspirin Given at Discharge	288	100%	100%	99%
Fibrinolytic Meds Within 30 Min. of Arrival[7]	-	-	20%	54%
PCI Within 90 Minutes of Arrival	106	97%	97%	96%
Statin Prescribed at Discharge	290	100%	99%	98%
Heart Failure Care				
ACE Inhibitor or ARB for LVSD	56	100%	97%	97%
Discharge Instructions Given	148	96%	93%	94%
Evaluation of LVS Function	201	100%	99%	99%
Medicare Spending				
Medicare Spending per Patient (ratio)	-	1.02	0.95	0.98

NOTE: Hospital profiles are in alphabetical order by state, then city, then hospital within the city; Rankings exclude hospitals with less than 25 cases except for patient surveys which excludes hospitals with less than 100 cases; (a) 100-299 cases; (1) The number of cases/patients is too few to report; (2) Data submitted were based on a sample of cases/patients; (3) Results are based on a shorter time period than required; (4) Data suppressed by CMS for one or more quarters; (5) Results are not available for this reporting period; (6) Fewer than 100 patients completed the HCAHPS survey; (7) No cases met the criteria for this measure; (8) The lower limit of the confidence interval cannot be calculated if the number of observed infections equals zero; (9) No data are available from the state/territory for this reporting period; (10) The scores shown reflect fewer than 50 completed surveys; (11) There were discrepancies in the data collection process; (12) This measure does not apply to this hospital for this reporting period; (13) Results cannot be calculated for this reporting period; (14) The results for this state are combined with nearby states to protect confidentiality; Please refer to the User's Guide for a full explanation of data.

Pneumonia Care				
Appropriate Initial Antibiotic Given[2]	93	100%	95%	95%
Blood Culture Timing[2]	137	96%	98%	98%
Pregnancy and Delivery Care				
Newborn Deliveries Scheduled Early[2,7]	-	-	2%	6%
Preventive Care				
Immunization for Influenza[2]	644	94%	92%	90%
Immunization for Pneumonia[2]	805	93%	92%	92%
Stroke Care				
Anticoagulation Therapy for Atrial Fibrillation	35	100%	97%	95%
Antithrombotic Therapy Timing	132	98%	98%	98%
Assessed for Rehabilitation	268	99%	98%	97%
Discharged on Antithrombotic Therapy	197	99%	100%	99%
Discharged on Statin Medication	123	93%	94%	94%
Thrombolytic Therapy Timing	50	40%	78%	66%
Venous Thromboembolism Prophylaxis	274	98%	96%	94%
Written Stroke Educational Materials Given	141	97%	87%	88%
Surgical Care Improvement Project				
Appropriate Beta Blocker Usage[2]	170	97%	98%	98%
Appropriate VTP Within 24 Hours[2]	337	98%	98%	98%
Controlled Postoperative Blood Glucose[2]	104	95%	96%	97%
Perioperative Temperature Management[2]	420	100%	99%	100%
Prophylactic Antibiotic Selection[2]	349	99%	99%	99%
Prophylactic Antibiotic Selection (Outpatient)	264	100%	98%	98%
Prophylactic Antibiotic Stopped[2]	336	97%	98%	98%
Prophylactic Antibiotic Timing[2]	349	99%	98%	99%
Prophylactic Antibiotic Timing (Outpatient)	266	96%	98%	98%
Urinary Catheter Removal[2]	307	96%	97%	97%
Survey of Patients' Hospital Experiences				
Area Around Room 'Always' Quiet at Night	300+	60%	64%	61%
Doctors 'Always' Communicated Well	300+	78%	81%	82%
Home Recovery Information Given	300+	88%	87%	85%
Hospital Given 9 or 10 on 10 Point Scale	300+	76%	75%	71%
Meds 'Always' Explained Before Given	300+	62%	67%	64%
Nurses 'Always' Communicated Well	300+	77%	79%	79%
Pain 'Always' Well Controlled	300+	70%	72%	71%
Room and Bathroom 'Always' Clean	300+	73%	74%	73%
Timely Help 'Always' Received	300+	64%	70%	68%
Would Definitely Recommend Hospital	300+	79%	76%	71%
Use of Medical Imaging				
Cardiac Imaging Stress Test before Surgery	136	9.6%	5%	5.3%
Combination Abdominal CT Scan	507	3.4%	10%	10.5%
Combination Brain/Sinus CT Scan[1]	-	-	2.1%	2.7%
Combination Chest CT Scan	255	1.2%	3.1%	2.7%
Follow-up Mammogram/Ultrasound	297	8.1%	8.7%	8.8%
Lumbar Spine MRI for Low Back Pain	59	42.4%	39.7%	37.2%

Orthocolorado Hospital at Saint Anthony Medical Campus

11650 W 2nd Place
Lakewood, CO 80228
Phone: 720-321-5000
URL: www.orthocolorado.org
Type: Acute Care Hospitals
Emergency Services: Yes
Ownership: Proprietary
Beds: 222

Key Personnel:

CEO .... Jude Torchia

Measure	Cases	This Hosp.	State Avg.	U.S. Avg.
Blood Clot Prevention and Treatment				
Anticoagulation Overlap Therapy[1,2]	-	-	97%	93%
ICU Venous Thromboembolism Prophylaxis[2,7]	-	-	95%	92%
Incidence of Potentially Preventable VTE[2,7]	-	-	8%	10%
UFH with Dosages/Platelet Monitoring[2,7]	-	-	97%	97%
Venous Thromboembolism Prophylaxis[2]	64	100%	90%	85%
Warfarin Therapy Discharge Instructions[1,2]	-	-	69%	75%
Chest Pain/Possible Heart Attack Care				
Aspirin Given Within 24 Hours of Arrival[5]	-	-	97%	96%
Fibrinolytic Meds Within 30 Min. of Arrival[5]	-	-	55%	58%
Average Time to ECG (minutes)[5]	-	-	8	7
Average Time to Transfer (minutes)[5]	-	-	74	60
Children's Asthma Care				
Received Home Management Plan of Care	-	-	-	88%
Received Reliever Medication	-	-	-	100%
Received Systemic Corticosteroids	-	-	-	100%
Emergency Department				
Admittance Decision Time (minutes)[2,7]	-	-	96	98
Head CT Results Within 45 Min. of Arrival[5]	-	-	67%	57%
Patients Who Left ER Before Being Seen[5]	-	-	2%	2%
Time from ER Arrival to Admit. (minutes)[2,7]	-	-	244	274
Time from ER Arrival to Discharge (minutes)[5]	-	-	139	134
Time in ER Before Being Evaluated (minutes)[5]	-	-	20	26
Time to Pain Meds for Fractures (minutes)[5]	-	-	45	57
Heart Attack Care				
Aspirin Given at Discharge[5]	-	-	100%	99%
Fibrinolytic Meds Within 30 Min. of Arrival[5]	-	-	20%	54%
PCI Within 90 Minutes of Arrival[5]	-	-	97%	96%
Statin Prescribed at Discharge[5]	-	-	99%	98%
Heart Failure Care				
ACE Inhibitor or ARB for LVSD[5]	-	-	97%	97%
Discharge Instructions Given[5]	-	-	93%	94%
Evaluation of LVS Function[5]	-	-	99%	99%
Medicare Spending				
Medicare Spending per Patient (ratio)	-	0.90	0.95	0.98
Pneumonia Care				
Appropriate Initial Antibiotic Given[5]	-	-	95%	95%
Blood Culture Timing[5]	-	-	98%	98%
Pregnancy and Delivery Care				
Newborn Deliveries Scheduled Early[2,7]	-	-	2%	6%
Preventive Care				
Immunization for Influenza[2]	358	78%	92%	90%
Immunization for Pneumonia[2]	456	84%	92%	92%
Stroke Care				
Anticoagulation Therapy for Atrial Fibrillation[5]	-	-	97%	95%
Antithrombotic Therapy Timing[5]	-	-	98%	98%
Assessed for Rehabilitation[5]	-	-	98%	97%
Discharged on Antithrombotic Therapy[5]	-	-	100%	99%
Discharged on Statin Medication[5]	-	-	94%	94%
Thrombolytic Therapy Timing[5]	-	-	78%	66%
Venous Thromboembolism Prophylaxis[5]	-	-	96%	94%
Written Stroke Educational Materials Given[5]	-	-	87%	88%
Surgical Care Improvement Project				
Appropriate Beta Blocker Usage[2]	82	96%	98%	98%
Appropriate VTP Within 24 Hours[2]	308	100%	98%	98%
Controlled Postoperative Blood Glucose[2,7]	-	-	96%	97%
Perioperative Temperature Management[2]	352	100%	99%	100%
Prophylactic Antibiotic Selection[2]	267	100%	99%	99%
Prophylactic Antibiotic Selection (Outpatient)	174	100%	98%	98%
Prophylactic Antibiotic Stopped[2]	266	100%	98%	98%
Prophylactic Antibiotic Timing[2]	267	99%	98%	99%
Prophylactic Antibiotic Timing (Outpatient)	174	99%	98%	98%
Urinary Catheter Removal[2]	325	100%	97%	97%
Survey of Patients' Hospital Experiences				
Area Around Room 'Always' Quiet at Night	300+	75%	64%	61%
Doctors 'Always' Communicated Well	300+	85%	81%	82%
Home Recovery Information Given	300+	91%	87%	85%
Hospital Given 9 or 10 on 10 Point Scale	300+	81%	75%	71%
Meds 'Always' Explained Before Given	300+	69%	67%	64%
Nurses 'Always' Communicated Well	300+	81%	79%	79%
Pain 'Always' Well Controlled	300+	73%	72%	71%
Room and Bathroom 'Always' Clean	300+	84%	74%	73%
Timely Help 'Always' Received	300+	66%	70%	68%
Would Definitely Recommend Hospital	300+	83%	76%	71%
Use of Medical Imaging				
Cardiac Imaging Stress Test before Surgery[7]	-	-	5%	5.3%
Combination Abdominal CT Scan[7]	-	-	10%	10.5%
Combination Brain/Sinus CT Scan[7]	-	-	2.1%	2.7%
Combination Chest CT Scan[7]	-	-	3.1%	2.7%
Follow-up Mammogram/Ultrasound[7]	-	-	8.7%	8.8%
Lumbar Spine MRI for Low Back Pain[7]	-	-	39.7%	37.2%

Prowers Medical Center

401 Kendall Drive
Lamar, CO 81052
Phone: 719-336-4343
Fax: 719-336-3805
E-mail: shawnah@lpmc.org
URL: www.prowersmedical.com
Type: Critical Access Hospitals
Emergency Services: Yes
Ownership: Govt - Hospital Dist/Auth
Beds: 28

Key Personnel:

Radiology.................. Maxwell Bret Abbott
Quality Assurance .... Karen Bryant
Chief of Medical Staff.......... Sam Downing
Pediatric Ambulatory Care ...... Gino Figlio, MD
Cardiology.................. George Gibson, MD
Pediatric In-Patient Care .... Nikki Hamilton
CEO .... Craig R. Loveless
Infection Control.............. Martha Thompson

Measure	Cases	This Hosp.	State Avg.	U.S. Avg.
Blood Clot Prevention and Treatment				
Anticoagulation Overlap Therapy[5]	-	-	97%	93%
ICU Venous Thromboembolism Prophylaxis[5]	-	-	95%	92%
Incidence of Potentially Preventable VTE[5]	-	-	8%	10%
UFH with Dosages/Platelet Monitoring[5]	-	-	97%	97%
Venous Thromboembolism Prophylaxis[5]	-	-	90%	85%
Warfarin Therapy Discharge Instructions[5]	-	-	69%	75%
Chest Pain/Possible Heart Attack Care				
Aspirin Given Within 24 Hours of Arrival	-	-	97%	96%
Fibrinolytic Meds Within 30 Min. of Arrival	-	-	55%	58%
Average Time to ECG (minutes)	-	-	8	7
Average Time to Transfer (minutes)	-	-	74	60
Children's Asthma Care				
Received Home Management Plan of Care	-	-	-	88%
Received Reliever Medication	-	-	-	100%
Received Systemic Corticosteroids	-	-	-	100%
Emergency Department				
Admittance Decision Time (minutes)[1,3]	-	-	96	98
Head CT Results Within 45 Min. of Arrival	-	-	67%	57%
Patients Who Left ER Before Being Seen	-	-	2%	2%
Time from ER Arrival to Admit. (minutes)[1,3]	-	-	244	274
Time from ER Arrival to Discharge (minutes)	-	-	139	134
Time in ER Before Being Evaluated (minutes)	-	-	20	26
Time to Pain Meds for Fractures (minutes)	-	-	45	57
Heart Attack Care				
Aspirin Given at Discharge[5]	-	-	100%	99%
Fibrinolytic Meds Within 30 Min. of Arrival[5]	-	-	20%	54%
PCI Within 90 Minutes of Arrival[5]	-	-	97%	96%
Statin Prescribed at Discharge[5]	-	-	99%	98%
Heart Failure Care				
ACE Inhibitor or ARB for LVSD[3,7]	-	-	97%	97%
Discharge Instructions Given[1,3]	-	-	93%	94%
Evaluation of LVS Function[1,3]	-	-	99%	99%
Medicare Spending				
Medicare Spending per Patient (ratio)	-	-	0.95	0.98
Pneumonia Care				
Appropriate Initial Antibiotic Given[1,3]	-	-	95%	95%
Blood Culture Timing[1,3]	-	-	98%	98%
Pregnancy and Delivery Care				
Newborn Deliveries Scheduled Early[5]	-	-	2%	6%
Preventive Care				
Immunization for Influenza[3]	21	52%	92%	90%
Immunization for Pneumonia[3]	20	50%	92%	92%
Stroke Care				
Anticoagulation Therapy for Atrial Fibrillation[5]	-	-	97%	95%
Antithrombotic Therapy Timing[5]	-	-	98%	98%
Assessed for Rehabilitation[5]	-	-	98%	97%
Discharged on Antithrombotic Therapy[5]	-	-	100%	99%
Discharged on Statin Medication[5]	-	-	94%	94%
Thrombolytic Therapy Timing[5]	-	-	78%	66%
Venous Thromboembolism Prophylaxis[5]	-	-	96%	94%
Written Stroke Educational Materials Given[5]	-	-	87%	88%
Surgical Care Improvement Project				
Appropriate Beta Blocker Usage[5]	-	-	98%	98%
Appropriate VTP Within 24 Hours[5]	-	-	98%	98%
Controlled Postoperative Blood Glucose[5]	-	-	96%	97%
Perioperative Temperature Management[5]	-	-	99%	100%

NOTE: Hospital profiles are in alphabetical order by state, then city, then hospital within the city; Rankings exclude hospitals with less than 25 cases except for patient surveys which excludes hospitals with less than 100 cases; (a) 100-299 cases; (1) The number of cases/patients is too few to report; (2) Data submitted were based on a sample of cases/patients; (3) Results are based on a shorter time period than required; (4) Data suppressed by CMS for one or more quarters; (5) Results are not available for this reporting period; (6) Fewer than 100 patients completed the HCAHPS survey; (7) No cases met the criteria for this measure; (8) The lower limit of the confidence interval cannot be calculated if the number of observed infections equals zero; (9) No data are available from the state/territory for this reporting period; (10) The scores shown reflect fewer than 50 completed surveys; (11) There were discrepancies in the data collection process; (12) This measure does not apply to this hospital for this reporting period; (13) Results cannot be calculated for this reporting period; (14) The results for this state are combined with nearby states to protect confidentiality; Please refer to the User's Guide for a full explanation of data.

Measure	Cases	This Hosp.	State Avg.	U.S. Avg.
Prophylactic Antibiotic Selection[5]	-	-	99%	99%
Prophylactic Antibiotic Selection (Outpatient)	-	-	98%	98%
Prophylactic Antibiotic Stopped[5]	-	-	98%	98%
Prophylactic Antibiotic Timing[5]	-	-	98%	99%
Prophylactic Antibiotic Timing (Outpatient)	-	-	98%	98%
Urinary Catheter Removal[5]	-	-	97%	97%
Survey of Patients' Hospital Experiences				
Area Around Room 'Always' Quiet at Night[5]	-	-	64%	61%
Doctors 'Always' Communicated Well[5]	-	-	81%	82%
Home Recovery Information Given[5]	-	-	87%	85%
Hospital Given 9 or 10 on 10 Point Scale[5]	-	-	75%	71%
Meds 'Always' Explained Before Given[5]	-	-	67%	64%
Nurses 'Always' Communicated Well[5]	-	-	79%	79%
Pain 'Always' Well Controlled[5]	-	-	72%	71%
Room and Bathroom 'Always' Clean[5]	-	-	74%	73%
Timely Help 'Always' Received[5]	-	-	70%	68%
Would Definitely Recommend Hospital[5]	-	-	76%	71%
Use of Medical Imaging				
Cardiac Imaging Stress Test before Surgery	-	-	5%	5.3%
Combination Abdominal CT Scan	-	-	10%	10.5%
Combination Brain/Sinus CT Scan	-	-	2.1%	2.7%
Combination Chest CT Scan	-	-	3.1%	2.7%
Follow-up Mammogram/Ultrasound	-	-	8.7%	8.8%
Lumbar Spine MRI for Low Back Pain	-	-	39.7%	37.2%

Saint Vincent Hospital General District

822 W 4th Street Phone: 719-486-0230
Leadville, CO 80461 Fax: 719-486-1077
E-mail: info@svghd.org
URL: www.svghd.org
Type: Critical Access Hospitals Emergency Services: Yes
Ownership: Govt - Hospital Dist/Auth Beds: 25

Key Personnel:
CEO . . . . Joyce Beck
Operating Room. . . . . Birgit Brilliot
Emergency Room . . . . Jone Fretz
Patient Relations . . . . Jo Johnson
Infection Control. . . . . Sarah Martin
Anesthesiology. . . . . Charles Moss, CRNA
Chief of Medical Staff . . . . Lisa Zwerdlinger, MD

Measure	Cases	This Hosp.	State Avg.	U.S. Avg.
Blood Clot Prevention and Treatment				
Anticoagulation Overlap Therapy[5]	-	-	97%	93%
ICU Venous Thromboembolism Prophylaxis[5]	-	-	95%	92%
Incidence of Potentially Preventable VTE[5]	-	-	8%	10%
UFH with Dosages/Platelet Monitoring[5]	-	-	97%	97%
Venous Thromboembolism Prophylaxis[5]	-	-	90%	85%
Warfarin Therapy Discharge Instructions[5]	-	-	69%	75%
Chest Pain/Possible Heart Attack Care				
Aspirin Given Within 24 Hours of Arrival	-	-	97%	96%
Fibrinolytic Meds Within 30 Min. of Arrival	-	-	55%	58%
Average Time to ECG (minutes)	-	-	8	7
Average Time to Transfer (minutes)	-	-	74	60
Children's Asthma Care				
Received Home Management Plan of Care	-	-	-	88%
Received Reliever Medication	-	-	-	100%
Received Systemic Corticosteroids	-	-	-	100%
Emergency Department				
Admittance Decision Time (minutes)[5]	-	-	96	98
Head CT Results Within 45 Min. of Arrival	-	-	67%	57%
Patients Who Left ER Before Being Seen	-	-	2%	2%
Time from ER Arrival to Admit. (minutes)[5]	-	-	244	274
Time from ER Arrival to Discharge (minutes)	-	-	139	134
Time in ER Before Being Evaluated (minutes)	-	-	20	26
Time to Pain Meds for Fractures (minutes)	-	-	45	57
Heart Attack Care				
Aspirin Given at Discharge[5]	-	-	100%	99%
Fibrinolytic Meds Within 30 Min. of Arrival[5]	-	-	20%	54%
PCI Within 90 Minutes of Arrival[5]	-	-	97%	96%
Statin Prescribed at Discharge[5]	-	-	99%	98%
Heart Failure Care				
ACE Inhibitor or ARB for LVSD[5]	-	-	97%	97%
Discharge Instructions Given[5]	-	-	93%	94%
Evaluation of LVS Function[5]	-	-	99%	99%
Medicare Spending				
Medicare Spending per Patient (ratio)	-	-	0.95	0.98
Pneumonia Care				
Appropriate Initial Antibiotic Given[2,3]	-	-	95%	95%
Blood Culture Timing[2,3]	-	-	98%	98%
Pregnancy and Delivery Care				
Newborn Deliveries Scheduled Early[5]	-	-	2%	6%
Preventive Care				
Immunization for Influenza[5]	-	-	92%	90%
Immunization for Pneumonia[5]	-	-	92%	92%
Stroke Care				
Anticoagulation Therapy for Atrial Fibrillation[5]	-	-	97%	95%
Antithrombotic Therapy Timing[5]	-	-	98%	98%
Assessed for Rehabilitation[5]	-	-	98%	97%
Discharged on Antithrombotic Therapy[5]	-	-	100%	99%
Discharged on Statin Medication[5]	-	-	94%	94%
Thrombolytic Therapy Timing[5]	-	-	78%	66%
Venous Thromboembolism Prophylaxis[5]	-	-	96%	94%
Written Stroke Educational Materials Given[5]	-	-	87%	88%
Surgical Care Improvement Project				
Appropriate Beta Blocker Usage[5]	-	-	98%	98%
Appropriate VTP Within 24 Hours[5]	-	-	98%	98%
Controlled Postoperative Blood Glucose[5]	-	-	96%	97%
Perioperative Temperature Management[5]	-	-	99%	100%
Prophylactic Antibiotic Selection[5]	-	-	99%	99%
Prophylactic Antibiotic Selection (Outpatient)	-	-	98%	98%
Prophylactic Antibiotic Stopped[5]	-	-	98%	98%
Prophylactic Antibiotic Timing[5]	-	-	98%	99%
Prophylactic Antibiotic Timing (Outpatient)	-	-	98%	98%
Urinary Catheter Removal[5]	-	-	97%	97%
Survey of Patients' Hospital Experiences				
Area Around Room 'Always' Quiet at Night[5]	-	-	64%	61%
Doctors 'Always' Communicated Well[5]	-	-	81%	82%
Home Recovery Information Given[5]	-	-	87%	85%
Hospital Given 9 or 10 on 10 Point Scale[5]	-	-	75%	71%
Meds 'Always' Explained Before Given[5]	-	-	67%	64%
Nurses 'Always' Communicated Well[5]	-	-	79%	79%
Pain 'Always' Well Controlled[5]	-	-	72%	71%
Room and Bathroom 'Always' Clean[5]	-	-	74%	73%
Timely Help 'Always' Received[5]	-	-	70%	68%
Would Definitely Recommend Hospital[5]	-	-	76%	71%
Use of Medical Imaging				
Cardiac Imaging Stress Test before Surgery	-	-	5%	5.3%
Combination Abdominal CT Scan	-	-	10%	10.5%
Combination Brain/Sinus CT Scan	-	-	2.1%	2.7%
Combination Chest CT Scan	-	-	3.1%	2.7%
Follow-up Mammogram/Ultrasound	-	-	8.7%	8.8%
Lumbar Spine MRI for Low Back Pain	-	-	39.7%	37.2%

Centura Health - Littleton Adventist Hospital

7700 S Broadway Phone: 303-730-5888
Littleton, CO 80122 Fax: 303-738-2688
URL: www.littletonhosp.org
Type: Acute Care Hospitals Emergency Services: Yes
Ownership: Voluntary non-profit - Church Beds: 237

Key Personnel:
Radiology. . . . . Simeon David Abramson
Emergency Room . . . . Stefen Ammon
CEO/President. . . . . Ken Bacon
Cardiac Laboratory. . . . . J Kern Buckner
Chief of Medical Staff . . . . Thomas Fawell

Measure	Cases	This Hosp.	State Avg.	U.S. Avg.
Blood Clot Prevention and Treatment				
Anticoagulation Overlap Therapy[2]	113	99%	97%	93%
ICU Venous Thromboembolism Prophylaxis[2]	81	98%	95%	92%
Incidence of Potentially Preventable VTE[2]	26	12%	8%	10%
UFH with Dosages/Platelet Monitoring[2]	120	96%	97%	97%
Venous Thromboembolism Prophylaxis[2]	336	88%	90%	85%
Warfarin Therapy Discharge Instructions[2]	92	30%	69%	75%
Chest Pain/Possible Heart Attack Care				
Aspirin Given Within 24 Hours of Arrival	99	99%	97%	96%
Fibrinolytic Meds Within 30 Min. of Arrival[3,7]	-	-	55%	58%
Average Time to ECG (minutes)	100	6	8	7
Average Time to Transfer (minutes)[3,7]	-	-	74	60
Children's Asthma Care				
Received Home Management Plan of Care	-	-	-	88%
Received Reliever Medication	-	-	-	100%
Received Systemic Corticosteroids	-	-	-	100%
Emergency Department				
Admittance Decision Time (minutes)[2]	653	135	96	98
Head CT Results Within 45 Min. of Arrival[1]	-	-	67%	57%
Patients Who Left ER Before Being Seen	35,786	1%	2%	2%
Time from ER Arrival to Admit. (minutes)[2]	701	294	244	274
Time from ER Arrival to Discharge (minutes)	435	161	139	134
Time in ER Before Being Evaluated (minutes)	447	14	20	26
Time to Pain Meds for Fractures (minutes)	196	44	45	57
Heart Attack Care				
Aspirin Given at Discharge	115	100%	100%	99%
Fibrinolytic Meds Within 30 Min. of Arrival[7]	-	-	20%	54%
PCI Within 90 Minutes of Arrival	59	100%	97%	96%
Statin Prescribed at Discharge	119	100%	99%	98%
Heart Failure Care				
ACE Inhibitor or ARB for LVSD	32	100%	97%	97%
Discharge Instructions Given	105	95%	93%	94%
Evaluation of LVS Function	133	100%	99%	99%
Medicare Spending				
Medicare Spending per Patient (ratio)	-	1.01	0.95	0.98
Pneumonia Care				
Appropriate Initial Antibiotic Given	124	97%	95%	95%
Blood Culture Timing	166	97%	98%	98%
Pregnancy and Delivery Care				
Newborn Deliveries Scheduled Early[2]	42	10%	2%	6%
Preventive Care				
Immunization for Influenza[2]	550	95%	92%	90%
Immunization for Pneumonia[2]	565	97%	92%	92%
Stroke Care				
Anticoagulation Therapy for Atrial Fibrillation	17	88%	97%	95%
Antithrombotic Therapy Timing	84	100%	98%	98%
Assessed for Rehabilitation	142	98%	98%	97%
Discharged on Antithrombotic Therapy	110	99%	100%	99%
Discharged on Statin Medication	83	99%	94%	94%
Thrombolytic Therapy Timing	21	90%	78%	66%
Venous Thromboembolism Prophylaxis	141	100%	96%	94%
Written Stroke Educational Materials Given	58	62%	87%	88%
Surgical Care Improvement Project				
Appropriate Beta Blocker Usage[2]	113	98%	98%	98%
Appropriate VTP Within 24 Hours[2]	418	99%	98%	98%
Controlled Postoperative Blood Glucose[2,7]	-	-	96%	97%
Perioperative Temperature Management[2]	470	100%	99%	100%
Prophylactic Antibiotic Selection[2]	301	99%	99%	99%
Prophylactic Antibiotic Selection (Outpatient)	368	96%	98%	98%
Prophylactic Antibiotic Stopped[2]	291	98%	98%	98%
Prophylactic Antibiotic Timing[2]	300	97%	98%	99%
Prophylactic Antibiotic Timing (Outpatient)	370	99%	98%	98%
Urinary Catheter Removal[2]	309	99%	97%	97%
Survey of Patients' Hospital Experiences				
Area Around Room 'Always' Quiet at Night	300+	54%	64%	61%
Doctors 'Always' Communicated Well	300+	79%	81%	82%
Home Recovery Information Given	300+	87%	87%	85%
Hospital Given 9 or 10 on 10 Point Scale	300+	73%	75%	71%
Meds 'Always' Explained Before Given	300+	61%	67%	64%
Nurses 'Always' Communicated Well	300+	77%	79%	79%
Pain 'Always' Well Controlled	300+	70%	72%	71%
Room and Bathroom 'Always' Clean	300+	69%	74%	73%
Timely Help 'Always' Received	300+	63%	70%	68%
Would Definitely Recommend Hospital	300+	77%	76%	71%
Use of Medical Imaging				
Cardiac Imaging Stress Test before Surgery	1,180	4.8%	5%	5.3%
Combination Abdominal CT Scan	582	15.5%	10%	10.5%
Combination Brain/Sinus CT Scan	542	2.4%	2.1%	2.7%
Combination Chest CT Scan	289	5.9%	3.1%	2.7%
Follow-up Mammogram/Ultrasound	633	9.8%	8.7%	8.8%
Lumbar Spine MRI for Low Back Pain	49	42.9%	39.7%	37.2%

NOTE: Hospital profiles are in alphabetical order by state, then city, then hospital within the city; Rankings exclude hospitals with less than 25 cases except for patient surveys which excludes hospitals with less than 100 cases; (a) 100-299 cases; (1) The number of cases/patients is too few to report; (2) Data submitted were based on a sample of cases/patients; (3) Results are based on a shorter time period than required; (4) Data suppressed by CMS for one or more quarters; (5) Results are not available for this reporting period; (6) Fewer than 100 patients completed the HCAHPS survey; (7) No cases met the criteria for this measure; (8) The lower limit of the confidence interval cannot be calculated if the number of observed infections equals zero; (9) No data are available from the state/territory for this reporting period; (10) The scores shown reflect fewer than 50 completed surveys; (11) There were discrepancies in the data collection process; (12) This measure does not apply to this hospital for this reporting period; (13) Results cannot be calculated for this reporting period; (14) The results for this state are combined with nearby states to protect confidentiality; Please refer to the User's Guide for a full explanation of data.

Sky Ridge Medical Center

10101 Ridge Gate Parkway Phone: 720-225-1000
Lone Tree, CO 80124 Fax: 720-225-1029
URL: www.skyridgemedcenter.com
Type: Acute Care Hospitals Emergency Services: Yes
Ownership: Proprietary Beds: 156

Key Personnel:
Chief of Medical Staff. . . . . Dr Brian Gill, MD
Emergency Room . . . . Dr Heinz
CEO . . . . Susan Hicks
Operating Room. . . . . Craig Hornbarger
CEO/President. . . . . Maureen Tarrant

Measure	Cases	This Hosp.	State Avg.	U.S. Avg.
Blood Clot Prevention and Treatment				
Anticoagulation Overlap Therapy[2]	114	99%	97%	93%
ICU Venous Thromboembolism Prophylaxis[2]	75	99%	95%	92%
Incidence of Potentially Preventable VTE[2]	15	0%	8%	10%
UFH with Dosages/Platelet Monitoring[2]	82	100%	97%	97%
Venous Thromboembolism Prophylaxis[2]	349	99%	90%	85%
Warfarin Therapy Discharge Instructions[2]	92	96%	69%	75%
Chest Pain/Possible Heart Attack Care				
Aspirin Given Within 24 Hours of Arrival[1,3]	-	-	97%	96%
Fibrinolytic Meds Within 30 Min. of Arrival[5]	-	-	55%	58%
Average Time to ECG (minutes)[1,3]	-	-	8	7
Average Time to Transfer (minutes)[5]	-	-	74	60
Children's Asthma Care				
Received Home Management Plan of Care	-	-	-	88%
Received Reliever Medication	-	-	-	100%
Received Systemic Corticosteroids	-	-	-	100%
Emergency Department				
Admittance Decision Time (minutes)[2]	379	119	96	98
Head CT Results Within 45 Min. of Arrival[1]	-	-	67%	57%
Patients Who Left ER Before Being Seen	36,596	0%	2%	2%
Time from ER Arrival to Admit. (minutes)[2]	379	219	244	274
Time from ER Arrival to Discharge (minutes)	445	149	139	134
Time in ER Before Being Evaluated (minutes)	523	15	20	26
Time to Pain Meds for Fractures (minutes)	184	35	45	57
Heart Attack Care				
Aspirin Given at Discharge	118	100%	100%	99%
Fibrinolytic Meds Within 30 Min. of Arrival[7]	-	-	20%	54%
PCI Within 90 Minutes of Arrival	38	100%	97%	96%
Statin Prescribed at Discharge	116	100%	99%	98%
Heart Failure Care				
ACE Inhibitor or ARB for LVSD	29	100%	97%	97%
Discharge Instructions Given	104	99%	93%	94%
Evaluation of LVS Function	129	100%	99%	99%
Medicare Spending				
Medicare Spending per Patient (ratio)	-	0.99	0.95	0.98
Pneumonia Care				
Appropriate Initial Antibiotic Given[2]	88	98%	95%	95%
Blood Culture Timing[2]	120	99%	98%	98%
Pregnancy and Delivery Care				
Newborn Deliveries Scheduled Early[2]	78	0%	2%	6%
Preventive Care				
Immunization for Influenza[2]	574	97%	92%	90%
Immunization for Pneumonia[2]	504	96%	92%	92%
Stroke Care				
Anticoagulation Therapy for Atrial Fibrillation[1,2]	-	-	97%	95%
Antithrombotic Therapy Timing[2]	46	100%	98%	98%
Assessed for Rehabilitation[2]	59	100%	98%	97%
Discharged on Antithrombotic Therapy[2]	52	100%	100%	99%
Discharged on Statin Medication[2]	41	100%	94%	94%
Thrombolytic Therapy Timing[1,2]	-	-	78%	66%
Venous Thromboembolism Prophylaxis[2]	59	100%	96%	94%
Written Stroke Educational Materials Given[2]	30	93%	87%	88%
Surgical Care Improvement Project				
Appropriate Beta Blocker Usage[2]	119	100%	98%	98%
Appropriate VTP Within 24 Hours[2]	443	100%	98%	98%
Controlled Postoperative Blood Glucose[2]	33	91%	96%	97%
Perioperative Temperature Management[2]	568	100%	99%	100%
Prophylactic Antibiotic Selection[2]	386	100%	99%	99%
Prophylactic Antibiotic Selection (Outpatient)	561	99%	98%	98%
Prophylactic Antibiotic Stopped[2]	375	100%	98%	98%
Prophylactic Antibiotic Timing[2]	387	100%	98%	99%
Prophylactic Antibiotic Timing (Outpatient)	561	100%	98%	98%
Urinary Catheter Removal[2]	175	99%	97%	97%
Survey of Patients' Hospital Experiences				
Area Around Room 'Always' Quiet at Night	300+	64%	64%	61%
Doctors 'Always' Communicated Well	300+	76%	81%	82%
Home Recovery Information Given	300+	88%	87%	85%
Hospital Given 9 or 10 on 10 Point Scale	300+	75%	75%	71%
Meds 'Always' Explained Before Given	300+	63%	67%	64%
Nurses 'Always' Communicated Well	300+	76%	79%	79%
Pain 'Always' Well Controlled	300+	68%	72%	71%
Room and Bathroom 'Always' Clean	300+	73%	74%	73%
Timely Help 'Always' Received	300+	64%	70%	68%
Would Definitely Recommend Hospital	300+	77%	76%	71%
Use of Medical Imaging				
Cardiac Imaging Stress Test before Surgery	237	4.2%	5%	5.3%
Combination Abdominal CT Scan	519	10.0%	10%	10.5%
Combination Brain/Sinus CT Scan[1]	-	-	2.1%	2.7%
Combination Chest CT Scan	380	0.5%	3.1%	2.7%
Follow-up Mammogram/Ultrasound[7]	-	-	8.7%	8.8%
Lumbar Spine MRI for Low Back Pain	104	54.8%	39.7%	37.2%

Longmont United Hospital

1950 Mountain View Avenue Phone: 303-651-5111
Longmont, CO 80501 Fax: 303-678-4050
URL: www.luhcares.org
Type: Acute Care Hospitals Emergency Services: Yes
Ownership: Voluntary non-profit - Other Beds: 143

Key Personnel:
Operating Room. . . . . Kevin R Berg
CEO/President. . . . . Michell C. Carson
Radiology. . . . . David G Goodbee, MD
Chief of Medical Staff. . . . . Amy Johnson, MD
Surgery . . . . Troy Malcom, DO
Quality Assurance . . . . Diana Norris
Pediatric Ambulatory Care . . . . . . Mark Shane, MD
Pediatric In-Patient Care . . . . Mark Shane, MD

Measure	Cases	This Hosp.	State Avg.	U.S. Avg.
Blood Clot Prevention and Treatment				
Anticoagulation Overlap Therapy[2]	81	99%	97%	93%
ICU Venous Thromboembolism Prophylaxis[2]	89	79%	95%	92%
Incidence of Potentially Preventable VTE[1,2]	-	-	8%	10%
UFH with Dosages/Platelet Monitoring[2]	79	100%	97%	97%
Venous Thromboembolism Prophylaxis[2]	297	77%	90%	85%
Warfarin Therapy Discharge Instructions[2]	70	44%	69%	75%
Chest Pain/Possible Heart Attack Care				
Aspirin Given Within 24 Hours of Arrival	15	100%	97%	96%
Fibrinolytic Meds Within 30 Min. of Arrival[3,7]	-	-	55%	58%
Average Time to ECG (minutes)	15	6	8	7
Average Time to Transfer (minutes)[3,7]	-	-	74	60
Children's Asthma Care				
Received Home Management Plan of Care	-	-	-	88%
Received Reliever Medication	-	-	-	100%
Received Systemic Corticosteroids	-	-	-	100%
Emergency Department				
Admittance Decision Time (minutes)[2]	701	75	96	98
Head CT Results Within 45 Min. of Arrival[1]	-	-	67%	57%
Patients Who Left ER Before Being Seen	16,486	1%	2%	2%
Time from ER Arrival to Admit. (minutes)[2]	701	194	244	274
Time from ER Arrival to Discharge (minutes)	363	138	139	134
Time in ER Before Being Evaluated (minutes)	368	32	20	26
Time to Pain Meds for Fractures (minutes)	118	32	45	57
Heart Attack Care				
Aspirin Given at Discharge	107	100%	100%	99%
Fibrinolytic Meds Within 30 Min. of Arrival[7]	-	-	20%	54%
PCI Within 90 Minutes of Arrival	44	100%	97%	96%
Statin Prescribed at Discharge	103	97%	99%	98%
Heart Failure Care				
ACE Inhibitor or ARB for LVSD	23	96%	97%	97%
Discharge Instructions Given	106	94%	93%	94%
Evaluation of LVS Function	141	99%	99%	99%
Medicare Spending				
Medicare Spending per Patient (ratio)	-	0.97	0.95	0.98
Pneumonia Care				
Appropriate Initial Antibiotic Given	83	94%	95%	95%
Blood Culture Timing	90	99%	98%	98%
Pregnancy and Delivery Care				
Newborn Deliveries Scheduled Early	106	1%	2%	6%
Preventive Care				
Immunization for Influenza[2]	544	94%	92%	90%
Immunization for Pneumonia[2]	624	92%	92%	92%
Stroke Care				
Anticoagulation Therapy for Atrial Fibrillation[1]	-	-	97%	95%
Antithrombotic Therapy Timing	59	95%	98%	98%
Assessed for Rehabilitation	65	97%	98%	97%
Discharged on Antithrombotic Therapy	60	98%	100%	99%
Discharged on Statin Medication	47	72%	94%	94%
Thrombolytic Therapy Timing	11	91%	78%	66%
Venous Thromboembolism Prophylaxis	78	77%	96%	94%
Written Stroke Educational Materials Given	37	76%	87%	88%
Surgical Care Improvement Project				
Appropriate Beta Blocker Usage	121	96%	98%	98%
Appropriate VTP Within 24 Hours	538	98%	98%	98%
Controlled Postoperative Blood Glucose[7]	-	-	96%	97%
Perioperative Temperature Management	612	100%	99%	100%
Prophylactic Antibiotic Selection	375	98%	99%	99%
Prophylactic Antibiotic Selection (Outpatient)	224	98%	98%	98%
Prophylactic Antibiotic Stopped	370	98%	98%	98%
Prophylactic Antibiotic Timing	375	99%	98%	99%
Prophylactic Antibiotic Timing (Outpatient)	225	99%	98%	98%
Urinary Catheter Removal	368	94%	97%	97%
Survey of Patients' Hospital Experiences				
Area Around Room 'Always' Quiet at Night	300+	68%	64%	61%
Doctors 'Always' Communicated Well	300+	78%	81%	82%
Home Recovery Information Given	300+	88%	87%	85%
Hospital Given 9 or 10 on 10 Point Scale	300+	76%	75%	71%
Meds 'Always' Explained Before Given	300+	62%	67%	64%
Nurses 'Always' Communicated Well	300+	79%	79%	79%
Pain 'Always' Well Controlled	300+	69%	72%	71%
Room and Bathroom 'Always' Clean	300+	72%	74%	73%
Timely Help 'Always' Received	300+	68%	70%	68%
Would Definitely Recommend Hospital	300+	74%	76%	71%
Use of Medical Imaging				
Cardiac Imaging Stress Test before Surgery	82	2.4%	5%	5.3%
Combination Abdominal CT Scan	336	11.6%	10%	10.5%
Combination Brain/Sinus CT Scan	425	1.6%	2.1%	2.7%
Combination Chest CT Scan	103	2.9%	3.1%	2.7%
Follow-up Mammogram/Ultrasound	1,035	4.6%	8.7%	8.8%
Lumbar Spine MRI for Low Back Pain	57	43.9%	39.7%	37.2%

Centura Health - Avista Adventist Hospital

100 Health Park Drive Phone: 303-673-1000
Louisville, CO 80027 Fax: 303-673-1283
URL: www.avistahosp.org
Type: Acute Care Hospitals Emergency Services: Yes
Ownership: Voluntary non-profit - Church Beds: 99

Key Personnel:
Radiology. . . . . Mitchell Dean Achee
CEO/President. . . . . Dennis Bart
Chief of Medical Staff. . . . . David Ehrenberger

Measure	Cases	This Hosp.	State Avg.	U.S. Avg.
Blood Clot Prevention and Treatment				
Anticoagulation Overlap Therapy[2]	39	95%	97%	93%
ICU Venous Thromboembolism Prophylaxis[2]	46	85%	95%	92%
Incidence of Potentially Preventable VTE[1,2]	-	-	8%	10%
UFH with Dosages/Platelet Monitoring[2]	19	100%	97%	97%
Venous Thromboembolism Prophylaxis[2]	140	81%	90%	85%
Warfarin Therapy Discharge Instructions[2]	32	28%	69%	75%
Chest Pain/Possible Heart Attack Care				
Aspirin Given Within 24 Hours of Arrival[1,3]	-	-	97%	96%
Fibrinolytic Meds Within 30 Min. of Arrival[5]	-	-	55%	58%
Average Time to ECG (minutes)[1,3]	-	-	8	7
Average Time to Transfer (minutes)[5]	-	-	74	60
Children's Asthma Care				
Received Home Management Plan of Care	-	-	-	88%
Received Reliever Medication	-	-	-	100%
Received Systemic Corticosteroids	-	-	-	100%

NOTE: Hospital profiles are in alphabetical order by state, then city, then hospital within the city; Rankings exclude hospitals with less than 25 cases except for patient surveys which excludes hospitals with less than 100 cases; (a) 100-299 cases; (1) The number of cases/patients is too few to report; (2) Data submitted were based on a sample of cases/patients; (3) Results are based on a shorter time period than required; (4) Data suppressed by CMS for one or more quarters; (5) Results are not available for this reporting period; (6) Fewer than 100 patients completed the HCAHPS survey; (7) No cases met the criteria for this measure; (8) The lower limit of the confidence interval cannot be calculated if the number of observed infections equals zero; (9) No data are available from the state/territory for this reporting period; (10) The scores shown reflect fewer than 50 completed surveys; (11) There were discrepancies in the data collection process; (12) This measure does not apply to this hospital for this reporting period; (13) Results cannot be calculated for this reporting period; (14) The results for this state are combined with nearby states to protect confidentiality; Please refer to the User's Guide for a full explanation of data.

Emergency Department				
Admittance Decision Time (minutes)[2]	194	92	96	98
Head CT Results Within 45 Min. of Arrival[1]	-	-	67%	57%
Patients Who Left ER Before Being Seen	11,999	0%	2%	2%
Time from ER Arrival to Admit. (minutes)[2]	196	222	244	274
Time from ER Arrival to Discharge (minutes)	420	136	139	134
Time in ER Before Being Evaluated (minutes)	499	12	20	26
Time to Pain Meds for Fractures (minutes)	51	57	45	57
Heart Attack Care				
Aspirin Given at Discharge	21	100%	100%	99%
Fibrinolytic Meds Within 30 Min. of Arrival[7]	-	-	20%	54%
PCI Within 90 Minutes of Arrival[1]	-	-	97%	96%
Statin Prescribed at Discharge	23	100%	99%	98%
Heart Failure Care				
ACE Inhibitor or ARB for LVSD[1]	-	-	97%	97%
Discharge Instructions Given	18	83%	93%	94%
Evaluation of LVS Function	24	100%	99%	99%
Medicare Spending				
Medicare Spending per Patient (ratio)	-	0.99	0.95	0.98
Pneumonia Care				
Appropriate Initial Antibiotic Given	57	96%	95%	95%
Blood Culture Timing	63	94%	98%	98%
Pregnancy and Delivery Care				
Newborn Deliveries Scheduled Early[2]	38	5%	2%	6%
Preventive Care				
Immunization for Influenza[2]	427	99%	92%	90%
Immunization for Pneumonia[2]	262	96%	92%	92%
Stroke Care				
Anticoagulation Therapy for Atrial Fibrillation[1]	-	-	97%	95%
Antithrombotic Therapy Timing[1]	-	-	98%	98%
Assessed for Rehabilitation	11	100%	98%	97%
Discharged on Antithrombotic Therapy	11	100%	100%	99%
Discharged on Statin Medication[1]	-	-	94%	94%
Thrombolytic Therapy Timing[7]	-	-	78%	66%
Venous Thromboembolism Prophylaxis[1]	-	-	96%	94%
Written Stroke Educational Materials Given[1]	-	-	87%	88%
Surgical Care Improvement Project				
Appropriate Beta Blocker Usage	67	100%	98%	98%
Appropriate VTP Within 24 Hours	227	97%	98%	98%
Controlled Postoperative Blood Glucose[7]	-	-	96%	97%
Perioperative Temperature Management	341	99%	99%	100%
Prophylactic Antibiotic Selection	247	100%	99%	99%
Prophylactic Antibiotic Selection (Outpatient)	129	100%	98%	98%
Prophylactic Antibiotic Stopped	243	100%	98%	98%
Prophylactic Antibiotic Timing	247	98%	98%	99%
Prophylactic Antibiotic Timing (Outpatient)	129	98%	98%	98%
Urinary Catheter Removal	179	99%	97%	97%
Survey of Patients' Hospital Experiences				
Area Around Room 'Always' Quiet at Night	300+	65%	64%	61%
Doctors 'Always' Communicated Well	300+	82%	81%	82%
Home Recovery Information Given	300+	90%	87%	85%
Hospital Given 9 or 10 on 10 Point Scale	300+	80%	75%	71%
Meds 'Always' Explained Before Given	300+	66%	67%	64%
Nurses 'Always' Communicated Well	300+	79%	79%	79%
Pain 'Always' Well Controlled	300+	72%	72%	71%
Room and Bathroom 'Always' Clean	300+	73%	74%	73%
Timely Help 'Always' Received	300+	71%	70%	68%
Would Definitely Recommend Hospital	300+	81%	76%	71%
Use of Medical Imaging				
Cardiac Imaging Stress Test before Surgery	83	8.4%	5%	5.3%
Combination Abdominal CT Scan	187	9.6%	10%	10.5%
Combination Brain/Sinus CT Scan[1]	-	-	2.1%	2.7%
Combination Chest CT Scan	56	1.8%	3.1%	2.7%
Follow-up Mammogram/Ultrasound	511	6.7%	8.7%	8.8%
Lumbar Spine MRI for Low Back Pain[1]	-	-	39.7%	37.2%

McKee Medical Center

2000 Boise Ave
Loveland, CO 80538
Phone: 970-669-4640
Fax: 970-635-4066
URL: www.bannerhealth.comkeyword:mckee
Type: Acute Care Hospitals
Emergency Services: Yes
Ownership: Voluntary non-profit - Private
Beds: 132

Key Personnel:

Chief of Medical Staff.......... William Culver
Emergency Room .... Teri Huffman
Hemotology Center .... Cindy McBlair
Intensive Care Unit.......... Pat McKinnon
Quality Assurance .... Penny Rollins
Infection Control............... Joan Strauch
CEO/President................ Richard O Sutton

Measure	Cases	This Hosp.	State Avg.	U.S. Avg.
Blood Clot Prevention and Treatment				
Anticoagulation Overlap Therapy[2]	31	100%	97%	93%
ICU Venous Thromboembolism Prophylaxis[2]	30	97%	95%	92%
Incidence of Potentially Preventable VTE[1,2]	-	-	8%	10%
UFH with Dosages/Platelet Monitoring[1,2]	-	-	97%	97%
Venous Thromboembolism Prophylaxis[2]	268	96%	90%	85%
Warfarin Therapy Discharge Instructions[2]	27	63%	69%	75%
Chest Pain/Possible Heart Attack Care				
Aspirin Given Within 24 Hours of Arrival[3,7]	-	-	97%	96%
Fibrinolytic Meds Within 30 Min. of Arrival[5]	-	-	55%	58%
Average Time to ECG (minutes)[3,7]	-	-	8	7
Average Time to Transfer (minutes)[5]	-	-	74	60
Children's Asthma Care				
Received Home Management Plan of Care	-	-	-	88%
Received Reliever Medication	-	-	-	100%
Received Systemic Corticosteroids	-	-	-	100%
Emergency Department				
Admittance Decision Time (minutes)[2]	559	64	96	98
Head CT Results Within 45 Min. of Arrival	11	64%	67%	57%
Patients Who Left ER Before Being Seen	27,515	1%	2%	2%
Time from ER Arrival to Admit. (minutes)[2]	578	226	244	274
Time from ER Arrival to Discharge (minutes)	337	128	139	134
Time in ER Before Being Evaluated (minutes)	349	18	20	26
Time to Pain Meds for Fractures (minutes)	106	48	45	57
Heart Attack Care				
Aspirin Given at Discharge	91	100%	100%	99%
Fibrinolytic Meds Within 30 Min. of Arrival[7]	-	-	20%	54%
PCI Within 90 Minutes of Arrival	22	100%	97%	96%
Statin Prescribed at Discharge	79	100%	99%	98%
Heart Failure Care				
ACE Inhibitor or ARB for LVSD[2]	14	100%	97%	97%
Discharge Instructions Given[2]	69	99%	93%	94%
Evaluation of LVS Function[2]	84	100%	99%	99%
Medicare Spending				
Medicare Spending per Patient (ratio)	-	0.93	0.95	0.98
Pneumonia Care				
Appropriate Initial Antibiotic Given[2]	73	99%	95%	95%
Blood Culture Timing[2]	131	100%	98%	98%
Pregnancy and Delivery Care				
Newborn Deliveries Scheduled Early[2]	32	16%	2%	6%
Preventive Care				
Immunization for Influenza[2]	519	98%	92%	90%
Immunization for Pneumonia[2]	619	94%	92%	92%
Stroke Care				
Anticoagulation Therapy for Atrial Fibrillation[1]	-	-	97%	95%
Antithrombotic Therapy Timing	44	98%	98%	98%
Assessed for Rehabilitation	60	100%	98%	97%
Discharged on Antithrombotic Therapy	58	98%	100%	99%
Discharged on Statin Medication	48	90%	94%	94%
Thrombolytic Therapy Timing[1]	-	-	78%	66%
Venous Thromboembolism Prophylaxis	46	98%	96%	94%
Written Stroke Educational Materials Given	33	70%	87%	88%
Surgical Care Improvement Project				
Appropriate Beta Blocker Usage[2]	82	98%	98%	98%
Appropriate VTP Within 24 Hours[2]	287	97%	98%	98%
Controlled Postoperative Blood Glucose[2,7]	-	-	96%	97%
Perioperative Temperature Management[2]	332	100%	99%	100%
Prophylactic Antibiotic Selection[2]	216	100%	99%	99%
Prophylactic Antibiotic Selection (Outpatient)	110	98%	98%	98%
Prophylactic Antibiotic Stopped[2]	212	98%	98%	98%
Prophylactic Antibiotic Timing[2]	216	100%	98%	99%
Prophylactic Antibiotic Timing (Outpatient)	112	97%	98%	98%
Urinary Catheter Removal[2]	117	96%	97%	97%
Survey of Patients' Hospital Experiences				
Area Around Room 'Always' Quiet at Night[11]	300+	64%	64%	61%
Doctors 'Always' Communicated Well[11]	300+	83%	81%	82%
Home Recovery Information Given[11]	300+	92%	87%	85%
Hospital Given 9 or 10 on 10 Point Scale[11]	300+	75%	75%	71%
Meds 'Always' Explained Before Given[11]	300+	70%	67%	64%
Nurses 'Always' Communicated Well[11]	300+	82%	79%	79%
Pain 'Always' Well Controlled[11]	300+	75%	72%	71%
Room and Bathroom 'Always' Clean[11]	300+	78%	74%	73%
Timely Help 'Always' Received[11]	300+	70%	70%	68%
Would Definitely Recommend Hospital[11]	300+	77%	76%	71%
Use of Medical Imaging				
Cardiac Imaging Stress Test before Surgery	185	5.4%	5%	5.3%
Combination Abdominal CT Scan	592	12.0%	10%	10.5%
Combination Brain/Sinus CT Scan[1]	-	-	2.1%	2.7%
Combination Chest CT Scan	235	6.4%	3.1%	2.7%
Follow-up Mammogram/Ultrasound	1,560	6.5%	8.7%	8.8%
Lumbar Spine MRI for Low Back Pain	116	38.8%	39.7%	37.2%

Medical Center of the Rockies

2500 Rocky Mountain Avenue
Loveland, CO 80538
Phone: 970-624-2500
URL: www.pvhs.org/mcr
Type: Acute Care Hospitals
Emergency Services: Yes
Ownership: Voluntary non-profit - Private
Beds: 136

Key Personnel:

Chief of Medical Staff.......... Troy Ford, MD
President/CEO............... Kevin Unger

Measure	Cases	This Hosp.	State Avg.	U.S. Avg.
Blood Clot Prevention and Treatment				
Anticoagulation Overlap Therapy[2]	93	81%	97%	93%
ICU Venous Thromboembolism Prophylaxis[2]	93	97%	95%	92%
Incidence of Potentially Preventable VTE[1,2]	-	-	8%	10%
UFH with Dosages/Platelet Monitoring[2]	48	90%	97%	97%
Venous Thromboembolism Prophylaxis[2]	294	85%	90%	85%
Warfarin Therapy Discharge Instructions[2]	77	56%	69%	75%
Chest Pain/Possible Heart Attack Care				
Aspirin Given Within 24 Hours of Arrival[1,3]	-	-	97%	96%
Fibrinolytic Meds Within 30 Min. of Arrival[5]	-	-	55%	58%
Average Time to ECG (minutes)[1,3]	-	-	8	7
Average Time to Transfer (minutes)[5]	-	-	74	60
Children's Asthma Care				
Received Home Management Plan of Care	-	-	-	88%
Received Reliever Medication	-	-	-	100%
Received Systemic Corticosteroids	-	-	-	100%
Emergency Department				
Admittance Decision Time (minutes)[2]	392	113	96	98
Head CT Results Within 45 Min. of Arrival	12	17%	67%	57%
Patients Who Left ER Before Being Seen	4,365	2%	2%	2%
Time from ER Arrival to Admit. (minutes)[2]	449	216	244	274
Time from ER Arrival to Discharge (minutes)	443	133	139	134
Time in ER Before Being Evaluated (minutes)	461	18	20	26
Time to Pain Meds for Fractures (minutes)	168	66	45	57
Heart Attack Care				
Aspirin Given at Discharge[2]	356	100%	100%	99%
Fibrinolytic Meds Within 30 Min. of Arrival[2,7]	-	-	20%	54%
PCI Within 90 Minutes of Arrival[2]	58	100%	97%	96%
Statin Prescribed at Discharge[2]	330	99%	99%	98%
Heart Failure Care				
ACE Inhibitor or ARB for LVSD	49	96%	97%	97%
Discharge Instructions Given	129	95%	93%	94%
Evaluation of LVS Function	148	100%	99%	99%
Medicare Spending				
Medicare Spending per Patient (ratio)	-	1.02	0.95	0.98
Pneumonia Care				
Appropriate Initial Antibiotic Given[2]	76	91%	95%	95%
Blood Culture Timing[2]	158	99%	98%	98%
Pregnancy and Delivery Care				
Newborn Deliveries Scheduled Early[2]	31	0%	2%	6%
Preventive Care				
Immunization for Influenza[2]	579	78%	92%	90%
Immunization for Pneumonia[2]	707	79%	92%	92%
Stroke Care				
Anticoagulation Therapy for Atrial Fibrillation[1]	-	-	97%	95%
Antithrombotic Therapy Timing	47	98%	98%	98%
Assessed for Rehabilitation	66	100%	98%	97%

NOTE: Hospital profiles are in alphabetical order by state, then city, then hospital within the city; Rankings exclude hospitals with less than 25 cases except for patient surveys which excludes hospitals with less than 100 cases; (a) 100-299 cases; (1) The number of cases/patients is too few to report; (2) Data submitted were based on a sample of cases/patients; (3) Results are based on a shorter time period than required; (4) Data suppressed by CMS for one or more quarters; (5) Results are not available for this reporting period; (6) Fewer than 100 patients completed the HCAHPS survey; (7) No cases met the criteria for this measure; (8) The lower limit of the confidence interval cannot be calculated if the number of observed infections equals zero; (9) No data are available from the state/territory for this reporting period; (10) The scores shown reflect fewer than 50 completed surveys; (11) There were discrepancies in the data collection process; (12) This measure does not apply to this hospital for this reporting period; (13) Results cannot be calculated for this reporting period; (14) The results for this state are combined with nearby states to protect confidentiality; Please refer to the User's Guide for a full explanation of data.

Measure	Cases	This Hosp.	State Avg.	U.S. Avg.
Discharged on Antithrombotic Therapy	54	100%	100%	99%
Discharged on Statin Medication	40	95%	94%	94%
Thrombolytic Therapy Timing[1]	-	-	78%	66%
Venous Thromboembolism Prophylaxis	65	92%	96%	94%
Written Stroke Educational Materials Given	32	81%	87%	88%
Surgical Care Improvement Project				
Appropriate Beta Blocker Usage[2]	209	100%	98%	98%
Appropriate VTP Within 24 Hours[2]	345	97%	98%	98%
Controlled Postoperative Blood Glucose[2]	211	97%	96%	97%
Perioperative Temperature Management[2]	454	100%	99%	100%
Prophylactic Antibiotic Selection[2]	434	99%	99%	99%
Prophylactic Antibiotic Selection (Outpatient)	367	99%	98%	98%
Prophylactic Antibiotic Stopped[2]	426	96%	98%	98%
Prophylactic Antibiotic Timing[2]	436	98%	98%	99%
Prophylactic Antibiotic Timing (Outpatient)	368	99%	98%	98%
Urinary Catheter Removal[2]	411	96%	97%	97%
Survey of Patients' Hospital Experiences				
Area Around Room 'Always' Quiet at Night	300+	67%	64%	61%
Doctors 'Always' Communicated Well	300+	79%	81%	82%
Home Recovery Information Given	300+	88%	87%	85%
Hospital Given 9 or 10 on 10 Point Scale	300+	82%	75%	71%
Meds 'Always' Explained Before Given	300+	66%	67%	64%
Nurses 'Always' Communicated Well	300+	79%	79%	79%
Pain 'Always' Well Controlled	300+	73%	72%	71%
Room and Bathroom 'Always' Clean	300+	80%	74%	73%
Timely Help 'Always' Received	300+	65%	70%	68%
Would Definitely Recommend Hospital	300+	83%	76%	71%
Use of Medical Imaging				
Cardiac Imaging Stress Test before Surgery	511	4.1%	5%	5.3%
Combination Abdominal CT Scan	877	9.1%	10%	10.5%
Combination Brain/Sinus CT Scan	492	1.2%	2.1%	2.7%
Combination Chest CT Scan	467	1.5%	3.1%	2.7%
Follow-up Mammogram/Ultrasound	1,065	5.7%	8.7%	8.8%
Lumbar Spine MRI for Low Back Pain	192	38.0%	39.7%	37.2%

Pioneers Medical Center

345 Cleveland Street
Meeker, CO 81641
Phone: 970-878-5047
Fax: 970-878-3285
E-mail: tmorgan@pioneershospital.com
URL: www.pioneershospital.org
Type: Critical Access Hospitals
Emergency Services: Yes
Ownership: Govt - Hospital Dist/Auth
Beds: 15

Key Personnel:
CEO . . . . Ken Harman
Radiology. . . . . Elizabeth Kulwi
Infection Control. . . . . Amy May, RN
Chief of Medical Staff. . . . . Victor Mihal, DO
Emergency Room . . . . Drew Varland

Measure	Cases	This Hosp.	State Avg.	U.S. Avg.
Blood Clot Prevention and Treatment				
Anticoagulation Overlap Therapy[5]	-	-	97%	93%
ICU Venous Thromboembolism Prophylaxis[5]	-	-	95%	92%
Incidence of Potentially Preventable VTE[5]	-	-	8%	10%
UFH with Dosages/Platelet Monitoring[5]	-	-	97%	97%
Venous Thromboembolism Prophylaxis[5]	-	-	90%	85%
Warfarin Therapy Discharge Instructions[5]	-	-	69%	75%
Chest Pain/Possible Heart Attack Care				
Aspirin Given Within 24 Hours of Arrival[5]	-	-	97%	96%
Fibrinolytic Meds Within 30 Min. of Arrival[5]	-	-	55%	58%
Average Time to ECG (minutes)[5]	-	-	8	7
Average Time to Transfer (minutes)[5]	-	-	74	60
Children's Asthma Care				
Received Home Management Plan of Care	-	-	-	88%
Received Reliever Medication	-	-	-	100%
Received Systemic Corticosteroids	-	-	-	100%
Emergency Department				
Admittance Decision Time (minutes)[5]	-	-	96	98
Head CT Results Within 45 Min. of Arrival[5]	-	-	67%	57%
Patients Who Left ER Before Being Seen[5]	-	-	2%	2%
Time from ER Arrival to Admit. (minutes)[5]	-	-	244	274
Time from ER Arrival to Discharge (minutes)[5]	-	-	139	134
Time in ER Before Being Evaluated (minutes)[5]	-	-	20	26
Time to Pain Meds for Fractures (minutes)[5]	-	-	45	57
Heart Attack Care				
Aspirin Given at Discharge[5]	-	-	100%	99%
Fibrinolytic Meds Within 30 Min. of Arrival[5]	-	-	20%	54%
PCI Within 90 Minutes of Arrival[5]	-	-	97%	96%
Statin Prescribed at Discharge[5]	-	-	99%	98%
Heart Failure Care				
ACE Inhibitor or ARB for LVSD[1,3]	-	-	97%	97%
Discharge Instructions Given[1,3]	-	-	93%	94%
Evaluation of LVS Function[1,3]	-	-	99%	99%
Medicare Spending				
Medicare Spending per Patient (ratio)	-	-	0.95	0.98
Pneumonia Care				
Appropriate Initial Antibiotic Given[1,3]	-	-	95%	95%
Blood Culture Timing[1,3]	-	-	98%	98%
Pregnancy and Delivery Care				
Newborn Deliveries Scheduled Early[5]	-	-	2%	6%
Preventive Care				
Immunization for Influenza[5]	-	-	92%	90%
Immunization for Pneumonia[5]	-	-	92%	92%
Stroke Care				
Anticoagulation Therapy for Atrial Fibrillation[5]	-	-	97%	95%
Antithrombotic Therapy Timing[5]	-	-	98%	98%
Assessed for Rehabilitation[5]	-	-	98%	97%
Discharged on Antithrombotic Therapy[5]	-	-	100%	99%
Discharged on Statin Medication[5]	-	-	94%	94%
Thrombolytic Therapy Timing[5]	-	-	78%	66%
Venous Thromboembolism Prophylaxis[5]	-	-	96%	94%
Written Stroke Educational Materials Given[5]	-	-	87%	88%
Surgical Care Improvement Project				
Appropriate Beta Blocker Usage[5]	-	-	98%	98%
Appropriate VTP Within 24 Hours[5]	-	-	98%	98%
Controlled Postoperative Blood Glucose[5]	-	-	96%	97%
Perioperative Temperature Management[5]	-	-	99%	100%
Prophylactic Antibiotic Selection[5]	-	-	99%	99%
Prophylactic Antibiotic Selection (Outpatient)[5]	-	-	98%	98%
Prophylactic Antibiotic Stopped[5]	-	-	98%	98%
Prophylactic Antibiotic Timing[5]	-	-	98%	99%
Prophylactic Antibiotic Timing (Outpatient)[5]	-	-	98%	98%
Urinary Catheter Removal[5]	-	-	97%	97%
Survey of Patients' Hospital Experiences				
Area Around Room 'Always' Quiet at Night[10]	<100	64%	64%	61%
Doctors 'Always' Communicated Well[10]	<100	90%	81%	82%
Home Recovery Information Given[10]	<100	91%	87%	85%
Hospital Given 9 or 10 on 10 Point Scale[10]	<100	78%	75%	71%
Meds 'Always' Explained Before Given[10]	<100	66%	67%	64%
Nurses 'Always' Communicated Well[10]	<100	83%	79%	79%
Pain 'Always' Well Controlled[10]	<100	74%	72%	71%
Room and Bathroom 'Always' Clean[10]	<100	71%	74%	73%
Timely Help 'Always' Received[10]	<100	77%	70%	68%
Would Definitely Recommend Hospital[10]	<100	71%	76%	71%
Use of Medical Imaging				
Cardiac Imaging Stress Test before Surgery[7]	-	-	5%	5.3%
Combination Abdominal CT Scan[1]	-	-	10%	10.5%
Combination Brain/Sinus CT Scan[1]	-	-	2.1%	2.7%
Combination Chest CT Scan[1]	-	-	3.1%	2.7%
Follow-up Mammogram/Ultrasound	64	6.3%	8.7%	8.8%
Lumbar Spine MRI for Low Back Pain[1]	-	-	39.7%	37.2%

Montrose Memorial Hospital

800 S 3rd St
Montrose, CO 81401
Phone: 970-249-2211
Fax: 970-252-2525
URL: www.montrosehospital.com
Type: Acute Care Hospitals
Emergency Services: Yes
Ownership: Government - Local
Beds: 75

Key Personnel:
Operating Room. . . . . Sharon Eshelman, RN
Chairman/CEO . . . . Debrah Harmon
Infection Control. . . . . Bert Hatter, RN
Quality Assurance . . . . Bert Hatter, RN
Cardiac Laboratory. . . . . Larry Peeters, RCVT
Radiology. . . . . Randall Raziano, MD
Chief of Medical Staff. . . . . Richard Shannon, MD

Measure	Cases	This Hosp.	State Avg.	U.S. Avg.
Blood Clot Prevention and Treatment				
Anticoagulation Overlap Therapy[2]	33	100%	97%	93%
ICU Venous Thromboembolism Prophylaxis[2]	43	95%	95%	92%
Incidence of Potentially Preventable VTE[1,2]	-	-	8%	10%
UFH with Dosages/Platelet Monitoring[1,2]	-	-	97%	97%
Venous Thromboembolism Prophylaxis[2]	147	95%	90%	85%
Warfarin Therapy Discharge Instructions[2]	35	83%	69%	75%
Chest Pain/Possible Heart Attack Care				
Aspirin Given Within 24 Hours of Arrival	20	90%	97%	96%
Fibrinolytic Meds Within 30 Min. of Arrival[1]	-	-	55%	58%
Average Time to ECG (minutes)	20	8	8	7
Average Time to Transfer (minutes)[7]	-	-	74	60
Children's Asthma Care				
Received Home Management Plan of Care	-	-	-	88%
Received Reliever Medication	-	-	-	100%
Received Systemic Corticosteroids	-	-	-	100%
Emergency Department				
Admittance Decision Time (minutes)[2]	304	116	96	98
Head CT Results Within 45 Min. of Arrival[1]	-	-	67%	57%
Patients Who Left ER Before Being Seen	16,650	1%	2%	2%
Time from ER Arrival to Admit. (minutes)[2]	304	223	244	274
Time from ER Arrival to Discharge (minutes)	428	102	139	134
Time in ER Before Being Evaluated (minutes)	472	15	20	26
Time to Pain Meds for Fractures (minutes)	36	38	45	57
Heart Attack Care				
Aspirin Given at Discharge	45	100%	100%	99%
Fibrinolytic Meds Within 30 Min. of Arrival[7]	-	-	20%	54%
PCI Within 90 Minutes of Arrival	18	94%	97%	96%
Statin Prescribed at Discharge	40	98%	99%	98%
Heart Failure Care				
ACE Inhibitor or ARB for LVSD	17	94%	97%	97%
Discharge Instructions Given	47	94%	93%	94%
Evaluation of LVS Function	54	100%	99%	99%
Medicare Spending				
Medicare Spending per Patient (ratio)	-	0.90	0.95	0.98
Pneumonia Care				
Appropriate Initial Antibiotic Given	54	96%	95%	95%
Blood Culture Timing	66	89%	98%	98%
Pregnancy and Delivery Care				
Newborn Deliveries Scheduled Early	37	8%	2%	6%
Preventive Care				
Immunization for Influenza[2]	279	96%	92%	90%
Immunization for Pneumonia[2]	310	95%	92%	92%
Stroke Care				
Anticoagulation Therapy for Atrial Fibrillation[1]	-	-	97%	95%
Antithrombotic Therapy Timing	21	100%	98%	98%
Assessed for Rehabilitation	28	100%	98%	97%
Discharged on Antithrombotic Therapy	27	100%	100%	99%
Discharged on Statin Medication	22	86%	94%	94%
Thrombolytic Therapy Timing[1]	-	-	78%	66%
Venous Thromboembolism Prophylaxis	21	100%	96%	94%
Written Stroke Educational Materials Given[1]	-	-	87%	88%
Surgical Care Improvement Project				
Appropriate Beta Blocker Usage[2]	67	97%	98%	98%
Appropriate VTP Within 24 Hours[2]	274	98%	98%	98%
Controlled Postoperative Blood Glucose[2,7]	-	-	96%	97%
Perioperative Temperature Management[2]	300	99%	99%	100%
Prophylactic Antibiotic Selection[2]	213	100%	99%	99%
Prophylactic Antibiotic Selection (Outpatient)	153	95%	98%	98%
Prophylactic Antibiotic Stopped[2]	212	99%	98%	98%
Prophylactic Antibiotic Timing[2]	214	95%	98%	99%
Prophylactic Antibiotic Timing (Outpatient)	156	95%	98%	98%
Urinary Catheter Removal[2]	238	96%	97%	97%
Survey of Patients' Hospital Experiences				
Area Around Room 'Always' Quiet at Night	300+	62%	64%	61%
Doctors 'Always' Communicated Well	300+	81%	81%	82%
Home Recovery Information Given	300+	84%	87%	85%
Hospital Given 9 or 10 on 10 Point Scale	300+	74%	75%	71%
Meds 'Always' Explained Before Given	300+	66%	67%	64%
Nurses 'Always' Communicated Well	300+	78%	79%	79%
Pain 'Always' Well Controlled	300+	69%	72%	71%
Room and Bathroom 'Always' Clean	300+	86%	74%	73%
Timely Help 'Always' Received	300+	73%	70%	68%
Would Definitely Recommend Hospital	300+	73%	76%	71%

NOTE: Hospital profiles are in alphabetical order by state, then city, then hospital within the city; Rankings exclude hospitals with less than 25 cases except for patient surveys which excludes hospitals with less than 100 cases; (a) 100-299 cases; (1) The number of cases/patients is too few to report; (2) Data submitted were based on a sample of cases/patients; (3) Results are based on a shorter time period than required; (4) Data suppressed by CMS for one or more quarters; (5) Results are not available for this reporting period; (6) Fewer than 100 patients completed the HCAHPS survey; (7) No cases met the criteria for this measure; (8) The lower limit of the confidence interval cannot be calculated if the number of observed infections equals zero; (9) No data are available from the state/territory for this reporting period; (10) The scores shown reflect fewer than 50 completed surveys; (11) There were discrepancies in the data collection process; (12) This measure does not apply to this hospital for this reporting period; (13) Results cannot be calculated for this reporting period; (14) The results for this state are combined with nearby states to protect confidentiality; Please refer to the User's Guide for a full explanation of data.

Use of Medical Imaging				
Cardiac Imaging Stress Test before Surgery	267	5.2%	5%	5.3%
Combination Abdominal CT Scan	462	20.6%	10%	10.5%
Combination Brain/Sinus CT Scan	265	1.1%	2.1%	2.7%
Combination Chest CT Scan	226	11.9%	3.1%	2.7%
Follow-up Mammogram/Ultrasound	956	10.0%	8.7%	8.8%
Lumbar Spine MRI for Low Back Pain	114	35.1%	39.7%	37.2%

Pagosa Springs Medical Center

95 South Pagosa Boulevard — Phone: 970-731-3700
Pagosa Springs, CO 81147
URL: www.pagosamountainhospital.com
Type: Critical Access Hospitals — Emergency Services: Yes
Ownership: Govt - Hospital Dist/Auth

Key Personnel:
CEO . . . . Bradley A Cochennet

Measure	Cases	This Hosp.	State Avg.	U.S. Avg.
Blood Clot Prevention and Treatment				
Anticoagulation Overlap Therapy[5]	-	-	97%	93%
ICU Venous Thromboembolism Prophylaxis[5]	-	-	95%	92%
Incidence of Potentially Preventable VTE[5]	-	-	8%	10%
UFH with Dosages/Platelet Monitoring[5]	-	-	97%	97%
Venous Thromboembolism Prophylaxis[5]	-	-	90%	85%
Warfarin Therapy Discharge Instructions[5]	-	-	69%	75%
Chest Pain/Possible Heart Attack Care				
Aspirin Given Within 24 Hours of Arrival	-	-	97%	96%
Fibrinolytic Meds Within 30 Min. of Arrival	-	-	55%	58%
Average Time to ECG (minutes)	-	-	8	7
Average Time to Transfer (minutes)	-	-	74	60
Children's Asthma Care				
Received Home Management Plan of Care	-	-	-	88%
Received Reliever Medication	-	-	-	100%
Received Systemic Corticosteroids	-	-	-	100%
Emergency Department				
Admittance Decision Time (minutes)[5]	-	-	96	98
Head CT Results Within 45 Min. of Arrival	-	-	67%	57%
Patients Who Left ER Before Being Seen	-	-	2%	2%
Time from ER Arrival to Admit. (minutes)[5]	-	-	244	274
Time from ER Arrival to Discharge (minutes)	-	-	139	134
Time in ER Before Being Evaluated (minutes)	-	-	20	26
Time to Pain Meds for Fractures (minutes)	-	-	45	57
Heart Attack Care				
Aspirin Given at Discharge[5]	-	-	100%	99%
Fibrinolytic Meds Within 30 Min. of Arrival[5]	-	-	20%	54%
PCI Within 90 Minutes of Arrival[5]	-	-	97%	96%
Statin Prescribed at Discharge[5]	-	-	99%	98%
Heart Failure Care				
ACE Inhibitor or ARB for LVSD[5]	-	-	97%	97%
Discharge Instructions Given[5]	-	-	93%	94%
Evaluation of LVS Function[5]	-	-	99%	99%
Medicare Spending				
Medicare Spending per Patient (ratio)	-	-	0.95	0.98
Pneumonia Care				
Appropriate Initial Antibiotic Given[5]	-	-	95%	95%
Blood Culture Timing[5]	-	-	98%	98%
Pregnancy and Delivery Care				
Newborn Deliveries Scheduled Early[5]	-	-	2%	6%
Preventive Care				
Immunization for Influenza[5]	-	-	92%	90%
Immunization for Pneumonia[5]	-	-	92%	92%
Stroke Care				
Anticoagulation Therapy for Atrial Fibrillation[5]	-	-	97%	95%
Antithrombotic Therapy Timing[5]	-	-	98%	98%
Assessed for Rehabilitation[5]	-	-	98%	97%
Discharged on Antithrombotic Therapy[5]	-	-	100%	99%
Discharged on Statin Medication[5]	-	-	94%	94%
Thrombolytic Therapy Timing[5]	-	-	78%	66%
Venous Thromboembolism Prophylaxis[5]	-	-	96%	94%
Written Stroke Educational Materials Given[5]	-	-	87%	88%
Surgical Care Improvement Project				
Appropriate Beta Blocker Usage[5]	-	-	98%	98%
Appropriate VTP Within 24 Hours[5]	-	-	98%	98%
Controlled Postoperative Blood Glucose[5]	-	-	96%	97%
Perioperative Temperature Management[5]	-	-	99%	100%
Prophylactic Antibiotic Selection[5]	-	-	99%	99%
Prophylactic Antibiotic Selection (Outpatient)	-	-	98%	98%
Prophylactic Antibiotic Stopped[5]	-	-	98%	98%
Prophylactic Antibiotic Timing[5]	-	-	98%	99%
Prophylactic Antibiotic Timing (Outpatient)	-	-	98%	98%
Urinary Catheter Removal[5]	-	-	97%	97%
Survey of Patients' Hospital Experiences				
Area Around Room 'Always' Quiet at Night[5]	-	-	64%	61%
Doctors 'Always' Communicated Well[5]	-	-	81%	82%
Home Recovery Information Given[5]	-	-	87%	85%
Hospital Given 9 or 10 on 10 Point Scale[5]	-	-	75%	71%
Meds 'Always' Explained Before Given[5]	-	-	67%	64%
Nurses 'Always' Communicated Well[5]	-	-	79%	79%
Pain 'Always' Well Controlled[5]	-	-	72%	71%
Room and Bathroom 'Always' Clean[5]	-	-	74%	73%
Timely Help 'Always' Received[5]	-	-	70%	68%
Would Definitely Recommend Hospital[5]	-	-	76%	71%
Use of Medical Imaging				
Cardiac Imaging Stress Test before Surgery	-	-	5%	5.3%
Combination Abdominal CT Scan	-	-	10%	10.5%
Combination Brain/Sinus CT Scan	-	-	2.1%	2.7%
Combination Chest CT Scan	-	-	3.1%	2.7%
Follow-up Mammogram/Ultrasound	-	-	8.7%	8.8%
Lumbar Spine MRI for Low Back Pain	-	-	39.7%	37.2%

Parker Adventist Hospital

9395 Crown Crest Blvd — Phone: 303-269-4000
Parker, CO 80138 — Fax: 303-269-4031
URL: www.parkerhospital.org
Type: Acute Care Hospitals — Emergency Services: Yes
Ownership: Voluntary non-profit - Private — Beds: 100

Key Personnel:
Radiology. . . . . Mitchell Dean Achee
CEO/President. . . . . Terry Forde
Chief of Medical Staff. . . . . Todd Mydler

Measure	Cases	This Hosp.	State Avg.	U.S. Avg.
Blood Clot Prevention and Treatment				
Anticoagulation Overlap Therapy[2]	60	95%	97%	93%
ICU Venous Thromboembolism Prophylaxis[2]	96	98%	95%	92%
Incidence of Potentially Preventable VTE[2]	14	21%	8%	10%
UFH with Dosages/Platelet Monitoring[2]	56	96%	97%	97%
Venous Thromboembolism Prophylaxis[2]	313	95%	90%	85%
Warfarin Therapy Discharge Instructions[2]	45	58%	69%	75%
Chest Pain/Possible Heart Attack Care				
Aspirin Given Within 24 Hours of Arrival	16	100%	97%	96%
Fibrinolytic Meds Within 30 Min. of Arrival[3,7]	-	-	55%	58%
Average Time to ECG (minutes)	17	6	8	7
Average Time to Transfer (minutes)[3,7]	-	-	74	60
Children's Asthma Care				
Received Home Management Plan of Care	-	-	-	88%
Received Reliever Medication	-	-	-	100%
Received Systemic Corticosteroids	-	-	-	100%
Emergency Department				
Admittance Decision Time (minutes)[2]	448	113	96	98
Head CT Results Within 45 Min. of Arrival[1]	-	-	67%	57%
Patients Who Left ER Before Being Seen	25,556	1%	2%	2%
Time from ER Arrival to Admit. (minutes)[2]	453	274	244	274
Time from ER Arrival to Discharge (minutes)	434	198	139	134
Time in ER Before Being Evaluated (minutes)	462	17	20	26
Time to Pain Meds for Fractures (minutes)	138	56	45	57
Heart Attack Care				
Aspirin Given at Discharge	63	100%	100%	99%
Fibrinolytic Meds Within 30 Min. of Arrival[7]	-	-	20%	54%
PCI Within 90 Minutes of Arrival	22	100%	97%	96%
Statin Prescribed at Discharge	59	100%	99%	98%
Heart Failure Care				
ACE Inhibitor or ARB for LVSD	21	95%	97%	97%
Discharge Instructions Given	72	92%	93%	94%
Evaluation of LVS Function	88	99%	99%	99%
Medicare Spending				
Medicare Spending per Patient (ratio)	-	0.96	0.95	0.98
Pneumonia Care				
Appropriate Initial Antibiotic Given	106	100%	95%	95%
Blood Culture Timing	117	98%	98%	98%
Pregnancy and Delivery Care				
Newborn Deliveries Scheduled Early[2]	32	3%	2%	6%
Preventive Care				
Immunization for Influenza[2]	524	88%	92%	90%
Immunization for Pneumonia[2]	475	86%	92%	92%
Stroke Care				
Anticoagulation Therapy for Atrial Fibrillation[1]	-	-	97%	95%
Antithrombotic Therapy Timing	43	100%	98%	98%
Assessed for Rehabilitation	65	98%	98%	97%
Discharged on Antithrombotic Therapy	59	100%	100%	99%
Discharged on Statin Medication	42	95%	94%	94%
Thrombolytic Therapy Timing	11	64%	78%	66%
Venous Thromboembolism Prophylaxis	56	100%	96%	94%
Written Stroke Educational Materials Given	39	67%	87%	88%
Surgical Care Improvement Project				
Appropriate Beta Blocker Usage	126	98%	98%	98%
Appropriate VTP Within 24 Hours	449	99%	98%	98%
Controlled Postoperative Blood Glucose[7]	-	-	96%	97%
Perioperative Temperature Management	656	100%	99%	100%
Prophylactic Antibiotic Selection	349	99%	99%	99%
Prophylactic Antibiotic Selection (Outpatient)	337	97%	98%	98%
Prophylactic Antibiotic Stopped	341	99%	98%	98%
Prophylactic Antibiotic Timing	350	99%	98%	99%
Prophylactic Antibiotic Timing (Outpatient)	338	99%	98%	98%
Urinary Catheter Removal	256	92%	97%	97%
Survey of Patients' Hospital Experiences				
Area Around Room 'Always' Quiet at Night	300+	64%	64%	61%
Doctors 'Always' Communicated Well	300+	80%	81%	82%
Home Recovery Information Given	300+	91%	87%	85%
Hospital Given 9 or 10 on 10 Point Scale	300+	76%	75%	71%
Meds 'Always' Explained Before Given	300+	64%	67%	64%
Nurses 'Always' Communicated Well	300+	79%	79%	79%
Pain 'Always' Well Controlled	300+	69%	72%	71%
Room and Bathroom 'Always' Clean	300+	72%	74%	73%
Timely Help 'Always' Received	300+	63%	70%	68%
Would Definitely Recommend Hospital	300+	79%	76%	71%
Use of Medical Imaging				
Cardiac Imaging Stress Test before Surgery	161	3.1%	5%	5.3%
Combination Abdominal CT Scan	458	12.2%	10%	10.5%
Combination Brain/Sinus CT Scan[1]	-	-	2.1%	2.7%
Combination Chest CT Scan	233	9.9%	3.1%	2.7%
Follow-up Mammogram/Ultrasound	422	11.6%	8.7%	8.8%
Lumbar Spine MRI for Low Back Pain	73	35.6%	39.7%	37.2%

Centura Health - Saint Mary Corwin Medical Center

1008 Minnequa Ave — Phone: 719-557-4000
Pueblo, CO 81004 — Fax: 719-557-5950
URL: www.stmarycorwin.org
Type: Acute Care Hospitals — Emergency Services: Yes
Ownership: Voluntary non-profit - Church — Beds: 408

Key Personnel:
Radiology. . . . . Louis Gregory Arvanetes
Intensive Care Unit. . . . . Donna Fisher
Infection Control. . . . . Sandra Gallegos
CEO/President. . . . . Brian Moore
Chief of Medical Staff . . . . Charles Raye, MD
Quality Assurance . . . . John Sanchez
Patient Relations . . . . Bryan Serena
Coronary Care . . . . Jodee Trainor

Measure	Cases	This Hosp.	State Avg.	U.S. Avg.
Blood Clot Prevention and Treatment				
Anticoagulation Overlap Therapy[2]	63	100%	97%	93%
ICU Venous Thromboembolism Prophylaxis[2]	84	96%	95%	92%
Incidence of Potentially Preventable VTE[1,2]	-	-	8%	10%
UFH with Dosages/Platelet Monitoring[1,2]	-	-	97%	97%
Venous Thromboembolism Prophylaxis[2]	347	88%	90%	85%
Warfarin Therapy Discharge Instructions[2]	52	96%	69%	75%
Chest Pain/Possible Heart Attack Care				
Aspirin Given Within 24 Hours of Arrival[1,3]	-	-	97%	96%
Fibrinolytic Meds Within 30 Min. of Arrival[3,7]	-	-	55%	58%
Average Time to ECG (minutes)[1,3]	-	-	8	7
Average Time to Transfer (minutes)[3,7]	-	-	74	60

NOTE: Hospital profiles are in alphabetical order by state, then city, then hospital within the city; Rankings exclude hospitals with less than 25 cases except for patient surveys which excludes hospitals with less than 100 cases; (a) 100-299 cases; (1) The number of cases/patients is too few to report; (2) Data submitted were based on a sample of cases/patients; (3) Results are based on a shorter time period than required; (4) Data suppressed by CMS for one or more quarters; (5) Results are not available for this reporting period; (6) Fewer than 100 patients completed the HCAHPS survey; (7) No cases met the criteria for this measure; (8) The lower limit of the confidence interval cannot be calculated if the number of observed infections equals zero; (9) No data are available from the state/territory for this reporting period; (10) The scores shown reflect fewer than 50 completed surveys; (11) There were discrepancies in the data collection process; (12) This measure does not apply to this hospital for this reporting period; (13) Results cannot be calculated for this reporting period; (14) The results for this state are combined with nearby states to protect confidentiality; Please refer to the User's Guide for a full explanation of data.

Measure	Cases	This Hosp.	State Avg.	U.S. Avg.
Children's Asthma Care				
Received Home Management Plan of Care	-	-	-	88%
Received Reliever Medication	-	-	-	100%
Received Systemic Corticosteroids	-	-	-	100%
Emergency Department				
Admittance Decision Time (minutes)[2]	486	146	96	98
Head CT Results Within 45 Min. of Arrival[1]	-	-	67%	57%
Patients Who Left ER Before Being Seen	35,223	1%	2%	2%
Time from ER Arrival to Admit. (minutes)[2]	499	272	244	274
Time from ER Arrival to Discharge (minutes)	466	116	139	134
Time in ER Before Being Evaluated (minutes)	496	36	20	26
Time to Pain Meds for Fractures (minutes)	100	58	45	57
Heart Attack Care				
Aspirin Given at Discharge	161	100%	100%	99%
Fibrinolytic Meds Within 30 Min. of Arrival[1]	-	-	20%	54%
PCI Within 90 Minutes of Arrival	33	100%	97%	96%
Statin Prescribed at Discharge	164	99%	99%	98%
Heart Failure Care				
ACE Inhibitor or ARB for LVSD	38	100%	97%	97%
Discharge Instructions Given	93	96%	93%	94%
Evaluation of LVS Function	116	100%	99%	99%
Medicare Spending				
Medicare Spending per Patient (ratio)	-	1.00	0.95	0.98
Pneumonia Care				
Appropriate Initial Antibiotic Given	76	99%	95%	95%
Blood Culture Timing	114	100%	98%	98%
Pregnancy and Delivery Care				
Newborn Deliveries Scheduled Early	58	2%	2%	6%
Preventive Care				
Immunization for Influenza[2]	588	97%	92%	90%
Immunization for Pneumonia[2]	748	97%	92%	92%
Stroke Care				
Anticoagulation Therapy for Atrial Fibrillation[1]	-	-	97%	95%
Antithrombotic Therapy Timing	59	100%	98%	98%
Assessed for Rehabilitation	83	100%	98%	97%
Discharged on Antithrombotic Therapy	70	99%	100%	99%
Discharged on Statin Medication	43	93%	94%	94%
Thrombolytic Therapy Timing	19	95%	78%	66%
Venous Thromboembolism Prophylaxis	90	97%	96%	94%
Written Stroke Educational Materials Given	37	97%	87%	88%
Surgical Care Improvement Project				
Appropriate Beta Blocker Usage	113	98%	98%	98%
Appropriate VTP Within 24 Hours	454	98%	98%	98%
Controlled Postoperative Blood Glucose[7]	-	-	96%	97%
Perioperative Temperature Management	493	100%	99%	100%
Prophylactic Antibiotic Selection	312	100%	99%	99%
Prophylactic Antibiotic Selection (Outpatient)	224	97%	98%	98%
Prophylactic Antibiotic Stopped	305	100%	98%	98%
Prophylactic Antibiotic Timing	312	100%	98%	99%
Prophylactic Antibiotic Timing (Outpatient)	224	100%	98%	98%
Urinary Catheter Removal	103	90%	97%	97%
Survey of Patients' Hospital Experiences				
Area Around Room 'Always' Quiet at Night	300+	56%	64%	61%
Doctors 'Always' Communicated Well	300+	80%	81%	82%
Home Recovery Information Given	300+	88%	87%	85%
Hospital Given 9 or 10 on 10 Point Scale	300+	71%	75%	71%
Meds 'Always' Explained Before Given	300+	68%	67%	64%
Nurses 'Always' Communicated Well	300+	77%	79%	79%
Pain 'Always' Well Controlled	300+	69%	72%	71%
Room and Bathroom 'Always' Clean	300+	71%	74%	73%
Timely Help 'Always' Received	300+	64%	70%	68%
Would Definitely Recommend Hospital	300+	74%	76%	71%
Use of Medical Imaging				
Cardiac Imaging Stress Test before Surgery	165	4.8%	5%	5.3%
Combination Abdominal CT Scan	652	11.7%	10%	10.5%
Combination Brain/Sinus CT Scan[1]	-	-	2.1%	2.7%
Combination Chest CT Scan	363	8.3%	3.1%	2.7%
Follow-up Mammogram/Ultrasound	1,836	9.2%	8.7%	8.8%
Lumbar Spine MRI for Low Back Pain	74	41.9%	39.7%	37.2%

Parkview Medical Center

400 W 16th Street
Pueblo, CO 81003
Phone: 719-584-4000
Fax: 719-544-6663
E-mail: info@parkviewmc.org
URL: www.parkviewmc.com
Type: Acute Care Hospitals
Emergency Services: Yes
Ownership: Voluntary non-profit - Private
Beds: 350

Key Personnel:
Chief of Medical Staff. . . . . Ernest Steinle, MD

Measure	Cases	This Hosp.	State Avg.	U.S. Avg.
Blood Clot Prevention and Treatment				
Anticoagulation Overlap Therapy[2]	167	94%	97%	93%
ICU Venous Thromboembolism Prophylaxis[2]	88	93%	95%	92%
Incidence of Potentially Preventable VTE[2]	21	0%	8%	10%
UFH with Dosages/Platelet Monitoring[2]	47	100%	97%	97%
Venous Thromboembolism Prophylaxis[2]	322	87%	90%	85%
Warfarin Therapy Discharge Instructions[2]	134	97%	69%	75%
Chest Pain/Possible Heart Attack Care				
Aspirin Given Within 24 Hours of Arrival[1,3]	-	-	97%	96%
Fibrinolytic Meds Within 30 Min. of Arrival[5]	-	-	55%	58%
Average Time to ECG (minutes)[1,3]	-	-	8	7
Average Time to Transfer (minutes)[5]	-	-	74	60
Children's Asthma Care				
Received Home Management Plan of Care	-	-	-	88%
Received Reliever Medication	-	-	-	100%
Received Systemic Corticosteroids	-	-	-	100%
Emergency Department				
Admittance Decision Time (minutes)[2]	464	118	96	98
Head CT Results Within 45 Min. of Arrival[1]	-	-	67%	57%
Patients Who Left ER Before Being Seen	60,705	3%	2%	2%
Time from ER Arrival to Admit. (minutes)[2]	468	250	244	274
Time from ER Arrival to Discharge (minutes)	349	147	139	134
Time in ER Before Being Evaluated (minutes)	392	37	20	26
Time to Pain Meds for Fractures (minutes)	217	47	45	57
Heart Attack Care				
Aspirin Given at Discharge	255	98%	100%	99%
Fibrinolytic Meds Within 30 Min. of Arrival[1]	-	-	20%	54%
PCI Within 90 Minutes of Arrival	50	98%	97%	96%
Statin Prescribed at Discharge	257	99%	99%	98%
Heart Failure Care				
ACE Inhibitor or ARB for LVSD	63	97%	97%	97%
Discharge Instructions Given	182	95%	93%	94%
Evaluation of LVS Function	219	100%	99%	99%
Medicare Spending				
Medicare Spending per Patient (ratio)	-	0.94	0.95	0.98
Pneumonia Care				
Appropriate Initial Antibiotic Given[2]	70	97%	95%	95%
Blood Culture Timing[2]	119	97%	98%	98%
Pregnancy and Delivery Care				
Newborn Deliveries Scheduled Early	173	2%	2%	6%
Preventive Care				
Immunization for Influenza[2]	524	92%	92%	90%
Immunization for Pneumonia[2]	594	85%	92%	92%
Stroke Care				
Anticoagulation Therapy for Atrial Fibrillation	22	95%	97%	95%
Antithrombotic Therapy Timing	115	100%	98%	98%
Assessed for Rehabilitation	134	97%	98%	97%
Discharged on Antithrombotic Therapy	125	98%	100%	99%
Discharged on Statin Medication	86	93%	94%	94%
Thrombolytic Therapy Timing	15	80%	78%	66%
Venous Thromboembolism Prophylaxis	139	94%	96%	94%
Written Stroke Educational Materials Given	85	99%	87%	88%
Surgical Care Improvement Project				
Appropriate Beta Blocker Usage[2]	146	97%	98%	98%
Appropriate VTP Within 24 Hours[2]	397	95%	98%	98%
Controlled Postoperative Blood Glucose[2]	51	90%	96%	97%
Perioperative Temperature Management[2]	437	100%	99%	100%
Prophylactic Antibiotic Selection[2]	326	99%	99%	99%
Prophylactic Antibiotic Selection (Outpatient)	483	98%	98%	98%
Prophylactic Antibiotic Stopped[2]	311	95%	98%	98%
Prophylactic Antibiotic Timing[2]	326	98%	98%	99%
Prophylactic Antibiotic Timing (Outpatient)	485	95%	98%	98%
Urinary Catheter Removal[2]	307	94%	97%	97%
Survey of Patients' Hospital Experiences				
Area Around Room 'Always' Quiet at Night	300+	58%	64%	61%
Doctors 'Always' Communicated Well	300+	76%	81%	82%
Home Recovery Information Given	300+	84%	87%	85%
Hospital Given 9 or 10 on 10 Point Scale	300+	76%	75%	71%
Meds 'Always' Explained Before Given	300+	62%	67%	64%
Nurses 'Always' Communicated Well	300+	78%	79%	79%
Pain 'Always' Well Controlled	300+	70%	72%	71%
Room and Bathroom 'Always' Clean	300+	81%	74%	73%
Timely Help 'Always' Received	300+	64%	70%	68%
Would Definitely Recommend Hospital	300+	80%	76%	71%
Use of Medical Imaging				
Cardiac Imaging Stress Test before Surgery	870	6.1%	5%	5.3%
Combination Abdominal CT Scan	1,526	5.6%	10%	10.5%
Combination Brain/Sinus CT Scan	1,156	2.2%	2.1%	2.7%
Combination Chest CT Scan	520	0.2%	3.1%	2.7%
Follow-up Mammogram/Ultrasound	605	12.2%	8.7%	8.8%
Lumbar Spine MRI for Low Back Pain	143	39.2%	39.7%	37.2%

Rangely District Hospital

225 Eaglecrest
Rangely, CO 81648
Phone: 970-675-5011
Fax: 970-675-5224
URL: www.rangelyhospital.com
Type: Critical Access Hospitals
Emergency Services: Yes
Ownership: Govt - Hospital Dist/Auth
Beds: 25

Key Personnel:
Radiology. . . . . Nancy Droste
CEO/President. . . . . Nick Goshe
Emergency Room . . . . Sheryl Sheley
Chief of Medical Staff. . . . . David Benjamin Udall

Measure	Cases	This Hosp.	State Avg.	U.S. Avg.
Blood Clot Prevention and Treatment				
Anticoagulation Overlap Therapy[5]	-	-	97%	93%
ICU Venous Thromboembolism Prophylaxis[5]	-	-	95%	92%
Incidence of Potentially Preventable VTE[5]	-	-	8%	10%
UFH with Dosages/Platelet Monitoring[5]	-	-	97%	97%
Venous Thromboembolism Prophylaxis[5]	-	-	90%	85%
Warfarin Therapy Discharge Instructions[5]	-	-	69%	75%
Chest Pain/Possible Heart Attack Care				
Aspirin Given Within 24 Hours of Arrival	-	-	97%	96%
Fibrinolytic Meds Within 30 Min. of Arrival	-	-	55%	58%
Average Time to ECG (minutes)	-	-	8	7
Average Time to Transfer (minutes)	-	-	74	60
Children's Asthma Care				
Received Home Management Plan of Care	-	-	-	88%
Received Reliever Medication	-	-	-	100%
Received Systemic Corticosteroids	-	-	-	100%
Emergency Department				
Admittance Decision Time (minutes)[5]	-	-	96	98
Head CT Results Within 45 Min. of Arrival	-	-	67%	57%
Patients Who Left ER Before Being Seen	-	-	2%	2%
Time from ER Arrival to Admit. (minutes)[5]	-	-	244	274
Time from ER Arrival to Discharge (minutes)	-	-	139	134
Time in ER Before Being Evaluated (minutes)	-	-	20	26
Time to Pain Meds for Fractures (minutes)	-	-	45	57
Heart Attack Care				
Aspirin Given at Discharge[5]	-	-	100%	99%
Fibrinolytic Meds Within 30 Min. of Arrival[5]	-	-	20%	54%
PCI Within 90 Minutes of Arrival[5]	-	-	97%	96%
Statin Prescribed at Discharge[5]	-	-	99%	98%
Heart Failure Care				
ACE Inhibitor or ARB for LVSD[5]	-	-	97%	97%
Discharge Instructions Given[5]	-	-	93%	94%
Evaluation of LVS Function[5]	-	-	99%	99%
Medicare Spending				
Medicare Spending per Patient (ratio)	-	-	0.95	0.98
Pneumonia Care				
Appropriate Initial Antibiotic Given[5]	-	-	95%	95%
Blood Culture Timing[5]	-	-	98%	98%
Pregnancy and Delivery Care				
Newborn Deliveries Scheduled Early[5]	-	-	2%	6%
Preventive Care				
Immunization for Influenza[5]	-	-	92%	90%

NOTE: Hospital profiles are in alphabetical order by state, then city, then hospital within the city; Rankings exclude hospitals with less than 25 cases except for patient surveys which excludes hospitals with less than 100 cases; (a) 100-299 cases; (1) The number of cases/patients is too few to report; (2) Data submitted were based on a sample of cases/patients; (3) Results are based on a shorter time period than required; (4) Data suppressed by CMS for one or more quarters; (5) Results are not available for this reporting period; (6) Fewer than 100 patients completed the HCAHPS survey; (7) No cases met the criteria for this measure; (8) The lower limit of the confidence interval cannot be calculated if the number of observed infections equals zero; (9) No data are available from the state/territory for this reporting period; (10) The scores shown reflect fewer than 50 completed surveys; (11) There were discrepancies in the data collection process; (12) This measure does not apply to this hospital for this reporting period; (13) Results cannot be calculated for this reporting period; (14) The results for this state are combined with nearby states to protect confidentiality; Please refer to the User's Guide for a full explanation of data.

Measure	Cases	This Hosp.	State Avg.	U.S. Avg.
Immunization for Pneumonia[5]	-	-	92%	92%
Stroke Care				
Anticoagulation Therapy for Atrial Fibrillation[5]	-	-	97%	95%
Antithrombotic Therapy Timing[5]	-	-	98%	98%
Assessed for Rehabilitation[5]	-	-	98%	97%
Discharged on Antithrombotic Therapy[5]	-	-	100%	99%
Discharged on Statin Medication[5]	-	-	94%	94%
Thrombolytic Therapy Timing[5]	-	-	78%	66%
Venous Thromboembolism Prophylaxis[5]	-	-	96%	94%
Written Stroke Educational Materials Given[5]	-	-	87%	88%
Surgical Care Improvement Project				
Appropriate Beta Blocker Usage[5]	-	-	98%	98%
Appropriate VTP Within 24 Hours[5]	-	-	98%	98%
Controlled Postoperative Blood Glucose[5]	-	-	96%	97%
Perioperative Temperature Management[5]	-	-	99%	100%
Prophylactic Antibiotic Selection[5]	-	-	99%	99%
Prophylactic Antibiotic Selection (Outpatient)	-	-	98%	98%
Prophylactic Antibiotic Stopped[5]	-	-	98%	98%
Prophylactic Antibiotic Timing[5]	-	-	98%	99%
Prophylactic Antibiotic Timing (Outpatient)	-	-	98%	98%
Urinary Catheter Removal[5]	-	-	97%	97%
Survey of Patients' Hospital Experiences				
Area Around Room 'Always' Quiet at Night[5]	-	-	64%	61%
Doctors 'Always' Communicated Well[5]	-	-	81%	82%
Home Recovery Information Given[5]	-	-	87%	85%
Hospital Given 9 or 10 on 10 Point Scale[5]	-	-	75%	71%
Meds 'Always' Explained Before Given[5]	-	-	67%	64%
Nurses 'Always' Communicated Well[5]	-	-	79%	79%
Pain 'Always' Well Controlled[5]	-	-	72%	71%
Room and Bathroom 'Always' Clean[5]	-	-	74%	73%
Timely Help 'Always' Received[5]	-	-	70%	68%
Would Definitely Recommend Hospital[5]	-	-	76%	71%
Use of Medical Imaging				
Cardiac Imaging Stress Test before Surgery	-	-	5%	5.3%
Combination Abdominal CT Scan	-	-	10%	10.5%
Combination Brain/Sinus CT Scan	-	-	2.1%	2.7%
Combination Chest CT Scan	-	-	3.1%	2.7%
Follow-up Mammogram/Ultrasound	-	-	8.7%	8.8%
Lumbar Spine MRI for Low Back Pain	-	-	39.7%	37.2%

Grand River Medical Center

501 Airport Road
Rifle, CO 81650
URL: www.grhd.org
Phone: 970-625-1510
Fax: 970-625-6486
Type: Critical Access Hospitals
Emergency Services: Yes
Ownership: Govt - Hospital Dist/Auth
Beds: 25

Key Personnel:
Operating Room. . . . . Linda Bessette
Chief of Medical Staff. . . . . Deborah Brown, MD
Emergency Room . . . . Yvette Burdick, RN
CEO . . . . Jim Coombs
Patient Relations . . . . Mary DesOrmeau
Radiology. . . . . Charles Fowler
Infection Control. . . . . Sara Jacobson
Quality Assurance . . . . Rusty Stevens

Measure	Cases	This Hosp.	State Avg.	U.S. Avg.
Blood Clot Prevention and Treatment				
Anticoagulation Overlap Therapy[1,2]	-	-	97%	93%
ICU Venous Thromboembolism Prophylaxis[2,7]	-	-	95%	92%
Incidence of Potentially Preventable VTE[1,2]	-	-	8%	10%
UFH with Dosages/Platelet Monitoring[2,7]	-	-	97%	97%
Venous Thromboembolism Prophylaxis[2]	83	77%	90%	85%
Warfarin Therapy Discharge Instructions[1,2]	-	-	69%	75%
Chest Pain/Possible Heart Attack Care				
Aspirin Given Within 24 Hours of Arrival	-	-	97%	96%
Fibrinolytic Meds Within 30 Min. of Arrival	-	-	55%	58%
Average Time to ECG (minutes)	-	-	8	7
Average Time to Transfer (minutes)	-	-	74	60
Children's Asthma Care				
Received Home Management Plan of Care	-	-	-	88%
Received Reliever Medication	-	-	-	100%
Received Systemic Corticosteroids	-	-	-	100%
Emergency Department				
Admittance Decision Time (minutes)[5]	-	-	96	98
Head CT Results Within 45 Min. of Arrival	-	-	67%	57%
Patients Who Left ER Before Being Seen	-	-	2%	2%
Time from ER Arrival to Admit. (minutes)[5]	-	-	244	274
Time from ER Arrival to Discharge (minutes)	-	-	139	134
Time in ER Before Being Evaluated (minutes)	-	-	20	26
Time to Pain Meds for Fractures (minutes)	-	-	45	57
Heart Attack Care				
Aspirin Given at Discharge[5]	-	-	100%	99%
Fibrinolytic Meds Within 30 Min. of Arrival[5]	-	-	20%	54%
PCI Within 90 Minutes of Arrival[5]	-	-	97%	96%
Statin Prescribed at Discharge[5]	-	-	99%	98%
Heart Failure Care				
ACE Inhibitor or ARB for LVSD[1]	-	-	97%	97%
Discharge Instructions Given[1]	-	-	93%	94%
Evaluation of LVS Function[1]	-	-	99%	99%
Medicare Spending				
Medicare Spending per Patient (ratio)	-	-	0.95	0.98
Pneumonia Care				
Appropriate Initial Antibiotic Given	19	89%	95%	95%
Blood Culture Timing	32	97%	98%	98%
Pregnancy and Delivery Care				
Newborn Deliveries Scheduled Early[5]	-	-	2%	6%
Preventive Care				
Immunization for Influenza[5]	-	-	92%	90%
Immunization for Pneumonia[5]	-	-	92%	92%
Stroke Care				
Anticoagulation Therapy for Atrial Fibrillation[1,3]	-	-	97%	95%
Antithrombotic Therapy Timing[1,3]	-	-	98%	98%
Assessed for Rehabilitation[1,3]	-	-	98%	97%
Discharged on Antithrombotic Therapy[1,3]	-	-	100%	99%
Discharged on Statin Medication[1,3]	-	-	94%	94%
Thrombolytic Therapy Timing[1,3]	-	-	78%	66%
Venous Thromboembolism Prophylaxis[1,3]	-	-	96%	94%
Written Stroke Educational Materials Given[1,3]	-	-	87%	88%
Surgical Care Improvement Project				
Appropriate Beta Blocker Usage[1,3]	-	-	98%	98%
Appropriate VTP Within 24 Hours[3]	23	91%	98%	98%
Controlled Postoperative Blood Glucose[3,7]	-	-	96%	97%
Perioperative Temperature Management[3]	31	100%	99%	100%
Prophylactic Antibiotic Selection[1,3]	-	-	99%	99%
Prophylactic Antibiotic Selection (Outpatient)	-	-	98%	98%
Prophylactic Antibiotic Stopped[1,3]	-	-	98%	98%
Prophylactic Antibiotic Timing[1,3]	-	-	98%	99%
Prophylactic Antibiotic Timing (Outpatient)	-	-	98%	98%
Urinary Catheter Removal[3]	13	100%	97%	97%
Survey of Patients' Hospital Experiences				
Area Around Room 'Always' Quiet at Night[5]	-	-	64%	61%
Doctors 'Always' Communicated Well[5]	-	-	81%	82%
Home Recovery Information Given[5]	-	-	87%	85%
Hospital Given 9 or 10 on 10 Point Scale[5]	-	-	75%	71%
Meds 'Always' Explained Before Given[5]	-	-	67%	64%
Nurses 'Always' Communicated Well[5]	-	-	79%	79%
Pain 'Always' Well Controlled[5]	-	-	72%	71%
Room and Bathroom 'Always' Clean[5]	-	-	74%	73%
Timely Help 'Always' Received[5]	-	-	70%	68%
Would Definitely Recommend Hospital[5]	-	-	76%	71%
Use of Medical Imaging				
Cardiac Imaging Stress Test before Surgery	-	-	5%	5.3%
Combination Abdominal CT Scan	-	-	10%	10.5%
Combination Brain/Sinus CT Scan	-	-	2.1%	2.7%
Combination Chest CT Scan	-	-	3.1%	2.7%
Follow-up Mammogram/Ultrasound	-	-	8.7%	8.8%
Lumbar Spine MRI for Low Back Pain	-	-	39.7%	37.2%

Heart of the Rockies Regional Medical Center

1000 Rush Drive
Salida, CO 81201
E-mail: info@hrrmc.net
URL: www.hrrmc.com
Phone: 719-530-2200
Type: Critical Access Hospitals
Emergency Services: Yes
Ownership: Govt - Hospital Dist/Auth
Beds: 25

Key Personnel:
Emergency Room . . . . Kenneth Eckstein, RN
Radiology. . . . . Deborah M Lince
CEO . . . . Bob Morasko, MBA, FACHE
Chief of Medical Staff. . . . . Carolyn Webb

Measure	Cases	This Hosp.	State Avg.	U.S. Avg.
Blood Clot Prevention and Treatment				
Anticoagulation Overlap Therapy[5]	-	-	97%	93%
ICU Venous Thromboembolism Prophylaxis[5]	-	-	95%	92%
Incidence of Potentially Preventable VTE[5]	-	-	8%	10%
UFH with Dosages/Platelet Monitoring[5]	-	-	97%	97%
Venous Thromboembolism Prophylaxis[5]	-	-	90%	85%
Warfarin Therapy Discharge Instructions[5]	-	-	69%	75%
Chest Pain/Possible Heart Attack Care				
Aspirin Given Within 24 Hours of Arrival	-	-	97%	96%
Fibrinolytic Meds Within 30 Min. of Arrival	-	-	55%	58%
Average Time to ECG (minutes)	-	-	8	7
Average Time to Transfer (minutes)	-	-	74	60
Children's Asthma Care				
Received Home Management Plan of Care	-	-	-	88%
Received Reliever Medication	-	-	-	100%
Received Systemic Corticosteroids	-	-	-	100%
Emergency Department				
Admittance Decision Time (minutes)[5]	-	-	96	98
Head CT Results Within 45 Min. of Arrival	-	-	67%	57%
Patients Who Left ER Before Being Seen	-	-	2%	2%
Time from ER Arrival to Admit. (minutes)[5]	-	-	244	274
Time from ER Arrival to Discharge (minutes)	-	-	139	134
Time in ER Before Being Evaluated (minutes)	-	-	20	26
Time to Pain Meds for Fractures (minutes)	-	-	45	57
Heart Attack Care				
Aspirin Given at Discharge[5]	-	-	100%	99%
Fibrinolytic Meds Within 30 Min. of Arrival[5]	-	-	20%	54%
PCI Within 90 Minutes of Arrival[5]	-	-	97%	96%
Statin Prescribed at Discharge[5]	-	-	99%	98%
Heart Failure Care				
ACE Inhibitor or ARB for LVSD[1]	-	-	97%	97%
Discharge Instructions Given	22	32%	93%	94%
Evaluation of LVS Function	25	84%	99%	99%
Medicare Spending				
Medicare Spending per Patient (ratio)	-	-	0.95	0.98
Pneumonia Care				
Appropriate Initial Antibiotic Given	24	62%	95%	95%
Blood Culture Timing	23	83%	98%	98%
Pregnancy and Delivery Care				
Newborn Deliveries Scheduled Early[5]	-	-	2%	6%
Preventive Care				
Immunization for Influenza[5]	-	-	92%	90%
Immunization for Pneumonia[5]	-	-	92%	92%
Stroke Care				
Anticoagulation Therapy for Atrial Fibrillation[5]	-	-	97%	95%
Antithrombotic Therapy Timing[5]	-	-	98%	98%
Assessed for Rehabilitation[5]	-	-	98%	97%
Discharged on Antithrombotic Therapy[5]	-	-	100%	99%
Discharged on Statin Medication[5]	-	-	94%	94%
Thrombolytic Therapy Timing[5]	-	-	78%	66%
Venous Thromboembolism Prophylaxis[5]	-	-	96%	94%
Written Stroke Educational Materials Given[5]	-	-	87%	88%
Surgical Care Improvement Project				
Appropriate Beta Blocker Usage[5]	-	-	98%	98%
Appropriate VTP Within 24 Hours[5]	-	-	98%	98%
Controlled Postoperative Blood Glucose[5]	-	-	96%	97%
Perioperative Temperature Management[5]	-	-	99%	100%
Prophylactic Antibiotic Selection[5]	-	-	99%	99%
Prophylactic Antibiotic Selection (Outpatient)	-	-	98%	98%
Prophylactic Antibiotic Stopped[5]	-	-	98%	98%
Prophylactic Antibiotic Timing[5]	-	-	98%	99%
Prophylactic Antibiotic Timing (Outpatient)	-	-	98%	98%
Urinary Catheter Removal[5]	-	-	97%	97%
Survey of Patients' Hospital Experiences				
Area Around Room 'Always' Quiet at Night	(a)	69%	64%	61%
Doctors 'Always' Communicated Well	(a)	85%	81%	82%
Home Recovery Information Given	(a)	89%	87%	85%
Hospital Given 9 or 10 on 10 Point Scale	(a)	82%	75%	71%
Meds 'Always' Explained Before Given	(a)	78%	67%	64%

NOTE: Hospital profiles are in alphabetical order by state, then city, then hospital within the city; Rankings exclude hospitals with less than 25 cases except for patient surveys which excludes hospitals with less than 100 cases; (a) 100-299 cases; (1) The number of cases/patients is too few to report; (2) Data submitted were based on a sample of cases/patients; (3) Results are based on a shorter time period than required; (4) Data suppressed by CMS for one or more quarters; (5) Results are not available for this reporting period; (6) Fewer than 100 patients completed the HCAHPS survey; (7) No cases met the criteria for this measure; (8) The lower limit of the confidence interval cannot be calculated if the number of observed infections equals zero; (9) No data are available from the state/territory for this reporting period; (10) The scores shown reflect fewer than 50 completed surveys; (11) There were discrepancies in the data collection process; (12) This measure does not apply to this hospital for this reporting period; (13) Results cannot be calculated for this reporting period; (14) The results for this state are combined with nearby states to protect confidentiality; Please refer to the User's Guide for a full explanation of data.

Measure	Cases	This Hosp.	State Avg.	U.S. Avg.
Nurses 'Always' Communicated Well	(a)	85%	79%	79%
Pain 'Always' Well Controlled	(a)	79%	72%	71%
Room and Bathroom 'Always' Clean	(a)	78%	74%	73%
Timely Help 'Always' Received	(a)	82%	70%	68%
Would Definitely Recommend Hospital	(a)	81%	76%	71%
Use of Medical Imaging				
Cardiac Imaging Stress Test before Surgery	-	-	5%	5.3%
Combination Abdominal CT Scan	-	-	10%	10.5%
Combination Brain/Sinus CT Scan	-	-	2.1%	2.7%
Combination Chest CT Scan	-	-	3.1%	2.7%
Follow-up Mammogram/Ultrasound	-	-	8.7%	8.8%
Lumbar Spine MRI for Low Back Pain	-	-	39.7%	37.2%

Southeast Colorado Hospital

373 E Tenth Ave
Springfield, CO 81073
Phone: 719-523-4501
Fax: 719-523-4763
E-mail: sechosp@sechosp.org
URL: www.sechosp.org
Type: Critical Access Hospitals
Emergency Services: Yes
Ownership: Govt - Hospital Dist/Auth
Beds: 81

Key Personnel:
Operating Room. . . . . Marla Baxter
Chief of Medical Staff . . . . Nagesh Chopra
CEO/President. . . . . Ty Shettron
Radiology. . . . . Kristy Turner, PT
Quality Assurance . . . . Sherrilyn Turner

Measure	Cases	This Hosp.	State Avg.	U.S. Avg.
Blood Clot Prevention and Treatment				
Anticoagulation Overlap Therapy[5]	-	-	97%	93%
ICU Venous Thromboembolism Prophylaxis[5]	-	-	95%	92%
Incidence of Potentially Preventable VTE[5]	-	-	8%	10%
UFH with Dosages/Platelet Monitoring[5]	-	-	97%	97%
Venous Thromboembolism Prophylaxis[5]	-	-	90%	85%
Warfarin Therapy Discharge Instructions[5]	-	-	69%	75%
Chest Pain/Possible Heart Attack Care				
Aspirin Given Within 24 Hours of Arrival	-	-	97%	96%
Fibrinolytic Meds Within 30 Min. of Arrival	-	-	55%	58%
Average Time to ECG (minutes)	-	-	8	7
Average Time to Transfer (minutes)	-	-	74	60
Children's Asthma Care				
Received Home Management Plan of Care	-	-	-	88%
Received Reliever Medication	-	-	-	100%
Received Systemic Corticosteroids	-	-	-	100%
Emergency Department				
Admittance Decision Time (minutes)	24	0	96	98
Head CT Results Within 45 Min. of Arrival	-	-	67%	57%
Patients Who Left ER Before Being Seen	-	-	2%	2%
Time from ER Arrival to Admit. (minutes)	86	122	244	274
Time from ER Arrival to Discharge (minutes)	-	-	139	134
Time in ER Before Being Evaluated (minutes)	-	-	20	26
Time to Pain Meds for Fractures (minutes)	-	-	45	57
Heart Attack Care				
Aspirin Given at Discharge[5]	-	-	100%	99%
Fibrinolytic Meds Within 30 Min. of Arrival[5]	-	-	20%	54%
PCI Within 90 Minutes of Arrival[5]	-	-	97%	96%
Statin Prescribed at Discharge[5]	-	-	99%	98%
Heart Failure Care				
ACE Inhibitor or ARB for LVSD[3,7]	-	-	97%	97%
Discharge Instructions Given[1,3]	-	-	93%	94%
Evaluation of LVS Function[1,3]	-	-	99%	99%
Medicare Spending				
Medicare Spending per Patient (ratio)	-	-	0.95	0.98
Pneumonia Care				
Appropriate Initial Antibiotic Given[1]	-	-	95%	95%
Blood Culture Timing[1]	-	-	98%	98%
Pregnancy and Delivery Care				
Newborn Deliveries Scheduled Early[5]	-	-	2%	6%
Preventive Care				
Immunization for Influenza[2]	34	32%	92%	90%
Immunization for Pneumonia[2]	62	76%	92%	92%
Stroke Care				
Anticoagulation Therapy for Atrial Fibrillation[5]	-	-	97%	95%
Antithrombotic Therapy Timing[5]	-	-	98%	98%
Assessed for Rehabilitation[5]	-	-	98%	97%
Discharged on Antithrombotic Therapy[5]	-	-	100%	99%
Discharged on Statin Medication[5]	-	-	94%	94%
Thrombolytic Therapy Timing[5]	-	-	78%	66%
Venous Thromboembolism Prophylaxis[5]	-	-	96%	94%
Written Stroke Educational Materials Given[5]	-	-	87%	88%
Surgical Care Improvement Project				
Appropriate Beta Blocker Usage[5]	-	-	98%	98%
Appropriate VTP Within 24 Hours[5]	-	-	98%	98%
Controlled Postoperative Blood Glucose[5]	-	-	96%	97%
Perioperative Temperature Management[5]	-	-	99%	100%
Prophylactic Antibiotic Selection[5]	-	-	99%	99%
Prophylactic Antibiotic Selection (Outpatient)	-	-	98%	98%
Prophylactic Antibiotic Stopped[5]	-	-	98%	98%
Prophylactic Antibiotic Timing[5]	-	-	98%	99%
Prophylactic Antibiotic Timing (Outpatient)	-	-	98%	98%
Urinary Catheter Removal[5]	-	-	97%	97%
Survey of Patients' Hospital Experiences				
Area Around Room 'Always' Quiet at Night[5]	-	-	64%	61%
Doctors 'Always' Communicated Well[5]	-	-	81%	82%
Home Recovery Information Given[5]	-	-	87%	85%
Hospital Given 9 or 10 on 10 Point Scale[5]	-	-	75%	71%
Meds 'Always' Explained Before Given[5]	-	-	67%	64%
Nurses 'Always' Communicated Well[5]	-	-	79%	79%
Pain 'Always' Well Controlled[5]	-	-	72%	71%
Room and Bathroom 'Always' Clean[5]	-	-	74%	73%
Timely Help 'Always' Received[5]	-	-	70%	68%
Would Definitely Recommend Hospital[5]	-	-	76%	71%
Use of Medical Imaging				
Cardiac Imaging Stress Test before Surgery	-	-	5%	5.3%
Combination Abdominal CT Scan	-	-	10%	10.5%
Combination Brain/Sinus CT Scan	-	-	2.1%	2.7%
Combination Chest CT Scan	-	-	3.1%	2.7%
Follow-up Mammogram/Ultrasound	-	-	8.7%	8.8%
Lumbar Spine MRI for Low Back Pain	-	-	39.7%	37.2%

Yampa Valley Medical Center

1024 Central Park Dr
Steamboat Springs, CO 80487
Phone: 970-879-1322
Fax: 970-870-1223
URL: www.yvmc.org
Type: Acute Care Hospitals
Emergency Services: Yes
Ownership: Voluntary non-profit - Private
Beds: 29

Key Personnel:
Operating Room. . . . . Allen Belshaw
Pediatric Ambulatory Care . . . . . . Ron Famiglietti, MD
Pediatric In-Patient Care . . . . Ron Famiglietti, MD
Radiology. . . . . J David Gilliland, MD
Chief of Medical Staff . . . . G Edward Kimm, MD
CEO . . . . Frank T May
Quality Assurance . . . . Judie Zuccone

Measure	Cases	This Hosp.	State Avg.	U.S. Avg.
Blood Clot Prevention and Treatment				
Anticoagulation Overlap Therapy[2]	16	94%	97%	93%
ICU Venous Thromboembolism Prophylaxis[2,7]	-	-	95%	92%
Incidence of Potentially Preventable VTE[1,2]	-	-	8%	10%
UFH with Dosages/Platelet Monitoring[2,7]	-	-	97%	97%
Venous Thromboembolism Prophylaxis[2]	83	96%	90%	85%
Warfarin Therapy Discharge Instructions[2]	15	60%	69%	75%
Chest Pain/Possible Heart Attack Care				
Aspirin Given Within 24 Hours of Arrival[3]	11	100%	97%	96%
Fibrinolytic Meds Within 30 Min. of Arrival[1,3]	-	-	55%	58%
Average Time to ECG (minutes)[3]	11	9	8	7
Average Time to Transfer (minutes)[3,7]	-	-	74	60
Children's Asthma Care				
Received Home Management Plan of Care	-	-	-	88%
Received Reliever Medication	-	-	-	100%
Received Systemic Corticosteroids	-	-	-	100%
Emergency Department				
Admittance Decision Time (minutes)[2]	191	71	96	98
Head CT Results Within 45 Min. of Arrival[7]	-	-	67%	57%
Patients Who Left ER Before Being Seen	8,028	1%	2%	2%
Time from ER Arrival to Admit. (minutes)[2]	208	181	244	274
Time from ER Arrival to Discharge (minutes)	361	94	139	134
Time in ER Before Being Evaluated (minutes)	392	14	20	26
Time to Pain Meds for Fractures (minutes)	103	39	45	57
Heart Attack Care				
Aspirin Given at Discharge[1]	-	-	100%	99%
Fibrinolytic Meds Within 30 Min. of Arrival[7]	-	-	20%	54%
PCI Within 90 Minutes of Arrival[7]	-	-	97%	96%
Statin Prescribed at Discharge[1]	-	-	99%	98%
Heart Failure Care				
ACE Inhibitor or ARB for LVSD[1]	-	-	97%	97%
Discharge Instructions Given	14	86%	93%	94%
Evaluation of LVS Function	17	100%	99%	99%
Medicare Spending				
Medicare Spending per Patient (ratio)	-	0.90	0.95	0.98
Pneumonia Care				
Appropriate Initial Antibiotic Given	13	92%	95%	95%
Blood Culture Timing	23	100%	98%	98%
Pregnancy and Delivery Care				
Newborn Deliveries Scheduled Early[2]	21	0%	2%	6%
Preventive Care				
Immunization for Influenza[2]	251	93%	92%	90%
Immunization for Pneumonia[2]	184	97%	92%	92%
Stroke Care				
Anticoagulation Therapy for Atrial Fibrillation[1]	-	-	97%	95%
Antithrombotic Therapy Timing[1]	-	-	98%	98%
Assessed for Rehabilitation[1]	-	-	98%	97%
Discharged on Antithrombotic Therapy[1]	-	-	100%	99%
Discharged on Statin Medication[1]	-	-	94%	94%
Thrombolytic Therapy Timing[7]	-	-	78%	66%
Venous Thromboembolism Prophylaxis[1]	-	-	96%	94%
Written Stroke Educational Materials Given[1]	-	-	87%	88%
Surgical Care Improvement Project				
Appropriate Beta Blocker Usage[2]	24	88%	98%	98%
Appropriate VTP Within 24 Hours[2]	140	97%	98%	98%
Controlled Postoperative Blood Glucose[2,7]	-	-	96%	97%
Perioperative Temperature Management[2]	155	100%	99%	100%
Prophylactic Antibiotic Selection[2]	111	99%	99%	99%
Prophylactic Antibiotic Selection (Outpatient)	113	98%	98%	98%
Prophylactic Antibiotic Stopped[2]	111	100%	98%	98%
Prophylactic Antibiotic Timing[2]	112	97%	98%	99%
Prophylactic Antibiotic Timing (Outpatient)	114	96%	98%	98%
Urinary Catheter Removal[2]	108	99%	97%	97%
Survey of Patients' Hospital Experiences				
Area Around Room 'Always' Quiet at Night	300+	70%	64%	61%
Doctors 'Always' Communicated Well	300+	85%	81%	82%
Home Recovery Information Given	300+	89%	87%	85%
Hospital Given 9 or 10 on 10 Point Scale	300+	83%	75%	71%
Meds 'Always' Explained Before Given	300+	69%	67%	64%
Nurses 'Always' Communicated Well	300+	81%	79%	79%
Pain 'Always' Well Controlled	300+	72%	72%	71%
Room and Bathroom 'Always' Clean	300+	79%	74%	73%
Timely Help 'Always' Received	300+	79%	70%	68%
Would Definitely Recommend Hospital	300+	85%	76%	71%
Use of Medical Imaging				
Cardiac Imaging Stress Test before Surgery	77	5.2%	5%	5.3%
Combination Abdominal CT Scan	156	7.7%	10%	10.5%
Combination Brain/Sinus CT Scan[1]	-	-	2.1%	2.7%
Combination Chest CT Scan	133	0.0%	3.1%	2.7%
Follow-up Mammogram/Ultrasound	332	7.2%	8.7%	8.8%
Lumbar Spine MRI for Low Back Pain	51	49.0%	39.7%	37.2%

Sterling Regional Medcenter

615 Fairhurst St
Sterling, CO 80751
Phone: 970-522-0122
Fax: 970-522-8532
URL: www.wphn.com/srmc_frm.htm
Type: Acute Care Hospitals
Emergency Services: Yes
Ownership: Voluntary non-profit - Other
Beds: 25

Key Personnel:
Infection Control. . . . . Janet Conner
Quality Assurance . . . . Rosemary Coody
Chief of Medical Staff . . . . Dan Elliff, MD
Anesthesiology. . . . . Daryl Harriman
CEO . . . . Julie Klein
Operating Room. . . . . Sonja Mueller
Emergency Room . . . . Jeanne Schuppe, RN

Measure	Cases	This Hosp.	State Avg.	U.S. Avg.
Blood Clot Prevention and Treatment				

NOTE: Hospital profiles are in alphabetical order by state, then city, then hospital within the city; Rankings exclude hospitals with less than 25 cases except for patient surveys which excludes hospitals with less than 100 cases; (a) 100-299 cases; (1) The number of cases/patients is too few to report; (2) Data submitted were based on a sample of cases/patients; (3) Results are based on a shorter time period than required; (4) Data suppressed by CMS for one or more quarters; (5) Results are not available for this reporting period; (6) Fewer than 100 patients completed the HCAHPS survey; (7) No cases met the criteria for this measure; (8) The lower limit of the confidence interval cannot be calculated if the number of observed infections equals zero; (9) No data are available from the state/territory for this reporting period; (10) The scores shown reflect fewer than 50 completed surveys; (11) There were discrepancies in the data collection process; (12) This measure does not apply to this hospital for this reporting period; (13) Results cannot be calculated for this reporting period; (14) The results for this state are combined with nearby states to protect confidentiality; Please refer to the User's Guide for a full explanation of data.

Measure	Cases	This Hosp.	State Avg.	U.S. Avg.
Anticoagulation Overlap Therapy[2]	12	92%	97%	93%
ICU Venous Thromboembolism Prophylaxis[2]	22	100%	95%	92%
Incidence of Potentially Preventable VTE[2,7]	-	-	8%	10%
UFH with Dosages/Platelet Monitoring[2,7]	-	-	97%	97%
Venous Thromboembolism Prophylaxis[2]	93	91%	90%	85%
Warfarin Therapy Discharge Instructions[2]	11	73%	69%	75%
Chest Pain/Possible Heart Attack Care				
Aspirin Given Within 24 Hours of Arrival	29	100%	97%	96%
Fibrinolytic Meds Within 30 Min. of Arrival[1]	-	-	55%	58%
Average Time to ECG (minutes)	29	6	8	7
Average Time to Transfer (minutes)[1]	-	-	74	60
Children's Asthma Care				
Received Home Management Plan of Care	-	-	-	88%
Received Reliever Medication	-	-	-	100%
Received Systemic Corticosteroids	-	-	-	100%
Emergency Department				
Admittance Decision Time (minutes)[2]	247	38	96	98
Head CT Results Within 45 Min. of Arrival[1]	-	-	67%	57%
Patients Who Left ER Before Being Seen	7,850	1%	2%	2%
Time from ER Arrival to Admit. (minutes)[2]	285	178	244	274
Time from ER Arrival to Discharge (minutes)	346	114	139	134
Time in ER Before Being Evaluated (minutes)	339	20	20	26
Time to Pain Meds for Fractures (minutes)	31	48	45	57
Heart Attack Care				
Aspirin Given at Discharge[1]	-	-	100%	99%
Fibrinolytic Meds Within 30 Min. of Arrival[7]	-	-	20%	54%
PCI Within 90 Minutes of Arrival[7]	-	-	97%	96%
Statin Prescribed at Discharge[1]	-	-	99%	98%
Heart Failure Care				
ACE Inhibitor or ARB for LVSD[1]	-	-	97%	97%
Discharge Instructions Given	26	100%	93%	94%
Evaluation of LVS Function	28	100%	99%	99%
Medicare Spending				
Medicare Spending per Patient (ratio)	-	0.92	0.95	0.98
Pneumonia Care				
Appropriate Initial Antibiotic Given	21	100%	95%	95%
Blood Culture Timing	31	97%	98%	98%
Pregnancy and Delivery Care				
Newborn Deliveries Scheduled Early[2]	17	6%	2%	6%
Preventive Care				
Immunization for Influenza[2]	229	96%	92%	90%
Immunization for Pneumonia[2]	306	95%	92%	92%
Stroke Care				
Anticoagulation Therapy for Atrial Fibrillation[1]	-	-	97%	95%
Antithrombotic Therapy Timing	11	91%	98%	98%
Assessed for Rehabilitation	12	100%	98%	97%
Discharged on Antithrombotic Therapy	12	100%	100%	99%
Discharged on Statin Medication[1]	-	-	94%	94%
Thrombolytic Therapy Timing[7]	-	-	78%	66%
Venous Thromboembolism Prophylaxis	12	92%	96%	94%
Written Stroke Educational Materials Given[1]	-	-	87%	88%
Surgical Care Improvement Project				
Appropriate Beta Blocker Usage	15	100%	98%	98%
Appropriate VTP Within 24 Hours	78	92%	98%	98%
Controlled Postoperative Blood Glucose[7]	-	-	96%	97%
Perioperative Temperature Management	85	100%	99%	100%
Prophylactic Antibiotic Selection	57	98%	99%	99%
Prophylactic Antibiotic Selection (Outpatient)[1,3]	-	-	98%	98%
Prophylactic Antibiotic Stopped	55	96%	98%	98%
Prophylactic Antibiotic Timing	57	100%	98%	99%
Prophylactic Antibiotic Timing (Outpatient)[1,3]	-	-	98%	98%
Urinary Catheter Removal	50	100%	97%	97%
Survey of Patients' Hospital Experiences				
Area Around Room 'Always' Quiet at Night[11]	(a)	67%	64%	61%
Doctors 'Always' Communicated Well[11]	(a)	84%	81%	82%
Home Recovery Information Given[11]	(a)	92%	87%	85%
Hospital Given 9 or 10 on 10 Point Scale[11]	(a)	77%	75%	71%
Meds 'Always' Explained Before Given[11]	(a)	69%	67%	64%
Nurses 'Always' Communicated Well[11]	(a)	84%	79%	79%
Pain 'Always' Well Controlled[11]	(a)	73%	72%	71%
Room and Bathroom 'Always' Clean[11]	(a)	76%	74%	73%
Timely Help 'Always' Received[11]	(a)	75%	70%	68%
Would Definitely Recommend Hospital[11]	(a)	69%	76%	71%
Use of Medical Imaging				
Cardiac Imaging Stress Test before Surgery	108	4.6%	5%	5.3%
Combination Abdominal CT Scan	253	20.6%	10%	10.5%
Combination Brain/Sinus CT Scan[1]	-	-	2.1%	2.7%
Combination Chest CT Scan	148	9.5%	3.1%	2.7%
Follow-up Mammogram/Ultrasound	649	15.4%	8.7%	8.8%
Lumbar Spine MRI for Low Back Pain	63	42.9%	39.7%	37.2%

North Suburban Medical Center

9191 Grant St
Thornton, CO 80229
Phone: 303-451-7800
Fax: 303-450-4458
URL: www.northsuburban.com
Type: Acute Care Hospitals
Emergency Services: No
Ownership: Voluntary non-profit - Private
Beds: 157

Key Personnel:
CEO/President. . . . . Todd Steward

Measure	Cases	This Hosp.	State Avg.	U.S. Avg.
Blood Clot Prevention and Treatment				
Anticoagulation Overlap Therapy[2]	49	100%	97%	93%
ICU Venous Thromboembolism Prophylaxis[2]	110	100%	95%	92%
Incidence of Potentially Preventable VTE[2,7]	-	-	8%	10%
UFH with Dosages/Platelet Monitoring[2]	27	100%	97%	97%
Venous Thromboembolism Prophylaxis[2]	307	98%	90%	85%
Warfarin Therapy Discharge Instructions[2]	45	91%	69%	75%
Chest Pain/Possible Heart Attack Care				
Aspirin Given Within 24 Hours of Arrival	15	100%	97%	96%
Fibrinolytic Meds Within 30 Min. of Arrival[3,7]	-	-	55%	58%
Average Time to ECG (minutes)	15	4	8	7
Average Time to Transfer (minutes)[3,7]	-	-	74	60
Children's Asthma Care				
Received Home Management Plan of Care	-	-	-	88%
Received Reliever Medication	-	-	-	100%
Received Systemic Corticosteroids	-	-	-	100%
Emergency Department				
Admittance Decision Time (minutes)[2]	508	85	96	98
Head CT Results Within 45 Min. of Arrival	33	88%	67%	57%
Patients Who Left ER Before Being Seen	56,259	1%	2%	2%
Time from ER Arrival to Admit. (minutes)[2]	508	228	244	274
Time from ER Arrival to Discharge (minutes)	477	129	139	134
Time in ER Before Being Evaluated (minutes)	529	15	20	26
Time to Pain Meds for Fractures (minutes)	212	33	45	57
Heart Attack Care				
Aspirin Given at Discharge[2]	115	100%	100%	99%
Fibrinolytic Meds Within 30 Min. of Arrival[2,7]	-	-	20%	54%
PCI Within 90 Minutes of Arrival[2]	34	100%	97%	96%
Statin Prescribed at Discharge[2]	110	100%	99%	98%
Heart Failure Care				
ACE Inhibitor or ARB for LVSD[2]	22	100%	97%	97%
Discharge Instructions Given[2]	56	100%	93%	94%
Evaluation of LVS Function[2]	69	100%	99%	99%
Medicare Spending				
Medicare Spending per Patient (ratio)	-	1.03	0.95	0.98
Pneumonia Care				
Appropriate Initial Antibiotic Given[2]	72	100%	95%	95%
Blood Culture Timing[2]	156	100%	98%	98%
Pregnancy and Delivery Care				
Newborn Deliveries Scheduled Early[2]	35	0%	2%	6%
Preventive Care				
Immunization for Influenza[2]	499	99%	92%	90%
Immunization for Pneumonia[2]	495	98%	92%	92%
Stroke Care				
Anticoagulation Therapy for Atrial Fibrillation[1,2]	-	-	97%	95%
Antithrombotic Therapy Timing[2]	38	100%	98%	98%
Assessed for Rehabilitation[2]	38	100%	98%	97%
Discharged on Antithrombotic Therapy[2]	36	100%	100%	99%
Discharged on Statin Medication[2]	25	100%	94%	94%
Thrombolytic Therapy Timing[2,7]	-	-	78%	66%
Venous Thromboembolism Prophylaxis[2]	34	100%	96%	94%
Written Stroke Educational Materials Given[2]	23	100%	87%	88%
Surgical Care Improvement Project				
Appropriate Beta Blocker Usage[2]	53	100%	98%	98%
Appropriate VTP Within 24 Hours[2]	280	100%	98%	98%
Controlled Postoperative Blood Glucose[2,7]	-	-	96%	97%
Perioperative Temperature Management[2]	310	100%	99%	100%
Prophylactic Antibiotic Selection[2]	180	100%	99%	99%
Prophylactic Antibiotic Selection (Outpatient)	178	100%	98%	98%
Prophylactic Antibiotic Stopped[2]	171	100%	98%	98%
Prophylactic Antibiotic Timing[2]	180	100%	98%	99%
Prophylactic Antibiotic Timing (Outpatient)	178	100%	98%	98%
Urinary Catheter Removal[2]	180	100%	97%	97%
Survey of Patients' Hospital Experiences				
Area Around Room 'Always' Quiet at Night	300+	56%	64%	61%
Doctors 'Always' Communicated Well	300+	76%	81%	82%
Home Recovery Information Given	300+	86%	87%	85%
Hospital Given 9 or 10 on 10 Point Scale	300+	66%	75%	71%
Meds 'Always' Explained Before Given	300+	63%	67%	64%
Nurses 'Always' Communicated Well	300+	75%	79%	79%
Pain 'Always' Well Controlled	300+	70%	72%	71%
Room and Bathroom 'Always' Clean	300+	72%	74%	73%
Timely Help 'Always' Received	300+	63%	70%	68%
Would Definitely Recommend Hospital	300+	65%	76%	71%
Use of Medical Imaging				
Cardiac Imaging Stress Test before Surgery	124	3.2%	5%	5.3%
Combination Abdominal CT Scan	371	3.5%	10%	10.5%
Combination Brain/Sinus CT Scan[1]	-	-	2.1%	2.7%
Combination Chest CT Scan	60	0.0%	3.1%	2.7%
Follow-up Mammogram/Ultrasound	412	10.4%	8.7%	8.8%
Lumbar Spine MRI for Low Back Pain[1]	-	-	39.7%	37.2%

Mount San Rafael Hospital

410 Benedicta Avenue
Trinidad, CO 81082
Phone: 719-846-9213
Fax: 719-846-2752
E-mail: hospital@msrhc.org
URL: www.msrhc.org
Type: Critical Access Hospitals
Emergency Services: Yes
Ownership: Voluntary non-profit - Private
Beds: 25

Key Personnel:
Pediatrics. Jun Flores, MD
Chief of Medical Staff. . . . . Thomas Goodell, MD
Emergency Room . . . . Clay Hart
CEO . . . . Bob Quist
Infection Control. . . . . Renee Walton

Measure	Cases	This Hosp.	State Avg.	U.S. Avg.
Blood Clot Prevention and Treatment				
Anticoagulation Overlap Therapy[5]	-	-	97%	93%
ICU Venous Thromboembolism Prophylaxis[5]	-	-	95%	92%
Incidence of Potentially Preventable VTE[5]	-	-	8%	10%
UFH with Dosages/Platelet Monitoring[5]	-	-	97%	97%
Venous Thromboembolism Prophylaxis[5]	-	-	90%	85%
Warfarin Therapy Discharge Instructions[5]	-	-	69%	75%
Chest Pain/Possible Heart Attack Care				
Aspirin Given Within 24 Hours of Arrival	-	-	97%	96%
Fibrinolytic Meds Within 30 Min. of Arrival	-	-	55%	58%
Average Time to ECG (minutes)	-	-	8	7
Average Time to Transfer (minutes)	-	-	74	60
Children's Asthma Care				
Received Home Management Plan of Care	-	-	-	88%
Received Reliever Medication	-	-	-	100%
Received Systemic Corticosteroids	-	-	-	100%
Emergency Department				
Admittance Decision Time (minutes)[5]	-	-	96	98
Head CT Results Within 45 Min. of Arrival	-	-	67%	57%
Patients Who Left ER Before Being Seen	-	-	2%	2%
Time from ER Arrival to Admit. (minutes)[5]	-	-	244	274
Time from ER Arrival to Discharge (minutes)	-	-	139	134
Time in ER Before Being Evaluated (minutes)	-	-	20	26
Time to Pain Meds for Fractures (minutes)	-	-	45	57
Heart Attack Care				
Aspirin Given at Discharge[5]	-	-	100%	99%
Fibrinolytic Meds Within 30 Min. of Arrival[5]	-	-	20%	54%
PCI Within 90 Minutes of Arrival[5]	-	-	97%	96%
Statin Prescribed at Discharge[5]	-	-	99%	98%
Heart Failure Care				
ACE Inhibitor or ARB for LVSD[5]	-	-	97%	97%
Discharge Instructions Given[5]	-	-	93%	94%
Evaluation of LVS Function[5]	-	-	99%	99%

NOTE: Hospital profiles are in alphabetical order by state, then city, then hospital within the city; Rankings exclude hospitals with less than 25 cases except for patient surveys which excludes hospitals with less than 100 cases; (a) 100-299 cases; (1) The number of cases/patients is too few to report; (2) Data submitted were based on a sample of cases/patients; (3) Results are based on a shorter time period than required; (4) Data suppressed by CMS for one or more quarters; (5) Results are not available for this reporting period; (6) Fewer than 100 patients completed the HCAHPS survey; (7) No cases met the criteria for this measure; (8) The lower limit of the confidence interval cannot be calculated if the number of observed infections equals zero; (9) No data are available from the state/territory for this reporting period; (10) The scores shown reflect fewer than 50 completed surveys; (11) There were discrepancies in the data collection process; (12) This measure does not apply to this hospital for this reporting period; (13) Results cannot be calculated for this reporting period; (14) The results for this state are combined with nearby states to protect confidentiality; Please refer to the User's Guide for a full explanation of data.

Measure	Cases	This Hosp.	State Avg.	U.S. Avg.
Medicare Spending				
Medicare Spending per Patient (ratio)	-	-	0.95	0.98
Pneumonia Care				
Appropriate Initial Antibiotic Given[1,3]	-	-	95%	95%
Blood Culture Timing[1,3]	-	-	98%	98%
Pregnancy and Delivery Care				
Newborn Deliveries Scheduled Early[5]	-	-	2%	6%
Preventive Care				
Immunization for Influenza[5]	-	-	92%	90%
Immunization for Pneumonia[5]	-	-	92%	92%
Stroke Care				
Anticoagulation Therapy for Atrial Fibrillation[5]	-	-	97%	95%
Antithrombotic Therapy Timing[5]	-	-	98%	98%
Assessed for Rehabilitation[5]	-	-	98%	97%
Discharged on Antithrombotic Therapy[5]	-	-	100%	99%
Discharged on Statin Medication[5]	-	-	94%	94%
Thrombolytic Therapy Timing[5]	-	-	78%	66%
Venous Thromboembolism Prophylaxis[5]	-	-	96%	94%
Written Stroke Educational Materials Given[5]	-	-	87%	88%
Surgical Care Improvement Project				
Appropriate Beta Blocker Usage[5]	-	-	98%	98%
Appropriate VTP Within 24 Hours[5]	-	-	98%	98%
Controlled Postoperative Blood Glucose[5]	-	-	96%	97%
Perioperative Temperature Management[5]	-	-	99%	100%
Prophylactic Antibiotic Selection[5]	-	-	99%	99%
Prophylactic Antibiotic Selection (Outpatient)	-	-	98%	98%
Prophylactic Antibiotic Stopped[5]	-	-	98%	98%
Prophylactic Antibiotic Timing[5]	-	-	98%	99%
Prophylactic Antibiotic Timing (Outpatient)	-	-	98%	98%
Urinary Catheter Removal[5]	-	-	97%	97%
Survey of Patients' Hospital Experiences				
Area Around Room 'Always' Quiet at Night	(a)	56%	64%	61%
Doctors 'Always' Communicated Well	(a)	83%	81%	82%
Home Recovery Information Given	(a)	84%	87%	85%
Hospital Given 9 or 10 on 10 Point Scale	(a)	66%	75%	71%
Meds 'Always' Explained Before Given	(a)	66%	67%	64%
Nurses 'Always' Communicated Well	(a)	72%	79%	79%
Pain 'Always' Well Controlled	(a)	62%	72%	71%
Room and Bathroom 'Always' Clean	(a)	84%	74%	73%
Timely Help 'Always' Received	(a)	68%	70%	68%
Would Definitely Recommend Hospital	(a)	60%	76%	71%
Use of Medical Imaging				
Cardiac Imaging Stress Test before Surgery	-	-	5%	5.3%
Combination Abdominal CT Scan	-	-	10%	10.5%
Combination Brain/Sinus CT Scan	-	-	2.1%	2.7%
Combination Chest CT Scan	-	-	3.1%	2.7%
Follow-up Mammogram/Ultrasound	-	-	8.7%	8.8%
Lumbar Spine MRI for Low Back Pain	-	-	39.7%	37.2%

Vail Valley Medical Center

181 W Meadow Drive — Phone: 970-476-2451
Vail, CO 81657 — Fax: 970-479-7192
URL: www.vvmc.com
Type: Acute Care Hospitals — Emergency Services: Yes
Ownership: Voluntary non-profit - Other — Beds: 58

Key Personnel:
Quality Assurance . . . . Linda Brophy, RN, MN
Anesthesiology. . . . . Steve Ellstrom, MD
Chairman/CEO . . . . Art Kelton
CEO/President. . . . . Doris Kirchner
Emergency Room . . . . Joyce Morgan, RN
Radiology. . . . . Janice Joyce Ugale
Chief of Medical Staff . . . . John B Woodland, MD

Measure	Cases	This Hosp.	State Avg.	U.S. Avg.
Blood Clot Prevention and Treatment				
Anticoagulation Overlap Therapy[1,2]	-	-	97%	93%
ICU Venous Thromboembolism Prophylaxis[2]	41	98%	95%	92%
Incidence of Potentially Preventable VTE[1,2]	-	-	8%	10%
UFH with Dosages/Platelet Monitoring[1,2]	-	-	97%	97%
Venous Thromboembolism Prophylaxis[2]	105	98%	90%	85%
Warfarin Therapy Discharge Instructions[1,2]	-	-	69%	75%
Chest Pain/Possible Heart Attack Care				
Aspirin Given Within 24 Hours of Arrival	76	100%	97%	96%
Fibrinolytic Meds Within 30 Min. of Arrival[1]	-	-	55%	58%
Average Time to ECG (minutes)	76	12	8	7
Average Time to Transfer (minutes)[1]	-	-	74	60
Children's Asthma Care				
Received Home Management Plan of Care	-	-	-	88%
Received Reliever Medication	-	-	-	100%
Received Systemic Corticosteroids	-	-	-	100%
Emergency Department				
Admittance Decision Time (minutes)[2]	99	70	96	98
Head CT Results Within 45 Min. of Arrival[1]	-	-	67%	57%
Patients Who Left ER Before Being Seen	11,610	1%	2%	2%
Time from ER Arrival to Admit. (minutes)[2]	116	223	244	274
Time from ER Arrival to Discharge (minutes)	574	101	139	134
Time in ER Before Being Evaluated (minutes)	592	25	20	26
Time to Pain Meds for Fractures (minutes)	102	48	45	57
Heart Attack Care				
Aspirin Given at Discharge[1,3]	-	-	100%	99%
Fibrinolytic Meds Within 30 Min. of Arrival[3,7]	-	-	20%	54%
PCI Within 90 Minutes of Arrival[3,7]	-	-	97%	96%
Statin Prescribed at Discharge[1,3]	-	-	99%	98%
Heart Failure Care				
ACE Inhibitor or ARB for LVSD[1,3]	-	-	97%	97%
Discharge Instructions Given[1,3]	-	-	93%	94%
Evaluation of LVS Function[1,3]	-	-	99%	99%
Medicare Spending				
Medicare Spending per Patient (ratio)	-	0.96	0.95	0.98
Pneumonia Care				
Appropriate Initial Antibiotic Given	15	93%	95%	95%
Blood Culture Timing	17	94%	98%	98%
Pregnancy and Delivery Care				
Newborn Deliveries Scheduled Early	48	4%	2%	6%
Preventive Care				
Immunization for Influenza[2]	249	96%	92%	90%
Immunization for Pneumonia[2]	153	91%	92%	92%
Stroke Care				
Anticoagulation Therapy for Atrial Fibrillation[1]	-	-	97%	95%
Antithrombotic Therapy Timing[1]	-	-	98%	98%
Assessed for Rehabilitation[1]	-	-	98%	97%
Discharged on Antithrombotic Therapy[1]	-	-	100%	99%
Discharged on Statin Medication[1]	-	-	94%	94%
Thrombolytic Therapy Timing[1]	-	-	78%	66%
Venous Thromboembolism Prophylaxis[1]	-	-	96%	94%
Written Stroke Educational Materials Given[1]	-	-	87%	88%
Surgical Care Improvement Project				
Appropriate Beta Blocker Usage	29	97%	98%	98%
Appropriate VTP Within 24 Hours	178	97%	98%	98%
Controlled Postoperative Blood Glucose[7]	-	-	96%	97%
Perioperative Temperature Management	183	99%	99%	100%
Prophylactic Antibiotic Selection	150	99%	99%	99%
Prophylactic Antibiotic Selection (Outpatient)	132	98%	98%	98%
Prophylactic Antibiotic Stopped	149	97%	98%	98%
Prophylactic Antibiotic Timing	150	95%	98%	99%
Prophylactic Antibiotic Timing (Outpatient)	132	95%	98%	98%
Urinary Catheter Removal	148	97%	97%	97%
Survey of Patients' Hospital Experiences				
Area Around Room 'Always' Quiet at Night	300+	67%	64%	61%
Doctors 'Always' Communicated Well	300+	83%	81%	82%
Home Recovery Information Given	300+	90%	87%	85%
Hospital Given 9 or 10 on 10 Point Scale	300+	79%	75%	71%
Meds 'Always' Explained Before Given	300+	66%	67%	64%
Nurses 'Always' Communicated Well	300+	82%	79%	79%
Pain 'Always' Well Controlled	300+	74%	72%	71%
Room and Bathroom 'Always' Clean	300+	85%	74%	73%
Timely Help 'Always' Received	300+	74%	70%	68%
Would Definitely Recommend Hospital	300+	82%	76%	71%
Use of Medical Imaging				
Cardiac Imaging Stress Test before Surgery	127	7.1%	5%	5.3%
Combination Abdominal CT Scan	173	11.0%	10%	10.5%
Combination Brain/Sinus CT Scan[1]	-	-	2.1%	2.7%
Combination Chest CT Scan	99	0.0%	3.1%	2.7%
Follow-up Mammogram/Ultrasound	509	7.3%	8.7%	8.8%
Lumbar Spine MRI for Low Back Pain[1]	-	-	39.7%	37.2%

Spanish Peaks Regional Health Center

23500 Us Hwy 160 — Phone: 719-738-5100
Walsenburg, CO 81089
URL: www.sprhc.org
Type: Critical Access Hospitals — Emergency Services: Yes
Ownership: Govt - Hospital Dist/Auth

Key Personnel:
CEO/President. . . . . Steven Perkins

Measure	Cases	This Hosp.	State Avg.	U.S. Avg.
Blood Clot Prevention and Treatment				
Anticoagulation Overlap Therapy[5]	-	-	97%	93%
ICU Venous Thromboembolism Prophylaxis[5]	-	-	95%	92%
Incidence of Potentially Preventable VTE[5]	-	-	8%	10%
UFH with Dosages/Platelet Monitoring[5]	-	-	97%	97%
Venous Thromboembolism Prophylaxis[5]	-	-	90%	85%
Warfarin Therapy Discharge Instructions[5]	-	-	69%	75%
Chest Pain/Possible Heart Attack Care				
Aspirin Given Within 24 Hours of Arrival[3]	13	92%	97%	96%
Fibrinolytic Meds Within 30 Min. of Arrival[1,3]	-	-	55%	58%
Average Time to ECG (minutes)[3]	14	9	8	7
Average Time to Transfer (minutes)[3,7]	-	-	74	60
Children's Asthma Care				
Received Home Management Plan of Care	-	-	-	88%
Received Reliever Medication	-	-	-	100%
Received Systemic Corticosteroids	-	-	-	100%
Emergency Department				
Admittance Decision Time (minutes)[5]	-	-	96	98
Head CT Results Within 45 Min. of Arrival[5]	-	-	67%	57%
Patients Who Left ER Before Being Seen[5]	-	-	2%	2%
Time from ER Arrival to Admit. (minutes)[5]	-	-	244	274
Time from ER Arrival to Discharge (minutes)[5]	-	-	139	134
Time in ER Before Being Evaluated (minutes)[5]	-	-	20	26
Time to Pain Meds for Fractures (minutes)[5]	-	-	45	57
Heart Attack Care				
Aspirin Given at Discharge[5]	-	-	100%	99%
Fibrinolytic Meds Within 30 Min. of Arrival[5]	-	-	20%	54%
PCI Within 90 Minutes of Arrival[5]	-	-	97%	96%
Statin Prescribed at Discharge[5]	-	-	99%	98%
Heart Failure Care				
ACE Inhibitor or ARB for LVSD[1,2]	-	-	97%	97%
Discharge Instructions Given[1,2]	-	-	93%	94%
Evaluation of LVS Function[2]	14	79%	99%	99%
Medicare Spending				
Medicare Spending per Patient (ratio)	-	-	0.95	0.98
Pneumonia Care				
Appropriate Initial Antibiotic Given	16	88%	95%	95%
Blood Culture Timing	29	93%	98%	98%
Pregnancy and Delivery Care				
Newborn Deliveries Scheduled Early[5]	-	-	2%	6%
Preventive Care				
Immunization for Influenza[5]	-	-	92%	90%
Immunization for Pneumonia[5]	-	-	92%	92%
Stroke Care				
Anticoagulation Therapy for Atrial Fibrillation[5]	-	-	97%	95%
Antithrombotic Therapy Timing[5]	-	-	98%	98%
Assessed for Rehabilitation[5]	-	-	98%	97%
Discharged on Antithrombotic Therapy[5]	-	-	100%	99%
Discharged on Statin Medication[5]	-	-	94%	94%
Thrombolytic Therapy Timing[5]	-	-	78%	66%
Venous Thromboembolism Prophylaxis[5]	-	-	96%	94%
Written Stroke Educational Materials Given[5]	-	-	87%	88%
Surgical Care Improvement Project				
Appropriate Beta Blocker Usage[5]	-	-	98%	98%
Appropriate VTP Within 24 Hours[5]	-	-	98%	98%
Controlled Postoperative Blood Glucose[5]	-	-	96%	97%
Perioperative Temperature Management[5]	-	-	99%	100%
Prophylactic Antibiotic Selection[5]	-	-	99%	99%
Prophylactic Antibiotic Selection (Outpatient)[5]	-	-	98%	98%
Prophylactic Antibiotic Stopped[5]	-	-	98%	98%
Prophylactic Antibiotic Timing[5]	-	-	98%	99%
Prophylactic Antibiotic Timing (Outpatient)[5]	-	-	98%	98%
Urinary Catheter Removal[5]	-	-	97%	97%
Survey of Patients' Hospital Experiences				

NOTE: Hospital profiles are in alphabetical order by state, then city, then hospital within the city; Rankings exclude hospitals with less than 25 cases except for patient surveys which excludes hospitals with less than 100 cases; (a) 100-299 cases; (1) The number of cases/patients is too few to report; (2) Data submitted were based on a sample of cases/patients; (3) Results are based on a shorter time period than required; (4) Data suppressed by CMS for one or more quarters; (5) Results are not available for this reporting period; (6) Fewer than 100 patients completed the HCAHPS survey; (7) No cases met the criteria for this measure; (8) The lower limit of the confidence interval cannot be calculated if the number of observed infections equals zero; (9) No data are available from the state/territory for this reporting period; (10) The scores shown reflect fewer than 50 completed surveys; (11) There were discrepancies in the data collection process; (12) This measure does not apply to this hospital for this reporting period; (13) Results cannot be calculated for this reporting period; (14) The results for this state are combined with nearby states to protect confidentiality; Please refer to the User's Guide for a full explanation of data.

Measure	Cases	This Hosp.	State Avg.	U.S. Avg.
Area Around Room 'Always' Quiet at Night[10]	<100	53%	64%	61%
Doctors 'Always' Communicated Well[10]	<100	78%	81%	82%
Home Recovery Information Given[10]	<100	82%	87%	85%
Hospital Given 9 or 10 on 10 Point Scale[10]	<100	58%	75%	71%
Meds 'Always' Explained Before Given[10]	<100	57%	67%	64%
Nurses 'Always' Communicated Well[10]	<100	77%	79%	79%
Pain 'Always' Well Controlled[10]	<100	58%	72%	71%
Room and Bathroom 'Always' Clean[10]	<100	76%	74%	73%
Timely Help 'Always' Received[10]	<100	79%	70%	68%
Would Definitely Recommend Hospital[10]	<100	60%	76%	71%
Use of Medical Imaging				
Cardiac Imaging Stress Test before Surgery[7]	-	-	5%	5.3%
Combination Abdominal CT Scan	116	10.3%	10%	10.5%
Combination Brain/Sinus CT Scan[1]	-	-	2.1%	2.7%
Combination Chest CT Scan	75	4.0%	3.1%	2.7%
Follow-up Mammogram/Ultrasound[7]	-	-	8.7%	8.8%
Lumbar Spine MRI for Low Back Pain[1]	-	-	39.7%	37.2%

Centura Health - Saint Anthony North Hospital

2551 W 84th Avenue Phone: 303-430-3201
Westminster, CO 80031 Fax: 303-426-2155
URL: www.stanthonyhosp.org
Type: Acute Care Hospitals Emergency Services: Yes
Ownership: Voluntary non-profit - Church Beds: 196

Key Personnel:
Infection Control.............. Chris Baumann
CEO/President.............. Jeff Brickman
Operating Room.............. James Charles Garlitz
Coronary Care.............. Cathy Laguardia
Intensive Care Unit.............. Cathy Laguardia
Radiology.............. Christopher Jos Leoni
Patient Relations.............. Marcus McCoy
Chief of Medical Staff.............. Christopher J. Ott, MD, FACEP

Measure	Cases	This Hosp.	State Avg.	U.S. Avg.
Blood Clot Prevention and Treatment				
Anticoagulation Overlap Therapy[2]	51	86%	97%	93%
ICU Venous Thromboembolism Prophylaxis[2]	54	98%	95%	92%
Incidence of Potentially Preventable VTE[1,2]	-	-	8%	10%
UFH with Dosages/Platelet Monitoring[2]	35	97%	97%	97%
Venous Thromboembolism Prophylaxis[2]	348	94%	90%	85%
Warfarin Therapy Discharge Instructions[2]	41	15%	69%	75%
Chest Pain/Possible Heart Attack Care				
Aspirin Given Within 24 Hours of Arrival	15	93%	97%	96%
Fibrinolytic Meds Within 30 Min. of Arrival[7]	-	-	55%	58%
Average Time to ECG (minutes)	14	4	8	7
Average Time to Transfer (minutes)[1]	-	-	74	60
Children's Asthma Care				
Received Home Management Plan of Care	-	-	-	88%
Received Reliever Medication	-	-	-	100%
Received Systemic Corticosteroids	-	-	-	100%
Emergency Department				
Admittance Decision Time (minutes)[2]	691	138	96	98
Head CT Results Within 45 Min. of Arrival	45	76%	67%	57%
Patients Who Left ER Before Being Seen	36,801	3%	2%	2%
Time from ER Arrival to Admit. (minutes)[2]	738	280	244	274
Time from ER Arrival to Discharge (minutes)	441	129	139	134
Time in ER Before Being Evaluated (minutes)	364	10	20	26
Time to Pain Meds for Fractures (minutes)	180	50	45	57
Heart Attack Care				
Aspirin Given at Discharge	163	99%	100%	99%
Fibrinolytic Meds Within 30 Min. of Arrival[7]	-	-	20%	54%
PCI Within 90 Minutes of Arrival	48	94%	97%	96%
Statin Prescribed at Discharge	159	99%	99%	98%
Heart Failure Care				
ACE Inhibitor or ARB for LVSD	43	100%	97%	97%
Discharge Instructions Given	141	95%	93%	94%
Evaluation of LVS Function	166	100%	99%	99%
Medicare Spending				
Medicare Spending per Patient (ratio)	-	0.99	0.95	0.98
Pneumonia Care				
Appropriate Initial Antibiotic Given	149	97%	95%	95%
Blood Culture Timing	114	100%	98%	98%
Pregnancy and Delivery Care				
Newborn Deliveries Scheduled Early[2]	17	6%	2%	6%
Preventive Care				
Immunization for Influenza[2]	542	96%	92%	90%
Immunization for Pneumonia[2]	719	99%	92%	92%
Stroke Care				
Anticoagulation Therapy for Atrial Fibrillation[1]	-	-	97%	95%
Antithrombotic Therapy Timing	41	98%	98%	98%
Assessed for Rehabilitation	42	100%	98%	97%
Discharged on Antithrombotic Therapy	41	100%	100%	99%
Discharged on Statin Medication	29	93%	94%	94%
Thrombolytic Therapy Timing[1]	-	-	78%	66%
Venous Thromboembolism Prophylaxis	39	97%	96%	94%
Written Stroke Educational Materials Given	24	79%	87%	88%
Surgical Care Improvement Project				
Appropriate Beta Blocker Usage	74	100%	98%	98%
Appropriate VTP Within 24 Hours	297	96%	98%	98%
Controlled Postoperative Blood Glucose[7]	-	-	96%	97%
Perioperative Temperature Management	327	100%	99%	100%
Prophylactic Antibiotic Selection	177	97%	99%	99%
Prophylactic Antibiotic Selection (Outpatient)	84	98%	98%	98%
Prophylactic Antibiotic Stopped	169	97%	98%	98%
Prophylactic Antibiotic Timing	177	99%	98%	99%
Prophylactic Antibiotic Timing (Outpatient)	84	99%	98%	98%
Urinary Catheter Removal	242	99%	97%	97%
Survey of Patients' Hospital Experiences				
Area Around Room 'Always' Quiet at Night	300+	54%	64%	61%
Doctors 'Always' Communicated Well	300+	77%	81%	82%
Home Recovery Information Given	300+	86%	87%	85%
Hospital Given 9 or 10 on 10 Point Scale	300+	68%	75%	71%
Meds 'Always' Explained Before Given	300+	64%	67%	64%
Nurses 'Always' Communicated Well	300+	76%	79%	79%
Pain 'Always' Well Controlled	300+	65%	72%	71%
Room and Bathroom 'Always' Clean	300+	66%	74%	73%
Timely Help 'Always' Received	300+	58%	70%	68%
Would Definitely Recommend Hospital	300+	68%	76%	71%
Use of Medical Imaging				
Cardiac Imaging Stress Test before Surgery	107	3.7%	5%	5.3%
Combination Abdominal CT Scan	413	3.6%	10%	10.5%
Combination Brain/Sinus CT Scan[1]	-	-	2.1%	2.7%
Combination Chest CT Scan	189	3.7%	3.1%	2.7%
Follow-up Mammogram/Ultrasound	641	8.3%	8.7%	8.8%
Lumbar Spine MRI for Low Back Pain[1]	-	-	39.7%	37.2%

Exempla Lutheran Medical Center

8300 W 38th Ave Phone: 303-425-4500
Wheat Ridge, CO 80033 Fax: 303-425-8198
URL: www.exemlpa.org
Type: Acute Care Hospitals Emergency Services: Yes
Ownership: Voluntary non-profit - Private Beds: 400

Key Personnel:
Chief of Medical Staff.............. Christina Johnson, MD, FACEP
Quality Assurance.............. Melanie McKee
Emergency Room.............. Jim Thompson, MD
Patient Relations.............. Colleen Whalen
CEO/President.............. Grant Wicklund

Measure	Cases	This Hosp.	State Avg.	U.S. Avg.
Blood Clot Prevention and Treatment				
Anticoagulation Overlap Therapy[2]	110	98%	97%	93%
ICU Venous Thromboembolism Prophylaxis[2]	83	93%	95%	92%
Incidence of Potentially Preventable VTE[2]	11	9%	8%	10%
UFH with Dosages/Platelet Monitoring[2]	71	99%	97%	97%
Venous Thromboembolism Prophylaxis[2]	365	88%	90%	85%
Warfarin Therapy Discharge Instructions[2]	90	74%	69%	75%
Chest Pain/Possible Heart Attack Care				
Aspirin Given Within 24 Hours of Arrival[1,3]	-	-	97%	96%
Fibrinolytic Meds Within 30 Min. of Arrival[5]	-	-	55%	58%
Average Time to ECG (minutes)[1,3]	-	-	8	7
Average Time to Transfer (minutes)[5]	-	-	74	60
Children's Asthma Care				
Received Home Management Plan of Care	-	-	-	88%
Received Reliever Medication	-	-	-	100%
Received Systemic Corticosteroids	-	-	-	100%
Emergency Department				
Admittance Decision Time (minutes)[2]	623	75	96	98
Head CT Results Within 45 Min. of Arrival[1]	-	-	67%	57%
Patients Who Left ER Before Being Seen	72,155	0%	2%	2%
Time from ER Arrival to Admit. (minutes)[2]	624	271	244	274
Time from ER Arrival to Discharge (minutes)	315	172	139	134
Time in ER Before Being Evaluated (minutes)	383	32	20	26
Time to Pain Meds for Fractures (minutes)	196	52	45	57
Heart Attack Care				
Aspirin Given at Discharge	257	100%	100%	99%
Fibrinolytic Meds Within 30 Min. of Arrival[7]	-	-	20%	54%
PCI Within 90 Minutes of Arrival	61	100%	97%	96%
Statin Prescribed at Discharge	248	99%	99%	98%
Heart Failure Care				
ACE Inhibitor or ARB for LVSD[2]	50	100%	97%	97%
Discharge Instructions Given[2]	154	99%	93%	94%
Evaluation of LVS Function[2]	189	99%	99%	99%
Medicare Spending				
Medicare Spending per Patient (ratio)	-	1.00	0.95	0.98
Pneumonia Care				
Appropriate Initial Antibiotic Given	192	100%	95%	95%
Blood Culture Timing	391	99%	98%	98%
Pregnancy and Delivery Care				
Newborn Deliveries Scheduled Early	208	0%	2%	6%
Preventive Care				
Immunization for Influenza[2]	487	91%	92%	90%
Immunization for Pneumonia[2]	534	92%	92%	92%
Stroke Care				
Anticoagulation Therapy for Atrial Fibrillation	33	100%	97%	95%
Antithrombotic Therapy Timing	104	96%	98%	98%
Assessed for Rehabilitation	158	99%	98%	97%
Discharged on Antithrombotic Therapy	134	100%	100%	99%
Discharged on Statin Medication	103	97%	94%	94%
Thrombolytic Therapy Timing	15	100%	78%	66%
Venous Thromboembolism Prophylaxis	156	97%	96%	94%
Written Stroke Educational Materials Given	81	93%	87%	88%
Surgical Care Improvement Project				
Appropriate Beta Blocker Usage[2]	138	100%	98%	98%
Appropriate VTP Within 24 Hours[2]	257	100%	98%	98%
Controlled Postoperative Blood Glucose[2]	106	98%	96%	97%
Perioperative Temperature Management[2]	330	100%	99%	100%
Prophylactic Antibiotic Selection[2]	296	100%	99%	99%
Prophylactic Antibiotic Selection (Outpatient)	533	99%	98%	98%
Prophylactic Antibiotic Stopped[2]	285	98%	98%	98%
Prophylactic Antibiotic Timing[2]	295	99%	98%	99%
Prophylactic Antibiotic Timing (Outpatient)	534	99%	98%	98%
Urinary Catheter Removal[2]	197	97%	97%	97%
Survey of Patients' Hospital Experiences				
Area Around Room 'Always' Quiet at Night	300+	60%	64%	61%
Doctors 'Always' Communicated Well	300+	78%	81%	82%
Home Recovery Information Given	300+	88%	87%	85%
Hospital Given 9 or 10 on 10 Point Scale	300+	75%	75%	71%
Meds 'Always' Explained Before Given	300+	62%	67%	64%
Nurses 'Always' Communicated Well	300+	78%	79%	79%
Pain 'Always' Well Controlled	300+	71%	72%	71%
Room and Bathroom 'Always' Clean	300+	70%	74%	73%
Timely Help 'Always' Received	300+	63%	70%	68%
Would Definitely Recommend Hospital	300+	76%	76%	71%
Use of Medical Imaging				
Cardiac Imaging Stress Test before Surgery	181	6.1%	5%	5.3%
Combination Abdominal CT Scan	901	3.4%	10%	10.5%
Combination Brain/Sinus CT Scan	810	1.6%	2.1%	2.7%
Combination Chest CT Scan	548	0.5%	3.1%	2.7%
Follow-up Mammogram/Ultrasound	2,197	11.6%	8.7%	8.8%
Lumbar Spine MRI for Low Back Pain	117	34.2%	39.7%	37.2%

Pikes Peak Regional Hospital

16420 Highway 24 Phone: 719-687-9999
Woodland Park, CO 80863
URL: www.pikespeakregionalhospital.com
Type: Critical Access Hospitals Emergency Services: Yes
Ownership: Voluntary non-profit - Private

Key Personnel:
CEO.............. Terry Buckner

Measure	Cases	This Hosp.	State Avg.	U.S. Avg.

NOTE: Hospital profiles are in alphabetical order by state, then city, then hospital within the city; Rankings exclude hospitals with less than 25 cases except for patient surveys which excludes hospitals with less than 100 cases; (a) 100-299 cases; (1) The number of cases/patients is too few to report; (2) Data submitted were based on a sample of cases/patients; (3) Results are based on a shorter time period than required; (4) Data suppressed by CMS for one or more quarters; (5) Results are not available for this reporting period; (6) Fewer than 100 patients completed the HCAHPS survey; (7) No cases met the criteria for this measure; (8) The lower limit of the confidence interval cannot be calculated if the number of observed infections equals zero; (9) No data are available from the state/territory for this reporting period; (10) The scores shown reflect fewer than 50 completed surveys; (11) There were discrepancies in the data collection process; (12) This measure does not apply to this hospital for this reporting period; (13) Results cannot be calculated for this reporting period; (14) The results for this state are combined with nearby states to protect confidentiality; Please refer to the User's Guide for a full explanation of data.

Measure	Cases	This Hosp.	State Avg.	U.S. Avg.
Blood Clot Prevention and Treatment				
Anticoagulation Overlap Therapy[2]	11	91%	97%	93%
ICU Venous Thromboembolism Prophylaxis[2,7]	-	-	95%	92%
Incidence of Potentially Preventable VTE[1,2]	-	-	8%	10%
UFH with Dosages/Platelet Monitoring[1,2]	-	-	97%	97%
Venous Thromboembolism Prophylaxis[2]	94	86%	90%	85%
Warfarin Therapy Discharge Instructions[1,2]	-	-	69%	75%
Chest Pain/Possible Heart Attack Care				
Aspirin Given Within 24 Hours of Arrival	-	-	97%	96%
Fibrinolytic Meds Within 30 Min. of Arrival	-	-	55%	58%
Average Time to ECG (minutes)	-	-	8	7
Average Time to Transfer (minutes)	-	-	74	60
Children's Asthma Care				
Received Home Management Plan of Care	-	-	-	88%
Received Reliever Medication	-	-	-	100%
Received Systemic Corticosteroids	-	-	-	100%
Emergency Department				
Admittance Decision Time (minutes)[5]	-	-	96	98
Head CT Results Within 45 Min. of Arrival	-	-	67%	57%
Patients Who Left ER Before Being Seen	-	-	2%	2%
Time from ER Arrival to Admit. (minutes)[5]	-	-	244	274
Time from ER Arrival to Discharge (minutes)	-	-	139	134
Time in ER Before Being Evaluated (minutes)	-	-	20	26
Time to Pain Meds for Fractures (minutes)	-	-	45	57
Heart Attack Care				
Aspirin Given at Discharge[3,7]	-	-	100%	99%
Fibrinolytic Meds Within 30 Min. of Arrival[3,7]	-	-	20%	54%
PCI Within 90 Minutes of Arrival[3,7]	-	-	97%	96%
Statin Prescribed at Discharge[3,7]	-	-	99%	98%
Heart Failure Care				
ACE Inhibitor or ARB for LVSD[1,3]	-	-	97%	97%
Discharge Instructions Given[1,3]	-	-	93%	94%
Evaluation of LVS Function[1,3]	-	-	99%	99%
Medicare Spending				
Medicare Spending per Patient (ratio)	-	-	0.95	0.98
Pneumonia Care				
Appropriate Initial Antibiotic Given	20	100%	95%	95%
Blood Culture Timing	18	100%	98%	98%
Pregnancy and Delivery Care				
Newborn Deliveries Scheduled Early[3,7]	-	-	2%	6%
Preventive Care				
Immunization for Influenza[5]	-	-	92%	90%
Immunization for Pneumonia[5]	-	-	92%	92%
Stroke Care				
Anticoagulation Therapy for Atrial Fibrillation[3,7]	-	-	97%	95%
Antithrombotic Therapy Timing[1,3]	-	-	98%	98%
Assessed for Rehabilitation[1,3]	-	-	98%	97%
Discharged on Antithrombotic Therapy[1,3]	-	-	100%	99%
Discharged on Statin Medication[1,3]	-	-	94%	94%
Thrombolytic Therapy Timing[3,7]	-	-	78%	66%
Venous Thromboembolism Prophylaxis[1,3]	-	-	96%	94%
Written Stroke Educational Materials Given[3,7]	-	-	87%	88%
Surgical Care Improvement Project				
Appropriate Beta Blocker Usage	12	100%	98%	98%
Appropriate VTP Within 24 Hours	44	100%	98%	98%
Controlled Postoperative Blood Glucose[3,7]	-	-	96%	97%
Perioperative Temperature Management	48	100%	99%	100%
Prophylactic Antibiotic Selection	40	98%	99%	99%
Prophylactic Antibiotic Selection (Outpatient)	-	-	98%	98%
Prophylactic Antibiotic Stopped	38	95%	98%	98%
Prophylactic Antibiotic Timing	40	98%	98%	99%
Prophylactic Antibiotic Timing (Outpatient)	-	-	98%	98%
Urinary Catheter Removal	44	98%	97%	97%
Survey of Patients' Hospital Experiences				
Area Around Room 'Always' Quiet at Night	(a)	76%	64%	61%
Doctors 'Always' Communicated Well	(a)	83%	81%	82%
Home Recovery Information Given	(a)	91%	87%	85%
Hospital Given 9 or 10 on 10 Point Scale	(a)	79%	75%	71%
Meds 'Always' Explained Before Given	(a)	69%	67%	64%
Nurses 'Always' Communicated Well	(a)	83%	79%	79%
Pain 'Always' Well Controlled	(a)	74%	72%	71%
Room and Bathroom 'Always' Clean	(a)	77%	74%	73%
Timely Help 'Always' Received	(a)	77%	70%	68%
Would Definitely Recommend Hospital	(a)	78%	76%	71%
Use of Medical Imaging				
Cardiac Imaging Stress Test before Surgery	-	-	5%	5.3%
Combination Abdominal CT Scan	-	-	10%	10.5%
Combination Brain/Sinus CT Scan	-	-	2.1%	2.7%
Combination Chest CT Scan	-	-	3.1%	2.7%
Follow-up Mammogram/Ultrasound	-	-	8.7%	8.8%
Lumbar Spine MRI for Low Back Pain	-	-	39.7%	37.2%

Wray Community District Hospital

1017 W 7th St
Wray, CO 80758
Phone: 970-332-4811
Fax: 970-332-4017
URL: www.wphn.com/wray_frm.htm
Type: Critical Access Hospitals
Emergency Services: Yes
Ownership: Govt - Hospital Dist/Auth
Beds: 15

Key Personnel:

Infection Control. . . . . Kathy Bard
CEO/President. . . . . Ed Finley
Cardiac Laboratory. . . . . Jennifer Kramer
Operating Room. . . . . Jodi Kramer, RN
Chief of Medical Staff . . . . Robert Loyd, MD
Emergency Room . . . . Christine Wall

Measure	Cases	This Hosp.	State Avg.	U.S. Avg.
Blood Clot Prevention and Treatment				
Anticoagulation Overlap Therapy[5]	-	-	97%	93%
ICU Venous Thromboembolism Prophylaxis[5]	-	-	95%	92%
Incidence of Potentially Preventable VTE[5]	-	-	8%	10%
UFH with Dosages/Platelet Monitoring[5]	-	-	97%	97%
Venous Thromboembolism Prophylaxis[5]	-	-	90%	85%
Warfarin Therapy Discharge Instructions[5]	-	-	69%	75%
Chest Pain/Possible Heart Attack Care				
Aspirin Given Within 24 Hours of Arrival	-	-	97%	96%
Fibrinolytic Meds Within 30 Min. of Arrival	-	-	55%	58%
Average Time to ECG (minutes)	-	-	8	7
Average Time to Transfer (minutes)	-	-	74	60
Children's Asthma Care				
Received Home Management Plan of Care	-	-	-	88%
Received Reliever Medication	-	-	-	100%
Received Systemic Corticosteroids	-	-	-	100%
Emergency Department				
Admittance Decision Time (minutes)[5]	-	-	96	98
Head CT Results Within 45 Min. of Arrival	-	-	67%	57%
Patients Who Left ER Before Being Seen	-	-	2%	2%
Time from ER Arrival to Admit. (minutes)[5]	-	-	244	274
Time from ER Arrival to Discharge (minutes)	-	-	139	134
Time in ER Before Being Evaluated (minutes)	-	-	20	26
Time to Pain Meds for Fractures (minutes)	-	-	45	57
Heart Attack Care				
Aspirin Given at Discharge[1,3]	-	-	100%	99%
Fibrinolytic Meds Within 30 Min. of Arrival[3,7]	-	-	20%	54%
PCI Within 90 Minutes of Arrival[3,7]	-	-	97%	96%
Statin Prescribed at Discharge[1,3]	-	-	99%	98%
Heart Failure Care				
ACE Inhibitor or ARB for LVSD[1]	-	-	97%	97%
Discharge Instructions Given[1]	-	-	93%	94%
Evaluation of LVS Function[1]	-	-	99%	99%
Medicare Spending				
Medicare Spending per Patient (ratio)	-	-	0.95	0.98
Pneumonia Care				
Appropriate Initial Antibiotic Given[1]	-	-	95%	95%
Blood Culture Timing[1]	-	-	98%	98%
Pregnancy and Delivery Care				
Newborn Deliveries Scheduled Early[5]	-	-	2%	6%
Preventive Care				
Immunization for Influenza	11	91%	92%	90%
Immunization for Pneumonia	12	83%	92%	92%
Stroke Care				
Anticoagulation Therapy for Atrial Fibrillation[3,7]	-	-	97%	95%
Antithrombotic Therapy Timing[3,7]	-	-	98%	98%
Assessed for Rehabilitation[3,7]	-	-	98%	97%
Discharged on Antithrombotic Therapy[3,7]	-	-	100%	99%
Discharged on Statin Medication[3,7]	-	-	94%	94%
Thrombolytic Therapy Timing[3,7]	-	-	78%	66%
Venous Thromboembolism Prophylaxis[3,7]	-	-	96%	94%
Written Stroke Educational Materials Given[3,7]	-	-	87%	88%
Surgical Care Improvement Project				
Appropriate Beta Blocker Usage[1]	-	-	98%	98%
Appropriate VTP Within 24 Hours	18	100%	98%	98%
Controlled Postoperative Blood Glucose[7]	-	-	96%	97%
Perioperative Temperature Management	26	100%	99%	100%
Prophylactic Antibiotic Selection	23	100%	99%	99%
Prophylactic Antibiotic Selection (Outpatient)	-	-	98%	98%
Prophylactic Antibiotic Stopped	23	100%	98%	98%
Prophylactic Antibiotic Timing	23	83%	98%	99%
Prophylactic Antibiotic Timing (Outpatient)	-	-	98%	98%
Urinary Catheter Removal	22	100%	97%	97%
Survey of Patients' Hospital Experiences				
Area Around Room 'Always' Quiet at Night[6]	<100	66%	64%	61%
Doctors 'Always' Communicated Well[6]	<100	88%	81%	82%
Home Recovery Information Given[6]	<100	85%	87%	85%
Hospital Given 9 or 10 on 10 Point Scale[6]	<100	77%	75%	71%
Meds 'Always' Explained Before Given[6]	<100	68%	67%	64%
Nurses 'Always' Communicated Well[6]	<100	85%	79%	79%
Pain 'Always' Well Controlled[6]	<100	80%	72%	71%
Room and Bathroom 'Always' Clean[6]	<100	78%	74%	73%
Timely Help 'Always' Received[6]	<100	81%	70%	68%
Would Definitely Recommend Hospital[6]	<100	84%	76%	71%
Use of Medical Imaging				
Cardiac Imaging Stress Test before Surgery	-	-	5%	5.3%
Combination Abdominal CT Scan	-	-	10%	10.5%
Combination Brain/Sinus CT Scan	-	-	2.1%	2.7%
Combination Chest CT Scan	-	-	3.1%	2.7%
Follow-up Mammogram/Ultrasound	-	-	8.7%	8.8%
Lumbar Spine MRI for Low Back Pain	-	-	39.7%	37.2%

Yuma District Hospital

1000 West 8th Avenue
Yuma, CO 80759
Phone: 970-848-5405
Fax: 970-848-2116
URL: www.yumahospital.org
Type: Critical Access Hospitals
Emergency Services: Yes
Ownership: Govt - Hospital Dist/Auth
Beds: 14

Key Personnel:

Chief of Medical Staff . . . . Douglas Everson, MD
Patient Relations . . . . Bev Funaro, RN
Quality Assurance . . . . Bev Funaro, RN
CEO . . . . John Gardner
Infection Control. . . . . Beth Saxton
Operating Room. . . . . John Wolz

Measure	Cases	This Hosp.	State Avg.	U.S. Avg.
Blood Clot Prevention and Treatment				
Anticoagulation Overlap Therapy[5]	-	-	97%	93%
ICU Venous Thromboembolism Prophylaxis[5]	-	-	95%	92%
Incidence of Potentially Preventable VTE[5]	-	-	8%	10%
UFH with Dosages/Platelet Monitoring[5]	-	-	97%	97%
Venous Thromboembolism Prophylaxis[5]	-	-	90%	85%
Warfarin Therapy Discharge Instructions[5]	-	-	69%	75%
Chest Pain/Possible Heart Attack Care				
Aspirin Given Within 24 Hours of Arrival[1,3]	-	-	97%	96%
Fibrinolytic Meds Within 30 Min. of Arrival[1,3]	-	-	55%	58%
Average Time to ECG (minutes)[1,3]	-	-	8	7
Average Time to Transfer (minutes)[3,7]	-	-	74	60
Children's Asthma Care				
Received Home Management Plan of Care	-	-	-	88%
Received Reliever Medication	-	-	-	100%
Received Systemic Corticosteroids	-	-	-	100%
Emergency Department				
Admittance Decision Time (minutes)	15	24	96	98
Head CT Results Within 45 Min. of Arrival[1,3]	-	-	67%	57%
Patients Who Left ER Before Being Seen[5]	-	-	2%	2%
Time from ER Arrival to Admit. (minutes)	98	120	244	274
Time from ER Arrival to Discharge (minutes)[5]	-	-	139	134
Time in ER Before Being Evaluated (minutes)[5]	-	-	20	26
Time to Pain Meds for Fractures (minutes)[1,3]	-	-	45	57
Heart Attack Care				
Aspirin Given at Discharge[1,3]	-	-	100%	99%
Fibrinolytic Meds Within 30 Min. of Arrival[3,7]	-	-	20%	54%
PCI Within 90 Minutes of Arrival[3,7]	-	-	97%	96%

NOTE: Hospital profiles are in alphabetical order by state, then city, then hospital within the city; Rankings exclude hospitals with less than 25 cases except for patient surveys which excludes hospitals with less than 100 cases; (a) 100-299 cases; (1) The number of cases/patients is too few to report; (2) Data submitted were based on a sample of cases/patients; (3) Results are based on a shorter time period than required; (4) Data suppressed by CMS for one or more quarters; (5) Results are not available for this reporting period; (6) Fewer than 100 patients completed the HCAHPS survey; (7) No cases met the criteria for this measure; (8) The lower limit of the confidence interval cannot be calculated if the number of observed infections equals zero; (9) No data are available from the state/territory for this reporting period; (10) The scores shown reflect fewer than 50 completed surveys; (11) There were discrepancies in the data collection process; (12) This measure does not apply to this hospital for this reporting period; (13) Results cannot be calculated for this reporting period; (14) The results for this state are combined with nearby states to protect confidentiality; Please refer to the User's Guide for a full explanation of data.

Statin Prescribed at Discharge[1,3]	-	-	99%	98%
Heart Failure Care				
ACE Inhibitor or ARB for LVSD[7]	-	-	97%	97%
Discharge Instructions Given[1]	-	-	93%	94%
Evaluation of LVS Function	11	100%	99%	99%
Medicare Spending				
Medicare Spending per Patient (ratio)	-	-	0.95	0.98
Pneumonia Care				
Appropriate Initial Antibiotic Given[1]	-	-	95%	95%
Blood Culture Timing[1]	-	-	98%	98%
Pregnancy and Delivery Care				
Newborn Deliveries Scheduled Early[5]	-	-	2%	6%
Preventive Care				
Immunization for Influenza	83	71%	92%	90%
Immunization for Pneumonia	159	77%	92%	92%
Stroke Care				
Anticoagulation Therapy for Atrial Fibrillation[3,7]	-	-	97%	95%
Antithrombotic Therapy Timing[3,7]	-	-	98%	98%
Assessed for Rehabilitation[3,7]	-	-	98%	97%
Discharged on Antithrombotic Therapy[3,7]	-	-	100%	99%
Discharged on Statin Medication[3,7]	-	-	94%	94%
Thrombolytic Therapy Timing[3,7]	-	-	78%	66%
Venous Thromboembolism Prophylaxis[1,3]	-	-	96%	94%
Written Stroke Educational Materials Given[3,7]	-	-	87%	88%
Surgical Care Improvement Project				
Appropriate Beta Blocker Usage[5]	-	-	98%	98%
Appropriate VTP Within 24 Hours[5]	-	-	98%	98%
Controlled Postoperative Blood Glucose[5]	-	-	96%	97%
Perioperative Temperature Management[5]	-	-	99%	100%
Prophylactic Antibiotic Selection[5]	-	-	99%	99%
Prophylactic Antibiotic Selection (Outpatient)[5]	-	-	98%	98%
Prophylactic Antibiotic Stopped[5]	-	-	98%	98%
Prophylactic Antibiotic Timing[5]	-	-	98%	99%
Prophylactic Antibiotic Timing (Outpatient)[5]	-	-	98%	98%
Urinary Catheter Removal[5]	-	-	97%	97%
Survey of Patients' Hospital Experiences				
Area Around Room 'Always' Quiet at Night[6]	<100	78%	64%	61%
Doctors 'Always' Communicated Well[6]	<100	83%	81%	82%
Home Recovery Information Given[6]	<100	87%	87%	85%
Hospital Given 9 or 10 on 10 Point Scale[6]	<100	78%	75%	71%
Meds 'Always' Explained Before Given[6]	<100	79%	67%	64%
Nurses 'Always' Communicated Well[6]	<100	88%	79%	79%
Pain 'Always' Well Controlled[6]	<100	86%	72%	71%
Room and Bathroom 'Always' Clean[6]	<100	88%	74%	73%
Timely Help 'Always' Received[6]	<100	87%	70%	68%
Would Definitely Recommend Hospital[6]	<100	71%	76%	71%
Use of Medical Imaging				
Cardiac Imaging Stress Test before Surgery[1]	-	-	5%	5.3%
Combination Abdominal CT Scan	98	5.1%	10%	10.5%
Combination Brain/Sinus CT Scan	69	8.7%	2.1%	2.7%
Combination Chest CT Scan	57	1.8%	3.1%	2.7%
Follow-up Mammogram/Ultrasound	165	8.5%	8.7%	8.8%
Lumbar Spine MRI for Low Back Pain[1]	-	-	39.7%	37.2%

NOTE: Hospital profiles are in alphabetical order by state, then city, then hospital within the city; Rankings exclude hospitals with less than 25 cases except for patient surveys which excludes hospitals with less than 100 cases; (a) 100-299 cases; (1) The number of cases/patients is too few to report; (2) Data submitted were based on a sample of cases/patients; (3) Results are based on a shorter time period than required; (4) Data suppressed by CMS for one or more quarters; (5) Results are not available for this reporting period; (6) Fewer than 100 patients completed the HCAHPS survey; (7) No cases met the criteria for this measure; (8) The lower limit of the confidence interval cannot be calculated if the number of observed infections equals zero; (9) No data are available from the state/territory for this reporting period; (10) The scores shown reflect fewer than 50 completed surveys; (11) There were discrepancies in the data collection process; (12) This measure does not apply to this hospital for this reporting period; (13) Results cannot be calculated for this reporting period; (14) The results for this state are combined with nearby states to protect confidentiality; Please refer to the User's Guide for a full explanation of data.

Blood Clot Prevention and Treatment

Anticoagulation Overlap Therapy

Hospital Name	City	Rate	Cases
Kaiser Foundation Hospital[2]	Honolulu	98%	55
Straub Clinic & Hospital[2]	Honolulu	97%	37
Hilo Medical Center[2]	Hilo	93%	27
The Queens Medical Center[2]	Honolulu	84%	92
Maui Memorial Medical Center[2]	Wailuku	75%	40

ICU Venous Thromboembolism Prophylaxis

Hospital Name	City	Rate	Cases
North Hawaii Community Hospital[2]	Kamuela	100%	35
Pali Momi Medical Center[2]	Aiea	100%	43
Straub Clinic & Hospital[2]	Honolulu	100%	70
Wilcox Memorial Hospital[2]	Lihue	100%	67
Hilo Medical Center[2]	Hilo	99%	73
Kuakini Medical Center[2]	Honolulu	97%	74
Maui Memorial Medical Center[2]	Wailuku	97%	98
Kona Community Hospital[2]	Kealakekua	95%	44
Kaiser Foundation Hospital[2]	Honolulu	93%	56
Kauai Veterans Memorial Hospital[2]	Waimea	93%	41
Wahiawa General Hospital[2]	Wahiawa	89%	45
Castle Medical Center[2]	Kailua	87%	47
The Queens Medical Center[2]	Honolulu	79%	63

Incidence of Potentially Preventable VTE

Hospital Name	City	Rate	Cases
The Queens Medical Center[2]	Honolulu	12%	33

UFH with Dosages/Platelet Count Monitoring

Hospital Name	City	Rate	Cases
The Queens Medical Center[2]	Honolulu	100%	45
Kaiser Foundation Hospital[2]	Honolulu	98%	53
Maui Memorial Medical Center[2]	Wailuku	83%	30

Venous Thromboembolism Prophylaxis

Hospital Name	City	Rate	Cases
Wilcox Memorial Hospital[2]	Lihue	100%	261
Pali Momi Medical Center[2]	Aiea	99%	387
Straub Clinic & Hospital[2]	Honolulu	99%	335
Hilo Medical Center[2]	Hilo	96%	366
Kaiser Foundation Hospital[2]	Honolulu	93%	336
North Hawaii Community Hospital[2]	Kamuela	93%	108
Kuakini Medical Center[2]	Honolulu	92%	386
Kauai Veterans Memorial Hospital[2]	Waimea	79%	76
Castle Medical Center[2]	Kailua	77%	327
Maui Memorial Medical Center[2]	Wailuku	73%	349
Kona Community Hospital[2]	Kealakekua	71%	199
The Queens Medical Center[2]	Honolulu	71%	375
Wahiawa General Hospital[2]	Wahiawa	70%	321

Warfarin Therapy Discharge Instructions

Hospital Name	City	Rate	Cases
Straub Clinic & Hospital[2]	Honolulu	100%	25
Kaiser Foundation Hospital[2]	Honolulu	98%	51
Hilo Medical Center[2]	Hilo	96%	26
Maui Memorial Medical Center[2]	Wailuku	19%	31
The Queens Medical Center[2]	Honolulu	0%	71

Chest Pain/Possible Heart Attack Care

Aspirin Given Within 24 Hours of Arrival

Hospital Name	City	Rate	Cases
North Hawaii Community Hospital	Kamuela	100%	40
Wilcox Memorial Hospital	Lihue	100%	35
Hilo Medical Center	Hilo	99%	153
Castle Medical Center	Kailua	98%	61
Kona Community Hospital	Kealakekua	97%	37
Pali Momi Medical Center	Aiea	97%	33
Wahiawa General Hospital	Wahiawa	93%	42

Average Time to ECG (minutes)

Hospital Name	City	Min.	Cases
Wahiawa General Hospital	Wahiawa	0	45
Castle Medical Center	Kailua	5	62
Kona Community Hospital	Kealakekua	6	38
Wilcox Memorial Hospital	Lihue	7	37
North Hawaii Community Hospital	Kamuela	8	51
Pali Momi Medical Center	Aiea	9	34
Hilo Medical Center	Hilo	12	157

Children's Asthma Care

No hospitals met the 25 case threshold.

Emergency Department

Admittance Decision Time (minutes)

Hospital Name	City	Min.	Cases
Wahiawa General Hospital[2]	Wahiawa	75	314
Kona Community Hospital[2]	Kealakekua	84	328
Straub Clinic & Hospital[2]	Honolulu	100	537
Castle Medical Center[2]	Kailua	101	602
Kaiser Foundation Hospital	Honolulu	102	5568
Kauai Veterans Memorial Hospital[2]	Waimea	110	189
The Queens Medical Center[2]	Honolulu	116	576
North Hawaii Community Hospital[2]	Kamuela	125	238
Wilcox Memorial Hospital[2]	Lihue	129	458
Kuakini Medical Center[2]	Honolulu	143	653
Maui Memorial Medical Center[2]	Wailuku	150	422
Hilo Medical Center[2]	Hilo	154	616
Pali Momi Medical Center[2]	Aiea	254	1006

Patients Who Left ER Before Being Seen

Hospital Name	City	Rate	Cases
Castle Medical Center	Kailua	0%	33251
Kahuku Medical Center	Kahuku	0%	5081
Pali Momi Medical Center	Aiea	0%	52027
Straub Clinic & Hospital	Honolulu	0%	28077
Wilcox Memorial Hospital	Lihue	0%	23916
Hilo Medical Center	Hilo	1%	41243
Kona Community Hospital	Kealakekua	1%	20483
Kuakini Medical Center	Honolulu	1%	16568
Maui Memorial Medical Center	Wailuku	1%	40589
North Hawaii Community Hospital	Kamuela	1%	12606
Wahiawa General Hospital	Wahiawa	1%	17929
The Queens Medical Center	Honolulu	2%	60567

Time from ER Arrival to Being Admitted (minutes)

Hospital Name	City	Min.	Cases
Wahiawa General Hospital[2]	Wahiawa	223	320
Castle Medical Center[2]	Kailua	237	610
Kauai Veterans Memorial Hospital[2]	Waimea	251	269
Straub Clinic & Hospital[2]	Honolulu	258	558
Wilcox Memorial Hospital[2]	Lihue	280	461
Kuakini Medical Center[2]	Honolulu	282	750
Maui Memorial Medical Center[2]	Wailuku	285	471
North Hawaii Community Hospital[2]	Kamuela	287	262
Kaiser Foundation Hospital	Honolulu	327	5568
Hilo Medical Center[2]	Hilo	341	624
Kona Community Hospital[2]	Kealakekua	342	332
The Queens Medical Center[2]	Honolulu	378	583
Pali Momi Medical Center[2]	Aiea	446	1029

Time from ER Arrival to Discharge (minutes)

Hospital Name	City	Min.	Cases
Wahiawa General Hospital	Wahiawa	91	425
Castle Medical Center	Kailua	105	353
North Hawaii Community Hospital	Kamuela	116	344
Straub Clinic & Hospital	Honolulu	124	365
Wilcox Memorial Hospital	Lihue	131	359
Pali Momi Medical Center	Aiea	137	369
Maui Memorial Medical Center	Wailuku	152	390
Hilo Medical Center	Hilo	156	473
Kona Community Hospital	Kealakekua	170	370
Kuakini Medical Center	Honolulu	190	357
The Queens Medical Center	Honolulu	197	346

Time in ER Before Being Evaluated (minutes)

Hospital Name	City	Min.	Cases
North Hawaii Community Hospital	Kamuela	13	161
Wahiawa General Hospital	Wahiawa	15	457
Castle Medical Center	Kailua	17	383
Wilcox Memorial Hospital	Lihue	17	383
Pali Momi Medical Center	Aiea	19	384
Hilo Medical Center	Hilo	21	503
Straub Clinic & Hospital	Honolulu	25	257
Kuakini Medical Center	Honolulu	30	396
Maui Memorial Medical Center	Wailuku	43	366
Kona Community Hospital	Kealakekua	48	418
The Queens Medical Center	Honolulu	50	431

Time to Pain Meds for Bone Fractures (minutes)

Hospital Name	City	Min.	Cases
Wahiawa General Hospital	Wahiawa	35	88
North Hawaii Community Hospital	Kamuela	40	75
Pali Momi Medical Center	Aiea	47	275
Castle Medical Center	Kailua	48	132
Kuakini Medical Center	Honolulu	48	27
Hilo Medical Center	Hilo	53	133
Straub Clinic & Hospital	Honolulu	54	64
Wilcox Memorial Hospital	Lihue	57	149
Maui Memorial Medical Center	Wailuku	59	275
Kona Community Hospital	Kealakekua	67	103
The Queens Medical Center	Honolulu	72	128

Heart Attack Care

Aspirin Given at Discharge

Hospital Name	City	Rate	Cases
Castle Medical Center	Kailua	100%	116
Kaiser Foundation Hospital	Honolulu	100%	302
Pali Momi Medical Center	Aiea	100%	222
The Queens Medical Center	Honolulu	100%	535
Straub Clinic & Hospital	Honolulu	99%	254
Wahiawa General Hospital	Wahiawa	99%	73
Maui Memorial Medical Center	Wailuku	98%	207
Hilo Medical Center	Hilo	96%	75
Kuakini Medical Center[2]	Honolulu	95%	135

PCI Within 90 Minutes of Arrival

Hospital Name	City	Rate	Cases
The Queens Medical Center	Honolulu	100%	44
Maui Memorial Medical Center	Wailuku	98%	40
Straub Clinic & Hospital	Honolulu	97%	38
Pali Momi Medical Center	Aiea	94%	54
Kuakini Medical Center[2]	Honolulu	79%	29

Statin Prescribed at Discharge

Hospital Name	City	Rate	Cases
Castle Medical Center	Kailua	100%	121
Kaiser Foundation Hospital	Honolulu	100%	299
Pali Momi Medical Center	Aiea	100%	228
The Queens Medical Center	Honolulu	100%	541
Maui Memorial Medical Center	Wailuku	99%	211
Straub Clinic & Hospital	Honolulu	99%	263
Wahiawa General Hospital	Wahiawa	99%	71
Hilo Medical Center	Hilo	97%	78
Kuakini Medical Center[2]	Honolulu	97%	145

Heart Failure Care

ACE Inhibitor or ARB for LVSD

Hospital Name	City	Rate	Cases
Castle Medical Center	Kailua	100%	46
Hilo Medical Center	Hilo	100%	66
Kaiser Foundation Hospital	Honolulu	100%	112
Maui Memorial Medical Center	Wailuku	100%	92
Pali Momi Medical Center	Aiea	100%	145
The Queens Medical Center	Honolulu	100%	279
Straub Clinic & Hospital	Honolulu	100%	103
Wilcox Memorial Hospital	Lihue	100%	40
Wahiawa General Hospital	Wahiawa	99%	72
Kuakini Medical Center[2]	Honolulu	90%	67
Kona Community Hospital	Kealakekua	85%	33

Discharge Instructions Given

Hospital Name	City	Rate	Cases
Castle Medical Center	Kailua	100%	114
Kaiser Foundation Hospital	Honolulu	100%	335
Kauai Veterans Memorial Hospital	Waimea	100%	30
Pali Momi Medical Center	Aiea	100%	292
Straub Clinic & Hospital	Honolulu	100%	260
Wilcox Memorial Hospital	Lihue	100%	98
Maui Memorial Medical Center	Wailuku	98%	183
The Queens Medical Center	Honolulu	97%	543
Hilo Medical Center	Hilo	93%	214
North Hawaii Community Hospital	Kamuela	91%	47
Kuakini Medical Center[2]	Honolulu	85%	180
Kona Community Hospital	Kealakekua	84%	69
Wahiawa General Hospital	Wahiawa	80%	176

Evaluation of LVS Function

Hospital Name	City	Rate	Cases
Castle Medical Center	Kailua	100%	124
Hilo Medical Center	Hilo	100%	241
Kaiser Foundation Hospital	Honolulu	100%	347
Kauai Veterans Memorial Hospital	Waimea	100%	37
Maui Memorial Medical Center	Wailuku	100%	191
North Hawaii Community Hospital	Kamuela	100%	48
Pali Momi Medical Center	Aiea	100%	317
The Queens Medical Center	Honolulu	100%	603
Straub Clinic & Hospital	Honolulu	100%	289
Wahiawa General Hospital	Wahiawa	100%	187
Wilcox Memorial Hospital	Lihue	100%	108
Kona Community Hospital	Kealakekua	99%	78
Kuakini Medical Center[2]	Honolulu	99%	204

NOTE: Hospital profiles are in alphabetical order by state, then city, then hospital within the city; Rankings exclude hospitals with less than 25 cases except for patient surveys which excludes hospitals with less than 100 cases; (a) 100-299 cases; (1) The number of cases/patients is too few to report; (2) Data submitted were based on a sample of cases/patients; (3) Results are based on a shorter time period than required; (4) Data suppressed by CMS for one or more quarters; (5) Results are not available for this reporting period; (6) Fewer than 100 patients completed the HCAHPS survey; (7) No cases met the criteria for this measure; (8) The lower limit of the confidence interval cannot be calculated if the number of observed infections equals zero; (9) No data are available from the state/territory for this reporting period; (10) The scores shown reflect fewer than 50 completed surveys; (11) There were discrepancies in the data collection process; (12) This measure does not apply to this hospital for this reporting period; (13) Results cannot be calculated for this reporting period; (14) The results for this state are combined with nearby states to protect confidentiality; Please refer to the User's Guide for a full explanation of data.

Medicare Spending

Medicare Spending per Patient (ratio)

Hospital Name	City	Ratio	Cases
Kona Community Hospital	Kealakekua	0.81	-
North Hawaii Community Hospital	Kamuela	0.81	-
Kaiser Foundation Hospital	Honolulu	0.82	-
Castle Medical Center	Kailua	0.85	-
The Queens Medical Center	Honolulu	0.85	-
Wilcox Memorial Hospital	Lihue	0.87	-
Maui Memorial Medical Center	Wailuku	0.89	-
Pali Momi Medical Center	Aiea	0.90	-
Wahiawa General Hospital	Wahiawa	0.90	-
Hilo Medical Center	Hilo	0.92	-
Kuakini Medical Center	Honolulu	0.92	-
Straub Clinic & Hospital	Honolulu	0.93	-

Pneumonia Care

Appropriate Initial Antibiotic Given

Hospital Name	City	Rate	Cases
Wilcox Memorial Hospital	Lihue	100%	73
Kaiser Foundation Hospital	Honolulu	99%	174
Straub Clinic & Hospital	Honolulu	99%	136
Kona Community Hospital	Kealakekua	98%	80
The Queens Medical Center	Honolulu	98%	294
Wahiawa General Hospital	Wahiawa	98%	84
Castle Medical Center	Kailua	97%	91
Kauai Veterans Memorial Hospital	Waimea	97%	33
Pali Momi Medical Center	Aiea	97%	233
Maui Memorial Medical Center	Wailuku	96%	137
Hilo Medical Center	Hilo	94%	118
Kuakini Medical Center[2]	Honolulu	84%	98

Blood Culture Timing

Hospital Name	City	Rate	Cases
Kauai Veterans Memorial Hospital	Waimea	100%	49
Kona Community Hospital	Kealakekua	100%	118
Straub Clinic & Hospital	Honolulu	100%	226
Wilcox Memorial Hospital	Lihue	100%	134
Castle Medical Center	Kailua	99%	178
Kaiser Foundation Hospital	Honolulu	99%	366
Pali Momi Medical Center	Aiea	98%	288
The Queens Medical Center	Honolulu	98%	486
Wahiawa General Hospital	Wahiawa	98%	211
Maui Memorial Medical Center	Wailuku	97%	223
Kuakini Medical Center[2]	Honolulu	96%	144
Hilo Medical Center	Hilo	95%	130
North Hawaii Community Hospital	Kamuela	94%	31

Pregnancy and Delivery Care

Newborns whose Deliveries were Scheduled Early

Hospital Name	City	Rate	Cases
Castle Medical Center[2]	Kailua	0%	30
Kauai Veterans Memorial Hospital	Waimea	0%	27
North Hawaii Community Hospital[2]	Kamuela	0%	49
The Queens Medical Center	Honolulu	1%	270
Wilcox Memorial Hospital[2]	Lihue	5%	55
Hilo Medical Center[2]	Hilo	14%	50
Kona Community Hospital[2]	Kealakekua	21%	58
Maui Memorial Medical Center[2]	Wailuku	53%	32

Preventive Care

Immunization for Influenza

Hospital Name	City	Rate	Cases
Pali Momi Medical Center[2]	Aiea	99%	574
Wilcox Memorial Hospital[2]	Lihue	99%	336
Hilo Medical Center[2]	Hilo	96%	552
Straub Clinic & Hospital[2]	Honolulu	95%	588
Wahiawa General Hospital[2]	Wahiawa	90%	357
Kona Community Hospital[2]	Kealakekua	85%	301
North Hawaii Community Hospital[2]	Kamuela	84%	228
Kauai Veterans Memorial Hospital[2]	Waimea	83%	242
The Queens Medical Center[2]	Honolulu	83%	577
Maui Memorial Medical Center[2]	Wailuku	79%	579
Kaiser Foundation Hospital	Honolulu	78%	5323
Kuakini Medical Center[2]	Honolulu	64%	506
Castle Medical Center[2]	Kailua	59%	528

Immunization for Pneumonia

Hospital Name	City	Rate	Cases
Pali Momi Medical Center[2]	Aiea	99%	863
Wilcox Memorial Hospital[2]	Lihue	99%	385
Hilo Medical Center[2]	Hilo	96%	623
Kauai Veterans Memorial Hospital[2]	Waimea	95%	249
Kaiser Foundation Hospital	Honolulu	93%	6778
North Hawaii Community Hospital[2]	Kamuela	93%	229
Straub Clinic & Hospital[2]	Honolulu	92%	867
Wahiawa General Hospital[2]	Wahiawa	90%	559
The Queens Medical Center[2]	Honolulu	84%	656
Kona Community Hospital[2]	Kealakekua	77%	243
Maui Memorial Medical Center[2]	Wailuku	76%	598
Castle Medical Center[2]	Kailua	70%	562
Kuakini Medical Center[2]	Honolulu	66%	812

Stroke Care

Anticoagulation Therapy for Atrial Fibrillation

Hospital Name	City	Rate	Cases
Kaiser Foundation Hospital	Honolulu	100%	27
The Queens Medical Center	Honolulu	100%	35

Antithrombotic Therapy Timing

Hospital Name	City	Rate	Cases
Kona Community Hospital	Kealakekua	100%	27
Maui Memorial Medical Center	Wailuku	100%	116
Pali Momi Medical Center	Aiea	100%	133
The Queens Medical Center	Honolulu	100%	238
Wilcox Memorial Hospital	Lihue	100%	55
Castle Medical Center	Kailua	99%	80
Hilo Medical Center	Hilo	99%	81
Kaiser Foundation Hospital	Honolulu	99%	144
Straub Clinic & Hospital	Honolulu	99%	142
Kuakini Medical Center[2]	Honolulu	98%	57
Wahiawa General Hospital	Wahiawa	89%	38

Assessed for Rehabilitation

Hospital Name	City	Rate	Cases
Maui Memorial Medical Center	Wailuku	100%	152
The Queens Medical Center	Honolulu	100%	384
Wahiawa General Hospital	Wahiawa	100%	39
Wilcox Memorial Hospital	Lihue	100%	78
Kaiser Foundation Hospital	Honolulu	99%	215
Pali Momi Medical Center	Aiea	99%	155
Hilo Medical Center	Hilo	98%	103
Straub Clinic & Hospital	Honolulu	98%	168
Castle Medical Center	Kailua	96%	90
Kuakini Medical Center[2]	Honolulu	96%	82
Kona Community Hospital	Kealakekua	94%	34

Discharged on Antithrombotic Therapy

Hospital Name	City	Rate	Cases
Hilo Medical Center	Hilo	100%	95
Kaiser Foundation Hospital	Honolulu	100%	166
Kuakini Medical Center[2]	Honolulu	100%	58
Maui Memorial Medical Center	Wailuku	100%	125
Pali Momi Medical Center	Aiea	100%	138
The Queens Medical Center	Honolulu	100%	277
Wahiawa General Hospital	Wahiawa	100%	34
Wilcox Memorial Hospital	Lihue	100%	64
Castle Medical Center	Kailua	99%	79
Straub Clinic & Hospital	Honolulu	99%	138
Kona Community Hospital	Kealakekua	97%	32

Discharged on Statin Medication

Hospital Name	City	Rate	Cases
Castle Medical Center	Kailua	100%	74
Pali Momi Medical Center	Aiea	100%	101
Wilcox Memorial Hospital	Lihue	100%	49
Kaiser Foundation Hospital	Honolulu	99%	137
Maui Memorial Medical Center	Wailuku	99%	104
The Queens Medical Center	Honolulu	99%	191
Straub Clinic & Hospital	Honolulu	99%	105
Kuakini Medical Center[2]	Honolulu	94%	52
Hilo Medical Center	Hilo	93%	81
Wahiawa General Hospital	Wahiawa	92%	25

Venous Thromboembolism (VTE) Prophylaxis

Hospital Name	City	Rate	Cases
Kaiser Foundation Hospital	Honolulu	100%	215
Maui Memorial Medical Center	Wailuku	100%	148
Wilcox Memorial Hospital	Lihue	100%	68
Pali Momi Medical Center	Aiea	99%	164
Hilo Medical Center	Hilo	98%	99
The Queens Medical Center	Honolulu	98%	393
Straub Clinic & Hospital	Honolulu	98%	174
Kona Community Hospital	Kealakekua	94%	31
Kuakini Medical Center[2]	Honolulu	93%	88
Castle Medical Center	Kailua	91%	100
Wahiawa General Hospital	Wahiawa	82%	40

Written Stroke Educational Materials Given

Hospital Name	City	Rate	Cases
Maui Memorial Medical Center	Wailuku	100%	121
Pali Momi Medical Center	Aiea	100%	95
Wilcox Memorial Hospital	Lihue	100%	57
Kaiser Foundation Hospital	Honolulu	98%	162
Straub Clinic & Hospital	Honolulu	97%	104
Castle Medical Center	Kailua	95%	56
Hilo Medical Center	Hilo	92%	50
The Queens Medical Center	Honolulu	92%	224
Kuakini Medical Center[2]	Honolulu	78%	36
Kona Community Hospital	Kealakekua	50%	28

Surgical Care Improvement Project

Appropriate Beta Blocker Usage

Hospital Name	City	Rate	Cases
Hilo Medical Center	Hilo	100%	56
Kaiser Foundation Hospital[2]	Honolulu	100%	319
Maui Memorial Medical Center[2]	Wailuku	99%	118
The Queens Medical Center[2]	Honolulu	99%	470
Straub Clinic & Hospital	Honolulu	99%	314
Kuakini Medical Center[2]	Honolulu	98%	99
Wilcox Memorial Hospital	Lihue	98%	43
Pali Momi Medical Center	Aiea	95%	74
Castle Medical Center[2]	Kailua	88%	52

Appropriate VTP Within 24 Hours

Hospital Name	City	Rate	Cases
Kaiser Foundation Hospital[2]	Honolulu	100%	793
The Queens Medical Center[2]	Honolulu	99%	930
Straub Clinic & Hospital	Honolulu	99%	757
Wilcox Memorial Hospital	Lihue	99%	194
Kuakini Medical Center[2]	Honolulu	98%	283
Pali Momi Medical Center	Aiea	98%	306
Hilo Medical Center	Hilo	97%	197
Maui Memorial Medical Center[2]	Wailuku	97%	222
North Hawaii Community Hospital	Kamuela	97%	79
Castle Medical Center[2]	Kailua	96%	270
Wahiawa General Hospital	Wahiawa	95%	38
Kona Community Hospital[2]	Kealakekua	89%	56

Controlled Postoperative Blood Glucose

Hospital Name	City	Rate	Cases
Kaiser Foundation Hospital[2]	Honolulu	99%	136
The Queens Medical Center[2]	Honolulu	99%	422
Straub Clinic & Hospital	Honolulu	99%	166
Maui Memorial Medical Center[2]	Wailuku	96%	95
Kuakini Medical Center[2]	Honolulu	91%	68

Perioperative Temperature Management

Hospital Name	City	Rate	Cases
Castle Medical Center[2]	Kailua	100%	310
Hilo Medical Center	Hilo	100%	257
Kaiser Foundation Hospital[2]	Honolulu	100%	908
Kuakini Medical Center[2]	Honolulu	100%	307
Maui Memorial Medical Center[2]	Wailuku	100%	275
Pali Momi Medical Center	Aiea	100%	367
The Queens Medical Center[2]	Honolulu	100%	1112
Straub Clinic & Hospital	Honolulu	100%	850
Wahiawa General Hospital	Wahiawa	100%	43
Wilcox Memorial Hospital	Lihue	100%	208
Kona Community Hospital[2]	Kealakekua	99%	78
North Hawaii Community Hospital	Kamuela	99%	94

Prophylactic Antibiotic Selection

Hospital Name	City	Rate	Cases
Kaiser Foundation Hospital[2]	Honolulu	100%	878
Kuakini Medical Center[2]	Honolulu	100%	253
Maui Memorial Medical Center[2]	Wailuku	100%	200
The Queens Medical Center[2]	Honolulu	100%	1155
Castle Medical Center[2]	Kailua	99%	196
Pali Momi Medical Center	Aiea	99%	147
Straub Clinic & Hospital	Honolulu	99%	689
Wilcox Memorial Hospital	Lihue	99%	139
Hilo Medical Center	Hilo	98%	156
North Hawaii Community Hospital	Kamuela	98%	47
Kona Community Hospital[2]	Kealakekua	94%	31

Prophylactic Antibiotic Selection (Outpatient)

Hospital Name	City	Rate	Cases
Kuakini Medical Center	Honolulu	99%	70
Maui Memorial Medical Center	Wailuku	99%	77
Pali Momi Medical Center	Aiea	99%	129
The Queens Medical Center	Honolulu	99%	835
Straub Clinic & Hospital	Honolulu	98%	356
North Hawaii Community Hospital	Kamuela	97%	37

NOTE: Hospital profiles are in alphabetical order by state, then city, then hospital within the city; Rankings exclude hospitals with less than 25 cases except for patient surveys which excludes hospitals with less than 100 cases; (a) 100-299 cases; (1) The number of cases/patients is too few to report; (2) Data submitted were based on a sample of cases/patients; (3) Results are based on a shorter time period than required; (4) Data suppressed by CMS for one or more quarters; (5) Results are not available for this reporting period; (6) Fewer than 100 patients completed the HCAHPS survey; (7) No cases met the criteria for this measure; (8) The lower limit of the confidence interval cannot be calculated if the number of observed infections equals zero; (9) No data are available from the state/territory for this reporting period; (10) The scores shown reflect fewer than 50 completed surveys; (11) There were discrepancies in the data collection process; (12) This measure does not apply to this hospital for this reporting period; (13) Results cannot be calculated for this reporting period; (14) The results for this state are combined with nearby states to protect confidentiality; Please refer to the User's Guide for a full explanation of data.

Hospital Name	City	Rate	Cases
Wilcox Memorial Hospital	Lihue	97%	39
Castle Medical Center	Kailua	96%	108
Hilo Medical Center	Hilo	95%	56

Prophylactic Antibiotic Stopped

Hospital Name	City	Rate	Cases
Kaiser Foundation Hospital[2]	Honolulu	100%	839
Maui Memorial Medical Center[2]	Wailuku	99%	193
The Queens Medical Center[2]	Honolulu	99%	1093
Straub Clinic & Hospital	Honolulu	99%	682
Wilcox Memorial Hospital	Lihue	99%	137
Castle Medical Center[2]	Kailua	98%	193
Kuakini Medical Center[2]	Honolulu	98%	242
Pali Momi Medical Center	Aiea	98%	145
Hilo Medical Center	Hilo	97%	150
Kona Community Hospital[2]	Kealakekua	93%	30
North Hawaii Community Hospital	Kamuela	93%	45

Prophylactic Antibiotic Timing

Hospital Name	City	Rate	Cases
Castle Medical Center[2]	Kailua	100%	196
Kaiser Foundation Hospital[2]	Honolulu	100%	878
Maui Memorial Medical Center[2]	Wailuku	100%	200
The Queens Medical Center[2]	Honolulu	100%	1159
Hilo Medical Center	Hilo	99%	156
Kuakini Medical Center[2]	Honolulu	99%	254
Pali Momi Medical Center	Aiea	99%	147
Straub Clinic & Hospital	Honolulu	99%	689
Wilcox Memorial Hospital	Lihue	99%	142
North Hawaii Community Hospital	Kamuela	98%	47
Kona Community Hospital[2]	Kealakekua	97%	31

Prophylactic Antibiotic Timing (Outpatient)

Hospital Name	City	Rate	Cases
North Hawaii Community Hospital	Kamuela	100%	37
Straub Clinic & Hospital	Honolulu	100%	310
Maui Memorial Medical Center	Wailuku	99%	77
The Queens Medical Center	Honolulu	99%	836
Pali Momi Medical Center	Aiea	98%	129
Wilcox Memorial Hospital	Lihue	97%	39
Castle Medical Center	Kailua	96%	110
Kuakini Medical Center	Honolulu	96%	71
Hilo Medical Center	Hilo	95%	56

Urinary Catheter Removal

Hospital Name	City	Rate	Cases
Kaiser Foundation Hospital[2]	Honolulu	100%	805
Pali Momi Medical Center	Aiea	100%	201
Wilcox Memorial Hospital	Lihue	100%	138
Maui Memorial Medical Center[2]	Wailuku	99%	268
The Queens Medical Center[2]	Honolulu	99%	1144
Kuakini Medical Center[2]	Honolulu	98%	284
North Hawaii Community Hospital	Kamuela	98%	58
Straub Clinic & Hospital	Honolulu	98%	854
Castle Medical Center[2]	Kailua	97%	217
Hilo Medical Center	Hilo	96%	135
Wahiawa General Hospital	Wahiawa	91%	32
Kona Community Hospital[2]	Kealakekua	86%	51

Survey of Patients' Hospital Experiences

Area Around Room 'Always' Quiet at Night

Hospital Name	City	Rate	Cases
Kauai Veterans Memorial Hospital	Waimea	71%	(a)
Castle Medical Center	Kailua	67%	300+
North Hawaii Community Hospital	Kamuela	65%	300+
Wilcox Memorial Hospital	Lihue	63%	300+
Pali Momi Medical Center	Aiea	60%	300+
Straub Clinic & Hospital	Honolulu	60%	300+
The Queens Medical Center	Honolulu	56%	300+
Kaiser Foundation Hospital	Honolulu	52%	300+
Maui Memorial Medical Center	Wailuku	52%	300+
Wahiawa General Hospital	Wahiawa	49%	300+
Hilo Medical Center	Hilo	44%	300+
Kuakini Medical Center	Honolulu	42%	300+

Doctors 'Always' Communicated Well

Hospital Name	City	Rate	Cases
Wilcox Memorial Hospital	Lihue	88%	300+
Kauai Veterans Memorial Hospital	Waimea	86%	(a)
Castle Medical Center	Kailua	84%	300+
Kaiser Foundation Hospital	Honolulu	84%	300+
Straub Clinic & Hospital	Honolulu	84%	300+
North Hawaii Community Hospital	Kamuela	83%	300+
Pali Momi Medical Center	Aiea	83%	300+
Hilo Medical Center	Hilo	79%	300+
Maui Memorial Medical Center	Wailuku	78%	300+
The Queens Medical Center	Honolulu	78%	300+

Hospital Name	City	Rate	Cases
Wahiawa General Hospital	Wahiawa	78%	300+
Kuakini Medical Center	Honolulu	77%	300+

Home Recovery Information Given

Hospital Name	City	Rate	Cases
Castle Medical Center	Kailua	90%	300+
Kauai Veterans Memorial Hospital	Waimea	90%	(a)
Kaiser Foundation Hospital	Honolulu	88%	300+
Pali Momi Medical Center	Aiea	87%	300+
Straub Clinic & Hospital	Honolulu	86%	300+
Wilcox Memorial Hospital	Lihue	86%	300+
The Queens Medical Center	Honolulu	84%	300+
Hilo Medical Center	Hilo	83%	300+
North Hawaii Community Hospital	Kamuela	83%	300+
Wahiawa General Hospital	Wahiawa	82%	300+
Maui Memorial Medical Center	Wailuku	81%	300+
Kuakini Medical Center	Honolulu	80%	300+

Hospital Given 9 or 10 on 10 Point Scale

Hospital Name	City	Rate	Cases
Straub Clinic & Hospital	Honolulu	82%	300+
North Hawaii Community Hospital	Kamuela	79%	300+
Castle Medical Center	Kailua	78%	300+
Kauai Veterans Memorial Hospital	Waimea	78%	(a)
The Queens Medical Center	Honolulu	78%	300+
Kaiser Foundation Hospital	Honolulu	77%	300+
Pali Momi Medical Center	Aiea	77%	300+
Wilcox Memorial Hospital	Lihue	77%	300+
Maui Memorial Medical Center	Wailuku	61%	300+
Hilo Medical Center	Hilo	57%	300+
Kuakini Medical Center	Honolulu	55%	300+
Wahiawa General Hospital	Wahiawa	50%	300+

Meds 'Always' Explained Before Given

Hospital Name	City	Rate	Cases
Wilcox Memorial Hospital	Lihue	72%	300+
Straub Clinic & Hospital	Honolulu	70%	300+
Castle Medical Center	Kailua	69%	300+
Kaiser Foundation Hospital	Honolulu	69%	300+
Pali Momi Medical Center	Aiea	69%	300+
North Hawaii Community Hospital	Kamuela	66%	300+
Kauai Veterans Memorial Hospital	Waimea	65%	(a)
The Queens Medical Center	Honolulu	65%	300+
Maui Memorial Medical Center	Wailuku	63%	300+
Wahiawa General Hospital	Wahiawa	59%	300+
Hilo Medical Center	Hilo	58%	300+
Kuakini Medical Center	Honolulu	57%	300+

Nurses 'Always' Communicated Well

Hospital Name	City	Rate	Cases
Straub Clinic & Hospital	Honolulu	84%	300+
Wilcox Memorial Hospital	Lihue	84%	300+
Castle Medical Center	Kailua	82%	300+
Kauai Veterans Memorial Hospital	Waimea	82%	(a)
Pali Momi Medical Center	Aiea	82%	300+
Kaiser Foundation Hospital	Honolulu	78%	300+
North Hawaii Community Hospital	Kamuela	78%	300+
The Queens Medical Center	Honolulu	78%	300+
Maui Memorial Medical Center	Wailuku	77%	300+
Hilo Medical Center	Hilo	76%	300+
Kuakini Medical Center	Honolulu	70%	300+
Wahiawa General Hospital	Wahiawa	70%	300+

Pain 'Always' Well Controlled

Hospital Name	City	Rate	Cases
Straub Clinic & Hospital	Honolulu	76%	300+
Kauai Veterans Memorial Hospital	Waimea	75%	(a)
Wilcox Memorial Hospital	Lihue	75%	300+
Pali Momi Medical Center	Aiea	73%	300+
Kaiser Foundation Hospital	Honolulu	72%	300+
North Hawaii Community Hospital	Kamuela	72%	300+
Castle Medical Center	Kailua	71%	300+
Maui Memorial Medical Center	Wailuku	71%	300+
Hilo Medical Center	Hilo	69%	300+
Kuakini Medical Center	Honolulu	67%	300+
The Queens Medical Center	Honolulu	67%	300+
Wahiawa General Hospital	Wahiawa	60%	300+

Room and Bathroom 'Always' Clean

Hospital Name	City	Rate	Cases
Castle Medical Center	Kailua	84%	300+
Straub Clinic & Hospital	Honolulu	81%	300+
Kauai Veterans Memorial Hospital	Waimea	80%	(a)
Wilcox Memorial Hospital	Lihue	80%	300+
Pali Momi Medical Center	Aiea	77%	300+
Maui Memorial Medical Center	Wailuku	76%	300+
North Hawaii Community Hospital	Kamuela	75%	300+
Kaiser Foundation Hospital	Honolulu	74%	300+

Hospital Name	City	Rate	Cases
Hilo Medical Center	Hilo	73%	300+
The Queens Medical Center	Honolulu	73%	300+
Kuakini Medical Center	Honolulu	67%	300+
Wahiawa General Hospital	Wahiawa	64%	300+

Timely Help 'Always' Received

Hospital Name	City	Rate	Cases
Kauai Veterans Memorial Hospital	Waimea	79%	(a)
Straub Clinic & Hospital	Honolulu	77%	300+
Castle Medical Center	Kailua	71%	300+
Wilcox Memorial Hospital	Lihue	70%	300+
Maui Memorial Medical Center	Wailuku	69%	300+
Kaiser Foundation Hospital	Honolulu	68%	300+
North Hawaii Community Hospital	Kamuela	68%	300+
Hilo Medical Center	Hilo	67%	300+
Pali Momi Medical Center	Aiea	67%	300+
The Queens Medical Center	Honolulu	60%	300+
Kuakini Medical Center	Honolulu	58%	300+
Wahiawa General Hospital	Wahiawa	58%	300+

Would Definitely Recommend Hospital

Hospital Name	City	Rate	Cases
Kauai Veterans Memorial Hospital	Waimea	85%	(a)
Straub Clinic & Hospital	Honolulu	84%	300+
North Hawaii Community Hospital	Kamuela	82%	300+
The Queens Medical Center	Honolulu	81%	300+
Castle Medical Center	Kailua	80%	300+
Wilcox Memorial Hospital	Lihue	80%	300+
Pali Momi Medical Center	Aiea	79%	300+
Kaiser Foundation Hospital	Honolulu	78%	300+
Maui Memorial Medical Center	Wailuku	63%	300+
Kuakini Medical Center	Honolulu	58%	300+
Hilo Medical Center	Hilo	57%	300+
Wahiawa General Hospital	Wahiawa	50%	300+

Use of Medical Imaging

Cardiac Imaging Stress Test before OP Surgery

Hospital Name	City	Rate	Cases
Castle Medical Center	Kailua	1.7%	119
Wahiawa General Hospital	Wahiawa	2.1%	94
North Hawaii Community Hospital	Kamuela	2.4%	167
Wilcox Memorial Hospital	Lihue	3.0%	336
Pali Momi Medical Center	Aiea	3.2%	412
The Queens Medical Center	Honolulu	3.3%	393
Straub Clinic & Hospital	Honolulu	4.3%	585
Maui Memorial Medical Center	Wailuku	4.5%	199
Hilo Medical Center	Hilo	5.7%	140
Kuakini Medical Center	Honolulu	6.3%	285

Combination Abdominal CT Scan

Hospital Name	City	Rate	Cases
Castle Medical Center	Kailua	0.6%	343
Wilcox Memorial Hospital	Lihue	1.3%	311
Maui Memorial Medical Center	Wailuku	1.8%	389
Wahiawa General Hospital	Wahiawa	2.3%	172
The Queens Medical Center	Honolulu	5.4%	1254
Pali Momi Medical Center	Aiea	5.9%	958
Straub Clinic & Hospital	Honolulu	6.7%	731
Kuakini Medical Center	Honolulu	8.1%	470
North Hawaii Community Hospital	Kamuela	8.3%	180
Kona Community Hospital	Kealakekua	45.6%	149
Hilo Medical Center	Hilo	52.0%	331

Combination Brain/Sinus CT Scan

Hospital Name	City	Rate	Cases
Kuakini Medical Center	Honolulu	1.1%	625
Pali Momi Medical Center	Aiea	1.1%	744
Maui Memorial Medical Center	Wailuku	1.3%	373
Hilo Medical Center	Hilo	2.0%	451
Straub Clinic & Hospital	Honolulu	2.9%	625
The Queens Medical Center	Honolulu	3.3%	729

Combination Chest CT Scan

Hospital Name	City	Rate	Cases
Castle Medical Center	Kailua	0.0%	166
Maui Memorial Medical Center	Wailuku	0.0%	165
Wilcox Memorial Hospital	Lihue	0.0%	208
The Queens Medical Center	Honolulu	0.1%	1072
Straub Clinic & Hospital	Honolulu	0.4%	538
Pali Momi Medical Center	Aiea	0.6%	798
Kuakini Medical Center	Honolulu	0.8%	477
North Hawaii Community Hospital	Kamuela	3.1%	128
Hilo Medical Center	Hilo	3.3%	91
Kona Community Hospital	Kealakekua	5.4%	130
Wahiawa General Hospital	Wahiawa	5.6%	90

NOTE: Hospital profiles are in alphabetical order by state, then city, then hospital within the city; Rankings exclude hospitals with less than 25 cases except for patient surveys which excludes hospitals with less than 100 cases; (a) 100-299 cases; (1) The number of cases/patients is too few to report; (2) Data submitted were based on a sample of cases/patients; (3) Results are based on a shorter time period than required; (4) Data suppressed by CMS for one or more quarters; (5) Results are not available for this reporting period; (6) Fewer than 100 patients completed the HCAHPS survey; (7) No cases met the criteria for this measure; (8) The lower limit of the confidence interval cannot be calculated if the number of observed infections equals zero; (9) No data are available from the state/territory for this reporting period; (10) The scores shown reflect fewer than 50 completed surveys; (11) There were discrepancies in the data collection process; (12) This measure does not apply to this hospital for this reporting period; (13) Results cannot be calculated for this reporting period; (14) The results for this state are combined with nearby states to protect confidentiality; Please refer to the User's Guide for a full explanation of data.

Follow-up Mammogram/Ultrasound

A follow-up rate near zero may indicate missed cancer; a rate higher than 14% may mean there is unnecessary follow up.

Hospital Name	City	Rate	Cases
Wilcox Memorial Hospital	Lihue	3.8%	943
The Queens Medical Center	Honolulu	5.8%	1659
Wahiawa General Hospital	Wahiawa	6.4%	425
Pali Momi Medical Center	Aiea	7.6%	2459
Kuakini Medical Center	Honolulu	9.1%	802
Straub Clinic & Hospital	Honolulu	9.8%	1523
North Hawaii Community Hospital	Kamuela	11.8%	195
Castle Medical Center	Kailua	21.7%	885

Lumbar Spine MRI for Low Back Pain

Hospital Name	City	Rate	Cases
Straub Clinic & Hospital	Honolulu	31.0%	100
Kuakini Medical Center	Honolulu	34.0%	47
Pali Momi Medical Center	Aiea	39.8%	118
Wilcox Memorial Hospital	Lihue	40.0%	45
The Queens Medical Center	Honolulu	40.2%	107

NOTE: Hospital profiles are in alphabetical order by state, then city, then hospital within the city; Rankings exclude hospitals with less than 25 cases except for patient surveys which excludes hospitals with less than 100 cases; (a) 100-299 cases; (1) The number of cases/patients is too few to report; (2) Data submitted were based on a sample of cases/patients; (3) Results are based on a shorter time period than required; (4) Data suppressed by CMS for one or more quarters; (5) Results are not available for this reporting period; (6) Fewer than 100 patients completed the HCAHPS survey; (7) No cases met the criteria for this measure; (8) The lower limit of the confidence interval cannot be calculated if the number of observed infections equals zero; (9) No data are available from the state/territory for this reporting period; (10) The scores shown reflect fewer than 50 completed surveys; (11) There were discrepancies in the data collection process; (12) This measure does not apply to this hospital for this reporting period; (13) Results cannot be calculated for this reporting period; (14) The results for this state are combined with nearby states to protect confidentiality; Please refer to the User's Guide for a full explanation of data.

Pali Momi Medical Center

98-1079 Moanalua Road
Aiea, HI 96701
URL: www.kapiolani.org
Type: Acute Care Hospitals
Ownership: Proprietary

Phone: 808-486-6000
Fax: 808-485-4400

Emergency Services: Yes
Beds: 116

Key Personnel:

Emergency Room . . . . Robert Canonico, MD
Intensive Care Unit. . . . . Shayne Castanera, MD
Chairman/CEO . . . . Mark Grief, MD
Quality Assurance . . . . Dani Kroll
Imaging . . . . Gordon W. Ng, MD
Anesthesiology. . . . . Mark Nishijo, MD
Chief of Medical Staff . . . . Eugene Tanabe, MD
CEO/President. . . . . Ray Vara

Measure	Cases	This Hosp.	State Avg.	U.S. Avg.
Blood Clot Prevention and Treatment				
Anticoagulation Overlap Therapy[2]	15	93%	89%	93%
ICU Venous Thromboembolism Prophylaxis[2]	43	100%	95%	92%
Incidence of Potentially Preventable VTE[2,7]	-	-	11%	10%
UFH with Dosages/Platelet Monitoring[1,2]	-	-	97%	97%
Venous Thromboembolism Prophylaxis[2]	387	99%	86%	85%
Warfarin Therapy Discharge Instructions[2]	11	100%	58%	75%
Chest Pain/Possible Heart Attack Care				
Aspirin Given Within 24 Hours of Arrival	33	97%	97%	96%
Fibrinolytic Meds Within 30 Min. of Arrival[7]	-	-	56%	58%
Average Time to ECG (minutes)	34	9	8	7
Average Time to Transfer (minutes)[7]	-	-	205	60
Children's Asthma Care				
Received Home Management Plan of Care	-	-	-	88%
Received Reliever Medication	-	-	-	100%
Received Systemic Corticosteroids	-	-	-	100%
Emergency Department				
Admittance Decision Time (minutes)[2]	1,006	254	113	98
Head CT Results Within 45 Min. of Arrival	14	64%	52%	57%
Patients Who Left ER Before Being Seen	52,027	0%	1%	2%
Time from ER Arrival to Admit. (minutes)[2]	1,029	446	311	274
Time from ER Arrival to Discharge (minutes)	369	137	125	134
Time in ER Before Being Evaluated (minutes)	384	19	21	26
Time to Pain Meds for Fractures (minutes)	275	47	51	57
Heart Attack Care				
Aspirin Given at Discharge	222	100%	99%	99%
Fibrinolytic Meds Within 30 Min. of Arrival[7]	-	-	-	54%
PCI Within 90 Minutes of Arrival	54	94%	94%	96%
Statin Prescribed at Discharge	228	100%	99%	98%
Heart Failure Care				
ACE Inhibitor or ARB for LVSD	145	100%	99%	97%
Discharge Instructions Given	292	100%	95%	94%
Evaluation of LVS Function	317	100%	100%	99%
Medicare Spending				
Medicare Spending per Patient (ratio)	-	0.90	0.87	0.98
Pneumonia Care				
Appropriate Initial Antibiotic Given	233	97%	96%	95%
Blood Culture Timing	288	98%	98%	98%
Pregnancy and Delivery Care				
Newborn Deliveries Scheduled Early[7]	-	-	7%	6%
Preventive Care				
Immunization for Influenza[2]	574	99%	81%	90%
Immunization for Pneumonia[2]	863	99%	89%	92%
Stroke Care				
Anticoagulation Therapy for Atrial Fibrillation	18	100%	97%	95%
Antithrombotic Therapy Timing	133	100%	99%	98%
Assessed for Rehabilitation	155	99%	99%	97%
Discharged on Antithrombotic Therapy	138	100%	100%	99%
Discharged on Statin Medication	101	100%	98%	94%
Thrombolytic Therapy Timing[1]	-	-	64%	66%
Venous Thromboembolism Prophylaxis	164	99%	98%	94%
Written Stroke Educational Materials Given	95	100%	94%	88%
Surgical Care Improvement Project				
Appropriate Beta Blocker Usage	74	95%	98%	98%
Appropriate VTP Within 24 Hours	306	98%	99%	98%
Controlled Postoperative Blood Glucose[7]	-	-	98%	97%
Perioperative Temperature Management	367	100%	100%	100%
Prophylactic Antibiotic Selection	147	99%	99%	99%
Prophylactic Antibiotic Selection (Outpatient)	129	99%	99%	98%
Prophylactic Antibiotic Stopped	145	98%	99%	98%
Prophylactic Antibiotic Timing	147	99%	99%	99%
Prophylactic Antibiotic Timing (Outpatient)	129	98%	99%	98%
Urinary Catheter Removal	201	100%	99%	97%
Survey of Patients' Hospital Experiences				
Area Around Room 'Always' Quiet at Night	300+	60%	57%	61%
Doctors 'Always' Communicated Well	300+	83%	82%	82%
Home Recovery Information Given	300+	87%	81%	85%
Hospital Given 9 or 10 on 10 Point Scale	300+	77%	66%	71%
Meds 'Always' Explained Before Given	300+	69%	66%	64%
Nurses 'Always' Communicated Well	300+	82%	80%	79%
Pain 'Always' Well Controlled	300+	73%	71%	71%
Room and Bathroom 'Always' Clean	300+	77%	74%	73%
Timely Help 'Always' Received	300+	67%	69%	68%
Would Definitely Recommend Hospital	300+	79%	69%	71%
Use of Medical Imaging				
Cardiac Imaging Stress Test before Surgery	412	3.2%	3.8%	5.3%
Combination Abdominal CT Scan	958	5.9%	8.9%	10.5%
Combination Brain/Sinus CT Scan	744	1.1%	2.1%	2.7%
Combination Chest CT Scan	798	0.6%	0.9%	2.7%
Follow-up Mammogram/Ultrasound	2,459	7.6%	9.4%	8.8%
Lumbar Spine MRI for Low Back Pain	118	39.8%	37.2%	37.2%

Hilo Medical Center

1190 Waianuenue Avenue
Hilo, HI 96720
E-mail: hhsc@hhsc.org
URL: www.hhsc.org
Type: Acute Care Hospitals
Ownership: Government - State

Phone: 808-974-4700
Fax: 808-974-4746

Emergency Services: Yes
Beds: 275

Key Personnel:

CEO/President. . . . . Dan Brinkman, RN, MPA
Operating Room. . . . . Dana Deranja, RN
Chief of Medical Staff . . . . Buddy Festerly
Infection Control. . . . . John Halloran, RN
Surgery . . . . Frederick Nitta, MD
Quality Assurance . . . . Steve Palmore, RN
Emergency Room . . . . Odetta Repoza-Pung, RN
Hemotology Center . . . . Noreen Silva

Measure	Cases	This Hosp.	State Avg.	U.S. Avg.
Blood Clot Prevention and Treatment				
Anticoagulation Overlap Therapy[2]	27	93%	89%	93%
ICU Venous Thromboembolism Prophylaxis[2]	73	99%	95%	92%
Incidence of Potentially Preventable VTE[1,2]	-	-	11%	10%
UFH with Dosages/Platelet Monitoring[1,2]	-	-	97%	97%
Venous Thromboembolism Prophylaxis[2]	366	96%	86%	85%
Warfarin Therapy Discharge Instructions[2]	26	96%	58%	75%
Chest Pain/Possible Heart Attack Care				
Aspirin Given Within 24 Hours of Arrival	153	99%	97%	96%
Fibrinolytic Meds Within 30 Min. of Arrival	15	60%	56%	58%
Average Time to ECG (minutes)	157	12	8	7
Average Time to Transfer (minutes)[1]	-	-	205	60
Children's Asthma Care				
Received Home Management Plan of Care	-	-	-	88%
Received Reliever Medication	-	-	-	100%
Received Systemic Corticosteroids	-	-	-	100%
Emergency Department				
Admittance Decision Time (minutes)[2]	616	154	113	98
Head CT Results Within 45 Min. of Arrival[1]	-	-	52%	57%
Patients Who Left ER Before Being Seen	41,243	1%	1%	2%
Time from ER Arrival to Admit. (minutes)[2]	624	341	311	274
Time from ER Arrival to Discharge (minutes)	473	156	125	134
Time in ER Before Being Evaluated (minutes)	503	21	21	26
Time to Pain Meds for Fractures (minutes)	133	53	51	57
Heart Attack Care				
Aspirin Given at Discharge	75	96%	99%	99%
Fibrinolytic Meds Within 30 Min. of Arrival[7]	-	-	-	54%
PCI Within 90 Minutes of Arrival[7]	-	-	94%	96%
Statin Prescribed at Discharge	78	97%	99%	98%
Heart Failure Care				
ACE Inhibitor or ARB for LVSD	66	100%	99%	97%
Discharge Instructions Given	214	93%	95%	94%
Evaluation of LVS Function	241	100%	100%	99%
Medicare Spending				
Medicare Spending per Patient (ratio)	-	0.92	0.87	0.98
Pneumonia Care				
Appropriate Initial Antibiotic Given	118	94%	96%	95%
Blood Culture Timing	130	95%	98%	98%
Pregnancy and Delivery Care				
Newborn Deliveries Scheduled Early[2]	50	14%	7%	6%
Preventive Care				
Immunization for Influenza[2]	552	96%	81%	90%
Immunization for Pneumonia[2]	623	96%	89%	92%
Stroke Care				
Anticoagulation Therapy for Atrial Fibrillation	14	93%	97%	95%
Antithrombotic Therapy Timing	81	99%	99%	98%
Assessed for Rehabilitation	103	98%	99%	97%
Discharged on Antithrombotic Therapy	95	100%	100%	99%
Discharged on Statin Medication	81	93%	98%	94%
Thrombolytic Therapy Timing	13	62%	64%	66%
Venous Thromboembolism Prophylaxis	99	98%	98%	94%
Written Stroke Educational Materials Given	50	92%	94%	88%
Surgical Care Improvement Project				
Appropriate Beta Blocker Usage	56	100%	98%	98%
Appropriate VTP Within 24 Hours	197	97%	99%	98%
Controlled Postoperative Blood Glucose[7]	-	-	98%	97%
Perioperative Temperature Management	257	100%	100%	100%
Prophylactic Antibiotic Selection	156	98%	99%	99%
Prophylactic Antibiotic Selection (Outpatient)	56	95%	99%	98%
Prophylactic Antibiotic Stopped	150	97%	99%	98%
Prophylactic Antibiotic Timing	156	99%	99%	99%
Prophylactic Antibiotic Timing (Outpatient)	56	95%	99%	98%
Urinary Catheter Removal	135	96%	99%	97%
Survey of Patients' Hospital Experiences				
Area Around Room 'Always' Quiet at Night	300+	44%	57%	61%
Doctors 'Always' Communicated Well	300+	79%	82%	82%
Home Recovery Information Given	300+	83%	81%	85%
Hospital Given 9 or 10 on 10 Point Scale	300+	57%	66%	71%
Meds 'Always' Explained Before Given	300+	58%	66%	64%
Nurses 'Always' Communicated Well	300+	76%	80%	79%
Pain 'Always' Well Controlled	300+	69%	71%	71%
Room and Bathroom 'Always' Clean	300+	73%	74%	73%
Timely Help 'Always' Received	300+	67%	69%	68%
Would Definitely Recommend Hospital	300+	57%	69%	71%
Use of Medical Imaging				
Cardiac Imaging Stress Test before Surgery	140	5.7%	3.8%	5.3%
Combination Abdominal CT Scan	331	52.0%	8.9%	10.5%
Combination Brain/Sinus CT Scan	451	2.0%	2.1%	2.7%
Combination Chest CT Scan	91	3.3%	0.9%	2.7%
Follow-up Mammogram/Ultrasound[7]	-	-	9.4%	8.8%
Lumbar Spine MRI for Low Back Pain[1]	-	-	37.2%	37.2%

Kaiser Foundation Hospital

3288 Moanalua Rd
Honolulu, HI 96819
URL: www.kaiserpermanente.com
Type: Acute Care Hospitals
Ownership: Voluntary non-profit - Private

Phone: 808-432-0000
Fax: 808-432-7736

Emergency Services: Yes
Beds: 202

Key Personnel:

Operating Room. . . . . Janet S Abadir, RN
Radiology. . . . . Peter Abcarian, MD
Pediatric Ambulatory Care . . . . . . Yi-Chuan Ching, MD
Pediatric In-Patient Care . . . . Yi-Chuan Ching, MD
Chief of Medical Staff . . . . Martin Leftik, MD
Quality Assurance . . . . Louise Samuels
Coronary Care . . . . Hazel Villegas

Measure	Cases	This Hosp.	State Avg.	U.S. Avg.
Blood Clot Prevention and Treatment				
Anticoagulation Overlap Therapy[2]	55	98%	89%	93%
ICU Venous Thromboembolism Prophylaxis[2]	56	93%	95%	92%
Incidence of Potentially Preventable VTE[1,2]	-	-	11%	10%
UFH with Dosages/Platelet Monitoring[2]	53	98%	97%	97%
Venous Thromboembolism Prophylaxis[2]	336	93%	86%	85%
Warfarin Therapy Discharge Instructions[2]	51	98%	58%	75%
Chest Pain/Possible Heart Attack Care				
Aspirin Given Within 24 Hours of Arrival	-	-	97%	96%
Fibrinolytic Meds Within 30 Min. of Arrival	-	-	56%	58%

NOTE: Hospital profiles are in alphabetical order by state, then city, then hospital within the city; Rankings exclude hospitals with less than 25 cases except for patient surveys which excludes hospitals with less than 100 cases; (a) 100-299 cases; (1) The number of cases/patients is too few to report; (2) Data submitted were based on a sample of cases/patients; (3) Results are based on a shorter time period than required; (4) Data suppressed by CMS for one or more quarters; (5) Results are not available for this reporting period; (6) Fewer than 100 patients completed the HCAHPS survey; (7) No cases met the criteria for this measure; (8) The lower limit of the confidence interval cannot be calculated if the number of observed infections equals zero; (9) No data are available from the state/territory for this reporting period; (10) The scores shown reflect fewer than 50 completed surveys; (11) There were discrepancies in the data collection process; (12) This measure does not apply to this hospital for this reporting period; (13) Results cannot be calculated for this reporting period; (14) The results for this state are combined with nearby states to protect confidentiality; Please refer to the User's Guide for a full explanation of data.

Measure	Cases	This Hosp.	State Avg.	U.S. Avg.
Average Time to ECG (minutes)	-	-	8	7
Average Time to Transfer (minutes)	-	-	205	60
Children's Asthma Care				
Received Home Management Plan of Care	-	-	-	88%
Received Reliever Medication	-	-	-	100%
Received Systemic Corticosteroids	-	-	-	100%
Emergency Department				
Admittance Decision Time (minutes)	5,568	102	113	98
Head CT Results Within 45 Min. of Arrival	-	-	52%	57%
Patients Who Left ER Before Being Seen	-	-	1%	2%
Time from ER Arrival to Admit. (minutes)	5,568	327	311	274
Time from ER Arrival to Discharge (minutes)	-	-	125	134
Time in ER Before Being Evaluated (minutes)	-	-	21	26
Time to Pain Meds for Fractures (minutes)	-	-	51	57
Heart Attack Care				
Aspirin Given at Discharge	302	100%	99%	99%
Fibrinolytic Meds Within 30 Min. of Arrival[7]	-	-	-	54%
PCI Within 90 Minutes of Arrival	24	96%	94%	96%
Statin Prescribed at Discharge	299	100%	99%	98%
Heart Failure Care				
ACE Inhibitor or ARB for LVSD	112	100%	99%	97%
Discharge Instructions Given	335	100%	95%	94%
Evaluation of LVS Function	347	100%	100%	99%
Medicare Spending				
Medicare Spending per Patient (ratio)	-	0.82	0.87	0.98
Pneumonia Care				
Appropriate Initial Antibiotic Given	174	99%	96%	95%
Blood Culture Timing	366	99%	98%	98%
Pregnancy and Delivery Care				
Newborn Deliveries Scheduled Early[2]	20	0%	7%	6%
Preventive Care				
Immunization for Influenza	5,323	78%	81%	90%
Immunization for Pneumonia	6,778	93%	89%	92%
Stroke Care				
Anticoagulation Therapy for Atrial Fibrillation	27	100%	97%	95%
Antithrombotic Therapy Timing	144	99%	99%	98%
Assessed for Rehabilitation	215	99%	99%	97%
Discharged on Antithrombotic Therapy	166	100%	100%	99%
Discharged on Statin Medication	137	99%	98%	94%
Thrombolytic Therapy Timing[1]	-	-	64%	66%
Venous Thromboembolism Prophylaxis	215	100%	98%	94%
Written Stroke Educational Materials Given	162	98%	94%	88%
Surgical Care Improvement Project				
Appropriate Beta Blocker Usage[2]	319	100%	98%	98%
Appropriate VTP Within 24 Hours[2]	793	100%	99%	98%
Controlled Postoperative Blood Glucose[2]	136	99%	98%	97%
Perioperative Temperature Management[2]	908	100%	100%	100%
Prophylactic Antibiotic Selection[2]	878	100%	99%	99%
Prophylactic Antibiotic Selection (Outpatient)	-	-	99%	98%
Prophylactic Antibiotic Stopped[2]	839	100%	99%	98%
Prophylactic Antibiotic Timing[2]	878	100%	99%	99%
Prophylactic Antibiotic Timing (Outpatient)	-	-	99%	98%
Urinary Catheter Removal[2]	805	100%	99%	97%
Survey of Patients' Hospital Experiences				
Area Around Room 'Always' Quiet at Night	300+	52%	57%	61%
Doctors 'Always' Communicated Well	300+	84%	82%	82%
Home Recovery Information Given	300+	88%	81%	85%
Hospital Given 9 or 10 on 10 Point Scale	300+	77%	66%	71%
Meds 'Always' Explained Before Given	300+	69%	66%	64%
Nurses 'Always' Communicated Well	300+	78%	80%	79%
Pain 'Always' Well Controlled	300+	72%	71%	71%
Room and Bathroom 'Always' Clean	300+	74%	74%	73%
Timely Help 'Always' Received	300+	68%	69%	68%
Would Definitely Recommend Hospital	300+	78%	69%	71%
Use of Medical Imaging				
Cardiac Imaging Stress Test before Surgery	-	-	3.8%	5.3%
Combination Abdominal CT Scan	-	-	8.9%	10.5%
Combination Brain/Sinus CT Scan	-	-	2.1%	2.7%
Combination Chest CT Scan	-	-	0.9%	2.7%
Follow-up Mammogram/Ultrasound	-	-	9.4%	8.8%
Lumbar Spine MRI for Low Back Pain	-	-	37.2%	37.2%

Kuakini Medical Center

347 North Kuakini Street Phone: 808-536-2236
Honolulu, HI 96817 Fax: 808-547-9547
E-mail: pr@kuakini.org
URL: www.kuakini.org
Type: Acute Care Hospitals Emergency Services: Yes
Ownership: Voluntary non-profit - Private Beds: 379
Key Personnel:
CEO/President. . . . . Gary K Kajiwara

Measure	Cases	This Hosp.	State Avg.	U.S. Avg.
Blood Clot Prevention and Treatment				
Anticoagulation Overlap Therapy[1,2]	-	-	89%	93%
ICU Venous Thromboembolism Prophylaxis[2]	74	97%	95%	92%
Incidence of Potentially Preventable VTE[2,7]	-	-	11%	10%
UFH with Dosages/Platelet Monitoring[1,2]	-	-	97%	97%
Venous Thromboembolism Prophylaxis[2]	386	92%	86%	85%
Warfarin Therapy Discharge Instructions[1,2]	-	-	58%	75%
Chest Pain/Possible Heart Attack Care				
Aspirin Given Within 24 Hours of Arrival[1,3]	-	-	97%	96%
Fibrinolytic Meds Within 30 Min. of Arrival[5]	-	-	56%	58%
Average Time to ECG (minutes)[1,3]	-	-	8	7
Average Time to Transfer (minutes)[5]	-	-	205	60
Children's Asthma Care				
Received Home Management Plan of Care	-	-	-	88%
Received Reliever Medication	-	-	-	100%
Received Systemic Corticosteroids	-	-	-	100%
Emergency Department				
Admittance Decision Time (minutes)[2]	653	143	113	98
Head CT Results Within 45 Min. of Arrival[1]	-	-	52%	57%
Patients Who Left ER Before Being Seen	16,568	1%	1%	2%
Time from ER Arrival to Admit. (minutes)[2]	750	282	311	274
Time from ER Arrival to Discharge (minutes)	357	190	125	134
Time in ER Before Being Evaluated (minutes)	396	30	21	26
Time to Pain Meds for Fractures (minutes)	27	48	51	57
Heart Attack Care				
Aspirin Given at Discharge[2]	135	95%	99%	99%
Fibrinolytic Meds Within 30 Min. of Arrival[2,7]	-	-	-	54%
PCI Within 90 Minutes of Arrival[2]	29	79%	94%	96%
Statin Prescribed at Discharge[2]	145	97%	99%	98%
Heart Failure Care				
ACE Inhibitor or ARB for LVSD[2]	67	90%	99%	97%
Discharge Instructions Given[2]	180	85%	95%	94%
Evaluation of LVS Function[2]	204	99%	100%	99%
Medicare Spending				
Medicare Spending per Patient (ratio)	-	0.92	0.87	0.98
Pneumonia Care				
Appropriate Initial Antibiotic Given[2]	98	84%	96%	95%
Blood Culture Timing[2]	144	96%	98%	98%
Pregnancy and Delivery Care				
Newborn Deliveries Scheduled Early[7]	-	-	7%	6%
Preventive Care				
Immunization for Influenza[2]	506	64%	81%	90%
Immunization for Pneumonia[2]	812	66%	89%	92%
Stroke Care				
Anticoagulation Therapy for Atrial Fibrillation[1,2]	-	-	97%	95%
Antithrombotic Therapy Timing[2]	57	98%	99%	98%
Assessed for Rehabilitation[2]	82	96%	99%	97%
Discharged on Antithrombotic Therapy[2]	58	100%	100%	99%
Discharged on Statin Medication[2]	52	94%	98%	94%
Thrombolytic Therapy Timing[2]	13	23%	64%	66%
Venous Thromboembolism Prophylaxis[2]	88	93%	98%	94%
Written Stroke Educational Materials Given[2]	36	78%	94%	88%
Surgical Care Improvement Project				
Appropriate Beta Blocker Usage[2]	99	98%	98%	98%
Appropriate VTP Within 24 Hours[2]	283	98%	99%	98%
Controlled Postoperative Blood Glucose[2]	68	91%	98%	97%
Perioperative Temperature Management[2]	307	100%	100%	100%
Prophylactic Antibiotic Selection[2]	253	100%	99%	99%
Prophylactic Antibiotic Selection (Outpatient)	70	99%	99%	98%
Prophylactic Antibiotic Stopped[2]	242	98%	99%	98%
Prophylactic Antibiotic Timing[2]	254	99%	99%	99%
Prophylactic Antibiotic Timing (Outpatient)	71	96%	99%	98%
Urinary Catheter Removal[2]	284	98%	99%	97%
Survey of Patients' Hospital Experiences				
Area Around Room 'Always' Quiet at Night	300+	42%	57%	61%
Doctors 'Always' Communicated Well	300+	77%	82%	82%
Home Recovery Information Given	300+	80%	81%	85%
Hospital Given 9 or 10 on 10 Point Scale	300+	55%	66%	71%
Meds 'Always' Explained Before Given	300+	57%	66%	64%
Nurses 'Always' Communicated Well	300+	70%	80%	79%
Pain 'Always' Well Controlled	300+	67%	71%	71%
Room and Bathroom 'Always' Clean	300+	67%	74%	73%
Timely Help 'Always' Received	300+	58%	69%	68%
Would Definitely Recommend Hospital	300+	58%	69%	71%
Use of Medical Imaging				
Cardiac Imaging Stress Test before Surgery	285	6.3%	3.8%	5.3%
Combination Abdominal CT Scan	470	8.1%	8.9%	10.5%
Combination Brain/Sinus CT Scan	625	1.1%	2.1%	2.7%
Combination Chest CT Scan	477	0.8%	0.9%	2.7%
Follow-up Mammogram/Ultrasound	802	9.1%	9.4%	8.8%
Lumbar Spine MRI for Low Back Pain	47	34.0%	37.2%	37.2%

The Queens Medical Center

1301 Punchbowl St Phone: 808-538-9011
Honolulu, HI 96813 Fax: 808-537-7887
URL: www.queens.org
Type: Acute Care Hospitals Emergency Services: Yes
Ownership: Voluntary non-profit - Private Beds: 533
Key Personnel:
Chief of Medical Staff . . . . Gerard Akaka
Patient Relations . . . . Darlena Chadwick, RN, MSN
Radiology. . . . . Stephen Holmes
CEO/President. . . . . Arthur Ushijima

Measure	Cases	This Hosp.	State Avg.	U.S. Avg.
Blood Clot Prevention and Treatment				
Anticoagulation Overlap Therapy[2]	92	84%	89%	93%
ICU Venous Thromboembolism Prophylaxis[2]	63	79%	95%	92%
Incidence of Potentially Preventable VTE[2]	33	12%	11%	10%
UFH with Dosages/Platelet Monitoring[2]	45	100%	97%	97%
Venous Thromboembolism Prophylaxis[2]	375	71%	86%	85%
Warfarin Therapy Discharge Instructions[2]	71	0%	58%	75%
Chest Pain/Possible Heart Attack Care				
Aspirin Given Within 24 Hours of Arrival[5]	-	-	97%	96%
Fibrinolytic Meds Within 30 Min. of Arrival[5]	-	-	56%	58%
Average Time to ECG (minutes)[5]	-	-	8	7
Average Time to Transfer (minutes)[5]	-	-	205	60
Children's Asthma Care				
Received Home Management Plan of Care	-	-	-	88%
Received Reliever Medication	-	-	-	100%
Received Systemic Corticosteroids	-	-	-	100%
Emergency Department				
Admittance Decision Time (minutes)[2]	576	116	113	98
Head CT Results Within 45 Min. of Arrival[1]	-	-	52%	57%
Patients Who Left ER Before Being Seen	60,567	2%	1%	2%
Time from ER Arrival to Admit. (minutes)[2]	583	378	311	274
Time from ER Arrival to Discharge (minutes)	346	197	125	134
Time in ER Before Being Evaluated (minutes)	431	50	21	26
Time to Pain Meds for Fractures (minutes)	128	72	51	57
Heart Attack Care				
Aspirin Given at Discharge	535	100%	99%	99%
Fibrinolytic Meds Within 30 Min. of Arrival[7]	-	-	-	54%
PCI Within 90 Minutes of Arrival	44	100%	94%	96%
Statin Prescribed at Discharge	541	100%	99%	98%
Heart Failure Care				
ACE Inhibitor or ARB for LVSD	279	100%	99%	97%
Discharge Instructions Given	543	97%	95%	94%
Evaluation of LVS Function	603	100%	100%	99%
Medicare Spending				
Medicare Spending per Patient (ratio)	-	0.85	0.87	0.98
Pneumonia Care				
Appropriate Initial Antibiotic Given	294	98%	96%	95%
Blood Culture Timing	486	98%	98%	98%
Pregnancy and Delivery Care				
Newborn Deliveries Scheduled Early	270	1%	7%	6%
Preventive Care				
Immunization for Influenza[2]	577	83%	81%	90%

NOTE: Hospital profiles are in alphabetical order by state, then city, then hospital within the city; Rankings exclude hospitals with less than 25 cases except for patient surveys which excludes hospitals with less than 100 cases; (a) 100-299 cases; (1) The number of cases/patients is too few to report; (2) Data submitted were based on a sample of cases/patients; (3) Results are based on a shorter time period than required; (4) Data suppressed by CMS for one or more quarters; (5) Results are not available for this reporting period; (6) Fewer than 100 patients completed the HCAHPS survey; (7) No cases met the criteria for this measure; (8) The lower limit of the confidence interval cannot be calculated if the number of observed infections equals zero; (9) No data are available from the state/territory for this reporting period; (10) The scores shown reflect fewer than 50 completed surveys; (11) There were discrepancies in the data collection process; (12) This measure does not apply to this hospital for this reporting period; (13) Results cannot be calculated for this reporting period; (14) The results for this state are combined with nearby states to protect confidentiality; Please refer to the User's Guide for a full explanation of data.

Measure	Cases	This Hosp.	State Avg.	U.S. Avg.
Immunization for Pneumonia[2]	656	84%	89%	92%
Stroke Care				
Anticoagulation Therapy for Atrial Fibrillation	35	100%	97%	95%
Antithrombotic Therapy Timing	238	100%	99%	98%
Assessed for Rehabilitation	384	100%	99%	97%
Discharged on Antithrombotic Therapy	277	100%	100%	99%
Discharged on Statin Medication	191	99%	98%	94%
Thrombolytic Therapy Timing	15	100%	64%	66%
Venous Thromboembolism Prophylaxis	393	98%	98%	94%
Written Stroke Educational Materials Given	224	92%	94%	88%
Surgical Care Improvement Project				
Appropriate Beta Blocker Usage[2]	470	99%	98%	98%
Appropriate VTP Within 24 Hours[2]	930	99%	99%	98%
Controlled Postoperative Blood Glucose[2]	422	99%	98%	97%
Perioperative Temperature Management[2]	1,112	100%	100%	100%
Prophylactic Antibiotic Selection[2]	1,155	100%	99%	99%
Prophylactic Antibiotic Selection (Outpatient)	835	99%	99%	98%
Prophylactic Antibiotic Stopped[2]	1,093	99%	99%	98%
Prophylactic Antibiotic Timing[2]	1,159	100%	99%	99%
Prophylactic Antibiotic Timing (Outpatient)	836	99%	99%	98%
Urinary Catheter Removal[2]	1,144	99%	99%	97%
Survey of Patients' Hospital Experiences				
Area Around Room 'Always' Quiet at Night	300+	56%	57%	61%
Doctors 'Always' Communicated Well	300+	78%	82%	82%
Home Recovery Information Given	300+	84%	81%	85%
Hospital Given 9 or 10 on 10 Point Scale	300+	78%	66%	71%
Meds 'Always' Explained Before Given	300+	65%	66%	64%
Nurses 'Always' Communicated Well	300+	78%	80%	79%
Pain 'Always' Well Controlled	300+	67%	71%	71%
Room and Bathroom 'Always' Clean	300+	73%	74%	73%
Timely Help 'Always' Received	300+	60%	69%	68%
Would Definitely Recommend Hospital	300+	81%	69%	71%
Use of Medical Imaging				
Cardiac Imaging Stress Test before Surgery	393	3.3%	3.8%	5.3%
Combination Abdominal CT Scan	1,254	5.4%	8.9%	10.5%
Combination Brain/Sinus CT Scan	729	3.3%	2.1%	2.7%
Combination Chest CT Scan	1,072	0.1%	0.9%	2.7%
Follow-up Mammogram/Ultrasound	1,659	5.8%	9.4%	8.8%
Lumbar Spine MRI for Low Back Pain	107	40.2%	37.2%	37.2%

Straub Clinic & Hospital

888 So King Street
Honolulu, HI 96813
Type: Acute Care Hospitals
Ownership: Proprietary
Phone: 808-522-4000
Fax: 808-522-4111
Emergency Services: Yes
Beds: 159

Key Personnel:
Radiology. Andrew Barger, MD
Quality Assurance . . . . John Berthiaume, MD
Infection Control. . . . . Diadema Bonnell
Pediatric Ambulatory Care . . . . . . Edgar CK Ho, MD
Pediatric In-Patient Care . . . . Edgar CK Ho, MD
Operating Room. . . . . George McPheeters, RN
CEO/President. . . . . Ray Vara
Chief of Medical Staff. . . . . Randy Yates, MD

Measure	Cases	This Hosp.	State Avg.	U.S. Avg.
Blood Clot Prevention and Treatment				
Anticoagulation Overlap Therapy[2]	37	97%	89%	93%
ICU Venous Thromboembolism Prophylaxis[2]	70	100%	95%	92%
Incidence of Potentially Preventable VTE[1,2]	-	-	11%	10%
UFH with Dosages/Platelet Monitoring[2]	24	100%	97%	97%
Venous Thromboembolism Prophylaxis[2]	335	99%	86%	85%
Warfarin Therapy Discharge Instructions[2]	25	100%	58%	75%
Chest Pain/Possible Heart Attack Care				
Aspirin Given Within 24 Hours of Arrival[1,3]	-	-	97%	96%
Fibrinolytic Meds Within 30 Min. of Arrival[3,7]	-	-	56%	58%
Average Time to ECG (minutes)[1,3]	-	-	8	7
Average Time to Transfer (minutes)[3,7]	-	-	205	60
Children's Asthma Care				
Received Home Management Plan of Care	-	-	-	88%
Received Reliever Medication	-	-	-	100%
Received Systemic Corticosteroids	-	-	-	100%
Emergency Department				
Admittance Decision Time (minutes)[2]	537	100	113	98
Head CT Results Within 45 Min. of Arrival[1]	-	-	52%	57%
Patients Who Left ER Before Being Seen	28,077	0%	1%	2%
Time from ER Arrival to Admit. (minutes)[2]	558	258	311	274
Time from ER Arrival to Discharge (minutes)	365	124	125	134
Time in ER Before Being Evaluated (minutes)	257	25	21	26
Time to Pain Meds for Fractures (minutes)	64	54	51	57
Heart Attack Care				
Aspirin Given at Discharge	254	99%	99%	99%
Fibrinolytic Meds Within 30 Min. of Arrival[1]	-	-	-	54%
PCI Within 90 Minutes of Arrival	38	97%	94%	96%
Statin Prescribed at Discharge	263	99%	99%	98%
Heart Failure Care				
ACE Inhibitor or ARB for LVSD	103	100%	99%	97%
Discharge Instructions Given	260	100%	95%	94%
Evaluation of LVS Function	289	100%	100%	99%
Medicare Spending				
Medicare Spending per Patient (ratio)	-	0.93	0.87	0.98
Pneumonia Care				
Appropriate Initial Antibiotic Given	136	99%	96%	95%
Blood Culture Timing	226	100%	98%	98%
Pregnancy and Delivery Care				
Newborn Deliveries Scheduled Early[7]	-	-	7%	6%
Preventive Care				
Immunization for Influenza[2]	588	95%	81%	90%
Immunization for Pneumonia[2]	867	92%	89%	92%
Stroke Care				
Anticoagulation Therapy for Atrial Fibrillation	12	100%	97%	95%
Antithrombotic Therapy Timing	142	99%	99%	98%
Assessed for Rehabilitation	168	98%	99%	97%
Discharged on Antithrombotic Therapy	138	99%	100%	99%
Discharged on Statin Medication	105	99%	98%	94%
Thrombolytic Therapy Timing[1]	-	-	64%	66%
Venous Thromboembolism Prophylaxis	174	98%	98%	94%
Written Stroke Educational Materials Given	104	97%	94%	88%
Surgical Care Improvement Project				
Appropriate Beta Blocker Usage	314	99%	98%	98%
Appropriate VTP Within 24 Hours	757	99%	99%	98%
Controlled Postoperative Blood Glucose	166	99%	98%	97%
Perioperative Temperature Management	850	100%	100%	100%
Prophylactic Antibiotic Selection	689	99%	99%	99%
Prophylactic Antibiotic Selection (Outpatient)	356	98%	99%	98%
Prophylactic Antibiotic Stopped	682	99%	99%	98%
Prophylactic Antibiotic Timing	689	99%	99%	99%
Prophylactic Antibiotic Timing (Outpatient)	310	100%	99%	98%
Urinary Catheter Removal	854	98%	99%	97%
Survey of Patients' Hospital Experiences				
Area Around Room 'Always' Quiet at Night	300+	60%	57%	61%
Doctors 'Always' Communicated Well	300+	84%	82%	82%
Home Recovery Information Given	300+	86%	81%	85%
Hospital Given 9 or 10 on 10 Point Scale	300+	82%	66%	71%
Meds 'Always' Explained Before Given	300+	70%	66%	64%
Nurses 'Always' Communicated Well	300+	84%	80%	79%
Pain 'Always' Well Controlled	300+	76%	71%	71%
Room and Bathroom 'Always' Clean	300+	81%	74%	73%
Timely Help 'Always' Received	300+	77%	69%	68%
Would Definitely Recommend Hospital	300+	84%	69%	71%
Use of Medical Imaging				
Cardiac Imaging Stress Test before Surgery	585	4.3%	3.8%	5.3%
Combination Abdominal CT Scan	731	6.7%	8.9%	10.5%
Combination Brain/Sinus CT Scan	625	2.9%	2.1%	2.7%
Combination Chest CT Scan	538	0.4%	0.9%	2.7%
Follow-up Mammogram/Ultrasound	1,523	9.8%	9.4%	8.8%
Lumbar Spine MRI for Low Back Pain	100	31.0%	37.2%	37.2%

Kahuku Medical Center

56-117 Pualalea Street
Kahuku, HI 96731
Type: Critical Access Hospitals
Ownership: Voluntary non-profit - Other
Phone: 808-293-9221
Fax: 808-293-2262
Emergency Services: Yes
Beds: 25

Key Personnel:
CEO . . . . Stephany Nihipali, Vaioleti
Quality Assurance . . . . Debbie Cabanilla
Chief of Medical Staff. . . . . Richard Price, MD
Operating Room. . . . . Nancy Solomans
Radiology. . . . . Jay White

Measure	Cases	This Hosp.	State Avg.	U.S. Avg.
Blood Clot Prevention and Treatment				
Anticoagulation Overlap Therapy[3,7]	-	-	89%	93%
ICU Venous Thromboembolism Prophylaxis[3,7]	-	-	95%	92%
Incidence of Potentially Preventable VTE[3,7]	-	-	11%	10%
UFH with Dosages/Platelet Monitoring[3,7]	-	-	97%	97%
Venous Thromboembolism Prophylaxis[1,3]	-	-	86%	85%
Warfarin Therapy Discharge Instructions[3,7]	-	-	58%	75%
Chest Pain/Possible Heart Attack Care				
Aspirin Given Within 24 Hours of Arrival[1,3]	-	-	97%	96%
Fibrinolytic Meds Within 30 Min. of Arrival[3,7]	-	-	56%	58%
Average Time to ECG (minutes)[1,3]	-	-	8	7
Average Time to Transfer (minutes)[3,7]	-	-	205	60
Children's Asthma Care				
Received Home Management Plan of Care	-	-	-	88%
Received Reliever Medication	-	-	-	100%
Received Systemic Corticosteroids	-	-	-	100%
Emergency Department				
Admittance Decision Time (minutes)[5]	-	-	113	98
Head CT Results Within 45 Min. of Arrival[5]	-	-	52%	57%
Patients Who Left ER Before Being Seen	5,081	0%	1%	2%
Time from ER Arrival to Admit. (minutes)[5]	-	-	311	274
Time from ER Arrival to Discharge (minutes)[1,3]	-	-	125	134
Time in ER Before Being Evaluated (minutes)[1,3]	-	-	21	26
Time to Pain Meds for Fractures (minutes)[5]	-	-	51	57
Heart Attack Care				
Aspirin Given at Discharge[5]	-	-	99%	99%
Fibrinolytic Meds Within 30 Min. of Arrival[5]	-	-	-	54%
PCI Within 90 Minutes of Arrival[5]	-	-	94%	96%
Statin Prescribed at Discharge[5]	-	-	99%	98%
Heart Failure Care				
ACE Inhibitor or ARB for LVSD[3,7]	-	-	99%	97%
Discharge Instructions Given[3,7]	-	-	95%	94%
Evaluation of LVS Function[3,7]	-	-	100%	99%
Medicare Spending				
Medicare Spending per Patient (ratio)	-	-	0.87	0.98
Pneumonia Care				
Appropriate Initial Antibiotic Given[1,3]	-	-	96%	95%
Blood Culture Timing[1,3]	-	-	98%	98%
Pregnancy and Delivery Care				
Newborn Deliveries Scheduled Early[5]	-	-	7%	6%
Preventive Care				
Immunization for Influenza[5]	-	-	81%	90%
Immunization for Pneumonia[5]	-	-	89%	92%
Stroke Care				
Anticoagulation Therapy for Atrial Fibrillation[5]	-	-	97%	95%
Antithrombotic Therapy Timing[5]	-	-	99%	98%
Assessed for Rehabilitation[5]	-	-	99%	97%
Discharged on Antithrombotic Therapy[5]	-	-	100%	99%
Discharged on Statin Medication[5]	-	-	98%	94%
Thrombolytic Therapy Timing[5]	-	-	64%	66%
Venous Thromboembolism Prophylaxis[5]	-	-	98%	94%
Written Stroke Educational Materials Given[5]	-	-	94%	88%
Surgical Care Improvement Project				
Appropriate Beta Blocker Usage[5]	-	-	98%	98%
Appropriate VTP Within 24 Hours[5]	-	-	99%	98%
Controlled Postoperative Blood Glucose[5]	-	-	98%	97%
Perioperative Temperature Management[5]	-	-	100%	100%
Prophylactic Antibiotic Selection[5]	-	-	99%	99%
Prophylactic Antibiotic Selection (Outpatient)[5]	-	-	99%	98%
Prophylactic Antibiotic Stopped[5]	-	-	99%	98%
Prophylactic Antibiotic Timing[5]	-	-	99%	99%
Prophylactic Antibiotic Timing (Outpatient)[5]	-	-	99%	98%
Urinary Catheter Removal[5]	-	-	99%	97%
Survey of Patients' Hospital Experiences				
Area Around Room 'Always' Quiet at Night[10]	<100	100%	57%	61%
Doctors 'Always' Communicated Well[10]	<100	100%	82%	82%
Home Recovery Information Given[10]	<100	29%	81%	85%
Hospital Given 9 or 10 on 10 Point Scale[10]	<100	53%	66%	71%
Meds 'Always' Explained Before Given[10]	<100	-	66%	64%
Nurses 'Always' Communicated Well[10]	<100	100%	80%	79%

NOTE: Hospital profiles are in alphabetical order by state, then city, then hospital within the city; Rankings exclude hospitals with less than 25 cases except for patient surveys which excludes hospitals with less than 100 cases; (a) 100-299 cases; (1) The number of cases/patients is too few to report; (2) Data submitted were based on a sample of cases/patients; (3) Results are based on a shorter time period than required; (4) Data suppressed by CMS for one or more quarters; (5) Results are not available for this reporting period; (6) Fewer than 100 patients completed the HCAHPS survey; (7) No cases met the criteria for this measure; (8) The lower limit of the confidence interval cannot be calculated if the number of observed infections equals zero; (9) No data are available from the state/territory for this reporting period; (10) The scores shown reflect fewer than 50 completed surveys; (11) There were discrepancies in the data collection process; (12) This measure does not apply to this hospital for this reporting period; (13) Results cannot be calculated for this reporting period; (14) The results for this state are combined with nearby states to protect confidentiality; Please refer to the User's Guide for a full explanation of data.

Measure	Cases	This Hosp.	State Avg.	U.S. Avg.
Pain 'Always' Well Controlled[10]	<100	-	71%	71%
Room and Bathroom 'Always' Clean[10]	<100	53%	74%	73%
Timely Help 'Always' Received[10]	<100	100%	69%	68%
Would Definitely Recommend Hospital[10]	<100	-	69%	71%
Use of Medical Imaging				
Cardiac Imaging Stress Test before Surgery[7]	-	-	3.8%	5.3%
Combination Abdominal CT Scan[7]	-	-	8.9%	10.5%
Combination Brain/Sinus CT Scan[7]	-	-	2.1%	2.7%
Combination Chest CT Scan[7]	-	-	0.9%	2.7%
Follow-up Mammogram/Ultrasound[7]	-	-	9.4%	8.8%
Lumbar Spine MRI for Low Back Pain[7]	-	-	37.2%	37.2%

Castle Medical Center

640 Ulukahiki St
Kailua, HI 96734
URL: www.castlemed.com
Phone: 808-263-5500
Fax: 808-263-5123
Type: Acute Care Hospitals
Emergency Services: Yes
Ownership: Voluntary non-profit - Church
Beds: 160

Key Personnel:
Chief of Medical Staff . . . . Virginia A Abshier
Quality Assurance . . . . Judith Correa, RN
CEO/President . . . . Kathryn Kathryn, FACHE
Patient Relations . . . . Kathryn Raethel
Chair/CEO . . . . Scott Reiner

Measure	Cases	This Hosp.	State Avg.	U.S. Avg.
Blood Clot Prevention and Treatment				
Anticoagulation Overlap Therapy[2]	13	100%	89%	93%
ICU Venous Thromboembolism Prophylaxis[2]	47	87%	95%	92%
Incidence of Potentially Preventable VTE[1,2]	-	-	11%	10%
UFH with Dosages/Platelet Monitoring[1,2]	-	-	97%	97%
Venous Thromboembolism Prophylaxis[2]	327	77%	86%	85%
Warfarin Therapy Discharge Instructions[1,2]	-	-	58%	75%
Chest Pain/Possible Heart Attack Care				
Aspirin Given Within 24 Hours of Arrival	61	98%	97%	96%
Fibrinolytic Meds Within 30 Min. of Arrival[7]	-	-	56%	58%
Average Time to ECG (minutes)	62	5	8	7
Average Time to Transfer (minutes)[7]	-	-	205	60
Children's Asthma Care				
Received Home Management Plan of Care	-	-	-	88%
Received Reliever Medication	-	-	-	100%
Received Systemic Corticosteroids	-	-	-	100%
Emergency Department				
Admittance Decision Time (minutes)[2]	602	101	113	98
Head CT Results Within 45 Min. of Arrival	24	50%	52%	57%
Patients Who Left ER Before Being Seen	33,251	0%	1%	2%
Time from ER Arrival to Admit. (minutes)[2]	610	237	311	274
Time from ER Arrival to Discharge (minutes)	353	105	125	134
Time in ER Before Being Evaluated (minutes)	383	17	21	26
Time to Pain Meds for Fractures (minutes)	132	48	51	57
Heart Attack Care				
Aspirin Given at Discharge	116	100%	99%	99%
Fibrinolytic Meds Within 30 Min. of Arrival[7]	-	-	-	54%
PCI Within 90 Minutes of Arrival	17	88%	94%	96%
Statin Prescribed at Discharge	121	100%	99%	98%
Heart Failure Care				
ACE Inhibitor or ARB for LVSD	46	100%	99%	97%
Discharge Instructions Given	114	100%	95%	94%
Evaluation of LVS Function	124	100%	100%	99%
Medicare Spending				
Medicare Spending per Patient (ratio)	-	0.85	0.87	0.98
Pneumonia Care				
Appropriate Initial Antibiotic Given	91	97%	96%	95%
Blood Culture Timing	178	99%	98%	98%
Pregnancy and Delivery Care				
Newborn Deliveries Scheduled Early[2]	30	0%	7%	6%
Preventive Care				
Immunization for Influenza[2]	528	59%	81%	90%
Immunization for Pneumonia[2]	562	70%	89%	92%
Stroke Care				
Anticoagulation Therapy for Atrial Fibrillation[1]	-	-	97%	95%
Antithrombotic Therapy Timing	80	99%	99%	98%
Assessed for Rehabilitation	90	96%	99%	97%
Discharged on Antithrombotic Therapy	79	99%	100%	99%
Discharged on Statin Medication	74	100%	98%	94%
Thrombolytic Therapy Timing	11	45%	64%	66%
Venous Thromboembolism Prophylaxis	100	91%	98%	94%
Written Stroke Educational Materials Given	56	95%	94%	88%
Surgical Care Improvement Project				
Appropriate Beta Blocker Usage[2]	52	88%	98%	98%
Appropriate VTP Within 24 Hours[2]	270	96%	99%	98%
Controlled Postoperative Blood Glucose[1,2]	-	-	98%	97%
Perioperative Temperature Management[2]	310	100%	100%	100%
Prophylactic Antibiotic Selection[2]	196	99%	99%	99%
Prophylactic Antibiotic Selection (Outpatient)	108	96%	99%	98%
Prophylactic Antibiotic Stopped[2]	193	98%	99%	98%
Prophylactic Antibiotic Timing[2]	196	100%	99%	99%
Prophylactic Antibiotic Timing (Outpatient)	110	96%	99%	98%
Urinary Catheter Removal[2]	217	97%	99%	97%
Survey of Patients' Hospital Experiences				
Area Around Room 'Always' Quiet at Night	300+	67%	57%	61%
Doctors 'Always' Communicated Well	300+	84%	82%	82%
Home Recovery Information Given	300+	90%	81%	85%
Hospital Given 9 or 10 on 10 Point Scale	300+	78%	66%	71%
Meds 'Always' Explained Before Given	300+	69%	66%	64%
Nurses 'Always' Communicated Well	300+	82%	80%	79%
Pain 'Always' Well Controlled	300+	71%	71%	71%
Room and Bathroom 'Always' Clean	300+	84%	74%	73%
Timely Help 'Always' Received	300+	71%	69%	68%
Would Definitely Recommend Hospital	300+	80%	69%	71%
Use of Medical Imaging				
Cardiac Imaging Stress Test before Surgery	119	1.7%	3.8%	5.3%
Combination Abdominal CT Scan	343	0.6%	8.9%	10.5%
Combination Brain/Sinus CT Scan[1]	-	-	2.1%	2.7%
Combination Chest CT Scan	166	0.0%	0.9%	2.7%
Follow-up Mammogram/Ultrasound	885	21.7%	9.4%	8.8%
Lumbar Spine MRI for Low Back Pain[1]	-	-	37.2%	37.2%

North Hawaii Community Hospital

67 1125 Mamalahoa Highway
Kamuela, HI 96743
URL: www.northhawaiicommunityhospital.org
Phone: 808-885-4444
Fax: 808-881-4415
Type: Acute Care Hospitals
Emergency Services: Yes
Ownership: Voluntary non-profit - Private
Beds: 40

Key Personnel:
Radiology. . . . . Indu Agarwal
Quality Assurance . . . . Lauraine DuPont, RN
CEO/President. . . . . Kenneth D. Graham
Pediatrics. . . . . Peter Gregg, MD
Surgery . . . . Lyn Lam, MD
Cardiology . . . . James Lucas, MD
Chairman/CEO . . . . Arthur A. Ushijima
Chief of Medical Staff . . . . Howard Wong, MD

Measure	Cases	This Hosp.	State Avg.	U.S. Avg.
Blood Clot Prevention and Treatment				
Anticoagulation Overlap Therapy[1,2]	-	-	89%	93%
ICU Venous Thromboembolism Prophylaxis[2]	35	100%	95%	92%
Incidence of Potentially Preventable VTE[2,7]	-	-	11%	10%
UFH with Dosages/Platelet Monitoring[1,2]	-	-	97%	97%
Venous Thromboembolism Prophylaxis[2]	108	93%	86%	85%
Warfarin Therapy Discharge Instructions[1,2]	-	-	58%	75%
Chest Pain/Possible Heart Attack Care				
Aspirin Given Within 24 Hours of Arrival	40	100%	97%	96%
Fibrinolytic Meds Within 30 Min. of Arrival[1]	-	-	56%	58%
Average Time to ECG (minutes)	51	8	8	7
Average Time to Transfer (minutes)[1]	-	-	205	60
Children's Asthma Care				
Received Home Management Plan of Care	-	-	-	88%
Received Reliever Medication	-	-	-	100%
Received Systemic Corticosteroids	-	-	-	100%
Emergency Department				
Admittance Decision Time (minutes)[2]	238	125	113	98
Head CT Results Within 45 Min. of Arrival[1]	-	-	52%	57%
Patients Who Left ER Before Being Seen	12,606	1%	1%	2%
Time from ER Arrival to Admit. (minutes)[2]	262	287	311	274
Time from ER Arrival to Discharge (minutes)	344	116	125	134
Time in ER Before Being Evaluated (minutes)	161	13	21	26
Time to Pain Meds for Fractures (minutes)	75	40	51	57
Heart Attack Care				
Aspirin Given at Discharge[1]	-	-	99%	99%
Fibrinolytic Meds Within 30 Min. of Arrival[7]	-	-	-	54%
PCI Within 90 Minutes of Arrival[7]	-	-	94%	96%
Statin Prescribed at Discharge[1]	-	-	99%	98%
Heart Failure Care				
ACE Inhibitor or ARB for LVSD	19	95%	99%	97%
Discharge Instructions Given	47	91%	95%	94%
Evaluation of LVS Function	48	100%	100%	99%
Medicare Spending				
Medicare Spending per Patient (ratio)	-	0.81	0.87	0.98
Pneumonia Care				
Appropriate Initial Antibiotic Given	24	88%	96%	95%
Blood Culture Timing	31	94%	98%	98%
Pregnancy and Delivery Care				
Newborn Deliveries Scheduled Early[2]	49	0%	7%	6%
Preventive Care				
Immunization for Influenza[2]	228	84%	81%	90%
Immunization for Pneumonia[2]	229	93%	89%	92%
Stroke Care				
Anticoagulation Therapy for Atrial Fibrillation[1]	-	-	97%	95%
Antithrombotic Therapy Timing	15	100%	99%	98%
Assessed for Rehabilitation	21	100%	99%	97%
Discharged on Antithrombotic Therapy	20	100%	100%	99%
Discharged on Statin Medication	15	100%	98%	94%
Thrombolytic Therapy Timing[1]	-	-	64%	66%
Venous Thromboembolism Prophylaxis	22	95%	98%	94%
Written Stroke Educational Materials Given	15	87%	94%	88%
Surgical Care Improvement Project				
Appropriate Beta Blocker Usage	17	94%	98%	98%
Appropriate VTP Within 24 Hours	79	97%	99%	98%
Controlled Postoperative Blood Glucose[7]	-	-	98%	97%
Perioperative Temperature Management	94	99%	100%	100%
Prophylactic Antibiotic Selection	47	98%	99%	99%
Prophylactic Antibiotic Selection (Outpatient)	37	97%	99%	98%
Prophylactic Antibiotic Stopped	45	93%	99%	98%
Prophylactic Antibiotic Timing	47	98%	99%	99%
Prophylactic Antibiotic Timing (Outpatient)	37	100%	99%	98%
Urinary Catheter Removal	58	98%	99%	97%
Survey of Patients' Hospital Experiences				
Area Around Room 'Always' Quiet at Night	300+	65%	57%	61%
Doctors 'Always' Communicated Well	300+	83%	82%	82%
Home Recovery Information Given	300+	83%	81%	85%
Hospital Given 9 or 10 on 10 Point Scale	300+	79%	66%	71%
Meds 'Always' Explained Before Given	300+	66%	66%	64%
Nurses 'Always' Communicated Well	300+	78%	80%	79%
Pain 'Always' Well Controlled	300+	72%	71%	71%
Room and Bathroom 'Always' Clean	300+	75%	74%	73%
Timely Help 'Always' Received	300+	68%	69%	68%
Would Definitely Recommend Hospital	300+	82%	69%	71%
Use of Medical Imaging				
Cardiac Imaging Stress Test before Surgery	167	2.4%	3.8%	5.3%
Combination Abdominal CT Scan	180	8.3%	8.9%	10.5%
Combination Brain/Sinus CT Scan[1]	-	-	2.1%	2.7%
Combination Chest CT Scan	128	3.1%	0.9%	2.7%
Follow-up Mammogram/Ultrasound	195	11.8%	9.4%	8.8%
Lumbar Spine MRI for Low Back Pain[1]	-	-	37.2%	37.2%

Samuel Mahelona Memorial Hospital

4800 Kawaihau Road
Kapaa, HI 96746
Phone: 808-822-4961
Type: Critical Access Hospitals
Emergency Services: No
Ownership: Government - State

Measure	Cases	This Hosp.	State Avg.	U.S. Avg.
Blood Clot Prevention and Treatment				
Anticoagulation Overlap Therapy[7]	-	-	89%	93%
ICU Venous Thromboembolism Prophylaxis[7]	-	-	95%	92%
Incidence of Potentially Preventable VTE[7]	-	-	11%	10%
UFH with Dosages/Platelet Monitoring[7]	-	-	97%	97%
Venous Thromboembolism Prophylaxis[1]	-	-	86%	85%
Warfarin Therapy Discharge Instructions[7]	-	-	58%	75%
Chest Pain/Possible Heart Attack Care				
Aspirin Given Within 24 Hours of Arrival	-	-	97%	96%

NOTE: Hospital profiles are in alphabetical order by state, then city, then hospital within the city; Rankings exclude hospitals with less than 25 cases except for patient surveys which excludes hospitals with less than 100 cases; (a) 100-299 cases; (1) The number of cases/patients is too few to report; (2) Data submitted were based on a sample of cases/patients; (3) Results are based on a shorter time period than required; (4) Data suppressed by CMS for one or more quarters; (5) Results are not available for this reporting period; (6) Fewer than 100 patients completed the HCAHPS survey; (7) No cases met the criteria for this measure; (8) The lower limit of the confidence interval cannot be calculated if the number of observed infections equals zero; (9) No data are available from the state/territory for this reporting period; (10) The scores shown reflect fewer than 50 completed surveys; (11) There were discrepancies in the data collection process; (12) This measure does not apply to this hospital for this reporting period; (13) Results cannot be calculated for this reporting period; (14) The results for this state are combined with nearby states to protect confidentiality; Please refer to the User's Guide for a full explanation of data.

Fibrinolytic Meds Within 30 Min. of Arrival	-	-	56%	58%
Average Time to ECG (minutes)	-	-	8	7
Average Time to Transfer (minutes)	-	-	205	60
Children's Asthma Care				
Received Home Management Plan of Care	-	-	-	88%
Received Reliever Medication	-	-	-	100%
Received Systemic Corticosteroids	-	-	-	100%
Emergency Department				
Admittance Decision Time (minutes)[1]	-	-	113	98
Head CT Results Within 45 Min. of Arrival	-	-	52%	57%
Patients Who Left ER Before Being Seen	-	-	1%	2%
Time from ER Arrival to Admit. (minutes)[1]	-	-	311	274
Time from ER Arrival to Discharge (minutes)	-	-	125	134
Time in ER Before Being Evaluated (minutes)	-	-	21	26
Time to Pain Meds for Fractures (minutes)	-	-	51	57
Heart Attack Care				
Aspirin Given at Discharge[5]	-	-	99%	99%
Fibrinolytic Meds Within 30 Min. of Arrival[5]	-	-	-	54%
PCI Within 90 Minutes of Arrival[5]	-	-	94%	96%
Statin Prescribed at Discharge[5]	-	-	99%	98%
Heart Failure Care				
ACE Inhibitor or ARB for LVSD[5]	-	-	99%	97%
Discharge Instructions Given[5]	-	-	95%	94%
Evaluation of LVS Function[5]	-	-	100%	99%
Medicare Spending				
Medicare Spending per Patient (ratio)	-	-	0.87	0.98
Pneumonia Care				
Appropriate Initial Antibiotic Given[1,3]	-	-	96%	95%
Blood Culture Timing[1,3]	-	-	98%	98%
Pregnancy and Delivery Care				
Newborn Deliveries Scheduled Early[3,7]	-	-	7%	6%
Preventive Care				
Immunization for Influenza[1]	-	-	81%	90%
Immunization for Pneumonia[1]	-	-	89%	92%
Stroke Care				
Anticoagulation Therapy for Atrial Fibrillation[5]	-	-	97%	95%
Antithrombotic Therapy Timing[5]	-	-	99%	98%
Assessed for Rehabilitation[5]	-	-	99%	97%
Discharged on Antithrombotic Therapy[5]	-	-	100%	99%
Discharged on Statin Medication[5]	-	-	98%	94%
Thrombolytic Therapy Timing[5]	-	-	64%	66%
Venous Thromboembolism Prophylaxis[5]	-	-	98%	94%
Written Stroke Educational Materials Given[5]	-	-	94%	88%
Surgical Care Improvement Project				
Appropriate Beta Blocker Usage[5]	-	-	98%	98%
Appropriate VTP Within 24 Hours[5]	-	-	99%	98%
Controlled Postoperative Blood Glucose[5]	-	-	98%	97%
Perioperative Temperature Management[5]	-	-	100%	100%
Prophylactic Antibiotic Selection[5]	-	-	99%	99%
Prophylactic Antibiotic Selection (Outpatient)	-	-	99%	98%
Prophylactic Antibiotic Stopped[5]	-	-	99%	98%
Prophylactic Antibiotic Timing[5]	-	-	99%	99%
Prophylactic Antibiotic Timing (Outpatient)	-	-	99%	98%
Urinary Catheter Removal[5]	-	-	99%	97%
Survey of Patients' Hospital Experiences				
Area Around Room 'Always' Quiet at Night[5]	-	-	57%	61%
Doctors 'Always' Communicated Well[5]	-	-	82%	82%
Home Recovery Information Given[5]	-	-	81%	85%
Hospital Given 9 or 10 on 10 Point Scale[5]	-	-	66%	71%
Meds 'Always' Explained Before Given[5]	-	-	66%	64%
Nurses 'Always' Communicated Well[5]	-	-	80%	79%
Pain 'Always' Well Controlled[5]	-	-	71%	71%
Room and Bathroom 'Always' Clean[5]	-	-	74%	73%
Timely Help 'Always' Received[5]	-	-	69%	68%
Would Definitely Recommend Hospital[5]	-	-	69%	71%
Use of Medical Imaging				
Cardiac Imaging Stress Test before Surgery	-	-	3.8%	5.3%
Combination Abdominal CT Scan	-	-	8.9%	10.5%
Combination Brain/Sinus CT Scan	-	-	2.1%	2.7%
Combination Chest CT Scan	-	-	0.9%	2.7%
Follow-up Mammogram/Ultrasound	-	-	9.4%	8.8%
Lumbar Spine MRI for Low Back Pain	-	-	37.2%	37.2%

Molokai General Hospital

280 Home Olu Place
Kaunakakai, HI 96748
Phone: 808-553-5331
Fax: 808-536-2224
URL: www.queens.org/qhs/mgh.htm
Type: Critical Access Hospitals
Emergency Services: Yes
Ownership: Voluntary non-profit - Private
Beds: 30

Key Personnel:

CEO/President. . . . . N Emmett Aluli, MD
Infection Control. . . . . Mary Anne Hill
Quality Assurance . . . . Mary Anne Hill
Chief of Medical Staff. . . . . Mark Schmalz, MD
Emergency Room . . . . Mark Schmalz, MD

Measure	Cases	This Hosp.	State Avg.	U.S. Avg.
Blood Clot Prevention and Treatment				
Anticoagulation Overlap Therapy[3,7]	-	-	89%	93%
ICU Venous Thromboembolism Prophylaxis[3,7]	-	-	95%	92%
Incidence of Potentially Preventable VTE[3,7]	-	-	11%	10%
UFH with Dosages/Platelet Monitoring[3,7]	-	-	97%	97%
Venous Thromboembolism Prophylaxis[1,3]	-	-	86%	85%
Warfarin Therapy Discharge Instructions[3,7]	-	-	58%	75%
Chest Pain/Possible Heart Attack Care				
Aspirin Given Within 24 Hours of Arrival	-	-	97%	96%
Fibrinolytic Meds Within 30 Min. of Arrival	-	-	56%	58%
Average Time to ECG (minutes)	-	-	8	7
Average Time to Transfer (minutes)	-	-	205	60
Children's Asthma Care				
Received Home Management Plan of Care	-	-	-	88%
Received Reliever Medication	-	-	-	100%
Received Systemic Corticosteroids	-	-	-	100%
Emergency Department				
Admittance Decision Time (minutes)[5]	-	-	113	98
Head CT Results Within 45 Min. of Arrival	-	-	52%	57%
Patients Who Left ER Before Being Seen	-	-	1%	2%
Time from ER Arrival to Admit. (minutes)[5]	-	-	311	274
Time from ER Arrival to Discharge (minutes)	-	-	125	134
Time in ER Before Being Evaluated (minutes)	-	-	21	26
Time to Pain Meds for Fractures (minutes)	-	-	51	57
Heart Attack Care				
Aspirin Given at Discharge[5]	-	-	99%	99%
Fibrinolytic Meds Within 30 Min. of Arrival[5]	-	-	-	54%
PCI Within 90 Minutes of Arrival[5]	-	-	94%	96%
Statin Prescribed at Discharge[5]	-	-	99%	98%
Heart Failure Care				
ACE Inhibitor or ARB for LVSD[1,3]	-	-	99%	97%
Discharge Instructions Given[1,3]	-	-	95%	94%
Evaluation of LVS Function[1,3]	-	-	100%	99%
Medicare Spending				
Medicare Spending per Patient (ratio)	-	-	0.87	0.98
Pneumonia Care				
Appropriate Initial Antibiotic Given[1]	-	-	96%	95%
Blood Culture Timing	11	100%	98%	98%
Pregnancy and Delivery Care				
Newborn Deliveries Scheduled Early[5]	-	-	7%	6%
Preventive Care				
Immunization for Influenza[5]	-	-	81%	90%
Immunization for Pneumonia[5]	-	-	89%	92%
Stroke Care				
Anticoagulation Therapy for Atrial Fibrillation[5]	-	-	97%	95%
Antithrombotic Therapy Timing[5]	-	-	99%	98%
Assessed for Rehabilitation[5]	-	-	99%	97%
Discharged on Antithrombotic Therapy[5]	-	-	100%	99%
Discharged on Statin Medication[5]	-	-	98%	94%
Thrombolytic Therapy Timing[5]	-	-	64%	66%
Venous Thromboembolism Prophylaxis[5]	-	-	98%	94%
Written Stroke Educational Materials Given[5]	-	-	94%	88%
Surgical Care Improvement Project				
Appropriate Beta Blocker Usage[5]	-	-	98%	98%
Appropriate VTP Within 24 Hours[5]	-	-	99%	98%
Controlled Postoperative Blood Glucose[5]	-	-	98%	97%
Perioperative Temperature Management[5]	-	-	100%	100%
Prophylactic Antibiotic Selection[5]	-	-	99%	99%
Prophylactic Antibiotic Selection (Outpatient)	-	-	99%	98%
Prophylactic Antibiotic Stopped[5]	-	-	99%	98%
Prophylactic Antibiotic Timing[5]	-	-	99%	99%
Prophylactic Antibiotic Timing (Outpatient)	-	-	99%	98%
Urinary Catheter Removal[5]	-	-	99%	97%
Survey of Patients' Hospital Experiences				
Area Around Room 'Always' Quiet at Night[10]	<100	66%	57%	61%
Doctors 'Always' Communicated Well[10]	<100	87%	82%	82%
Home Recovery Information Given[10]	<100	86%	81%	85%
Hospital Given 9 or 10 on 10 Point Scale[10]	<100	70%	66%	71%
Meds 'Always' Explained Before Given[10]	<100	79%	66%	64%
Nurses 'Always' Communicated Well[10]	<100	76%	80%	79%
Pain 'Always' Well Controlled[10]	<100	73%	71%	71%
Room and Bathroom 'Always' Clean[10]	<100	92%	74%	73%
Timely Help 'Always' Received[10]	<100	64%	69%	68%
Would Definitely Recommend Hospital[10]	<100	77%	69%	71%
Use of Medical Imaging				
Cardiac Imaging Stress Test before Surgery	-	-	3.8%	5.3%
Combination Abdominal CT Scan	-	-	8.9%	10.5%
Combination Brain/Sinus CT Scan	-	-	2.1%	2.7%
Combination Chest CT Scan	-	-	0.9%	2.7%
Follow-up Mammogram/Ultrasound	-	-	9.4%	8.8%
Lumbar Spine MRI for Low Back Pain	-	-	37.2%	37.2%

Kona Community Hospital

79-1019 Haukapila Street
Kealakekua, HI 96750
Phone: 808-322-9311
Fax: 808-322-4488
URL: www.kch.hhsc.org
Type: Acute Care Hospitals
Emergency Services: Yes
Ownership: Government - State
Beds: 94

Key Personnel:

Operating Room. . . . . Dawn Brewer
Infection Control. . . . . Lisa Downing
CEO/President. . . . . Earl Greenia
Chief of Medical Staff. . . . . Eddie Herd
Emergency Room . . . . Richard McDowell, MD
Quality Assurance . . . . Marcy Rogers

Measure	Cases	This Hosp.	State Avg.	U.S. Avg.
Blood Clot Prevention and Treatment				
Anticoagulation Overlap Therapy[1,2]	-	-	89%	93%
ICU Venous Thromboembolism Prophylaxis[2]	44	95%	95%	92%
Incidence of Potentially Preventable VTE[1,2]	-	-	11%	10%
UFH with Dosages/Platelet Monitoring[1,2]	-	-	97%	97%
Venous Thromboembolism Prophylaxis[2]	199	71%	86%	85%
Warfarin Therapy Discharge Instructions[2]	13	38%	58%	75%
Chest Pain/Possible Heart Attack Care				
Aspirin Given Within 24 Hours of Arrival	37	97%	97%	96%
Fibrinolytic Meds Within 30 Min. of Arrival[1,3]	-	-	56%	58%
Average Time to ECG (minutes)	38	6	8	7
Average Time to Transfer (minutes)[3,7]	-	-	205	60
Children's Asthma Care				
Received Home Management Plan of Care	-	-	-	88%
Received Reliever Medication	-	-	-	100%
Received Systemic Corticosteroids	-	-	-	100%
Emergency Department				
Admittance Decision Time (minutes)[2]	328	84	113	98
Head CT Results Within 45 Min. of Arrival[1]	-	-	52%	57%
Patients Who Left ER Before Being Seen	20,483	1%	1%	2%
Time from ER Arrival to Admit. (minutes)[2]	332	342	311	274
Time from ER Arrival to Discharge (minutes)	370	170	125	134
Time in ER Before Being Evaluated (minutes)	418	48	21	26
Time to Pain Meds for Fractures (minutes)	103	67	51	57
Heart Attack Care				
Aspirin Given at Discharge[1]	-	-	99%	99%
Fibrinolytic Meds Within 30 Min. of Arrival[1]	-	-	-	54%
PCI Within 90 Minutes of Arrival[7]	-	-	94%	96%
Statin Prescribed at Discharge[1]	-	-	99%	98%
Heart Failure Care				
ACE Inhibitor or ARB for LVSD	33	85%	99%	97%
Discharge Instructions Given	69	84%	95%	94%
Evaluation of LVS Function	78	99%	100%	99%
Medicare Spending				
Medicare Spending per Patient (ratio)	-	0.81	0.87	0.98
Pneumonia Care				
Appropriate Initial Antibiotic Given	80	98%	96%	95%
Blood Culture Timing	118	100%	98%	98%

NOTE: Hospital profiles are in alphabetical order by state, then city, then hospital within the city; Rankings exclude hospitals with less than 25 cases except for patient surveys which excludes hospitals with less than 100 cases; (a) 100-299 cases; (1) The number of cases/patients is too few to report; (2) Data submitted were based on a sample of cases/patients; (3) Results are based on a shorter time period than required; (4) Data suppressed by CMS for one or more quarters; (5) Results are not available for this reporting period; (6) Fewer than 100 patients completed the HCAHPS survey; (7) No cases met the criteria for this measure; (8) The lower limit of the confidence interval cannot be calculated if the number of observed infections equals zero; (9) No data are available from the state/territory for this reporting period; (10) The scores shown reflect fewer than 50 completed surveys; (11) There were discrepancies in the data collection process; (12) This measure does not apply to this hospital for this reporting period; (13) Results cannot be calculated for this reporting period; (14) The results for this state are combined with nearby states to protect confidentiality; Please refer to the User's Guide for a full explanation of data.

Measure	Cases	This Hosp.	State Avg.	U.S. Avg.
Pregnancy and Delivery Care				
Newborn Deliveries Scheduled Early[2]	58	21%	7%	6%
Preventive Care				
Immunization for Influenza[2]	301	85%	81%	90%
Immunization for Pneumonia[2]	243	77%	89%	92%
Stroke Care				
Anticoagulation Therapy for Atrial Fibrillation[1]	-	-	97%	95%
Antithrombotic Therapy Timing	27	100%	99%	98%
Assessed for Rehabilitation	34	94%	99%	97%
Discharged on Antithrombotic Therapy	32	97%	100%	99%
Discharged on Statin Medication	23	100%	98%	94%
Thrombolytic Therapy Timing[1]	-	-	64%	66%
Venous Thromboembolism Prophylaxis	31	94%	98%	94%
Written Stroke Educational Materials Given	28	50%	94%	88%
Surgical Care Improvement Project				
Appropriate Beta Blocker Usage[1,2]	-	-	98%	98%
Appropriate VTP Within 24 Hours[2]	56	89%	99%	98%
Controlled Postoperative Blood Glucose[2,7]	-	-	98%	97%
Perioperative Temperature Management[2]	78	99%	100%	100%
Prophylactic Antibiotic Selection[2]	31	94%	99%	99%
Prophylactic Antibiotic Selection (Outpatient)[1,3]	-	-	99%	98%
Prophylactic Antibiotic Stopped[2]	30	93%	99%	98%
Prophylactic Antibiotic Timing[2]	31	97%	99%	99%
Prophylactic Antibiotic Timing (Outpatient)[1,3]	-	-	99%	98%
Urinary Catheter Removal[2]	51	86%	99%	97%
Survey of Patients' Hospital Experiences				
Area Around Room 'Always' Quiet at Night[5]	-	-	57%	61%
Doctors 'Always' Communicated Well[5]	-	-	82%	82%
Home Recovery Information Given[5]	-	-	81%	85%
Hospital Given 9 or 10 on 10 Point Scale[5]	-	-	66%	71%
Meds 'Always' Explained Before Given[5]	-	-	66%	64%
Nurses 'Always' Communicated Well[5]	-	-	80%	79%
Pain 'Always' Well Controlled[5]	-	-	71%	71%
Room and Bathroom 'Always' Clean[5]	-	-	74%	73%
Timely Help 'Always' Received[5]	-	-	69%	68%
Would Definitely Recommend Hospital[5]	-	-	69%	71%
Use of Medical Imaging				
Cardiac Imaging Stress Test before Surgery[1]	-	-	3.8%	5.3%
Combination Abdominal CT Scan	149	45.6%	8.9%	10.5%
Combination Brain/Sinus CT Scan[1]	-	-	2.1%	2.7%
Combination Chest CT Scan	130	5.4%	0.9%	2.7%
Follow-up Mammogram/Ultrasound[7]	-	-	9.4%	8.8%
Lumbar Spine MRI for Low Back Pain[1]	-	-	37.2%	37.2%

Kula Hospital

100 Kokea Place
Kula, HI 96790
Phone: 808-878-1221
Fax: 808-878-1791
URL: www.kula.hhsc.org
Type: Critical Access Hospitals
Emergency Services: Yes
Ownership: Government - State
Beds: 115

Key Personnel:
Chief of Medical Staff.......... Nicole Apolopna, MD
Quality Assurance .... Mary Lou Carter
CEO .... Wesley Lo

Measure	Cases	This Hosp.	State Avg.	U.S. Avg.
Blood Clot Prevention and Treatment				
Anticoagulation Overlap Therapy[5]	-	-	89%	93%
ICU Venous Thromboembolism Prophylaxis[5]	-	-	95%	92%
Incidence of Potentially Preventable VTE[5]	-	-	11%	10%
UFH with Dosages/Platelet Monitoring[5]	-	-	97%	97%
Venous Thromboembolism Prophylaxis[5]	-	-	86%	85%
Warfarin Therapy Discharge Instructions[5]	-	-	58%	75%
Chest Pain/Possible Heart Attack Care				
Aspirin Given Within 24 Hours of Arrival	-	-	97%	96%
Fibrinolytic Meds Within 30 Min. of Arrival	-	-	56%	58%
Average Time to ECG (minutes)	-	-	8	7
Average Time to Transfer (minutes)	-	-	205	60
Children's Asthma Care				
Received Home Management Plan of Care	-	-	-	88%
Received Reliever Medication	-	-	-	100%
Received Systemic Corticosteroids	-	-	-	100%
Emergency Department				
Admittance Decision Time (minutes)[5]	-	-	113	98
Head CT Results Within 45 Min. of Arrival	-	-	52%	57%
Patients Who Left ER Before Being Seen	-	-	1%	2%
Time from ER Arrival to Admit. (minutes)[5]	-	-	311	274
Time from ER Arrival to Discharge (minutes)	-	-	125	134
Time in ER Before Being Evaluated (minutes)	-	-	21	26
Time to Pain Meds for Fractures (minutes)	-	-	51	57
Heart Attack Care				
Aspirin Given at Discharge[5]	-	-	99%	99%
Fibrinolytic Meds Within 30 Min. of Arrival[5]	-	-	-	54%
PCI Within 90 Minutes of Arrival[5]	-	-	94%	96%
Statin Prescribed at Discharge[5]	-	-	99%	98%
Heart Failure Care				
ACE Inhibitor or ARB for LVSD[5]	-	-	99%	97%
Discharge Instructions Given[5]	-	-	95%	94%
Evaluation of LVS Function[5]	-	-	100%	99%
Medicare Spending				
Medicare Spending per Patient (ratio)	-	-	0.87	0.98
Pneumonia Care				
Appropriate Initial Antibiotic Given[5]	-	-	96%	95%
Blood Culture Timing[5]	-	-	98%	98%
Pregnancy and Delivery Care				
Newborn Deliveries Scheduled Early[5]	-	-	7%	6%
Preventive Care				
Immunization for Influenza[5]	-	-	81%	90%
Immunization for Pneumonia[5]	-	-	89%	92%
Stroke Care				
Anticoagulation Therapy for Atrial Fibrillation[5]	-	-	97%	95%
Antithrombotic Therapy Timing[5]	-	-	99%	98%
Assessed for Rehabilitation[5]	-	-	99%	97%
Discharged on Antithrombotic Therapy[5]	-	-	100%	99%
Discharged on Statin Medication[5]	-	-	98%	94%
Thrombolytic Therapy Timing[5]	-	-	64%	66%
Venous Thromboembolism Prophylaxis[5]	-	-	98%	94%
Written Stroke Educational Materials Given[5]	-	-	94%	88%
Surgical Care Improvement Project				
Appropriate Beta Blocker Usage[5]	-	-	98%	98%
Appropriate VTP Within 24 Hours[5]	-	-	99%	98%
Controlled Postoperative Blood Glucose[5]	-	-	98%	97%
Perioperative Temperature Management[5]	-	-	100%	100%
Prophylactic Antibiotic Selection[5]	-	-	99%	99%
Prophylactic Antibiotic Selection (Outpatient)	-	-	99%	98%
Prophylactic Antibiotic Stopped[5]	-	-	99%	98%
Prophylactic Antibiotic Timing[5]	-	-	99%	99%
Prophylactic Antibiotic Timing (Outpatient)	-	-	99%	98%
Urinary Catheter Removal[5]	-	-	99%	97%
Survey of Patients' Hospital Experiences				
Area Around Room 'Always' Quiet at Night[5]	-	-	57%	61%
Doctors 'Always' Communicated Well[5]	-	-	82%	82%
Home Recovery Information Given[5]	-	-	81%	85%
Hospital Given 9 or 10 on 10 Point Scale[5]	-	-	66%	71%
Meds 'Always' Explained Before Given[5]	-	-	66%	64%
Nurses 'Always' Communicated Well[5]	-	-	80%	79%
Pain 'Always' Well Controlled[5]	-	-	71%	71%
Room and Bathroom 'Always' Clean[5]	-	-	74%	73%
Timely Help 'Always' Received[5]	-	-	69%	68%
Would Definitely Recommend Hospital[5]	-	-	69%	71%
Use of Medical Imaging				
Cardiac Imaging Stress Test before Surgery	-	-	3.8%	5.3%
Combination Abdominal CT Scan	-	-	8.9%	10.5%
Combination Brain/Sinus CT Scan	-	-	2.1%	2.7%
Combination Chest CT Scan	-	-	0.9%	2.7%
Follow-up Mammogram/Ultrasound	-	-	9.4%	8.8%
Lumbar Spine MRI for Low Back Pain	-	-	37.2%	37.2%

Wilcox Memorial Hospital

3-3420 Kuhio Highway
Lihue, HI 96766
Phone: 808-245-1103
Fax: 808-245-1211
URL: www.wilcoxhealth.org
Type: Acute Care Hospitals
Emergency Services: Yes
Ownership: Government - Federal
Beds: 86

Key Personnel:
Pediatric Ambulatory Care ...... Terrence Carolan
Pediatric In-Patient Care .... Terrence Carolan
Radiology.................. Allen Johnson, MD
Emergency Room .... Linda Leavitt, RN
Quality Assurance .... Teresa Ramey, RN
Chief of Medical Staff .... Kenneth B Robbins, MD
CEO/President............... Raymond Vara

Measure	Cases	This Hosp.	State Avg.	U.S. Avg.
Blood Clot Prevention and Treatment				
Anticoagulation Overlap Therapy[2]	12	100%	89%	93%
ICU Venous Thromboembolism Prophylaxis[2]	67	100%	95%	92%
Incidence of Potentially Preventable VTE[1,2]	-	-	11%	10%
UFH with Dosages/Platelet Monitoring[1,2]	-	-	97%	97%
Venous Thromboembolism Prophylaxis[2]	261	100%	86%	85%
Warfarin Therapy Discharge Instructions[1,2]	-	-	58%	75%
Chest Pain/Possible Heart Attack Care				
Aspirin Given Within 24 Hours of Arrival	35	100%	97%	96%
Fibrinolytic Meds Within 30 Min. of Arrival[7]	-	-	56%	58%
Average Time to ECG (minutes)	37	7	8	7
Average Time to Transfer (minutes)[7]	-	-	205	60
Children's Asthma Care				
Received Home Management Plan of Care	-	-	-	88%
Received Reliever Medication	-	-	-	100%
Received Systemic Corticosteroids	-	-	-	100%
Emergency Department				
Admittance Decision Time (minutes)[2]	458	129	113	98
Head CT Results Within 45 Min. of Arrival[1]	-	-	52%	57%
Patients Who Left ER Before Being Seen	23,916	0%	1%	2%
Time from ER Arrival to Admit. (minutes)[2]	461	280	311	274
Time from ER Arrival to Discharge (minutes)	359	131	125	134
Time in ER Before Being Evaluated (minutes)	383	17	21	26
Time to Pain Meds for Fractures (minutes)	149	57	51	57
Heart Attack Care				
Aspirin Given at Discharge	15	100%	99%	99%
Fibrinolytic Meds Within 30 Min. of Arrival[7]	-	-	-	54%
PCI Within 90 Minutes of Arrival[7]	-	-	94%	96%
Statin Prescribed at Discharge	16	100%	99%	98%
Heart Failure Care				
ACE Inhibitor or ARB for LVSD	40	100%	99%	97%
Discharge Instructions Given	98	100%	95%	94%
Evaluation of LVS Function	108	100%	100%	99%
Medicare Spending				
Medicare Spending per Patient (ratio)	-	0.87	0.87	0.98
Pneumonia Care				
Appropriate Initial Antibiotic Given	73	100%	96%	95%
Blood Culture Timing	134	100%	98%	98%
Pregnancy and Delivery Care				
Newborn Deliveries Scheduled Early[2]	55	5%	7%	6%
Preventive Care				
Immunization for Influenza[2]	336	99%	81%	90%
Immunization for Pneumonia[2]	385	99%	89%	92%
Stroke Care				
Anticoagulation Therapy for Atrial Fibrillation	13	100%	97%	95%
Antithrombotic Therapy Timing	55	100%	99%	98%
Assessed for Rehabilitation	78	100%	99%	97%
Discharged on Antithrombotic Therapy	64	100%	100%	99%
Discharged on Statin Medication	49	100%	98%	94%
Thrombolytic Therapy Timing[1]	-	-	64%	66%
Venous Thromboembolism Prophylaxis	68	100%	98%	94%
Written Stroke Educational Materials Given	57	100%	94%	88%
Surgical Care Improvement Project				
Appropriate Beta Blocker Usage	43	98%	98%	98%
Appropriate VTP Within 24 Hours	194	99%	99%	98%
Controlled Postoperative Blood Glucose[7]	-	-	98%	97%
Perioperative Temperature Management	208	100%	100%	100%
Prophylactic Antibiotic Selection	139	99%	99%	99%
Prophylactic Antibiotic Selection (Outpatient)	39	97%	99%	98%
Prophylactic Antibiotic Stopped	137	99%	99%	98%
Prophylactic Antibiotic Timing	142	99%	99%	99%
Prophylactic Antibiotic Timing (Outpatient)	39	97%	99%	98%
Urinary Catheter Removal	138	100%	99%	97%
Survey of Patients' Hospital Experiences				
Area Around Room 'Always' Quiet at Night	300+	63%	57%	61%
Doctors 'Always' Communicated Well	300+	88%	82%	82%
Home Recovery Information Given	300+	86%	81%	85%

NOTE: Hospital profiles are in alphabetical order by state, then city, then hospital within the city; Rankings exclude hospitals with less than 25 cases except for patient surveys which excludes hospitals with less than 100 cases; (a) 100-299 cases; (1) The number of cases/patients is too few to report; (2) Data submitted were based on a sample of cases/patients; (3) Results are based on a shorter time period than required; (4) Data suppressed by CMS for one or more quarters; (5) Results are not available for this reporting period; (6) Fewer than 100 patients completed the HCAHPS survey; (7) No cases met the criteria for this measure; (8) The lower limit of the confidence interval cannot be calculated if the number of observed infections equals zero; (9) No data are available from the state/territory for this reporting period; (10) The scores shown reflect fewer than 50 completed surveys; (11) There were discrepancies in the data collection process; (12) This measure does not apply to this hospital for this reporting period; (13) Results cannot be calculated for this reporting period; (14) The results for this state are combined with nearby states to protect confidentiality; Please refer to the User's Guide for a full explanation of data.

Hospital Given 9 or 10 on 10 Point Scale	300+	77%	66%	71%
Meds 'Always' Explained Before Given	300+	72%	66%	64%
Nurses 'Always' Communicated Well	300+	84%	80%	79%
Pain 'Always' Well Controlled	300+	75%	71%	71%
Room and Bathroom 'Always' Clean	300+	80%	74%	73%
Timely Help 'Always' Received	300+	70%	69%	68%
Would Definitely Recommend Hospital	300+	80%	69%	71%
Use of Medical Imaging				
Cardiac Imaging Stress Test before Surgery	336	3.0%	3.8%	5.3%
Combination Abdominal CT Scan	311	1.3%	8.9%	10.5%
Combination Brain/Sinus CT Scan[1]	-	-	2.1%	2.7%
Combination Chest CT Scan	208	0.0%	0.9%	2.7%
Follow-up Mammogram/Ultrasound	943	3.8%	9.4%	8.8%
Lumbar Spine MRI for Low Back Pain	45	40.0%	37.2%	37.2%

Kau Hospital

1 Kamani Street
Pahala, HI 96777
Phone: 808-928-8331
Type: Critical Access Hospitals
Emergency Services: Yes
Ownership: Government - State

Measure	Cases	This Hosp.	State Avg.	U.S. Avg.
Blood Clot Prevention and Treatment				
Anticoagulation Overlap Therapy[5]	-	-	89%	93%
ICU Venous Thromboembolism Prophylaxis[5]	-	-	95%	92%
Incidence of Potentially Preventable VTE[5]	-	-	11%	10%
UFH with Dosages/Platelet Monitoring[5]	-	-	97%	97%
Venous Thromboembolism Prophylaxis[5]	-	-	86%	85%
Warfarin Therapy Discharge Instructions[5]	-	-	58%	75%
Chest Pain/Possible Heart Attack Care				
Aspirin Given Within 24 Hours of Arrival[1,3]	-	-	97%	96%
Fibrinolytic Meds Within 30 Min. of Arrival[1,3]	-	-	56%	58%
Average Time to ECG (minutes)[1,3]	-	-	8	7
Average Time to Transfer (minutes)[3,7]	-	-	205	60
Children's Asthma Care				
Received Home Management Plan of Care	-	-	-	88%
Received Reliever Medication	-	-	-	100%
Received Systemic Corticosteroids	-	-	-	100%
Emergency Department				
Admittance Decision Time (minutes)[5]	-	-	113	98
Head CT Results Within 45 Min. of Arrival[5]	-	-	52%	57%
Patients Who Left ER Before Being Seen[5]	-	-	1%	2%
Time from ER Arrival to Admit. (minutes)[5]	-	-	311	274
Time from ER Arrival to Discharge (minutes)[5]	-	-	125	134
Time in ER Before Being Evaluated (minutes)[5]	-	-	21	26
Time to Pain Meds for Fractures (minutes)[1,3]	-	-	51	57
Heart Attack Care				
Aspirin Given at Discharge[5]	-	-	99%	99%
Fibrinolytic Meds Within 30 Min. of Arrival[5]	-	-	-	54%
PCI Within 90 Minutes of Arrival[5]	-	-	94%	96%
Statin Prescribed at Discharge[5]	-	-	99%	98%
Heart Failure Care				
ACE Inhibitor or ARB for LVSD[5]	-	-	99%	97%
Discharge Instructions Given[5]	-	-	95%	94%
Evaluation of LVS Function[5]	-	-	100%	99%
Medicare Spending				
Medicare Spending per Patient (ratio)	-	-	0.87	0.98
Pneumonia Care				
Appropriate Initial Antibiotic Given[1,3]	-	-	96%	95%
Blood Culture Timing[1,3]	-	-	98%	98%
Pregnancy and Delivery Care				
Newborn Deliveries Scheduled Early[5]	-	-	7%	6%
Preventive Care				
Immunization for Influenza[5]	-	-	81%	90%
Immunization for Pneumonia[5]	-	-	89%	92%
Stroke Care				
Anticoagulation Therapy for Atrial Fibrillation[5]	-	-	97%	95%
Antithrombotic Therapy Timing[5]	-	-	99%	98%
Assessed for Rehabilitation[5]	-	-	99%	97%
Discharged on Antithrombotic Therapy[5]	-	-	100%	99%
Discharged on Statin Medication[5]	-	-	98%	94%
Thrombolytic Therapy Timing[5]	-	-	64%	66%
Venous Thromboembolism Prophylaxis[5]	-	-	98%	94%
Written Stroke Educational Materials Given[5]	-	-	94%	88%
Surgical Care Improvement Project				
Appropriate Beta Blocker Usage[5]	-	-	98%	98%
Appropriate VTP Within 24 Hours[5]	-	-	99%	98%
Controlled Postoperative Blood Glucose[5]	-	-	98%	97%
Perioperative Temperature Management[5]	-	-	100%	100%
Prophylactic Antibiotic Selection[5]	-	-	99%	99%
Prophylactic Antibiotic Selection (Outpatient)[5]	-	-	99%	98%
Prophylactic Antibiotic Stopped[5]	-	-	99%	98%
Prophylactic Antibiotic Timing[5]	-	-	99%	99%
Prophylactic Antibiotic Timing (Outpatient)[5]	-	-	99%	98%
Urinary Catheter Removal[5]	-	-	99%	97%
Survey of Patients' Hospital Experiences				
Area Around Room 'Always' Quiet at Night[5]	-	-	57%	61%
Doctors 'Always' Communicated Well[5]	-	-	82%	82%
Home Recovery Information Given[5]	-	-	81%	85%
Hospital Given 9 or 10 on 10 Point Scale[5]	-	-	66%	71%
Meds 'Always' Explained Before Given[5]	-	-	66%	64%
Nurses 'Always' Communicated Well[5]	-	-	80%	79%
Pain 'Always' Well Controlled[5]	-	-	71%	71%
Room and Bathroom 'Always' Clean[5]	-	-	74%	73%
Timely Help 'Always' Received[5]	-	-	69%	68%
Would Definitely Recommend Hospital[5]	-	-	69%	71%
Use of Medical Imaging				
Cardiac Imaging Stress Test before Surgery[5]	-	-	3.8%	5.3%
Combination Abdominal CT Scan[5]	-	-	8.9%	10.5%
Combination Brain/Sinus CT Scan[5]	-	-	2.1%	2.7%
Combination Chest CT Scan[5]	-	-	0.9%	2.7%
Follow-up Mammogram/Ultrasound[5]	-	-	9.4%	8.8%
Lumbar Spine MRI for Low Back Pain[5]	-	-	37.2%	37.2%

Wahiawa General Hospital

128 Lehua Street
Wahiawa, HI 96786
Phone: 808-621-8411
Fax: 808-621-4451
E-mail: contactus@wahiawageneral.org
URL: www.wahiawageneral.org
Type: Acute Care Hospitals
Emergency Services: Yes
Ownership: Voluntary non-profit - Private
Beds: 162

Key Personnel:
Operating Room. . . . . Pat Gregor, RN
CEO/President. . . . . Jack Julius
Quality Assurance . . . . Linda Markt
Chief of Medical Staff. . . . . Leo Pastua

Measure	Cases	This Hosp.	State Avg.	U.S. Avg.
Blood Clot Prevention and Treatment				
Anticoagulation Overlap Therapy[2]	17	71%	89%	93%
ICU Venous Thromboembolism Prophylaxis[2]	45	89%	95%	92%
Incidence of Potentially Preventable VTE[1,2]	-	-	11%	10%
UFH with Dosages/Platelet Monitoring[1,2]	-	-	97%	97%
Venous Thromboembolism Prophylaxis[2]	321	70%	86%	85%
Warfarin Therapy Discharge Instructions[2]	12	25%	58%	75%
Chest Pain/Possible Heart Attack Care				
Aspirin Given Within 24 Hours of Arrival	42	93%	97%	96%
Fibrinolytic Meds Within 30 Min. of Arrival[7]	-	-	56%	58%
Average Time to ECG (minutes)	45	0	8	7
Average Time to Transfer (minutes)[1]	-	-	205	60
Children's Asthma Care				
Received Home Management Plan of Care	-	-	-	88%
Received Reliever Medication	-	-	-	100%
Received Systemic Corticosteroids	-	-	-	100%
Emergency Department				
Admittance Decision Time (minutes)[2]	314	75	113	98
Head CT Results Within 45 Min. of Arrival	12	67%	52%	57%
Patients Who Left ER Before Being Seen	17,929	1%	1%	2%
Time from ER Arrival to Admit. (minutes)[2]	320	223	311	274
Time from ER Arrival to Discharge (minutes)	425	91	125	134
Time in ER Before Being Evaluated (minutes)	457	15	21	26
Time to Pain Meds for Fractures (minutes)	88	35	51	57
Heart Attack Care				
Aspirin Given at Discharge	73	99%	99%	99%
Fibrinolytic Meds Within 30 Min. of Arrival[7]	-	-	-	54%
PCI Within 90 Minutes of Arrival[7]	-	-	94%	96%
Statin Prescribed at Discharge	71	99%	99%	98%
Heart Failure Care				
ACE Inhibitor or ARB for LVSD	72	99%	99%	97%
Discharge Instructions Given	176	80%	95%	94%
Evaluation of LVS Function	187	100%	100%	99%
Medicare Spending				
Medicare Spending per Patient (ratio)	-	0.90	0.87	0.98
Pneumonia Care				
Appropriate Initial Antibiotic Given	84	98%	96%	95%
Blood Culture Timing	211	98%	98%	98%
Pregnancy and Delivery Care				
Newborn Deliveries Scheduled Early[7]	-	-	7%	6%
Preventive Care				
Immunization for Influenza[2]	357	90%	81%	90%
Immunization for Pneumonia[2]	559	90%	89%	92%
Stroke Care				
Anticoagulation Therapy for Atrial Fibrillation[1]	-	-	97%	95%
Antithrombotic Therapy Timing	38	89%	99%	98%
Assessed for Rehabilitation	39	100%	99%	97%
Discharged on Antithrombotic Therapy	34	100%	100%	99%
Discharged on Statin Medication	25	92%	98%	94%
Thrombolytic Therapy Timing[1]	-	-	64%	66%
Venous Thromboembolism Prophylaxis	40	82%	98%	94%
Written Stroke Educational Materials Given	16	75%	94%	88%
Surgical Care Improvement Project				
Appropriate Beta Blocker Usage[1]	-	-	98%	98%
Appropriate VTP Within 24 Hours	38	95%	99%	98%
Controlled Postoperative Blood Glucose[7]	-	-	98%	97%
Perioperative Temperature Management	43	100%	100%	100%
Prophylactic Antibiotic Selection	24	100%	99%	99%
Prophylactic Antibiotic Selection (Outpatient)[1,3]	-	-	99%	98%
Prophylactic Antibiotic Stopped	23	96%	99%	98%
Prophylactic Antibiotic Timing	24	96%	99%	99%
Prophylactic Antibiotic Timing (Outpatient)[1,3]	-	-	99%	98%
Urinary Catheter Removal	32	91%	99%	97%
Survey of Patients' Hospital Experiences				
Area Around Room 'Always' Quiet at Night	300+	49%	57%	61%
Doctors 'Always' Communicated Well	300+	78%	82%	82%
Home Recovery Information Given	300+	82%	81%	85%
Hospital Given 9 or 10 on 10 Point Scale	300+	50%	66%	71%
Meds 'Always' Explained Before Given	300+	59%	66%	64%
Nurses 'Always' Communicated Well	300+	70%	80%	79%
Pain 'Always' Well Controlled	300+	60%	71%	71%
Room and Bathroom 'Always' Clean	300+	64%	74%	73%
Timely Help 'Always' Received	300+	58%	69%	68%
Would Definitely Recommend Hospital	300+	50%	69%	71%
Use of Medical Imaging				
Cardiac Imaging Stress Test before Surgery	94	2.1%	3.8%	5.3%
Combination Abdominal CT Scan	172	2.3%	8.9%	10.5%
Combination Brain/Sinus CT Scan[1]	-	-	2.1%	2.7%
Combination Chest CT Scan	90	5.6%	0.9%	2.7%
Follow-up Mammogram/Ultrasound	425	6.4%	9.4%	8.8%
Lumbar Spine MRI for Low Back Pain[7]	-	-	37.2%	37.2%

Maui Memorial Medical Center

221 Mahalani Street
Wailuku, HI 96793
Phone: 808-442-5101
Fax: 808-243-4628
URL: www.mauimemorialmedical.org
Type: Acute Care Hospitals
Emergency Services: Yes
Ownership: Government - State
Beds: 191

Key Personnel:
Radiology. . . . . Bobby Baker, MD
Operating Room. . . . . Lorraine Borsum
Chief of Medical Staff. . . . . Darren Egamia, MD
Quality Assurance . . . . Carolyn Joyo
Pediatric Ambulatory Care . . . . . . Pierre Langeron, MD
Pediatric In-Patient Care . . . . Pierre Langeron, MD
CEO . . . . Wesley P. Lo
Cardiac Laboratory. . . . . Mark Schwak, MD

Measure	Cases	This Hosp.	State Avg.	U.S. Avg.
Blood Clot Prevention and Treatment				
Anticoagulation Overlap Therapy[2]	40	75%	89%	93%
ICU Venous Thromboembolism Prophylaxis[2]	98	97%	95%	92%
Incidence of Potentially Preventable VTE[1,2]	-	-	11%	10%
UFH with Dosages/Platelet Monitoring[2]	30	83%	97%	97%

NOTE: Hospital profiles are in alphabetical order by state, then city, then hospital within the city; Rankings exclude hospitals with less than 25 cases except for patient surveys which excludes hospitals with less than 100 cases; (a) 100-299 cases; (1) The number of cases/patients is too few to report; (2) Data submitted were based on a sample of cases/patients; (3) Results are based on a shorter time period than required; (4) Data suppressed by CMS for one or more quarters; (5) Results are not available for this reporting period; (6) Fewer than 100 patients completed the HCAHPS survey; (7) No cases met the criteria for this measure; (8) The lower limit of the confidence interval cannot be calculated if the number of observed infections equals zero; (9) No data are available from the state/territory for this reporting period; (10) The scores shown reflect fewer than 50 completed surveys; (11) There were discrepancies in the data collection process; (12) This measure does not apply to this hospital for this reporting period; (13) Results cannot be calculated for this reporting period; (14) The results for this state are combined with nearby states to protect confidentiality; Please refer to the User's Guide for a full explanation of data.

Venous Thromboembolism Prophylaxis[2]	349	73%	86%	85%
Warfarin Therapy Discharge Instructions[2]	31	19%	58%	75%
Chest Pain/Possible Heart Attack Care				
Aspirin Given Within 24 Hours of Arrival[1]	-	-	97%	96%
Fibrinolytic Meds Within 30 Min. of Arrival[3,7]	-	-	56%	58%
Average Time to ECG (minutes)[1]	-	-	8	7
Average Time to Transfer (minutes)[3,7]	-	-	205	60
Children's Asthma Care				
Received Home Management Plan of Care	-	-	-	88%
Received Reliever Medication	-	-	-	100%
Received Systemic Corticosteroids	-	-	-	100%
Emergency Department				
Admittance Decision Time (minutes)[2]	422	150	113	98
Head CT Results Within 45 Min. of Arrival[1]	-	-	52%	57%
Patients Who Left ER Before Being Seen	40,589	1%	1%	2%
Time from ER Arrival to Admit. (minutes)[2]	471	285	311	274
Time from ER Arrival to Discharge (minutes)	390	152	125	134
Time in ER Before Being Evaluated (minutes)	366	43	21	26
Time to Pain Meds for Fractures (minutes)	275	59	51	57
Heart Attack Care				
Aspirin Given at Discharge	207	98%	99%	99%
Fibrinolytic Meds Within 30 Min. of Arrival[7]	-	-	-	54%
PCI Within 90 Minutes of Arrival	40	98%	94%	96%
Statin Prescribed at Discharge	211	99%	99%	98%
Heart Failure Care				
ACE Inhibitor or ARB for LVSD	92	100%	99%	97%
Discharge Instructions Given	183	98%	95%	94%
Evaluation of LVS Function	191	100%	100%	99%
Medicare Spending				
Medicare Spending per Patient (ratio)	-	0.89	0.87	0.98
Pneumonia Care				
Appropriate Initial Antibiotic Given	137	96%	96%	95%
Blood Culture Timing	223	97%	98%	98%
Pregnancy and Delivery Care				
Newborn Deliveries Scheduled Early[2]	32	53%	7%	6%
Preventive Care				
Immunization for Influenza[2]	579	79%	81%	90%
Immunization for Pneumonia[2]	598	76%	89%	92%
Stroke Care				
Anticoagulation Therapy for Atrial Fibrillation	13	100%	97%	95%
Antithrombotic Therapy Timing	116	100%	99%	98%
Assessed for Rehabilitation	152	100%	99%	97%
Discharged on Antithrombotic Therapy	125	100%	100%	99%
Discharged on Statin Medication	104	99%	98%	94%
Thrombolytic Therapy Timing	14	64%	64%	66%
Venous Thromboembolism Prophylaxis	148	100%	98%	94%
Written Stroke Educational Materials Given	121	100%	94%	88%
Surgical Care Improvement Project				
Appropriate Beta Blocker Usage[2]	118	99%	98%	98%
Appropriate VTP Within 24 Hours[2]	222	97%	99%	98%
Controlled Postoperative Blood Glucose[2]	95	96%	98%	97%
Perioperative Temperature Management[2]	275	100%	100%	100%
Prophylactic Antibiotic Selection[2]	200	100%	99%	99%
Prophylactic Antibiotic Selection (Outpatient)	77	99%	99%	98%
Prophylactic Antibiotic Stopped[2]	193	99%	99%	98%
Prophylactic Antibiotic Timing[2]	200	100%	99%	99%
Prophylactic Antibiotic Timing (Outpatient)	77	99%	99%	98%
Urinary Catheter Removal[2]	268	99%	99%	97%
Survey of Patients' Hospital Experiences				
Area Around Room 'Always' Quiet at Night	300+	52%	57%	61%
Doctors 'Always' Communicated Well	300+	78%	82%	82%
Home Recovery Information Given	300+	81%	81%	85%
Hospital Given 9 or 10 on 10 Point Scale	300+	61%	66%	71%
Meds 'Always' Explained Before Given	300+	63%	66%	64%
Nurses 'Always' Communicated Well	300+	77%	80%	79%
Pain 'Always' Well Controlled	300+	71%	71%	71%
Room and Bathroom 'Always' Clean	300+	76%	74%	73%
Timely Help 'Always' Received	300+	69%	69%	68%
Would Definitely Recommend Hospital	300+	63%	69%	71%
Use of Medical Imaging				
Cardiac Imaging Stress Test before Surgery	199	4.5%	3.8%	5.3%
Combination Abdominal CT Scan	389	1.8%	8.9%	10.5%
Combination Brain/Sinus CT Scan	373	1.3%	2.1%	2.7%
Combination Chest CT Scan	165	0.0%	0.9%	2.7%
Follow-up Mammogram/Ultrasound[1]	-	-	9.4%	8.8%
Lumbar Spine MRI for Low Back Pain[1]	-	-	37.2%	37.2%

Kauai Veterans Memorial Hospital

4643 Waimea Canyon Drive
Waimea, HI 96796
Phone: 808-338-9248
Type: Critical Access Hospitals
Emergency Services: Yes
Ownership: Government - State

Measure	Cases	This Hosp.	State Avg.	U.S. Avg.
Blood Clot Prevention and Treatment				
Anticoagulation Overlap Therapy[2,7]	-	-	89%	93%
ICU Venous Thromboembolism Prophylaxis[2]	41	93%	95%	92%
Incidence of Potentially Preventable VTE[1,2]	-	-	11%	10%
UFH with Dosages/Platelet Monitoring[2,7]	-	-	97%	97%
Venous Thromboembolism Prophylaxis[2]	76	79%	86%	85%
Warfarin Therapy Discharge Instructions[2,7]	-	-	58%	75%
Chest Pain/Possible Heart Attack Care				
Aspirin Given Within 24 Hours of Arrival	-	-	97%	96%
Fibrinolytic Meds Within 30 Min. of Arrival	-	-	56%	58%
Average Time to ECG (minutes)	-	-	8	7
Average Time to Transfer (minutes)	-	-	205	60
Children's Asthma Care				
Received Home Management Plan of Care	-	-	-	88%
Received Reliever Medication	-	-	-	100%
Received Systemic Corticosteroids	-	-	-	100%
Emergency Department				
Admittance Decision Time (minutes)[2]	189	110	113	98
Head CT Results Within 45 Min. of Arrival	-	-	52%	57%
Patients Who Left ER Before Being Seen	-	-	1%	2%
Time from ER Arrival to Admit. (minutes)[2]	269	251	311	274
Time from ER Arrival to Discharge (minutes)	-	-	125	134
Time in ER Before Being Evaluated (minutes)	-	-	21	26
Time to Pain Meds for Fractures (minutes)	-	-	51	57
Heart Attack Care				
Aspirin Given at Discharge[1,3]	-	-	99%	99%
Fibrinolytic Meds Within 30 Min. of Arrival[3,7]	-	-	-	54%
PCI Within 90 Minutes of Arrival[3,7]	-	-	94%	96%
Statin Prescribed at Discharge[1,3]	-	-	99%	98%
Heart Failure Care				
ACE Inhibitor or ARB for LVSD	13	100%	99%	97%
Discharge Instructions Given	30	100%	95%	94%
Evaluation of LVS Function	37	100%	100%	99%
Medicare Spending				
Medicare Spending per Patient (ratio)	-	-	0.87	0.98
Pneumonia Care				
Appropriate Initial Antibiotic Given	33	97%	96%	95%
Blood Culture Timing	49	100%	98%	98%
Pregnancy and Delivery Care				
Newborn Deliveries Scheduled Early	27	0%	7%	6%
Preventive Care				
Immunization for Influenza[2]	242	83%	81%	90%
Immunization for Pneumonia[2]	249	95%	89%	92%
Stroke Care				
Anticoagulation Therapy for Atrial Fibrillation[5]	-	-	97%	95%
Antithrombotic Therapy Timing[5]	-	-	99%	98%
Assessed for Rehabilitation[5]	-	-	99%	97%
Discharged on Antithrombotic Therapy[5]	-	-	100%	99%
Discharged on Statin Medication[5]	-	-	98%	94%
Thrombolytic Therapy Timing[5]	-	-	64%	66%
Venous Thromboembolism Prophylaxis[5]	-	-	98%	94%
Written Stroke Educational Materials Given[5]	-	-	94%	88%
Surgical Care Improvement Project				
Appropriate Beta Blocker Usage[5]	-	-	98%	98%
Appropriate VTP Within 24 Hours[5]	-	-	99%	98%
Controlled Postoperative Blood Glucose[5]	-	-	98%	97%
Perioperative Temperature Management[5]	-	-	100%	100%
Prophylactic Antibiotic Selection[5]	-	-	99%	99%
Prophylactic Antibiotic Selection (Outpatient)	-	-	99%	98%
Prophylactic Antibiotic Stopped[5]	-	-	99%	98%
Prophylactic Antibiotic Timing[5]	-	-	99%	99%
Prophylactic Antibiotic Timing (Outpatient)	-	-	99%	98%
Urinary Catheter Removal[5]	-	-	99%	97%
Survey of Patients' Hospital Experiences				
Area Around Room 'Always' Quiet at Night	(a)	71%	57%	61%
Doctors 'Always' Communicated Well	(a)	86%	82%	82%
Home Recovery Information Given	(a)	90%	81%	85%
Hospital Given 9 or 10 on 10 Point Scale	(a)	78%	66%	71%
Meds 'Always' Explained Before Given	(a)	65%	66%	64%
Nurses 'Always' Communicated Well	(a)	82%	80%	79%
Pain 'Always' Well Controlled	(a)	75%	71%	71%
Room and Bathroom 'Always' Clean	(a)	80%	74%	73%
Timely Help 'Always' Received	(a)	79%	69%	68%
Would Definitely Recommend Hospital	(a)	85%	69%	71%
Use of Medical Imaging				
Cardiac Imaging Stress Test before Surgery	-	-	3.8%	5.3%
Combination Abdominal CT Scan	-	-	8.9%	10.5%
Combination Brain/Sinus CT Scan	-	-	2.1%	2.7%
Combination Chest CT Scan	-	-	0.9%	2.7%
Follow-up Mammogram/Ultrasound	-	-	9.4%	8.8%
Lumbar Spine MRI for Low Back Pain	-	-	37.2%	37.2%

NOTE: Hospital profiles are in alphabetical order by state, then city, then hospital within the city; Rankings exclude hospitals with less than 25 cases except for patient surveys which excludes hospitals with less than 100 cases; (a) 100-299 cases; (1) The number of cases/patients is too few to report; (2) Data submitted were based on a sample of cases/patients; (3) Results are based on a shorter time period than required; (4) Data suppressed by CMS for one or more quarters; (5) Results are not available for this reporting period; (6) Fewer than 100 patients completed the HCAHPS survey; (7) No cases met the criteria for this measure; (8) The lower limit of the confidence interval cannot be calculated if the number of observed infections equals zero; (9) No data are available from the state/territory for this reporting period; (10) The scores shown reflect fewer than 50 completed surveys; (11) There were discrepancies in the data collection process; (12) This measure does not apply to this hospital for this reporting period; (13) Results cannot be calculated for this reporting period; (14) The results for this state are combined with nearby states to protect confidentiality; Please refer to the User's Guide for a full explanation of data.

Blood Clot Prevention and Treatment

Anticoagulation Overlap Therapy

Hospital Name	City	Rate	Cases
Eastern Idaho Regional Medical Center[2]	Idaho Falls	100%	92
Saint Alphonsus Regional Medical Center[2]	Boise	100%	125
West Valley Medical Center[2]	Caldwell	100%	33
Saint Luke's Regional Medical Center[2]	Boise	99%	208
Portneuf Medical Center[2]	Pocatello	97%	73
Saint Alphonsus Medical Center - Nampa[2]	Nampa	95%	41
Saint Luke's Magic Valley Rmc[2]	Twin Falls	94%	65
Saint Joseph Regional Medical Center[2]	Lewiston	85%	27
Kootenai Medical Center[2]	Coeur D'alene	83%	69

ICU Venous Thromboembolism Prophylaxis

Hospital Name	City	Rate	Cases
West Valley Medical Center[2]	Caldwell	100%	67
Saint Luke's Regional Medical Center[2]	Boise	99%	80
Saint Alphonsus Regional Medical Center[2]	Boise	94%	89
Bingham Memorial Hospital[3]	Blackfoot	93%	71
Portneuf Medical Center[2]	Pocatello	93%	98
Saint Alphonsus Medical Center - Nampa[2]	Nampa	93%	104
Eastern Idaho Regional Medical Center[2]	Idaho Falls	92%	85
Cassia Regional Medical Center[2]	Burley	91%	45
Saint Joseph Regional Medical Center[2]	Lewiston	90%	99
Madison Memorial Hospital[2]	Rexburg	88%	34
Kootenai Medical Center[2]	Coeur D'alene	87%	67
Saint Luke's Magic Valley Rmc[2]	Twin Falls	84%	68

Incidence of Potentially Preventable VTE

Hospital Name	City	Rate	Cases
Saint Alphonsus Regional Medical Center[2]	Boise	0%	51
Saint Luke's Regional Medical Center[2]	Boise	3%	34

UFH with Dosages/Platelet Count Monitoring

Hospital Name	City	Rate	Cases
Portneuf Medical Center[2]	Pocatello	100%	37
Saint Luke's Regional Medical Center[2]	Boise	100%	67
Eastern Idaho Regional Medical Center[2]	Idaho Falls	98%	46
Saint Alphonsus Regional Medical Center[2]	Boise	98%	50

Venous Thromboembolism Prophylaxis

Hospital Name	City	Rate	Cases
Idaho Doctors Hospital	Blackfoot	100%	37
Treasure Valley Hospital	Boise	100%	159
West Valley Medical Center[2]	Caldwell	98%	232
Northwest Specialty Hospital[2]	Post Falls	97%	68
Portneuf Medical Center[2]	Pocatello	95%	279
Saint Luke's Regional Medical Center[2]	Boise	91%	270
Bingham Memorial Hospital[3]	Blackfoot	90%	263
Saint Alphonsus Regional Medical Center[2]	Boise	90%	216
Saint Alphonsus Medical Center - Nampa[2]	Nampa	88%	241
Saint Luke's Magic Valley Rmc[2]	Twin Falls	85%	310
Cassia Regional Medical Center[2]	Burley	83%	70
Kootenai Medical Center[2]	Coeur D'alene	82%	238
Eastern Idaho Regional Medical Center[2]	Idaho Falls	77%	341
Saint Joseph Regional Medical Center[2]	Lewiston	77%	268
Madison Memorial Hospital[2]	Rexburg	72%	120

Warfarin Therapy Discharge Instructions

Hospital Name	City	Rate	Cases
West Valley Medical Center[2]	Caldwell	100%	29
Eastern Idaho Regional Medical Center[2]	Idaho Falls	97%	78
Portneuf Medical Center[2]	Pocatello	97%	60
Saint Luke's Regional Medical Center[2]	Boise	88%	176
Saint Alphonsus Medical Center - Nampa[2]	Nampa	79%	29
Saint Luke's Magic Valley Rmc[2]	Twin Falls	53%	49
Kootenai Medical Center[2]	Coeur D'alene	50%	48
Saint Alphonsus Regional Medical Center[2]	Boise	44%	101

Chest Pain/Possible Heart Attack Care

Aspirin Given Within 24 Hours of Arrival

Hospital Name	City	Rate	Cases
West Valley Medical Center[3]	Caldwell	100%	30
Bonner General Hospital	Sandpoint	98%	43
Cassia Regional Medical Center	Burley	96%	45
Madison Memorial Hospital	Rexburg	91%	47

Average Time to ECG (minutes)

Hospital Name	City	Min.	Cases
Bonner General Hospital	Sandpoint	4	45
West Valley Medical Center[3]	Caldwell	8	31
Madison Memorial Hospital	Rexburg	14	48
Cassia Regional Medical Center	Burley	15	44

Children's Asthma Care

Received Home Management Plan of Care

Hospital Name	City	Rate	Cases
Saint Luke's Regional Medical Center	Boise	93%	72

Received Reliever Medication

Hospital Name	City	Rate	Cases
Saint Luke's Regional Medical Center	Boise	100%	73

Received Systemic Corticosteroids

Hospital Name	City	Rate	Cases
Saint Luke's Regional Medical Center	Boise	100%	72

Emergency Department

Admittance Decision Time (minutes)

Hospital Name	City	Min.	Cases
Saint Joseph Regional Medical Center[2]	Lewiston	42	138
Bingham Memorial Hospital[2]	Blackfoot	45	126
Madison Memorial Hospital[2]	Rexburg	51	87
Gritman Medical Center[2]	Moscow	54	371
Bonner General Hospital[2]	Sandpoint	55	329
Eastern Idaho Regional Medical Center[2]	Idaho Falls	62	672
Saint Alphonsus Medical Center - Nampa[2]	Nampa	70	405
West Valley Medical Center[2]	Caldwell	70	547
Cassia Regional Medical Center[2]	Burley	77	119
Saint Luke's Regional Medical Center[2]	Boise	86	413
Portneuf Medical Center[2]	Pocatello	91	472
Kootenai Medical Center[2]	Coeur D'alene	94	420
Saint Luke's Magic Valley Rmc[2]	Twin Falls	95	478
Saint Alphonsus Regional Medical Center[2]	Boise	118	474

Patients Who Left ER Before Being Seen

Hospital Name	City	Rate	Cases
Benewah Community Hospital	Saint Maries	0%	2960
Eastern Idaho Regional Medical Center	Idaho Falls	0%	40412
Madison Memorial Hospital	Rexburg	0%	10487
Portneuf Medical Center	Pocatello	0%	34537
Syringa General Hospital	Grangeville	0%	2335
West Valley Medical Center	Caldwell	0%	34563
Cassia Regional Medical Center	Burley	1%	11770
Saint Alphonsus Medical Center - Nampa	Nampa	1%	36065
Saint Alphonsus Regional Medical Center	Boise	1%	54071
Saint Joseph Regional Medical Center	Lewiston	1%	10112
Saint Luke's Magic Valley Rmc	Twin Falls	1%	38143
Saint Luke's Regional Medical Center	Boise	1%	99053
Kootenai Medical Center	Coeur D'alene	2%	47985

Time from ER Arrival to Being Admitted (minutes)

Hospital Name	City	Min.	Cases
Madison Memorial Hospital[2]	Rexburg	164	121
Gritman Medical Center[2]	Moscow	196	376
Bonner General Hospital[2]	Sandpoint	202	340
Bingham Memorial Hospital[2]	Blackfoot	206	144
Portneuf Medical Center[2]	Pocatello	220	472
Eastern Idaho Regional Medical Center[2]	Idaho Falls	227	672
West Valley Medical Center[2]	Caldwell	227	547
Saint Alphonsus Medical Center - Nampa[2]	Nampa	237	483
Saint Luke's Magic Valley Rmc[2]	Twin Falls	237	515
Kootenai Medical Center[2]	Coeur D'alene	240	428
Saint Joseph Regional Medical Center[2]	Lewiston	246	495
Cassia Regional Medical Center[2]	Burley	253	153
Saint Luke's Regional Medical Center[2]	Boise	254	415
Saint Alphonsus Regional Medical Center[2]	Boise	279	474

Time from ER Arrival to Discharge (minutes)

Hospital Name	City	Min.	Cases
Madison Memorial Hospital	Rexburg	99	1465
Portneuf Medical Center	Pocatello	106	356
Eastern Idaho Regional Medical Center	Idaho Falls	120	539
Saint Alphonsus Medical Center - Nampa	Nampa	120	358
Saint Luke's Regional Medical Center	Boise	120	420
Saint Luke's Magic Valley Rmc	Twin Falls	128	298
Bonner General Hospital	Sandpoint	130	368
Cassia Regional Medical Center	Burley	130	384
West Valley Medical Center	Caldwell	130	463
Saint Alphonsus Regional Medical Center	Boise	132	338
Kootenai Medical Center	Coeur D'alene	146	348
Saint Joseph Regional Medical Center	Lewiston	163	354

Time in ER Before Being Evaluated (minutes)

Hospital Name	City	Min.	Cases
Portneuf Medical Center	Pocatello	9	312
Eastern Idaho Regional Medical Center	Idaho Falls	12	564
West Valley Medical Center	Caldwell	16	497
Saint Alphonsus Medical Center - Nampa	Nampa	17	348
Madison Memorial Hospital	Rexburg	21	1378
Cassia Regional Medical Center	Burley	23	381
Saint Alphonsus Regional Medical Center	Boise	27	80
Saint Luke's Magic Valley Rmc	Twin Falls	28	225
Saint Luke's Regional Medical Center	Boise	28	441
Bonner General Hospital	Sandpoint	33	362
Saint Joseph Regional Medical Center	Lewiston	40	27
Kootenai Medical Center	Coeur D'alene	44	307

Time to Pain Meds for Bone Fractures (minutes)

Hospital Name	City	Min.	Cases
Portneuf Medical Center	Pocatello	37	137
Madison Memorial Hospital	Rexburg	38	98
Saint Alphonsus Medical Center - Nampa	Nampa	38	131
Saint Luke's Regional Medical Center	Boise	42	381
Eastern Idaho Regional Medical Center	Idaho Falls	44	183
Saint Luke's Magic Valley Rmc	Twin Falls	45	119
Cassia Regional Medical Center	Burley	46	61
Saint Alphonsus Regional Medical Center	Boise	46	232
West Valley Medical Center	Caldwell	50	127
Bonner General Hospital	Sandpoint	51	64
Kootenai Medical Center	Coeur D'alene	60	151
Saint Joseph Regional Medical Center	Lewiston	66	61

Heart Attack Care

Aspirin Given at Discharge

Hospital Name	City	Rate	Cases
Eastern Idaho Regional Medical Center	Idaho Falls	100%	234
Kootenai Medical Center	Coeur D'alene	100%	268
Portneuf Medical Center	Pocatello	100%	149
Saint Alphonsus Medical Center - Nampa	Nampa	100%	66
Saint Luke's Magic Valley Rmc	Twin Falls	100%	147
Saint Luke's Regional Medical Center[2]	Boise	100%	368
West Valley Medical Center	Caldwell	100%	27
Saint Alphonsus Regional Medical Center	Boise	99%	335
Saint Joseph Regional Medical Center	Lewiston	99%	102

PCI Within 90 Minutes of Arrival

Hospital Name	City	Rate	Cases
Eastern Idaho Regional Medical Center	Idaho Falls	100%	52
Saint Luke's Magic Valley Rmc	Twin Falls	100%	29
Saint Alphonsus Regional Medical Center	Boise	98%	49
Saint Luke's Regional Medical Center[2]	Boise	98%	61
Kootenai Medical Center	Coeur D'alene	97%	72

Statin Prescribed at Discharge

Hospital Name	City	Rate	Cases
Eastern Idaho Regional Medical Center	Idaho Falls	100%	215
Kootenai Medical Center	Coeur D'alene	100%	267
Portneuf Medical Center	Pocatello	100%	140
Saint Alphonsus Medical Center - Nampa	Nampa	100%	70
Saint Luke's Magic Valley Rmc	Twin Falls	100%	140
Saint Luke's Regional Medical Center[2]	Boise	100%	356
Saint Alphonsus Regional Medical Center	Boise	99%	324
Saint Joseph Regional Medical Center	Lewiston	96%	98

Heart Failure Care

ACE Inhibitor or ARB for LVSD

Hospital Name	City	Rate	Cases
Boise VA Medical Center	Boise	100%	31
Eastern Idaho Regional Medical Center	Idaho Falls	100%	33
Portneuf Medical Center	Pocatello	100%	35
Saint Alphonsus Medical Center - Nampa	Nampa	100%	44
Saint Joseph Regional Medical Center	Lewiston	100%	35
Saint Luke's Magic Valley Rmc	Twin Falls	100%	54
Saint Luke's Regional Medical Center[2]	Boise	100%	96
Kootenai Medical Center	Coeur D'alene	99%	67
Saint Alphonsus Regional Medical Center	Boise	98%	47

Discharge Instructions Given

Hospital Name	City	Rate	Cases
Eastern Idaho Regional Medical Center	Idaho Falls	100%	108
Kootenai Medical Center	Coeur D'alene	100%	205
Saint Joseph Regional Medical Center	Lewiston	100%	76
Saint Luke's Magic Valley Rmc	Twin Falls	100%	121
West Valley Medical Center	Caldwell	99%	70
Saint Alphonsus Regional Medical Center	Boise	98%	162
Saint Luke's Regional Medical Center[2]	Boise	97%	317
Portneuf Medical Center	Pocatello	93%	86
Boise VA Medical Center	Boise	89%	96
Saint Alphonsus Medical Center - Nampa	Nampa	89%	105
Bingham Memorial Hospital	Blackfoot	19%	26

NOTE: Hospital profiles are in alphabetical order by state, then city, then hospital within the city; Rankings exclude hospitals with less than 25 cases except for patient surveys which excludes hospitals with less than 100 cases; (a) 100-299 cases; (1) The number of cases/patients is too few to report; (2) Data submitted were based on a sample of cases/patients; (3) Results are based on a shorter time period than required; (4) Data suppressed by CMS for one or more quarters; (5) Results are not available for this reporting period; (6) Fewer than 100 patients completed the HCAHPS survey; (7) No cases met the criteria for this measure; (8) The lower limit of the confidence interval cannot be calculated if the number of observed infections equals zero; (9) No data are available from the state/territory for this reporting period; (10) The scores shown reflect fewer than 50 completed surveys; (11) There were discrepancies in the data collection process; (12) This measure does not apply to this hospital for this reporting period; (13) Results cannot be calculated for this reporting period; (14) The results for this state are combined with nearby states to protect confidentiality; Please refer to the User's Guide for a full explanation of data.

Evaluation of LVS Function

Hospital Name	City	Rate	Cases
Boise VA Medical Center	Boise	100%	112
Eastern Idaho Regional Medical Center	Idaho Falls	100%	126
Gritman Medical Center	Moscow	100%	30
Kootenai Medical Center	Coeur D'alene	100%	253
Portneuf Medical Center	Pocatello	100%	100
Saint Alphonsus Medical Center - Nampa	Nampa	100%	119
Saint Joseph Regional Medical Center	Lewiston	100%	105
Saint Luke's Magic Valley Rmc	Twin Falls	100%	164
Saint Luke's Regional Medical Center[2]	Boise	100%	380
West Valley Medical Center	Caldwell	100%	77
Saint Alphonsus Regional Medical Center	Boise	99%	201
Bonner General Hospital[2]	Sandpoint	96%	26
Bingham Memorial Hospital	Blackfoot	74%	35

Medicare Spending

Medicare Spending per Patient (ratio)

Hospital Name	City	Ratio	Cases
Treasure Valley Hospital	Boise	0.83	-
Madison Memorial Hospital	Rexburg	0.89	-
West Valley Medical Center	Caldwell	0.90	-
Mountain View Hospital	Idaho Falls	0.91	-
Northwest Specialty Hospital	Post Falls	0.92	-
Saint Joseph Regional Medical Center	Lewiston	0.93	-
Saint Alphonsus Regional Medical Center	Boise	0.94	-
Portneuf Medical Center	Pocatello	0.95	-
Saint Alphonsus Medical Center - Nampa	Nampa	0.95	-
Eastern Idaho Regional Medical Center	Idaho Falls	0.96	-
Saint Luke's Magic Valley Rmc	Twin Falls	0.96	-
Saint Luke's Regional Medical Center	Boise	0.96	-
Kootenai Medical Center	Coeur D'alene	0.99	-

Pneumonia Care

Appropriate Initial Antibiotic Given

Hospital Name	City	Rate	Cases
Bonner General Hospital[2]	Sandpoint	100%	30
Eastern Idaho Regional Medical Center	Idaho Falls	100%	153
Saint Luke's Magic Valley Rmc	Twin Falls	100%	142
Portneuf Medical Center	Pocatello	99%	123
Saint Luke's Regional Medical Center[2]	Boise	99%	127
West Valley Medical Center	Caldwell	99%	93
Kootenai Medical Center	Coeur D'alene	97%	176
Madison Memorial Hospital	Rexburg	97%	36
Saint Alphonsus Regional Medical Center	Boise	97%	144
Saint Alphonsus Medical Center - Nampa	Nampa	96%	125
Clearwater Valley Hospital & Clinics	Orofino	94%	34
Boise VA Medical Center	Boise	92%	37
Saint Mary's Hospital[2]	Cottonwood	92%	26
Saint Joseph Regional Medical Center	Lewiston	90%	86
Bingham Memorial Hospital	Blackfoot	87%	45
Gritman Medical Center	Moscow	85%	26

Blood Culture Timing

Hospital Name	City	Rate	Cases
Bonner General Hospital[2]	Sandpoint	100%	27
Cassia Regional Medical Center	Burley	100%	36
Clearwater Valley Hospital & Clinics[3]	Orofino	100%	25
Eastern Idaho Regional Medical Center	Idaho Falls	100%	233
Portneuf Medical Center	Pocatello	100%	252
Saint Alphonsus Regional Medical Center	Boise	100%	258
Saint Luke's Magic Valley Rmc	Twin Falls	100%	241
Saint Luke's Regional Medical Center[2]	Boise	100%	213
West Valley Medical Center	Caldwell	100%	128
Boise VA Medical Center	Boise	99%	89
Gritman Medical Center	Moscow	98%	44
Kootenai Medical Center	Coeur D'alene	98%	246
Madison Memorial Hospital	Rexburg	97%	37
Saint Alphonsus Medical Center - Nampa	Nampa	97%	185
North Canyon Medical Center	Gooding	93%	45
Saint Joseph Regional Medical Center	Lewiston	84%	134
Bingham Memorial Hospital	Blackfoot	81%	37

Pregnancy and Delivery Care

Newborns whose Deliveries were Scheduled Early

Hospital Name	City	Rate	Cases
Mountain View Hospital[2]	Idaho Falls	0%	29
Saint Alphonsus Regional Medical Center[2]	Boise	1%	104
Kootenai Medical Center[2]	Coeur D'alene	4%	187
Saint Luke's Regional Medical Center[2]	Boise	4%	75
West Valley Medical Center	Caldwell	4%	70
Portneuf Medical Center	Pocatello	5%	152
Eastern Idaho Regional Medical Center[2]	Idaho Falls	9%	34
Madison Memorial Hospital[2]	Rexburg	9%	88
Saint Joseph Regional Medical Center[2]	Lewiston	11%	28
Saint Luke's Magic Valley Rmc[2]	Twin Falls	15%	47
Saint Alphonsus Medical Center - Nampa[2]	Nampa	32%	40

Preventive Care

Immunization for Influenza

Hospital Name	City	Rate	Cases
Mountain View Hospital[2]	Idaho Falls	100%	234
Saint Luke's Regional Medical Center[2]	Boise	97%	639
Saint Alphonsus Regional Medical Center[2]	Boise	95%	553
Cassia Regional Medical Center[2]	Burley	94%	223
Saint Luke's Magic Valley Rmc[2]	Twin Falls	92%	494
West Valley Medical Center[2]	Caldwell	92%	440
Portneuf Medical Center[2]	Pocatello	91%	489
Eastern Idaho Regional Medical Center[2]	Idaho Falls	87%	543
Saint Joseph Regional Medical Center[2]	Lewiston	84%	428
Bonner General Hospital[2]	Sandpoint	83%	297
Northwest Specialty Hospital[2]	Post Falls	82%	341
Kootenai Medical Center[2]	Coeur D'alene	81%	522
Saint Alphonsus Medical Center - Nampa[2]	Nampa	80%	479
Gritman Medical Center[2]	Moscow	74%	487
Madison Memorial Hospital[2]	Rexburg	68%	276
Treasure Valley Hospital	Boise	55%	194
Idaho Doctors Hospital	Blackfoot	33%	54
Bingham Memorial Hospital[2]	Blackfoot	31%	306

Immunization for Pneumonia

Hospital Name	City	Rate	Cases
Mountain View Hospital[2]	Idaho Falls	100%	118
West Valley Medical Center[2]	Caldwell	97%	560
Saint Luke's Magic Valley Rmc[2]	Twin Falls	95%	546
Saint Luke's Regional Medical Center[2]	Boise	95%	611
Saint Joseph Regional Medical Center[2]	Lewiston	94%	547
Eastern Idaho Regional Medical Center[2]	Idaho Falls	93%	615
Northwest Specialty Hospital[2]	Post Falls	93%	352
Saint Alphonsus Medical Center - Nampa[2]	Nampa	93%	543
Portneuf Medical Center[2]	Pocatello	90%	541
Saint Alphonsus Regional Medical Center[2]	Boise	88%	593
Gritman Medical Center[2]	Moscow	87%	367
Cassia Regional Medical Center[2]	Burley	86%	175
Kootenai Medical Center[2]	Coeur D'alene	83%	544
Bonner General Hospital[2]	Sandpoint	82%	559
Bingham Memorial Hospital[2]	Blackfoot	73%	354
Treasure Valley Hospital	Boise	71%	196
Madison Memorial Hospital[2]	Rexburg	63%	143

Stroke Care

Anticoagulation Therapy for Atrial Fibrillation

Hospital Name	City	Rate	Cases
Saint Luke's Regional Medical Center	Boise	100%	26

Antithrombotic Therapy Timing

Hospital Name	City	Rate	Cases
Eastern Idaho Regional Medical Center	Idaho Falls	100%	78
Kootenai Medical Center	Coeur D'alene	100%	102
Portneuf Medical Center	Pocatello	100%	58
Saint Alphonsus Medical Center - Nampa	Nampa	100%	38
Saint Alphonsus Regional Medical Center[2]	Boise	100%	114
Saint Luke's Regional Medical Center	Boise	100%	190
Saint Luke's Magic Valley Rmc	Twin Falls	90%	80
Saint Joseph Regional Medical Center[2]	Lewiston	89%	57

Assessed for Rehabilitation

Hospital Name	City	Rate	Cases
Eastern Idaho Regional Medical Center	Idaho Falls	100%	118
Portneuf Medical Center	Pocatello	100%	68
Saint Alphonsus Regional Medical Center[2]	Boise	100%	180
West Valley Medical Center[2]	Caldwell	100%	29
Kootenai Medical Center	Coeur D'alene	99%	143
Saint Luke's Regional Medical Center	Boise	99%	270
Saint Luke's Magic Valley Rmc	Twin Falls	97%	99
Saint Alphonsus Medical Center - Nampa	Nampa	95%	42
Saint Joseph Regional Medical Center[2]	Lewiston	89%	72

Discharged on Antithrombotic Therapy

Hospital Name	City	Rate	Cases
Eastern Idaho Regional Medical Center	Idaho Falls	100%	99
Portneuf Medical Center	Pocatello	100%	62
Saint Alphonsus Medical Center - Nampa	Nampa	100%	40
Saint Alphonsus Regional Medical Center[2]	Boise	100%	150
Saint Luke's Regional Medical Center	Boise	100%	239
West Valley Medical Center[2]	Caldwell	100%	28
Kootenai Medical Center	Coeur D'alene	98%	124
Saint Joseph Regional Medical Center[2]	Lewiston	97%	64
Saint Luke's Magic Valley Rmc	Twin Falls	94%	93

Discharged on Statin Medication

Hospital Name	City	Rate	Cases
Saint Luke's Regional Medical Center	Boise	98%	183
Saint Alphonsus Regional Medical Center[2]	Boise	97%	118
Saint Alphonsus Medical Center - Nampa	Nampa	94%	33
Eastern Idaho Regional Medical Center	Idaho Falls	92%	63
Portneuf Medical Center	Pocatello	92%	38
Saint Luke's Magic Valley Rmc	Twin Falls	91%	79
Kootenai Medical Center	Coeur D'alene	85%	97
Saint Joseph Regional Medical Center[2]	Lewiston	73%	60

Thrombolytic Therapy Timing

Hospital Name	City	Rate	Cases
Saint Joseph Regional Medical Center[2]	Lewiston	7%	29

Venous Thromboembolism (VTE) Prophylaxis

Hospital Name	City	Rate	Cases
Saint Alphonsus Regional Medical Center[2]	Boise	99%	183
Saint Luke's Regional Medical Center	Boise	98%	252
Portneuf Medical Center	Pocatello	95%	65
Saint Alphonsus Medical Center - Nampa	Nampa	95%	40
Eastern Idaho Regional Medical Center	Idaho Falls	93%	116
Kootenai Medical Center	Coeur D'alene	90%	127
Saint Luke's Magic Valley Rmc	Twin Falls	88%	99
Saint Joseph Regional Medical Center[2]	Lewiston	81%	69

Written Stroke Educational Materials Given

Hospital Name	City	Rate	Cases
Eastern Idaho Regional Medical Center	Idaho Falls	99%	69
Saint Luke's Regional Medical Center	Boise	93%	162
Saint Joseph Regional Medical Center[2]	Lewiston	90%	41
Kootenai Medical Center	Coeur D'alene	85%	78
Saint Alphonsus Regional Medical Center[2]	Boise	84%	92
Saint Luke's Magic Valley Rmc	Twin Falls	82%	55
Portneuf Medical Center	Pocatello	68%	28
Saint Alphonsus Medical Center - Nampa	Nampa	48%	29

Surgical Care Improvement Project

Appropriate Beta Blocker Usage

Hospital Name	City	Rate	Cases
Mountain View Hospital[2]	Idaho Falls	100%	52
Northwest Specialty Hospital[2]	Post Falls	100%	54
Saint Alphonsus Medical Center - Nampa	Nampa	100%	113
West Valley Medical Center[2]	Caldwell	100%	70
Eastern Idaho Regional Medical Center[2]	Idaho Falls	99%	140
Portneuf Medical Center	Pocatello	99%	254
Saint Alphonsus Regional Medical Center[2]	Boise	99%	325
Saint Luke's Regional Medical Center[2]	Boise	99%	224
Saint Joseph Regional Medical Center[2]	Lewiston	98%	102
Kootenai Medical Center[2]	Coeur D'alene	97%	316
Saint Luke's Magic Valley Rmc[2]	Twin Falls	97%	117
Boise VA Medical Center[2]	Boise	96%	70
Madison Memorial Hospital	Rexburg	96%	47
Gritman Medical Center	Moscow	91%	35
Bonner General Hospital[2]	Sandpoint	90%	41
Bingham Memorial Hospital	Blackfoot	89%	38

Appropriate VTP Within 24 Hours

Hospital Name	City	Rate	Cases
Saint Luke's Magic Valley Rmc[2]	Twin Falls	100%	384
Saint Luke's Mccall	Mc Call	100%	77
Weiser Memorial Hospital	Weiser	100%	57
Eastern Idaho Regional Medical Center[2]	Idaho Falls	99%	337
Mountain View Hospital[2]	Idaho Falls	99%	345
Portneuf Medical Center	Pocatello	99%	827
Saint Alphonsus Medical Center - Nampa	Nampa	99%	426
West Valley Medical Center[2]	Caldwell	99%	278
Saint Luke's Regional Medical Center[2]	Boise	98%	458
Cassia Regional Medical Center[2]	Burley	97%	101
Gritman Medical Center	Moscow	97%	124
Kootenai Medical Center[2]	Coeur D'alene	97%	632
Northwest Specialty Hospital[2]	Post Falls	97%	261
Saint Alphonsus Regional Medical Center[2]	Boise	97%	922
Saint Joseph Regional Medical Center[2]	Lewiston	97%	449
Madison Memorial Hospital	Rexburg	96%	195
Treasure Valley Hospital	Boise	96%	26
Bonner General Hospital[2]	Sandpoint	94%	181
Bingham Memorial Hospital	Blackfoot	92%	187
Boise VA Medical Center[2]	Boise	90%	182

Controlled Postoperative Blood Glucose

Hospital Name	City	Rate	Cases
Eastern Idaho Regional Medical Center[2]	Idaho Falls	100%	83
Saint Alphonsus Regional Medical Center[2]	Boise	100%	136
Saint Luke's Regional Medical Center[2]	Boise	99%	150
Kootenai Medical Center[2]	Coeur D'alene	98%	186

NOTE: Hospital profiles are in alphabetical order by state, then city, then hospital within the city; Rankings exclude hospitals with less than 25 cases except for patient surveys which excludes hospitals with less than 100 cases; (a) 100-299 cases; (1) The number of cases/patients is too few to report; (2) Data submitted were based on a sample of cases/patients; (3) Results are based on a shorter time period than required; (4) Data suppressed by CMS for one or more quarters; (5) Results are not available for this reporting period; (6) Fewer than 100 patients completed the HCAHPS survey; (7) No cases met the criteria for this measure; (8) The lower limit of the confidence interval cannot be calculated if the number of observed infections equals zero; (9) No data are available from the state/territory for this reporting period; (10) The scores shown reflect fewer than 50 completed surveys; (11) There were discrepancies in the data collection process; (12) This measure does not apply to this hospital for this reporting period; (13) Results cannot be calculated for this reporting period; (14) The results for this state are combined with nearby states to protect confidentiality; Please refer to the User's Guide for a full explanation of data.

Hospital Name	City	Rate	Cases
Portneuf Medical Center	Pocatello	94%	67

Perioperative Temperature Management

Hospital Name	City	Rate	Cases
Bingham Memorial Hospital	Blackfoot	100%	218
Boise VA Medical Center[2]	Boise	100%	219
Eastern Idaho Regional Medical Center[2]	Idaho Falls	100%	445
Gritman Medical Center	Moscow	100%	142
Kootenai Medical Center[2]	Coeur D'alene	100%	766
Madison Memorial Hospital	Rexburg	100%	212
Mountain View Hospital[2]	Idaho Falls	100%	368
Portneuf Medical Center	Pocatello	100%	981
Saint Joseph Regional Medical Center[2]	Lewiston	100%	499
Saint Luke's Magic Valley Rmc[2]	Twin Falls	100%	539
Saint Luke's Mccall	Mc Call	100%	86
Saint Luke's Regional Medical Center[2]	Boise	100%	623
Treasure Valley Hospital	Boise	100%	38
West Valley Medical Center[2]	Caldwell	100%	315
Bonner General Hospital[2]	Sandpoint	99%	208
Cassia Regional Medical Center[2]	Burley	99%	116
Saint Alphonsus Regional Medical Center[2]	Boise	99%	1170
Saint Alphonsus Medical Center - Nampa	Nampa	98%	473
Northwest Specialty Hospital[2]	Post Falls	97%	304
Weiser Memorial Hospital	Weiser	92%	60

Prophylactic Antibiotic Selection

Hospital Name	City	Rate	Cases
Boise VA Medical Center	Boise	100%	131
Northwest Specialty Hospital[2]	Post Falls	100%	274
Portneuf Medical Center	Pocatello	100%	731
Saint Alphonsus Medical Center - Nampa	Nampa	100%	332
Saint Luke's Magic Valley Rmc[2]	Twin Falls	100%	350
Saint Luke's Mccall	Mc Call	100%	81
Weiser Memorial Hospital	Weiser	100%	51
Bonner General Hospital[2]	Sandpoint	99%	173
Cassia Regional Medical Center[2]	Burley	99%	98
Gritman Medical Center	Moscow	99%	118
Madison Memorial Hospital	Rexburg	99%	161
Mountain View Hospital[2]	Idaho Falls	99%	299
Saint Alphonsus Regional Medical Center[2]	Boise	99%	1131
Saint Joseph Regional Medical Center[2]	Lewiston	99%	384
Saint Luke's Regional Medical Center[2]	Boise	99%	521
West Valley Medical Center[2]	Caldwell	99%	204
Eastern Idaho Regional Medical Center[2]	Idaho Falls	98%	294
Kootenai Medical Center[2]	Coeur D'alene	98%	787
Bingham Memorial Hospital	Blackfoot	97%	166
Treasure Valley Hospital	Boise	89%	35

Prophylactic Antibiotic Selection (Outpatient)

Hospital Name	City	Rate	Cases
Madison Memorial Hospital	Rexburg	100%	62
Mountain View Hospital	Idaho Falls	100%	445
Northwest Specialty Hospital[3]	Post Falls	100%	44
Eastern Idaho Regional Medical Center	Idaho Falls	99%	380
Portneuf Medical Center	Pocatello	99%	351
Saint Luke's Magic Valley Rmc	Twin Falls	99%	316
Saint Luke's Regional Medical Center	Boise	99%	959
Treasure Valley Hospital	Boise	99%	153
Kootenai Medical Center	Coeur D'alene	98%	360
Saint Alphonsus Medical Center - Nampa	Nampa	98%	97
Saint Alphonsus Regional Medical Center	Boise	98%	950
West Valley Medical Center	Caldwell	98%	190
Saint Joseph Regional Medical Center	Lewiston	90%	426
Idaho Doctors Hospital	Blackfoot	88%	72

Prophylactic Antibiotic Stopped

Hospital Name	City	Rate	Cases
Mountain View Hospital[2]	Idaho Falls	100%	298
Saint Luke's Mccall	Mc Call	100%	81
Boise VA Medical Center	Boise	99%	129
Eastern Idaho Regional Medical Center[2]	Idaho Falls	99%	290
Kootenai Medical Center[2]	Coeur D'alene	99%	778
Northwest Specialty Hospital[2]	Post Falls	99%	273
Portneuf Medical Center	Pocatello	99%	717
Saint Alphonsus Medical Center - Nampa	Nampa	99%	321
Saint Alphonsus Regional Medical Center[2]	Boise	99%	1120
Saint Luke's Magic Valley Rmc[2]	Twin Falls	99%	340
Saint Luke's Regional Medical Center[2]	Boise	99%	518
Bonner General Hospital[2]	Sandpoint	98%	172
Bingham Memorial Hospital	Blackfoot	97%	163
Gritman Medical Center	Moscow	97%	116
Madison Memorial Hospital	Rexburg	97%	161
West Valley Medical Center[2]	Caldwell	97%	203
Saint Joseph Regional Medical Center[2]	Lewiston	96%	376
Cassia Regional Medical Center[2]	Burley	91%	98
Treasure Valley Hospital	Boise	91%	35
Weiser Memorial Hospital	Weiser	51%	51

Prophylactic Antibiotic Timing

Hospital Name	City	Rate	Cases
Mountain View Hospital[2]	Idaho Falls	100%	299
West Valley Medical Center[2]	Caldwell	100%	204
Boise VA Medical Center	Boise	99%	131
Cassia Regional Medical Center[2]	Burley	99%	98
Eastern Idaho Regional Medical Center[2]	Idaho Falls	99%	294
Gritman Medical Center	Moscow	99%	117
Madison Memorial Hospital	Rexburg	99%	161
Portneuf Medical Center	Pocatello	99%	732
Saint Alphonsus Regional Medical Center[2]	Boise	99%	1132
Saint Luke's Magic Valley Rmc[2]	Twin Falls	99%	350
Saint Luke's Mccall	Mc Call	99%	81
Saint Luke's Regional Medical Center[2]	Boise	99%	521
Bonner General Hospital[2]	Sandpoint	98%	173
Saint Alphonsus Medical Center - Nampa	Nampa	98%	332
Saint Joseph Regional Medical Center[2]	Lewiston	97%	384
Treasure Valley Hospital	Boise	97%	35
Kootenai Medical Center[2]	Coeur D'alene	96%	788
Northwest Specialty Hospital[2]	Post Falls	96%	274
Bingham Memorial Hospital	Blackfoot	90%	166
Weiser Memorial Hospital	Weiser	45%	51

Prophylactic Antibiotic Timing (Outpatient)

Hospital Name	City	Rate	Cases
Mountain View Hospital	Idaho Falls	100%	445
Northwest Specialty Hospital[3]	Post Falls	100%	44
Portneuf Medical Center	Pocatello	100%	351
Eastern Idaho Regional Medical Center	Idaho Falls	99%	380
Saint Alphonsus Regional Medical Center	Boise	99%	953
Saint Luke's Magic Valley Rmc	Twin Falls	99%	217
West Valley Medical Center	Caldwell	99%	134
Saint Luke's Regional Medical Center	Boise	97%	849
Treasure Valley Hospital	Boise	97%	153
Madison Memorial Hospital	Rexburg	94%	65
Saint Joseph Regional Medical Center	Lewiston	93%	357
Saint Alphonsus Medical Center - Nampa	Nampa	90%	101
Kootenai Medical Center	Coeur D'alene	89%	378
Idaho Doctors Hospital	Blackfoot	86%	72

Urinary Catheter Removal

Hospital Name	City	Rate	Cases
Saint Luke's Mccall	Mc Call	100%	83
Mountain View Hospital[2]	Idaho Falls	99%	79
Northwest Specialty Hospital[2]	Post Falls	99%	156
Portneuf Medical Center	Pocatello	99%	791
Saint Luke's Magic Valley Rmc[2]	Twin Falls	99%	284
West Valley Medical Center[2]	Caldwell	99%	213
Saint Alphonsus Medical Center - Nampa	Nampa	98%	351
Saint Alphonsus Regional Medical Center[2]	Boise	98%	968
Saint Luke's Regional Medical Center[2]	Boise	98%	521
Weiser Memorial Hospital	Weiser	98%	59
Boise VA Medical Center[2]	Boise	96%	127
Eastern Idaho Regional Medical Center[2]	Idaho Falls	95%	166
Gritman Medical Center	Moscow	95%	97
Saint Joseph Regional Medical Center[2]	Lewiston	95%	407
Bonner General Hospital[2]	Sandpoint	94%	167
Bingham Memorial Hospital	Blackfoot	89%	140
Kootenai Medical Center[2]	Coeur D'alene	89%	358
Madison Memorial Hospital	Rexburg	89%	145
Cassia Regional Medical Center[2]	Burley	84%	69

Survey of Patients' Hospital Experiences

Area Around Room 'Always' Quiet at Night

Hospital Name	City	Rate	Cases
Treasure Valley Hospital	Boise	78%	300+
Saint Luke's Wood River Medical Center	Ketchum	72%	300+
Northwest Specialty Hospital	Post Falls	71%	300+
North Canyon Medical Center	Gooding	70%	(a)
Benewah Community Hospital	Saint Maries	68%	(a)
Bonner General Hospital	Sandpoint	64%	300+
Gritman Medical Center	Moscow	64%	300+
West Valley Medical Center	Caldwell	64%	300+
Saint Luke's Mccall	Mc Call	62%	(a)
Saint Luke's Magic Valley Rmc	Twin Falls	60%	300+
Mountain View Hospital	Idaho Falls	59%	300+
Portneuf Medical Center	Pocatello	59%	300+
Saint Luke's Regional Medical Center	Boise	59%	300+
Cassia Regional Medical Center	Burley	58%	(a)
Saint Alphonsus Regional Medical Center	Boise	58%	300+
Saint Luke's Elmore Medical Center	Mountain Home	57%	(a)
Saint Joseph Regional Medical Center	Lewiston	56%	300+
Madison Memorial Hospital	Rexburg	55%	300+
Saint Alphonsus Medical Center - Nampa	Nampa	51%	300+
Saint Mary's Hospital[11]	Cottonwood	51%	300+
Eastern Idaho Regional Medical Center	Idaho Falls	50%	300+
Clearwater Valley Hospital & Clinics[11]	Orofino	48%	300+
Bingham Memorial Hospital	Blackfoot	47%	300+
Kootenai Medical Center	Coeur D'alene	44%	300+

Doctors 'Always' Communicated Well

Hospital Name	City	Rate	Cases
Northwest Specialty Hospital	Post Falls	88%	300+
Saint Mary's Hospital[11]	Cottonwood	88%	300+
North Canyon Medical Center	Gooding	87%	(a)
Saint Luke's Wood River Medical Center	Ketchum	86%	300+
Cassia Regional Medical Center	Burley	85%	(a)
Clearwater Valley Hospital & Clinics[11]	Orofino	83%	300+
Saint Luke's Regional Medical Center	Boise	83%	300+
Gritman Medical Center	Moscow	82%	300+
Mountain View Hospital	Idaho Falls	82%	300+
Saint Luke's Magic Valley Rmc	Twin Falls	82%	300+
Saint Luke's Mccall	Mc Call	82%	(a)
Benewah Community Hospital	Saint Maries	81%	(a)
Bingham Memorial Hospital	Blackfoot	81%	300+
Saint Alphonsus Medical Center - Nampa	Nampa	81%	300+
Treasure Valley Hospital	Boise	81%	300+
West Valley Medical Center	Caldwell	81%	300+
Saint Joseph Regional Medical Center	Lewiston	80%	300+
Bonner General Hospital	Sandpoint	79%	300+
Saint Alphonsus Regional Medical Center	Boise	79%	300+
Madison Memorial Hospital	Rexburg	78%	300+
Portneuf Medical Center	Pocatello	78%	300+
Kootenai Medical Center	Coeur D'alene	77%	300+
Saint Luke's Elmore Medical Center	Mountain Home	77%	(a)
Eastern Idaho Regional Medical Center	Idaho Falls	76%	300+

Home Recovery Information Given

Hospital Name	City	Rate	Cases
Cassia Regional Medical Center	Burley	91%	(a)
Gritman Medical Center	Moscow	91%	300+
Saint Luke's Wood River Medical Center	Ketchum	91%	300+
Northwest Specialty Hospital	Post Falls	90%	300+
Saint Joseph Regional Medical Center	Lewiston	90%	300+
Treasure Valley Hospital	Boise	90%	300+
Saint Luke's Regional Medical Center	Boise	89%	300+
Bingham Memorial Hospital	Blackfoot	88%	300+
Saint Alphonsus Medical Center - Nampa	Nampa	88%	300+
Saint Alphonsus Regional Medical Center	Boise	88%	300+
Kootenai Medical Center	Coeur D'alene	87%	300+
North Canyon Medical Center	Gooding	87%	(a)
Portneuf Medical Center	Pocatello	87%	300+
Saint Luke's Magic Valley Rmc	Twin Falls	87%	300+
West Valley Medical Center	Caldwell	87%	300+
Bonner General Hospital	Sandpoint	86%	300+
Clearwater Valley Hospital & Clinics[11]	Orofino	86%	300+
Mountain View Hospital	Idaho Falls	86%	300+
Saint Luke's Mccall	Mc Call	86%	(a)
Eastern Idaho Regional Medical Center	Idaho Falls	85%	300+
Benewah Community Hospital	Saint Maries	84%	(a)
Madison Memorial Hospital	Rexburg	84%	300+
Saint Luke's Elmore Medical Center	Mountain Home	82%	(a)
Saint Mary's Hospital[11]	Cottonwood	82%	300+

Hospital Given 9 or 10 on 10 Point Scale

Hospital Name	City	Rate	Cases
Treasure Valley Hospital	Boise	87%	300+
Northwest Specialty Hospital	Post Falls	85%	300+
Saint Luke's Wood River Medical Center	Ketchum	83%	300+
Saint Luke's Mccall	Mc Call	81%	(a)
Gritman Medical Center	Moscow	80%	300+
North Canyon Medical Center	Gooding	80%	(a)
Saint Luke's Regional Medical Center	Boise	77%	300+
Benewah Community Hospital	Saint Maries	74%	(a)
Bonner General Hospital	Sandpoint	73%	300+
Cassia Regional Medical Center	Burley	72%	(a)
Saint Luke's Magic Valley Rmc	Twin Falls	72%	300+
West Valley Medical Center	Caldwell	72%	300+
Saint Alphonsus Regional Medical Center	Boise	71%	300+
Saint Mary's Hospital[11]	Cottonwood	71%	300+
Bingham Memorial Hospital	Blackfoot	70%	300+
Clearwater Valley Hospital & Clinics[11]	Orofino	69%	300+
Mountain View Hospital	Idaho Falls	69%	300+
Saint Joseph Regional Medical Center	Lewiston	69%	300+
Portneuf Medical Center	Pocatello	68%	300+
Saint Alphonsus Medical Center - Nampa	Nampa	68%	300+
Madison Memorial Hospital	Rexburg	67%	300+
Kootenai Medical Center	Coeur D'alene	65%	300+
Eastern Idaho Regional Medical Center	Idaho Falls	61%	300+
Saint Luke's Elmore Medical Center	Mountain Home	54%	(a)

Meds 'Always' Explained Before Given

Hospital Name	City	Rate	Cases
Treasure Valley Hospital	Boise	75%	300+
Northwest Specialty Hospital	Post Falls	73%	300+
Saint Luke's Wood River Medical Center	Ketchum	71%	300+
Cassia Regional Medical Center	Burley	70%	(a)

NOTE: Hospital profiles are in alphabetical order by state, then city, then hospital within the city; Rankings exclude hospitals with less than 25 cases except for patient surveys which excludes hospitals with less than 100 cases; (a) 100-299 cases; (1) The number of cases/patients is too few to report; (2) Data submitted were based on a sample of cases/patients; (3) Results are based on a shorter time period than required; (4) Data suppressed by CMS for one or more quarters; (5) Results are not available for this reporting period; (6) Fewer than 100 patients completed the HCAHPS survey; (7) No cases met the criteria for this measure; (8) The lower limit of the confidence interval cannot be calculated if the number of observed infections equals zero; (9) No data are available from the state/territory for this reporting period; (10) The scores shown reflect fewer than 50 completed surveys; (11) There were discrepancies in the data collection process; (12) This measure does not apply to this hospital for this reporting period; (13) Results cannot be calculated for this reporting period; (14) The results for this state are combined with nearby states to protect confidentiality; Please refer to the User's Guide for a full explanation of data.

Gritman Medical Center	Moscow	69%	300+
Saint Luke's Mccall	Mc Call	69%	(a)
Bonner General Hospital	Sandpoint	68%	300+
North Canyon Medical Center	Gooding	67%	(a)
Saint Luke's Regional Medical Center	Boise	67%	300+
Saint Luke's Elmore Medical Center	Mountain Home	66%	(a)
Saint Luke's Magic Valley Rmc	Twin Falls	66%	300+
Mountain View Hospital	Idaho Falls	65%	300+
Saint Joseph Regional Medical Center	Lewiston	65%	300+
Bingham Memorial Hospital	Blackfoot	64%	300+
West Valley Medical Center	Caldwell	64%	300+
Benewah Community Hospital	Saint Maries	63%	(a)
Kootenai Medical Center	Coeur D'alene	61%	300+
Madison Memorial Hospital	Rexburg	61%	300+
Portneuf Medical Center	Pocatello	60%	300+
Saint Mary's Hospital[11]	Cottonwood	60%	300+
Clearwater Valley Hospital & Clinics[11]	Orofino	58%	300+
Saint Alphonsus Regional Medical Center	Boise	58%	300+
Saint Alphonsus Medical Center - Nampa	Nampa	57%	300+
Eastern Idaho Regional Medical Center	Idaho Falls	56%	300+

Nurses 'Always' Communicated Well

Hospital Name	City	Rate	Cases
Northwest Specialty Hospital	Post Falls	88%	300+
Treasure Valley Hospital	Boise	88%	300+
Saint Luke's Wood River Medical Center	Ketchum	86%	300+
Saint Luke's Mccall	Mc Call	84%	(a)
Benewah Community Hospital	Saint Maries	83%	(a)
Gritman Medical Center	Moscow	81%	300+
North Canyon Medical Center	Gooding	80%	(a)
Saint Luke's Regional Medical Center	Boise	80%	300+
Bonner General Hospital	Sandpoint	79%	300+
Cassia Regional Medical Center	Burley	79%	(a)
Clearwater Valley Hospital & Clinics[11]	Orofino	79%	300+
Saint Luke's Magic Valley Rmc	Twin Falls	79%	300+
West Valley Medical Center	Caldwell	78%	300+
Bingham Memorial Hospital	Blackfoot	77%	300+
Mountain View Hospital	Idaho Falls	77%	300+
Saint Joseph Regional Medical Center	Lewiston	77%	300+
Saint Mary's Hospital[11]	Cottonwood	76%	300+
Portneuf Medical Center	Pocatello	75%	300+
Saint Alphonsus Medical Center - Nampa	Nampa	74%	300+
Saint Luke's Elmore Medical Center	Mountain Home	74%	(a)
Kootenai Medical Center	Coeur D'alene	73%	300+
Eastern Idaho Regional Medical Center	Idaho Falls	72%	300+
Saint Alphonsus Regional Medical Center	Boise	72%	300+
Madison Memorial Hospital	Rexburg	69%	300+

Pain 'Always' Well Controlled

Hospital Name	City	Rate	Cases
Treasure Valley Hospital	Boise	84%	300+
North Canyon Medical Center	Gooding	81%	(a)
Northwest Specialty Hospital	Post Falls	79%	300+
Saint Luke's Wood River Medical Center	Ketchum	79%	300+
Saint Luke's Mccall	Mc Call	78%	(a)
Bonner General Hospital	Sandpoint	76%	300+
Cassia Regional Medical Center	Burley	75%	(a)
Saint Luke's Regional Medical Center	Boise	74%	300+
Saint Luke's Magic Valley Rmc	Twin Falls	73%	300+
Gritman Medical Center	Moscow	72%	300+
Mountain View Hospital	Idaho Falls	72%	300+
Bingham Memorial Hospital	Blackfoot	71%	300+
Saint Mary's Hospital[11]	Cottonwood	71%	300+
West Valley Medical Center	Caldwell	70%	300+
Clearwater Valley Hospital & Clinics[11]	Orofino	69%	300+
Benewah Community Hospital	Saint Maries	68%	(a)
Kootenai Medical Center	Coeur D'alene	68%	300+
Portneuf Medical Center	Pocatello	67%	300+
Saint Alphonsus Medical Center - Nampa	Nampa	67%	300+
Saint Alphonsus Regional Medical Center	Boise	67%	300+
Saint Luke's Elmore Medical Center	Mountain Home	67%	(a)
Saint Joseph Regional Medical Center	Lewiston	66%	300+
Eastern Idaho Regional Medical Center	Idaho Falls	64%	300+
Madison Memorial Hospital	Rexburg	60%	300+

Room and Bathroom 'Always' Clean

Hospital Name	City	Rate	Cases
North Canyon Medical Center	Gooding	92%	(a)
Benewah Community Hospital	Saint Maries	90%	(a)
Saint Luke's Magic Valley Rmc	Twin Falls	85%	300+
Saint Luke's Elmore Medical Center	Mountain Home	82%	(a)
Saint Luke's Wood River Medical Center	Ketchum	82%	300+
Treasure Valley Hospital	Boise	82%	300+
Bonner General Hospital	Sandpoint	81%	300+
Madison Memorial Hospital	Rexburg	79%	300+
Clearwater Valley Hospital & Clinics[11]	Orofino	78%	300+
Northwest Specialty Hospital	Post Falls	78%	300+
Saint Mary's Hospital[11]	Cottonwood	78%	300+
Gritman Medical Center	Moscow	77%	300+
Saint Luke's Regional Medical Center	Boise	77%	300+
Saint Luke's Mccall	Mc Call	76%	(a)
Bingham Memorial Hospital	Blackfoot	73%	300+
West Valley Medical Center	Caldwell	72%	300+
Cassia Regional Medical Center	Burley	70%	(a)
Mountain View Hospital	Idaho Falls	70%	300+
Portneuf Medical Center	Pocatello	70%	300+
Saint Joseph Regional Medical Center	Lewiston	69%	300+
Kootenai Medical Center	Coeur D'alene	68%	300+
Saint Alphonsus Regional Medical Center	Boise	68%	300+
Saint Alphonsus Medical Center - Nampa	Nampa	66%	300+
Eastern Idaho Regional Medical Center	Idaho Falls	63%	300+

Timely Help 'Always' Received

Hospital Name	City	Rate	Cases
Treasure Valley Hospital	Boise	88%	300+
Northwest Specialty Hospital	Post Falls	85%	300+
Benewah Community Hospital	Saint Maries	84%	(a)
Saint Luke's Mccall	Mc Call	83%	(a)
Saint Luke's Wood River Medical Center	Ketchum	81%	300+
Bonner General Hospital	Sandpoint	78%	300+
North Canyon Medical Center	Gooding	77%	(a)
Gritman Medical Center	Moscow	72%	300+
Saint Luke's Magic Valley Rmc	Twin Falls	72%	300+
Cassia Regional Medical Center	Burley	71%	(a)
Clearwater Valley Hospital & Clinics[11]	Orofino	70%	300+
Bingham Memorial Hospital	Blackfoot	69%	300+
Saint Luke's Elmore Medical Center	Mountain Home	69%	(a)
Saint Joseph Regional Medical Center	Lewiston	68%	300+
Saint Luke's Regional Medical Center	Boise	68%	300+
Mountain View Hospital	Idaho Falls	67%	300+
Saint Mary's Hospital[11]	Cottonwood	66%	300+
West Valley Medical Center	Caldwell	66%	300+
Portneuf Medical Center	Pocatello	64%	300+
Madison Memorial Hospital	Rexburg	63%	300+
Saint Alphonsus Medical Center - Nampa	Nampa	60%	300+
Saint Alphonsus Regional Medical Center	Boise	60%	300+
Kootenai Medical Center	Coeur D'alene	58%	300+
Eastern Idaho Regional Medical Center	Idaho Falls	57%	300+

Would Definitely Recommend Hospital

Hospital Name	City	Rate	Cases
Northwest Specialty Hospital	Post Falls	91%	300+
Saint Luke's Wood River Medical Center	Ketchum	88%	300+
Treasure Valley Hospital	Boise	87%	300+
Saint Luke's Regional Medical Center	Boise	84%	300+
Saint Luke's Mccall	Mc Call	81%	(a)
Mountain View Hospital	Idaho Falls	80%	300+
Saint Mary's Hospital[11]	Cottonwood	80%	300+
Gritman Medical Center	Moscow	77%	300+
North Canyon Medical Center	Gooding	76%	(a)
Benewah Community Hospital	Saint Maries	75%	(a)
Saint Alphonsus Regional Medical Center	Boise	74%	300+
Bonner General Hospital	Sandpoint	72%	300+
Saint Luke's Magic Valley Rmc	Twin Falls	72%	300+
Cassia Regional Medical Center	Burley	70%	(a)
Saint Joseph Regional Medical Center	Lewiston	70%	300+
Kootenai Medical Center	Coeur D'alene	69%	300+
West Valley Medical Center	Caldwell	69%	300+
Portneuf Medical Center	Pocatello	68%	300+
Madison Memorial Hospital	Rexburg	67%	300+
Bingham Memorial Hospital	Blackfoot	66%	300+
Saint Alphonsus Medical Center - Nampa	Nampa	65%	300+
Clearwater Valley Hospital & Clinics[11]	Orofino	64%	300+
Eastern Idaho Regional Medical Center	Idaho Falls	63%	300+
Saint Luke's Elmore Medical Center	Mountain Home	50%	(a)

Use of Medical Imaging

Cardiac Imaging Stress Test before OP Surgery

Hospital Name	City	Rate	Cases
Madison Memorial Hospital	Rexburg	2.0%	50
Saint Joseph Regional Medical Center	Lewiston	4.1%	193
Kootenai Medical Center	Coeur D'alene	4.3%	1445
Bonner General Hospital	Sandpoint	4.4%	226
Eastern Idaho Regional Medical Center	Idaho Falls	4.5%	111
Saint Alphonsus Medical Center - Nampa	Nampa	4.6%	87
Portneuf Medical Center	Pocatello	4.8%	462
Saint Alphonsus Regional Medical Center	Boise	4.8%	722
Saint Luke's Regional Medical Center	Boise	4.8%	727
West Valley Medical Center	Caldwell	5.1%	196
Saint Luke's Magic Valley Rmc	Twin Falls	6.1%	545
Cassia Regional Medical Center	Burley	7.5%	67

Combination Abdominal CT Scan

Hospital Name	City	Rate	Cases
Saint Alphonsus Medical Center - Nampa	Nampa	1.6%	384
Madison Memorial Hospital	Rexburg	1.8%	171
Eastern Idaho Regional Medical Center	Idaho Falls	2.3%	524
Steele Memorial Medical Center	Salmon	2.3%	133
Saint Joseph Regional Medical Center	Lewiston	3.1%	712
Saint Alphonsus Regional Medical Center	Boise	3.5%	885
Northwest Specialty Hospital	Post Falls	4.1%	73
Mountain View Hospital	Idaho Falls	4.3%	185
Cassia Regional Medical Center	Burley	4.5%	178
West Valley Medical Center	Caldwell	4.6%	413
Walter Knox Memorial Hospital	Emmett	4.7%	150
Bonner General Hospital	Sandpoint	4.8%	394
Saint Luke's Magic Valley Rmc	Twin Falls	7.5%	1216
Saint Luke's Regional Medical Center	Boise	7.5%	2383
Portneuf Medical Center	Pocatello	7.9%	544
Kootenai Medical Center	Coeur D'alene	9.0%	1356
Benewah Community Hospital	Saint Maries	9.1%	99
Syringa General Hospital	Grangeville	15.0%	80

Combination Brain/Sinus CT Scan

Hospital Name	City	Rate	Cases
Benewah Community Hospital	Saint Maries	0.0%	56
Walter Knox Memorial Hospital	Emmett	0.0%	135
Saint Alphonsus Regional Medical Center	Boise	0.2%	471
West Valley Medical Center	Caldwell	0.4%	237
Saint Luke's Magic Valley Rmc	Twin Falls	0.9%	527
Bonner General Hospital	Sandpoint	1.0%	200
Saint Luke's Regional Medical Center	Boise	1.6%	950
Portneuf Medical Center	Pocatello	1.8%	488
Eastern Idaho Regional Medical Center	Idaho Falls	2.0%	461
Kootenai Medical Center	Coeur D'alene	2.6%	853

Combination Chest CT Scan

Hospital Name	City	Rate	Cases
Eastern Idaho Regional Medical Center	Idaho Falls	0.0%	153
Mountain View Hospital	Idaho Falls	0.0%	254
Saint Joseph Regional Medical Center	Lewiston	0.0%	429
Steele Memorial Medical Center	Salmon	0.0%	69
West Valley Medical Center	Caldwell	0.0%	140
Saint Luke's Magic Valley Rmc	Twin Falls	0.2%	566
Bonner General Hospital	Sandpoint	0.4%	253
Kootenai Medical Center	Coeur D'alene	0.4%	1043
Saint Alphonsus Medical Center - Nampa	Nampa	0.6%	155
Saint Luke's Regional Medical Center	Boise	0.9%	1646
Cassia Regional Medical Center	Burley	1.2%	86
Benewah Community Hospital	Saint Maries	1.3%	80
Northwest Specialty Hospital	Post Falls	1.7%	58
Saint Alphonsus Regional Medical Center	Boise	1.7%	605
Walter Knox Memorial Hospital	Emmett	1.8%	57
Madison Memorial Hospital	Rexburg	2.7%	73
Portneuf Medical Center	Pocatello	3.8%	209

Follow-up Mammogram/Ultrasound

A follow-up rate near zero may indicate missed cancer; a rate higher than 14% may mean there is unnecessary follow up.

Hospital Name	City	Rate	Cases
Benewah Community Hospital	Saint Maries	4.7%	128
Eastern Idaho Regional Medical Center	Idaho Falls	5.8%	906
Teton Valley Hospital	Victor	6.3%	80
Kootenai Medical Center	Coeur D'alene	6.7%	2838
Mountain View Hospital	Idaho Falls	6.9%	333
Portneuf Medical Center	Pocatello	7.1%	1624
Saint Luke's Magic Valley Rmc	Twin Falls	7.1%	2082
Steele Memorial Medical Center	Salmon	8.0%	212
Saint Luke's Regional Medical Center	Boise	8.4%	5826
Saint Alphonsus Regional Medical Center	Boise	8.9%	1860
Saint Alphonsus Medical Center - Nampa	Nampa	9.2%	888
West Valley Medical Center	Caldwell	10.5%	446
Saint Joseph Regional Medical Center	Lewiston	10.6%	1074
Cassia Regional Medical Center	Burley	14.2%	339
Bonner General Hospital	Sandpoint	14.8%	520

Lumbar Spine MRI for Low Back Pain

Hospital Name	City	Rate	Cases
Northwest Specialty Hospital	Post Falls	32.9%	76
Saint Joseph Regional Medical Center	Lewiston	34.5%	139
Kootenai Medical Center	Coeur D'alene	35.8%	240
Saint Luke's Magic Valley Rmc	Twin Falls	37.2%	172
Saint Luke's Regional Medical Center	Boise	37.3%	303
Cassia Regional Medical Center	Burley	40.8%	71
Portneuf Medical Center	Pocatello	41.2%	318
Mountain View Hospital	Idaho Falls	41.3%	160
Eastern Idaho Regional Medical Center	Idaho Falls	42.4%	85
Bonner General Hospital	Sandpoint	45.2%	84

NOTE: Hospital profiles are in alphabetical order by state, then city, then hospital within the city; Rankings exclude hospitals with less than 25 cases except for patient surveys which excludes hospitals with less than 100 cases; (a) 100-299 cases; (1) The number of cases/patients is too few to report; (2) Data submitted were based on a sample of cases/patients; (3) Results are based on a shorter time period than required; (4) Data suppressed by CMS for one or more quarters; (5) Results are not available for this reporting period; (6) Fewer than 100 patients completed the HCAHPS survey; (7) No cases met the criteria for this measure; (8) The lower limit of the confidence interval cannot be calculated if the number of observed infections equals zero; (9) No data are available from the state/territory for this reporting period; (10) The scores shown reflect fewer than 50 completed surveys; (11) There were discrepancies in the data collection process; (12) This measure does not apply to this hospital for this reporting period; (13) Results cannot be calculated for this reporting period; (14) The results for this state are combined with nearby states to protect confidentiality; Please refer to the User's Guide for a full explanation of data.

Harms Memorial Hospital

510 Roosevelt Street
American Falls, ID 83211
Phone: 208-226-3200
Type: Critical Access Hospitals
Emergency Services: Yes
Ownership: Govt - Hospital Dist/Auth

Measure	Cases	This Hosp.	State Avg.	U.S. Avg.
Blood Clot Prevention and Treatment				
Anticoagulation Overlap Therapy[5]	-	-	95%	93%
ICU Venous Thromboembolism Prophylaxis[5]	-	-	92%	92%
Incidence of Potentially Preventable VTE[5]	-	-	11%	10%
UFH with Dosages/Platelet Monitoring[5]	-	-	99%	97%
Venous Thromboembolism Prophylaxis[5]	-	-	87%	85%
Warfarin Therapy Discharge Instructions[5]	-	-	75%	75%
Chest Pain/Possible Heart Attack Care				
Aspirin Given Within 24 Hours of Arrival	-	-	96%	96%
Fibrinolytic Meds Within 30 Min. of Arrival	-	-	55%	58%
Average Time to ECG (minutes)	-	-	9	7
Average Time to Transfer (minutes)	-	-	62	60
Children's Asthma Care				
Received Home Management Plan of Care	-	-	-	88%
Received Reliever Medication	-	-	-	100%
Received Systemic Corticosteroids	-	-	-	100%
Emergency Department				
Admittance Decision Time (minutes)[5]	-	-	76	98
Head CT Results Within 45 Min. of Arrival	-	-	38%	57%
Patients Who Left ER Before Being Seen	-	-	1%	2%
Time from ER Arrival to Admit. (minutes)[5]	-	-	232	274
Time from ER Arrival to Discharge (minutes)	-	-	121	134
Time in ER Before Being Evaluated (minutes)	-	-	21	26
Time to Pain Meds for Fractures (minutes)	-	-	46	57
Heart Attack Care				
Aspirin Given at Discharge[5]	-	-	100%	99%
Fibrinolytic Meds Within 30 Min. of Arrival[5]	-	-	-	54%
PCI Within 90 Minutes of Arrival[5]	-	-	98%	96%
Statin Prescribed at Discharge[5]	-	-	99%	98%
Heart Failure Care				
ACE Inhibitor or ARB for LVSD[5]	-	-	98%	97%
Discharge Instructions Given[5]	-	-	94%	94%
Evaluation of LVS Function[5]	-	-	97%	99%
Medicare Spending				
Medicare Spending per Patient (ratio)	-	-	0.91	0.98
Pneumonia Care				
Appropriate Initial Antibiotic Given[1,2]	-	-	94%	95%
Blood Culture Timing[2,3]	-	-	98%	98%
Pregnancy and Delivery Care				
Newborn Deliveries Scheduled Early[5]	-	-	6%	6%
Preventive Care				
Immunization for Influenza[5]	-	-	83%	90%
Immunization for Pneumonia[5]	-	-	89%	92%
Stroke Care				
Anticoagulation Therapy for Atrial Fibrillation[5]	-	-	97%	95%
Antithrombotic Therapy Timing[5]	-	-	98%	98%
Assessed for Rehabilitation[5]	-	-	98%	97%
Discharged on Antithrombotic Therapy[5]	-	-	99%	99%
Discharged on Statin Medication[5]	-	-	91%	94%
Thrombolytic Therapy Timing[5]	-	-	55%	66%
Venous Thromboembolism Prophylaxis[5]	-	-	93%	94%
Written Stroke Educational Materials Given[5]	-	-	84%	88%
Surgical Care Improvement Project				
Appropriate Beta Blocker Usage[5]	-	-	98%	98%
Appropriate VTP Within 24 Hours[5]	-	-	98%	98%
Controlled Postoperative Blood Glucose[5]	-	-	99%	97%
Perioperative Temperature Management[5]	-	-	99%	100%
Prophylactic Antibiotic Selection[5]	-	-	99%	99%
Prophylactic Antibiotic Selection (Outpatient)	-	-	98%	98%
Prophylactic Antibiotic Stopped[5]	-	-	98%	98%
Prophylactic Antibiotic Timing[5]	-	-	98%	99%
Prophylactic Antibiotic Timing (Outpatient)	-	-	97%	98%
Urinary Catheter Removal[5]	-	-	96%	97%
Survey of Patients' Hospital Experiences				
Area Around Room 'Always' Quiet at Night[5]	-	-	61%	61%
Doctors 'Always' Communicated Well[5]	-	-	83%	82%
Home Recovery Information Given[5]	-	-	88%	85%
Hospital Given 9 or 10 on 10 Point Scale[5]	-	-	73%	71%
Meds 'Always' Explained Before Given[5]	-	-	66%	64%
Nurses 'Always' Communicated Well[5]	-	-	80%	79%
Pain 'Always' Well Controlled[5]	-	-	72%	71%
Room and Bathroom 'Always' Clean[5]	-	-	77%	73%
Timely Help 'Always' Received[5]	-	-	73%	68%
Would Definitely Recommend Hospital[5]	-	-	74%	71%
Use of Medical Imaging				
Cardiac Imaging Stress Test before Surgery	-	-	4.6%	5.3%
Combination Abdominal CT Scan	-	-	7.3%	10.5%
Combination Brain/Sinus CT Scan	-	-	1.7%	2.7%
Combination Chest CT Scan	-	-	1.8%	2.7%
Follow-up Mammogram/Ultrasound	-	-	8.2%	8.8%
Lumbar Spine MRI for Low Back Pain	-	-	40.3%	37.2%

Lost Rivers Medical Center

551 Highland Drive
Arco, ID 83213
Phone: 208-527-8206
Type: Critical Access Hospitals
Emergency Services: Yes
Ownership: Govt - Hospital Dist/Auth

Measure	Cases	This Hosp.	State Avg.	U.S. Avg.
Blood Clot Prevention and Treatment				
Anticoagulation Overlap Therapy[5]	-	-	95%	93%
ICU Venous Thromboembolism Prophylaxis[5]	-	-	92%	92%
Incidence of Potentially Preventable VTE[5]	-	-	11%	10%
UFH with Dosages/Platelet Monitoring[5]	-	-	99%	97%
Venous Thromboembolism Prophylaxis[5]	-	-	87%	85%
Warfarin Therapy Discharge Instructions[5]	-	-	75%	75%
Chest Pain/Possible Heart Attack Care				
Aspirin Given Within 24 Hours of Arrival[1,3]	-	-	96%	96%
Fibrinolytic Meds Within 30 Min. of Arrival[3,7]	-	-	55%	58%
Average Time to ECG (minutes)[1,3]	-	-	9	7
Average Time to Transfer (minutes)[3,7]	-	-	62	60
Children's Asthma Care				
Received Home Management Plan of Care	-	-	-	88%
Received Reliever Medication	-	-	-	100%
Received Systemic Corticosteroids	-	-	-	100%
Emergency Department				
Admittance Decision Time (minutes)[5]	-	-	76	98
Head CT Results Within 45 Min. of Arrival[5]	-	-	38%	57%
Patients Who Left ER Before Being Seen[5]	-	-	1%	2%
Time from ER Arrival to Admit. (minutes)[5]	-	-	232	274
Time from ER Arrival to Discharge (minutes)[5]	-	-	121	134
Time in ER Before Being Evaluated (minutes)[5]	-	-	21	26
Time to Pain Meds for Fractures (minutes)[5]	-	-	46	57
Heart Attack Care				
Aspirin Given at Discharge[5]	-	-	100%	99%
Fibrinolytic Meds Within 30 Min. of Arrival[5]	-	-	-	54%
PCI Within 90 Minutes of Arrival[5]	-	-	98%	96%
Statin Prescribed at Discharge[5]	-	-	99%	98%
Heart Failure Care				
ACE Inhibitor or ARB for LVSD[3,7]	-	-	98%	97%
Discharge Instructions Given[1,3]	-	-	94%	94%
Evaluation of LVS Function[1,3]	-	-	97%	99%
Medicare Spending				
Medicare Spending per Patient (ratio)	-	-	0.91	0.98
Pneumonia Care				
Appropriate Initial Antibiotic Given[1]	-	-	94%	95%
Blood Culture Timing[1]	-	-	98%	98%
Pregnancy and Delivery Care				
Newborn Deliveries Scheduled Early[5]	-	-	6%	6%
Preventive Care				
Immunization for Influenza[1]	-	-	83%	90%
Immunization for Pneumonia	17	88%	89%	92%
Stroke Care				
Anticoagulation Therapy for Atrial Fibrillation[5]	-	-	97%	95%
Antithrombotic Therapy Timing[5]	-	-	98%	98%
Assessed for Rehabilitation[5]	-	-	98%	97%
Discharged on Antithrombotic Therapy[5]	-	-	99%	99%
Discharged on Statin Medication[5]	-	-	91%	94%
Thrombolytic Therapy Timing[5]	-	-	55%	66%
Venous Thromboembolism Prophylaxis[5]	-	-	93%	94%
Written Stroke Educational Materials Given[5]	-	-	84%	88%
Surgical Care Improvement Project				
Appropriate Beta Blocker Usage[5]	-	-	98%	98%
Appropriate VTP Within 24 Hours[5]	-	-	98%	98%
Controlled Postoperative Blood Glucose[5]	-	-	99%	97%
Perioperative Temperature Management[5]	-	-	99%	100%
Prophylactic Antibiotic Selection[5]	-	-	99%	99%
Prophylactic Antibiotic Selection (Outpatient)[5]	-	-	98%	98%
Prophylactic Antibiotic Stopped[5]	-	-	98%	98%
Prophylactic Antibiotic Timing[5]	-	-	98%	99%
Prophylactic Antibiotic Timing (Outpatient)[5]	-	-	97%	98%
Urinary Catheter Removal[5]	-	-	96%	97%
Survey of Patients' Hospital Experiences				
Area Around Room 'Always' Quiet at Night[5]	-	-	61%	61%
Doctors 'Always' Communicated Well[5]	-	-	83%	82%
Home Recovery Information Given[5]	-	-	88%	85%
Hospital Given 9 or 10 on 10 Point Scale[5]	-	-	73%	71%
Meds 'Always' Explained Before Given[5]	-	-	66%	64%
Nurses 'Always' Communicated Well[5]	-	-	80%	79%
Pain 'Always' Well Controlled[5]	-	-	72%	71%
Room and Bathroom 'Always' Clean[5]	-	-	77%	73%
Timely Help 'Always' Received[5]	-	-	73%	68%
Would Definitely Recommend Hospital[5]	-	-	74%	71%
Use of Medical Imaging				
Cardiac Imaging Stress Test before Surgery[7]	-	-	4.6%	5.3%
Combination Abdominal CT Scan[1]	-	-	7.3%	10.5%
Combination Brain/Sinus CT Scan[1]	-	-	1.7%	2.7%
Combination Chest CT Scan[1]	-	-	1.8%	2.7%
Follow-up Mammogram/Ultrasound[7]	-	-	8.2%	8.8%
Lumbar Spine MRI for Low Back Pain[1]	-	-	40.3%	37.2%

Bingham Memorial Hospital

98 Poplar Street
Blackfoot, ID 83221
Phone: 208-785-3804
Type: Critical Access Hospitals
Emergency Services: Yes
Ownership: Voluntary non-profit - Private

Measure	Cases	This Hosp.	State Avg.	U.S. Avg.
Blood Clot Prevention and Treatment				
Anticoagulation Overlap Therapy[1,3]	-	-	95%	93%
ICU Venous Thromboembolism Prophylaxis[3]	71	93%	92%	92%
Incidence of Potentially Preventable VTE[1,3]	-	-	11%	10%
UFH with Dosages/Platelet Monitoring[3,7]	-	-	99%	97%
Venous Thromboembolism Prophylaxis[3]	263	90%	87%	85%
Warfarin Therapy Discharge Instructions[1,3]	-	-	75%	75%
Chest Pain/Possible Heart Attack Care				
Aspirin Given Within 24 Hours of Arrival	-	-	96%	96%
Fibrinolytic Meds Within 30 Min. of Arrival	-	-	55%	58%
Average Time to ECG (minutes)	-	-	9	7
Average Time to Transfer (minutes)	-	-	62	60
Children's Asthma Care				
Received Home Management Plan of Care	-	-	-	88%
Received Reliever Medication	-	-	-	100%
Received Systemic Corticosteroids	-	-	-	100%
Emergency Department				
Admittance Decision Time (minutes)[2]	126	45	76	98
Head CT Results Within 45 Min. of Arrival	-	-	38%	57%
Patients Who Left ER Before Being Seen	-	-	1%	2%
Time from ER Arrival to Admit. (minutes)[2]	144	206	232	274
Time from ER Arrival to Discharge (minutes)	-	-	121	134
Time in ER Before Being Evaluated (minutes)	-	-	21	26
Time to Pain Meds for Fractures (minutes)	-	-	46	57
Heart Attack Care				
Aspirin Given at Discharge[5]	-	-	100%	99%
Fibrinolytic Meds Within 30 Min. of Arrival[5]	-	-	-	54%
PCI Within 90 Minutes of Arrival[5]	-	-	98%	96%
Statin Prescribed at Discharge[5]	-	-	99%	98%
Heart Failure Care				
ACE Inhibitor or ARB for LVSD[1]	-	-	98%	97%
Discharge Instructions Given	26	19%	94%	94%
Evaluation of LVS Function	35	74%	97%	99%
Medicare Spending				

NOTE: Hospital profiles are in alphabetical order by state, then city, then hospital within the city; Rankings exclude hospitals with less than 25 cases except for patient surveys which excludes hospitals with less than 100 cases; (a) 100-299 cases; (1) The number of cases/patients is too few to report; (2) Data submitted were based on a sample of cases/patients; (3) Results are based on a shorter time period than required; (4) Data suppressed by CMS for one or more quarters; (5) Results are not available for this reporting period; (6) Fewer than 100 patients completed the HCAHPS survey; (7) No cases met the criteria for this measure; (8) The lower limit of the confidence interval cannot be calculated if the number of observed infections equals zero; (9) No data are available from the state/territory for this reporting period; (10) The scores shown reflect fewer than 50 completed surveys; (11) There were discrepancies in the data collection process; (12) This measure does not apply to this hospital for this reporting period; (13) Results cannot be calculated for this reporting period; (14) The results for this state are combined with nearby states to protect confidentiality; Please refer to the User's Guide for a full explanation of data.

Measure	Cases	This Hosp.	State Avg.	U.S. Avg.
Medicare Spending per Patient (ratio)	-	-	0.91	0.98
Pneumonia Care				
Appropriate Initial Antibiotic Given	45	87%	94%	95%
Blood Culture Timing	37	81%	98%	98%
Pregnancy and Delivery Care				
Newborn Deliveries Scheduled Early[5]	-	-	6%	6%
Preventive Care				
Immunization for Influenza[2]	306	31%	83%	90%
Immunization for Pneumonia[2]	354	73%	89%	92%
Stroke Care				
Anticoagulation Therapy for Atrial Fibrillation[5]	-	-	97%	95%
Antithrombotic Therapy Timing[5]	-	-	98%	98%
Assessed for Rehabilitation[5]	-	-	98%	97%
Discharged on Antithrombotic Therapy[5]	-	-	99%	99%
Discharged on Statin Medication[5]	-	-	91%	94%
Thrombolytic Therapy Timing[5]	-	-	55%	66%
Venous Thromboembolism Prophylaxis[5]	-	-	93%	94%
Written Stroke Educational Materials Given[5]	-	-	84%	88%
Surgical Care Improvement Project				
Appropriate Beta Blocker Usage	38	89%	98%	98%
Appropriate VTP Within 24 Hours	187	92%	98%	98%
Controlled Postoperative Blood Glucose[7]	-	-	99%	97%
Perioperative Temperature Management	218	100%	99%	100%
Prophylactic Antibiotic Selection	166	97%	99%	99%
Prophylactic Antibiotic Selection (Outpatient)	-	-	98%	98%
Prophylactic Antibiotic Stopped	163	97%	98%	98%
Prophylactic Antibiotic Timing	166	90%	98%	99%
Prophylactic Antibiotic Timing (Outpatient)	-	-	97%	98%
Urinary Catheter Removal	140	89%	96%	97%
Survey of Patients' Hospital Experiences				
Area Around Room 'Always' Quiet at Night	300+	47%	61%	61%
Doctors 'Always' Communicated Well	300+	81%	83%	82%
Home Recovery Information Given	300+	88%	88%	85%
Hospital Given 9 or 10 on 10 Point Scale	300+	70%	73%	71%
Meds 'Always' Explained Before Given	300+	64%	66%	64%
Nurses 'Always' Communicated Well	300+	77%	80%	79%
Pain 'Always' Well Controlled	300+	71%	72%	71%
Room and Bathroom 'Always' Clean	300+	73%	77%	73%
Timely Help 'Always' Received	300+	69%	73%	68%
Would Definitely Recommend Hospital	300+	66%	74%	71%
Use of Medical Imaging				
Cardiac Imaging Stress Test before Surgery	-	-	4.6%	5.3%
Combination Abdominal CT Scan	-	-	7.3%	10.5%
Combination Brain/Sinus CT Scan	-	-	1.7%	2.7%
Combination Chest CT Scan	-	-	1.8%	2.7%
Follow-up Mammogram/Ultrasound	-	-	8.2%	8.8%
Lumbar Spine MRI for Low Back Pain	-	-	40.3%	37.2%

Idaho Doctors Hospital

350 North Meridian Street
Blackfoot, ID 83221
Type: Acute Care Hospitals
Ownership: Proprietary
Phone: 208-782-2900
Emergency Services: No

Measure	Cases	This Hosp.	State Avg.	U.S. Avg.
Blood Clot Prevention and Treatment				
Anticoagulation Overlap Therapy[7]	-	-	95%	93%
ICU Venous Thromboembolism Prophylaxis[7]	-	-	92%	92%
Incidence of Potentially Preventable VTE[7]	-	-	11%	10%
UFH with Dosages/Platelet Monitoring[7]	-	-	99%	97%
Venous Thromboembolism Prophylaxis	37	100%	87%	85%
Warfarin Therapy Discharge Instructions[7]	-	-	75%	75%
Chest Pain/Possible Heart Attack Care				
Aspirin Given Within 24 Hours of Arrival[5]	-	-	96%	96%
Fibrinolytic Meds Within 30 Min. of Arrival[5]	-	-	55%	58%
Average Time to ECG (minutes)[5]	-	-	9	7
Average Time to Transfer (minutes)[5]	-	-	62	60
Children's Asthma Care				
Received Home Management Plan of Care	-	-	-	88%
Received Reliever Medication	-	-	-	100%
Received Systemic Corticosteroids	-	-	-	100%
Emergency Department				
Admittance Decision Time (minutes)[7]	-	-	76	98
Head CT Results Within 45 Min. of Arrival[5]	-	-	38%	57%
Patients Who Left ER Before Being Seen[5]	-	-	1%	2%
Time from ER Arrival to Admit. (minutes)[7]	-	-	232	274
Time from ER Arrival to Discharge (minutes)[5]	-	-	121	134
Time in ER Before Being Evaluated (minutes)[5]	-	-	21	26
Time to Pain Meds for Fractures (minutes)[5]	-	-	46	57
Heart Attack Care				
Aspirin Given at Discharge[5]	-	-	100%	99%
Fibrinolytic Meds Within 30 Min. of Arrival[5]	-	-	-	54%
PCI Within 90 Minutes of Arrival[5]	-	-	98%	96%
Statin Prescribed at Discharge[5]	-	-	99%	98%
Heart Failure Care				
ACE Inhibitor or ARB for LVSD[5]	-	-	98%	97%
Discharge Instructions Given[5]	-	-	94%	94%
Evaluation of LVS Function[5]	-	-	97%	99%
Medicare Spending				
Medicare Spending per Patient (ratio)[1]	-	-	0.91	0.98
Pneumonia Care				
Appropriate Initial Antibiotic Given[5]	-	-	94%	95%
Blood Culture Timing[5]	-	-	98%	98%
Pregnancy and Delivery Care				
Newborn Deliveries Scheduled Early[7]	-	-	6%	6%
Preventive Care				
Immunization for Influenza	54	33%	83%	90%
Immunization for Pneumonia	20	90%	89%	92%
Stroke Care				
Anticoagulation Therapy for Atrial Fibrillation[5]	-	-	97%	95%
Antithrombotic Therapy Timing[5]	-	-	98%	98%
Assessed for Rehabilitation[5]	-	-	98%	97%
Discharged on Antithrombotic Therapy[5]	-	-	99%	99%
Discharged on Statin Medication[5]	-	-	91%	94%
Thrombolytic Therapy Timing[5]	-	-	55%	66%
Venous Thromboembolism Prophylaxis[5]	-	-	93%	94%
Written Stroke Educational Materials Given[5]	-	-	84%	88%
Surgical Care Improvement Project				
Appropriate Beta Blocker Usage[5]	-	-	98%	98%
Appropriate VTP Within 24 Hours[5]	-	-	98%	98%
Controlled Postoperative Blood Glucose[5]	-	-	99%	97%
Perioperative Temperature Management[5]	-	-	99%	100%
Prophylactic Antibiotic Selection[5]	-	-	99%	99%
Prophylactic Antibiotic Selection (Outpatient)	72	88%	98%	98%
Prophylactic Antibiotic Stopped[5]	-	-	98%	98%
Prophylactic Antibiotic Timing[5]	-	-	98%	99%
Prophylactic Antibiotic Timing (Outpatient)	72	86%	97%	98%
Urinary Catheter Removal[5]	-	-	96%	97%
Survey of Patients' Hospital Experiences				
Area Around Room 'Always' Quiet at Night[6]	<100	96%	61%	61%
Doctors 'Always' Communicated Well[6]	<100	90%	83%	82%
Home Recovery Information Given[6]	<100	88%	88%	85%
Hospital Given 9 or 10 on 10 Point Scale[6]	<100	99%	73%	71%
Meds 'Always' Explained Before Given[6]	<100	77%	66%	64%
Nurses 'Always' Communicated Well[6]	<100	97%	80%	79%
Pain 'Always' Well Controlled[6]	<100	85%	72%	71%
Room and Bathroom 'Always' Clean[6]	<100	90%	77%	73%
Timely Help 'Always' Received[6]	<100	97%	73%	68%
Would Definitely Recommend Hospital[6]	<100	100%	74%	71%
Use of Medical Imaging				
Cardiac Imaging Stress Test before Surgery[7]	-	-	4.6%	5.3%
Combination Abdominal CT Scan[7]	-	-	7.3%	10.5%
Combination Brain/Sinus CT Scan[7]	-	-	1.7%	2.7%
Combination Chest CT Scan[7]	-	-	1.8%	2.7%
Follow-up Mammogram/Ultrasound[7]	-	-	8.2%	8.8%
Lumbar Spine MRI for Low Back Pain[7]	-	-	40.3%	37.2%

Boise VA Medical Center

500 W. Fort Street
Boise, ID 83702
Type: Acute Care - VA
Ownership: Government Federal
Phone: 208-422-1000
Fax: 208-422-1326
Emergency Services: No
Beds: 176

Key Personnel:
Chief of Medical Staff.......... Paul M Lambert, MD
Emergency Room .... Anne Palma, MD
CEO/President............... Wayne C Tipets

Measure	Cases	This Hosp.	State Avg.	U.S. Avg.
Blood Clot Prevention and Treatment				
Anticoagulation Overlap Therapy	-	-	95%	93%
ICU Venous Thromboembolism Prophylaxis	-	-	92%	92%
Incidence of Potentially Preventable VTE	-	-	11%	10%
UFH with Dosages/Platelet Monitoring	-	-	99%	97%
Venous Thromboembolism Prophylaxis	-	-	87%	85%
Warfarin Therapy Discharge Instructions	-	-	75%	75%
Chest Pain/Possible Heart Attack Care				
Aspirin Given Within 24 Hours of Arrival	-	-	96%	96%
Fibrinolytic Meds Within 30 Min. of Arrival	-	-	55%	58%
Average Time to ECG (minutes)	-	-	9	7
Average Time to Transfer (minutes)	-	-	62	60
Children's Asthma Care				
Received Home Management Plan of Care	-	-	-	88%
Received Reliever Medication	-	-	-	100%
Received Systemic Corticosteroids	-	-	-	100%
Emergency Department				
Admittance Decision Time (minutes)	-	-	76	98
Head CT Results Within 45 Min. of Arrival	-	-	38%	57%
Patients Who Left ER Before Being Seen	-	-	1%	2%
Time from ER Arrival to Admit. (minutes)	-	-	232	274
Time from ER Arrival to Discharge (minutes)	-	-	121	134
Time in ER Before Being Evaluated (minutes)	-	-	21	26
Time to Pain Meds for Fractures (minutes)	-	-	46	57
Heart Attack Care				
Aspirin Given at Discharge[1]	15	100%	100%	99%
Fibrinolytic Meds Within 30 Min. of Arrival[5]	-	-	-	54%
PCI Within 90 Minutes of Arrival[5]	-	-	98%	96%
Statin Prescribed at Discharge[1]	16	100%	99%	98%
Heart Failure Care				
ACE Inhibitor or ARB for LVSD	31	100%	98%	97%
Discharge Instructions Given	96	89%	94%	94%
Evaluation of LVS Function	112	100%	97%	99%
Medicare Spending				
Medicare Spending per Patient (ratio)	-	-	0.91	0.98
Pneumonia Care				
Appropriate Initial Antibiotic Given	37	92%	94%	95%
Blood Culture Timing	89	99%	98%	98%
Pregnancy and Delivery Care				
Newborn Deliveries Scheduled Early	-	-	6%	6%
Preventive Care				
Immunization for Influenza[5]	-	-	83%	90%
Immunization for Pneumonia[5]	-	-	89%	92%
Stroke Care				
Anticoagulation Therapy for Atrial Fibrillation	-	-	97%	95%
Antithrombotic Therapy Timing	-	-	98%	98%
Assessed for Rehabilitation	-	-	98%	97%
Discharged on Antithrombotic Therapy	-	-	99%	99%
Discharged on Statin Medication	-	-	91%	94%
Thrombolytic Therapy Timing	-	-	55%	66%
Venous Thromboembolism Prophylaxis	-	-	93%	94%
Written Stroke Educational Materials Given	-	-	84%	88%
Surgical Care Improvement Project				
Appropriate Beta Blocker Usage[2]	70	96%	98%	98%
Appropriate VTP Within 24 Hours[2]	182	90%	98%	98%
Controlled Postoperative Blood Glucose[5]	-	-	99%	97%
Perioperative Temperature Management[2]	219	100%	99%	100%
Prophylactic Antibiotic Selection	131	100%	99%	99%
Prophylactic Antibiotic Selection (Outpatient)	-	-	98%	98%
Prophylactic Antibiotic Stopped	129	99%	98%	98%
Prophylactic Antibiotic Timing	131	99%	98%	99%
Prophylactic Antibiotic Timing (Outpatient)	-	-	97%	98%
Urinary Catheter Removal[2]	127	96%	96%	97%
Survey of Patients' Hospital Experiences				
Area Around Room 'Always' Quiet at Night	-	-	61%	61%
Doctors 'Always' Communicated Well	-	-	83%	82%
Home Recovery Information Given	-	-	88%	85%
Hospital Given 9 or 10 on 10 Point Scale	-	-	73%	71%
Meds 'Always' Explained Before Given	-	-	66%	64%
Nurses 'Always' Communicated Well	-	-	80%	79%
Pain 'Always' Well Controlled	-	-	72%	71%

NOTE: Hospital profiles are in alphabetical order by state, then city, then hospital within the city; Rankings exclude hospitals with less than 25 cases except for patient surveys which excludes hospitals with less than 100 cases; (a) 100-299 cases; (1) The number of cases/patients is too few to report; (2) Data submitted were based on a sample of cases/patients; (3) Results are based on a shorter time period than required; (4) Data suppressed by CMS for one or more quarters; (5) Results are not available for this reporting period; (6) Fewer than 100 patients completed the HCAHPS survey; (7) No cases met the criteria for this measure; (8) The lower limit of the confidence interval cannot be calculated if the number of observed infections equals zero; (9) No data are available from the state/territory for this reporting period; (10) The scores shown reflect fewer than 50 completed surveys; (11) There were discrepancies in the data collection process; (12) This measure does not apply to this hospital for this reporting period; (13) Results cannot be calculated for this reporting period; (14) The results for this state are combined with nearby states to protect confidentiality; Please refer to the User's Guide for a full explanation of data.

Measure	Cases	This Hosp.	State Avg.	U.S. Avg.
Room and Bathroom 'Always' Clean	-	-	77%	73%
Timely Help 'Always' Received	-	-	73%	68%
Would Definitely Recommend Hospital	-	-	74%	71%
Use of Medical Imaging				
Cardiac Imaging Stress Test before Surgery	-	-	4.6%	5.3%
Combination Abdominal CT Scan	-	-	7.3%	10.5%
Combination Brain/Sinus CT Scan	-	-	1.7%	2.7%
Combination Chest CT Scan	-	-	1.8%	2.7%
Follow-up Mammogram/Ultrasound	-	-	8.2%	8.8%
Lumbar Spine MRI for Low Back Pain	-	-	40.3%	37.2%

Saint Alphonsus Regional Medical Center

1055 North Curtis Road Phone: 208-367-2121
Boise, ID 83706 Fax: 208-367-3123
E-mail: inquiries@sarmc.org
URL: www.saintalphonsus.org
Type: Acute Care Hospitals Emergency Services: Yes
Ownership: Voluntary non-profit - Church Beds: 381

Key Personnel:
CEO/President. . . . . Sandra Bennett Bruce
Radiology. . . . . Carolyn E Coffman
Chief of Medical Staff. . . . . Gary Goldberg

Measure	Cases	This Hosp.	State Avg.	U.S. Avg.
Blood Clot Prevention and Treatment				
Anticoagulation Overlap Therapy[2]	125	100%	95%	93%
ICU Venous Thromboembolism Prophylaxis[2]	89	94%	92%	92%
Incidence of Potentially Preventable VTE[2]	51	0%	11%	10%
UFH with Dosages/Platelet Monitoring[2]	50	98%	99%	97%
Venous Thromboembolism Prophylaxis[2]	216	90%	87%	85%
Warfarin Therapy Discharge Instructions[2]	101	44%	75%	75%
Chest Pain/Possible Heart Attack Care				
Aspirin Given Within 24 Hours of Arrival[1]	-	-	96%	96%
Fibrinolytic Meds Within 30 Min. of Arrival[3,7]	-	-	55%	58%
Average Time to ECG (minutes)[1]	-	-	9	7
Average Time to Transfer (minutes)[3,7]	-	-	62	60
Children's Asthma Care				
Received Home Management Plan of Care	-	-	-	88%
Received Reliever Medication	-	-	-	100%
Received Systemic Corticosteroids	-	-	-	100%
Emergency Department				
Admittance Decision Time (minutes)[2]	474	118	76	98
Head CT Results Within 45 Min. of Arrival[1]	-	-	38%	57%
Patients Who Left ER Before Being Seen	54,071	1%	1%	2%
Time from ER Arrival to Admit. (minutes)[2]	474	279	232	274
Time from ER Arrival to Discharge (minutes)	338	132	121	134
Time in ER Before Being Evaluated (minutes)	80	27	21	26
Time to Pain Meds for Fractures (minutes)	232	46	46	57
Heart Attack Care				
Aspirin Given at Discharge	335	99%	100%	99%
Fibrinolytic Meds Within 30 Min. of Arrival[7]	-	-	-	54%
PCI Within 90 Minutes of Arrival	49	98%	98%	96%
Statin Prescribed at Discharge	324	99%	99%	98%
Heart Failure Care				
ACE Inhibitor or ARB for LVSD	47	98%	98%	97%
Discharge Instructions Given	162	98%	94%	94%
Evaluation of LVS Function	201	99%	97%	99%
Medicare Spending				
Medicare Spending per Patient (ratio)	-	0.94	0.91	0.98
Pneumonia Care				
Appropriate Initial Antibiotic Given	144	97%	94%	95%
Blood Culture Timing	258	100%	98%	98%
Pregnancy and Delivery Care				
Newborn Deliveries Scheduled Early[2]	104	1%	6%	6%
Preventive Care				
Immunization for Influenza[2]	553	95%	83%	90%
Immunization for Pneumonia[2]	593	88%	89%	92%
Stroke Care				
Anticoagulation Therapy for Atrial Fibrillation[2]	22	100%	97%	95%
Antithrombotic Therapy Timing[2]	114	100%	98%	98%
Assessed for Rehabilitation[2]	180	100%	98%	97%
Discharged on Antithrombotic Therapy[2]	150	100%	99%	99%
Discharged on Statin Medication[2]	118	97%	91%	94%
Thrombolytic Therapy Timing[1,2]	-	-	55%	66%
Venous Thromboembolism Prophylaxis[2]	183	99%	93%	94%
Written Stroke Educational Materials Given[2]	92	84%	84%	88%
Surgical Care Improvement Project				
Appropriate Beta Blocker Usage[2]	325	99%	98%	98%
Appropriate VTP Within 24 Hours[2]	922	97%	98%	98%
Controlled Postoperative Blood Glucose[2]	136	100%	99%	97%
Perioperative Temperature Management[2]	1,170	99%	99%	100%
Prophylactic Antibiotic Selection[2]	1,131	99%	99%	99%
Prophylactic Antibiotic Selection (Outpatient)	950	98%	98%	98%
Prophylactic Antibiotic Stopped[2]	1,120	99%	98%	98%
Prophylactic Antibiotic Timing[2]	1,132	99%	98%	99%
Prophylactic Antibiotic Timing (Outpatient)	953	99%	97%	98%
Urinary Catheter Removal[2]	968	98%	96%	97%
Survey of Patients' Hospital Experiences				
Area Around Room 'Always' Quiet at Night	300+	58%	61%	61%
Doctors 'Always' Communicated Well	300+	79%	83%	82%
Home Recovery Information Given	300+	88%	88%	85%
Hospital Given 9 or 10 on 10 Point Scale	300+	71%	73%	71%
Meds 'Always' Explained Before Given	300+	58%	66%	64%
Nurses 'Always' Communicated Well	300+	72%	80%	79%
Pain 'Always' Well Controlled	300+	67%	72%	71%
Room and Bathroom 'Always' Clean	300+	68%	77%	73%
Timely Help 'Always' Received	300+	60%	73%	68%
Would Definitely Recommend Hospital	300+	74%	74%	71%
Use of Medical Imaging				
Cardiac Imaging Stress Test before Surgery	722	4.8%	4.6%	5.3%
Combination Abdominal CT Scan	885	3.5%	7.3%	10.5%
Combination Brain/Sinus CT Scan	471	0.2%	1.7%	2.7%
Combination Chest CT Scan	605	1.7%	1.8%	2.7%
Follow-up Mammogram/Ultrasound	1,860	8.9%	8.2%	8.8%
Lumbar Spine MRI for Low Back Pain[1]	-	-	40.3%	37.2%

Saint Luke's Regional Medical Center

190 East Bannock Street Phone: 208-381-2222
Boise, ID 83712 Fax: 208-381-2861
URL: www.slrmc.org
Type: Acute Care Hospitals Emergency Services: Yes
Ownership: Voluntary non-profit - Private Beds: 403

Key Personnel:
Operating Room. . . . . Sherry Daniels-Boyer, RN
CEO/President. . . . . Gary Fletcher
Cardiac Laboratory. . . . . Stefanie Fry, MD
Pediatrics. . . . . Susan Kim, MD
Radiology. . . . . Peter Langhus, MD
Chief of Medical Staff. . . . . Leslie Nona, MD
Quality Assurance . . . . Brian Schreek
Surgery . . . . Mark Szentes, MD

Measure	Cases	This Hosp.	State Avg.	U.S. Avg.
Blood Clot Prevention and Treatment				
Anticoagulation Overlap Therapy[2]	208	99%	95%	93%
ICU Venous Thromboembolism Prophylaxis[2]	80	99%	92%	92%
Incidence of Potentially Preventable VTE[2]	34	3%	11%	10%
UFH with Dosages/Platelet Monitoring[2]	67	100%	99%	97%
Venous Thromboembolism Prophylaxis[2]	270	91%	87%	85%
Warfarin Therapy Discharge Instructions[2]	176	88%	75%	75%
Chest Pain/Possible Heart Attack Care				
Aspirin Given Within 24 Hours of Arrival[1]	-	-	96%	96%
Fibrinolytic Meds Within 30 Min. of Arrival[5]	-	-	55%	58%
Average Time to ECG (minutes)[1]	-	-	9	7
Average Time to Transfer (minutes)[5]	-	-	62	60
Children's Asthma Care				
Received Home Management Plan of Care	72	93%	-	88%
Received Reliever Medication	73	100%	-	100%
Received Systemic Corticosteroids	72	100%	-	100%
Emergency Department				
Admittance Decision Time (minutes)[2]	413	86	76	98
Head CT Results Within 45 Min. of Arrival[1]	-	-	38%	57%
Patients Who Left ER Before Being Seen	99,053	1%	1%	2%
Time from ER Arrival to Admit. (minutes)[2]	415	254	232	274
Time from ER Arrival to Discharge (minutes)	420	120	121	134
Time in ER Before Being Evaluated (minutes)	441	28	21	26
Time to Pain Meds for Fractures (minutes)	381	42	46	57
Heart Attack Care				
Aspirin Given at Discharge[2]	368	100%	100%	99%
Fibrinolytic Meds Within 30 Min. of Arrival[2,7]	-	-	-	54%
PCI Within 90 Minutes of Arrival[2]	61	98%	98%	96%
Statin Prescribed at Discharge[2]	356	100%	99%	98%
Heart Failure Care				
ACE Inhibitor or ARB for LVSD[2]	96	100%	98%	97%
Discharge Instructions Given[2]	317	97%	94%	94%
Evaluation of LVS Function[2]	380	100%	97%	99%
Medicare Spending				
Medicare Spending per Patient (ratio)	-	0.96	0.91	0.98
Pneumonia Care				
Appropriate Initial Antibiotic Given[2]	127	99%	94%	95%
Blood Culture Timing[2]	213	100%	98%	98%
Pregnancy and Delivery Care				
Newborn Deliveries Scheduled Early[2]	75	4%	6%	6%
Preventive Care				
Immunization for Influenza[2]	639	97%	83%	90%
Immunization for Pneumonia[2]	611	95%	89%	92%
Stroke Care				
Anticoagulation Therapy for Atrial Fibrillation	26	100%	97%	95%
Antithrombotic Therapy Timing	190	100%	98%	98%
Assessed for Rehabilitation	270	99%	98%	97%
Discharged on Antithrombotic Therapy	239	100%	99%	99%
Discharged on Statin Medication	183	98%	91%	94%
Thrombolytic Therapy Timing	17	88%	55%	66%
Venous Thromboembolism Prophylaxis	252	98%	93%	94%
Written Stroke Educational Materials Given	162	93%	84%	88%
Surgical Care Improvement Project				
Appropriate Beta Blocker Usage[2]	224	99%	98%	98%
Appropriate VTP Within 24 Hours[2]	458	98%	98%	98%
Controlled Postoperative Blood Glucose[2]	150	99%	99%	97%
Perioperative Temperature Management[2]	623	100%	99%	100%
Prophylactic Antibiotic Selection[2]	521	99%	99%	99%
Prophylactic Antibiotic Selection (Outpatient)	959	99%	98%	98%
Prophylactic Antibiotic Stopped[2]	518	99%	98%	98%
Prophylactic Antibiotic Timing[2]	521	99%	98%	99%
Prophylactic Antibiotic Timing (Outpatient)	849	97%	97%	98%
Urinary Catheter Removal[2]	521	98%	96%	97%
Survey of Patients' Hospital Experiences				
Area Around Room 'Always' Quiet at Night	300+	59%	61%	61%
Doctors 'Always' Communicated Well	300+	83%	83%	82%
Home Recovery Information Given	300+	89%	88%	85%
Hospital Given 9 or 10 on 10 Point Scale	300+	77%	73%	71%
Meds 'Always' Explained Before Given	300+	67%	66%	64%
Nurses 'Always' Communicated Well	300+	80%	80%	79%
Pain 'Always' Well Controlled	300+	74%	72%	71%
Room and Bathroom 'Always' Clean	300+	77%	77%	73%
Timely Help 'Always' Received	300+	68%	73%	68%
Would Definitely Recommend Hospital	300+	84%	74%	71%
Use of Medical Imaging				
Cardiac Imaging Stress Test before Surgery	727	4.8%	4.6%	5.3%
Combination Abdominal CT Scan	2,383	7.5%	7.3%	10.5%
Combination Brain/Sinus CT Scan	950	1.6%	1.7%	2.7%
Combination Chest CT Scan	1,646	0.9%	1.8%	2.7%
Follow-up Mammogram/Ultrasound	5,826	8.4%	8.2%	8.8%
Lumbar Spine MRI for Low Back Pain	303	37.3%	40.3%	37.2%

Treasure Valley Hospital

8800 West Emerald Street Phone: 208-373-5000
Boise, ID 83704
URL: www.treasurevalleyhospital.com
Type: Acute Care Hospitals Emergency Services: No
Ownership: Proprietary

Key Personnel:
Administrator . . . . Michael Long

Measure	Cases	This Hosp.	State Avg.	U.S. Avg.
Blood Clot Prevention and Treatment				
Anticoagulation Overlap Therapy[7]	-	-	95%	93%
ICU Venous Thromboembolism Prophylaxis[7]	-	-	92%	92%
Incidence of Potentially Preventable VTE[7]	-	-	11%	10%
UFH with Dosages/Platelet Monitoring[7]	-	-	99%	97%
Venous Thromboembolism Prophylaxis	159	100%	87%	85%
Warfarin Therapy Discharge Instructions[7]	-	-	75%	75%
Chest Pain/Possible Heart Attack Care				

NOTE: Hospital profiles are in alphabetical order by state, then city, then hospital within the city; Rankings exclude hospitals with less than 25 cases except for patient surveys which excludes hospitals with less than 100 cases; (a) 100-299 cases; (1) The number of cases/patients is too few to report; (2) Data submitted were based on a sample of cases/patients; (3) Results are based on a shorter time period than required; (4) Data suppressed by CMS for one or more quarters; (5) Results are not available for this reporting period; (6) Fewer than 100 patients completed the HCAHPS survey; (7) No cases met the criteria for this measure; (8) The lower limit of the confidence interval cannot be calculated if the number of observed infections equals zero; (9) No data are available from the state/territory for this reporting period; (10) The scores shown reflect fewer than 50 completed surveys; (11) There were discrepancies in the data collection process; (12) This measure does not apply to this hospital for this reporting period; (13) Results cannot be calculated for this reporting period; (14) The results for this state are combined with nearby states to protect confidentiality; Please refer to the User's Guide for a full explanation of data.

Measure	Cases	This Hosp.	State Avg.	U.S. Avg.
Aspirin Given Within 24 Hours of Arrival[5]	-	-	96%	96%
Fibrinolytic Meds Within 30 Min. of Arrival[5]	-	-	55%	58%
Average Time to ECG (minutes)[5]	-	-	9	7
Average Time to Transfer (minutes)[5]	-	-	62	60
Children's Asthma Care				
Received Home Management Plan of Care	-	-	-	88%
Received Reliever Medication	-	-	-	100%
Received Systemic Corticosteroids	-	-	-	100%
Emergency Department				
Admittance Decision Time (minutes)[7]	-	-	76	98
Head CT Results Within 45 Min. of Arrival[5]	-	-	38%	57%
Patients Who Left ER Before Being Seen[5]	-	-	1%	2%
Time from ER Arrival to Admit. (minutes)[7]	-	-	232	274
Time from ER Arrival to Discharge (minutes)[5]	-	-	121	134
Time in ER Before Being Evaluated (minutes)[5]	-	-	21	26
Time to Pain Meds for Fractures (minutes)[5]	-	-	46	57
Heart Attack Care				
Aspirin Given at Discharge[5]	-	-	100%	99%
Fibrinolytic Meds Within 30 Min. of Arrival[5]	-	-	-	54%
PCI Within 90 Minutes of Arrival[5]	-	-	98%	96%
Statin Prescribed at Discharge[5]	-	-	99%	98%
Heart Failure Care				
ACE Inhibitor or ARB for LVSD[5]	-	-	98%	97%
Discharge Instructions Given[5]	-	-	94%	94%
Evaluation of LVS Function[5]	-	-	97%	99%
Medicare Spending				
Medicare Spending per Patient (ratio)	-	0.83	0.91	0.98
Pneumonia Care				
Appropriate Initial Antibiotic Given[5]	-	-	94%	95%
Blood Culture Timing[5]	-	-	98%	98%
Pregnancy and Delivery Care				
Newborn Deliveries Scheduled Early[7]	-	-	6%	6%
Preventive Care				
Immunization for Influenza	194	55%	83%	90%
Immunization for Pneumonia	196	71%	89%	92%
Stroke Care				
Anticoagulation Therapy for Atrial Fibrillation[5]	-	-	97%	95%
Antithrombotic Therapy Timing[5]	-	-	98%	98%
Assessed for Rehabilitation[5]	-	-	98%	97%
Discharged on Antithrombotic Therapy[5]	-	-	99%	99%
Discharged on Statin Medication[5]	-	-	91%	94%
Thrombolytic Therapy Timing[5]	-	-	55%	66%
Venous Thromboembolism Prophylaxis[5]	-	-	93%	94%
Written Stroke Educational Materials Given[5]	-	-	84%	88%
Surgical Care Improvement Project				
Appropriate Beta Blocker Usage[1]	-	-	98%	98%
Appropriate VTP Within 24 Hours	26	96%	98%	98%
Controlled Postoperative Blood Glucose[7]	-	-	99%	97%
Perioperative Temperature Management	38	100%	99%	100%
Prophylactic Antibiotic Selection	35	89%	99%	99%
Prophylactic Antibiotic Selection (Outpatient)	153	99%	98%	98%
Prophylactic Antibiotic Stopped	35	91%	98%	98%
Prophylactic Antibiotic Timing	35	97%	98%	99%
Prophylactic Antibiotic Timing (Outpatient)	153	97%	97%	98%
Urinary Catheter Removal	14	100%	96%	97%
Survey of Patients' Hospital Experiences				
Area Around Room 'Always' Quiet at Night	300+	78%	61%	61%
Doctors 'Always' Communicated Well	300+	81%	83%	82%
Home Recovery Information Given	300+	90%	88%	85%
Hospital Given 9 or 10 on 10 Point Scale	300+	87%	73%	71%
Meds 'Always' Explained Before Given	300+	75%	66%	64%
Nurses 'Always' Communicated Well	300+	88%	80%	79%
Pain 'Always' Well Controlled	300+	84%	72%	71%
Room and Bathroom 'Always' Clean	300+	82%	77%	73%
Timely Help 'Always' Received	300+	88%	73%	68%
Would Definitely Recommend Hospital	300+	87%	74%	71%
Use of Medical Imaging				
Cardiac Imaging Stress Test before Surgery[7]	-	-	4.6%	5.3%
Combination Abdominal CT Scan[7]	-	-	7.3%	10.5%
Combination Brain/Sinus CT Scan[7]	-	-	1.7%	2.7%
Combination Chest CT Scan[7]	-	-	1.8%	2.7%
Follow-up Mammogram/Ultrasound[7]	-	-	8.2%	8.8%
Lumbar Spine MRI for Low Back Pain[1]	-	-	40.3%	37.2%

Boundary Community Hospital

6640 Kaniksu Street Phone: 208-267-4850
Bonners Ferry, ID 83805
Type: Critical Access Hospitals Emergency Services: Yes
Ownership: Voluntary non-profit - Other

Measure	Cases	This Hosp.	State Avg.	U.S. Avg.
Blood Clot Prevention and Treatment				
Anticoagulation Overlap Therapy[5]	-	-	95%	93%
ICU Venous Thromboembolism Prophylaxis[5]	-	-	92%	92%
Incidence of Potentially Preventable VTE[5]	-	-	11%	10%
UFH with Dosages/Platelet Monitoring[5]	-	-	99%	97%
Venous Thromboembolism Prophylaxis[5]	-	-	87%	85%
Warfarin Therapy Discharge Instructions[5]	-	-	75%	75%
Chest Pain/Possible Heart Attack Care				
Aspirin Given Within 24 Hours of Arrival	-	-	96%	96%
Fibrinolytic Meds Within 30 Min. of Arrival	-	-	55%	58%
Average Time to ECG (minutes)	-	-	9	7
Average Time to Transfer (minutes)	-	-	62	60
Children's Asthma Care				
Received Home Management Plan of Care	-	-	-	88%
Received Reliever Medication	-	-	-	100%
Received Systemic Corticosteroids	-	-	-	100%
Emergency Department				
Admittance Decision Time (minutes)[5]	-	-	76	98
Head CT Results Within 45 Min. of Arrival	-	-	38%	57%
Patients Who Left ER Before Being Seen	-	-	1%	2%
Time from ER Arrival to Admit. (minutes)[5]	-	-	232	274
Time from ER Arrival to Discharge (minutes)	-	-	121	134
Time in ER Before Being Evaluated (minutes)	-	-	21	26
Time to Pain Meds for Fractures (minutes)	-	-	46	57
Heart Attack Care				
Aspirin Given at Discharge[5]	-	-	100%	99%
Fibrinolytic Meds Within 30 Min. of Arrival[5]	-	-	-	54%
PCI Within 90 Minutes of Arrival[5]	-	-	98%	96%
Statin Prescribed at Discharge[5]	-	-	99%	98%
Heart Failure Care				
ACE Inhibitor or ARB for LVSD[5]	-	-	98%	97%
Discharge Instructions Given[5]	-	-	94%	94%
Evaluation of LVS Function[5]	-	-	97%	99%
Medicare Spending				
Medicare Spending per Patient (ratio)	-	-	0.91	0.98
Pneumonia Care				
Appropriate Initial Antibiotic Given[1,3]	-	-	94%	95%
Blood Culture Timing[1,3]	-	-	98%	98%
Pregnancy and Delivery Care				
Newborn Deliveries Scheduled Early[5]	-	-	6%	6%
Preventive Care				
Immunization for Influenza[5]	-	-	83%	90%
Immunization for Pneumonia[5]	-	-	89%	92%
Stroke Care				
Anticoagulation Therapy for Atrial Fibrillation[5]	-	-	97%	95%
Antithrombotic Therapy Timing[5]	-	-	98%	98%
Assessed for Rehabilitation[5]	-	-	98%	97%
Discharged on Antithrombotic Therapy[5]	-	-	99%	99%
Discharged on Statin Medication[5]	-	-	91%	94%
Thrombolytic Therapy Timing[5]	-	-	55%	66%
Venous Thromboembolism Prophylaxis[5]	-	-	93%	94%
Written Stroke Educational Materials Given[5]	-	-	84%	88%
Surgical Care Improvement Project				
Appropriate Beta Blocker Usage[5]	-	-	98%	98%
Appropriate VTP Within 24 Hours[5]	-	-	98%	98%
Controlled Postoperative Blood Glucose[5]	-	-	99%	97%
Perioperative Temperature Management[5]	-	-	99%	100%
Prophylactic Antibiotic Selection[5]	-	-	99%	99%
Prophylactic Antibiotic Selection (Outpatient)	-	-	98%	98%
Prophylactic Antibiotic Stopped[5]	-	-	98%	98%
Prophylactic Antibiotic Timing[5]	-	-	98%	99%
Prophylactic Antibiotic Timing (Outpatient)	-	-	97%	98%
Urinary Catheter Removal[5]	-	-	96%	97%
Survey of Patients' Hospital Experiences				
Area Around Room 'Always' Quiet at Night[5]	-	-	61%	61%
Doctors 'Always' Communicated Well[5]	-	-	83%	82%
Home Recovery Information Given[5]	-	-	88%	85%
Hospital Given 9 or 10 on 10 Point Scale[5]	-	-	73%	71%
Meds 'Always' Explained Before Given[5]	-	-	66%	64%
Nurses 'Always' Communicated Well[5]	-	-	80%	79%
Pain 'Always' Well Controlled[5]	-	-	72%	71%
Room and Bathroom 'Always' Clean[5]	-	-	77%	73%
Timely Help 'Always' Received[5]	-	-	73%	68%
Would Definitely Recommend Hospital[5]	-	-	74%	71%
Use of Medical Imaging				
Cardiac Imaging Stress Test before Surgery	-	-	4.6%	5.3%
Combination Abdominal CT Scan	-	-	7.3%	10.5%
Combination Brain/Sinus CT Scan	-	-	1.7%	2.7%
Combination Chest CT Scan	-	-	1.8%	2.7%
Follow-up Mammogram/Ultrasound	-	-	8.2%	8.8%
Lumbar Spine MRI for Low Back Pain	-	-	40.3%	37.2%

Cassia Regional Medical Center

1501 Hiland Avenue Phone: 208-678-4444
Burley, ID 83318 Fax: 208-677-6555
URL: www.ihc.com
Type: Critical Access Hospitals Emergency Services: Yes
Ownership: Voluntary non-profit - Private Beds: 38

Key Personnel:
Radiology. . . . . Wayne D Adams, MD
Emergency Room . . . . Matthew Ahern
Administrator . . . . Rod Barton
Quality Assurance . . . . Nancy Gerrard
Chair/CEO. . . . . Clay Handy
Operating Room. . . . . Victor Varela, RN
Chief of Medical Staff . . . . Frederick Wood

Measure	Cases	This Hosp.	State Avg.	U.S. Avg.
Blood Clot Prevention and Treatment				
Anticoagulation Overlap Therapy[2]	19	74%	95%	93%
ICU Venous Thromboembolism Prophylaxis[2]	45	91%	92%	92%
Incidence of Potentially Preventable VTE[1,2]	-	-	11%	10%
UFH with Dosages/Platelet Monitoring[2]	18	100%	99%	97%
Venous Thromboembolism Prophylaxis[2]	70	83%	87%	85%
Warfarin Therapy Discharge Instructions[2]	14	57%	75%	75%
Chest Pain/Possible Heart Attack Care				
Aspirin Given Within 24 Hours of Arrival	45	96%	96%	96%
Fibrinolytic Meds Within 30 Min. of Arrival[7]	-	-	55%	58%
Average Time to ECG (minutes)	44	15	9	7
Average Time to Transfer (minutes)[1]	-	-	62	60
Children's Asthma Care				
Received Home Management Plan of Care	-	-	-	88%
Received Reliever Medication	-	-	-	100%
Received Systemic Corticosteroids	-	-	-	100%
Emergency Department				
Admittance Decision Time (minutes)[2]	119	77	76	98
Head CT Results Within 45 Min. of Arrival[1]	-	-	38%	57%
Patients Who Left ER Before Being Seen	11,770	1%	1%	2%
Time from ER Arrival to Admit. (minutes)[2]	153	253	232	274
Time from ER Arrival to Discharge (minutes)	384	130	121	134
Time in ER Before Being Evaluated (minutes)	381	23	21	26
Time to Pain Meds for Fractures (minutes)	61	46	46	57
Heart Attack Care				
Aspirin Given at Discharge[1,3]	-	-	100%	99%
Fibrinolytic Meds Within 30 Min. of Arrival[3,7]	-	-	-	54%
PCI Within 90 Minutes of Arrival[3,7]	-	-	98%	96%
Statin Prescribed at Discharge[1,3]	-	-	99%	98%
Heart Failure Care				
ACE Inhibitor or ARB for LVSD[1]	-	-	98%	97%
Discharge Instructions Given	17	88%	94%	94%
Evaluation of LVS Function	22	100%	97%	99%
Medicare Spending				
Medicare Spending per Patient (ratio)	-	-	0.91	0.98
Pneumonia Care				
Appropriate Initial Antibiotic Given	21	81%	94%	95%
Blood Culture Timing	36	100%	98%	98%
Pregnancy and Delivery Care				
Newborn Deliveries Scheduled Early[2,3]	16	0%	6%	6%
Preventive Care				

NOTE: Hospital profiles are in alphabetical order by state, then city, then hospital within the city; Rankings exclude hospitals with less than 25 cases except for patient surveys which excludes hospitals with less than 100 cases; (a) 100-299 cases; (1) The number of cases/patients is too few to report; (2) Data submitted were based on a sample of cases/patients; (3) Results are based on a shorter time period than required; (4) Data suppressed by CMS for one or more quarters; (5) Results are not available for this reporting period; (6) Fewer than 100 patients completed the HCAHPS survey; (7) No cases met the criteria for this measure; (8) The lower limit of the confidence interval cannot be calculated if the number of observed infections equals zero; (9) No data are available from the state/territory for this reporting period; (10) The scores shown reflect fewer than 50 completed surveys; (11) There were discrepancies in the data collection process; (12) This measure does not apply to this hospital for this reporting period; (13) Results cannot be calculated for this reporting period; (14) The results for this state are combined with nearby states to protect confidentiality; Please refer to the User's Guide for a full explanation of data.

Immunization for Influenza[2]	223	94%	83%	90%
Immunization for Pneumonia[2]	175	86%	89%	92%
Stroke Care				
Anticoagulation Therapy for Atrial Fibrillation[1]	-	-	97%	95%
Antithrombotic Therapy Timing[1]	-	-	98%	98%
Assessed for Rehabilitation[1]	-	-	98%	97%
Discharged on Antithrombotic Therapy[1]	-	-	99%	99%
Discharged on Statin Medication[1]	-	-	91%	94%
Thrombolytic Therapy Timing[7]	-	-	55%	66%
Venous Thromboembolism Prophylaxis[1]	-	-	93%	94%
Written Stroke Educational Materials Given[1]	-	-	84%	88%
Surgical Care Improvement Project				
Appropriate Beta Blocker Usage[2]	22	95%	98%	98%
Appropriate VTP Within 24 Hours[2]	101	97%	98%	98%
Controlled Postoperative Blood Glucose[2,7]	-	-	99%	97%
Perioperative Temperature Management[2]	116	99%	99%	100%
Prophylactic Antibiotic Selection[2]	98	99%	99%	99%
Prophylactic Antibiotic Selection (Outpatient)	16	94%	98%	98%
Prophylactic Antibiotic Stopped[2]	98	91%	98%	98%
Prophylactic Antibiotic Timing[2]	98	99%	98%	99%
Prophylactic Antibiotic Timing (Outpatient)	20	75%	97%	98%
Urinary Catheter Removal[2]	69	84%	96%	97%
Survey of Patients' Hospital Experiences				
Area Around Room 'Always' Quiet at Night	(a)	58%	61%	61%
Doctors 'Always' Communicated Well	(a)	85%	83%	82%
Home Recovery Information Given	(a)	91%	88%	85%
Hospital Given 9 or 10 on 10 Point Scale	(a)	72%	73%	71%
Meds 'Always' Explained Before Given	(a)	70%	66%	64%
Nurses 'Always' Communicated Well	(a)	79%	80%	79%
Pain 'Always' Well Controlled	(a)	75%	72%	71%
Room and Bathroom 'Always' Clean	(a)	70%	77%	73%
Timely Help 'Always' Received	(a)	71%	73%	68%
Would Definitely Recommend Hospital	(a)	70%	74%	71%
Use of Medical Imaging				
Cardiac Imaging Stress Test before Surgery	67	7.5%	4.6%	5.3%
Combination Abdominal CT Scan	178	4.5%	7.3%	10.5%
Combination Brain/Sinus CT Scan[1]	-	-	1.7%	2.7%
Combination Chest CT Scan	86	1.2%	1.8%	2.7%
Follow-up Mammogram/Ultrasound	339	14.2%	8.2%	8.8%
Lumbar Spine MRI for Low Back Pain	71	40.8%	40.3%	37.2%

West Valley Medical Center

1717 Arlington Street
Caldwell, ID 83605
Phone: 208-459-4641
Fax: 208-455-3717
URL: www.westvalleymedctr.com
Type: Acute Care Hospitals
Emergency Services: Yes
Ownership: Proprietary
Beds: 150

Key Personnel:
Operating Room. . . . . Jon Agee
Radiology. . . . . Carolyn Coffman
CEO/President. . . . . Kathy D Moore
Emergency Room . . . . J Mullins, MD
Quality Assurance . . . . Jana Willis

Measure	Cases	This Hosp.	State Avg.	U.S. Avg.
Blood Clot Prevention and Treatment				
Anticoagulation Overlap Therapy[2]	33	100%	95%	93%
ICU Venous Thromboembolism Prophylaxis[2]	67	100%	92%	92%
Incidence of Potentially Preventable VTE[1,2]	-	-	11%	10%
UFH with Dosages/Platelet Monitoring[2]	12	100%	99%	97%
Venous Thromboembolism Prophylaxis[2]	232	98%	87%	85%
Warfarin Therapy Discharge Instructions[2]	29	100%	75%	75%
Chest Pain/Possible Heart Attack Care				
Aspirin Given Within 24 Hours of Arrival[3]	30	100%	96%	96%
Fibrinolytic Meds Within 30 Min. of Arrival[3,7]	-	-	55%	58%
Average Time to ECG (minutes)[3]	31	8	9	7
Average Time to Transfer (minutes)[3]	11	35	62	60
Children's Asthma Care				
Received Home Management Plan of Care	-	-	-	88%
Received Reliever Medication	-	-	-	100%
Received Systemic Corticosteroids	-	-	-	100%
Emergency Department				
Admittance Decision Time (minutes)[2]	547	70	76	98
Head CT Results Within 45 Min. of Arrival	12	50%	38%	57%
Patients Who Left ER Before Being Seen	34,563	0%	1%	2%
Time from ER Arrival to Admit. (minutes)[2]	547	227	232	274
Time from ER Arrival to Discharge (minutes)	463	130	121	134
Time in ER Before Being Evaluated (minutes)	497	16	21	26
Time to Pain Meds for Fractures (minutes)	127	50	46	57
Heart Attack Care				
Aspirin Given at Discharge	27	100%	100%	99%
Fibrinolytic Meds Within 30 Min. of Arrival[7]	-	-	-	54%
PCI Within 90 Minutes of Arrival[7]	-	-	98%	96%
Statin Prescribed at Discharge	23	100%	99%	98%
Heart Failure Care				
ACE Inhibitor or ARB for LVSD	14	100%	98%	97%
Discharge Instructions Given	70	99%	94%	94%
Evaluation of LVS Function	77	100%	97%	99%
Medicare Spending				
Medicare Spending per Patient (ratio)	-	0.90	0.91	0.98
Pneumonia Care				
Appropriate Initial Antibiotic Given	93	99%	94%	95%
Blood Culture Timing	128	100%	98%	98%
Pregnancy and Delivery Care				
Newborn Deliveries Scheduled Early	70	4%	6%	6%
Preventive Care				
Immunization for Influenza[2]	440	92%	83%	90%
Immunization for Pneumonia[2]	560	97%	89%	92%
Stroke Care				
Anticoagulation Therapy for Atrial Fibrillation[2,7]	-	-	97%	95%
Antithrombotic Therapy Timing[2]	19	100%	98%	98%
Assessed for Rehabilitation[2]	29	100%	98%	97%
Discharged on Antithrombotic Therapy[2]	28	100%	99%	99%
Discharged on Statin Medication[2]	18	94%	91%	94%
Thrombolytic Therapy Timing[2,7]	-	-	55%	66%
Venous Thromboembolism Prophylaxis[2]	18	100%	93%	94%
Written Stroke Educational Materials Given[2]	24	100%	84%	88%
Surgical Care Improvement Project				
Appropriate Beta Blocker Usage[2]	70	100%	98%	98%
Appropriate VTP Within 24 Hours[2]	278	99%	98%	98%
Controlled Postoperative Blood Glucose[2,7]	-	-	99%	97%
Perioperative Temperature Management[2]	315	100%	99%	100%
Prophylactic Antibiotic Selection[2]	204	99%	99%	99%
Prophylactic Antibiotic Selection (Outpatient)	190	98%	98%	98%
Prophylactic Antibiotic Stopped[2]	203	97%	98%	98%
Prophylactic Antibiotic Timing[2]	204	100%	98%	99%
Prophylactic Antibiotic Timing (Outpatient)	134	99%	97%	98%
Urinary Catheter Removal[2]	213	99%	96%	97%
Survey of Patients' Hospital Experiences				
Area Around Room 'Always' Quiet at Night	300+	64%	61%	61%
Doctors 'Always' Communicated Well	300+	81%	83%	82%
Home Recovery Information Given	300+	87%	88%	85%
Hospital Given 9 or 10 on 10 Point Scale	300+	72%	73%	71%
Meds 'Always' Explained Before Given	300+	64%	66%	64%
Nurses 'Always' Communicated Well	300+	78%	80%	79%
Pain 'Always' Well Controlled	300+	70%	72%	71%
Room and Bathroom 'Always' Clean	300+	72%	77%	73%
Timely Help 'Always' Received	300+	66%	73%	68%
Would Definitely Recommend Hospital	300+	69%	74%	71%
Use of Medical Imaging				
Cardiac Imaging Stress Test before Surgery	196	5.1%	4.6%	5.3%
Combination Abdominal CT Scan	413	4.6%	7.3%	10.5%
Combination Brain/Sinus CT Scan	237	0.4%	1.7%	2.7%
Combination Chest CT Scan	140	0.0%	1.8%	2.7%
Follow-up Mammogram/Ultrasound	446	10.5%	8.2%	8.8%
Lumbar Spine MRI for Low Back Pain[1]	-	-	40.3%	37.2%

Cascade Medical Center

402 Lake Cascade Parkway
Cascade, ID 83611
Phone: 208-382-4242
Type: Critical Access Hospitals
Emergency Services: Yes
Ownership: Govt - Hospital Dist/Auth

Measure	Cases	This Hosp.	State Avg.	U.S. Avg.
Blood Clot Prevention and Treatment				
Anticoagulation Overlap Therapy[5]	-	-	95%	93%
ICU Venous Thromboembolism Prophylaxis[5]	-	-	92%	92%
Incidence of Potentially Preventable VTE[5]	-	-	11%	10%
UFH with Dosages/Platelet Monitoring[5]	-	-	99%	97%
Venous Thromboembolism Prophylaxis[5]	-	-	87%	85%
Warfarin Therapy Discharge Instructions[5]	-	-	75%	75%
Chest Pain/Possible Heart Attack Care				
Aspirin Given Within 24 Hours of Arrival	-	-	96%	96%
Fibrinolytic Meds Within 30 Min. of Arrival	-	-	55%	58%
Average Time to ECG (minutes)	-	-	9	7
Average Time to Transfer (minutes)	-	-	62	60
Children's Asthma Care				
Received Home Management Plan of Care	-	-	-	88%
Received Reliever Medication	-	-	-	100%
Received Systemic Corticosteroids	-	-	-	100%
Emergency Department				
Admittance Decision Time (minutes)[5]	-	-	76	98
Head CT Results Within 45 Min. of Arrival	-	-	38%	57%
Patients Who Left ER Before Being Seen	-	-	1%	2%
Time from ER Arrival to Admit. (minutes)[5]	-	-	232	274
Time from ER Arrival to Discharge (minutes)	-	-	121	134
Time in ER Before Being Evaluated (minutes)	-	-	21	26
Time to Pain Meds for Fractures (minutes)	-	-	46	57
Heart Attack Care				
Aspirin Given at Discharge[5]	-	-	100%	99%
Fibrinolytic Meds Within 30 Min. of Arrival[5]	-	-	-	54%
PCI Within 90 Minutes of Arrival[5]	-	-	98%	96%
Statin Prescribed at Discharge[5]	-	-	99%	98%
Heart Failure Care				
ACE Inhibitor or ARB for LVSD[5]	-	-	98%	97%
Discharge Instructions Given[5]	-	-	94%	94%
Evaluation of LVS Function[5]	-	-	97%	99%
Medicare Spending				
Medicare Spending per Patient (ratio)	-	-	0.91	0.98
Pneumonia Care				
Appropriate Initial Antibiotic Given[5]	-	-	94%	95%
Blood Culture Timing[5]	-	-	98%	98%
Pregnancy and Delivery Care				
Newborn Deliveries Scheduled Early[5]	-	-	6%	6%
Preventive Care				
Immunization for Influenza[5]	-	-	83%	90%
Immunization for Pneumonia[5]	-	-	89%	92%
Stroke Care				
Anticoagulation Therapy for Atrial Fibrillation[5]	-	-	97%	95%
Antithrombotic Therapy Timing[5]	-	-	98%	98%
Assessed for Rehabilitation[5]	-	-	98%	97%
Discharged on Antithrombotic Therapy[5]	-	-	99%	99%
Discharged on Statin Medication[5]	-	-	91%	94%
Thrombolytic Therapy Timing[5]	-	-	55%	66%
Venous Thromboembolism Prophylaxis[5]	-	-	93%	94%
Written Stroke Educational Materials Given[5]	-	-	84%	88%
Surgical Care Improvement Project				
Appropriate Beta Blocker Usage[5]	-	-	98%	98%
Appropriate VTP Within 24 Hours[5]	-	-	98%	98%
Controlled Postoperative Blood Glucose[5]	-	-	99%	97%
Perioperative Temperature Management[5]	-	-	99%	100%
Prophylactic Antibiotic Selection[5]	-	-	99%	99%
Prophylactic Antibiotic Selection (Outpatient)	-	-	98%	98%
Prophylactic Antibiotic Stopped[5]	-	-	98%	98%
Prophylactic Antibiotic Timing[5]	-	-	98%	99%
Prophylactic Antibiotic Timing (Outpatient)	-	-	97%	98%
Urinary Catheter Removal[5]	-	-	96%	97%
Survey of Patients' Hospital Experiences				
Area Around Room 'Always' Quiet at Night[5]	-	-	61%	61%
Doctors 'Always' Communicated Well[5]	-	-	83%	82%
Home Recovery Information Given[5]	-	-	88%	85%
Hospital Given 9 or 10 on 10 Point Scale[5]	-	-	73%	71%
Meds 'Always' Explained Before Given[5]	-	-	66%	64%
Nurses 'Always' Communicated Well[5]	-	-	80%	79%
Pain 'Always' Well Controlled[5]	-	-	72%	71%
Room and Bathroom 'Always' Clean[5]	-	-	77%	73%
Timely Help 'Always' Received[5]	-	-	73%	68%
Would Definitely Recommend Hospital[5]	-	-	74%	71%
Use of Medical Imaging				

NOTE: Hospital profiles are in alphabetical order by state, then city, then hospital within the city; Rankings exclude hospitals with less than 25 cases except for patient surveys which excludes hospitals with less than 100 cases; (a) 100-299 cases; (1) The number of cases/patients is too few to report; (2) Data submitted were based on a sample of cases/patients; (3) Results are based on a shorter time period than required; (4) Data suppressed by CMS for one or more quarters; (5) Results are not available for this reporting period; (6) Fewer than 100 patients completed the HCAHPS survey; (7) No cases met the criteria for this measure; (8) The lower limit of the confidence interval cannot be calculated if the number of observed infections equals zero; (9) No data are available from the state/territory for this reporting period; (10) The scores shown reflect fewer than 50 completed surveys; (11) There were discrepancies in the data collection process; (12) This measure does not apply to this hospital for this reporting period; (13) Results cannot be calculated for this reporting period; (14) The results for this state are combined with nearby states to protect confidentiality; Please refer to the User's Guide for a full explanation of data.

Cardiac Imaging Stress Test before Surgery	-	-	4.6%	5.3%
Combination Abdominal CT Scan	-	-	7.3%	10.5%
Combination Brain/Sinus CT Scan	-	-	1.7%	2.7%
Combination Chest CT Scan	-	-	1.8%	2.7%
Follow-up Mammogram/Ultrasound	-	-	8.2%	8.8%
Lumbar Spine MRI for Low Back Pain	-	-	40.3%	37.2%

Kootenai Medical Center

2003 Kootenai Health Way
Coeur D'alene, ID 83814
Phone: 208-625-4001
Fax: 208-666-3299
URL: www.kootenaihealth.org
Type: Acute Care Hospitals
Emergency Services: Yes
Ownership: Govt - Hospital Dist/Auth
Beds: 337

Key Personnel:
Operating Room. . . . . Frederick Ambrose
Patient Relations . . . . Carmen Brochu
Radiology. . . . . Nicole Burbank
Infection Control. . . . . Marty Fallon
Intensive Care Unit. . . . . Sandy Lascuola
CEO/President. . . . . Jon Ness
Pediatric Ambulatory Care . . . . . . Lori Schneider
Pediatric In-Patient Care . . . . Lori Schneider

Measure	Cases	This Hosp.	State Avg.	U.S. Avg.
Blood Clot Prevention and Treatment				
Anticoagulation Overlap Therapy[2]	69	83%	95%	93%
ICU Venous Thromboembolism Prophylaxis[2]	67	87%	92%	92%
Incidence of Potentially Preventable VTE[2]	13	23%	11%	10%
UFH with Dosages/Platelet Monitoring[2]	17	100%	99%	97%
Venous Thromboembolism Prophylaxis[2]	238	82%	87%	85%
Warfarin Therapy Discharge Instructions[2]	48	50%	75%	75%
Chest Pain/Possible Heart Attack Care				
Aspirin Given Within 24 Hours of Arrival[5]	-	-	96%	96%
Fibrinolytic Meds Within 30 Min. of Arrival[5]	-	-	55%	58%
Average Time to ECG (minutes)[5]	-	-	9	7
Average Time to Transfer (minutes)[5]	-	-	62	60
Children's Asthma Care				
Received Home Management Plan of Care	-	-	-	88%
Received Reliever Medication	-	-	-	100%
Received Systemic Corticosteroids	-	-	-	100%
Emergency Department				
Admittance Decision Time (minutes)[2]	420	94	76	98
Head CT Results Within 45 Min. of Arrival[1]	-	-	38%	57%
Patients Who Left ER Before Being Seen	47,985	2%	1%	2%
Time from ER Arrival to Admit. (minutes)[2]	428	240	232	274
Time from ER Arrival to Discharge (minutes)	348	146	121	134
Time in ER Before Being Evaluated (minutes)	307	44	21	26
Time to Pain Meds for Fractures (minutes)	151	60	46	57
Heart Attack Care				
Aspirin Given at Discharge	268	100%	100%	99%
Fibrinolytic Meds Within 30 Min. of Arrival[7]	-	-	-	54%
PCI Within 90 Minutes of Arrival	72	97%	98%	96%
Statin Prescribed at Discharge	267	100%	99%	98%
Heart Failure Care				
ACE Inhibitor or ARB for LVSD	67	99%	98%	97%
Discharge Instructions Given	205	100%	94%	94%
Evaluation of LVS Function	253	100%	97%	99%
Medicare Spending				
Medicare Spending per Patient (ratio)	-	0.99	0.91	0.98
Pneumonia Care				
Appropriate Initial Antibiotic Given	176	97%	94%	95%
Blood Culture Timing	246	98%	98%	98%
Pregnancy and Delivery Care				
Newborn Deliveries Scheduled Early[2]	187	4%	6%	6%
Preventive Care				
Immunization for Influenza[2]	522	81%	83%	90%
Immunization for Pneumonia[2]	544	83%	89%	92%
Stroke Care				
Anticoagulation Therapy for Atrial Fibrillation	22	100%	97%	95%
Antithrombotic Therapy Timing	102	100%	98%	98%
Assessed for Rehabilitation	143	99%	98%	97%
Discharged on Antithrombotic Therapy	124	98%	99%	99%
Discharged on Statin Medication	97	85%	91%	94%
Thrombolytic Therapy Timing	11	73%	55%	66%
Venous Thromboembolism Prophylaxis	127	90%	93%	94%
Written Stroke Educational Materials Given	78	85%	84%	88%
Surgical Care Improvement Project				
Appropriate Beta Blocker Usage[2]	316	97%	98%	98%
Appropriate VTP Within 24 Hours[2]	632	97%	98%	98%
Controlled Postoperative Blood Glucose[2]	186	98%	99%	97%
Perioperative Temperature Management[2]	766	100%	99%	100%
Prophylactic Antibiotic Selection[2]	787	98%	99%	99%
Prophylactic Antibiotic Selection (Outpatient)	360	98%	98%	98%
Prophylactic Antibiotic Stopped[2]	778	99%	98%	98%
Prophylactic Antibiotic Timing[2]	788	96%	98%	99%
Prophylactic Antibiotic Timing (Outpatient)	378	89%	97%	98%
Urinary Catheter Removal[2]	358	89%	96%	97%
Survey of Patients' Hospital Experiences				
Area Around Room 'Always' Quiet at Night	300+	44%	61%	61%
Doctors 'Always' Communicated Well	300+	77%	83%	82%
Home Recovery Information Given	300+	87%	88%	85%
Hospital Given 9 or 10 on 10 Point Scale	300+	65%	73%	71%
Meds 'Always' Explained Before Given	300+	61%	66%	64%
Nurses 'Always' Communicated Well	300+	73%	80%	79%
Pain 'Always' Well Controlled	300+	68%	72%	71%
Room and Bathroom 'Always' Clean	300+	68%	77%	73%
Timely Help 'Always' Received	300+	58%	73%	68%
Would Definitely Recommend Hospital	300+	69%	74%	71%
Use of Medical Imaging				
Cardiac Imaging Stress Test before Surgery	1,445	4.3%	4.6%	5.3%
Combination Abdominal CT Scan	1,356	9.0%	7.3%	10.5%
Combination Brain/Sinus CT Scan	853	2.6%	1.7%	2.7%
Combination Chest CT Scan	1,043	0.4%	1.8%	2.7%
Follow-up Mammogram/Ultrasound	2,838	6.7%	8.2%	8.8%
Lumbar Spine MRI for Low Back Pain	240	35.8%	40.3%	37.2%

Saint Mary's Hospital

701 Lewiston St
Cottonwood, ID 83522
Phone: 208-962-3251
Fax: 208-962-3722
E-mail: stmarys@camasnet.com
Type: Critical Access Hospitals
Emergency Services: Yes
Ownership: Voluntary non-profit - Private
Beds: 28

Key Personnel:
Quality Assurance . . . . Iris Hawley
CEO/President. . . . . Casey Meza
Operating Room. . . . . Barb Michels
Emergency Room . . . . Susan Nau
Chief of Medical Staff. . . . . Ronald Sigler

Measure	Cases	This Hosp.	State Avg.	U.S. Avg.
Blood Clot Prevention and Treatment				
Anticoagulation Overlap Therapy[5]	-	-	95%	93%
ICU Venous Thromboembolism Prophylaxis[5]	-	-	92%	92%
Incidence of Potentially Preventable VTE[5]	-	-	11%	10%
UFH with Dosages/Platelet Monitoring[5]	-	-	99%	97%
Venous Thromboembolism Prophylaxis[5]	-	-	87%	85%
Warfarin Therapy Discharge Instructions[5]	-	-	75%	75%
Chest Pain/Possible Heart Attack Care				
Aspirin Given Within 24 Hours of Arrival	-	-	96%	96%
Fibrinolytic Meds Within 30 Min. of Arrival	-	-	55%	58%
Average Time to ECG (minutes)	-	-	9	7
Average Time to Transfer (minutes)	-	-	62	60
Children's Asthma Care				
Received Home Management Plan of Care	-	-	-	88%
Received Reliever Medication	-	-	-	100%
Received Systemic Corticosteroids	-	-	-	100%
Emergency Department				
Admittance Decision Time (minutes)[5]	-	-	76	98
Head CT Results Within 45 Min. of Arrival	-	-	38%	57%
Patients Who Left ER Before Being Seen	-	-	1%	2%
Time from ER Arrival to Admit. (minutes)[5]	-	-	232	274
Time from ER Arrival to Discharge (minutes)	-	-	121	134
Time in ER Before Being Evaluated (minutes)	-	-	21	26
Time to Pain Meds for Fractures (minutes)	-	-	46	57
Heart Attack Care				
Aspirin Given at Discharge[5]	-	-	100%	99%
Fibrinolytic Meds Within 30 Min. of Arrival[5]	-	-	-	54%
PCI Within 90 Minutes of Arrival[5]	-	-	98%	96%
Statin Prescribed at Discharge[5]	-	-	99%	98%
Heart Failure Care				
ACE Inhibitor or ARB for LVSD[1]	-	-	98%	97%
Discharge Instructions Given[1]	-	-	94%	94%
Evaluation of LVS Function[1]	-	-	97%	99%
Medicare Spending				
Medicare Spending per Patient (ratio)	-	-	0.91	0.98
Pneumonia Care				
Appropriate Initial Antibiotic Given[2]	26	92%	94%	95%
Blood Culture Timing[2,3]	14	100%	98%	98%
Pregnancy and Delivery Care				
Newborn Deliveries Scheduled Early[5]	-	-	6%	6%
Preventive Care				
Immunization for Influenza[5]	-	-	83%	90%
Immunization for Pneumonia[5]	-	-	89%	92%
Stroke Care				
Anticoagulation Therapy for Atrial Fibrillation[1]	-	-	97%	95%
Antithrombotic Therapy Timing[7]	-	-	98%	98%
Assessed for Rehabilitation[1]	-	-	98%	97%
Discharged on Antithrombotic Therapy[1]	-	-	99%	99%
Discharged on Statin Medication[1]	-	-	91%	94%
Thrombolytic Therapy Timing[7]	-	-	55%	66%
Venous Thromboembolism Prophylaxis[1]	-	-	93%	94%
Written Stroke Educational Materials Given[1]	-	-	84%	88%
Surgical Care Improvement Project				
Appropriate Beta Blocker Usage[3,7]	-	-	98%	98%
Appropriate VTP Within 24 Hours[1,3]	-	-	98%	98%
Controlled Postoperative Blood Glucose[5]	-	-	99%	97%
Perioperative Temperature Management[1,3]	-	-	99%	100%
Prophylactic Antibiotic Selection[1,3]	-	-	99%	99%
Prophylactic Antibiotic Selection (Outpatient)	-	-	98%	98%
Prophylactic Antibiotic Stopped[1,3]	-	-	98%	98%
Prophylactic Antibiotic Timing[1,3]	-	-	98%	99%
Prophylactic Antibiotic Timing (Outpatient)	-	-	97%	98%
Urinary Catheter Removal[3,7]	-	-	96%	97%
Survey of Patients' Hospital Experiences				
Area Around Room 'Always' Quiet at Night[11]	300+	51%	61%	61%
Doctors 'Always' Communicated Well[11]	300+	88%	83%	82%
Home Recovery Information Given[11]	300+	82%	88%	85%
Hospital Given 9 or 10 on 10 Point Scale[11]	300+	71%	73%	71%
Meds 'Always' Explained Before Given[11]	300+	60%	66%	64%
Nurses 'Always' Communicated Well[11]	300+	76%	80%	79%
Pain 'Always' Well Controlled[11]	300+	71%	72%	71%
Room and Bathroom 'Always' Clean[11]	300+	78%	77%	73%
Timely Help 'Always' Received[11]	300+	66%	73%	68%
Would Definitely Recommend Hospital[11]	300+	80%	74%	71%
Use of Medical Imaging				
Cardiac Imaging Stress Test before Surgery	-	-	4.6%	5.3%
Combination Abdominal CT Scan	-	-	7.3%	10.5%
Combination Brain/Sinus CT Scan	-	-	1.7%	2.7%
Combination Chest CT Scan	-	-	1.8%	2.7%
Follow-up Mammogram/Ultrasound	-	-	8.2%	8.8%
Lumbar Spine MRI for Low Back Pain	-	-	40.3%	37.2%

Walter Knox Memorial Hospital

1202 East Locust Street
Emmett, ID 83617
Phone: 208-365-3561
Type: Critical Access Hospitals
Emergency Services: Yes
Ownership: Government - Local

Measure	Cases	This Hosp.	State Avg.	U.S. Avg.
Blood Clot Prevention and Treatment				
Anticoagulation Overlap Therapy[5]	-	-	95%	93%
ICU Venous Thromboembolism Prophylaxis[5]	-	-	92%	92%
Incidence of Potentially Preventable VTE[5]	-	-	11%	10%
UFH with Dosages/Platelet Monitoring[5]	-	-	99%	97%
Venous Thromboembolism Prophylaxis[5]	-	-	87%	85%
Warfarin Therapy Discharge Instructions[5]	-	-	75%	75%
Chest Pain/Possible Heart Attack Care				
Aspirin Given Within 24 Hours of Arrival[1,3]	-	-	96%	96%
Fibrinolytic Meds Within 30 Min. of Arrival[3,7]	-	-	55%	58%
Average Time to ECG (minutes)[1,3]	-	-	9	7
Average Time to Transfer (minutes)[1,3]	-	-	62	60
Children's Asthma Care				

NOTE: Hospital profiles are in alphabetical order by state, then city, then hospital within the city; Rankings exclude hospitals with less than 25 cases except for patient surveys which excludes hospitals with less than 100 cases; (a) 100-299 cases; (1) The number of cases/patients is too few to report; (2) Data submitted were based on a sample of cases/patients; (3) Results are based on a shorter time period than required; (4) Data suppressed by CMS for one or more quarters; (5) Results are not available for this reporting period; (6) Fewer than 100 patients completed the HCAHPS survey; (7) No cases met the criteria for this measure; (8) The lower limit of the confidence interval cannot be calculated if the number of observed infections equals zero; (9) No data are available from the state/territory for this reporting period; (10) The scores shown reflect fewer than 50 completed surveys; (11) There were discrepancies in the data collection process; (12) This measure does not apply to this hospital for this reporting period; (13) Results cannot be calculated for this reporting period; (14) The results for this state are combined with nearby states to protect confidentiality; Please refer to the User's Guide for a full explanation of data.

Measure	Cases	This Hosp.	State Avg.	U.S. Avg.
Received Home Management Plan of Care	-	-	-	88%
Received Reliever Medication	-	-	-	100%
Received Systemic Corticosteroids	-	-	-	100%
Emergency Department				
Admittance Decision Time (minutes)[5]	-	-	76	98
Head CT Results Within 45 Min. of Arrival[5]	-	-	38%	57%
Patients Who Left ER Before Being Seen[5]	-	-	1%	2%
Time from ER Arrival to Admit. (minutes)[5]	-	-	232	274
Time from ER Arrival to Discharge (minutes)[5]	-	-	121	134
Time in ER Before Being Evaluated (minutes)[5]	-	-	21	26
Time to Pain Meds for Fractures (minutes)[5]	-	-	46	57
Heart Attack Care				
Aspirin Given at Discharge[5]	-	-	100%	99%
Fibrinolytic Meds Within 30 Min. of Arrival[5]	-	-	-	54%
PCI Within 90 Minutes of Arrival[5]	-	-	98%	96%
Statin Prescribed at Discharge[5]	-	-	99%	98%
Heart Failure Care				
ACE Inhibitor or ARB for LVSD[3,7]	-	-	98%	97%
Discharge Instructions Given[1,3]	-	-	94%	94%
Evaluation of LVS Function[1,3]	-	-	97%	99%
Medicare Spending				
Medicare Spending per Patient (ratio)	-	-	0.91	0.98
Pneumonia Care				
Appropriate Initial Antibiotic Given[1,3]	-	-	94%	95%
Blood Culture Timing[1,3]	-	-	98%	98%
Pregnancy and Delivery Care				
Newborn Deliveries Scheduled Early[5]	-	-	6%	6%
Preventive Care				
Immunization for Influenza[5]	-	-	83%	90%
Immunization for Pneumonia[5]	-	-	89%	92%
Stroke Care				
Anticoagulation Therapy for Atrial Fibrillation[5]	-	-	97%	95%
Antithrombotic Therapy Timing[5]	-	-	98%	98%
Assessed for Rehabilitation[5]	-	-	98%	97%
Discharged on Antithrombotic Therapy[5]	-	-	99%	99%
Discharged on Statin Medication[5]	-	-	91%	94%
Thrombolytic Therapy Timing[5]	-	-	55%	66%
Venous Thromboembolism Prophylaxis[5]	-	-	93%	94%
Written Stroke Educational Materials Given[5]	-	-	84%	88%
Surgical Care Improvement Project				
Appropriate Beta Blocker Usage[5]	-	-	98%	98%
Appropriate VTP Within 24 Hours[5]	-	-	98%	98%
Controlled Postoperative Blood Glucose[5]	-	-	99%	97%
Perioperative Temperature Management[5]	-	-	99%	100%
Prophylactic Antibiotic Selection[5]	-	-	99%	99%
Prophylactic Antibiotic Selection (Outpatient)[1,3]	-	-	98%	98%
Prophylactic Antibiotic Stopped[5]	-	-	98%	98%
Prophylactic Antibiotic Timing[5]	-	-	98%	99%
Prophylactic Antibiotic Timing (Outpatient)[1,3]	-	-	97%	98%
Urinary Catheter Removal[5]	-	-	96%	97%
Survey of Patients' Hospital Experiences				
Area Around Room 'Always' Quiet at Night[5]	-	-	61%	61%
Doctors 'Always' Communicated Well[5]	-	-	83%	82%
Home Recovery Information Given[5]	-	-	88%	85%
Hospital Given 9 or 10 on 10 Point Scale[5]	-	-	73%	71%
Meds 'Always' Explained Before Given[5]	-	-	66%	64%
Nurses 'Always' Communicated Well[5]	-	-	80%	79%
Pain 'Always' Well Controlled[5]	-	-	72%	71%
Room and Bathroom 'Always' Clean[5]	-	-	77%	73%
Timely Help 'Always' Received[5]	-	-	73%	68%
Would Definitely Recommend Hospital[5]	-	-	74%	71%
Use of Medical Imaging				
Cardiac Imaging Stress Test before Surgery[7]	-	-	4.6%	5.3%
Combination Abdominal CT Scan	150	4.7%	7.3%	10.5%
Combination Brain/Sinus CT Scan	135	0.0%	1.7%	2.7%
Combination Chest CT Scan	57	1.8%	1.8%	2.7%
Follow-up Mammogram/Ultrasound[7]	-	-	8.2%	8.8%
Lumbar Spine MRI for Low Back Pain[1]	-	-	40.3%	37.2%

North Canyon Medical Center

267 North Canyon Dr
Gooding, ID 83330
Phone: 208-934-4433
Type: Critical Access Hospitals
Emergency Services: Yes
Ownership: Voluntary non-profit - Other

Measure	Cases	This Hosp.	State Avg.	U.S. Avg.
Blood Clot Prevention and Treatment				
Anticoagulation Overlap Therapy[5]	-	-	95%	93%
ICU Venous Thromboembolism Prophylaxis[5]	-	-	92%	92%
Incidence of Potentially Preventable VTE[5]	-	-	11%	10%
UFH with Dosages/Platelet Monitoring[5]	-	-	99%	97%
Venous Thromboembolism Prophylaxis[5]	-	-	87%	85%
Warfarin Therapy Discharge Instructions[5]	-	-	75%	75%
Chest Pain/Possible Heart Attack Care				
Aspirin Given Within 24 Hours of Arrival	-	-	96%	96%
Fibrinolytic Meds Within 30 Min. of Arrival	-	-	55%	58%
Average Time to ECG (minutes)	-	-	9	7
Average Time to Transfer (minutes)	-	-	62	60
Children's Asthma Care				
Received Home Management Plan of Care	-	-	-	88%
Received Reliever Medication	-	-	-	100%
Received Systemic Corticosteroids	-	-	-	100%
Emergency Department				
Admittance Decision Time (minutes)[5]	-	-	76	98
Head CT Results Within 45 Min. of Arrival	-	-	38%	57%
Patients Who Left ER Before Being Seen	-	-	1%	2%
Time from ER Arrival to Admit. (minutes)[5]	-	-	232	274
Time from ER Arrival to Discharge (minutes)	-	-	121	134
Time in ER Before Being Evaluated (minutes)	-	-	21	26
Time to Pain Meds for Fractures (minutes)	-	-	46	57
Heart Attack Care				
Aspirin Given at Discharge[5]	-	-	100%	99%
Fibrinolytic Meds Within 30 Min. of Arrival[5]	-	-	-	54%
PCI Within 90 Minutes of Arrival[5]	-	-	98%	96%
Statin Prescribed at Discharge[5]	-	-	99%	98%
Heart Failure Care				
ACE Inhibitor or ARB for LVSD[1]	-	-	98%	97%
Discharge Instructions Given	11	100%	94%	94%
Evaluation of LVS Function	16	69%	97%	99%
Medicare Spending				
Medicare Spending per Patient (ratio)	-	-	0.91	0.98
Pneumonia Care				
Appropriate Initial Antibiotic Given	24	67%	94%	95%
Blood Culture Timing	45	93%	98%	98%
Pregnancy and Delivery Care				
Newborn Deliveries Scheduled Early[5]	-	-	6%	6%
Preventive Care				
Immunization for Influenza[5]	-	-	83%	90%
Immunization for Pneumonia[5]	-	-	89%	92%
Stroke Care				
Anticoagulation Therapy for Atrial Fibrillation[5]	-	-	97%	95%
Antithrombotic Therapy Timing[5]	-	-	98%	98%
Assessed for Rehabilitation[5]	-	-	98%	97%
Discharged on Antithrombotic Therapy[5]	-	-	99%	99%
Discharged on Statin Medication[5]	-	-	91%	94%
Thrombolytic Therapy Timing[5]	-	-	55%	66%
Venous Thromboembolism Prophylaxis[5]	-	-	93%	94%
Written Stroke Educational Materials Given[5]	-	-	84%	88%
Surgical Care Improvement Project				
Appropriate Beta Blocker Usage[5]	-	-	98%	98%
Appropriate VTP Within 24 Hours[5]	-	-	98%	98%
Controlled Postoperative Blood Glucose[5]	-	-	99%	97%
Perioperative Temperature Management[5]	-	-	99%	100%
Prophylactic Antibiotic Selection[5]	-	-	99%	99%
Prophylactic Antibiotic Selection (Outpatient)	-	-	98%	98%
Prophylactic Antibiotic Stopped[5]	-	-	98%	98%
Prophylactic Antibiotic Timing[5]	-	-	98%	99%
Prophylactic Antibiotic Timing (Outpatient)	-	-	97%	98%
Urinary Catheter Removal[5]	-	-	96%	97%
Survey of Patients' Hospital Experiences				
Area Around Room 'Always' Quiet at Night	(a)	70%	61%	61%
Doctors 'Always' Communicated Well	(a)	87%	83%	82%
Home Recovery Information Given	(a)	87%	88%	85%
Hospital Given 9 or 10 on 10 Point Scale	(a)	80%	73%	71%
Meds 'Always' Explained Before Given	(a)	67%	66%	64%
Nurses 'Always' Communicated Well	(a)	80%	80%	79%
Pain 'Always' Well Controlled	(a)	81%	72%	71%
Room and Bathroom 'Always' Clean	(a)	92%	77%	73%
Timely Help 'Always' Received	(a)	77%	73%	68%
Would Definitely Recommend Hospital	(a)	76%	74%	71%
Use of Medical Imaging				
Cardiac Imaging Stress Test before Surgery	-	-	4.6%	5.3%
Combination Abdominal CT Scan	-	-	7.3%	10.5%
Combination Brain/Sinus CT Scan	-	-	1.7%	2.7%
Combination Chest CT Scan	-	-	1.8%	2.7%
Follow-up Mammogram/Ultrasound	-	-	8.2%	8.8%
Lumbar Spine MRI for Low Back Pain	-	-	40.3%	37.2%

Syringa General Hospital

607 W Main Street
Grangeville, ID 83530
Phone: 208-983-1700
Type: Critical Access Hospitals
Emergency Services: Yes
Ownership: Govt - Hospital Dist/Auth

Measure	Cases	This Hosp.	State Avg.	U.S. Avg.
Blood Clot Prevention and Treatment				
Anticoagulation Overlap Therapy[5]	-	-	95%	93%
ICU Venous Thromboembolism Prophylaxis[5]	-	-	92%	92%
Incidence of Potentially Preventable VTE[5]	-	-	11%	10%
UFH with Dosages/Platelet Monitoring[5]	-	-	99%	97%
Venous Thromboembolism Prophylaxis[5]	-	-	87%	85%
Warfarin Therapy Discharge Instructions[5]	-	-	75%	75%
Chest Pain/Possible Heart Attack Care				
Aspirin Given Within 24 Hours of Arrival	16	100%	96%	96%
Fibrinolytic Meds Within 30 Min. of Arrival[1]	-	-	55%	58%
Average Time to ECG (minutes)	16	1	9	7
Average Time to Transfer (minutes)[1]	-	-	62	60
Children's Asthma Care				
Received Home Management Plan of Care	-	-	-	88%
Received Reliever Medication	-	-	-	100%
Received Systemic Corticosteroids	-	-	-	100%
Emergency Department				
Admittance Decision Time (minutes)[5]	-	-	76	98
Head CT Results Within 45 Min. of Arrival[5]	-	-	38%	57%
Patients Who Left ER Before Being Seen	2,335	0%	1%	2%
Time from ER Arrival to Admit. (minutes)[5]	-	-	232	274
Time from ER Arrival to Discharge (minutes)[5]	-	-	121	134
Time in ER Before Being Evaluated (minutes)[5]	-	-	21	26
Time to Pain Meds for Fractures (minutes)[5]	-	-	46	57
Heart Attack Care				
Aspirin Given at Discharge[5]	-	-	100%	99%
Fibrinolytic Meds Within 30 Min. of Arrival[5]	-	-	-	54%
PCI Within 90 Minutes of Arrival[5]	-	-	98%	96%
Statin Prescribed at Discharge[5]	-	-	99%	98%
Heart Failure Care				
ACE Inhibitor or ARB for LVSD[1]	-	-	98%	97%
Discharge Instructions Given[1]	-	-	94%	94%
Evaluation of LVS Function[1]	-	-	97%	99%
Medicare Spending				
Medicare Spending per Patient (ratio)	-	-	0.91	0.98
Pneumonia Care				
Appropriate Initial Antibiotic Given[2]	20	95%	94%	95%
Blood Culture Timing[2]	12	100%	98%	98%
Pregnancy and Delivery Care				
Newborn Deliveries Scheduled Early[5]	-	-	6%	6%
Preventive Care				
Immunization for Influenza[5]	-	-	83%	90%
Immunization for Pneumonia[5]	-	-	89%	92%
Stroke Care				
Anticoagulation Therapy for Atrial Fibrillation[5]	-	-	97%	95%
Antithrombotic Therapy Timing[5]	-	-	98%	98%
Assessed for Rehabilitation[5]	-	-	98%	97%
Discharged on Antithrombotic Therapy[5]	-	-	99%	99%
Discharged on Statin Medication[5]	-	-	91%	94%
Thrombolytic Therapy Timing[5]	-	-	55%	66%

NOTE: Hospital profiles are in alphabetical order by state, then city, then hospital within the city; Rankings exclude hospitals with less than 25 cases except for patient surveys which excludes hospitals with less than 100 cases; (a) 100-299 cases; (1) The number of cases/patients is too few to report; (2) Data submitted were based on a sample of cases/patients; (3) Results are based on a shorter time period than required; (4) Data suppressed by CMS for one or more quarters; (5) Results are not available for this reporting period; (6) Fewer than 100 patients completed the HCAHPS survey; (7) No cases met the criteria for this measure; (8) The lower limit of the confidence interval cannot be calculated if the number of observed infections equals zero; (9) No data are available from the state/territory for this reporting period; (10) The scores shown reflect fewer than 50 completed surveys; (11) There were discrepancies in the data collection process; (12) This measure does not apply to this hospital for this reporting period; (13) Results cannot be calculated for this reporting period; (14) The results for this state are combined with nearby states to protect confidentiality; Please refer to the User's Guide for a full explanation of data.

Measure	Cases	This Hosp.	State Avg.	U.S. Avg.
Venous Thromboembolism Prophylaxis[5]	-	-	93%	94%
Written Stroke Educational Materials Given[5]	-	-	84%	88%
Surgical Care Improvement Project				
Appropriate Beta Blocker Usage[5]	-	-	98%	98%
Appropriate VTP Within 24 Hours[5]	-	-	98%	98%
Controlled Postoperative Blood Glucose[5]	-	-	99%	97%
Perioperative Temperature Management[5]	-	-	99%	100%
Prophylactic Antibiotic Selection[5]	-	-	99%	99%
Prophylactic Antibiotic Selection (Outpatient)[5]	-	-	98%	98%
Prophylactic Antibiotic Stopped[5]	-	-	98%	98%
Prophylactic Antibiotic Timing[5]	-	-	98%	99%
Prophylactic Antibiotic Timing (Outpatient)[5]	-	-	97%	98%
Urinary Catheter Removal[5]	-	-	96%	97%
Survey of Patients' Hospital Experiences				
Area Around Room 'Always' Quiet at Night[6]	<100	65%	61%	61%
Doctors 'Always' Communicated Well[6]	<100	87%	83%	82%
Home Recovery Information Given[6]	<100	92%	88%	85%
Hospital Given 9 or 10 on 10 Point Scale[6]	<100	74%	73%	71%
Meds 'Always' Explained Before Given[6]	<100	58%	66%	64%
Nurses 'Always' Communicated Well[6]	<100	82%	80%	79%
Pain 'Always' Well Controlled[6]	<100	71%	72%	71%
Room and Bathroom 'Always' Clean[6]	<100	81%	77%	73%
Timely Help 'Always' Received[6]	<100	83%	73%	68%
Would Definitely Recommend Hospital[6]	<100	76%	74%	71%
Use of Medical Imaging				
Cardiac Imaging Stress Test before Surgery[7]	-	-	4.6%	5.3%
Combination Abdominal CT Scan	80	15.0%	7.3%	10.5%
Combination Brain/Sinus CT Scan[1]	-	-	1.7%	2.7%
Combination Chest CT Scan[1]	-	-	1.8%	2.7%
Follow-up Mammogram/Ultrasound[7]	-	-	8.2%	8.8%
Lumbar Spine MRI for Low Back Pain[1]	-	-	40.3%	37.2%

Eastern Idaho Regional Medical Center

3100 Channing Way
Idaho Falls, ID 83404
Phone: 208-529-6111
Fax: 208-529-7090
URL: www.eirmc.org
Type: Acute Care Hospitals
Ownership: Proprietary
Emergency Services: Yes
Beds: 242

Key Personnel:
Infection Control. . . . . Barb Brown
Quality Assurance . . . . Loui Fatkin
Emergency Room . . . . Brad Hobbs
Chief of Medical Staff. . . . . Calvin J McAllister, MD
Pediatric In-Patient Care . . . . Robert Pettit
Hemotology Center . . . . Jim State
Intensive Care Unit. . . . . Greg Trosper
Radiology. . . . . David Warden

Measure	Cases	This Hosp.	State Avg.	U.S. Avg.
Blood Clot Prevention and Treatment				
Anticoagulation Overlap Therapy[2]	92	100%	95%	93%
ICU Venous Thromboembolism Prophylaxis[2]	85	92%	92%	92%
Incidence of Potentially Preventable VTE[2]	12	33%	11%	10%
UFH with Dosages/Platelet Monitoring[2]	46	98%	99%	97%
Venous Thromboembolism Prophylaxis[2]	341	77%	87%	85%
Warfarin Therapy Discharge Instructions[2]	78	97%	75%	75%
Chest Pain/Possible Heart Attack Care				
Aspirin Given Within 24 Hours of Arrival[5]	-	-	96%	96%
Fibrinolytic Meds Within 30 Min. of Arrival[5]	-	-	55%	58%
Average Time to ECG (minutes)[5]	-	-	9	7
Average Time to Transfer (minutes)[5]	-	-	62	60
Children's Asthma Care				
Received Home Management Plan of Care	-	-	-	88%
Received Reliever Medication	-	-	-	100%
Received Systemic Corticosteroids	-	-	-	100%
Emergency Department				
Admittance Decision Time (minutes)[2]	672	62	76	98
Head CT Results Within 45 Min. of Arrival[7]	-	-	38%	57%
Patients Who Left ER Before Being Seen	40,412	0%	1%	2%
Time from ER Arrival to Admit. (minutes)[2]	672	227	232	274
Time from ER Arrival to Discharge (minutes)	539	120	121	134
Time in ER Before Being Evaluated (minutes)	564	12	21	26
Time to Pain Meds for Fractures (minutes)	183	44	46	57
Heart Attack Care				
Aspirin Given at Discharge	234	100%	100%	99%
Fibrinolytic Meds Within 30 Min. of Arrival[7]	-	-	-	54%
PCI Within 90 Minutes of Arrival	52	100%	98%	96%
Statin Prescribed at Discharge	215	100%	99%	98%
Heart Failure Care				
ACE Inhibitor or ARB for LVSD	33	100%	98%	97%
Discharge Instructions Given	108	100%	94%	94%
Evaluation of LVS Function	126	100%	97%	99%
Medicare Spending				
Medicare Spending per Patient (ratio)	-	0.96	0.91	0.98
Pneumonia Care				
Appropriate Initial Antibiotic Given	153	100%	94%	95%
Blood Culture Timing	233	100%	98%	98%
Pregnancy and Delivery Care				
Newborn Deliveries Scheduled Early[2]	34	9%	6%	6%
Preventive Care				
Immunization for Influenza[2]	543	87%	83%	90%
Immunization for Pneumonia[2]	615	93%	89%	92%
Stroke Care				
Anticoagulation Therapy for Atrial Fibrillation	20	100%	97%	95%
Antithrombotic Therapy Timing	78	100%	98%	98%
Assessed for Rehabilitation	118	100%	98%	97%
Discharged on Antithrombotic Therapy	99	100%	99%	99%
Discharged on Statin Medication	63	92%	91%	94%
Thrombolytic Therapy Timing[1]	-	-	55%	66%
Venous Thromboembolism Prophylaxis	116	93%	93%	94%
Written Stroke Educational Materials Given	69	99%	84%	88%
Surgical Care Improvement Project				
Appropriate Beta Blocker Usage[2]	140	99%	98%	98%
Appropriate VTP Within 24 Hours[2]	337	99%	98%	98%
Controlled Postoperative Blood Glucose[2]	83	100%	99%	97%
Perioperative Temperature Management[2]	445	100%	99%	100%
Prophylactic Antibiotic Selection[2]	294	98%	99%	99%
Prophylactic Antibiotic Selection (Outpatient)	380	99%	98%	98%
Prophylactic Antibiotic Stopped[2]	290	99%	98%	98%
Prophylactic Antibiotic Timing[2]	294	99%	98%	99%
Prophylactic Antibiotic Timing (Outpatient)	380	99%	97%	98%
Urinary Catheter Removal[2]	166	95%	96%	97%
Survey of Patients' Hospital Experiences				
Area Around Room 'Always' Quiet at Night	300+	50%	61%	61%
Doctors 'Always' Communicated Well	300+	76%	83%	82%
Home Recovery Information Given	300+	85%	88%	85%
Hospital Given 9 or 10 on 10 Point Scale	300+	61%	73%	71%
Meds 'Always' Explained Before Given	300+	56%	66%	64%
Nurses 'Always' Communicated Well	300+	72%	80%	79%
Pain 'Always' Well Controlled	300+	64%	72%	71%
Room and Bathroom 'Always' Clean	300+	63%	77%	73%
Timely Help 'Always' Received	300+	57%	73%	68%
Would Definitely Recommend Hospital	300+	63%	74%	71%
Use of Medical Imaging				
Cardiac Imaging Stress Test before Surgery	111	4.5%	4.6%	5.3%
Combination Abdominal CT Scan	524	2.3%	7.3%	10.5%
Combination Brain/Sinus CT Scan	461	2.0%	1.7%	2.7%
Combination Chest CT Scan	153	0.0%	1.8%	2.7%
Follow-up Mammogram/Ultrasound	906	5.8%	8.2%	8.8%
Lumbar Spine MRI for Low Back Pain	85	42.4%	40.3%	37.2%

Mountain View Hospital

2325 Coronado Street
Idaho Falls, ID 83404
Phone: 208-557-2899
URL: www.mountainviewhospital.org
Type: Acute Care Hospitals
Ownership: Proprietary
Emergency Services: Yes
Beds: 25

Measure	Cases	This Hosp.	State Avg.	U.S. Avg.
Blood Clot Prevention and Treatment				
Anticoagulation Overlap Therapy[1,2]	-	-	95%	93%
ICU Venous Thromboembolism Prophylaxis[2,7]	-	-	92%	92%
Incidence of Potentially Preventable VTE[1,2]	-	-	11%	10%
UFH with Dosages/Platelet Monitoring[2,7]	-	-	99%	97%
Venous Thromboembolism Prophylaxis[2]	15	100%	87%	85%
Warfarin Therapy Discharge Instructions[1,2]	-	-	75%	75%
Chest Pain/Possible Heart Attack Care				
Aspirin Given Within 24 Hours of Arrival[5]	-	-	96%	96%
Fibrinolytic Meds Within 30 Min. of Arrival[5]	-	-	55%	58%
Average Time to ECG (minutes)[5]	-	-	9	7
Average Time to Transfer (minutes)[5]	-	-	62	60
Children's Asthma Care				
Received Home Management Plan of Care	-	-	-	88%
Received Reliever Medication	-	-	-	100%
Received Systemic Corticosteroids	-	-	-	100%
Emergency Department				
Admittance Decision Time (minutes)[2,7]	-	-	76	98
Head CT Results Within 45 Min. of Arrival[5]	-	-	38%	57%
Patients Who Left ER Before Being Seen[5]	-	-	1%	2%
Time from ER Arrival to Admit. (minutes)[2,7]	-	-	232	274
Time from ER Arrival to Discharge (minutes)[5]	-	-	121	134
Time in ER Before Being Evaluated (minutes)[5]	-	-	21	26
Time to Pain Meds for Fractures (minutes)[5]	-	-	46	57
Heart Attack Care				
Aspirin Given at Discharge[5]	-	-	100%	99%
Fibrinolytic Meds Within 30 Min. of Arrival[5]	-	-	-	54%
PCI Within 90 Minutes of Arrival[5]	-	-	98%	96%
Statin Prescribed at Discharge[5]	-	-	99%	98%
Heart Failure Care				
ACE Inhibitor or ARB for LVSD[5]	-	-	98%	97%
Discharge Instructions Given[5]	-	-	94%	94%
Evaluation of LVS Function[5]	-	-	97%	99%
Medicare Spending				
Medicare Spending per Patient (ratio)	-	0.91	0.91	0.98
Pneumonia Care				
Appropriate Initial Antibiotic Given[5]	-	-	94%	95%
Blood Culture Timing[5]	-	-	98%	98%
Pregnancy and Delivery Care				
Newborn Deliveries Scheduled Early[2]	29	0%	6%	6%
Preventive Care				
Immunization for Influenza[2]	234	100%	83%	90%
Immunization for Pneumonia[2]	118	100%	89%	92%
Stroke Care				
Anticoagulation Therapy for Atrial Fibrillation[5]	-	-	97%	95%
Antithrombotic Therapy Timing[5]	-	-	98%	98%
Assessed for Rehabilitation[5]	-	-	98%	97%
Discharged on Antithrombotic Therapy[5]	-	-	99%	99%
Discharged on Statin Medication[5]	-	-	91%	94%
Thrombolytic Therapy Timing[5]	-	-	55%	66%
Venous Thromboembolism Prophylaxis[5]	-	-	93%	94%
Written Stroke Educational Materials Given[5]	-	-	84%	88%
Surgical Care Improvement Project				
Appropriate Beta Blocker Usage[2]	52	100%	98%	98%
Appropriate VTP Within 24 Hours[2]	345	99%	98%	98%
Controlled Postoperative Blood Glucose[2,7]	-	-	99%	97%
Perioperative Temperature Management[2]	368	100%	99%	100%
Prophylactic Antibiotic Selection[2]	299	99%	99%	99%
Prophylactic Antibiotic Selection (Outpatient)	445	100%	98%	98%
Prophylactic Antibiotic Stopped[2]	298	100%	98%	98%
Prophylactic Antibiotic Timing[2]	299	100%	98%	99%
Prophylactic Antibiotic Timing (Outpatient)	445	100%	97%	98%
Urinary Catheter Removal[2]	79	99%	96%	97%
Survey of Patients' Hospital Experiences				
Area Around Room 'Always' Quiet at Night	300+	59%	61%	61%
Doctors 'Always' Communicated Well	300+	82%	83%	82%
Home Recovery Information Given	300+	86%	88%	85%
Hospital Given 9 or 10 on 10 Point Scale	300+	69%	73%	71%
Meds 'Always' Explained Before Given	300+	65%	66%	64%
Nurses 'Always' Communicated Well	300+	77%	80%	79%
Pain 'Always' Well Controlled	300+	72%	72%	71%
Room and Bathroom 'Always' Clean	300+	70%	77%	73%
Timely Help 'Always' Received	300+	67%	73%	68%
Would Definitely Recommend Hospital	300+	80%	74%	71%
Use of Medical Imaging				
Cardiac Imaging Stress Test before Surgery[7]	-	-	4.6%	5.3%
Combination Abdominal CT Scan	185	4.3%	7.3%	10.5%
Combination Brain/Sinus CT Scan[1]	-	-	1.7%	2.7%
Combination Chest CT Scan	254	0.0%	1.8%	2.7%
Follow-up Mammogram/Ultrasound	333	6.9%	8.2%	8.8%
Lumbar Spine MRI for Low Back Pain	160	41.3%	40.3%	37.2%

NOTE: Hospital profiles are in alphabetical order by state, then city, then hospital within the city; Rankings exclude hospitals with less than 25 cases except for patient surveys which excludes hospitals with less than 100 cases; (a) 100-299 cases; (1) The number of cases/patients is too few to report; (2) Data submitted were based on a sample of cases/patients; (3) Results are based on a shorter time period than required; (4) Data suppressed by CMS for one or more quarters; (5) Results are not available for this reporting period; (6) Fewer than 100 patients completed the HCAHPS survey; (7) No cases met the criteria for this measure; (8) The lower limit of the confidence interval cannot be calculated if the number of observed infections equals zero; (9) No data are available from the state/territory for this reporting period; (10) The scores shown reflect fewer than 50 completed surveys; (11) There were discrepancies in the data collection process; (12) This measure does not apply to this hospital for this reporting period; (13) Results cannot be calculated for this reporting period; (14) The results for this state are combined with nearby states to protect confidentiality; Please refer to the User's Guide for a full explanation of data.

Saint Luke's Jerome

709 North Lincoln Avenue Phone: 208-324-4301
Jerome, ID 83338
Type: Critical Access Hospitals Emergency Services: Yes
Ownership: Voluntary non-profit - Church

Measure	Cases	This Hosp.	State Avg.	U.S. Avg.
Blood Clot Prevention and Treatment				
Anticoagulation Overlap Therapy[5]	-	-	95%	93%
ICU Venous Thromboembolism Prophylaxis[5]	-	-	92%	92%
Incidence of Potentially Preventable VTE[5]	-	-	11%	10%
UFH with Dosages/Platelet Monitoring[5]	-	-	99%	97%
Venous Thromboembolism Prophylaxis[5]	-	-	87%	85%
Warfarin Therapy Discharge Instructions[5]	-	-	75%	75%
Chest Pain/Possible Heart Attack Care				
Aspirin Given Within 24 Hours of Arrival	-	-	96%	96%
Fibrinolytic Meds Within 30 Min. of Arrival	-	-	55%	58%
Average Time to ECG (minutes)	-	-	9	7
Average Time to Transfer (minutes)	-	-	62	60
Children's Asthma Care				
Received Home Management Plan of Care	-	-	-	88%
Received Reliever Medication	-	-	-	100%
Received Systemic Corticosteroids	-	-	-	100%
Emergency Department				
Admittance Decision Time (minutes)[5]	-	-	76	98
Head CT Results Within 45 Min. of Arrival	-	-	38%	57%
Patients Who Left ER Before Being Seen	-	-	1%	2%
Time from ER Arrival to Admit. (minutes)[5]	-	-	232	274
Time from ER Arrival to Discharge (minutes)	-	-	121	134
Time in ER Before Being Evaluated (minutes)	-	-	21	26
Time to Pain Meds for Fractures (minutes)	-	-	46	57
Heart Attack Care				
Aspirin Given at Discharge[5]	-	-	100%	99%
Fibrinolytic Meds Within 30 Min. of Arrival[5]	-	-	-	54%
PCI Within 90 Minutes of Arrival[5]	-	-	98%	96%
Statin Prescribed at Discharge[5]	-	-	99%	98%
Heart Failure Care				
ACE Inhibitor or ARB for LVSD[2,3]	-	-	98%	97%
Discharge Instructions Given[1,2]	-	-	94%	94%
Evaluation of LVS Function[1,2]	-	-	97%	99%
Medicare Spending				
Medicare Spending per Patient (ratio)	-	-	0.91	0.98
Pneumonia Care				
Appropriate Initial Antibiotic Given[1,2]	-	-	94%	95%
Blood Culture Timing[1,2]	-	-	98%	98%
Pregnancy and Delivery Care				
Newborn Deliveries Scheduled Early[5]	-	-	6%	6%
Preventive Care				
Immunization for Influenza[5]	-	-	83%	90%
Immunization for Pneumonia[5]	-	-	89%	92%
Stroke Care				
Anticoagulation Therapy for Atrial Fibrillation[5]	-	-	97%	95%
Antithrombotic Therapy Timing[5]	-	-	98%	98%
Assessed for Rehabilitation[5]	-	-	98%	97%
Discharged on Antithrombotic Therapy[5]	-	-	99%	99%
Discharged on Statin Medication[5]	-	-	91%	94%
Thrombolytic Therapy Timing[5]	-	-	55%	66%
Venous Thromboembolism Prophylaxis[5]	-	-	93%	94%
Written Stroke Educational Materials Given[5]	-	-	84%	88%
Surgical Care Improvement Project				
Appropriate Beta Blocker Usage[5]	-	-	98%	98%
Appropriate VTP Within 24 Hours[5]	-	-	98%	98%
Controlled Postoperative Blood Glucose[5]	-	-	99%	97%
Perioperative Temperature Management[5]	-	-	99%	100%
Prophylactic Antibiotic Selection[5]	-	-	99%	99%
Prophylactic Antibiotic Selection (Outpatient)	-	-	98%	98%
Prophylactic Antibiotic Stopped[5]	-	-	98%	98%
Prophylactic Antibiotic Timing[5]	-	-	98%	99%
Prophylactic Antibiotic Timing (Outpatient)	-	-	97%	98%
Urinary Catheter Removal[5]	-	-	96%	97%
Survey of Patients' Hospital Experiences				
Area Around Room 'Always' Quiet at Night[6]	<100	58%	61%	61%
Doctors 'Always' Communicated Well[6]	<100	88%	83%	82%
Home Recovery Information Given[6]	<100	88%	88%	85%
Hospital Given 9 or 10 on 10 Point Scale[6]	<100	69%	73%	71%
Meds 'Always' Explained Before Given[6]	<100	76%	66%	64%
Nurses 'Always' Communicated Well[6]	<100	87%	80%	79%
Pain 'Always' Well Controlled[6]	<100	73%	72%	71%
Room and Bathroom 'Always' Clean[6]	<100	77%	77%	73%
Timely Help 'Always' Received[6]	<100	82%	73%	68%
Would Definitely Recommend Hospital[6]	<100	71%	74%	71%
Use of Medical Imaging				
Cardiac Imaging Stress Test before Surgery	-	-	4.6%	5.3%
Combination Abdominal CT Scan	-	-	7.3%	10.5%
Combination Brain/Sinus CT Scan	-	-	1.7%	2.7%
Combination Chest CT Scan	-	-	1.8%	2.7%
Follow-up Mammogram/Ultrasound	-	-	8.2%	8.8%
Lumbar Spine MRI for Low Back Pain	-	-	40.3%	37.2%

Shoshone Medical Center

25 Jacobs Gulch Road Phone: 208-784-1221
Kellogg, ID 83837
Type: Critical Access Hospitals Emergency Services: Yes
Ownership: Govt - Hospital Dist/Auth

Measure	Cases	This Hosp.	State Avg.	U.S. Avg.
Blood Clot Prevention and Treatment				
Anticoagulation Overlap Therapy[5]	-	-	95%	93%
ICU Venous Thromboembolism Prophylaxis[5]	-	-	92%	92%
Incidence of Potentially Preventable VTE[5]	-	-	11%	10%
UFH with Dosages/Platelet Monitoring[5]	-	-	99%	97%
Venous Thromboembolism Prophylaxis[5]	-	-	87%	85%
Warfarin Therapy Discharge Instructions[5]	-	-	75%	75%
Chest Pain/Possible Heart Attack Care				
Aspirin Given Within 24 Hours of Arrival	-	-	96%	96%
Fibrinolytic Meds Within 30 Min. of Arrival	-	-	55%	58%
Average Time to ECG (minutes)	-	-	9	7
Average Time to Transfer (minutes)	-	-	62	60
Children's Asthma Care				
Received Home Management Plan of Care	-	-	-	88%
Received Reliever Medication	-	-	-	100%
Received Systemic Corticosteroids	-	-	-	100%
Emergency Department				
Admittance Decision Time (minutes)[5]	-	-	76	98
Head CT Results Within 45 Min. of Arrival	-	-	38%	57%
Patients Who Left ER Before Being Seen	-	-	1%	2%
Time from ER Arrival to Admit. (minutes)[5]	-	-	232	274
Time from ER Arrival to Discharge (minutes)	-	-	121	134
Time in ER Before Being Evaluated (minutes)	-	-	21	26
Time to Pain Meds for Fractures (minutes)	-	-	46	57
Heart Attack Care				
Aspirin Given at Discharge[5]	-	-	100%	99%
Fibrinolytic Meds Within 30 Min. of Arrival[5]	-	-	-	54%
PCI Within 90 Minutes of Arrival[5]	-	-	98%	96%
Statin Prescribed at Discharge[5]	-	-	99%	98%
Heart Failure Care				
ACE Inhibitor or ARB for LVSD[1]	-	-	98%	97%
Discharge Instructions Given[1]	-	-	94%	94%
Evaluation of LVS Function[1]	-	-	97%	99%
Medicare Spending				
Medicare Spending per Patient (ratio)	-	-	0.91	0.98
Pneumonia Care				
Appropriate Initial Antibiotic Given[1]	-	-	94%	95%
Blood Culture Timing[1]	-	-	98%	98%
Pregnancy and Delivery Care				
Newborn Deliveries Scheduled Early[5]	-	-	6%	6%
Preventive Care				
Immunization for Influenza[5]	-	-	83%	90%
Immunization for Pneumonia[5]	-	-	89%	92%
Stroke Care				
Anticoagulation Therapy for Atrial Fibrillation[5]	-	-	97%	95%
Antithrombotic Therapy Timing[5]	-	-	98%	98%
Assessed for Rehabilitation[5]	-	-	98%	97%
Discharged on Antithrombotic Therapy[5]	-	-	99%	99%
Discharged on Statin Medication[5]	-	-	91%	94%
Thrombolytic Therapy Timing[5]	-	-	55%	66%
Venous Thromboembolism Prophylaxis[5]	-	-	93%	94%
Written Stroke Educational Materials Given[5]	-	-	84%	88%
Surgical Care Improvement Project				
Appropriate Beta Blocker Usage[5]	-	-	98%	98%
Appropriate VTP Within 24 Hours[5]	-	-	98%	98%
Controlled Postoperative Blood Glucose[5]	-	-	99%	97%
Perioperative Temperature Management[5]	-	-	99%	100%
Prophylactic Antibiotic Selection[5]	-	-	99%	99%
Prophylactic Antibiotic Selection (Outpatient)	-	-	98%	98%
Prophylactic Antibiotic Stopped[5]	-	-	98%	98%
Prophylactic Antibiotic Timing[5]	-	-	98%	99%
Prophylactic Antibiotic Timing (Outpatient)	-	-	97%	98%
Urinary Catheter Removal[5]	-	-	96%	97%
Survey of Patients' Hospital Experiences				
Area Around Room 'Always' Quiet at Night[5]	-	-	61%	61%
Doctors 'Always' Communicated Well[5]	-	-	83%	82%
Home Recovery Information Given[5]	-	-	88%	85%
Hospital Given 9 or 10 on 10 Point Scale[5]	-	-	73%	71%
Meds 'Always' Explained Before Given[5]	-	-	66%	64%
Nurses 'Always' Communicated Well[5]	-	-	80%	79%
Pain 'Always' Well Controlled[5]	-	-	72%	71%
Room and Bathroom 'Always' Clean[5]	-	-	77%	73%
Timely Help 'Always' Received[5]	-	-	73%	68%
Would Definitely Recommend Hospital[5]	-	-	74%	71%
Use of Medical Imaging				
Cardiac Imaging Stress Test before Surgery	-	-	4.6%	5.3%
Combination Abdominal CT Scan	-	-	7.3%	10.5%
Combination Brain/Sinus CT Scan	-	-	1.7%	2.7%
Combination Chest CT Scan	-	-	1.8%	2.7%
Follow-up Mammogram/Ultrasound	-	-	8.2%	8.8%
Lumbar Spine MRI for Low Back Pain	-	-	40.3%	37.2%

Saint Luke's Wood River Medical Center

100 Hospital Drive Phone: 208-727-8800
Ketchum, ID 83340 Fax: 208-727-8412
URL: www.stlukesonline.org/wood_river
Type: Critical Access Hospitals Emergency Services: Yes
Ownership: Voluntary non-profit - Private Beds: 39

Key Personnel:

Chief of Medical Staff . . . . Herb Alexander, MD
Infection Control. . . . . Jodie Alverson
Radiology. . . . . Dennis Davis, MD
CEO/President. . . . . Cody Langbehn
Patient Relations . . . . Kathleen Loughney
Operating Room. . . . . Ed Rotttengill
Emergency Room . . . . Keith Sivertson
Quality Assurance . . . . Genie Swyers

Measure	Cases	This Hosp.	State Avg.	U.S. Avg.
Blood Clot Prevention and Treatment				
Anticoagulation Overlap Therapy[5]	-	-	95%	93%
ICU Venous Thromboembolism Prophylaxis[5]	-	-	92%	92%
Incidence of Potentially Preventable VTE[5]	-	-	11%	10%
UFH with Dosages/Platelet Monitoring[5]	-	-	99%	97%
Venous Thromboembolism Prophylaxis[5]	-	-	87%	85%
Warfarin Therapy Discharge Instructions[5]	-	-	75%	75%
Chest Pain/Possible Heart Attack Care				
Aspirin Given Within 24 Hours of Arrival	-	-	96%	96%
Fibrinolytic Meds Within 30 Min. of Arrival	-	-	55%	58%
Average Time to ECG (minutes)	-	-	9	7
Average Time to Transfer (minutes)	-	-	62	60
Children's Asthma Care				
Received Home Management Plan of Care	-	-	-	88%
Received Reliever Medication	-	-	-	100%
Received Systemic Corticosteroids	-	-	-	100%
Emergency Department				
Admittance Decision Time (minutes)[5]	-	-	76	98
Head CT Results Within 45 Min. of Arrival	-	-	38%	57%
Patients Who Left ER Before Being Seen	-	-	1%	2%
Time from ER Arrival to Admit. (minutes)[5]	-	-	232	274
Time from ER Arrival to Discharge (minutes)	-	-	121	134
Time in ER Before Being Evaluated (minutes)	-	-	21	26
Time to Pain Meds for Fractures (minutes)	-	-	46	57
Heart Attack Care				
Aspirin Given at Discharge[5]	-	-	100%	99%

NOTE: Hospital profiles are in alphabetical order by state, then city, then hospital within the city; Rankings exclude hospitals with less than 25 cases except for patient surveys which excludes hospitals with less than 100 cases; (a) 100-299 cases; (1) The number of cases/patients is too few to report; (2) Data submitted were based on a sample of cases/patients; (3) Results are based on a shorter time period than required; (4) Data suppressed by CMS for one or more quarters; (5) Results are not available for this reporting period; (6) Fewer than 100 patients completed the HCAHPS survey; (7) No cases met the criteria for this measure; (8) The lower limit of the confidence interval cannot be calculated if the number of observed infections equals zero; (9) No data are available from the state/territory for this reporting period; (10) The scores shown reflect fewer than 50 completed surveys; (11) There were discrepancies in the data collection process; (12) This measure does not apply to this hospital for this reporting period; (13) Results cannot be calculated for this reporting period; (14) The results for this state are combined with nearby states to protect confidentiality; Please refer to the User's Guide for a full explanation of data.

Measure	Cases	This Hosp.	State Avg.	U.S. Avg.
Fibrinolytic Meds Within 30 Min. of Arrival[5]	-	-	-	54%
PCI Within 90 Minutes of Arrival[5]	-	-	98%	96%
Statin Prescribed at Discharge[5]	-	-	99%	98%
Heart Failure Care				
ACE Inhibitor or ARB for LVSD[1]	-	-	98%	97%
Discharge Instructions Given[1]	-	-	94%	94%
Evaluation of LVS Function[1]	-	-	97%	99%
Medicare Spending				
Medicare Spending per Patient (ratio)	-	-	0.91	0.98
Pneumonia Care				
Appropriate Initial Antibiotic Given[1]	-	-	94%	95%
Blood Culture Timing	14	100%	98%	98%
Pregnancy and Delivery Care				
Newborn Deliveries Scheduled Early[5]	-	-	6%	6%
Preventive Care				
Immunization for Influenza[5]	-	-	83%	90%
Immunization for Pneumonia[5]	-	-	89%	92%
Stroke Care				
Anticoagulation Therapy for Atrial Fibrillation[5]	-	-	97%	95%
Antithrombotic Therapy Timing[5]	-	-	98%	98%
Assessed for Rehabilitation[5]	-	-	98%	97%
Discharged on Antithrombotic Therapy[5]	-	-	99%	99%
Discharged on Statin Medication[5]	-	-	91%	94%
Thrombolytic Therapy Timing[5]	-	-	55%	66%
Venous Thromboembolism Prophylaxis[5]	-	-	93%	94%
Written Stroke Educational Materials Given[5]	-	-	84%	88%
Surgical Care Improvement Project				
Appropriate Beta Blocker Usage[5]	-	-	98%	98%
Appropriate VTP Within 24 Hours[5]	-	-	98%	98%
Controlled Postoperative Blood Glucose[5]	-	-	99%	97%
Perioperative Temperature Management[5]	-	-	99%	100%
Prophylactic Antibiotic Selection[5]	-	-	99%	99%
Prophylactic Antibiotic Selection (Outpatient)	-	-	98%	98%
Prophylactic Antibiotic Stopped[5]	-	-	98%	98%
Prophylactic Antibiotic Timing[5]	-	-	98%	99%
Prophylactic Antibiotic Timing (Outpatient)	-	-	97%	98%
Urinary Catheter Removal[5]	-	-	96%	97%
Survey of Patients' Hospital Experiences				
Area Around Room 'Always' Quiet at Night	300+	72%	61%	61%
Doctors 'Always' Communicated Well	300+	86%	83%	82%
Home Recovery Information Given	300+	91%	88%	85%
Hospital Given 9 or 10 on 10 Point Scale	300+	83%	73%	71%
Meds 'Always' Explained Before Given	300+	71%	66%	64%
Nurses 'Always' Communicated Well	300+	86%	80%	79%
Pain 'Always' Well Controlled	300+	79%	72%	71%
Room and Bathroom 'Always' Clean	300+	82%	77%	73%
Timely Help 'Always' Received	300+	81%	73%	68%
Would Definitely Recommend Hospital	300+	88%	74%	71%
Use of Medical Imaging				
Cardiac Imaging Stress Test before Surgery	-	-	4.6%	5.3%
Combination Abdominal CT Scan	-	-	7.3%	10.5%
Combination Brain/Sinus CT Scan	-	-	1.7%	2.7%
Combination Chest CT Scan	-	-	1.8%	2.7%
Follow-up Mammogram/Ultrasound	-	-	8.2%	8.8%
Lumbar Spine MRI for Low Back Pain	-	-	40.3%	37.2%

Saint Joseph Regional Medical Center

415 Sixth Street | Phone: 208-743-2511
Lewiston, ID 83501 | Fax: 208-799-6508
URL: www.sjrmc.org
Type: Acute Care Hospitals | Emergency Services: Yes
Ownership: Voluntary non-profit - Private | Beds: 160

Key Personnel:
Emergency Room . . . . Nancy Berkheiser
Radiology. . . . . Jeffrey C Bickel
Chief of Medical Staff . . . . Christina Bjornstad
Quality Assurance . . . . Jill Carlson-Balmer
Operating Room. . . . . Scott Gardner
CEO/President. . . . . Howard A Hayes
Pediatric In-Patient Care . . . . Earlene Pedersen
Chair/CEO . . . . Mike Thomason

Measure	Cases	This Hosp.	State Avg.	U.S. Avg.
Blood Clot Prevention and Treatment				
Anticoagulation Overlap Therapy[2]	27	85%	95%	93%
ICU Venous Thromboembolism Prophylaxis[2]	99	90%	92%	92%
Incidence of Potentially Preventable VTE[1,2]	-	-	11%	10%
UFH with Dosages/Platelet Monitoring[2]	11	100%	99%	97%
Venous Thromboembolism Prophylaxis[2]	268	77%	87%	85%
Warfarin Therapy Discharge Instructions[2]	23	61%	75%	75%
Chest Pain/Possible Heart Attack Care				
Aspirin Given Within 24 Hours of Arrival[1,3]	-	-	96%	96%
Fibrinolytic Meds Within 30 Min. of Arrival[1,3]	-	-	55%	58%
Average Time to ECG (minutes)[1,3]	-	-	9	7
Average Time to Transfer (minutes)[1,3]	-	-	62	60
Children's Asthma Care				
Received Home Management Plan of Care	-	-	-	88%
Received Reliever Medication	-	-	-	100%
Received Systemic Corticosteroids	-	-	-	100%
Emergency Department				
Admittance Decision Time (minutes)[2]	138	42	76	98
Head CT Results Within 45 Min. of Arrival[1]	-	-	38%	57%
Patients Who Left ER Before Being Seen	10,112	1%	1%	2%
Time from ER Arrival to Admit. (minutes)[2]	495	246	232	274
Time from ER Arrival to Discharge (minutes)	354	163	121	134
Time in ER Before Being Evaluated (minutes)	27	40	21	26
Time to Pain Meds for Fractures (minutes)	61	66	46	57
Heart Attack Care				
Aspirin Given at Discharge	102	99%	100%	99%
Fibrinolytic Meds Within 30 Min. of Arrival[7]	-	-	-	54%
PCI Within 90 Minutes of Arrival	17	100%	98%	96%
Statin Prescribed at Discharge	98	96%	99%	98%
Heart Failure Care				
ACE Inhibitor or ARB for LVSD	35	100%	98%	97%
Discharge Instructions Given	76	100%	94%	94%
Evaluation of LVS Function	105	100%	97%	99%
Medicare Spending				
Medicare Spending per Patient (ratio)	-	0.93	0.91	0.98
Pneumonia Care				
Appropriate Initial Antibiotic Given	86	90%	94%	95%
Blood Culture Timing	134	84%	98%	98%
Pregnancy and Delivery Care				
Newborn Deliveries Scheduled Early[2]	28	11%	6%	6%
Preventive Care				
Immunization for Influenza[2]	428	84%	83%	90%
Immunization for Pneumonia[2]	547	94%	89%	92%
Stroke Care				
Anticoagulation Therapy for Atrial Fibrillation[2]	16	94%	97%	95%
Antithrombotic Therapy Timing[2]	57	89%	98%	98%
Assessed for Rehabilitation[2]	72	89%	98%	97%
Discharged on Antithrombotic Therapy[2]	64	97%	99%	99%
Discharged on Statin Medication[2]	60	73%	91%	94%
Thrombolytic Therapy Timing[2]	29	7%	55%	66%
Venous Thromboembolism Prophylaxis[2]	69	81%	93%	94%
Written Stroke Educational Materials Given[2]	41	90%	84%	88%
Surgical Care Improvement Project				
Appropriate Beta Blocker Usage[2]	102	98%	98%	98%
Appropriate VTP Within 24 Hours[2]	449	97%	98%	98%
Controlled Postoperative Blood Glucose[2,7]	-	-	99%	97%
Perioperative Temperature Management[2]	499	100%	99%	100%
Prophylactic Antibiotic Selection[2]	384	99%	99%	99%
Prophylactic Antibiotic Selection (Outpatient)	426	90%	98%	98%
Prophylactic Antibiotic Stopped[2]	376	96%	98%	98%
Prophylactic Antibiotic Timing[2]	384	97%	98%	99%
Prophylactic Antibiotic Timing (Outpatient)	357	93%	97%	98%
Urinary Catheter Removal[2]	407	95%	96%	97%
Survey of Patients' Hospital Experiences				
Area Around Room 'Always' Quiet at Night	300+	56%	61%	61%
Doctors 'Always' Communicated Well	300+	80%	83%	82%
Home Recovery Information Given	300+	90%	88%	85%
Hospital Given 9 or 10 on 10 Point Scale	300+	69%	73%	71%
Meds 'Always' Explained Before Given	300+	65%	66%	64%
Nurses 'Always' Communicated Well	300+	77%	80%	79%
Pain 'Always' Well Controlled	300+	66%	72%	71%
Room and Bathroom 'Always' Clean	300+	69%	77%	73%
Timely Help 'Always' Received	300+	68%	73%	68%
Would Definitely Recommend Hospital	300+	70%	74%	71%
Use of Medical Imaging				
Cardiac Imaging Stress Test before Surgery	193	4.1%	4.6%	5.3%
Combination Abdominal CT Scan	712	3.1%	7.3%	10.5%
Combination Brain/Sinus CT Scan[1]	-	-	1.7%	2.7%
Combination Chest CT Scan	429	0.0%	1.8%	2.7%
Follow-up Mammogram/Ultrasound	1,074	10.6%	8.2%	8.8%
Lumbar Spine MRI for Low Back Pain	139	34.5%	40.3%	37.2%

Oneida County Hospital

150 North 200 West | Phone: 208-766-2231
Malad City, ID 83252
Type: Critical Access Hospitals | Emergency Services: Yes
Ownership: Government - Local

Measure	Cases	This Hosp.	State Avg.	U.S. Avg.
Blood Clot Prevention and Treatment				
Anticoagulation Overlap Therapy[5]	-	-	95%	93%
ICU Venous Thromboembolism Prophylaxis[5]	-	-	92%	92%
Incidence of Potentially Preventable VTE[5]	-	-	11%	10%
UFH with Dosages/Platelet Monitoring[5]	-	-	99%	97%
Venous Thromboembolism Prophylaxis[5]	-	-	87%	85%
Warfarin Therapy Discharge Instructions[5]	-	-	75%	75%
Chest Pain/Possible Heart Attack Care				
Aspirin Given Within 24 Hours of Arrival	-	-	96%	96%
Fibrinolytic Meds Within 30 Min. of Arrival	-	-	55%	58%
Average Time to ECG (minutes)	-	-	9	7
Average Time to Transfer (minutes)	-	-	62	60
Children's Asthma Care				
Received Home Management Plan of Care	-	-	-	88%
Received Reliever Medication	-	-	-	100%
Received Systemic Corticosteroids	-	-	-	100%
Emergency Department				
Admittance Decision Time (minutes)[5]	-	-	76	98
Head CT Results Within 45 Min. of Arrival	-	-	38%	57%
Patients Who Left ER Before Being Seen	-	-	1%	2%
Time from ER Arrival to Admit. (minutes)[5]	-	-	232	274
Time from ER Arrival to Discharge (minutes)	-	-	121	134
Time in ER Before Being Evaluated (minutes)	-	-	21	26
Time to Pain Meds for Fractures (minutes)	-	-	46	57
Heart Attack Care				
Aspirin Given at Discharge[5]	-	-	100%	99%
Fibrinolytic Meds Within 30 Min. of Arrival[5]	-	-	-	54%
PCI Within 90 Minutes of Arrival[5]	-	-	98%	96%
Statin Prescribed at Discharge[5]	-	-	99%	98%
Heart Failure Care				
ACE Inhibitor or ARB for LVSD[5]	-	-	98%	97%
Discharge Instructions Given[5]	-	-	94%	94%
Evaluation of LVS Function[5]	-	-	97%	99%
Medicare Spending				
Medicare Spending per Patient (ratio)	-	-	0.91	0.98
Pneumonia Care				
Appropriate Initial Antibiotic Given[1,3]	-	-	94%	95%
Blood Culture Timing[1,3]	-	-	98%	98%
Pregnancy and Delivery Care				
Newborn Deliveries Scheduled Early[5]	-	-	6%	6%
Preventive Care				
Immunization for Influenza[5]	-	-	83%	90%
Immunization for Pneumonia[5]	-	-	89%	92%
Stroke Care				
Anticoagulation Therapy for Atrial Fibrillation[5]	-	-	97%	95%
Antithrombotic Therapy Timing[5]	-	-	98%	98%
Assessed for Rehabilitation[5]	-	-	98%	97%
Discharged on Antithrombotic Therapy[5]	-	-	99%	99%
Discharged on Statin Medication[5]	-	-	91%	94%
Thrombolytic Therapy Timing[5]	-	-	55%	66%
Venous Thromboembolism Prophylaxis[5]	-	-	93%	94%
Written Stroke Educational Materials Given[5]	-	-	84%	88%
Surgical Care Improvement Project				
Appropriate Beta Blocker Usage[5]	-	-	98%	98%
Appropriate VTP Within 24 Hours[5]	-	-	98%	98%
Controlled Postoperative Blood Glucose[5]	-	-	99%	97%
Perioperative Temperature Management[5]	-	-	99%	100%
Prophylactic Antibiotic Selection[5]	-	-	99%	99%

NOTE: Hospital profiles are in alphabetical order by state, then city, then hospital within the city; Rankings exclude hospitals with less than 25 cases except for patient surveys which excludes hospitals with less than 100 cases; (a) 100-299 cases; (1) The number of cases/patients is too few to report; (2) Data submitted were based on a sample of cases/patients; (3) Results are based on a shorter time period than required; (4) Data suppressed by CMS for one or more quarters; (5) Results are not available for this reporting period; (6) Fewer than 100 patients completed the HCAHPS survey; (7) No cases met the criteria for this measure; (8) The lower limit of the confidence interval cannot be calculated if the number of observed infections equals zero; (9) No data are available from the state/territory for this reporting period; (10) The scores shown reflect fewer than 50 completed surveys; (11) There were discrepancies in the data collection process; (12) This measure does not apply to this hospital for this reporting period; (13) Results cannot be calculated for this reporting period; (14) The results for this state are combined with nearby states to protect confidentiality; Please refer to the User's Guide for a full explanation of data.

Measure	Cases	This Hosp.	State Avg.	U.S. Avg.
Prophylactic Antibiotic Selection (Outpatient)	-	-	98%	98%
Prophylactic Antibiotic Stopped[5]	-	-	98%	98%
Prophylactic Antibiotic Timing[5]	-	-	98%	99%
Prophylactic Antibiotic Timing (Outpatient)	-	-	97%	98%
Urinary Catheter Removal[5]	-	-	96%	97%
Survey of Patients' Hospital Experiences				
Area Around Room 'Always' Quiet at Night[5]	-	-	61%	61%
Doctors 'Always' Communicated Well[5]	-	-	83%	82%
Home Recovery Information Given[5]	-	-	88%	85%
Hospital Given 9 or 10 on 10 Point Scale[5]	-	-	73%	71%
Meds 'Always' Explained Before Given[5]	-	-	66%	64%
Nurses 'Always' Communicated Well[5]	-	-	80%	79%
Pain 'Always' Well Controlled[5]	-	-	72%	71%
Room and Bathroom 'Always' Clean[5]	-	-	77%	73%
Timely Help 'Always' Received[5]	-	-	73%	68%
Would Definitely Recommend Hospital[5]	-	-	74%	71%
Use of Medical Imaging				
Cardiac Imaging Stress Test before Surgery	-	-	4.6%	5.3%
Combination Abdominal CT Scan	-	-	7.3%	10.5%
Combination Brain/Sinus CT Scan	-	-	1.7%	2.7%
Combination Chest CT Scan	-	-	1.8%	2.7%
Follow-up Mammogram/Ultrasound	-	-	8.2%	8.8%
Lumbar Spine MRI for Low Back Pain	-	-	40.3%	37.2%

Saint Luke's Mccall

1000 State Street
Mc Call, ID 83638
Phone: 208-634-2221
Type: Critical Access Hospitals
Emergency Services: Yes
Ownership: Voluntary non-profit - Private

Measure	Cases	This Hosp.	State Avg.	U.S. Avg.
Blood Clot Prevention and Treatment				
Anticoagulation Overlap Therapy[5]	-	-	95%	93%
ICU Venous Thromboembolism Prophylaxis[5]	-	-	92%	92%
Incidence of Potentially Preventable VTE[5]	-	-	11%	10%
UFH with Dosages/Platelet Monitoring[5]	-	-	99%	97%
Venous Thromboembolism Prophylaxis[5]	-	-	87%	85%
Warfarin Therapy Discharge Instructions[5]	-	-	75%	75%
Chest Pain/Possible Heart Attack Care				
Aspirin Given Within 24 Hours of Arrival	-	-	96%	96%
Fibrinolytic Meds Within 30 Min. of Arrival	-	-	55%	58%
Average Time to ECG (minutes)	-	-	9	7
Average Time to Transfer (minutes)	-	-	62	60
Children's Asthma Care				
Received Home Management Plan of Care	-	-	-	88%
Received Reliever Medication	-	-	-	100%
Received Systemic Corticosteroids	-	-	-	100%
Emergency Department				
Admittance Decision Time (minutes)[5]	-	-	76	98
Head CT Results Within 45 Min. of Arrival	-	-	38%	57%
Patients Who Left ER Before Being Seen	-	-	1%	2%
Time from ER Arrival to Admit. (minutes)[5]	-	-	232	274
Time from ER Arrival to Discharge (minutes)	-	-	121	134
Time in ER Before Being Evaluated (minutes)	-	-	21	26
Time to Pain Meds for Fractures (minutes)	-	-	46	57
Heart Attack Care				
Aspirin Given at Discharge[5]	-	-	100%	99%
Fibrinolytic Meds Within 30 Min. of Arrival[5]	-	-	-	54%
PCI Within 90 Minutes of Arrival[5]	-	-	98%	96%
Statin Prescribed at Discharge[5]	-	-	99%	98%
Heart Failure Care				
ACE Inhibitor or ARB for LVSD[1]	-	-	98%	97%
Discharge Instructions Given[1]	-	-	94%	94%
Evaluation of LVS Function[1]	-	-	97%	99%
Medicare Spending				
Medicare Spending per Patient (ratio)	-	-	0.91	0.98
Pneumonia Care				
Appropriate Initial Antibiotic Given	13	100%	94%	95%
Blood Culture Timing	15	100%	98%	98%
Pregnancy and Delivery Care				
Newborn Deliveries Scheduled Early[5]	-	-	6%	6%
Preventive Care				
Immunization for Influenza[5]	-	-	83%	90%
Immunization for Pneumonia[5]	-	-	89%	92%
Stroke Care				
Anticoagulation Therapy for Atrial Fibrillation[5]	-	-	97%	95%
Antithrombotic Therapy Timing[5]	-	-	98%	98%
Assessed for Rehabilitation[5]	-	-	98%	97%
Discharged on Antithrombotic Therapy[5]	-	-	99%	99%
Discharged on Statin Medication[5]	-	-	91%	94%
Thrombolytic Therapy Timing[5]	-	-	55%	66%
Venous Thromboembolism Prophylaxis[5]	-	-	93%	94%
Written Stroke Educational Materials Given[5]	-	-	84%	88%
Surgical Care Improvement Project				
Appropriate Beta Blocker Usage	18	100%	98%	98%
Appropriate VTP Within 24 Hours	77	100%	98%	98%
Controlled Postoperative Blood Glucose[7]	-	-	99%	97%
Perioperative Temperature Management	86	100%	99%	100%
Prophylactic Antibiotic Selection	81	100%	99%	99%
Prophylactic Antibiotic Selection (Outpatient)	-	-	98%	98%
Prophylactic Antibiotic Stopped	81	100%	98%	98%
Prophylactic Antibiotic Timing	81	99%	98%	99%
Prophylactic Antibiotic Timing (Outpatient)	-	-	97%	98%
Urinary Catheter Removal	83	100%	96%	97%
Survey of Patients' Hospital Experiences				
Area Around Room 'Always' Quiet at Night	(a)	62%	61%	61%
Doctors 'Always' Communicated Well	(a)	82%	83%	82%
Home Recovery Information Given	(a)	86%	88%	85%
Hospital Given 9 or 10 on 10 Point Scale	(a)	81%	73%	71%
Meds 'Always' Explained Before Given	(a)	69%	66%	64%
Nurses 'Always' Communicated Well	(a)	84%	80%	79%
Pain 'Always' Well Controlled	(a)	78%	72%	71%
Room and Bathroom 'Always' Clean	(a)	76%	77%	73%
Timely Help 'Always' Received	(a)	83%	73%	68%
Would Definitely Recommend Hospital	(a)	81%	74%	71%
Use of Medical Imaging				
Cardiac Imaging Stress Test before Surgery	-	-	4.6%	5.3%
Combination Abdominal CT Scan	-	-	7.3%	10.5%
Combination Brain/Sinus CT Scan	-	-	1.7%	2.7%
Combination Chest CT Scan	-	-	1.8%	2.7%
Follow-up Mammogram/Ultrasound	-	-	8.2%	8.8%
Lumbar Spine MRI for Low Back Pain	-	-	40.3%	37.2%

Bear Lake Memorial Hospital

164 South Fifth Street
Montpelier, ID 83254
Phone: 208-847-1630
Type: Critical Access Hospitals
Emergency Services: Yes
Ownership: Government - Local

Measure	Cases	This Hosp.	State Avg.	U.S. Avg.
Blood Clot Prevention and Treatment				
Anticoagulation Overlap Therapy[3,7]	-	-	95%	93%
ICU Venous Thromboembolism Prophylaxis[3,7]	-	-	92%	92%
Incidence of Potentially Preventable VTE[3,7]	-	-	11%	10%
UFH with Dosages/Platelet Monitoring[3,7]	-	-	99%	97%
Venous Thromboembolism Prophylaxis[1,3]	-	-	87%	85%
Warfarin Therapy Discharge Instructions[3,7]	-	-	75%	75%
Chest Pain/Possible Heart Attack Care				
Aspirin Given Within 24 Hours of Arrival	-	-	96%	96%
Fibrinolytic Meds Within 30 Min. of Arrival	-	-	55%	58%
Average Time to ECG (minutes)	-	-	9	7
Average Time to Transfer (minutes)	-	-	62	60
Children's Asthma Care				
Received Home Management Plan of Care	-	-	-	88%
Received Reliever Medication	-	-	-	100%
Received Systemic Corticosteroids	-	-	-	100%
Emergency Department				
Admittance Decision Time (minutes)[5]	-	-	76	98
Head CT Results Within 45 Min. of Arrival	-	-	38%	57%
Patients Who Left ER Before Being Seen	-	-	1%	2%
Time from ER Arrival to Admit. (minutes)[5]	-	-	232	274
Time from ER Arrival to Discharge (minutes)	-	-	121	134
Time in ER Before Being Evaluated (minutes)	-	-	21	26
Time to Pain Meds for Fractures (minutes)	-	-	46	57
Heart Attack Care				
Aspirin Given at Discharge[5]	-	-	100%	99%
Fibrinolytic Meds Within 30 Min. of Arrival[5]	-	-	-	54%
PCI Within 90 Minutes of Arrival[5]	-	-	98%	96%
Statin Prescribed at Discharge[5]	-	-	99%	98%
Heart Failure Care				
ACE Inhibitor or ARB for LVSD[3,7]	-	-	98%	97%
Discharge Instructions Given[1,3]	-	-	94%	94%
Evaluation of LVS Function[1,3]	-	-	97%	99%
Medicare Spending				
Medicare Spending per Patient (ratio)	-	-	0.91	0.98
Pneumonia Care				
Appropriate Initial Antibiotic Given[1]	-	-	94%	95%
Blood Culture Timing[1]	-	-	98%	98%
Pregnancy and Delivery Care				
Newborn Deliveries Scheduled Early[5]	-	-	6%	6%
Preventive Care				
Immunization for Influenza[5]	-	-	83%	90%
Immunization for Pneumonia[5]	-	-	89%	92%
Stroke Care				
Anticoagulation Therapy for Atrial Fibrillation[5]	-	-	97%	95%
Antithrombotic Therapy Timing[5]	-	-	98%	98%
Assessed for Rehabilitation[5]	-	-	98%	97%
Discharged on Antithrombotic Therapy[5]	-	-	99%	99%
Discharged on Statin Medication[5]	-	-	91%	94%
Thrombolytic Therapy Timing[5]	-	-	55%	66%
Venous Thromboembolism Prophylaxis[5]	-	-	93%	94%
Written Stroke Educational Materials Given[5]	-	-	84%	88%
Surgical Care Improvement Project				
Appropriate Beta Blocker Usage[5]	-	-	98%	98%
Appropriate VTP Within 24 Hours[5]	-	-	98%	98%
Controlled Postoperative Blood Glucose[5]	-	-	99%	97%
Perioperative Temperature Management[5]	-	-	99%	100%
Prophylactic Antibiotic Selection[5]	-	-	99%	99%
Prophylactic Antibiotic Selection (Outpatient)	-	-	98%	98%
Prophylactic Antibiotic Stopped[5]	-	-	98%	98%
Prophylactic Antibiotic Timing[5]	-	-	98%	99%
Prophylactic Antibiotic Timing (Outpatient)	-	-	97%	98%
Urinary Catheter Removal[5]	-	-	96%	97%
Survey of Patients' Hospital Experiences				
Area Around Room 'Always' Quiet at Night[5]	-	-	61%	61%
Doctors 'Always' Communicated Well[5]	-	-	83%	82%
Home Recovery Information Given[5]	-	-	88%	85%
Hospital Given 9 or 10 on 10 Point Scale[5]	-	-	73%	71%
Meds 'Always' Explained Before Given[5]	-	-	66%	64%
Nurses 'Always' Communicated Well[5]	-	-	80%	79%
Pain 'Always' Well Controlled[5]	-	-	72%	71%
Room and Bathroom 'Always' Clean[5]	-	-	77%	73%
Timely Help 'Always' Received[5]	-	-	73%	68%
Would Definitely Recommend Hospital[5]	-	-	74%	71%
Use of Medical Imaging				
Cardiac Imaging Stress Test before Surgery	-	-	4.6%	5.3%
Combination Abdominal CT Scan	-	-	7.3%	10.5%
Combination Brain/Sinus CT Scan	-	-	1.7%	2.7%
Combination Chest CT Scan	-	-	1.8%	2.7%
Follow-up Mammogram/Ultrasound	-	-	8.2%	8.8%
Lumbar Spine MRI for Low Back Pain	-	-	40.3%	37.2%

Gritman Medical Center

700 South Main Street
Moscow, ID 83843
Phone: 208-882-4511
Fax: 208-883-6571
E-mail: valerie.strong@gritman.org
URL: www.gritman.org
Type: Critical Access Hospitals
Emergency Services: Yes
Ownership: Voluntary non-profit - Private
Beds: 40

Key Personnel:

Radiology. . . . . Mark H Bechtel
Chief of Medical Staff . . . . John Brown, MD
Patient Relations . . . . Debi Dockinsn
CEO/President. . . . . Jeffrey W Martin
Infection Control. . . . . Sue Rand
Quality Assurance . . . . Sue Rand
Intensive Care Unit. . . . . Pat Riley
Operating Room. . . . . David Vanek

Measure	Cases	This Hosp.	State Avg.	U.S. Avg.
Blood Clot Prevention and Treatment				

NOTE: Hospital profiles are in alphabetical order by state, then city, then hospital within the city; Rankings exclude hospitals with less than 25 cases except for patient surveys which excludes hospitals with less than 100 cases; (a) 100-299 cases; (1) The number of cases/patients is too few to report; (2) Data submitted were based on a sample of cases/patients; (3) Results are based on a shorter time period than required; (4) Data suppressed by CMS for one or more quarters; (5) Results are not available for this reporting period; (6) Fewer than 100 patients completed the HCAHPS survey; (7) No cases met the criteria for this measure; (8) The lower limit of the confidence interval cannot be calculated if the number of observed infections equals zero; (9) No data are available from the state/territory for this reporting period; (10) The scores shown reflect fewer than 50 completed surveys; (11) There were discrepancies in the data collection process; (12) This measure does not apply to this hospital for this reporting period; (13) Results cannot be calculated for this reporting period; (14) The results for this state are combined with nearby states to protect confidentiality; Please refer to the User's Guide for a full explanation of data.

Anticoagulation Overlap Therapy[5]	-	-	95%	93%
ICU Venous Thromboembolism Prophylaxis[5]	-	-	92%	92%
Incidence of Potentially Preventable VTE[5]	-	-	11%	10%
UFH with Dosages/Platelet Monitoring[5]	-	-	99%	97%
Venous Thromboembolism Prophylaxis[5]	-	-	87%	85%
Warfarin Therapy Discharge Instructions[5]	-	-	75%	75%
Chest Pain/Possible Heart Attack Care				
Aspirin Given Within 24 Hours of Arrival	-	-	96%	96%
Fibrinolytic Meds Within 30 Min. of Arrival	-	-	55%	58%
Average Time to ECG (minutes)	-	-	9	7
Average Time to Transfer (minutes)	-	-	62	60
Children's Asthma Care				
Received Home Management Plan of Care	-	-	-	88%
Received Reliever Medication	-	-	-	100%
Received Systemic Corticosteroids	-	-	-	100%
Emergency Department				
Admittance Decision Time (minutes)[2]	371	54	76	98
Head CT Results Within 45 Min. of Arrival	-	-	38%	57%
Patients Who Left ER Before Being Seen	-	-	1%	2%
Time from ER Arrival to Admit. (minutes)[2]	376	196	232	274
Time from ER Arrival to Discharge (minutes)	-	-	121	134
Time in ER Before Being Evaluated (minutes)	-	-	21	26
Time to Pain Meds for Fractures (minutes)	-	-	46	57
Heart Attack Care				
Aspirin Given at Discharge[1]	-	-	100%	99%
Fibrinolytic Meds Within 30 Min. of Arrival[7]	-	-	-	54%
PCI Within 90 Minutes of Arrival[3,7]	-	-	98%	96%
Statin Prescribed at Discharge[1]	-	-	99%	98%
Heart Failure Care				
ACE Inhibitor or ARB for LVSD[1]	-	-	98%	97%
Discharge Instructions Given	21	90%	94%	94%
Evaluation of LVS Function	30	100%	97%	99%
Medicare Spending				
Medicare Spending per Patient (ratio)	-	-	0.91	0.98
Pneumonia Care				
Appropriate Initial Antibiotic Given	26	85%	94%	95%
Blood Culture Timing	44	98%	98%	98%
Pregnancy and Delivery Care				
Newborn Deliveries Scheduled Early[5]	-	-	6%	6%
Preventive Care				
Immunization for Influenza[2]	487	74%	83%	90%
Immunization for Pneumonia[2]	367	87%	89%	92%
Stroke Care				
Anticoagulation Therapy for Atrial Fibrillation[5]	-	-	97%	95%
Antithrombotic Therapy Timing[5]	-	-	98%	98%
Assessed for Rehabilitation[5]	-	-	98%	97%
Discharged on Antithrombotic Therapy[5]	-	-	99%	99%
Discharged on Statin Medication[5]	-	-	91%	94%
Thrombolytic Therapy Timing[5]	-	-	55%	66%
Venous Thromboembolism Prophylaxis[5]	-	-	93%	94%
Written Stroke Educational Materials Given[5]	-	-	84%	88%
Surgical Care Improvement Project				
Appropriate Beta Blocker Usage	35	91%	98%	98%
Appropriate VTP Within 24 Hours	124	97%	98%	98%
Controlled Postoperative Blood Glucose[7]	-	-	99%	97%
Perioperative Temperature Management	142	100%	99%	100%
Prophylactic Antibiotic Selection	118	99%	99%	99%
Prophylactic Antibiotic Selection (Outpatient)	-	-	98%	98%
Prophylactic Antibiotic Stopped	116	97%	98%	98%
Prophylactic Antibiotic Timing	117	99%	98%	99%
Prophylactic Antibiotic Timing (Outpatient)	-	-	97%	98%
Urinary Catheter Removal	97	95%	96%	97%
Survey of Patients' Hospital Experiences				
Area Around Room 'Always' Quiet at Night	300+	64%	61%	61%
Doctors 'Always' Communicated Well	300+	82%	83%	82%
Home Recovery Information Given	300+	91%	88%	85%
Hospital Given 9 or 10 on 10 Point Scale	300+	80%	73%	71%
Meds 'Always' Explained Before Given	300+	69%	66%	64%
Nurses 'Always' Communicated Well	300+	81%	80%	79%
Pain 'Always' Well Controlled	300+	72%	72%	71%
Room and Bathroom 'Always' Clean	300+	77%	77%	73%
Timely Help 'Always' Received	300+	72%	73%	68%
Would Definitely Recommend Hospital	300+	77%	74%	71%
Use of Medical Imaging				
Cardiac Imaging Stress Test before Surgery	-	-	4.6%	5.3%
Combination Abdominal CT Scan	-	-	7.3%	10.5%
Combination Brain/Sinus CT Scan	-	-	1.7%	2.7%
Combination Chest CT Scan	-	-	1.8%	2.7%
Follow-up Mammogram/Ultrasound	-	-	8.2%	8.8%
Lumbar Spine MRI for Low Back Pain	-	-	40.3%	37.2%

Saint Luke's Elmore Medical Center

895 North 6th East Phone: 208-587-8401
Mountain Home, ID 83647
Type: Critical Access Hospitals Emergency Services: Yes
Ownership: Govt - Hospital Dist/Auth

Measure	Cases	This Hosp.	State Avg.	U.S. Avg.
Blood Clot Prevention and Treatment				
Anticoagulation Overlap Therapy[5]	-	-	95%	93%
ICU Venous Thromboembolism Prophylaxis[5]	-	-	92%	92%
Incidence of Potentially Preventable VTE[5]	-	-	11%	10%
UFH with Dosages/Platelet Monitoring[5]	-	-	99%	97%
Venous Thromboembolism Prophylaxis[5]	-	-	87%	85%
Warfarin Therapy Discharge Instructions[5]	-	-	75%	75%
Chest Pain/Possible Heart Attack Care				
Aspirin Given Within 24 Hours of Arrival	-	-	96%	96%
Fibrinolytic Meds Within 30 Min. of Arrival	-	-	55%	58%
Average Time to ECG (minutes)	-	-	9	7
Average Time to Transfer (minutes)	-	-	62	60
Children's Asthma Care				
Received Home Management Plan of Care	-	-	-	88%
Received Reliever Medication	-	-	-	100%
Received Systemic Corticosteroids	-	-	-	100%
Emergency Department				
Admittance Decision Time (minutes)[5]	-	-	76	98
Head CT Results Within 45 Min. of Arrival	-	-	38%	57%
Patients Who Left ER Before Being Seen	-	-	1%	2%
Time from ER Arrival to Admit. (minutes)[5]	-	-	232	274
Time from ER Arrival to Discharge (minutes)	-	-	121	134
Time in ER Before Being Evaluated (minutes)	-	-	21	26
Time to Pain Meds for Fractures (minutes)	-	-	46	57
Heart Attack Care				
Aspirin Given at Discharge[5]	-	-	100%	99%
Fibrinolytic Meds Within 30 Min. of Arrival[5]	-	-	-	54%
PCI Within 90 Minutes of Arrival[5]	-	-	98%	96%
Statin Prescribed at Discharge[5]	-	-	99%	98%
Heart Failure Care				
ACE Inhibitor or ARB for LVSD[1,3]	-	-	98%	97%
Discharge Instructions Given[1,3]	-	-	94%	94%
Evaluation of LVS Function[1,3]	-	-	97%	99%
Medicare Spending				
Medicare Spending per Patient (ratio)	-	-	0.91	0.98
Pneumonia Care				
Appropriate Initial Antibiotic Given[3,7]	-	-	94%	95%
Blood Culture Timing[3,7]	-	-	98%	98%
Pregnancy and Delivery Care				
Newborn Deliveries Scheduled Early[5]	-	-	6%	6%
Preventive Care				
Immunization for Influenza[5]	-	-	83%	90%
Immunization for Pneumonia[5]	-	-	89%	92%
Stroke Care				
Anticoagulation Therapy for Atrial Fibrillation[5]	-	-	97%	95%
Antithrombotic Therapy Timing[5]	-	-	98%	98%
Assessed for Rehabilitation[5]	-	-	98%	97%
Discharged on Antithrombotic Therapy[5]	-	-	99%	99%
Discharged on Statin Medication[5]	-	-	91%	94%
Thrombolytic Therapy Timing[5]	-	-	55%	66%
Venous Thromboembolism Prophylaxis[5]	-	-	93%	94%
Written Stroke Educational Materials Given[5]	-	-	84%	88%
Surgical Care Improvement Project				
Appropriate Beta Blocker Usage[5]	-	-	98%	98%
Appropriate VTP Within 24 Hours[5]	-	-	98%	98%
Controlled Postoperative Blood Glucose[5]	-	-	99%	97%
Perioperative Temperature Management[5]	-	-	99%	100%
Prophylactic Antibiotic Selection[5]	-	-	99%	99%
Prophylactic Antibiotic Selection (Outpatient)	-	-	98%	98%
Prophylactic Antibiotic Stopped[5]	-	-	98%	98%
Prophylactic Antibiotic Timing[5]	-	-	98%	99%
Prophylactic Antibiotic Timing (Outpatient)	-	-	97%	98%
Urinary Catheter Removal[5]	-	-	96%	97%
Survey of Patients' Hospital Experiences				
Area Around Room 'Always' Quiet at Night	(a)	57%	61%	61%
Doctors 'Always' Communicated Well	(a)	77%	83%	82%
Home Recovery Information Given	(a)	82%	88%	85%
Hospital Given 9 or 10 on 10 Point Scale	(a)	54%	73%	71%
Meds 'Always' Explained Before Given	(a)	66%	66%	64%
Nurses 'Always' Communicated Well	(a)	74%	80%	79%
Pain 'Always' Well Controlled	(a)	67%	72%	71%
Room and Bathroom 'Always' Clean	(a)	82%	77%	73%
Timely Help 'Always' Received	(a)	69%	73%	68%
Would Definitely Recommend Hospital	(a)	50%	74%	71%
Use of Medical Imaging				
Cardiac Imaging Stress Test before Surgery	-	-	4.6%	5.3%
Combination Abdominal CT Scan	-	-	7.3%	10.5%
Combination Brain/Sinus CT Scan	-	-	1.7%	2.7%
Combination Chest CT Scan	-	-	1.8%	2.7%
Follow-up Mammogram/Ultrasound	-	-	8.2%	8.8%
Lumbar Spine MRI for Low Back Pain	-	-	40.3%	37.2%

Saint Alphonsus Medical Center - Nampa

1512 Twelfth Avenue Road Phone: 208-463-5000
Nampa, ID 83686 Fax: 208-463-5775
URL: www.mercyoftoday.com
Type: Acute Care Hospitals Emergency Services: Yes
Ownership: Voluntary non-profit - Church Beds: 152

Key Personnel:
Radiology. . . . . Dirk E Bigler
Operating Room. . . . . Joanne Cruson
Intensive Care Unit. . . . . Kathy Grzeskiewicz
Chief of Medical Staff . . . . Joseph Kronz, MD
CEO/President. . . . . Joseph Messmer
Infection Control. . . . . Karen Otter

Measure	Cases	This Hosp.	State Avg.	U.S. Avg.
Blood Clot Prevention and Treatment				
Anticoagulation Overlap Therapy[2]	41	95%	95%	93%
ICU Venous Thromboembolism Prophylaxis[2]	104	93%	92%	92%
Incidence of Potentially Preventable VTE[1,2]	-	-	11%	10%
UFH with Dosages/Platelet Monitoring[2]	21	100%	99%	97%
Venous Thromboembolism Prophylaxis[2]	241	88%	87%	85%
Warfarin Therapy Discharge Instructions[2]	29	79%	75%	75%
Chest Pain/Possible Heart Attack Care				
Aspirin Given Within 24 Hours of Arrival[1]	-	-	96%	96%
Fibrinolytic Meds Within 30 Min. of Arrival[3,7]	-	-	55%	58%
Average Time to ECG (minutes)	11	13	9	7
Average Time to Transfer (minutes)[3,7]	-	-	62	60
Children's Asthma Care				
Received Home Management Plan of Care	-	-	-	88%
Received Reliever Medication	-	-	-	100%
Received Systemic Corticosteroids	-	-	-	100%
Emergency Department				
Admittance Decision Time (minutes)[2]	405	70	76	98
Head CT Results Within 45 Min. of Arrival[1]	-	-	38%	57%
Patients Who Left ER Before Being Seen	36,065	1%	1%	2%
Time from ER Arrival to Admit. (minutes)[2]	483	237	232	274
Time from ER Arrival to Discharge (minutes)	358	120	121	134
Time in ER Before Being Evaluated (minutes)	348	17	21	26
Time to Pain Meds for Fractures (minutes)	131	38	46	57
Heart Attack Care				
Aspirin Given at Discharge	66	100%	100%	99%
Fibrinolytic Meds Within 30 Min. of Arrival[7]	-	-	-	54%
PCI Within 90 Minutes of Arrival	22	95%	98%	96%
Statin Prescribed at Discharge	70	100%	99%	98%
Heart Failure Care				
ACE Inhibitor or ARB for LVSD	44	100%	98%	97%
Discharge Instructions Given	105	89%	94%	94%
Evaluation of LVS Function	119	100%	97%	99%
Medicare Spending				
Medicare Spending per Patient (ratio)	-	0.95	0.91	0.98

NOTE: Hospital profiles are in alphabetical order by state, then city, then hospital within the city; Rankings exclude hospitals with less than 25 cases except for patient surveys which excludes hospitals with less than 100 cases; (a) 100-299 cases; (1) The number of cases/patients is too few to report; (2) Data submitted were based on a sample of cases/patients; (3) Results are based on a shorter time period than required; (4) Data suppressed by CMS for one or more quarters; (5) Results are not available for this reporting period; (6) Fewer than 100 patients completed the HCAHPS survey; (7) No cases met the criteria for this measure; (8) The lower limit of the confidence interval cannot be calculated if the number of observed infections equals zero; (9) No data are available from the state/territory for this reporting period; (10) The scores shown reflect fewer than 50 completed surveys; (11) There were discrepancies in the data collection process; (12) This measure does not apply to this hospital for this reporting period; (13) Results cannot be calculated for this reporting period; (14) The results for this state are combined with nearby states to protect confidentiality; Please refer to the User's Guide for a full explanation of data.

Measure	Cases	This Hosp.	State Avg.	U.S. Avg.
Pneumonia Care				
Appropriate Initial Antibiotic Given	125	96%	94%	95%
Blood Culture Timing	185	97%	98%	98%
Pregnancy and Delivery Care				
Newborn Deliveries Scheduled Early[2]	40	32%	6%	6%
Preventive Care				
Immunization for Influenza[2]	479	80%	83%	90%
Immunization for Pneumonia[2]	543	93%	89%	92%
Stroke Care				
Anticoagulation Therapy for Atrial Fibrillation	13	100%	97%	95%
Antithrombotic Therapy Timing	38	100%	98%	98%
Assessed for Rehabilitation	42	95%	98%	97%
Discharged on Antithrombotic Therapy	40	100%	99%	99%
Discharged on Statin Medication	33	94%	91%	94%
Thrombolytic Therapy Timing[7]	-	-	55%	66%
Venous Thromboembolism Prophylaxis	40	95%	93%	94%
Written Stroke Educational Materials Given	29	48%	84%	88%
Surgical Care Improvement Project				
Appropriate Beta Blocker Usage	113	100%	98%	98%
Appropriate VTP Within 24 Hours	426	99%	98%	98%
Controlled Postoperative Blood Glucose[7]	-	-	99%	97%
Perioperative Temperature Management	473	98%	99%	100%
Prophylactic Antibiotic Selection	332	100%	99%	99%
Prophylactic Antibiotic Selection (Outpatient)	97	98%	98%	98%
Prophylactic Antibiotic Stopped	321	99%	98%	98%
Prophylactic Antibiotic Timing	332	98%	98%	99%
Prophylactic Antibiotic Timing (Outpatient)	101	90%	97%	98%
Urinary Catheter Removal	351	98%	96%	97%
Survey of Patients' Hospital Experiences				
Area Around Room 'Always' Quiet at Night	300+	51%	61%	61%
Doctors 'Always' Communicated Well	300+	81%	83%	82%
Home Recovery Information Given	300+	88%	88%	85%
Hospital Given 9 or 10 on 10 Point Scale	300+	68%	73%	71%
Meds 'Always' Explained Before Given	300+	57%	66%	64%
Nurses 'Always' Communicated Well	300+	74%	80%	79%
Pain 'Always' Well Controlled	300+	67%	72%	71%
Room and Bathroom 'Always' Clean	300+	66%	77%	73%
Timely Help 'Always' Received	300+	60%	73%	68%
Would Definitely Recommend Hospital	300+	65%	74%	71%
Use of Medical Imaging				
Cardiac Imaging Stress Test before Surgery	87	4.6%	4.6%	5.3%
Combination Abdominal CT Scan	384	1.6%	7.3%	10.5%
Combination Brain/Sinus CT Scan[1]	-	-	1.7%	2.7%
Combination Chest CT Scan	155	0.6%	1.8%	2.7%
Follow-up Mammogram/Ultrasound	888	9.2%	8.2%	8.8%
Lumbar Spine MRI for Low Back Pain[1]	-	-	40.3%	37.2%

Clearwater Valley Hospital & Clinics

301 Cedar Street
Orofino, ID 83544
Phone: 208-476-4555
Fax: 208-476-5385
URL: www.cvh-clrwater.com
Type: Critical Access Hospitals
Emergency Services: Yes
Ownership: Voluntary non-profit - Private
Beds: 23

Key Personnel:
Quality Assurance . . . . Jean Albers, RN
Emergency Room . . . . William Caldwell, MD
CEO/President. . . . . Casey Meza
Chief of Medical Staff . . . . Michael Meza

Measure	Cases	This Hosp.	State Avg.	U.S. Avg.
Blood Clot Prevention and Treatment				
Anticoagulation Overlap Therapy[5]	-	-	95%	93%
ICU Venous Thromboembolism Prophylaxis[5]	-	-	92%	92%
Incidence of Potentially Preventable VTE[5]	-	-	11%	10%
UFH with Dosages/Platelet Monitoring[5]	-	-	99%	97%
Venous Thromboembolism Prophylaxis[5]	-	-	87%	85%
Warfarin Therapy Discharge Instructions[5]	-	-	75%	75%
Chest Pain/Possible Heart Attack Care				
Aspirin Given Within 24 Hours of Arrival	-	-	96%	96%
Fibrinolytic Meds Within 30 Min. of Arrival	-	-	55%	58%
Average Time to ECG (minutes)	-	-	9	7
Average Time to Transfer (minutes)	-	-	62	60
Children's Asthma Care				
Received Home Management Plan of Care	-	-	-	88%
Received Reliever Medication	-	-	-	100%
Received Systemic Corticosteroids	-	-	-	100%
Emergency Department				
Admittance Decision Time (minutes)[5]	-	-	76	98
Head CT Results Within 45 Min. of Arrival	-	-	38%	57%
Patients Who Left ER Before Being Seen	-	-	1%	2%
Time from ER Arrival to Admit. (minutes)[5]	-	-	232	274
Time from ER Arrival to Discharge (minutes)	-	-	121	134
Time in ER Before Being Evaluated (minutes)	-	-	21	26
Time to Pain Meds for Fractures (minutes)	-	-	46	57
Heart Attack Care				
Aspirin Given at Discharge[5]	-	-	100%	99%
Fibrinolytic Meds Within 30 Min. of Arrival[5]	-	-	-	54%
PCI Within 90 Minutes of Arrival[5]	-	-	98%	96%
Statin Prescribed at Discharge[5]	-	-	99%	98%
Heart Failure Care				
ACE Inhibitor or ARB for LVSD	11	91%	98%	97%
Discharge Instructions Given	15	93%	94%	94%
Evaluation of LVS Function	22	91%	97%	99%
Medicare Spending				
Medicare Spending per Patient (ratio)	-	-	0.91	0.98
Pneumonia Care				
Appropriate Initial Antibiotic Given	34	94%	94%	95%
Blood Culture Timing[3]	25	100%	98%	98%
Pregnancy and Delivery Care				
Newborn Deliveries Scheduled Early[5]	-	-	6%	6%
Preventive Care				
Immunization for Influenza[5]	-	-	83%	90%
Immunization for Pneumonia[5]	-	-	89%	92%
Stroke Care				
Anticoagulation Therapy for Atrial Fibrillation[3,7]	-	-	97%	95%
Antithrombotic Therapy Timing[1,3]	-	-	98%	98%
Assessed for Rehabilitation[1,3]	-	-	98%	97%
Discharged on Antithrombotic Therapy[1,3]	-	-	99%	99%
Discharged on Statin Medication[1,3]	-	-	91%	94%
Thrombolytic Therapy Timing[1,3]	-	-	55%	66%
Venous Thromboembolism Prophylaxis[1,3]	-	-	93%	94%
Written Stroke Educational Materials Given[1,3]	-	-	84%	88%
Surgical Care Improvement Project				
Appropriate Beta Blocker Usage[5]	-	-	98%	98%
Appropriate VTP Within 24 Hours[5]	-	-	98%	98%
Controlled Postoperative Blood Glucose[5]	-	-	99%	97%
Perioperative Temperature Management[5]	-	-	99%	100%
Prophylactic Antibiotic Selection[5]	-	-	99%	99%
Prophylactic Antibiotic Selection (Outpatient)	-	-	98%	98%
Prophylactic Antibiotic Stopped[5]	-	-	98%	98%
Prophylactic Antibiotic Timing[5]	-	-	98%	99%
Prophylactic Antibiotic Timing (Outpatient)	-	-	97%	98%
Urinary Catheter Removal[5]	-	-	96%	97%
Survey of Patients' Hospital Experiences				
Area Around Room 'Always' Quiet at Night[11]	300+	48%	61%	61%
Doctors 'Always' Communicated Well[11]	300+	83%	83%	82%
Home Recovery Information Given[11]	300+	86%	88%	85%
Hospital Given 9 or 10 on 10 Point Scale[11]	300+	69%	73%	71%
Meds 'Always' Explained Before Given[11]	300+	58%	66%	64%
Nurses 'Always' Communicated Well[11]	300+	79%	80%	79%
Pain 'Always' Well Controlled[11]	300+	69%	72%	71%
Room and Bathroom 'Always' Clean[11]	300+	78%	77%	73%
Timely Help 'Always' Received[11]	300+	70%	73%	68%
Would Definitely Recommend Hospital[11]	300+	64%	74%	71%
Use of Medical Imaging				
Cardiac Imaging Stress Test before Surgery	-	-	4.6%	5.3%
Combination Abdominal CT Scan	-	-	7.3%	10.5%
Combination Brain/Sinus CT Scan	-	-	1.7%	2.7%
Combination Chest CT Scan	-	-	1.8%	2.7%
Follow-up Mammogram/Ultrasound	-	-	8.2%	8.8%
Lumbar Spine MRI for Low Back Pain	-	-	40.3%	37.2%

Portneuf Medical Center

777 Hospital Way
Pocatello, ID 83201
Phone: 208-239-1000
Fax: 208-239-1993
URL: www.portmed.org
Type: Acute Care Hospitals
Emergency Services: Yes
Ownership: Proprietary
Beds: 367

Key Personnel:
Chairman/CEO . . . . Mark Buckalew
Chief of Medical Staff . . . . Mike Callaghan, MD
Operating Room. . . . . Terry Elquist, RN
Pediatric Ambulatory Care . . . . . . Lloyd Jensen, MD
CEO/President. . . . . Dan Orydna
Quality Assurance . . . . Debbie Shell
Radiology. . . . . George Stephens, MD

Measure	Cases	This Hosp.	State Avg.	U.S. Avg.
Blood Clot Prevention and Treatment				
Anticoagulation Overlap Therapy[2]	73	97%	95%	93%
ICU Venous Thromboembolism Prophylaxis[2]	98	93%	92%	92%
Incidence of Potentially Preventable VTE[1,2]	-	-	11%	10%
UFH with Dosages/Platelet Monitoring[2]	37	100%	99%	97%
Venous Thromboembolism Prophylaxis[2]	279	95%	87%	85%
Warfarin Therapy Discharge Instructions[2]	60	97%	75%	75%
Chest Pain/Possible Heart Attack Care				
Aspirin Given Within 24 Hours of Arrival[1,3]	-	-	96%	96%
Fibrinolytic Meds Within 30 Min. of Arrival[3,7]	-	-	55%	58%
Average Time to ECG (minutes)[1,3]	-	-	9	7
Average Time to Transfer (minutes)[3,7]	-	-	62	60
Children's Asthma Care				
Received Home Management Plan of Care	-	-	-	88%
Received Reliever Medication	-	-	-	100%
Received Systemic Corticosteroids	-	-	-	100%
Emergency Department				
Admittance Decision Time (minutes)[2]	472	91	76	98
Head CT Results Within 45 Min. of Arrival[1]	-	-	38%	57%
Patients Who Left ER Before Being Seen	34,537	0%	1%	2%
Time from ER Arrival to Admit. (minutes)[2]	472	220	232	274
Time from ER Arrival to Discharge (minutes)	356	106	121	134
Time in ER Before Being Evaluated (minutes)	312	9	21	26
Time to Pain Meds for Fractures (minutes)	137	37	46	57
Heart Attack Care				
Aspirin Given at Discharge	149	100%	100%	99%
Fibrinolytic Meds Within 30 Min. of Arrival[7]	-	-	-	54%
PCI Within 90 Minutes of Arrival	19	95%	98%	96%
Statin Prescribed at Discharge	140	100%	99%	98%
Heart Failure Care				
ACE Inhibitor or ARB for LVSD	35	100%	98%	97%
Discharge Instructions Given	86	93%	94%	94%
Evaluation of LVS Function	100	100%	97%	99%
Medicare Spending				
Medicare Spending per Patient (ratio)	-	0.95	0.91	0.98
Pneumonia Care				
Appropriate Initial Antibiotic Given	123	99%	94%	95%
Blood Culture Timing	252	100%	98%	98%
Pregnancy and Delivery Care				
Newborn Deliveries Scheduled Early	152	5%	6%	6%
Preventive Care				
Immunization for Influenza[2]	489	91%	83%	90%
Immunization for Pneumonia[2]	541	90%	89%	92%
Stroke Care				
Anticoagulation Therapy for Atrial Fibrillation	11	100%	97%	95%
Antithrombotic Therapy Timing	58	100%	98%	98%
Assessed for Rehabilitation	68	100%	98%	97%
Discharged on Antithrombotic Therapy	62	100%	99%	99%
Discharged on Statin Medication	38	92%	91%	94%
Thrombolytic Therapy Timing[1]	-	-	55%	66%
Venous Thromboembolism Prophylaxis	65	95%	93%	94%
Written Stroke Educational Materials Given	28	68%	84%	88%
Surgical Care Improvement Project				
Appropriate Beta Blocker Usage	254	99%	98%	98%
Appropriate VTP Within 24 Hours	827	99%	98%	98%
Controlled Postoperative Blood Glucose	67	94%	99%	97%
Perioperative Temperature Management	981	100%	99%	100%
Prophylactic Antibiotic Selection	731	100%	99%	99%
Prophylactic Antibiotic Selection (Outpatient)	351	99%	98%	98%

NOTE: Hospital profiles are in alphabetical order by state, then city, then hospital within the city; Rankings exclude hospitals with less than 25 cases except for patient surveys which excludes hospitals with less than 100 cases; (a) 100-299 cases; (1) The number of cases/patients is too few to report; (2) Data submitted were based on a sample of cases/patients; (3) Results are based on a shorter time period than required; (4) Data suppressed by CMS for one or more quarters; (5) Results are not available for this reporting period; (6) Fewer than 100 patients completed the HCAHPS survey; (7) No cases met the criteria for this measure; (8) The lower limit of the confidence interval cannot be calculated if the number of observed infections equals zero; (9) No data are available from the state/territory for this reporting period; (10) The scores shown reflect fewer than 50 completed surveys; (11) There were discrepancies in the data collection process; (12) This measure does not apply to this hospital for this reporting period; (13) Results cannot be calculated for this reporting period; (14) The results for this state are combined with nearby states to protect confidentiality; Please refer to the User's Guide for a full explanation of data.

Prophylactic Antibiotic Stopped	717	99%	98%	98%
Prophylactic Antibiotic Timing	732	99%	98%	99%
Prophylactic Antibiotic Timing (Outpatient)	351	100%	97%	98%
Urinary Catheter Removal	791	99%	96%	97%
Survey of Patients' Hospital Experiences				
Area Around Room 'Always' Quiet at Night	300+	59%	61%	61%
Doctors 'Always' Communicated Well	300+	78%	83%	82%
Home Recovery Information Given	300+	87%	88%	85%
Hospital Given 9 or 10 on 10 Point Scale	300+	68%	73%	71%
Meds 'Always' Explained Before Given	300+	60%	66%	64%
Nurses 'Always' Communicated Well	300+	75%	80%	79%
Pain 'Always' Well Controlled	300+	67%	72%	71%
Room and Bathroom 'Always' Clean	300+	70%	77%	73%
Timely Help 'Always' Received	300+	64%	73%	68%
Would Definitely Recommend Hospital	300+	68%	74%	71%
Use of Medical Imaging				
Cardiac Imaging Stress Test before Surgery	462	4.8%	4.6%	5.3%
Combination Abdominal CT Scan	544	7.9%	7.3%	10.5%
Combination Brain/Sinus CT Scan	488	1.8%	1.7%	2.7%
Combination Chest CT Scan	209	3.8%	1.8%	2.7%
Follow-up Mammogram/Ultrasound	1,624	7.1%	8.2%	8.8%
Lumbar Spine MRI for Low Back Pain	318	41.2%	40.3%	37.2%
Preventive Care				
Immunization for Influenza[2]	341	82%	83%	90%
Immunization for Pneumonia[2]	352	93%	89%	92%
Stroke Care				
Anticoagulation Therapy for Atrial Fibrillation[5]	-	-	97%	95%
Antithrombotic Therapy Timing[5]	-	-	98%	98%
Assessed for Rehabilitation[5]	-	-	98%	97%
Discharged on Antithrombotic Therapy[5]	-	-	99%	99%
Discharged on Statin Medication[5]	-	-	91%	94%
Thrombolytic Therapy Timing[5]	-	-	55%	66%
Venous Thromboembolism Prophylaxis[5]	-	-	93%	94%
Written Stroke Educational Materials Given[5]	-	-	84%	88%
Surgical Care Improvement Project				
Appropriate Beta Blocker Usage[2]	54	100%	98%	98%
Appropriate VTP Within 24 Hours[2]	261	97%	98%	98%
Controlled Postoperative Blood Glucose[2,7]	-	-	99%	97%
Perioperative Temperature Management[2]	304	97%	99%	100%
Prophylactic Antibiotic Selection[2]	274	100%	99%	99%
Prophylactic Antibiotic Selection (Outpatient)[3]	44	100%	98%	98%
Prophylactic Antibiotic Stopped[2]	273	99%	98%	98%
Prophylactic Antibiotic Timing[2]	274	96%	98%	99%
Prophylactic Antibiotic Timing (Outpatient)[3]	44	100%	97%	98%
Urinary Catheter Removal[2]	156	99%	96%	97%
Survey of Patients' Hospital Experiences				
Area Around Room 'Always' Quiet at Night	300+	71%	61%	61%
Doctors 'Always' Communicated Well	300+	88%	83%	82%
Home Recovery Information Given	300+	90%	88%	85%
Hospital Given 9 or 10 on 10 Point Scale	300+	85%	73%	71%
Meds 'Always' Explained Before Given	300+	73%	66%	64%
Nurses 'Always' Communicated Well	300+	88%	80%	79%
Pain 'Always' Well Controlled	300+	79%	72%	71%
Room and Bathroom 'Always' Clean	300+	78%	77%	73%
Timely Help 'Always' Received	300+	85%	73%	68%
Would Definitely Recommend Hospital	300+	91%	74%	71%
Use of Medical Imaging				
Cardiac Imaging Stress Test before Surgery[7]	-	-	4.6%	5.3%
Combination Abdominal CT Scan	73	4.1%	7.3%	10.5%
Combination Brain/Sinus CT Scan[1]	-	-	1.7%	2.7%
Combination Chest CT Scan	58	1.7%	1.8%	2.7%
Follow-up Mammogram/Ultrasound[7]	-	-	8.2%	8.8%
Lumbar Spine MRI for Low Back Pain	76	32.9%	40.3%	37.2%

Northwest Specialty Hospital

1593 East Polston Avenue — Phone: 208-262-2300
Post Falls, ID 83854
URL: www.northwestspecialtyhospital.com
Type: Acute Care Hospitals — Emergency Services: No
Ownership: Proprietary — Beds: 22

Key Personnel:
Radiology. . . . . Lisa Schuler
CEO . . . . Vaughn Ward

Measure	Cases	This Hosp.	State Avg.	U.S. Avg.
Blood Clot Prevention and Treatment				
Anticoagulation Overlap Therapy[1,2]	-	-	95%	93%
ICU Venous Thromboembolism Prophylaxis[2,7]	-	-	92%	92%
Incidence of Potentially Preventable VTE[2,7]	-	-	11%	10%
UFH with Dosages/Platelet Monitoring[2,7]	-	-	99%	97%
Venous Thromboembolism Prophylaxis[2]	68	97%	87%	85%
Warfarin Therapy Discharge Instructions[2,7]	-	-	75%	75%
Chest Pain/Possible Heart Attack Care				
Aspirin Given Within 24 Hours of Arrival[5]	-	-	96%	96%
Fibrinolytic Meds Within 30 Min. of Arrival[5]	-	-	55%	58%
Average Time to ECG (minutes)[5]	-	-	9	7
Average Time to Transfer (minutes)[5]	-	-	62	60
Children's Asthma Care				
Received Home Management Plan of Care	-	-	-	88%
Received Reliever Medication	-	-	-	100%
Received Systemic Corticosteroids	-	-	-	100%
Emergency Department				
Admittance Decision Time (minutes)[2,7]	-	-	76	98
Head CT Results Within 45 Min. of Arrival[5]	-	-	38%	57%
Patients Who Left ER Before Being Seen[5]	-	-	1%	2%
Time from ER Arrival to Admit. (minutes)[2,7]	-	-	232	274
Time from ER Arrival to Discharge (minutes)[5]	-	-	121	134
Time in ER Before Being Evaluated (minutes)[5]	-	-	21	26
Time to Pain Meds for Fractures (minutes)[5]	-	-	46	57
Heart Attack Care				
Aspirin Given at Discharge[5]	-	-	100%	99%
Fibrinolytic Meds Within 30 Min. of Arrival[5]	-	-	-	54%
PCI Within 90 Minutes of Arrival[5]	-	-	98%	96%
Statin Prescribed at Discharge[5]	-	-	99%	98%
Heart Failure Care				
ACE Inhibitor or ARB for LVSD[5]	-	-	98%	97%
Discharge Instructions Given[5]	-	-	94%	94%
Evaluation of LVS Function[5]	-	-	97%	99%
Medicare Spending				
Medicare Spending per Patient (ratio)	-	0.92	0.91	0.98
Pneumonia Care				
Appropriate Initial Antibiotic Given[5]	-	-	94%	95%
Blood Culture Timing[5]	-	-	98%	98%
Pregnancy and Delivery Care				
Newborn Deliveries Scheduled Early[7]	-	-	6%	6%

Franklin County Medical Center

44 North First East — Phone: 208-852-0137
Preston, ID 83263
Type: Critical Access Hospitals — Emergency Services: Yes
Ownership: Government - Local

Measure	Cases	This Hosp.	State Avg.	U.S. Avg.
Blood Clot Prevention and Treatment				
Anticoagulation Overlap Therapy[5]	-	-	95%	93%
ICU Venous Thromboembolism Prophylaxis[5]	-	-	92%	92%
Incidence of Potentially Preventable VTE[5]	-	-	11%	10%
UFH with Dosages/Platelet Monitoring[5]	-	-	99%	97%
Venous Thromboembolism Prophylaxis[5]	-	-	87%	85%
Warfarin Therapy Discharge Instructions[5]	-	-	75%	75%
Chest Pain/Possible Heart Attack Care				
Aspirin Given Within 24 Hours of Arrival	-	-	96%	96%
Fibrinolytic Meds Within 30 Min. of Arrival	-	-	55%	58%
Average Time to ECG (minutes)	-	-	9	7
Average Time to Transfer (minutes)	-	-	62	60
Children's Asthma Care				
Received Home Management Plan of Care	-	-	-	88%
Received Reliever Medication	-	-	-	100%
Received Systemic Corticosteroids	-	-	-	100%
Emergency Department				
Admittance Decision Time (minutes)[5]	-	-	76	98
Head CT Results Within 45 Min. of Arrival	-	-	38%	57%
Patients Who Left ER Before Being Seen	-	-	1%	2%
Time from ER Arrival to Admit. (minutes)[5]	-	-	232	274
Time from ER Arrival to Discharge (minutes)	-	-	121	134
Time in ER Before Being Evaluated (minutes)	-	-	21	26
Time to Pain Meds for Fractures (minutes)	-	-	46	57
Heart Attack Care				
Aspirin Given at Discharge[5]	-	-	100%	99%
Fibrinolytic Meds Within 30 Min. of Arrival[5]	-	-	-	54%
PCI Within 90 Minutes of Arrival[5]	-	-	98%	96%
Statin Prescribed at Discharge[3,7]	-	-	99%	98%
Heart Failure Care				
ACE Inhibitor or ARB for LVSD[3,7]	-	-	98%	97%
Discharge Instructions Given[1,3]	-	-	94%	94%
Evaluation of LVS Function[1,3]	-	-	97%	99%
Medicare Spending				
Medicare Spending per Patient (ratio)	-	-	0.91	0.98
Pneumonia Care				
Appropriate Initial Antibiotic Given	15	47%	94%	95%
Blood Culture Timing[1]	-	-	98%	98%
Pregnancy and Delivery Care				
Newborn Deliveries Scheduled Early[5]	-	-	6%	6%
Preventive Care				
Immunization for Influenza[5]	-	-	83%	90%
Immunization for Pneumonia[5]	-	-	89%	92%
Stroke Care				
Anticoagulation Therapy for Atrial Fibrillation[5]	-	-	97%	95%
Antithrombotic Therapy Timing[5]	-	-	98%	98%
Assessed for Rehabilitation[5]	-	-	98%	97%
Discharged on Antithrombotic Therapy[5]	-	-	99%	99%
Discharged on Statin Medication[5]	-	-	91%	94%
Thrombolytic Therapy Timing[5]	-	-	55%	66%
Venous Thromboembolism Prophylaxis[5]	-	-	93%	94%
Written Stroke Educational Materials Given[5]	-	-	84%	88%
Surgical Care Improvement Project				
Appropriate Beta Blocker Usage[5]	-	-	98%	98%
Appropriate VTP Within 24 Hours[5]	-	-	98%	98%
Controlled Postoperative Blood Glucose[5]	-	-	99%	97%
Perioperative Temperature Management[5]	-	-	99%	100%
Prophylactic Antibiotic Selection[5]	-	-	99%	99%
Prophylactic Antibiotic Selection (Outpatient)	-	-	98%	98%
Prophylactic Antibiotic Stopped[5]	-	-	98%	98%
Prophylactic Antibiotic Timing[5]	-	-	98%	99%
Prophylactic Antibiotic Timing (Outpatient)	-	-	97%	98%
Urinary Catheter Removal[5]	-	-	96%	97%
Survey of Patients' Hospital Experiences				
Area Around Room 'Always' Quiet at Night[5]	-	-	61%	61%
Doctors 'Always' Communicated Well[5]	-	-	83%	82%
Home Recovery Information Given[5]	-	-	88%	85%
Hospital Given 9 or 10 on 10 Point Scale[5]	-	-	73%	71%
Meds 'Always' Explained Before Given[5]	-	-	66%	64%
Nurses 'Always' Communicated Well[5]	-	-	80%	79%
Pain 'Always' Well Controlled[5]	-	-	72%	71%
Room and Bathroom 'Always' Clean[5]	-	-	77%	73%
Timely Help 'Always' Received[5]	-	-	73%	68%
Would Definitely Recommend Hospital[5]	-	-	74%	71%
Use of Medical Imaging				
Cardiac Imaging Stress Test before Surgery	-	-	4.6%	5.3%
Combination Abdominal CT Scan	-	-	7.3%	10.5%
Combination Brain/Sinus CT Scan	-	-	1.7%	2.7%
Combination Chest CT Scan	-	-	1.8%	2.7%
Follow-up Mammogram/Ultrasound	-	-	8.2%	8.8%
Lumbar Spine MRI for Low Back Pain	-	-	40.3%	37.2%

Madison Memorial Hospital

450 East Main Street — Phone: 208-359-6900
Rexburg, ID 83440 — Fax: 208-359-6454
URL: www.madisonhospital.org
Type: Acute Care Hospitals — Emergency Services: Yes
Ownership: Government - Local — Beds: 51

Key Personnel:
Radiology. . . . . Dr Barry Birkin
Cardiac Laboratory. . . . . Kirt Crittenden
Hemotology Center . . . . Dane J Dickson, MD
Chief of Medical Staff . . . . David V Hansen, MD
Infection Control. . . . . Chris Hobbs
Operating Room. . . . . Lowell Nygaard
CEO/President. . . . . David Rowe
Emergency Room . . . . Mary Zollinger, RN

Measure	Cases	This Hosp.	State Avg.	U.S. Avg.

NOTE: Hospital profiles are in alphabetical order by state, then city, then hospital within the city; Rankings exclude hospitals with less than 25 cases except for patient surveys which excludes hospitals with less than 100 cases; (a) 100-299 cases; (1) The number of cases/patients is too few to report; (2) Data submitted were based on a sample of cases/patients; (3) Results are based on a shorter time period than required; (4) Data suppressed by CMS for one or more quarters; (5) Results are not available for this reporting period; (6) Fewer than 100 patients completed the HCAHPS survey; (7) No cases met the criteria for this measure; (8) The lower limit of the confidence interval cannot be calculated if the number of observed infections equals zero; (9) No data are available from the state/territory for this reporting period; (10) The scores shown reflect fewer than 50 completed surveys; (11) There were discrepancies in the data collection process; (12) This measure does not apply to this hospital for this reporting period; (13) Results cannot be calculated for this reporting period; (14) The results for this state are combined with nearby states to protect confidentiality; Please refer to the User's Guide for a full explanation of data.

Measure	Cases	This Hosp.	State Avg.	U.S. Avg.
Blood Clot Prevention and Treatment				
Anticoagulation Overlap Therapy[2]	15	80%	95%	93%
ICU Venous Thromboembolism Prophylaxis[2]	34	88%	92%	92%
Incidence of Potentially Preventable VTE[1,2]	-	-	11%	10%
UFH with Dosages/Platelet Monitoring[1,2]	-	-	99%	97%
Venous Thromboembolism Prophylaxis[2]	120	72%	87%	85%
Warfarin Therapy Discharge Instructions[1,2]	-	-	75%	75%
Chest Pain/Possible Heart Attack Care				
Aspirin Given Within 24 Hours of Arrival	47	91%	96%	96%
Fibrinolytic Meds Within 30 Min. of Arrival[1]	-	-	55%	58%
Average Time to ECG (minutes)	48	14	9	7
Average Time to Transfer (minutes)	12	62	62	60
Children's Asthma Care				
Received Home Management Plan of Care	-	-	-	88%
Received Reliever Medication	-	-	-	100%
Received Systemic Corticosteroids	-	-	-	100%
Emergency Department				
Admittance Decision Time (minutes)[2]	87	51	76	98
Head CT Results Within 45 Min. of Arrival[1]	-	-	38%	57%
Patients Who Left ER Before Being Seen	10,487	0%	1%	2%
Time from ER Arrival to Admit. (minutes)[2]	121	164	232	274
Time from ER Arrival to Discharge (minutes)	1,465	99	121	134
Time in ER Before Being Evaluated (minutes)	1,378	21	21	26
Time to Pain Meds for Fractures (minutes)	98	38	46	57
Heart Attack Care				
Aspirin Given at Discharge[1,3]	-	-	100%	99%
Fibrinolytic Meds Within 30 Min. of Arrival[3,7]	-	-	-	54%
PCI Within 90 Minutes of Arrival[3,7]	-	-	98%	96%
Statin Prescribed at Discharge[1,3]	-	-	99%	98%
Heart Failure Care				
ACE Inhibitor or ARB for LVSD[7]	-	-	98%	97%
Discharge Instructions Given	12	92%	94%	94%
Evaluation of LVS Function	19	95%	97%	99%
Medicare Spending				
Medicare Spending per Patient (ratio)	-	0.89	0.91	0.98
Pneumonia Care				
Appropriate Initial Antibiotic Given	36	97%	94%	95%
Blood Culture Timing	37	97%	98%	98%
Pregnancy and Delivery Care				
Newborn Deliveries Scheduled Early[2]	88	9%	6%	6%
Preventive Care				
Immunization for Influenza[2]	276	68%	83%	90%
Immunization for Pneumonia[2]	143	63%	89%	92%
Stroke Care				
Anticoagulation Therapy for Atrial Fibrillation[3,7]	-	-	97%	95%
Antithrombotic Therapy Timing[1,3]	-	-	98%	98%
Assessed for Rehabilitation[1,3]	-	-	98%	97%
Discharged on Antithrombotic Therapy[1,3]	-	-	99%	99%
Discharged on Statin Medication[1,3]	-	-	91%	94%
Thrombolytic Therapy Timing[3,7]	-	-	55%	66%
Venous Thromboembolism Prophylaxis[1,3]	-	-	93%	94%
Written Stroke Educational Materials Given[1,3]	-	-	84%	88%
Surgical Care Improvement Project				
Appropriate Beta Blocker Usage	47	96%	98%	98%
Appropriate VTP Within 24 Hours	195	96%	98%	98%
Controlled Postoperative Blood Glucose[7]	-	-	99%	97%
Perioperative Temperature Management	212	100%	99%	100%
Prophylactic Antibiotic Selection	161	99%	99%	99%
Prophylactic Antibiotic Selection (Outpatient)	62	100%	98%	98%
Prophylactic Antibiotic Stopped	161	97%	98%	98%
Prophylactic Antibiotic Timing	161	99%	98%	99%
Prophylactic Antibiotic Timing (Outpatient)	65	94%	97%	98%
Urinary Catheter Removal	145	89%	96%	97%
Survey of Patients' Hospital Experiences				
Area Around Room 'Always' Quiet at Night	300+	55%	61%	61%
Doctors 'Always' Communicated Well	300+	78%	83%	82%
Home Recovery Information Given	300+	84%	88%	85%
Hospital Given 9 or 10 on 10 Point Scale	300+	67%	73%	71%
Meds 'Always' Explained Before Given	300+	61%	66%	64%
Nurses 'Always' Communicated Well	300+	69%	80%	79%
Pain 'Always' Well Controlled	300+	60%	72%	71%
Room and Bathroom 'Always' Clean	300+	79%	77%	73%
Timely Help 'Always' Received	300+	63%	73%	68%
Would Definitely Recommend Hospital	300+	67%	74%	71%
Use of Medical Imaging				
Cardiac Imaging Stress Test before Surgery	50	2.0%	4.6%	5.3%
Combination Abdominal CT Scan	171	1.8%	7.3%	10.5%
Combination Brain/Sinus CT Scan[1]	-	-	1.7%	2.7%
Combination Chest CT Scan	73	2.7%	1.8%	2.7%
Follow-up Mammogram/Ultrasound[7]	-	-	8.2%	8.8%
Lumbar Spine MRI for Low Back Pain[1]	-	-	40.3%	37.2%

Minidoka Memorial Hospital

1224 Eighth Street
Rupert, ID 83350
Phone: 208-436-0481
Type: Critical Access Hospitals
Emergency Services: Yes
Ownership: Government - Local

Measure	Cases	This Hosp.	State Avg.	U.S. Avg.
Blood Clot Prevention and Treatment				
Anticoagulation Overlap Therapy[5]	-	-	95%	93%
ICU Venous Thromboembolism Prophylaxis[5]	-	-	92%	92%
Incidence of Potentially Preventable VTE[5]	-	-	11%	10%
UFH with Dosages/Platelet Monitoring[5]	-	-	99%	97%
Venous Thromboembolism Prophylaxis[5]	-	-	87%	85%
Warfarin Therapy Discharge Instructions[5]	-	-	75%	75%
Chest Pain/Possible Heart Attack Care				
Aspirin Given Within 24 Hours of Arrival	-	-	96%	96%
Fibrinolytic Meds Within 30 Min. of Arrival	-	-	55%	58%
Average Time to ECG (minutes)	-	-	9	7
Average Time to Transfer (minutes)	-	-	62	60
Children's Asthma Care				
Received Home Management Plan of Care	-	-	-	88%
Received Reliever Medication	-	-	-	100%
Received Systemic Corticosteroids	-	-	-	100%
Emergency Department				
Admittance Decision Time (minutes)[5]	-	-	76	98
Head CT Results Within 45 Min. of Arrival	-	-	38%	57%
Patients Who Left ER Before Being Seen	-	-	1%	2%
Time from ER Arrival to Admit. (minutes)[5]	-	-	232	274
Time from ER Arrival to Discharge (minutes)	-	-	121	134
Time in ER Before Being Evaluated (minutes)	-	-	21	26
Time to Pain Meds for Fractures (minutes)	-	-	46	57
Heart Attack Care				
Aspirin Given at Discharge[5]	-	-	100%	99%
Fibrinolytic Meds Within 30 Min. of Arrival[5]	-	-	-	54%
PCI Within 90 Minutes of Arrival[5]	-	-	98%	96%
Statin Prescribed at Discharge[5]	-	-	99%	98%
Heart Failure Care				
ACE Inhibitor or ARB for LVSD[5]	-	-	98%	97%
Discharge Instructions Given[5]	-	-	94%	94%
Evaluation of LVS Function[5]	-	-	97%	99%
Medicare Spending				
Medicare Spending per Patient (ratio)	-	-	0.91	0.98
Pneumonia Care				
Appropriate Initial Antibiotic Given[5]	-	-	94%	95%
Blood Culture Timing[5]	-	-	98%	98%
Pregnancy and Delivery Care				
Newborn Deliveries Scheduled Early[5]	-	-	6%	6%
Preventive Care				
Immunization for Influenza[5]	-	-	83%	90%
Immunization for Pneumonia[5]	-	-	89%	92%
Stroke Care				
Anticoagulation Therapy for Atrial Fibrillation[5]	-	-	97%	95%
Antithrombotic Therapy Timing[5]	-	-	98%	98%
Assessed for Rehabilitation[5]	-	-	98%	97%
Discharged on Antithrombotic Therapy[5]	-	-	99%	99%
Discharged on Statin Medication[5]	-	-	91%	94%
Thrombolytic Therapy Timing[5]	-	-	55%	66%
Venous Thromboembolism Prophylaxis[5]	-	-	93%	94%
Written Stroke Educational Materials Given[5]	-	-	84%	88%
Surgical Care Improvement Project				
Appropriate Beta Blocker Usage[5]	-	-	98%	98%
Appropriate VTP Within 24 Hours[5]	-	-	98%	98%
Controlled Postoperative Blood Glucose[5]	-	-	99%	97%
Perioperative Temperature Management[5]	-	-	99%	100%
Prophylactic Antibiotic Selection[5]	-	-	99%	99%
Prophylactic Antibiotic Selection (Outpatient)	-	-	98%	98%
Prophylactic Antibiotic Stopped[5]	-	-	98%	98%
Prophylactic Antibiotic Timing[5]	-	-	98%	99%
Prophylactic Antibiotic Timing (Outpatient)	-	-	97%	98%
Urinary Catheter Removal[5]	-	-	96%	97%
Survey of Patients' Hospital Experiences				
Area Around Room 'Always' Quiet at Night[5]	-	-	61%	61%
Doctors 'Always' Communicated Well[5]	-	-	83%	82%
Home Recovery Information Given[5]	-	-	88%	85%
Hospital Given 9 or 10 on 10 Point Scale[5]	-	-	73%	71%
Meds 'Always' Explained Before Given[5]	-	-	66%	64%
Nurses 'Always' Communicated Well[5]	-	-	80%	79%
Pain 'Always' Well Controlled[5]	-	-	72%	71%
Room and Bathroom 'Always' Clean[5]	-	-	77%	73%
Timely Help 'Always' Received[5]	-	-	73%	68%
Would Definitely Recommend Hospital[5]	-	-	74%	71%
Use of Medical Imaging				
Cardiac Imaging Stress Test before Surgery	-	-	4.6%	5.3%
Combination Abdominal CT Scan	-	-	7.3%	10.5%
Combination Brain/Sinus CT Scan	-	-	1.7%	2.7%
Combination Chest CT Scan	-	-	1.8%	2.7%
Follow-up Mammogram/Ultrasound	-	-	8.2%	8.8%
Lumbar Spine MRI for Low Back Pain	-	-	40.3%	37.2%

Benewah Community Hospital

229 South 7th Street
Saint Maries, ID 83861
Phone: 208-245-7614
Type: Critical Access Hospitals
Emergency Services: Yes
Ownership: Government - Local

Measure	Cases	This Hosp.	State Avg.	U.S. Avg.
Blood Clot Prevention and Treatment				
Anticoagulation Overlap Therapy[5]	-	-	95%	93%
ICU Venous Thromboembolism Prophylaxis[5]	-	-	92%	92%
Incidence of Potentially Preventable VTE[5]	-	-	11%	10%
UFH with Dosages/Platelet Monitoring[5]	-	-	99%	97%
Venous Thromboembolism Prophylaxis[5]	-	-	87%	85%
Warfarin Therapy Discharge Instructions[5]	-	-	75%	75%
Chest Pain/Possible Heart Attack Care				
Aspirin Given Within 24 Hours of Arrival	20	100%	96%	96%
Fibrinolytic Meds Within 30 Min. of Arrival[1]	-	-	55%	58%
Average Time to ECG (minutes)	21	13	9	7
Average Time to Transfer (minutes)[1]	-	-	62	60
Children's Asthma Care				
Received Home Management Plan of Care	-	-	-	88%
Received Reliever Medication	-	-	-	100%
Received Systemic Corticosteroids	-	-	-	100%
Emergency Department				
Admittance Decision Time (minutes)[5]	-	-	76	98
Head CT Results Within 45 Min. of Arrival[1]	-	-	38%	57%
Patients Who Left ER Before Being Seen	2,960	0%	1%	2%
Time from ER Arrival to Admit. (minutes)[5]	-	-	232	274
Time from ER Arrival to Discharge (minutes)[5]	-	-	121	134
Time in ER Before Being Evaluated (minutes)[5]	-	-	21	26
Time to Pain Meds for Fractures (minutes)[1,3]	-	-	46	57
Heart Attack Care				
Aspirin Given at Discharge[5]	-	-	100%	99%
Fibrinolytic Meds Within 30 Min. of Arrival[5]	-	-	-	54%
PCI Within 90 Minutes of Arrival[5]	-	-	98%	96%
Statin Prescribed at Discharge[5]	-	-	99%	98%
Heart Failure Care				
ACE Inhibitor or ARB for LVSD[3,7]	-	-	98%	97%
Discharge Instructions Given[1,3]	-	-	94%	94%
Evaluation of LVS Function[1,3]	-	-	97%	99%
Medicare Spending				
Medicare Spending per Patient (ratio)	-	-	0.91	0.98
Pneumonia Care				
Appropriate Initial Antibiotic Given[1]	-	-	94%	95%
Blood Culture Timing[1]	-	-	98%	98%
Pregnancy and Delivery Care				
Newborn Deliveries Scheduled Early[1,3]	-	-	6%	6%

NOTE: Hospital profiles are in alphabetical order by state, then city, then hospital within the city; Rankings exclude hospitals with less than 25 cases except for patient surveys which excludes hospitals with less than 100 cases; (a) 100-299 cases; (1) The number of cases/patients is too few to report; (2) Data submitted were based on a sample of cases/patients; (3) Results are based on a shorter time period than required; (4) Data suppressed by CMS for one or more quarters; (5) Results are not available for this reporting period; (6) Fewer than 100 patients completed the HCAHPS survey; (7) No cases met the criteria for this measure; (8) The lower limit of the confidence interval cannot be calculated if the number of observed infections equals zero; (9) No data are available from the state/territory for this reporting period; (10) The scores shown reflect fewer than 50 completed surveys; (11) There were discrepancies in the data collection process; (12) This measure does not apply to this hospital for this reporting period; (13) Results cannot be calculated for this reporting period; (14) The results for this state are combined with nearby states to protect confidentiality; Please refer to the User's Guide for a full explanation of data.

Measure	Cases	This Hosp.	State Avg.	U.S. Avg.
Preventive Care				
Immunization for Influenza[5]	-	-	83%	90%
Immunization for Pneumonia[5]	-	-	89%	92%
Stroke Care				
Anticoagulation Therapy for Atrial Fibrillation[5]	-	-	97%	95%
Antithrombotic Therapy Timing[5]	-	-	98%	98%
Assessed for Rehabilitation[5]	-	-	98%	97%
Discharged on Antithrombotic Therapy[5]	-	-	99%	99%
Discharged on Statin Medication[5]	-	-	91%	94%
Thrombolytic Therapy Timing[5]	-	-	55%	66%
Venous Thromboembolism Prophylaxis[5]	-	-	93%	94%
Written Stroke Educational Materials Given[5]	-	-	84%	88%
Surgical Care Improvement Project				
Appropriate Beta Blocker Usage[5]	-	-	98%	98%
Appropriate VTP Within 24 Hours[5]	-	-	98%	98%
Controlled Postoperative Blood Glucose[5]	-	-	99%	97%
Perioperative Temperature Management[5]	-	-	99%	100%
Prophylactic Antibiotic Selection[5]	-	-	99%	99%
Prophylactic Antibiotic Selection (Outpatient)[1,3]	-	-	98%	98%
Prophylactic Antibiotic Stopped[5]	-	-	98%	98%
Prophylactic Antibiotic Timing[5]	-	-	98%	99%
Prophylactic Antibiotic Timing (Outpatient)[1,3]	-	-	97%	98%
Urinary Catheter Removal[5]	-	-	96%	97%
Survey of Patients' Hospital Experiences				
Area Around Room 'Always' Quiet at Night	(a)	68%	61%	61%
Doctors 'Always' Communicated Well	(a)	81%	83%	82%
Home Recovery Information Given	(a)	84%	88%	85%
Hospital Given 9 or 10 on 10 Point Scale	(a)	74%	73%	71%
Meds 'Always' Explained Before Given	(a)	63%	66%	64%
Nurses 'Always' Communicated Well	(a)	83%	80%	79%
Pain 'Always' Well Controlled	(a)	68%	72%	71%
Room and Bathroom 'Always' Clean	(a)	90%	77%	73%
Timely Help 'Always' Received	(a)	84%	73%	68%
Would Definitely Recommend Hospital	(a)	75%	74%	71%
Use of Medical Imaging				
Cardiac Imaging Stress Test before Surgery[7]	-	-	4.6%	5.3%
Combination Abdominal CT Scan	99	9.1%	7.3%	10.5%
Combination Brain/Sinus CT Scan	56	0.0%	1.7%	2.7%
Combination Chest CT Scan	80	1.3%	1.8%	2.7%
Follow-up Mammogram/Ultrasound	128	4.7%	8.2%	8.8%
Lumbar Spine MRI for Low Back Pain[1]	-	-	40.3%	37.2%

Steele Memorial Medical Center

203 South Daisy Street
Salmon, ID 83467
Phone: 208-756-5600
Fax: 208-756-4169
E-mail: admin@steelemh.org
URL: www.steelemh.org
Type: Critical Access Hospitals
Emergency Services: Yes
Ownership: Voluntary non-profit - Other
Beds: 35

Key Personnel:

Operating Room. . . . . Adam Deutchman, RN
Quality Assurance . . . . Donna Hayden
CEO . . . . Jeff Hill
Chief of Medical Staff. . . . . Diane Zavotsky

Measure	Cases	This Hosp.	State Avg.	U.S. Avg.
Blood Clot Prevention and Treatment				
Anticoagulation Overlap Therapy[5]	-	-	95%	93%
ICU Venous Thromboembolism Prophylaxis[5]	-	-	92%	92%
Incidence of Potentially Preventable VTE[5]	-	-	11%	10%
UFH with Dosages/Platelet Monitoring[5]	-	-	99%	97%
Venous Thromboembolism Prophylaxis[5]	-	-	87%	85%
Warfarin Therapy Discharge Instructions[5]	-	-	75%	75%
Chest Pain/Possible Heart Attack Care				
Aspirin Given Within 24 Hours of Arrival[1,3]	-	-	96%	96%
Fibrinolytic Meds Within 30 Min. of Arrival[1,3]	-	-	55%	58%
Average Time to ECG (minutes)[1,3]	-	-	9	7
Average Time to Transfer (minutes)[1,3]	-	-	62	60
Children's Asthma Care				
Received Home Management Plan of Care	-	-	-	88%
Received Reliever Medication	-	-	-	100%
Received Systemic Corticosteroids	-	-	-	100%
Emergency Department				
Admittance Decision Time (minutes)[5]	-	-	76	98
Head CT Results Within 45 Min. of Arrival[5]	-	-	38%	57%
Patients Who Left ER Before Being Seen[5]	-	-	1%	2%
Time from ER Arrival to Admit. (minutes)[5]	-	-	232	274
Time from ER Arrival to Discharge (minutes)[5]	-	-	121	134
Time in ER Before Being Evaluated (minutes)[5]	-	-	21	26
Time to Pain Meds for Fractures (minutes)[5]	-	-	46	57
Heart Attack Care				
Aspirin Given at Discharge[5]	-	-	100%	99%
Fibrinolytic Meds Within 30 Min. of Arrival[5]	-	-	-	54%
PCI Within 90 Minutes of Arrival[5]	-	-	98%	96%
Statin Prescribed at Discharge[5]	-	-	99%	98%
Heart Failure Care				
ACE Inhibitor or ARB for LVSD[3,7]	-	-	98%	97%
Discharge Instructions Given[1,3]	-	-	94%	94%
Evaluation of LVS Function[1,3]	-	-	97%	99%
Medicare Spending				
Medicare Spending per Patient (ratio)	-	-	0.91	0.98
Pneumonia Care				
Appropriate Initial Antibiotic Given[3,7]	-	-	94%	95%
Blood Culture Timing[1,3]	-	-	98%	98%
Pregnancy and Delivery Care				
Newborn Deliveries Scheduled Early[5]	-	-	6%	6%
Preventive Care				
Immunization for Influenza[5]	-	-	83%	90%
Immunization for Pneumonia[5]	-	-	89%	92%
Stroke Care				
Anticoagulation Therapy for Atrial Fibrillation[5]	-	-	97%	95%
Antithrombotic Therapy Timing[5]	-	-	98%	98%
Assessed for Rehabilitation[5]	-	-	98%	97%
Discharged on Antithrombotic Therapy[5]	-	-	99%	99%
Discharged on Statin Medication[5]	-	-	91%	94%
Thrombolytic Therapy Timing[5]	-	-	55%	66%
Venous Thromboembolism Prophylaxis[5]	-	-	93%	94%
Written Stroke Educational Materials Given[5]	-	-	84%	88%
Surgical Care Improvement Project				
Appropriate Beta Blocker Usage[5]	-	-	98%	98%
Appropriate VTP Within 24 Hours[5]	-	-	98%	98%
Controlled Postoperative Blood Glucose[5]	-	-	99%	97%
Perioperative Temperature Management[5]	-	-	99%	100%
Prophylactic Antibiotic Selection[5]	-	-	99%	99%
Prophylactic Antibiotic Selection (Outpatient)[5]	-	-	98%	98%
Prophylactic Antibiotic Stopped[5]	-	-	98%	98%
Prophylactic Antibiotic Timing[5]	-	-	98%	99%
Prophylactic Antibiotic Timing (Outpatient)[5]	-	-	97%	98%
Urinary Catheter Removal[5]	-	-	96%	97%
Survey of Patients' Hospital Experiences				
Area Around Room 'Always' Quiet at Night[6]	<100	64%	61%	61%
Doctors 'Always' Communicated Well[6]	<100	89%	83%	82%
Home Recovery Information Given[6]	<100	91%	88%	85%
Hospital Given 9 or 10 on 10 Point Scale[6]	<100	73%	73%	71%
Meds 'Always' Explained Before Given[6]	<100	70%	66%	64%
Nurses 'Always' Communicated Well[6]	<100	83%	80%	79%
Pain 'Always' Well Controlled[6]	<100	74%	72%	71%
Room and Bathroom 'Always' Clean[6]	<100	83%	77%	73%
Timely Help 'Always' Received[6]	<100	82%	73%	68%
Would Definitely Recommend Hospital[6]	<100	77%	74%	71%
Use of Medical Imaging				
Cardiac Imaging Stress Test before Surgery[1]	-	-	4.6%	5.3%
Combination Abdominal CT Scan	133	2.3%	7.3%	10.5%
Combination Brain/Sinus CT Scan[1]	-	-	1.7%	2.7%
Combination Chest CT Scan	69	0.0%	1.8%	2.7%
Follow-up Mammogram/Ultrasound	212	8.0%	8.2%	8.8%
Lumbar Spine MRI for Low Back Pain[1]	-	-	40.3%	37.2%

Bonner General Hospital

520 North Third Avenue
Sandpoint, ID 83864
Phone: 208-263-1441
URL: www.bonnergeneral.org
Type: Critical Access Hospitals
Emergency Services: Yes
Ownership: Voluntary non-profit - Private

Measure	Cases	This Hosp.	State Avg.	U.S. Avg.
Blood Clot Prevention and Treatment				
Anticoagulation Overlap Therapy[5]	-	-	95%	93%
ICU Venous Thromboembolism Prophylaxis[5]	-	-	92%	92%
Incidence of Potentially Preventable VTE[5]	-	-	11%	10%
UFH with Dosages/Platelet Monitoring[5]	-	-	99%	97%
Venous Thromboembolism Prophylaxis[5]	-	-	87%	85%
Warfarin Therapy Discharge Instructions[5]	-	-	75%	75%
Chest Pain/Possible Heart Attack Care				
Aspirin Given Within 24 Hours of Arrival	43	98%	96%	96%
Fibrinolytic Meds Within 30 Min. of Arrival[7]	-	-	55%	58%
Average Time to ECG (minutes)	45	4	9	7
Average Time to Transfer (minutes)[1]	-	-	62	60
Children's Asthma Care				
Received Home Management Plan of Care	-	-	-	88%
Received Reliever Medication	-	-	-	100%
Received Systemic Corticosteroids	-	-	-	100%
Emergency Department				
Admittance Decision Time (minutes)[2]	329	55	76	98
Head CT Results Within 45 Min. of Arrival[1]	-	-	38%	57%
Patients Who Left ER Before Being Seen[5]	-	-	1%	2%
Time from ER Arrival to Admit. (minutes)[2]	340	202	232	274
Time from ER Arrival to Discharge (minutes)	368	130	121	134
Time in ER Before Being Evaluated (minutes)	362	33	21	26
Time to Pain Meds for Fractures (minutes)	64	51	46	57
Heart Attack Care				
Aspirin Given at Discharge[1]	-	-	100%	99%
Fibrinolytic Meds Within 30 Min. of Arrival[7]	-	-	-	54%
PCI Within 90 Minutes of Arrival[7]	-	-	98%	96%
Statin Prescribed at Discharge[1]	-	-	99%	98%
Heart Failure Care				
ACE Inhibitor or ARB for LVSD[1,2]	-	-	98%	97%
Discharge Instructions Given[2]	16	94%	94%	94%
Evaluation of LVS Function[2]	26	96%	97%	99%
Medicare Spending				
Medicare Spending per Patient (ratio)	-	-	0.91	0.98
Pneumonia Care				
Appropriate Initial Antibiotic Given[2]	30	100%	94%	95%
Blood Culture Timing[2]	27	100%	98%	98%
Pregnancy and Delivery Care				
Newborn Deliveries Scheduled Early[5]	-	-	6%	6%
Preventive Care				
Immunization for Influenza[2]	297	83%	83%	90%
Immunization for Pneumonia[2]	559	82%	89%	92%
Stroke Care				
Anticoagulation Therapy for Atrial Fibrillation[1]	-	-	97%	95%
Antithrombotic Therapy Timing	13	92%	98%	98%
Assessed for Rehabilitation	23	96%	98%	97%
Discharged on Antithrombotic Therapy	18	89%	99%	99%
Discharged on Statin Medication	19	63%	91%	94%
Thrombolytic Therapy Timing[7]	-	-	55%	66%
Venous Thromboembolism Prophylaxis	20	65%	93%	94%
Written Stroke Educational Materials Given	11	36%	84%	88%
Surgical Care Improvement Project				
Appropriate Beta Blocker Usage[2]	41	90%	98%	98%
Appropriate VTP Within 24 Hours[2]	181	94%	98%	98%
Controlled Postoperative Blood Glucose[2,7]	-	-	99%	97%
Perioperative Temperature Management[2]	208	99%	99%	100%
Prophylactic Antibiotic Selection[2]	173	99%	99%	99%
Prophylactic Antibiotic Selection (Outpatient)	24	96%	98%	98%
Prophylactic Antibiotic Stopped[2]	172	98%	98%	98%
Prophylactic Antibiotic Timing[2]	173	98%	98%	99%
Prophylactic Antibiotic Timing (Outpatient)	24	96%	97%	98%
Urinary Catheter Removal[2]	167	94%	96%	97%
Survey of Patients' Hospital Experiences				
Area Around Room 'Always' Quiet at Night	300+	64%	61%	61%
Doctors 'Always' Communicated Well	300+	79%	83%	82%
Home Recovery Information Given	300+	86%	88%	85%
Hospital Given 9 or 10 on 10 Point Scale	300+	73%	73%	71%
Meds 'Always' Explained Before Given	300+	68%	66%	64%
Nurses 'Always' Communicated Well	300+	79%	80%	79%
Pain 'Always' Well Controlled	300+	76%	72%	71%
Room and Bathroom 'Always' Clean	300+	81%	77%	73%
Timely Help 'Always' Received	300+	78%	73%	68%

NOTE: Hospital profiles are in alphabetical order by state, then city, then hospital within the city; Rankings exclude hospitals with less than 25 cases except for patient surveys which excludes hospitals with less than 100 cases; (a) 100-299 cases; (1) The number of cases/patients is too few to report; (2) Data submitted were based on a sample of cases/patients; (3) Results are based on a shorter time period than required; (4) Data suppressed by CMS for one or more quarters; (5) Results are not available for this reporting period; (6) Fewer than 100 patients completed the HCAHPS survey; (7) No cases met the criteria for this measure; (8) The lower limit of the confidence interval cannot be calculated if the number of observed infections equals zero; (9) No data are available from the state/territory for this reporting period; (10) The scores shown reflect fewer than 50 completed surveys; (11) There were discrepancies in the data collection process; (12) This measure does not apply to this hospital for this reporting period; (13) Results cannot be calculated for this reporting period; (14) The results for this state are combined with nearby states to protect confidentiality; Please refer to the User's Guide for a full explanation of data.

Measure	Cases	This Hosp.	State Avg.	U.S. Avg.
Would Definitely Recommend Hospital	300+	72%	74%	71%
Use of Medical Imaging				
Cardiac Imaging Stress Test before Surgery	226	4.4%	4.6%	5.3%
Combination Abdominal CT Scan	394	4.8%	7.3%	10.5%
Combination Brain/Sinus CT Scan	200	1.0%	1.7%	2.7%
Combination Chest CT Scan	253	0.4%	1.8%	2.7%
Follow-up Mammogram/Ultrasound	520	14.8%	8.2%	8.8%
Lumbar Spine MRI for Low Back Pain	84	45.2%	40.3%	37.2%

Caribou Memorial Hospital

300 South 3rd West Phone: 208-547-3341
Soda Springs, ID 83276
Type: Critical Access Hospitals Emergency Services: No
Ownership: Government - Local

Measure	Cases	This Hosp.	State Avg.	U.S. Avg.
Blood Clot Prevention and Treatment				
Anticoagulation Overlap Therapy[5]	-	-	95%	93%
ICU Venous Thromboembolism Prophylaxis[5]	-	-	92%	92%
Incidence of Potentially Preventable VTE[5]	-	-	11%	10%
UFH with Dosages/Platelet Monitoring[5]	-	-	99%	97%
Venous Thromboembolism Prophylaxis[5]	-	-	87%	85%
Warfarin Therapy Discharge Instructions[5]	-	-	75%	75%
Chest Pain/Possible Heart Attack Care				
Aspirin Given Within 24 Hours of Arrival	-	-	96%	96%
Fibrinolytic Meds Within 30 Min. of Arrival	-	-	55%	58%
Average Time to ECG (minutes)	-	-	9	7
Average Time to Transfer (minutes)	-	-	62	60
Children's Asthma Care				
Received Home Management Plan of Care	-	-	-	88%
Received Reliever Medication	-	-	-	100%
Received Systemic Corticosteroids	-	-	-	100%
Emergency Department				
Admittance Decision Time (minutes)[5]	-	-	76	98
Head CT Results Within 45 Min. of Arrival	-	-	38%	57%
Patients Who Left ER Before Being Seen	-	-	1%	2%
Time from ER Arrival to Admit. (minutes)[5]	-	-	232	274
Time from ER Arrival to Discharge (minutes)	-	-	121	134
Time in ER Before Being Evaluated (minutes)	-	-	21	26
Time to Pain Meds for Fractures (minutes)	-	-	46	57
Heart Attack Care				
Aspirin Given at Discharge[5]	-	-	100%	99%
Fibrinolytic Meds Within 30 Min. of Arrival[5]	-	-	-	54%
PCI Within 90 Minutes of Arrival[5]	-	-	98%	96%
Statin Prescribed at Discharge[5]	-	-	99%	98%
Heart Failure Care				
ACE Inhibitor or ARB for LVSD[5]	-	-	98%	97%
Discharge Instructions Given[5]	-	-	94%	94%
Evaluation of LVS Function[5]	-	-	97%	99%
Medicare Spending				
Medicare Spending per Patient (ratio)	-	-	0.91	0.98
Pneumonia Care				
Appropriate Initial Antibiotic Given[1,3]	-	-	94%	95%
Blood Culture Timing[1,3]	-	-	98%	98%
Pregnancy and Delivery Care				
Newborn Deliveries Scheduled Early[5]	-	-	6%	6%
Preventive Care				
Immunization for Influenza[5]	-	-	83%	90%
Immunization for Pneumonia[5]	-	-	89%	92%
Stroke Care				
Anticoagulation Therapy for Atrial Fibrillation[5]	-	-	97%	95%
Antithrombotic Therapy Timing[5]	-	-	98%	98%
Assessed for Rehabilitation[5]	-	-	98%	97%
Discharged on Antithrombotic Therapy[5]	-	-	99%	99%
Discharged on Statin Medication[5]	-	-	91%	94%
Thrombolytic Therapy Timing[5]	-	-	55%	66%
Venous Thromboembolism Prophylaxis[5]	-	-	93%	94%
Written Stroke Educational Materials Given[5]	-	-	84%	88%
Surgical Care Improvement Project				
Appropriate Beta Blocker Usage[5]	-	-	98%	98%
Appropriate VTP Within 24 Hours[5]	-	-	98%	98%
Controlled Postoperative Blood Glucose[5]	-	-	99%	97%
Perioperative Temperature Management[5]	-	-	99%	100%
Prophylactic Antibiotic Selection[5]	-	-	99%	99%
Prophylactic Antibiotic Selection (Outpatient)	-	-	98%	98%
Prophylactic Antibiotic Stopped[5]	-	-	98%	98%
Prophylactic Antibiotic Timing[5]	-	-	98%	99%
Prophylactic Antibiotic Timing (Outpatient)	-	-	97%	98%
Urinary Catheter Removal[5]	-	-	96%	97%
Survey of Patients' Hospital Experiences				
Area Around Room 'Always' Quiet at Night[5]	-	-	61%	61%
Doctors 'Always' Communicated Well[5]	-	-	83%	82%
Home Recovery Information Given[5]	-	-	88%	85%
Hospital Given 9 or 10 on 10 Point Scale[5]	-	-	73%	71%
Meds 'Always' Explained Before Given[5]	-	-	66%	64%
Nurses 'Always' Communicated Well[5]	-	-	80%	79%
Pain 'Always' Well Controlled[5]	-	-	72%	71%
Room and Bathroom 'Always' Clean[5]	-	-	77%	73%
Timely Help 'Always' Received[5]	-	-	73%	68%
Would Definitely Recommend Hospital[5]	-	-	74%	71%
Use of Medical Imaging				
Cardiac Imaging Stress Test before Surgery	-	-	4.6%	5.3%
Combination Abdominal CT Scan	-	-	7.3%	10.5%
Combination Brain/Sinus CT Scan	-	-	1.7%	2.7%
Combination Chest CT Scan	-	-	1.8%	2.7%
Follow-up Mammogram/Ultrasound	-	-	8.2%	8.8%
Lumbar Spine MRI for Low Back Pain	-	-	40.3%	37.2%

Saint Luke's Magic Valley Rmc

801 Pole Line Road West Phone: 208-814-1000
Twin Falls, ID 83301 Fax: 208-737-2786
URL: www.stlukesonline.org/magic_valley
Type: Acute Care Hospitals Emergency Services: Yes
Ownership: Voluntary non-profit - Private Beds: 204

Key Personnel:

Pediatric Ambulatory Care . . . . . . Barton Adrian, MD
Pediatric In-Patient Care . . . . Barton Adrian, MD
Radiology. . . . . Dan Alder
CEO . . . . James L. Angle, FACHE
Quality Assurance . . . . Sharon Fischer
Emergency Room . . . . Marlys Massey
President/CEO. . . . . David C. Pate, MD, JD
Operating Room. . . . . Jo Riter, RN

Measure	Cases	This Hosp.	State Avg.	U.S. Avg.
Blood Clot Prevention and Treatment				
Anticoagulation Overlap Therapy[2]	65	94%	95%	93%
ICU Venous Thromboembolism Prophylaxis[2]	68	84%	92%	92%
Incidence of Potentially Preventable VTE[1,2]	-	-	11%	10%
UFH with Dosages/Platelet Monitoring[1,2]	-	-	99%	97%
Venous Thromboembolism Prophylaxis[2]	310	85%	87%	85%
Warfarin Therapy Discharge Instructions[2]	49	53%	75%	75%
Chest Pain/Possible Heart Attack Care				
Aspirin Given Within 24 Hours of Arrival[1,3]	-	-	96%	96%
Fibrinolytic Meds Within 30 Min. of Arrival[5]	-	-	55%	58%
Average Time to ECG (minutes)[1,3]	-	-	9	7
Average Time to Transfer (minutes)[5]	-	-	62	60
Children's Asthma Care				
Received Home Management Plan of Care	-	-	-	88%
Received Reliever Medication	-	-	-	100%
Received Systemic Corticosteroids	-	-	-	100%
Emergency Department				
Admittance Decision Time (minutes)[2]	478	95	76	98
Head CT Results Within 45 Min. of Arrival[1]	-	-	38%	57%
Patients Who Left ER Before Being Seen	38,143	1%	1%	2%
Time from ER Arrival to Admit. (minutes)[2]	515	237	232	274
Time from ER Arrival to Discharge (minutes)	298	128	121	134
Time in ER Before Being Evaluated (minutes)	225	28	21	26
Time to Pain Meds for Fractures (minutes)	119	45	46	57
Heart Attack Care				
Aspirin Given at Discharge	147	100%	100%	99%
Fibrinolytic Meds Within 30 Min. of Arrival[7]	-	-	-	54%
PCI Within 90 Minutes of Arrival	29	100%	98%	96%
Statin Prescribed at Discharge	140	100%	99%	98%
Heart Failure Care				
ACE Inhibitor or ARB for LVSD	54	100%	98%	97%
Discharge Instructions Given	121	100%	94%	94%
Evaluation of LVS Function	164	100%	97%	99%
Medicare Spending				
Medicare Spending per Patient (ratio)	-	0.96	0.91	0.98
Pneumonia Care				
Appropriate Initial Antibiotic Given	142	100%	94%	95%
Blood Culture Timing	241	100%	98%	98%
Pregnancy and Delivery Care				
Newborn Deliveries Scheduled Early[2]	47	15%	6%	6%
Preventive Care				
Immunization for Influenza[2]	494	92%	83%	90%
Immunization for Pneumonia[2]	546	95%	89%	92%
Stroke Care				
Anticoagulation Therapy for Atrial Fibrillation	19	84%	97%	95%
Antithrombotic Therapy Timing	80	90%	98%	98%
Assessed for Rehabilitation	99	97%	98%	97%
Discharged on Antithrombotic Therapy	93	94%	99%	99%
Discharged on Statin Medication	79	91%	91%	94%
Thrombolytic Therapy Timing	15	80%	55%	66%
Venous Thromboembolism Prophylaxis	99	88%	93%	94%
Written Stroke Educational Materials Given	55	82%	84%	88%
Surgical Care Improvement Project				
Appropriate Beta Blocker Usage[2]	117	97%	98%	98%
Appropriate VTP Within 24 Hours[2]	384	100%	98%	98%
Controlled Postoperative Blood Glucose[2,7]	-	-	99%	97%
Perioperative Temperature Management[2]	539	100%	99%	100%
Prophylactic Antibiotic Selection[2]	350	100%	99%	99%
Prophylactic Antibiotic Selection (Outpatient)	316	99%	98%	98%
Prophylactic Antibiotic Stopped[2]	340	99%	98%	98%
Prophylactic Antibiotic Timing[2]	350	99%	98%	99%
Prophylactic Antibiotic Timing (Outpatient)	217	99%	97%	98%
Urinary Catheter Removal[2]	284	99%	96%	97%
Survey of Patients' Hospital Experiences				
Area Around Room 'Always' Quiet at Night	300+	60%	61%	61%
Doctors 'Always' Communicated Well	300+	82%	83%	82%
Home Recovery Information Given	300+	87%	88%	85%
Hospital Given 9 or 10 on 10 Point Scale	300+	72%	73%	71%
Meds 'Always' Explained Before Given	300+	66%	66%	64%
Nurses 'Always' Communicated Well	300+	79%	80%	79%
Pain 'Always' Well Controlled	300+	73%	72%	71%
Room and Bathroom 'Always' Clean	300+	85%	77%	73%
Timely Help 'Always' Received	300+	72%	73%	68%
Would Definitely Recommend Hospital	300+	72%	74%	71%
Use of Medical Imaging				
Cardiac Imaging Stress Test before Surgery	545	6.1%	4.6%	5.3%
Combination Abdominal CT Scan	1,216	7.5%	7.3%	10.5%
Combination Brain/Sinus CT Scan	527	0.9%	1.7%	2.7%
Combination Chest CT Scan	566	0.2%	1.8%	2.7%
Follow-up Mammogram/Ultrasound	2,082	7.1%	8.2%	8.8%
Lumbar Spine MRI for Low Back Pain	172	37.2%	40.3%	37.2%

Teton Valley Hospital

252 South Main Street Phone: 208-354-2383
Victor, ID 83455
Type: Critical Access Hospitals Emergency Services: Yes
Ownership: Voluntary non-profit - Private

Measure	Cases	This Hosp.	State Avg.	U.S. Avg.
Blood Clot Prevention and Treatment				
Anticoagulation Overlap Therapy	-	-	95%	93%
ICU Venous Thromboembolism Prophylaxis	-	-	92%	92%
Incidence of Potentially Preventable VTE	-	-	11%	10%
UFH with Dosages/Platelet Monitoring	-	-	99%	97%
Venous Thromboembolism Prophylaxis	-	-	87%	85%
Warfarin Therapy Discharge Instructions	-	-	75%	75%
Chest Pain/Possible Heart Attack Care				
Aspirin Given Within 24 Hours of Arrival[5]	-	-	96%	96%
Fibrinolytic Meds Within 30 Min. of Arrival[5]	-	-	55%	58%
Average Time to ECG (minutes)[5]	-	-	9	7
Average Time to Transfer (minutes)[5]	-	-	62	60
Children's Asthma Care				
Received Home Management Plan of Care	-	-	-	88%
Received Reliever Medication	-	-	-	100%
Received Systemic Corticosteroids	-	-	-	100%
Emergency Department				

NOTE: Hospital profiles are in alphabetical order by state, then city, then hospital within the city; Rankings exclude hospitals with less than 25 cases except for patient surveys which excludes hospitals with less than 100 cases; (a) 100-299 cases; (1) The number of cases/patients is too few to report; (2) Data submitted were based on a sample of cases/patients; (3) Results are based on a shorter time period than required; (4) Data suppressed by CMS for one or more quarters; (5) Results are not available for this reporting period; (6) Fewer than 100 patients completed the HCAHPS survey; (7) No cases met the criteria for this measure; (8) The lower limit of the confidence interval cannot be calculated if the number of observed infections equals zero; (9) No data are available from the state/territory for this reporting period; (10) The scores shown reflect fewer than 50 completed surveys; (11) There were discrepancies in the data collection process; (12) This measure does not apply to this hospital for this reporting period; (13) Results cannot be calculated for this reporting period; (14) The results for this state are combined with nearby states to protect confidentiality; Please refer to the User's Guide for a full explanation of data.

Measure	Cases	This Hosp.	State Avg.	U.S. Avg.
Admittance Decision Time (minutes)	-	-	76	98
Head CT Results Within 45 Min. of Arrival[5]	-	-	38%	57%
Patients Who Left ER Before Being Seen[5]	-	-	1%	2%
Time from ER Arrival to Admit. (minutes)	-	-	232	274
Time from ER Arrival to Discharge (minutes)[5]	-	-	121	134
Time in ER Before Being Evaluated (minutes)[5]	-	-	21	26
Time to Pain Meds for Fractures (minutes)[5]	-	-	46	57
Heart Attack Care				
Aspirin Given at Discharge	-	-	100%	99%
Fibrinolytic Meds Within 30 Min. of Arrival	-	-	-	54%
PCI Within 90 Minutes of Arrival	-	-	98%	96%
Statin Prescribed at Discharge	-	-	99%	98%
Heart Failure Care				
ACE Inhibitor or ARB for LVSD	-	-	98%	97%
Discharge Instructions Given	-	-	94%	94%
Evaluation of LVS Function	-	-	97%	99%
Medicare Spending				
Medicare Spending per Patient (ratio)	-	-	0.91	0.98
Pneumonia Care				
Appropriate Initial Antibiotic Given	-	-	94%	95%
Blood Culture Timing	-	-	98%	98%
Pregnancy and Delivery Care				
Newborn Deliveries Scheduled Early	-	-	6%	6%
Preventive Care				
Immunization for Influenza	-	-	83%	90%
Immunization for Pneumonia	-	-	89%	92%
Stroke Care				
Anticoagulation Therapy for Atrial Fibrillation	-	-	97%	95%
Antithrombotic Therapy Timing	-	-	98%	98%
Assessed for Rehabilitation	-	-	98%	97%
Discharged on Antithrombotic Therapy	-	-	99%	99%
Discharged on Statin Medication	-	-	91%	94%
Thrombolytic Therapy Timing	-	-	55%	66%
Venous Thromboembolism Prophylaxis	-	-	93%	94%
Written Stroke Educational Materials Given	-	-	84%	88%
Surgical Care Improvement Project				
Appropriate Beta Blocker Usage	-	-	98%	98%
Appropriate VTP Within 24 Hours	-	-	98%	98%
Controlled Postoperative Blood Glucose	-	-	99%	97%
Perioperative Temperature Management	-	-	99%	100%
Prophylactic Antibiotic Selection	-	-	99%	99%
Prophylactic Antibiotic Selection (Outpatient)[5]	-	-	98%	98%
Prophylactic Antibiotic Stopped	-	-	98%	98%
Prophylactic Antibiotic Timing	-	-	98%	99%
Prophylactic Antibiotic Timing (Outpatient)[5]	-	-	97%	98%
Urinary Catheter Removal	-	-	96%	97%
Survey of Patients' Hospital Experiences				
Area Around Room 'Always' Quiet at Night	-	-	61%	61%
Doctors 'Always' Communicated Well	-	-	83%	82%
Home Recovery Information Given	-	-	88%	85%
Hospital Given 9 or 10 on 10 Point Scale	-	-	73%	71%
Meds 'Always' Explained Before Given	-	-	66%	64%
Nurses 'Always' Communicated Well	-	-	80%	79%
Pain 'Always' Well Controlled	-	-	72%	71%
Room and Bathroom 'Always' Clean	-	-	77%	73%
Timely Help 'Always' Received	-	-	73%	68%
Would Definitely Recommend Hospital	-	-	74%	71%
Use of Medical Imaging				
Cardiac Imaging Stress Test before Surgery[1]	-	-	4.6%	5.3%
Combination Abdominal CT Scan[1]	-	-	7.3%	10.5%
Combination Brain/Sinus CT Scan[1]	-	-	1.7%	2.7%
Combination Chest CT Scan[1]	-	-	1.8%	2.7%
Follow-up Mammogram/Ultrasound	80	6.3%	8.2%	8.8%
Lumbar Spine MRI for Low Back Pain[1]	-	-	40.3%	37.2%

Weiser Memorial Hospital

645 East 5th Street
Weiser, ID 83672
Type: Critical Access Hospitals
Ownership: Govt - Hospital Dist/Auth

Phone: 208-549-0370
Emergency Services: Yes

Measure	Cases	This Hosp.	State Avg.	U.S. Avg.
Blood Clot Prevention and Treatment				
Anticoagulation Overlap Therapy[5]	-	-	95%	93%
ICU Venous Thromboembolism Prophylaxis[5]	-	-	92%	92%
Incidence of Potentially Preventable VTE[5]	-	-	11%	10%
UFH with Dosages/Platelet Monitoring[5]	-	-	99%	97%
Venous Thromboembolism Prophylaxis[5]	-	-	87%	85%
Warfarin Therapy Discharge Instructions[5]	-	-	75%	75%
Chest Pain/Possible Heart Attack Care				
Aspirin Given Within 24 Hours of Arrival	-	-	96%	96%
Fibrinolytic Meds Within 30 Min. of Arrival	-	-	55%	58%
Average Time to ECG (minutes)	-	-	9	7
Average Time to Transfer (minutes)	-	-	62	60
Children's Asthma Care				
Received Home Management Plan of Care	-	-	-	88%
Received Reliever Medication	-	-	-	100%
Received Systemic Corticosteroids	-	-	-	100%
Emergency Department				
Admittance Decision Time (minutes)[5]	-	-	76	98
Head CT Results Within 45 Min. of Arrival	-	-	38%	57%
Patients Who Left ER Before Being Seen	-	-	1%	2%
Time from ER Arrival to Admit. (minutes)[5]	-	-	232	274
Time from ER Arrival to Discharge (minutes)	-	-	121	134
Time in ER Before Being Evaluated (minutes)	-	-	21	26
Time to Pain Meds for Fractures (minutes)	-	-	46	57
Heart Attack Care				
Aspirin Given at Discharge[5]	-	-	100%	99%
Fibrinolytic Meds Within 30 Min. of Arrival[5]	-	-	-	54%
PCI Within 90 Minutes of Arrival[5]	-	-	98%	96%
Statin Prescribed at Discharge[5]	-	-	99%	98%
Heart Failure Care				
ACE Inhibitor or ARB for LVSD[1]	-	-	98%	97%
Discharge Instructions Given[1]	-	-	94%	94%
Evaluation of LVS Function	14	71%	97%	99%
Medicare Spending				
Medicare Spending per Patient (ratio)	-	-	0.91	0.98
Pneumonia Care				
Appropriate Initial Antibiotic Given	17	82%	94%	95%
Blood Culture Timing	13	92%	98%	98%
Pregnancy and Delivery Care				
Newborn Deliveries Scheduled Early[5]	-	-	6%	6%
Preventive Care				
Immunization for Influenza[5]	-	-	83%	90%
Immunization for Pneumonia[5]	-	-	89%	92%
Stroke Care				
Anticoagulation Therapy for Atrial Fibrillation[5]	-	-	97%	95%
Antithrombotic Therapy Timing[5]	-	-	98%	98%
Assessed for Rehabilitation[5]	-	-	98%	97%
Discharged on Antithrombotic Therapy[5]	-	-	99%	99%
Discharged on Statin Medication[5]	-	-	91%	94%
Thrombolytic Therapy Timing[5]	-	-	55%	66%
Venous Thromboembolism Prophylaxis[5]	-	-	93%	94%
Written Stroke Educational Materials Given[5]	-	-	84%	88%
Surgical Care Improvement Project				
Appropriate Beta Blocker Usage	14	79%	98%	98%
Appropriate VTP Within 24 Hours	57	100%	98%	98%
Controlled Postoperative Blood Glucose[7]	-	-	99%	97%
Perioperative Temperature Management	60	92%	99%	100%
Prophylactic Antibiotic Selection	51	100%	99%	99%
Prophylactic Antibiotic Selection (Outpatient)	-	-	98%	98%
Prophylactic Antibiotic Stopped	51	51%	98%	98%
Prophylactic Antibiotic Timing	51	45%	98%	99%
Prophylactic Antibiotic Timing (Outpatient)	-	-	97%	98%
Urinary Catheter Removal	59	98%	96%	97%
Survey of Patients' Hospital Experiences				
Area Around Room 'Always' Quiet at Night[5]	-	-	61%	61%
Doctors 'Always' Communicated Well[5]	-	-	83%	82%
Home Recovery Information Given[5]	-	-	88%	85%
Hospital Given 9 or 10 on 10 Point Scale[5]	-	-	73%	71%
Meds 'Always' Explained Before Given[5]	-	-	66%	64%
Nurses 'Always' Communicated Well[5]	-	-	80%	79%
Pain 'Always' Well Controlled[5]	-	-	72%	71%
Room and Bathroom 'Always' Clean[5]	-	-	77%	73%
Timely Help 'Always' Received[5]	-	-	73%	68%
Would Definitely Recommend Hospital[5]	-	-	74%	71%
Use of Medical Imaging				
Cardiac Imaging Stress Test before Surgery	-	-	4.6%	5.3%
Combination Abdominal CT Scan	-	-	7.3%	10.5%
Combination Brain/Sinus CT Scan	-	-	1.7%	2.7%
Combination Chest CT Scan	-	-	1.8%	2.7%
Follow-up Mammogram/Ultrasound	-	-	8.2%	8.8%
Lumbar Spine MRI for Low Back Pain	-	-	40.3%	37.2%

NOTE: Hospital profiles are in alphabetical order by state, then city, then hospital within the city; Rankings exclude hospitals with less than 25 cases except for patient surveys which excludes hospitals with less than 100 cases; (a) 100-299 cases; (1) The number of cases/patients is too few to report; (2) Data submitted were based on a sample of cases/patients; (3) Results are based on a shorter time period than required; (4) Data suppressed by CMS for one or more quarters; (5) Results are not available for this reporting period; (6) Fewer than 100 patients completed the HCAHPS survey; (7) No cases met the criteria for this measure; (8) The lower limit of the confidence interval cannot be calculated if the number of observed infections equals zero; (9) No data are available from the state/territory for this reporting period; (10) The scores shown reflect fewer than 50 completed surveys; (11) There were discrepancies in the data collection process; (12) This measure does not apply to this hospital for this reporting period; (13) Results cannot be calculated for this reporting period; (14) The results for this state are combined with nearby states to protect confidentiality; Please refer to the User's Guide for a full explanation of data.

Blood Clot Prevention and Treatment

Anticoagulation Overlap Therapy

Hospital Name	City	Rate	Cases
Benefis Hospitals[2]	Great Falls	100%	63
Bozeman Deaconess Hospital[2]	Bozeman	100%	65
Community Medical Center[2]	Missoula	100%	29
Saint Peter's Hospital[2]	Helena	100%	38
Billings Clinic Hospital[2]	Billings	99%	89
Kalispell Regional Medical Center[2]	Kalispell	98%	50
Saint Vincent Healthcare[2]	Billings	98%	54
Saint Patrick Hospital[2]	Missoula	95%	87
Saint James Healthcare[2]	Butte	94%	34

ICU Venous Thromboembolism Prophylaxis

Hospital Name	City	Rate	Cases
Benefis Hospitals[2]	Great Falls	100%	47
Community Medical Center[2]	Missoula	100%	30
Kalispell Regional Medical Center[2]	Kalispell	100%	54
Holy Rosary Healthcare	Miles City	98%	113
Saint Peter's Hospital[2]	Helena	94%	79
Billings Clinic Hospital[2]	Billings	92%	83
Saint Vincent Healthcare[2]	Billings	92%	89
Sidney Health Center[2]	Sidney	92%	25
Bozeman Deaconess Hospital[2]	Bozeman	88%	48
Saint James Healthcare[2]	Butte	88%	91
Saint Patrick Hospital[2]	Missoula	87%	63
Northern Montana Hospital[2]	Havre	73%	41

UFH with Dosages/Platelet Count Monitoring

Hospital Name	City	Rate	Cases
Billings Clinic Hospital[2]	Billings	100%	57
Saint Patrick Hospital[2]	Missoula	100%	39

Venous Thromboembolism Prophylaxis

Hospital Name	City	Rate	Cases
Benefis Hospitals[2]	Great Falls	97%	344
Community Medical Center[2]	Missoula	97%	232
Holy Rosary Healthcare	Miles City	95%	278
Kalispell Regional Medical Center[2]	Kalispell	95%	311
Saint James Healthcare[2]	Butte	92%	256
Bozeman Deaconess Hospital[2]	Bozeman	91%	257
Saint Patrick Hospital[2]	Missoula	89%	298
Saint Vincent Healthcare[2]	Billings	88%	322
Health Center Northwest[2]	Kalispell	87%	38
Great Falls Clinic Medical Center	Great Falls	85%	146
Providence Saint Joseph Medical Center[2]	Polson	85%	82
Rosebud Health Care Center[2]	Forsyth	83%	69
Sidney Health Center[2]	Sidney	82%	94
Saint Peter's Hospital[2]	Helena	80%	334
Billings Clinic Hospital[2]	Billings	79%	247
Northern Montana Hospital[2]	Havre	78%	85
Roundup Memorial Healthcare	Roundup	56%	25
Central Montana Medical Center[2,3]	Lewistown	31%	86
Northern Rockies Medical Center[3]	Cut Bank	29%	28
PHS Indian Hosp at Browning-Blackfeet	Browning	20%	193

Warfarin Therapy Discharge Instructions

Hospital Name	City	Rate	Cases
Kalispell Regional Medical Center[2]	Kalispell	100%	30
Saint Vincent Healthcare[2]	Billings	98%	41
Billings Clinic Hospital[2]	Billings	97%	74
Saint Peter's Hospital[2]	Helena	94%	31
Bozeman Deaconess Hospital[2]	Bozeman	93%	54
Benefis Hospitals[2]	Great Falls	90%	52
Saint James Healthcare[2]	Butte	64%	25
Saint Patrick Hospital[2]	Missoula	47%	76

Chest Pain/Possible Heart Attack Care

No hospitals met the 25 case threshold.

Children's Asthma Care

No hospitals met the 25 case threshold.

Emergency Department

Admittance Decision Time (minutes)

Hospital Name	City	Min.	Cases
Clark Fork Valley Hospital[2]	Plains	22	48
Sidney Health Center[2]	Sidney	25	195
PHS Indian Hosp at Browning-Blackfeet	Browning	29	293
Central Montana Medical Center[2]	Lewistown	30	325
Northern Montana Hospital[2]	Havre	39	357
Saint James Healthcare[2]	Butte	43	384
PHS Indian Hosp Crow/Northern Cheyenne[3]	Crow Agency	44	33
Holy Rosary Healthcare[2]	Miles City	52	216
Saint Vincent Healthcare[2]	Billings	74	358
Kalispell Regional Medical Center[2]	Kalispell	82	615
Benefis Hospitals[2]	Great Falls	84	598
Community Medical Center[2]	Missoula	88	278
Saint Peter's Hospital[2]	Helena	96	450
Saint Patrick Hospital[2]	Missoula	101	510
Bozeman Deaconess Hospital[2]	Bozeman	139	511
Billings Clinic Hospital[2]	Billings	156	453

Patients Who Left ER Before Being Seen

Hospital Name	City	Rate	Cases
Barrett Memorial Hospital	Dillon	0%	4019
Cabinet Peaks Medical Center	Libby	0%	6353
Community Medical Center	Missoula	0%	17062
Saint Vincent Healthcare	Billings	0%	56624
Billings Clinic Hospital	Billings	1%	40808
Bozeman Deaconess Hospital	Bozeman	1%	23901
North Valley Hospital	Whitefish	1%	7478
Saint James Healthcare	Butte	1%	13724
Saint Peter's Hospital	Helena	1%	22671
Sidney Health Center	Sidney	1%	6971
Central Montana Medical Center	Lewistown	2%	1670
Kalispell Regional Medical Center	Kalispell	2%	22634
Northern Montana Hospital	Havre	2%	8680
Benefis Hospitals	Great Falls	3%	35949
Saint Patrick Hospital	Missoula	4%	28071

Time from ER Arrival to Being Admitted (minutes)

Hospital Name	City	Min.	Cases
Central Montana Medical Center[2]	Lewistown	135	373
Clark Fork Valley Hospital[2]	Plains	154	48
Sidney Health Center[2]	Sidney	155	209
Northern Montana Hospital[2]	Havre	172	471
Holy Rosary Healthcare[2]	Miles City	174	219
PHS Indian Hosp at Browning-Blackfeet	Browning	176	294
Saint James Healthcare[2]	Butte	181	410
Saint Vincent Healthcare[2]	Billings	203	375
PHS Indian Hosp Crow/Northern Cheyenne[3]	Crow Agency	212	40
Kalispell Regional Medical Center[2]	Kalispell	233	621
Community Medical Center[2]	Missoula	234	295
Saint Patrick Hospital[2]	Missoula	249	589
Saint Peter's Hospital[2]	Helena	262	556
Benefis Hospitals[2]	Great Falls	273	598
Bozeman Deaconess Hospital[2]	Bozeman	288	548
Billings Clinic Hospital[2]	Billings	290	460

Time from ER Arrival to Discharge (minutes)

Hospital Name	City	Min.	Cases
Central Montana Medical Center	Lewistown	70	306
Holy Rosary Healthcare	Miles City	85	336
Northern Montana Hospital	Havre	100	374
Providence Saint Joseph Medical Center	Polson	101	304
Saint James Healthcare	Butte	101	395
Community Medical Center	Missoula	125	394
Billings Clinic Hospital	Billings	126	367
Benefis Hospitals	Great Falls	132	394
Saint Peter's Hospital	Helena	137	354
Kalispell Regional Medical Center	Kalispell	138	376
Saint Vincent Healthcare	Billings	141	389
Saint Patrick Hospital	Missoula	143	357
Bozeman Deaconess Hospital	Bozeman	155	457

Time in ER Before Being Evaluated (minutes)

Hospital Name	City	Min.	Cases
Central Montana Medical Center	Lewistown	10	326
Saint James Healthcare	Butte	12	106
Providence Saint Joseph Medical Center	Polson	14	382
Billings Clinic Hospital	Billings	15	383
Holy Rosary Healthcare	Miles City	17	377
Kalispell Regional Medical Center	Kalispell	18	391
Saint Vincent Healthcare	Billings	21	373
Saint Peter's Hospital	Helena	22	278
Bozeman Deaconess Hospital	Bozeman	30	501
Community Medical Center	Missoula	33	389
Northern Montana Hospital	Havre	34	361
Saint Patrick Hospital	Missoula	40	342
Benefis Hospitals	Great Falls	41	382

Time to Pain Meds for Bone Fractures (minutes)

Hospital Name	City	Min.	Cases
Providence Saint Joseph Medical Center	Polson	28	48
Barrett Memorial Hospital	Dillon	31	27
Holy Rosary Healthcare	Miles City	32	28
Kalispell Regional Medical Center	Kalispell	36	122
Sidney Health Center	Sidney	38	42
Saint James Healthcare	Butte	41	59
Community Medical Center	Missoula	44	84
Saint Peter's Hospital	Helena	44	124
Saint Vincent Healthcare	Billings	46	106
North Valley Hospital	Whitefish	49	91
Saint Patrick Hospital	Missoula	53	85
Billings Clinic Hospital	Billings	56	162
Bozeman Deaconess Hospital	Bozeman	56	161
Northern Montana Hospital	Havre	56	38
Benefis Hospitals	Great Falls	63	94

Heart Attack Care

Aspirin Given at Discharge

Hospital Name	City	Rate	Cases
Benefis Hospitals	Great Falls	100%	189
Billings Clinic Hospital	Billings	100%	305
Bozeman Deaconess Hospital	Bozeman	100%	84
Community Medical Center	Missoula	100%	35
Kalispell Regional Medical Center	Kalispell	100%	172
Saint James Healthcare	Butte	100%	47
Saint Patrick Hospital	Missoula	100%	348
Saint Peter's Hospital	Helena	100%	96
Saint Vincent Healthcare	Billings	100%	249

PCI Within 90 Minutes of Arrival

Hospital Name	City	Rate	Cases
Billings Clinic Hospital	Billings	100%	51
Saint Vincent Healthcare	Billings	100%	28
Benefis Hospitals	Great Falls	98%	41
Kalispell Regional Medical Center	Kalispell	97%	32
Saint Peter's Hospital	Helena	94%	31
Saint Patrick Hospital	Missoula	90%	30

Statin Prescribed at Discharge

Hospital Name	City	Rate	Cases
Billings Clinic Hospital	Billings	100%	295
Bozeman Deaconess Hospital	Bozeman	100%	80
Community Medical Center	Missoula	100%	32
Saint Patrick Hospital	Missoula	100%	339
Saint Peter's Hospital	Helena	100%	95
Saint Vincent Healthcare	Billings	100%	234
Benefis Hospitals	Great Falls	99%	182
Kalispell Regional Medical Center	Kalispell	97%	157
Saint James Healthcare	Butte	93%	46

Heart Failure Care

ACE Inhibitor or ARB for LVSD

Hospital Name	City	Rate	Cases
Kalispell Regional Medical Center	Kalispell	100%	41
Saint Patrick Hospital	Missoula	100%	62
Saint Peter's Hospital	Helena	100%	30
Saint Vincent Healthcare	Billings	100%	65
Billings Clinic Hospital	Billings	99%	70
Benefis Hospitals	Great Falls	92%	50

Discharge Instructions Given

Hospital Name	City	Rate	Cases
Livingston Healthcare	Livingston	100%	25
VA Montana Healthcare System	Fort Harrison	100%	42
Kalispell Regional Medical Center	Kalispell	99%	119
Benefis Hospitals	Great Falls	98%	180
Billings Clinic Hospital	Billings	98%	205
Bozeman Deaconess Hospital	Bozeman	97%	64
Saint Vincent Healthcare	Billings	97%	188
Saint Patrick Hospital	Missoula	96%	154
Saint James Healthcare	Butte	95%	65
Marcus Daly Memorial Hospital	Hamilton	93%	41
Saint Peter's Hospital	Helena	86%	78
Community Medical Center	Missoula	84%	38

Evaluation of LVS Function

Hospital Name	City	Rate	Cases
Billings Clinic Hospital	Billings	100%	246
Bozeman Deaconess Hospital	Bozeman	100%	84
Community Medical Center	Missoula	100%	59
Kalispell Regional Medical Center	Kalispell	100%	149
Marcus Daly Memorial Hospital	Hamilton	100%	53
Saint Patrick Hospital	Missoula	100%	177
Saint Peter's Hospital	Helena	100%	86
Saint Vincent Healthcare	Billings	100%	241
Saint James Healthcare	Butte	99%	87
Benefis Hospitals	Great Falls	98%	220
VA Montana Healthcare System	Fort Harrison	98%	43
Livingston Healthcare	Livingston	97%	34
Central Montana Medical Center	Lewistown	80%	30

NOTE: Hospital profiles are in alphabetical order by state, then city, then hospital within the city; Rankings exclude hospitals with less than 25 cases except for patient surveys which excludes hospitals with less than 100 cases; (a) 100-299 cases; (1) The number of cases/patients is too few to report; (2) Data submitted were based on a sample of cases/patients; (3) Results are based on a shorter time period than required; (4) Data suppressed by CMS for one or more quarters; (5) Results are not available for this reporting period; (6) Fewer than 100 patients completed the HCAHPS survey; (7) No cases met the criteria for this measure; (8) The lower limit of the confidence interval cannot be calculated if the number of observed infections equals zero; (9) No data are available from the state/territory for this reporting period; (10) The scores shown reflect fewer than 50 completed surveys; (11) There were discrepancies in the data collection process; (12) This measure does not apply to this hospital for this reporting period; (13) Results cannot be calculated for this reporting period; (14) The results for this state are combined with nearby states to protect confidentiality; Please refer to the User's Guide for a full explanation of data.

Medicare Spending

Medicare Spending per Patient (ratio)

Hospital Name	City	Ratio	Cases
PHS Indian Hosp at Browning-Blackfeet	Browning	0.72	-
Northern Montana Hospital	Havre	0.80	-
Great Falls Clinic Medical Center	Great Falls	0.85	-
Saint Peter's Hospital	Helena	0.85	-
Health Center Northwest	Kalispell	0.88	-
Billings Clinic Hospital	Billings	0.90	-
Community Medical Center	Missoula	0.90	-
Saint Patrick Hospital	Missoula	0.90	-
Bozeman Deaconess Hospital	Bozeman	0.92	-
Saint Vincent Healthcare	Billings	0.93	-
Kalispell Regional Medical Center	Kalispell	0.94	-
Benefis Hospitals	Great Falls	0.96	-
Saint James Healthcare	Butte	1.01	-

Pneumonia Care

Appropriate Initial Antibiotic Given

Hospital Name	City	Rate	Cases
Billings Clinic Hospital	Billings	100%	151
North Valley Hospital	Whitefish	100%	25
Benefis Hospitals	Great Falls	99%	151
Kalispell Regional Medical Center	Kalispell	99%	94
Saint Peter's Hospital	Helena	99%	73
Saint Vincent Healthcare	Billings	99%	195
Community Medical Center	Missoula	98%	41
Central Montana Medical Center	Lewistown	97%	32
Saint Patrick Hospital	Missoula	97%	119
VA Montana Healthcare System	Fort Harrison	97%	33
Marcus Daly Memorial Hospital[2]	Hamilton	95%	41
Northern Montana Hospital[2]	Havre	95%	42
Saint Luke Community Hospital[2]	Ronan	94%	47
Frances Mahon Deaconess Hospital	Glasgow	93%	28
Holy Rosary Healthcare	Miles City	93%	41
Livingston Healthcare	Livingston	93%	27
Saint James Healthcare	Butte	92%	66
Bozeman Deaconess Hospital	Bozeman	91%	66

Blood Culture Timing

Hospital Name	City	Rate	Cases
Central Montana Medical Center	Lewistown	100%	33
Community Medical Center	Missoula	100%	53
Holy Rosary Healthcare	Miles City	100%	67
Marcus Daly Memorial Hospital[2]	Hamilton	100%	58
Northern Montana Hospital[2]	Havre	100%	43
Saint Luke Community Hospital[2]	Ronan	100%	49
VA Montana Healthcare System	Fort Harrison	100%	41
Billings Clinic Hospital	Billings	99%	281
Saint Vincent Healthcare	Billings	99%	335
Benefis Hospitals	Great Falls	98%	229
Kalispell Regional Medical Center	Kalispell	97%	175
North Valley Hospital	Whitefish	97%	33
Saint Patrick Hospital	Missoula	97%	187
Cabinet Peaks Medical Center	Libby	96%	25
Bozeman Deaconess Hospital	Bozeman	94%	98
Saint James Healthcare	Butte	94%	101
Saint Peter's Hospital	Helena	94%	137
PHS Indian Hosp at Browning-Blackfeet	Browning	92%	25

Pregnancy and Delivery Care

Newborns whose Deliveries were Scheduled Early

Hospital Name	City	Rate	Cases
Billings Clinic Hospital	Billings	3%	119
Benefis Hospitals[2]	Great Falls	4%	27
Saint Peter's Hospital	Helena	6%	83
Saint Vincent Healthcare[2]	Billings	6%	35
Kalispell Regional Medical Center	Kalispell	8%	36
Bozeman Deaconess Hospital[2]	Bozeman	15%	34
Northern Montana Hospital	Havre	19%	52

Preventive Care

Immunization for Influenza

Hospital Name	City	Rate	Cases
Barrett Memorial Hospital[3]	Dillon	100%	42
Billings Clinic Hospital[2]	Billings	95%	559
Saint Luke Community Hospital[2]	Ronan	94%	50
Benefis Hospitals[2]	Great Falls	93%	535
Saint Peter's Hospital[2]	Helena	93%	534
Bozeman Deaconess Hospital[2]	Bozeman	92%	525
Kalispell Regional Medical Center[2]	Kalispell	92%	576
Community Medical Center[2]	Missoula	91%	457
Rosebud Health Care Center	Forsyth	90%	70
Saint Patrick Hospital[2]	Missoula	89%	616
Sidney Health Center[2]	Sidney	89%	245
Saint Vincent Healthcare[2]	Billings	88%	543
Saint James Healthcare[2]	Butte	87%	357
PHS Indian Hosp at Browning-Blackfeet	Browning	85%	271
Central Montana Medical Center[2]	Lewistown	81%	213
Northern Montana Hospital[2]	Havre	79%	275
Great Falls Clinic Medical Center	Great Falls	76%	290
Holy Rosary Healthcare[2]	Miles City	68%	225
Providence Saint Joseph Medical Center[2]	Polson	65%	240
Health Center Northwest[2]	Kalispell	58%	293
Roundup Memorial Healthcare	Roundup	48%	27

Immunization for Pneumonia

Hospital Name	City	Rate	Cases
Rosebud Health Care Center	Forsyth	98%	92
Barrett Memorial Hospital[2,3]	Dillon	97%	146
Billings Clinic Hospital[2]	Billings	97%	640
Bozeman Deaconess Hospital[2]	Bozeman	97%	495
Kalispell Regional Medical Center[2]	Kalispell	96%	693
PHS Indian Hosp at Browning-Blackfeet	Browning	96%	170
Saint Luke Community Hospital[2]	Ronan	96%	73
Sidney Health Center[2]	Sidney	94%	283
Clark Fork Valley Hospital[2]	Plains	93%	44
Community Medical Center[2]	Missoula	93%	369
Saint Vincent Healthcare[2]	Billings	93%	633
Saint Peter's Hospital[2]	Helena	90%	576
Benefis Hospitals[2]	Great Falls	89%	613
Great Falls Clinic Medical Center	Great Falls	88%	335
Central Montana Medical Center[2]	Lewistown	87%	400
Saint James Healthcare[2]	Butte	86%	454
Saint Patrick Hospital[2]	Missoula	84%	831
PHS Indian Hosp Crow/Northern Cheyenne[3]	Crow Agency	80%	30
Holy Rosary Healthcare[2]	Miles City	79%	228
Northern Montana Hospital[2]	Havre	75%	298
Providence Saint Joseph Medical Center[2]	Polson	74%	249
Health Center Northwest[2]	Kalispell	72%	293
Roundup Memorial Healthcare	Roundup	56%	36
Northern Rockies Medical Center[6]	Cut Bank	51%	37

Stroke Care

Antithrombotic Therapy Timing

Hospital Name	City	Rate	Cases
Billings Clinic Hospital	Billings	100%	112
Bozeman Deaconess Hospital	Bozeman	100%	37
Kalispell Regional Medical Center	Kalispell	100%	56
Saint Patrick Hospital[2]	Missoula	100%	58
Saint Vincent Healthcare	Billings	100%	88
Benefis Hospitals[2]	Great Falls	98%	58
Saint Peter's Hospital	Helena	98%	59
Saint James Healthcare	Butte	96%	25

Assessed for Rehabilitation

Hospital Name	City	Rate	Cases
Billings Clinic Hospital	Billings	100%	157
Kalispell Regional Medical Center	Kalispell	100%	89
Saint Peter's Hospital	Helena	100%	63
Saint Vincent Healthcare	Billings	100%	120
Saint Patrick Hospital[2]	Missoula	99%	88
Bozeman Deaconess Hospital	Bozeman	98%	48
Saint James Healthcare	Butte	97%	30
Benefis Hospitals[2]	Great Falls	95%	77

Discharged on Antithrombotic Therapy

Hospital Name	City	Rate	Cases
Billings Clinic Hospital	Billings	100%	118
Bozeman Deaconess Hospital	Bozeman	100%	45
Kalispell Regional Medical Center	Kalispell	100%	81
Saint James Healthcare	Butte	100%	28
Saint Patrick Hospital[2]	Missoula	100%	74
Saint Peter's Hospital	Helena	100%	60
Saint Vincent Healthcare	Billings	100%	102
Benefis Hospitals[2]	Great Falls	98%	66

Discharged on Statin Medication

Hospital Name	City	Rate	Cases
Saint Vincent Healthcare	Billings	100%	76
Saint Patrick Hospital[2]	Missoula	98%	52
Benefis Hospitals[2]	Great Falls	96%	54
Billings Clinic Hospital	Billings	96%	93
Kalispell Regional Medical Center	Kalispell	94%	63
Saint Peter's Hospital	Helena	94%	49
Bozeman Deaconess Hospital	Bozeman	86%	35
Saint James Healthcare	Butte	81%	26

Venous Thromboembolism (VTE) Prophylaxis

Hospital Name	City	Rate	Cases
Benefis Hospitals[2]	Great Falls	100%	81
Kalispell Regional Medical Center	Kalispell	100%	76
Saint Vincent Healthcare	Billings	100%	119
Billings Clinic Hospital	Billings	95%	158
Saint James Healthcare	Butte	93%	27
Saint Patrick Hospital[2]	Missoula	93%	86
Saint Peter's Hospital	Helena	92%	63
Bozeman Deaconess Hospital	Bozeman	89%	38

Written Stroke Educational Materials Given

Hospital Name	City	Rate	Cases
Kalispell Regional Medical Center	Kalispell	98%	47
Saint Vincent Healthcare	Billings	97%	69
Billings Clinic Hospital	Billings	93%	109
Benefis Hospitals[2]	Great Falls	88%	40
Saint Patrick Hospital[2]	Missoula	86%	56
Bozeman Deaconess Hospital	Bozeman	58%	33
Saint Peter's Hospital	Helena	56%	36

Surgical Care Improvement Project

Appropriate Beta Blocker Usage

Hospital Name	City	Rate	Cases
Billings Clinic Hospital	Billings	100%	509
Saint Patrick Hospital[2]	Missoula	100%	159
Saint Vincent Healthcare[2]	Billings	100%	483
Community Medical Center[2]	Missoula	99%	81
Kalispell Regional Medical Center[2]	Kalispell	99%	167
Bozeman Deaconess Hospital[2]	Bozeman	98%	66
Benefis Hospitals[2]	Great Falls	97%	215
Saint Peter's Hospital[2]	Helena	97%	97
Health Center Northwest	Kalispell	96%	50
Saint James Healthcare	Butte	96%	47
VA Montana Healthcare System[2]	Fort Harrison	96%	26
Great Falls Clinic Medical Center	Great Falls	94%	83
North Valley Hospital	Whitefish	94%	49

Appropriate VTP Within 24 Hours

Hospital Name	City	Rate	Cases
Barrett Memorial Hospital	Dillon	100%	38
Billings Clinic Hospital	Billings	100%	1321
Bozeman Deaconess Hospital[2]	Bozeman	100%	341
Holy Rosary Healthcare	Miles City	100%	106
Saint Vincent Healthcare[2]	Billings	100%	979
Sidney Health Center[2]	Sidney	100%	73
Community Hospital of Anaconda	Anaconda	99%	79
Frances Mahon Deaconess Hospital[2]	Glasgow	99%	78
Great Falls Clinic Medical Center	Great Falls	99%	265
Health Center Northwest	Kalispell	99%	206
Saint James Healthcare	Butte	99%	217
Saint Peter's Hospital[2]	Helena	99%	361
Marcus Daly Memorial Hospital	Hamilton	98%	54
Saint Patrick Hospital[2]	Missoula	97%	278
Community Medical Center[2]	Missoula	96%	347
Kalispell Regional Medical Center[2]	Kalispell	96%	606
Livingston Healthcare	Livingston	96%	46
North Valley Hospital	Whitefish	96%	219
Benefis Hospitals[2]	Great Falls	95%	394
VA Montana Healthcare System[2]	Fort Harrison	94%	97
Northern Montana Hospital	Havre	92%	48

Controlled Postoperative Blood Glucose

Hospital Name	City	Rate	Cases
Saint Vincent Healthcare[2]	Billings	99%	219
Saint Patrick Hospital[2]	Missoula	97%	150
Billings Clinic Hospital	Billings	96%	223
Benefis Hospitals[2]	Great Falls	94%	116
Kalispell Regional Medical Center[2]	Kalispell	89%	88

Perioperative Temperature Management

Hospital Name	City	Rate	Cases
Barrett Memorial Hospital	Dillon	100%	52
Benefis Hospitals[2]	Great Falls	100%	486
Billings Clinic Hospital	Billings	100%	1549
Bozeman Deaconess Hospital[2]	Bozeman	100%	390
Cabinet Peaks Medical Center[2,3]	Libby	100%	26
Community Hospital of Anaconda	Anaconda	100%	87
Community Medical Center[2]	Missoula	100%	400
Frances Mahon Deaconess Hospital[2]	Glasgow	100%	81
Great Falls Clinic Medical Center	Great Falls	100%	297
Health Center Northwest	Kalispell	100%	232
Holy Rosary Healthcare	Miles City	100%	117
Kalispell Regional Medical Center[2]	Kalispell	100%	743
Livingston Healthcare	Livingston	100%	49
Marcus Daly Memorial Hospital	Hamilton	100%	63
North Valley Hospital	Whitefish	100%	267
Northern Montana Hospital	Havre	100%	67
Providence Saint Joseph Medical Center	Polson	100%	30
Saint James Healthcare	Butte	100%	239

NOTE: Hospital profiles are in alphabetical order by state, then city, then hospital within the city; Rankings exclude hospitals with less than 25 cases except for patient surveys which excludes hospitals with less than 100 cases; (a) 100-299 cases; (1) The number of cases/patients is too few to report; (2) Data submitted were based on a sample of cases/patients; (3) Results are based on a shorter time period than required; (4) Data suppressed by CMS for one or more quarters; (5) Results are not available for this reporting period; (6) Fewer than 100 patients completed the HCAHPS survey; (7) No cases met the criteria for this measure; (8) The lower limit of the confidence interval cannot be calculated if the number of observed infections equals zero; (9) No data are available from the state/territory for this reporting period; (10) The scores shown reflect fewer than 50 completed surveys; (11) There were discrepancies in the data collection process; (12) This measure does not apply to this hospital for this reporting period; (13) Results cannot be calculated for this reporting period; (14) The results for this state are combined with nearby states to protect confidentiality; Please refer to the User's Guide for a full explanation of data.

Hospital Name	City	Rate	Cases
Saint Patrick Hospital[2]	Missoula	100%	322
Saint Peter's Hospital[2]	Helena	100%	402
Saint Vincent Healthcare[2]	Billings	100%	1230
Sidney Health Center[2]	Sidney	100%	80
VA Montana Healthcare System[2]	Fort Harrison	100%	107

Prophylactic Antibiotic Selection

Hospital Name	City	Rate	Cases
Bozeman Deaconess Hospital[2]	Bozeman	100%	273
Community Hospital of Anaconda	Anaconda	100%	64
Great Falls Clinic Medical Center	Great Falls	100%	254
Health Center Northwest	Kalispell	100%	208
Holy Rosary Healthcare	Miles City	100%	90
Kalispell Regional Medical Center[2]	Kalispell	100%	571
North Valley Hospital	Whitefish	100%	203
Saint Peter's Hospital[2]	Helena	100%	278
Saint Vincent Healthcare[2]	Billings	100%	1202
Sidney Health Center[2]	Sidney	100%	67
VA Montana Healthcare System	Fort Harrison	100%	74
Benefis Hospitals[2]	Great Falls	99%	404
Billings Clinic Hospital	Billings	99%	1106
Community Medical Center[2]	Missoula	99%	274
Saint James Healthcare	Butte	99%	138
Saint Patrick Hospital[2]	Missoula	99%	331
Barrett Memorial Hospital	Dillon	98%	49
Frances Mahon Deaconess Hospital[2]	Glasgow	98%	81
Livingston Healthcare	Livingston	98%	46
Marcus Daly Memorial Hospital	Hamilton	97%	35
Northern Montana Hospital	Havre	96%	55

Prophylactic Antibiotic Selection (Outpatient)

Hospital Name	City	Rate	Cases
Saint James Healthcare	Butte	100%	161
Benefis Hospitals	Great Falls	99%	472
Bozeman Deaconess Hospital	Bozeman	99%	344
Community Medical Center	Missoula	99%	267
Health Center Northwest	Kalispell	99%	267
Saint Vincent Healthcare	Billings	99%	739
Billings Clinic Hospital	Billings	98%	808
Kalispell Regional Medical Center	Kalispell	98%	300
Great Falls Clinic Medical Center	Great Falls	97%	38
North Valley Hospital	Whitefish	95%	38
Saint Patrick Hospital	Missoula	93%	397
Saint Peter's Hospital	Helena	92%	237

Prophylactic Antibiotic Stopped

Hospital Name	City	Rate	Cases
Barrett Memorial Hospital	Dillon	100%	49
Billings Clinic Hospital	Billings	100%	1103
Bozeman Deaconess Hospital[2]	Bozeman	100%	268
Community Hospital of Anaconda	Anaconda	100%	64
Frances Mahon Deaconess Hospital[2]	Glasgow	100%	81
Kalispell Regional Medical Center[2]	Kalispell	100%	564
Saint James Healthcare	Butte	100%	130
Sidney Health Center[2]	Sidney	100%	66
Health Center Northwest	Kalispell	99%	208
Holy Rosary Healthcare	Miles City	99%	88
Saint Vincent Healthcare[2]	Billings	99%	1183
Benefis Hospitals[2]	Great Falls	98%	383
Community Medical Center[2]	Missoula	98%	270
Great Falls Clinic Medical Center	Great Falls	98%	252
Livingston Healthcare	Livingston	98%	46
North Valley Hospital	Whitefish	98%	198
Saint Patrick Hospital[2]	Missoula	98%	324
Marcus Daly Memorial Hospital	Hamilton	97%	30
Saint Peter's Hospital[2]	Helena	97%	274
VA Montana Healthcare System	Fort Harrison	97%	73
Northern Montana Hospital	Havre	96%	53

Prophylactic Antibiotic Timing

Hospital Name	City	Rate	Cases
Benefis Hospitals[2]	Great Falls	100%	406
Billings Clinic Hospital	Billings	100%	1109
Community Hospital of Anaconda	Anaconda	100%	65
Community Medical Center[2]	Missoula	100%	274
Health Center Northwest	Kalispell	100%	208
Holy Rosary Healthcare	Miles City	100%	91
Kalispell Regional Medical Center[2]	Kalispell	100%	574
Marcus Daly Memorial Hospital	Hamilton	100%	35
Saint Vincent Healthcare[2]	Billings	100%	1204
Bozeman Deaconess Hospital[2]	Bozeman	99%	273
Frances Mahon Deaconess Hospital[2]	Glasgow	99%	81
Saint James Healthcare	Butte	99%	138
Sidney Health Center[2]	Sidney	99%	67
Great Falls Clinic Medical Center	Great Falls	98%	254
Livingston Healthcare	Livingston	98%	46
Northern Montana Hospital	Havre	98%	55
Saint Peter's Hospital[2]	Helena	98%	278
Saint Patrick Hospital[2]	Missoula	96%	331
North Valley Hospital	Whitefish	95%	203
VA Montana Healthcare System	Fort Harrison	95%	74
Barrett Memorial Hospital	Dillon	92%	49

Prophylactic Antibiotic Timing (Outpatient)

Hospital Name	City	Rate	Cases
Community Medical Center	Missoula	100%	267
Saint Vincent Healthcare	Billings	100%	740
Benefis Hospitals	Great Falls	99%	471
Health Center Northwest	Kalispell	99%	207
Kalispell Regional Medical Center	Kalispell	99%	301
Bozeman Deaconess Hospital	Bozeman	98%	169
Billings Clinic Hospital	Billings	97%	531
Great Falls Clinic Medical Center	Great Falls	97%	38
Saint Patrick Hospital	Missoula	97%	404
Saint James Healthcare	Butte	93%	164
North Valley Hospital	Whitefish	92%	38
Saint Peter's Hospital	Helena	91%	211

Urinary Catheter Removal

Hospital Name	City	Rate	Cases
Billings Clinic Hospital	Billings	100%	1137
Community Hospital of Anaconda	Anaconda	100%	62
Frances Mahon Deaconess Hospital[2]	Glasgow	100%	41
Health Center Northwest	Kalispell	100%	63
Saint Vincent Healthcare[2]	Billings	100%	866
Sidney Health Center[2]	Sidney	100%	67
Holy Rosary Healthcare	Miles City	99%	86
Kalispell Regional Medical Center[2]	Kalispell	99%	525
Great Falls Clinic Medical Center	Great Falls	98%	257
North Valley Hospital	Whitefish	98%	123
Barrett Memorial Hospital	Dillon	97%	34
Benefis Hospitals[2]	Great Falls	97%	448
Northern Montana Hospital	Havre	97%	37
Saint Patrick Hospital[2]	Missoula	97%	244
Saint Peter's Hospital[2]	Helena	97%	107
Bozeman Deaconess Hospital[2]	Bozeman	96%	253
Saint James Healthcare	Butte	96%	73
VA Montana Healthcare System[2]	Fort Harrison	94%	47
Community Medical Center[2]	Missoula	93%	43

Survey of Patients' Hospital Experiences

Area Around Room 'Always' Quiet at Night

Hospital Name	City	Rate	Cases
Barrett Memorial Hospital	Dillon	81%	(a)
Great Falls Clinic Medical Center	Great Falls	78%	(a)
North Valley Hospital	Whitefish	66%	300+
Central Montana Medical Center	Lewistown	65%	(a)
Health Center Northwest	Kalispell	65%	(a)
Frances Mahon Deaconess Hospital	Glasgow	64%	(a)
Northern Montana Hospital	Havre	63%	(a)
Saint Luke Community Hospital	Ronan	60%	(a)
Sidney Health Center	Sidney	60%	(a)
Community Medical Center	Missoula	59%	300+
Marcus Daly Memorial Hospital	Hamilton	59%	(a)
Holy Rosary Healthcare	Miles City	58%	(a)
Saint Patrick Hospital	Missoula	58%	300+
Saint Peter's Hospital	Helena	58%	300+
Cabinet Peaks Medical Center	Libby	57%	(a)
Saint Vincent Healthcare	Billings	57%	300+
Benefis Hospitals	Great Falls	56%	300+
Billings Clinic Hospital	Billings	54%	300+
Providence Saint Joseph Medical Center	Polson	54%	(a)
Saint James Healthcare	Butte	54%	300+
Bozeman Deaconess Hospital	Bozeman	52%	300+
Community Hospital of Anaconda	Anaconda	52%	(a)
Livingston Healthcare	Livingston	52%	(a)
Kalispell Regional Medical Center	Kalispell	46%	300+

Doctors 'Always' Communicated Well

Hospital Name	City	Rate	Cases
Barrett Memorial Hospital	Dillon	89%	(a)
Great Falls Clinic Medical Center	Great Falls	88%	(a)
Community Hospital of Anaconda	Anaconda	86%	(a)
Central Montana Medical Center	Lewistown	85%	(a)
Health Center Northwest	Kalispell	85%	(a)
Livingston Healthcare	Livingston	85%	(a)
Frances Mahon Deaconess Hospital	Glasgow	84%	(a)
Saint Peter's Hospital	Helena	84%	300+
Cabinet Peaks Medical Center	Libby	83%	(a)
Providence Saint Joseph Medical Center	Polson	83%	(a)
Marcus Daly Memorial Hospital	Hamilton	82%	(a)
North Valley Hospital	Whitefish	82%	300+
Community Medical Center	Missoula	81%	300+
Saint Patrick Hospital	Missoula	81%	300+
Saint Vincent Healthcare	Billings	81%	300+
Billings Clinic Hospital	Billings	80%	300+
Bozeman Deaconess Hospital	Bozeman	80%	300+
Saint James Healthcare	Butte	80%	300+
Saint Luke Community Hospital	Ronan	79%	(a)
Holy Rosary Healthcare	Miles City	78%	(a)
Kalispell Regional Medical Center	Kalispell	77%	300+
Northern Montana Hospital	Havre	77%	(a)
Sidney Health Center	Sidney	77%	(a)
Benefis Hospitals	Great Falls	74%	300+

Home Recovery Information Given

Hospital Name	City	Rate	Cases
Barrett Memorial Hospital	Dillon	91%	(a)
Great Falls Clinic Medical Center	Great Falls	91%	(a)
Health Center Northwest	Kalispell	90%	(a)
North Valley Hospital	Whitefish	90%	300+
Saint Vincent Healthcare	Billings	89%	300+
Community Hospital of Anaconda	Anaconda	88%	(a)
Providence Saint Joseph Medical Center	Polson	88%	(a)
Billings Clinic Hospital	Billings	87%	300+
Community Medical Center	Missoula	87%	300+
Frances Mahon Deaconess Hospital	Glasgow	87%	(a)
Holy Rosary Healthcare	Miles City	87%	(a)
Saint Patrick Hospital	Missoula	87%	300+
Bozeman Deaconess Hospital	Bozeman	86%	300+
Kalispell Regional Medical Center	Kalispell	86%	300+
Saint James Healthcare	Butte	86%	300+
Saint Peter's Hospital	Helena	85%	300+
Central Montana Medical Center	Lewistown	83%	(a)
Livingston Healthcare	Livingston	83%	(a)
Sidney Health Center	Sidney	83%	(a)
Cabinet Peaks Medical Center	Libby	82%	(a)
Northern Montana Hospital	Havre	82%	(a)
Marcus Daly Memorial Hospital	Hamilton	81%	(a)
Benefis Hospitals	Great Falls	80%	300+
Saint Luke Community Hospital	Ronan	73%	(a)

Hospital Given 9 or 10 on 10 Point Scale

Hospital Name	City	Rate	Cases
Great Falls Clinic Medical Center	Great Falls	84%	(a)
North Valley Hospital	Whitefish	81%	300+
Barrett Memorial Hospital	Dillon	79%	(a)
Billings Clinic Hospital	Billings	79%	300+
Health Center Northwest	Kalispell	77%	(a)
Saint Patrick Hospital	Missoula	77%	300+
Community Medical Center	Missoula	75%	300+
Saint Vincent Healthcare	Billings	75%	300+
Bozeman Deaconess Hospital	Bozeman	71%	300+
Community Hospital of Anaconda	Anaconda	69%	(a)
Frances Mahon Deaconess Hospital	Glasgow	69%	(a)
Providence Saint Joseph Medical Center	Polson	69%	(a)
Holy Rosary Healthcare	Miles City	68%	(a)
Kalispell Regional Medical Center	Kalispell	68%	300+
Central Montana Medical Center	Lewistown	67%	(a)
Sidney Health Center	Sidney	67%	(a)
Saint James Healthcare	Butte	65%	300+
Cabinet Peaks Medical Center	Libby	64%	(a)
Livingston Healthcare	Livingston	64%	(a)
Saint Peter's Hospital	Helena	63%	300+
Benefis Hospitals	Great Falls	61%	300+
Marcus Daly Memorial Hospital	Hamilton	61%	(a)
Saint Luke Community Hospital	Ronan	57%	(a)
Northern Montana Hospital	Havre	51%	(a)

Meds 'Always' Explained Before Given

Hospital Name	City	Rate	Cases
Great Falls Clinic Medical Center	Great Falls	74%	(a)
Barrett Memorial Hospital	Dillon	72%	(a)
Frances Mahon Deaconess Hospital	Glasgow	71%	(a)
Community Hospital of Anaconda	Anaconda	69%	(a)
North Valley Hospital	Whitefish	68%	300+
Livingston Healthcare	Livingston	67%	(a)
Saint Patrick Hospital	Missoula	66%	300+
Health Center Northwest	Kalispell	65%	(a)
Central Montana Medical Center	Lewistown	64%	(a)
Holy Rosary Healthcare	Miles City	64%	(a)
Saint Peter's Hospital	Helena	64%	300+
Saint Vincent Healthcare	Billings	64%	300+
Billings Clinic Hospital	Billings	63%	300+
Saint Luke Community Hospital	Ronan	62%	(a)
Community Medical Center	Missoula	61%	300+
Marcus Daly Memorial Hospital	Hamilton	61%	(a)
Benefis Hospitals	Great Falls	60%	300+
Bozeman Deaconess Hospital	Bozeman	60%	300+
Cabinet Peaks Medical Center	Libby	60%	(a)
Providence Saint Joseph Medical Center	Polson	60%	(a)
Saint James Healthcare	Butte	59%	300+
Sidney Health Center	Sidney	59%	(a)
Kalispell Regional Medical Center	Kalispell	58%	300+
Northern Montana Hospital	Havre	58%	(a)

NOTE: Hospital profiles are in alphabetical order by state, then city, then hospital within the city; Rankings exclude hospitals with less than 25 cases except for patient surveys which excludes hospitals with less than 100 cases; (a) 100-299 cases; (1) The number of cases/patients is too few to report; (2) Data submitted were based on a sample of cases/patients; (3) Results are based on a shorter time period than required; (4) Data suppressed by CMS for one or more quarters; (5) Results are not available for this reporting period; (6) Fewer than 100 patients completed the HCAHPS survey; (7) No cases met the criteria for this measure; (8) The lower limit of the confidence interval cannot be calculated if the number of observed infections equals zero; (9) No data are available from the state/territory for this reporting period; (10) The scores shown reflect fewer than 50 completed surveys; (11) There were discrepancies in the data collection process; (12) This measure does not apply to this hospital for this reporting period; (13) Results cannot be calculated for this reporting period; (14) The results for this state are combined with nearby states to protect confidentiality; Please refer to the User's Guide for a full explanation of data.

Nurses 'Always' Communicated Well

Hospital Name	City	Rate	Cases
North Valley Hospital	Whitefish	83%	300+
Central Montana Medical Center	Lewistown	82%	(a)
Great Falls Clinic Medical Center	Great Falls	82%	(a)
Livingston Healthcare	Livingston	82%	(a)
Barrett Memorial Hospital	Dillon	81%	(a)
Frances Mahon Deaconess Hospital	Glasgow	81%	(a)
Health Center Northwest	Kalispell	81%	(a)
Holy Rosary Healthcare	Miles City	81%	(a)
Community Hospital of Anaconda	Anaconda	79%	(a)
Billings Clinic Hospital	Billings	78%	300+
Bozeman Deaconess Hospital	Bozeman	78%	300+
Marcus Daly Memorial Hospital	Hamilton	78%	(a)
Providence Saint Joseph Medical Center	Polson	78%	(a)
Saint Patrick Hospital	Missoula	78%	300+
Saint Peter's Hospital	Helena	78%	300+
Saint Vincent Healthcare	Billings	78%	300+
Community Medical Center	Missoula	77%	300+
Saint James Healthcare	Butte	76%	300+
Sidney Health Center	Sidney	76%	(a)
Kalispell Regional Medical Center	Kalispell	75%	300+
Northern Montana Hospital	Havre	74%	(a)
Cabinet Peaks Medical Center	Libby	73%	(a)
Benefis Hospitals	Great Falls	71%	300+
Saint Luke Community Hospital	Ronan	67%	(a)

Pain 'Always' Well Controlled

Hospital Name	City	Rate	Cases
North Valley Hospital	Whitefish	79%	300+
Great Falls Clinic Medical Center	Great Falls	78%	(a)
Holy Rosary Healthcare	Miles City	76%	(a)
Health Center Northwest	Kalispell	75%	(a)
Livingston Healthcare	Livingston	73%	(a)
Saint Peter's Hospital	Helena	73%	300+
Barrett Memorial Hospital	Dillon	72%	(a)
Providence Saint Joseph Medical Center	Polson	72%	(a)
Billings Clinic Hospital	Billings	71%	300+
Saint Patrick Hospital	Missoula	71%	300+
Sidney Health Center	Sidney	71%	(a)
Community Medical Center	Missoula	70%	300+
Saint James Healthcare	Butte	70%	300+
Benefis Hospitals	Great Falls	69%	300+
Bozeman Deaconess Hospital	Bozeman	69%	300+
Central Montana Medical Center	Lewistown	69%	(a)
Saint Luke Community Hospital	Ronan	69%	(a)
Saint Vincent Healthcare	Billings	69%	300+
Cabinet Peaks Medical Center	Libby	68%	(a)
Frances Mahon Deaconess Hospital	Glasgow	67%	(a)
Northern Montana Hospital	Havre	67%	(a)
Community Hospital of Anaconda	Anaconda	66%	(a)
Kalispell Regional Medical Center	Kalispell	66%	300+
Marcus Daly Memorial Hospital	Hamilton	65%	(a)

Room and Bathroom 'Always' Clean

Hospital Name	City	Rate	Cases
North Valley Hospital	Whitefish	82%	300+
Livingston Healthcare	Livingston	81%	(a)
Frances Mahon Deaconess Hospital	Glasgow	80%	(a)
Barrett Memorial Hospital	Dillon	79%	(a)
Great Falls Clinic Medical Center	Great Falls	79%	(a)
Marcus Daly Memorial Hospital	Hamilton	78%	(a)
Saint Peter's Hospital	Helena	77%	300+
Kalispell Regional Medical Center	Kalispell	75%	300+
Community Medical Center	Missoula	74%	300+
Saint Patrick Hospital	Missoula	74%	300+
Billings Clinic Hospital	Billings	73%	300+
Health Center Northwest	Kalispell	73%	(a)
Community Hospital of Anaconda	Anaconda	71%	(a)
Benefis Hospitals	Great Falls	70%	300+
Bozeman Deaconess Hospital	Bozeman	69%	300+
Providence Saint Joseph Medical Center	Polson	69%	(a)
Saint Vincent Healthcare	Billings	69%	300+
Cabinet Peaks Medical Center	Libby	68%	(a)
Holy Rosary Healthcare	Miles City	67%	(a)
Saint Luke Community Hospital	Ronan	67%	(a)
Saint James Healthcare	Butte	65%	300+
Northern Montana Hospital	Havre	64%	(a)
Sidney Health Center	Sidney	62%	(a)
Central Montana Medical Center	Lewistown	58%	(a)

Timely Help 'Always' Received

Hospital Name	City	Rate	Cases
Great Falls Clinic Medical Center	Great Falls	84%	(a)
Barrett Memorial Hospital	Dillon	82%	(a)
North Valley Hospital	Whitefish	78%	300+
Livingston Healthcare	Livingston	77%	(a)
Providence Saint Joseph Medical Center	Polson	77%	(a)
Frances Mahon Deaconess Hospital	Glasgow	73%	(a)
Health Center Northwest	Kalispell	73%	(a)
Central Montana Medical Center	Lewistown	71%	(a)
Community Hospital of Anaconda	Anaconda	70%	(a)
Billings Clinic Hospital	Billings	69%	300+
Cabinet Peaks Medical Center	Libby	69%	(a)
Northern Montana Hospital	Havre	69%	(a)
Sidney Health Center	Sidney	69%	(a)
Holy Rosary Healthcare	Miles City	68%	(a)
Saint Peter's Hospital	Helena	67%	300+
Saint Vincent Healthcare	Billings	67%	300+
Bozeman Deaconess Hospital	Bozeman	66%	300+
Marcus Daly Memorial Hospital	Hamilton	66%	(a)
Saint Patrick Hospital	Missoula	66%	300+
Saint James Healthcare	Butte	65%	300+
Community Medical Center	Missoula	64%	300+
Saint Luke Community Hospital	Ronan	64%	(a)
Kalispell Regional Medical Center	Kalispell	63%	300+
Benefis Hospitals	Great Falls	61%	300+

Would Definitely Recommend Hospital

Hospital Name	City	Rate	Cases
Great Falls Clinic Medical Center	Great Falls	87%	(a)
North Valley Hospital	Whitefish	83%	300+
Saint Patrick Hospital	Missoula	83%	300+
Billings Clinic Hospital	Billings	82%	300+
Health Center Northwest	Kalispell	82%	(a)
Saint Vincent Healthcare	Billings	80%	300+
Community Medical Center	Missoula	77%	300+
Frances Mahon Deaconess Hospital	Glasgow	76%	(a)
Barrett Memorial Hospital	Dillon	75%	(a)
Kalispell Regional Medical Center	Kalispell	75%	300+
Community Hospital of Anaconda	Anaconda	73%	(a)
Bozeman Deaconess Hospital	Bozeman	71%	300+
Providence Saint Joseph Medical Center	Polson	70%	(a)
Holy Rosary Healthcare	Miles City	69%	(a)
Central Montana Medical Center	Lewistown	66%	(a)
Livingston Healthcare	Livingston	63%	(a)
Saint Luke Community Hospital	Ronan	63%	(a)
Sidney Health Center	Sidney	63%	(a)
Marcus Daly Memorial Hospital	Hamilton	62%	(a)
Benefis Hospitals	Great Falls	61%	300+
Saint Peter's Hospital	Helena	61%	300+
Cabinet Peaks Medical Center	Libby	59%	(a)
Saint James Healthcare	Butte	57%	300+
Northern Montana Hospital	Havre	46%	(a)

Use of Medical Imaging

Cardiac Imaging Stress Test before OP Surgery

Hospital Name	City	Rate	Cases
Northern Montana Hospital	Havre	1.7%	58
Saint Vincent Healthcare	Billings	1.7%	60
Saint Patrick Hospital	Missoula	3.8%	788
Saint Peter's Hospital	Helena	3.9%	205
Saint James Healthcare	Butte	4.0%	99
Cabinet Peaks Medical Center	Libby	4.3%	46
Bozeman Deaconess Hospital	Bozeman	4.6%	499
Kalispell Regional Medical Center	Kalispell	4.8%	730
Frances Mahon Deaconess Hospital	Glasgow	4.9%	61
Benefis Hospitals	Great Falls	5.2%	556
Billings Clinic Hospital	Billings	5.9%	936
North Valley Hospital	Whitefish	7.8%	64
Community Medical Center	Missoula	8.3%	120

Combination Abdominal CT Scan

Hospital Name	City	Rate	Cases
Sidney Health Center	Sidney	0.5%	203
Kalispell Regional Medical Center	Kalispell	4.5%	243
Big Horn Co Memorial Hospital	Hardin	4.6%	65
Barrett Memorial Hospital	Dillon	5.0%	222
Billings Clinic Hospital	Billings	5.0%	1332
Benefis Hospitals	Great Falls	5.2%	899
Bozeman Deaconess Hospital	Bozeman	5.2%	446
Saint James Healthcare	Butte	5.5%	272
Saint Vincent Healthcare	Billings	5.6%	752
Providence Saint Joseph Medical Center	Polson	6.2%	145
Northern Montana Hospital	Havre	6.8%	162
Saint Peter's Hospital	Helena	8.2%	646
Saint Patrick Hospital	Missoula	8.5%	1003
Holy Rosary Healthcare	Miles City	9.9%	121
North Valley Hospital	Whitefish	12.9%	271
Community Medical Center	Missoula	15.2%	466
Cabinet Peaks Medical Center	Libby	15.8%	146
Health Center Northwest	Kalispell	18.7%	852
Central Montana Medical Center	Lewistown	38.2%	89
Saint Luke Community Hospital	Ronan	53.8%	160
Frances Mahon Deaconess Hospital	Glasgow	61.9%	105

Combination Brain/Sinus CT Scan

Hospital Name	City	Rate	Cases
Big Horn Co Memorial Hospital	Hardin	0.0%	81
Providence Saint Joseph Medical Center	Polson	0.0%	114
Roundup Memorial Healthcare	Roundup	0.0%	47
Community Medical Center	Missoula	0.4%	252
Saint Patrick Hospital	Missoula	0.8%	530
Bozeman Deaconess Hospital	Bozeman	1.3%	446
Billings Clinic Hospital	Billings	1.4%	721
Saint Vincent Healthcare	Billings	1.9%	623
Saint Peter's Hospital	Helena	2.2%	453

Combination Chest CT Scan

Hospital Name	City	Rate	Cases
Saint Patrick Hospital	Missoula	0.0%	720
Billings Clinic Hospital	Billings	0.2%	1035
Benefis Hospitals	Great Falls	0.4%	897
Community Medical Center	Missoula	0.4%	267
Saint Vincent Healthcare	Billings	0.5%	428
Barrett Memorial Hospital	Dillon	0.7%	150
Health Center Northwest	Kalispell	0.7%	744
Central Montana Medical Center	Lewistown	0.9%	111
Providence Saint Joseph Medical Center	Polson	1.2%	83
Sidney Health Center	Sidney	1.2%	168
Holy Rosary Healthcare	Miles City	1.4%	73
Saint James Healthcare	Butte	1.6%	125
North Valley Hospital	Whitefish	2.6%	117
Bozeman Deaconess Hospital	Bozeman	2.8%	212
Kalispell Regional Medical Center	Kalispell	3.2%	62
Saint Peter's Hospital	Helena	4.6%	461
Northern Montana Hospital	Havre	6.5%	77
Cabinet Peaks Medical Center	Libby	7.9%	203
Frances Mahon Deaconess Hospital	Glasgow	13.4%	67
Saint Luke Community Hospital	Ronan	44.6%	65

Follow-up Mammogram/Ultrasound

A follow-up rate near zero may indicate missed cancer; a rate higher than 14% may mean there is unnecessary follow up.

Hospital Name	City	Rate	Cases
Kalispell Regional Medical Center	Kalispell	3.7%	161
Billings Clinic Hospital	Billings	4.3%	2617
Central Montana Medical Center	Lewistown	4.7%	379
Saint Vincent Healthcare	Billings	4.9%	2182
Health Center Northwest	Kalispell	5.8%	1991
Big Horn Co Memorial Hospital	Hardin	6.0%	134
Cabinet Peaks Medical Center	Libby	6.3%	254
Providence Saint Joseph Medical Center	Polson	6.7%	298
Saint Patrick Hospital	Missoula	6.8%	2083
Northern Montana Hospital	Havre	7.0%	342
Holy Rosary Healthcare	Miles City	8.2%	170
Community Medical Center	Missoula	8.3%	1333
Barrett Memorial Hospital	Dillon	8.6%	339
Saint Peter's Hospital	Helena	8.6%	1546
Benefis Hospitals	Great Falls	8.8%	1291
North Valley Hospital	Whitefish	9.3%	473
Saint James Healthcare	Butte	10.9%	603
Frances Mahon Deaconess Hospital	Glasgow	13.7%	262
Saint Luke Community Hospital	Ronan	15.1%	212
Sidney Health Center	Sidney	17.2%	209

Lumbar Spine MRI for Low Back Pain

Hospital Name	City	Rate	Cases
Health Center Northwest	Kalispell	33.6%	268
Community Medical Center	Missoula	35.9%	156
Bozeman Deaconess Hospital	Bozeman	36.1%	72
Billings Clinic Hospital	Billings	37.7%	220
Saint Patrick Hospital	Missoula	37.7%	276
Benefis Hospitals	Great Falls	40.4%	146
Saint Peter's Hospital	Helena	40.6%	143
Holy Rosary Healthcare	Miles City	47.6%	42
Saint James Healthcare	Butte	48.1%	52
Saint Vincent Healthcare	Billings	50.3%	147
Frances Mahon Deaconess Hospital	Glasgow	61.0%	59

NOTE: Hospital profiles are in alphabetical order by state, then city, then hospital within the city; Rankings exclude hospitals with less than 25 cases except for patient surveys which excludes hospitals with less than 100 cases; (a) 100-299 cases; (1) The number of cases/patients is too few to report; (2) Data submitted were based on a sample of cases/patients; (3) Results are based on a shorter time period than required; (4) Data suppressed by CMS for one or more quarters; (5) Results are not available for this reporting period; (6) Fewer than 100 patients completed the HCAHPS survey; (7) No cases met the criteria for this measure; (8) The lower limit of the confidence interval cannot be calculated if the number of observed infections equals zero; (9) No data are available from the state/territory for this reporting period; (10) The scores shown reflect fewer than 50 completed surveys; (11) There were discrepancies in the data collection process; (12) This measure does not apply to this hospital for this reporting period; (13) Results cannot be calculated for this reporting period; (14) The results for this state are combined with nearby states to protect confidentiality; Please refer to the User's Guide for a full explanation of data.

Community Hospital of Anaconda

401 W Pennsylvania Phone: 406-563-8500
Anaconda, MT 59711 Fax: 406-563-8565
URL: www.communityhospitalofanaconda.org
Type: Critical Access Hospitals Emergency Services: Yes
Ownership: Voluntary non-profit - Private Beds: 40

Key Personnel:
Emergency Room . . . . Meg Bryan
Radiology. . . . . Jesse Cole
CEO . . . . Steve S McNeece
Operating Room. . . . . Patty Stanberry
Chief of Medical Staff . . . . Robyn Toles

Measure	Cases	This Hosp.	State Avg.	U.S. Avg.
Blood Clot Prevention and Treatment				
Anticoagulation Overlap Therapy[5]	-	-	97%	93%
ICU Venous Thromboembolism Prophylaxis[5]	-	-	92%	92%
Incidence of Potentially Preventable VTE[5]	-	-	4%	10%
UFH with Dosages/Platelet Monitoring[5]	-	-	97%	97%
Venous Thromboembolism Prophylaxis[5]	-	-	83%	85%
Warfarin Therapy Discharge Instructions[5]	-	-	84%	75%
Chest Pain/Possible Heart Attack Care				
Aspirin Given Within 24 Hours of Arrival	-	-	97%	96%
Fibrinolytic Meds Within 30 Min. of Arrival	-	-	43%	58%
Average Time to ECG (minutes)	-	-	10	7
Average Time to Transfer (minutes)	-	-	78	60
Children's Asthma Care				
Received Home Management Plan of Care	-	-	-	88%
Received Reliever Medication	-	-	-	100%
Received Systemic Corticosteroids	-	-	-	100%
Emergency Department				
Admittance Decision Time (minutes)[5]	-	-	72	98
Head CT Results Within 45 Min. of Arrival	-	-	26%	57%
Patients Who Left ER Before Being Seen	-	-	2%	2%
Time from ER Arrival to Admit. (minutes)[5]	-	-	220	274
Time from ER Arrival to Discharge (minutes)	-	-	120	134
Time in ER Before Being Evaluated (minutes)	-	-	23	26
Time to Pain Meds for Fractures (minutes)	-	-	47	57
Heart Attack Care				
Aspirin Given at Discharge[1]	-	-	100%	99%
Fibrinolytic Meds Within 30 Min. of Arrival[7]	-	-	50%	54%
PCI Within 90 Minutes of Arrival[7]	-	-	96%	96%
Statin Prescribed at Discharge[1]	-	-	99%	98%
Heart Failure Care				
ACE Inhibitor or ARB for LVSD[1]	-	-	97%	97%
Discharge Instructions Given[1]	-	-	92%	94%
Evaluation of LVS Function	11	100%	94%	99%
Medicare Spending				
Medicare Spending per Patient (ratio)	-	-	0.89	0.98
Pneumonia Care				
Appropriate Initial Antibiotic Given	16	100%	94%	95%
Blood Culture Timing	18	100%	97%	98%
Pregnancy and Delivery Care				
Newborn Deliveries Scheduled Early[5]	-	-	7%	6%
Preventive Care				
Immunization for Influenza[5]	-	-	86%	90%
Immunization for Pneumonia[5]	-	-	89%	92%
Stroke Care				
Anticoagulation Therapy for Atrial Fibrillation[5]	-	-	98%	95%
Antithrombotic Therapy Timing[5]	-	-	99%	98%
Assessed for Rehabilitation[5]	-	-	99%	97%
Discharged on Antithrombotic Therapy[5]	-	-	100%	99%
Discharged on Statin Medication[5]	-	-	94%	94%
Thrombolytic Therapy Timing[5]	-	-	67%	66%
Venous Thromboembolism Prophylaxis[5]	-	-	96%	94%
Written Stroke Educational Materials Given[5]	-	-	85%	88%
Surgical Care Improvement Project				
Appropriate Beta Blocker Usage	15	93%	98%	98%
Appropriate VTP Within 24 Hours	79	99%	98%	98%
Controlled Postoperative Blood Glucose[7]	-	-	96%	97%
Perioperative Temperature Management	87	100%	100%	100%
Prophylactic Antibiotic Selection	64	100%	99%	99%
Prophylactic Antibiotic Selection (Outpatient)	-	-	98%	98%
Prophylactic Antibiotic Stopped	64	100%	99%	98%
Prophylactic Antibiotic Timing	65	100%	99%	99%
Prophylactic Antibiotic Timing (Outpatient)	-	-	98%	98%
Urinary Catheter Removal	62	100%	99%	97%
Survey of Patients' Hospital Experiences				
Area Around Room 'Always' Quiet at Night	(a)	52%	60%	61%
Doctors 'Always' Communicated Well	(a)	86%	81%	82%
Home Recovery Information Given	(a)	88%	83%	85%
Hospital Given 9 or 10 on 10 Point Scale	(a)	69%	68%	71%
Meds 'Always' Explained Before Given	(a)	69%	63%	64%
Nurses 'Always' Communicated Well	(a)	79%	77%	79%
Pain 'Always' Well Controlled	(a)	66%	70%	71%
Room and Bathroom 'Always' Clean	(a)	71%	72%	73%
Timely Help 'Always' Received	(a)	70%	69%	68%
Would Definitely Recommend Hospital	(a)	73%	67%	71%
Use of Medical Imaging				
Cardiac Imaging Stress Test before Surgery	-	-	4.9%	5.3%
Combination Abdominal CT Scan	-	-	10.6%	10.5%
Combination Brain/Sinus CT Scan	-	-	1.9%	2.7%
Combination Chest CT Scan	-	-	2.4%	2.7%
Follow-up Mammogram/Ultrasound	-	-	6.9%	8.8%
Lumbar Spine MRI for Low Back Pain	-	-	41.5%	37.2%

Big Sandy Medical Center

166 Montana Ave E Phone: 406-378-2188
Big Sandy, MT 59520
Type: Critical Access Hospitals Emergency Services: Yes
Ownership: Govt - Hospital Dist/Auth

Measure	Cases	This Hosp.	State Avg.	U.S. Avg.
Blood Clot Prevention and Treatment				
Anticoagulation Overlap Therapy[3,7]	-	-	97%	93%
ICU Venous Thromboembolism Prophylaxis[3,7]	-	-	92%	92%
Incidence of Potentially Preventable VTE[3,7]	-	-	4%	10%
UFH with Dosages/Platelet Monitoring[3,7]	-	-	97%	97%
Venous Thromboembolism Prophylaxis[1,3]	-	-	83%	85%
Warfarin Therapy Discharge Instructions[3,7]	-	-	84%	75%
Chest Pain/Possible Heart Attack Care				
Aspirin Given Within 24 Hours of Arrival	-	-	97%	96%
Fibrinolytic Meds Within 30 Min. of Arrival	-	-	43%	58%
Average Time to ECG (minutes)	-	-	10	7
Average Time to Transfer (minutes)	-	-	78	60
Children's Asthma Care				
Received Home Management Plan of Care	-	-	-	88%
Received Reliever Medication	-	-	-	100%
Received Systemic Corticosteroids	-	-	-	100%
Emergency Department				
Admittance Decision Time (minutes)[5]	-	-	72	98
Head CT Results Within 45 Min. of Arrival	-	-	26%	57%
Patients Who Left ER Before Being Seen	-	-	2%	2%
Time from ER Arrival to Admit. (minutes)[5]	-	-	220	274
Time from ER Arrival to Discharge (minutes)	-	-	120	134
Time in ER Before Being Evaluated (minutes)	-	-	23	26
Time to Pain Meds for Fractures (minutes)	-	-	47	57
Heart Attack Care				
Aspirin Given at Discharge[5]	-	-	100%	99%
Fibrinolytic Meds Within 30 Min. of Arrival[5]	-	-	50%	54%
PCI Within 90 Minutes of Arrival[5]	-	-	96%	96%
Statin Prescribed at Discharge[5]	-	-	99%	98%
Heart Failure Care				
ACE Inhibitor or ARB for LVSD[5]	-	-	97%	97%
Discharge Instructions Given[5]	-	-	92%	94%
Evaluation of LVS Function[5]	-	-	94%	99%
Medicare Spending				
Medicare Spending per Patient (ratio)	-	-	0.89	0.98
Pneumonia Care				
Appropriate Initial Antibiotic Given[3,7]	-	-	94%	95%
Blood Culture Timing[3,7]	-	-	97%	98%
Pregnancy and Delivery Care				
Newborn Deliveries Scheduled Early[5]	-	-	7%	6%
Preventive Care				
Immunization for Influenza[5]	-	-	86%	90%
Immunization for Pneumonia[5]	-	-	89%	92%
Stroke Care				
Anticoagulation Therapy for Atrial Fibrillation[5]	-	-	98%	95%
Antithrombotic Therapy Timing[5]	-	-	99%	98%
Assessed for Rehabilitation[5]	-	-	99%	97%
Discharged on Antithrombotic Therapy[5]	-	-	100%	99%
Discharged on Statin Medication[5]	-	-	94%	94%
Thrombolytic Therapy Timing[5]	-	-	67%	66%
Venous Thromboembolism Prophylaxis[5]	-	-	96%	94%
Written Stroke Educational Materials Given[5]	-	-	85%	88%
Surgical Care Improvement Project				
Appropriate Beta Blocker Usage[5]	-	-	98%	98%
Appropriate VTP Within 24 Hours[5]	-	-	98%	98%
Controlled Postoperative Blood Glucose[5]	-	-	96%	97%
Perioperative Temperature Management[5]	-	-	100%	100%
Prophylactic Antibiotic Selection[5]	-	-	99%	99%
Prophylactic Antibiotic Selection (Outpatient)	-	-	98%	98%
Prophylactic Antibiotic Stopped[5]	-	-	99%	98%
Prophylactic Antibiotic Timing[5]	-	-	99%	99%
Prophylactic Antibiotic Timing (Outpatient)	-	-	98%	98%
Urinary Catheter Removal[5]	-	-	99%	97%
Survey of Patients' Hospital Experiences				
Area Around Room 'Always' Quiet at Night[6]	-	-	60%	61%
Doctors 'Always' Communicated Well[5]	-	-	81%	82%
Home Recovery Information Given[5]	-	-	83%	85%
Hospital Given 9 or 10 on 10 Point Scale[5]	-	-	68%	71%
Meds 'Always' Explained Before Given[5]	-	-	63%	64%
Nurses 'Always' Communicated Well[5]	-	-	77%	79%
Pain 'Always' Well Controlled[5]	-	-	70%	71%
Room and Bathroom 'Always' Clean[5]	-	-	72%	73%
Timely Help 'Always' Received[5]	-	-	69%	68%
Would Definitely Recommend Hospital[5]	-	-	67%	71%
Use of Medical Imaging				
Cardiac Imaging Stress Test before Surgery	-	-	4.9%	5.3%
Combination Abdominal CT Scan	-	-	10.6%	10.5%
Combination Brain/Sinus CT Scan	-	-	1.9%	2.7%
Combination Chest CT Scan	-	-	2.4%	2.7%
Follow-up Mammogram/Ultrasound	-	-	6.9%	8.8%
Lumbar Spine MRI for Low Back Pain	-	-	41.5%	37.2%

Pioneer Medical Center

301 W 7th Ave Phone: 406-932-4603
Big Timber, MT 59011
URL: www.billingsclinic.com
Type: Critical Access Hospitals Emergency Services: Yes
Ownership: Government - Local Beds: 60

Key Personnel:
Chairman/CEO . . . . J. Scott Millikan, MD, FACS
Chief of Medical Staff. . . . . Mark Rumans
CEO/President. . . . . Nicholas Wolter, MD

Measure	Cases	This Hosp.	State Avg.	U.S. Avg.
Blood Clot Prevention and Treatment				
Anticoagulation Overlap Therapy[5]	-	-	97%	93%
ICU Venous Thromboembolism Prophylaxis[5]	-	-	92%	92%
Incidence of Potentially Preventable VTE[5]	-	-	4%	10%
UFH with Dosages/Platelet Monitoring[5]	-	-	97%	97%
Venous Thromboembolism Prophylaxis[5]	-	-	83%	85%
Warfarin Therapy Discharge Instructions[5]	-	-	84%	75%
Chest Pain/Possible Heart Attack Care				
Aspirin Given Within 24 Hours of Arrival	-	-	97%	96%
Fibrinolytic Meds Within 30 Min. of Arrival	-	-	43%	58%
Average Time to ECG (minutes)	-	-	10	7
Average Time to Transfer (minutes)	-	-	78	60
Children's Asthma Care				
Received Home Management Plan of Care	-	-	-	88%
Received Reliever Medication	-	-	-	100%
Received Systemic Corticosteroids	-	-	-	100%
Emergency Department				
Admittance Decision Time (minutes)[5]	-	-	72	98
Head CT Results Within 45 Min. of Arrival	-	-	26%	57%
Patients Who Left ER Before Being Seen	-	-	2%	2%
Time from ER Arrival to Admit. (minutes)[5]	-	-	220	274
Time from ER Arrival to Discharge (minutes)	-	-	120	134
Time in ER Before Being Evaluated (minutes)	-	-	23	26
Time to Pain Meds for Fractures (minutes)	-	-	47	57

NOTE: Hospital profiles are in alphabetical order by state, then city, then hospital within the city; Rankings exclude hospitals with less than 25 cases except for patient surveys which excludes hospitals with less than 100 cases; (a) 100-299 cases; (1) The number of cases/patients is too few to report; (2) Data submitted were based on a sample of cases/patients; (3) Results are based on a shorter time period than required; (4) Data suppressed by CMS for one or more quarters; (5) Results are not available for this reporting period; (6) Fewer than 100 patients completed the HCAHPS survey; (7) No cases met the criteria for this measure; (8) The lower limit of the confidence interval cannot be calculated if the number of observed infections equals zero; (9) No data are available from the state/territory for this reporting period; (10) The scores shown reflect fewer than 50 completed surveys; (11) There were discrepancies in the data collection process; (12) This measure does not apply to this hospital for this reporting period; (13) Results cannot be calculated for this reporting period; (14) The results for this state are combined with nearby states to protect confidentiality; Please refer to the User's Guide for a full explanation of data.

Measure	Cases	This Hosp.	State Avg.	U.S. Avg.
Heart Attack Care				
Aspirin Given at Discharge[3,7]	-	-	100%	99%
Fibrinolytic Meds Within 30 Min. of Arrival[3,7]	-	-	50%	54%
PCI Within 90 Minutes of Arrival[3,7]	-	-	96%	96%
Statin Prescribed at Discharge[3,7]	-	-	99%	98%
Heart Failure Care				
ACE Inhibitor or ARB for LVSD[1,3]	-	-	97%	97%
Discharge Instructions Given[1,3]	-	-	92%	94%
Evaluation of LVS Function[1,3]	-	-	94%	99%
Medicare Spending				
Medicare Spending per Patient (ratio)	-	-	0.89	0.98
Pneumonia Care				
Appropriate Initial Antibiotic Given[1]	-	-	94%	95%
Blood Culture Timing[7]	-	-	97%	98%
Pregnancy and Delivery Care				
Newborn Deliveries Scheduled Early[5]	-	-	7%	6%
Preventive Care				
Immunization for Influenza[1]	-	-	86%	90%
Immunization for Pneumonia	14	86%	89%	92%
Stroke Care				
Anticoagulation Therapy for Atrial Fibrillation[5]	-	-	98%	95%
Antithrombotic Therapy Timing[5]	-	-	99%	98%
Assessed for Rehabilitation[5]	-	-	99%	97%
Discharged on Antithrombotic Therapy[5]	-	-	100%	99%
Discharged on Statin Medication[5]	-	-	94%	94%
Thrombolytic Therapy Timing[5]	-	-	67%	66%
Venous Thromboembolism Prophylaxis[5]	-	-	96%	94%
Written Stroke Educational Materials Given[5]	-	-	85%	88%
Surgical Care Improvement Project				
Appropriate Beta Blocker Usage[5]	-	-	98%	98%
Appropriate VTP Within 24 Hours[5]	-	-	98%	98%
Controlled Postoperative Blood Glucose[5]	-	-	96%	97%
Perioperative Temperature Management[5]	-	-	100%	100%
Prophylactic Antibiotic Selection[5]	-	-	99%	99%
Prophylactic Antibiotic Selection (Outpatient)	-	-	98%	98%
Prophylactic Antibiotic Stopped[5]	-	-	99%	98%
Prophylactic Antibiotic Timing[5]	-	-	99%	99%
Prophylactic Antibiotic Timing (Outpatient)	-	-	98%	98%
Urinary Catheter Removal[5]	-	-	99%	97%
Survey of Patients' Hospital Experiences				
Area Around Room 'Always' Quiet at Night[5]	-	-	60%	61%
Doctors 'Always' Communicated Well[5]	-	-	81%	82%
Home Recovery Information Given[5]	-	-	83%	85%
Hospital Given 9 or 10 on 10 Point Scale[5]	-	-	68%	71%
Meds 'Always' Explained Before Given[5]	-	-	63%	64%
Nurses 'Always' Communicated Well[5]	-	-	77%	79%
Pain 'Always' Well Controlled[5]	-	-	70%	71%
Room and Bathroom 'Always' Clean[5]	-	-	72%	73%
Timely Help 'Always' Received[5]	-	-	69%	68%
Would Definitely Recommend Hospital[5]	-	-	67%	71%
Use of Medical Imaging				
Cardiac Imaging Stress Test before Surgery	-	-	4.9%	5.3%
Combination Abdominal CT Scan	-	-	10.6%	10.5%
Combination Brain/Sinus CT Scan	-	-	1.9%	2.7%
Combination Chest CT Scan	-	-	2.4%	2.7%
Follow-up Mammogram/Ultrasound	-	-	6.9%	8.8%
Lumbar Spine MRI for Low Back Pain	-	-	41.5%	37.2%

Billings Clinic Hospital

2800 10th Ave N
Billings, MT 59101
URL: www.billingsclinic.com
Phone: 406-657-4000
Fax: 406-238-2355
Type: Acute Care Hospitals
Emergency Services: Yes
Ownership: Voluntary non-profit - Private
Beds: 285

Key Personnel:
Radiology. . . . . Douglas Bell
Chairman/CEO . . . . J. Scott Millikan, MD, FACS
Chief of Medical Staff. . . . . Mark C Rumans
CEO/President. . . . . Nicholas J Wolter, MD

Measure	Cases	This Hosp.	State Avg.	U.S. Avg.
Blood Clot Prevention and Treatment				
Anticoagulation Overlap Therapy[2]	89	99%	97%	93%
ICU Venous Thromboembolism Prophylaxis[2]	83	92%	92%	92%
Incidence of Potentially Preventable VTE[2]	16	0%	4%	10%
UFH with Dosages/Platelet Monitoring[2]	57	100%	97%	97%
Venous Thromboembolism Prophylaxis[2]	247	79%	83%	85%
Warfarin Therapy Discharge Instructions[2]	74	97%	84%	75%
Chest Pain/Possible Heart Attack Care				
Aspirin Given Within 24 Hours of Arrival[5]	-	-	97%	96%
Fibrinolytic Meds Within 30 Min. of Arrival[5]	-	-	43%	58%
Average Time to ECG (minutes)[5]	-	-	10	7
Average Time to Transfer (minutes)[5]	-	-	78	60
Children's Asthma Care				
Received Home Management Plan of Care	-	-	-	88%
Received Reliever Medication	-	-	-	100%
Received Systemic Corticosteroids	-	-	-	100%
Emergency Department				
Admittance Decision Time (minutes)[2]	453	156	72	98
Head CT Results Within 45 Min. of Arrival[1]	-	-	26%	57%
Patients Who Left ER Before Being Seen	40,808	1%	2%	2%
Time from ER Arrival to Admit. (minutes)[2]	460	290	220	274
Time from ER Arrival to Discharge (minutes)	367	126	120	134
Time in ER Before Being Evaluated (minutes)	383	15	23	26
Time to Pain Meds for Fractures (minutes)	162	56	47	57
Heart Attack Care				
Aspirin Given at Discharge	305	100%	100%	99%
Fibrinolytic Meds Within 30 Min. of Arrival[7]	-	-	50%	54%
PCI Within 90 Minutes of Arrival	51	100%	96%	96%
Statin Prescribed at Discharge	295	100%	99%	98%
Heart Failure Care				
ACE Inhibitor or ARB for LVSD	70	99%	97%	97%
Discharge Instructions Given	205	98%	92%	94%
Evaluation of LVS Function	246	100%	94%	99%
Medicare Spending				
Medicare Spending per Patient (ratio)	-	0.90	0.89	0.98
Pneumonia Care				
Appropriate Initial Antibiotic Given	151	100%	94%	95%
Blood Culture Timing	281	99%	97%	98%
Pregnancy and Delivery Care				
Newborn Deliveries Scheduled Early	119	3%	7%	6%
Preventive Care				
Immunization for Influenza[2]	559	95%	86%	90%
Immunization for Pneumonia[2]	640	97%	89%	92%
Stroke Care				
Anticoagulation Therapy for Atrial Fibrillation	13	100%	98%	95%
Antithrombotic Therapy Timing	112	100%	99%	98%
Assessed for Rehabilitation	157	100%	99%	97%
Discharged on Antithrombotic Therapy	118	100%	100%	99%
Discharged on Statin Medication	93	96%	94%	94%
Thrombolytic Therapy Timing[1]	-	-	67%	66%
Venous Thromboembolism Prophylaxis	158	95%	96%	94%
Written Stroke Educational Materials Given	109	93%	85%	88%
Surgical Care Improvement Project				
Appropriate Beta Blocker Usage	509	100%	98%	98%
Appropriate VTP Within 24 Hours	1,321	100%	98%	98%
Controlled Postoperative Blood Glucose	223	96%	96%	97%
Perioperative Temperature Management	1,549	100%	100%	100%
Prophylactic Antibiotic Selection	1,106	99%	99%	99%
Prophylactic Antibiotic Selection (Outpatient)	808	98%	98%	98%
Prophylactic Antibiotic Stopped	1,103	100%	99%	98%
Prophylactic Antibiotic Timing	1,109	100%	99%	99%
Prophylactic Antibiotic Timing (Outpatient)	531	97%	98%	98%
Urinary Catheter Removal	1,137	100%	99%	97%
Survey of Patients' Hospital Experiences				
Area Around Room 'Always' Quiet at Night	300+	54%	60%	61%
Doctors 'Always' Communicated Well	300+	80%	81%	82%
Home Recovery Information Given	300+	87%	83%	85%
Hospital Given 9 or 10 on 10 Point Scale	300+	79%	68%	71%
Meds 'Always' Explained Before Given	300+	63%	63%	64%
Nurses 'Always' Communicated Well	300+	78%	77%	79%
Pain 'Always' Well Controlled	300+	71%	70%	71%
Room and Bathroom 'Always' Clean	300+	73%	72%	73%
Timely Help 'Always' Received	300+	69%	69%	68%
Would Definitely Recommend Hospital	300+	82%	67%	71%
Use of Medical Imaging				
Cardiac Imaging Stress Test before Surgery	936	5.9%	4.9%	5.3%
Combination Abdominal CT Scan	1,332	5.0%	10.6%	10.5%
Combination Brain/Sinus CT Scan	721	1.4%	1.9%	2.7%
Combination Chest CT Scan	1,035	0.2%	2.4%	2.7%
Follow-up Mammogram/Ultrasound	2,617	4.3%	6.9%	8.8%
Lumbar Spine MRI for Low Back Pain	220	37.7%	41.5%	37.2%

Saint Vincent Healthcare

1233 N 30th St
Billings, MT 59107
Phone: 406-657-7000
Fax: 406-237-3078
E-mail: web-rn@svh-mt.org
URL: www.svh-mt.org
Type: Acute Care Hospitals
Emergency Services: Yes
Ownership: Voluntary non-profit - Church
Beds: 300

Key Personnel:
Operating Room. . . . . Bonnie Bickler
Chief of Medical Staff. . . . . Michael Bush, MD
Radiology. . . . . Mitchell Gallagher, MD
CEO/President. . . . . David Irion
Pediatric In-Patient Care . . . . Marian Kummer, MD
CEO . . . . Steve Loveless
Quality Assurance . . . . Irene McCall

Measure	Cases	This Hosp.	State Avg.	U.S. Avg.
Blood Clot Prevention and Treatment				
Anticoagulation Overlap Therapy[2]	54	98%	97%	93%
ICU Venous Thromboembolism Prophylaxis[2]	89	92%	92%	92%
Incidence of Potentially Preventable VTE[2]	11	9%	4%	10%
UFH with Dosages/Platelet Monitoring[1,2]	-	-	97%	97%
Venous Thromboembolism Prophylaxis[2]	322	88%	83%	85%
Warfarin Therapy Discharge Instructions[2]	41	98%	84%	75%
Chest Pain/Possible Heart Attack Care				
Aspirin Given Within 24 Hours of Arrival[1,3]	-	-	97%	96%
Fibrinolytic Meds Within 30 Min. of Arrival[5]	-	-	43%	58%
Average Time to ECG (minutes)[1,3]	-	-	10	7
Average Time to Transfer (minutes)[5]	-	-	78	60
Children's Asthma Care				
Received Home Management Plan of Care	-	-	-	88%
Received Reliever Medication	-	-	-	100%
Received Systemic Corticosteroids	-	-	-	100%
Emergency Department				
Admittance Decision Time (minutes)[2]	358	74	72	98
Head CT Results Within 45 Min. of Arrival[1]	-	-	26%	57%
Patients Who Left ER Before Being Seen	56,624	0%	2%	2%
Time from ER Arrival to Admit. (minutes)[2]	375	203	220	274
Time from ER Arrival to Discharge (minutes)	389	141	120	134
Time in ER Before Being Evaluated (minutes)	373	21	23	26
Time to Pain Meds for Fractures (minutes)	106	46	47	57
Heart Attack Care				
Aspirin Given at Discharge	249	100%	100%	99%
Fibrinolytic Meds Within 30 Min. of Arrival[7]	-	-	50%	54%
PCI Within 90 Minutes of Arrival	28	100%	96%	96%
Statin Prescribed at Discharge	234	100%	99%	98%
Heart Failure Care				
ACE Inhibitor or ARB for LVSD	65	100%	97%	97%
Discharge Instructions Given	188	97%	92%	94%
Evaluation of LVS Function	241	100%	94%	99%
Medicare Spending				
Medicare Spending per Patient (ratio)	-	0.93	0.89	0.98
Pneumonia Care				
Appropriate Initial Antibiotic Given	195	99%	94%	95%
Blood Culture Timing	335	99%	97%	98%
Pregnancy and Delivery Care				
Newborn Deliveries Scheduled Early[2]	35	6%	7%	6%
Preventive Care				
Immunization for Influenza[2]	543	88%	86%	90%
Immunization for Pneumonia[2]	633	93%	89%	92%
Stroke Care				
Anticoagulation Therapy for Atrial Fibrillation	13	100%	98%	95%
Antithrombotic Therapy Timing	88	100%	99%	98%
Assessed for Rehabilitation	120	100%	99%	97%
Discharged on Antithrombotic Therapy	102	100%	100%	99%
Discharged on Statin Medication	76	100%	94%	94%
Thrombolytic Therapy Timing[1]	-	-	67%	66%
Venous Thromboembolism Prophylaxis	119	100%	96%	94%

NOTE: Hospital profiles are in alphabetical order by state, then city, then hospital within the city; Rankings exclude hospitals with less than 25 cases except for patient surveys which excludes hospitals with less than 100 cases; (a) 100-299 cases; (1) The number of cases/patients is too few to report; (2) Data submitted were based on a sample of cases/patients; (3) Results are based on a shorter time period than required; (4) Data suppressed by CMS for one or more quarters; (5) Results are not available for this reporting period; (6) Fewer than 100 patients completed the HCAHPS survey; (7) No cases met the criteria for this measure; (8) The lower limit of the confidence interval cannot be calculated if the number of observed infections equals zero; (9) No data are available from the state/territory for this reporting period; (10) The scores shown reflect fewer than 50 completed surveys; (11) There were discrepancies in the data collection process; (12) This measure does not apply to this hospital for this reporting period; (13) Results cannot be calculated for this reporting period; (14) The results for this state are combined with nearby states to protect confidentiality; Please refer to the User's Guide for a full explanation of data.

Measure	Cases	This Hosp.	State Avg.	U.S. Avg.
Written Stroke Educational Materials Given	69	97%	85%	88%
Surgical Care Improvement Project				
Appropriate Beta Blocker Usage[2]	483	100%	98%	98%
Appropriate VTP Within 24 Hours[2]	979	100%	98%	98%
Controlled Postoperative Blood Glucose[2]	219	99%	96%	97%
Perioperative Temperature Management[2]	1,230	100%	100%	100%
Prophylactic Antibiotic Selection[2]	1,202	100%	99%	99%
Prophylactic Antibiotic Selection (Outpatient)	739	99%	98%	98%
Prophylactic Antibiotic Stopped[2]	1,183	99%	99%	98%
Prophylactic Antibiotic Timing[2]	1,204	100%	99%	99%
Prophylactic Antibiotic Timing (Outpatient)	740	100%	98%	98%
Urinary Catheter Removal[2]	866	100%	99%	97%
Survey of Patients' Hospital Experiences				
Area Around Room 'Always' Quiet at Night	300+	57%	60%	61%
Doctors 'Always' Communicated Well	300+	81%	81%	82%
Home Recovery Information Given	300+	89%	83%	85%
Hospital Given 9 or 10 on 10 Point Scale	300+	75%	68%	71%
Meds 'Always' Explained Before Given	300+	64%	63%	64%
Nurses 'Always' Communicated Well	300+	78%	77%	79%
Pain 'Always' Well Controlled	300+	69%	70%	71%
Room and Bathroom 'Always' Clean	300+	69%	72%	73%
Timely Help 'Always' Received	300+	67%	69%	68%
Would Definitely Recommend Hospital	300+	80%	67%	71%
Use of Medical Imaging				
Cardiac Imaging Stress Test before Surgery	60	1.7%	4.9%	5.3%
Combination Abdominal CT Scan	752	5.6%	10.6%	10.5%
Combination Brain/Sinus CT Scan	623	1.9%	1.9%	2.7%
Combination Chest CT Scan	428	0.5%	2.4%	2.7%
Follow-up Mammogram/Ultrasound	2,182	4.9%	6.9%	8.8%
Lumbar Spine MRI for Low Back Pain	147	50.3%	41.5%	37.2%

Bozeman Deaconess Hospital

915 Highland Blvd
Bozeman, MT 59715
Phone: 406-585-5000
Fax: 406-585-1071
Type: Acute Care Hospitals
Emergency Services: Yes
Ownership: Voluntary non-profit - Private
Beds: 86

Key Personnel:
Chief of Medical Staff.......... Stephen Ley, MD
CEO/President............... John Nordwick

Measure	Cases	This Hosp.	State Avg.	U.S. Avg.
Blood Clot Prevention and Treatment				
Anticoagulation Overlap Therapy[2]	65	100%	97%	93%
ICU Venous Thromboembolism Prophylaxis[2]	48	88%	92%	92%
Incidence of Potentially Preventable VTE[1,2]	-	-	4%	10%
UFH with Dosages/Platelet Monitoring[2]	17	100%	97%	97%
Venous Thromboembolism Prophylaxis[2]	257	91%	83%	85%
Warfarin Therapy Discharge Instructions[2]	54	93%	84%	75%
Chest Pain/Possible Heart Attack Care				
Aspirin Given Within 24 Hours of Arrival[1,3]	-	-	97%	96%
Fibrinolytic Meds Within 30 Min. of Arrival[3,7]	-	-	43%	58%
Average Time to ECG (minutes)[1,3]	-	-	10	7
Average Time to Transfer (minutes)[3,7]	-	-	78	60
Children's Asthma Care				
Received Home Management Plan of Care	-	-	-	88%
Received Reliever Medication	-	-	-	100%
Received Systemic Corticosteroids	-	-	-	100%
Emergency Department				
Admittance Decision Time (minutes)[2]	511	139	72	98
Head CT Results Within 45 Min. of Arrival[1]	-	-	26%	57%
Patients Who Left ER Before Being Seen	23,901	1%	2%	2%
Time from ER Arrival to Admit. (minutes)[2]	548	288	220	274
Time from ER Arrival to Discharge (minutes)	457	155	120	134
Time in ER Before Being Evaluated (minutes)	501	30	23	26
Time to Pain Meds for Fractures (minutes)	161	56	47	57
Heart Attack Care				
Aspirin Given at Discharge	84	100%	100%	99%
Fibrinolytic Meds Within 30 Min. of Arrival[7]	-	-	50%	54%
PCI Within 90 Minutes of Arrival	18	100%	96%	96%
Statin Prescribed at Discharge	80	100%	99%	98%
Heart Failure Care				
ACE Inhibitor or ARB for LVSD	15	100%	97%	97%
Discharge Instructions Given	64	97%	92%	94%
Evaluation of LVS Function	84	100%	94%	99%
Medicare Spending				
Medicare Spending per Patient (ratio)	-	0.92	0.89	0.98
Pneumonia Care				
Appropriate Initial Antibiotic Given	66	91%	94%	95%
Blood Culture Timing	98	94%	97%	98%
Pregnancy and Delivery Care				
Newborn Deliveries Scheduled Early[2]	34	15%	7%	6%
Preventive Care				
Immunization for Influenza[2]	525	92%	86%	90%
Immunization for Pneumonia[2]	495	97%	89%	92%
Stroke Care				
Anticoagulation Therapy for Atrial Fibrillation[1]	-	-	98%	95%
Antithrombotic Therapy Timing	37	100%	99%	98%
Assessed for Rehabilitation	48	98%	99%	97%
Discharged on Antithrombotic Therapy	45	100%	100%	99%
Discharged on Statin Medication	35	86%	94%	94%
Thrombolytic Therapy Timing[7]	-	-	67%	66%
Venous Thromboembolism Prophylaxis	38	89%	96%	94%
Written Stroke Educational Materials Given	33	58%	85%	88%
Surgical Care Improvement Project				
Appropriate Beta Blocker Usage[2]	66	98%	98%	98%
Appropriate VTP Within 24 Hours[2]	341	100%	98%	98%
Controlled Postoperative Blood Glucose[2,7]	-	-	96%	97%
Perioperative Temperature Management[2]	390	100%	100%	100%
Prophylactic Antibiotic Selection[2]	273	100%	99%	99%
Prophylactic Antibiotic Selection (Outpatient)	344	99%	98%	98%
Prophylactic Antibiotic Stopped[2]	268	100%	99%	98%
Prophylactic Antibiotic Timing[2]	273	99%	99%	99%
Prophylactic Antibiotic Timing (Outpatient)	169	98%	98%	98%
Urinary Catheter Removal[2]	253	96%	99%	97%
Survey of Patients' Hospital Experiences				
Area Around Room 'Always' Quiet at Night	300+	52%	60%	61%
Doctors 'Always' Communicated Well	300+	80%	81%	82%
Home Recovery Information Given	300+	86%	83%	85%
Hospital Given 9 or 10 on 10 Point Scale	300+	71%	68%	71%
Meds 'Always' Explained Before Given	300+	60%	63%	64%
Nurses 'Always' Communicated Well	300+	78%	77%	79%
Pain 'Always' Well Controlled	300+	69%	70%	71%
Room and Bathroom 'Always' Clean	300+	69%	72%	73%
Timely Help 'Always' Received	300+	66%	69%	68%
Would Definitely Recommend Hospital	300+	71%	67%	71%
Use of Medical Imaging				
Cardiac Imaging Stress Test before Surgery	499	4.6%	4.9%	5.3%
Combination Abdominal CT Scan	446	5.2%	10.6%	10.5%
Combination Brain/Sinus CT Scan	446	1.3%	1.9%	2.7%
Combination Chest CT Scan	212	2.8%	2.4%	2.7%
Follow-up Mammogram/Ultrasound[7]	-	-	6.9%	8.8%
Lumbar Spine MRI for Low Back Pain	72	36.1%	41.5%	37.2%

P H S Indian Hospital at Browning - Blackfeet

760 Hospital Circle, Post Office Box 760
Browning, MT 59417
Phone: 406-338-6157
Fax: 406-338-2959
URL: www.ihs.gov
Type: Acute Care Hospitals
Emergency Services: Yes
Ownership: Government - Federal
Beds: 27

Measure	Cases	This Hosp.	State Avg.	U.S. Avg.
Blood Clot Prevention and Treatment				
Anticoagulation Overlap Therapy[1]	-	-	97%	93%
ICU Venous Thromboembolism Prophylaxis[7]	-	-	92%	92%
Incidence of Potentially Preventable VTE[1]	-	-	4%	10%
UFH with Dosages/Platelet Monitoring[7]	-	-	97%	97%
Venous Thromboembolism Prophylaxis	193	20%	83%	85%
Warfarin Therapy Discharge Instructions[1]	-	-	84%	75%
Chest Pain/Possible Heart Attack Care				
Aspirin Given Within 24 Hours of Arrival	-	-	97%	96%
Fibrinolytic Meds Within 30 Min. of Arrival	-	-	43%	58%
Average Time to ECG (minutes)	-	-	10	7
Average Time to Transfer (minutes)	-	-	78	60
Children's Asthma Care				
Received Home Management Plan of Care	-	-	-	88%
Received Reliever Medication	-	-	-	100%
Received Systemic Corticosteroids	-	-	-	100%
Emergency Department				
Admittance Decision Time (minutes)	293	29	72	98
Head CT Results Within 45 Min. of Arrival	-	-	26%	57%
Patients Who Left ER Before Being Seen	-	-	2%	2%
Time from ER Arrival to Admit. (minutes)	294	176	220	274
Time from ER Arrival to Discharge (minutes)	-	-	120	134
Time in ER Before Being Evaluated (minutes)	-	-	23	26
Time to Pain Meds for Fractures (minutes)	-	-	47	57
Heart Attack Care				
Aspirin Given at Discharge[5]	-	-	100%	99%
Fibrinolytic Meds Within 30 Min. of Arrival[5]	-	-	50%	54%
PCI Within 90 Minutes of Arrival[5]	-	-	96%	96%
Statin Prescribed at Discharge[5]	-	-	99%	98%
Heart Failure Care				
ACE Inhibitor or ARB for LVSD[5]	-	-	97%	97%
Discharge Instructions Given[5]	-	-	92%	94%
Evaluation of LVS Function[5]	-	-	94%	99%
Medicare Spending				
Medicare Spending per Patient (ratio)	-	0.72	0.89	0.98
Pneumonia Care				
Appropriate Initial Antibiotic Given	22	82%	94%	95%
Blood Culture Timing	25	92%	97%	98%
Pregnancy and Delivery Care				
Newborn Deliveries Scheduled Early[1]	-	-	7%	6%
Preventive Care				
Immunization for Influenza	271	85%	86%	90%
Immunization for Pneumonia	170	96%	89%	92%
Stroke Care				
Anticoagulation Therapy for Atrial Fibrillation[5]	-	-	98%	95%
Antithrombotic Therapy Timing[5]	-	-	99%	98%
Assessed for Rehabilitation[5]	-	-	99%	97%
Discharged on Antithrombotic Therapy[5]	-	-	100%	99%
Discharged on Statin Medication[5]	-	-	94%	94%
Thrombolytic Therapy Timing[5]	-	-	67%	66%
Venous Thromboembolism Prophylaxis[5]	-	-	96%	94%
Written Stroke Educational Materials Given[5]	-	-	85%	88%
Surgical Care Improvement Project				
Appropriate Beta Blocker Usage[5]	-	-	98%	98%
Appropriate VTP Within 24 Hours[5]	-	-	98%	98%
Controlled Postoperative Blood Glucose[5]	-	-	96%	97%
Perioperative Temperature Management[5]	-	-	100%	100%
Prophylactic Antibiotic Selection[5]	-	-	99%	99%
Prophylactic Antibiotic Selection (Outpatient)	-	-	98%	98%
Prophylactic Antibiotic Stopped[5]	-	-	99%	98%
Prophylactic Antibiotic Timing[5]	-	-	99%	99%
Prophylactic Antibiotic Timing (Outpatient)	-	-	98%	98%
Urinary Catheter Removal[5]	-	-	99%	97%
Survey of Patients' Hospital Experiences				
Area Around Room 'Always' Quiet at Night[6]	<100	63%	60%	61%
Doctors 'Always' Communicated Well[6]	<100	71%	81%	82%
Home Recovery Information Given[6]	<100	68%	83%	85%
Hospital Given 9 or 10 on 10 Point Scale[6]	<100	43%	68%	71%
Meds 'Always' Explained Before Given[6]	<100	51%	63%	64%
Nurses 'Always' Communicated Well[6]	<100	59%	77%	79%
Pain 'Always' Well Controlled[6]	<100	55%	70%	71%
Room and Bathroom 'Always' Clean[6]	<100	58%	72%	73%
Timely Help 'Always' Received[6]	<100	35%	69%	68%
Would Definitely Recommend Hospital[6]	<100	41%	67%	71%
Use of Medical Imaging				
Cardiac Imaging Stress Test before Surgery	-	-	4.9%	5.3%
Combination Abdominal CT Scan	-	-	10.6%	10.5%
Combination Brain/Sinus CT Scan	-	-	1.9%	2.7%
Combination Chest CT Scan	-	-	2.4%	2.7%
Follow-up Mammogram/Ultrasound	-	-	6.9%	8.8%
Lumbar Spine MRI for Low Back Pain	-	-	41.5%	37.2%

NOTE: Hospital profiles are in alphabetical order by state, then city, then hospital within the city; Rankings exclude hospitals with less than 25 cases except for patient surveys which excludes hospitals with less than 100 cases; (a) 100-299 cases; (1) The number of cases/patients is too few to report; (2) Data submitted were based on a sample of cases/patients; (3) Results are based on a shorter time period than required; (4) Data suppressed by CMS for one or more quarters; (5) Results are not available for this reporting period; (6) Fewer than 100 patients completed the HCAHPS survey; (7) No cases met the criteria for this measure; (8) The lower limit of the confidence interval cannot be calculated if the number of observed infections equals zero; (9) No data are available from the state/territory for this reporting period; (10) The scores shown reflect fewer than 50 completed surveys; (11) There were discrepancies in the data collection process; (12) This measure does not apply to this hospital for this reporting period; (13) Results cannot be calculated for this reporting period; (14) The results for this state are combined with nearby states to protect confidentiality; Please refer to the User's Guide for a full explanation of data.

Saint James Healthcare

400 S Clark St
Butte, MT 59701
E-mail: info@sjch.org
URL: www.stjameshealthcare.org
Phone: 406-723-2500
Fax: 406-723-2534
Type: Acute Care Hospitals
Emergency Services: Yes
Ownership: Voluntary non-profit - Private
Beds: 164

Key Personnel:
Chief of Medical Staff.......... Jeremy Blanchard, MD
Quality Assurance .... Patrick Dudley
Cardiac Laboratory............ Dave Kelso
Radiology.................... Rashmikant Shah, MD
Pediatric Ambulatory Care ...... Elaine Stasny, MD
Pediatric In-Patient Care .... Elaine Stasny, MD
Emergency Room .... Richard Thorne
CEO/President............... Chuck Wright

Measure	Cases	This Hosp.	State Avg.	U.S. Avg.
Blood Clot Prevention and Treatment				
Anticoagulation Overlap Therapy[2]	34	94%	97%	93%
ICU Venous Thromboembolism Prophylaxis[2]	91	88%	92%	92%
Incidence of Potentially Preventable VTE[1,2]	-	-	4%	10%
UFH with Dosages/Platelet Monitoring[1,2]	-	-	97%	97%
Venous Thromboembolism Prophylaxis[2]	256	92%	83%	85%
Warfarin Therapy Discharge Instructions[2]	25	64%	84%	75%
Chest Pain/Possible Heart Attack Care				
Aspirin Given Within 24 Hours of Arrival[1,3]	-	-	97%	96%
Fibrinolytic Meds Within 30 Min. of Arrival[1,3]	-	-	43%	58%
Average Time to ECG (minutes)[3]	11	14	10	7
Average Time to Transfer (minutes)[3,7]	-	-	78	60
Children's Asthma Care				
Received Home Management Plan of Care	-	-	-	88%
Received Reliever Medication	-	-	-	100%
Received Systemic Corticosteroids	-	-	-	100%
Emergency Department				
Admittance Decision Time (minutes)[2]	384	43	72	98
Head CT Results Within 45 Min. of Arrival[7]	-	-	26%	57%
Patients Who Left ER Before Being Seen	13,724	1%	2%	2%
Time from ER Arrival to Admit. (minutes)[2]	410	181	220	274
Time from ER Arrival to Discharge (minutes)	395	101	120	134
Time in ER Before Being Evaluated (minutes)	106	12	23	26
Time to Pain Meds for Fractures (minutes)	59	41	47	57
Heart Attack Care				
Aspirin Given at Discharge	47	100%	100%	99%
Fibrinolytic Meds Within 30 Min. of Arrival[7]	-	-	50%	54%
PCI Within 90 Minutes of Arrival[1]	-	-	96%	96%
Statin Prescribed at Discharge	46	93%	99%	98%
Heart Failure Care				
ACE Inhibitor or ARB for LVSD	11	91%	97%	97%
Discharge Instructions Given	65	95%	92%	94%
Evaluation of LVS Function	87	99%	94%	99%
Medicare Spending				
Medicare Spending per Patient (ratio)	-	1.01	0.89	0.98
Pneumonia Care				
Appropriate Initial Antibiotic Given	66	92%	94%	95%
Blood Culture Timing	101	94%	97%	98%
Pregnancy and Delivery Care				
Newborn Deliveries Scheduled Early[2]	23	4%	7%	6%
Preventive Care				
Immunization for Influenza[2]	357	87%	86%	90%
Immunization for Pneumonia[2]	454	86%	89%	92%
Stroke Care				
Anticoagulation Therapy for Atrial Fibrillation[1]	-	-	98%	95%
Antithrombotic Therapy Timing	25	96%	99%	98%
Assessed for Rehabilitation	30	97%	99%	97%
Discharged on Antithrombotic Therapy	28	100%	100%	99%
Discharged on Statin Medication	26	81%	94%	94%
Thrombolytic Therapy Timing[1]	-	-	67%	66%
Venous Thromboembolism Prophylaxis	27	93%	96%	94%
Written Stroke Educational Materials Given	14	71%	85%	88%
Surgical Care Improvement Project				
Appropriate Beta Blocker Usage	47	96%	98%	98%
Appropriate VTP Within 24 Hours	217	99%	98%	98%
Controlled Postoperative Blood Glucose[7]	-	-	96%	97%
Perioperative Temperature Management	239	100%	100%	100%
Prophylactic Antibiotic Selection	138	99%	99%	99%
Prophylactic Antibiotic Selection (Outpatient)	161	100%	98%	98%
Prophylactic Antibiotic Stopped	130	100%	99%	98%
Prophylactic Antibiotic Timing	138	99%	99%	99%
Prophylactic Antibiotic Timing (Outpatient)	164	93%	98%	98%
Urinary Catheter Removal	73	96%	99%	97%
Survey of Patients' Hospital Experiences				
Area Around Room 'Always' Quiet at Night	300+	54%	60%	61%
Doctors 'Always' Communicated Well	300+	80%	81%	82%
Home Recovery Information Given	300+	86%	83%	85%
Hospital Given 9 or 10 on 10 Point Scale	300+	65%	68%	71%
Meds 'Always' Explained Before Given	300+	59%	63%	64%
Nurses 'Always' Communicated Well	300+	76%	77%	79%
Pain 'Always' Well Controlled	300+	70%	70%	71%
Room and Bathroom 'Always' Clean	300+	65%	72%	73%
Timely Help 'Always' Received	300+	65%	69%	68%
Would Definitely Recommend Hospital	300+	57%	67%	71%
Use of Medical Imaging				
Cardiac Imaging Stress Test before Surgery	99	4.0%	4.9%	5.3%
Combination Abdominal CT Scan	272	5.5%	10.6%	10.5%
Combination Brain/Sinus CT Scan[1]	-	-	1.9%	2.7%
Combination Chest CT Scan	125	1.6%	2.4%	2.7%
Follow-up Mammogram/Ultrasound	603	10.9%	6.9%	8.8%
Lumbar Spine MRI for Low Back Pain	52	48.1%	41.5%	37.2%

Liberty Medical Center

315 W Madison Ave
Chester, MT 59522
URL: www.lchnh.org
Phone: 406-759-5181
Fax: 406-759-5799
Type: Critical Access Hospitals
Emergency Services: Yes
Ownership: Voluntary non-profit - Private
Beds: 11

Key Personnel:
CEO .... Derek Daly
Emergency Room .... Anna Earl
Patient Relations .... Glenda Hanson
Chief of Medical Staff.......... Natalie Mattson
Radiology.................. Natalie Mattson
Administrator .... Karen Shaw, RN

Measure	Cases	This Hosp.	State Avg.	U.S. Avg.
Blood Clot Prevention and Treatment				
Anticoagulation Overlap Therapy[5]	-	-	97%	93%
ICU Venous Thromboembolism Prophylaxis[5]	-	-	92%	92%
Incidence of Potentially Preventable VTE[5]	-	-	4%	10%
UFH with Dosages/Platelet Monitoring[5]	-	-	97%	97%
Venous Thromboembolism Prophylaxis[5]	-	-	83%	85%
Warfarin Therapy Discharge Instructions[5]	-	-	84%	75%
Chest Pain/Possible Heart Attack Care				
Aspirin Given Within 24 Hours of Arrival	-	-	97%	96%
Fibrinolytic Meds Within 30 Min. of Arrival	-	-	43%	58%
Average Time to ECG (minutes)	-	-	10	7
Average Time to Transfer (minutes)	-	-	78	60
Children's Asthma Care				
Received Home Management Plan of Care	-	-	-	88%
Received Reliever Medication	-	-	-	100%
Received Systemic Corticosteroids	-	-	-	100%
Emergency Department				
Admittance Decision Time (minutes)[5]	-	-	72	98
Head CT Results Within 45 Min. of Arrival	-	-	26%	57%
Patients Who Left ER Before Being Seen	-	-	2%	2%
Time from ER Arrival to Admit. (minutes)[5]	-	-	220	274
Time from ER Arrival to Discharge (minutes)	-	-	120	134
Time in ER Before Being Evaluated (minutes)	-	-	23	26
Time to Pain Meds for Fractures (minutes)	-	-	47	57
Heart Attack Care				
Aspirin Given at Discharge[3,7]	-	-	100%	99%
Fibrinolytic Meds Within 30 Min. of Arrival[3,7]	-	-	50%	54%
PCI Within 90 Minutes of Arrival[3,7]	-	-	96%	96%
Statin Prescribed at Discharge[3,7]	-	-	99%	98%
Heart Failure Care				
ACE Inhibitor or ARB for LVSD[3,7]	-	-	97%	97%
Discharge Instructions Given[1,3]	-	-	92%	94%
Evaluation of LVS Function[1,3]	-	-	94%	99%
Medicare Spending				
Medicare Spending per Patient (ratio)	-	-	0.89	0.98
Pneumonia Care				
Appropriate Initial Antibiotic Given[1]	-	-	94%	95%
Blood Culture Timing[1]	-	-	97%	98%
Pregnancy and Delivery Care				
Newborn Deliveries Scheduled Early[5]	-	-	7%	6%
Preventive Care				
Immunization for Influenza[5]	-	-	86%	90%
Immunization for Pneumonia[5]	-	-	89%	92%
Stroke Care				
Anticoagulation Therapy for Atrial Fibrillation[5]	-	-	98%	95%
Antithrombotic Therapy Timing[5]	-	-	99%	98%
Assessed for Rehabilitation[5]	-	-	99%	97%
Discharged on Antithrombotic Therapy[5]	-	-	100%	99%
Discharged on Statin Medication[5]	-	-	94%	94%
Thrombolytic Therapy Timing[5]	-	-	67%	66%
Venous Thromboembolism Prophylaxis[5]	-	-	96%	94%
Written Stroke Educational Materials Given[5]	-	-	85%	88%
Surgical Care Improvement Project				
Appropriate Beta Blocker Usage[5]	-	-	98%	98%
Appropriate VTP Within 24 Hours[5]	-	-	98%	98%
Controlled Postoperative Blood Glucose[5]	-	-	96%	97%
Perioperative Temperature Management[5]	-	-	100%	100%
Prophylactic Antibiotic Selection[5]	-	-	99%	99%
Prophylactic Antibiotic Selection (Outpatient)	-	-	98%	98%
Prophylactic Antibiotic Stopped[5]	-	-	99%	98%
Prophylactic Antibiotic Timing[5]	-	-	99%	99%
Prophylactic Antibiotic Timing (Outpatient)	-	-	98%	98%
Urinary Catheter Removal[5]	-	-	99%	97%
Survey of Patients' Hospital Experiences				
Area Around Room 'Always' Quiet at Night[5]	-	-	60%	61%
Doctors 'Always' Communicated Well[5]	-	-	81%	82%
Home Recovery Information Given[5]	-	-	83%	85%
Hospital Given 9 or 10 on 10 Point Scale[5]	-	-	68%	71%
Meds 'Always' Explained Before Given[5]	-	-	63%	64%
Nurses 'Always' Communicated Well[5]	-	-	77%	79%
Pain 'Always' Well Controlled[5]	-	-	70%	71%
Room and Bathroom 'Always' Clean[5]	-	-	72%	73%
Timely Help 'Always' Received[5]	-	-	69%	68%
Would Definitely Recommend Hospital[5]	-	-	67%	71%
Use of Medical Imaging				
Cardiac Imaging Stress Test before Surgery	-	-	4.9%	5.3%
Combination Abdominal CT Scan	-	-	10.6%	10.5%
Combination Brain/Sinus CT Scan	-	-	1.9%	2.7%
Combination Chest CT Scan	-	-	2.4%	2.7%
Follow-up Mammogram/Ultrasound	-	-	6.9%	8.8%
Lumbar Spine MRI for Low Back Pain	-	-	41.5%	37.2%

Teton Medical Center

915 4th Saint Nw
Choteau, MT 59422
E-mail: tetonmc@tetonmedicalcenter.net
URL: www.tetonmedicalcenter.net
Phone: 406-466-5763
Fax: 406-466-5852
Type: Critical Access Hospitals
Emergency Services: Yes
Ownership: Govt - Hospital Dist/Auth
Beds: 7

Key Personnel:
CEO .... Louie King
Quality Assurance .... Susan Murphy, RHIT
Chief of Medical Staff.......... Laura Shelton, MD
Patient Relations .... Dina Vansetten

Measure	Cases	This Hosp.	State Avg.	U.S. Avg.
Blood Clot Prevention and Treatment				
Anticoagulation Overlap Therapy[5]	-	-	97%	93%
ICU Venous Thromboembolism Prophylaxis[5]	-	-	92%	92%
Incidence of Potentially Preventable VTE[5]	-	-	4%	10%
UFH with Dosages/Platelet Monitoring[5]	-	-	97%	97%
Venous Thromboembolism Prophylaxis[5]	-	-	83%	85%
Warfarin Therapy Discharge Instructions[5]	-	-	84%	75%
Chest Pain/Possible Heart Attack Care				
Aspirin Given Within 24 Hours of Arrival	-	-	97%	96%
Fibrinolytic Meds Within 30 Min. of Arrival	-	-	43%	58%
Average Time to ECG (minutes)	-	-	10	7
Average Time to Transfer (minutes)	-	-	78	60
Children's Asthma Care				

NOTE: Hospital profiles are in alphabetical order by state, then city, then hospital within the city; Rankings exclude hospitals with less than 25 cases except for patient surveys which excludes hospitals with less than 100 cases; (a) 100-299 cases; (1) The number of cases/patients is too few to report; (2) Data submitted were based on a sample of cases/patients; (3) Results are based on a shorter time period than required; (4) Data suppressed by CMS for one or more quarters; (5) Results are not available for this reporting period; (6) Fewer than 100 patients completed the HCAHPS survey; (7) No cases met the criteria for this measure; (8) The lower limit of the confidence interval cannot be calculated if the number of observed infections equals zero; (9) No data are available from the state/territory for this reporting period; (10) The scores shown reflect fewer than 50 completed surveys; (11) There were discrepancies in the data collection process; (12) This measure does not apply to this hospital for this reporting period; (13) Results cannot be calculated for this reporting period; (14) The results for this state are combined with nearby states to protect confidentiality; Please refer to the User's Guide for a full explanation of data.

Received Home Management Plan of Care	-	-	-	88%
Received Reliever Medication	-	-	-	100%
Received Systemic Corticosteroids	-	-	-	100%
Emergency Department				
Admittance Decision Time (minutes)[5]	-	-	72	98
Head CT Results Within 45 Min. of Arrival	-	-	26%	57%
Patients Who Left ER Before Being Seen	-	-	2%	2%
Time from ER Arrival to Admit. (minutes)[5]	-	-	220	274
Time from ER Arrival to Discharge (minutes)	-	-	120	134
Time in ER Before Being Evaluated (minutes)	-	-	23	26
Time to Pain Meds for Fractures (minutes)	-	-	47	57
Heart Attack Care				
Aspirin Given at Discharge[5]	-	-	100%	99%
Fibrinolytic Meds Within 30 Min. of Arrival[5]	-	-	50%	54%
PCI Within 90 Minutes of Arrival[5]	-	-	96%	96%
Statin Prescribed at Discharge[5]	-	-	99%	98%
Heart Failure Care				
ACE Inhibitor or ARB for LVSD[3,7]	-	-	97%	97%
Discharge Instructions Given[1,3]	-	-	92%	94%
Evaluation of LVS Function[1,3]	-	-	94%	99%
Medicare Spending				
Medicare Spending per Patient (ratio)	-	-	0.89	0.98
Pneumonia Care				
Appropriate Initial Antibiotic Given[1]	-	-	94%	95%
Blood Culture Timing[1]	-	-	97%	98%
Pregnancy and Delivery Care				
Newborn Deliveries Scheduled Early[5]	-	-	7%	6%
Preventive Care				
Immunization for Influenza[5]	-	-	86%	90%
Immunization for Pneumonia[5]	-	-	89%	92%
Stroke Care				
Anticoagulation Therapy for Atrial Fibrillation[5]	-	-	98%	95%
Antithrombotic Therapy Timing[5]	-	-	99%	98%
Assessed for Rehabilitation[5]	-	-	99%	97%
Discharged on Antithrombotic Therapy[5]	-	-	100%	99%
Discharged on Statin Medication[5]	-	-	94%	94%
Thrombolytic Therapy Timing[5]	-	-	67%	66%
Venous Thromboembolism Prophylaxis[5]	-	-	96%	94%
Written Stroke Educational Materials Given[5]	-	-	85%	88%
Surgical Care Improvement Project				
Appropriate Beta Blocker Usage[5]	-	-	98%	98%
Appropriate VTP Within 24 Hours[5]	-	-	98%	98%
Controlled Postoperative Blood Glucose[5]	-	-	96%	97%
Perioperative Temperature Management[5]	-	-	100%	100%
Prophylactic Antibiotic Selection[5]	-	-	99%	99%
Prophylactic Antibiotic Selection (Outpatient)	-	-	98%	98%
Prophylactic Antibiotic Stopped[5]	-	-	99%	98%
Prophylactic Antibiotic Timing[5]	-	-	99%	99%
Prophylactic Antibiotic Timing (Outpatient)	-	-	98%	98%
Urinary Catheter Removal[5]	-	-	99%	97%
Survey of Patients' Hospital Experiences				
Area Around Room 'Always' Quiet at Night[5]	-	-	60%	61%
Doctors 'Always' Communicated Well[5]	-	-	81%	82%
Home Recovery Information Given[5]	-	-	83%	85%
Hospital Given 9 or 10 on 10 Point Scale[5]	-	-	68%	71%
Meds 'Always' Explained Before Given[5]	-	-	63%	64%
Nurses 'Always' Communicated Well[5]	-	-	77%	79%
Pain 'Always' Well Controlled[5]	-	-	70%	71%
Room and Bathroom 'Always' Clean[5]	-	-	72%	73%
Timely Help 'Always' Received[5]	-	-	69%	68%
Would Definitely Recommend Hospital[5]	-	-	67%	71%
Use of Medical Imaging				
Cardiac Imaging Stress Test before Surgery	-	-	4.9%	5.3%
Combination Abdominal CT Scan	-	-	10.6%	10.5%
Combination Brain/Sinus CT Scan	-	-	1.9%	2.7%
Combination Chest CT Scan	-	-	2.4%	2.7%
Follow-up Mammogram/Ultrasound	-	-	6.9%	8.8%
Lumbar Spine MRI for Low Back Pain	-	-	41.5%	37.2%

McCone County Health Center

605 Sullivan Ave
Circle, MT 59215
Phone: 406-485-3381
URL: www.mcconehealth.org
Type: Critical Access Hospitals
Emergency Services: Yes
Ownership: Voluntary non-profit - Private
Key Personnel:
CEO/President. . . . . Nancy Hansen

Measure	Cases	This Hosp.	State Avg.	U.S. Avg.
Blood Clot Prevention and Treatment				
Anticoagulation Overlap Therapy[3,7]	-	-	97%	93%
ICU Venous Thromboembolism Prophylaxis[3,7]	-	-	92%	92%
Incidence of Potentially Preventable VTE[3,7]	-	-	4%	10%
UFH with Dosages/Platelet Monitoring[3,7]	-	-	97%	97%
Venous Thromboembolism Prophylaxis[1,3]	-	-	83%	85%
Warfarin Therapy Discharge Instructions[3,7]	-	-	84%	75%
Chest Pain/Possible Heart Attack Care				
Aspirin Given Within 24 Hours of Arrival[5]	-	-	97%	96%
Fibrinolytic Meds Within 30 Min. of Arrival[5]	-	-	43%	58%
Average Time to ECG (minutes)[5]	-	-	10	7
Average Time to Transfer (minutes)[5]	-	-	78	60
Children's Asthma Care				
Received Home Management Plan of Care	-	-	-	88%
Received Reliever Medication	-	-	-	100%
Received Systemic Corticosteroids	-	-	-	100%
Emergency Department				
Admittance Decision Time (minutes)[5]	-	-	72	98
Head CT Results Within 45 Min. of Arrival[5]	-	-	26%	57%
Patients Who Left ER Before Being Seen[5]	-	-	2%	2%
Time from ER Arrival to Admit. (minutes)[5]	-	-	220	274
Time from ER Arrival to Discharge (minutes)[5]	-	-	120	134
Time in ER Before Being Evaluated (minutes)[5]	-	-	23	26
Time to Pain Meds for Fractures (minutes)[5]	-	-	47	57
Heart Attack Care				
Aspirin Given at Discharge[5]	-	-	100%	99%
Fibrinolytic Meds Within 30 Min. of Arrival[5]	-	-	50%	54%
PCI Within 90 Minutes of Arrival[5]	-	-	96%	96%
Statin Prescribed at Discharge[5]	-	-	99%	98%
Heart Failure Care				
ACE Inhibitor or ARB for LVSD[5]	-	-	97%	97%
Discharge Instructions Given[5]	-	-	92%	94%
Evaluation of LVS Function[5]	-	-	94%	99%
Medicare Spending				
Medicare Spending per Patient (ratio)	-	-	0.89	0.98
Pneumonia Care				
Appropriate Initial Antibiotic Given[5]	-	-	94%	95%
Blood Culture Timing[5]	-	-	97%	98%
Pregnancy and Delivery Care				
Newborn Deliveries Scheduled Early[5]	-	-	7%	6%
Preventive Care				
Immunization for Influenza[5]	-	-	86%	90%
Immunization for Pneumonia[5]	-	-	89%	92%
Stroke Care				
Anticoagulation Therapy for Atrial Fibrillation[5]	-	-	98%	95%
Antithrombotic Therapy Timing[5]	-	-	99%	98%
Assessed for Rehabilitation[5]	-	-	99%	97%
Discharged on Antithrombotic Therapy[5]	-	-	100%	99%
Discharged on Statin Medication[5]	-	-	94%	94%
Thrombolytic Therapy Timing[5]	-	-	67%	66%
Venous Thromboembolism Prophylaxis[5]	-	-	96%	94%
Written Stroke Educational Materials Given[5]	-	-	85%	88%
Surgical Care Improvement Project				
Appropriate Beta Blocker Usage[5]	-	-	98%	98%
Appropriate VTP Within 24 Hours[5]	-	-	98%	98%
Controlled Postoperative Blood Glucose[5]	-	-	96%	97%
Perioperative Temperature Management[5]	-	-	100%	100%
Prophylactic Antibiotic Selection[5]	-	-	99%	99%
Prophylactic Antibiotic Selection (Outpatient)[5]	-	-	98%	98%
Prophylactic Antibiotic Stopped[5]	-	-	99%	98%
Prophylactic Antibiotic Timing[5]	-	-	99%	99%
Prophylactic Antibiotic Timing (Outpatient)[5]	-	-	98%	98%
Urinary Catheter Removal[5]	-	-	99%	97%
Survey of Patients' Hospital Experiences				
Area Around Room 'Always' Quiet at Night[5]	-	-	60%	61%
Doctors 'Always' Communicated Well[5]	-	-	81%	82%
Home Recovery Information Given[5]	-	-	83%	85%
Hospital Given 9 or 10 on 10 Point Scale[5]	-	-	68%	71%
Meds 'Always' Explained Before Given[5]	-	-	63%	64%
Nurses 'Always' Communicated Well[5]	-	-	77%	79%
Pain 'Always' Well Controlled[5]	-	-	70%	71%
Room and Bathroom 'Always' Clean[5]	-	-	72%	73%
Timely Help 'Always' Received[5]	-	-	69%	68%
Would Definitely Recommend Hospital[5]	-	-	67%	71%
Use of Medical Imaging				
Cardiac Imaging Stress Test before Surgery[7]	-	-	4.9%	5.3%
Combination Abdominal CT Scan[7]	-	-	10.6%	10.5%
Combination Brain/Sinus CT Scan[7]	-	-	1.9%	2.7%
Combination Chest CT Scan[7]	-	-	2.4%	2.7%
Follow-up Mammogram/Ultrasound[7]	-	-	6.9%	8.8%
Lumbar Spine MRI for Low Back Pain[7]	-	-	41.5%	37.2%

Stillwater Billings Clinic

710 N 11th St
Columbus, MT 59019
Phone: 406-322-5316
Fax: 406-322-5207
Type: Critical Access Hospitals
Emergency Services: Yes
Ownership: Voluntary non-profit - Private
Beds: 23
Key Personnel:
Infection Control. . . . . Denise Donohue
President . . . . John Hungerford
CEO . . . . Tim Russell

Measure	Cases	This Hosp.	State Avg.	U.S. Avg.
Blood Clot Prevention and Treatment				
Anticoagulation Overlap Therapy[5]	-	-	97%	93%
ICU Venous Thromboembolism Prophylaxis[5]	-	-	92%	92%
Incidence of Potentially Preventable VTE[5]	-	-	4%	10%
UFH with Dosages/Platelet Monitoring[5]	-	-	97%	97%
Venous Thromboembolism Prophylaxis[5]	-	-	83%	85%
Warfarin Therapy Discharge Instructions[5]	-	-	84%	75%
Chest Pain/Possible Heart Attack Care				
Aspirin Given Within 24 Hours of Arrival	-	-	97%	96%
Fibrinolytic Meds Within 30 Min. of Arrival	-	-	43%	58%
Average Time to ECG (minutes)	-	-	10	7
Average Time to Transfer (minutes)	-	-	78	60
Children's Asthma Care				
Received Home Management Plan of Care	-	-	-	88%
Received Reliever Medication	-	-	-	100%
Received Systemic Corticosteroids	-	-	-	100%
Emergency Department				
Admittance Decision Time (minutes)[5]	-	-	72	98
Head CT Results Within 45 Min. of Arrival	-	-	26%	57%
Patients Who Left ER Before Being Seen	-	-	2%	2%
Time from ER Arrival to Admit. (minutes)[5]	-	-	220	274
Time from ER Arrival to Discharge (minutes)	-	-	120	134
Time in ER Before Being Evaluated (minutes)	-	-	23	26
Time to Pain Meds for Fractures (minutes)	-	-	47	57
Heart Attack Care				
Aspirin Given at Discharge[3,7]	-	-	100%	99%
Fibrinolytic Meds Within 30 Min. of Arrival[3,7]	-	-	50%	54%
PCI Within 90 Minutes of Arrival[3,7]	-	-	96%	96%
Statin Prescribed at Discharge[3,7]	-	-	99%	98%
Heart Failure Care				
ACE Inhibitor or ARB for LVSD[7]	-	-	97%	97%
Discharge Instructions Given[1]	-	-	92%	94%
Evaluation of LVS Function[1]	-	-	94%	99%
Medicare Spending				
Medicare Spending per Patient (ratio)	-	-	0.89	0.98
Pneumonia Care				
Appropriate Initial Antibiotic Given[1]	-	-	94%	95%
Blood Culture Timing[1]	-	-	97%	98%
Pregnancy and Delivery Care				
Newborn Deliveries Scheduled Early[5]	-	-	7%	6%
Preventive Care				
Immunization for Influenza[5]	-	-	86%	90%
Immunization for Pneumonia[5]	-	-	89%	92%
Stroke Care				
Anticoagulation Therapy for Atrial Fibrillation[7]	-	-	98%	95%

NOTE: Hospital profiles are in alphabetical order by state, then city, then hospital within the city; Rankings exclude hospitals with less than 25 cases except for patient surveys which excludes hospitals with less than 100 cases; (a) 100-299 cases; (1) The number of cases/patients is too few to report; (2) Data submitted were based on a sample of cases/patients; (3) Results are based on a shorter time period than required; (4) Data suppressed by CMS for one or more quarters; (5) Results are not available for this reporting period; (6) Fewer than 100 patients completed the HCAHPS survey; (7) No cases met the criteria for this measure; (8) The lower limit of the confidence interval cannot be calculated if the number of observed infections equals zero; (9) No data are available from the state/territory for this reporting period; (10) The scores shown reflect fewer than 50 completed surveys; (11) There were discrepancies in the data collection process; (12) This measure does not apply to this hospital for this reporting period; (13) Results cannot be calculated for this reporting period; (14) The results for this state are combined with nearby states to protect confidentiality; Please refer to the User's Guide for a full explanation of data.

Measure	Cases	This Hosp.	State Avg.	U.S. Avg.
Antithrombotic Therapy Timing[7]	-	-	99%	98%
Assessed for Rehabilitation[1]	-	-	99%	97%
Discharged on Antithrombotic Therapy[1]	-	-	100%	99%
Discharged on Statin Medication[7]	-	-	94%	94%
Thrombolytic Therapy Timing[7]	-	-	67%	66%
Venous Thromboembolism Prophylaxis[7]	-	-	96%	94%
Written Stroke Educational Materials Given[1]	-	-	85%	88%
Surgical Care Improvement Project				
Appropriate Beta Blocker Usage[5]	-	-	98%	98%
Appropriate VTP Within 24 Hours[5]	-	-	98%	98%
Controlled Postoperative Blood Glucose[5]	-	-	96%	97%
Perioperative Temperature Management[5]	-	-	100%	100%
Prophylactic Antibiotic Selection[5]	-	-	99%	99%
Prophylactic Antibiotic Selection (Outpatient)	-	-	98%	98%
Prophylactic Antibiotic Stopped[5]	-	-	99%	98%
Prophylactic Antibiotic Timing[5]	-	-	99%	99%
Prophylactic Antibiotic Timing (Outpatient)	-	-	98%	98%
Urinary Catheter Removal[5]	-	-	99%	97%
Survey of Patients' Hospital Experiences				
Area Around Room 'Always' Quiet at Night[5]	-	-	60%	61%
Doctors 'Always' Communicated Well[5]	-	-	81%	82%
Home Recovery Information Given[5]	-	-	83%	85%
Hospital Given 9 or 10 on 10 Point Scale[5]	-	-	68%	71%
Meds 'Always' Explained Before Given[5]	-	-	63%	64%
Nurses 'Always' Communicated Well[5]	-	-	77%	79%
Pain 'Always' Well Controlled[5]	-	-	70%	71%
Room and Bathroom 'Always' Clean[5]	-	-	72%	73%
Timely Help 'Always' Received[5]	-	-	69%	68%
Would Definitely Recommend Hospital[5]	-	-	67%	71%
Use of Medical Imaging				
Cardiac Imaging Stress Test before Surgery	-	-	4.9%	5.3%
Combination Abdominal CT Scan	-	-	10.6%	10.5%
Combination Brain/Sinus CT Scan	-	-	1.9%	2.7%
Combination Chest CT Scan	-	-	2.4%	2.7%
Follow-up Mammogram/Ultrasound	-	-	6.9%	8.8%
Lumbar Spine MRI for Low Back Pain	-	-	41.5%	37.2%

Pondera Medical Center

805 Sunset Blvd
Conrad, MT 59425
Phone: 406-271-3211
Fax: 406-271-3917
URL: www.ponderamedical.com
Type: Critical Access Hospitals
Emergency Services: Yes
Ownership: Voluntary non-profit - Private
Beds: 20

Key Personnel:
Quality Assurance .... Wayne Ashworth
Radiology.................... Lisa Hanson
Chief of Medical Staff.......... Dennis Lott
CEO/President................ Bill O'Leary

Measure	Cases	This Hosp.	State Avg.	U.S. Avg.
Blood Clot Prevention and Treatment				
Anticoagulation Overlap Therapy[5]	-	-	97%	93%
ICU Venous Thromboembolism Prophylaxis[5]	-	-	92%	92%
Incidence of Potentially Preventable VTE[5]	-	-	4%	10%
UFH with Dosages/Platelet Monitoring[5]	-	-	97%	97%
Venous Thromboembolism Prophylaxis[5]	-	-	83%	85%
Warfarin Therapy Discharge Instructions[5]	-	-	84%	75%
Chest Pain/Possible Heart Attack Care				
Aspirin Given Within 24 Hours of Arrival	-	-	97%	96%
Fibrinolytic Meds Within 30 Min. of Arrival	-	-	43%	58%
Average Time to ECG (minutes)	-	-	10	7
Average Time to Transfer (minutes)	-	-	78	60
Children's Asthma Care				
Received Home Management Plan of Care	-	-	-	88%
Received Reliever Medication	-	-	-	100%
Received Systemic Corticosteroids	-	-	-	100%
Emergency Department				
Admittance Decision Time (minutes)[5]	-	-	72	98
Head CT Results Within 45 Min. of Arrival	-	-	26%	57%
Patients Who Left ER Before Being Seen	-	-	2%	2%
Time from ER Arrival to Admit. (minutes)[5]	-	-	220	274
Time from ER Arrival to Discharge (minutes)	-	-	120	134
Time in ER Before Being Evaluated (minutes)	-	-	23	26
Time to Pain Meds for Fractures (minutes)	-	-	47	57
Heart Attack Care				
Aspirin Given at Discharge[1,3]	-	-	100%	99%
Fibrinolytic Meds Within 30 Min. of Arrival[3,7]	-	-	50%	54%
PCI Within 90 Minutes of Arrival[3,7]	-	-	96%	96%
Statin Prescribed at Discharge[1,3]	-	-	99%	98%
Heart Failure Care				
ACE Inhibitor or ARB for LVSD[3,7]	-	-	97%	97%
Discharge Instructions Given[3,7]	-	-	92%	94%
Evaluation of LVS Function[1,3]	-	-	94%	99%
Medicare Spending				
Medicare Spending per Patient (ratio)	-	-	0.89	0.98
Pneumonia Care				
Appropriate Initial Antibiotic Given[1]	-	-	94%	95%
Blood Culture Timing[1]	-	-	97%	98%
Pregnancy and Delivery Care				
Newborn Deliveries Scheduled Early[5]	-	-	7%	6%
Preventive Care				
Immunization for Influenza[5]	-	-	86%	90%
Immunization for Pneumonia[5]	-	-	89%	92%
Stroke Care				
Anticoagulation Therapy for Atrial Fibrillation[5]	-	-	98%	95%
Antithrombotic Therapy Timing[5]	-	-	99%	98%
Assessed for Rehabilitation[5]	-	-	99%	97%
Discharged on Antithrombotic Therapy[5]	-	-	100%	99%
Discharged on Statin Medication[5]	-	-	94%	94%
Thrombolytic Therapy Timing[5]	-	-	67%	66%
Venous Thromboembolism Prophylaxis[5]	-	-	96%	94%
Written Stroke Educational Materials Given[5]	-	-	85%	88%
Surgical Care Improvement Project				
Appropriate Beta Blocker Usage[5]	-	-	98%	98%
Appropriate VTP Within 24 Hours[5]	-	-	98%	98%
Controlled Postoperative Blood Glucose[5]	-	-	96%	97%
Perioperative Temperature Management[5]	-	-	100%	100%
Prophylactic Antibiotic Selection[5]	-	-	99%	99%
Prophylactic Antibiotic Selection (Outpatient)	-	-	98%	98%
Prophylactic Antibiotic Stopped[5]	-	-	99%	98%
Prophylactic Antibiotic Timing[5]	-	-	99%	99%
Prophylactic Antibiotic Timing (Outpatient)	-	-	98%	98%
Urinary Catheter Removal[5]	-	-	99%	97%
Survey of Patients' Hospital Experiences				
Area Around Room 'Always' Quiet at Night[10]	<100	60%	60%	61%
Doctors 'Always' Communicated Well[10]	<100	94%	81%	82%
Home Recovery Information Given[10]	<100	99%	83%	85%
Hospital Given 9 or 10 on 10 Point Scale[10]	<100	86%	68%	71%
Meds 'Always' Explained Before Given[10]	<100	86%	63%	64%
Nurses 'Always' Communicated Well[10]	<100	90%	77%	79%
Pain 'Always' Well Controlled[10]	<100	82%	70%	71%
Room and Bathroom 'Always' Clean[10]	<100	77%	72%	73%
Timely Help 'Always' Received[10]	<100	96%	69%	68%
Would Definitely Recommend Hospital[10]	<100	62%	67%	71%
Use of Medical Imaging				
Cardiac Imaging Stress Test before Surgery	-	-	4.9%	5.3%
Combination Abdominal CT Scan	-	-	10.6%	10.5%
Combination Brain/Sinus CT Scan	-	-	1.9%	2.7%
Combination Chest CT Scan	-	-	2.4%	2.7%
Follow-up Mammogram/Ultrasound	-	-	6.9%	8.8%
Lumbar Spine MRI for Low Back Pain	-	-	41.5%	37.2%

P H S Indian Hospital Crow/Northern Cheyenne

1010 South 7650 East, Post Office Box 9
Crow Agency, MT 59022
Phone: 406-638-2626
Fax: 406-638-3569
Type: Critical Access Hospitals
Emergency Services: Yes
Ownership: Government - Federal
Beds: 24

Key Personnel:
Emergency Room .... Clayton Bunt, MD
Cardiac Laboratory............ Rob Diron
CEO/President................ Kevin Ftiffarm
Quality Assurance .... Mary Wan Leven
Chief of Medical Staff.......... David Mark

Measure	Cases	This Hosp.	State Avg.	U.S. Avg.
Blood Clot Prevention and Treatment				
Anticoagulation Overlap Therapy[3,7]	-	-	97%	93%
ICU Venous Thromboembolism Prophylaxis[3,7]	-	-	92%	92%
Incidence of Potentially Preventable VTE[3,7]	-	-	4%	10%
UFH with Dosages/Platelet Monitoring[3,7]	-	-	97%	97%
Venous Thromboembolism Prophylaxis[1,3]	-	-	83%	85%
Warfarin Therapy Discharge Instructions[3,7]	-	-	84%	75%
Chest Pain/Possible Heart Attack Care				
Aspirin Given Within 24 Hours of Arrival	-	-	97%	96%
Fibrinolytic Meds Within 30 Min. of Arrival	-	-	43%	58%
Average Time to ECG (minutes)	-	-	10	7
Average Time to Transfer (minutes)	-	-	78	60
Children's Asthma Care				
Received Home Management Plan of Care	-	-	-	88%
Received Reliever Medication	-	-	-	100%
Received Systemic Corticosteroids	-	-	-	100%
Emergency Department				
Admittance Decision Time (minutes)[3]	33	44	72	98
Head CT Results Within 45 Min. of Arrival	-	-	26%	57%
Patients Who Left ER Before Being Seen	-	-	2%	2%
Time from ER Arrival to Admit. (minutes)[3]	40	212	220	274
Time from ER Arrival to Discharge (minutes)	-	-	120	134
Time in ER Before Being Evaluated (minutes)	-	-	23	26
Time to Pain Meds for Fractures (minutes)	-	-	47	57
Heart Attack Care				
Aspirin Given at Discharge[5]	-	-	100%	99%
Fibrinolytic Meds Within 30 Min. of Arrival[5]	-	-	50%	54%
PCI Within 90 Minutes of Arrival[5]	-	-	96%	96%
Statin Prescribed at Discharge[5]	-	-	99%	98%
Heart Failure Care				
ACE Inhibitor or ARB for LVSD[3,7]	-	-	97%	97%
Discharge Instructions Given[1,3]	-	-	92%	94%
Evaluation of LVS Function[1,3]	-	-	94%	99%
Medicare Spending				
Medicare Spending per Patient (ratio)	-	-	0.89	0.98
Pneumonia Care				
Appropriate Initial Antibiotic Given[1,3]	-	-	94%	95%
Blood Culture Timing[1,3]	-	-	97%	98%
Pregnancy and Delivery Care				
Newborn Deliveries Scheduled Early[5]	-	-	7%	6%
Preventive Care				
Immunization for Influenza[5]	-	-	86%	90%
Immunization for Pneumonia[3]	30	80%	89%	92%
Stroke Care				
Anticoagulation Therapy for Atrial Fibrillation[5]	-	-	98%	95%
Antithrombotic Therapy Timing[5]	-	-	99%	98%
Assessed for Rehabilitation[5]	-	-	99%	97%
Discharged on Antithrombotic Therapy[5]	-	-	100%	99%
Discharged on Statin Medication[5]	-	-	94%	94%
Thrombolytic Therapy Timing[5]	-	-	67%	66%
Venous Thromboembolism Prophylaxis[5]	-	-	96%	94%
Written Stroke Educational Materials Given[5]	-	-	85%	88%
Surgical Care Improvement Project				
Appropriate Beta Blocker Usage[5]	-	-	98%	98%
Appropriate VTP Within 24 Hours[5]	-	-	98%	98%
Controlled Postoperative Blood Glucose[5]	-	-	96%	97%
Perioperative Temperature Management[5]	-	-	100%	100%
Prophylactic Antibiotic Selection[5]	-	-	99%	99%
Prophylactic Antibiotic Selection (Outpatient)	-	-	98%	98%
Prophylactic Antibiotic Stopped[5]	-	-	99%	98%
Prophylactic Antibiotic Timing[5]	-	-	99%	99%
Prophylactic Antibiotic Timing (Outpatient)	-	-	98%	98%
Urinary Catheter Removal[5]	-	-	99%	97%
Survey of Patients' Hospital Experiences				
Area Around Room 'Always' Quiet at Night[5]	-	-	60%	61%
Doctors 'Always' Communicated Well[5]	-	-	81%	82%
Home Recovery Information Given[5]	-	-	83%	85%
Hospital Given 9 or 10 on 10 Point Scale[5]	-	-	68%	71%
Meds 'Always' Explained Before Given[5]	-	-	63%	64%
Nurses 'Always' Communicated Well[5]	-	-	77%	79%
Pain 'Always' Well Controlled[5]	-	-	70%	71%
Room and Bathroom 'Always' Clean[5]	-	-	72%	73%
Timely Help 'Always' Received[5]	-	-	69%	68%
Would Definitely Recommend Hospital[5]	-	-	67%	71%
Use of Medical Imaging				

NOTE: Hospital profiles are in alphabetical order by state, then city, then hospital within the city; Rankings exclude hospitals with less than 25 cases except for patient surveys which excludes hospitals with less than 100 cases; (a) 100-299 cases; (1) The number of cases/patients is too few to report; (2) Data submitted were based on a sample of cases/patients; (3) Results are based on a shorter time period than required; (4) Data suppressed by CMS for one or more quarters; (5) Results are not available for this reporting period; (6) Fewer than 100 patients completed the HCAHPS survey; (7) No cases met the criteria for this measure; (8) The lower limit of the confidence interval cannot be calculated if the number of observed infections equals zero; (9) No data are available from the state/territory for this reporting period; (10) The scores shown reflect fewer than 50 completed surveys; (11) There were discrepancies in the data collection process; (12) This measure does not apply to this hospital for this reporting period; (13) Results cannot be calculated for this reporting period; (14) The results for this state are combined with nearby states to protect confidentiality; Please refer to the User's Guide for a full explanation of data.

Measure	Cases	This Hosp.	State Avg.	U.S. Avg.
Cardiac Imaging Stress Test before Surgery	-	-	4.9%	5.3%
Combination Abdominal CT Scan	-	-	10.6%	10.5%
Combination Brain/Sinus CT Scan	-	-	1.9%	2.7%
Combination Chest CT Scan	-	-	2.4%	2.7%
Follow-up Mammogram/Ultrasound	-	-	6.9%	8.8%
Lumbar Spine MRI for Low Back Pain	-	-	41.5%	37.2%

Roosevelt Medical Center

818 2nd Ave E
Culbertson, MT 59218
Phone: 406-787-6401
Fax: 406-787-6461
E-mail: astromberg@roosmem.org
URL: www.roosmem.org
Type: Critical Access Hospitals
Emergency Services: Yes
Ownership: Voluntary non-profit - Private
Beds: 42

Measure	Cases	This Hosp.	State Avg.	U.S. Avg.
Blood Clot Prevention and Treatment				
Anticoagulation Overlap Therapy[5]	-	-	97%	93%
ICU Venous Thromboembolism Prophylaxis[5]	-	-	92%	92%
Incidence of Potentially Preventable VTE[5]	-	-	4%	10%
UFH with Dosages/Platelet Monitoring[5]	-	-	97%	97%
Venous Thromboembolism Prophylaxis[5]	-	-	83%	85%
Warfarin Therapy Discharge Instructions[5]	-	-	84%	75%
Chest Pain/Possible Heart Attack Care				
Aspirin Given Within 24 Hours of Arrival	-	-	97%	96%
Fibrinolytic Meds Within 30 Min. of Arrival	-	-	43%	58%
Average Time to ECG (minutes)	-	-	10	7
Average Time to Transfer (minutes)	-	-	78	60
Children's Asthma Care				
Received Home Management Plan of Care	-	-	-	88%
Received Reliever Medication	-	-	-	100%
Received Systemic Corticosteroids	-	-	-	100%
Emergency Department				
Admittance Decision Time (minutes)[5]	-	-	72	98
Head CT Results Within 45 Min. of Arrival	-	-	26%	57%
Patients Who Left ER Before Being Seen	-	-	2%	2%
Time from ER Arrival to Admit. (minutes)[5]	-	-	220	274
Time from ER Arrival to Discharge (minutes)	-	-	120	134
Time in ER Before Being Evaluated (minutes)	-	-	23	26
Time to Pain Meds for Fractures (minutes)	-	-	47	57
Heart Attack Care				
Aspirin Given at Discharge[5]	-	-	100%	99%
Fibrinolytic Meds Within 30 Min. of Arrival[5]	-	-	50%	54%
PCI Within 90 Minutes of Arrival[5]	-	-	96%	96%
Statin Prescribed at Discharge[5]	-	-	99%	98%
Heart Failure Care				
ACE Inhibitor or ARB for LVSD[5]	-	-	97%	97%
Discharge Instructions Given[5]	-	-	92%	94%
Evaluation of LVS Function[5]	-	-	94%	99%
Medicare Spending				
Medicare Spending per Patient (ratio)	-	-	0.89	0.98
Pneumonia Care				
Appropriate Initial Antibiotic Given[3,7]	-	-	94%	95%
Blood Culture Timing[3,7]	-	-	97%	98%
Pregnancy and Delivery Care				
Newborn Deliveries Scheduled Early[5]	-	-	7%	6%
Preventive Care				
Immunization for Influenza[5]	-	-	86%	90%
Immunization for Pneumonia[5]	-	-	89%	92%
Stroke Care				
Anticoagulation Therapy for Atrial Fibrillation[5]	-	-	98%	95%
Antithrombotic Therapy Timing[5]	-	-	99%	98%
Assessed for Rehabilitation[5]	-	-	99%	97%
Discharged on Antithrombotic Therapy[5]	-	-	100%	99%
Discharged on Statin Medication[5]	-	-	94%	94%
Thrombolytic Therapy Timing[5]	-	-	67%	66%
Venous Thromboembolism Prophylaxis[5]	-	-	96%	94%
Written Stroke Educational Materials Given[5]	-	-	85%	88%
Surgical Care Improvement Project				
Appropriate Beta Blocker Usage[5]	-	-	98%	98%
Appropriate VTP Within 24 Hours[5]	-	-	98%	98%
Controlled Postoperative Blood Glucose[5]	-	-	96%	97%
Perioperative Temperature Management[5]	-	-	100%	100%
Prophylactic Antibiotic Selection[5]	-	-	99%	99%
Prophylactic Antibiotic Selection (Outpatient)	-	-	98%	98%
Prophylactic Antibiotic Stopped[5]	-	-	99%	98%
Prophylactic Antibiotic Timing[5]	-	-	99%	99%
Prophylactic Antibiotic Timing (Outpatient)	-	-	98%	98%
Urinary Catheter Removal[5]	-	-	99%	97%
Survey of Patients' Hospital Experiences				
Area Around Room 'Always' Quiet at Night[5]	-	-	60%	61%
Doctors 'Always' Communicated Well[5]	-	-	81%	82%
Home Recovery Information Given[5]	-	-	83%	85%
Hospital Given 9 or 10 on 10 Point Scale[5]	-	-	68%	71%
Meds 'Always' Explained Before Given[5]	-	-	63%	64%
Nurses 'Always' Communicated Well[5]	-	-	77%	79%
Pain 'Always' Well Controlled[5]	-	-	70%	71%
Room and Bathroom 'Always' Clean[5]	-	-	72%	73%
Timely Help 'Always' Received[5]	-	-	69%	68%
Would Definitely Recommend Hospital[5]	-	-	67%	71%
Use of Medical Imaging				
Cardiac Imaging Stress Test before Surgery	-	-	4.9%	5.3%
Combination Abdominal CT Scan	-	-	10.6%	10.5%
Combination Brain/Sinus CT Scan	-	-	1.9%	2.7%
Combination Chest CT Scan	-	-	2.4%	2.7%
Follow-up Mammogram/Ultrasound	-	-	6.9%	8.8%
Lumbar Spine MRI for Low Back Pain	-	-	41.5%	37.2%

Northern Rockies Medical Center

802 2nd Saint Se
Cut Bank, MT 59427
Phone: 406-873-2251
Fax: 406-873-4861
Type: Critical Access Hospitals
Emergency Services: Yes
Ownership: Voluntary non-profit - Private
Beds: 20

Key Personnel:

CEO/President. . . . . Cherie Taylor
Chief of Medical Staff. . . . . Randy Webb

Measure	Cases	This Hosp.	State Avg.	U.S. Avg.
Blood Clot Prevention and Treatment				
Anticoagulation Overlap Therapy[3,7]	-	-	97%	93%
ICU Venous Thromboembolism Prophylaxis[3,7]	-	-	92%	92%
Incidence of Potentially Preventable VTE[3,7]	-	-	4%	10%
UFH with Dosages/Platelet Monitoring[3,7]	-	-	97%	97%
Venous Thromboembolism Prophylaxis[3]	28	29%	83%	85%
Warfarin Therapy Discharge Instructions[3,7]	-	-	84%	75%
Chest Pain/Possible Heart Attack Care				
Aspirin Given Within 24 Hours of Arrival	-	-	97%	96%
Fibrinolytic Meds Within 30 Min. of Arrival	-	-	43%	58%
Average Time to ECG (minutes)	-	-	10	7
Average Time to Transfer (minutes)	-	-	78	60
Children's Asthma Care				
Received Home Management Plan of Care	-	-	-	88%
Received Reliever Medication	-	-	-	100%
Received Systemic Corticosteroids	-	-	-	100%
Emergency Department				
Admittance Decision Time (minutes)[3]	13	0	72	98
Head CT Results Within 45 Min. of Arrival	-	-	26%	57%
Patients Who Left ER Before Being Seen	-	-	2%	2%
Time from ER Arrival to Admit. (minutes)[3]	13	0	220	274
Time from ER Arrival to Discharge (minutes)	-	-	120	134
Time in ER Before Being Evaluated (minutes)	-	-	23	26
Time to Pain Meds for Fractures (minutes)	-	-	47	57
Heart Attack Care				
Aspirin Given at Discharge[5]	-	-	100%	99%
Fibrinolytic Meds Within 30 Min. of Arrival[5]	-	-	50%	54%
PCI Within 90 Minutes of Arrival[5]	-	-	96%	96%
Statin Prescribed at Discharge[5]	-	-	99%	98%
Heart Failure Care				
ACE Inhibitor or ARB for LVSD[1,3]	-	-	97%	97%
Discharge Instructions Given[1,3]	-	-	92%	94%
Evaluation of LVS Function[1,3]	-	-	94%	99%
Medicare Spending				
Medicare Spending per Patient (ratio)	-	-	0.89	0.98
Pneumonia Care				
Appropriate Initial Antibiotic Given[1]	-	-	94%	95%
Blood Culture Timing[1]	-	-	97%	98%
Pregnancy and Delivery Care				
Newborn Deliveries Scheduled Early[5]	-	-	7%	6%
Preventive Care				
Immunization for Influenza[3]	12	67%	86%	90%
Immunization for Pneumonia[3]	37	51%	89%	92%
Stroke Care				
Anticoagulation Therapy for Atrial Fibrillation[3,7]	-	-	98%	95%
Antithrombotic Therapy Timing[1,3]	-	-	99%	98%
Assessed for Rehabilitation[3,7]	-	-	99%	97%
Discharged on Antithrombotic Therapy[3,7]	-	-	100%	99%
Discharged on Statin Medication[3,7]	-	-	94%	94%
Thrombolytic Therapy Timing[1,3]	-	-	67%	66%
Venous Thromboembolism Prophylaxis[1,3]	-	-	96%	94%
Written Stroke Educational Materials Given[3,7]	-	-	85%	88%
Surgical Care Improvement Project				
Appropriate Beta Blocker Usage[5]	-	-	98%	98%
Appropriate VTP Within 24 Hours[5]	-	-	98%	98%
Controlled Postoperative Blood Glucose[5]	-	-	96%	97%
Perioperative Temperature Management[5]	-	-	100%	100%
Prophylactic Antibiotic Selection[5]	-	-	99%	99%
Prophylactic Antibiotic Selection (Outpatient)	-	-	98%	98%
Prophylactic Antibiotic Stopped[5]	-	-	99%	98%
Prophylactic Antibiotic Timing[5]	-	-	99%	99%
Prophylactic Antibiotic Timing (Outpatient)	-	-	98%	98%
Urinary Catheter Removal[5]	-	-	99%	97%
Survey of Patients' Hospital Experiences				
Area Around Room 'Always' Quiet at Night[5]	-	-	60%	61%
Doctors 'Always' Communicated Well[5]	-	-	81%	82%
Home Recovery Information Given[5]	-	-	83%	85%
Hospital Given 9 or 10 on 10 Point Scale[5]	-	-	68%	71%
Meds 'Always' Explained Before Given[5]	-	-	63%	64%
Nurses 'Always' Communicated Well[5]	-	-	77%	79%
Pain 'Always' Well Controlled[5]	-	-	70%	71%
Room and Bathroom 'Always' Clean[5]	-	-	72%	73%
Timely Help 'Always' Received[5]	-	-	69%	68%
Would Definitely Recommend Hospital[5]	-	-	67%	71%
Use of Medical Imaging				
Cardiac Imaging Stress Test before Surgery	-	-	4.9%	5.3%
Combination Abdominal CT Scan	-	-	10.6%	10.5%
Combination Brain/Sinus CT Scan	-	-	1.9%	2.7%
Combination Chest CT Scan	-	-	2.4%	2.7%
Follow-up Mammogram/Ultrasound	-	-	6.9%	8.8%
Lumbar Spine MRI for Low Back Pain	-	-	41.5%	37.2%

Barrett Memorial Hospital

600 Mt Hwy 91 S
Dillon, MT 59725
Phone: 406-683-3000
Fax: 406-683-3011
URL: www.barretthospital.org
Type: Critical Access Hospitals
Emergency Services: Yes
Ownership: Govt - Hospital Dist/Auth
Beds: 20

Key Personnel:

Chief of Medical Staff. . . . . Mick Lifson, MD, FACOG
President . . . . Patti Mitchell
CEO . . . . Ken Westman

Measure	Cases	This Hosp.	State Avg.	U.S. Avg.
Blood Clot Prevention and Treatment				
Anticoagulation Overlap Therapy[3,7]	-	-	97%	93%
ICU Venous Thromboembolism Prophylaxis[3,7]	-	-	92%	92%
Incidence of Potentially Preventable VTE[3,7]	-	-	4%	10%
UFH with Dosages/Platelet Monitoring[3,7]	-	-	97%	97%
Venous Thromboembolism Prophylaxis[1,3]	-	-	83%	85%
Warfarin Therapy Discharge Instructions[3,7]	-	-	84%	75%
Chest Pain/Possible Heart Attack Care				
Aspirin Given Within 24 Hours of Arrival	21	100%	97%	96%
Fibrinolytic Meds Within 30 Min. of Arrival[1]	-	-	43%	58%
Average Time to ECG (minutes)	21	6	10	7
Average Time to Transfer (minutes)[1]	-	-	78	60
Children's Asthma Care				
Received Home Management Plan of Care	-	-	-	88%
Received Reliever Medication	-	-	-	100%
Received Systemic Corticosteroids	-	-	-	100%
Emergency Department				
Admittance Decision Time (minutes)[5]	-	-	72	98
Head CT Results Within 45 Min. of Arrival[1]	-	-	26%	57%
Patients Who Left ER Before Being Seen	4,019	0%	2%	2%

NOTE: Hospital profiles are in alphabetical order by state, then city, then hospital within the city; Rankings exclude hospitals with less than 25 cases except for patient surveys which excludes hospitals with less than 100 cases; (a) 100-299 cases; (1) The number of cases/patients is too few to report; (2) Data submitted were based on a sample of cases/patients; (3) Results are based on a shorter time period than required; (4) Data suppressed by CMS for one or more quarters; (5) Results are not available for this reporting period; (6) Fewer than 100 patients completed the HCAHPS survey; (7) No cases met the criteria for this measure; (8) The lower limit of the confidence interval cannot be calculated if the number of observed infections equals zero; (9) No data are available from the state/territory for this reporting period; (10) The scores shown reflect fewer than 50 completed surveys; (11) There were discrepancies in the data collection process; (12) This measure does not apply to this hospital for this reporting period; (13) Results cannot be calculated for this reporting period; (14) The results for this state are combined with nearby states to protect confidentiality; Please refer to the User's Guide for a full explanation of data.

Measure	Cases	This Hosp.	State Avg.	U.S. Avg.
Time from ER Arrival to Admit. (minutes)[5]	-	-	220	274
Time from ER Arrival to Discharge (minutes)[5]	-	-	120	134
Time in ER Before Being Evaluated (minutes)[5]	-	-	23	26
Time to Pain Meds for Fractures (minutes)	27	31	47	57
Heart Attack Care				
Aspirin Given at Discharge[1,3]	-	-	100%	99%
Fibrinolytic Meds Within 30 Min. of Arrival[1,3]	-	-	50%	54%
PCI Within 90 Minutes of Arrival[3,7]	-	-	96%	96%
Statin Prescribed at Discharge[1,3]	-	-	99%	98%
Heart Failure Care				
ACE Inhibitor or ARB for LVSD[1]	-	-	97%	97%
Discharge Instructions Given	14	93%	92%	94%
Evaluation of LVS Function	16	100%	94%	99%
Medicare Spending				
Medicare Spending per Patient (ratio)	-	-	0.89	0.98
Pneumonia Care				
Appropriate Initial Antibiotic Given	19	95%	94%	95%
Blood Culture Timing	23	100%	97%	98%
Pregnancy and Delivery Care				
Newborn Deliveries Scheduled Early[5]	-	-	7%	6%
Preventive Care				
Immunization for Influenza[3]	42	100%	86%	90%
Immunization for Pneumonia[2,3]	146	97%	89%	92%
Stroke Care				
Anticoagulation Therapy for Atrial Fibrillation[1]	-	-	98%	95%
Antithrombotic Therapy Timing[1]	-	-	99%	98%
Assessed for Rehabilitation[1]	-	-	99%	97%
Discharged on Antithrombotic Therapy[1]	-	-	100%	99%
Discharged on Statin Medication[1]	-	-	94%	94%
Thrombolytic Therapy Timing[7]	-	-	67%	66%
Venous Thromboembolism Prophylaxis[1]	-	-	96%	94%
Written Stroke Educational Materials Given[1]	-	-	85%	88%
Surgical Care Improvement Project				
Appropriate Beta Blocker Usage[1]	-	-	98%	98%
Appropriate VTP Within 24 Hours	38	100%	98%	98%
Controlled Postoperative Blood Glucose[3,7]	-	-	96%	97%
Perioperative Temperature Management	52	100%	100%	100%
Prophylactic Antibiotic Selection	49	98%	99%	99%
Prophylactic Antibiotic Selection (Outpatient)[3]	18	100%	98%	98%
Prophylactic Antibiotic Stopped	49	100%	99%	98%
Prophylactic Antibiotic Timing	49	92%	99%	99%
Prophylactic Antibiotic Timing (Outpatient)[3]	18	94%	98%	98%
Urinary Catheter Removal	34	97%	99%	97%
Survey of Patients' Hospital Experiences				
Area Around Room 'Always' Quiet at Night	(a)	81%	60%	61%
Doctors 'Always' Communicated Well	(a)	89%	81%	82%
Home Recovery Information Given	(a)	91%	83%	85%
Hospital Given 9 or 10 on 10 Point Scale	(a)	79%	68%	71%
Meds 'Always' Explained Before Given	(a)	72%	63%	64%
Nurses 'Always' Communicated Well	(a)	81%	77%	79%
Pain 'Always' Well Controlled	(a)	72%	70%	71%
Room and Bathroom 'Always' Clean	(a)	79%	72%	73%
Timely Help 'Always' Received	(a)	82%	69%	68%
Would Definitely Recommend Hospital	(a)	75%	67%	71%
Use of Medical Imaging				
Cardiac Imaging Stress Test before Surgery[1]	-	-	4.9%	5.3%
Combination Abdominal CT Scan	222	5.0%	10.6%	10.5%
Combination Brain/Sinus CT Scan[1]	-	-	1.9%	2.7%
Combination Chest CT Scan	150	0.7%	2.4%	2.7%
Follow-up Mammogram/Ultrasound	339	8.6%	6.9%	8.8%
Lumbar Spine MRI for Low Back Pain[1]	-	-	41.5%	37.2%

Dahl Memorial Healthcare Assoc

215 Sandy St
Ekalaka, MT 59324
Phone: 406-775-8739
Fax: 406-775-6706
E-mail: dahl@midrivers.com
Type: Critical Access Hospitals
Emergency Services: Yes
Ownership: Voluntary non-profit - Private
Beds: 10

Measure	Cases	This Hosp.	State Avg.	U.S. Avg.
Blood Clot Prevention and Treatment				
Anticoagulation Overlap Therapy[7]	-	-	97%	93%
ICU Venous Thromboembolism Prophylaxis[7]	-	-	92%	92%
Incidence of Potentially Preventable VTE[7]	-	-	4%	10%
UFH with Dosages/Platelet Monitoring[7]	-	-	97%	97%
Venous Thromboembolism Prophylaxis[1]	-	-	83%	85%
Warfarin Therapy Discharge Instructions[7]	-	-	84%	75%
Chest Pain/Possible Heart Attack Care				
Aspirin Given Within 24 Hours of Arrival[5]	-	-	97%	96%
Fibrinolytic Meds Within 30 Min. of Arrival[5]	-	-	43%	58%
Average Time to ECG (minutes)[5]	-	-	10	7
Average Time to Transfer (minutes)[5]	-	-	78	60
Children's Asthma Care				
Received Home Management Plan of Care	-	-	-	88%
Received Reliever Medication	-	-	-	100%
Received Systemic Corticosteroids	-	-	-	100%
Emergency Department				
Admittance Decision Time (minutes)[5]	-	-	72	98
Head CT Results Within 45 Min. of Arrival[5]	-	-	26%	57%
Patients Who Left ER Before Being Seen[5]	-	-	2%	2%
Time from ER Arrival to Admit. (minutes)[5]	-	-	220	274
Time from ER Arrival to Discharge (minutes)[1,3]	-	-	120	134
Time in ER Before Being Evaluated (minutes)[1,3]	-	-	23	26
Time to Pain Meds for Fractures (minutes)[5]	-	-	47	57
Heart Attack Care				
Aspirin Given at Discharge[5]	-	-	100%	99%
Fibrinolytic Meds Within 30 Min. of Arrival[5]	-	-	50%	54%
PCI Within 90 Minutes of Arrival[5]	-	-	96%	96%
Statin Prescribed at Discharge[5]	-	-	99%	98%
Heart Failure Care				
ACE Inhibitor or ARB for LVSD[5]	-	-	97%	97%
Discharge Instructions Given[5]	-	-	92%	94%
Evaluation of LVS Function[5]	-	-	94%	99%
Medicare Spending				
Medicare Spending per Patient (ratio)	-	-	0.89	0.98
Pneumonia Care				
Appropriate Initial Antibiotic Given[5]	-	-	94%	95%
Blood Culture Timing[5]	-	-	97%	98%
Pregnancy and Delivery Care				
Newborn Deliveries Scheduled Early[5]	-	-	7%	6%
Preventive Care				
Immunization for Influenza[5]	-	-	86%	90%
Immunization for Pneumonia[5]	-	-	89%	92%
Stroke Care				
Anticoagulation Therapy for Atrial Fibrillation[5]	-	-	98%	95%
Antithrombotic Therapy Timing[5]	-	-	99%	98%
Assessed for Rehabilitation[5]	-	-	99%	97%
Discharged on Antithrombotic Therapy[5]	-	-	100%	99%
Discharged on Statin Medication[5]	-	-	94%	94%
Thrombolytic Therapy Timing[5]	-	-	67%	66%
Venous Thromboembolism Prophylaxis[5]	-	-	96%	94%
Written Stroke Educational Materials Given[5]	-	-	85%	88%
Surgical Care Improvement Project				
Appropriate Beta Blocker Usage[5]	-	-	98%	98%
Appropriate VTP Within 24 Hours[5]	-	-	98%	98%
Controlled Postoperative Blood Glucose[5]	-	-	96%	97%
Perioperative Temperature Management[5]	-	-	100%	100%
Prophylactic Antibiotic Selection[5]	-	-	99%	99%
Prophylactic Antibiotic Selection (Outpatient)[5]	-	-	98%	98%
Prophylactic Antibiotic Stopped[5]	-	-	99%	98%
Prophylactic Antibiotic Timing[5]	-	-	99%	99%
Prophylactic Antibiotic Timing (Outpatient)[5]	-	-	98%	98%
Urinary Catheter Removal[5]	-	-	99%	97%
Survey of Patients' Hospital Experiences				
Area Around Room 'Always' Quiet at Night[5]	-	-	60%	61%
Doctors 'Always' Communicated Well[5]	-	-	81%	82%
Home Recovery Information Given[5]	-	-	83%	85%
Hospital Given 9 or 10 on 10 Point Scale[5]	-	-	68%	71%
Meds 'Always' Explained Before Given[5]	-	-	63%	64%
Nurses 'Always' Communicated Well[5]	-	-	77%	79%
Pain 'Always' Well Controlled[5]	-	-	70%	71%
Room and Bathroom 'Always' Clean[5]	-	-	72%	73%
Timely Help 'Always' Received[5]	-	-	69%	68%
Would Definitely Recommend Hospital[5]	-	-	67%	71%
Use of Medical Imaging				
Cardiac Imaging Stress Test before Surgery[7]	-	-	4.9%	5.3%
Combination Abdominal CT Scan[7]	-	-	10.6%	10.5%
Combination Brain/Sinus CT Scan[7]	-	-	1.9%	2.7%
Combination Chest CT Scan[7]	-	-	2.4%	2.7%
Follow-up Mammogram/Ultrasound[7]	-	-	6.9%	8.8%
Lumbar Spine MRI for Low Back Pain[7]	-	-	41.5%	37.2%

Rosebud Health Care Center

383 N 17th Av
Phone: 406-346-2161
Forsyth, MT 59327
Type: Critical Access Hospitals
Emergency Services: Yes
Ownership: Voluntary non-profit - Private

Measure	Cases	This Hosp.	State Avg.	U.S. Avg.
Blood Clot Prevention and Treatment				
Anticoagulation Overlap Therapy[1,2]	-	-	97%	93%
ICU Venous Thromboembolism Prophylaxis[1,2]	-	-	92%	92%
Incidence of Potentially Preventable VTE[2,7]	-	-	4%	10%
UFH with Dosages/Platelet Monitoring[2,7]	-	-	97%	97%
Venous Thromboembolism Prophylaxis[2]	69	83%	83%	85%
Warfarin Therapy Discharge Instructions[2,7]	-	-	84%	75%
Chest Pain/Possible Heart Attack Care				
Aspirin Given Within 24 Hours of Arrival	-	-	97%	96%
Fibrinolytic Meds Within 30 Min. of Arrival	-	-	43%	58%
Average Time to ECG (minutes)	-	-	10	7
Average Time to Transfer (minutes)	-	-	78	60
Children's Asthma Care				
Received Home Management Plan of Care	-	-	-	88%
Received Reliever Medication	-	-	-	100%
Received Systemic Corticosteroids	-	-	-	100%
Emergency Department				
Admittance Decision Time (minutes)[5]	-	-	72	98
Head CT Results Within 45 Min. of Arrival	-	-	26%	57%
Patients Who Left ER Before Being Seen	-	-	2%	2%
Time from ER Arrival to Admit. (minutes)[5]	-	-	220	274
Time from ER Arrival to Discharge (minutes)	-	-	120	134
Time in ER Before Being Evaluated (minutes)	-	-	23	26
Time to Pain Meds for Fractures (minutes)	-	-	47	57
Heart Attack Care				
Aspirin Given at Discharge[5]	-	-	100%	99%
Fibrinolytic Meds Within 30 Min. of Arrival[5]	-	-	50%	54%
PCI Within 90 Minutes of Arrival[5]	-	-	96%	96%
Statin Prescribed at Discharge[5]	-	-	99%	98%
Heart Failure Care				
ACE Inhibitor or ARB for LVSD[1]	-	-	97%	97%
Discharge Instructions Given[1]	-	-	92%	94%
Evaluation of LVS Function[1]	-	-	94%	99%
Medicare Spending				
Medicare Spending per Patient (ratio)	-	-	0.89	0.98
Pneumonia Care				
Appropriate Initial Antibiotic Given[1]	-	-	94%	95%
Blood Culture Timing[1]	-	-	97%	98%
Pregnancy and Delivery Care				
Newborn Deliveries Scheduled Early[5]	-	-	7%	6%
Preventive Care				
Immunization for Influenza	70	90%	86%	90%
Immunization for Pneumonia	92	98%	89%	92%
Stroke Care				
Anticoagulation Therapy for Atrial Fibrillation[3,7]	-	-	98%	95%
Antithrombotic Therapy Timing[1,3]	-	-	99%	98%
Assessed for Rehabilitation[1,3]	-	-	99%	97%
Discharged on Antithrombotic Therapy[1,3]	-	-	100%	99%
Discharged on Statin Medication[1,3]	-	-	94%	94%
Thrombolytic Therapy Timing[3,7]	-	-	67%	66%
Venous Thromboembolism Prophylaxis[1,3]	-	-	96%	94%
Written Stroke Educational Materials Given[3,7]	-	-	85%	88%
Surgical Care Improvement Project				
Appropriate Beta Blocker Usage[5]	-	-	98%	98%
Appropriate VTP Within 24 Hours[5]	-	-	98%	98%
Controlled Postoperative Blood Glucose[5]	-	-	96%	97%
Perioperative Temperature Management[5]	-	-	100%	100%
Prophylactic Antibiotic Selection[5]	-	-	99%	99%
Prophylactic Antibiotic Selection (Outpatient)	-	-	98%	98%

NOTE: Hospital profiles are in alphabetical order by state, then city, then hospital within the city; Rankings exclude hospitals with less than 25 cases except for patient surveys which excludes hospitals with less than 100 cases; (a) 100-299 cases; (1) The number of cases/patients is too few to report; (2) Data submitted were based on a sample of cases/patients; (3) Results are based on a shorter time period than required; (4) Data suppressed by CMS for one or more quarters; (5) Results are not available for this reporting period; (6) Fewer than 100 patients completed the HCAHPS survey; (7) No cases met the criteria for this measure; (8) The lower limit of the confidence interval cannot be calculated if the number of observed infections equals zero; (9) No data are available from the state/territory for this reporting period; (10) The scores shown reflect fewer than 50 completed surveys; (11) There were discrepancies in the data collection process; (12) This measure does not apply to this hospital for this reporting period; (13) Results cannot be calculated for this reporting period; (14) The results for this state are combined with nearby states to protect confidentiality; Please refer to the User's Guide for a full explanation of data.

Measure	Cases	This Hosp.	State Avg.	U.S. Avg.
Prophylactic Antibiotic Stopped[5]	-	-	99%	98%
Prophylactic Antibiotic Timing[5]	-	-	99%	99%
Prophylactic Antibiotic Timing (Outpatient)	-	-	98%	98%
Urinary Catheter Removal[5]	-	-	99%	97%
Survey of Patients' Hospital Experiences				
Area Around Room 'Always' Quiet at Night[5]	-	-	60%	61%
Doctors 'Always' Communicated Well[5]	-	-	81%	82%
Home Recovery Information Given[5]	-	-	83%	85%
Hospital Given 9 or 10 on 10 Point Scale[5]	-	-	68%	71%
Meds 'Always' Explained Before Given[5]	-	-	63%	64%
Nurses 'Always' Communicated Well[5]	-	-	77%	79%
Pain 'Always' Well Controlled[5]	-	-	70%	71%
Room and Bathroom 'Always' Clean[5]	-	-	72%	73%
Timely Help 'Always' Received[5]	-	-	69%	68%
Would Definitely Recommend Hospital[5]	-	-	67%	71%
Use of Medical Imaging				
Cardiac Imaging Stress Test before Surgery	-	-	4.9%	5.3%
Combination Abdominal CT Scan	-	-	10.6%	10.5%
Combination Brain/Sinus CT Scan	-	-	1.9%	2.7%
Combination Chest CT Scan	-	-	2.4%	2.7%
Follow-up Mammogram/Ultrasound	-	-	6.9%	8.8%
Lumbar Spine MRI for Low Back Pain	-	-	41.5%	37.2%

Missouri River Medical Center

1501 Saint Charles St
Fort Benton, MT 59442
Phone: 406-622-3331
Fax: 406-622-5670
E-mail: mrmc@mtintouch.net
URL: www.mrmcfb.org
Type: Critical Access Hospitals
Emergency Services: Yes
Ownership: Govt - Hospital Dist/Auth
Beds: 52

Key Personnel:
Quality Assurance . . . . Wendy Brandt
Chief of Medical Staff . . . . Mark Buck, MD

Measure	Cases	This Hosp.	State Avg.	U.S. Avg.
Blood Clot Prevention and Treatment				
Anticoagulation Overlap Therapy[5]	-	-	97%	93%
ICU Venous Thromboembolism Prophylaxis[5]	-	-	92%	92%
Incidence of Potentially Preventable VTE[5]	-	-	4%	10%
UFH with Dosages/Platelet Monitoring[5]	-	-	97%	97%
Venous Thromboembolism Prophylaxis[5]	-	-	83%	85%
Warfarin Therapy Discharge Instructions[5]	-	-	84%	75%
Chest Pain/Possible Heart Attack Care				
Aspirin Given Within 24 Hours of Arrival	-	-	97%	96%
Fibrinolytic Meds Within 30 Min. of Arrival	-	-	43%	58%
Average Time to ECG (minutes)	-	-	10	7
Average Time to Transfer (minutes)	-	-	78	60
Children's Asthma Care				
Received Home Management Plan of Care	-	-	-	88%
Received Reliever Medication	-	-	-	100%
Received Systemic Corticosteroids	-	-	-	100%
Emergency Department				
Admittance Decision Time (minutes)[5]	-	-	72	98
Head CT Results Within 45 Min. of Arrival	-	-	26%	57%
Patients Who Left ER Before Being Seen	-	-	2%	2%
Time from ER Arrival to Admit. (minutes)[5]	-	-	220	274
Time from ER Arrival to Discharge (minutes)	-	-	120	134
Time in ER Before Being Evaluated (minutes)	-	-	23	26
Time to Pain Meds for Fractures (minutes)	-	-	47	57
Heart Attack Care				
Aspirin Given at Discharge[5]	-	-	100%	99%
Fibrinolytic Meds Within 30 Min. of Arrival[5]	-	-	50%	54%
PCI Within 90 Minutes of Arrival[5]	-	-	96%	96%
Statin Prescribed at Discharge[5]	-	-	99%	98%
Heart Failure Care				
ACE Inhibitor or ARB for LVSD[3,7]	-	-	97%	97%
Discharge Instructions Given[1,3]	-	-	92%	94%
Evaluation of LVS Function[1,3]	-	-	94%	99%
Medicare Spending				
Medicare Spending per Patient (ratio)	-	-	0.89	0.98
Pneumonia Care				
Appropriate Initial Antibiotic Given[1,3]	-	-	94%	95%
Blood Culture Timing[3,7]	-	-	97%	98%
Pregnancy and Delivery Care				
Newborn Deliveries Scheduled Early[5]	-	-	7%	6%
Preventive Care				
Immunization for Influenza[5]	-	-	86%	90%
Immunization for Pneumonia[5]	-	-	89%	92%
Stroke Care				
Anticoagulation Therapy for Atrial Fibrillation[3,7]	-	-	98%	95%
Antithrombotic Therapy Timing[3,7]	-	-	99%	98%
Assessed for Rehabilitation[3,7]	-	-	99%	97%
Discharged on Antithrombotic Therapy[3,7]	-	-	100%	99%
Discharged on Statin Medication[3,7]	-	-	94%	94%
Thrombolytic Therapy Timing[3,7]	-	-	67%	66%
Venous Thromboembolism Prophylaxis[3,7]	-	-	96%	94%
Written Stroke Educational Materials Given[3,7]	-	-	85%	88%
Surgical Care Improvement Project				
Appropriate Beta Blocker Usage[5]	-	-	98%	98%
Appropriate VTP Within 24 Hours[5]	-	-	98%	98%
Controlled Postoperative Blood Glucose[5]	-	-	96%	97%
Perioperative Temperature Management[5]	-	-	100%	100%
Prophylactic Antibiotic Selection[5]	-	-	99%	99%
Prophylactic Antibiotic Selection (Outpatient)	-	-	98%	98%
Prophylactic Antibiotic Stopped[5]	-	-	99%	98%
Prophylactic Antibiotic Timing[5]	-	-	99%	99%
Prophylactic Antibiotic Timing (Outpatient)	-	-	98%	98%
Urinary Catheter Removal[5]	-	-	99%	97%
Survey of Patients' Hospital Experiences				
Area Around Room 'Always' Quiet at Night[5]	-	-	60%	61%
Doctors 'Always' Communicated Well[5]	-	-	81%	82%
Home Recovery Information Given[5]	-	-	83%	85%
Hospital Given 9 or 10 on 10 Point Scale[5]	-	-	68%	71%
Meds 'Always' Explained Before Given[5]	-	-	63%	64%
Nurses 'Always' Communicated Well[5]	-	-	77%	79%
Pain 'Always' Well Controlled[5]	-	-	70%	71%
Room and Bathroom 'Always' Clean[5]	-	-	72%	73%
Timely Help 'Always' Received[5]	-	-	69%	68%
Would Definitely Recommend Hospital[5]	-	-	67%	71%
Use of Medical Imaging				
Cardiac Imaging Stress Test before Surgery	-	-	4.9%	5.3%
Combination Abdominal CT Scan	-	-	10.6%	10.5%
Combination Brain/Sinus CT Scan	-	-	1.9%	2.7%
Combination Chest CT Scan	-	-	2.4%	2.7%
Follow-up Mammogram/Ultrasound	-	-	6.9%	8.8%
Lumbar Spine MRI for Low Back Pain	-	-	41.5%	37.2%

VA Montana Healthcare System

1892 Williams Street
Fort Harrison, MT 59636
Phone: 406-447-7900
Fax: 406-447-7916
URL: www.va.gov
Type: Acute Care - VA
Emergency Services: No
Ownership: Government Federal
Beds: 50

Key Personnel:
Quality Assurance . . . . Maryann Hamman
Chief of Medical Staff . . . . Jose D. Riojas
CEO/President . . . . Joseph M Underkofler

Measure	Cases	This Hosp.	State Avg.	U.S. Avg.
Blood Clot Prevention and Treatment				
Anticoagulation Overlap Therapy	-	-	97%	93%
ICU Venous Thromboembolism Prophylaxis	-	-	92%	92%
Incidence of Potentially Preventable VTE	-	-	4%	10%
UFH with Dosages/Platelet Monitoring	-	-	97%	97%
Venous Thromboembolism Prophylaxis	-	-	83%	85%
Warfarin Therapy Discharge Instructions	-	-	84%	75%
Chest Pain/Possible Heart Attack Care				
Aspirin Given Within 24 Hours of Arrival	-	-	97%	96%
Fibrinolytic Meds Within 30 Min. of Arrival	-	-	43%	58%
Average Time to ECG (minutes)	-	-	10	7
Average Time to Transfer (minutes)	-	-	78	60
Children's Asthma Care				
Received Home Management Plan of Care	-	-	-	88%
Received Reliever Medication	-	-	-	100%
Received Systemic Corticosteroids	-	-	-	100%
Emergency Department				
Admittance Decision Time (minutes)	-	-	72	98
Head CT Results Within 45 Min. of Arrival	-	-	26%	57%
Patients Who Left ER Before Being Seen	-	-	2%	2%
Time from ER Arrival to Admit. (minutes)	-	-	220	274
Time from ER Arrival to Discharge (minutes)	-	-	120	134
Time in ER Before Being Evaluated (minutes)	-	-	23	26
Time to Pain Meds for Fractures (minutes)	-	-	47	57
Heart Attack Care				
Aspirin Given at Discharge[5]	-	-	100%	99%
Fibrinolytic Meds Within 30 Min. of Arrival[5]	-	-	50%	54%
PCI Within 90 Minutes of Arrival[5]	-	-	96%	96%
Statin Prescribed at Discharge[5]	-	-	99%	98%
Heart Failure Care				
ACE Inhibitor or ARB for LVSD[1]	16	100%	97%	97%
Discharge Instructions Given	42	100%	92%	94%
Evaluation of LVS Function	43	98%	94%	99%
Medicare Spending				
Medicare Spending per Patient (ratio)	-	-	0.89	0.98
Pneumonia Care				
Appropriate Initial Antibiotic Given	33	97%	94%	95%
Blood Culture Timing	41	100%	97%	98%
Pregnancy and Delivery Care				
Newborn Deliveries Scheduled Early	-	-	7%	6%
Preventive Care				
Immunization for Influenza[5]	-	-	86%	90%
Immunization for Pneumonia[5]	-	-	89%	92%
Stroke Care				
Anticoagulation Therapy for Atrial Fibrillation	-	-	98%	95%
Antithrombotic Therapy Timing	-	-	99%	98%
Assessed for Rehabilitation	-	-	99%	97%
Discharged on Antithrombotic Therapy	-	-	100%	99%
Discharged on Statin Medication	-	-	94%	94%
Thrombolytic Therapy Timing	-	-	67%	66%
Venous Thromboembolism Prophylaxis	-	-	96%	94%
Written Stroke Educational Materials Given	-	-	85%	88%
Surgical Care Improvement Project				
Appropriate Beta Blocker Usage[2]	26	96%	98%	98%
Appropriate VTP Within 24 Hours[2]	97	94%	98%	98%
Controlled Postoperative Blood Glucose[5]	-	-	96%	97%
Perioperative Temperature Management[2]	107	100%	100%	100%
Prophylactic Antibiotic Selection	74	100%	99%	99%
Prophylactic Antibiotic Selection (Outpatient)	-	-	98%	98%
Prophylactic Antibiotic Stopped	73	97%	99%	98%
Prophylactic Antibiotic Timing	74	95%	99%	99%
Prophylactic Antibiotic Timing (Outpatient)	-	-	98%	98%
Urinary Catheter Removal[2]	47	94%	99%	97%
Survey of Patients' Hospital Experiences				
Area Around Room 'Always' Quiet at Night	-	-	60%	61%
Doctors 'Always' Communicated Well	-	-	81%	82%
Home Recovery Information Given	-	-	83%	85%
Hospital Given 9 or 10 on 10 Point Scale	-	-	68%	71%
Meds 'Always' Explained Before Given	-	-	63%	64%
Nurses 'Always' Communicated Well	-	-	77%	79%
Pain 'Always' Well Controlled	-	-	70%	71%
Room and Bathroom 'Always' Clean	-	-	72%	73%
Timely Help 'Always' Received	-	-	69%	68%
Would Definitely Recommend Hospital	-	-	67%	71%
Use of Medical Imaging				
Cardiac Imaging Stress Test before Surgery	-	-	4.9%	5.3%
Combination Abdominal CT Scan	-	-	10.6%	10.5%
Combination Brain/Sinus CT Scan	-	-	1.9%	2.7%
Combination Chest CT Scan	-	-	2.4%	2.7%
Follow-up Mammogram/Ultrasound	-	-	6.9%	8.8%
Lumbar Spine MRI for Low Back Pain	-	-	41.5%	37.2%

Frances Mahon Deaconess Hospital

621 3rd Saint S
Glasgow, MT 59230
Phone: 406-228-3500
Fax: 406-228-3535
E-mail: fmdh@fmdh.org
URL: www.fmdh.org/contact
Type: Critical Access Hospitals
Emergency Services: Yes
Ownership: Voluntary non-profit - Private
Beds: 25

Key Personnel:
Chief of Medical Staff . . . . Gordon Bell, MD
Cardiac Laboratory . . . . Bev Falcon
President . . . . Pat Gunderson
CEO/President . . . . Randall Holom, CEO

NOTE: Hospital profiles are in alphabetical order by state, then city, then hospital within the city; Rankings exclude hospitals with less than 25 cases except for patient surveys which excludes hospitals with less than 100 cases; (a) 100-299 cases; (1) The number of cases/patients is too few to report; (2) Data submitted were based on a sample of cases/patients; (3) Results are based on a shorter time period than required; (4) Data suppressed by CMS for one or more quarters; (5) Results are not available for this reporting period; (6) Fewer than 100 patients completed the HCAHPS survey; (7) No cases met the criteria for this measure; (8) The lower limit of the confidence interval cannot be calculated if the number of observed infections equals zero; (9) No data are available from the state/territory for this reporting period; (10) The scores shown reflect fewer than 50 completed surveys; (11) There were discrepancies in the data collection process; (12) This measure does not apply to this hospital for this reporting period; (13) Results cannot be calculated for this reporting period; (14) The results for this state are combined with nearby states to protect confidentiality; Please refer to the User's Guide for a full explanation of data.

Operating Room. . . . . Jill Meiers, RN
Infection Control. . . . . Saralyn Potter
Radiology. . . . . Walter Smith, MD
Quality Assurance . . . . Shelly Vanburen

Measure	Cases	This Hosp.	State Avg.	U.S. Avg.
Blood Clot Prevention and Treatment				
Anticoagulation Overlap Therapy[5]	-	-	97%	93%
ICU Venous Thromboembolism Prophylaxis[5]	-	-	92%	92%
Incidence of Potentially Preventable VTE[5]	-	-	4%	10%
UFH with Dosages/Platelet Monitoring[5]	-	-	97%	97%
Venous Thromboembolism Prophylaxis[5]	-	-	83%	85%
Warfarin Therapy Discharge Instructions[5]	-	-	84%	75%
Chest Pain/Possible Heart Attack Care				
Aspirin Given Within 24 Hours of Arrival[1,3]	-	-	97%	96%
Fibrinolytic Meds Within 30 Min. of Arrival[1,3]	-	-	43%	58%
Average Time to ECG (minutes)[1,3]	-	-	10	7
Average Time to Transfer (minutes)[3,7]	-	-	78	60
Children's Asthma Care				
Received Home Management Plan of Care	-	-	-	88%
Received Reliever Medication	-	-	-	100%
Received Systemic Corticosteroids	-	-	-	100%
Emergency Department				
Admittance Decision Time (minutes)[5]	-	-	72	98
Head CT Results Within 45 Min. of Arrival[5]	-	-	26%	57%
Patients Who Left ER Before Being Seen[5]	-	-	2%	2%
Time from ER Arrival to Admit. (minutes)[5]	-	-	220	274
Time from ER Arrival to Discharge (minutes)[5]	-	-	120	134
Time in ER Before Being Evaluated (minutes)[5]	-	-	23	26
Time to Pain Meds for Fractures (minutes)[5]	-	-	47	57
Heart Attack Care				
Aspirin Given at Discharge[1,3]	-	-	100%	99%
Fibrinolytic Meds Within 30 Min. of Arrival[3,7]	-	-	50%	54%
PCI Within 90 Minutes of Arrival[3,7]	-	-	96%	96%
Statin Prescribed at Discharge[1,3]	-	-	99%	98%
Heart Failure Care				
ACE Inhibitor or ARB for LVSD[1]	-	-	97%	97%
Discharge Instructions Given[1]	-	-	92%	94%
Evaluation of LVS Function[1]	-	-	94%	99%
Medicare Spending				
Medicare Spending per Patient (ratio)	-	-	0.89	0.98
Pneumonia Care				
Appropriate Initial Antibiotic Given	28	93%	94%	95%
Blood Culture Timing[1]	-	-	97%	98%
Pregnancy and Delivery Care				
Newborn Deliveries Scheduled Early[5]	-	-	7%	6%
Preventive Care				
Immunization for Influenza[5]	-	-	86%	90%
Immunization for Pneumonia[5]	-	-	89%	92%
Stroke Care				
Anticoagulation Therapy for Atrial Fibrillation[3,7]	-	-	98%	95%
Antithrombotic Therapy Timing[3,7]	-	-	99%	98%
Assessed for Rehabilitation[3,7]	-	-	99%	97%
Discharged on Antithrombotic Therapy[3,7]	-	-	100%	99%
Discharged on Statin Medication[3,7]	-	-	94%	94%
Thrombolytic Therapy Timing[3,7]	-	-	67%	66%
Venous Thromboembolism Prophylaxis[3,7]	-	-	96%	94%
Written Stroke Educational Materials Given[3,7]	-	-	85%	88%
Surgical Care Improvement Project				
Appropriate Beta Blocker Usage[2]	18	94%	98%	98%
Appropriate VTP Within 24 Hours[2]	78	99%	98%	98%
Controlled Postoperative Blood Glucose[2,7]	-	-	96%	97%
Perioperative Temperature Management[2]	81	100%	100%	100%
Prophylactic Antibiotic Selection[2]	81	98%	99%	99%
Prophylactic Antibiotic Selection (Outpatient)[5]	-	-	98%	98%
Prophylactic Antibiotic Stopped[2]	81	100%	99%	98%
Prophylactic Antibiotic Timing[2]	81	99%	99%	99%
Prophylactic Antibiotic Timing (Outpatient)[5]	-	-	98%	98%
Urinary Catheter Removal[2]	41	100%	99%	97%
Survey of Patients' Hospital Experiences				
Area Around Room 'Always' Quiet at Night	(a)	64%	60%	61%
Doctors 'Always' Communicated Well	(a)	84%	81%	82%
Home Recovery Information Given	(a)	87%	83%	85%
Hospital Given 9 or 10 on 10 Point Scale	(a)	69%	68%	71%
Meds 'Always' Explained Before Given	(a)	71%	63%	64%
Nurses 'Always' Communicated Well	(a)	81%	77%	79%
Pain 'Always' Well Controlled	(a)	67%	70%	71%
Room and Bathroom 'Always' Clean	(a)	80%	72%	73%
Timely Help 'Always' Received	(a)	73%	69%	68%
Would Definitely Recommend Hospital	(a)	76%	67%	71%
Use of Medical Imaging				
Cardiac Imaging Stress Test before Surgery	61	4.9%	4.9%	5.3%
Combination Abdominal CT Scan	105	61.9%	10.6%	10.5%
Combination Brain/Sinus CT Scan[1]	-	-	1.9%	2.7%
Combination Chest CT Scan	67	13.4%	2.4%	2.7%
Follow-up Mammogram/Ultrasound	262	13.7%	6.9%	8.8%
Lumbar Spine MRI for Low Back Pain	59	61.0%	41.5%	37.2%

Glendive Medical Center

202 Prospect Dr
Glendive, MT 59330
Phone: 406-345-3306
Fax: 406-345-3318
URL: www.gmc.org
Type: Critical Access Hospitals
Emergency Services: Yes
Ownership: Voluntary non-profit - Private
Beds: 25

Key Personnel:
Operating Room. . . . . Shawna Dorwart
Radiology. . . . . Deborah Dougless
CEO/President. . . . . Scott A Duke, CEO
Chief of Medical Staff . . . . Arthur K Fink, DO
Infection Control. . . . . Jamie Heyen
Quality Assurance . . . . Mona Humphry
Pediatric Ambulatory Care . . . . . . Sonja Samsoondar, MD
Pediatric In-Patient Care . . . . Sonja Samsoondar, MD

Measure	Cases	This Hosp.	State Avg.	U.S. Avg.
Blood Clot Prevention and Treatment				
Anticoagulation Overlap Therapy[5]	-	-	97%	93%
ICU Venous Thromboembolism Prophylaxis[5]	-	-	92%	92%
Incidence of Potentially Preventable VTE[5]	-	-	4%	10%
UFH with Dosages/Platelet Monitoring[5]	-	-	97%	97%
Venous Thromboembolism Prophylaxis[5]	-	-	83%	85%
Warfarin Therapy Discharge Instructions[5]	-	-	84%	75%
Chest Pain/Possible Heart Attack Care				
Aspirin Given Within 24 Hours of Arrival	-	-	97%	96%
Fibrinolytic Meds Within 30 Min. of Arrival	-	-	43%	58%
Average Time to ECG (minutes)	-	-	10	7
Average Time to Transfer (minutes)	-	-	78	60
Children's Asthma Care				
Received Home Management Plan of Care	-	-	-	88%
Received Reliever Medication	-	-	-	100%
Received Systemic Corticosteroids	-	-	-	100%
Emergency Department				
Admittance Decision Time (minutes)[5]	-	-	72	98
Head CT Results Within 45 Min. of Arrival	-	-	26%	57%
Patients Who Left ER Before Being Seen	-	-	2%	2%
Time from ER Arrival to Admit. (minutes)[5]	-	-	220	274
Time from ER Arrival to Discharge (minutes)	-	-	120	134
Time in ER Before Being Evaluated (minutes)	-	-	23	26
Time to Pain Meds for Fractures (minutes)	-	-	47	57
Heart Attack Care				
Aspirin Given at Discharge[1,3]	-	-	100%	99%
Fibrinolytic Meds Within 30 Min. of Arrival[3,7]	-	-	50%	54%
PCI Within 90 Minutes of Arrival[3,7]	-	-	96%	96%
Statin Prescribed at Discharge[1,3]	-	-	99%	98%
Heart Failure Care				
ACE Inhibitor or ARB for LVSD[7]	-	-	97%	97%
Discharge Instructions Given	14	36%	92%	94%
Evaluation of LVS Function	19	11%	94%	99%
Medicare Spending				
Medicare Spending per Patient (ratio)	-	-	0.89	0.98
Pneumonia Care				
Appropriate Initial Antibiotic Given[2]	21	81%	94%	95%
Blood Culture Timing[2]	22	64%	97%	98%
Pregnancy and Delivery Care				
Newborn Deliveries Scheduled Early[5]	-	-	7%	6%
Preventive Care				
Immunization for Influenza[5]	-	-	86%	90%
Immunization for Pneumonia[5]	-	-	89%	92%
Stroke Care				
Anticoagulation Therapy for Atrial Fibrillation[5]	-	-	98%	95%
Antithrombotic Therapy Timing[5]	-	-	99%	98%
Assessed for Rehabilitation[5]	-	-	99%	97%
Discharged on Antithrombotic Therapy[5]	-	-	100%	99%
Discharged on Statin Medication[5]	-	-	94%	94%
Thrombolytic Therapy Timing[5]	-	-	67%	66%
Venous Thromboembolism Prophylaxis[5]	-	-	96%	94%
Written Stroke Educational Materials Given[5]	-	-	85%	88%
Surgical Care Improvement Project				
Appropriate Beta Blocker Usage[1]	-	-	98%	98%
Appropriate VTP Within 24 Hours[1]	-	-	98%	98%
Controlled Postoperative Blood Glucose[7]	-	-	96%	97%
Perioperative Temperature Management[1]	-	-	100%	100%
Prophylactic Antibiotic Selection[1]	-	-	99%	99%
Prophylactic Antibiotic Selection (Outpatient)	-	-	98%	98%
Prophylactic Antibiotic Stopped[1]	-	-	99%	98%
Prophylactic Antibiotic Timing[1]	-	-	99%	99%
Prophylactic Antibiotic Timing (Outpatient)	-	-	98%	98%
Urinary Catheter Removal[1]	-	-	99%	97%
Survey of Patients' Hospital Experiences				
Area Around Room 'Always' Quiet at Night[6]	<100	55%	60%	61%
Doctors 'Always' Communicated Well[6]	<100	68%	81%	82%
Home Recovery Information Given[6]	<100	81%	83%	85%
Hospital Given 9 or 10 on 10 Point Scale[6]	<100	55%	68%	71%
Meds 'Always' Explained Before Given[6]	<100	62%	63%	64%
Nurses 'Always' Communicated Well[6]	<100	75%	77%	79%
Pain 'Always' Well Controlled[6]	<100	68%	70%	71%
Room and Bathroom 'Always' Clean[6]	<100	73%	72%	73%
Timely Help 'Always' Received[6]	<100	54%	69%	68%
Would Definitely Recommend Hospital[6]	<100	49%	67%	71%
Use of Medical Imaging				
Cardiac Imaging Stress Test before Surgery	-	-	4.9%	5.3%
Combination Abdominal CT Scan	-	-	10.6%	10.5%
Combination Brain/Sinus CT Scan	-	-	1.9%	2.7%
Combination Chest CT Scan	-	-	2.4%	2.7%
Follow-up Mammogram/Ultrasound	-	-	6.9%	8.8%
Lumbar Spine MRI for Low Back Pain	-	-	41.5%	37.2%

Benefis Hospitals

1101 26th Saint S
Great Falls, MT 59405
Phone: 406-455-5000
Fax: 406-455-4995
E-mail: benefis@benefis.org
URL: www.benefis.org
Type: Acute Care Hospitals
Emergency Services: Yes
Ownership: Voluntary non-profit - Private
Beds: 326

Key Personnel:
Chief of Medical Staff . . . . Paul Dolan, MD
CEO/President. . . . . John Goodnow
Chair/CEO . . . . Susan Humble
Quality Assurance . . . . Deb McCracken

Measure	Cases	This Hosp.	State Avg.	U.S. Avg.
Blood Clot Prevention and Treatment				
Anticoagulation Overlap Therapy[2]	63	100%	97%	93%
ICU Venous Thromboembolism Prophylaxis[2]	47	100%	92%	92%
Incidence of Potentially Preventable VTE[2]	16	0%	4%	10%
UFH with Dosages/Platelet Monitoring[2]	24	100%	97%	97%
Venous Thromboembolism Prophylaxis[2]	344	97%	83%	85%
Warfarin Therapy Discharge Instructions[2]	52	90%	84%	75%
Chest Pain/Possible Heart Attack Care				
Aspirin Given Within 24 Hours of Arrival[5]	-	-	97%	96%
Fibrinolytic Meds Within 30 Min. of Arrival[5]	-	-	43%	58%
Average Time to ECG (minutes)[5]	-	-	10	7
Average Time to Transfer (minutes)[5]	-	-	78	60
Children's Asthma Care				
Received Home Management Plan of Care	-	-	-	88%
Received Reliever Medication	-	-	-	100%
Received Systemic Corticosteroids	-	-	-	100%
Emergency Department				
Admittance Decision Time (minutes)[2]	598	84	72	98
Head CT Results Within 45 Min. of Arrival[5]	-	-	26%	57%
Patients Who Left ER Before Being Seen	35,949	3%	2%	2%
Time from ER Arrival to Admit. (minutes)[2]	598	273	220	274

NOTE: Hospital profiles are in alphabetical order by state, then city, then hospital within the city; Rankings exclude hospitals with less than 25 cases except for patient surveys which excludes hospitals with less than 100 cases; (a) 100-299 cases; (1) The number of cases/patients is too few to report; (2) Data submitted were based on a sample of cases/patients; (3) Results are based on a shorter time period than required; (4) Data suppressed by CMS for one or more quarters; (5) Results are not available for this reporting period; (6) Fewer than 100 patients completed the HCAHPS survey; (7) No cases met the criteria for this measure; (8) The lower limit of the confidence interval cannot be calculated if the number of observed infections equals zero; (9) No data are available from the state/territory for this reporting period; (10) The scores shown reflect fewer than 50 completed surveys; (11) There were discrepancies in the data collection process; (12) This measure does not apply to this hospital for this reporting period; (13) Results cannot be calculated for this reporting period; (14) The results for this state are combined with nearby states to protect confidentiality; Please refer to the User's Guide for a full explanation of data.

Measure	Cases	This Hosp.	State Avg.	U.S. Avg.
Time from ER Arrival to Discharge (minutes)	394	132	120	134
Time in ER Before Being Evaluated (minutes)	382	41	23	26
Time to Pain Meds for Fractures (minutes)	94	63	47	57
Heart Attack Care				
Aspirin Given at Discharge	189	100%	100%	99%
Fibrinolytic Meds Within 30 Min. of Arrival[7]	-	-	50%	54%
PCI Within 90 Minutes of Arrival	41	98%	96%	96%
Statin Prescribed at Discharge	182	99%	99%	98%
Heart Failure Care				
ACE Inhibitor or ARB for LVSD	50	92%	97%	97%
Discharge Instructions Given	180	98%	92%	94%
Evaluation of LVS Function	220	98%	94%	99%
Medicare Spending				
Medicare Spending per Patient (ratio)	-	0.96	0.89	0.98
Pneumonia Care				
Appropriate Initial Antibiotic Given	151	99%	94%	95%
Blood Culture Timing	229	98%	97%	98%
Pregnancy and Delivery Care				
Newborn Deliveries Scheduled Early[2]	27	4%	7%	6%
Preventive Care				
Immunization for Influenza[2]	535	93%	86%	90%
Immunization for Pneumonia[2]	613	89%	89%	92%
Stroke Care				
Anticoagulation Therapy for Atrial Fibrillation[2]	12	100%	98%	95%
Antithrombotic Therapy Timing[2]	58	98%	99%	98%
Assessed for Rehabilitation[2]	77	95%	99%	97%
Discharged on Antithrombotic Therapy[2]	66	98%	100%	99%
Discharged on Statin Medication[2]	54	96%	94%	94%
Thrombolytic Therapy Timing[1,2]	-	-	67%	66%
Venous Thromboembolism Prophylaxis[2]	81	100%	96%	94%
Written Stroke Educational Materials Given[2]	40	88%	85%	88%
Surgical Care Improvement Project				
Appropriate Beta Blocker Usage[2]	215	97%	98%	98%
Appropriate VTP Within 24 Hours[2]	394	95%	98%	98%
Controlled Postoperative Blood Glucose[2]	116	94%	96%	97%
Perioperative Temperature Management[2]	486	100%	100%	100%
Prophylactic Antibiotic Selection[2]	404	99%	99%	99%
Prophylactic Antibiotic Selection (Outpatient)	472	99%	98%	98%
Prophylactic Antibiotic Stopped[2]	383	98%	99%	98%
Prophylactic Antibiotic Timing[2]	406	100%	99%	99%
Prophylactic Antibiotic Timing (Outpatient)	471	99%	98%	98%
Urinary Catheter Removal[2]	448	97%	99%	97%
Survey of Patients' Hospital Experiences				
Area Around Room 'Always' Quiet at Night	300+	56%	60%	61%
Doctors 'Always' Communicated Well	300+	74%	81%	82%
Home Recovery Information Given	300+	80%	83%	85%
Hospital Given 9 or 10 on 10 Point Scale	300+	61%	68%	71%
Meds 'Always' Explained Before Given	300+	60%	63%	64%
Nurses 'Always' Communicated Well	300+	71%	77%	79%
Pain 'Always' Well Controlled	300+	69%	70%	71%
Room and Bathroom 'Always' Clean	300+	70%	72%	73%
Timely Help 'Always' Received	300+	61%	69%	68%
Would Definitely Recommend Hospital	300+	61%	67%	71%
Use of Medical Imaging				
Cardiac Imaging Stress Test before Surgery	556	5.2%	4.9%	5.3%
Combination Abdominal CT Scan	899	5.2%	10.6%	10.5%
Combination Brain/Sinus CT Scan[1]	-	-	1.9%	2.7%
Combination Chest CT Scan	897	0.4%	2.4%	2.7%
Follow-up Mammogram/Ultrasound	1,291	8.8%	6.9%	8.8%
Lumbar Spine MRI for Low Back Pain	146	40.4%	41.5%	37.2%

Great Falls Clinic Medical Center

1411 9th Saint S
Great Falls, MT 59405
Phone: 406-216-8000
URL: www.gfclinic.com
Type: Acute Care Hospitals
Emergency Services: No
Ownership: Proprietary

Measure	Cases	This Hosp.	State Avg.	U.S. Avg.
Blood Clot Prevention and Treatment				
Anticoagulation Overlap Therapy[1]	-	-	97%	93%
ICU Venous Thromboembolism Prophylaxis[7]	-	-	92%	92%
Incidence of Potentially Preventable VTE[1]	-	-	4%	10%
UFH with Dosages/Platelet Monitoring[1]	-	-	97%	97%
Venous Thromboembolism Prophylaxis	146	85%	83%	85%
Warfarin Therapy Discharge Instructions[1]	-	-	84%	75%
Chest Pain/Possible Heart Attack Care				
Aspirin Given Within 24 Hours of Arrival[5]	-	-	97%	96%
Fibrinolytic Meds Within 30 Min. of Arrival[5]	-	-	43%	58%
Average Time to ECG (minutes)[5]	-	-	10	7
Average Time to Transfer (minutes)[5]	-	-	78	60
Children's Asthma Care				
Received Home Management Plan of Care	-	-	-	88%
Received Reliever Medication	-	-	-	100%
Received Systemic Corticosteroids	-	-	-	100%
Emergency Department				
Admittance Decision Time (minutes)[7]	-	-	72	98
Head CT Results Within 45 Min. of Arrival[5]	-	-	26%	57%
Patients Who Left ER Before Being Seen[5]	-	-	2%	2%
Time from ER Arrival to Admit. (minutes)[7]	-	-	220	274
Time from ER Arrival to Discharge (minutes)[5]	-	-	120	134
Time in ER Before Being Evaluated (minutes)[5]	-	-	23	26
Time to Pain Meds for Fractures (minutes)[5]	-	-	47	57
Heart Attack Care				
Aspirin Given at Discharge[5]	-	-	100%	99%
Fibrinolytic Meds Within 30 Min. of Arrival[5]	-	-	50%	54%
PCI Within 90 Minutes of Arrival[5]	-	-	96%	96%
Statin Prescribed at Discharge[5]	-	-	99%	98%
Heart Failure Care				
ACE Inhibitor or ARB for LVSD[5]	-	-	97%	97%
Discharge Instructions Given[5]	-	-	92%	94%
Evaluation of LVS Function[5]	-	-	94%	99%
Medicare Spending				
Medicare Spending per Patient (ratio)	-	0.85	0.89	0.98
Pneumonia Care				
Appropriate Initial Antibiotic Given[1,3]	-	-	94%	95%
Blood Culture Timing[3,7]	-	-	97%	98%
Pregnancy and Delivery Care				
Newborn Deliveries Scheduled Early[7]	-	-	7%	6%
Preventive Care				
Immunization for Influenza	290	76%	86%	90%
Immunization for Pneumonia	335	88%	89%	92%
Stroke Care				
Anticoagulation Therapy for Atrial Fibrillation[5]	-	-	98%	95%
Antithrombotic Therapy Timing[5]	-	-	99%	98%
Assessed for Rehabilitation[5]	-	-	99%	97%
Discharged on Antithrombotic Therapy[5]	-	-	100%	99%
Discharged on Statin Medication[5]	-	-	94%	94%
Thrombolytic Therapy Timing[5]	-	-	67%	66%
Venous Thromboembolism Prophylaxis[5]	-	-	96%	94%
Written Stroke Educational Materials Given[5]	-	-	85%	88%
Surgical Care Improvement Project				
Appropriate Beta Blocker Usage	83	94%	98%	98%
Appropriate VTP Within 24 Hours	265	99%	98%	98%
Controlled Postoperative Blood Glucose[7]	-	-	96%	97%
Perioperative Temperature Management	297	100%	100%	100%
Prophylactic Antibiotic Selection	254	100%	99%	99%
Prophylactic Antibiotic Selection (Outpatient)	38	97%	98%	98%
Prophylactic Antibiotic Stopped	252	98%	99%	98%
Prophylactic Antibiotic Timing	254	98%	99%	99%
Prophylactic Antibiotic Timing (Outpatient)	38	97%	98%	98%
Urinary Catheter Removal	257	98%	99%	97%
Survey of Patients' Hospital Experiences				
Area Around Room 'Always' Quiet at Night	(a)	78%	60%	61%
Doctors 'Always' Communicated Well	(a)	88%	81%	82%
Home Recovery Information Given	(a)	91%	83%	85%
Hospital Given 9 or 10 on 10 Point Scale	(a)	84%	68%	71%
Meds 'Always' Explained Before Given	(a)	74%	63%	64%
Nurses 'Always' Communicated Well	(a)	82%	77%	79%
Pain 'Always' Well Controlled	(a)	78%	70%	71%
Room and Bathroom 'Always' Clean	(a)	79%	72%	73%
Timely Help 'Always' Received	(a)	84%	69%	68%
Would Definitely Recommend Hospital	(a)	87%	67%	71%
Use of Medical Imaging				
Cardiac Imaging Stress Test before Surgery[7]	-	-	4.9%	5.3%
Combination Abdominal CT Scan[1]	-	-	10.6%	10.5%
Combination Brain/Sinus CT Scan[1]	-	-	1.9%	2.7%
Combination Chest CT Scan[7]	-	-	2.4%	2.7%
Follow-up Mammogram/Ultrasound[7]	-	-	6.9%	8.8%
Lumbar Spine MRI for Low Back Pain[1]	-	-	41.5%	37.2%

Marcus Daly Memorial Hospital

1200 Westwood Dr
Hamilton, MT 59840
Phone: 406-375-4408
Fax: 406-363-6536
E-mail: info@mdmh.org
URL: www.mdmh.org
Type: Critical Access Hospitals
Emergency Services: Yes
Ownership: Voluntary non-profit - Private
Beds: 48

Key Personnel:

Quality Assurance . . . . John Bargus
CEO . . . . John Bartos
CEO/President . . . . John Bartos
Emergency Room . . . . James Hansen, MD
Chief of Medical Staff . . . . Brian Kelleher, MD, MHA
Chairman/CEO . . . . Don Lodmell, PhD
Radiology . . . . Lance Pysher
President . . . . Bill Rummel

Measure	Cases	This Hosp.	State Avg.	U.S. Avg.
Blood Clot Prevention and Treatment				
Anticoagulation Overlap Therapy[5]	-	-	97%	93%
ICU Venous Thromboembolism Prophylaxis[5]	-	-	92%	92%
Incidence of Potentially Preventable VTE[5]	-	-	4%	10%
UFH with Dosages/Platelet Monitoring[5]	-	-	97%	97%
Venous Thromboembolism Prophylaxis[5]	-	-	83%	85%
Warfarin Therapy Discharge Instructions[5]	-	-	84%	75%
Chest Pain/Possible Heart Attack Care				
Aspirin Given Within 24 Hours of Arrival	-	-	97%	96%
Fibrinolytic Meds Within 30 Min. of Arrival	-	-	43%	58%
Average Time to ECG (minutes)	-	-	10	7
Average Time to Transfer (minutes)	-	-	78	60
Children's Asthma Care				
Received Home Management Plan of Care	-	-	-	88%
Received Reliever Medication	-	-	-	100%
Received Systemic Corticosteroids	-	-	-	100%
Emergency Department				
Admittance Decision Time (minutes)[5]	-	-	72	98
Head CT Results Within 45 Min. of Arrival	-	-	26%	57%
Patients Who Left ER Before Being Seen	-	-	2%	2%
Time from ER Arrival to Admit. (minutes)[5]	-	-	220	274
Time from ER Arrival to Discharge (minutes)	-	-	120	134
Time in ER Before Being Evaluated (minutes)	-	-	23	26
Time to Pain Meds for Fractures (minutes)	-	-	47	57
Heart Attack Care				
Aspirin Given at Discharge[1]	-	-	100%	99%
Fibrinolytic Meds Within 30 Min. of Arrival[7]	-	-	50%	54%
PCI Within 90 Minutes of Arrival[3,7]	-	-	96%	96%
Statin Prescribed at Discharge[1]	-	-	99%	98%
Heart Failure Care				
ACE Inhibitor or ARB for LVSD	12	100%	97%	97%
Discharge Instructions Given	41	93%	92%	94%
Evaluation of LVS Function	53	100%	94%	99%
Medicare Spending				
Medicare Spending per Patient (ratio)		-	0.89	0.98
Pneumonia Care				
Appropriate Initial Antibiotic Given[2]	41	95%	94%	95%
Blood Culture Timing[2]	58	100%	97%	98%
Pregnancy and Delivery Care				
Newborn Deliveries Scheduled Early[5]	-	-	7%	6%
Preventive Care				
Immunization for Influenza[5]	-	-	86%	90%
Immunization for Pneumonia[5]	-	-	89%	92%
Stroke Care				
Anticoagulation Therapy for Atrial Fibrillation[5]	-	-	98%	95%
Antithrombotic Therapy Timing[5]	-	-	99%	98%
Assessed for Rehabilitation[5]	-	-	99%	97%
Discharged on Antithrombotic Therapy[5]	-	-	100%	99%
Discharged on Statin Medication[5]	-	-	94%	94%
Thrombolytic Therapy Timing[5]	-	-	67%	66%
Venous Thromboembolism Prophylaxis[5]	-	-	96%	94%

NOTE: Hospital profiles are in alphabetical order by state, then city, then hospital within the city; Rankings exclude hospitals with less than 25 cases except for patient surveys which excludes hospitals with less than 100 cases; (a) 100-299 cases; (1) The number of cases/patients is too few to report; (2) Data submitted were based on a sample of cases/patients; (3) Results are based on a shorter time period than required; (4) Data suppressed by CMS for one or more quarters; (5) Results are not available for this reporting period; (6) Fewer than 100 patients completed the HCAHPS survey; (7) No cases met the criteria for this measure; (8) The lower limit of the confidence interval cannot be calculated if the number of observed infections equals zero; (9) No data are available from the state/territory for this reporting period; (10) The scores shown reflect fewer than 50 completed surveys; (11) There were discrepancies in the data collection process; (12) This measure does not apply to this hospital for this reporting period; (13) Results cannot be calculated for this reporting period; (14) The results for this state are combined with nearby states to protect confidentiality; Please refer to the User's Guide for a full explanation of data.

Measure	Cases	This Hosp.	State Avg.	U.S. Avg.
Written Stroke Educational Materials Given[5]	-	-	85%	88%
Surgical Care Improvement Project				
Appropriate Beta Blocker Usage[1]	-	-	98%	98%
Appropriate VTP Within 24 Hours	54	98%	98%	98%
Controlled Postoperative Blood Glucose[3,7]	-	-	96%	97%
Perioperative Temperature Management	63	100%	100%	100%
Prophylactic Antibiotic Selection	35	97%	99%	99%
Prophylactic Antibiotic Selection (Outpatient)	-	-	98%	98%
Prophylactic Antibiotic Stopped	30	97%	99%	98%
Prophylactic Antibiotic Timing	35	100%	99%	99%
Prophylactic Antibiotic Timing (Outpatient)	-	-	98%	98%
Urinary Catheter Removal	20	100%	99%	97%
Survey of Patients' Hospital Experiences				
Area Around Room 'Always' Quiet at Night	(a)	59%	60%	61%
Doctors 'Always' Communicated Well	(a)	82%	81%	82%
Home Recovery Information Given	(a)	81%	83%	85%
Hospital Given 9 or 10 on 10 Point Scale	(a)	61%	68%	71%
Meds 'Always' Explained Before Given	(a)	61%	63%	64%
Nurses 'Always' Communicated Well	(a)	78%	77%	79%
Pain 'Always' Well Controlled	(a)	65%	70%	71%
Room and Bathroom 'Always' Clean	(a)	78%	72%	73%
Timely Help 'Always' Received	(a)	66%	69%	68%
Would Definitely Recommend Hospital	(a)	62%	67%	71%
Use of Medical Imaging				
Cardiac Imaging Stress Test before Surgery	-	-	4.9%	5.3%
Combination Abdominal CT Scan	-	-	10.6%	10.5%
Combination Brain/Sinus CT Scan	-	-	1.9%	2.7%
Combination Chest CT Scan	-	-	2.4%	2.7%
Follow-up Mammogram/Ultrasound	-	-	6.9%	8.8%
Lumbar Spine MRI for Low Back Pain	-	-	41.5%	37.2%

Big Horn Co Memorial Hospital

17 N Miles Phone: 406-665-2310
Hardin, MT 59034 Fax: 406-665-9238
URL: www.bighornhospital.org
Type: Critical Access Hospitals Emergency Services: Yes
Ownership: Government - Local Beds: 16
Key Personnel:
CEO/President. . . . . Robert Notarianni

Measure	Cases	This Hosp.	State Avg.	U.S. Avg.
Blood Clot Prevention and Treatment				
Anticoagulation Overlap Therapy[5]	-	-	97%	93%
ICU Venous Thromboembolism Prophylaxis[5]	-	-	92%	92%
Incidence of Potentially Preventable VTE[5]	-	-	4%	10%
UFH with Dosages/Platelet Monitoring[5]	-	-	97%	97%
Venous Thromboembolism Prophylaxis[5]	-	-	83%	85%
Warfarin Therapy Discharge Instructions[5]	-	-	84%	75%
Chest Pain/Possible Heart Attack Care				
Aspirin Given Within 24 Hours of Arrival[1,3]	-	-	97%	96%
Fibrinolytic Meds Within 30 Min. of Arrival[5]	-	-	43%	58%
Average Time to ECG (minutes)[1,3]	-	-	10	7
Average Time to Transfer (minutes)[5]	-	-	78	60
Children's Asthma Care				
Received Home Management Plan of Care	-	-	-	88%
Received Reliever Medication	-	-	-	100%
Received Systemic Corticosteroids	-	-	-	100%
Emergency Department				
Admittance Decision Time (minutes)[5]	-	-	72	98
Head CT Results Within 45 Min. of Arrival[1,3]	-	-	26%	57%
Patients Who Left ER Before Being Seen[5]	-	-	2%	2%
Time from ER Arrival to Admit. (minutes)[5]	-	-	220	274
Time from ER Arrival to Discharge (minutes)[5]	-	-	120	134
Time in ER Before Being Evaluated (minutes)[5]	-	-	23	26
Time to Pain Meds for Fractures (minutes)[5]	-	-	47	57
Heart Attack Care				
Aspirin Given at Discharge[5]	-	-	100%	99%
Fibrinolytic Meds Within 30 Min. of Arrival[5]	-	-	50%	54%
PCI Within 90 Minutes of Arrival[5]	-	-	96%	96%
Statin Prescribed at Discharge[5]	-	-	99%	98%
Heart Failure Care				
ACE Inhibitor or ARB for LVSD[3,7]	-	-	97%	97%
Discharge Instructions Given[1,3]	-	-	92%	94%
Evaluation of LVS Function[1,3]	-	-	94%	99%
Medicare Spending				
Medicare Spending per Patient (ratio)	-	-	0.89	0.98
Pneumonia Care				
Appropriate Initial Antibiotic Given[1]	-	-	94%	95%
Blood Culture Timing[1]	-	-	97%	98%
Pregnancy and Delivery Care				
Newborn Deliveries Scheduled Early[5]	-	-	7%	6%
Preventive Care				
Immunization for Influenza[5]	-	-	86%	90%
Immunization for Pneumonia[5]	-	-	89%	92%
Stroke Care				
Anticoagulation Therapy for Atrial Fibrillation[5]	-	-	98%	95%
Antithrombotic Therapy Timing[5]	-	-	99%	98%
Assessed for Rehabilitation[5]	-	-	99%	97%
Discharged on Antithrombotic Therapy[5]	-	-	100%	99%
Discharged on Statin Medication[5]	-	-	94%	94%
Thrombolytic Therapy Timing[5]	-	-	67%	66%
Venous Thromboembolism Prophylaxis[5]	-	-	96%	94%
Written Stroke Educational Materials Given[5]	-	-	85%	88%
Surgical Care Improvement Project				
Appropriate Beta Blocker Usage[5]	-	-	98%	98%
Appropriate VTP Within 24 Hours[5]	-	-	98%	98%
Controlled Postoperative Blood Glucose[5]	-	-	96%	97%
Perioperative Temperature Management[5]	-	-	100%	100%
Prophylactic Antibiotic Selection[5]	-	-	99%	99%
Prophylactic Antibiotic Selection (Outpatient)[5]	-	-	98%	98%
Prophylactic Antibiotic Stopped[5]	-	-	99%	98%
Prophylactic Antibiotic Timing[5]	-	-	99%	99%
Prophylactic Antibiotic Timing (Outpatient)[5]	-	-	98%	98%
Urinary Catheter Removal[5]	-	-	99%	97%
Survey of Patients' Hospital Experiences				
Area Around Room 'Always' Quiet at Night[5]	-	-	60%	61%
Doctors 'Always' Communicated Well[5]	-	-	81%	82%
Home Recovery Information Given[5]	-	-	83%	85%
Hospital Given 9 or 10 on 10 Point Scale[5]	-	-	68%	71%
Meds 'Always' Explained Before Given[5]	-	-	63%	64%
Nurses 'Always' Communicated Well[5]	-	-	77%	79%
Pain 'Always' Well Controlled[5]	-	-	70%	71%
Room and Bathroom 'Always' Clean[5]	-	-	72%	73%
Timely Help 'Always' Received[5]	-	-	69%	68%
Would Definitely Recommend Hospital[5]	-	-	67%	71%
Use of Medical Imaging				
Cardiac Imaging Stress Test before Surgery[7]	-	-	4.9%	5.3%
Combination Abdominal CT Scan	65	4.6%	10.6%	10.5%
Combination Brain/Sinus CT Scan	81	0.0%	1.9%	2.7%
Combination Chest CT Scan[1]	-	-	2.4%	2.7%
Follow-up Mammogram/Ultrasound	134	6.0%	6.9%	8.8%
Lumbar Spine MRI for Low Back Pain[1]	-	-	41.5%	37.2%

Wheatland Memorial Hospital

530 3rd Saint Nw Phone: 406-632-4351
Harlowton, MT 59036 Fax: 406-632-3172
URL: www.wheatlandmemorial.org
Type: Critical Access Hospitals Emergency Services: Yes
Ownership: Voluntary non-profit - Private Beds: 25
Key Personnel:
Radiology. Sharlett Dale
CEO . . . . Mike Zwicker

Measure	Cases	This Hosp.	State Avg.	U.S. Avg.
Blood Clot Prevention and Treatment				
Anticoagulation Overlap Therapy	-	-	97%	93%
ICU Venous Thromboembolism Prophylaxis	-	-	92%	92%
Incidence of Potentially Preventable VTE	-	-	4%	10%
UFH with Dosages/Platelet Monitoring	-	-	97%	97%
Venous Thromboembolism Prophylaxis	-	-	83%	85%
Warfarin Therapy Discharge Instructions	-	-	84%	75%
Chest Pain/Possible Heart Attack Care				
Aspirin Given Within 24 Hours of Arrival[5]	-	-	97%	96%
Fibrinolytic Meds Within 30 Min. of Arrival[5]	-	-	43%	58%
Average Time to ECG (minutes)[5]	-	-	10	7
Average Time to Transfer (minutes)[5]	-	-	78	60
Children's Asthma Care				
Received Home Management Plan of Care	-	-	-	88%
Received Reliever Medication	-	-	-	100%
Received Systemic Corticosteroids	-	-	-	100%
Emergency Department				
Admittance Decision Time (minutes)	-	-	72	98
Head CT Results Within 45 Min. of Arrival[5]	-	-	26%	57%
Patients Who Left ER Before Being Seen[5]	-	-	2%	2%
Time from ER Arrival to Admit. (minutes)	-	-	220	274
Time from ER Arrival to Discharge (minutes)[5]	-	-	120	134
Time in ER Before Being Evaluated (minutes)[5]	-	-	23	26
Time to Pain Meds for Fractures (minutes)[5]	-	-	47	57
Heart Attack Care				
Aspirin Given at Discharge	-	-	100%	99%
Fibrinolytic Meds Within 30 Min. of Arrival	-	-	50%	54%
PCI Within 90 Minutes of Arrival	-	-	96%	96%
Statin Prescribed at Discharge	-	-	99%	98%
Heart Failure Care				
ACE Inhibitor or ARB for LVSD	-	-	97%	97%
Discharge Instructions Given	-	-	92%	94%
Evaluation of LVS Function	-	-	94%	99%
Medicare Spending				
Medicare Spending per Patient (ratio)	-	-	0.89	0.98
Pneumonia Care				
Appropriate Initial Antibiotic Given	-	-	94%	95%
Blood Culture Timing	-	-	97%	98%
Pregnancy and Delivery Care				
Newborn Deliveries Scheduled Early	-	-	7%	6%
Preventive Care				
Immunization for Influenza	-	-	86%	90%
Immunization for Pneumonia	-	-	89%	92%
Stroke Care				
Anticoagulation Therapy for Atrial Fibrillation	-	-	98%	95%
Antithrombotic Therapy Timing	-	-	99%	98%
Assessed for Rehabilitation	-	-	99%	97%
Discharged on Antithrombotic Therapy	-	-	100%	99%
Discharged on Statin Medication	-	-	94%	94%
Thrombolytic Therapy Timing	-	-	67%	66%
Venous Thromboembolism Prophylaxis	-	-	96%	94%
Written Stroke Educational Materials Given	-	-	85%	88%
Surgical Care Improvement Project				
Appropriate Beta Blocker Usage	-	-	98%	98%
Appropriate VTP Within 24 Hours	-	-	98%	98%
Controlled Postoperative Blood Glucose	-	-	96%	97%
Perioperative Temperature Management	-	-	100%	100%
Prophylactic Antibiotic Selection	-	-	99%	99%
Prophylactic Antibiotic Selection (Outpatient)[5]	-	-	98%	98%
Prophylactic Antibiotic Stopped	-	-	99%	98%
Prophylactic Antibiotic Timing	-	-	99%	99%
Prophylactic Antibiotic Timing (Outpatient)[5]	-	-	98%	98%
Urinary Catheter Removal	-	-	99%	97%
Survey of Patients' Hospital Experiences				
Area Around Room 'Always' Quiet at Night	-	-	60%	61%
Doctors 'Always' Communicated Well	-	-	81%	82%
Home Recovery Information Given	-	-	83%	85%
Hospital Given 9 or 10 on 10 Point Scale	-	-	68%	71%
Meds 'Always' Explained Before Given	-	-	63%	64%
Nurses 'Always' Communicated Well	-	-	77%	79%
Pain 'Always' Well Controlled	-	-	70%	71%
Room and Bathroom 'Always' Clean	-	-	72%	73%
Timely Help 'Always' Received	-	-	69%	68%
Would Definitely Recommend Hospital	-	-	67%	71%
Use of Medical Imaging				
Cardiac Imaging Stress Test before Surgery[1]	-	-	4.9%	5.3%
Combination Abdominal CT Scan[1]	-	-	10.6%	10.5%
Combination Brain/Sinus CT Scan[1]	-	-	1.9%	2.7%
Combination Chest CT Scan[1]	-	-	2.4%	2.7%
Follow-up Mammogram/Ultrasound[1]	-	-	6.9%	8.8%
Lumbar Spine MRI for Low Back Pain[7]	-	-	41.5%	37.2%

NOTE: Hospital profiles are in alphabetical order by state, then city, then hospital within the city; Rankings exclude hospitals with less than 25 cases except for patient surveys which excludes hospitals with less than 100 cases; (a) 100-299 cases; (1) The number of cases/patients is too few to report; (2) Data submitted were based on a sample of cases/patients; (3) Results are based on a shorter time period than required; (4) Data suppressed by CMS for one or more quarters; (5) Results are not available for this reporting period; (6) Fewer than 100 patients completed the HCAHPS survey; (7) No cases met the criteria for this measure; (8) The lower limit of the confidence interval cannot be calculated if the number of observed infections equals zero; (9) No data are available from the state/territory for this reporting period; (10) The scores shown reflect fewer than 50 completed surveys; (11) There were discrepancies in the data collection process; (12) This measure does not apply to this hospital for this reporting period; (13) Results cannot be calculated for this reporting period; (14) The results for this state are combined with nearby states to protect confidentiality; Please refer to the User's Guide for a full explanation of data.

Northern Montana Hospital

30 13th St
Havre, MT 59501
Phone: 406-265-2211
Fax: 406-265-1651
URL: www.nmhcare.com
Type: Acute Care Hospitals
Emergency Services: Yes
Ownership: Voluntary non-profit - Private
Beds: 49

Key Personnel:
Chairman/CEO . . . . Miles Hamilton
Radiology. . . . . Earl Harrison
CEO/President. . . . . Dave Henry
Emergency Room . . . . Kathy Lataty
Chief of Medical Staff. . . . . Dr. Steven Liston, MD

Measure	Cases	This Hosp.	State Avg.	U.S. Avg.
Blood Clot Prevention and Treatment				
Anticoagulation Overlap Therapy[1,2]	-	-	97%	93%
ICU Venous Thromboembolism Prophylaxis[2]	41	73%	92%	92%
Incidence of Potentially Preventable VTE[1,2]	-	-	4%	10%
UFH with Dosages/Platelet Monitoring[1,2]	-	-	97%	97%
Venous Thromboembolism Prophylaxis[2]	85	78%	83%	85%
Warfarin Therapy Discharge Instructions[1,2]	-	-	84%	75%
Chest Pain/Possible Heart Attack Care				
Aspirin Given Within 24 Hours of Arrival[3]	23	100%	97%	96%
Fibrinolytic Meds Within 30 Min. of Arrival[1,3]	-	-	43%	58%
Average Time to ECG (minutes)[3]	22	16	10	7
Average Time to Transfer (minutes)[1,3]	-	-	78	60
Children's Asthma Care				
Received Home Management Plan of Care	-	-	-	88%
Received Reliever Medication	-	-	-	100%
Received Systemic Corticosteroids	-	-	-	100%
Emergency Department				
Admittance Decision Time (minutes)[2]	357	39	72	98
Head CT Results Within 45 Min. of Arrival[1,3]	-	-	26%	57%
Patients Who Left ER Before Being Seen	8,680	2%	2%	2%
Time from ER Arrival to Admit. (minutes)[2]	471	172	220	274
Time from ER Arrival to Discharge (minutes)	374	100	120	134
Time in ER Before Being Evaluated (minutes)	361	34	23	26
Time to Pain Meds for Fractures (minutes)	38	56	47	57
Heart Attack Care				
Aspirin Given at Discharge[5]	-	-	100%	99%
Fibrinolytic Meds Within 30 Min. of Arrival[5]	-	-	50%	54%
PCI Within 90 Minutes of Arrival[5]	-	-	96%	96%
Statin Prescribed at Discharge[5]	-	-	99%	98%
Heart Failure Care				
ACE Inhibitor or ARB for LVSD[1,2]	-	-	97%	97%
Discharge Instructions Given[2,3]	14	79%	92%	94%
Evaluation of LVS Function[2,3]	23	87%	94%	99%
Medicare Spending				
Medicare Spending per Patient (ratio)	-	0.80	0.89	0.98
Pneumonia Care				
Appropriate Initial Antibiotic Given[2]	42	95%	94%	95%
Blood Culture Timing[2]	43	100%	97%	98%
Pregnancy and Delivery Care				
Newborn Deliveries Scheduled Early	52	19%	7%	6%
Preventive Care				
Immunization for Influenza[2]	275	79%	86%	90%
Immunization for Pneumonia[2]	298	75%	89%	92%
Stroke Care				
Anticoagulation Therapy for Atrial Fibrillation[1,3]	-	-	98%	95%
Antithrombotic Therapy Timing[1,3]	-	-	99%	98%
Assessed for Rehabilitation[1,3]	-	-	99%	97%
Discharged on Antithrombotic Therapy[1,3]	-	-	100%	99%
Discharged on Statin Medication[1,3]	-	-	94%	94%
Thrombolytic Therapy Timing[1,3]	-	-	67%	66%
Venous Thromboembolism Prophylaxis[1,3]	-	-	96%	94%
Written Stroke Educational Materials Given[1,3]	-	-	85%	88%
Surgical Care Improvement Project				
Appropriate Beta Blocker Usage	17	94%	98%	98%
Appropriate VTP Within 24 Hours	48	92%	98%	98%
Controlled Postoperative Blood Glucose[7]	-	-	96%	97%
Perioperative Temperature Management	67	100%	100%	100%
Prophylactic Antibiotic Selection	55	96%	99%	99%
Prophylactic Antibiotic Selection (Outpatient)	22	100%	98%	98%
Prophylactic Antibiotic Stopped	53	96%	99%	98%
Prophylactic Antibiotic Timing	55	98%	99%	99%
Prophylactic Antibiotic Timing (Outpatient)	22	100%	98%	98%
Urinary Catheter Removal	37	97%	99%	97%
Survey of Patients' Hospital Experiences				
Area Around Room 'Always' Quiet at Night	(a)	63%	60%	61%
Doctors 'Always' Communicated Well	(a)	77%	81%	82%
Home Recovery Information Given	(a)	82%	83%	85%
Hospital Given 9 or 10 on 10 Point Scale	(a)	51%	68%	71%
Meds 'Always' Explained Before Given	(a)	58%	63%	64%
Nurses 'Always' Communicated Well	(a)	74%	77%	79%
Pain 'Always' Well Controlled	(a)	67%	70%	71%
Room and Bathroom 'Always' Clean	(a)	64%	72%	73%
Timely Help 'Always' Received	(a)	69%	69%	68%
Would Definitely Recommend Hospital	(a)	46%	67%	71%
Use of Medical Imaging				
Cardiac Imaging Stress Test before Surgery	58	1.7%	4.9%	5.3%
Combination Abdominal CT Scan	162	6.8%	10.6%	10.5%
Combination Brain/Sinus CT Scan[1]	-	-	1.9%	2.7%
Combination Chest CT Scan	77	6.5%	2.4%	2.7%
Follow-up Mammogram/Ultrasound	342	7.0%	6.9%	8.8%
Lumbar Spine MRI for Low Back Pain[1]	-	-	41.5%	37.2%

Saint Peter's Hospital

2475 Broadway
Helena, MT 59601
Phone: 406-442-2480
Fax: 406-444-2389
URL: www.stpetes.org
Type: Acute Care Hospitals
Emergency Services: Yes
Ownership: Voluntary non-profit - Private
Beds: 99

Key Personnel:
Radiology. . . . . Keith Edwards
Chief of Medical Staff. . . . . Jim Haley
Emergency Room . . . . Doug Kuntzweiler, RN
CEO/President. . . . . John Solheim
Quality Assurance . . . . Lisa Strom
Operating Room. . . . . Kathleen Zarndt

Measure	Cases	This Hosp.	State Avg.	U.S. Avg.
Blood Clot Prevention and Treatment				
Anticoagulation Overlap Therapy[2]	38	100%	97%	93%
ICU Venous Thromboembolism Prophylaxis[2]	79	94%	92%	92%
Incidence of Potentially Preventable VTE[1,2]	-	-	4%	10%
UFH with Dosages/Platelet Monitoring[1,2]	-	-	97%	97%
Venous Thromboembolism Prophylaxis[2]	334	80%	83%	85%
Warfarin Therapy Discharge Instructions[2]	31	94%	84%	75%
Chest Pain/Possible Heart Attack Care				
Aspirin Given Within 24 Hours of Arrival[1,3]	-	-	97%	96%
Fibrinolytic Meds Within 30 Min. of Arrival[5]	-	-	43%	58%
Average Time to ECG (minutes)[1,3]	-	-	10	7
Average Time to Transfer (minutes)[5]	-	-	78	60
Children's Asthma Care				
Received Home Management Plan of Care	-	-	-	88%
Received Reliever Medication	-	-	-	100%
Received Systemic Corticosteroids	-	-	-	100%
Emergency Department				
Admittance Decision Time (minutes)[2]	450	96	72	98
Head CT Results Within 45 Min. of Arrival[1]	-	-	26%	57%
Patients Who Left ER Before Being Seen	22,671	1%	2%	2%
Time from ER Arrival to Admit. (minutes)[2]	556	262	220	274
Time from ER Arrival to Discharge (minutes)	354	137	120	134
Time in ER Before Being Evaluated (minutes)	278	22	23	26
Time to Pain Meds for Fractures (minutes)	124	44	47	57
Heart Attack Care				
Aspirin Given at Discharge	96	100%	100%	99%
Fibrinolytic Meds Within 30 Min. of Arrival[7]	-	-	50%	54%
PCI Within 90 Minutes of Arrival	31	94%	96%	96%
Statin Prescribed at Discharge	95	100%	99%	98%
Heart Failure Care				
ACE Inhibitor or ARB for LVSD	30	100%	97%	97%
Discharge Instructions Given	78	86%	92%	94%
Evaluation of LVS Function	86	100%	94%	99%
Medicare Spending				
Medicare Spending per Patient (ratio)	-	0.85	0.89	0.98
Pneumonia Care				
Appropriate Initial Antibiotic Given	73	99%	94%	95%
Blood Culture Timing	137	94%	97%	98%
Pregnancy and Delivery Care				
Newborn Deliveries Scheduled Early	83	6%	7%	6%
Preventive Care				
Immunization for Influenza[2]	534	93%	86%	90%
Immunization for Pneumonia[2]	576	90%	89%	92%
Stroke Care				
Anticoagulation Therapy for Atrial Fibrillation	11	100%	98%	95%
Antithrombotic Therapy Timing	59	98%	99%	98%
Assessed for Rehabilitation	63	100%	99%	97%
Discharged on Antithrombotic Therapy	60	100%	100%	99%
Discharged on Statin Medication	49	94%	94%	94%
Thrombolytic Therapy Timing[1]	-	-	67%	66%
Venous Thromboembolism Prophylaxis	63	92%	96%	94%
Written Stroke Educational Materials Given	36	56%	85%	88%
Surgical Care Improvement Project				
Appropriate Beta Blocker Usage[2]	97	97%	98%	98%
Appropriate VTP Within 24 Hours[2]	361	99%	98%	98%
Controlled Postoperative Blood Glucose[2,7]	-	-	96%	97%
Perioperative Temperature Management[2]	402	100%	100%	100%
Prophylactic Antibiotic Selection[2]	278	100%	99%	99%
Prophylactic Antibiotic Selection (Outpatient)	237	92%	98%	98%
Prophylactic Antibiotic Stopped[2]	274	97%	99%	98%
Prophylactic Antibiotic Timing[2]	278	98%	99%	99%
Prophylactic Antibiotic Timing (Outpatient)	211	91%	98%	98%
Urinary Catheter Removal[2]	107	97%	99%	97%
Survey of Patients' Hospital Experiences				
Area Around Room 'Always' Quiet at Night	300+	58%	60%	61%
Doctors 'Always' Communicated Well	300+	84%	81%	82%
Home Recovery Information Given	300+	85%	83%	85%
Hospital Given 9 or 10 on 10 Point Scale	300+	63%	68%	71%
Meds 'Always' Explained Before Given	300+	64%	63%	64%
Nurses 'Always' Communicated Well	300+	78%	77%	79%
Pain 'Always' Well Controlled	300+	73%	70%	71%
Room and Bathroom 'Always' Clean	300+	77%	72%	73%
Timely Help 'Always' Received	300+	67%	69%	68%
Would Definitely Recommend Hospital	300+	61%	67%	71%
Use of Medical Imaging				
Cardiac Imaging Stress Test before Surgery	205	3.9%	4.9%	5.3%
Combination Abdominal CT Scan	646	8.2%	10.6%	10.5%
Combination Brain/Sinus CT Scan	453	2.2%	1.9%	2.7%
Combination Chest CT Scan	461	4.6%	2.4%	2.7%
Follow-up Mammogram/Ultrasound	1,546	8.6%	6.9%	8.8%
Lumbar Spine MRI for Low Back Pain	143	40.6%	41.5%	37.2%

Garfield County Health Center

332 Leavitt Ave
Jordan, MT 59337
Phone: 406-557-2500
Type: Critical Access Hospitals
Emergency Services: Yes
Ownership: Government - Local

Measure	Cases	This Hosp.	State Avg.	U.S. Avg.
Blood Clot Prevention and Treatment				
Anticoagulation Overlap Therapy[5]	-	-	97%	93%
ICU Venous Thromboembolism Prophylaxis[5]	-	-	92%	92%
Incidence of Potentially Preventable VTE[5]	-	-	4%	10%
UFH with Dosages/Platelet Monitoring[5]	-	-	97%	97%
Venous Thromboembolism Prophylaxis[5]	-	-	83%	85%
Warfarin Therapy Discharge Instructions[5]	-	-	84%	75%
Chest Pain/Possible Heart Attack Care				
Aspirin Given Within 24 Hours of Arrival	-	-	97%	96%
Fibrinolytic Meds Within 30 Min. of Arrival	-	-	43%	58%
Average Time to ECG (minutes)	-	-	10	7
Average Time to Transfer (minutes)	-	-	78	60
Children's Asthma Care				
Received Home Management Plan of Care	-	-	-	88%
Received Reliever Medication	-	-	-	100%
Received Systemic Corticosteroids	-	-	-	100%
Emergency Department				
Admittance Decision Time (minutes)[5]	-	-	72	98
Head CT Results Within 45 Min. of Arrival	-	-	26%	57%
Patients Who Left ER Before Being Seen	-	-	2%	2%
Time from ER Arrival to Admit. (minutes)[5]	-	-	220	274
Time from ER Arrival to Discharge (minutes)	-	-	120	134

NOTE: Hospital profiles are in alphabetical order by state, then city, then hospital within the city; Rankings exclude hospitals with less than 25 cases except for patient surveys which excludes hospitals with less than 100 cases; (a) 100-299 cases; (1) The number of cases/patients is too few to report; (2) Data submitted were based on a sample of cases/patients; (3) Results are based on a shorter time period than required; (4) Data suppressed by CMS for one or more quarters; (5) Results are not available for this reporting period; (6) Fewer than 100 patients completed the HCAHPS survey; (7) No cases met the criteria for this measure; (8) The lower limit of the confidence interval cannot be calculated if the number of observed infections equals zero; (9) No data are available from the state/territory for this reporting period; (10) The scores shown reflect fewer than 50 completed surveys; (11) There were discrepancies in the data collection process; (12) This measure does not apply to this hospital for this reporting period; (13) Results cannot be calculated for this reporting period; (14) The results for this state are combined with nearby states to protect confidentiality; Please refer to the User's Guide for a full explanation of data.

Measure	Cases	This Hosp.	State Avg.	U.S. Avg.
Time in ER Before Being Evaluated (minutes)	-	-	23	26
Time to Pain Meds for Fractures (minutes)	-	-	47	57
Heart Attack Care				
Aspirin Given at Discharge[5]	-	-	100%	99%
Fibrinolytic Meds Within 30 Min. of Arrival[5]	-	-	50%	54%
PCI Within 90 Minutes of Arrival[5]	-	-	96%	96%
Statin Prescribed at Discharge[5]	-	-	99%	98%
Heart Failure Care				
ACE Inhibitor or ARB for LVSD[5]	-	-	97%	97%
Discharge Instructions Given[5]	-	-	92%	94%
Evaluation of LVS Function[5]	-	-	94%	99%
Medicare Spending				
Medicare Spending per Patient (ratio)	-	-	0.89	0.98
Pneumonia Care				
Appropriate Initial Antibiotic Given[5]	-	-	94%	95%
Blood Culture Timing[5]	-	-	97%	98%
Pregnancy and Delivery Care				
Newborn Deliveries Scheduled Early[5]	-	-	7%	6%
Preventive Care				
Immunization for Influenza[5]	-	-	86%	90%
Immunization for Pneumonia[5]	-	-	89%	92%
Stroke Care				
Anticoagulation Therapy for Atrial Fibrillation[5]	-	-	98%	95%
Antithrombotic Therapy Timing[5]	-	-	99%	98%
Assessed for Rehabilitation[5]	-	-	99%	97%
Discharged on Antithrombotic Therapy[5]	-	-	100%	99%
Discharged on Statin Medication[5]	-	-	94%	94%
Thrombolytic Therapy Timing[5]	-	-	67%	66%
Venous Thromboembolism Prophylaxis[5]	-	-	96%	94%
Written Stroke Educational Materials Given[5]	-	-	85%	88%
Surgical Care Improvement Project				
Appropriate Beta Blocker Usage[5]	-	-	98%	98%
Appropriate VTP Within 24 Hours[5]	-	-	98%	98%
Controlled Postoperative Blood Glucose[5]	-	-	96%	97%
Perioperative Temperature Management[5]	-	-	100%	100%
Prophylactic Antibiotic Selection[5]	-	-	99%	99%
Prophylactic Antibiotic Selection (Outpatient)	-	-	98%	98%
Prophylactic Antibiotic Stopped[5]	-	-	99%	98%
Prophylactic Antibiotic Timing[5]	-	-	99%	99%
Prophylactic Antibiotic Timing (Outpatient)	-	-	98%	98%
Urinary Catheter Removal[5]	-	-	99%	97%
Survey of Patients' Hospital Experiences				
Area Around Room 'Always' Quiet at Night[5]	-	-	60%	61%
Doctors 'Always' Communicated Well[5]	-	-	81%	82%
Home Recovery Information Given[5]	-	-	83%	85%
Hospital Given 9 or 10 on 10 Point Scale[5]	-	-	68%	71%
Meds 'Always' Explained Before Given[5]	-	-	63%	64%
Nurses 'Always' Communicated Well[5]	-	-	77%	79%
Pain 'Always' Well Controlled[5]	-	-	70%	71%
Room and Bathroom 'Always' Clean[5]	-	-	72%	73%
Timely Help 'Always' Received[5]	-	-	69%	68%
Would Definitely Recommend Hospital[5]	-	-	67%	71%
Use of Medical Imaging				
Cardiac Imaging Stress Test before Surgery	-	-	4.9%	5.3%
Combination Abdominal CT Scan	-	-	10.6%	10.5%
Combination Brain/Sinus CT Scan	-	-	1.9%	2.7%
Combination Chest CT Scan	-	-	2.4%	2.7%
Follow-up Mammogram/Ultrasound	-	-	6.9%	8.8%
Lumbar Spine MRI for Low Back Pain	-	-	41.5%	37.2%

Health Center Northwest

320 Sunnyview Lane
Kalispell, MT 59901
Phone: 406-751-7550
Type: Acute Care Hospitals
Emergency Services: No
Ownership: Proprietary

Measure	Cases	This Hosp.	State Avg.	U.S. Avg.
Blood Clot Prevention and Treatment				
Anticoagulation Overlap Therapy[2,7]	-	-	97%	93%
ICU Venous Thromboembolism Prophylaxis[2,7]	-	-	92%	92%
Incidence of Potentially Preventable VTE[2,7]	-	-	4%	10%
UFH with Dosages/Platelet Monitoring[2,7]	-	-	97%	97%
Venous Thromboembolism Prophylaxis[2]	38	87%	83%	85%
Warfarin Therapy Discharge Instructions[2,7]	-	-	84%	75%
Chest Pain/Possible Heart Attack Care				
Aspirin Given Within 24 Hours of Arrival[5]	-	-	97%	96%
Fibrinolytic Meds Within 30 Min. of Arrival[5]	-	-	43%	58%
Average Time to ECG (minutes)[5]	-	-	10	7
Average Time to Transfer (minutes)[5]	-	-	78	60
Children's Asthma Care				
Received Home Management Plan of Care	-	-	-	88%
Received Reliever Medication	-	-	-	100%
Received Systemic Corticosteroids	-	-	-	100%
Emergency Department				
Admittance Decision Time (minutes)[2,7]	-	-	72	98
Head CT Results Within 45 Min. of Arrival[5]	-	-	26%	57%
Patients Who Left ER Before Being Seen[5]	-	-	2%	2%
Time from ER Arrival to Admit. (minutes)[2,7]	-	-	220	274
Time from ER Arrival to Discharge (minutes)[5]	-	-	120	134
Time in ER Before Being Evaluated (minutes)[5]	-	-	23	26
Time to Pain Meds for Fractures (minutes)[5]	-	-	47	57
Heart Attack Care				
Aspirin Given at Discharge[5]	-	-	100%	99%
Fibrinolytic Meds Within 30 Min. of Arrival[5]	-	-	50%	54%
PCI Within 90 Minutes of Arrival[5]	-	-	96%	96%
Statin Prescribed at Discharge[5]	-	-	99%	98%
Heart Failure Care				
ACE Inhibitor or ARB for LVSD[3,7]	-	-	97%	97%
Discharge Instructions Given[3,7]	-	-	92%	94%
Evaluation of LVS Function[1,3]	-	-	94%	99%
Medicare Spending				
Medicare Spending per Patient (ratio)	-	0.88	0.89	0.98
Pneumonia Care				
Appropriate Initial Antibiotic Given[5]	-	-	94%	95%
Blood Culture Timing[5]	-	-	97%	98%
Pregnancy and Delivery Care				
Newborn Deliveries Scheduled Early[7]	-	-	7%	6%
Preventive Care				
Immunization for Influenza[2]	293	58%	86%	90%
Immunization for Pneumonia[2]	293	72%	89%	92%
Stroke Care				
Anticoagulation Therapy for Atrial Fibrillation[3,7]	-	-	98%	95%
Antithrombotic Therapy Timing[1,3]	-	-	99%	98%
Assessed for Rehabilitation[1,3]	-	-	99%	97%
Discharged on Antithrombotic Therapy[1,3]	-	-	100%	99%
Discharged on Statin Medication[1,3]	-	-	94%	94%
Thrombolytic Therapy Timing[3,7]	-	-	67%	66%
Venous Thromboembolism Prophylaxis[1,3]	-	-	96%	94%
Written Stroke Educational Materials Given[1,3]	-	-	85%	88%
Surgical Care Improvement Project				
Appropriate Beta Blocker Usage	50	96%	98%	98%
Appropriate VTP Within 24 Hours	206	99%	98%	98%
Controlled Postoperative Blood Glucose[7]	-	-	96%	97%
Perioperative Temperature Management	232	100%	100%	100%
Prophylactic Antibiotic Selection	208	100%	99%	99%
Prophylactic Antibiotic Selection (Outpatient)	267	99%	98%	98%
Prophylactic Antibiotic Stopped	208	99%	99%	98%
Prophylactic Antibiotic Timing	208	100%	99%	99%
Prophylactic Antibiotic Timing (Outpatient)	207	99%	98%	98%
Urinary Catheter Removal	63	100%	99%	97%
Survey of Patients' Hospital Experiences				
Area Around Room 'Always' Quiet at Night	(a)	65%	60%	61%
Doctors 'Always' Communicated Well	(a)	85%	81%	82%
Home Recovery Information Given	(a)	90%	83%	85%
Hospital Given 9 or 10 on 10 Point Scale	(a)	77%	68%	71%
Meds 'Always' Explained Before Given	(a)	65%	63%	64%
Nurses 'Always' Communicated Well	(a)	81%	77%	79%
Pain 'Always' Well Controlled	(a)	75%	70%	71%
Room and Bathroom 'Always' Clean	(a)	73%	72%	73%
Timely Help 'Always' Received	(a)	73%	69%	68%
Would Definitely Recommend Hospital	(a)	82%	67%	71%
Use of Medical Imaging				
Cardiac Imaging Stress Test before Surgery[7]	-	-	4.9%	5.3%
Combination Abdominal CT Scan	852	18.7%	10.6%	10.5%
Combination Brain/Sinus CT Scan[1]	-	-	1.9%	2.7%
Combination Chest CT Scan	744	0.7%	2.4%	2.7%
Follow-up Mammogram/Ultrasound	1,991	5.8%	6.9%	8.8%
Lumbar Spine MRI for Low Back Pain	268	33.6%	41.5%	37.2%

Kalispell Regional Medical Center

310 Sunnyview Lane
Kalispell, MT 59901
Phone: 406-752-5111
Fax: 406-756-2703
E-mail: jolive@krmc.orgrg
URL: www.krmc.org
Type: Acute Care Hospitals
Emergency Services: Yes
Ownership: Voluntary non-profit - Private
Beds: 143

Key Personnel:

Patient Relations . . . . Lori Alsbary
Radiology. . . . . William R Benedetto
Infection Control. . . . . Tereal Dammell
Operating Room. . . . . Bev Dowling
Chief of Medical Staff . . . . Gwen Jonds
Intensive Care Unit. . . . . Jeannie Laleah
Cardiac Laboratory. . . . . Renae Solum
CEO/President. . . . . Velinda Stevens

Measure	Cases	This Hosp.	State Avg.	U.S. Avg.
Blood Clot Prevention and Treatment				
Anticoagulation Overlap Therapy[2]	50	98%	97%	93%
ICU Venous Thromboembolism Prophylaxis[2]	54	100%	92%	92%
Incidence of Potentially Preventable VTE[1,2]	-	-	4%	10%
UFH with Dosages/Platelet Monitoring[2]	14	100%	97%	97%
Venous Thromboembolism Prophylaxis[2]	311	95%	83%	85%
Warfarin Therapy Discharge Instructions[2]	30	100%	84%	75%
Chest Pain/Possible Heart Attack Care				
Aspirin Given Within 24 Hours of Arrival[3,7]	-	-	97%	96%
Fibrinolytic Meds Within 30 Min. of Arrival[5]	-	-	43%	58%
Average Time to ECG (minutes)[3,7]	-	-	10	7
Average Time to Transfer (minutes)[5]	-	-	78	60
Children's Asthma Care				
Received Home Management Plan of Care	-	-	-	88%
Received Reliever Medication	-	-	-	100%
Received Systemic Corticosteroids	-	-	-	100%
Emergency Department				
Admittance Decision Time (minutes)[2]	615	82	72	98
Head CT Results Within 45 Min. of Arrival[1]	-	-	26%	57%
Patients Who Left ER Before Being Seen	22,634	2%	2%	2%
Time from ER Arrival to Admit. (minutes)[2]	621	233	220	274
Time from ER Arrival to Discharge (minutes)	376	138	120	134
Time in ER Before Being Evaluated (minutes)	391	18	23	26
Time to Pain Meds for Fractures (minutes)	122	36	47	57
Heart Attack Care				
Aspirin Given at Discharge	172	100%	100%	99%
Fibrinolytic Meds Within 30 Min. of Arrival[7]	-	-	50%	54%
PCI Within 90 Minutes of Arrival	32	97%	96%	96%
Statin Prescribed at Discharge	157	97%	99%	98%
Heart Failure Care				
ACE Inhibitor or ARB for LVSD	41	100%	97%	97%
Discharge Instructions Given	119	99%	92%	94%
Evaluation of LVS Function	149	100%	94%	99%
Medicare Spending				
Medicare Spending per Patient (ratio)	-	0.94	0.89	0.98
Pneumonia Care				
Appropriate Initial Antibiotic Given	94	99%	94%	95%
Blood Culture Timing	175	97%	97%	98%
Pregnancy and Delivery Care				
Newborn Deliveries Scheduled Early	36	8%	7%	6%
Preventive Care				
Immunization for Influenza[2]	576	92%	86%	90%
Immunization for Pneumonia[2]	693	96%	89%	92%
Stroke Care				
Anticoagulation Therapy for Atrial Fibrillation	18	100%	98%	95%
Antithrombotic Therapy Timing	56	100%	99%	98%
Assessed for Rehabilitation	89	100%	99%	97%
Discharged on Antithrombotic Therapy	81	100%	100%	99%
Discharged on Statin Medication	63	94%	94%	94%
Thrombolytic Therapy Timing[1]	-	-	67%	66%
Venous Thromboembolism Prophylaxis	76	100%	96%	94%
Written Stroke Educational Materials Given	47	98%	85%	88%
Surgical Care Improvement Project				

NOTE: Hospital profiles are in alphabetical order by state, then city, then hospital within the city; Rankings exclude hospitals with less than 25 cases except for patient surveys which excludes hospitals with less than 100 cases; (a) 100-299 cases; (1) The number of cases/patients is too few to report; (2) Data submitted were based on a sample of cases/patients; (3) Results are based on a shorter time period than required; (4) Data suppressed by CMS for one or more quarters; (5) Results are not available for this reporting period; (6) Fewer than 100 patients completed the HCAHPS survey; (7) No cases met the criteria for this measure; (8) The lower limit of the confidence interval cannot be calculated if the number of observed infections equals zero; (9) No data are available from the state/territory for this reporting period; (10) The scores shown reflect fewer than 50 completed surveys; (11) There were discrepancies in the data collection process; (12) This measure does not apply to this hospital for this reporting period; (13) Results cannot be calculated for this reporting period; (14) The results for this state are combined with nearby states to protect confidentiality; Please refer to the User's Guide for a full explanation of data.

Measure	Cases	This Hosp.	State Avg.	U.S. Avg.
Appropriate Beta Blocker Usage[2]	167	99%	98%	98%
Appropriate VTP Within 24 Hours[2]	606	96%	98%	98%
Controlled Postoperative Blood Glucose[2]	88	89%	96%	97%
Perioperative Temperature Management[2]	743	100%	100%	100%
Prophylactic Antibiotic Selection[2]	571	100%	99%	99%
Prophylactic Antibiotic Selection (Outpatient)	300	98%	98%	98%
Prophylactic Antibiotic Stopped[2]	564	100%	99%	98%
Prophylactic Antibiotic Timing[2]	574	100%	99%	99%
Prophylactic Antibiotic Timing (Outpatient)	301	99%	98%	98%
Urinary Catheter Removal[2]	525	99%	99%	97%
Survey of Patients' Hospital Experiences				
Area Around Room 'Always' Quiet at Night	300+	46%	60%	61%
Doctors 'Always' Communicated Well	300+	77%	81%	82%
Home Recovery Information Given	300+	86%	83%	85%
Hospital Given 9 or 10 on 10 Point Scale	300+	68%	68%	71%
Meds 'Always' Explained Before Given	300+	58%	63%	64%
Nurses 'Always' Communicated Well	300+	75%	77%	79%
Pain 'Always' Well Controlled	300+	66%	70%	71%
Room and Bathroom 'Always' Clean	300+	75%	72%	73%
Timely Help 'Always' Received	300+	63%	69%	68%
Would Definitely Recommend Hospital	300+	75%	67%	71%
Use of Medical Imaging				
Cardiac Imaging Stress Test before Surgery	730	4.8%	4.9%	5.3%
Combination Abdominal CT Scan	243	4.5%	10.6%	10.5%
Combination Brain/Sinus CT Scan[1]	-	-	1.9%	2.7%
Combination Chest CT Scan	62	3.2%	2.4%	2.7%
Follow-up Mammogram/Ultrasound	161	3.7%	6.9%	8.8%
Lumbar Spine MRI for Low Back Pain[1]	-	-	41.5%	37.2%

Central Montana Medical Center

408 Wendell Ave
Lewistown, MT 59457
Phone: 406-535-7711
Fax: 406-538-6392
URL: www.cmmccares.com
Type: Critical Access Hospitals
Emergency Services: Yes
Ownership: Voluntary non-profit - Private
Beds: 47

Key Personnel:
CEO/President. . . . . Wayne Edwards
Radiology. . . . . V Anne Hingle
Cardiac Laboratory. . . . . Debbie Lee
Intensive Care Unit. . . . . Dianne Scotten
Quality Assurance . . . . Marilyn Sparks
Chief of Medical Staff . . . . Thomas Troop, MD
Chairman/CEO . . . . Mike Zacher

Measure	Cases	This Hosp.	State Avg.	U.S. Avg.
Blood Clot Prevention and Treatment				
Anticoagulation Overlap Therapy[1,2]	-	-	97%	93%
ICU Venous Thromboembolism Prophylaxis[1,2]	-	-	92%	92%
Incidence of Potentially Preventable VTE[2,3]	-	-	4%	10%
UFH with Dosages/Platelet Monitoring[2,3]	-	-	97%	97%
Venous Thromboembolism Prophylaxis[2,3]	86	31%	83%	85%
Warfarin Therapy Discharge Instructions[1,2]	-	-	84%	75%
Chest Pain/Possible Heart Attack Care				
Aspirin Given Within 24 Hours of Arrival	23	96%	97%	96%
Fibrinolytic Meds Within 30 Min. of Arrival[1]	-	-	43%	58%
Average Time to ECG (minutes)	23	13	10	7
Average Time to Transfer (minutes)[7]	-	-	78	60
Children's Asthma Care				
Received Home Management Plan of Care	-	-	-	88%
Received Reliever Medication	-	-	-	100%
Received Systemic Corticosteroids	-	-	-	100%
Emergency Department				
Admittance Decision Time (minutes)[2]	325	30	72	98
Head CT Results Within 45 Min. of Arrival[1,3]	-	-	26%	57%
Patients Who Left ER Before Being Seen	1,670	2%	2%	2%
Time from ER Arrival to Admit. (minutes)[2]	373	135	220	274
Time from ER Arrival to Discharge (minutes)	306	70	120	134
Time in ER Before Being Evaluated (minutes)	326	10	23	26
Time to Pain Meds for Fractures (minutes)	24	18	47	57
Heart Attack Care				
Aspirin Given at Discharge[1,3]	-	-	100%	99%
Fibrinolytic Meds Within 30 Min. of Arrival[3,7]	-	-	50%	54%
PCI Within 90 Minutes of Arrival[3,7]	-	-	96%	96%
Statin Prescribed at Discharge[1,3]	-	-	99%	98%
Heart Failure Care				
ACE Inhibitor or ARB for LVSD	11	91%	97%	97%
Discharge Instructions Given	23	87%	92%	94%
Evaluation of LVS Function	30	80%	94%	99%
Medicare Spending				
Medicare Spending per Patient (ratio)	-	-	0.89	0.98
Pneumonia Care				
Appropriate Initial Antibiotic Given	32	97%	94%	95%
Blood Culture Timing	33	100%	97%	98%
Pregnancy and Delivery Care				
Newborn Deliveries Scheduled Early[5]	-	-	7%	6%
Preventive Care				
Immunization for Influenza[2]	213	81%	86%	90%
Immunization for Pneumonia[2]	400	87%	89%	92%
Stroke Care				
Anticoagulation Therapy for Atrial Fibrillation[3,7]	-	-	98%	95%
Antithrombotic Therapy Timing[1,3]	-	-	99%	98%
Assessed for Rehabilitation[1,3]	-	-	99%	97%
Discharged on Antithrombotic Therapy[1,3]	-	-	100%	99%
Discharged on Statin Medication[1,3]	-	-	94%	94%
Thrombolytic Therapy Timing[1,3]	-	-	67%	66%
Venous Thromboembolism Prophylaxis[1,3]	-	-	96%	94%
Written Stroke Educational Materials Given[1,3]	-	-	85%	88%
Surgical Care Improvement Project				
Appropriate Beta Blocker Usage[1]	-	-	98%	98%
Appropriate VTP Within 24 Hours	18	94%	98%	98%
Controlled Postoperative Blood Glucose[7]	-	-	96%	97%
Perioperative Temperature Management	21	100%	100%	100%
Prophylactic Antibiotic Selection	18	100%	99%	99%
Prophylactic Antibiotic Selection (Outpatient)[1,3]	-	-	98%	98%
Prophylactic Antibiotic Stopped	17	88%	99%	98%
Prophylactic Antibiotic Timing	18	100%	99%	99%
Prophylactic Antibiotic Timing (Outpatient)[1,3]	-	-	98%	98%
Urinary Catheter Removal	19	89%	99%	97%
Survey of Patients' Hospital Experiences				
Area Around Room 'Always' Quiet at Night	(a)	65%	60%	61%
Doctors 'Always' Communicated Well	(a)	85%	81%	82%
Home Recovery Information Given	(a)	83%	83%	85%
Hospital Given 9 or 10 on 10 Point Scale	(a)	67%	68%	71%
Meds 'Always' Explained Before Given	(a)	64%	63%	64%
Nurses 'Always' Communicated Well	(a)	82%	77%	79%
Pain 'Always' Well Controlled	(a)	69%	70%	71%
Room and Bathroom 'Always' Clean	(a)	58%	72%	73%
Timely Help 'Always' Received	(a)	71%	69%	68%
Would Definitely Recommend Hospital	(a)	66%	67%	71%
Use of Medical Imaging				
Cardiac Imaging Stress Test before Surgery[1]	-	-	4.9%	5.3%
Combination Abdominal CT Scan	89	38.2%	10.6%	10.5%
Combination Brain/Sinus CT Scan[1]	-	-	1.9%	2.7%
Combination Chest CT Scan	111	0.9%	2.4%	2.7%
Follow-up Mammogram/Ultrasound	379	4.7%	6.9%	8.8%
Lumbar Spine MRI for Low Back Pain[1]	-	-	41.5%	37.2%

Cabinet Peaks Medical Center

209 Health Park Dr
Libby, MT 59923
Phone: 406-293-0100
Fax: 406-293-7931
URL: www.sjlh.com
Type: Critical Access Hospitals
Emergency Services: Yes
Ownership: Voluntary non-profit - Private
Beds: 25

Key Personnel:
Radiology. . . . . Stephen Becker
Quality Assurance . . . . Barb Dumont
Chief of Medical Staff. . . . . Lance Ercanbrack, MD
Surgery . . . . Lance L. Ercanbrack, MD
CEO/President. . . . . Bill Patten
Infection Control. . . . . Clarice Thompson
Operating Room. . . . . Clarice Thompson

Measure	Cases	This Hosp.	State Avg.	U.S. Avg.
Blood Clot Prevention and Treatment				
Anticoagulation Overlap Therapy[5]	-	-	97%	93%
ICU Venous Thromboembolism Prophylaxis[5]	-	-	92%	92%
Incidence of Potentially Preventable VTE[5]	-	-	4%	10%
UFH with Dosages/Platelet Monitoring[5]	-	-	97%	97%
Venous Thromboembolism Prophylaxis[5]	-	-	83%	85%
Warfarin Therapy Discharge Instructions[5]	-	-	84%	75%
Chest Pain/Possible Heart Attack Care				
Aspirin Given Within 24 Hours of Arrival	17	100%	97%	96%
Fibrinolytic Meds Within 30 Min. of Arrival[1,3]	-	-	43%	58%
Average Time to ECG (minutes)	21	13	10	7
Average Time to Transfer (minutes)[1,3]	-	-	78	60
Children's Asthma Care				
Received Home Management Plan of Care	-	-	-	88%
Received Reliever Medication	-	-	-	100%
Received Systemic Corticosteroids	-	-	-	100%
Emergency Department				
Admittance Decision Time (minutes)[5]	-	-	72	98
Head CT Results Within 45 Min. of Arrival[1,3]	-	-	26%	57%
Patients Who Left ER Before Being Seen	6,353	0%	2%	2%
Time from ER Arrival to Admit. (minutes)[5]	-	-	220	274
Time from ER Arrival to Discharge (minutes)[5]	-	-	120	134
Time in ER Before Being Evaluated (minutes)[5]	-	-	23	26
Time to Pain Meds for Fractures (minutes)[5]	-	-	47	57
Heart Attack Care				
Aspirin Given at Discharge[3,7]	-	-	100%	99%
Fibrinolytic Meds Within 30 Min. of Arrival[3,7]	-	-	50%	54%
PCI Within 90 Minutes of Arrival[3,7]	-	-	96%	96%
Statin Prescribed at Discharge[3,7]	-	-	99%	98%
Heart Failure Care				
ACE Inhibitor or ARB for LVSD[1]	-	-	97%	97%
Discharge Instructions Given	14	100%	92%	94%
Evaluation of LVS Function	18	94%	94%	99%
Medicare Spending				
Medicare Spending per Patient (ratio)	-	-	0.89	0.98
Pneumonia Care				
Appropriate Initial Antibiotic Given	20	85%	94%	95%
Blood Culture Timing	25	96%	97%	98%
Pregnancy and Delivery Care				
Newborn Deliveries Scheduled Early[5]	-	-	7%	6%
Preventive Care				
Immunization for Influenza[5]	-	-	86%	90%
Immunization for Pneumonia[5]	-	-	89%	92%
Stroke Care				
Anticoagulation Therapy for Atrial Fibrillation[1]	-	-	98%	95%
Antithrombotic Therapy Timing[1]	-	-	99%	98%
Assessed for Rehabilitation[1]	-	-	99%	97%
Discharged on Antithrombotic Therapy[1]	-	-	100%	99%
Discharged on Statin Medication[1]	-	-	94%	94%
Thrombolytic Therapy Timing[1]	-	-	67%	66%
Venous Thromboembolism Prophylaxis[1]	-	-	96%	94%
Written Stroke Educational Materials Given[1]	-	-	85%	88%
Surgical Care Improvement Project				
Appropriate Beta Blocker Usage[1,2]	-	-	98%	98%
Appropriate VTP Within 24 Hours[2,3]	21	90%	98%	98%
Controlled Postoperative Blood Glucose[2,3]	-	-	96%	97%
Perioperative Temperature Management[2,3]	26	100%	100%	100%
Prophylactic Antibiotic Selection[2,3]	14	100%	99%	99%
Prophylactic Antibiotic Selection (Outpatient)	16	100%	98%	98%
Prophylactic Antibiotic Stopped[2,3]	14	86%	99%	98%
Prophylactic Antibiotic Timing[2,3]	14	100%	99%	99%
Prophylactic Antibiotic Timing (Outpatient)	16	100%	98%	98%
Urinary Catheter Removal[2,3]	12	100%	99%	97%
Survey of Patients' Hospital Experiences				
Area Around Room 'Always' Quiet at Night	(a)	57%	60%	61%
Doctors 'Always' Communicated Well	(a)	83%	81%	82%
Home Recovery Information Given	(a)	82%	83%	85%
Hospital Given 9 or 10 on 10 Point Scale	(a)	64%	68%	71%
Meds 'Always' Explained Before Given	(a)	60%	63%	64%
Nurses 'Always' Communicated Well	(a)	73%	77%	79%
Pain 'Always' Well Controlled	(a)	68%	70%	71%
Room and Bathroom 'Always' Clean	(a)	68%	72%	73%
Timely Help 'Always' Received	(a)	69%	69%	68%
Would Definitely Recommend Hospital	(a)	59%	67%	71%
Use of Medical Imaging				
Cardiac Imaging Stress Test before Surgery	46	4.3%	4.9%	5.3%
Combination Abdominal CT Scan	146	15.8%	10.6%	10.5%
Combination Brain/Sinus CT Scan[1]	-	-	1.9%	2.7%
Combination Chest CT Scan	203	7.9%	2.4%	2.7%

NOTE: Hospital profiles are in alphabetical order by state, then city, then hospital within the city; Rankings exclude hospitals with less than 25 cases except for patient surveys which excludes hospitals with less than 100 cases; (a) 100-299 cases; (1) The number of cases/patients is too few to report; (2) Data submitted were based on a sample of cases/patients; (3) Results are based on a shorter time period than required; (4) Data suppressed by CMS for one or more quarters; (5) Results are not available for this reporting period; (6) Fewer than 100 patients completed the HCAHPS survey; (7) No cases met the criteria for this measure; (8) The lower limit of the confidence interval cannot be calculated if the number of observed infections equals zero; (9) No data are available from the state/territory for this reporting period; (10) The scores shown reflect fewer than 50 completed surveys; (11) There were discrepancies in the data collection process; (12) This measure does not apply to this hospital for this reporting period; (13) Results cannot be calculated for this reporting period; (14) The results for this state are combined with nearby states to protect confidentiality; Please refer to the User's Guide for a full explanation of data.

Follow-up Mammogram/Ultrasound	254	6.3%	6.9%	8.8%
Lumbar Spine MRI for Low Back Pain[1]	-	-	41.5%	37.2%

Livingston Healthcare

504 S 13th St
Livingston, MT 59047
Type: Critical Access Hospitals
Ownership: Voluntary non-profit - Private
Phone: 406-222-3541
Fax: 406-222-5099
Emergency Services: Yes
Beds: 45

Key Personnel:
President . . . . Michelle Becker
CEO/President. . . . . Richard Brown
CEO . . . . Bren Lowe

Measure	Cases	This Hosp.	State Avg.	U.S. Avg.
Blood Clot Prevention and Treatment				
Anticoagulation Overlap Therapy[5]	-	-	97%	93%
ICU Venous Thromboembolism Prophylaxis[5]	-	-	92%	92%
Incidence of Potentially Preventable VTE[5]	-	-	4%	10%
UFH with Dosages/Platelet Monitoring[5]	-	-	97%	97%
Venous Thromboembolism Prophylaxis[5]	-	-	83%	85%
Warfarin Therapy Discharge Instructions[5]	-	-	84%	75%
Chest Pain/Possible Heart Attack Care				
Aspirin Given Within 24 Hours of Arrival	-	-	97%	96%
Fibrinolytic Meds Within 30 Min. of Arrival	-	-	43%	58%
Average Time to ECG (minutes)	-	-	10	7
Average Time to Transfer (minutes)	-	-	78	60
Children's Asthma Care				
Received Home Management Plan of Care	-	-	-	88%
Received Reliever Medication	-	-	-	100%
Received Systemic Corticosteroids	-	-	-	100%
Emergency Department				
Admittance Decision Time (minutes)[5]	-	-	72	98
Head CT Results Within 45 Min. of Arrival	-	-	26%	57%
Patients Who Left ER Before Being Seen	-	-	2%	2%
Time from ER Arrival to Admit. (minutes)[5]	-	-	220	274
Time from ER Arrival to Discharge (minutes)	-	-	120	134
Time in ER Before Being Evaluated (minutes)	-	-	23	26
Time to Pain Meds for Fractures (minutes)	-	-	47	57
Heart Attack Care				
Aspirin Given at Discharge[3,7]	-	-	100%	99%
Fibrinolytic Meds Within 30 Min. of Arrival[3,7]	-	-	50%	54%
PCI Within 90 Minutes of Arrival[5]	-	-	96%	96%
Statin Prescribed at Discharge[3,7]	-	-	99%	98%
Heart Failure Care				
ACE Inhibitor or ARB for LVSD[1]	-	-	97%	97%
Discharge Instructions Given	25	100%	92%	94%
Evaluation of LVS Function	34	97%	94%	99%
Medicare Spending				
Medicare Spending per Patient (ratio)	-	-	0.89	0.98
Pneumonia Care				
Appropriate Initial Antibiotic Given	27	93%	94%	95%
Blood Culture Timing	21	100%	97%	98%
Pregnancy and Delivery Care				
Newborn Deliveries Scheduled Early[5]	-	-	7%	6%
Preventive Care				
Immunization for Influenza[5]	-	-	86%	90%
Immunization for Pneumonia[5]	-	-	89%	92%
Stroke Care				
Anticoagulation Therapy for Atrial Fibrillation[1,3]	-	-	98%	95%
Antithrombotic Therapy Timing[1,3]	-	-	99%	98%
Assessed for Rehabilitation[1,3]	-	-	99%	97%
Discharged on Antithrombotic Therapy[1,3]	-	-	100%	99%
Discharged on Statin Medication[1,3]	-	-	94%	94%
Thrombolytic Therapy Timing[3,7]	-	-	67%	66%
Venous Thromboembolism Prophylaxis[1,3]	-	-	96%	94%
Written Stroke Educational Materials Given[1,3]	-	-	85%	88%
Surgical Care Improvement Project				
Appropriate Beta Blocker Usage	12	100%	98%	98%
Appropriate VTP Within 24 Hours	46	96%	98%	98%
Controlled Postoperative Blood Glucose[7]	-	-	96%	97%
Perioperative Temperature Management	49	100%	100%	100%
Prophylactic Antibiotic Selection	46	98%	99%	99%
Prophylactic Antibiotic Selection (Outpatient)	-	-	98%	98%
Prophylactic Antibiotic Stopped	46	98%	99%	98%
Prophylactic Antibiotic Timing	46	98%	99%	99%
Prophylactic Antibiotic Timing (Outpatient)	-	-	98%	98%
Urinary Catheter Removal	18	94%	99%	97%
Survey of Patients' Hospital Experiences				
Area Around Room 'Always' Quiet at Night	(a)	52%	60%	61%
Doctors 'Always' Communicated Well	(a)	85%	81%	82%
Home Recovery Information Given	(a)	83%	83%	85%
Hospital Given 9 or 10 on 10 Point Scale	(a)	64%	68%	71%
Meds 'Always' Explained Before Given	(a)	67%	63%	64%
Nurses 'Always' Communicated Well	(a)	82%	77%	79%
Pain 'Always' Well Controlled	(a)	73%	70%	71%
Room and Bathroom 'Always' Clean	(a)	81%	72%	73%
Timely Help 'Always' Received	(a)	77%	69%	68%
Would Definitely Recommend Hospital	(a)	63%	67%	71%
Use of Medical Imaging				
Cardiac Imaging Stress Test before Surgery	-	-	4.9%	5.3%
Combination Abdominal CT Scan	-	-	10.6%	10.5%
Combination Brain/Sinus CT Scan	-	-	1.9%	2.7%
Combination Chest CT Scan	-	-	2.4%	2.7%
Follow-up Mammogram/Ultrasound	-	-	6.9%	8.8%
Lumbar Spine MRI for Low Back Pain	-	-	41.5%	37.2%

Phillips County Medical Center

311 S 8th Ave E
Malta, MT 59538
Type: Critical Access Hospitals
Ownership: Voluntary non-profit - Private
Phone: 406-654-1100
Fax: 406-654-2876
Emergency Services: Yes
Beds: 14

Key Personnel:
CEO/President. . . . . Larry Putnam

Measure	Cases	This Hosp.	State Avg.	U.S. Avg.
Blood Clot Prevention and Treatment				
Anticoagulation Overlap Therapy[5]	-	-	97%	93%
ICU Venous Thromboembolism Prophylaxis[5]	-	-	92%	92%
Incidence of Potentially Preventable VTE[5]	-	-	4%	10%
UFH with Dosages/Platelet Monitoring[5]	-	-	97%	97%
Venous Thromboembolism Prophylaxis[5]	-	-	83%	85%
Warfarin Therapy Discharge Instructions[5]	-	-	84%	75%
Chest Pain/Possible Heart Attack Care				
Aspirin Given Within 24 Hours of Arrival	-	-	97%	96%
Fibrinolytic Meds Within 30 Min. of Arrival	-	-	43%	58%
Average Time to ECG (minutes)	-	-	10	7
Average Time to Transfer (minutes)	-	-	78	60
Children's Asthma Care				
Received Home Management Plan of Care	-	-	-	88%
Received Reliever Medication	-	-	-	100%
Received Systemic Corticosteroids	-	-	-	100%
Emergency Department				
Admittance Decision Time (minutes)[5]	-	-	72	98
Head CT Results Within 45 Min. of Arrival	-	-	26%	57%
Patients Who Left ER Before Being Seen	-	-	2%	2%
Time from ER Arrival to Admit. (minutes)[5]	-	-	220	274
Time from ER Arrival to Discharge (minutes)	-	-	120	134
Time in ER Before Being Evaluated (minutes)	-	-	23	26
Time to Pain Meds for Fractures (minutes)	-	-	47	57
Heart Attack Care				
Aspirin Given at Discharge[5]	-	-	100%	99%
Fibrinolytic Meds Within 30 Min. of Arrival[5]	-	-	50%	54%
PCI Within 90 Minutes of Arrival[5]	-	-	96%	96%
Statin Prescribed at Discharge[5]	-	-	99%	98%
Heart Failure Care				
ACE Inhibitor or ARB for LVSD[3,7]	-	-	97%	97%
Discharge Instructions Given[1,3]	-	-	92%	94%
Evaluation of LVS Function[1,3]	-	-	94%	99%
Medicare Spending				
Medicare Spending per Patient (ratio)	-	-	0.89	0.98
Pneumonia Care				
Appropriate Initial Antibiotic Given[1,3]	-	-	94%	95%
Blood Culture Timing[1,3]	-	-	97%	98%
Pregnancy and Delivery Care				
Newborn Deliveries Scheduled Early[5]	-	-	7%	6%
Preventive Care				
Immunization for Influenza[5]	-	-	86%	90%
Immunization for Pneumonia[5]	-	-	89%	92%
Stroke Care				
Anticoagulation Therapy for Atrial Fibrillation[5]	-	-	98%	95%
Antithrombotic Therapy Timing[5]	-	-	99%	98%
Assessed for Rehabilitation[5]	-	-	99%	97%
Discharged on Antithrombotic Therapy[5]	-	-	100%	99%
Discharged on Statin Medication[5]	-	-	94%	94%
Thrombolytic Therapy Timing[5]	-	-	67%	66%
Venous Thromboembolism Prophylaxis[5]	-	-	96%	94%
Written Stroke Educational Materials Given[5]	-	-	85%	88%
Surgical Care Improvement Project				
Appropriate Beta Blocker Usage[5]	-	-	98%	98%
Appropriate VTP Within 24 Hours[5]	-	-	98%	98%
Controlled Postoperative Blood Glucose[5]	-	-	96%	97%
Perioperative Temperature Management[5]	-	-	100%	100%
Prophylactic Antibiotic Selection[5]	-	-	99%	99%
Prophylactic Antibiotic Selection (Outpatient)	-	-	98%	98%
Prophylactic Antibiotic Stopped[5]	-	-	99%	98%
Prophylactic Antibiotic Timing[5]	-	-	99%	99%
Prophylactic Antibiotic Timing (Outpatient)	-	-	98%	98%
Urinary Catheter Removal[5]	-	-	99%	97%
Survey of Patients' Hospital Experiences				
Area Around Room 'Always' Quiet at Night[5]	-	-	60%	61%
Doctors 'Always' Communicated Well[5]	-	-	81%	82%
Home Recovery Information Given[5]	-	-	83%	85%
Hospital Given 9 or 10 on 10 Point Scale[5]	-	-	68%	71%
Meds 'Always' Explained Before Given[5]	-	-	63%	64%
Nurses 'Always' Communicated Well[5]	-	-	77%	79%
Pain 'Always' Well Controlled[5]	-	-	70%	71%
Room and Bathroom 'Always' Clean[5]	-	-	72%	73%
Timely Help 'Always' Received[5]	-	-	69%	68%
Would Definitely Recommend Hospital[5]	-	-	67%	71%
Use of Medical Imaging				
Cardiac Imaging Stress Test before Surgery	-	-	4.9%	5.3%
Combination Abdominal CT Scan	-	-	10.6%	10.5%
Combination Brain/Sinus CT Scan	-	-	1.9%	2.7%
Combination Chest CT Scan	-	-	2.4%	2.7%
Follow-up Mammogram/Ultrasound	-	-	6.9%	8.8%
Lumbar Spine MRI for Low Back Pain	-	-	41.5%	37.2%

Holy Rosary Healthcare

2600 Wilson St
Miles City, MT 59301
Type: Critical Access Hospitals
Ownership: Voluntary non-profit - Church
Phone: 406-233-2600
Emergency Services: Yes

Measure	Cases	This Hosp.	State Avg.	U.S. Avg.
Blood Clot Prevention and Treatment				
Anticoagulation Overlap Therapy[1]	-	-	97%	93%
ICU Venous Thromboembolism Prophylaxis	113	98%	92%	92%
Incidence of Potentially Preventable VTE[1]	-	-	4%	10%
UFH with Dosages/Platelet Monitoring[7]	-	-	97%	97%
Venous Thromboembolism Prophylaxis	278	95%	83%	85%
Warfarin Therapy Discharge Instructions[1]	-	-	84%	75%
Chest Pain/Possible Heart Attack Care				
Aspirin Given Within 24 Hours of Arrival	14	100%	97%	96%
Fibrinolytic Meds Within 30 Min. of Arrival[1,3]	-	-	43%	58%
Average Time to ECG (minutes)	16	34	10	7
Average Time to Transfer (minutes)[3,7]	-	-	78	60
Children's Asthma Care				
Received Home Management Plan of Care	-	-	-	88%
Received Reliever Medication	-	-	-	100%
Received Systemic Corticosteroids	-	-	-	100%
Emergency Department				
Admittance Decision Time (minutes)[2]	216	52	72	98
Head CT Results Within 45 Min. of Arrival[1]	-	-	26%	57%
Patients Who Left ER Before Being Seen[5]	-	-	2%	2%
Time from ER Arrival to Admit. (minutes)[2]	219	174	220	274
Time from ER Arrival to Discharge (minutes)	336	85	120	134
Time in ER Before Being Evaluated (minutes)	377	17	23	26
Time to Pain Meds for Fractures (minutes)	28	32	47	57
Heart Attack Care				
Aspirin Given at Discharge[1,3]	-	-	100%	99%
Fibrinolytic Meds Within 30 Min. of Arrival[3,7]	-	-	50%	54%

NOTE: Hospital profiles are in alphabetical order by state, then city, then hospital within the city; Rankings exclude hospitals with less than 25 cases except for patient surveys which excludes hospitals with less than 100 cases; (a) 100-299 cases; (1) The number of cases/patients is too few to report; (2) Data submitted were based on a sample of cases/patients; (3) Results are based on a shorter time period than required; (4) Data suppressed by CMS for one or more quarters; (5) Results are not available for this reporting period; (6) Fewer than 100 patients completed the HCAHPS survey; (7) No cases met the criteria for this measure; (8) The lower limit of the confidence interval cannot be calculated if the number of observed infections equals zero; (9) No data are available from the state/territory for this reporting period; (10) The scores shown reflect fewer than 50 completed surveys; (11) There were discrepancies in the data collection process; (12) This measure does not apply to this hospital for this reporting period; (13) Results cannot be calculated for this reporting period; (14) The results for this state are combined with nearby states to protect confidentiality; Please refer to the User's Guide for a full explanation of data.

Measure	Cases	This Hosp.	State Avg.	U.S. Avg.
PCI Within 90 Minutes of Arrival[3,7]	-	-	96%	96%
Statin Prescribed at Discharge[1,3]	-	-	99%	98%
Heart Failure Care				
ACE Inhibitor or ARB for LVSD	11	100%	97%	97%
Discharge Instructions Given	18	100%	92%	94%
Evaluation of LVS Function	23	100%	94%	99%
Medicare Spending				
Medicare Spending per Patient (ratio)	-	-	0.89	0.98
Pneumonia Care				
Appropriate Initial Antibiotic Given	41	93%	94%	95%
Blood Culture Timing	67	100%	97%	98%
Pregnancy and Delivery Care				
Newborn Deliveries Scheduled Early[5]	-	-	7%	6%
Preventive Care				
Immunization for Influenza[2]	225	68%	86%	90%
Immunization for Pneumonia[2]	228	79%	89%	92%
Stroke Care				
Anticoagulation Therapy for Atrial Fibrillation[1]	-	-	98%	95%
Antithrombotic Therapy Timing	12	100%	99%	98%
Assessed for Rehabilitation	12	100%	99%	97%
Discharged on Antithrombotic Therapy[1]	-	-	100%	99%
Discharged on Statin Medication[1]	-	-	94%	94%
Thrombolytic Therapy Timing[1]	-	-	67%	66%
Venous Thromboembolism Prophylaxis	16	100%	96%	94%
Written Stroke Educational Materials Given[1]	-	-	85%	88%
Surgical Care Improvement Project				
Appropriate Beta Blocker Usage	13	100%	98%	98%
Appropriate VTP Within 24 Hours	106	100%	98%	98%
Controlled Postoperative Blood Glucose[7]	-	-	96%	97%
Perioperative Temperature Management	117	100%	100%	100%
Prophylactic Antibiotic Selection	90	100%	99%	99%
Prophylactic Antibiotic Selection (Outpatient)	12	75%	98%	98%
Prophylactic Antibiotic Stopped	88	99%	99%	98%
Prophylactic Antibiotic Timing	91	100%	99%	99%
Prophylactic Antibiotic Timing (Outpatient)	23	48%	98%	98%
Urinary Catheter Removal	86	99%	99%	97%
Survey of Patients' Hospital Experiences				
Area Around Room 'Always' Quiet at Night	(a)	58%	60%	61%
Doctors 'Always' Communicated Well	(a)	78%	81%	82%
Home Recovery Information Given	(a)	87%	83%	85%
Hospital Given 9 or 10 on 10 Point Scale	(a)	68%	68%	71%
Meds 'Always' Explained Before Given	(a)	64%	63%	64%
Nurses 'Always' Communicated Well	(a)	81%	77%	79%
Pain 'Always' Well Controlled	(a)	76%	70%	71%
Room and Bathroom 'Always' Clean	(a)	67%	72%	73%
Timely Help 'Always' Received	(a)	68%	69%	68%
Would Definitely Recommend Hospital	(a)	69%	67%	71%
Use of Medical Imaging				
Cardiac Imaging Stress Test before Surgery[1]	-	-	4.9%	5.3%
Combination Abdominal CT Scan	121	9.9%	10.6%	10.5%
Combination Brain/Sinus CT Scan[1]	-	-	1.9%	2.7%
Combination Chest CT Scan	73	1.4%	2.4%	2.7%
Follow-up Mammogram/Ultrasound	170	8.2%	6.9%	8.8%
Lumbar Spine MRI for Low Back Pain	42	47.6%	41.5%	37.2%

Community Medical Center

2827 Fort Missoula Rd
Missoula, MT 59804
Phone: 406-728-4100
Fax: 406-327-4580
Type: Acute Care Hospitals
Emergency Services: Yes
Ownership: Voluntary non-profit - Private
Beds: 125

Key Personnel:
Emergency Room . . . . Jessica Bayless
Radiology. . . . . Adam Benson
CEO/President. . . . . Steve Carlson
Cardiac Laboratory. . . . . John Dague
CEO . . . . Christine Noguera
Chief of Medical Staff . . . . Tom Randall

Measure	Cases	This Hosp.	State Avg.	U.S. Avg.
Blood Clot Prevention and Treatment				
Anticoagulation Overlap Therapy[2]	29	100%	97%	93%
ICU Venous Thromboembolism Prophylaxis[2]	30	100%	92%	92%
Incidence of Potentially Preventable VTE[1,2]	-	-	4%	10%
UFH with Dosages/Platelet Monitoring[1,2]	-	-	97%	97%
Venous Thromboembolism Prophylaxis[2]	232	97%	83%	85%
Warfarin Therapy Discharge Instructions[2]	24	100%	84%	75%
Chest Pain/Possible Heart Attack Care				
Aspirin Given Within 24 Hours of Arrival[1,3]	-	-	97%	96%
Fibrinolytic Meds Within 30 Min. of Arrival[5]	-	-	43%	58%
Average Time to ECG (minutes)[1,3]	-	-	10	7
Average Time to Transfer (minutes)[5]	-	-	78	60
Children's Asthma Care				
Received Home Management Plan of Care	-	-	-	88%
Received Reliever Medication	-	-	-	100%
Received Systemic Corticosteroids	-	-	-	100%
Emergency Department				
Admittance Decision Time (minutes)[2]	278	88	72	98
Head CT Results Within 45 Min. of Arrival[1]	-	-	26%	57%
Patients Who Left ER Before Being Seen	17,062	0%	2%	2%
Time from ER Arrival to Admit. (minutes)[2]	295	234	220	274
Time from ER Arrival to Discharge (minutes)	394	125	120	134
Time in ER Before Being Evaluated (minutes)	389	33	23	26
Time to Pain Meds for Fractures (minutes)	84	44	47	57
Heart Attack Care				
Aspirin Given at Discharge	35	100%	100%	99%
Fibrinolytic Meds Within 30 Min. of Arrival[7]	-	-	50%	54%
PCI Within 90 Minutes of Arrival[1]	-	-	96%	96%
Statin Prescribed at Discharge	32	100%	99%	98%
Heart Failure Care				
ACE Inhibitor or ARB for LVSD	16	100%	97%	97%
Discharge Instructions Given	38	84%	92%	94%
Evaluation of LVS Function	59	100%	94%	99%
Medicare Spending				
Medicare Spending per Patient (ratio)	-	0.90	0.89	0.98
Pneumonia Care				
Appropriate Initial Antibiotic Given	41	98%	94%	95%
Blood Culture Timing	53	100%	97%	98%
Pregnancy and Delivery Care				
Newborn Deliveries Scheduled Early[2]	24	4%	7%	6%
Preventive Care				
Immunization for Influenza[2]	457	91%	86%	90%
Immunization for Pneumonia[2]	369	93%	89%	92%
Stroke Care				
Anticoagulation Therapy for Atrial Fibrillation[1]	-	-	98%	95%
Antithrombotic Therapy Timing	20	100%	99%	98%
Assessed for Rehabilitation	23	100%	99%	97%
Discharged on Antithrombotic Therapy	20	100%	100%	99%
Discharged on Statin Medication	16	100%	94%	94%
Thrombolytic Therapy Timing[7]	-	-	67%	66%
Venous Thromboembolism Prophylaxis	23	100%	96%	94%
Written Stroke Educational Materials Given[1]	-	-	85%	88%
Surgical Care Improvement Project				
Appropriate Beta Blocker Usage[2]	81	99%	98%	98%
Appropriate VTP Within 24 Hours[2]	347	96%	98%	98%
Controlled Postoperative Blood Glucose[2,7]	-	-	96%	97%
Perioperative Temperature Management[2]	400	100%	100%	100%
Prophylactic Antibiotic Selection[2]	274	99%	99%	99%
Prophylactic Antibiotic Selection (Outpatient)	267	99%	98%	98%
Prophylactic Antibiotic Stopped[2]	270	98%	99%	98%
Prophylactic Antibiotic Timing[2]	274	100%	99%	99%
Prophylactic Antibiotic Timing (Outpatient)	267	100%	98%	98%
Urinary Catheter Removal[2]	43	93%	99%	97%
Survey of Patients' Hospital Experiences				
Area Around Room 'Always' Quiet at Night	300+	59%	60%	61%
Doctors 'Always' Communicated Well	300+	81%	81%	82%
Home Recovery Information Given	300+	87%	83%	85%
Hospital Given 9 or 10 on 10 Point Scale	300+	75%	68%	71%
Meds 'Always' Explained Before Given	300+	61%	63%	64%
Nurses 'Always' Communicated Well	300+	77%	77%	79%
Pain 'Always' Well Controlled	300+	70%	70%	71%
Room and Bathroom 'Always' Clean	300+	74%	72%	73%
Timely Help 'Always' Received	300+	64%	69%	68%
Would Definitely Recommend Hospital	300+	77%	67%	71%
Use of Medical Imaging				
Cardiac Imaging Stress Test before Surgery	120	8.3%	4.9%	5.3%
Combination Abdominal CT Scan	466	15.2%	10.6%	10.5%
Combination Brain/Sinus CT Scan	252	0.4%	1.9%	2.7%
Combination Chest CT Scan	267	0.4%	2.4%	2.7%
Follow-up Mammogram/Ultrasound	1,333	8.3%	6.9%	8.8%
Lumbar Spine MRI for Low Back Pain	156	35.9%	41.5%	37.2%

Saint Patrick Hospital

500 W Broadway
Missoula, MT 59806
Phone: 406-543-7271
Fax: 406-329-5693
URL: www.saintpatrick.org
Type: Acute Care Hospitals
Emergency Services: Yes
Ownership: Voluntary non-profit - Church
Beds: 213

Key Personnel:
Quality Assurance . . . . Lou Corts
CEO/President. . . . . Jeff Fee
Chief of Medical Staff . . . . Matt Maxwell, MD
Operating Room. . . . . Matt Maxwell, MD
Radiology. . . . . James McKay, MD
Pediatric Ambulatory Care . . . . . . Kathleen S Rogers, MD
Pediatric In-Patient Care . . . . Kathleen S Rogers, MD

Measure	Cases	This Hosp.	State Avg.	U.S. Avg.
Blood Clot Prevention and Treatment				
Anticoagulation Overlap Therapy[2]	87	95%	97%	93%
ICU Venous Thromboembolism Prophylaxis[2]	63	87%	92%	92%
Incidence of Potentially Preventable VTE[2]	16	6%	4%	10%
UFH with Dosages/Platelet Monitoring[2]	39	100%	97%	97%
Venous Thromboembolism Prophylaxis[2]	298	89%	83%	85%
Warfarin Therapy Discharge Instructions[2]	76	47%	84%	75%
Chest Pain/Possible Heart Attack Care				
Aspirin Given Within 24 Hours of Arrival[3,7]	-	-	97%	96%
Fibrinolytic Meds Within 30 Min. of Arrival[5]	-	-	43%	58%
Average Time to ECG (minutes)[3,7]	-	-	10	7
Average Time to Transfer (minutes)[5]	-	-	78	60
Children's Asthma Care				
Received Home Management Plan of Care	-	-	-	88%
Received Reliever Medication	-	-	-	100%
Received Systemic Corticosteroids	-	-	-	100%
Emergency Department				
Admittance Decision Time (minutes)[2]	510	101	72	98
Head CT Results Within 45 Min. of Arrival[1]	-	-	26%	57%
Patients Who Left ER Before Being Seen	28,071	4%	2%	2%
Time from ER Arrival to Admit. (minutes)[2]	589	249	220	274
Time from ER Arrival to Discharge (minutes)	357	143	120	134
Time in ER Before Being Evaluated (minutes)	342	40	23	26
Time to Pain Meds for Fractures (minutes)	85	53	47	57
Heart Attack Care				
Aspirin Given at Discharge	348	100%	100%	99%
Fibrinolytic Meds Within 30 Min. of Arrival[7]	-	-	50%	54%
PCI Within 90 Minutes of Arrival	30	90%	96%	96%
Statin Prescribed at Discharge	339	100%	99%	98%
Heart Failure Care				
ACE Inhibitor or ARB for LVSD	62	100%	97%	97%
Discharge Instructions Given	154	96%	92%	94%
Evaluation of LVS Function	177	100%	94%	99%
Medicare Spending				
Medicare Spending per Patient (ratio)	-	0.90	0.89	0.98
Pneumonia Care				
Appropriate Initial Antibiotic Given	119	97%	94%	95%
Blood Culture Timing	187	97%	97%	98%
Pregnancy and Delivery Care				
Newborn Deliveries Scheduled Early[2,7]	-	-	7%	6%
Preventive Care				
Immunization for Influenza[2]	616	89%	86%	90%
Immunization for Pneumonia[2]	831	84%	89%	92%
Stroke Care				
Anticoagulation Therapy for Atrial Fibrillation[1,2]	-	-	98%	95%
Antithrombotic Therapy Timing[2]	58	100%	99%	98%
Assessed for Rehabilitation[2]	88	99%	99%	97%
Discharged on Antithrombotic Therapy[2]	74	100%	100%	99%
Discharged on Statin Medication[2]	52	98%	94%	94%
Thrombolytic Therapy Timing[1,2]	-	-	67%	66%
Venous Thromboembolism Prophylaxis[2]	86	93%	96%	94%
Written Stroke Educational Materials Given[2]	56	86%	85%	88%
Surgical Care Improvement Project				
Appropriate Beta Blocker Usage[2]	159	100%	98%	98%

NOTE: Hospital profiles are in alphabetical order by state, then city, then hospital within the city; Rankings exclude hospitals with less than 25 cases except for patient surveys which excludes hospitals with less than 100 cases; (a) 100-299 cases; (1) The number of cases/patients is too few to report; (2) Data submitted were based on a sample of cases/patients; (3) Results are based on a shorter time period than required; (4) Data suppressed by CMS for one or more quarters; (5) Results are not available for this reporting period; (6) Fewer than 100 patients completed the HCAHPS survey; (7) No cases met the criteria for this measure; (8) The lower limit of the confidence interval cannot be calculated if the number of observed infections equals zero; (9) No data are available from the state/territory for this reporting period; (10) The scores shown reflect fewer than 50 completed surveys; (11) There were discrepancies in the data collection process; (12) This measure does not apply to this hospital for this reporting period; (13) Results cannot be calculated for this reporting period; (14) The results for this state are combined with nearby states to protect confidentiality; Please refer to the User's Guide for a full explanation of data.

Measure	Cases	This Hosp.	State Avg.	U.S. Avg.
Appropriate VTP Within 24 Hours[2]	278	97%	98%	98%
Controlled Postoperative Blood Glucose[2]	150	97%	96%	97%
Perioperative Temperature Management[2]	322	100%	100%	100%
Prophylactic Antibiotic Selection[2]	331	99%	99%	99%
Prophylactic Antibiotic Selection (Outpatient)	397	93%	98%	98%
Prophylactic Antibiotic Stopped[2]	324	98%	99%	98%
Prophylactic Antibiotic Timing[2]	331	96%	99%	99%
Prophylactic Antibiotic Timing (Outpatient)	404	97%	98%	98%
Urinary Catheter Removal[2]	244	97%	99%	97%
Survey of Patients' Hospital Experiences				
Area Around Room 'Always' Quiet at Night	300+	58%	60%	61%
Doctors 'Always' Communicated Well	300+	81%	81%	82%
Home Recovery Information Given	300+	87%	83%	85%
Hospital Given 9 or 10 on 10 Point Scale	300+	77%	68%	71%
Meds 'Always' Explained Before Given	300+	66%	63%	64%
Nurses 'Always' Communicated Well	300+	78%	77%	79%
Pain 'Always' Well Controlled	300+	71%	70%	71%
Room and Bathroom 'Always' Clean	300+	74%	72%	73%
Timely Help 'Always' Received	300+	66%	69%	68%
Would Definitely Recommend Hospital	300+	83%	67%	71%
Use of Medical Imaging				
Cardiac Imaging Stress Test before Surgery	788	3.8%	4.9%	5.3%
Combination Abdominal CT Scan	1,003	8.5%	10.6%	10.5%
Combination Brain/Sinus CT Scan	530	0.8%	1.9%	2.7%
Combination Chest CT Scan	720	0.0%	2.4%	2.7%
Follow-up Mammogram/Ultrasound	2,083	6.8%	6.9%	8.8%
Lumbar Spine MRI for Low Back Pain	276	37.7%	41.5%	37.2%

Granite County Medical Center

310 Sansome St
Philipsburg, MT 59858
Phone: 406-859-3271
Type: Critical Access Hospitals
Emergency Services: Yes
Ownership: Govt - Hospital Dist/Auth

Measure	Cases	This Hosp.	State Avg.	U.S. Avg.
Blood Clot Prevention and Treatment				
Anticoagulation Overlap Therapy[5]	-	-	97%	93%
ICU Venous Thromboembolism Prophylaxis[5]	-	-	92%	92%
Incidence of Potentially Preventable VTE[5]	-	-	4%	10%
UFH with Dosages/Platelet Monitoring[5]	-	-	97%	97%
Venous Thromboembolism Prophylaxis[5]	-	-	83%	85%
Warfarin Therapy Discharge Instructions[5]	-	-	84%	75%
Chest Pain/Possible Heart Attack Care				
Aspirin Given Within 24 Hours of Arrival	-	-	97%	96%
Fibrinolytic Meds Within 30 Min. of Arrival	-	-	43%	58%
Average Time to ECG (minutes)	-	-	10	7
Average Time to Transfer (minutes)	-	-	78	60
Children's Asthma Care				
Received Home Management Plan of Care	-	-	-	88%
Received Reliever Medication	-	-	-	100%
Received Systemic Corticosteroids	-	-	-	100%
Emergency Department				
Admittance Decision Time (minutes)[5]	-	-	72	98
Head CT Results Within 45 Min. of Arrival	-	-	26%	57%
Patients Who Left ER Before Being Seen	-	-	2%	2%
Time from ER Arrival to Admit. (minutes)[5]	-	-	220	274
Time from ER Arrival to Discharge (minutes)	-	-	120	134
Time in ER Before Being Evaluated (minutes)	-	-	23	26
Time to Pain Meds for Fractures (minutes)	-	-	47	57
Heart Attack Care				
Aspirin Given at Discharge[5]	-	-	100%	99%
Fibrinolytic Meds Within 30 Min. of Arrival[5]	-	-	50%	54%
PCI Within 90 Minutes of Arrival[5]	-	-	96%	96%
Statin Prescribed at Discharge[5]	-	-	99%	98%
Heart Failure Care				
ACE Inhibitor or ARB for LVSD[3,7]	-	-	97%	97%
Discharge Instructions Given[3,7]	-	-	92%	94%
Evaluation of LVS Function[3,7]	-	-	94%	99%
Medicare Spending				
Medicare Spending per Patient (ratio)	-	-	0.89	0.98
Pneumonia Care				
Appropriate Initial Antibiotic Given[3,7]	-	-	94%	95%
Blood Culture Timing[3,7]	-	-	97%	98%
Pregnancy and Delivery Care				
Newborn Deliveries Scheduled Early[5]	-	-	7%	6%
Preventive Care				
Immunization for Influenza[5]	-	-	86%	90%
Immunization for Pneumonia[5]	-	-	89%	92%
Stroke Care				
Anticoagulation Therapy for Atrial Fibrillation[5]	-	-	98%	95%
Antithrombotic Therapy Timing[5]	-	-	99%	98%
Assessed for Rehabilitation[5]	-	-	99%	97%
Discharged on Antithrombotic Therapy[5]	-	-	100%	99%
Discharged on Statin Medication[5]	-	-	94%	94%
Thrombolytic Therapy Timing[5]	-	-	67%	66%
Venous Thromboembolism Prophylaxis[5]	-	-	96%	94%
Written Stroke Educational Materials Given[5]	-	-	85%	88%
Surgical Care Improvement Project				
Appropriate Beta Blocker Usage[5]	-	-	98%	98%
Appropriate VTP Within 24 Hours[5]	-	-	98%	98%
Controlled Postoperative Blood Glucose[5]	-	-	96%	97%
Perioperative Temperature Management[5]	-	-	100%	100%
Prophylactic Antibiotic Selection[5]	-	-	99%	99%
Prophylactic Antibiotic Selection (Outpatient)	-	-	98%	98%
Prophylactic Antibiotic Stopped[5]	-	-	99%	98%
Prophylactic Antibiotic Timing[5]	-	-	99%	99%
Prophylactic Antibiotic Timing (Outpatient)	-	-	98%	98%
Urinary Catheter Removal[5]	-	-	99%	97%
Survey of Patients' Hospital Experiences				
Area Around Room 'Always' Quiet at Night[5]	-	-	60%	61%
Doctors 'Always' Communicated Well[5]	-	-	81%	82%
Home Recovery Information Given[5]	-	-	83%	85%
Hospital Given 9 or 10 on 10 Point Scale[5]	-	-	68%	71%
Meds 'Always' Explained Before Given[5]	-	-	63%	64%
Nurses 'Always' Communicated Well[5]	-	-	77%	79%
Pain 'Always' Well Controlled[5]	-	-	70%	71%
Room and Bathroom 'Always' Clean[5]	-	-	72%	73%
Timely Help 'Always' Received[5]	-	-	69%	68%
Would Definitely Recommend Hospital[5]	-	-	67%	71%
Use of Medical Imaging				
Cardiac Imaging Stress Test before Surgery	-	-	4.9%	5.3%
Combination Abdominal CT Scan	-	-	10.6%	10.5%
Combination Brain/Sinus CT Scan	-	-	1.9%	2.7%
Combination Chest CT Scan	-	-	2.4%	2.7%
Follow-up Mammogram/Ultrasound	-	-	6.9%	8.8%
Lumbar Spine MRI for Low Back Pain	-	-	41.5%	37.2%

Clark Fork Valley Hospital

10 Kruger Rd
Plains, MT 59859
Phone: 406-826-4800
Fax: 406-826-4880
E-mail: clarkc@st.patrick.org
Type: Critical Access Hospitals
Emergency Services: Yes
Ownership: Voluntary non-profit - Private
Beds: 16

Key Personnel:

Anesthesiology. . . . . David Boharski, CRNA
Quality Assurance . . . . Carla Eneiman
Chief of Medical Staff. . . . . Deb Green
CEO/President. . . . . Gregory Hanson
Emergency Room . . . . Linda Sund

Measure	Cases	This Hosp.	State Avg.	U.S. Avg.
Blood Clot Prevention and Treatment				
Anticoagulation Overlap Therapy[5]	-	-	97%	93%
ICU Venous Thromboembolism Prophylaxis[5]	-	-	92%	92%
Incidence of Potentially Preventable VTE[5]	-	-	4%	10%
UFH with Dosages/Platelet Monitoring[5]	-	-	97%	97%
Venous Thromboembolism Prophylaxis[5]	-	-	83%	85%
Warfarin Therapy Discharge Instructions[5]	-	-	84%	75%
Chest Pain/Possible Heart Attack Care				
Aspirin Given Within 24 Hours of Arrival	-	-	97%	96%
Fibrinolytic Meds Within 30 Min. of Arrival	-	-	43%	58%
Average Time to ECG (minutes)	-	-	10	7
Average Time to Transfer (minutes)	-	-	78	60
Children's Asthma Care				
Received Home Management Plan of Care	-	-	-	88%
Received Reliever Medication	-	-	-	100%
Received Systemic Corticosteroids	-	-	-	100%
Emergency Department				
Admittance Decision Time (minutes)[2]	48	22	72	98
Head CT Results Within 45 Min. of Arrival	-	-	26%	57%
Patients Who Left ER Before Being Seen	-	-	2%	2%
Time from ER Arrival to Admit. (minutes)[2]	48	154	220	274
Time from ER Arrival to Discharge (minutes)	-	-	120	134
Time in ER Before Being Evaluated (minutes)	-	-	23	26
Time to Pain Meds for Fractures (minutes)	-	-	47	57
Heart Attack Care				
Aspirin Given at Discharge[1,3]	-	-	100%	99%
Fibrinolytic Meds Within 30 Min. of Arrival[3,7]	-	-	50%	54%
PCI Within 90 Minutes of Arrival[3,7]	-	-	96%	96%
Statin Prescribed at Discharge[1,3]	-	-	99%	98%
Heart Failure Care				
ACE Inhibitor or ARB for LVSD[1]	-	-	97%	97%
Discharge Instructions Given[1]	-	-	92%	94%
Evaluation of LVS Function	12	100%	94%	99%
Medicare Spending				
Medicare Spending per Patient (ratio)	-	-	0.89	0.98
Pneumonia Care				
Appropriate Initial Antibiotic Given	22	95%	94%	95%
Blood Culture Timing	22	100%	97%	98%
Pregnancy and Delivery Care				
Newborn Deliveries Scheduled Early[5]	-	-	7%	6%
Preventive Care				
Immunization for Influenza[2]	23	100%	86%	90%
Immunization for Pneumonia[2]	44	93%	89%	92%
Stroke Care				
Anticoagulation Therapy for Atrial Fibrillation[5]	-	-	98%	95%
Antithrombotic Therapy Timing[5]	-	-	99%	98%
Assessed for Rehabilitation[5]	-	-	99%	97%
Discharged on Antithrombotic Therapy[5]	-	-	100%	99%
Discharged on Statin Medication[5]	-	-	94%	94%
Thrombolytic Therapy Timing[5]	-	-	67%	66%
Venous Thromboembolism Prophylaxis[5]	-	-	96%	94%
Written Stroke Educational Materials Given[5]	-	-	85%	88%
Surgical Care Improvement Project				
Appropriate Beta Blocker Usage[5]	-	-	98%	98%
Appropriate VTP Within 24 Hours[5]	-	-	98%	98%
Controlled Postoperative Blood Glucose[5]	-	-	96%	97%
Perioperative Temperature Management[5]	-	-	100%	100%
Prophylactic Antibiotic Selection[5]	-	-	99%	99%
Prophylactic Antibiotic Selection (Outpatient)	-	-	98%	98%
Prophylactic Antibiotic Stopped[5]	-	-	99%	98%
Prophylactic Antibiotic Timing[5]	-	-	99%	99%
Prophylactic Antibiotic Timing (Outpatient)	-	-	98%	98%
Urinary Catheter Removal[5]	-	-	99%	97%
Survey of Patients' Hospital Experiences				
Area Around Room 'Always' Quiet at Night[6]	<100	50%	60%	61%
Doctors 'Always' Communicated Well[6]	<100	77%	81%	82%
Home Recovery Information Given[6]	<100	77%	83%	85%
Hospital Given 9 or 10 on 10 Point Scale[6]	<100	63%	68%	71%
Meds 'Always' Explained Before Given[6]	<100	62%	63%	64%
Nurses 'Always' Communicated Well[6]	<100	73%	77%	79%
Pain 'Always' Well Controlled[6]	<100	65%	70%	71%
Room and Bathroom 'Always' Clean[6]	<100	71%	72%	73%
Timely Help 'Always' Received[6]	<100	68%	69%	68%
Would Definitely Recommend Hospital[6]	<100	64%	67%	71%
Use of Medical Imaging				
Cardiac Imaging Stress Test before Surgery	-	-	4.9%	5.3%
Combination Abdominal CT Scan	-	-	10.6%	10.5%
Combination Brain/Sinus CT Scan	-	-	1.9%	2.7%
Combination Chest CT Scan	-	-	2.4%	2.7%
Follow-up Mammogram/Ultrasound	-	-	6.9%	8.8%
Lumbar Spine MRI for Low Back Pain	-	-	41.5%	37.2%

Sheridan Memorial Hosptial

440 W Laurel Ave
Plentywood, MT 59254
Phone: 406-765-3700
Fax: 406-765-3800
URL: www.sheridanmemorial.net
Type: Critical Access Hospitals
Emergency Services: Yes
Ownership: Voluntary non-profit - Other
Beds: 96

Key Personnel:

Chair/CEO. . . . . Jake Fladager

NOTE: Hospital profiles are in alphabetical order by state, then city, then hospital within the city; Rankings exclude hospitals with less than 25 cases except for patient surveys which excludes hospitals with less than 100 cases; (a) 100-299 cases; (1) The number of cases/patients is too few to report; (2) Data submitted were based on a sample of cases/patients; (3) Results are based on a shorter time period than required; (4) Data suppressed by CMS for one or more quarters; (5) Results are not available for this reporting period; (6) Fewer than 100 patients completed the HCAHPS survey; (7) No cases met the criteria for this measure; (8) The lower limit of the confidence interval cannot be calculated if the number of observed infections equals zero; (9) No data are available from the state/territory for this reporting period; (10) The scores shown reflect fewer than 50 completed surveys; (11) There were discrepancies in the data collection process; (12) This measure does not apply to this hospital for this reporting period; (13) Results cannot be calculated for this reporting period; (14) The results for this state are combined with nearby states to protect confidentiality; Please refer to the User's Guide for a full explanation of data.

CEO . . . . Rob Brandt
Infection Control. . . . . Debbie Somppi
Chief of Medical Staff . . . . Kirk Stoner, MD

Measure	Cases	This Hosp.	State Avg.	U.S. Avg.
Blood Clot Prevention and Treatment				
Anticoagulation Overlap Therapy[5]	-	-	97%	93%
ICU Venous Thromboembolism Prophylaxis[5]	-	-	92%	92%
Incidence of Potentially Preventable VTE[5]	-	-	4%	10%
UFH with Dosages/Platelet Monitoring[5]	-	-	97%	97%
Venous Thromboembolism Prophylaxis[5]	-	-	83%	85%
Warfarin Therapy Discharge Instructions[5]	-	-	84%	75%
Chest Pain/Possible Heart Attack Care				
Aspirin Given Within 24 Hours of Arrival	-	-	97%	96%
Fibrinolytic Meds Within 30 Min. of Arrival	-	-	43%	58%
Average Time to ECG (minutes)	-	-	10	7
Average Time to Transfer (minutes)	-	-	78	60
Children's Asthma Care				
Received Home Management Plan of Care	-	-	-	88%
Received Reliever Medication	-	-	-	100%
Received Systemic Corticosteroids	-	-	-	100%
Emergency Department				
Admittance Decision Time (minutes)[5]	-	-	72	98
Head CT Results Within 45 Min. of Arrival	-	-	26%	57%
Patients Who Left ER Before Being Seen	-	-	2%	2%
Time from ER Arrival to Admit. (minutes)[5]	-	-	220	274
Time from ER Arrival to Discharge (minutes)	-	-	120	134
Time in ER Before Being Evaluated (minutes)	-	-	23	26
Time to Pain Meds for Fractures (minutes)	-	-	47	57
Heart Attack Care				
Aspirin Given at Discharge[1,3]	-	-	100%	99%
Fibrinolytic Meds Within 30 Min. of Arrival[3,7]	-	-	50%	54%
PCI Within 90 Minutes of Arrival[3,7]	-	-	96%	96%
Statin Prescribed at Discharge[1,3]	-	-	99%	98%
Heart Failure Care				
ACE Inhibitor or ARB for LVSD[1,3]	-	-	97%	97%
Discharge Instructions Given[1,3]	-	-	92%	94%
Evaluation of LVS Function[1,3]	-	-	94%	99%
Medicare Spending				
Medicare Spending per Patient (ratio)	-	-	0.89	0.98
Pneumonia Care				
Appropriate Initial Antibiotic Given[3]	19	53%	94%	95%
Blood Culture Timing[1,3]	-	-	97%	98%
Pregnancy and Delivery Care				
Newborn Deliveries Scheduled Early[5]	-	-	7%	6%
Preventive Care				
Immunization for Influenza[5]	-	-	86%	90%
Immunization for Pneumonia[5]	-	-	89%	92%
Stroke Care				
Anticoagulation Therapy for Atrial Fibrillation[5]	-	-	98%	95%
Antithrombotic Therapy Timing[5]	-	-	99%	98%
Assessed for Rehabilitation[5]	-	-	99%	97%
Discharged on Antithrombotic Therapy[5]	-	-	100%	99%
Discharged on Statin Medication[5]	-	-	94%	94%
Thrombolytic Therapy Timing[5]	-	-	67%	66%
Venous Thromboembolism Prophylaxis[5]	-	-	96%	94%
Written Stroke Educational Materials Given[5]	-	-	85%	88%
Surgical Care Improvement Project				
Appropriate Beta Blocker Usage[5]	-	-	98%	98%
Appropriate VTP Within 24 Hours[5]	-	-	98%	98%
Controlled Postoperative Blood Glucose[5]	-	-	96%	97%
Perioperative Temperature Management[5]	-	-	100%	100%
Prophylactic Antibiotic Selection[5]	-	-	99%	99%
Prophylactic Antibiotic Selection (Outpatient)	-	-	98%	98%
Prophylactic Antibiotic Stopped[5]	-	-	99%	98%
Prophylactic Antibiotic Timing[5]	-	-	99%	99%
Prophylactic Antibiotic Timing (Outpatient)	-	-	98%	98%
Urinary Catheter Removal[5]	-	-	99%	97%
Survey of Patients' Hospital Experiences				
Area Around Room 'Always' Quiet at Night[5]	-	-	60%	61%
Doctors 'Always' Communicated Well[5]	-	-	81%	82%
Home Recovery Information Given[5]	-	-	83%	85%
Hospital Given 9 or 10 on 10 Point Scale[5]	-	-	68%	71%
Meds 'Always' Explained Before Given[5]	-	-	63%	64%
Nurses 'Always' Communicated Well[5]	-	-	77%	79%
Pain 'Always' Well Controlled[5]	-	-	70%	71%
Room and Bathroom 'Always' Clean[5]	-	-	72%	73%
Timely Help 'Always' Received[5]	-	-	69%	68%
Would Definitely Recommend Hospital[5]	-	-	67%	71%
Use of Medical Imaging				
Cardiac Imaging Stress Test before Surgery	-	-	4.9%	5.3%
Combination Abdominal CT Scan	-	-	10.6%	10.5%
Combination Brain/Sinus CT Scan	-	-	1.9%	2.7%
Combination Chest CT Scan	-	-	2.4%	2.7%
Follow-up Mammogram/Ultrasound	-	-	6.9%	8.8%
Lumbar Spine MRI for Low Back Pain	-	-	41.5%	37.2%

Providence Saint Joseph Medical Center

6 13th Ave E
Polson, MT 59860
Phone: 406-883-5377
Fax: 406-883-8439
Type: Critical Access Hospitals
Emergency Services: Yes
Ownership: Voluntary non-profit - Private
Beds: 40

Key Personnel:
Chairman/CEO . . . . William Beck, Jr.
Cardiac Laboratory. . . . . Darleen Cooper
CEO/President. . . . . James Kiser
Chief of Medical Staff . . . . Karen Lund

Measure	Cases	This Hosp.	State Avg.	U.S. Avg.
Blood Clot Prevention and Treatment				
Anticoagulation Overlap Therapy[1,2]	-	-	97%	93%
ICU Venous Thromboembolism Prophylaxis[1,2]	-	-	92%	92%
Incidence of Potentially Preventable VTE[2,7]	-	-	4%	10%
UFH with Dosages/Platelet Monitoring[1,2]	-	-	97%	97%
Venous Thromboembolism Prophylaxis[2]	82	85%	83%	85%
Warfarin Therapy Discharge Instructions[1,2]	-	-	84%	75%
Chest Pain/Possible Heart Attack Care				
Aspirin Given Within 24 Hours of Arrival[5]	-	-	97%	96%
Fibrinolytic Meds Within 30 Min. of Arrival[5]	-	-	43%	58%
Average Time to ECG (minutes)[5]	-	-	10	7
Average Time to Transfer (minutes)[5]	-	-	78	60
Children's Asthma Care				
Received Home Management Plan of Care	-	-	-	88%
Received Reliever Medication	-	-	-	100%
Received Systemic Corticosteroids	-	-	-	100%
Emergency Department				
Admittance Decision Time (minutes)[2,7]	-	-	72	98
Head CT Results Within 45 Min. of Arrival[1]	-	-	26%	57%
Patients Who Left ER Before Being Seen[5]	-	-	2%	2%
Time from ER Arrival to Admit. (minutes)[2,7]	-	-	220	274
Time from ER Arrival to Discharge (minutes)	304	101	120	134
Time in ER Before Being Evaluated (minutes)	382	14	23	26
Time to Pain Meds for Fractures (minutes)	48	28	47	57
Heart Attack Care				
Aspirin Given at Discharge[3,7]	-	-	100%	99%
Fibrinolytic Meds Within 30 Min. of Arrival[3,7]	-	-	50%	54%
PCI Within 90 Minutes of Arrival[3,7]	-	-	96%	96%
Statin Prescribed at Discharge[3,7]	-	-	99%	98%
Heart Failure Care				
ACE Inhibitor or ARB for LVSD[1,3]	-	-	97%	97%
Discharge Instructions Given[1,3]	-	-	92%	94%
Evaluation of LVS Function[1,3]	-	-	94%	99%
Medicare Spending				
Medicare Spending per Patient (ratio)	-	-	0.89	0.98
Pneumonia Care				
Appropriate Initial Antibiotic Given[1]	-	-	94%	95%
Blood Culture Timing	12	100%	97%	98%
Pregnancy and Delivery Care				
Newborn Deliveries Scheduled Early[5]	-	-	7%	6%
Preventive Care				
Immunization for Influenza[2]	240	65%	86%	90%
Immunization for Pneumonia[2]	249	74%	89%	92%
Stroke Care				
Anticoagulation Therapy for Atrial Fibrillation[3,7]	-	-	98%	95%
Antithrombotic Therapy Timing[3,7]	-	-	99%	98%
Assessed for Rehabilitation[1,3]	-	-	99%	97%
Discharged on Antithrombotic Therapy[1,3]	-	-	100%	99%
Discharged on Statin Medication[1,3]	-	-	94%	94%
Thrombolytic Therapy Timing[1,3]	-	-	67%	66%
Venous Thromboembolism Prophylaxis[1,3]	-	-	96%	94%
Written Stroke Educational Materials Given[1,3]	-	-	85%	88%
Surgical Care Improvement Project				
Appropriate Beta Blocker Usage[1]	-	-	98%	98%
Appropriate VTP Within 24 Hours[1]	23	100%	98%	98%
Controlled Postoperative Blood Glucose[7]	-	-	96%	97%
Perioperative Temperature Management	30	100%	100%	100%
Prophylactic Antibiotic Selection	19	100%	99%	99%
Prophylactic Antibiotic Selection (Outpatient)[5]	-	-	98%	98%
Prophylactic Antibiotic Stopped	19	100%	99%	98%
Prophylactic Antibiotic Timing	19	100%	99%	99%
Prophylactic Antibiotic Timing (Outpatient)[5]	-	-	98%	98%
Urinary Catheter Removal	13	100%	99%	97%
Survey of Patients' Hospital Experiences				
Area Around Room 'Always' Quiet at Night	(a)	54%	60%	61%
Doctors 'Always' Communicated Well	(a)	83%	81%	82%
Home Recovery Information Given	(a)	88%	83%	85%
Hospital Given 9 or 10 on 10 Point Scale	(a)	69%	68%	71%
Meds 'Always' Explained Before Given	(a)	60%	63%	64%
Nurses 'Always' Communicated Well	(a)	78%	77%	79%
Pain 'Always' Well Controlled	(a)	72%	70%	71%
Room and Bathroom 'Always' Clean	(a)	69%	72%	73%
Timely Help 'Always' Received	(a)	77%	69%	68%
Would Definitely Recommend Hospital	(a)	70%	67%	71%
Use of Medical Imaging				
Cardiac Imaging Stress Test before Surgery[1]	-	-	4.9%	5.3%
Combination Abdominal CT Scan	145	6.2%	10.6%	10.5%
Combination Brain/Sinus CT Scan	114	0.0%	1.9%	2.7%
Combination Chest CT Scan	83	1.2%	2.4%	2.7%
Follow-up Mammogram/Ultrasound	298	6.7%	6.9%	8.8%
Lumbar Spine MRI for Low Back Pain[1]	-	-	41.5%	37.2%

Poplar Community Hospital

211 H Saint E
Poplar, MT 59255
Phone: 406-768-6100
Fax: 406-768-6160
URL: www.nemhs.net
Type: Critical Access Hospitals
Emergency Services: Yes
Ownership: Voluntary non-profit - Private
Beds: 22

Key Personnel:
CEO/President. . . . . Peg Norgaard, MD

Measure	Cases	This Hosp.	State Avg.	U.S. Avg.
Blood Clot Prevention and Treatment				
Anticoagulation Overlap Therapy[5]	-	-	97%	93%
ICU Venous Thromboembolism Prophylaxis[5]	-	-	92%	92%
Incidence of Potentially Preventable VTE[5]	-	-	4%	10%
UFH with Dosages/Platelet Monitoring[5]	-	-	97%	97%
Venous Thromboembolism Prophylaxis[5]	-	-	83%	85%
Warfarin Therapy Discharge Instructions[5]	-	-	84%	75%
Chest Pain/Possible Heart Attack Care				
Aspirin Given Within 24 Hours of Arrival	-	-	97%	96%
Fibrinolytic Meds Within 30 Min. of Arrival	-	-	43%	58%
Average Time to ECG (minutes)	-	-	10	7
Average Time to Transfer (minutes)	-	-	78	60
Children's Asthma Care				
Received Home Management Plan of Care	-	-	-	88%
Received Reliever Medication	-	-	-	100%
Received Systemic Corticosteroids	-	-	-	100%
Emergency Department				
Admittance Decision Time (minutes)[5]	-	-	72	98
Head CT Results Within 45 Min. of Arrival	-	-	26%	57%
Patients Who Left ER Before Being Seen	-	-	2%	2%
Time from ER Arrival to Admit. (minutes)[5]	-	-	220	274
Time from ER Arrival to Discharge (minutes)	-	-	120	134
Time in ER Before Being Evaluated (minutes)	-	-	23	26
Time to Pain Meds for Fractures (minutes)	-	-	47	57
Heart Attack Care				
Aspirin Given at Discharge[5]	-	-	100%	99%
Fibrinolytic Meds Within 30 Min. of Arrival[5]	-	-	50%	54%
PCI Within 90 Minutes of Arrival[5]	-	-	96%	96%
Statin Prescribed at Discharge[5]	-	-	99%	98%
Heart Failure Care				

NOTE: Hospital profiles are in alphabetical order by state, then city, then hospital within the city; Rankings exclude hospitals with less than 25 cases except for patient surveys which excludes hospitals with less than 100 cases; (a) 100-299 cases; (1) The number of cases/patients is too few to report; (2) Data submitted were based on a sample of cases/patients; (3) Results are based on a shorter time period than required; (4) Data suppressed by CMS for one or more quarters; (5) Results are not available for this reporting period; (6) Fewer than 100 patients completed the HCAHPS survey; (7) No cases met the criteria for this measure; (8) The lower limit of the confidence interval cannot be calculated if the number of observed infections equals zero; (9) No data are available from the state/territory for this reporting period; (10) The scores shown reflect fewer than 50 completed surveys; (11) There were discrepancies in the data collection process; (12) This measure does not apply to this hospital for this reporting period; (13) Results cannot be calculated for this reporting period; (14) The results for this state are combined with nearby states to protect confidentiality; Please refer to the User's Guide for a full explanation of data.

Measure	Cases	This Hosp.	State Avg.	U.S. Avg.
ACE Inhibitor or ARB for LVSD[3,7]	-	-	97%	97%
Discharge Instructions Given[1,3]	-	-	92%	94%
Evaluation of LVS Function[1,3]	-	-	94%	99%
Medicare Spending				
Medicare Spending per Patient (ratio)	-	-	0.89	0.98
Pneumonia Care				
Appropriate Initial Antibiotic Given[1]	-	-	94%	95%
Blood Culture Timing[7]	-	-	97%	98%
Pregnancy and Delivery Care				
Newborn Deliveries Scheduled Early[5]	-	-	7%	6%
Preventive Care				
Immunization for Influenza[5]	-	-	86%	90%
Immunization for Pneumonia[5]	-	-	89%	92%
Stroke Care				
Anticoagulation Therapy for Atrial Fibrillation[5]	-	-	98%	95%
Antithrombotic Therapy Timing[5]	-	-	99%	98%
Assessed for Rehabilitation[5]	-	-	99%	97%
Discharged on Antithrombotic Therapy[5]	-	-	100%	99%
Discharged on Statin Medication[5]	-	-	94%	94%
Thrombolytic Therapy Timing[5]	-	-	67%	66%
Venous Thromboembolism Prophylaxis[5]	-	-	96%	94%
Written Stroke Educational Materials Given[5]	-	-	85%	88%
Surgical Care Improvement Project				
Appropriate Beta Blocker Usage[5]	-	-	98%	98%
Appropriate VTP Within 24 Hours[5]	-	-	98%	98%
Controlled Postoperative Blood Glucose[5]	-	-	96%	97%
Perioperative Temperature Management[5]	-	-	100%	100%
Prophylactic Antibiotic Selection[5]	-	-	99%	99%
Prophylactic Antibiotic Selection (Outpatient)	-	-	98%	98%
Prophylactic Antibiotic Stopped[5]	-	-	99%	98%
Prophylactic Antibiotic Timing[5]	-	-	99%	99%
Prophylactic Antibiotic Timing (Outpatient)	-	-	98%	98%
Urinary Catheter Removal[5]	-	-	99%	97%
Survey of Patients' Hospital Experiences				
Area Around Room 'Always' Quiet at Night[5]	-	-	60%	61%
Doctors 'Always' Communicated Well[5]	-	-	81%	82%
Home Recovery Information Given[5]	-	-	83%	85%
Hospital Given 9 or 10 on 10 Point Scale[5]	-	-	68%	71%
Meds 'Always' Explained Before Given[5]	-	-	63%	64%
Nurses 'Always' Communicated Well[5]	-	-	77%	79%
Pain 'Always' Well Controlled[5]	-	-	70%	71%
Room and Bathroom 'Always' Clean[5]	-	-	72%	73%
Timely Help 'Always' Received[5]	-	-	69%	68%
Would Definitely Recommend Hospital[5]	-	-	67%	71%
Use of Medical Imaging				
Cardiac Imaging Stress Test before Surgery	-	-	4.9%	5.3%
Combination Abdominal CT Scan	-	-	10.6%	10.5%
Combination Brain/Sinus CT Scan	-	-	1.9%	2.7%
Combination Chest CT Scan	-	-	2.4%	2.7%
Follow-up Mammogram/Ultrasound	-	-	6.9%	8.8%
Lumbar Spine MRI for Low Back Pain	-	-	41.5%	37.2%

Beartooth Billings Clinic

2525 N Broadway
Red Lodge, MT 59068
Phone: 406-446-2345
Type: Critical Access Hospitals
Emergency Services: Yes
Ownership: Voluntary non-profit - Private

Measure	Cases	This Hosp.	State Avg.	U.S. Avg.
Blood Clot Prevention and Treatment				
Anticoagulation Overlap Therapy[5]	-	-	97%	93%
ICU Venous Thromboembolism Prophylaxis[5]	-	-	92%	92%
Incidence of Potentially Preventable VTE[5]	-	-	4%	10%
UFH with Dosages/Platelet Monitoring[5]	-	-	97%	97%
Venous Thromboembolism Prophylaxis[5]	-	-	83%	85%
Warfarin Therapy Discharge Instructions[5]	-	-	84%	75%
Chest Pain/Possible Heart Attack Care				
Aspirin Given Within 24 Hours of Arrival	-	-	97%	96%
Fibrinolytic Meds Within 30 Min. of Arrival	-	-	43%	58%
Average Time to ECG (minutes)	-	-	10	7
Average Time to Transfer (minutes)	-	-	78	60
Children's Asthma Care				
Received Home Management Plan of Care	-	-	-	88%
Received Reliever Medication	-	-	-	100%
Received Systemic Corticosteroids	-	-	-	100%
Emergency Department				
Admittance Decision Time (minutes)[5]	-	-	72	98
Head CT Results Within 45 Min. of Arrival	-	-	26%	57%
Patients Who Left ER Before Being Seen	-	-	2%	2%
Time from ER Arrival to Admit. (minutes)[5]	-	-	220	274
Time from ER Arrival to Discharge (minutes)	-	-	120	134
Time in ER Before Being Evaluated (minutes)	-	-	23	26
Time to Pain Meds for Fractures (minutes)	-	-	47	57
Heart Attack Care				
Aspirin Given at Discharge[5]	-	-	100%	99%
Fibrinolytic Meds Within 30 Min. of Arrival[5]	-	-	50%	54%
PCI Within 90 Minutes of Arrival[5]	-	-	96%	96%
Statin Prescribed at Discharge[5]	-	-	99%	98%
Heart Failure Care				
ACE Inhibitor or ARB for LVSD[1]	-	-	97%	97%
Discharge Instructions Given[1]	-	-	92%	94%
Evaluation of LVS Function[1]	-	-	94%	99%
Medicare Spending				
Medicare Spending per Patient (ratio)	-	-	0.89	0.98
Pneumonia Care				
Appropriate Initial Antibiotic Given	15	73%	94%	95%
Blood Culture Timing[1]	-	-	97%	98%
Pregnancy and Delivery Care				
Newborn Deliveries Scheduled Early[5]	-	-	7%	6%
Preventive Care				
Immunization for Influenza[5]	-	-	86%	90%
Immunization for Pneumonia[5]	-	-	89%	92%
Stroke Care				
Anticoagulation Therapy for Atrial Fibrillation[5]	-	-	98%	95%
Antithrombotic Therapy Timing[5]	-	-	99%	98%
Assessed for Rehabilitation[5]	-	-	99%	97%
Discharged on Antithrombotic Therapy[5]	-	-	100%	99%
Discharged on Statin Medication[5]	-	-	94%	94%
Thrombolytic Therapy Timing[5]	-	-	67%	66%
Venous Thromboembolism Prophylaxis[5]	-	-	96%	94%
Written Stroke Educational Materials Given[5]	-	-	85%	88%
Surgical Care Improvement Project				
Appropriate Beta Blocker Usage[5]	-	-	98%	98%
Appropriate VTP Within 24 Hours[5]	-	-	98%	98%
Controlled Postoperative Blood Glucose[5]	-	-	96%	97%
Perioperative Temperature Management[5]	-	-	100%	100%
Prophylactic Antibiotic Selection[5]	-	-	99%	99%
Prophylactic Antibiotic Selection (Outpatient)	-	-	98%	98%
Prophylactic Antibiotic Stopped[5]	-	-	99%	98%
Prophylactic Antibiotic Timing[5]	-	-	99%	99%
Prophylactic Antibiotic Timing (Outpatient)	-	-	98%	98%
Urinary Catheter Removal[5]	-	-	99%	97%
Survey of Patients' Hospital Experiences				
Area Around Room 'Always' Quiet at Night[5]	-	-	60%	61%
Doctors 'Always' Communicated Well[5]	-	-	81%	82%
Home Recovery Information Given[5]	-	-	83%	85%
Hospital Given 9 or 10 on 10 Point Scale[5]	-	-	68%	71%
Meds 'Always' Explained Before Given[5]	-	-	63%	64%
Nurses 'Always' Communicated Well[5]	-	-	77%	79%
Pain 'Always' Well Controlled[5]	-	-	70%	71%
Room and Bathroom 'Always' Clean[5]	-	-	72%	73%
Timely Help 'Always' Received[5]	-	-	69%	68%
Would Definitely Recommend Hospital[5]	-	-	67%	71%
Use of Medical Imaging				
Cardiac Imaging Stress Test before Surgery	-	-	4.9%	5.3%
Combination Abdominal CT Scan	-	-	10.6%	10.5%
Combination Brain/Sinus CT Scan	-	-	1.9%	2.7%
Combination Chest CT Scan	-	-	2.4%	2.7%
Follow-up Mammogram/Ultrasound	-	-	6.9%	8.8%
Lumbar Spine MRI for Low Back Pain	-	-	41.5%	37.2%

Saint Luke Community Hospital

107 6th Ave Sw
Ronan, MT 59864
Phone: 406-676-4441
Fax: 406-676-0835
URL: www.stlukehealthnet.org
Type: Critical Access Hospitals
Emergency Services: Yes
Ownership: Voluntary non-profit - Private
Beds: 25

Key Personnel:
Emergency Room . . . . Leah Amerson
Quality Assurance . . . . Leah Emerson
Operating Room. . . . . Larry Scott
CEO . . . . Steve Todd

Measure	Cases	This Hosp.	State Avg.	U.S. Avg.
Blood Clot Prevention and Treatment				
Anticoagulation Overlap Therapy[5]	-	-	97%	93%
ICU Venous Thromboembolism Prophylaxis[5]	-	-	92%	92%
Incidence of Potentially Preventable VTE[5]	-	-	4%	10%
UFH with Dosages/Platelet Monitoring[5]	-	-	97%	97%
Venous Thromboembolism Prophylaxis[5]	-	-	83%	85%
Warfarin Therapy Discharge Instructions[5]	-	-	84%	75%
Chest Pain/Possible Heart Attack Care				
Aspirin Given Within 24 Hours of Arrival	22	100%	97%	96%
Fibrinolytic Meds Within 30 Min. of Arrival[1,3]	-	-	43%	58%
Average Time to ECG (minutes)	22	8	10	7
Average Time to Transfer (minutes)[1,3]	-	-	78	60
Children's Asthma Care				
Received Home Management Plan of Care	-	-	-	88%
Received Reliever Medication	-	-	-	100%
Received Systemic Corticosteroids	-	-	-	100%
Emergency Department				
Admittance Decision Time (minutes)[5]	-	-	72	98
Head CT Results Within 45 Min. of Arrival[3,7]	-	-	26%	57%
Patients Who Left ER Before Being Seen[5]	-	-	2%	2%
Time from ER Arrival to Admit. (minutes)[5]	-	-	220	274
Time from ER Arrival to Discharge (minutes)[5]	-	-	120	134
Time in ER Before Being Evaluated (minutes)[5]	-	-	23	26
Time to Pain Meds for Fractures (minutes)[1,3]	-	-	47	57
Heart Attack Care				
Aspirin Given at Discharge[1,3]	-	-	100%	99%
Fibrinolytic Meds Within 30 Min. of Arrival[3,7]	-	-	50%	54%
PCI Within 90 Minutes of Arrival[3,7]	-	-	96%	96%
Statin Prescribed at Discharge[1,3]	-	-	99%	98%
Heart Failure Care				
ACE Inhibitor or ARB for LVSD[1]	-	-	97%	97%
Discharge Instructions Given	14	93%	92%	94%
Evaluation of LVS Function	19	89%	94%	99%
Medicare Spending				
Medicare Spending per Patient (ratio)	-	-	0.89	0.98
Pneumonia Care				
Appropriate Initial Antibiotic Given[2]	47	94%	94%	95%
Blood Culture Timing[2]	49	100%	97%	98%
Pregnancy and Delivery Care				
Newborn Deliveries Scheduled Early[5]	-	-	7%	6%
Preventive Care				
Immunization for Influenza[2]	50	94%	86%	90%
Immunization for Pneumonia[2]	73	96%	89%	92%
Stroke Care				
Anticoagulation Therapy for Atrial Fibrillation[5]	-	-	98%	95%
Antithrombotic Therapy Timing[5]	-	-	99%	98%
Assessed for Rehabilitation[5]	-	-	99%	97%
Discharged on Antithrombotic Therapy[5]	-	-	100%	99%
Discharged on Statin Medication[5]	-	-	94%	94%
Thrombolytic Therapy Timing[5]	-	-	67%	66%
Venous Thromboembolism Prophylaxis[5]	-	-	96%	94%
Written Stroke Educational Materials Given[5]	-	-	85%	88%
Surgical Care Improvement Project				
Appropriate Beta Blocker Usage[3,7]	-	-	98%	98%
Appropriate VTP Within 24 Hours[1,3]	-	-	98%	98%
Controlled Postoperative Blood Glucose[3,7]	-	-	96%	97%
Perioperative Temperature Management[1,3]	-	-	100%	100%
Prophylactic Antibiotic Selection[1,3]	-	-	99%	99%
Prophylactic Antibiotic Selection (Outpatient)[1,3]	-	-	98%	98%
Prophylactic Antibiotic Stopped[1,3]	-	-	99%	98%
Prophylactic Antibiotic Timing[1,3]	-	-	99%	99%

NOTE: Hospital profiles are in alphabetical order by state, then city, then hospital within the city; Rankings exclude hospitals with less than 25 cases except for patient surveys which excludes hospitals with less than 100 cases; (a) 100-299 cases; (1) The number of cases/patients is too few to report; (2) Data submitted were based on a sample of cases/patients; (3) Results are based on a shorter time period than required; (4) Data suppressed by CMS for one or more quarters; (5) Results are not available for this reporting period; (6) Fewer than 100 patients completed the HCAHPS survey; (7) No cases met the criteria for this measure; (8) The lower limit of the confidence interval cannot be calculated if the number of observed infections equals zero; (9) No data are available from the state/territory for this reporting period; (10) The scores shown reflect fewer than 50 completed surveys; (11) There were discrepancies in the data collection process; (12) This measure does not apply to this hospital for this reporting period; (13) Results cannot be calculated for this reporting period; (14) The results for this state are combined with nearby states to protect confidentiality; Please refer to the User's Guide for a full explanation of data.

Measure	Cases	This Hosp.	State Avg.	U.S. Avg.
Prophylactic Antibiotic Timing (Outpatient)[1,3]	-	-	98%	98%
Urinary Catheter Removal[1,3]	-	-	99%	97%
Survey of Patients' Hospital Experiences				
Area Around Room 'Always' Quiet at Night	(a)	60%	60%	61%
Doctors 'Always' Communicated Well	(a)	79%	81%	82%
Home Recovery Information Given	(a)	73%	83%	85%
Hospital Given 9 or 10 on 10 Point Scale	(a)	57%	68%	71%
Meds 'Always' Explained Before Given	(a)	62%	63%	64%
Nurses 'Always' Communicated Well	(a)	67%	77%	79%
Pain 'Always' Well Controlled	(a)	69%	70%	71%
Room and Bathroom 'Always' Clean	(a)	67%	72%	73%
Timely Help 'Always' Received	(a)	64%	69%	68%
Would Definitely Recommend Hospital	(a)	63%	67%	71%
Use of Medical Imaging				
Cardiac Imaging Stress Test before Surgery[1]	-	-	4.9%	5.3%
Combination Abdominal CT Scan	160	53.8%	10.6%	10.5%
Combination Brain/Sinus CT Scan[1]	-	-	1.9%	2.7%
Combination Chest CT Scan	65	44.6%	2.4%	2.7%
Follow-up Mammogram/Ultrasound	212	15.1%	6.9%	8.8%
Lumbar Spine MRI for Low Back Pain[1]	-	-	41.5%	37.2%

Roundup Memorial Healthcare

1202 3rd Saint W
Roundup, MT 59072
Phone: 406-323-2301
Fax: 406-323-1170
E-mail: rmhclnh@midrivers.com
Type: Critical Access Hospitals
Emergency Services: Yes
Ownership: Govt - Hospital Dist/Auth
Beds: 48

Key Personnel:
Emergency Room . . . . Brenda Dagley
CEO . . . . Brad Howell
Chair/CEO . . . . Gordon Kilby
Chief of Medical Staff . . . . Sunny Lageschulte
President . . . . John Pfister
CEO/President . . . . Lee Rhodes

Measure	Cases	This Hosp.	State Avg.	U.S. Avg.
Blood Clot Prevention and Treatment				
Anticoagulation Overlap Therapy[1]	-	-	97%	93%
ICU Venous Thromboembolism Prophylaxis[7]	-	-	92%	92%
Incidence of Potentially Preventable VTE[7]	-	-	4%	10%
UFH with Dosages/Platelet Monitoring[7]	-	-	97%	97%
Venous Thromboembolism Prophylaxis	25	56%	83%	85%
Warfarin Therapy Discharge Instructions[7]	-	-	84%	75%
Chest Pain/Possible Heart Attack Care				
Aspirin Given Within 24 Hours of Arrival[1]	-	-	97%	96%
Fibrinolytic Meds Within 30 Min. of Arrival[1,3]	-	-	43%	58%
Average Time to ECG (minutes)	11	9	10	7
Average Time to Transfer (minutes)[1,3]	-	-	78	60
Children's Asthma Care				
Received Home Management Plan of Care	-	-	-	88%
Received Reliever Medication	-	-	-	100%
Received Systemic Corticosteroids	-	-	-	100%
Emergency Department				
Admittance Decision Time (minutes)	12	12	72	98
Head CT Results Within 45 Min. of Arrival[1,3]	-	-	26%	57%
Patients Who Left ER Before Being Seen[5]	-	-	2%	2%
Time from ER Arrival to Admit. (minutes)	21	110	220	274
Time from ER Arrival to Discharge (minutes)[5]	-	-	120	134
Time in ER Before Being Evaluated (minutes)[5]	-	-	23	26
Time to Pain Meds for Fractures (minutes)	13	30	47	57
Heart Attack Care				
Aspirin Given at Discharge[5]	-	-	100%	99%
Fibrinolytic Meds Within 30 Min. of Arrival[5]	-	-	50%	54%
PCI Within 90 Minutes of Arrival[5]	-	-	96%	96%
Statin Prescribed at Discharge[5]	-	-	99%	98%
Heart Failure Care				
ACE Inhibitor or ARB for LVSD[1]	-	-	97%	97%
Discharge Instructions Given[1]	-	-	92%	94%
Evaluation of LVS Function	12	83%	94%	99%
Medicare Spending				
Medicare Spending per Patient (ratio)	-	-	0.89	0.98
Pneumonia Care				
Appropriate Initial Antibiotic Given	17	100%	94%	95%
Blood Culture Timing[1]	-	-	97%	98%
Pregnancy and Delivery Care				
Newborn Deliveries Scheduled Early[5]	-	-	7%	6%
Preventive Care				
Immunization for Influenza	27	48%	86%	90%
Immunization for Pneumonia	36	56%	89%	92%
Stroke Care				
Anticoagulation Therapy for Atrial Fibrillation[5]	-	-	98%	95%
Antithrombotic Therapy Timing[5]	-	-	99%	98%
Assessed for Rehabilitation[5]	-	-	99%	97%
Discharged on Antithrombotic Therapy[5]	-	-	100%	99%
Discharged on Statin Medication[5]	-	-	94%	94%
Thrombolytic Therapy Timing[5]	-	-	67%	66%
Venous Thromboembolism Prophylaxis[5]	-	-	96%	94%
Written Stroke Educational Materials Given[5]	-	-	85%	88%
Surgical Care Improvement Project				
Appropriate Beta Blocker Usage[5]	-	-	98%	98%
Appropriate VTP Within 24 Hours[5]	-	-	98%	98%
Controlled Postoperative Blood Glucose[5]	-	-	96%	97%
Perioperative Temperature Management[5]	-	-	100%	100%
Prophylactic Antibiotic Selection[5]	-	-	99%	99%
Prophylactic Antibiotic Selection (Outpatient)[5]	-	-	98%	98%
Prophylactic Antibiotic Stopped[5]	-	-	99%	98%
Prophylactic Antibiotic Timing[5]	-	-	99%	99%
Prophylactic Antibiotic Timing (Outpatient)[5]	-	-	98%	98%
Urinary Catheter Removal[5]	-	-	99%	97%
Survey of Patients' Hospital Experiences				
Area Around Room 'Always' Quiet at Night[10]	<100	74%	60%	61%
Doctors 'Always' Communicated Well[10]	<100	81%	81%	82%
Home Recovery Information Given[10]	<100	72%	83%	85%
Hospital Given 9 or 10 on 10 Point Scale[10]	<100	69%	68%	71%
Meds 'Always' Explained Before Given[10]	<100	53%	63%	64%
Nurses 'Always' Communicated Well[10]	<100	74%	77%	79%
Pain 'Always' Well Controlled[10]	<100	61%	70%	71%
Room and Bathroom 'Always' Clean[10]	<100	93%	72%	73%
Timely Help 'Always' Received[10]	<100	68%	69%	68%
Would Definitely Recommend Hospital[10]	<100	61%	67%	71%
Use of Medical Imaging				
Cardiac Imaging Stress Test before Surgery[7]	-	-	4.9%	5.3%
Combination Abdominal CT Scan[1]	-	-	10.6%	10.5%
Combination Brain/Sinus CT Scan	47	0.0%	1.9%	2.7%
Combination Chest CT Scan[1]	-	-	2.4%	2.7%
Follow-up Mammogram/Ultrasound[7]	-	-	6.9%	8.8%
Lumbar Spine MRI for Low Back Pain[7]	-	-	41.5%	37.2%

Daniels Memorial Hospital

105 5th Ave E
Scobey, MT 59263
Phone: 406-487-2296
Fax: 406-487-2471
Type: Critical Access Hospitals
Emergency Services: Yes
Ownership: Govt - Hospital Dist/Auth
Beds: 54

Key Personnel:
Chief of Medical Staff . . . . William Escoffery, MD
Quality Assurance . . . . Karla Hansen, RN
CEO/President . . . . Davie Lloyd
Infection Control . . . . Naomi Reed, RN

Measure	Cases	This Hosp.	State Avg.	U.S. Avg.
Blood Clot Prevention and Treatment				
Anticoagulation Overlap Therapy[3,7]	-	-	97%	93%
ICU Venous Thromboembolism Prophylaxis[3,7]	-	-	92%	92%
Incidence of Potentially Preventable VTE[3,7]	-	-	4%	10%
UFH with Dosages/Platelet Monitoring[3,7]	-	-	97%	97%
Venous Thromboembolism Prophylaxis[3,7]	-	-	83%	85%
Warfarin Therapy Discharge Instructions[3,7]	-	-	84%	75%
Chest Pain/Possible Heart Attack Care				
Aspirin Given Within 24 Hours of Arrival[5]	-	-	97%	96%
Fibrinolytic Meds Within 30 Min. of Arrival[5]	-	-	43%	58%
Average Time to ECG (minutes)[5]	-	-	10	7
Average Time to Transfer (minutes)[5]	-	-	78	60
Children's Asthma Care				
Received Home Management Plan of Care	-	-	-	88%
Received Reliever Medication	-	-	-	100%
Received Systemic Corticosteroids	-	-	-	100%
Emergency Department				
Admittance Decision Time (minutes)[5]	-	-	72	98
Head CT Results Within 45 Min. of Arrival[1,3]	-	-	26%	57%
Patients Who Left ER Before Being Seen[5]	-	-	2%	2%
Time from ER Arrival to Admit. (minutes)[5]	-	-	220	274
Time from ER Arrival to Discharge (minutes)[5]	-	-	120	134
Time in ER Before Being Evaluated (minutes)[5]	-	-	23	26
Time to Pain Meds for Fractures (minutes)[1,3]	-	-	47	57
Heart Attack Care				
Aspirin Given at Discharge[5]	-	-	100%	99%
Fibrinolytic Meds Within 30 Min. of Arrival[5]	-	-	50%	54%
PCI Within 90 Minutes of Arrival[5]	-	-	96%	96%
Statin Prescribed at Discharge[5]	-	-	99%	98%
Heart Failure Care				
ACE Inhibitor or ARB for LVSD[3,7]	-	-	97%	97%
Discharge Instructions Given[1,3]	-	-	92%	94%
Evaluation of LVS Function[1,3]	-	-	94%	99%
Medicare Spending				
Medicare Spending per Patient (ratio)	-	-	0.89	0.98
Pneumonia Care				
Appropriate Initial Antibiotic Given[3,7]	-	-	94%	95%
Blood Culture Timing[3,7]	-	-	97%	98%
Pregnancy and Delivery Care				
Newborn Deliveries Scheduled Early[5]	-	-	7%	6%
Preventive Care				
Immunization for Influenza[5]	-	-	86%	90%
Immunization for Pneumonia[5]	-	-	89%	92%
Stroke Care				
Anticoagulation Therapy for Atrial Fibrillation[3,7]	-	-	98%	95%
Antithrombotic Therapy Timing[1,3]	-	-	99%	98%
Assessed for Rehabilitation[3,7]	-	-	99%	97%
Discharged on Antithrombotic Therapy[3,7]	-	-	100%	99%
Discharged on Statin Medication[3,7]	-	-	94%	94%
Thrombolytic Therapy Timing[3,7]	-	-	67%	66%
Venous Thromboembolism Prophylaxis[1,3]	-	-	96%	94%
Written Stroke Educational Materials Given[3,7]	-	-	85%	88%
Surgical Care Improvement Project				
Appropriate Beta Blocker Usage[5]	-	-	98%	98%
Appropriate VTP Within 24 Hours[5]	-	-	98%	98%
Controlled Postoperative Blood Glucose[5]	-	-	96%	97%
Perioperative Temperature Management[5]	-	-	100%	100%
Prophylactic Antibiotic Selection[5]	-	-	99%	99%
Prophylactic Antibiotic Selection (Outpatient)[5]	-	-	98%	98%
Prophylactic Antibiotic Stopped[5]	-	-	99%	98%
Prophylactic Antibiotic Timing[5]	-	-	99%	99%
Prophylactic Antibiotic Timing (Outpatient)[5]	-	-	98%	98%
Urinary Catheter Removal[5]	-	-	99%	97%
Survey of Patients' Hospital Experiences				
Area Around Room 'Always' Quiet at Night[5]	-	-	60%	61%
Doctors 'Always' Communicated Well[5]	-	-	81%	82%
Home Recovery Information Given[5]	-	-	83%	85%
Hospital Given 9 or 10 on 10 Point Scale[5]	-	-	68%	71%
Meds 'Always' Explained Before Given[5]	-	-	63%	64%
Nurses 'Always' Communicated Well[5]	-	-	77%	79%
Pain 'Always' Well Controlled[5]	-	-	70%	71%
Room and Bathroom 'Always' Clean[5]	-	-	72%	73%
Timely Help 'Always' Received[5]	-	-	69%	68%
Would Definitely Recommend Hospital[5]	-	-	67%	71%
Use of Medical Imaging				
Cardiac Imaging Stress Test before Surgery[5]	-	-	4.9%	5.3%
Combination Abdominal CT Scan[5]	-	-	10.6%	10.5%
Combination Brain/Sinus CT Scan[5]	-	-	1.9%	2.7%
Combination Chest CT Scan[5]	-	-	2.4%	2.7%
Follow-up Mammogram/Ultrasound[5]	-	-	6.9%	8.8%
Lumbar Spine MRI for Low Back Pain[5]	-	-	41.5%	37.2%

Marias Medical Center

640 Park Dr
Shelby, MT 59474
Phone: 406-434-3200
Fax: 406-434-3213
URL: www.mmcmt.org
Type: Critical Access Hospitals
Emergency Services: Yes
Ownership: Government - Local
Beds: 20

Key Personnel:
Radiology. . . . . Tom Carter
Emergency Room . . . . Julia Drishenski, RN
Intensive Care Unit. . . . . Julia Drishenski, RN
Operating Room. . . . . Julia Drishinski, RN
CEO . . . . Bill Hartley

NOTE: Hospital profiles are in alphabetical order by state, then city, then hospital within the city; Rankings exclude hospitals with less than 25 cases except for patient surveys which excludes hospitals with less than 100 cases; (a) 100-299 cases; (1) The number of cases/patients is too few to report; (2) Data submitted were based on a sample of cases/patients; (3) Results are based on a shorter time period than required; (4) Data suppressed by CMS for one or more quarters; (5) Results are not available for this reporting period; (6) Fewer than 100 patients completed the HCAHPS survey; (7) No cases met the criteria for this measure; (8) The lower limit of the confidence interval cannot be calculated if the number of observed infections equals zero; (9) No data are available from the state/territory for this reporting period; (10) The scores shown reflect fewer than 50 completed surveys; (11) There were discrepancies in the data collection process; (12) This measure does not apply to this hospital for this reporting period; (13) Results cannot be calculated for this reporting period; (14) The results for this state are combined with nearby states to protect confidentiality; Please refer to the User's Guide for a full explanation of data.

Infection Control . . . . Nancy Hiartarson, RN
Quality Assurance . . . . Bonnie Weigand

Measure	Cases	This Hosp.	State Avg.	U.S. Avg.
Blood Clot Prevention and Treatment				
Anticoagulation Overlap Therapy[5]	-	-	97%	93%
ICU Venous Thromboembolism Prophylaxis[5]	-	-	92%	92%
Incidence of Potentially Preventable VTE[5]	-	-	4%	10%
UFH with Dosages/Platelet Monitoring[5]	-	-	97%	97%
Venous Thromboembolism Prophylaxis[5]	-	-	83%	85%
Warfarin Therapy Discharge Instructions[5]	-	-	84%	75%
Chest Pain/Possible Heart Attack Care				
Aspirin Given Within 24 Hours of Arrival	-	-	97%	96%
Fibrinolytic Meds Within 30 Min. of Arrival	-	-	43%	58%
Average Time to ECG (minutes)	-	-	10	7
Average Time to Transfer (minutes)	-	-	78	60
Children's Asthma Care				
Received Home Management Plan of Care	-	-	-	88%
Received Reliever Medication	-	-	-	100%
Received Systemic Corticosteroids	-	-	-	100%
Emergency Department				
Admittance Decision Time (minutes)[5]	-	-	72	98
Head CT Results Within 45 Min. of Arrival	-	-	26%	57%
Patients Who Left ER Before Being Seen	-	-	2%	2%
Time from ER Arrival to Admit. (minutes)[5]	-	-	220	274
Time from ER Arrival to Discharge (minutes)	-	-	120	134
Time in ER Before Being Evaluated (minutes)	-	-	23	26
Time to Pain Meds for Fractures (minutes)	-	-	47	57
Heart Attack Care				
Aspirin Given at Discharge[1,3]	-	-	100%	99%
Fibrinolytic Meds Within 30 Min. of Arrival[3,7]	-	-	50%	54%
PCI Within 90 Minutes of Arrival[3,7]	-	-	96%	96%
Statin Prescribed at Discharge[1,3]	-	-	99%	98%
Heart Failure Care				
ACE Inhibitor or ARB for LVSD[1]	-	-	97%	97%
Discharge Instructions Given[1]	-	-	92%	94%
Evaluation of LVS Function[1]	-	-	94%	99%
Medicare Spending				
Medicare Spending per Patient (ratio)	-	-	0.89	0.98
Pneumonia Care				
Appropriate Initial Antibiotic Given	17	76%	94%	95%
Blood Culture Timing[7]	-	-	97%	98%
Pregnancy and Delivery Care				
Newborn Deliveries Scheduled Early[5]	-	-	7%	6%
Preventive Care				
Immunization for Influenza[2,3]	20	90%	86%	90%
Immunization for Pneumonia[2,3]	17	100%	89%	92%
Stroke Care				
Anticoagulation Therapy for Atrial Fibrillation[5]	-	-	98%	95%
Antithrombotic Therapy Timing[5]	-	-	99%	98%
Assessed for Rehabilitation[5]	-	-	99%	97%
Discharged on Antithrombotic Therapy[5]	-	-	100%	99%
Discharged on Statin Medication[5]	-	-	94%	94%
Thrombolytic Therapy Timing[5]	-	-	67%	66%
Venous Thromboembolism Prophylaxis[5]	-	-	96%	94%
Written Stroke Educational Materials Given[5]	-	-	85%	88%
Surgical Care Improvement Project				
Appropriate Beta Blocker Usage[5]	-	-	98%	98%
Appropriate VTP Within 24 Hours[5]	-	-	98%	98%
Controlled Postoperative Blood Glucose[5]	-	-	96%	97%
Perioperative Temperature Management[5]	-	-	100%	100%
Prophylactic Antibiotic Selection[5]	-	-	99%	99%
Prophylactic Antibiotic Selection (Outpatient)	-	-	98%	98%
Prophylactic Antibiotic Stopped[5]	-	-	99%	98%
Prophylactic Antibiotic Timing[5]	-	-	99%	99%
Prophylactic Antibiotic Timing (Outpatient)	-	-	98%	98%
Urinary Catheter Removal[5]	-	-	99%	97%
Survey of Patients' Hospital Experiences				
Area Around Room 'Always' Quiet at Night[5]	-	-	60%	61%
Doctors 'Always' Communicated Well[5]	-	-	81%	82%
Home Recovery Information Given[5]	-	-	83%	85%
Hospital Given 9 or 10 on 10 Point Scale[5]	-	-	68%	71%
Meds 'Always' Explained Before Given[5]	-	-	63%	64%
Nurses 'Always' Communicated Well[5]	-	-	77%	79%
Pain 'Always' Well Controlled[5]	-	-	70%	71%
Room and Bathroom 'Always' Clean[5]	-	-	72%	73%
Timely Help 'Always' Received[5]	-	-	69%	68%
Would Definitely Recommend Hospital[5]	-	-	67%	71%
Use of Medical Imaging				
Cardiac Imaging Stress Test before Surgery	-	-	4.9%	5.3%
Combination Abdominal CT Scan	-	-	10.6%	10.5%
Combination Brain/Sinus CT Scan	-	-	1.9%	2.7%
Combination Chest CT Scan	-	-	2.4%	2.7%
Follow-up Mammogram/Ultrasound	-	-	6.9%	8.8%
Lumbar Spine MRI for Low Back Pain	-	-	41.5%	37.2%

Ruby Valley Hospital

220 E Crofoot
Sheridan, MT 59749
Phone: 406-842-5453
Fax: 406-842-5455
Type: Critical Access Hospitals
Emergency Services: Yes
Ownership: Govt - Hospital Dist/Auth
Beds: 20

Key Personnel:

Chief of Medical Staff . . . . Gail Leary
Radiology . . . . Linda Parsons
CEO . . . . John Semingson

Measure	Cases	This Hosp.	State Avg.	U.S. Avg.
Blood Clot Prevention and Treatment				
Anticoagulation Overlap Therapy[5]	-	-	97%	93%
ICU Venous Thromboembolism Prophylaxis[5]	-	-	92%	92%
Incidence of Potentially Preventable VTE[5]	-	-	4%	10%
UFH with Dosages/Platelet Monitoring[5]	-	-	97%	97%
Venous Thromboembolism Prophylaxis[5]	-	-	83%	85%
Warfarin Therapy Discharge Instructions[5]	-	-	84%	75%
Chest Pain/Possible Heart Attack Care				
Aspirin Given Within 24 Hours of Arrival	-	-	97%	96%
Fibrinolytic Meds Within 30 Min. of Arrival	-	-	43%	58%
Average Time to ECG (minutes)	-	-	10	7
Average Time to Transfer (minutes)	-	-	78	60
Children's Asthma Care				
Received Home Management Plan of Care	-	-	-	88%
Received Reliever Medication	-	-	-	100%
Received Systemic Corticosteroids	-	-	-	100%
Emergency Department				
Admittance Decision Time (minutes)[5]	-	-	72	98
Head CT Results Within 45 Min. of Arrival	-	-	26%	57%
Patients Who Left ER Before Being Seen	-	-	2%	2%
Time from ER Arrival to Admit. (minutes)[5]	-	-	220	274
Time from ER Arrival to Discharge (minutes)	-	-	120	134
Time in ER Before Being Evaluated (minutes)	-	-	23	26
Time to Pain Meds for Fractures (minutes)	-	-	47	57
Heart Attack Care				
Aspirin Given at Discharge[5]	-	-	100%	99%
Fibrinolytic Meds Within 30 Min. of Arrival[5]	-	-	50%	54%
PCI Within 90 Minutes of Arrival[5]	-	-	96%	96%
Statin Prescribed at Discharge[5]	-	-	99%	98%
Heart Failure Care				
ACE Inhibitor or ARB for LVSD[7]	-	-	97%	97%
Discharge Instructions Given[1]	-	-	92%	94%
Evaluation of LVS Function[1]	-	-	94%	99%
Medicare Spending				
Medicare Spending per Patient (ratio)	-	-	0.89	0.98
Pneumonia Care				
Appropriate Initial Antibiotic Given[7]	-	-	94%	95%
Blood Culture Timing[1]	-	-	97%	98%
Pregnancy and Delivery Care				
Newborn Deliveries Scheduled Early[5]	-	-	7%	6%
Preventive Care				
Immunization for Influenza[5]	-	-	86%	90%
Immunization for Pneumonia[5]	-	-	89%	92%
Stroke Care				
Anticoagulation Therapy for Atrial Fibrillation[5]	-	-	98%	95%
Antithrombotic Therapy Timing[5]	-	-	99%	98%
Assessed for Rehabilitation[5]	-	-	99%	97%
Discharged on Antithrombotic Therapy[5]	-	-	100%	99%
Discharged on Statin Medication[5]	-	-	94%	94%
Thrombolytic Therapy Timing[5]	-	-	67%	66%
Venous Thromboembolism Prophylaxis[5]	-	-	96%	94%
Written Stroke Educational Materials Given[5]	-	-	85%	88%
Surgical Care Improvement Project				
Appropriate Beta Blocker Usage[5]	-	-	98%	98%
Appropriate VTP Within 24 Hours[5]	-	-	98%	98%
Controlled Postoperative Blood Glucose[5]	-	-	96%	97%
Perioperative Temperature Management[5]	-	-	100%	100%
Prophylactic Antibiotic Selection[5]	-	-	99%	99%
Prophylactic Antibiotic Selection (Outpatient)	-	-	98%	98%
Prophylactic Antibiotic Stopped[5]	-	-	99%	98%
Prophylactic Antibiotic Timing[5]	-	-	99%	99%
Prophylactic Antibiotic Timing (Outpatient)	-	-	98%	98%
Urinary Catheter Removal[5]	-	-	99%	97%
Survey of Patients' Hospital Experiences				
Area Around Room 'Always' Quiet at Night[5]	-	-	60%	61%
Doctors 'Always' Communicated Well[5]	-	-	81%	82%
Home Recovery Information Given[5]	-	-	83%	85%
Hospital Given 9 or 10 on 10 Point Scale[5]	-	-	68%	71%
Meds 'Always' Explained Before Given[5]	-	-	63%	64%
Nurses 'Always' Communicated Well[5]	-	-	77%	79%
Pain 'Always' Well Controlled[5]	-	-	70%	71%
Room and Bathroom 'Always' Clean[5]	-	-	72%	73%
Timely Help 'Always' Received[5]	-	-	69%	68%
Would Definitely Recommend Hospital[5]	-	-	67%	71%
Use of Medical Imaging				
Cardiac Imaging Stress Test before Surgery	-	-	4.9%	5.3%
Combination Abdominal CT Scan	-	-	10.6%	10.5%
Combination Brain/Sinus CT Scan	-	-	1.9%	2.7%
Combination Chest CT Scan	-	-	2.4%	2.7%
Follow-up Mammogram/Ultrasound	-	-	6.9%	8.8%
Lumbar Spine MRI for Low Back Pain	-	-	41.5%	37.2%

Sidney Health Center

216 14th Ave Sw
Sidney, MT 59270
Phone: 406-488-2100
Fax: 406-488-2115
URL: www.sidneyhealth.org
Type: Critical Access Hospitals
Emergency Services: Yes
Ownership: Voluntary non-profit - Private
Beds: 118

Key Personnel:

CEO . . . . Rick Haraldson
Radiology . . . . Rance Haralson
Operating Room . . . . Judy Jensen
President . . . . Randy Johnson
Quality Assurance . . . . Peggy Kopp
Chief of Medical Staff . . . . Carlos Trevino, MD

Measure	Cases	This Hosp.	State Avg.	U.S. Avg.
Blood Clot Prevention and Treatment				
Anticoagulation Overlap Therapy[1,2]	-	-	97%	93%
ICU Venous Thromboembolism Prophylaxis[2]	25	92%	92%	92%
Incidence of Potentially Preventable VTE[1,2]	-	-	4%	10%
UFH with Dosages/Platelet Monitoring[2,7]	-	-	97%	97%
Venous Thromboembolism Prophylaxis[2]	94	82%	83%	85%
Warfarin Therapy Discharge Instructions[1,2]	-	-	84%	75%
Chest Pain/Possible Heart Attack Care				
Aspirin Given Within 24 Hours of Arrival[1]	-	-	97%	96%
Fibrinolytic Meds Within 30 Min. of Arrival[1]	-	-	43%	58%
Average Time to ECG (minutes)[1]	-	-	10	7
Average Time to Transfer (minutes)[7]	-	-	78	60
Children's Asthma Care				
Received Home Management Plan of Care	-	-	-	88%
Received Reliever Medication	-	-	-	100%
Received Systemic Corticosteroids	-	-	-	100%
Emergency Department				
Admittance Decision Time (minutes)[2]	195	25	72	98
Head CT Results Within 45 Min. of Arrival[1]	-	-	26%	57%
Patients Who Left ER Before Being Seen	6,971	1%	2%	2%
Time from ER Arrival to Admit. (minutes)[2]	209	155	220	274
Time from ER Arrival to Discharge (minutes)[5]	-	-	120	134
Time in ER Before Being Evaluated (minutes)[5]	-	-	23	26
Time to Pain Meds for Fractures (minutes)	42	38	47	57
Heart Attack Care				
Aspirin Given at Discharge[1,3]	-	-	100%	99%
Fibrinolytic Meds Within 30 Min. of Arrival[3,7]	-	-	50%	54%
PCI Within 90 Minutes of Arrival[3,7]	-	-	96%	96%

NOTE: Hospital profiles are in alphabetical order by state, then city, then hospital within the city; Rankings exclude hospitals with less than 25 cases except for patient surveys which excludes hospitals with less than 100 cases; (a) 100-299 cases; (1) The number of cases/patients is too few to report; (2) Data submitted were based on a sample of cases/patients; (3) Results are based on a shorter time period than required; (4) Data suppressed by CMS for one or more quarters; (5) Results are not available for this reporting period; (6) Fewer than 100 patients completed the HCAHPS survey; (7) No cases met the criteria for this measure; (8) The lower limit of the confidence interval cannot be calculated if the number of observed infections equals zero; (9) No data are available from the state/territory for this reporting period; (10) The scores shown reflect fewer than 50 completed surveys; (11) There were discrepancies in the data collection process; (12) This measure does not apply to this hospital for this reporting period; (13) Results cannot be calculated for this reporting period; (14) The results for this state are combined with nearby states to protect confidentiality; Please refer to the User's Guide for a full explanation of data.

Measure	Cases	This Hosp.	State Avg.	U.S. Avg.
Statin Prescribed at Discharge[1,3]	-	-	99%	98%
Heart Failure Care				
ACE Inhibitor or ARB for LVSD[1]	-	-	97%	97%
Discharge Instructions Given	16	81%	92%	94%
Evaluation of LVS Function	21	90%	94%	99%
Medicare Spending				
Medicare Spending per Patient (ratio)	-	-	0.89	0.98
Pneumonia Care				
Appropriate Initial Antibiotic Given[2]	21	100%	94%	95%
Blood Culture Timing[2]	16	88%	97%	98%
Pregnancy and Delivery Care				
Newborn Deliveries Scheduled Early[5]	-	-	7%	6%
Preventive Care				
Immunization for Influenza[2]	245	89%	86%	90%
Immunization for Pneumonia[2]	283	94%	89%	92%
Stroke Care				
Anticoagulation Therapy for Atrial Fibrillation[1,3]	-	-	98%	95%
Antithrombotic Therapy Timing[1,3]	-	-	99%	98%
Assessed for Rehabilitation[1,3]	-	-	99%	97%
Discharged on Antithrombotic Therapy[1,3]	-	-	100%	99%
Discharged on Statin Medication[1,3]	-	-	94%	94%
Thrombolytic Therapy Timing[3,7]	-	-	67%	66%
Venous Thromboembolism Prophylaxis[1,3]	-	-	96%	94%
Written Stroke Educational Materials Given[1,3]	-	-	85%	88%
Surgical Care Improvement Project				
Appropriate Beta Blocker Usage[2]	19	95%	98%	98%
Appropriate VTP Within 24 Hours[2]	73	100%	98%	98%
Controlled Postoperative Blood Glucose[2,3]	-	-	96%	97%
Perioperative Temperature Management[2]	80	100%	100%	100%
Prophylactic Antibiotic Selection[2]	67	100%	99%	99%
Prophylactic Antibiotic Selection (Outpatient)	13	100%	98%	98%
Prophylactic Antibiotic Stopped[2]	66	100%	99%	98%
Prophylactic Antibiotic Timing[2]	67	99%	99%	99%
Prophylactic Antibiotic Timing (Outpatient)	13	100%	98%	98%
Urinary Catheter Removal[2]	67	100%	99%	97%
Survey of Patients' Hospital Experiences				
Area Around Room 'Always' Quiet at Night	(a)	60%	60%	61%
Doctors 'Always' Communicated Well	(a)	77%	81%	82%
Home Recovery Information Given	(a)	83%	83%	85%
Hospital Given 9 or 10 on 10 Point Scale	(a)	67%	68%	71%
Meds 'Always' Explained Before Given	(a)	59%	63%	64%
Nurses 'Always' Communicated Well	(a)	76%	77%	79%
Pain 'Always' Well Controlled	(a)	71%	70%	71%
Room and Bathroom 'Always' Clean	(a)	62%	72%	73%
Timely Help 'Always' Received	(a)	69%	69%	68%
Would Definitely Recommend Hospital	(a)	63%	67%	71%
Use of Medical Imaging				
Cardiac Imaging Stress Test before Surgery[1]	-	-	4.9%	5.3%
Combination Abdominal CT Scan	203	0.5%	10.6%	10.5%
Combination Brain/Sinus CT Scan[1]	-	-	1.9%	2.7%
Combination Chest CT Scan	168	1.2%	2.4%	2.7%
Follow-up Mammogram/Ultrasound	209	17.2%	6.9%	8.8%
Lumbar Spine MRI for Low Back Pain[1]	-	-	41.5%	37.2%

Mineral Community Hospital

1208 6th Ave E
Superior, MT 59872
Phone: 406-822-4841
Type: Critical Access Hospitals
Emergency Services: Yes
Ownership: Voluntary non-profit - Private

Measure	Cases	This Hosp.	State Avg.	U.S. Avg.
Blood Clot Prevention and Treatment				
Anticoagulation Overlap Therapy[5]	-	-	97%	93%
ICU Venous Thromboembolism Prophylaxis[5]	-	-	92%	92%
Incidence of Potentially Preventable VTE[5]	-	-	4%	10%
UFH with Dosages/Platelet Monitoring[5]	-	-	97%	97%
Venous Thromboembolism Prophylaxis[5]	-	-	83%	85%
Warfarin Therapy Discharge Instructions[5]	-	-	84%	75%
Chest Pain/Possible Heart Attack Care				
Aspirin Given Within 24 Hours of Arrival	-	-	97%	96%
Fibrinolytic Meds Within 30 Min. of Arrival	-	-	43%	58%
Average Time to ECG (minutes)	-	-	10	7
Average Time to Transfer (minutes)	-	-	78	60
Children's Asthma Care				
Received Home Management Plan of Care	-	-	-	88%
Received Reliever Medication	-	-	-	100%
Received Systemic Corticosteroids	-	-	-	100%
Emergency Department				
Admittance Decision Time (minutes)[5]	-	-	72	98
Head CT Results Within 45 Min. of Arrival	-	-	26%	57%
Patients Who Left ER Before Being Seen	-	-	2%	2%
Time from ER Arrival to Admit. (minutes)[5]	-	-	220	274
Time from ER Arrival to Discharge (minutes)	-	-	120	134
Time in ER Before Being Evaluated (minutes)	-	-	23	26
Time to Pain Meds for Fractures (minutes)	-	-	47	57
Heart Attack Care				
Aspirin Given at Discharge[5]	-	-	100%	99%
Fibrinolytic Meds Within 30 Min. of Arrival[5]	-	-	50%	54%
PCI Within 90 Minutes of Arrival[5]	-	-	96%	96%
Statin Prescribed at Discharge[5]	-	-	99%	98%
Heart Failure Care				
ACE Inhibitor or ARB for LVSD[3,7]	-	-	97%	97%
Discharge Instructions Given[1,3]	-	-	92%	94%
Evaluation of LVS Function[1,3]	-	-	94%	99%
Medicare Spending				
Medicare Spending per Patient (ratio)	-	-	0.89	0.98
Pneumonia Care				
Appropriate Initial Antibiotic Given[1]	-	-	94%	95%
Blood Culture Timing[1]	-	-	97%	98%
Pregnancy and Delivery Care				
Newborn Deliveries Scheduled Early[5]	-	-	7%	6%
Preventive Care				
Immunization for Influenza[5]	-	-	86%	90%
Immunization for Pneumonia[5]	-	-	89%	92%
Stroke Care				
Anticoagulation Therapy for Atrial Fibrillation[5]	-	-	98%	95%
Antithrombotic Therapy Timing[5]	-	-	99%	98%
Assessed for Rehabilitation[5]	-	-	99%	97%
Discharged on Antithrombotic Therapy[5]	-	-	100%	99%
Discharged on Statin Medication[5]	-	-	94%	94%
Thrombolytic Therapy Timing[5]	-	-	67%	66%
Venous Thromboembolism Prophylaxis[5]	-	-	96%	94%
Written Stroke Educational Materials Given[5]	-	-	85%	88%
Surgical Care Improvement Project				
Appropriate Beta Blocker Usage[5]	-	-	98%	98%
Appropriate VTP Within 24 Hours[5]	-	-	98%	98%
Controlled Postoperative Blood Glucose[5]	-	-	96%	97%
Perioperative Temperature Management[5]	-	-	100%	100%
Prophylactic Antibiotic Selection[5]	-	-	99%	99%
Prophylactic Antibiotic Selection (Outpatient)	-	-	98%	98%
Prophylactic Antibiotic Stopped[5]	-	-	99%	98%
Prophylactic Antibiotic Timing[5]	-	-	99%	99%
Prophylactic Antibiotic Timing (Outpatient)	-	-	98%	98%
Urinary Catheter Removal[5]	-	-	99%	97%
Survey of Patients' Hospital Experiences				
Area Around Room 'Always' Quiet at Night[5]	-	-	60%	61%
Doctors 'Always' Communicated Well[5]	-	-	81%	82%
Home Recovery Information Given[5]	-	-	83%	85%
Hospital Given 9 or 10 on 10 Point Scale[5]	-	-	68%	71%
Meds 'Always' Explained Before Given[5]	-	-	63%	64%
Nurses 'Always' Communicated Well[5]	-	-	77%	79%
Pain 'Always' Well Controlled[5]	-	-	70%	71%
Room and Bathroom 'Always' Clean[5]	-	-	72%	73%
Timely Help 'Always' Received[5]	-	-	69%	68%
Would Definitely Recommend Hospital[5]	-	-	67%	71%
Use of Medical Imaging				
Cardiac Imaging Stress Test before Surgery	-	-	4.9%	5.3%
Combination Abdominal CT Scan	-	-	10.6%	10.5%
Combination Brain/Sinus CT Scan	-	-	1.9%	2.7%
Combination Chest CT Scan	-	-	2.4%	2.7%
Follow-up Mammogram/Ultrasound	-	-	6.9%	8.8%
Lumbar Spine MRI for Low Back Pain	-	-	41.5%	37.2%

Prairie Community Hospital

312 S Adams
Terry, MT 59349
Phone: 406-635-5511
Fax: 406-635-5510
Type: Critical Access Hospitals
Emergency Services: Yes
Ownership: Govt - Hospital Dist/Auth
Beds: 21
Key Personnel:
CEO/President. . . . . James Mantz

Measure	Cases	This Hosp.	State Avg.	U.S. Avg.
Blood Clot Prevention and Treatment				
Anticoagulation Overlap Therapy[3,7]	-	-	97%	93%
ICU Venous Thromboembolism Prophylaxis[3,7]	-	-	92%	92%
Incidence of Potentially Preventable VTE[3,7]	-	-	4%	10%
UFH with Dosages/Platelet Monitoring[3,7]	-	-	97%	97%
Venous Thromboembolism Prophylaxis[1,3]	-	-	83%	85%
Warfarin Therapy Discharge Instructions[3,7]	-	-	84%	75%
Chest Pain/Possible Heart Attack Care				
Aspirin Given Within 24 Hours of Arrival	-	-	97%	96%
Fibrinolytic Meds Within 30 Min. of Arrival	-	-	43%	58%
Average Time to ECG (minutes)	-	-	10	7
Average Time to Transfer (minutes)	-	-	78	60
Children's Asthma Care				
Received Home Management Plan of Care	-	-	-	88%
Received Reliever Medication	-	-	-	100%
Received Systemic Corticosteroids	-	-	-	100%
Emergency Department				
Admittance Decision Time (minutes)[5]	-	-	72	98
Head CT Results Within 45 Min. of Arrival	-	-	26%	57%
Patients Who Left ER Before Being Seen	-	-	2%	2%
Time from ER Arrival to Admit. (minutes)[5]	-	-	220	274
Time from ER Arrival to Discharge (minutes)	-	-	120	134
Time in ER Before Being Evaluated (minutes)	-	-	23	26
Time to Pain Meds for Fractures (minutes)	-	-	47	57
Heart Attack Care				
Aspirin Given at Discharge[5]	-	-	100%	99%
Fibrinolytic Meds Within 30 Min. of Arrival[5]	-	-	50%	54%
PCI Within 90 Minutes of Arrival[5]	-	-	96%	96%
Statin Prescribed at Discharge[5]	-	-	99%	98%
Heart Failure Care				
ACE Inhibitor or ARB for LVSD[5]	-	-	97%	97%
Discharge Instructions Given[5]	-	-	92%	94%
Evaluation of LVS Function[5]	-	-	94%	99%
Medicare Spending				
Medicare Spending per Patient (ratio)	-	-	0.89	0.98
Pneumonia Care				
Appropriate Initial Antibiotic Given[5]	-	-	94%	95%
Blood Culture Timing[5]	-	-	97%	98%
Pregnancy and Delivery Care				
Newborn Deliveries Scheduled Early[5]	-	-	7%	6%
Preventive Care				
Immunization for Influenza[5]	-	-	86%	90%
Immunization for Pneumonia[5]	-	-	89%	92%
Stroke Care				
Anticoagulation Therapy for Atrial Fibrillation[5]	-	-	98%	95%
Antithrombotic Therapy Timing[5]	-	-	99%	98%
Assessed for Rehabilitation[5]	-	-	99%	97%
Discharged on Antithrombotic Therapy[5]	-	-	100%	99%
Discharged on Statin Medication[5]	-	-	94%	94%
Thrombolytic Therapy Timing[5]	-	-	67%	66%
Venous Thromboembolism Prophylaxis[5]	-	-	96%	94%
Written Stroke Educational Materials Given[5]	-	-	85%	88%
Surgical Care Improvement Project				
Appropriate Beta Blocker Usage[5]	-	-	98%	98%
Appropriate VTP Within 24 Hours[5]	-	-	98%	98%
Controlled Postoperative Blood Glucose[5]	-	-	96%	97%
Perioperative Temperature Management[5]	-	-	100%	100%
Prophylactic Antibiotic Selection[5]	-	-	99%	99%
Prophylactic Antibiotic Selection (Outpatient)	-	-	98%	98%
Prophylactic Antibiotic Stopped[5]	-	-	99%	98%
Prophylactic Antibiotic Timing[5]	-	-	99%	99%
Prophylactic Antibiotic Timing (Outpatient)	-	-	98%	98%
Urinary Catheter Removal[5]	-	-	99%	97%
Survey of Patients' Hospital Experiences				

NOTE: Hospital profiles are in alphabetical order by state, then city, then hospital within the city; Rankings exclude hospitals with less than 25 cases except for patient surveys which excludes hospitals with less than 100 cases; (a) 100-299 cases; (1) The number of cases/patients is too few to report; (2) Data submitted were based on a sample of cases/patients; (3) Results are based on a shorter time period than required; (4) Data suppressed by CMS for one or more quarters; (5) Results are not available for this reporting period; (6) Fewer than 100 patients completed the HCAHPS survey; (7) No cases met the criteria for this measure; (8) The lower limit of the confidence interval cannot be calculated if the number of observed infections equals zero; (9) No data are available from the state/territory for this reporting period; (10) The scores shown reflect fewer than 50 completed surveys; (11) There were discrepancies in the data collection process; (12) This measure does not apply to this hospital for this reporting period; (13) Results cannot be calculated for this reporting period; (14) The results for this state are combined with nearby states to protect confidentiality; Please refer to the User's Guide for a full explanation of data.

Measure	Cases	This Hosp.	State Avg.	U.S. Avg.
Area Around Room 'Always' Quiet at Night[5]	-	-	60%	61%
Doctors 'Always' Communicated Well[5]	-	-	81%	82%
Home Recovery Information Given[5]	-	-	83%	85%
Hospital Given 9 or 10 on 10 Point Scale[5]	-	-	68%	71%
Meds 'Always' Explained Before Given[5]	-	-	63%	64%
Nurses 'Always' Communicated Well[5]	-	-	77%	79%
Pain 'Always' Well Controlled[5]	-	-	70%	71%
Room and Bathroom 'Always' Clean[5]	-	-	72%	73%
Timely Help 'Always' Received[5]	-	-	69%	68%
Would Definitely Recommend Hospital[5]	-	-	67%	71%
Use of Medical Imaging				
Cardiac Imaging Stress Test before Surgery	-	-	4.9%	5.3%
Combination Abdominal CT Scan	-	-	10.6%	10.5%
Combination Brain/Sinus CT Scan	-	-	1.9%	2.7%
Combination Chest CT Scan	-	-	2.4%	2.7%
Follow-up Mammogram/Ultrasound	-	-	6.9%	8.8%
Lumbar Spine MRI for Low Back Pain	-	-	41.5%	37.2%

Broadwater Health Center

110 N Oak St Phone: 406-266-3186
Townsend, MT 59644
Type: Critical Access Hospitals Emergency Services: Yes
Ownership: Voluntary non-profit - Private

Measure	Cases	This Hosp.	State Avg.	U.S. Avg.
Blood Clot Prevention and Treatment				
Anticoagulation Overlap Therapy[5]	-	-	97%	93%
ICU Venous Thromboembolism Prophylaxis[5]	-	-	92%	92%
Incidence of Potentially Preventable VTE[5]	-	-	4%	10%
UFH with Dosages/Platelet Monitoring[5]	-	-	97%	97%
Venous Thromboembolism Prophylaxis[5]	-	-	83%	85%
Warfarin Therapy Discharge Instructions[5]	-	-	84%	75%
Chest Pain/Possible Heart Attack Care				
Aspirin Given Within 24 Hours of Arrival	-	-	97%	96%
Fibrinolytic Meds Within 30 Min. of Arrival	-	-	43%	58%
Average Time to ECG (minutes)	-	-	10	7
Average Time to Transfer (minutes)	-	-	78	60
Children's Asthma Care				
Received Home Management Plan of Care	-	-	-	88%
Received Reliever Medication	-	-	-	100%
Received Systemic Corticosteroids	-	-	-	100%
Emergency Department				
Admittance Decision Time (minutes)[5]	-	-	72	98
Head CT Results Within 45 Min. of Arrival	-	-	26%	57%
Patients Who Left ER Before Being Seen	-	-	2%	2%
Time from ER Arrival to Admit. (minutes)[5]	-	-	220	274
Time from ER Arrival to Discharge (minutes)	-	-	120	134
Time in ER Before Being Evaluated (minutes)	-	-	23	26
Time to Pain Meds for Fractures (minutes)	-	-	47	57
Heart Attack Care				
Aspirin Given at Discharge[5]	-	-	100%	99%
Fibrinolytic Meds Within 30 Min. of Arrival[5]	-	-	50%	54%
PCI Within 90 Minutes of Arrival[5]	-	-	96%	96%
Statin Prescribed at Discharge[5]	-	-	99%	98%
Heart Failure Care				
ACE Inhibitor or ARB for LVSD[3,7]	-	-	97%	97%
Discharge Instructions Given[3,7]	-	-	92%	94%
Evaluation of LVS Function[3,7]	-	-	94%	99%
Medicare Spending				
Medicare Spending per Patient (ratio)	-	-	0.89	0.98
Pneumonia Care				
Appropriate Initial Antibiotic Given[3,7]	-	-	94%	95%
Blood Culture Timing[1,3]	-	-	97%	98%
Pregnancy and Delivery Care				
Newborn Deliveries Scheduled Early[5]	-	-	7%	6%
Preventive Care				
Immunization for Influenza[5]	-	-	86%	90%
Immunization for Pneumonia[5]	-	-	89%	92%
Stroke Care				
Anticoagulation Therapy for Atrial Fibrillation[5]	-	-	98%	95%
Antithrombotic Therapy Timing[5]	-	-	99%	98%
Assessed for Rehabilitation[5]	-	-	99%	97%
Discharged on Antithrombotic Therapy[5]	-	-	100%	99%
Discharged on Statin Medication[5]	-	-	94%	94%
Thrombolytic Therapy Timing[5]	-	-	67%	66%
Venous Thromboembolism Prophylaxis[5]	-	-	96%	94%
Written Stroke Educational Materials Given[5]	-	-	85%	88%
Surgical Care Improvement Project				
Appropriate Beta Blocker Usage[5]	-	-	98%	98%
Appropriate VTP Within 24 Hours[5]	-	-	98%	98%
Controlled Postoperative Blood Glucose[5]	-	-	96%	97%
Perioperative Temperature Management[5]	-	-	100%	100%
Prophylactic Antibiotic Selection[5]	-	-	99%	99%
Prophylactic Antibiotic Selection (Outpatient)	-	-	98%	98%
Prophylactic Antibiotic Stopped[5]	-	-	99%	98%
Prophylactic Antibiotic Timing[5]	-	-	99%	99%
Prophylactic Antibiotic Timing (Outpatient)	-	-	98%	98%
Urinary Catheter Removal[5]	-	-	99%	97%
Survey of Patients' Hospital Experiences				
Area Around Room 'Always' Quiet at Night[5]	-	-	60%	61%
Doctors 'Always' Communicated Well[5]	-	-	81%	82%
Home Recovery Information Given[5]	-	-	83%	85%
Hospital Given 9 or 10 on 10 Point Scale[5]	-	-	68%	71%
Meds 'Always' Explained Before Given[5]	-	-	63%	64%
Nurses 'Always' Communicated Well[5]	-	-	77%	79%
Pain 'Always' Well Controlled[5]	-	-	70%	71%
Room and Bathroom 'Always' Clean[5]	-	-	72%	73%
Timely Help 'Always' Received[5]	-	-	69%	68%
Would Definitely Recommend Hospital[5]	-	-	67%	71%
Use of Medical Imaging				
Cardiac Imaging Stress Test before Surgery	-	-	4.9%	5.3%
Combination Abdominal CT Scan	-	-	10.6%	10.5%
Combination Brain/Sinus CT Scan	-	-	1.9%	2.7%
Combination Chest CT Scan	-	-	2.4%	2.7%
Follow-up Mammogram/Ultrasound	-	-	6.9%	8.8%
Lumbar Spine MRI for Low Back Pain	-	-	41.5%	37.2%

Mountainview Medical Center

16 W Main St Phone: 406-547-3321
White Sulphur Spring, MT 59645 Fax: 406-547-3589
E-mail: info@mvmc.org
URL: www.mvmc.org
Type: Critical Access Hospitals Emergency Services: Yes
Ownership: Voluntary non-profit - Private Beds: 6
Key Personnel:
Quality Assurance . . . . Jane Atkins
Chief of Medical Staff . . . . David Kidder
CEO/President. . . . . Aaron Rogers, CHE
Emergency Room . . . . Bev Zehntner, RN

Measure	Cases	This Hosp.	State Avg.	U.S. Avg.
Blood Clot Prevention and Treatment				
Anticoagulation Overlap Therapy[5]	-	-	97%	93%
ICU Venous Thromboembolism Prophylaxis[5]	-	-	92%	92%
Incidence of Potentially Preventable VTE[5]	-	-	4%	10%
UFH with Dosages/Platelet Monitoring[5]	-	-	97%	97%
Venous Thromboembolism Prophylaxis[5]	-	-	83%	85%
Warfarin Therapy Discharge Instructions[5]	-	-	84%	75%
Chest Pain/Possible Heart Attack Care				
Aspirin Given Within 24 Hours of Arrival	-	-	97%	96%
Fibrinolytic Meds Within 30 Min. of Arrival	-	-	43%	58%
Average Time to ECG (minutes)	-	-	10	7
Average Time to Transfer (minutes)	-	-	78	60
Children's Asthma Care				
Received Home Management Plan of Care	-	-	-	88%
Received Reliever Medication	-	-	-	100%
Received Systemic Corticosteroids	-	-	-	100%
Emergency Department				
Admittance Decision Time (minutes)[5]	-	-	72	98
Head CT Results Within 45 Min. of Arrival	-	-	26%	57%
Patients Who Left ER Before Being Seen	-	-	2%	2%
Time from ER Arrival to Admit. (minutes)[5]	-	-	220	274
Time from ER Arrival to Discharge (minutes)	-	-	120	134
Time in ER Before Being Evaluated (minutes)	-	-	23	26
Time to Pain Meds for Fractures (minutes)	-	-	47	57
Heart Attack Care				
Aspirin Given at Discharge[5]	-	-	100%	99%
Fibrinolytic Meds Within 30 Min. of Arrival[5]	-	-	50%	54%
PCI Within 90 Minutes of Arrival[5]	-	-	96%	96%
Statin Prescribed at Discharge[5]	-	-	99%	98%
Heart Failure Care				
ACE Inhibitor or ARB for LVSD[1,3]	-	-	97%	97%
Discharge Instructions Given[1,3]	-	-	92%	94%
Evaluation of LVS Function[1,3]	-	-	94%	99%
Medicare Spending				
Medicare Spending per Patient (ratio)	-	-	0.89	0.98
Pneumonia Care				
Appropriate Initial Antibiotic Given[3,7]	-	-	94%	95%
Blood Culture Timing[3,7]	-	-	97%	98%
Pregnancy and Delivery Care				
Newborn Deliveries Scheduled Early[5]	-	-	7%	6%
Preventive Care				
Immunization for Influenza[5]	-	-	86%	90%
Immunization for Pneumonia[5]	-	-	89%	92%
Stroke Care				
Anticoagulation Therapy for Atrial Fibrillation[5]	-	-	98%	95%
Antithrombotic Therapy Timing[5]	-	-	99%	98%
Assessed for Rehabilitation[5]	-	-	99%	97%
Discharged on Antithrombotic Therapy[5]	-	-	100%	99%
Discharged on Statin Medication[5]	-	-	94%	94%
Thrombolytic Therapy Timing[5]	-	-	67%	66%
Venous Thromboembolism Prophylaxis[5]	-	-	96%	94%
Written Stroke Educational Materials Given[5]	-	-	85%	88%
Surgical Care Improvement Project				
Appropriate Beta Blocker Usage[5]	-	-	98%	98%
Appropriate VTP Within 24 Hours[5]	-	-	98%	98%
Controlled Postoperative Blood Glucose[5]	-	-	96%	97%
Perioperative Temperature Management[5]	-	-	100%	100%
Prophylactic Antibiotic Selection[5]	-	-	99%	99%
Prophylactic Antibiotic Selection (Outpatient)	-	-	98%	98%
Prophylactic Antibiotic Stopped[5]	-	-	99%	98%
Prophylactic Antibiotic Timing[5]	-	-	99%	99%
Prophylactic Antibiotic Timing (Outpatient)	-	-	98%	98%
Urinary Catheter Removal[5]	-	-	99%	97%
Survey of Patients' Hospital Experiences				
Area Around Room 'Always' Quiet at Night[5]	-	-	60%	61%
Doctors 'Always' Communicated Well[5]	-	-	81%	82%
Home Recovery Information Given[5]	-	-	83%	85%
Hospital Given 9 or 10 on 10 Point Scale[5]	-	-	68%	71%
Meds 'Always' Explained Before Given[5]	-	-	63%	64%
Nurses 'Always' Communicated Well[5]	-	-	77%	79%
Pain 'Always' Well Controlled[5]	-	-	70%	71%
Room and Bathroom 'Always' Clean[5]	-	-	72%	73%
Timely Help 'Always' Received[5]	-	-	69%	68%
Would Definitely Recommend Hospital[5]	-	-	67%	71%
Use of Medical Imaging				
Cardiac Imaging Stress Test before Surgery	-	-	4.9%	5.3%
Combination Abdominal CT Scan	-	-	10.6%	10.5%
Combination Brain/Sinus CT Scan	-	-	1.9%	2.7%
Combination Chest CT Scan	-	-	2.4%	2.7%
Follow-up Mammogram/Ultrasound	-	-	6.9%	8.8%
Lumbar Spine MRI for Low Back Pain	-	-	41.5%	37.2%

North Valley Hospital

1600 Hospital Way Phone: 406-863-3550
Whitefish, MT 59937 Fax: 406-862-2532
E-mail: nvhosp@nvhosp.org
URL: www.nvhosp.org
Type: Critical Access Hospitals Emergency Services: Yes
Ownership: Voluntary non-profit - Private Beds: 25
Key Personnel:
Operating Room. . . . . Donna Holland, RN
Emergency Room . . . . Ken McFadden, MD
Patient Relations . . . . Laurie Pierce
CEO/President. . . . . Jason A Spring
Radiology. . . . . Doug Wehrli

Measure	Cases	This Hosp.	State Avg.	U.S. Avg.
Blood Clot Prevention and Treatment				
Anticoagulation Overlap Therapy[5]	-	-	97%	93%
ICU Venous Thromboembolism Prophylaxis[5]	-	-	92%	92%
Incidence of Potentially Preventable VTE[5]	-	-	4%	10%

NOTE: Hospital profiles are in alphabetical order by state, then city, then hospital within the city; Rankings exclude hospitals with less than 25 cases except for patient surveys which excludes hospitals with less than 100 cases; (a) 100-299 cases; (1) The number of cases/patients is too few to report; (2) Data submitted were based on a sample of cases/patients; (3) Results are based on a shorter time period than required; (4) Data suppressed by CMS for one or more quarters; (5) Results are not available for this reporting period; (6) Fewer than 100 patients completed the HCAHPS survey; (7) No cases met the criteria for this measure; (8) The lower limit of the confidence interval cannot be calculated if the number of observed infections equals zero; (9) No data are available from the state/territory for this reporting period; (10) The scores shown reflect fewer than 50 completed surveys; (11) There were discrepancies in the data collection process; (12) This measure does not apply to this hospital for this reporting period; (13) Results cannot be calculated for this reporting period; (14) The results for this state are combined with nearby states to protect confidentiality; Please refer to the User's Guide for a full explanation of data.

UFH with Dosages/Platelet Monitoring[5]	-	-	97%	97%
Venous Thromboembolism Prophylaxis[5]	-	-	83%	85%
Warfarin Therapy Discharge Instructions[5]	-	-	84%	75%
Chest Pain/Possible Heart Attack Care				
Aspirin Given Within 24 Hours of Arrival	21	90%	97%	96%
Fibrinolytic Meds Within 30 Min. of Arrival[7]	-	-	43%	58%
Average Time to ECG (minutes)	21	10	10	7
Average Time to Transfer (minutes)[1]	-	-	78	60
Children's Asthma Care				
Received Home Management Plan of Care	-	-	-	88%
Received Reliever Medication	-	-	-	100%
Received Systemic Corticosteroids	-	-	-	100%
Emergency Department				
Admittance Decision Time (minutes)[5]	-	-	72	98
Head CT Results Within 45 Min. of Arrival[5]	-	-	26%	57%
Patients Who Left ER Before Being Seen	7,478	1%	2%	2%
Time from ER Arrival to Admit. (minutes)[5]	-	-	220	274
Time from ER Arrival to Discharge (minutes)[5]	-	-	120	134
Time in ER Before Being Evaluated (minutes)[5]	-	-	23	26
Time to Pain Meds for Fractures (minutes)	91	49	47	57
Heart Attack Care				
Aspirin Given at Discharge[1,3]	-	-	100%	99%
Fibrinolytic Meds Within 30 Min. of Arrival[3,7]	-	-	50%	54%
PCI Within 90 Minutes of Arrival[3,7]	-	-	96%	96%
Statin Prescribed at Discharge[3,7]	-	-	99%	98%
Heart Failure Care				
ACE Inhibitor or ARB for LVSD[1]	-	-	97%	97%
Discharge Instructions Given	15	80%	92%	94%
Evaluation of LVS Function	21	100%	94%	99%
Medicare Spending				
Medicare Spending per Patient (ratio)	-	-	0.89	0.98
Pneumonia Care				
Appropriate Initial Antibiotic Given	25	100%	94%	95%
Blood Culture Timing	33	97%	97%	98%
Pregnancy and Delivery Care				
Newborn Deliveries Scheduled Early[5]	-	-	7%	6%
Preventive Care				
Immunization for Influenza[5]	-	-	86%	90%
Immunization for Pneumonia[5]	-	-	89%	92%
Stroke Care				
Anticoagulation Therapy for Atrial Fibrillation[5]	-	-	98%	95%
Antithrombotic Therapy Timing[5]	-	-	99%	98%
Assessed for Rehabilitation[5]	-	-	99%	97%
Discharged on Antithrombotic Therapy[5]	-	-	100%	99%
Discharged on Statin Medication[5]	-	-	94%	94%
Thrombolytic Therapy Timing[5]	-	-	67%	66%
Venous Thromboembolism Prophylaxis[5]	-	-	96%	94%
Written Stroke Educational Materials Given[5]	-	-	85%	88%
Surgical Care Improvement Project				
Appropriate Beta Blocker Usage	49	94%	98%	98%
Appropriate VTP Within 24 Hours	219	96%	98%	98%
Controlled Postoperative Blood Glucose[3,7]	-	-	96%	97%
Perioperative Temperature Management	267	100%	100%	100%
Prophylactic Antibiotic Selection	203	100%	99%	99%
Prophylactic Antibiotic Selection (Outpatient)	38	95%	98%	98%
Prophylactic Antibiotic Stopped	198	98%	99%	98%
Prophylactic Antibiotic Timing	203	95%	99%	99%
Prophylactic Antibiotic Timing (Outpatient)	38	92%	98%	98%
Urinary Catheter Removal	123	98%	99%	97%
Survey of Patients' Hospital Experiences				
Area Around Room 'Always' Quiet at Night	300+	66%	60%	61%
Doctors 'Always' Communicated Well	300+	82%	81%	82%
Home Recovery Information Given	300+	90%	83%	85%
Hospital Given 9 or 10 on 10 Point Scale	300+	81%	68%	71%
Meds 'Always' Explained Before Given	300+	68%	63%	64%
Nurses 'Always' Communicated Well	300+	83%	77%	79%
Pain 'Always' Well Controlled	300+	79%	70%	71%
Room and Bathroom 'Always' Clean	300+	82%	72%	73%
Timely Help 'Always' Received	300+	78%	69%	68%
Would Definitely Recommend Hospital	300+	83%	67%	71%
Use of Medical Imaging				
Cardiac Imaging Stress Test before Surgery	64	7.8%	4.9%	5.3%
Combination Abdominal CT Scan	271	12.9%	10.6%	10.5%
Combination Brain/Sinus CT Scan[1]	-	-	1.9%	2.7%
Combination Chest CT Scan	117	2.6%	2.4%	2.7%
Follow-up Mammogram/Ultrasound	473	9.3%	6.9%	8.8%
Lumbar Spine MRI for Low Back Pain[1]	-	-	41.5%	37.2%

Trinity Hospital

315 Knapp St
Wolf Point, MT 59201
URL: www.nemhs.net
Type: Critical Access Hospitals
Ownership: Voluntary non-profit - Private
Phone: 406-653-6500
Fax: 406-653-6592
Emergency Services: Yes
Beds: 20

Key Personnel:
CEO/President. . . . . Peg Norgaard
Emergency Room . . . . Lee Robertson, DON
Chief of Medical Staff. . . . . Mark Zilkoski

Measure	Cases	This Hosp.	State Avg.	U.S. Avg.
Blood Clot Prevention and Treatment				
Anticoagulation Overlap Therapy[5]	-	-	97%	93%
ICU Venous Thromboembolism Prophylaxis[5]	-	-	92%	92%
Incidence of Potentially Preventable VTE[5]	-	-	4%	10%
UFH with Dosages/Platelet Monitoring[5]	-	-	97%	97%
Venous Thromboembolism Prophylaxis[5]	-	-	83%	85%
Warfarin Therapy Discharge Instructions[5]	-	-	84%	75%
Chest Pain/Possible Heart Attack Care				
Aspirin Given Within 24 Hours of Arrival	-	-	97%	96%
Fibrinolytic Meds Within 30 Min. of Arrival	-	-	43%	58%
Average Time to ECG (minutes)	-	-	10	7
Average Time to Transfer (minutes)	-	-	78	60
Children's Asthma Care				
Received Home Management Plan of Care	-	-	-	88%
Received Reliever Medication	-	-	-	100%
Received Systemic Corticosteroids	-	-	-	100%
Emergency Department				
Admittance Decision Time (minutes)[5]	-	-	72	98
Head CT Results Within 45 Min. of Arrival	-	-	26%	57%
Patients Who Left ER Before Being Seen	-	-	2%	2%
Time from ER Arrival to Admit. (minutes)[5]	-	-	220	274
Time from ER Arrival to Discharge (minutes)	-	-	120	134
Time in ER Before Being Evaluated (minutes)	-	-	23	26
Time to Pain Meds for Fractures (minutes)	-	-	47	57
Heart Attack Care				
Aspirin Given at Discharge[5]	-	-	100%	99%
Fibrinolytic Meds Within 30 Min. of Arrival[5]	-	-	50%	54%
PCI Within 90 Minutes of Arrival[5]	-	-	96%	96%
Statin Prescribed at Discharge[5]	-	-	99%	98%
Heart Failure Care				
ACE Inhibitor or ARB for LVSD[3,7]	-	-	97%	97%
Discharge Instructions Given[1,3]	-	-	92%	94%
Evaluation of LVS Function[1,3]	-	-	94%	99%
Medicare Spending				
Medicare Spending per Patient (ratio)	-	-	0.89	0.98
Pneumonia Care				
Appropriate Initial Antibiotic Given	12	67%	94%	95%
Blood Culture Timing[1]	-	-	97%	98%
Pregnancy and Delivery Care				
Newborn Deliveries Scheduled Early[5]	-	-	7%	6%
Preventive Care				
Immunization for Influenza[5]	-	-	86%	90%
Immunization for Pneumonia[5]	-	-	89%	92%
Stroke Care				
Anticoagulation Therapy for Atrial Fibrillation[5]	-	-	98%	95%
Antithrombotic Therapy Timing[5]	-	-	99%	98%
Assessed for Rehabilitation[5]	-	-	99%	97%
Discharged on Antithrombotic Therapy[5]	-	-	100%	99%
Discharged on Statin Medication[5]	-	-	94%	94%
Thrombolytic Therapy Timing[5]	-	-	67%	66%
Venous Thromboembolism Prophylaxis[5]	-	-	96%	94%
Written Stroke Educational Materials Given[5]	-	-	85%	88%
Surgical Care Improvement Project				
Appropriate Beta Blocker Usage[5]	-	-	98%	98%
Appropriate VTP Within 24 Hours[5]	-	-	98%	98%
Controlled Postoperative Blood Glucose[5]	-	-	96%	97%
Perioperative Temperature Management[5]	-	-	100%	100%
Prophylactic Antibiotic Selection[5]	-	-	99%	99%
Prophylactic Antibiotic Selection (Outpatient)	-	-	98%	98%
Prophylactic Antibiotic Stopped[5]	-	-	99%	98%
Prophylactic Antibiotic Timing[5]	-	-	99%	99%
Prophylactic Antibiotic Timing (Outpatient)	-	-	98%	98%
Urinary Catheter Removal[5]	-	-	99%	97%
Survey of Patients' Hospital Experiences				
Area Around Room 'Always' Quiet at Night[5]	-	-	60%	61%
Doctors 'Always' Communicated Well[5]	-	-	81%	82%
Home Recovery Information Given[5]	-	-	83%	85%
Hospital Given 9 or 10 on 10 Point Scale[5]	-	-	68%	71%
Meds 'Always' Explained Before Given[5]	-	-	63%	64%
Nurses 'Always' Communicated Well[5]	-	-	77%	79%
Pain 'Always' Well Controlled[5]	-	-	70%	71%
Room and Bathroom 'Always' Clean[5]	-	-	72%	73%
Timely Help 'Always' Received[5]	-	-	69%	68%
Would Definitely Recommend Hospital[5]	-	-	67%	71%
Use of Medical Imaging				
Cardiac Imaging Stress Test before Surgery	-	-	4.9%	5.3%
Combination Abdominal CT Scan	-	-	10.6%	10.5%
Combination Brain/Sinus CT Scan	-	-	1.9%	2.7%
Combination Chest CT Scan	-	-	2.4%	2.7%
Follow-up Mammogram/Ultrasound	-	-	6.9%	8.8%
Lumbar Spine MRI for Low Back Pain	-	-	41.5%	37.2%

NOTE: Hospital profiles are in alphabetical order by state, then city, then hospital within the city; Rankings exclude hospitals with less than 25 cases except for patient surveys which excludes hospitals with less than 100 cases; (a) 100-299 cases; (1) The number of cases/patients is too few to report; (2) Data submitted were based on a sample of cases/patients; (3) Results are based on a shorter time period than required; (4) Data suppressed by CMS for one or more quarters; (5) Results are not available for this reporting period; (6) Fewer than 100 patients completed the HCAHPS survey; (7) No cases met the criteria for this measure; (8) The lower limit of the confidence interval cannot be calculated if the number of observed infections equals zero; (9) No data are available from the state/territory for this reporting period; (10) The scores shown reflect fewer than 50 completed surveys; (11) There were discrepancies in the data collection process; (12) This measure does not apply to this hospital for this reporting period; (13) Results cannot be calculated for this reporting period; (14) The results for this state are combined with nearby states to protect confidentiality; Please refer to the User's Guide for a full explanation of data.

Blood Clot Prevention and Treatment

Anticoagulation Overlap Therapy

Hospital Name	City	Rate	Cases
Renown South Meadows Medical Center[2]	Reno	100%	32
St Rose Dominican Hosps-Rose De Lima[2]	Henderson	100%	60
Carson Tahoe Regional Medical Center[2]	Carson City	99%	87
St Rose Dominican Hosps-Siena[2]	Henderson	99%	149
Mountainview Hospital[2]	Las Vegas	98%	162
North Vista Hospital[2]	North Las Vegas	98%	58
Southern Hills Hospital & Medical Center[2]	Las Vegas	98%	61
Centennial Hills Hospital Medical Center[2]	Las Vegas	97%	87
St Rose Dominican Hosps-San Martin[2]	Las Vegas	97%	76
Sunrise Hospital & Medical Center[2]	Las Vegas	97%	142
Saint Mary's Regional Medical Center[2]	Reno	96%	121
Spring Valley Hospital Medical Center[2]	Las Vegas	96%	96
Summerlin Hospital Medical Center[2]	Las Vegas	96%	103
Renown Regional Medical Center[2]	Reno	95%	197
Desert Springs Hospital[2]	Las Vegas	94%	36
UMC of Southern Nevada[2]	Las Vegas	94%	113
Valley Hospital Medical Center[2]	Las Vegas	94%	50
Northern Nevada Medical Center[2]	Sparks	88%	32

ICU Venous Thromboembolism Prophylaxis

Hospital Name	City	Rate	Cases
Mesa View Regional Hospital[2]	Mesquite	100%	33
North Vista Hospital[2]	North Las Vegas	100%	201
Northern Nevada Medical Center[2]	Sparks	100%	30
Renown South Meadows Medical Center[2]	Reno	100%	34
Southern Hills Hospital & Medical Center[2]	Las Vegas	99%	108
St Rose Dominican Hosps-San Martin[2]	Las Vegas	97%	63
Sunrise Hospital & Medical Center[2]	Las Vegas	97%	148
Renown Regional Medical Center[2]	Reno	96%	123
Valley Hospital Medical Center[2]	Las Vegas	96%	114
Saint Mary's Regional Medical Center[2]	Reno	95%	59
St Rose Dominican Hosps-Siena[2]	Henderson	94%	54
St Rose Dominican Hosps-Rose De Lima[2]	Henderson	91%	70
Mountainview Hospital[2]	Las Vegas	87%	102
Desert Springs Hospital[2]	Las Vegas	86%	98
Carson Tahoe Regional Medical Center[2]	Carson City	85%	53
UMC of Southern Nevada[2]	Las Vegas	81%	110
Centennial Hills Hospital Medical Center[2]	Las Vegas	79%	57
Northeastern Nevada Regional Hospital[2]	Elko	79%	47
Spring Valley Hospital Medical Center[2]	Las Vegas	79%	62
Summerlin Hospital Medical Center[2]	Las Vegas	74%	72

Incidence of Potentially Preventable VTE

Hospital Name	City	Rate	Cases
Mountainview Hospital[2]	Las Vegas	3%	32
Renown Regional Medical Center[2]	Reno	3%	37
St Rose Dominican Hosps-Siena[2]	Henderson	3%	33
UMC of Southern Nevada[2]	Las Vegas	16%	38
Spring Valley Hospital Medical Center[2]	Las Vegas	28%	25

UFH with Dosages/Platelet Count Monitoring

Hospital Name	City	Rate	Cases
Desert Springs Hospital[2]	Las Vegas	100%	29
North Vista Hospital[2]	North Las Vegas	100%	33
Renown Regional Medical Center[2]	Reno	100%	99
Saint Mary's Regional Medical Center[2]	Reno	100%	97
St Rose Dominican Hosps-Rose De Lima[2]	Henderson	100%	43
St Rose Dominican Hosps-San Martin[2]	Las Vegas	100%	56
Southern Hills Hospital & Medical Center[2]	Las Vegas	100%	55
Spring Valley Hospital Medical Center[2]	Las Vegas	100%	54
Summerlin Hospital Medical Center[2]	Las Vegas	100%	82
Sunrise Hospital & Medical Center[2]	Las Vegas	100%	99
UMC of Southern Nevada[2]	Las Vegas	100%	85
Valley Hospital Medical Center[2]	Las Vegas	100%	57
Centennial Hills Hospital Medical Center[2]	Las Vegas	99%	70
Mountainview Hospital[2]	Las Vegas	99%	112
St Rose Dominican Hosps-Siena[2]	Henderson	99%	119
Carson Tahoe Regional Medical Center[2]	Carson City	98%	43

Venous Thromboembolism Prophylaxis

Hospital Name	City	Rate	Cases
Renown South Meadows Medical Center[2]	Reno	100%	226
Sierra Surgery Hospital[2]	Carson City	100%	41
Southern Hills Hospital & Medical Center[2]	Las Vegas	100%	254
Mesa View Regional Hospital[2]	Mesquite	99%	207
Northern Nevada Medical Center[2]	Sparks	97%	238
Saint Mary's Regional Medical Center[2]	Reno	97%	322
Banner Churchill Community Hospital[2]	Fallon	96%	134
North Vista Hospital[2]	North Las Vegas	96%	497
Renown Regional Medical Center[2]	Reno	94%	332
St Rose Dominican Hosps-San Martin[2]	Las Vegas	93%	363
St Rose Dominican Hosps-Siena[2]	Henderson	93%	313
Carson Tahoe Regional Medical Center[2]	Carson City	90%	324
St Rose Dominican Hosps-Rose De Lima[2]	Henderson	90%	354
Mountainview Hospital[2]	Las Vegas	80%	365
Centennial Hills Hospital Medical Center[2]	Las Vegas	77%	292
Desert Springs Hospital[2]	Las Vegas	77%	342
Sunrise Hospital & Medical Center[2]	Las Vegas	76%	323
UMC of Southern Nevada[2]	Las Vegas	73%	283
Valley Hospital Medical Center[2]	Las Vegas	70%	292
Spring Valley Hospital Medical Center[2]	Las Vegas	60%	289
Summerlin Hospital Medical Center[2]	Las Vegas	58%	329
Northeastern Nevada Regional Hospital[2]	Elko	52%	161

Warfarin Therapy Discharge Instructions

Hospital Name	City	Rate	Cases
Renown South Meadows Medical Center[2]	Reno	100%	31
Southern Hills Hospital & Medical Center[2]	Las Vegas	100%	41
Sunrise Hospital & Medical Center[2]	Las Vegas	100%	99
Saint Mary's Regional Medical Center[2]	Reno	98%	102
Carson Tahoe Regional Medical Center[2]	Carson City	95%	75
Centennial Hills Hospital Medical Center[2]	Las Vegas	95%	59
Spring Valley Hospital Medical Center[2]	Las Vegas	94%	70
Renown Regional Medical Center[2]	Reno	93%	154
St Rose Dominican Hosps-San Martin[2]	Las Vegas	90%	51
Summerlin Hospital Medical Center[2]	Las Vegas	90%	67
Mountainview Hospital[2]	Las Vegas	88%	120
UMC of Southern Nevada[2]	Las Vegas	88%	82
St Rose Dominican Hosps-Rose De Lima[2]	Henderson	78%	36
St Rose Dominican Hosps-Siena[2]	Henderson	77%	97

Chest Pain/Possible Heart Attack Care

Aspirin Given Within 24 Hours of Arrival

Hospital Name	City	Rate	Cases
Banner Churchill Community Hospital	Fallon	100%	43
Mesa View Regional Hospital	Mesquite	100%	45
St Rose Dominican Hosps-Siena	Henderson	100%	42
St Rose Dominican Hosps-Rose De Lima	Henderson	98%	40
Carson Valley Medical Center	Gardnerville	97%	34
Humboldt General Hospital	Winnemucca	94%	35

Average Time to ECG (minutes)

Hospital Name	City	Min.	Cases
Mesa View Regional Hospital	Mesquite	4	44
Humboldt General Hospital	Winnemucca	6	37
Northeastern Nevada Regional Hospital	Elko	6	25
Banner Churchill Community Hospital	Fallon	8	43
Carson Valley Medical Center	Gardnerville	10	31
St Rose Dominican Hosps-Rose De Lima	Henderson	10	44
St Rose Dominican Hosps-Siena	Henderson	12	42

Average Time to Transfer (minutes)

Hospital Name	City	Min.	Cases
St Rose Dominican Hosps-Rose De Lima	Henderson	60	25

Children's Asthma Care

Received Home Management Plan of Care

Hospital Name	City	Rate	Cases
Renown Regional Medical Center	Reno	99%	73

Received Reliever Medication

Hospital Name	City	Rate	Cases
Renown Regional Medical Center	Reno	100%	75

Received Systemic Corticosteroids

Hospital Name	City	Rate	Cases
Renown Regional Medical Center	Reno	100%	75

Emergency Department

Admittance Decision Time (minutes)

Hospital Name	City	Min.	Cases
Mesa View Regional Hospital[2]	Mesquite	45	369
Banner Churchill Community Hospital[2]	Fallon	51	409
Renown South Meadows Medical Center[2]	Reno	53	488
Renown Regional Medical Center[2]	Reno	58	614
Humboldt General Hospital[2]	Winnemucca	65	235
Northeastern Nevada Regional Hospital[2]	Elko	88	275
Carson Tahoe Regional Medical Center[2]	Carson City	96	599
Northern Nevada Medical Center[2]	Sparks	101	408
Saint Mary's Regional Medical Center[2]	Reno	115	661
St Rose Dominican Hosps-San Martin[2]	Las Vegas	116	575
UMC of Southern Nevada[2]	Las Vegas	162	545
Summerlin Hospital Medical Center[2]	Las Vegas	164	547
Southern Hills Hospital & Medical Center[2]	Las Vegas	165	584
Centennial Hills Hospital Medical Center[2]	Las Vegas	176	686
North Vista Hospital[2]	North Las Vegas	180	701
Sunrise Hospital & Medical Center[2]	Las Vegas	194	574
Mountainview Hospital[2]	Las Vegas	210	835
St Rose Dominican Hosps-Siena[2]	Henderson	242	492
St Rose Dominican Hosps-Rose De Lima[2]	Henderson	253	898
Valley Hospital Medical Center[2]	Las Vegas	278	755
Spring Valley Hospital Medical Center[2]	Las Vegas	298	541
Desert Springs Hospital[2]	Las Vegas	405	980

Patients Who Left ER Before Being Seen

Hospital Name	City	Rate	Cases
Mesa View Regional Hospital	Mesquite	0%	8150
Mountainview Hospital	Las Vegas	0%	49073
Nye Regional Medical Center	Tonopah	0%	2683
St Rose Dominican Hosps-Rose De Lima	Henderson	0%	38522
Sunrise Hospital & Medical Center	Las Vegas	0%	114432
Banner Churchill Community Hospital	Fallon	1%	17090
Carson Valley Medical Center	Gardnerville	1%	9441
Grover C Dils Medical Center	Caliente	1%	890
North Vista Hospital	North Las Vegas	1%	35333
Renown South Meadows Medical Center	Reno	1%	20251
Saint Mary's Regional Medical Center	Reno	1%	53801
St Rose Dominican Hosps-San Martin	Las Vegas	1%	26449
St Rose Dominican Hosps-Siena	Henderson	1%	64545
Southern Hills Hospital & Medical Center	Las Vegas	1%	23464
Carson Tahoe Regional Medical Center	Carson City	2%	25944
Desert View Regional Medical Center	Pahrump	2%	14234
Mount Grant General Hospital	Hawthorne	2%	2085
Northeastern Nevada Regional Hospital	Elko	2%	25123
Northern Nevada Medical Center	Sparks	2%	19444
Renown Regional Medical Center	Reno	2%	84092
Spring Valley Hospital Medical Center	Las Vegas	2%	43972
Summerlin Hospital Medical Center	Las Vegas	2%	44997
Valley Hospital Medical Center	Las Vegas	2%	39185
Desert Springs Hospital	Las Vegas	3%	37077
William Bee Ririe Hospital	Ely	3%	5428
Centennial Hills Hospital Medical Center	Las Vegas	4%	39474
UMC of Southern Nevada	Las Vegas	5%	83395

Time from ER Arrival to Being Admitted (minutes)

Hospital Name	City	Min.	Cases
Mesa View Regional Hospital[2]	Mesquite	196	371
Banner Churchill Community Hospital[2]	Fallon	218	410
Humboldt General Hospital[2]	Winnemucca	231	259
Renown South Meadows Medical Center[2]	Reno	238	488
Southern Hills Hospital & Medical Center[2]	Las Vegas	244	584
Northern Nevada Medical Center[2]	Sparks	254	481
Saint Mary's Regional Medical Center[2]	Reno	268	661
Northeastern Nevada Regional Hospital[2]	Elko	269	277
Carson Tahoe Regional Medical Center[2]	Carson City	274	618
Renown Regional Medical Center[2]	Reno	277	623
St Rose Dominican Hosps-San Martin[2]	Las Vegas	283	632
Sunrise Hospital & Medical Center[2]	Las Vegas	340	575
Mountainview Hospital[2]	Las Vegas	350	835
North Vista Hospital[2]	North Las Vegas	360	700
Summerlin Hospital Medical Center[2]	Las Vegas	380	554
Centennial Hills Hospital Medical Center[2]	Las Vegas	392	690
St Rose Dominican Hosps-Siena[2]	Henderson	450	528
St Rose Dominican Hosps-Rose De Lima[2]	Henderson	453	938
UMC of Southern Nevada[2]	Las Vegas	463	545
Valley Hospital Medical Center[2]	Las Vegas	494	758
Spring Valley Hospital Medical Center[2]	Las Vegas	524	542
Desert Springs Hospital[2]	Las Vegas	637	983

Time from ER Arrival to Discharge (minutes)

Hospital Name	City	Min.	Cases
Humboldt General Hospital	Winnemucca	99	365
Mesa View Regional Hospital	Mesquite	112	344
Banner Churchill Community Hospital	Fallon	115	321
Nye Regional Medical Center	Tonopah	119	242
Northeastern Nevada Regional Hospital	Elko	122	387
North Vista Hospital	North Las Vegas	129	933
St Rose Dominican Hosps-San Martin	Las Vegas	129	376
Southern Hills Hospital & Medical Center	Las Vegas	134	392
Renown South Meadows Medical Center	Reno	136	416
Northern Nevada Medical Center	Sparks	140	365
St Rose Dominican Hosps-Rose De Lima	Henderson	145	359
Saint Mary's Regional Medical Center	Reno	153	385
Sunrise Hospital & Medical Center	Las Vegas	156	403
St Rose Dominican Hosps-Siena	Henderson	162	360
Renown Regional Medical Center	Reno	164	376
Carson Tahoe Regional Medical Center	Carson City	167	361
Summerlin Hospital Medical Center	Las Vegas	174	351
Centennial Hills Hospital Medical Center	Las Vegas	178	350
Mountainview Hospital	Las Vegas	180	371
Spring Valley Hospital Medical Center	Las Vegas	205	344
Valley Hospital Medical Center	Las Vegas	214	338
Desert Springs Hospital	Las Vegas	228	330
UMC of Southern Nevada	Las Vegas	253	327

NOTE: Hospital profiles are in alphabetical order by state, then city, then hospital within the city; Rankings exclude hospitals with less than 25 cases except for patient surveys which excludes hospitals with less than 100 cases; (a) 100-299 cases; (1) The number of cases/patients is too few to report; (2) Data submitted were based on a sample of cases/patients; (3) Results are based on a shorter time period than required; (4) Data suppressed by CMS for one or more quarters; (5) Results are not available for this reporting period; (6) Fewer than 100 patients completed the HCAHPS survey; (7) No cases met the criteria for this measure; (8) The lower limit of the confidence interval cannot be calculated if the number of observed infections equals zero; (9) No data are available from the state/territory for this reporting period; (10) The scores shown reflect fewer than 50 completed surveys; (11) There were discrepancies in the data collection process; (12) This measure does not apply to this hospital for this reporting period; (13) Results cannot be calculated for this reporting period; (14) The results for this state are combined with nearby states to protect confidentiality; Please refer to the User's Guide for a full explanation of data.

Time in ER Before Being Evaluated (minutes)

Hospital Name	City	Min.	Cases
Southern Hills Hospital & Medical Center	Las Vegas	10	443
Sunrise Hospital & Medical Center	Las Vegas	11	494
Northeastern Nevada Regional Hospital	Elko	12	414
Mesa View Regional Hospital	Mesquite	14	418
St Rose Dominican Hosps-San Martin	Las Vegas	14	432
Mountainview Hospital	Las Vegas	15	463
Banner Churchill Community Hospital	Fallon	17	384
North Vista Hospital	North Las Vegas	20	1052
St Rose Dominican Hosps-Rose De Lima	Henderson	20	410
Humboldt General Hospital	Winnemucca	21	356
Northern Nevada Medical Center	Sparks	23	361
Renown South Meadows Medical Center	Reno	23	454
St Rose Dominican Hosps-Siena	Henderson	24	415
Nye Regional Medical Center	Tonopah	26	242
Summerlin Hospital Medical Center	Las Vegas	28	383
Saint Mary's Regional Medical Center	Reno	29	405
Spring Valley Hospital Medical Center	Las Vegas	33	391
Valley Hospital Medical Center	Las Vegas	34	404
Centennial Hills Hospital Medical Center	Las Vegas	36	400
Desert Springs Hospital	Las Vegas	42	407
Renown Regional Medical Center	Reno	42	432
Carson Tahoe Regional Medical Center	Carson City	44	362
UMC of Southern Nevada	Las Vegas	73	343

Time to Pain Meds for Bone Fractures (minutes)

Hospital Name	City	Min.	Cases
Mesa View Regional Hospital	Mesquite	28	59
UMC of Southern Nevada	Las Vegas	31	209
Southern Hills Hospital & Medical Center	Las Vegas	32	85
St Rose Dominican Hosps-San Martin	Las Vegas	39	90
Humboldt General Hospital	Winnemucca	40	27
Sunrise Hospital & Medical Center	Las Vegas	41	351
Northeastern Nevada Regional Hospital	Elko	43	119
St Rose Dominican Hosps-Rose De Lima	Henderson	44	139
Renown South Meadows Medical Center	Reno	50	92
Banner Churchill Community Hospital	Fallon	54	54
Saint Mary's Regional Medical Center	Reno	54	157
Mountainview Hospital	Las Vegas	56	122
St Rose Dominican Hosps-Siena	Henderson	57	251
Summerlin Hospital Medical Center	Las Vegas	59	211
Renown Regional Medical Center	Reno	60	236
North Vista Hospital	North Las Vegas	62	116
Valley Hospital Medical Center	Las Vegas	66	69
Centennial Hills Hospital Medical Center	Las Vegas	70	170
Spring Valley Hospital Medical Center	Las Vegas	73	135
Carson Tahoe Regional Medical Center	Carson City	74	151
Northern Nevada Medical Center	Sparks	74	64
Desert Springs Hospital	Las Vegas	88	88

Heart Attack Care

Aspirin Given at Discharge

Hospital Name	City	Rate	Cases
Desert Springs Hospital[2]	Las Vegas	100%	258
Mountainview Hospital	Las Vegas	100%	257
Northern Nevada Medical Center	Sparks	100%	67
Renown Regional Medical Center[2]	Reno	100%	302
Saint Mary's Regional Medical Center	Reno	100%	231
St Rose Dominican Hosps-Rose De Lima	Henderson	100%	68
Southern Hills Hospital & Medical Center	Las Vegas	100%	47
Summerlin Hospital Medical Center[2]	Las Vegas	100%	208
Sunrise Hospital & Medical Center[2]	Las Vegas	100%	290
VA Sierra Nevada Healthcare System	Reno	100%	26
Valley Hospital Medical Center[2]	Las Vegas	100%	276
Carson Tahoe Regional Medical Center[2]	Carson City	99%	257
Centennial Hills Hospital Medical Center[2]	Las Vegas	99%	145
St Rose Dominican Hosps-Siena[2]	Henderson	99%	295
Spring Valley Hospital Medical Center[2]	Las Vegas	99%	272
North Vista Hospital	North Las Vegas	98%	65
St Rose Dominican Hosps-San Martin	Las Vegas	98%	87
UMC of Southern Nevada[2]	Las Vegas	96%	208

PCI Within 90 Minutes of Arrival

Hospital Name	City	Rate	Cases
Renown Regional Medical Center[2]	Reno	100%	51
Saint Mary's Regional Medical Center	Reno	100%	45
Summerlin Hospital Medical Center[2]	Las Vegas	100%	36
Sunrise Hospital & Medical Center[2]	Las Vegas	100%	51
UMC of Southern Nevada[2]	Las Vegas	100%	41
Spring Valley Hospital Medical Center[2]	Las Vegas	98%	65
Carson Tahoe Regional Medical Center[2]	Carson City	97%	37
St Rose Dominican Hosps-Siena[2]	Henderson	97%	93
Desert Springs Hospital[2]	Las Vegas	96%	51
Mountainview Hospital	Las Vegas	95%	57
Centennial Hills Hospital Medical Center[2]	Las Vegas	94%	34
Valley Hospital Medical Center[2]	Las Vegas	93%	42

Statin Prescribed at Discharge

Hospital Name	City	Rate	Cases
Carson Tahoe Regional Medical Center[2]	Carson City	100%	242
Northern Nevada Medical Center	Sparks	100%	67
Renown Regional Medical Center[2]	Reno	100%	297
St Rose Dominican Hosps-Rose De Lima	Henderson	100%	65
Southern Hills Hospital & Medical Center	Las Vegas	100%	48
VA Sierra Nevada Healthcare System	Reno	100%	26
Mountainview Hospital	Las Vegas	99%	252
Saint Mary's Regional Medical Center	Reno	99%	225
St Rose Dominican Hosps-San Martin	Las Vegas	99%	83
St Rose Dominican Hosps-Siena[2]	Henderson	99%	290
Spring Valley Hospital Medical Center[2]	Las Vegas	99%	268
Sunrise Hospital & Medical Center[2]	Las Vegas	99%	286
Desert Springs Hospital[2]	Las Vegas	98%	259
North Vista Hospital	North Las Vegas	97%	62
Summerlin Hospital Medical Center[2]	Las Vegas	97%	210
UMC of Southern Nevada[2]	Las Vegas	97%	209
Valley Hospital Medical Center[2]	Las Vegas	97%	276
Centennial Hills Hospital Medical Center[2]	Las Vegas	94%	144

Heart Failure Care

ACE Inhibitor or ARB for LVSD

Hospital Name	City	Rate	Cases
Carson Tahoe Regional Medical Center[2]	Carson City	100%	71
Northern Nevada Medical Center	Sparks	100%	25
Renown Regional Medical Center[2]	Reno	100%	141
Saint Mary's Regional Medical Center[2]	Reno	100%	112
Southern Hills Hospital & Medical Center	Las Vegas	100%	36
Sunrise Hospital & Medical Center[2]	Las Vegas	100%	140
VA Sierra Nevada Healthcare System	Reno	100%	41
Mountainview Hospital[2]	Las Vegas	99%	150
St Rose Dominican Hosps-Rose De Lima	Henderson	98%	65
Centennial Hills Hospital Medical Center	Las Vegas	97%	68
North Vista Hospital	North Las Vegas	97%	103
Spring Valley Hospital Medical Center[2]	Las Vegas	97%	92
Desert Springs Hospital[2]	Las Vegas	96%	109
St Rose Dominican Hosps-Siena[2]	Henderson	96%	105
UMC of Southern Nevada[2]	Las Vegas	96%	171
Valley Hospital Medical Center[2]	Las Vegas	95%	136
Summerlin Hospital Medical Center[2]	Las Vegas	94%	103
St Rose Dominican Hosps-San Martin	Las Vegas	91%	65

Discharge Instructions Given

Hospital Name	City	Rate	Cases
Banner Churchill Community Hospital[2]	Fallon	100%	34
Renown South Meadows Medical Center	Reno	100%	50
Southern Hills Hospital & Medical Center	Las Vegas	100%	88
Renown Regional Medical Center[2]	Reno	97%	279
Saint Mary's Regional Medical Center[2]	Reno	97%	251
St Rose Dominican Hosps-San Martin	Las Vegas	97%	147
Sunrise Hospital & Medical Center[2]	Las Vegas	97%	255
Mountainview Hospital[2]	Las Vegas	96%	352
North Vista Hospital	North Las Vegas	96%	210
St Rose Dominican Hosps-Rose De Lima	Henderson	96%	113
VA Sierra Nevada Healthcare System	Reno	96%	81
Desert Springs Hospital[2]	Las Vegas	92%	226
St Rose Dominican Hosps-Siena[2]	Henderson	92%	252
Valley Hospital Medical Center[2]	Las Vegas	92%	247
Northeastern Nevada Regional Hospital	Elko	90%	50
Northern Nevada Medical Center	Sparks	89%	47
Summerlin Hospital Medical Center[2]	Las Vegas	87%	255
Carson Tahoe Regional Medical Center[2]	Carson City	85%	215
Centennial Hills Hospital Medical Center	Las Vegas	85%	173
Spring Valley Hospital Medical Center[2]	Las Vegas	84%	210
UMC of Southern Nevada[2]	Las Vegas	74%	278

Evaluation of LVS Function

Hospital Name	City	Rate	Cases
Banner Churchill Community Hospital[2]	Fallon	100%	38
Carson Tahoe Regional Medical Center[2]	Carson City	100%	260
Centennial Hills Hospital Medical Center	Las Vegas	100%	208
Desert Springs Hospital[2]	Las Vegas	100%	290
Mountainview Hospital[2]	Las Vegas	100%	438
North Vista Hospital	North Las Vegas	100%	240
Northern Nevada Medical Center	Sparks	100%	53
Renown Regional Medical Center[2]	Reno	100%	327
Renown South Meadows Medical Center	Reno	100%	54
Saint Mary's Regional Medical Center[2]	Reno	100%	288
St Rose Dominican Hosps-Siena[2]	Henderson	100%	322
Southern Hills Hospital & Medical Center	Las Vegas	100%	106
Spring Valley Hospital Medical Center[2]	Las Vegas	100%	252
Summerlin Hospital Medical Center[2]	Las Vegas	100%	322
Sunrise Hospital & Medical Center[2]	Las Vegas	100%	301
VA Sierra Nevada Healthcare System	Reno	100%	88
Valley Hospital Medical Center[2]	Las Vegas	100%	292
St Rose Dominican Hosps-Rose De Lima	Henderson	99%	168
St Rose Dominican Hosps-San Martin	Las Vegas	99%	184
UMC of Southern Nevada[2]	Las Vegas	99%	300
Northeastern Nevada Regional Hospital	Elko	89%	62

Medicare Spending

Medicare Spending per Patient (ratio)

Hospital Name	City	Ratio	Cases
South Lyon Medical Center	Yerington	0.72	-
Nye Regional Medical Center	Tonopah	0.86	-
Banner Churchill Community Hospital	Fallon	0.88	-
Renown South Meadows Medical Center	Reno	0.89	-
Sierra Surgery Hospital	Carson City	0.89	-
Northern Nevada Medical Center	Sparks	0.94	-
Saint Mary's Regional Medical Center	Reno	0.94	-
Northeastern Nevada Regional Hospital	Elko	0.95	-
Carson Tahoe Regional Medical Center	Carson City	0.98	-
Renown Regional Medical Center	Reno	0.98	-
UMC of Southern Nevada	Las Vegas	1.05	-
Southern Hills Hospital & Medical Center	Las Vegas	1.08	-
Mountainview Hospital	Las Vegas	1.09	-
St Rose Dominican Hosps-Siena	Henderson	1.09	-
Centennial Hills Hospital Medical Center	Las Vegas	1.10	-
Summerlin Hospital Medical Center	Las Vegas	1.12	-
Desert Springs Hospital	Las Vegas	1.14	-
Sunrise Hospital & Medical Center	Las Vegas	1.16	-
Spring Valley Hospital Medical Center	Las Vegas	1.17	-
Valley Hospital Medical Center	Las Vegas	1.17	-
St Rose Dominican Hosps-Rose De Lima	Henderson	1.18	-
St Rose Dominican Hosps-San Martin	Las Vegas	1.18	-
North Vista Hospital	North Las Vegas	1.19	-

Pneumonia Care

Appropriate Initial Antibiotic Given

Hospital Name	City	Rate	Cases
Mountainview Hospital[2]	Las Vegas	100%	59
Northern Nevada Medical Center	Sparks	100%	61
Renown South Meadows Medical Center	Reno	100%	78
VA Sierra Nevada Healthcare System	Reno	100%	47
Valley Hospital Medical Center[2]	Las Vegas	100%	77
Carson Tahoe Regional Medical Center[2]	Carson City	99%	99
Sunrise Hospital & Medical Center[2]	Las Vegas	99%	74
Desert Springs Hospital[2]	Las Vegas	98%	84
Renown Regional Medical Center[2]	Reno	98%	80
St Rose Dominican Hosps-Siena[2]	Henderson	98%	86
Southern Hills Hospital & Medical Center	Las Vegas	98%	63
Banner Churchill Community Hospital[2]	Fallon	97%	71
Centennial Hills Hospital Medical Center[2]	Las Vegas	97%	105
Summerlin Hospital Medical Center[2]	Las Vegas	97%	77
North Vista Hospital	North Las Vegas	96%	68
Saint Mary's Regional Medical Center[2]	Reno	96%	72
UMC of Southern Nevada[2]	Las Vegas	95%	95
Spring Valley Hospital Medical Center[2]	Las Vegas	94%	79
St Rose Dominican Hosps-Rose De Lima[2]	Henderson	93%	75
Carson Valley Medical Center[3]	Gardnerville	92%	26
St Rose Dominican Hosps-San Martin[2]	Las Vegas	92%	73
Northeastern Nevada Regional Hospital	Elko	91%	100
William Bee Ririe Hospital	Ely	89%	27

Blood Culture Timing

Hospital Name	City	Rate	Cases
Mesa View Regional Hospital	Mesquite	100%	30
North Vista Hospital	North Las Vegas	100%	134
Renown South Meadows Medical Center	Reno	100%	115
Southern Hills Hospital & Medical Center	Las Vegas	100%	135
Mountainview Hospital[2]	Las Vegas	99%	157
Northern Nevada Medical Center	Sparks	99%	95
Saint Mary's Regional Medical Center[2]	Reno	99%	150
Sunrise Hospital & Medical Center[2]	Las Vegas	99%	167
VA Sierra Nevada Healthcare System	Reno	99%	128
Centennial Hills Hospital Medical Center[2]	Las Vegas	98%	113
Renown Regional Medical Center[2]	Reno	98%	153
Banner Churchill Community Hospital[2]	Fallon	97%	102
Carson Tahoe Regional Medical Center[2]	Carson City	97%	131
Northeastern Nevada Regional Hospital	Elko	96%	139
St Rose Dominican Hosps-Rose De Lima[2]	Henderson	96%	151
St Rose Dominican Hosps-San Martin[2]	Las Vegas	96%	155
St Rose Dominican Hosps-Siena[2]	Henderson	96%	178
Valley Hospital Medical Center[2]	Las Vegas	96%	100
Desert Springs Hospital[2]	Las Vegas	93%	69
Carson Valley Medical Center[3]	Gardnerville	92%	26
Summerlin Hospital Medical Center[2]	Las Vegas	91%	97
UMC of Southern Nevada[2]	Las Vegas	91%	148
Spring Valley Hospital Medical Center[2]	Las Vegas	90%	97

NOTE: Hospital profiles are in alphabetical order by state, then city, then hospital within the city; Rankings exclude hospitals with less than 25 cases except for patient surveys which excludes hospitals with less than 100 cases; (a) 100-299 cases; (1) The number of cases/patients is too few to report; (2) Data submitted were based on a sample of cases/patients; (3) Results are based on a shorter time period than required; (4) Data suppressed by CMS for one or more quarters; (5) Results are not available for this reporting period; (6) Fewer than 100 patients completed the HCAHPS survey; (7) No cases met the criteria for this measure; (8) The lower limit of the confidence interval cannot be calculated if the number of observed infections equals zero; (9) No data are available from the state/territory for this reporting period; (10) The scores shown reflect fewer than 50 completed surveys; (11) There were discrepancies in the data collection process; (12) This measure does not apply to this hospital for this reporting period; (13) Results cannot be calculated for this reporting period; (14) The results for this state are combined with nearby states to protect confidentiality; Please refer to the User's Guide for a full explanation of data.

Pregnancy and Delivery Care

Newborns whose Deliveries were Scheduled Early

Hospital Name	City	Rate	Cases
Carson Tahoe Regional Medical Center	Carson City	0%	77
Saint Mary's Regional Medical Center[2]	Reno	2%	45
Spring Valley Hospital Medical Center[2]	Las Vegas	2%	43
Sunrise Hospital & Medical Center[2]	Las Vegas	2%	108
UMC of Southern Nevada[2]	Las Vegas	2%	56
Mountainview Hospital[2]	Las Vegas	3%	37
Southern Hills Hospital & Medical Center	Las Vegas	4%	112
Valley Hospital Medical Center[2]	Las Vegas	4%	55
Centennial Hills Hospital Medical Center[2]	Las Vegas	5%	41
St Rose Dominican Hosps-Siena[2]	Henderson	6%	68
Renown Regional Medical Center[2]	Reno	10%	30
Summerlin Hospital Medical Center[2]	Las Vegas	12%	77
St Rose Dominican Hosps-San Martin[2]	Las Vegas	15%	46
Northeastern Nevada Regional Hospital[2]	Elko	22%	40

Preventive Care

Immunization for Influenza

Hospital Name	City	Rate	Cases
Mountainview Hospital[2]	Las Vegas	100%	642
Renown South Meadows Medical Center[2]	Reno	100%	338
North Vista Hospital[2]	North Las Vegas	99%	419
Renown Regional Medical Center[2]	Reno	99%	537
Southern Hills Hospital & Medical Center[2]	Las Vegas	99%	528
Northern Nevada Medical Center[2]	Sparks	98%	330
St Rose Dominican Hosps-San Martin[2]	Las Vegas	98%	548
Carson Tahoe Regional Medical Center[2]	Carson City	97%	528
Desert Springs Hospital[2]	Las Vegas	97%	605
Banner Churchill Community Hospital[2]	Fallon	96%	262
St Rose Dominican Hosps-Rose De Lima[2]	Henderson	95%	526
St Rose Dominican Hosps-Siena[2]	Henderson	95%	506
Saint Mary's Regional Medical Center[2]	Reno	93%	523
Sunrise Hospital & Medical Center[2]	Las Vegas	93%	547
Mesa View Regional Hospital[2]	Mesquite	92%	293
Valley Hospital Medical Center[2]	Las Vegas	90%	536
Centennial Hills Hospital Medical Center[2]	Las Vegas	89%	550
Sierra Surgery Hospital[2]	Carson City	88%	348
Spring Valley Hospital Medical Center[2]	Las Vegas	88%	526
Summerlin Hospital Medical Center[2]	Las Vegas	85%	514
Northeastern Nevada Regional Hospital[2]	Elko	82%	243
Humboldt General Hospital[2]	Winnemucca	78%	251
UMC of Southern Nevada[2]	Las Vegas	74%	499

Immunization for Pneumonia

Hospital Name	City	Rate	Cases
Renown South Meadows Medical Center[2]	Reno	100%	434
Mountainview Hospital[2]	Las Vegas	99%	887
North Vista Hospital[2]	North Las Vegas	99%	653
Northern Nevada Medical Center[2]	Sparks	99%	456
Southern Hills Hospital & Medical Center[2]	Las Vegas	99%	583
Renown Regional Medical Center[2]	Reno	98%	562
Banner Churchill Community Hospital[2]	Fallon	97%	344
Carson Tahoe Regional Medical Center[2]	Carson City	97%	701
Mesa View Regional Hospital[2]	Mesquite	97%	379
St Rose Dominican Hosps-Siena[2]	Henderson	97%	527
Desert Springs Hospital[2]	Las Vegas	96%	864
Saint Mary's Regional Medical Center[2]	Reno	96%	524
St Rose Dominican Hosps-Rose De Lima[2]	Henderson	96%	757
Sunrise Hospital & Medical Center[2]	Las Vegas	96%	538
St Rose Dominican Hosps-San Martin[2]	Las Vegas	95%	630
Summerlin Hospital Medical Center[2]	Las Vegas	93%	483
Centennial Hills Hospital Medical Center[2]	Las Vegas	92%	550
Valley Hospital Medical Center[2]	Las Vegas	91%	644
Sierra Surgery Hospital[2]	Carson City	85%	428
Northeastern Nevada Regional Hospital[2]	Elko	84%	200
Spring Valley Hospital Medical Center[2]	Las Vegas	83%	532
UMC of Southern Nevada[2]	Las Vegas	82%	453
Humboldt General Hospital[2]	Winnemucca	54%	188

Stroke Care

Anticoagulation Therapy for Atrial Fibrillation

Hospital Name	City	Rate	Cases
Saint Mary's Regional Medical Center	Reno	96%	27

Antithrombotic Therapy Timing

Hospital Name	City	Rate	Cases
Carson Tahoe Regional Medical Center[2]	Carson City	100%	91
Southern Hills Hospital & Medical Center[2]	Las Vegas	100%	34
UMC of Southern Nevada	Las Vegas	100%	114
St Rose Dominican Hosps-Siena	Henderson	99%	141
Summerlin Hospital Medical Center[2]	Las Vegas	99%	90
Sunrise Hospital & Medical Center[2]	Las Vegas	99%	73
Renown Regional Medical Center[2]	Reno	98%	86
Centennial Hills Hospital Medical Center	Las Vegas	97%	63
Mountainview Hospital[2]	Las Vegas	97%	104
Saint Mary's Regional Medical Center	Reno	97%	97
Northern Nevada Medical Center	Sparks	96%	25
St Rose Dominican Hosps-Rose De Lima	Henderson	96%	50
St Rose Dominican Hosps-San Martin	Las Vegas	96%	47
Desert Springs Hospital[2]	Las Vegas	95%	92
Spring Valley Hospital Medical Center[2]	Las Vegas	93%	81
Valley Hospital Medical Center[2]	Las Vegas	92%	74

Assessed for Rehabilitation

Hospital Name	City	Rate	Cases
Northern Nevada Medical Center	Sparks	100%	37
Renown Regional Medical Center[2]	Reno	100%	130
Southern Hills Hospital & Medical Center[2]	Las Vegas	100%	40
Sunrise Hospital & Medical Center[2]	Las Vegas	99%	105
UMC of Southern Nevada	Las Vegas	99%	162
Desert Springs Hospital[2]	Las Vegas	98%	107
St Rose Dominican Hosps-San Martin	Las Vegas	98%	48
Carson Tahoe Regional Medical Center[2]	Carson City	97%	103
Mountainview Hospital[2]	Las Vegas	97%	118
Saint Mary's Regional Medical Center	Reno	97%	128
St Rose Dominican Hosps-Rose De Lima	Henderson	96%	67
Summerlin Hospital Medical Center[2]	Las Vegas	96%	98
Spring Valley Hospital Medical Center[2]	Las Vegas	94%	126
Valley Hospital Medical Center[2]	Las Vegas	94%	107
St Rose Dominican Hosps-Siena	Henderson	93%	187
Centennial Hills Hospital Medical Center	Las Vegas	88%	68

Discharged on Antithrombotic Therapy

Hospital Name	City	Rate	Cases
Centennial Hills Hospital Medical Center	Las Vegas	100%	60
Mountainview Hospital[2]	Las Vegas	100%	108
Northern Nevada Medical Center	Sparks	100%	36
Saint Mary's Regional Medical Center	Reno	100%	110
St Rose Dominican Hosps-San Martin	Las Vegas	100%	46
St Rose Dominican Hosps-Siena	Henderson	100%	156
Southern Hills Hospital & Medical Center[2]	Las Vegas	100%	39
Spring Valley Hospital Medical Center[2]	Las Vegas	100%	90
Summerlin Hospital Medical Center[2]	Las Vegas	100%	98
Sunrise Hospital & Medical Center[2]	Las Vegas	100%	86
UMC of Southern Nevada	Las Vegas	100%	128
Carson Tahoe Regional Medical Center[2]	Carson City	99%	100
Renown Regional Medical Center[2]	Reno	99%	104
Desert Springs Hospital[2]	Las Vegas	98%	103
St Rose Dominican Hosps-Rose De Lima	Henderson	98%	64
Valley Hospital Medical Center[2]	Las Vegas	98%	80

Discharged on Statin Medication

Hospital Name	City	Rate	Cases
Centennial Hills Hospital Medical Center	Las Vegas	100%	43
Sunrise Hospital & Medical Center[2]	Las Vegas	100%	57
UMC of Southern Nevada	Las Vegas	100%	91
Saint Mary's Regional Medical Center	Reno	98%	82
Southern Hills Hospital & Medical Center[2]	Las Vegas	97%	32
Carson Tahoe Regional Medical Center[2]	Carson City	96%	80
Desert Springs Hospital[2]	Las Vegas	96%	78
Mountainview Hospital[2]	Las Vegas	96%	84
Renown Regional Medical Center[2]	Reno	96%	77
St Rose Dominican Hosps-Siena	Henderson	94%	114
Spring Valley Hospital Medical Center[2]	Las Vegas	93%	75
Valley Hospital Medical Center[2]	Las Vegas	93%	75
St Rose Dominican Hosps-San Martin	Las Vegas	90%	40
Summerlin Hospital Medical Center[2]	Las Vegas	90%	80
St Rose Dominican Hosps-Rose De Lima	Henderson	89%	54

Venous Thromboembolism (VTE) Prophylaxis

Hospital Name	City	Rate	Cases
St Rose Dominican Hosps-San Martin	Las Vegas	100%	46
Southern Hills Hospital & Medical Center[2]	Las Vegas	100%	41
Sunrise Hospital & Medical Center[2]	Las Vegas	100%	122
Renown Regional Medical Center[2]	Reno	99%	131
Mountainview Hospital[2]	Las Vegas	98%	122
St Rose Dominican Hosps-Siena	Henderson	94%	175
UMC of Southern Nevada	Las Vegas	94%	172
Carson Tahoe Regional Medical Center[2]	Carson City	93%	92
Saint Mary's Regional Medical Center	Reno	93%	134
St Rose Dominican Hosps-Rose De Lima	Henderson	92%	53
Summerlin Hospital Medical Center[2]	Las Vegas	84%	89
Spring Valley Hospital Medical Center[2]	Las Vegas	82%	120
Centennial Hills Hospital Medical Center	Las Vegas	81%	68
Desert Springs Hospital[2]	Las Vegas	77%	109
Valley Hospital Medical Center[2]	Las Vegas	74%	133

Written Stroke Educational Materials Given

Hospital Name	City	Rate	Cases
Mountainview Hospital[2]	Las Vegas	100%	68
Southern Hills Hospital & Medical Center[2]	Las Vegas	100%	30
Sunrise Hospital & Medical Center[2]	Las Vegas	100%	53
Saint Mary's Regional Medical Center	Reno	98%	80
St Rose Dominican Hosps-Siena	Henderson	98%	99
Renown Regional Medical Center[2]	Reno	96%	69
St Rose Dominican Hosps-Rose De Lima	Henderson	95%	41
Summerlin Hospital Medical Center[2]	Las Vegas	91%	57
UMC of Southern Nevada	Las Vegas	91%	131
Carson Tahoe Regional Medical Center[2]	Carson City	79%	52
Centennial Hills Hospital Medical Center	Las Vegas	69%	42
Desert Springs Hospital[2]	Las Vegas	67%	63
Spring Valley Hospital Medical Center[2]	Las Vegas	65%	69
Valley Hospital Medical Center[2]	Las Vegas	53%	49

Surgical Care Improvement Project

Appropriate Beta Blocker Usage

Hospital Name	City	Rate	Cases
Mountainview Hospital[2]	Las Vegas	100%	205
Renown South Meadows Medical Center	Reno	100%	99
Saint Mary's Regional Medical Center[2]	Reno	100%	110
Centennial Hills Hospital Medical Center[2]	Las Vegas	99%	91
Desert Springs Hospital[2]	Las Vegas	99%	173
Renown Regional Medical Center[2]	Reno	99%	245
Sunrise Hospital & Medical Center[2]	Las Vegas	99%	233
VA Sierra Nevada Healthcare System[2]	Reno	99%	72
Southern Hills Hospital & Medical Center[2]	Las Vegas	98%	85
Carson Tahoe Regional Medical Center[2]	Carson City	97%	143
Northern Nevada Medical Center[2]	Sparks	97%	65
St Rose Dominican Hosps-San Martin[2]	Las Vegas	97%	169
Valley Hospital Medical Center[2]	Las Vegas	96%	163
Sierra Surgery Hospital[2]	Carson City	95%	39
St Rose Dominican Hosps-Siena[2]	Henderson	94%	219
Summerlin Hospital Medical Center[2]	Las Vegas	92%	180
Spring Valley Hospital Medical Center[2]	Las Vegas	91%	140
UMC of Southern Nevada[2]	Las Vegas	87%	98
St Rose Dominican Hosps-Rose De Lima[2]	Henderson	83%	65

Appropriate VTP Within 24 Hours

Hospital Name	City	Rate	Cases
Mesa View Regional Hospital	Mesquite	100%	68
Mountainview Hospital[2]	Las Vegas	100%	446
Northern Nevada Medical Center[2]	Sparks	100%	218
Renown Regional Medical Center[2]	Reno	100%	553
Renown South Meadows Medical Center	Reno	100%	314
Saint Mary's Regional Medical Center[2]	Reno	100%	341
Southern Hills Hospital & Medical Center[2]	Las Vegas	100%	328
Sunrise Hospital & Medical Center[2]	Las Vegas	100%	407
Desert Springs Hospital[2]	Las Vegas	99%	232
St Rose Dominican Hosps-Siena[2]	Henderson	99%	401
Spring Valley Hospital Medical Center[2]	Las Vegas	99%	452
Banner Churchill Community Hospital	Fallon	98%	60
Carson Tahoe Regional Medical Center[2]	Carson City	98%	260
Centennial Hills Hospital Medical Center[2]	Las Vegas	98%	336
Northeastern Nevada Regional Hospital	Elko	98%	105
Carson Valley Medical Center[3]	Gardnerville	97%	31
Summerlin Hospital Medical Center[2]	Las Vegas	97%	379
VA Sierra Nevada Healthcare System[2]	Reno	97%	128
Valley Hospital Medical Center[2]	Las Vegas	96%	341
St Rose Dominican Hosps-Rose De Lima[2]	Henderson	95%	246
St Rose Dominican Hosps-San Martin[2]	Las Vegas	95%	278
Sierra Surgery Hospital[2]	Carson City	95%	283
North Vista Hospital	North Las Vegas	94%	96
UMC of Southern Nevada[2]	Las Vegas	93%	256

Controlled Postoperative Blood Glucose

Hospital Name	City	Rate	Cases
Mountainview Hospital[2]	Las Vegas	100%	130
St Rose Dominican Hosps-Siena[2]	Henderson	99%	147
Summerlin Hospital Medical Center[2]	Las Vegas	99%	105
Valley Hospital Medical Center[2]	Las Vegas	99%	99
Desert Springs Hospital[2]	Las Vegas	98%	124
Renown Regional Medical Center[2]	Reno	98%	225
Carson Tahoe Regional Medical Center[2]	Carson City	97%	74
St Rose Dominican Hosps-San Martin[2]	Las Vegas	97%	146
Sunrise Hospital & Medical Center[2]	Las Vegas	97%	160
Saint Mary's Regional Medical Center[2]	Reno	96%	97
UMC of Southern Nevada[2]	Las Vegas	93%	97
Spring Valley Hospital Medical Center[2]	Las Vegas	91%	54

Perioperative Temperature Management

Hospital Name	City	Rate	Cases
Carson Tahoe Regional Medical Center[2]	Carson City	100%	342
Carson Valley Medical Center[3]	Gardnerville	100%	37
Centennial Hills Hospital Medical Center[2]	Las Vegas	100%	387
Desert Springs Hospital[2]	Las Vegas	100%	315
Mesa View Regional Hospital	Mesquite	100%	79
Mountainview Hospital[2]	Las Vegas	100%	615
North Vista Hospital	North Las Vegas	100%	119
Northeastern Nevada Regional Hospital	Elko	100%	124
Northern Nevada Medical Center[2]	Sparks	100%	281

NOTE: Hospital profiles are in alphabetical order by state, then city, then hospital within the city; Rankings exclude hospitals with less than 25 cases except for patient surveys which excludes hospitals with less than 100 cases; (a) 100-299 cases; (1) The number of cases/patients is too few to report; (2) Data submitted were based on a sample of cases/patients; (3) Results are based on a shorter time period than required; (4) Data suppressed by CMS for one or more quarters; (5) Results are not available for this reporting period; (6) Fewer than 100 patients completed the HCAHPS survey; (7) No cases met the criteria for this measure; (8) The lower limit of the confidence interval cannot be calculated if the number of observed infections equals zero; (9) No data are available from the state/territory for this reporting period; (10) The scores shown reflect fewer than 50 completed surveys; (11) There were discrepancies in the data collection process; (12) This measure does not apply to this hospital for this reporting period; (13) Results cannot be calculated for this reporting period; (14) The results for this state are combined with nearby states to protect confidentiality; Please refer to the User's Guide for a full explanation of data.

Renown Regional Medical Center[2]	Reno	100%	741
Renown South Meadows Medical Center	Reno	100%	490
Saint Mary's Regional Medical Center[2]	Reno	100%	514
St Rose Dominican Hosps-Rose De Lima[2]	Henderson	100%	263
St Rose Dominican Hosps-San Martin[2]	Las Vegas	100%	426
St Rose Dominican Hosps-Siena[2]	Henderson	100%	531
Sierra Surgery Hospital[2]	Carson City	100%	302
Southern Hills Hospital & Medical Center[2]	Las Vegas	100%	402
Spring Valley Hospital Medical Center[2]	Las Vegas	100%	516
Summerlin Hospital Medical Center[2]	Las Vegas	100%	489
Sunrise Hospital & Medical Center[2]	Las Vegas	100%	575
UMC of Southern Nevada[2]	Las Vegas	100%	374
VA Sierra Nevada Healthcare System[2]	Reno	100%	190
Valley Hospital Medical Center[2]	Las Vegas	100%	474
Banner Churchill Community Hospital	Fallon	99%	71

Prophylactic Antibiotic Selection

Hospital Name	City	Rate	Cases
Banner Churchill Community Hospital	Fallon	100%	52
Desert Springs Hospital[2]	Las Vegas	100%	274
Mountainview Hospital[2]	Las Vegas	100%	449
Renown Regional Medical Center[2]	Reno	100%	670
Renown South Meadows Medical Center	Reno	100%	382
Saint Mary's Regional Medical Center[2]	Reno	100%	452
VA Sierra Nevada Healthcare System	Reno	100%	119
Carson Tahoe Regional Medical Center[2]	Carson City	99%	281
Northern Nevada Medical Center[2]	Sparks	99%	196
St Rose Dominican Hosps-San Martin[2]	Las Vegas	99%	357
Sunrise Hospital & Medical Center[2]	Las Vegas	99%	480
Northeastern Nevada Regional Hospital	Elko	98%	109
St Rose Dominican Hosps-Rose De Lima[2]	Henderson	98%	153
St Rose Dominican Hosps-Siena[2]	Henderson	98%	393
Southern Hills Hospital & Medical Center[2]	Las Vegas	98%	261
Spring Valley Hospital Medical Center[2]	Las Vegas	98%	419
Summerlin Hospital Medical Center[2]	Las Vegas	98%	419
Valley Hospital Medical Center[2]	Las Vegas	98%	347
Mesa View Regional Hospital	Mesquite	97%	63
North Vista Hospital	North Las Vegas	97%	39
UMC of Southern Nevada[2]	Las Vegas	97%	284
Carson Valley Medical Center[3]	Gardnerville	96%	26
Centennial Hills Hospital Medical Center[2]	Las Vegas	96%	221
Sierra Surgery Hospital[2]	Carson City	94%	233

Prophylactic Antibiotic Selection (Outpatient)

Hospital Name	City	Rate	Cases
Carson Valley Medical Center	Gardnerville	100%	27
Mountainview Hospital	Las Vegas	100%	484
Northeastern Nevada Regional Hospital	Elko	100%	67
Northern Nevada Medical Center	Sparks	100%	78
Renown Regional Medical Center	Reno	100%	481
Renown South Meadows Medical Center	Reno	100%	28
Sunrise Hospital & Medical Center	Las Vegas	100%	408
Desert Springs Hospital	Las Vegas	99%	240
St Rose Dominican Hosps-Rose De Lima	Henderson	99%	90
St Rose Dominican Hosps-Siena	Henderson	99%	625
Southern Hills Hospital & Medical Center	Las Vegas	99%	156
Valley Hospital Medical Center	Las Vegas	99%	285
Carson Tahoe Regional Medical Center	Carson City	98%	213
Saint Mary's Regional Medical Center	Reno	98%	431
St Rose Dominican Hosps-San Martin	Las Vegas	98%	278
UMC of Southern Nevada	Las Vegas	98%	292
Summerlin Hospital Medical Center	Las Vegas	97%	434
Spring Valley Hospital Medical Center	Las Vegas	96%	345
Centennial Hills Hospital Medical Center	Las Vegas	94%	255
North Vista Hospital	North Las Vegas	94%	34
Sierra Surgery Hospital	Carson City	93%	175

Prophylactic Antibiotic Stopped

Hospital Name	City	Rate	Cases
Banner Churchill Community Hospital	Fallon	100%	48
Carson Valley Medical Center[3]	Gardnerville	100%	26
Mountainview Hospital[2]	Las Vegas	100%	426
North Vista Hospital	North Las Vegas	100%	39
Renown Regional Medical Center[2]	Reno	100%	628
Renown South Meadows Medical Center	Reno	100%	377
Sierra Surgery Hospital[2]	Carson City	100%	232
Southern Hills Hospital & Medical Center[2]	Las Vegas	100%	256
Sunrise Hospital & Medical Center[2]	Las Vegas	100%	456
Carson Tahoe Regional Medical Center[2]	Carson City	99%	269
Northeastern Nevada Regional Hospital	Elko	99%	108
Saint Mary's Regional Medical Center[2]	Reno	99%	443
St Rose Dominican Hosps-Rose De Lima[2]	Henderson	99%	145
Centennial Hills Hospital Medical Center[2]	Las Vegas	98%	219
Mesa View Regional Hospital	Mesquite	98%	62
St Rose Dominican Hosps-Siena[2]	Henderson	98%	379
Valley Hospital Medical Center[2]	Las Vegas	98%	340
Northern Nevada Medical Center[2]	Sparks	97%	194
St Rose Dominican Hosps-San Martin[2]	Las Vegas	97%	335
VA Sierra Nevada Healthcare System	Reno	97%	116
Desert Springs Hospital[2]	Las Vegas	96%	260
Spring Valley Hospital Medical Center[2]	Las Vegas	95%	408
Summerlin Hospital Medical Center[2]	Las Vegas	94%	403
UMC of Southern Nevada[2]	Las Vegas	94%	273

Prophylactic Antibiotic Timing

Hospital Name	City	Rate	Cases
Mesa View Regional Hospital	Mesquite	100%	63
Mountainview Hospital[2]	Las Vegas	100%	449
North Vista Hospital	North Las Vegas	100%	41
Renown South Meadows Medical Center	Reno	100%	382
St Rose Dominican Hosps-Rose De Lima[2]	Henderson	100%	153
Southern Hills Hospital & Medical Center[2]	Las Vegas	100%	261
Sunrise Hospital & Medical Center[2]	Las Vegas	100%	480
VA Sierra Nevada Healthcare System	Reno	100%	119
Carson Tahoe Regional Medical Center[2]	Carson City	99%	284
Centennial Hills Hospital Medical Center[2]	Las Vegas	99%	221
Desert Springs Hospital[2]	Las Vegas	99%	275
Renown Regional Medical Center[2]	Reno	99%	673
St Rose Dominican Hosps-San Martin[2]	Las Vegas	99%	357
Sierra Surgery Hospital[2]	Carson City	99%	233
Summerlin Hospital Medical Center[2]	Las Vegas	99%	419
Valley Hospital Medical Center[2]	Las Vegas	99%	347
Northern Nevada Medical Center[2]	Sparks	98%	196
St Rose Dominican Hosps-Siena[2]	Henderson	98%	393
Spring Valley Hospital Medical Center[2]	Las Vegas	98%	421
Northeastern Nevada Regional Hospital	Elko	97%	109
Saint Mary's Regional Medical Center[2]	Reno	97%	452
Banner Churchill Community Hospital	Fallon	96%	52
UMC of Southern Nevada[2]	Las Vegas	93%	288
Carson Valley Medical Center[3]	Gardnerville	92%	26

Prophylactic Antibiotic Timing (Outpatient)

Hospital Name	City	Rate	Cases
Mountainview Hospital	Las Vegas	100%	484
North Vista Hospital	North Las Vegas	100%	34
Northeastern Nevada Regional Hospital	Elko	100%	67
Northern Nevada Medical Center	Sparks	100%	78
Renown South Meadows Medical Center	Reno	100%	28
Sunrise Hospital & Medical Center	Las Vegas	100%	408
Desert Springs Hospital	Las Vegas	99%	243
Renown Regional Medical Center	Reno	99%	482
St Rose Dominican Hosps-Siena	Henderson	99%	629
Valley Hospital Medical Center	Las Vegas	99%	285
Centennial Hills Hospital Medical Center	Las Vegas	98%	258
Saint Mary's Regional Medical Center	Reno	98%	434
Southern Hills Hospital & Medical Center	Las Vegas	98%	160
Spring Valley Hospital Medical Center	Las Vegas	98%	348
Summerlin Hospital Medical Center	Las Vegas	98%	437
Carson Tahoe Regional Medical Center	Carson City	97%	212
St Rose Dominican Hosps-San Martin	Las Vegas	97%	279
Carson Valley Medical Center	Gardnerville	96%	27
Mesa View Regional Hospital	Mesquite	96%	25
Sierra Surgery Hospital	Carson City	96%	176
St Rose Dominican Hosps-Rose De Lima	Henderson	94%	94
UMC of Southern Nevada	Las Vegas	91%	299

Urinary Catheter Removal

Hospital Name	City	Rate	Cases
Desert Springs Hospital[2]	Las Vegas	100%	221
Mesa View Regional Hospital	Mesquite	100%	49
Mountainview Hospital[2]	Las Vegas	100%	308
Renown Regional Medical Center[2]	Reno	100%	459
Renown South Meadows Medical Center	Reno	100%	99
Saint Mary's Regional Medical Center[2]	Reno	100%	232
Southern Hills Hospital & Medical Center[2]	Las Vegas	100%	260
Sunrise Hospital & Medical Center[2]	Las Vegas	100%	400
Carson Tahoe Regional Medical Center[2]	Carson City	99%	301
Sierra Surgery Hospital[2]	Carson City	99%	228
VA Sierra Nevada Healthcare System[2]	Reno	99%	133
Northern Nevada Medical Center[2]	Sparks	98%	93
St Rose Dominican Hosps-San Martin[2]	Las Vegas	98%	311
St Rose Dominican Hosps-Siena[2]	Henderson	97%	377
Spring Valley Hospital Medical Center[2]	Las Vegas	96%	328
Summerlin Hospital Medical Center[2]	Las Vegas	96%	273
Centennial Hills Hospital Medical Center[2]	Las Vegas	95%	178
Northeastern Nevada Regional Hospital	Elko	94%	98
Valley Hospital Medical Center[2]	Las Vegas	94%	265
St Rose Dominican Hosps-Rose De Lima[2]	Henderson	93%	164
UMC of Southern Nevada[2]	Las Vegas	89%	172
North Vista Hospital	North Las Vegas	88%	33

Survey of Patients' Hospital Experiences

Area Around Room 'Always' Quiet at Night

Hospital Name	City	Rate	Cases
Mesa View Regional Hospital	Mesquite	71%	(a)
Sierra Surgery Hospital	Carson City	68%	300+
St Rose Dominican Hosps-San Martin	Las Vegas	64%	300+
Southern Hills Hospital & Medical Center	Las Vegas	63%	300+
Banner Churchill Community Hospital[11]	Fallon	62%	300+
Centennial Hills Hospital Medical Center	Las Vegas	62%	300+
Northeastern Nevada Regional Hospital	Elko	60%	300+
St Rose Dominican Hosps-Siena	Henderson	60%	300+
Mountainview Hospital	Las Vegas	59%	300+
North Vista Hospital	North Las Vegas	59%	300+
Summerlin Hospital Medical Center	Las Vegas	56%	300+
Spring Valley Hospital Medical Center	Las Vegas	55%	300+
Carson Tahoe Regional Medical Center	Carson City	54%	300+
Sunrise Hospital & Medical Center	Las Vegas	54%	300+
Desert Springs Hospital	Las Vegas	51%	300+
Saint Mary's Regional Medical Center	Reno	51%	300+
Northern Nevada Medical Center	Sparks	50%	300+
Renown South Meadows Medical Center	Reno	50%	300+
Valley Hospital Medical Center	Las Vegas	49%	300+
Renown Regional Medical Center	Reno	47%	300+
St Rose Dominican Hosps-Rose De Lima	Henderson	46%	300+

Doctors 'Always' Communicated Well

Hospital Name	City	Rate	Cases
Banner Churchill Community Hospital[11]	Fallon	84%	300+
Mesa View Regional Hospital	Mesquite	81%	(a)
Northern Nevada Medical Center	Sparks	80%	300+
Sierra Surgery Hospital	Carson City	80%	300+
North Vista Hospital	North Las Vegas	79%	300+
Carson Tahoe Regional Medical Center	Carson City	77%	300+
Saint Mary's Regional Medical Center	Reno	77%	300+
Northeastern Nevada Regional Hospital	Elko	76%	300+
Renown South Meadows Medical Center	Reno	76%	300+
St Rose Dominican Hosps-San Martin	Las Vegas	76%	300+
St Rose Dominican Hosps-Siena	Henderson	76%	300+
Southern Hills Hospital & Medical Center	Las Vegas	74%	300+
Renown Regional Medical Center	Reno	73%	300+
Summerlin Hospital Medical Center	Las Vegas	73%	300+
Valley Hospital Medical Center	Las Vegas	73%	300+
Centennial Hills Hospital Medical Center	Las Vegas	71%	300+
Mountainview Hospital	Las Vegas	71%	300+
Desert Springs Hospital	Las Vegas	70%	300+
Spring Valley Hospital Medical Center	Las Vegas	70%	300+
Sunrise Hospital & Medical Center	Las Vegas	70%	300+
St Rose Dominican Hosps-Rose De Lima	Henderson	66%	300+

Home Recovery Information Given

Hospital Name	City	Rate	Cases
Sierra Surgery Hospital	Carson City	90%	300+
Banner Churchill Community Hospital[11]	Fallon	88%	300+
Northern Nevada Medical Center	Sparks	87%	300+
Renown Regional Medical Center	Reno	87%	300+
Saint Mary's Regional Medical Center	Reno	87%	300+
St Rose Dominican Hosps-San Martin	Las Vegas	86%	300+
St Rose Dominican Hosps-Siena	Henderson	86%	300+
Carson Tahoe Regional Medical Center	Carson City	85%	300+
Renown South Meadows Medical Center	Reno	85%	300+
St Rose Dominican Hosps-Rose De Lima	Henderson	85%	300+
Southern Hills Hospital & Medical Center	Las Vegas	85%	300+
Mesa View Regional Hospital	Mesquite	84%	(a)
North Vista Hospital	North Las Vegas	84%	300+
Summerlin Hospital Medical Center	Las Vegas	84%	300+
Centennial Hills Hospital Medical Center	Las Vegas	83%	300+
Mountainview Hospital	Las Vegas	83%	300+
Northeastern Nevada Regional Hospital	Elko	83%	300+
Spring Valley Hospital Medical Center	Las Vegas	82%	300+
Valley Hospital Medical Center	Las Vegas	82%	300+
Desert Springs Hospital	Las Vegas	81%	300+
Sunrise Hospital & Medical Center	Las Vegas	78%	300+

Hospital Given 9 or 10 on 10 Point Scale

Hospital Name	City	Rate	Cases
Sierra Surgery Hospital	Carson City	77%	300+
St Rose Dominican Hosps-San Martin	Las Vegas	76%	300+
Banner Churchill Community Hospital[11]	Fallon	75%	300+
St Rose Dominican Hosps-Siena	Henderson	75%	300+
Mesa View Regional Hospital	Mesquite	73%	(a)
Renown South Meadows Medical Center	Reno	73%	300+
Northern Nevada Medical Center	Sparks	69%	300+
Carson Tahoe Regional Medical Center	Carson City	68%	300+
Renown Regional Medical Center	Reno	67%	300+
Southern Hills Hospital & Medical Center	Las Vegas	67%	300+
North Vista Hospital	North Las Vegas	66%	300+
Centennial Hills Hospital Medical Center	Las Vegas	64%	300+
Mountainview Hospital	Las Vegas	64%	300+
Saint Mary's Regional Medical Center	Reno	64%	300+
Spring Valley Hospital Medical Center	Las Vegas	62%	300+
Summerlin Hospital Medical Center	Las Vegas	61%	300+
Sunrise Hospital & Medical Center	Las Vegas	61%	300+
St Rose Dominican Hosps-Rose De Lima	Henderson	60%	300+
Valley Hospital Medical Center	Las Vegas	60%	300+
Desert Springs Hospital	Las Vegas	57%	300+
Northeastern Nevada Regional Hospital	Elko	56%	300+

NOTE: Hospital profiles are in alphabetical order by state, then city, then hospital within the city; Rankings exclude hospitals with less than 25 cases except for patient surveys which excludes hospitals with less than 100 cases; (a) 100-299 cases; (1) The number of cases/patients is too few to report; (2) Data submitted were based on a sample of cases/patients; (3) Results are based on a shorter time period than required; (4) Data suppressed by CMS for one or more quarters; (5) Results are not available for this reporting period; (6) Fewer than 100 patients completed the HCAHPS survey; (7) No cases met the criteria for this measure; (8) The lower limit of the confidence interval cannot be calculated if the number of observed infections equals zero; (9) No data are available from the state/territory for this reporting period; (10) The scores shown reflect fewer than 50 completed surveys; (11) There were discrepancies in the data collection process; (12) This measure does not apply to this hospital for this reporting period; (13) Results cannot be calculated for this reporting period; (14) The results for this state are combined with nearby states to protect confidentiality; Please refer to the User's Guide for a full explanation of data.

Meds 'Always' Explained Before Given

Hospital Name	City	Rate	Cases
Banner Churchill Community Hospital[11]	Fallon	70%	300+
Mesa View Regional Hospital	Mesquite	68%	(a)
Sierra Surgery Hospital	Carson City	68%	300+
Northern Nevada Medical Center	Sparks	67%	300+
Renown South Meadows Medical Center	Reno	65%	300+
St Rose Dominican Hosps-Siena	Henderson	65%	300+
Carson Tahoe Regional Medical Center	Carson City	64%	300+
North Vista Hospital	North Las Vegas	61%	300+
Saint Mary's Regional Medical Center	Reno	61%	300+
Northeastern Nevada Regional Hospital	Elko	60%	300+
Renown Regional Medical Center	Reno	60%	300+
St Rose Dominican Hosps-San Martin	Las Vegas	60%	300+
Mountainview Hospital	Las Vegas	57%	300+
St Rose Dominican Hosps-Rose De Lima	Henderson	57%	300+
Southern Hills Hospital & Medical Center	Las Vegas	57%	300+
Spring Valley Hospital Medical Center	Las Vegas	56%	300+
Summerlin Hospital Medical Center	Las Vegas	54%	300+
Sunrise Hospital & Medical Center	Las Vegas	54%	300+
Valley Hospital Medical Center	Las Vegas	52%	300+
Centennial Hills Hospital Medical Center	Las Vegas	50%	300+
Desert Springs Hospital	Las Vegas	49%	300+

Nurses 'Always' Communicated Well

Hospital Name	City	Rate	Cases
Banner Churchill Community Hospital[11]	Fallon	82%	300+
Renown South Meadows Medical Center	Reno	80%	300+
Sierra Surgery Hospital	Carson City	78%	300+
Mesa View Regional Hospital	Mesquite	76%	(a)
Northern Nevada Medical Center	Sparks	75%	300+
St Rose Dominican Hosps-Siena	Henderson	75%	300+
Carson Tahoe Regional Medical Center	Carson City	74%	300+
Renown Regional Medical Center	Reno	74%	300+
Saint Mary's Regional Medical Center	Reno	74%	300+
North Vista Hospital	North Las Vegas	73%	300+
St Rose Dominican Hosps-San Martin	Las Vegas	73%	300+
Mountainview Hospital	Las Vegas	71%	300+
Southern Hills Hospital & Medical Center	Las Vegas	71%	300+
Northeastern Nevada Regional Hospital	Elko	70%	300+
Summerlin Hospital Medical Center	Las Vegas	70%	300+
Valley Hospital Medical Center	Las Vegas	69%	300+
Centennial Hills Hospital Medical Center	Las Vegas	68%	300+
Desert Springs Hospital	Las Vegas	68%	300+
Spring Valley Hospital Medical Center	Las Vegas	68%	300+
St Rose Dominican Hosps-Rose De Lima	Henderson	66%	300+
Sunrise Hospital & Medical Center	Las Vegas	66%	300+

Pain 'Always' Well Controlled

Hospital Name	City	Rate	Cases
Sierra Surgery Hospital	Carson City	74%	300+
Banner Churchill Community Hospital[11]	Fallon	73%	300+
Renown South Meadows Medical Center	Reno	71%	300+
Renown Regional Medical Center	Reno	70%	300+
Mesa View Regional Hospital	Mesquite	69%	(a)
Saint Mary's Regional Medical Center	Reno	69%	300+
St Rose Dominican Hosps-San Martin	Las Vegas	69%	300+
St Rose Dominican Hosps-Siena	Henderson	69%	300+
North Vista Hospital	North Las Vegas	68%	300+
Northern Nevada Medical Center	Sparks	68%	300+
Southern Hills Hospital & Medical Center	Las Vegas	67%	300+
Carson Tahoe Regional Medical Center	Carson City	66%	300+
Desert Springs Hospital	Las Vegas	66%	300+
Mountainview Hospital	Las Vegas	66%	300+
Centennial Hills Hospital Medical Center	Las Vegas	64%	300+
St Rose Dominican Hosps-Rose De Lima	Henderson	64%	300+
Spring Valley Hospital Medical Center	Las Vegas	64%	300+
Valley Hospital Medical Center	Las Vegas	64%	300+
Summerlin Hospital Medical Center	Las Vegas	63%	300+
Sunrise Hospital & Medical Center	Las Vegas	63%	300+
Northeastern Nevada Regional Hospital	Elko	62%	300+

Room and Bathroom 'Always' Clean

Hospital Name	City	Rate	Cases
Sierra Surgery Hospital	Carson City	80%	300+
Mesa View Regional Hospital	Mesquite	75%	(a)
St Rose Dominican Hosps-Siena	Henderson	75%	300+
Renown South Meadows Medical Center	Reno	72%	300+
Banner Churchill Community Hospital[11]	Fallon	70%	300+
Mountainview Hospital	Las Vegas	70%	300+
Northern Nevada Medical Center	Sparks	70%	300+
Saint Mary's Regional Medical Center	Reno	70%	300+
St Rose Dominican Hosps-San Martin	Las Vegas	70%	300+
Southern Hills Hospital & Medical Center	Las Vegas	70%	300+
Northeastern Nevada Regional Hospital	Elko	69%	300+
Carson Tahoe Regional Medical Center	Carson City	67%	300+
North Vista Hospital	North Las Vegas	67%	300+
Renown Regional Medical Center	Reno	66%	300+
St Rose Dominican Hosps-Rose De Lima	Henderson	66%	300+
Sunrise Hospital & Medical Center	Las Vegas	64%	300+
Centennial Hills Hospital Medical Center	Las Vegas	63%	300+
Desert Springs Hospital	Las Vegas	63%	300+
Summerlin Hospital Medical Center	Las Vegas	63%	300+
Spring Valley Hospital Medical Center	Las Vegas	61%	300+
Valley Hospital Medical Center	Las Vegas	61%	300+

Timely Help 'Always' Received

Hospital Name	City	Rate	Cases
Banner Churchill Community Hospital[11]	Fallon	74%	300+
Sierra Surgery Hospital	Carson City	72%	300+
Mesa View Regional Hospital	Mesquite	68%	(a)
Renown South Meadows Medical Center	Reno	68%	300+
Northern Nevada Medical Center	Sparks	64%	300+
St Rose Dominican Hosps-Siena	Henderson	62%	300+
North Vista Hospital	North Las Vegas	60%	300+
Carson Tahoe Regional Medical Center	Carson City	59%	300+
Mountainview Hospital	Las Vegas	59%	300+
Southern Hills Hospital & Medical Center	Las Vegas	59%	300+
Renown Regional Medical Center	Reno	58%	300+
St Rose Dominican Hosps-San Martin	Las Vegas	58%	300+
Northeastern Nevada Regional Hospital	Elko	57%	300+
Saint Mary's Regional Medical Center	Reno	56%	300+
Centennial Hills Hospital Medical Center	Las Vegas	54%	300+
Desert Springs Hospital	Las Vegas	53%	300+
Summerlin Hospital Medical Center	Las Vegas	53%	300+
Sunrise Hospital & Medical Center	Las Vegas	53%	300+
Spring Valley Hospital Medical Center	Las Vegas	52%	300+
Valley Hospital Medical Center	Las Vegas	52%	300+
St Rose Dominican Hosps-Rose De Lima	Henderson	50%	300+

Would Definitely Recommend Hospital

Hospital Name	City	Rate	Cases
Sierra Surgery Hospital	Carson City	82%	300+
Renown South Meadows Medical Center	Reno	80%	300+
St Rose Dominican Hosps-Siena	Henderson	80%	300+
St Rose Dominican Hosps-San Martin	Las Vegas	78%	300+
Saint Mary's Regional Medical Center	Reno	73%	300+
Banner Churchill Community Hospital[11]	Fallon	72%	300+
Mesa View Regional Hospital	Mesquite	72%	(a)
Northern Nevada Medical Center	Sparks	72%	300+
Carson Tahoe Regional Medical Center	Carson City	71%	300+
Renown Regional Medical Center	Reno	71%	300+
Centennial Hills Hospital Medical Center	Las Vegas	69%	300+
Southern Hills Hospital & Medical Center	Las Vegas	69%	300+
Mountainview Hospital	Las Vegas	68%	300+
Spring Valley Hospital Medical Center	Las Vegas	67%	300+
North Vista Hospital	North Las Vegas	66%	300+
Summerlin Hospital Medical Center	Las Vegas	66%	300+
St Rose Dominican Hosps-Rose De Lima	Henderson	63%	300+
Sunrise Hospital & Medical Center	Las Vegas	62%	300+
Valley Hospital Medical Center	Las Vegas	61%	300+
Desert Springs Hospital	Las Vegas	60%	300+
Northeastern Nevada Regional Hospital	Elko	53%	300+

Use of Medical Imaging

Cardiac Imaging Stress Test before OP Surgery

Hospital Name	City	Rate	Cases
Humboldt General Hospital	Winnemucca	0.0%	64
Banner Churchill Community Hospital	Fallon	1.0%	105
Carson Valley Medical Center	Gardnerville	2.7%	149
North Vista Hospital	North Las Vegas	2.9%	104
Southern Hills Hospital & Medical Center	Las Vegas	3.2%	94
Spring Valley Hospital Medical Center	Las Vegas	3.2%	124
Mesa View Regional Hospital	Mesquite	3.6%	83
UMC of Southern Nevada	Las Vegas	3.7%	241
Sunrise Hospital & Medical Center	Las Vegas	4.0%	346
Renown Regional Medical Center	Reno	4.6%	1388
Saint Mary's Regional Medical Center	Reno	4.7%	278
Valley Hospital Medical Center	Las Vegas	4.9%	163
Renown South Meadows Medical Center	Reno	5.0%	199
Carson Tahoe Regional Medical Center	Carson City	5.2%	1041
Mountainview Hospital	Las Vegas	5.3%	188
Northern Nevada Medical Center	Sparks	5.6%	248
Desert Springs Hospital	Las Vegas	5.8%	171
St Rose Dominican Hosps-Rose De Lima	Henderson	5.8%	171
St Rose Dominican Hosps-Siena	Henderson	6.0%	332
Summerlin Hospital Medical Center	Las Vegas	6.3%	176
Centennial Hills Hospital Medical Center	Las Vegas	7.1%	155
St Rose Dominican Hosps-San Martin	Las Vegas	7.5%	226

Combination Abdominal CT Scan

Hospital Name	City	Rate	Cases
Incline Village Health Center	Incline Village	1.6%	61
William Bee Ririe Hospital	Ely	1.6%	125
Southern Hills Hospital & Medical Center	Las Vegas	1.8%	226
Valley Hospital Medical Center	Las Vegas	2.2%	325
North Vista Hospital	North Las Vegas	2.4%	211
Desert Springs Hospital	Las Vegas	2.8%	363
Spring Valley Hospital Medical Center	Las Vegas	2.8%	391
Centennial Hills Hospital Medical Center	Las Vegas	3.7%	383
Northern Nevada Medical Center	Sparks	3.8%	287
Mountainview Hospital	Las Vegas	4.4%	662
St Rose Dominican Hosps-San Martin	Las Vegas	4.4%	338
Summerlin Hospital Medical Center	Las Vegas	5.0%	479
St Rose Dominican Hosps-Rose De Lima	Henderson	5.1%	468
Renown Regional Medical Center	Reno	5.2%	944
Sunrise Hospital & Medical Center	Las Vegas	5.4%	664
Saint Mary's Regional Medical Center	Reno	5.6%	623
Humboldt General Hospital	Winnemucca	6.0%	117
St Rose Dominican Hosps-Siena	Henderson	6.0%	822
UMC of Southern Nevada	Las Vegas	6.2%	385
Carson Valley Medical Center	Gardnerville	6.4%	450
Banner Churchill Community Hospital	Fallon	7.4%	296
Renown South Meadows Medical Center	Reno	8.1%	520
Carson Tahoe Regional Medical Center	Carson City	10.6%	1041
Boulder City Hospital	Boulder City	12.8%	149
Mesa View Regional Hospital	Mesquite	14.2%	310
Desert View Regional Medical Center	Pahrump	15.3%	320
Sierra Surgery Hospital	Carson City	19.0%	195
Northeastern Nevada Regional Hospital	Elko	33.1%	248

Combination Brain/Sinus CT Scan

Hospital Name	City	Rate	Cases
Battle Mountain General Hospital	Batte Mtn	0.0%	31
Grover C Dils Medical Center	Caliente	0.0%	41
Carson Valley Medical Center	Gardnerville	0.9%	443
Desert View Regional Medical Center	Pahrump	1.0%	387
Spring Valley Hospital Medical Center	Las Vegas	1.4%	483
Centennial Hills Hospital Medical Center	Las Vegas	1.5%	395
Carson Tahoe Regional Medical Center	Carson City	1.8%	906
St Rose Dominican Hosps-Siena	Henderson	2.5%	951
Renown Regional Medical Center	Reno	2.8%	950
Valley Hospital Medical Center	Las Vegas	3.0%	604
Mountainview Hospital	Las Vegas	3.4%	756
St Rose Dominican Hosps-Rose De Lima	Henderson	4.1%	458
Sunrise Hospital & Medical Center	Las Vegas	4.4%	838
St Rose Dominican Hosps-San Martin	Las Vegas	5.3%	319
Northeastern Nevada Regional Hospital	Elko	5.7%	211

Combination Chest CT Scan

Hospital Name	City	Rate	Cases
Northern Nevada Medical Center	Sparks	0.0%	149
Renown Regional Medical Center	Reno	0.0%	736
Renown South Meadows Medical Center	Reno	0.0%	357
Saint Mary's Regional Medical Center	Reno	0.0%	493
St Rose Dominican Hosps-Rose De Lima	Henderson	0.0%	57
William Bee Ririe Hospital	Ely	0.0%	116
Sierra Surgery Hospital	Carson City	0.6%	163
Banner Churchill Community Hospital	Fallon	1.8%	165
Carson Tahoe Regional Medical Center	Carson City	1.8%	1160
Mountainview Hospital	Las Vegas	1.9%	372
Northeastern Nevada Regional Hospital	Elko	2.8%	106
Southern Hills Hospital & Medical Center	Las Vegas	3.1%	128
Humboldt General Hospital	Winnemucca	4.6%	87
Carson Valley Medical Center	Gardnerville	4.9%	368
Sunrise Hospital & Medical Center	Las Vegas	5.3%	207
St Rose Dominican Hosps-Siena	Henderson	5.4%	149
Summerlin Hospital Medical Center	Las Vegas	10.7%	103
Desert View Regional Medical Center	Pahrump	13.4%	313
UMC of Southern Nevada	Las Vegas	15.1%	126
Mesa View Regional Hospital	Mesquite	19.2%	104
Boulder City Hospital	Boulder City	34.0%	53

Follow-up Mammogram/Ultrasound

A follow-up rate near zero may indicate missed cancer; a rate higher than 14% may mean there is unnecessary follow up.

Hospital Name	City	Rate	Cases
Humboldt General Hospital	Winnemucca	2.0%	150
William Bee Ririe Hospital	Ely	3.8%	133
Banner Churchill Community Hospital	Fallon	4.1%	615
Northern Nevada Medical Center	Sparks	4.8%	480
Carson Valley Medical Center	Gardnerville	6.1%	495
Sierra Surgery Hospital	Carson City	6.2%	501
St Rose Dominican Hosps-Siena	Henderson	6.7%	104
Desert View Regional Medical Center	Pahrump	6.9%	173
Carson Tahoe Regional Medical Center	Carson City	7.2%	2995
Summerlin Hospital Medical Center	Las Vegas	7.5%	186
Mesa View Regional Hospital	Mesquite	8.0%	561
Sunrise Hospital & Medical Center	Las Vegas	8.7%	393
Saint Mary's Regional Medical Center	Reno	9.1%	724
Centennial Hills Hospital Medical Center	Las Vegas	9.7%	93
Mountainview Hospital	Las Vegas	10.1%	358
St Rose Dominican Hosps-Rose De Lima	Henderson	10.1%	99
Northeastern Nevada Regional Hospital	Elko	14.9%	295

NOTE: Hospital profiles are in alphabetical order by state, then city, then hospital within the city; Rankings exclude hospitals with less than 25 cases except for patient surveys which excludes hospitals with less than 100 cases; (a) 100-299 cases; (1) The number of cases/patients is too few to report; (2) Data submitted were based on a sample of cases/patients; (3) Results are based on a shorter time period than required; (4) Data suppressed by CMS for one or more quarters; (5) Results are not available for this reporting period; (6) Fewer than 100 patients completed the HCAHPS survey; (7) No cases met the criteria for this measure; (8) The lower limit of the confidence interval cannot be calculated if the number of observed infections equals zero; (9) No data are available from the state/territory for this reporting period; (10) The scores shown reflect fewer than 50 completed surveys; (11) There were discrepancies in the data collection process; (12) This measure does not apply to this hospital for this reporting period; (13) Results cannot be calculated for this reporting period; (14) The results for this state are combined with nearby states to protect confidentiality; Please refer to the User's Guide for a full explanation of data.

Lumbar Spine MRI for Low Back Pain

Hospital Name	City	Rate	Cases
Renown Regional Medical Center	Reno	29.9%	164
Carson Valley Medical Center	Gardnerville	32.2%	59
Sierra Surgery Hospital	Carson City	33.1%	121
Mesa View Regional Hospital	Mesquite	35.3%	51
Renown South Meadows Medical Center	Reno	35.8%	95
Carson Tahoe Regional Medical Center	Carson City	38.1%	310
Northeastern Nevada Regional Hospital	Elko	40.0%	60
Saint Mary's Regional Medical Center	Reno	40.2%	82
Banner Churchill Community Hospital	Fallon	42.9%	56

NOTE: Hospital profiles are in alphabetical order by state, then city, then hospital within the city; Rankings exclude hospitals with less than 25 cases except for patient surveys which excludes hospitals with less than 100 cases; (a) 100-299 cases; (1) The number of cases/patients is too few to report; (2) Data submitted were based on a sample of cases/patients; (3) Results are based on a shorter time period than required; (4) Data suppressed by CMS for one or more quarters; (5) Results are not available for this reporting period; (6) Fewer than 100 patients completed the HCAHPS survey; (7) No cases met the criteria for this measure; (8) The lower limit of the confidence interval cannot be calculated if the number of observed infections equals zero; (9) No data are available from the state/territory for this reporting period; (10) The scores shown reflect fewer than 50 completed surveys; (11) There were discrepancies in the data collection process; (12) This measure does not apply to this hospital for this reporting period; (13) Results cannot be calculated for this reporting period; (14) The results for this state are combined with nearby states to protect confidentiality; Please refer to the User's Guide for a full explanation of data.

Battle Mountain General Hospital

535 South Humboldt Street Phone: 775-635-2550
Batte Mtn, NV 89820
Type: Critical Access Hospitals Emergency Services: Yes
Ownership: Govt - Hospital Dist/Auth

Measure	Cases	This Hosp.	State Avg.	U.S. Avg.
Blood Clot Prevention and Treatment				
Anticoagulation Overlap Therapy[5]	-	-	96%	93%
ICU Venous Thromboembolism Prophylaxis[5]	-	-	91%	92%
Incidence of Potentially Preventable VTE[5]	-	-	10%	10%
UFH with Dosages/Platelet Monitoring[5]	-	-	99%	97%
Venous Thromboembolism Prophylaxis[5]	-	-	84%	85%
Warfarin Therapy Discharge Instructions[5]	-	-	90%	75%
Chest Pain/Possible Heart Attack Care				
Aspirin Given Within 24 Hours of Arrival[1,3]	-	-	98%	96%
Fibrinolytic Meds Within 30 Min. of Arrival[3,7]	-	-	40%	58%
Average Time to ECG (minutes)[1,3]	-	-	9	7
Average Time to Transfer (minutes)[3,7]	-	-	66	60
Children's Asthma Care				
Received Home Management Plan of Care	-	-	-	88%
Received Reliever Medication	-	-	-	100%
Received Systemic Corticosteroids	-	-	-	100%
Emergency Department				
Admittance Decision Time (minutes)[5]	-	-	151	98
Head CT Results Within 45 Min. of Arrival[5]	-	-	44%	57%
Patients Who Left ER Before Being Seen[5]	-	-	2%	2%
Time from ER Arrival to Admit. (minutes)[5]	-	-	337	274
Time from ER Arrival to Discharge (minutes)[5]	-	-	150	134
Time in ER Before Being Evaluated (minutes)[5]	-	-	22	26
Time to Pain Meds for Fractures (minutes)[5]	-	-	54	57
Heart Attack Care				
Aspirin Given at Discharge[5]	-	-	99%	99%
Fibrinolytic Meds Within 30 Min. of Arrival[5]	-	-	67%	54%
PCI Within 90 Minutes of Arrival[5]	-	-	97%	96%
Statin Prescribed at Discharge[5]	-	-	98%	98%
Heart Failure Care				
ACE Inhibitor or ARB for LVSD[3,7]	-	-	97%	97%
Discharge Instructions Given[3,7]	-	-	91%	94%
Evaluation of LVS Function[3,7]	-	-	99%	99%
Medicare Spending				
Medicare Spending per Patient (ratio)	-	-	1.04	0.98
Pneumonia Care				
Appropriate Initial Antibiotic Given[1,3]	-	-	96%	95%
Blood Culture Timing[1,3]	-	-	96%	98%
Pregnancy and Delivery Care				
Newborn Deliveries Scheduled Early[5]	-	-	6%	6%
Preventive Care				
Immunization for Influenza[5]	-	-	93%	90%
Immunization for Pneumonia[5]	-	-	94%	92%
Stroke Care				
Anticoagulation Therapy for Atrial Fibrillation[5]	-	-	92%	95%
Antithrombotic Therapy Timing[5]	-	-	97%	98%
Assessed for Rehabilitation[5]	-	-	96%	97%
Discharged on Antithrombotic Therapy[5]	-	-	99%	99%
Discharged on Statin Medication[5]	-	-	95%	94%
Thrombolytic Therapy Timing[5]	-	-	80%	66%
Venous Thromboembolism Prophylaxis[5]	-	-	91%	94%
Written Stroke Educational Materials Given[5]	-	-	87%	88%
Surgical Care Improvement Project				
Appropriate Beta Blocker Usage[5]	-	-	96%	98%
Appropriate VTP Within 24 Hours[5]	-	-	98%	98%
Controlled Postoperative Blood Glucose[5]	-	-	97%	97%
Perioperative Temperature Management[5]	-	-	100%	100%
Prophylactic Antibiotic Selection[5]	-	-	99%	99%
Prophylactic Antibiotic Selection (Outpatient)[5]	-	-	98%	98%
Prophylactic Antibiotic Stopped[5]	-	-	98%	98%
Prophylactic Antibiotic Timing[5]	-	-	99%	99%
Prophylactic Antibiotic Timing (Outpatient)[5]	-	-	98%	98%
Urinary Catheter Removal[5]	-	-	98%	97%
Survey of Patients' Hospital Experiences				
Area Around Room 'Always' Quiet at Night[5]	-	-	57%	61%
Doctors 'Always' Communicated Well[5]	-	-	75%	82%
Home Recovery Information Given[5]	-	-	85%	85%
Hospital Given 9 or 10 on 10 Point Scale[5]	-	-	66%	71%
Meds 'Always' Explained Before Given[5]	-	-	60%	64%
Nurses 'Always' Communicated Well[5]	-	-	72%	79%
Pain 'Always' Well Controlled[5]	-	-	67%	71%
Room and Bathroom 'Always' Clean[5]	-	-	68%	73%
Timely Help 'Always' Received[5]	-	-	59%	68%
Would Definitely Recommend Hospital[5]	-	-	69%	71%
Use of Medical Imaging				
Cardiac Imaging Stress Test before Surgery[7]	-	-	4.8%	5.3%
Combination Abdominal CT Scan[1]	-	-	6.9%	10.5%
Combination Brain/Sinus CT Scan	31	0.0%	2.7%	2.7%
Combination Chest CT Scan[1]	-	-	3.7%	2.7%
Follow-up Mammogram/Ultrasound[7]	-	-	7.3%	8.8%
Lumbar Spine MRI for Low Back Pain[1]	-	-	36.8%	37.2%

Boulder City Hospital

901 Adams Blvd Phone: 702-293-4111
Boulder City, NV 89005 Fax: 702-293-0430
E-mail: info@bouldercityhospital.org
URL: www.bouldercityhospital.org
Type: Critical Access Hospitals Emergency Services: Yes
Ownership: Voluntary non-profit - Private Beds: 67

Key Personnel:
Operating Room. . . . . Leslie Buchanan
Emergency Room . . . . David Daitch, DO
Infection Control. . . . . Kim Falco
Intensive Care Unit. . . . . Maryann Hanson
Radiology. . . . . Kathy Kahler
Chief of Medical Staff. . . . . Derek Meeks
CEO/President. . . . . Christine Milburn

Measure	Cases	This Hosp.	State Avg.	U.S. Avg.
Blood Clot Prevention and Treatment				
Anticoagulation Overlap Therapy[5]	-	-	96%	93%
ICU Venous Thromboembolism Prophylaxis[5]	-	-	91%	92%
Incidence of Potentially Preventable VTE[5]	-	-	10%	10%
UFH with Dosages/Platelet Monitoring[5]	-	-	99%	97%
Venous Thromboembolism Prophylaxis[5]	-	-	84%	85%
Warfarin Therapy Discharge Instructions[5]	-	-	90%	75%
Chest Pain/Possible Heart Attack Care				
Aspirin Given Within 24 Hours of Arrival[3]	14	100%	98%	96%
Fibrinolytic Meds Within 30 Min. of Arrival[3,7]	-	-	40%	58%
Average Time to ECG (minutes)[3]	14	10	9	7
Average Time to Transfer (minutes)[1,3]	-	-	66	60
Children's Asthma Care				
Received Home Management Plan of Care	-	-	-	88%
Received Reliever Medication	-	-	-	100%
Received Systemic Corticosteroids	-	-	-	100%
Emergency Department				
Admittance Decision Time (minutes)[5]	-	-	151	98
Head CT Results Within 45 Min. of Arrival[5]	-	-	44%	57%
Patients Who Left ER Before Being Seen[5]	-	-	2%	2%
Time from ER Arrival to Admit. (minutes)[5]	-	-	337	274
Time from ER Arrival to Discharge (minutes)[5]	-	-	150	134
Time in ER Before Being Evaluated (minutes)[5]	-	-	22	26
Time to Pain Meds for Fractures (minutes)[5]	-	-	54	57
Heart Attack Care				
Aspirin Given at Discharge[5]	-	-	99%	99%
Fibrinolytic Meds Within 30 Min. of Arrival[5]	-	-	67%	54%
PCI Within 90 Minutes of Arrival[5]	-	-	97%	96%
Statin Prescribed at Discharge[5]	-	-	98%	98%
Heart Failure Care				
ACE Inhibitor or ARB for LVSD[1,3]	-	-	97%	97%
Discharge Instructions Given[3]	11	91%	91%	94%
Evaluation of LVS Function[3]	12	58%	99%	99%
Medicare Spending				
Medicare Spending per Patient (ratio)	-	-	1.04	0.98
Pneumonia Care				
Appropriate Initial Antibiotic Given[1,3]	-	-	96%	95%
Blood Culture Timing[1,3]	-	-	96%	98%
Pregnancy and Delivery Care				
Newborn Deliveries Scheduled Early[5]	-	-	6%	6%
Preventive Care				
Immunization for Influenza[5]	-	-	93%	90%
Immunization for Pneumonia[5]	-	-	94%	92%
Stroke Care				
Anticoagulation Therapy for Atrial Fibrillation[5]	-	-	92%	95%
Antithrombotic Therapy Timing[5]	-	-	97%	98%
Assessed for Rehabilitation[5]	-	-	96%	97%
Discharged on Antithrombotic Therapy[5]	-	-	99%	99%
Discharged on Statin Medication[5]	-	-	95%	94%
Thrombolytic Therapy Timing[5]	-	-	80%	66%
Venous Thromboembolism Prophylaxis[5]	-	-	91%	94%
Written Stroke Educational Materials Given[5]	-	-	87%	88%
Surgical Care Improvement Project				
Appropriate Beta Blocker Usage[5]	-	-	96%	98%
Appropriate VTP Within 24 Hours[5]	-	-	98%	98%
Controlled Postoperative Blood Glucose[5]	-	-	97%	97%
Perioperative Temperature Management[5]	-	-	100%	100%
Prophylactic Antibiotic Selection[5]	-	-	99%	99%
Prophylactic Antibiotic Selection (Outpatient)[5]	-	-	98%	98%
Prophylactic Antibiotic Stopped[5]	-	-	98%	98%
Prophylactic Antibiotic Timing[5]	-	-	99%	99%
Prophylactic Antibiotic Timing (Outpatient)[5]	-	-	98%	98%
Urinary Catheter Removal[5]	-	-	98%	97%
Survey of Patients' Hospital Experiences				
Area Around Room 'Always' Quiet at Night[5]	-	-	57%	61%
Doctors 'Always' Communicated Well[5]	-	-	75%	82%
Home Recovery Information Given[5]	-	-	85%	85%
Hospital Given 9 or 10 on 10 Point Scale[5]	-	-	66%	71%
Meds 'Always' Explained Before Given[5]	-	-	60%	64%
Nurses 'Always' Communicated Well[5]	-	-	72%	79%
Pain 'Always' Well Controlled[5]	-	-	67%	71%
Room and Bathroom 'Always' Clean[5]	-	-	68%	73%
Timely Help 'Always' Received[5]	-	-	59%	68%
Would Definitely Recommend Hospital[5]	-	-	69%	71%
Use of Medical Imaging				
Cardiac Imaging Stress Test before Surgery[1]	-	-	4.8%	5.3%
Combination Abdominal CT Scan	149	12.8%	6.9%	10.5%
Combination Brain/Sinus CT Scan[1]	-	-	2.7%	2.7%
Combination Chest CT Scan	53	34.0%	3.7%	2.7%
Follow-up Mammogram/Ultrasound[1]	-	-	7.3%	8.8%
Lumbar Spine MRI for Low Back Pain[1]	-	-	36.8%	37.2%

Grover C Dils Medical Center

700 N Spring St, Box 1010 - C - Adm Bldg Phone: 775-726-3171
Caliente, NV 89008
Type: Critical Access Hospitals Emergency Services: Yes
Ownership: Govt - Hospital Dist/Auth

Measure	Cases	This Hosp.	State Avg.	U.S. Avg.
Blood Clot Prevention and Treatment				
Anticoagulation Overlap Therapy[5]	-	-	96%	93%
ICU Venous Thromboembolism Prophylaxis[5]	-	-	91%	92%
Incidence of Potentially Preventable VTE[5]	-	-	10%	10%
UFH with Dosages/Platelet Monitoring[5]	-	-	99%	97%
Venous Thromboembolism Prophylaxis[5]	-	-	84%	85%
Warfarin Therapy Discharge Instructions[5]	-	-	90%	75%
Chest Pain/Possible Heart Attack Care				
Aspirin Given Within 24 Hours of Arrival[1,3]	-	-	98%	96%
Fibrinolytic Meds Within 30 Min. of Arrival[3,7]	-	-	40%	58%
Average Time to ECG (minutes)[3,7]	-	-	9	7
Average Time to Transfer (minutes)[1,3]	-	-	66	60
Children's Asthma Care				
Received Home Management Plan of Care	-	-	-	88%
Received Reliever Medication	-	-	-	100%
Received Systemic Corticosteroids	-	-	-	100%
Emergency Department				
Admittance Decision Time (minutes)[5]	-	-	151	98
Head CT Results Within 45 Min. of Arrival[5]	-	-	44%	57%
Patients Who Left ER Before Being Seen	890	1%	2%	2%
Time from ER Arrival to Admit. (minutes)[5]	-	-	337	274
Time from ER Arrival to Discharge (minutes)[5]	-	-	150	134
Time in ER Before Being Evaluated (minutes)[5]	-	-	22	26
Time to Pain Meds for Fractures (minutes)[5]	-	-	54	57
Heart Attack Care				
Aspirin Given at Discharge[5]	-	-	99%	99%

NOTE: Hospital profiles are in alphabetical order by state, then city, then hospital within the city; Rankings exclude hospitals with less than 25 cases except for patient surveys which excludes hospitals with less than 100 cases; (a) 100-299 cases; (1) The number of cases/patients is too few to report; (2) Data submitted were based on a sample of cases/patients; (3) Results are based on a shorter time period than required; (4) Data suppressed by CMS for one or more quarters; (5) Results are not available for this reporting period; (6) Fewer than 100 patients completed the HCAHPS survey; (7) No cases met the criteria for this measure; (8) The lower limit of the confidence interval cannot be calculated if the number of observed infections equals zero; (9) No data are available from the state/territory for this reporting period; (10) The scores shown reflect fewer than 50 completed surveys; (11) There were discrepancies in the data collection process; (12) This measure does not apply to this hospital for this reporting period; (13) Results cannot be calculated for this reporting period; (14) The results for this state are combined with nearby states to protect confidentiality; Please refer to the User's Guide for a full explanation of data.

Measure	Cases	This Hosp.	State Avg.	U.S. Avg.
Fibrinolytic Meds Within 30 Min. of Arrival[5]	-	-	67%	54%
PCI Within 90 Minutes of Arrival[5]	-	-	97%	96%
Statin Prescribed at Discharge[5]	-	-	98%	98%
Heart Failure Care				
ACE Inhibitor or ARB for LVSD[2,3]	-	-	97%	97%
Discharge Instructions Given[2,3]	-	-	91%	94%
Evaluation of LVS Function[2,3]	-	-	99%	99%
Medicare Spending				
Medicare Spending per Patient (ratio)	-	-	1.04	0.98
Pneumonia Care				
Appropriate Initial Antibiotic Given[2,3]	-	-	96%	95%
Blood Culture Timing[2,3]	-	-	96%	98%
Pregnancy and Delivery Care				
Newborn Deliveries Scheduled Early[5]	-	-	6%	6%
Preventive Care				
Immunization for Influenza[5]	-	-	93%	90%
Immunization for Pneumonia[5]	-	-	94%	92%
Stroke Care				
Anticoagulation Therapy for Atrial Fibrillation[5]	-	-	92%	95%
Antithrombotic Therapy Timing[5]	-	-	97%	98%
Assessed for Rehabilitation[5]	-	-	96%	97%
Discharged on Antithrombotic Therapy[5]	-	-	99%	99%
Discharged on Statin Medication[5]	-	-	95%	94%
Thrombolytic Therapy Timing[5]	-	-	80%	66%
Venous Thromboembolism Prophylaxis[5]	-	-	91%	94%
Written Stroke Educational Materials Given[5]	-	-	87%	88%
Surgical Care Improvement Project				
Appropriate Beta Blocker Usage[5]	-	-	96%	98%
Appropriate VTP Within 24 Hours[5]	-	-	98%	98%
Controlled Postoperative Blood Glucose[5]	-	-	97%	97%
Perioperative Temperature Management[5]	-	-	100%	100%
Prophylactic Antibiotic Selection[5]	-	-	99%	99%
Prophylactic Antibiotic Selection (Outpatient)[5]	-	-	98%	98%
Prophylactic Antibiotic Stopped[5]	-	-	98%	98%
Prophylactic Antibiotic Timing[5]	-	-	99%	99%
Prophylactic Antibiotic Timing (Outpatient)[5]	-	-	98%	98%
Urinary Catheter Removal[5]	-	-	98%	97%
Survey of Patients' Hospital Experiences				
Area Around Room 'Always' Quiet at Night[5]	-	-	57%	61%
Doctors 'Always' Communicated Well[5]	-	-	75%	82%
Home Recovery Information Given[5]	-	-	85%	85%
Hospital Given 9 or 10 on 10 Point Scale[5]	-	-	66%	71%
Meds 'Always' Explained Before Given[5]	-	-	60%	64%
Nurses 'Always' Communicated Well[5]	-	-	72%	79%
Pain 'Always' Well Controlled[5]	-	-	67%	71%
Room and Bathroom 'Always' Clean[5]	-	-	68%	73%
Timely Help 'Always' Received[5]	-	-	59%	68%
Would Definitely Recommend Hospital[5]	-	-	69%	71%
Use of Medical Imaging				
Cardiac Imaging Stress Test before Surgery[7]	-	-	4.8%	5.3%
Combination Abdominal CT Scan[1]	-	-	6.9%	10.5%
Combination Brain/Sinus CT Scan	41	0.0%	2.7%	2.7%
Combination Chest CT Scan[1]	-	-	3.7%	2.7%
Follow-up Mammogram/Ultrasound[7]	-	-	7.3%	8.8%
Lumbar Spine MRI for Low Back Pain[7]	-	-	36.8%	37.2%

Carson Tahoe Regional Medical Center

1600 Medical Parkway
Carson City, NV 89703
Phone: 775-445-8000
Fax: 775-885-4447
E-mail: info@c-th.com
URL: www.carsontahoehospital.com
Type: Acute Care Hospitals
Emergency Services: Yes
Ownership: Voluntary non-profit - Private
Beds: 128

Key Personnel:
CEO/President . . . . Ed Epperson
Quality Assurance . . . . Gordon Hutting
Emergency Room . . . . Deena McKenzie
Chair/CEO . . . . Jonathan Miller
Infection Control. . . . . Kim Neiman
Operating Room. . . . . Annette Patellos, RN
Chief of Medical Staff . . . . Richard P. Rodriguez, MD

Measure	Cases	This Hosp.	State Avg.	U.S. Avg.
Blood Clot Prevention and Treatment				
Anticoagulation Overlap Therapy[2]	87	99%	96%	93%
ICU Venous Thromboembolism Prophylaxis[2]	53	85%	91%	92%
Incidence of Potentially Preventable VTE[2]	15	20%	10%	10%
UFH with Dosages/Platelet Monitoring[2]	43	98%	99%	97%
Venous Thromboembolism Prophylaxis[2]	324	90%	84%	85%
Warfarin Therapy Discharge Instructions[2]	75	95%	90%	75%
Chest Pain/Possible Heart Attack Care				
Aspirin Given Within 24 Hours of Arrival[1,3]	-	-	98%	96%
Fibrinolytic Meds Within 30 Min. of Arrival[3,7]	-	-	40%	58%
Average Time to ECG (minutes)[1,3]	-	-	9	7
Average Time to Transfer (minutes)[3,7]	-	-	66	60
Children's Asthma Care				
Received Home Management Plan of Care	-	-	-	88%
Received Reliever Medication	-	-	-	100%
Received Systemic Corticosteroids	-	-	-	100%
Emergency Department				
Admittance Decision Time (minutes)[2]	599	96	151	98
Head CT Results Within 45 Min. of Arrival	15	40%	44%	57%
Patients Who Left ER Before Being Seen	25,944	2%	2%	2%
Time from ER Arrival to Admit. (minutes)[2]	618	274	337	274
Time from ER Arrival to Discharge (minutes)	361	167	150	134
Time in ER Before Being Evaluated (minutes)	362	44	22	26
Time to Pain Meds for Fractures (minutes)	151	74	54	57
Heart Attack Care				
Aspirin Given at Discharge[2]	257	99%	99%	99%
Fibrinolytic Meds Within 30 Min. of Arrival[2,7]	-	-	67%	54%
PCI Within 90 Minutes of Arrival[2]	37	97%	97%	96%
Statin Prescribed at Discharge[2]	242	100%	98%	98%
Heart Failure Care				
ACE Inhibitor or ARB for LVSD[2]	71	100%	97%	97%
Discharge Instructions Given[2]	215	85%	91%	94%
Evaluation of LVS Function[2]	260	100%	99%	99%
Medicare Spending				
Medicare Spending per Patient (ratio)	-	0.98	1.04	0.98
Pneumonia Care				
Appropriate Initial Antibiotic Given[2]	99	99%	96%	95%
Blood Culture Timing[2]	131	97%	96%	98%
Pregnancy and Delivery Care				
Newborn Deliveries Scheduled Early	77	0%	6%	6%
Preventive Care				
Immunization for Influenza[2]	528	97%	93%	90%
Immunization for Pneumonia[2]	701	97%	94%	92%
Stroke Care				
Anticoagulation Therapy for Atrial Fibrillation[2]	17	100%	92%	95%
Antithrombotic Therapy Timing[2]	91	100%	97%	98%
Assessed for Rehabilitation[2]	103	97%	96%	97%
Discharged on Antithrombotic Therapy[2]	100	99%	99%	99%
Discharged on Statin Medication[2]	80	96%	95%	94%
Thrombolytic Therapy Timing[1,2]	-	-	80%	66%
Venous Thromboembolism Prophylaxis[2]	92	93%	91%	94%
Written Stroke Educational Materials Given[2]	52	79%	87%	88%
Surgical Care Improvement Project				
Appropriate Beta Blocker Usage[2]	143	97%	96%	98%
Appropriate VTP Within 24 Hours[2]	260	98%	98%	98%
Controlled Postoperative Blood Glucose[2]	74	97%	97%	97%
Perioperative Temperature Management[2]	342	100%	100%	100%
Prophylactic Antibiotic Selection[2]	281	99%	99%	99%
Prophylactic Antibiotic Selection (Outpatient)	213	98%	98%	98%
Prophylactic Antibiotic Stopped[2]	269	99%	98%	98%
Prophylactic Antibiotic Timing[2]	284	99%	99%	99%
Prophylactic Antibiotic Timing (Outpatient)	212	97%	98%	98%
Urinary Catheter Removal[2]	301	99%	98%	97%
Survey of Patients' Hospital Experiences				
Area Around Room 'Always' Quiet at Night	300+	54%	57%	61%
Doctors 'Always' Communicated Well	300+	77%	75%	82%
Home Recovery Information Given	300+	85%	85%	85%
Hospital Given 9 or 10 on 10 Point Scale	300+	68%	66%	71%
Meds 'Always' Explained Before Given	300+	64%	60%	64%
Nurses 'Always' Communicated Well	300+	74%	72%	79%
Pain 'Always' Well Controlled	300+	66%	67%	71%
Room and Bathroom 'Always' Clean	300+	67%	68%	73%
Timely Help 'Always' Received	300+	59%	59%	68%
Would Definitely Recommend Hospital	300+	71%	69%	71%
Use of Medical Imaging				
Cardiac Imaging Stress Test before Surgery	1,041	5.2%	4.8%	5.3%
Combination Abdominal CT Scan	1,041	10.6%	6.9%	10.5%
Combination Brain/Sinus CT Scan	906	1.8%	2.7%	2.7%
Combination Chest CT Scan	1,160	1.8%	3.7%	2.7%
Follow-up Mammogram/Ultrasound	2,995	7.2%	7.3%	8.8%
Lumbar Spine MRI for Low Back Pain	310	38.1%	36.8%	37.2%

Sierra Surgery Hospital

1400 Medical Pkwy
Carson City, NV 89703
Phone: 775-883-1700
Fax: 775-883-8905
URL: www.sierrasurgery.com
Type: Acute Care Hospitals
Emergency Services: No
Ownership: Proprietary
Beds: 15

Key Personnel:
CEO/President . . . . Ed Epperson
Administrator . . . . Jan Hewitt
Chief of Medical Staff . . . . Richard P. Rodriguez, MD

Measure	Cases	This Hosp.	State Avg.	U.S. Avg.
Blood Clot Prevention and Treatment				
Anticoagulation Overlap Therapy[2,7]	-	-	96%	93%
ICU Venous Thromboembolism Prophylaxis[2,7]	-	-	91%	92%
Incidence of Potentially Preventable VTE[2,7]	-	-	10%	10%
UFH with Dosages/Platelet Monitoring[2,7]	-	-	99%	97%
Venous Thromboembolism Prophylaxis[2]	41	100%	84%	85%
Warfarin Therapy Discharge Instructions[2,7]	-	-	90%	75%
Chest Pain/Possible Heart Attack Care				
Aspirin Given Within 24 Hours of Arrival[5]	-	-	98%	96%
Fibrinolytic Meds Within 30 Min. of Arrival[5]	-	-	40%	58%
Average Time to ECG (minutes)[5]	-	-	9	7
Average Time to Transfer (minutes)[5]	-	-	66	60
Children's Asthma Care				
Received Home Management Plan of Care	-	-	-	88%
Received Reliever Medication	-	-	-	100%
Received Systemic Corticosteroids	-	-	-	100%
Emergency Department				
Admittance Decision Time (minutes)[2,7]	-	-	151	98
Head CT Results Within 45 Min. of Arrival[5]	-	-	44%	57%
Patients Who Left ER Before Being Seen[5]	-	-	2%	2%
Time from ER Arrival to Admit. (minutes)[2,7]	-	-	337	274
Time from ER Arrival to Discharge (minutes)[5]	-	-	150	134
Time in ER Before Being Evaluated (minutes)[5]	-	-	22	26
Time to Pain Meds for Fractures (minutes)[5]	-	-	54	57
Heart Attack Care				
Aspirin Given at Discharge[5]	-	-	99%	99%
Fibrinolytic Meds Within 30 Min. of Arrival[5]	-	-	67%	54%
PCI Within 90 Minutes of Arrival[5]	-	-	97%	96%
Statin Prescribed at Discharge[5]	-	-	98%	98%
Heart Failure Care				
ACE Inhibitor or ARB for LVSD[5]	-	-	97%	97%
Discharge Instructions Given[5]	-	-	91%	94%
Evaluation of LVS Function[5]	-	-	99%	99%
Medicare Spending				
Medicare Spending per Patient (ratio)	-	0.89	1.04	0.98
Pneumonia Care				
Appropriate Initial Antibiotic Given[5]	-	-	96%	95%
Blood Culture Timing[5]	-	-	96%	98%
Pregnancy and Delivery Care				
Newborn Deliveries Scheduled Early[7]	-	-	6%	6%
Preventive Care				
Immunization for Influenza[2]	348	88%	93%	90%
Immunization for Pneumonia[2]	428	85%	94%	92%
Stroke Care				
Anticoagulation Therapy for Atrial Fibrillation[5]	-	-	92%	95%
Antithrombotic Therapy Timing[5]	-	-	97%	98%
Assessed for Rehabilitation[5]	-	-	96%	97%
Discharged on Antithrombotic Therapy[5]	-	-	99%	99%
Discharged on Statin Medication[5]	-	-	95%	94%
Thrombolytic Therapy Timing[5]	-	-	80%	66%
Venous Thromboembolism Prophylaxis[5]	-	-	91%	94%
Written Stroke Educational Materials Given[5]	-	-	87%	88%
Surgical Care Improvement Project				
Appropriate Beta Blocker Usage[2]	39	95%	96%	98%

NOTE: Hospital profiles are in alphabetical order by state, then city, then hospital within the city; Rankings exclude hospitals with less than 25 cases except for patient surveys which excludes hospitals with less than 100 cases; (a) 100-299 cases; (1) The number of cases/patients is too few to report; (2) Data submitted were based on a sample of cases/patients; (3) Results are based on a shorter time period than required; (4) Data suppressed by CMS for one or more quarters; (5) Results are not available for this reporting period; (6) Fewer than 100 patients completed the HCAHPS survey; (7) No cases met the criteria for this measure; (8) The lower limit of the confidence interval cannot be calculated if the number of observed infections equals zero; (9) No data are available from the state/territory for this reporting period; (10) The scores shown reflect fewer than 50 completed surveys; (11) There were discrepancies in the data collection process; (12) This measure does not apply to this hospital for this reporting period; (13) Results cannot be calculated for this reporting period; (14) The results for this state are combined with nearby states to protect confidentiality; Please refer to the User's Guide for a full explanation of data.

Measure	Cases	This Hosp.	State Avg.	U.S. Avg.
Appropriate VTP Within 24 Hours[2]	283	95%	98%	98%
Controlled Postoperative Blood Glucose[2,7]	-	-	97%	97%
Perioperative Temperature Management[2]	302	100%	100%	100%
Prophylactic Antibiotic Selection[2]	233	94%	99%	99%
Prophylactic Antibiotic Selection (Outpatient)	175	93%	98%	98%
Prophylactic Antibiotic Stopped[2]	232	100%	98%	98%
Prophylactic Antibiotic Timing[2]	233	99%	99%	99%
Prophylactic Antibiotic Timing (Outpatient)	176	96%	98%	98%
Urinary Catheter Removal[2]	228	99%	98%	97%
Survey of Patients' Hospital Experiences				
Area Around Room 'Always' Quiet at Night	300+	68%	57%	61%
Doctors 'Always' Communicated Well	300+	80%	75%	82%
Home Recovery Information Given	300+	90%	85%	85%
Hospital Given 9 or 10 on 10 Point Scale	300+	77%	66%	71%
Meds 'Always' Explained Before Given	300+	68%	60%	64%
Nurses 'Always' Communicated Well	300+	78%	72%	79%
Pain 'Always' Well Controlled	300+	74%	67%	71%
Room and Bathroom 'Always' Clean	300+	80%	68%	73%
Timely Help 'Always' Received	300+	72%	59%	68%
Would Definitely Recommend Hospital	300+	82%	69%	71%
Use of Medical Imaging				
Cardiac Imaging Stress Test before Surgery[7]	-	-	4.8%	5.3%
Combination Abdominal CT Scan	195	19.0%	6.9%	10.5%
Combination Brain/Sinus CT Scan[1]	-	-	2.7%	2.7%
Combination Chest CT Scan	163	0.6%	3.7%	2.7%
Follow-up Mammogram/Ultrasound	501	6.2%	7.3%	8.8%
Lumbar Spine MRI for Low Back Pain	121	33.1%	36.8%	37.2%

Northeastern Nevada Regional Hospital

2001 Errecart Blvd
Elko, NV 89801
Phone: 775-738-5151
Fax: 775-748-2002
URL: www.nnrhospital.com
Type: Acute Care Hospitals
Emergency Services: Yes
Ownership: Proprietary
Beds: 75

Key Personnel:

Radiology. . . . . Troy Belle
Operating Room. . . . . Kurt Doggwiler
Infection Control. . . . . Lynn Gauthier
Quality Assurance . . . . Lynn Gauthier
Intensive Care Unit. . . . . Raquel Guerrero
CEO . . . . Gene Miller
Chief of Medical Staff. . . . . Mitchell Miller, MD
Emergency Room . . . . Robert Stefanko, MD

Measure	Cases	This Hosp.	State Avg.	U.S. Avg.
Blood Clot Prevention and Treatment				
Anticoagulation Overlap Therapy[2]	20	65%	96%	93%
ICU Venous Thromboembolism Prophylaxis[2]	47	79%	91%	92%
Incidence of Potentially Preventable VTE[1,2]	-	-	10%	10%
UFH with Dosages/Platelet Monitoring[1,2]	-	-	99%	97%
Venous Thromboembolism Prophylaxis[2]	161	52%	84%	85%
Warfarin Therapy Discharge Instructions[2]	18	89%	90%	75%
Chest Pain/Possible Heart Attack Care				
Aspirin Given Within 24 Hours of Arrival	22	100%	98%	96%
Fibrinolytic Meds Within 30 Min. of Arrival[1,3]	-	-	40%	58%
Average Time to ECG (minutes)	25	6	9	7
Average Time to Transfer (minutes)[1,3]	-	-	66	60
Children's Asthma Care				
Received Home Management Plan of Care	-	-	-	88%
Received Reliever Medication	-	-	-	100%
Received Systemic Corticosteroids	-	-	-	100%
Emergency Department				
Admittance Decision Time (minutes)[2]	275	88	151	98
Head CT Results Within 45 Min. of Arrival[1]	-	-	44%	57%
Patients Who Left ER Before Being Seen	25,123	2%	2%	2%
Time from ER Arrival to Admit. (minutes)[2]	277	269	337	274
Time from ER Arrival to Discharge (minutes)	387	122	150	134
Time in ER Before Being Evaluated (minutes)	414	12	22	26
Time to Pain Meds for Fractures (minutes)	119	43	54	57
Heart Attack Care				
Aspirin Given at Discharge	16	88%	99%	99%
Fibrinolytic Meds Within 30 Min. of Arrival[7]	-	-	67%	54%
PCI Within 90 Minutes of Arrival[7]	-	-	97%	96%
Statin Prescribed at Discharge	16	94%	98%	98%
Heart Failure Care				
ACE Inhibitor or ARB for LVSD[1]	-	-	97%	97%
Discharge Instructions Given	50	90%	91%	94%
Evaluation of LVS Function	62	89%	99%	99%
Medicare Spending				
Medicare Spending per Patient (ratio)	-	0.95	1.04	0.98
Pneumonia Care				
Appropriate Initial Antibiotic Given	100	91%	96%	95%
Blood Culture Timing	139	96%	96%	98%
Pregnancy and Delivery Care				
Newborn Deliveries Scheduled Early[2]	40	22%	6%	6%
Preventive Care				
Immunization for Influenza[2]	243	82%	93%	90%
Immunization for Pneumonia[2]	200	84%	94%	92%
Stroke Care				
Anticoagulation Therapy for Atrial Fibrillation[1]	-	-	92%	95%
Antithrombotic Therapy Timing	16	100%	97%	98%
Assessed for Rehabilitation	19	100%	96%	97%
Discharged on Antithrombotic Therapy	17	94%	99%	99%
Discharged on Statin Medication	12	92%	95%	94%
Thrombolytic Therapy Timing[1]	-	-	80%	66%
Venous Thromboembolism Prophylaxis	18	72%	91%	94%
Written Stroke Educational Materials Given[1]	-	-	87%	88%
Surgical Care Improvement Project				
Appropriate Beta Blocker Usage	16	100%	96%	98%
Appropriate VTP Within 24 Hours	105	98%	98%	98%
Controlled Postoperative Blood Glucose[7]	-	-	97%	97%
Perioperative Temperature Management	124	100%	100%	100%
Prophylactic Antibiotic Selection	109	98%	99%	99%
Prophylactic Antibiotic Selection (Outpatient)	67	100%	98%	98%
Prophylactic Antibiotic Stopped	108	99%	98%	98%
Prophylactic Antibiotic Timing	109	97%	99%	99%
Prophylactic Antibiotic Timing (Outpatient)	67	100%	98%	98%
Urinary Catheter Removal	98	94%	98%	97%
Survey of Patients' Hospital Experiences				
Area Around Room 'Always' Quiet at Night	300+	60%	57%	61%
Doctors 'Always' Communicated Well	300+	76%	75%	82%
Home Recovery Information Given	300+	83%	85%	85%
Hospital Given 9 or 10 on 10 Point Scale	300+	56%	66%	71%
Meds 'Always' Explained Before Given	300+	60%	60%	64%
Nurses 'Always' Communicated Well	300+	70%	72%	79%
Pain 'Always' Well Controlled	300+	62%	67%	71%
Room and Bathroom 'Always' Clean	300+	69%	68%	73%
Timely Help 'Always' Received	300+	57%	59%	68%
Would Definitely Recommend Hospital	300+	53%	69%	71%
Use of Medical Imaging				
Cardiac Imaging Stress Test before Surgery[1]	-	-	4.8%	5.3%
Combination Abdominal CT Scan	248	33.1%	6.9%	10.5%
Combination Brain/Sinus CT Scan	211	5.7%	2.7%	2.7%
Combination Chest CT Scan	106	2.8%	3.7%	2.7%
Follow-up Mammogram/Ultrasound	295	14.9%	7.3%	8.8%
Lumbar Spine MRI for Low Back Pain	60	40.0%	36.8%	37.2%

William Bee Ririe Hospital

1500 Avenue H
Ely, NV 89301
Phone: 775-289-3001
Type: Critical Access Hospitals
Emergency Services: Yes
Ownership: Govt - Hospital Dist/Auth

Measure	Cases	This Hosp.	State Avg.	U.S. Avg.
Blood Clot Prevention and Treatment				
Anticoagulation Overlap Therapy[5]	-	-	96%	93%
ICU Venous Thromboembolism Prophylaxis[5]	-	-	91%	92%
Incidence of Potentially Preventable VTE[5]	-	-	10%	10%
UFH with Dosages/Platelet Monitoring[5]	-	-	99%	97%
Venous Thromboembolism Prophylaxis[5]	-	-	84%	85%
Warfarin Therapy Discharge Instructions[5]	-	-	90%	75%
Chest Pain/Possible Heart Attack Care				
Aspirin Given Within 24 Hours of Arrival	24	88%	98%	96%
Fibrinolytic Meds Within 30 Min. of Arrival[1]	-	-	40%	58%
Average Time to ECG (minutes)	24	30	9	7
Average Time to Transfer (minutes)[7]	-	-	66	60
Children's Asthma Care				
Received Home Management Plan of Care	-	-	-	88%
Received Reliever Medication	-	-	-	100%
Received Systemic Corticosteroids	-	-	-	100%
Emergency Department				
Admittance Decision Time (minutes)[5]	-	-	151	98
Head CT Results Within 45 Min. of Arrival[5]	-	-	44%	57%
Patients Who Left ER Before Being Seen	5,428	3%	2%	2%
Time from ER Arrival to Admit. (minutes)[5]	-	-	337	274
Time from ER Arrival to Discharge (minutes)[5]	-	-	150	134
Time in ER Before Being Evaluated (minutes)[5]	-	-	22	26
Time to Pain Meds for Fractures (minutes)[5]	-	-	54	57
Heart Attack Care				
Aspirin Given at Discharge[5]	-	-	99%	99%
Fibrinolytic Meds Within 30 Min. of Arrival[5]	-	-	67%	54%
PCI Within 90 Minutes of Arrival[5]	-	-	97%	96%
Statin Prescribed at Discharge[5]	-	-	98%	98%
Heart Failure Care				
ACE Inhibitor or ARB for LVSD[1]	-	-	97%	97%
Discharge Instructions Given[1]	-	-	91%	94%
Evaluation of LVS Function	11	73%	99%	99%
Medicare Spending				
Medicare Spending per Patient (ratio)	-	-	1.04	0.98
Pneumonia Care				
Appropriate Initial Antibiotic Given	27	89%	96%	95%
Blood Culture Timing	14	64%	96%	98%
Pregnancy and Delivery Care				
Newborn Deliveries Scheduled Early[5]	-	-	6%	6%
Preventive Care				
Immunization for Influenza[5]	-	-	93%	90%
Immunization for Pneumonia[5]	-	-	94%	92%
Stroke Care				
Anticoagulation Therapy for Atrial Fibrillation[5]	-	-	92%	95%
Antithrombotic Therapy Timing[5]	-	-	97%	98%
Assessed for Rehabilitation[5]	-	-	96%	97%
Discharged on Antithrombotic Therapy[5]	-	-	99%	99%
Discharged on Statin Medication[5]	-	-	95%	94%
Thrombolytic Therapy Timing[5]	-	-	80%	66%
Venous Thromboembolism Prophylaxis[5]	-	-	91%	94%
Written Stroke Educational Materials Given[5]	-	-	87%	88%
Surgical Care Improvement Project				
Appropriate Beta Blocker Usage[5]	-	-	96%	98%
Appropriate VTP Within 24 Hours[5]	-	-	98%	98%
Controlled Postoperative Blood Glucose[5]	-	-	97%	97%
Perioperative Temperature Management[5]	-	-	100%	100%
Prophylactic Antibiotic Selection[5]	-	-	99%	99%
Prophylactic Antibiotic Selection (Outpatient)	14	100%	98%	98%
Prophylactic Antibiotic Stopped[5]	-	-	98%	98%
Prophylactic Antibiotic Timing[5]	-	-	99%	99%
Prophylactic Antibiotic Timing (Outpatient)	16	88%	98%	98%
Urinary Catheter Removal[5]	-	-	98%	97%
Survey of Patients' Hospital Experiences				
Area Around Room 'Always' Quiet at Night[5]	-	-	57%	61%
Doctors 'Always' Communicated Well[5]	-	-	75%	82%
Home Recovery Information Given[5]	-	-	85%	85%
Hospital Given 9 or 10 on 10 Point Scale[5]	-	-	66%	71%
Meds 'Always' Explained Before Given[5]	-	-	60%	64%
Nurses 'Always' Communicated Well[5]	-	-	72%	79%
Pain 'Always' Well Controlled[5]	-	-	67%	71%
Room and Bathroom 'Always' Clean[5]	-	-	68%	73%
Timely Help 'Always' Received[5]	-	-	59%	68%
Would Definitely Recommend Hospital[5]	-	-	69%	71%
Use of Medical Imaging				
Cardiac Imaging Stress Test before Surgery[1]	-	-	4.8%	5.3%
Combination Abdominal CT Scan	125	1.6%	6.9%	10.5%
Combination Brain/Sinus CT Scan[1]	-	-	2.7%	2.7%
Combination Chest CT Scan	116	0.0%	3.7%	2.7%
Follow-up Mammogram/Ultrasound	133	3.8%	7.3%	8.8%
Lumbar Spine MRI for Low Back Pain[1]	-	-	36.8%	37.2%

NOTE: Hospital profiles are in alphabetical order by state, then city, then hospital within the city; Rankings exclude hospitals with less than 25 cases except for patient surveys which excludes hospitals with less than 100 cases; (a) 100-299 cases; (1) The number of cases/patients is too few to report; (2) Data submitted were based on a sample of cases/patients; (3) Results are based on a shorter time period than required; (4) Data suppressed by CMS for one or more quarters; (5) Results are not available for this reporting period; (6) Fewer than 100 patients completed the HCAHPS survey; (7) No cases met the criteria for this measure; (8) The lower limit of the confidence interval cannot be calculated if the number of observed infections equals zero; (9) No data are available from the state/territory for this reporting period; (10) The scores shown reflect fewer than 50 completed surveys; (11) There were discrepancies in the data collection process; (12) This measure does not apply to this hospital for this reporting period; (13) Results cannot be calculated for this reporting period; (14) The results for this state are combined with nearby states to protect confidentiality; Please refer to the User's Guide for a full explanation of data.

Banner Churchill Community Hospital

801 East Williams Avenue Phone: 775-423-3151
Fallon, NV 89406 Fax: 775-423-3793
Type: Acute Care Hospitals Emergency Services: Yes
Ownership: Voluntary non-profit - Private Beds: 40

Key Personnel:
Emergency Room . . . . Laura Carter, MD
Chief of Medical Staff . . . . Erick Herzog, MD
Operating Room. . . . . Thomas V McCormick
Quality Assurance . . . . Arlene McDonell, RN
Infection Control. . . . . Arlene McDonnel, RN
CEO/President. . . . . Charles Myers

Measure	Cases	This Hosp.	State Avg.	U.S. Avg.
Blood Clot Prevention and Treatment				
Anticoagulation Overlap Therapy[1,2]	-	-	96%	93%
ICU Venous Thromboembolism Prophylaxis[2]	24	96%	91%	92%
Incidence of Potentially Preventable VTE[2,7]	-	-	10%	10%
UFH with Dosages/Platelet Monitoring[2,7]	-	-	99%	97%
Venous Thromboembolism Prophylaxis[2]	134	96%	84%	85%
Warfarin Therapy Discharge Instructions[2]	11	55%	90%	75%
Chest Pain/Possible Heart Attack Care				
Aspirin Given Within 24 Hours of Arrival	43	100%	98%	96%
Fibrinolytic Meds Within 30 Min. of Arrival[1]	-	-	40%	58%
Average Time to ECG (minutes)	43	8	9	7
Average Time to Transfer (minutes)[7]	-	-	66	60
Children's Asthma Care				
Received Home Management Plan of Care	-	-	-	88%
Received Reliever Medication	-	-	-	100%
Received Systemic Corticosteroids	-	-	-	100%
Emergency Department				
Admittance Decision Time (minutes)[2]	409	51	151	98
Head CT Results Within 45 Min. of Arrival	12	33%	44%	57%
Patients Who Left ER Before Being Seen	17,090	1%	2%	2%
Time from ER Arrival to Admit. (minutes)[2]	410	218	337	274
Time from ER Arrival to Discharge (minutes)	321	115	150	134
Time in ER Before Being Evaluated (minutes)	384	17	22	26
Time to Pain Meds for Fractures (minutes)	54	54	54	57
Heart Attack Care				
Aspirin Given at Discharge[1,3]	-	-	99%	99%
Fibrinolytic Meds Within 30 Min. of Arrival[3,7]	-	-	67%	54%
PCI Within 90 Minutes of Arrival[3,7]	-	-	97%	96%
Statin Prescribed at Discharge[1,3]	-	-	98%	98%
Heart Failure Care				
ACE Inhibitor or ARB for LVSD[1,2]	-	-	97%	97%
Discharge Instructions Given[2]	34	100%	91%	94%
Evaluation of LVS Function[2]	38	100%	99%	99%
Medicare Spending				
Medicare Spending per Patient (ratio)	-	0.88	1.04	0.98
Pneumonia Care				
Appropriate Initial Antibiotic Given[2]	71	97%	96%	95%
Blood Culture Timing[2]	102	97%	96%	98%
Pregnancy and Delivery Care				
Newborn Deliveries Scheduled Early[2]	23	17%	6%	6%
Preventive Care				
Immunization for Influenza[2]	262	96%	93%	90%
Immunization for Pneumonia[2]	344	97%	94%	92%
Stroke Care				
Anticoagulation Therapy for Atrial Fibrillation[1]	-	-	92%	95%
Antithrombotic Therapy Timing[1]	-	-	97%	98%
Assessed for Rehabilitation[1]	-	-	96%	97%
Discharged on Antithrombotic Therapy[1]	-	-	99%	99%
Discharged on Statin Medication[1]	-	-	95%	94%
Thrombolytic Therapy Timing[7]	-	-	80%	66%
Venous Thromboembolism Prophylaxis[1]	-	-	91%	94%
Written Stroke Educational Materials Given[1]	-	-	87%	88%
Surgical Care Improvement Project				
Appropriate Beta Blocker Usage	16	94%	96%	98%
Appropriate VTP Within 24 Hours	60	98%	98%	98%
Controlled Postoperative Blood Glucose[7]	-	-	97%	97%
Perioperative Temperature Management	71	99%	100%	100%
Prophylactic Antibiotic Selection	52	100%	99%	99%
Prophylactic Antibiotic Selection (Outpatient)	18	94%	98%	98%
Prophylactic Antibiotic Stopped	48	100%	98%	98%
Prophylactic Antibiotic Timing	52	96%	99%	99%
Prophylactic Antibiotic Timing (Outpatient)	18	89%	98%	98%
Urinary Catheter Removal	18	94%	98%	97%
Survey of Patients' Hospital Experiences				
Area Around Room 'Always' Quiet at Night[11]	300+	62%	57%	61%
Doctors 'Always' Communicated Well[11]	300+	84%	75%	82%
Home Recovery Information Given[11]	300+	88%	85%	85%
Hospital Given 9 or 10 on 10 Point Scale[11]	300+	75%	66%	71%
Meds 'Always' Explained Before Given[11]	300+	70%	60%	64%
Nurses 'Always' Communicated Well[11]	300+	82%	72%	79%
Pain 'Always' Well Controlled[11]	300+	73%	67%	71%
Room and Bathroom 'Always' Clean[11]	300+	70%	68%	73%
Timely Help 'Always' Received[11]	300+	74%	59%	68%
Would Definitely Recommend Hospital[11]	300+	72%	69%	71%
Use of Medical Imaging				
Cardiac Imaging Stress Test before Surgery	105	1.0%	4.8%	5.3%
Combination Abdominal CT Scan	296	7.4%	6.9%	10.5%
Combination Brain/Sinus CT Scan[1]	-	-	2.7%	2.7%
Combination Chest CT Scan	165	1.8%	3.7%	2.7%
Follow-up Mammogram/Ultrasound	615	4.1%	7.3%	8.8%
Lumbar Spine MRI for Low Back Pain	56	42.9%	36.8%	37.2%

Carson Valley Medical Center

1107 Highway 395 Phone: 775-782-1500
Gardnerville, NV 89410
Type: Critical Access Hospitals Emergency Services: Yes
Ownership: Proprietary

Measure	Cases	This Hosp.	State Avg.	U.S. Avg.
Blood Clot Prevention and Treatment				
Anticoagulation Overlap Therapy[5]	-	-	96%	93%
ICU Venous Thromboembolism Prophylaxis[5]	-	-	91%	92%
Incidence of Potentially Preventable VTE[5]	-	-	10%	10%
UFH with Dosages/Platelet Monitoring[5]	-	-	99%	97%
Venous Thromboembolism Prophylaxis[5]	-	-	84%	85%
Warfarin Therapy Discharge Instructions[5]	-	-	90%	75%
Chest Pain/Possible Heart Attack Care				
Aspirin Given Within 24 Hours of Arrival	34	97%	98%	96%
Fibrinolytic Meds Within 30 Min. of Arrival[7]	-	-	40%	58%
Average Time to ECG (minutes)	31	10	9	7
Average Time to Transfer (minutes)[1]	-	-	66	60
Children's Asthma Care				
Received Home Management Plan of Care	-	-	-	88%
Received Reliever Medication	-	-	-	100%
Received Systemic Corticosteroids	-	-	-	100%
Emergency Department				
Admittance Decision Time (minutes)[5]	-	-	151	98
Head CT Results Within 45 Min. of Arrival[5]	-	-	44%	57%
Patients Who Left ER Before Being Seen	9,441	1%	2%	2%
Time from ER Arrival to Admit. (minutes)[5]	-	-	337	274
Time from ER Arrival to Discharge (minutes)[5]	-	-	150	134
Time in ER Before Being Evaluated (minutes)[5]	-	-	22	26
Time to Pain Meds for Fractures (minutes)[5]	-	-	54	57
Heart Attack Care				
Aspirin Given at Discharge[3,7]	-	-	99%	99%
Fibrinolytic Meds Within 30 Min. of Arrival[3,7]	-	-	67%	54%
PCI Within 90 Minutes of Arrival[3,7]	-	-	97%	96%
Statin Prescribed at Discharge[1,3]	-	-	98%	98%
Heart Failure Care				
ACE Inhibitor or ARB for LVSD[1,3]	-	-	97%	97%
Discharge Instructions Given[3]	15	93%	91%	94%
Evaluation of LVS Function[3]	15	100%	99%	99%
Medicare Spending				
Medicare Spending per Patient (ratio)	-	-	1.04	0.98
Pneumonia Care				
Appropriate Initial Antibiotic Given[3]	26	92%	96%	95%
Blood Culture Timing[3]	26	92%	96%	98%
Pregnancy and Delivery Care				
Newborn Deliveries Scheduled Early[5]	-	-	6%	6%
Preventive Care				
Immunization for Influenza[5]	-	-	93%	90%
Immunization for Pneumonia[5]	-	-	94%	92%
Stroke Care				
Anticoagulation Therapy for Atrial Fibrillation[5]	-	-	92%	95%
Antithrombotic Therapy Timing[5]	-	-	97%	98%
Assessed for Rehabilitation[5]	-	-	96%	97%
Discharged on Antithrombotic Therapy[5]	-	-	99%	99%
Discharged on Statin Medication[5]	-	-	95%	94%
Thrombolytic Therapy Timing[5]	-	-	80%	66%
Venous Thromboembolism Prophylaxis[5]	-	-	91%	94%
Written Stroke Educational Materials Given[5]	-	-	87%	88%
Surgical Care Improvement Project				
Appropriate Beta Blocker Usage[1,3]	-	-	96%	98%
Appropriate VTP Within 24 Hours[3]	31	97%	98%	98%
Controlled Postoperative Blood Glucose[3,7]	-	-	97%	97%
Perioperative Temperature Management[3]	37	100%	100%	100%
Prophylactic Antibiotic Selection[3]	26	96%	99%	99%
Prophylactic Antibiotic Selection (Outpatient)	27	100%	98%	98%
Prophylactic Antibiotic Stopped[3]	26	100%	98%	98%
Prophylactic Antibiotic Timing[3]	26	92%	99%	99%
Prophylactic Antibiotic Timing (Outpatient)	27	96%	98%	98%
Urinary Catheter Removal[3]	22	95%	98%	97%
Survey of Patients' Hospital Experiences				
Area Around Room 'Always' Quiet at Night[5]	-	-	57%	61%
Doctors 'Always' Communicated Well[5]	-	-	75%	82%
Home Recovery Information Given[5]	-	-	85%	85%
Hospital Given 9 or 10 on 10 Point Scale[5]	-	-	66%	71%
Meds 'Always' Explained Before Given[5]	-	-	60%	64%
Nurses 'Always' Communicated Well[5]	-	-	72%	79%
Pain 'Always' Well Controlled[5]	-	-	67%	71%
Room and Bathroom 'Always' Clean[5]	-	-	68%	73%
Timely Help 'Always' Received[5]	-	-	59%	68%
Would Definitely Recommend Hospital[5]	-	-	69%	71%
Use of Medical Imaging				
Cardiac Imaging Stress Test before Surgery	149	2.7%	4.8%	5.3%
Combination Abdominal CT Scan	450	6.4%	6.9%	10.5%
Combination Brain/Sinus CT Scan	443	0.9%	2.7%	2.7%
Combination Chest CT Scan	368	4.9%	3.7%	2.7%
Follow-up Mammogram/Ultrasound	495	6.1%	7.3%	8.8%
Lumbar Spine MRI for Low Back Pain	59	32.2%	36.8%	37.2%

Mount Grant General Hospital

First & A Streets Phone: 702-945-2461
Hawthorne, NV 89415
Type: Critical Access Hospitals Emergency Services: Yes
Ownership: Govt - Hospital Dist/Auth

Measure	Cases	This Hosp.	State Avg.	U.S. Avg.
Blood Clot Prevention and Treatment				
Anticoagulation Overlap Therapy[5]	-	-	96%	93%
ICU Venous Thromboembolism Prophylaxis[5]	-	-	91%	92%
Incidence of Potentially Preventable VTE[5]	-	-	10%	10%
UFH with Dosages/Platelet Monitoring[5]	-	-	99%	97%
Venous Thromboembolism Prophylaxis[5]	-	-	84%	85%
Warfarin Therapy Discharge Instructions[5]	-	-	90%	75%
Chest Pain/Possible Heart Attack Care				
Aspirin Given Within 24 Hours of Arrival[1,3]	-	-	98%	96%
Fibrinolytic Meds Within 30 Min. of Arrival[1,3]	-	-	40%	58%
Average Time to ECG (minutes)[1,3]	-	-	9	7
Average Time to Transfer (minutes)[3,7]	-	-	66	60
Children's Asthma Care				
Received Home Management Plan of Care	-	-	-	88%
Received Reliever Medication	-	-	-	100%
Received Systemic Corticosteroids	-	-	-	100%
Emergency Department				
Admittance Decision Time (minutes)[5]	-	-	151	98
Head CT Results Within 45 Min. of Arrival[5]	-	-	44%	57%
Patients Who Left ER Before Being Seen	2,085	2%	2%	2%
Time from ER Arrival to Admit. (minutes)[5]	-	-	337	274
Time from ER Arrival to Discharge (minutes)[5]	-	-	150	134
Time in ER Before Being Evaluated (minutes)[5]	-	-	22	26
Time to Pain Meds for Fractures (minutes)[5]	-	-	54	57
Heart Attack Care				
Aspirin Given at Discharge[5]	-	-	99%	99%
Fibrinolytic Meds Within 30 Min. of Arrival[5]	-	-	67%	54%
PCI Within 90 Minutes of Arrival[5]	-	-	97%	96%

NOTE: Hospital profiles are in alphabetical order by state, then city, then hospital within the city; Rankings exclude hospitals with less than 25 cases except for patient surveys which excludes hospitals with less than 100 cases; (a) 100-299 cases; (1) The number of cases/patients is too few to report; (2) Data submitted were based on a sample of cases/patients; (3) Results are based on a shorter time period than required; (4) Data suppressed by CMS for one or more quarters; (5) Results are not available for this reporting period; (6) Fewer than 100 patients completed the HCAHPS survey; (7) No cases met the criteria for this measure; (8) The lower limit of the confidence interval cannot be calculated if the number of observed infections equals zero; (9) No data are available from the state/territory for this reporting period; (10) The scores shown reflect fewer than 50 completed surveys; (11) There were discrepancies in the data collection process; (12) This measure does not apply to this hospital for this reporting period; (13) Results cannot be calculated for this reporting period; (14) The results for this state are combined with nearby states to protect confidentiality; Please refer to the User's Guide for a full explanation of data.

Measure	Cases	This Hosp.	State Avg.	U.S. Avg.
Statin Prescribed at Discharge[5]	-	-	98%	98%
Heart Failure Care				
ACE Inhibitor or ARB for LVSD[1]	-	-	97%	97%
Discharge Instructions Given[1]	-	-	91%	94%
Evaluation of LVS Function	11	55%	99%	99%
Medicare Spending				
Medicare Spending per Patient (ratio)	-	-	1.04	0.98
Pneumonia Care				
Appropriate Initial Antibiotic Given[1]	-	-	96%	95%
Blood Culture Timing[1]	-	-	96%	98%
Pregnancy and Delivery Care				
Newborn Deliveries Scheduled Early[5]	-	-	6%	6%
Preventive Care				
Immunization for Influenza[5]	-	-	93%	90%
Immunization for Pneumonia[5]	-	-	94%	92%
Stroke Care				
Anticoagulation Therapy for Atrial Fibrillation[5]	-	-	92%	95%
Antithrombotic Therapy Timing[5]	-	-	97%	98%
Assessed for Rehabilitation[5]	-	-	96%	97%
Discharged on Antithrombotic Therapy[5]	-	-	99%	99%
Discharged on Statin Medication[5]	-	-	95%	94%
Thrombolytic Therapy Timing[5]	-	-	80%	66%
Venous Thromboembolism Prophylaxis[5]	-	-	91%	94%
Written Stroke Educational Materials Given[5]	-	-	87%	88%
Surgical Care Improvement Project				
Appropriate Beta Blocker Usage[5]	-	-	96%	98%
Appropriate VTP Within 24 Hours[5]	-	-	98%	98%
Controlled Postoperative Blood Glucose[5]	-	-	97%	97%
Perioperative Temperature Management[5]	-	-	100%	100%
Prophylactic Antibiotic Selection[5]	-	-	99%	99%
Prophylactic Antibiotic Selection (Outpatient)[5]	-	-	98%	98%
Prophylactic Antibiotic Stopped[5]	-	-	98%	98%
Prophylactic Antibiotic Timing[5]	-	-	99%	99%
Prophylactic Antibiotic Timing (Outpatient)[5]	-	-	98%	98%
Urinary Catheter Removal[5]	-	-	98%	97%
Survey of Patients' Hospital Experiences				
Area Around Room 'Always' Quiet at Night[5]	-	-	57%	61%
Doctors 'Always' Communicated Well[5]	-	-	75%	82%
Home Recovery Information Given[5]	-	-	85%	85%
Hospital Given 9 or 10 on 10 Point Scale[5]	-	-	66%	71%
Meds 'Always' Explained Before Given[5]	-	-	60%	64%
Nurses 'Always' Communicated Well[5]	-	-	72%	79%
Pain 'Always' Well Controlled[5]	-	-	67%	71%
Room and Bathroom 'Always' Clean[5]	-	-	68%	73%
Timely Help 'Always' Received[5]	-	-	59%	68%
Would Definitely Recommend Hospital[5]	-	-	69%	71%
Use of Medical Imaging				
Cardiac Imaging Stress Test before Surgery[7]	-	-	4.8%	5.3%
Combination Abdominal CT Scan[1]	-	-	6.9%	10.5%
Combination Brain/Sinus CT Scan[1]	-	-	2.7%	2.7%
Combination Chest CT Scan[1]	-	-	3.7%	2.7%
Follow-up Mammogram/Ultrasound[7]	-	-	7.3%	8.8%
Lumbar Spine MRI for Low Back Pain[1]	-	-	36.8%	37.2%

Saint Rose Dominican Hospitals - Rose De Lima Campus

102 E Lake Mead Dr
Henderson, NV 89015
Phone: 702-616-5000
Fax: 702-616-4820
URL: www.dignityhealth.org/las-vegas
Type: Acute Care Hospitals
Emergency Services: Yes
Ownership: Voluntary non-profit - Church
Beds: 143

Key Personnel:

Radiology. . . . . Steven C Bessen, MD
CEO/President. . . . . Rod A Davis
Operating Room. . . . . Kevin Fradkin
Infection Control. . . . . Ann Jenkins
Quality Assurance . . . . Maureen Kopecky
Intensive Care Unit. . . . . Linda Mayland, RN
Chief of Medical Staff . . . . Matt McMahon, DO
Pediatric In-Patient Care . . . . Hesham A Sirsy, MD

Measure	Cases	This Hosp.	State Avg.	U.S. Avg.
Blood Clot Prevention and Treatment				
Anticoagulation Overlap Therapy[2]	60	100%	96%	93%
ICU Venous Thromboembolism Prophylaxis[2]	70	91%	91%	92%
Incidence of Potentially Preventable VTE[1,2]	-	-	10%	10%
UFH with Dosages/Platelet Monitoring[2]	43	100%	99%	97%
Venous Thromboembolism Prophylaxis[2]	354	90%	84%	85%
Warfarin Therapy Discharge Instructions[2]	36	78%	90%	75%
Chest Pain/Possible Heart Attack Care				
Aspirin Given Within 24 Hours of Arrival	40	98%	98%	96%
Fibrinolytic Meds Within 30 Min. of Arrival[7]	-	-	40%	58%
Average Time to ECG (minutes)	44	10	9	7
Average Time to Transfer (minutes)	25	60	66	60
Children's Asthma Care				
Received Home Management Plan of Care	-	-	-	88%
Received Reliever Medication	-	-	-	100%
Received Systemic Corticosteroids	-	-	-	100%
Emergency Department				
Admittance Decision Time (minutes)[2]	898	253	151	98
Head CT Results Within 45 Min. of Arrival[1]	-	-	44%	57%
Patients Who Left ER Before Being Seen	38,522	0%	2%	2%
Time from ER Arrival to Admit. (minutes)[2]	938	453	337	274
Time from ER Arrival to Discharge (minutes)	359	145	150	134
Time in ER Before Being Evaluated (minutes)	410	20	22	26
Time to Pain Meds for Fractures (minutes)	139	44	54	57
Heart Attack Care				
Aspirin Given at Discharge	68	100%	99%	99%
Fibrinolytic Meds Within 30 Min. of Arrival[7]	-	-	67%	54%
PCI Within 90 Minutes of Arrival[1]	-	-	97%	96%
Statin Prescribed at Discharge	65	100%	98%	98%
Heart Failure Care				
ACE Inhibitor or ARB for LVSD	65	98%	97%	97%
Discharge Instructions Given	113	96%	91%	94%
Evaluation of LVS Function	168	99%	99%	99%
Medicare Spending				
Medicare Spending per Patient (ratio)	-	1.18	1.04	0.98
Pneumonia Care				
Appropriate Initial Antibiotic Given[2]	75	93%	96%	95%
Blood Culture Timing[2]	151	96%	96%	98%
Pregnancy and Delivery Care				
Newborn Deliveries Scheduled Early[7]	-	-	6%	6%
Preventive Care				
Immunization for Influenza[2]	526	95%	93%	90%
Immunization for Pneumonia[2]	757	96%	94%	92%
Stroke Care				
Anticoagulation Therapy for Atrial Fibrillation[1]	-	-	92%	95%
Antithrombotic Therapy Timing	50	96%	97%	98%
Assessed for Rehabilitation	67	96%	96%	97%
Discharged on Antithrombotic Therapy	64	98%	99%	99%
Discharged on Statin Medication	54	89%	95%	94%
Thrombolytic Therapy Timing[1]	-	-	80%	66%
Venous Thromboembolism Prophylaxis	53	92%	91%	94%
Written Stroke Educational Materials Given	41	95%	87%	88%
Surgical Care Improvement Project				
Appropriate Beta Blocker Usage[2]	65	83%	96%	98%
Appropriate VTP Within 24 Hours[2]	246	95%	98%	98%
Controlled Postoperative Blood Glucose[2,7]	-	-	97%	97%
Perioperative Temperature Management[2]	263	100%	100%	100%
Prophylactic Antibiotic Selection[2]	153	98%	99%	99%
Prophylactic Antibiotic Selection (Outpatient)	90	99%	98%	98%
Prophylactic Antibiotic Stopped[2]	145	99%	98%	98%
Prophylactic Antibiotic Timing[2]	153	100%	99%	99%
Prophylactic Antibiotic Timing (Outpatient)	94	94%	98%	98%
Urinary Catheter Removal[2]	164	93%	98%	97%
Survey of Patients' Hospital Experiences				
Area Around Room 'Always' Quiet at Night	300+	46%	57%	61%
Doctors 'Always' Communicated Well	300+	66%	75%	82%
Home Recovery Information Given	300+	85%	85%	85%
Hospital Given 9 or 10 on 10 Point Scale	300+	60%	66%	71%
Meds 'Always' Explained Before Given	300+	57%	60%	64%
Nurses 'Always' Communicated Well	300+	66%	72%	79%
Pain 'Always' Well Controlled	300+	64%	67%	71%
Room and Bathroom 'Always' Clean	300+	66%	68%	73%
Timely Help 'Always' Received	300+	50%	59%	68%
Would Definitely Recommend Hospital	300+	63%	69%	71%
Use of Medical Imaging				
Cardiac Imaging Stress Test before Surgery	171	5.8%	4.8%	5.3%
Combination Abdominal CT Scan	468	5.1%	6.9%	10.5%
Combination Brain/Sinus CT Scan	458	4.1%	2.7%	2.7%
Combination Chest CT Scan	57	0.0%	3.7%	2.7%
Follow-up Mammogram/Ultrasound	99	10.1%	7.3%	8.8%
Lumbar Spine MRI for Low Back Pain[1]	-	-	36.8%	37.2%

Saint Rose Dominican Hospitals - Siena Campus

3001 Saint Rose Parkway
Henderson, NV 89052
Phone: 702-616-5000
URL: www.strosehospitals.org
Type: Acute Care Hospitals
Emergency Services: Yes
Ownership: Proprietary
Beds: 219

Key Personnel:

CEO . . . . James Barrett, Jr
Chief of Medical Staff . . . . Stephen Jones, MD

Measure	Cases	This Hosp.	State Avg.	U.S. Avg.
Blood Clot Prevention and Treatment				
Anticoagulation Overlap Therapy[2]	149	99%	96%	93%
ICU Venous Thromboembolism Prophylaxis[2]	54	94%	91%	92%
Incidence of Potentially Preventable VTE[2]	33	3%	10%	10%
UFH with Dosages/Platelet Monitoring[2]	119	99%	99%	97%
Venous Thromboembolism Prophylaxis[2]	313	93%	84%	85%
Warfarin Therapy Discharge Instructions[2]	97	77%	90%	75%
Chest Pain/Possible Heart Attack Care				
Aspirin Given Within 24 Hours of Arrival	42	100%	98%	96%
Fibrinolytic Meds Within 30 Min. of Arrival[3,7]	-	-	40%	58%
Average Time to ECG (minutes)	42	12	9	7
Average Time to Transfer (minutes)[3,7]	-	-	66	60
Children's Asthma Care				
Received Home Management Plan of Care	-	-	-	88%
Received Reliever Medication	-	-	-	100%
Received Systemic Corticosteroids	-	-	-	100%
Emergency Department				
Admittance Decision Time (minutes)[2]	492	242	151	98
Head CT Results Within 45 Min. of Arrival[1]	-	-	44%	57%
Patients Who Left ER Before Being Seen	64,545	1%	2%	2%
Time from ER Arrival to Admit. (minutes)[2]	528	450	337	274
Time from ER Arrival to Discharge (minutes)	360	162	150	134
Time in ER Before Being Evaluated (minutes)	415	24	22	26
Time to Pain Meds for Fractures (minutes)	251	57	54	57
Heart Attack Care				
Aspirin Given at Discharge[2]	295	99%	99%	99%
Fibrinolytic Meds Within 30 Min. of Arrival[1,2]	-	-	67%	54%
PCI Within 90 Minutes of Arrival[2]	93	97%	97%	96%
Statin Prescribed at Discharge[2]	290	99%	98%	98%
Heart Failure Care				
ACE Inhibitor or ARB for LVSD[2]	105	96%	97%	97%
Discharge Instructions Given[2]	252	92%	91%	94%
Evaluation of LVS Function[2]	322	100%	99%	99%
Medicare Spending				
Medicare Spending per Patient (ratio)	-	1.09	1.04	0.98
Pneumonia Care				
Appropriate Initial Antibiotic Given[2]	86	98%	96%	95%
Blood Culture Timing[2]	178	96%	96%	98%
Pregnancy and Delivery Care				
Newborn Deliveries Scheduled Early[2]	68	6%	6%	6%
Preventive Care				
Immunization for Influenza[2]	506	95%	93%	90%
Immunization for Pneumonia[2]	527	97%	94%	92%
Stroke Care				
Anticoagulation Therapy for Atrial Fibrillation	17	100%	92%	95%
Antithrombotic Therapy Timing	141	99%	97%	98%
Assessed for Rehabilitation	187	93%	96%	97%
Discharged on Antithrombotic Therapy	156	100%	99%	99%
Discharged on Statin Medication	114	94%	95%	94%
Thrombolytic Therapy Timing	14	79%	80%	66%
Venous Thromboembolism Prophylaxis	175	94%	91%	94%
Written Stroke Educational Materials Given	99	98%	87%	88%
Surgical Care Improvement Project				
Appropriate Beta Blocker Usage[2]	219	94%	96%	98%
Appropriate VTP Within 24 Hours[2]	401	99%	98%	98%
Controlled Postoperative Blood Glucose[2]	147	99%	97%	97%

NOTE: Hospital profiles are in alphabetical order by state, then city, then hospital within the city; Rankings exclude hospitals with less than 25 cases except for patient surveys which excludes hospitals with less than 100 cases; (a) 100-299 cases; (1) The number of cases/patients is too few to report; (2) Data submitted were based on a sample of cases/patients; (3) Results are based on a shorter time period than required; (4) Data suppressed by CMS for one or more quarters; (5) Results are not available for this reporting period; (6) Fewer than 100 patients completed the HCAHPS survey; (7) No cases met the criteria for this measure; (8) The lower limit of the confidence interval cannot be calculated if the number of observed infections equals zero; (9) No data are available from the state/territory for this reporting period; (10) The scores shown reflect fewer than 50 completed surveys; (11) There were discrepancies in the data collection process; (12) This measure does not apply to this hospital for this reporting period; (13) Results cannot be calculated for this reporting period; (14) The results for this state are combined with nearby states to protect confidentiality; Please refer to the User's Guide for a full explanation of data.

Measure	Cases	This Hosp.	State Avg.	U.S. Avg.
Perioperative Temperature Management[2]	531	100%	100%	100%
Prophylactic Antibiotic Selection[2]	393	98%	99%	99%
Prophylactic Antibiotic Selection (Outpatient)	625	99%	98%	98%
Prophylactic Antibiotic Stopped[2]	379	98%	98%	98%
Prophylactic Antibiotic Timing[2]	393	98%	99%	99%
Prophylactic Antibiotic Timing (Outpatient)	629	99%	98%	98%
Urinary Catheter Removal[2]	377	97%	98%	97%
Survey of Patients' Hospital Experiences				
Area Around Room 'Always' Quiet at Night	300+	60%	57%	61%
Doctors 'Always' Communicated Well	300+	76%	75%	82%
Home Recovery Information Given	300+	86%	85%	85%
Hospital Given 9 or 10 on 10 Point Scale	300+	75%	66%	71%
Meds 'Always' Explained Before Given	300+	65%	60%	64%
Nurses 'Always' Communicated Well	300+	75%	72%	79%
Pain 'Always' Well Controlled	300+	69%	67%	71%
Room and Bathroom 'Always' Clean	300+	75%	68%	73%
Timely Help 'Always' Received	300+	62%	59%	68%
Would Definitely Recommend Hospital	300+	80%	69%	71%
Use of Medical Imaging				
Cardiac Imaging Stress Test before Surgery	332	6.0%	4.8%	5.3%
Combination Abdominal CT Scan	822	6.0%	6.9%	10.5%
Combination Brain/Sinus CT Scan	951	2.5%	2.7%	2.7%
Combination Chest CT Scan	149	5.4%	3.7%	2.7%
Follow-up Mammogram/Ultrasound	104	6.7%	7.3%	8.8%
Lumbar Spine MRI for Low Back Pain[1]	-	-	36.8%	37.2%

Incline Village Health Center

880 Alder Street
Incline Village, NV 89451
Phone: 775-833-4100
Type: Critical Access Hospitals
Emergency Services: Yes
Ownership: Govt - Hospital Dist/Auth

Measure	Cases	This Hosp.	State Avg.	U.S. Avg.
Blood Clot Prevention and Treatment				
Anticoagulation Overlap Therapy[5]	-	-	96%	93%
ICU Venous Thromboembolism Prophylaxis[5]	-	-	91%	92%
Incidence of Potentially Preventable VTE[5]	-	-	10%	10%
UFH with Dosages/Platelet Monitoring[5]	-	-	99%	97%
Venous Thromboembolism Prophylaxis[5]	-	-	84%	85%
Warfarin Therapy Discharge Instructions[5]	-	-	90%	75%
Chest Pain/Possible Heart Attack Care				
Aspirin Given Within 24 Hours of Arrival[5]	-	-	98%	96%
Fibrinolytic Meds Within 30 Min. of Arrival[5]	-	-	40%	58%
Average Time to ECG (minutes)[5]	-	-	9	7
Average Time to Transfer (minutes)[5]	-	-	66	60
Children's Asthma Care				
Received Home Management Plan of Care	-	-	-	88%
Received Reliever Medication	-	-	-	100%
Received Systemic Corticosteroids	-	-	-	100%
Emergency Department				
Admittance Decision Time (minutes)[1,3]	-	-	151	98
Head CT Results Within 45 Min. of Arrival[5]	-	-	44%	57%
Patients Who Left ER Before Being Seen[5]	-	-	2%	2%
Time from ER Arrival to Admit. (minutes)[1,3]	-	-	337	274
Time from ER Arrival to Discharge (minutes)[5]	-	-	150	134
Time in ER Before Being Evaluated (minutes)[5]	-	-	22	26
Time to Pain Meds for Fractures (minutes)[5]	-	-	54	57
Heart Attack Care				
Aspirin Given at Discharge[5]	-	-	99%	99%
Fibrinolytic Meds Within 30 Min. of Arrival[5]	-	-	67%	54%
PCI Within 90 Minutes of Arrival[5]	-	-	97%	96%
Statin Prescribed at Discharge[5]	-	-	98%	98%
Heart Failure Care				
ACE Inhibitor or ARB for LVSD[5]	-	-	97%	97%
Discharge Instructions Given[5]	-	-	91%	94%
Evaluation of LVS Function[5]	-	-	99%	99%
Medicare Spending				
Medicare Spending per Patient (ratio)	-	-	1.04	0.98
Pneumonia Care				
Appropriate Initial Antibiotic Given[5]	-	-	96%	95%
Blood Culture Timing[5]	-	-	96%	98%
Pregnancy and Delivery Care				
Newborn Deliveries Scheduled Early[5]	-	-	6%	6%
Preventive Care				
Immunization for Influenza[1,3]	-	-	93%	90%
Immunization for Pneumonia[1,3]	-	-	94%	92%
Stroke Care				
Anticoagulation Therapy for Atrial Fibrillation[5]	-	-	92%	95%
Antithrombotic Therapy Timing[5]	-	-	97%	98%
Assessed for Rehabilitation[5]	-	-	96%	97%
Discharged on Antithrombotic Therapy[5]	-	-	99%	99%
Discharged on Statin Medication[5]	-	-	95%	94%
Thrombolytic Therapy Timing[5]	-	-	80%	66%
Venous Thromboembolism Prophylaxis[5]	-	-	91%	94%
Written Stroke Educational Materials Given[5]	-	-	87%	88%
Surgical Care Improvement Project				
Appropriate Beta Blocker Usage[5]	-	-	96%	98%
Appropriate VTP Within 24 Hours[5]	-	-	98%	98%
Controlled Postoperative Blood Glucose[5]	-	-	97%	97%
Perioperative Temperature Management[5]	-	-	100%	100%
Prophylactic Antibiotic Selection[5]	-	-	99%	99%
Prophylactic Antibiotic Selection (Outpatient)[5]	-	-	98%	98%
Prophylactic Antibiotic Stopped[5]	-	-	98%	98%
Prophylactic Antibiotic Timing[5]	-	-	99%	99%
Prophylactic Antibiotic Timing (Outpatient)[5]	-	-	98%	98%
Urinary Catheter Removal[5]	-	-	98%	97%
Survey of Patients' Hospital Experiences				
Area Around Room 'Always' Quiet at Night[5]	-	-	57%	61%
Doctors 'Always' Communicated Well[5]	-	-	75%	82%
Home Recovery Information Given[5]	-	-	85%	85%
Hospital Given 9 or 10 on 10 Point Scale[5]	-	-	66%	71%
Meds 'Always' Explained Before Given[5]	-	-	60%	64%
Nurses 'Always' Communicated Well[5]	-	-	72%	79%
Pain 'Always' Well Controlled[5]	-	-	67%	71%
Room and Bathroom 'Always' Clean[5]	-	-	68%	73%
Timely Help 'Always' Received[5]	-	-	59%	68%
Would Definitely Recommend Hospital[5]	-	-	69%	71%
Use of Medical Imaging				
Cardiac Imaging Stress Test before Surgery[7]	-	-	4.8%	5.3%
Combination Abdominal CT Scan	61	1.6%	6.9%	10.5%
Combination Brain/Sinus CT Scan[1]	-	-	2.7%	2.7%
Combination Chest CT Scan[1]	-	-	3.7%	2.7%
Follow-up Mammogram/Ultrasound[7]	-	-	7.3%	8.8%
Lumbar Spine MRI for Low Back Pain[7]	-	-	36.8%	37.2%

Centennial Hills Hospital Medical Center

6900 N Durango Dr
Las Vegas, NV 89149
Phone: 702-835-9700
URL: www.centennialhillshospital.com
Type: Acute Care Hospitals
Emergency Services: Yes
Ownership: Voluntary non-profit - Private
Beds: 171
Key Personnel:
CEO . . . . Sajit Pullarkat

Measure	Cases	This Hosp.	State Avg.	U.S. Avg.
Blood Clot Prevention and Treatment				
Anticoagulation Overlap Therapy[2]	87	97%	96%	93%
ICU Venous Thromboembolism Prophylaxis[2]	57	79%	91%	92%
Incidence of Potentially Preventable VTE[2]	11	9%	10%	10%
UFH with Dosages/Platelet Monitoring[2]	70	99%	99%	97%
Venous Thromboembolism Prophylaxis[2]	292	77%	84%	85%
Warfarin Therapy Discharge Instructions[2]	59	95%	90%	75%
Chest Pain/Possible Heart Attack Care				
Aspirin Given Within 24 Hours of Arrival[1,3]	-	-	98%	96%
Fibrinolytic Meds Within 30 Min. of Arrival[5]	-	-	40%	58%
Average Time to ECG (minutes)[1,3]	-	-	9	7
Average Time to Transfer (minutes)[5]	-	-	66	60
Children's Asthma Care				
Received Home Management Plan of Care	-	-	-	88%
Received Reliever Medication	-	-	-	100%
Received Systemic Corticosteroids	-	-	-	100%
Emergency Department				
Admittance Decision Time (minutes)[2]	686	176	151	98
Head CT Results Within 45 Min. of Arrival	16	50%	44%	57%
Patients Who Left ER Before Being Seen	39,474	4%	2%	2%
Time from ER Arrival to Admit. (minutes)[2]	690	392	337	274
Time from ER Arrival to Discharge (minutes)	350	178	150	134
Time in ER Before Being Evaluated (minutes)	400	36	22	26
Time to Pain Meds for Fractures (minutes)	170	70	54	57
Heart Attack Care				
Aspirin Given at Discharge[2]	145	99%	99%	99%
Fibrinolytic Meds Within 30 Min. of Arrival[2,7]	-	-	67%	54%
PCI Within 90 Minutes of Arrival[2]	34	94%	97%	96%
Statin Prescribed at Discharge[2]	144	94%	98%	98%
Heart Failure Care				
ACE Inhibitor or ARB for LVSD	68	97%	97%	97%
Discharge Instructions Given	173	85%	91%	94%
Evaluation of LVS Function	208	100%	99%	99%
Medicare Spending				
Medicare Spending per Patient (ratio)	-	1.10	1.04	0.98
Pneumonia Care				
Appropriate Initial Antibiotic Given[2]	105	97%	96%	95%
Blood Culture Timing[2]	113	98%	96%	98%
Pregnancy and Delivery Care				
Newborn Deliveries Scheduled Early[2]	41	5%	6%	6%
Preventive Care				
Immunization for Influenza[2]	550	89%	93%	90%
Immunization for Pneumonia[2]	550	92%	94%	92%
Stroke Care				
Anticoagulation Therapy for Atrial Fibrillation[1]	-	-	92%	95%
Antithrombotic Therapy Timing	63	97%	97%	98%
Assessed for Rehabilitation	68	88%	96%	97%
Discharged on Antithrombotic Therapy	60	100%	99%	99%
Discharged on Statin Medication	43	100%	95%	94%
Thrombolytic Therapy Timing[1]	-	-	80%	66%
Venous Thromboembolism Prophylaxis	68	81%	91%	94%
Written Stroke Educational Materials Given	42	69%	87%	88%
Surgical Care Improvement Project				
Appropriate Beta Blocker Usage[2]	91	99%	96%	98%
Appropriate VTP Within 24 Hours[2]	336	98%	98%	98%
Controlled Postoperative Blood Glucose[2,7]	-	-	97%	97%
Perioperative Temperature Management[2]	387	100%	100%	100%
Prophylactic Antibiotic Selection[2]	221	96%	99%	99%
Prophylactic Antibiotic Selection (Outpatient)	255	94%	98%	98%
Prophylactic Antibiotic Stopped[2]	219	98%	98%	98%
Prophylactic Antibiotic Timing[2]	221	99%	99%	99%
Prophylactic Antibiotic Timing (Outpatient)	258	98%	98%	98%
Urinary Catheter Removal[2]	178	95%	98%	97%
Survey of Patients' Hospital Experiences				
Area Around Room 'Always' Quiet at Night	300+	62%	57%	61%
Doctors 'Always' Communicated Well	300+	71%	75%	82%
Home Recovery Information Given	300+	83%	85%	85%
Hospital Given 9 or 10 on 10 Point Scale	300+	64%	66%	71%
Meds 'Always' Explained Before Given	300+	50%	60%	64%
Nurses 'Always' Communicated Well	300+	68%	72%	79%
Pain 'Always' Well Controlled	300+	64%	67%	71%
Room and Bathroom 'Always' Clean	300+	63%	68%	73%
Timely Help 'Always' Received	300+	54%	59%	68%
Would Definitely Recommend Hospital	300+	69%	69%	71%
Use of Medical Imaging				
Cardiac Imaging Stress Test before Surgery	155	7.1%	4.8%	5.3%
Combination Abdominal CT Scan	383	3.7%	6.9%	10.5%
Combination Brain/Sinus CT Scan	395	1.5%	2.7%	2.7%
Combination Chest CT Scan[1]	-	-	3.7%	2.7%
Follow-up Mammogram/Ultrasound	93	9.7%	7.3%	8.8%
Lumbar Spine MRI for Low Back Pain[1]	-	-	36.8%	37.2%

Desert Springs Hospital

2075 East Flamingo Road
Las Vegas, NV 89119
Phone: 702-369-7600
Fax: 702-894-5654
URL: www.desertspringshospital.net/p12.html
Type: Acute Care Hospitals
Emergency Services: Yes
Ownership: Proprietary
Beds: 286

Measure	Cases	This Hosp.	State Avg.	U.S. Avg.
Blood Clot Prevention and Treatment				
Anticoagulation Overlap Therapy[2]	36	94%	96%	93%
ICU Venous Thromboembolism Prophylaxis[2]	98	86%	91%	92%
Incidence of Potentially Preventable VTE[1,2]	-	-	10%	10%
UFH with Dosages/Platelet Monitoring[2]	29	100%	99%	97%

NOTE: Hospital profiles are in alphabetical order by state, then city, then hospital within the city; Rankings exclude hospitals with less than 25 cases except for patient surveys which excludes hospitals with less than 100 cases; (a) 100-299 cases; (1) The number of cases/patients is too few to report; (2) Data submitted were based on a sample of cases/patients; (3) Results are based on a shorter time period than required; (4) Data suppressed by CMS for one or more quarters; (5) Results are not available for this reporting period; (6) Fewer than 100 patients completed the HCAHPS survey; (7) No cases met the criteria for this measure; (8) The lower limit of the confidence interval cannot be calculated if the number of observed infections equals zero; (9) No data are available from the state/territory for this reporting period; (10) The scores shown reflect fewer than 50 completed surveys; (11) There were discrepancies in the data collection process; (12) This measure does not apply to this hospital for this reporting period; (13) Results cannot be calculated for this reporting period; (14) The results for this state are combined with nearby states to protect confidentiality; Please refer to the User's Guide for a full explanation of data.

Measure	Cases	This Hosp.	State Avg.	U.S. Avg.
Venous Thromboembolism Prophylaxis[2]	342	77%	84%	85%
Warfarin Therapy Discharge Instructions[2]	18	83%	90%	75%
Chest Pain/Possible Heart Attack Care				
Aspirin Given Within 24 Hours of Arrival[1,3]	-	-	98%	96%
Fibrinolytic Meds Within 30 Min. of Arrival[5]	-	-	40%	58%
Average Time to ECG (minutes)[1,3]	-	-	9	7
Average Time to Transfer (minutes)[5]	-	-	66	60
Children's Asthma Care				
Received Home Management Plan of Care	-	-	-	88%
Received Reliever Medication	-	-	-	100%
Received Systemic Corticosteroids	-	-	-	100%
Emergency Department				
Admittance Decision Time (minutes)[2]	980	405	151	98
Head CT Results Within 45 Min. of Arrival	20	50%	44%	57%
Patients Who Left ER Before Being Seen	37,077	3%	2%	2%
Time from ER Arrival to Admit. (minutes)[2]	983	637	337	274
Time from ER Arrival to Discharge (minutes)	330	228	150	134
Time in ER Before Being Evaluated (minutes)	407	42	22	26
Time to Pain Meds for Fractures (minutes)	88	88	54	57
Heart Attack Care				
Aspirin Given at Discharge[2]	258	100%	99%	99%
Fibrinolytic Meds Within 30 Min. of Arrival[2,7]	-	-	67%	54%
PCI Within 90 Minutes of Arrival[2]	51	96%	97%	96%
Statin Prescribed at Discharge[2]	259	98%	98%	98%
Heart Failure Care				
ACE Inhibitor or ARB for LVSD[2]	109	96%	97%	97%
Discharge Instructions Given[2]	226	92%	91%	94%
Evaluation of LVS Function[2]	290	100%	99%	99%
Medicare Spending				
Medicare Spending per Patient (ratio)	-	1.14	1.04	0.98
Pneumonia Care				
Appropriate Initial Antibiotic Given[2]	84	98%	96%	95%
Blood Culture Timing[2]	69	93%	96%	98%
Pregnancy and Delivery Care				
Newborn Deliveries Scheduled Early[7]	-	-	6%	6%
Preventive Care				
Immunization for Influenza[2]	605	97%	93%	90%
Immunization for Pneumonia[2]	864	96%	94%	92%
Stroke Care				
Anticoagulation Therapy for Atrial Fibrillation[2]	14	86%	92%	95%
Antithrombotic Therapy Timing[2]	92	95%	97%	98%
Assessed for Rehabilitation[2]	107	98%	96%	97%
Discharged on Antithrombotic Therapy[2]	103	98%	99%	99%
Discharged on Statin Medication[2]	78	96%	95%	94%
Thrombolytic Therapy Timing[2]	15	100%	80%	66%
Venous Thromboembolism Prophylaxis[2]	109	77%	91%	94%
Written Stroke Educational Materials Given[2]	63	67%	87%	88%
Surgical Care Improvement Project				
Appropriate Beta Blocker Usage[2]	173	99%	96%	98%
Appropriate VTP Within 24 Hours[2]	232	99%	98%	98%
Controlled Postoperative Blood Glucose[2]	124	98%	97%	97%
Perioperative Temperature Management[2]	315	100%	100%	100%
Prophylactic Antibiotic Selection[2]	274	100%	99%	99%
Prophylactic Antibiotic Selection (Outpatient)	240	99%	98%	98%
Prophylactic Antibiotic Stopped[2]	260	96%	98%	98%
Prophylactic Antibiotic Timing[2]	275	99%	99%	99%
Prophylactic Antibiotic Timing (Outpatient)	243	99%	98%	98%
Urinary Catheter Removal[2]	221	100%	98%	97%
Survey of Patients' Hospital Experiences				
Area Around Room 'Always' Quiet at Night	300+	51%	57%	61%
Doctors 'Always' Communicated Well	300+	70%	75%	82%
Home Recovery Information Given	300+	81%	85%	85%
Hospital Given 9 or 10 on 10 Point Scale	300+	57%	66%	71%
Meds 'Always' Explained Before Given	300+	49%	60%	64%
Nurses 'Always' Communicated Well	300+	68%	72%	79%
Pain 'Always' Well Controlled	300+	66%	67%	71%
Room and Bathroom 'Always' Clean	300+	63%	68%	73%
Timely Help 'Always' Received	300+	53%	59%	68%
Would Definitely Recommend Hospital	300+	60%	69%	71%
Use of Medical Imaging				
Cardiac Imaging Stress Test before Surgery	171	5.8%	4.8%	5.3%
Combination Abdominal CT Scan	363	2.8%	6.9%	10.5%
Combination Brain/Sinus CT Scan[1]	-	-	2.7%	2.7%
Combination Chest CT Scan[1]	-	-	3.7%	2.7%
Follow-up Mammogram/Ultrasound[7]	-	-	7.3%	8.8%
Lumbar Spine MRI for Low Back Pain[7]	-	-	36.8%	37.2%

Mountainview Hospital

3100 N Tenaya Way
Las Vegas, NV 89128
Phone: 702-255-5065
Fax: 702-255-5074
URL: www.mountainview-hospital.com
Type: Acute Care Hospitals
Emergency Services: Yes
Ownership: Proprietary
Beds: 235
Key Personnel:
Chief of Medical Staff. . . . . Elvira B Acosta
Radiology. . . . . Troy Belle
Coronary Care . . . . Dena Dzierbicki
CEO/President. . . . . Mark J Howard

Measure	Cases	This Hosp.	State Avg.	U.S. Avg.
Blood Clot Prevention and Treatment				
Anticoagulation Overlap Therapy[2]	162	98%	96%	93%
ICU Venous Thromboembolism Prophylaxis[2]	102	87%	91%	92%
Incidence of Potentially Preventable VTE[2]	32	3%	10%	10%
UFH with Dosages/Platelet Monitoring[2]	112	99%	99%	97%
Venous Thromboembolism Prophylaxis[2]	365	80%	84%	85%
Warfarin Therapy Discharge Instructions[2]	120	88%	90%	75%
Chest Pain/Possible Heart Attack Care				
Aspirin Given Within 24 Hours of Arrival	20	100%	98%	96%
Fibrinolytic Meds Within 30 Min. of Arrival[7]	-	-	40%	58%
Average Time to ECG (minutes)	20	6	9	7
Average Time to Transfer (minutes)[7]	-	-	66	60
Children's Asthma Care				
Received Home Management Plan of Care	-	-	-	88%
Received Reliever Medication	-	-	-	100%
Received Systemic Corticosteroids	-	-	-	100%
Emergency Department				
Admittance Decision Time (minutes)[2]	835	210	151	98
Head CT Results Within 45 Min. of Arrival[1]	-	-	44%	57%
Patients Who Left ER Before Being Seen	49,073	0%	2%	2%
Time from ER Arrival to Admit. (minutes)[2]	835	350	337	274
Time from ER Arrival to Discharge (minutes)	371	180	150	134
Time in ER Before Being Evaluated (minutes)	463	15	22	26
Time to Pain Meds for Fractures (minutes)	122	56	54	57
Heart Attack Care				
Aspirin Given at Discharge	257	100%	99%	99%
Fibrinolytic Meds Within 30 Min. of Arrival[7]	-	-	67%	54%
PCI Within 90 Minutes of Arrival	57	95%	97%	96%
Statin Prescribed at Discharge	252	99%	98%	98%
Heart Failure Care				
ACE Inhibitor or ARB for LVSD[2]	150	99%	97%	97%
Discharge Instructions Given[2]	352	96%	91%	94%
Evaluation of LVS Function[2]	438	100%	99%	99%
Medicare Spending				
Medicare Spending per Patient (ratio)	-	1.09	1.04	0.98
Pneumonia Care				
Appropriate Initial Antibiotic Given[2]	59	100%	96%	95%
Blood Culture Timing[2]	157	99%	96%	98%
Pregnancy and Delivery Care				
Newborn Deliveries Scheduled Early[2]	37	3%	6%	6%
Preventive Care				
Immunization for Influenza[2]	642	100%	93%	90%
Immunization for Pneumonia[2]	887	99%	94%	92%
Stroke Care				
Anticoagulation Therapy for Atrial Fibrillation[2]	14	100%	92%	95%
Antithrombotic Therapy Timing[2]	104	97%	97%	98%
Assessed for Rehabilitation[2]	118	97%	96%	97%
Discharged on Antithrombotic Therapy[2]	108	100%	99%	99%
Discharged on Statin Medication[2]	84	96%	95%	94%
Thrombolytic Therapy Timing[1,2]	-	-	80%	66%
Venous Thromboembolism Prophylaxis[2]	122	98%	91%	94%
Written Stroke Educational Materials Given[2]	68	100%	87%	88%
Surgical Care Improvement Project				
Appropriate Beta Blocker Usage[2]	205	100%	96%	98%
Appropriate VTP Within 24 Hours[2]	446	100%	98%	98%
Controlled Postoperative Blood Glucose[2]	130	100%	97%	97%
Perioperative Temperature Management[2]	615	100%	100%	100%
Prophylactic Antibiotic Selection[2]	449	100%	99%	99%
Prophylactic Antibiotic Selection (Outpatient)	484	100%	98%	98%
Prophylactic Antibiotic Stopped[2]	426	100%	98%	98%
Prophylactic Antibiotic Timing[2]	449	100%	99%	99%
Prophylactic Antibiotic Timing (Outpatient)	484	100%	98%	98%
Urinary Catheter Removal[2]	308	100%	98%	97%
Survey of Patients' Hospital Experiences				
Area Around Room 'Always' Quiet at Night	300+	59%	57%	61%
Doctors 'Always' Communicated Well	300+	71%	75%	82%
Home Recovery Information Given	300+	83%	85%	85%
Hospital Given 9 or 10 on 10 Point Scale	300+	64%	66%	71%
Meds 'Always' Explained Before Given	300+	57%	60%	64%
Nurses 'Always' Communicated Well	300+	71%	72%	79%
Pain 'Always' Well Controlled	300+	66%	67%	71%
Room and Bathroom 'Always' Clean	300+	70%	68%	73%
Timely Help 'Always' Received	300+	59%	59%	68%
Would Definitely Recommend Hospital	300+	68%	69%	71%
Use of Medical Imaging				
Cardiac Imaging Stress Test before Surgery	188	5.3%	4.8%	5.3%
Combination Abdominal CT Scan	662	4.4%	6.9%	10.5%
Combination Brain/Sinus CT Scan	756	3.4%	2.7%	2.7%
Combination Chest CT Scan	372	1.9%	3.7%	2.7%
Follow-up Mammogram/Ultrasound	358	10.1%	7.3%	8.8%
Lumbar Spine MRI for Low Back Pain[1]	-	-	36.8%	37.2%

Saint Rose Dominican Hospitals - San Martin Campus

8280 W Warm Springs Road
Las Vegas, NV 89113
Phone: 702-616-5509
URL: www.strosehospitals.org
Type: Acute Care Hospitals
Emergency Services: Yes
Ownership: Voluntary non-profit - Church
Beds: 147
Key Personnel:
President/CEO. . . . . Rod Davis

Measure	Cases	This Hosp.	State Avg.	U.S. Avg.
Blood Clot Prevention and Treatment				
Anticoagulation Overlap Therapy[2]	76	97%	96%	93%
ICU Venous Thromboembolism Prophylaxis[2]	63	97%	91%	92%
Incidence of Potentially Preventable VTE[2]	11	0%	10%	10%
UFH with Dosages/Platelet Monitoring[2]	56	100%	99%	97%
Venous Thromboembolism Prophylaxis[2]	363	93%	84%	85%
Warfarin Therapy Discharge Instructions[2]	51	90%	90%	75%
Chest Pain/Possible Heart Attack Care				
Aspirin Given Within 24 Hours of Arrival[1,3]	-	-	98%	96%
Fibrinolytic Meds Within 30 Min. of Arrival[5]	-	-	40%	58%
Average Time to ECG (minutes)[1,3]	-	-	9	7
Average Time to Transfer (minutes)[5]	-	-	66	60
Children's Asthma Care				
Received Home Management Plan of Care	-	-	-	88%
Received Reliever Medication	-	-	-	100%
Received Systemic Corticosteroids	-	-	-	100%
Emergency Department				
Admittance Decision Time (minutes)[2]	575	116	151	98
Head CT Results Within 45 Min. of Arrival[1]	-	-	44%	57%
Patients Who Left ER Before Being Seen	26,449	1%	2%	2%
Time from ER Arrival to Admit. (minutes)[2]	632	283	337	274
Time from ER Arrival to Discharge (minutes)	376	129	150	134
Time in ER Before Being Evaluated (minutes)	432	14	22	26
Time to Pain Meds for Fractures (minutes)	90	39	54	57
Heart Attack Care				
Aspirin Given at Discharge	87	98%	99%	99%
Fibrinolytic Meds Within 30 Min. of Arrival[7]	-	-	67%	54%
PCI Within 90 Minutes of Arrival	16	100%	97%	96%
Statin Prescribed at Discharge	83	99%	98%	98%
Heart Failure Care				
ACE Inhibitor or ARB for LVSD	65	91%	97%	97%
Discharge Instructions Given	147	97%	91%	94%
Evaluation of LVS Function	184	99%	99%	99%
Medicare Spending				
Medicare Spending per Patient (ratio)	-	1.18	1.04	0.98
Pneumonia Care				
Appropriate Initial Antibiotic Given[2]	73	92%	96%	95%

NOTE: Hospital profiles are in alphabetical order by state, then city, then hospital within the city; Rankings exclude hospitals with less than 25 cases except for patient surveys which excludes hospitals with less than 100 cases; (a) 100-299 cases; (1) The number of cases/patients is too few to report; (2) Data submitted were based on a sample of cases/patients; (3) Results are based on a shorter time period than required; (4) Data suppressed by CMS for one or more quarters; (5) Results are not available for this reporting period; (6) Fewer than 100 patients completed the HCAHPS survey; (7) No cases met the criteria for this measure; (8) The lower limit of the confidence interval cannot be calculated if the number of observed infections equals zero; (9) No data are available from the state/territory for this reporting period; (10) The scores shown reflect fewer than 50 completed surveys; (11) There were discrepancies in the data collection process; (12) This measure does not apply to this hospital for this reporting period; (13) Results cannot be calculated for this reporting period; (14) The results for this state are combined with nearby states to protect confidentiality; Please refer to the User's Guide for a full explanation of data.

Measure	Cases	This Hosp.	State Avg.	U.S. Avg.
Blood Culture Timing[2]	155	96%	96%	98%
Pregnancy and Delivery Care				
Newborn Deliveries Scheduled Early[2]	46	15%	6%	6%
Preventive Care				
Immunization for Influenza[2]	548	98%	93%	90%
Immunization for Pneumonia[2]	630	95%	94%	92%
Stroke Care				
Anticoagulation Therapy for Atrial Fibrillation[1]	-	-	92%	95%
Antithrombotic Therapy Timing	47	96%	97%	98%
Assessed for Rehabilitation	48	98%	96%	97%
Discharged on Antithrombotic Therapy	46	100%	99%	99%
Discharged on Statin Medication	40	90%	95%	94%
Thrombolytic Therapy Timing[1]	-	-	80%	66%
Venous Thromboembolism Prophylaxis	46	100%	91%	94%
Written Stroke Educational Materials Given	17	94%	87%	88%
Surgical Care Improvement Project				
Appropriate Beta Blocker Usage[2]	169	97%	96%	98%
Appropriate VTP Within 24 Hours[2]	278	95%	98%	98%
Controlled Postoperative Blood Glucose[2]	146	97%	97%	97%
Perioperative Temperature Management[2]	426	100%	100%	100%
Prophylactic Antibiotic Selection[2]	357	99%	99%	99%
Prophylactic Antibiotic Selection (Outpatient)	278	98%	98%	98%
Prophylactic Antibiotic Stopped[2]	335	97%	98%	98%
Prophylactic Antibiotic Timing[2]	357	99%	99%	99%
Prophylactic Antibiotic Timing (Outpatient)	279	97%	98%	98%
Urinary Catheter Removal[2]	311	98%	98%	97%
Survey of Patients' Hospital Experiences				
Area Around Room 'Always' Quiet at Night	300+	64%	57%	61%
Doctors 'Always' Communicated Well	300+	76%	75%	82%
Home Recovery Information Given	300+	86%	85%	85%
Hospital Given 9 or 10 on 10 Point Scale	300+	76%	66%	71%
Meds 'Always' Explained Before Given	300+	60%	60%	64%
Nurses 'Always' Communicated Well	300+	73%	72%	79%
Pain 'Always' Well Controlled	300+	69%	67%	71%
Room and Bathroom 'Always' Clean	300+	70%	68%	73%
Timely Help 'Always' Received	300+	58%	59%	68%
Would Definitely Recommend Hospital	300+	78%	69%	71%
Use of Medical Imaging				
Cardiac Imaging Stress Test before Surgery	226	7.5%	4.8%	5.3%
Combination Abdominal CT Scan	338	4.4%	6.9%	10.5%
Combination Brain/Sinus CT Scan	319	5.3%	2.7%	2.7%
Combination Chest CT Scan[1]	-	-	3.7%	2.7%
Follow-up Mammogram/Ultrasound[1]	-	-	7.3%	8.8%
Lumbar Spine MRI for Low Back Pain[1]	-	-	36.8%	37.2%

Southern Hills Hospital & Medical Center

9300 West Sunset Rd
Las Vegas, NV 89148
Phone: 702-880-2100
Fax: 702-880-2961
URL: www.southernhillshospital.com
Type: Acute Care Hospitals
Emergency Services: Yes
Ownership: Voluntary non-profit - Private
Beds: 139

Key Personnel:
CEO/President. . . . . Michael Johnson
Chief of Medical Staff . . . . Timothy Trainor

Measure	Cases	This Hosp.	State Avg.	U.S. Avg.
Blood Clot Prevention and Treatment				
Anticoagulation Overlap Therapy[2]	61	98%	96%	93%
ICU Venous Thromboembolism Prophylaxis[2]	108	99%	91%	92%
Incidence of Potentially Preventable VTE[2]	11	9%	10%	10%
UFH with Dosages/Platelet Monitoring[2]	55	100%	99%	97%
Venous Thromboembolism Prophylaxis[2]	254	100%	84%	85%
Warfarin Therapy Discharge Instructions[2]	41	100%	90%	75%
Chest Pain/Possible Heart Attack Care				
Aspirin Given Within 24 Hours of Arrival	19	95%	98%	96%
Fibrinolytic Meds Within 30 Min. of Arrival[3,7]	-	-	40%	58%
Average Time to ECG (minutes)	20	8	9	7
Average Time to Transfer (minutes)[3,7]	-	-	66	60
Children's Asthma Care				
Received Home Management Plan of Care	-	-	-	88%
Received Reliever Medication	-	-	-	100%
Received Systemic Corticosteroids	-	-	-	100%
Emergency Department				
Admittance Decision Time (minutes)[2]	584	165	151	98
Head CT Results Within 45 Min. of Arrival[1]	-	-	44%	57%
Patients Who Left ER Before Being Seen	23,464	1%	2%	2%
Time from ER Arrival to Admit. (minutes)[2]	584	244	337	274
Time from ER Arrival to Discharge (minutes)	392	134	150	134
Time in ER Before Being Evaluated (minutes)	443	10	22	26
Time to Pain Meds for Fractures (minutes)	85	32	54	57
Heart Attack Care				
Aspirin Given at Discharge	47	100%	99%	99%
Fibrinolytic Meds Within 30 Min. of Arrival[7]	-	-	67%	54%
PCI Within 90 Minutes of Arrival	19	100%	97%	96%
Statin Prescribed at Discharge	48	100%	98%	98%
Heart Failure Care				
ACE Inhibitor or ARB for LVSD	36	100%	97%	97%
Discharge Instructions Given	88	100%	91%	94%
Evaluation of LVS Function	106	100%	99%	99%
Medicare Spending				
Medicare Spending per Patient (ratio)	-	1.08	1.04	0.98
Pneumonia Care				
Appropriate Initial Antibiotic Given	63	98%	96%	95%
Blood Culture Timing	135	100%	96%	98%
Pregnancy and Delivery Care				
Newborn Deliveries Scheduled Early	112	4%	6%	6%
Preventive Care				
Immunization for Influenza[2]	528	99%	93%	90%
Immunization for Pneumonia[2]	583	99%	94%	92%
Stroke Care				
Anticoagulation Therapy for Atrial Fibrillation[1,2]	-	-	92%	95%
Antithrombotic Therapy Timing[2]	34	100%	97%	98%
Assessed for Rehabilitation[2]	40	100%	96%	97%
Discharged on Antithrombotic Therapy[2]	39	100%	99%	99%
Discharged on Statin Medication[2]	32	97%	95%	94%
Thrombolytic Therapy Timing[1,2]	-	-	80%	66%
Venous Thromboembolism Prophylaxis[2]	41	100%	91%	94%
Written Stroke Educational Materials Given[2]	30	100%	87%	88%
Surgical Care Improvement Project				
Appropriate Beta Blocker Usage[2]	85	98%	96%	98%
Appropriate VTP Within 24 Hours[2]	328	100%	98%	98%
Controlled Postoperative Blood Glucose[2,7]	-	-	97%	97%
Perioperative Temperature Management[2]	402	100%	100%	100%
Prophylactic Antibiotic Selection[2]	261	98%	99%	99%
Prophylactic Antibiotic Selection (Outpatient)	156	99%	98%	98%
Prophylactic Antibiotic Stopped[2]	256	100%	98%	98%
Prophylactic Antibiotic Timing[2]	261	100%	99%	99%
Prophylactic Antibiotic Timing (Outpatient)	160	98%	98%	98%
Urinary Catheter Removal[2]	260	100%	98%	97%
Survey of Patients' Hospital Experiences				
Area Around Room 'Always' Quiet at Night	300+	63%	57%	61%
Doctors 'Always' Communicated Well	300+	74%	75%	82%
Home Recovery Information Given	300+	85%	85%	85%
Hospital Given 9 or 10 on 10 Point Scale	300+	67%	66%	71%
Meds 'Always' Explained Before Given	300+	57%	60%	64%
Nurses 'Always' Communicated Well	300+	71%	72%	79%
Pain 'Always' Well Controlled	300+	67%	67%	71%
Room and Bathroom 'Always' Clean	300+	70%	68%	73%
Timely Help 'Always' Received	300+	59%	59%	68%
Would Definitely Recommend Hospital	300+	69%	69%	71%
Use of Medical Imaging				
Cardiac Imaging Stress Test before Surgery	94	3.2%	4.8%	5.3%
Combination Abdominal CT Scan	226	1.8%	6.9%	10.5%
Combination Brain/Sinus CT Scan[1]	-	-	2.7%	2.7%
Combination Chest CT Scan	128	3.1%	3.7%	2.7%
Follow-up Mammogram/Ultrasound[1]	-	-	7.3%	8.8%
Lumbar Spine MRI for Low Back Pain[1]	-	-	36.8%	37.2%

Spring Valley Hospital Medical Center

5400 South Rainbow Blvd
Las Vegas, NV 89118
Phone: 702-853-3000
Fax: 702-853-3340
URL: www.springvalleyhospital.com
Type: Acute Care Hospitals
Emergency Services: Yes
Ownership: Proprietary
Beds: 210

Key Personnel:
Radiology. . . . . Rajneesh Agrawal, MD
Anesthesiology. . . . . John Brouwers, MD
Emergency Room . . . . Kathleen Cornia, DO
CEO . . . . Leonard Freehof, MD
Administrator . . . . Matthew Frye
Pediatric Ambulatory Care . . . . . . Marc Leitner, MD
Chief of Medical Staff. . . . . S Daniel McBride, MD
Operating Room. . . . . Randal Peoples, MD

Measure	Cases	This Hosp.	State Avg.	U.S. Avg.
Blood Clot Prevention and Treatment				
Anticoagulation Overlap Therapy[2]	96	96%	96%	93%
ICU Venous Thromboembolism Prophylaxis[2]	62	79%	91%	92%
Incidence of Potentially Preventable VTE[2]	25	28%	10%	10%
UFH with Dosages/Platelet Monitoring[2]	54	100%	99%	97%
Venous Thromboembolism Prophylaxis[2]	289	60%	84%	85%
Warfarin Therapy Discharge Instructions[2]	70	94%	90%	75%
Chest Pain/Possible Heart Attack Care				
Aspirin Given Within 24 Hours of Arrival[1,3]	-	-	98%	96%
Fibrinolytic Meds Within 30 Min. of Arrival[3,7]	-	-	40%	58%
Average Time to ECG (minutes)[1,3]	-	-	9	7
Average Time to Transfer (minutes)[3,7]	-	-	66	60
Children's Asthma Care				
Received Home Management Plan of Care	-	-	-	88%
Received Reliever Medication	-	-	-	100%
Received Systemic Corticosteroids	-	-	-	100%
Emergency Department				
Admittance Decision Time (minutes)[2]	541	298	151	98
Head CT Results Within 45 Min. of Arrival[1]	-	-	44%	57%
Patients Who Left ER Before Being Seen	43,972	2%	2%	2%
Time from ER Arrival to Admit. (minutes)[2]	542	524	337	274
Time from ER Arrival to Discharge (minutes)	344	205	150	134
Time in ER Before Being Evaluated (minutes)	391	33	22	26
Time to Pain Meds for Fractures (minutes)	135	73	54	57
Heart Attack Care				
Aspirin Given at Discharge[2]	272	99%	99%	99%
Fibrinolytic Meds Within 30 Min. of Arrival[2,7]	-	-	67%	54%
PCI Within 90 Minutes of Arrival[2]	65	98%	97%	96%
Statin Prescribed at Discharge[2]	268	99%	98%	98%
Heart Failure Care				
ACE Inhibitor or ARB for LVSD[2]	92	97%	97%	97%
Discharge Instructions Given[2]	210	84%	91%	94%
Evaluation of LVS Function[2]	252	100%	99%	99%
Medicare Spending				
Medicare Spending per Patient (ratio)	-	1.17	1.04	0.98
Pneumonia Care				
Appropriate Initial Antibiotic Given[2]	79	94%	96%	95%
Blood Culture Timing[2]	97	90%	96%	98%
Pregnancy and Delivery Care				
Newborn Deliveries Scheduled Early[2]	43	2%	6%	6%
Preventive Care				
Immunization for Influenza[2]	526	88%	93%	90%
Immunization for Pneumonia[2]	532	83%	94%	92%
Stroke Care				
Anticoagulation Therapy for Atrial Fibrillation[2]	13	100%	92%	95%
Antithrombotic Therapy Timing[2]	81	93%	97%	98%
Assessed for Rehabilitation[2]	126	94%	96%	97%
Discharged on Antithrombotic Therapy[2]	90	100%	99%	99%
Discharged on Statin Medication[2]	75	93%	95%	94%
Thrombolytic Therapy Timing[1,2]	-	-	80%	66%
Venous Thromboembolism Prophylaxis[2]	120	82%	91%	94%
Written Stroke Educational Materials Given[2]	69	65%	87%	88%
Surgical Care Improvement Project				
Appropriate Beta Blocker Usage[2]	140	91%	96%	98%
Appropriate VTP Within 24 Hours[2]	452	99%	98%	98%
Controlled Postoperative Blood Glucose[2]	54	91%	97%	97%
Perioperative Temperature Management[2]	516	100%	100%	100%
Prophylactic Antibiotic Selection[2]	419	98%	99%	99%
Prophylactic Antibiotic Selection (Outpatient)	345	96%	98%	98%
Prophylactic Antibiotic Stopped[2]	408	95%	98%	98%
Prophylactic Antibiotic Timing[2]	421	98%	99%	99%
Prophylactic Antibiotic Timing (Outpatient)	348	98%	98%	98%
Urinary Catheter Removal[2]	328	96%	98%	97%
Survey of Patients' Hospital Experiences				
Area Around Room 'Always' Quiet at Night	300+	55%	57%	61%
Doctors 'Always' Communicated Well	300+	70%	75%	82%

NOTE: Hospital profiles are in alphabetical order by state, then city, then hospital within the city; Rankings exclude hospitals with less than 25 cases except for patient surveys which excludes hospitals with less than 100 cases; (a) 100-299 cases; (1) The number of cases/patients is too few to report; (2) Data submitted were based on a sample of cases/patients; (3) Results are based on a shorter time period than required; (4) Data suppressed by CMS for one or more quarters; (5) Results are not available for this reporting period; (6) Fewer than 100 patients completed the HCAHPS survey; (7) No cases met the criteria for this measure; (8) The lower limit of the confidence interval cannot be calculated if the number of observed infections equals zero; (9) No data are available from the state/territory for this reporting period; (10) The scores shown reflect fewer than 50 completed surveys; (11) There were discrepancies in the data collection process; (12) This measure does not apply to this hospital for this reporting period; (13) Results cannot be calculated for this reporting period; (14) The results for this state are combined with nearby states to protect confidentiality; Please refer to the User's Guide for a full explanation of data.

Measure	Cases	This Hosp.	State Avg.	U.S. Avg.
Home Recovery Information Given	300+	82%	85%	85%
Hospital Given 9 or 10 on 10 Point Scale	300+	62%	66%	71%
Meds 'Always' Explained Before Given	300+	56%	60%	64%
Nurses 'Always' Communicated Well	300+	68%	72%	79%
Pain 'Always' Well Controlled	300+	64%	67%	71%
Room and Bathroom 'Always' Clean	300+	61%	68%	73%
Timely Help 'Always' Received	300+	52%	59%	68%
Would Definitely Recommend Hospital	300+	67%	69%	71%
Use of Medical Imaging				
Cardiac Imaging Stress Test before Surgery	124	3.2%	4.8%	5.3%
Combination Abdominal CT Scan	391	2.8%	6.9%	10.5%
Combination Brain/Sinus CT Scan	483	1.4%	2.7%	2.7%
Combination Chest CT Scan[1]	-	-	3.7%	2.7%
Follow-up Mammogram/Ultrasound[1]	-	-	7.3%	8.8%
Lumbar Spine MRI for Low Back Pain[1]	-	-	36.8%	37.2%

Summerlin Hospital Medical Center

657 Town Center Drive
Las Vegas, NV 89144
Phone: 702-233-7500
Fax: 702-233-7599
URL: www.summerlinhospital.org
Type: Acute Care Hospitals
Emergency Services: Yes
Ownership: Proprietary
Beds: 274
Key Personnel:
Cardiac Laboratory. . . . . Nancy Donahoe, MD
CEO/President. . . . . Robert Freymuller
Pediatric In-Patient Care . . . . Marc Leitner, MD
Chief of Medical Staff. . . . . Roxanne Terrase

Measure	Cases	This Hosp.	State Avg.	U.S. Avg.
Blood Clot Prevention and Treatment				
Anticoagulation Overlap Therapy[2]	103	96%	96%	93%
ICU Venous Thromboembolism Prophylaxis[2]	72	74%	91%	92%
Incidence of Potentially Preventable VTE[2]	20	25%	10%	10%
UFH with Dosages/Platelet Monitoring[2]	82	100%	99%	97%
Venous Thromboembolism Prophylaxis[2]	329	58%	84%	85%
Warfarin Therapy Discharge Instructions[2]	67	90%	90%	75%
Chest Pain/Possible Heart Attack Care				
Aspirin Given Within 24 Hours of Arrival[3,7]	-	-	98%	96%
Fibrinolytic Meds Within 30 Min. of Arrival[5]	-	-	40%	58%
Average Time to ECG (minutes)[3,7]	-	-	9	7
Average Time to Transfer (minutes)[5]	-	-	66	60
Children's Asthma Care				
Received Home Management Plan of Care	-	-	-	88%
Received Reliever Medication	-	-	-	100%
Received Systemic Corticosteroids	-	-	-	100%
Emergency Department				
Admittance Decision Time (minutes)[2]	547	164	151	98
Head CT Results Within 45 Min. of Arrival	13	46%	44%	57%
Patients Who Left ER Before Being Seen	44,997	2%	2%	2%
Time from ER Arrival to Admit. (minutes)[2]	554	380	337	274
Time from ER Arrival to Discharge (minutes)	351	174	150	134
Time in ER Before Being Evaluated (minutes)	383	28	22	26
Time to Pain Meds for Fractures (minutes)	211	59	54	57
Heart Attack Care				
Aspirin Given at Discharge[2]	208	100%	99%	99%
Fibrinolytic Meds Within 30 Min. of Arrival[2,7]	-	-	67%	54%
PCI Within 90 Minutes of Arrival[2]	36	100%	97%	96%
Statin Prescribed at Discharge[2]	210	97%	98%	98%
Heart Failure Care				
ACE Inhibitor or ARB for LVSD[2]	103	94%	97%	97%
Discharge Instructions Given[2]	255	87%	91%	94%
Evaluation of LVS Function[2]	322	100%	99%	99%
Medicare Spending				
Medicare Spending per Patient (ratio)	-	1.12	1.04	0.98
Pneumonia Care				
Appropriate Initial Antibiotic Given[2]	77	97%	96%	95%
Blood Culture Timing[2]	97	91%	96%	98%
Pregnancy and Delivery Care				
Newborn Deliveries Scheduled Early[2]	77	12%	6%	6%
Preventive Care				
Immunization for Influenza[2]	514	85%	93%	90%
Immunization for Pneumonia[2]	483	93%	94%	92%
Stroke Care				
Anticoagulation Therapy for Atrial Fibrillation[2]	20	85%	92%	95%
Antithrombotic Therapy Timing[2]	90	99%	97%	98%
Assessed for Rehabilitation[2]	98	96%	96%	97%
Discharged on Antithrombotic Therapy[2]	98	100%	99%	99%
Discharged on Statin Medication[2]	80	90%	95%	94%
Thrombolytic Therapy Timing[1,2]	-	-	80%	66%
Venous Thromboembolism Prophylaxis[2]	89	84%	91%	94%
Written Stroke Educational Materials Given[2]	57	91%	87%	88%
Surgical Care Improvement Project				
Appropriate Beta Blocker Usage[2]	180	92%	96%	98%
Appropriate VTP Within 24 Hours[2]	379	97%	98%	98%
Controlled Postoperative Blood Glucose[2]	105	99%	97%	97%
Perioperative Temperature Management[2]	489	100%	100%	100%
Prophylactic Antibiotic Selection[2]	419	98%	99%	99%
Prophylactic Antibiotic Selection (Outpatient)	434	97%	98%	98%
Prophylactic Antibiotic Stopped[2]	403	94%	98%	98%
Prophylactic Antibiotic Timing[2]	419	99%	99%	99%
Prophylactic Antibiotic Timing (Outpatient)	437	98%	98%	98%
Urinary Catheter Removal[2]	273	96%	98%	97%
Survey of Patients' Hospital Experiences				
Area Around Room 'Always' Quiet at Night	300+	56%	57%	61%
Doctors 'Always' Communicated Well	300+	73%	75%	82%
Home Recovery Information Given	300+	84%	85%	85%
Hospital Given 9 or 10 on 10 Point Scale	300+	61%	66%	71%
Meds 'Always' Explained Before Given	300+	54%	60%	64%
Nurses 'Always' Communicated Well	300+	70%	72%	79%
Pain 'Always' Well Controlled	300+	63%	67%	71%
Room and Bathroom 'Always' Clean	300+	63%	68%	73%
Timely Help 'Always' Received	300+	53%	59%	68%
Would Definitely Recommend Hospital	300+	66%	69%	71%
Use of Medical Imaging				
Cardiac Imaging Stress Test before Surgery	176	6.3%	4.8%	5.3%
Combination Abdominal CT Scan	479	5.0%	6.9%	10.5%
Combination Brain/Sinus CT Scan[1]	-	-	2.7%	2.7%
Combination Chest CT Scan	103	10.7%	3.7%	2.7%
Follow-up Mammogram/Ultrasound	186	7.5%	7.3%	8.8%
Lumbar Spine MRI for Low Back Pain[1]	-	-	36.8%	37.2%

Sunrise Hospital & Medical Center

3186 S Maryland Pkwy
Las Vegas, NV 89109
Phone: 702-731-8000
Fax: 702-731-8668
URL: www.sunrisehospital.com
Type: Acute Care Hospitals
Emergency Services: Yes
Ownership: Proprietary
Beds: 701
Key Personnel:
Pediatric In-Patient Care . . . . Todd Sklamberg
CEO/President. . . . . Sylvia Young

Measure	Cases	This Hosp.	State Avg.	U.S. Avg.
Blood Clot Prevention and Treatment				
Anticoagulation Overlap Therapy[2]	142	97%	96%	93%
ICU Venous Thromboembolism Prophylaxis[2]	148	97%	91%	92%
Incidence of Potentially Preventable VTE[2]	21	0%	10%	10%
UFH with Dosages/Platelet Monitoring[2]	99	100%	99%	97%
Venous Thromboembolism Prophylaxis[2]	323	76%	84%	85%
Warfarin Therapy Discharge Instructions[2]	99	100%	90%	75%
Chest Pain/Possible Heart Attack Care				
Aspirin Given Within 24 Hours of Arrival	15	93%	98%	96%
Fibrinolytic Meds Within 30 Min. of Arrival[5]	-	-	40%	58%
Average Time to ECG (minutes)	14	13	9	7
Average Time to Transfer (minutes)[5]	-	-	66	60
Children's Asthma Care				
Received Home Management Plan of Care	-	-	-	88%
Received Reliever Medication	-	-	-	100%
Received Systemic Corticosteroids	-	-	-	100%
Emergency Department				
Admittance Decision Time (minutes)[2]	574	194	151	98
Head CT Results Within 45 Min. of Arrival[1]	-	-	44%	57%
Patients Who Left ER Before Being Seen	>100k	0%	2%	2%
Time from ER Arrival to Admit. (minutes)[2]	575	340	337	274
Time from ER Arrival to Discharge (minutes)	403	156	150	134
Time in ER Before Being Evaluated (minutes)	494	11	22	26
Time to Pain Meds for Fractures (minutes)	351	41	54	57
Heart Attack Care				
Aspirin Given at Discharge[2]	290	100%	99%	99%
Fibrinolytic Meds Within 30 Min. of Arrival[2,7]	-	-	67%	54%
PCI Within 90 Minutes of Arrival[2]	51	100%	97%	96%
Statin Prescribed at Discharge[2]	286	99%	98%	98%
Heart Failure Care				
ACE Inhibitor or ARB for LVSD[2]	140	100%	97%	97%
Discharge Instructions Given[2]	255	97%	91%	94%
Evaluation of LVS Function[2]	301	100%	99%	99%
Medicare Spending				
Medicare Spending per Patient (ratio)	-	1.16	1.04	0.98
Pneumonia Care				
Appropriate Initial Antibiotic Given[2]	74	99%	96%	95%
Blood Culture Timing[2]	167	99%	96%	98%
Pregnancy and Delivery Care				
Newborn Deliveries Scheduled Early[2]	108	2%	6%	6%
Preventive Care				
Immunization for Influenza[2]	547	93%	93%	90%
Immunization for Pneumonia[2]	538	96%	94%	92%
Stroke Care				
Anticoagulation Therapy for Atrial Fibrillation[1,2]	-	-	92%	95%
Antithrombotic Therapy Timing[2]	73	99%	97%	98%
Assessed for Rehabilitation[2]	105	99%	96%	97%
Discharged on Antithrombotic Therapy[2]	86	100%	99%	99%
Discharged on Statin Medication[2]	57	100%	95%	94%
Thrombolytic Therapy Timing[2]	12	100%	80%	66%
Venous Thromboembolism Prophylaxis[2]	122	100%	91%	94%
Written Stroke Educational Materials Given[2]	53	100%	87%	88%
Surgical Care Improvement Project				
Appropriate Beta Blocker Usage[2]	233	99%	96%	98%
Appropriate VTP Within 24 Hours[2]	407	100%	98%	98%
Controlled Postoperative Blood Glucose[2]	160	97%	97%	97%
Perioperative Temperature Management[2]	575	100%	100%	100%
Prophylactic Antibiotic Selection[2]	480	99%	99%	99%
Prophylactic Antibiotic Selection (Outpatient)	408	100%	98%	98%
Prophylactic Antibiotic Stopped[2]	456	100%	98%	98%
Prophylactic Antibiotic Timing[2]	480	100%	99%	99%
Prophylactic Antibiotic Timing (Outpatient)	408	100%	98%	98%
Urinary Catheter Removal[2]	400	100%	98%	97%
Survey of Patients' Hospital Experiences				
Area Around Room 'Always' Quiet at Night	300+	54%	57%	61%
Doctors 'Always' Communicated Well	300+	70%	75%	82%
Home Recovery Information Given	300+	78%	85%	85%
Hospital Given 9 or 10 on 10 Point Scale	300+	61%	66%	71%
Meds 'Always' Explained Before Given	300+	54%	60%	64%
Nurses 'Always' Communicated Well	300+	66%	72%	79%
Pain 'Always' Well Controlled	300+	63%	67%	71%
Room and Bathroom 'Always' Clean	300+	64%	68%	73%
Timely Help 'Always' Received	300+	53%	59%	68%
Would Definitely Recommend Hospital	300+	62%	69%	71%
Use of Medical Imaging				
Cardiac Imaging Stress Test before Surgery	346	4.0%	4.8%	5.3%
Combination Abdominal CT Scan	664	5.4%	6.9%	10.5%
Combination Brain/Sinus CT Scan	838	4.4%	2.7%	2.7%
Combination Chest CT Scan	207	5.3%	3.7%	2.7%
Follow-up Mammogram/Ultrasound	393	8.7%	7.3%	8.8%
Lumbar Spine MRI for Low Back Pain[1]	-	-	36.8%	37.2%

UMC of Southern Nevada

1800 W Charleston Blvd
Las Vegas, NV 89102
Phone: 702-383-2000
Fax: 702-383-2067
URL: www.umc-cares.org
Type: Acute Care Hospitals
Emergency Services: Yes
Ownership: Government - Local
Beds: 541
Key Personnel:
Quality Assurance . . . . Annette Bradley
Chief of Medical Staff. . . . . Dale Carrison, DO
Radiology. . . . . George Cervantes
Pediatric Ambulatory Care . . . . . . Sandra Gain
Coronary Care . . . . Joy Guideng
Infection Control. . . . . Tracy Puckett
Pediatric In-Patient Care . . . . Cindy Roybal
CEO/President. . . . . Kathleen Silver

Measure	Cases	This Hosp.	State Avg.	U.S. Avg.
Blood Clot Prevention and Treatment				
Anticoagulation Overlap Therapy[2]	113	94%	96%	93%

NOTE: Hospital profiles are in alphabetical order by state, then city, then hospital within the city; Rankings exclude hospitals with less than 25 cases except for patient surveys which excludes hospitals with less than 100 cases; (a) 100-299 cases; (1) The number of cases/patients is too few to report; (2) Data submitted were based on a sample of cases/patients; (3) Results are based on a shorter time period than required; (4) Data suppressed by CMS for one or more quarters; (5) Results are not available for this reporting period; (6) Fewer than 100 patients completed the HCAHPS survey; (7) No cases met the criteria for this measure; (8) The lower limit of the confidence interval cannot be calculated if the number of observed infections equals zero; (9) No data are available from the state/territory for this reporting period; (10) The scores shown reflect fewer than 50 completed surveys; (11) There were discrepancies in the data collection process; (12) This measure does not apply to this hospital for this reporting period; (13) Results cannot be calculated for this reporting period; (14) The results for this state are combined with nearby states to protect confidentiality; Please refer to the User's Guide for a full explanation of data.

Measure	Cases	This Hosp.	State Avg.	U.S. Avg.
ICU Venous Thromboembolism Prophylaxis[2]	110	81%	91%	92%
Incidence of Potentially Preventable VTE[2]	38	16%	10%	10%
UFH with Dosages/Platelet Monitoring[2]	85	100%	99%	97%
Venous Thromboembolism Prophylaxis[2]	283	73%	84%	85%
Warfarin Therapy Discharge Instructions[2]	82	88%	90%	75%
Chest Pain/Possible Heart Attack Care				
Aspirin Given Within 24 Hours of Arrival[5]	-	-	98%	96%
Fibrinolytic Meds Within 30 Min. of Arrival[5]	-	-	40%	58%
Average Time to ECG (minutes)[5]	-	-	9	7
Average Time to Transfer (minutes)[5]	-	-	66	60
Children's Asthma Care				
Received Home Management Plan of Care	-	-	-	88%
Received Reliever Medication	-	-	-	100%
Received Systemic Corticosteroids	-	-	-	100%
Emergency Department				
Admittance Decision Time (minutes)[2]	545	162	151	98
Head CT Results Within 45 Min. of Arrival[1]	-	-	44%	57%
Patients Who Left ER Before Being Seen	83,395	5%	2%	2%
Time from ER Arrival to Admit. (minutes)[2]	545	463	337	274
Time from ER Arrival to Discharge (minutes)	327	253	150	134
Time in ER Before Being Evaluated (minutes)	343	73	22	26
Time to Pain Meds for Fractures (minutes)	209	31	54	57
Heart Attack Care				
Aspirin Given at Discharge[2]	208	96%	99%	99%
Fibrinolytic Meds Within 30 Min. of Arrival[2,7]	-	-	67%	54%
PCI Within 90 Minutes of Arrival[2]	41	100%	97%	96%
Statin Prescribed at Discharge[2]	209	97%	98%	98%
Heart Failure Care				
ACE Inhibitor or ARB for LVSD[2]	171	96%	97%	97%
Discharge Instructions Given[2]	278	74%	91%	94%
Evaluation of LVS Function[2]	300	99%	99%	99%
Medicare Spending				
Medicare Spending per Patient (ratio)	-	1.05	1.04	0.98
Pneumonia Care				
Appropriate Initial Antibiotic Given[2]	95	95%	96%	95%
Blood Culture Timing[2]	148	91%	96%	98%
Pregnancy and Delivery Care				
Newborn Deliveries Scheduled Early[2]	56	2%	6%	6%
Preventive Care				
Immunization for Influenza[2]	499	74%	93%	90%
Immunization for Pneumonia[2]	453	82%	94%	92%
Stroke Care				
Anticoagulation Therapy for Atrial Fibrillation	11	91%	92%	95%
Antithrombotic Therapy Timing	114	100%	97%	98%
Assessed for Rehabilitation	162	99%	96%	97%
Discharged on Antithrombotic Therapy	128	100%	99%	99%
Discharged on Statin Medication	91	100%	95%	94%
Thrombolytic Therapy Timing	11	91%	80%	66%
Venous Thromboembolism Prophylaxis	172	94%	91%	94%
Written Stroke Educational Materials Given	131	91%	87%	88%
Surgical Care Improvement Project				
Appropriate Beta Blocker Usage[2]	98	87%	96%	98%
Appropriate VTP Within 24 Hours[2]	256	93%	98%	98%
Controlled Postoperative Blood Glucose[2]	97	93%	97%	97%
Perioperative Temperature Management[2]	374	100%	100%	100%
Prophylactic Antibiotic Selection[2]	284	97%	99%	99%
Prophylactic Antibiotic Selection (Outpatient)	292	98%	98%	98%
Prophylactic Antibiotic Stopped[2]	273	94%	98%	98%
Prophylactic Antibiotic Timing[2]	288	93%	99%	99%
Prophylactic Antibiotic Timing (Outpatient)	299	91%	98%	98%
Urinary Catheter Removal[2]	172	89%	98%	97%
Survey of Patients' Hospital Experiences				
Area Around Room 'Always' Quiet at Night[5]	-	-	57%	61%
Doctors 'Always' Communicated Well[5]	-	-	75%	82%
Home Recovery Information Given[5]	-	-	85%	85%
Hospital Given 9 or 10 on 10 Point Scale[5]	-	-	66%	71%
Meds 'Always' Explained Before Given[5]	-	-	60%	64%
Nurses 'Always' Communicated Well[5]	-	-	72%	79%
Pain 'Always' Well Controlled[5]	-	-	67%	71%
Room and Bathroom 'Always' Clean[5]	-	-	68%	73%
Timely Help 'Always' Received[5]	-	-	59%	68%
Would Definitely Recommend Hospital[5]	-	-	69%	71%
Use of Medical Imaging				
Cardiac Imaging Stress Test before Surgery	241	3.7%	4.8%	5.3%
Combination Abdominal CT Scan	385	6.2%	6.9%	10.5%
Combination Brain/Sinus CT Scan[1]	-	-	2.7%	2.7%
Combination Chest CT Scan	126	15.1%	3.7%	2.7%
Follow-up Mammogram/Ultrasound[7]	-	-	7.3%	8.8%
Lumbar Spine MRI for Low Back Pain[1]	-	-	36.8%	37.2%

Valley Hospital Medical Center

620 Shadow Lane
Las Vegas, NV 89106
URL: www.valleyhealthsystem.org
Type: Acute Care Hospitals
Ownership: Proprietary
Phone: 702-388-4000
Fax: 702-388-4618
Emergency Services: Yes
Beds: 409

Key Personnel:
Operating Room. . . . . Jose Berlanga, RN
CEO/President. . . . . Gregory E Boyer
Quality Assurance . . . . Karen Faulis, RN
Chief of Medical Staff. . . . . Paul Heeren, MD
Radiology. . . . . Christopher Jones
Pediatric In-Patient Care . . . . Martha Knutsen, MD
Cardiac Laboratory. . . . . Diane Rybko

Measure	Cases	This Hosp.	State Avg.	U.S. Avg.
Blood Clot Prevention and Treatment				
Anticoagulation Overlap Therapy[2]	50	94%	96%	93%
ICU Venous Thromboembolism Prophylaxis[2]	114	96%	91%	92%
Incidence of Potentially Preventable VTE[1,2]	-	-	10%	10%
UFH with Dosages/Platelet Monitoring[2]	57	100%	99%	97%
Venous Thromboembolism Prophylaxis[2]	292	70%	84%	85%
Warfarin Therapy Discharge Instructions[2]	17	94%	90%	75%
Chest Pain/Possible Heart Attack Care				
Aspirin Given Within 24 Hours of Arrival[1,3]	-	-	98%	96%
Fibrinolytic Meds Within 30 Min. of Arrival[5]	-	-	40%	58%
Average Time to ECG (minutes)[1,3]	-	-	9	7
Average Time to Transfer (minutes)[5]	-	-	66	60
Children's Asthma Care				
Received Home Management Plan of Care	-	-	-	88%
Received Reliever Medication	-	-	-	100%
Received Systemic Corticosteroids	-	-	-	100%
Emergency Department				
Admittance Decision Time (minutes)[2]	755	278	151	98
Head CT Results Within 45 Min. of Arrival[1]	-	-	44%	57%
Patients Who Left ER Before Being Seen	39,185	2%	2%	2%
Time from ER Arrival to Admit. (minutes)[2]	758	494	337	274
Time from ER Arrival to Discharge (minutes)	338	214	150	134
Time in ER Before Being Evaluated (minutes)	404	34	22	26
Time to Pain Meds for Fractures (minutes)	69	66	54	57
Heart Attack Care				
Aspirin Given at Discharge[2]	276	100%	99%	99%
Fibrinolytic Meds Within 30 Min. of Arrival[2,7]	-	-	67%	54%
PCI Within 90 Minutes of Arrival[2]	42	93%	97%	96%
Statin Prescribed at Discharge[2]	276	97%	98%	98%
Heart Failure Care				
ACE Inhibitor or ARB for LVSD[2]	136	95%	97%	97%
Discharge Instructions Given[2]	247	92%	91%	94%
Evaluation of LVS Function[2]	292	100%	99%	99%
Medicare Spending				
Medicare Spending per Patient (ratio)	-	1.17	1.04	0.98
Pneumonia Care				
Appropriate Initial Antibiotic Given[2]	77	100%	96%	95%
Blood Culture Timing[2]	100	96%	96%	98%
Pregnancy and Delivery Care				
Newborn Deliveries Scheduled Early[2]	55	4%	6%	6%
Preventive Care				
Immunization for Influenza[2]	536	90%	93%	90%
Immunization for Pneumonia[2]	644	91%	94%	92%
Stroke Care				
Anticoagulation Therapy for Atrial Fibrillation[2]	12	92%	92%	95%
Antithrombotic Therapy Timing[2]	74	92%	97%	98%
Assessed for Rehabilitation[2]	107	94%	96%	97%
Discharged on Antithrombotic Therapy[2]	80	98%	99%	99%
Discharged on Statin Medication[2]	75	93%	95%	94%
Thrombolytic Therapy Timing[1,2]	-	-	80%	66%
Venous Thromboembolism Prophylaxis[2]	133	74%	91%	94%
Written Stroke Educational Materials Given[2]	49	53%	87%	88%
Surgical Care Improvement Project				
Appropriate Beta Blocker Usage[2]	163	96%	96%	98%
Appropriate VTP Within 24 Hours[2]	341	96%	98%	98%
Controlled Postoperative Blood Glucose[2]	99	99%	97%	97%
Perioperative Temperature Management[2]	474	100%	100%	100%
Prophylactic Antibiotic Selection[2]	347	98%	99%	99%
Prophylactic Antibiotic Selection (Outpatient)	285	99%	98%	98%
Prophylactic Antibiotic Stopped[2]	340	98%	98%	98%
Prophylactic Antibiotic Timing[2]	347	99%	99%	99%
Prophylactic Antibiotic Timing (Outpatient)	285	99%	98%	98%
Urinary Catheter Removal[2]	265	94%	98%	97%
Survey of Patients' Hospital Experiences				
Area Around Room 'Always' Quiet at Night	300+	49%	57%	61%
Doctors 'Always' Communicated Well	300+	73%	75%	82%
Home Recovery Information Given	300+	82%	85%	85%
Hospital Given 9 or 10 on 10 Point Scale	300+	60%	66%	71%
Meds 'Always' Explained Before Given	300+	52%	60%	64%
Nurses 'Always' Communicated Well	300+	69%	72%	79%
Pain 'Always' Well Controlled	300+	64%	67%	71%
Room and Bathroom 'Always' Clean	300+	61%	68%	73%
Timely Help 'Always' Received	300+	52%	59%	68%
Would Definitely Recommend Hospital	300+	61%	69%	71%
Use of Medical Imaging				
Cardiac Imaging Stress Test before Surgery	163	4.9%	4.8%	5.3%
Combination Abdominal CT Scan	325	2.2%	6.9%	10.5%
Combination Brain/Sinus CT Scan	604	3.0%	2.7%	2.7%
Combination Chest CT Scan[1]	-	-	3.7%	2.7%
Follow-up Mammogram/Ultrasound[1]	-	-	7.3%	8.8%
Lumbar Spine MRI for Low Back Pain[1]	-	-	36.8%	37.2%

Pershing General Hospital

855 6th Street/po Box 661
Lovelock, NV 89419
Type: Critical Access Hospitals
Ownership: Govt - Hospital Dist/Auth
Phone: 775-273-2621
Emergency Services: Yes

Measure	Cases	This Hosp.	State Avg.	U.S. Avg.
Blood Clot Prevention and Treatment				
Anticoagulation Overlap Therapy[5]	-	-	96%	93%
ICU Venous Thromboembolism Prophylaxis[5]	-	-	91%	92%
Incidence of Potentially Preventable VTE[5]	-	-	10%	10%
UFH with Dosages/Platelet Monitoring[5]	-	-	99%	97%
Venous Thromboembolism Prophylaxis[5]	-	-	84%	85%
Warfarin Therapy Discharge Instructions[5]	-	-	90%	75%
Chest Pain/Possible Heart Attack Care				
Aspirin Given Within 24 Hours of Arrival[1,3]	-	-	98%	96%
Fibrinolytic Meds Within 30 Min. of Arrival[1,3]	-	-	40%	58%
Average Time to ECG (minutes)[1,3]	-	-	9	7
Average Time to Transfer (minutes)[3,7]	-	-	66	60
Children's Asthma Care				
Received Home Management Plan of Care	-	-	-	88%
Received Reliever Medication	-	-	-	100%
Received Systemic Corticosteroids	-	-	-	100%
Emergency Department				
Admittance Decision Time (minutes)[5]	-	-	151	98
Head CT Results Within 45 Min. of Arrival[5]	-	-	44%	57%
Patients Who Left ER Before Being Seen[5]	-	-	2%	2%
Time from ER Arrival to Admit. (minutes)[5]	-	-	337	274
Time from ER Arrival to Discharge (minutes)[5]	-	-	150	134
Time in ER Before Being Evaluated (minutes)[5]	-	-	22	26
Time to Pain Meds for Fractures (minutes)[5]	-	-	54	57
Heart Attack Care				
Aspirin Given at Discharge[5]	-	-	99%	99%
Fibrinolytic Meds Within 30 Min. of Arrival[5]	-	-	67%	54%
PCI Within 90 Minutes of Arrival[5]	-	-	97%	96%
Statin Prescribed at Discharge[5]	-	-	98%	98%
Heart Failure Care				
ACE Inhibitor or ARB for LVSD[5]	-	-	97%	97%
Discharge Instructions Given[5]	-	-	91%	94%
Evaluation of LVS Function[5]	-	-	99%	99%
Medicare Spending				
Medicare Spending per Patient (ratio)	-	-	1.04	0.98

NOTE: Hospital profiles are in alphabetical order by state, then city, then hospital within the city; Rankings exclude hospitals with less than 25 cases except for patient surveys which excludes hospitals with less than 100 cases; (a) 100-299 cases; (1) The number of cases/patients is too few to report; (2) Data submitted were based on a sample of cases/patients; (3) Results are based on a shorter time period than required; (4) Data suppressed by CMS for one or more quarters; (5) Results are not available for this reporting period; (6) Fewer than 100 patients completed the HCAHPS survey; (7) No cases met the criteria for this measure; (8) The lower limit of the confidence interval cannot be calculated if the number of observed infections equals zero; (9) No data are available from the state/territory for this reporting period; (10) The scores shown reflect fewer than 50 completed surveys; (11) There were discrepancies in the data collection process; (12) This measure does not apply to this hospital for this reporting period; (13) Results cannot be calculated for this reporting period; (14) The results for this state are combined with nearby states to protect confidentiality; Please refer to the User's Guide for a full explanation of data.

Measure	Cases	This Hosp.	State Avg.	U.S. Avg.
Pneumonia Care				
Appropriate Initial Antibiotic Given[3,7]	-	-	96%	95%
Blood Culture Timing[3,7]	-	-	96%	98%
Pregnancy and Delivery Care				
Newborn Deliveries Scheduled Early[5]	-	-	6%	6%
Preventive Care				
Immunization for Influenza[5]	-	-	93%	90%
Immunization for Pneumonia[5]	-	-	94%	92%
Stroke Care				
Anticoagulation Therapy for Atrial Fibrillation[5]	-	-	92%	95%
Antithrombotic Therapy Timing[5]	-	-	97%	98%
Assessed for Rehabilitation[5]	-	-	96%	97%
Discharged on Antithrombotic Therapy[5]	-	-	99%	99%
Discharged on Statin Medication[5]	-	-	95%	94%
Thrombolytic Therapy Timing[5]	-	-	80%	66%
Venous Thromboembolism Prophylaxis[5]	-	-	91%	94%
Written Stroke Educational Materials Given[5]	-	-	87%	88%
Surgical Care Improvement Project				
Appropriate Beta Blocker Usage[5]	-	-	96%	98%
Appropriate VTP Within 24 Hours[5]	-	-	98%	98%
Controlled Postoperative Blood Glucose[5]	-	-	97%	97%
Perioperative Temperature Management[5]	-	-	100%	100%
Prophylactic Antibiotic Selection[5]	-	-	99%	99%
Prophylactic Antibiotic Selection (Outpatient)[5]	-	-	98%	98%
Prophylactic Antibiotic Stopped[5]	-	-	98%	98%
Prophylactic Antibiotic Timing[5]	-	-	99%	99%
Prophylactic Antibiotic Timing (Outpatient)[5]	-	-	98%	98%
Urinary Catheter Removal[5]	-	-	98%	97%
Survey of Patients' Hospital Experiences				
Area Around Room 'Always' Quiet at Night[5]	-	-	57%	61%
Doctors 'Always' Communicated Well[5]	-	-	75%	82%
Home Recovery Information Given[5]	-	-	85%	85%
Hospital Given 9 or 10 on 10 Point Scale[5]	-	-	66%	71%
Meds 'Always' Explained Before Given[5]	-	-	60%	64%
Nurses 'Always' Communicated Well[5]	-	-	72%	79%
Pain 'Always' Well Controlled[5]	-	-	67%	71%
Room and Bathroom 'Always' Clean[5]	-	-	68%	73%
Timely Help 'Always' Received[5]	-	-	59%	68%
Would Definitely Recommend Hospital[5]	-	-	69%	71%
Use of Medical Imaging				
Cardiac Imaging Stress Test before Surgery[7]	-	-	4.8%	5.3%
Combination Abdominal CT Scan[1]	-	-	6.9%	10.5%
Combination Brain/Sinus CT Scan[1]	-	-	2.7%	2.7%
Combination Chest CT Scan[1]	-	-	3.7%	2.7%
Follow-up Mammogram/Ultrasound[7]	-	-	7.3%	8.8%
Lumbar Spine MRI for Low Back Pain[1]	-	-	36.8%	37.2%

Mesa View Regional Hospital

1299 Bertha Howe Avenue
Mesquite, NV 89027
Phone: 702-346-8040
URL: www.mesaviewhospital.com
Type: Critical Access Hospitals
Emergency Services: Yes
Ownership: Voluntary non-profit - Private
Key Personnel:
Chief of Medical Staff.......... Enrique Alfaro, MD

Measure	Cases	This Hosp.	State Avg.	U.S. Avg.
Blood Clot Prevention and Treatment				
Anticoagulation Overlap Therapy[1,2]	-	-	96%	93%
ICU Venous Thromboembolism Prophylaxis[2]	33	100%	91%	92%
Incidence of Potentially Preventable VTE[1,2]	-	-	10%	10%
UFH with Dosages/Platelet Monitoring[1,2]	-	-	99%	97%
Venous Thromboembolism Prophylaxis[2]	207	99%	84%	85%
Warfarin Therapy Discharge Instructions[1,2]	-	-	90%	75%
Chest Pain/Possible Heart Attack Care				
Aspirin Given Within 24 Hours of Arrival	45	100%	98%	96%
Fibrinolytic Meds Within 30 Min. of Arrival[1]	-	-	40%	58%
Average Time to ECG (minutes)	44	4	9	7
Average Time to Transfer (minutes)[1]	-	-	66	60
Children's Asthma Care				
Received Home Management Plan of Care	-	-	-	88%
Received Reliever Medication	-	-	-	100%
Received Systemic Corticosteroids	-	-	-	100%
Emergency Department				
Admittance Decision Time (minutes)[2]	369	45	151	98
Head CT Results Within 45 Min. of Arrival	22	36%	44%	57%
Patients Who Left ER Before Being Seen	8,150	0%	2%	2%
Time from ER Arrival to Admit. (minutes)[2]	371	196	337	274
Time from ER Arrival to Discharge (minutes)	344	112	150	134
Time in ER Before Being Evaluated (minutes)	418	14	22	26
Time to Pain Meds for Fractures (minutes)	59	28	54	57
Heart Attack Care				
Aspirin Given at Discharge[3,7]	-	-	99%	99%
Fibrinolytic Meds Within 30 Min. of Arrival[3,7]	-	-	67%	54%
PCI Within 90 Minutes of Arrival[3,7]	-	-	97%	96%
Statin Prescribed at Discharge[3,7]	-	-	98%	98%
Heart Failure Care				
ACE Inhibitor or ARB for LVSD[1]	-	-	97%	97%
Discharge Instructions Given	17	100%	91%	94%
Evaluation of LVS Function	21	100%	99%	99%
Medicare Spending				
Medicare Spending per Patient (ratio)	-		1.04	0.98
Pneumonia Care				
Appropriate Initial Antibiotic Given	19	95%	96%	95%
Blood Culture Timing	30	100%	96%	98%
Pregnancy and Delivery Care				
Newborn Deliveries Scheduled Early[1,2]	-	-	6%	6%
Preventive Care				
Immunization for Influenza[2]	293	92%	93%	90%
Immunization for Pneumonia[2]	379	97%	94%	92%
Stroke Care				
Anticoagulation Therapy for Atrial Fibrillation[7]	-	-	92%	95%
Antithrombotic Therapy Timing[1]	-	-	97%	98%
Assessed for Rehabilitation[1]	-	-	96%	97%
Discharged on Antithrombotic Therapy[1]	-	-	99%	99%
Discharged on Statin Medication[7]	-	-	95%	94%
Thrombolytic Therapy Timing[1]	-	-	80%	66%
Venous Thromboembolism Prophylaxis[1]	-	-	91%	94%
Written Stroke Educational Materials Given[1]	-	-	87%	88%
Surgical Care Improvement Project				
Appropriate Beta Blocker Usage	19	100%	96%	98%
Appropriate VTP Within 24 Hours	68	100%	98%	98%
Controlled Postoperative Blood Glucose[7]	-	-	97%	97%
Perioperative Temperature Management	79	100%	100%	100%
Prophylactic Antibiotic Selection	63	97%	99%	99%
Prophylactic Antibiotic Selection (Outpatient)	24	96%	98%	98%
Prophylactic Antibiotic Stopped	62	98%	98%	98%
Prophylactic Antibiotic Timing	63	100%	99%	99%
Prophylactic Antibiotic Timing (Outpatient)	25	96%	98%	98%
Urinary Catheter Removal	49	100%	98%	97%
Survey of Patients' Hospital Experiences				
Area Around Room 'Always' Quiet at Night	(a)	71%	57%	61%
Doctors 'Always' Communicated Well	(a)	81%	75%	82%
Home Recovery Information Given	(a)	84%	85%	85%
Hospital Given 9 or 10 on 10 Point Scale	(a)	73%	66%	71%
Meds 'Always' Explained Before Given	(a)	68%	60%	64%
Nurses 'Always' Communicated Well	(a)	76%	72%	79%
Pain 'Always' Well Controlled	(a)	69%	67%	71%
Room and Bathroom 'Always' Clean	(a)	75%	68%	73%
Timely Help 'Always' Received	(a)	68%	59%	68%
Would Definitely Recommend Hospital	(a)	72%	69%	71%
Use of Medical Imaging				
Cardiac Imaging Stress Test before Surgery	83	3.6%	4.8%	5.3%
Combination Abdominal CT Scan	310	14.2%	6.9%	10.5%
Combination Brain/Sinus CT Scan[1]	-	-	2.7%	2.7%
Combination Chest CT Scan	104	19.2%	3.7%	2.7%
Follow-up Mammogram/Ultrasound	561	8.0%	7.3%	8.8%
Lumbar Spine MRI for Low Back Pain	51	35.3%	36.8%	37.2%

North Vista Hospital

1409 East Lake Mead Blvd
North Las Vegas, NV 89030
Phone: 702-657-5504
Fax: 702-657-5605
URL: www.northvistahospital.com
Type: Acute Care Hospitals
Emergency Services: Yes
Ownership: Proprietary
Beds: 185
Key Personnel:
CEO/President............... Tony Marinello

Measure	Cases	This Hosp.	State Avg.	U.S. Avg.
Blood Clot Prevention and Treatment				
Anticoagulation Overlap Therapy[2]	58	98%	96%	93%
ICU Venous Thromboembolism Prophylaxis[2]	201	100%	91%	92%
Incidence of Potentially Preventable VTE[2]	23	0%	10%	10%
UFH with Dosages/Platelet Monitoring[2]	33	100%	99%	97%
Venous Thromboembolism Prophylaxis[2]	497	96%	84%	85%
Warfarin Therapy Discharge Instructions[2]	24	100%	90%	75%
Chest Pain/Possible Heart Attack Care				
Aspirin Given Within 24 Hours of Arrival[1,3]	-	-	98%	96%
Fibrinolytic Meds Within 30 Min. of Arrival[3,7]	-	-	40%	58%
Average Time to ECG (minutes)[1,3]	-	-	9	7
Average Time to Transfer (minutes)[3,7]	-	-	66	60
Children's Asthma Care				
Received Home Management Plan of Care	-	-	-	88%
Received Reliever Medication	-	-	-	100%
Received Systemic Corticosteroids	-	-	-	100%
Emergency Department				
Admittance Decision Time (minutes)[2]	701	180	151	98
Head CT Results Within 45 Min. of Arrival[3,7]	-	-	44%	57%
Patients Who Left ER Before Being Seen	35,333	1%	2%	2%
Time from ER Arrival to Admit. (minutes)[2]	700	360	337	274
Time from ER Arrival to Discharge (minutes)	933	129	150	134
Time in ER Before Being Evaluated (minutes)	1,052	20	22	26
Time to Pain Meds for Fractures (minutes)	116	62	54	57
Heart Attack Care				
Aspirin Given at Discharge	65	98%	99%	99%
Fibrinolytic Meds Within 30 Min. of Arrival[7]	-	-	67%	54%
PCI Within 90 Minutes of Arrival[1]	-	-	97%	96%
Statin Prescribed at Discharge	62	97%	98%	98%
Heart Failure Care				
ACE Inhibitor or ARB for LVSD	103	97%	97%	97%
Discharge Instructions Given	210	96%	91%	94%
Evaluation of LVS Function	240	100%	99%	99%
Medicare Spending				
Medicare Spending per Patient (ratio)	-	1.19	1.04	0.98
Pneumonia Care				
Appropriate Initial Antibiotic Given	68	96%	96%	95%
Blood Culture Timing	134	100%	96%	98%
Pregnancy and Delivery Care				
Newborn Deliveries Scheduled Early[7]	-	-	6%	6%
Preventive Care				
Immunization for Influenza[2]	419	99%	93%	90%
Immunization for Pneumonia[2]	653	99%	94%	92%
Stroke Care				
Anticoagulation Therapy for Atrial Fibrillation[1]	-	-	92%	95%
Antithrombotic Therapy Timing	21	100%	97%	98%
Assessed for Rehabilitation	22	100%	96%	97%
Discharged on Antithrombotic Therapy	22	95%	99%	99%
Discharged on Statin Medication	16	100%	95%	94%
Thrombolytic Therapy Timing[7]	-	-	80%	66%
Venous Thromboembolism Prophylaxis	23	100%	91%	94%
Written Stroke Educational Materials Given[1]	-	-	87%	88%
Surgical Care Improvement Project				
Appropriate Beta Blocker Usage	24	100%	96%	98%
Appropriate VTP Within 24 Hours	96	94%	98%	98%
Controlled Postoperative Blood Glucose[7]	-	-	97%	97%
Perioperative Temperature Management	119	100%	100%	100%
Prophylactic Antibiotic Selection	39	97%	99%	99%
Prophylactic Antibiotic Selection (Outpatient)	34	94%	98%	98%
Prophylactic Antibiotic Stopped	39	100%	98%	98%
Prophylactic Antibiotic Timing	41	100%	99%	99%
Prophylactic Antibiotic Timing (Outpatient)	34	100%	98%	98%
Urinary Catheter Removal	33	88%	98%	97%
Survey of Patients' Hospital Experiences				
Area Around Room 'Always' Quiet at Night	300+	59%	57%	61%
Doctors 'Always' Communicated Well	300+	79%	75%	82%
Home Recovery Information Given	300+	84%	85%	85%
Hospital Given 9 or 10 on 10 Point Scale	300+	66%	66%	71%
Meds 'Always' Explained Before Given	300+	61%	60%	64%
Nurses 'Always' Communicated Well	300+	73%	72%	79%
Pain 'Always' Well Controlled	300+	68%	67%	71%

NOTE: Hospital profiles are in alphabetical order by state, then city, then hospital within the city; Rankings exclude hospitals with less than 25 cases except for patient surveys which excludes hospitals with less than 100 cases; (a) 100-299 cases; (1) The number of cases/patients is too few to report; (2) Data submitted were based on a sample of cases/patients; (3) Results are based on a shorter time period than required; (4) Data suppressed by CMS for one or more quarters; (5) Results are not available for this reporting period; (6) Fewer than 100 patients completed the HCAHPS survey; (7) No cases met the criteria for this measure; (8) The lower limit of the confidence interval cannot be calculated if the number of observed infections equals zero; (9) No data are available from the state/territory for this reporting period; (10) The scores shown reflect fewer than 50 completed surveys; (11) There were discrepancies in the data collection process; (12) This measure does not apply to this hospital for this reporting period; (13) Results cannot be calculated for this reporting period; (14) The results for this state are combined with nearby states to protect confidentiality; Please refer to the User's Guide for a full explanation of data.

Measure	Cases	This Hosp.	State Avg.	U.S. Avg.
Room and Bathroom 'Always' Clean	300+	67%	68%	73%
Timely Help 'Always' Received	300+	60%	59%	68%
Would Definitely Recommend Hospital	300+	66%	69%	71%
Use of Medical Imaging				
Cardiac Imaging Stress Test before Surgery	104	2.9%	4.8%	5.3%
Combination Abdominal CT Scan	211	2.4%	6.9%	10.5%
Combination Brain/Sinus CT Scan[1]	-	-	2.7%	2.7%
Combination Chest CT Scan[1]	-	-	3.7%	2.7%
Follow-up Mammogram/Ultrasound[1]	-	-	7.3%	8.8%
Lumbar Spine MRI for Low Back Pain[1]	-	-	36.8%	37.2%

Desert View Regional Medical Center

360 South Lola Lane Phone: 775-751-7500
Pahrump, NV 89048
Type: Critical Access Hospitals Emergency Services: Yes
Ownership: Proprietary

Measure	Cases	This Hosp.	State Avg.	U.S. Avg.
Blood Clot Prevention and Treatment				
Anticoagulation Overlap Therapy[5]	-	-	96%	93%
ICU Venous Thromboembolism Prophylaxis[5]	-	-	91%	92%
Incidence of Potentially Preventable VTE[5]	-	-	10%	10%
UFH with Dosages/Platelet Monitoring[5]	-	-	99%	97%
Venous Thromboembolism Prophylaxis[5]	-	-	84%	85%
Warfarin Therapy Discharge Instructions[5]	-	-	90%	75%
Chest Pain/Possible Heart Attack Care				
Aspirin Given Within 24 Hours of Arrival[1,3]	-	-	98%	96%
Fibrinolytic Meds Within 30 Min. of Arrival[5]	-	-	40%	58%
Average Time to ECG (minutes)[1,3]	-	-	9	7
Average Time to Transfer (minutes)[5]	-	-	66	60
Children's Asthma Care				
Received Home Management Plan of Care	-	-	-	88%
Received Reliever Medication	-	-	-	100%
Received Systemic Corticosteroids	-	-	-	100%
Emergency Department				
Admittance Decision Time (minutes)[5]	-	-	151	98
Head CT Results Within 45 Min. of Arrival[5]	-	-	44%	57%
Patients Who Left ER Before Being Seen	14,234	2%	2%	2%
Time from ER Arrival to Admit. (minutes)[5]	-	-	337	274
Time from ER Arrival to Discharge (minutes)[5]	-	-	150	134
Time in ER Before Being Evaluated (minutes)[5]	-	-	22	26
Time to Pain Meds for Fractures (minutes)[5]	-	-	54	57
Heart Attack Care				
Aspirin Given at Discharge[5]	-	-	99%	99%
Fibrinolytic Meds Within 30 Min. of Arrival[5]	-	-	67%	54%
PCI Within 90 Minutes of Arrival[5]	-	-	97%	96%
Statin Prescribed at Discharge[5]	-	-	98%	98%
Heart Failure Care				
ACE Inhibitor or ARB for LVSD[5]	-	-	97%	97%
Discharge Instructions Given[3]	17	100%	91%	94%
Evaluation of LVS Function[5]	-	-	99%	99%
Medicare Spending				
Medicare Spending per Patient (ratio)	-	-	1.04	0.98
Pneumonia Care				
Appropriate Initial Antibiotic Given[1,3]	-	-	96%	95%
Blood Culture Timing[5]	-	-	96%	98%
Pregnancy and Delivery Care				
Newborn Deliveries Scheduled Early[5]	-	-	6%	6%
Preventive Care				
Immunization for Influenza[5]	-	-	93%	90%
Immunization for Pneumonia[5]	-	-	94%	92%
Stroke Care				
Anticoagulation Therapy for Atrial Fibrillation[5]	-	-	92%	95%
Antithrombotic Therapy Timing[5]	-	-	97%	98%
Assessed for Rehabilitation[5]	-	-	96%	97%
Discharged on Antithrombotic Therapy[5]	-	-	99%	99%
Discharged on Statin Medication[5]	-	-	95%	94%
Thrombolytic Therapy Timing[5]	-	-	80%	66%
Venous Thromboembolism Prophylaxis[5]	-	-	91%	94%
Written Stroke Educational Materials Given[5]	-	-	87%	88%
Surgical Care Improvement Project				
Appropriate Beta Blocker Usage[5]	-	-	96%	98%
Appropriate VTP Within 24 Hours[5]	-	-	98%	98%
Controlled Postoperative Blood Glucose[5]	-	-	97%	97%
Perioperative Temperature Management[5]	-	-	100%	100%
Prophylactic Antibiotic Selection[5]	-	-	99%	99%
Prophylactic Antibiotic Selection (Outpatient)[5]	-	-	98%	98%
Prophylactic Antibiotic Stopped[5]	-	-	98%	98%
Prophylactic Antibiotic Timing[5]	-	-	99%	99%
Prophylactic Antibiotic Timing (Outpatient)[5]	-	-	98%	98%
Urinary Catheter Removal[5]	-	-	98%	97%
Survey of Patients' Hospital Experiences				
Area Around Room 'Always' Quiet at Night[5]	-	-	57%	61%
Doctors 'Always' Communicated Well[5]	-	-	75%	82%
Home Recovery Information Given[5]	-	-	85%	85%
Hospital Given 9 or 10 on 10 Point Scale[5]	-	-	66%	71%
Meds 'Always' Explained Before Given[5]	-	-	60%	64%
Nurses 'Always' Communicated Well[5]	-	-	72%	79%
Pain 'Always' Well Controlled[5]	-	-	67%	71%
Room and Bathroom 'Always' Clean[5]	-	-	68%	73%
Timely Help 'Always' Received[5]	-	-	59%	68%
Would Definitely Recommend Hospital[5]	-	-	69%	71%
Use of Medical Imaging				
Cardiac Imaging Stress Test before Surgery[1]	-	-	4.8%	5.3%
Combination Abdominal CT Scan	320	15.3%	6.9%	10.5%
Combination Brain/Sinus CT Scan	387	1.0%	2.7%	2.7%
Combination Chest CT Scan	313	13.4%	3.7%	2.7%
Follow-up Mammogram/Ultrasound	173	6.9%	7.3%	8.8%
Lumbar Spine MRI for Low Back Pain[1]	-	-	36.8%	37.2%

Renown Regional Medical Center

1155 Mill Street Phone: 775-982-4100
Reno, NV 89502
URL: www.renown.org
Type: Acute Care Hospitals Emergency Services: Yes
Ownership: Voluntary non-profit - Other
Key Personnel:
Chief of Medical Staff. . . . . Max Jackson
CEO/President. . . . . Anthony D. Slonim, MD, DrPH

Measure	Cases	This Hosp.	State Avg.	U.S. Avg.
Blood Clot Prevention and Treatment				
Anticoagulation Overlap Therapy[2]	197	95%	96%	93%
ICU Venous Thromboembolism Prophylaxis[2]	123	96%	91%	92%
Incidence of Potentially Preventable VTE[2]	37	3%	10%	10%
UFH with Dosages/Platelet Monitoring[2]	99	100%	99%	97%
Venous Thromboembolism Prophylaxis[2]	332	94%	84%	85%
Warfarin Therapy Discharge Instructions[2]	154	93%	90%	75%
Chest Pain/Possible Heart Attack Care				
Aspirin Given Within 24 Hours of Arrival[5]	-	-	98%	96%
Fibrinolytic Meds Within 30 Min. of Arrival[5]	-	-	40%	58%
Average Time to ECG (minutes)[5]	-	-	9	7
Average Time to Transfer (minutes)[5]	-	-	66	60
Children's Asthma Care				
Received Home Management Plan of Care	73	99%	-	88%
Received Reliever Medication	75	100%	-	100%
Received Systemic Corticosteroids	75	100%	-	100%
Emergency Department				
Admittance Decision Time (minutes)[2]	614	58	151	98
Head CT Results Within 45 Min. of Arrival[1]	-	-	44%	57%
Patients Who Left ER Before Being Seen	84,092	2%	2%	2%
Time from ER Arrival to Admit. (minutes)[2]	623	277	337	274
Time from ER Arrival to Discharge (minutes)	376	164	150	134
Time in ER Before Being Evaluated (minutes)	432	42	22	26
Time to Pain Meds for Fractures (minutes)	236	60	54	57
Heart Attack Care				
Aspirin Given at Discharge[2]	302	100%	99%	99%
Fibrinolytic Meds Within 30 Min. of Arrival[2,7]	-	-	67%	54%
PCI Within 90 Minutes of Arrival[2]	51	100%	97%	96%
Statin Prescribed at Discharge[2]	297	100%	98%	98%
Heart Failure Care				
ACE Inhibitor or ARB for LVSD[2]	141	100%	97%	97%
Discharge Instructions Given[2]	279	97%	91%	94%
Evaluation of LVS Function[2]	327	100%	99%	99%
Medicare Spending				
Medicare Spending per Patient (ratio)	-	0.98	1.04	0.98
Pneumonia Care				
Appropriate Initial Antibiotic Given[2]	80	98%	96%	95%
Blood Culture Timing[2]	153	98%	96%	98%
Pregnancy and Delivery Care				
Newborn Deliveries Scheduled Early[2]	30	10%	6%	6%
Preventive Care				
Immunization for Influenza[2]	537	99%	93%	90%
Immunization for Pneumonia[2]	562	98%	94%	92%
Stroke Care				
Anticoagulation Therapy for Atrial Fibrillation[2]	19	100%	92%	95%
Antithrombotic Therapy Timing[2]	86	98%	97%	98%
Assessed for Rehabilitation[2]	130	100%	96%	97%
Discharged on Antithrombotic Therapy[2]	104	99%	99%	99%
Discharged on Statin Medication[2]	77	96%	95%	94%
Thrombolytic Therapy Timing[2]	12	58%	80%	66%
Venous Thromboembolism Prophylaxis[2]	131	99%	91%	94%
Written Stroke Educational Materials Given[2]	69	96%	87%	88%
Surgical Care Improvement Project				
Appropriate Beta Blocker Usage[2]	245	99%	96%	98%
Appropriate VTP Within 24 Hours[2]	553	100%	98%	98%
Controlled Postoperative Blood Glucose[2]	225	98%	97%	97%
Perioperative Temperature Management[2]	741	100%	100%	100%
Prophylactic Antibiotic Selection[2]	670	100%	99%	99%
Prophylactic Antibiotic Selection (Outpatient)	481	100%	98%	98%
Prophylactic Antibiotic Stopped[2]	628	100%	98%	98%
Prophylactic Antibiotic Timing[2]	673	99%	99%	99%
Prophylactic Antibiotic Timing (Outpatient)	482	99%	98%	98%
Urinary Catheter Removal[2]	459	100%	98%	97%
Survey of Patients' Hospital Experiences				
Area Around Room 'Always' Quiet at Night	300+	47%	57%	61%
Doctors 'Always' Communicated Well	300+	73%	75%	82%
Home Recovery Information Given	300+	87%	85%	85%
Hospital Given 9 or 10 on 10 Point Scale	300+	67%	66%	71%
Meds 'Always' Explained Before Given	300+	60%	60%	64%
Nurses 'Always' Communicated Well	300+	74%	72%	79%
Pain 'Always' Well Controlled	300+	70%	67%	71%
Room and Bathroom 'Always' Clean	300+	66%	68%	73%
Timely Help 'Always' Received	300+	58%	59%	68%
Would Definitely Recommend Hospital	300+	71%	69%	71%
Use of Medical Imaging				
Cardiac Imaging Stress Test before Surgery	1,388	4.6%	4.8%	5.3%
Combination Abdominal CT Scan	944	5.2%	6.9%	10.5%
Combination Brain/Sinus CT Scan	950	2.8%	2.7%	2.7%
Combination Chest CT Scan	736	0.0%	3.7%	2.7%
Follow-up Mammogram/Ultrasound[7]	-	-	7.3%	8.8%
Lumbar Spine MRI for Low Back Pain	164	29.9%	36.8%	37.2%

Renown South Meadows Medical Center

10101 Double R Blvd Phone: 775-982-7000
Reno, NV 89521
URL: www.renown.org
Type: Acute Care Hospitals Emergency Services: Yes
Ownership: Voluntary non-profit - Private
Key Personnel:
CEO/President. . . . . Alan Olive
Ambulatory Care . . . . Larry Trilops

Measure	Cases	This Hosp.	State Avg.	U.S. Avg.
Blood Clot Prevention and Treatment				
Anticoagulation Overlap Therapy[2]	32	100%	96%	93%
ICU Venous Thromboembolism Prophylaxis[2]	34	100%	91%	92%
Incidence of Potentially Preventable VTE[2,7]	-	-	10%	10%
UFH with Dosages/Platelet Monitoring[1,2]	-	-	99%	97%
Venous Thromboembolism Prophylaxis[2]	226	100%	84%	85%
Warfarin Therapy Discharge Instructions[2]	31	100%	90%	75%
Chest Pain/Possible Heart Attack Care				
Aspirin Given Within 24 Hours of Arrival	18	100%	98%	96%
Fibrinolytic Meds Within 30 Min. of Arrival[7]	-	-	40%	58%
Average Time to ECG (minutes)	18	7	9	7
Average Time to Transfer (minutes)[7]	-	-	66	60
Children's Asthma Care				
Received Home Management Plan of Care	-	-	-	88%
Received Reliever Medication	-	-	-	100%
Received Systemic Corticosteroids	-	-	-	100%
Emergency Department				

NOTE: Hospital profiles are in alphabetical order by state, then city, then hospital within the city; Rankings exclude hospitals with less than 25 cases except for patient surveys which excludes hospitals with less than 100 cases; (a) 100-299 cases; (1) The number of cases/patients is too few to report; (2) Data submitted were based on a sample of cases/patients; (3) Results are based on a shorter time period than required; (4) Data suppressed by CMS for one or more quarters; (5) Results are not available for this reporting period; (6) Fewer than 100 patients completed the HCAHPS survey; (7) No cases met the criteria for this measure; (8) The lower limit of the confidence interval cannot be calculated if the number of observed infections equals zero; (9) No data are available from the state/territory for this reporting period; (10) The scores shown reflect fewer than 50 completed surveys; (11) There were discrepancies in the data collection process; (12) This measure does not apply to this hospital for this reporting period; (13) Results cannot be calculated for this reporting period; (14) The results for this state are combined with nearby states to protect confidentiality; Please refer to the User's Guide for a full explanation of data.

Admittance Decision Time (minutes)[2]	488	53	151	98
Head CT Results Within 45 Min. of Arrival[1]	-	-	44%	57%
Patients Who Left ER Before Being Seen	20,251	1%	2%	2%
Time from ER Arrival to Admit. (minutes)[2]	488	238	337	274
Time from ER Arrival to Discharge (minutes)	416	136	150	134
Time in ER Before Being Evaluated (minutes)	454	23	22	26
Time to Pain Meds for Fractures (minutes)	92	50	54	57
Heart Attack Care				
Aspirin Given at Discharge[1]	-	-	99%	99%
Fibrinolytic Meds Within 30 Min. of Arrival[7]	-	-	67%	54%
PCI Within 90 Minutes of Arrival[7]	-	-	97%	96%
Statin Prescribed at Discharge[1]	-	-	98%	98%
Heart Failure Care				
ACE Inhibitor or ARB for LVSD	16	100%	97%	97%
Discharge Instructions Given	50	100%	91%	94%
Evaluation of LVS Function	54	100%	99%	99%
Medicare Spending				
Medicare Spending per Patient (ratio)	-	0.89	1.04	0.98
Pneumonia Care				
Appropriate Initial Antibiotic Given	78	100%	96%	95%
Blood Culture Timing	115	100%	96%	98%
Pregnancy and Delivery Care				
Newborn Deliveries Scheduled Early[7]	-	-	6%	6%
Preventive Care				
Immunization for Influenza[2]	338	100%	93%	90%
Immunization for Pneumonia[2]	434	100%	94%	92%
Stroke Care				
Anticoagulation Therapy for Atrial Fibrillation[1]	-	-	92%	95%
Antithrombotic Therapy Timing[1]	-	-	97%	98%
Assessed for Rehabilitation[1]	-	-	96%	97%
Discharged on Antithrombotic Therapy[1]	-	-	99%	99%
Discharged on Statin Medication[1]	-	-	95%	94%
Thrombolytic Therapy Timing[7]	-	-	80%	66%
Venous Thromboembolism Prophylaxis[1]	-	-	91%	94%
Written Stroke Educational Materials Given[1]	-	-	87%	88%
Surgical Care Improvement Project				
Appropriate Beta Blocker Usage	99	100%	96%	98%
Appropriate VTP Within 24 Hours	314	100%	98%	98%
Controlled Postoperative Blood Glucose[7]	-	-	97%	97%
Perioperative Temperature Management	490	100%	100%	100%
Prophylactic Antibiotic Selection	382	100%	99%	99%
Prophylactic Antibiotic Selection (Outpatient)	28	100%	98%	98%
Prophylactic Antibiotic Stopped	377	100%	98%	98%
Prophylactic Antibiotic Timing	382	100%	99%	99%
Prophylactic Antibiotic Timing (Outpatient)	28	100%	98%	98%
Urinary Catheter Removal	99	100%	98%	97%
Survey of Patients' Hospital Experiences				
Area Around Room 'Always' Quiet at Night	300+	50%	57%	61%
Doctors 'Always' Communicated Well	300+	76%	75%	82%
Home Recovery Information Given	300+	85%	85%	85%
Hospital Given 9 or 10 on 10 Point Scale	300+	73%	66%	71%
Meds 'Always' Explained Before Given	300+	65%	60%	64%
Nurses 'Always' Communicated Well	300+	80%	72%	79%
Pain 'Always' Well Controlled	300+	71%	67%	71%
Room and Bathroom 'Always' Clean	300+	72%	68%	73%
Timely Help 'Always' Received	300+	68%	59%	68%
Would Definitely Recommend Hospital	300+	80%	69%	71%
Use of Medical Imaging				
Cardiac Imaging Stress Test before Surgery	199	5.0%	4.8%	5.3%
Combination Abdominal CT Scan	520	8.1%	6.9%	10.5%
Combination Brain/Sinus CT Scan[1]	-	-	2.7%	2.7%
Combination Chest CT Scan	357	0.0%	3.7%	2.7%
Follow-up Mammogram/Ultrasound[7]	-	-	7.3%	8.8%
Lumbar Spine MRI for Low Back Pain	95	35.8%	36.8%	37.2%

Saint Mary's Regional Medical Center

235 W 6th St
Reno, NV 89503
Phone: 775-770-3000
Fax: 775-770-3963
URL: www.saintmarysreno.com
Type: Acute Care Hospitals
Emergency Services: Yes
Ownership: Voluntary non-profit - Private
Beds: 408

Key Personnel:

CEO/President. . . . . Jeff K Bills
Radiology. . . . . George Cervantes, MD
Quality Assurance . . . . Linda Charlebois, RN
Infection Control. . . . . Cyndie Kern, RN
Operating Room. . . . . Kit Landis, RN
Pediatric Ambulatory Care . . . . . . Terri Mishlr, RN
Chief of Medical Staff . . . . John Williamson, MD

Measure	Cases	This Hosp.	State Avg.	U.S. Avg.
Blood Clot Prevention and Treatment				
Anticoagulation Overlap Therapy[2]	121	96%	96%	93%
ICU Venous Thromboembolism Prophylaxis[2]	59	95%	91%	92%
Incidence of Potentially Preventable VTE[2]	15	7%	10%	10%
UFH with Dosages/Platelet Monitoring[2]	97	100%	99%	97%
Venous Thromboembolism Prophylaxis[2]	322	97%	84%	85%
Warfarin Therapy Discharge Instructions[2]	102	98%	90%	75%
Chest Pain/Possible Heart Attack Care				
Aspirin Given Within 24 Hours of Arrival[5]	-	-	98%	96%
Fibrinolytic Meds Within 30 Min. of Arrival[5]	-	-	40%	58%
Average Time to ECG (minutes)[1]	-	-	9	7
Average Time to Transfer (minutes)[5]	-	-	66	60
Children's Asthma Care				
Received Home Management Plan of Care	-	-	-	88%
Received Reliever Medication	-	-	-	100%
Received Systemic Corticosteroids	-	-	-	100%
Emergency Department				
Admittance Decision Time (minutes)[2]	661	115	151	98
Head CT Results Within 45 Min. of Arrival[1]	-	-	44%	57%
Patients Who Left ER Before Being Seen	53,801	1%	2%	2%
Time from ER Arrival to Admit. (minutes)[2]	661	268	337	274
Time from ER Arrival to Discharge (minutes)	385	153	150	134
Time in ER Before Being Evaluated (minutes)	405	29	22	26
Time to Pain Meds for Fractures (minutes)	157	54	54	57
Heart Attack Care				
Aspirin Given at Discharge	231	100%	99%	99%
Fibrinolytic Meds Within 30 Min. of Arrival[7]	-	-	67%	54%
PCI Within 90 Minutes of Arrival	45	100%	97%	96%
Statin Prescribed at Discharge	225	99%	98%	98%
Heart Failure Care				
ACE Inhibitor or ARB for LVSD[2]	112	100%	97%	97%
Discharge Instructions Given[2]	251	97%	91%	94%
Evaluation of LVS Function[2]	288	100%	99%	99%
Medicare Spending				
Medicare Spending per Patient (ratio)	-	0.94	1.04	0.98
Pneumonia Care				
Appropriate Initial Antibiotic Given[2]	72	96%	96%	95%
Blood Culture Timing[2]	150	99%	96%	98%
Pregnancy and Delivery Care				
Newborn Deliveries Scheduled Early[2]	45	2%	6%	6%
Preventive Care				
Immunization for Influenza[2]	523	93%	93%	90%
Immunization for Pneumonia[2]	524	96%	94%	92%
Stroke Care				
Anticoagulation Therapy for Atrial Fibrillation	27	96%	92%	95%
Antithrombotic Therapy Timing	97	97%	97%	98%
Assessed for Rehabilitation	128	97%	96%	97%
Discharged on Antithrombotic Therapy	110	100%	99%	99%
Discharged on Statin Medication	82	98%	95%	94%
Thrombolytic Therapy Timing	11	64%	80%	66%
Venous Thromboembolism Prophylaxis	134	93%	91%	94%
Written Stroke Educational Materials Given	80	98%	87%	88%
Surgical Care Improvement Project				
Appropriate Beta Blocker Usage[2]	110	100%	96%	98%
Appropriate VTP Within 24 Hours[2]	341	100%	98%	98%
Controlled Postoperative Blood Glucose[2]	97	96%	97%	97%
Perioperative Temperature Management[2]	514	100%	100%	100%
Prophylactic Antibiotic Selection[2]	452	100%	99%	99%
Prophylactic Antibiotic Selection (Outpatient)	431	98%	98%	98%
Prophylactic Antibiotic Stopped[2]	443	99%	98%	98%
Prophylactic Antibiotic Timing[2]	452	97%	99%	99%
Prophylactic Antibiotic Timing (Outpatient)	434	98%	98%	98%
Urinary Catheter Removal[2]	232	100%	98%	97%
Survey of Patients' Hospital Experiences				
Area Around Room 'Always' Quiet at Night	300+	51%	57%	61%
Doctors 'Always' Communicated Well	300+	77%	75%	82%
Home Recovery Information Given	300+	87%	85%	85%
Hospital Given 9 or 10 on 10 Point Scale	300+	64%	66%	71%
Meds 'Always' Explained Before Given	300+	61%	60%	64%
Nurses 'Always' Communicated Well	300+	74%	72%	79%
Pain 'Always' Well Controlled	300+	69%	67%	71%
Room and Bathroom 'Always' Clean	300+	70%	68%	73%
Timely Help 'Always' Received	300+	56%	59%	68%
Would Definitely Recommend Hospital	300+	73%	69%	71%
Use of Medical Imaging				
Cardiac Imaging Stress Test before Surgery	278	4.7%	4.8%	5.3%
Combination Abdominal CT Scan	623	5.6%	6.9%	10.5%
Combination Brain/Sinus CT Scan[1]	-	-	2.7%	2.7%
Combination Chest CT Scan	493	0.0%	3.7%	2.7%
Follow-up Mammogram/Ultrasound	724	9.1%	7.3%	8.8%
Lumbar Spine MRI for Low Back Pain	82	40.2%	36.8%	37.2%

VA Sierra Nevada Healthcare System

1000 Locust Street
Reno, NV 89502
Phone: 775-328-1263
Fax: 775-328-1464
URL: www.reno.va.gov
Type: Acute Care - VA
Emergency Services: No
Ownership: Government Federal
Beds: 228

Key Personnel:

Anesthesiology. . . . . Joseph Bovill, MD
Chief of Medical Staff . . . . Steven E Brilliant, MD
Cardiac Laboratory. . . . . Dr William Graettinger
Intensive Care Unit. . . . . Nancy Johnson, RN
Operating Room. . . . . Dr Phillip Lisagor
Infection Control. . . . . Theresa Rucker, RN
Emergency Room . . . . Bonnie Rudolph, RN

Measure	Cases	This Hosp.	State Avg.	U.S. Avg.
Blood Clot Prevention and Treatment				
Anticoagulation Overlap Therapy	-	-	96%	93%
ICU Venous Thromboembolism Prophylaxis	-	-	91%	92%
Incidence of Potentially Preventable VTE	-	-	10%	10%
UFH with Dosages/Platelet Monitoring	-	-	99%	97%
Venous Thromboembolism Prophylaxis	-	-	84%	85%
Warfarin Therapy Discharge Instructions	-	-	90%	75%
Chest Pain/Possible Heart Attack Care				
Aspirin Given Within 24 Hours of Arrival	-	-	98%	96%
Fibrinolytic Meds Within 30 Min. of Arrival	-	-	40%	58%
Average Time to ECG (minutes)	-	-	9	7
Average Time to Transfer (minutes)	-	-	66	60
Children's Asthma Care				
Received Home Management Plan of Care	-	-	-	88%
Received Reliever Medication	-	-	-	100%
Received Systemic Corticosteroids	-	-	-	100%
Emergency Department				
Admittance Decision Time (minutes)	-	-	151	98
Head CT Results Within 45 Min. of Arrival	-	-	44%	57%
Patients Who Left ER Before Being Seen	-	-	2%	2%
Time from ER Arrival to Admit. (minutes)	-	-	337	274
Time from ER Arrival to Discharge (minutes)	-	-	150	134
Time in ER Before Being Evaluated (minutes)	-	-	22	26
Time to Pain Meds for Fractures (minutes)	-	-	54	57
Heart Attack Care				
Aspirin Given at Discharge	26	100%	99%	99%
Fibrinolytic Meds Within 30 Min. of Arrival[5]	-	-	67%	54%
PCI Within 90 Minutes of Arrival[5]	-	-	97%	96%
Statin Prescribed at Discharge	26	100%	98%	98%
Heart Failure Care				
ACE Inhibitor or ARB for LVSD	41	100%	97%	97%
Discharge Instructions Given	81	96%	91%	94%
Evaluation of LVS Function	88	100%	99%	99%
Medicare Spending				
Medicare Spending per Patient (ratio)	-	-	1.04	0.98
Pneumonia Care				
Appropriate Initial Antibiotic Given	47	100%	96%	95%
Blood Culture Timing	128	99%	96%	98%
Pregnancy and Delivery Care				
Newborn Deliveries Scheduled Early	-	-	6%	6%
Preventive Care				
Immunization for Influenza[5]	-	-	93%	90%
Immunization for Pneumonia[5]	-	-	94%	92%

NOTE: Hospital profiles are in alphabetical order by state, then city, then hospital within the city; Rankings exclude hospitals with less than 25 cases except for patient surveys which excludes hospitals with less than 100 cases; (a) 100-299 cases; (1) The number of cases/patients is too few to report; (2) Data submitted were based on a sample of cases/patients; (3) Results are based on a shorter time period than required; (4) Data suppressed by CMS for one or more quarters; (5) Results are not available for this reporting period; (6) Fewer than 100 patients completed the HCAHPS survey; (7) No cases met the criteria for this measure; (8) The lower limit of the confidence interval cannot be calculated if the number of observed infections equals zero; (9) No data are available from the state/territory for this reporting period; (10) The scores shown reflect fewer than 50 completed surveys; (11) There were discrepancies in the data collection process; (12) This measure does not apply to this hospital for this reporting period; (13) Results cannot be calculated for this reporting period; (14) The results for this state are combined with nearby states to protect confidentiality; Please refer to the User's Guide for a full explanation of data.

Measure	Cases	This Hosp.	State Avg.	U.S. Avg.
Stroke Care				
Anticoagulation Therapy for Atrial Fibrillation	-	-	92%	95%
Antithrombotic Therapy Timing	-	-	97%	98%
Assessed for Rehabilitation	-	-	96%	97%
Discharged on Antithrombotic Therapy	-	-	99%	99%
Discharged on Statin Medication	-	-	95%	94%
Thrombolytic Therapy Timing	-	-	80%	66%
Venous Thromboembolism Prophylaxis	-	-	91%	94%
Written Stroke Educational Materials Given	-	-	87%	88%
Surgical Care Improvement Project				
Appropriate Beta Blocker Usage[2]	72	99%	96%	98%
Appropriate VTP Within 24 Hours[2]	128	97%	98%	98%
Controlled Postoperative Blood Glucose[5]	-	-	97%	97%
Perioperative Temperature Management[2]	190	100%	100%	100%
Prophylactic Antibiotic Selection	119	100%	99%	99%
Prophylactic Antibiotic Selection (Outpatient)	-	-	98%	98%
Prophylactic Antibiotic Stopped	116	97%	98%	98%
Prophylactic Antibiotic Timing	119	100%	99%	99%
Prophylactic Antibiotic Timing (Outpatient)	-	-	98%	98%
Urinary Catheter Removal[2]	133	99%	98%	97%
Survey of Patients' Hospital Experiences				
Area Around Room 'Always' Quiet at Night	-	-	57%	61%
Doctors 'Always' Communicated Well	-	-	75%	82%
Home Recovery Information Given	-	-	85%	85%
Hospital Given 9 or 10 on 10 Point Scale	-	-	66%	71%
Meds 'Always' Explained Before Given	-	-	60%	64%
Nurses 'Always' Communicated Well	-	-	72%	79%
Pain 'Always' Well Controlled	-	-	67%	71%
Room and Bathroom 'Always' Clean	-	-	68%	73%
Timely Help 'Always' Received	-	-	59%	68%
Would Definitely Recommend Hospital	-	-	69%	71%
Use of Medical Imaging				
Cardiac Imaging Stress Test before Surgery	-	-	4.8%	5.3%
Combination Abdominal CT Scan	-	-	6.9%	10.5%
Combination Brain/Sinus CT Scan	-	-	2.7%	2.7%
Combination Chest CT Scan	-	-	3.7%	2.7%
Follow-up Mammogram/Ultrasound	-	-	7.3%	8.8%
Lumbar Spine MRI for Low Back Pain	-	-	36.8%	37.2%

Northern Nevada Medical Center

2375 Prater Way
Sparks, NV 89434
Phone: 775-331-7000
Fax: 775-356-4901
URL: www.northernnvmed.com
Type: Acute Care Hospitals
Emergency Services: Yes
Ownership: Proprietary
Beds: 100

Key Personnel:
CEO/President. . . . . Mark W Crawford
Operating Room. . . . . William Ford, MD
Emergency Room . . . . Lisa Nelson, DO
Anesthesiology. . . . . Scott Parkhill, MD
Chief of Medical Staff . . . . Randall Pierce, MD
Quality Assurance . . . . Nancy Whitney

Measure	Cases	This Hosp.	State Avg.	U.S. Avg.
Blood Clot Prevention and Treatment				
Anticoagulation Overlap Therapy[2]	32	88%	96%	93%
ICU Venous Thromboembolism Prophylaxis[2]	30	100%	91%	92%
Incidence of Potentially Preventable VTE[1,2]	-	-	10%	10%
UFH with Dosages/Platelet Monitoring[2]	11	100%	99%	97%
Venous Thromboembolism Prophylaxis[2]	238	97%	84%	85%
Warfarin Therapy Discharge Instructions[2]	23	22%	90%	75%
Chest Pain/Possible Heart Attack Care				
Aspirin Given Within 24 Hours of Arrival[1,3]	-	-	98%	96%
Fibrinolytic Meds Within 30 Min. of Arrival[5]	-	-	40%	58%
Average Time to ECG (minutes)[1,3]	-	-	9	7
Average Time to Transfer (minutes)[5]	-	-	66	60
Children's Asthma Care				
Received Home Management Plan of Care	-	-	-	88%
Received Reliever Medication	-	-	-	100%
Received Systemic Corticosteroids	-	-	-	100%
Emergency Department				
Admittance Decision Time (minutes)[2]	408	101	151	98
Head CT Results Within 45 Min. of Arrival[1]	-	-	44%	57%
Patients Who Left ER Before Being Seen	19,444	2%	2%	2%
Time from ER Arrival to Admit. (minutes)[2]	481	254	337	274
Time from ER Arrival to Discharge (minutes)	365	140	150	134
Time in ER Before Being Evaluated (minutes)	361	23	22	26
Time to Pain Meds for Fractures (minutes)	64	74	54	57
Heart Attack Care				
Aspirin Given at Discharge	67	100%	99%	99%
Fibrinolytic Meds Within 30 Min. of Arrival[7]	-	-	67%	54%
PCI Within 90 Minutes of Arrival	20	70%	97%	96%
Statin Prescribed at Discharge	67	100%	98%	98%
Heart Failure Care				
ACE Inhibitor or ARB for LVSD	25	100%	97%	97%
Discharge Instructions Given	47	89%	91%	94%
Evaluation of LVS Function	53	100%	99%	99%
Medicare Spending				
Medicare Spending per Patient (ratio)	-	0.94	1.04	0.98
Pneumonia Care				
Appropriate Initial Antibiotic Given	61	100%	96%	95%
Blood Culture Timing	95	99%	96%	98%
Pregnancy and Delivery Care				
Newborn Deliveries Scheduled Early[7]	-	-	6%	6%
Preventive Care				
Immunization for Influenza[2]	330	98%	93%	90%
Immunization for Pneumonia[2]	456	99%	94%	92%
Stroke Care				
Anticoagulation Therapy for Atrial Fibrillation[1]	-	-	92%	95%
Antithrombotic Therapy Timing	25	96%	97%	98%
Assessed for Rehabilitation	37	100%	96%	97%
Discharged on Antithrombotic Therapy	36	100%	99%	99%
Discharged on Statin Medication	24	100%	95%	94%
Thrombolytic Therapy Timing[1]	-	-	80%	66%
Venous Thromboembolism Prophylaxis	23	96%	91%	94%
Written Stroke Educational Materials Given	23	91%	87%	88%
Surgical Care Improvement Project				
Appropriate Beta Blocker Usage[2]	65	97%	96%	98%
Appropriate VTP Within 24 Hours[2]	218	100%	98%	98%
Controlled Postoperative Blood Glucose[2,7]	-	-	97%	97%
Perioperative Temperature Management[2]	281	100%	100%	100%
Prophylactic Antibiotic Selection[2]	196	99%	99%	99%
Prophylactic Antibiotic Selection (Outpatient)	78	100%	98%	98%
Prophylactic Antibiotic Stopped[2]	194	97%	98%	98%
Prophylactic Antibiotic Timing[2]	196	98%	99%	99%
Prophylactic Antibiotic Timing (Outpatient)	78	100%	98%	98%
Urinary Catheter Removal[2]	93	98%	98%	97%
Survey of Patients' Hospital Experiences				
Area Around Room 'Always' Quiet at Night	300+	50%	57%	61%
Doctors 'Always' Communicated Well	300+	80%	75%	82%
Home Recovery Information Given	300+	87%	85%	85%
Hospital Given 9 or 10 on 10 Point Scale	300+	69%	66%	71%
Meds 'Always' Explained Before Given	300+	67%	60%	64%
Nurses 'Always' Communicated Well	300+	75%	72%	79%
Pain 'Always' Well Controlled	300+	68%	67%	71%
Room and Bathroom 'Always' Clean	300+	70%	68%	73%
Timely Help 'Always' Received	300+	64%	59%	68%
Would Definitely Recommend Hospital	300+	72%	69%	71%
Use of Medical Imaging				
Cardiac Imaging Stress Test before Surgery	248	5.6%	4.8%	5.3%
Combination Abdominal CT Scan	287	3.8%	6.9%	10.5%
Combination Brain/Sinus CT Scan[1]	-	-	2.7%	2.7%
Combination Chest CT Scan	149	0.0%	3.7%	2.7%
Follow-up Mammogram/Ultrasound	480	4.8%	7.3%	8.8%
Lumbar Spine MRI for Low Back Pain[1]	-	-	36.8%	37.2%

Nye Regional Medical Center

825 Erie Main Saint (aka South Main)
Tonopah, NV 89049
Phone: 775-482-6233
Fax: 775-482-8272
Type: Acute Care Hospitals
Emergency Services: Yes
Ownership: Voluntary non-profit - Other
Beds: 44

Key Personnel:
CEO/President. . . . . Rick Kilburn
Chief of Medical Staff . . . . Vincent Scoccia
Patient Relations . . . . Vincent Scoccia
Radiology. . . . . Vincent Scoccia
Chair/CEO . . . . Warren Setnan
Emergency Room . . . . Pat Steffens
Infection Control. . . . . Jessica Thompson

Measure	Cases	This Hosp.	State Avg.	U.S. Avg.
Blood Clot Prevention and Treatment				
Anticoagulation Overlap Therapy[5]	-	-	96%	93%
ICU Venous Thromboembolism Prophylaxis[5]	-	-	91%	92%
Incidence of Potentially Preventable VTE[5]	-	-	10%	10%
UFH with Dosages/Platelet Monitoring[5]	-	-	99%	97%
Venous Thromboembolism Prophylaxis[5]	-	-	84%	85%
Warfarin Therapy Discharge Instructions[5]	-	-	90%	75%
Chest Pain/Possible Heart Attack Care				
Aspirin Given Within 24 Hours of Arrival[5]	-	-	98%	96%
Fibrinolytic Meds Within 30 Min. of Arrival[5]	-	-	40%	58%
Average Time to ECG (minutes)[5]	-	-	9	7
Average Time to Transfer (minutes)[5]	-	-	66	60
Children's Asthma Care				
Received Home Management Plan of Care	-	-	-	88%
Received Reliever Medication	-	-	-	100%
Received Systemic Corticosteroids	-	-	-	100%
Emergency Department				
Admittance Decision Time (minutes)[5]	-	-	151	98
Head CT Results Within 45 Min. of Arrival[5]	-	-	44%	57%
Patients Who Left ER Before Being Seen	2,683	0%	2%	2%
Time from ER Arrival to Admit. (minutes)[5]	-	-	337	274
Time from ER Arrival to Discharge (minutes)	242	119	150	134
Time in ER Before Being Evaluated (minutes)	242	26	22	26
Time to Pain Meds for Fractures (minutes)[1,3]	-	-	54	57
Heart Attack Care				
Aspirin Given at Discharge[5]	-	-	99%	99%
Fibrinolytic Meds Within 30 Min. of Arrival[5]	-	-	67%	54%
PCI Within 90 Minutes of Arrival[5]	-	-	97%	96%
Statin Prescribed at Discharge[5]	-	-	98%	98%
Heart Failure Care				
ACE Inhibitor or ARB for LVSD[5]	-	-	97%	97%
Discharge Instructions Given[5]	-	-	91%	94%
Evaluation of LVS Function[5]	-	-	99%	99%
Medicare Spending				
Medicare Spending per Patient (ratio)	-	0.86	1.04	0.98
Pneumonia Care				
Appropriate Initial Antibiotic Given[5]	-	-	96%	95%
Blood Culture Timing[5]	-	-	96%	98%
Pregnancy and Delivery Care				
Newborn Deliveries Scheduled Early[5]	-	-	6%	6%
Preventive Care				
Immunization for Influenza[5]	-	-	93%	90%
Immunization for Pneumonia[5]	-	-	94%	92%
Stroke Care				
Anticoagulation Therapy for Atrial Fibrillation[5]	-	-	92%	95%
Antithrombotic Therapy Timing[5]	-	-	97%	98%
Assessed for Rehabilitation[5]	-	-	96%	97%
Discharged on Antithrombotic Therapy[5]	-	-	99%	99%
Discharged on Statin Medication[5]	-	-	95%	94%
Thrombolytic Therapy Timing[5]	-	-	80%	66%
Venous Thromboembolism Prophylaxis[5]	-	-	91%	94%
Written Stroke Educational Materials Given[5]	-	-	87%	88%
Surgical Care Improvement Project				
Appropriate Beta Blocker Usage[5]	-	-	96%	98%
Appropriate VTP Within 24 Hours[5]	-	-	98%	98%
Controlled Postoperative Blood Glucose[5]	-	-	97%	97%
Perioperative Temperature Management[5]	-	-	100%	100%
Prophylactic Antibiotic Selection[5]	-	-	99%	99%
Prophylactic Antibiotic Selection (Outpatient)[5]	-	-	98%	98%
Prophylactic Antibiotic Stopped[5]	-	-	98%	98%
Prophylactic Antibiotic Timing[5]	-	-	99%	99%
Prophylactic Antibiotic Timing (Outpatient)[5]	-	-	98%	98%
Urinary Catheter Removal[5]	-	-	98%	97%
Survey of Patients' Hospital Experiences				
Area Around Room 'Always' Quiet at Night[5]	-	-	57%	61%
Doctors 'Always' Communicated Well[5]	-	-	75%	82%
Home Recovery Information Given[5]	-	-	85%	85%
Hospital Given 9 or 10 on 10 Point Scale[5]	-	-	66%	71%
Meds 'Always' Explained Before Given[5]	-	-	60%	64%
Nurses 'Always' Communicated Well[5]	-	-	72%	79%
Pain 'Always' Well Controlled[5]	-	-	67%	71%

NOTE: Hospital profiles are in alphabetical order by state, then city, then hospital within the city; Rankings exclude hospitals with less than 25 cases except for patient surveys which excludes hospitals with less than 100 cases; (a) 100-299 cases; (1) The number of cases/patients is too few to report; (2) Data submitted were based on a sample of cases/patients; (3) Results are based on a shorter time period than required; (4) Data suppressed by CMS for one or more quarters; (5) Results are not available for this reporting period; (6) Fewer than 100 patients completed the HCAHPS survey; (7) No cases met the criteria for this measure; (8) The lower limit of the confidence interval cannot be calculated if the number of observed infections equals zero; (9) No data are available from the state/territory for this reporting period; (10) The scores shown reflect fewer than 50 completed surveys; (11) There were discrepancies in the data collection process; (12) This measure does not apply to this hospital for this reporting period; (13) Results cannot be calculated for this reporting period; (14) The results for this state are combined with nearby states to protect confidentiality; Please refer to the User's Guide for a full explanation of data.

Measure	Cases	This Hosp.	State Avg.	U.S. Avg.
Room and Bathroom 'Always' Clean[5]	-	-	68%	73%
Timely Help 'Always' Received[5]	-	-	59%	68%
Would Definitely Recommend Hospital[5]	-	-	69%	71%
Use of Medical Imaging				
Cardiac Imaging Stress Test before Surgery[1]	-	-	4.8%	5.3%
Combination Abdominal CT Scan[1]	-	-	6.9%	10.5%
Combination Brain/Sinus CT Scan[1]	-	-	2.7%	2.7%
Combination Chest CT Scan[1]	-	-	3.7%	2.7%
Follow-up Mammogram/Ultrasound[7]	-	-	7.3%	8.8%
Lumbar Spine MRI for Low Back Pain[1]	-	-	36.8%	37.2%

Humboldt General Hospital

118 East Haskell Street
Winnemucca, NV 89445
URL: www.hghospital.ws
Type: Critical Access Hospitals
Ownership: Govt - Hospital Dist/Auth
Phone: 775-623-5222
Fax: 775-623-5904
Emergency Services: Yes
Beds: 52

Key Personnel:

Anesthesiology. . . . . Carole Cain, CRNA
Operating Room. . . . . Kathy Gillihan, RN
Infection Control. . . . . Robin Gillis, RN
Quality Assurance . . . . Erika Gratwohl, RN
Chief of Medical Staff. . . . . Richard Ingle
Radiology. . . . . Leon Jackson
CEO/President. . . . . James Parrish
Emergency Room . . . . Pat Songer, RN

Measure	Cases	This Hosp.	State Avg.	U.S. Avg.
Blood Clot Prevention and Treatment				
Anticoagulation Overlap Therapy[5]	-	-	96%	93%
ICU Venous Thromboembolism Prophylaxis[5]	-	-	91%	92%
Incidence of Potentially Preventable VTE[5]	-	-	10%	10%
UFH with Dosages/Platelet Monitoring[5]	-	-	99%	97%
Venous Thromboembolism Prophylaxis[5]	-	-	84%	85%
Warfarin Therapy Discharge Instructions[5]	-	-	90%	75%
Chest Pain/Possible Heart Attack Care				
Aspirin Given Within 24 Hours of Arrival	35	94%	98%	96%
Fibrinolytic Meds Within 30 Min. of Arrival[1,3]	-	-	40%	58%
Average Time to ECG (minutes)	37	6	9	7
Average Time to Transfer (minutes)[3,7]	-	-	66	60
Children's Asthma Care				
Received Home Management Plan of Care	-	-	-	88%
Received Reliever Medication	-	-	-	100%
Received Systemic Corticosteroids	-	-	-	100%
Emergency Department				
Admittance Decision Time (minutes)[2]	235	65	151	98
Head CT Results Within 45 Min. of Arrival[1]	-	-	44%	57%
Patients Who Left ER Before Being Seen[5]	-	-	2%	2%
Time from ER Arrival to Admit. (minutes)[2]	259	231	337	274
Time from ER Arrival to Discharge (minutes)	365	99	150	134
Time in ER Before Being Evaluated (minutes)	356	21	22	26
Time to Pain Meds for Fractures (minutes)	27	40	54	57
Heart Attack Care				
Aspirin Given at Discharge[1,3]	-	-	99%	99%
Fibrinolytic Meds Within 30 Min. of Arrival[3,7]	-	-	67%	54%
PCI Within 90 Minutes of Arrival[3,7]	-	-	97%	96%
Statin Prescribed at Discharge[1,3]	-	-	98%	98%
Heart Failure Care				
ACE Inhibitor or ARB for LVSD[1]	-	-	97%	97%
Discharge Instructions Given[1]	-	-	91%	94%
Evaluation of LVS Function[1]	-	-	99%	99%
Medicare Spending				
Medicare Spending per Patient (ratio)	-	-	1.04	0.98
Pneumonia Care				
Appropriate Initial Antibiotic Given	15	87%	96%	95%
Blood Culture Timing	17	65%	96%	98%
Pregnancy and Delivery Care				
Newborn Deliveries Scheduled Early[5]	-	-	6%	6%
Preventive Care				
Immunization for Influenza[2]	251	78%	93%	90%
Immunization for Pneumonia[2]	188	54%	94%	92%
Stroke Care				
Anticoagulation Therapy for Atrial Fibrillation[5]	-	-	92%	95%
Antithrombotic Therapy Timing[5]	-	-	97%	98%
Assessed for Rehabilitation[5]	-	-	96%	97%
Discharged on Antithrombotic Therapy[5]	-	-	99%	99%
Discharged on Statin Medication[5]	-	-	95%	94%
Thrombolytic Therapy Timing[5]	-	-	80%	66%
Venous Thromboembolism Prophylaxis[5]	-	-	91%	94%
Written Stroke Educational Materials Given[5]	-	-	87%	88%
Surgical Care Improvement Project				
Appropriate Beta Blocker Usage[1,3]	-	-	96%	98%
Appropriate VTP Within 24 Hours[1,3]	-	-	98%	98%
Controlled Postoperative Blood Glucose[3,7]	-	-	97%	97%
Perioperative Temperature Management[1,3]	-	-	100%	100%
Prophylactic Antibiotic Selection[1,3]	-	-	99%	99%
Prophylactic Antibiotic Selection (Outpatient)[5]	-	-	98%	98%
Prophylactic Antibiotic Stopped[1,3]	-	-	98%	98%
Prophylactic Antibiotic Timing[1,3]	-	-	99%	99%
Prophylactic Antibiotic Timing (Outpatient)[5]	-	-	98%	98%
Urinary Catheter Removal[1,3]	-	-	98%	97%
Survey of Patients' Hospital Experiences				
Area Around Room 'Always' Quiet at Night[5]	-	-	57%	61%
Doctors 'Always' Communicated Well[5]	-	-	75%	82%
Home Recovery Information Given[5]	-	-	85%	85%
Hospital Given 9 or 10 on 10 Point Scale[5]	-	-	66%	71%
Meds 'Always' Explained Before Given[5]	-	-	60%	64%
Nurses 'Always' Communicated Well[5]	-	-	72%	79%
Pain 'Always' Well Controlled[5]	-	-	67%	71%
Room and Bathroom 'Always' Clean[5]	-	-	68%	73%
Timely Help 'Always' Received[5]	-	-	59%	68%
Would Definitely Recommend Hospital[5]	-	-	69%	71%
Use of Medical Imaging				
Cardiac Imaging Stress Test before Surgery	64	0.0%	4.8%	5.3%
Combination Abdominal CT Scan	117	6.0%	6.9%	10.5%
Combination Brain/Sinus CT Scan[1]	-	-	2.7%	2.7%
Combination Chest CT Scan	87	4.6%	3.7%	2.7%
Follow-up Mammogram/Ultrasound	150	2.0%	7.3%	8.8%
Lumbar Spine MRI for Low Back Pain[1]	-	-	36.8%	37.2%

South Lyon Medical Center

213 S Whitacre/po Box 940
Yerington, NV 89447
Type: Acute Care Hospitals
Ownership: Govt - Hospital Dist/Auth
Phone: 775-781-3761
Emergency Services: Yes

Measure	Cases	This Hosp.	State Avg.	U.S. Avg.
Blood Clot Prevention and Treatment				
Anticoagulation Overlap Therapy[5]	-	-	96%	93%
ICU Venous Thromboembolism Prophylaxis[5]	-	-	91%	92%
Incidence of Potentially Preventable VTE[5]	-	-	10%	10%
UFH with Dosages/Platelet Monitoring[5]	-	-	99%	97%
Venous Thromboembolism Prophylaxis[5]	-	-	84%	85%
Warfarin Therapy Discharge Instructions[5]	-	-	90%	75%
Chest Pain/Possible Heart Attack Care				
Aspirin Given Within 24 Hours of Arrival	-	-	98%	96%
Fibrinolytic Meds Within 30 Min. of Arrival	-	-	40%	58%
Average Time to ECG (minutes)	-	-	9	7
Average Time to Transfer (minutes)	-	-	66	60
Children's Asthma Care				
Received Home Management Plan of Care	-	-	-	88%
Received Reliever Medication	-	-	-	100%
Received Systemic Corticosteroids	-	-	-	100%
Emergency Department				
Admittance Decision Time (minutes)[5]	-	-	151	98
Head CT Results Within 45 Min. of Arrival	-	-	44%	57%
Patients Who Left ER Before Being Seen	-	-	2%	2%
Time from ER Arrival to Admit. (minutes)[5]	-	-	337	274
Time from ER Arrival to Discharge (minutes)	-	-	150	134
Time in ER Before Being Evaluated (minutes)	-	-	22	26
Time to Pain Meds for Fractures (minutes)	-	-	54	57
Heart Attack Care				
Aspirin Given at Discharge[5]	-	-	99%	99%
Fibrinolytic Meds Within 30 Min. of Arrival[5]	-	-	67%	54%
PCI Within 90 Minutes of Arrival[5]	-	-	97%	96%
Statin Prescribed at Discharge[5]	-	-	98%	98%
Heart Failure Care				
ACE Inhibitor or ARB for LVSD[3,7]	-	-	97%	97%
Discharge Instructions Given[1,3]	-	-	91%	94%
Evaluation of LVS Function[1,3]	-	-	99%	99%
Medicare Spending				
Medicare Spending per Patient (ratio)	-	0.72	1.04	0.98
Pneumonia Care				
Appropriate Initial Antibiotic Given[3,7]	-	-	96%	95%
Blood Culture Timing[3,7]	-	-	96%	98%
Pregnancy and Delivery Care				
Newborn Deliveries Scheduled Early[5]	-	-	6%	6%
Preventive Care				
Immunization for Influenza[5]	-	-	93%	90%
Immunization for Pneumonia[5]	-	-	94%	92%
Stroke Care				
Anticoagulation Therapy for Atrial Fibrillation[5]	-	-	92%	95%
Antithrombotic Therapy Timing[5]	-	-	97%	98%
Assessed for Rehabilitation[5]	-	-	96%	97%
Discharged on Antithrombotic Therapy[5]	-	-	99%	99%
Discharged on Statin Medication[5]	-	-	95%	94%
Thrombolytic Therapy Timing[5]	-	-	80%	66%
Venous Thromboembolism Prophylaxis[5]	-	-	91%	94%
Written Stroke Educational Materials Given[5]	-	-	87%	88%
Surgical Care Improvement Project				
Appropriate Beta Blocker Usage[5]	-	-	96%	98%
Appropriate VTP Within 24 Hours[5]	-	-	98%	98%
Controlled Postoperative Blood Glucose[5]	-	-	97%	97%
Perioperative Temperature Management[5]	-	-	100%	100%
Prophylactic Antibiotic Selection[5]	-	-	99%	99%
Prophylactic Antibiotic Selection (Outpatient)	-	-	98%	98%
Prophylactic Antibiotic Stopped[5]	-	-	98%	98%
Prophylactic Antibiotic Timing[5]	-	-	99%	99%
Prophylactic Antibiotic Timing (Outpatient)	-	-	98%	98%
Urinary Catheter Removal[5]	-	-	98%	97%
Survey of Patients' Hospital Experiences				
Area Around Room 'Always' Quiet at Night[5]	-	-	57%	61%
Doctors 'Always' Communicated Well[5]	-	-	75%	82%
Home Recovery Information Given[5]	-	-	85%	85%
Hospital Given 9 or 10 on 10 Point Scale[5]	-	-	66%	71%
Meds 'Always' Explained Before Given[5]	-	-	60%	64%
Nurses 'Always' Communicated Well[5]	-	-	72%	79%
Pain 'Always' Well Controlled[5]	-	-	67%	71%
Room and Bathroom 'Always' Clean[5]	-	-	68%	73%
Timely Help 'Always' Received[5]	-	-	59%	68%
Would Definitely Recommend Hospital[5]	-	-	69%	71%
Use of Medical Imaging				
Cardiac Imaging Stress Test before Surgery	-	-	4.8%	5.3%
Combination Abdominal CT Scan	-	-	6.9%	10.5%
Combination Brain/Sinus CT Scan	-	-	2.7%	2.7%
Combination Chest CT Scan	-	-	3.7%	2.7%
Follow-up Mammogram/Ultrasound	-	-	7.3%	8.8%
Lumbar Spine MRI for Low Back Pain	-	-	36.8%	37.2%

NOTE: Hospital profiles are in alphabetical order by state, then city, then hospital within the city; Rankings exclude hospitals with less than 25 cases except for patient surveys which excludes hospitals with less than 100 cases; (a) 100-299 cases; (1) The number of cases/patients is too few to report; (2) Data submitted were based on a sample of cases/patients; (3) Results are based on a shorter time period than required; (4) Data suppressed by CMS for one or more quarters; (5) Results are not available for this reporting period; (6) Fewer than 100 patients completed the HCAHPS survey; (7) No cases met the criteria for this measure; (8) The lower limit of the confidence interval cannot be calculated if the number of observed infections equals zero; (9) No data are available from the state/territory for this reporting period; (10) The scores shown reflect fewer than 50 completed surveys; (11) There were discrepancies in the data collection process; (12) This measure does not apply to this hospital for this reporting period; (13) Results cannot be calculated for this reporting period; (14) The results for this state are combined with nearby states to protect confidentiality; Please refer to the User's Guide for a full explanation of data.

Blood Clot Prevention and Treatment

Anticoagulation Overlap Therapy

Hospital Name	City	Rate	Cases
Mimbres Memorial Hospital[2]	Deming	100%	50
Mountain View Regional Medical Center[2]	Las Cruces	100%	66
Presbyterian Hospital[2]	Albuquerque	100%	332
UNM Hospital[2]	Albuquerque	100%	132
Lovelace Medical Center[2]	Albuquerque	99%	159
Memorial Medical Center[2]	Las Cruces	99%	68
Eastern New Mexico Medical Center[2]	Roswell	98%	45
Carlsbad Medical Center[2]	Carlsbad	96%	25
Gerald Champion Regional Medical Center[2]	Alamogordo	96%	25
Saint Vincent Hospital[2]	Santa Fe	95%	107
Plains Regional Medical Center[2]	Clovis	93%	27
San Juan Regional Medical Center[2]	Farmington	93%	75
Gila Regional Medical Center[2]	Silver City	61%	44

ICU Venous Thromboembolism Prophylaxis

Hospital Name	City	Rate	Cases
Lovelace Medical Center[2]	Albuquerque	100%	83
Lovelace Westside Hospital[2]	Albuquerque	100%	34
Lovelace Women's Hospital[2]	Albuquerque	100%	41
Presbyterian Hospital[2]	Albuquerque	100%	25
San Juan Regional Medical Center[2]	Farmington	100%	40
Alta Vista Regional Hospital[2]	Las Vegas	99%	94
Memorial Medical Center[2]	Las Cruces	99%	69
Mountain View Regional Medical Center[2]	Las Cruces	99%	163
UNM Hospital[2]	Albuquerque	99%	90
Carlsbad Medical Center[2]	Carlsbad	97%	73
Eastern New Mexico Medical Center[2]	Roswell	94%	70
Lea Regional Medical Center[2]	Hobbs	94%	83
Saint Vincent Hospital[2]	Santa Fe	94%	52
Holy Cross Hospital[2]	Taos	91%	79
Presbyterian Espanola Hospital[2]	Espanola	89%	44
Plains Regional Medical Center[2]	Clovis	87%	71
Gila Regional Medical Center[2]	Silver City	86%	50
Gerald Champion Regional Medical Center[2]	Alamogordo	84%	37
UNM Sandoval Regional Medical Center[2]	Rio Rancho	81%	26
Rehoboth Mckinley Christian HCS[2]	Gallup	53%	51

Incidence of Potentially Preventable VTE

Hospital Name	City	Rate	Cases
Lovelace Medical Center[2]	Albuquerque	0%	41
Presbyterian Hospital[2]	Albuquerque	2%	55
UNM Hospital[2]	Albuquerque	2%	45

UFH with Dosages/Platelet Count Monitoring

Hospital Name	City	Rate	Cases
Lovelace Medical Center[2]	Albuquerque	100%	93
Mountain View Regional Medical Center[2]	Las Cruces	100%	32
Presbyterian Hospital[2]	Albuquerque	100%	84
Saint Vincent Hospital[2]	Santa Fe	100%	44
UNM Hospital[2]	Albuquerque	100%	108
Memorial Medical Center[2]	Las Cruces	97%	35
San Juan Regional Medical Center[2]	Farmington	96%	53

Venous Thromboembolism Prophylaxis

Hospital Name	City	Rate	Cases
Lovelace Medical Center[2]	Albuquerque	100%	353
Lovelace Women's Hospital[2]	Albuquerque	100%	216
Mountain View Regional Medical Center[2]	Las Cruces	100%	362
Carlsbad Medical Center[2]	Carlsbad	99%	247
Lovelace Westside Hospital[2]	Albuquerque	98%	173
Memorial Medical Center[2]	Las Cruces	98%	356
Alta Vista Regional Hospital[2]	Las Vegas	97%	147
Eastern New Mexico Medical Center[2]	Roswell	94%	296
Lea Regional Medical Center[2]	Hobbs	94%	140
UNM Hospital[2]	Albuquerque	94%	326
Plains Regional Medical Center[2]	Clovis	92%	258
Gerald Champion Regional Medical Center[2]	Alamogordo	90%	299
Mimbres Memorial Hospital[2]	Deming	90%	251
Guadalupe County Hospital[2]	Santa Rosa	89%	82
Holy Cross Hospital[2]	Taos	89%	204
San Juan Regional Medical Center[2]	Farmington	86%	333
Los Alamos Medical Center[2]	Los Alamos	84%	86
Lovelace Regional Hospital - Roswell[2]	Roswell	82%	114
Presbyterian Hospital[2]	Albuquerque	82%	374
Saint Vincent Hospital[2]	Santa Fe	81%	345
Presbyterian Espanola Hospital[2]	Espanola	77%	173
Roosevelt General Hospital[2]	Portales	77%	206
Northern Navajo Medical Center	Shiprock	76%	99
UNM Sandoval Regional Medical Center[2]	Rio Rancho	76%	186
Zuni Comprehensive Comm Health Ctr[2]	Zuni	76%	119
Gallup Indian Medical Center[2]	Gallup	69%	80
Rehoboth Mckinley Christian HCS[2]	Gallup	68%	181
Gila Regional Medical Center[2]	Silver City	67%	144
Crownpoint Healthcare Facility[2]	Crownpoint	41%	108
Artesia General Hospital[2]	Artesia	37%	76
Santa Fe Phs Indian Hospital[2]	Santa Fe	26%	50
Nor-Lea Hospital District[2,3]	Lovington	11%	27
Dhhs Usphs Indian Health Services[2]	San Fidel	8%	101
Mescalero PHS Indian Hospital[2,3]	Mescalero	1%	71

Warfarin Therapy Discharge Instructions

Hospital Name	City	Rate	Cases
Eastern New Mexico Medical Center[2]	Roswell	100%	34
Mimbres Memorial Hospital[2]	Deming	100%	38
Mountain View Regional Medical Center[2]	Las Cruces	100%	49
Lovelace Medical Center[2]	Albuquerque	99%	128
Presbyterian Hospital[2]	Albuquerque	99%	245
Memorial Medical Center[2]	Las Cruces	96%	47
Saint Vincent Hospital[2]	Santa Fe	89%	90
UNM Hospital[2]	Albuquerque	85%	91
Gila Regional Medical Center[2]	Silver City	59%	39
San Juan Regional Medical Center[2]	Farmington	0%	63

Chest Pain/Possible Heart Attack Care

Aspirin Given Within 24 Hours of Arrival

Hospital Name	City	Rate	Cases
Alta Vista Regional Hospital	Las Vegas	100%	31
Carlsbad Medical Center	Carlsbad	100%	87
Holy Cross Hospital	Taos	100%	84
Lea Regional Medical Center	Hobbs	100%	109
Lovelace Women's Hospital	Albuquerque	100%	46
Mimbres Memorial Hospital	Deming	100%	129
Presbyterian Hospital	Albuquerque	100%	155
Presbyterian Espanola Hospital	Espanola	99%	72
Lovelace Westside Hospital	Albuquerque	98%	59
Artesia General Hospital	Artesia	96%	26
Roosevelt General Hospital	Portales	96%	47
Cibola General Hospital	Grants	95%	56
Gila Regional Medical Center	Silver City	95%	78
Plains Regional Medical Center	Clovis	95%	84
Lovelace Regional Hospital - Roswell	Roswell	88%	26
Gerald Champion Regional Medical Center	Alamogordo	83%	60
Nor-Lea Hospital District	Lovington	77%	31

Average Time to ECG (minutes)

Hospital Name	City	Min.	Cases
Alta Vista Regional Hospital	Las Vegas	4	33
Artesia General Hospital	Artesia	5	27
Carlsbad Medical Center	Carlsbad	5	91
Lea Regional Medical Center	Hobbs	6	111
Lovelace Westside Hospital	Albuquerque	6	59
Gila Regional Medical Center	Silver City	8	80
Lovelace Regional Hospital - Roswell	Roswell	8	26
Mimbres Memorial Hospital	Deming	8	135
Plains Regional Medical Center	Clovis	8	101
Presbyterian Hospital	Albuquerque	9	163
Lovelace Women's Hospital	Albuquerque	10	45
Roosevelt General Hospital	Portales	11	49
Holy Cross Hospital	Taos	13	85
Nor-Lea Hospital District	Lovington	13	29
Cibola General Hospital	Grants	14	58
Presbyterian Espanola Hospital	Espanola	14	70
Gerald Champion Regional Medical Center	Alamogordo	16	61

Children's Asthma Care

Received Home Management Plan of Care

Hospital Name	City	Rate	Cases
Memorial Medical Center	Las Cruces	96%	27
UNM Hospital[2]	Albuquerque	93%	144

Received Reliever Medication

Hospital Name	City	Rate	Cases
Memorial Medical Center	Las Cruces	100%	27
UNM Hospital	Albuquerque	100%	146

Received Systemic Corticosteroids

Hospital Name	City	Rate	Cases
Memorial Medical Center	Las Cruces	100%	27
UNM Hospital	Albuquerque	100%	146

Emergency Department

Admittance Decision Time (minutes)

Hospital Name	City	Min.	Cases
Guadalupe County Hospital[2]	Santa Rosa	1	61
Miners' Colfax Medical Center[2]	Raton	45	187
Los Alamos Medical Center[2]	Los Alamos	50	322
Roosevelt General Hospital[2]	Portales	52	276
Sierra Vista Hospital[3]	T Or C	54	112
Artesia General Hospital[2]	Artesia	55	218
Presbyterian Espanola Hospital[2]	Espanola	67	282
Dhhs Usphs Indian Health Services	San Fidel	70	150
Lovelace Regional Hospital - Roswell[2]	Roswell	80	162
Nor-Lea Hospital District[2]	Lovington	80	145
Northern Navajo Medical Center[2]	Shiprock	85	525
Carlsbad Medical Center[2]	Carlsbad	86	500
Gerald Champion Regional Medical Center[2]	Alamogordo	92	288
Lovelace Westside Hospital[2]	Albuquerque	92	423
Lovelace Women's Hospital[2]	Albuquerque	96	226
Mimbres Memorial Hospital[2]	Deming	100	320
Alta Vista Regional Hospital[2]	Las Vegas	101	420
Eastern New Mexico Medical Center[2]	Roswell	110	520
Presbyterian Hospital[2]	Albuquerque	110	311
Rehoboth Mckinley Christian HCS[2]	Gallup	112	235
Lea Regional Medical Center[2]	Hobbs	114	402
Gila Regional Medical Center[2]	Silver City	116	244
Mountain View Regional Medical Center[2]	Las Cruces	117	631
Lovelace Medical Center[2]	Albuquerque	123	740
UNM Sandoval Regional Medical Center[2,3]	Rio Rancho	126	248
Gallup Indian Medical Center[2]	Gallup	135	563
Plains Regional Medical Center[2]	Clovis	138	342
San Juan Regional Medical Center[2]	Farmington	139	580
Holy Cross Hospital[2]	Taos	158	361
Memorial Medical Center[2]	Las Cruces	170	441
Saint Vincent Hospital[2]	Santa Fe	206	671
UNM Hospital[2]	Albuquerque	371	270

Head CT Results Within 45 Minutes of Arrival

Hospital Name	City	Rate	Cases
Presbyterian Hospital	Albuquerque	70%	30

Patients Who Left ER Before Being Seen

Hospital Name	City	Rate	Cases
Los Alamos Medical Center	Los Alamos	0%	8515
Alta Vista Regional Hospital	Las Vegas	1%	13661
Artesia General Hospital	Artesia	1%	11547
Eastern New Mexico Medical Center	Roswell	1%	23318
Lovelace Medical Center	Albuquerque	1%	38326
Lovelace Westside Hospital	Albuquerque	1%	20485
Mimbres Memorial Hospital	Deming	1%	10875
Miners' Colfax Medical Center	Raton	1%	5588
Saint Vincent Hospital	Santa Fe	1%	54253
San Juan Regional Medical Center	Farmington	1%	48074
UNM Sandoval Regional Medical Center	Rio Rancho	1%	3864
Holy Cross Hospital	Taos	2%	15821
Mountain View Regional Medical Center	Las Cruces	2%	15099
Nor-Lea Hospital District	Lovington	2%	10169
Plains Regional Medical Center	Clovis	2%	30470
Presbyterian Espanola Hospital	Espanola	2%	20544
Carlsbad Medical Center	Carlsbad	3%	24279
Gerald Champion Regional Medical Center	Alamogordo	3%	28019
Gila Regional Medical Center	Silver City	3%	18621
Lea Regional Medical Center	Hobbs	3%	21123
Memorial Medical Center	Las Cruces	3%	42060
Cibola General Hospital	Grants	4%	9290
Lovelace Women's Hospital	Albuquerque	4%	27455
Rehoboth Mckinley Christian HCS	Gallup	4%	21850
Lovelace Regional Hospital - Roswell	Roswell	5%	10544
Presbyterian Hospital	Albuquerque	5%	130733
Roosevelt General Hospital	Portales	7%	7478
UNM Hospital	Albuquerque	12%	103444

Time from ER Arrival to Being Admitted (minutes)

Hospital Name	City	Min.	Cases
Guadalupe County Hospital[2]	Santa Rosa	106	61
Miners' Colfax Medical Center[2]	Raton	200	207
Roosevelt General Hospital[2]	Portales	214	352
Presbyterian Espanola Hospital[2]	Espanola	227	292
Los Alamos Medical Center[2]	Los Alamos	233	324
Carlsbad Medical Center[2]	Carlsbad	247	513
Sierra Vista Hospital[3]	T Or C	247	113
Northern Navajo Medical Center[2]	Shiprock	248	535
Artesia General Hospital[2]	Artesia	250	346
Dhhs Usphs Indian Health Services	San Fidel	254	150
Alta Vista Regional Hospital[2]	Las Vegas	260	441
Lovelace Westside Hospital[2]	Albuquerque	266	423
Zuni Comprehensive Comm Health Ctr[2]	Zuni	270	34
UNM Sandoval Regional Medical Center[2,3]	Rio Rancho	272	258
Mountain View Regional Medical Center[2]	Las Cruces	277	635
Lea Regional Medical Center[2]	Hobbs	279	407
Nor-Lea Hospital District[2]	Lovington	280	153
Eastern New Mexico Medical Center[2]	Roswell	282	529
Rehoboth Mckinley Christian HCS[2]	Gallup	285	242
San Juan Regional Medical Center[2]	Farmington	286	587
Mimbres Memorial Hospital[2]	Deming	288	326
Lovelace Regional Hospital - Roswell[2]	Roswell	298	190
Gila Regional Medical Center[2]	Silver City	300	251
Gerald Champion Regional Medical Center[2]	Alamogordo	304	317
Gallup Indian Medical Center[2]	Gallup	315	563

NOTE: Hospital profiles are in alphabetical order by state, then city, then hospital within the city; Rankings exclude hospitals with less than 25 cases except for patient surveys which excludes hospitals with less than 100 cases; (a) 100-299 cases; (1) The number of cases/patients is too few to report; (2) Data submitted were based on a sample of cases/patients; (3) Results are based on a shorter time period than required; (4) Data suppressed by CMS for one or more quarters; (5) Results are not available for this reporting period; (6) Fewer than 100 patients completed the HCAHPS survey; (7) No cases met the criteria for this measure; (8) The lower limit of the confidence interval cannot be calculated if the number of observed infections equals zero; (9) No data are available from the state/territory for this reporting period; (10) The scores shown reflect fewer than 50 completed surveys; (11) There were discrepancies in the data collection process; (12) This measure does not apply to this hospital for this reporting period; (13) Results cannot be calculated for this reporting period; (14) The results for this state are combined with nearby states to protect confidentiality; Please refer to the User's Guide for a full explanation of data.

Presbyterian Hospital[2]	Albuquerque	320	398
Lovelace Medical Center[2]	Albuquerque	324	749
Crownpoint Healthcare Facility[2]	Crownpoint	326	188
Lovelace Women's Hospital[2]	Albuquerque	327	227
Holy Cross Hospital[2]	Taos	334	374
Plains Regional Medical Center[2]	Clovis	361	359
Memorial Medical Center[2]	Las Cruces	364	504
Saint Vincent Hospital[2]	Santa Fe	437	747
UNM Hospital[2]	Albuquerque	778	274

Time from ER Arrival to Discharge (minutes)

Hospital Name	City	Min.	Cases
Artesia General Hospital	Artesia	102	362
Rehoboth Mckinley Christian HCS	Gallup	112	384
Roosevelt General Hospital	Portales	114	324
Presbyterian Espanola Hospital	Espanola	117	387
Cibola General Hospital	Grants	118	372
Los Alamos Medical Center	Los Alamos	119	395
Lea Regional Medical Center	Hobbs	120	381
Guadalupe County Hospital	Santa Rosa	123	255
Mountain View Regional Medical Center	Las Cruces	124	390
Carlsbad Medical Center	Carlsbad	128	367
Mimbres Memorial Hospital	Deming	128	323
Nor-Lea Hospital District	Lovington	134	1423
San Juan Regional Medical Center	Farmington	136	354
Lovelace Westside Hospital	Albuquerque	140	389
Miners' Colfax Medical Center[3]	Raton	141	221
Gila Regional Medical Center	Silver City	144	382
Alta Vista Regional Hospital	Las Vegas	150	374
Holy Cross Hospital	Taos	152	374
Lovelace Regional Hospital - Roswell	Roswell	152	372
Eastern New Mexico Medical Center	Roswell	153	355
Gerald Champion Regional Medical Center	Alamogordo	153	360
Plains Regional Medical Center	Clovis	160	366
Lovelace Women's Hospital	Albuquerque	161	363
UNM Sandoval Regional Medical Center[3]	Rio Rancho	166	316
Saint Vincent Hospital	Santa Fe	172	372
Memorial Medical Center	Las Cruces	194	418
Lovelace Medical Center	Albuquerque	197	369
Presbyterian Hospital	Albuquerque	209	380
UNM Hospital	Albuquerque	326	328

Time in ER Before Being Evaluated (minutes)

Hospital Name	City	Min.	Cases
Lea Regional Medical Center	Hobbs	14	396
Mimbres Memorial Hospital	Deming	15	414
Eastern New Mexico Medical Center	Roswell	16	416
Miners' Colfax Medical Center[3]	Raton	16	280
Alta Vista Regional Hospital	Las Vegas	17	422
Gila Regional Medical Center	Silver City	17	400
Roosevelt General Hospital	Portales	18	397
San Juan Regional Medical Center	Farmington	19	383
Los Alamos Medical Center	Los Alamos	20	418
Cibola General Hospital	Grants	21	404
Lovelace Westside Hospital	Albuquerque	22	418
Carlsbad Medical Center	Carlsbad	23	417
Mountain View Regional Medical Center	Las Cruces	23	422
Lovelace Medical Center	Albuquerque	27	426
Artesia General Hospital	Artesia	28	359
Holy Cross Hospital	Taos	29	396
Memorial Medical Center	Las Cruces	31	393
Gerald Champion Regional Medical Center	Alamogordo	32	392
Presbyterian Espanola Hospital	Espanola	33	378
Saint Vincent Hospital	Santa Fe	34	412
Guadalupe County Hospital	Santa Rosa	35	320
Plains Regional Medical Center	Clovis	35	405
Nor-Lea Hospital District	Lovington	36	1763
Lovelace Regional Hospital - Roswell	Roswell	38	408
Lovelace Women's Hospital	Albuquerque	38	404
Rehoboth Mckinley Christian HCS	Gallup	41	391
Presbyterian Hospital	Albuquerque	49	431
UNM Sandoval Regional Medical Center[3]	Rio Rancho	50	361
UNM Hospital	Albuquerque	112	296

Time to Pain Meds for Bone Fractures (minutes)

Hospital Name	City	Min.	Cases
Roosevelt General Hospital	Portales	30	40
Gila Regional Medical Center	Silver City	40	71
Lovelace Westside Hospital	Albuquerque	42	86
Lea Regional Medical Center	Hobbs	43	141
Eastern New Mexico Medical Center	Roswell	44	67
San Juan Regional Medical Center	Farmington	45	210
Artesia General Hospital	Artesia	46	61
Mountain View Regional Medical Center	Las Cruces	48	158
UNM Sandoval Regional Medical Center[3]	Rio Rancho	50	31
Holy Cross Hospital	Taos	54	98
Carlsbad Medical Center	Carlsbad	56	106
Cibola General Hospital	Grants	56	43
Alta Vista Regional Hospital	Las Vegas	58	67
Mimbres Memorial Hospital	Deming	58	62
Lovelace Women's Hospital	Albuquerque	59	101
Memorial Medical Center	Las Cruces	59	128
Rehoboth Mckinley Christian HCS	Gallup	59	71
Presbyterian Espanola Hospital	Espanola	63	87
Lovelace Regional Hospital - Roswell	Roswell	67	52
Los Alamos Medical Center	Los Alamos	68	65
Nor-Lea Hospital District	Lovington	70	32
Lovelace Medical Center	Albuquerque	73	136
Gerald Champion Regional Medical Center	Alamogordo	76	108
Plains Regional Medical Center	Clovis	76	142
Saint Vincent Hospital	Santa Fe	76	201
Presbyterian Hospital	Albuquerque	78	311
UNM Hospital	Albuquerque	79	225

Heart Attack Care

Aspirin Given at Discharge

Hospital Name	City	Rate	Cases
Lovelace Medical Center[2]	Albuquerque	100%	322
Memorial Medical Center	Las Cruces	100%	151
Presbyterian Hospital	Albuquerque	100%	666
Saint Vincent Hospital	Santa Fe	100%	219
UNM Hospital[2]	Albuquerque	100%	270
Mountain View Regional Medical Center	Las Cruces	99%	247
San Juan Regional Medical Center	Farmington	99%	160
VA New Mexico Healthcare System	Albuquerque	99%	122
Eastern New Mexico Medical Center	Roswell	97%	89

PCI Within 90 Minutes of Arrival

Hospital Name	City	Rate	Cases
Presbyterian Hospital	Albuquerque	98%	86
UNM Hospital[2]	Albuquerque	98%	57
Lovelace Medical Center[2]	Albuquerque	97%	39
San Juan Regional Medical Center	Farmington	95%	42
Mountain View Regional Medical Center	Las Cruces	93%	29
Memorial Medical Center	Las Cruces	90%	31
Saint Vincent Hospital	Santa Fe	89%	47

Statin Prescribed at Discharge

Hospital Name	City	Rate	Cases
Mountain View Regional Medical Center	Las Cruces	100%	218
Presbyterian Hospital	Albuquerque	100%	632
Saint Vincent Hospital	Santa Fe	100%	220
Lovelace Medical Center[2]	Albuquerque	99%	312
Memorial Medical Center	Las Cruces	99%	148
UNM Hospital[2]	Albuquerque	99%	268
Eastern New Mexico Medical Center	Roswell	98%	87
San Juan Regional Medical Center	Farmington	96%	151
VA New Mexico Healthcare System	Albuquerque	95%	121

Heart Failure Care

ACE Inhibitor or ARB for LVSD

Hospital Name	City	Rate	Cases
Eastern New Mexico Medical Center	Roswell	100%	31
Presbyterian Hospital[2]	Albuquerque	100%	123
UNM Hospital[2]	Albuquerque	99%	126
Carlsbad Medical Center	Carlsbad	98%	42
Lovelace Medical Center[2]	Albuquerque	98%	93
Mountain View Regional Medical Center	Las Cruces	97%	71
Saint Vincent Hospital	Santa Fe	97%	79
Memorial Medical Center	Las Cruces	95%	88
San Juan Regional Medical Center	Farmington	93%	58
VA New Mexico Healthcare System	Albuquerque	92%	99
Rehoboth Mckinley Christian HCS	Gallup	75%	28

Discharge Instructions Given

Hospital Name	City	Rate	Cases
Holy Cross Hospital	Taos	100%	44
Lea Regional Medical Center	Hobbs	100%	33
Lovelace Medical Center[2]	Albuquerque	100%	253
Lovelace Regional Hospital - Roswell	Roswell	100%	55
Mimbres Memorial Hospital	Deming	100%	59
Mountain View Regional Medical Center	Las Cruces	99%	148
UNM Hospital[2]	Albuquerque	99%	232
Alta Vista Regional Hospital	Las Vegas	98%	60
Lovelace Women's Hospital	Albuquerque	98%	46
Saint Vincent Hospital	Santa Fe	98%	167
Lovelace Westside Hospital	Albuquerque	96%	47
Rehoboth Mckinley Christian HCS	Gallup	96%	79
Carlsbad Medical Center	Carlsbad	95%	88
Eastern New Mexico Medical Center	Roswell	95%	84
Lincoln County Medical Center	Ruidoso	94%	34
Presbyterian Hospital[2]	Albuquerque	94%	282
VA New Mexico Healthcare System	Albuquerque	92%	208
Plains Regional Medical Center	Clovis	91%	66
Memorial Medical Center	Las Cruces	85%	164
Gerald Champion Regional Medical Center	Alamogordo	83%	60
Northern Navajo Medical Center	Shiprock	80%	40
San Juan Regional Medical Center	Farmington	73%	161
Gallup Indian Medical Center[2]	Gallup	69%	29
Nor-Lea Hospital District[2]	Lovington	65%	31
Gila Regional Medical Center	Silver City	63%	52
UNM Sandoval Regional Medical Center[3]	Rio Rancho	38%	29
Roosevelt General Hospital[2]	Portales	7%	46

Evaluation of LVS Function

Hospital Name	City	Rate	Cases
Alta Vista Regional Hospital	Las Vegas	100%	72
Carlsbad Medical Center	Carlsbad	100%	98
Holy Cross Hospital	Taos	100%	52
Lea Regional Medical Center	Hobbs	100%	45
Lincoln County Medical Center	Ruidoso	100%	37
Lovelace Women's Hospital	Albuquerque	100%	54
Memorial Medical Center	Las Cruces	100%	200
Mimbres Memorial Hospital	Deming	100%	62
Mountain View Regional Medical Center	Las Cruces	100%	169
Presbyterian Hospital[2]	Albuquerque	100%	339
UNM Hospital[2]	Albuquerque	100%	258
UNM Sandoval Regional Medical Center[3]	Rio Rancho	100%	32
Eastern New Mexico Medical Center	Roswell	99%	107
Lovelace Medical Center[2]	Albuquerque	99%	310
Plains Regional Medical Center	Clovis	99%	71
VA New Mexico Healthcare System	Albuquerque	99%	222
Lovelace Westside Hospital	Albuquerque	98%	58
Northern Navajo Medical Center	Shiprock	98%	47
Saint Vincent Hospital	Santa Fe	98%	175
San Juan Regional Medical Center	Farmington	98%	197
Lovelace Regional Hospital - Roswell	Roswell	97%	58
Gerald Champion Regional Medical Center	Alamogordo	95%	64
Los Alamos Medical Center	Los Alamos	93%	27
Gallup Indian Medical Center[2]	Gallup	91%	32
Gila Regional Medical Center	Silver City	89%	53
Rehoboth Mckinley Christian HCS	Gallup	81%	78
Nor-Lea Hospital District[2]	Lovington	76%	34
Roosevelt General Hospital[2]	Portales	55%	51

Medicare Spending

Medicare Spending per Patient (ratio)

Hospital Name	City	Ratio	Cases
Dhhs Usphs Indian Health Services	San Fidel	0.53	-
Crownpoint Healthcare Facility	Crownpoint	0.59	-
Zuni Comprehensive Comm Health Ctr	Zuni	0.60	-
Guadalupe County Hospital	Santa Rosa	0.69	-
Gallup Indian Medical Center	Gallup	0.74	-
Northern Navajo Medical Center	Shiprock	0.76	-
Roosevelt General Hospital	Portales	0.78	-
Alta Vista Regional Hospital	Las Vegas	0.79	-
Presbyterian Espanola Hospital	Espanola	0.81	-
Rehoboth Mckinley Christian HCS	Gallup	0.81	-
Holy Cross Hospital	Taos	0.83	-
Artesia General Hospital	Artesia	0.87	-
Carlsbad Medical Center	Carlsbad	0.90	-
Lovelace Women's Hospital	Albuquerque	0.90	-
Gerald Champion Regional Medical Center	Alamogordo	0.91	-
Gila Regional Medical Center	Silver City	0.91	-
Lovelace Regional Hospital - Roswell	Roswell	0.92	-
Saint Vincent Hospital	Santa Fe	0.92	-
San Juan Regional Medical Center	Farmington	0.92	-
Lea Regional Medical Center	Hobbs	0.93	-
Los Alamos Medical Center	Los Alamos	0.93	-
Plains Regional Medical Center	Clovis	0.93	-
Eastern New Mexico Medical Center	Roswell	0.96	-
Lovelace Westside Hospital	Albuquerque	0.97	-
UNM Hospital	Albuquerque	0.97	-
Lovelace Medical Center	Albuquerque	0.99	-
Presbyterian Hospital	Albuquerque	0.99	-
Memorial Medical Center	Las Cruces	1.01	-
Mountain View Regional Medical Center	Las Cruces	1.01	-

Pneumonia Care

Appropriate Initial Antibiotic Given

Hospital Name	City	Rate	Cases
Alta Vista Regional Hospital	Las Vegas	100%	44
Lea Regional Medical Center	Hobbs	100%	44
Mimbres Memorial Hospital	Deming	100%	53
Mountain View Regional Medical Center	Las Cruces	100%	130
Eastern New Mexico Medical Center	Roswell	99%	106
Holy Cross Hospital	Taos	99%	82
Lovelace Westside Hospital[2]	Albuquerque	98%	87
Presbyterian Hospital[2]	Albuquerque	98%	93
Carlsbad Medical Center	Carlsbad	97%	112
Lovelace Medical Center[2]	Albuquerque	97%	91
Plains Regional Medical Center	Clovis	97%	75
San Juan Regional Medical Center	Farmington	97%	149

NOTE: Hospital profiles are in alphabetical order by state, then city, then hospital within the city; Rankings exclude hospitals with less than 25 cases except for patient surveys which excludes hospitals with less than 100 cases; (a) 100-299 cases; (1) The number of cases/patients is too few to report; (2) Data submitted were based on a sample of cases/patients; (3) Results are based on a shorter time period than required; (4) Data suppressed by CMS for one or more quarters; (5) Results are not available for this reporting period; (6) Fewer than 100 patients completed the HCAHPS survey; (7) No cases met the criteria for this measure; (8) The lower limit of the confidence interval cannot be calculated if the number of observed infections equals zero; (9) No data are available from the state/territory for this reporting period; (10) The scores shown reflect fewer than 50 completed surveys; (11) There were discrepancies in the data collection process; (12) This measure does not apply to this hospital for this reporting period; (13) Results cannot be calculated for this reporting period; (14) The results for this state are combined with nearby states to protect confidentiality; Please refer to the User's Guide for a full explanation of data.

Hospital Name	City	Rate	Cases
UNM Sandoval Regional Medical Center[3]	Rio Rancho	97%	30
Lovelace Regional Hospital - Roswell	Roswell	96%	27
Memorial Medical Center	Las Cruces	96%	141
UNM Hospital[2]	Albuquerque	96%	55
Lovelace Women's Hospital	Albuquerque	94%	67
Saint Vincent Hospital[2]	Santa Fe	94%	93
Presbyterian Espanola Hospital	Espanola	93%	55
Artesia General Hospital	Artesia	92%	38
Gila Regional Medical Center	Silver City	90%	48
Roosevelt General Hospital	Portales	90%	29
VA New Mexico Healthcare System	Albuquerque	90%	87
Gallup Indian Medical Center[2]	Gallup	87%	45
Gerald Champion Regional Medical Center	Alamogordo	86%	97
Sierra Vista Hospital[2]	T Or C	84%	31
Rehoboth Mckinley Christian HCS[2]	Gallup	79%	48
Los Alamos Medical Center	Los Alamos	74%	27
Nor-Lea Hospital District[2]	Lovington	67%	33
Northern Navajo Medical Center	Shiprock	66%	62

Blood Culture Timing

Hospital Name	City	Rate	Cases
Holy Cross Hospital	Taos	100%	116
Lovelace Westside Hospital[2]	Albuquerque	100%	107
Mountain View Regional Medical Center	Las Cruces	100%	203
Presbyterian Hospital[2]	Albuquerque	100%	125
Alta Vista Regional Hospital	Las Vegas	99%	76
Lovelace Women's Hospital	Albuquerque	99%	82
San Juan Regional Medical Center	Farmington	99%	300
Artesia General Hospital	Artesia	98%	44
Carlsbad Medical Center	Carlsbad	98%	166
Eastern New Mexico Medical Center	Roswell	98%	149
Gila Regional Medical Center	Silver City	98%	82
Lincoln County Medical Center	Ruidoso	98%	41
Lovelace Regional Hospital - Roswell	Roswell	98%	41
Memorial Medical Center	Las Cruces	98%	208
Plains Regional Medical Center	Clovis	98%	164
Presbyterian Espanola Hospital	Espanola	98%	62
UNM Hospital[2]	Albuquerque	98%	106
Los Alamos Medical Center	Los Alamos	97%	37
Lovelace Medical Center[2]	Albuquerque	97%	160
Mimbres Memorial Hospital	Deming	97%	63
VA New Mexico Healthcare System	Albuquerque	97%	156
Lea Regional Medical Center	Hobbs	96%	68
Nor-Lea Hospital District[2]	Lovington	96%	26
Saint Vincent Hospital[2]	Santa Fe	96%	136
Northern Navajo Medical Center	Shiprock	95%	38
Cibola General Hospital	Grants	94%	31
Gallup Indian Medical Center[2]	Gallup	94%	50
Gerald Champion Regional Medical Center	Alamogordo	90%	111
Roosevelt General Hospital[2]	Portales	90%	31
Sierra Vista Hospital[2]	T Or C	90%	31
Rehoboth Mckinley Christian HCS[2]	Gallup	85%	86
UNM Sandoval Regional Medical Center[3]	Rio Rancho	83%	42
Crownpoint Healthcare Facility[2]	Crownpoint	79%	28

Pregnancy and Delivery Care

Newborns whose Deliveries were Scheduled Early

Hospital Name	City	Rate	Cases
Alta Vista Regional Hospital[2]	Las Vegas	0%	34
Carlsbad Medical Center[2]	Carlsbad	0%	34
Gallup Indian Medical Center[2]	Gallup	0%	190
Memorial Medical Center[2]	Las Cruces	0%	27
Northern Navajo Medical Center	Shiprock	0%	117
Presbyterian Espanola Hospital[2]	Espanola	0%	27
Lovelace Women's Hospital[2]	Albuquerque	1%	240
Miners' Colfax Medical Center	Raton	2%	41
Presbyterian Hospital[2]	Albuquerque	2%	80
Rehoboth Mckinley Christian HCS[2]	Gallup	2%	44
Plains Regional Medical Center[2]	Clovis	3%	38
Gila Regional Medical Center	Silver City	4%	69
Lovelace Regional Hospital - Roswell	Roswell	4%	134
Mountain View Regional Medical Center[2]	Las Cruces	4%	27
Saint Vincent Hospital[2]	Santa Fe	4%	103
San Juan Regional Medical Center	Farmington	4%	301
Lea Regional Medical Center[2]	Hobbs	5%	44
Eastern New Mexico Medical Center[2]	Roswell	8%	25
UNM Hospital[2]	Albuquerque	10%	42
Gerald Champion Regional Medical Center[2]	Alamogordo	11%	36

Preventive Care

Immunization for Influenza

Hospital Name	City	Rate	Cases
Lovelace Women's Hospital[2]	Albuquerque	100%	436
Mimbres Memorial Hospital[2]	Deming	100%	299
Mountain View Regional Medical Center[2]	Las Cruces	100%	618
Eastern New Mexico Medical Center[2]	Roswell	99%	356
Lovelace Westside Hospital[2]	Albuquerque	99%	278
Alta Vista Regional Hospital[2]	Las Vegas	98%	304
Holy Cross Hospital[2]	Taos	97%	271
Carlsbad Medical Center[2]	Carlsbad	96%	389
Lovelace Medical Center[2]	Albuquerque	96%	621
Memorial Medical Center[2]	Las Cruces	95%	514
Lea Regional Medical Center[2]	Hobbs	94%	366
Miners' Colfax Medical Center[2]	Raton	94%	126
Presbyterian Hospital[2]	Albuquerque	94%	549
Lovelace Regional Hospital - Roswell[2]	Roswell	92%	274
Presbyterian Espanola Hospital[2]	Espanola	91%	268
UNM Sandoval Regional Medical Center[2,3]	Rio Rancho	90%	135
Gerald Champion Regional Medical Center[2]	Alamogordo	86%	293
San Juan Regional Medical Center[2]	Farmington	85%	515
Gila Regional Medical Center[2]	Silver City	84%	268
Los Alamos Medical Center[2]	Los Alamos	84%	265
Artesia General Hospital[2]	Artesia	81%	287
Northern Navajo Medical Center	Shiprock	81%	465
Santa Fe Phs Indian Hospital[2]	Santa Fe	80%	76
Rehoboth Mckinley Christian HCS[2]	Gallup	77%	297
Dhhs Usphs Indian Health Services	San Fidel	76%	99
Saint Vincent Hospital[2]	Santa Fe	75%	568
Crownpoint Healthcare Facility[2]	Crownpoint	74%	276
Mescalero PHS Indian Hospital	Mescalero	71%	124
Nor-Lea Hospital District[2]	Lovington	71%	66
Gallup Indian Medical Center[2]	Gallup	69%	298
Roosevelt General Hospital[2]	Portales	66%	299
UNM Hospital[2]	Albuquerque	64%	502
Plains Regional Medical Center[2]	Clovis	63%	515
Zuni Comprehensive Comm Health Ctr[2]	Zuni	54%	190
Guadalupe County Hospital[2]	Santa Rosa	50%	94

Immunization for Pneumonia

Hospital Name	City	Rate	Cases
Mimbres Memorial Hospital[2]	Deming	100%	388
Mountain View Regional Medical Center[2]	Las Cruces	100%	746
Alta Vista Regional Hospital[2]	Las Vegas	99%	341
Carlsbad Medical Center[2]	Carlsbad	99%	391
Eastern New Mexico Medical Center[2]	Roswell	99%	484
Holy Cross Hospital[2]	Taos	99%	307
Lovelace Women's Hospital[2]	Albuquerque	99%	251
Memorial Medical Center[2]	Las Cruces	99%	550
Lea Regional Medical Center[2]	Hobbs	98%	272
Lovelace Medical Center[2]	Albuquerque	98%	975
Lovelace Regional Hospital - Roswell[2]	Roswell	96%	304
Lovelace Westside Hospital[2]	Albuquerque	96%	341
Presbyterian Espanola Hospital[2]	Espanola	95%	267
Presbyterian Hospital[2]	Albuquerque	95%	597
Gila Regional Medical Center[2]	Silver City	94%	282
Mescalero PHS Indian Hospital	Mescalero	94%	50
Northern Navajo Medical Center	Shiprock	91%	564
Dhhs Usphs Indian Health Services	San Fidel	90%	172
Gerald Champion Regional Medical Center[2]	Alamogordo	90%	305
Los Alamos Medical Center[2]	Los Alamos	88%	290
Santa Fe Phs Indian Hospital[2]	Santa Fe	88%	90
Miners' Colfax Medical Center[2]	Raton	86%	175
San Juan Regional Medical Center[2]	Farmington	84%	553
Plains Regional Medical Center[2]	Clovis	82%	407
Gallup Indian Medical Center[2]	Gallup	81%	496
Zuni Comprehensive Comm Health Ctr[2]	Zuni	81%	183
Crownpoint Healthcare Facility[2]	Crownpoint	80%	217
Artesia General Hospital[2]	Artesia	78%	396
Rehoboth Mckinley Christian HCS[2]	Gallup	78%	273
Sierra Vista Hospital[3]	T Or C	75%	89
Roosevelt General Hospital[2]	Portales	74%	427
Saint Vincent Hospital[2]	Santa Fe	74%	636
Nor-Lea Hospital District[2]	Lovington	70%	150
UNM Hospital[2]	Albuquerque	68%	367
UNM Sandoval Regional Medical Center[2,3]	Rio Rancho	66%	258
Guadalupe County Hospital[2]	Santa Rosa	54%	104

Stroke Care

Antithrombotic Therapy Timing

Hospital Name	City	Rate	Cases
Carlsbad Medical Center	Carlsbad	100%	31
Lovelace Medical Center[2]	Albuquerque	100%	79
Mountain View Regional Medical Center	Las Cruces	100%	59
Presbyterian Hospital[2]	Albuquerque	100%	94
Memorial Medical Center	Las Cruces	97%	68
San Juan Regional Medical Center	Farmington	92%	65
Saint Vincent Hospital	Santa Fe	90%	81
UNM Hospital[2]	Albuquerque	90%	49
Gerald Champion Regional Medical Center	Alamogordo	89%	37

Assessed for Rehabilitation

Hospital Name	City	Rate	Cases
Lovelace Medical Center[2]	Albuquerque	100%	102
Memorial Medical Center	Las Cruces	100%	77
Gerald Champion Regional Medical Center	Alamogordo	98%	43
Mountain View Regional Medical Center	Las Cruces	98%	82
Saint Vincent Hospital	Santa Fe	98%	119
Carlsbad Medical Center	Carlsbad	97%	34
Presbyterian Hospital[2]	Albuquerque	97%	127
UNM Hospital[2]	Albuquerque	93%	96
San Juan Regional Medical Center	Farmington	85%	84

Discharged on Antithrombotic Therapy

Hospital Name	City	Rate	Cases
Carlsbad Medical Center	Carlsbad	100%	34
Gerald Champion Regional Medical Center	Alamogordo	100%	43
Lovelace Medical Center[2]	Albuquerque	100%	93
Mountain View Regional Medical Center	Las Cruces	100%	68
Memorial Medical Center	Las Cruces	99%	73
Presbyterian Hospital[2]	Albuquerque	99%	122
Saint Vincent Hospital	Santa Fe	98%	91
UNM Hospital[2]	Albuquerque	96%	52
San Juan Regional Medical Center	Farmington	94%	72

Discharged on Statin Medication

Hospital Name	City	Rate	Cases
Lovelace Medical Center[2]	Albuquerque	100%	62
Mountain View Regional Medical Center	Las Cruces	98%	46
Memorial Medical Center	Las Cruces	97%	61
Gerald Champion Regional Medical Center	Alamogordo	89%	37
Saint Vincent Hospital	Santa Fe	88%	68
San Juan Regional Medical Center	Farmington	88%	49
Presbyterian Hospital[2]	Albuquerque	87%	87
UNM Hospital[2]	Albuquerque	87%	38

Venous Thromboembolism (VTE) Prophylaxis

Hospital Name	City	Rate	Cases
Carlsbad Medical Center	Carlsbad	100%	35
Lovelace Medical Center[2]	Albuquerque	99%	96
Memorial Medical Center	Las Cruces	99%	76
UNM Hospital[2]	Albuquerque	97%	109
Mountain View Regional Medical Center	Las Cruces	95%	87
Presbyterian Hospital[2]	Albuquerque	93%	113
Gerald Champion Regional Medical Center	Alamogordo	92%	39
Eastern New Mexico Medical Center	Roswell	85%	27
San Juan Regional Medical Center	Farmington	84%	81
Saint Vincent Hospital	Santa Fe	78%	116

Written Stroke Educational Materials Given

Hospital Name	City	Rate	Cases
Lovelace Medical Center[2]	Albuquerque	100%	43
Memorial Medical Center	Las Cruces	89%	38
Gerald Champion Regional Medical Center	Alamogordo	88%	25
Mountain View Regional Medical Center	Las Cruces	88%	34
UNM Hospital[2]	Albuquerque	79%	53
Saint Vincent Hospital	Santa Fe	78%	67
San Juan Regional Medical Center	Farmington	52%	56
Presbyterian Hospital[2]	Albuquerque	42%	66

Surgical Care Improvement Project

Appropriate Beta Blocker Usage

Hospital Name	City	Rate	Cases
Carlsbad Medical Center	Carlsbad	100%	25
Mountain View Regional Medical Center	Las Cruces	100%	164
Lovelace Medical Center[2]	Albuquerque	99%	209
Presbyterian Hospital[2]	Albuquerque	99%	220
Lovelace Westside Hospital[2]	Albuquerque	98%	42
Lovelace Women's Hospital[2]	Albuquerque	98%	57
Plains Regional Medical Center	Clovis	98%	47
Memorial Medical Center[2]	Las Cruces	97%	119
San Juan Regional Medical Center[2]	Farmington	97%	110
Eastern New Mexico Medical Center	Roswell	96%	49
Gila Regional Medical Center	Silver City	95%	58
VA New Mexico Healthcare System[2]	Albuquerque	94%	146
Lovelace Regional Hospital - Roswell[2]	Roswell	93%	55
UNM Hospital[2]	Albuquerque	93%	123
Gerald Champion Regional Medical Center	Alamogordo	88%	93
Saint Vincent Hospital[2]	Santa Fe	83%	53
UNM Sandoval Regional Medical Center[2,3]	Rio Rancho	69%	29
Artesia General Hospital[2]	Artesia	66%	29

Appropriate VTP Within 24 Hours

Hospital Name	City	Rate	Cases
Alta Vista Regional Hospital	Las Vegas	100%	59
Carlsbad Medical Center	Carlsbad	100%	82
Holy Cross Hospital	Taos	100%	120
Lea Regional Medical Center	Hobbs	100%	91
Lincoln County Medical Center	Ruidoso	100%	34
Lovelace Westside Hospital[2]	Albuquerque	100%	198
Memorial Medical Center[2]	Las Cruces	100%	364
Mimbres Memorial Hospital	Deming	100%	25
Lovelace Regional Hospital - Roswell[2]	Roswell	99%	185

NOTE: Hospital profiles are in alphabetical order by state, then city, then hospital within the city; Rankings exclude hospitals with less than 25 cases except for patient surveys which excludes hospitals with less than 100 cases; (a) 100-299 cases; (1) The number of cases/patients is too few to report; (2) Data submitted were based on a sample of cases/patients; (3) Results are based on a shorter time period than required; (4) Data suppressed by CMS for one or more quarters; (5) Results are not available for this reporting period; (6) Fewer than 100 patients completed the HCAHPS survey; (7) No cases met the criteria for this measure; (8) The lower limit of the confidence interval cannot be calculated if the number of observed infections equals zero; (9) No data are available from the state/territory for this reporting period; (10) The scores shown reflect fewer than 50 completed surveys; (11) There were discrepancies in the data collection process; (12) This measure does not apply to this hospital for this reporting period; (13) Results cannot be calculated for this reporting period; (14) The results for this state are combined with nearby states to protect confidentiality; Please refer to the User's Guide for a full explanation of data.

Hospital Name	City	Rate	Cases
Lovelace Women's Hospital[2]	Albuquerque	99%	314
Mountain View Regional Medical Center	Las Cruces	99%	359
Plains Regional Medical Center	Clovis	99%	220
Gila Regional Medical Center	Silver City	98%	282
Los Alamos Medical Center	Los Alamos	98%	111
Presbyterian Hospital[2]	Albuquerque	98%	547
Saint Vincent Hospital[2]	Santa Fe	98%	330
Eastern New Mexico Medical Center	Roswell	97%	169
UNM Hospital[2]	Albuquerque	97%	327
UNM Sandoval Regional Medical Center[2,3]	Rio Rancho	97%	187
Lovelace Medical Center[2]	Albuquerque	96%	402
Presbyterian Espanola Hospital	Espanola	96%	144
San Juan Regional Medical Center[2]	Farmington	95%	402
VA New Mexico Healthcare System[2]	Albuquerque	95%	305
Gerald Champion Regional Medical Center	Alamogordo	94%	232
Artesia General Hospital[2]	Artesia	92%	124
Gallup Indian Medical Center[2]	Gallup	80%	30
Northern Navajo Medical Center	Shiprock	75%	36
Rehoboth Mckinley Christian HCS	Gallup	48%	27

Controlled Postoperative Blood Glucose

Hospital Name	City	Rate	Cases
Mountain View Regional Medical Center	Las Cruces	100%	84
Lovelace Medical Center[2]	Albuquerque	98%	191
Memorial Medical Center[2]	Las Cruces	97%	75
UNM Hospital[2]	Albuquerque	96%	105
Presbyterian Hospital[2]	Albuquerque	95%	175
VA New Mexico Healthcare System[2]	Albuquerque	94%	51

Perioperative Temperature Management

Hospital Name	City	Rate	Cases
Alta Vista Regional Hospital	Las Vegas	100%	69
Artesia General Hospital[2]	Artesia	100%	130
Carlsbad Medical Center	Carlsbad	100%	144
Eastern New Mexico Medical Center	Roswell	100%	184
Gerald Champion Regional Medical Center	Alamogordo	100%	277
Gila Regional Medical Center	Silver City	100%	303
Holy Cross Hospital	Taos	100%	125
Lea Regional Medical Center	Hobbs	100%	120
Lincoln County Medical Center	Ruidoso	100%	46
Los Alamos Medical Center	Los Alamos	100%	121
Lovelace Medical Center[2]	Albuquerque	100%	623
Lovelace Regional Hospital - Roswell[2]	Roswell	100%	222
Lovelace Westside Hospital[2]	Albuquerque	100%	215
Lovelace Women's Hospital[2]	Albuquerque	100%	389
Memorial Medical Center[2]	Las Cruces	100%	432
Mimbres Memorial Hospital	Deming	100%	36
Mountain View Regional Medical Center	Las Cruces	100%	489
Northern Navajo Medical Center	Shiprock	100%	41
Plains Regional Medical Center	Clovis	100%	240
Presbyterian Espanola Hospital	Espanola	100%	153
Presbyterian Hospital[2]	Albuquerque	100%	663
Rehoboth Mckinley Christian HCS	Gallup	100%	39
Saint Vincent Hospital[2]	Santa Fe	100%	412
San Juan Regional Medical Center[2]	Farmington	100%	441
UNM Hospital[2]	Albuquerque	99%	469
VA New Mexico Healthcare System[2]	Albuquerque	93%	366
Gallup Indian Medical Center[2]	Gallup	92%	63
UNM Sandoval Regional Medical Center[2,3]	Rio Rancho	88%	216

Prophylactic Antibiotic Selection

Hospital Name	City	Rate	Cases
Alta Vista Regional Hospital	Las Vegas	100%	43
Carlsbad Medical Center	Carlsbad	100%	96
Eastern New Mexico Medical Center	Roswell	100%	51
Holy Cross Hospital	Taos	100%	84
Lea Regional Medical Center	Hobbs	100%	86
Lincoln County Medical Center	Ruidoso	100%	32
Lovelace Women's Hospital[2]	Albuquerque	100%	258
Memorial Medical Center[2]	Las Cruces	100%	342
Presbyterian Espanola Hospital	Espanola	100%	115
Presbyterian Hospital[2]	Albuquerque	100%	641
Artesia General Hospital[2]	Artesia	99%	96
Los Alamos Medical Center	Los Alamos	99%	103
Lovelace Regional Hospital - Roswell[2]	Roswell	99%	187
Lovelace Westside Hospital[2]	Albuquerque	99%	157
Mountain View Regional Medical Center	Las Cruces	99%	344
Saint Vincent Hospital[2]	Santa Fe	99%	271
VA New Mexico Healthcare System	Albuquerque	99%	271
Gerald Champion Regional Medical Center	Alamogordo	98%	220
Lovelace Medical Center[2]	Albuquerque	98%	444
Plains Regional Medical Center	Clovis	98%	193
San Juan Regional Medical Center[2]	Farmington	98%	260
UNM Hospital[2]	Albuquerque	98%	367
UNM Sandoval Regional Medical Center[2,3]	Rio Rancho	95%	121
Rehoboth Mckinley Christian HCS	Gallup	92%	26
Gallup Indian Medical Center[2]	Gallup	89%	28
Gila Regional Medical Center	Silver City	87%	255

Prophylactic Antibiotic Selection (Outpatient)

Hospital Name	City	Rate	Cases
Eastern New Mexico Medical Center	Roswell	100%	36
Holy Cross Hospital	Taos	100%	47
Los Alamos Medical Center	Los Alamos	100%	42
Lovelace Medical Center	Albuquerque	100%	470
Lovelace Regional Hospital - Roswell	Roswell	100%	154
Mountain View Regional Medical Center	Las Cruces	99%	322
Presbyterian Hospital	Albuquerque	99%	682
UNM Hospital	Albuquerque	98%	151
Lovelace Women's Hospital	Albuquerque	97%	282
Memorial Medical Center	Las Cruces	97%	142
Plains Regional Medical Center	Clovis	97%	134
Saint Vincent Hospital	Santa Fe	96%	159
San Juan Regional Medical Center	Farmington	95%	212
Carlsbad Medical Center	Carlsbad	91%	54
Gila Regional Medical Center	Silver City	89%	36

Prophylactic Antibiotic Stopped

Hospital Name	City	Rate	Cases
Gerald Champion Regional Medical Center	Alamogordo	100%	220
Holy Cross Hospital	Taos	100%	82
Lea Regional Medical Center	Hobbs	100%	85
Lovelace Westside Hospital[2]	Albuquerque	100%	156
Mountain View Regional Medical Center	Las Cruces	100%	341
Carlsbad Medical Center	Carlsbad	99%	93
Lovelace Medical Center[2]	Albuquerque	99%	437
Lovelace Regional Hospital - Roswell[2]	Roswell	99%	187
Lovelace Women's Hospital[2]	Albuquerque	99%	250
Memorial Medical Center[2]	Las Cruces	99%	331
Eastern New Mexico Medical Center	Roswell	98%	50
Presbyterian Espanola Hospital	Espanola	98%	115
Presbyterian Hospital[2]	Albuquerque	98%	615
UNM Hospital[2]	Albuquerque	98%	362
Gila Regional Medical Center	Silver City	97%	242
Lincoln County Medical Center	Ruidoso	97%	32
Saint Vincent Hospital[2]	Santa Fe	97%	267
Plains Regional Medical Center	Clovis	96%	183
Rehoboth Mckinley Christian HCS	Gallup	96%	25
San Juan Regional Medical Center[2]	Farmington	96%	255
VA New Mexico Healthcare System	Albuquerque	96%	268
Alta Vista Regional Hospital	Las Vegas	95%	43
Los Alamos Medical Center	Los Alamos	94%	100
UNM Sandoval Regional Medical Center[2,3]	Rio Rancho	93%	120
Gallup Indian Medical Center[2]	Gallup	89%	28
Artesia General Hospital[2]	Artesia	80%	95

Prophylactic Antibiotic Timing

Hospital Name	City	Rate	Cases
Alta Vista Regional Hospital	Las Vegas	100%	44
Carlsbad Medical Center	Carlsbad	100%	96
Eastern New Mexico Medical Center	Roswell	100%	51
Lea Regional Medical Center	Hobbs	100%	86
Lincoln County Medical Center	Ruidoso	100%	32
Lovelace Regional Hospital - Roswell[2]	Roswell	100%	187
Lovelace Westside Hospital[2]	Albuquerque	100%	157
Lovelace Women's Hospital[2]	Albuquerque	100%	258
Mountain View Regional Medical Center	Las Cruces	100%	345
VA New Mexico Healthcare System	Albuquerque	100%	272
Holy Cross Hospital	Taos	99%	84
Memorial Medical Center[2]	Las Cruces	99%	343
Plains Regional Medical Center	Clovis	99%	193
Presbyterian Hospital[2]	Albuquerque	99%	642
Saint Vincent Hospital[2]	Santa Fe	99%	274
San Juan Regional Medical Center[2]	Farmington	99%	261
Gila Regional Medical Center	Silver City	98%	255
Los Alamos Medical Center	Los Alamos	98%	103
Presbyterian Espanola Hospital	Espanola	98%	115
UNM Hospital[2]	Albuquerque	98%	369
Lovelace Medical Center[2]	Albuquerque	97%	445
Artesia General Hospital[2]	Artesia	96%	96
Gerald Champion Regional Medical Center	Alamogordo	94%	220
UNM Sandoval Regional Medical Center[2,3]	Rio Rancho	85%	123
Rehoboth Mckinley Christian HCS	Gallup	80%	30
Gallup Indian Medical Center[2]	Gallup	67%	30

Prophylactic Antibiotic Timing (Outpatient)

Hospital Name	City	Rate	Cases
Carlsbad Medical Center	Carlsbad	100%	54
Eastern New Mexico Medical Center	Roswell	100%	36
Holy Cross Hospital	Taos	100%	31
Los Alamos Medical Center	Los Alamos	100%	42
Lovelace Women's Hospital	Albuquerque	100%	282
Mountain View Regional Medical Center	Las Cruces	100%	321
Presbyterian Hospital	Albuquerque	99%	684
Lovelace Medical Center	Albuquerque	98%	474
Memorial Medical Center	Las Cruces	98%	141
Gila Regional Medical Center	Silver City	97%	36
Lovelace Regional Hospital - Roswell	Roswell	97%	156
Plains Regional Medical Center	Clovis	96%	137
San Juan Regional Medical Center	Farmington	91%	171
Saint Vincent Hospital	Santa Fe	87%	176
UNM Hospital	Albuquerque	66%	86

Urinary Catheter Removal

Hospital Name	City	Rate	Cases
Holy Cross Hospital	Taos	100%	51
Lovelace Women's Hospital[2]	Albuquerque	100%	206
Mountain View Regional Medical Center	Las Cruces	100%	318
Presbyterian Hospital[2]	Albuquerque	100%	532
Lovelace Regional Hospital - Roswell[2]	Roswell	99%	153
Plains Regional Medical Center	Clovis	99%	152
Presbyterian Espanola Hospital	Espanola	99%	127
Gila Regional Medical Center	Silver City	98%	195
Memorial Medical Center[2]	Las Cruces	98%	298
Eastern New Mexico Medical Center	Roswell	97%	143
Lea Regional Medical Center	Hobbs	97%	32
Los Alamos Medical Center	Los Alamos	97%	97
Lovelace Medical Center[2]	Albuquerque	97%	470
Lovelace Westside Hospital[2]	Albuquerque	97%	190
Saint Vincent Hospital[2]	Santa Fe	97%	260
Carlsbad Medical Center	Carlsbad	96%	46
UNM Sandoval Regional Medical Center[2,3]	Rio Rancho	96%	182
VA New Mexico Healthcare System[2]	Albuquerque	96%	229
San Juan Regional Medical Center[2]	Farmington	95%	311
UNM Hospital[2]	Albuquerque	95%	321
Artesia General Hospital[2]	Artesia	89%	90

Survey of Patients' Hospital Experiences

Area Around Room 'Always' Quiet at Night

Hospital Name	City	Rate	Cases
Lincoln County Medical Center	Ruidoso	70%	(a)
UNM Sandoval Regional Medical Center	Rio Rancho	69%	300+
Nor-Lea Hospital District	Lovington	68%	(a)
Artesia General Hospital	Artesia	67%	(a)
Lovelace Regional Hospital - Roswell	Roswell	63%	300+
Lovelace Westside Hospital	Albuquerque	62%	300+
Cibola General Hospital	Grants	61%	(a)
Holy Cross Hospital	Taos	61%	300+
Presbyterian Espanola Hospital	Espanola	61%	300+
San Juan Regional Medical Center	Farmington	61%	300+
Los Alamos Medical Center	Los Alamos	60%	(a)
Mountain View Regional Medical Center	Las Cruces	60%	300+
Alta Vista Regional Hospital	Las Vegas	59%	300+
Lea Regional Medical Center	Hobbs	59%	300+
Presbyterian Hospital	Albuquerque	59%	300+
Miners' Colfax Medical Center	Raton	58%	(a)
Plains Regional Medical Center	Clovis	58%	300+
Carlsbad Medical Center	Carlsbad	56%	300+
Gerald Champion Regional Medical Center	Alamogordo	56%	300+
Gila Regional Medical Center	Silver City	56%	300+
Lovelace Medical Center	Albuquerque	55%	300+
Lovelace Women's Hospital	Albuquerque	55%	300+
Rehoboth Mckinley Christian HCS	Gallup	55%	300+
Eastern New Mexico Medical Center	Roswell	54%	300+
Memorial Medical Center	Las Cruces	54%	300+
Mimbres Memorial Hospital	Deming	53%	300+
Gallup Indian Medical Center	Gallup	47%	300+
UNM Hospital	Albuquerque	47%	300+
Northern Navajo Medical Center	Shiprock	43%	(a)
Saint Vincent Hospital	Santa Fe	40%	300+

Doctors 'Always' Communicated Well

Hospital Name	City	Rate	Cases
Lincoln County Medical Center	Ruidoso	88%	(a)
Nor-Lea Hospital District	Lovington	87%	(a)
UNM Sandoval Regional Medical Center	Rio Rancho	85%	300+
Lovelace Regional Hospital - Roswell	Roswell	84%	300+
Artesia General Hospital	Artesia	83%	(a)
Alta Vista Regional Hospital	Las Vegas	81%	300+
Cibola General Hospital	Grants	81%	(a)
Mountain View Regional Medical Center	Las Cruces	81%	300+
Gila Regional Medical Center	Silver City	80%	300+
Los Alamos Medical Center	Los Alamos	80%	(a)
Miners' Colfax Medical Center	Raton	80%	(a)
Holy Cross Hospital	Taos	79%	300+
Lea Regional Medical Center	Hobbs	79%	300+
Presbyterian Hospital	Albuquerque	79%	300+
Lovelace Westside Hospital	Albuquerque	78%	300+
San Juan Regional Medical Center	Farmington	78%	300+
Carlsbad Medical Center	Carlsbad	77%	300+
Eastern New Mexico Medical Center	Roswell	77%	300+
Mimbres Memorial Hospital	Deming	77%	300+
Memorial Medical Center	Las Cruces	76%	300+
Plains Regional Medical Center	Clovis	76%	300+
Saint Vincent Hospital	Santa Fe	76%	300+
Lovelace Medical Center	Albuquerque	75%	300+

NOTE: Hospital profiles are in alphabetical order by state, then city, then hospital within the city; Rankings exclude hospitals with less than 25 cases except for patient surveys which excludes hospitals with less than 100 cases; (a) 100-299 cases; (1) The number of cases/patients is too few to report; (2) Data submitted were based on a sample of cases/patients; (3) Results are based on a shorter time period than required; (4) Data suppressed by CMS for one or more quarters; (5) Results are not available for this reporting period; (6) Fewer than 100 patients completed the HCAHPS survey; (7) No cases met the criteria for this measure; (8) The lower limit of the confidence interval cannot be calculated if the number of observed infections equals zero; (9) No data are available from the state/territory for this reporting period; (10) The scores shown reflect fewer than 50 completed surveys; (11) There were discrepancies in the data collection process; (12) This measure does not apply to this hospital for this reporting period; (13) Results cannot be calculated for this reporting period; (14) The results for this state are combined with nearby states to protect confidentiality; Please refer to the User's Guide for a full explanation of data.

Hospital Name	City	Rate	Cases
Lovelace Women's Hospital	Albuquerque	75%	300+
UNM Hospital	Albuquerque	75%	300+
Gallup Indian Medical Center	Gallup	73%	300+
Rehoboth Mckinley Christian HCS	Gallup	73%	300+
Gerald Champion Regional Medical Center	Alamogordo	72%	300+
Presbyterian Espanola Hospital	Espanola	72%	300+
Northern Navajo Medical Center	Shiprock	69%	(a)

Home Recovery Information Given

Hospital Name	City	Rate	Cases
Lovelace Westside Hospital	Albuquerque	89%	300+
Gila Regional Medical Center	Silver City	87%	300+
Lincoln County Medical Center	Ruidoso	87%	(a)
Mountain View Regional Medical Center	Las Cruces	87%	300+
Nor-Lea Hospital District	Lovington	87%	(a)
Los Alamos Medical Center	Los Alamos	86%	(a)
Lovelace Women's Hospital	Albuquerque	86%	300+
Mimbres Memorial Hospital	Deming	86%	300+
UNM Hospital	Albuquerque	86%	300+
Artesia General Hospital	Artesia	85%	(a)
Cibola General Hospital	Grants	85%	(a)
Lovelace Medical Center	Albuquerque	85%	300+
Memorial Medical Center	Las Cruces	85%	300+
Presbyterian Hospital	Albuquerque	85%	300+
San Juan Regional Medical Center	Farmington	85%	300+
Carlsbad Medical Center	Carlsbad	84%	300+
Eastern New Mexico Medical Center	Roswell	84%	300+
Alta Vista Regional Hospital	Las Vegas	83%	300+
Lea Regional Medical Center	Hobbs	83%	300+
Lovelace Regional Hospital - Roswell	Roswell	83%	300+
Northern Navajo Medical Center	Shiprock	83%	(a)
Plains Regional Medical Center	Clovis	83%	300+
UNM Sandoval Regional Medical Center	Rio Rancho	83%	300+
Presbyterian Espanola Hospital	Espanola	82%	300+
Rehoboth Mckinley Christian HCS	Gallup	82%	300+
Gerald Champion Regional Medical Center	Alamogordo	81%	300+
Miners' Colfax Medical Center	Raton	81%	(a)
Saint Vincent Hospital	Santa Fe	81%	300+
Holy Cross Hospital	Taos	80%	300+
Gallup Indian Medical Center	Gallup	79%	300+

Hospital Given 9 or 10 on 10 Point Scale

Hospital Name	City	Rate	Cases
UNM Sandoval Regional Medical Center	Rio Rancho	82%	300+
Lincoln County Medical Center	Ruidoso	78%	(a)
Lovelace Regional Hospital - Roswell	Roswell	74%	300+
Lovelace Westside Hospital	Albuquerque	74%	300+
Nor-Lea Hospital District	Lovington	74%	(a)
Mountain View Regional Medical Center	Las Cruces	72%	300+
Cibola General Hospital	Grants	71%	(a)
Presbyterian Hospital	Albuquerque	70%	300+
Holy Cross Hospital	Taos	69%	300+
Los Alamos Medical Center	Los Alamos	69%	(a)
Miners' Colfax Medical Center	Raton	69%	(a)
Artesia General Hospital	Artesia	67%	(a)
Lovelace Women's Hospital	Albuquerque	67%	300+
Presbyterian Espanola Hospital	Espanola	67%	300+
Gila Regional Medical Center	Silver City	65%	300+
San Juan Regional Medical Center	Farmington	65%	300+
UNM Hospital	Albuquerque	65%	300+
Lovelace Medical Center	Albuquerque	63%	300+
Memorial Medical Center	Las Cruces	63%	300+
Carlsbad Medical Center	Carlsbad	62%	300+
Mimbres Memorial Hospital	Deming	61%	300+
Rehoboth Mckinley Christian HCS	Gallup	60%	300+
Eastern New Mexico Medical Center	Roswell	59%	300+
Lea Regional Medical Center	Hobbs	59%	300+
Plains Regional Medical Center	Clovis	59%	300+
Alta Vista Regional Hospital	Las Vegas	58%	300+
Gerald Champion Regional Medical Center	Alamogordo	58%	300+
Saint Vincent Hospital	Santa Fe	50%	300+
Northern Navajo Medical Center	Shiprock	48%	(a)
Gallup Indian Medical Center	Gallup	47%	300+

Meds 'Always' Explained Before Given

Hospital Name	City	Rate	Cases
Lincoln County Medical Center	Ruidoso	75%	(a)
Nor-Lea Hospital District	Lovington	71%	(a)
San Juan Regional Medical Center	Farmington	69%	300+
Carlsbad Medical Center	Carlsbad	65%	300+
Cibola General Hospital	Grants	65%	(a)
Gila Regional Medical Center	Silver City	65%	300+
Lovelace Westside Hospital	Albuquerque	64%	300+
Plains Regional Medical Center	Clovis	64%	300+
Alta Vista Regional Hospital	Las Vegas	63%	300+
Lovelace Regional Hospital - Roswell	Roswell	63%	300+
Presbyterian Hospital	Albuquerque	63%	300+
Rehoboth Mckinley Christian HCS	Gallup	62%	300+
UNM Sandoval Regional Medical Center	Rio Rancho	62%	300+
Artesia General Hospital	Artesia	61%	(a)
Lovelace Women's Hospital	Albuquerque	61%	300+
Miners' Colfax Medical Center	Raton	61%	(a)
Northern Navajo Medical Center	Shiprock	61%	(a)
Holy Cross Hospital	Taos	60%	300+
Mimbres Memorial Hospital	Deming	60%	300+
UNM Hospital	Albuquerque	60%	300+
Eastern New Mexico Medical Center	Roswell	59%	300+
Los Alamos Medical Center	Los Alamos	59%	(a)
Gallup Indian Medical Center	Gallup	58%	300+
Mountain View Regional Medical Center	Las Cruces	58%	300+
Presbyterian Espanola Hospital	Espanola	58%	300+
Lea Regional Medical Center	Hobbs	57%	300+
Memorial Medical Center	Las Cruces	56%	300+
Saint Vincent Hospital	Santa Fe	55%	300+
Gerald Champion Regional Medical Center	Alamogordo	54%	300+
Lovelace Medical Center	Albuquerque	53%	300+

Nurses 'Always' Communicated Well

Hospital Name	City	Rate	Cases
Lincoln County Medical Center	Ruidoso	88%	(a)
Miners' Colfax Medical Center	Raton	82%	(a)
UNM Sandoval Regional Medical Center	Rio Rancho	81%	300+
Lovelace Westside Hospital	Albuquerque	80%	300+
Nor-Lea Hospital District	Lovington	80%	(a)
Gila Regional Medical Center	Silver City	79%	300+
Lovelace Regional Hospital - Roswell	Roswell	79%	300+
Plains Regional Medical Center	Clovis	79%	300+
San Juan Regional Medical Center	Farmington	78%	300+
Holy Cross Hospital	Taos	77%	300+
Mountain View Regional Medical Center	Las Cruces	77%	300+
Carlsbad Medical Center	Carlsbad	76%	300+
Cibola General Hospital	Grants	76%	(a)
Los Alamos Medical Center	Los Alamos	76%	(a)
Presbyterian Hospital	Albuquerque	76%	300+
Alta Vista Regional Hospital	Las Vegas	75%	300+
Artesia General Hospital	Artesia	75%	(a)
Lovelace Women's Hospital	Albuquerque	74%	300+
Mimbres Memorial Hospital	Deming	74%	300+
Presbyterian Espanola Hospital	Espanola	74%	300+
UNM Hospital	Albuquerque	74%	300+
Lovelace Medical Center	Albuquerque	72%	300+
Northern Navajo Medical Center	Shiprock	72%	(a)
Rehoboth Mckinley Christian HCS	Gallup	72%	300+
Lea Regional Medical Center	Hobbs	71%	300+
Memorial Medical Center	Las Cruces	71%	300+
Eastern New Mexico Medical Center	Roswell	70%	300+
Gerald Champion Regional Medical Center	Alamogordo	70%	300+
Saint Vincent Hospital	Santa Fe	68%	300+
Gallup Indian Medical Center	Gallup	65%	300+

Pain 'Always' Well Controlled

Hospital Name	City	Rate	Cases
Lincoln County Medical Center	Ruidoso	80%	(a)
Lovelace Regional Hospital - Roswell	Roswell	76%	300+
UNM Sandoval Regional Medical Center	Rio Rancho	76%	300+
Lovelace Westside Hospital	Albuquerque	75%	300+
Miners' Colfax Medical Center	Raton	74%	(a)
Nor-Lea Hospital District	Lovington	71%	(a)
Mountain View Regional Medical Center	Las Cruces	70%	300+
Plains Regional Medical Center	Clovis	70%	300+
Los Alamos Medical Center	Los Alamos	69%	(a)
Mimbres Memorial Hospital	Deming	69%	300+
Presbyterian Hospital	Albuquerque	69%	300+
Rehoboth Mckinley Christian HCS	Gallup	69%	300+
Artesia General Hospital	Artesia	68%	(a)
Carlsbad Medical Center	Carlsbad	68%	300+
Cibola General Hospital	Grants	68%	(a)
Holy Cross Hospital	Taos	68%	300+
San Juan Regional Medical Center	Farmington	68%	300+
Gila Regional Medical Center	Silver City	67%	300+
Lovelace Women's Hospital	Albuquerque	67%	300+
Lovelace Medical Center	Albuquerque	66%	300+
Memorial Medical Center	Las Cruces	66%	300+
Presbyterian Espanola Hospital	Espanola	66%	300+
UNM Hospital	Albuquerque	66%	300+
Eastern New Mexico Medical Center	Roswell	65%	300+
Gallup Indian Medical Center	Gallup	65%	300+
Gerald Champion Regional Medical Center	Alamogordo	64%	300+
Northern Navajo Medical Center	Shiprock	64%	(a)
Lea Regional Medical Center	Hobbs	63%	300+
Alta Vista Regional Hospital	Las Vegas	62%	300+
Saint Vincent Hospital	Santa Fe	62%	300+

Room and Bathroom 'Always' Clean

Hospital Name	City	Rate	Cases
Nor-Lea Hospital District	Lovington	82%	(a)
Miners' Colfax Medical Center	Raton	80%	(a)
Lincoln County Medical Center	Ruidoso	77%	(a)
UNM Sandoval Regional Medical Center	Rio Rancho	76%	300+
Lovelace Regional Hospital - Roswell	Roswell	75%	300+
Presbyterian Espanola Hospital	Espanola	75%	300+
Mimbres Memorial Hospital	Deming	73%	300+
Carlsbad Medical Center	Carlsbad	72%	300+
Gila Regional Medical Center	Silver City	72%	300+
Cibola General Hospital	Grants	71%	(a)
Gerald Champion Regional Medical Center	Alamogordo	71%	300+
Lovelace Westside Hospital	Albuquerque	71%	300+
Holy Cross Hospital	Taos	70%	300+
Lovelace Women's Hospital	Albuquerque	70%	300+
Rehoboth Mckinley Christian HCS	Gallup	70%	300+
Artesia General Hospital	Artesia	68%	(a)
Mountain View Regional Medical Center	Las Cruces	68%	300+
Plains Regional Medical Center	Clovis	68%	300+
Presbyterian Hospital	Albuquerque	68%	300+
San Juan Regional Medical Center	Farmington	67%	300+
Lovelace Medical Center	Albuquerque	66%	300+
Eastern New Mexico Medical Center	Roswell	65%	300+
Lea Regional Medical Center	Hobbs	64%	300+
UNM Hospital	Albuquerque	64%	300+
Alta Vista Regional Hospital	Las Vegas	62%	300+
Los Alamos Medical Center	Los Alamos	62%	(a)
Memorial Medical Center	Las Cruces	62%	300+
Gallup Indian Medical Center	Gallup	60%	300+
Northern Navajo Medical Center	Shiprock	55%	(a)
Saint Vincent Hospital	Santa Fe	53%	300+

Timely Help 'Always' Received

Hospital Name	City	Rate	Cases
Lincoln County Medical Center	Ruidoso	81%	(a)
Miners' Colfax Medical Center	Raton	79%	(a)
Cibola General Hospital	Grants	76%	(a)
Lovelace Westside Hospital	Albuquerque	74%	300+
UNM Sandoval Regional Medical Center	Rio Rancho	73%	300+
Nor-Lea Hospital District	Lovington	72%	(a)
Gila Regional Medical Center	Silver City	71%	300+
Lovelace Regional Hospital - Roswell	Roswell	69%	300+
Los Alamos Medical Center	Los Alamos	68%	(a)
Plains Regional Medical Center	Clovis	68%	300+
Holy Cross Hospital	Taos	67%	300+
Mountain View Regional Medical Center	Las Cruces	66%	300+
Gerald Champion Regional Medical Center	Alamogordo	65%	300+
Lovelace Women's Hospital	Albuquerque	64%	300+
Presbyterian Espanola Hospital	Espanola	64%	300+
Rehoboth Mckinley Christian HCS	Gallup	64%	300+
San Juan Regional Medical Center	Farmington	64%	300+
Carlsbad Medical Center	Carlsbad	63%	300+
Mimbres Memorial Hospital	Deming	63%	300+
Presbyterian Hospital	Albuquerque	63%	300+
UNM Hospital	Albuquerque	63%	300+
Artesia General Hospital	Artesia	62%	(a)
Alta Vista Regional Hospital	Las Vegas	61%	300+
Lea Regional Medical Center	Hobbs	56%	300+
Lovelace Medical Center	Albuquerque	56%	300+
Northern Navajo Medical Center	Shiprock	56%	(a)
Memorial Medical Center	Las Cruces	55%	300+
Gallup Indian Medical Center	Gallup	52%	300+
Saint Vincent Hospital	Santa Fe	51%	300+
Eastern New Mexico Medical Center	Roswell	50%	300+

Would Definitely Recommend Hospital

Hospital Name	City	Rate	Cases
UNM Sandoval Regional Medical Center	Rio Rancho	84%	300+
Nor-Lea Hospital District	Lovington	81%	(a)
Presbyterian Hospital	Albuquerque	78%	300+
Lovelace Regional Hospital - Roswell	Roswell	77%	300+
Mountain View Regional Medical Center	Las Cruces	77%	300+
Lovelace Westside Hospital	Albuquerque	76%	300+
Lincoln County Medical Center	Ruidoso	74%	(a)
Los Alamos Medical Center	Los Alamos	73%	(a)
Lovelace Women's Hospital	Albuquerque	72%	300+
Presbyterian Espanola Hospital	Espanola	71%	300+
Cibola General Hospital	Grants	70%	(a)
Holy Cross Hospital	Taos	70%	300+
UNM Hospital	Albuquerque	68%	300+
Artesia General Hospital	Artesia	67%	(a)
Lovelace Medical Center	Albuquerque	67%	300+
San Juan Regional Medical Center	Farmington	67%	300+
Gila Regional Medical Center	Silver City	66%	300+
Memorial Medical Center	Las Cruces	64%	300+
Miners' Colfax Medical Center	Raton	64%	(a)
Eastern New Mexico Medical Center	Roswell	60%	300+
Rehoboth Mckinley Christian HCS	Gallup	58%	300+
Mimbres Memorial Hospital	Deming	56%	300+
Carlsbad Medical Center	Carlsbad	55%	300+
Lea Regional Medical Center	Hobbs	55%	300+
Alta Vista Regional Hospital	Las Vegas	54%	300+
Plains Regional Medical Center	Clovis	53%	300+
Saint Vincent Hospital	Santa Fe	53%	300+
Gerald Champion Regional Medical Center	Alamogordo	52%	300+
Northern Navajo Medical Center	Shiprock	49%	(a)

NOTE: Hospital profiles are in alphabetical order by state, then city, then hospital within the city; Rankings exclude hospitals with less than 25 cases except for patient surveys which excludes hospitals with less than 100 cases; (a) 100-299 cases; (1) The number of cases/patients is too few to report; (2) Data submitted were based on a sample of cases/patients; (3) Results are based on a shorter time period than required; (4) Data suppressed by CMS for one or more quarters; (5) Results are not available for this reporting period; (6) Fewer than 100 patients completed the HCAHPS survey; (7) No cases met the criteria for this measure; (8) The lower limit of the confidence interval cannot be calculated if the number of observed infections equals zero; (9) No data are available from the state/territory for this reporting period; (10) The scores shown reflect fewer than 50 completed surveys; (11) There were discrepancies in the data collection process; (12) This measure does not apply to this hospital for this reporting period; (13) Results cannot be calculated for this reporting period; (14) The results for this state are combined with nearby states to protect confidentiality; Please refer to the User's Guide for a full explanation of data.

Gallup Indian Medical Center	Gallup	36%	300+

Use of Medical Imaging

Cardiac Imaging Stress Test before OP Surgery

Hospital Name	City	Rate	Cases
Lovelace Women's Hospital	Albuquerque	2.1%	48
Mountain View Regional Medical Center	Las Cruces	2.2%	278
Lovelace Medical Center	Albuquerque	3.1%	162
Presbyterian Hospital	Albuquerque	3.1%	580
San Juan Regional Medical Center	Farmington	3.3%	600
UNM Hospital	Albuquerque	3.4%	294
Holy Cross Hospital	Taos	3.7%	189
Memorial Medical Center	Las Cruces	3.8%	212
Carlsbad Medical Center	Carlsbad	4.1%	122
Saint Vincent Hospital	Santa Fe	4.8%	372
Alta Vista Regional Hospital	Las Vegas	4.9%	163
Lea Regional Medical Center	Hobbs	5.4%	111
Gerald Champion Regional Medical Center	Alamogordo	5.5%	272
Artesia General Hospital	Artesia	6.3%	63
Mimbres Memorial Hospital	Deming	6.3%	64
Nor-Lea Hospital District	Lovington	6.8%	205

Combination Abdominal CT Scan

Hospital Name	City	Rate	Cases
Roosevelt General Hospital	Portales	1.8%	166
Mimbres Memorial Hospital	Deming	2.5%	322
Holy Cross Hospital	Taos	3.2%	279
Lovelace Women's Hospital	Albuquerque	3.2%	278
San Juan Regional Medical Center	Farmington	3.4%	1041
Gerald Champion Regional Medical Center	Alamogordo	3.7%	458
Carlsbad Medical Center	Carlsbad	4.3%	486
Saint Vincent Hospital	Santa Fe	4.6%	587
Lovelace Medical Center	Albuquerque	4.9%	487
Lea Regional Medical Center	Hobbs	5.0%	282
Lovelace Westside Hospital	Albuquerque	5.1%	195
Lovelace Regional Hospital - Roswell	Roswell	5.2%	385
Cibola General Hospital	Grants	5.5%	165
Presbyterian Espanola Hospital	Espanola	5.9%	320
Rehoboth Mckinley Christian HCS	Gallup	6.6%	243
Artesia General Hospital	Artesia	6.7%	193
Gila Regional Medical Center	Silver City	7.5%	442
Presbyterian Hospital	Albuquerque	8.2%	1753
Mountain View Regional Medical Center	Las Cruces	8.4%	415
Plains Regional Medical Center	Clovis	8.8%	512
Los Alamos Medical Center	Los Alamos	11.2%	233
Alta Vista Regional Hospital	Las Vegas	11.8%	381
UNM Hospital	Albuquerque	11.8%	1113
Miners' Colfax Medical Center	Raton	13.4%	134
Eastern New Mexico Medical Center	Roswell	15.9%	497
Nor-Lea Hospital District	Lovington	30.4%	382
Memorial Medical Center	Las Cruces	40.8%	595

Combination Brain/Sinus CT Scan

Hospital Name	City	Rate	Cases
Saint Vincent Hospital	Santa Fe	0.8%	732
Gila Regional Medical Center	Silver City	0.9%	350
Los Alamos Medical Center	Los Alamos	1.1%	175
UNM Hospital	Albuquerque	1.2%	583
San Juan Regional Medical Center	Farmington	1.4%	642
Plains Regional Medical Center	Clovis	1.5%	478
Carlsbad Medical Center	Carlsbad	1.6%	383
Lovelace Medical Center	Albuquerque	1.7%	521
Memorial Medical Center	Las Cruces	2.1%	528
Eastern New Mexico Medical Center	Roswell	2.7%	524
Presbyterian Hospital	Albuquerque	2.9%	1434
Gerald Champion Regional Medical Center	Alamogordo	4.1%	468
Lea Regional Medical Center	Hobbs	4.3%	372
Rehoboth Mckinley Christian HCS	Gallup	6.1%	163

Combination Chest CT Scan

Hospital Name	City	Rate	Cases
Holy Cross Hospital	Taos	0.0%	118
Saint Vincent Hospital	Santa Fe	0.0%	220
San Juan Regional Medical Center	Farmington	0.0%	537
Lovelace Regional Hospital - Roswell	Roswell	0.5%	217
UNM Hospital	Albuquerque	0.6%	994
Gila Regional Medical Center	Silver City	0.8%	254
Los Alamos Medical Center	Los Alamos	0.9%	109
Lovelace Medical Center	Albuquerque	0.9%	116
Cibola General Hospital	Grants	1.1%	89
Carlsbad Medical Center	Carlsbad	1.3%	233
Artesia General Hospital	Artesia	2.2%	93
Mimbres Memorial Hospital	Deming	2.3%	132
Gerald Champion Regional Medical Center	Alamogordo	3.4%	232
Rehoboth Mckinley Christian HCS	Gallup	3.9%	77
Presbyterian Espanola Hospital	Espanola	4.0%	149
Alta Vista Regional Hospital	Las Vegas	5.1%	215
Plains Regional Medical Center	Clovis	7.3%	245
Mountain View Regional Medical Center	Las Cruces	7.6%	131
Memorial Medical Center	Las Cruces	8.2%	425
Miners' Colfax Medical Center	Raton	8.6%	81
Lea Regional Medical Center	Hobbs	9.7%	113
Presbyterian Hospital	Albuquerque	9.9%	738
Eastern New Mexico Medical Center	Roswell	18.4%	228
Nor-Lea Hospital District	Lovington	23.7%	299

Follow-up Mammogram/Ultrasound

A follow-up rate near zero may indicate missed cancer; a rate higher than 14% may mean there is unnecessary follow up.

Hospital Name	City	Rate	Cases
Lovelace Women's Hospital	Albuquerque	5.4%	555
Mountain View Regional Medical Center	Las Cruces	5.6%	177
Lea Regional Medical Center	Hobbs	5.9%	476
Rehoboth Mckinley Christian HCS	Gallup	6.5%	262
Roosevelt General Hospital	Portales	6.9%	159
Artesia General Hospital	Artesia	7.1%	184
Lovelace Westside Hospital	Albuquerque	7.1%	127
Los Alamos Medical Center	Los Alamos	7.2%	530
San Juan Regional Medical Center	Farmington	7.3%	1410
Memorial Medical Center	Las Cruces	7.7%	587
Gila Regional Medical Center	Silver City	8.5%	717
Presbyterian Espanola Hospital	Espanola	8.5%	331
Eastern New Mexico Medical Center	Roswell	8.6%	672
UNM Hospital	Albuquerque	8.8%	1202
Nor-Lea Hospital District	Lovington	9.0%	310
Plains Regional Medical Center	Clovis	9.0%	733
Cibola General Hospital	Grants	9.8%	275
Holy Cross Hospital	Taos	11.2%	546
Carlsbad Medical Center	Carlsbad	13.6%	711
Alta Vista Regional Hospital	Las Vegas	15.1%	305
Mimbres Memorial Hospital	Deming	17.3%	294

Lumbar Spine MRI for Low Back Pain

Hospital Name	City	Rate	Cases
Mountain View Regional Medical Center	Las Cruces	26.7%	60
UNM Hospital	Albuquerque	29.4%	153
Eastern New Mexico Medical Center	Roswell	30.9%	149
Gila Regional Medical Center	Silver City	32.4%	68
Presbyterian Hospital	Albuquerque	34.1%	211
Saint Vincent Hospital	Santa Fe	35.7%	56
Rehoboth Mckinley Christian HCS	Gallup	38.1%	42
San Juan Regional Medical Center	Farmington	38.5%	192
Presbyterian Espanola Hospital	Espanola	39.6%	48
Gerald Champion Regional Medical Center	Alamogordo	44.0%	50
Roosevelt General Hospital	Portales	58.5%	41
Nor-Lea Hospital District	Lovington	59.6%	57

NOTE: Hospital profiles are in alphabetical order by state, then city, then hospital within the city; Rankings exclude hospitals with less than 25 cases except for patient surveys which excludes hospitals with less than 100 cases; (a) 100-299 cases; (1) The number of cases/patients is too few to report; (2) Data submitted were based on a sample of cases/patients; (3) Results are based on a shorter time period than required; (4) Data suppressed by CMS for one or more quarters; (5) Results are not available for this reporting period; (6) Fewer than 100 patients completed the HCAHPS survey; (7) No cases met the criteria for this measure; (8) The lower limit of the confidence interval cannot be calculated if the number of observed infections equals zero; (9) No data are available from the state/territory for this reporting period; (10) The scores shown reflect fewer than 50 completed surveys; (11) There were discrepancies in the data collection process; (12) This measure does not apply to this hospital for this reporting period; (13) Results cannot be calculated for this reporting period; (14) The results for this state are combined with nearby states to protect confidentiality; Please refer to the User's Guide for a full explanation of data.

Gerald Champion Regional Medical Center

2669 North Scenic Drive Phone: 575-439-6100
Alamogordo, NM 88310 Fax: 505-443-7858
URL: www.gcrmc.org
Type: Acute Care Hospitals Emergency Services: Yes
Ownership: Voluntary non-profit - Private
Key Personnel:
Chief of Medical Staff . . . . Arthur Austin, MD
Radiology. . . . . Christopher Creel
CEO . . . . Jim Heckert

Measure	Cases	This Hosp.	State Avg.	U.S. Avg.
Blood Clot Prevention and Treatment				
Anticoagulation Overlap Therapy[2]	25	96%	96%	93%
ICU Venous Thromboembolism Prophylaxis[2]	37	84%	92%	92%
Incidence of Potentially Preventable VTE[1,2]	-	-	3%	10%
UFH with Dosages/Platelet Monitoring[1,2]	-	-	99%	97%
Venous Thromboembolism Prophylaxis[2]	299	90%	84%	85%
Warfarin Therapy Discharge Instructions[2]	18	72%	85%	75%
Chest Pain/Possible Heart Attack Care				
Aspirin Given Within 24 Hours of Arrival	60	83%	97%	96%
Fibrinolytic Meds Within 30 Min. of Arrival[1]	-	-	62%	58%
Average Time to ECG (minutes)	61	16	9	7
Average Time to Transfer (minutes)[1]	-	-	99	60
Children's Asthma Care				
Received Home Management Plan of Care	-	-	-	88%
Received Reliever Medication	-	-	-	100%
Received Systemic Corticosteroids	-	-	-	100%
Emergency Department				
Admittance Decision Time (minutes)[2]	288	92	108	98
Head CT Results Within 45 Min. of Arrival[1]	-	-	46%	57%
Patients Who Left ER Before Being Seen	28,019	3%	4%	2%
Time from ER Arrival to Admit. (minutes)[2]	317	304	290	274
Time from ER Arrival to Discharge (minutes)	360	153	143	134
Time in ER Before Being Evaluated (minutes)	392	32	28	26
Time to Pain Meds for Fractures (minutes)	108	76	57	57
Heart Attack Care				
Aspirin Given at Discharge[1]	-	-	99%	99%
Fibrinolytic Meds Within 30 Min. of Arrival[7]	-	-	75%	54%
PCI Within 90 Minutes of Arrival[7]	-	-	95%	96%
Statin Prescribed at Discharge[1]	-	-	99%	98%
Heart Failure Care				
ACE Inhibitor or ARB for LVSD	19	89%	97%	97%
Discharge Instructions Given	60	83%	89%	94%
Evaluation of LVS Function	64	95%	96%	99%
Medicare Spending				
Medicare Spending per Patient (ratio)	-	0.91	0.85	0.98
Pneumonia Care				
Appropriate Initial Antibiotic Given	97	86%	93%	95%
Blood Culture Timing	111	90%	97%	98%
Pregnancy and Delivery Care				
Newborn Deliveries Scheduled Early[2]	36	11%	3%	6%
Preventive Care				
Immunization for Influenza[2]	293	86%	86%	90%
Immunization for Pneumonia[2]	305	90%	89%	92%
Stroke Care				
Anticoagulation Therapy for Atrial Fibrillation[1]	-	-	96%	95%
Antithrombotic Therapy Timing	37	89%	94%	98%
Assessed for Rehabilitation	43	98%	95%	97%
Discharged on Antithrombotic Therapy	43	100%	97%	99%
Discharged on Statin Medication	37	89%	89%	94%
Thrombolytic Therapy Timing[7]	-	-	61%	66%
Venous Thromboembolism Prophylaxis	39	92%	91%	94%
Written Stroke Educational Materials Given	25	88%	73%	88%
Surgical Care Improvement Project				
Appropriate Beta Blocker Usage	93	88%	94%	98%
Appropriate VTP Within 24 Hours	232	94%	97%	98%
Controlled Postoperative Blood Glucose[7]	-	-	97%	97%
Perioperative Temperature Management	277	100%	99%	100%
Prophylactic Antibiotic Selection	220	98%	98%	99%
Prophylactic Antibiotic Selection (Outpatient)[1]	-	-	98%	98%
Prophylactic Antibiotic Stopped	220	100%	98%	98%
Prophylactic Antibiotic Timing	220	94%	98%	99%
Prophylactic Antibiotic Timing (Outpatient)[1]	-	-	96%	98%
Urinary Catheter Removal	24	67%	97%	97%
Survey of Patients' Hospital Experiences				
Area Around Room 'Always' Quiet at Night	300+	56%	61%	61%
Doctors 'Always' Communicated Well	300+	72%	78%	82%
Home Recovery Information Given	300+	81%	83%	85%
Hospital Given 9 or 10 on 10 Point Scale	300+	58%	65%	71%
Meds 'Always' Explained Before Given	300+	54%	63%	64%
Nurses 'Always' Communicated Well	300+	70%	76%	79%
Pain 'Always' Well Controlled	300+	64%	68%	71%
Room and Bathroom 'Always' Clean	300+	71%	70%	73%
Timely Help 'Always' Received	300+	65%	66%	68%
Would Definitely Recommend Hospital	300+	52%	63%	71%
Use of Medical Imaging				
Cardiac Imaging Stress Test before Surgery	272	5.5%	4.2%	5.3%
Combination Abdominal CT Scan	458	3.7%	9.6%	10.5%
Combination Brain/Sinus CT Scan	468	4.1%	2.3%	2.7%
Combination Chest CT Scan	232	3.4%	5.6%	2.7%
Follow-up Mammogram/Ultrasound[7]	-	-	8.6%	8.8%
Lumbar Spine MRI for Low Back Pain	50	44.0%	36.9%	37.2%

Lovelace Medical Center

601 Dr Martin Luther King Jr Ave Ne Phone: 505-727-8000
Albuquerque, NM 87102 Fax: 505-727-8162
URL: www.lovelace.com
Type: Acute Care Hospitals Emergency Services: Yes
Ownership: Voluntary non-profit - Private Beds: 254
Key Personnel:
Chief of Medical Staff . . . . John Cruickshank
CEO . . . . Troy Greer
Emergency Room . . . . Erica Hamilton
President/CEO. . . . . Ron Stern

Measure	Cases	This Hosp.	State Avg.	U.S. Avg.
Blood Clot Prevention and Treatment				
Anticoagulation Overlap Therapy[2]	159	99%	96%	93%
ICU Venous Thromboembolism Prophylaxis[2]	83	100%	92%	92%
Incidence of Potentially Preventable VTE[2]	41	0%	3%	10%
UFH with Dosages/Platelet Monitoring[2]	93	100%	99%	97%
Venous Thromboembolism Prophylaxis[2]	353	100%	84%	85%
Warfarin Therapy Discharge Instructions[2]	128	99%	85%	75%
Chest Pain/Possible Heart Attack Care				
Aspirin Given Within 24 Hours of Arrival	14	100%	97%	96%
Fibrinolytic Meds Within 30 Min. of Arrival[3,7]	-	-	62%	58%
Average Time to ECG (minutes)	15	8	9	7
Average Time to Transfer (minutes)[3,7]	-	-	99	60
Children's Asthma Care				
Received Home Management Plan of Care	-	-	-	88%
Received Reliever Medication	-	-	-	100%
Received Systemic Corticosteroids	-	-	-	100%
Emergency Department				
Admittance Decision Time (minutes)[2]	740	123	108	98
Head CT Results Within 45 Min. of Arrival	20	45%	46%	57%
Patients Who Left ER Before Being Seen	38,326	1%	4%	2%
Time from ER Arrival to Admit. (minutes)[2]	749	324	290	274
Time from ER Arrival to Discharge (minutes)	369	197	143	134
Time in ER Before Being Evaluated (minutes)	426	27	28	26
Time to Pain Meds for Fractures (minutes)	136	73	57	57
Heart Attack Care				
Aspirin Given at Discharge[2]	322	100%	99%	99%
Fibrinolytic Meds Within 30 Min. of Arrival[2,7]	-	-	75%	54%
PCI Within 90 Minutes of Arrival[2]	39	97%	95%	96%
Statin Prescribed at Discharge[2]	312	99%	99%	98%
Heart Failure Care				
ACE Inhibitor or ARB for LVSD[2]	93	98%	97%	97%
Discharge Instructions Given[2]	253	100%	89%	94%
Evaluation of LVS Function[2]	310	99%	96%	99%
Medicare Spending				
Medicare Spending per Patient (ratio)	-	0.99	0.85	0.98
Pneumonia Care				
Appropriate Initial Antibiotic Given[2]	91	97%	93%	95%
Blood Culture Timing[2]	160	97%	97%	98%
Pregnancy and Delivery Care				
Newborn Deliveries Scheduled Early[7]	-	-	3%	6%
Preventive Care				
Immunization for Influenza[2]	621	96%	86%	90%
Immunization for Pneumonia[2]	975	98%	89%	92%
Stroke Care				
Anticoagulation Therapy for Atrial Fibrillation[2]	14	100%	96%	95%
Antithrombotic Therapy Timing[2]	79	100%	94%	98%
Assessed for Rehabilitation[2]	102	100%	95%	97%
Discharged on Antithrombotic Therapy[2]	93	100%	97%	99%
Discharged on Statin Medication[2]	62	100%	89%	94%
Thrombolytic Therapy Timing[1,2]	-	-	61%	66%
Venous Thromboembolism Prophylaxis[2]	96	99%	91%	94%
Written Stroke Educational Materials Given[2]	43	100%	73%	88%
Surgical Care Improvement Project				
Appropriate Beta Blocker Usage[2]	209	99%	94%	98%
Appropriate VTP Within 24 Hours[2]	402	96%	97%	98%
Controlled Postoperative Blood Glucose[2]	191	98%	97%	97%
Perioperative Temperature Management[2]	623	100%	99%	100%
Prophylactic Antibiotic Selection[2]	444	98%	98%	99%
Prophylactic Antibiotic Selection (Outpatient)	470	100%	98%	98%
Prophylactic Antibiotic Stopped[2]	437	99%	98%	98%
Prophylactic Antibiotic Timing[2]	445	97%	98%	99%
Prophylactic Antibiotic Timing (Outpatient)	474	98%	96%	98%
Urinary Catheter Removal[2]	470	97%	97%	97%
Survey of Patients' Hospital Experiences				
Area Around Room 'Always' Quiet at Night	300+	55%	61%	61%
Doctors 'Always' Communicated Well	300+	75%	78%	82%
Home Recovery Information Given	300+	85%	83%	85%
Hospital Given 9 or 10 on 10 Point Scale	300+	63%	65%	71%
Meds 'Always' Explained Before Given	300+	53%	63%	64%
Nurses 'Always' Communicated Well	300+	72%	76%	79%
Pain 'Always' Well Controlled	300+	66%	68%	71%
Room and Bathroom 'Always' Clean	300+	66%	70%	73%
Timely Help 'Always' Received	300+	56%	66%	68%
Would Definitely Recommend Hospital	300+	67%	63%	71%
Use of Medical Imaging				
Cardiac Imaging Stress Test before Surgery	162	3.1%	4.2%	5.3%
Combination Abdominal CT Scan	487	4.9%	9.6%	10.5%
Combination Brain/Sinus CT Scan	521	1.7%	2.3%	2.7%
Combination Chest CT Scan	116	0.9%	5.6%	2.7%
Follow-up Mammogram/Ultrasound[7]	-	-	8.6%	8.8%
Lumbar Spine MRI for Low Back Pain[1]	-	-	36.9%	37.2%

Lovelace Westside Hospital

10501 Golfcourse Road Nw Phone: 505-727-2001
Albuquerque, NM 87114
URL: www.lovelace.com/content/westsidehospital.htm
Type: Acute Care Hospitals Emergency Services: Yes
Ownership: Government - Federal Beds: 95
Key Personnel:
Chief of Medical Staff . . . . Cindy Bullock DPM
CEO/President. . . . . Troy Greer

Measure	Cases	This Hosp.	State Avg.	U.S. Avg.
Blood Clot Prevention and Treatment				
Anticoagulation Overlap Therapy[2]	17	94%	96%	93%
ICU Venous Thromboembolism Prophylaxis[2]	34	100%	92%	92%
Incidence of Potentially Preventable VTE[1,2]	-	-	3%	10%
UFH with Dosages/Platelet Monitoring[1,2]	-	-	99%	97%
Venous Thromboembolism Prophylaxis[2]	173	98%	84%	85%
Warfarin Therapy Discharge Instructions[2]	12	83%	85%	75%
Chest Pain/Possible Heart Attack Care				
Aspirin Given Within 24 Hours of Arrival	59	98%	97%	96%
Fibrinolytic Meds Within 30 Min. of Arrival[7]	-	-	62%	58%
Average Time to ECG (minutes)	59	6	9	7
Average Time to Transfer (minutes)[1]	-	-	99	60
Children's Asthma Care				
Received Home Management Plan of Care	-	-	-	88%
Received Reliever Medication	-	-	-	100%
Received Systemic Corticosteroids	-	-	-	100%
Emergency Department				
Admittance Decision Time (minutes)[2]	423	92	108	98
Head CT Results Within 45 Min. of Arrival[1]	-	-	46%	57%
Patients Who Left ER Before Being Seen	20,485	1%	4%	2%
Time from ER Arrival to Admit. (minutes)[2]	423	266	290	274
Time from ER Arrival to Discharge (minutes)	389	140	143	134

NOTE: Hospital profiles are in alphabetical order by state, then city, then hospital within the city; Rankings exclude hospitals with less than 25 cases except for patient surveys which excludes hospitals with less than 100 cases; (a) 100-299 cases; (1) The number of cases/patients is too few to report; (2) Data submitted were based on a sample of cases/patients; (3) Results are based on a shorter time period than required; (4) Data suppressed by CMS for one or more quarters; (5) Results are not available for this reporting period; (6) Fewer than 100 patients completed the HCAHPS survey; (7) No cases met the criteria for this measure; (8) The lower limit of the confidence interval cannot be calculated if the number of observed infections equals zero; (9) No data are available from the state/territory for this reporting period; (10) The scores shown reflect fewer than 50 completed surveys; (11) There were discrepancies in the data collection process; (12) This measure does not apply to this hospital for this reporting period; (13) Results cannot be calculated for this reporting period; (14) The results for this state are combined with nearby states to protect confidentiality; Please refer to the User's Guide for a full explanation of data.

Measure	Cases	This Hosp.	State Avg.	U.S. Avg.
Time in ER Before Being Evaluated (minutes)	418	22	28	26
Time to Pain Meds for Fractures (minutes)	86	42	57	57
Heart Attack Care				
Aspirin Given at Discharge[1]	-	-	99%	99%
Fibrinolytic Meds Within 30 Min. of Arrival[7]	-	-	75%	54%
PCI Within 90 Minutes of Arrival[7]	-	-	95%	96%
Statin Prescribed at Discharge[1]	-	-	99%	98%
Heart Failure Care				
ACE Inhibitor or ARB for LVSD[1]	-	-	97%	97%
Discharge Instructions Given	47	96%	89%	94%
Evaluation of LVS Function	58	98%	96%	99%
Medicare Spending				
Medicare Spending per Patient (ratio)	-	0.97	0.85	0.98
Pneumonia Care				
Appropriate Initial Antibiotic Given[2]	87	98%	93%	95%
Blood Culture Timing[2]	107	100%	97%	98%
Pregnancy and Delivery Care				
Newborn Deliveries Scheduled Early	20	0%	3%	6%
Preventive Care				
Immunization for Influenza[2]	278	99%	86%	90%
Immunization for Pneumonia[2]	341	96%	89%	92%
Stroke Care				
Anticoagulation Therapy for Atrial Fibrillation[3,7]	-	-	96%	95%
Antithrombotic Therapy Timing[1,3]	-	-	94%	98%
Assessed for Rehabilitation[1,3]	-	-	95%	97%
Discharged on Antithrombotic Therapy[1,3]	-	-	97%	99%
Discharged on Statin Medication[1,3]	-	-	89%	94%
Thrombolytic Therapy Timing[3,7]	-	-	61%	66%
Venous Thromboembolism Prophylaxis[1,3]	-	-	91%	94%
Written Stroke Educational Materials Given[1,3]	-	-	73%	88%
Surgical Care Improvement Project				
Appropriate Beta Blocker Usage[2]	42	98%	94%	98%
Appropriate VTP Within 24 Hours[2]	198	100%	97%	98%
Controlled Postoperative Blood Glucose[2,7]	-	-	97%	97%
Perioperative Temperature Management[2]	215	100%	99%	100%
Prophylactic Antibiotic Selection[2]	157	99%	98%	99%
Prophylactic Antibiotic Selection (Outpatient)	15	100%	98%	98%
Prophylactic Antibiotic Stopped[2]	156	100%	98%	98%
Prophylactic Antibiotic Timing[2]	157	100%	98%	99%
Prophylactic Antibiotic Timing (Outpatient)	15	100%	96%	98%
Urinary Catheter Removal[2]	190	97%	97%	97%
Survey of Patients' Hospital Experiences				
Area Around Room 'Always' Quiet at Night	300+	62%	61%	61%
Doctors 'Always' Communicated Well	300+	78%	78%	82%
Home Recovery Information Given	300+	89%	83%	85%
Hospital Given 9 or 10 on 10 Point Scale	300+	74%	65%	71%
Meds 'Always' Explained Before Given	300+	64%	63%	64%
Nurses 'Always' Communicated Well	300+	80%	76%	79%
Pain 'Always' Well Controlled	300+	75%	68%	71%
Room and Bathroom 'Always' Clean	300+	71%	70%	73%
Timely Help 'Always' Received	300+	74%	66%	68%
Would Definitely Recommend Hospital	300+	76%	63%	71%
Use of Medical Imaging				
Cardiac Imaging Stress Test before Surgery[1]	-	-	4.2%	5.3%
Combination Abdominal CT Scan	195	5.1%	9.6%	10.5%
Combination Brain/Sinus CT Scan[1]	-	-	2.3%	2.7%
Combination Chest CT Scan[1]	-	-	5.6%	2.7%
Follow-up Mammogram/Ultrasound	127	7.1%	8.6%	8.8%
Lumbar Spine MRI for Low Back Pain[1]	-	-	36.9%	37.2%

Lovelace Women's Hospital

4701 Montgomery Boulevard Ne
Albuquerque, NM 87109
Phone: 505-727-7805
Fax: 505-727-7888
Type: Acute Care Hospitals
Emergency Services: Yes
Ownership: Government - State
Beds: 112

Measure	Cases	This Hosp.	State Avg.	U.S. Avg.
Blood Clot Prevention and Treatment				
Anticoagulation Overlap Therapy[2]	22	100%	96%	93%
ICU Venous Thromboembolism Prophylaxis[2]	41	100%	92%	92%
Incidence of Potentially Preventable VTE[1,2]	-	-	3%	10%
UFH with Dosages/Platelet Monitoring[1,2]	-	-	99%	97%
Venous Thromboembolism Prophylaxis[2]	216	100%	84%	85%
Warfarin Therapy Discharge Instructions[2]	20	100%	85%	75%
Chest Pain/Possible Heart Attack Care				
Aspirin Given Within 24 Hours of Arrival	46	100%	97%	96%
Fibrinolytic Meds Within 30 Min. of Arrival[7]	-	-	62%	58%
Average Time to ECG (minutes)	45	10	9	7
Average Time to Transfer (minutes)[1]	-	-	99	60
Children's Asthma Care				
Received Home Management Plan of Care	-	-	-	88%
Received Reliever Medication	-	-	-	100%
Received Systemic Corticosteroids	-	-	-	100%
Emergency Department				
Admittance Decision Time (minutes)[2]	226	96	108	98
Head CT Results Within 45 Min. of Arrival[1]	-	-	46%	57%
Patients Who Left ER Before Being Seen	27,455	4%	4%	2%
Time from ER Arrival to Admit. (minutes)[2]	227	327	290	274
Time from ER Arrival to Discharge (minutes)	363	161	143	134
Time in ER Before Being Evaluated (minutes)	404	38	28	26
Time to Pain Meds for Fractures (minutes)	101	59	57	57
Heart Attack Care				
Aspirin Given at Discharge[1]	-	-	99%	99%
Fibrinolytic Meds Within 30 Min. of Arrival[7]	-	-	75%	54%
PCI Within 90 Minutes of Arrival[7]	-	-	95%	96%
Statin Prescribed at Discharge[1]	-	-	99%	98%
Heart Failure Care				
ACE Inhibitor or ARB for LVSD[1]	-	-	97%	97%
Discharge Instructions Given	46	98%	89%	94%
Evaluation of LVS Function	54	100%	96%	99%
Medicare Spending				
Medicare Spending per Patient (ratio)	-	0.90	0.85	0.98
Pneumonia Care				
Appropriate Initial Antibiotic Given	67	94%	93%	95%
Blood Culture Timing	82	99%	97%	98%
Pregnancy and Delivery Care				
Newborn Deliveries Scheduled Early[2]	240	1%	3%	6%
Preventive Care				
Immunization for Influenza[2]	436	100%	86%	90%
Immunization for Pneumonia[2]	251	99%	89%	92%
Stroke Care				
Anticoagulation Therapy for Atrial Fibrillation[1,3]	-	-	96%	95%
Antithrombotic Therapy Timing[3,7]	-	-	94%	98%
Assessed for Rehabilitation[1,3]	-	-	95%	97%
Discharged on Antithrombotic Therapy[1,3]	-	-	97%	99%
Discharged on Statin Medication[1,3]	-	-	89%	94%
Thrombolytic Therapy Timing[3,7]	-	-	61%	66%
Venous Thromboembolism Prophylaxis[3,7]	-	-	91%	94%
Written Stroke Educational Materials Given[1,3]	-	-	73%	88%
Surgical Care Improvement Project				
Appropriate Beta Blocker Usage[2]	57	98%	94%	98%
Appropriate VTP Within 24 Hours[2]	314	99%	97%	98%
Controlled Postoperative Blood Glucose[2,7]	-	-	97%	97%
Perioperative Temperature Management[2]	389	100%	99%	100%
Prophylactic Antibiotic Selection[2]	258	100%	98%	99%
Prophylactic Antibiotic Selection (Outpatient)	282	97%	98%	98%
Prophylactic Antibiotic Stopped[2]	250	99%	98%	98%
Prophylactic Antibiotic Timing[2]	258	100%	98%	99%
Prophylactic Antibiotic Timing (Outpatient)	282	100%	96%	98%
Urinary Catheter Removal[2]	206	100%	97%	97%
Survey of Patients' Hospital Experiences				
Area Around Room 'Always' Quiet at Night	300+	55%	61%	61%
Doctors 'Always' Communicated Well	300+	75%	78%	82%
Home Recovery Information Given	300+	86%	83%	85%
Hospital Given 9 or 10 on 10 Point Scale	300+	67%	65%	71%
Meds 'Always' Explained Before Given	300+	61%	63%	64%
Nurses 'Always' Communicated Well	300+	74%	76%	79%
Pain 'Always' Well Controlled	300+	67%	68%	71%
Room and Bathroom 'Always' Clean	300+	70%	70%	73%
Timely Help 'Always' Received	300+	64%	66%	68%
Would Definitely Recommend Hospital	300+	72%	63%	71%
Use of Medical Imaging				
Cardiac Imaging Stress Test before Surgery	48	2.1%	4.2%	5.3%
Combination Abdominal CT Scan	278	3.2%	9.6%	10.5%
Combination Brain/Sinus CT Scan[1]	-	-	2.3%	2.7%
Combination Chest CT Scan[1]	-	-	5.6%	2.7%
Follow-up Mammogram/Ultrasound	555	5.4%	8.6%	8.8%
Lumbar Spine MRI for Low Back Pain[1]	-	-	36.9%	37.2%

Presbyterian Hospital

1100 Central Avenue Se
Phone: 505-724-8386
Albuquerque, NM 87106
URL: www.phs.org
Type: Acute Care Hospitals
Emergency Services: Yes
Ownership: Govt - Hospital Dist/Auth
Beds: 453
Key Personnel:
Administrator . . . . Doyle Boykin

Measure	Cases	This Hosp.	State Avg.	U.S. Avg.
Blood Clot Prevention and Treatment				
Anticoagulation Overlap Therapy[2]	332	100%	96%	93%
ICU Venous Thromboembolism Prophylaxis[2]	25	100%	92%	92%
Incidence of Potentially Preventable VTE[2]	55	2%	3%	10%
UFH with Dosages/Platelet Monitoring[2]	84	100%	99%	97%
Venous Thromboembolism Prophylaxis[2]	374	82%	84%	85%
Warfarin Therapy Discharge Instructions[2]	245	99%	85%	75%
Chest Pain/Possible Heart Attack Care				
Aspirin Given Within 24 Hours of Arrival	155	100%	97%	96%
Fibrinolytic Meds Within 30 Min. of Arrival[7]	-	-	62%	58%
Average Time to ECG (minutes)	163	9	9	7
Average Time to Transfer (minutes)	13	48	99	60
Children's Asthma Care				
Received Home Management Plan of Care	-	-	-	88%
Received Reliever Medication	-	-	-	100%
Received Systemic Corticosteroids	-	-	-	100%
Emergency Department				
Admittance Decision Time (minutes)[2]	311	110	108	98
Head CT Results Within 45 Min. of Arrival	30	70%	46%	57%
Patients Who Left ER Before Being Seen	>100k	5%	4%	2%
Time from ER Arrival to Admit. (minutes)[2]	398	320	290	274
Time from ER Arrival to Discharge (minutes)	380	209	143	134
Time in ER Before Being Evaluated (minutes)	431	49	28	26
Time to Pain Meds for Fractures (minutes)	311	78	57	57
Heart Attack Care				
Aspirin Given at Discharge	666	100%	99%	99%
Fibrinolytic Meds Within 30 Min. of Arrival[7]	-	-	75%	54%
PCI Within 90 Minutes of Arrival	86	98%	95%	96%
Statin Prescribed at Discharge	632	100%	99%	98%
Heart Failure Care				
ACE Inhibitor or ARB for LVSD[2]	123	100%	97%	97%
Discharge Instructions Given[2]	282	94%	89%	94%
Evaluation of LVS Function[2]	339	100%	96%	99%
Medicare Spending				
Medicare Spending per Patient (ratio)	-	0.99	0.85	0.98
Pneumonia Care				
Appropriate Initial Antibiotic Given[2]	93	98%	93%	95%
Blood Culture Timing[2]	125	100%	97%	98%
Pregnancy and Delivery Care				
Newborn Deliveries Scheduled Early[2]	80	2%	3%	6%
Preventive Care				
Immunization for Influenza[2]	549	94%	86%	90%
Immunization for Pneumonia[2]	597	95%	89%	92%
Stroke Care				
Anticoagulation Therapy for Atrial Fibrillation[2]	15	93%	96%	95%
Antithrombotic Therapy Timing[2]	94	100%	94%	98%
Assessed for Rehabilitation[2]	127	97%	95%	97%
Discharged on Antithrombotic Therapy[2]	122	99%	97%	99%
Discharged on Statin Medication[2]	87	87%	89%	94%
Thrombolytic Therapy Timing[2]	13	69%	61%	66%
Venous Thromboembolism Prophylaxis[2]	113	93%	91%	94%
Written Stroke Educational Materials Given[2]	66	42%	73%	88%
Surgical Care Improvement Project				
Appropriate Beta Blocker Usage[2]	220	99%	94%	98%
Appropriate VTP Within 24 Hours[2]	547	98%	97%	98%
Controlled Postoperative Blood Glucose[2]	175	95%	97%	97%
Perioperative Temperature Management[2]	663	100%	99%	100%
Prophylactic Antibiotic Selection[2]	641	100%	98%	99%
Prophylactic Antibiotic Selection (Outpatient)	682	99%	98%	98%
Prophylactic Antibiotic Stopped[2]	615	98%	98%	98%

NOTE: Hospital profiles are in alphabetical order by state, then city, then hospital within the city; Rankings exclude hospitals with less than 25 cases except for patient surveys which excludes hospitals with less than 100 cases; (a) 100-299 cases; (1) The number of cases/patients is too few to report; (2) Data submitted were based on a sample of cases/patients; (3) Results are based on a shorter time period than required; (4) Data suppressed by CMS for one or more quarters; (5) Results are not available for this reporting period; (6) Fewer than 100 patients completed the HCAHPS survey; (7) No cases met the criteria for this measure; (8) The lower limit of the confidence interval cannot be calculated if the number of observed infections equals zero; (9) No data are available from the state/territory for this reporting period; (10) The scores shown reflect fewer than 50 completed surveys; (11) There were discrepancies in the data collection process; (12) This measure does not apply to this hospital for this reporting period; (13) Results cannot be calculated for this reporting period; (14) The results for this state are combined with nearby states to protect confidentiality; Please refer to the User's Guide for a full explanation of data.

Prophylactic Antibiotic Timing[2]	642	99%	98%	99%
Prophylactic Antibiotic Timing (Outpatient)	684	99%	96%	98%
Urinary Catheter Removal[2]	532	100%	97%	97%
Survey of Patients' Hospital Experiences				
Area Around Room 'Always' Quiet at Night	300+	59%	61%	61%
Doctors 'Always' Communicated Well	300+	79%	78%	82%
Home Recovery Information Given	300+	85%	83%	85%
Hospital Given 9 or 10 on 10 Point Scale	300+	70%	65%	71%
Meds 'Always' Explained Before Given	300+	63%	63%	64%
Nurses 'Always' Communicated Well	300+	76%	76%	79%
Pain 'Always' Well Controlled	300+	69%	68%	71%
Room and Bathroom 'Always' Clean	300+	68%	70%	73%
Timely Help 'Always' Received	300+	63%	66%	68%
Would Definitely Recommend Hospital	300+	78%	63%	71%
Use of Medical Imaging				
Cardiac Imaging Stress Test before Surgery	580	3.1%	4.2%	5.3%
Combination Abdominal CT Scan	1,753	8.2%	9.6%	10.5%
Combination Brain/Sinus CT Scan	1,434	2.9%	2.3%	2.7%
Combination Chest CT Scan	738	9.9%	5.6%	2.7%
Follow-up Mammogram/Ultrasound[7]	-	-	8.6%	8.8%
Lumbar Spine MRI for Low Back Pain	211	34.1%	36.9%	37.2%

UNM Hospital

2211 Lomas Boulevard Ne
Albuquerque, NM 87106
Phone: 505-272-2111
Fax: 505-272-0940
E-mail: montiveros@salud.unm.edu
URL: www.hospitals.unm.edu/unmh
Type: Acute Care Hospitals
Emergency Services: Yes
Ownership: Voluntary non-profit - Other
Beds: 333

Key Personnel:
Emergency Room . . . . Michael Chicarelli
Ambulatory Care . . . . Karen Ellingboe
Pediatric Ambulatory Care . . . . . . John D Johnson, MD
Pediatric In-Patient Care . . . . John D Johnson, MD
Quality Assurance . . . . Kathy Karnaze
CEO/President. . . . . Steve McKernan
Chief of Medical Staff. . . . . David Pitcher
Radiology. . . . . Gordon Weimer

Measure	Cases	This Hosp.	State Avg.	U.S. Avg.
Blood Clot Prevention and Treatment				
Anticoagulation Overlap Therapy[2]	132	100%	96%	93%
ICU Venous Thromboembolism Prophylaxis[2]	90	99%	92%	92%
Incidence of Potentially Preventable VTE[2]	45	2%	3%	10%
UFH with Dosages/Platelet Monitoring[2]	108	100%	99%	97%
Venous Thromboembolism Prophylaxis[2]	326	94%	84%	85%
Warfarin Therapy Discharge Instructions[2]	91	85%	85%	75%
Chest Pain/Possible Heart Attack Care				
Aspirin Given Within 24 Hours of Arrival[5]	-	-	97%	96%
Fibrinolytic Meds Within 30 Min. of Arrival[5]	-	-	62%	58%
Average Time to ECG (minutes)[5]	-	-	9	7
Average Time to Transfer (minutes)[5]	-	-	99	60
Children's Asthma Care				
Received Home Management Plan of Care[2]	144	93%	-	88%
Received Reliever Medication	146	100%	-	100%
Received Systemic Corticosteroids	146	100%	-	100%
Emergency Department				
Admittance Decision Time (minutes)[2]	270	371	108	98
Head CT Results Within 45 Min. of Arrival[1]	-	-	46%	57%
Patients Who Left ER Before Being Seen	>100k	12%	4%	2%
Time from ER Arrival to Admit. (minutes)[2]	274	778	290	274
Time from ER Arrival to Discharge (minutes)	328	326	143	134
Time in ER Before Being Evaluated (minutes)	296	112	28	26
Time to Pain Meds for Fractures (minutes)	225	79	57	57
Heart Attack Care				
Aspirin Given at Discharge[2]	270	100%	99%	99%
Fibrinolytic Meds Within 30 Min. of Arrival[2,7]	-	-	75%	54%
PCI Within 90 Minutes of Arrival[2]	57	98%	95%	96%
Statin Prescribed at Discharge[2]	268	99%	99%	98%
Heart Failure Care				
ACE Inhibitor or ARB for LVSD[2]	126	99%	97%	97%
Discharge Instructions Given[2]	232	99%	89%	94%
Evaluation of LVS Function[2]	258	100%	96%	99%
Medicare Spending				
Medicare Spending per Patient (ratio)	-	0.97	0.85	0.98
Pneumonia Care				
Appropriate Initial Antibiotic Given[2]	55	96%	93%	95%
Blood Culture Timing[2]	106	98%	97%	98%
Pregnancy and Delivery Care				
Newborn Deliveries Scheduled Early[2]	42	10%	3%	6%
Preventive Care				
Immunization for Influenza[2]	502	64%	86%	90%
Immunization for Pneumonia[2]	367	68%	89%	92%
Stroke Care				
Anticoagulation Therapy for Atrial Fibrillation[1,2]	-	-	96%	95%
Antithrombotic Therapy Timing[2]	49	90%	94%	98%
Assessed for Rehabilitation[2]	96	93%	95%	97%
Discharged on Antithrombotic Therapy[2]	52	96%	97%	99%
Discharged on Statin Medication[2]	38	87%	89%	94%
Thrombolytic Therapy Timing[1,2]	-	-	61%	66%
Venous Thromboembolism Prophylaxis[2]	109	97%	91%	94%
Written Stroke Educational Materials Given[2]	53	79%	73%	88%
Surgical Care Improvement Project				
Appropriate Beta Blocker Usage[2]	123	93%	94%	98%
Appropriate VTP Within 24 Hours[2]	327	97%	97%	98%
Controlled Postoperative Blood Glucose[2]	105	96%	97%	97%
Perioperative Temperature Management[2]	469	99%	99%	100%
Prophylactic Antibiotic Selection[2]	367	98%	98%	99%
Prophylactic Antibiotic Selection (Outpatient)	151	98%	98%	98%
Prophylactic Antibiotic Stopped[2]	362	98%	98%	98%
Prophylactic Antibiotic Timing[2]	369	98%	98%	99%
Prophylactic Antibiotic Timing (Outpatient)	86	66%	96%	98%
Urinary Catheter Removal[2]	321	95%	97%	97%
Survey of Patients' Hospital Experiences				
Area Around Room 'Always' Quiet at Night	300+	47%	61%	61%
Doctors 'Always' Communicated Well	300+	75%	78%	82%
Home Recovery Information Given	300+	86%	83%	85%
Hospital Given 9 or 10 on 10 Point Scale	300+	65%	65%	71%
Meds 'Always' Explained Before Given	300+	60%	63%	64%
Nurses 'Always' Communicated Well	300+	74%	76%	79%
Pain 'Always' Well Controlled	300+	66%	68%	71%
Room and Bathroom 'Always' Clean	300+	64%	70%	73%
Timely Help 'Always' Received	300+	63%	66%	68%
Would Definitely Recommend Hospital	300+	68%	63%	71%
Use of Medical Imaging				
Cardiac Imaging Stress Test before Surgery	294	3.4%	4.2%	5.3%
Combination Abdominal CT Scan	1,113	11.8%	9.6%	10.5%
Combination Brain/Sinus CT Scan	583	1.2%	2.3%	2.7%
Combination Chest CT Scan	994	0.6%	5.6%	2.7%
Follow-up Mammogram/Ultrasound	1,202	8.8%	8.6%	8.8%
Lumbar Spine MRI for Low Back Pain	153	29.4%	36.9%	37.2%

VA New Mexico Healthcare System

1501 San Pedro Drive Se
Albuquerque, NM 87108
Phone: 505-256-2889
Fax: 505-256-2855
URL: www.southwest.va.gov/albuquerque
Type: Acute Care - VA
Emergency Services: No
Ownership: Government Federal
Beds: 217

Key Personnel:
CEO/President. . . . . Mary Bowling
Quality Assurance . . . . Rene Lameka, RN
Chief of Medical Staff. . . . . Joseph Saiers, MD

Measure	Cases	This Hosp.	State Avg.	U.S. Avg.
Blood Clot Prevention and Treatment				
Anticoagulation Overlap Therapy	-	-	96%	93%
ICU Venous Thromboembolism Prophylaxis	-	-	92%	92%
Incidence of Potentially Preventable VTE	-	-	3%	10%
UFH with Dosages/Platelet Monitoring	-	-	99%	97%
Venous Thromboembolism Prophylaxis	-	-	84%	85%
Warfarin Therapy Discharge Instructions	-	-	85%	75%
Chest Pain/Possible Heart Attack Care				
Aspirin Given Within 24 Hours of Arrival	-	-	97%	96%
Fibrinolytic Meds Within 30 Min. of Arrival	-	-	62%	58%
Average Time to ECG (minutes)	-	-	9	7
Average Time to Transfer (minutes)	-	-	99	60
Children's Asthma Care				
Received Home Management Plan of Care	-	-	-	88%
Received Reliever Medication	-	-	-	100%
Received Systemic Corticosteroids	-	-	-	100%
Emergency Department				
Admittance Decision Time (minutes)	-	-	108	98
Head CT Results Within 45 Min. of Arrival	-	-	46%	57%
Patients Who Left ER Before Being Seen	-	-	4%	2%
Time from ER Arrival to Admit. (minutes)	-	-	290	274
Time from ER Arrival to Discharge (minutes)	-	-	143	134
Time in ER Before Being Evaluated (minutes)	-	-	28	26
Time to Pain Meds for Fractures (minutes)	-	-	57	57
Heart Attack Care				
Aspirin Given at Discharge	122	99%	99%	99%
Fibrinolytic Meds Within 30 Min. of Arrival[5]	-	-	75%	54%
PCI Within 90 Minutes of Arrival[1]	24	79%	95%	96%
Statin Prescribed at Discharge	121	95%	99%	98%
Heart Failure Care				
ACE Inhibitor or ARB for LVSD	99	92%	97%	97%
Discharge Instructions Given	208	92%	89%	94%
Evaluation of LVS Function	222	99%	96%	99%
Medicare Spending				
Medicare Spending per Patient (ratio)	-	-	0.85	0.98
Pneumonia Care				
Appropriate Initial Antibiotic Given	87	90%	93%	95%
Blood Culture Timing	156	97%	97%	98%
Pregnancy and Delivery Care				
Newborn Deliveries Scheduled Early	-	-	3%	6%
Preventive Care				
Immunization for Influenza[5]	-	-	86%	90%
Immunization for Pneumonia[5]	-	-	89%	92%
Stroke Care				
Anticoagulation Therapy for Atrial Fibrillation	-	-	96%	95%
Antithrombotic Therapy Timing	-	-	94%	98%
Assessed for Rehabilitation	-	-	95%	97%
Discharged on Antithrombotic Therapy	-	-	97%	99%
Discharged on Statin Medication	-	-	89%	94%
Thrombolytic Therapy Timing	-	-	61%	66%
Venous Thromboembolism Prophylaxis	-	-	91%	94%
Written Stroke Educational Materials Given	-	-	73%	88%
Surgical Care Improvement Project				
Appropriate Beta Blocker Usage[2]	146	94%	94%	98%
Appropriate VTP Within 24 Hours[2]	305	95%	97%	98%
Controlled Postoperative Blood Glucose[2]	51	94%	97%	97%
Perioperative Temperature Management[2]	366	93%	99%	100%
Prophylactic Antibiotic Selection	271	99%	98%	99%
Prophylactic Antibiotic Selection (Outpatient)	-	-	98%	98%
Prophylactic Antibiotic Stopped	268	96%	98%	98%
Prophylactic Antibiotic Timing	272	100%	98%	99%
Prophylactic Antibiotic Timing (Outpatient)	-	-	96%	98%
Urinary Catheter Removal[2]	229	96%	97%	97%
Survey of Patients' Hospital Experiences				
Area Around Room 'Always' Quiet at Night	-	-	61%	61%
Doctors 'Always' Communicated Well	-	-	78%	82%
Home Recovery Information Given	-	-	83%	85%
Hospital Given 9 or 10 on 10 Point Scale	-	-	65%	71%
Meds 'Always' Explained Before Given	-	-	63%	64%
Nurses 'Always' Communicated Well	-	-	76%	79%
Pain 'Always' Well Controlled	-	-	68%	71%
Room and Bathroom 'Always' Clean	-	-	70%	73%
Timely Help 'Always' Received	-	-	66%	68%
Would Definitely Recommend Hospital	-	-	63%	71%
Use of Medical Imaging				
Cardiac Imaging Stress Test before Surgery	-	-	4.2%	5.3%
Combination Abdominal CT Scan	-	-	9.6%	10.5%
Combination Brain/Sinus CT Scan	-	-	2.3%	2.7%
Combination Chest CT Scan	-	-	5.6%	2.7%
Follow-up Mammogram/Ultrasound	-	-	8.6%	8.8%
Lumbar Spine MRI for Low Back Pain	-	-	36.9%	37.2%

NOTE: Hospital profiles are in alphabetical order by state, then city, then hospital within the city; Rankings exclude hospitals with less than 25 cases except for patient surveys which excludes hospitals with less than 100 cases; (a) 100-299 cases; (1) The number of cases/patients is too few to report; (2) Data submitted were based on a sample of cases/patients; (3) Results are based on a shorter time period than required; (4) Data suppressed by CMS for one or more quarters; (5) Results are not available for this reporting period; (6) Fewer than 100 patients completed the HCAHPS survey; (7) No cases met the criteria for this measure; (8) The lower limit of the confidence interval cannot be calculated if the number of observed infections equals zero; (9) No data are available from the state/territory for this reporting period; (10) The scores shown reflect fewer than 50 completed surveys; (11) There were discrepancies in the data collection process; (12) This measure does not apply to this hospital for this reporting period; (13) Results cannot be calculated for this reporting period; (14) The results for this state are combined with nearby states to protect confidentiality; Please refer to the User's Guide for a full explanation of data.

Artesia General Hospital

702 N 13th Street Phone: 575-748-3333
Artesia, NM 88210 Fax: 505-748-8377
E-mail: info@artesiageneral.com
URL: www.artesiageneral.com
Type: Acute Care Hospitals Emergency Services: Yes
Ownership: Govt - Hospital Dist/Auth Beds: 34
Key Personnel:
Surgery . . . . Shahriar Anoushfar, DO, FACOS
Cardiology . . . . John Batty, MD, FACC
CEO . . . . Kenneth W Randall
Radiology. . . . . Jon Spar, MD
Emergency Room . . . . Kelli Suto

Measure	Cases	This Hosp.	State Avg.	U.S. Avg.
Blood Clot Prevention and Treatment				
Anticoagulation Overlap Therapy[1,2]	-	-	96%	93%
ICU Venous Thromboembolism Prophylaxis[2]	23	35%	92%	92%
Incidence of Potentially Preventable VTE[1,2]	-	-	3%	10%
UFH with Dosages/Platelet Monitoring[2,7]	-	-	99%	97%
Venous Thromboembolism Prophylaxis[2]	76	37%	84%	85%
Warfarin Therapy Discharge Instructions[1,2]	-	-	85%	75%
Chest Pain/Possible Heart Attack Care				
Aspirin Given Within 24 Hours of Arrival	26	96%	97%	96%
Fibrinolytic Meds Within 30 Min. of Arrival[1]	-	-	62%	58%
Average Time to ECG (minutes)	27	5	9	7
Average Time to Transfer (minutes)[7]	-	-	99	60
Children's Asthma Care				
Received Home Management Plan of Care	-	-	-	88%
Received Reliever Medication	-	-	-	100%
Received Systemic Corticosteroids	-	-	-	100%
Emergency Department				
Admittance Decision Time (minutes)[2]	218	55	108	98
Head CT Results Within 45 Min. of Arrival[1,3]	-	-	46%	57%
Patients Who Left ER Before Being Seen	11,547	1%	4%	2%
Time from ER Arrival to Admit. (minutes)[2]	346	250	290	274
Time from ER Arrival to Discharge (minutes)	362	102	143	134
Time in ER Before Being Evaluated (minutes)	359	28	28	26
Time to Pain Meds for Fractures (minutes)	61	46	57	57
Heart Attack Care				
Aspirin Given at Discharge[1,3]	-	-	99%	99%
Fibrinolytic Meds Within 30 Min. of Arrival[3,7]	-	-	75%	54%
PCI Within 90 Minutes of Arrival[3,7]	-	-	95%	96%
Statin Prescribed at Discharge[1,3]	-	-	99%	98%
Heart Failure Care				
ACE Inhibitor or ARB for LVSD[1,2]	-	-	97%	97%
Discharge Instructions Given[2]	15	80%	89%	94%
Evaluation of LVS Function[2]	17	76%	96%	99%
Medicare Spending				
Medicare Spending per Patient (ratio)	-	0.87	0.85	0.98
Pneumonia Care				
Appropriate Initial Antibiotic Given	38	92%	93%	95%
Blood Culture Timing	44	98%	97%	98%
Pregnancy and Delivery Care				
Newborn Deliveries Scheduled Early[7]	-	-	3%	6%
Preventive Care				
Immunization for Influenza[2]	287	81%	86%	90%
Immunization for Pneumonia[2]	396	78%	89%	92%
Stroke Care				
Anticoagulation Therapy for Atrial Fibrillation[1]	-	-	96%	95%
Antithrombotic Therapy Timing	13	85%	94%	98%
Assessed for Rehabilitation	11	91%	95%	97%
Discharged on Antithrombotic Therapy	11	64%	97%	99%
Discharged on Statin Medication	11	45%	89%	94%
Thrombolytic Therapy Timing[1]	-	-	61%	66%
Venous Thromboembolism Prophylaxis	13	15%	91%	94%
Written Stroke Educational Materials Given[1]	-	-	73%	88%
Surgical Care Improvement Project				
Appropriate Beta Blocker Usage[2]	29	66%	94%	98%
Appropriate VTP Within 24 Hours[2]	124	92%	97%	98%
Controlled Postoperative Blood Glucose[2,7]	-	-	97%	97%
Perioperative Temperature Management[2]	130	100%	99%	100%
Prophylactic Antibiotic Selection[2]	96	99%	98%	99%
Prophylactic Antibiotic Selection (Outpatient)[3,7]	-	-	98%	98%
Prophylactic Antibiotic Stopped[2]	95	80%	98%	98%
Prophylactic Antibiotic Timing[2]	96	96%	98%	99%
Prophylactic Antibiotic Timing (Outpatient)[3,7]	-	-	96%	98%
Urinary Catheter Removal[2]	90	89%	97%	97%
Survey of Patients' Hospital Experiences				
Area Around Room 'Always' Quiet at Night	(a)	67%	61%	61%
Doctors 'Always' Communicated Well	(a)	83%	78%	82%
Home Recovery Information Given	(a)	85%	83%	85%
Hospital Given 9 or 10 on 10 Point Scale	(a)	67%	65%	71%
Meds 'Always' Explained Before Given	(a)	61%	63%	64%
Nurses 'Always' Communicated Well	(a)	75%	76%	79%
Pain 'Always' Well Controlled	(a)	68%	68%	71%
Room and Bathroom 'Always' Clean	(a)	68%	70%	73%
Timely Help 'Always' Received	(a)	62%	66%	68%
Would Definitely Recommend Hospital	(a)	67%	63%	71%
Use of Medical Imaging				
Cardiac Imaging Stress Test before Surgery	63	6.3%	4.2%	5.3%
Combination Abdominal CT Scan	193	6.7%	9.6%	10.5%
Combination Brain/Sinus CT Scan[1]	-	-	2.3%	2.7%
Combination Chest CT Scan	93	2.2%	5.6%	2.7%
Follow-up Mammogram/Ultrasound	184	7.1%	8.6%	8.8%
Lumbar Spine MRI for Low Back Pain[1]	-	-	36.9%	37.2%

Carlsbad Medical Center

2430 West Pierce Street Phone: 575-887-4570
Carlsbad, NM 88220 Fax: 505-887-4256
URL: www.carlsbadmedicalcenter.com
Type: Acute Care Hospitals Emergency Services: Yes
Ownership: Proprietary Beds: 127
Key Personnel:
Operating Room. . . . . Murugan Athigaman, RN
CEO/President . . . . Janet Carbary
Intensive Care Unit. . . . . Elizabeth Madison, RN
Chief of Medical Staff. . . . . Michael Sims, MD
Quality Assurance . . . . Shelda Strahan
Radiology. . . . . Lawrence Wayburn
Emergency Room . . . . James Wells
Infection Control. . . . . Marcia Westfall, RN

Measure	Cases	This Hosp.	State Avg.	U.S. Avg.
Blood Clot Prevention and Treatment				
Anticoagulation Overlap Therapy[2]	25	96%	96%	93%
ICU Venous Thromboembolism Prophylaxis[2]	73	97%	92%	92%
Incidence of Potentially Preventable VTE[1,2]	-	-	3%	10%
UFH with Dosages/Platelet Monitoring[1,2]	-	-	99%	97%
Venous Thromboembolism Prophylaxis[2]	247	99%	84%	85%
Warfarin Therapy Discharge Instructions[2]	22	91%	85%	75%
Chest Pain/Possible Heart Attack Care				
Aspirin Given Within 24 Hours of Arrival	87	100%	97%	96%
Fibrinolytic Meds Within 30 Min. of Arrival	16	75%	62%	58%
Average Time to ECG (minutes)	91	5	9	7
Average Time to Transfer (minutes)[7]	-	-	99	60
Children's Asthma Care				
Received Home Management Plan of Care	-	-	-	88%
Received Reliever Medication	-	-	-	100%
Received Systemic Corticosteroids	-	-	-	100%
Emergency Department				
Admittance Decision Time (minutes)[2]	500	86	108	98
Head CT Results Within 45 Min. of Arrival[1]	-	-	46%	57%
Patients Who Left ER Before Being Seen	24,279	3%	4%	2%
Time from ER Arrival to Admit. (minutes)[2]	513	247	290	274
Time from ER Arrival to Discharge (minutes)	367	128	143	134
Time in ER Before Being Evaluated (minutes)	417	23	28	26
Time to Pain Meds for Fractures (minutes)	106	56	57	57
Heart Attack Care				
Aspirin Given at Discharge[1]	-	-	99%	99%
Fibrinolytic Meds Within 30 Min. of Arrival[7]	-	-	75%	54%
PCI Within 90 Minutes of Arrival[7]	-	-	95%	96%
Statin Prescribed at Discharge[7]	-	-	99%	98%
Heart Failure Care				
ACE Inhibitor or ARB for LVSD	42	98%	97%	97%
Discharge Instructions Given	88	95%	89%	94%
Evaluation of LVS Function	98	100%	96%	99%
Medicare Spending				
Medicare Spending per Patient (ratio)	-	0.90	0.85	0.98
Pneumonia Care				
Appropriate Initial Antibiotic Given	112	97%	93%	95%
Blood Culture Timing	166	98%	97%	98%
Pregnancy and Delivery Care				
Newborn Deliveries Scheduled Early[2]	34	0%	3%	6%
Preventive Care				
Immunization for Influenza[2]	389	96%	86%	90%
Immunization for Pneumonia[2]	391	99%	89%	92%
Stroke Care				
Anticoagulation Therapy for Atrial Fibrillation[1]	-	-	96%	95%
Antithrombotic Therapy Timing	31	100%	94%	98%
Assessed for Rehabilitation	34	97%	95%	97%
Discharged on Antithrombotic Therapy	34	100%	97%	99%
Discharged on Statin Medication	21	95%	89%	94%
Thrombolytic Therapy Timing[1]	-	-	61%	66%
Venous Thromboembolism Prophylaxis	35	100%	91%	94%
Written Stroke Educational Materials Given	13	92%	73%	88%
Surgical Care Improvement Project				
Appropriate Beta Blocker Usage	25	100%	94%	98%
Appropriate VTP Within 24 Hours	82	100%	97%	98%
Controlled Postoperative Blood Glucose[7]	-	-	97%	97%
Perioperative Temperature Management	144	100%	99%	100%
Prophylactic Antibiotic Selection	96	100%	98%	99%
Prophylactic Antibiotic Selection (Outpatient)	54	91%	98%	98%
Prophylactic Antibiotic Stopped	93	99%	98%	98%
Prophylactic Antibiotic Timing	96	100%	98%	99%
Prophylactic Antibiotic Timing (Outpatient)	54	100%	96%	98%
Urinary Catheter Removal	46	96%	97%	97%
Survey of Patients' Hospital Experiences				
Area Around Room 'Always' Quiet at Night	300+	56%	61%	61%
Doctors 'Always' Communicated Well	300+	77%	78%	82%
Home Recovery Information Given	300+	84%	83%	85%
Hospital Given 9 or 10 on 10 Point Scale	300+	62%	65%	71%
Meds 'Always' Explained Before Given	300+	65%	63%	64%
Nurses 'Always' Communicated Well	300+	76%	76%	79%
Pain 'Always' Well Controlled	300+	68%	68%	71%
Room and Bathroom 'Always' Clean	300+	72%	70%	73%
Timely Help 'Always' Received	300+	63%	66%	68%
Would Definitely Recommend Hospital	300+	55%	63%	71%
Use of Medical Imaging				
Cardiac Imaging Stress Test before Surgery	122	4.1%	4.2%	5.3%
Combination Abdominal CT Scan	486	4.3%	9.6%	10.5%
Combination Brain/Sinus CT Scan	383	1.6%	2.3%	2.7%
Combination Chest CT Scan	233	1.3%	5.6%	2.7%
Follow-up Mammogram/Ultrasound	711	13.6%	8.6%	8.8%
Lumbar Spine MRI for Low Back Pain[1]	-	-	36.9%	37.2%

Union County General Hospital

300 Wilson Street Phone: 575-374-2585
Clayton, NM 88415 Fax: 505-374-8146
URL: www.unioncountygeneral.com
Type: Critical Access Hospitals Emergency Services: Yes
Ownership: Voluntary non-profit - Private Beds: 25
Key Personnel:
Quality Assurance . . . . Loretta Butler
CEO/President. . . . . Steve Campbell
Chief of Medical Staff. . . . . Michael Jenkins

Measure	Cases	This Hosp.	State Avg.	U.S. Avg.
Blood Clot Prevention and Treatment				
Anticoagulation Overlap Therapy[1,2]	-	-	96%	93%
ICU Venous Thromboembolism Prophylaxis[2,3]	-	-	92%	92%
Incidence of Potentially Preventable VTE[2,3]	-	-	3%	10%
UFH with Dosages/Platelet Monitoring[1,2]	-	-	99%	97%
Venous Thromboembolism Prophylaxis[2,3]	-	-	84%	85%
Warfarin Therapy Discharge Instructions[1,2]	-	-	85%	75%
Chest Pain/Possible Heart Attack Care				
Aspirin Given Within 24 Hours of Arrival	-	-	97%	96%
Fibrinolytic Meds Within 30 Min. of Arrival	-	-	62%	58%
Average Time to ECG (minutes)	-	-	9	7
Average Time to Transfer (minutes)	-	-	99	60
Children's Asthma Care				
Received Home Management Plan of Care	-	-	-	88%
Received Reliever Medication	-	-	-	100%
Received Systemic Corticosteroids	-	-	-	100%

NOTE: Hospital profiles are in alphabetical order by state, then city, then hospital within the city; Rankings exclude hospitals with less than 25 cases except for patient surveys which excludes hospitals with less than 100 cases; (a) 100-299 cases; (1) The number of cases/patients is too few to report; (2) Data submitted were based on a sample of cases/patients; (3) Results are based on a shorter time period than required; (4) Data suppressed by CMS for one or more quarters; (5) Results are not available for this reporting period; (6) Fewer than 100 patients completed the HCAHPS survey; (7) No cases met the criteria for this measure; (8) The lower limit of the confidence interval cannot be calculated if the number of observed infections equals zero; (9) No data are available from the state/territory for this reporting period; (10) The scores shown reflect fewer than 50 completed surveys; (11) There were discrepancies in the data collection process; (12) This measure does not apply to this hospital for this reporting period; (13) Results cannot be calculated for this reporting period; (14) The results for this state are combined with nearby states to protect confidentiality; Please refer to the User's Guide for a full explanation of data.

Measure	Cases	This Hosp.	State Avg.	U.S. Avg.
Emergency Department				
Admittance Decision Time (minutes)[5]	-	-	108	98
Head CT Results Within 45 Min. of Arrival	-	-	46%	57%
Patients Who Left ER Before Being Seen	-	-	4%	2%
Time from ER Arrival to Admit. (minutes)[5]	-	-	290	274
Time from ER Arrival to Discharge (minutes)	-	-	143	134
Time in ER Before Being Evaluated (minutes)	-	-	28	26
Time to Pain Meds for Fractures (minutes)	-	-	57	57
Heart Attack Care				
Aspirin Given at Discharge[5]	-	-	99%	99%
Fibrinolytic Meds Within 30 Min. of Arrival[5]	-	-	75%	54%
PCI Within 90 Minutes of Arrival[5]	-	-	95%	96%
Statin Prescribed at Discharge[5]	-	-	99%	98%
Heart Failure Care				
ACE Inhibitor or ARB for LVSD[2,3]	-	-	97%	97%
Discharge Instructions Given[1,2]	-	-	89%	94%
Evaluation of LVS Function[1,2]	-	-	96%	99%
Medicare Spending				
Medicare Spending per Patient (ratio)	-	-	0.85	0.98
Pneumonia Care				
Appropriate Initial Antibiotic Given[2]	11	100%	93%	95%
Blood Culture Timing[1,2]	-	-	97%	98%
Pregnancy and Delivery Care				
Newborn Deliveries Scheduled Early[1,2]	-	-	3%	6%
Preventive Care				
Immunization for Influenza[5]	-	-	86%	90%
Immunization for Pneumonia[5]	-	-	89%	92%
Stroke Care				
Anticoagulation Therapy for Atrial Fibrillation[5]	-	-	96%	95%
Antithrombotic Therapy Timing[5]	-	-	94%	98%
Assessed for Rehabilitation[5]	-	-	95%	97%
Discharged on Antithrombotic Therapy[5]	-	-	97%	99%
Discharged on Statin Medication[5]	-	-	89%	94%
Thrombolytic Therapy Timing[5]	-	-	61%	66%
Venous Thromboembolism Prophylaxis[5]	-	-	91%	94%
Written Stroke Educational Materials Given[5]	-	-	73%	88%
Surgical Care Improvement Project				
Appropriate Beta Blocker Usage[5]	-	-	94%	98%
Appropriate VTP Within 24 Hours[5]	-	-	97%	98%
Controlled Postoperative Blood Glucose[5]	-	-	97%	97%
Perioperative Temperature Management[5]	-	-	99%	100%
Prophylactic Antibiotic Selection[5]	-	-	98%	99%
Prophylactic Antibiotic Selection (Outpatient)	-	-	98%	98%
Prophylactic Antibiotic Stopped[5]	-	-	98%	98%
Prophylactic Antibiotic Timing[5]	-	-	98%	99%
Prophylactic Antibiotic Timing (Outpatient)	-	-	96%	98%
Urinary Catheter Removal[5]	-	-	97%	97%
Survey of Patients' Hospital Experiences				
Area Around Room 'Always' Quiet at Night[6]	<100	72%	61%	61%
Doctors 'Always' Communicated Well[6]	<100	83%	78%	82%
Home Recovery Information Given[6]	<100	84%	83%	85%
Hospital Given 9 or 10 on 10 Point Scale[6]	<100	62%	65%	71%
Meds 'Always' Explained Before Given[6]	<100	63%	63%	64%
Nurses 'Always' Communicated Well[6]	<100	82%	76%	79%
Pain 'Always' Well Controlled[6]	<100	75%	68%	71%
Room and Bathroom 'Always' Clean[6]	<100	76%	70%	73%
Timely Help 'Always' Received[6]	<100	72%	66%	68%
Would Definitely Recommend Hospital[6]	<100	68%	63%	71%
Use of Medical Imaging				
Cardiac Imaging Stress Test before Surgery	-	-	4.2%	5.3%
Combination Abdominal CT Scan	-	-	9.6%	10.5%
Combination Brain/Sinus CT Scan	-	-	2.3%	2.7%
Combination Chest CT Scan	-	-	5.6%	2.7%
Follow-up Mammogram/Ultrasound	-	-	8.6%	8.8%
Lumbar Spine MRI for Low Back Pain	-	-	36.9%	37.2%

Plains Regional Medical Center

2100 N Martin Luther King, Jr, Blvd
Clovis, NM 88101
Phone: 575-769-7155
Fax: 505-769-7526
URL: www.phs.org/facilities/clovis
Type: Acute Care Hospitals
Emergency Services: Yes
Ownership: Government - Federal
Beds: 106

Key Personnel:

Infection Control. . . . . Donna Chartien
President . . . . Albert Kwan, MD, F.A.C.S.
Quality Assurance . . . . Terry Marney
CEO . . . . Tom Phelps
Chief of Medical Staff. . . . . Cynthia Smithnd

Measure	Cases	This Hosp.	State Avg.	U.S. Avg.
Blood Clot Prevention and Treatment				
Anticoagulation Overlap Therapy[2]	27	93%	96%	93%
ICU Venous Thromboembolism Prophylaxis[2]	71	87%	92%	92%
Incidence of Potentially Preventable VTE[1,2]	-	-	3%	10%
UFH with Dosages/Platelet Monitoring[1,2]	-	-	99%	97%
Venous Thromboembolism Prophylaxis[2]	258	92%	84%	85%
Warfarin Therapy Discharge Instructions[2]	22	82%	85%	75%
Chest Pain/Possible Heart Attack Care				
Aspirin Given Within 24 Hours of Arrival	84	95%	97%	96%
Fibrinolytic Meds Within 30 Min. of Arrival[1]	-	-	62%	58%
Average Time to ECG (minutes)	101	8	9	7
Average Time to Transfer (minutes)[1]	-	-	99	60
Children's Asthma Care				
Received Home Management Plan of Care	-	-	-	88%
Received Reliever Medication	-	-	-	100%
Received Systemic Corticosteroids	-	-	-	100%
Emergency Department				
Admittance Decision Time (minutes)[2]	342	138	108	98
Head CT Results Within 45 Min. of Arrival	13	31%	46%	57%
Patients Who Left ER Before Being Seen	30,470	2%	4%	2%
Time from ER Arrival to Admit. (minutes)[2]	359	361	290	274
Time from ER Arrival to Discharge (minutes)	366	160	143	134
Time in ER Before Being Evaluated (minutes)	405	35	28	26
Time to Pain Meds for Fractures (minutes)	142	76	57	57
Heart Attack Care				
Aspirin Given at Discharge	19	84%	99%	99%
Fibrinolytic Meds Within 30 Min. of Arrival[7]	-	-	75%	54%
PCI Within 90 Minutes of Arrival[7]	-	-	95%	96%
Statin Prescribed at Discharge	16	94%	99%	98%
Heart Failure Care				
ACE Inhibitor or ARB for LVSD	20	100%	97%	97%
Discharge Instructions Given	66	91%	89%	94%
Evaluation of LVS Function	71	99%	96%	99%
Medicare Spending				
Medicare Spending per Patient (ratio)	-	0.93	0.85	0.98
Pneumonia Care				
Appropriate Initial Antibiotic Given	75	97%	93%	95%
Blood Culture Timing	164	98%	97%	98%
Pregnancy and Delivery Care				
Newborn Deliveries Scheduled Early[2]	38	3%	3%	6%
Preventive Care				
Immunization for Influenza[2]	515	63%	86%	90%
Immunization for Pneumonia[2]	407	82%	89%	92%
Stroke Care				
Anticoagulation Therapy for Atrial Fibrillation[7]	-	-	96%	95%
Antithrombotic Therapy Timing[1]	-	-	94%	98%
Assessed for Rehabilitation[1]	-	-	95%	97%
Discharged on Antithrombotic Therapy[1]	-	-	97%	99%
Discharged on Statin Medication[1]	-	-	89%	94%
Thrombolytic Therapy Timing[1]	-	-	61%	66%
Venous Thromboembolism Prophylaxis[1]	-	-	91%	94%
Written Stroke Educational Materials Given[1]	-	-	73%	88%
Surgical Care Improvement Project				
Appropriate Beta Blocker Usage	47	98%	94%	98%
Appropriate VTP Within 24 Hours	220	99%	97%	98%
Controlled Postoperative Blood Glucose[7]	-	-	97%	97%
Perioperative Temperature Management	240	100%	99%	100%
Prophylactic Antibiotic Selection	193	98%	98%	99%
Prophylactic Antibiotic Selection (Outpatient)	134	97%	98%	98%
Prophylactic Antibiotic Stopped	183	96%	98%	98%
Prophylactic Antibiotic Timing	193	99%	98%	99%
Prophylactic Antibiotic Timing (Outpatient)	137	96%	96%	98%
Urinary Catheter Removal	152	99%	97%	97%
Survey of Patients' Hospital Experiences				
Area Around Room 'Always' Quiet at Night	300+	58%	61%	61%
Doctors 'Always' Communicated Well	300+	76%	78%	82%
Home Recovery Information Given	300+	83%	83%	85%
Hospital Given 9 or 10 on 10 Point Scale	300+	59%	65%	71%
Meds 'Always' Explained Before Given	300+	64%	63%	64%
Nurses 'Always' Communicated Well	300+	79%	76%	79%
Pain 'Always' Well Controlled	300+	70%	68%	71%
Room and Bathroom 'Always' Clean	300+	68%	70%	73%
Timely Help 'Always' Received	300+	68%	66%	68%
Would Definitely Recommend Hospital	300+	53%	63%	71%
Use of Medical Imaging				
Cardiac Imaging Stress Test before Surgery[1]	-	-	4.2%	5.3%
Combination Abdominal CT Scan	512	8.8%	9.6%	10.5%
Combination Brain/Sinus CT Scan	478	1.5%	2.3%	2.7%
Combination Chest CT Scan	245	7.3%	5.6%	2.7%
Follow-up Mammogram/Ultrasound	733	9.0%	8.6%	8.8%
Lumbar Spine MRI for Low Back Pain[1]	-	-	36.9%	37.2%

Crownpoint Healthcare Facility

Junction of Hwy 371
Crownpoint, NM 87313
Phone: 505-786-5291
Fax: 928-729-8269
URL: www.ihs.gov
Type: Acute Care Hospitals
Emergency Services: Yes
Ownership: Government - Federal
Beds: 39

Key Personnel:

CEO/President. . . . . Anita Nuneta
Chief of Medical Staff. . . . . Mary Lou Stanton

Measure	Cases	This Hosp.	State Avg.	U.S. Avg.
Blood Clot Prevention and Treatment				
Anticoagulation Overlap Therapy[2,7]	-	-	96%	93%
ICU Venous Thromboembolism Prophylaxis[1,2]	-	-	92%	92%
Incidence of Potentially Preventable VTE[2,7]	-	-	3%	10%
UFH with Dosages/Platelet Monitoring[2,7]	-	-	99%	97%
Venous Thromboembolism Prophylaxis[2]	108	41%	84%	85%
Warfarin Therapy Discharge Instructions[2,7]	-	-	85%	75%
Chest Pain/Possible Heart Attack Care				
Aspirin Given Within 24 Hours of Arrival	-	-	97%	96%
Fibrinolytic Meds Within 30 Min. of Arrival	-	-	62%	58%
Average Time to ECG (minutes)	-	-	9	7
Average Time to Transfer (minutes)	-	-	99	60
Children's Asthma Care				
Received Home Management Plan of Care	-	-	-	88%
Received Reliever Medication	-	-	-	100%
Received Systemic Corticosteroids	-	-	-	100%
Emergency Department				
Admittance Decision Time (minutes)[2]	22	123	108	98
Head CT Results Within 45 Min. of Arrival	-	-	46%	57%
Patients Who Left ER Before Being Seen	-	-	4%	2%
Time from ER Arrival to Admit. (minutes)[2]	188	326	290	274
Time from ER Arrival to Discharge (minutes)	-	-	143	134
Time in ER Before Being Evaluated (minutes)	-	-	28	26
Time to Pain Meds for Fractures (minutes)	-	-	57	57
Heart Attack Care				
Aspirin Given at Discharge[5]	-	-	99%	99%
Fibrinolytic Meds Within 30 Min. of Arrival[5]	-	-	75%	54%
PCI Within 90 Minutes of Arrival[5]	-	-	95%	96%
Statin Prescribed at Discharge[5]	-	-	99%	98%
Heart Failure Care				
ACE Inhibitor or ARB for LVSD[2,7]	-	-	97%	97%
Discharge Instructions Given[1,2]	-	-	89%	94%
Evaluation of LVS Function[1,2]	-	-	96%	99%
Medicare Spending				
Medicare Spending per Patient (ratio)	-	0.59	0.85	0.98
Pneumonia Care				
Appropriate Initial Antibiotic Given[2]	11	55%	93%	95%
Blood Culture Timing[2]	28	79%	97%	98%
Pregnancy and Delivery Care				
Newborn Deliveries Scheduled Early[2]	13	0%	3%	6%
Preventive Care				
Immunization for Influenza[2]	276	74%	86%	90%
Immunization for Pneumonia[2]	217	80%	89%	92%
Stroke Care				
Anticoagulation Therapy for Atrial Fibrillation[5]	-	-	96%	95%
Antithrombotic Therapy Timing[5]	-	-	94%	98%
Assessed for Rehabilitation[5]	-	-	95%	97%
Discharged on Antithrombotic Therapy[5]	-	-	97%	99%

NOTE: Hospital profiles are in alphabetical order by state, then city, then hospital within the city; Rankings exclude hospitals with less than 25 cases except for patient surveys which excludes hospitals with less than 100 cases; (a) 100-299 cases; (1) The number of cases/patients is too few to report; (2) Data submitted were based on a sample of cases/patients; (3) Results are based on a shorter time period than required; (4) Data suppressed by CMS for one or more quarters; (5) Results are not available for this reporting period; (6) Fewer than 100 patients completed the HCAHPS survey; (7) No cases met the criteria for this measure; (8) The lower limit of the confidence interval cannot be calculated if the number of observed infections equals zero; (9) No data are available from the state/territory for this reporting period; (10) The scores shown reflect fewer than 50 completed surveys; (11) There were discrepancies in the data collection process; (12) This measure does not apply to this hospital for this reporting period; (13) Results cannot be calculated for this reporting period; (14) The results for this state are combined with nearby states to protect confidentiality; Please refer to the User's Guide for a full explanation of data.

Measure	Cases	This Hosp.	State Avg.	U.S. Avg.
Discharged on Statin Medication[5]	-	-	89%	94%
Thrombolytic Therapy Timing[5]	-	-	61%	66%
Venous Thromboembolism Prophylaxis[5]	-	-	91%	94%
Written Stroke Educational Materials Given[5]	-	-	73%	88%
Surgical Care Improvement Project				
Appropriate Beta Blocker Usage[5]	-	-	94%	98%
Appropriate VTP Within 24 Hours[5]	-	-	97%	98%
Controlled Postoperative Blood Glucose[5]	-	-	97%	97%
Perioperative Temperature Management[5]	-	-	99%	100%
Prophylactic Antibiotic Selection[5]	-	-	98%	99%
Prophylactic Antibiotic Selection (Outpatient)	-	-	98%	98%
Prophylactic Antibiotic Stopped[5]	-	-	98%	98%
Prophylactic Antibiotic Timing[5]	-	-	98%	99%
Prophylactic Antibiotic Timing (Outpatient)	-	-	96%	98%
Urinary Catheter Removal[5]	-	-	97%	97%
Survey of Patients' Hospital Experiences				
Area Around Room 'Always' Quiet at Night[3,10]	<100	67%	61%	61%
Doctors 'Always' Communicated Well[3,10]	<100	67%	78%	82%
Home Recovery Information Given[3,10]	<100	77%	83%	85%
Hospital Given 9 or 10 on 10 Point Scale[3,10]	<100	49%	65%	71%
Meds 'Always' Explained Before Given[3,10]	<100	53%	63%	64%
Nurses 'Always' Communicated Well[3,10]	<100	65%	76%	79%
Pain 'Always' Well Controlled[3,10]	<100	43%	68%	71%
Room and Bathroom 'Always' Clean[3,10]	<100	54%	70%	73%
Timely Help 'Always' Received[3,10]	<100	52%	66%	68%
Would Definitely Recommend Hospital[3,10]	<100	32%	63%	71%
Use of Medical Imaging				
Cardiac Imaging Stress Test before Surgery	-	-	4.2%	5.3%
Combination Abdominal CT Scan	-	-	9.6%	10.5%
Combination Brain/Sinus CT Scan	-	-	2.3%	2.7%
Combination Chest CT Scan	-	-	5.6%	2.7%
Follow-up Mammogram/Ultrasound	-	-	8.6%	8.8%
Lumbar Spine MRI for Low Back Pain	-	-	36.9%	37.2%

Mimbres Memorial Hospital

900 W Ash
Deming, NM 88031
Phone: 575-546-5803
URL: www.mimbresmemorial.com
Type: Critical Access Hospitals
Emergency Services: Yes
Ownership: Proprietary

Measure	Cases	This Hosp.	State Avg.	U.S. Avg.
Blood Clot Prevention and Treatment				
Anticoagulation Overlap Therapy[2]	50	100%	96%	93%
ICU Venous Thromboembolism Prophylaxis[2]	16	94%	92%	92%
Incidence of Potentially Preventable VTE[1,2]	-	-	3%	10%
UFH with Dosages/Platelet Monitoring[1,2]	-	-	99%	97%
Venous Thromboembolism Prophylaxis[2]	251	90%	84%	85%
Warfarin Therapy Discharge Instructions[2]	38	100%	85%	75%
Chest Pain/Possible Heart Attack Care				
Aspirin Given Within 24 Hours of Arrival	129	100%	97%	96%
Fibrinolytic Meds Within 30 Min. of Arrival	15	67%	62%	58%
Average Time to ECG (minutes)	135	8	9	7
Average Time to Transfer (minutes)[1]	-	-	99	60
Children's Asthma Care				
Received Home Management Plan of Care	-	-	-	88%
Received Reliever Medication	-	-	-	100%
Received Systemic Corticosteroids	-	-	-	100%
Emergency Department				
Admittance Decision Time (minutes)[2]	320	100	108	98
Head CT Results Within 45 Min. of Arrival[1]	-	-	46%	57%
Patients Who Left ER Before Being Seen	10,875	1%	4%	2%
Time from ER Arrival to Admit. (minutes)[2]	326	288	290	274
Time from ER Arrival to Discharge (minutes)	323	128	143	134
Time in ER Before Being Evaluated (minutes)	414	15	28	26
Time to Pain Meds for Fractures (minutes)	62	58	57	57
Heart Attack Care				
Aspirin Given at Discharge[3,7]	-	-	99%	99%
Fibrinolytic Meds Within 30 Min. of Arrival[3,7]	-	-	75%	54%
PCI Within 90 Minutes of Arrival[3,7]	-	-	95%	96%
Statin Prescribed at Discharge[3,7]	-	-	99%	98%
Heart Failure Care				
ACE Inhibitor or ARB for LVSD	11	100%	97%	97%
Discharge Instructions Given	59	100%	89%	94%
Evaluation of LVS Function	62	100%	96%	99%
Medicare Spending				
Medicare Spending per Patient (ratio)	-	-	0.85	0.98
Pneumonia Care				
Appropriate Initial Antibiotic Given	53	100%	93%	95%
Blood Culture Timing	63	97%	97%	98%
Pregnancy and Delivery Care				
Newborn Deliveries Scheduled Early[2,3]	15	0%	3%	6%
Preventive Care				
Immunization for Influenza[2]	299	100%	86%	90%
Immunization for Pneumonia[2]	388	100%	89%	92%
Stroke Care				
Anticoagulation Therapy for Atrial Fibrillation[1]	-	-	96%	95%
Antithrombotic Therapy Timing[1]	-	-	94%	98%
Assessed for Rehabilitation[1]	-	-	95%	97%
Discharged on Antithrombotic Therapy[1]	-	-	97%	99%
Discharged on Statin Medication[1]	-	-	89%	94%
Thrombolytic Therapy Timing[7]	-	-	61%	66%
Venous Thromboembolism Prophylaxis[1]	-	-	91%	94%
Written Stroke Educational Materials Given[1]	-	-	73%	88%
Surgical Care Improvement Project				
Appropriate Beta Blocker Usage[1]	-	-	94%	98%
Appropriate VTP Within 24 Hours	25	100%	97%	98%
Controlled Postoperative Blood Glucose[7]	-	-	97%	97%
Perioperative Temperature Management	36	100%	99%	100%
Prophylactic Antibiotic Selection	14	100%	98%	99%
Prophylactic Antibiotic Selection (Outpatient)[1,3]	-	-	98%	98%
Prophylactic Antibiotic Stopped	14	100%	98%	98%
Prophylactic Antibiotic Timing	14	100%	98%	99%
Prophylactic Antibiotic Timing (Outpatient)[1,3]	-	-	96%	98%
Urinary Catheter Removal	21	100%	97%	97%
Survey of Patients' Hospital Experiences				
Area Around Room 'Always' Quiet at Night	300+	53%	61%	61%
Doctors 'Always' Communicated Well	300+	77%	78%	82%
Home Recovery Information Given	300+	86%	83%	85%
Hospital Given 9 or 10 on 10 Point Scale	300+	61%	65%	71%
Meds 'Always' Explained Before Given	300+	60%	63%	64%
Nurses 'Always' Communicated Well	300+	74%	76%	79%
Pain 'Always' Well Controlled	300+	69%	68%	71%
Room and Bathroom 'Always' Clean	300+	73%	70%	73%
Timely Help 'Always' Received	300+	63%	66%	68%
Would Definitely Recommend Hospital	300+	56%	63%	71%
Use of Medical Imaging				
Cardiac Imaging Stress Test before Surgery	64	6.3%	4.2%	5.3%
Combination Abdominal CT Scan	322	2.5%	9.6%	10.5%
Combination Brain/Sinus CT Scan[1]	-	-	2.3%	2.7%
Combination Chest CT Scan	132	2.3%	5.6%	2.7%
Follow-up Mammogram/Ultrasound	294	17.3%	8.6%	8.8%
Lumbar Spine MRI for Low Back Pain[1]	-	-	36.9%	37.2%

Presbyterian Espanola Hospital

1010 Spruce Street
Espanola, NM 87532
Phone: 505-753-7111
Fax: 505-753-1536
URL: www.phs.org
Type: Acute Care Hospitals
Emergency Services: Yes
Ownership: Voluntary non-profit - Private
Beds: 180

Key Personnel:
Quality Assurance . . . . Barbara Garcia, RN
Infection Control. . . . . Susan Wagner, RN

Measure	Cases	This Hosp.	State Avg.	U.S. Avg.
Blood Clot Prevention and Treatment				
Anticoagulation Overlap Therapy[2]	15	100%	96%	93%
ICU Venous Thromboembolism Prophylaxis[2]	44	89%	92%	92%
Incidence of Potentially Preventable VTE[2,7]	-	-	3%	10%
UFH with Dosages/Platelet Monitoring[1,2]	-	-	99%	97%
Venous Thromboembolism Prophylaxis[2]	173	77%	84%	85%
Warfarin Therapy Discharge Instructions[2]	15	100%	85%	75%
Chest Pain/Possible Heart Attack Care				
Aspirin Given Within 24 Hours of Arrival	72	99%	97%	96%
Fibrinolytic Meds Within 30 Min. of Arrival[7]	-	-	62%	58%
Average Time to ECG (minutes)	70	14	9	7
Average Time to Transfer (minutes)	11	58	99	60
Children's Asthma Care				
Received Home Management Plan of Care	-	-	-	88%
Received Reliever Medication	-	-	-	100%
Received Systemic Corticosteroids	-	-	-	100%
Emergency Department				
Admittance Decision Time (minutes)[2]	282	67	108	98
Head CT Results Within 45 Min. of Arrival[1,3]	-	-	46%	57%
Patients Who Left ER Before Being Seen	20,544	2%	4%	2%
Time from ER Arrival to Admit. (minutes)[2]	292	227	290	274
Time from ER Arrival to Discharge (minutes)	387	117	143	134
Time in ER Before Being Evaluated (minutes)	378	33	28	26
Time to Pain Meds for Fractures (minutes)	87	63	57	57
Heart Attack Care				
Aspirin Given at Discharge[3,7]	-	-	99%	99%
Fibrinolytic Meds Within 30 Min. of Arrival[3,7]	-	-	75%	54%
PCI Within 90 Minutes of Arrival[3,7]	-	-	95%	96%
Statin Prescribed at Discharge[3,7]	-	-	99%	98%
Heart Failure Care				
ACE Inhibitor or ARB for LVSD[1]	-	-	97%	97%
Discharge Instructions Given	22	77%	89%	94%
Evaluation of LVS Function	24	100%	96%	99%
Medicare Spending				
Medicare Spending per Patient (ratio)	-	0.81	0.85	0.98
Pneumonia Care				
Appropriate Initial Antibiotic Given	55	93%	93%	95%
Blood Culture Timing	62	98%	97%	98%
Pregnancy and Delivery Care				
Newborn Deliveries Scheduled Early[2]	27	0%	3%	6%
Preventive Care				
Immunization for Influenza[2]	268	91%	86%	90%
Immunization for Pneumonia[2]	267	95%	89%	92%
Stroke Care				
Anticoagulation Therapy for Atrial Fibrillation[1]	-	-	96%	95%
Antithrombotic Therapy Timing	11	82%	94%	98%
Assessed for Rehabilitation	15	73%	95%	97%
Discharged on Antithrombotic Therapy	14	93%	97%	99%
Discharged on Statin Medication	13	62%	89%	94%
Thrombolytic Therapy Timing[7]	-	-	61%	66%
Venous Thromboembolism Prophylaxis	11	64%	91%	94%
Written Stroke Educational Materials Given[1]	-	-	73%	88%
Surgical Care Improvement Project				
Appropriate Beta Blocker Usage	23	87%	94%	98%
Appropriate VTP Within 24 Hours	144	96%	97%	98%
Controlled Postoperative Blood Glucose[7]	-	-	97%	97%
Perioperative Temperature Management	153	100%	99%	100%
Prophylactic Antibiotic Selection	115	100%	98%	99%
Prophylactic Antibiotic Selection (Outpatient)[1,3]	-	-	98%	98%
Prophylactic Antibiotic Stopped	115	98%	98%	98%
Prophylactic Antibiotic Timing	115	98%	98%	99%
Prophylactic Antibiotic Timing (Outpatient)[1,3]	-	-	96%	98%
Urinary Catheter Removal	127	99%	97%	97%
Survey of Patients' Hospital Experiences				
Area Around Room 'Always' Quiet at Night	300+	61%	61%	61%
Doctors 'Always' Communicated Well	300+	72%	78%	82%
Home Recovery Information Given	300+	82%	83%	85%
Hospital Given 9 or 10 on 10 Point Scale	300+	67%	65%	71%
Meds 'Always' Explained Before Given	300+	58%	63%	64%
Nurses 'Always' Communicated Well	300+	74%	76%	79%
Pain 'Always' Well Controlled	300+	66%	68%	71%
Room and Bathroom 'Always' Clean	300+	75%	70%	73%
Timely Help 'Always' Received	300+	64%	66%	68%
Would Definitely Recommend Hospital	300+	71%	63%	71%
Use of Medical Imaging				
Cardiac Imaging Stress Test before Surgery[7]	-	-	4.2%	5.3%
Combination Abdominal CT Scan	320	5.9%	9.6%	10.5%
Combination Brain/Sinus CT Scan[1]	-	-	2.3%	2.7%
Combination Chest CT Scan	149	4.0%	5.6%	2.7%
Follow-up Mammogram/Ultrasound	331	8.5%	8.6%	8.8%
Lumbar Spine MRI for Low Back Pain	48	39.6%	36.9%	37.2%

NOTE: Hospital profiles are in alphabetical order by state, then city, then hospital within the city; Rankings exclude hospitals with less than 25 cases except for patient surveys which excludes hospitals with less than 100 cases; (a) 100-299 cases; (1) The number of cases/patients is too few to report; (2) Data submitted were based on a sample of cases/patients; (3) Results are based on a shorter time period than required; (4) Data suppressed by CMS for one or more quarters; (5) Results are not available for this reporting period; (6) Fewer than 100 patients completed the HCAHPS survey; (7) No cases met the criteria for this measure; (8) The lower limit of the confidence interval cannot be calculated if the number of observed infections equals zero; (9) No data are available from the state/territory for this reporting period; (10) The scores shown reflect fewer than 50 completed surveys; (11) There were discrepancies in the data collection process; (12) This measure does not apply to this hospital for this reporting period; (13) Results cannot be calculated for this reporting period; (14) The results for this state are combined with nearby states to protect confidentiality; Please refer to the User's Guide for a full explanation of data.

San Juan Regional Medical Center

801 West Maple Street Phone: 505-609-2000
Farmington, NM 87401 Fax: 505-599-6249
URL: www.sanjuanregional.com
Type: Acute Care Hospitals Emergency Services: Yes
Ownership: Voluntary non-profit - Private Beds: 240

Key Personnel:
Radiology. . . . . Alan Alarcon
Patient Relations . . . . Teresa Becker
Emergency Room . . . . Mike Berve
Intensive Care Unit. . . . . Kris Cuthair
Infection Control. . . . . Penny Hill
Operating Room. . . . . Donna Kline
Quality Assurance . . . . Gary Nielson
CEO/President. . . . . Linda Thompson

Measure	Cases	This Hosp.	State Avg.	U.S. Avg.
Blood Clot Prevention and Treatment				
Anticoagulation Overlap Therapy[2]	75	93%	96%	93%
ICU Venous Thromboembolism Prophylaxis[2]	40	100%	92%	92%
Incidence of Potentially Preventable VTE[2]	11	9%	3%	10%
UFH with Dosages/Platelet Monitoring[2]	53	96%	99%	97%
Venous Thromboembolism Prophylaxis[2]	333	86%	84%	85%
Warfarin Therapy Discharge Instructions[2]	63	0%	85%	75%
Chest Pain/Possible Heart Attack Care				
Aspirin Given Within 24 Hours of Arrival[1]	-	-	97%	96%
Fibrinolytic Meds Within 30 Min. of Arrival[3,7]	-	-	62%	58%
Average Time to ECG (minutes)[1]	-	-	9	7
Average Time to Transfer (minutes)[3,7]	-	-	99	60
Children's Asthma Care				
Received Home Management Plan of Care	-	-	-	88%
Received Reliever Medication	-	-	-	100%
Received Systemic Corticosteroids	-	-	-	100%
Emergency Department				
Admittance Decision Time (minutes)[2]	580	139	108	98
Head CT Results Within 45 Min. of Arrival[1,3]	-	-	46%	57%
Patients Who Left ER Before Being Seen	48,074	1%	4%	2%
Time from ER Arrival to Admit. (minutes)[2]	587	286	290	274
Time from ER Arrival to Discharge (minutes)	354	136	143	134
Time in ER Before Being Evaluated (minutes)	383	19	28	26
Time to Pain Meds for Fractures (minutes)	210	45	57	57
Heart Attack Care				
Aspirin Given at Discharge	160	99%	99%	99%
Fibrinolytic Meds Within 30 Min. of Arrival[7]	-	-	75%	54%
PCI Within 90 Minutes of Arrival	42	95%	95%	96%
Statin Prescribed at Discharge	151	96%	99%	98%
Heart Failure Care				
ACE Inhibitor or ARB for LVSD	58	93%	97%	97%
Discharge Instructions Given	161	73%	89%	94%
Evaluation of LVS Function	197	98%	96%	99%
Medicare Spending				
Medicare Spending per Patient (ratio)	-	0.92	0.85	0.98
Pneumonia Care				
Appropriate Initial Antibiotic Given	149	97%	93%	95%
Blood Culture Timing	300	99%	97%	98%
Pregnancy and Delivery Care				
Newborn Deliveries Scheduled Early	301	4%	3%	6%
Preventive Care				
Immunization for Influenza[2]	515	85%	86%	90%
Immunization for Pneumonia[2]	553	84%	89%	92%
Stroke Care				
Anticoagulation Therapy for Atrial Fibrillation[1]	-	-	96%	95%
Antithrombotic Therapy Timing	65	92%	94%	98%
Assessed for Rehabilitation	84	85%	95%	97%
Discharged on Antithrombotic Therapy	72	94%	97%	99%
Discharged on Statin Medication	49	88%	89%	94%
Thrombolytic Therapy Timing[1]	-	-	61%	66%
Venous Thromboembolism Prophylaxis	81	84%	91%	94%
Written Stroke Educational Materials Given	56	52%	73%	88%
Surgical Care Improvement Project				
Appropriate Beta Blocker Usage[2]	110	97%	94%	98%
Appropriate VTP Within 24 Hours[2]	402	95%	97%	98%
Controlled Postoperative Blood Glucose[2,7]	-	-	97%	97%
Perioperative Temperature Management[2]	441	100%	99%	100%
Prophylactic Antibiotic Selection[2]	260	98%	98%	99%
Prophylactic Antibiotic Selection (Outpatient)	212	95%	98%	98%
Prophylactic Antibiotic Stopped[2]	255	96%	98%	98%
Prophylactic Antibiotic Timing[2]	261	99%	98%	99%
Prophylactic Antibiotic Timing (Outpatient)	171	91%	96%	98%
Urinary Catheter Removal[2]	311	95%	97%	97%
Survey of Patients' Hospital Experiences				
Area Around Room 'Always' Quiet at Night	300+	61%	61%	61%
Doctors 'Always' Communicated Well	300+	78%	78%	82%
Home Recovery Information Given	300+	85%	83%	85%
Hospital Given 9 or 10 on 10 Point Scale	300+	65%	65%	71%
Meds 'Always' Explained Before Given	300+	69%	63%	64%
Nurses 'Always' Communicated Well	300+	78%	76%	79%
Pain 'Always' Well Controlled	300+	68%	68%	71%
Room and Bathroom 'Always' Clean	300+	67%	70%	73%
Timely Help 'Always' Received	300+	64%	66%	68%
Would Definitely Recommend Hospital	300+	67%	63%	71%
Use of Medical Imaging				
Cardiac Imaging Stress Test before Surgery	600	3.3%	4.2%	5.3%
Combination Abdominal CT Scan	1,041	3.4%	9.6%	10.5%
Combination Brain/Sinus CT Scan	642	1.4%	2.3%	2.7%
Combination Chest CT Scan	537	0.0%	5.6%	2.7%
Follow-up Mammogram/Ultrasound	1,410	7.3%	8.6%	8.8%
Lumbar Spine MRI for Low Back Pain	192	38.5%	36.9%	37.2%

Gallup Indian Medical Center

516 E Nizhoni Blvd Phone: 505-722-1000
Gallup, NM 87301 Fax: 505-722-1386
URL: www.ihs.gov/facilitiesservices
Type: Acute Care Hospitals Emergency Services: Yes
Ownership: Government - Federal Beds: 99

Key Personnel:
Chief of Medical Staff. . . . . Jerome Alford, DDS
Quality Assurance . . . . Sandra Becenti
Pediatric In-Patient Care . . . . Lorelia Booqua
Operating Room. . . . . Donna Huber
Infection Control. . . . . Richard Nauman
Pediatric Ambulatory Care . . . . . . Evelyn Pena
CEO/President. . . . . Floyd Thompson

Measure	Cases	This Hosp.	State Avg.	U.S. Avg.
Blood Clot Prevention and Treatment				
Anticoagulation Overlap Therapy[1,2]	-	-	96%	93%
ICU Venous Thromboembolism Prophylaxis[2]	24	75%	92%	92%
Incidence of Potentially Preventable VTE[2,7]	-	-	3%	10%
UFH with Dosages/Platelet Monitoring[2,7]	-	-	99%	97%
Venous Thromboembolism Prophylaxis[2]	80	69%	84%	85%
Warfarin Therapy Discharge Instructions[1,2]	-	-	85%	75%
Chest Pain/Possible Heart Attack Care				
Aspirin Given Within 24 Hours of Arrival	-	-	97%	96%
Fibrinolytic Meds Within 30 Min. of Arrival	-	-	62%	58%
Average Time to ECG (minutes)	-	-	9	7
Average Time to Transfer (minutes)	-	-	99	60
Children's Asthma Care				
Received Home Management Plan of Care	-	-	-	88%
Received Reliever Medication	-	-	-	100%
Received Systemic Corticosteroids	-	-	-	100%
Emergency Department				
Admittance Decision Time (minutes)[2]	563	135	108	98
Head CT Results Within 45 Min. of Arrival	-	-	46%	57%
Patients Who Left ER Before Being Seen	-	-	4%	2%
Time from ER Arrival to Admit. (minutes)[2]	563	315	290	274
Time from ER Arrival to Discharge (minutes)	-	-	143	134
Time in ER Before Being Evaluated (minutes)	-	-	28	26
Time to Pain Meds for Fractures (minutes)	-	-	57	57
Heart Attack Care				
Aspirin Given at Discharge[5]	-	-	99%	99%
Fibrinolytic Meds Within 30 Min. of Arrival[5]	-	-	75%	54%
PCI Within 90 Minutes of Arrival[5]	-	-	95%	96%
Statin Prescribed at Discharge[5]	-	-	99%	98%
Heart Failure Care				
ACE Inhibitor or ARB for LVSD[2]	21	90%	97%	97%
Discharge Instructions Given[2]	29	69%	89%	94%
Evaluation of LVS Function[2]	32	91%	96%	99%
Medicare Spending				
Medicare Spending per Patient (ratio)	-	0.74	0.85	0.98
Pneumonia Care				
Appropriate Initial Antibiotic Given[2]	45	87%	93%	95%
Blood Culture Timing[2]	50	94%	97%	98%
Pregnancy and Delivery Care				
Newborn Deliveries Scheduled Early[2]	190	0%	3%	6%
Preventive Care				
Immunization for Influenza[2]	298	69%	86%	90%
Immunization for Pneumonia[2]	496	81%	89%	92%
Stroke Care				
Anticoagulation Therapy for Atrial Fibrillation[5]	-	-	96%	95%
Antithrombotic Therapy Timing[5]	-	-	94%	98%
Assessed for Rehabilitation[5]	-	-	95%	97%
Discharged on Antithrombotic Therapy[5]	-	-	97%	99%
Discharged on Statin Medication[5]	-	-	89%	94%
Thrombolytic Therapy Timing[5]	-	-	61%	66%
Venous Thromboembolism Prophylaxis[5]	-	-	91%	94%
Written Stroke Educational Materials Given[5]	-	-	73%	88%
Surgical Care Improvement Project				
Appropriate Beta Blocker Usage[1,2]	-	-	94%	98%
Appropriate VTP Within 24 Hours[2]	30	80%	97%	98%
Controlled Postoperative Blood Glucose[2,7]	-	-	97%	97%
Perioperative Temperature Management[2]	63	92%	99%	100%
Prophylactic Antibiotic Selection[2]	28	89%	98%	99%
Prophylactic Antibiotic Selection (Outpatient)	-	-	98%	98%
Prophylactic Antibiotic Stopped[2]	28	89%	98%	98%
Prophylactic Antibiotic Timing[2]	30	67%	98%	99%
Prophylactic Antibiotic Timing (Outpatient)	-	-	96%	98%
Urinary Catheter Removal[2]	20	90%	97%	97%
Survey of Patients' Hospital Experiences				
Area Around Room 'Always' Quiet at Night	300+	47%	61%	61%
Doctors 'Always' Communicated Well	300+	73%	78%	82%
Home Recovery Information Given	300+	79%	83%	85%
Hospital Given 9 or 10 on 10 Point Scale	300+	47%	65%	71%
Meds 'Always' Explained Before Given	300+	58%	63%	64%
Nurses 'Always' Communicated Well	300+	65%	76%	79%
Pain 'Always' Well Controlled	300+	65%	68%	71%
Room and Bathroom 'Always' Clean	300+	60%	70%	73%
Timely Help 'Always' Received	300+	52%	66%	68%
Would Definitely Recommend Hospital	300+	36%	63%	71%
Use of Medical Imaging				
Cardiac Imaging Stress Test before Surgery	-	-	4.2%	5.3%
Combination Abdominal CT Scan	-	-	9.6%	10.5%
Combination Brain/Sinus CT Scan	-	-	2.3%	2.7%
Combination Chest CT Scan	-	-	5.6%	2.7%
Follow-up Mammogram/Ultrasound	-	-	8.6%	8.8%
Lumbar Spine MRI for Low Back Pain	-	-	36.9%	37.2%

Rehoboth Mckinley Christian Health Care Services

1901 Red Rock Drive Phone: 505-863-7000
Gallup, NM 87301 Fax: 505-863-8920
URL: www.rmch.org
Type: Acute Care Hospitals Emergency Services: Yes
Ownership: Voluntary non-profit - Private Beds: 69

Key Personnel:
Emergency Room . . . . Alan Beamsley
Intensive Care Unit. . . . . Donna Corley
Radiology. . . . . Pierre Lanthiez
CEO . . . . Barry L. Mousa, FACHE
Chief of Medical Staff. . . . . Mary Poel
Quality Assurance . . . . Sherri Shuman
Infection Control. . . . . Jay Vink

Measure	Cases	This Hosp.	State Avg.	U.S. Avg.
Blood Clot Prevention and Treatment				
Anticoagulation Overlap Therapy[1,2]	-	-	96%	93%
ICU Venous Thromboembolism Prophylaxis[2]	51	53%	92%	92%
Incidence of Potentially Preventable VTE[1,2]	-	-	3%	10%
UFH with Dosages/Platelet Monitoring[1,2]	-	-	99%	97%
Venous Thromboembolism Prophylaxis[2]	181	68%	84%	85%
Warfarin Therapy Discharge Instructions[1,2]	-	-	85%	75%
Chest Pain/Possible Heart Attack Care				
Aspirin Given Within 24 Hours of Arrival[1,3]	-	-	97%	96%
Fibrinolytic Meds Within 30 Min. of Arrival[1,3]	-	-	62%	58%
Average Time to ECG (minutes)[1,3]	-	-	9	7
Average Time to Transfer (minutes)[3,7]	-	-	99	60

NOTE: Hospital profiles are in alphabetical order by state, then city, then hospital within the city; Rankings exclude hospitals with less than 25 cases except for patient surveys which excludes hospitals with less than 100 cases; (a) 100-299 cases; (1) The number of cases/patients is too few to report; (2) Data submitted were based on a sample of cases/patients; (3) Results are based on a shorter time period than required; (4) Data suppressed by CMS for one or more quarters; (5) Results are not available for this reporting period; (6) Fewer than 100 patients completed the HCAHPS survey; (7) No cases met the criteria for this measure; (8) The lower limit of the confidence interval cannot be calculated if the number of observed infections equals zero; (9) No data are available from the state/territory for this reporting period; (10) The scores shown reflect fewer than 50 completed surveys; (11) There were discrepancies in the data collection process; (12) This measure does not apply to this hospital for this reporting period; (13) Results cannot be calculated for this reporting period; (14) The results for this state are combined with nearby states to protect confidentiality; Please refer to the User's Guide for a full explanation of data.

Measure	Cases	This Hosp.	State Avg.	U.S. Avg.
Children's Asthma Care				
Received Home Management Plan of Care	-	-	-	88%
Received Reliever Medication	-	-	-	100%
Received Systemic Corticosteroids	-	-	-	100%
Emergency Department				
Admittance Decision Time (minutes)[2]	235	112	108	98
Head CT Results Within 45 Min. of Arrival[1]	-	-	46%	57%
Patients Who Left ER Before Being Seen	21,850	4%	4%	2%
Time from ER Arrival to Admit. (minutes)[2]	242	285	290	274
Time from ER Arrival to Discharge (minutes)	384	112	143	134
Time in ER Before Being Evaluated (minutes)	391	41	28	26
Time to Pain Meds for Fractures (minutes)	71	59	57	57
Heart Attack Care				
Aspirin Given at Discharge[1]	-	-	99%	99%
Fibrinolytic Meds Within 30 Min. of Arrival[7]	-	-	75%	54%
PCI Within 90 Minutes of Arrival[7]	-	-	95%	96%
Statin Prescribed at Discharge[1]	-	-	99%	98%
Heart Failure Care				
ACE Inhibitor or ARB for LVSD	28	75%	97%	97%
Discharge Instructions Given	79	96%	89%	94%
Evaluation of LVS Function	78	81%	96%	99%
Medicare Spending				
Medicare Spending per Patient (ratio)	-	0.81	0.85	0.98
Pneumonia Care				
Appropriate Initial Antibiotic Given[2]	48	79%	93%	95%
Blood Culture Timing[2]	86	85%	97%	98%
Pregnancy and Delivery Care				
Newborn Deliveries Scheduled Early[2]	44	2%	3%	6%
Preventive Care				
Immunization for Influenza[2]	297	77%	86%	90%
Immunization for Pneumonia[2]	273	78%	89%	92%
Stroke Care				
Anticoagulation Therapy for Atrial Fibrillation[7]	-	-	96%	95%
Antithrombotic Therapy Timing	15	87%	94%	98%
Assessed for Rehabilitation[1]	-	-	95%	97%
Discharged on Antithrombotic Therapy[1]	-	-	97%	99%
Discharged on Statin Medication[1]	-	-	89%	94%
Thrombolytic Therapy Timing[1]	-	-	61%	66%
Venous Thromboembolism Prophylaxis	13	69%	91%	94%
Written Stroke Educational Materials Given[1]	-	-	73%	88%
Surgical Care Improvement Project				
Appropriate Beta Blocker Usage[1]	-	-	94%	98%
Appropriate VTP Within 24 Hours	27	48%	97%	98%
Controlled Postoperative Blood Glucose[7]	-	-	97%	97%
Perioperative Temperature Management	39	100%	99%	100%
Prophylactic Antibiotic Selection	26	92%	98%	99%
Prophylactic Antibiotic Selection (Outpatient)	16	100%	98%	98%
Prophylactic Antibiotic Stopped	25	96%	98%	98%
Prophylactic Antibiotic Timing	30	80%	98%	99%
Prophylactic Antibiotic Timing (Outpatient)	16	88%	96%	98%
Urinary Catheter Removal[1]	-	-	97%	97%
Survey of Patients' Hospital Experiences				
Area Around Room 'Always' Quiet at Night	300+	55%	61%	61%
Doctors 'Always' Communicated Well	300+	73%	78%	82%
Home Recovery Information Given	300+	82%	83%	85%
Hospital Given 9 or 10 on 10 Point Scale	300+	60%	65%	71%
Meds 'Always' Explained Before Given	300+	62%	63%	64%
Nurses 'Always' Communicated Well	300+	72%	76%	79%
Pain 'Always' Well Controlled	300+	69%	68%	71%
Room and Bathroom 'Always' Clean	300+	70%	70%	73%
Timely Help 'Always' Received	300+	64%	66%	68%
Would Definitely Recommend Hospital	300+	58%	63%	71%
Use of Medical Imaging				
Cardiac Imaging Stress Test before Surgery[1]	-	-	4.2%	5.3%
Combination Abdominal CT Scan	243	6.6%	9.6%	10.5%
Combination Brain/Sinus CT Scan	163	6.1%	2.3%	2.7%
Combination Chest CT Scan	77	3.9%	5.6%	2.7%
Follow-up Mammogram/Ultrasound	262	6.5%	8.6%	8.8%
Lumbar Spine MRI for Low Back Pain	42	38.1%	36.9%	37.2%

Cibola General Hospital

1016 Roosevelt Avenue — Phone: 505-287-4446
Grants, NM 87020
Type: Critical Access Hospitals — Emergency Services: Yes
Ownership: Voluntary non-profit - Private

Measure	Cases	This Hosp.	State Avg.	U.S. Avg.
Blood Clot Prevention and Treatment				
Anticoagulation Overlap Therapy[5]	-	-	96%	93%
ICU Venous Thromboembolism Prophylaxis[5]	-	-	92%	92%
Incidence of Potentially Preventable VTE[5]	-	-	3%	10%
UFH with Dosages/Platelet Monitoring[5]	-	-	99%	97%
Venous Thromboembolism Prophylaxis[5]	-	-	84%	85%
Warfarin Therapy Discharge Instructions[5]	-	-	85%	75%
Chest Pain/Possible Heart Attack Care				
Aspirin Given Within 24 Hours of Arrival	56	95%	97%	96%
Fibrinolytic Meds Within 30 Min. of Arrival[1]	-	-	62%	58%
Average Time to ECG (minutes)	58	14	9	7
Average Time to Transfer (minutes)[1]	-	-	99	60
Children's Asthma Care				
Received Home Management Plan of Care	-	-	-	88%
Received Reliever Medication	-	-	-	100%
Received Systemic Corticosteroids	-	-	-	100%
Emergency Department				
Admittance Decision Time (minutes)[5]	-	-	108	98
Head CT Results Within 45 Min. of Arrival[1,3]	-	-	46%	57%
Patients Who Left ER Before Being Seen	9,290	4%	4%	2%
Time from ER Arrival to Admit. (minutes)[5]	-	-	290	274
Time from ER Arrival to Discharge (minutes)	372	118	143	134
Time in ER Before Being Evaluated (minutes)	404	21	28	26
Time to Pain Meds for Fractures (minutes)	43	56	57	57
Heart Attack Care				
Aspirin Given at Discharge[5]	-	-	99%	99%
Fibrinolytic Meds Within 30 Min. of Arrival[5]	-	-	75%	54%
PCI Within 90 Minutes of Arrival[5]	-	-	95%	96%
Statin Prescribed at Discharge[5]	-	-	99%	98%
Heart Failure Care				
ACE Inhibitor or ARB for LVSD[7]	-	-	97%	97%
Discharge Instructions Given[1]	-	-	89%	94%
Evaluation of LVS Function[1]	-	-	96%	99%
Medicare Spending				
Medicare Spending per Patient (ratio)	-	-	0.85	0.98
Pneumonia Care				
Appropriate Initial Antibiotic Given	19	58%	93%	95%
Blood Culture Timing	31	94%	97%	98%
Pregnancy and Delivery Care				
Newborn Deliveries Scheduled Early[2]	21	10%	3%	6%
Preventive Care				
Immunization for Influenza[5]	-	-	86%	90%
Immunization for Pneumonia[5]	-	-	89%	92%
Stroke Care				
Anticoagulation Therapy for Atrial Fibrillation[5]	-	-	96%	95%
Antithrombotic Therapy Timing[5]	-	-	94%	98%
Assessed for Rehabilitation[5]	-	-	95%	97%
Discharged on Antithrombotic Therapy[5]	-	-	97%	99%
Discharged on Statin Medication[5]	-	-	89%	94%
Thrombolytic Therapy Timing[5]	-	-	61%	66%
Venous Thromboembolism Prophylaxis[5]	-	-	91%	94%
Written Stroke Educational Materials Given[5]	-	-	73%	88%
Surgical Care Improvement Project				
Appropriate Beta Blocker Usage[1]	-	-	94%	98%
Appropriate VTP Within 24 Hours	24	71%	97%	98%
Controlled Postoperative Blood Glucose[7]	-	-	97%	97%
Perioperative Temperature Management	24	100%	99%	100%
Prophylactic Antibiotic Selection[1]	-	-	98%	99%
Prophylactic Antibiotic Selection (Outpatient)[1,3]	-	-	98%	98%
Prophylactic Antibiotic Stopped[1]	-	-	98%	98%
Prophylactic Antibiotic Timing[1]	-	-	98%	99%
Prophylactic Antibiotic Timing (Outpatient)[1,3]	-	-	96%	98%
Urinary Catheter Removal[1]	-	-	97%	97%
Survey of Patients' Hospital Experiences				
Area Around Room 'Always' Quiet at Night	(a)	61%	61%	61%
Doctors 'Always' Communicated Well	(a)	81%	78%	82%
Home Recovery Information Given	(a)	85%	83%	85%
Hospital Given 9 or 10 on 10 Point Scale	(a)	71%	65%	71%
Meds 'Always' Explained Before Given	(a)	65%	63%	64%
Nurses 'Always' Communicated Well	(a)	76%	76%	79%
Pain 'Always' Well Controlled	(a)	68%	68%	71%
Room and Bathroom 'Always' Clean	(a)	71%	70%	73%
Timely Help 'Always' Received	(a)	76%	66%	68%
Would Definitely Recommend Hospital	(a)	70%	63%	71%
Use of Medical Imaging				
Cardiac Imaging Stress Test before Surgery[7]	-	-	4.2%	5.3%
Combination Abdominal CT Scan	165	5.5%	9.6%	10.5%
Combination Brain/Sinus CT Scan[1]	-	-	2.3%	2.7%
Combination Chest CT Scan	89	1.1%	5.6%	2.7%
Follow-up Mammogram/Ultrasound	275	9.8%	8.6%	8.8%
Lumbar Spine MRI for Low Back Pain[1]	-	-	36.9%	37.2%

Lea Regional Medical Center

5419 N Lovington Highway — Phone: 575-492-5000
Hobbs, NM 88240 — Fax: 505-492-5393
URL: www.learegionalmedical.com
Type: Acute Care Hospitals — Emergency Services: Yes
Ownership: Proprietary — Beds: 250

Key Personnel:
CEO/President. . . . . Larry Bozeman
Chief of Medical Staff. . . . . Andre Feria, MD
Quality Assurance . . . . Sandi Henley
Radiology. . . . . Howard Nunn, MD
Emergency Room . . . . Jamie Todd, RN
Operating Room. . . . . Sarah Vickers, RN

Measure	Cases	This Hosp.	State Avg.	U.S. Avg.
Blood Clot Prevention and Treatment				
Anticoagulation Overlap Therapy[2]	23	91%	96%	93%
ICU Venous Thromboembolism Prophylaxis[2]	83	94%	92%	92%
Incidence of Potentially Preventable VTE[1,2]	-	-	3%	10%
UFH with Dosages/Platelet Monitoring[2,7]	-	-	99%	97%
Venous Thromboembolism Prophylaxis[2]	140	94%	84%	85%
Warfarin Therapy Discharge Instructions[2]	14	93%	85%	75%
Chest Pain/Possible Heart Attack Care				
Aspirin Given Within 24 Hours of Arrival	109	100%	97%	96%
Fibrinolytic Meds Within 30 Min. of Arrival	13	85%	62%	58%
Average Time to ECG (minutes)	111	6	9	7
Average Time to Transfer (minutes)[7]	-	-	99	60
Children's Asthma Care				
Received Home Management Plan of Care	-	-	-	88%
Received Reliever Medication	-	-	-	100%
Received Systemic Corticosteroids	-	-	-	100%
Emergency Department				
Admittance Decision Time (minutes)[2]	402	114	108	98
Head CT Results Within 45 Min. of Arrival[1]	-	-	46%	57%
Patients Who Left ER Before Being Seen	21,123	3%	4%	2%
Time from ER Arrival to Admit. (minutes)[2]	407	279	290	274
Time from ER Arrival to Discharge (minutes)	381	120	143	134
Time in ER Before Being Evaluated (minutes)	396	14	28	26
Time to Pain Meds for Fractures (minutes)	141	43	57	57
Heart Attack Care				
Aspirin Given at Discharge[1]	-	-	99%	99%
Fibrinolytic Meds Within 30 Min. of Arrival[7]	-	-	75%	54%
PCI Within 90 Minutes of Arrival[7]	-	-	95%	96%
Statin Prescribed at Discharge[1]	-	-	99%	98%
Heart Failure Care				
ACE Inhibitor or ARB for LVSD	24	100%	97%	97%
Discharge Instructions Given	33	100%	89%	94%
Evaluation of LVS Function	45	100%	96%	99%
Medicare Spending				
Medicare Spending per Patient (ratio)	-	0.93	0.85	0.98
Pneumonia Care				
Appropriate Initial Antibiotic Given	44	100%	93%	95%
Blood Culture Timing	68	96%	97%	98%
Pregnancy and Delivery Care				
Newborn Deliveries Scheduled Early[2]	44	5%	3%	6%
Preventive Care				
Immunization for Influenza[2]	366	94%	86%	90%
Immunization for Pneumonia[2]	272	98%	89%	92%
Stroke Care				

NOTE: Hospital profiles are in alphabetical order by state, then city, then hospital within the city; Rankings exclude hospitals with less than 25 cases except for patient surveys which excludes hospitals with less than 100 cases; (a) 100-299 cases; (1) The number of cases/patients is too few to report; (2) Data submitted were based on a sample of cases/patients; (3) Results are based on a shorter time period than required; (4) Data suppressed by CMS for one or more quarters; (5) Results are not available for this reporting period; (6) Fewer than 100 patients completed the HCAHPS survey; (7) No cases met the criteria for this measure; (8) The lower limit of the confidence interval cannot be calculated if the number of observed infections equals zero; (9) No data are available from the state/territory for this reporting period; (10) The scores shown reflect fewer than 50 completed surveys; (11) There were discrepancies in the data collection process; (12) This measure does not apply to this hospital for this reporting period; (13) Results cannot be calculated for this reporting period; (14) The results for this state are combined with nearby states to protect confidentiality; Please refer to the User's Guide for a full explanation of data.

Measure	Cases	This Hosp.	State Avg.	U.S. Avg.
Anticoagulation Therapy for Atrial Fibrillation[1]	-	-	96%	95%
Antithrombotic Therapy Timing	20	100%	94%	98%
Assessed for Rehabilitation	19	95%	95%	97%
Discharged on Antithrombotic Therapy	18	100%	97%	99%
Discharged on Statin Medication	14	100%	89%	94%
Thrombolytic Therapy Timing[1]	-	-	61%	66%
Venous Thromboembolism Prophylaxis	20	95%	91%	94%
Written Stroke Educational Materials Given[1]	-	-	73%	88%
Surgical Care Improvement Project				
Appropriate Beta Blocker Usage	20	90%	94%	98%
Appropriate VTP Within 24 Hours	91	100%	97%	98%
Controlled Postoperative Blood Glucose[7]	-	-	97%	97%
Perioperative Temperature Management	120	100%	99%	100%
Prophylactic Antibiotic Selection	86	100%	98%	99%
Prophylactic Antibiotic Selection (Outpatient)[1]	-	-	98%	98%
Prophylactic Antibiotic Stopped	85	100%	98%	98%
Prophylactic Antibiotic Timing	86	100%	98%	99%
Prophylactic Antibiotic Timing (Outpatient)	11	82%	96%	98%
Urinary Catheter Removal	32	97%	97%	97%
Survey of Patients' Hospital Experiences				
Area Around Room 'Always' Quiet at Night	300+	59%	61%	61%
Doctors 'Always' Communicated Well	300+	79%	78%	82%
Home Recovery Information Given	300+	83%	83%	85%
Hospital Given 9 or 10 on 10 Point Scale	300+	59%	65%	71%
Meds 'Always' Explained Before Given	300+	57%	63%	64%
Nurses 'Always' Communicated Well	300+	71%	76%	79%
Pain 'Always' Well Controlled	300+	63%	68%	71%
Room and Bathroom 'Always' Clean	300+	64%	70%	73%
Timely Help 'Always' Received	300+	56%	66%	68%
Would Definitely Recommend Hospital	300+	55%	63%	71%
Use of Medical Imaging				
Cardiac Imaging Stress Test before Surgery	111	5.4%	4.2%	5.3%
Combination Abdominal CT Scan	282	5.0%	9.6%	10.5%
Combination Brain/Sinus CT Scan	372	4.3%	2.3%	2.7%
Combination Chest CT Scan	113	9.7%	5.6%	2.7%
Follow-up Mammogram/Ultrasound	476	5.9%	8.6%	8.8%
Lumbar Spine MRI for Low Back Pain[1]	-	-	36.9%	37.2%

Memorial Medical Center

2450 South Telshor Blvd
Las Cruces, NM 88011
Phone: 575-522-8641
Fax: 505-556-5837
URL: www.mmclc.org
Type: Acute Care Hospitals
Emergency Services: Yes
Ownership: Proprietary
Beds: 286

Key Personnel:

Chair/CEO . . . . William Einig, MD
CEO/President. . . . . John Harris
Chief of Medical Staff . . . . Bruce D. San Filippo, MD

Measure	Cases	This Hosp.	State Avg.	U.S. Avg.
Blood Clot Prevention and Treatment				
Anticoagulation Overlap Therapy[2]	68	99%	96%	93%
ICU Venous Thromboembolism Prophylaxis[2]	69	99%	92%	92%
Incidence of Potentially Preventable VTE[2]	11	9%	3%	10%
UFH with Dosages/Platelet Monitoring[2]	35	97%	99%	97%
Venous Thromboembolism Prophylaxis[2]	356	98%	84%	85%
Warfarin Therapy Discharge Instructions[2]	47	96%	85%	75%
Chest Pain/Possible Heart Attack Care				
Aspirin Given Within 24 Hours of Arrival[5]	-	-	97%	96%
Fibrinolytic Meds Within 30 Min. of Arrival[5]	-	-	62%	58%
Average Time to ECG (minutes)[5]	-	-	9	7
Average Time to Transfer (minutes)[5]	-	-	99	60
Children's Asthma Care				
Received Home Management Plan of Care	27	96%	-	88%
Received Reliever Medication	27	100%	-	100%
Received Systemic Corticosteroids	27	100%	-	100%
Emergency Department				
Admittance Decision Time (minutes)[2]	441	170	108	98
Head CT Results Within 45 Min. of Arrival[1]	-	-	46%	57%
Patients Who Left ER Before Being Seen	42,060	3%	4%	2%
Time from ER Arrival to Admit. (minutes)[2]	504	364	290	274
Time from ER Arrival to Discharge (minutes)	418	194	143	134
Time in ER Before Being Evaluated (minutes)	393	31	28	26
Time to Pain Meds for Fractures (minutes)	128	59	57	57
Heart Attack Care				
Aspirin Given at Discharge	151	100%	99%	99%
Fibrinolytic Meds Within 30 Min. of Arrival[7]	-	-	75%	54%
PCI Within 90 Minutes of Arrival	31	90%	95%	96%
Statin Prescribed at Discharge	148	99%	99%	98%
Heart Failure Care				
ACE Inhibitor or ARB for LVSD	88	95%	97%	97%
Discharge Instructions Given	164	85%	89%	94%
Evaluation of LVS Function	200	100%	96%	99%
Medicare Spending				
Medicare Spending per Patient (ratio)	-	1.01	0.85	0.98
Pneumonia Care				
Appropriate Initial Antibiotic Given	141	96%	93%	95%
Blood Culture Timing	208	98%	97%	98%
Pregnancy and Delivery Care				
Newborn Deliveries Scheduled Early[2]	27	0%	3%	6%
Preventive Care				
Immunization for Influenza[2]	514	95%	86%	90%
Immunization for Pneumonia[2]	550	99%	89%	92%
Stroke Care				
Anticoagulation Therapy for Atrial Fibrillation	14	100%	96%	95%
Antithrombotic Therapy Timing	68	97%	94%	98%
Assessed for Rehabilitation	77	100%	95%	97%
Discharged on Antithrombotic Therapy	73	99%	97%	99%
Discharged on Statin Medication	61	97%	89%	94%
Thrombolytic Therapy Timing[1]	-	-	61%	66%
Venous Thromboembolism Prophylaxis	76	99%	91%	94%
Written Stroke Educational Materials Given	38	89%	73%	88%
Surgical Care Improvement Project				
Appropriate Beta Blocker Usage[2]	119	97%	94%	98%
Appropriate VTP Within 24 Hours[2]	364	100%	97%	98%
Controlled Postoperative Blood Glucose[2]	75	97%	97%	97%
Perioperative Temperature Management[2]	432	100%	99%	100%
Prophylactic Antibiotic Selection[2]	342	100%	98%	99%
Prophylactic Antibiotic Selection (Outpatient)	142	97%	98%	98%
Prophylactic Antibiotic Stopped[2]	331	99%	98%	98%
Prophylactic Antibiotic Timing[2]	343	99%	98%	99%
Prophylactic Antibiotic Timing (Outpatient)	141	98%	96%	98%
Urinary Catheter Removal[2]	298	98%	97%	97%
Survey of Patients' Hospital Experiences				
Area Around Room 'Always' Quiet at Night	300+	54%	61%	61%
Doctors 'Always' Communicated Well	300+	76%	78%	82%
Home Recovery Information Given	300+	85%	83%	85%
Hospital Given 9 or 10 on 10 Point Scale	300+	63%	65%	71%
Meds 'Always' Explained Before Given	300+	56%	63%	64%
Nurses 'Always' Communicated Well	300+	71%	76%	79%
Pain 'Always' Well Controlled	300+	66%	68%	71%
Room and Bathroom 'Always' Clean	300+	62%	70%	73%
Timely Help 'Always' Received	300+	55%	66%	68%
Would Definitely Recommend Hospital	300+	64%	63%	71%
Use of Medical Imaging				
Cardiac Imaging Stress Test before Surgery	212	3.8%	4.2%	5.3%
Combination Abdominal CT Scan	595	40.8%	9.6%	10.5%
Combination Brain/Sinus CT Scan	528	2.1%	2.3%	2.7%
Combination Chest CT Scan	425	8.2%	5.6%	2.7%
Follow-up Mammogram/Ultrasound	587	7.7%	8.6%	8.8%
Lumbar Spine MRI for Low Back Pain[1]	-	-	36.9%	37.2%

Mountain View Regional Medical Center

4311 East Lohman Avenue
Las Cruces, NM 88011
Phone: 575-556-7600
Fax: 505-556-7619
URL: www.mountainviewregional.com
Type: Acute Care Hospitals
Emergency Services: Yes
Ownership: Proprietary
Beds: 168

Key Personnel:

Chief of Medical Staff . . . . Laura Enn
Radiology. Joseph W Fischer
Pediatrics. . . . . El Maragaghy Hala, MD
CEO/President. . . . . Karen Springer
Cardiac Laboratory. . . . . Jose Tutierrev

Measure	Cases	This Hosp.	State Avg.	U.S. Avg.
Blood Clot Prevention and Treatment				
Anticoagulation Overlap Therapy[2]	66	100%	96%	93%
ICU Venous Thromboembolism Prophylaxis[2]	163	99%	92%	92%
Incidence of Potentially Preventable VTE[2]	17	0%	3%	10%
UFH with Dosages/Platelet Monitoring[2]	32	100%	99%	97%
Venous Thromboembolism Prophylaxis[2]	362	100%	84%	85%
Warfarin Therapy Discharge Instructions[2]	49	100%	85%	75%
Chest Pain/Possible Heart Attack Care				
Aspirin Given Within 24 Hours of Arrival[3,7]	-	-	97%	96%
Fibrinolytic Meds Within 30 Min. of Arrival[5]	-	-	62%	58%
Average Time to ECG (minutes)[1,3]	-	-	9	7
Average Time to Transfer (minutes)[5]	-	-	99	60
Children's Asthma Care				
Received Home Management Plan of Care	-	-	-	88%
Received Reliever Medication	-	-	-	100%
Received Systemic Corticosteroids	-	-	-	100%
Emergency Department				
Admittance Decision Time (minutes)[2]	631	117	108	98
Head CT Results Within 45 Min. of Arrival[1]	-	-	46%	57%
Patients Who Left ER Before Being Seen	15,099	2%	4%	2%
Time from ER Arrival to Admit. (minutes)[2]	635	277	290	274
Time from ER Arrival to Discharge (minutes)	390	124	143	134
Time in ER Before Being Evaluated (minutes)	422	23	28	26
Time to Pain Meds for Fractures (minutes)	158	48	57	57
Heart Attack Care				
Aspirin Given at Discharge	247	99%	99%	99%
Fibrinolytic Meds Within 30 Min. of Arrival[1]	-	-	75%	54%
PCI Within 90 Minutes of Arrival	29	93%	95%	96%
Statin Prescribed at Discharge	218	100%	99%	98%
Heart Failure Care				
ACE Inhibitor or ARB for LVSD	71	97%	97%	97%
Discharge Instructions Given	148	99%	89%	94%
Evaluation of LVS Function	169	100%	96%	99%
Medicare Spending				
Medicare Spending per Patient (ratio)	-	1.01	0.85	0.98
Pneumonia Care				
Appropriate Initial Antibiotic Given	130	100%	93%	95%
Blood Culture Timing	203	100%	97%	98%
Pregnancy and Delivery Care				
Newborn Deliveries Scheduled Early[2]	27	4%	3%	6%
Preventive Care				
Immunization for Influenza[2]	618	100%	86%	90%
Immunization for Pneumonia[2]	746	100%	89%	92%
Stroke Care				
Anticoagulation Therapy for Atrial Fibrillation[1]	-	-	96%	95%
Antithrombotic Therapy Timing	59	100%	94%	98%
Assessed for Rehabilitation	82	98%	95%	97%
Discharged on Antithrombotic Therapy	68	100%	97%	99%
Discharged on Statin Medication	46	98%	89%	94%
Thrombolytic Therapy Timing[1]	-	-	61%	66%
Venous Thromboembolism Prophylaxis	87	95%	91%	94%
Written Stroke Educational Materials Given	34	88%	73%	88%
Surgical Care Improvement Project				
Appropriate Beta Blocker Usage	164	100%	94%	98%
Appropriate VTP Within 24 Hours	359	99%	97%	98%
Controlled Postoperative Blood Glucose	84	100%	97%	97%
Perioperative Temperature Management	489	100%	99%	100%
Prophylactic Antibiotic Selection	344	99%	98%	99%
Prophylactic Antibiotic Selection (Outpatient)	322	99%	98%	98%
Prophylactic Antibiotic Stopped	341	100%	98%	98%
Prophylactic Antibiotic Timing	345	100%	98%	99%
Prophylactic Antibiotic Timing (Outpatient)	321	100%	96%	98%
Urinary Catheter Removal	318	100%	97%	97%
Survey of Patients' Hospital Experiences				
Area Around Room 'Always' Quiet at Night	300+	60%	61%	61%
Doctors 'Always' Communicated Well	300+	81%	78%	82%
Home Recovery Information Given	300+	87%	83%	85%
Hospital Given 9 or 10 on 10 Point Scale	300+	72%	65%	71%
Meds 'Always' Explained Before Given	300+	58%	63%	64%
Nurses 'Always' Communicated Well	300+	77%	76%	79%
Pain 'Always' Well Controlled	300+	70%	68%	71%
Room and Bathroom 'Always' Clean	300+	68%	70%	73%
Timely Help 'Always' Received	300+	66%	66%	68%
Would Definitely Recommend Hospital	300+	77%	63%	71%
Use of Medical Imaging				

NOTE: Hospital profiles are in alphabetical order by state, then city, then hospital within the city; Rankings exclude hospitals with less than 25 cases except for patient surveys which excludes hospitals with less than 100 cases; (a) 100-299 cases; (1) The number of cases/patients is too few to report; (2) Data submitted were based on a sample of cases/patients; (3) Results are based on a shorter time period than required; (4) Data suppressed by CMS for one or more quarters; (5) Results are not available for this reporting period; (6) Fewer than 100 patients completed the HCAHPS survey; (7) No cases met the criteria for this measure; (8) The lower limit of the confidence interval cannot be calculated if the number of observed infections equals zero; (9) No data are available from the state/territory for this reporting period; (10) The scores shown reflect fewer than 50 completed surveys; (11) There were discrepancies in the data collection process; (12) This measure does not apply to this hospital for this reporting period; (13) Results cannot be calculated for this reporting period; (14) The results for this state are combined with nearby states to protect confidentiality; Please refer to the User's Guide for a full explanation of data.

Measure	Cases	This Hosp.	State Avg.	U.S. Avg.
Cardiac Imaging Stress Test before Surgery	278	2.2%	4.2%	5.3%
Combination Abdominal CT Scan	415	8.4%	9.6%	10.5%
Combination Brain/Sinus CT Scan[1]	-	-	2.3%	2.7%
Combination Chest CT Scan	131	7.6%	5.6%	2.7%
Follow-up Mammogram/Ultrasound	177	5.6%	8.6%	8.8%
Lumbar Spine MRI for Low Back Pain	60	26.7%	36.9%	37.2%

Alta Vista Regional Hospital

104 Legion Drive
Las Vegas, NM 87701
Phone: 505-426-3930
Fax: 505-426-3611
URL: www.altavistaregioanlhospital.com
Type: Acute Care Hospitals
Emergency Services: Yes
Ownership: Govt - Hospital Dist/Auth
Beds: 54

Key Personnel:
Emergency Room . . . . Bradford Cambron
CEO/President. . . . . Brian Gibbons
Cardiac Laboratory. . . . . Barbara Travis

Measure	Cases	This Hosp.	State Avg.	U.S. Avg.
Blood Clot Prevention and Treatment				
Anticoagulation Overlap Therapy[2]	11	91%	96%	93%
ICU Venous Thromboembolism Prophylaxis[2]	94	99%	92%	92%
Incidence of Potentially Preventable VTE[2,7]	-	-	3%	10%
UFH with Dosages/Platelet Monitoring[1,2]	-	-	99%	97%
Venous Thromboembolism Prophylaxis[2]	147	97%	84%	85%
Warfarin Therapy Discharge Instructions[1,2]	-	-	85%	75%
Chest Pain/Possible Heart Attack Care				
Aspirin Given Within 24 Hours of Arrival	31	100%	97%	96%
Fibrinolytic Meds Within 30 Min. of Arrival[1]	-	-	62%	58%
Average Time to ECG (minutes)	33	4	9	7
Average Time to Transfer (minutes)[1]	-	-	99	60
Children's Asthma Care				
Received Home Management Plan of Care	-	-	-	88%
Received Reliever Medication	-	-	-	100%
Received Systemic Corticosteroids	-	-	-	100%
Emergency Department				
Admittance Decision Time (minutes)[2]	420	101	108	98
Head CT Results Within 45 Min. of Arrival[1,3]	-	-	46%	57%
Patients Who Left ER Before Being Seen	13,661	1%	4%	2%
Time from ER Arrival to Admit. (minutes)[2]	441	260	290	274
Time from ER Arrival to Discharge (minutes)	374	150	143	134
Time in ER Before Being Evaluated (minutes)	422	17	28	26
Time to Pain Meds for Fractures (minutes)	67	58	57	57
Heart Attack Care				
Aspirin Given at Discharge[7]	-	-	99%	99%
Fibrinolytic Meds Within 30 Min. of Arrival[7]	-	-	75%	54%
PCI Within 90 Minutes of Arrival[7]	-	-	95%	96%
Statin Prescribed at Discharge[1]	-	-	99%	98%
Heart Failure Care				
ACE Inhibitor or ARB for LVSD	13	100%	97%	97%
Discharge Instructions Given	60	98%	89%	94%
Evaluation of LVS Function	72	100%	96%	99%
Medicare Spending				
Medicare Spending per Patient (ratio)	-	0.79	0.85	0.98
Pneumonia Care				
Appropriate Initial Antibiotic Given	44	100%	93%	95%
Blood Culture Timing	76	99%	97%	98%
Pregnancy and Delivery Care				
Newborn Deliveries Scheduled Early[2]	34	0%	3%	6%
Preventive Care				
Immunization for Influenza[2]	304	98%	86%	90%
Immunization for Pneumonia[2]	341	99%	89%	92%
Stroke Care				
Anticoagulation Therapy for Atrial Fibrillation[1]	-	-	96%	95%
Antithrombotic Therapy Timing[1]	-	-	94%	98%
Assessed for Rehabilitation	18	100%	95%	97%
Discharged on Antithrombotic Therapy	16	100%	97%	99%
Discharged on Statin Medication	16	88%	89%	94%
Thrombolytic Therapy Timing[1]	-	-	61%	66%
Venous Thromboembolism Prophylaxis	11	100%	91%	94%
Written Stroke Educational Materials Given	13	77%	73%	88%
Surgical Care Improvement Project				
Appropriate Beta Blocker Usage[1]	-	-	94%	98%
Appropriate VTP Within 24 Hours	59	100%	97%	98%
Controlled Postoperative Blood Glucose[7]	-	-	97%	97%
Perioperative Temperature Management	69	100%	99%	100%
Prophylactic Antibiotic Selection	43	100%	98%	99%
Prophylactic Antibiotic Selection (Outpatient)[1,3]	-	-	98%	98%
Prophylactic Antibiotic Stopped	43	95%	98%	98%
Prophylactic Antibiotic Timing	44	100%	98%	99%
Prophylactic Antibiotic Timing (Outpatient)[1,3]	-	-	96%	98%
Urinary Catheter Removal	16	94%	97%	97%
Survey of Patients' Hospital Experiences				
Area Around Room 'Always' Quiet at Night	300+	59%	61%	61%
Doctors 'Always' Communicated Well	300+	81%	78%	82%
Home Recovery Information Given	300+	83%	83%	85%
Hospital Given 9 or 10 on 10 Point Scale	300+	58%	65%	71%
Meds 'Always' Explained Before Given	300+	63%	63%	64%
Nurses 'Always' Communicated Well	300+	75%	76%	79%
Pain 'Always' Well Controlled	300+	62%	68%	71%
Room and Bathroom 'Always' Clean	300+	62%	70%	73%
Timely Help 'Always' Received	300+	61%	66%	68%
Would Definitely Recommend Hospital	300+	54%	63%	71%
Use of Medical Imaging				
Cardiac Imaging Stress Test before Surgery	163	4.9%	4.2%	5.3%
Combination Abdominal CT Scan	381	11.8%	9.6%	10.5%
Combination Brain/Sinus CT Scan[1]	-	-	2.3%	2.7%
Combination Chest CT Scan	215	5.1%	5.6%	2.7%
Follow-up Mammogram/Ultrasound	305	15.1%	8.6%	8.8%
Lumbar Spine MRI for Low Back Pain[1]	-	-	36.9%	37.2%

Los Alamos Medical Center

3917 West Road
Los Alamos, NM 87544
Phone: 505-662-4201
Fax: 505-661-9598
URL: www.losalamosmedicalcenter.com
Type: Acute Care Hospitals
Emergency Services: Yes
Ownership: Proprietary
Beds: 47

Key Personnel:
Chief of Medical Staff. . . . . Marylen Chanodi
Emergency Room . . . . Vickie Davy
Quality Assurance . . . . Nancy Eckerson
CEO . . . . Feliciano Jiron
CEO/President. . . . . Gary Nichols

Measure	Cases	This Hosp.	State Avg.	U.S. Avg.
Blood Clot Prevention and Treatment				
Anticoagulation Overlap Therapy[2]	13	85%	96%	93%
ICU Venous Thromboembolism Prophylaxis[2]	17	94%	92%	92%
Incidence of Potentially Preventable VTE[1,2]	-	-	3%	10%
UFH with Dosages/Platelet Monitoring[2,7]	-	-	99%	97%
Venous Thromboembolism Prophylaxis[2]	86	84%	84%	85%
Warfarin Therapy Discharge Instructions[2]	11	100%	85%	75%
Chest Pain/Possible Heart Attack Care				
Aspirin Given Within 24 Hours of Arrival	20	100%	97%	96%
Fibrinolytic Meds Within 30 Min. of Arrival[1,3]	-	-	62%	58%
Average Time to ECG (minutes)	20	8	9	7
Average Time to Transfer (minutes)[1,3]	-	-	99	60
Children's Asthma Care				
Received Home Management Plan of Care	-	-	-	88%
Received Reliever Medication	-	-	-	100%
Received Systemic Corticosteroids	-	-	-	100%
Emergency Department				
Admittance Decision Time (minutes)[2]	322	50	108	98
Head CT Results Within 45 Min. of Arrival[1]	-	-	46%	57%
Patients Who Left ER Before Being Seen	8,515	0%	4%	2%
Time from ER Arrival to Admit. (minutes)[2]	324	233	290	274
Time from ER Arrival to Discharge (minutes)	395	119	143	134
Time in ER Before Being Evaluated (minutes)	418	20	28	26
Time to Pain Meds for Fractures (minutes)	65	68	57	57
Heart Attack Care				
Aspirin Given at Discharge[1,3]	-	-	99%	99%
Fibrinolytic Meds Within 30 Min. of Arrival[3,7]	-	-	75%	54%
PCI Within 90 Minutes of Arrival[3,7]	-	-	95%	96%
Statin Prescribed at Discharge[1,3]	-	-	99%	98%
Heart Failure Care				
ACE Inhibitor or ARB for LVSD[1]	-	-	97%	97%
Discharge Instructions Given	21	90%	89%	94%
Evaluation of LVS Function	27	93%	96%	99%
Medicare Spending				
Medicare Spending per Patient (ratio)	-	0.93	0.85	0.98
Pneumonia Care				
Appropriate Initial Antibiotic Given	27	74%	93%	95%
Blood Culture Timing	37	97%	97%	98%
Pregnancy and Delivery Care				
Newborn Deliveries Scheduled Early[2]	14	7%	3%	6%
Preventive Care				
Immunization for Influenza[2]	265	84%	86%	90%
Immunization for Pneumonia[2]	290	88%	89%	92%
Stroke Care				
Anticoagulation Therapy for Atrial Fibrillation[7]	-	-	96%	95%
Antithrombotic Therapy Timing[1]	-	-	94%	98%
Assessed for Rehabilitation[1]	-	-	95%	97%
Discharged on Antithrombotic Therapy[1]	-	-	97%	99%
Discharged on Statin Medication[1]	-	-	89%	94%
Thrombolytic Therapy Timing[7]	-	-	61%	66%
Venous Thromboembolism Prophylaxis[1]	-	-	91%	94%
Written Stroke Educational Materials Given[1]	-	-	73%	88%
Surgical Care Improvement Project				
Appropriate Beta Blocker Usage	11	64%	94%	98%
Appropriate VTP Within 24 Hours	111	98%	97%	98%
Controlled Postoperative Blood Glucose[7]	-	-	97%	97%
Perioperative Temperature Management	121	100%	99%	100%
Prophylactic Antibiotic Selection	103	99%	98%	99%
Prophylactic Antibiotic Selection (Outpatient)	42	100%	98%	98%
Prophylactic Antibiotic Stopped	100	94%	98%	98%
Prophylactic Antibiotic Timing	103	98%	98%	99%
Prophylactic Antibiotic Timing (Outpatient)	42	100%	96%	98%
Urinary Catheter Removal	97	97%	97%	97%
Survey of Patients' Hospital Experiences				
Area Around Room 'Always' Quiet at Night	(a)	60%	61%	61%
Doctors 'Always' Communicated Well	(a)	80%	78%	82%
Home Recovery Information Given	(a)	86%	83%	85%
Hospital Given 9 or 10 on 10 Point Scale	(a)	69%	65%	71%
Meds 'Always' Explained Before Given	(a)	59%	63%	64%
Nurses 'Always' Communicated Well	(a)	76%	76%	79%
Pain 'Always' Well Controlled	(a)	69%	68%	71%
Room and Bathroom 'Always' Clean	(a)	62%	70%	73%
Timely Help 'Always' Received	(a)	68%	66%	68%
Would Definitely Recommend Hospital	(a)	73%	63%	71%
Use of Medical Imaging				
Cardiac Imaging Stress Test before Surgery[1]	-	-	4.2%	5.3%
Combination Abdominal CT Scan	233	11.2%	9.6%	10.5%
Combination Brain/Sinus CT Scan	175	1.1%	2.3%	2.7%
Combination Chest CT Scan	109	0.9%	5.6%	2.7%
Follow-up Mammogram/Ultrasound	530	7.2%	8.6%	8.8%
Lumbar Spine MRI for Low Back Pain[1]	-	-	36.9%	37.2%

Nor-Lea Hospital District

1600 North Main
Lovington, NM 88260
Phone: 575-396-6611
Fax: 505-396-0938
E-mail: john.mcculloch@nlgh.org
URL: www.nlgh.org
Type: Critical Access Hospitals
Emergency Services: Yes
Ownership: Govt - Hospital Dist/Auth
Beds: 28

Key Personnel:
Quality Assurance . . . . Dan Hamilton
Chief of Medical Staff. . . . . Ronald D Hopkins, DO
Operating Room. . . . . Katy Sandoval
Infection Control. . . . . Katie Sandovil
CEO/President. . . . . David Shaw
Radiology. . . . . Dean Shippey

Measure	Cases	This Hosp.	State Avg.	U.S. Avg.
Blood Clot Prevention and Treatment				
Anticoagulation Overlap Therapy[1,2]	-	-	96%	93%
ICU Venous Thromboembolism Prophylaxis[2,3]	-	-	92%	92%
Incidence of Potentially Preventable VTE[2,3]	-	-	3%	10%
UFH with Dosages/Platelet Monitoring[2,3]	-	-	99%	97%
Venous Thromboembolism Prophylaxis[2,3]	27	11%	84%	85%
Warfarin Therapy Discharge Instructions[1,2]	-	-	85%	75%
Chest Pain/Possible Heart Attack Care				
Aspirin Given Within 24 Hours of Arrival	31	77%	97%	96%
Fibrinolytic Meds Within 30 Min. of Arrival[1]	-	-	62%	58%

NOTE: Hospital profiles are in alphabetical order by state, then city, then hospital within the city; Rankings exclude hospitals with less than 25 cases except for patient surveys which excludes hospitals with less than 100 cases; (a) 100-299 cases; (1) The number of cases/patients is too few to report; (2) Data submitted were based on a sample of cases/patients; (3) Results are based on a shorter time period than required; (4) Data suppressed by CMS for one or more quarters; (5) Results are not available for this reporting period; (6) Fewer than 100 patients completed the HCAHPS survey; (7) No cases met the criteria for this measure; (8) The lower limit of the confidence interval cannot be calculated if the number of observed infections equals zero; (9) No data are available from the state/territory for this reporting period; (10) The scores shown reflect fewer than 50 completed surveys; (11) There were discrepancies in the data collection process; (12) This measure does not apply to this hospital for this reporting period; (13) Results cannot be calculated for this reporting period; (14) The results for this state are combined with nearby states to protect confidentiality; Please refer to the User's Guide for a full explanation of data.

Measure	Cases	This Hosp.	State Avg.	U.S. Avg.
Average Time to ECG (minutes)	29	13	9	7
Average Time to Transfer (minutes)[1]	-	-	99	60
Children's Asthma Care				
Received Home Management Plan of Care	-	-	-	88%
Received Reliever Medication	-	-	-	100%
Received Systemic Corticosteroids	-	-	-	100%
Emergency Department				
Admittance Decision Time (minutes)[2]	145	80	108	98
Head CT Results Within 45 Min. of Arrival[1,3]	-	-	46%	57%
Patients Who Left ER Before Being Seen	10,169	2%	4%	2%
Time from ER Arrival to Admit. (minutes)[2]	153	280	290	274
Time from ER Arrival to Discharge (minutes)	1,423	134	143	134
Time in ER Before Being Evaluated (minutes)	1,763	36	28	26
Time to Pain Meds for Fractures (minutes)	32	70	57	57
Heart Attack Care				
Aspirin Given at Discharge[2,3]	-	-	99%	99%
Fibrinolytic Meds Within 30 Min. of Arrival[2,3]	-	-	75%	54%
PCI Within 90 Minutes of Arrival[2,3]	-	-	95%	96%
Statin Prescribed at Discharge[2,3]	-	-	99%	98%
Heart Failure Care				
ACE Inhibitor or ARB for LVSD[1,2]	-	-	97%	97%
Discharge Instructions Given[2]	31	65%	89%	94%
Evaluation of LVS Function[2]	34	76%	96%	99%
Medicare Spending				
Medicare Spending per Patient (ratio)	-	-	0.85	0.98
Pneumonia Care				
Appropriate Initial Antibiotic Given[2]	33	67%	93%	95%
Blood Culture Timing[2]	26	96%	97%	98%
Pregnancy and Delivery Care				
Newborn Deliveries Scheduled Early[3,7]	-	-	3%	6%
Preventive Care				
Immunization for Influenza[2]	66	71%	86%	90%
Immunization for Pneumonia[2]	150	70%	89%	92%
Stroke Care				
Anticoagulation Therapy for Atrial Fibrillation[1,3]	-	-	96%	95%
Antithrombotic Therapy Timing[1,3]	-	-	94%	98%
Assessed for Rehabilitation[1,3]	-	-	95%	97%
Discharged on Antithrombotic Therapy[1,3]	-	-	97%	99%
Discharged on Statin Medication[1,3]	-	-	89%	94%
Thrombolytic Therapy Timing[1,3]	-	-	61%	66%
Venous Thromboembolism Prophylaxis[1,3]	-	-	91%	94%
Written Stroke Educational Materials Given[1,3]	-	-	73%	88%
Surgical Care Improvement Project				
Appropriate Beta Blocker Usage[5]	-	-	94%	98%
Appropriate VTP Within 24 Hours[5]	-	-	97%	98%
Controlled Postoperative Blood Glucose[5]	-	-	97%	97%
Perioperative Temperature Management[5]	-	-	99%	100%
Prophylactic Antibiotic Selection[5]	-	-	98%	99%
Prophylactic Antibiotic Selection (Outpatient)[5]	-	-	98%	98%
Prophylactic Antibiotic Stopped[5]	-	-	98%	98%
Prophylactic Antibiotic Timing[5]	-	-	98%	99%
Prophylactic Antibiotic Timing (Outpatient)[5]	-	-	96%	98%
Urinary Catheter Removal[5]	-	-	97%	97%
Survey of Patients' Hospital Experiences				
Area Around Room 'Always' Quiet at Night	(a)	68%	61%	61%
Doctors 'Always' Communicated Well	(a)	87%	78%	82%
Home Recovery Information Given	(a)	87%	83%	85%
Hospital Given 9 or 10 on 10 Point Scale	(a)	74%	65%	71%
Meds 'Always' Explained Before Given	(a)	71%	63%	64%
Nurses 'Always' Communicated Well	(a)	80%	76%	79%
Pain 'Always' Well Controlled	(a)	71%	68%	71%
Room and Bathroom 'Always' Clean	(a)	82%	70%	73%
Timely Help 'Always' Received	(a)	72%	66%	68%
Would Definitely Recommend Hospital	(a)	81%	63%	71%
Use of Medical Imaging				
Cardiac Imaging Stress Test before Surgery	205	6.8%	4.2%	5.3%
Combination Abdominal CT Scan	382	30.4%	9.6%	10.5%
Combination Brain/Sinus CT Scan[1]	-	-	2.3%	2.7%
Combination Chest CT Scan	299	23.7%	5.6%	2.7%
Follow-up Mammogram/Ultrasound	310	9.0%	8.6%	8.8%
Lumbar Spine MRI for Low Back Pain	57	59.6%	36.9%	37.2%

Mescalero PHS Indian Hospital

PO Box 210 Phone: 505-464-4441
Mescalero, NM 88340
Type: Acute Care Hospitals Emergency Services: No
Ownership: Government - Federal
Key Personnel:
Quality Assurance . . . . Greg Powers

Measure	Cases	This Hosp.	State Avg.	U.S. Avg.
Blood Clot Prevention and Treatment				
Anticoagulation Overlap Therapy[2,3]	-	-	96%	93%
ICU Venous Thromboembolism Prophylaxis[2,3]	-	-	92%	92%
Incidence of Potentially Preventable VTE[2,3]	-	-	3%	10%
UFH with Dosages/Platelet Monitoring[2,3]	-	-	99%	97%
Venous Thromboembolism Prophylaxis[2,3]	71	1%	84%	85%
Warfarin Therapy Discharge Instructions[2,3]	-	-	85%	75%
Chest Pain/Possible Heart Attack Care				
Aspirin Given Within 24 Hours of Arrival	-	-	97%	96%
Fibrinolytic Meds Within 30 Min. of Arrival	-	-	62%	58%
Average Time to ECG (minutes)	-	-	9	7
Average Time to Transfer (minutes)	-	-	99	60
Children's Asthma Care				
Received Home Management Plan of Care	-	-	-	88%
Received Reliever Medication	-	-	-	100%
Received Systemic Corticosteroids	-	-	-	100%
Emergency Department				
Admittance Decision Time (minutes)[7]	-	-	108	98
Head CT Results Within 45 Min. of Arrival	-	-	46%	57%
Patients Who Left ER Before Being Seen	-	-	4%	2%
Time from ER Arrival to Admit. (minutes)[7]	-	-	290	274
Time from ER Arrival to Discharge (minutes)	-	-	143	134
Time in ER Before Being Evaluated (minutes)	-	-	28	26
Time to Pain Meds for Fractures (minutes)	-	-	57	57
Heart Attack Care				
Aspirin Given at Discharge[5]	-	-	99%	99%
Fibrinolytic Meds Within 30 Min. of Arrival[5]	-	-	75%	54%
PCI Within 90 Minutes of Arrival[5]	-	-	95%	96%
Statin Prescribed at Discharge[5]	-	-	99%	98%
Heart Failure Care				
ACE Inhibitor or ARB for LVSD[3,7]	-	-	97%	97%
Discharge Instructions Given[1,3]	-	-	89%	94%
Evaluation of LVS Function[1,3]	-	-	96%	99%
Medicare Spending				
Medicare Spending per Patient (ratio)[1]	-	-	0.85	0.98
Pneumonia Care				
Appropriate Initial Antibiotic Given[1]	-	-	93%	95%
Blood Culture Timing[1]	-	-	97%	98%
Pregnancy and Delivery Care				
Newborn Deliveries Scheduled Early[7]	-	-	3%	6%
Preventive Care				
Immunization for Influenza	124	71%	86%	90%
Immunization for Pneumonia	50	94%	89%	92%
Stroke Care				
Anticoagulation Therapy for Atrial Fibrillation[5]	-	-	96%	95%
Antithrombotic Therapy Timing[5]	-	-	94%	98%
Assessed for Rehabilitation[5]	-	-	95%	97%
Discharged on Antithrombotic Therapy[5]	-	-	97%	99%
Discharged on Statin Medication[5]	-	-	89%	94%
Thrombolytic Therapy Timing[5]	-	-	61%	66%
Venous Thromboembolism Prophylaxis[5]	-	-	91%	94%
Written Stroke Educational Materials Given[5]	-	-	73%	88%
Surgical Care Improvement Project				
Appropriate Beta Blocker Usage[5]	-	-	94%	98%
Appropriate VTP Within 24 Hours[5]	-	-	97%	98%
Controlled Postoperative Blood Glucose[5]	-	-	97%	97%
Perioperative Temperature Management[5]	-	-	99%	100%
Prophylactic Antibiotic Selection[5]	-	-	98%	99%
Prophylactic Antibiotic Selection (Outpatient)	-	-	98%	98%
Prophylactic Antibiotic Stopped[5]	-	-	98%	98%
Prophylactic Antibiotic Timing[5]	-	-	98%	99%
Prophylactic Antibiotic Timing (Outpatient)	-	-	96%	98%
Urinary Catheter Removal[5]	-	-	97%	97%
Survey of Patients' Hospital Experiences				
Area Around Room 'Always' Quiet at Night[10]	<100	80%	61%	61%
Doctors 'Always' Communicated Well[10]	<100	68%	78%	82%
Home Recovery Information Given[10]	<100	71%	83%	85%
Hospital Given 9 or 10 on 10 Point Scale[10]	<100	52%	65%	71%
Meds 'Always' Explained Before Given[10]	<100	49%	63%	64%
Nurses 'Always' Communicated Well[10]	<100	68%	76%	79%
Pain 'Always' Well Controlled[10]	<100	46%	68%	71%
Room and Bathroom 'Always' Clean[10]	<100	56%	70%	73%
Timely Help 'Always' Received[10]	<100	67%	66%	68%
Would Definitely Recommend Hospital[10]	<100	45%	63%	71%
Use of Medical Imaging				
Cardiac Imaging Stress Test before Surgery	-	-	4.2%	5.3%
Combination Abdominal CT Scan	-	-	9.6%	10.5%
Combination Brain/Sinus CT Scan	-	-	2.3%	2.7%
Combination Chest CT Scan	-	-	5.6%	2.7%
Follow-up Mammogram/Ultrasound	-	-	8.6%	8.8%
Lumbar Spine MRI for Low Back Pain	-	-	36.9%	37.2%

Roosevelt General Hospital

42121 Us Highway 70 Phone: 575-356-3412
Portales, NM 88130
URL: www.covenanthealth.org
Type: Acute Care Hospitals Emergency Services: Yes
Ownership: Govt - Hospital Dist/Auth
Key Personnel:
CEO/President. . . . . James D'Agostino

Measure	Cases	This Hosp.	State Avg.	U.S. Avg.
Blood Clot Prevention and Treatment				
Anticoagulation Overlap Therapy[1,2]	-	-	96%	93%
ICU Venous Thromboembolism Prophylaxis[2,7]	-	-	92%	92%
Incidence of Potentially Preventable VTE[2,7]	-	-	3%	10%
UFH with Dosages/Platelet Monitoring[1,2]	-	-	99%	97%
Venous Thromboembolism Prophylaxis[2]	206	77%	84%	85%
Warfarin Therapy Discharge Instructions[1,2]	-	-	85%	75%
Chest Pain/Possible Heart Attack Care				
Aspirin Given Within 24 Hours of Arrival	47	96%	97%	96%
Fibrinolytic Meds Within 30 Min. of Arrival[1]	-	-	62%	58%
Average Time to ECG (minutes)	49	11	9	7
Average Time to Transfer (minutes)[1]	-	-	99	60
Children's Asthma Care				
Received Home Management Plan of Care	-	-	-	88%
Received Reliever Medication	-	-	-	100%
Received Systemic Corticosteroids	-	-	-	100%
Emergency Department				
Admittance Decision Time (minutes)[2]	276	52	108	98
Head CT Results Within 45 Min. of Arrival[1]	-	-	46%	57%
Patients Who Left ER Before Being Seen	7,478	7%	4%	2%
Time from ER Arrival to Admit. (minutes)[2]	352	214	290	274
Time from ER Arrival to Discharge (minutes)	324	114	143	134
Time in ER Before Being Evaluated (minutes)	397	18	28	26
Time to Pain Meds for Fractures (minutes)	40	30	57	57
Heart Attack Care				
Aspirin Given at Discharge[1,3]	-	-	99%	99%
Fibrinolytic Meds Within 30 Min. of Arrival[3,7]	-	-	75%	54%
PCI Within 90 Minutes of Arrival[3,7]	-	-	95%	96%
Statin Prescribed at Discharge[1,3]	-	-	99%	98%
Heart Failure Care				
ACE Inhibitor or ARB for LVSD[1,2]	-	-	97%	97%
Discharge Instructions Given[2]	46	7%	89%	94%
Evaluation of LVS Function[2]	51	55%	96%	99%
Medicare Spending				
Medicare Spending per Patient (ratio)	-	0.78	0.85	0.98
Pneumonia Care				
Appropriate Initial Antibiotic Given[2]	29	90%	93%	95%
Blood Culture Timing[2]	31	90%	97%	98%
Pregnancy and Delivery Care				
Newborn Deliveries Scheduled Early[7]	-	-	3%	6%
Preventive Care				
Immunization for Influenza[2]	299	66%	86%	90%
Immunization for Pneumonia[2]	427	74%	89%	92%
Stroke Care				
Anticoagulation Therapy for Atrial Fibrillation[3,7]	-	-	96%	95%
Antithrombotic Therapy Timing[1,3]	-	-	94%	98%

NOTE: Hospital profiles are in alphabetical order by state, then city, then hospital within the city; Rankings exclude hospitals with less than 25 cases except for patient surveys which excludes hospitals with less than 100 cases; (a) 100-299 cases; (1) The number of cases/patients is too few to report; (2) Data submitted were based on a sample of cases/patients; (3) Results are based on a shorter time period than required; (4) Data suppressed by CMS for one or more quarters; (5) Results are not available for this reporting period; (6) Fewer than 100 patients completed the HCAHPS survey; (7) No cases met the criteria for this measure; (8) The lower limit of the confidence interval cannot be calculated if the number of observed infections equals zero; (9) No data are available from the state/territory for this reporting period; (10) The scores shown reflect fewer than 50 completed surveys; (11) There were discrepancies in the data collection process; (12) This measure does not apply to this hospital for this reporting period; (13) Results cannot be calculated for this reporting period; (14) The results for this state are combined with nearby states to protect confidentiality; Please refer to the User's Guide for a full explanation of data.

Measure	Cases	This Hosp.	State Avg.	U.S. Avg.
Assessed for Rehabilitation[1,3]	-	-	95%	97%
Discharged on Antithrombotic Therapy[1,3]	-	-	97%	99%
Discharged on Statin Medication[1,3]	-	-	89%	94%
Thrombolytic Therapy Timing[3,7]	-	-	61%	66%
Venous Thromboembolism Prophylaxis[1,3]	-	-	91%	94%
Written Stroke Educational Materials Given[1,3]	-	-	73%	88%
Surgical Care Improvement Project				
Appropriate Beta Blocker Usage[5]	-	-	94%	98%
Appropriate VTP Within 24 Hours[5]	-	-	97%	98%
Controlled Postoperative Blood Glucose[5]	-	-	97%	97%
Perioperative Temperature Management[5]	-	-	99%	100%
Prophylactic Antibiotic Selection[5]	-	-	98%	99%
Prophylactic Antibiotic Selection (Outpatient)[5]	-	-	98%	98%
Prophylactic Antibiotic Stopped[5]	-	-	98%	98%
Prophylactic Antibiotic Timing[5]	-	-	98%	99%
Prophylactic Antibiotic Timing (Outpatient)[5]	-	-	96%	98%
Urinary Catheter Removal[5]	-	-	97%	97%
Survey of Patients' Hospital Experiences				
Area Around Room 'Always' Quiet at Night[6]	<100	73%	61%	61%
Doctors 'Always' Communicated Well[6]	<100	74%	78%	82%
Home Recovery Information Given[6]	<100	76%	83%	85%
Hospital Given 9 or 10 on 10 Point Scale[6]	<100	73%	65%	71%
Meds 'Always' Explained Before Given[6]	<100	66%	63%	64%
Nurses 'Always' Communicated Well[6]	<100	82%	76%	79%
Pain 'Always' Well Controlled[6]	<100	75%	68%	71%
Room and Bathroom 'Always' Clean[6]	<100	71%	70%	73%
Timely Help 'Always' Received[6]	<100	70%	66%	68%
Would Definitely Recommend Hospital[6]	<100	63%	63%	71%
Use of Medical Imaging				
Cardiac Imaging Stress Test before Surgery[1]	-	-	4.2%	5.3%
Combination Abdominal CT Scan	166	1.8%	9.6%	10.5%
Combination Brain/Sinus CT Scan[1]	-	-	2.3%	2.7%
Combination Chest CT Scan[1]	-	-	5.6%	2.7%
Follow-up Mammogram/Ultrasound	159	6.9%	8.6%	8.8%
Lumbar Spine MRI for Low Back Pain	41	58.5%	36.9%	37.2%

Miners' Colfax Medical Center

203 Hospital Drive Phone: 575-445-3661
Raton, NM 87740
Type: Critical Access Hospitals Emergency Services: Yes
Ownership: Government - Local

Measure	Cases	This Hosp.	State Avg.	U.S. Avg.
Blood Clot Prevention and Treatment				
Anticoagulation Overlap Therapy[5]	-	-	96%	93%
ICU Venous Thromboembolism Prophylaxis[5]	-	-	92%	92%
Incidence of Potentially Preventable VTE[5]	-	-	3%	10%
UFH with Dosages/Platelet Monitoring[5]	-	-	99%	97%
Venous Thromboembolism Prophylaxis[5]	-	-	84%	85%
Warfarin Therapy Discharge Instructions[5]	-	-	85%	75%
Chest Pain/Possible Heart Attack Care				
Aspirin Given Within 24 Hours of Arrival[3]	12	100%	97%	96%
Fibrinolytic Meds Within 30 Min. of Arrival[1,3]	-	-	62%	58%
Average Time to ECG (minutes)[3]	15	9	9	7
Average Time to Transfer (minutes)[3,7]	-	-	99	60
Children's Asthma Care				
Received Home Management Plan of Care	-	-	-	88%
Received Reliever Medication	-	-	-	100%
Received Systemic Corticosteroids	-	-	-	100%
Emergency Department				
Admittance Decision Time (minutes)[2]	187	45	108	98
Head CT Results Within 45 Min. of Arrival[5]	-	-	46%	57%
Patients Who Left ER Before Being Seen	5,588	1%	4%	2%
Time from ER Arrival to Admit. (minutes)[2]	207	200	290	274
Time from ER Arrival to Discharge (minutes)[3]	221	141	143	134
Time in ER Before Being Evaluated (minutes)[3]	280	16	28	26
Time to Pain Meds for Fractures (minutes)[5]	-	-	57	57
Heart Attack Care				
Aspirin Given at Discharge[1,3]	-	-	99%	99%
Fibrinolytic Meds Within 30 Min. of Arrival[3,7]	-	-	75%	54%
PCI Within 90 Minutes of Arrival[3,7]	-	-	95%	96%
Statin Prescribed at Discharge[1,3]	-	-	99%	98%
Heart Failure Care				
ACE Inhibitor or ARB for LVSD[1]	-	-	97%	97%
Discharge Instructions Given[1]	-	-	89%	94%
Evaluation of LVS Function	16	38%	96%	99%
Medicare Spending				
Medicare Spending per Patient (ratio)	-	-	0.85	0.98
Pneumonia Care				
Appropriate Initial Antibiotic Given	16	56%	93%	95%
Blood Culture Timing	18	94%	97%	98%
Pregnancy and Delivery Care				
Newborn Deliveries Scheduled Early	41	2%	3%	6%
Preventive Care				
Immunization for Influenza[2]	126	94%	86%	90%
Immunization for Pneumonia[2]	175	86%	89%	92%
Stroke Care				
Anticoagulation Therapy for Atrial Fibrillation[5]	-	-	96%	95%
Antithrombotic Therapy Timing[5]	-	-	94%	98%
Assessed for Rehabilitation[5]	-	-	95%	97%
Discharged on Antithrombotic Therapy[5]	-	-	97%	99%
Discharged on Statin Medication[5]	-	-	89%	94%
Thrombolytic Therapy Timing[5]	-	-	61%	66%
Venous Thromboembolism Prophylaxis[5]	-	-	91%	94%
Written Stroke Educational Materials Given[5]	-	-	73%	88%
Surgical Care Improvement Project				
Appropriate Beta Blocker Usage[1]	-	-	94%	98%
Appropriate VTP Within 24 Hours	11	82%	97%	98%
Controlled Postoperative Blood Glucose[7]	-	-	97%	97%
Perioperative Temperature Management	15	93%	99%	100%
Prophylactic Antibiotic Selection[1]	-	-	98%	99%
Prophylactic Antibiotic Selection (Outpatient)[5]	-	-	98%	98%
Prophylactic Antibiotic Stopped[1]	-	-	98%	98%
Prophylactic Antibiotic Timing[1]	-	-	98%	99%
Prophylactic Antibiotic Timing (Outpatient)[5]	-	-	96%	98%
Urinary Catheter Removal[1]	-	-	97%	97%
Survey of Patients' Hospital Experiences				
Area Around Room 'Always' Quiet at Night	(a)	58%	61%	61%
Doctors 'Always' Communicated Well	(a)	80%	78%	82%
Home Recovery Information Given	(a)	81%	83%	85%
Hospital Given 9 or 10 on 10 Point Scale	(a)	69%	65%	71%
Meds 'Always' Explained Before Given	(a)	61%	63%	64%
Nurses 'Always' Communicated Well	(a)	82%	76%	79%
Pain 'Always' Well Controlled	(a)	74%	68%	71%
Room and Bathroom 'Always' Clean	(a)	80%	70%	73%
Timely Help 'Always' Received	(a)	79%	66%	68%
Would Definitely Recommend Hospital	(a)	64%	63%	71%
Use of Medical Imaging				
Cardiac Imaging Stress Test before Surgery[1]	-	-	4.2%	5.3%
Combination Abdominal CT Scan	134	13.4%	9.6%	10.5%
Combination Brain/Sinus CT Scan[1]	-	-	2.3%	2.7%
Combination Chest CT Scan	81	8.6%	5.6%	2.7%
Follow-up Mammogram/Ultrasound[7]	-	-	8.6%	8.8%
Lumbar Spine MRI for Low Back Pain[1]	-	-	36.9%	37.2%

UNM Sandoval Regional Medical Center

3001 Broadmoor Blvd Ne Phone: 505-272-8087
Rio Rancho, NM 87144
Type: Acute Care Hospitals Emergency Services: Yes
Ownership: Voluntary non-profit - Private

Measure	Cases	This Hosp.	State Avg.	U.S. Avg.
Blood Clot Prevention and Treatment				
Anticoagulation Overlap Therapy[2]	15	100%	96%	93%
ICU Venous Thromboembolism Prophylaxis[2]	26	81%	92%	92%
Incidence of Potentially Preventable VTE[2,7]	-	-	3%	10%
UFH with Dosages/Platelet Monitoring[1,2]	-	-	99%	97%
Venous Thromboembolism Prophylaxis[2]	186	76%	84%	85%
Warfarin Therapy Discharge Instructions[2]	16	56%	85%	75%
Chest Pain/Possible Heart Attack Care				
Aspirin Given Within 24 Hours of Arrival[5]	-	-	97%	96%
Fibrinolytic Meds Within 30 Min. of Arrival[5]	-	-	62%	58%
Average Time to ECG (minutes)[5]	-	-	9	7
Average Time to Transfer (minutes)[5]	-	-	99	60
Children's Asthma Care				
Received Home Management Plan of Care	-	-	-	88%
Received Reliever Medication	-	-	-	100%
Received Systemic Corticosteroids	-	-	-	100%
Emergency Department				
Admittance Decision Time (minutes)[2,3]	248	126	108	98
Head CT Results Within 45 Min. of Arrival[1,3]	-	-	46%	57%
Patients Who Left ER Before Being Seen	3,864	1%	4%	2%
Time from ER Arrival to Admit. (minutes)[2,3]	258	272	290	274
Time from ER Arrival to Discharge (minutes)[3]	316	166	143	134
Time in ER Before Being Evaluated (minutes)[3]	361	50	28	26
Time to Pain Meds for Fractures (minutes)[3]	31	50	57	57
Heart Attack Care				
Aspirin Given at Discharge[1,3]	-	-	99%	99%
Fibrinolytic Meds Within 30 Min. of Arrival[3,7]	-	-	75%	54%
PCI Within 90 Minutes of Arrival[3,7]	-	-	95%	96%
Statin Prescribed at Discharge[1,3]	-	-	99%	98%
Heart Failure Care				
ACE Inhibitor or ARB for LVSD[3]	11	91%	97%	97%
Discharge Instructions Given[3]	29	38%	89%	94%
Evaluation of LVS Function[3]	32	100%	96%	99%
Medicare Spending				
Medicare Spending per Patient (ratio)	-	-	0.85	0.98
Pneumonia Care				
Appropriate Initial Antibiotic Given[3]	30	97%	93%	95%
Blood Culture Timing[3]	42	83%	97%	98%
Pregnancy and Delivery Care				
Newborn Deliveries Scheduled Early[7]	-	-	3%	6%
Preventive Care				
Immunization for Influenza[2,3]	135	90%	86%	90%
Immunization for Pneumonia[2,3]	258	66%	89%	92%
Stroke Care				
Anticoagulation Therapy for Atrial Fibrillation[1]	-	-	96%	95%
Antithrombotic Therapy Timing[1]	-	-	94%	98%
Assessed for Rehabilitation[1]	-	-	95%	97%
Discharged on Antithrombotic Therapy[1]	-	-	97%	99%
Discharged on Statin Medication[1]	-	-	89%	94%
Thrombolytic Therapy Timing[7]	-	-	61%	66%
Venous Thromboembolism Prophylaxis[1]	-	-	91%	94%
Written Stroke Educational Materials Given[1]	-	-	73%	88%
Surgical Care Improvement Project				
Appropriate Beta Blocker Usage[2,3]	29	69%	94%	98%
Appropriate VTP Within 24 Hours[2,3]	187	97%	97%	98%
Controlled Postoperative Blood Glucose[2,3]	-	-	97%	97%
Perioperative Temperature Management[2,3]	216	88%	99%	100%
Prophylactic Antibiotic Selection[2,3]	121	95%	98%	99%
Prophylactic Antibiotic Selection (Outpatient)[5]	-	-	98%	98%
Prophylactic Antibiotic Stopped[2,3]	120	93%	98%	98%
Prophylactic Antibiotic Timing[2,3]	123	85%	98%	99%
Prophylactic Antibiotic Timing (Outpatient)[5]	-	-	96%	98%
Urinary Catheter Removal[2,3]	182	96%	97%	97%
Survey of Patients' Hospital Experiences				
Area Around Room 'Always' Quiet at Night	300+	69%	61%	61%
Doctors 'Always' Communicated Well	300+	85%	78%	82%
Home Recovery Information Given	300+	83%	83%	85%
Hospital Given 9 or 10 on 10 Point Scale	300+	82%	65%	71%
Meds 'Always' Explained Before Given	300+	62%	63%	64%
Nurses 'Always' Communicated Well	300+	81%	76%	79%
Pain 'Always' Well Controlled	300+	76%	68%	71%
Room and Bathroom 'Always' Clean	300+	76%	70%	73%
Timely Help 'Always' Received	300+	73%	66%	68%
Would Definitely Recommend Hospital	300+	84%	63%	71%
Use of Medical Imaging				
Cardiac Imaging Stress Test before Surgery[1]	-	-	4.2%	5.3%
Combination Abdominal CT Scan[1]	-	-	9.6%	10.5%
Combination Brain/Sinus CT Scan[1]	-	-	2.3%	2.7%
Combination Chest CT Scan[1]	-	-	5.6%	2.7%
Follow-up Mammogram/Ultrasound[1]	-	-	8.6%	8.8%
Lumbar Spine MRI for Low Back Pain[1]	-	-	36.9%	37.2%

NOTE: Hospital profiles are in alphabetical order by state, then city, then hospital within the city; Rankings exclude hospitals with less than 25 cases except for patient surveys which excludes hospitals with less than 100 cases; (a) 100-299 cases; (1) The number of cases/patients is too few to report; (2) Data submitted were based on a sample of cases/patients; (3) Results are based on a shorter time period than required; (4) Data suppressed by CMS for one or more quarters; (5) Results are not available for this reporting period; (6) Fewer than 100 patients completed the HCAHPS survey; (7) No cases met the criteria for this measure; (8) The lower limit of the confidence interval cannot be calculated if the number of observed infections equals zero; (9) No data are available from the state/territory for this reporting period; (10) The scores shown reflect fewer than 50 completed surveys; (11) There were discrepancies in the data collection process; (12) This measure does not apply to this hospital for this reporting period; (13) Results cannot be calculated for this reporting period; (14) The results for this state are combined with nearby states to protect confidentiality; Please refer to the User's Guide for a full explanation of data.

Eastern New Mexico Medical Center

405 W Country Club Road
Roswell, NM 88201
E-mail: enmmc@enmmc.com
URL: www.enmmc.com
Phone: 575-624-8722
Fax: 505-624-8726

Type: Acute Care Hospitals
Ownership: Proprietary
Emergency Services: Yes
Beds: 162

Key Personnel:

Operating Room. . . . . Akbar Ali, RN
Quality Assurance . . . . Tammie Chavez
Pediatric In-Patient Care . . . . Beverley Elliot, MD
Infection Control. . . . . Susan Esparsen
CEO/President. . . . . Brian Gibbons
Radiology. . . . . Joseph Orzel
Chief of Medical Staff . . . . Madhu Sasidhar, MD

Measure	Cases	This Hosp.	State Avg.	U.S. Avg.
Blood Clot Prevention and Treatment				
Anticoagulation Overlap Therapy[2]	45	98%	96%	93%
ICU Venous Thromboembolism Prophylaxis[2]	70	94%	92%	92%
Incidence of Potentially Preventable VTE[1,2]	-	-	3%	10%
UFH with Dosages/Platelet Monitoring[2]	14	100%	99%	97%
Venous Thromboembolism Prophylaxis[2]	296	94%	84%	85%
Warfarin Therapy Discharge Instructions[2]	34	100%	85%	75%
Chest Pain/Possible Heart Attack Care				
Aspirin Given Within 24 Hours of Arrival[1]	-	-	97%	96%
Fibrinolytic Meds Within 30 Min. of Arrival[1,3]	-	-	62%	58%
Average Time to ECG (minutes)	11	7	9	7
Average Time to Transfer (minutes)[3,7]	-	-	99	60
Children's Asthma Care				
Received Home Management Plan of Care	-	-	-	88%
Received Reliever Medication	-	-	-	100%
Received Systemic Corticosteroids	-	-	-	100%
Emergency Department				
Admittance Decision Time (minutes)[2]	520	110	108	98
Head CT Results Within 45 Min. of Arrival[1]	-	-	46%	57%
Patients Who Left ER Before Being Seen	23,318	1%	4%	2%
Time from ER Arrival to Admit. (minutes)[2]	529	282	290	274
Time from ER Arrival to Discharge (minutes)	355	153	143	134
Time in ER Before Being Evaluated (minutes)	416	16	28	26
Time to Pain Meds for Fractures (minutes)	67	44	57	57
Heart Attack Care				
Aspirin Given at Discharge	89	97%	99%	99%
Fibrinolytic Meds Within 30 Min. of Arrival[1]	-	-	75%	54%
PCI Within 90 Minutes of Arrival[1]	-	-	95%	96%
Statin Prescribed at Discharge	87	98%	99%	98%
Heart Failure Care				
ACE Inhibitor or ARB for LVSD	31	100%	97%	97%
Discharge Instructions Given	84	95%	89%	94%
Evaluation of LVS Function	107	99%	96%	99%
Medicare Spending				
Medicare Spending per Patient (ratio)	-	0.96	0.85	0.98
Pneumonia Care				
Appropriate Initial Antibiotic Given	106	99%	93%	95%
Blood Culture Timing	149	98%	97%	98%
Pregnancy and Delivery Care				
Newborn Deliveries Scheduled Early[2]	25	8%	3%	6%
Preventive Care				
Immunization for Influenza[2]	356	99%	86%	90%
Immunization for Pneumonia[2]	484	99%	89%	92%
Stroke Care				
Anticoagulation Therapy for Atrial Fibrillation[1]	-	-	96%	95%
Antithrombotic Therapy Timing	13	92%	94%	98%
Assessed for Rehabilitation	21	95%	95%	97%
Discharged on Antithrombotic Therapy	15	93%	97%	99%
Discharged on Statin Medication	17	88%	89%	94%
Thrombolytic Therapy Timing[1]	-	-	61%	66%
Venous Thromboembolism Prophylaxis	27	85%	91%	94%
Written Stroke Educational Materials Given	11	100%	73%	88%
Surgical Care Improvement Project				
Appropriate Beta Blocker Usage	49	96%	94%	98%
Appropriate VTP Within 24 Hours	169	97%	97%	98%
Controlled Postoperative Blood Glucose[7]	-	-	97%	97%
Perioperative Temperature Management	184	100%	99%	100%
Prophylactic Antibiotic Selection	51	100%	98%	99%
Prophylactic Antibiotic Selection (Outpatient)	36	100%	98%	98%
Prophylactic Antibiotic Stopped	50	98%	98%	98%
Prophylactic Antibiotic Timing	51	100%	98%	99%
Prophylactic Antibiotic Timing (Outpatient)	36	100%	96%	98%
Urinary Catheter Removal	143	97%	97%	97%
Survey of Patients' Hospital Experiences				
Area Around Room 'Always' Quiet at Night	300+	54%	61%	61%
Doctors 'Always' Communicated Well	300+	77%	78%	82%
Home Recovery Information Given	300+	84%	83%	85%
Hospital Given 9 or 10 on 10 Point Scale	300+	59%	65%	71%
Meds 'Always' Explained Before Given	300+	59%	63%	64%
Nurses 'Always' Communicated Well	300+	70%	76%	79%
Pain 'Always' Well Controlled	300+	65%	68%	71%
Room and Bathroom 'Always' Clean	300+	65%	70%	73%
Timely Help 'Always' Received	300+	50%	66%	68%
Would Definitely Recommend Hospital	300+	60%	63%	71%
Use of Medical Imaging				
Cardiac Imaging Stress Test before Surgery[1]	-	-	4.2%	5.3%
Combination Abdominal CT Scan	497	15.9%	9.6%	10.5%
Combination Brain/Sinus CT Scan	524	2.7%	2.3%	2.7%
Combination Chest CT Scan	228	18.4%	5.6%	2.7%
Follow-up Mammogram/Ultrasound	672	8.6%	8.6%	8.8%
Lumbar Spine MRI for Low Back Pain	149	30.9%	36.9%	37.2%

Lovelace Regional Hospital - Roswell

117 East 19th Street
Roswell, NM 88201
URL: www.roswellregional.com
Phone: 575-627-7000

Type: Acute Care Hospitals
Ownership: Physician
Emergency Services: Yes
Beds: 26

Measure	Cases	This Hosp.	State Avg.	U.S. Avg.
Blood Clot Prevention and Treatment				
Anticoagulation Overlap Therapy[1,2]	-	-	96%	93%
ICU Venous Thromboembolism Prophylaxis[2]	22	91%	92%	92%
Incidence of Potentially Preventable VTE[1,2]	-	-	3%	10%
UFH with Dosages/Platelet Monitoring[1,2]	-	-	99%	97%
Venous Thromboembolism Prophylaxis[2]	114	82%	84%	85%
Warfarin Therapy Discharge Instructions[1,2]	-	-	85%	75%
Chest Pain/Possible Heart Attack Care				
Aspirin Given Within 24 Hours of Arrival	26	88%	97%	96%
Fibrinolytic Meds Within 30 Min. of Arrival[1,3]	-	-	62%	58%
Average Time to ECG (minutes)	26	8	9	7
Average Time to Transfer (minutes)[1,3]	-	-	99	60
Children's Asthma Care				
Received Home Management Plan of Care	-	-	-	88%
Received Reliever Medication	-	-	-	100%
Received Systemic Corticosteroids	-	-	-	100%
Emergency Department				
Admittance Decision Time (minutes)[2]	162	80	108	98
Head CT Results Within 45 Min. of Arrival[1]	-	-	46%	57%
Patients Who Left ER Before Being Seen	10,544	5%	4%	2%
Time from ER Arrival to Admit. (minutes)[2]	190	298	290	274
Time from ER Arrival to Discharge (minutes)	372	152	143	134
Time in ER Before Being Evaluated (minutes)	408	38	28	26
Time to Pain Meds for Fractures (minutes)	52	67	57	57
Heart Attack Care				
Aspirin Given at Discharge	22	95%	99%	99%
Fibrinolytic Meds Within 30 Min. of Arrival[7]	-	-	75%	54%
PCI Within 90 Minutes of Arrival[7]	-	-	95%	96%
Statin Prescribed at Discharge	20	95%	99%	98%
Heart Failure Care				
ACE Inhibitor or ARB for LVSD	17	100%	97%	97%
Discharge Instructions Given	55	100%	89%	94%
Evaluation of LVS Function	58	97%	96%	99%
Medicare Spending				
Medicare Spending per Patient (ratio)	-	0.92	0.85	0.98
Pneumonia Care				
Appropriate Initial Antibiotic Given	27	96%	93%	95%
Blood Culture Timing	41	98%	97%	98%
Pregnancy and Delivery Care				
Newborn Deliveries Scheduled Early	134	4%	3%	6%
Preventive Care				
Immunization for Influenza[2]	274	92%	86%	90%
Immunization for Pneumonia[2]	304	96%	89%	92%
Stroke Care				
Anticoagulation Therapy for Atrial Fibrillation[1]	-	-	96%	95%
Antithrombotic Therapy Timing	11	100%	94%	98%
Assessed for Rehabilitation	11	100%	95%	97%
Discharged on Antithrombotic Therapy[1]	-	-	97%	99%
Discharged on Statin Medication[1]	-	-	89%	94%
Thrombolytic Therapy Timing[1]	-	-	61%	66%
Venous Thromboembolism Prophylaxis[1]	-	-	91%	94%
Written Stroke Educational Materials Given[1]	-	-	73%	88%
Surgical Care Improvement Project				
Appropriate Beta Blocker Usage[2]	55	93%	94%	98%
Appropriate VTP Within 24 Hours[2]	185	99%	97%	98%
Controlled Postoperative Blood Glucose[2,7]	-	-	97%	97%
Perioperative Temperature Management[2]	222	100%	99%	100%
Prophylactic Antibiotic Selection[2]	187	99%	98%	99%
Prophylactic Antibiotic Selection (Outpatient)	154	100%	98%	98%
Prophylactic Antibiotic Stopped[2]	187	99%	98%	98%
Prophylactic Antibiotic Timing[2]	187	100%	98%	99%
Prophylactic Antibiotic Timing (Outpatient)	156	97%	96%	98%
Urinary Catheter Removal[2]	153	99%	97%	97%
Survey of Patients' Hospital Experiences				
Area Around Room 'Always' Quiet at Night	300+	63%	61%	61%
Doctors 'Always' Communicated Well	300+	84%	78%	82%
Home Recovery Information Given	300+	83%	83%	85%
Hospital Given 9 or 10 on 10 Point Scale	300+	74%	65%	71%
Meds 'Always' Explained Before Given	300+	63%	63%	64%
Nurses 'Always' Communicated Well	300+	79%	76%	79%
Pain 'Always' Well Controlled	300+	76%	68%	71%
Room and Bathroom 'Always' Clean	300+	75%	70%	73%
Timely Help 'Always' Received	300+	69%	66%	68%
Would Definitely Recommend Hospital	300+	77%	63%	71%
Use of Medical Imaging				
Cardiac Imaging Stress Test before Surgery[7]	-	-	4.2%	5.3%
Combination Abdominal CT Scan	385	5.2%	9.6%	10.5%
Combination Brain/Sinus CT Scan[1]	-	-	2.3%	2.7%
Combination Chest CT Scan	217	0.5%	5.6%	2.7%
Follow-up Mammogram/Ultrasound[7]	-	-	8.6%	8.8%
Lumbar Spine MRI for Low Back Pain[1]	-	-	36.9%	37.2%

Lincoln County Medical Center

211 Sudderth Drive
Ruidoso, NM 88345
URL: www.phs.org/facilities/lcmc
Phone: 575-257-8250
Fax: 505-630-4233

Type: Critical Access Hospitals
Ownership: Voluntary non-profit - Private
Emergency Services: Yes
Beds: 22

Key Personnel:

Radiology. . . . . Farooq P Agha
Chief of Medical Staff . . . . Eddie Benge, DO
CEO/President. . . . . Jim Gibson

Measure	Cases	This Hosp.	State Avg.	U.S. Avg.
Blood Clot Prevention and Treatment				
Anticoagulation Overlap Therapy[5]	-	-	96%	93%
ICU Venous Thromboembolism Prophylaxis[5]	-	-	92%	92%
Incidence of Potentially Preventable VTE[5]	-	-	3%	10%
UFH with Dosages/Platelet Monitoring[5]	-	-	99%	97%
Venous Thromboembolism Prophylaxis[5]	-	-	84%	85%
Warfarin Therapy Discharge Instructions[5]	-	-	85%	75%
Chest Pain/Possible Heart Attack Care				
Aspirin Given Within 24 Hours of Arrival	-	-	97%	96%
Fibrinolytic Meds Within 30 Min. of Arrival	-	-	62%	58%
Average Time to ECG (minutes)	-	-	9	7
Average Time to Transfer (minutes)	-	-	99	60
Children's Asthma Care				
Received Home Management Plan of Care	-	-	-	88%
Received Reliever Medication	-	-	-	100%
Received Systemic Corticosteroids	-	-	-	100%
Emergency Department				
Admittance Decision Time (minutes)[5]	-	-	108	98
Head CT Results Within 45 Min. of Arrival	-	-	46%	57%
Patients Who Left ER Before Being Seen	-	-	4%	2%
Time from ER Arrival to Admit. (minutes)[5]	-	-	290	274

NOTE: Hospital profiles are in alphabetical order by state, then city, then hospital within the city; Rankings exclude hospitals with less than 25 cases except for patient surveys which excludes hospitals with less than 100 cases; (a) 100-299 cases; (1) The number of cases/patients is too few to report; (2) Data submitted were based on a sample of cases/patients; (3) Results are based on a shorter time period than required; (4) Data suppressed by CMS for one or more quarters; (5) Results are not available for this reporting period; (6) Fewer than 100 patients completed the HCAHPS survey; (7) No cases met the criteria for this measure; (8) The lower limit of the confidence interval cannot be calculated if the number of observed infections equals zero; (9) No data are available from the state/territory for this reporting period; (10) The scores shown reflect fewer than 50 completed surveys; (11) There were discrepancies in the data collection process; (12) This measure does not apply to this hospital for this reporting period; (13) Results cannot be calculated for this reporting period; (14) The results for this state are combined with nearby states to protect confidentiality; Please refer to the User's Guide for a full explanation of data.

Measure	Cases	This Hosp.	State Avg.	U.S. Avg.
Time from ER Arrival to Discharge (minutes)	-	-	143	134
Time in ER Before Being Evaluated (minutes)	-	-	28	26
Time to Pain Meds for Fractures (minutes)	-	-	57	57
Heart Attack Care				
Aspirin Given at Discharge[5]	-	-	99%	99%
Fibrinolytic Meds Within 30 Min. of Arrival[5]	-	-	75%	54%
PCI Within 90 Minutes of Arrival[5]	-	-	95%	96%
Statin Prescribed at Discharge[5]	-	-	99%	98%
Heart Failure Care				
ACE Inhibitor or ARB for LVSD[1]	-	-	97%	97%
Discharge Instructions Given	34	94%	89%	94%
Evaluation of LVS Function	37	100%	96%	99%
Medicare Spending				
Medicare Spending per Patient (ratio)	-	-	0.85	0.98
Pneumonia Care				
Appropriate Initial Antibiotic Given	21	100%	93%	95%
Blood Culture Timing	41	98%	97%	98%
Pregnancy and Delivery Care				
Newborn Deliveries Scheduled Early[5]	-	-	3%	6%
Preventive Care				
Immunization for Influenza[5]	-	-	86%	90%
Immunization for Pneumonia[5]	-	-	89%	92%
Stroke Care				
Anticoagulation Therapy for Atrial Fibrillation[5]	-	-	96%	95%
Antithrombotic Therapy Timing[5]	-	-	94%	98%
Assessed for Rehabilitation[5]	-	-	95%	97%
Discharged on Antithrombotic Therapy[5]	-	-	97%	99%
Discharged on Statin Medication[5]	-	-	89%	94%
Thrombolytic Therapy Timing[5]	-	-	61%	66%
Venous Thromboembolism Prophylaxis[5]	-	-	91%	94%
Written Stroke Educational Materials Given[5]	-	-	73%	88%
Surgical Care Improvement Project				
Appropriate Beta Blocker Usage[1]	-	-	94%	98%
Appropriate VTP Within 24 Hours	34	100%	97%	98%
Controlled Postoperative Blood Glucose[7]	-	-	97%	97%
Perioperative Temperature Management	46	100%	99%	100%
Prophylactic Antibiotic Selection	32	100%	98%	99%
Prophylactic Antibiotic Selection (Outpatient)	-	-	98%	98%
Prophylactic Antibiotic Stopped	32	97%	98%	98%
Prophylactic Antibiotic Timing	32	100%	98%	99%
Prophylactic Antibiotic Timing (Outpatient)	-	-	96%	98%
Urinary Catheter Removal[1]	-	-	97%	97%
Survey of Patients' Hospital Experiences				
Area Around Room 'Always' Quiet at Night	(a)	70%	61%	61%
Doctors 'Always' Communicated Well	(a)	88%	78%	82%
Home Recovery Information Given	(a)	87%	83%	85%
Hospital Given 9 or 10 on 10 Point Scale	(a)	78%	65%	71%
Meds 'Always' Explained Before Given	(a)	75%	63%	64%
Nurses 'Always' Communicated Well	(a)	88%	76%	79%
Pain 'Always' Well Controlled	(a)	80%	68%	71%
Room and Bathroom 'Always' Clean	(a)	77%	70%	73%
Timely Help 'Always' Received	(a)	81%	66%	68%
Would Definitely Recommend Hospital	(a)	74%	63%	71%
Use of Medical Imaging				
Cardiac Imaging Stress Test before Surgery	-	-	4.2%	5.3%
Combination Abdominal CT Scan	-	-	9.6%	10.5%
Combination Brain/Sinus CT Scan	-	-	2.3%	2.7%
Combination Chest CT Scan	-	-	5.6%	2.7%
Follow-up Mammogram/Ultrasound	-	-	8.6%	8.8%
Lumbar Spine MRI for Low Back Pain	-	-	36.9%	37.2%

Dhhs Usphs Indian Health Services

Exit #102 Off I-40 1/2 Mile South
San Fidel, NM 87049
Phone: 505-552-5300
Fax: 505-552-5490
URL: www.ihs.gov
Type: Acute Care Hospitals
Emergency Services: Yes
Ownership: Government - Federal
Beds: 25

Key Personnel:
Quality Assurance . . . . Lydia Bequy
CEO/President. . . . . William Thorne Jr

Measure	Cases	This Hosp.	State Avg.	U.S. Avg.
Blood Clot Prevention and Treatment				
Anticoagulation Overlap Therapy[2,7]	-	-	96%	93%
ICU Venous Thromboembolism Prophylaxis[1,2]	-	-	92%	92%
Incidence of Potentially Preventable VTE[2,7]	-	-	3%	10%
UFH with Dosages/Platelet Monitoring[2,7]	-	-	99%	97%
Venous Thromboembolism Prophylaxis[2]	101	8%	84%	85%
Warfarin Therapy Discharge Instructions[2,7]	-	-	85%	75%
Chest Pain/Possible Heart Attack Care				
Aspirin Given Within 24 Hours of Arrival	-	-	97%	96%
Fibrinolytic Meds Within 30 Min. of Arrival	-	-	62%	58%
Average Time to ECG (minutes)	-	-	9	7
Average Time to Transfer (minutes)	-	-	99	60
Children's Asthma Care				
Received Home Management Plan of Care	-	-	-	88%
Received Reliever Medication	-	-	-	100%
Received Systemic Corticosteroids	-	-	-	100%
Emergency Department				
Admittance Decision Time (minutes)	150	70	108	98
Head CT Results Within 45 Min. of Arrival	-	-	46%	57%
Patients Who Left ER Before Being Seen	-	-	4%	2%
Time from ER Arrival to Admit. (minutes)	150	254	290	274
Time from ER Arrival to Discharge (minutes)	-	-	143	134
Time in ER Before Being Evaluated (minutes)	-	-	28	26
Time to Pain Meds for Fractures (minutes)	-	-	57	57
Heart Attack Care				
Aspirin Given at Discharge[5]	-	-	99%	99%
Fibrinolytic Meds Within 30 Min. of Arrival[5]	-	-	75%	54%
PCI Within 90 Minutes of Arrival[5]	-	-	95%	96%
Statin Prescribed at Discharge[5]	-	-	99%	98%
Heart Failure Care				
ACE Inhibitor or ARB for LVSD[1,3]	-	-	97%	97%
Discharge Instructions Given[1,3]	-	-	89%	94%
Evaluation of LVS Function[1,3]	-	-	96%	99%
Medicare Spending				
Medicare Spending per Patient (ratio)	-	0.53	0.85	0.98
Pneumonia Care				
Appropriate Initial Antibiotic Given[1]	-	-	93%	95%
Blood Culture Timing	15	100%	97%	98%
Pregnancy and Delivery Care				
Newborn Deliveries Scheduled Early[7]	-	-	3%	6%
Preventive Care				
Immunization for Influenza	99	76%	86%	90%
Immunization for Pneumonia	172	90%	89%	92%
Stroke Care				
Anticoagulation Therapy for Atrial Fibrillation[5]	-	-	96%	95%
Antithrombotic Therapy Timing[5]	-	-	94%	98%
Assessed for Rehabilitation[5]	-	-	95%	97%
Discharged on Antithrombotic Therapy[5]	-	-	97%	99%
Discharged on Statin Medication[5]	-	-	89%	94%
Thrombolytic Therapy Timing[5]	-	-	61%	66%
Venous Thromboembolism Prophylaxis[5]	-	-	91%	94%
Written Stroke Educational Materials Given[5]	-	-	73%	88%
Surgical Care Improvement Project				
Appropriate Beta Blocker Usage[5]	-	-	94%	98%
Appropriate VTP Within 24 Hours[5]	-	-	97%	98%
Controlled Postoperative Blood Glucose[5]	-	-	97%	97%
Perioperative Temperature Management[5]	-	-	99%	100%
Prophylactic Antibiotic Selection[5]	-	-	98%	99%
Prophylactic Antibiotic Selection (Outpatient)	-	-	98%	98%
Prophylactic Antibiotic Stopped[5]	-	-	98%	98%
Prophylactic Antibiotic Timing[5]	-	-	98%	99%
Prophylactic Antibiotic Timing (Outpatient)	-	-	96%	98%
Urinary Catheter Removal[5]	-	-	97%	97%
Survey of Patients' Hospital Experiences				
Area Around Room 'Always' Quiet at Night[6]	<100	78%	61%	61%
Doctors 'Always' Communicated Well[6]	<100	81%	78%	82%
Home Recovery Information Given[6]	<100	80%	83%	85%
Hospital Given 9 or 10 on 10 Point Scale[6]	<100	50%	65%	71%
Meds 'Always' Explained Before Given[6]	<100	75%	63%	64%
Nurses 'Always' Communicated Well[6]	<100	72%	76%	79%
Pain 'Always' Well Controlled[6]	<100	67%	68%	71%
Room and Bathroom 'Always' Clean[6]	<100	72%	70%	73%
Timely Help 'Always' Received[6]	<100	66%	66%	68%
Would Definitely Recommend Hospital[6]	<100	34%	63%	71%
Use of Medical Imaging				
Cardiac Imaging Stress Test before Surgery	-	-	4.2%	5.3%
Combination Abdominal CT Scan	-	-	9.6%	10.5%
Combination Brain/Sinus CT Scan	-	-	2.3%	2.7%
Combination Chest CT Scan	-	-	5.6%	2.7%
Follow-up Mammogram/Ultrasound	-	-	8.6%	8.8%
Lumbar Spine MRI for Low Back Pain	-	-	36.9%	37.2%

Saint Vincent Hospital

455 Saint Michael's Drive
Santa Fe, NM 87505
Phone: 505-913-5201
Fax: 505-989-6408
E-mail: contactus@stvin.org
URL: www.stvin.org
Type: Acute Care Hospitals
Emergency Services: Yes
Ownership: Voluntary non-profit - Private
Beds: 268

Key Personnel:
Chief of Medical Staff . . . . John Beeson, MD
Chair/CEO . . . . Dave Delgado
Pediatric Ambulatory Care . . . . . . Lucinda Dyke, MD
Pediatric In-Patient Care . . . . Lucinda Dyke, MD
CEO/President. . . . . Bruce Tassin
Quality Assurance . . . . Leslie Urquhart

Measure	Cases	This Hosp.	State Avg.	U.S. Avg.
Blood Clot Prevention and Treatment				
Anticoagulation Overlap Therapy[2]	107	95%	96%	93%
ICU Venous Thromboembolism Prophylaxis[2]	52	94%	92%	92%
Incidence of Potentially Preventable VTE[2]	12	0%	3%	10%
UFH with Dosages/Platelet Monitoring[2]	44	100%	99%	97%
Venous Thromboembolism Prophylaxis[2]	345	81%	84%	85%
Warfarin Therapy Discharge Instructions[2]	90	89%	85%	75%
Chest Pain/Possible Heart Attack Care				
Aspirin Given Within 24 Hours of Arrival[1,3]	-	-	97%	96%
Fibrinolytic Meds Within 30 Min. of Arrival[1,3]	-	-	62%	58%
Average Time to ECG (minutes)[1,3]	-	-	9	7
Average Time to Transfer (minutes)[1,3]	-	-	99	60
Children's Asthma Care				
Received Home Management Plan of Care	-	-	-	88%
Received Reliever Medication	-	-	-	100%
Received Systemic Corticosteroids	-	-	-	100%
Emergency Department				
Admittance Decision Time (minutes)[2]	671	206	108	98
Head CT Results Within 45 Min. of Arrival[1]	-	-	46%	57%
Patients Who Left ER Before Being Seen	54,253	1%	4%	2%
Time from ER Arrival to Admit. (minutes)[2]	747	437	290	274
Time from ER Arrival to Discharge (minutes)	372	172	143	134
Time in ER Before Being Evaluated (minutes)	412	34	28	26
Time to Pain Meds for Fractures (minutes)	201	76	57	57
Heart Attack Care				
Aspirin Given at Discharge	219	100%	99%	99%
Fibrinolytic Meds Within 30 Min. of Arrival[7]	-	-	75%	54%
PCI Within 90 Minutes of Arrival	47	89%	95%	96%
Statin Prescribed at Discharge	220	100%	99%	98%
Heart Failure Care				
ACE Inhibitor or ARB for LVSD	79	97%	97%	97%
Discharge Instructions Given	167	98%	89%	94%
Evaluation of LVS Function	175	98%	96%	99%
Medicare Spending				
Medicare Spending per Patient (ratio)	-	0.92	0.85	0.98
Pneumonia Care				
Appropriate Initial Antibiotic Given[2]	93	94%	93%	95%
Blood Culture Timing[2]	136	96%	97%	98%
Pregnancy and Delivery Care				
Newborn Deliveries Scheduled Early[2]	103	4%	3%	6%
Preventive Care				
Immunization for Influenza[2]	568	75%	86%	90%
Immunization for Pneumonia[2]	636	74%	89%	92%
Stroke Care				
Anticoagulation Therapy for Atrial Fibrillation	15	100%	96%	95%
Antithrombotic Therapy Timing	81	90%	94%	98%
Assessed for Rehabilitation	119	98%	95%	97%
Discharged on Antithrombotic Therapy	91	98%	97%	99%
Discharged on Statin Medication	68	88%	89%	94%
Thrombolytic Therapy Timing	15	53%	61%	66%
Venous Thromboembolism Prophylaxis	116	78%	91%	94%

NOTE: Hospital profiles are in alphabetical order by state, then city, then hospital within the city; Rankings exclude hospitals with less than 25 cases except for patient surveys which excludes hospitals with less than 100 cases; (a) 100-299 cases; (1) The number of cases/patients is too few to report; (2) Data submitted were based on a sample of cases/patients; (3) Results are based on a shorter time period than required; (4) Data suppressed by CMS for one or more quarters; (5) Results are not available for this reporting period; (6) Fewer than 100 patients completed the HCAHPS survey; (7) No cases met the criteria for this measure; (8) The lower limit of the confidence interval cannot be calculated if the number of observed infections equals zero; (9) No data are available from the state/territory for this reporting period; (10) The scores shown reflect fewer than 50 completed surveys; (11) There were discrepancies in the data collection process; (12) This measure does not apply to this hospital for this reporting period; (13) Results cannot be calculated for this reporting period; (14) The results for this state are combined with nearby states to protect confidentiality; Please refer to the User's Guide for a full explanation of data.

Measure	Cases	This Hosp.	State Avg.	U.S. Avg.
Written Stroke Educational Materials Given	67	78%	73%	88%
Surgical Care Improvement Project				
Appropriate Beta Blocker Usage[2]	53	83%	94%	98%
Appropriate VTP Within 24 Hours[2]	330	98%	97%	98%
Controlled Postoperative Blood Glucose[2,7]	-	-	97%	97%
Perioperative Temperature Management[2]	412	100%	99%	100%
Prophylactic Antibiotic Selection[2]	271	99%	98%	99%
Prophylactic Antibiotic Selection (Outpatient)	159	96%	98%	98%
Prophylactic Antibiotic Stopped[2]	267	97%	98%	98%
Prophylactic Antibiotic Timing[2]	274	99%	98%	99%
Prophylactic Antibiotic Timing (Outpatient)	176	87%	96%	98%
Urinary Catheter Removal[2]	260	97%	97%	97%
Survey of Patients' Hospital Experiences				
Area Around Room 'Always' Quiet at Night	300+	40%	61%	61%
Doctors 'Always' Communicated Well	300+	76%	78%	82%
Home Recovery Information Given	300+	81%	83%	85%
Hospital Given 9 or 10 on 10 Point Scale	300+	50%	65%	71%
Meds 'Always' Explained Before Given	300+	55%	63%	64%
Nurses 'Always' Communicated Well	300+	68%	76%	79%
Pain 'Always' Well Controlled	300+	62%	68%	71%
Room and Bathroom 'Always' Clean	300+	53%	70%	73%
Timely Help 'Always' Received	300+	51%	66%	68%
Would Definitely Recommend Hospital	300+	53%	63%	71%
Use of Medical Imaging				
Cardiac Imaging Stress Test before Surgery	372	4.8%	4.2%	5.3%
Combination Abdominal CT Scan	587	4.6%	9.6%	10.5%
Combination Brain/Sinus CT Scan	732	0.8%	2.3%	2.7%
Combination Chest CT Scan	220	0.0%	5.6%	2.7%
Follow-up Mammogram/Ultrasound[7]	-	-	8.6%	8.8%
Lumbar Spine MRI for Low Back Pain	56	35.7%	36.9%	37.2%

Santa Fe Phs Indian Hospital

1700 Cerrillos Road
Santa Fe, NM 87501
Phone: 505-988-9821
Fax: 505-986-0751
URL: www.ihs.gov
Type: Acute Care Hospitals
Emergency Services: No
Ownership: Government - Federal
Beds: 39

Key Personnel:
CEO/President . . . . Richard Zethier

Measure	Cases	This Hosp.	State Avg.	U.S. Avg.
Blood Clot Prevention and Treatment				
Anticoagulation Overlap Therapy[2,7]	-	-	96%	93%
ICU Venous Thromboembolism Prophylaxis[2,7]	-	-	92%	92%
Incidence of Potentially Preventable VTE[2,7]	-	-	3%	10%
UFH with Dosages/Platelet Monitoring[2,7]	-	-	99%	97%
Venous Thromboembolism Prophylaxis[2]	50	26%	84%	85%
Warfarin Therapy Discharge Instructions[2,7]	-	-	85%	75%
Chest Pain/Possible Heart Attack Care				
Aspirin Given Within 24 Hours of Arrival	-	-	97%	96%
Fibrinolytic Meds Within 30 Min. of Arrival	-	-	62%	58%
Average Time to ECG (minutes)	-	-	9	7
Average Time to Transfer (minutes)	-	-	99	60
Children's Asthma Care				
Received Home Management Plan of Care	-	-	-	88%
Received Reliever Medication	-	-	-	100%
Received Systemic Corticosteroids	-	-	-	100%
Emergency Department				
Admittance Decision Time (minutes)[2,7]	-	-	108	98
Head CT Results Within 45 Min. of Arrival	-	-	46%	57%
Patients Who Left ER Before Being Seen	-	-	4%	2%
Time from ER Arrival to Admit. (minutes)[2,7]	-	-	290	274
Time from ER Arrival to Discharge (minutes)	-	-	143	134
Time in ER Before Being Evaluated (minutes)	-	-	28	26
Time to Pain Meds for Fractures (minutes)	-	-	57	57
Heart Attack Care				
Aspirin Given at Discharge[5]	-	-	99%	99%
Fibrinolytic Meds Within 30 Min. of Arrival[5]	-	-	75%	54%
PCI Within 90 Minutes of Arrival[5]	-	-	95%	96%
Statin Prescribed at Discharge[5]	-	-	99%	98%
Heart Failure Care				
ACE Inhibitor or ARB for LVSD[2,3]	-	-	97%	97%
Discharge Instructions Given[1,2]	-	-	89%	94%
Evaluation of LVS Function[1,2]	-	-	96%	99%
Medicare Spending				
Medicare Spending per Patient (ratio)[1]	-	-	0.85	0.98
Pneumonia Care				
Appropriate Initial Antibiotic Given[2,3]	-	-	93%	95%
Blood Culture Timing[1,2]	-	-	97%	98%
Pregnancy and Delivery Care				
Newborn Deliveries Scheduled Early[2,7]	-	-	3%	6%
Preventive Care				
Immunization for Influenza[2]	76	80%	86%	90%
Immunization for Pneumonia[2]	90	88%	89%	92%
Stroke Care				
Anticoagulation Therapy for Atrial Fibrillation[5]	-	-	96%	95%
Antithrombotic Therapy Timing[5]	-	-	94%	98%
Assessed for Rehabilitation[5]	-	-	95%	97%
Discharged on Antithrombotic Therapy[5]	-	-	97%	99%
Discharged on Statin Medication[5]	-	-	89%	94%
Thrombolytic Therapy Timing[5]	-	-	61%	66%
Venous Thromboembolism Prophylaxis[5]	-	-	91%	94%
Written Stroke Educational Materials Given[5]	-	-	73%	88%
Surgical Care Improvement Project				
Appropriate Beta Blocker Usage[5]	-	-	94%	98%
Appropriate VTP Within 24 Hours[5]	-	-	97%	98%
Controlled Postoperative Blood Glucose[5]	-	-	97%	97%
Perioperative Temperature Management[5]	-	-	99%	100%
Prophylactic Antibiotic Selection[5]	-	-	98%	99%
Prophylactic Antibiotic Selection (Outpatient)	-	-	98%	98%
Prophylactic Antibiotic Stopped[5]	-	-	98%	98%
Prophylactic Antibiotic Timing[5]	-	-	98%	99%
Prophylactic Antibiotic Timing (Outpatient)	-	-	96%	98%
Urinary Catheter Removal[5]	-	-	97%	97%
Survey of Patients' Hospital Experiences				
Area Around Room 'Always' Quiet at Night[10]	<100	67%	61%	61%
Doctors 'Always' Communicated Well[10]	<100	96%	78%	82%
Home Recovery Information Given[10]	<100	89%	83%	85%
Hospital Given 9 or 10 on 10 Point Scale[10]	<100	64%	65%	71%
Meds 'Always' Explained Before Given[10]	<100	85%	63%	64%
Nurses 'Always' Communicated Well[10]	<100	81%	76%	79%
Pain 'Always' Well Controlled[10]	<100	76%	68%	71%
Room and Bathroom 'Always' Clean[10]	<100	77%	70%	73%
Timely Help 'Always' Received[10]	<100	70%	66%	68%
Would Definitely Recommend Hospital[10]	<100	59%	63%	71%
Use of Medical Imaging				
Cardiac Imaging Stress Test before Surgery	-	-	4.2%	5.3%
Combination Abdominal CT Scan	-	-	9.6%	10.5%
Combination Brain/Sinus CT Scan	-	-	2.3%	2.7%
Combination Chest CT Scan	-	-	5.6%	2.7%
Follow-up Mammogram/Ultrasound	-	-	8.6%	8.8%
Lumbar Spine MRI for Low Back Pain	-	-	36.9%	37.2%

Guadalupe County Hospital

117 Camino De Vida, Suite 100
Santa Rosa, NM 88435
Phone: 575-472-3417
Fax: 505-472-4587
Type: Acute Care Hospitals
Emergency Services: No
Ownership: Government - Local
Beds: 12

Key Personnel:
Chief of Medical Staff . . . . Mubarak Khawaja
CEO/President . . . . Christina Tampos

Measure	Cases	This Hosp.	State Avg.	U.S. Avg.
Blood Clot Prevention and Treatment				
Anticoagulation Overlap Therapy[1,2]	-	-	96%	93%
ICU Venous Thromboembolism Prophylaxis[2,7]	-	-	92%	92%
Incidence of Potentially Preventable VTE[2,7]	-	-	3%	10%
UFH with Dosages/Platelet Monitoring[2,7]	-	-	99%	97%
Venous Thromboembolism Prophylaxis[2]	82	89%	84%	85%
Warfarin Therapy Discharge Instructions[1,2]	-	-	85%	75%
Chest Pain/Possible Heart Attack Care				
Aspirin Given Within 24 Hours of Arrival[1,3]	-	-	97%	96%
Fibrinolytic Meds Within 30 Min. of Arrival[1,3]	-	-	62%	58%
Average Time to ECG (minutes)[1,3]	-	-	9	7
Average Time to Transfer (minutes)[1,3]	-	-	99	60
Children's Asthma Care				
Received Home Management Plan of Care	-	-	-	88%
Received Reliever Medication	-	-	-	100%
Received Systemic Corticosteroids	-	-	-	100%
Emergency Department				
Admittance Decision Time (minutes)[2]	61	1	108	98
Head CT Results Within 45 Min. of Arrival[3,7]	-	-	46%	57%
Patients Who Left ER Before Being Seen[1]	-	-	4%	2%
Time from ER Arrival to Admit. (minutes)[2]	61	106	290	274
Time from ER Arrival to Discharge (minutes)	255	123	143	134
Time in ER Before Being Evaluated (minutes)	320	35	28	26
Time to Pain Meds for Fractures (minutes)[1,3]	-	-	57	57
Heart Attack Care				
Aspirin Given at Discharge[2,3]	-	-	99%	99%
Fibrinolytic Meds Within 30 Min. of Arrival[2,3]	-	-	75%	54%
PCI Within 90 Minutes of Arrival[2,3]	-	-	95%	96%
Statin Prescribed at Discharge[2,3]	-	-	99%	98%
Heart Failure Care				
ACE Inhibitor or ARB for LVSD[2,3]	-	-	97%	97%
Discharge Instructions Given[1,2]	-	-	89%	94%
Evaluation of LVS Function[1,2]	-	-	96%	99%
Medicare Spending				
Medicare Spending per Patient (ratio)	-	0.69	0.85	0.98
Pneumonia Care				
Appropriate Initial Antibiotic Given[2]	20	75%	93%	95%
Blood Culture Timing[1,2]	-	-	97%	98%
Pregnancy and Delivery Care				
Newborn Deliveries Scheduled Early[7]	-	-	3%	6%
Preventive Care				
Immunization for Influenza[2]	94	50%	86%	90%
Immunization for Pneumonia[2]	104	54%	89%	92%
Stroke Care				
Anticoagulation Therapy for Atrial Fibrillation[2,3]	-	-	96%	95%
Antithrombotic Therapy Timing[1,2]	-	-	94%	98%
Assessed for Rehabilitation[1,2]	-	-	95%	97%
Discharged on Antithrombotic Therapy[1,2]	-	-	97%	99%
Discharged on Statin Medication[2,3]	-	-	89%	94%
Thrombolytic Therapy Timing[2,3]	-	-	61%	66%
Venous Thromboembolism Prophylaxis[1,2]	-	-	91%	94%
Written Stroke Educational Materials Given[1,2]	-	-	73%	88%
Surgical Care Improvement Project				
Appropriate Beta Blocker Usage[5]	-	-	94%	98%
Appropriate VTP Within 24 Hours[5]	-	-	97%	98%
Controlled Postoperative Blood Glucose[5]	-	-	97%	97%
Perioperative Temperature Management[5]	-	-	99%	100%
Prophylactic Antibiotic Selection[5]	-	-	98%	99%
Prophylactic Antibiotic Selection (Outpatient)[5]	-	-	98%	98%
Prophylactic Antibiotic Stopped[5]	-	-	98%	98%
Prophylactic Antibiotic Timing[5]	-	-	98%	99%
Prophylactic Antibiotic Timing (Outpatient)[5]	-	-	96%	98%
Urinary Catheter Removal[5]	-	-	97%	97%
Survey of Patients' Hospital Experiences				
Area Around Room 'Always' Quiet at Night[10]	<100	74%	61%	61%
Doctors 'Always' Communicated Well[10]	<100	88%	78%	82%
Home Recovery Information Given[10]	<100	83%	83%	85%
Hospital Given 9 or 10 on 10 Point Scale[10]	<100	90%	65%	71%
Meds 'Always' Explained Before Given[10]	<100	78%	63%	64%
Nurses 'Always' Communicated Well[10]	<100	90%	76%	79%
Pain 'Always' Well Controlled[10]	<100	77%	68%	71%
Room and Bathroom 'Always' Clean[10]	<100	73%	70%	73%
Timely Help 'Always' Received[10]	<100	70%	66%	68%
Would Definitely Recommend Hospital[10]	<100	88%	63%	71%
Use of Medical Imaging				
Cardiac Imaging Stress Test before Surgery[7]	-	-	4.2%	5.3%
Combination Abdominal CT Scan[1]	-	-	9.6%	10.5%
Combination Brain/Sinus CT Scan[1]	-	-	2.3%	2.7%
Combination Chest CT Scan[1]	-	-	5.6%	2.7%
Follow-up Mammogram/Ultrasound[7]	-	-	8.6%	8.8%
Lumbar Spine MRI for Low Back Pain[1]	-	-	36.9%	37.2%

NOTE: Hospital profiles are in alphabetical order by state, then city, then hospital within the city; Rankings exclude hospitals with less than 25 cases except for patient surveys which excludes hospitals with less than 100 cases; (a) 100-299 cases; (1) The number of cases/patients is too few to report; (2) Data submitted were based on a sample of cases/patients; (3) Results are based on a shorter time period than required; (4) Data suppressed by CMS for one or more quarters; (5) Results are not available for this reporting period; (6) Fewer than 100 patients completed the HCAHPS survey; (7) No cases met the criteria for this measure; (8) The lower limit of the confidence interval cannot be calculated if the number of observed infections equals zero; (9) No data are available from the state/territory for this reporting period; (10) The scores shown reflect fewer than 50 completed surveys; (11) There were discrepancies in the data collection process; (12) This measure does not apply to this hospital for this reporting period; (13) Results cannot be calculated for this reporting period; (14) The results for this state are combined with nearby states to protect confidentiality; Please refer to the User's Guide for a full explanation of data.

Northern Navajo Medical Center

Us Hwy 491 North
Shiprock, NM 87420
Phone: 505-368-6001
Fax: 505-368-6260
URL: www.ihs.gov
Type: Acute Care Hospitals
Emergency Services: Yes
Ownership: Government - Federal
Beds: 55

Key Personnel:

CEO/President. . . . . Carla Baha-Al-Chesay
Emergency Room . . . . Steve Bowers
Operating Room. . . . . Sandy Collins
Anesthesiology. . . . . Donna Hausken, MD
Chief of Medical Staff . . . . John Mohs
Infection Control. . . . . Linda Schweigman, RN
Quality Assurance . . . . Pauline Stubberud
Pediatric In-Patient Care . . . . Donald Vasser

Measure	Cases	This Hosp.	State Avg.	U.S. Avg.
Blood Clot Prevention and Treatment				
Anticoagulation Overlap Therapy[1]	-	-	96%	93%
ICU Venous Thromboembolism Prophylaxis	11	100%	92%	92%
Incidence of Potentially Preventable VTE[1]	-	-	3%	10%
UFH with Dosages/Platelet Monitoring[7]	-	-	99%	97%
Venous Thromboembolism Prophylaxis	99	76%	84%	85%
Warfarin Therapy Discharge Instructions[1]	-	-	85%	75%
Chest Pain/Possible Heart Attack Care				
Aspirin Given Within 24 Hours of Arrival	-	-	97%	96%
Fibrinolytic Meds Within 30 Min. of Arrival	-	-	62%	58%
Average Time to ECG (minutes)	-	-	9	7
Average Time to Transfer (minutes)	-	-	99	60
Children's Asthma Care				
Received Home Management Plan of Care	-	-	-	88%
Received Reliever Medication	-	-	-	100%
Received Systemic Corticosteroids	-	-	-	100%
Emergency Department				
Admittance Decision Time (minutes)[2]	525	85	108	98
Head CT Results Within 45 Min. of Arrival	-	-	46%	57%
Patients Who Left ER Before Being Seen	-	-	4%	2%
Time from ER Arrival to Admit. (minutes)[2]	535	248	290	274
Time from ER Arrival to Discharge (minutes)	-	-	143	134
Time in ER Before Being Evaluated (minutes)	-	-	28	26
Time to Pain Meds for Fractures (minutes)	-	-	57	57
Heart Attack Care				
Aspirin Given at Discharge[5]	-	-	99%	99%
Fibrinolytic Meds Within 30 Min. of Arrival[5]	-	-	75%	54%
PCI Within 90 Minutes of Arrival[5]	-	-	95%	96%
Statin Prescribed at Discharge[5]	-	-	99%	98%
Heart Failure Care				
ACE Inhibitor or ARB for LVSD	15	100%	97%	97%
Discharge Instructions Given	40	80%	89%	94%
Evaluation of LVS Function	47	98%	96%	99%
Medicare Spending				
Medicare Spending per Patient (ratio)	-	0.76	0.85	0.98
Pneumonia Care				
Appropriate Initial Antibiotic Given	62	66%	93%	95%
Blood Culture Timing	38	95%	97%	98%
Pregnancy and Delivery Care				
Newborn Deliveries Scheduled Early	117	0%	3%	6%
Preventive Care				
Immunization for Influenza	465	81%	86%	90%
Immunization for Pneumonia	564	91%	89%	92%
Stroke Care				
Anticoagulation Therapy for Atrial Fibrillation[5]	-	-	96%	95%
Antithrombotic Therapy Timing[5]	-	-	94%	98%
Assessed for Rehabilitation[5]	-	-	95%	97%
Discharged on Antithrombotic Therapy[5]	-	-	97%	99%
Discharged on Statin Medication[5]	-	-	89%	94%
Thrombolytic Therapy Timing[5]	-	-	61%	66%
Venous Thromboembolism Prophylaxis[5]	-	-	91%	94%
Written Stroke Educational Materials Given[5]	-	-	73%	88%
Surgical Care Improvement Project				
Appropriate Beta Blocker Usage[1]	-	-	94%	98%
Appropriate VTP Within 24 Hours	36	75%	97%	98%
Controlled Postoperative Blood Glucose[7]	-	-	97%	97%
Perioperative Temperature Management	41	100%	99%	100%
Prophylactic Antibiotic Selection	14	86%	98%	99%
Prophylactic Antibiotic Selection (Outpatient)	-	-	98%	98%
Prophylactic Antibiotic Stopped	14	100%	98%	98%
Prophylactic Antibiotic Timing	14	100%	98%	99%
Prophylactic Antibiotic Timing (Outpatient)	-	-	96%	98%
Urinary Catheter Removal	13	92%	97%	97%
Survey of Patients' Hospital Experiences				
Area Around Room 'Always' Quiet at Night	(a)	43%	61%	61%
Doctors 'Always' Communicated Well	(a)	69%	78%	82%
Home Recovery Information Given	(a)	83%	83%	85%
Hospital Given 9 or 10 on 10 Point Scale	(a)	48%	65%	71%
Meds 'Always' Explained Before Given	(a)	61%	63%	64%
Nurses 'Always' Communicated Well	(a)	72%	76%	79%
Pain 'Always' Well Controlled	(a)	64%	68%	71%
Room and Bathroom 'Always' Clean	(a)	55%	70%	73%
Timely Help 'Always' Received	(a)	56%	66%	68%
Would Definitely Recommend Hospital	(a)	49%	63%	71%
Use of Medical Imaging				
Cardiac Imaging Stress Test before Surgery	-	-	4.2%	5.3%
Combination Abdominal CT Scan	-	-	9.6%	10.5%
Combination Brain/Sinus CT Scan	-	-	2.3%	2.7%
Combination Chest CT Scan	-	-	5.6%	2.7%
Follow-up Mammogram/Ultrasound	-	-	8.6%	8.8%
Lumbar Spine MRI for Low Back Pain	-	-	36.9%	37.2%

Gila Regional Medical Center

1313 E 32nd St
Silver City, NM 88061
Phone: 575-538-4000
Fax: 505-538-9714
URL: www.grmc.org
Type: Acute Care Hospitals
Emergency Services: Yes
Ownership: Govt - Hospital Dist/Auth
Beds: 68

Key Personnel:

Emergency Room . . . . Christine Brickley, MD
Radiology. . . . . James Burke
Quality Assurance . . . . Scott Campbell
CEO/President. . . . . John Rossfeld
Chief of Medical Staff . . . . Robert Wilcox, MD

Measure	Cases	This Hosp.	State Avg.	U.S. Avg.
Blood Clot Prevention and Treatment				
Anticoagulation Overlap Therapy[2]	44	61%	96%	93%
ICU Venous Thromboembolism Prophylaxis[2]	50	86%	92%	92%
Incidence of Potentially Preventable VTE[1,2]	-	-	3%	10%
UFH with Dosages/Platelet Monitoring[1,2]	-	-	99%	97%
Venous Thromboembolism Prophylaxis[2]	144	67%	84%	85%
Warfarin Therapy Discharge Instructions[2]	39	59%	85%	75%
Chest Pain/Possible Heart Attack Care				
Aspirin Given Within 24 Hours of Arrival	78	95%	97%	96%
Fibrinolytic Meds Within 30 Min. of Arrival	14	36%	62%	58%
Average Time to ECG (minutes)	80	8	9	7
Average Time to Transfer (minutes)[1]	-	-	99	60
Children's Asthma Care				
Received Home Management Plan of Care	-	-	-	88%
Received Reliever Medication	-	-	-	100%
Received Systemic Corticosteroids	-	-	-	100%
Emergency Department				
Admittance Decision Time (minutes)[2]	244	116	108	98
Head CT Results Within 45 Min. of Arrival[1]	-	-	46%	57%
Patients Who Left ER Before Being Seen	18,621	3%	4%	2%
Time from ER Arrival to Admit. (minutes)[2]	251	300	290	274
Time from ER Arrival to Discharge (minutes)	382	144	143	134
Time in ER Before Being Evaluated (minutes)	400	17	28	26
Time to Pain Meds for Fractures (minutes)	71	40	57	57
Heart Attack Care				
Aspirin Given at Discharge[1,3]	-	-	99%	99%
Fibrinolytic Meds Within 30 Min. of Arrival[3,7]	-	-	75%	54%
PCI Within 90 Minutes of Arrival[3,7]	-	-	95%	96%
Statin Prescribed at Discharge[1,3]	-	-	99%	98%
Heart Failure Care				
ACE Inhibitor or ARB for LVSD	17	100%	97%	97%
Discharge Instructions Given	52	63%	89%	94%
Evaluation of LVS Function	53	89%	96%	99%
Medicare Spending				
Medicare Spending per Patient (ratio)	-	0.91	0.85	0.98
Pneumonia Care				
Appropriate Initial Antibiotic Given	48	90%	93%	95%
Blood Culture Timing	82	98%	97%	98%
Pregnancy and Delivery Care				
Newborn Deliveries Scheduled Early	69	4%	3%	6%
Preventive Care				
Immunization for Influenza[2]	268	84%	86%	90%
Immunization for Pneumonia[2]	282	94%	89%	92%
Stroke Care				
Anticoagulation Therapy for Atrial Fibrillation[1]	-	-	96%	95%
Antithrombotic Therapy Timing	12	92%	94%	98%
Assessed for Rehabilitation[1]	-	-	95%	97%
Discharged on Antithrombotic Therapy[1]	-	-	97%	99%
Discharged on Statin Medication[1]	-	-	89%	94%
Thrombolytic Therapy Timing[7]	-	-	61%	66%
Venous Thromboembolism Prophylaxis	13	100%	91%	94%
Written Stroke Educational Materials Given[1]	-	-	73%	88%
Surgical Care Improvement Project				
Appropriate Beta Blocker Usage	58	95%	94%	98%
Appropriate VTP Within 24 Hours	282	98%	97%	98%
Controlled Postoperative Blood Glucose[7]	-	-	97%	97%
Perioperative Temperature Management	303	100%	99%	100%
Prophylactic Antibiotic Selection	255	87%	98%	99%
Prophylactic Antibiotic Selection (Outpatient)	36	89%	98%	98%
Prophylactic Antibiotic Stopped	242	97%	98%	98%
Prophylactic Antibiotic Timing	255	98%	98%	99%
Prophylactic Antibiotic Timing (Outpatient)	36	97%	96%	98%
Urinary Catheter Removal	195	98%	97%	97%
Survey of Patients' Hospital Experiences				
Area Around Room 'Always' Quiet at Night	300+	56%	61%	61%
Doctors 'Always' Communicated Well	300+	80%	78%	82%
Home Recovery Information Given	300+	87%	83%	85%
Hospital Given 9 or 10 on 10 Point Scale	300+	65%	65%	71%
Meds 'Always' Explained Before Given	300+	65%	63%	64%
Nurses 'Always' Communicated Well	300+	79%	76%	79%
Pain 'Always' Well Controlled	300+	67%	68%	71%
Room and Bathroom 'Always' Clean	300+	72%	70%	73%
Timely Help 'Always' Received	300+	71%	66%	68%
Would Definitely Recommend Hospital	300+	66%	63%	71%
Use of Medical Imaging				
Cardiac Imaging Stress Test before Surgery[1]	-	-	4.2%	5.3%
Combination Abdominal CT Scan	442	7.5%	9.6%	10.5%
Combination Brain/Sinus CT Scan	350	0.9%	2.3%	2.7%
Combination Chest CT Scan	254	0.8%	5.6%	2.7%
Follow-up Mammogram/Ultrasound	717	8.5%	8.6%	8.8%
Lumbar Spine MRI for Low Back Pain	68	32.4%	36.9%	37.2%

Socorro General Hospital

1202 Highway 60 West
Socorro, NM 87801
Phone: 575-835-1140
Fax: 505-835-8703
URL: www.phs.org
Type: Critical Access Hospitals
Emergency Services: Yes
Ownership: Proprietary

Key Personnel:

CEO/President. . . . . Bo Beames

Measure	Cases	This Hosp.	State Avg.	U.S. Avg.
Blood Clot Prevention and Treatment				
Anticoagulation Overlap Therapy[5]	-	-	96%	93%
ICU Venous Thromboembolism Prophylaxis[5]	-	-	92%	92%
Incidence of Potentially Preventable VTE[5]	-	-	3%	10%
UFH with Dosages/Platelet Monitoring[5]	-	-	99%	97%
Venous Thromboembolism Prophylaxis[5]	-	-	84%	85%
Warfarin Therapy Discharge Instructions[5]	-	-	85%	75%
Chest Pain/Possible Heart Attack Care				
Aspirin Given Within 24 Hours of Arrival	-	-	97%	96%
Fibrinolytic Meds Within 30 Min. of Arrival	-	-	62%	58%
Average Time to ECG (minutes)	-	-	9	7
Average Time to Transfer (minutes)	-	-	99	60
Children's Asthma Care				
Received Home Management Plan of Care	-	-	-	88%
Received Reliever Medication	-	-	-	100%
Received Systemic Corticosteroids	-	-	-	100%
Emergency Department				
Admittance Decision Time (minutes)[5]	-	-	108	98

NOTE: Hospital profiles are in alphabetical order by state, then city, then hospital within the city; Rankings exclude hospitals with less than 25 cases except for patient surveys which excludes hospitals with less than 100 cases; (a) 100-299 cases; (1) The number of cases/patients is too few to report; (2) Data submitted were based on a sample of cases/patients; (3) Results are based on a shorter time period than required; (4) Data suppressed by CMS for one or more quarters; (5) Results are not available for this reporting period; (6) Fewer than 100 patients completed the HCAHPS survey; (7) No cases met the criteria for this measure; (8) The lower limit of the confidence interval cannot be calculated if the number of observed infections equals zero; (9) No data are available from the state/territory for this reporting period; (10) The scores shown reflect fewer than 50 completed surveys; (11) There were discrepancies in the data collection process; (12) This measure does not apply to this hospital for this reporting period; (13) Results cannot be calculated for this reporting period; (14) The results for this state are combined with nearby states to protect confidentiality; Please refer to the User's Guide for a full explanation of data.

Measure	Cases	This Hosp.	State Avg.	U.S. Avg.
Head CT Results Within 45 Min. of Arrival	-	-	46%	57%
Patients Who Left ER Before Being Seen	-	-	4%	2%
Time from ER Arrival to Admit. (minutes)[5]	-	-	290	274
Time from ER Arrival to Discharge (minutes)	-	-	143	134
Time in ER Before Being Evaluated (minutes)	-	-	28	26
Time to Pain Meds for Fractures (minutes)	-	-	57	57
Heart Attack Care				
Aspirin Given at Discharge[5]	-	-	99%	99%
Fibrinolytic Meds Within 30 Min. of Arrival[5]	-	-	75%	54%
PCI Within 90 Minutes of Arrival[5]	-	-	95%	96%
Statin Prescribed at Discharge[5]	-	-	99%	98%
Heart Failure Care				
ACE Inhibitor or ARB for LVSD[1]	-	-	97%	97%
Discharge Instructions Given	14	100%	89%	94%
Evaluation of LVS Function	14	100%	96%	99%
Medicare Spending				
Medicare Spending per Patient (ratio)	-	-	0.85	0.98
Pneumonia Care				
Appropriate Initial Antibiotic Given	17	100%	93%	95%
Blood Culture Timing	17	100%	97%	98%
Pregnancy and Delivery Care				
Newborn Deliveries Scheduled Early[5]	-	-	3%	6%
Preventive Care				
Immunization for Influenza[5]	-	-	86%	90%
Immunization for Pneumonia[5]	-	-	89%	92%
Stroke Care				
Anticoagulation Therapy for Atrial Fibrillation[5]	-	-	96%	95%
Antithrombotic Therapy Timing[5]	-	-	94%	98%
Assessed for Rehabilitation[5]	-	-	95%	97%
Discharged on Antithrombotic Therapy[5]	-	-	97%	99%
Discharged on Statin Medication[5]	-	-	89%	94%
Thrombolytic Therapy Timing[5]	-	-	61%	66%
Venous Thromboembolism Prophylaxis[5]	-	-	91%	94%
Written Stroke Educational Materials Given[5]	-	-	73%	88%
Surgical Care Improvement Project				
Appropriate Beta Blocker Usage[7]	-	-	94%	98%
Appropriate VTP Within 24 Hours[1]	-	-	97%	98%
Controlled Postoperative Blood Glucose[7]	-	-	97%	97%
Perioperative Temperature Management	11	100%	99%	100%
Prophylactic Antibiotic Selection[1]	-	-	98%	99%
Prophylactic Antibiotic Selection (Outpatient)	-	-	98%	98%
Prophylactic Antibiotic Stopped[1]	-	-	98%	98%
Prophylactic Antibiotic Timing[1]	-	-	98%	99%
Prophylactic Antibiotic Timing (Outpatient)	-	-	96%	98%
Urinary Catheter Removal[7]	-	-	97%	97%
Survey of Patients' Hospital Experiences				
Area Around Room 'Always' Quiet at Night[6]	<100	67%	61%	61%
Doctors 'Always' Communicated Well[6]	<100	89%	78%	82%
Home Recovery Information Given[6]	<100	88%	83%	85%
Hospital Given 9 or 10 on 10 Point Scale[6]	<100	85%	65%	71%
Meds 'Always' Explained Before Given[6]	<100	77%	63%	64%
Nurses 'Always' Communicated Well[6]	<100	92%	76%	79%
Pain 'Always' Well Controlled[6]	<100	82%	68%	71%
Room and Bathroom 'Always' Clean[6]	<100	89%	70%	73%
Timely Help 'Always' Received[6]	<100	89%	66%	68%
Would Definitely Recommend Hospital[6]	<100	83%	63%	71%
Use of Medical Imaging				
Cardiac Imaging Stress Test before Surgery	-	-	4.2%	5.3%
Combination Abdominal CT Scan	-	-	9.6%	10.5%
Combination Brain/Sinus CT Scan	-	-	2.3%	2.7%
Combination Chest CT Scan	-	-	5.6%	2.7%
Follow-up Mammogram/Ultrasound	-	-	8.6%	8.8%
Lumbar Spine MRI for Low Back Pain	-	-	36.9%	37.2%

Sierra Vista Hospital

800 E Ninth Avenue
T Or C, NM 87901
Phone: 575-894-2111
Fax: 505-894-7659
Type: Critical Access Hospitals
Emergency Services: Yes
Ownership: Government - Local
Beds: 25

Key Personnel:

Emergency Room . . . . Dolly Creller, RN
Chief of Medical Staff. . . . . Mario Herrera
Infection Control. . . . . Mary Hubble, RN
Radiology. . . . . Paul Johnson
CEO/President. . . . . Domenica Rush, JR
Quality Assurance . . . . Sue Wortman, RN

Measure	Cases	This Hosp.	State Avg.	U.S. Avg.
Blood Clot Prevention and Treatment				
Anticoagulation Overlap Therapy[5]	-	-	96%	93%
ICU Venous Thromboembolism Prophylaxis[5]	-	-	92%	92%
Incidence of Potentially Preventable VTE[5]	-	-	3%	10%
UFH with Dosages/Platelet Monitoring[5]	-	-	99%	97%
Venous Thromboembolism Prophylaxis[5]	-	-	84%	85%
Warfarin Therapy Discharge Instructions[5]	-	-	85%	75%
Chest Pain/Possible Heart Attack Care				
Aspirin Given Within 24 Hours of Arrival	-	-	97%	96%
Fibrinolytic Meds Within 30 Min. of Arrival	-	-	62%	58%
Average Time to ECG (minutes)	-	-	9	7
Average Time to Transfer (minutes)	-	-	99	60
Children's Asthma Care				
Received Home Management Plan of Care	-	-	-	88%
Received Reliever Medication	-	-	-	100%
Received Systemic Corticosteroids	-	-	-	100%
Emergency Department				
Admittance Decision Time (minutes)[3]	112	54	108	98
Head CT Results Within 45 Min. of Arrival	-	-	46%	57%
Patients Who Left ER Before Being Seen	-	-	4%	2%
Time from ER Arrival to Admit. (minutes)[3]	113	247	290	274
Time from ER Arrival to Discharge (minutes)	-	-	143	134
Time in ER Before Being Evaluated (minutes)	-	-	28	26
Time to Pain Meds for Fractures (minutes)	-	-	57	57
Heart Attack Care				
Aspirin Given at Discharge[3,7]	-	-	99%	99%
Fibrinolytic Meds Within 30 Min. of Arrival[3,7]	-	-	75%	54%
PCI Within 90 Minutes of Arrival[3,7]	-	-	95%	96%
Statin Prescribed at Discharge[3,7]	-	-	99%	98%
Heart Failure Care				
ACE Inhibitor or ARB for LVSD[1]	-	-	97%	97%
Discharge Instructions Given[1]	-	-	89%	94%
Evaluation of LVS Function[1]	-	-	96%	99%
Medicare Spending				
Medicare Spending per Patient (ratio)	-	-	0.85	0.98
Pneumonia Care				
Appropriate Initial Antibiotic Given[2]	31	84%	93%	95%
Blood Culture Timing[2]	31	90%	97%	98%
Pregnancy and Delivery Care				
Newborn Deliveries Scheduled Early[3,7]	-	-	3%	6%
Preventive Care				
Immunization for Influenza[1,3]	-	-	86%	90%
Immunization for Pneumonia[3]	89	75%	89%	92%
Stroke Care				
Anticoagulation Therapy for Atrial Fibrillation[5]	-	-	96%	95%
Antithrombotic Therapy Timing[5]	-	-	94%	98%
Assessed for Rehabilitation[5]	-	-	95%	97%
Discharged on Antithrombotic Therapy[5]	-	-	97%	99%
Discharged on Statin Medication[5]	-	-	89%	94%
Thrombolytic Therapy Timing[5]	-	-	61%	66%
Venous Thromboembolism Prophylaxis[5]	-	-	91%	94%
Written Stroke Educational Materials Given[5]	-	-	73%	88%
Surgical Care Improvement Project				
Appropriate Beta Blocker Usage[5]	-	-	94%	98%
Appropriate VTP Within 24 Hours[5]	-	-	97%	98%
Controlled Postoperative Blood Glucose[5]	-	-	97%	97%
Perioperative Temperature Management[5]	-	-	99%	100%
Prophylactic Antibiotic Selection[5]	-	-	98%	99%
Prophylactic Antibiotic Selection (Outpatient)	-	-	98%	98%
Prophylactic Antibiotic Stopped[5]	-	-	98%	98%
Prophylactic Antibiotic Timing[5]	-	-	98%	99%
Prophylactic Antibiotic Timing (Outpatient)	-	-	96%	98%
Urinary Catheter Removal[5]	-	-	97%	97%
Survey of Patients' Hospital Experiences				
Area Around Room 'Always' Quiet at Night[5]	-	-	61%	61%
Doctors 'Always' Communicated Well[5]	-	-	78%	82%
Home Recovery Information Given[5]	-	-	83%	85%
Hospital Given 9 or 10 on 10 Point Scale[5]	-	-	65%	71%
Meds 'Always' Explained Before Given[5]	-	-	63%	64%
Nurses 'Always' Communicated Well[5]	-	-	76%	79%
Pain 'Always' Well Controlled[5]	-	-	68%	71%
Room and Bathroom 'Always' Clean[5]	-	-	70%	73%
Timely Help 'Always' Received[5]	-	-	66%	68%
Would Definitely Recommend Hospital[5]	-	-	63%	71%
Use of Medical Imaging				
Cardiac Imaging Stress Test before Surgery	-	-	4.2%	5.3%
Combination Abdominal CT Scan	-	-	9.6%	10.5%
Combination Brain/Sinus CT Scan	-	-	2.3%	2.7%
Combination Chest CT Scan	-	-	5.6%	2.7%
Follow-up Mammogram/Ultrasound	-	-	8.6%	8.8%
Lumbar Spine MRI for Low Back Pain	-	-	36.9%	37.2%

Holy Cross Hospital

1397 Weimer Road
Taos, NM 87571
Phone: 575-758-8883
Fax: 505-751-5719
E-mail: mcornum@taoshospital.org
URL: www.taoshospital.org
Type: Acute Care Hospitals
Emergency Services: Yes
Ownership: Voluntary non-profit - Private
Beds: 49

Key Personnel:

Operating Room. . . . . Linda Chase, RN
Quality Assurance . . . . Linda Chase
Emergency Room . . . . Lesa Fraker
Radiology. . . . . Paul Johnson
Anesthesiology. . . . . Jim Jones
Chief of Medical Staff . . . . Loretta Ortiz y Pino
Intensive Care Unit. . . . . Ashley Pond, MD
CEO/President. . . . . Warren K Spellman

Measure	Cases	This Hosp.	State Avg.	U.S. Avg.
Blood Clot Prevention and Treatment				
Anticoagulation Overlap Therapy[2]	14	100%	96%	93%
ICU Venous Thromboembolism Prophylaxis[2]	79	91%	92%	92%
Incidence of Potentially Preventable VTE[2,7]	-	-	3%	10%
UFH with Dosages/Platelet Monitoring[1,2]	-	-	99%	97%
Venous Thromboembolism Prophylaxis[2]	204	89%	84%	85%
Warfarin Therapy Discharge Instructions[2]	14	93%	85%	75%
Chest Pain/Possible Heart Attack Care				
Aspirin Given Within 24 Hours of Arrival	84	100%	97%	96%
Fibrinolytic Meds Within 30 Min. of Arrival[1]	-	-	62%	58%
Average Time to ECG (minutes)	85	13	9	7
Average Time to Transfer (minutes)[7]	-	-	99	60
Children's Asthma Care				
Received Home Management Plan of Care	-	-	-	88%
Received Reliever Medication	-	-	-	100%
Received Systemic Corticosteroids	-	-	-	100%
Emergency Department				
Admittance Decision Time (minutes)[2]	361	158	108	98
Head CT Results Within 45 Min. of Arrival[1]	-	-	46%	57%
Patients Who Left ER Before Being Seen	15,821	2%	4%	2%
Time from ER Arrival to Admit. (minutes)[2]	374	334	290	274
Time from ER Arrival to Discharge (minutes)	374	152	143	134
Time in ER Before Being Evaluated (minutes)	396	29	28	26
Time to Pain Meds for Fractures (minutes)	98	54	57	57
Heart Attack Care				
Aspirin Given at Discharge[1,3]	-	-	99%	99%
Fibrinolytic Meds Within 30 Min. of Arrival[3,7]	-	-	75%	54%
PCI Within 90 Minutes of Arrival[3,7]	-	-	95%	96%
Statin Prescribed at Discharge[3,7]	-	-	99%	98%
Heart Failure Care				
ACE Inhibitor or ARB for LVSD	14	100%	97%	97%
Discharge Instructions Given	44	100%	89%	94%
Evaluation of LVS Function	52	100%	96%	99%
Medicare Spending				
Medicare Spending per Patient (ratio)	-	0.83	0.85	0.98
Pneumonia Care				
Appropriate Initial Antibiotic Given	82	99%	93%	95%
Blood Culture Timing	116	100%	97%	98%
Pregnancy and Delivery Care				
Newborn Deliveries Scheduled Early	23	0%	3%	6%
Preventive Care				
Immunization for Influenza[2]	271	97%	86%	90%
Immunization for Pneumonia[2]	307	99%	89%	92%
Stroke Care				

NOTE: Hospital profiles are in alphabetical order by state, then city, then hospital within the city; Rankings exclude hospitals with less than 25 cases except for patient surveys which excludes hospitals with less than 100 cases; (a) 100-299 cases; (1) The number of cases/patients is too few to report; (2) Data submitted were based on a sample of cases/patients; (3) Results are based on a shorter time period than required; (4) Data suppressed by CMS for one or more quarters; (5) Results are not available for this reporting period; (6) Fewer than 100 patients completed the HCAHPS survey; (7) No cases met the criteria for this measure; (8) The lower limit of the confidence interval cannot be calculated if the number of observed infections equals zero; (9) No data are available from the state/territory for this reporting period; (10) The scores shown reflect fewer than 50 completed surveys; (11) There were discrepancies in the data collection process; (12) This measure does not apply to this hospital for this reporting period; (13) Results cannot be calculated for this reporting period; (14) The results for this state are combined with nearby states to protect confidentiality; Please refer to the User's Guide for a full explanation of data.

Measure	Cases	This Hosp.	State Avg.	U.S. Avg.
Anticoagulation Therapy for Atrial Fibrillation[1]	-	-	96%	95%
Antithrombotic Therapy Timing	17	100%	94%	98%
Assessed for Rehabilitation	17	100%	95%	97%
Discharged on Antithrombotic Therapy	17	100%	97%	99%
Discharged on Statin Medication	13	100%	89%	94%
Thrombolytic Therapy Timing[7]	-	-	61%	66%
Venous Thromboembolism Prophylaxis	18	100%	91%	94%
Written Stroke Educational Materials Given[1]	-	-	73%	88%
Surgical Care Improvement Project				
Appropriate Beta Blocker Usage	18	94%	94%	98%
Appropriate VTP Within 24 Hours	120	100%	97%	98%
Controlled Postoperative Blood Glucose[7]	-	-	97%	97%
Perioperative Temperature Management	125	100%	99%	100%
Prophylactic Antibiotic Selection	84	100%	98%	99%
Prophylactic Antibiotic Selection (Outpatient)	47	100%	98%	98%
Prophylactic Antibiotic Stopped	82	100%	98%	98%
Prophylactic Antibiotic Timing	84	99%	98%	99%
Prophylactic Antibiotic Timing (Outpatient)	31	100%	96%	98%
Urinary Catheter Removal	51	100%	97%	97%
Survey of Patients' Hospital Experiences				
Area Around Room 'Always' Quiet at Night	300+	61%	61%	61%
Doctors 'Always' Communicated Well	300+	79%	78%	82%
Home Recovery Information Given	300+	80%	83%	85%
Hospital Given 9 or 10 on 10 Point Scale	300+	69%	65%	71%
Meds 'Always' Explained Before Given	300+	60%	63%	64%
Nurses 'Always' Communicated Well	300+	77%	76%	79%
Pain 'Always' Well Controlled	300+	68%	68%	71%
Room and Bathroom 'Always' Clean	300+	70%	70%	73%
Timely Help 'Always' Received	300+	67%	66%	68%
Would Definitely Recommend Hospital	300+	70%	63%	71%
Use of Medical Imaging				
Cardiac Imaging Stress Test before Surgery	189	3.7%	4.2%	5.3%
Combination Abdominal CT Scan	279	3.2%	9.6%	10.5%
Combination Brain/Sinus CT Scan[1]	-	-	2.3%	2.7%
Combination Chest CT Scan	118	0.0%	5.6%	2.7%
Follow-up Mammogram/Ultrasound	546	11.2%	8.6%	8.8%
Lumbar Spine MRI for Low Back Pain[1]	-	-	36.9%	37.2%

Doctor Dan C Trigg Memorial Hospital

301 East Miel De Luna Avenue Phone: 575-461-7007
Tucumcari, NM 88401 Fax: 505-461-7272
URL: www.phs.org/facilities/tucumcari
Type: Critical Access Hospitals Emergency Services: Yes
Ownership: Voluntary non-profit - Private Beds: 25

Key Personnel:
CEO/President. . . . . Bo Beames
Chief of Medical Staff. . . . . John Faith
Emergency Room . . . . Twila Loudder
Quality Assurance . . . . Linda Marquez

Measure	Cases	This Hosp.	State Avg.	U.S. Avg.
Blood Clot Prevention and Treatment				
Anticoagulation Overlap Therapy[5]	-	-	96%	93%
ICU Venous Thromboembolism Prophylaxis[5]	-	-	92%	92%
Incidence of Potentially Preventable VTE[5]	-	-	3%	10%
UFH with Dosages/Platelet Monitoring[5]	-	-	99%	97%
Venous Thromboembolism Prophylaxis[5]	-	-	84%	85%
Warfarin Therapy Discharge Instructions[5]	-	-	85%	75%
Chest Pain/Possible Heart Attack Care				
Aspirin Given Within 24 Hours of Arrival	-	-	97%	96%
Fibrinolytic Meds Within 30 Min. of Arrival	-	-	62%	58%
Average Time to ECG (minutes)	-	-	9	7
Average Time to Transfer (minutes)	-	-	99	60
Children's Asthma Care				
Received Home Management Plan of Care	-	-	-	88%
Received Reliever Medication	-	-	-	100%
Received Systemic Corticosteroids	-	-	-	100%
Emergency Department				
Admittance Decision Time (minutes)[5]	-	-	108	98
Head CT Results Within 45 Min. of Arrival	-	-	46%	57%
Patients Who Left ER Before Being Seen	-	-	4%	2%
Time from ER Arrival to Admit. (minutes)[5]	-	-	290	274
Time from ER Arrival to Discharge (minutes)	-	-	143	134
Time in ER Before Being Evaluated (minutes)	-	-	28	26
Time to Pain Meds for Fractures (minutes)	-	-	57	57
Heart Attack Care				
Aspirin Given at Discharge[5]	-	-	99%	99%
Fibrinolytic Meds Within 30 Min. of Arrival[5]	-	-	75%	54%
PCI Within 90 Minutes of Arrival[5]	-	-	95%	96%
Statin Prescribed at Discharge[5]	-	-	99%	98%
Heart Failure Care				
ACE Inhibitor or ARB for LVSD[7]	-	-	97%	97%
Discharge Instructions Given[1]	-	-	89%	94%
Evaluation of LVS Function[1]	-	-	96%	99%
Medicare Spending				
Medicare Spending per Patient (ratio)	-	-	0.85	0.98
Pneumonia Care				
Appropriate Initial Antibiotic Given	15	100%	93%	95%
Blood Culture Timing	18	100%	97%	98%
Pregnancy and Delivery Care				
Newborn Deliveries Scheduled Early[5]	-	-	3%	6%
Preventive Care				
Immunization for Influenza[5]	-	-	86%	90%
Immunization for Pneumonia[5]	-	-	89%	92%
Stroke Care				
Anticoagulation Therapy for Atrial Fibrillation[5]	-	-	96%	95%
Antithrombotic Therapy Timing[5]	-	-	94%	98%
Assessed for Rehabilitation[5]	-	-	95%	97%
Discharged on Antithrombotic Therapy[5]	-	-	97%	99%
Discharged on Statin Medication[5]	-	-	89%	94%
Thrombolytic Therapy Timing[5]	-	-	61%	66%
Venous Thromboembolism Prophylaxis[5]	-	-	91%	94%
Written Stroke Educational Materials Given[5]	-	-	73%	88%
Surgical Care Improvement Project				
Appropriate Beta Blocker Usage[5]	-	-	94%	98%
Appropriate VTP Within 24 Hours[5]	-	-	97%	98%
Controlled Postoperative Blood Glucose[5]	-	-	97%	97%
Perioperative Temperature Management[5]	-	-	99%	100%
Prophylactic Antibiotic Selection[5]	-	-	98%	99%
Prophylactic Antibiotic Selection (Outpatient)	-	-	98%	98%
Prophylactic Antibiotic Stopped[5]	-	-	98%	98%
Prophylactic Antibiotic Timing[5]	-	-	98%	99%
Prophylactic Antibiotic Timing (Outpatient)	-	-	96%	98%
Urinary Catheter Removal[5]	-	-	97%	97%
Survey of Patients' Hospital Experiences				
Area Around Room 'Always' Quiet at Night[6]	<100	62%	61%	61%
Doctors 'Always' Communicated Well[6]	<100	80%	78%	82%
Home Recovery Information Given[6]	<100	79%	83%	85%
Hospital Given 9 or 10 on 10 Point Scale[6]	<100	69%	65%	71%
Meds 'Always' Explained Before Given[6]	<100	62%	63%	64%
Nurses 'Always' Communicated Well[6]	<100	84%	76%	79%
Pain 'Always' Well Controlled[6]	<100	70%	68%	71%
Room and Bathroom 'Always' Clean[6]	<100	77%	70%	73%
Timely Help 'Always' Received[6]	<100	81%	66%	68%
Would Definitely Recommend Hospital[6]	<100	59%	63%	71%
Use of Medical Imaging				
Cardiac Imaging Stress Test before Surgery	-	-	4.2%	5.3%
Combination Abdominal CT Scan	-	-	9.6%	10.5%
Combination Brain/Sinus CT Scan	-	-	2.3%	2.7%
Combination Chest CT Scan	-	-	5.6%	2.7%
Follow-up Mammogram/Ultrasound	-	-	8.6%	8.8%
Lumbar Spine MRI for Low Back Pain	-	-	36.9%	37.2%

Zuni Comprehensive Community Health Center

Route 301 North B Street Phone: 505-782-4431
Zuni, NM 87327 Fax: 505-782-7405
URL: www.ihs.gov
Type: Acute Care Hospitals Emergency Services: Yes
Ownership: Government - Federal Beds: 45

Key Personnel:
Chief of Medical Staff. . . . . Robert DeMartino, MD
Quality Assurance . . . . Rebecca Grizzle

Measure	Cases	This Hosp.	State Avg.	U.S. Avg.
Blood Clot Prevention and Treatment				
Anticoagulation Overlap Therapy[2,7]	-	-	96%	93%
ICU Venous Thromboembolism Prophylaxis[1,2]	-	-	92%	92%
Incidence of Potentially Preventable VTE[2,7]	-	-	3%	10%
UFH with Dosages/Platelet Monitoring[2,7]	-	-	99%	97%
Venous Thromboembolism Prophylaxis[2]	119	76%	84%	85%
Warfarin Therapy Discharge Instructions[2,7]	-	-	85%	75%
Chest Pain/Possible Heart Attack Care				
Aspirin Given Within 24 Hours of Arrival[5]	-	-	97%	96%
Fibrinolytic Meds Within 30 Min. of Arrival[5]	-	-	62%	58%
Average Time to ECG (minutes)[5]	-	-	9	7
Average Time to Transfer (minutes)[5]	-	-	99	60
Children's Asthma Care				
Received Home Management Plan of Care	-	-	-	88%
Received Reliever Medication	-	-	-	100%
Received Systemic Corticosteroids	-	-	-	100%
Emergency Department				
Admittance Decision Time (minutes)[2]	23	72	108	98
Head CT Results Within 45 Min. of Arrival[5]	-	-	46%	57%
Patients Who Left ER Before Being Seen[5]	-	-	4%	2%
Time from ER Arrival to Admit. (minutes)[2]	34	270	290	274
Time from ER Arrival to Discharge (minutes)[5]	-	-	143	134
Time in ER Before Being Evaluated (minutes)[5]	-	-	28	26
Time to Pain Meds for Fractures (minutes)[5]	-	-	57	57
Heart Attack Care				
Aspirin Given at Discharge[5]	-	-	99%	99%
Fibrinolytic Meds Within 30 Min. of Arrival[5]	-	-	75%	54%
PCI Within 90 Minutes of Arrival[5]	-	-	95%	96%
Statin Prescribed at Discharge[5]	-	-	99%	98%
Heart Failure Care				
ACE Inhibitor or ARB for LVSD[1,2]	-	-	97%	97%
Discharge Instructions Given[1,2]	-	-	89%	94%
Evaluation of LVS Function[1,2]	-	-	96%	99%
Medicare Spending				
Medicare Spending per Patient (ratio)	-	0.60	0.85	0.98
Pneumonia Care				
Appropriate Initial Antibiotic Given[2,7]	-	-	93%	95%
Blood Culture Timing[1,2]	-	-	97%	98%
Pregnancy and Delivery Care				
Newborn Deliveries Scheduled Early[2]	12	75%	3%	6%
Preventive Care				
Immunization for Influenza[2]	190	54%	86%	90%
Immunization for Pneumonia[2]	183	81%	89%	92%
Stroke Care				
Anticoagulation Therapy for Atrial Fibrillation[2,3]	-	-	96%	95%
Antithrombotic Therapy Timing[2,3]	-	-	94%	98%
Assessed for Rehabilitation[1,2]	-	-	95%	97%
Discharged on Antithrombotic Therapy[2,3]	-	-	97%	99%
Discharged on Statin Medication[2,3]	-	-	89%	94%
Thrombolytic Therapy Timing[2,3]	-	-	61%	66%
Venous Thromboembolism Prophylaxis[1,2]	-	-	91%	94%
Written Stroke Educational Materials Given[2,3]	-	-	73%	88%
Surgical Care Improvement Project				
Appropriate Beta Blocker Usage[5]	-	-	94%	98%
Appropriate VTP Within 24 Hours[5]	-	-	97%	98%
Controlled Postoperative Blood Glucose[5]	-	-	97%	97%
Perioperative Temperature Management[5]	-	-	99%	100%
Prophylactic Antibiotic Selection[5]	-	-	98%	99%
Prophylactic Antibiotic Selection (Outpatient)[5]	-	-	98%	98%
Prophylactic Antibiotic Stopped[5]	-	-	98%	98%
Prophylactic Antibiotic Timing[5]	-	-	98%	99%
Prophylactic Antibiotic Timing (Outpatient)[5]	-	-	96%	98%
Urinary Catheter Removal[5]	-	-	97%	97%
Survey of Patients' Hospital Experiences				
Area Around Room 'Always' Quiet at Night[6]	<100	53%	61%	61%
Doctors 'Always' Communicated Well[6]	<100	67%	78%	82%
Home Recovery Information Given[6]	<100	86%	83%	85%
Hospital Given 9 or 10 on 10 Point Scale[6]	<100	67%	65%	71%
Meds 'Always' Explained Before Given[6]	<100	53%	63%	64%
Nurses 'Always' Communicated Well[6]	<100	65%	76%	79%
Pain 'Always' Well Controlled[6]	<100	57%	68%	71%
Room and Bathroom 'Always' Clean[6]	<100	78%	70%	73%
Timely Help 'Always' Received[6]	<100	71%	66%	68%
Would Definitely Recommend Hospital[6]	<100	40%	63%	71%
Use of Medical Imaging				
Cardiac Imaging Stress Test before Surgery[7]	-	-	4.2%	5.3%

NOTE: Hospital profiles are in alphabetical order by state, then city, then hospital within the city; Rankings exclude hospitals with less than 25 cases except for patient surveys which excludes hospitals with less than 100 cases; (a) 100-299 cases; (1) The number of cases/patients is too few to report; (2) Data submitted were based on a sample of cases/patients; (3) Results are based on a shorter time period than required; (4) Data suppressed by CMS for one or more quarters; (5) Results are not available for this reporting period; (6) Fewer than 100 patients completed the HCAHPS survey; (7) No cases met the criteria for this measure; (8) The lower limit of the confidence interval cannot be calculated if the number of observed infections equals zero; (9) No data are available from the state/territory for this reporting period; (10) The scores shown reflect fewer than 50 completed surveys; (11) There were discrepancies in the data collection process; (12) This measure does not apply to this hospital for this reporting period; (13) Results cannot be calculated for this reporting period; (14) The results for this state are combined with nearby states to protect confidentiality; Please refer to the User's Guide for a full explanation of data.

Combination Abdominal CT Scan[7]	-	-	9.6%	10.5%
Combination Brain/Sinus CT Scan[7]	-	-	2.3%	2.7%
Combination Chest CT Scan[7]	-	-	5.6%	2.7%
Follow-up Mammogram/Ultrasound[7]	-	-	8.6%	8.8%
Lumbar Spine MRI for Low Back Pain[7]	-	-	36.9%	37.2%

NOTE: Hospital profiles are in alphabetical order by state, then city, then hospital within the city; Rankings exclude hospitals with less than 25 cases except for patient surveys which excludes hospitals with less than 100 cases; (a) 100-299 cases; (1) The number of cases/patients is too few to report; (2) Data submitted were based on a sample of cases/patients; (3) Results are based on a shorter time period than required; (4) Data suppressed by CMS for one or more quarters; (5) Results are not available for this reporting period; (6) Fewer than 100 patients completed the HCAHPS survey; (7) No cases met the criteria for this measure; (8) The lower limit of the confidence interval cannot be calculated if the number of observed infections equals zero; (9) No data are available from the state/territory for this reporting period; (10) The scores shown reflect fewer than 50 completed surveys; (11) There were discrepancies in the data collection process; (12) This measure does not apply to this hospital for this reporting period; (13) Results cannot be calculated for this reporting period; (14) The results for this state are combined with nearby states to protect confidentiality; Please refer to the User's Guide for a full explanation of data.

Blood Clot Prevention and Treatment

Anticoagulation Overlap Therapy

Hospital Name	City	Rate	Cases
Asante Three Rivers Medical Center[2]	Grants Pass	100%	44
Legacy Emanuel Medical Center[2]	Portland	100%	71
Legacy Good Samaritan Medical Center[2]	Portland	100%	45
Legacy Meridian Park Medical Center[2]	Tualatin	100%	38
Saint Alphonsus Medical Center - Ontario[2]	Ontario	100%	25
Tuality Community Hospital[2]	Hillsboro	100%	25
Willamette Valley Medical Center[2]	Mcminnville	100%	28
Asante Rogue Regional Medical Center[2]	Medford	99%	120
Kaiser Sunnyside Medical Center[2]	Clackamas	98%	117
Providence Medford Medical Center[2]	Medford	98%	59
Providence Saint Vincent Medical Center[2]	Portland	98%	128
Saint Charles Medical Center - Bend[2]	Bend	98%	55
Adventist Medical Center[2]	Portland	97%	62
Bay Area Hospital[2]	Coos Bay	97%	30
Sacred Heart Medical Center - Riverbend[2]	Springfield	97%	128
Good Samaritan Regional Medical Center[2]	Corvallis	96%	54
Saint Charles Medical Center - Redmond[2]	Redmond	96%	25
Salem Hospital[2]	Salem	96%	153
OHSU Hospital & Clinics[2]	Portland	94%	69
Providence Portland Medical Center[2]	Portland	93%	138
Sky Lakes Medical Center[2]	Klamath Falls	89%	75
Providence Milwaukie Hospital[2]	Milwaukie	85%	27
Mercy Medical Center[2]	Roseburg	80%	56

ICU Venous Thromboembolism Prophylaxis

Hospital Name	City	Rate	Cases
McKenzie - Willamette Medical Center[2]	Springfield	100%	121
Mid - Columbia Medical Center[2]	The Dalles	100%	26
Peace Harbor Medical Center[2]	Florence	100%	52
Willamette Valley Medical Center[2]	Mcminnville	100%	53
Legacy Mount Hood Medical Center[2]	Gresham	97%	66
Sky Lakes Medical Center[2]	Klamath Falls	97%	36
Good Shepherd Medical Center[2]	Hermiston	96%	47
Kaiser Sunnyside Medical Center[2]	Clackamas	96%	55
Saint Alphonsus Medical Center - Ontario[2]	Ontario	96%	47
Salem Hospital[2]	Salem	96%	133
Samaritan Lebanon Community Hospital[2]	Lebanon	96%	45
Legacy Meridian Park Medical Center[2]	Tualatin	95%	60
Legacy Emanuel Medical Center[2]	Portland	94%	155
Providence Saint Vincent Medical Center[2]	Portland	94%	308
Legacy Good Samaritan Medical Center[2]	Portland	93%	87
Sacred Heart Medical Center - Riverbend[2]	Springfield	92%	53
Saint Charles Medical Center - Bend[2]	Bend	92%	63
Asante Rogue Regional Medical Center[2]	Medford	90%	113
Tuality Community Hospital[2]	Hillsboro	90%	48
Samaritan Pacific Communities Hospital[2]	Newport	89%	27
OHSU Hospital & Clinics[2]	Portland	88%	139
Providence Willamette Falls Med Ctr[2]	Oregon City	88%	174
Mercy Medical Center[2]	Roseburg	85%	84
Providence Newberg Medical Center[2]	Newberg	85%	158
Saint Charles Medical Center - Redmond[2]	Redmond	85%	27
Samaritan Albany General Hospital[2]	Albany	85%	54
Providence Medford Medical Center[2]	Medford	84%	400
Adventist Medical Center[2]	Portland	83%	59
Providence Seaside Hospital[2]	Seaside	82%	103
Good Samaritan Regional Medical Center[2]	Corvallis	81%	53
Providence Portland Medical Center[2]	Portland	79%	419
Asante Three Rivers Medical Center[2]	Grants Pass	78%	73
Providence Hood River Memorial Hospital[2]	Hood River	73%	67
Providence Milwaukie Hospital[2]	Milwaukie	70%	177
Samaritan North Lincoln Hospital[2]	Lincoln City	69%	36
Bay Area Hospital[2]	Coos Bay	56%	55

Incidence of Potentially Preventable VTE

Hospital Name	City	Rate	Cases
Legacy Emanuel Medical Center[2]	Portland	3%	37
OHSU Hospital & Clinics[2]	Portland	5%	66
Providence Portland Medical Center[2]	Portland	13%	30
Providence Saint Vincent Medical Center[2]	Portland	24%	41
Kaiser Sunnyside Medical Center[2]	Clackamas	36%	25

UFH with Dosages/Platelet Count Monitoring

Hospital Name	City	Rate	Cases
Kaiser Sunnyside Medical Center[2]	Clackamas	100%	59
Legacy Emanuel Medical Center[2]	Portland	100%	26
Mercy Medical Center[2]	Roseburg	100%	28
OHSU Hospital & Clinics[2]	Portland	100%	42
Providence Medford Medical Center[2]	Medford	100%	25
Providence Portland Medical Center[2]	Portland	100%	30
Providence Saint Vincent Medical Center[2]	Portland	100%	54
Sacred Heart Medical Center - Riverbend[2]	Springfield	100%	48
Salem Hospital[2]	Salem	100%	130
Sky Lakes Medical Center[2]	Klamath Falls	100%	28
Good Samaritan Regional Medical Center[2]	Corvallis	98%	50

Venous Thromboembolism Prophylaxis

Hospital Name	City	Rate	Cases
Asante Ashland Community Hospital[2]	Ashland	100%	86
Willamette Valley Medical Center[2]	Mcminnville	100%	255
McKenzie - Willamette Medical Center[2]	Springfield	98%	331
Peace Harbor Medical Center[2]	Florence	98%	64
Mid - Columbia Medical Center[2]	The Dalles	97%	151
Samaritan Lebanon Community Hospital[2]	Lebanon	96%	94
Sky Lakes Medical Center[2]	Klamath Falls	96%	388
Sacred Heart University District[2]	Eugene	93%	103
Saint Charles Medical Center - Redmond[2]	Redmond	93%	107
Tillamook Regional Medical Center[2]	Tillamook	93%	68
Good Shepherd Medical Center[2]	Hermiston	92%	132
Legacy Good Samaritan Medical Center[2]	Portland	92%	283
Samaritan Pacific Communities Hospital[2]	Newport	92%	93
Kaiser Sunnyside Medical Center[2]	Clackamas	91%	266
Legacy Meridian Park Medical Center[2]	Tualatin	89%	270
Salem Hospital[2]	Salem	89%	384
Legacy Mount Hood Medical Center[2]	Gresham	86%	265
Sacred Heart Medical Center - Riverbend[2]	Springfield	86%	298
Saint Alphonsus Medical Center - Ontario[2]	Ontario	86%	111
Santiam Memorial Hospital[2]	Stayton	86%	98
Providence Medford Medical Center[2]	Medford	85%	105
Providence Saint Vincent Medical Center[2]	Portland	85%	190
Good Samaritan Regional Medical Center[2]	Corvallis	84%	313
Providence Willamette Falls Med Ctr[2]	Oregon City	84%	147
Providence Newberg Medical Center[2]	Newberg	83%	52
Samaritan Albany General Hospital[2]	Albany	83%	180
Providence Portland Medical Center[2]	Portland	82%	115
Saint Charles Medical Center - Bend[2]	Bend	82%	248
Asante Rogue Regional Medical Center[2]	Medford	81%	281
Legacy Emanuel Medical Center[2]	Portland	80%	234
Tuality Community Hospital[2]	Hillsboro	80%	311
Adventist Medical Center[2]	Portland	78%	262
Silverton Hospital[2]	Silverton	77%	95
OHSU Hospital & Clinics[2]	Portland	76%	269
Samaritan North Lincoln Hospital[2]	Lincoln City	73%	62
Peacehealth Cottage Grove Comm Med Ctr[2]	Cottage Grove	68%	120
Asante Three Rivers Medical Center[2]	Grants Pass	65%	279
Providence Milwaukie Hospital[2]	Milwaukie	61%	121
Mercy Medical Center[2]	Roseburg	60%	311
Bay Area Hospital[2]	Coos Bay	59%	290
Providence Hood River Memorial Hospital[2]	Hood River	57%	42
Lake District Hospital[2]	Lakeview	32%	153

Warfarin Therapy Discharge Instructions

Hospital Name	City	Rate	Cases
Asante Three Rivers Medical Center[2]	Grants Pass	100%	29
OHSU Hospital & Clinics[2]	Portland	100%	40
Legacy Emanuel Medical Center[2]	Portland	98%	50
Legacy Good Samaritan Medical Center[2]	Portland	95%	41
Legacy Mount Hood Medical Center[2]	Gresham	92%	25
Sky Lakes Medical Center[2]	Klamath Falls	90%	60
Asante Rogue Regional Medical Center[2]	Medford	89%	98
Legacy Meridian Park Medical Center[2]	Tualatin	85%	34
Saint Charles Medical Center - Bend[2]	Bend	81%	42
Adventist Medical Center[2]	Portland	79%	53
Sacred Heart Medical Center - Riverbend[2]	Springfield	78%	103
Good Samaritan Regional Medical Center[2]	Corvallis	76%	45
Salem Hospital[2]	Salem	25%	126
Providence Saint Vincent Medical Center[2]	Portland	13%	102
Providence Medford Medical Center[2]	Medford	9%	58
Kaiser Sunnyside Medical Center[2]	Clackamas	6%	100
Providence Portland Medical Center[2]	Portland	4%	108
Mercy Medical Center[2]	Roseburg	2%	48

Chest Pain/Possible Heart Attack Care

Aspirin Given Within 24 Hours of Arrival

Hospital Name	City	Rate	Cases
Coquille Valley Hospital District	Coquille	100%	30
Legacy Mount Hood Medical Center	Gresham	100%	58
Peace Harbor Medical Center	Florence	100%	50
Peacehealth Cottage Grove Comm Med Ctr	Cottage Grove	100%	31
Providence Hood River Memorial Hospital	Hood River	100%	25
Providence Newberg Medical Center	Newberg	100%	45
Providence Seaside Hospital	Seaside	100%	36
Sacred Heart University District	Eugene	100%	32
Samaritan Albany General Hospital	Albany	100%	37
West Valley Hospital	Dallas	100%	49
Asante Three Rivers Medical Center	Grants Pass	99%	82
Providence Willamette Falls Med Ctr	Oregon City	98%	53
Mid - Columbia Medical Center	The Dalles	97%	77
Providence Milwaukie Hospital	Milwaukie	97%	72
Providence Saint Vincent Medical Center	Portland	97%	32
Saint Alphonsus Medical Center - Ontario	Ontario	97%	67
Bay Area Hospital	Coos Bay	96%	54
Salem Hospital	Salem	94%	36
Silverton Hospital	Silverton	93%	76
Saint Charles Medical Center - Redmond	Redmond	84%	32
Santiam Memorial Hospital	Stayton	81%	27

Average Time to ECG (minutes)

Hospital Name	City	Min.	Cases
Providence Saint Vincent Medical Center	Portland	3	32
Mid - Columbia Medical Center	The Dalles	5	78
Providence Newberg Medical Center	Newberg	5	45
Providence Seaside Hospital	Seaside	6	36
West Valley Hospital	Dallas	6	51
Bay Area Hospital	Coos Bay	7	56
Providence Willamette Falls Med Ctr	Oregon City	7	56
Peace Harbor Medical Center	Florence	8	51
Providence Hood River Memorial Hospital	Hood River	8	25
Providence Milwaukie Hospital	Milwaukie	8	73
Coquille Valley Hospital District	Coquille	9	32
Legacy Mount Hood Medical Center	Gresham	9	60
Peacehealth Cottage Grove Comm Med Ctr	Cottage Grove	9	32
Saint Alphonsus Medical Center - Ontario	Ontario	9	70
Silverton Hospital	Silverton	9	82
Saint Charles Medical Center - Redmond	Redmond	10	32
Santiam Memorial Hospital	Stayton	10	29
Sacred Heart University District	Eugene	12	34
Salem Hospital	Salem	12	38
Samaritan Albany General Hospital	Albany	15	39
Asante Three Rivers Medical Center	Grants Pass	18	85

Average Time to Transfer (minutes)

Hospital Name	City	Min.	Cases
Legacy Mount Hood Medical Center	Gresham	51	29
Asante Three Rivers Medical Center	Grants Pass	53	30

Children's Asthma Care

Received Home Management Plan of Care

Hospital Name	City	Rate	Cases
Legacy Emanuel Medical Center	Portland	88%	184

Received Reliever Medication

Hospital Name	City	Rate	Cases
Legacy Emanuel Medical Center	Portland	100%	184

Received Systemic Corticosteroids

Hospital Name	City	Rate	Cases
Legacy Emanuel Medical Center	Portland	100%	184

Emergency Department

Admittance Decision Time (minutes)

Hospital Name	City	Min.	Cases
Lake District Hospital[2]	Lakeview	26	144
Samaritan Albany General Hospital[2]	Albany	44	196
Tuality Community Hospital[2]	Hillsboro	45	422
Bay Area Hospital[2]	Coos Bay	48	496
Peace Harbor Medical Center[2]	Florence	48	387
Harney District Hospital[2]	Burns	50	121
Peacehealth Cottage Grove Comm Med Ctr[2]	Cottage Grove	50	270
Silverton Hospital[2]	Silverton	55	180
Samaritan North Lincoln Hospital[2]	Lincoln City	61	220
Good Samaritan Regional Medical Center[2]	Corvallis	63	434
Pioneer Memorial Hospital[2]	Prineville	65	279
Sacred Heart University District[2]	Eugene	65	427
Providence Willamette Falls Med Ctr[2]	Oregon City	70	274
Saint Charles Medical Center - Redmond[2]	Redmond	71	260
Samaritan Pacific Communities Hospital[2]	Newport	74	260
Santiam Memorial Hospital[2]	Stayton	75	269
Mercy Medical Center[2]	Roseburg	79	738
Sacred Heart Medical Center - Riverbend[2]	Springfield	79	467
Kaiser Sunnyside Medical Center[2]	Clackamas	81	406
Providence Milwaukie Hospital[2]	Milwaukie	81	432
Asante Ashland Community Hospital[2]	Ashland	82	249
Asante Three Rivers Medical Center[2]	Grants Pass	82	378
Legacy Mount Hood Medical Center[2]	Gresham	85	706
Providence Saint Vincent Medical Center[2]	Portland	86	521
Providence Portland Medical Center[2]	Portland	87	378
Adventist Medical Center[2]	Portland	89	523
Legacy Meridian Park Medical Center[2]	Tualatin	89	675
Legacy Emanuel Medical Center[2]	Portland	90	600
McKenzie - Willamette Medical Center[2]	Springfield	90	481
Providence Newberg Medical Center[2]	Newberg	91	293
Saint Charles Medical Center - Bend[2]	Bend	92	376
Samaritan Lebanon Community Hospital[2]	Lebanon	94	242
Good Shepherd Medical Center[2]	Hermiston	96	392
Providence Seaside Hospital[2]	Seaside	96	311
Willamette Valley Medical Center[2]	Mcminnville	100	455
Salem Hospital[2]	Salem	101	517
Saint Alphonsus Medical Center - Ontario[2]	Ontario	104	189
Providence Hood River Memorial Hospital[2]	Hood River	106	170

NOTE: Hospital profiles are in alphabetical order by state, then city, then hospital within the city; Rankings exclude hospitals with less than 25 cases except for patient surveys which excludes hospitals with less than 100 cases; (a) 100-299 cases; (1) The number of cases/patients is too few to report; (2) Data submitted were based on a sample of cases/patients; (3) Results are based on a shorter time period than required; (4) Data suppressed by CMS for one or more quarters; (5) Results are not available for this reporting period; (6) Fewer than 100 patients completed the HCAHPS survey; (7) No cases met the criteria for this measure; (8) The lower limit of the confidence interval cannot be calculated if the number of observed infections equals zero; (9) No data are available from the state/territory for this reporting period; (10) The scores shown reflect fewer than 50 completed surveys; (11) There were discrepancies in the data collection process; (12) This measure does not apply to this hospital for this reporting period; (13) Results cannot be calculated for this reporting period; (14) The results for this state are combined with nearby states to protect confidentiality; Please refer to the User's Guide for a full explanation of data.

OHSU Hospital & Clinics[2]	Portland	109	232
Legacy Good Samaritan Medical Center[2]	Portland	112	560
Mid - Columbia Medical Center[2]	The Dalles	129	353
Asante Rogue Regional Medical Center[2]	Medford	133	339
Providence Medford Medical Center[2]	Medford	170	669
Sky Lakes Medical Center[2]	Klamath Falls	220	600

Head CT Results Within 45 Minutes of Arrival

Hospital Name	City	Rate	Cases
Salem Hospital	Salem	29%	35

Patients Who Left ER Before Being Seen

Hospital Name	City	Rate	Cases
Legacy Meridian Park Medical Center	Tualatin	0%	34762
Pioneer Memorial Hospital	Heppner	0%	839
Providence Newberg Medical Center	Newberg	0%	19191
Saint Charles Medical Center - Bend	Bend	0%	29737
Saint Charles Medical Center - Redmond	Redmond	0%	15667
Samaritan Albany General Hospital	Albany	0%	22039
Santiam Memorial Hospital	Stayton	0%	10340
Silverton Hospital	Silverton	0%	23249
Adventist Medical Center	Portland	1%	50418
Asante Ashland Community Hospital	Ashland	1%	8261
Good Samaritan Regional Medical Center	Corvallis	1%	18752
Legacy Good Samaritan Medical Center	Portland	1%	30576
Legacy Mount Hood Medical Center	Gresham	1%	46956
McKenzie - Willamette Medical Center	Springfield	1%	32262
Mercy Medical Center	Roseburg	1%	45813
Providence Hood River Memorial Hospital	Hood River	1%	9342
Providence Medford Medical Center	Medford	1%	32904
Providence Milwaukie Hospital	Milwaukie	1%	33412
Providence Seaside Hospital	Seaside	1%	9289
Willamette Valley Medical Center	Mcminnville	1%	25242
Legacy Emanuel Medical Center	Portland	2%	60696
Mid - Columbia Medical Center	The Dalles	2%	15968
OHSU Hospital & Clinics	Portland	2%	46782
Peace Harbor Medical Center	Florence	2%	8131
Peacehealth Cottage Grove Comm Med Ctr	Cottage Grove	2%	10957
Providence Portland Medical Center	Portland	2%	66877
Providence Saint Vincent Medical Center	Portland	2%	86558
Providence Willamette Falls Med Ctr	Oregon City	2%	29858
Sacred Heart Medical Center - Riverbend	Springfield	2%	54061
Asante Rogue Regional Medical Center	Medford	3%	39108
Asante Three Rivers Medical Center	Grants Pass	3%	38864
Bay Area Hospital	Coos Bay	3%	26600
Sacred Heart University District	Eugene	3%	25522
Saint Alphonsus Medical Center - Ontario	Ontario	3%	20467
Salem Hospital	Salem	3%	93387
Tuality Community Hospital	Hillsboro	3%	41868
Sky Lakes Medical Center	Klamath Falls	4%	19588

Time from ER Arrival to Being Admitted (minutes)

Hospital Name	City	Min.	Cases
Lake District Hospital[2]	Lakeview	135	212
Samaritan Albany General Hospital[2]	Albany	151	393
Harney District Hospital[2]	Burns	155	151
Lower Umpqua Hospital District[2,3]	Reedsport	173	30
Silverton Hospital[2]	Silverton	183	186
Peacehealth Cottage Grove Comm Med Ctr[2]	Cottage Grove	187	273
Mercy Medical Center[2]	Roseburg	194	755
Samaritan North Lincoln Hospital[2]	Lincoln City	194	332
McKenzie - Willamette Medical Center[2]	Springfield	196	664
Legacy Emanuel Medical Center[2]	Portland	197	606
Peace Harbor Medical Center[2]	Florence	205	390
Providence Seaside Hospital[2]	Seaside	206	316
Legacy Meridian Park Medical Center[2]	Tualatin	207	681
Samaritan Pacific Communities Hospital[2]	Newport	208	394
Adventist Medical Center[2]	Portland	211	528
Bay Area Hospital[2]	Coos Bay	215	550
Providence Hood River Memorial Hospital[2]	Hood River	217	215
Pioneer Memorial Hospital[2]	Prineville	225	290
Providence Newberg Medical Center[2]	Newberg	227	309
Good Samaritan Regional Medical Center[2]	Corvallis	228	448
Legacy Good Samaritan Medical Center[2]	Portland	228	561
Saint Charles Medical Center - Redmond[2]	Redmond	229	262
Providence Milwaukie Hospital[2]	Milwaukie	230	439
Sacred Heart University District[2]	Eugene	235	449
Legacy Mount Hood Medical Center[2]	Gresham	237	706
Sacred Heart Medical Center - Riverbend[2]	Springfield	239	472
Willamette Valley Medical Center[2]	Mcminnville	240	455
Tuality Community Hospital[2]	Hillsboro	242	422
Saint Charles Medical Center - Bend[2]	Bend	243	392
Santiam Memorial Hospital[2]	Stayton	244	284
Mid - Columbia Medical Center[2]	The Dalles	248	368
Samaritan Lebanon Community Hospital[2]	Lebanon	250	331
Providence Portland Medical Center[2]	Portland	254	399
Good Shepherd Medical Center[2]	Hermiston	255	404
OHSU Hospital & Clinics[2]	Portland	257	233
Providence Willamette Falls Med Ctr[2]	Oregon City	265	285
Providence Saint Vincent Medical Center[2]	Portland	268	522
Salem Hospital[2]	Salem	269	521
Asante Three Rivers Medical Center[2]	Grants Pass	278	427
Asante Rogue Regional Medical Center[2]	Medford	282	350
Saint Alphonsus Medical Center - Ontario[2]	Ontario	295	212
Asante Ashland Community Hospital[2]	Ashland	310	264
Providence Medford Medical Center[2]	Medford	318	728
Kaiser Sunnyside Medical Center[2]	Clackamas	320	437
Sky Lakes Medical Center[2]	Klamath Falls	429	716

Time from ER Arrival to Discharge (minutes)

Hospital Name	City	Min.	Cases
Samaritan Albany General Hospital	Albany	82	391
Harney District Hospital[3]	Burns	84	302
Peacehealth Cottage Grove Comm Med Ctr	Cottage Grove	85	373
Silverton Hospital	Silverton	86	359
Lake District Hospital[3]	Lakeview	90	49
McKenzie - Willamette Medical Center	Springfield	91	394
Mercy Medical Center	Roseburg	93	441
Peace Harbor Medical Center	Florence	94	410
Providence Hood River Memorial Hospital	Hood River	97	271
Lower Umpqua Hospital District[3]	Reedsport	112	117
Providence Seaside Hospital	Seaside	112	134
Santiam Memorial Hospital	Stayton	112	373
Pioneer Memorial Hospital	Prineville	113	372
Bay Area Hospital	Coos Bay	116	384
Asante Ashland Community Hospital	Ashland	120	351
Sacred Heart University District	Eugene	123	364
Mid - Columbia Medical Center	The Dalles	125	345
Providence Milwaukie Hospital	Milwaukie	126	198
Saint Charles Medical Center - Redmond	Redmond	128	369
Tuality Community Hospital	Hillsboro	136	386
Good Samaritan Regional Medical Center	Corvallis	140	356
Legacy Emanuel Medical Center	Portland	141	346
Providence Newberg Medical Center	Newberg	143	245
Saint Alphonsus Medical Center - Ontario	Ontario	143	350
Providence Willamette Falls Med Ctr	Oregon City	150	345
Legacy Meridian Park Medical Center	Tualatin	154	356
Saint Charles Medical Center - Bend	Bend	156	366
Willamette Valley Medical Center	Mcminnville	156	477
Adventist Medical Center	Portland	162	345
Legacy Good Samaritan Medical Center	Portland	167	325
Providence Medford Medical Center	Medford	167	176
Legacy Mount Hood Medical Center	Gresham	172	360
Sacred Heart Medical Center - Riverbend	Springfield	173	371
Providence Portland Medical Center	Portland	177	333
Asante Three Rivers Medical Center	Grants Pass	178	339
Providence Saint Vincent Medical Center	Portland	185	345
Asante Rogue Regional Medical Center	Medford	186	332
Salem Hospital	Salem	188	430
OHSU Hospital & Clinics	Portland	204	358
Sky Lakes Medical Center	Klamath Falls	218	559

Time in ER Before Being Evaluated (minutes)

Hospital Name	City	Min.	Cases
Harney District Hospital[3]	Burns	6	300
Providence Seaside Hospital	Seaside	9	46
Mercy Medical Center	Roseburg	12	472
Silverton Hospital	Silverton	13	193
Peace Harbor Medical Center	Florence	15	440
McKenzie - Willamette Medical Center	Springfield	18	335
Pioneer Memorial Hospital	Prineville	18	398
Providence Newberg Medical Center	Newberg	19	246
Legacy Good Samaritan Medical Center	Portland	20	392
Providence Milwaukie Hospital	Milwaukie	20	56
Saint Charles Medical Center - Redmond	Redmond	21	367
Tuality Community Hospital	Hillsboro	21	417
Providence Hood River Memorial Hospital	Hood River	22	280
Samaritan Albany General Hospital	Albany	22	80
Legacy Meridian Park Medical Center	Tualatin	23	381
Peacehealth Cottage Grove Comm Med Ctr	Cottage Grove	25	396
Saint Alphonsus Medical Center - Ontario	Ontario	25	267
Santiam Memorial Hospital	Stayton	25	375
Lower Umpqua Hospital District[3]	Reedsport	27	99
Willamette Valley Medical Center	Mcminnville	27	506
Mid - Columbia Medical Center	The Dalles	28	386
Asante Ashland Community Hospital	Ashland	30	381
Adventist Medical Center	Portland	32	326
Good Samaritan Regional Medical Center	Corvallis	32	346
Legacy Mount Hood Medical Center	Gresham	35	395
Saint Charles Medical Center - Bend	Bend	35	389
Bay Area Hospital	Coos Bay	36	389
Legacy Emanuel Medical Center	Portland	36	367
Sacred Heart Medical Center - Riverbend	Springfield	36	389
OHSU Hospital & Clinics	Portland	37	383
Providence Willamette Falls Med Ctr	Oregon City	39	120
Asante Rogue Regional Medical Center	Medford	40	202
Lake District Hospital[3]	Lakeview	40	127
Sacred Heart University District	Eugene	41	425
Providence Medford Medical Center	Medford	42	61
Providence Saint Vincent Medical Center	Portland	46	73
Salem Hospital	Salem	48	474
Asante Three Rivers Medical Center	Grants Pass	50	62
Providence Portland Medical Center	Portland	67	119
Sky Lakes Medical Center	Klamath Falls	67	597

Time to Pain Meds for Bone Fractures (minutes)

Hospital Name	City	Min.	Cases
Mercy Medical Center	Roseburg	26	184
Providence Seaside Hospital	Seaside	30	37
Legacy Emanuel Medical Center	Portland	34	194
West Valley Hospital	Dallas	34	64
Silverton Hospital	Silverton	41	99
Peacehealth Cottage Grove Comm Med Ctr	Cottage Grove	42	26
Providence Hood River Memorial Hospital	Hood River	42	52
Providence Newberg Medical Center	Newberg	42	85
Willamette Valley Medical Center	Mcminnville	43	81
Legacy Meridian Park Medical Center	Tualatin	45	144
Samaritan Albany General Hospital	Albany	45	91
Mid - Columbia Medical Center	The Dalles	46	49
Adventist Medical Center	Portland	47	135
McKenzie - Willamette Medical Center	Springfield	49	125
Providence Milwaukie Hospital	Milwaukie	50	120
Saint Charles Medical Center - Redmond	Redmond	51	76
Peace Harbor Medical Center	Florence	52	45
Pioneer Memorial Hospital	Prineville	53	47
Sacred Heart University District	Eugene	53	49
Saint Alphonsus Medical Center - Ontario	Ontario	54	102
Santiam Memorial Hospital	Stayton	56	58
Legacy Mount Hood Medical Center	Gresham	58	138
Legacy Good Samaritan Medical Center	Portland	59	53
Asante Ashland Community Hospital	Ashland	60	68
Good Samaritan Regional Medical Center	Corvallis	60	106
Providence Medford Medical Center	Medford	60	110
Salem Hospital	Salem	61	259
Sacred Heart Medical Center - Riverbend	Springfield	63	183
Bay Area Hospital	Coos Bay	64	73
Asante Rogue Regional Medical Center	Medford	65	158
OHSU Hospital & Clinics	Portland	66	141
Providence Willamette Falls Med Ctr	Oregon City	67	134
Providence Portland Medical Center	Portland	68	146
Providence Saint Vincent Medical Center	Portland	68	267
Tuality Community Hospital	Hillsboro	69	175
Saint Charles Medical Center - Bend	Bend	72	172
Asante Three Rivers Medical Center	Grants Pass	82	152
Sky Lakes Medical Center	Klamath Falls	116	138

Heart Attack Care

Aspirin Given at Discharge

Hospital Name	City	Rate	Cases
Adventist Medical Center	Portland	100%	261
Kaiser Sunnyside Medical Center	Clackamas	100%	409
Legacy Good Samaritan Medical Center	Portland	100%	216
Legacy Meridian Park Medical Center	Tualatin	100%	174
McKenzie - Willamette Medical Center	Springfield	100%	140
OHSU Hospital & Clinics[2]	Portland	100%	218
Portland VA Medical Center	Portland	100%	72
Providence Medford Medical Center[2]	Medford	100%	86
Providence Saint Vincent Medical Center[2]	Portland	100%	539
Saint Charles Medical Center - Bend	Bend	100%	235
Tuality Community Hospital	Hillsboro	100%	124
Good Samaritan Regional Medical Center	Corvallis	99%	302
Legacy Emanuel Medical Center	Portland	99%	148
Mercy Medical Center[2]	Roseburg	99%	144
Providence Portland Medical Center[2]	Portland	99%	388
Sacred Heart Medical Center - Riverbend	Springfield	99%	579
Salem Hospital[2]	Salem	99%	297
Asante Rogue Regional Medical Center[2]	Medford	98%	281
Asante Three Rivers Medical Center	Grants Pass	98%	47
Bay Area Hospital	Coos Bay	97%	62
Sky Lakes Medical Center	Klamath Falls	96%	113

PCI Within 90 Minutes of Arrival

Hospital Name	City	Rate	Cases
Salem Hospital[2]	Salem	98%	64
Adventist Medical Center	Portland	97%	66
Asante Rogue Regional Medical Center[2]	Medford	97%	30
Legacy Meridian Park Medical Center	Tualatin	96%	56
Mercy Medical Center[2]	Roseburg	96%	28
Sacred Heart Medical Center - Riverbend	Springfield	96%	79
Good Samaritan Regional Medical Center	Corvallis	95%	40
Providence Saint Vincent Medical Center[2]	Portland	95%	95
Providence Portland Medical Center[2]	Portland	94%	34
Kaiser Sunnyside Medical Center	Clackamas	91%	34
Legacy Emanuel Medical Center	Portland	91%	33
Sky Lakes Medical Center	Klamath Falls	90%	30
Tuality Community Hospital	Hillsboro	85%	26
Saint Charles Medical Center - Bend	Bend	71%	41

NOTE: Hospital profiles are in alphabetical order by state, then city, then hospital within the city; Rankings exclude hospitals with less than 25 cases except for patient surveys which excludes hospitals with less than 100 cases; (a) 100-299 cases; (1) The number of cases/patients is too few to report; (2) Data submitted were based on a sample of cases/patients; (3) Results are based on a shorter time period than required; (4) Data suppressed by CMS for one or more quarters; (5) Results are not available for this reporting period; (6) Fewer than 100 patients completed the HCAHPS survey; (7) No cases met the criteria for this measure; (8) The lower limit of the confidence interval cannot be calculated if the number of observed infections equals zero; (9) No data are available from the state/territory for this reporting period; (10) The scores shown reflect fewer than 50 completed surveys; (11) There were discrepancies in the data collection process; (12) This measure does not apply to this hospital for this reporting period; (13) Results cannot be calculated for this reporting period; (14) The results for this state are combined with nearby states to protect confidentiality; Please refer to the User's Guide for a full explanation of data.

Statin Prescribed at Discharge

Hospital Name	City	Rate	Cases
Kaiser Sunnyside Medical Center	Clackamas	100%	402
Legacy Good Samaritan Medical Center	Portland	100%	212
McKenzie - Willamette Medical Center	Springfield	100%	140
OHSU Hospital & Clinics[2]	Portland	100%	217
Portland VA Medical Center	Portland	100%	68
Asante Rogue Regional Medical Center[2]	Medford	99%	223
Good Samaritan Regional Medical Center	Corvallis	99%	302
Legacy Emanuel Medical Center	Portland	99%	141
Providence Portland Medical Center[2]	Portland	99%	375
Sacred Heart Medical Center - Riverbend	Springfield	99%	566
Adventist Medical Center	Portland	98%	255
Legacy Meridian Park Medical Center	Tualatin	98%	171
Mercy Medical Center[2]	Roseburg	98%	143
Providence Medford Medical Center[2]	Medford	98%	84
Providence Saint Vincent Medical Center[2]	Portland	98%	517
Salem Hospital[2]	Salem	98%	266
Tuality Community Hospital	Hillsboro	98%	109
Saint Charles Medical Center - Bend	Bend	97%	228
Asante Three Rivers Medical Center	Grants Pass	95%	38
Sky Lakes Medical Center	Klamath Falls	91%	101
Bay Area Hospital	Coos Bay	85%	62

Heart Failure Care

ACE Inhibitor or ARB for LVSD

Hospital Name	City	Rate	Cases
Good Samaritan Regional Medical Center	Corvallis	100%	62
Kaiser Sunnyside Medical Center	Clackamas	100%	96
Legacy Emanuel Medical Center	Portland	100%	72
Legacy Mount Hood Medical Center	Gresham	100%	43
OHSU Hospital & Clinics[2]	Portland	100%	103
Providence Milwaukie Hospital[2]	Milwaukie	100%	37
Providence Willamette Falls Med Ctr[2]	Oregon City	100%	39
Sacred Heart Medical Center - Riverbend	Springfield	100%	120
Salem Hospital[2]	Salem	100%	77
Adventist Medical Center	Portland	99%	79
Asante Rogue Regional Medical Center[2]	Medford	99%	87
Sky Lakes Medical Center	Klamath Falls	98%	50
Portland VA Medical Center	Portland	97%	138
Saint Charles Medical Center - Bend	Bend	97%	58
Legacy Good Samaritan Medical Center	Portland	96%	77
McKenzie - Willamette Medical Center	Springfield	96%	46
Legacy Meridian Park Medical Center	Tualatin	95%	64
Mercy Medical Center[2]	Roseburg	95%	39
Providence Portland Medical Center[2]	Portland	92%	63
Asante Three Rivers Medical Center	Grants Pass	90%	50
Providence Medford Medical Center[2]	Medford	90%	48
Providence Saint Vincent Medical Center[2]	Portland	90%	84
Tuality Community Hospital	Hillsboro	87%	30
Bay Area Hospital	Coos Bay	86%	56

Discharge Instructions Given

Hospital Name	City	Rate	Cases
Good Shepherd Medical Center[2]	Hermiston	100%	27
Saint Alphonsus Medical Center - Ontario	Ontario	100%	49
Samaritan Lebanon Community Hospital	Lebanon	100%	66
Willamette Valley Medical Center	Mcminnville	100%	138
Asante Three Rivers Medical Center	Grants Pass	99%	110
Good Samaritan Regional Medical Center	Corvallis	99%	157
Legacy Mount Hood Medical Center	Gresham	99%	154
Portland VA Medical Center	Portland	99%	386
Salem Hospital[2]	Salem	99%	265
Adventist Medical Center	Portland	98%	275
Legacy Good Samaritan Medical Center	Portland	98%	202
Legacy Meridian Park Medical Center	Tualatin	98%	172
McKenzie - Willamette Medical Center	Springfield	98%	166
Mid - Columbia Medical Center	The Dalles	98%	52
Kaiser Sunnyside Medical Center	Clackamas	97%	383
Legacy Emanuel Medical Center	Portland	97%	187
Mercy Medical Center[2]	Roseburg	96%	160
OHSU Hospital & Clinics[2]	Portland	96%	239
Providence Hood River Memorial Hospital[2]	Hood River	96%	28
Providence Milwaukie Hospital[2]	Milwaukie	95%	101
Asante Rogue Regional Medical Center[2]	Medford	94%	307
Providence Medford Medical Center[2]	Medford	94%	158
Providence Newberg Medical Center[2]	Newberg	94%	84
Providence Portland Medical Center[2]	Portland	94%	236
Sacred Heart Medical Center - Riverbend	Springfield	94%	364
Tuality Community Hospital	Hillsboro	93%	111
Grande Ronde Hospital	La Grande	91%	32
Bay Area Hospital	Coos Bay	89%	116
Providence Saint Vincent Medical Center[2]	Portland	89%	227
Providence Willamette Falls Med Ctr[2]	Oregon City	88%	88
Sacred Heart University District	Eugene	88%	25
Sky Lakes Medical Center	Klamath Falls	87%	128
Saint Charles Medical Center - Redmond	Redmond	86%	42
Samaritan Albany General Hospital	Albany	84%	62
Samaritan Pacific Communities Hospital	Newport	84%	44
Samaritan North Lincoln Hospital	Lincoln City	81%	26
Coquille Valley Hospital District	Coquille	79%	28
Saint Charles Medical Center - Bend	Bend	76%	190
Silverton Hospital	Silverton	49%	35

Evaluation of LVS Function

Hospital Name	City	Rate	Cases
Adventist Medical Center	Portland	100%	308
Asante Rogue Regional Medical Center[2]	Medford	100%	332
Asante Three Rivers Medical Center	Grants Pass	100%	145
Good Samaritan Regional Medical Center	Corvallis	100%	176
Good Shepherd Medical Center[2]	Hermiston	100%	30
Kaiser Sunnyside Medical Center	Clackamas	100%	438
Legacy Emanuel Medical Center	Portland	100%	201
Legacy Good Samaritan Medical Center	Portland	100%	245
Legacy Meridian Park Medical Center	Tualatin	100%	225
Legacy Mount Hood Medical Center	Gresham	100%	163
McKenzie - Willamette Medical Center	Springfield	100%	208
Mercy Medical Center[2]	Roseburg	100%	184
OHSU Hospital & Clinics[2]	Portland	100%	270
Portland VA Medical Center	Portland	100%	421
Providence Hood River Memorial Hospital[2]	Hood River	100%	35
Providence Milwaukie Hospital[2]	Milwaukie	100%	121
Providence Portland Medical Center[2]	Portland	100%	268
Providence Willamette Falls Med Ctr[2]	Oregon City	100%	102
Sacred Heart Medical Center - Riverbend	Springfield	100%	433
Sacred Heart University District	Eugene	100%	33
Salem Hospital[2]	Salem	100%	303
Samaritan Albany General Hospital	Albany	100%	71
Samaritan Lebanon Community Hospital	Lebanon	100%	83
Samaritan North Lincoln Hospital	Lincoln City	100%	29
Tuality Community Hospital	Hillsboro	100%	138
Willamette Valley Medical Center	Mcminnville	100%	167
Bay Area Hospital	Coos Bay	99%	145
Providence Medford Medical Center[2]	Medford	99%	181
Providence Newberg Medical Center[2]	Newberg	99%	96
Providence Saint Vincent Medical Center[2]	Portland	99%	269
Mid - Columbia Medical Center	The Dalles	98%	60
Saint Alphonsus Medical Center - Ontario	Ontario	98%	62
Saint Charles Medical Center - Bend	Bend	98%	209
Silverton Hospital	Silverton	98%	44
Sky Lakes Medical Center	Klamath Falls	98%	149
Grande Ronde Hospital	La Grande	97%	39
VA Roseburg Healthcare System	Roseburg	97%	29
Saint Charles Medical Center - Redmond	Redmond	96%	46
Samaritan Pacific Communities Hospital	Newport	94%	47
Coquille Valley Hospital District	Coquille	88%	33
Saint Charles - Madras	Madras	58%	26

Medicare Spending

Medicare Spending per Patient (ratio)

Hospital Name	City	Ratio	Cases
Sacred Heart University District	Eugene	0.72	-
Kaiser Sunnyside Medical Center	Clackamas	0.73	-
Providence Newberg Medical Center	Newberg	0.80	-
Samaritan Albany General Hospital	Albany	0.82	-
Santiam Memorial Hospital	Stayton	0.82	-
Silverton Hospital	Silverton	0.83	-
Adventist Medical Center	Portland	0.85	-
Legacy Mount Hood Medical Center	Gresham	0.86	-
Mercy Medical Center	Roseburg	0.86	-
Mid - Columbia Medical Center	The Dalles	0.87	-
Providence Milwaukie Hospital	Milwaukie	0.87	-
Sacred Heart Medical Center - Riverbend	Springfield	0.87	-
Saint Charles Medical Center - Redmond	Redmond	0.87	-
Sky Lakes Medical Center	Klamath Falls	0.87	-
Providence Willamette Falls Med Ctr	Oregon City	0.88	-
Asante Three Rivers Medical Center	Grants Pass	0.89	-
Providence Saint Vincent Medical Center	Portland	0.89	-
Asante Rogue Regional Medical Center	Medford	0.90	-
Good Samaritan Regional Medical Center	Corvallis	0.90	-
Legacy Meridian Park Medical Center	Tualatin	0.90	-
McKenzie - Willamette Medical Center	Springfield	0.90	-
Providence Medford Medical Center	Medford	0.90	-
Saint Charles Medical Center - Bend	Bend	0.90	-
Willamette Valley Medical Center	Mcminnville	0.90	-
Bay Area Hospital	Coos Bay	0.91	-
Legacy Emanuel Medical Center	Portland	0.91	-
Asante Ashland Community Hospital	Ashland	0.92	-
Providence Portland Medical Center	Portland	0.92	-
Salem Hospital	Salem	0.92	-
Legacy Good Samaritan Medical Center	Portland	0.93	-
OHSU Hospital & Clinics	Portland	0.93	-
Saint Alphonsus Medical Center - Ontario	Ontario	0.93	-
Tuality Community Hospital	Hillsboro	0.93	-

Pneumonia Care

Appropriate Initial Antibiotic Given

Hospital Name	City	Rate	Cases
Asante Ashland Community Hospital[2]	Ashland	100%	38
Asante Rogue Regional Medical Center[2]	Medford	100%	83
Legacy Emanuel Medical Center	Portland	100%	73
OHSU Hospital & Clinics[2]	Portland	100%	39
Providence Saint Vincent Medical Center[2]	Portland	100%	109
Silverton Hospital	Silverton	100%	56
McKenzie - Willamette Medical Center	Springfield	99%	147
Providence Medford Medical Center[2]	Medford	99%	123
Tuality Community Hospital	Hillsboro	99%	74
Willamette Valley Medical Center	Mcminnville	99%	127
Adventist Medical Center	Portland	98%	129
Legacy Mount Hood Medical Center	Gresham	98%	127
Mid - Columbia Medical Center	The Dalles	98%	54
Portland VA Medical Center	Portland	98%	93
Saint Alphonsus Medical Center - Ontario	Ontario	98%	62
Samaritan Lebanon Community Hospital	Lebanon	98%	82
Asante Three Rivers Medical Center[2]	Grants Pass	97%	108
Kaiser Sunnyside Medical Center[2]	Clackamas	97%	107
Legacy Meridian Park Medical Center	Tualatin	97%	104
Providence Newberg Medical Center[2]	Newberg	97%	30
Sacred Heart Medical Center - Riverbend	Springfield	97%	259
Providence Milwaukie Hospital[2]	Milwaukie	96%	74
Providence Seaside Hospital[2]	Seaside	96%	27
Providence Willamette Falls Med Ctr[2]	Oregon City	96%	89
Sacred Heart University District	Eugene	96%	57
Bay Area Hospital	Coos Bay	95%	80
Legacy Good Samaritan Medical Center	Portland	95%	76
Mercy Medical Center[2]	Roseburg	95%	105
Providence Hood River Memorial Hospital[2]	Hood River	95%	41
Providence Portland Medical Center[2]	Portland	95%	104
Salem Hospital[2]	Salem	95%	101
Sky Lakes Medical Center	Klamath Falls	94%	110
Samaritan Pacific Communities Hospital	Newport	93%	43
Samaritan Albany General Hospital	Albany	92%	79
Samaritan North Lincoln Hospital	Lincoln City	92%	26
Good Samaritan Regional Medical Center	Corvallis	91%	93
Saint Charles Medical Center - Redmond	Redmond	89%	28
Santiam Memorial Hospital	Stayton	89%	45
VA Roseburg Healthcare System	Roseburg	89%	27
Coquille Valley Hospital District	Coquille	88%	25
Good Shepherd Medical Center[2]	Hermiston	88%	41
St Alphonsus Med Ctr-Baker City[2,3]	Baker City	88%	32
Saint Charles Medical Center - Bend	Bend	88%	82
Grande Ronde Hospital	La Grande	87%	75
Tillamook Regional Medical Center	Tillamook	85%	27

Blood Culture Timing

Hospital Name	City	Rate	Cases
Adventist Medical Center	Portland	100%	259
Asante Ashland Community Hospital[2]	Ashland	100%	47
Asante Rogue Regional Medical Center[2]	Medford	100%	119
Columbia Memorial Hospital[3]	Astoria	100%	26
McKenzie - Willamette Medical Center	Springfield	100%	141
OHSU Hospital & Clinics[2]	Portland	100%	94
Peace Harbor Medical Center	Florence	100%	42
Providence Hood River Memorial Hospital[2]	Hood River	100%	46
Providence Medford Medical Center[2]	Medford	100%	168
Providence Seaside Hospital[2]	Seaside	100%	60
Providence Willamette Falls Med Ctr[2]	Oregon City	100%	129
St Alphonsus Med Ctr-Baker City[2,3]	Baker City	100%	28
Saint Charles Medical Center - Redmond	Redmond	100%	64
Samaritan North Lincoln Hospital	Lincoln City	100%	34
Silverton Hospital	Silverton	100%	75
VA Roseburg Healthcare System	Roseburg	100%	28
Legacy Good Samaritan Medical Center	Portland	99%	143
Legacy Meridian Park Medical Center	Tualatin	99%	178
Portland VA Medical Center	Portland	99%	166
Providence Portland Medical Center[2]	Portland	99%	173
Providence Saint Vincent Medical Center[2]	Portland	99%	152
Saint Alphonsus Medical Center - Ontario	Ontario	99%	75
Willamette Valley Medical Center	Mcminnville	99%	198
Legacy Emanuel Medical Center	Portland	98%	111
Legacy Mount Hood Medical Center	Gresham	98%	217
Mercy Medical Center[2]	Roseburg	98%	90
Mid - Columbia Medical Center	The Dalles	98%	104
Providence Milwaukie Hospital[2]	Milwaukie	98%	95
Providence Newberg Medical Center[2]	Newberg	98%	61
Sacred Heart Medical Center - Riverbend	Springfield	98%	377
Saint Charles Medical Center - Bend	Bend	98%	132
Tillamook Regional Medical Center	Tillamook	98%	43
Asante Three Rivers Medical Center[2]	Grants Pass	97%	165
Good Shepherd Medical Center[2]	Hermiston	97%	68
Grande Ronde Hospital	La Grande	97%	97
Kaiser Sunnyside Medical Center[2]	Clackamas	97%	202
Pioneer Memorial Hospital	Prineville	97%	29
Salem Hospital[2]	Salem	97%	193

NOTE: Hospital profiles are in alphabetical order by state, then city, then hospital within the city; Rankings exclude hospitals with less than 25 cases except for patient surveys which excludes hospitals with less than 100 cases; (a) 100-299 cases; (1) The number of cases/patients is too few to report; (2) Data submitted were based on a sample of cases/patients; (3) Results are based on a shorter time period than required; (4) Data suppressed by CMS for one or more quarters; (5) Results are not available for this reporting period; (6) Fewer than 100 patients completed the HCAHPS survey; (7) No cases met the criteria for this measure; (8) The lower limit of the confidence interval cannot be calculated if the number of observed infections equals zero; (9) No data are available from the state/territory for this reporting period; (10) The scores shown reflect fewer than 50 completed surveys; (11) There were discrepancies in the data collection process; (12) This measure does not apply to this hospital for this reporting period; (13) Results cannot be calculated for this reporting period; (14) The results for this state are combined with nearby states to protect confidentiality; Please refer to the User's Guide for a full explanation of data.

Tuality Community Hospital	Hillsboro	96%	127
Samaritan Lebanon Community Hospital	Lebanon	95%	131
Sky Lakes Medical Center	Klamath Falls	95%	151
Good Samaritan Regional Medical Center	Corvallis	94%	176
Sacred Heart University District	Eugene	94%	65
Bay Area Hospital	Coos Bay	93%	106
Samaritan Pacific Communities Hospital	Newport	93%	61
Samaritan Albany General Hospital	Albany	92%	133
Santiam Memorial Hospital	Stayton	86%	56
Saint Charles - Madras	Madras	85%	26

Pregnancy and Delivery Care

Newborns whose Deliveries were Scheduled Early

Hospital Name	City	Rate	Cases
Asante Three Rivers Medical Center[2]	Grants Pass	0%	31
Bay Area Hospital[2]	Coos Bay	0%	40
Legacy Mount Hood Medical Center[2]	Gresham	0%	28
Providence Hood River Memorial Hospital	Hood River	0%	26
Providence Newberg Medical Center	Newberg	0%	41
Saint Alphonsus Medical Center - Ontario[2]	Ontario	0%	122
Silverton Hospital[2]	Silverton	0%	26
Kaiser Sunnyside Medical Center[2]	Clackamas	1%	280
Sacred Heart Medical Center - Riverbend	Springfield	1%	159
Providence Saint Vincent Medical Center	Portland	2%	312
Providence Willamette Falls Med Ctr	Oregon City	2%	88
Sky Lakes Medical Center	Klamath Falls	2%	64
McKenzie - Willamette Medical Center[2]	Springfield	3%	30
Willamette Valley Medical Center[2]	Mcminnville	3%	37
Asante Rogue Regional Medical Center[2]	Medford	4%	48
Providence Medford Medical Center	Medford	4%	28
Salem Hospital[2]	Salem	4%	57
Samaritan Albany General Hospital	Albany	4%	53
Providence Portland Medical Center	Portland	6%	159
Tuality Community Hospital	Hillsboro	6%	69
Legacy Good Samaritan Medical Center[2]	Portland	7%	30
Asante Ashland Community Hospital	Ashland	8%	25
Mercy Medical Center[2]	Roseburg	9%	33
Saint Charles Medical Center - Bend[2]	Bend	21%	28
Saint Charles Medical Center - Redmond	Redmond	29%	34

Preventive Care

Immunization for Influenza

Hospital Name	City	Rate	Cases
Asante Ashland Community Hospital[2]	Ashland	100%	245
McKenzie - Willamette Medical Center[2]	Springfield	99%	642
Peace Harbor Medical Center[2]	Florence	99%	279
Mercy Medical Center[2]	Roseburg	96%	540
Willamette Valley Medical Center[2]	Mcminnville	96%	370
Kaiser Sunnyside Medical Center[2]	Clackamas	95%	595
Asante Rogue Regional Medical Center[2]	Medford	94%	489
Asante Three Rivers Medical Center[2]	Grants Pass	94%	480
Legacy Meridian Park Medical Center[2]	Tualatin	94%	562
Legacy Good Samaritan Medical Center[2]	Portland	93%	578
Peacehealth Cottage Grove Comm Med Ctr[2]	Cottage Grove	93%	157
Sacred Heart University District[2]	Eugene	93%	284
Providence Milwaukie Hospital[2]	Milwaukie	91%	331
Samaritan Lebanon Community Hospital[2]	Lebanon	91%	244
Legacy Mount Hood Medical Center[2]	Gresham	90%	519
Pioneer Memorial Hospital[2]	Prineville	90%	278
West Valley Hospital	Dallas	90%	72
Saint Charles Medical Center - Redmond[2]	Redmond	89%	247
Salem Hospital[2]	Salem	89%	579
Providence Hood River Memorial Hospital[2]	Hood River	88%	241
Adventist Medical Center[2]	Portland	87%	532
Mid - Columbia Medical Center[2]	The Dalles	87%	260
Providence Newberg Medical Center[2]	Newberg	87%	267
Providence Seaside Hospital[2]	Seaside	87%	273
Providence Willamette Falls Med Ctr[2]	Oregon City	87%	456
Samaritan Albany General Hospital[2]	Albany	86%	320
Samaritan Pacific Communities Hospital[2]	Newport	86%	260
Santiam Memorial Hospital[2]	Stayton	84%	296
Good Shepherd Medical Center[2]	Hermiston	83%	343
OHSU Hospital & Clinics[2]	Portland	83%	548
Sky Lakes Medical Center[2]	Klamath Falls	83%	574
Bay Area Hospital[2]	Coos Bay	82%	524
Providence Medford Medical Center[2]	Medford	82%	605
Saint Charles Medical Center - Bend[2]	Bend	81%	568
Lower Umpqua Hospital District[2]	Reedsport	80%	44
Good Samaritan Regional Medical Center[2]	Corvallis	79%	559
Legacy Emanuel Medical Center[2]	Portland	76%	520
Samaritan North Lincoln Hospital[2]	Lincoln City	75%	271
Sacred Heart Medical Center - Riverbend[2]	Springfield	74%	546
Tuality Community Hospital[2]	Hillsboro	74%	424
Providence Portland Medical Center[2]	Portland	73%	538
Providence Saint Vincent Medical Center[2]	Portland	73%	642
Saint Alphonsus Medical Center - Ontario[2]	Ontario	73%	260
Lake District Hospital[2]	Lakeview	68%	142
Silverton Hospital[2]	Silverton	59%	312
Harney District Hospital[2,3]	Burns	37%	35

Immunization for Pneumonia

Hospital Name	City	Rate	Cases
Peace Harbor Medical Center[2]	Florence	99%	450
Willamette Valley Medical Center[2]	Mcminnville	99%	456
Asante Ashland Community Hospital[2]	Ashland	98%	261
McKenzie - Willamette Medical Center[2]	Springfield	98%	851
Mercy Medical Center[2]	Roseburg	97%	758
West Valley Hospital	Dallas	97%	124
Kaiser Sunnyside Medical Center[2]	Clackamas	96%	759
Legacy Good Samaritan Medical Center[2]	Portland	96%	717
Legacy Meridian Park Medical Center[2]	Tualatin	95%	692
Asante Three Rivers Medical Center[2]	Grants Pass	94%	656
Harney District Hospital[2,3]	Burns	94%	35
Legacy Mount Hood Medical Center[2]	Gresham	94%	562
Sacred Heart University District[2]	Eugene	94%	429
Samaritan Lebanon Community Hospital[2]	Lebanon	94%	323
Salem Hospital[2]	Salem	93%	749
Peacehealth Cottage Grove Comm Med Ctr[2]	Cottage Grove	92%	253
Sky Lakes Medical Center[2]	Klamath Falls	92%	765
Mid - Columbia Medical Center[2]	The Dalles	91%	335
Pioneer Memorial Hospital[2]	Prineville	91%	450
Asante Rogue Regional Medical Center[2]	Medford	90%	667
Providence Seaside Hospital[2]	Seaside	90%	366
Providence Hood River Memorial Hospital[2]	Hood River	89%	242
Providence Milwaukie Hospital[2]	Milwaukie	89%	445
Bay Area Hospital[2]	Coos Bay	88%	621
Saint Alphonsus Medical Center - Ontario[2]	Ontario	88%	273
Saint Charles Medical Center - Redmond[2]	Redmond	88%	302
Good Shepherd Medical Center[2]	Hermiston	87%	414
Providence Medford Medical Center[2]	Medford	86%	845
Saint Charles Medical Center - Bend[2]	Bend	86%	657
Providence Newberg Medical Center[2]	Newberg	85%	304
Lake District Hospital[2]	Lakeview	82%	171
Adventist Medical Center[2]	Portland	81%	653
Legacy Emanuel Medical Center[2]	Portland	81%	345
Providence Willamette Falls Med Ctr[2]	Oregon City	81%	458
Santiam Memorial Hospital[2]	Stayton	81%	365
Tuality Community Hospital[2]	Hillsboro	81%	457
OHSU Hospital & Clinics[2]	Portland	80%	429
Good Samaritan Regional Medical Center[2]	Corvallis	79%	698
Silverton Hospital[2]	Silverton	77%	207
Samaritan North Lincoln Hospital[2]	Lincoln City	76%	355
Samaritan Pacific Communities Hospital[2]	Newport	76%	334
Providence Portland Medical Center[2]	Portland	75%	672
Samaritan Albany General Hospital[2]	Albany	74%	403
Providence Saint Vincent Medical Center[2]	Portland	73%	660
Sacred Heart Medical Center - Riverbend[2]	Springfield	73%	628
Lower Umpqua Hospital District[2]	Reedsport	67%	76

Stroke Care

Anticoagulation Therapy for Atrial Fibrillation

Hospital Name	City	Rate	Cases
Kaiser Sunnyside Medical Center	Clackamas	100%	28
Legacy Emanuel Medical Center	Portland	100%	25
Legacy Meridian Park Medical Center	Tualatin	100%	31
Saint Charles Medical Center - Bend	Bend	100%	27
Salem Hospital[2]	Salem	82%	28

Antithrombotic Therapy Timing

Hospital Name	City	Rate	Cases
Asante Rogue Regional Medical Center[2]	Medford	100%	109
Legacy Mount Hood Medical Center	Gresham	100%	51
McKenzie - Willamette Medical Center	Springfield	100%	33
Providence Saint Vincent Medical Center[2]	Portland	100%	73
Providence Willamette Falls Med Ctr[2]	Oregon City	100%	30
Samaritan Albany General Hospital	Albany	100%	26
Samaritan Lebanon Community Hospital	Lebanon	100%	26
Sky Lakes Medical Center	Klamath Falls	100%	46
Tuality Community Hospital	Hillsboro	100%	51
Adventist Medical Center	Portland	99%	81
Providence Portland Medical Center[2]	Portland	99%	76
Bay Area Hospital	Coos Bay	98%	61
Kaiser Sunnyside Medical Center	Clackamas	98%	121
Legacy Good Samaritan Medical Center	Portland	98%	63
Legacy Meridian Park Medical Center	Tualatin	98%	100
Mercy Medical Center[2]	Roseburg	98%	81
Providence Medford Medical Center[2]	Medford	98%	61
Willamette Valley Medical Center	Mcminnville	98%	41
Good Samaritan Regional Medical Center	Corvallis	97%	104
OHSU Hospital & Clinics[2]	Portland	97%	30
Providence Milwaukie Hospital[2]	Milwaukie	97%	35
Sacred Heart Medical Center - Riverbend[2]	Springfield	97%	77
Asante Three Rivers Medical Center[2]	Grants Pass	96%	77
Saint Charles Medical Center - Bend	Bend	96%	104
Salem Hospital[2]	Salem	95%	171
Legacy Emanuel Medical Center	Portland	91%	66

Assessed for Rehabilitation

Hospital Name	City	Rate	Cases
Asante Rogue Regional Medical Center[2]	Medford	100%	135
Kaiser Sunnyside Medical Center	Clackamas	100%	212
McKenzie - Willamette Medical Center	Springfield	100%	42
OHSU Hospital & Clinics[2]	Portland	100%	90
Providence Medford Medical Center[2]	Medford	100%	72
Samaritan Lebanon Community Hospital	Lebanon	100%	26
Sky Lakes Medical Center	Klamath Falls	100%	48
Tuality Community Hospital	Hillsboro	100%	69
Willamette Valley Medical Center	Mcminnville	100%	48
Adventist Medical Center	Portland	98%	111
Asante Three Rivers Medical Center[2]	Grants Pass	98%	84
Good Samaritan Regional Medical Center	Corvallis	97%	146
Legacy Good Samaritan Medical Center	Portland	97%	90
Mercy Medical Center[2]	Roseburg	97%	78
Providence Portland Medical Center[2]	Portland	97%	115
Sacred Heart Medical Center - Riverbend[2]	Springfield	97%	115
Salem Hospital[2]	Salem	97%	188
Samaritan Albany General Hospital	Albany	97%	30
Legacy Emanuel Medical Center	Portland	96%	134
Legacy Mount Hood Medical Center	Gresham	96%	73
Providence Newberg Medical Center[2]	Newberg	96%	25
Providence Milwaukie Hospital[2]	Milwaukie	95%	38
Legacy Meridian Park Medical Center	Tualatin	93%	130
Providence Saint Vincent Medical Center[2]	Portland	93%	113
Bay Area Hospital	Coos Bay	92%	75
Providence Willamette Falls Med Ctr[2]	Oregon City	92%	40
Saint Charles Medical Center - Bend	Bend	90%	145

Discharged on Antithrombotic Therapy

Hospital Name	City	Rate	Cases
Kaiser Sunnyside Medical Center	Clackamas	100%	187
Legacy Good Samaritan Medical Center	Portland	100%	79
Legacy Meridian Park Medical Center	Tualatin	100%	119
Legacy Mount Hood Medical Center	Gresham	100%	68
McKenzie - Willamette Medical Center	Springfield	100%	39
Mercy Medical Center[2]	Roseburg	100%	78
OHSU Hospital & Clinics[2]	Portland	100%	51
Providence Milwaukie Hospital[2]	Milwaukie	100%	38
Providence Newberg Medical Center[2]	Newberg	100%	25
Providence Willamette Falls Med Ctr[2]	Oregon City	100%	40
Sacred Heart Medical Center - Riverbend[2]	Springfield	100%	88
Samaritan Albany General Hospital	Albany	100%	29
Sky Lakes Medical Center	Klamath Falls	100%	44
Tuality Community Hospital	Hillsboro	100%	59
Willamette Valley Medical Center	Mcminnville	100%	47
Asante Three Rivers Medical Center[2]	Grants Pass	99%	78
Bay Area Hospital	Coos Bay	99%	72
Legacy Emanuel Medical Center	Portland	99%	105
Providence Portland Medical Center[2]	Portland	99%	104
Providence Saint Vincent Medical Center[2]	Portland	99%	96
Saint Charles Medical Center - Bend	Bend	99%	120
Salem Hospital[2]	Salem	99%	183
Adventist Medical Center	Portland	98%	109
Asante Rogue Regional Medical Center[2]	Medford	98%	120
Good Samaritan Regional Medical Center	Corvallis	98%	128
Providence Medford Medical Center[2]	Medford	96%	68

Discharged on Statin Medication

Hospital Name	City	Rate	Cases
Adventist Medical Center	Portland	100%	80
McKenzie - Willamette Medical Center	Springfield	100%	28
Tuality Community Hospital	Hillsboro	100%	44
Asante Rogue Regional Medical Center[2]	Medford	99%	79
Kaiser Sunnyside Medical Center	Clackamas	99%	144
Legacy Mount Hood Medical Center	Gresham	98%	51
Providence Saint Vincent Medical Center[2]	Portland	97%	79
Providence Willamette Falls Med Ctr[2]	Oregon City	97%	31
Sacred Heart Medical Center - Riverbend[2]	Springfield	97%	65
Willamette Valley Medical Center	Mcminnville	97%	33
Legacy Good Samaritan Medical Center	Portland	96%	56
Good Samaritan Regional Medical Center	Corvallis	95%	105
Legacy Emanuel Medical Center	Portland	95%	78
Legacy Meridian Park Medical Center	Tualatin	95%	96
Providence Portland Medical Center[2]	Portland	95%	75
Salem Hospital[2]	Salem	95%	146
Sky Lakes Medical Center	Klamath Falls	93%	29
OHSU Hospital & Clinics[2]	Portland	92%	38
Providence Milwaukie Hospital[2]	Milwaukie	91%	32
Saint Charles Medical Center - Bend	Bend	88%	89
Mercy Medical Center[2]	Roseburg	87%	60
Providence Medford Medical Center[2]	Medford	86%	57
Asante Three Rivers Medical Center[2]	Grants Pass	85%	55
Bay Area Hospital	Coos Bay	68%	66

Thrombolytic Therapy Timing

Hospital Name	City	Rate	Cases
Legacy Emanuel Medical Center	Portland	97%	29

NOTE: Hospital profiles are in alphabetical order by state, then city, then hospital within the city; Rankings exclude hospitals with less than 25 cases except for patient surveys which excludes hospitals with less than 100 cases; (a) 100-299 cases; (1) The number of cases/patients is too few to report; (2) Data submitted were based on a sample of cases/patients; (3) Results are based on a shorter time period than required; (4) Data suppressed by CMS for one or more quarters; (5) Results are not available for this reporting period; (6) Fewer than 100 patients completed the HCAHPS survey; (7) No cases met the criteria for this measure; (8) The lower limit of the confidence interval cannot be calculated if the number of observed infections equals zero; (9) No data are available from the state/territory for this reporting period; (10) The scores shown reflect fewer than 50 completed surveys; (11) There were discrepancies in the data collection process; (12) This measure does not apply to this hospital for this reporting period; (13) Results cannot be calculated for this reporting period; (14) The results for this state are combined with nearby states to protect confidentiality; Please refer to the User's Guide for a full explanation of data.

Venous Thromboembolism (VTE) Prophylaxis

Hospital Name	City	Rate	Cases
McKenzie - Willamette Medical Center	Springfield	100%	34
Samaritan Albany General Hospital	Albany	100%	27
Samaritan Lebanon Community Hospital	Lebanon	100%	27
Willamette Valley Medical Center	Mcminnville	100%	39
Legacy Mount Hood Medical Center	Gresham	99%	67
OHSU Hospital & Clinics[2]	Portland	99%	89
Kaiser Sunnyside Medical Center	Clackamas	98%	166
Adventist Medical Center	Portland	97%	87
Tuality Community Hospital	Hillsboro	97%	69
Salem Hospital[2]	Salem	96%	181
Sky Lakes Medical Center	Klamath Falls	96%	52
Asante Rogue Regional Medical Center[2]	Medford	95%	131
Legacy Good Samaritan Medical Center	Portland	95%	85
Good Samaritan Regional Medical Center	Corvallis	93%	149
Sacred Heart Medical Center - Riverbend[2]	Springfield	93%	118
Legacy Meridian Park Medical Center	Tualatin	92%	121
Saint Charles Medical Center - Bend	Bend	91%	134
Legacy Emanuel Medical Center	Portland	90%	147
Providence Saint Vincent Medical Center[2]	Portland	88%	100
Providence Willamette Falls Med Ctr[2]	Oregon City	86%	29
Providence Medford Medical Center[2]	Medford	82%	74
Providence Portland Medical Center[2]	Portland	77%	115
Asante Three Rivers Medical Center[2]	Grants Pass	71%	89
Mercy Medical Center[2]	Roseburg	71%	79
Providence Milwaukie Hospital[2]	Milwaukie	63%	35
Bay Area Hospital	Coos Bay	62%	65

Written Stroke Educational Materials Given

Hospital Name	City	Rate	Cases
Asante Three Rivers Medical Center[2]	Grants Pass	100%	51
Good Samaritan Regional Medical Center	Corvallis	98%	92
Legacy Good Samaritan Medical Center	Portland	98%	54
Legacy Mount Hood Medical Center	Gresham	98%	52
Tuality Community Hospital	Hillsboro	97%	31
Willamette Valley Medical Center	Mcminnville	97%	32
Adventist Medical Center	Portland	96%	70
McKenzie - Willamette Medical Center	Springfield	96%	26
Salem Hospital[2]	Salem	96%	101
Kaiser Sunnyside Medical Center	Clackamas	93%	120
Asante Rogue Regional Medical Center[2]	Medford	92%	84
Legacy Meridian Park Medical Center	Tualatin	91%	68
OHSU Hospital & Clinics[2]	Portland	90%	58
Sacred Heart Medical Center - Riverbend[2]	Springfield	89%	70
Legacy Emanuel Medical Center	Portland	88%	78
Sky Lakes Medical Center	Klamath Falls	81%	32
Providence Saint Vincent Medical Center[2]	Portland	79%	73
Providence Willamette Falls Med Ctr[2]	Oregon City	71%	28
Saint Charles Medical Center - Bend	Bend	67%	81
Providence Medford Medical Center[2]	Medford	54%	41
Providence Portland Medical Center[2]	Portland	52%	60
Bay Area Hospital	Coos Bay	51%	49
Mercy Medical Center[2]	Roseburg	0%	50

Surgical Care Improvement Project

Appropriate Beta Blocker Usage

Hospital Name	City	Rate	Cases
Asante Rogue Regional Medical Center[2]	Medford	100%	230
Legacy Good Samaritan Medical Center[2]	Portland	100%	182
Legacy Meridian Park Medical Center[2]	Tualatin	100%	62
Legacy Mount Hood Medical Center[2]	Gresham	100%	71
McKenzie - Willamette Medical Center	Springfield	100%	245
Mercy Medical Center	Roseburg	100%	115
Peace Harbor Medical Center	Florence	100%	26
Portland VA Medical Center[2]	Portland	100%	267
Providence Hood River Memorial Hospital[2]	Hood River	100%	30
Providence Newberg Medical Center[2]	Newberg	100%	42
Sacred Heart Medical Center - Riverbend[2]	Springfield	100%	271
Saint Anthony Hospital[2]	Pendleton	100%	25
Good Samaritan Regional Medical Center[2]	Corvallis	99%	290
Legacy Emanuel Medical Center[2]	Portland	99%	119
Providence Medford Medical Center[2]	Medford	99%	94
Asante Three Rivers Medical Center[2]	Grants Pass	98%	103
Kaiser Sunnyside Medical Center[2]	Clackamas	98%	294
Mid - Columbia Medical Center	The Dalles	98%	55
OHSU Hospital & Clinics[2]	Portland	98%	186
Providence Portland Medical Center[2]	Portland	98%	259
Tuality Community Hospital[2]	Hillsboro	98%	106
Adventist Medical Center[2]	Portland	97%	259
Asante Ashland Community Hospital[2]	Ashland	97%	33
Providence Saint Vincent Medical Center[2]	Portland	97%	233
Saint Alphonsus Medical Center - Ontario	Ontario	97%	58
Salem Hospital[2]	Salem	97%	219
Samaritan Albany General Hospital[2]	Albany	97%	103
Sky Lakes Medical Center	Klamath Falls	97%	127
Saint Charles Medical Center - Bend[2]	Bend	96%	274
Providence Willamette Falls Med Ctr[2]	Oregon City	95%	76
Saint Charles Medical Center - Redmond	Redmond	95%	42
Willamette Valley Medical Center	Mcminnville	95%	65
Providence Milwaukie Hospital[2]	Milwaukie	94%	52
Silverton Hospital[2]	Silverton	94%	53
Bay Area Hospital	Coos Bay	91%	144

Appropriate VTP Within 24 Hours

Hospital Name	City	Rate	Cases
Asante Ashland Community Hospital[2]	Ashland	100%	133
McKenzie - Willamette Medical Center	Springfield	100%	625
Mercy Medical Center	Roseburg	100%	328
Peace Harbor Medical Center	Florence	100%	74
Providence Medford Medical Center[2]	Medford	100%	280
Saint Anthony Hospital[2]	Pendleton	100%	102
Tillamook Regional Medical Center	Tillamook	100%	49
Asante Rogue Regional Medical Center[2]	Medford	99%	356
Coquille Valley Hospital District	Coquille	99%	74
Legacy Good Samaritan Medical Center[2]	Portland	99%	344
Legacy Meridian Park Medical Center[2]	Tualatin	99%	280
Providence Newberg Medical Center[2]	Newberg	99%	161
Providence Portland Medical Center[2]	Portland	99%	396
Sacred Heart Medical Center - Riverbend[2]	Springfield	99%	408
Saint Alphonsus Medical Center - Ontario	Ontario	99%	280
Willamette Valley Medical Center	Mcminnville	99%	212
Kaiser Sunnyside Medical Center[2]	Clackamas	98%	394
Legacy Emanuel Medical Center[2]	Portland	98%	164
Sky Lakes Medical Center	Klamath Falls	98%	475
Adventist Medical Center[2]	Portland	97%	544
Good Samaritan Regional Medical Center[2]	Corvallis	97%	604
Mid - Columbia Medical Center	The Dalles	97%	190
Columbia Memorial Hospital[3]	Astoria	96%	26
Good Shepherd Medical Center	Hermiston	96%	198
Grande Ronde Hospital	La Grande	96%	81
Legacy Mount Hood Medical Center[2]	Gresham	96%	243
Providence Hood River Memorial Hospital[2]	Hood River	96%	142
Providence Milwaukie Hospital[2]	Milwaukie	96%	213
Salem Hospital[2]	Salem	96%	385
Samaritan Albany General Hospital[2]	Albany	96%	290
Samaritan North Lincoln Hospital	Lincoln City	96%	56
Silverton Hospital[2]	Silverton	96%	257
Asante Three Rivers Medical Center[2]	Grants Pass	95%	236
Bay Area Hospital	Coos Bay	95%	458
OHSU Hospital & Clinics[2]	Portland	95%	356
Santiam Memorial Hospital	Stayton	95%	62
Providence Saint Vincent Medical Center[2]	Portland	94%	347
Saint Charles Medical Center - Bend[2]	Bend	94%	730
Portland VA Medical Center[2]	Portland	93%	254
Providence Willamette Falls Med Ctr[2]	Oregon City	93%	286
Tuality Community Hospital[2]	Hillsboro	93%	318
Samaritan Lebanon Community Hospital	Lebanon	87%	45
Saint Charles Medical Center - Redmond	Redmond	86%	172
Samaritan Pacific Communities Hospital	Newport	84%	58

Controlled Postoperative Blood Glucose

Hospital Name	City	Rate	Cases
Kaiser Sunnyside Medical Center[2]	Clackamas	100%	151
McKenzie - Willamette Medical Center	Springfield	100%	112
Saint Charles Medical Center - Bend[2]	Bend	100%	212
Salem Hospital[2]	Salem	100%	160
Tuality Community Hospital[2]	Hillsboro	100%	33
Adventist Medical Center[2]	Portland	98%	136
Asante Rogue Regional Medical Center[2]	Medford	98%	160
Providence Portland Medical Center[2]	Portland	98%	166
Providence Saint Vincent Medical Center[2]	Portland	98%	172
Legacy Good Samaritan Medical Center[2]	Portland	97%	148
Sacred Heart Medical Center - Riverbend[2]	Springfield	97%	170
Good Samaritan Regional Medical Center[2]	Corvallis	96%	156
OHSU Hospital & Clinics[2]	Portland	96%	119
Portland VA Medical Center[2]	Portland	95%	177
Legacy Emanuel Medical Center[2]	Portland	89%	63

Perioperative Temperature Management

Hospital Name	City	Rate	Cases
Adventist Medical Center[2]	Portland	100%	726
Asante Ashland Community Hospital[2]	Ashland	100%	139
Asante Rogue Regional Medical Center[2]	Medford	100%	543
Asante Three Rivers Medical Center[2]	Grants Pass	100%	438
Bay Area Hospital	Coos Bay	100%	515
Columbia Memorial Hospital[3]	Astoria	100%	30
Coquille Valley Hospital District	Coquille	100%	82
Good Samaritan Regional Medical Center[2]	Corvallis	100%	770
Good Shepherd Medical Center	Hermiston	100%	218
Grande Ronde Hospital	La Grande	100%	106
Kaiser Sunnyside Medical Center[2]	Clackamas	100%	570
Legacy Emanuel Medical Center[2]	Portland	100%	312
Legacy Good Samaritan Medical Center[2]	Portland	100%	415
Legacy Meridian Park Medical Center[2]	Tualatin	100%	345
Legacy Mount Hood Medical Center[2]	Gresham	100%	297
McKenzie - Willamette Medical Center	Springfield	100%	756
Mercy Medical Center	Roseburg	100%	377
Mid - Columbia Medical Center	The Dalles	100%	217
Providence Hood River Memorial Hospital[2]	Hood River	100%	175
Providence Medford Medical Center[2]	Medford	100%	355
Providence Milwaukie Hospital[2]	Milwaukie	100%	228
Providence Newberg Medical Center[2]	Newberg	100%	175
Providence Portland Medical Center[2]	Portland	100%	581
Providence Saint Vincent Medical Center[2]	Portland	100%	610
Providence Seaside Hospital[2]	Seaside	100%	26
Providence Willamette Falls Med Ctr[2]	Oregon City	100%	347
Sacred Heart Medical Center - Riverbend[2]	Springfield	100%	552
Saint Alphonsus Medical Center - Ontario	Ontario	100%	322
Saint Anthony Hospital[2,3]	Pendleton	100%	31
Saint Charles Medical Center - Redmond	Redmond	100%	210
Salem Hospital[2]	Salem	100%	531
Samaritan Albany General Hospital[2]	Albany	100%	324
Samaritan Lebanon Community Hospital	Lebanon	100%	59
Samaritan North Lincoln Hospital	Lincoln City	100%	62
Samaritan Pacific Communities Hospital	Newport	100%	72
Santiam Memorial Hospital	Stayton	100%	72
Silverton Hospital[2]	Silverton	100%	283
Sky Lakes Medical Center	Klamath Falls	100%	509
Tillamook Regional Medical Center	Tillamook	100%	71
Tuality Community Hospital[2]	Hillsboro	100%	402
Willamette Valley Medical Center	Mcminnville	100%	295
OHSU Hospital & Clinics[2]	Portland	99%	529
Peace Harbor Medical Center	Florence	99%	93
Saint Charles Medical Center - Bend[2]	Bend	99%	889
Portland VA Medical Center[2]	Portland	98%	332

Prophylactic Antibiotic Selection

Hospital Name	City	Rate	Cases
Adventist Medical Center[2]	Portland	100%	588
Asante Ashland Community Hospital[2]	Ashland	100%	108
Legacy Meridian Park Medical Center[2]	Tualatin	100%	234
McKenzie - Willamette Medical Center	Springfield	100%	632
Mercy Medical Center	Roseburg	100%	262
Mid - Columbia Medical Center	The Dalles	100%	175
Providence Hood River Memorial Hospital[2]	Hood River	100%	127
Providence Newberg Medical Center[2]	Newberg	100%	118
Sacred Heart Medical Center - Riverbend[2]	Springfield	100%	505
St Alphonsus Med Ctr-Baker City[3]	Baker City	100%	49
Samaritan Lebanon Community Hospital	Lebanon	100%	29
Samaritan North Lincoln Hospital	Lincoln City	100%	48
Sky Lakes Medical Center	Klamath Falls	100%	412
Tillamook Regional Medical Center	Tillamook	100%	46
Tuality Community Hospital[2]	Hillsboro	100%	292
Willamette Valley Medical Center	Mcminnville	100%	217
Asante Rogue Regional Medical Center[2]	Medford	99%	493
Asante Three Rivers Medical Center[2]	Grants Pass	99%	298
Coquille Valley Hospital District	Coquille	99%	69
Good Samaritan Regional Medical Center[2]	Corvallis	99%	716
Kaiser Sunnyside Medical Center[2]	Clackamas	99%	499
Legacy Emanuel Medical Center[2]	Portland	99%	222
Legacy Good Samaritan Medical Center[2]	Portland	99%	400
Legacy Mount Hood Medical Center[2]	Gresham	99%	177
OHSU Hospital & Clinics[2]	Portland	99%	374
Peace Harbor Medical Center	Florence	99%	68
Portland VA Medical Center	Portland	99%	353
Providence Medford Medical Center[2]	Medford	99%	222
Providence Milwaukie Hospital[2]	Milwaukie	99%	156
Providence Portland Medical Center[2]	Portland	99%	521
Providence Saint Vincent Medical Center[2]	Portland	99%	535
Providence Willamette Falls Med Ctr[2]	Oregon City	99%	239
Saint Charles Medical Center - Bend[2]	Bend	99%	904
Saint Charles Medical Center - Redmond	Redmond	99%	135
Salem Hospital[2]	Salem	99%	495
Samaritan Albany General Hospital[2]	Albany	99%	228
Good Shepherd Medical Center	Hermiston	98%	181
Saint Alphonsus Medical Center - Ontario	Ontario	98%	248
Bay Area Hospital	Coos Bay	97%	345
Grande Ronde Hospital	La Grande	97%	77
Saint Anthony Hospital[2]	Pendleton	97%	97
Santiam Memorial Hospital	Stayton	97%	30
Silverton Hospital[2]	Silverton	95%	193
Columbia Memorial Hospital[3]	Astoria	90%	29
Samaritan Pacific Communities Hospital	Newport	85%	34

Prophylactic Antibiotic Selection (Outpatient)

Hospital Name	City	Rate	Cases
Asante Ashland Community Hospital	Ashland	100%	33
McKenzie - Willamette Medical Center	Springfield	100%	316
Tuality Community Hospital	Hillsboro	100%	115
Willamette Valley Medical Center	Mcminnville	100%	106
Asante Rogue Regional Medical Center	Medford	99%	503
Asante Three Rivers Medical Center	Grants Pass	99%	82
Good Samaritan Regional Medical Center	Corvallis	99%	521
Legacy Meridian Park Medical Center	Tualatin	99%	461
Mercy Medical Center	Roseburg	99%	322
Sacred Heart Medical Center - Riverbend	Springfield	99%	894
Salem Hospital	Salem	99%	714

NOTE: Hospital profiles are in alphabetical order by state, then city, then hospital within the city; Rankings exclude hospitals with less than 25 cases except for patient surveys which excludes hospitals with less than 100 cases; (a) 100-299 cases; (1) The number of cases/patients is too few to report; (2) Data submitted were based on a sample of cases/patients; (3) Results are based on a shorter time period than required; (4) Data suppressed by CMS for one or more quarters; (5) Results are not available for this reporting period; (6) Fewer than 100 patients completed the HCAHPS survey; (7) No cases met the criteria for this measure; (8) The lower limit of the confidence interval cannot be calculated if the number of observed infections equals zero; (9) No data are available from the state/territory for this reporting period; (10) The scores shown reflect fewer than 50 completed surveys; (11) There were discrepancies in the data collection process; (12) This measure does not apply to this hospital for this reporting period; (13) Results cannot be calculated for this reporting period; (14) The results for this state are combined with nearby states to protect confidentiality; Please refer to the User's Guide for a full explanation of data.

Hospital Name	City	Rate	Cases
Adventist Medical Center	Portland	98%	261
Legacy Good Samaritan Medical Center	Portland	98%	437
Providence Hood River Memorial Hospital	Hood River	98%	49
Providence Newberg Medical Center	Newberg	98%	40
Providence Portland Medical Center	Portland	98%	546
OHSU Hospital & Clinics	Portland	97%	399
Providence Medford Medical Center	Medford	97%	372
Providence Saint Vincent Medical Center	Portland	97%	636
Legacy Emanuel Medical Center	Portland	96%	173
Mid - Columbia Medical Center	The Dalles	96%	46
Legacy Mount Hood Medical Center	Gresham	95%	168
Providence Willamette Falls Med Ctr	Oregon City	95%	116
Saint Charles Medical Center - Bend	Bend	95%	385
Silverton Hospital	Silverton	95%	81
Sky Lakes Medical Center	Klamath Falls	95%	185
Samaritan Albany General Hospital	Albany	94%	50
Bay Area Hospital	Coos Bay	90%	92

Prophylactic Antibiotic Stopped

Hospital Name	City	Rate	Cases
Kaiser Sunnyside Medical Center[2]	Clackamas	100%	489
McKenzie - Willamette Medical Center	Springfield	100%	616
Mercy Medical Center	Roseburg	100%	257
Peace Harbor Medical Center	Florence	100%	67
Providence Medford Medical Center[2]	Medford	100%	218
Providence Milwaukie Hospital[2]	Milwaukie	100%	151
Providence Newberg Medical Center[2]	Newberg	100%	115
Samaritan North Lincoln Hospital	Lincoln City	100%	48
Tillamook Regional Medical Center	Tillamook	100%	46
Willamette Valley Medical Center	Mcminnville	100%	212
Asante Ashland Community Hospital[2]	Ashland	99%	107
Asante Rogue Regional Medical Center[2]	Medford	99%	486
Asante Three Rivers Medical Center[2]	Grants Pass	99%	296
Good Samaritan Regional Medical Center[2]	Corvallis	99%	702
Good Shepherd Medical Center	Hermiston	99%	181
Legacy Good Samaritan Medical Center[2]	Portland	99%	390
Legacy Meridian Park Medical Center[2]	Tualatin	99%	233
Mid - Columbia Medical Center	The Dalles	99%	176
Providence Saint Vincent Medical Center[2]	Portland	99%	530
Providence Willamette Falls Med Ctr[2]	Oregon City	99%	237
Salem Hospital[2]	Salem	99%	494
Tuality Community Hospital[2]	Hillsboro	99%	288
Adventist Medical Center[2]	Portland	98%	588
Legacy Mount Hood Medical Center[2]	Gresham	98%	175
Portland VA Medical Center	Portland	98%	349
Providence Hood River Memorial Hospital[2]	Hood River	98%	104
Providence Portland Medical Center[2]	Portland	98%	508
Sacred Heart Medical Center - Riverbend[2]	Springfield	98%	483
Silverton Hospital[2]	Silverton	98%	189
Sky Lakes Medical Center	Klamath Falls	98%	404
OHSU Hospital & Clinics[2]	Portland	97%	366
Saint Alphonsus Medical Center - Ontario	Ontario	97%	241
Saint Charles Medical Center - Bend[2]	Bend	97%	898
Santiam Memorial Hospital	Stayton	97%	29
Coquille Valley Hospital District	Coquille	96%	69
Legacy Emanuel Medical Center[2]	Portland	96%	220
St Alphonsus Med Ctr-Baker City[3]	Baker City	96%	49
Samaritan Albany General Hospital[2]	Albany	96%	223
Bay Area Hospital	Coos Bay	93%	336
Columbia Memorial Hospital[3]	Astoria	93%	29
Grande Ronde Hospital	La Grande	92%	73
Saint Charles Medical Center - Redmond	Redmond	90%	131
Samaritan Pacific Communities Hospital	Newport	90%	31
Saint Anthony Hospital[2]	Pendleton	89%	95
Samaritan Lebanon Community Hospital	Lebanon	85%	27

Prophylactic Antibiotic Timing

Hospital Name	City	Rate	Cases
Asante Three Rivers Medical Center[2]	Grants Pass	100%	298
McKenzie - Willamette Medical Center	Springfield	100%	632
Mercy Medical Center	Roseburg	100%	262
Providence Hood River Memorial Hospital[2]	Hood River	100%	127
Sacred Heart Medical Center - Riverbend[2]	Springfield	100%	507
Saint Alphonsus Medical Center - Ontario	Ontario	100%	248
Willamette Valley Medical Center	Mcminnville	100%	217
Adventist Medical Center[2]	Portland	99%	588
Asante Ashland Community Hospital[2]	Ashland	99%	108
Asante Rogue Regional Medical Center[2]	Medford	99%	496
Kaiser Sunnyside Medical Center[2]	Clackamas	99%	499
Legacy Emanuel Medical Center[2]	Portland	99%	222
Mid - Columbia Medical Center	The Dalles	99%	175
Portland VA Medical Center	Portland	99%	353
Sky Lakes Medical Center	Klamath Falls	99%	412
Legacy Meridian Park Medical Center[2]	Tualatin	98%	234
OHSU Hospital & Clinics[2]	Portland	98%	374
Providence Medford Medical Center[2]	Medford	98%	222
Providence Portland Medical Center[2]	Portland	98%	521
Samaritan North Lincoln Hospital	Lincoln City	98%	49
Good Samaritan Regional Medical Center[2]	Corvallis	97%	717
Legacy Good Samaritan Medical Center[2]	Portland	97%	404
Peace Harbor Medical Center	Florence	97%	68
Providence Newberg Medical Center[2]	Newberg	97%	118
Providence Saint Vincent Medical Center[2]	Portland	97%	537
Providence Willamette Falls Med Ctr[2]	Oregon City	97%	239
Salem Hospital[2]	Salem	97%	504
Samaritan Lebanon Community Hospital	Lebanon	97%	29
Tuality Community Hospital[2]	Hillsboro	97%	293
Coquille Valley Hospital District	Coquille	96%	70
Providence Milwaukie Hospital[2]	Milwaukie	96%	157
Saint Anthony Hospital[2]	Pendleton	96%	97
Saint Charles Medical Center - Bend[2]	Bend	96%	906
Samaritan Albany General Hospital[2]	Albany	96%	228
Silverton Hospital[2]	Silverton	96%	195
Tillamook Regional Medical Center	Tillamook	96%	46
Bay Area Hospital	Coos Bay	94%	348
Saint Charles Medical Center - Redmond	Redmond	94%	135
Samaritan Pacific Communities Hospital	Newport	94%	34
Columbia Memorial Hospital[3]	Astoria	93%	29
Good Shepherd Medical Center	Hermiston	93%	181
Legacy Mount Hood Medical Center[2]	Gresham	93%	180
Grande Ronde Hospital	La Grande	91%	79
St Alphonsus Med Ctr-Baker City[3]	Baker City	90%	49
Santiam Memorial Hospital	Stayton	71%	31

Prophylactic Antibiotic Timing (Outpatient)

Hospital Name	City	Rate	Cases
McKenzie - Willamette Medical Center	Springfield	100%	316
Mercy Medical Center	Roseburg	100%	322
Mid - Columbia Medical Center	The Dalles	100%	46
Providence Hood River Memorial Hospital	Hood River	100%	49
Willamette Valley Medical Center	Mcminnville	100%	106
Legacy Meridian Park Medical Center	Tualatin	99%	461
Sacred Heart Medical Center - Riverbend	Springfield	99%	891
Asante Rogue Regional Medical Center	Medford	98%	506
Good Samaritan Regional Medical Center	Corvallis	98%	526
Legacy Good Samaritan Medical Center	Portland	98%	437
Silverton Hospital	Silverton	98%	82
Providence Saint Vincent Medical Center	Portland	97%	641
OHSU Hospital & Clinics	Portland	96%	401
Providence Willamette Falls Med Ctr	Oregon City	96%	117
Tuality Community Hospital	Hillsboro	96%	116
Adventist Medical Center	Portland	95%	266
Saint Charles Medical Center - Bend	Bend	95%	392
Salem Hospital	Salem	95%	727
Asante Three Rivers Medical Center	Grants Pass	94%	80
Legacy Emanuel Medical Center	Portland	94%	173
Legacy Mount Hood Medical Center	Gresham	93%	169
Asante Ashland Community Hospital	Ashland	92%	36
Providence Medford Medical Center	Medford	92%	366
Providence Portland Medical Center	Portland	92%	543
Samaritan Albany General Hospital	Albany	91%	53
Bay Area Hospital	Coos Bay	89%	97
Providence Newberg Medical Center	Newberg	89%	44
Sky Lakes Medical Center	Klamath Falls	73%	184

Urinary Catheter Removal

Hospital Name	City	Rate	Cases
Adventist Medical Center[2]	Portland	100%	568
Coquille Valley Hospital District	Coquille	100%	77
McKenzie - Willamette Medical Center	Springfield	100%	516
Mercy Medical Center	Roseburg	100%	256
Saint Alphonsus Medical Center - Ontario	Ontario	100%	204
Kaiser Sunnyside Medical Center[2]	Clackamas	99%	442
Legacy Good Samaritan Medical Center[2]	Portland	99%	380
Legacy Meridian Park Medical Center[2]	Tualatin	99%	148
Providence Newberg Medical Center[2]	Newberg	99%	129
Sacred Heart Medical Center - Riverbend[2]	Springfield	99%	256
Willamette Valley Medical Center	Mcminnville	99%	191
Good Samaritan Regional Medical Center[2]	Corvallis	98%	682
Grande Ronde Hospital	La Grande	98%	49
OHSU Hospital & Clinics[2]	Portland	98%	315
Providence Portland Medical Center[2]	Portland	98%	437
Sky Lakes Medical Center	Klamath Falls	98%	396
Asante Rogue Regional Medical Center[2]	Medford	97%	261
Legacy Mount Hood Medical Center[2]	Gresham	97%	145
Portland VA Medical Center[2]	Portland	97%	231
Providence Saint Vincent Medical Center[2]	Portland	97%	313
Saint Charles Medical Center - Bend[2]	Bend	97%	833
Salem Hospital[2]	Salem	97%	455
Tuality Community Hospital[2]	Hillsboro	97%	234
Bay Area Hospital	Coos Bay	96%	367
Providence Hood River Memorial Hospital[2]	Hood River	96%	47
Samaritan Albany General Hospital[2]	Albany	96%	236
Good Shepherd Medical Center	Hermiston	95%	184
Providence Milwaukie Hospital[2]	Milwaukie	95%	171
Asante Ashland Community Hospital[2]	Ashland	94%	36
Asante Three Rivers Medical Center[2]	Grants Pass	94%	111
Legacy Emanuel Medical Center[2]	Portland	94%	207
Providence Medford Medical Center[2]	Medford	94%	47
Samaritan North Lincoln Hospital	Lincoln City	93%	45
Samaritan Pacific Communities Hospital	Newport	93%	45
Mid - Columbia Medical Center	The Dalles	91%	96
Santiam Memorial Hospital	Stayton	91%	46
Silverton Hospital[2]	Silverton	91%	188
Providence Willamette Falls Med Ctr[2]	Oregon City	89%	62
Saint Charles Medical Center - Redmond	Redmond	88%	137
Samaritan Lebanon Community Hospital	Lebanon	85%	33

Survey of Patients' Hospital Experiences

Area Around Room 'Always' Quiet at Night

Hospital Name	City	Rate	Cases
Wallowa Memorial Hospital	Enterprise	74%	(a)
Providence Hood River Memorial Hospital	Hood River	67%	300+
Providence Newberg Medical Center	Newberg	66%	300+
Willamette Valley Medical Center	Mcminnville	65%	300+
Tillamook Regional Medical Center	Tillamook	64%	(a)
St Alphonsus Med Ctr-Baker City	Baker City	62%	(a)
Columbia Memorial Hospital	Astoria	60%	300+
Good Shepherd Medical Center	Hermiston	60%	300+
Sacred Heart Medical Center - Riverbend	Springfield	60%	300+
Silverton Hospital	Silverton	60%	300+
Kaiser Sunnyside Medical Center	Clackamas	59%	300+
Saint Alphonsus Medical Center - Ontario	Ontario	59%	300+
Samaritan Albany General Hospital	Albany	59%	300+
Samaritan Pacific Communities Hospital	Newport	59%	300+
Legacy Meridian Park Medical Center	Tualatin	58%	300+
Legacy Mount Hood Medical Center	Gresham	58%	300+
Saint Charles Medical Center - Redmond	Redmond	58%	300+
Samaritan North Lincoln Hospital	Lincoln City	58%	(a)
Adventist Medical Center	Portland	57%	300+
Asante Ashland Community Hospital	Ashland	57%	300+
Coquille Valley Hospital District	Coquille	57%	(a)
Legacy Emanuel Medical Center	Portland	57%	300+
Legacy Good Samaritan Medical Center	Portland	57%	300+
Providence Portland Medical Center	Portland	57%	300+
McKenzie - Willamette Medical Center	Springfield	56%	300+
Santiam Memorial Hospital	Stayton	56%	(a)
Tuality Community Hospital	Hillsboro	56%	300+
Providence Saint Vincent Medical Center	Portland	55%	300+
OHSU Hospital & Clinics	Portland	54%	300+
Saint Charles - Madras	Madras	54%	(a)
Mid - Columbia Medical Center	The Dalles	53%	300+
Peace Harbor Medical Center	Florence	53%	(a)
Pioneer Memorial Hospital	Prineville	53%	(a)
Providence Milwaukie Hospital	Milwaukie	53%	300+
Providence Seaside Hospital	Seaside	53%	(a)
Providence Willamette Falls Med Ctr	Oregon City	53%	300+
Saint Charles Medical Center - Bend	Bend	53%	300+
Salem Hospital	Salem	53%	300+
Asante Three Rivers Medical Center	Grants Pass	52%	300+
Mercy Medical Center	Roseburg	52%	300+
Sacred Heart University District	Eugene	52%	(a)
Sky Lakes Medical Center	Klamath Falls	52%	300+
Asante Rogue Regional Medical Center	Medford	51%	300+
Bay Area Hospital	Coos Bay	50%	300+
Samaritan Lebanon Community Hospital	Lebanon	49%	300+
Providence Medford Medical Center	Medford	48%	300+
Good Samaritan Regional Medical Center	Corvallis	39%	300+

Doctors 'Always' Communicated Well

Hospital Name	City	Rate	Cases
Coquille Valley Hospital District	Coquille	90%	(a)
Wallowa Memorial Hospital	Enterprise	89%	(a)
Providence Hood River Memorial Hospital	Hood River	87%	300+
St Alphonsus Med Ctr-Baker City	Baker City	87%	(a)
Asante Ashland Community Hospital	Ashland	85%	300+
Pioneer Memorial Hospital	Prineville	85%	(a)
Silverton Hospital	Silverton	84%	300+
Providence Newberg Medical Center	Newberg	83%	300+
Saint Alphonsus Medical Center - Ontario	Ontario	83%	300+
Samaritan Albany General Hospital	Albany	83%	300+
Samaritan Pacific Communities Hospital	Newport	83%	300+
Willamette Valley Medical Center	Mcminnville	83%	300+
Providence Willamette Falls Med Ctr	Oregon City	82%	300+
Kaiser Sunnyside Medical Center	Clackamas	81%	300+
Legacy Meridian Park Medical Center	Tualatin	81%	300+
McKenzie - Willamette Medical Center	Springfield	81%	300+
Mid - Columbia Medical Center	The Dalles	81%	300+
Peace Harbor Medical Center	Florence	81%	(a)
Providence Milwaukie Hospital	Milwaukie	81%	300+
Santiam Memorial Hospital	Stayton	81%	(a)
Adventist Medical Center	Portland	80%	300+
Asante Three Rivers Medical Center	Grants Pass	80%	300+
Columbia Memorial Hospital	Astoria	80%	300+
Legacy Mount Hood Medical Center	Gresham	80%	300+
Providence Portland Medical Center	Portland	80%	300+
Providence Saint Vincent Medical Center	Portland	80%	300+
Salem Hospital	Salem	80%	300+
Samaritan North Lincoln Hospital	Lincoln City	80%	(a)

NOTE: Hospital profiles are in alphabetical order by state, then city, then hospital within the city; Rankings exclude hospitals with less than 25 cases except for patient surveys which excludes hospitals with less than 100 cases; (a) 100-299 cases; (1) The number of cases/patients is too few to report; (2) Data submitted were based on a sample of cases/patients; (3) Results are based on a shorter time period than required; (4) Data suppressed by CMS for one or more quarters; (5) Results are not available for this reporting period; (6) Fewer than 100 patients completed the HCAHPS survey; (7) No cases met the criteria for this measure; (8) The lower limit of the confidence interval cannot be calculated if the number of observed infections equals zero; (9) No data are available from the state/territory for this reporting period; (10) The scores shown reflect fewer than 50 completed surveys; (11) There were discrepancies in the data collection process; (12) This measure does not apply to this hospital for this reporting period; (13) Results cannot be calculated for this reporting period; (14) The results for this state are combined with nearby states to protect confidentiality; Please refer to the User's Guide for a full explanation of data.

Sky Lakes Medical Center	Klamath Falls	80%	300+
Tuality Community Hospital	Hillsboro	80%	300+
Asante Rogue Regional Medical Center	Medford	79%	300+
Good Shepherd Medical Center	Hermiston	79%	300+
Legacy Good Samaritan Medical Center	Portland	79%	300+
Providence Seaside Hospital	Seaside	79%	(a)
Saint Charles Medical Center - Redmond	Redmond	79%	300+
Tillamook Regional Medical Center	Tillamook	79%	(a)
Mercy Medical Center	Roseburg	78%	300+
OHSU Hospital & Clinics	Portland	78%	300+
Sacred Heart Medical Center - Riverbend	Springfield	78%	300+
Saint Charles Medical Center - Bend	Bend	78%	300+
Legacy Emanuel Medical Center	Portland	77%	300+
Saint Charles - Madras	Madras	77%	(a)
Bay Area Hospital	Coos Bay	76%	300+
Good Samaritan Regional Medical Center	Corvallis	76%	300+
Sacred Heart University District	Eugene	76%	(a)
Providence Medford Medical Center	Medford	75%	300+
Samaritan Lebanon Community Hospital	Lebanon	75%	300+

Home Recovery Information Given

Hospital Name	City	Rate	Cases
St Alphonsus Med Ctr-Baker City	Baker City	92%	(a)
Good Shepherd Medical Center	Hermiston	91%	300+
Peace Harbor Medical Center	Florence	91%	(a)
Asante Ashland Community Hospital	Ashland	90%	300+
Coquille Valley Hospital District	Coquille	90%	(a)
Kaiser Sunnyside Medical Center	Clackamas	89%	300+
Legacy Emanuel Medical Center	Portland	89%	300+
Saint Alphonsus Medical Center - Ontario	Ontario	89%	300+
Willamette Valley Medical Center	Mcminnville	89%	300+
Adventist Medical Center	Portland	88%	300+
Columbia Memorial Hospital	Astoria	88%	300+
Legacy Mount Hood Medical Center	Gresham	88%	300+
McKenzie - Willamette Medical Center	Springfield	88%	300+
Mid - Columbia Medical Center	The Dalles	88%	300+
OHSU Hospital & Clinics	Portland	88%	300+
Providence Hood River Memorial Hospital	Hood River	88%	300+
Sacred Heart Medical Center - Riverbend	Springfield	88%	300+
Tillamook Regional Medical Center	Tillamook	88%	(a)
Tuality Community Hospital	Hillsboro	88%	300+
Wallowa Memorial Hospital	Enterprise	88%	(a)
Bay Area Hospital	Coos Bay	87%	300+
Legacy Good Samaritan Medical Center	Portland	87%	300+
Legacy Meridian Park Medical Center	Tualatin	87%	300+
Providence Newberg Medical Center	Newberg	87%	300+
Providence Portland Medical Center	Portland	87%	300+
Providence Saint Vincent Medical Center	Portland	87%	300+
Saint Charles Medical Center - Bend	Bend	87%	300+
Saint Charles Medical Center - Redmond	Redmond	87%	300+
Samaritan Albany General Hospital	Albany	87%	300+
Silverton Hospital	Silverton	87%	300+
Providence Milwaukie Hospital	Milwaukie	86%	300+
Providence Willamette Falls Med Ctr	Oregon City	86%	300+
Salem Hospital	Salem	86%	300+
Sky Lakes Medical Center	Klamath Falls	86%	300+
Asante Three Rivers Medical Center	Grants Pass	84%	300+
Good Samaritan Regional Medical Center	Corvallis	84%	300+
Providence Medford Medical Center	Medford	84%	300+
Samaritan Lebanon Community Hospital	Lebanon	84%	300+
Samaritan Pacific Communities Hospital	Newport	84%	300+
Santiam Memorial Hospital	Stayton	84%	(a)
Saint Charles - Madras	Madras	83%	(a)
Asante Rogue Regional Medical Center	Medford	82%	300+
Mercy Medical Center	Roseburg	82%	300+
Pioneer Memorial Hospital	Prineville	82%	(a)
Sacred Heart University District	Eugene	82%	(a)
Providence Seaside Hospital	Seaside	81%	(a)
Samaritan North Lincoln Hospital	Lincoln City	81%	(a)

Hospital Given 9 or 10 on 10 Point Scale

Hospital Name	City	Rate	Cases
Silverton Hospital	Silverton	82%	300+
Coquille Valley Hospital District	Coquille	81%	(a)
Legacy Meridian Park Medical Center	Tualatin	78%	300+
Providence Hood River Memorial Hospital	Hood River	77%	300+
Providence Newberg Medical Center	Newberg	77%	300+
Providence Milwaukie Hospital	Milwaukie	76%	300+
Providence Portland Medical Center	Portland	76%	300+
Sacred Heart Medical Center - Riverbend	Springfield	76%	300+
St Alphonsus Med Ctr-Baker City	Baker City	76%	(a)
OHSU Hospital & Clinics	Portland	75%	300+
Wallowa Memorial Hospital	Enterprise	75%	(a)
Willamette Valley Medical Center	Mcminnville	75%	300+
Asante Ashland Community Hospital	Ashland	74%	300+
Asante Rogue Regional Medical Center	Medford	74%	300+
Kaiser Sunnyside Medical Center	Clackamas	74%	300+
Legacy Good Samaritan Medical Center	Portland	74%	300+
Providence Saint Vincent Medical Center	Portland	74%	300+
Saint Charles Medical Center - Redmond	Redmond	74%	300+
Salem Hospital	Salem	74%	300+
Santiam Memorial Hospital	Stayton	74%	(a)
McKenzie - Willamette Medical Center	Springfield	73%	300+
Legacy Emanuel Medical Center	Portland	72%	300+
Providence Seaside Hospital	Seaside	72%	(a)
Columbia Memorial Hospital	Astoria	71%	300+
Peace Harbor Medical Center	Florence	71%	(a)
Saint Charles Medical Center - Bend	Bend	71%	300+
Samaritan Albany General Hospital	Albany	71%	300+
Legacy Mount Hood Medical Center	Gresham	70%	300+
Pioneer Memorial Hospital	Prineville	70%	(a)
Adventist Medical Center	Portland	69%	300+
Mid - Columbia Medical Center	The Dalles	69%	300+
Samaritan Pacific Communities Hospital	Newport	69%	300+
Providence Medford Medical Center	Medford	68%	300+
Saint Alphonsus Medical Center - Ontario	Ontario	68%	300+
Good Shepherd Medical Center	Hermiston	67%	300+
Tillamook Regional Medical Center	Tillamook	66%	(a)
Asante Three Rivers Medical Center	Grants Pass	65%	300+
Providence Willamette Falls Med Ctr	Oregon City	65%	300+
Saint Charles - Madras	Madras	65%	(a)
Tuality Community Hospital	Hillsboro	65%	300+
Bay Area Hospital	Coos Bay	64%	300+
Good Samaritan Regional Medical Center	Corvallis	64%	300+
Mercy Medical Center	Roseburg	63%	300+
Samaritan North Lincoln Hospital	Lincoln City	62%	(a)
Sky Lakes Medical Center	Klamath Falls	62%	300+
Sacred Heart University District	Eugene	61%	(a)
Samaritan Lebanon Community Hospital	Lebanon	61%	300+

Meds 'Always' Explained Before Given

Hospital Name	City	Rate	Cases
Pioneer Memorial Hospital	Prineville	75%	(a)
Coquille Valley Hospital District	Coquille	73%	(a)
St Alphonsus Med Ctr-Baker City	Baker City	73%	(a)
Samaritan Pacific Communities Hospital	Newport	70%	300+
Providence Hood River Memorial Hospital	Hood River	69%	300+
Silverton Hospital	Silverton	69%	300+
Asante Ashland Community Hospital	Ashland	68%	300+
Mid - Columbia Medical Center	The Dalles	68%	300+
Providence Willamette Falls Med Ctr	Oregon City	68%	300+
Wallowa Memorial Hospital	Enterprise	68%	(a)
Columbia Memorial Hospital	Astoria	67%	300+
McKenzie - Willamette Medical Center	Springfield	67%	300+
Samaritan North Lincoln Hospital	Lincoln City	67%	(a)
Providence Milwaukie Hospital	Milwaukie	66%	300+
Adventist Medical Center	Portland	65%	300+
Good Shepherd Medical Center	Hermiston	65%	300+
Kaiser Sunnyside Medical Center	Clackamas	65%	300+
Peace Harbor Medical Center	Florence	65%	(a)
Providence Portland Medical Center	Portland	65%	300+
Saint Charles - Madras	Madras	65%	(a)
Saint Charles Medical Center - Redmond	Redmond	65%	300+
Sky Lakes Medical Center	Klamath Falls	65%	300+
Providence Newberg Medical Center	Newberg	64%	300+
Providence Saint Vincent Medical Center	Portland	64%	300+
Samaritan Albany General Hospital	Albany	64%	300+
Willamette Valley Medical Center	Mcminnville	64%	300+
Legacy Good Samaritan Medical Center	Portland	63%	300+
Legacy Meridian Park Medical Center	Tualatin	63%	300+
Legacy Mount Hood Medical Center	Gresham	63%	300+
OHSU Hospital & Clinics	Portland	63%	300+
Tillamook Regional Medical Center	Tillamook	63%	(a)
Asante Rogue Regional Medical Center	Medford	62%	300+
Good Samaritan Regional Medical Center	Corvallis	62%	300+
Legacy Emanuel Medical Center	Portland	62%	300+
Providence Seaside Hospital	Seaside	61%	(a)
Saint Alphonsus Medical Center - Ontario	Ontario	61%	300+
Saint Charles Medical Center - Bend	Bend	61%	300+
Salem Hospital	Salem	61%	300+
Samaritan Lebanon Community Hospital	Lebanon	61%	300+
Tuality Community Hospital	Hillsboro	60%	300+
Asante Three Rivers Medical Center	Grants Pass	59%	300+
Providence Medford Medical Center	Medford	59%	300+
Bay Area Hospital	Coos Bay	58%	300+
Mercy Medical Center	Roseburg	57%	300+
Sacred Heart Medical Center - Riverbend	Springfield	57%	300+
Santiam Memorial Hospital	Stayton	57%	(a)
Sacred Heart University District	Eugene	56%	(a)

Nurses 'Always' Communicated Well

Hospital Name	City	Rate	Cases
Providence Seaside Hospital	Seaside	84%	(a)
Pioneer Memorial Hospital	Prineville	83%	(a)
Asante Ashland Community Hospital	Ashland	82%	300+
Coquille Valley Hospital District	Coquille	82%	(a)
Providence Hood River Memorial Hospital	Hood River	82%	300+
Samaritan Pacific Communities Hospital	Newport	82%	300+
Silverton Hospital	Silverton	82%	300+
Wallowa Memorial Hospital	Enterprise	82%	(a)
Willamette Valley Medical Center	Mcminnville	82%	300+
Providence Milwaukie Hospital	Milwaukie	81%	300+
Providence Newberg Medical Center	Newberg	81%	300+
Santiam Memorial Hospital	Stayton	81%	(a)
Columbia Memorial Hospital	Astoria	80%	300+
Legacy Meridian Park Medical Center	Tualatin	80%	300+
Mid - Columbia Medical Center	The Dalles	80%	300+
Peace Harbor Medical Center	Florence	80%	(a)
St Alphonsus Med Ctr-Baker City	Baker City	80%	(a)
Adventist Medical Center	Portland	79%	300+
Asante Rogue Regional Medical Center	Medford	79%	300+
Good Shepherd Medical Center	Hermiston	79%	300+
McKenzie - Willamette Medical Center	Springfield	79%	300+
Salem Hospital	Salem	79%	300+
Tillamook Regional Medical Center	Tillamook	79%	(a)
Kaiser Sunnyside Medical Center	Clackamas	78%	300+
Providence Portland Medical Center	Portland	78%	300+
Providence Saint Vincent Medical Center	Portland	78%	300+
Providence Willamette Falls Med Ctr	Oregon City	78%	300+
Saint Alphonsus Medical Center - Ontario	Ontario	78%	300+
Saint Charles Medical Center - Redmond	Redmond	78%	300+
Samaritan Albany General Hospital	Albany	78%	300+
Samaritan Lebanon Community Hospital	Lebanon	78%	300+
Legacy Good Samaritan Medical Center	Portland	77%	300+
Legacy Mount Hood Medical Center	Gresham	77%	300+
Saint Charles - Madras	Madras	77%	(a)
Saint Charles Medical Center - Bend	Bend	77%	300+
Samaritan North Lincoln Hospital	Lincoln City	77%	(a)
Asante Three Rivers Medical Center	Grants Pass	76%	300+
Bay Area Hospital	Coos Bay	76%	300+
Legacy Emanuel Medical Center	Portland	76%	300+
Mercy Medical Center	Roseburg	76%	300+
OHSU Hospital & Clinics	Portland	76%	300+
Good Samaritan Regional Medical Center	Corvallis	75%	300+
Providence Medford Medical Center	Medford	75%	300+
Sacred Heart University District	Eugene	74%	(a)
Sacred Heart Medical Center - Riverbend	Springfield	73%	300+
Sky Lakes Medical Center	Klamath Falls	73%	300+
Tuality Community Hospital	Hillsboro	73%	300+

Pain 'Always' Well Controlled

Hospital Name	City	Rate	Cases
Pioneer Memorial Hospital	Prineville	77%	(a)
Samaritan North Lincoln Hospital	Lincoln City	76%	(a)
Willamette Valley Medical Center	Mcminnville	76%	300+
Asante Ashland Community Hospital	Ashland	75%	300+
Coquille Valley Hospital District	Coquille	75%	(a)
Peace Harbor Medical Center	Florence	75%	(a)
St Alphonsus Med Ctr-Baker City	Baker City	75%	(a)
Bay Area Hospital	Coos Bay	74%	300+
Providence Portland Medical Center	Portland	74%	300+
Columbia Memorial Hospital	Astoria	73%	300+
Legacy Meridian Park Medical Center	Tualatin	73%	300+
Samaritan Albany General Hospital	Albany	73%	300+
Santiam Memorial Hospital	Stayton	73%	(a)
Adventist Medical Center	Portland	72%	300+
Kaiser Sunnyside Medical Center	Clackamas	72%	300+
McKenzie - Willamette Medical Center	Springfield	72%	300+
Providence Hood River Memorial Hospital	Hood River	72%	300+
Providence Newberg Medical Center	Newberg	72%	300+
Providence Seaside Hospital	Seaside	72%	(a)
Saint Alphonsus Medical Center - Ontario	Ontario	72%	300+
Saint Charles Medical Center - Redmond	Redmond	72%	300+
Silverton Hospital	Silverton	72%	300+
Asante Three Rivers Medical Center	Grants Pass	71%	300+
Providence Saint Vincent Medical Center	Portland	71%	300+
Saint Charles Medical Center - Bend	Bend	71%	300+
Salem Hospital	Salem	71%	300+
Samaritan Pacific Communities Hospital	Newport	71%	300+
Tillamook Regional Medical Center	Tillamook	71%	(a)
Tuality Community Hospital	Hillsboro	71%	300+
Wallowa Memorial Hospital	Enterprise	71%	(a)
Asante Rogue Regional Medical Center	Medford	70%	300+
Legacy Emanuel Medical Center	Portland	70%	300+
Legacy Good Samaritan Medical Center	Portland	70%	300+
Providence Medford Medical Center	Medford	70%	300+
Providence Milwaukie Hospital	Milwaukie	70%	300+
Good Shepherd Medical Center	Hermiston	69%	300+
Legacy Mount Hood Medical Center	Gresham	69%	300+
Mercy Medical Center	Roseburg	69%	300+
Mid - Columbia Medical Center	The Dalles	69%	300+
OHSU Hospital & Clinics	Portland	69%	300+
Providence Willamette Falls Med Ctr	Oregon City	68%	300+
Sacred Heart Medical Center - Riverbend	Springfield	68%	300+
Samaritan Lebanon Community Hospital	Lebanon	68%	300+
Good Samaritan Regional Medical Center	Corvallis	67%	300+
Saint Charles - Madras	Madras	67%	(a)
Sacred Heart University District	Eugene	66%	(a)
Sky Lakes Medical Center	Klamath Falls	65%	300+

NOTE: Hospital profiles are in alphabetical order by state, then city, then hospital within the city; Rankings exclude hospitals with less than 25 cases except for patient surveys which excludes hospitals with less than 100 cases; (a) 100-299 cases; (1) The number of cases/patients is too few to report; (2) Data submitted were based on a sample of cases/patients; (3) Results are based on a shorter time period than required; (4) Data suppressed by CMS for one or more quarters; (5) Results are not available for this reporting period; (6) Fewer than 100 patients completed the HCAHPS survey; (7) No cases met the criteria for this measure; (8) The lower limit of the confidence interval cannot be calculated if the number of observed infections equals zero; (9) No data are available from the state/territory for this reporting period; (10) The scores shown reflect fewer than 50 completed surveys; (11) There were discrepancies in the data collection process; (12) This measure does not apply to this hospital for this reporting period; (13) Results cannot be calculated for this reporting period; (14) The results for this state are combined with nearby states to protect confidentiality; Please refer to the User's Guide for a full explanation of data.

Room and Bathroom 'Always' Clean

Hospital Name	City	Rate	Cases
Providence Seaside Hospital	Seaside	85%	(a)
Coquille Valley Hospital District	Coquille	82%	(a)
Saint Charles - Madras	Madras	82%	(a)
Santiam Memorial Hospital	Stayton	82%	(a)
Peace Harbor Medical Center	Florence	80%	(a)
Providence Hood River Memorial Hospital	Hood River	80%	300+
Samaritan Albany General Hospital	Albany	80%	300+
Providence Milwaukie Hospital	Milwaukie	79%	300+
Silverton Hospital	Silverton	79%	300+
Wallowa Memorial Hospital	Enterprise	78%	(a)
Providence Newberg Medical Center	Newberg	77%	300+
St Alphonsus Med Ctr-Baker City	Baker City	76%	(a)
Samaritan Lebanon Community Hospital	Lebanon	76%	300+
Samaritan Pacific Communities Hospital	Newport	76%	300+
Columbia Memorial Hospital	Astoria	75%	300+
Sacred Heart University District	Eugene	75%	(a)
Asante Ashland Community Hospital	Ashland	74%	300+
Mid - Columbia Medical Center	The Dalles	74%	300+
Salem Hospital	Salem	74%	300+
Samaritan North Lincoln Hospital	Lincoln City	74%	(a)
Asante Three Rivers Medical Center	Grants Pass	73%	300+
Kaiser Sunnyside Medical Center	Clackamas	73%	300+
Saint Charles Medical Center - Redmond	Redmond	73%	300+
Tillamook Regional Medical Center	Tillamook	73%	(a)
Good Shepherd Medical Center	Hermiston	72%	300+
Pioneer Memorial Hospital	Prineville	72%	(a)
Providence Saint Vincent Medical Center	Portland	72%	300+
Sky Lakes Medical Center	Klamath Falls	72%	300+
Asante Rogue Regional Medical Center	Medford	71%	300+
Legacy Good Samaritan Medical Center	Portland	71%	300+
McKenzie - Willamette Medical Center	Springfield	71%	300+
Saint Alphonsus Medical Center - Ontario	Ontario	71%	300+
Adventist Medical Center	Portland	70%	300+
Legacy Emanuel Medical Center	Portland	70%	300+
Legacy Meridian Park Medical Center	Tualatin	70%	300+
Mercy Medical Center	Roseburg	70%	300+
OHSU Hospital & Clinics	Portland	70%	300+
Providence Portland Medical Center	Portland	70%	300+
Providence Willamette Falls Med Ctr	Oregon City	70%	300+
Bay Area Hospital	Coos Bay	69%	300+
Providence Medford Medical Center	Medford	69%	300+
Sacred Heart Medical Center - Riverbend	Springfield	67%	300+
Good Samaritan Regional Medical Center	Corvallis	66%	300+
Legacy Mount Hood Medical Center	Gresham	66%	300+
Saint Charles Medical Center - Bend	Bend	66%	300+
Tuality Community Hospital	Hillsboro	66%	300+
Willamette Valley Medical Center	Mcminnville	64%	300+

Timely Help 'Always' Received

Hospital Name	City	Rate	Cases
Samaritan Pacific Communities Hospital	Newport	82%	300+
St Alphonsus Med Ctr-Baker City	Baker City	80%	(a)
Coquille Valley Hospital District	Coquille	76%	(a)
Good Shepherd Medical Center	Hermiston	75%	300+
Providence Seaside Hospital	Seaside	75%	(a)
Samaritan North Lincoln Hospital	Lincoln City	75%	(a)
Columbia Memorial Hospital	Astoria	74%	300+
Peace Harbor Medical Center	Florence	74%	(a)
Samaritan Lebanon Community Hospital	Lebanon	74%	300+
Mid - Columbia Medical Center	The Dalles	72%	300+
Providence Hood River Memorial Hospital	Hood River	72%	300+
Saint Alphonsus Medical Center - Ontario	Ontario	72%	300+
Tillamook Regional Medical Center	Tillamook	72%	(a)
Wallowa Memorial Hospital	Enterprise	71%	(a)
Legacy Meridian Park Medical Center	Tualatin	70%	300+
Pioneer Memorial Hospital	Prineville	69%	(a)
Providence Milwaukie Hospital	Milwaukie	69%	300+
Saint Charles Medical Center - Redmond	Redmond	69%	300+
Asante Ashland Community Hospital	Ashland	68%	300+
Tuality Community Hospital	Hillsboro	68%	300+
Willamette Valley Medical Center	Mcminnville	68%	300+
Adventist Medical Center	Portland	67%	300+
Bay Area Hospital	Coos Bay	67%	300+
Saint Charles - Madras	Madras	67%	(a)
Silverton Hospital	Silverton	66%	300+
McKenzie - Willamette Medical Center	Springfield	65%	300+
Providence Newberg Medical Center	Newberg	65%	300+
Providence Portland Medical Center	Portland	65%	300+
Saint Charles Medical Center - Bend	Bend	65%	300+
Salem Hospital	Salem	65%	300+
Samaritan Albany General Hospital	Albany	65%	300+
Santiam Memorial Hospital	Stayton	65%	(a)
Good Samaritan Regional Medical Center	Corvallis	64%	300+
Kaiser Sunnyside Medical Center	Clackamas	63%	300+
Legacy Good Samaritan Medical Center	Portland	63%	300+
Providence Saint Vincent Medical Center	Portland	63%	300+
Asante Three Rivers Medical Center	Grants Pass	62%	300+
Sky Lakes Medical Center	Klamath Falls	62%	300+
Legacy Mount Hood Medical Center	Gresham	61%	300+
OHSU Hospital & Clinics	Portland	61%	300+
Providence Medford Medical Center	Medford	61%	300+
Asante Rogue Regional Medical Center	Medford	60%	300+
Legacy Emanuel Medical Center	Portland	60%	300+
Sacred Heart Medical Center - Riverbend	Springfield	60%	300+
Sacred Heart University District	Eugene	59%	(a)
Providence Willamette Falls Med Ctr	Oregon City	58%	300+
Mercy Medical Center	Roseburg	55%	300+

Would Definitely Recommend Hospital

Hospital Name	City	Rate	Cases
Silverton Hospital	Silverton	84%	300+
Providence Newberg Medical Center	Newberg	83%	300+
Providence Milwaukie Hospital	Milwaukie	82%	300+
Asante Ashland Community Hospital	Ashland	81%	300+
Asante Rogue Regional Medical Center	Medford	81%	300+
Coquille Valley Hospital District	Coquille	81%	(a)
Legacy Meridian Park Medical Center	Tualatin	81%	300+
OHSU Hospital & Clinics	Portland	81%	300+
Providence Hood River Memorial Hospital	Hood River	81%	300+
Providence Saint Vincent Medical Center	Portland	81%	300+
Providence Portland Medical Center	Portland	79%	300+
Legacy Emanuel Medical Center	Portland	78%	300+
Sacred Heart Medical Center - Riverbend	Springfield	78%	300+
Saint Charles Medical Center - Bend	Bend	78%	300+
Salem Hospital	Salem	78%	300+
Wallowa Memorial Hospital	Enterprise	78%	(a)
Legacy Good Samaritan Medical Center	Portland	77%	300+
McKenzie - Willamette Medical Center	Springfield	76%	300+
Saint Charles Medical Center - Redmond	Redmond	76%	300+
Adventist Medical Center	Portland	75%	300+
Kaiser Sunnyside Medical Center	Clackamas	75%	300+
Legacy Mount Hood Medical Center	Gresham	75%	300+
Columbia Memorial Hospital	Astoria	74%	300+
Providence Medford Medical Center	Medford	74%	300+
Samaritan Albany General Hospital	Albany	74%	300+
Providence Willamette Falls Med Ctr	Oregon City	72%	300+
Willamette Valley Medical Center	Mcminnville	72%	300+
Peace Harbor Medical Center	Florence	71%	(a)
Samaritan Pacific Communities Hospital	Newport	71%	300+
Santiam Memorial Hospital	Stayton	71%	(a)
Good Samaritan Regional Medical Center	Corvallis	70%	300+
Providence Seaside Hospital	Seaside	70%	(a)
St Alphonsus Med Ctr-Baker City	Baker City	70%	(a)
Mid - Columbia Medical Center	The Dalles	69%	300+
Tuality Community Hospital	Hillsboro	69%	300+
Bay Area Hospital	Coos Bay	68%	300+
Asante Three Rivers Medical Center	Grants Pass	66%	300+
Sacred Heart University District	Eugene	66%	(a)
Saint Charles - Madras	Madras	65%	(a)
Pioneer Memorial Hospital	Prineville	64%	(a)
Samaritan North Lincoln Hospital	Lincoln City	63%	(a)
Mercy Medical Center	Roseburg	62%	300+
Saint Alphonsus Medical Center - Ontario	Ontario	62%	300+
Samaritan Lebanon Community Hospital	Lebanon	62%	300+
Sky Lakes Medical Center	Klamath Falls	60%	300+
Tillamook Regional Medical Center	Tillamook	60%	(a)
Good Shepherd Medical Center	Hermiston	58%	300+

Use of Medical Imaging

Cardiac Imaging Stress Test before OP Surgery

Hospital Name	City	Rate	Cases
Santiam Memorial Hospital	Stayton	0.0%	53
Sky Lakes Medical Center	Klamath Falls	0.9%	107
Legacy Meridian Park Medical Center	Tualatin	1.6%	61
Lower Umpqua Hospital District	Reedsport	1.9%	53
Peace Harbor Medical Center	Florence	1.9%	103
McKenzie - Willamette Medical Center	Springfield	2.2%	91
Salem Hospital	Salem	3.1%	64
Providence Medford Medical Center	Medford	3.3%	214
Samaritan Albany General Hospital	Albany	3.3%	61
Curry General Hospital	Gold Beach	3.6%	137
Saint Alphonsus Medical Center - Ontario	Ontario	3.8%	183
Grande Ronde Hospital	La Grande	4.0%	149
Willamette Valley Medical Center	Mcminnville	4.2%	96
Asante Rogue Regional Medical Center	Medford	4.3%	820
Providence Saint Vincent Medical Center	Portland	4.7%	532
Good Samaritan Regional Medical Center	Corvallis	4.9%	283
OHSU Hospital & Clinics	Portland	4.9%	429
Sacred Heart Medical Center - Riverbend	Springfield	4.9%	668
Silverton Hospital	Silverton	4.9%	61
Adventist Medical Center	Portland	5.0%	121
Mercy Medical Center	Roseburg	5.0%	337
Providence Portland Medical Center	Portland	5.0%	359
Mid - Columbia Medical Center	The Dalles	5.4%	184
Asante Three Rivers Medical Center	Grants Pass	6.0%	367
Bay Area Hospital	Coos Bay	6.6%	288
Providence Hood River Memorial Hospital	Hood River	7.1%	99
Providence Newberg Medical Center	Newberg	7.4%	95
Legacy Mount Hood Medical Center	Gresham	9.4%	64

Combination Abdominal CT Scan

Hospital Name	City	Rate	Cases
Sacred Heart University District	Eugene	0.0%	82
Saint Charles Medical Center - Redmond	Redmond	0.0%	186
Saint Charles Medical Center - Bend	Bend	0.5%	375
McKenzie - Willamette Medical Center	Springfield	0.9%	211
Lake District Hospital	Lakeview	1.2%	83
Sacred Heart Medical Center - Riverbend	Springfield	1.4%	363
Santiam Memorial Hospital	Stayton	1.4%	141
Bay Area Hospital	Coos Bay	2.1%	577
Tuality Community Hospital	Hillsboro	2.5%	438
Providence Willamette Falls Med Ctr	Oregon City	3.4%	293
Asante Ashland Community Hospital	Ashland	3.5%	143
Coquille Valley Hospital District	Coquille	3.5%	143
Legacy Meridian Park Medical Center	Tualatin	3.6%	603
Salem Hospital	Salem	3.6%	915
West Valley Hospital	Dallas	3.8%	132
Willamette Valley Medical Center	Mcminnville	3.8%	447
Sky Lakes Medical Center	Klamath Falls	4.0%	793
Harney District Hospital	Burns	4.1%	98
Providence Milwaukie Hospital	Milwaukie	4.2%	265
Providence Seaside Hospital	Seaside	4.3%	230
Asante Three Rivers Medical Center	Grants Pass	4.6%	715
Curry General Hospital	Gold Beach	4.8%	294
Peacehealth Cottage Grove Comm Med Ctr	Cottage Grove	5.2%	134
Silverton Hospital	Silverton	5.2%	233
Saint Alphonsus Medical Center - Ontario	Ontario	5.3%	551
Saint Charles - Madras	Madras	5.6%	126
Legacy Good Samaritan Medical Center	Portland	6.0%	562
Samaritan Albany General Hospital	Albany	6.0%	332
Peace Harbor Medical Center	Florence	6.3%	301
Legacy Emanuel Medical Center	Portland	6.4%	250
Asante Rogue Regional Medical Center	Medford	6.5%	649
Providence Saint Vincent Medical Center	Portland	6.7%	867
Pioneer Memorial Hospital	Prineville	7.0%	227
Providence Portland Medical Center	Portland	7.4%	835
Grande Ronde Hospital	La Grande	7.8%	459
Lower Umpqua Hospital District	Reedsport	7.8%	102
Good Samaritan Regional Medical Center	Corvallis	7.9%	365
Providence Newberg Medical Center	Newberg	9.6%	281
Providence Hood River Memorial Hospital	Hood River	10.0%	259
Mercy Medical Center	Roseburg	10.1%	953
Mid - Columbia Medical Center	The Dalles	11.0%	409
Legacy Mount Hood Medical Center	Gresham	11.7%	418
Adventist Medical Center	Portland	11.8%	594
Providence Medford Medical Center	Medford	12.9%	660
OHSU Hospital & Clinics	Portland	15.4%	1742

Combination Brain/Sinus CT Scan

Hospital Name	City	Rate	Cases
Peacehealth Cottage Grove Comm Med Ctr	Cottage Grove	0.0%	131
Pioneer Memorial Hospital	Heppner	0.0%	34
Providence Seaside Hospital	Seaside	0.0%	165
Providence Portland Medical Center	Portland	0.4%	457
Mercy Medical Center	Roseburg	0.7%	609
Santiam Memorial Hospital	Stayton	0.7%	141
Providence Medford Medical Center	Medford	0.8%	354
Legacy Meridian Park Medical Center	Tualatin	0.9%	456
Providence Milwaukie Hospital	Milwaukie	0.9%	220
Tuality Community Hospital	Hillsboro	1.0%	384
Mid - Columbia Medical Center	The Dalles	1.1%	267
Asante Rogue Regional Medical Center	Medford	1.5%	659
Saint Alphonsus Medical Center - Ontario	Ontario	1.5%	469
Sky Lakes Medical Center	Klamath Falls	1.9%	593
Sacred Heart Medical Center - Riverbend	Springfield	2.0%	590
Providence Saint Vincent Medical Center	Portland	2.5%	647
Adventist Medical Center	Portland	2.6%	500
Salem Hospital	Salem	2.8%	757
Bay Area Hospital	Coos Bay	3.8%	424
Legacy Emanuel Medical Center	Portland	4.8%	315
McKenzie - Willamette Medical Center	Springfield	5.0%	219

Combination Chest CT Scan

Hospital Name	City	Rate	Cases
Asante Ashland Community Hospital	Ashland	0.0%	54
Coquille Valley Hospital District	Coquille	0.0%	61
Lake District Hospital	Lakeview	0.0%	53
McKenzie - Willamette Medical Center	Springfield	0.0%	51
Mercy Medical Center	Roseburg	0.0%	802
Peace Harbor Medical Center	Florence	0.0%	178
Peacehealth Cottage Grove Comm Med Ctr	Cottage Grove	0.0%	84
Providence Milwaukie Hospital	Milwaukie	0.0%	162
Providence Portland Medical Center	Portland	0.0%	643
Providence Saint Vincent Medical Center	Portland	0.0%	578
Providence Willamette Falls Med Ctr	Oregon City	0.0%	149
Samaritan Albany General Hospital	Albany	0.0%	219
Santiam Memorial Hospital	Stayton	0.0%	91

NOTE: Hospital profiles are in alphabetical order by state, then city, then hospital within the city; Rankings exclude hospitals with less than 25 cases except for patient surveys which excludes hospitals with less than 100 cases; (a) 100-299 cases; (1) The number of cases/patients is too few to report; (2) Data submitted were based on a sample of cases/patients; (3) Results are based on a shorter time period than required; (4) Data suppressed by CMS for one or more quarters; (5) Results are not available for this reporting period; (6) Fewer than 100 patients completed the HCAHPS survey; (7) No cases met the criteria for this measure; (8) The lower limit of the confidence interval cannot be calculated if the number of observed infections equals zero; (9) No data are available from the state/territory for this reporting period; (10) The scores shown reflect fewer than 50 completed surveys; (11) There were discrepancies in the data collection process; (12) This measure does not apply to this hospital for this reporting period; (13) Results cannot be calculated for this reporting period; (14) The results for this state are combined with nearby states to protect confidentiality; Please refer to the User's Guide for a full explanation of data.

Silverton Hospital	Silverton	0.0%	84
Tuality Community Hospital	Hillsboro	0.0%	243
West Valley Hospital	Dallas	0.0%	68
Willamette Valley Medical Center	Mcminnville	0.0%	302
Sky Lakes Medical Center	Klamath Falls	0.2%	604
Bay Area Hospital	Coos Bay	0.3%	352
Providence Medford Medical Center	Medford	0.4%	262
Curry General Hospital	Gold Beach	0.5%	216
Legacy Mount Hood Medical Center	Gresham	0.5%	214
Saint Alphonsus Medical Center - Ontario	Ontario	0.5%	207
Asante Three Rivers Medical Center	Grants Pass	0.6%	510
Legacy Good Samaritan Medical Center	Portland	0.7%	440
Legacy Emanuel Medical Center	Portland	0.8%	131
Legacy Meridian Park Medical Center	Tualatin	1.0%	487
OHSU Hospital & Clinics	Portland	1.0%	1589
Providence Newberg Medical Center	Newberg	1.1%	175
Salem Hospital	Salem	1.2%	491
Saint Charles - Madras	Madras	1.4%	74
Asante Rogue Regional Medical Center	Medford	1.5%	399
Harney District Hospital	Burns	1.7%	58
Providence Seaside Hospital	Seaside	1.8%	111
Grande Ronde Hospital	La Grande	2.0%	306
Good Samaritan Regional Medical Center	Corvallis	2.2%	225
Mid - Columbia Medical Center	The Dalles	2.3%	305
Providence Hood River Memorial Hospital	Hood River	2.6%	155
Saint Charles Medical Center - Redmond	Redmond	3.1%	131
Lower Umpqua Hospital District	Reedsport	3.8%	53
Pioneer Memorial Hospital	Prineville	3.9%	178
Adventist Medical Center	Portland	5.2%	326
Saint Charles Medical Center - Bend	Bend	8.1%	272
Providence Willamette Falls Med Ctr	Oregon City	41.9%	74
Mercy Medical Center	Roseburg	42.3%	182
Legacy Good Samaritan Medical Center	Portland	43.1%	65
Adventist Medical Center	Portland	46.1%	154
Peace Harbor Medical Center	Florence	48.0%	50
Providence Saint Vincent Medical Center	Portland	50.6%	83
Legacy Mount Hood Medical Center	Gresham	54.3%	46
Mid - Columbia Medical Center	The Dalles	56.0%	84

Follow-up Mammogram/Ultrasound

A follow-up rate near zero may indicate missed cancer; a rate higher than 14% may mean there is unnecessary follow up.

Hospital Name	City	Rate	Cases
Curry General Hospital	Gold Beach	3.2%	564
Coquille Valley Hospital District	Coquille	3.3%	272
Lower Umpqua Hospital District	Reedsport	3.9%	152
Asante Three Rivers Medical Center	Grants Pass	4.5%	2242
Peace Harbor Medical Center	Florence	4.9%	649
Adventist Medical Center	Portland	5.6%	1086
Good Samaritan Regional Medical Center	Corvallis	5.6%	1301
Tuality Community Hospital	Hillsboro	5.6%	1031
Mercy Medical Center	Roseburg	5.8%	2794
Lake District Hospital	Lakeview	6.6%	211
Peacehealth Cottage Grove Comm Med Ctr	Cottage Grove	6.6%	317
Saint Alphonsus Medical Center - Ontario	Ontario	6.8%	863
Providence Saint Vincent Medical Center	Portland	7.3%	1811
Samaritan Albany General Hospital	Albany	7.8%	978
Willamette Valley Medical Center	Mcminnville	7.8%	806
OHSU Hospital & Clinics	Portland	8.0%	960
Bay Area Hospital	Coos Bay	8.2%	2061
Providence Hood River Memorial Hospital	Hood River	8.7%	551
Providence Portland Medical Center	Portland	8.8%	1142
Providence Newberg Medical Center	Newberg	8.9%	531
Legacy Good Samaritan Medical Center	Portland	9.1%	1311
Legacy Meridian Park Medical Center	Tualatin	9.2%	1211
Legacy Emanuel Medical Center	Portland	10.3%	272
Salem Hospital	Salem	10.3%	174
Providence Seaside Hospital	Seaside	10.4%	366
Asante Rogue Regional Medical Center	Medford	10.5%	2857
Santiam Memorial Hospital	Stayton	10.7%	205
Pioneer Memorial Hospital	Prineville	10.8%	435
Asante Ashland Community Hospital	Ashland	11.4%	699
Legacy Mount Hood Medical Center	Gresham	11.7%	487
Providence Medford Medical Center	Medford	12.1%	1606
Providence Milwaukie Hospital	Milwaukie	12.1%	601
Saint Charles - Madras	Madras	12.1%	207
Mid - Columbia Medical Center	The Dalles	12.2%	770
Harney District Hospital	Burns	12.6%	198
West Valley Hospital	Dallas	12.6%	206
Providence Willamette Falls Med Ctr	Oregon City	15.1%	617
Grande Ronde Hospital	La Grande	16.6%	620
Silverton Hospital	Silverton	17.2%	551
Sky Lakes Medical Center	Klamath Falls	20.6%	1039

Lumbar Spine MRI for Low Back Pain

Hospital Name	City	Rate	Cases
Samaritan Albany General Hospital	Albany	30.9%	81
Asante Three Rivers Medical Center	Grants Pass	31.0%	145
OHSU Hospital & Clinics	Portland	33.7%	163
Sky Lakes Medical Center	Klamath Falls	33.9%	224
Providence Portland Medical Center	Portland	34.5%	58
Tuality Community Hospital	Hillsboro	34.6%	104
Grande Ronde Hospital	La Grande	35.3%	116
Willamette Valley Medical Center	Mcminnville	36.7%	49
Legacy Meridian Park Medical Center	Tualatin	37.9%	174
Salem Hospital	Salem	38.5%	117
Bay Area Hospital	Coos Bay	41.0%	61
Curry General Hospital	Gold Beach	41.7%	60

NOTE: Hospital profiles are in alphabetical order by state, then city, then hospital within the city; Rankings exclude hospitals with less than 25 cases except for patient surveys which excludes hospitals with less than 100 cases; (a) 100-299 cases; (1) The number of cases/patients is too few to report; (2) Data submitted were based on a sample of cases/patients; (3) Results are based on a shorter time period than required; (4) Data suppressed by CMS for one or more quarters; (5) Results are not available for this reporting period; (6) Fewer than 100 patients completed the HCAHPS survey; (7) No cases met the criteria for this measure; (8) The lower limit of the confidence interval cannot be calculated if the number of observed infections equals zero; (9) No data are available from the state/territory for this reporting period; (10) The scores shown reflect fewer than 50 completed surveys; (11) There were discrepancies in the data collection process; (12) This measure does not apply to this hospital for this reporting period; (13) Results cannot be calculated for this reporting period; (14) The results for this state are combined with nearby states to protect confidentiality; Please refer to the User's Guide for a full explanation of data.

Samaritan Albany General Hospital

1046 6th Avenue Sw
Albany, OR 97321
Phone: 541-812-4000
Fax: 541-812-4126
E-mail: saghrecruiters@samhealth.org
URL: www.samhealth.org/shs_facilities
Type: Acute Care Hospitals
Emergency Services: Yes
Ownership: Voluntary non-profit - Church
Beds: 76

Key Personnel:
Emergency Room . . . . Harry Adamo
Operating Room. . . . . Myrna Butler, RN
Infection Control. . . . . Kim Forrester, RN
Pediatric In-Patient Care . . . . Douglas Gamet, MD
Anesthesiology. . . . . Oren Leong, MD
CEO/President. . . . . Larry A Mullins, DHA
Chief of Medical Staff. . . . . Thomas Rafalski, MD
Quality Assurance . . . . Petra Shane

Measure	Cases	This Hosp.	State Avg.	U.S. Avg.
Blood Clot Prevention and Treatment				
Anticoagulation Overlap Therapy[2]	24	100%	95%	93%
ICU Venous Thromboembolism Prophylaxis[2]	54	85%	87%	92%
Incidence of Potentially Preventable VTE[2,7]	-	-	13%	10%
UFH with Dosages/Platelet Monitoring[1,2]	-	-	100%	97%
Venous Thromboembolism Prophylaxis[2]	180	83%	83%	85%
Warfarin Therapy Discharge Instructions[2]	21	29%	54%	75%
Chest Pain/Possible Heart Attack Care				
Aspirin Given Within 24 Hours of Arrival	37	100%	97%	96%
Fibrinolytic Meds Within 30 Min. of Arrival[7]	-	-	57%	58%
Average Time to ECG (minutes)	39	15	9	7
Average Time to Transfer (minutes)	11	53	52	60
Children's Asthma Care				
Received Home Management Plan of Care	-	-	-	88%
Received Reliever Medication	-	-	-	100%
Received Systemic Corticosteroids	-	-	-	100%
Emergency Department				
Admittance Decision Time (minutes)[2]	196	44	85	98
Head CT Results Within 45 Min. of Arrival	16	50%	45%	57%
Patients Who Left ER Before Being Seen	22,039	0%	2%	2%
Time from ER Arrival to Admit. (minutes)[2]	393	151	235	274
Time from ER Arrival to Discharge (minutes)	391	82	136	134
Time in ER Before Being Evaluated (minutes)	80	22	27	26
Time to Pain Meds for Fractures (minutes)	91	45	56	57
Heart Attack Care				
Aspirin Given at Discharge[1]	-	-	99%	99%
Fibrinolytic Meds Within 30 Min. of Arrival[7]	-	-	57%	54%
PCI Within 90 Minutes of Arrival[7]	-	-	93%	96%
Statin Prescribed at Discharge[1]	-	-	98%	98%
Heart Failure Care				
ACE Inhibitor or ARB for LVSD	15	93%	96%	97%
Discharge Instructions Given	62	84%	93%	94%
Evaluation of LVS Function	71	100%	99%	99%
Medicare Spending				
Medicare Spending per Patient (ratio)	-	0.82	0.88	0.98
Pneumonia Care				
Appropriate Initial Antibiotic Given	79	92%	96%	95%
Blood Culture Timing	133	92%	98%	98%
Pregnancy and Delivery Care				
Newborn Deliveries Scheduled Early	53	4%	3%	6%
Preventive Care				
Immunization for Influenza[2]	320	86%	86%	90%
Immunization for Pneumonia[2]	403	74%	88%	92%
Stroke Care				
Anticoagulation Therapy for Atrial Fibrillation[1]	-	-	94%	95%
Antithrombotic Therapy Timing	26	100%	97%	98%
Assessed for Rehabilitation	30	97%	96%	97%
Discharged on Antithrombotic Therapy	29	100%	99%	99%
Discharged on Statin Medication	23	100%	93%	94%
Thrombolytic Therapy Timing[1]	-	-	55%	66%
Venous Thromboembolism Prophylaxis	27	100%	90%	94%
Written Stroke Educational Materials Given	19	84%	81%	88%
Surgical Care Improvement Project				
Appropriate Beta Blocker Usage[2]	103	97%	98%	98%
Appropriate VTP Within 24 Hours[2]	290	96%	97%	98%
Controlled Postoperative Blood Glucose[2,7]	-	-	98%	97%
Perioperative Temperature Management[2]	324	100%	100%	100%
Prophylactic Antibiotic Selection[2]	228	99%	99%	99%
Prophylactic Antibiotic Selection (Outpatient)	50	94%	98%	98%
Prophylactic Antibiotic Stopped[2]	223	96%	98%	98%
Prophylactic Antibiotic Timing[2]	228	96%	98%	99%
Prophylactic Antibiotic Timing (Outpatient)	53	91%	96%	98%
Urinary Catheter Removal[2]	236	96%	97%	97%
Survey of Patients' Hospital Experiences				
Area Around Room 'Always' Quiet at Night	300+	59%	57%	61%
Doctors 'Always' Communicated Well	300+	83%	81%	82%
Home Recovery Information Given	300+	87%	86%	85%
Hospital Given 9 or 10 on 10 Point Scale	300+	71%	70%	71%
Meds 'Always' Explained Before Given	300+	64%	65%	64%
Nurses 'Always' Communicated Well	300+	78%	79%	79%
Pain 'Always' Well Controlled	300+	73%	71%	71%
Room and Bathroom 'Always' Clean	300+	80%	74%	73%
Timely Help 'Always' Received	300+	65%	68%	68%
Would Definitely Recommend Hospital	300+	74%	72%	71%
Use of Medical Imaging				
Cardiac Imaging Stress Test before Surgery	61	3.3%	4.7%	5.3%
Combination Abdominal CT Scan	332	6.0%	6.6%	10.5%
Combination Brain/Sinus CT Scan[1]	-	-	2.1%	2.7%
Combination Chest CT Scan	219	0.0%	1.1%	2.7%
Follow-up Mammogram/Ultrasound	978	7.8%	8.9%	8.8%
Lumbar Spine MRI for Low Back Pain	81	30.9%	41.7%	37.2%

Asante Ashland Community Hospital

280 Maple Street
Ashland, OR 97520
Phone: 541-201-4001
Fax: 541-488-7417
E-mail: bhamlett@ashlandhospital.org
URL: www.ashlandhospital.org
Type: Acute Care Hospitals
Emergency Services: Yes
Ownership: Government - Local
Beds: 49

Key Personnel:
Radiology. . . . . Mack Bandler, MD
Quality Assurance . . . . Midge Black, RN
Infection Control. . . . . Erin Coke
Emergency Room . . . . Carl Griesser, MD
Intensive Care Unit. . . . . Cindy Lilley, RN
Operating Room. . . . . T Marcoulier, RN
Chief of Medical Staff. . . . . Thomas Marguilies, MD
CEO/President. . . . . Roy Vinyard

Measure	Cases	This Hosp.	State Avg.	U.S. Avg.
Blood Clot Prevention and Treatment				
Anticoagulation Overlap Therapy[2]	14	93%	95%	93%
ICU Venous Thromboembolism Prophylaxis[2]	14	93%	87%	92%
Incidence of Potentially Preventable VTE[2,7]	-	-	13%	10%
UFH with Dosages/Platelet Monitoring[2,7]	-	-	100%	97%
Venous Thromboembolism Prophylaxis[2]	86	100%	83%	85%
Warfarin Therapy Discharge Instructions[1,2]	-	-	54%	75%
Chest Pain/Possible Heart Attack Care				
Aspirin Given Within 24 Hours of Arrival	15	93%	97%	96%
Fibrinolytic Meds Within 30 Min. of Arrival[3,7]	-	-	57%	58%
Average Time to ECG (minutes)	16	26	9	7
Average Time to Transfer (minutes)[1,3]	-	-	52	60
Children's Asthma Care				
Received Home Management Plan of Care	-	-	-	88%
Received Reliever Medication	-	-	-	100%
Received Systemic Corticosteroids	-	-	-	100%
Emergency Department				
Admittance Decision Time (minutes)[2]	249	82	85	98
Head CT Results Within 45 Min. of Arrival[3,7]	-	-	45%	57%
Patients Who Left ER Before Being Seen	8,261	1%	2%	2%
Time from ER Arrival to Admit. (minutes)[2]	264	310	235	274
Time from ER Arrival to Discharge (minutes)	351	120	136	134
Time in ER Before Being Evaluated (minutes)	381	30	27	26
Time to Pain Meds for Fractures (minutes)	68	60	56	57
Heart Attack Care				
Aspirin Given at Discharge[1,2]	-	-	99%	99%
Fibrinolytic Meds Within 30 Min. of Arrival[2,7]	-	-	57%	54%
PCI Within 90 Minutes of Arrival[2,7]	-	-	93%	96%
Statin Prescribed at Discharge[1,2]	-	-	98%	98%
Heart Failure Care				
ACE Inhibitor or ARB for LVSD[1]	-	-	96%	97%
Discharge Instructions Given	11	100%	93%	94%
Evaluation of LVS Function	15	100%	99%	99%
Medicare Spending				
Medicare Spending per Patient (ratio)	-	0.92	0.88	0.98
Pneumonia Care				
Appropriate Initial Antibiotic Given[2]	38	100%	96%	95%
Blood Culture Timing[2]	47	100%	98%	98%
Pregnancy and Delivery Care				
Newborn Deliveries Scheduled Early	25	8%	3%	6%
Preventive Care				
Immunization for Influenza[2]	245	100%	86%	90%
Immunization for Pneumonia[2]	261	98%	88%	92%
Stroke Care				
Anticoagulation Therapy for Atrial Fibrillation[7]	-	-	94%	95%
Antithrombotic Therapy Timing[1]	-	-	97%	98%
Assessed for Rehabilitation[1]	-	-	96%	97%
Discharged on Antithrombotic Therapy[1]	-	-	99%	99%
Discharged on Statin Medication[1]	-	-	93%	94%
Thrombolytic Therapy Timing[7]	-	-	55%	66%
Venous Thromboembolism Prophylaxis[1]	-	-	90%	94%
Written Stroke Educational Materials Given[1]	-	-	81%	88%
Surgical Care Improvement Project				
Appropriate Beta Blocker Usage[2]	33	97%	98%	98%
Appropriate VTP Within 24 Hours[2]	133	100%	97%	98%
Controlled Postoperative Blood Glucose[2,7]	-	-	98%	97%
Perioperative Temperature Management[2]	139	100%	100%	100%
Prophylactic Antibiotic Selection[2]	108	100%	99%	99%
Prophylactic Antibiotic Selection (Outpatient)	33	100%	98%	98%
Prophylactic Antibiotic Stopped[2]	107	99%	98%	98%
Prophylactic Antibiotic Timing[2]	108	99%	98%	99%
Prophylactic Antibiotic Timing (Outpatient)	36	92%	96%	98%
Urinary Catheter Removal[2]	36	94%	97%	97%
Survey of Patients' Hospital Experiences				
Area Around Room 'Always' Quiet at Night	300+	57%	57%	61%
Doctors 'Always' Communicated Well	300+	85%	81%	82%
Home Recovery Information Given	300+	90%	86%	85%
Hospital Given 9 or 10 on 10 Point Scale	300+	74%	70%	71%
Meds 'Always' Explained Before Given	300+	68%	65%	64%
Nurses 'Always' Communicated Well	300+	82%	79%	79%
Pain 'Always' Well Controlled	300+	75%	71%	71%
Room and Bathroom 'Always' Clean	300+	74%	74%	73%
Timely Help 'Always' Received	300+	68%	68%	68%
Would Definitely Recommend Hospital	300+	81%	72%	71%
Use of Medical Imaging				
Cardiac Imaging Stress Test before Surgery[7]	-	-	4.7%	5.3%
Combination Abdominal CT Scan	143	3.5%	6.6%	10.5%
Combination Brain/Sinus CT Scan[1]	-	-	2.1%	2.7%
Combination Chest CT Scan	54	0.0%	1.1%	2.7%
Follow-up Mammogram/Ultrasound	699	11.4%	8.9%	8.8%
Lumbar Spine MRI for Low Back Pain[7]	-	-	41.7%	37.2%

Columbia Memorial Hospital

2111 Exchange Street
Astoria, OR 97103
Phone: 503-325-4321
Type: Critical Access Hospitals
Emergency Services: Yes
Ownership: Proprietary

Key Personnel:
President . . . . Bill Lind
Chief of Medical Staff . . . . Houman Sabahi, MD
CEO . . . . Erik Thorsen

Measure	Cases	This Hosp.	State Avg.	U.S. Avg.
Blood Clot Prevention and Treatment				
Anticoagulation Overlap Therapy[5]	-	-	95%	93%
ICU Venous Thromboembolism Prophylaxis[5]	-	-	87%	92%
Incidence of Potentially Preventable VTE[5]	-	-	13%	10%
UFH with Dosages/Platelet Monitoring[5]	-	-	100%	97%
Venous Thromboembolism Prophylaxis[5]	-	-	83%	85%
Warfarin Therapy Discharge Instructions[5]	-	-	54%	75%
Chest Pain/Possible Heart Attack Care				
Aspirin Given Within 24 Hours of Arrival	-	-	97%	96%
Fibrinolytic Meds Within 30 Min. of Arrival	-	-	57%	58%
Average Time to ECG (minutes)	-	-	9	7
Average Time to Transfer (minutes)	-	-	52	60
Children's Asthma Care				

NOTE: Hospital profiles are in alphabetical order by state, then city, then hospital within the city; Rankings exclude hospitals with less than 25 cases except for patient surveys which excludes hospitals with less than 100 cases; (a) 100-299 cases; (1) The number of cases/patients is too few to report; (2) Data submitted were based on a sample of cases/patients; (3) Results are based on a shorter time period than required; (4) Data suppressed by CMS for one or more quarters; (5) Results are not available for this reporting period; (6) Fewer than 100 patients completed the HCAHPS survey; (7) No cases met the criteria for this measure; (8) The lower limit of the confidence interval cannot be calculated if the number of observed infections equals zero; (9) No data are available from the state/territory for this reporting period; (10) The scores shown reflect fewer than 50 completed surveys; (11) There were discrepancies in the data collection process; (12) This measure does not apply to this hospital for this reporting period; (13) Results cannot be calculated for this reporting period; (14) The results for this state are combined with nearby states to protect confidentiality; Please refer to the User's Guide for a full explanation of data.

Measure	Cases	This Hosp.	State Avg.	U.S. Avg.
Received Home Management Plan of Care	-	-	-	88%
Received Reliever Medication	-	-	-	100%
Received Systemic Corticosteroids	-	-	-	100%
Emergency Department				
Admittance Decision Time (minutes)[5]	-	-	85	98
Head CT Results Within 45 Min. of Arrival	-	-	45%	57%
Patients Who Left ER Before Being Seen	-	-	2%	2%
Time from ER Arrival to Admit. (minutes)[5]	-	-	235	274
Time from ER Arrival to Discharge (minutes)	-	-	136	134
Time in ER Before Being Evaluated (minutes)	-	-	27	26
Time to Pain Meds for Fractures (minutes)	-	-	56	57
Heart Attack Care				
Aspirin Given at Discharge[3,7]	-	-	99%	99%
Fibrinolytic Meds Within 30 Min. of Arrival[3,7]	-	-	57%	54%
PCI Within 90 Minutes of Arrival[3,7]	-	-	93%	96%
Statin Prescribed at Discharge[3,7]	-	-	98%	98%
Heart Failure Care				
ACE Inhibitor or ARB for LVSD[1,3]	-	-	96%	97%
Discharge Instructions Given[1,3]	-	-	93%	94%
Evaluation of LVS Function[1,3]	-	-	99%	99%
Medicare Spending				
Medicare Spending per Patient (ratio)	-	-	0.88	0.98
Pneumonia Care				
Appropriate Initial Antibiotic Given[3]	17	88%	96%	95%
Blood Culture Timing[3]	26	100%	98%	98%
Pregnancy and Delivery Care				
Newborn Deliveries Scheduled Early[5]	-	-	3%	6%
Preventive Care				
Immunization for Influenza[5]	-	-	86%	90%
Immunization for Pneumonia[5]	-	-	88%	92%
Stroke Care				
Anticoagulation Therapy for Atrial Fibrillation[5]	-	-	94%	95%
Antithrombotic Therapy Timing[5]	-	-	97%	98%
Assessed for Rehabilitation[5]	-	-	96%	97%
Discharged on Antithrombotic Therapy[5]	-	-	99%	99%
Discharged on Statin Medication[5]	-	-	93%	94%
Thrombolytic Therapy Timing[5]	-	-	55%	66%
Venous Thromboembolism Prophylaxis[5]	-	-	90%	94%
Written Stroke Educational Materials Given[5]	-	-	81%	88%
Surgical Care Improvement Project				
Appropriate Beta Blocker Usage[1,3]	-	-	98%	98%
Appropriate VTP Within 24 Hours[3]	26	96%	97%	98%
Controlled Postoperative Blood Glucose[3,7]	-	-	98%	97%
Perioperative Temperature Management[3]	30	100%	100%	100%
Prophylactic Antibiotic Selection[3]	29	90%	99%	99%
Prophylactic Antibiotic Selection (Outpatient)	-	-	98%	98%
Prophylactic Antibiotic Stopped[3]	29	93%	98%	98%
Prophylactic Antibiotic Timing[3]	29	93%	98%	99%
Prophylactic Antibiotic Timing (Outpatient)	-	-	96%	98%
Urinary Catheter Removal[3]	22	95%	97%	97%
Survey of Patients' Hospital Experiences				
Area Around Room 'Always' Quiet at Night	300+	60%	57%	61%
Doctors 'Always' Communicated Well	300+	80%	81%	82%
Home Recovery Information Given	300+	88%	86%	85%
Hospital Given 9 or 10 on 10 Point Scale	300+	71%	70%	71%
Meds 'Always' Explained Before Given	300+	67%	65%	64%
Nurses 'Always' Communicated Well	300+	80%	79%	79%
Pain 'Always' Well Controlled	300+	73%	71%	71%
Room and Bathroom 'Always' Clean	300+	75%	74%	73%
Timely Help 'Always' Received	300+	74%	68%	68%
Would Definitely Recommend Hospital	300+	74%	72%	71%
Use of Medical Imaging				
Cardiac Imaging Stress Test before Surgery	-	-	4.7%	5.3%
Combination Abdominal CT Scan	-	-	6.6%	10.5%
Combination Brain/Sinus CT Scan	-	-	2.1%	2.7%
Combination Chest CT Scan	-	-	1.1%	2.7%
Follow-up Mammogram/Ultrasound	-	-	8.9%	8.8%
Lumbar Spine MRI for Low Back Pain	-	-	41.7%	37.2%

Saint Alphonsus Medical Center - Baker City

3325 Pocahontas Road — Phone: 541-523-6461
Baker City, OR 97814 — Fax: 541-523-8151
URL: www.stelizabethhealth.com
Type: Critical Access Hospitals — Emergency Services: Yes
Ownership: Voluntary non-profit - Church — Beds: 96

Key Personnel:
Chief of Medical Staff.......... Neal Jacobson
Anesthesiology.............. David Loper
Intensive Care Unit........... Dave McCloskey
Emergency Room .... David Richards, RN
Operating Room............. Maxine Sundman
Radiology.................. Brent Wilson
CEO/President............... George Winn

Measure	Cases	This Hosp.	State Avg.	U.S. Avg.
Blood Clot Prevention and Treatment				
Anticoagulation Overlap Therapy[5]	-	-	95%	93%
ICU Venous Thromboembolism Prophylaxis[5]	-	-	87%	92%
Incidence of Potentially Preventable VTE[5]	-	-	13%	10%
UFH with Dosages/Platelet Monitoring[5]	-	-	100%	97%
Venous Thromboembolism Prophylaxis[5]	-	-	83%	85%
Warfarin Therapy Discharge Instructions[5]	-	-	54%	75%
Chest Pain/Possible Heart Attack Care				
Aspirin Given Within 24 Hours of Arrival	-	-	97%	96%
Fibrinolytic Meds Within 30 Min. of Arrival	-	-	57%	58%
Average Time to ECG (minutes)	-	-	9	7
Average Time to Transfer (minutes)	-	-	52	60
Children's Asthma Care				
Received Home Management Plan of Care	-	-	-	88%
Received Reliever Medication	-	-	-	100%
Received Systemic Corticosteroids	-	-	-	100%
Emergency Department				
Admittance Decision Time (minutes)[5]	-	-	85	98
Head CT Results Within 45 Min. of Arrival	-	-	45%	57%
Patients Who Left ER Before Being Seen	-	-	2%	2%
Time from ER Arrival to Admit. (minutes)[5]	-	-	235	274
Time from ER Arrival to Discharge (minutes)	-	-	136	134
Time in ER Before Being Evaluated (minutes)	-	-	27	26
Time to Pain Meds for Fractures (minutes)	-	-	56	57
Heart Attack Care				
Aspirin Given at Discharge[5]	-	-	99%	99%
Fibrinolytic Meds Within 30 Min. of Arrival[5]	-	-	57%	54%
PCI Within 90 Minutes of Arrival[5]	-	-	93%	96%
Statin Prescribed at Discharge[5]	-	-	98%	98%
Heart Failure Care				
ACE Inhibitor or ARB for LVSD[1,3]	-	-	96%	97%
Discharge Instructions Given[1,3]	-	-	93%	94%
Evaluation of LVS Function[1,3]	-	-	99%	99%
Medicare Spending				
Medicare Spending per Patient (ratio)	-	-	0.88	0.98
Pneumonia Care				
Appropriate Initial Antibiotic Given[2,3]	32	88%	96%	95%
Blood Culture Timing[2,3]	28	100%	98%	98%
Pregnancy and Delivery Care				
Newborn Deliveries Scheduled Early[5]	-	-	3%	6%
Preventive Care				
Immunization for Influenza[5]	-	-	86%	90%
Immunization for Pneumonia[5]	-	-	88%	92%
Stroke Care				
Anticoagulation Therapy for Atrial Fibrillation[5]	-	-	94%	95%
Antithrombotic Therapy Timing[5]	-	-	97%	98%
Assessed for Rehabilitation[5]	-	-	96%	97%
Discharged on Antithrombotic Therapy[5]	-	-	99%	99%
Discharged on Statin Medication[5]	-	-	93%	94%
Thrombolytic Therapy Timing[5]	-	-	55%	66%
Venous Thromboembolism Prophylaxis[5]	-	-	90%	94%
Written Stroke Educational Materials Given[5]	-	-	81%	88%
Surgical Care Improvement Project				
Appropriate Beta Blocker Usage[1,3]	-	-	98%	98%
Appropriate VTP Within 24 Hours[5]	-	-	97%	98%
Controlled Postoperative Blood Glucose[5]	-	-	98%	97%
Perioperative Temperature Management[5]	-	-	100%	100%
Prophylactic Antibiotic Selection[3]	49	100%	99%	99%
Prophylactic Antibiotic Selection (Outpatient)	-	-	98%	98%
Prophylactic Antibiotic Stopped[3]	49	96%	98%	98%
Prophylactic Antibiotic Timing[3]	49	90%	98%	99%
Prophylactic Antibiotic Timing (Outpatient)	-	-	96%	98%
Urinary Catheter Removal[5]	-	-	97%	97%
Survey of Patients' Hospital Experiences				
Area Around Room 'Always' Quiet at Night	(a)	62%	57%	61%
Doctors 'Always' Communicated Well	(a)	87%	81%	82%
Home Recovery Information Given	(a)	92%	86%	85%
Hospital Given 9 or 10 on 10 Point Scale	(a)	76%	70%	71%
Meds 'Always' Explained Before Given	(a)	73%	65%	64%
Nurses 'Always' Communicated Well	(a)	80%	79%	79%
Pain 'Always' Well Controlled	(a)	75%	71%	71%
Room and Bathroom 'Always' Clean	(a)	76%	74%	73%
Timely Help 'Always' Received	(a)	80%	68%	68%
Would Definitely Recommend Hospital	(a)	70%	72%	71%
Use of Medical Imaging				
Cardiac Imaging Stress Test before Surgery	-	-	4.7%	5.3%
Combination Abdominal CT Scan	-	-	6.6%	10.5%
Combination Brain/Sinus CT Scan	-	-	2.1%	2.7%
Combination Chest CT Scan	-	-	1.1%	2.7%
Follow-up Mammogram/Ultrasound	-	-	8.9%	8.8%
Lumbar Spine MRI for Low Back Pain	-	-	41.7%	37.2%

Southern Coos Hospital & Health Center

900 11th Street Se — Phone: 541-347-2426
Bandon, OR 97411 — Fax: 541-347-3923
URL: www.southerncoos.com
Type: Critical Access Hospitals — Emergency Services: Yes
Ownership: Govt - Hospital Dist/Auth — Beds: 21

Key Personnel:
CEO/President............... James A Wathen

Measure	Cases	This Hosp.	State Avg.	U.S. Avg.
Blood Clot Prevention and Treatment				
Anticoagulation Overlap Therapy[5]	-	-	95%	93%
ICU Venous Thromboembolism Prophylaxis[5]	-	-	87%	92%
Incidence of Potentially Preventable VTE[5]	-	-	13%	10%
UFH with Dosages/Platelet Monitoring[5]	-	-	100%	97%
Venous Thromboembolism Prophylaxis[5]	-	-	83%	85%
Warfarin Therapy Discharge Instructions[5]	-	-	54%	75%
Chest Pain/Possible Heart Attack Care				
Aspirin Given Within 24 Hours of Arrival	-	-	97%	96%
Fibrinolytic Meds Within 30 Min. of Arrival	-	-	57%	58%
Average Time to ECG (minutes)	-	-	9	7
Average Time to Transfer (minutes)	-	-	52	60
Children's Asthma Care				
Received Home Management Plan of Care	-	-	-	88%
Received Reliever Medication	-	-	-	100%
Received Systemic Corticosteroids	-	-	-	100%
Emergency Department				
Admittance Decision Time (minutes)[5]	-	-	85	98
Head CT Results Within 45 Min. of Arrival	-	-	45%	57%
Patients Who Left ER Before Being Seen	-	-	2%	2%
Time from ER Arrival to Admit. (minutes)[5]	-	-	235	274
Time from ER Arrival to Discharge (minutes)	-	-	136	134
Time in ER Before Being Evaluated (minutes)	-	-	27	26
Time to Pain Meds for Fractures (minutes)	-	-	56	57
Heart Attack Care				
Aspirin Given at Discharge[3,7]	-	-	99%	99%
Fibrinolytic Meds Within 30 Min. of Arrival[3,7]	-	-	57%	54%
PCI Within 90 Minutes of Arrival[5]	-	-	93%	96%
Statin Prescribed at Discharge[5]	-	-	98%	98%
Heart Failure Care				
ACE Inhibitor or ARB for LVSD[3,7]	-	-	96%	97%
Discharge Instructions Given[3]	12	50%	93%	94%
Evaluation of LVS Function[3]	13	15%	99%	99%
Medicare Spending				
Medicare Spending per Patient (ratio)	-	-	0.88	0.98
Pneumonia Care				
Appropriate Initial Antibiotic Given	17	88%	96%	95%
Blood Culture Timing	15	100%	98%	98%
Pregnancy and Delivery Care				
Newborn Deliveries Scheduled Early[5]	-	-	3%	6%
Preventive Care				

NOTE: Hospital profiles are in alphabetical order by state, then city, then hospital within the city; Rankings exclude hospitals with less than 25 cases except for patient surveys which excludes hospitals with less than 100 cases; (a) 100-299 cases; (1) The number of cases/patients is too few to report; (2) Data submitted were based on a sample of cases/patients; (3) Results are based on a shorter time period than required; (4) Data suppressed by CMS for one or more quarters; (5) Results are not available for this reporting period; (6) Fewer than 100 patients completed the HCAHPS survey; (7) No cases met the criteria for this measure; (8) The lower limit of the confidence interval cannot be calculated if the number of observed infections equals zero; (9) No data are available from the state/territory for this reporting period; (10) The scores shown reflect fewer than 50 completed surveys; (11) There were discrepancies in the data collection process; (12) This measure does not apply to this hospital for this reporting period; (13) Results cannot be calculated for this reporting period; (14) The results for this state are combined with nearby states to protect confidentiality; Please refer to the User's Guide for a full explanation of data.

Measure	Cases	This Hosp.	State Avg.	U.S. Avg.
Immunization for Influenza[5]	-	-	86%	90%
Immunization for Pneumonia[5]	-	-	88%	92%
Stroke Care				
Anticoagulation Therapy for Atrial Fibrillation[5]	-	-	94%	95%
Antithrombotic Therapy Timing[5]	-	-	97%	98%
Assessed for Rehabilitation[5]	-	-	96%	97%
Discharged on Antithrombotic Therapy[5]	-	-	99%	99%
Discharged on Statin Medication[5]	-	-	93%	94%
Thrombolytic Therapy Timing[5]	-	-	55%	66%
Venous Thromboembolism Prophylaxis[5]	-	-	90%	94%
Written Stroke Educational Materials Given[5]	-	-	81%	88%
Surgical Care Improvement Project				
Appropriate Beta Blocker Usage[3,7]	-	-	98%	98%
Appropriate VTP Within 24 Hours[1,3]	-	-	97%	98%
Controlled Postoperative Blood Glucose[3,7]	-	-	98%	97%
Perioperative Temperature Management[1,3]	-	-	100%	100%
Prophylactic Antibiotic Selection[1,3]	-	-	99%	99%
Prophylactic Antibiotic Selection (Outpatient)	-	-	98%	98%
Prophylactic Antibiotic Stopped[1,3]	-	-	98%	98%
Prophylactic Antibiotic Timing[1,3]	-	-	98%	99%
Prophylactic Antibiotic Timing (Outpatient)	-	-	96%	98%
Urinary Catheter Removal[1,3]	-	-	97%	97%
Survey of Patients' Hospital Experiences				
Area Around Room 'Always' Quiet at Night[6]	<100	66%	57%	61%
Doctors 'Always' Communicated Well[6]	<100	81%	81%	82%
Home Recovery Information Given[6]	<100	86%	86%	85%
Hospital Given 9 or 10 on 10 Point Scale[6]	<100	61%	70%	71%
Meds 'Always' Explained Before Given[6]	<100	69%	65%	64%
Nurses 'Always' Communicated Well[6]	<100	80%	79%	79%
Pain 'Always' Well Controlled[6]	<100	75%	71%	71%
Room and Bathroom 'Always' Clean[6]	<100	79%	74%	73%
Timely Help 'Always' Received[6]	<100	84%	68%	68%
Would Definitely Recommend Hospital[6]	<100	63%	72%	71%
Use of Medical Imaging				
Cardiac Imaging Stress Test before Surgery	-	-	4.7%	5.3%
Combination Abdominal CT Scan	-	-	6.6%	10.5%
Combination Brain/Sinus CT Scan	-	-	2.1%	2.7%
Combination Chest CT Scan	-	-	1.1%	2.7%
Follow-up Mammogram/Ultrasound	-	-	8.9%	8.8%
Lumbar Spine MRI for Low Back Pain	-	-	41.7%	37.2%

Saint Charles Medical Center - Bend

2500 Ne Neff Road
Bend, OR 97701
Phone: 541-382-4321
Fax: 541-388-7791
E-mail: scmc@scmc.org
URL: www.scmc.org
Type: Acute Care Hospitals
Emergency Services: Yes
Ownership: Voluntary non-profit - Private
Beds: 220

Key Personnel:
Chief of Medical Staff. . . . . Gary Buchholz
Radiology. . . . . Peggy Carey
President/CEO. . . . . Jim Diegel
Quality Assurance . . . . Claudia MacDonald
Pediatric In-Patient Care . . . . . . Allen Merritt, MD
Infection Control. . . . . Merlene Morris
Operating Room. . . . . Tom Solitz

Measure	Cases	This Hosp.	State Avg.	U.S. Avg.
Blood Clot Prevention and Treatment				
Anticoagulation Overlap Therapy[2]	55	98%	95%	93%
ICU Venous Thromboembolism Prophylaxis[2]	63	92%	87%	92%
Incidence of Potentially Preventable VTE[2]	13	8%	13%	10%
UFH with Dosages/Platelet Monitoring[2]	17	100%	100%	97%
Venous Thromboembolism Prophylaxis[2]	248	82%	83%	85%
Warfarin Therapy Discharge Instructions[2]	42	81%	54%	75%
Chest Pain/Possible Heart Attack Care				
Aspirin Given Within 24 Hours of Arrival[5]	-	-	97%	96%
Fibrinolytic Meds Within 30 Min. of Arrival[5]	-	-	57%	58%
Average Time to ECG (minutes)[5]	-	-	9	7
Average Time to Transfer (minutes)[5]	-	-	52	60
Children's Asthma Care				
Received Home Management Plan of Care	-	-	-	88%
Received Reliever Medication	-	-	-	100%
Received Systemic Corticosteroids	-	-	-	100%
Emergency Department				
Admittance Decision Time (minutes)[2]	376	92	85	98
Head CT Results Within 45 Min. of Arrival[1]	-	-	45%	57%
Patients Who Left ER Before Being Seen	29,737	0%	2%	2%
Time from ER Arrival to Admit. (minutes)[2]	392	243	235	274
Time from ER Arrival to Discharge (minutes)	366	156	136	134
Time in ER Before Being Evaluated (minutes)	389	35	27	26
Time to Pain Meds for Fractures (minutes)	172	72	56	57
Heart Attack Care				
Aspirin Given at Discharge	235	100%	99%	99%
Fibrinolytic Meds Within 30 Min. of Arrival[1]	-	-	57%	54%
PCI Within 90 Minutes of Arrival	41	71%	93%	96%
Statin Prescribed at Discharge	228	97%	98%	98%
Heart Failure Care				
ACE Inhibitor or ARB for LVSD	58	97%	96%	97%
Discharge Instructions Given	190	76%	93%	94%
Evaluation of LVS Function	209	98%	99%	99%
Medicare Spending				
Medicare Spending per Patient (ratio)	-	0.90	0.88	0.98
Pneumonia Care				
Appropriate Initial Antibiotic Given	82	88%	96%	95%
Blood Culture Timing	132	98%	98%	98%
Pregnancy and Delivery Care				
Newborn Deliveries Scheduled Early[2]	28	21%	3%	6%
Preventive Care				
Immunization for Influenza[2]	568	81%	86%	90%
Immunization for Pneumonia[2]	657	86%	88%	92%
Stroke Care				
Anticoagulation Therapy for Atrial Fibrillation	27	100%	94%	95%
Antithrombotic Therapy Timing	104	96%	97%	98%
Assessed for Rehabilitation	145	90%	96%	97%
Discharged on Antithrombotic Therapy	120	99%	99%	99%
Discharged on Statin Medication	89	88%	93%	94%
Thrombolytic Therapy Timing	15	13%	55%	66%
Venous Thromboembolism Prophylaxis	134	91%	90%	94%
Written Stroke Educational Materials Given	81	67%	81%	88%
Surgical Care Improvement Project				
Appropriate Beta Blocker Usage[2]	274	96%	98%	98%
Appropriate VTP Within 24 Hours[2]	730	94%	97%	98%
Controlled Postoperative Blood Glucose[2]	212	100%	98%	97%
Perioperative Temperature Management[2]	889	99%	100%	100%
Prophylactic Antibiotic Selection[2]	904	99%	99%	99%
Prophylactic Antibiotic Selection (Outpatient)	385	95%	98%	98%
Prophylactic Antibiotic Stopped[2]	898	97%	98%	98%
Prophylactic Antibiotic Timing[2]	906	96%	98%	99%
Prophylactic Antibiotic Timing (Outpatient)	392	95%	96%	98%
Urinary Catheter Removal[2]	833	97%	97%	97%
Survey of Patients' Hospital Experiences				
Area Around Room 'Always' Quiet at Night	300+	53%	57%	61%
Doctors 'Always' Communicated Well	300+	78%	81%	82%
Home Recovery Information Given	300+	87%	86%	85%
Hospital Given 9 or 10 on 10 Point Scale	300+	71%	70%	71%
Meds 'Always' Explained Before Given	300+	61%	65%	64%
Nurses 'Always' Communicated Well	300+	77%	79%	79%
Pain 'Always' Well Controlled	300+	71%	71%	71%
Room and Bathroom 'Always' Clean	300+	66%	74%	73%
Timely Help 'Always' Received	300+	65%	68%	68%
Would Definitely Recommend Hospital	300+	78%	72%	71%
Use of Medical Imaging				
Cardiac Imaging Stress Test before Surgery[1]	-	-	4.7%	5.3%
Combination Abdominal CT Scan	375	0.5%	6.6%	10.5%
Combination Brain/Sinus CT Scan[1]	-	-	2.1%	2.7%
Combination Chest CT Scan	272	8.1%	1.1%	2.7%
Follow-up Mammogram/Ultrasound[7]	-	-	8.9%	8.8%
Lumbar Spine MRI for Low Back Pain[1]	-	-	41.7%	37.2%

Harney District Hospital

557 W Washington Street
Burns, OR 97720
Phone: 541-573-7281
Fax: 541-573-8353
URL: www.harneydh.com
Type: Critical Access Hospitals
Emergency Services: Yes
Ownership: Govt - Hospital Dist/Auth
Beds: 22

Key Personnel:
CEO/President. . . . . Nick Bottom
Chief of Medical Staff. . . . . Tom Fitzpatrick, MD
Operating Room. . . . . Jackie Hurd, RN
Anesthesiology. . . . . Harley Kelley, MD
Emergency Room . . . . Tim Peck, EMS
Intensive Care Unit. . . . . Thomas Wendel, MD
Pediatric In-Patient Care . . . . . . Thomas Wendel, MD
Quality Assurance . . . . Beth Williams, RN

Measure	Cases	This Hosp.	State Avg.	U.S. Avg.
Blood Clot Prevention and Treatment				
Anticoagulation Overlap Therapy[5]	-	-	95%	93%
ICU Venous Thromboembolism Prophylaxis[5]	-	-	87%	92%
Incidence of Potentially Preventable VTE[5]	-	-	13%	10%
UFH with Dosages/Platelet Monitoring[5]	-	-	100%	97%
Venous Thromboembolism Prophylaxis[5]	-	-	83%	85%
Warfarin Therapy Discharge Instructions[5]	-	-	54%	75%
Chest Pain/Possible Heart Attack Care				
Aspirin Given Within 24 Hours of Arrival[1,3]	-	-	97%	96%
Fibrinolytic Meds Within 30 Min. of Arrival[1,3]	-	-	57%	58%
Average Time to ECG (minutes)[1,3]	-	-	9	7
Average Time to Transfer (minutes)[3,7]	-	-	52	60
Children's Asthma Care				
Received Home Management Plan of Care	-	-	-	88%
Received Reliever Medication	-	-	-	100%
Received Systemic Corticosteroids	-	-	-	100%
Emergency Department				
Admittance Decision Time (minutes)[2]	121	50	85	98
Head CT Results Within 45 Min. of Arrival[3,7]	-	-	45%	57%
Patients Who Left ER Before Being Seen[5]	-	-	2%	2%
Time from ER Arrival to Admit. (minutes)[2]	151	155	235	274
Time from ER Arrival to Discharge (minutes)[3]	302	84	136	134
Time in ER Before Being Evaluated (minutes)[3]	300	6	27	26
Time to Pain Meds for Fractures (minutes)[5]	-	-	56	57
Heart Attack Care				
Aspirin Given at Discharge[5]	-	-	99%	99%
Fibrinolytic Meds Within 30 Min. of Arrival[5]	-	-	57%	54%
PCI Within 90 Minutes of Arrival[5]	-	-	93%	96%
Statin Prescribed at Discharge[5]	-	-	98%	98%
Heart Failure Care				
ACE Inhibitor or ARB for LVSD[3,7]	-	-	96%	97%
Discharge Instructions Given[1,3]	-	-	93%	94%
Evaluation of LVS Function[1,3]	-	-	99%	99%
Medicare Spending				
Medicare Spending per Patient (ratio)	-	-	0.88	0.98
Pneumonia Care				
Appropriate Initial Antibiotic Given[5]	-	-	96%	95%
Blood Culture Timing[5]	-	-	98%	98%
Pregnancy and Delivery Care				
Newborn Deliveries Scheduled Early[5]	-	-	3%	6%
Preventive Care				
Immunization for Influenza[2,3]	35	37%	86%	90%
Immunization for Pneumonia[2,3]	35	94%	88%	92%
Stroke Care				
Anticoagulation Therapy for Atrial Fibrillation[3,7]	-	-	94%	95%
Antithrombotic Therapy Timing[3,7]	-	-	97%	98%
Assessed for Rehabilitation[1,3]	-	-	96%	97%
Discharged on Antithrombotic Therapy[1,3]	-	-	99%	99%
Discharged on Statin Medication[1,3]	-	-	93%	94%
Thrombolytic Therapy Timing[3,7]	-	-	55%	66%
Venous Thromboembolism Prophylaxis[3,7]	-	-	90%	94%
Written Stroke Educational Materials Given[1,3]	-	-	81%	88%
Surgical Care Improvement Project				
Appropriate Beta Blocker Usage[5]	-	-	98%	98%
Appropriate VTP Within 24 Hours[5]	-	-	97%	98%
Controlled Postoperative Blood Glucose[5]	-	-	98%	97%
Perioperative Temperature Management[5]	-	-	100%	100%
Prophylactic Antibiotic Selection[5]	-	-	99%	99%
Prophylactic Antibiotic Selection (Outpatient)[5]	-	-	98%	98%
Prophylactic Antibiotic Stopped[5]	-	-	98%	98%
Prophylactic Antibiotic Timing[5]	-	-	98%	99%
Prophylactic Antibiotic Timing (Outpatient)[5]	-	-	96%	98%
Urinary Catheter Removal[5]	-	-	97%	97%
Survey of Patients' Hospital Experiences				
Area Around Room 'Always' Quiet at Night[5]	-	-	57%	61%
Doctors 'Always' Communicated Well[5]	-	-	81%	82%

NOTE: Hospital profiles are in alphabetical order by state, then city, then hospital within the city; Rankings exclude hospitals with less than 25 cases except for patient surveys which excludes hospitals with less than 100 cases; (a) 100-299 cases; (1) The number of cases/patients is too few to report; (2) Data submitted were based on a sample of cases/patients; (3) Results are based on a shorter time period than required; (4) Data suppressed by CMS for one or more quarters; (5) Results are not available for this reporting period; (6) Fewer than 100 patients completed the HCAHPS survey; (7) No cases met the criteria for this measure; (8) The lower limit of the confidence interval cannot be calculated if the number of observed infections equals zero; (9) No data are available from the state/territory for this reporting period; (10) The scores shown reflect fewer than 50 completed surveys; (11) There were discrepancies in the data collection process; (12) This measure does not apply to this hospital for this reporting period; (13) Results cannot be calculated for this reporting period; (14) The results for this state are combined with nearby states to protect confidentiality; Please refer to the User's Guide for a full explanation of data.

Measure	Cases	This Hosp.	State Avg.	U.S. Avg.
Home Recovery Information Given[5]	-	-	86%	85%
Hospital Given 9 or 10 on 10 Point Scale[5]	-	-	70%	71%
Meds 'Always' Explained Before Given[5]	-	-	65%	64%
Nurses 'Always' Communicated Well[5]	-	-	79%	79%
Pain 'Always' Well Controlled[5]	-	-	71%	71%
Room and Bathroom 'Always' Clean[5]	-	-	74%	73%
Timely Help 'Always' Received[5]	-	-	68%	68%
Would Definitely Recommend Hospital[5]	-	-	72%	71%
Use of Medical Imaging				
Cardiac Imaging Stress Test before Surgery[1]	-	-	4.7%	5.3%
Combination Abdominal CT Scan	98	4.1%	6.6%	10.5%
Combination Brain/Sinus CT Scan[1]	-	-	2.1%	2.7%
Combination Chest CT Scan	58	1.7%	1.1%	2.7%
Follow-up Mammogram/Ultrasound	198	12.6%	8.9%	8.8%
Lumbar Spine MRI for Low Back Pain[1]	-	-	41.7%	37.2%

Kaiser Sunnyside Medical Center

10180 Se Sunnyside Road Phone: 503-571-2880
Clackamas, OR 97015 Fax: 503-571-2671
URL: www.members.kaiserpermanente.org
Type: Acute Care Hospitals Emergency Services: Yes
Ownership: Voluntary non-profit - Other Beds: 196

Key Personnel:
Radiology. . . . . Kenneth H Bookstein, MD
Chief of Medical Staff . . . . Tom Harburg, MD
CEO/President. . . . . Sharon M Higgins, MD
Infection Control. . . . . Joseph Kane, MD
Pediatric In-Patient Care . . . . John Pearson, MD
Operating Room. . . . . Neen Pernard, RN
Quality Assurance . . . . Pam Smith

Measure	Cases	This Hosp.	State Avg.	U.S. Avg.
Blood Clot Prevention and Treatment				
Anticoagulation Overlap Therapy[2]	117	98%	95%	93%
ICU Venous Thromboembolism Prophylaxis[2]	55	96%	87%	92%
Incidence of Potentially Preventable VTE[2]	25	36%	13%	10%
UFH with Dosages/Platelet Monitoring[2]	59	100%	100%	97%
Venous Thromboembolism Prophylaxis[2]	266	91%	83%	85%
Warfarin Therapy Discharge Instructions[2]	100	6%	54%	75%
Chest Pain/Possible Heart Attack Care				
Aspirin Given Within 24 Hours of Arrival	-	-	97%	96%
Fibrinolytic Meds Within 30 Min. of Arrival	-	-	57%	58%
Average Time to ECG (minutes)	-	-	9	7
Average Time to Transfer (minutes)	-	-	52	60
Children's Asthma Care				
Received Home Management Plan of Care	-	-	-	88%
Received Reliever Medication	-	-	-	100%
Received Systemic Corticosteroids	-	-	-	100%
Emergency Department				
Admittance Decision Time (minutes)[2]	406	81	85	98
Head CT Results Within 45 Min. of Arrival	-	-	45%	57%
Patients Who Left ER Before Being Seen	-	-	2%	2%
Time from ER Arrival to Admit. (minutes)[2]	437	320	235	274
Time from ER Arrival to Discharge (minutes)	-	-	136	134
Time in ER Before Being Evaluated (minutes)	-	-	27	26
Time to Pain Meds for Fractures (minutes)	-	-	56	57
Heart Attack Care				
Aspirin Given at Discharge	409	100%	99%	99%
Fibrinolytic Meds Within 30 Min. of Arrival[7]	-	-	57%	54%
PCI Within 90 Minutes of Arrival	34	91%	93%	96%
Statin Prescribed at Discharge	402	100%	98%	98%
Heart Failure Care				
ACE Inhibitor or ARB for LVSD	96	100%	96%	97%
Discharge Instructions Given	383	97%	93%	94%
Evaluation of LVS Function	438	100%	99%	99%
Medicare Spending				
Medicare Spending per Patient (ratio)	-	0.73	0.88	0.98
Pneumonia Care				
Appropriate Initial Antibiotic Given[2]	107	97%	96%	95%
Blood Culture Timing[2]	202	97%	98%	98%
Pregnancy and Delivery Care				
Newborn Deliveries Scheduled Early[2]	280	1%	3%	6%
Preventive Care				
Immunization for Influenza[2]	595	95%	86%	90%
Immunization for Pneumonia[2]	759	96%	88%	92%
Stroke Care				
Anticoagulation Therapy for Atrial Fibrillation	28	100%	94%	95%
Antithrombotic Therapy Timing	121	98%	97%	98%
Assessed for Rehabilitation	212	100%	96%	97%
Discharged on Antithrombotic Therapy	187	100%	99%	99%
Discharged on Statin Medication	144	99%	93%	94%
Thrombolytic Therapy Timing[1]	-	-	55%	66%
Venous Thromboembolism Prophylaxis	166	98%	90%	94%
Written Stroke Educational Materials Given	120	93%	81%	88%
Surgical Care Improvement Project				
Appropriate Beta Blocker Usage[2]	294	98%	98%	98%
Appropriate VTP Within 24 Hours[2]	394	98%	97%	98%
Controlled Postoperative Blood Glucose[2]	151	100%	98%	97%
Perioperative Temperature Management[2]	570	100%	100%	100%
Prophylactic Antibiotic Selection[2]	499	99%	99%	99%
Prophylactic Antibiotic Selection (Outpatient)	-	-	98%	98%
Prophylactic Antibiotic Stopped[2]	489	100%	98%	98%
Prophylactic Antibiotic Timing[2]	499	99%	98%	99%
Prophylactic Antibiotic Timing (Outpatient)	-	-	96%	98%
Urinary Catheter Removal[2]	442	99%	97%	97%
Survey of Patients' Hospital Experiences				
Area Around Room 'Always' Quiet at Night	300+	59%	57%	61%
Doctors 'Always' Communicated Well	300+	81%	81%	82%
Home Recovery Information Given	300+	89%	86%	85%
Hospital Given 9 or 10 on 10 Point Scale	300+	74%	70%	71%
Meds 'Always' Explained Before Given	300+	65%	65%	64%
Nurses 'Always' Communicated Well	300+	78%	79%	79%
Pain 'Always' Well Controlled	300+	72%	71%	71%
Room and Bathroom 'Always' Clean	300+	73%	74%	73%
Timely Help 'Always' Received	300+	63%	68%	68%
Would Definitely Recommend Hospital	300+	75%	72%	71%
Use of Medical Imaging				
Cardiac Imaging Stress Test before Surgery	-	-	4.7%	5.3%
Combination Abdominal CT Scan	-	-	6.6%	10.5%
Combination Brain/Sinus CT Scan	-	-	2.1%	2.7%
Combination Chest CT Scan	-	-	1.1%	2.7%
Follow-up Mammogram/Ultrasound	-	-	8.9%	8.8%
Lumbar Spine MRI for Low Back Pain	-	-	41.7%	37.2%

Bay Area Hospital

1775 Thompson Road Phone: 541-269-8111
Coos Bay, OR 97420 Fax: 541-267-7057
E-mail: cacace@bayareahospital.org
URL: www.bayareahospital.org
Type: Acute Care Hospitals Emergency Services: Yes
Ownership: Govt - Hospital Dist/Auth Beds: 172

Key Personnel:
Radiology. . . . . Cathryn Chicola
Cardiac Laboratory. . . . . Anne Ericckson
Emergency Room . . . . Clyde Hill
Chief of Medical Staff. . . . . Shaun Hobson
CEO/President. . . . . Paul Janke
Operating Room. . . . . Lori Krenos
Quality Assurance . . . . Tam Laurie

Measure	Cases	This Hosp.	State Avg.	U.S. Avg.
Blood Clot Prevention and Treatment				
Anticoagulation Overlap Therapy[2]	30	97%	95%	93%
ICU Venous Thromboembolism Prophylaxis[2]	55	56%	87%	92%
Incidence of Potentially Preventable VTE[2]	11	45%	13%	10%
UFH with Dosages/Platelet Monitoring[1,2]	-	-	100%	97%
Venous Thromboembolism Prophylaxis[2]	290	59%	83%	85%
Warfarin Therapy Discharge Instructions[2]	17	35%	54%	75%
Chest Pain/Possible Heart Attack Care				
Aspirin Given Within 24 Hours of Arrival	54	96%	97%	96%
Fibrinolytic Meds Within 30 Min. of Arrival[1]	-	-	57%	58%
Average Time to ECG (minutes)	56	7	9	7
Average Time to Transfer (minutes)[7]	-	-	52	60
Children's Asthma Care				
Received Home Management Plan of Care	-	-	-	88%
Received Reliever Medication	-	-	-	100%
Received Systemic Corticosteroids	-	-	-	100%
Emergency Department				
Admittance Decision Time (minutes)[2]	496	48	85	98
Head CT Results Within 45 Min. of Arrival[1]	-	-	45%	57%
Patients Who Left ER Before Being Seen	26,600	3%	2%	2%
Time from ER Arrival to Admit. (minutes)[2]	550	215	235	274
Time from ER Arrival to Discharge (minutes)	384	116	136	134
Time in ER Before Being Evaluated (minutes)	389	36	27	26
Time to Pain Meds for Fractures (minutes)	73	64	56	57
Heart Attack Care				
Aspirin Given at Discharge	62	97%	99%	99%
Fibrinolytic Meds Within 30 Min. of Arrival[1]	-	-	57%	54%
PCI Within 90 Minutes of Arrival[1]	-	-	93%	96%
Statin Prescribed at Discharge	62	85%	98%	98%
Heart Failure Care				
ACE Inhibitor or ARB for LVSD	56	86%	96%	97%
Discharge Instructions Given	116	89%	93%	94%
Evaluation of LVS Function	145	99%	99%	99%
Medicare Spending				
Medicare Spending per Patient (ratio)	-	0.91	0.88	0.98
Pneumonia Care				
Appropriate Initial Antibiotic Given	80	95%	96%	95%
Blood Culture Timing	106	93%	98%	98%
Pregnancy and Delivery Care				
Newborn Deliveries Scheduled Early[2]	40	0%	3%	6%
Preventive Care				
Immunization for Influenza[2]	524	82%	86%	90%
Immunization for Pneumonia[2]	621	88%	88%	92%
Stroke Care				
Anticoagulation Therapy for Atrial Fibrillation	11	100%	94%	95%
Antithrombotic Therapy Timing	61	98%	97%	98%
Assessed for Rehabilitation	75	92%	96%	97%
Discharged on Antithrombotic Therapy	72	99%	99%	99%
Discharged on Statin Medication	66	68%	93%	94%
Thrombolytic Therapy Timing[1]	-	-	55%	66%
Venous Thromboembolism Prophylaxis	65	62%	90%	94%
Written Stroke Educational Materials Given	49	51%	81%	88%
Surgical Care Improvement Project				
Appropriate Beta Blocker Usage	144	91%	98%	98%
Appropriate VTP Within 24 Hours	458	95%	97%	98%
Controlled Postoperative Blood Glucose[7]	-	-	98%	97%
Perioperative Temperature Management	515	100%	100%	100%
Prophylactic Antibiotic Selection	345	97%	99%	99%
Prophylactic Antibiotic Selection (Outpatient)	92	90%	98%	98%
Prophylactic Antibiotic Stopped	336	93%	98%	98%
Prophylactic Antibiotic Timing	348	94%	98%	99%
Prophylactic Antibiotic Timing (Outpatient)	97	89%	96%	98%
Urinary Catheter Removal	367	96%	97%	97%
Survey of Patients' Hospital Experiences				
Area Around Room 'Always' Quiet at Night	300+	50%	57%	61%
Doctors 'Always' Communicated Well	300+	76%	81%	82%
Home Recovery Information Given	300+	87%	86%	85%
Hospital Given 9 or 10 on 10 Point Scale	300+	64%	70%	71%
Meds 'Always' Explained Before Given	300+	58%	65%	64%
Nurses 'Always' Communicated Well	300+	76%	79%	79%
Pain 'Always' Well Controlled	300+	74%	71%	71%
Room and Bathroom 'Always' Clean	300+	69%	74%	73%
Timely Help 'Always' Received	300+	67%	68%	68%
Would Definitely Recommend Hospital	300+	68%	72%	71%
Use of Medical Imaging				
Cardiac Imaging Stress Test before Surgery	288	6.6%	4.7%	5.3%
Combination Abdominal CT Scan	577	2.1%	6.6%	10.5%
Combination Brain/Sinus CT Scan	424	3.8%	2.1%	2.7%
Combination Chest CT Scan	352	0.3%	1.1%	2.7%
Follow-up Mammogram/Ultrasound	2,061	8.2%	8.9%	8.8%
Lumbar Spine MRI for Low Back Pain	61	41.0%	41.7%	37.2%

Coquille Valley Hospital District

940 East 5th Street Phone: 541-396-3101
Coquille, OR 97423 Fax: 541-396-5760
URL: www.cvhospital.org
Type: Critical Access Hospitals Emergency Services: Yes
Ownership: Govt - Hospital Dist/Auth Beds: 25

Key Personnel:
Infection Control. . . . . Renee Marineau
Emergency Room . . . . James Sinnott
Chief of Medical Staff . . . . James J Sinnott
Anesthesiology. . . . . Richard E Todd
CEO/President. . . . . Dennis Zielinski

NOTE: Hospital profiles are in alphabetical order by state, then city, then hospital within the city; Rankings exclude hospitals with less than 25 cases except for patient surveys which excludes hospitals with less than 100 cases; (a) 100-299 cases; (1) The number of cases/patients is too few to report; (2) Data submitted were based on a sample of cases/patients; (3) Results are based on a shorter time period than required; (4) Data suppressed by CMS for one or more quarters; (5) Results are not available for this reporting period; (6) Fewer than 100 patients completed the HCAHPS survey; (7) No cases met the criteria for this measure; (8) The lower limit of the confidence interval cannot be calculated if the number of observed infections equals zero; (9) No data are available from the state/territory for this reporting period; (10) The scores shown reflect fewer than 50 completed surveys; (11) There were discrepancies in the data collection process; (12) This measure does not apply to this hospital for this reporting period; (13) Results cannot be calculated for this reporting period; (14) The results for this state are combined with nearby states to protect confidentiality; Please refer to the User's Guide for a full explanation of data.

Measure	Cases	This Hosp.	State Avg.	U.S. Avg.
Blood Clot Prevention and Treatment				
Anticoagulation Overlap Therapy[5]	-	-	95%	93%
ICU Venous Thromboembolism Prophylaxis[5]	-	-	87%	92%
Incidence of Potentially Preventable VTE[5]	-	-	13%	10%
UFH with Dosages/Platelet Monitoring[5]	-	-	100%	97%
Venous Thromboembolism Prophylaxis[5]	-	-	83%	85%
Warfarin Therapy Discharge Instructions[5]	-	-	54%	75%
Chest Pain/Possible Heart Attack Care				
Aspirin Given Within 24 Hours of Arrival	30	100%	97%	96%
Fibrinolytic Meds Within 30 Min. of Arrival[1]	-	-	57%	58%
Average Time to ECG (minutes)	32	9	9	7
Average Time to Transfer (minutes)[1]	-	-	52	60
Children's Asthma Care				
Received Home Management Plan of Care	-	-	-	88%
Received Reliever Medication	-	-	-	100%
Received Systemic Corticosteroids	-	-	-	100%
Emergency Department				
Admittance Decision Time (minutes)[5]	-	-	85	98
Head CT Results Within 45 Min. of Arrival[5]	-	-	45%	57%
Patients Who Left ER Before Being Seen[5]	-	-	2%	2%
Time from ER Arrival to Admit. (minutes)[5]	-	-	235	274
Time from ER Arrival to Discharge (minutes)[5]	-	-	136	134
Time in ER Before Being Evaluated (minutes)[5]	-	-	27	26
Time to Pain Meds for Fractures (minutes)[5]	-	-	56	57
Heart Attack Care				
Aspirin Given at Discharge[1]	-	-	99%	99%
Fibrinolytic Meds Within 30 Min. of Arrival[7]	-	-	57%	54%
PCI Within 90 Minutes of Arrival[3,7]	-	-	93%	96%
Statin Prescribed at Discharge[1,3]	-	-	98%	98%
Heart Failure Care				
ACE Inhibitor or ARB for LVSD[1]	-	-	96%	97%
Discharge Instructions Given	28	79%	93%	94%
Evaluation of LVS Function	33	88%	99%	99%
Medicare Spending				
Medicare Spending per Patient (ratio)	-	-	0.88	0.98
Pneumonia Care				
Appropriate Initial Antibiotic Given	25	88%	96%	95%
Blood Culture Timing	16	88%	98%	98%
Pregnancy and Delivery Care				
Newborn Deliveries Scheduled Early[5]	-	-	3%	6%
Preventive Care				
Immunization for Influenza[5]	-	-	86%	90%
Immunization for Pneumonia[5]	-	-	88%	92%
Stroke Care				
Anticoagulation Therapy for Atrial Fibrillation[5]	-	-	94%	95%
Antithrombotic Therapy Timing[5]	-	-	97%	98%
Assessed for Rehabilitation[5]	-	-	96%	97%
Discharged on Antithrombotic Therapy[5]	-	-	99%	99%
Discharged on Statin Medication[5]	-	-	93%	94%
Thrombolytic Therapy Timing[5]	-	-	55%	66%
Venous Thromboembolism Prophylaxis[5]	-	-	90%	94%
Written Stroke Educational Materials Given[5]	-	-	81%	88%
Surgical Care Improvement Project				
Appropriate Beta Blocker Usage	23	100%	98%	98%
Appropriate VTP Within 24 Hours	74	99%	97%	98%
Controlled Postoperative Blood Glucose[3,7]	-	-	98%	97%
Perioperative Temperature Management	82	100%	100%	100%
Prophylactic Antibiotic Selection	69	99%	99%	99%
Prophylactic Antibiotic Selection (Outpatient)[3,7]	-	-	98%	98%
Prophylactic Antibiotic Stopped	69	96%	98%	98%
Prophylactic Antibiotic Timing	70	96%	98%	99%
Prophylactic Antibiotic Timing (Outpatient)[1,3]	-	-	96%	98%
Urinary Catheter Removal	77	100%	97%	97%
Survey of Patients' Hospital Experiences				
Area Around Room 'Always' Quiet at Night	(a)	57%	57%	61%
Doctors 'Always' Communicated Well	(a)	90%	81%	82%
Home Recovery Information Given	(a)	90%	86%	85%
Hospital Given 9 or 10 on 10 Point Scale	(a)	81%	70%	71%
Meds 'Always' Explained Before Given	(a)	73%	65%	64%
Nurses 'Always' Communicated Well	(a)	82%	79%	79%
Pain 'Always' Well Controlled	(a)	75%	71%	71%
Room and Bathroom 'Always' Clean	(a)	82%	74%	73%
Timely Help 'Always' Received	(a)	76%	68%	68%
Would Definitely Recommend Hospital	(a)	81%	72%	71%
Use of Medical Imaging				
Cardiac Imaging Stress Test before Surgery[7]	-	-	4.7%	5.3%
Combination Abdominal CT Scan	143	3.5%	6.6%	10.5%
Combination Brain/Sinus CT Scan[1]	-	-	2.1%	2.7%
Combination Chest CT Scan	61	0.0%	1.1%	2.7%
Follow-up Mammogram/Ultrasound	272	3.3%	8.9%	8.8%
Lumbar Spine MRI for Low Back Pain[1]	-	-	41.7%	37.2%

Good Samaritan Regional Medical Center

3600 Nw Samaritan Drive Phone: 541-768-5111
Corvallis, OR 97330 Fax: 541-768-6400
URL: www.samhealth.org/shs_facilities
Type: Acute Care Hospitals Emergency Services: Yes
Ownership: Voluntary non-profit - Private Beds: 188
Key Personnel:
Chief of Medical Staff.......... Steven Athay, MD
Operating Room.............. Scott Barlow, PA-C
Emergency Room .... P Daniel Dale
Radiology................... Jeff Hamlin, MD

Measure	Cases	This Hosp.	State Avg.	U.S. Avg.
Blood Clot Prevention and Treatment				
Anticoagulation Overlap Therapy[2]	54	96%	95%	93%
ICU Venous Thromboembolism Prophylaxis[2]	53	81%	87%	92%
Incidence of Potentially Preventable VTE[1,2]	-	-	13%	10%
UFH with Dosages/Platelet Monitoring[2]	50	98%	100%	97%
Venous Thromboembolism Prophylaxis[2]	313	84%	83%	85%
Warfarin Therapy Discharge Instructions[2]	45	76%	54%	75%
Chest Pain/Possible Heart Attack Care				
Aspirin Given Within 24 Hours of Arrival[1,3]	-	-	97%	96%
Fibrinolytic Meds Within 30 Min. of Arrival[5]	-	-	57%	58%
Average Time to ECG (minutes)[1,3]	-	-	9	7
Average Time to Transfer (minutes)[5]	-	-	52	60
Children's Asthma Care				
Received Home Management Plan of Care	-	-	-	88%
Received Reliever Medication	-	-	-	100%
Received Systemic Corticosteroids	-	-	-	100%
Emergency Department				
Admittance Decision Time (minutes)[2]	434	63	85	98
Head CT Results Within 45 Min. of Arrival[1]	-	-	45%	57%
Patients Who Left ER Before Being Seen	18,752	1%	2%	2%
Time from ER Arrival to Admit. (minutes)[2]	448	228	235	274
Time from ER Arrival to Discharge (minutes)	356	140	136	134
Time in ER Before Being Evaluated (minutes)	346	32	27	26
Time to Pain Meds for Fractures (minutes)	106	60	56	57
Heart Attack Care				
Aspirin Given at Discharge	302	99%	99%	99%
Fibrinolytic Meds Within 30 Min. of Arrival[7]	-	-	57%	54%
PCI Within 90 Minutes of Arrival	40	95%	93%	96%
Statin Prescribed at Discharge	302	99%	98%	98%
Heart Failure Care				
ACE Inhibitor or ARB for LVSD	62	100%	96%	97%
Discharge Instructions Given	157	99%	93%	94%
Evaluation of LVS Function	176	100%	99%	99%
Medicare Spending				
Medicare Spending per Patient (ratio)	-	0.90	0.88	0.98
Pneumonia Care				
Appropriate Initial Antibiotic Given	93	91%	96%	95%
Blood Culture Timing	176	94%	98%	98%
Pregnancy and Delivery Care				
Newborn Deliveries Scheduled Early[2]	14	7%	3%	6%
Preventive Care				
Immunization for Influenza[2]	559	79%	86%	90%
Immunization for Pneumonia[2]	698	79%	88%	92%
Stroke Care				
Anticoagulation Therapy for Atrial Fibrillation	24	100%	94%	95%
Antithrombotic Therapy Timing	104	97%	97%	98%
Assessed for Rehabilitation	146	97%	96%	97%
Discharged on Antithrombotic Therapy	128	98%	99%	99%
Discharged on Statin Medication	105	95%	93%	94%
Thrombolytic Therapy Timing	16	81%	55%	66%
Venous Thromboembolism Prophylaxis	149	93%	90%	94%
Written Stroke Educational Materials Given	92	98%	81%	88%
Surgical Care Improvement Project				
Appropriate Beta Blocker Usage[2]	290	99%	98%	98%
Appropriate VTP Within 24 Hours[2]	604	97%	97%	98%
Controlled Postoperative Blood Glucose[2]	156	96%	98%	97%
Perioperative Temperature Management[2]	770	100%	100%	100%
Prophylactic Antibiotic Selection[2]	716	99%	99%	99%
Prophylactic Antibiotic Selection (Outpatient)	521	99%	98%	98%
Prophylactic Antibiotic Stopped[2]	702	99%	98%	98%
Prophylactic Antibiotic Timing[2]	717	97%	98%	99%
Prophylactic Antibiotic Timing (Outpatient)	526	98%	96%	98%
Urinary Catheter Removal[2]	682	98%	97%	97%
Survey of Patients' Hospital Experiences				
Area Around Room 'Always' Quiet at Night	300+	39%	57%	61%
Doctors 'Always' Communicated Well	300+	76%	81%	82%
Home Recovery Information Given	300+	84%	86%	85%
Hospital Given 9 or 10 on 10 Point Scale	300+	64%	70%	71%
Meds 'Always' Explained Before Given	300+	62%	65%	64%
Nurses 'Always' Communicated Well	300+	75%	79%	79%
Pain 'Always' Well Controlled	300+	67%	71%	71%
Room and Bathroom 'Always' Clean	300+	66%	74%	73%
Timely Help 'Always' Received	300+	64%	68%	68%
Would Definitely Recommend Hospital	300+	70%	72%	71%
Use of Medical Imaging				
Cardiac Imaging Stress Test before Surgery	283	4.9%	4.7%	5.3%
Combination Abdominal CT Scan	365	7.9%	6.6%	10.5%
Combination Brain/Sinus CT Scan[1]	-	-	2.1%	2.7%
Combination Chest CT Scan	225	2.2%	1.1%	2.7%
Follow-up Mammogram/Ultrasound	1,301	5.6%	8.9%	8.8%
Lumbar Spine MRI for Low Back Pain[1]	-	-	41.7%	37.2%

Peacehealth Cottage Grove Community Medical Center

1515 Village Drive Phone: 541-767-5500
Cottage Grove, OR 97424 Fax: 541-942-0353
URL: www.peacehealth.org/oregon
Type: Critical Access Hospitals Emergency Services: Yes
Ownership: Voluntary non-profit - Private Beds: 14
Key Personnel:
Chief of Medical Staff.......... David DeHass
CEO/President............... Mary Anne McMurren
Operating Room............. Sheila Pratt, RN
Quality Assurance .... Warren Reddick

Measure	Cases	This Hosp.	State Avg.	U.S. Avg.
Blood Clot Prevention and Treatment				
Anticoagulation Overlap Therapy[1,2]	-	-	95%	93%
ICU Venous Thromboembolism Prophylaxis[2,7]	-	-	87%	92%
Incidence of Potentially Preventable VTE[2,7]	-	-	13%	10%
UFH with Dosages/Platelet Monitoring[1,2]	-	-	100%	97%
Venous Thromboembolism Prophylaxis[2]	120	68%	83%	85%
Warfarin Therapy Discharge Instructions[1,2]	-	-	54%	75%
Chest Pain/Possible Heart Attack Care				
Aspirin Given Within 24 Hours of Arrival	31	100%	97%	96%
Fibrinolytic Meds Within 30 Min. of Arrival[7]	-	-	57%	58%
Average Time to ECG (minutes)	32	9	9	7
Average Time to Transfer (minutes)[1]	-	-	52	60
Children's Asthma Care				
Received Home Management Plan of Care	-	-	-	88%
Received Reliever Medication	-	-	-	100%
Received Systemic Corticosteroids	-	-	-	100%
Emergency Department				
Admittance Decision Time (minutes)[2]	270	50	85	98
Head CT Results Within 45 Min. of Arrival[1]	-	-	45%	57%
Patients Who Left ER Before Being Seen	10,957	2%	2%	2%
Time from ER Arrival to Admit. (minutes)[2]	273	187	235	274
Time from ER Arrival to Discharge (minutes)	373	85	136	134
Time in ER Before Being Evaluated (minutes)	396	25	27	26
Time to Pain Meds for Fractures (minutes)	26	42	56	57
Heart Attack Care				
Aspirin Given at Discharge[5]	-	-	99%	99%
Fibrinolytic Meds Within 30 Min. of Arrival[5]	-	-	57%	54%
PCI Within 90 Minutes of Arrival[5]	-	-	93%	96%

NOTE: Hospital profiles are in alphabetical order by state, then city, then hospital within the city; Rankings exclude hospitals with less than 25 cases except for patient surveys which excludes hospitals with less than 100 cases; (a) 100-299 cases; (1) The number of cases/patients is too few to report; (2) Data submitted were based on a sample of cases/patients; (3) Results are based on a shorter time period than required; (4) Data suppressed by CMS for one or more quarters; (5) Results are not available for this reporting period; (6) Fewer than 100 patients completed the HCAHPS survey; (7) No cases met the criteria for this measure; (8) The lower limit of the confidence interval cannot be calculated if the number of observed infections equals zero; (9) No data are available from the state/territory for this reporting period; (10) The scores shown reflect fewer than 50 completed surveys; (11) There were discrepancies in the data collection process; (12) This measure does not apply to this hospital for this reporting period; (13) Results cannot be calculated for this reporting period; (14) The results for this state are combined with nearby states to protect confidentiality; Please refer to the User's Guide for a full explanation of data.

Measure	Cases	This Hosp.	State Avg.	U.S. Avg.
Statin Prescribed at Discharge[5]	-	-	98%	98%
Heart Failure Care				
ACE Inhibitor or ARB for LVSD[1]	-	-	96%	97%
Discharge Instructions Given	16	81%	93%	94%
Evaluation of LVS Function	17	100%	99%	99%
Medicare Spending				
Medicare Spending per Patient (ratio)	-	-	0.88	0.98
Pneumonia Care				
Appropriate Initial Antibiotic Given	14	100%	96%	95%
Blood Culture Timing	21	95%	98%	98%
Pregnancy and Delivery Care				
Newborn Deliveries Scheduled Early[3,7]	-	-	3%	6%
Preventive Care				
Immunization for Influenza[2]	157	93%	86%	90%
Immunization for Pneumonia[2]	253	92%	88%	92%
Stroke Care				
Anticoagulation Therapy for Atrial Fibrillation[3,7]	-	-	94%	95%
Antithrombotic Therapy Timing[3,7]	-	-	97%	98%
Assessed for Rehabilitation[3,7]	-	-	96%	97%
Discharged on Antithrombotic Therapy[3,7]	-	-	99%	99%
Discharged on Statin Medication[3,7]	-	-	93%	94%
Thrombolytic Therapy Timing[3,7]	-	-	55%	66%
Venous Thromboembolism Prophylaxis[3,7]	-	-	90%	94%
Written Stroke Educational Materials Given[3,7]	-	-	81%	88%
Surgical Care Improvement Project				
Appropriate Beta Blocker Usage[5]	-	-	98%	98%
Appropriate VTP Within 24 Hours[5]	-	-	97%	98%
Controlled Postoperative Blood Glucose[5]	-	-	98%	97%
Perioperative Temperature Management[5]	-	-	100%	100%
Prophylactic Antibiotic Selection[5]	-	-	99%	99%
Prophylactic Antibiotic Selection (Outpatient)[5]	-	-	98%	98%
Prophylactic Antibiotic Stopped[5]	-	-	98%	98%
Prophylactic Antibiotic Timing[5]	-	-	98%	99%
Prophylactic Antibiotic Timing (Outpatient)[5]	-	-	96%	98%
Urinary Catheter Removal[5]	-	-	97%	97%
Survey of Patients' Hospital Experiences				
Area Around Room 'Always' Quiet at Night[6]	<100	63%	57%	61%
Doctors 'Always' Communicated Well[6]	<100	87%	81%	82%
Home Recovery Information Given[6]	<100	91%	86%	85%
Hospital Given 9 or 10 on 10 Point Scale[6]	<100	88%	70%	71%
Meds 'Always' Explained Before Given[6]	<100	77%	65%	64%
Nurses 'Always' Communicated Well[6]	<100	88%	79%	79%
Pain 'Always' Well Controlled[6]	<100	77%	71%	71%
Room and Bathroom 'Always' Clean[6]	<100	89%	74%	73%
Timely Help 'Always' Received[6]	<100	80%	68%	68%
Would Definitely Recommend Hospital[6]	<100	80%	72%	71%
Use of Medical Imaging				
Cardiac Imaging Stress Test before Surgery[7]	-	-	4.7%	5.3%
Combination Abdominal CT Scan	134	5.2%	6.6%	10.5%
Combination Brain/Sinus CT Scan	131	0.0%	2.1%	2.7%
Combination Chest CT Scan	84	0.0%	1.1%	2.7%
Follow-up Mammogram/Ultrasound	317	6.6%	8.9%	8.8%
Lumbar Spine MRI for Low Back Pain[7]	-	-	41.7%	37.2%

West Valley Hospital

525 Se Washington Street
Dallas, OR 97338
Phone: 503-623-8301
Fax: 503-623-7337
URL: www.westvalleyhospital.org
Type: Critical Access Hospitals
Emergency Services: Yes
Ownership: Voluntary non-profit - Private
Beds: 15

Key Personnel:

Quality Assurance . . . . Linda Beck
Emergency Room . . . . Tampanela Beffoer
Radiology. . . . . John Borris
CEO/President. . . . . Norm Gruber
Chief of Medical Staff. . . . . Melinda Seibert

Measure	Cases	This Hosp.	State Avg.	U.S. Avg.
Blood Clot Prevention and Treatment				
Anticoagulation Overlap Therapy[5]	-	-	95%	93%
ICU Venous Thromboembolism Prophylaxis[5]	-	-	87%	92%
Incidence of Potentially Preventable VTE[5]	-	-	13%	10%
UFH with Dosages/Platelet Monitoring[5]	-	-	100%	97%
Venous Thromboembolism Prophylaxis[5]	-	-	83%	85%
Warfarin Therapy Discharge Instructions[5]	-	-	54%	75%
Chest Pain/Possible Heart Attack Care				
Aspirin Given Within 24 Hours of Arrival	49	100%	97%	96%
Fibrinolytic Meds Within 30 Min. of Arrival[7]	-	-	57%	58%
Average Time to ECG (minutes)	51	6	9	7
Average Time to Transfer (minutes)	11	51	52	60
Children's Asthma Care				
Received Home Management Plan of Care	-	-	-	88%
Received Reliever Medication	-	-	-	100%
Received Systemic Corticosteroids	-	-	-	100%
Emergency Department				
Admittance Decision Time (minutes)[5]	-	-	85	98
Head CT Results Within 45 Min. of Arrival[3,7]	-	-	45%	57%
Patients Who Left ER Before Being Seen[5]	-	-	2%	2%
Time from ER Arrival to Admit. (minutes)[5]	-	-	235	274
Time from ER Arrival to Discharge (minutes)[5]	-	-	136	134
Time in ER Before Being Evaluated (minutes)[5]	-	-	27	26
Time to Pain Meds for Fractures (minutes)	64	34	56	57
Heart Attack Care				
Aspirin Given at Discharge[5]	-	-	99%	99%
Fibrinolytic Meds Within 30 Min. of Arrival[5]	-	-	57%	54%
PCI Within 90 Minutes of Arrival[5]	-	-	93%	96%
Statin Prescribed at Discharge[5]	-	-	98%	98%
Heart Failure Care				
ACE Inhibitor or ARB for LVSD[3,7]	-	-	96%	97%
Discharge Instructions Given[1,3]	-	-	93%	94%
Evaluation of LVS Function[1,3]	-	-	99%	99%
Medicare Spending				
Medicare Spending per Patient (ratio)	-	-	0.88	0.98
Pneumonia Care				
Appropriate Initial Antibiotic Given	13	85%	96%	95%
Blood Culture Timing	16	100%	98%	98%
Pregnancy and Delivery Care				
Newborn Deliveries Scheduled Early[3,7]	-	-	3%	6%
Preventive Care				
Immunization for Influenza	72	90%	86%	90%
Immunization for Pneumonia	124	97%	88%	92%
Stroke Care				
Anticoagulation Therapy for Atrial Fibrillation[5]	-	-	94%	95%
Antithrombotic Therapy Timing[5]	-	-	97%	98%
Assessed for Rehabilitation[5]	-	-	96%	97%
Discharged on Antithrombotic Therapy[5]	-	-	99%	99%
Discharged on Statin Medication[5]	-	-	93%	94%
Thrombolytic Therapy Timing[5]	-	-	55%	66%
Venous Thromboembolism Prophylaxis[5]	-	-	90%	94%
Written Stroke Educational Materials Given[5]	-	-	81%	88%
Surgical Care Improvement Project				
Appropriate Beta Blocker Usage[5]	-	-	98%	98%
Appropriate VTP Within 24 Hours[5]	-	-	97%	98%
Controlled Postoperative Blood Glucose[5]	-	-	98%	97%
Perioperative Temperature Management[5]	-	-	100%	100%
Prophylactic Antibiotic Selection[5]	-	-	99%	99%
Prophylactic Antibiotic Selection (Outpatient)[5]	-	-	98%	98%
Prophylactic Antibiotic Stopped[5]	-	-	98%	98%
Prophylactic Antibiotic Timing[5]	-	-	98%	99%
Prophylactic Antibiotic Timing (Outpatient)[5]	-	-	96%	98%
Urinary Catheter Removal[5]	-	-	97%	97%
Survey of Patients' Hospital Experiences				
Area Around Room 'Always' Quiet at Night[5]	-	-	57%	61%
Doctors 'Always' Communicated Well[5]	-	-	81%	82%
Home Recovery Information Given[5]	-	-	86%	85%
Hospital Given 9 or 10 on 10 Point Scale[5]	-	-	70%	71%
Meds 'Always' Explained Before Given[5]	-	-	65%	64%
Nurses 'Always' Communicated Well[5]	-	-	79%	79%
Pain 'Always' Well Controlled[5]	-	-	71%	71%
Room and Bathroom 'Always' Clean[5]	-	-	74%	73%
Timely Help 'Always' Received[5]	-	-	68%	68%
Would Definitely Recommend Hospital[5]	-	-	72%	71%
Use of Medical Imaging				
Cardiac Imaging Stress Test before Surgery[7]	-	-	4.7%	5.3%
Combination Abdominal CT Scan	132	3.8%	6.6%	10.5%
Combination Brain/Sinus CT Scan[1]	-	-	2.1%	2.7%
Combination Chest CT Scan	68	0.0%	1.1%	2.7%
Follow-up Mammogram/Ultrasound	206	12.6%	8.9%	8.8%
Lumbar Spine MRI for Low Back Pain[1]	-	-	41.7%	37.2%

Wallowa Memorial Hospital

601 Medical Parkway
Enterprise, OR 97828
Phone: 541-426-3111
Fax: 541-426-4095
E-mail: ceo@wchcd.org
URL: www.wchcd.org
Type: Critical Access Hospitals
Emergency Services: Yes
Ownership: Govt - Hospital Dist/Auth
Beds: 57

Key Personnel:

CEO/President. . . . . Larry Davy
Emergency Room . . . . Lowell E Euhus, MD
Surgery . . . . Kenneth D. Rose, MD
Chief of Medical Staff . . . . Scott Sebde
Chairman/CEO . . . . Robert Williams
Quality Assurance . . . . Cathy Wobster

Measure	Cases	This Hosp.	State Avg.	U.S. Avg.
Blood Clot Prevention and Treatment				
Anticoagulation Overlap Therapy[5]	-	-	95%	93%
ICU Venous Thromboembolism Prophylaxis[5]	-	-	87%	92%
Incidence of Potentially Preventable VTE[5]	-	-	13%	10%
UFH with Dosages/Platelet Monitoring[5]	-	-	100%	97%
Venous Thromboembolism Prophylaxis[5]	-	-	83%	85%
Warfarin Therapy Discharge Instructions[5]	-	-	54%	75%
Chest Pain/Possible Heart Attack Care				
Aspirin Given Within 24 Hours of Arrival	-	-	97%	96%
Fibrinolytic Meds Within 30 Min. of Arrival	-	-	57%	58%
Average Time to ECG (minutes)	-	-	9	7
Average Time to Transfer (minutes)	-	-	52	60
Children's Asthma Care				
Received Home Management Plan of Care	-	-	-	88%
Received Reliever Medication	-	-	-	100%
Received Systemic Corticosteroids	-	-	-	100%
Emergency Department				
Admittance Decision Time (minutes)[5]	-	-	85	98
Head CT Results Within 45 Min. of Arrival	-	-	45%	57%
Patients Who Left ER Before Being Seen	-	-	2%	2%
Time from ER Arrival to Admit. (minutes)[5]	-	-	235	274
Time from ER Arrival to Discharge (minutes)	-	-	136	134
Time in ER Before Being Evaluated (minutes)	-	-	27	26
Time to Pain Meds for Fractures (minutes)	-	-	56	57
Heart Attack Care				
Aspirin Given at Discharge[5]	-	-	99%	99%
Fibrinolytic Meds Within 30 Min. of Arrival[5]	-	-	57%	54%
PCI Within 90 Minutes of Arrival[5]	-	-	93%	96%
Statin Prescribed at Discharge[5]	-	-	98%	98%
Heart Failure Care				
ACE Inhibitor or ARB for LVSD[1,3]	-	-	96%	97%
Discharge Instructions Given[3]	11	55%	93%	94%
Evaluation of LVS Function[3]	17	76%	99%	99%
Medicare Spending				
Medicare Spending per Patient (ratio)	-	-	0.88	0.98
Pneumonia Care				
Appropriate Initial Antibiotic Given[3]	13	92%	96%	95%
Blood Culture Timing[3]	11	73%	98%	98%
Pregnancy and Delivery Care				
Newborn Deliveries Scheduled Early[5]	-	-	3%	6%
Preventive Care				
Immunization for Influenza[5]	-	-	86%	90%
Immunization for Pneumonia[5]	-	-	88%	92%
Stroke Care				
Anticoagulation Therapy for Atrial Fibrillation[5]	-	-	94%	95%
Antithrombotic Therapy Timing[5]	-	-	97%	98%
Assessed for Rehabilitation[5]	-	-	96%	97%
Discharged on Antithrombotic Therapy[5]	-	-	99%	99%
Discharged on Statin Medication[5]	-	-	93%	94%
Thrombolytic Therapy Timing[5]	-	-	55%	66%
Venous Thromboembolism Prophylaxis[5]	-	-	90%	94%
Written Stroke Educational Materials Given[5]	-	-	81%	88%
Surgical Care Improvement Project				
Appropriate Beta Blocker Usage[5]	-	-	98%	98%
Appropriate VTP Within 24 Hours[5]	-	-	97%	98%

NOTE: Hospital profiles are in alphabetical order by state, then city, then hospital within the city; Rankings exclude hospitals with less than 25 cases except for patient surveys which excludes hospitals with less than 100 cases; (a) 100-299 cases; (1) The number of cases/patients is too few to report; (2) Data submitted were based on a sample of cases/patients; (3) Results are based on a shorter time period than required; (4) Data suppressed by CMS for one or more quarters; (5) Results are not available for this reporting period; (6) Fewer than 100 patients completed the HCAHPS survey; (7) No cases met the criteria for this measure; (8) The lower limit of the confidence interval cannot be calculated if the number of observed infections equals zero; (9) No data are available from the state/territory for this reporting period; (10) The scores shown reflect fewer than 50 completed surveys; (11) There were discrepancies in the data collection process; (12) This measure does not apply to this hospital for this reporting period; (13) Results cannot be calculated for this reporting period; (14) The results for this state are combined with nearby states to protect confidentiality; Please refer to the User's Guide for a full explanation of data.

Measure	Cases	This Hosp.	State Avg.	U.S. Avg.
Controlled Postoperative Blood Glucose[5]	-	-	98%	97%
Perioperative Temperature Management[5]	-	-	100%	100%
Prophylactic Antibiotic Selection[5]	-	-	99%	99%
Prophylactic Antibiotic Selection (Outpatient)	-	-	98%	98%
Prophylactic Antibiotic Stopped[5]	-	-	98%	98%
Prophylactic Antibiotic Timing[5]	-	-	98%	99%
Prophylactic Antibiotic Timing (Outpatient)	-	-	96%	98%
Urinary Catheter Removal[5]	-	-	97%	97%
Survey of Patients' Hospital Experiences				
Area Around Room 'Always' Quiet at Night	(a)	74%	57%	61%
Doctors 'Always' Communicated Well	(a)	89%	81%	82%
Home Recovery Information Given	(a)	88%	86%	85%
Hospital Given 9 or 10 on 10 Point Scale	(a)	75%	70%	71%
Meds 'Always' Explained Before Given	(a)	68%	65%	64%
Nurses 'Always' Communicated Well	(a)	82%	79%	79%
Pain 'Always' Well Controlled	(a)	71%	71%	71%
Room and Bathroom 'Always' Clean	(a)	78%	74%	73%
Timely Help 'Always' Received	(a)	71%	68%	68%
Would Definitely Recommend Hospital	(a)	78%	72%	71%
Use of Medical Imaging				
Cardiac Imaging Stress Test before Surgery	-	-	4.7%	5.3%
Combination Abdominal CT Scan	-	-	6.6%	10.5%
Combination Brain/Sinus CT Scan	-	-	2.1%	2.7%
Combination Chest CT Scan	-	-	1.1%	2.7%
Follow-up Mammogram/Ultrasound	-	-	8.9%	8.8%
Lumbar Spine MRI for Low Back Pain	-	-	41.7%	37.2%

Sacred Heart University District

1255 Hilyard Street
Eugene, OR 97401
Phone: 541-686-7300
Fax: 541-686-7005
URL: www.peacehealth.org
Type: Acute Care Hospitals
Emergency Services: Yes
Ownership: Voluntary non-profit - Private
Beds: 432

Key Personnel:

Coronary Care . . . . Angela Christensen
Pediatric In-Patient Care . . . . Sally Cochrane, RN
Radiology. . . . . Carol Doyle
CEO/President. . . . . John Hill
Infection Control. . . . . Susan Kline
Quality Assurance . . . . Jim Lemieux, RN
Chief of Medical Staff. . . . . Michael Menen, MD
Operating Room. . . . . Hedy Scheft

Measure	Cases	This Hosp.	State Avg.	U.S. Avg.
Blood Clot Prevention and Treatment				
Anticoagulation Overlap Therapy[1,2]	-	-	95%	93%
ICU Venous Thromboembolism Prophylaxis[2,7]	-	-	87%	92%
Incidence of Potentially Preventable VTE[2,7]	-	-	13%	10%
UFH with Dosages/Platelet Monitoring[1,2]	-	-	100%	97%
Venous Thromboembolism Prophylaxis[2]	103	93%	83%	85%
Warfarin Therapy Discharge Instructions[1,2]	-	-	54%	75%
Chest Pain/Possible Heart Attack Care				
Aspirin Given Within 24 Hours of Arrival	32	100%	97%	96%
Fibrinolytic Meds Within 30 Min. of Arrival[7]	-	-	57%	58%
Average Time to ECG (minutes)	34	12	9	7
Average Time to Transfer (minutes)[1]	-	-	52	60
Children's Asthma Care				
Received Home Management Plan of Care	-	-	-	88%
Received Reliever Medication	-	-	-	100%
Received Systemic Corticosteroids	-	-	-	100%
Emergency Department				
Admittance Decision Time (minutes)[2]	427	65	85	98
Head CT Results Within 45 Min. of Arrival[1]	-	-	45%	57%
Patients Who Left ER Before Being Seen	25,522	3%	2%	2%
Time from ER Arrival to Admit. (minutes)[2]	449	235	235	274
Time from ER Arrival to Discharge (minutes)	364	123	136	134
Time in ER Before Being Evaluated (minutes)	425	41	27	26
Time to Pain Meds for Fractures (minutes)	49	53	56	57
Heart Attack Care				
Aspirin Given at Discharge[1]	-	-	99%	99%
Fibrinolytic Meds Within 30 Min. of Arrival[7]	-	-	57%	54%
PCI Within 90 Minutes of Arrival[7]	-	-	93%	96%
Statin Prescribed at Discharge[1]	-	-	98%	98%
Heart Failure Care				
ACE Inhibitor or ARB for LVSD[1]	-	-	96%	97%
Discharge Instructions Given	25	88%	93%	94%
Evaluation of LVS Function	33	100%	99%	99%
Medicare Spending				
Medicare Spending per Patient (ratio)	-	0.72	0.88	0.98
Pneumonia Care				
Appropriate Initial Antibiotic Given	57	96%	96%	95%
Blood Culture Timing	65	94%	98%	98%
Pregnancy and Delivery Care				
Newborn Deliveries Scheduled Early[7]	-	-	3%	6%
Preventive Care				
Immunization for Influenza[2]	284	93%	86%	90%
Immunization for Pneumonia[2]	429	94%	88%	92%
Stroke Care				
Anticoagulation Therapy for Atrial Fibrillation[1]	-	-	94%	95%
Antithrombotic Therapy Timing	11	100%	97%	98%
Assessed for Rehabilitation[1]	-	-	96%	97%
Discharged on Antithrombotic Therapy[1]	-	-	99%	99%
Discharged on Statin Medication[1]	-	-	93%	94%
Thrombolytic Therapy Timing[7]	-	-	55%	66%
Venous Thromboembolism Prophylaxis	12	100%	90%	94%
Written Stroke Educational Materials Given[1]	-	-	81%	88%
Surgical Care Improvement Project				
Appropriate Beta Blocker Usage[5]	-	-	98%	98%
Appropriate VTP Within 24 Hours[5]	-	-	97%	98%
Controlled Postoperative Blood Glucose[5]	-	-	98%	97%
Perioperative Temperature Management[5]	-	-	100%	100%
Prophylactic Antibiotic Selection[5]	-	-	99%	99%
Prophylactic Antibiotic Selection (Outpatient)[5]	-	-	98%	98%
Prophylactic Antibiotic Stopped[5]	-	-	98%	98%
Prophylactic Antibiotic Timing[5]	-	-	98%	99%
Prophylactic Antibiotic Timing (Outpatient)[5]	-	-	96%	98%
Urinary Catheter Removal[5]	-	-	97%	97%
Survey of Patients' Hospital Experiences				
Area Around Room 'Always' Quiet at Night	(a)	52%	57%	61%
Doctors 'Always' Communicated Well	(a)	76%	81%	82%
Home Recovery Information Given	(a)	82%	86%	85%
Hospital Given 9 or 10 on 10 Point Scale	(a)	61%	70%	71%
Meds 'Always' Explained Before Given	(a)	56%	65%	64%
Nurses 'Always' Communicated Well	(a)	74%	79%	79%
Pain 'Always' Well Controlled	(a)	66%	71%	71%
Room and Bathroom 'Always' Clean	(a)	75%	74%	73%
Timely Help 'Always' Received	(a)	59%	68%	68%
Would Definitely Recommend Hospital	(a)	66%	72%	71%
Use of Medical Imaging				
Cardiac Imaging Stress Test before Surgery[7]	-	-	4.7%	5.3%
Combination Abdominal CT Scan	82	0.0%	6.6%	10.5%
Combination Brain/Sinus CT Scan[1]	-	-	2.1%	2.7%
Combination Chest CT Scan[1]	-	-	1.1%	2.7%
Follow-up Mammogram/Ultrasound[7]	-	-	8.9%	8.8%
Lumbar Spine MRI for Low Back Pain[1]	-	-	41.7%	37.2%

Peace Harbor Medical Center

400 9th Street
Florence, OR 97439
Phone: 541-997-8412
Fax: 541-997-9155
URL: www.peacehealth.org/siuslaw
Type: Critical Access Hospitals
Emergency Services: Yes
Ownership: Voluntary non-profit - Church
Beds: 21

Key Personnel:

Anesthesiology. . . . . Ed Geers
Operating Room. . . . . Linda Gould, RN
Chief of Medical Staff . . . . Ronald Shearer
Emergency Room . . . . Mathew Valentine
Infection Control. . . . . Leslie Weaver
CEO . . . . Rick Yecny

Measure	Cases	This Hosp.	State Avg.	U.S. Avg.
Blood Clot Prevention and Treatment				
Anticoagulation Overlap Therapy[1,2]	-	-	95%	93%
ICU Venous Thromboembolism Prophylaxis[2]	52	100%	87%	92%
Incidence of Potentially Preventable VTE[2,7]	-	-	13%	10%
UFH with Dosages/Platelet Monitoring[1,2]	-	-	100%	97%
Venous Thromboembolism Prophylaxis[2]	64	98%	83%	85%
Warfarin Therapy Discharge Instructions[1,2]	-	-	54%	75%
Chest Pain/Possible Heart Attack Care				
Aspirin Given Within 24 Hours of Arrival	50	100%	97%	96%
Fibrinolytic Meds Within 30 Min. of Arrival[1]	-	-	57%	58%
Average Time to ECG (minutes)	51	8	9	7
Average Time to Transfer (minutes)[7]	-	-	52	60
Children's Asthma Care				
Received Home Management Plan of Care	-	-	-	88%
Received Reliever Medication	-	-	-	100%
Received Systemic Corticosteroids	-	-	-	100%
Emergency Department				
Admittance Decision Time (minutes)[2]	387	48	85	98
Head CT Results Within 45 Min. of Arrival[1]	-	-	45%	57%
Patients Who Left ER Before Being Seen	8,131	2%	2%	2%
Time from ER Arrival to Admit. (minutes)[2]	390	205	235	274
Time from ER Arrival to Discharge (minutes)	410	94	136	134
Time in ER Before Being Evaluated (minutes)	440	15	27	26
Time to Pain Meds for Fractures (minutes)	45	52	56	57
Heart Attack Care				
Aspirin Given at Discharge[1]	-	-	99%	99%
Fibrinolytic Meds Within 30 Min. of Arrival[7]	-	-	57%	54%
PCI Within 90 Minutes of Arrival[7]	-	-	93%	96%
Statin Prescribed at Discharge[1]	-	-	98%	98%
Heart Failure Care				
ACE Inhibitor or ARB for LVSD[1]	-	-	96%	97%
Discharge Instructions Given	17	100%	93%	94%
Evaluation of LVS Function	22	100%	99%	99%
Medicare Spending				
Medicare Spending per Patient (ratio)	-	-	0.88	0.98
Pneumonia Care				
Appropriate Initial Antibiotic Given	17	100%	96%	95%
Blood Culture Timing	42	100%	98%	98%
Pregnancy and Delivery Care				
Newborn Deliveries Scheduled Early[1]	-	-	3%	6%
Preventive Care				
Immunization for Influenza[2]	279	99%	86%	90%
Immunization for Pneumonia[2]	450	99%	88%	92%
Stroke Care				
Anticoagulation Therapy for Atrial Fibrillation[1]	-	-	94%	95%
Antithrombotic Therapy Timing	14	100%	97%	98%
Assessed for Rehabilitation	16	100%	96%	97%
Discharged on Antithrombotic Therapy	15	100%	99%	99%
Discharged on Statin Medication[1]	-	-	93%	94%
Thrombolytic Therapy Timing[7]	-	-	55%	66%
Venous Thromboembolism Prophylaxis	14	93%	90%	94%
Written Stroke Educational Materials Given[1]	-	-	81%	88%
Surgical Care Improvement Project				
Appropriate Beta Blocker Usage	26	100%	98%	98%
Appropriate VTP Within 24 Hours	74	100%	97%	98%
Controlled Postoperative Blood Glucose[7]	-	-	98%	97%
Perioperative Temperature Management	93	99%	100%	100%
Prophylactic Antibiotic Selection	68	99%	99%	99%
Prophylactic Antibiotic Selection (Outpatient)[3,7]	-	-	98%	98%
Prophylactic Antibiotic Stopped	67	100%	98%	98%
Prophylactic Antibiotic Timing	68	97%	98%	99%
Prophylactic Antibiotic Timing (Outpatient)[1,3]	-	-	96%	98%
Urinary Catheter Removal	20	100%	97%	97%
Survey of Patients' Hospital Experiences				
Area Around Room 'Always' Quiet at Night	(a)	53%	57%	61%
Doctors 'Always' Communicated Well	(a)	81%	81%	82%
Home Recovery Information Given	(a)	91%	86%	85%
Hospital Given 9 or 10 on 10 Point Scale	(a)	71%	70%	71%
Meds 'Always' Explained Before Given	(a)	65%	65%	64%
Nurses 'Always' Communicated Well	(a)	80%	79%	79%
Pain 'Always' Well Controlled	(a)	75%	71%	71%
Room and Bathroom 'Always' Clean	(a)	80%	74%	73%
Timely Help 'Always' Received	(a)	74%	68%	68%
Would Definitely Recommend Hospital	(a)	71%	72%	71%
Use of Medical Imaging				
Cardiac Imaging Stress Test before Surgery	103	1.9%	4.7%	5.3%
Combination Abdominal CT Scan	301	6.3%	6.6%	10.5%
Combination Brain/Sinus CT Scan[1]	-	-	2.1%	2.7%
Combination Chest CT Scan	178	0.0%	1.1%	2.7%
Follow-up Mammogram/Ultrasound	649	4.9%	8.9%	8.8%
Lumbar Spine MRI for Low Back Pain	50	48.0%	41.7%	37.2%

NOTE: Hospital profiles are in alphabetical order by state, then city, then hospital within the city; Rankings exclude hospitals with less than 25 cases except for patient surveys which excludes hospitals with less than 100 cases; (a) 100-299 cases; (1) The number of cases/patients is too few to report; (2) Data submitted were based on a sample of cases/patients; (3) Results are based on a shorter time period than required; (4) Data suppressed by CMS for one or more quarters; (5) Results are not available for this reporting period; (6) Fewer than 100 patients completed the HCAHPS survey; (7) No cases met the criteria for this measure; (8) The lower limit of the confidence interval cannot be calculated if the number of observed infections equals zero; (9) No data are available from the state/territory for this reporting period; (10) The scores shown reflect fewer than 50 completed surveys; (11) There were discrepancies in the data collection process; (12) This measure does not apply to this hospital for this reporting period; (13) Results cannot be calculated for this reporting period; (14) The results for this state are combined with nearby states to protect confidentiality; Please refer to the User's Guide for a full explanation of data.

Curry General Hospital

94220 Fourth Street
Gold Beach, OR 97444
Phone: 541-247-3000
Fax: 541-247-2012
E-mail: info@curryhealthnetwork.com
URL: www.currygeneralhospital.com
Type: Critical Access Hospitals
Emergency Services: Yes
Ownership: Govt - Hospital Dist/Auth
Beds: 24

Key Personnel:
Infection Control . . . . Kelly Anderson, RN
CEO . . . . Andrew P. Bair, RN, MBA
Quality Assurance . . . . Pam Brown
Emergency Room . . . . Virginia Hochberg
Operating Room. . . . . Kelli McKinny, RN
Anesthesiology. . . . . Donelle Schacher, CRNA
Chief of Medical Staff . . . . RG Williams, MD

Measure	Cases	This Hosp.	State Avg.	U.S. Avg.
Blood Clot Prevention and Treatment				
Anticoagulation Overlap Therapy[5]	-	-	95%	93%
ICU Venous Thromboembolism Prophylaxis[5]	-	-	87%	92%
Incidence of Potentially Preventable VTE[5]	-	-	13%	10%
UFH with Dosages/Platelet Monitoring[5]	-	-	100%	97%
Venous Thromboembolism Prophylaxis[5]	-	-	83%	85%
Warfarin Therapy Discharge Instructions[5]	-	-	54%	75%
Chest Pain/Possible Heart Attack Care				
Aspirin Given Within 24 Hours of Arrival[5]	-	-	97%	96%
Fibrinolytic Meds Within 30 Min. of Arrival[5]	-	-	57%	58%
Average Time to ECG (minutes)[5]	-	-	9	7
Average Time to Transfer (minutes)[5]	-	-	52	60
Children's Asthma Care				
Received Home Management Plan of Care	-	-	-	88%
Received Reliever Medication	-	-	-	100%
Received Systemic Corticosteroids	-	-	-	100%
Emergency Department				
Admittance Decision Time (minutes)[5]	-	-	85	98
Head CT Results Within 45 Min. of Arrival[5]	-	-	45%	57%
Patients Who Left ER Before Being Seen[5]	-	-	2%	2%
Time from ER Arrival to Admit. (minutes)[5]	-	-	235	274
Time from ER Arrival to Discharge (minutes)[5]	-	-	136	134
Time in ER Before Being Evaluated (minutes)[5]	-	-	27	26
Time to Pain Meds for Fractures (minutes)[5]	-	-	56	57
Heart Attack Care				
Aspirin Given at Discharge[5]	-	-	99%	99%
Fibrinolytic Meds Within 30 Min. of Arrival[5]	-	-	57%	54%
PCI Within 90 Minutes of Arrival[5]	-	-	93%	96%
Statin Prescribed at Discharge[5]	-	-	98%	98%
Heart Failure Care				
ACE Inhibitor or ARB for LVSD[5]	-	-	96%	97%
Discharge Instructions Given[5]	-	-	93%	94%
Evaluation of LVS Function[5]	-	-	99%	99%
Medicare Spending				
Medicare Spending per Patient (ratio)	-	-	0.88	0.98
Pneumonia Care				
Appropriate Initial Antibiotic Given[5]	-	-	96%	95%
Blood Culture Timing[5]	-	-	98%	98%
Pregnancy and Delivery Care				
Newborn Deliveries Scheduled Early[5]	-	-	3%	6%
Preventive Care				
Immunization for Influenza[5]	-	-	86%	90%
Immunization for Pneumonia[5]	-	-	88%	92%
Stroke Care				
Anticoagulation Therapy for Atrial Fibrillation[5]	-	-	94%	95%
Antithrombotic Therapy Timing[5]	-	-	97%	98%
Assessed for Rehabilitation[5]	-	-	96%	97%
Discharged on Antithrombotic Therapy[5]	-	-	99%	99%
Discharged on Statin Medication[5]	-	-	93%	94%
Thrombolytic Therapy Timing[5]	-	-	55%	66%
Venous Thromboembolism Prophylaxis[5]	-	-	90%	94%
Written Stroke Educational Materials Given[5]	-	-	81%	88%
Surgical Care Improvement Project				
Appropriate Beta Blocker Usage[5]	-	-	98%	98%
Appropriate VTP Within 24 Hours[5]	-	-	97%	98%
Controlled Postoperative Blood Glucose[5]	-	-	98%	97%
Perioperative Temperature Management[5]	-	-	100%	100%
Prophylactic Antibiotic Selection[5]	-	-	99%	99%
Prophylactic Antibiotic Selection (Outpatient)[5]	-	-	98%	98%
Prophylactic Antibiotic Stopped[5]	-	-	98%	98%
Prophylactic Antibiotic Timing[5]	-	-	98%	99%
Prophylactic Antibiotic Timing (Outpatient)[5]	-	-	96%	98%
Urinary Catheter Removal[5]	-	-	97%	97%
Survey of Patients' Hospital Experiences				
Area Around Room 'Always' Quiet at Night[6]	<100	41%	57%	61%
Doctors 'Always' Communicated Well[6]	<100	77%	81%	82%
Home Recovery Information Given[6]	<100	70%	86%	85%
Hospital Given 9 or 10 on 10 Point Scale[6]	<100	50%	70%	71%
Meds 'Always' Explained Before Given[6]	<100	67%	65%	64%
Nurses 'Always' Communicated Well[6]	<100	76%	79%	79%
Pain 'Always' Well Controlled[6]	<100	64%	71%	71%
Room and Bathroom 'Always' Clean[6]	<100	82%	74%	73%
Timely Help 'Always' Received[6]	<100	65%	68%	68%
Would Definitely Recommend Hospital[6]	<100	42%	72%	71%
Use of Medical Imaging				
Cardiac Imaging Stress Test before Surgery	137	3.6%	4.7%	5.3%
Combination Abdominal CT Scan	294	4.8%	6.6%	10.5%
Combination Brain/Sinus CT Scan[1]	-	-	2.1%	2.7%
Combination Chest CT Scan	216	0.5%	1.1%	2.7%
Follow-up Mammogram/Ultrasound	564	3.2%	8.9%	8.8%
Lumbar Spine MRI for Low Back Pain	60	41.7%	41.7%	37.2%

Asante Three Rivers Medical Center

500 Sw Ramsey Avenue
Grants Pass, OR 97527
Phone: 541-472-7000
Fax: 541-472-7381
E-mail: pmckeen@asante.org
URL: www.asante.org
Type: Acute Care Hospitals
Emergency Services: Yes
Ownership: Voluntary non-profit - Other
Beds: 150

Key Personnel:
Emergency Room . . . . Ken Buccino, MD
Chief of Medical Staff. . . . . Kelley Burnett
Intensive Care Unit. . . . . Sherri Dague, RN
Operating Room. . . . . T Marcoulier, RN
Quality Assurance . . . . Terri Scott
Patient Relations . . . . Diana Sheldon, RN
Infection Control. . . . . Sheri Thomson, RN
CEO/President. . . . . Roy Vinyard

Measure	Cases	This Hosp.	State Avg.	U.S. Avg.
Blood Clot Prevention and Treatment				
Anticoagulation Overlap Therapy[2]	44	100%	95%	93%
ICU Venous Thromboembolism Prophylaxis[2]	73	78%	87%	92%
Incidence of Potentially Preventable VTE[1,2]	-	-	13%	10%
UFH with Dosages/Platelet Monitoring[1,2]	-	-	100%	97%
Venous Thromboembolism Prophylaxis[2]	279	65%	83%	85%
Warfarin Therapy Discharge Instructions[2]	29	100%	54%	75%
Chest Pain/Possible Heart Attack Care				
Aspirin Given Within 24 Hours of Arrival	82	99%	97%	96%
Fibrinolytic Meds Within 30 Min. of Arrival[7]	-	-	57%	58%
Average Time to ECG (minutes)	85	18	9	7
Average Time to Transfer (minutes)	30	53	52	60
Children's Asthma Care				
Received Home Management Plan of Care	-	-	-	88%
Received Reliever Medication	-	-	-	100%
Received Systemic Corticosteroids	-	-	-	100%
Emergency Department				
Admittance Decision Time (minutes)[2]	378	82	85	98
Head CT Results Within 45 Min. of Arrival[1]	-	-	45%	57%
Patients Who Left ER Before Being Seen	38,864	3%	2%	2%
Time from ER Arrival to Admit. (minutes)[2]	427	278	235	274
Time from ER Arrival to Discharge (minutes)	339	178	136	134
Time in ER Before Being Evaluated (minutes)	62	50	27	26
Time to Pain Meds for Fractures (minutes)	152	82	56	57
Heart Attack Care				
Aspirin Given at Discharge	47	98%	99%	99%
Fibrinolytic Meds Within 30 Min. of Arrival[7]	-	-	57%	54%
PCI Within 90 Minutes of Arrival[7]	-	-	93%	96%
Statin Prescribed at Discharge	38	95%	98%	98%
Heart Failure Care				
ACE Inhibitor or ARB for LVSD	50	90%	96%	97%
Discharge Instructions Given	110	99%	93%	94%
Evaluation of LVS Function	145	100%	99%	99%
Medicare Spending				
Medicare Spending per Patient (ratio)	-	0.89	0.88	0.98
Pneumonia Care				
Appropriate Initial Antibiotic Given[2]	108	97%	96%	95%
Blood Culture Timing[2]	165	97%	98%	98%
Pregnancy and Delivery Care				
Newborn Deliveries Scheduled Early[2]	31	0%	3%	6%
Preventive Care				
Immunization for Influenza[2]	480	94%	86%	90%
Immunization for Pneumonia[2]	656	94%	88%	92%
Stroke Care				
Anticoagulation Therapy for Atrial Fibrillation[2]	13	85%	94%	95%
Antithrombotic Therapy Timing[2]	77	96%	97%	98%
Assessed for Rehabilitation[2]	84	98%	96%	97%
Discharged on Antithrombotic Therapy[2]	78	99%	99%	99%
Discharged on Statin Medication[2]	55	85%	93%	94%
Thrombolytic Therapy Timing[1,2]	-	-	55%	66%
Venous Thromboembolism Prophylaxis[2]	89	71%	90%	94%
Written Stroke Educational Materials Given[2]	51	100%	81%	88%
Surgical Care Improvement Project				
Appropriate Beta Blocker Usage[2]	103	98%	98%	98%
Appropriate VTP Within 24 Hours[2]	236	95%	97%	98%
Controlled Postoperative Blood Glucose[2,7]	-	-	98%	97%
Perioperative Temperature Management[2]	438	100%	100%	100%
Prophylactic Antibiotic Selection[2]	298	99%	99%	99%
Prophylactic Antibiotic Selection (Outpatient)	82	99%	98%	98%
Prophylactic Antibiotic Stopped[2]	296	99%	98%	98%
Prophylactic Antibiotic Timing[2]	298	100%	98%	99%
Prophylactic Antibiotic Timing (Outpatient)	80	94%	96%	98%
Urinary Catheter Removal[2]	111	94%	97%	97%
Survey of Patients' Hospital Experiences				
Area Around Room 'Always' Quiet at Night	300+	52%	57%	61%
Doctors 'Always' Communicated Well	300+	80%	81%	82%
Home Recovery Information Given	300+	84%	86%	85%
Hospital Given 9 or 10 on 10 Point Scale	300+	65%	70%	71%
Meds 'Always' Explained Before Given	300+	59%	65%	64%
Nurses 'Always' Communicated Well	300+	76%	79%	79%
Pain 'Always' Well Controlled	300+	71%	71%	71%
Room and Bathroom 'Always' Clean	300+	73%	74%	73%
Timely Help 'Always' Received	300+	62%	68%	68%
Would Definitely Recommend Hospital	300+	66%	72%	71%
Use of Medical Imaging				
Cardiac Imaging Stress Test before Surgery	367	6.0%	4.7%	5.3%
Combination Abdominal CT Scan	715	4.6%	6.6%	10.5%
Combination Brain/Sinus CT Scan[1]	-	-	2.1%	2.7%
Combination Chest CT Scan	510	0.6%	1.1%	2.7%
Follow-up Mammogram/Ultrasound	2,242	4.5%	8.9%	8.8%
Lumbar Spine MRI for Low Back Pain	145	31.0%	41.7%	37.2%

Legacy Mount Hood Medical Center

24800 Se Stark Street
Gresham, OR 97030
Phone: 503-674-1122
Fax: 503-415-5954
URL: www.legacyhealth.org
Type: Acute Care Hospitals
Emergency Services: Yes
Ownership: Voluntary non-profit - Private
Beds: 81

Key Personnel:
Emergency Room . . . . Joel Brenner
CEO/President. . . . . George J Brown
Chief of Medical Staff . . . . Jack Cioffi, MD
Infection Control. . . . . Kelly Eagan
Intensive Care Unit. . . . . Shannon Muse
Radiology. . . . . Steven M Urman
Quality Assurance . . . . Barb Wheatley

Measure	Cases	This Hosp.	State Avg.	U.S. Avg.
Blood Clot Prevention and Treatment				
Anticoagulation Overlap Therapy[2]	24	100%	95%	93%
ICU Venous Thromboembolism Prophylaxis[2]	66	97%	87%	92%
Incidence of Potentially Preventable VTE[1,2]	-	-	13%	10%
UFH with Dosages/Platelet Monitoring[1,2]	-	-	100%	97%
Venous Thromboembolism Prophylaxis[2]	265	86%	83%	85%
Warfarin Therapy Discharge Instructions[2]	25	92%	54%	75%
Chest Pain/Possible Heart Attack Care				
Aspirin Given Within 24 Hours of Arrival	58	100%	97%	96%
Fibrinolytic Meds Within 30 Min. of Arrival[7]	-	-	57%	58%

NOTE: Hospital profiles are in alphabetical order by state, then city, then hospital within the city; Rankings exclude hospitals with less than 25 cases except for patient surveys which excludes hospitals with less than 100 cases; (a) 100-299 cases; (1) The number of cases/patients is too few to report; (2) Data submitted were based on a sample of cases/patients; (3) Results are based on a shorter time period than required; (4) Data suppressed by CMS for one or more quarters; (5) Results are not available for this reporting period; (6) Fewer than 100 patients completed the HCAHPS survey; (7) No cases met the criteria for this measure; (8) The lower limit of the confidence interval cannot be calculated if the number of observed infections equals zero; (9) No data are available from the state/territory for this reporting period; (10) The scores shown reflect fewer than 50 completed surveys; (11) There were discrepancies in the data collection process; (12) This measure does not apply to this hospital for this reporting period; (13) Results cannot be calculated for this reporting period; (14) The results for this state are combined with nearby states to protect confidentiality; Please refer to the User's Guide for a full explanation of data.

Measure	Cases	This Hosp.	State Avg.	U.S. Avg.
Average Time to ECG (minutes)	60	9	9	7
Average Time to Transfer (minutes)	29	51	52	60
Children's Asthma Care				
Received Home Management Plan of Care	-	-	-	88%
Received Reliever Medication	-	-	-	100%
Received Systemic Corticosteroids	-	-	-	100%
Emergency Department				
Admittance Decision Time (minutes)[2]	706	85	85	98
Head CT Results Within 45 Min. of Arrival[1]	-	-	45%	57%
Patients Who Left ER Before Being Seen	46,956	1%	2%	2%
Time from ER Arrival to Admit. (minutes)[2]	706	237	235	274
Time from ER Arrival to Discharge (minutes)	360	172	136	134
Time in ER Before Being Evaluated (minutes)	395	35	27	26
Time to Pain Meds for Fractures (minutes)	138	58	56	57
Heart Attack Care				
Aspirin Given at Discharge	23	100%	99%	99%
Fibrinolytic Meds Within 30 Min. of Arrival[7]	-	-	57%	54%
PCI Within 90 Minutes of Arrival[7]	-	-	93%	96%
Statin Prescribed at Discharge	22	100%	98%	98%
Heart Failure Care				
ACE Inhibitor or ARB for LVSD	43	100%	96%	97%
Discharge Instructions Given	154	99%	93%	94%
Evaluation of LVS Function	163	100%	99%	99%
Medicare Spending				
Medicare Spending per Patient (ratio)	-	0.86	0.88	0.98
Pneumonia Care				
Appropriate Initial Antibiotic Given	127	98%	96%	95%
Blood Culture Timing	217	98%	98%	98%
Pregnancy and Delivery Care				
Newborn Deliveries Scheduled Early[2]	28	0%	3%	6%
Preventive Care				
Immunization for Influenza[2]	519	90%	86%	90%
Immunization for Pneumonia[2]	562	94%	88%	92%
Stroke Care				
Anticoagulation Therapy for Atrial Fibrillation	15	93%	94%	95%
Antithrombotic Therapy Timing	51	100%	97%	98%
Assessed for Rehabilitation	73	96%	96%	97%
Discharged on Antithrombotic Therapy	68	100%	99%	99%
Discharged on Statin Medication	51	98%	93%	94%
Thrombolytic Therapy Timing	12	75%	55%	66%
Venous Thromboembolism Prophylaxis	67	99%	90%	94%
Written Stroke Educational Materials Given	52	98%	81%	88%
Surgical Care Improvement Project				
Appropriate Beta Blocker Usage[2]	71	100%	98%	98%
Appropriate VTP Within 24 Hours[2]	243	96%	97%	98%
Controlled Postoperative Blood Glucose[2,7]	-	-	98%	97%
Perioperative Temperature Management[2]	297	100%	100%	100%
Prophylactic Antibiotic Selection[2]	177	99%	99%	99%
Prophylactic Antibiotic Selection (Outpatient)	168	95%	98%	98%
Prophylactic Antibiotic Stopped[2]	175	98%	98%	98%
Prophylactic Antibiotic Timing[2]	180	93%	98%	99%
Prophylactic Antibiotic Timing (Outpatient)	169	93%	96%	98%
Urinary Catheter Removal[2]	145	97%	97%	97%
Survey of Patients' Hospital Experiences				
Area Around Room 'Always' Quiet at Night	300+	58%	57%	61%
Doctors 'Always' Communicated Well	300+	80%	81%	82%
Home Recovery Information Given	300+	88%	86%	85%
Hospital Given 9 or 10 on 10 Point Scale	300+	70%	70%	71%
Meds 'Always' Explained Before Given	300+	63%	65%	64%
Nurses 'Always' Communicated Well	300+	77%	79%	79%
Pain 'Always' Well Controlled	300+	69%	71%	71%
Room and Bathroom 'Always' Clean	300+	66%	74%	73%
Timely Help 'Always' Received	300+	61%	68%	68%
Would Definitely Recommend Hospital	300+	75%	72%	71%
Use of Medical Imaging				
Cardiac Imaging Stress Test before Surgery	64	9.4%	4.7%	5.3%
Combination Abdominal CT Scan	418	11.7%	6.6%	10.5%
Combination Brain/Sinus CT Scan[1]	-	-	2.1%	2.7%
Combination Chest CT Scan	214	0.5%	1.1%	2.7%
Follow-up Mammogram/Ultrasound	487	11.7%	8.9%	8.8%
Lumbar Spine MRI for Low Back Pain	46	54.3%	41.7%	37.2%

Pioneer Memorial Hospital

564 E Pioneer Drive
Heppner, OR 97836
Type: Critical Access Hospitals
Ownership: Govt - Hospital Dist/Auth
Phone: 541-676-9133
Fax: 541-676-2900
Emergency Services: Yes
Beds: 44

Key Personnel:
Radiology . . . . Melissa Pederse, RT
Intensive Care Unit. . . . . Molly Rhea, RN
Infection Control . . . . Jay Straley
Chief of Medical Staff . . . . Kenneth F Wenberg, MD
Emergency Room . . . . Kenneth F Wenberg, MD

Measure	Cases	This Hosp.	State Avg.	U.S. Avg.
Blood Clot Prevention and Treatment				
Anticoagulation Overlap Therapy[5]	-	-	95%	93%
ICU Venous Thromboembolism Prophylaxis[5]	-	-	87%	92%
Incidence of Potentially Preventable VTE[5]	-	-	13%	10%
UFH with Dosages/Platelet Monitoring[5]	-	-	100%	97%
Venous Thromboembolism Prophylaxis[5]	-	-	83%	85%
Warfarin Therapy Discharge Instructions[5]	-	-	54%	75%
Chest Pain/Possible Heart Attack Care				
Aspirin Given Within 24 Hours of Arrival[1,3]	-	-	97%	96%
Fibrinolytic Meds Within 30 Min. of Arrival[3,7]	-	-	57%	58%
Average Time to ECG (minutes)[1,3]	-	-	9	7
Average Time to Transfer (minutes)[3,7]	-	-	52	60
Children's Asthma Care				
Received Home Management Plan of Care	-	-	-	88%
Received Reliever Medication	-	-	-	100%
Received Systemic Corticosteroids	-	-	-	100%
Emergency Department				
Admittance Decision Time (minutes)[5]	-	-	85	98
Head CT Results Within 45 Min. of Arrival[1,3]	-	-	45%	57%
Patients Who Left ER Before Being Seen	839	0%	2%	2%
Time from ER Arrival to Admit. (minutes)[5]	-	-	235	274
Time from ER Arrival to Discharge (minutes)[5]	-	-	136	134
Time in ER Before Being Evaluated (minutes)[5]	-	-	27	26
Time to Pain Meds for Fractures (minutes)[3,7]	-	-	56	57
Heart Attack Care				
Aspirin Given at Discharge[1,3]	-	-	99%	99%
Fibrinolytic Meds Within 30 Min. of Arrival[3,7]	-	-	57%	54%
PCI Within 90 Minutes of Arrival[5]	-	-	93%	96%
Statin Prescribed at Discharge[1,3]	-	-	98%	98%
Heart Failure Care				
ACE Inhibitor or ARB for LVSD[5]	-	-	96%	97%
Discharge Instructions Given[5]	-	-	93%	94%
Evaluation of LVS Function[5]	-	-	99%	99%
Medicare Spending				
Medicare Spending per Patient (ratio)	-	-	0.88	0.98
Pneumonia Care				
Appropriate Initial Antibiotic Given[1,3]	-	-	96%	95%
Blood Culture Timing[1,3]	-	-	98%	98%
Pregnancy and Delivery Care				
Newborn Deliveries Scheduled Early[5]	-	-	3%	6%
Preventive Care				
Immunization for Influenza[5]	-	-	86%	90%
Immunization for Pneumonia[5]	-	-	88%	92%
Stroke Care				
Anticoagulation Therapy for Atrial Fibrillation[3,7]	-	-	94%	95%
Antithrombotic Therapy Timing[1,3]	-	-	97%	98%
Assessed for Rehabilitation[1,3]	-	-	96%	97%
Discharged on Antithrombotic Therapy[1,3]	-	-	99%	99%
Discharged on Statin Medication[1,3]	-	-	93%	94%
Thrombolytic Therapy Timing[3,7]	-	-	55%	66%
Venous Thromboembolism Prophylaxis[1,3]	-	-	90%	94%
Written Stroke Educational Materials Given[1,3]	-	-	81%	88%
Surgical Care Improvement Project				
Appropriate Beta Blocker Usage[5]	-	-	98%	98%
Appropriate VTP Within 24 Hours[5]	-	-	97%	98%
Controlled Postoperative Blood Glucose[5]	-	-	98%	97%
Perioperative Temperature Management[5]	-	-	100%	100%
Prophylactic Antibiotic Selection[5]	-	-	99%	99%
Prophylactic Antibiotic Selection (Outpatient)[5]	-	-	98%	98%
Prophylactic Antibiotic Stopped[5]	-	-	98%	98%
Prophylactic Antibiotic Timing[5]	-	-	98%	99%
Prophylactic Antibiotic Timing (Outpatient)[5]	-	-	96%	98%
Urinary Catheter Removal[5]	-	-	97%	97%
Survey of Patients' Hospital Experiences				
Area Around Room 'Always' Quiet at Night[5]	-	-	57%	61%
Doctors 'Always' Communicated Well[5]	-	-	81%	82%
Home Recovery Information Given[5]	-	-	86%	85%
Hospital Given 9 or 10 on 10 Point Scale[5]	-	-	70%	71%
Meds 'Always' Explained Before Given[5]	-	-	65%	64%
Nurses 'Always' Communicated Well[5]	-	-	79%	79%
Pain 'Always' Well Controlled[5]	-	-	71%	71%
Room and Bathroom 'Always' Clean[5]	-	-	74%	73%
Timely Help 'Always' Received[5]	-	-	68%	68%
Would Definitely Recommend Hospital[5]	-	-	72%	71%
Use of Medical Imaging				
Cardiac Imaging Stress Test before Surgery[7]	-	-	4.7%	5.3%
Combination Abdominal CT Scan[1]	-	-	6.6%	10.5%
Combination Brain/Sinus CT Scan	34	0.0%	2.1%	2.7%
Combination Chest CT Scan[1]	-	-	1.1%	2.7%
Follow-up Mammogram/Ultrasound[7]	-	-	8.9%	8.8%
Lumbar Spine MRI for Low Back Pain[7]	-	-	41.7%	37.2%

Good Shepherd Medical Center

610 Nw 11th Street
Hermiston, OR 97838
URL: www.gshealth.org
Type: Critical Access Hospitals
Ownership: Voluntary non-profit - Private
Phone: 541-667-3400
Fax: 541-667-3414
Emergency Services: Yes
Beds: 25

Key Personnel:
Cardiology . . . . Naveen Acharya, MD
Surgery . . . . Robert Berecz, MD, FACS
Emergency Room . . . . Steven Blackthorne, MD
CEO/President. . . . . Dennis Eurke
Chief of Medical Staff . . . . Winn Gregory
Cardiac Laboratory. . . . . E Ricketts

Measure	Cases	This Hosp.	State Avg.	U.S. Avg.
Blood Clot Prevention and Treatment				
Anticoagulation Overlap Therapy[2]	18	89%	95%	93%
ICU Venous Thromboembolism Prophylaxis[2]	47	96%	87%	92%
Incidence of Potentially Preventable VTE[1,2]	-	-	13%	10%
UFH with Dosages/Platelet Monitoring[1,2]	-	-	100%	97%
Venous Thromboembolism Prophylaxis[2]	132	92%	83%	85%
Warfarin Therapy Discharge Instructions[2]	17	100%	54%	75%
Chest Pain/Possible Heart Attack Care				
Aspirin Given Within 24 Hours of Arrival	-	-	97%	96%
Fibrinolytic Meds Within 30 Min. of Arrival	-	-	57%	58%
Average Time to ECG (minutes)	-	-	9	7
Average Time to Transfer (minutes)	-	-	52	60
Children's Asthma Care				
Received Home Management Plan of Care	-	-	-	88%
Received Reliever Medication	-	-	-	100%
Received Systemic Corticosteroids	-	-	-	100%
Emergency Department				
Admittance Decision Time (minutes)[2]	392	96	85	98
Head CT Results Within 45 Min. of Arrival	-	-	45%	57%
Patients Who Left ER Before Being Seen	-	-	2%	2%
Time from ER Arrival to Admit. (minutes)[2]	404	255	235	274
Time from ER Arrival to Discharge (minutes)	-	-	136	134
Time in ER Before Being Evaluated (minutes)	-	-	27	26
Time to Pain Meds for Fractures (minutes)	-	-	56	57
Heart Attack Care				
Aspirin Given at Discharge[1]	-	-	99%	99%
Fibrinolytic Meds Within 30 Min. of Arrival[3,7]	-	-	57%	54%
PCI Within 90 Minutes of Arrival[3,7]	-	-	93%	96%
Statin Prescribed at Discharge[1,3]	-	-	98%	98%
Heart Failure Care				
ACE Inhibitor or ARB for LVSD[2]	11	100%	96%	97%
Discharge Instructions Given[2]	27	100%	93%	94%
Evaluation of LVS Function[2]	30	100%	99%	99%
Medicare Spending				
Medicare Spending per Patient (ratio)	-	-	0.88	0.98
Pneumonia Care				
Appropriate Initial Antibiotic Given[2]	41	88%	96%	95%
Blood Culture Timing[2]	68	97%	98%	98%
Pregnancy and Delivery Care				

NOTE: Hospital profiles are in alphabetical order by state, then city, then hospital within the city; Rankings exclude hospitals with less than 25 cases except for patient surveys which excludes hospitals with less than 100 cases; (a) 100-299 cases; (1) The number of cases/patients is too few to report; (2) Data submitted were based on a sample of cases/patients; (3) Results are based on a shorter time period than required; (4) Data suppressed by CMS for one or more quarters; (5) Results are not available for this reporting period; (6) Fewer than 100 patients completed the HCAHPS survey; (7) No cases met the criteria for this measure; (8) The lower limit of the confidence interval cannot be calculated if the number of observed infections equals zero; (9) No data are available from the state/territory for this reporting period; (10) The scores shown reflect fewer than 50 completed surveys; (11) There were discrepancies in the data collection process; (12) This measure does not apply to this hospital for this reporting period; (13) Results cannot be calculated for this reporting period; (14) The results for this state are combined with nearby states to protect confidentiality; Please refer to the User's Guide for a full explanation of data.

Measure	Cases	This Hosp.	State Avg.	U.S. Avg.
Newborn Deliveries Scheduled Early[5]	-	-	3%	6%
Preventive Care				
Immunization for Influenza[2]	343	83%	86%	90%
Immunization for Pneumonia[2]	414	87%	88%	92%
Stroke Care				
Anticoagulation Therapy for Atrial Fibrillation[1,2]	-	-	94%	95%
Antithrombotic Therapy Timing[2]	13	100%	97%	98%
Assessed for Rehabilitation[2]	14	71%	96%	97%
Discharged on Antithrombotic Therapy[2]	14	100%	99%	99%
Discharged on Statin Medication[2]	11	100%	93%	94%
Thrombolytic Therapy Timing[1,2]	-	-	55%	66%
Venous Thromboembolism Prophylaxis[2]	14	100%	90%	94%
Written Stroke Educational Materials Given[2]	11	73%	81%	88%
Surgical Care Improvement Project				
Appropriate Beta Blocker Usage[3]	22	100%	98%	98%
Appropriate VTP Within 24 Hours	198	96%	97%	98%
Controlled Postoperative Blood Glucose[3,7]	-	-	98%	97%
Perioperative Temperature Management	218	100%	100%	100%
Prophylactic Antibiotic Selection	181	98%	99%	99%
Prophylactic Antibiotic Selection (Outpatient)	-	-	98%	98%
Prophylactic Antibiotic Stopped	181	99%	98%	98%
Prophylactic Antibiotic Timing	181	93%	98%	99%
Prophylactic Antibiotic Timing (Outpatient)	-	-	96%	98%
Urinary Catheter Removal	184	95%	97%	97%
Survey of Patients' Hospital Experiences				
Area Around Room 'Always' Quiet at Night	300+	60%	57%	61%
Doctors 'Always' Communicated Well	300+	79%	81%	82%
Home Recovery Information Given	300+	91%	86%	85%
Hospital Given 9 or 10 on 10 Point Scale	300+	67%	70%	71%
Meds 'Always' Explained Before Given	300+	65%	65%	64%
Nurses 'Always' Communicated Well	300+	79%	79%	79%
Pain 'Always' Well Controlled	300+	69%	71%	71%
Room and Bathroom 'Always' Clean	300+	72%	74%	73%
Timely Help 'Always' Received	300+	75%	68%	68%
Would Definitely Recommend Hospital	300+	58%	72%	71%
Use of Medical Imaging				
Cardiac Imaging Stress Test before Surgery	-	-	4.7%	5.3%
Combination Abdominal CT Scan	-	-	6.6%	10.5%
Combination Brain/Sinus CT Scan	-	-	2.1%	2.7%
Combination Chest CT Scan	-	-	1.1%	2.7%
Follow-up Mammogram/Ultrasound	-	-	8.9%	8.8%
Lumbar Spine MRI for Low Back Pain	-	-	41.7%	37.2%

Kaiser Foundation Hospital - Westside

2875 Nw Stucki Ave Phone: 971-310-5700
Hillsboro, OR 97124
Type: Acute Care Hospitals Emergency Services: Yes
Ownership: Voluntary non-profit - Private

Measure	Cases	This Hosp.	State Avg.	U.S. Avg.
Blood Clot Prevention and Treatment				
Anticoagulation Overlap Therapy[5]	-	-	95%	93%
ICU Venous Thromboembolism Prophylaxis[5]	-	-	87%	92%
Incidence of Potentially Preventable VTE[5]	-	-	13%	10%
UFH with Dosages/Platelet Monitoring[5]	-	-	100%	97%
Venous Thromboembolism Prophylaxis[5]	-	-	83%	85%
Warfarin Therapy Discharge Instructions[5]	-	-	54%	75%
Chest Pain/Possible Heart Attack Care				
Aspirin Given Within 24 Hours of Arrival	-	-	97%	96%
Fibrinolytic Meds Within 30 Min. of Arrival	-	-	57%	58%
Average Time to ECG (minutes)	-	-	9	7
Average Time to Transfer (minutes)	-	-	52	60
Children's Asthma Care				
Received Home Management Plan of Care	-	-	-	88%
Received Reliever Medication	-	-	-	100%
Received Systemic Corticosteroids	-	-	-	100%
Emergency Department				
Admittance Decision Time (minutes)[5]	-	-	85	98
Head CT Results Within 45 Min. of Arrival	-	-	45%	57%
Patients Who Left ER Before Being Seen	-	-	2%	2%
Time from ER Arrival to Admit. (minutes)[5]	-	-	235	274
Time from ER Arrival to Discharge (minutes)	-	-	136	134
Time in ER Before Being Evaluated (minutes)	-	-	27	26
Time to Pain Meds for Fractures (minutes)	-	-	56	57
Heart Attack Care				
Aspirin Given at Discharge[5]	-	-	99%	99%
Fibrinolytic Meds Within 30 Min. of Arrival[5]	-	-	57%	54%
PCI Within 90 Minutes of Arrival[5]	-	-	93%	96%
Statin Prescribed at Discharge[5]	-	-	98%	98%
Heart Failure Care				
ACE Inhibitor or ARB for LVSD[5]	-	-	96%	97%
Discharge Instructions Given[5]	-	-	93%	94%
Evaluation of LVS Function[5]	-	-	99%	99%
Medicare Spending				
Medicare Spending per Patient (ratio)	-	-	0.88	0.98
Pneumonia Care				
Appropriate Initial Antibiotic Given[5]	-	-	96%	95%
Blood Culture Timing[5]	-	-	98%	98%
Pregnancy and Delivery Care				
Newborn Deliveries Scheduled Early[5]	-	-	3%	6%
Preventive Care				
Immunization for Influenza[5]	-	-	86%	90%
Immunization for Pneumonia[5]	-	-	88%	92%
Stroke Care				
Anticoagulation Therapy for Atrial Fibrillation[5]	-	-	94%	95%
Antithrombotic Therapy Timing[5]	-	-	97%	98%
Assessed for Rehabilitation[5]	-	-	96%	97%
Discharged on Antithrombotic Therapy[5]	-	-	99%	99%
Discharged on Statin Medication[5]	-	-	93%	94%
Thrombolytic Therapy Timing[5]	-	-	55%	66%
Venous Thromboembolism Prophylaxis[5]	-	-	90%	94%
Written Stroke Educational Materials Given[5]	-	-	81%	88%
Surgical Care Improvement Project				
Appropriate Beta Blocker Usage[5]	-	-	98%	98%
Appropriate VTP Within 24 Hours[5]	-	-	97%	98%
Controlled Postoperative Blood Glucose[5]	-	-	98%	97%
Perioperative Temperature Management[5]	-	-	100%	100%
Prophylactic Antibiotic Selection[5]	-	-	99%	99%
Prophylactic Antibiotic Selection (Outpatient)	-	-	98%	98%
Prophylactic Antibiotic Stopped[5]	-	-	98%	98%
Prophylactic Antibiotic Timing[5]	-	-	98%	99%
Prophylactic Antibiotic Timing (Outpatient)	-	-	96%	98%
Urinary Catheter Removal[5]	-	-	97%	97%
Survey of Patients' Hospital Experiences				
Area Around Room 'Always' Quiet at Night[5]	-	-	57%	61%
Doctors 'Always' Communicated Well[5]	-	-	81%	82%
Home Recovery Information Given[5]	-	-	86%	85%
Hospital Given 9 or 10 on 10 Point Scale[5]	-	-	70%	71%
Meds 'Always' Explained Before Given[5]	-	-	65%	64%
Nurses 'Always' Communicated Well[5]	-	-	79%	79%
Pain 'Always' Well Controlled[5]	-	-	71%	71%
Room and Bathroom 'Always' Clean[5]	-	-	74%	73%
Timely Help 'Always' Received[5]	-	-	68%	68%
Would Definitely Recommend Hospital[5]	-	-	72%	71%
Use of Medical Imaging				
Cardiac Imaging Stress Test before Surgery	-	-	4.7%	5.3%
Combination Abdominal CT Scan	-	-	6.6%	10.5%
Combination Brain/Sinus CT Scan	-	-	2.1%	2.7%
Combination Chest CT Scan	-	-	1.1%	2.7%
Follow-up Mammogram/Ultrasound	-	-	8.9%	8.8%
Lumbar Spine MRI for Low Back Pain	-	-	41.7%	37.2%

Tuality Community Hospital

335 Se 8th Avenue Phone: 503-681-1111
Hillsboro, OR 97123 Fax: 503-681-1695
URL: www.tuality.com
Type: Acute Care Hospitals Emergency Services: Yes
Ownership: Voluntary non-profit - Private Beds: 167
Key Personnel:
CEO/President. . . . . Manuel Berman, FACHE
Anesthesiology. . . . . Steven Eyler, MD
Chief of Medical Staff. . . . . Thomas Gilberts, MD
Radiology. . . . . Geoffrey M Gullo
Emergency Room . . . . David Miller, MD
Quality Assurance . . . . Sharon Saty
Operating Room. . . . . Susan Terry

Measure	Cases	This Hosp.	State Avg.	U.S. Avg.
Blood Clot Prevention and Treatment				
Anticoagulation Overlap Therapy[2]	25	100%	95%	93%
ICU Venous Thromboembolism Prophylaxis[2]	48	90%	87%	92%
Incidence of Potentially Preventable VTE[1,2]	-	-	13%	10%
UFH with Dosages/Platelet Monitoring[1,2]	-	-	100%	97%
Venous Thromboembolism Prophylaxis[2]	311	80%	83%	85%
Warfarin Therapy Discharge Instructions[2]	17	76%	54%	75%
Chest Pain/Possible Heart Attack Care				
Aspirin Given Within 24 Hours of Arrival[1]	-	-	97%	96%
Fibrinolytic Meds Within 30 Min. of Arrival[3,7]	-	-	57%	58%
Average Time to ECG (minutes)[1]	-	-	9	7
Average Time to Transfer (minutes)[1,3]	-	-	52	60
Children's Asthma Care				
Received Home Management Plan of Care	-	-	-	88%
Received Reliever Medication	-	-	-	100%
Received Systemic Corticosteroids	-	-	-	100%
Emergency Department				
Admittance Decision Time (minutes)[2]	422	45	85	98
Head CT Results Within 45 Min. of Arrival[1]	-	-	45%	57%
Patients Who Left ER Before Being Seen	41,868	3%	2%	2%
Time from ER Arrival to Admit. (minutes)[2]	422	242	235	274
Time from ER Arrival to Discharge (minutes)	386	136	136	134
Time in ER Before Being Evaluated (minutes)	417	21	27	26
Time to Pain Meds for Fractures (minutes)	175	69	56	57
Heart Attack Care				
Aspirin Given at Discharge	124	100%	99%	99%
Fibrinolytic Meds Within 30 Min. of Arrival[7]	-	-	57%	54%
PCI Within 90 Minutes of Arrival	26	85%	93%	96%
Statin Prescribed at Discharge	109	98%	98%	98%
Heart Failure Care				
ACE Inhibitor or ARB for LVSD	30	87%	96%	97%
Discharge Instructions Given	111	93%	93%	94%
Evaluation of LVS Function	138	100%	99%	99%
Medicare Spending				
Medicare Spending per Patient (ratio)	-	0.93	0.88	0.98
Pneumonia Care				
Appropriate Initial Antibiotic Given	74	99%	96%	95%
Blood Culture Timing	127	96%	98%	98%
Pregnancy and Delivery Care				
Newborn Deliveries Scheduled Early	69	6%	3%	6%
Preventive Care				
Immunization for Influenza[2]	424	74%	86%	90%
Immunization for Pneumonia[2]	457	81%	88%	92%
Stroke Care				
Anticoagulation Therapy for Atrial Fibrillation[1]	-	-	94%	95%
Antithrombotic Therapy Timing	51	100%	97%	98%
Assessed for Rehabilitation	69	100%	96%	97%
Discharged on Antithrombotic Therapy	59	100%	99%	99%
Discharged on Statin Medication	44	100%	93%	94%
Thrombolytic Therapy Timing[1]	-	-	55%	66%
Venous Thromboembolism Prophylaxis	69	97%	90%	94%
Written Stroke Educational Materials Given	31	97%	81%	88%
Surgical Care Improvement Project				
Appropriate Beta Blocker Usage[2]	106	98%	98%	98%
Appropriate VTP Within 24 Hours[2]	318	93%	97%	98%
Controlled Postoperative Blood Glucose[2]	33	100%	98%	97%
Perioperative Temperature Management[2]	402	100%	100%	100%
Prophylactic Antibiotic Selection[2]	292	100%	99%	99%
Prophylactic Antibiotic Selection (Outpatient)	115	100%	98%	98%
Prophylactic Antibiotic Stopped[2]	288	99%	98%	98%
Prophylactic Antibiotic Timing[2]	293	97%	98%	99%
Prophylactic Antibiotic Timing (Outpatient)	116	96%	96%	98%
Urinary Catheter Removal[2]	234	97%	97%	97%
Survey of Patients' Hospital Experiences				
Area Around Room 'Always' Quiet at Night	300+	56%	57%	61%
Doctors 'Always' Communicated Well	300+	80%	81%	82%
Home Recovery Information Given	300+	88%	86%	85%
Hospital Given 9 or 10 on 10 Point Scale	300+	65%	70%	71%
Meds 'Always' Explained Before Given	300+	60%	65%	64%
Nurses 'Always' Communicated Well	300+	73%	79%	79%
Pain 'Always' Well Controlled	300+	71%	71%	71%
Room and Bathroom 'Always' Clean	300+	66%	74%	73%

NOTE: Hospital profiles are in alphabetical order by state, then city, then hospital within the city; Rankings exclude hospitals with less than 25 cases except for patient surveys which excludes hospitals with less than 100 cases; (a) 100-299 cases; (1) The number of cases/patients is too few to report; (2) Data submitted were based on a sample of cases/patients; (3) Results are based on a shorter time period than required; (4) Data suppressed by CMS for one or more quarters; (5) Results are not available for this reporting period; (6) Fewer than 100 patients completed the HCAHPS survey; (7) No cases met the criteria for this measure; (8) The lower limit of the confidence interval cannot be calculated if the number of observed infections equals zero; (9) No data are available from the state/territory for this reporting period; (10) The scores shown reflect fewer than 50 completed surveys; (11) There were discrepancies in the data collection process; (12) This measure does not apply to this hospital for this reporting period; (13) Results cannot be calculated for this reporting period; (14) The results for this state are combined with nearby states to protect confidentiality; Please refer to the User's Guide for a full explanation of data.

Measure	Cases	This Hosp.	State Avg.	U.S. Avg.
Timely Help 'Always' Received	300+	68%	68%	68%
Would Definitely Recommend Hospital	300+	69%	72%	71%
Use of Medical Imaging				
Cardiac Imaging Stress Test before Surgery[1]	-	-	4.7%	5.3%
Combination Abdominal CT Scan	438	2.5%	6.6%	10.5%
Combination Brain/Sinus CT Scan	384	1.0%	2.1%	2.7%
Combination Chest CT Scan	243	0.0%	1.1%	2.7%
Follow-up Mammogram/Ultrasound	1,031	5.6%	8.9%	8.8%
Lumbar Spine MRI for Low Back Pain	104	34.6%	41.7%	37.2%

Providence Hood River Memorial Hospital

810 12th Street
Hood River, OR 97031
Phone: 541-386-3911
Fax: 541-387-6462
E-mail: elizabethsettje@providence.org
URL: www.providence.org/hoodriver
Type: Critical Access Hospitals
Emergency Services: Yes
Ownership: Voluntary non-profit - Private
Beds: 25

Key Personnel:
CEO/President. . . . . Larry Beth
Emergency Room . . . . Philip Chadwick

Measure	Cases	This Hosp.	State Avg.	U.S. Avg.
Blood Clot Prevention and Treatment				
Anticoagulation Overlap Therapy[1,2]	-	-	95%	93%
ICU Venous Thromboembolism Prophylaxis[2]	67	73%	87%	92%
Incidence of Potentially Preventable VTE[1,2]	-	-	13%	10%
UFH with Dosages/Platelet Monitoring[2,7]	-	-	100%	97%
Venous Thromboembolism Prophylaxis[2]	42	57%	83%	85%
Warfarin Therapy Discharge Instructions[1,2]	-	-	54%	75%
Chest Pain/Possible Heart Attack Care				
Aspirin Given Within 24 Hours of Arrival	25	100%	97%	96%
Fibrinolytic Meds Within 30 Min. of Arrival[1]	-	-	57%	58%
Average Time to ECG (minutes)	25	8	9	7
Average Time to Transfer (minutes)[1]	-	-	52	60
Children's Asthma Care				
Received Home Management Plan of Care	-	-	-	88%
Received Reliever Medication	-	-	-	100%
Received Systemic Corticosteroids	-	-	-	100%
Emergency Department				
Admittance Decision Time (minutes)[2]	170	106	85	98
Head CT Results Within 45 Min. of Arrival	13	46%	45%	57%
Patients Who Left ER Before Being Seen	9,342	1%	2%	2%
Time from ER Arrival to Admit. (minutes)[2]	215	217	235	274
Time from ER Arrival to Discharge (minutes)	271	97	136	134
Time in ER Before Being Evaluated (minutes)	280	22	27	26
Time to Pain Meds for Fractures (minutes)	52	42	56	57
Heart Attack Care				
Aspirin Given at Discharge[1,2]	-	-	99%	99%
Fibrinolytic Meds Within 30 Min. of Arrival[2,7]	-	-	57%	54%
PCI Within 90 Minutes of Arrival[2,7]	-	-	93%	96%
Statin Prescribed at Discharge[1,2]	-	-	98%	98%
Heart Failure Care				
ACE Inhibitor or ARB for LVSD[1,2]	-	-	96%	97%
Discharge Instructions Given[2]	28	96%	93%	94%
Evaluation of LVS Function[2]	35	100%	99%	99%
Medicare Spending				
Medicare Spending per Patient (ratio)	-	-	0.88	0.98
Pneumonia Care				
Appropriate Initial Antibiotic Given[2]	41	95%	96%	95%
Blood Culture Timing[2]	46	100%	98%	98%
Pregnancy and Delivery Care				
Newborn Deliveries Scheduled Early	26	0%	3%	6%
Preventive Care				
Immunization for Influenza[2]	241	88%	86%	90%
Immunization for Pneumonia[2]	242	89%	88%	92%
Stroke Care				
Anticoagulation Therapy for Atrial Fibrillation[1,2]	-	-	94%	95%
Antithrombotic Therapy Timing[1,2]	-	-	97%	98%
Assessed for Rehabilitation[2]	14	86%	96%	97%
Discharged on Antithrombotic Therapy[2]	14	100%	99%	99%
Discharged on Statin Medication[2]	13	62%	93%	94%
Thrombolytic Therapy Timing[2,7]	-	-	55%	66%
Venous Thromboembolism Prophylaxis[1,2]	-	-	90%	94%
Written Stroke Educational Materials Given[1,2]	-	-	81%	88%
Surgical Care Improvement Project				
Appropriate Beta Blocker Usage[2]	30	100%	98%	98%
Appropriate VTP Within 24 Hours[2]	142	96%	97%	98%
Controlled Postoperative Blood Glucose[2,7]	-	-	98%	97%
Perioperative Temperature Management[2]	175	100%	100%	100%
Prophylactic Antibiotic Selection[2]	127	100%	99%	99%
Prophylactic Antibiotic Selection (Outpatient)	49	98%	98%	98%
Prophylactic Antibiotic Stopped[2]	126	98%	98%	98%
Prophylactic Antibiotic Timing[2]	127	100%	98%	99%
Prophylactic Antibiotic Timing (Outpatient)	49	100%	96%	98%
Urinary Catheter Removal[2]	47	96%	97%	97%
Survey of Patients' Hospital Experiences				
Area Around Room 'Always' Quiet at Night	300+	67%	57%	61%
Doctors 'Always' Communicated Well	300+	87%	81%	82%
Home Recovery Information Given	300+	88%	86%	85%
Hospital Given 9 or 10 on 10 Point Scale	300+	77%	70%	71%
Meds 'Always' Explained Before Given	300+	69%	65%	64%
Nurses 'Always' Communicated Well	300+	82%	79%	79%
Pain 'Always' Well Controlled	300+	72%	71%	71%
Room and Bathroom 'Always' Clean	300+	80%	74%	73%
Timely Help 'Always' Received	300+	72%	68%	68%
Would Definitely Recommend Hospital	300+	81%	72%	71%
Use of Medical Imaging				
Cardiac Imaging Stress Test before Surgery	99	7.1%	4.7%	5.3%
Combination Abdominal CT Scan	259	10.0%	6.6%	10.5%
Combination Brain/Sinus CT Scan[1]	-	-	2.1%	2.7%
Combination Chest CT Scan	155	2.6%	1.1%	2.7%
Follow-up Mammogram/Ultrasound	551	8.7%	8.9%	8.8%
Lumbar Spine MRI for Low Back Pain[1]	-	-	41.7%	37.2%

Blue Mountain Hospital

170 Ford Road
John Day, OR 97845
Phone: 541-575-1311
Type: Critical Access Hospitals
Emergency Services: Yes
Ownership: Govt - Hospital Dist/Auth

Measure	Cases	This Hosp.	State Avg.	U.S. Avg.
Blood Clot Prevention and Treatment				
Anticoagulation Overlap Therapy[5]	-	-	95%	93%
ICU Venous Thromboembolism Prophylaxis[5]	-	-	87%	92%
Incidence of Potentially Preventable VTE[5]	-	-	13%	10%
UFH with Dosages/Platelet Monitoring[5]	-	-	100%	97%
Venous Thromboembolism Prophylaxis[5]	-	-	83%	85%
Warfarin Therapy Discharge Instructions[5]	-	-	54%	75%
Chest Pain/Possible Heart Attack Care				
Aspirin Given Within 24 Hours of Arrival	-	-	97%	96%
Fibrinolytic Meds Within 30 Min. of Arrival	-	-	57%	58%
Average Time to ECG (minutes)	-	-	9	7
Average Time to Transfer (minutes)	-	-	52	60
Children's Asthma Care				
Received Home Management Plan of Care	-	-	-	88%
Received Reliever Medication	-	-	-	100%
Received Systemic Corticosteroids	-	-	-	100%
Emergency Department				
Admittance Decision Time (minutes)[5]	-	-	85	98
Head CT Results Within 45 Min. of Arrival	-	-	45%	57%
Patients Who Left ER Before Being Seen	-	-	2%	2%
Time from ER Arrival to Admit. (minutes)[5]	-	-	235	274
Time from ER Arrival to Discharge (minutes)	-	-	136	134
Time in ER Before Being Evaluated (minutes)	-	-	27	26
Time to Pain Meds for Fractures (minutes)	-	-	56	57
Heart Attack Care				
Aspirin Given at Discharge[1,3]	-	-	99%	99%
Fibrinolytic Meds Within 30 Min. of Arrival[3,7]	-	-	57%	54%
PCI Within 90 Minutes of Arrival[3,7]	-	-	93%	96%
Statin Prescribed at Discharge[1,3]	-	-	98%	98%
Heart Failure Care				
ACE Inhibitor or ARB for LVSD[1,3]	-	-	96%	97%
Discharge Instructions Given[1,3]	-	-	93%	94%
Evaluation of LVS Function[1,3]	-	-	99%	99%
Medicare Spending				
Medicare Spending per Patient (ratio)	-	-	0.88	0.98
Pneumonia Care				
Appropriate Initial Antibiotic Given[3]	14	93%	96%	95%
Blood Culture Timing[1,3]	-	-	98%	98%
Pregnancy and Delivery Care				
Newborn Deliveries Scheduled Early[1,3]	-	-	3%	6%
Preventive Care				
Immunization for Influenza[5]	-	-	86%	90%
Immunization for Pneumonia[5]	-	-	88%	92%
Stroke Care				
Anticoagulation Therapy for Atrial Fibrillation[5]	-	-	94%	95%
Antithrombotic Therapy Timing[5]	-	-	97%	98%
Assessed for Rehabilitation[5]	-	-	96%	97%
Discharged on Antithrombotic Therapy[5]	-	-	99%	99%
Discharged on Statin Medication[5]	-	-	93%	94%
Thrombolytic Therapy Timing[5]	-	-	55%	66%
Venous Thromboembolism Prophylaxis[5]	-	-	90%	94%
Written Stroke Educational Materials Given[5]	-	-	81%	88%
Surgical Care Improvement Project				
Appropriate Beta Blocker Usage[1,3]	-	-	98%	98%
Appropriate VTP Within 24 Hours[1,3]	-	-	97%	98%
Controlled Postoperative Blood Glucose[3,7]	-	-	98%	97%
Perioperative Temperature Management[1,3]	-	-	100%	100%
Prophylactic Antibiotic Selection[1,3]	-	-	99%	99%
Prophylactic Antibiotic Selection (Outpatient)	-	-	98%	98%
Prophylactic Antibiotic Stopped[1,3]	-	-	98%	98%
Prophylactic Antibiotic Timing[1,3]	-	-	98%	99%
Prophylactic Antibiotic Timing (Outpatient)	-	-	96%	98%
Urinary Catheter Removal[1,3]	-	-	97%	97%
Survey of Patients' Hospital Experiences				
Area Around Room 'Always' Quiet at Night[6]	<100	60%	57%	61%
Doctors 'Always' Communicated Well[6]	<100	82%	81%	82%
Home Recovery Information Given[6]	<100	84%	86%	85%
Hospital Given 9 or 10 on 10 Point Scale[6]	<100	62%	70%	71%
Meds 'Always' Explained Before Given[6]	<100	68%	65%	64%
Nurses 'Always' Communicated Well[6]	<100	82%	79%	79%
Pain 'Always' Well Controlled[6]	<100	79%	71%	71%
Room and Bathroom 'Always' Clean[6]	<100	68%	74%	73%
Timely Help 'Always' Received[6]	<100	71%	68%	68%
Would Definitely Recommend Hospital[6]	<100	67%	72%	71%
Use of Medical Imaging				
Cardiac Imaging Stress Test before Surgery	-	-	4.7%	5.3%
Combination Abdominal CT Scan	-	-	6.6%	10.5%
Combination Brain/Sinus CT Scan	-	-	2.1%	2.7%
Combination Chest CT Scan	-	-	1.1%	2.7%
Follow-up Mammogram/Ultrasound	-	-	8.9%	8.8%
Lumbar Spine MRI for Low Back Pain	-	-	41.7%	37.2%

Sky Lakes Medical Center

2865 Daggett Avenue
Klamath Falls, OR 97601
Phone: 541-274-6150
Fax: 541-274-6725
URL: www.skylakes.org
Type: Acute Care Hospitals
Emergency Services: Yes
Ownership: Voluntary non-profit - Private
Beds: 243

Key Personnel:
Chief of Medical Staff. . . . . Kathy Bakke
Infection Control. . . . . Laurie Gerskey, RN
Pediatric In-Patient Care . . . . Jan Gilmore, RN
Quality Assurance . . . . Larry Howard
Coronary Care. . . . . Don Hundley
Operating Room. . . . . Don Hundley
CEO/President. . . . . Paul R Stewart
Pediatric Ambulatory Care . . . . . . John Wilson, MD

Measure	Cases	This Hosp.	State Avg.	U.S. Avg.
Blood Clot Prevention and Treatment				
Anticoagulation Overlap Therapy[2]	75	89%	95%	93%
ICU Venous Thromboembolism Prophylaxis[2]	36	97%	87%	92%
Incidence of Potentially Preventable VTE[1,2]	-	-	13%	10%
UFH with Dosages/Platelet Monitoring[2]	28	100%	100%	97%
Venous Thromboembolism Prophylaxis[2]	388	96%	83%	85%
Warfarin Therapy Discharge Instructions[2]	60	90%	54%	75%
Chest Pain/Possible Heart Attack Care				
Aspirin Given Within 24 Hours of Arrival[1,3]	-	-	97%	96%
Fibrinolytic Meds Within 30 Min. of Arrival[3,7]	-	-	57%	58%
Average Time to ECG (minutes)[1,3]	-	-	9	7
Average Time to Transfer (minutes)[1,3]	-	-	52	60

NOTE: Hospital profiles are in alphabetical order by state, then city, then hospital within the city; Rankings exclude hospitals with less than 25 cases except for patient surveys which excludes hospitals with less than 100 cases; (a) 100-299 cases; (1) The number of cases/patients is too few to report; (2) Data submitted were based on a sample of cases/patients; (3) Results are based on a shorter time period than required; (4) Data suppressed by CMS for one or more quarters; (5) Results are not available for this reporting period; (6) Fewer than 100 patients completed the HCAHPS survey; (7) No cases met the criteria for this measure; (8) The lower limit of the confidence interval cannot be calculated if the number of observed infections equals zero; (9) No data are available from the state/territory for this reporting period; (10) The scores shown reflect fewer than 50 completed surveys; (11) There were discrepancies in the data collection process; (12) This measure does not apply to this hospital for this reporting period; (13) Results cannot be calculated for this reporting period; (14) The results for this state are combined with nearby states to protect confidentiality; Please refer to the User's Guide for a full explanation of data.

Children's Asthma Care				
Received Home Management Plan of Care	-	-	-	88%
Received Reliever Medication	-	-	-	100%
Received Systemic Corticosteroids	-	-	-	100%
Emergency Department				
Admittance Decision Time (minutes)[2]	600	220	85	98
Head CT Results Within 45 Min. of Arrival[1]	-	-	45%	57%
Patients Who Left ER Before Being Seen	19,588	4%	2%	2%
Time from ER Arrival to Admit. (minutes)[2]	716	429	235	274
Time from ER Arrival to Discharge (minutes)	559	218	136	134
Time in ER Before Being Evaluated (minutes)	597	67	27	26
Time to Pain Meds for Fractures (minutes)	138	116	56	57
Heart Attack Care				
Aspirin Given at Discharge	113	96%	99%	99%
Fibrinolytic Meds Within 30 Min. of Arrival[7]	-	-	57%	54%
PCI Within 90 Minutes of Arrival	30	90%	93%	96%
Statin Prescribed at Discharge	101	91%	98%	98%
Heart Failure Care				
ACE Inhibitor or ARB for LVSD	50	98%	96%	97%
Discharge Instructions Given	128	87%	93%	94%
Evaluation of LVS Function	149	98%	99%	99%
Medicare Spending				
Medicare Spending per Patient (ratio)	-	0.87	0.88	0.98
Pneumonia Care				
Appropriate Initial Antibiotic Given	110	94%	96%	95%
Blood Culture Timing	151	95%	98%	98%
Pregnancy and Delivery Care				
Newborn Deliveries Scheduled Early	64	2%	3%	6%
Preventive Care				
Immunization for Influenza[2]	574	83%	86%	90%
Immunization for Pneumonia[2]	765	92%	88%	92%
Stroke Care				
Anticoagulation Therapy for Atrial Fibrillation[1]	-	-	94%	95%
Antithrombotic Therapy Timing	46	100%	97%	98%
Assessed for Rehabilitation	48	100%	96%	97%
Discharged on Antithrombotic Therapy	44	100%	99%	99%
Discharged on Statin Medication	29	93%	93%	94%
Thrombolytic Therapy Timing[1]	-	-	55%	66%
Venous Thromboembolism Prophylaxis	52	96%	90%	94%
Written Stroke Educational Materials Given	32	81%	81%	88%
Surgical Care Improvement Project				
Appropriate Beta Blocker Usage	127	97%	98%	98%
Appropriate VTP Within 24 Hours	475	98%	97%	98%
Controlled Postoperative Blood Glucose[7]	-	-	98%	97%
Perioperative Temperature Management	509	100%	100%	100%
Prophylactic Antibiotic Selection	412	100%	99%	99%
Prophylactic Antibiotic Selection (Outpatient)	185	95%	98%	98%
Prophylactic Antibiotic Stopped	404	98%	98%	98%
Prophylactic Antibiotic Timing	412	99%	98%	99%
Prophylactic Antibiotic Timing (Outpatient)	184	73%	96%	98%
Urinary Catheter Removal	396	98%	97%	97%
Survey of Patients' Hospital Experiences				
Area Around Room 'Always' Quiet at Night	300+	52%	57%	61%
Doctors 'Always' Communicated Well	300+	80%	81%	82%
Home Recovery Information Given	300+	86%	86%	85%
Hospital Given 9 or 10 on 10 Point Scale	300+	62%	70%	71%
Meds 'Always' Explained Before Given	300+	65%	65%	64%
Nurses 'Always' Communicated Well	300+	73%	79%	79%
Pain 'Always' Well Controlled	300+	65%	71%	71%
Room and Bathroom 'Always' Clean	300+	72%	74%	73%
Timely Help 'Always' Received	300+	62%	68%	68%
Would Definitely Recommend Hospital	300+	60%	72%	71%
Use of Medical Imaging				
Cardiac Imaging Stress Test before Surgery	107	0.9%	4.7%	5.3%
Combination Abdominal CT Scan	793	4.0%	6.6%	10.5%
Combination Brain/Sinus CT Scan	593	1.9%	2.1%	2.7%
Combination Chest CT Scan	604	0.2%	1.1%	2.7%
Follow-up Mammogram/Ultrasound	1,039	20.6%	8.9%	8.8%
Lumbar Spine MRI for Low Back Pain	224	33.9%	41.7%	37.2%

Grande Ronde Hospital

900 Sunset Drive
La Grande, OR 97850
E-mail: wkr0@grh.org
URL: www.grh.org
Phone: 541-963-8421
Fax: 541-963-1485
Type: Critical Access Hospitals
Ownership: Voluntary non-profit - Private
Emergency Services: Yes
Beds: 49

Key Personnel:
Infection Control . . . . Vicki Hill-Brown, RN
Intensive Care Unit. . . . . Nena Jones, RN
Quality Assurance . . . . Jori Journigan
CEO/President. . . . . James A Mattes
Radiology. . . . . Allen Matthew
Operating Room. . . . . Terja Shodin, RN
Chief of Medical Staff . . . . Randy Siltanen, MD
Patient Relations . . . . Janet Wright, RN

Measure	Cases	This Hosp.	State Avg.	U.S. Avg.
Blood Clot Prevention and Treatment				
Anticoagulation Overlap Therapy[5]	-	-	95%	93%
ICU Venous Thromboembolism Prophylaxis[5]	-	-	87%	92%
Incidence of Potentially Preventable VTE[5]	-	-	13%	10%
UFH with Dosages/Platelet Monitoring[5]	-	-	100%	97%
Venous Thromboembolism Prophylaxis[5]	-	-	83%	85%
Warfarin Therapy Discharge Instructions[5]	-	-	54%	75%
Chest Pain/Possible Heart Attack Care				
Aspirin Given Within 24 Hours of Arrival[5]	-	-	97%	96%
Fibrinolytic Meds Within 30 Min. of Arrival[5]	-	-	57%	58%
Average Time to ECG (minutes)[5]	-	-	9	7
Average Time to Transfer (minutes)[5]	-	-	52	60
Children's Asthma Care				
Received Home Management Plan of Care	-	-	-	88%
Received Reliever Medication	-	-	-	100%
Received Systemic Corticosteroids	-	-	-	100%
Emergency Department				
Admittance Decision Time (minutes)[5]	-	-	85	98
Head CT Results Within 45 Min. of Arrival[5]	-	-	45%	57%
Patients Who Left ER Before Being Seen[5]	-	-	2%	2%
Time from ER Arrival to Admit. (minutes)[5]	-	-	235	274
Time from ER Arrival to Discharge (minutes)[5]	-	-	136	134
Time in ER Before Being Evaluated (minutes)[5]	-	-	27	26
Time to Pain Meds for Fractures (minutes)[5]	-	-	56	57
Heart Attack Care				
Aspirin Given at Discharge[5]	-	-	99%	99%
Fibrinolytic Meds Within 30 Min. of Arrival[5]	-	-	57%	54%
PCI Within 90 Minutes of Arrival[5]	-	-	93%	96%
Statin Prescribed at Discharge[5]	-	-	98%	98%
Heart Failure Care				
ACE Inhibitor or ARB for LVSD[1]	-	-	96%	97%
Discharge Instructions Given	32	91%	93%	94%
Evaluation of LVS Function	39	97%	99%	99%
Medicare Spending				
Medicare Spending per Patient (ratio)	-	-	0.88	0.98
Pneumonia Care				
Appropriate Initial Antibiotic Given	75	87%	96%	95%
Blood Culture Timing	97	97%	98%	98%
Pregnancy and Delivery Care				
Newborn Deliveries Scheduled Early[5]	-	-	3%	6%
Preventive Care				
Immunization for Influenza[5]	-	-	86%	90%
Immunization for Pneumonia[5]	-	-	88%	92%
Stroke Care				
Anticoagulation Therapy for Atrial Fibrillation[5]	-	-	94%	95%
Antithrombotic Therapy Timing[5]	-	-	97%	98%
Assessed for Rehabilitation[5]	-	-	96%	97%
Discharged on Antithrombotic Therapy[5]	-	-	99%	99%
Discharged on Statin Medication[5]	-	-	93%	94%
Thrombolytic Therapy Timing[5]	-	-	55%	66%
Venous Thromboembolism Prophylaxis[5]	-	-	90%	94%
Written Stroke Educational Materials Given[5]	-	-	81%	88%
Surgical Care Improvement Project				
Appropriate Beta Blocker Usage	18	100%	98%	98%
Appropriate VTP Within 24 Hours	81	96%	97%	98%
Controlled Postoperative Blood Glucose[7]	-	-	98%	97%
Perioperative Temperature Management	106	100%	100%	100%
Prophylactic Antibiotic Selection	77	97%	99%	99%
Prophylactic Antibiotic Selection (Outpatient)[5]	-	-	98%	98%
Prophylactic Antibiotic Stopped	73	92%	98%	98%
Prophylactic Antibiotic Timing	79	91%	98%	99%
Prophylactic Antibiotic Timing (Outpatient)[5]	-	-	96%	98%
Urinary Catheter Removal	49	98%	97%	97%
Survey of Patients' Hospital Experiences				
Area Around Room 'Always' Quiet at Night[5]	-	-	57%	61%
Doctors 'Always' Communicated Well[5]	-	-	81%	82%
Home Recovery Information Given[5]	-	-	86%	85%
Hospital Given 9 or 10 on 10 Point Scale[5]	-	-	70%	71%
Meds 'Always' Explained Before Given[5]	-	-	65%	64%
Nurses 'Always' Communicated Well[5]	-	-	79%	79%
Pain 'Always' Well Controlled[5]	-	-	71%	71%
Room and Bathroom 'Always' Clean[5]	-	-	74%	73%
Timely Help 'Always' Received[5]	-	-	68%	68%
Would Definitely Recommend Hospital[5]	-	-	72%	71%
Use of Medical Imaging				
Cardiac Imaging Stress Test before Surgery	149	4.0%	4.7%	5.3%
Combination Abdominal CT Scan	459	7.8%	6.6%	10.5%
Combination Brain/Sinus CT Scan[1]	-	-	2.1%	2.7%
Combination Chest CT Scan	306	2.0%	1.1%	2.7%
Follow-up Mammogram/Ultrasound	620	16.6%	8.9%	8.8%
Lumbar Spine MRI for Low Back Pain	116	35.3%	41.7%	37.2%

Lake District Hospital

700 South J Street
Lakeview, OR 97630
Phone: 541-947-2114
Type: Critical Access Hospitals
Ownership: Govt - Hospital Dist/Auth
Emergency Services: Yes

Key Personnel:
CEO . . . . Charlie Tveit

Measure	Cases	This Hosp.	State Avg.	U.S. Avg.
Blood Clot Prevention and Treatment				
Anticoagulation Overlap Therapy[2,7]	-	-	95%	93%
ICU Venous Thromboembolism Prophylaxis[5]	-	-	87%	92%
Incidence of Potentially Preventable VTE[2,7]	-	-	13%	10%
UFH with Dosages/Platelet Monitoring[1,2]	-	-	100%	97%
Venous Thromboembolism Prophylaxis[2]	153	32%	83%	85%
Warfarin Therapy Discharge Instructions[1,2]	-	-	54%	75%
Chest Pain/Possible Heart Attack Care				
Aspirin Given Within 24 Hours of Arrival[1,3]	-	-	97%	96%
Fibrinolytic Meds Within 30 Min. of Arrival[1,3]	-	-	57%	58%
Average Time to ECG (minutes)[1,3]	-	-	9	7
Average Time to Transfer (minutes)[3,7]	-	-	52	60
Children's Asthma Care				
Received Home Management Plan of Care	-	-	-	88%
Received Reliever Medication	-	-	-	100%
Received Systemic Corticosteroids	-	-	-	100%
Emergency Department				
Admittance Decision Time (minutes)[2]	144	26	85	98
Head CT Results Within 45 Min. of Arrival[3,7]	-	-	45%	57%
Patients Who Left ER Before Being Seen[5]	-	-	2%	2%
Time from ER Arrival to Admit. (minutes)[2]	212	135	235	274
Time from ER Arrival to Discharge (minutes)[3]	49	90	136	134
Time in ER Before Being Evaluated (minutes)[3]	127	40	27	26
Time to Pain Meds for Fractures (minutes)[1,3]	-	-	56	57
Heart Attack Care				
Aspirin Given at Discharge[5]	-	-	99%	99%
Fibrinolytic Meds Within 30 Min. of Arrival[5]	-	-	57%	54%
PCI Within 90 Minutes of Arrival[5]	-	-	93%	96%
Statin Prescribed at Discharge[5]	-	-	98%	98%
Heart Failure Care				
ACE Inhibitor or ARB for LVSD[1]	-	-	96%	97%
Discharge Instructions Given	16	81%	93%	94%
Evaluation of LVS Function	19	89%	99%	99%
Medicare Spending				
Medicare Spending per Patient (ratio)	-	-	0.88	0.98
Pneumonia Care				
Appropriate Initial Antibiotic Given	15	100%	96%	95%
Blood Culture Timing[1]	-	-	98%	98%
Pregnancy and Delivery Care				

NOTE: Hospital profiles are in alphabetical order by state, then city, then hospital within the city; Rankings exclude hospitals with less than 25 cases except for patient surveys which excludes hospitals with less than 100 cases; (a) 100-299 cases; (1) The number of cases/patients is too few to report; (2) Data submitted were based on a sample of cases/patients; (3) Results are based on a shorter time period than required; (4) Data suppressed by CMS for one or more quarters; (5) Results are not available for this reporting period; (6) Fewer than 100 patients completed the HCAHPS survey; (7) No cases met the criteria for this measure; (8) The lower limit of the confidence interval cannot be calculated if the number of observed infections equals zero; (9) No data are available from the state/territory for this reporting period; (10) The scores shown reflect fewer than 50 completed surveys; (11) There were discrepancies in the data collection process; (12) This measure does not apply to this hospital for this reporting period; (13) Results cannot be calculated for this reporting period; (14) The results for this state are combined with nearby states to protect confidentiality; Please refer to the User's Guide for a full explanation of data.

Measure	Cases	This Hosp.	State Avg.	U.S. Avg.
Newborn Deliveries Scheduled Early	11	9%	3%	6%
Preventive Care				
Immunization for Influenza[2]	142	68%	86%	90%
Immunization for Pneumonia[2]	171	82%	88%	92%
Stroke Care				
Anticoagulation Therapy for Atrial Fibrillation[3,7]	-	-	94%	95%
Antithrombotic Therapy Timing[3,7]	-	-	97%	98%
Assessed for Rehabilitation[1,3]	-	-	96%	97%
Discharged on Antithrombotic Therapy[1,3]	-	-	99%	99%
Discharged on Statin Medication[1,3]	-	-	93%	94%
Thrombolytic Therapy Timing[3,7]	-	-	55%	66%
Venous Thromboembolism Prophylaxis[1,3]	-	-	90%	94%
Written Stroke Educational Materials Given[1,3]	-	-	81%	88%
Surgical Care Improvement Project				
Appropriate Beta Blocker Usage[3,7]	-	-	98%	98%
Appropriate VTP Within 24 Hours[1]	-	-	97%	98%
Controlled Postoperative Blood Glucose[3,7]	-	-	98%	97%
Perioperative Temperature Management[1]	-	-	100%	100%
Prophylactic Antibiotic Selection[1]	-	-	99%	99%
Prophylactic Antibiotic Selection (Outpatient)[1,3]	-	-	98%	98%
Prophylactic Antibiotic Stopped[1]	-	-	98%	98%
Prophylactic Antibiotic Timing[1]	-	-	98%	99%
Prophylactic Antibiotic Timing (Outpatient)[1,3]	-	-	96%	98%
Urinary Catheter Removal[1]	-	-	97%	97%
Survey of Patients' Hospital Experiences				
Area Around Room 'Always' Quiet at Night[6]	<100	56%	57%	61%
Doctors 'Always' Communicated Well[6]	<100	90%	81%	82%
Home Recovery Information Given[6]	<100	80%	86%	85%
Hospital Given 9 or 10 on 10 Point Scale[6]	<100	81%	70%	71%
Meds 'Always' Explained Before Given[6]	<100	67%	65%	64%
Nurses 'Always' Communicated Well[6]	<100	82%	79%	79%
Pain 'Always' Well Controlled[6]	<100	69%	71%	71%
Room and Bathroom 'Always' Clean[6]	<100	78%	74%	73%
Timely Help 'Always' Received[6]	<100	84%	68%	68%
Would Definitely Recommend Hospital[6]	<100	79%	72%	71%
Use of Medical Imaging				
Cardiac Imaging Stress Test before Surgery[7]	-	-	4.7%	5.3%
Combination Abdominal CT Scan	83	1.2%	6.6%	10.5%
Combination Brain/Sinus CT Scan[1]	-	-	2.1%	2.7%
Combination Chest CT Scan	53	0.0%	1.1%	2.7%
Follow-up Mammogram/Ultrasound	211	6.6%	8.9%	8.8%
Lumbar Spine MRI for Low Back Pain[1]	-	-	41.7%	37.2%

Samaritan Lebanon Community Hospital

525 N Santiam Highway
Lebanon, OR 97355
Phone: 541-258-2101
Fax: 541-768-5124
URL: www.samhealth.org
Type: Critical Access Hospitals
Emergency Services: Yes
Ownership: Voluntary non-profit - Church
Beds: 49

Key Personnel:

Chief of Medical Staff.......... Dorothy Albrecht
Cardiac Laboratory............ Randy Cox
CEO/President................ Larry A Mullins
Radiology.................... Stephen Quinn

Measure	Cases	This Hosp.	State Avg.	U.S. Avg.
Blood Clot Prevention and Treatment				
Anticoagulation Overlap Therapy[1,2]	-	-	95%	93%
ICU Venous Thromboembolism Prophylaxis[2]	45	96%	87%	92%
Incidence of Potentially Preventable VTE[2,7]	-	-	13%	10%
UFH with Dosages/Platelet Monitoring[1,2]	-	-	100%	97%
Venous Thromboembolism Prophylaxis[2]	94	96%	83%	85%
Warfarin Therapy Discharge Instructions[1,2]	-	-	54%	75%
Chest Pain/Possible Heart Attack Care				
Aspirin Given Within 24 Hours of Arrival	-	-	97%	96%
Fibrinolytic Meds Within 30 Min. of Arrival	-	-	57%	58%
Average Time to ECG (minutes)	-	-	9	7
Average Time to Transfer (minutes)	-	-	52	60
Children's Asthma Care				
Received Home Management Plan of Care	-	-	-	88%
Received Reliever Medication	-	-	-	100%
Received Systemic Corticosteroids	-	-	-	100%
Emergency Department				
Admittance Decision Time (minutes)[2]	242	94	85	98
Head CT Results Within 45 Min. of Arrival	-	-	45%	57%
Patients Who Left ER Before Being Seen	-	-	2%	2%
Time from ER Arrival to Admit. (minutes)[2]	331	250	235	274
Time from ER Arrival to Discharge (minutes)	-	-	136	134
Time in ER Before Being Evaluated (minutes)	-	-	27	26
Time to Pain Meds for Fractures (minutes)	-	-	56	57
Heart Attack Care				
Aspirin Given at Discharge[5]	-	-	99%	99%
Fibrinolytic Meds Within 30 Min. of Arrival[5]	-	-	57%	54%
PCI Within 90 Minutes of Arrival[5]	-	-	93%	96%
Statin Prescribed at Discharge[5]	-	-	98%	98%
Heart Failure Care				
ACE Inhibitor or ARB for LVSD	21	100%	96%	97%
Discharge Instructions Given	66	100%	93%	94%
Evaluation of LVS Function	83	100%	99%	99%
Medicare Spending				
Medicare Spending per Patient (ratio)	-	-	0.88	0.98
Pneumonia Care				
Appropriate Initial Antibiotic Given	82	98%	96%	95%
Blood Culture Timing	131	95%	98%	98%
Pregnancy and Delivery Care				
Newborn Deliveries Scheduled Early[3]	12	0%	3%	6%
Preventive Care				
Immunization for Influenza[2]	244	91%	86%	90%
Immunization for Pneumonia[2]	323	94%	88%	92%
Stroke Care				
Anticoagulation Therapy for Atrial Fibrillation[1]	-	-	94%	95%
Antithrombotic Therapy Timing	26	100%	97%	98%
Assessed for Rehabilitation	26	100%	96%	97%
Discharged on Antithrombotic Therapy	23	100%	99%	99%
Discharged on Statin Medication	15	100%	93%	94%
Thrombolytic Therapy Timing[7]	-	-	55%	66%
Venous Thromboembolism Prophylaxis	27	100%	90%	94%
Written Stroke Educational Materials Given[1]	-	-	81%	88%
Surgical Care Improvement Project				
Appropriate Beta Blocker Usage	12	100%	98%	98%
Appropriate VTP Within 24 Hours	45	87%	97%	98%
Controlled Postoperative Blood Glucose[7]	-	-	98%	97%
Perioperative Temperature Management	59	100%	100%	100%
Prophylactic Antibiotic Selection	29	100%	99%	99%
Prophylactic Antibiotic Selection (Outpatient)	-	-	98%	98%
Prophylactic Antibiotic Stopped	27	85%	98%	98%
Prophylactic Antibiotic Timing	29	97%	98%	99%
Prophylactic Antibiotic Timing (Outpatient)	-	-	96%	98%
Urinary Catheter Removal	33	85%	97%	97%
Survey of Patients' Hospital Experiences				
Area Around Room 'Always' Quiet at Night	300+	49%	57%	61%
Doctors 'Always' Communicated Well	300+	75%	81%	82%
Home Recovery Information Given	300+	84%	86%	85%
Hospital Given 9 or 10 on 10 Point Scale	300+	61%	70%	71%
Meds 'Always' Explained Before Given	300+	61%	65%	64%
Nurses 'Always' Communicated Well	300+	78%	79%	79%
Pain 'Always' Well Controlled	300+	68%	71%	71%
Room and Bathroom 'Always' Clean	300+	76%	74%	73%
Timely Help 'Always' Received	300+	74%	68%	68%
Would Definitely Recommend Hospital	300+	62%	72%	71%
Use of Medical Imaging				
Cardiac Imaging Stress Test before Surgery	-	-	4.7%	5.3%
Combination Abdominal CT Scan	-	-	6.6%	10.5%
Combination Brain/Sinus CT Scan	-	-	2.1%	2.7%
Combination Chest CT Scan	-	-	1.1%	2.7%
Follow-up Mammogram/Ultrasound	-	-	8.9%	8.8%
Lumbar Spine MRI for Low Back Pain	-	-	41.7%	37.2%

Samaritan North Lincoln Hospital

3043 Ne 28th Street
Lincoln City, OR 97367
Phone: 541-994-3661
Fax: 541-996-7386
URL: www.samhealth.org/shs_facilities
Type: Critical Access Hospitals
Emergency Services: Yes
Ownership: Voluntary non-profit - Private
Beds: 25

Key Personnel:

Infection Control.............. Leah Baker-Fones, RN
Intensive Care Unit............ Willa Espinoza, RN
CEO/President.............. Jack Flaig
Operating Room.............. Ladonna Love, RN
Chief of Medical Staff.......... David Rosencrentz

Measure	Cases	This Hosp.	State Avg.	U.S. Avg.
Blood Clot Prevention and Treatment				
Anticoagulation Overlap Therapy[1,2]	-	-	95%	93%
ICU Venous Thromboembolism Prophylaxis[2]	36	69%	87%	92%
Incidence of Potentially Preventable VTE[1,2]	-	-	13%	10%
UFH with Dosages/Platelet Monitoring[1,2]	-	-	100%	97%
Venous Thromboembolism Prophylaxis[2]	62	73%	83%	85%
Warfarin Therapy Discharge Instructions[1,2]	-	-	54%	75%
Chest Pain/Possible Heart Attack Care				
Aspirin Given Within 24 Hours of Arrival[5]	-	-	97%	96%
Fibrinolytic Meds Within 30 Min. of Arrival[5]	-	-	57%	58%
Average Time to ECG (minutes)[5]	-	-	9	7
Average Time to Transfer (minutes)[5]	-	-	52	60
Children's Asthma Care				
Received Home Management Plan of Care	-	-	-	88%
Received Reliever Medication	-	-	-	100%
Received Systemic Corticosteroids	-	-	-	100%
Emergency Department				
Admittance Decision Time (minutes)[2]	220	61	85	98
Head CT Results Within 45 Min. of Arrival[5]	-	-	45%	57%
Patients Who Left ER Before Being Seen[5]	-	-	2%	2%
Time from ER Arrival to Admit. (minutes)[2]	332	194	235	274
Time from ER Arrival to Discharge (minutes)[5]	-	-	136	134
Time in ER Before Being Evaluated (minutes)[5]	-	-	27	26
Time to Pain Meds for Fractures (minutes)[5]	-	-	56	57
Heart Attack Care				
Aspirin Given at Discharge[5]	-	-	99%	99%
Fibrinolytic Meds Within 30 Min. of Arrival[5]	-	-	57%	54%
PCI Within 90 Minutes of Arrival[5]	-	-	93%	96%
Statin Prescribed at Discharge[5]	-	-	98%	98%
Heart Failure Care				
ACE Inhibitor or ARB for LVSD[1]	-	-	96%	97%
Discharge Instructions Given	26	81%	93%	94%
Evaluation of LVS Function	29	100%	99%	99%
Medicare Spending				
Medicare Spending per Patient (ratio)	-	-	0.88	0.98
Pneumonia Care				
Appropriate Initial Antibiotic Given	26	92%	96%	95%
Blood Culture Timing	34	100%	98%	98%
Pregnancy and Delivery Care				
Newborn Deliveries Scheduled Early[1,3]	-	-	3%	6%
Preventive Care				
Immunization for Influenza[2]	271	75%	86%	90%
Immunization for Pneumonia[2]	355	76%	88%	92%
Stroke Care				
Anticoagulation Therapy for Atrial Fibrillation[1]	-	-	94%	95%
Antithrombotic Therapy Timing	15	93%	97%	98%
Assessed for Rehabilitation	21	95%	96%	97%
Discharged on Antithrombotic Therapy	21	100%	99%	99%
Discharged on Statin Medication	16	62%	93%	94%
Thrombolytic Therapy Timing[7]	-	-	55%	66%
Venous Thromboembolism Prophylaxis	19	47%	90%	94%
Written Stroke Educational Materials Given[1]	-	-	81%	88%
Surgical Care Improvement Project				
Appropriate Beta Blocker Usage	21	100%	98%	98%
Appropriate VTP Within 24 Hours	56	96%	97%	98%
Controlled Postoperative Blood Glucose[7]	-	-	98%	97%
Perioperative Temperature Management	62	100%	100%	100%
Prophylactic Antibiotic Selection	48	100%	99%	99%
Prophylactic Antibiotic Selection (Outpatient)[5]	-	-	98%	98%
Prophylactic Antibiotic Stopped	48	100%	98%	98%
Prophylactic Antibiotic Timing	48	98%	98%	99%
Prophylactic Antibiotic Timing (Outpatient)[5]	-	-	96%	98%
Urinary Catheter Removal	45	93%	97%	97%
Survey of Patients' Hospital Experiences				
Area Around Room 'Always' Quiet at Night	(a)	58%	57%	61%
Doctors 'Always' Communicated Well	(a)	80%	81%	82%
Home Recovery Information Given	(a)	81%	86%	85%
Hospital Given 9 or 10 on 10 Point Scale	(a)	62%	70%	71%
Meds 'Always' Explained Before Given	(a)	67%	65%	64%

NOTE: Hospital profiles are in alphabetical order by state, then city, then hospital within the city; Rankings exclude hospitals with less than 25 cases except for patient surveys which excludes hospitals with less than 100 cases; (a) 100-299 cases; (1) The number of cases/patients is too few to report; (2) Data submitted were based on a sample of cases/patients; (3) Results are based on a shorter time period than required; (4) Data suppressed by CMS for one or more quarters; (5) Results are not available for this reporting period; (6) Fewer than 100 patients completed the HCAHPS survey; (7) No cases met the criteria for this measure; (8) The lower limit of the confidence interval cannot be calculated if the number of observed infections equals zero; (9) No data are available from the state/territory for this reporting period; (10) The scores shown reflect fewer than 50 completed surveys; (11) There were discrepancies in the data collection process; (12) This measure does not apply to this hospital for this reporting period; (13) Results cannot be calculated for this reporting period; (14) The results for this state are combined with nearby states to protect confidentiality; Please refer to the User's Guide for a full explanation of data.

Nurses 'Always' Communicated Well	(a)	77%	79%	79%
Pain 'Always' Well Controlled	(a)	76%	71%	71%
Room and Bathroom 'Always' Clean	(a)	74%	74%	73%
Timely Help 'Always' Received	(a)	75%	68%	68%
Would Definitely Recommend Hospital	(a)	63%	72%	71%
Use of Medical Imaging				
Cardiac Imaging Stress Test before Surgery[5]	-	-	4.7%	5.3%
Combination Abdominal CT Scan[5]	-	-	6.6%	10.5%
Combination Brain/Sinus CT Scan[5]	-	-	2.1%	2.7%
Combination Chest CT Scan[5]	-	-	1.1%	2.7%
Follow-up Mammogram/Ultrasound[5]	-	-	8.9%	8.8%
Lumbar Spine MRI for Low Back Pain[5]	-	-	41.7%	37.2%

Saint Charles - Madras

470 Ne A Street | Phone: 541-460-4200
Madras, OR 97741 | Fax: 541-475-0615
E-mail: mvhd@mvhd.org
URL: www.mvhd.org
Type: Critical Access Hospitals | Emergency Services: Yes
Ownership: Govt - Hospital Dist/Auth | Beds: 60

Measure	Cases	This Hosp.	State Avg.	U.S. Avg.
Blood Clot Prevention and Treatment				
Anticoagulation Overlap Therapy[5]	-	-	95%	93%
ICU Venous Thromboembolism Prophylaxis[5]	-	-	87%	92%
Incidence of Potentially Preventable VTE[5]	-	-	13%	10%
UFH with Dosages/Platelet Monitoring[5]	-	-	100%	97%
Venous Thromboembolism Prophylaxis[5]	-	-	83%	85%
Warfarin Therapy Discharge Instructions[5]	-	-	54%	75%
Chest Pain/Possible Heart Attack Care				
Aspirin Given Within 24 Hours of Arrival[5]	-	-	97%	96%
Fibrinolytic Meds Within 30 Min. of Arrival[5]	-	-	57%	58%
Average Time to ECG (minutes)[5]	-	-	9	7
Average Time to Transfer (minutes)[5]	-	-	52	60
Children's Asthma Care				
Received Home Management Plan of Care	-	-	-	88%
Received Reliever Medication	-	-	-	100%
Received Systemic Corticosteroids	-	-	-	100%
Emergency Department				
Admittance Decision Time (minutes)[5]	-	-	85	98
Head CT Results Within 45 Min. of Arrival[5]	-	-	45%	57%
Patients Who Left ER Before Being Seen[5]	-	-	2%	2%
Time from ER Arrival to Admit. (minutes)[5]	-	-	235	274
Time from ER Arrival to Discharge (minutes)[5]	-	-	136	134
Time in ER Before Being Evaluated (minutes)[5]	-	-	27	26
Time to Pain Meds for Fractures (minutes)[5]	-	-	56	57
Heart Attack Care				
Aspirin Given at Discharge[1,3]	-	-	99%	99%
Fibrinolytic Meds Within 30 Min. of Arrival[3,7]	-	-	57%	54%
PCI Within 90 Minutes of Arrival[5]	-	-	93%	96%
Statin Prescribed at Discharge[1,3]	-	-	98%	98%
Heart Failure Care				
ACE Inhibitor or ARB for LVSD[1]	-	-	96%	97%
Discharge Instructions Given	23	65%	93%	94%
Evaluation of LVS Function	26	58%	99%	99%
Medicare Spending				
Medicare Spending per Patient (ratio)	-	-	0.88	0.98
Pneumonia Care				
Appropriate Initial Antibiotic Given	18	100%	96%	95%
Blood Culture Timing	26	85%	98%	98%
Pregnancy and Delivery Care				
Newborn Deliveries Scheduled Early[5]	-	-	3%	6%
Preventive Care				
Immunization for Influenza[5]	-	-	86%	90%
Immunization for Pneumonia[5]	-	-	88%	92%
Stroke Care				
Anticoagulation Therapy for Atrial Fibrillation[5]	-	-	94%	95%
Antithrombotic Therapy Timing[5]	-	-	97%	98%
Assessed for Rehabilitation[5]	-	-	96%	97%
Discharged on Antithrombotic Therapy[5]	-	-	99%	99%
Discharged on Statin Medication[5]	-	-	93%	94%
Thrombolytic Therapy Timing[5]	-	-	55%	66%
Venous Thromboembolism Prophylaxis[5]	-	-	90%	94%
Written Stroke Educational Materials Given[5]	-	-	81%	88%
Surgical Care Improvement Project				
Appropriate Beta Blocker Usage[7]	-	-	98%	98%
Appropriate VTP Within 24 Hours	14	79%	97%	98%
Controlled Postoperative Blood Glucose[3,7]	-	-	98%	97%
Perioperative Temperature Management[7]	-	-	100%	100%
Prophylactic Antibiotic Selection	13	100%	99%	99%
Prophylactic Antibiotic Selection (Outpatient)[5]	-	-	98%	98%
Prophylactic Antibiotic Stopped	13	92%	98%	98%
Prophylactic Antibiotic Timing	13	85%	98%	99%
Prophylactic Antibiotic Timing (Outpatient)[5]	-	-	96%	98%
Urinary Catheter Removal	14	100%	97%	97%
Survey of Patients' Hospital Experiences				
Area Around Room 'Always' Quiet at Night	(a)	54%	57%	61%
Doctors 'Always' Communicated Well	(a)	77%	81%	82%
Home Recovery Information Given	(a)	83%	86%	85%
Hospital Given 9 or 10 on 10 Point Scale	(a)	65%	70%	71%
Meds 'Always' Explained Before Given	(a)	65%	65%	64%
Nurses 'Always' Communicated Well	(a)	77%	79%	79%
Pain 'Always' Well Controlled	(a)	67%	71%	71%
Room and Bathroom 'Always' Clean	(a)	82%	74%	73%
Timely Help 'Always' Received	(a)	67%	68%	68%
Would Definitely Recommend Hospital	(a)	65%	72%	71%
Use of Medical Imaging				
Cardiac Imaging Stress Test before Surgery[7]	-	-	4.7%	5.3%
Combination Abdominal CT Scan	126	5.6%	6.6%	10.5%
Combination Brain/Sinus CT Scan[1]	-	-	2.1%	2.7%
Combination Chest CT Scan	74	1.4%	1.1%	2.7%
Follow-up Mammogram/Ultrasound	207	12.1%	8.9%	8.8%
Lumbar Spine MRI for Low Back Pain[1]	-	-	41.7%	37.2%

Willamette Valley Medical Center

2700 Se Stratus Ave. | Phone: 503-472-6131
Mcminnville, OR 97128 | Fax: 503-472-8691
URL: www.wvmcweb.com
Type: Acute Care Hospitals | Emergency Services: Yes
Ownership: Voluntary non-profit - Private | Beds: 55

Key Personnel:
CEO/President. . . . . Rosemari Davis
Radiology. . . . . Steven Edelman, MD
Emergency Room . . . . Mary Harbor, MD
Cardiology . . . . A. Wayne Hurty, MD
Emergency Room . . . . John Jacobson, MD
Anesthesiology. . . . . Andrew Madden, CRNA
Operating Room. . . . . Margaret Meyer
Chief of Medical Staff. . . . . John Topping

Measure	Cases	This Hosp.	State Avg.	U.S. Avg.
Blood Clot Prevention and Treatment				
Anticoagulation Overlap Therapy[2]	28	100%	95%	93%
ICU Venous Thromboembolism Prophylaxis[2]	53	100%	87%	92%
Incidence of Potentially Preventable VTE[1,2]	-	-	13%	10%
UFH with Dosages/Platelet Monitoring[1,2]	-	-	100%	97%
Venous Thromboembolism Prophylaxis[2]	255	100%	83%	85%
Warfarin Therapy Discharge Instructions[2]	21	95%	54%	75%
Chest Pain/Possible Heart Attack Care				
Aspirin Given Within 24 Hours of Arrival	21	100%	97%	96%
Fibrinolytic Meds Within 30 Min. of Arrival[1]	-	-	57%	58%
Average Time to ECG (minutes)	21	9	9	7
Average Time to Transfer (minutes)[1]	-	-	52	60
Children's Asthma Care				
Received Home Management Plan of Care	-	-	-	88%
Received Reliever Medication	-	-	-	100%
Received Systemic Corticosteroids	-	-	-	100%
Emergency Department				
Admittance Decision Time (minutes)[2]	455	100	85	98
Head CT Results Within 45 Min. of Arrival	16	69%	45%	57%
Patients Who Left ER Before Being Seen	25,242	1%	2%	2%
Time from ER Arrival to Admit. (minutes)[2]	455	240	235	274
Time from ER Arrival to Discharge (minutes)	477	156	136	134
Time in ER Before Being Evaluated (minutes)	506	27	27	26
Time to Pain Meds for Fractures (minutes)	81	43	56	57
Heart Attack Care				
Aspirin Given at Discharge	17	100%	99%	99%
Fibrinolytic Meds Within 30 Min. of Arrival[7]	-	-	57%	54%
PCI Within 90 Minutes of Arrival[7]	-	-	93%	96%
Statin Prescribed at Discharge	18	100%	98%	98%
Heart Failure Care				
ACE Inhibitor or ARB for LVSD	16	100%	96%	97%
Discharge Instructions Given	138	100%	93%	94%
Evaluation of LVS Function	167	100%	99%	99%
Medicare Spending				
Medicare Spending per Patient (ratio)	-	0.90	0.88	0.98
Pneumonia Care				
Appropriate Initial Antibiotic Given	127	99%	96%	95%
Blood Culture Timing	198	99%	98%	98%
Pregnancy and Delivery Care				
Newborn Deliveries Scheduled Early[2]	37	3%	3%	6%
Preventive Care				
Immunization for Influenza[2]	370	96%	86%	90%
Immunization for Pneumonia[2]	456	99%	88%	92%
Stroke Care				
Anticoagulation Therapy for Atrial Fibrillation[1]	-	-	94%	95%
Antithrombotic Therapy Timing	41	98%	97%	98%
Assessed for Rehabilitation	48	100%	96%	97%
Discharged on Antithrombotic Therapy	47	100%	99%	99%
Discharged on Statin Medication	33	97%	93%	94%
Thrombolytic Therapy Timing[1]	-	-	55%	66%
Venous Thromboembolism Prophylaxis	39	100%	90%	94%
Written Stroke Educational Materials Given	32	97%	81%	88%
Surgical Care Improvement Project				
Appropriate Beta Blocker Usage	65	95%	98%	98%
Appropriate VTP Within 24 Hours	212	99%	97%	98%
Controlled Postoperative Blood Glucose[7]	-	-	98%	97%
Perioperative Temperature Management	295	100%	100%	100%
Prophylactic Antibiotic Selection	217	100%	99%	99%
Prophylactic Antibiotic Selection (Outpatient)	106	100%	98%	98%
Prophylactic Antibiotic Stopped	212	100%	98%	98%
Prophylactic Antibiotic Timing	217	100%	98%	99%
Prophylactic Antibiotic Timing (Outpatient)	106	100%	96%	98%
Urinary Catheter Removal	191	99%	97%	97%
Survey of Patients' Hospital Experiences				
Area Around Room 'Always' Quiet at Night	300+	65%	57%	61%
Doctors 'Always' Communicated Well	300+	83%	81%	82%
Home Recovery Information Given	300+	89%	86%	85%
Hospital Given 9 or 10 on 10 Point Scale	300+	75%	70%	71%
Meds 'Always' Explained Before Given	300+	64%	65%	64%
Nurses 'Always' Communicated Well	300+	82%	79%	79%
Pain 'Always' Well Controlled	300+	76%	71%	71%
Room and Bathroom 'Always' Clean	300+	64%	74%	73%
Timely Help 'Always' Received	300+	68%	68%	68%
Would Definitely Recommend Hospital	300+	72%	72%	71%
Use of Medical Imaging				
Cardiac Imaging Stress Test before Surgery	96	4.2%	4.7%	5.3%
Combination Abdominal CT Scan	447	3.8%	6.6%	10.5%
Combination Brain/Sinus CT Scan[1]	-	-	2.1%	2.7%
Combination Chest CT Scan	302	0.0%	1.1%	2.7%
Follow-up Mammogram/Ultrasound	806	7.8%	8.9%	8.8%
Lumbar Spine MRI for Low Back Pain	49	36.7%	41.7%	37.2%

Asante Rogue Regional Medical Center

2825 E Barnett Road | Phone: 541-789-7000
Medford, OR 97504 | Fax: 541-789-5870
URL: www.asante.org
Type: Acute Care Hospitals | Emergency Services: Yes
Ownership: Voluntary non-profit - Private | Beds: 378

Key Personnel:
Quality Assurance . . . . Roberta Bowsher
Chief of Medical Staff. . . . . Lee Harker, MD
Radiology. . . . . Bob James
CEO/President. . . . . Scott Kelly
Emergency Room . . . . Ken Rhee
Pediatric Ambulatory Care . . . . . . Barbara Roberts
Pediatric In-Patient Care . . . . Barbara Roberts

Measure	Cases	This Hosp.	State Avg.	U.S. Avg.
Blood Clot Prevention and Treatment				
Anticoagulation Overlap Therapy[2]	120	99%	95%	93%
ICU Venous Thromboembolism Prophylaxis[2]	113	90%	87%	92%
Incidence of Potentially Preventable VTE[2]	15	0%	13%	10%
UFH with Dosages/Platelet Monitoring[2]	22	100%	100%	97%

NOTE: Hospital profiles are in alphabetical order by state, then city, then hospital within the city; Rankings exclude hospitals with less than 25 cases except for patient surveys which excludes hospitals with less than 100 cases; (a) 100-299 cases; (1) The number of cases/patients is too few to report; (2) Data submitted were based on a sample of cases/patients; (3) Results are based on a shorter time period than required; (4) Data suppressed by CMS for one or more quarters; (5) Results are not available for this reporting period; (6) Fewer than 100 patients completed the HCAHPS survey; (7) No cases met the criteria for this measure; (8) The lower limit of the confidence interval cannot be calculated if the number of observed infections equals zero; (9) No data are available from the state/territory for this reporting period; (10) The scores shown reflect fewer than 50 completed surveys; (11) There were discrepancies in the data collection process; (12) This measure does not apply to this hospital for this reporting period; (13) Results cannot be calculated for this reporting period; (14) The results for this state are combined with nearby states to protect confidentiality; Please refer to the User's Guide for a full explanation of data.

Measure	Cases	This Hosp.	State Avg.	U.S. Avg.
Venous Thromboembolism Prophylaxis[2]	281	81%	83%	85%
Warfarin Therapy Discharge Instructions[2]	98	89%	54%	75%
Chest Pain/Possible Heart Attack Care				
Aspirin Given Within 24 Hours of Arrival[1,3]	-	-	97%	96%
Fibrinolytic Meds Within 30 Min. of Arrival[5]	-	-	57%	58%
Average Time to ECG (minutes)[1,3]	-	-	9	7
Average Time to Transfer (minutes)[5]	-	-	52	60
Children's Asthma Care				
Received Home Management Plan of Care	-	-	-	88%
Received Reliever Medication	-	-	-	100%
Received Systemic Corticosteroids	-	-	-	100%
Emergency Department				
Admittance Decision Time (minutes)[2]	339	133	85	98
Head CT Results Within 45 Min. of Arrival	17	47%	45%	57%
Patients Who Left ER Before Being Seen	39,108	3%	2%	2%
Time from ER Arrival to Admit. (minutes)[2]	350	282	235	274
Time from ER Arrival to Discharge (minutes)	332	186	136	134
Time in ER Before Being Evaluated (minutes)	202	40	27	26
Time to Pain Meds for Fractures (minutes)	158	65	56	57
Heart Attack Care				
Aspirin Given at Discharge[2]	281	98%	99%	99%
Fibrinolytic Meds Within 30 Min. of Arrival[2,7]	-	-	57%	54%
PCI Within 90 Minutes of Arrival[2]	30	97%	93%	96%
Statin Prescribed at Discharge[2]	223	99%	98%	98%
Heart Failure Care				
ACE Inhibitor or ARB for LVSD[2]	87	99%	96%	97%
Discharge Instructions Given[2]	307	94%	93%	94%
Evaluation of LVS Function[2]	332	100%	99%	99%
Medicare Spending				
Medicare Spending per Patient (ratio)	-	0.90	0.88	0.98
Pneumonia Care				
Appropriate Initial Antibiotic Given[2]	83	100%	96%	95%
Blood Culture Timing[2]	119	100%	98%	98%
Pregnancy and Delivery Care				
Newborn Deliveries Scheduled Early[2]	48	4%	3%	6%
Preventive Care				
Immunization for Influenza[2]	489	94%	86%	90%
Immunization for Pneumonia[2]	667	90%	88%	92%
Stroke Care				
Anticoagulation Therapy for Atrial Fibrillation[2]	18	100%	94%	95%
Antithrombotic Therapy Timing[2]	109	100%	97%	98%
Assessed for Rehabilitation[2]	135	100%	96%	97%
Discharged on Antithrombotic Therapy[2]	120	98%	99%	99%
Discharged on Statin Medication[2]	79	99%	93%	94%
Thrombolytic Therapy Timing[1,2]	-	-	55%	66%
Venous Thromboembolism Prophylaxis[2]	131	95%	90%	94%
Written Stroke Educational Materials Given[2]	84	92%	81%	88%
Surgical Care Improvement Project				
Appropriate Beta Blocker Usage[2]	230	100%	98%	98%
Appropriate VTP Within 24 Hours[2]	356	99%	97%	98%
Controlled Postoperative Blood Glucose[2]	160	98%	98%	97%
Perioperative Temperature Management[2]	543	100%	100%	100%
Prophylactic Antibiotic Selection[2]	493	99%	99%	99%
Prophylactic Antibiotic Selection (Outpatient)	503	99%	98%	98%
Prophylactic Antibiotic Stopped[2]	486	99%	98%	98%
Prophylactic Antibiotic Timing[2]	496	99%	98%	99%
Prophylactic Antibiotic Timing (Outpatient)	506	98%	96%	98%
Urinary Catheter Removal[2]	261	97%	97%	97%
Survey of Patients' Hospital Experiences				
Area Around Room 'Always' Quiet at Night	300+	51%	57%	61%
Doctors 'Always' Communicated Well	300+	79%	81%	82%
Home Recovery Information Given	300+	82%	86%	85%
Hospital Given 9 or 10 on 10 Point Scale	300+	74%	70%	71%
Meds 'Always' Explained Before Given	300+	62%	65%	64%
Nurses 'Always' Communicated Well	300+	79%	79%	79%
Pain 'Always' Well Controlled	300+	70%	71%	71%
Room and Bathroom 'Always' Clean	300+	71%	74%	73%
Timely Help 'Always' Received	300+	60%	68%	68%
Would Definitely Recommend Hospital	300+	81%	72%	71%
Use of Medical Imaging				
Cardiac Imaging Stress Test before Surgery	820	4.3%	4.7%	5.3%
Combination Abdominal CT Scan	649	6.5%	6.6%	10.5%
Combination Brain/Sinus CT Scan	659	1.5%	2.1%	2.7%
Combination Chest CT Scan	399	1.5%	1.1%	2.7%
Follow-up Mammogram/Ultrasound	2,857	10.5%	8.9%	8.8%
Lumbar Spine MRI for Low Back Pain[1]	-	-	41.7%	37.2%

Providence Medford Medical Center

1111 Crater Lake Avenue
Medford, OR 97504
Phone: 541-732-5196
Fax: 541-732-5872
URL: www.providence.org/medford
Type: Acute Care Hospitals
Emergency Services: Yes
Ownership: Voluntary non-profit - Church
Beds: 168

Key Personnel:

Emergency Room . . . . Gordon Everett
Operating Room. . . . . Tracy Haley
Infection Control. . . . . Carleen Lawence
Chief of Medical Staff. . . . . Erich Weber, MD
CEO/President. . . . . Charles T Wright

Measure	Cases	This Hosp.	State Avg.	U.S. Avg.
Blood Clot Prevention and Treatment				
Anticoagulation Overlap Therapy[2]	59	98%	95%	93%
ICU Venous Thromboembolism Prophylaxis[2]	400	84%	87%	92%
Incidence of Potentially Preventable VTE[1,2]	-	-	13%	10%
UFH with Dosages/Platelet Monitoring[2]	25	100%	100%	97%
Venous Thromboembolism Prophylaxis[2]	105	85%	83%	85%
Warfarin Therapy Discharge Instructions[2]	58	9%	54%	75%
Chest Pain/Possible Heart Attack Care				
Aspirin Given Within 24 Hours of Arrival[1,3]	-	-	97%	96%
Fibrinolytic Meds Within 30 Min. of Arrival[5]	-	-	57%	58%
Average Time to ECG (minutes)[1,3]	-	-	9	7
Average Time to Transfer (minutes)[5]	-	-	52	60
Children's Asthma Care				
Received Home Management Plan of Care	-	-	-	88%
Received Reliever Medication	-	-	-	100%
Received Systemic Corticosteroids	-	-	-	100%
Emergency Department				
Admittance Decision Time (minutes)[2]	669	170	85	98
Head CT Results Within 45 Min. of Arrival[1]	-	-	45%	57%
Patients Who Left ER Before Being Seen	32,904	1%	2%	2%
Time from ER Arrival to Admit. (minutes)[2]	728	318	235	274
Time from ER Arrival to Discharge (minutes)	176	167	136	134
Time in ER Before Being Evaluated (minutes)	61	42	27	26
Time to Pain Meds for Fractures (minutes)	110	60	56	57
Heart Attack Care				
Aspirin Given at Discharge[2]	86	100%	99%	99%
Fibrinolytic Meds Within 30 Min. of Arrival[2,7]	-	-	57%	54%
PCI Within 90 Minutes of Arrival[2]	16	100%	93%	96%
Statin Prescribed at Discharge[2]	84	98%	98%	98%
Heart Failure Care				
ACE Inhibitor or ARB for LVSD[2]	48	90%	96%	97%
Discharge Instructions Given[2]	158	94%	93%	94%
Evaluation of LVS Function[2]	181	99%	99%	99%
Medicare Spending				
Medicare Spending per Patient (ratio)	-	0.90	0.88	0.98
Pneumonia Care				
Appropriate Initial Antibiotic Given[2]	123	99%	96%	95%
Blood Culture Timing[2]	168	100%	98%	98%
Pregnancy and Delivery Care				
Newborn Deliveries Scheduled Early	28	4%	3%	6%
Preventive Care				
Immunization for Influenza[2]	605	82%	86%	90%
Immunization for Pneumonia[2]	845	86%	88%	92%
Stroke Care				
Anticoagulation Therapy for Atrial Fibrillation[2]	16	94%	94%	95%
Antithrombotic Therapy Timing[2]	61	98%	97%	98%
Assessed for Rehabilitation[2]	72	100%	96%	97%
Discharged on Antithrombotic Therapy[2]	68	96%	99%	99%
Discharged on Statin Medication[2]	57	86%	93%	94%
Thrombolytic Therapy Timing[1,2]	-	-	55%	66%
Venous Thromboembolism Prophylaxis[2]	74	82%	90%	94%
Written Stroke Educational Materials Given[2]	41	54%	81%	88%
Surgical Care Improvement Project				
Appropriate Beta Blocker Usage[2]	94	99%	98%	98%
Appropriate VTP Within 24 Hours[2]	280	100%	97%	98%
Controlled Postoperative Blood Glucose[2,7]	-	-	98%	97%
Perioperative Temperature Management[2]	355	100%	100%	100%
Prophylactic Antibiotic Selection[2]	222	99%	99%	99%
Prophylactic Antibiotic Selection (Outpatient)	372	97%	98%	98%
Prophylactic Antibiotic Stopped[2]	218	100%	98%	98%
Prophylactic Antibiotic Timing[2]	222	98%	98%	99%
Prophylactic Antibiotic Timing (Outpatient)	366	92%	96%	98%
Urinary Catheter Removal[2]	47	94%	97%	97%
Survey of Patients' Hospital Experiences				
Area Around Room 'Always' Quiet at Night	300+	48%	57%	61%
Doctors 'Always' Communicated Well	300+	75%	81%	82%
Home Recovery Information Given	300+	84%	86%	85%
Hospital Given 9 or 10 on 10 Point Scale	300+	68%	70%	71%
Meds 'Always' Explained Before Given	300+	59%	65%	64%
Nurses 'Always' Communicated Well	300+	75%	79%	79%
Pain 'Always' Well Controlled	300+	70%	71%	71%
Room and Bathroom 'Always' Clean	300+	69%	74%	73%
Timely Help 'Always' Received	300+	61%	68%	68%
Would Definitely Recommend Hospital	300+	74%	72%	71%
Use of Medical Imaging				
Cardiac Imaging Stress Test before Surgery	214	3.3%	4.7%	5.3%
Combination Abdominal CT Scan	660	12.9%	6.6%	10.5%
Combination Brain/Sinus CT Scan	354	0.8%	2.1%	2.7%
Combination Chest CT Scan	262	0.4%	1.1%	2.7%
Follow-up Mammogram/Ultrasound	1,606	12.1%	8.9%	8.8%
Lumbar Spine MRI for Low Back Pain[1]	-	-	41.7%	37.2%

Providence Milwaukie Hospital

10150 Se 32nd Avenue
Milwaukie, OR 97222
Phone: 503-513-8336
Fax: 503-513-8463
URL: www.providence.org/oregon
Type: Acute Care Hospitals
Emergency Services: Yes
Ownership: Voluntary non-profit - Church
Beds: 77

Key Personnel:

Chief of Medical Staff. . . . . Scott Browning, MD
Emergency Room . . . . Fred Underwood

Measure	Cases	This Hosp.	State Avg.	U.S. Avg.
Blood Clot Prevention and Treatment				
Anticoagulation Overlap Therapy[2]	27	85%	95%	93%
ICU Venous Thromboembolism Prophylaxis[2]	177	70%	87%	92%
Incidence of Potentially Preventable VTE[1,2]	-	-	13%	10%
UFH with Dosages/Platelet Monitoring[1,2]	-	-	100%	97%
Venous Thromboembolism Prophylaxis[2]	121	61%	83%	85%
Warfarin Therapy Discharge Instructions[2]	21	0%	54%	75%
Chest Pain/Possible Heart Attack Care				
Aspirin Given Within 24 Hours of Arrival	72	97%	97%	96%
Fibrinolytic Meds Within 30 Min. of Arrival[1]	-	-	57%	58%
Average Time to ECG (minutes)	73	8	9	7
Average Time to Transfer (minutes)	20	32	52	60
Children's Asthma Care				
Received Home Management Plan of Care	-	-	-	88%
Received Reliever Medication	-	-	-	100%
Received Systemic Corticosteroids	-	-	-	100%
Emergency Department				
Admittance Decision Time (minutes)[2]	432	81	85	98
Head CT Results Within 45 Min. of Arrival	12	58%	45%	57%
Patients Who Left ER Before Being Seen	33,412	1%	2%	2%
Time from ER Arrival to Admit. (minutes)[2]	439	230	235	274
Time from ER Arrival to Discharge (minutes)	198	126	136	134
Time in ER Before Being Evaluated (minutes)	56	20	27	26
Time to Pain Meds for Fractures (minutes)	120	50	56	57
Heart Attack Care				
Aspirin Given at Discharge[1,2]	-	-	99%	99%
Fibrinolytic Meds Within 30 Min. of Arrival[2,7]	-	-	57%	54%
PCI Within 90 Minutes of Arrival[2,7]	-	-	93%	96%
Statin Prescribed at Discharge[1,2]	-	-	98%	98%
Heart Failure Care				
ACE Inhibitor or ARB for LVSD[2]	37	100%	96%	97%
Discharge Instructions Given[2]	101	95%	93%	94%
Evaluation of LVS Function[2]	121	100%	99%	99%
Medicare Spending				
Medicare Spending per Patient (ratio)	-	0.87	0.88	0.98
Pneumonia Care				
Appropriate Initial Antibiotic Given[2]	74	96%	96%	95%

NOTE: Hospital profiles are in alphabetical order by state, then city, then hospital within the city; Rankings exclude hospitals with less than 25 cases except for patient surveys which excludes hospitals with less than 100 cases; (a) 100-299 cases; (1) The number of cases/patients is too few to report; (2) Data submitted were based on a sample of cases/patients; (3) Results are based on a shorter time period than required; (4) Data suppressed by CMS for one or more quarters; (5) Results are not available for this reporting period; (6) Fewer than 100 patients completed the HCAHPS survey; (7) No cases met the criteria for this measure; (8) The lower limit of the confidence interval cannot be calculated if the number of observed infections equals zero; (9) No data are available from the state/territory for this reporting period; (10) The scores shown reflect fewer than 50 completed surveys; (11) There were discrepancies in the data collection process; (12) This measure does not apply to this hospital for this reporting period; (13) Results cannot be calculated for this reporting period; (14) The results for this state are combined with nearby states to protect confidentiality; Please refer to the User's Guide for a full explanation of data.

Blood Culture Timing[2]	95	98%	98%	98%
Pregnancy and Delivery Care				
Newborn Deliveries Scheduled Early	17	0%	3%	6%
Preventive Care				
Immunization for Influenza[2]	331	91%	86%	90%
Immunization for Pneumonia[2]	445	89%	88%	92%
Stroke Care				
Anticoagulation Therapy for Atrial Fibrillation[1,2]	-	-	94%	95%
Antithrombotic Therapy Timing[2]	35	97%	97%	98%
Assessed for Rehabilitation[2]	38	95%	96%	97%
Discharged on Antithrombotic Therapy[2]	38	100%	99%	99%
Discharged on Statin Medication[2]	32	91%	93%	94%
Thrombolytic Therapy Timing[1,2]	-	-	55%	66%
Venous Thromboembolism Prophylaxis[2]	35	63%	90%	94%
Written Stroke Educational Materials Given[2]	22	36%	81%	88%
Surgical Care Improvement Project				
Appropriate Beta Blocker Usage[2]	52	94%	98%	98%
Appropriate VTP Within 24 Hours[2]	213	96%	97%	98%
Controlled Postoperative Blood Glucose[2,7]	-	-	98%	97%
Perioperative Temperature Management[2]	228	100%	100%	100%
Prophylactic Antibiotic Selection[2]	156	99%	99%	99%
Prophylactic Antibiotic Selection (Outpatient)	22	91%	98%	98%
Prophylactic Antibiotic Stopped[2]	151	100%	98%	98%
Prophylactic Antibiotic Timing[2]	157	96%	98%	99%
Prophylactic Antibiotic Timing (Outpatient)	22	95%	96%	98%
Urinary Catheter Removal[2]	171	95%	97%	97%
Survey of Patients' Hospital Experiences				
Area Around Room 'Always' Quiet at Night	300+	53%	57%	61%
Doctors 'Always' Communicated Well	300+	81%	81%	82%
Home Recovery Information Given	300+	86%	86%	85%
Hospital Given 9 or 10 on 10 Point Scale	300+	76%	70%	71%
Meds 'Always' Explained Before Given	300+	66%	65%	64%
Nurses 'Always' Communicated Well	300+	81%	79%	79%
Pain 'Always' Well Controlled	300+	70%	71%	71%
Room and Bathroom 'Always' Clean	300+	79%	74%	73%
Timely Help 'Always' Received	300+	69%	68%	68%
Would Definitely Recommend Hospital	300+	82%	72%	71%
Use of Medical Imaging				
Cardiac Imaging Stress Test before Surgery[1]	-	-	4.7%	5.3%
Combination Abdominal CT Scan	265	4.2%	6.6%	10.5%
Combination Brain/Sinus CT Scan	220	0.9%	2.1%	2.7%
Combination Chest CT Scan	162	0.0%	1.1%	2.7%
Follow-up Mammogram/Ultrasound	601	12.1%	8.9%	8.8%
Lumbar Spine MRI for Low Back Pain[1]	-	-	41.7%	37.2%

Providence Newberg Medical Center

1001 Providence Drive Phone: 503-537-1555
Newberg, OR 97132 Fax: 503-537-1815
URL: www.providence.org/yamhill
Type: Acute Care Hospitals Emergency Services: Yes
Ownership: Voluntary non-profit - Church Beds: 40

Key Personnel:
Quality Assurance . . . . Lee Anne Chandler
CEO/President. . . . . Mark W Meinert
Chief of Medical Staff. . . . . Steve Townsend, MD
Emergency Room . . . . John Van Eaton, MD

Measure	Cases	This Hosp.	State Avg.	U.S. Avg.
Blood Clot Prevention and Treatment				
Anticoagulation Overlap Therapy[1,2]	-	-	95%	93%
ICU Venous Thromboembolism Prophylaxis[2]	158	85%	87%	92%
Incidence of Potentially Preventable VTE[1,2]	-	-	13%	10%
UFH with Dosages/Platelet Monitoring[1,2]	-	-	100%	97%
Venous Thromboembolism Prophylaxis[2]	52	83%	83%	85%
Warfarin Therapy Discharge Instructions[2]	13	8%	54%	75%
Chest Pain/Possible Heart Attack Care				
Aspirin Given Within 24 Hours of Arrival	45	100%	97%	96%
Fibrinolytic Meds Within 30 Min. of Arrival[7]	-	-	57%	58%
Average Time to ECG (minutes)	45	5	9	7
Average Time to Transfer (minutes)	11	36	52	60
Children's Asthma Care				
Received Home Management Plan of Care	-	-	-	88%
Received Reliever Medication	-	-	-	100%
Received Systemic Corticosteroids	-	-	-	100%
Emergency Department				
Admittance Decision Time (minutes)[2]	293	91	85	98
Head CT Results Within 45 Min. of Arrival[1]	-	-	45%	57%
Patients Who Left ER Before Being Seen	19,191	0%	2%	2%
Time from ER Arrival to Admit. (minutes)[2]	309	227	235	274
Time from ER Arrival to Discharge (minutes)	245	143	136	134
Time in ER Before Being Evaluated (minutes)	246	19	27	26
Time to Pain Meds for Fractures (minutes)	85	42	56	57
Heart Attack Care				
Aspirin Given at Discharge[2]	13	100%	99%	99%
Fibrinolytic Meds Within 30 Min. of Arrival[2,7]	-	-	57%	54%
PCI Within 90 Minutes of Arrival[2,7]	-	-	93%	96%
Statin Prescribed at Discharge[2]	15	100%	98%	98%
Heart Failure Care				
ACE Inhibitor or ARB for LVSD[2]	11	73%	96%	97%
Discharge Instructions Given[2]	84	94%	93%	94%
Evaluation of LVS Function[2]	96	99%	99%	99%
Medicare Spending				
Medicare Spending per Patient (ratio)	-	0.80	0.88	0.98
Pneumonia Care				
Appropriate Initial Antibiotic Given[2]	30	97%	96%	95%
Blood Culture Timing[2]	61	98%	98%	98%
Pregnancy and Delivery Care				
Newborn Deliveries Scheduled Early	41	0%	3%	6%
Preventive Care				
Immunization for Influenza[2]	267	87%	86%	90%
Immunization for Pneumonia[2]	304	85%	88%	92%
Stroke Care				
Anticoagulation Therapy for Atrial Fibrillation[1,2]	-	-	94%	95%
Antithrombotic Therapy Timing[2]	17	100%	97%	98%
Assessed for Rehabilitation[2]	25	96%	96%	97%
Discharged on Antithrombotic Therapy[2]	25	100%	99%	99%
Discharged on Statin Medication[2]	22	91%	93%	94%
Thrombolytic Therapy Timing[1,2]	-	-	55%	66%
Venous Thromboembolism Prophylaxis[2]	17	94%	90%	94%
Written Stroke Educational Materials Given[2]	22	14%	81%	88%
Surgical Care Improvement Project				
Appropriate Beta Blocker Usage[2]	42	100%	98%	98%
Appropriate VTP Within 24 Hours[2]	161	99%	97%	98%
Controlled Postoperative Blood Glucose[2,7]	-	-	98%	97%
Perioperative Temperature Management[2]	175	100%	100%	100%
Prophylactic Antibiotic Selection[2]	118	100%	99%	99%
Prophylactic Antibiotic Selection (Outpatient)	40	98%	98%	98%
Prophylactic Antibiotic Stopped[2]	115	100%	98%	98%
Prophylactic Antibiotic Timing[2]	118	97%	98%	99%
Prophylactic Antibiotic Timing (Outpatient)	44	89%	96%	98%
Urinary Catheter Removal[2]	129	99%	97%	97%
Survey of Patients' Hospital Experiences				
Area Around Room 'Always' Quiet at Night	300+	66%	57%	61%
Doctors 'Always' Communicated Well	300+	83%	81%	82%
Home Recovery Information Given	300+	87%	86%	85%
Hospital Given 9 or 10 on 10 Point Scale	300+	77%	70%	71%
Meds 'Always' Explained Before Given	300+	64%	65%	64%
Nurses 'Always' Communicated Well	300+	81%	79%	79%
Pain 'Always' Well Controlled	300+	72%	71%	71%
Room and Bathroom 'Always' Clean	300+	77%	74%	73%
Timely Help 'Always' Received	300+	65%	68%	68%
Would Definitely Recommend Hospital	300+	83%	72%	71%
Use of Medical Imaging				
Cardiac Imaging Stress Test before Surgery	95	7.4%	4.7%	5.3%
Combination Abdominal CT Scan	281	9.6%	6.6%	10.5%
Combination Brain/Sinus CT Scan[1]	-	-	2.1%	2.7%
Combination Chest CT Scan	175	1.1%	1.1%	2.7%
Follow-up Mammogram/Ultrasound	531	8.9%	8.9%	8.8%
Lumbar Spine MRI for Low Back Pain[1]	-	-	41.7%	37.2%

Samaritan Pacific Communities Hospital

930 Sw Abbey Street Phone: 541-265-2244
Newport, OR 97365 Fax: 541-574-4664
URL: www.samhealth.org
Type: Critical Access Hospitals Emergency Services: Yes
Ownership: Voluntary non-profit - Private Beds: 48

Key Personnel:
CEO/President. . . . . David C Bigelow

Measure	Cases	This Hosp.	State Avg.	U.S. Avg.
Blood Clot Prevention and Treatment				
Anticoagulation Overlap Therapy[1,2]	-	-	95%	93%
ICU Venous Thromboembolism Prophylaxis[2]	27	89%	87%	92%
Incidence of Potentially Preventable VTE[2,7]	-	-	13%	10%
UFH with Dosages/Platelet Monitoring[1,2]	-	-	100%	97%
Venous Thromboembolism Prophylaxis[2]	93	92%	83%	85%
Warfarin Therapy Discharge Instructions[1,2]	-	-	54%	75%
Chest Pain/Possible Heart Attack Care				
Aspirin Given Within 24 Hours of Arrival	-	-	97%	96%
Fibrinolytic Meds Within 30 Min. of Arrival	-	-	57%	58%
Average Time to ECG (minutes)	-	-	9	7
Average Time to Transfer (minutes)	-	-	52	60
Children's Asthma Care				
Received Home Management Plan of Care	-	-	-	88%
Received Reliever Medication	-	-	-	100%
Received Systemic Corticosteroids	-	-	-	100%
Emergency Department				
Admittance Decision Time (minutes)[2]	260	74	85	98
Head CT Results Within 45 Min. of Arrival	-	-	45%	57%
Patients Who Left ER Before Being Seen	-	-	2%	2%
Time from ER Arrival to Admit. (minutes)[2]	394	208	235	274
Time from ER Arrival to Discharge (minutes)	-	-	136	134
Time in ER Before Being Evaluated (minutes)	-	-	27	26
Time to Pain Meds for Fractures (minutes)	-	-	56	57
Heart Attack Care				
Aspirin Given at Discharge[1]	-	-	99%	99%
Fibrinolytic Meds Within 30 Min. of Arrival[7]	-	-	57%	54%
PCI Within 90 Minutes of Arrival[7]	-	-	93%	96%
Statin Prescribed at Discharge[1]	-	-	98%	98%
Heart Failure Care				
ACE Inhibitor or ARB for LVSD	13	92%	96%	97%
Discharge Instructions Given	44	84%	93%	94%
Evaluation of LVS Function	47	94%	99%	99%
Medicare Spending				
Medicare Spending per Patient (ratio)	-	-	0.88	0.98
Pneumonia Care				
Appropriate Initial Antibiotic Given	43	93%	96%	95%
Blood Culture Timing	61	93%	98%	98%
Pregnancy and Delivery Care				
Newborn Deliveries Scheduled Early[1,3]	-	-	3%	6%
Preventive Care				
Immunization for Influenza[2]	260	86%	86%	90%
Immunization for Pneumonia[2]	334	76%	88%	92%
Stroke Care				
Anticoagulation Therapy for Atrial Fibrillation[1]	-	-	94%	95%
Antithrombotic Therapy Timing[1]	-	-	97%	98%
Assessed for Rehabilitation	19	89%	96%	97%
Discharged on Antithrombotic Therapy	17	100%	99%	99%
Discharged on Statin Medication	13	85%	93%	94%
Thrombolytic Therapy Timing[1]	-	-	55%	66%
Venous Thromboembolism Prophylaxis	15	100%	90%	94%
Written Stroke Educational Materials Given	11	100%	81%	88%
Surgical Care Improvement Project				
Appropriate Beta Blocker Usage	12	92%	98%	98%
Appropriate VTP Within 24 Hours	58	84%	97%	98%
Controlled Postoperative Blood Glucose[7]	-	-	98%	97%
Perioperative Temperature Management	72	100%	100%	100%
Prophylactic Antibiotic Selection	34	85%	99%	99%
Prophylactic Antibiotic Selection (Outpatient)	-	-	98%	98%
Prophylactic Antibiotic Stopped	31	90%	98%	98%
Prophylactic Antibiotic Timing	34	94%	98%	99%
Prophylactic Antibiotic Timing (Outpatient)	-	-	96%	98%
Urinary Catheter Removal	45	93%	97%	97%
Survey of Patients' Hospital Experiences				
Area Around Room 'Always' Quiet at Night	300+	59%	57%	61%
Doctors 'Always' Communicated Well	300+	83%	81%	82%
Home Recovery Information Given	300+	84%	86%	85%
Hospital Given 9 or 10 on 10 Point Scale	300+	69%	70%	71%
Meds 'Always' Explained Before Given	300+	70%	65%	64%
Nurses 'Always' Communicated Well	300+	82%	79%	79%
Pain 'Always' Well Controlled	300+	71%	71%	71%

NOTE: Hospital profiles are in alphabetical order by state, then city, then hospital within the city; Rankings exclude hospitals with less than 25 cases except for patient surveys which excludes hospitals with less than 100 cases; (a) 100-299 cases; (1) The number of cases/patients is too few to report; (2) Data submitted were based on a sample of cases/patients; (3) Results are based on a shorter time period than required; (4) Data suppressed by CMS for one or more quarters; (5) Results are not available for this reporting period; (6) Fewer than 100 patients completed the HCAHPS survey; (7) No cases met the criteria for this measure; (8) The lower limit of the confidence interval cannot be calculated if the number of observed infections equals zero; (9) No data are available from the state/territory for this reporting period; (10) The scores shown reflect fewer than 50 completed surveys; (11) There were discrepancies in the data collection process; (12) This measure does not apply to this hospital for this reporting period; (13) Results cannot be calculated for this reporting period; (14) The results for this state are combined with nearby states to protect confidentiality; Please refer to the User's Guide for a full explanation of data.

Room and Bathroom 'Always' Clean	300+	76%	74%	73%
Timely Help 'Always' Received	300+	82%	68%	68%
Would Definitely Recommend Hospital	300+	71%	72%	71%
Use of Medical Imaging				
Cardiac Imaging Stress Test before Surgery	-	-	4.7%	5.3%
Combination Abdominal CT Scan	-	-	6.6%	10.5%
Combination Brain/Sinus CT Scan	-	-	2.1%	2.7%
Combination Chest CT Scan	-	-	1.1%	2.7%
Follow-up Mammogram/Ultrasound	-	-	8.9%	8.8%
Lumbar Spine MRI for Low Back Pain	-	-	41.7%	37.2%

Saint Alphonsus Medical Center - Ontario

351 Sw 9th Street
Ontario, OR 97914
Phone: 541-881-7000
Fax: 541-881-7184
URL: www.holyrosary-ontario.org
Type: Acute Care Hospitals
Emergency Services: Yes
Ownership: Voluntary non-profit - Church
Beds: 49

Key Personnel:
Chief of Medical Staff. . . . . Pamela Bruce, MD
CEO/President. . . . . Mark Dalley
Pediatric In-Patient Care . . . . Sandra Dunbrasky, MD
CEO . . . . Karl Keeler
Radiology. . . . . Fred Oyer, MD
Infection Control. . . . . Patrick Plummer, MD
Quality Assurance . . . . Morris Smith, MD
Operating Room. . . . . Frank Spokas, MD

Measure	Cases	This Hosp.	State Avg.	U.S. Avg.
Blood Clot Prevention and Treatment				
Anticoagulation Overlap Therapy[2]	25	100%	95%	93%
ICU Venous Thromboembolism Prophylaxis[2]	47	96%	87%	92%
Incidence of Potentially Preventable VTE[1,2]	-	-	13%	10%
UFH with Dosages/Platelet Monitoring[2]	22	100%	100%	97%
Venous Thromboembolism Prophylaxis[2]	111	86%	83%	85%
Warfarin Therapy Discharge Instructions[2]	21	95%	54%	75%
Chest Pain/Possible Heart Attack Care				
Aspirin Given Within 24 Hours of Arrival	67	97%	97%	96%
Fibrinolytic Meds Within 30 Min. of Arrival[1]	-	-	57%	58%
Average Time to ECG (minutes)	70	9	9	7
Average Time to Transfer (minutes)[1]	-	-	52	60
Children's Asthma Care				
Received Home Management Plan of Care	-	-	-	88%
Received Reliever Medication	-	-	-	100%
Received Systemic Corticosteroids	-	-	-	100%
Emergency Department				
Admittance Decision Time (minutes)[2]	189	104	85	98
Head CT Results Within 45 Min. of Arrival	20	35%	45%	57%
Patients Who Left ER Before Being Seen	20,467	3%	2%	2%
Time from ER Arrival to Admit. (minutes)[2]	212	295	235	274
Time from ER Arrival to Discharge (minutes)	350	143	136	134
Time in ER Before Being Evaluated (minutes)	267	25	27	26
Time to Pain Meds for Fractures (minutes)	102	54	56	57
Heart Attack Care				
Aspirin Given at Discharge[1,3]	-	-	99%	99%
Fibrinolytic Meds Within 30 Min. of Arrival[3,7]	-	-	57%	54%
PCI Within 90 Minutes of Arrival[3,7]	-	-	93%	96%
Statin Prescribed at Discharge[1,3]	-	-	98%	98%
Heart Failure Care				
ACE Inhibitor or ARB for LVSD	21	100%	96%	97%
Discharge Instructions Given	49	100%	93%	94%
Evaluation of LVS Function	62	98%	99%	99%
Medicare Spending				
Medicare Spending per Patient (ratio)	-	0.93	0.88	0.98
Pneumonia Care				
Appropriate Initial Antibiotic Given	62	98%	96%	95%
Blood Culture Timing	75	99%	98%	98%
Pregnancy and Delivery Care				
Newborn Deliveries Scheduled Early[2]	122	0%	3%	6%
Preventive Care				
Immunization for Influenza[2]	260	73%	86%	90%
Immunization for Pneumonia[2]	273	88%	88%	92%
Stroke Care				
Anticoagulation Therapy for Atrial Fibrillation[1]	-	-	94%	95%
Antithrombotic Therapy Timing	20	100%	97%	98%
Assessed for Rehabilitation	24	100%	96%	97%
Discharged on Antithrombotic Therapy	18	100%	99%	99%
Discharged on Statin Medication	14	93%	93%	94%
Thrombolytic Therapy Timing	12	0%	55%	66%
Venous Thromboembolism Prophylaxis	22	100%	90%	94%
Written Stroke Educational Materials Given	11	82%	81%	88%
Surgical Care Improvement Project				
Appropriate Beta Blocker Usage	58	97%	98%	98%
Appropriate VTP Within 24 Hours	280	99%	97%	98%
Controlled Postoperative Blood Glucose[7]	-	-	98%	97%
Perioperative Temperature Management	322	100%	100%	100%
Prophylactic Antibiotic Selection	248	98%	99%	99%
Prophylactic Antibiotic Selection (Outpatient)	14	86%	98%	98%
Prophylactic Antibiotic Stopped	241	97%	98%	98%
Prophylactic Antibiotic Timing	248	100%	98%	99%
Prophylactic Antibiotic Timing (Outpatient)	14	100%	96%	98%
Urinary Catheter Removal	204	100%	97%	97%
Survey of Patients' Hospital Experiences				
Area Around Room 'Always' Quiet at Night	300+	59%	57%	61%
Doctors 'Always' Communicated Well	300+	83%	81%	82%
Home Recovery Information Given	300+	89%	86%	85%
Hospital Given 9 or 10 on 10 Point Scale	300+	68%	70%	71%
Meds 'Always' Explained Before Given	300+	61%	65%	64%
Nurses 'Always' Communicated Well	300+	78%	79%	79%
Pain 'Always' Well Controlled	300+	72%	71%	71%
Room and Bathroom 'Always' Clean	300+	71%	74%	73%
Timely Help 'Always' Received	300+	72%	68%	68%
Would Definitely Recommend Hospital	300+	62%	72%	71%
Use of Medical Imaging				
Cardiac Imaging Stress Test before Surgery	183	3.8%	4.7%	5.3%
Combination Abdominal CT Scan	551	5.3%	6.6%	10.5%
Combination Brain/Sinus CT Scan	469	1.5%	2.1%	2.7%
Combination Chest CT Scan	207	0.5%	1.1%	2.7%
Follow-up Mammogram/Ultrasound	863	6.8%	8.9%	8.8%
Lumbar Spine MRI for Low Back Pain[1]	-	-	41.7%	37.2%

Providence Willamette Falls Medical Center

1500 Division Street
Oregon City, OR 97045
Phone: 503-657-6915
Fax: 503-557-2101
E-mail: wfh@wfhonline.org
URL: www.willamettefallshospital.org
Type: Acute Care Hospitals
Emergency Services: Yes
Ownership: Voluntary non-profit - Private
Beds: 143

Key Personnel:
Anesthesiology. . . . . Michael Bespaly, MD
CEO/President. . . . . Russ Reinhard

Measure	Cases	This Hosp.	State Avg.	U.S. Avg.
Blood Clot Prevention and Treatment				
Anticoagulation Overlap Therapy[2]	22	86%	95%	93%
ICU Venous Thromboembolism Prophylaxis[2]	174	88%	87%	92%
Incidence of Potentially Preventable VTE[1,2]	-	-	13%	10%
UFH with Dosages/Platelet Monitoring[1,2]	-	-	100%	97%
Venous Thromboembolism Prophylaxis[2]	147	84%	83%	85%
Warfarin Therapy Discharge Instructions[2]	21	5%	54%	75%
Chest Pain/Possible Heart Attack Care				
Aspirin Given Within 24 Hours of Arrival	53	98%	97%	96%
Fibrinolytic Meds Within 30 Min. of Arrival[7]	-	-	57%	58%
Average Time to ECG (minutes)	56	7	9	7
Average Time to Transfer (minutes)	19	45	52	60
Children's Asthma Care				
Received Home Management Plan of Care	-	-	-	88%
Received Reliever Medication	-	-	-	100%
Received Systemic Corticosteroids	-	-	-	100%
Emergency Department				
Admittance Decision Time (minutes)[2]	274	70	85	98
Head CT Results Within 45 Min. of Arrival[1]	-	-	45%	57%
Patients Who Left ER Before Being Seen	29,858	2%	2%	2%
Time from ER Arrival to Admit. (minutes)[2]	285	265	235	274
Time from ER Arrival to Discharge (minutes)	345	150	136	134
Time in ER Before Being Evaluated (minutes)	120	39	27	26
Time to Pain Meds for Fractures (minutes)	134	67	56	57
Heart Attack Care				
Aspirin Given at Discharge[2]	11	100%	99%	99%
Fibrinolytic Meds Within 30 Min. of Arrival[2,7]	-	-	57%	54%
PCI Within 90 Minutes of Arrival[2,7]	-	-	93%	96%
Statin Prescribed at Discharge[1,2]	-	-	98%	98%
Heart Failure Care				
ACE Inhibitor or ARB for LVSD[2]	39	100%	96%	97%
Discharge Instructions Given[2]	88	88%	93%	94%
Evaluation of LVS Function[2]	102	100%	99%	99%
Medicare Spending				
Medicare Spending per Patient (ratio)	-	0.88	0.88	0.98
Pneumonia Care				
Appropriate Initial Antibiotic Given[2]	89	96%	96%	95%
Blood Culture Timing[2]	129	100%	98%	98%
Pregnancy and Delivery Care				
Newborn Deliveries Scheduled Early	88	2%	3%	6%
Preventive Care				
Immunization for Influenza[2]	456	87%	86%	90%
Immunization for Pneumonia[2]	458	81%	88%	92%
Stroke Care				
Anticoagulation Therapy for Atrial Fibrillation[1,2]	-	-	94%	95%
Antithrombotic Therapy Timing[2]	30	100%	97%	98%
Assessed for Rehabilitation[2]	40	92%	96%	97%
Discharged on Antithrombotic Therapy[2]	40	100%	99%	99%
Discharged on Statin Medication[2]	31	97%	93%	94%
Thrombolytic Therapy Timing[1,2]	-	-	55%	66%
Venous Thromboembolism Prophylaxis[2]	29	86%	90%	94%
Written Stroke Educational Materials Given[2]	28	71%	81%	88%
Surgical Care Improvement Project				
Appropriate Beta Blocker Usage[2]	76	95%	98%	98%
Appropriate VTP Within 24 Hours[2]	286	93%	97%	98%
Controlled Postoperative Blood Glucose[2,7]	-	-	98%	97%
Perioperative Temperature Management[2]	347	100%	100%	100%
Prophylactic Antibiotic Selection[2]	239	99%	99%	99%
Prophylactic Antibiotic Selection (Outpatient)	116	95%	98%	98%
Prophylactic Antibiotic Stopped[2]	237	99%	98%	98%
Prophylactic Antibiotic Timing[2]	239	97%	98%	99%
Prophylactic Antibiotic Timing (Outpatient)	117	96%	96%	98%
Urinary Catheter Removal[2]	62	89%	97%	97%
Survey of Patients' Hospital Experiences				
Area Around Room 'Always' Quiet at Night	300+	53%	57%	61%
Doctors 'Always' Communicated Well	300+	82%	81%	82%
Home Recovery Information Given	300+	86%	86%	85%
Hospital Given 9 or 10 on 10 Point Scale	300+	65%	70%	71%
Meds 'Always' Explained Before Given	300+	68%	65%	64%
Nurses 'Always' Communicated Well	300+	78%	79%	79%
Pain 'Always' Well Controlled	300+	68%	71%	71%
Room and Bathroom 'Always' Clean	300+	70%	74%	73%
Timely Help 'Always' Received	300+	58%	68%	68%
Would Definitely Recommend Hospital	300+	72%	72%	71%
Use of Medical Imaging				
Cardiac Imaging Stress Test before Surgery[1]	-	-	4.7%	5.3%
Combination Abdominal CT Scan	293	3.4%	6.6%	10.5%
Combination Brain/Sinus CT Scan[1]	-	-	2.1%	2.7%
Combination Chest CT Scan	149	0.0%	1.1%	2.7%
Follow-up Mammogram/Ultrasound	617	15.1%	8.9%	8.8%
Lumbar Spine MRI for Low Back Pain	74	41.9%	41.7%	37.2%

Saint Anthony Hospital

2801 Saint Anthony Way
Pendleton, OR 97801
Phone: 541-276-5121
Fax: 541-278-3227
URL: www.sahpendleton.org
Type: Critical Access Hospitals
Emergency Services: Yes
Ownership: Voluntary non-profit - Church
Beds: 49

Key Personnel:
Chairman/CEO . . . . Robert J. Blanc
Operating Room. . . . . Thom Clarke, RN
President . . . . Harry Geller
Infection Control. . . . . Dean Kindle, RN
Quality Assurance . . . . Dean Kindle, RN
Emergency Room . . . . Kathy Stein, DO
Chief of Medical Staff . . . . Malcolm Townsley

Measure	Cases	This Hosp.	State Avg.	U.S. Avg.
Blood Clot Prevention and Treatment				
Anticoagulation Overlap Therapy[1,2]	-	-	95%	93%
ICU Venous Thromboembolism Prophylaxis[2]	12	92%	87%	92%
Incidence of Potentially Preventable VTE[2,7]	-	-	13%	10%

NOTE: Hospital profiles are in alphabetical order by state, then city, then hospital within the city; Rankings exclude hospitals with less than 25 cases except for patient surveys which excludes hospitals with less than 100 cases; (a) 100-299 cases; (1) The number of cases/patients is too few to report; (2) Data submitted were based on a sample of cases/patients; (3) Results are based on a shorter time period than required; (4) Data suppressed by CMS for one or more quarters; (5) Results are not available for this reporting period; (6) Fewer than 100 patients completed the HCAHPS survey; (7) No cases met the criteria for this measure; (8) The lower limit of the confidence interval cannot be calculated if the number of observed infections equals zero; (9) No data are available from the state/territory for this reporting period; (10) The scores shown reflect fewer than 50 completed surveys; (11) There were discrepancies in the data collection process; (12) This measure does not apply to this hospital for this reporting period; (13) Results cannot be calculated for this reporting period; (14) The results for this state are combined with nearby states to protect confidentiality; Please refer to the User's Guide for a full explanation of data.

Measure	Cases	This Hosp.	State Avg.	U.S. Avg.
UFH with Dosages/Platelet Monitoring[1,2]	-	-	100%	97%
Venous Thromboembolism Prophylaxis[2]	24	92%	83%	85%
Warfarin Therapy Discharge Instructions[1,2]	-	-	54%	75%
Chest Pain/Possible Heart Attack Care				
Aspirin Given Within 24 Hours of Arrival	-	-	97%	96%
Fibrinolytic Meds Within 30 Min. of Arrival	-	-	57%	58%
Average Time to ECG (minutes)	-	-	9	7
Average Time to Transfer (minutes)	-	-	52	60
Children's Asthma Care				
Received Home Management Plan of Care	-	-	-	88%
Received Reliever Medication	-	-	-	100%
Received Systemic Corticosteroids	-	-	-	100%
Emergency Department				
Admittance Decision Time (minutes)[5]	-	-	85	98
Head CT Results Within 45 Min. of Arrival	-	-	45%	57%
Patients Who Left ER Before Being Seen	-	-	2%	2%
Time from ER Arrival to Admit. (minutes)[5]	-	-	235	274
Time from ER Arrival to Discharge (minutes)	-	-	136	134
Time in ER Before Being Evaluated (minutes)	-	-	27	26
Time to Pain Meds for Fractures (minutes)	-	-	56	57
Heart Attack Care				
Aspirin Given at Discharge[1,2]	-	-	99%	99%
Fibrinolytic Meds Within 30 Min. of Arrival[2,3]	-	-	57%	54%
PCI Within 90 Minutes of Arrival[2,3]	-	-	93%	96%
Statin Prescribed at Discharge[1,2]	-	-	98%	98%
Heart Failure Care				
ACE Inhibitor or ARB for LVSD[1,2]	-	-	96%	97%
Discharge Instructions Given[2]	19	53%	93%	94%
Evaluation of LVS Function[2]	22	100%	99%	99%
Medicare Spending				
Medicare Spending per Patient (ratio)	-	-	0.88	0.98
Pneumonia Care				
Appropriate Initial Antibiotic Given[1,2]	-	-	96%	95%
Blood Culture Timing[2]	22	95%	98%	98%
Pregnancy and Delivery Care				
Newborn Deliveries Scheduled Early[5]	-	-	3%	6%
Preventive Care				
Immunization for Influenza[5]	-	-	86%	90%
Immunization for Pneumonia[5]	-	-	88%	92%
Stroke Care				
Anticoagulation Therapy for Atrial Fibrillation[1,2]	-	-	94%	95%
Antithrombotic Therapy Timing[2]	12	100%	97%	98%
Assessed for Rehabilitation[2]	12	100%	96%	97%
Discharged on Antithrombotic Therapy[2]	12	100%	99%	99%
Discharged on Statin Medication[1,2]	-	-	93%	94%
Thrombolytic Therapy Timing[1,2]	-	-	55%	66%
Venous Thromboembolism Prophylaxis[2]	13	100%	90%	94%
Written Stroke Educational Materials Given[1,2]	-	-	81%	88%
Surgical Care Improvement Project				
Appropriate Beta Blocker Usage[2]	25	100%	98%	98%
Appropriate VTP Within 24 Hours[2]	102	100%	97%	98%
Controlled Postoperative Blood Glucose[2,3]	-	-	98%	97%
Perioperative Temperature Management[2,3]	31	100%	100%	100%
Prophylactic Antibiotic Selection[2]	97	97%	99%	99%
Prophylactic Antibiotic Selection (Outpatient)	-	-	98%	98%
Prophylactic Antibiotic Stopped[2]	95	89%	98%	98%
Prophylactic Antibiotic Timing[2]	97	96%	98%	99%
Prophylactic Antibiotic Timing (Outpatient)	-	-	96%	98%
Urinary Catheter Removal[1,2]	-	-	97%	97%
Survey of Patients' Hospital Experiences				
Area Around Room 'Always' Quiet at Night[5]	-	-	57%	61%
Doctors 'Always' Communicated Well[5]	-	-	81%	82%
Home Recovery Information Given[5]	-	-	86%	85%
Hospital Given 9 or 10 on 10 Point Scale[5]	-	-	70%	71%
Meds 'Always' Explained Before Given[5]	-	-	65%	64%
Nurses 'Always' Communicated Well[5]	-	-	79%	79%
Pain 'Always' Well Controlled[5]	-	-	71%	71%
Room and Bathroom 'Always' Clean[5]	-	-	74%	73%
Timely Help 'Always' Received[5]	-	-	68%	68%
Would Definitely Recommend Hospital[5]	-	-	72%	71%
Use of Medical Imaging				
Cardiac Imaging Stress Test before Surgery	-	-	4.7%	5.3%
Combination Abdominal CT Scan	-	-	6.6%	10.5%
Combination Brain/Sinus CT Scan	-	-	2.1%	2.7%
Combination Chest CT Scan	-	-	1.1%	2.7%
Follow-up Mammogram/Ultrasound	-	-	8.9%	8.8%
Lumbar Spine MRI for Low Back Pain	-	-	41.7%	37.2%

Adventist Medical Center

10123 Se Market Street
Portland, OR 97216
Phone: 503-257-2500
Fax: 503-251-6318
URL: www.adventisthealth.com
Type: Acute Care Hospitals
Emergency Services: Yes
Ownership: Voluntary non-profit - Church
Beds: 302

Key Personnel:
Emergency Room . . . . Joyce Goitein
Radiology. . . . . Scott Israel, MD
Quality Assurance . . . . Carolyn Kozik
Anesthesiology. . . . . Robert S Lovitz, MD
CEO/President. . . . . Joyce Newmyer
Cardiac Laboratory. . . . . Larry Popplewell
Chief of Medical Staff . . . . Wesley Rippeys, MD

Measure	Cases	This Hosp.	State Avg.	U.S. Avg.
Blood Clot Prevention and Treatment				
Anticoagulation Overlap Therapy[2]	62	97%	95%	93%
ICU Venous Thromboembolism Prophylaxis[2]	59	83%	87%	92%
Incidence of Potentially Preventable VTE[1,2]	-	-	13%	10%
UFH with Dosages/Platelet Monitoring[2]	15	100%	100%	97%
Venous Thromboembolism Prophylaxis[2]	262	78%	83%	85%
Warfarin Therapy Discharge Instructions[2]	53	79%	54%	75%
Chest Pain/Possible Heart Attack Care				
Aspirin Given Within 24 Hours of Arrival[1]	-	-	97%	96%
Fibrinolytic Meds Within 30 Min. of Arrival[7]	-	-	57%	58%
Average Time to ECG (minutes)[1]	-	-	9	7
Average Time to Transfer (minutes)[7]	-	-	52	60
Children's Asthma Care				
Received Home Management Plan of Care	-	-	-	88%
Received Reliever Medication	-	-	-	100%
Received Systemic Corticosteroids	-	-	-	100%
Emergency Department				
Admittance Decision Time (minutes)[2]	523	89	85	98
Head CT Results Within 45 Min. of Arrival	16	81%	45%	57%
Patients Who Left ER Before Being Seen	50,418	1%	2%	2%
Time from ER Arrival to Admit. (minutes)[2]	528	211	235	274
Time from ER Arrival to Discharge (minutes)	345	162	136	134
Time in ER Before Being Evaluated (minutes)	326	32	27	26
Time to Pain Meds for Fractures (minutes)	135	47	56	57
Heart Attack Care				
Aspirin Given at Discharge	261	100%	99%	99%
Fibrinolytic Meds Within 30 Min. of Arrival[7]	-	-	57%	54%
PCI Within 90 Minutes of Arrival	66	97%	93%	96%
Statin Prescribed at Discharge	255	98%	98%	98%
Heart Failure Care				
ACE Inhibitor or ARB for LVSD	79	99%	96%	97%
Discharge Instructions Given	275	98%	93%	94%
Evaluation of LVS Function	308	100%	99%	99%
Medicare Spending				
Medicare Spending per Patient (ratio)	-	0.85	0.88	0.98
Pneumonia Care				
Appropriate Initial Antibiotic Given	129	98%	96%	95%
Blood Culture Timing	259	100%	98%	98%
Pregnancy and Delivery Care				
Newborn Deliveries Scheduled Early[2]	19	5%	3%	6%
Preventive Care				
Immunization for Influenza[2]	532	87%	86%	90%
Immunization for Pneumonia[2]	653	81%	88%	92%
Stroke Care				
Anticoagulation Therapy for Atrial Fibrillation	16	100%	94%	95%
Antithrombotic Therapy Timing	81	99%	97%	98%
Assessed for Rehabilitation	111	98%	96%	97%
Discharged on Antithrombotic Therapy	109	98%	99%	99%
Discharged on Statin Medication	80	100%	93%	94%
Thrombolytic Therapy Timing[1]	-	-	55%	66%
Venous Thromboembolism Prophylaxis	87	97%	90%	94%
Written Stroke Educational Materials Given	70	96%	81%	88%
Surgical Care Improvement Project				
Appropriate Beta Blocker Usage[2]	259	97%	98%	98%
Appropriate VTP Within 24 Hours[2]	544	97%	97%	98%
Controlled Postoperative Blood Glucose[2]	136	98%	98%	97%
Perioperative Temperature Management[2]	726	100%	100%	100%
Prophylactic Antibiotic Selection[2]	588	100%	99%	99%
Prophylactic Antibiotic Selection (Outpatient)	261	98%	98%	98%
Prophylactic Antibiotic Stopped[2]	588	98%	98%	98%
Prophylactic Antibiotic Timing[2]	588	99%	98%	99%
Prophylactic Antibiotic Timing (Outpatient)	266	95%	96%	98%
Urinary Catheter Removal[2]	568	100%	97%	97%
Survey of Patients' Hospital Experiences				
Area Around Room 'Always' Quiet at Night	300+	57%	57%	61%
Doctors 'Always' Communicated Well	300+	80%	81%	82%
Home Recovery Information Given	300+	88%	86%	85%
Hospital Given 9 or 10 on 10 Point Scale	300+	69%	70%	71%
Meds 'Always' Explained Before Given	300+	65%	65%	64%
Nurses 'Always' Communicated Well	300+	79%	79%	79%
Pain 'Always' Well Controlled	300+	72%	71%	71%
Room and Bathroom 'Always' Clean	300+	70%	74%	73%
Timely Help 'Always' Received	300+	67%	68%	68%
Would Definitely Recommend Hospital	300+	75%	72%	71%
Use of Medical Imaging				
Cardiac Imaging Stress Test before Surgery	121	5.0%	4.7%	5.3%
Combination Abdominal CT Scan	594	11.8%	6.6%	10.5%
Combination Brain/Sinus CT Scan	500	2.6%	2.1%	2.7%
Combination Chest CT Scan	326	5.2%	1.1%	2.7%
Follow-up Mammogram/Ultrasound	1,086	5.6%	8.9%	8.8%
Lumbar Spine MRI for Low Back Pain	154	46.1%	41.7%	37.2%

Legacy Emanuel Medical Center

2801 N Gantenbein Avenue
Portland, OR 97227
Phone: 503-413-2200
Fax: 503-415-5777
URL: www.legacyhealth.org
Type: Acute Care Hospitals
Emergency Services: Yes
Ownership: Voluntary non-profit - Private
Beds: 554

Key Personnel:
CEO/President. . . . . George J Brown, MD

Measure	Cases	This Hosp.	State Avg.	U.S. Avg.
Blood Clot Prevention and Treatment				
Anticoagulation Overlap Therapy[2]	71	100%	95%	93%
ICU Venous Thromboembolism Prophylaxis[2]	155	94%	87%	92%
Incidence of Potentially Preventable VTE[2]	37	3%	13%	10%
UFH with Dosages/Platelet Monitoring[2]	26	100%	100%	97%
Venous Thromboembolism Prophylaxis[2]	234	80%	83%	85%
Warfarin Therapy Discharge Instructions[2]	50	98%	54%	75%
Chest Pain/Possible Heart Attack Care				
Aspirin Given Within 24 Hours of Arrival	12	100%	97%	96%
Fibrinolytic Meds Within 30 Min. of Arrival[3,7]	-	-	57%	58%
Average Time to ECG (minutes)	12	2	9	7
Average Time to Transfer (minutes)[3,7]	-	-	52	60
Children's Asthma Care				
Received Home Management Plan of Care	184	88%	-	88%
Received Reliever Medication	184	100%	-	100%
Received Systemic Corticosteroids	184	100%	-	100%
Emergency Department				
Admittance Decision Time (minutes)[2]	600	90	85	98
Head CT Results Within 45 Min. of Arrival[1]	-	-	45%	57%
Patients Who Left ER Before Being Seen	60,696	2%	2%	2%
Time from ER Arrival to Admit. (minutes)[2]	606	197	235	274
Time from ER Arrival to Discharge (minutes)	346	141	136	134
Time in ER Before Being Evaluated (minutes)	367	36	27	26
Time to Pain Meds for Fractures (minutes)	194	34	56	57
Heart Attack Care				
Aspirin Given at Discharge	148	99%	99%	99%
Fibrinolytic Meds Within 30 Min. of Arrival[7]	-	-	57%	54%
PCI Within 90 Minutes of Arrival	33	91%	93%	96%
Statin Prescribed at Discharge	141	99%	98%	98%
Heart Failure Care				
ACE Inhibitor or ARB for LVSD	72	100%	96%	97%
Discharge Instructions Given	187	97%	93%	94%
Evaluation of LVS Function	201	100%	99%	99%
Medicare Spending				
Medicare Spending per Patient (ratio)	-	0.91	0.88	0.98

NOTE: Hospital profiles are in alphabetical order by state, then city, then hospital within the city; Rankings exclude hospitals with less than 25 cases except for patient surveys which excludes hospitals with less than 100 cases; (a) 100-299 cases; (1) The number of cases/patients is too few to report; (2) Data submitted were based on a sample of cases/patients; (3) Results are based on a shorter time period than required; (4) Data suppressed by CMS for one or more quarters; (5) Results are not available for this reporting period; (6) Fewer than 100 patients completed the HCAHPS survey; (7) No cases met the criteria for this measure; (8) The lower limit of the confidence interval cannot be calculated if the number of observed infections equals zero; (9) No data are available from the state/territory for this reporting period; (10) The scores shown reflect fewer than 50 completed surveys; (11) There were discrepancies in the data collection process; (12) This measure does not apply to this hospital for this reporting period; (13) Results cannot be calculated for this reporting period; (14) The results for this state are combined with nearby states to protect confidentiality; Please refer to the User's Guide for a full explanation of data.

Measure	Cases	This Hosp.	State Avg.	U.S. Avg.
Pneumonia Care				
Appropriate Initial Antibiotic Given	73	100%	96%	95%
Blood Culture Timing	111	98%	98%	98%
Pregnancy and Delivery Care				
Newborn Deliveries Scheduled Early[2]	24	4%	3%	6%
Preventive Care				
Immunization for Influenza[2]	520	76%	86%	90%
Immunization for Pneumonia[2]	345	81%	88%	92%
Stroke Care				
Anticoagulation Therapy for Atrial Fibrillation	25	100%	94%	95%
Antithrombotic Therapy Timing	66	91%	97%	98%
Assessed for Rehabilitation	134	96%	96%	97%
Discharged on Antithrombotic Therapy	105	99%	99%	99%
Discharged on Statin Medication	78	95%	93%	94%
Thrombolytic Therapy Timing	29	97%	55%	66%
Venous Thromboembolism Prophylaxis	147	90%	90%	94%
Written Stroke Educational Materials Given	78	88%	81%	88%
Surgical Care Improvement Project				
Appropriate Beta Blocker Usage[2]	119	99%	98%	98%
Appropriate VTP Within 24 Hours[2]	164	98%	97%	98%
Controlled Postoperative Blood Glucose[2]	63	89%	98%	97%
Perioperative Temperature Management[2]	312	100%	100%	100%
Prophylactic Antibiotic Selection[2]	222	99%	99%	99%
Prophylactic Antibiotic Selection (Outpatient)	173	96%	98%	98%
Prophylactic Antibiotic Stopped[2]	220	96%	98%	98%
Prophylactic Antibiotic Timing[2]	222	99%	98%	99%
Prophylactic Antibiotic Timing (Outpatient)	173	94%	96%	98%
Urinary Catheter Removal[2]	207	94%	97%	97%
Survey of Patients' Hospital Experiences				
Area Around Room 'Always' Quiet at Night	300+	57%	57%	61%
Doctors 'Always' Communicated Well	300+	77%	81%	82%
Home Recovery Information Given	300+	89%	86%	85%
Hospital Given 9 or 10 on 10 Point Scale	300+	72%	70%	71%
Meds 'Always' Explained Before Given	300+	62%	65%	64%
Nurses 'Always' Communicated Well	300+	76%	79%	79%
Pain 'Always' Well Controlled	300+	70%	71%	71%
Room and Bathroom 'Always' Clean	300+	70%	74%	73%
Timely Help 'Always' Received	300+	60%	68%	68%
Would Definitely Recommend Hospital	300+	78%	72%	71%
Use of Medical Imaging				
Cardiac Imaging Stress Test before Surgery[1]	-	-	4.7%	5.3%
Combination Abdominal CT Scan	250	6.4%	6.6%	10.5%
Combination Brain/Sinus CT Scan	315	4.8%	2.1%	2.7%
Combination Chest CT Scan	131	0.8%	1.1%	2.7%
Follow-up Mammogram/Ultrasound	272	10.3%	8.9%	8.8%
Lumbar Spine MRI for Low Back Pain[1]	-	-	41.7%	37.2%

Legacy Good Samaritan Medical Center

1015 Nw 22nd Avenue, W121
Portland, OR 97210
Phone: 503-413-7682
Fax: 503-413-6347
URL: www.legacyhealth.org
Type: Acute Care Hospitals
Emergency Services: Yes
Ownership: Voluntary non-profit - Private
Beds: 539

Key Personnel:
Cardiac Laboratory. . . . . Margaret Allee
Radiology. . . . . Diane Bueit-Anderson
CEO/President. . . . . Lee Domanico
Coronary Care . . . . P Campbell Groner, III
Infection Control. . . . . Julia Marcotte
Quality Assurance . . . . Nancy McKean
Chief of Medical Staff . . . . Ted Schreck

Measure	Cases	This Hosp.	State Avg.	U.S. Avg.
Blood Clot Prevention and Treatment				
Anticoagulation Overlap Therapy[2]	45	100%	95%	93%
ICU Venous Thromboembolism Prophylaxis[2]	87	93%	87%	92%
Incidence of Potentially Preventable VTE[1,2]	-	-	13%	10%
UFH with Dosages/Platelet Monitoring[2]	16	100%	100%	97%
Venous Thromboembolism Prophylaxis[2]	283	92%	83%	85%
Warfarin Therapy Discharge Instructions[2]	41	95%	54%	75%
Chest Pain/Possible Heart Attack Care				
Aspirin Given Within 24 Hours of Arrival[1,3]	-	-	97%	96%
Fibrinolytic Meds Within 30 Min. of Arrival[5]	-	-	57%	58%
Average Time to ECG (minutes)[1,3]	-	-	9	7
Average Time to Transfer (minutes)[5]	-	-	52	60
Children's Asthma Care				
Received Home Management Plan of Care	-	-	-	88%
Received Reliever Medication	-	-	-	100%
Received Systemic Corticosteroids	-	-	-	100%
Emergency Department				
Admittance Decision Time (minutes)[2]	560	112	85	98
Head CT Results Within 45 Min. of Arrival[1]	-	-	45%	57%
Patients Who Left ER Before Being Seen	30,576	1%	2%	2%
Time from ER Arrival to Admit. (minutes)[2]	561	228	235	274
Time from ER Arrival to Discharge (minutes)	325	167	136	134
Time in ER Before Being Evaluated (minutes)	392	20	27	26
Time to Pain Meds for Fractures (minutes)	53	59	56	57
Heart Attack Care				
Aspirin Given at Discharge	216	100%	99%	99%
Fibrinolytic Meds Within 30 Min. of Arrival[7]	-	-	57%	54%
PCI Within 90 Minutes of Arrival	17	94%	93%	96%
Statin Prescribed at Discharge	212	100%	98%	98%
Heart Failure Care				
ACE Inhibitor or ARB for LVSD	77	96%	96%	97%
Discharge Instructions Given	202	98%	93%	94%
Evaluation of LVS Function	245	100%	99%	99%
Medicare Spending				
Medicare Spending per Patient (ratio)	-	0.93	0.88	0.98
Pneumonia Care				
Appropriate Initial Antibiotic Given	76	95%	96%	95%
Blood Culture Timing	143	99%	98%	98%
Pregnancy and Delivery Care				
Newborn Deliveries Scheduled Early[2]	30	7%	3%	6%
Preventive Care				
Immunization for Influenza[2]	578	93%	86%	90%
Immunization for Pneumonia[2]	717	96%	88%	92%
Stroke Care				
Anticoagulation Therapy for Atrial Fibrillation	12	100%	94%	95%
Antithrombotic Therapy Timing	63	98%	97%	98%
Assessed for Rehabilitation	90	97%	96%	97%
Discharged on Antithrombotic Therapy	79	100%	99%	99%
Discharged on Statin Medication	56	96%	93%	94%
Thrombolytic Therapy Timing	12	83%	55%	66%
Venous Thromboembolism Prophylaxis	85	95%	90%	94%
Written Stroke Educational Materials Given	54	98%	81%	88%
Surgical Care Improvement Project				
Appropriate Beta Blocker Usage[2]	182	100%	98%	98%
Appropriate VTP Within 24 Hours[2]	344	99%	97%	98%
Controlled Postoperative Blood Glucose[2]	148	97%	98%	97%
Perioperative Temperature Management[2]	415	100%	100%	100%
Prophylactic Antibiotic Selection[2]	400	99%	99%	99%
Prophylactic Antibiotic Selection (Outpatient)	437	98%	98%	98%
Prophylactic Antibiotic Stopped[2]	390	99%	98%	98%
Prophylactic Antibiotic Timing[2]	404	97%	98%	99%
Prophylactic Antibiotic Timing (Outpatient)	437	98%	96%	98%
Urinary Catheter Removal[2]	380	99%	97%	97%
Survey of Patients' Hospital Experiences				
Area Around Room 'Always' Quiet at Night	300+	57%	57%	61%
Doctors 'Always' Communicated Well	300+	79%	81%	82%
Home Recovery Information Given	300+	87%	86%	85%
Hospital Given 9 or 10 on 10 Point Scale	300+	74%	70%	71%
Meds 'Always' Explained Before Given	300+	63%	65%	64%
Nurses 'Always' Communicated Well	300+	77%	79%	79%
Pain 'Always' Well Controlled	300+	70%	71%	71%
Room and Bathroom 'Always' Clean	300+	71%	74%	73%
Timely Help 'Always' Received	300+	63%	68%	68%
Would Definitely Recommend Hospital	300+	77%	72%	71%
Use of Medical Imaging				
Cardiac Imaging Stress Test before Surgery[1]	-	-	4.7%	5.3%
Combination Abdominal CT Scan	562	6.0%	6.6%	10.5%
Combination Brain/Sinus CT Scan[1]	-	-	2.1%	2.7%
Combination Chest CT Scan	440	0.7%	1.1%	2.7%
Follow-up Mammogram/Ultrasound	1,311	9.1%	8.9%	8.8%
Lumbar Spine MRI for Low Back Pain	65	43.1%	41.7%	37.2%

OHSU Hospital & Clinics

3181 Sw Sam Jackson Park Road
Portland, OR 97239
Phone: 503-494-4036
Fax: 503-494-6469
URL: www.ohsu.edu
Type: Acute Care Hospitals
Emergency Services: Yes
Ownership: Voluntary non-profit - Other
Beds: 572

Key Personnel:
Quality Assurance . . . . Sue Gerberding
Radiology. . . . . Fred Keller, MD
Infection Control. . . . . Paul Lewis, MD
Operating Room. . . . . Margaret Montgomery
CEO/President. . . . . Joseph Robertson, MD, MBA
Pediatric Ambulatory Care . . . . . . Ron Rosenfeld, MD
Pediatric In-Patient Care . . . . Ron Rosenfeld, MD

Measure	Cases	This Hosp.	State Avg.	U.S. Avg.
Blood Clot Prevention and Treatment				
Anticoagulation Overlap Therapy[2]	69	94%	95%	93%
ICU Venous Thromboembolism Prophylaxis[2]	139	88%	87%	92%
Incidence of Potentially Preventable VTE[2]	66	5%	13%	10%
UFH with Dosages/Platelet Monitoring[2]	42	100%	100%	97%
Venous Thromboembolism Prophylaxis[2]	269	76%	83%	85%
Warfarin Therapy Discharge Instructions[2]	40	100%	54%	75%
Chest Pain/Possible Heart Attack Care				
Aspirin Given Within 24 Hours of Arrival[5]	-	-	97%	96%
Fibrinolytic Meds Within 30 Min. of Arrival[5]	-	-	57%	58%
Average Time to ECG (minutes)[5]	-	-	9	7
Average Time to Transfer (minutes)[5]	-	-	52	60
Children's Asthma Care				
Received Home Management Plan of Care	-	-	-	88%
Received Reliever Medication	-	-	-	100%
Received Systemic Corticosteroids	-	-	-	100%
Emergency Department				
Admittance Decision Time (minutes)[2]	232	109	85	98
Head CT Results Within 45 Min. of Arrival[1]	-	-	45%	57%
Patients Who Left ER Before Being Seen	46,782	2%	2%	2%
Time from ER Arrival to Admit. (minutes)[2]	233	257	235	274
Time from ER Arrival to Discharge (minutes)	358	204	136	134
Time in ER Before Being Evaluated (minutes)	383	37	27	26
Time to Pain Meds for Fractures (minutes)	141	66	56	57
Heart Attack Care				
Aspirin Given at Discharge[2]	218	100%	99%	99%
Fibrinolytic Meds Within 30 Min. of Arrival[2,7]	-	-	57%	54%
PCI Within 90 Minutes of Arrival[2]	21	95%	93%	96%
Statin Prescribed at Discharge[2]	217	100%	98%	98%
Heart Failure Care				
ACE Inhibitor or ARB for LVSD[2]	103	100%	96%	97%
Discharge Instructions Given[2]	239	96%	93%	94%
Evaluation of LVS Function[2]	270	100%	99%	99%
Medicare Spending				
Medicare Spending per Patient (ratio)	-	0.93	0.88	0.98
Pneumonia Care				
Appropriate Initial Antibiotic Given[2]	39	100%	96%	95%
Blood Culture Timing[2]	94	100%	98%	98%
Pregnancy and Delivery Care				
Newborn Deliveries Scheduled Early[2]	23	9%	3%	6%
Preventive Care				
Immunization for Influenza[2]	548	83%	86%	90%
Immunization for Pneumonia[2]	429	80%	88%	92%
Stroke Care				
Anticoagulation Therapy for Atrial Fibrillation[1,2]	-	-	94%	95%
Antithrombotic Therapy Timing[2]	30	97%	97%	98%
Assessed for Rehabilitation[2]	90	100%	96%	97%
Discharged on Antithrombotic Therapy[2]	51	100%	99%	99%
Discharged on Statin Medication[2]	38	92%	93%	94%
Thrombolytic Therapy Timing[1,2]	-	-	55%	66%
Venous Thromboembolism Prophylaxis[2]	89	99%	90%	94%
Written Stroke Educational Materials Given[2]	58	90%	81%	88%
Surgical Care Improvement Project				
Appropriate Beta Blocker Usage[2]	186	98%	98%	98%
Appropriate VTP Within 24 Hours[2]	356	95%	97%	98%
Controlled Postoperative Blood Glucose[2]	119	96%	98%	97%
Perioperative Temperature Management[2]	529	99%	100%	100%
Prophylactic Antibiotic Selection[2]	374	99%	99%	99%
Prophylactic Antibiotic Selection (Outpatient)	399	97%	98%	98%

NOTE: Hospital profiles are in alphabetical order by state, then city, then hospital within the city; Rankings exclude hospitals with less than 25 cases except for patient surveys which excludes hospitals with less than 100 cases; (a) 100-299 cases; (1) The number of cases/patients is too few to report; (2) Data submitted were based on a sample of cases/patients; (3) Results are based on a shorter time period than required; (4) Data suppressed by CMS for one or more quarters; (5) Results are not available for this reporting period; (6) Fewer than 100 patients completed the HCAHPS survey; (7) No cases met the criteria for this measure; (8) The lower limit of the confidence interval cannot be calculated if the number of observed infections equals zero; (9) No data are available from the state/territory for this reporting period; (10) The scores shown reflect fewer than 50 completed surveys; (11) There were discrepancies in the data collection process; (12) This measure does not apply to this hospital for this reporting period; (13) Results cannot be calculated for this reporting period; (14) The results for this state are combined with nearby states to protect confidentiality; Please refer to the User's Guide for a full explanation of data.

Measure	Cases	This Hosp.	State Avg.	U.S. Avg.
Prophylactic Antibiotic Stopped[2]	366	97%	98%	98%
Prophylactic Antibiotic Timing[2]	374	98%	98%	99%
Prophylactic Antibiotic Timing (Outpatient)	401	96%	96%	98%
Urinary Catheter Removal[2]	315	98%	97%	97%
Survey of Patients' Hospital Experiences				
Area Around Room 'Always' Quiet at Night	300+	54%	57%	61%
Doctors 'Always' Communicated Well	300+	78%	81%	82%
Home Recovery Information Given	300+	88%	86%	85%
Hospital Given 9 or 10 on 10 Point Scale	300+	75%	70%	71%
Meds 'Always' Explained Before Given	300+	63%	65%	64%
Nurses 'Always' Communicated Well	300+	76%	79%	79%
Pain 'Always' Well Controlled	300+	69%	71%	71%
Room and Bathroom 'Always' Clean	300+	70%	74%	73%
Timely Help 'Always' Received	300+	61%	68%	68%
Would Definitely Recommend Hospital	300+	81%	72%	71%
Use of Medical Imaging				
Cardiac Imaging Stress Test before Surgery	429	4.9%	4.7%	5.3%
Combination Abdominal CT Scan	1,742	15.4%	6.6%	10.5%
Combination Brain/Sinus CT Scan[1]	-	-	2.1%	2.7%
Combination Chest CT Scan	1,589	1.0%	1.1%	2.7%
Follow-up Mammogram/Ultrasound	960	8.0%	8.9%	8.8%
Lumbar Spine MRI for Low Back Pain	163	33.7%	41.7%	37.2%

Portland VA Medical Center

3710 Sw Us Veterans Hospital
Portland, OR 97239
Phone: 503-220-8262
Fax: 503-273-5319
E-mail: kim.winn@med.va.gov
URL: www.va.gov/portland/index.asp
Type: Acute Care - VA
Emergency Services: No
Ownership: Government Federal
Beds: 622

Key Personnel:
Hemotology Center . . . . Grover Bagby, MD
Patient Relations . . . . Kathleen M Chapman, RN, MN
Chief of Medical Staff . . . . John D Dryden, MD
Operating Room. . . . . James Edwards
Quality Assurance . . . . Beth Keeth
Radiology. . . . . Kathryn Morton, MD
Infection Control. . . . . Thomas Ward

Measure	Cases	This Hosp.	State Avg.	U.S. Avg.
Blood Clot Prevention and Treatment				
Anticoagulation Overlap Therapy	-	-	95%	93%
ICU Venous Thromboembolism Prophylaxis	-	-	87%	92%
Incidence of Potentially Preventable VTE	-	-	13%	10%
UFH with Dosages/Platelet Monitoring	-	-	100%	97%
Venous Thromboembolism Prophylaxis	-	-	83%	85%
Warfarin Therapy Discharge Instructions	-	-	54%	75%
Chest Pain/Possible Heart Attack Care				
Aspirin Given Within 24 Hours of Arrival	-	-	97%	96%
Fibrinolytic Meds Within 30 Min. of Arrival	-	-	57%	58%
Average Time to ECG (minutes)	-	-	9	7
Average Time to Transfer (minutes)	-	-	52	60
Children's Asthma Care				
Received Home Management Plan of Care	-	-	-	88%
Received Reliever Medication	-	-	-	100%
Received Systemic Corticosteroids	-	-	-	100%
Emergency Department				
Admittance Decision Time (minutes)	-	-	85	98
Head CT Results Within 45 Min. of Arrival	-	-	45%	57%
Patients Who Left ER Before Being Seen	-	-	2%	2%
Time from ER Arrival to Admit. (minutes)	-	-	235	274
Time from ER Arrival to Discharge (minutes)	-	-	136	134
Time in ER Before Being Evaluated (minutes)	-	-	27	26
Time to Pain Meds for Fractures (minutes)	-	-	56	57
Heart Attack Care				
Aspirin Given at Discharge	72	100%	99%	99%
Fibrinolytic Meds Within 30 Min. of Arrival[5]	-	-	57%	54%
PCI Within 90 Minutes of Arrival[1]	-	-	93%	96%
Statin Prescribed at Discharge	68	100%	98%	98%
Heart Failure Care				
ACE Inhibitor or ARB for LVSD	138	97%	96%	97%
Discharge Instructions Given	386	99%	93%	94%
Evaluation of LVS Function	421	100%	99%	99%
Medicare Spending				
Medicare Spending per Patient (ratio)	-	-	0.88	0.98
Pneumonia Care				
Appropriate Initial Antibiotic Given	93	98%	96%	95%
Blood Culture Timing	166	99%	98%	98%
Pregnancy and Delivery Care				
Newborn Deliveries Scheduled Early	-	-	3%	6%
Preventive Care				
Immunization for Influenza[5]	-	-	86%	90%
Immunization for Pneumonia[5]	-	-	88%	92%
Stroke Care				
Anticoagulation Therapy for Atrial Fibrillation	-	-	94%	95%
Antithrombotic Therapy Timing	-	-	97%	98%
Assessed for Rehabilitation	-	-	96%	97%
Discharged on Antithrombotic Therapy	-	-	99%	99%
Discharged on Statin Medication	-	-	93%	94%
Thrombolytic Therapy Timing	-	-	55%	66%
Venous Thromboembolism Prophylaxis	-	-	90%	94%
Written Stroke Educational Materials Given	-	-	81%	88%
Surgical Care Improvement Project				
Appropriate Beta Blocker Usage[2]	267	100%	98%	98%
Appropriate VTP Within 24 Hours[2]	254	93%	97%	98%
Controlled Postoperative Blood Glucose[2]	177	95%	98%	97%
Perioperative Temperature Management[2]	332	98%	100%	100%
Prophylactic Antibiotic Selection	353	99%	99%	99%
Prophylactic Antibiotic Selection (Outpatient)	-	-	98%	98%
Prophylactic Antibiotic Stopped	349	98%	98%	98%
Prophylactic Antibiotic Timing	353	99%	98%	99%
Prophylactic Antibiotic Timing (Outpatient)	-	-	96%	98%
Urinary Catheter Removal[2]	231	97%	97%	97%
Survey of Patients' Hospital Experiences				
Area Around Room 'Always' Quiet at Night	-	-	57%	61%
Doctors 'Always' Communicated Well	-	-	81%	82%
Home Recovery Information Given	-	-	86%	85%
Hospital Given 9 or 10 on 10 Point Scale	-	-	70%	71%
Meds 'Always' Explained Before Given	-	-	65%	64%
Nurses 'Always' Communicated Well	-	-	79%	79%
Pain 'Always' Well Controlled	-	-	71%	71%
Room and Bathroom 'Always' Clean	-	-	74%	73%
Timely Help 'Always' Received	-	-	68%	68%
Would Definitely Recommend Hospital	-	-	72%	71%
Use of Medical Imaging				
Cardiac Imaging Stress Test before Surgery	-	-	4.7%	5.3%
Combination Abdominal CT Scan	-	-	6.6%	10.5%
Combination Brain/Sinus CT Scan	-	-	2.1%	2.7%
Combination Chest CT Scan	-	-	1.1%	2.7%
Follow-up Mammogram/Ultrasound	-	-	8.9%	8.8%
Lumbar Spine MRI for Low Back Pain	-	-	41.7%	37.2%

Providence Portland Medical Center

4805 Ne Glisan Street
Portland, OR 97213
Phone: 503-215-1111
Fax: 503-215-0431
URL: www.providence.org/oregon
Type: Acute Care Hospitals
Emergency Services: Yes
Ownership: Voluntary non-profit - Church
Beds: 483

Key Personnel:
Operating Room. . . . . Arlene Austinson, RN
Infection Control. . . . . Joanne Jackson
Patient Relations . . . . Karen Logsdon
Emergency Room . . . . Jene Williamson

Measure	Cases	This Hosp.	State Avg.	U.S. Avg.
Blood Clot Prevention and Treatment				
Anticoagulation Overlap Therapy[2]	138	93%	95%	93%
ICU Venous Thromboembolism Prophylaxis[2]	419	79%	87%	92%
Incidence of Potentially Preventable VTE[2]	30	13%	13%	10%
UFH with Dosages/Platelet Monitoring[2]	30	100%	100%	97%
Venous Thromboembolism Prophylaxis[2]	115	82%	83%	85%
Warfarin Therapy Discharge Instructions[2]	108	4%	54%	75%
Chest Pain/Possible Heart Attack Care				
Aspirin Given Within 24 Hours of Arrival[1]	-	-	97%	96%
Fibrinolytic Meds Within 30 Min. of Arrival[5]	-	-	57%	58%
Average Time to ECG (minutes)[1]	-	-	9	7
Average Time to Transfer (minutes)[5]	-	-	52	60
Children's Asthma Care				
Received Home Management Plan of Care	-	-	-	88%
Received Reliever Medication	-	-	-	100%
Received Systemic Corticosteroids	-	-	-	100%
Emergency Department				
Admittance Decision Time (minutes)[2]	378	87	85	98
Head CT Results Within 45 Min. of Arrival[1]	-	-	45%	57%
Patients Who Left ER Before Being Seen	66,877	2%	2%	2%
Time from ER Arrival to Admit. (minutes)[2]	399	254	235	274
Time from ER Arrival to Discharge (minutes)	333	177	136	134
Time in ER Before Being Evaluated (minutes)	119	67	27	26
Time to Pain Meds for Fractures (minutes)	146	68	56	57
Heart Attack Care				
Aspirin Given at Discharge[2]	388	99%	99%	99%
Fibrinolytic Meds Within 30 Min. of Arrival[2,7]	-	-	57%	54%
PCI Within 90 Minutes of Arrival[2]	34	94%	93%	96%
Statin Prescribed at Discharge[2]	375	99%	98%	98%
Heart Failure Care				
ACE Inhibitor or ARB for LVSD[2]	63	92%	96%	97%
Discharge Instructions Given[2]	236	94%	93%	94%
Evaluation of LVS Function[2]	268	100%	99%	99%
Medicare Spending				
Medicare Spending per Patient (ratio)	-	0.92	0.88	0.98
Pneumonia Care				
Appropriate Initial Antibiotic Given[2]	104	95%	96%	95%
Blood Culture Timing[2]	173	99%	98%	98%
Pregnancy and Delivery Care				
Newborn Deliveries Scheduled Early	159	6%	3%	6%
Preventive Care				
Immunization for Influenza[2]	538	73%	86%	90%
Immunization for Pneumonia[2]	672	75%	88%	92%
Stroke Care				
Anticoagulation Therapy for Atrial Fibrillation[2]	18	72%	94%	95%
Antithrombotic Therapy Timing[2]	76	99%	97%	98%
Assessed for Rehabilitation[2]	115	97%	96%	97%
Discharged on Antithrombotic Therapy[2]	104	99%	99%	99%
Discharged on Statin Medication[2]	75	95%	93%	94%
Thrombolytic Therapy Timing[2]	15	80%	55%	66%
Venous Thromboembolism Prophylaxis[2]	115	77%	90%	94%
Written Stroke Educational Materials Given[2]	60	52%	81%	88%
Surgical Care Improvement Project				
Appropriate Beta Blocker Usage[2]	259	98%	98%	98%
Appropriate VTP Within 24 Hours[2]	396	99%	97%	98%
Controlled Postoperative Blood Glucose[2]	166	98%	98%	97%
Perioperative Temperature Management[2]	581	100%	100%	100%
Prophylactic Antibiotic Selection[2]	521	99%	99%	99%
Prophylactic Antibiotic Selection (Outpatient)	546	98%	98%	98%
Prophylactic Antibiotic Stopped[2]	508	98%	98%	98%
Prophylactic Antibiotic Timing[2]	521	98%	98%	99%
Prophylactic Antibiotic Timing (Outpatient)	543	92%	96%	98%
Urinary Catheter Removal[2]	437	98%	97%	97%
Survey of Patients' Hospital Experiences				
Area Around Room 'Always' Quiet at Night	300+	57%	57%	61%
Doctors 'Always' Communicated Well	300+	80%	81%	82%
Home Recovery Information Given	300+	87%	86%	85%
Hospital Given 9 or 10 on 10 Point Scale	300+	76%	70%	71%
Meds 'Always' Explained Before Given	300+	65%	65%	64%
Nurses 'Always' Communicated Well	300+	78%	79%	79%
Pain 'Always' Well Controlled	300+	74%	71%	71%
Room and Bathroom 'Always' Clean	300+	70%	74%	73%
Timely Help 'Always' Received	300+	65%	68%	68%
Would Definitely Recommend Hospital	300+	79%	72%	71%
Use of Medical Imaging				
Cardiac Imaging Stress Test before Surgery	359	5.0%	4.7%	5.3%
Combination Abdominal CT Scan	835	7.4%	6.6%	10.5%
Combination Brain/Sinus CT Scan	457	0.4%	2.1%	2.7%
Combination Chest CT Scan	643	0.0%	1.1%	2.7%
Follow-up Mammogram/Ultrasound	1,142	8.8%	8.9%	8.8%
Lumbar Spine MRI for Low Back Pain	58	34.5%	41.7%	37.2%

NOTE: Hospital profiles are in alphabetical order by state, then city, then hospital within the city; Rankings exclude hospitals with less than 25 cases except for patient surveys which excludes hospitals with less than 100 cases; (a) 100-299 cases; (1) The number of cases/patients is too few to report; (2) Data submitted were based on a sample of cases/patients; (3) Results are based on a shorter time period than required; (4) Data suppressed by CMS for one or more quarters; (5) Results are not available for this reporting period; (6) Fewer than 100 patients completed the HCAHPS survey; (7) No cases met the criteria for this measure; (8) The lower limit of the confidence interval cannot be calculated if the number of observed infections equals zero; (9) No data are available from the state/territory for this reporting period; (10) The scores shown reflect fewer than 50 completed surveys; (11) There were discrepancies in the data collection process; (12) This measure does not apply to this hospital for this reporting period; (13) Results cannot be calculated for this reporting period; (14) The results for this state are combined with nearby states to protect confidentiality; Please refer to the User's Guide for a full explanation of data.

Providence Saint Vincent Medical Center

9205 Sw Barnes Road Phone: 503-216-1234
Portland, OR 97225 Fax: 503-216-4659
URL: www.providence.org
Type: Acute Care Hospitals Emergency Services: Yes
Ownership: Voluntary non-profit - Other Beds: 523

Key Personnel:
Operating Room. . . . . Gay Adams, RN
CEO/President. . . . . Janice Burger
Emergency Room . . . . Daniel Craig, MD
Infection Control. . . . . Woodruff English, MD
Anesthesiology. . . . . John Evans, MD
Chief of Medical Staff. . . . . Fred Ey, MD
Intensive Care Unit. . . . . Joyce Rountree, RN
Quality Assurance . . . . Lynette Savage, RN

Measure	Cases	This Hosp.	State Avg.	U.S. Avg.
Blood Clot Prevention and Treatment				
Anticoagulation Overlap Therapy[2]	128	98%	95%	93%
ICU Venous Thromboembolism Prophylaxis[2]	308	94%	87%	92%
Incidence of Potentially Preventable VTE[2]	41	24%	13%	10%
UFH with Dosages/Platelet Monitoring[2]	54	100%	100%	97%
Venous Thromboembolism Prophylaxis[2]	190	85%	83%	85%
Warfarin Therapy Discharge Instructions[2]	102	13%	54%	75%
Chest Pain/Possible Heart Attack Care				
Aspirin Given Within 24 Hours of Arrival	32	97%	97%	96%
Fibrinolytic Meds Within 30 Min. of Arrival[7]	-	-	57%	58%
Average Time to ECG (minutes)	32	3	9	7
Average Time to Transfer (minutes)[7]	-	-	52	60
Children's Asthma Care				
Received Home Management Plan of Care	-	-	-	88%
Received Reliever Medication	-	-	-	100%
Received Systemic Corticosteroids	-	-	-	100%
Emergency Department				
Admittance Decision Time (minutes)[2]	521	86	85	98
Head CT Results Within 45 Min. of Arrival[1]	-	-	45%	57%
Patients Who Left ER Before Being Seen	86,558	2%	2%	2%
Time from ER Arrival to Admit. (minutes)[2]	522	268	235	274
Time from ER Arrival to Discharge (minutes)	345	185	136	134
Time in ER Before Being Evaluated (minutes)	73	46	27	26
Time to Pain Meds for Fractures (minutes)	267	68	56	57
Heart Attack Care				
Aspirin Given at Discharge[2]	539	100%	99%	99%
Fibrinolytic Meds Within 30 Min. of Arrival[2,7]	-	-	57%	54%
PCI Within 90 Minutes of Arrival[2]	95	95%	93%	96%
Statin Prescribed at Discharge[2]	517	98%	98%	98%
Heart Failure Care				
ACE Inhibitor or ARB for LVSD[2]	84	90%	96%	97%
Discharge Instructions Given[2]	227	89%	93%	94%
Evaluation of LVS Function[2]	269	99%	99%	99%
Medicare Spending				
Medicare Spending per Patient (ratio)	-	0.89	0.88	0.98
Pneumonia Care				
Appropriate Initial Antibiotic Given[2]	109	100%	96%	95%
Blood Culture Timing[2]	152	99%	98%	98%
Pregnancy and Delivery Care				
Newborn Deliveries Scheduled Early	312	2%	3%	6%
Preventive Care				
Immunization for Influenza[2]	642	73%	86%	90%
Immunization for Pneumonia[2]	660	73%	88%	92%
Stroke Care				
Anticoagulation Therapy for Atrial Fibrillation[2]	22	91%	94%	95%
Antithrombotic Therapy Timing[2]	73	100%	97%	98%
Assessed for Rehabilitation[2]	113	93%	96%	97%
Discharged on Antithrombotic Therapy[2]	96	99%	99%	99%
Discharged on Statin Medication[2]	79	97%	93%	94%
Thrombolytic Therapy Timing[1,2]	-	-	55%	66%
Venous Thromboembolism Prophylaxis[2]	100	88%	90%	94%
Written Stroke Educational Materials Given[2]	73	79%	81%	88%
Surgical Care Improvement Project				
Appropriate Beta Blocker Usage[2]	233	97%	98%	98%
Appropriate VTP Within 24 Hours[2]	347	94%	97%	98%
Controlled Postoperative Blood Glucose[2]	172	98%	98%	97%
Perioperative Temperature Management[2]	610	100%	100%	100%
Prophylactic Antibiotic Selection[2]	535	99%	99%	99%
Prophylactic Antibiotic Selection (Outpatient)	636	97%	98%	98%
Prophylactic Antibiotic Stopped[2]	530	99%	98%	98%
Prophylactic Antibiotic Timing[2]	537	97%	98%	99%
Prophylactic Antibiotic Timing (Outpatient)	641	97%	96%	98%
Urinary Catheter Removal[2]	313	97%	97%	97%
Survey of Patients' Hospital Experiences				
Area Around Room 'Always' Quiet at Night	300+	55%	57%	61%
Doctors 'Always' Communicated Well	300+	80%	81%	82%
Home Recovery Information Given	300+	87%	86%	85%
Hospital Given 9 or 10 on 10 Point Scale	300+	74%	70%	71%
Meds 'Always' Explained Before Given	300+	64%	65%	64%
Nurses 'Always' Communicated Well	300+	78%	79%	79%
Pain 'Always' Well Controlled	300+	71%	71%	71%
Room and Bathroom 'Always' Clean	300+	72%	74%	73%
Timely Help 'Always' Received	300+	63%	68%	68%
Would Definitely Recommend Hospital	300+	81%	72%	71%
Use of Medical Imaging				
Cardiac Imaging Stress Test before Surgery	532	4.7%	4.7%	5.3%
Combination Abdominal CT Scan	867	6.7%	6.6%	10.5%
Combination Brain/Sinus CT Scan	647	2.5%	2.1%	2.7%
Combination Chest CT Scan	578	0.0%	1.1%	2.7%
Follow-up Mammogram/Ultrasound	1,811	7.3%	8.9%	8.8%
Lumbar Spine MRI for Low Back Pain	83	50.6%	41.7%	37.2%

Pioneer Memorial Hospital

1201 Ne Elm Street Phone: 541-447-6254
Prineville, OR 97754 Fax: 541-447-6705
URL: www.pmhprineville.org
Type: Critical Access Hospitals Emergency Services: Yes
Ownership: Voluntary non-profit - Private Beds: 35

Key Personnel:
Quality Assurance . . . . Virginia Cannon
CEO/President. . . . . Don Wee

Measure	Cases	This Hosp.	State Avg.	U.S. Avg.
Blood Clot Prevention and Treatment				
Anticoagulation Overlap Therapy[5]	-	-	95%	93%
ICU Venous Thromboembolism Prophylaxis[5]	-	-	87%	92%
Incidence of Potentially Preventable VTE[5]	-	-	13%	10%
UFH with Dosages/Platelet Monitoring[5]	-	-	100%	97%
Venous Thromboembolism Prophylaxis[5]	-	-	83%	85%
Warfarin Therapy Discharge Instructions[5]	-	-	54%	75%
Chest Pain/Possible Heart Attack Care				
Aspirin Given Within 24 Hours of Arrival	17	100%	97%	96%
Fibrinolytic Meds Within 30 Min. of Arrival[7]	-	-	57%	58%
Average Time to ECG (minutes)	18	10	9	7
Average Time to Transfer (minutes)[1]	-	-	52	60
Children's Asthma Care				
Received Home Management Plan of Care	-	-	-	88%
Received Reliever Medication	-	-	-	100%
Received Systemic Corticosteroids	-	-	-	100%
Emergency Department				
Admittance Decision Time (minutes)[2]	279	65	85	98
Head CT Results Within 45 Min. of Arrival[1]	-	-	45%	57%
Patients Who Left ER Before Being Seen[5]	-	-	2%	2%
Time from ER Arrival to Admit. (minutes)[2]	290	225	235	274
Time from ER Arrival to Discharge (minutes)	372	113	136	134
Time in ER Before Being Evaluated (minutes)	398	18	27	26
Time to Pain Meds for Fractures (minutes)	47	53	56	57
Heart Attack Care				
Aspirin Given at Discharge[3,7]	-	-	99%	99%
Fibrinolytic Meds Within 30 Min. of Arrival[3,7]	-	-	57%	54%
PCI Within 90 Minutes of Arrival[3,7]	-	-	93%	96%
Statin Prescribed at Discharge[3,7]	-	-	98%	98%
Heart Failure Care				
ACE Inhibitor or ARB for LVSD[1]	-	-	96%	97%
Discharge Instructions Given	12	75%	93%	94%
Evaluation of LVS Function	14	100%	99%	99%
Medicare Spending				
Medicare Spending per Patient (ratio)	-	-	0.88	0.98
Pneumonia Care				
Appropriate Initial Antibiotic Given	22	82%	96%	95%
Blood Culture Timing	29	97%	98%	98%
Pregnancy and Delivery Care				
Newborn Deliveries Scheduled Early[3,7]	-	-	3%	6%
Preventive Care				
Immunization for Influenza[2]	278	90%	86%	90%
Immunization for Pneumonia[2]	450	91%	88%	92%
Stroke Care				
Anticoagulation Therapy for Atrial Fibrillation[5]	-	-	94%	95%
Antithrombotic Therapy Timing[5]	-	-	97%	98%
Assessed for Rehabilitation[5]	-	-	96%	97%
Discharged on Antithrombotic Therapy[5]	-	-	99%	99%
Discharged on Statin Medication[5]	-	-	93%	94%
Thrombolytic Therapy Timing[5]	-	-	55%	66%
Venous Thromboembolism Prophylaxis[5]	-	-	90%	94%
Written Stroke Educational Materials Given[5]	-	-	81%	88%
Surgical Care Improvement Project				
Appropriate Beta Blocker Usage[1]	-	-	98%	98%
Appropriate VTP Within 24 Hours	13	69%	97%	98%
Controlled Postoperative Blood Glucose[3,7]	-	-	98%	97%
Perioperative Temperature Management	17	100%	100%	100%
Prophylactic Antibiotic Selection[1]	-	-	99%	99%
Prophylactic Antibiotic Selection (Outpatient)[1,3]	-	-	98%	98%
Prophylactic Antibiotic Stopped[1]	-	-	98%	98%
Prophylactic Antibiotic Timing[1]	-	-	98%	99%
Prophylactic Antibiotic Timing (Outpatient)[1,3]	-	-	96%	98%
Urinary Catheter Removal	11	100%	97%	97%
Survey of Patients' Hospital Experiences				
Area Around Room 'Always' Quiet at Night	(a)	53%	57%	61%
Doctors 'Always' Communicated Well	(a)	85%	81%	82%
Home Recovery Information Given	(a)	82%	86%	85%
Hospital Given 9 or 10 on 10 Point Scale	(a)	70%	70%	71%
Meds 'Always' Explained Before Given	(a)	75%	65%	64%
Nurses 'Always' Communicated Well	(a)	83%	79%	79%
Pain 'Always' Well Controlled	(a)	77%	71%	71%
Room and Bathroom 'Always' Clean	(a)	72%	74%	73%
Timely Help 'Always' Received	(a)	69%	68%	68%
Would Definitely Recommend Hospital	(a)	64%	72%	71%
Use of Medical Imaging				
Cardiac Imaging Stress Test before Surgery[7]	-	-	4.7%	5.3%
Combination Abdominal CT Scan	227	7.0%	6.6%	10.5%
Combination Brain/Sinus CT Scan[1]	-	-	2.1%	2.7%
Combination Chest CT Scan	178	3.9%	1.1%	2.7%
Follow-up Mammogram/Ultrasound	435	10.8%	8.9%	8.8%
Lumbar Spine MRI for Low Back Pain[1]	-	-	41.7%	37.2%

Saint Charles Medical Center - Redmond

1253 N Canal Blvd Phone: 541-548-8131
Redmond, OR 97756 Fax: 541-388-7791
URL: www.scmc.org
Type: Acute Care Hospitals Emergency Services: Yes
Ownership: Voluntary non-profit - Private Beds: 48

Measure	Cases	This Hosp.	State Avg.	U.S. Avg.
Blood Clot Prevention and Treatment				
Anticoagulation Overlap Therapy[2]	25	96%	95%	93%
ICU Venous Thromboembolism Prophylaxis[2]	27	85%	87%	92%
Incidence of Potentially Preventable VTE[1,2]	-	-	13%	10%
UFH with Dosages/Platelet Monitoring[1,2]	-	-	100%	97%
Venous Thromboembolism Prophylaxis[2]	107	93%	83%	85%
Warfarin Therapy Discharge Instructions[2]	22	86%	54%	75%
Chest Pain/Possible Heart Attack Care				
Aspirin Given Within 24 Hours of Arrival	32	84%	97%	96%
Fibrinolytic Meds Within 30 Min. of Arrival[7]	-	-	57%	58%
Average Time to ECG (minutes)	32	10	9	7
Average Time to Transfer (minutes)[1]	-	-	52	60
Children's Asthma Care				
Received Home Management Plan of Care	-	-	-	88%
Received Reliever Medication	-	-	-	100%
Received Systemic Corticosteroids	-	-	-	100%
Emergency Department				
Admittance Decision Time (minutes)[2]	260	71	85	98
Head CT Results Within 45 Min. of Arrival[1]	-	-	45%	57%
Patients Who Left ER Before Being Seen	15,667	0%	2%	2%
Time from ER Arrival to Admit. (minutes)[2]	262	229	235	274
Time from ER Arrival to Discharge (minutes)	369	128	136	134

NOTE: Hospital profiles are in alphabetical order by state, then city, then hospital within the city; Rankings exclude hospitals with less than 25 cases except for patient surveys which excludes hospitals with less than 100 cases; (a) 100-299 cases; (1) The number of cases/patients is too few to report; (2) Data submitted were based on a sample of cases/patients; (3) Results are based on a shorter time period than required; (4) Data suppressed by CMS for one or more quarters; (5) Results are not available for this reporting period; (6) Fewer than 100 patients completed the HCAHPS survey; (7) No cases met the criteria for this measure; (8) The lower limit of the confidence interval cannot be calculated if the number of observed infections equals zero; (9) No data are available from the state/territory for this reporting period; (10) The scores shown reflect fewer than 50 completed surveys; (11) There were discrepancies in the data collection process; (12) This measure does not apply to this hospital for this reporting period; (13) Results cannot be calculated for this reporting period; (14) The results for this state are combined with nearby states to protect confidentiality; Please refer to the User's Guide for a full explanation of data.

Measure	Cases	This Hosp.	State Avg.	U.S. Avg.
Time in ER Before Being Evaluated (minutes)	367	21	27	26
Time to Pain Meds for Fractures (minutes)	76	51	56	57
Heart Attack Care				
Aspirin Given at Discharge[1]	-	-	99%	99%
Fibrinolytic Meds Within 30 Min. of Arrival[7]	-	-	57%	54%
PCI Within 90 Minutes of Arrival[7]	-	-	93%	96%
Statin Prescribed at Discharge[1]	-	-	98%	98%
Heart Failure Care				
ACE Inhibitor or ARB for LVSD[1]	-	-	96%	97%
Discharge Instructions Given	42	86%	93%	94%
Evaluation of LVS Function	46	96%	99%	99%
Medicare Spending				
Medicare Spending per Patient (ratio)	-	0.87	0.88	0.98
Pneumonia Care				
Appropriate Initial Antibiotic Given	28	89%	96%	95%
Blood Culture Timing	64	100%	98%	98%
Pregnancy and Delivery Care				
Newborn Deliveries Scheduled Early	34	29%	3%	6%
Preventive Care				
Immunization for Influenza[2]	247	89%	86%	90%
Immunization for Pneumonia[2]	302	88%	88%	92%
Stroke Care				
Anticoagulation Therapy for Atrial Fibrillation[1]	-	-	94%	95%
Antithrombotic Therapy Timing	13	100%	97%	98%
Assessed for Rehabilitation	16	100%	96%	97%
Discharged on Antithrombotic Therapy	16	100%	99%	99%
Discharged on Statin Medication	13	100%	93%	94%
Thrombolytic Therapy Timing[1]	-	-	55%	66%
Venous Thromboembolism Prophylaxis	12	83%	90%	94%
Written Stroke Educational Materials Given[1]	-	-	81%	88%
Surgical Care Improvement Project				
Appropriate Beta Blocker Usage	42	95%	98%	98%
Appropriate VTP Within 24 Hours	172	86%	97%	98%
Controlled Postoperative Blood Glucose[7]	-	-	98%	97%
Perioperative Temperature Management	210	100%	100%	100%
Prophylactic Antibiotic Selection	135	99%	99%	99%
Prophylactic Antibiotic Selection (Outpatient)	13	100%	98%	98%
Prophylactic Antibiotic Stopped	131	90%	98%	98%
Prophylactic Antibiotic Timing	135	94%	98%	99%
Prophylactic Antibiotic Timing (Outpatient)	14	93%	96%	98%
Urinary Catheter Removal	137	88%	97%	97%
Survey of Patients' Hospital Experiences				
Area Around Room 'Always' Quiet at Night	300+	58%	57%	61%
Doctors 'Always' Communicated Well	300+	79%	81%	82%
Home Recovery Information Given	300+	87%	86%	85%
Hospital Given 9 or 10 on 10 Point Scale	300+	74%	70%	71%
Meds 'Always' Explained Before Given	300+	65%	65%	64%
Nurses 'Always' Communicated Well	300+	78%	79%	79%
Pain 'Always' Well Controlled	300+	72%	71%	71%
Room and Bathroom 'Always' Clean	300+	73%	74%	73%
Timely Help 'Always' Received	300+	69%	68%	68%
Would Definitely Recommend Hospital	300+	76%	72%	71%
Use of Medical Imaging				
Cardiac Imaging Stress Test before Surgery[7]	-	-	4.7%	5.3%
Combination Abdominal CT Scan	186	0.0%	6.6%	10.5%
Combination Brain/Sinus CT Scan[1]	-	-	2.1%	2.7%
Combination Chest CT Scan	131	3.1%	1.1%	2.7%
Follow-up Mammogram/Ultrasound[7]	-	-	8.9%	8.8%
Lumbar Spine MRI for Low Back Pain[1]	-	-	41.7%	37.2%

Lower Umpqua Hospital District

600 Ranch Road
Reedsport, OR 97467
Phone: 541-271-2171
Fax: 541-271-2941
Type: Critical Access Hospitals
Emergency Services: Yes
Ownership: Govt - Hospital Dist/Auth
Beds: 40

Key Personnel:

Infection Control. . . . . Judie Carey, RN
Emergency Room . . . . John Crocker, MD
President . . . . Dorothy Denman
Chief of Medical Staff. . . . . Michael Ivanitsky, MD
Anesthesiology. . . . . Greg Pigeon, CRNA
Quality Assurance . . . . John Quinlan, RN
Operating Room. . . . . Jeffery Snyder

Measure	Cases	This Hosp.	State Avg.	U.S. Avg.
Blood Clot Prevention and Treatment				
Anticoagulation Overlap Therapy[1,2]	-	-	95%	93%
ICU Venous Thromboembolism Prophylaxis[2,7]	-	-	87%	92%
Incidence of Potentially Preventable VTE[2,7]	-	-	13%	10%
UFH with Dosages/Platelet Monitoring[2,7]	-	-	100%	97%
Venous Thromboembolism Prophylaxis[2,7]	-	-	83%	85%
Warfarin Therapy Discharge Instructions[1,2]	-	-	54%	75%
Chest Pain/Possible Heart Attack Care				
Aspirin Given Within 24 Hours of Arrival[3,7]	-	-	97%	96%
Fibrinolytic Meds Within 30 Min. of Arrival[1,3]	-	-	57%	58%
Average Time to ECG (minutes)[1,3]	-	-	9	7
Average Time to Transfer (minutes)[3,7]	-	-	52	60
Children's Asthma Care				
Received Home Management Plan of Care	-	-	-	88%
Received Reliever Medication	-	-	-	100%
Received Systemic Corticosteroids	-	-	-	100%
Emergency Department				
Admittance Decision Time (minutes)[2,3]	19	35	85	98
Head CT Results Within 45 Min. of Arrival[1,3]	-	-	45%	57%
Patients Who Left ER Before Being Seen[5]	-	-	2%	2%
Time from ER Arrival to Admit. (minutes)[2,3]	30	173	235	274
Time from ER Arrival to Discharge (minutes)[3]	117	112	136	134
Time in ER Before Being Evaluated (minutes)[3]	99	27	27	26
Time to Pain Meds for Fractures (minutes)[5]	-	-	56	57
Heart Attack Care				
Aspirin Given at Discharge[2,3]	-	-	99%	99%
Fibrinolytic Meds Within 30 Min. of Arrival[2,3]	-	-	57%	54%
PCI Within 90 Minutes of Arrival[2,3]	-	-	93%	96%
Statin Prescribed at Discharge[1,2]	-	-	98%	98%
Heart Failure Care				
ACE Inhibitor or ARB for LVSD[1,2]	-	-	96%	97%
Discharge Instructions Given[1,2]	-	-	93%	94%
Evaluation of LVS Function[1,2]	-	-	99%	99%
Medicare Spending				
Medicare Spending per Patient (ratio)	-	-	0.88	0.98
Pneumonia Care				
Appropriate Initial Antibiotic Given[1,2]	-	-	96%	95%
Blood Culture Timing[1,2]	-	-	98%	98%
Pregnancy and Delivery Care				
Newborn Deliveries Scheduled Early[5]	-	-	3%	6%
Preventive Care				
Immunization for Influenza[2]	44	80%	86%	90%
Immunization for Pneumonia[2]	76	67%	88%	92%
Stroke Care				
Anticoagulation Therapy for Atrial Fibrillation[2,7]	-	-	94%	95%
Antithrombotic Therapy Timing[1,2]	-	-	97%	98%
Assessed for Rehabilitation[1,2]	-	-	96%	97%
Discharged on Antithrombotic Therapy[1,2]	-	-	99%	99%
Discharged on Statin Medication[1,2]	-	-	93%	94%
Thrombolytic Therapy Timing[1,2]	-	-	55%	66%
Venous Thromboembolism Prophylaxis[1,2]	-	-	90%	94%
Written Stroke Educational Materials Given[1,2]	-	-	81%	88%
Surgical Care Improvement Project				
Appropriate Beta Blocker Usage[1,2]	-	-	98%	98%
Appropriate VTP Within 24 Hours[5]	-	-	97%	98%
Controlled Postoperative Blood Glucose[5]	-	-	98%	97%
Perioperative Temperature Management[1,2]	-	-	100%	100%
Prophylactic Antibiotic Selection[5]	-	-	99%	99%
Prophylactic Antibiotic Selection (Outpatient)[5]	-	-	98%	98%
Prophylactic Antibiotic Stopped[5]	-	-	98%	98%
Prophylactic Antibiotic Timing[5]	-	-	98%	99%
Prophylactic Antibiotic Timing (Outpatient)[5]	-	-	96%	98%
Urinary Catheter Removal[1,2]	-	-	97%	97%
Survey of Patients' Hospital Experiences				
Area Around Room 'Always' Quiet at Night[6]	<100	66%	57%	61%
Doctors 'Always' Communicated Well[6]	<100	81%	81%	82%
Home Recovery Information Given[6]	<100	83%	86%	85%
Hospital Given 9 or 10 on 10 Point Scale[6]	<100	58%	70%	71%
Meds 'Always' Explained Before Given[6]	<100	63%	65%	64%
Nurses 'Always' Communicated Well[6]	<100	75%	79%	79%
Pain 'Always' Well Controlled[6]	<100	71%	71%	71%
Room and Bathroom 'Always' Clean[6]	<100	71%	74%	73%
Timely Help 'Always' Received[6]	<100	77%	68%	68%
Would Definitely Recommend Hospital[6]	<100	59%	72%	71%
Use of Medical Imaging				
Cardiac Imaging Stress Test before Surgery	53	1.9%	4.7%	5.3%
Combination Abdominal CT Scan	102	7.8%	6.6%	10.5%
Combination Brain/Sinus CT Scan[1]	-	-	2.1%	2.7%
Combination Chest CT Scan	53	3.8%	1.1%	2.7%
Follow-up Mammogram/Ultrasound	152	3.9%	8.9%	8.8%
Lumbar Spine MRI for Low Back Pain[1]	-	-	41.7%	37.2%

Mercy Medical Center

2700 Nw Stewart Parkway
Roseburg, OR 97471
Phone: 541-673-0611
Fax: 541-677-4830
URL: www.mercyrose.org
Type: Acute Care Hospitals
Emergency Services: Yes
Ownership: Govt - Hospital Dist/Auth
Beds: 153

Key Personnel:

Radiology. . . . . Ed Cox
CEO/President. . . . . Victor J Fresolone, FACHE
Pediatric In-Patient Care . . . . Ann Fuller
Quality Assurance . . . . Ruth Galster
Operating Room. . . . . Laurie Hayes
Chief of Medical Staff . . . . Timothy McCarter, MD
Coronary Care . . . . Cheryl Palmer
Infection Control. . . . . Sharon Standiford

Measure	Cases	This Hosp.	State Avg.	U.S. Avg.
Blood Clot Prevention and Treatment				
Anticoagulation Overlap Therapy[2]	56	80%	95%	93%
ICU Venous Thromboembolism Prophylaxis[2]	84	85%	87%	92%
Incidence of Potentially Preventable VTE[1,2]	-	-	13%	10%
UFH with Dosages/Platelet Monitoring[2]	28	100%	100%	97%
Venous Thromboembolism Prophylaxis[2]	311	60%	83%	85%
Warfarin Therapy Discharge Instructions[2]	48	2%	54%	75%
Chest Pain/Possible Heart Attack Care				
Aspirin Given Within 24 Hours of Arrival[1,3]	-	-	97%	96%
Fibrinolytic Meds Within 30 Min. of Arrival[1,3]	-	-	57%	58%
Average Time to ECG (minutes)[1,3]	-	-	9	7
Average Time to Transfer (minutes)[1,3]	-	-	52	60
Children's Asthma Care				
Received Home Management Plan of Care	-	-	-	88%
Received Reliever Medication	-	-	-	100%
Received Systemic Corticosteroids	-	-	-	100%
Emergency Department				
Admittance Decision Time (minutes)[2]	738	79	85	98
Head CT Results Within 45 Min. of Arrival	12	50%	45%	57%
Patients Who Left ER Before Being Seen	45,813	1%	2%	2%
Time from ER Arrival to Admit. (minutes)[2]	755	194	235	274
Time from ER Arrival to Discharge (minutes)	441	93	136	134
Time in ER Before Being Evaluated (minutes)	472	12	27	26
Time to Pain Meds for Fractures (minutes)	184	26	56	57
Heart Attack Care				
Aspirin Given at Discharge[2]	144	99%	99%	99%
Fibrinolytic Meds Within 30 Min. of Arrival[2,7]	-	-	57%	54%
PCI Within 90 Minutes of Arrival[2]	28	96%	93%	96%
Statin Prescribed at Discharge[2]	143	98%	98%	98%
Heart Failure Care				
ACE Inhibitor or ARB for LVSD[2]	39	95%	96%	97%
Discharge Instructions Given[2]	160	96%	93%	94%
Evaluation of LVS Function[2]	184	100%	99%	99%
Medicare Spending				
Medicare Spending per Patient (ratio)	-	0.86	0.88	0.98
Pneumonia Care				
Appropriate Initial Antibiotic Given[2]	105	95%	96%	95%
Blood Culture Timing[2]	90	98%	98%	98%
Pregnancy and Delivery Care				
Newborn Deliveries Scheduled Early[2]	33	9%	3%	6%
Preventive Care				
Immunization for Influenza[2]	540	96%	86%	90%
Immunization for Pneumonia[2]	758	97%	88%	92%
Stroke Care				
Anticoagulation Therapy for Atrial Fibrillation[2]	11	91%	94%	95%
Antithrombotic Therapy Timing[2]	81	98%	97%	98%
Assessed for Rehabilitation[2]	78	97%	96%	97%
Discharged on Antithrombotic Therapy[2]	78	100%	99%	99%

NOTE: Hospital profiles are in alphabetical order by state, then city, then hospital within the city; Rankings exclude hospitals with less than 25 cases except for patient surveys which excludes hospitals with less than 100 cases; (a) 100-299 cases; (1) The number of cases/patients is too few to report; (2) Data submitted were based on a sample of cases/patients; (3) Results are based on a shorter time period than required; (4) Data suppressed by CMS for one or more quarters; (5) Results are not available for this reporting period; (6) Fewer than 100 patients completed the HCAHPS survey; (7) No cases met the criteria for this measure; (8) The lower limit of the confidence interval cannot be calculated if the number of observed infections equals zero; (9) No data are available from the state/territory for this reporting period; (10) The scores shown reflect fewer than 50 completed surveys; (11) There were discrepancies in the data collection process; (12) This measure does not apply to this hospital for this reporting period; (13) Results cannot be calculated for this reporting period; (14) The results for this state are combined with nearby states to protect confidentiality; Please refer to the User's Guide for a full explanation of data.

Discharged on Statin Medication[2]	60	87%	93%	94%
Thrombolytic Therapy Timing[1,2]	-	-	55%	66%
Venous Thromboembolism Prophylaxis[2]	79	71%	90%	94%
Written Stroke Educational Materials Given[2]	50	0%	81%	88%
Surgical Care Improvement Project				
Appropriate Beta Blocker Usage	115	100%	98%	98%
Appropriate VTP Within 24 Hours	328	100%	97%	98%
Controlled Postoperative Blood Glucose[7]	-	-	98%	97%
Perioperative Temperature Management	377	100%	100%	100%
Prophylactic Antibiotic Selection	262	100%	99%	99%
Prophylactic Antibiotic Selection (Outpatient)	322	99%	98%	98%
Prophylactic Antibiotic Stopped	257	100%	98%	98%
Prophylactic Antibiotic Timing	262	100%	98%	99%
Prophylactic Antibiotic Timing (Outpatient)	322	100%	96%	98%
Urinary Catheter Removal	256	100%	97%	97%
Survey of Patients' Hospital Experiences				
Area Around Room 'Always' Quiet at Night	300+	52%	57%	61%
Doctors 'Always' Communicated Well	300+	78%	81%	82%
Home Recovery Information Given	300+	82%	86%	85%
Hospital Given 9 or 10 on 10 Point Scale	300+	63%	70%	71%
Meds 'Always' Explained Before Given	300+	57%	65%	64%
Nurses 'Always' Communicated Well	300+	76%	79%	79%
Pain 'Always' Well Controlled	300+	69%	71%	71%
Room and Bathroom 'Always' Clean	300+	70%	74%	73%
Timely Help 'Always' Received	300+	55%	68%	68%
Would Definitely Recommend Hospital	300+	62%	72%	71%
Use of Medical Imaging				
Cardiac Imaging Stress Test before Surgery	337	5.0%	4.7%	5.3%
Combination Abdominal CT Scan	953	10.1%	6.6%	10.5%
Combination Brain/Sinus CT Scan	609	0.7%	2.1%	2.7%
Combination Chest CT Scan	802	0.0%	1.1%	2.7%
Follow-up Mammogram/Ultrasound	2,794	5.8%	8.9%	8.8%
Lumbar Spine MRI for Low Back Pain	182	42.3%	41.7%	37.2%

VA Roseburg Healthcare System

913 Nw Garden Valley Blvd.
Roseburg, OR 97470
Phone: 541-440-1000
Fax: 541-440-1225
Type: Acute Care - VA
Emergency Services: No
Ownership: Government Federal
Beds: 342

Key Personnel:
Quality Assurance .... Paul Brunner
Chief of Medical Staff .... Steven Gibsom, MD
Emergency Room .... Phillip Hunter, MD
Radiology.................. Adolph Morlang, MD
Operating Room.............. Fred Wilkins, RN

Measure	Cases	This Hosp.	State Avg.	U.S. Avg.
Blood Clot Prevention and Treatment				
Anticoagulation Overlap Therapy	-	-	95%	93%
ICU Venous Thromboembolism Prophylaxis	-	-	87%	92%
Incidence of Potentially Preventable VTE	-	-	13%	10%
UFH with Dosages/Platelet Monitoring	-	-	100%	97%
Venous Thromboembolism Prophylaxis	-	-	83%	85%
Warfarin Therapy Discharge Instructions	-	-	54%	75%
Chest Pain/Possible Heart Attack Care				
Aspirin Given Within 24 Hours of Arrival	-	-	97%	96%
Fibrinolytic Meds Within 30 Min. of Arrival	-	-	57%	58%
Average Time to ECG (minutes)	-	-	9	7
Average Time to Transfer (minutes)	-	-	52	60
Children's Asthma Care				
Received Home Management Plan of Care	-	-	-	88%
Received Reliever Medication	-	-	-	100%
Received Systemic Corticosteroids	-	-	-	100%
Emergency Department				
Admittance Decision Time (minutes)	-	-	85	98
Head CT Results Within 45 Min. of Arrival	-	-	45%	57%
Patients Who Left ER Before Being Seen	-	-	2%	2%
Time from ER Arrival to Admit. (minutes)	-	-	235	274
Time from ER Arrival to Discharge (minutes)	-	-	136	134
Time in ER Before Being Evaluated (minutes)	-	-	27	26
Time to Pain Meds for Fractures (minutes)	-	-	56	57
Heart Attack Care				
Aspirin Given at Discharge[5]	-	-	99%	99%
Fibrinolytic Meds Within 30 Min. of Arrival[5]	-	-	57%	54%
PCI Within 90 Minutes of Arrival[5]	-	-	93%	96%
Statin Prescribed at Discharge[1]	-	-	98%	98%
Heart Failure Care				
ACE Inhibitor or ARB for LVSD[1]	-	-	96%	97%
Discharge Instructions Given[1]	22	95%	93%	94%
Evaluation of LVS Function	29	97%	99%	99%
Medicare Spending				
Medicare Spending per Patient (ratio)	-	-	0.88	0.98
Pneumonia Care				
Appropriate Initial Antibiotic Given	27	89%	96%	95%
Blood Culture Timing	28	100%	98%	98%
Pregnancy and Delivery Care				
Newborn Deliveries Scheduled Early	-	-	3%	6%
Preventive Care				
Immunization for Influenza[5]	-	-	86%	90%
Immunization for Pneumonia[5]	-	-	88%	92%
Stroke Care				
Anticoagulation Therapy for Atrial Fibrillation	-	-	94%	95%
Antithrombotic Therapy Timing	-	-	97%	98%
Assessed for Rehabilitation	-	-	96%	97%
Discharged on Antithrombotic Therapy	-	-	99%	99%
Discharged on Statin Medication	-	-	93%	94%
Thrombolytic Therapy Timing	-	-	55%	66%
Venous Thromboembolism Prophylaxis	-	-	90%	94%
Written Stroke Educational Materials Given	-	-	81%	88%
Surgical Care Improvement Project				
Appropriate Beta Blocker Usage[5]	-	-	98%	98%
Appropriate VTP Within 24 Hours[1,2]	-	-	97%	98%
Controlled Postoperative Blood Glucose[5]	-	-	98%	97%
Perioperative Temperature Management[1,2]	-	-	100%	100%
Prophylactic Antibiotic Selection[5]	-	-	99%	99%
Prophylactic Antibiotic Selection (Outpatient)	-	-	98%	98%
Prophylactic Antibiotic Stopped[5]	-	-	98%	98%
Prophylactic Antibiotic Timing[5]	-	-	98%	99%
Prophylactic Antibiotic Timing (Outpatient)	-	-	96%	98%
Urinary Catheter Removal[1,2]	-	-	97%	97%
Survey of Patients' Hospital Experiences				
Area Around Room 'Always' Quiet at Night	-	-	57%	61%
Doctors 'Always' Communicated Well	-	-	81%	82%
Home Recovery Information Given	-	-	86%	85%
Hospital Given 9 or 10 on 10 Point Scale	-	-	70%	71%
Meds 'Always' Explained Before Given	-	-	65%	64%
Nurses 'Always' Communicated Well	-	-	79%	79%
Pain 'Always' Well Controlled	-	-	71%	71%
Room and Bathroom 'Always' Clean	-	-	74%	73%
Timely Help 'Always' Received	-	-	68%	68%
Would Definitely Recommend Hospital	-	-	72%	71%
Use of Medical Imaging				
Cardiac Imaging Stress Test before Surgery	-	-	4.7%	5.3%
Combination Abdominal CT Scan	-	-	6.6%	10.5%
Combination Brain/Sinus CT Scan	-	-	2.1%	2.7%
Combination Chest CT Scan	-	-	1.1%	2.7%
Follow-up Mammogram/Ultrasound	-	-	8.9%	8.8%
Lumbar Spine MRI for Low Back Pain	-	-	41.7%	37.2%

Salem Hospital

890 Oak Street, Se
Salem, OR 97301
Phone: 503-561-5200
E-mail: cr@salemhospital.org
URL: www.salemhospital.org
Type: Acute Care Hospitals
Emergency Services: Yes
Ownership: Voluntary non-profit - Other
Beds: 454

Key Personnel:
Intensive Care Unit............ Cindy Armstrong
Chief of Medical Staff.......... Cort Garrison, MD, MBA
Chair/CEO.................. Kathy Gordon
CEO/President.............. Norman Gruber
President.................. Michael Hanslits, MD
Infection Control............. Pat Mason, RN
Emergency Room .... Susie Mendoza

Measure	Cases	This Hosp.	State Avg.	U.S. Avg.
Blood Clot Prevention and Treatment				
Anticoagulation Overlap Therapy[2]	153	96%	95%	93%
ICU Venous Thromboembolism Prophylaxis[2]	133	96%	87%	92%
Incidence of Potentially Preventable VTE[2]	24	17%	13%	10%
UFH with Dosages/Platelet Monitoring[2]	130	100%	100%	97%
Venous Thromboembolism Prophylaxis[2]	384	89%	83%	85%
Warfarin Therapy Discharge Instructions[2]	126	25%	54%	75%
Chest Pain/Possible Heart Attack Care				
Aspirin Given Within 24 Hours of Arrival	36	94%	97%	96%
Fibrinolytic Meds Within 30 Min. of Arrival[7]	-	-	57%	58%
Average Time to ECG (minutes)	38	`12	9	7
Average Time to Transfer (minutes)[7]	-	-	52	60
Children's Asthma Care				
Received Home Management Plan of Care	-	-	-	88%
Received Reliever Medication	-	-	-	100%
Received Systemic Corticosteroids	-	-	-	100%
Emergency Department				
Admittance Decision Time (minutes)[2]	517	101	85	98
Head CT Results Within 45 Min. of Arrival	35	29%	45%	57%
Patients Who Left ER Before Being Seen	93,387	3%	2%	2%
Time from ER Arrival to Admit. (minutes)[2]	521	269	235	274
Time from ER Arrival to Discharge (minutes)	430	188	136	134
Time in ER Before Being Evaluated (minutes)	474	48	27	26
Time to Pain Meds for Fractures (minutes)	259	61	56	57
Heart Attack Care				
Aspirin Given at Discharge[2]	297	99%	99%	99%
Fibrinolytic Meds Within 30 Min. of Arrival[1,2]	-	-	57%	54%
PCI Within 90 Minutes of Arrival[2]	64	98%	93%	96%
Statin Prescribed at Discharge[2]	266	98%	98%	98%
Heart Failure Care				
ACE Inhibitor or ARB for LVSD[2]	77	100%	96%	97%
Discharge Instructions Given[2]	265	99%	93%	94%
Evaluation of LVS Function[2]	303	100%	99%	99%
Medicare Spending				
Medicare Spending per Patient (ratio)	-	0.92	0.88	0.98
Pneumonia Care				
Appropriate Initial Antibiotic Given[2]	101	95%	96%	95%
Blood Culture Timing[2]	193	97%	98%	98%
Pregnancy and Delivery Care				
Newborn Deliveries Scheduled Early[2]	57	4%	3%	6%
Preventive Care				
Immunization for Influenza[2]	579	89%	86%	90%
Immunization for Pneumonia[2]	749	93%	88%	92%
Stroke Care				
Anticoagulation Therapy for Atrial Fibrillation[2]	28	82%	94%	95%
Antithrombotic Therapy Timing[2]	171	95%	97%	98%
Assessed for Rehabilitation[2]	188	97%	96%	97%
Discharged on Antithrombotic Therapy[2]	183	99%	99%	99%
Discharged on Statin Medication[2]	146	95%	93%	94%
Thrombolytic Therapy Timing[2]	23	22%	55%	66%
Venous Thromboembolism Prophylaxis[2]	181	96%	90%	94%
Written Stroke Educational Materials Given[2]	101	96%	81%	88%
Surgical Care Improvement Project				
Appropriate Beta Blocker Usage[2]	219	97%	98%	98%
Appropriate VTP Within 24 Hours[2]	385	96%	97%	98%
Controlled Postoperative Blood Glucose[2]	160	100%	98%	97%
Perioperative Temperature Management[2]	531	100%	100%	100%
Prophylactic Antibiotic Selection[2]	495	99%	99%	99%
Prophylactic Antibiotic Selection (Outpatient)	714	99%	98%	98%
Prophylactic Antibiotic Stopped[2]	494	99%	98%	98%
Prophylactic Antibiotic Timing[2]	504	97%	98%	99%
Prophylactic Antibiotic Timing (Outpatient)	727	95%	96%	98%
Urinary Catheter Removal[2]	455	97%	97%	97%
Survey of Patients' Hospital Experiences				
Area Around Room 'Always' Quiet at Night	300+	53%	57%	61%
Doctors 'Always' Communicated Well	300+	80%	81%	82%
Home Recovery Information Given	300+	86%	86%	85%
Hospital Given 9 or 10 on 10 Point Scale	300+	74%	70%	71%
Meds 'Always' Explained Before Given	300+	61%	65%	64%
Nurses 'Always' Communicated Well	300+	79%	79%	79%
Pain 'Always' Well Controlled	300+	71%	71%	71%
Room and Bathroom 'Always' Clean	300+	74%	74%	73%
Timely Help 'Always' Received	300+	65%	68%	68%
Would Definitely Recommend Hospital	300+	78%	72%	71%
Use of Medical Imaging				

NOTE: Hospital profiles are in alphabetical order by state, then city, then hospital within the city; Rankings exclude hospitals with less than 25 cases except for patient surveys which excludes hospitals with less than 100 cases; (a) 100-299 cases; (1) The number of cases/patients is too few to report; (2) Data submitted were based on a sample of cases/patients; (3) Results are based on a shorter time period than required; (4) Data suppressed by CMS for one or more quarters; (5) Results are not available for this reporting period; (6) Fewer than 100 patients completed the HCAHPS survey; (7) No cases met the criteria for this measure; (8) The lower limit of the confidence interval cannot be calculated if the number of observed infections equals zero; (9) No data are available from the state/territory for this reporting period; (10) The scores shown reflect fewer than 50 completed surveys; (11) There were discrepancies in the data collection process; (12) This measure does not apply to this hospital for this reporting period; (13) Results cannot be calculated for this reporting period; (14) The results for this state are combined with nearby states to protect confidentiality; Please refer to the User's Guide for a full explanation of data.

Cardiac Imaging Stress Test before Surgery	64	3.1%	4.7%	5.3%
Combination Abdominal CT Scan	915	3.6%	6.6%	10.5%
Combination Brain/Sinus CT Scan	757	2.8%	2.1%	2.7%
Combination Chest CT Scan	491	1.2%	1.1%	2.7%
Follow-up Mammogram/Ultrasound	174	10.3%	8.9%	8.8%
Lumbar Spine MRI for Low Back Pain	117	38.5%	41.7%	37.2%

Providence Seaside Hospital

725 S Wahanna Road Phone: 503-717-7000
Seaside, OR 97138 Fax: 503-717-7505
URL: www.providence.org/northcoast
Type: Critical Access Hospitals Emergency Services: Yes
Ownership: Voluntary non-profit - Church Beds: 27
Key Personnel:
Patient Relations . . . . Vickie Condon
Chief of Medical Staff . . . . Dominique Greco, MD
Emergency Room . . . . Jim Sisk, MD

Measure	Cases	This Hosp.	State Avg.	U.S. Avg.
Blood Clot Prevention and Treatment				
Anticoagulation Overlap Therapy[1,2]	-	-	95%	93%
ICU Venous Thromboembolism Prophylaxis[2]	103	82%	87%	92%
Incidence of Potentially Preventable VTE[1,2]	-	-	13%	10%
UFH with Dosages/Platelet Monitoring[1,2]	-	-	100%	97%
Venous Thromboembolism Prophylaxis[2]	19	53%	83%	85%
Warfarin Therapy Discharge Instructions[1,2]	-	-	54%	75%
Chest Pain/Possible Heart Attack Care				
Aspirin Given Within 24 Hours of Arrival	36	100%	97%	96%
Fibrinolytic Meds Within 30 Min. of Arrival[1]	-	-	57%	58%
Average Time to ECG (minutes)	36	6	9	7
Average Time to Transfer (minutes)[1]	-	-	52	60
Children's Asthma Care				
Received Home Management Plan of Care	-	-	-	88%
Received Reliever Medication	-	-	-	100%
Received Systemic Corticosteroids	-	-	-	100%
Emergency Department				
Admittance Decision Time (minutes)[2]	311	96	85	98
Head CT Results Within 45 Min. of Arrival[1]	-	-	45%	57%
Patients Who Left ER Before Being Seen	9,289	1%	2%	2%
Time from ER Arrival to Admit. (minutes)[2]	316	206	235	274
Time from ER Arrival to Discharge (minutes)	134	112	136	134
Time in ER Before Being Evaluated (minutes)	46	9	27	26
Time to Pain Meds for Fractures (minutes)	37	30	56	57
Heart Attack Care				
Aspirin Given at Discharge[1,2]	-	-	99%	99%
Fibrinolytic Meds Within 30 Min. of Arrival[2,3]	-	-	57%	54%
PCI Within 90 Minutes of Arrival[2,3]	-	-	93%	96%
Statin Prescribed at Discharge[1,2]	-	-	98%	98%
Heart Failure Care				
ACE Inhibitor or ARB for LVSD[1,2]	-	-	96%	97%
Discharge Instructions Given[2]	21	86%	93%	94%
Evaluation of LVS Function[2]	24	92%	99%	99%
Medicare Spending				
Medicare Spending per Patient (ratio)	-	-	0.88	0.98
Pneumonia Care				
Appropriate Initial Antibiotic Given[2]	27	96%	96%	95%
Blood Culture Timing[2]	60	100%	98%	98%
Pregnancy and Delivery Care				
Newborn Deliveries Scheduled Early[1]	-	-	3%	6%
Preventive Care				
Immunization for Influenza[2]	273	87%	86%	90%
Immunization for Pneumonia[2]	366	90%	88%	92%
Stroke Care				
Anticoagulation Therapy for Atrial Fibrillation[1,2]	-	-	94%	95%
Antithrombotic Therapy Timing[2]	11	82%	97%	98%
Assessed for Rehabilitation[2]	12	92%	96%	97%
Discharged on Antithrombotic Therapy[2]	12	100%	99%	99%
Discharged on Statin Medication[2]	11	82%	93%	94%
Thrombolytic Therapy Timing[2,7]	-	-	55%	66%
Venous Thromboembolism Prophylaxis[2]	12	58%	90%	94%
Written Stroke Educational Materials Given[1,2]	-	-	81%	88%
Surgical Care Improvement Project				
Appropriate Beta Blocker Usage[1,2]	-	-	98%	98%
Appropriate VTP Within 24 Hours[2]	23	96%	97%	98%
Controlled Postoperative Blood Glucose[2,7]	-	-	98%	97%
Perioperative Temperature Management[2]	26	100%	100%	100%
Prophylactic Antibiotic Selection[2]	22	100%	99%	99%
Prophylactic Antibiotic Selection (Outpatient)	15	73%	98%	98%
Prophylactic Antibiotic Stopped[2]	22	95%	98%	98%
Prophylactic Antibiotic Timing[2]	22	100%	98%	99%
Prophylactic Antibiotic Timing (Outpatient)	15	73%	96%	98%
Urinary Catheter Removal[2]	13	100%	97%	97%
Survey of Patients' Hospital Experiences				
Area Around Room 'Always' Quiet at Night	(a)	53%	57%	61%
Doctors 'Always' Communicated Well	(a)	79%	81%	82%
Home Recovery Information Given	(a)	81%	86%	85%
Hospital Given 9 or 10 on 10 Point Scale	(a)	72%	70%	71%
Meds 'Always' Explained Before Given	(a)	61%	65%	64%
Nurses 'Always' Communicated Well	(a)	84%	79%	79%
Pain 'Always' Well Controlled	(a)	72%	71%	71%
Room and Bathroom 'Always' Clean	(a)	85%	74%	73%
Timely Help 'Always' Received	(a)	75%	68%	68%
Would Definitely Recommend Hospital	(a)	70%	72%	71%
Use of Medical Imaging				
Cardiac Imaging Stress Test before Surgery[1]	-	-	4.7%	5.3%
Combination Abdominal CT Scan	230	4.3%	6.6%	10.5%
Combination Brain/Sinus CT Scan	165	0.0%	2.1%	2.7%
Combination Chest CT Scan	111	1.8%	1.1%	2.7%
Follow-up Mammogram/Ultrasound	366	10.4%	8.9%	8.8%
Lumbar Spine MRI for Low Back Pain[1]	-	-	41.7%	37.2%

Silverton Hospital

342 Fairview Street Phone: 503-873-1500
Silverton, OR 97381 Fax: 503-873-1534
E-mail: wwsilver@open.org
URL: www.silvertonhospital.org
Type: Acute Care Hospitals Emergency Services: Yes
Ownership: Voluntary non-profit - Private Beds: 48
Key Personnel:
Cardiac Laboratory . . . . Glen Cunningham
Quality Assurance . . . . Kathy Fluery
Chief of Medical Staff . . . . John Gilliam
Radiology . . . . Christopher D Groeser
Infection Control . . . . Becci Hopper
Operating Room . . . . Pam Kloft, RN
Emergency Room . . . . Frank Lord
Intensive Care Unit . . . . Maureen Murphy, RN

Measure	Cases	This Hosp.	State Avg.	U.S. Avg.
Blood Clot Prevention and Treatment				
Anticoagulation Overlap Therapy[2]	16	81%	95%	93%
ICU Venous Thromboembolism Prophylaxis[2]	16	75%	87%	92%
Incidence of Potentially Preventable VTE[1,2]	-	-	13%	10%
UFH with Dosages/Platelet Monitoring[1,2]	-	-	100%	97%
Venous Thromboembolism Prophylaxis[2]	95	77%	83%	85%
Warfarin Therapy Discharge Instructions[2]	15	0%	54%	75%
Chest Pain/Possible Heart Attack Care				
Aspirin Given Within 24 Hours of Arrival	76	93%	97%	96%
Fibrinolytic Meds Within 30 Min. of Arrival[1]	-	-	57%	58%
Average Time to ECG (minutes)	82	9	9	7
Average Time to Transfer (minutes)[1]	-	-	52	60
Children's Asthma Care				
Received Home Management Plan of Care	-	-	-	88%
Received Reliever Medication	-	-	-	100%
Received Systemic Corticosteroids	-	-	-	100%
Emergency Department				
Admittance Decision Time (minutes)[2]	180	55	85	98
Head CT Results Within 45 Min. of Arrival[1]	-	-	45%	57%
Patients Who Left ER Before Being Seen	23,249	0%	2%	2%
Time from ER Arrival to Admit. (minutes)[2]	186	183	235	274
Time from ER Arrival to Discharge (minutes)	359	86	136	134
Time in ER Before Being Evaluated (minutes)	193	13	27	26
Time to Pain Meds for Fractures (minutes)	99	41	56	57
Heart Attack Care				
Aspirin Given at Discharge	16	100%	99%	99%
Fibrinolytic Meds Within 30 Min. of Arrival[7]	-	-	57%	54%
PCI Within 90 Minutes of Arrival[7]	-	-	93%	96%
Statin Prescribed at Discharge	15	87%	98%	98%
Heart Failure Care				
ACE Inhibitor or ARB for LVSD[1]	-	-	96%	97%
Discharge Instructions Given	35	49%	93%	94%
Evaluation of LVS Function	44	98%	99%	99%
Medicare Spending				
Medicare Spending per Patient (ratio)	-	0.83	0.88	0.98
Pneumonia Care				
Appropriate Initial Antibiotic Given	56	100%	96%	95%
Blood Culture Timing	75	100%	98%	98%
Pregnancy and Delivery Care				
Newborn Deliveries Scheduled Early[2]	26	0%	3%	6%
Preventive Care				
Immunization for Influenza[2]	312	59%	86%	90%
Immunization for Pneumonia[2]	207	77%	88%	92%
Stroke Care				
Anticoagulation Therapy for Atrial Fibrillation[1,2]	-	-	94%	95%
Antithrombotic Therapy Timing[2]	20	100%	97%	98%
Assessed for Rehabilitation[2]	20	95%	96%	97%
Discharged on Antithrombotic Therapy[2]	19	95%	99%	99%
Discharged on Statin Medication[2]	15	80%	93%	94%
Thrombolytic Therapy Timing[1,2]	-	-	55%	66%
Venous Thromboembolism Prophylaxis[2]	18	94%	90%	94%
Written Stroke Educational Materials Given[1,2]	-	-	81%	88%
Surgical Care Improvement Project				
Appropriate Beta Blocker Usage[2]	53	94%	98%	98%
Appropriate VTP Within 24 Hours[2]	257	96%	97%	98%
Controlled Postoperative Blood Glucose[2,7]	-	-	98%	97%
Perioperative Temperature Management[2]	283	100%	100%	100%
Prophylactic Antibiotic Selection[2]	193	95%	99%	99%
Prophylactic Antibiotic Selection (Outpatient)	81	95%	98%	98%
Prophylactic Antibiotic Stopped[2]	189	98%	98%	98%
Prophylactic Antibiotic Timing[2]	195	96%	98%	99%
Prophylactic Antibiotic Timing (Outpatient)	82	98%	96%	98%
Urinary Catheter Removal[2]	188	91%	97%	97%
Survey of Patients' Hospital Experiences				
Area Around Room 'Always' Quiet at Night	300+	60%	57%	61%
Doctors 'Always' Communicated Well	300+	84%	81%	82%
Home Recovery Information Given	300+	87%	86%	85%
Hospital Given 9 or 10 on 10 Point Scale	300+	82%	70%	71%
Meds 'Always' Explained Before Given	300+	69%	65%	64%
Nurses 'Always' Communicated Well	300+	82%	79%	79%
Pain 'Always' Well Controlled	300+	72%	71%	71%
Room and Bathroom 'Always' Clean	300+	79%	74%	73%
Timely Help 'Always' Received	300+	66%	68%	68%
Would Definitely Recommend Hospital	300+	84%	72%	71%
Use of Medical Imaging				
Cardiac Imaging Stress Test before Surgery	61	4.9%	4.7%	5.3%
Combination Abdominal CT Scan	233	5.2%	6.6%	10.5%
Combination Brain/Sinus CT Scan[1]	-	-	2.1%	2.7%
Combination Chest CT Scan	84	0.0%	1.1%	2.7%
Follow-up Mammogram/Ultrasound	551	17.2%	8.9%	8.8%
Lumbar Spine MRI for Low Back Pain[1]	-	-	41.7%	37.2%

McKenzie - Willamette Medical Center

1460 G Street Phone: 541-726-4400
Springfield, OR 97477 Fax: 541-726-4540
E-mail: royorr@mckweb.com
URL: www.mckweb.com
Type: Acute Care Hospitals Emergency Services: Yes
Ownership: Voluntary non-profit - Private Beds: 114
Key Personnel:
Operating Room . . . . Thomas Bascom, RN
Quality Assurance . . . . Margaret Beals
Radiology . . . . David Board, MD
Intensive Care Unit . . . . Joe Kintz, MD
Emergency Room . . . . Alex Morley, MD
CEO/President . . . . Roy J Orr
Infection Control . . . . Cathy Stone
Chief of Medical Staff . . . . Larry Vinis, MD

Measure	Cases	This Hosp.	State Avg.	U.S. Avg.
Blood Clot Prevention and Treatment				
Anticoagulation Overlap Therapy[2]	24	100%	95%	93%
ICU Venous Thromboembolism Prophylaxis[2]	121	100%	87%	92%
Incidence of Potentially Preventable VTE[1,2]	-	-	13%	10%
UFH with Dosages/Platelet Monitoring[2]	14	100%	100%	97%

NOTE: Hospital profiles are in alphabetical order by state, then city, then hospital within the city; Rankings exclude hospitals with less than 25 cases except for patient surveys which excludes hospitals with less than 100 cases; (a) 100-299 cases; (1) The number of cases/patients is too few to report; (2) Data submitted were based on a sample of cases/patients; (3) Results are based on a shorter time period than required; (4) Data suppressed by CMS for one or more quarters; (5) Results are not available for this reporting period; (6) Fewer than 100 patients completed the HCAHPS survey; (7) No cases met the criteria for this measure; (8) The lower limit of the confidence interval cannot be calculated if the number of observed infections equals zero; (9) No data are available from the state/territory for this reporting period; (10) The scores shown reflect fewer than 50 completed surveys; (11) There were discrepancies in the data collection process; (12) This measure does not apply to this hospital for this reporting period; (13) Results cannot be calculated for this reporting period; (14) The results for this state are combined with nearby states to protect confidentiality; Please refer to the User's Guide for a full explanation of data.

Venous Thromboembolism Prophylaxis[2]	331	98%	83%	85%
Warfarin Therapy Discharge Instructions[2]	21	100%	54%	75%
Chest Pain/Possible Heart Attack Care				
Aspirin Given Within 24 Hours of Arrival[5]	-	-	97%	96%
Fibrinolytic Meds Within 30 Min. of Arrival[5]	-	-	57%	58%
Average Time to ECG (minutes)[5]	-	-	9	7
Average Time to Transfer (minutes)[5]	-	-	52	60
Children's Asthma Care				
Received Home Management Plan of Care	-	-	-	88%
Received Reliever Medication	-	-	-	100%
Received Systemic Corticosteroids	-	-	-	100%
Emergency Department				
Admittance Decision Time (minutes)[2]	481	90	85	98
Head CT Results Within 45 Min. of Arrival[1]	-	-	45%	57%
Patients Who Left ER Before Being Seen	32,262	1%	2%	2%
Time from ER Arrival to Admit. (minutes)[2]	664	196	235	274
Time from ER Arrival to Discharge (minutes)	394	91	136	134
Time in ER Before Being Evaluated (minutes)	335	18	27	26
Time to Pain Meds for Fractures (minutes)	125	49	56	57
Heart Attack Care				
Aspirin Given at Discharge	140	100%	99%	99%
Fibrinolytic Meds Within 30 Min. of Arrival[7]	-	-	57%	54%
PCI Within 90 Minutes of Arrival	20	100%	93%	96%
Statin Prescribed at Discharge	140	100%	98%	98%
Heart Failure Care				
ACE Inhibitor or ARB for LVSD	46	96%	96%	97%
Discharge Instructions Given	166	98%	93%	94%
Evaluation of LVS Function	208	100%	99%	99%
Medicare Spending				
Medicare Spending per Patient (ratio)	-	0.90	0.88	0.98
Pneumonia Care				
Appropriate Initial Antibiotic Given	147	99%	96%	95%
Blood Culture Timing	141	100%	98%	98%
Pregnancy and Delivery Care				
Newborn Deliveries Scheduled Early[2]	30	3%	3%	6%
Preventive Care				
Immunization for Influenza[2]	642	99%	86%	90%
Immunization for Pneumonia[2]	851	98%	88%	92%
Stroke Care				
Anticoagulation Therapy for Atrial Fibrillation[1]	-	-	94%	95%
Antithrombotic Therapy Timing	33	100%	97%	98%
Assessed for Rehabilitation	42	100%	96%	97%
Discharged on Antithrombotic Therapy	39	100%	99%	99%
Discharged on Statin Medication	28	100%	93%	94%
Thrombolytic Therapy Timing[1]	-	-	55%	66%
Venous Thromboembolism Prophylaxis	34	100%	90%	94%
Written Stroke Educational Materials Given	26	96%	81%	88%
Surgical Care Improvement Project				
Appropriate Beta Blocker Usage	245	100%	98%	98%
Appropriate VTP Within 24 Hours	625	100%	97%	98%
Controlled Postoperative Blood Glucose	112	100%	98%	97%
Perioperative Temperature Management	756	100%	100%	100%
Prophylactic Antibiotic Selection	632	100%	99%	99%
Prophylactic Antibiotic Selection (Outpatient)	316	100%	98%	98%
Prophylactic Antibiotic Stopped	616	100%	98%	98%
Prophylactic Antibiotic Timing	632	100%	98%	99%
Prophylactic Antibiotic Timing (Outpatient)	316	100%	96%	98%
Urinary Catheter Removal	516	100%	97%	97%
Survey of Patients' Hospital Experiences				
Area Around Room 'Always' Quiet at Night	300+	56%	57%	61%
Doctors 'Always' Communicated Well	300+	81%	81%	82%
Home Recovery Information Given	300+	88%	86%	85%
Hospital Given 9 or 10 on 10 Point Scale	300+	73%	70%	71%
Meds 'Always' Explained Before Given	300+	67%	65%	64%
Nurses 'Always' Communicated Well	300+	79%	79%	79%
Pain 'Always' Well Controlled	300+	72%	71%	71%
Room and Bathroom 'Always' Clean	300+	71%	74%	73%
Timely Help 'Always' Received	300+	65%	68%	68%
Would Definitely Recommend Hospital	300+	76%	72%	71%
Use of Medical Imaging				
Cardiac Imaging Stress Test before Surgery	91	2.2%	4.7%	5.3%
Combination Abdominal CT Scan	211	0.9%	6.6%	10.5%
Combination Brain/Sinus CT Scan	219	5.0%	2.1%	2.7%
Combination Chest CT Scan	51	0.0%	1.1%	2.7%
Follow-up Mammogram/Ultrasound[7]	-	-	8.9%	8.8%
Lumbar Spine MRI for Low Back Pain[1]	-	-	41.7%	37.2%

Sacred Heart Medical Center - Riverbend

3333 Riverbend Drive — Phone: 541-222-7300
Springfield, OR 97477
URL: www.peacehealth.org/sacred-heart-riverbend
Type: Acute Care Hospitals — Emergency Services: Yes
Ownership: Voluntary non-profit - Private

Measure	Cases	This Hosp.	State Avg.	U.S. Avg.
Blood Clot Prevention and Treatment				
Anticoagulation Overlap Therapy[2]	128	97%	95%	93%
ICU Venous Thromboembolism Prophylaxis[2]	53	92%	87%	92%
Incidence of Potentially Preventable VTE[2]	17	6%	13%	10%
UFH with Dosages/Platelet Monitoring[2]	48	100%	100%	97%
Venous Thromboembolism Prophylaxis[2]	298	86%	83%	85%
Warfarin Therapy Discharge Instructions[2]	103	78%	54%	75%
Chest Pain/Possible Heart Attack Care				
Aspirin Given Within 24 Hours of Arrival[1,3]	-	-	97%	96%
Fibrinolytic Meds Within 30 Min. of Arrival[3,7]	-	-	57%	58%
Average Time to ECG (minutes)[1,3]	-	-	9	7
Average Time to Transfer (minutes)[3,7]	-	-	52	60
Children's Asthma Care				
Received Home Management Plan of Care	-	-	-	88%
Received Reliever Medication	-	-	-	100%
Received Systemic Corticosteroids	-	-	-	100%
Emergency Department				
Admittance Decision Time (minutes)[2]	467	79	85	98
Head CT Results Within 45 Min. of Arrival[1]	-	-	45%	57%
Patients Who Left ER Before Being Seen	54,061	2%	2%	2%
Time from ER Arrival to Admit. (minutes)[2]	472	239	235	274
Time from ER Arrival to Discharge (minutes)	371	173	136	134
Time in ER Before Being Evaluated (minutes)	389	36	27	26
Time to Pain Meds for Fractures (minutes)	183	63	56	57
Heart Attack Care				
Aspirin Given at Discharge	579	99%	99%	99%
Fibrinolytic Meds Within 30 Min. of Arrival[7]	-	-	57%	54%
PCI Within 90 Minutes of Arrival	79	96%	93%	96%
Statin Prescribed at Discharge	566	99%	98%	98%
Heart Failure Care				
ACE Inhibitor or ARB for LVSD	120	100%	96%	97%
Discharge Instructions Given	364	94%	93%	94%
Evaluation of LVS Function	433	100%	99%	99%
Medicare Spending				
Medicare Spending per Patient (ratio)	-	0.87	0.88	0.98
Pneumonia Care				
Appropriate Initial Antibiotic Given	259	97%	96%	95%
Blood Culture Timing	377	98%	98%	98%
Pregnancy and Delivery Care				
Newborn Deliveries Scheduled Early	159	1%	3%	6%
Preventive Care				
Immunization for Influenza[2]	546	74%	86%	90%
Immunization for Pneumonia[2]	628	73%	88%	92%
Stroke Care				
Anticoagulation Therapy for Atrial Fibrillation[2]	15	93%	94%	95%
Antithrombotic Therapy Timing[2]	77	97%	97%	98%
Assessed for Rehabilitation[2]	115	97%	96%	97%
Discharged on Antithrombotic Therapy[2]	88	100%	99%	99%
Discharged on Statin Medication[2]	65	97%	93%	94%
Thrombolytic Therapy Timing[1,2]	-	-	55%	66%
Venous Thromboembolism Prophylaxis[2]	118	93%	90%	94%
Written Stroke Educational Materials Given[2]	70	89%	81%	88%
Surgical Care Improvement Project				
Appropriate Beta Blocker Usage[2]	271	100%	98%	98%
Appropriate VTP Within 24 Hours[2]	408	99%	97%	98%
Controlled Postoperative Blood Glucose[2]	170	97%	98%	97%
Perioperative Temperature Management[2]	552	100%	100%	100%
Prophylactic Antibiotic Selection[2]	505	100%	99%	99%
Prophylactic Antibiotic Selection (Outpatient)	894	99%	98%	98%
Prophylactic Antibiotic Stopped[2]	483	98%	98%	98%
Prophylactic Antibiotic Timing[2]	507	100%	98%	99%
Prophylactic Antibiotic Timing (Outpatient)	891	99%	96%	98%
Urinary Catheter Removal[2]	256	99%	97%	97%
Survey of Patients' Hospital Experiences				
Area Around Room 'Always' Quiet at Night	300+	60%	57%	61%
Doctors 'Always' Communicated Well	300+	78%	81%	82%
Home Recovery Information Given	300+	88%	86%	85%
Hospital Given 9 or 10 on 10 Point Scale	300+	76%	70%	71%
Meds 'Always' Explained Before Given	300+	57%	65%	64%
Nurses 'Always' Communicated Well	300+	73%	79%	79%
Pain 'Always' Well Controlled	300+	68%	71%	71%
Room and Bathroom 'Always' Clean	300+	67%	74%	73%
Timely Help 'Always' Received	300+	60%	68%	68%
Would Definitely Recommend Hospital	300+	78%	72%	71%
Use of Medical Imaging				
Cardiac Imaging Stress Test before Surgery	668	4.9%	4.7%	5.3%
Combination Abdominal CT Scan	363	1.4%	6.6%	10.5%
Combination Brain/Sinus CT Scan	590	2.0%	2.1%	2.7%
Combination Chest CT Scan[1]	-	-	1.1%	2.7%
Follow-up Mammogram/Ultrasound[7]	-	-	8.9%	8.8%
Lumbar Spine MRI for Low Back Pain[1]	-	-	41.7%	37.2%

Santiam Memorial Hospital

1401 N 10th Avenue — Phone: 503-769-2175
Stayton, OR 97383 — Fax: 503-769-5877
URL: www.santiamhospital.com
Type: Acute Care Hospitals — Emergency Services: Yes
Ownership: Voluntary non-profit - Private — Beds: 40

Key Personnel:
Anesthesiology. . . . . Frederick Carlock, MD
CEO/President. . . . . Terry Fletchall
Radiology. . . . . John Hoffman, MD
Chief of Medical Staff . . . . Thomas Vanveen
Emergency Room . . . . Steven Vets, DO
Cardiology . . . . James Wasenmiller, MD
Surgery . . . . Clark Yoder

Measure	Cases	This Hosp.	State Avg.	U.S. Avg.
Blood Clot Prevention and Treatment				
Anticoagulation Overlap Therapy[2]	14	50%	95%	93%
ICU Venous Thromboembolism Prophylaxis[1,2]	-	-	87%	92%
Incidence of Potentially Preventable VTE[1,2]	-	-	13%	10%
UFH with Dosages/Platelet Monitoring[1,2]	-	-	100%	97%
Venous Thromboembolism Prophylaxis[2]	98	86%	83%	85%
Warfarin Therapy Discharge Instructions[2]	11	100%	54%	75%
Chest Pain/Possible Heart Attack Care				
Aspirin Given Within 24 Hours of Arrival	27	81%	97%	96%
Fibrinolytic Meds Within 30 Min. of Arrival[7]	-	-	57%	58%
Average Time to ECG (minutes)	29	10	9	7
Average Time to Transfer (minutes)[1]	-	-	52	60
Children's Asthma Care				
Received Home Management Plan of Care	-	-	-	88%
Received Reliever Medication	-	-	-	100%
Received Systemic Corticosteroids	-	-	-	100%
Emergency Department				
Admittance Decision Time (minutes)[2]	269	75	85	98
Head CT Results Within 45 Min. of Arrival[1]	-	-	45%	57%
Patients Who Left ER Before Being Seen	10,340	0%	2%	2%
Time from ER Arrival to Admit. (minutes)[2]	284	244	235	274
Time from ER Arrival to Discharge (minutes)	373	112	136	134
Time in ER Before Being Evaluated (minutes)	375	25	27	26
Time to Pain Meds for Fractures (minutes)	58	56	56	57
Heart Attack Care				
Aspirin Given at Discharge[3,7]	-	-	99%	99%
Fibrinolytic Meds Within 30 Min. of Arrival[3,7]	-	-	57%	54%
PCI Within 90 Minutes of Arrival[3,7]	-	-	93%	96%
Statin Prescribed at Discharge[3,7]	-	-	98%	98%
Heart Failure Care				
ACE Inhibitor or ARB for LVSD[1]	-	-	96%	97%
Discharge Instructions Given[1]	-	-	93%	94%
Evaluation of LVS Function	13	100%	99%	99%
Medicare Spending				
Medicare Spending per Patient (ratio)	-	0.82	0.88	0.98
Pneumonia Care				
Appropriate Initial Antibiotic Given	45	89%	96%	95%

NOTE: Hospital profiles are in alphabetical order by state, then city, then hospital within the city; Rankings exclude hospitals with less than 25 cases except for patient surveys which excludes hospitals with less than 100 cases; (a) 100-299 cases; (1) The number of cases/patients is too few to report; (2) Data submitted were based on a sample of cases/patients; (3) Results are based on a shorter time period than required; (4) Data suppressed by CMS for one or more quarters; (5) Results are not available for this reporting period; (6) Fewer than 100 patients completed the HCAHPS survey; (7) No cases met the criteria for this measure; (8) The lower limit of the confidence interval cannot be calculated if the number of observed infections equals zero; (9) No data are available from the state/territory for this reporting period; (10) The scores shown reflect fewer than 50 completed surveys; (11) There were discrepancies in the data collection process; (12) This measure does not apply to this hospital for this reporting period; (13) Results cannot be calculated for this reporting period; (14) The results for this state are combined with nearby states to protect confidentiality; Please refer to the User's Guide for a full explanation of data.

Measure	Cases	This Hosp.	State Avg.	U.S. Avg.
Blood Culture Timing	56	86%	98%	98%
Pregnancy and Delivery Care				
Newborn Deliveries Scheduled Early	11	9%	3%	6%
Preventive Care				
Immunization for Influenza[2]	296	84%	86%	90%
Immunization for Pneumonia[2]	365	81%	88%	92%
Stroke Care				
Anticoagulation Therapy for Atrial Fibrillation[1]	-	-	94%	95%
Antithrombotic Therapy Timing[1]	-	-	97%	98%
Assessed for Rehabilitation	12	100%	96%	97%
Discharged on Antithrombotic Therapy	11	91%	99%	99%
Discharged on Statin Medication	11	27%	93%	94%
Thrombolytic Therapy Timing[1]	-	-	55%	66%
Venous Thromboembolism Prophylaxis	13	92%	90%	94%
Written Stroke Educational Materials Given[1]	-	-	81%	88%
Surgical Care Improvement Project				
Appropriate Beta Blocker Usage	11	91%	98%	98%
Appropriate VTP Within 24 Hours	62	95%	97%	98%
Controlled Postoperative Blood Glucose[7]	-	-	98%	97%
Perioperative Temperature Management	72	100%	100%	100%
Prophylactic Antibiotic Selection	30	97%	99%	99%
Prophylactic Antibiotic Selection (Outpatient)[1,3]	-	-	98%	98%
Prophylactic Antibiotic Stopped	29	97%	98%	98%
Prophylactic Antibiotic Timing	31	71%	98%	99%
Prophylactic Antibiotic Timing (Outpatient)[1,3]	-	-	96%	98%
Urinary Catheter Removal	46	91%	97%	97%
Survey of Patients' Hospital Experiences				
Area Around Room 'Always' Quiet at Night	(a)	56%	57%	61%
Doctors 'Always' Communicated Well	(a)	81%	81%	82%
Home Recovery Information Given	(a)	84%	86%	85%
Hospital Given 9 or 10 on 10 Point Scale	(a)	74%	70%	71%
Meds 'Always' Explained Before Given	(a)	57%	65%	64%
Nurses 'Always' Communicated Well	(a)	81%	79%	79%
Pain 'Always' Well Controlled	(a)	73%	71%	71%
Room and Bathroom 'Always' Clean	(a)	82%	74%	73%
Timely Help 'Always' Received	(a)	65%	68%	68%
Would Definitely Recommend Hospital	(a)	71%	72%	71%
Use of Medical Imaging				
Cardiac Imaging Stress Test before Surgery	53	0.0%	4.7%	5.3%
Combination Abdominal CT Scan	141	1.4%	6.6%	10.5%
Combination Brain/Sinus CT Scan	141	0.7%	2.1%	2.7%
Combination Chest CT Scan	91	0.0%	1.1%	2.7%
Follow-up Mammogram/Ultrasound	205	10.7%	8.9%	8.8%
Lumbar Spine MRI for Low Back Pain[1]	-	-	41.7%	37.2%

Mid - Columbia Medical Center

1700 E 19th Street
The Dalles, OR 97058
Phone: 541-296-1111
Fax: 541-296-7600
URL: www.mcmc.net
Type: Acute Care Hospitals
Emergency Services: Yes
Ownership: Voluntary non-profit - Other
Beds: 49

Key Personnel:
Chief of Medical Staff.......... Changes Annually
Anesthesiology............... A Keith Burns, MD
Radiology................... Michael Capek, MD
Emergency Room .... John Jacobson, MD
Quality Assurance .... Barbara Larsen
Operating Room.............. Dick Ohnemus
Intensive Care Unit............ Shelley Reynolds-Wacker
Infection Control.............. Catherine Sessions

Measure	Cases	This Hosp.	State Avg.	U.S. Avg.
Blood Clot Prevention and Treatment				
Anticoagulation Overlap Therapy[1,2]	-	-	95%	93%
ICU Venous Thromboembolism Prophylaxis[2]	26	100%	87%	92%
Incidence of Potentially Preventable VTE[1,2]	-	-	13%	10%
UFH with Dosages/Platelet Monitoring[2,7]	-	-	100%	97%
Venous Thromboembolism Prophylaxis[2]	151	97%	83%	85%
Warfarin Therapy Discharge Instructions[1,2]	-	-	54%	75%
Chest Pain/Possible Heart Attack Care				
Aspirin Given Within 24 Hours of Arrival	77	97%	97%	96%
Fibrinolytic Meds Within 30 Min. of Arrival[1]	-	-	57%	58%
Average Time to ECG (minutes)	78	5	9	7
Average Time to Transfer (minutes)[1]	-	-	52	60
Children's Asthma Care				
Received Home Management Plan of Care	-	-	-	88%
Received Reliever Medication	-	-	-	100%
Received Systemic Corticosteroids	-	-	-	100%
Emergency Department				
Admittance Decision Time (minutes)[2]	353	129	85	98
Head CT Results Within 45 Min. of Arrival[1]	-	-	45%	57%
Patients Who Left ER Before Being Seen	15,968	2%	2%	2%
Time from ER Arrival to Admit. (minutes)[2]	368	248	235	274
Time from ER Arrival to Discharge (minutes)	345	125	136	134
Time in ER Before Being Evaluated (minutes)	386	28	27	26
Time to Pain Meds for Fractures (minutes)	49	46	56	57
Heart Attack Care				
Aspirin Given at Discharge	12	100%	99%	99%
Fibrinolytic Meds Within 30 Min. of Arrival[7]	-	-	57%	54%
PCI Within 90 Minutes of Arrival[7]	-	-	93%	96%
Statin Prescribed at Discharge[1]	-	-	98%	98%
Heart Failure Care				
ACE Inhibitor or ARB for LVSD	20	85%	96%	97%
Discharge Instructions Given	52	98%	93%	94%
Evaluation of LVS Function	60	98%	99%	99%
Medicare Spending				
Medicare Spending per Patient (ratio)	-	0.87	0.88	0.98
Pneumonia Care				
Appropriate Initial Antibiotic Given	54	98%	96%	95%
Blood Culture Timing	104	98%	98%	98%
Pregnancy and Delivery Care				
Newborn Deliveries Scheduled Early	12	0%	3%	6%
Preventive Care				
Immunization for Influenza[2]	260	87%	86%	90%
Immunization for Pneumonia[2]	335	91%	88%	92%
Stroke Care				
Anticoagulation Therapy for Atrial Fibrillation[1]	-	-	94%	95%
Antithrombotic Therapy Timing	17	100%	97%	98%
Assessed for Rehabilitation	24	100%	96%	97%
Discharged on Antithrombotic Therapy	24	100%	99%	99%
Discharged on Statin Medication	18	94%	93%	94%
Thrombolytic Therapy Timing[1]	-	-	55%	66%
Venous Thromboembolism Prophylaxis	17	100%	90%	94%
Written Stroke Educational Materials Given	19	100%	81%	88%
Surgical Care Improvement Project				
Appropriate Beta Blocker Usage	55	98%	98%	98%
Appropriate VTP Within 24 Hours	190	97%	97%	98%
Controlled Postoperative Blood Glucose[7]	-	-	98%	97%
Perioperative Temperature Management	217	100%	100%	100%
Prophylactic Antibiotic Selection	175	100%	99%	99%
Prophylactic Antibiotic Selection (Outpatient)	46	96%	98%	98%
Prophylactic Antibiotic Stopped	174	99%	98%	98%
Prophylactic Antibiotic Timing	175	99%	98%	99%
Prophylactic Antibiotic Timing (Outpatient)	46	100%	96%	98%
Urinary Catheter Removal	96	91%	97%	97%
Survey of Patients' Hospital Experiences				
Area Around Room 'Always' Quiet at Night	300+	53%	57%	61%
Doctors 'Always' Communicated Well	300+	81%	81%	82%
Home Recovery Information Given	300+	88%	86%	85%
Hospital Given 9 or 10 on 10 Point Scale	300+	69%	70%	71%
Meds 'Always' Explained Before Given	300+	68%	65%	64%
Nurses 'Always' Communicated Well	300+	80%	79%	79%
Pain 'Always' Well Controlled	300+	69%	71%	71%
Room and Bathroom 'Always' Clean	300+	74%	74%	73%
Timely Help 'Always' Received	300+	72%	68%	68%
Would Definitely Recommend Hospital	300+	69%	72%	71%
Use of Medical Imaging				
Cardiac Imaging Stress Test before Surgery	184	5.4%	4.7%	5.3%
Combination Abdominal CT Scan	409	11.0%	6.6%	10.5%
Combination Brain/Sinus CT Scan	267	1.1%	2.1%	2.7%
Combination Chest CT Scan	305	2.3%	1.1%	2.7%
Follow-up Mammogram/Ultrasound	770	12.2%	8.9%	8.8%
Lumbar Spine MRI for Low Back Pain	84	56.0%	41.7%	37.2%

Tillamook Regional Medical Center

1000 Third Street
Tillamook, OR 97141
Phone: 503-842-4444
Fax: 503-842-3062
E-mail: morrispa@ah.org
URL: www.tcgh.com
Type: Critical Access Hospitals
Emergency Services: Yes
Ownership: Voluntary non-profit - Church
Beds: 49

Key Personnel:
Radiology................... Randall L Bivens, MD
CEO/President............... David Butler
Emergency Room .... Larry Hamelton, RN
Operating Room.............. Lyle R Mohr, RN
Quality Assurance .... Gina Seufert
Chief of Medical Staff.......... Matt Turney
Infection Control.............. Pat Valenti

Measure	Cases	This Hosp.	State Avg.	U.S. Avg.
Blood Clot Prevention and Treatment				
Anticoagulation Overlap Therapy[1,2]	-	-	95%	93%
ICU Venous Thromboembolism Prophylaxis[2]	12	83%	87%	92%
Incidence of Potentially Preventable VTE[2,7]	-	-	13%	10%
UFH with Dosages/Platelet Monitoring[2,7]	-	-	100%	97%
Venous Thromboembolism Prophylaxis[2]	68	93%	83%	85%
Warfarin Therapy Discharge Instructions[1,2]	-	-	54%	75%
Chest Pain/Possible Heart Attack Care				
Aspirin Given Within 24 Hours of Arrival	-	-	97%	96%
Fibrinolytic Meds Within 30 Min. of Arrival	-	-	57%	58%
Average Time to ECG (minutes)	-	-	9	7
Average Time to Transfer (minutes)	-	-	52	60
Children's Asthma Care				
Received Home Management Plan of Care	-	-	-	88%
Received Reliever Medication	-	-	-	100%
Received Systemic Corticosteroids	-	-	-	100%
Emergency Department				
Admittance Decision Time (minutes)[5]	-	-	85	98
Head CT Results Within 45 Min. of Arrival	-	-	45%	57%
Patients Who Left ER Before Being Seen	-	-	2%	2%
Time from ER Arrival to Admit. (minutes)[5]	-	-	235	274
Time from ER Arrival to Discharge (minutes)	-	-	136	134
Time in ER Before Being Evaluated (minutes)	-	-	27	26
Time to Pain Meds for Fractures (minutes)	-	-	56	57
Heart Attack Care				
Aspirin Given at Discharge[1]	-	-	99%	99%
Fibrinolytic Meds Within 30 Min. of Arrival[7]	-	-	57%	54%
PCI Within 90 Minutes of Arrival[7]	-	-	93%	96%
Statin Prescribed at Discharge[1]	-	-	98%	98%
Heart Failure Care				
ACE Inhibitor or ARB for LVSD[1]	-	-	96%	97%
Discharge Instructions Given	14	100%	93%	94%
Evaluation of LVS Function	16	100%	99%	99%
Medicare Spending				
Medicare Spending per Patient (ratio)	-	-	0.88	0.98
Pneumonia Care				
Appropriate Initial Antibiotic Given	27	85%	96%	95%
Blood Culture Timing	43	98%	98%	98%
Pregnancy and Delivery Care				
Newborn Deliveries Scheduled Early[5]	-	-	3%	6%
Preventive Care				
Immunization for Influenza[5]	-	-	86%	90%
Immunization for Pneumonia[5]	-	-	88%	92%
Stroke Care				
Anticoagulation Therapy for Atrial Fibrillation[5]	-	-	94%	95%
Antithrombotic Therapy Timing[5]	-	-	97%	98%
Assessed for Rehabilitation[5]	-	-	96%	97%
Discharged on Antithrombotic Therapy[5]	-	-	99%	99%
Discharged on Statin Medication[5]	-	-	93%	94%
Thrombolytic Therapy Timing[5]	-	-	55%	66%
Venous Thromboembolism Prophylaxis[5]	-	-	90%	94%
Written Stroke Educational Materials Given[5]	-	-	81%	88%
Surgical Care Improvement Project				
Appropriate Beta Blocker Usage	15	100%	98%	98%
Appropriate VTP Within 24 Hours	49	100%	97%	98%
Controlled Postoperative Blood Glucose[7]	-	-	98%	97%
Perioperative Temperature Management	71	100%	100%	100%
Prophylactic Antibiotic Selection	46	100%	99%	99%

NOTE: Hospital profiles are in alphabetical order by state, then city, then hospital within the city; Rankings exclude hospitals with less than 25 cases except for patient surveys which excludes hospitals with less than 100 cases; (a) 100-299 cases; (1) The number of cases/patients is too few to report; (2) Data submitted were based on a sample of cases/patients; (3) Results are based on a shorter time period than required; (4) Data suppressed by CMS for one or more quarters; (5) Results are not available for this reporting period; (6) Fewer than 100 patients completed the HCAHPS survey; (7) No cases met the criteria for this measure; (8) The lower limit of the confidence interval cannot be calculated if the number of observed infections equals zero; (9) No data are available from the state/territory for this reporting period; (10) The scores shown reflect fewer than 50 completed surveys; (11) There were discrepancies in the data collection process; (12) This measure does not apply to this hospital for this reporting period; (13) Results cannot be calculated for this reporting period; (14) The results for this state are combined with nearby states to protect confidentiality; Please refer to the User's Guide for a full explanation of data.

Measure	Cases	This Hosp.	State Avg.	U.S. Avg.
Prophylactic Antibiotic Selection (Outpatient)	-	-	98%	98%
Prophylactic Antibiotic Stopped	46	100%	98%	98%
Prophylactic Antibiotic Timing	46	96%	98%	99%
Prophylactic Antibiotic Timing (Outpatient)	-	-	96%	98%
Urinary Catheter Removal[1]	-	-	97%	97%
Survey of Patients' Hospital Experiences				
Area Around Room 'Always' Quiet at Night	(a)	64%	57%	61%
Doctors 'Always' Communicated Well	(a)	79%	81%	82%
Home Recovery Information Given	(a)	88%	86%	85%
Hospital Given 9 or 10 on 10 Point Scale	(a)	66%	70%	71%
Meds 'Always' Explained Before Given	(a)	63%	65%	64%
Nurses 'Always' Communicated Well	(a)	79%	79%	79%
Pain 'Always' Well Controlled	(a)	71%	71%	71%
Room and Bathroom 'Always' Clean	(a)	73%	74%	73%
Timely Help 'Always' Received	(a)	72%	68%	68%
Would Definitely Recommend Hospital	(a)	60%	72%	71%
Use of Medical Imaging				
Cardiac Imaging Stress Test before Surgery	-	-	4.7%	5.3%
Combination Abdominal CT Scan	-	-	6.6%	10.5%
Combination Brain/Sinus CT Scan	-	-	2.1%	2.7%
Combination Chest CT Scan	-	-	1.1%	2.7%
Follow-up Mammogram/Ultrasound	-	-	8.9%	8.8%
Lumbar Spine MRI for Low Back Pain	-	-	41.7%	37.2%

Legacy Meridian Park Medical Center

19300 Sw 65th Avenue
Tualatin, OR 97062
Phone: 503-692-2182
Fax: 503-691-0919
URL: www.legacyhealth.org
Type: Acute Care Hospitals
Emergency Services: Yes
Ownership: Voluntary non-profit - Private
Beds: 133

Key Personnel:
Chief of Medical Staff. . . . . Jack Cioffi, MD
CEO/President. . . . . Lee Domanico
Intensive Care Unit. . . . . Sue Ellison, RN
Emergency Room . . . . M Scott Miller, MD
Operating Room. . . . . Rick Sexton, RN
Infection Control. . . . . Mary Shanks, RN

Measure	Cases	This Hosp.	State Avg.	U.S. Avg.
Blood Clot Prevention and Treatment				
Anticoagulation Overlap Therapy[2]	38	100%	95%	93%
ICU Venous Thromboembolism Prophylaxis[2]	60	95%	87%	92%
Incidence of Potentially Preventable VTE[1,2]	-	-	13%	10%
UFH with Dosages/Platelet Monitoring[2]	12	100%	100%	97%
Venous Thromboembolism Prophylaxis[2]	270	89%	83%	85%
Warfarin Therapy Discharge Instructions[2]	34	85%	54%	75%
Chest Pain/Possible Heart Attack Care				
Aspirin Given Within 24 Hours of Arrival	12	100%	97%	96%
Fibrinolytic Meds Within 30 Min. of Arrival[3,7]	-	-	57%	58%
Average Time to ECG (minutes)	12	0	9	7
Average Time to Transfer (minutes)[3,7]	-	-	52	60
Children's Asthma Care				
Received Home Management Plan of Care	-	-	-	88%
Received Reliever Medication	-	-	-	100%
Received Systemic Corticosteroids	-	-	-	100%
Emergency Department				
Admittance Decision Time (minutes)[2]	675	89	85	98
Head CT Results Within 45 Min. of Arrival[1]	-	-	45%	57%
Patients Who Left ER Before Being Seen	34,762	0%	2%	2%
Time from ER Arrival to Admit. (minutes)[2]	681	207	235	274
Time from ER Arrival to Discharge (minutes)	356	154	136	134
Time in ER Before Being Evaluated (minutes)	381	23	27	26
Time to Pain Meds for Fractures (minutes)	144	45	56	57
Heart Attack Care				
Aspirin Given at Discharge	174	100%	99%	99%
Fibrinolytic Meds Within 30 Min. of Arrival[7]	-	-	57%	54%
PCI Within 90 Minutes of Arrival	56	96%	93%	96%
Statin Prescribed at Discharge	171	98%	98%	98%
Heart Failure Care				
ACE Inhibitor or ARB for LVSD	64	95%	96%	97%
Discharge Instructions Given	172	98%	93%	94%
Evaluation of LVS Function	225	100%	99%	99%
Medicare Spending				
Medicare Spending per Patient (ratio)	-	0.90	0.88	0.98
Pneumonia Care				
Appropriate Initial Antibiotic Given	104	97%	96%	95%
Blood Culture Timing	178	99%	98%	98%
Pregnancy and Delivery Care				
Newborn Deliveries Scheduled Early[2]	14	14%	3%	6%
Preventive Care				
Immunization for Influenza[2]	562	94%	86%	90%
Immunization for Pneumonia[2]	692	95%	88%	92%
Stroke Care				
Anticoagulation Therapy for Atrial Fibrillation	31	100%	94%	95%
Antithrombotic Therapy Timing	100	98%	97%	98%
Assessed for Rehabilitation	130	93%	96%	97%
Discharged on Antithrombotic Therapy	119	100%	99%	99%
Discharged on Statin Medication	96	95%	93%	94%
Thrombolytic Therapy Timing[1]	-	-	55%	66%
Venous Thromboembolism Prophylaxis	121	92%	90%	94%
Written Stroke Educational Materials Given	68	91%	81%	88%
Surgical Care Improvement Project				
Appropriate Beta Blocker Usage[2]	62	100%	98%	98%
Appropriate VTP Within 24 Hours[2]	280	99%	97%	98%
Controlled Postoperative Blood Glucose[2,7]	-	-	98%	97%
Perioperative Temperature Management[2]	345	100%	100%	100%
Prophylactic Antibiotic Selection[2]	234	100%	99%	99%
Prophylactic Antibiotic Selection (Outpatient)	461	99%	98%	98%
Prophylactic Antibiotic Stopped[2]	233	99%	98%	98%
Prophylactic Antibiotic Timing[2]	234	98%	98%	99%
Prophylactic Antibiotic Timing (Outpatient)	461	99%	96%	98%
Urinary Catheter Removal[2]	148	99%	97%	97%
Survey of Patients' Hospital Experiences				
Area Around Room 'Always' Quiet at Night	300+	58%	57%	61%
Doctors 'Always' Communicated Well	300+	81%	81%	82%
Home Recovery Information Given	300+	87%	86%	85%
Hospital Given 9 or 10 on 10 Point Scale	300+	78%	70%	71%
Meds 'Always' Explained Before Given	300+	63%	65%	64%
Nurses 'Always' Communicated Well	300+	80%	79%	79%
Pain 'Always' Well Controlled	300+	73%	71%	71%
Room and Bathroom 'Always' Clean	300+	70%	74%	73%
Timely Help 'Always' Received	300+	70%	68%	68%
Would Definitely Recommend Hospital	300+	81%	72%	71%
Use of Medical Imaging				
Cardiac Imaging Stress Test before Surgery	61	1.6%	4.7%	5.3%
Combination Abdominal CT Scan	603	3.6%	6.6%	10.5%
Combination Brain/Sinus CT Scan	456	0.9%	2.1%	2.7%
Combination Chest CT Scan	487	1.0%	1.1%	2.7%
Follow-up Mammogram/Ultrasound	1,211	9.2%	8.9%	8.8%
Lumbar Spine MRI for Low Back Pain	174	37.9%	41.7%	37.2%

NOTE: Hospital profiles are in alphabetical order by state, then city, then hospital within the city; Rankings exclude hospitals with less than 25 cases except for patient surveys which excludes hospitals with less than 100 cases; (a) 100-299 cases; (1) The number of cases/patients is too few to report; (2) Data submitted were based on a sample of cases/patients; (3) Results are based on a shorter time period than required; (4) Data suppressed by CMS for one or more quarters; (5) Results are not available for this reporting period; (6) Fewer than 100 patients completed the HCAHPS survey; (7) No cases met the criteria for this measure; (8) The lower limit of the confidence interval cannot be calculated if the number of observed infections equals zero; (9) No data are available from the state/territory for this reporting period; (10) The scores shown reflect fewer than 50 completed surveys; (11) There were discrepancies in the data collection process; (12) This measure does not apply to this hospital for this reporting period; (13) Results cannot be calculated for this reporting period; (14) The results for this state are combined with nearby states to protect confidentiality; Please refer to the User's Guide for a full explanation of data.

Blood Clot Prevention and Treatment

Anticoagulation Overlap Therapy

Hospital Name	City	Rate	Cases
Alta View Hospital[2]	Sandy	100%	43
Lakeview Hospital[2]	Bountiful	100%	48
Mountain View Hospital[2]	Payson	100%	32
Valley View Medical Center[2]	Cedar City	100%	36
Dixie Regional Medical Center[2]	Saint George	99%	139
Saint Marks Hospital[2]	Salt Lake City	99%	187
Logan Regional Hospital[2]	Logan	98%	45
Ogden Regional Medical Center[2]	Ogden	98%	49
Davis Hospital & Medical Center[2]	Layton	97%	35
Jordan Valley Medical Center[2]	West Jordan	97%	74
Riverton Hospital[2]	Riverton	97%	29
Intermountain Medical Center[2]	Murray	96%	257
McKay Dee Hospital[2]	Ogden	96%	198
Univ Health Care/Univ Hosps[2]	Salt Lake City	92%	145
American Fork Hospital[2]	American Fork	90%	41
LDS Hospital[2]	Salt Lake City	89%	56
Timpanogos Regional Hospital[2]	Orem	89%	27
Castleview Hospital[2]	Price	88%	32
Utah Valley Regional Medical Center[2]	Provo	88%	141

ICU Venous Thromboembolism Prophylaxis

Hospital Name	City	Rate	Cases
McKay Dee Hospital[2]	Ogden	100%	45
Mountain View Hospital[2]	Payson	100%	49
Mountain West Medical Center[2]	Tooele	100%	39
Ogden Regional Medical Center[2]	Ogden	100%	74
Saint Marks Hospital[2]	Salt Lake City	99%	80
Univ Health Care/Univ Hosps[2]	Salt Lake City	96%	82
Intermountain Medical Center[2]	Murray	95%	129
Jordan Valley Medical Center[2]	West Jordan	95%	177
Timpanogos Regional Hospital[2]	Orem	94%	51
Dixie Regional Medical Center[2]	Saint George	93%	70
Alta View Hospital[2]	Sandy	92%	26
American Fork Hospital[2]	American Fork	91%	44
Ashley Regional Medical Center[2]	Vernal	91%	34
Lakeview Hospital[2]	Bountiful	90%	40
LDS Hospital[2]	Salt Lake City	90%	58
Castleview Hospital[2]	Price	89%	45
Davis Hospital & Medical Center[2]	Layton	89%	66
Logan Regional Hospital[2]	Logan	89%	46
Salt Lake Regional Medical Center[2]	Salt Lake City	88%	76
Valley View Medical Center[2]	Cedar City	85%	33
Utah Valley Regional Medical Center[2]	Provo	84%	135

Incidence of Potentially Preventable VTE

Hospital Name	City	Rate	Cases
Intermountain Medical Center[2]	Murray	0%	48
Saint Marks Hospital[2]	Salt Lake City	0%	26
Univ Health Care/Univ Hosps[2]	Salt Lake City	4%	47
Utah Valley Regional Medical Center[2]	Provo	8%	40

UFH with Dosages/Platelet Count Monitoring

Hospital Name	City	Rate	Cases
Dixie Regional Medical Center[2]	Saint George	100%	143
Ogden Regional Medical Center[2]	Ogden	100%	39
Saint Marks Hospital[2]	Salt Lake City	100%	52
Univ Health Care/Univ Hosps[2]	Salt Lake City	100%	116
McKay Dee Hospital[2]	Ogden	96%	107
Utah Valley Regional Medical Center[2]	Provo	94%	35
Intermountain Medical Center[2]	Murray	91%	144

Venous Thromboembolism Prophylaxis

Hospital Name	City	Rate	Cases
Mountain View Hospital[2]	Payson	100%	137
The Orthopedic Specialty Hospital[2]	Murray	100%	46
Mountain West Medical Center[2]	Tooele	98%	127
Saint Marks Hospital[2]	Salt Lake City	97%	289
Jordan Valley Medical Center[2]	West Jordan	95%	526
Park City Medical Center[2]	Park City	95%	42
Timpanogos Regional Hospital[2]	Orem	95%	198
Lakeview Hospital[2]	Bountiful	94%	238
Ogden Regional Medical Center[2]	Ogden	94%	283
Riverton Hospital[2]	Riverton	94%	112
Davis Hospital & Medical Center[2]	Layton	93%	270
Castleview Hospital[2]	Price	92%	106
Salt Lake Regional Medical Center[2]	Salt Lake City	91%	150
McKay Dee Hospital[2]	Ogden	90%	283
Intermountain Medical Center[2]	Murray	88%	238
Alta View Hospital[2]	Sandy	87%	138
Univ Health Care/Univ Hosps[2]	Salt Lake City	86%	318
Dixie Regional Medical Center[2]	Saint George	84%	274
Utah Valley Regional Medical Center[2]	Provo	84%	237
American Fork Hospital[2]	American Fork	83%	192
Cache Valley Speciality Hospital[2]	North Logan	83%	66
Logan Regional Hospital[2]	Logan	83%	226
LDS Hospital[2]	Salt Lake City	82%	271
Brigham City Community Hospital[2]	Brigham City	81%	74
Ashley Regional Medical Center[2]	Vernal	77%	101
Bear River Valley Hospital[2]	Tremonton	75%	60
Delta Community Medical Center	Delta	71%	59
Valley View Medical Center[2]	Cedar City	71%	115
Sanpete Valley Hospital[2]	Mount Pleasant	68%	82
Heber Valley Medical Center[2]	Heber City	67%	79
Uintah Basin Medical Center[2]	Roosevelt	66%	68
Fillmore Community Medical Center	Fillmore	65%	51
Garfield Memorial Hospital[2]	Panguitch	62%	99
Sevier Valley Medical Center[2]	Richfield	51%	97
Beaver Valley Hospital[2]	Beaver	29%	102

Warfarin Therapy Discharge Instructions

Hospital Name	City	Rate	Cases
Lakeview Hospital[2]	Bountiful	100%	25
Saint Marks Hospital[2]	Salt Lake City	98%	131
American Fork Hospital[2]	American Fork	97%	31
Davis Hospital & Medical Center[2]	Layton	93%	30
Univ Health Care/Univ Hosps[2]	Salt Lake City	93%	107
Ogden Regional Medical Center[2]	Ogden	91%	32
Logan Regional Hospital[2]	Logan	89%	36
McKay Dee Hospital[2]	Ogden	88%	159
Jordan Valley Medical Center[2]	West Jordan	80%	54
Utah Valley Regional Medical Center[2]	Provo	76%	116
Intermountain Medical Center[2]	Murray	60%	209
Valley View Medical Center[2]	Cedar City	31%	29
LDS Hospital[2]	Salt Lake City	30%	53
Dixie Regional Medical Center[2]	Saint George	26%	116
Alta View Hospital[2]	Sandy	21%	39

Chest Pain/Possible Heart Attack Care

Aspirin Given Within 24 Hours of Arrival

Hospital Name	City	Rate	Cases
American Fork Hospital	American Fork	100%	68
Ashley Regional Medical Center	Vernal	100%	29
Mountain West Medical Center	Tooele	100%	34
Riverton Hospital	Riverton	100%	65
Alta View Hospital	Sandy	98%	81
Brigham City Community Hospital	Brigham City	98%	40
Park City Medical Center	Park City	98%	54
Uintah Basin Medical Center	Roosevelt	98%	56
Valley View Medical Center	Cedar City	98%	44
Bear River Valley Hospital	Tremonton	97%	32
Castleview Hospital	Price	97%	72
Logan Regional Hospital	Logan	96%	26
Sevier Valley Medical Center	Richfield	95%	38
LDS Hospital	Salt Lake City	92%	39

Average Time to ECG (minutes)

Hospital Name	City	Min.	Cases
Riverton Hospital	Riverton	3	66
Alta View Hospital	Sandy	5	84
Ashley Regional Medical Center	Vernal	5	30
American Fork Hospital	American Fork	6	71
Logan Regional Hospital	Logan	6	26
Mountain West Medical Center	Tooele	6	36
Park City Medical Center	Park City	6	56
Bear River Valley Hospital	Tremonton	8	34
LDS Hospital	Salt Lake City	8	37
Sevier Valley Medical Center	Richfield	8	37
Uintah Basin Medical Center	Roosevelt	8	59
Valley View Medical Center	Cedar City	8	44
Castleview Hospital	Price	10	73
Brigham City Community Hospital	Brigham City	11	41

Children's Asthma Care

Received Home Management Plan of Care

Hospital Name	City	Rate	Cases
Primary Childrens Hospital	Salt Lake City	96%	410

Received Reliever Medication

Hospital Name	City	Rate	Cases
Primary Childrens Hospital	Salt Lake City	100%	411

Received Systemic Corticosteroids

Hospital Name	City	Rate	Cases
Primary Childrens Hospital	Salt Lake City	100%	410

Emergency Department

Admittance Decision Time (minutes)

Hospital Name	City	Min.	Cases
Beaver Valley Hospital[2]	Beaver	0	129
Delta Community Medical Center	Delta	15	75
Brigham City Community Hospital[2]	Brigham City	26	204
Sanpete Valley Hospital	Mount Pleasant	32	133
Sevier Valley Medical Center[2]	Richfield	34	127
Fillmore Community Medical Center	Fillmore	35	49
Castleview Hospital[2]	Price	38	305
Garfield Memorial Hospital	Panguitch	41	150
Uintah Basin Medical Center[2]	Roosevelt	49	601
Heber Valley Medical Center[2]	Heber City	50	157
Mountain View Hospital[2]	Payson	53	357
Cache Valley Speciality Hospital[2]	North Logan	55	103
Ashley Regional Medical Center[2]	Vernal	59	251
Davis Hospital & Medical Center[2]	Layton	60	596
Timpanogos Regional Hospital[2]	Orem	60	231
American Fork Hospital[2]	American Fork	62	305
Bear River Valley Hospital[2]	Tremonton	62	156
Valley View Medical Center[2]	Cedar City	62	264
Dixie Regional Medical Center[2]	Saint George	63	510
Jordan Valley Medical Center[2]	West Jordan	70	759
Ogden Regional Medical Center[2]	Ogden	70	376
Alta View Hospital[2]	Sandy	75	303
Lakeview Hospital[2]	Bountiful	76	360
McKay Dee Hospital[2]	Ogden	76	480
LDS Hospital[2]	Salt Lake City	77	288
Riverton Hospital[2]	Riverton	77	272
Intermountain Medical Center[2]	Murray	83	484
Park City Medical Center[2]	Park City	84	145
Logan Regional Hospital[2]	Logan	85	251
Mountain West Medical Center[2]	Tooele	85	349
Utah Valley Regional Medical Center[2]	Provo	85	387
Saint Marks Hospital[2]	Salt Lake City	94	488
Univ Health Care/Univ Hosps[2]	Salt Lake City	100	118
Salt Lake Regional Medical Center[2]	Salt Lake City	150	166

Patients Who Left ER Before Being Seen

Hospital Name	City	Rate	Cases
American Fork Hospital	American Fork	0%	28218
Bear River Valley Hospital	Tremonton	0%	5899
Beaver Valley Hospital	Beaver	0%	2234
Brigham City Community Hospital	Brigham City	0%	8501
Cache Valley Speciality Hospital	North Logan	0%	3695
Central Valley Medical Center	Nephi	0%	4167
Garfield Memorial Hospital	Panguitch	0%	2202
Heber Valley Medical Center	Heber City	0%	5471
Lakeview Hospital	Bountiful	0%	16525
Logan Regional Hospital	Logan	0%	24546
Mountain View Hospital	Payson	0%	17399
Ogden Regional Medical Center	Ogden	0%	25713
Park City Medical Center	Park City	0%	9801
Saint Marks Hospital	Salt Lake City	0%	49893
San Juan Hospital	Monticello	0%	1822
Timpanogos Regional Hospital	Orem	0%	16342
Alta View Hospital	Sandy	1%	24431
Ashley Regional Medical Center	Vernal	1%	11343
Davis Hospital & Medical Center	Layton	1%	31099
Dixie Regional Medical Center	Saint George	1%	42809
Jordan Valley Medical Center	West Jordan	1%	57229
LDS Hospital	Salt Lake City	1%	24082
McKay Dee Hospital	Ogden	1%	64435
Mountain West Medical Center	Tooele	1%	15535
Orem Community Hospital	Orem	1%	7256
Riverton Hospital	Riverton	1%	25598
Salt Lake Regional Medical Center	Salt Lake City	1%	10789
Sevier Valley Medical Center	Richfield	1%	6852
Uintah Basin Medical Center	Roosevelt	1%	10708
Univ Health Care/Univ Hosps	Salt Lake City	1%	42688
Utah Valley Regional Medical Center	Provo	1%	46924
Valley View Medical Center	Cedar City	1%	15489
Castleview Hospital	Price	2%	11931
Gunnison Valley Hospital	Gunnison	2%	3691
Intermountain Medical Center	Murray	2%	86341

Time from ER Arrival to Being Admitted (minutes)

Hospital Name	City	Min.	Cases
Beaver Valley Hospital[2]	Beaver	101	129
Delta Community Medical Center	Delta	130	102
Fillmore Community Medical Center	Fillmore	143	59
Sevier Valley Medical Center[2]	Richfield	156	270
Garfield Memorial Hospital	Panguitch	161	158
Mountain View Hospital[2]	Payson	179	357
Uintah Basin Medical Center[2]	Roosevelt	180	602
Cache Valley Speciality Hospital[2]	North Logan	192	105
Brigham City Community Hospital[2]	Brigham City	198	204
Ogden Regional Medical Center[2]	Ogden	200	377
Sanpete Valley Hospital	Mount Pleasant	201	184

NOTE: Hospital profiles are in alphabetical order by state, then city, then hospital within the city; Rankings exclude hospitals with less than 25 cases except for patient surveys which excludes hospitals with less than 100 cases; (a) 100-299 cases; (1) The number of cases/patients is too few to report; (2) Data submitted were based on a sample of cases/patients; (3) Results are based on a shorter time period than required; (4) Data suppressed by CMS for one or more quarters; (5) Results are not available for this reporting period; (6) Fewer than 100 patients completed the HCAHPS survey; (7) No cases met the criteria for this measure; (8) The lower limit of the confidence interval cannot be calculated if the number of observed infections equals zero; (9) No data are available from the state/territory for this reporting period; (10) The scores shown reflect fewer than 50 completed surveys; (11) There were discrepancies in the data collection process; (12) This measure does not apply to this hospital for this reporting period; (13) Results cannot be calculated for this reporting period; (14) The results for this state are combined with nearby states to protect confidentiality; Please refer to the User's Guide for a full explanation of data.

Lakeview Hospital[2]	Bountiful	204	360
Timpanogos Regional Hospital[2]	Orem	204	231
Dixie Regional Medical Center[2]	Saint George	205	518
American Fork Hospital[2]	American Fork	206	307
Davis Hospital & Medical Center[2]	Layton	208	600
Valley View Medical Center[2]	Cedar City	208	266
Park City Medical Center[2]	Park City	210	152
Bear River Valley Hospital[2]	Tremonton	213	175
Heber Valley Medical Center[2]	Heber City	218	173
Castleview Hospital[2]	Price	221	309
McKay Dee Hospital[2]	Ogden	228	491
Utah Valley Regional Medical Center[2]	Provo	234	387
Logan Regional Hospital[2]	Logan	239	267
Ashley Regional Medical Center[2]	Vernal	241	251
Mountain West Medical Center[2]	Tooele	241	349
Jordan Valley Medical Center[2]	West Jordan	242	769
Saint Marks Hospital[2]	Salt Lake City	245	492
LDS Hospital[2]	Salt Lake City	248	294
Riverton Hospital[2]	Riverton	252	284
Alta View Hospital[2]	Sandy	266	307
Intermountain Medical Center[2]	Murray	273	491
Univ Health Care/Univ Hosps[2]	Salt Lake City	296	278
Salt Lake Regional Medical Center[2]	Salt Lake City	312	178

Time from ER Arrival to Discharge (minutes)

Hospital Name	City	Min.	Cases
Delta Community Medical Center	Delta	81	252
Brigham City Community Hospital	Brigham City	86	408
Orem Community Hospital	Orem	86	393
Uintah Basin Medical Center	Roosevelt	86	384
Cache Valley Speciality Hospital	North Logan	92	201
Heber Valley Medical Center	Heber City	94	393
Sanpete Valley Hospital	Mount Pleasant	94	357
Bear River Valley Hospital	Tremonton	97	368
Garfield Memorial Hospital	Panguitch	101	239
Sevier Valley Medical Center	Richfield	101	392
Fillmore Community Medical Center	Fillmore	102	244
Park City Medical Center	Park City	102	384
Beaver Valley Hospital	Beaver	105	616
Mountain View Hospital	Payson	111	435
Timpanogos Regional Hospital	Orem	112	444
Ogden Regional Medical Center	Ogden	116	492
Ashley Regional Medical Center	Vernal	118	394
Valley View Medical Center	Cedar City	118	385
American Fork Hospital	American Fork	121	406
Mountain West Medical Center	Tooele	125	375
Lakeview Hospital	Bountiful	129	430
Dixie Regional Medical Center	Saint George	130	387
Davis Hospital & Medical Center	Layton	132	761
Castleview Hospital	Price	137	373
Logan Regional Hospital	Logan	140	271
McKay Dee Hospital	Ogden	140	382
Salt Lake Regional Medical Center	Salt Lake City	140	402
Utah Valley Regional Medical Center	Provo	142	399
Jordan Valley Medical Center	West Jordan	145	1343
Saint Marks Hospital	Salt Lake City	146	498
LDS Hospital	Salt Lake City	156	374
Riverton Hospital	Riverton	156	395
Alta View Hospital	Sandy	166	387
Univ Health Care/Univ Hosps	Salt Lake City	172	329
Intermountain Medical Center	Murray	206	416

Time in ER Before Being Evaluated (minutes)

Hospital Name	City	Min.	Cases
Park City Medical Center	Park City	3	458
Bear River Valley Hospital	Tremonton	4	394
Cache Valley Speciality Hospital	North Logan	10	252
Brigham City Community Hospital	Brigham City	11	462
Ashley Regional Medical Center	Vernal	12	437
Lakeview Hospital	Bountiful	12	498
Logan Regional Hospital	Logan	12	279
Mountain View Hospital	Payson	13	467
Sanpete Valley Hospital	Mount Pleasant	13	399
Saint Marks Hospital	Salt Lake City	14	543
Timpanogos Regional Hospital	Orem	14	475
Garfield Memorial Hospital	Panguitch	15	217
Ogden Regional Medical Center	Ogden	15	507
Orem Community Hospital	Orem	15	423
American Fork Hospital	American Fork	16	426
Heber Valley Medical Center	Heber City	16	376
Mountain West Medical Center	Tooele	16	418
Valley View Medical Center	Cedar City	17	369
Alta View Hospital	Sandy	20	421
Beaver Valley Hospital	Beaver	20	588
Castleview Hospital	Price	20	415
Jordan Valley Medical Center	West Jordan	20	1461
LDS Hospital	Salt Lake City	20	411
Uintah Basin Medical Center	Roosevelt	20	401
McKay Dee Hospital	Ogden	21	404
Dixie Regional Medical Center	Saint George	22	420

Fillmore Community Medical Center	Fillmore	22	269
Riverton Hospital	Riverton	22	420
Sevier Valley Medical Center	Richfield	22	417
Utah Valley Regional Medical Center	Provo	25	426
Delta Community Medical Center	Delta	26	235
Intermountain Medical Center	Murray	28	443
Univ Health Care/Univ Hosps	Salt Lake City	28	365
Davis Hospital & Medical Center	Layton	31	762
Salt Lake Regional Medical Center	Salt Lake City	41	441

Time to Pain Meds for Bone Fractures (minutes)

Hospital Name	City	Min.	Cases
Cache Valley Speciality Hospital	North Logan	24	40
Mountain View Hospital	Payson	27	100
Park City Medical Center	Park City	28	142
Bear River Valley Hospital	Tremonton	30	54
Orem Community Hospital	Orem	30	36
Heber Valley Medical Center	Heber City	34	54
American Fork Hospital	American Fork	35	203
Alta View Hospital	Sandy	38	138
Lakeview Hospital	Bountiful	39	79
Jordan Valley Medical Center	West Jordan	40	322
Ogden Regional Medical Center	Ogden	40	110
Logan Regional Hospital	Logan	41	185
Riverton Hospital	Riverton	42	196
LDS Hospital	Salt Lake City	43	57
Sanpete Valley Hospital	Mount Pleasant	43	34
Uintah Basin Medical Center	Roosevelt	43	63
Ashley Regional Medical Center	Vernal	44	86
Sevier Valley Medical Center	Richfield	44	40
Timpanogos Regional Hospital	Orem	46	102
Davis Hospital & Medical Center	Layton	47	206
Valley View Medical Center	Cedar City	47	77
Castleview Hospital	Price	48	71
McKay Dee Hospital	Ogden	50	308
Saint Marks Hospital	Salt Lake City	50	146
Univ Health Care/Univ Hosps	Salt Lake City	50	123
Mountain West Medical Center	Tooele	51	105
Brigham City Community Hospital	Brigham City	53	41
Dixie Regional Medical Center	Saint George	53	198
Utah Valley Regional Medical Center	Provo	53	184
Intermountain Medical Center	Murray	58	200

Heart Attack Care

Aspirin Given at Discharge

Hospital Name	City	Rate	Cases
Davis Hospital & Medical Center	Layton	100%	66
Intermountain Medical Center[2]	Murray	100%	564
Jordan Valley Medical Center	West Jordan	100%	147
Lakeview Hospital	Bountiful	100%	74
Logan Regional Hospital	Logan	100%	51
McKay Dee Hospital	Ogden	100%	193
Salt Lake Regional Medical Center	Salt Lake City	100%	65
Timpanogos Regional Hospital	Orem	100%	52
Univ Health Care/Univ Hosps	Salt Lake City	100%	241
VA Salt Lake City Healthcare	Salt Lake City	100%	61
Dixie Regional Medical Center	Saint George	99%	360
Ogden Regional Medical Center[2]	Ogden	99%	92
Saint Marks Hospital	Salt Lake City	99%	183
Utah Valley Regional Medical Center	Provo	99%	389
Mountain View Hospital[2]	Payson	95%	39

PCI Within 90 Minutes of Arrival

Hospital Name	City	Rate	Cases
Intermountain Medical Center[2]	Murray	100%	100
Lakeview Hospital	Bountiful	100%	28
Saint Marks Hospital	Salt Lake City	100%	34
Jordan Valley Medical Center	West Jordan	98%	60
McKay Dee Hospital	Ogden	98%	54
Utah Valley Regional Medical Center	Provo	98%	53
Univ Health Care/Univ Hosps	Salt Lake City	96%	26
Dixie Regional Medical Center	Saint George	90%	50

Statin Prescribed at Discharge

Hospital Name	City	Rate	Cases
Intermountain Medical Center[2]	Murray	100%	555
Jordan Valley Medical Center	West Jordan	100%	141
Lakeview Hospital	Bountiful	100%	65
Logan Regional Hospital	Logan	100%	52
McKay Dee Hospital	Ogden	100%	194
Mountain View Hospital[2]	Payson	100%	41
Ogden Regional Medical Center[2]	Ogden	100%	89
Salt Lake Regional Medical Center	Salt Lake City	100%	65
Timpanogos Regional Hospital	Orem	100%	53
Univ Health Care/Univ Hosps	Salt Lake City	100%	246
VA Salt Lake City Healthcare	Salt Lake City	100%	66
Dixie Regional Medical Center	Saint George	99%	340
Saint Marks Hospital	Salt Lake City	99%	170

Utah Valley Regional Medical Center	Provo	99%	399
Davis Hospital & Medical Center	Layton	98%	65

Heart Failure Care

ACE Inhibitor or ARB for LVSD

Hospital Name	City	Rate	Cases
Davis Hospital & Medical Center	Layton	100%	31
Jordan Valley Medical Center	West Jordan	100%	40
Ogden Regional Medical Center[2]	Ogden	100%	28
Saint Marks Hospital	Salt Lake City	100%	102
Univ Health Care/Univ Hosps	Salt Lake City	100%	111
Intermountain Medical Center	Murray	99%	209
VA Salt Lake City Healthcare	Salt Lake City	99%	92
Utah Valley Regional Medical Center	Provo	97%	66
Dixie Regional Medical Center	Saint George	96%	46
McKay Dee Hospital	Ogden	95%	88

Discharge Instructions Given

Hospital Name	City	Rate	Cases
Alta View Hospital	Sandy	100%	26
Davis Hospital & Medical Center	Layton	100%	60
Lakeview Hospital	Bountiful	100%	46
McKay Dee Hospital	Ogden	100%	210
Saint Marks Hospital	Salt Lake City	100%	223
VA Salt Lake City Healthcare	Salt Lake City	100%	214
Dixie Regional Medical Center	Saint George	99%	189
Ogden Regional Medical Center[2]	Ogden	99%	69
Univ Health Care/Univ Hosps	Salt Lake City	99%	280
Intermountain Medical Center	Murray	98%	499
LDS Hospital	Salt Lake City	98%	52
Mountain View Hospital[2]	Payson	98%	40
Salt Lake Regional Medical Center	Salt Lake City	98%	52
American Fork Hospital	American Fork	97%	39
Logan Regional Hospital	Logan	97%	37
Valley View Medical Center	Cedar City	94%	31
Utah Valley Regional Medical Center	Provo	92%	165
Jordan Valley Medical Center	West Jordan	91%	102

Evaluation of LVS Function

Hospital Name	City	Rate	Cases
Alta View Hospital	Sandy	100%	35
American Fork Hospital	American Fork	100%	47
Davis Hospital & Medical Center	Layton	100%	90
Dixie Regional Medical Center	Saint George	100%	233
Intermountain Medical Center	Murray	100%	572
Jordan Valley Medical Center	West Jordan	100%	128
Lakeview Hospital	Bountiful	100%	75
LDS Hospital	Salt Lake City	100%	61
Logan Regional Hospital	Logan	100%	44
McKay Dee Hospital	Ogden	100%	259
Mountain View Hospital[2]	Payson	100%	54
Mountain West Medical Center	Tooele	100%	31
Ogden Regional Medical Center[2]	Ogden	100%	90
Saint Marks Hospital	Salt Lake City	100%	296
Salt Lake Regional Medical Center	Salt Lake City	100%	70
Timpanogos Regional Hospital	Orem	100%	26
Univ Health Care/Univ Hosps	Salt Lake City	100%	308
Utah Valley Regional Medical Center	Provo	100%	208
VA Salt Lake City Healthcare	Salt Lake City	100%	228
Valley View Medical Center	Cedar City	100%	32
Uintah Basin Medical Center	Roosevelt	71%	28

Medicare Spending

Medicare Spending per Patient (ratio)

Hospital Name	City	Ratio	Cases
Beaver Valley Hospital	Beaver	0.72	-
Bear River Valley Hospital	Tremonton	0.76	-
Ashley Regional Medical Center	Vernal	0.81	-
Garfield Memorial Hospital	Panguitch	0.84	-
Uintah Basin Medical Center	Roosevelt	0.85	-
Logan Regional Hospital	Logan	0.88	-
Valley View Medical Center	Cedar City	0.91	-
Castleview Hospital	Price	0.93	-
Dixie Regional Medical Center	Saint George	0.93	-
Riverton Hospital	Riverton	0.93	-
Alta View Hospital	Sandy	0.95	-
Brigham City Community Hospital	Brigham City	0.95	-
American Fork Hospital	American Fork	0.96	-
LDS Hospital	Salt Lake City	0.96	-
McKay Dee Hospital	Ogden	0.96	-
The Orthopedic Specialty Hospital	Murray	0.96	-
Park City Medical Center	Park City	0.96	-
Cache Valley Speciality Hospital	North Logan	0.97	-
Intermountain Medical Center	Murray	0.97	-
Mountain West Medical Center	Tooele	0.98	-
Mountain View Hospital	Payson	0.99	-
Ogden Regional Medical Center	Ogden	1.00	-

NOTE: Hospital profiles are in alphabetical order by state, then city, then hospital within the city; Rankings exclude hospitals with less than 25 cases except for patient surveys which excludes hospitals with less than 100 cases; (a) 100-299 cases; (1) The number of cases/patients is too few to report; (2) Data submitted were based on a sample of cases/patients; (3) Results are based on a shorter time period than required; (4) Data suppressed by CMS for one or more quarters; (5) Results are not available for this reporting period; (6) Fewer than 100 patients completed the HCAHPS survey; (7) No cases met the criteria for this measure; (8) The lower limit of the confidence interval cannot be calculated if the number of observed infections equals zero; (9) No data are available from the state/territory for this reporting period; (10) The scores shown reflect fewer than 50 completed surveys; (11) There were discrepancies in the data collection process; (12) This measure does not apply to this hospital for this reporting period; (13) Results cannot be calculated for this reporting period; (14) The results for this state are combined with nearby states to protect confidentiality; Please refer to the User's Guide for a full explanation of data.

Univ Health Care/Univ Hosps	Salt Lake City	1.00	-
Lakeview Hospital	Bountiful	1.01	-
Utah Valley Regional Medical Center	Provo	1.02	-
Saint Marks Hospital	Salt Lake City	1.04	-
Timpanogos Regional Hospital	Orem	1.04	-
Jordan Valley Medical Center	West Jordan	1.07	-
Salt Lake Regional Medical Center	Salt Lake City	1.09	-
Davis Hospital & Medical Center	Layton	1.11	-
Sevier Valley Medical Center	Richfield	1.11	-

Pneumonia Care

Appropriate Initial Antibiotic Given

Hospital Name	City	Rate	Cases
Alta View Hospital[2]	Sandy	100%	81
Ashley Regional Medical Center	Vernal	100%	41
Davis Hospital & Medical Center	Layton	100%	68
Intermountain Medical Center[2]	Murray	100%	83
Lakeview Hospital	Bountiful	100%	71
Logan Regional Hospital[2]	Logan	100%	81
Mountain View Hospital[2]	Payson	100%	56
Timpanogos Regional Hospital	Orem	100%	56
VA Salt Lake City Healthcare	Salt Lake City	100%	58
American Fork Hospital[2]	American Fork	99%	83
Univ Health Care/Univ Hosps	Salt Lake City	99%	84
Jordan Valley Medical Center	West Jordan	98%	161
LDS Hospital[2]	Salt Lake City	98%	115
Mountain West Medical Center	Tooele	98%	56
Ogden Regional Medical Center[2]	Ogden	98%	84
Riverton Hospital	Riverton	98%	63
Valley View Medical Center	Cedar City	98%	46
Salt Lake Regional Medical Center	Salt Lake City	97%	35
Utah Valley Regional Medical Center[2]	Provo	97%	73
Saint Marks Hospital[2]	Salt Lake City	96%	113
Dixie Regional Medical Center[2]	Saint George	95%	87
McKay Dee Hospital[2]	Ogden	94%	116
Beaver Valley Hospital[2]	Beaver	91%	34
Castleview Hospital	Price	86%	49
Sevier Valley Medical Center	Richfield	86%	29
Central Valley Medical Center	Nephi	84%	57
Uintah Basin Medical Center	Roosevelt	83%	30
Gunnison Valley Hospital[2]	Gunnison	81%	36

Blood Culture Timing

Hospital Name	City	Rate	Cases
Davis Hospital & Medical Center	Layton	100%	91
Dixie Regional Medical Center[2]	Saint George	100%	116
Intermountain Medical Center[2]	Murray	100%	123
LDS Hospital[2]	Salt Lake City	100%	131
Mountain View Hospital[2]	Payson	100%	90
Ogden Regional Medical Center[2]	Ogden	100%	114
Park City Medical Center	Park City	100%	32
Riverton Hospital	Riverton	100%	53
Sevier Valley Medical Center	Richfield	100%	37
Utah Valley Regional Medical Center[2]	Provo	100%	163
American Fork Hospital[2]	American Fork	99%	111
Castleview Hospital	Price	99%	86
Jordan Valley Medical Center	West Jordan	99%	218
Lakeview Hospital	Bountiful	99%	128
Logan Regional Hospital[2]	Logan	99%	130
Timpanogos Regional Hospital	Orem	99%	77
VA Salt Lake City Healthcare	Salt Lake City	99%	105
Valley View Medical Center	Cedar City	99%	68
Ashley Regional Medical Center	Vernal	98%	49
McKay Dee Hospital[2]	Ogden	98%	184
Saint Marks Hospital[2]	Salt Lake City	98%	154
Salt Lake Regional Medical Center	Salt Lake City	98%	46
Alta View Hospital[2]	Sandy	97%	90
Mountain West Medical Center	Tooele	96%	72
Univ Health Care/Univ Hosps	Salt Lake City	96%	130
Uintah Basin Medical Center	Roosevelt	94%	36
Central Valley Medical Center	Nephi	91%	35

Pregnancy and Delivery Care

Newborns whose Deliveries were Scheduled Early

Hospital Name	City	Rate	Cases
Davis Hospital & Medical Center[2]	Layton	0%	55
Mountain West Medical Center[2]	Tooele	0%	39
Ogden Regional Medical Center[2]	Ogden	0%	52
Sevier Valley Medical Center	Richfield	0%	36
Uintah Basin Medical Center	Roosevelt	0%	48
Dixie Regional Medical Center[2]	Saint George	1%	80
McKay Dee Hospital[2]	Ogden	1%	87
American Fork Hospital[2]	American Fork	2%	64
Alta View Hospital[2]	Sandy	3%	32
Univ Health Care/Univ Hosps[2]	Salt Lake City	3%	59
Utah Valley Regional Medical Center[2]	Provo	4%	81
Valley View Medical Center[2]	Cedar City	4%	46
Mountain View Hospital[2]	Payson	5%	43
Orem Community Hospital[2]	Orem	5%	39
Riverton Hospital[2]	Riverton	5%	66
Timpanogos Regional Hospital[2]	Orem	5%	65
Intermountain Medical Center[2]	Murray	6%	87
Saint Marks Hospital[2]	Salt Lake City	6%	66
Lakeview Hospital	Bountiful	7%	83
LDS Hospital[2]	Salt Lake City	7%	58
Logan Regional Hospital[2]	Logan	7%	76
Jordan Valley Medical Center[2]	West Jordan	8%	87
Brigham City Community Hospital[2]	Brigham City	10%	42
Ashley Regional Medical Center[2]	Vernal	12%	50
Castleview Hospital[2]	Price	12%	41
Park City Medical Center[2]	Park City	13%	39
Salt Lake Regional Medical Center[2]	Salt Lake City	31%	39

Preventive Care

Immunization for Influenza

Hospital Name	City	Rate	Cases
Bear River Valley Hospital[2]	Tremonton	100%	200
Davis Hospital & Medical Center[2]	Layton	99%	707
Mountain View Hospital[2]	Payson	99%	359
Alta View Hospital[2]	Sandy	98%	367
Dixie Regional Medical Center[2]	Saint George	98%	535
Jordan Valley Medical Center[2]	West Jordan	98%	843
Lakeview Hospital[2]	Bountiful	98%	416
Orem Community Hospital[2]	Orem	98%	168
The Orthopedic Specialty Hospital[2]	Murray	98%	319
Salt Lake Regional Medical Center[2]	Salt Lake City	98%	329
Mountain West Medical Center[2]	Tooele	97%	287
Sevier Valley Medical Center[2]	Richfield	97%	250
McKay Dee Hospital[2]	Ogden	96%	508
Valley View Medical Center[2]	Cedar City	96%	276
Ashley Regional Medical Center[2]	Vernal	94%	252
Castleview Hospital[2]	Price	94%	252
Riverton Hospital[2]	Riverton	94%	407
LDS Hospital[2]	Salt Lake City	93%	468
Saint Marks Hospital[2]	Salt Lake City	93%	572
Univ Health Care/Univ Hosps[2]	Salt Lake City	93%	500
Brigham City Community Hospital[2]	Brigham City	92%	259
Garfield Memorial Hospital	Panguitch	92%	112
Intermountain Medical Center[2]	Murray	92%	521
Logan Regional Hospital[2]	Logan	92%	431
Timpanogos Regional Hospital[2]	Orem	92%	420
American Fork Hospital[2]	American Fork	90%	422
Cache Valley Speciality Hospital[2]	North Logan	89%	312
Park City Medical Center[2]	Park City	87%	292
Sanpete Valley Hospital	Mount Pleasant	87%	196
Utah Valley Regional Medical Center[2]	Provo	86%	508
Fillmore Community Medical Center	Fillmore	85%	74
Ogden Regional Medical Center[2]	Ogden	85%	485
Heber Valley Medical Center[2]	Heber City	83%	209
Delta Community Medical Center	Delta	78%	117
Uintah Basin Medical Center[2]	Roosevelt	75%	287
Beaver Valley Hospital[2]	Beaver	9%	138

Immunization for Pneumonia

Hospital Name	City	Rate	Cases
Bear River Valley Hospital[2]	Tremonton	99%	161
Castleview Hospital[2]	Price	98%	264
Jordan Valley Medical Center[2]	West Jordan	98%	684
Mountain View Hospital[2]	Payson	98%	375
Mountain West Medical Center[2]	Tooele	98%	267
Salt Lake Regional Medical Center[2]	Salt Lake City	98%	369
Lakeview Hospital[2]	Bountiful	97%	544
Timpanogos Regional Hospital[2]	Orem	97%	270
Brigham City Community Hospital[2]	Brigham City	96%	225
Davis Hospital & Medical Center[2]	Layton	96%	592
Alta View Hospital[2]	Sandy	95%	305
The Orthopedic Specialty Hospital[2]	Murray	95%	371
Saint Marks Hospital[2]	Salt Lake City	95%	630
Riverton Hospital[2]	Riverton	94%	176
Dixie Regional Medical Center[2]	Saint George	93%	629
McKay Dee Hospital[2]	Ogden	93%	464
Valley View Medical Center[2]	Cedar City	93%	209
Garfield Memorial Hospital	Panguitch	91%	157
Ogden Regional Medical Center[2]	Ogden	90%	404
Univ Health Care/Univ Hosps[2]	Salt Lake City	89%	437
Utah Valley Regional Medical Center[2]	Provo	89%	461
Sevier Valley Medical Center[2]	Richfield	88%	236
Intermountain Medical Center[2]	Murray	87%	542
American Fork Hospital[2]	American Fork	86%	272
Ashley Regional Medical Center[2]	Vernal	86%	187
Sanpete Valley Hospital	Mount Pleasant	86%	168
Fillmore Community Medical Center	Fillmore	85%	59
LDS Hospital[2]	Salt Lake City	84%	371
Delta Community Medical Center	Delta	82%	79
Heber Valley Medical Center[2]	Heber City	82%	136
Uintah Basin Medical Center[2]	Roosevelt	81%	339
Logan Regional Hospital[2]	Logan	79%	291
Park City Medical Center[2]	Park City	79%	213
Cache Valley Speciality Hospital[2]	North Logan	77%	385
Beaver Valley Hospital[2]	Beaver	18%	110

Stroke Care

Anticoagulation Therapy for Atrial Fibrillation

Hospital Name	City	Rate	Cases
Dixie Regional Medical Center	Saint George	100%	32
Intermountain Medical Center	Murray	98%	57
Saint Marks Hospital[2]	Salt Lake City	96%	25

Antithrombotic Therapy Timing

Hospital Name	City	Rate	Cases
Intermountain Medical Center	Murray	100%	232
Jordan Valley Medical Center	West Jordan	100%	50
Lakeview Hospital[2]	Bountiful	100%	41
Ogden Regional Medical Center[2]	Ogden	100%	51
Saint Marks Hospital[2]	Salt Lake City	100%	65
Dixie Regional Medical Center	Saint George	99%	112
Utah Valley Regional Medical Center	Provo	99%	119
McKay Dee Hospital	Ogden	98%	92
Univ Health Care/Univ Hosps[2]	Salt Lake City	98%	46
Davis Hospital & Medical Center	Layton	96%	28

Assessed for Rehabilitation

Hospital Name	City	Rate	Cases
Davis Hospital & Medical Center	Layton	100%	30
Intermountain Medical Center	Murray	100%	430
Lakeview Hospital[2]	Bountiful	100%	50
Ogden Regional Medical Center[2]	Ogden	100%	64
Saint Marks Hospital[2]	Salt Lake City	100%	100
Univ Health Care/Univ Hosps[2]	Salt Lake City	100%	100
Dixie Regional Medical Center	Saint George	99%	160
McKay Dee Hospital	Ogden	97%	154
Logan Regional Hospital	Logan	96%	25
Utah Valley Regional Medical Center	Provo	96%	204
Jordan Valley Medical Center	West Jordan	94%	63

Discharged on Antithrombotic Therapy

Hospital Name	City	Rate	Cases
Davis Hospital & Medical Center	Layton	100%	30
Intermountain Medical Center	Murray	100%	346
Jordan Valley Medical Center	West Jordan	100%	60
Lakeview Hospital[2]	Bountiful	100%	47
Ogden Regional Medical Center[2]	Ogden	100%	56
Saint Marks Hospital[2]	Salt Lake City	100%	93
Dixie Regional Medical Center	Saint George	99%	150
McKay Dee Hospital	Ogden	99%	136
Univ Health Care/Univ Hosps[2]	Salt Lake City	99%	78
Utah Valley Regional Medical Center	Provo	98%	166

Discharged on Statin Medication

Hospital Name	City	Rate	Cases
Intermountain Medical Center	Murray	99%	218
Saint Marks Hospital[2]	Salt Lake City	99%	69
Jordan Valley Medical Center	West Jordan	98%	51
McKay Dee Hospital	Ogden	98%	101
Ogden Regional Medical Center[2]	Ogden	98%	41
Univ Health Care/Univ Hosps[2]	Salt Lake City	98%	53
Dixie Regional Medical Center	Saint George	97%	117
Lakeview Hospital[2]	Bountiful	97%	37
Utah Valley Regional Medical Center	Provo	95%	121

Thrombolytic Therapy Timing

Hospital Name	City	Rate	Cases
Intermountain Medical Center	Murray	98%	50

Venous Thromboembolism (VTE) Prophylaxis

Hospital Name	City	Rate	Cases
Ogden Regional Medical Center[2]	Ogden	100%	66
Saint Marks Hospital[2]	Salt Lake City	100%	86
Univ Health Care/Univ Hosps[2]	Salt Lake City	99%	104
Dixie Regional Medical Center	Saint George	98%	122
Davis Hospital & Medical Center	Layton	97%	29
Intermountain Medical Center	Murray	97%	395
Lakeview Hospital[2]	Bountiful	95%	41
Utah Valley Regional Medical Center	Provo	94%	205
Jordan Valley Medical Center	West Jordan	93%	57
McKay Dee Hospital	Ogden	91%	116

Written Stroke Educational Materials Given

Hospital Name	City	Rate	Cases
McKay Dee Hospital	Ogden	98%	82
Dixie Regional Medical Center	Saint George	96%	91
Saint Marks Hospital[2]	Salt Lake City	96%	48

NOTE: Hospital profiles are in alphabetical order by state, then city, then hospital within the city; Rankings exclude hospitals with less than 25 cases except for patient surveys which excludes hospitals with less than 100 cases; (a) 100-299 cases; (1) The number of cases/patients is too few to report; (2) Data submitted were based on a sample of cases/patients; (3) Results are based on a shorter time period than required; (4) Data suppressed by CMS for one or more quarters; (5) Results are not available for this reporting period; (6) Fewer than 100 patients completed the HCAHPS survey; (7) No cases met the criteria for this measure; (8) The lower limit of the confidence interval cannot be calculated if the number of observed infections equals zero; (9) No data are available from the state/territory for this reporting period; (10) The scores shown reflect fewer than 50 completed surveys; (11) There were discrepancies in the data collection process; (12) This measure does not apply to this hospital for this reporting period; (13) Results cannot be calculated for this reporting period; (14) The results for this state are combined with nearby states to protect confidentiality; Please refer to the User's Guide for a full explanation of data.

Hospital Name	City	Rate	Cases
Ogden Regional Medical Center[2]	Ogden	94%	31
Intermountain Medical Center	Murray	92%	288
Lakeview Hospital[2]	Bountiful	91%	32
Jordan Valley Medical Center	West Jordan	85%	48
Univ Health Care/Univ Hosps[2]	Salt Lake City	84%	56
Utah Valley Regional Medical Center	Provo	83%	115

Surgical Care Improvement Project

Appropriate Beta Blocker Usage

Hospital Name	City	Rate	Cases
Cache Valley Speciality Hospital[2]	North Logan	100%	27
Intermountain Medical Center[2]	Murray	100%	195
Jordan Valley Medical Center	West Jordan	100%	84
Logan Regional Hospital[2]	Logan	100%	55
Mountain View Hospital[2]	Payson	100%	67
The Orthopedic Specialty Hospital[2]	Murray	100%	81
Timpanogos Regional Hospital[2]	Orem	100%	70
Lakeview Hospital[2]	Bountiful	99%	68
McKay Dee Hospital[2]	Ogden	99%	162
American Fork Hospital[2]	American Fork	98%	54
Dixie Regional Medical Center[2]	Saint George	98%	247
LDS Hospital[2]	Salt Lake City	98%	61
Saint Marks Hospital[2]	Salt Lake City	98%	185
Salt Lake Regional Medical Center	Salt Lake City	98%	181
Utah Valley Regional Medical Center[2]	Provo	98%	165
VA Salt Lake City Healthcare[2]	Salt Lake City	98%	56
Alta View Hospital[2]	Sandy	97%	60
Ogden Regional Medical Center[2]	Ogden	97%	106
Park City Medical Center[2]	Park City	97%	34
Riverton Hospital[2]	Riverton	97%	32
Univ Health Care/Univ Hosps[2]	Salt Lake City	96%	151
Davis Hospital & Medical Center	Layton	95%	41
Valley View Medical Center[2]	Cedar City	95%	62
Castleview Hospital	Price	92%	25

Appropriate VTP Within 24 Hours

Hospital Name	City	Rate	Cases
Bear River Valley Hospital	Tremonton	100%	27
Dixie Regional Medical Center[2]	Saint George	100%	403
Heber Valley Medical Center	Heber City	100%	28
Lakeview Hospital[2]	Bountiful	100%	226
Logan Regional Hospital[2]	Logan	100%	306
Mountain View Hospital[2]	Payson	100%	297
The Orthopedic Specialty Hospital[2]	Murray	100%	409
Park City Medical Center[2]	Park City	100%	275
Sevier Valley Medical Center[2]	Richfield	100%	59
VA Salt Lake City Healthcare[2]	Salt Lake City	100%	163
Alta View Hospital[2]	Sandy	99%	326
Brigham City Community Hospital	Brigham City	99%	165
Davis Hospital & Medical Center	Layton	99%	362
Intermountain Medical Center[2]	Murray	99%	426
Jordan Valley Medical Center	West Jordan	99%	557
McKay Dee Hospital[2]	Ogden	99%	384
Ogden Regional Medical Center[2]	Ogden	99%	341
Riverton Hospital[2]	Riverton	99%	234
Saint Marks Hospital[2]	Salt Lake City	99%	511
Salt Lake Regional Medical Center	Salt Lake City	99%	768
Timpanogos Regional Hospital[2]	Orem	99%	301
American Fork Hospital[2]	American Fork	98%	290
Cache Valley Speciality Hospital[2]	North Logan	98%	271
LDS Hospital[2]	Salt Lake City	98%	371
Mountain West Medical Center	Tooele	98%	133
Valley View Medical Center[2]	Cedar City	98%	198
Castleview Hospital	Price	97%	116
Central Valley Medical Center	Nephi	97%	67
Utah Valley Regional Medical Center[2]	Provo	97%	451
Univ Health Care/Univ Hosps[2]	Salt Lake City	96%	388
Uintah Basin Medical Center[2]	Roosevelt	94%	90
Ashley Regional Medical Center	Vernal	92%	50

Controlled Postoperative Blood Glucose

Hospital Name	City	Rate	Cases
Utah Valley Regional Medical Center[2]	Provo	100%	139
Dixie Regional Medical Center[2]	Saint George	99%	183
Saint Marks Hospital[2]	Salt Lake City	99%	158
McKay Dee Hospital[2]	Ogden	98%	160
VA Salt Lake City Healthcare[2]	Salt Lake City	97%	32
Intermountain Medical Center[2]	Murray	96%	201
Salt Lake Regional Medical Center	Salt Lake City	95%	79
Timpanogos Regional Hospital[2]	Orem	95%	40
Ogden Regional Medical Center[2]	Ogden	91%	75
Univ Health Care/Univ Hosps[2]	Salt Lake City	91%	126

Perioperative Temperature Management

Hospital Name	City	Rate	Cases
Alta View Hospital[2]	Sandy	100%	405
American Fork Hospital[2]	American Fork	100%	356
Ashley Regional Medical Center	Vernal	100%	62
Bear River Valley Hospital	Tremonton	100%	33
Brigham City Community Hospital	Brigham City	100%	212
Cache Valley Speciality Hospital[2]	North Logan	100%	298
Davis Hospital & Medical Center	Layton	100%	426
Dixie Regional Medical Center[2]	Saint George	100%	492
Intermountain Medical Center[2]	Murray	100%	590
Jordan Valley Medical Center	West Jordan	100%	643
Lakeview Hospital[2]	Bountiful	100%	352
LDS Hospital[2]	Salt Lake City	100%	508
Logan Regional Hospital[2]	Logan	100%	353
McKay Dee Hospital[2]	Ogden	100%	479
Mountain View Hospital[2]	Payson	100%	363
Mountain West Medical Center	Tooele	100%	170
Ogden Regional Medical Center[2]	Ogden	100%	391
Orem Community Hospital[2]	Orem	100%	48
The Orthopedic Specialty Hospital[2]	Murray	100%	486
Park City Medical Center[2]	Park City	100%	293
Riverton Hospital[2]	Riverton	100%	279
Saint Marks Hospital[2]	Salt Lake City	100%	661
Salt Lake Regional Medical Center	Salt Lake City	100%	851
Sevier Valley Medical Center[2]	Richfield	100%	62
Timpanogos Regional Hospital[2]	Orem	100%	365
Univ Health Care/Univ Hosps[2]	Salt Lake City	100%	490
Utah Valley Regional Medical Center[2]	Provo	100%	564
VA Salt Lake City Healthcare[2]	Salt Lake City	100%	220
Valley View Medical Center[2]	Cedar City	100%	234
Castleview Hospital	Price	99%	130
Central Valley Medical Center	Nephi	97%	78
Heber Valley Medical Center	Heber City	96%	28
Uintah Basin Medical Center[2]	Roosevelt	94%	127

Prophylactic Antibiotic Selection

Hospital Name	City	Rate	Cases
Bear River Valley Hospital	Tremonton	100%	27
Cache Valley Speciality Hospital[2]	North Logan	100%	230
Davis Hospital & Medical Center	Layton	100%	317
Lakeview Hospital[2]	Bountiful	100%	227
LDS Hospital[2]	Salt Lake City	100%	312
Logan Regional Hospital[2]	Logan	100%	232
McKay Dee Hospital[2]	Ogden	100%	441
Mountain View Hospital[2]	Payson	100%	237
The Orthopedic Specialty Hospital[2]	Murray	100%	355
Park City Medical Center[2]	Park City	100%	254
Riverton Hospital[2]	Riverton	100%	196
Salt Lake Regional Medical Center	Salt Lake City	100%	524
Timpanogos Regional Hospital[2]	Orem	100%	275
VA Salt Lake City Healthcare	Salt Lake City	100%	116
Alta View Hospital[2]	Sandy	99%	302
American Fork Hospital[2]	American Fork	99%	242
Brigham City Community Hospital	Brigham City	99%	164
Dixie Regional Medical Center[2]	Saint George	99%	497
Intermountain Medical Center[2]	Murray	99%	505
Jordan Valley Medical Center	West Jordan	99%	454
Mountain West Medical Center	Tooele	99%	126
Ogden Regional Medical Center[2]	Ogden	99%	298
Saint Marks Hospital[2]	Salt Lake City	99%	569
Univ Health Care/Univ Hosps[2]	Salt Lake City	99%	387
Utah Valley Regional Medical Center[2]	Provo	99%	464
Valley View Medical Center[2]	Cedar City	99%	171
Central Valley Medical Center	Nephi	98%	65
Uintah Basin Medical Center[2]	Roosevelt	98%	113
Castleview Hospital	Price	97%	88
Ashley Regional Medical Center	Vernal	96%	46
Sevier Valley Medical Center[2]	Richfield	96%	50
Orem Community Hospital[2]	Orem	94%	36

Prophylactic Antibiotic Selection (Outpatient)

Hospital Name	City	Rate	Cases
Cache Valley Speciality Hospital	North Logan	100%	67
Orem Community Hospital	Orem	100%	42
The Orthopedic Specialty Hospital	Murray	100%	436
Valley View Medical Center	Cedar City	100%	77
Alta View Hospital	Sandy	99%	208
American Fork Hospital	American Fork	99%	145
Davis Hospital & Medical Center	Layton	99%	579
Dixie Regional Medical Center	Saint George	99%	467
Jordan Valley Medical Center	West Jordan	99%	296
LDS Hospital	Salt Lake City	99%	379
Logan Regional Hospital	Logan	99%	336
McKay Dee Hospital	Ogden	99%	505
Riverton Hospital	Riverton	99%	267
Intermountain Medical Center	Murray	98%	729
Mountain West Medical Center	Tooele	98%	44
Ogden Regional Medical Center	Ogden	98%	428
Park City Medical Center	Park City	98%	95
Salt Lake Regional Medical Center	Salt Lake City	98%	277
Timpanogos Regional Hospital	Orem	98%	227
Castleview Hospital	Price	97%	34
Lakeview Hospital	Bountiful	97%	132
Mountain View Hospital	Payson	97%	33
Saint Marks Hospital	Salt Lake City	97%	560
Univ Health Care/Univ Hosps	Salt Lake City	95%	494
Ashley Regional Medical Center	Vernal	93%	43
Utah Valley Regional Medical Center	Provo	84%	366

Prophylactic Antibiotic Stopped

Hospital Name	City	Rate	Cases
Alta View Hospital[2]	Sandy	100%	298
Bear River Valley Hospital	Tremonton	100%	27
Brigham City Community Hospital	Brigham City	100%	154
Lakeview Hospital[2]	Bountiful	100%	226
Logan Regional Hospital[2]	Logan	100%	222
Mountain View Hospital[2]	Payson	100%	232
Orem Community Hospital[2]	Orem	100%	36
Salt Lake Regional Medical Center	Salt Lake City	100%	517
American Fork Hospital[2]	American Fork	99%	231
Castleview Hospital	Price	99%	88
Davis Hospital & Medical Center	Layton	99%	296
Dixie Regional Medical Center[2]	Saint George	99%	482
Jordan Valley Medical Center	West Jordan	99%	449
McKay Dee Hospital[2]	Ogden	99%	428
Ogden Regional Medical Center[2]	Ogden	99%	284
The Orthopedic Specialty Hospital[2]	Murray	99%	351
Park City Medical Center[2]	Park City	99%	253
Saint Marks Hospital[2]	Salt Lake City	99%	553
Timpanogos Regional Hospital[2]	Orem	99%	264
Utah Valley Regional Medical Center[2]	Provo	99%	439
Central Valley Medical Center	Nephi	98%	64
Intermountain Medical Center[2]	Murray	98%	487
Mountain West Medical Center	Tooele	98%	125
Riverton Hospital[2]	Riverton	98%	193
VA Salt Lake City Healthcare	Salt Lake City	98%	113
Cache Valley Speciality Hospital[2]	North Logan	97%	228
LDS Hospital[2]	Salt Lake City	97%	308
Sevier Valley Medical Center[2]	Richfield	96%	50
Valley View Medical Center[2]	Cedar City	96%	169
Univ Health Care/Univ Hosps[2]	Salt Lake City	94%	378
Ashley Regional Medical Center	Vernal	93%	46
Uintah Basin Medical Center[2]	Roosevelt	89%	109

Prophylactic Antibiotic Timing

Hospital Name	City	Rate	Cases
Alta View Hospital[2]	Sandy	100%	302
American Fork Hospital[2]	American Fork	100%	242
Bear River Valley Hospital	Tremonton	100%	27
Davis Hospital & Medical Center	Layton	100%	320
Dixie Regional Medical Center[2]	Saint George	100%	497
Jordan Valley Medical Center	West Jordan	100%	454
Lakeview Hospital[2]	Bountiful	100%	228
Logan Regional Hospital[2]	Logan	100%	232
Mountain View Hospital[2]	Payson	100%	237
Mountain West Medical Center	Tooele	100%	126
Ogden Regional Medical Center[2]	Ogden	100%	298
Park City Medical Center[2]	Park City	100%	254
Riverton Hospital[2]	Riverton	100%	196
Salt Lake Regional Medical Center	Salt Lake City	100%	525
Sevier Valley Medical Center[2]	Richfield	100%	50
Timpanogos Regional Hospital[2]	Orem	100%	275
Brigham City Community Hospital	Brigham City	99%	164
Cache Valley Speciality Hospital[2]	North Logan	99%	230
Castleview Hospital	Price	99%	88
Intermountain Medical Center[2]	Murray	99%	504
McKay Dee Hospital[2]	Ogden	99%	444
The Orthopedic Specialty Hospital[2]	Murray	99%	355
Saint Marks Hospital[2]	Salt Lake City	99%	571
Univ Health Care/Univ Hosps[2]	Salt Lake City	99%	388
Utah Valley Regional Medical Center[2]	Provo	99%	465
VA Salt Lake City Healthcare	Salt Lake City	99%	116
Ashley Regional Medical Center	Vernal	98%	46
LDS Hospital[2]	Salt Lake City	98%	312
Central Valley Medical Center	Nephi	97%	65
Orem Community Hospital[2]	Orem	97%	37
Valley View Medical Center[2]	Cedar City	95%	171
Uintah Basin Medical Center[2]	Roosevelt	92%	113

Prophylactic Antibiotic Timing (Outpatient)

Hospital Name	City	Rate	Cases
Castleview Hospital	Price	100%	34
Lakeview Hospital	Bountiful	100%	132
Salt Lake Regional Medical Center	Salt Lake City	100%	277
Davis Hospital & Medical Center	Layton	99%	580
Intermountain Medical Center	Murray	99%	729
LDS Hospital	Salt Lake City	99%	379
The Orthopedic Specialty Hospital	Murray	99%	436
Riverton Hospital	Riverton	99%	269
Saint Marks Hospital	Salt Lake City	99%	562
Timpanogos Regional Hospital	Orem	99%	227
Alta View Hospital	Sandy	98%	209
Ashley Regional Medical Center	Vernal	98%	43
Dixie Regional Medical Center	Saint George	98%	468

NOTE: Hospital profiles are in alphabetical order by state, then city, then hospital within the city; Rankings exclude hospitals with less than 25 cases except for patient surveys which excludes hospitals with less than 100 cases; (a) 100-299 cases; (1) The number of cases/patients is too few to report; (2) Data submitted were based on a sample of cases/patients; (3) Results are based on a shorter time period than required; (4) Data suppressed by CMS for one or more quarters; (5) Results are not available for this reporting period; (6) Fewer than 100 patients completed the HCAHPS survey; (7) No cases met the criteria for this measure; (8) The lower limit of the confidence interval cannot be calculated if the number of observed infections equals zero; (9) No data are available from the state/territory for this reporting period; (10) The scores shown reflect fewer than 50 completed surveys; (11) There were discrepancies in the data collection process; (12) This measure does not apply to this hospital for this reporting period; (13) Results cannot be calculated for this reporting period; (14) The results for this state are combined with nearby states to protect confidentiality; Please refer to the User's Guide for a full explanation of data.

Hospital Name	City	Rate	Cases
Jordan Valley Medical Center	West Jordan	98%	268
Logan Regional Hospital	Logan	98%	339
McKay Dee Hospital	Ogden	98%	506
Ogden Regional Medical Center	Ogden	98%	430
Park City Medical Center	Park City	98%	96
Mountain View Hospital	Payson	97%	32
Cache Valley Specialty Hospital	North Logan	96%	69
Orem Community Hospital	Orem	95%	42
American Fork Hospital	American Fork	94%	152
Univ Health Care/Univ Hosps	Salt Lake City	93%	429
Utah Valley Regional Medical Center	Provo	93%	368
Valley View Medical Center	Cedar City	92%	80

Urinary Catheter Removal

Hospital Name	City	Rate	Cases
Logan Regional Hospital[2]	Logan	100%	198
Mountain View Hospital[2]	Payson	100%	237
The Orthopedic Specialty Hospital[2]	Murray	100%	230
Park City Medical Center[2]	Park City	100%	143
Riverton Hospital[2]	Riverton	100%	155
Salt Lake Regional Medical Center	Salt Lake City	100%	52
Sevier Valley Medical Center[2]	Richfield	100%	37
VA Salt Lake City Healthcare[2]	Salt Lake City	100%	98
American Fork Hospital[2]	American Fork	99%	96
Cache Valley Specialty Hospital[2]	North Logan	99%	254
Davis Hospital & Medical Center	Layton	99%	175
Valley View Medical Center[2]	Cedar City	99%	182
Ashley Regional Medical Center	Vernal	98%	40
Jordan Valley Medical Center	West Jordan	98%	358
Lakeview Hospital[2]	Bountiful	98%	65
McKay Dee Hospital[2]	Ogden	98%	379
Ogden Regional Medical Center[2]	Ogden	98%	294
Utah Valley Regional Medical Center[2]	Provo	98%	383
Alta View Hospital[2]	Sandy	97%	235
Castleview Hospital	Price	97%	94
Intermountain Medical Center[2]	Murray	97%	366
Saint Marks Hospital[2]	Salt Lake City	97%	464
Timpanogos Regional Hospital[2]	Orem	97%	229
Uintah Basin Medical Center[2]	Roosevelt	97%	37
Dixie Regional Medical Center[2]	Saint George	96%	369
LDS Hospital[2]	Salt Lake City	96%	73
Mountain West Medical Center	Tooele	96%	113
Brigham City Community Hospital	Brigham City	95%	99
Central Valley Medical Center	Nephi	95%	64
Univ Health Care/Univ Hosps[2]	Salt Lake City	93%	325

Survey of Patients' Hospital Experiences

Area Around Room 'Always' Quiet at Night

Hospital Name	City	Rate	Cases
Bear River Valley Hospital	Tremonton	74%	(a)
Park City Medical Center	Park City	74%	300+
Heber Valley Medical Center	Heber City	71%	(a)
Cache Valley Specialty Hospital	North Logan	70%	300+
The Orthopedic Specialty Hospital	Murray	69%	300+
Central Valley Medical Center	Nephi	67%	(a)
Sevier Valley Medical Center	Richfield	64%	(a)
Mountain West Medical Center	Tooele	63%	300+
Timpanogos Regional Hospital	Orem	63%	300+
Univ Health Care/Univ Hosps	Salt Lake City	62%	300+
Brigham City Community Hospital	Brigham City	61%	(a)
Sanpete Valley Hospital	Mount Pleasant	61%	(a)
Alta View Hospital	Sandy	60%	300+
Jordan Valley Medical Center	West Jordan	60%	300+
LDS Hospital	Salt Lake City	60%	300+
Dixie Regional Medical Center	Saint George	59%	300+
Logan Regional Hospital	Logan	59%	300+
Salt Lake Regional Medical Center	Salt Lake City	59%	300+
Orem Community Hospital	Orem	58%	300+
Uintah Basin Medical Center	Roosevelt	58%	(a)
Castleview Hospital	Price	57%	300+
Intermountain Medical Center	Murray	56%	300+
Riverton Hospital	Riverton	56%	300+
Ashley Regional Medical Center	Vernal	55%	300+
Mountain View Hospital	Payson	55%	300+
Davis Hospital & Medical Center	Layton	54%	300+
Lakeview Hospital	Bountiful	54%	300+
Utah Valley Regional Medical Center	Provo	54%	300+
Valley View Medical Center	Cedar City	54%	300+
McKay Dee Hospital	Ogden	53%	300+
Saint Marks Hospital	Salt Lake City	53%	300+
Ogden Regional Medical Center	Ogden	51%	300+
American Fork Hospital	American Fork	49%	300+

Doctors 'Always' Communicated Well

Hospital Name	City	Rate	Cases
Central Valley Medical Center	Nephi	94%	(a)
Sevier Valley Medical Center	Richfield	89%	(a)
Sanpete Valley Hospital	Mount Pleasant	88%	(a)
Heber Valley Medical Center	Heber City	87%	(a)
The Orthopedic Specialty Hospital	Murray	87%	300+
Bear River Valley Hospital	Tremonton	86%	(a)
Park City Medical Center	Park City	86%	300+
Alta View Hospital	Sandy	84%	300+
Davis Hospital & Medical Center	Layton	84%	300+
Dixie Regional Medical Center	Saint George	84%	300+
Riverton Hospital	Riverton	84%	300+
Valley View Medical Center	Cedar City	84%	300+
Lakeview Hospital	Bountiful	83%	300+
LDS Hospital	Salt Lake City	83%	300+
Logan Regional Hospital	Logan	83%	300+
American Fork Hospital	American Fork	82%	300+
Orem Community Hospital	Orem	82%	300+
Salt Lake Regional Medical Center	Salt Lake City	82%	300+
Brigham City Community Hospital	Brigham City	81%	(a)
Cache Valley Specialty Hospital	North Logan	81%	300+
Intermountain Medical Center	Murray	81%	300+
McKay Dee Hospital	Ogden	81%	300+
Utah Valley Regional Medical Center	Provo	81%	300+
Castleview Hospital	Price	80%	300+
Jordan Valley Medical Center	West Jordan	80%	300+
Mountain View Hospital	Payson	80%	300+
Mountain West Medical Center	Tooele	80%	300+
Ashley Regional Medical Center	Vernal	79%	300+
Timpanogos Regional Hospital	Orem	78%	300+
Univ Health Care/Univ Hosps	Salt Lake City	78%	300+
Ogden Regional Medical Center	Ogden	77%	300+
Saint Marks Hospital	Salt Lake City	77%	300+
Uintah Basin Medical Center	Roosevelt	77%	(a)

Home Recovery Information Given

Hospital Name	City	Rate	Cases
Heber Valley Medical Center	Heber City	94%	(a)
Orem Community Hospital	Orem	94%	300+
Bear River Valley Hospital	Tremonton	93%	(a)
Sanpete Valley Hospital	Mount Pleasant	93%	(a)
Alta View Hospital	Sandy	92%	300+
American Fork Hospital	American Fork	92%	300+
Park City Medical Center	Park City	92%	300+
Valley View Medical Center	Cedar City	92%	300+
Cache Valley Specialty Hospital	North Logan	91%	300+
Dixie Regional Medical Center	Saint George	91%	300+
Logan Regional Hospital	Logan	91%	300+
The Orthopedic Specialty Hospital	Murray	91%	300+
Sevier Valley Medical Center	Richfield	91%	(a)
Central Valley Medical Center	Nephi	90%	(a)
Intermountain Medical Center	Murray	90%	300+
Lakeview Hospital	Bountiful	90%	300+
LDS Hospital	Salt Lake City	90%	300+
McKay Dee Hospital	Ogden	90%	300+
Riverton Hospital	Riverton	90%	300+
Utah Valley Regional Medical Center	Provo	90%	300+
Castleview Hospital	Price	89%	300+
Davis Hospital & Medical Center	Layton	89%	300+
Salt Lake Regional Medical Center	Salt Lake City	89%	300+
Jordan Valley Medical Center	West Jordan	88%	300+
Mountain View Hospital	Payson	88%	300+
Ogden Regional Medical Center	Ogden	88%	300+
Univ Health Care/Univ Hosps	Salt Lake City	88%	300+
Mountain West Medical Center	Tooele	87%	300+
Timpanogos Regional Hospital	Orem	87%	300+
Ashley Regional Medical Center	Vernal	86%	300+
Saint Marks Hospital	Salt Lake City	86%	300+
Brigham City Community Hospital	Brigham City	85%	(a)
Uintah Basin Medical Center	Roosevelt	81%	(a)

Hospital Given 9 or 10 on 10 Point Scale

Hospital Name	City	Rate	Cases
Orem Community Hospital	Orem	86%	300+
Bear River Valley Hospital	Tremonton	85%	(a)
Park City Medical Center	Park City	83%	300+
Sevier Valley Medical Center	Richfield	83%	(a)
Heber Valley Medical Center	Heber City	82%	(a)
Dixie Regional Medical Center	Saint George	79%	300+
Valley View Medical Center	Cedar City	79%	300+
The Orthopedic Specialty Hospital	Murray	78%	300+
LDS Hospital	Salt Lake City	77%	300+
McKay Dee Hospital	Ogden	77%	300+
Riverton Hospital	Riverton	77%	300+
Logan Regional Hospital	Logan	76%	300+
Sanpete Valley Hospital	Mount Pleasant	76%	(a)
Univ Health Care/Univ Hosps	Salt Lake City	76%	300+
Alta View Hospital	Sandy	75%	300+
American Fork Hospital	American Fork	75%	300+
Utah Valley Regional Medical Center	Provo	75%	300+
Central Valley Medical Center	Nephi	74%	(a)
Intermountain Medical Center	Murray	74%	300+
Cache Valley Specialty Hospital	North Logan	71%	300+
Timpanogos Regional Hospital	Orem	71%	300+
Lakeview Hospital	Bountiful	70%	300+
Mountain View Hospital	Payson	70%	300+
Mountain West Medical Center	Tooele	69%	300+
Davis Hospital & Medical Center	Layton	68%	300+
Salt Lake Regional Medical Center	Salt Lake City	68%	300+
Brigham City Community Hospital	Brigham City	67%	(a)
Jordan Valley Medical Center	West Jordan	67%	300+
Ogden Regional Medical Center	Ogden	67%	300+
Saint Marks Hospital	Salt Lake City	66%	300+
Uintah Basin Medical Center	Roosevelt	64%	(a)
Castleview Hospital	Price	63%	300+
Ashley Regional Medical Center	Vernal	60%	300+

Meds 'Always' Explained Before Given

Hospital Name	City	Rate	Cases
Bear River Valley Hospital	Tremonton	88%	(a)
Sevier Valley Medical Center	Richfield	80%	(a)
Sanpete Valley Hospital	Mount Pleasant	78%	(a)
Heber Valley Medical Center	Heber City	75%	(a)
Park City Medical Center	Park City	75%	300+
Dixie Regional Medical Center	Saint George	74%	300+
American Fork Hospital	American Fork	73%	300+
Orem Community Hospital	Orem	73%	300+
The Orthopedic Specialty Hospital	Murray	72%	300+
Central Valley Medical Center	Nephi	71%	(a)
Logan Regional Hospital	Logan	71%	300+
Valley View Medical Center	Cedar City	71%	300+
Cache Valley Specialty Hospital	North Logan	70%	300+
LDS Hospital	Salt Lake City	70%	300+
McKay Dee Hospital	Ogden	70%	300+
Utah Valley Regional Medical Center	Provo	70%	300+
Riverton Hospital	Riverton	69%	300+
Alta View Hospital	Sandy	68%	300+
Intermountain Medical Center	Murray	68%	300+
Ashley Regional Medical Center	Vernal	64%	300+
Lakeview Hospital	Bountiful	64%	300+
Davis Hospital & Medical Center	Layton	63%	300+
Jordan Valley Medical Center	West Jordan	63%	300+
Salt Lake Regional Medical Center	Salt Lake City	63%	300+
Univ Health Care/Univ Hosps	Salt Lake City	63%	300+
Castleview Hospital	Price	62%	300+
Mountain West Medical Center	Tooele	62%	300+
Mountain View Hospital	Payson	60%	300+
Uintah Basin Medical Center	Roosevelt	60%	(a)
Ogden Regional Medical Center	Ogden	59%	300+
Timpanogos Regional Hospital	Orem	58%	300+
Saint Marks Hospital	Salt Lake City	54%	300+
Brigham City Community Hospital	Brigham City	52%	(a)

Nurses 'Always' Communicated Well

Hospital Name	City	Rate	Cases
Bear River Valley Hospital	Tremonton	86%	(a)
Sevier Valley Medical Center	Richfield	85%	(a)
Park City Medical Center	Park City	84%	300+
Sanpete Valley Hospital	Mount Pleasant	84%	(a)
Heber Valley Medical Center	Heber City	83%	(a)
Orem Community Hospital	Orem	82%	300+
Valley View Medical Center	Cedar City	82%	300+
Central Valley Medical Center	Nephi	81%	(a)
Cache Valley Specialty Hospital	North Logan	80%	300+
Dixie Regional Medical Center	Saint George	80%	300+
LDS Hospital	Salt Lake City	80%	300+
Logan Regional Hospital	Logan	80%	300+
McKay Dee Hospital	Ogden	79%	300+
The Orthopedic Specialty Hospital	Murray	79%	300+
Alta View Hospital	Sandy	78%	300+
American Fork Hospital	American Fork	78%	300+
Mountain West Medical Center	Tooele	78%	300+
Riverton Hospital	Riverton	78%	300+
Utah Valley Regional Medical Center	Provo	78%	300+
Intermountain Medical Center	Murray	77%	300+
Lakeview Hospital	Bountiful	77%	300+
Timpanogos Regional Hospital	Orem	76%	300+
Univ Health Care/Univ Hosps	Salt Lake City	76%	300+
Uintah Basin Medical Center	Roosevelt	75%	(a)
Ashley Regional Medical Center	Vernal	74%	300+
Brigham City Community Hospital	Brigham City	74%	(a)
Castleview Hospital	Price	74%	300+
Davis Hospital & Medical Center	Layton	74%	300+
Salt Lake Regional Medical Center	Salt Lake City	74%	300+
Jordan Valley Medical Center	West Jordan	73%	300+
Mountain View Hospital	Payson	73%	300+
Ogden Regional Medical Center	Ogden	70%	300+
Saint Marks Hospital	Salt Lake City	69%	300+

Pain 'Always' Well Controlled

Hospital Name	City	Rate	Cases
Bear River Valley Hospital	Tremonton	82%	(a)
Central Valley Medical Center	Nephi	81%	(a)
Sanpete Valley Hospital	Mount Pleasant	78%	(a)

NOTE: Hospital profiles are in alphabetical order by state, then city, then hospital within the city; Rankings exclude hospitals with less than 25 cases except for patient surveys which excludes hospitals with less than 100 cases; (a) 100-299 cases; (1) The number of cases/patients is too few to report; (2) Data submitted were based on a sample of cases/patients; (3) Results are based on a shorter time period than required; (4) Data suppressed by CMS for one or more quarters; (5) Results are not available for this reporting period; (6) Fewer than 100 patients completed the HCAHPS survey; (7) No cases met the criteria for this measure; (8) The lower limit of the confidence interval cannot be calculated if the number of observed infections equals zero; (9) No data are available from the state/territory for this reporting period; (10) The scores shown reflect fewer than 50 completed surveys; (11) There were discrepancies in the data collection process; (12) This measure does not apply to this hospital for this reporting period; (13) Results cannot be calculated for this reporting period; (14) The results for this state are combined with nearby states to protect confidentiality; Please refer to the User's Guide for a full explanation of data.

LDS Hospital	Salt Lake City	77%	300+
Park City Medical Center	Park City	77%	300+
Sevier Valley Medical Center	Richfield	77%	(a)
Logan Regional Hospital	Logan	76%	300+
Orem Community Hospital	Orem	76%	300+
Valley View Medical Center	Cedar City	76%	300+
Dixie Regional Medical Center	Saint George	75%	300+
American Fork Hospital	American Fork	73%	300+
Heber Valley Medical Center	Heber City	73%	(a)
Intermountain Medical Center	Murray	73%	300+
Mountain West Medical Center	Tooele	73%	300+
The Orthopedic Specialty Hospital	Murray	73%	300+
Utah Valley Regional Medical Center	Provo	73%	300+
Riverton Hospital	Riverton	72%	300+
Alta View Hospital	Sandy	71%	300+
Cache Valley Speciality Hospital	North Logan	71%	300+
McKay Dee Hospital	Ogden	71%	300+
Timpanogos Regional Hospital	Orem	70%	300+
Brigham City Community Hospital	Brigham City	69%	(a)
Castleview Hospital	Price	69%	300+
Davis Hospital & Medical Center	Layton	69%	300+
Lakeview Hospital	Bountiful	68%	300+
Mountain View Hospital	Payson	68%	300+
Univ Health Care/Univ Hosps	Salt Lake City	68%	300+
Jordan Valley Medical Center	West Jordan	67%	300+
Saint Marks Hospital	Salt Lake City	67%	300+
Salt Lake Regional Medical Center	Salt Lake City	67%	300+
Ogden Regional Medical Center	Ogden	65%	300+
Uintah Basin Medical Center	Roosevelt	65%	(a)
Ashley Regional Medical Center	Vernal	64%	300+

Room and Bathroom 'Always' Clean

Hospital Name	City	Rate	Cases
Bear River Valley Hospital	Tremonton	83%	(a)
Sevier Valley Medical Center	Richfield	83%	(a)
Central Valley Medical Center	Nephi	81%	(a)
The Orthopedic Specialty Hospital	Murray	77%	300+
Univ Health Care/Univ Hosps	Salt Lake City	77%	300+
Cache Valley Speciality Hospital	North Logan	76%	300+
Orem Community Hospital	Orem	76%	300+
Timpanogos Regional Hospital	Orem	76%	300+
Dixie Regional Medical Center	Saint George	75%	300+
Park City Medical Center	Park City	75%	300+
LDS Hospital	Salt Lake City	74%	300+
Logan Regional Hospital	Logan	74%	300+
Mountain West Medical Center	Tooele	74%	300+
American Fork Hospital	American Fork	73%	300+
Sanpete Valley Hospital	Mount Pleasant	73%	(a)
Utah Valley Regional Medical Center	Provo	73%	300+
Valley View Medical Center	Cedar City	73%	300+
Alta View Hospital	Sandy	72%	300+
Davis Hospital & Medical Center	Layton	72%	300+
Intermountain Medical Center	Murray	72%	300+
Lakeview Hospital	Bountiful	72%	300+
McKay Dee Hospital	Ogden	72%	300+
Riverton Hospital	Riverton	72%	300+
Salt Lake Regional Medical Center	Salt Lake City	72%	300+
Brigham City Community Hospital	Brigham City	71%	(a)
Castleview Hospital	Price	70%	300+
Heber Valley Medical Center	Heber City	70%	(a)
Jordan Valley Medical Center	West Jordan	69%	300+
Uintah Basin Medical Center	Roosevelt	68%	(a)
Mountain View Hospital	Payson	67%	300+
Saint Marks Hospital	Salt Lake City	66%	300+
Ashley Regional Medical Center	Vernal	64%	300+
Ogden Regional Medical Center	Ogden	59%	300+

Timely Help 'Always' Received

Hospital Name	City	Rate	Cases
Sanpete Valley Hospital	Mount Pleasant	86%	(a)
Bear River Valley Hospital	Tremonton	83%	(a)
Sevier Valley Medical Center	Richfield	83%	(a)
Cache Valley Speciality Hospital	North Logan	75%	300+
Park City Medical Center	Park City	75%	300+
Central Valley Medical Center	Nephi	74%	(a)
Heber Valley Medical Center	Heber City	72%	(a)
The Orthopedic Specialty Hospital	Murray	71%	300+
Dixie Regional Medical Center	Saint George	70%	300+
LDS Hospital	Salt Lake City	69%	300+
Logan Regional Hospital	Logan	69%	300+
Mountain West Medical Center	Tooele	69%	300+
Orem Community Hospital	Orem	69%	300+
Alta View Hospital	Sandy	68%	300+
Valley View Medical Center	Cedar City	68%	300+
American Fork Hospital	American Fork	67%	300+
Brigham City Community Hospital	Brigham City	67%	(a)
Castleview Hospital	Price	67%	300+
Utah Valley Regional Medical Center	Provo	67%	300+
McKay Dee Hospital	Ogden	66%	300+
Uintah Basin Medical Center	Roosevelt	65%	(a)

Ashley Regional Medical Center	Vernal	64%	300+
Intermountain Medical Center	Murray	64%	300+
Mountain View Hospital	Payson	64%	300+
Timpanogos Regional Hospital	Orem	64%	300+
Lakeview Hospital	Bountiful	63%	300+
Riverton Hospital	Riverton	63%	300+
Salt Lake Regional Medical Center	Salt Lake City	63%	300+
Davis Hospital & Medical Center	Layton	62%	300+
Univ Health Care/Univ Hosps	Salt Lake City	62%	300+
Jordan Valley Medical Center	West Jordan	58%	300+
Ogden Regional Medical Center	Ogden	58%	300+
Saint Marks Hospital	Salt Lake City	56%	300+

Would Definitely Recommend Hospital

Hospital Name	City	Rate	Cases
Central Valley Medical Center	Nephi	88%	(a)
Orem Community Hospital	Orem	86%	300+
Park City Medical Center	Park City	86%	300+
Dixie Regional Medical Center	Saint George	84%	300+
The Orthopedic Specialty Hospital	Murray	84%	300+
Bear River Valley Hospital	Tremonton	83%	(a)
LDS Hospital	Salt Lake City	81%	300+
McKay Dee Hospital	Ogden	81%	300+
Univ Health Care/Univ Hosps	Salt Lake City	81%	300+
Intermountain Medical Center	Murray	80%	300+
Riverton Hospital	Riverton	80%	300+
American Fork Hospital	American Fork	79%	300+
Valley View Medical Center	Cedar City	79%	300+
Utah Valley Regional Medical Center	Provo	78%	300+
Heber Valley Medical Center	Heber City	77%	(a)
Logan Regional Hospital	Logan	77%	300+
Alta View Hospital	Sandy	76%	300+
Cache Valley Speciality Hospital	North Logan	75%	300+
Sanpete Valley Hospital	Mount Pleasant	74%	(a)
Sevier Valley Medical Center	Richfield	72%	(a)
Timpanogos Regional Hospital	Orem	72%	300+
Lakeview Hospital	Bountiful	70%	300+
Ogden Regional Medical Center	Ogden	70%	300+
Salt Lake Regional Medical Center	Salt Lake City	69%	300+
Saint Marks Hospital	Salt Lake City	68%	300+
Uintah Basin Medical Center	Roosevelt	68%	(a)
Davis Hospital & Medical Center	Layton	67%	300+
Jordan Valley Medical Center	West Jordan	67%	300+
Mountain View Hospital	Payson	67%	300+
Brigham City Community Hospital	Brigham City	66%	(a)
Mountain West Medical Center	Tooele	63%	300+
Castleview Hospital	Price	58%	300+
Ashley Regional Medical Center	Vernal	56%	300+

Use of Medical Imaging

Cardiac Imaging Stress Test before OP Surgery

Hospital Name	City	Rate	Cases
Ashley Regional Medical Center	Vernal	1.6%	64
American Fork Hospital	American Fork	2.2%	45
Jordan Valley Medical Center	West Jordan	2.7%	333
Sevier Valley Medical Center	Richfield	3.0%	67
Logan Regional Hospital	Logan	3.2%	311
Intermountain Medical Center	Murray	3.3%	845
Mountain View Hospital	Payson	3.4%	116
Mountain West Medical Center	Tooele	3.4%	59
Uintah Basin Medical Center	Roosevelt	3.4%	88
Riverton Hospital	Riverton	4.4%	113
LDS Hospital	Salt Lake City	4.5%	155
Castleview Hospital	Price	4.7%	106
Saint Marks Hospital	Salt Lake City	4.7%	576
Ogden Regional Medical Center	Ogden	5.0%	238
Valley View Medical Center	Cedar City	5.2%	290
Alta View Hospital	Sandy	5.3%	133
McKay Dee Hospital	Ogden	5.3%	831
Dixie Regional Medical Center	Saint George	5.4%	687
Utah Valley Regional Medical Center	Provo	5.4%	186
Lakeview Hospital	Bountiful	5.6%	72
Univ Health Care/Univ Hosps	Salt Lake City	6.4%	707
Davis Hospital & Medical Center	Layton	6.6%	106
Park City Medical Center	Park City	6.7%	90
Salt Lake Regional Medical Center	Salt Lake City	7.8%	167
Brigham City Community Hospital	Brigham City	9.0%	100
Timpanogos Regional Hospital	Orem	9.4%	64

Combination Abdominal CT Scan

Hospital Name	City	Rate	Cases
Garfield Memorial Hospital	Panguitch	0.0%	46
Kane County Hospital	Kanab	1.0%	102
Moab Regional Hospital	Moab	1.1%	93
Davis Hospital & Medical Center	Layton	1.3%	311
Uintah Basin Medical Center	Roosevelt	1.3%	149
Bear River Valley Hospital	Tremonton	1.4%	73
Beaver Valley Hospital	Beaver	1.4%	74

Central Valley Medical Center	Nephi	1.6%	129
Castleview Hospital	Price	2.3%	353
Gunnison Valley Hospital	Gunnison	2.5%	122
Jordan Valley Medical Center	West Jordan	2.7%	446
McKay Dee Hospital	Ogden	2.7%	1129
Ashley Regional Medical Center	Vernal	2.8%	143
Univ Health Care/Univ Hosps	Salt Lake City	3.1%	1867
Saint Marks Hospital	Salt Lake City	3.3%	871
Valley View Medical Center	Cedar City	3.6%	359
Intermountain Medical Center	Murray	3.8%	1023
Lakeview Hospital	Bountiful	3.8%	344
Alta View Hospital	Sandy	4.1%	438
Cache Valley Speciality Hospital	North Logan	4.3%	47
LDS Hospital	Salt Lake City	4.6%	372
Heber Valley Medical Center	Heber City	4.9%	61
Utah Valley Regional Medical Center	Provo	4.9%	800
Sanpete Valley Hospital	Mount Pleasant	5.2%	97
Ogden Regional Medical Center	Ogden	5.5%	311
Salt Lake Regional Medical Center	Salt Lake City	5.5%	181
Riverton Hospital	Riverton	5.8%	242
Sevier Valley Medical Center	Richfield	5.8%	137
Park City Medical Center	Park City	6.3%	158
Mountain West Medical Center	Tooele	6.7%	163
Logan Regional Hospital	Logan	6.8%	414
American Fork Hospital	American Fork	7.0%	430
Dixie Regional Medical Center	Saint George	8.4%	1458
The Orthopedic Specialty Hospital	Murray	8.9%	157
Mountain View Hospital	Payson	9.2%	184
Timpanogos Regional Hospital	Orem	9.4%	128
Orem Community Hospital	Orem	12.6%	87
Brigham City Community Hospital	Brigham City	38.7%	150

Combination Brain/Sinus CT Scan

Hospital Name	City	Rate	Cases
Blue Mountain Hospital	Blanding	0.0%	36
Fillmore Community Medical Center	Fillmore	0.0%	37
San Juan Hospital	Monticello	0.0%	30
Alta View Hospital	Sandy	0.9%	224
Jordan Valley Medical Center	West Jordan	1.2%	347
Univ Health Care/Univ Hosps	Salt Lake City	2.0%	546
McKay Dee Hospital	Ogden	2.4%	797
Utah Valley Regional Medical Center	Provo	2.4%	500
Intermountain Medical Center	Murray	2.7%	820
Saint Marks Hospital	Salt Lake City	3.1%	608
Dixie Regional Medical Center	Saint George	3.6%	828
Lakeview Hospital	Bountiful	5.0%	300
Valley View Medical Center	Cedar City	9.2%	163
Garfield Memorial Hospital	Panguitch	9.4%	53
Beaver Valley Hospital	Beaver	16.7%	60

Combination Chest CT Scan

Hospital Name	City	Rate	Cases
American Fork Hospital	American Fork	0.0%	158
Bear River Valley Hospital	Tremonton	0.0%	45
Brigham City Community Hospital	Brigham City	0.0%	45
Central Valley Medical Center	Nephi	0.0%	55
Davis Hospital & Medical Center	Layton	0.0%	131
Gunnison Valley Hospital	Gunnison	0.0%	67
Jordan Valley Medical Center	West Jordan	0.0%	92
Kane County Hospital	Kanab	0.0%	70
Mountain View Hospital	Payson	0.0%	107
Ogden Regional Medical Center	Ogden	0.0%	142
The Orthopedic Specialty Hospital	Murray	0.0%	96
Riverton Hospital	Riverton	0.0%	54
Univ Health Care/Univ Hosps	Salt Lake City	0.1%	2067
Saint Marks Hospital	Salt Lake City	0.4%	243
Dixie Regional Medical Center	Saint George	0.5%	841
LDS Hospital	Salt Lake City	0.6%	181
Utah Valley Regional Medical Center	Provo	0.6%	528
Castleview Hospital	Price	0.7%	144
Intermountain Medical Center	Murray	0.7%	540
McKay Dee Hospital	Ogden	0.7%	595
Park City Medical Center	Park City	1.4%	69
Alta View Hospital	Sandy	1.9%	156
Logan Regional Hospital	Logan	1.9%	264
Valley View Medical Center	Cedar City	2.5%	161
Sevier Valley Medical Center	Richfield	3.2%	63
Lakeview Hospital	Bountiful	7.2%	97

Follow-up Mammogram/Ultrasound

A follow-up rate near zero may indicate missed cancer; a rate higher than 14% may mean there is unnecessary follow up.

Hospital Name	City	Rate	Cases
San Juan Hospital	Monticello	4.4%	45
Valley View Medical Center	Cedar City	4.6%	692
Mountain West Medical Center	Tooele	4.7%	342
Park City Medical Center	Park City	5.1%	158
Uintah Basin Medical Center	Roosevelt	5.3%	188
Heber Valley Medical Center	Heber City	5.7%	194
Dixie Regional Medical Center	Saint George	6.0%	3472

NOTE: Hospital profiles are in alphabetical order by state, then city, then hospital within the city; Rankings exclude hospitals with less than 25 cases except for patient surveys which excludes hospitals with less than 100 cases; (a) 100-299 cases; (1) The number of cases/patients is too few to report; (2) Data submitted were based on a sample of cases/patients; (3) Results are based on a shorter time period than required; (4) Data suppressed by CMS for one or more quarters; (5) Results are not available for this reporting period; (6) Fewer than 100 patients completed the HCAHPS survey; (7) No cases met the criteria for this measure; (8) The lower limit of the confidence interval cannot be calculated if the number of observed infections equals zero; (9) No data are available from the state/territory for this reporting period; (10) The scores shown reflect fewer than 50 completed surveys; (11) There were discrepancies in the data collection process; (12) This measure does not apply to this hospital for this reporting period; (13) Results cannot be calculated for this reporting period; (14) The results for this state are combined with nearby states to protect confidentiality; Please refer to the User's Guide for a full explanation of data.

Saint Marks Hospital	Salt Lake City	6.0%	2040
Sanpete Valley Hospital	Mount Pleasant	6.1%	165
Utah Valley Regional Medical Center	Provo	6.1%	958
Alta View Hospital	Sandy	6.5%	967
Ashley Regional Medical Center	Vernal	6.7%	195
Orem Community Hospital	Orem	6.8%	205
Garfield Memorial Hospital	Panguitch	6.9%	288
McKay Dee Hospital	Ogden	6.9%	2676
Logan Regional Hospital	Logan	7.0%	971
Univ Health Care/Univ Hosps	Salt Lake City	7.4%	1866
Delta Community Medical Center	Delta	7.6%	66
American Fork Hospital	American Fork	7.8%	962
Intermountain Medical Center	Murray	8.0%	2125
Moab Regional Hospital	Moab	8.5%	106
Sevier Valley Medical Center	Richfield	8.7%	366
Ogden Regional Medical Center	Ogden	8.9%	654
Jordan Valley Medical Center	West Jordan	9.0%	733
Riverton Hospital	Riverton	9.1%	340
Davis Hospital & Medical Center	Layton	9.4%	1100
Brigham City Community Hospital	Brigham City	9.7%	340
LDS Hospital	Salt Lake City	9.7%	853
Bear River Valley Hospital	Tremonton	10.6%	132
Salt Lake Regional Medical Center	Salt Lake City	11.2%	473
Castleview Hospital	Price	13.2%	515
Cache Valley Speciality Hospital	North Logan	13.3%	120
Mountain View Hospital	Payson	17.6%	347
Gunnison Valley Hospital	Gunnison	18.3%	197
Timpanogos Regional Hospital	Orem	22.4%	125
Central Valley Medical Center	Nephi	24.4%	156
Lakeview Hospital	Bountiful	31.2%	783

Lumbar Spine MRI for Low Back Pain

Hospital Name	City	Rate	Cases
Brigham City Community Hospital	Brigham City	33.9%	59
Univ Health Care/Univ Hosps	Salt Lake City	36.1%	277
Logan Regional Hospital	Logan	38.8%	129
Riverton Hospital	Riverton	39.5%	43
Cache Valley Speciality Hospital	North Logan	39.7%	73
Dixie Regional Medical Center	Saint George	41.4%	442
Lakeview Hospital	Bountiful	41.7%	84
Intermountain Medical Center	Murray	45.0%	109
Ogden Regional Medical Center	Ogden	45.9%	61
American Fork Hospital	American Fork	46.8%	77
Alta View Hospital	Sandy	46.9%	49
Valley View Medical Center	Cedar City	47.0%	100
McKay Dee Hospital	Ogden	47.2%	375
The Orthopedic Specialty Hospital	Murray	47.3%	110
Salt Lake Regional Medical Center	Salt Lake City	47.9%	48
Castleview Hospital	Price	48.4%	91
Mountain View Hospital	Payson	50.0%	42
Jordan Valley Medical Center	West Jordan	50.7%	69
Saint Marks Hospital	Salt Lake City	51.1%	131
Utah Valley Regional Medical Center	Provo	51.3%	150
Davis Hospital & Medical Center	Layton	53.3%	60
LDS Hospital	Salt Lake City	54.1%	61

NOTE: Hospital profiles are in alphabetical order by state, then city, then hospital within the city; Rankings exclude hospitals with less than 25 cases except for patient surveys which excludes hospitals with less than 100 cases; (a) 100-299 cases; (1) The number of cases/patients is too few to report; (2) Data submitted were based on a sample of cases/patients; (3) Results are based on a shorter time period than required; (4) Data suppressed by CMS for one or more quarters; (5) Results are not available for this reporting period; (6) Fewer than 100 patients completed the HCAHPS survey; (7) No cases met the criteria for this measure; (8) The lower limit of the confidence interval cannot be calculated if the number of observed infections equals zero; (9) No data are available from the state/territory for this reporting period; (10) The scores shown reflect fewer than 50 completed surveys; (11) There were discrepancies in the data collection process; (12) This measure does not apply to this hospital for this reporting period; (13) Results cannot be calculated for this reporting period; (14) The results for this state are combined with nearby states to protect confidentiality; Please refer to the User's Guide for a full explanation of data.

American Fork Hospital

170 North 1100 East Phone: 801-855-3305
American Fork, UT 84003 Fax: 801-855-3586
URL: www.ihc.com/facility/facilityresults.jsp
Type: Acute Care Hospitals Emergency Services: Yes
Ownership: Voluntary non-profit - Private Beds: 117

Key Personnel:
Radiology. . . . . Dan Hatch
CEO/President. . . . . Michael R Olson

Measure	Cases	This Hosp.	State Avg.	U.S. Avg.
Blood Clot Prevention and Treatment				
Anticoagulation Overlap Therapy[2]	41	90%	95%	93%
ICU Venous Thromboembolism Prophylaxis[2]	44	91%	93%	92%
Incidence of Potentially Preventable VTE[1,2]	-	-	5%	10%
UFH with Dosages/Platelet Monitoring[1,2]	-	-	95%	97%
Venous Thromboembolism Prophylaxis[2]	192	83%	86%	85%
Warfarin Therapy Discharge Instructions[2]	31	97%	73%	75%
Chest Pain/Possible Heart Attack Care				
Aspirin Given Within 24 Hours of Arrival	68	100%	97%	96%
Fibrinolytic Meds Within 30 Min. of Arrival[7]	-	-	52%	58%
Average Time to ECG (minutes)	71	6	7	7
Average Time to Transfer (minutes)	12	28	36	60
Children's Asthma Care				
Received Home Management Plan of Care	-	-	-	88%
Received Reliever Medication	-	-	-	100%
Received Systemic Corticosteroids	-	-	-	100%
Emergency Department				
Admittance Decision Time (minutes)[2]	305	62	66	98
Head CT Results Within 45 Min. of Arrival	15	67%	60%	57%
Patients Who Left ER Before Being Seen	28,218	0%	1%	2%
Time from ER Arrival to Admit. (minutes)[2]	307	206	217	274
Time from ER Arrival to Discharge (minutes)	406	121	123	134
Time in ER Before Being Evaluated (minutes)	426	16	17	26
Time to Pain Meds for Fractures (minutes)	203	35	43	57
Heart Attack Care				
Aspirin Given at Discharge[1]	-	-	99%	99%
Fibrinolytic Meds Within 30 Min. of Arrival[7]	-	-	100%	54%
PCI Within 90 Minutes of Arrival[7]	-	-	98%	96%
Statin Prescribed at Discharge[7]	-	-	100%	98%
Heart Failure Care				
ACE Inhibitor or ARB for LVSD	12	100%	98%	97%
Discharge Instructions Given	39	97%	96%	94%
Evaluation of LVS Function	47	100%	98%	99%
Medicare Spending				
Medicare Spending per Patient (ratio)	-	0.96	0.98	0.98
Pneumonia Care				
Appropriate Initial Antibiotic Given[2]	83	99%	96%	95%
Blood Culture Timing[2]	111	99%	99%	98%
Pregnancy and Delivery Care				
Newborn Deliveries Scheduled Early[2]	64	2%	6%	6%
Preventive Care				
Immunization for Influenza[2]	422	90%	92%	90%
Immunization for Pneumonia[2]	272	86%	91%	92%
Stroke Care				
Anticoagulation Therapy for Atrial Fibrillation[1]	-	-	95%	95%
Antithrombotic Therapy Timing	11	91%	99%	98%
Assessed for Rehabilitation	13	100%	98%	97%
Discharged on Antithrombotic Therapy	11	82%	99%	99%
Discharged on Statin Medication[1]	-	-	96%	94%
Thrombolytic Therapy Timing[1]	-	-	89%	66%
Venous Thromboembolism Prophylaxis	12	75%	95%	94%
Written Stroke Educational Materials Given[1]	-	-	89%	88%
Surgical Care Improvement Project				
Appropriate Beta Blocker Usage[2]	54	98%	98%	98%
Appropriate VTP Within 24 Hours[2]	290	98%	99%	98%
Controlled Postoperative Blood Glucose[2,7]	-	-	97%	97%
Perioperative Temperature Management[2]	356	100%	100%	100%
Prophylactic Antibiotic Selection[2]	242	99%	99%	99%
Prophylactic Antibiotic Selection (Outpatient)	145	99%	98%	98%
Prophylactic Antibiotic Stopped[2]	231	99%	98%	98%
Prophylactic Antibiotic Timing[2]	242	100%	99%	99%
Prophylactic Antibiotic Timing (Outpatient)	152	94%	98%	98%
Urinary Catheter Removal[2]	96	99%	98%	97%
Survey of Patients' Hospital Experiences				
Area Around Room 'Always' Quiet at Night	300+	49%	60%	61%
Doctors 'Always' Communicated Well	300+	82%	83%	82%
Home Recovery Information Given	300+	92%	90%	85%
Hospital Given 9 or 10 on 10 Point Scale	300+	75%	74%	71%
Meds 'Always' Explained Before Given	300+	73%	68%	64%
Nurses 'Always' Communicated Well	300+	78%	79%	79%
Pain 'Always' Well Controlled	300+	73%	73%	71%
Room and Bathroom 'Always' Clean	300+	73%	74%	73%
Timely Help 'Always' Received	300+	67%	69%	68%
Would Definitely Recommend Hospital	300+	79%	76%	71%
Use of Medical Imaging				
Cardiac Imaging Stress Test before Surgery	45	2.2%	4.9%	5.3%
Combination Abdominal CT Scan	430	7.0%	4.9%	10.5%
Combination Brain/Sinus CT Scan[1]	-	-	3%	2.7%
Combination Chest CT Scan	158	0.0%	0.8%	2.7%
Follow-up Mammogram/Ultrasound	962	7.8%	8.5%	8.8%
Lumbar Spine MRI for Low Back Pain	77	46.8%	43.8%	37.2%

Beaver Valley Hospital

1109 North 100 West Phone: 435-438-7102
Beaver, UT 84713
Type: Acute Care Hospitals Emergency Services: Yes
Ownership: Government - Local

Measure	Cases	This Hosp.	State Avg.	U.S. Avg.
Blood Clot Prevention and Treatment				
Anticoagulation Overlap Therapy[1,2]	-	-	95%	93%
ICU Venous Thromboembolism Prophylaxis[2,7]	-	-	93%	92%
Incidence of Potentially Preventable VTE[2,7]	-	-	5%	10%
UFH with Dosages/Platelet Monitoring[1,2]	-	-	95%	97%
Venous Thromboembolism Prophylaxis[2]	102	29%	86%	85%
Warfarin Therapy Discharge Instructions[1,2]	-	-	73%	75%
Chest Pain/Possible Heart Attack Care				
Aspirin Given Within 24 Hours of Arrival	11	82%	97%	96%
Fibrinolytic Meds Within 30 Min. of Arrival[1]	-	-	52%	58%
Average Time to ECG (minutes)[1]	-	-	7	7
Average Time to Transfer (minutes)[1]	-	-	36	60
Children's Asthma Care				
Received Home Management Plan of Care	-	-	-	88%
Received Reliever Medication	-	-	-	100%
Received Systemic Corticosteroids	-	-	-	100%
Emergency Department				
Admittance Decision Time (minutes)[2]	129	0	66	98
Head CT Results Within 45 Min. of Arrival[1,3]	-	-	60%	57%
Patients Who Left ER Before Being Seen	2,234	0%	1%	2%
Time from ER Arrival to Admit. (minutes)[2]	129	101	217	274
Time from ER Arrival to Discharge (minutes)	616	105	123	134
Time in ER Before Being Evaluated (minutes)	588	20	17	26
Time to Pain Meds for Fractures (minutes)	13	66	43	57
Heart Attack Care				
Aspirin Given at Discharge[5]	-	-	99%	99%
Fibrinolytic Meds Within 30 Min. of Arrival[5]	-	-	100%	54%
PCI Within 90 Minutes of Arrival[5]	-	-	98%	96%
Statin Prescribed at Discharge[5]	-	-	100%	98%
Heart Failure Care				
ACE Inhibitor or ARB for LVSD[7]	-	-	98%	97%
Discharge Instructions Given[1]	-	-	96%	94%
Evaluation of LVS Function[1]	-	-	98%	99%
Medicare Spending				
Medicare Spending per Patient (ratio)	-	0.72	0.98	0.98
Pneumonia Care				
Appropriate Initial Antibiotic Given[2]	34	91%	96%	95%
Blood Culture Timing[1,2]	-	-	99%	98%
Pregnancy and Delivery Care				
Newborn Deliveries Scheduled Early[2]	18	72%	6%	6%
Preventive Care				
Immunization for Influenza[2]	138	9%	92%	90%
Immunization for Pneumonia[2]	110	18%	91%	92%
Stroke Care				
Anticoagulation Therapy for Atrial Fibrillation[1,3]	-	-	95%	95%
Antithrombotic Therapy Timing[1,3]	-	-	99%	98%
Assessed for Rehabilitation[1,3]	-	-	98%	97%
Discharged on Antithrombotic Therapy[1,3]	-	-	99%	99%
Discharged on Statin Medication[1,3]	-	-	96%	94%
Thrombolytic Therapy Timing[3,7]	-	-	89%	66%
Venous Thromboembolism Prophylaxis[1,3]	-	-	95%	94%
Written Stroke Educational Materials Given[1,3]	-	-	89%	88%
Surgical Care Improvement Project				
Appropriate Beta Blocker Usage[3,7]	-	-	98%	98%
Appropriate VTP Within 24 Hours[3,7]	-	-	99%	98%
Controlled Postoperative Blood Glucose[3,7]	-	-	97%	97%
Perioperative Temperature Management[1,3]	-	-	100%	100%
Prophylactic Antibiotic Selection[3,7]	-	-	99%	99%
Prophylactic Antibiotic Selection (Outpatient)[5]	-	-	98%	98%
Prophylactic Antibiotic Stopped[3,7]	-	-	98%	98%
Prophylactic Antibiotic Timing[1,3]	-	-	99%	99%
Prophylactic Antibiotic Timing (Outpatient)[5]	-	-	98%	98%
Urinary Catheter Removal[3,7]	-	-	98%	97%
Survey of Patients' Hospital Experiences				
Area Around Room 'Always' Quiet at Night[6]	<100	64%	60%	61%
Doctors 'Always' Communicated Well[6]	<100	90%	83%	82%
Home Recovery Information Given[6]	<100	91%	90%	85%
Hospital Given 9 or 10 on 10 Point Scale[6]	<100	80%	74%	71%
Meds 'Always' Explained Before Given[6]	<100	55%	68%	64%
Nurses 'Always' Communicated Well[6]	<100	79%	79%	79%
Pain 'Always' Well Controlled[6]	<100	74%	73%	71%
Room and Bathroom 'Always' Clean[6]	<100	83%	74%	73%
Timely Help 'Always' Received[6]	<100	75%	69%	68%
Would Definitely Recommend Hospital[6]	<100	79%	76%	71%
Use of Medical Imaging				
Cardiac Imaging Stress Test before Surgery[7]	-	-	4.9%	5.3%
Combination Abdominal CT Scan	74	1.4%	4.9%	10.5%
Combination Brain/Sinus CT Scan	60	16.7%	3%	2.7%
Combination Chest CT Scan[1]	-	-	0.8%	2.7%
Follow-up Mammogram/Ultrasound[7]	-	-	8.5%	8.8%
Lumbar Spine MRI for Low Back Pain[1]	-	-	43.8%	37.2%

Blue Mountain Hospital

802 South 200 West Phone: 435-678-3993
Blanding, UT 84511
URL: www.bluemountainhospital.org
Type: Critical Access Hospitals Emergency Services: Yes
Ownership: Voluntary non-profit - Private

Key Personnel:
CEO . . . . Robert Houser

Measure	Cases	This Hosp.	State Avg.	U.S. Avg.
Blood Clot Prevention and Treatment				
Anticoagulation Overlap Therapy[5]	-	-	95%	93%
ICU Venous Thromboembolism Prophylaxis[5]	-	-	93%	92%
Incidence of Potentially Preventable VTE[5]	-	-	5%	10%
UFH with Dosages/Platelet Monitoring[5]	-	-	95%	97%
Venous Thromboembolism Prophylaxis[5]	-	-	86%	85%
Warfarin Therapy Discharge Instructions[5]	-	-	73%	75%
Chest Pain/Possible Heart Attack Care				
Aspirin Given Within 24 Hours of Arrival[1,3]	-	-	97%	96%
Fibrinolytic Meds Within 30 Min. of Arrival[3,7]	-	-	52%	58%
Average Time to ECG (minutes)[1,3]	-	-	7	7
Average Time to Transfer (minutes)[3,7]	-	-	36	60
Children's Asthma Care				
Received Home Management Plan of Care	-	-	-	88%
Received Reliever Medication	-	-	-	100%
Received Systemic Corticosteroids	-	-	-	100%
Emergency Department				
Admittance Decision Time (minutes)[3]	17	29	66	98
Head CT Results Within 45 Min. of Arrival[5]	-	-	60%	57%
Patients Who Left ER Before Being Seen[5]	-	-	1%	2%
Time from ER Arrival to Admit. (minutes)[3]	17	184	217	274
Time from ER Arrival to Discharge (minutes)[5]	-	-	123	134
Time in ER Before Being Evaluated (minutes)[5]	-	-	17	26
Time to Pain Meds for Fractures (minutes)[1,3]	-	-	43	57
Heart Attack Care				
Aspirin Given at Discharge[5]	-	-	99%	99%
Fibrinolytic Meds Within 30 Min. of Arrival[5]	-	-	100%	54%
PCI Within 90 Minutes of Arrival[5]	-	-	98%	96%
Statin Prescribed at Discharge[5]	-	-	100%	98%

NOTE: Hospital profiles are in alphabetical order by state, then city, then hospital within the city; Rankings exclude hospitals with less than 25 cases except for patient surveys which excludes hospitals with less than 100 cases; (a) 100-299 cases; (1) The number of cases/patients is too few to report; (2) Data submitted were based on a sample of cases/patients; (3) Results are based on a shorter time period than required; (4) Data suppressed by CMS for one or more quarters; (5) Results are not available for this reporting period; (6) Fewer than 100 patients completed the HCAHPS survey; (7) No cases met the criteria for this measure; (8) The lower limit of the confidence interval cannot be calculated if the number of observed infections equals zero; (9) No data are available from the state/territory for this reporting period; (10) The scores shown reflect fewer than 50 completed surveys; (11) There were discrepancies in the data collection process; (12) This measure does not apply to this hospital for this reporting period; (13) Results cannot be calculated for this reporting period; (14) The results for this state are combined with nearby states to protect confidentiality; Please refer to the User's Guide for a full explanation of data.

Heart Failure Care				
ACE Inhibitor or ARB for LVSD[3,7]	-	-	98%	97%
Discharge Instructions Given[1,3]	-	-	96%	94%
Evaluation of LVS Function[1,3]	-	-	98%	99%
Medicare Spending				
Medicare Spending per Patient (ratio)	-	-	0.98	0.98
Pneumonia Care				
Appropriate Initial Antibiotic Given[1,3]	-	-	96%	95%
Blood Culture Timing[1,3]	-	-	99%	98%
Pregnancy and Delivery Care				
Newborn Deliveries Scheduled Early[5]	-	-	6%	6%
Preventive Care				
Immunization for Influenza[5]	-	-	92%	90%
Immunization for Pneumonia[5]	-	-	91%	92%
Stroke Care				
Anticoagulation Therapy for Atrial Fibrillation[5]	-	-	95%	95%
Antithrombotic Therapy Timing[5]	-	-	99%	98%
Assessed for Rehabilitation[5]	-	-	98%	97%
Discharged on Antithrombotic Therapy[5]	-	-	99%	99%
Discharged on Statin Medication[5]	-	-	96%	94%
Thrombolytic Therapy Timing[5]	-	-	89%	66%
Venous Thromboembolism Prophylaxis[5]	-	-	95%	94%
Written Stroke Educational Materials Given[5]	-	-	89%	88%
Surgical Care Improvement Project				
Appropriate Beta Blocker Usage[5]	-	-	98%	98%
Appropriate VTP Within 24 Hours[5]	-	-	99%	98%
Controlled Postoperative Blood Glucose[5]	-	-	97%	97%
Perioperative Temperature Management[5]	-	-	100%	100%
Prophylactic Antibiotic Selection[5]	-	-	99%	99%
Prophylactic Antibiotic Selection (Outpatient)[5]	-	-	98%	98%
Prophylactic Antibiotic Stopped[5]	-	-	98%	98%
Prophylactic Antibiotic Timing[5]	-	-	99%	99%
Prophylactic Antibiotic Timing (Outpatient)[5]	-	-	98%	98%
Urinary Catheter Removal[5]	-	-	98%	97%
Survey of Patients' Hospital Experiences				
Area Around Room 'Always' Quiet at Night[5]	-	-	60%	61%
Doctors 'Always' Communicated Well[5]	-	-	83%	82%
Home Recovery Information Given[5]	-	-	90%	85%
Hospital Given 9 or 10 on 10 Point Scale[5]	-	-	74%	71%
Meds 'Always' Explained Before Given[5]	-	-	68%	64%
Nurses 'Always' Communicated Well[5]	-	-	79%	79%
Pain 'Always' Well Controlled[5]	-	-	73%	71%
Room and Bathroom 'Always' Clean[5]	-	-	74%	73%
Timely Help 'Always' Received[5]	-	-	69%	68%
Would Definitely Recommend Hospital[5]	-	-	76%	71%
Use of Medical Imaging				
Cardiac Imaging Stress Test before Surgery[7]	-	-	4.9%	5.3%
Combination Abdominal CT Scan[1]	-	-	4.9%	10.5%
Combination Brain/Sinus CT Scan	36	0.0%	3%	2.7%
Combination Chest CT Scan[1]	-	-	0.8%	2.7%
Follow-up Mammogram/Ultrasound[1]	-	-	8.5%	8.8%
Lumbar Spine MRI for Low Back Pain[1]	-	-	43.8%	37.2%

Lakeview Hospital

630 East Medical Drive
Bountiful, UT 84010
Phone: 801-299-2211
Fax: 801-299-2511
URL: www.lakeviewhospital.com
Type: Acute Care Hospitals
Emergency Services: Yes
Ownership: Proprietary
Beds: 128

Key Personnel:

Intensive Care Unit. . . . . Jolene Casper
Operating Room. . . . . Kevin N Clark
Infection Control. . . . . Pam Clark
Emergency Room . . . . Mark Flammer, MD
Radiology. . . . . Richard Hartvigsen, MD
CEO/President. . . . . Rand Kerr
Quality Assurance . . . . Elaine Shutt
Pediatric In-Patient Care . . . . . . Jacqueline Tinnini

Measure	Cases	This Hosp.	State Avg.	U.S. Avg.
Blood Clot Prevention and Treatment				
Anticoagulation Overlap Therapy[2]	48	100%	95%	93%
ICU Venous Thromboembolism Prophylaxis[2]	40	90%	93%	92%
Incidence of Potentially Preventable VTE[1,2]	-	-	5%	10%
UFH with Dosages/Platelet Monitoring[1,2]	-	-	95%	97%
Venous Thromboembolism Prophylaxis[2]	238	94%	86%	85%
Warfarin Therapy Discharge Instructions[2]	25	100%	73%	75%
Chest Pain/Possible Heart Attack Care				
Aspirin Given Within 24 Hours of Arrival[1]	-	-	97%	96%
Fibrinolytic Meds Within 30 Min. of Arrival[3,7]	-	-	52%	58%
Average Time to ECG (minutes)[1]	-	-	7	7
Average Time to Transfer (minutes)[1,3]	-	-	36	60
Children's Asthma Care				
Received Home Management Plan of Care	-	-	-	88%
Received Reliever Medication	-	-	-	100%
Received Systemic Corticosteroids	-	-	-	100%
Emergency Department				
Admittance Decision Time (minutes)[2]	360	76	66	98
Head CT Results Within 45 Min. of Arrival	13	92%	60%	57%
Patients Who Left ER Before Being Seen	16,525	0%	1%	2%
Time from ER Arrival to Admit. (minutes)[2]	360	204	217	274
Time from ER Arrival to Discharge (minutes)	430	129	123	134
Time in ER Before Being Evaluated (minutes)	498	12	17	26
Time to Pain Meds for Fractures (minutes)	79	39	43	57
Heart Attack Care				
Aspirin Given at Discharge	74	100%	99%	99%
Fibrinolytic Meds Within 30 Min. of Arrival[7]	-	-	100%	54%
PCI Within 90 Minutes of Arrival	28	100%	98%	96%
Statin Prescribed at Discharge	65	100%	100%	98%
Heart Failure Care				
ACE Inhibitor or ARB for LVSD	20	100%	98%	97%
Discharge Instructions Given	46	100%	96%	94%
Evaluation of LVS Function	75	100%	98%	99%
Medicare Spending				
Medicare Spending per Patient (ratio)	-	1.01	0.98	0.98
Pneumonia Care				
Appropriate Initial Antibiotic Given	71	100%	96%	95%
Blood Culture Timing	128	99%	99%	98%
Pregnancy and Delivery Care				
Newborn Deliveries Scheduled Early	83	7%	6%	6%
Preventive Care				
Immunization for Influenza[2]	416	98%	92%	90%
Immunization for Pneumonia[2]	544	97%	91%	92%
Stroke Care				
Anticoagulation Therapy for Atrial Fibrillation[1,2]	-	-	95%	95%
Antithrombotic Therapy Timing[2]	41	100%	99%	98%
Assessed for Rehabilitation[2]	50	100%	98%	97%
Discharged on Antithrombotic Therapy[2]	47	100%	99%	99%
Discharged on Statin Medication[2]	37	97%	96%	94%
Thrombolytic Therapy Timing[1,2]	-	-	89%	66%
Venous Thromboembolism Prophylaxis[2]	41	95%	95%	94%
Written Stroke Educational Materials Given[2]	32	91%	89%	88%
Surgical Care Improvement Project				
Appropriate Beta Blocker Usage[2]	68	99%	98%	98%
Appropriate VTP Within 24 Hours[2]	226	100%	99%	98%
Controlled Postoperative Blood Glucose[2,7]	-	-	97%	97%
Perioperative Temperature Management[2]	352	100%	100%	100%
Prophylactic Antibiotic Selection[2]	227	100%	99%	99%
Prophylactic Antibiotic Selection (Outpatient)	132	97%	98%	98%
Prophylactic Antibiotic Stopped[2]	226	100%	98%	98%
Prophylactic Antibiotic Timing[2]	228	100%	99%	99%
Prophylactic Antibiotic Timing (Outpatient)	132	100%	98%	98%
Urinary Catheter Removal[2]	65	98%	98%	97%
Survey of Patients' Hospital Experiences				
Area Around Room 'Always' Quiet at Night	300+	54%	60%	61%
Doctors 'Always' Communicated Well	300+	83%	83%	82%
Home Recovery Information Given	300+	90%	90%	85%
Hospital Given 9 or 10 on 10 Point Scale	300+	70%	74%	71%
Meds 'Always' Explained Before Given	300+	64%	68%	64%
Nurses 'Always' Communicated Well	300+	77%	79%	79%
Pain 'Always' Well Controlled	300+	68%	73%	71%
Room and Bathroom 'Always' Clean	300+	72%	74%	73%
Timely Help 'Always' Received	300+	63%	69%	68%
Would Definitely Recommend Hospital	300+	70%	76%	71%
Use of Medical Imaging				
Cardiac Imaging Stress Test before Surgery	72	5.6%	4.9%	5.3%
Combination Abdominal CT Scan	344	3.8%	4.9%	10.5%
Combination Brain/Sinus CT Scan	300	5.0%	3%	2.7%
Combination Chest CT Scan	97	7.2%	0.8%	2.7%
Follow-up Mammogram/Ultrasound	783	31.2%	8.5%	8.8%
Lumbar Spine MRI for Low Back Pain	84	41.7%	43.8%	37.2%

Brigham City Community Hospital

950 South Medical Drive
Brigham City, UT 84302
Phone: 435-734-9471
Fax: 435-723-5085
URL: www.brighamcityhospital.com
Type: Acute Care Hospitals
Emergency Services: Yes
Ownership: Proprietary
Beds: 49

Key Personnel:

CEO/President. . . . . Steven B Bateman
Infection Control. . . . . Kelli Cox, RN
Quality Assurance . . . . Kelli Cox, RN
Radiology. . . . . Richard Dunn
Emergency Room . . . . Corey Johnson, MD
Anesthesiology. . . . . Kent Johnson, MD
Chief of Medical Staff . . . . Michael Sumko, DO
Intensive Care Unit. . . . . Susan Thompson, RN

Measure	Cases	This Hosp.	State Avg.	U.S. Avg.
Blood Clot Prevention and Treatment				
Anticoagulation Overlap Therapy[2]	19	95%	95%	93%
ICU Venous Thromboembolism Prophylaxis[1,2]	-	-	93%	92%
Incidence of Potentially Preventable VTE[1,2]	-	-	5%	10%
UFH with Dosages/Platelet Monitoring[1,2]	-	-	95%	97%
Venous Thromboembolism Prophylaxis[2]	74	81%	86%	85%
Warfarin Therapy Discharge Instructions[2]	14	86%	73%	75%
Chest Pain/Possible Heart Attack Care				
Aspirin Given Within 24 Hours of Arrival	40	98%	97%	96%
Fibrinolytic Meds Within 30 Min. of Arrival[7]	-	-	52%	58%
Average Time to ECG (minutes)	41	11	7	7
Average Time to Transfer (minutes)[1]	-	-	36	60
Children's Asthma Care				
Received Home Management Plan of Care	-	-	-	88%
Received Reliever Medication	-	-	-	100%
Received Systemic Corticosteroids	-	-	-	100%
Emergency Department				
Admittance Decision Time (minutes)[2]	204	26	66	98
Head CT Results Within 45 Min. of Arrival[1]	-	-	60%	57%
Patients Who Left ER Before Being Seen	8,501	0%	1%	2%
Time from ER Arrival to Admit. (minutes)[2]	204	198	217	274
Time from ER Arrival to Discharge (minutes)	408	86	123	134
Time in ER Before Being Evaluated (minutes)	462	11	17	26
Time to Pain Meds for Fractures (minutes)	41	53	43	57
Heart Attack Care				
Aspirin Given at Discharge[1,3]	-	-	99%	99%
Fibrinolytic Meds Within 30 Min. of Arrival[3,7]	-	-	100%	54%
PCI Within 90 Minutes of Arrival[3,7]	-	-	98%	96%
Statin Prescribed at Discharge[1,3]	-	-	100%	98%
Heart Failure Care				
ACE Inhibitor or ARB for LVSD[1,3]	-	-	98%	97%
Discharge Instructions Given[1,3]	-	-	96%	94%
Evaluation of LVS Function[1,3]	-	-	98%	99%
Medicare Spending				
Medicare Spending per Patient (ratio)	-	0.95	0.98	0.98
Pneumonia Care				
Appropriate Initial Antibiotic Given	15	87%	96%	95%
Blood Culture Timing	21	100%	99%	98%
Pregnancy and Delivery Care				
Newborn Deliveries Scheduled Early[2]	42	10%	6%	6%
Preventive Care				
Immunization for Influenza[2]	259	92%	92%	90%
Immunization for Pneumonia[2]	225	96%	91%	92%
Stroke Care				
Anticoagulation Therapy for Atrial Fibrillation[1,2]	-	-	95%	95%
Antithrombotic Therapy Timing[2]	11	100%	99%	98%
Assessed for Rehabilitation[2]	11	100%	98%	97%
Discharged on Antithrombotic Therapy[2]	11	100%	99%	99%
Discharged on Statin Medication[1,2]	-	-	96%	94%
Thrombolytic Therapy Timing[1,2]	-	-	89%	66%
Venous Thromboembolism Prophylaxis[2]	11	91%	95%	94%
Written Stroke Educational Materials Given[1,2]	-	-	89%	88%
Surgical Care Improvement Project				

NOTE: Hospital profiles are in alphabetical order by state, then city, then hospital within the city; Rankings exclude hospitals with less than 25 cases except for patient surveys which excludes hospitals with less than 100 cases; (a) 100-299 cases; (1) The number of cases/patients is too few to report; (2) Data submitted were based on a sample of cases/patients; (3) Results are based on a shorter time period than required; (4) Data suppressed by CMS for one or more quarters; (5) Results are not available for this reporting period; (6) Fewer than 100 patients completed the HCAHPS survey; (7) No cases met the criteria for this measure; (8) The lower limit of the confidence interval cannot be calculated if the number of observed infections equals zero; (9) No data are available from the state/territory for this reporting period; (10) The scores shown reflect fewer than 50 completed surveys; (11) There were discrepancies in the data collection process; (12) This measure does not apply to this hospital for this reporting period; (13) Results cannot be calculated for this reporting period; (14) The results for this state are combined with nearby states to protect confidentiality; Please refer to the User's Guide for a full explanation of data.

Appropriate Beta Blocker Usage	20	100%	98%	98%
Appropriate VTP Within 24 Hours	165	99%	99%	98%
Controlled Postoperative Blood Glucose[7]	-	-	97%	97%
Perioperative Temperature Management	212	100%	100%	100%
Prophylactic Antibiotic Selection	164	99%	99%	99%
Prophylactic Antibiotic Selection (Outpatient)	13	92%	98%	98%
Prophylactic Antibiotic Stopped	154	100%	98%	98%
Prophylactic Antibiotic Timing	164	99%	99%	99%
Prophylactic Antibiotic Timing (Outpatient)	13	100%	98%	98%
Urinary Catheter Removal	99	95%	98%	97%
Survey of Patients' Hospital Experiences				
Area Around Room 'Always' Quiet at Night	(a)	61%	60%	61%
Doctors 'Always' Communicated Well	(a)	81%	83%	82%
Home Recovery Information Given	(a)	85%	90%	85%
Hospital Given 9 or 10 on 10 Point Scale	(a)	67%	74%	71%
Meds 'Always' Explained Before Given	(a)	52%	68%	64%
Nurses 'Always' Communicated Well	(a)	74%	79%	79%
Pain 'Always' Well Controlled	(a)	69%	73%	71%
Room and Bathroom 'Always' Clean	(a)	71%	74%	73%
Timely Help 'Always' Received	(a)	67%	69%	68%
Would Definitely Recommend Hospital	(a)	66%	76%	71%
Use of Medical Imaging				
Cardiac Imaging Stress Test before Surgery	100	9.0%	4.9%	5.3%
Combination Abdominal CT Scan	150	38.7%	4.9%	10.5%
Combination Brain/Sinus CT Scan[1]	-	-	3%	2.7%
Combination Chest CT Scan	45	0.0%	0.8%	2.7%
Follow-up Mammogram/Ultrasound	340	9.7%	8.5%	8.8%
Lumbar Spine MRI for Low Back Pain	59	33.9%	43.8%	37.2%

Valley View Medical Center

1303 North Main Street
Cedar City, UT 84721
Phone: 435-868-5800
Fax: 435-868-5814
URL: www.intermountainhealthcare.org
Type: Acute Care Hospitals
Emergency Services: Yes
Ownership: Voluntary non-profit - Private
Beds: 42

Key Personnel:
Chief of Medical Staff . . . . E Alfaro, MD
Radiology. . . . . Shane A Baker, MD
Quality Assurance . . . . Renee Burkley, RN
Anesthesiology. . . . . Bill Dancer, CRNA
Operating Room. . . . . Debbie Esplin, RN
Pediatric In-Patient Care . . . . Kourosh Ghaffari, MD
Emergency Room . . . . G Kim Rowland, MD

Measure	Cases	This Hosp.	State Avg.	U.S. Avg.
Blood Clot Prevention and Treatment				
Anticoagulation Overlap Therapy[2]	36	100%	95%	93%
ICU Venous Thromboembolism Prophylaxis[2]	33	85%	93%	92%
Incidence of Potentially Preventable VTE[1,2]	-	-	5%	10%
UFH with Dosages/Platelet Monitoring[2]	12	100%	95%	97%
Venous Thromboembolism Prophylaxis[2]	115	71%	86%	85%
Warfarin Therapy Discharge Instructions[2]	29	31%	73%	75%
Chest Pain/Possible Heart Attack Care				
Aspirin Given Within 24 Hours of Arrival	44	98%	97%	96%
Fibrinolytic Meds Within 30 Min. of Arrival[1]	-	-	52%	58%
Average Time to ECG (minutes)	44	8	7	7
Average Time to Transfer (minutes)[1]	-	-	36	60
Children's Asthma Care				
Received Home Management Plan of Care	-	-	-	88%
Received Reliever Medication	-	-	-	100%
Received Systemic Corticosteroids	-	-	-	100%
Emergency Department				
Admittance Decision Time (minutes)[2]	264	62	66	98
Head CT Results Within 45 Min. of Arrival[1]	-	-	60%	57%
Patients Who Left ER Before Being Seen	15,489	1%	1%	2%
Time from ER Arrival to Admit. (minutes)[2]	266	208	217	274
Time from ER Arrival to Discharge (minutes)	385	118	123	134
Time in ER Before Being Evaluated (minutes)	369	17	17	26
Time to Pain Meds for Fractures (minutes)	77	47	43	57
Heart Attack Care				
Aspirin Given at Discharge[1]	-	-	99%	99%
Fibrinolytic Meds Within 30 Min. of Arrival[7]	-	-	100%	54%
PCI Within 90 Minutes of Arrival[7]	-	-	98%	96%
Statin Prescribed at Discharge[1]	-	-	100%	98%
Heart Failure Care				
ACE Inhibitor or ARB for LVSD	11	91%	98%	97%
Discharge Instructions Given	31	94%	96%	94%
Evaluation of LVS Function	32	100%	98%	99%
Medicare Spending				
Medicare Spending per Patient (ratio)	-	0.91	0.98	0.98
Pneumonia Care				
Appropriate Initial Antibiotic Given	46	98%	96%	95%
Blood Culture Timing	68	99%	99%	98%
Pregnancy and Delivery Care				
Newborn Deliveries Scheduled Early[2]	46	4%	6%	6%
Preventive Care				
Immunization for Influenza[2]	276	96%	92%	90%
Immunization for Pneumonia[2]	209	93%	91%	92%
Stroke Care				
Anticoagulation Therapy for Atrial Fibrillation[1]	-	-	95%	95%
Antithrombotic Therapy Timing	18	100%	99%	98%
Assessed for Rehabilitation	23	100%	98%	97%
Discharged on Antithrombotic Therapy	23	100%	99%	99%
Discharged on Statin Medication	20	75%	96%	94%
Thrombolytic Therapy Timing[7]	-	-	89%	66%
Venous Thromboembolism Prophylaxis	19	58%	95%	94%
Written Stroke Educational Materials Given	13	77%	89%	88%
Surgical Care Improvement Project				
Appropriate Beta Blocker Usage[2]	62	95%	98%	98%
Appropriate VTP Within 24 Hours[2]	198	98%	99%	98%
Controlled Postoperative Blood Glucose[2,7]	-	-	97%	97%
Perioperative Temperature Management[2]	234	100%	100%	100%
Prophylactic Antibiotic Selection[2]	171	99%	99%	99%
Prophylactic Antibiotic Selection (Outpatient)	77	100%	98%	98%
Prophylactic Antibiotic Stopped[2]	169	96%	98%	98%
Prophylactic Antibiotic Timing[2]	171	95%	99%	99%
Prophylactic Antibiotic Timing (Outpatient)	80	92%	98%	98%
Urinary Catheter Removal[2]	182	99%	98%	97%
Survey of Patients' Hospital Experiences				
Area Around Room 'Always' Quiet at Night	300+	54%	60%	61%
Doctors 'Always' Communicated Well	300+	84%	83%	82%
Home Recovery Information Given	300+	92%	90%	85%
Hospital Given 9 or 10 on 10 Point Scale	300+	79%	74%	71%
Meds 'Always' Explained Before Given	300+	71%	68%	64%
Nurses 'Always' Communicated Well	300+	82%	79%	79%
Pain 'Always' Well Controlled	300+	76%	73%	71%
Room and Bathroom 'Always' Clean	300+	73%	74%	73%
Timely Help 'Always' Received	300+	68%	69%	68%
Would Definitely Recommend Hospital	300+	79%	76%	71%
Use of Medical Imaging				
Cardiac Imaging Stress Test before Surgery	290	5.2%	4.9%	5.3%
Combination Abdominal CT Scan	359	3.6%	4.9%	10.5%
Combination Brain/Sinus CT Scan	163	9.2%	3%	2.7%
Combination Chest CT Scan	161	2.5%	0.8%	2.7%
Follow-up Mammogram/Ultrasound	692	4.6%	8.5%	8.8%
Lumbar Spine MRI for Low Back Pain	100	47.0%	43.8%	37.2%

Delta Community Medical Center

126 South White Sage Avenue
Delta, UT 84624
Phone: 435-864-5591
Fax: 435-864-4186
URL: www.ihc.com/delta
Type: Critical Access Hospitals
Emergency Services: Yes
Ownership: Voluntary non-profit - Private
Beds: 20

Key Personnel:
Radiology. . . . . Mark S Asay
CEO/President. . . . . James Beckstrand
Administrator . . . . James E. Beckstrand
Chief of Medical Staff. . . . . Steven W Shamo

Measure	Cases	This Hosp.	State Avg.	U.S. Avg.
Blood Clot Prevention and Treatment				
Anticoagulation Overlap Therapy[1]	-	-	95%	93%
ICU Venous Thromboembolism Prophylaxis[7]	-	-	93%	92%
Incidence of Potentially Preventable VTE[7]	-	-	5%	10%
UFH with Dosages/Platelet Monitoring[7]	-	-	95%	97%
Venous Thromboembolism Prophylaxis	59	71%	86%	85%
Warfarin Therapy Discharge Instructions[1]	-	-	73%	75%
Chest Pain/Possible Heart Attack Care				
Aspirin Given Within 24 Hours of Arrival	15	100%	97%	96%
Fibrinolytic Meds Within 30 Min. of Arrival[1,3]	-	-	52%	58%
Average Time to ECG (minutes)	15	11	7	7
Average Time to Transfer (minutes)[3,7]	-	-	36	60
Children's Asthma Care				
Received Home Management Plan of Care	-	-	-	88%
Received Reliever Medication	-	-	-	100%
Received Systemic Corticosteroids	-	-	-	100%
Emergency Department				
Admittance Decision Time (minutes)	75	15	66	98
Head CT Results Within 45 Min. of Arrival[1]	-	-	60%	57%
Patients Who Left ER Before Being Seen[5]	-	-	1%	2%
Time from ER Arrival to Admit. (minutes)	102	130	217	274
Time from ER Arrival to Discharge (minutes)	252	81	123	134
Time in ER Before Being Evaluated (minutes)	235	26	17	26
Time to Pain Meds for Fractures (minutes)	20	59	43	57
Heart Attack Care				
Aspirin Given at Discharge[1,3]	-	-	99%	99%
Fibrinolytic Meds Within 30 Min. of Arrival[3,7]	-	-	100%	54%
PCI Within 90 Minutes of Arrival[3,7]	-	-	98%	96%
Statin Prescribed at Discharge[1,3]	-	-	100%	98%
Heart Failure Care				
ACE Inhibitor or ARB for LVSD[3,7]	-	-	98%	97%
Discharge Instructions Given[1,3]	-	-	96%	94%
Evaluation of LVS Function[3,7]	-	-	98%	99%
Medicare Spending				
Medicare Spending per Patient (ratio)	-	-	0.98	0.98
Pneumonia Care				
Appropriate Initial Antibiotic Given	12	92%	96%	95%
Blood Culture Timing[1]	-	-	99%	98%
Pregnancy and Delivery Care				
Newborn Deliveries Scheduled Early[1,3]	-	-	6%	6%
Preventive Care				
Immunization for Influenza	117	78%	92%	90%
Immunization for Pneumonia	79	82%	91%	92%
Stroke Care				
Anticoagulation Therapy for Atrial Fibrillation[3,7]	-	-	95%	95%
Antithrombotic Therapy Timing[1,3]	-	-	99%	98%
Assessed for Rehabilitation[1,3]	-	-	98%	97%
Discharged on Antithrombotic Therapy[1,3]	-	-	99%	99%
Discharged on Statin Medication[1,3]	-	-	96%	94%
Thrombolytic Therapy Timing[3,7]	-	-	89%	66%
Venous Thromboembolism Prophylaxis[1,3]	-	-	95%	94%
Written Stroke Educational Materials Given[3,7]	-	-	89%	88%
Surgical Care Improvement Project				
Appropriate Beta Blocker Usage[5]	-	-	98%	98%
Appropriate VTP Within 24 Hours[5]	-	-	99%	98%
Controlled Postoperative Blood Glucose[5]	-	-	97%	97%
Perioperative Temperature Management[5]	-	-	100%	100%
Prophylactic Antibiotic Selection[5]	-	-	99%	99%
Prophylactic Antibiotic Selection (Outpatient)[5]	-	-	98%	98%
Prophylactic Antibiotic Stopped[5]	-	-	98%	98%
Prophylactic Antibiotic Timing[5]	-	-	99%	99%
Prophylactic Antibiotic Timing (Outpatient)[5]	-	-	98%	98%
Urinary Catheter Removal[5]	-	-	98%	97%
Survey of Patients' Hospital Experiences				
Area Around Room 'Always' Quiet at Night[6]	<100	69%	60%	61%
Doctors 'Always' Communicated Well[6]	<100	91%	83%	82%
Home Recovery Information Given[6]	<100	91%	90%	85%
Hospital Given 9 or 10 on 10 Point Scale[6]	<100	80%	74%	71%
Meds 'Always' Explained Before Given[6]	<100	71%	68%	64%
Nurses 'Always' Communicated Well[6]	<100	82%	79%	79%
Pain 'Always' Well Controlled[6]	<100	79%	73%	71%
Room and Bathroom 'Always' Clean[6]	<100	90%	74%	73%
Timely Help 'Always' Received[6]	<100	71%	69%	68%
Would Definitely Recommend Hospital[6]	<100	82%	76%	71%
Use of Medical Imaging				
Cardiac Imaging Stress Test before Surgery[7]	-	-	4.9%	5.3%
Combination Abdominal CT Scan[1]	-	-	4.9%	10.5%
Combination Brain/Sinus CT Scan[1]	-	-	3%	2.7%
Combination Chest CT Scan[1]	-	-	0.8%	2.7%
Follow-up Mammogram/Ultrasound	66	7.6%	8.5%	8.8%
Lumbar Spine MRI for Low Back Pain[1]	-	-	43.8%	37.2%

NOTE: Hospital profiles are in alphabetical order by state, then city, then hospital within the city; Rankings exclude hospitals with less than 25 cases except for patient surveys which excludes hospitals with less than 100 cases; (a) 100-299 cases; (1) The number of cases/patients is too few to report; (2) Data submitted were based on a sample of cases/patients; (3) Results are based on a shorter time period than required; (4) Data suppressed by CMS for one or more quarters; (5) Results are not available for this reporting period; (6) Fewer than 100 patients completed the HCAHPS survey; (7) No cases met the criteria for this measure; (8) The lower limit of the confidence interval cannot be calculated if the number of observed infections equals zero; (9) No data are available from the state/territory for this reporting period; (10) The scores shown reflect fewer than 50 completed surveys; (11) There were discrepancies in the data collection process; (12) This measure does not apply to this hospital for this reporting period; (13) Results cannot be calculated for this reporting period; (14) The results for this state are combined with nearby states to protect confidentiality; Please refer to the User's Guide for a full explanation of data.

Lone Peak Hospital

11925 S State Street
Draper, UT 84020
Phone: 801-545-8001
Type: Acute Care Hospitals
Emergency Services: Yes
Ownership: Proprietary

Measure	Cases	This Hosp.	State Avg.	U.S. Avg.
Blood Clot Prevention and Treatment				
Anticoagulation Overlap Therapy[5]	-	-	95%	93%
ICU Venous Thromboembolism Prophylaxis[5]	-	-	93%	92%
Incidence of Potentially Preventable VTE[5]	-	-	5%	10%
UFH with Dosages/Platelet Monitoring[5]	-	-	95%	97%
Venous Thromboembolism Prophylaxis[5]	-	-	86%	85%
Warfarin Therapy Discharge Instructions[5]	-	-	73%	75%
Chest Pain/Possible Heart Attack Care				
Aspirin Given Within 24 Hours of Arrival[5]	-	-	97%	96%
Fibrinolytic Meds Within 30 Min. of Arrival[5]	-	-	52%	58%
Average Time to ECG (minutes)[5]	-	-	7	7
Average Time to Transfer (minutes)[5]	-	-	36	60
Children's Asthma Care				
Received Home Management Plan of Care	-	-	-	88%
Received Reliever Medication	-	-	-	100%
Received Systemic Corticosteroids	-	-	-	100%
Emergency Department				
Admittance Decision Time (minutes)[5]	-	-	66	98
Head CT Results Within 45 Min. of Arrival[5]	-	-	60%	57%
Patients Who Left ER Before Being Seen[5]	-	-	1%	2%
Time from ER Arrival to Admit. (minutes)[5]	-	-	217	274
Time from ER Arrival to Discharge (minutes)[5]	-	-	123	134
Time in ER Before Being Evaluated (minutes)[5]	-	-	17	26
Time to Pain Meds for Fractures (minutes)[5]	-	-	43	57
Heart Attack Care				
Aspirin Given at Discharge[5]	-	-	99%	99%
Fibrinolytic Meds Within 30 Min. of Arrival[5]	-	-	100%	54%
PCI Within 90 Minutes of Arrival[5]	-	-	98%	96%
Statin Prescribed at Discharge[5]	-	-	100%	98%
Heart Failure Care				
ACE Inhibitor or ARB for LVSD[5]	-	-	98%	97%
Discharge Instructions Given[5]	-	-	96%	94%
Evaluation of LVS Function[5]	-	-	98%	99%
Medicare Spending				
Medicare Spending per Patient (ratio)	-	-	0.98	0.98
Pneumonia Care				
Appropriate Initial Antibiotic Given[5]	-	-	96%	95%
Blood Culture Timing[5]	-	-	99%	98%
Pregnancy and Delivery Care				
Newborn Deliveries Scheduled Early[5]	-	-	6%	6%
Preventive Care				
Immunization for Influenza[5]	-	-	92%	90%
Immunization for Pneumonia[5]	-	-	91%	92%
Stroke Care				
Anticoagulation Therapy for Atrial Fibrillation[5]	-	-	95%	95%
Antithrombotic Therapy Timing[5]	-	-	99%	98%
Assessed for Rehabilitation[5]	-	-	98%	97%
Discharged on Antithrombotic Therapy[5]	-	-	99%	99%
Discharged on Statin Medication[5]	-	-	96%	94%
Thrombolytic Therapy Timing[5]	-	-	89%	66%
Venous Thromboembolism Prophylaxis[5]	-	-	95%	94%
Written Stroke Educational Materials Given[5]	-	-	89%	88%
Surgical Care Improvement Project				
Appropriate Beta Blocker Usage[5]	-	-	98%	98%
Appropriate VTP Within 24 Hours[5]	-	-	99%	98%
Controlled Postoperative Blood Glucose[5]	-	-	97%	97%
Perioperative Temperature Management[5]	-	-	100%	100%
Prophylactic Antibiotic Selection[5]	-	-	99%	99%
Prophylactic Antibiotic Selection (Outpatient)[5]	-	-	98%	98%
Prophylactic Antibiotic Stopped[5]	-	-	98%	98%
Prophylactic Antibiotic Timing[5]	-	-	99%	99%
Prophylactic Antibiotic Timing (Outpatient)[5]	-	-	98%	98%
Urinary Catheter Removal[5]	-	-	98%	97%
Survey of Patients' Hospital Experiences				
Area Around Room 'Always' Quiet at Night[5]	-	-	60%	61%
Doctors 'Always' Communicated Well[5]	-	-	83%	82%
Home Recovery Information Given[5]	-	-	90%	85%
Hospital Given 9 or 10 on 10 Point Scale[5]	-	-	74%	71%
Meds 'Always' Explained Before Given[5]	-	-	68%	64%
Nurses 'Always' Communicated Well[5]	-	-	79%	79%
Pain 'Always' Well Controlled[5]	-	-	73%	71%
Room and Bathroom 'Always' Clean[5]	-	-	74%	73%
Timely Help 'Always' Received[5]	-	-	69%	68%
Would Definitely Recommend Hospital[5]	-	-	76%	71%
Use of Medical Imaging				
Cardiac Imaging Stress Test before Surgery[5]	-	-	4.9%	5.3%
Combination Abdominal CT Scan[5]	-	-	4.9%	10.5%
Combination Brain/Sinus CT Scan[5]	-	-	3%	2.7%
Combination Chest CT Scan[5]	-	-	0.8%	2.7%
Follow-up Mammogram/Ultrasound[5]	-	-	8.5%	8.8%
Lumbar Spine MRI for Low Back Pain[5]	-	-	43.8%	37.2%

Fillmore Community Medical Center

674 South Highway 99
Fillmore, UT 84631
Phone: 435-743-5591
Fax: 435-743-6312
URL: www.ihc.com
Type: Critical Access Hospitals
Emergency Services: Yes
Ownership: Voluntary non-profit - Private
Beds: 20

Key Personnel:

Quality Assurance . . . . James Beckstrand
Radiology. . . . . Carl M Black
Emergency Room . . . . Paul Blad
Anesthesiology. . . . . Ron Draper
CEO/President. . . . . Charles W. Sorenson, MD

Measure	Cases	This Hosp.	State Avg.	U.S. Avg.
Blood Clot Prevention and Treatment				
Anticoagulation Overlap Therapy[7]	-	-	95%	93%
ICU Venous Thromboembolism Prophylaxis[7]	-	-	93%	92%
Incidence of Potentially Preventable VTE[7]	-	-	5%	10%
UFH with Dosages/Platelet Monitoring[7]	-	-	95%	97%
Venous Thromboembolism Prophylaxis	51	65%	86%	85%
Warfarin Therapy Discharge Instructions[7]	-	-	73%	75%
Chest Pain/Possible Heart Attack Care				
Aspirin Given Within 24 Hours of Arrival	13	100%	97%	96%
Fibrinolytic Meds Within 30 Min. of Arrival[1]	-	-	52%	58%
Average Time to ECG (minutes)	13	10	7	7
Average Time to Transfer (minutes)[7]	-	-	36	60
Children's Asthma Care				
Received Home Management Plan of Care	-	-	-	88%
Received Reliever Medication	-	-	-	100%
Received Systemic Corticosteroids	-	-	-	100%
Emergency Department				
Admittance Decision Time (minutes)	49	35	66	98
Head CT Results Within 45 Min. of Arrival[3,7]	-	-	60%	57%
Patients Who Left ER Before Being Seen[5]	-	-	1%	2%
Time from ER Arrival to Admit. (minutes)	59	143	217	274
Time from ER Arrival to Discharge (minutes)	244	102	123	134
Time in ER Before Being Evaluated (minutes)	269	22	17	26
Time to Pain Meds for Fractures (minutes)	12	54	43	57
Heart Attack Care				
Aspirin Given at Discharge[5]	-	-	99%	99%
Fibrinolytic Meds Within 30 Min. of Arrival[5]	-	-	100%	54%
PCI Within 90 Minutes of Arrival[5]	-	-	98%	96%
Statin Prescribed at Discharge[5]	-	-	100%	98%
Heart Failure Care				
ACE Inhibitor or ARB for LVSD[1,3]	-	-	98%	97%
Discharge Instructions Given[3,7]	-	-	96%	94%
Evaluation of LVS Function[1,3]	-	-	98%	99%
Medicare Spending				
Medicare Spending per Patient (ratio)	-	-	0.98	0.98
Pneumonia Care				
Appropriate Initial Antibiotic Given[1]	-	-	96%	95%
Blood Culture Timing[1]	-	-	99%	98%
Pregnancy and Delivery Care				
Newborn Deliveries Scheduled Early[1,3]	-	-	6%	6%
Preventive Care				
Immunization for Influenza	74	85%	92%	90%
Immunization for Pneumonia	59	85%	91%	92%
Stroke Care				
Anticoagulation Therapy for Atrial Fibrillation[3,7]	-	-	95%	95%
Antithrombotic Therapy Timing[3,7]	-	-	99%	98%
Assessed for Rehabilitation[1,3]	-	-	98%	97%
Discharged on Antithrombotic Therapy[3,7]	-	-	99%	99%
Discharged on Statin Medication[3,7]	-	-	96%	94%
Thrombolytic Therapy Timing[3,7]	-	-	89%	66%
Venous Thromboembolism Prophylaxis[3,7]	-	-	95%	94%
Written Stroke Educational Materials Given[1,3]	-	-	89%	88%
Surgical Care Improvement Project				
Appropriate Beta Blocker Usage[5]	-	-	98%	98%
Appropriate VTP Within 24 Hours[5]	-	-	99%	98%
Controlled Postoperative Blood Glucose[5]	-	-	97%	97%
Perioperative Temperature Management[5]	-	-	100%	100%
Prophylactic Antibiotic Selection[5]	-	-	99%	99%
Prophylactic Antibiotic Selection (Outpatient)[3,7]	-	-	98%	98%
Prophylactic Antibiotic Stopped[5]	-	-	98%	98%
Prophylactic Antibiotic Timing[5]	-	-	99%	99%
Prophylactic Antibiotic Timing (Outpatient)[1,3]	-	-	98%	98%
Urinary Catheter Removal[5]	-	-	98%	97%
Survey of Patients' Hospital Experiences				
Area Around Room 'Always' Quiet at Night[10]	<100	52%	60%	61%
Doctors 'Always' Communicated Well[10]	<100	91%	83%	82%
Home Recovery Information Given[10]	<100	97%	90%	85%
Hospital Given 9 or 10 on 10 Point Scale[10]	<100	87%	74%	71%
Meds 'Always' Explained Before Given[10]	<100	75%	68%	64%
Nurses 'Always' Communicated Well[10]	<100	84%	79%	79%
Pain 'Always' Well Controlled[10]	<100	78%	73%	71%
Room and Bathroom 'Always' Clean[10]	<100	68%	74%	73%
Timely Help 'Always' Received[10]	<100	74%	69%	68%
Would Definitely Recommend Hospital[10]	<100	88%	76%	71%
Use of Medical Imaging				
Cardiac Imaging Stress Test before Surgery[7]	-	-	4.9%	5.3%
Combination Abdominal CT Scan[1]	-	-	4.9%	10.5%
Combination Brain/Sinus CT Scan	37	0.0%	3%	2.7%
Combination Chest CT Scan[1]	-	-	0.8%	2.7%
Follow-up Mammogram/Ultrasound[1]	-	-	8.5%	8.8%
Lumbar Spine MRI for Low Back Pain[1]	-	-	43.8%	37.2%

Gunnison Valley Hospital

64 East 100 North
Gunnison, UT 84634
Phone: 435-528-7246
Fax: 435-528-2190
E-mail: greg.rosenvall@utahtelehealth.net
URL: www.gvhomecare.org
Type: Critical Access Hospitals
Emergency Services: Yes
Ownership: Voluntary non-profit - Other
Beds: 25

Key Personnel:

Chief of Medical Staff . . . . Richard Anderson, MD
Radiology. . . . . Richard Cutshal
Operating Room. . . . . Shara Peterson, RN
CEO/President. . . . . Greg Rosenvall
Quality Assurance . . . . Nicki Stewart

Measure	Cases	This Hosp.	State Avg.	U.S. Avg.
Blood Clot Prevention and Treatment				
Anticoagulation Overlap Therapy[5]	-	-	95%	93%
ICU Venous Thromboembolism Prophylaxis[5]	-	-	93%	92%
Incidence of Potentially Preventable VTE[5]	-	-	5%	10%
UFH with Dosages/Platelet Monitoring[5]	-	-	95%	97%
Venous Thromboembolism Prophylaxis[5]	-	-	86%	85%
Warfarin Therapy Discharge Instructions[5]	-	-	73%	75%
Chest Pain/Possible Heart Attack Care				
Aspirin Given Within 24 Hours of Arrival	18	89%	97%	96%
Fibrinolytic Meds Within 30 Min. of Arrival[1]	-	-	52%	58%
Average Time to ECG (minutes)	18	4	7	7
Average Time to Transfer (minutes)[7]	-	-	36	60
Children's Asthma Care				
Received Home Management Plan of Care	-	-	-	88%
Received Reliever Medication	-	-	-	100%
Received Systemic Corticosteroids	-	-	-	100%
Emergency Department				
Admittance Decision Time (minutes)[5]	-	-	66	98
Head CT Results Within 45 Min. of Arrival[3,7]	-	-	60%	57%
Patients Who Left ER Before Being Seen	3,691	2%	1%	2%
Time from ER Arrival to Admit. (minutes)[5]	-	-	217	274
Time from ER Arrival to Discharge (minutes)[5]	-	-	123	134
Time in ER Before Being Evaluated (minutes)[5]	-	-	17	26

NOTE: Hospital profiles are in alphabetical order by state, then city, then hospital within the city; Rankings exclude hospitals with less than 25 cases except for patient surveys which excludes hospitals with less than 100 cases; (a) 100-299 cases; (1) The number of cases/patients is too few to report; (2) Data submitted were based on a sample of cases/patients; (3) Results are based on a shorter time period than required; (4) Data suppressed by CMS for one or more quarters; (5) Results are not available for this reporting period; (6) Fewer than 100 patients completed the HCAHPS survey; (7) No cases met the criteria for this measure; (8) The lower limit of the confidence interval cannot be calculated if the number of observed infections equals zero; (9) No data are available from the state/territory for this reporting period; (10) The scores shown reflect fewer than 50 completed surveys; (11) There were discrepancies in the data collection process; (12) This measure does not apply to this hospital for this reporting period; (13) Results cannot be calculated for this reporting period; (14) The results for this state are combined with nearby states to protect confidentiality; Please refer to the User's Guide for a full explanation of data.

Measure	Cases	This Hosp.	State Avg.	U.S. Avg.
Time to Pain Meds for Fractures (minutes)[5]	-	-	43	57
Heart Attack Care				
Aspirin Given at Discharge[3,7]	-	-	99%	99%
Fibrinolytic Meds Within 30 Min. of Arrival[3,7]	-	-	100%	54%
PCI Within 90 Minutes of Arrival[3,7]	-	-	98%	96%
Statin Prescribed at Discharge[3,7]	-	-	100%	98%
Heart Failure Care				
ACE Inhibitor or ARB for LVSD[7]	-	-	98%	97%
Discharge Instructions Given[1]	-	-	96%	94%
Evaluation of LVS Function	11	73%	98%	99%
Medicare Spending				
Medicare Spending per Patient (ratio)	-	-	0.98	0.98
Pneumonia Care				
Appropriate Initial Antibiotic Given[2]	36	81%	96%	95%
Blood Culture Timing[1,2]	-	-	99%	98%
Pregnancy and Delivery Care				
Newborn Deliveries Scheduled Early[5]	-	-	6%	6%
Preventive Care				
Immunization for Influenza[5]	-	-	92%	90%
Immunization for Pneumonia[5]	-	-	91%	92%
Stroke Care				
Anticoagulation Therapy for Atrial Fibrillation[5]	-	-	95%	95%
Antithrombotic Therapy Timing[5]	-	-	99%	98%
Assessed for Rehabilitation[5]	-	-	98%	97%
Discharged on Antithrombotic Therapy[5]	-	-	99%	99%
Discharged on Statin Medication[5]	-	-	96%	94%
Thrombolytic Therapy Timing[5]	-	-	89%	66%
Venous Thromboembolism Prophylaxis[5]	-	-	95%	94%
Written Stroke Educational Materials Given[5]	-	-	89%	88%
Surgical Care Improvement Project				
Appropriate Beta Blocker Usage[3,7]	-	-	98%	98%
Appropriate VTP Within 24 Hours[1,3]	-	-	99%	98%
Controlled Postoperative Blood Glucose[3,7]	-	-	97%	97%
Perioperative Temperature Management[1,3]	-	-	100%	100%
Prophylactic Antibiotic Selection[1,3]	-	-	99%	99%
Prophylactic Antibiotic Selection (Outpatient)[5]	-	-	98%	98%
Prophylactic Antibiotic Stopped[1,3]	-	-	98%	98%
Prophylactic Antibiotic Timing[1,3]	-	-	99%	99%
Prophylactic Antibiotic Timing (Outpatient)[5]	-	-	98%	98%
Urinary Catheter Removal[1,3]	-	-	98%	97%
Survey of Patients' Hospital Experiences				
Area Around Room 'Always' Quiet at Night[5]	-	-	60%	61%
Doctors 'Always' Communicated Well[5]	-	-	83%	82%
Home Recovery Information Given[5]	-	-	90%	85%
Hospital Given 9 or 10 on 10 Point Scale[5]	-	-	74%	71%
Meds 'Always' Explained Before Given[5]	-	-	68%	64%
Nurses 'Always' Communicated Well[5]	-	-	79%	79%
Pain 'Always' Well Controlled[5]	-	-	73%	71%
Room and Bathroom 'Always' Clean[5]	-	-	74%	73%
Timely Help 'Always' Received[5]	-	-	69%	68%
Would Definitely Recommend Hospital[5]	-	-	76%	71%
Use of Medical Imaging				
Cardiac Imaging Stress Test before Surgery[7]	-	-	4.9%	5.3%
Combination Abdominal CT Scan	122	2.5%	4.9%	10.5%
Combination Brain/Sinus CT Scan[1]	-	-	3%	2.7%
Combination Chest CT Scan	67	0.0%	0.8%	2.7%
Follow-up Mammogram/Ultrasound	197	18.3%	8.5%	8.8%
Lumbar Spine MRI for Low Back Pain[1]	-	-	43.8%	37.2%

Heber Valley Medical Center

1485 South Highway 40
Heber City, UT 84032
Phone: 435-654-2500
URL: www.intermountainhealthcare.org
Type: Critical Access Hospitals
Emergency Services: Yes
Ownership: Voluntary non-profit - Private

Measure	Cases	This Hosp.	State Avg.	U.S. Avg.
Blood Clot Prevention and Treatment				
Anticoagulation Overlap Therapy[1,2]	-	-	95%	93%
ICU Venous Thromboembolism Prophylaxis[2,7]	-	-	93%	92%
Incidence of Potentially Preventable VTE[1,2]	-	-	5%	10%
UFH with Dosages/Platelet Monitoring[2,7]	-	-	95%	97%
Venous Thromboembolism Prophylaxis[2]	79	67%	86%	85%
Warfarin Therapy Discharge Instructions[1,2]	-	-	73%	75%
Chest Pain/Possible Heart Attack Care				
Aspirin Given Within 24 Hours of Arrival	14	100%	97%	96%
Fibrinolytic Meds Within 30 Min. of Arrival[7]	-	-	52%	58%
Average Time to ECG (minutes)	14	6	7	7
Average Time to Transfer (minutes)[1]	-	-	36	60
Children's Asthma Care				
Received Home Management Plan of Care	-	-	-	88%
Received Reliever Medication	-	-	-	100%
Received Systemic Corticosteroids	-	-	-	100%
Emergency Department				
Admittance Decision Time (minutes)[2]	157	50	66	98
Head CT Results Within 45 Min. of Arrival[1]	-	-	60%	57%
Patients Who Left ER Before Being Seen	5,471	0%	1%	2%
Time from ER Arrival to Admit. (minutes)[2]	173	218	217	274
Time from ER Arrival to Discharge (minutes)	393	94	123	134
Time in ER Before Being Evaluated (minutes)	376	16	17	26
Time to Pain Meds for Fractures (minutes)	54	34	43	57
Heart Attack Care				
Aspirin Given at Discharge[1,3]	-	-	99%	99%
Fibrinolytic Meds Within 30 Min. of Arrival[3,7]	-	-	100%	54%
PCI Within 90 Minutes of Arrival[3,7]	-	-	98%	96%
Statin Prescribed at Discharge[1,3]	-	-	100%	98%
Heart Failure Care				
ACE Inhibitor or ARB for LVSD[3,7]	-	-	98%	97%
Discharge Instructions Given[3,7]	-	-	96%	94%
Evaluation of LVS Function[1,3]	-	-	98%	99%
Medicare Spending				
Medicare Spending per Patient (ratio)	-	-	0.98	0.98
Pneumonia Care				
Appropriate Initial Antibiotic Given	17	94%	96%	95%
Blood Culture Timing	14	100%	99%	98%
Pregnancy and Delivery Care				
Newborn Deliveries Scheduled Early[3]	13	0%	6%	6%
Preventive Care				
Immunization for Influenza[2]	209	83%	92%	90%
Immunization for Pneumonia[2]	136	82%	91%	92%
Stroke Care				
Anticoagulation Therapy for Atrial Fibrillation[1,3]	-	-	95%	95%
Antithrombotic Therapy Timing[1,3]	-	-	99%	98%
Assessed for Rehabilitation[1,3]	-	-	98%	97%
Discharged on Antithrombotic Therapy[1,3]	-	-	99%	99%
Discharged on Statin Medication[1,3]	-	-	96%	94%
Thrombolytic Therapy Timing[3,7]	-	-	89%	66%
Venous Thromboembolism Prophylaxis[1,3]	-	-	95%	94%
Written Stroke Educational Materials Given[1,3]	-	-	89%	88%
Surgical Care Improvement Project				
Appropriate Beta Blocker Usage[1]	-	-	98%	98%
Appropriate VTP Within 24 Hours	28	100%	99%	98%
Controlled Postoperative Blood Glucose[7]	-	-	97%	97%
Perioperative Temperature Management	28	96%	100%	100%
Prophylactic Antibiotic Selection	21	95%	99%	99%
Prophylactic Antibiotic Selection (Outpatient)	16	100%	98%	98%
Prophylactic Antibiotic Stopped	21	100%	98%	98%
Prophylactic Antibiotic Timing	21	95%	99%	99%
Prophylactic Antibiotic Timing (Outpatient)	17	94%	98%	98%
Urinary Catheter Removal	11	91%	98%	97%
Survey of Patients' Hospital Experiences				
Area Around Room 'Always' Quiet at Night	(a)	71%	60%	61%
Doctors 'Always' Communicated Well	(a)	87%	83%	82%
Home Recovery Information Given	(a)	94%	90%	85%
Hospital Given 9 or 10 on 10 Point Scale	(a)	82%	74%	71%
Meds 'Always' Explained Before Given	(a)	75%	68%	64%
Nurses 'Always' Communicated Well	(a)	83%	79%	79%
Pain 'Always' Well Controlled	(a)	73%	73%	71%
Room and Bathroom 'Always' Clean	(a)	70%	74%	73%
Timely Help 'Always' Received	(a)	72%	69%	68%
Would Definitely Recommend Hospital	(a)	77%	76%	71%
Use of Medical Imaging				
Cardiac Imaging Stress Test before Surgery[7]	-	-	4.9%	5.3%
Combination Abdominal CT Scan	61	4.9%	4.9%	10.5%
Combination Brain/Sinus CT Scan[1]	-	-	3%	2.7%
Combination Chest CT Scan[1]	-	-	0.8%	2.7%
Follow-up Mammogram/Ultrasound	194	5.7%	8.5%	8.8%
Lumbar Spine MRI for Low Back Pain[1]	-	-	43.8%	37.2%

Kane County Hospital

355 North Main Street
Kanab, UT 84741
Phone: 435-644-5811
Fax: 435-644-4140
Type: Critical Access Hospitals
Emergency Services: Yes
Ownership: Govt - Hospital Dist/Auth
Beds: 38

Key Personnel:

Operating Room. . . . . Rosalie Esplin
Quality Assurance . . . . Jamie Mackelprang
Anesthesiology. . . . . Lou Ann Marocchi
Emergency Room . . . . K Mortenson, MD
Chief of Medical Staff . . . . Avnish P Pandyah, MD
Radiology. . . . . Lori Ramsay

Measure	Cases	This Hosp.	State Avg.	U.S. Avg.
Blood Clot Prevention and Treatment				
Anticoagulation Overlap Therapy[5]	-	-	95%	93%
ICU Venous Thromboembolism Prophylaxis[5]	-	-	93%	92%
Incidence of Potentially Preventable VTE[5]	-	-	5%	10%
UFH with Dosages/Platelet Monitoring[5]	-	-	95%	97%
Venous Thromboembolism Prophylaxis[5]	-	-	86%	85%
Warfarin Therapy Discharge Instructions[5]	-	-	73%	75%
Chest Pain/Possible Heart Attack Care				
Aspirin Given Within 24 Hours of Arrival[5]	-	-	97%	96%
Fibrinolytic Meds Within 30 Min. of Arrival[5]	-	-	52%	58%
Average Time to ECG (minutes)[5]	-	-	7	7
Average Time to Transfer (minutes)[5]	-	-	36	60
Children's Asthma Care				
Received Home Management Plan of Care	-	-	-	88%
Received Reliever Medication	-	-	-	100%
Received Systemic Corticosteroids	-	-	-	100%
Emergency Department				
Admittance Decision Time (minutes)[5]	-	-	66	98
Head CT Results Within 45 Min. of Arrival[5]	-	-	60%	57%
Patients Who Left ER Before Being Seen[5]	-	-	1%	2%
Time from ER Arrival to Admit. (minutes)[5]	-	-	217	274
Time from ER Arrival to Discharge (minutes)[5]	-	-	123	134
Time in ER Before Being Evaluated (minutes)[5]	-	-	17	26
Time to Pain Meds for Fractures (minutes)[5]	-	-	43	57
Heart Attack Care				
Aspirin Given at Discharge[5]	-	-	99%	99%
Fibrinolytic Meds Within 30 Min. of Arrival[5]	-	-	100%	54%
PCI Within 90 Minutes of Arrival[5]	-	-	98%	96%
Statin Prescribed at Discharge[5]	-	-	100%	98%
Heart Failure Care				
ACE Inhibitor or ARB for LVSD[2,3]	-	-	98%	97%
Discharge Instructions Given[1,2]	-	-	96%	94%
Evaluation of LVS Function[1,2]	-	-	98%	99%
Medicare Spending				
Medicare Spending per Patient (ratio)	-	-	0.98	0.98
Pneumonia Care				
Appropriate Initial Antibiotic Given[1,2]	-	-	96%	95%
Blood Culture Timing[1,2]	-	-	99%	98%
Pregnancy and Delivery Care				
Newborn Deliveries Scheduled Early[5]	-	-	6%	6%
Preventive Care				
Immunization for Influenza[5]	-	-	92%	90%
Immunization for Pneumonia[5]	-	-	91%	92%
Stroke Care				
Anticoagulation Therapy for Atrial Fibrillation[5]	-	-	95%	95%
Antithrombotic Therapy Timing[5]	-	-	99%	98%
Assessed for Rehabilitation[5]	-	-	98%	97%
Discharged on Antithrombotic Therapy[5]	-	-	99%	99%
Discharged on Statin Medication[5]	-	-	96%	94%
Thrombolytic Therapy Timing[5]	-	-	89%	66%
Venous Thromboembolism Prophylaxis[5]	-	-	95%	94%
Written Stroke Educational Materials Given[5]	-	-	89%	88%
Surgical Care Improvement Project				
Appropriate Beta Blocker Usage[5]	-	-	98%	98%
Appropriate VTP Within 24 Hours[5]	-	-	99%	98%
Controlled Postoperative Blood Glucose[5]	-	-	97%	97%
Perioperative Temperature Management[5]	-	-	100%	100%

NOTE: Hospital profiles are in alphabetical order by state, then city, then hospital within the city; Rankings exclude hospitals with less than 25 cases except for patient surveys which excludes hospitals with less than 100 cases; (a) 100-299 cases; (1) The number of cases/patients is too few to report; (2) Data submitted were based on a sample of cases/patients; (3) Results are based on a shorter time period than required; (4) Data suppressed by CMS for one or more quarters; (5) Results are not available for this reporting period; (6) Fewer than 100 patients completed the HCAHPS survey; (7) No cases met the criteria for this measure; (8) The lower limit of the confidence interval cannot be calculated if the number of observed infections equals zero; (9) No data are available from the state/territory for this reporting period; (10) The scores shown reflect fewer than 50 completed surveys; (11) There were discrepancies in the data collection process; (12) This measure does not apply to this hospital for this reporting period; (13) Results cannot be calculated for this reporting period; (14) The results for this state are combined with nearby states to protect confidentiality; Please refer to the User's Guide for a full explanation of data.

Measure	Cases	This Hosp.	State Avg.	U.S. Avg.
Prophylactic Antibiotic Selection[5]	-	-	99%	99%
Prophylactic Antibiotic Selection (Outpatient)[5]	-	-	98%	98%
Prophylactic Antibiotic Stopped[5]	-	-	98%	98%
Prophylactic Antibiotic Timing[5]	-	-	99%	99%
Prophylactic Antibiotic Timing (Outpatient)[5]	-	-	98%	98%
Urinary Catheter Removal[5]	-	-	98%	97%
Survey of Patients' Hospital Experiences				
Area Around Room 'Always' Quiet at Night[5]	-	-	60%	61%
Doctors 'Always' Communicated Well[5]	-	-	83%	82%
Home Recovery Information Given[5]	-	-	90%	85%
Hospital Given 9 or 10 on 10 Point Scale[5]	-	-	74%	71%
Meds 'Always' Explained Before Given[5]	-	-	68%	64%
Nurses 'Always' Communicated Well[5]	-	-	79%	79%
Pain 'Always' Well Controlled[5]	-	-	73%	71%
Room and Bathroom 'Always' Clean[5]	-	-	74%	73%
Timely Help 'Always' Received[5]	-	-	69%	68%
Would Definitely Recommend Hospital[5]	-	-	76%	71%
Use of Medical Imaging				
Cardiac Imaging Stress Test before Surgery[7]	-	-	4.9%	5.3%
Combination Abdominal CT Scan	102	1.0%	4.9%	10.5%
Combination Brain/Sinus CT Scan[1]	-	-	3%	2.7%
Combination Chest CT Scan	70	0.0%	0.8%	2.7%
Follow-up Mammogram/Ultrasound[7]	-	-	8.5%	8.8%
Lumbar Spine MRI for Low Back Pain[7]	-	-	43.8%	37.2%

Davis Hospital & Medical Center

1600 West Antelope Drive
Layton, UT 84041
URL: www.davishospital.com
Type: Acute Care Hospitals
Ownership: Proprietary
Phone: 801-807-1000
Fax: 801-774-7045
Emergency Services: Yes
Beds: 126

Key Personnel:

Anesthesiology. . . . . Blake Brown, MD
Quality Assurance . . . . Da Nece Fickett
CEO . . . . Mike Jensen
Infection Control. . . . . Cindy Johnston
Emergency Room . . . . Bart Nilson
Pediatric Ambulatory Care . . . . . . Mic Schaelling, MD
Pediatric In-Patient Care . . . . . . Mic Schaelling, MD
Chief of Medical Staff. . . . . Stephen Tucker, MD

Measure	Cases	This Hosp.	State Avg.	U.S. Avg.
Blood Clot Prevention and Treatment				
Anticoagulation Overlap Therapy[2]	35	97%	95%	93%
ICU Venous Thromboembolism Prophylaxis[2]	66	89%	93%	92%
Incidence of Potentially Preventable VTE[2,7]	-	-	5%	10%
UFH with Dosages/Platelet Monitoring[2]	16	100%	95%	97%
Venous Thromboembolism Prophylaxis[2]	270	93%	86%	85%
Warfarin Therapy Discharge Instructions[2]	30	93%	73%	75%
Chest Pain/Possible Heart Attack Care				
Aspirin Given Within 24 Hours of Arrival[1,3]	-	-	97%	96%
Fibrinolytic Meds Within 30 Min. of Arrival[5]	-	-	52%	58%
Average Time to ECG (minutes)[1,3]	-	-	7	7
Average Time to Transfer (minutes)[5]	-	-	36	60
Children's Asthma Care				
Received Home Management Plan of Care	-	-	-	88%
Received Reliever Medication	-	-	-	100%
Received Systemic Corticosteroids	-	-	-	100%
Emergency Department				
Admittance Decision Time (minutes)[2]	596	60	66	98
Head CT Results Within 45 Min. of Arrival	12	100%	60%	57%
Patients Who Left ER Before Being Seen	31,099	1%	1%	2%
Time from ER Arrival to Admit. (minutes)[2]	600	208	217	274
Time from ER Arrival to Discharge (minutes)	761	132	123	134
Time in ER Before Being Evaluated (minutes)	762	31	17	26
Time to Pain Meds for Fractures (minutes)	206	47	43	57
Heart Attack Care				
Aspirin Given at Discharge	66	100%	99%	99%
Fibrinolytic Meds Within 30 Min. of Arrival[7]	-	-	100%	54%
PCI Within 90 Minutes of Arrival	24	100%	98%	96%
Statin Prescribed at Discharge	65	98%	100%	98%
Heart Failure Care				
ACE Inhibitor or ARB for LVSD	31	100%	98%	97%
Discharge Instructions Given	60	100%	96%	94%
Evaluation of LVS Function	90	100%	98%	99%
Medicare Spending				
Medicare Spending per Patient (ratio)	-	1.11	0.98	0.98
Pneumonia Care				
Appropriate Initial Antibiotic Given	68	100%	96%	95%
Blood Culture Timing	91	100%	99%	98%
Pregnancy and Delivery Care				
Newborn Deliveries Scheduled Early[2]	55	0%	6%	6%
Preventive Care				
Immunization for Influenza[2]	707	99%	92%	90%
Immunization for Pneumonia[2]	592	96%	91%	92%
Stroke Care				
Anticoagulation Therapy for Atrial Fibrillation[1]	-	-	95%	95%
Antithrombotic Therapy Timing	28	96%	99%	98%
Assessed for Rehabilitation	30	100%	98%	97%
Discharged on Antithrombotic Therapy	30	100%	99%	99%
Discharged on Statin Medication	22	95%	96%	94%
Thrombolytic Therapy Timing[7]	-	-	89%	66%
Venous Thromboembolism Prophylaxis	29	97%	95%	94%
Written Stroke Educational Materials Given	13	92%	89%	88%
Surgical Care Improvement Project				
Appropriate Beta Blocker Usage	41	95%	98%	98%
Appropriate VTP Within 24 Hours	362	99%	99%	98%
Controlled Postoperative Blood Glucose[7]	-	-	97%	97%
Perioperative Temperature Management	426	100%	100%	100%
Prophylactic Antibiotic Selection	317	100%	99%	99%
Prophylactic Antibiotic Selection (Outpatient)	579	99%	98%	98%
Prophylactic Antibiotic Stopped	296	99%	98%	98%
Prophylactic Antibiotic Timing	320	100%	99%	99%
Prophylactic Antibiotic Timing (Outpatient)	580	99%	98%	98%
Urinary Catheter Removal	175	99%	98%	97%
Survey of Patients' Hospital Experiences				
Area Around Room 'Always' Quiet at Night	300+	54%	60%	61%
Doctors 'Always' Communicated Well	300+	84%	83%	82%
Home Recovery Information Given	300+	89%	90%	85%
Hospital Given 9 or 10 on 10 Point Scale	300+	68%	74%	71%
Meds 'Always' Explained Before Given	300+	63%	68%	64%
Nurses 'Always' Communicated Well	300+	74%	79%	79%
Pain 'Always' Well Controlled	300+	69%	73%	71%
Room and Bathroom 'Always' Clean	300+	72%	74%	73%
Timely Help 'Always' Received	300+	62%	69%	68%
Would Definitely Recommend Hospital	300+	67%	76%	71%
Use of Medical Imaging				
Cardiac Imaging Stress Test before Surgery	106	6.6%	4.9%	5.3%
Combination Abdominal CT Scan	311	1.3%	4.9%	10.5%
Combination Brain/Sinus CT Scan[1]	-	-	3%	2.7%
Combination Chest CT Scan	131	0.0%	0.8%	2.7%
Follow-up Mammogram/Ultrasound	1,100	9.4%	8.5%	8.8%
Lumbar Spine MRI for Low Back Pain	60	53.3%	43.8%	37.2%

Logan Regional Hospital

500 East 1400 North
Logan, UT 84341
URL: www.intermountainhealthcare.org
Type: Acute Care Hospitals
Ownership: Voluntary non-profit - Private
Phone: 435-716-1000
Fax: 435-716-5409
Emergency Services: Yes
Beds: 148

Key Personnel:

Chief of Medical Staff. . . . . Todd Brown
Radiology. . . . . Terry Buccambuso
Quality Assurance . . . . Teri Chase-Dunn
Pediatric In-Patient Care . . . . Derrel W Clarke
Emergency Room . . . . James Davis
Operating Room. . . . . Pat DePietro
Infection Control. . . . . Debbi Moore
Intensive Care Unit. . . . . William Saul

Measure	Cases	This Hosp.	State Avg.	U.S. Avg.
Blood Clot Prevention and Treatment				
Anticoagulation Overlap Therapy[2]	45	98%	95%	93%
ICU Venous Thromboembolism Prophylaxis[2]	46	89%	93%	92%
Incidence of Potentially Preventable VTE[1,2]	-	-	5%	10%
UFH with Dosages/Platelet Monitoring[1,2]	-	-	95%	97%
Venous Thromboembolism Prophylaxis[2]	226	83%	86%	85%
Warfarin Therapy Discharge Instructions[2]	36	89%	73%	75%
Chest Pain/Possible Heart Attack Care				
Aspirin Given Within 24 Hours of Arrival	26	96%	97%	96%
Fibrinolytic Meds Within 30 Min. of Arrival[1]	-	-	52%	58%
Average Time to ECG (minutes)	26	6	7	7
Average Time to Transfer (minutes)[7]	-	-	36	60
Children's Asthma Care				
Received Home Management Plan of Care	-	-	-	88%
Received Reliever Medication	-	-	-	100%
Received Systemic Corticosteroids	-	-	-	100%
Emergency Department				
Admittance Decision Time (minutes)[2]	251	85	66	98
Head CT Results Within 45 Min. of Arrival	14	71%	60%	57%
Patients Who Left ER Before Being Seen	24,546	0%	1%	2%
Time from ER Arrival to Admit. (minutes)[2]	267	239	217	274
Time from ER Arrival to Discharge (minutes)	271	140	123	134
Time in ER Before Being Evaluated (minutes)	279	12	17	26
Time to Pain Meds for Fractures (minutes)	185	41	43	57
Heart Attack Care				
Aspirin Given at Discharge	51	100%	99%	99%
Fibrinolytic Meds Within 30 Min. of Arrival[7]	-	-	100%	54%
PCI Within 90 Minutes of Arrival[1]	-	-	98%	96%
Statin Prescribed at Discharge	52	100%	100%	98%
Heart Failure Care				
ACE Inhibitor or ARB for LVSD	12	100%	98%	97%
Discharge Instructions Given	37	97%	96%	94%
Evaluation of LVS Function	44	100%	98%	99%
Medicare Spending				
Medicare Spending per Patient (ratio)	-	0.88	0.98	0.98
Pneumonia Care				
Appropriate Initial Antibiotic Given[2]	81	100%	96%	95%
Blood Culture Timing[2]	130	99%	99%	98%
Pregnancy and Delivery Care				
Newborn Deliveries Scheduled Early[2]	76	7%	6%	6%
Preventive Care				
Immunization for Influenza[2]	431	92%	92%	90%
Immunization for Pneumonia[2]	291	79%	91%	92%
Stroke Care				
Anticoagulation Therapy for Atrial Fibrillation[1]	-	-	95%	95%
Antithrombotic Therapy Timing	19	100%	99%	98%
Assessed for Rehabilitation	25	96%	98%	97%
Discharged on Antithrombotic Therapy	22	100%	99%	99%
Discharged on Statin Medication	15	93%	96%	94%
Thrombolytic Therapy Timing[7]	-	-	89%	66%
Venous Thromboembolism Prophylaxis	19	84%	95%	94%
Written Stroke Educational Materials Given	17	76%	89%	88%
Surgical Care Improvement Project				
Appropriate Beta Blocker Usage[2]	55	100%	98%	98%
Appropriate VTP Within 24 Hours[2]	306	100%	99%	98%
Controlled Postoperative Blood Glucose[2,7]	-	-	97%	97%
Perioperative Temperature Management[2]	353	100%	100%	100%
Prophylactic Antibiotic Selection[2]	232	100%	99%	99%
Prophylactic Antibiotic Selection (Outpatient)	336	99%	98%	98%
Prophylactic Antibiotic Stopped[2]	222	100%	98%	98%
Prophylactic Antibiotic Timing[2]	232	100%	99%	99%
Prophylactic Antibiotic Timing (Outpatient)	339	98%	98%	98%
Urinary Catheter Removal[2]	198	100%	98%	97%
Survey of Patients' Hospital Experiences				
Area Around Room 'Always' Quiet at Night	300+	59%	60%	61%
Doctors 'Always' Communicated Well	300+	83%	83%	82%
Home Recovery Information Given	300+	91%	90%	85%
Hospital Given 9 or 10 on 10 Point Scale	300+	76%	74%	71%
Meds 'Always' Explained Before Given	300+	71%	68%	64%
Nurses 'Always' Communicated Well	300+	80%	79%	79%
Pain 'Always' Well Controlled	300+	76%	73%	71%
Room and Bathroom 'Always' Clean	300+	74%	74%	73%
Timely Help 'Always' Received	300+	69%	69%	68%
Would Definitely Recommend Hospital	300+	77%	76%	71%
Use of Medical Imaging				
Cardiac Imaging Stress Test before Surgery	311	3.2%	4.9%	5.3%
Combination Abdominal CT Scan	414	6.8%	4.9%	10.5%
Combination Brain/Sinus CT Scan[1]	-	-	3%	2.7%
Combination Chest CT Scan	264	1.9%	0.8%	2.7%
Follow-up Mammogram/Ultrasound	971	7.0%	8.5%	8.8%
Lumbar Spine MRI for Low Back Pain	129	38.8%	43.8%	37.2%

NOTE: Hospital profiles are in alphabetical order by state, then city, then hospital within the city; Rankings exclude hospitals with less than 25 cases except for patient surveys which excludes hospitals with less than 100 cases; (a) 100-299 cases; (1) The number of cases/patients is too few to report; (2) Data submitted were based on a sample of cases/patients; (3) Results are based on a shorter time period than required; (4) Data suppressed by CMS for one or more quarters; (5) Results are not available for this reporting period; (6) Fewer than 100 patients completed the HCAHPS survey; (7) No cases met the criteria for this measure; (8) The lower limit of the confidence interval cannot be calculated if the number of observed infections equals zero; (9) No data are available from the state/territory for this reporting period; (10) The scores shown reflect fewer than 50 completed surveys; (11) There were discrepancies in the data collection process; (12) This measure does not apply to this hospital for this reporting period; (13) Results cannot be calculated for this reporting period; (14) The results for this state are combined with nearby states to protect confidentiality; Please refer to the User's Guide for a full explanation of data.

Milford Valley Memorial Hospital

850 North Main Street Phone: 435-387-2411
Milford, UT 84751
Type: Critical Access Hospitals Emergency Services: Yes
Ownership: Govt - Hospital Dist/Auth

Measure	Cases	This Hosp.	State Avg.	U.S. Avg.
Blood Clot Prevention and Treatment				
Anticoagulation Overlap Therapy[5]	-	-	95%	93%
ICU Venous Thromboembolism Prophylaxis[5]	-	-	93%	92%
Incidence of Potentially Preventable VTE[5]	-	-	5%	10%
UFH with Dosages/Platelet Monitoring[5]	-	-	95%	97%
Venous Thromboembolism Prophylaxis[5]	-	-	86%	85%
Warfarin Therapy Discharge Instructions[5]	-	-	73%	75%
Chest Pain/Possible Heart Attack Care				
Aspirin Given Within 24 Hours of Arrival	-	-	97%	96%
Fibrinolytic Meds Within 30 Min. of Arrival	-	-	52%	58%
Average Time to ECG (minutes)	-	-	7	7
Average Time to Transfer (minutes)	-	-	36	60
Children's Asthma Care				
Received Home Management Plan of Care	-	-	-	88%
Received Reliever Medication	-	-	-	100%
Received Systemic Corticosteroids	-	-	-	100%
Emergency Department				
Admittance Decision Time (minutes)[5]	-	-	66	98
Head CT Results Within 45 Min. of Arrival	-	-	60%	57%
Patients Who Left ER Before Being Seen	-	-	1%	2%
Time from ER Arrival to Admit. (minutes)[5]	-	-	217	274
Time from ER Arrival to Discharge (minutes)	-	-	123	134
Time in ER Before Being Evaluated (minutes)	-	-	17	26
Time to Pain Meds for Fractures (minutes)	-	-	43	57
Heart Attack Care				
Aspirin Given at Discharge[5]	-	-	99%	99%
Fibrinolytic Meds Within 30 Min. of Arrival[5]	-	-	100%	54%
PCI Within 90 Minutes of Arrival[5]	-	-	98%	96%
Statin Prescribed at Discharge[5]	-	-	100%	98%
Heart Failure Care				
ACE Inhibitor or ARB for LVSD[5]	-	-	98%	97%
Discharge Instructions Given[5]	-	-	96%	94%
Evaluation of LVS Function[5]	-	-	98%	99%
Medicare Spending				
Medicare Spending per Patient (ratio)	-	-	0.98	0.98
Pneumonia Care				
Appropriate Initial Antibiotic Given[1,3]	-	-	96%	95%
Blood Culture Timing[3,7]	-	-	99%	98%
Pregnancy and Delivery Care				
Newborn Deliveries Scheduled Early[5]	-	-	6%	6%
Preventive Care				
Immunization for Influenza[5]	-	-	92%	90%
Immunization for Pneumonia[5]	-	-	91%	92%
Stroke Care				
Anticoagulation Therapy for Atrial Fibrillation[5]	-	-	95%	95%
Antithrombotic Therapy Timing[5]	-	-	99%	98%
Assessed for Rehabilitation[5]	-	-	98%	97%
Discharged on Antithrombotic Therapy[5]	-	-	99%	99%
Discharged on Statin Medication[5]	-	-	96%	94%
Thrombolytic Therapy Timing[5]	-	-	89%	66%
Venous Thromboembolism Prophylaxis[5]	-	-	95%	94%
Written Stroke Educational Materials Given[5]	-	-	89%	88%
Surgical Care Improvement Project				
Appropriate Beta Blocker Usage[5]	-	-	98%	98%
Appropriate VTP Within 24 Hours[5]	-	-	99%	98%
Controlled Postoperative Blood Glucose[5]	-	-	97%	97%
Perioperative Temperature Management[5]	-	-	100%	100%
Prophylactic Antibiotic Selection[5]	-	-	99%	99%
Prophylactic Antibiotic Selection (Outpatient)	-	-	98%	98%
Prophylactic Antibiotic Stopped[5]	-	-	98%	98%
Prophylactic Antibiotic Timing[5]	-	-	99%	99%
Prophylactic Antibiotic Timing (Outpatient)	-	-	98%	98%
Urinary Catheter Removal[5]	-	-	98%	97%
Survey of Patients' Hospital Experiences				
Area Around Room 'Always' Quiet at Night[5]	-	-	60%	61%
Doctors 'Always' Communicated Well[5]	-	-	83%	82%
Home Recovery Information Given[5]	-	-	90%	85%
Hospital Given 9 or 10 on 10 Point Scale[5]	-	-	74%	71%
Meds 'Always' Explained Before Given[5]	-	-	68%	64%
Nurses 'Always' Communicated Well[5]	-	-	79%	79%
Pain 'Always' Well Controlled[5]	-	-	73%	71%
Room and Bathroom 'Always' Clean[5]	-	-	74%	73%
Timely Help 'Always' Received[5]	-	-	69%	68%
Would Definitely Recommend Hospital[5]	-	-	76%	71%
Use of Medical Imaging				
Cardiac Imaging Stress Test before Surgery	-	-	4.9%	5.3%
Combination Abdominal CT Scan	-	-	4.9%	10.5%
Combination Brain/Sinus CT Scan	-	-	3%	2.7%
Combination Chest CT Scan	-	-	0.8%	2.7%
Follow-up Mammogram/Ultrasound	-	-	8.5%	8.8%
Lumbar Spine MRI for Low Back Pain	-	-	43.8%	37.2%

Moab Regional Hospital

450 West Williams Way Phone: 435-719-3501
Moab, UT 84532
Type: Critical Access Hospitals Emergency Services: Yes
Ownership: Voluntary non-profit - Private

Measure	Cases	This Hosp.	State Avg.	U.S. Avg.
Blood Clot Prevention and Treatment				
Anticoagulation Overlap Therapy[5]	-	-	95%	93%
ICU Venous Thromboembolism Prophylaxis[5]	-	-	93%	92%
Incidence of Potentially Preventable VTE[5]	-	-	5%	10%
UFH with Dosages/Platelet Monitoring[5]	-	-	95%	97%
Venous Thromboembolism Prophylaxis[5]	-	-	86%	85%
Warfarin Therapy Discharge Instructions[5]	-	-	73%	75%
Chest Pain/Possible Heart Attack Care				
Aspirin Given Within 24 Hours of Arrival[1,3]	-	-	97%	96%
Fibrinolytic Meds Within 30 Min. of Arrival[1,3]	-	-	52%	58%
Average Time to ECG (minutes)[1,3]	-	-	7	7
Average Time to Transfer (minutes)[3,7]	-	-	36	60
Children's Asthma Care				
Received Home Management Plan of Care	-	-	-	88%
Received Reliever Medication	-	-	-	100%
Received Systemic Corticosteroids	-	-	-	100%
Emergency Department				
Admittance Decision Time (minutes)[5]	-	-	66	98
Head CT Results Within 45 Min. of Arrival[5]	-	-	60%	57%
Patients Who Left ER Before Being Seen[5]	-	-	1%	2%
Time from ER Arrival to Admit. (minutes)[5]	-	-	217	274
Time from ER Arrival to Discharge (minutes)[5]	-	-	123	134
Time in ER Before Being Evaluated (minutes)[5]	-	-	17	26
Time to Pain Meds for Fractures (minutes)[5]	-	-	43	57
Heart Attack Care				
Aspirin Given at Discharge[5]	-	-	99%	99%
Fibrinolytic Meds Within 30 Min. of Arrival[5]	-	-	100%	54%
PCI Within 90 Minutes of Arrival[5]	-	-	98%	96%
Statin Prescribed at Discharge[5]	-	-	100%	98%
Heart Failure Care				
ACE Inhibitor or ARB for LVSD[2,3]	-	-	98%	97%
Discharge Instructions Given[1,2]	-	-	96%	94%
Evaluation of LVS Function[1,2]	-	-	98%	99%
Medicare Spending				
Medicare Spending per Patient (ratio)	-	-	0.98	0.98
Pneumonia Care				
Appropriate Initial Antibiotic Given[1,2]	-	-	96%	95%
Blood Culture Timing[1,2]	-	-	99%	98%
Pregnancy and Delivery Care				
Newborn Deliveries Scheduled Early[5]	-	-	6%	6%
Preventive Care				
Immunization for Influenza[5]	-	-	92%	90%
Immunization for Pneumonia[5]	-	-	91%	92%
Stroke Care				
Anticoagulation Therapy for Atrial Fibrillation[5]	-	-	95%	95%
Antithrombotic Therapy Timing[5]	-	-	99%	98%
Assessed for Rehabilitation[5]	-	-	98%	97%
Discharged on Antithrombotic Therapy[5]	-	-	99%	99%
Discharged on Statin Medication[5]	-	-	96%	94%
Thrombolytic Therapy Timing[5]	-	-	89%	66%
Venous Thromboembolism Prophylaxis[5]	-	-	95%	94%
Written Stroke Educational Materials Given[5]	-	-	89%	88%
Surgical Care Improvement Project				
Appropriate Beta Blocker Usage[1,3]	-	-	98%	98%
Appropriate VTP Within 24 Hours[3]	19	84%	99%	98%
Controlled Postoperative Blood Glucose[3,7]	-	-	97%	97%
Perioperative Temperature Management[3]	19	84%	100%	100%
Prophylactic Antibiotic Selection[1,3]	-	-	99%	99%
Prophylactic Antibiotic Selection (Outpatient)[5]	-	-	98%	98%
Prophylactic Antibiotic Stopped[1,3]	-	-	98%	98%
Prophylactic Antibiotic Timing[1,3]	-	-	99%	99%
Prophylactic Antibiotic Timing (Outpatient)[5]	-	-	98%	98%
Urinary Catheter Removal[1,3]	-	-	98%	97%
Survey of Patients' Hospital Experiences				
Area Around Room 'Always' Quiet at Night[5]	-	-	60%	61%
Doctors 'Always' Communicated Well[5]	-	-	83%	82%
Home Recovery Information Given[5]	-	-	90%	85%
Hospital Given 9 or 10 on 10 Point Scale[5]	-	-	74%	71%
Meds 'Always' Explained Before Given[5]	-	-	68%	64%
Nurses 'Always' Communicated Well[5]	-	-	79%	79%
Pain 'Always' Well Controlled[5]	-	-	73%	71%
Room and Bathroom 'Always' Clean[5]	-	-	74%	73%
Timely Help 'Always' Received[5]	-	-	69%	68%
Would Definitely Recommend Hospital[5]	-	-	76%	71%
Use of Medical Imaging				
Cardiac Imaging Stress Test before Surgery[7]	-	-	4.9%	5.3%
Combination Abdominal CT Scan	93	1.1%	4.9%	10.5%
Combination Brain/Sinus CT Scan[1]	-	-	3%	2.7%
Combination Chest CT Scan[1]	-	-	0.8%	2.7%
Follow-up Mammogram/Ultrasound	106	8.5%	8.5%	8.8%
Lumbar Spine MRI for Low Back Pain[1]	-	-	43.8%	37.2%

San Juan Hospital

380 West 100 North Phone: 435-587-2116
Monticello, UT 84535 Fax: 435-587-2061
Type: Critical Access Hospitals Emergency Services: Yes
Ownership: Govt - Hospital Dist/Auth Beds: 25

Key Personnel:
Operating Room. . . . . Julie Bronson
CEO/President. . . . . Phillip Lowe
Chief of Medical Staff . . . . Paul Reau
Emergency Room . . . . Laurie Schafer
Quality Assurance . . . . Laurie Schafer
Infection Control. . . . . Debbie Slade
Anesthesiology. . . . . Brad Young

Measure	Cases	This Hosp.	State Avg.	U.S. Avg.
Blood Clot Prevention and Treatment				
Anticoagulation Overlap Therapy[5]	-	-	95%	93%
ICU Venous Thromboembolism Prophylaxis[5]	-	-	93%	92%
Incidence of Potentially Preventable VTE[5]	-	-	5%	10%
UFH with Dosages/Platelet Monitoring[5]	-	-	95%	97%
Venous Thromboembolism Prophylaxis[5]	-	-	86%	85%
Warfarin Therapy Discharge Instructions[5]	-	-	73%	75%
Chest Pain/Possible Heart Attack Care				
Aspirin Given Within 24 Hours of Arrival[1,3]	-	-	97%	96%
Fibrinolytic Meds Within 30 Min. of Arrival[3,7]	-	-	52%	58%
Average Time to ECG (minutes)[1,3]	-	-	7	7
Average Time to Transfer (minutes)[3,7]	-	-	36	60
Children's Asthma Care				
Received Home Management Plan of Care	-	-	-	88%
Received Reliever Medication	-	-	-	100%
Received Systemic Corticosteroids	-	-	-	100%
Emergency Department				
Admittance Decision Time (minutes)[5]	-	-	66	98
Head CT Results Within 45 Min. of Arrival[5]	-	-	60%	57%
Patients Who Left ER Before Being Seen	1,822	0%	1%	2%
Time from ER Arrival to Admit. (minutes)[5]	-	-	217	274
Time from ER Arrival to Discharge (minutes)[5]	-	-	123	134
Time in ER Before Being Evaluated (minutes)[5]	-	-	17	26
Time to Pain Meds for Fractures (minutes)[5]	-	-	43	57
Heart Attack Care				
Aspirin Given at Discharge[5]	-	-	99%	99%
Fibrinolytic Meds Within 30 Min. of Arrival[5]	-	-	100%	54%
PCI Within 90 Minutes of Arrival[5]	-	-	98%	96%

NOTE: Hospital profiles are in alphabetical order by state, then city, then hospital within the city; Rankings exclude hospitals with less than 25 cases except for patient surveys which excludes hospitals with less than 100 cases; (a) 100-299 cases; (1) The number of cases/patients is too few to report; (2) Data submitted were based on a sample of cases/patients; (3) Results are based on a shorter time period than required; (4) Data suppressed by CMS for one or more quarters; (5) Results are not available for this reporting period; (6) Fewer than 100 patients completed the HCAHPS survey; (7) No cases met the criteria for this measure; (8) The lower limit of the confidence interval cannot be calculated if the number of observed infections equals zero; (9) No data are available from the state/territory for this reporting period; (10) The scores shown reflect fewer than 50 completed surveys; (11) There were discrepancies in the data collection process; (12) This measure does not apply to this hospital for this reporting period; (13) Results cannot be calculated for this reporting period; (14) The results for this state are combined with nearby states to protect confidentiality; Please refer to the User's Guide for a full explanation of data.

Measure	Cases	This Hosp.	State Avg.	U.S. Avg.
Statin Prescribed at Discharge[5]	-	-	100%	98%
Heart Failure Care				
ACE Inhibitor or ARB for LVSD[1,2]	-	-	98%	97%
Discharge Instructions Given[1,2]	-	-	96%	94%
Evaluation of LVS Function[2,3]	11	18%	98%	99%
Medicare Spending				
Medicare Spending per Patient (ratio)	-	-	0.98	0.98
Pneumonia Care				
Appropriate Initial Antibiotic Given[2,3]	16	75%	96%	95%
Blood Culture Timing[1,2]	-	-	99%	98%
Pregnancy and Delivery Care				
Newborn Deliveries Scheduled Early[5]	-	-	6%	6%
Preventive Care				
Immunization for Influenza[5]	-	-	92%	90%
Immunization for Pneumonia[5]	-	-	91%	92%
Stroke Care				
Anticoagulation Therapy for Atrial Fibrillation[5]	-	-	95%	95%
Antithrombotic Therapy Timing[5]	-	-	99%	98%
Assessed for Rehabilitation[5]	-	-	98%	97%
Discharged on Antithrombotic Therapy[5]	-	-	99%	99%
Discharged on Statin Medication[5]	-	-	96%	94%
Thrombolytic Therapy Timing[5]	-	-	89%	66%
Venous Thromboembolism Prophylaxis[5]	-	-	95%	94%
Written Stroke Educational Materials Given[5]	-	-	89%	88%
Surgical Care Improvement Project				
Appropriate Beta Blocker Usage[5]	-	-	98%	98%
Appropriate VTP Within 24 Hours[5]	-	-	99%	98%
Controlled Postoperative Blood Glucose[5]	-	-	97%	97%
Perioperative Temperature Management[5]	-	-	100%	100%
Prophylactic Antibiotic Selection[5]	-	-	99%	99%
Prophylactic Antibiotic Selection (Outpatient)[5]	-	-	98%	98%
Prophylactic Antibiotic Stopped[5]	-	-	98%	98%
Prophylactic Antibiotic Timing[5]	-	-	99%	99%
Prophylactic Antibiotic Timing (Outpatient)[5]	-	-	98%	98%
Urinary Catheter Removal[5]	-	-	98%	97%
Survey of Patients' Hospital Experiences				
Area Around Room 'Always' Quiet at Night[5]	-	-	60%	61%
Doctors 'Always' Communicated Well[5]	-	-	83%	82%
Home Recovery Information Given[5]	-	-	90%	85%
Hospital Given 9 or 10 on 10 Point Scale[5]	-	-	74%	71%
Meds 'Always' Explained Before Given[5]	-	-	68%	64%
Nurses 'Always' Communicated Well[5]	-	-	79%	79%
Pain 'Always' Well Controlled[5]	-	-	73%	71%
Room and Bathroom 'Always' Clean[5]	-	-	74%	73%
Timely Help 'Always' Received[5]	-	-	69%	68%
Would Definitely Recommend Hospital[5]	-	-	76%	71%
Use of Medical Imaging				
Cardiac Imaging Stress Test before Surgery[7]	-	-	4.9%	5.3%
Combination Abdominal CT Scan[1]	-	-	4.9%	10.5%
Combination Brain/Sinus CT Scan	30	0.0%	3%	2.7%
Combination Chest CT Scan[1]	-	-	0.8%	2.7%
Follow-up Mammogram/Ultrasound	45	4.4%	8.5%	8.8%
Lumbar Spine MRI for Low Back Pain[1]	-	-	43.8%	37.2%

Sanpete Valley Hospital

1100 South Medical Drive — Phone: 435-762-2441
Mount Pleasant, UT 84647 — Fax: 435-462-2609
URL: www.ihc.com
Type: Critical Access Hospitals — Emergency Services: Yes
Ownership: Voluntary non-profit - Private — Beds: 20

Key Personnel:
Chief of Medical Staff. . . . . Robert Amstrong, MD
Radiology. . . . . Carl M Black
Operating Room. . . . . Michael S Frischknecht, RN
Quality Assurance . . . . Ned Hill
Infection Control. . . . . Suana Olsen, RN
CEO/President. . . . . Charles W. Sorenson, MD

Measure	Cases	This Hosp.	State Avg.	U.S. Avg.
Blood Clot Prevention and Treatment				
Anticoagulation Overlap Therapy[1,2]	-	-	95%	93%
ICU Venous Thromboembolism Prophylaxis[2,7]	-	-	93%	92%
Incidence of Potentially Preventable VTE[2,7]	-	-	5%	10%
UFH with Dosages/Platelet Monitoring[2,7]	-	-	95%	97%
Venous Thromboembolism Prophylaxis[2]	82	68%	86%	85%
Warfarin Therapy Discharge Instructions[1,2]	-	-	73%	75%
Chest Pain/Possible Heart Attack Care				
Aspirin Given Within 24 Hours of Arrival	19	89%	97%	96%
Fibrinolytic Meds Within 30 Min. of Arrival[1,3]	-	-	52%	58%
Average Time to ECG (minutes)	20	4	7	7
Average Time to Transfer (minutes)[1,3]	-	-	36	60
Children's Asthma Care				
Received Home Management Plan of Care	-	-	-	88%
Received Reliever Medication	-	-	-	100%
Received Systemic Corticosteroids	-	-	-	100%
Emergency Department				
Admittance Decision Time (minutes)	133	32	66	98
Head CT Results Within 45 Min. of Arrival[1]	-	-	60%	57%
Patients Who Left ER Before Being Seen[5]	-	-	1%	2%
Time from ER Arrival to Admit. (minutes)	184	201	217	274
Time from ER Arrival to Discharge (minutes)	357	94	123	134
Time in ER Before Being Evaluated (minutes)	399	13	17	26
Time to Pain Meds for Fractures (minutes)	34	43	43	57
Heart Attack Care				
Aspirin Given at Discharge[5]	-	-	99%	99%
Fibrinolytic Meds Within 30 Min. of Arrival[5]	-	-	100%	54%
PCI Within 90 Minutes of Arrival[5]	-	-	98%	96%
Statin Prescribed at Discharge[5]	-	-	100%	98%
Heart Failure Care				
ACE Inhibitor or ARB for LVSD[1,3]	-	-	98%	97%
Discharge Instructions Given[1,3]	-	-	96%	94%
Evaluation of LVS Function[1,3]	-	-	98%	99%
Medicare Spending				
Medicare Spending per Patient (ratio)	-	-	0.98	0.98
Pneumonia Care				
Appropriate Initial Antibiotic Given	18	100%	96%	95%
Blood Culture Timing	18	94%	99%	98%
Pregnancy and Delivery Care				
Newborn Deliveries Scheduled Early[1,3]	-	-	6%	6%
Preventive Care				
Immunization for Influenza	196	87%	92%	90%
Immunization for Pneumonia	168	86%	91%	92%
Stroke Care				
Anticoagulation Therapy for Atrial Fibrillation[3,7]	-	-	95%	95%
Antithrombotic Therapy Timing[1,3]	-	-	99%	98%
Assessed for Rehabilitation[1,3]	-	-	98%	97%
Discharged on Antithrombotic Therapy[1,3]	-	-	99%	99%
Discharged on Statin Medication[1,3]	-	-	96%	94%
Thrombolytic Therapy Timing[1,3]	-	-	89%	66%
Venous Thromboembolism Prophylaxis[1,3]	-	-	95%	94%
Written Stroke Educational Materials Given[3,7]	-	-	89%	88%
Surgical Care Improvement Project				
Appropriate Beta Blocker Usage[7]	-	-	98%	98%
Appropriate VTP Within 24 Hours[1]	-	-	99%	98%
Controlled Postoperative Blood Glucose[7]	-	-	97%	97%
Perioperative Temperature Management[1]	-	-	100%	100%
Prophylactic Antibiotic Selection[1]	-	-	99%	99%
Prophylactic Antibiotic Selection (Outpatient)[1,3]	-	-	98%	98%
Prophylactic Antibiotic Stopped[1]	-	-	98%	98%
Prophylactic Antibiotic Timing[1]	-	-	99%	99%
Prophylactic Antibiotic Timing (Outpatient)[1,3]	-	-	98%	98%
Urinary Catheter Removal[1]	-	-	98%	97%
Survey of Patients' Hospital Experiences				
Area Around Room 'Always' Quiet at Night	(a)	61%	60%	61%
Doctors 'Always' Communicated Well	(a)	88%	83%	82%
Home Recovery Information Given	(a)	93%	90%	85%
Hospital Given 9 or 10 on 10 Point Scale	(a)	76%	74%	71%
Meds 'Always' Explained Before Given	(a)	78%	68%	64%
Nurses 'Always' Communicated Well	(a)	84%	79%	79%
Pain 'Always' Well Controlled	(a)	78%	73%	71%
Room and Bathroom 'Always' Clean	(a)	73%	74%	73%
Timely Help 'Always' Received	(a)	86%	69%	68%
Would Definitely Recommend Hospital	(a)	74%	76%	71%
Use of Medical Imaging				
Cardiac Imaging Stress Test before Surgery[7]	-	-	4.9%	5.3%
Combination Abdominal CT Scan	97	5.2%	4.9%	10.5%
Combination Brain/Sinus CT Scan[1]	-	-	3%	2.7%
Combination Chest CT Scan[1]	-	-	0.8%	2.7%
Follow-up Mammogram/Ultrasound	165	6.1%	8.5%	8.8%
Lumbar Spine MRI for Low Back Pain[1]	-	-	43.8%	37.2%

Intermountain Medical Center

5121 South Cottonwood Street — Phone: 801-507-7000
Murray, UT 84107
URL: www.intermountainhealthcare.org
Type: Acute Care Hospitals — Emergency Services: Yes
Ownership: Voluntary non-profit - Private

Key Personnel:
CEO/President. . . . . Charles W. Sorenson, MD

Measure	Cases	This Hosp.	State Avg.	U.S. Avg.
Blood Clot Prevention and Treatment				
Anticoagulation Overlap Therapy[2]	257	96%	95%	93%
ICU Venous Thromboembolism Prophylaxis[2]	129	95%	93%	92%
Incidence of Potentially Preventable VTE[2]	48	0%	5%	10%
UFH with Dosages/Platelet Monitoring[2]	144	91%	95%	97%
Venous Thromboembolism Prophylaxis[2]	238	88%	86%	85%
Warfarin Therapy Discharge Instructions[2]	209	60%	73%	75%
Chest Pain/Possible Heart Attack Care				
Aspirin Given Within 24 Hours of Arrival[1,3]	-	-	97%	96%
Fibrinolytic Meds Within 30 Min. of Arrival[5]	-	-	52%	58%
Average Time to ECG (minutes)[1,3]	-	-	7	7
Average Time to Transfer (minutes)[5]	-	-	36	60
Children's Asthma Care				
Received Home Management Plan of Care	-	-	-	88%
Received Reliever Medication	-	-	-	100%
Received Systemic Corticosteroids	-	-	-	100%
Emergency Department				
Admittance Decision Time (minutes)[2]	484	83	66	98
Head CT Results Within 45 Min. of Arrival[7]	-	-	60%	57%
Patients Who Left ER Before Being Seen	86,341	2%	1%	2%
Time from ER Arrival to Admit. (minutes)[2]	491	273	217	274
Time from ER Arrival to Discharge (minutes)	416	206	123	134
Time in ER Before Being Evaluated (minutes)	443	28	17	26
Time to Pain Meds for Fractures (minutes)	200	58	43	57
Heart Attack Care				
Aspirin Given at Discharge[2]	564	100%	99%	99%
Fibrinolytic Meds Within 30 Min. of Arrival[1,2]	-	-	100%	54%
PCI Within 90 Minutes of Arrival[2]	100	100%	98%	96%
Statin Prescribed at Discharge[2]	555	100%	100%	98%
Heart Failure Care				
ACE Inhibitor or ARB for LVSD	209	99%	98%	97%
Discharge Instructions Given	499	98%	96%	94%
Evaluation of LVS Function	572	100%	98%	99%
Medicare Spending				
Medicare Spending per Patient (ratio)	-	0.97	0.98	0.98
Pneumonia Care				
Appropriate Initial Antibiotic Given[2]	83	100%	96%	95%
Blood Culture Timing[2]	123	100%	99%	98%
Pregnancy and Delivery Care				
Newborn Deliveries Scheduled Early[2]	87	6%	6%	6%
Preventive Care				
Immunization for Influenza[2]	521	92%	92%	90%
Immunization for Pneumonia[2]	542	87%	91%	92%
Stroke Care				
Anticoagulation Therapy for Atrial Fibrillation	57	98%	95%	95%
Antithrombotic Therapy Timing	232	100%	99%	98%
Assessed for Rehabilitation	430	100%	98%	97%
Discharged on Antithrombotic Therapy	346	100%	99%	99%
Discharged on Statin Medication	218	99%	96%	94%
Thrombolytic Therapy Timing	50	98%	89%	66%
Venous Thromboembolism Prophylaxis	395	97%	95%	94%
Written Stroke Educational Materials Given	288	92%	89%	88%
Surgical Care Improvement Project				
Appropriate Beta Blocker Usage[2]	195	100%	98%	98%
Appropriate VTP Within 24 Hours[2]	426	99%	99%	98%
Controlled Postoperative Blood Glucose[2]	201	96%	97%	97%
Perioperative Temperature Management[2]	590	100%	100%	100%
Prophylactic Antibiotic Selection[2]	505	99%	99%	99%
Prophylactic Antibiotic Selection (Outpatient)	729	98%	98%	98%
Prophylactic Antibiotic Stopped[2]	487	98%	98%	98%

NOTE: Hospital profiles are in alphabetical order by state, then city, then hospital within the city; Rankings exclude hospitals with less than 25 cases except for patient surveys which excludes hospitals with less than 100 cases; (a) 100-299 cases; (1) The number of cases/patients is too few to report; (2) Data submitted were based on a sample of cases/patients; (3) Results are based on a shorter time period than required; (4) Data suppressed by CMS for one or more quarters; (5) Results are not available for this reporting period; (6) Fewer than 100 patients completed the HCAHPS survey; (7) No cases met the criteria for this measure; (8) The lower limit of the confidence interval cannot be calculated if the number of observed infections equals zero; (9) No data are available from the state/territory for this reporting period; (10) The scores shown reflect fewer than 50 completed surveys; (11) There were discrepancies in the data collection process; (12) This measure does not apply to this hospital for this reporting period; (13) Results cannot be calculated for this reporting period; (14) The results for this state are combined with nearby states to protect confidentiality; Please refer to the User's Guide for a full explanation of data.

Measure	Cases	This Hosp.	State Avg.	U.S. Avg.
Prophylactic Antibiotic Timing[2]	504	99%	99%	99%
Prophylactic Antibiotic Timing (Outpatient)	729	99%	98%	98%
Urinary Catheter Removal[2]	366	97%	98%	97%
Survey of Patients' Hospital Experiences				
Area Around Room 'Always' Quiet at Night	300+	56%	60%	61%
Doctors 'Always' Communicated Well	300+	81%	83%	82%
Home Recovery Information Given	300+	90%	90%	85%
Hospital Given 9 or 10 on 10 Point Scale	300+	74%	74%	71%
Meds 'Always' Explained Before Given	300+	68%	68%	64%
Nurses 'Always' Communicated Well	300+	77%	79%	79%
Pain 'Always' Well Controlled	300+	73%	73%	71%
Room and Bathroom 'Always' Clean	300+	72%	74%	73%
Timely Help 'Always' Received	300+	64%	69%	68%
Would Definitely Recommend Hospital	300+	80%	76%	71%
Use of Medical Imaging				
Cardiac Imaging Stress Test before Surgery	845	3.3%	4.9%	5.3%
Combination Abdominal CT Scan	1,023	3.8%	4.9%	10.5%
Combination Brain/Sinus CT Scan	820	2.7%	3%	2.7%
Combination Chest CT Scan	540	0.7%	0.8%	2.7%
Follow-up Mammogram/Ultrasound	2,125	8.0%	8.5%	8.8%
Lumbar Spine MRI for Low Back Pain	109	45.0%	43.8%	37.2%

Landmark Hospital of Salt Lake City

4252 S Birkhill Blvd
Murray, UT 84107
Phone: 801-268-5400
Type: Acute Care Hospitals
Emergency Services: No
Ownership: Proprietary

Measure	Cases	This Hosp.	State Avg.	U.S. Avg.
Blood Clot Prevention and Treatment				
Anticoagulation Overlap Therapy[5]	-	-	95%	93%
ICU Venous Thromboembolism Prophylaxis[5]	-	-	93%	92%
Incidence of Potentially Preventable VTE[5]	-	-	5%	10%
UFH with Dosages/Platelet Monitoring[5]	-	-	95%	97%
Venous Thromboembolism Prophylaxis[5]	-	-	86%	85%
Warfarin Therapy Discharge Instructions[5]	-	-	73%	75%
Chest Pain/Possible Heart Attack Care				
Aspirin Given Within 24 Hours of Arrival[5]	-	-	97%	96%
Fibrinolytic Meds Within 30 Min. of Arrival[5]	-	-	52%	58%
Average Time to ECG (minutes)[5]	-	-	7	7
Average Time to Transfer (minutes)[5]	-	-	36	60
Children's Asthma Care				
Received Home Management Plan of Care	-	-	-	88%
Received Reliever Medication	-	-	-	100%
Received Systemic Corticosteroids	-	-	-	100%
Emergency Department				
Admittance Decision Time (minutes)[5]	-	-	66	98
Head CT Results Within 45 Min. of Arrival[5]	-	-	60%	57%
Patients Who Left ER Before Being Seen[5]	-	-	1%	2%
Time from ER Arrival to Admit. (minutes)[5]	-	-	217	274
Time from ER Arrival to Discharge (minutes)[5]	-	-	123	134
Time in ER Before Being Evaluated (minutes)[5]	-	-	17	26
Time to Pain Meds for Fractures (minutes)[5]	-	-	43	57
Heart Attack Care				
Aspirin Given at Discharge[5]	-	-	99%	99%
Fibrinolytic Meds Within 30 Min. of Arrival[5]	-	-	100%	54%
PCI Within 90 Minutes of Arrival[5]	-	-	98%	96%
Statin Prescribed at Discharge[5]	-	-	100%	98%
Heart Failure Care				
ACE Inhibitor or ARB for LVSD[5]	-	-	98%	97%
Discharge Instructions Given[5]	-	-	96%	94%
Evaluation of LVS Function[5]	-	-	98%	99%
Medicare Spending				
Medicare Spending per Patient (ratio)	-	-	0.98	0.98
Pneumonia Care				
Appropriate Initial Antibiotic Given[5]	-	-	96%	95%
Blood Culture Timing[5]	-	-	99%	98%
Pregnancy and Delivery Care				
Newborn Deliveries Scheduled Early[5]	-	-	6%	6%
Preventive Care				
Immunization for Influenza[5]	-	-	92%	90%
Immunization for Pneumonia[5]	-	-	91%	92%
Stroke Care				
Anticoagulation Therapy for Atrial Fibrillation[5]	-	-	95%	95%
Antithrombotic Therapy Timing[5]	-	-	99%	98%
Assessed for Rehabilitation[5]	-	-	98%	97%
Discharged on Antithrombotic Therapy[5]	-	-	99%	99%
Discharged on Statin Medication[5]	-	-	96%	94%
Thrombolytic Therapy Timing[5]	-	-	89%	66%
Venous Thromboembolism Prophylaxis[5]	-	-	95%	94%
Written Stroke Educational Materials Given[5]	-	-	89%	88%
Surgical Care Improvement Project				
Appropriate Beta Blocker Usage[5]	-	-	98%	98%
Appropriate VTP Within 24 Hours[5]	-	-	99%	98%
Controlled Postoperative Blood Glucose[5]	-	-	97%	97%
Perioperative Temperature Management[5]	-	-	100%	100%
Prophylactic Antibiotic Selection[5]	-	-	99%	99%
Prophylactic Antibiotic Selection (Outpatient)[5]	-	-	98%	98%
Prophylactic Antibiotic Stopped[5]	-	-	98%	98%
Prophylactic Antibiotic Timing[5]	-	-	99%	99%
Prophylactic Antibiotic Timing (Outpatient)[5]	-	-	98%	98%
Urinary Catheter Removal[5]	-	-	98%	97%
Survey of Patients' Hospital Experiences				
Area Around Room 'Always' Quiet at Night[5]	-	-	60%	61%
Doctors 'Always' Communicated Well[5]	-	-	83%	82%
Home Recovery Information Given[5]	-	-	90%	85%
Hospital Given 9 or 10 on 10 Point Scale[5]	-	-	74%	71%
Meds 'Always' Explained Before Given[5]	-	-	68%	64%
Nurses 'Always' Communicated Well[5]	-	-	79%	79%
Pain 'Always' Well Controlled[5]	-	-	73%	71%
Room and Bathroom 'Always' Clean[5]	-	-	74%	73%
Timely Help 'Always' Received[5]	-	-	69%	68%
Would Definitely Recommend Hospital[5]	-	-	76%	71%
Use of Medical Imaging				
Cardiac Imaging Stress Test before Surgery[5]	-	-	4.9%	5.3%
Combination Abdominal CT Scan[5]	-	-	4.9%	10.5%
Combination Brain/Sinus CT Scan[5]	-	-	3%	2.7%
Combination Chest CT Scan[5]	-	-	0.8%	2.7%
Follow-up Mammogram/Ultrasound[5]	-	-	8.5%	8.8%
Lumbar Spine MRI for Low Back Pain[5]	-	-	43.8%	37.2%

The Orthopedic Specialty Hospital

5848 South 300 East
Murray, UT 84107
Phone: 801-314-4100
URL: www.intermountainhealthcare.org
Type: Acute Care Hospitals
Emergency Services: No
Ownership: Voluntary non-profit - Private
Key Personnel:
CEO/President. . . . . Bryan Johnson

Measure	Cases	This Hosp.	State Avg.	U.S. Avg.
Blood Clot Prevention and Treatment				
Anticoagulation Overlap Therapy[2,7]	-	-	95%	93%
ICU Venous Thromboembolism Prophylaxis[2,7]	-	-	93%	92%
Incidence of Potentially Preventable VTE[1,2]	-	-	5%	10%
UFH with Dosages/Platelet Monitoring[2,7]	-	-	95%	97%
Venous Thromboembolism Prophylaxis[2]	46	100%	86%	85%
Warfarin Therapy Discharge Instructions[2,7]	-	-	73%	75%
Chest Pain/Possible Heart Attack Care				
Aspirin Given Within 24 Hours of Arrival[5]	-	-	97%	96%
Fibrinolytic Meds Within 30 Min. of Arrival[5]	-	-	52%	58%
Average Time to ECG (minutes)[5]	-	-	7	7
Average Time to Transfer (minutes)[5]	-	-	36	60
Children's Asthma Care				
Received Home Management Plan of Care	-	-	-	88%
Received Reliever Medication	-	-	-	100%
Received Systemic Corticosteroids	-	-	-	100%
Emergency Department				
Admittance Decision Time (minutes)[2,7]	-	-	66	98
Head CT Results Within 45 Min. of Arrival[5]	-	-	60%	57%
Patients Who Left ER Before Being Seen[5]	-	-	1%	2%
Time from ER Arrival to Admit. (minutes)[2,7]	-	-	217	274
Time from ER Arrival to Discharge (minutes)[5]	-	-	123	134
Time in ER Before Being Evaluated (minutes)[5]	-	-	17	26
Time to Pain Meds for Fractures (minutes)[5]	-	-	43	57
Heart Attack Care				
Aspirin Given at Discharge[5]	-	-	99%	99%
Fibrinolytic Meds Within 30 Min. of Arrival[5]	-	-	100%	54%
PCI Within 90 Minutes of Arrival[5]	-	-	98%	96%
Statin Prescribed at Discharge[5]	-	-	100%	98%
Heart Failure Care				
ACE Inhibitor or ARB for LVSD[5]	-	-	98%	97%
Discharge Instructions Given[5]	-	-	96%	94%
Evaluation of LVS Function[5]	-	-	98%	99%
Medicare Spending				
Medicare Spending per Patient (ratio)	-	0.96	0.98	0.98
Pneumonia Care				
Appropriate Initial Antibiotic Given[5]	-	-	96%	95%
Blood Culture Timing[5]	-	-	99%	98%
Pregnancy and Delivery Care				
Newborn Deliveries Scheduled Early[7]	-	-	6%	6%
Preventive Care				
Immunization for Influenza[2]	319	98%	92%	90%
Immunization for Pneumonia[2]	371	95%	91%	92%
Stroke Care				
Anticoagulation Therapy for Atrial Fibrillation[5]	-	-	95%	95%
Antithrombotic Therapy Timing[5]	-	-	99%	98%
Assessed for Rehabilitation[5]	-	-	98%	97%
Discharged on Antithrombotic Therapy[5]	-	-	99%	99%
Discharged on Statin Medication[5]	-	-	96%	94%
Thrombolytic Therapy Timing[5]	-	-	89%	66%
Venous Thromboembolism Prophylaxis[5]	-	-	95%	94%
Written Stroke Educational Materials Given[5]	-	-	89%	88%
Surgical Care Improvement Project				
Appropriate Beta Blocker Usage[2]	81	100%	98%	98%
Appropriate VTP Within 24 Hours[2]	409	100%	99%	98%
Controlled Postoperative Blood Glucose[2,7]	-	-	97%	97%
Perioperative Temperature Management[2]	486	100%	100%	100%
Prophylactic Antibiotic Selection[2]	355	100%	99%	99%
Prophylactic Antibiotic Selection (Outpatient)	436	100%	98%	98%
Prophylactic Antibiotic Stopped[2]	351	99%	98%	98%
Prophylactic Antibiotic Timing[2]	355	99%	99%	99%
Prophylactic Antibiotic Timing (Outpatient)	436	99%	98%	98%
Urinary Catheter Removal[2]	230	100%	98%	97%
Survey of Patients' Hospital Experiences				
Area Around Room 'Always' Quiet at Night	300+	69%	60%	61%
Doctors 'Always' Communicated Well	300+	87%	83%	82%
Home Recovery Information Given	300+	91%	90%	85%
Hospital Given 9 or 10 on 10 Point Scale	300+	78%	74%	71%
Meds 'Always' Explained Before Given	300+	72%	68%	64%
Nurses 'Always' Communicated Well	300+	79%	79%	79%
Pain 'Always' Well Controlled	300+	73%	73%	71%
Room and Bathroom 'Always' Clean	300+	77%	74%	73%
Timely Help 'Always' Received	300+	71%	69%	68%
Would Definitely Recommend Hospital	300+	84%	76%	71%
Use of Medical Imaging				
Cardiac Imaging Stress Test before Surgery[7]	-	-	4.9%	5.3%
Combination Abdominal CT Scan	157	8.9%	4.9%	10.5%
Combination Brain/Sinus CT Scan[1]	-	-	3%	2.7%
Combination Chest CT Scan	96	0.0%	0.8%	2.7%
Follow-up Mammogram/Ultrasound[7]	-	-	8.5%	8.8%
Lumbar Spine MRI for Low Back Pain	110	47.3%	43.8%	37.2%

Central Valley Medical Center

48 West 1500 North
Nephi, UT 84648
Phone: 435-623-3000
Fax: 435-623-3290
URL: www.cvmed.net
Type: Critical Access Hospitals
Emergency Services: Yes
Ownership: Voluntary non-profit - Private
Beds: 25
Key Personnel:
Anesthesiology. . . . . Craig Hitchcock, CRDA
Radiology. . . . . Shelith Jacobson
Chief of Medical Staff. . . . . Mark Jones, DO
Infection Control. . . . . Yvette Larson
Emergency Room . . . . Tammy Scott, RN
CEO/President. . . . . Mark Stoddard
Quality Assurance . . . . Mindia Turpin, RN
Operating Room. . . . . Patricia Wahlberg, RN

Measure	Cases	This Hosp.	State Avg.	U.S. Avg.
Blood Clot Prevention and Treatment				
Anticoagulation Overlap Therapy[5]	-	-	95%	93%

NOTE: Hospital profiles are in alphabetical order by state, then city, then hospital within the city; Rankings exclude hospitals with less than 25 cases except for patient surveys which excludes hospitals with less than 100 cases; (a) 100-299 cases; (1) The number of cases/patients is too few to report; (2) Data submitted were based on a sample of cases/patients; (3) Results are based on a shorter time period than required; (4) Data suppressed by CMS for one or more quarters; (5) Results are not available for this reporting period; (6) Fewer than 100 patients completed the HCAHPS survey; (7) No cases met the criteria for this measure; (8) The lower limit of the confidence interval cannot be calculated if the number of observed infections equals zero; (9) No data are available from the state/territory for this reporting period; (10) The scores shown reflect fewer than 50 completed surveys; (11) There were discrepancies in the data collection process; (12) This measure does not apply to this hospital for this reporting period; (13) Results cannot be calculated for this reporting period; (14) The results for this state are combined with nearby states to protect confidentiality; Please refer to the User's Guide for a full explanation of data.

Measure	Cases	This Hosp.	State Avg.	U.S. Avg.
ICU Venous Thromboembolism Prophylaxis[5]	-	-	93%	92%
Incidence of Potentially Preventable VTE[5]	-	-	5%	10%
UFH with Dosages/Platelet Monitoring[5]	-	-	95%	97%
Venous Thromboembolism Prophylaxis[5]	-	-	86%	85%
Warfarin Therapy Discharge Instructions[5]	-	-	73%	75%
Chest Pain/Possible Heart Attack Care				
Aspirin Given Within 24 Hours of Arrival[3,7]	-	-	97%	96%
Fibrinolytic Meds Within 30 Min. of Arrival[5]	-	-	52%	58%
Average Time to ECG (minutes)[3,7]	-	-	7	7
Average Time to Transfer (minutes)[5]	-	-	36	60
Children's Asthma Care				
Received Home Management Plan of Care	-	-	-	88%
Received Reliever Medication	-	-	-	100%
Received Systemic Corticosteroids	-	-	-	100%
Emergency Department				
Admittance Decision Time (minutes)[5]	-	-	66	98
Head CT Results Within 45 Min. of Arrival[1,3]	-	-	60%	57%
Patients Who Left ER Before Being Seen	4,167	0%	1%	2%
Time from ER Arrival to Admit. (minutes)[5]	-	-	217	274
Time from ER Arrival to Discharge (minutes)[5]	-	-	123	134
Time in ER Before Being Evaluated (minutes)[5]	-	-	17	26
Time to Pain Meds for Fractures (minutes)[3]	18	46	43	57
Heart Attack Care				
Aspirin Given at Discharge[5]	-	-	99%	99%
Fibrinolytic Meds Within 30 Min. of Arrival[5]	-	-	100%	54%
PCI Within 90 Minutes of Arrival[5]	-	-	98%	96%
Statin Prescribed at Discharge[5]	-	-	100%	98%
Heart Failure Care				
ACE Inhibitor or ARB for LVSD[1,2]	-	-	98%	97%
Discharge Instructions Given[2]	14	71%	96%	94%
Evaluation of LVS Function[2]	15	73%	98%	99%
Medicare Spending				
Medicare Spending per Patient (ratio)	-	-	0.98	0.98
Pneumonia Care				
Appropriate Initial Antibiotic Given	57	84%	96%	95%
Blood Culture Timing	35	91%	99%	98%
Pregnancy and Delivery Care				
Newborn Deliveries Scheduled Early[5]	-	-	6%	6%
Preventive Care				
Immunization for Influenza[5]	-	-	92%	90%
Immunization for Pneumonia[5]	-	-	91%	92%
Stroke Care				
Anticoagulation Therapy for Atrial Fibrillation[5]	-	-	95%	95%
Antithrombotic Therapy Timing[5]	-	-	99%	98%
Assessed for Rehabilitation[5]	-	-	98%	97%
Discharged on Antithrombotic Therapy[5]	-	-	99%	99%
Discharged on Statin Medication[5]	-	-	96%	94%
Thrombolytic Therapy Timing[5]	-	-	89%	66%
Venous Thromboembolism Prophylaxis[5]	-	-	95%	94%
Written Stroke Educational Materials Given[5]	-	-	89%	88%
Surgical Care Improvement Project				
Appropriate Beta Blocker Usage	20	85%	98%	98%
Appropriate VTP Within 24 Hours	67	97%	99%	98%
Controlled Postoperative Blood Glucose[7]	-	-	97%	97%
Perioperative Temperature Management	78	97%	100%	100%
Prophylactic Antibiotic Selection	65	98%	99%	99%
Prophylactic Antibiotic Selection (Outpatient)[5]	-	-	98%	98%
Prophylactic Antibiotic Stopped	64	98%	98%	98%
Prophylactic Antibiotic Timing	65	97%	99%	99%
Prophylactic Antibiotic Timing (Outpatient)[5]	-	-	98%	98%
Urinary Catheter Removal	64	95%	98%	97%
Survey of Patients' Hospital Experiences				
Area Around Room 'Always' Quiet at Night	(a)	67%	60%	61%
Doctors 'Always' Communicated Well	(a)	94%	83%	82%
Home Recovery Information Given	(a)	90%	90%	85%
Hospital Given 9 or 10 on 10 Point Scale	(a)	74%	74%	71%
Meds 'Always' Explained Before Given	(a)	71%	68%	64%
Nurses 'Always' Communicated Well	(a)	81%	79%	79%
Pain 'Always' Well Controlled	(a)	81%	73%	71%
Room and Bathroom 'Always' Clean	(a)	81%	74%	73%
Timely Help 'Always' Received	(a)	74%	69%	68%
Would Definitely Recommend Hospital	(a)	88%	76%	71%
Use of Medical Imaging				
Cardiac Imaging Stress Test before Surgery[7]	-	-	4.9%	5.3%
Combination Abdominal CT Scan	129	1.6%	4.9%	10.5%
Combination Brain/Sinus CT Scan[1]	-	-	3%	2.7%
Combination Chest CT Scan	55	0.0%	0.8%	2.7%
Follow-up Mammogram/Ultrasound	156	24.4%	8.5%	8.8%
Lumbar Spine MRI for Low Back Pain[1]	-	-	43.8%	37.2%

Cache Valley Speciality Hospital

2380 North 400 East Phone: 435-713-9700
North Logan, UT 84341
URL: www.cachevalleyhospital.com
Type: Acute Care Hospitals Emergency Services: Yes
Ownership: Proprietary

Measure	Cases	This Hosp.	State Avg.	U.S. Avg.
Blood Clot Prevention and Treatment				
Anticoagulation Overlap Therapy[1,2]	-	-	95%	93%
ICU Venous Thromboembolism Prophylaxis[2,7]	-	-	93%	92%
Incidence of Potentially Preventable VTE[2,7]	-	-	5%	10%
UFH with Dosages/Platelet Monitoring[2,7]	-	-	95%	97%
Venous Thromboembolism Prophylaxis[2]	66	83%	86%	85%
Warfarin Therapy Discharge Instructions[1,2]	-	-	73%	75%
Chest Pain/Possible Heart Attack Care				
Aspirin Given Within 24 Hours of Arrival[5]	-	-	97%	96%
Fibrinolytic Meds Within 30 Min. of Arrival[5]	-	-	52%	58%
Average Time to ECG (minutes)[5]	-	-	7	7
Average Time to Transfer (minutes)[5]	-	-	36	60
Children's Asthma Care				
Received Home Management Plan of Care	-	-	-	88%
Received Reliever Medication	-	-	-	100%
Received Systemic Corticosteroids	-	-	-	100%
Emergency Department				
Admittance Decision Time (minutes)[2]	103	55	66	98
Head CT Results Within 45 Min. of Arrival[5]	-	-	60%	57%
Patients Who Left ER Before Being Seen	3,695	0%	1%	2%
Time from ER Arrival to Admit. (minutes)[2]	105	192	217	274
Time from ER Arrival to Discharge (minutes)	201	92	123	134
Time in ER Before Being Evaluated (minutes)	252	10	17	26
Time to Pain Meds for Fractures (minutes)	40	24	43	57
Heart Attack Care				
Aspirin Given at Discharge[5]	-	-	99%	99%
Fibrinolytic Meds Within 30 Min. of Arrival[5]	-	-	100%	54%
PCI Within 90 Minutes of Arrival[5]	-	-	98%	96%
Statin Prescribed at Discharge[5]	-	-	100%	98%
Heart Failure Care				
ACE Inhibitor or ARB for LVSD[5]	-	-	98%	97%
Discharge Instructions Given[5]	-	-	96%	94%
Evaluation of LVS Function[5]	-	-	98%	99%
Medicare Spending				
Medicare Spending per Patient (ratio)	-	0.97	0.98	0.98
Pneumonia Care				
Appropriate Initial Antibiotic Given[5]	-	-	96%	95%
Blood Culture Timing[5]	-	-	99%	98%
Pregnancy and Delivery Care				
Newborn Deliveries Scheduled Early[7]	-	-	6%	6%
Preventive Care				
Immunization for Influenza[2]	312	89%	92%	90%
Immunization for Pneumonia[2]	385	77%	91%	92%
Stroke Care				
Anticoagulation Therapy for Atrial Fibrillation[5]	-	-	95%	95%
Antithrombotic Therapy Timing[5]	-	-	99%	98%
Assessed for Rehabilitation[5]	-	-	98%	97%
Discharged on Antithrombotic Therapy[5]	-	-	99%	99%
Discharged on Statin Medication[5]	-	-	96%	94%
Thrombolytic Therapy Timing[5]	-	-	89%	66%
Venous Thromboembolism Prophylaxis[5]	-	-	95%	94%
Written Stroke Educational Materials Given[5]	-	-	89%	88%
Surgical Care Improvement Project				
Appropriate Beta Blocker Usage[2]	27	100%	98%	98%
Appropriate VTP Within 24 Hours[2]	271	98%	99%	98%
Controlled Postoperative Blood Glucose[2,7]	-	-	97%	97%
Perioperative Temperature Management[2]	298	100%	100%	100%
Prophylactic Antibiotic Selection[2]	230	100%	99%	99%
Prophylactic Antibiotic Selection (Outpatient)	67	100%	98%	98%
Prophylactic Antibiotic Stopped[2]	228	97%	98%	98%
Prophylactic Antibiotic Timing[2]	230	99%	99%	99%
Prophylactic Antibiotic Timing (Outpatient)	69	96%	98%	98%
Urinary Catheter Removal[2]	254	99%	98%	97%
Survey of Patients' Hospital Experiences				
Area Around Room 'Always' Quiet at Night	300+	70%	60%	61%
Doctors 'Always' Communicated Well	300+	81%	83%	82%
Home Recovery Information Given	300+	91%	90%	85%
Hospital Given 9 or 10 on 10 Point Scale	300+	71%	74%	71%
Meds 'Always' Explained Before Given	300+	70%	68%	64%
Nurses 'Always' Communicated Well	300+	80%	79%	79%
Pain 'Always' Well Controlled	300+	71%	73%	71%
Room and Bathroom 'Always' Clean	300+	76%	74%	73%
Timely Help 'Always' Received	300+	75%	69%	68%
Would Definitely Recommend Hospital	300+	75%	76%	71%
Use of Medical Imaging				
Cardiac Imaging Stress Test before Surgery[7]	-	-	4.9%	5.3%
Combination Abdominal CT Scan	47	4.3%	4.9%	10.5%
Combination Brain/Sinus CT Scan[1]	-	-	3%	2.7%
Combination Chest CT Scan[1]	-	-	0.8%	2.7%
Follow-up Mammogram/Ultrasound	120	13.3%	8.5%	8.8%
Lumbar Spine MRI for Low Back Pain	73	39.7%	43.8%	37.2%

McKay Dee Hospital

4401 Harrison Boulevard Phone: 801-387-2800
Ogden, UT 84403 Fax: 801-387-7755
URL: www.intermountainhealthcare.org
Type: Acute Care Hospitals Emergency Services: Yes
Ownership: Voluntary non-profit - Private Beds: 317
Key Personnel:
Chief of Medical Staff . . . . Richard Arbogast, MD
Intensive Care Unit. . . . . Bette Becker
Operating Room. . . . . Sandy Eghert
Cardiac Laboratory. . . . . Jim Hoellein
Infection Control . . . . Dot Kley
Quality Assurance . . . . Julie McIntire
CEO/President. . . . . Timothy T Pehrson
Radiology. . . . . Richard Taylor

Measure	Cases	This Hosp.	State Avg.	U.S. Avg.
Blood Clot Prevention and Treatment				
Anticoagulation Overlap Therapy[2]	198	96%	95%	93%
ICU Venous Thromboembolism Prophylaxis[2]	45	100%	93%	92%
Incidence of Potentially Preventable VTE[2]	22	0%	5%	10%
UFH with Dosages/Platelet Monitoring[2]	107	96%	95%	97%
Venous Thromboembolism Prophylaxis[2]	283	90%	86%	85%
Warfarin Therapy Discharge Instructions[2]	159	88%	73%	75%
Chest Pain/Possible Heart Attack Care				
Aspirin Given Within 24 Hours of Arrival[5]	-	-	97%	96%
Fibrinolytic Meds Within 30 Min. of Arrival[5]	-	-	52%	58%
Average Time to ECG (minutes)[5]	-	-	7	7
Average Time to Transfer (minutes)[5]	-	-	36	60
Children's Asthma Care				
Received Home Management Plan of Care	-	-	-	88%
Received Reliever Medication	-	-	-	100%
Received Systemic Corticosteroids	-	-	-	100%
Emergency Department				
Admittance Decision Time (minutes)[2]	480	76	66	98
Head CT Results Within 45 Min. of Arrival[1]	-	-	60%	57%
Patients Who Left ER Before Being Seen	64,435	1%	1%	2%
Time from ER Arrival to Admit. (minutes)[2]	491	228	217	274
Time from ER Arrival to Discharge (minutes)	382	140	123	134
Time in ER Before Being Evaluated (minutes)	404	21	17	26
Time to Pain Meds for Fractures (minutes)	308	50	43	57
Heart Attack Care				
Aspirin Given at Discharge	193	100%	99%	99%
Fibrinolytic Meds Within 30 Min. of Arrival[1]	-	-	100%	54%
PCI Within 90 Minutes of Arrival	54	98%	98%	96%
Statin Prescribed at Discharge	194	100%	100%	98%
Heart Failure Care				
ACE Inhibitor or ARB for LVSD	88	95%	98%	97%
Discharge Instructions Given	210	100%	96%	94%
Evaluation of LVS Function	259	100%	98%	99%

NOTE: Hospital profiles are in alphabetical order by state, then city, then hospital within the city; Rankings exclude hospitals with less than 25 cases except for patient surveys which excludes hospitals with less than 100 cases; (a) 100-299 cases; (1) The number of cases/patients is too few to report; (2) Data submitted were based on a sample of cases/patients; (3) Results are based on a shorter time period than required; (4) Data suppressed by CMS for one or more quarters; (5) Results are not available for this reporting period; (6) Fewer than 100 patients completed the HCAHPS survey; (7) No cases met the criteria for this measure; (8) The lower limit of the confidence interval cannot be calculated if the number of observed infections equals zero; (9) No data are available from the state/territory for this reporting period; (10) The scores shown reflect fewer than 50 completed surveys; (11) There were discrepancies in the data collection process; (12) This measure does not apply to this hospital for this reporting period; (13) Results cannot be calculated for this reporting period; (14) The results for this state are combined with nearby states to protect confidentiality; Please refer to the User's Guide for a full explanation of data.

Measure	Cases	This Hosp.	State Avg.	U.S. Avg.
Medicare Spending				
Medicare Spending per Patient (ratio)	-	0.96	0.98	0.98
Pneumonia Care				
Appropriate Initial Antibiotic Given[2]	116	94%	96%	95%
Blood Culture Timing[2]	184	98%	99%	98%
Pregnancy and Delivery Care				
Newborn Deliveries Scheduled Early[2]	87	1%	6%	6%
Preventive Care				
Immunization for Influenza[2]	508	96%	92%	90%
Immunization for Pneumonia[2]	464	93%	91%	92%
Stroke Care				
Anticoagulation Therapy for Atrial Fibrillation	15	87%	95%	95%
Antithrombotic Therapy Timing	92	98%	99%	98%
Assessed for Rehabilitation	154	97%	98%	97%
Discharged on Antithrombotic Therapy	136	99%	99%	99%
Discharged on Statin Medication	101	98%	96%	94%
Thrombolytic Therapy Timing	11	100%	89%	66%
Venous Thromboembolism Prophylaxis	116	91%	95%	94%
Written Stroke Educational Materials Given	82	98%	89%	88%
Surgical Care Improvement Project				
Appropriate Beta Blocker Usage[2]	162	99%	98%	98%
Appropriate VTP Within 24 Hours[2]	384	99%	99%	98%
Controlled Postoperative Blood Glucose[2]	160	98%	97%	97%
Perioperative Temperature Management[2]	479	100%	100%	100%
Prophylactic Antibiotic Selection[2]	441	100%	99%	99%
Prophylactic Antibiotic Selection (Outpatient)	505	99%	98%	98%
Prophylactic Antibiotic Stopped[2]	428	99%	98%	98%
Prophylactic Antibiotic Timing[2]	444	99%	99%	99%
Prophylactic Antibiotic Timing (Outpatient)	506	98%	98%	98%
Urinary Catheter Removal[2]	379	98%	98%	97%
Survey of Patients' Hospital Experiences				
Area Around Room 'Always' Quiet at Night	300+	53%	60%	61%
Doctors 'Always' Communicated Well	300+	81%	83%	82%
Home Recovery Information Given	300+	90%	90%	85%
Hospital Given 9 or 10 on 10 Point Scale	300+	77%	74%	71%
Meds 'Always' Explained Before Given	300+	70%	68%	64%
Nurses 'Always' Communicated Well	300+	79%	79%	79%
Pain 'Always' Well Controlled	300+	71%	73%	71%
Room and Bathroom 'Always' Clean	300+	72%	74%	73%
Timely Help 'Always' Received	300+	66%	69%	68%
Would Definitely Recommend Hospital	300+	81%	76%	71%
Use of Medical Imaging				
Cardiac Imaging Stress Test before Surgery	831	5.3%	4.9%	5.3%
Combination Abdominal CT Scan	1,129	2.7%	4.9%	10.5%
Combination Brain/Sinus CT Scan	797	2.4%	3%	2.7%
Combination Chest CT Scan	595	0.7%	0.8%	2.7%
Follow-up Mammogram/Ultrasound	2,676	6.9%	8.5%	8.8%
Lumbar Spine MRI for Low Back Pain	375	47.2%	43.8%	37.2%

Ogden Regional Medical Center

5475 South 500 East
Ogden, UT 84405
Phone: 801-479-2111
Type: Acute Care Hospitals
Emergency Services: Yes
Ownership: Proprietary
Beds: 227

Key Personnel:

Chief of Medical Staff.......... Michael Diehl, MD
Operating Room.............. Lori Gordon
President..................... Billy Parish
Cardiac Laboratory............ Doug Passey
Quality Assurance .... Marilyn Peterson
Radiology.................... Anthony Rodebush
Infection Control.............. Jeanette Smyth
Pediatric In-Patient Care .... Kim Tyler

Measure	Cases	This Hosp.	State Avg.	U.S. Avg.
Blood Clot Prevention and Treatment				
Anticoagulation Overlap Therapy[2]	49	98%	95%	93%
ICU Venous Thromboembolism Prophylaxis[2]	74	100%	93%	92%
Incidence of Potentially Preventable VTE[1,2]	-	-	5%	10%
UFH with Dosages/Platelet Monitoring[2]	39	100%	95%	97%
Venous Thromboembolism Prophylaxis[2]	283	94%	86%	85%
Warfarin Therapy Discharge Instructions[2]	32	91%	73%	75%
Chest Pain/Possible Heart Attack Care				
Aspirin Given Within 24 Hours of Arrival[1,3]	-	-	97%	96%
Fibrinolytic Meds Within 30 Min. of Arrival[5]	-	-	52%	58%
Average Time to ECG (minutes)[1,3]	-	-	7	7
Average Time to Transfer (minutes)[5]	-	-	36	60
Children's Asthma Care				
Received Home Management Plan of Care	-	-	-	88%
Received Reliever Medication	-	-	-	100%
Received Systemic Corticosteroids	-	-	-	100%
Emergency Department				
Admittance Decision Time (minutes)[2]	376	70	66	98
Head CT Results Within 45 Min. of Arrival[3,7]	-	-	60%	57%
Patients Who Left ER Before Being Seen	25,713	0%	1%	2%
Time from ER Arrival to Admit. (minutes)[2]	377	200	217	274
Time from ER Arrival to Discharge (minutes)	492	116	123	134
Time in ER Before Being Evaluated (minutes)	507	15	17	26
Time to Pain Meds for Fractures (minutes)	110	40	43	57
Heart Attack Care				
Aspirin Given at Discharge[2]	92	99%	99%	99%
Fibrinolytic Meds Within 30 Min. of Arrival[1,2]	-	-	100%	54%
PCI Within 90 Minutes of Arrival[1,2]	-	-	98%	96%
Statin Prescribed at Discharge[2]	89	100%	100%	98%
Heart Failure Care				
ACE Inhibitor or ARB for LVSD[2]	28	100%	98%	97%
Discharge Instructions Given[2]	69	99%	96%	94%
Evaluation of LVS Function[2]	90	100%	98%	99%
Medicare Spending				
Medicare Spending per Patient (ratio)	-	1.00	0.98	0.98
Pneumonia Care				
Appropriate Initial Antibiotic Given[2]	84	98%	96%	95%
Blood Culture Timing[2]	114	100%	99%	98%
Pregnancy and Delivery Care				
Newborn Deliveries Scheduled Early[2]	52	0%	6%	6%
Preventive Care				
Immunization for Influenza[2]	485	85%	92%	90%
Immunization for Pneumonia[2]	404	90%	91%	92%
Stroke Care				
Anticoagulation Therapy for Atrial Fibrillation[1,2]	-	-	95%	95%
Antithrombotic Therapy Timing[2]	51	100%	99%	98%
Assessed for Rehabilitation[2]	64	100%	98%	97%
Discharged on Antithrombotic Therapy[2]	56	100%	99%	99%
Discharged on Statin Medication[2]	41	98%	96%	94%
Thrombolytic Therapy Timing[1,2]	-	-	89%	66%
Venous Thromboembolism Prophylaxis[2]	66	100%	95%	94%
Written Stroke Educational Materials Given[2]	31	94%	89%	88%
Surgical Care Improvement Project				
Appropriate Beta Blocker Usage[2]	106	97%	98%	98%
Appropriate VTP Within 24 Hours[2]	341	99%	99%	98%
Controlled Postoperative Blood Glucose[2]	75	91%	97%	97%
Perioperative Temperature Management[2]	391	100%	100%	100%
Prophylactic Antibiotic Selection[2]	298	99%	99%	99%
Prophylactic Antibiotic Selection (Outpatient)	428	98%	98%	98%
Prophylactic Antibiotic Stopped[2]	284	99%	98%	98%
Prophylactic Antibiotic Timing[2]	298	100%	99%	99%
Prophylactic Antibiotic Timing (Outpatient)	430	98%	98%	98%
Urinary Catheter Removal[2]	294	98%	98%	97%
Survey of Patients' Hospital Experiences				
Area Around Room 'Always' Quiet at Night	300+	51%	60%	61%
Doctors 'Always' Communicated Well	300+	77%	83%	82%
Home Recovery Information Given	300+	88%	90%	85%
Hospital Given 9 or 10 on 10 Point Scale	300+	67%	74%	71%
Meds 'Always' Explained Before Given	300+	59%	68%	64%
Nurses 'Always' Communicated Well	300+	70%	79%	79%
Pain 'Always' Well Controlled	300+	65%	73%	71%
Room and Bathroom 'Always' Clean	300+	59%	74%	73%
Timely Help 'Always' Received	300+	58%	69%	68%
Would Definitely Recommend Hospital	300+	70%	76%	71%
Use of Medical Imaging				
Cardiac Imaging Stress Test before Surgery	238	5.0%	4.9%	5.3%
Combination Abdominal CT Scan	311	5.5%	4.9%	10.5%
Combination Brain/Sinus CT Scan[1]	-	-	3%	2.7%
Combination Chest CT Scan	142	0.0%	0.8%	2.7%
Follow-up Mammogram/Ultrasound	654	8.9%	8.5%	8.8%
Lumbar Spine MRI for Low Back Pain	61	45.9%	43.8%	37.2%

Orem Community Hospital

331 North 400 West
Orem, UT 84057
Phone: 801-714-3307
Fax: 801-714-3227
URL: www.ihc.com/och
Type: Acute Care Hospitals
Emergency Services: Yes
Ownership: Voluntary non-profit - Private
Beds: 20

Key Personnel:

Radiology.................. Fred Bandley, MD
Operating Room............ Cynthia Capel
Infection Control............. Steve Freestone, MD
Pediatric Ambulatory Care ...... Ronald C Jones, MD
Pediatric In-Patient Care .... Ronald C Jones, MD
Quality Assurance .... Karie Minager-Miya
Chief of Medical Staff.......... Todd Nielson, MD
CEO/President............... Charles W. Sorenson, MD

Measure	Cases	This Hosp.	State Avg.	U.S. Avg.
Blood Clot Prevention and Treatment				
Anticoagulation Overlap Therapy[7]	-	-	95%	93%
ICU Venous Thromboembolism Prophylaxis[7]	-	-	93%	92%
Incidence of Potentially Preventable VTE[7]	-	-	5%	10%
UFH with Dosages/Platelet Monitoring[7]	-	-	95%	97%
Venous Thromboembolism Prophylaxis	15	80%	86%	85%
Warfarin Therapy Discharge Instructions[7]	-	-	73%	75%
Chest Pain/Possible Heart Attack Care				
Aspirin Given Within 24 Hours of Arrival	20	70%	97%	96%
Fibrinolytic Meds Within 30 Min. of Arrival[7]	-	-	52%	58%
Average Time to ECG (minutes)	20	14	7	7
Average Time to Transfer (minutes)[1]	-	-	36	60
Children's Asthma Care				
Received Home Management Plan of Care	-	-	-	88%
Received Reliever Medication	-	-	-	100%
Received Systemic Corticosteroids	-	-	-	100%
Emergency Department				
Admittance Decision Time (minutes)[2,7]	-	-	66	98
Head CT Results Within 45 Min. of Arrival[3,7]	-	-	60%	57%
Patients Who Left ER Before Being Seen	7,256	1%	1%	2%
Time from ER Arrival to Admit. (minutes)[2,7]	-	-	217	274
Time from ER Arrival to Discharge (minutes)	393	86	123	134
Time in ER Before Being Evaluated (minutes)	423	15	17	26
Time to Pain Meds for Fractures (minutes)	36	30	43	57
Heart Attack Care				
Aspirin Given at Discharge[5]	-	-	99%	99%
Fibrinolytic Meds Within 30 Min. of Arrival[5]	-	-	100%	54%
PCI Within 90 Minutes of Arrival[5]	-	-	98%	96%
Statin Prescribed at Discharge[5]	-	-	100%	98%
Heart Failure Care				
ACE Inhibitor or ARB for LVSD[5]	-	-	98%	97%
Discharge Instructions Given[5]	-	-	96%	94%
Evaluation of LVS Function[5]	-	-	98%	99%
Medicare Spending				
Medicare Spending per Patient (ratio)[1]	-	-	0.98	0.98
Pneumonia Care				
Appropriate Initial Antibiotic Given[5]	-	-	96%	95%
Blood Culture Timing[5]	-	-	99%	98%
Pregnancy and Delivery Care				
Newborn Deliveries Scheduled Early[2]	39	5%	6%	6%
Preventive Care				
Immunization for Influenza[2]	168	98%	92%	90%
Immunization for Pneumonia[2]	16	69%	91%	92%
Stroke Care				
Anticoagulation Therapy for Atrial Fibrillation[5]	-	-	95%	95%
Antithrombotic Therapy Timing[5]	-	-	99%	98%
Assessed for Rehabilitation[5]	-	-	98%	97%
Discharged on Antithrombotic Therapy[5]	-	-	99%	99%
Discharged on Statin Medication[5]	-	-	96%	94%
Thrombolytic Therapy Timing[5]	-	-	89%	66%
Venous Thromboembolism Prophylaxis[5]	-	-	95%	94%
Written Stroke Educational Materials Given[5]	-	-	89%	88%
Surgical Care Improvement Project				
Appropriate Beta Blocker Usage[1,2]	-	-	98%	98%
Appropriate VTP Within 24 Hours[2]	13	100%	99%	98%
Controlled Postoperative Blood Glucose[2,7]	-	-	97%	97%
Perioperative Temperature Management[2]	48	100%	100%	100%
Prophylactic Antibiotic Selection[2]	36	94%	99%	99%

NOTE: Hospital profiles are in alphabetical order by state, then city, then hospital within the city; Rankings exclude hospitals with less than 25 cases except for patient surveys which excludes hospitals with less than 100 cases; (a) 100-299 cases; (1) The number of cases/patients is too few to report; (2) Data submitted were based on a sample of cases/patients; (3) Results are based on a shorter time period than required; (4) Data suppressed by CMS for one or more quarters; (5) Results are not available for this reporting period; (6) Fewer than 100 patients completed the HCAHPS survey; (7) No cases met the criteria for this measure; (8) The lower limit of the confidence interval cannot be calculated if the number of observed infections equals zero; (9) No data are available from the state/territory for this reporting period; (10) The scores shown reflect fewer than 50 completed surveys; (11) There were discrepancies in the data collection process; (12) This measure does not apply to this hospital for this reporting period; (13) Results cannot be calculated for this reporting period; (14) The results for this state are combined with nearby states to protect confidentiality; Please refer to the User's Guide for a full explanation of data.

Measure	Cases	This Hosp.	State Avg.	U.S. Avg.
Prophylactic Antibiotic Selection (Outpatient)	42	100%	98%	98%
Prophylactic Antibiotic Stopped[2]	36	100%	98%	98%
Prophylactic Antibiotic Timing[2]	37	97%	99%	99%
Prophylactic Antibiotic Timing (Outpatient)	42	95%	98%	98%
Urinary Catheter Removal[2,7]	-	-	98%	97%
Survey of Patients' Hospital Experiences				
Area Around Room 'Always' Quiet at Night	300+	58%	60%	61%
Doctors 'Always' Communicated Well	300+	82%	83%	82%
Home Recovery Information Given	300+	94%	90%	85%
Hospital Given 9 or 10 on 10 Point Scale	300+	86%	74%	71%
Meds 'Always' Explained Before Given	300+	73%	68%	64%
Nurses 'Always' Communicated Well	300+	82%	79%	79%
Pain 'Always' Well Controlled	300+	76%	73%	71%
Room and Bathroom 'Always' Clean	300+	76%	74%	73%
Timely Help 'Always' Received	300+	69%	69%	68%
Would Definitely Recommend Hospital	300+	86%	76%	71%
Use of Medical Imaging				
Cardiac Imaging Stress Test before Surgery[7]	-	-	4.9%	5.3%
Combination Abdominal CT Scan	87	12.6%	4.9%	10.5%
Combination Brain/Sinus CT Scan[1]	-	-	3%	2.7%
Combination Chest CT Scan[1]	-	-	0.8%	2.7%
Follow-up Mammogram/Ultrasound	205	6.8%	8.5%	8.8%
Lumbar Spine MRI for Low Back Pain[1]	-	-	43.8%	37.2%

Timpanogos Regional Hospital

750 West 800 North Phone: 801-714-6800
Orem, UT 84057 Fax: 801-714-6597
URL: www.timpanogosregionalhospital.com
Type: Acute Care Hospitals Emergency Services: Yes
Ownership: Proprietary Beds: 59
Key Personnel:
Radiology. . . . . Mark S Asay
CEO/President. . . . . Keith D Tintle

Measure	Cases	This Hosp.	State Avg.	U.S. Avg.
Blood Clot Prevention and Treatment				
Anticoagulation Overlap Therapy[2]	27	89%	95%	93%
ICU Venous Thromboembolism Prophylaxis[2]	51	94%	93%	92%
Incidence of Potentially Preventable VTE[1,2]	-	-	5%	10%
UFH with Dosages/Platelet Monitoring[1,2]	-	-	95%	97%
Venous Thromboembolism Prophylaxis[2]	198	95%	86%	85%
Warfarin Therapy Discharge Instructions[2]	21	90%	73%	75%
Chest Pain/Possible Heart Attack Care				
Aspirin Given Within 24 Hours of Arrival[1,3]	-	-	97%	96%
Fibrinolytic Meds Within 30 Min. of Arrival[5]	-	-	52%	58%
Average Time to ECG (minutes)[1,3]	-	-	7	7
Average Time to Transfer (minutes)[5]	-	-	36	60
Children's Asthma Care				
Received Home Management Plan of Care	-	-	-	88%
Received Reliever Medication	-	-	-	100%
Received Systemic Corticosteroids	-	-	-	100%
Emergency Department				
Admittance Decision Time (minutes)[2]	231	60	66	98
Head CT Results Within 45 Min. of Arrival[1]	-	-	60%	57%
Patients Who Left ER Before Being Seen	16,342	0%	1%	2%
Time from ER Arrival to Admit. (minutes)[2]	231	204	217	274
Time from ER Arrival to Discharge (minutes)	444	112	123	134
Time in ER Before Being Evaluated (minutes)	475	14	17	26
Time to Pain Meds for Fractures (minutes)	102	46	43	57
Heart Attack Care				
Aspirin Given at Discharge	52	100%	99%	99%
Fibrinolytic Meds Within 30 Min. of Arrival[7]	-	-	100%	54%
PCI Within 90 Minutes of Arrival	16	94%	98%	96%
Statin Prescribed at Discharge	53	100%	100%	98%
Heart Failure Care				
ACE Inhibitor or ARB for LVSD[1]	-	-	98%	97%
Discharge Instructions Given	17	100%	96%	94%
Evaluation of LVS Function	26	100%	98%	99%
Medicare Spending				
Medicare Spending per Patient (ratio)	-	1.04	0.98	0.98
Pneumonia Care				
Appropriate Initial Antibiotic Given	56	100%	96%	95%
Blood Culture Timing	77	99%	99%	98%
Pregnancy and Delivery Care				
Newborn Deliveries Scheduled Early[2]	65	5%	6%	6%
Preventive Care				
Immunization for Influenza[2]	420	92%	92%	90%
Immunization for Pneumonia[2]	270	97%	91%	92%
Stroke Care				
Anticoagulation Therapy for Atrial Fibrillation[1]	-	-	95%	95%
Antithrombotic Therapy Timing	17	100%	99%	98%
Assessed for Rehabilitation	17	94%	98%	97%
Discharged on Antithrombotic Therapy	17	94%	99%	99%
Discharged on Statin Medication	13	92%	96%	94%
Thrombolytic Therapy Timing[7]	-	-	89%	66%
Venous Thromboembolism Prophylaxis	16	100%	95%	94%
Written Stroke Educational Materials Given[1]	-	-	89%	88%
Surgical Care Improvement Project				
Appropriate Beta Blocker Usage[2]	70	100%	98%	98%
Appropriate VTP Within 24 Hours[2]	301	99%	99%	98%
Controlled Postoperative Blood Glucose[2]	40	95%	97%	97%
Perioperative Temperature Management[2]	365	100%	100%	100%
Prophylactic Antibiotic Selection[2]	275	100%	99%	99%
Prophylactic Antibiotic Selection (Outpatient)	227	98%	98%	98%
Prophylactic Antibiotic Stopped[2]	264	99%	98%	98%
Prophylactic Antibiotic Timing[2]	275	100%	99%	99%
Prophylactic Antibiotic Timing (Outpatient)	227	99%	98%	98%
Urinary Catheter Removal[2]	229	97%	98%	97%
Survey of Patients' Hospital Experiences				
Area Around Room 'Always' Quiet at Night	300+	63%	60%	61%
Doctors 'Always' Communicated Well	300+	78%	83%	82%
Home Recovery Information Given	300+	87%	90%	85%
Hospital Given 9 or 10 on 10 Point Scale	300+	71%	74%	71%
Meds 'Always' Explained Before Given	300+	58%	68%	64%
Nurses 'Always' Communicated Well	300+	76%	79%	79%
Pain 'Always' Well Controlled	300+	70%	73%	71%
Room and Bathroom 'Always' Clean	300+	76%	74%	73%
Timely Help 'Always' Received	300+	64%	69%	68%
Would Definitely Recommend Hospital	300+	72%	76%	71%
Use of Medical Imaging				
Cardiac Imaging Stress Test before Surgery	64	9.4%	4.9%	5.3%
Combination Abdominal CT Scan	128	9.4%	4.9%	10.5%
Combination Brain/Sinus CT Scan[1]	-	-	3%	2.7%
Combination Chest CT Scan[1]	-	-	0.8%	2.7%
Follow-up Mammogram/Ultrasound	125	22.4%	8.5%	8.8%
Lumbar Spine MRI for Low Back Pain[1]	-	-	43.8%	37.2%

Garfield Memorial Hospital

200 North 400 East Phone: 435-676-8811
Panguitch, UT 84759 Fax: 435-676-2679
URL: www.intermountainhealthcare.org
Type: Acute Care Hospitals Emergency Services: Yes
Ownership: Government - Local Beds: 44
Key Personnel:
Chair/CEO. . . . . A. Scott Anderson
Chief of Medical Staff. . . . . Shaun Shurtliff
CEO/President. . . . . Charles W. Sorenson, MD

Measure	Cases	This Hosp.	State Avg.	U.S. Avg.
Blood Clot Prevention and Treatment				
Anticoagulation Overlap Therapy[1,2]	-	-	95%	93%
ICU Venous Thromboembolism Prophylaxis[2,7]	-	-	93%	92%
Incidence of Potentially Preventable VTE[1,2]	-	-	5%	10%
UFH with Dosages/Platelet Monitoring[2,7]	-	-	95%	97%
Venous Thromboembolism Prophylaxis[2]	99	62%	86%	85%
Warfarin Therapy Discharge Instructions[1,2]	-	-	73%	75%
Chest Pain/Possible Heart Attack Care				
Aspirin Given Within 24 Hours of Arrival	20	100%	97%	96%
Fibrinolytic Meds Within 30 Min. of Arrival[1]	-	-	52%	58%
Average Time to ECG (minutes)	20	6	7	7
Average Time to Transfer (minutes)[7]	-	-	36	60
Children's Asthma Care				
Received Home Management Plan of Care	-	-	-	88%
Received Reliever Medication	-	-	-	100%
Received Systemic Corticosteroids	-	-	-	100%
Emergency Department				
Admittance Decision Time (minutes)	150	41	66	98
Head CT Results Within 45 Min. of Arrival[1,3]	-	-	60%	57%
Patients Who Left ER Before Being Seen	2,202	0%	1%	2%
Time from ER Arrival to Admit. (minutes)	158	161	217	274
Time from ER Arrival to Discharge (minutes)	239	101	123	134
Time in ER Before Being Evaluated (minutes)	217	15	17	26
Time to Pain Meds for Fractures (minutes)	19	35	43	57
Heart Attack Care				
Aspirin Given at Discharge[1,3]	-	-	99%	99%
Fibrinolytic Meds Within 30 Min. of Arrival[3,7]	-	-	100%	54%
PCI Within 90 Minutes of Arrival[3,7]	-	-	98%	96%
Statin Prescribed at Discharge[1,3]	-	-	100%	98%
Heart Failure Care				
ACE Inhibitor or ARB for LVSD[1]	-	-	98%	97%
Discharge Instructions Given	11	100%	96%	94%
Evaluation of LVS Function	11	100%	98%	99%
Medicare Spending				
Medicare Spending per Patient (ratio)	-	0.84	0.98	0.98
Pneumonia Care				
Appropriate Initial Antibiotic Given	15	100%	96%	95%
Blood Culture Timing	12	100%	99%	98%
Pregnancy and Delivery Care				
Newborn Deliveries Scheduled Early[1]	-	-	6%	6%
Preventive Care				
Immunization for Influenza	112	92%	92%	90%
Immunization for Pneumonia	157	91%	91%	92%
Stroke Care				
Anticoagulation Therapy for Atrial Fibrillation[1,3]	-	-	95%	95%
Antithrombotic Therapy Timing[1,3]	-	-	99%	98%
Assessed for Rehabilitation[1,3]	-	-	98%	97%
Discharged on Antithrombotic Therapy[1,3]	-	-	99%	99%
Discharged on Statin Medication[1,3]	-	-	96%	94%
Thrombolytic Therapy Timing[3,7]	-	-	89%	66%
Venous Thromboembolism Prophylaxis[1,3]	-	-	95%	94%
Written Stroke Educational Materials Given[1,3]	-	-	89%	88%
Surgical Care Improvement Project				
Appropriate Beta Blocker Usage[5]	-	-	98%	98%
Appropriate VTP Within 24 Hours[5]	-	-	99%	98%
Controlled Postoperative Blood Glucose[5]	-	-	97%	97%
Perioperative Temperature Management[5]	-	-	100%	100%
Prophylactic Antibiotic Selection[5]	-	-	99%	99%
Prophylactic Antibiotic Selection (Outpatient)[5]	-	-	98%	98%
Prophylactic Antibiotic Stopped[5]	-	-	98%	98%
Prophylactic Antibiotic Timing[5]	-	-	99%	99%
Prophylactic Antibiotic Timing (Outpatient)[5]	-	-	98%	98%
Urinary Catheter Removal[5]	-	-	98%	97%
Survey of Patients' Hospital Experiences				
Area Around Room 'Always' Quiet at Night[6]	<100	58%	60%	61%
Doctors 'Always' Communicated Well[6]	<100	89%	83%	82%
Home Recovery Information Given[6]	<100	95%	90%	85%
Hospital Given 9 or 10 on 10 Point Scale[6]	<100	81%	74%	71%
Meds 'Always' Explained Before Given[6]	<100	88%	68%	64%
Nurses 'Always' Communicated Well[6]	<100	90%	79%	79%
Pain 'Always' Well Controlled[6]	<100	79%	73%	71%
Room and Bathroom 'Always' Clean[6]	<100	80%	74%	73%
Timely Help 'Always' Received[6]	<100	82%	69%	68%
Would Definitely Recommend Hospital[6]	<100	84%	76%	71%
Use of Medical Imaging				
Cardiac Imaging Stress Test before Surgery[7]	-	-	4.9%	5.3%
Combination Abdominal CT Scan	46	0.0%	4.9%	10.5%
Combination Brain/Sinus CT Scan	53	9.4%	3%	2.7%
Combination Chest CT Scan[1]	-	-	0.8%	2.7%
Follow-up Mammogram/Ultrasound	288	6.9%	8.5%	8.8%
Lumbar Spine MRI for Low Back Pain[7]	-	-	43.8%	37.2%

Park City Medical Center

900 Round Valley Drive Phone: 435-658-7000
Park City, UT 84060
URL: www.intermountainhealthcare.org
Type: Acute Care Hospitals Emergency Services: Yes
Ownership: Proprietary
Key Personnel:
CEO/President. . . . . Charles W. Sorenson, MD

Measure	Cases	This Hosp.	State Avg.	U.S. Avg.
Blood Clot Prevention and Treatment				

NOTE: Hospital profiles are in alphabetical order by state, then city, then hospital within the city; Rankings exclude hospitals with less than 25 cases except for patient surveys which excludes hospitals with less than 100 cases; (a) 100-299 cases; (1) The number of cases/patients is too few to report; (2) Data submitted were based on a sample of cases/patients; (3) Results are based on a shorter time period than required; (4) Data suppressed by CMS for one or more quarters; (5) Results are not available for this reporting period; (6) Fewer than 100 patients completed the HCAHPS survey; (7) No cases met the criteria for this measure; (8) The lower limit of the confidence interval cannot be calculated if the number of observed infections equals zero; (9) No data are available from the state/territory for this reporting period; (10) The scores shown reflect fewer than 50 completed surveys; (11) There were discrepancies in the data collection process; (12) This measure does not apply to this hospital for this reporting period; (13) Results cannot be calculated for this reporting period; (14) The results for this state are combined with nearby states to protect confidentiality; Please refer to the User's Guide for a full explanation of data.

Anticoagulation Overlap Therapy[2]	19	89%	95%	93%
ICU Venous Thromboembolism Prophylaxis[1,2]	-	-	93%	92%
Incidence of Potentially Preventable VTE[1,2]	-	-	5%	10%
UFH with Dosages/Platelet Monitoring[1,2]	-	-	95%	97%
Venous Thromboembolism Prophylaxis[2]	42	95%	86%	85%
Warfarin Therapy Discharge Instructions[2]	18	33%	73%	75%
Chest Pain/Possible Heart Attack Care				
Aspirin Given Within 24 Hours of Arrival	54	98%	97%	96%
Fibrinolytic Meds Within 30 Min. of Arrival[7]	-	-	52%	58%
Average Time to ECG (minutes)	56	6	7	7
Average Time to Transfer (minutes)[1]	-	-	36	60
Children's Asthma Care				
Received Home Management Plan of Care	-	-	-	88%
Received Reliever Medication	-	-	-	100%
Received Systemic Corticosteroids	-	-	-	100%
Emergency Department				
Admittance Decision Time (minutes)[2]	145	84	66	98
Head CT Results Within 45 Min. of Arrival[1]	-	-	60%	57%
Patients Who Left ER Before Being Seen	9,801	0%	1%	2%
Time from ER Arrival to Admit. (minutes)[2]	152	210	217	274
Time from ER Arrival to Discharge (minutes)	384	102	123	134
Time in ER Before Being Evaluated (minutes)	458	3	17	26
Time to Pain Meds for Fractures (minutes)	142	28	43	57
Heart Attack Care				
Aspirin Given at Discharge[3,7]	-	-	99%	99%
Fibrinolytic Meds Within 30 Min. of Arrival[3,7]	-	-	100%	54%
PCI Within 90 Minutes of Arrival[3,7]	-	-	98%	96%
Statin Prescribed at Discharge[3,7]	-	-	100%	98%
Heart Failure Care				
ACE Inhibitor or ARB for LVSD[1]	-	-	98%	97%
Discharge Instructions Given[1]	-	-	96%	94%
Evaluation of LVS Function[1]	-	-	98%	99%
Medicare Spending				
Medicare Spending per Patient (ratio)	-	0.96	0.98	0.98
Pneumonia Care				
Appropriate Initial Antibiotic Given	21	95%	96%	95%
Blood Culture Timing	32	100%	99%	98%
Pregnancy and Delivery Care				
Newborn Deliveries Scheduled Early[2]	39	13%	6%	6%
Preventive Care				
Immunization for Influenza[2]	292	87%	92%	90%
Immunization for Pneumonia[2]	213	79%	91%	92%
Stroke Care				
Anticoagulation Therapy for Atrial Fibrillation[3,7]	-	-	95%	95%
Antithrombotic Therapy Timing[1,3]	-	-	99%	98%
Assessed for Rehabilitation[1,3]	-	-	98%	97%
Discharged on Antithrombotic Therapy[1,3]	-	-	99%	99%
Discharged on Statin Medication[1,3]	-	-	96%	94%
Thrombolytic Therapy Timing[3,7]	-	-	89%	66%
Venous Thromboembolism Prophylaxis[1,3]	-	-	95%	94%
Written Stroke Educational Materials Given[1,3]	-	-	89%	88%
Surgical Care Improvement Project				
Appropriate Beta Blocker Usage[2]	34	97%	98%	98%
Appropriate VTP Within 24 Hours[2]	275	100%	99%	98%
Controlled Postoperative Blood Glucose[2,7]	-	-	97%	97%
Perioperative Temperature Management[2]	293	100%	100%	100%
Prophylactic Antibiotic Selection[2]	254	100%	99%	99%
Prophylactic Antibiotic Selection (Outpatient)	95	98%	98%	98%
Prophylactic Antibiotic Stopped[2]	253	99%	98%	98%
Prophylactic Antibiotic Timing[2]	254	100%	99%	99%
Prophylactic Antibiotic Timing (Outpatient)	96	98%	98%	98%
Urinary Catheter Removal[2]	143	100%	98%	97%
Survey of Patients' Hospital Experiences				
Area Around Room 'Always' Quiet at Night	300+	74%	60%	61%
Doctors 'Always' Communicated Well	300+	86%	83%	82%
Home Recovery Information Given	300+	92%	90%	85%
Hospital Given 9 or 10 on 10 Point Scale	300+	83%	74%	71%
Meds 'Always' Explained Before Given	300+	75%	68%	64%
Nurses 'Always' Communicated Well	300+	84%	79%	79%
Pain 'Always' Well Controlled	300+	77%	73%	71%
Room and Bathroom 'Always' Clean	300+	75%	74%	73%
Timely Help 'Always' Received	300+	75%	69%	68%
Would Definitely Recommend Hospital	300+	86%	76%	71%
Use of Medical Imaging				
Cardiac Imaging Stress Test before Surgery	90	6.7%	4.9%	5.3%
Combination Abdominal CT Scan	158	6.3%	4.9%	10.5%
Combination Brain/Sinus CT Scan[1]	-	-	3%	2.7%
Combination Chest CT Scan	69	1.4%	0.8%	2.7%
Follow-up Mammogram/Ultrasound	158	5.1%	8.5%	8.8%
Lumbar Spine MRI for Low Back Pain[1]	-	-	43.8%	37.2%

Mountain View Hospital

1000 East 100 North
Payson, UT 84651
Phone: 801-465-7100
Fax: 801-465-7170
E-mail: kevin.johnson@columbia.net
URL: www.mvhpayson.com
Type: Acute Care Hospitals
Emergency Services: Yes
Ownership: Proprietary
Beds: 136

Key Personnel:
Emergency Room . . . . Cimby Ford
Quality Assurance . . . . Anna Lee Johnson
CEO/President . . . . Kevin Johnson
Radiology. . . . . Ric Johnson
Operating Room. . . . . Carey Lundell, RN
Infection Control. . . . . Pauline Smith
Intensive Care Unit. . . . . Lisa Topham, RN

Measure	Cases	This Hosp.	State Avg.	U.S. Avg.
Blood Clot Prevention and Treatment				
Anticoagulation Overlap Therapy[2]	32	100%	95%	93%
ICU Venous Thromboembolism Prophylaxis[2]	49	100%	93%	92%
Incidence of Potentially Preventable VTE[1,2]	-	-	5%	10%
UFH with Dosages/Platelet Monitoring[1,2]	-	-	95%	97%
Venous Thromboembolism Prophylaxis[2]	137	100%	86%	85%
Warfarin Therapy Discharge Instructions[2]	23	96%	73%	75%
Chest Pain/Possible Heart Attack Care				
Aspirin Given Within 24 Hours of Arrival[1]	-	-	97%	96%
Fibrinolytic Meds Within 30 Min. of Arrival[3,7]	-	-	52%	58%
Average Time to ECG (minutes)[1]	-	-	7	7
Average Time to Transfer (minutes)[3,7]	-	-	36	60
Children's Asthma Care				
Received Home Management Plan of Care	-	-	-	88%
Received Reliever Medication	-	-	-	100%
Received Systemic Corticosteroids	-	-	-	100%
Emergency Department				
Admittance Decision Time (minutes)[2]	357	53	66	98
Head CT Results Within 45 Min. of Arrival[1]	-	-	60%	57%
Patients Who Left ER Before Being Seen	17,399	0%	1%	2%
Time from ER Arrival to Admit. (minutes)[2]	357	179	217	274
Time from ER Arrival to Discharge (minutes)	435	111	123	134
Time in ER Before Being Evaluated (minutes)	467	13	17	26
Time to Pain Meds for Fractures (minutes)	100	27	43	57
Heart Attack Care				
Aspirin Given at Discharge[2]	39	95%	99%	99%
Fibrinolytic Meds Within 30 Min. of Arrival[2,7]	-	-	100%	54%
PCI Within 90 Minutes of Arrival[2]	16	100%	98%	96%
Statin Prescribed at Discharge[2]	41	100%	100%	98%
Heart Failure Care				
ACE Inhibitor or ARB for LVSD[2]	15	100%	98%	97%
Discharge Instructions Given[2]	40	98%	96%	94%
Evaluation of LVS Function[2]	54	100%	98%	99%
Medicare Spending				
Medicare Spending per Patient (ratio)	-	0.99	0.98	0.98
Pneumonia Care				
Appropriate Initial Antibiotic Given[2]	56	100%	96%	95%
Blood Culture Timing[2]	90	100%	99%	98%
Pregnancy and Delivery Care				
Newborn Deliveries Scheduled Early[2]	43	5%	6%	6%
Preventive Care				
Immunization for Influenza[2]	359	99%	92%	90%
Immunization for Pneumonia[2]	375	98%	91%	92%
Stroke Care				
Anticoagulation Therapy for Atrial Fibrillation[1,2]	-	-	95%	95%
Antithrombotic Therapy Timing[1,2]	-	-	99%	98%
Assessed for Rehabilitation[1,2]	-	-	98%	97%
Discharged on Antithrombotic Therapy[1,2]	-	-	99%	99%
Discharged on Statin Medication[1,2]	-	-	96%	94%
Thrombolytic Therapy Timing[2,7]	-	-	89%	66%
Venous Thromboembolism Prophylaxis[1,2]	-	-	95%	94%
Written Stroke Educational Materials Given[1,2]	-	-	89%	88%
Surgical Care Improvement Project				
Appropriate Beta Blocker Usage[2]	67	100%	98%	98%
Appropriate VTP Within 24 Hours[2]	297	100%	99%	98%
Controlled Postoperative Blood Glucose[2,7]	-	-	97%	97%
Perioperative Temperature Management[2]	363	100%	100%	100%
Prophylactic Antibiotic Selection[2]	237	100%	99%	99%
Prophylactic Antibiotic Selection (Outpatient)	33	97%	98%	98%
Prophylactic Antibiotic Stopped[2]	232	100%	98%	98%
Prophylactic Antibiotic Timing[2]	237	100%	99%	99%
Prophylactic Antibiotic Timing (Outpatient)	32	97%	98%	98%
Urinary Catheter Removal[2]	237	100%	98%	97%
Survey of Patients' Hospital Experiences				
Area Around Room 'Always' Quiet at Night	300+	55%	60%	61%
Doctors 'Always' Communicated Well	300+	80%	83%	82%
Home Recovery Information Given	300+	88%	90%	85%
Hospital Given 9 or 10 on 10 Point Scale	300+	70%	74%	71%
Meds 'Always' Explained Before Given	300+	60%	68%	64%
Nurses 'Always' Communicated Well	300+	73%	79%	79%
Pain 'Always' Well Controlled	300+	68%	73%	71%
Room and Bathroom 'Always' Clean	300+	67%	74%	73%
Timely Help 'Always' Received	300+	64%	69%	68%
Would Definitely Recommend Hospital	300+	67%	76%	71%
Use of Medical Imaging				
Cardiac Imaging Stress Test before Surgery	116	3.4%	4.9%	5.3%
Combination Abdominal CT Scan	184	9.2%	4.9%	10.5%
Combination Brain/Sinus CT Scan[1]	-	-	3%	2.7%
Combination Chest CT Scan	107	0.0%	0.8%	2.7%
Follow-up Mammogram/Ultrasound	347	17.6%	8.5%	8.8%
Lumbar Spine MRI for Low Back Pain	42	50.0%	43.8%	37.2%

Castleview Hospital

300 North Hospital Drive
Price, UT 84501
Phone: 435-637-4800
Fax: 435-637-9513
URL: www.castleviewhospital.net/index2.php
Type: Acute Care Hospitals
Emergency Services: Yes
Ownership: Proprietary
Beds: 88

Key Personnel:
Operating Room. . . . . Wayne E Cox
Radiology. . . . . Roy C Hammond
Chief of Medical Staff . . . . Kurt King, MD
Infection Control. . . . . Pam Konakis
Pediatric Ambulatory Care . . . . . . EK Madsen
Pediatric In-Patient Care . . . . EK Madsen
CEO/President. . . . . Ryan Moynier
Emergency Room . . . . Terry Watkins

Measure	Cases	This Hosp.	State Avg.	U.S. Avg.
Blood Clot Prevention and Treatment				
Anticoagulation Overlap Therapy[2]	32	88%	95%	93%
ICU Venous Thromboembolism Prophylaxis[2]	45	89%	93%	92%
Incidence of Potentially Preventable VTE[1,2]	-	-	5%	10%
UFH with Dosages/Platelet Monitoring[1,2]	-	-	95%	97%
Venous Thromboembolism Prophylaxis[2]	106	92%	86%	85%
Warfarin Therapy Discharge Instructions[2]	24	96%	73%	75%
Chest Pain/Possible Heart Attack Care				
Aspirin Given Within 24 Hours of Arrival	72	97%	97%	96%
Fibrinolytic Meds Within 30 Min. of Arrival[1]	-	-	52%	58%
Average Time to ECG (minutes)	73	10	7	7
Average Time to Transfer (minutes)[1]	-	-	36	60
Children's Asthma Care				
Received Home Management Plan of Care	-	-	-	88%
Received Reliever Medication	-	-	-	100%
Received Systemic Corticosteroids	-	-	-	100%
Emergency Department				
Admittance Decision Time (minutes)[2]	305	38	66	98
Head CT Results Within 45 Min. of Arrival[1,3]	-	-	60%	57%
Patients Who Left ER Before Being Seen	11,931	2%	1%	2%
Time from ER Arrival to Admit. (minutes)[2]	309	221	217	274
Time from ER Arrival to Discharge (minutes)	373	137	123	134
Time in ER Before Being Evaluated (minutes)	415	20	17	26
Time to Pain Meds for Fractures (minutes)	71	48	43	57
Heart Attack Care				

NOTE: Hospital profiles are in alphabetical order by state, then city, then hospital within the city; Rankings exclude hospitals with less than 25 cases except for patient surveys which excludes hospitals with less than 100 cases; (a) 100-299 cases; (1) The number of cases/patients is too few to report; (2) Data submitted were based on a sample of cases/patients; (3) Results are based on a shorter time period than required; (4) Data suppressed by CMS for one or more quarters; (5) Results are not available for this reporting period; (6) Fewer than 100 patients completed the HCAHPS survey; (7) No cases met the criteria for this measure; (8) The lower limit of the confidence interval cannot be calculated if the number of observed infections equals zero; (9) No data are available from the state/territory for this reporting period; (10) The scores shown reflect fewer than 50 completed surveys; (11) There were discrepancies in the data collection process; (12) This measure does not apply to this hospital for this reporting period; (13) Results cannot be calculated for this reporting period; (14) The results for this state are combined with nearby states to protect confidentiality; Please refer to the User's Guide for a full explanation of data.

Measure	Cases	This Hosp.	State Avg.	U.S. Avg.
Aspirin Given at Discharge[3,7]	-	-	99%	99%
Fibrinolytic Meds Within 30 Min. of Arrival[3,7]	-	-	100%	54%
PCI Within 90 Minutes of Arrival[3,7]	-	-	98%	96%
Statin Prescribed at Discharge[1,3]	-	-	100%	98%
Heart Failure Care				
ACE Inhibitor or ARB for LVSD[1]	-	-	98%	97%
Discharge Instructions Given	13	92%	96%	94%
Evaluation of LVS Function	17	100%	98%	99%
Medicare Spending				
Medicare Spending per Patient (ratio)	-	0.93	0.98	0.98
Pneumonia Care				
Appropriate Initial Antibiotic Given	49	86%	96%	95%
Blood Culture Timing	86	99%	99%	98%
Pregnancy and Delivery Care				
Newborn Deliveries Scheduled Early[2]	41	12%	6%	6%
Preventive Care				
Immunization for Influenza[2]	252	94%	92%	90%
Immunization for Pneumonia[2]	264	98%	91%	92%
Stroke Care				
Anticoagulation Therapy for Atrial Fibrillation[1]	-	-	95%	95%
Antithrombotic Therapy Timing	13	100%	99%	98%
Assessed for Rehabilitation	13	92%	98%	97%
Discharged on Antithrombotic Therapy	12	100%	99%	99%
Discharged on Statin Medication	11	91%	96%	94%
Thrombolytic Therapy Timing[1]	-	-	89%	66%
Venous Thromboembolism Prophylaxis	13	77%	95%	94%
Written Stroke Educational Materials Given[1]	-	-	89%	88%
Surgical Care Improvement Project				
Appropriate Beta Blocker Usage	25	92%	98%	98%
Appropriate VTP Within 24 Hours	116	97%	99%	98%
Controlled Postoperative Blood Glucose[7]	-	-	97%	97%
Perioperative Temperature Management	130	99%	100%	100%
Prophylactic Antibiotic Selection	88	97%	99%	99%
Prophylactic Antibiotic Selection (Outpatient)	34	97%	98%	98%
Prophylactic Antibiotic Stopped	88	99%	98%	98%
Prophylactic Antibiotic Timing	88	99%	99%	99%
Prophylactic Antibiotic Timing (Outpatient)	34	100%	98%	98%
Urinary Catheter Removal	94	97%	98%	97%
Survey of Patients' Hospital Experiences				
Area Around Room 'Always' Quiet at Night	300+	57%	60%	61%
Doctors 'Always' Communicated Well	300+	80%	83%	82%
Home Recovery Information Given	300+	89%	90%	85%
Hospital Given 9 or 10 on 10 Point Scale	300+	63%	74%	71%
Meds 'Always' Explained Before Given	300+	62%	68%	64%
Nurses 'Always' Communicated Well	300+	74%	79%	79%
Pain 'Always' Well Controlled	300+	69%	73%	71%
Room and Bathroom 'Always' Clean	300+	70%	74%	73%
Timely Help 'Always' Received	300+	67%	69%	68%
Would Definitely Recommend Hospital	300+	58%	76%	71%
Use of Medical Imaging				
Cardiac Imaging Stress Test before Surgery	106	4.7%	4.9%	5.3%
Combination Abdominal CT Scan	353	2.3%	4.9%	10.5%
Combination Brain/Sinus CT Scan[1]	-	-	3%	2.7%
Combination Chest CT Scan	144	0.7%	0.8%	2.7%
Follow-up Mammogram/Ultrasound	515	13.2%	8.5%	8.8%
Lumbar Spine MRI for Low Back Pain	91	48.4%	43.8%	37.2%

Utah Valley Regional Medical Center

1034 North 500 West Phone: 801-373-7850
Provo, UT 84604 Fax: 801-357-7590
URL: www.intermountainhealthcare.org/hospitals/uvrmc
Type: Acute Care Hospitals Emergency Services: Yes
Ownership: Voluntary non-profit - Private Beds: 409

Key Personnel:
Chief of Medical Staff.......... Clark Bishop, MD
Infection Control.............. Joan Golden
Intensive Care Unit............ Kim Henrickson
Operating Room............... Jan Johnson
CEO/President................ Mary Nann Young
Quality Assurance .... Merlene Sanders
Administrator .... Steve Smoot
Emergency Room .... Wayne Watson, RN

Measure	Cases	This Hosp.	State Avg.	U.S. Avg.
Blood Clot Prevention and Treatment				
Anticoagulation Overlap Therapy[2]	141	88%	95%	93%
ICU Venous Thromboembolism Prophylaxis[2]	135	84%	93%	92%
Incidence of Potentially Preventable VTE[2]	40	8%	5%	10%
UFH with Dosages/Platelet Monitoring[2]	35	94%	95%	97%
Venous Thromboembolism Prophylaxis[2]	237	84%	86%	85%
Warfarin Therapy Discharge Instructions[2]	116	76%	73%	75%
Chest Pain/Possible Heart Attack Care				
Aspirin Given Within 24 Hours of Arrival[1,3]	-	-	97%	96%
Fibrinolytic Meds Within 30 Min. of Arrival[5]	-	-	52%	58%
Average Time to ECG (minutes)[1,3]	-	-	7	7
Average Time to Transfer (minutes)[5]	-	-	36	60
Children's Asthma Care				
Received Home Management Plan of Care	-	-	-	88%
Received Reliever Medication	-	-	-	100%
Received Systemic Corticosteroids	-	-	-	100%
Emergency Department				
Admittance Decision Time (minutes)[2]	387	85	66	98
Head CT Results Within 45 Min. of Arrival[1]	-	-	60%	57%
Patients Who Left ER Before Being Seen	46,924	1%	1%	2%
Time from ER Arrival to Admit. (minutes)[2]	387	234	217	274
Time from ER Arrival to Discharge (minutes)	399	142	123	134
Time in ER Before Being Evaluated (minutes)	426	25	17	26
Time to Pain Meds for Fractures (minutes)	184	53	43	57
Heart Attack Care				
Aspirin Given at Discharge	389	99%	99%	99%
Fibrinolytic Meds Within 30 Min. of Arrival[7]	-	-	100%	54%
PCI Within 90 Minutes of Arrival	53	98%	98%	96%
Statin Prescribed at Discharge	399	99%	100%	98%
Heart Failure Care				
ACE Inhibitor or ARB for LVSD	66	97%	98%	97%
Discharge Instructions Given	165	92%	96%	94%
Evaluation of LVS Function	208	100%	98%	99%
Medicare Spending				
Medicare Spending per Patient (ratio)	-	1.02	0.98	0.98
Pneumonia Care				
Appropriate Initial Antibiotic Given[2]	73	97%	96%	95%
Blood Culture Timing[2]	163	100%	99%	98%
Pregnancy and Delivery Care				
Newborn Deliveries Scheduled Early[2]	81	4%	6%	6%
Preventive Care				
Immunization for Influenza[2]	508	86%	92%	90%
Immunization for Pneumonia[2]	461	89%	91%	92%
Stroke Care				
Anticoagulation Therapy for Atrial Fibrillation	23	91%	95%	95%
Antithrombotic Therapy Timing	119	99%	99%	98%
Assessed for Rehabilitation	204	96%	98%	97%
Discharged on Antithrombotic Therapy	166	98%	99%	99%
Discharged on Statin Medication	121	95%	96%	94%
Thrombolytic Therapy Timing	20	95%	89%	66%
Venous Thromboembolism Prophylaxis	205	94%	95%	94%
Written Stroke Educational Materials Given	115	83%	89%	88%
Surgical Care Improvement Project				
Appropriate Beta Blocker Usage[2]	165	98%	98%	98%
Appropriate VTP Within 24 Hours[2]	451	97%	99%	98%
Controlled Postoperative Blood Glucose[2]	139	100%	97%	97%
Perioperative Temperature Management[2]	564	100%	100%	100%
Prophylactic Antibiotic Selection[2]	464	99%	99%	99%
Prophylactic Antibiotic Selection (Outpatient)	366	84%	98%	98%
Prophylactic Antibiotic Stopped[2]	439	99%	98%	98%
Prophylactic Antibiotic Timing[2]	465	99%	99%	99%
Prophylactic Antibiotic Timing (Outpatient)	368	93%	98%	98%
Urinary Catheter Removal[2]	383	98%	98%	97%
Survey of Patients' Hospital Experiences				
Area Around Room 'Always' Quiet at Night	300+	54%	60%	61%
Doctors 'Always' Communicated Well	300+	81%	83%	82%
Home Recovery Information Given	300+	90%	90%	85%
Hospital Given 9 or 10 on 10 Point Scale	300+	75%	74%	71%
Meds 'Always' Explained Before Given	300+	70%	68%	64%
Nurses 'Always' Communicated Well	300+	78%	79%	79%
Pain 'Always' Well Controlled	300+	73%	73%	71%
Room and Bathroom 'Always' Clean	300+	73%	74%	73%
Timely Help 'Always' Received	300+	67%	69%	68%
Would Definitely Recommend Hospital	300+	78%	76%	71%
Use of Medical Imaging				
Cardiac Imaging Stress Test before Surgery	186	5.4%	4.9%	5.3%
Combination Abdominal CT Scan	800	4.9%	4.9%	10.5%
Combination Brain/Sinus CT Scan	500	2.4%	3%	2.7%
Combination Chest CT Scan	528	0.6%	0.8%	2.7%
Follow-up Mammogram/Ultrasound	958	6.1%	8.5%	8.8%
Lumbar Spine MRI for Low Back Pain	150	51.3%	43.8%	37.2%

Sevier Valley Medical Center

1000 North Main Street Phone: 435-893-4100
Richfield, UT 84701 Fax: 435-896-9449
URL: www.intermountainhealthcare.org
Type: Acute Care Hospitals Emergency Services: Yes
Ownership: Voluntary non-profit - Private Beds: 42

Key Personnel:
Surgery .... Brent J. Allen, DO
Chairman/CEO .... Eugene Beck
Administrator .... Gary E. Beck
Cardiology.................. Scott E. Bingham, MD
Radiology.................. Roger D Blomquist
Chief of Medical Staff.......... Mark Robert Greenwoo, MD
CEO/President............... Chris Thompson, MD

Measure	Cases	This Hosp.	State Avg.	U.S. Avg.
Blood Clot Prevention and Treatment				
Anticoagulation Overlap Therapy[1,2]	-	-	95%	93%
ICU Venous Thromboembolism Prophylaxis[2,7]	-	-	93%	92%
Incidence of Potentially Preventable VTE[1,2]	-	-	5%	10%
UFH with Dosages/Platelet Monitoring[1,2]	-	-	95%	97%
Venous Thromboembolism Prophylaxis[2]	97	51%	86%	85%
Warfarin Therapy Discharge Instructions[1,2]	-	-	73%	75%
Chest Pain/Possible Heart Attack Care				
Aspirin Given Within 24 Hours of Arrival	38	95%	97%	96%
Fibrinolytic Meds Within 30 Min. of Arrival[1]	-	-	52%	58%
Average Time to ECG (minutes)	37	8	7	7
Average Time to Transfer (minutes)[7]	-	-	36	60
Children's Asthma Care				
Received Home Management Plan of Care	-	-	-	88%
Received Reliever Medication	-	-	-	100%
Received Systemic Corticosteroids	-	-	-	100%
Emergency Department				
Admittance Decision Time (minutes)[2]	127	34	66	98
Head CT Results Within 45 Min. of Arrival[1]	-	-	60%	57%
Patients Who Left ER Before Being Seen	6,852	1%	1%	2%
Time from ER Arrival to Admit. (minutes)[2]	270	156	217	274
Time from ER Arrival to Discharge (minutes)	392	101	123	134
Time in ER Before Being Evaluated (minutes)	417	22	17	26
Time to Pain Meds for Fractures (minutes)	40	44	43	57
Heart Attack Care				
Aspirin Given at Discharge[3,7]	-	-	99%	99%
Fibrinolytic Meds Within 30 Min. of Arrival[3,7]	-	-	100%	54%
PCI Within 90 Minutes of Arrival[3,7]	-	-	98%	96%
Statin Prescribed at Discharge[3,7]	-	-	100%	98%
Heart Failure Care				
ACE Inhibitor or ARB for LVSD[1]	-	-	98%	97%
Discharge Instructions Given[1]	-	-	96%	94%
Evaluation of LVS Function	12	92%	98%	99%
Medicare Spending				
Medicare Spending per Patient (ratio)	-	1.11	0.98	0.98
Pneumonia Care				
Appropriate Initial Antibiotic Given	29	86%	96%	95%
Blood Culture Timing	37	100%	99%	98%
Pregnancy and Delivery Care				
Newborn Deliveries Scheduled Early	36	0%	6%	6%
Preventive Care				
Immunization for Influenza[2]	250	97%	92%	90%
Immunization for Pneumonia[2]	236	88%	91%	92%
Stroke Care				
Anticoagulation Therapy for Atrial Fibrillation[1,3]	-	-	95%	95%
Antithrombotic Therapy Timing[1,3]	-	-	99%	98%
Assessed for Rehabilitation[1,3]	-	-	98%	97%
Discharged on Antithrombotic Therapy[1,3]	-	-	99%	99%
Discharged on Statin Medication[1,3]	-	-	96%	94%
Thrombolytic Therapy Timing[3,7]	-	-	89%	66%

NOTE: Hospital profiles are in alphabetical order by state, then city, then hospital within the city; Rankings exclude hospitals with less than 25 cases except for patient surveys which excludes hospitals with less than 100 cases; (a) 100-299 cases; (1) The number of cases/patients is too few to report; (2) Data submitted were based on a sample of cases/patients; (3) Results are based on a shorter time period than required; (4) Data suppressed by CMS for one or more quarters; (5) Results are not available for this reporting period; (6) Fewer than 100 patients completed the HCAHPS survey; (7) No cases met the criteria for this measure; (8) The lower limit of the confidence interval cannot be calculated if the number of observed infections equals zero; (9) No data are available from the state/territory for this reporting period; (10) The scores shown reflect fewer than 50 completed surveys; (11) There were discrepancies in the data collection process; (12) This measure does not apply to this hospital for this reporting period; (13) Results cannot be calculated for this reporting period; (14) The results for this state are combined with nearby states to protect confidentiality; Please refer to the User's Guide for a full explanation of data.

Venous Thromboembolism Prophylaxis[1,3]	-	-	95%	94%
Written Stroke Educational Materials Given[1,3]	-	-	89%	88%
Surgical Care Improvement Project				
Appropriate Beta Blocker Usage[1,2]	-	-	98%	98%
Appropriate VTP Within 24 Hours[2]	59	100%	99%	98%
Controlled Postoperative Blood Glucose[2,7]	-	-	97%	97%
Perioperative Temperature Management[2]	62	100%	100%	100%
Prophylactic Antibiotic Selection[2]	50	96%	99%	99%
Prophylactic Antibiotic Selection (Outpatient)[1]	-	-	98%	98%
Prophylactic Antibiotic Stopped[2]	50	96%	98%	98%
Prophylactic Antibiotic Timing[2]	50	100%	99%	99%
Prophylactic Antibiotic Timing (Outpatient)	11	91%	98%	98%
Urinary Catheter Removal[2]	37	100%	98%	97%
Survey of Patients' Hospital Experiences				
Area Around Room 'Always' Quiet at Night	(a)	64%	60%	61%
Doctors 'Always' Communicated Well	(a)	89%	83%	82%
Home Recovery Information Given	(a)	91%	90%	85%
Hospital Given 9 or 10 on 10 Point Scale	(a)	83%	74%	71%
Meds 'Always' Explained Before Given	(a)	80%	68%	64%
Nurses 'Always' Communicated Well	(a)	85%	79%	79%
Pain 'Always' Well Controlled	(a)	77%	73%	71%
Room and Bathroom 'Always' Clean	(a)	83%	74%	73%
Timely Help 'Always' Received	(a)	83%	69%	68%
Would Definitely Recommend Hospital	(a)	72%	76%	71%
Use of Medical Imaging				
Cardiac Imaging Stress Test before Surgery	67	3.0%	4.9%	5.3%
Combination Abdominal CT Scan	137	5.8%	4.9%	10.5%
Combination Brain/Sinus CT Scan[1]	-	-	3%	2.7%
Combination Chest CT Scan	63	3.2%	0.8%	2.7%
Follow-up Mammogram/Ultrasound	366	8.7%	8.5%	8.8%
Lumbar Spine MRI for Low Back Pain[1]	-	-	43.8%	37.2%

Riverton Hospital

3741 West 12600 South Phone: 801-285-4000
Riverton, UT 84065
URL: www.intermountainhealthcare.org
Type: Acute Care Hospitals Emergency Services: Yes
Ownership: Voluntary non-profit - Private
Key Personnel:
CEO .... Blair Kent

Measure	Cases	This Hosp.	State Avg.	U.S. Avg.
Blood Clot Prevention and Treatment				
Anticoagulation Overlap Therapy[2]	29	97%	95%	93%
ICU Venous Thromboembolism Prophylaxis[2]	24	92%	93%	92%
Incidence of Potentially Preventable VTE[1,2]	-	-	5%	10%
UFH with Dosages/Platelet Monitoring[1,2]	-	-	95%	97%
Venous Thromboembolism Prophylaxis[2]	112	94%	86%	85%
Warfarin Therapy Discharge Instructions[2]	24	92%	73%	75%
Chest Pain/Possible Heart Attack Care				
Aspirin Given Within 24 Hours of Arrival	65	100%	97%	96%
Fibrinolytic Meds Within 30 Min. of Arrival[1]	-	-	52%	58%
Average Time to ECG (minutes)	66	3	7	7
Average Time to Transfer (minutes)	17	28	36	60
Children's Asthma Care				
Received Home Management Plan of Care	-	-	-	88%
Received Reliever Medication	-	-	-	100%
Received Systemic Corticosteroids	-	-	-	100%
Emergency Department				
Admittance Decision Time (minutes)[2]	272	77	66	98
Head CT Results Within 45 Min. of Arrival[1]	-	-	60%	57%
Patients Who Left ER Before Being Seen	25,598	1%	1%	2%
Time from ER Arrival to Admit. (minutes)[2]	284	252	217	274
Time from ER Arrival to Discharge (minutes)	395	156	123	134
Time in ER Before Being Evaluated (minutes)	420	22	17	26
Time to Pain Meds for Fractures (minutes)	196	42	43	57
Heart Attack Care				
Aspirin Given at Discharge[5]	-	-	99%	99%
Fibrinolytic Meds Within 30 Min. of Arrival[5]	-	-	100%	54%
PCI Within 90 Minutes of Arrival[5]	-	-	98%	96%
Statin Prescribed at Discharge[5]	-	-	100%	98%
Heart Failure Care				
ACE Inhibitor or ARB for LVSD[1]	-	-	98%	97%
Discharge Instructions Given	23	100%	96%	94%
Evaluation of LVS Function	24	100%	98%	99%
Medicare Spending				
Medicare Spending per Patient (ratio)	-	0.93	0.98	0.98
Pneumonia Care				
Appropriate Initial Antibiotic Given	63	98%	96%	95%
Blood Culture Timing	53	100%	99%	98%
Pregnancy and Delivery Care				
Newborn Deliveries Scheduled Early[2]	66	5%	6%	6%
Preventive Care				
Immunization for Influenza[2]	407	94%	92%	90%
Immunization for Pneumonia[2]	176	94%	91%	92%
Stroke Care				
Anticoagulation Therapy for Atrial Fibrillation[7]	-	-	95%	95%
Antithrombotic Therapy Timing[1]	-	-	99%	98%
Assessed for Rehabilitation[7]	-	-	98%	97%
Discharged on Antithrombotic Therapy[7]	-	-	99%	99%
Discharged on Statin Medication[7]	-	-	96%	94%
Thrombolytic Therapy Timing[7]	-	-	89%	66%
Venous Thromboembolism Prophylaxis[1]	-	-	95%	94%
Written Stroke Educational Materials Given[7]	-	-	89%	88%
Surgical Care Improvement Project				
Appropriate Beta Blocker Usage[2]	32	97%	98%	98%
Appropriate VTP Within 24 Hours[2]	234	99%	99%	98%
Controlled Postoperative Blood Glucose[2,7]	-	-	97%	97%
Perioperative Temperature Management[2]	279	100%	100%	100%
Prophylactic Antibiotic Selection[2]	196	100%	99%	99%
Prophylactic Antibiotic Selection (Outpatient)	267	99%	98%	98%
Prophylactic Antibiotic Stopped[2]	193	98%	98%	98%
Prophylactic Antibiotic Timing[2]	196	100%	99%	99%
Prophylactic Antibiotic Timing (Outpatient)	269	99%	98%	98%
Urinary Catheter Removal[2]	155	100%	98%	97%
Survey of Patients' Hospital Experiences				
Area Around Room 'Always' Quiet at Night	300+	56%	60%	61%
Doctors 'Always' Communicated Well	300+	84%	83%	82%
Home Recovery Information Given	300+	90%	90%	85%
Hospital Given 9 or 10 on 10 Point Scale	300+	77%	74%	71%
Meds 'Always' Explained Before Given	300+	69%	68%	64%
Nurses 'Always' Communicated Well	300+	78%	79%	79%
Pain 'Always' Well Controlled	300+	72%	73%	71%
Room and Bathroom 'Always' Clean	300+	72%	74%	73%
Timely Help 'Always' Received	300+	63%	69%	68%
Would Definitely Recommend Hospital	300+	80%	76%	71%
Use of Medical Imaging				
Cardiac Imaging Stress Test before Surgery	113	4.4%	4.9%	5.3%
Combination Abdominal CT Scan	242	5.8%	4.9%	10.5%
Combination Brain/Sinus CT Scan[1]	-	-	3%	2.7%
Combination Chest CT Scan	54	0.0%	0.8%	2.7%
Follow-up Mammogram/Ultrasound	340	9.1%	8.5%	8.8%
Lumbar Spine MRI for Low Back Pain	43	39.5%	43.8%	37.2%

Uintah Basin Medical Center

250 West 300 North (75-2) Phone: 435-722-6163
Roosevelt, UT 84066 Fax: 435-722-9291
Type: Acute Care Hospitals Emergency Services: Yes
Ownership: Government - Local Beds: 49
Key Personnel:
Infection Control.............. Lisa Evans
Operating Room............. Aliesha Foster
Radiology................... Jason Kelly
CEO/President............... Jim Marshall
Quality Assurance .... Roger Pourton
Pediatric Ambulatory Care ...... Christie Thacker, MD
Pediatric In-Patient Care .... Christie Thacker, MD
Chief of Medical Staff.......... Gary White

Measure	Cases	This Hosp.	State Avg.	U.S. Avg.
Blood Clot Prevention and Treatment				
Anticoagulation Overlap Therapy[1,2]	-	-	95%	93%
ICU Venous Thromboembolism Prophylaxis[2]	17	53%	93%	92%
Incidence of Potentially Preventable VTE[2,7]	-	-	5%	10%
UFH with Dosages/Platelet Monitoring[1,2]	-	-	95%	97%
Venous Thromboembolism Prophylaxis[2]	68	66%	86%	85%
Warfarin Therapy Discharge Instructions[1,2]	-	-	73%	75%
Chest Pain/Possible Heart Attack Care				
Aspirin Given Within 24 Hours of Arrival	56	98%	97%	96%
Fibrinolytic Meds Within 30 Min. of Arrival	11	64%	52%	58%
Average Time to ECG (minutes)	59	8	7	7
Average Time to Transfer (minutes)[7]	-	-	36	60
Children's Asthma Care				
Received Home Management Plan of Care	-	-	-	88%
Received Reliever Medication	-	-	-	100%
Received Systemic Corticosteroids	-	-	-	100%
Emergency Department				
Admittance Decision Time (minutes)[2]	601	49	66	98
Head CT Results Within 45 Min. of Arrival[1,3]	-	-	60%	57%
Patients Who Left ER Before Being Seen	10,708	1%	1%	2%
Time from ER Arrival to Admit. (minutes)[2]	602	180	217	274
Time from ER Arrival to Discharge (minutes)	384	86	123	134
Time in ER Before Being Evaluated (minutes)	401	20	17	26
Time to Pain Meds for Fractures (minutes)	63	43	43	57
Heart Attack Care				
Aspirin Given at Discharge[5]	-	-	99%	99%
Fibrinolytic Meds Within 30 Min. of Arrival[5]	-	-	100%	54%
PCI Within 90 Minutes of Arrival[5]	-	-	98%	96%
Statin Prescribed at Discharge[5]	-	-	100%	98%
Heart Failure Care				
ACE Inhibitor or ARB for LVSD[1]	-	-	98%	97%
Discharge Instructions Given	24	58%	96%	94%
Evaluation of LVS Function	28	71%	98%	99%
Medicare Spending				
Medicare Spending per Patient (ratio)	-	0.85	0.98	0.98
Pneumonia Care				
Appropriate Initial Antibiotic Given	30	83%	96%	95%
Blood Culture Timing	36	94%	99%	98%
Pregnancy and Delivery Care				
Newborn Deliveries Scheduled Early	48	0%	6%	6%
Preventive Care				
Immunization for Influenza[2]	287	75%	92%	90%
Immunization for Pneumonia[2]	339	81%	91%	92%
Stroke Care				
Anticoagulation Therapy for Atrial Fibrillation[5]	-	-	95%	95%
Antithrombotic Therapy Timing[5]	-	-	99%	98%
Assessed for Rehabilitation[5]	-	-	98%	97%
Discharged on Antithrombotic Therapy[5]	-	-	99%	99%
Discharged on Statin Medication[5]	-	-	96%	94%
Thrombolytic Therapy Timing[5]	-	-	89%	66%
Venous Thromboembolism Prophylaxis[5]	-	-	95%	94%
Written Stroke Educational Materials Given[5]	-	-	89%	88%
Surgical Care Improvement Project				
Appropriate Beta Blocker Usage[1,2]	-	-	98%	98%
Appropriate VTP Within 24 Hours[2]	90	94%	99%	98%
Controlled Postoperative Blood Glucose[2,7]	-	-	97%	97%
Perioperative Temperature Management[2]	127	94%	100%	100%
Prophylactic Antibiotic Selection[2]	113	98%	99%	99%
Prophylactic Antibiotic Selection (Outpatient)[5]	-	-	98%	98%
Prophylactic Antibiotic Stopped[2]	109	89%	98%	98%
Prophylactic Antibiotic Timing[2]	113	92%	99%	99%
Prophylactic Antibiotic Timing (Outpatient)[5]	-	-	98%	98%
Urinary Catheter Removal[2]	37	97%	98%	97%
Survey of Patients' Hospital Experiences				
Area Around Room 'Always' Quiet at Night	(a)	58%	60%	61%
Doctors 'Always' Communicated Well	(a)	77%	83%	82%
Home Recovery Information Given	(a)	81%	90%	85%
Hospital Given 9 or 10 on 10 Point Scale	(a)	64%	74%	71%
Meds 'Always' Explained Before Given	(a)	60%	68%	64%
Nurses 'Always' Communicated Well	(a)	75%	79%	79%
Pain 'Always' Well Controlled	(a)	65%	73%	71%
Room and Bathroom 'Always' Clean	(a)	68%	74%	73%
Timely Help 'Always' Received	(a)	65%	69%	68%
Would Definitely Recommend Hospital	(a)	68%	76%	71%
Use of Medical Imaging				
Cardiac Imaging Stress Test before Surgery	88	3.4%	4.9%	5.3%
Combination Abdominal CT Scan	149	1.3%	4.9%	10.5%
Combination Brain/Sinus CT Scan[1]	-	-	3%	2.7%
Combination Chest CT Scan[1]	-	-	0.8%	2.7%
Follow-up Mammogram/Ultrasound	188	5.3%	8.5%	8.8%
Lumbar Spine MRI for Low Back Pain[1]	-	-	43.8%	37.2%

NOTE: Hospital profiles are in alphabetical order by state, then city, then hospital within the city; Rankings exclude hospitals with less than 25 cases except for patient surveys which excludes hospitals with less than 100 cases; (a) 100-299 cases; (1) The number of cases/patients is too few to report; (2) Data submitted were based on a sample of cases/patients; (3) Results are based on a shorter time period than required; (4) Data suppressed by CMS for one or more quarters; (5) Results are not available for this reporting period; (6) Fewer than 100 patients completed the HCAHPS survey; (7) No cases met the criteria for this measure; (8) The lower limit of the confidence interval cannot be calculated if the number of observed infections equals zero; (9) No data are available from the state/territory for this reporting period; (10) The scores shown reflect fewer than 50 completed surveys; (11) There were discrepancies in the data collection process; (12) This measure does not apply to this hospital for this reporting period; (13) Results cannot be calculated for this reporting period; (14) The results for this state are combined with nearby states to protect confidentiality; Please refer to the User's Guide for a full explanation of data.

Dixie Regional Medical Center

1380 East Medical Center Drive Phone: 435-251-2100
Saint George, UT 84790 Fax: 435-688-4002
E-mail: dxllinds@ihc.com
URL: www.intermountainhealthcare.org
Type: Acute Care Hospitals Emergency Services: Yes
Ownership: Voluntary non-profit - Private Beds: 245

Key Personnel:
Patient Relations . . . . Kathy Andrus, RN
Radiology. . . . . Blake W Arnold
Anesthesiology. . . . . Eric Evans, MD
Chief of Medical Staff . . . . Jerry Hagen, MD
Intensive Care Unit. . . . . Vickie Howley, RN
Operating Room. . . . . Ryan L Lewis, RN
Infection Control. . . . . Linda Rider, RN
Emergency Room . . . . Steve Van Norman, MD

Measure	Cases	This Hosp.	State Avg.	U.S. Avg.
Blood Clot Prevention and Treatment				
Anticoagulation Overlap Therapy[2]	139	99%	95%	93%
ICU Venous Thromboembolism Prophylaxis[2]	70	93%	93%	92%
Incidence of Potentially Preventable VTE[1,2]	-	-	5%	10%
UFH with Dosages/Platelet Monitoring[2]	143	100%	95%	97%
Venous Thromboembolism Prophylaxis[2]	274	84%	86%	85%
Warfarin Therapy Discharge Instructions[2]	116	26%	73%	75%
Chest Pain/Possible Heart Attack Care				
Aspirin Given Within 24 Hours of Arrival[3,7]	-	-	97%	96%
Fibrinolytic Meds Within 30 Min. of Arrival[5]	-	-	52%	58%
Average Time to ECG (minutes)[1,3]	-	-	7	7
Average Time to Transfer (minutes)[5]	-	-	36	60
Children's Asthma Care				
Received Home Management Plan of Care	-	-	-	88%
Received Reliever Medication	-	-	-	100%
Received Systemic Corticosteroids	-	-	-	100%
Emergency Department				
Admittance Decision Time (minutes)[2]	510	63	66	98
Head CT Results Within 45 Min. of Arrival[1]	-	-	60%	57%
Patients Who Left ER Before Being Seen	42,809	1%	1%	2%
Time from ER Arrival to Admit. (minutes)[2]	518	205	217	274
Time from ER Arrival to Discharge (minutes)'	387	130	123	134
Time in ER Before Being Evaluated (minutes)	420	22	17	26
Time to Pain Meds for Fractures (minutes)	198	53	43	57
Heart Attack Care				
Aspirin Given at Discharge	360	99%	99%	99%
Fibrinolytic Meds Within 30 Min. of Arrival[7]	-	-	100%	54%
PCI Within 90 Minutes of Arrival	50	90%	98%	96%
Statin Prescribed at Discharge	340	99%	100%	98%
Heart Failure Care				
ACE Inhibitor or ARB for LVSD	46	96%	98%	97%
Discharge Instructions Given	189	99%	96%	94%
Evaluation of LVS Function	233	100%	98%	99%
Medicare Spending				
Medicare Spending per Patient (ratio)	-	0.93	0.98	0.98
Pneumonia Care				
Appropriate Initial Antibiotic Given[2]	87	95%	96%	95%
Blood Culture Timing[2]	116	100%	99%	98%
Pregnancy and Delivery Care				
Newborn Deliveries Scheduled Early[2]	80	1%	6%	6%
Preventive Care				
Immunization for Influenza[2]	535	98%	92%	90%
Immunization for Pneumonia[2]	629	93%	91%	92%
Stroke Care				
Anticoagulation Therapy for Atrial Fibrillation	32	100%	95%	95%
Antithrombotic Therapy Timing	112	99%	99%	98%
Assessed for Rehabilitation	160	99%	98%	97%
Discharged on Antithrombotic Therapy	150	99%	99%	99%
Discharged on Statin Medication	117	97%	96%	94%
Thrombolytic Therapy Timing[1]	-	-	89%	66%
Venous Thromboembolism Prophylaxis	122	98%	95%	94%
Written Stroke Educational Materials Given	91	96%	89%	88%
Surgical Care Improvement Project				
Appropriate Beta Blocker Usage[2]	247	98%	98%	98%
Appropriate VTP Within 24 Hours[2]	403	100%	99%	98%
Controlled Postoperative Blood Glucose[2]	183	99%	97%	97%
Perioperative Temperature Management[2]	492	100%	100%	100%
Prophylactic Antibiotic Selection[2]	497	99%	99%	99%
Prophylactic Antibiotic Selection (Outpatient)	467	99%	98%	98%
Prophylactic Antibiotic Stopped[2]	482	99%	98%	98%
Prophylactic Antibiotic Timing[2]	497	100%	99%	99%
Prophylactic Antibiotic Timing (Outpatient)	468	98%	98%	98%
Urinary Catheter Removal[2]	369	96%	98%	97%
Survey of Patients' Hospital Experiences				
Area Around Room 'Always' Quiet at Night	300+	59%	60%	61%
Doctors 'Always' Communicated Well	300+	84%	83%	82%
Home Recovery Information Given	300+	91%	90%	85%
Hospital Given 9 or 10 on 10 Point Scale	300+	79%	74%	71%
Meds 'Always' Explained Before Given	300+	74%	68%	64%
Nurses 'Always' Communicated Well	300+	80%	79%	79%
Pain 'Always' Well Controlled	300+	75%	73%	71%
Room and Bathroom 'Always' Clean	300+	75%	74%	73%
Timely Help 'Always' Received	300+	70%	69%	68%
Would Definitely Recommend Hospital	300+	84%	76%	71%
Use of Medical Imaging				
Cardiac Imaging Stress Test before Surgery	687	5.4%	4.9%	5.3%
Combination Abdominal CT Scan	1,458	8.4%	4.9%	10.5%
Combination Brain/Sinus CT Scan	828	3.6%	3%	2.7%
Combination Chest CT Scan	841	0.5%	0.8%	2.7%
Follow-up Mammogram/Ultrasound	3,472	6.0%	8.5%	8.8%
Lumbar Spine MRI for Low Back Pain	442	41.4%	43.8%	37.2%

LDS Hospital

8th Avenue & C Street Phone: 801-408-1100
Salt Lake City, UT 84143 Fax: 801-408-1663
URL: www.intermountainhealthcare.org
Type: Acute Care Hospitals Emergency Services: Yes
Ownership: Voluntary non-profit - Private Beds: 520

Key Personnel:
Operating Room. . . . . Dusty Clegg, RN
CEO/President. . . . . Mikelle D Moore
Quality Assurance . . . . Kendell Nelson
Administrator . . . . Jim Sheets

Measure	Cases	This Hosp.	State Avg.	U.S. Avg.
Blood Clot Prevention and Treatment				
Anticoagulation Overlap Therapy[2]	56	89%	95%	93%
ICU Venous Thromboembolism Prophylaxis[2]	58	90%	93%	92%
Incidence of Potentially Preventable VTE[1,2]	-	-	5%	10%
UFH with Dosages/Platelet Monitoring[2]	23	57%	95%	97%
Venous Thromboembolism Prophylaxis[2]	271	82%	86%	85%
Warfarin Therapy Discharge Instructions[2]	53	30%	73%	75%
Chest Pain/Possible Heart Attack Care				
Aspirin Given Within 24 Hours of Arrival	39	92%	97%	96%
Fibrinolytic Meds Within 30 Min. of Arrival[7]	-	-	52%	58%
Average Time to ECG (minutes)	37	8	7	7
Average Time to Transfer (minutes)	11	30	36	60
Children's Asthma Care				
Received Home Management Plan of Care	-	-	-	88%
Received Reliever Medication	-	-	-	100%
Received Systemic Corticosteroids	-	-	-	100%
Emergency Department				
Admittance Decision Time (minutes)[2]	288	77	66	98
Head CT Results Within 45 Min. of Arrival[1]	-	-	60%	57%
Patients Who Left ER Before Being Seen	24,082	1%	1%	2%
Time from ER Arrival to Admit. (minutes)[2]	294	248	217	274
Time from ER Arrival to Discharge (minutes)	374	156	123	134
Time in ER Before Being Evaluated (minutes)	411	20	17	26
Time to Pain Meds for Fractures (minutes)	57	43	43	57
Heart Attack Care				
Aspirin Given at Discharge[3,7]	-	-	99%	99%
Fibrinolytic Meds Within 30 Min. of Arrival[3,7]	-	-	100%	54%
PCI Within 90 Minutes of Arrival[3,7]	-	-	98%	96%
Statin Prescribed at Discharge[3,7]	-	-	100%	98%
Heart Failure Care				
ACE Inhibitor or ARB for LVSD	12	100%	98%	97%
Discharge Instructions Given	52	98%	96%	94%
Evaluation of LVS Function	61	100%	98%	99%
Medicare Spending				
Medicare Spending per Patient (ratio)	-	0.96	0.98	0.98
Pneumonia Care				
Appropriate Initial Antibiotic Given[2]	115	98%	96%	95%
Blood Culture Timing[2]	131	100%	99%	98%
Pregnancy and Delivery Care				
Newborn Deliveries Scheduled Early[2]	58	7%	6%	6%
Preventive Care				
Immunization for Influenza[2]	468	93%	92%	90%
Immunization for Pneumonia[2]	371	84%	91%	92%
Stroke Care				
Anticoagulation Therapy for Atrial Fibrillation[1]	-	-	95%	95%
Antithrombotic Therapy Timing	12	100%	99%	98%
Assessed for Rehabilitation	18	100%	98%	97%
Discharged on Antithrombotic Therapy	18	100%	99%	99%
Discharged on Statin Medication	14	100%	96%	94%
Thrombolytic Therapy Timing[7]	-	-	89%	66%
Venous Thromboembolism Prophylaxis	12	92%	95%	94%
Written Stroke Educational Materials Given[1]	-	-	89%	88%
Surgical Care Improvement Project				
Appropriate Beta Blocker Usage[2]	61	98%	98%	98%
Appropriate VTP Within 24 Hours[2]	371	98%	99%	98%
Controlled Postoperative Blood Glucose[2,7]	-	-	97%	97%
Perioperative Temperature Management[2]	508	100%	100%	100%
Prophylactic Antibiotic Selection[2]	312	100%	99%	99%
Prophylactic Antibiotic Selection (Outpatient)	379	99%	98%	98%
Prophylactic Antibiotic Stopped[2]	308	97%	98%	98%
Prophylactic Antibiotic Timing[2]	312	98%	99%	99%
Prophylactic Antibiotic Timing (Outpatient)	379	99%	98%	98%
Urinary Catheter Removal[2]	73	96%	98%	97%
Survey of Patients' Hospital Experiences				
Area Around Room 'Always' Quiet at Night	300+	60%	60%	61%
Doctors 'Always' Communicated Well	300+	83%	83%	82%
Home Recovery Information Given	300+	90%	90%	85%
Hospital Given 9 or 10 on 10 Point Scale	300+	77%	74%	71%
Meds 'Always' Explained Before Given	300+	70%	68%	64%
Nurses 'Always' Communicated Well	300+	80%	79%	79%
Pain 'Always' Well Controlled	300+	77%	73%	71%
Room and Bathroom 'Always' Clean	300+	74%	74%	73%
Timely Help 'Always' Received	300+	69%	69%	68%
Would Definitely Recommend Hospital	300+	81%	76%	71%
Use of Medical Imaging				
Cardiac Imaging Stress Test before Surgery	155	4.5%	4.9%	5.3%
Combination Abdominal CT Scan	372	4.6%	4.9%	10.5%
Combination Brain/Sinus CT Scan[1]	-	-	3%	2.7%
Combination Chest CT Scan	181	0.6%	0.8%	2.7%
Follow-up Mammogram/Ultrasound	853	9.7%	8.5%	8.8%
Lumbar Spine MRI for Low Back Pain	61	54.1%	43.8%	37.2%

Primary Childrens Hospital

100 North Mario Capecchi Drive Phone: 801-662-6200
Salt Lake City, UT 84113 Fax: 801-662-6247
Type: Childrens Emergency Services: Yes
Ownership: Voluntary non-profit - Private Beds: 232

Key Personnel:
Quality Assurance . . . . Susan Adams
Radiology. . . . . William C Andolsek
Chief of Medical Staff . . . . Richard F Black, MD
Infection Control. . . . . John Christianson, MD
Pediatric Ambulatory Care . . . . . . Edward Clark
Pediatric In-Patient Care . . . . Edward Clark
Operating Room. . . . . Sally McQueen
CEO/President. . . . . Joseph Mott

Measure	Cases	This Hosp.	State Avg.	U.S. Avg.
Blood Clot Prevention and Treatment				
Anticoagulation Overlap Therapy[5]	-	-	95%	93%
ICU Venous Thromboembolism Prophylaxis[5]	-	-	93%	92%
Incidence of Potentially Preventable VTE[5]	-	-	5%	10%
UFH with Dosages/Platelet Monitoring[5]	-	-	95%	97%
Venous Thromboembolism Prophylaxis[5]	-	-	86%	85%
Warfarin Therapy Discharge Instructions[5]	-	-	73%	75%
Chest Pain/Possible Heart Attack Care				
Aspirin Given Within 24 Hours of Arrival	-	-	97%	96%
Fibrinolytic Meds Within 30 Min. of Arrival	-	-	52%	58%
Average Time to ECG (minutes)	-	-	7	7
Average Time to Transfer (minutes)	-	-	36	60
Children's Asthma Care				

NOTE: Hospital profiles are in alphabetical order by state, then city, then hospital within the city; Rankings exclude hospitals with less than 25 cases except for patient surveys which excludes hospitals with less than 100 cases; (a) 100-299 cases; (1) The number of cases/patients is too few to report; (2) Data submitted were based on a sample of cases/patients; (3) Results are based on a shorter time period than required; (4) Data suppressed by CMS for one or more quarters; (5) Results are not available for this reporting period; (6) Fewer than 100 patients completed the HCAHPS survey; (7) No cases met the criteria for this measure; (8) The lower limit of the confidence interval cannot be calculated if the number of observed infections equals zero; (9) No data are available from the state/territory for this reporting period; (10) The scores shown reflect fewer than 50 completed surveys; (11) There were discrepancies in the data collection process; (12) This measure does not apply to this hospital for this reporting period; (13) Results cannot be calculated for this reporting period; (14) The results for this state are combined with nearby states to protect confidentiality; Please refer to the User's Guide for a full explanation of data.

Measure	Cases	This Hosp.	State Avg.	U.S. Avg.
Received Home Management Plan of Care	410	96%	-	88%
Received Reliever Medication	411	100%	-	100%
Received Systemic Corticosteroids	410	100%	-	100%
Emergency Department				
Admittance Decision Time (minutes)[5]	-	-	66	98
Head CT Results Within 45 Min. of Arrival	-	-	60%	57%
Patients Who Left ER Before Being Seen	-	-	1%	2%
Time from ER Arrival to Admit. (minutes)[5]	-	-	217	274
Time from ER Arrival to Discharge (minutes)	-	-	123	134
Time in ER Before Being Evaluated (minutes)	-	-	17	26
Time to Pain Meds for Fractures (minutes)	-	-	43	57
Heart Attack Care				
Aspirin Given at Discharge[5]	-	-	99%	99%
Fibrinolytic Meds Within 30 Min. of Arrival[5]	-	-	100%	54%
PCI Within 90 Minutes of Arrival[5]	-	-	98%	96%
Statin Prescribed at Discharge[5]	-	-	100%	98%
Heart Failure Care				
ACE Inhibitor or ARB for LVSD[5]	-	-	98%	97%
Discharge Instructions Given[5]	-	-	96%	94%
Evaluation of LVS Function[5]	-	-	98%	99%
Medicare Spending				
Medicare Spending per Patient (ratio)	-	-	0.98	0.98
Pneumonia Care				
Appropriate Initial Antibiotic Given[5]	-	-	96%	95%
Blood Culture Timing[5]	-	-	99%	98%
Pregnancy and Delivery Care				
Newborn Deliveries Scheduled Early[5]	-	-	6%	6%
Preventive Care				
Immunization for Influenza[5]	-	-	92%	90%
Immunization for Pneumonia[5]	-	-	91%	92%
Stroke Care				
Anticoagulation Therapy for Atrial Fibrillation[5]	-	-	95%	95%
Antithrombotic Therapy Timing[5]	-	-	99%	98%
Assessed for Rehabilitation[5]	-	-	98%	97%
Discharged on Antithrombotic Therapy[5]	-	-	99%	99%
Discharged on Statin Medication[5]	-	-	96%	94%
Thrombolytic Therapy Timing[5]	-	-	89%	66%
Venous Thromboembolism Prophylaxis[5]	-	-	95%	94%
Written Stroke Educational Materials Given[5]	-	-	89%	88%
Surgical Care Improvement Project				
Appropriate Beta Blocker Usage[5]	-	-	98%	98%
Appropriate VTP Within 24 Hours[5]	-	-	99%	98%
Controlled Postoperative Blood Glucose[5]	-	-	97%	97%
Perioperative Temperature Management[5]	-	-	100%	100%
Prophylactic Antibiotic Selection[5]	-	-	99%	99%
Prophylactic Antibiotic Selection (Outpatient)	-	-	98%	98%
Prophylactic Antibiotic Stopped[5]	-	-	98%	98%
Prophylactic Antibiotic Timing[5]	-	-	99%	99%
Prophylactic Antibiotic Timing (Outpatient)	-	-	98%	98%
Urinary Catheter Removal[5]	-	-	98%	97%
Survey of Patients' Hospital Experiences				
Area Around Room 'Always' Quiet at Night[5]	-	-	60%	61%
Doctors 'Always' Communicated Well[5]	-	-	83%	82%
Home Recovery Information Given[5]	-	-	90%	85%
Hospital Given 9 or 10 on 10 Point Scale[5]	-	-	74%	71%
Meds 'Always' Explained Before Given[5]	-	-	68%	64%
Nurses 'Always' Communicated Well[5]	-	-	79%	79%
Pain 'Always' Well Controlled[5]	-	-	73%	71%
Room and Bathroom 'Always' Clean[5]	-	-	74%	73%
Timely Help 'Always' Received[5]	-	-	69%	68%
Would Definitely Recommend Hospital[5]	-	-	76%	71%
Use of Medical Imaging				
Cardiac Imaging Stress Test before Surgery	-	-	4.9%	5.3%
Combination Abdominal CT Scan	-	-	4.9%	10.5%
Combination Brain/Sinus CT Scan	-	-	3%	2.7%
Combination Chest CT Scan	-	-	0.8%	2.7%
Follow-up Mammogram/Ultrasound	-	-	8.5%	8.8%
Lumbar Spine MRI for Low Back Pain	-	-	43.8%	37.2%

Saint Marks Hospital

1200 East 3900 South
Salt Lake City, UT 84124
URL: www.stmarkshospital.com
Type: Acute Care Hospitals
Ownership: Proprietary
Phone: 801-268-7700
Fax: 801-270-3353
Emergency Services: Yes
Beds: 317

Key Personnel:
Operating Room. . . . . Phyllis Abbott
Coronary Care. . . . . CJ Cooper
Infection Control. . . . . Lorie Gilette
CEO/President. . . . . John Hanshaw
Radiology. . . . . Craig Pendleton
Quality Assurance . . . . Louise Swensen

Measure	Cases	This Hosp.	State Avg.	U.S. Avg.
Blood Clot Prevention and Treatment				
Anticoagulation Overlap Therapy[2]	187	99%	95%	93%
ICU Venous Thromboembolism Prophylaxis[2]	80	99%	93%	92%
Incidence of Potentially Preventable VTE[2]	26	0%	5%	10%
UFH with Dosages/Platelet Monitoring[2]	52	100%	95%	97%
Venous Thromboembolism Prophylaxis[2]	289	97%	86%	85%
Warfarin Therapy Discharge Instructions[2]	131	98%	73%	75%
Chest Pain/Possible Heart Attack Care				
Aspirin Given Within 24 Hours of Arrival[1,3]	-	-	97%	96%
Fibrinolytic Meds Within 30 Min. of Arrival[5]	-	-	52%	58%
Average Time to ECG (minutes)[1,3]	-	-	7	7
Average Time to Transfer (minutes)[5]	-	-	36	60
Children's Asthma Care				
Received Home Management Plan of Care	-	-	-	88%
Received Reliever Medication	-	-	-	100%
Received Systemic Corticosteroids	-	-	-	100%
Emergency Department				
Admittance Decision Time (minutes)[2]	488	94	66	98
Head CT Results Within 45 Min. of Arrival[1]	-	-	60%	57%
Patients Who Left ER Before Being Seen	49,893	0%	1%	2%
Time from ER Arrival to Admit. (minutes)[2]	492	245	217	274
Time from ER Arrival to Discharge (minutes)	498	146	123	134
Time in ER Before Being Evaluated (minutes)	543	14	17	26
Time to Pain Meds for Fractures (minutes)	146	50	43	57
Heart Attack Care				
Aspirin Given at Discharge	183	99%	99%	99%
Fibrinolytic Meds Within 30 Min. of Arrival[7]	-	-	100%	54%
PCI Within 90 Minutes of Arrival	34	100%	98%	96%
Statin Prescribed at Discharge	170	99%	100%	98%
Heart Failure Care				
ACE Inhibitor or ARB for LVSD	102	100%	98%	97%
Discharge Instructions Given	223	100%	96%	94%
Evaluation of LVS Function	296	100%	98%	99%
Medicare Spending				
Medicare Spending per Patient (ratio)	-	1.04	0.98	0.98
Pneumonia Care				
Appropriate Initial Antibiotic Given[2]	113	96%	96%	95%
Blood Culture Timing[2]	154	98%	99%	98%
Pregnancy and Delivery Care				
Newborn Deliveries Scheduled Early[2]	66	6%	6%	6%
Preventive Care				
Immunization for Influenza[2]	572	93%	92%	90%
Immunization for Pneumonia[2]	630	95%	91%	92%
Stroke Care				
Anticoagulation Therapy for Atrial Fibrillation[2]	25	96%	95%	95%
Antithrombotic Therapy Timing[2]	65	100%	99%	98%
Assessed for Rehabilitation[2]	100	100%	98%	97%
Discharged on Antithrombotic Therapy[2]	93	100%	99%	99%
Discharged on Statin Medication[2]	69	99%	96%	94%
Thrombolytic Therapy Timing[1,2]	-	-	89%	66%
Venous Thromboembolism Prophylaxis[2]	86	100%	95%	94%
Written Stroke Educational Materials Given[2]	48	96%	89%	88%
Surgical Care Improvement Project				
Appropriate Beta Blocker Usage[2]	185	98%	98%	98%
Appropriate VTP Within 24 Hours[2]	511	99%	99%	98%
Controlled Postoperative Blood Glucose[2]	158	99%	97%	97%
Perioperative Temperature Management[2]	661	100%	100%	100%
Prophylactic Antibiotic Selection[2]	569	99%	99%	99%
Prophylactic Antibiotic Selection (Outpatient)	560	97%	98%	98%
Prophylactic Antibiotic Stopped[2]	553	99%	98%	98%
Prophylactic Antibiotic Timing[2]	571	99%	99%	99%
Prophylactic Antibiotic Timing (Outpatient)	562	99%	98%	98%
Urinary Catheter Removal[2]	464	97%	98%	97%
Survey of Patients' Hospital Experiences				
Area Around Room 'Always' Quiet at Night	300+	53%	60%	61%
Doctors 'Always' Communicated Well	300+	77%	83%	82%
Home Recovery Information Given	300+	86%	90%	85%
Hospital Given 9 or 10 on 10 Point Scale	300+	66%	74%	71%
Meds 'Always' Explained Before Given	300+	54%	68%	64%
Nurses 'Always' Communicated Well	300+	69%	79%	79%
Pain 'Always' Well Controlled	300+	67%	73%	71%
Room and Bathroom 'Always' Clean	300+	66%	74%	73%
Timely Help 'Always' Received	300+	56%	69%	68%
Would Definitely Recommend Hospital	300+	68%	76%	71%
Use of Medical Imaging				
Cardiac Imaging Stress Test before Surgery	576	4.7%	4.9%	5.3%
Combination Abdominal CT Scan	871	3.3%	4.9%	10.5%
Combination Brain/Sinus CT Scan	608	3.1%	3%	2.7%
Combination Chest CT Scan	243	0.4%	0.8%	2.7%
Follow-up Mammogram/Ultrasound	2,040	6.0%	8.5%	8.8%
Lumbar Spine MRI for Low Back Pain	131	51.1%	43.8%	37.2%

Salt Lake Regional Medical Center

1050 East South Temple
Salt Lake City, UT 84102
E-mail: saltlakeregional@iasishealthcare.com
URL: www.saltlakeregional.com
Type: Acute Care Hospitals
Ownership: Proprietary
Phone: 801-350-4111
Fax: 801-350-4323
Emergency Services: Yes
Beds: 200

Key Personnel:
Radiology. . . . . W Robert Brinton, MD
CEO/President. . . . . Brian E Dunn
Cardiac Laboratory. . . . . Sarah Evans
Infection Control. . . . . Chris Martin
Chief of Medical Staff. . . . . Kevin McKuster, MD
Quality Assurance . . . . Sara Phillips
Patient Relations . . . . Linda Wright

Measure	Cases	This Hosp.	State Avg.	U.S. Avg.
Blood Clot Prevention and Treatment				
Anticoagulation Overlap Therapy[2]	16	100%	95%	93%
ICU Venous Thromboembolism Prophylaxis[2]	76	88%	93%	92%
Incidence of Potentially Preventable VTE[1,2]	-	-	5%	10%
UFH with Dosages/Platelet Monitoring[1,2]	-	-	95%	97%
Venous Thromboembolism Prophylaxis[2]	150	91%	86%	85%
Warfarin Therapy Discharge Instructions[2]	11	91%	73%	75%
Chest Pain/Possible Heart Attack Care				
Aspirin Given Within 24 Hours of Arrival[5]	-	-	97%	96%
Fibrinolytic Meds Within 30 Min. of Arrival[5]	-	-	52%	58%
Average Time to ECG (minutes)[5]	-	-	7	7
Average Time to Transfer (minutes)[5]	-	-	36	60
Children's Asthma Care				
Received Home Management Plan of Care	-	-	-	88%
Received Reliever Medication	-	-	-	100%
Received Systemic Corticosteroids	-	-	-	100%
Emergency Department				
Admittance Decision Time (minutes)[2]	166	150	66	98
Head CT Results Within 45 Min. of Arrival[1,3]	-	-	60%	57%
Patients Who Left ER Before Being Seen	10,789	1%	1%	2%
Time from ER Arrival to Admit. (minutes)[2]	178	312	217	274
Time from ER Arrival to Discharge (minutes)	402	140	123	134
Time in ER Before Being Evaluated (minutes)	441	41	17	26
Time to Pain Meds for Fractures (minutes)	18	48	43	57
Heart Attack Care				
Aspirin Given at Discharge	65	100%	99%	99%
Fibrinolytic Meds Within 30 Min. of Arrival[7]	-	-	100%	54%
PCI Within 90 Minutes of Arrival[1]	-	-	98%	96%
Statin Prescribed at Discharge	65	100%	100%	98%
Heart Failure Care				
ACE Inhibitor or ARB for LVSD	22	100%	98%	97%
Discharge Instructions Given	52	98%	96%	94%
Evaluation of LVS Function	70	100%	98%	99%
Medicare Spending				
Medicare Spending per Patient (ratio)	-	1.09	0.98	0.98
Pneumonia Care				

NOTE: *Hospital profiles are in alphabetical order by state, then city, then hospital within the city; Rankings exclude hospitals with less than 25 cases except for patient surveys which excludes hospitals with less than 100 cases; (a) 100-299 cases; (1) The number of cases/patients is too few to report; (2) Data submitted were based on a sample of cases/patients; (3) Results are based on a shorter time period than required; (4) Data suppressed by CMS for one or more quarters; (5) Results are not available for this reporting period; (6) Fewer than 100 patients completed the HCAHPS survey; (7) No cases met the criteria for this measure; (8) The lower limit of the confidence interval cannot be calculated if the number of observed infections equals zero; (9) No data are available from the state/territory for this reporting period; (10) The scores shown reflect fewer than 50 completed surveys; (11) There were discrepancies in the data collection process; (12) This measure does not apply to this hospital for this reporting period; (13) Results cannot be calculated for this reporting period; (14) The results for this state are combined with nearby states to protect confidentiality; Please refer to the User's Guide for a full explanation of data.*

Measure	Cases	This Hosp.	State Avg.	U.S. Avg.
Appropriate Initial Antibiotic Given	35	97%	96%	95%
Blood Culture Timing	46	98%	99%	98%
Pregnancy and Delivery Care				
Newborn Deliveries Scheduled Early[2]	39	31%	6%	6%
Preventive Care				
Immunization for Influenza[2]	329	98%	92%	90%
Immunization for Pneumonia[2]	369	98%	91%	92%
Stroke Care				
Anticoagulation Therapy for Atrial Fibrillation[7]	-	-	95%	95%
Antithrombotic Therapy Timing[1]	-	-	99%	98%
Assessed for Rehabilitation[1]	-	-	98%	97%
Discharged on Antithrombotic Therapy[1]	-	-	99%	99%
Discharged on Statin Medication[1]	-	-	96%	94%
Thrombolytic Therapy Timing[7]	-	-	89%	66%
Venous Thromboembolism Prophylaxis	11	91%	95%	94%
Written Stroke Educational Materials Given[1]	-	-	89%	88%
Surgical Care Improvement Project				
Appropriate Beta Blocker Usage	181	98%	98%	98%
Appropriate VTP Within 24 Hours	768	99%	99%	98%
Controlled Postoperative Blood Glucose	79	95%	97%	97%
Perioperative Temperature Management	851	100%	100%	100%
Prophylactic Antibiotic Selection	524	100%	99%	99%
Prophylactic Antibiotic Selection (Outpatient)	277	98%	98%	98%
Prophylactic Antibiotic Stopped	517	100%	98%	98%
Prophylactic Antibiotic Timing	525	100%	99%	99%
Prophylactic Antibiotic Timing (Outpatient)	277	100%	98%	98%
Urinary Catheter Removal	52	100%	98%	97%
Survey of Patients' Hospital Experiences				
Area Around Room 'Always' Quiet at Night	300+	59%	60%	61%
Doctors 'Always' Communicated Well	300+	82%	83%	82%
Home Recovery Information Given	300+	89%	90%	85%
Hospital Given 9 or 10 on 10 Point Scale	300+	68%	74%	71%
Meds 'Always' Explained Before Given	300+	63%	68%	64%
Nurses 'Always' Communicated Well	300+	74%	79%	79%
Pain 'Always' Well Controlled	300+	67%	73%	71%
Room and Bathroom 'Always' Clean	300+	72%	74%	73%
Timely Help 'Always' Received	300+	63%	69%	68%
Would Definitely Recommend Hospital	300+	69%	76%	71%
Use of Medical Imaging				
Cardiac Imaging Stress Test before Surgery	167	7.8%	4.9%	5.3%
Combination Abdominal CT Scan	181	5.5%	4.9%	10.5%
Combination Brain/Sinus CT Scan[1]	-	-	3%	2.7%
Combination Chest CT Scan[1]	-	-	0.8%	2.7%
Follow-up Mammogram/Ultrasound	473	11.2%	8.5%	8.8%
Lumbar Spine MRI for Low Back Pain	48	47.9%	43.8%	37.2%

University Health Care/University Hospitals & Clinics

50 North Medical Drive Phone: 801-581-2121
Salt Lake City, UT 84132
URL: www.healthcare.utah.edu
Type: Acute Care Hospitals Emergency Services: Yes
Ownership: Government - State
Key Personnel:
CEO/President. . . . . David Entwistle
Ambulatory Care . . . . Rob Lloyd
Chief of Medical Staff. . . . . Tom Miller

Measure	Cases	This Hosp.	State Avg.	U.S. Avg.
Blood Clot Prevention and Treatment				
Anticoagulation Overlap Therapy[2]	145	92%	95%	93%
ICU Venous Thromboembolism Prophylaxis[2]	82	96%	93%	92%
Incidence of Potentially Preventable VTE[2]	47	4%	5%	10%
UFH with Dosages/Platelet Monitoring[2]	116	100%	95%	97%
Venous Thromboembolism Prophylaxis[2]	318	86%	86%	85%
Warfarin Therapy Discharge Instructions[2]	107	93%	73%	75%
Chest Pain/Possible Heart Attack Care				
Aspirin Given Within 24 Hours of Arrival[5]	-	-	97%	96%
Fibrinolytic Meds Within 30 Min. of Arrival[5]	-	-	52%	58%
Average Time to ECG (minutes)[5]	-	-	7	7
Average Time to Transfer (minutes)[5]	-	-	36	60
Children's Asthma Care				
Received Home Management Plan of Care	-	-	-	88%
Received Reliever Medication	-	-	-	100%
Received Systemic Corticosteroids	-	-	-	100%
Emergency Department				
Admittance Decision Time (minutes)[2]	118	100	66	98
Head CT Results Within 45 Min. of Arrival	11	18%	60%	57%
Patients Who Left ER Before Being Seen	42,688	1%	1%	2%
Time from ER Arrival to Admit. (minutes)[2]	278	296	217	274
Time from ER Arrival to Discharge (minutes)	329	172	123	134
Time in ER Before Being Evaluated (minutes)	365	28	17	26
Time to Pain Meds for Fractures (minutes)	123	50	43	57
Heart Attack Care				
Aspirin Given at Discharge	241	100%	99%	99%
Fibrinolytic Meds Within 30 Min. of Arrival[7]	-	-	100%	54%
PCI Within 90 Minutes of Arrival	26	96%	98%	96%
Statin Prescribed at Discharge	246	100%	100%	98%
Heart Failure Care				
ACE Inhibitor or ARB for LVSD	111	100%	98%	97%
Discharge Instructions Given	280	99%	96%	94%
Evaluation of LVS Function	308	100%	98%	99%
Medicare Spending				
Medicare Spending per Patient (ratio)	-	1.00	0.98	0.98
Pneumonia Care				
Appropriate Initial Antibiotic Given	84	99%	96%	95%
Blood Culture Timing	130	96%	99%	98%
Pregnancy and Delivery Care				
Newborn Deliveries Scheduled Early[2]	59	3%	6%	6%
Preventive Care				
Immunization for Influenza[2]	500	93%	92%	90%
Immunization for Pneumonia[2]	437	89%	91%	92%
Stroke Care				
Anticoagulation Therapy for Atrial Fibrillation[2]	11	91%	95%	95%
Antithrombotic Therapy Timing[2]	46	98%	99%	98%
Assessed for Rehabilitation[2]	100	100%	98%	97%
Discharged on Antithrombotic Therapy[2]	78	99%	99%	99%
Discharged on Statin Medication[2]	53	98%	96%	94%
Thrombolytic Therapy Timing[1,2]	-	-	89%	66%
Venous Thromboembolism Prophylaxis[2]	104	99%	95%	94%
Written Stroke Educational Materials Given[2]	56	84%	89%	88%
Surgical Care Improvement Project				
Appropriate Beta Blocker Usage[2]	151	96%	98%	98%
Appropriate VTP Within 24 Hours[2]	388	96%	99%	98%
Controlled Postoperative Blood Glucose[2]	126	91%	97%	97%
Perioperative Temperature Management[2]	490	100%	100%	100%
Prophylactic Antibiotic Selection[2]	387	99%	99%	99%
Prophylactic Antibiotic Selection (Outpatient)	494	95%	98%	98%
Prophylactic Antibiotic Stopped[2]	378	94%	98%	98%
Prophylactic Antibiotic Timing[2]	388	99%	99%	99%
Prophylactic Antibiotic Timing (Outpatient)	429	93%	98%	98%
Urinary Catheter Removal[2]	325	93%	98%	97%
Survey of Patients' Hospital Experiences				
Area Around Room 'Always' Quiet at Night	300+	62%	60%	61%
Doctors 'Always' Communicated Well	300+	78%	83%	82%
Home Recovery Information Given	300+	88%	90%	85%
Hospital Given 9 or 10 on 10 Point Scale	300+	76%	74%	71%
Meds 'Always' Explained Before Given	300+	63%	68%	64%
Nurses 'Always' Communicated Well	300+	76%	79%	79%
Pain 'Always' Well Controlled	300+	68%	73%	71%
Room and Bathroom 'Always' Clean	300+	77%	74%	73%
Timely Help 'Always' Received	300+	62%	69%	68%
Would Definitely Recommend Hospital	300+	81%	76%	71%
Use of Medical Imaging				
Cardiac Imaging Stress Test before Surgery	707	6.4%	4.9%	5.3%
Combination Abdominal CT Scan	1,867	3.1%	4.9%	10.5%
Combination Brain/Sinus CT Scan	546	2.0%	3%	2.7%
Combination Chest CT Scan	2,067	0.1%	0.8%	2.7%
Follow-up Mammogram/Ultrasound	1,866	7.4%	8.5%	8.8%
Lumbar Spine MRI for Low Back Pain	277	36.1%	43.8%	37.2%

VA Salt Lake City Healthcare - George E. Wahlen VA

500 Foothill Blvd. Phone: 801-584-1211
Salt Lake City, UT 84148 Fax: 801-584-1289
URL: www1.va.gov/directory/guide/facility.asp?
Type: Acute Care - VA Emergency Services: No
Ownership: Government Federal Beds: 121
Key Personnel:
Chief of Medical Staff . . . . Karen H. Gribbin, MD
Cardiac Laboratory. . . . . Charles Lui, MD
Quality Assurance . . . . Susan Meyers, RN
Infection Control. . . . . Susan O'Connor-Wright
Radiology. . . . . Donald Pifer
Operating Room. . . . . Margaret Riddle, MD
CEO/President. . . . . Steve Young, FACHE

Measure	Cases	This Hosp.	State Avg.	U.S. Avg.
Blood Clot Prevention and Treatment				
Anticoagulation Overlap Therapy	-	-	95%	93%
ICU Venous Thromboembolism Prophylaxis	-	-	93%	92%
Incidence of Potentially Preventable VTE	-	-	5%	10%
UFH with Dosages/Platelet Monitoring	-	-	95%	97%
Venous Thromboembolism Prophylaxis	-	-	86%	85%
Warfarin Therapy Discharge Instructions	-	-	73%	75%
Chest Pain/Possible Heart Attack Care				
Aspirin Given Within 24 Hours of Arrival	-	-	97%	96%
Fibrinolytic Meds Within 30 Min. of Arrival	-	-	52%	58%
Average Time to ECG (minutes)	-	-	7	7
Average Time to Transfer (minutes)	-	-	36	60
Children's Asthma Care				
Received Home Management Plan of Care	-	-	-	88%
Received Reliever Medication	-	-	-	100%
Received Systemic Corticosteroids	-	-	-	100%
Emergency Department				
Admittance Decision Time (minutes)	-	-	66	98
Head CT Results Within 45 Min. of Arrival	-	-	60%	57%
Patients Who Left ER Before Being Seen	-	-	1%	2%
Time from ER Arrival to Admit. (minutes)	-	-	217	274
Time from ER Arrival to Discharge (minutes)	-	-	123	134
Time in ER Before Being Evaluated (minutes)	-	-	17	26
Time to Pain Meds for Fractures (minutes)	-	-	43	57
Heart Attack Care				
Aspirin Given at Discharge	61	100%	99%	99%
Fibrinolytic Meds Within 30 Min. of Arrival[5]	-	-	100%	54%
PCI Within 90 Minutes of Arrival[1]	-	-	98%	96%
Statin Prescribed at Discharge	66	100%	100%	98%
Heart Failure Care				
ACE Inhibitor or ARB for LVSD	92	99%	98%	97%
Discharge Instructions Given	214	100%	96%	94%
Evaluation of LVS Function	228	100%	98%	99%
Medicare Spending				
Medicare Spending per Patient (ratio)	-	-	0.98	0.98
Pneumonia Care				
Appropriate Initial Antibiotic Given	58	100%	96%	95%
Blood Culture Timing	105	99%	99%	98%
Pregnancy and Delivery Care				
Newborn Deliveries Scheduled Early	-	-	6%	6%
Preventive Care				
Immunization for Influenza[5]	-	-	92%	90%
Immunization for Pneumonia[5]	-	-	91%	92%
Stroke Care				
Anticoagulation Therapy for Atrial Fibrillation	-	-	95%	95%
Antithrombotic Therapy Timing	-	-	99%	98%
Assessed for Rehabilitation	-	-	98%	97%
Discharged on Antithrombotic Therapy	-	-	99%	99%
Discharged on Statin Medication	-	-	96%	94%
Thrombolytic Therapy Timing	-	-	89%	66%
Venous Thromboembolism Prophylaxis	-	-	95%	94%
Written Stroke Educational Materials Given	-	-	89%	88%
Surgical Care Improvement Project				
Appropriate Beta Blocker Usage[2]	56	98%	98%	98%
Appropriate VTP Within 24 Hours[2]	163	100%	99%	98%
Controlled Postoperative Blood Glucose[2]	32	97%	97%	97%
Perioperative Temperature Management[2]	220	100%	100%	100%
Prophylactic Antibiotic Selection	116	100%	99%	99%
Prophylactic Antibiotic Selection (Outpatient)	-	-	98%	98%

NOTE: Hospital profiles are in alphabetical order by state, then city, then hospital within the city; Rankings exclude hospitals with less than 25 cases except for patient surveys which excludes hospitals with less than 100 cases; (a) 100-299 cases; (1) The number of cases/patients is too few to report; (2) Data submitted were based on a sample of cases/patients; (3) Results are based on a shorter time period than required; (4) Data suppressed by CMS for one or more quarters; (5) Results are not available for this reporting period; (6) Fewer than 100 patients completed the HCAHPS survey; (7) No cases met the criteria for this measure; (8) The lower limit of the confidence interval cannot be calculated if the number of observed infections equals zero; (9) No data are available from the state/territory for this reporting period; (10) The scores shown reflect fewer than 50 completed surveys; (11) There were discrepancies in the data collection process; (12) This measure does not apply to this hospital for this reporting period; (13) Results cannot be calculated for this reporting period; (14) The results for this state are combined with nearby states to protect confidentiality; Please refer to the User's Guide for a full explanation of data.

Prophylactic Antibiotic Stopped	113	98%	98%	98%
Prophylactic Antibiotic Timing	116	99%	99%	99%
Prophylactic Antibiotic Timing (Outpatient)	-	-	98%	98%
Urinary Catheter Removal[2]	98	100%	98%	97%
Survey of Patients' Hospital Experiences				
Area Around Room 'Always' Quiet at Night	-	-	60%	61%
Doctors 'Always' Communicated Well	-	-	83%	82%
Home Recovery Information Given	-	-	90%	85%
Hospital Given 9 or 10 on 10 Point Scale	-	-	74%	71%
Meds 'Always' Explained Before Given	-	-	68%	64%
Nurses 'Always' Communicated Well	-	-	79%	79%
Pain 'Always' Well Controlled	-	-	73%	71%
Room and Bathroom 'Always' Clean	-	-	74%	73%
Timely Help 'Always' Received	-	-	69%	68%
Would Definitely Recommend Hospital	-	-	76%	71%
Use of Medical Imaging				
Cardiac Imaging Stress Test before Surgery	-	-	4.9%	5.3%
Combination Abdominal CT Scan	-	-	4.9%	10.5%
Combination Brain/Sinus CT Scan	-	-	3%	2.7%
Combination Chest CT Scan	-	-	0.8%	2.7%
Follow-up Mammogram/Ultrasound	-	-	8.5%	8.8%
Lumbar Spine MRI for Low Back Pain	-	-	43.8%	37.2%

Alta View Hospital

9660 South 1300 East Phone: 801-501-2600
Sandy, UT 84094 Fax: 801-501-2043
URL: www.intermountainhealthcare.org
Type: Acute Care Hospitals Emergency Services: Yes
Ownership: Voluntary non-profit - Private Beds: 72

Key Personnel:
Radiology. . . . . Dale P Harris
CEO/President. . . . . Becky Kapp
Chief of Medical Staff . . . . Paul W Winterton

Measure	Cases	This Hosp.	State Avg.	U.S. Avg.
Blood Clot Prevention and Treatment				
Anticoagulation Overlap Therapy[2]	43	100%	95%	93%
ICU Venous Thromboembolism Prophylaxis[2]	26	92%	93%	92%
Incidence of Potentially Preventable VTE[1,2]	-	-	5%	10%
UFH with Dosages/Platelet Monitoring[1,2]	-	-	95%	97%
Venous Thromboembolism Prophylaxis[2]	138	87%	86%	85%
Warfarin Therapy Discharge Instructions[2]	39	21%	73%	75%
Chest Pain/Possible Heart Attack Care				
Aspirin Given Within 24 Hours of Arrival	81	98%	97%	96%
Fibrinolytic Meds Within 30 Min. of Arrival[7]	-	-	52%	58%
Average Time to ECG (minutes)	84	5	7	7
Average Time to Transfer (minutes)	13	35	36	60
Children's Asthma Care				
Received Home Management Plan of Care	-	-	-	88%
Received Reliever Medication	-	-	-	100%
Received Systemic Corticosteroids	-	-	-	100%
Emergency Department				
Admittance Decision Time (minutes)[2]	303	75	66	98
Head CT Results Within 45 Min. of Arrival[1]	-	-	60%	57%
Patients Who Left ER Before Being Seen	24,431	1%	1%	2%
Time from ER Arrival to Admit. (minutes)[2]	307	266	217	274
Time from ER Arrival to Discharge (minutes)	387	166	123	134
Time in ER Before Being Evaluated (minutes)	421	20	17	26
Time to Pain Meds for Fractures (minutes)	138	38	43	57
Heart Attack Care				
Aspirin Given at Discharge[1,3]	-	-	99%	99%
Fibrinolytic Meds Within 30 Min. of Arrival[3,7]	-	-	100%	54%
PCI Within 90 Minutes of Arrival[3,7]	-	-	98%	96%
Statin Prescribed at Discharge[1,3]	-	-	100%	98%
Heart Failure Care				
ACE Inhibitor or ARB for LVSD[1]	-	-	98%	97%
Discharge Instructions Given	26	100%	96%	94%
Evaluation of LVS Function	35	100%	98%	99%
Medicare Spending				
Medicare Spending per Patient (ratio)	-	0.95	0.98	0.98
Pneumonia Care				
Appropriate Initial Antibiotic Given[2]	81	100%	96%	95%
Blood Culture Timing[2]	90	97%	99%	98%
Pregnancy and Delivery Care				
Newborn Deliveries Scheduled Early[2]	32	3%	6%	6%
Preventive Care				
Immunization for Influenza[2]	367	98%	92%	90%
Immunization for Pneumonia[2]	305	95%	91%	92%
Stroke Care				
Anticoagulation Therapy for Atrial Fibrillation[1]	-	-	95%	95%
Antithrombotic Therapy Timing[1]	-	-	99%	98%
Assessed for Rehabilitation[1]	-	-	98%	97%
Discharged on Antithrombotic Therapy[1]	-	-	99%	99%
Discharged on Statin Medication[1]	-	-	96%	94%
Thrombolytic Therapy Timing[7]	-	-	89%	66%
Venous Thromboembolism Prophylaxis[1]	-	-	95%	94%
Written Stroke Educational Materials Given[1]	-	-	89%	88%
Surgical Care Improvement Project				
Appropriate Beta Blocker Usage[2]	60	97%	98%	98%
Appropriate VTP Within 24 Hours[2]	326	99%	99%	98%
Controlled Postoperative Blood Glucose[2,7]	-	-	97%	97%
Perioperative Temperature Management[2]	405	100%	100%	100%
Prophylactic Antibiotic Selection[2]	302	99%	99%	99%
Prophylactic Antibiotic Selection (Outpatient)	208	99%	98%	98%
Prophylactic Antibiotic Stopped[2]	298	100%	98%	98%
Prophylactic Antibiotic Timing[2]	302	100%	99%	99%
Prophylactic Antibiotic Timing (Outpatient)	209	98%	98%	98%
Urinary Catheter Removal[2]	235	97%	98%	97%
Survey of Patients' Hospital Experiences				
Area Around Room 'Always' Quiet at Night	300+	60%	60%	61%
Doctors 'Always' Communicated Well	300+	84%	83%	82%
Home Recovery Information Given	300+	92%	90%	85%
Hospital Given 9 or 10 on 10 Point Scale	300+	75%	74%	71%
Meds 'Always' Explained Before Given	300+	68%	68%	64%
Nurses 'Always' Communicated Well	300+	78%	79%	79%
Pain 'Always' Well Controlled	300+	71%	73%	71%
Room and Bathroom 'Always' Clean	300+	72%	74%	73%
Timely Help 'Always' Received	300+	68%	69%	68%
Would Definitely Recommend Hospital	300+	76%	76%	71%
Use of Medical Imaging				
Cardiac Imaging Stress Test before Surgery	133	5.3%	4.9%	5.3%
Combination Abdominal CT Scan	438	4.1%	4.9%	10.5%
Combination Brain/Sinus CT Scan	224	0.9%	3%	2.7%
Combination Chest CT Scan	156	1.9%	0.8%	2.7%
Follow-up Mammogram/Ultrasound	967	6.5%	8.5%	8.8%
Lumbar Spine MRI for Low Back Pain	49	46.9%	43.8%	37.2%

Mountain West Medical Center

2055 North Main Street Phone: 435-843-3700
Tooele, UT 84074 Fax: 435-843-3753
URL: www.mountainwestmc.com
Type: Acute Care Hospitals Emergency Services: Yes
Ownership: Proprietary Beds: 38

Key Personnel:
CEO/President. . . . . Denten Park
Radiology. . . . . James Webber, MD

Measure	Cases	This Hosp.	State Avg.	U.S. Avg.
Blood Clot Prevention and Treatment				
Anticoagulation Overlap Therapy[2]	19	100%	95%	93%
ICU Venous Thromboembolism Prophylaxis[2]	39	100%	93%	92%
Incidence of Potentially Preventable VTE[1,2]	-	-	5%	10%
UFH with Dosages/Platelet Monitoring[1,2]	-	-	95%	97%
Venous Thromboembolism Prophylaxis[2]	127	98%	86%	85%
Warfarin Therapy Discharge Instructions[2]	13	92%	73%	75%
Chest Pain/Possible Heart Attack Care				
Aspirin Given Within 24 Hours of Arrival	34	100%	97%	96%
Fibrinolytic Meds Within 30 Min. of Arrival[1]	-	-	52%	58%
Average Time to ECG (minutes)	36	6	7	7
Average Time to Transfer (minutes)[1]	-	-	36	60
Children's Asthma Care				
Received Home Management Plan of Care	-	-	-	88%
Received Reliever Medication	-	-	-	100%
Received Systemic Corticosteroids	-	-	-	100%
Emergency Department				
Admittance Decision Time (minutes)[2]	349	85	66	98
Head CT Results Within 45 Min. of Arrival	15	67%	60%	57%
Patients Who Left ER Before Being Seen	15,535	1%	1%	2%
Time from ER Arrival to Admit. (minutes)[2]	349	241	217	274
Time from ER Arrival to Discharge (minutes)	375	125	123	134
Time in ER Before Being Evaluated (minutes)	418	16	17	26
Time to Pain Meds for Fractures (minutes)	105	51	43	57
Heart Attack Care				
Aspirin Given at Discharge[1]	-	-	99%	99%
Fibrinolytic Meds Within 30 Min. of Arrival[7]	-	-	100%	54%
PCI Within 90 Minutes of Arrival[7]	-	-	98%	96%
Statin Prescribed at Discharge[1]	-	-	100%	98%
Heart Failure Care				
ACE Inhibitor or ARB for LVSD[1]	-	-	98%	97%
Discharge Instructions Given	21	76%	96%	94%
Evaluation of LVS Function	31	100%	98%	99%
Medicare Spending				
Medicare Spending per Patient (ratio)	-	0.98	0.98	0.98
Pneumonia Care				
Appropriate Initial Antibiotic Given	56	98%	96%	95%
Blood Culture Timing	72	96%	99%	98%
Pregnancy and Delivery Care				
Newborn Deliveries Scheduled Early[2]	39	0%	6%	6%
Preventive Care				
Immunization for Influenza[2]	287	97%	92%	90%
Immunization for Pneumonia[2]	267	98%	91%	92%
Stroke Care				
Anticoagulation Therapy for Atrial Fibrillation[1]	-	-	95%	95%
Antithrombotic Therapy Timing[1]	-	-	99%	98%
Assessed for Rehabilitation	11	100%	98%	97%
Discharged on Antithrombotic Therapy[1]	-	-	99%	99%
Discharged on Statin Medication[1]	-	-	96%	94%
Thrombolytic Therapy Timing[7]	-	-	89%	66%
Venous Thromboembolism Prophylaxis[1]	-	-	95%	94%
Written Stroke Educational Materials Given[1]	-	-	89%	88%
Surgical Care Improvement Project				
Appropriate Beta Blocker Usage	20	95%	98%	98%
Appropriate VTP Within 24 Hours	133	98%	99%	98%
Controlled Postoperative Blood Glucose[7]	-	-	97%	97%
Perioperative Temperature Management	170	100%	100%	100%
Prophylactic Antibiotic Selection	126	99%	99%	99%
Prophylactic Antibiotic Selection (Outpatient)	44	98%	98%	98%
Prophylactic Antibiotic Stopped	125	98%	98%	98%
Prophylactic Antibiotic Timing	126	100%	99%	99%
Prophylactic Antibiotic Timing (Outpatient)	15	87%	98%	98%
Urinary Catheter Removal	113	96%	98%	97%
Survey of Patients' Hospital Experiences				
Area Around Room 'Always' Quiet at Night	300+	63%	60%	61%
Doctors 'Always' Communicated Well	300+	80%	83%	82%
Home Recovery Information Given	300+	87%	90%	85%
Hospital Given 9 or 10 on 10 Point Scale	300+	69%	74%	71%
Meds 'Always' Explained Before Given	300+	62%	68%	64%
Nurses 'Always' Communicated Well	300+	78%	79%	79%
Pain 'Always' Well Controlled	300+	73%	73%	71%
Room and Bathroom 'Always' Clean	300+	74%	74%	73%
Timely Help 'Always' Received	300+	69%	69%	68%
Would Definitely Recommend Hospital	300+	63%	76%	71%
Use of Medical Imaging				
Cardiac Imaging Stress Test before Surgery	59	3.4%	4.9%	5.3%
Combination Abdominal CT Scan	163	6.7%	4.9%	10.5%
Combination Brain/Sinus CT Scan[1]	-	-	3%	2.7%
Combination Chest CT Scan[1]	-	-	0.8%	2.7%
Follow-up Mammogram/Ultrasound	342	4.7%	8.5%	8.8%
Lumbar Spine MRI for Low Back Pain[1]	-	-	43.8%	37.2%

Bear River Valley Hospital

905 North 1000 West Phone: 435-207-4708
Tremonton, UT 84337 Fax: 435-257-4386
URL: www.intermountainhealthcare.org
Type: Acute Care Hospitals Emergency Services: Yes
Ownership: Voluntary non-profit - Private Beds: 20

Key Personnel:
Radiology. . . . . Mark D Anderson
Anesthesiology. . . . . Jay Argyle
Operating Room. . . . . Jan M Ashdown
Emergency Room . . . . Rod Merrell, MD

NOTE: Hospital profiles are in alphabetical order by state, then city, then hospital within the city; Rankings exclude hospitals with less than 25 cases except for patient surveys which excludes hospitals with less than 100 cases; (a) 100-299 cases; (1) The number of cases/patients is too few to report; (2) Data submitted were based on a sample of cases/patients; (3) Results are based on a shorter time period than required; (4) Data suppressed by CMS for one or more quarters; (5) Results are not available for this reporting period; (6) Fewer than 100 patients completed the HCAHPS survey; (7) No cases met the criteria for this measure; (8) The lower limit of the confidence interval cannot be calculated if the number of observed infections equals zero; (9) No data are available from the state/territory for this reporting period; (10) The scores shown reflect fewer than 50 completed surveys; (11) There were discrepancies in the data collection process; (12) This measure does not apply to this hospital for this reporting period; (13) Results cannot be calculated for this reporting period; (14) The results for this state are combined with nearby states to protect confidentiality; Please refer to the User's Guide for a full explanation of data.

Measure	Cases	This Hosp.	State Avg.	U.S. Avg.
Blood Clot Prevention and Treatment				
Anticoagulation Overlap Therapy[1,2]	-	-	95%	93%
ICU Venous Thromboembolism Prophylaxis[2,7]	-	-	93%	92%
Incidence of Potentially Preventable VTE[1,2]	-	-	5%	10%
UFH with Dosages/Platelet Monitoring[2,7]	-	-	95%	97%
Venous Thromboembolism Prophylaxis[2]	60	75%	86%	85%
Warfarin Therapy Discharge Instructions[1,2]	-	-	73%	75%
Chest Pain/Possible Heart Attack Care				
Aspirin Given Within 24 Hours of Arrival	32	97%	97%	96%
Fibrinolytic Meds Within 30 Min. of Arrival[1]	-	-	52%	58%
Average Time to ECG (minutes)	34	8	7	7
Average Time to Transfer (minutes)[1]	-	-	36	60
Children's Asthma Care				
Received Home Management Plan of Care	-	-	-	88%
Received Reliever Medication	-	-	-	100%
Received Systemic Corticosteroids	-	-	-	100%
Emergency Department				
Admittance Decision Time (minutes)[2]	156	62	66	98
Head CT Results Within 45 Min. of Arrival[1]	-	-	60%	57%
Patients Who Left ER Before Being Seen	5,899	0%	1%	2%
Time from ER Arrival to Admit. (minutes)[2]	175	213	217	274
Time from ER Arrival to Discharge (minutes)	368	97	123	134
Time in ER Before Being Evaluated (minutes)	394	4	17	26
Time to Pain Meds for Fractures (minutes)	54	30	43	57
Heart Attack Care				
Aspirin Given at Discharge[3,7]	-	-	99%	99%
Fibrinolytic Meds Within 30 Min. of Arrival[3,7]	-	-	100%	54%
PCI Within 90 Minutes of Arrival[3,7]	-	-	98%	96%
Statin Prescribed at Discharge[3,7]	-	-	100%	98%
Heart Failure Care				
ACE Inhibitor or ARB for LVSD[1,3]	-	-	98%	97%
Discharge Instructions Given[1,3]	-	-	96%	94%
Evaluation of LVS Function[1,3]	-	-	98%	99%
Medicare Spending				
Medicare Spending per Patient (ratio)	-	0.76	0.98	0.98
Pneumonia Care				
Appropriate Initial Antibiotic Given[2]	16	94%	96%	95%
Blood Culture Timing[2]	16	100%	99%	98%
Pregnancy and Delivery Care				
Newborn Deliveries Scheduled Early	23	0%	6%	6%
Preventive Care				
Immunization for Influenza[2]	200	100%	92%	90%
Immunization for Pneumonia[2]	161	99%	91%	92%
Stroke Care				
Anticoagulation Therapy for Atrial Fibrillation[3,7]	-	-	95%	95%
Antithrombotic Therapy Timing[3,7]	-	-	99%	98%
Assessed for Rehabilitation[1,3]	-	-	98%	97%
Discharged on Antithrombotic Therapy[1,3]	-	-	99%	99%
Discharged on Statin Medication[3,7]	-	-	96%	94%
Thrombolytic Therapy Timing[3,7]	-	-	89%	66%
Venous Thromboembolism Prophylaxis[3,7]	-	-	95%	94%
Written Stroke Educational Materials Given[1,3]	-	-	89%	88%
Surgical Care Improvement Project				
Appropriate Beta Blocker Usage[1]	-	-	98%	98%
Appropriate VTP Within 24 Hours	27	100%	99%	98%
Controlled Postoperative Blood Glucose[7]	-	-	97%	97%
Perioperative Temperature Management	33	100%	100%	100%
Prophylactic Antibiotic Selection	27	100%	99%	99%
Prophylactic Antibiotic Selection (Outpatient)[1,3]	-	-	98%	98%
Prophylactic Antibiotic Stopped	27	100%	98%	98%
Prophylactic Antibiotic Timing	27	100%	99%	99%
Prophylactic Antibiotic Timing (Outpatient)[1,3]	-	-	98%	98%
Urinary Catheter Removal	17	100%	98%	97%
Survey of Patients' Hospital Experiences				
Area Around Room 'Always' Quiet at Night	(a)	74%	60%	61%
Doctors 'Always' Communicated Well	(a)	86%	83%	82%
Home Recovery Information Given	(a)	93%	90%	85%
Hospital Given 9 or 10 on 10 Point Scale	(a)	85%	74%	71%
Meds 'Always' Explained Before Given	(a)	88%	68%	64%
Nurses 'Always' Communicated Well	(a)	86%	79%	79%
Pain 'Always' Well Controlled	(a)	82%	73%	71%
Room and Bathroom 'Always' Clean	(a)	83%	74%	73%
Timely Help 'Always' Received	(a)	83%	69%	68%
Would Definitely Recommend Hospital	(a)	83%	76%	71%
Use of Medical Imaging				
Cardiac Imaging Stress Test before Surgery[7]	-	-	4.9%	5.3%
Combination Abdominal CT Scan	73	1.4%	4.9%	10.5%
Combination Brain/Sinus CT Scan[1]	-	-	3%	2.7%
Combination Chest CT Scan	45	0.0%	0.8%	2.7%
Follow-up Mammogram/Ultrasound	132	10.6%	8.5%	8.8%
Lumbar Spine MRI for Low Back Pain[1]	-	-	43.8%	37.2%

Ashley Regional Medical Center

150 West 100 North
Vernal, UT 84078
URL: www.ashleyregional.com
Type: Acute Care Hospitals
Ownership: Proprietary
Phone: 435-789-3342
Fax: 435-789-1314
Emergency Services: Yes
Beds: 39

Key Personnel:
Infection Control. . . . . Ruth Christensen
Chief of Medical Staff. . . . . Jon Griffith, MD
Radiology. . . . . Jeff Hanberg
Operating Room. . . . . Carol Hinschi
Pediatric Ambulatory Care . . . . . . Carol Hirschi
CEO/President. . . . . Si Hutt
Pediatric In-Patient Care . . . . Daniel Kwak, MD
Quality Assurance . . . . Debbie Spafford

Measure	Cases	This Hosp.	State Avg.	U.S. Avg.
Blood Clot Prevention and Treatment				
Anticoagulation Overlap Therapy[2]	13	92%	95%	93%
ICU Venous Thromboembolism Prophylaxis[2]	34	91%	93%	92%
Incidence of Potentially Preventable VTE[1,2]	-	-	5%	10%
UFH with Dosages/Platelet Monitoring[1,2]	-	-	95%	97%
Venous Thromboembolism Prophylaxis[2]	101	77%	86%	85%
Warfarin Therapy Discharge Instructions[2]	11	100%	73%	75%
Chest Pain/Possible Heart Attack Care				
Aspirin Given Within 24 Hours of Arrival	29	100%	97%	96%
Fibrinolytic Meds Within 30 Min. of Arrival[1]	-	-	52%	58%
Average Time to ECG (minutes)	30	5	7	7
Average Time to Transfer (minutes)[7]	-	-	36	60
Children's Asthma Care				
Received Home Management Plan of Care	-	-	-	88%
Received Reliever Medication	-	-	-	100%
Received Systemic Corticosteroids	-	-	-	100%
Emergency Department				
Admittance Decision Time (minutes)[2]	251	59	66	98
Head CT Results Within 45 Min. of Arrival	11	91%	60%	57%
Patients Who Left ER Before Being Seen	11,343	1%	1%	2%
Time from ER Arrival to Admit. (minutes)[2]	251	241	217	274
Time from ER Arrival to Discharge (minutes)	394	118	123	134
Time in ER Before Being Evaluated (minutes)	437	12	17	26
Time to Pain Meds for Fractures (minutes)	86	44	43	57
Heart Attack Care				
Aspirin Given at Discharge[3,7]	-	-	99%	99%
Fibrinolytic Meds Within 30 Min. of Arrival[3,7]	-	-	100%	54%
PCI Within 90 Minutes of Arrival[3,7]	-	-	98%	96%
Statin Prescribed at Discharge[3,7]	-	-	100%	98%
Heart Failure Care				
ACE Inhibitor or ARB for LVSD[1]	-	-	98%	97%
Discharge Instructions Given	15	87%	96%	94%
Evaluation of LVS Function	19	100%	98%	99%
Medicare Spending				
Medicare Spending per Patient (ratio)	-	0.81	0.98	0.98
Pneumonia Care				
Appropriate Initial Antibiotic Given	41	100%	96%	95%
Blood Culture Timing	49	98%	99%	98%
Pregnancy and Delivery Care				
Newborn Deliveries Scheduled Early[2]	50	12%	6%	6%
Preventive Care				
Immunization for Influenza[2]	252	94%	92%	90%
Immunization for Pneumonia[2]	187	86%	91%	92%
Stroke Care				
Anticoagulation Therapy for Atrial Fibrillation[1,3]	-	-	95%	95%
Antithrombotic Therapy Timing[1,3]	-	-	99%	98%
Assessed for Rehabilitation[1,3]	-	-	98%	97%
Discharged on Antithrombotic Therapy[1,3]	-	-	99%	99%
Discharged on Statin Medication[1,3]	-	-	96%	94%
Thrombolytic Therapy Timing[3,7]	-	-	89%	66%
Venous Thromboembolism Prophylaxis[1,3]	-	-	95%	94%
Written Stroke Educational Materials Given[1,3]	-	-	89%	88%
Surgical Care Improvement Project				
Appropriate Beta Blocker Usage[1]	-	-	98%	98%
Appropriate VTP Within 24 Hours	50	92%	99%	98%
Controlled Postoperative Blood Glucose[7]	-	-	97%	97%
Perioperative Temperature Management	62	100%	100%	100%
Prophylactic Antibiotic Selection	46	96%	99%	99%
Prophylactic Antibiotic Selection (Outpatient)	43	93%	98%	98%
Prophylactic Antibiotic Stopped	46	93%	98%	98%
Prophylactic Antibiotic Timing	46	98%	99%	99%
Prophylactic Antibiotic Timing (Outpatient)	43	98%	98%	98%
Urinary Catheter Removal	40	98%	98%	97%
Survey of Patients' Hospital Experiences				
Area Around Room 'Always' Quiet at Night	300+	55%	60%	61%
Doctors 'Always' Communicated Well	300+	79%	83%	82%
Home Recovery Information Given	300+	86%	90%	85%
Hospital Given 9 or 10 on 10 Point Scale	300+	60%	74%	71%
Meds 'Always' Explained Before Given	300+	64%	68%	64%
Nurses 'Always' Communicated Well	300+	74%	79%	79%
Pain 'Always' Well Controlled	300+	64%	73%	71%
Room and Bathroom 'Always' Clean	300+	64%	74%	73%
Timely Help 'Always' Received	300+	64%	69%	68%
Would Definitely Recommend Hospital	300+	56%	76%	71%
Use of Medical Imaging				
Cardiac Imaging Stress Test before Surgery	64	1.6%	4.9%	5.3%
Combination Abdominal CT Scan	143	2.8%	4.9%	10.5%
Combination Brain/Sinus CT Scan[1]	-	-	3%	2.7%
Combination Chest CT Scan[1]	-	-	0.8%	2.7%
Follow-up Mammogram/Ultrasound	195	6.7%	8.5%	8.8%
Lumbar Spine MRI for Low Back Pain[1]	-	-	43.8%	37.2%

Jordan Valley Medical Center

3580 West 9000 South
West Jordan, UT 84088
E-mail: info@iasishealthcare.com
URL: www.jordanvalleymc.com
Type: Acute Care Hospitals
Ownership: Voluntary non-profit - Other
Phone: 801-561-8888
Fax: 801-569-8723
Emergency Services: Yes
Beds: 172

Key Personnel:
Emergency Room . . . . Holly Burke, RN
Operating Room. . . . . Kelly Jackson
Quality Assurance . . . . Pat Lamuth
Radiology. . . . . Doug Madsen
Patient Relations . . . . Danielle Pate
CEO/President. . . . . Bryanie E Swilley
Chief of Medical Staff. . . . . Christopher B Valentine, MD
Intensive Care Unit. . . . . Jeff Weddle

Measure	Cases	This Hosp.	State Avg.	U.S. Avg.
Blood Clot Prevention and Treatment				
Anticoagulation Overlap Therapy[2]	74	97%	95%	93%
ICU Venous Thromboembolism Prophylaxis[2]	177	95%	93%	92%
Incidence of Potentially Preventable VTE[2]	11	0%	5%	10%
UFH with Dosages/Platelet Monitoring[2]	16	100%	95%	97%
Venous Thromboembolism Prophylaxis[2]	526	95%	86%	85%
Warfarin Therapy Discharge Instructions[2]	54	80%	73%	75%
Chest Pain/Possible Heart Attack Care				
Aspirin Given Within 24 Hours of Arrival	20	100%	97%	96%
Fibrinolytic Meds Within 30 Min. of Arrival[7]	-	-	52%	58%
Average Time to ECG (minutes)	22	2	7	7
Average Time to Transfer (minutes)[1]	-	-	36	60
Children's Asthma Care				
Received Home Management Plan of Care	-	-	-	88%
Received Reliever Medication	-	-	-	100%
Received Systemic Corticosteroids	-	-	-	100%
Emergency Department				
Admittance Decision Time (minutes)[2]	759	70	66	98
Head CT Results Within 45 Min. of Arrival	17	65%	60%	57%
Patients Who Left ER Before Being Seen	57,229	1%	1%	2%
Time from ER Arrival to Admit. (minutes)[2]	769	242	217	274
Time from ER Arrival to Discharge (minutes)	1,343	145	123	134

NOTE: Hospital profiles are in alphabetical order by state, then city, then hospital within the city; Rankings exclude hospitals with less than 25 cases except for patient surveys which excludes hospitals with less than 100 cases; (a) 100-299 cases; (1) The number of cases/patients is too few to report; (2) Data submitted were based on a sample of cases/patients; (3) Results are based on a shorter time period than required; (4) Data suppressed by CMS for one or more quarters; (5) Results are not available for this reporting period; (6) Fewer than 100 patients completed the HCAHPS survey; (7) No cases met the criteria for this measure; (8) The lower limit of the confidence interval cannot be calculated if the number of observed infections equals zero; (9) No data are available from the state/territory for this reporting period; (10) The scores shown reflect fewer than 50 completed surveys; (11) There were discrepancies in the data collection process; (12) This measure does not apply to this hospital for this reporting period; (13) Results cannot be calculated for this reporting period; (14) The results for this state are combined with nearby states to protect confidentiality; Please refer to the User's Guide for a full explanation of data.

Time in ER Before Being Evaluated (minutes)	1,461	20	17	26
Time to Pain Meds for Fractures (minutes)	322	40	43	57
Heart Attack Care				
Aspirin Given at Discharge	147	100%	99%	99%
Fibrinolytic Meds Within 30 Min. of Arrival[7]	-	-	100%	54%
PCI Within 90 Minutes of Arrival	60	98%	98%	96%
Statin Prescribed at Discharge	141	100%	100%	98%
Heart Failure Care				
ACE Inhibitor or ARB for LVSD	40	100%	98%	97%
Discharge Instructions Given	102	91%	96%	94%
Evaluation of LVS Function	128	100%	98%	99%
Medicare Spending				
Medicare Spending per Patient (ratio)	-	1.07	0.98	0.98
Pneumonia Care				
Appropriate Initial Antibiotic Given	161	98%	96%	95%
Blood Culture Timing	218	99%	99%	98%
Pregnancy and Delivery Care				
Newborn Deliveries Scheduled Early[2]	87	8%	6%	6%
Preventive Care				
Immunization for Influenza[2]	843	98%	92%	90%
Immunization for Pneumonia[2]	684	98%	91%	92%
Stroke Care				
Anticoagulation Therapy for Atrial Fibrillation[1]	-	-	95%	95%
Antithrombotic Therapy Timing	50	100%	99%	98%
Assessed for Rehabilitation	63	94%	98%	97%
Discharged on Antithrombotic Therapy	60	100%	99%	99%
Discharged on Statin Medication	51	98%	96%	94%
Thrombolytic Therapy Timing[1]	-	-	89%	66%
Venous Thromboembolism Prophylaxis	57	93%	95%	94%
Written Stroke Educational Materials Given	48	85%	89%	88%
Surgical Care Improvement Project				
Appropriate Beta Blocker Usage	84	100%	98%	98%
Appropriate VTP Within 24 Hours	557	99%	99%	98%
Controlled Postoperative Blood Glucose[7]	-	-	97%	97%
Perioperative Temperature Management	643	100%	100%	100%
Prophylactic Antibiotic Selection	454	99%	99%	99%
Prophylactic Antibiotic Selection (Outpatient)	296	99%	98%	98%
Prophylactic Antibiotic Stopped	449	99%	98%	98%
Prophylactic Antibiotic Timing	454	100%	99%	99%
Prophylactic Antibiotic Timing (Outpatient)	268	98%	98%	98%
Urinary Catheter Removal	358	98%	98%	97%
Survey of Patients' Hospital Experiences				
Area Around Room 'Always' Quiet at Night	300+	60%	60%	61%
Doctors 'Always' Communicated Well	300+	80%	83%	82%
Home Recovery Information Given	300+	88%	90%	85%
Hospital Given 9 or 10 on 10 Point Scale	300+	67%	74%	71%
Meds 'Always' Explained Before Given	300+	63%	68%	64%
Nurses 'Always' Communicated Well	300+	73%	79%	79%
Pain 'Always' Well Controlled	300+	67%	73%	71%
Room and Bathroom 'Always' Clean	300+	69%	74%	73%
Timely Help 'Always' Received	300+	58%	69%	68%
Would Definitely Recommend Hospital	300+	67%	76%	71%
Use of Medical Imaging				
Cardiac Imaging Stress Test before Surgery	333	2.7%	4.9%	5.3%
Combination Abdominal CT Scan	446	2.7%	4.9%	10.5%
Combination Brain/Sinus CT Scan	347	1.2%	3%	2.7%
Combination Chest CT Scan	92	0.0%	0.8%	2.7%
Follow-up Mammogram/Ultrasound	733	9.0%	8.5%	8.8%
Lumbar Spine MRI for Low Back Pain	69	50.7%	43.8%	37.2%

NOTE: Hospital profiles are in alphabetical order by state, then city, then hospital within the city; Rankings exclude hospitals with less than 25 cases except for patient surveys which excludes hospitals with less than 100 cases; (a) 100-299 cases; (1) The number of cases/patients is too few to report; (2) Data submitted were based on a sample of cases/patients; (3) Results are based on a shorter time period than required; (4) Data suppressed by CMS for one or more quarters; (5) Results are not available for this reporting period; (6) Fewer than 100 patients completed the HCAHPS survey; (7) No cases met the criteria for this measure; (8) The lower limit of the confidence interval cannot be calculated if the number of observed infections equals zero; (9) No data are available from the state/territory for this reporting period; (10) The scores shown reflect fewer than 50 completed surveys; (11) There were discrepancies in the data collection process; (12) This measure does not apply to this hospital for this reporting period; (13) Results cannot be calculated for this reporting period; (14) The results for this state are combined with nearby states to protect confidentiality; Please refer to the User's Guide for a full explanation of data.

Blood Clot Prevention and Treatment

Anticoagulation Overlap Therapy

Hospital Name	City	Rate	Cases
Central Washington Hospital[2]	Wenatchee	100%	54
Evergreen Hospital Medical Center[2]	Kirkland	100%	130
Highline Medical Center[2]	Burien	100%	52
Kennewick General Hospital[2]	Kennewick	100%	27
Legacy Salmon Creek Medical Center[2]	Vancouver	100%	62
Northwest Hospital[2]	Seattle	100%	73
Peacehealth Southwest Medical Center[2]	Vancouver	100%	161
Swedish Issaquah[2]	Issaquah	100%	28
Tacoma General Allenmore Hospital[2]	Tacoma	100%	131
University of Washington Medical Center[2]	Seattle	100%	51
Valley Hospital[2]	Spokane	100%	60
Kadlec Regional Medical Center[2]	Richland	99%	117
Multicare Good Samaritan Hospital[2]	Puyallup	99%	123
Providence Holy Family Hospital[2]	Spokane	99%	96
Providence Reg Med Ctr Everett[2]	Everett	99%	235
Providence Sacred Heart Medical Center[2]	Spokane	99%	119
Valley Medical Center[2]	Renton	99%	104
Deaconess Hospital[2]	Spokane	98%	63
Harrison Memorial Center[2]	Bremerton	98%	138
Multicare Auburn Medical Center[2]	Auburn	98%	59
Peacehealth Saint Joseph Medical Center[2]	Bellingham	98%	89
Swedish Medical Center[2]	Seattle	98%	87
Skagit Valley Hospital[2]	Mount Vernon	97%	39
Harborview Medical Center[2]	Seattle	96%	93
Providence Saint Peter Hospital[2]	Olympia	96%	141
Swedish Medical Center - Cherry Hill[2]	Seattle	96%	45
Virginia Mason Medical Center[2]	Seattle	96%	131
Peacehealth Saint John Medical Center[2]	Longview	95%	60
Swedish Edmonds Hospital[2]	Edmonds	95%	64
Providence Centralia Hospital[2]	Centralia	94%	31
Yakima Valley Memorial Hospital[2]	Yakima	94%	63
Overlake Hospital Medical Center[2]	Bellevue	93%	105
Saint Joseph Medical Center[2]	Tacoma	93%	138
Saint Anthony Hospital[2]	Gig Harbor	92%	52
Saint Clare Hospital[2]	Lakewood	92%	52
Saint Francis Community Hospital[2]	Federal Way	91%	69
Yakima Regional Medical & Cardiac Center[2]	Yakima	81%	42

ICU Venous Thromboembolism Prophylaxis

Hospital Name	City	Rate	Cases
Capital Medical Center[2]	Olympia	100%	74
Multicare Auburn Medical Center[2]	Auburn	100%	73
Swedish Medical Center[2]	Seattle	100%	61
Valley Hospital[2]	Spokane	100%	62
Harborview Medical Center[2]	Seattle	98%	184
Kennewick General Hospital[2]	Kennewick	98%	48
Peacehealth Southwest Medical Center[2]	Vancouver	98%	104
Peacehealth Saint John Medical Center[2]	Longview	98%	90
Saint Joseph Medical Center[2]	Tacoma	98%	53
University of Washington Medical Center[2]	Seattle	98%	102
Swedish Medical Center - Cherry Hill[2]	Seattle	97%	153
Tacoma General Allenmore Hospital[2]	Tacoma	97%	122
Virginia Mason Medical Center[2]	Seattle	97%	71
Cascade Valley Hospital[2]	Arlington	96%	27
Deaconess Hospital[2]	Spokane	96%	76
Legacy Salmon Creek Medical Center[2]	Vancouver	96%	68
Providence Holy Family Hospital[2]	Spokane	96%	56
Providence Saint Peter Hospital[2]	Olympia	96%	45
Harrison Memorial Center[2]	Bremerton	95%	58
Multicare Good Samaritan Hospital[2]	Puyallup	94%	32
Providence Reg Med Ctr Everett[2]	Everett	94%	50
Providence Sacred Heart Medical Center[2]	Spokane	94%	103
Olympic Medical Center[2]	Port Angeles	93%	75
Providence Centralia Hospital[2]	Centralia	93%	46
Saint Clare Hospital[2]	Lakewood	93%	27
Whidbey General Hospital[2]	Coupeville	92%	48
Providence Saint Mary Medical Center[2]	Walla Walla	91%	44
Skagit Valley Hospital[2]	Mount Vernon	91%	64
Valley Medical Center[2]	Renton	90%	51
Central Washington Hospital[2]	Wenatchee	89%	89
Overlake Hospital Medical Center[2]	Bellevue	89%	54
Swedish Edmonds Hospital[2]	Edmonds	89%	45
Evergreen Hospital Medical Center[2]	Kirkland	88%	69
Peacehealth Saint Joseph Medical Center[2]	Bellingham	88%	82
Northwest Hospital[2]	Seattle	87%	63
Saint Francis Community Hospital[2]	Federal Way	87%	38
Grays Harbor Community Hospital[2]	Aberdeen	86%	242
Swedish Issaquah[2]	Issaquah	86%	37
Highline Medical Center[2]	Burien	83%	47
Island Hospital[2]	Anacortes	81%	43
Kadlec Regional Medical Center[2]	Richland	80%	101
Yakima Valley Memorial Hospital[2]	Yakima	80%	51
Toppenish Community Hospital[2]	Toppenish	72%	40
Yakima Regional Medical & Cardiac Center[2]	Yakima	65%	69

Incidence of Potentially Preventable VTE

Hospital Name	City	Rate	Cases
Harborview Medical Center[2]	Seattle	0%	58
Virginia Mason Medical Center[2]	Seattle	2%	51
Saint Joseph Medical Center[2]	Tacoma	8%	25
Tacoma General Allenmore Hospital[2]	Tacoma	10%	30
University of Washington Medical Center[2]	Seattle	18%	34

UFH with Dosages/Platelet Count Monitoring

Hospital Name	City	Rate	Cases
Central Washington Hospital[2]	Wenatchee	100%	46
Deaconess Hospital[2]	Spokane	100%	46
Evergreen Hospital Medical Center[2]	Kirkland	100%	84
Harborview Medical Center[2]	Seattle	100%	78
Harrison Memorial Center[2]	Bremerton	100%	114
Highline Medical Center[2]	Burien	100%	45
Kadlec Regional Medical Center[2]	Richland	100%	90
Legacy Salmon Creek Medical Center[2]	Vancouver	100%	31
Multicare Auburn Medical Center[2]	Auburn	100%	38
Multicare Good Samaritan Hospital[2]	Puyallup	100%	98
Northwest Hospital[2]	Seattle	100%	31
Overlake Hospital Medical Center[2]	Bellevue	100%	56
Peacehealth Southwest Medical Center[2]	Vancouver	100%	141
Peacehealth Saint John Medical Center[2]	Longview	100%	28
Providence Holy Family Hospital[2]	Spokane	100%	86
Providence Reg Med Ctr Everett[2]	Everett	100%	133
Providence Saint Peter Hospital[2]	Olympia	100%	48
Saint Anthony Hospital[2]	Gig Harbor	100%	51
Saint Clare Hospital[2]	Lakewood	100%	47
Saint Francis Community Hospital[2]	Federal Way	100%	55
Saint Joseph Medical Center[2]	Tacoma	100%	126
Skagit Valley Hospital[2]	Mount Vernon	100%	29
Swedish Edmonds Hospital[2]	Edmonds	100%	38
Swedish Medical Center[2]	Seattle	100%	53
Swedish Medical Center - Cherry Hill[2]	Seattle	100%	38
Tacoma General Allenmore Hospital[2]	Tacoma	100%	77
University of Washington Medical Center[2]	Seattle	100%	69
Valley Hospital[2]	Spokane	100%	50
Valley Medical Center[2]	Renton	100%	49
Virginia Mason Medical Center[2]	Seattle	100%	115
Yakima Regional Medical & Cardiac Center[2]	Yakima	100%	44
Yakima Valley Memorial Hospital[2]	Yakima	100%	57
Peacehealth Saint Joseph Medical Center[2]	Bellingham	99%	82
Providence Sacred Heart Medical Center[2]	Spokane	99%	110

Venous Thromboembolism Prophylaxis

Hospital Name	City	Rate	Cases
Multicare Auburn Medical Center[2]	Auburn	98%	339
Providence Reg Med Ctr Everett[2]	Everett	98%	296
Skagit Valley Hospital[2]	Mount Vernon	98%	336
Capital Medical Center[2]	Olympia	97%	240
Legacy Salmon Creek Medical Center[2]	Vancouver	97%	239
Deaconess Hospital[2]	Spokane	96%	372
Cascade Valley Hospital[2]	Arlington	95%	117
Valley Hospital[2]	Spokane	95%	317
Walla Walla General Hospital[2]	Walla Walla	95%	64
Whidbey General Hospital[2]	Coupeville	95%	131
Kadlec Regional Medical Center[2]	Richland	94%	414
Peacehealth Southwest Medical Center[2]	Vancouver	94%	310
Virginia Mason Medical Center[2]	Seattle	94%	294
Swedish Issaquah[2]	Issaquah	93%	227
Saint Clare Hospital[2]	Lakewood	92%	324
Harborview Medical Center[2]	Seattle	91%	223
Harrison Memorial Center[2]	Bremerton	91%	314
Northwest Hospital[2]	Seattle	91%	296
Saint Anthony Hospital[2]	Gig Harbor	91%	336
Kittitas Valley Community Hospital[2]	Ellensburg	90%	170
Saint Joseph Medical Center[2]	Tacoma	90%	314
Providence Holy Family Hospital[2]	Spokane	89%	291
Skyline Hospital[3]	White Salmon	89%	28
Tacoma General Allenmore Hospital[2]	Tacoma	89%	628
Valley Medical Center[2]	Renton	89%	292
Kennewick General Hospital[2]	Kennewick	88%	343
Olympic Medical Center[2]	Port Angeles	88%	287
Saint Francis Community Hospital[2]	Federal Way	88%	326
Multicare Good Samaritan Hospital[2]	Puyallup	87%	383
Swedish Edmonds Hospital[2]	Edmonds	87%	296
Highline Medical Center[2]	Burien	86%	332
Evergreen Hospital Medical Center[2]	Kirkland	85%	312
Overlake Hospital Medical Center[2]	Bellevue	85%	259
Providence Saint Peter Hospital[2]	Olympia	85%	262
Valley General Hospital[2]	Monroe	85%	80
Peacehealth Saint John Medical Center[2]	Longview	84%	329
Providence Sacred Heart Medical Center[2]	Spokane	84%	264
Saint Elizabeth Hospital[2]	Enumclaw	84%	101
Lourdes Medical Center[2]	Pasco	83%	65
Providence Saint Mary Medical Center[2]	Walla Walla	83%	235
Swedish Medical Center - Cherry Hill[2]	Seattle	83%	211
Providence Centralia Hospital[2]	Centralia	82%	313
Central Washington Hospital[2]	Wenatchee	81%	267
Samaritan Hospital[2]	Moses Lake	81%	102
Swedish Medical Center[2]	Seattle	80%	400
University of Washington Medical Center[2]	Seattle	80%	350
Grays Harbor Community Hospital[2]	Aberdeen	78%	1181
Peacehealth Saint Joseph Medical Center[2]	Bellingham	76%	289
Island Hospital[2]	Anacortes	74%	246
Toppenish Community Hospital[2]	Toppenish	74%	145
Yakima Valley Memorial Hospital[2]	Yakima	72%	310
Yakima Regional Medical & Cardiac Center[2]	Yakima	61%	296
Confluence Hlth-Wenatchee Valley Hosp	Wenatchee	46%	74
Klickitat Valley Hospital	Goldendale	12%	80

Warfarin Therapy Discharge Instructions

Hospital Name	City	Rate	Cases
Kadlec Regional Medical Center[2]	Richland	100%	106
Multicare Good Samaritan Hospital[2]	Puyallup	96%	100
Tacoma General Allenmore Hospital[2]	Tacoma	94%	96
Evergreen Hospital Medical Center[2]	Kirkland	91%	100
Providence Sacred Heart Medical Center[2]	Spokane	91%	92
Valley Hospital[2]	Spokane	91%	58
Deaconess Hospital[2]	Spokane	90%	51
Harborview Medical Center[2]	Seattle	90%	51
Legacy Salmon Creek Medical Center[2]	Vancouver	90%	52
Northwest Hospital[2]	Seattle	90%	51
Multicare Auburn Medical Center[2]	Auburn	89%	44
Skagit Valley Hospital[2]	Mount Vernon	87%	31
Valley Medical Center[2]	Renton	87%	83
Providence Reg Med Ctr Everett[2]	Everett	86%	196
Virginia Mason Medical Center[2]	Seattle	86%	111
Peacehealth Saint John Medical Center[2]	Longview	83%	47
Saint Francis Community Hospital[2]	Federal Way	83%	52
Yakima Valley Memorial Hospital[2]	Yakima	82%	51
Providence Holy Family Hospital[2]	Spokane	75%	79
Overlake Hospital Medical Center[2]	Bellevue	74%	91
Peacehealth Saint Joseph Medical Center[2]	Bellingham	74%	69
Harrison Memorial Center[2]	Bremerton	70%	114
Saint Anthony Hospital[2]	Gig Harbor	70%	40
Saint Joseph Medical Center[2]	Tacoma	69%	116
Central Washington Hospital[2]	Wenatchee	68%	40
Providence Centralia Hospital[2]	Centralia	61%	31
Saint Clare Hospital[2]	Lakewood	61%	41
Peacehealth Southwest Medical Center[2]	Vancouver	57%	134
Highline Medical Center[2]	Burien	40%	45
Yakima Regional Medical & Cardiac Center[2]	Yakima	40%	35
University of Washington Medical Center[2]	Seattle	38%	40
Providence Saint Peter Hospital[2]	Olympia	25%	116
Swedish Medical Center - Cherry Hill[2]	Seattle	24%	25
Swedish Medical Center[2]	Seattle	11%	63
Swedish Edmonds Hospital[2]	Edmonds	0%	53

Chest Pain/Possible Heart Attack Care

Aspirin Given Within 24 Hours of Arrival

Hospital Name	City	Rate	Cases
Cascade Valley Hospital	Arlington	100%	37
Kennewick General Hospital	Kennewick	100%	33
Kittitas Valley Community Hospital	Ellensburg	100%	34
North Valley Hospital	Tonasket	100%	26
Peacehealth United General Medical Center	Sedro Woolley	100%	91
Providence Mount Carmel Hospital	Colville	100%	41
Providence Saint Mary Medical Center	Walla Walla	100%	45
Saint Anthony Hospital	Gig Harbor	100%	31
Valley General Hospital	Monroe	100%	36
Valley Hospital	Spokane	100%	107
Legacy Salmon Creek Medical Center	Vancouver	99%	79
Olympic Medical Center	Port Angeles	98%	100
Peacehealth Saint John Medical Center	Longview	98%	148
Saint Clare Hospital	Lakewood	98%	63
Saint Elizabeth Hospital	Enumclaw	98%	40
Tacoma General Allenmore Hospital	Tacoma	98%	59
Tri - State Memorial Hospital	Clarkston	98%	41
Island Hospital	Anacortes	97%	69
Samaritan Hospital	Moses Lake	97%	135
Toppenish Community Hospital	Toppenish	97%	34
Jefferson Healthcare Hospital[3]	Port Townsend	96%	28
Mid Valley Hospital	Omak	96%	28
Grays Harbor Community Hospital	Aberdeen	94%	50
Swedish Medical Center	Seattle	94%	181
Providence Holy Family Hospital	Spokane	93%	104
Providence Centralia Hospital	Centralia	92%	103

Average Time to ECG (minutes)

Hospital Name	City	Min.	Cases
Multicare Good Samaritan Hospital	Puyallup	0	25
Olympic Medical Center	Port Angeles	2	100
Kittitas Valley Community Hospital	Ellensburg	3	37
Providence Mount Carmel Hospital	Colville	3	46
Tri - State Memorial Hospital	Clarkston	3	45

NOTE: Hospital profiles are in alphabetical order by state, then city, then hospital within the city; Rankings exclude hospitals with less than 25 cases except for patient surveys which excludes hospitals with less than 100 cases; (a) 100-299 cases; (1) The number of cases/patients is too few to report; (2) Data submitted were based on a sample of cases/patients; (3) Results are based on a shorter time period than required; (4) Data suppressed by CMS for one or more quarters; (5) Results are not available for this reporting period; (6) Fewer than 100 patients completed the HCAHPS survey; (7) No cases met the criteria for this measure; (8) The lower limit of the confidence interval cannot be calculated if the number of observed infections equals zero; (9) No data are available from the state/territory for this reporting period; (10) The scores shown reflect fewer than 50 completed surveys; (11) There were discrepancies in the data collection process; (12) This measure does not apply to this hospital for this reporting period; (13) Results cannot be calculated for this reporting period; (14) The results for this state are combined with nearby states to protect confidentiality; Please refer to the User's Guide for a full explanation of data.

North Valley Hospital	Tonasket	5	28
Valley Hospital	Spokane	5	108
Peacehealth Saint John Medical Center	Longview	6	156
Saint Anthony Hospital	Gig Harbor	6	31
Jefferson Healthcare Hospital[3]	Port Townsend	7	32
Tacoma General Allenmore Hospital	Tacoma	8	63
Providence Centralia Hospital	Centralia	9	109
Providence Saint Mary Medical Center	Walla Walla	9	46
Swedish Medical Center	Seattle	9	190
Toppenish Community Hospital	Toppenish	9	37
Peacehealth United General Medical Center	Sedro Woolley	10	92
Cascade Valley Hospital	Arlington	11	37
Kennewick General Hospital	Kennewick	11	34
Providence Holy Family Hospital	Spokane	12	110
Saint Clare Hospital	Lakewood	12	40
Saint Elizabeth Hospital	Enumclaw	12	40
Valley General Hospital	Monroe	12	41
Island Hospital	Anacortes	13	69
Legacy Salmon Creek Medical Center	Vancouver	13	79
Sunnyside Community Hospital	Sunnyside	14	27
Grays Harbor Community Hospital	Aberdeen	15	59
Mid Valley Hospital	Omak	15	31
Samaritan Hospital	Moses Lake	15	140

Average Time to Transfer (minutes)

Hospital Name	City	Min.	Cases
Swedish Medical Center	Seattle	39	27
Legacy Salmon Creek Medical Center	Vancouver	45	26
Providence Holy Family Hospital	Spokane	47	25
Providence Centralia Hospital	Centralia	54	28
Peacehealth United General Medical Center	Sedro Woolley	196	37

Children's Asthma Care

Received Home Management Plan of Care

Hospital Name	City	Rate	Cases
Providence Saint Peter Hospital	Olympia	76%	33
Providence Sacred Heart Medical Center	Spokane	65%	48

Received Reliever Medication

Hospital Name	City	Rate	Cases
Providence Sacred Heart Medical Center	Spokane	100%	48
Providence Saint Peter Hospital	Olympia	100%	37

Received Systemic Corticosteroids

Hospital Name	City	Rate	Cases
Providence Sacred Heart Medical Center	Spokane	100%	48
Providence Saint Peter Hospital	Olympia	97%	37

Emergency Department

Admittance Decision Time (minutes)

Hospital Name	City	Min.	Cases
Skyline Hospital[3]	White Salmon	8	28
Providence Saint Joseph Hospital	Chewelah	36	180
Providence Mount Carmel Hospital[2]	Colville	43	253
Valley General Hospital[2]	Monroe	50	426
Providence Saint Mary Medical Center[2]	Walla Walla	51	428
Providence Sacred Heart Medical Center[2]	Spokane	53	293
Klickitat Valley Hospital[3]	Goldendale	59	50
Deaconess Hospital[2]	Spokane	61	377
Walla Walla General Hospital[2]	Walla Walla	62	126
Toppenish Community Hospital[2]	Toppenish	63	420
Island Hospital[2]	Anacortes	65	319
Samaritan Hospital[2]	Moses Lake	65	269
Cascade Valley Hospital[2]	Arlington	72	288
Swedish Issaquah[2]	Issaquah	72	490
Yakima Valley Memorial Hospital[2]	Yakima	74	516
Olympic Medical Center[2]	Port Angeles	75	514
Saint Elizabeth Hospital[2]	Enumclaw	75	286
Capital Medical Center[2]	Olympia	76	288
Central Washington Hospital[2]	Wenatchee	76	355
Skagit Valley Hospital[2]	Mount Vernon	78	358
Swedish Medical Center[2]	Seattle	79	438
Swedish Medical Center - Cherry Hill[2]	Seattle	79	332
Whidbey General Hospital[2]	Coupeville	81	429
Peacehealth Southwest Medical Center[2]	Vancouver	85	689
Peacehealth Saint John Medical Center[2]	Longview	85	704
Tacoma General Allenmore Hospital[2]	Tacoma	86	1037
Virginia Mason Medical Center[2]	Seattle	91	317
Grays Harbor Community Hospital[2]	Aberdeen	92	434
Legacy Salmon Creek Medical Center[2]	Vancouver	92	572
Valley Medical Center[2]	Renton	93	501
Kennewick General Hospital[2]	Kennewick	100	487
Providence Saint Peter Hospital[2]	Olympia	100	552
Northwest Hospital[2]	Seattle	102	591
Valley Hospital[2]	Spokane	102	686
Harrison Memorial Center[2]	Bremerton	103	546
Providence Centralia Hospital[2]	Centralia	103	731
Evergreen Hospital Medical Center[2]	Kirkland	105	564
Providence Reg Med Ctr Everett[2]	Everett	105	593
Multicare Auburn Medical Center[2]	Auburn	106	725
Yakima Regional Medical & Cardiac Center[2]	Yakima	108	554
Multicare Good Samaritan Hospital[2]	Puyallup	118	712
Providence Holy Family Hospital[2]	Spokane	129	593
Swedish Edmonds Hospital[2]	Edmonds	129	548
Highline Medical Center[2]	Burien	132	692
Peacehealth Saint Joseph Medical Center[2]	Bellingham	139	565
Overlake Hospital Medical Center[2]	Bellevue	140	381
Saint Anthony Hospital[2]	Gig Harbor	140	766
Kadlec Regional Medical Center[2]	Richland	142	421
Saint Francis Community Hospital[2]	Federal Way	147	683
Saint Clare Hospital[2]	Lakewood	151	945
Saint Joseph Medical Center[2]	Tacoma	168	365
University of Washington Medical Center[2]	Seattle	176	277
Harborview Medical Center[2]	Seattle	229	199

Head CT Results Within 45 Minutes of Arrival

Hospital Name	City	Rate	Cases
Peachealth Saint John Medical Center	Longview	88%	40
Grays Harbor Community Hospital	Aberdeen	84%	25
Saint Francis Community Hospital	Federal Way	78%	41
Multicare Auburn Medical Center	Auburn	62%	26
Providence Reg Med Ctr Everett	Everett	34%	32

Patients Who Left ER Before Being Seen

Hospital Name	City	Rate	Cases
Cascade Valley Hospital	Arlington	0%	19575
Saint Anthony Hospital	Gig Harbor	0%	22418
Saint Elizabeth Hospital	Enumclaw	0%	13730
Swedish Issaquah	Issaquah	0%	22789
Swedish Medical Center	Seattle	0%	96621
Swedish Medical Center - Cherry Hill	Seattle	0%	18916
Toppenish Community Hospital	Toppenish	0%	17320
Walla Walla General Hospital	Walla Walla	0%	10711
Central Washington Hospital	Wenatchee	1%	26513
Confluence Hlth-Wenatchee Valley Hosp	Wenatchee	1%	8747
Evergreen Hospital Medical Center	Kirkland	1%	44797
Highline Medical Center	Burien	1%	58095
Island Hospital	Anacortes	1%	12324
Kadlec Regional Medical Center	Richland	1%	59572
Kittitas Valley Community Hospital	Ellensburg	1%	11935
Legacy Salmon Creek Medical Center	Vancouver	1%	50602
Multicare Good Samaritan Hospital	Puyallup	1%	68228
Northwest Hospital	Seattle	1%	34150
Overlake Hospital Medical Center	Bellevue	1%	43750
Providence Reg Med Ctr Everett	Everett	1%	92075
Providence Saint Mary Medical Center	Walla Walla	1%	19814
Saint Francis Community Hospital	Federal Way	1%	47896
Saint Joseph Medical Center	Tacoma	1%	53136
Swedish Edmonds Hospital	Edmonds	1%	41092
Tacoma General Allenmore Hospital	Tacoma	1%	78161
Valley General Hospital	Monroe	1%	15017
Valley Medical Center	Renton	1%	76771
Yakima Valley Memorial Hospital	Yakima	1%	69471
Capital Medical Center	Olympia	2%	17286
Deaconess Hospital	Spokane	2%	25694
Grays Harbor Community Hospital	Aberdeen	2%	31869
Harrison Memorial Center	Bremerton	2%	71744
Kennewick General Hospital	Kennewick	2%	32458
Olympic Medical Center	Port Angeles	2%	22633
Peacehealth Southwest Medical Center	Vancouver	2%	79277
Peachealth Saint John Medical Center	Longview	2%	50432
Providence Saint Peter Hospital	Olympia	2%	66867
Saint Clare Hospital	Lakewood	2%	46048
Samaritan Hospital	Moses Lake	2%	13032
Skagit Valley Hospital	Mount Vernon	2%	29720
Valley Hospital	Spokane	2%	41280
Virginia Mason Medical Center	Seattle	2%	22978
Yakima Regional Medical & Cardiac Center	Yakima	2%	31900
Peacehealth Saint Joseph Medical Center	Bellingham	3%	57109
Providence Holy Family Hospital	Spokane	3%	64776
Providence Sacred Heart Medical Center	Spokane	3%	71543
University of Washington Medical Center	Seattle	3%	24221
Providence Centralia Hospital	Centralia	4%	30424
Harborview Medical Center	Seattle	5%	68534

Time from ER Arrival to Being Admitted (minutes)

Hospital Name	City	Min.	Cases
Swedish Issaquah[2]	Issaquah	154	490
Providence Saint Joseph Hospital	Chewelah	158	205
Island Hospital[2]	Anacortes	186	374
Providence Mount Carmel Hospital[2]	Colville	186	263
Swedish Medical Center - Cherry Hill[2]	Seattle	186	334
Toppenish Community Hospital[2]	Toppenish	188	420
Walla Walla General Hospital[2]	Walla Walla	194	178
Yakima Valley Memorial Hospital[2]	Yakima	203	516
Skyline Hospital[3]	White Salmon	204	41
Providence Sacred Heart Medical Center[2]	Spokane	211	422
Swedish Medical Center[2]	Seattle	211	440
Deaconess Hospital[2]	Spokane	222	495
Central Washington Hospital[2]	Wenatchee	227	359
Peacehealth Southwest Medical Center[2]	Vancouver	230	701
Peachealth Saint John Medical Center[2]	Longview	231	713
Kennewick General Hospital[2]	Kennewick	232	526
Saint Elizabeth Hospital[2]	Enumclaw	235	332
Cascade Valley Hospital[2]	Arlington	236	325
Samaritan Hospital[2]	Moses Lake	236	285
Valley General Hospital[2]	Monroe	236	465
Olympic Medical Center[2]	Port Angeles	239	554
Yakima Regional Medical & Cardiac Center[2]	Yakima	244	626
Virginia Mason Medical Center[2]	Seattle	246	322
Grays Harbor Community Hospital[2]	Aberdeen	248	502
Providence Saint Mary Medical Center[2]	Walla Walla	249	429
Legacy Salmon Creek Medical Center[2]	Vancouver	250	572
Overlake Hospital Medical Center[2]	Bellevue	251	408
Capital Medical Center[2]	Olympia	252	291
Whidbey General Hospital[2]	Coupeville	252	475
Evergreen Hospital Medical Center[2]	Kirkland	256	568
Skagit Valley Hospital[2]	Mount Vernon	258	563
Klickitat Valley Hospital[3]	Goldendale	259	76
Harrison Memorial Center[2]	Bremerton	262	605
Providence Saint Peter Hospital[2]	Olympia	263	578
Highline Medical Center[2]	Burien	264	695
Northwest Hospital[2]	Seattle	265	591
Valley Hospital[2]	Spokane	275	767
Providence Centralia Hospital[2]	Centralia	281	734
Peacehealth Saint Joseph Medical Center[2]	Bellingham	286	566
Swedish Edmonds Hospital[2]	Edmonds	287	549
Kadlec Regional Medical Center[2]	Richland	291	437
Tacoma General Allenmore Hospital[2]	Tacoma	294	1046
Multicare Auburn Medical Center[2]	Auburn	298	758
Saint Anthony Hospital[2]	Gig Harbor	298	782
Multicare Good Samaritan Hospital[2]	Puyallup	300	749
Valley Medical Center[2]	Renton	303	501
Providence Reg Med Ctr Everett[2]	Everett	307	593
Providence Holy Family Hospital[2]	Spokane	323	646
Saint Francis Community Hospital[2]	Federal Way	328	708
Saint Clare Hospital[2]	Lakewood	330	966
Saint Joseph Medical Center[2]	Tacoma	330	387
Harborview Medical Center[2]	Seattle	402	564
University of Washington Medical Center[2]	Seattle	423	285

Time from ER Arrival to Discharge (minutes)

Hospital Name	City	Min.	Cases
Toppenish Community Hospital	Toppenish	83	915
Swedish Issaquah	Issaquah	86	406
Cascade Valley Hospital	Arlington	90	401
Peacehealth Peace Island Medical Center[3]	Friday Harbor	91	68
Swedish Medical Center	Seattle	92	1572
Klickitat Valley Hospital[3]	Goldendale	93	169
Yakima Valley Memorial Hospital	Yakima	93	386
Providence Saint Mary Medical Center	Walla Walla	95	357
Walla Walla General Hospital	Walla Walla	100	353
Highline Medical Center	Burien	109	360
Island Hospital	Anacortes	112	466
Kennewick General Hospital	Kennewick	114	358
Providence Saint Joseph Hospital	Chewelah	114	299
Grays Harbor Community Hospital	Aberdeen	125	553
Peachealth Saint John Medical Center	Longview	126	399
Providence Mount Carmel Hospital	Colville	127	329
Saint Elizabeth Hospital	Enumclaw	127	407
Yakima Regional Medical & Cardiac Center	Yakima	127	351
Swedish Medical Center - Cherry Hill	Seattle	130	346
Kadlec Regional Medical Center	Richland	133	365
Central Washington Hospital	Wenatchee	134	877
Samaritan Hospital	Moses Lake	136	426
Swedish Edmonds Hospital	Edmonds	138	371
Evergreen Hospital Medical Center	Kirkland	139	385
Deaconess Hospital	Spokane	140	388
Valley General Hospital	Monroe	142	350
Olympic Medical Center	Port Angeles	150	449
Saint Francis Community Hospital	Federal Way	150	400
Northwest Hospital	Seattle	151	379
Saint Joseph Medical Center	Tacoma	151	347
Harrison Memorial Center	Bremerton	152	375
Providence Holy Family Hospital	Spokane	152	366
Capital Medical Center	Olympia	155	474
Peacehealth Southwest Medical Center	Vancouver	156	353
Valley Medical Center	Renton	156	360
Virginia Mason Medical Center	Seattle	156	410
Legacy Salmon Creek Medical Center	Vancouver	157	359
Skyline Hospital	White Salmon	158	70
Skagit Valley Hospital	Mount Vernon	159	361
Valley Hospital	Spokane	159	366
Multicare Auburn Medical Center	Auburn	160	385
Overlake Hospital Medical Center	Bellevue	161	377
Providence Centralia Hospital	Centralia	162	353
Peacehealth Saint Joseph Medical Center	Bellingham	164	332

NOTE: Hospital profiles are in alphabetical order by state, then city, then hospital within the city; Rankings exclude hospitals with less than 25 cases except for patient surveys which excludes hospitals with less than 100 cases; (a) 100-299 cases; (1) The number of cases/patients is too few to report; (2) Data submitted were based on a sample of cases/patients; (3) Results are based on a shorter time period than required; (4) Data suppressed by CMS for one or more quarters; (5) Results are not available for this reporting period; (6) Fewer than 100 patients completed the HCAHPS survey; (7) No cases met the criteria for this measure; (8) The lower limit of the confidence interval cannot be calculated if the number of observed infections equals zero; (9) No data are available from the state/territory for this reporting period; (10) The scores shown reflect fewer than 50 completed surveys; (11) There were discrepancies in the data collection process; (12) This measure does not apply to this hospital for this reporting period; (13) Results cannot be calculated for this reporting period; (14) The results for this state are combined with nearby states to protect confidentiality; Please refer to the User's Guide for a full explanation of data.

Saint Anthony Hospital	Gig Harbor	165	376
Saint Clare Hospital	Lakewood	165	380
Providence Saint Peter Hospital	Olympia	166	357
Providence Sacred Heart Medical Center	Spokane	176	328
Tacoma General Allenmore Hospital	Tacoma	177	1225
Multicare Good Samaritan Hospital	Puyallup	185	382
Providence Reg Med Ctr Everett	Everett	186	398
Harborview Medical Center	Seattle	222	297
University of Washington Medical Center	Seattle	231	357

Time in ER Before Being Evaluated (minutes)

Hospital Name	City	Min.	Cases
Swedish Issaquah	Issaquah	7	412
Saint Anthony Hospital	Gig Harbor	8	424
Swedish Medical Center	Seattle	8	1659
Lake Chelan Community Hospital	Chelan	11	90
Swedish Edmonds Hospital	Edmonds	11	279
Swedish Medical Center - Cherry Hill	Seattle	11	416
Peacehealth Peace Island Medical Center[3]	Friday Harbor	12	84
Providence Mount Carmel Hospital	Colville	13	364
Saint Elizabeth Hospital	Enumclaw	13	428
Toppenish Community Hospital	Toppenish	13	958
Walla Walla General Hospital	Walla Walla	15	381
Island Hospital	Anacortes	17	416
Klickitat Valley Hospital[3]	Goldendale	17	98
Evergreen Hospital Medical Center	Kirkland	19	282
Highline Medical Center	Burien	20	382
Overlake Hospital Medical Center	Bellevue	20	298
Providence Saint Mary Medical Center	Walla Walla	21	379
Yakima Valley Memorial Hospital	Yakima	21	408
Capital Medical Center	Olympia	22	497
Cascade Valley Hospital	Arlington	22	424
Grays Harbor Community Hospital	Aberdeen	22	636
Kadlec Regional Medical Center	Richland	22	343
Saint Clare Hospital	Lakewood	22	410
Providence Reg Med Ctr Everett	Everett	23	430
Skyline Hospital	White Salmon	23	78
Valley Medical Center	Renton	23	363
University of Washington Medical Center	Seattle	24	402
Harrison Memorial Center	Bremerton	25	415
Saint Francis Community Hospital	Federal Way	25	438
Deaconess Hospital	Spokane	26	369
Yakima Regional Medical & Cardiac Center	Yakima	26	397
Harborview Medical Center	Seattle	27	375
Valley General Hospital	Monroe	27	353
Virginia Mason Medical Center	Seattle	27	129
Providence Saint Joseph Hospital	Chewelah	29	288
Saint Joseph Medical Center	Tacoma	29	407
Samaritan Hospital	Moses Lake	29	451
Kennewick General Hospital	Kennewick	30	378
Legacy Salmon Creek Medical Center	Vancouver	30	388
Northwest Hospital	Seattle	30	408
Peacehealth Saint John Medical Center	Longview	31	398
Providence Holy Family Hospital	Spokane	31	383
Skagit Valley Hospital	Mount Vernon	34	358
Central Washington Hospital	Wenatchee	36	441
Multicare Auburn Medical Center	Auburn	36	296
Peacehealth Saint Joseph Medical Center	Bellingham	36	384
Valley Hospital	Spokane	41	293
Olympic Medical Center	Port Angeles	43	408
Peacehealth Southwest Medical Center	Vancouver	45	395
Providence Centralia Hospital	Centralia	45	284
Tacoma General Allenmore Hospital	Tacoma	46	459
Providence Sacred Heart Medical Center	Spokane	54	260
Multicare Good Samaritan Hospital	Puyallup	62	94
Providence Saint Peter Hospital	Olympia	64	99

Time to Pain Meds for Bone Fractures (minutes)

Hospital Name	City	Min.	Cases
Saint Anthony Hospital	Gig Harbor	28	107
Swedish Edmonds Hospital	Edmonds	34	167
Swedish Medical Center	Seattle	34	284
Kennewick General Hospital	Kennewick	35	97
Walla Walla General Hospital	Walla Walla	37	36
Saint Elizabeth Hospital	Enumclaw	38	93
Swedish Issaquah	Issaquah	38	111
Legacy Salmon Creek Medical Center	Vancouver	41	230
Skyline Hospital	White Salmon	41	27
Providence Saint Mary Medical Center	Walla Walla	42	88
Kadlec Regional Medical Center	Richland	43	273
Kittitas Valley Community Hospital	Ellensburg	44	73
Providence Saint Joseph Hospital	Chewelah	44	26
Yakima Valley Memorial Hospital	Yakima	44	249
Overlake Hospital Medical Center	Bellevue	46	354
Valley General Hospital	Monroe	46	46
Evergreen Hospital Medical Center	Kirkland	47	269
Highline Medical Center	Burien	47	136
Providence Mount Carmel Hospital	Colville	47	54
Saint Clare Hospital	Lakewood	47	81
Providence Sacred Heart Medical Center	Spokane	48	204
Saint Joseph Medical Center	Tacoma	48	66
Toppenish Community Hospital	Toppenish	48	91
Central Washington Hospital	Wenatchee	50	148
Valley Hospital	Spokane	50	145
Skagit Valley Hospital	Mount Vernon	51	125
Deaconess Hospital	Spokane	52	49
Harrison Memorial Center	Bremerton	52	167
Yakima Regional Medical & Cardiac Center	Yakima	52	72
Peacehealth Saint John Medical Center	Longview	53	189
Samaritan Hospital	Moses Lake	53	82
Island Hospital	Anacortes	54	80
Saint Francis Community Hospital	Federal Way	54	188
Valley Medical Center	Renton	54	212
Capital Medical Center	Olympia	55	44
Swedish Medical Center - Cherry Hill	Seattle	55	40
Cascade Valley Hospital	Arlington	57	74
Peacehealth Southwest Medical Center	Vancouver	58	202
Providence Centralia Hospital	Centralia	58	144
Multicare Auburn Medical Center	Auburn	59	126
Northwest Hospital	Seattle	59	100
Harborview Medical Center	Seattle	61	79
Virginia Mason Medical Center	Seattle	61	121
Providence Reg Med Ctr Everett	Everett	62	387
Tacoma General Allenmore Hospital	Tacoma	62	172
University of Washington Medical Center	Seattle	65	61
Providence Saint Peter Hospital	Olympia	66	234
Providence Holy Family Hospital	Spokane	67	193
Olympic Medical Center	Port Angeles	68	81
Peacehealth Saint Joseph Medical Center	Bellingham	73	263
Grays Harbor Community Hospital	Aberdeen	74	163
Multicare Good Samaritan Hospital	Puyallup	92	231

Heart Attack Care

Aspirin Given at Discharge

Hospital Name	City	Rate	Cases
Capital Medical Center	Olympia	100%	75
Central Washington Hospital	Wenatchee	100%	323
Deaconess Hospital	Spokane	100%	246
Evergreen Hospital Medical Center	Kirkland	100%	217
Harborview Medical Center	Seattle	100%	73
Legacy Salmon Creek Medical Center	Vancouver	100%	34
Overlake Hospital Medical Center	Bellevue	100%	246
Providence Holy Family Hospital	Spokane	100%	28
Providence Sacred Heart Medical Center	Spokane	100%	674
Providence Saint Mary Medical Center	Walla Walla	100%	30
Saint Anthony Hospital	Gig Harbor	100%	49
Saint Joseph Medical Center[2]	Tacoma	100%	452
Seattle VA Med Ctr-VA Pugit Sound	Seattle	100%	64
Swedish Issaquah	Issaquah	100%	67
Tacoma General Allenmore Hospital	Tacoma	100%	322
University of Washington Medical Center	Seattle	100%	107
Virginia Mason Medical Center	Seattle	100%	225
Walla Walla General Hospital	Walla Walla	100%	30
Yakima Valley Memorial Hospital	Yakima	100%	163
Harrison Memorial Center	Bremerton	99%	360
Kadlec Regional Medical Center	Richland	99%	412
Multicare Auburn Medical Center	Auburn	99%	116
Multicare Good Samaritan Hospital	Puyallup	99%	280
Northwest Hospital	Seattle	99%	156
Peacehealth Saint Joseph Medical Center	Bellingham	99%	347
Peacehealth Southwest Medical Center	Vancouver	99%	565
Peacehealth Saint John Medical Center	Longview	99%	144
Providence Reg Med Ctr Everett[2]	Everett	99%	348
Providence Saint Peter Hospital	Olympia	99%	564
Saint Francis Community Hospital	Federal Way	99%	148
Skagit Valley Hospital	Mount Vernon	99%	195
Swedish Medical Center - Cherry Hill	Seattle	99%	359
Valley Medical Center	Renton	99%	249
Yakima Regional Medical & Cardiac Center	Yakima	99%	265
Highline Medical Center	Burien	97%	131
Swedish Edmonds Hospital	Edmonds	95%	182

PCI Within 90 Minutes of Arrival

Hospital Name	City	Rate	Cases
Harrison Memorial Center	Bremerton	100%	60
Kadlec Regional Medical Center	Richland	100%	60
Multicare Auburn Medical Center	Auburn	100%	36
Multicare Good Samaritan Hospital	Puyallup	100%	70
Northwest Hospital	Seattle	100%	44
Providence Reg Med Ctr Everett[2]	Everett	100%	61
Swedish Medical Center - Cherry Hill	Seattle	100%	60
Tacoma General Allenmore Hospital	Tacoma	100%	36
Yakima Regional Medical & Cardiac Center	Yakima	100%	25
Providence Saint Peter Hospital	Olympia	99%	79
Overlake Hospital Medical Center	Bellevue	98%	58
Providence Sacred Heart Medical Center	Spokane	98%	92
Evergreen Hospital Medical Center	Kirkland	97%	63
Skagit Valley Hospital	Mount Vernon	97%	39
Highline Medical Center	Burien	96%	28
Saint Francis Community Hospital	Federal Way	96%	26
Valley Medical Center	Renton	96%	55
Saint Joseph Medical Center[2]	Tacoma	95%	59
Swedish Edmonds Hospital	Edmonds	95%	58
Virginia Mason Medical Center	Seattle	93%	29
Peacehealth Saint Joseph Medical Center	Bellingham	92%	73
Peacehealth Southwest Medical Center	Vancouver	90%	78

Statin Prescribed at Discharge

Hospital Name	City	Rate	Cases
Deaconess Hospital	Spokane	100%	235
Harborview Medical Center	Seattle	100%	70
Legacy Salmon Creek Medical Center	Vancouver	100%	30
Multicare Auburn Medical Center	Auburn	100%	118
Multicare Good Samaritan Hospital	Puyallup	100%	272
Providence Sacred Heart Medical Center	Spokane	100%	649
Providence Saint Mary Medical Center	Walla Walla	100%	27
Tacoma General Allenmore Hospital	Tacoma	100%	300
Virginia Mason Medical Center	Seattle	100%	230
Walla Walla General Hospital	Walla Walla	100%	28
Yakima Valley Memorial Hospital	Yakima	100%	164
Central Washington Hospital	Wenatchee	99%	317
Harrison Memorial Center	Bremerton	99%	347
Kadlec Regional Medical Center	Richland	99%	393
Overlake Hospital Medical Center	Bellevue	99%	246
Peacehealth Southwest Medical Center	Vancouver	99%	540
Providence Saint Peter Hospital	Olympia	99%	547
Saint Francis Community Hospital	Federal Way	99%	145
Saint Joseph Medical Center[2]	Tacoma	99%	451
Skagit Valley Hospital	Mount Vernon	99%	184
University of Washington Medical Center	Seattle	99%	108
Evergreen Hospital Medical Center	Kirkland	98%	205
Providence Reg Med Ctr Everett[2]	Everett	98%	333
Saint Anthony Hospital	Gig Harbor	98%	45
Valley Medical Center	Renton	98%	242
Yakima Regional Medical & Cardiac Center	Yakima	98%	257
Highline Medical Center	Burien	97%	119
Seattle VA Med Ctr-VA Pugit Sound	Seattle	97%	64
Swedish Issaquah	Issaquah	97%	63
Swedish Medical Center - Cherry Hill	Seattle	97%	357
Capital Medical Center	Olympia	96%	69
Northwest Hospital	Seattle	96%	150
Peacehealth Saint Joseph Medical Center	Bellingham	95%	333
Peacehealth Saint John Medical Center	Longview	95%	148
Swedish Edmonds Hospital	Edmonds	93%	175
Providence Holy Family Hospital	Spokane	89%	28

Heart Failure Care

ACE Inhibitor or ARB for LVSD

Hospital Name	City	Rate	Cases
Evergreen Hospital Medical Center	Kirkland	100%	51
Harborview Medical Center	Seattle	100%	72
Highline Medical Center	Burien	100%	47
Legacy Salmon Creek Medical Center	Vancouver	100%	65
Multicare Good Samaritan Hospital[2]	Puyallup	100%	103
Overlake Hospital Medical Center	Bellevue	100%	82
Providence Reg Med Ctr Everett[2]	Everett	100%	105
Saint Clare Hospital	Lakewood	100%	66
Seattle VA Med Ctr-VA Pugit Sound	Seattle	100%	55
Skagit Valley Hospital	Mount Vernon	100%	55
Swedish Medical Center	Seattle	100%	47
Tacoma General Allenmore Hospital[2]	Tacoma	100%	102
University of Washington Medical Center	Seattle	100%	148
Valley Hospital	Spokane	100%	26
Valley Medical Center[2]	Renton	100%	106
Yakima Valley Memorial Hospital	Yakima	100%	53
Deaconess Hospital	Spokane	99%	87
Kadlec Regional Medical Center	Richland	99%	88
Saint Francis Community Hospital	Federal Way	99%	72
Saint Joseph Medical Center[2]	Tacoma	99%	136
Virginia Mason Medical Center	Seattle	99%	79
Central Washington Hospital	Wenatchee	98%	62
Kennewick General Hospital	Kennewick	98%	43
Olympic Medical Center	Port Angeles	98%	43
Yakima Regional Medical & Cardiac Center	Yakima	98%	80
Harrison Memorial Center	Bremerton	97%	115
Providence Centralia Hospital[2]	Centralia	97%	59
Providence Sacred Heart Medical Center	Spokane	97%	160
Providence Saint Peter Hospital	Olympia	97%	154
Swedish Edmonds Hospital	Edmonds	97%	77
Peacehealth Southwest Medical Center	Vancouver	96%	195
Swedish Medical Center - Cherry Hill	Seattle	96%	128
Northwest Hospital	Seattle	95%	63
Peacehealth Saint John Medical Center	Longview	95%	77
Saint Anthony Hospital	Gig Harbor	95%	42
Multicare Auburn Medical Center[2]	Auburn	94%	80
Providence Holy Family Hospital	Spokane	93%	54
Peacehealth Saint Joseph Medical Center	Bellingham	90%	87
Grays Harbor Community Hospital	Aberdeen	83%	59

NOTE: Hospital profiles are in alphabetical order by state, then city, then hospital within the city; Rankings exclude hospitals with less than 25 cases except for patient surveys which excludes hospitals with less than 100 cases; (a) 100-299 cases; (1) The number of cases/patients is too few to report; (2) Data submitted were based on a sample of cases/patients; (3) Results are based on a shorter time period than required; (4) Data suppressed by CMS for one or more quarters; (5) Results are not available for this reporting period; (6) Fewer than 100 patients completed the HCAHPS survey; (7) No cases met the criteria for this measure; (8) The lower limit of the confidence interval cannot be calculated if the number of observed infections equals zero; (9) No data are available from the state/territory for this reporting period; (10) The scores shown reflect fewer than 50 completed surveys; (11) There were discrepancies in the data collection process; (12) This measure does not apply to this hospital for this reporting period; (13) Results cannot be calculated for this reporting period; (14) The results for this state are combined with nearby states to protect confidentiality; Please refer to the User's Guide for a full explanation of data.

Discharge Instructions Given

Hospital Name	City	Rate	Cases
Kennewick General Hospital	Kennewick	100%	153
Mason General Hospital	Shelton	100%	39
Providence Saint Mary Medical Center	Walla Walla	100%	74
Swedish Medical Center - Cherry Hill	Seattle	100%	290
Evergreen Hospital Medical Center	Kirkland	99%	202
Kadlec Regional Medical Center	Richland	99%	246
Multicare Good Samaritan Hospital[2]	Puyallup	99%	274
Swedish Issaquah	Issaquah	99%	67
University of Washington Medical Center	Seattle	99%	260
Highline Medical Center	Burien	98%	134
Legacy Salmon Creek Medical Center	Vancouver	98%	180
Walla Walla General Hospital	Walla Walla	98%	40
Yakima Valley Memorial Hospital	Yakima	98%	203
Cascade Valley Hospital	Arlington	97%	34
Harborview Medical Center	Seattle	97%	120
Peacehealth Southwest Medical Center	Vancouver	97%	587
Seattle VA Med Ctr-VA Pugit Sound	Seattle	97%	153
Skagit Valley Hospital	Mount Vernon	97%	138
Tacoma General Allenmore Hospital[2]	Tacoma	97%	345
Toppenish Community Hospital	Toppenish	97%	37
Virginia Mason Medical Center	Seattle	97%	306
Deaconess Hospital	Spokane	96%	187
Northwest Hospital	Seattle	96%	147
Providence Centralia Hospital[2]	Centralia	95%	153
Providence Saint Peter Hospital	Olympia	95%	382
Swedish Medical Center	Seattle	95%	167
Overlake Hospital Medical Center	Bellevue	94%	273
Peachealth Saint John Medical Center	Longview	94%	177
Saint Clare Hospital	Lakewood	94%	145
Grays Harbor Community Hospital	Aberdeen	93%	147
Island Hospital	Anacortes	93%	29
Providence Mount Carmel Hospital	Colville	93%	27
Yakima Regional Medical & Cardiac Center	Yakima	93%	156
Providence Holy Family Hospital	Spokane	92%	130
Providence Sacred Heart Medical Center	Spokane	92%	342
Olympic Medical Center	Port Angeles	91%	102
Peacehealth Saint Joseph Medical Center	Bellingham	90%	274
Samaritan Hospital[2]	Moses Lake	90%	31
Valley Hospital	Spokane	90%	92
Providence Reg Med Ctr Everett[2]	Everett	89%	279
Capital Medical Center	Olympia	88%	64
Harrison Memorial Center	Bremerton	88%	265
Saint Francis Community Hospital	Federal Way	88%	163
Tri - State Memorial Hospital	Clarkston	88%	25
Saint Anthony Hospital	Gig Harbor	87%	118
Valley Medical Center[2]	Renton	87%	225
Spokane VA Medical Center	Spokane	86%	36
Central Washington Hospital	Wenatchee	85%	201
Saint Elizabeth Hospital[2]	Enumclaw	85%	34
Saint Joseph Medical Center[2]	Tacoma	85%	330
Swedish Edmonds Hospital	Edmonds	82%	147
Sunnyside Community Hospital[2]	Sunnyside	81%	43
Multicare Auburn Medical Center[2]	Auburn	79%	206
Whidbey General Hospital	Coupeville	79%	39
Jefferson Healthcare Hospital	Port Townsend	76%	25

Evaluation of LVS Function

Hospital Name	City	Rate	Cases
Capital Medical Center	Olympia	100%	82
Cascade Valley Hospital	Arlington	100%	38
Central Washington Hospital	Wenatchee	100%	219
Deaconess Hospital	Spokane	100%	224
Evergreen Hospital Medical Center	Kirkland	100%	248
Harborview Medical Center	Seattle	100%	144
Harrison Memorial Center	Bremerton	100%	361
Highline Medical Center	Burien	100%	170
Island Hospital	Anacortes	100%	41
Jefferson Healthcare Hospital	Port Townsend	100%	27
Kadlec Regional Medical Center	Richland	100%	300
Legacy Salmon Creek Medical Center	Vancouver	100%	213
Mason General Hospital	Shelton	100%	52
Multicare Good Samaritan Hospital[2]	Puyallup	100%	315
Northwest Hospital	Seattle	100%	201
Overlake Hospital Medical Center	Bellevue	100%	331
Peacehealth Southwest Medical Center	Vancouver	100%	716
Peachealth Saint John Medical Center	Longview	100%	198
Providence Mount Carmel Hospital	Colville	100%	34
Providence Reg Med Ctr Everett[2]	Everett	100%	343
Providence Sacred Heart Medical Center	Spokane	100%	426
Providence Saint Peter Hospital	Olympia	100%	483
Saint Anthony Hospital	Gig Harbor	100%	134
Saint Clare Hospital	Lakewood	100%	174
Saint Elizabeth Hospital[2]	Enumclaw	100%	43
Saint Joseph Medical Center[2]	Tacoma	100%	382
Seattle VA Med Ctr-VA Pugit Sound	Seattle	100%	181
Skagit Valley Hospital	Mount Vernon	100%	165
Spokane VA Medical Center	Spokane	100%	39
Swedish Edmonds Hospital	Edmonds	100%	170
Swedish Issaquah	Issaquah	100%	81
Swedish Medical Center	Seattle	100%	227
Swedish Medical Center - Cherry Hill	Seattle	100%	344
Tacoma General Allenmore Hospital[2]	Tacoma	100%	402
Toppenish Community Hospital	Toppenish	100%	42
University of Washington Medical Center	Seattle	100%	297
Valley Hospital	Spokane	100%	109
Virginia Mason Medical Center	Seattle	100%	398
Walla Walla General Hospital	Walla Walla	100%	54
Yakima Valley Memorial Hospital	Yakima	100%	274
Multicare Auburn Medical Center[2]	Auburn	99%	240
Olympic Medical Center	Port Angeles	99%	122
Peacehealth Saint Joseph Medical Center	Bellingham	99%	337
Providence Centralia Hospital[2]	Centralia	99%	179
Providence Holy Family Hospital	Spokane	99%	169
Saint Francis Community Hospital	Federal Way	99%	185
Valley Medical Center[2]	Renton	99%	283
Yakima Regional Medical & Cardiac Center	Yakima	99%	193
Grays Harbor Community Hospital	Aberdeen	98%	188
Providence Saint Mary Medical Center	Walla Walla	98%	99
Kennewick General Hospital	Kennewick	96%	180
Samaritan Hospital[2]	Moses Lake	95%	40
Sunnyside Community Hospital[2]	Sunnyside	95%	61
Tri - State Memorial Hospital	Clarkston	92%	38
Whidbey General Hospital	Coupeville	92%	50
Valley General Hospital	Monroe	88%	25

Medicare Spending

Medicare Spending per Patient (ratio)

Hospital Name	City	Ratio	Cases
Confluence Hlth-Wenatchee Valley Hosp	Wenatchee	0.82	-
Valley General Hospital	Monroe	0.82	-
Samaritan Hospital	Moses Lake	0.85	-
Toppenish Community Hospital	Toppenish	0.86	-
Peacehealth Southwest Medical Center	Vancouver	0.88	-
Central Washington Hospital	Wenatchee	0.89	-
Legacy Salmon Creek Medical Center	Vancouver	0.89	-
Walla Walla General Hospital	Walla Walla	0.89	-
Providence Centralia Hospital	Centralia	0.90	-
Yakima Valley Memorial Hospital	Yakima	0.90	-
Grays Harbor Community Hospital	Aberdeen	0.91	-
Peachealth Saint John Medical Center	Longview	0.91	-
Providence Saint Peter Hospital	Olympia	0.91	-
Swedish Medical Center	Seattle	0.91	-
Multicare Good Samaritan Hospital	Puyallup	0.92	-
Peacehealth Saint Joseph Medical Center	Bellingham	0.92	-
Swedish Issaquah	Issaquah	0.92	-
Cascade Valley Hospital	Arlington	0.93	-
Evergreen Hospital Medical Center	Kirkland	0.93	-
Island Hospital	Anacortes	0.93	-
Kennewick General Hospital	Kennewick	0.93	-
Providence Reg Med Ctr Everett	Everett	0.93	-
Tacoma General Allenmore Hospital	Tacoma	0.93	-
Overlake Hospital Medical Center	Bellevue	0.94	-
Providence Sacred Heart Medical Center	Spokane	0.94	-
Providence Saint Mary Medical Center	Walla Walla	0.94	-
Virginia Mason Medical Center	Seattle	0.94	-
Highline Medical Center	Burien	0.95	-
Northwest Hospital	Seattle	0.95	-
Saint Clare Hospital	Lakewood	0.95	-
University of Washington Medical Center	Seattle	0.95	-
Valley Medical Center	Renton	0.95	-
Capital Medical Center	Olympia	0.96	-
Harrison Memorial Center	Bremerton	0.96	-
Skagit Valley Hospital	Mount Vernon	0.96	-
Harborview Medical Center	Seattle	0.97	-
Olympic Medical Center	Port Angeles	0.97	-
Providence Holy Family Hospital	Spokane	0.97	-
Saint Anthony Hospital	Gig Harbor	0.97	-
Saint Joseph Medical Center	Tacoma	0.97	-
Yakima Regional Medical & Cardiac Center	Yakima	0.97	-
Kadlec Regional Medical Center	Richland	0.98	-
Swedish Edmonds Hospital	Edmonds	0.98	-
Swedish Medical Center - Cherry Hill	Seattle	0.98	-
Deaconess Hospital	Spokane	0.99	-
Saint Francis Community Hospital	Federal Way	0.99	-
Valley Hospital	Spokane	0.99	-
Multicare Auburn Medical Center	Auburn	1.00	-

Pneumonia Care

Appropriate Initial Antibiotic Given

Hospital Name	City	Rate	Cases
Kadlec Regional Medical Center[2]	Richland	100%	79
Kennewick General Hospital	Kennewick	100%	64
Northwest Hospital[2]	Seattle	100%	77
Peachealth Saint John Medical Center	Longview	100%	152
Providence Saint Mary Medical Center	Walla Walla	100%	54
Saint Francis Community Hospital[2]	Federal Way	100%	114
Samaritan Hospital[2]	Moses Lake	100%	45
Spokane VA Medical Center	Spokane	100%	27
Toppenish Community Hospital	Toppenish	100%	43
Valley Medical Center[2]	Renton	100%	98
Overlake Hospital Medical Center	Bellevue	99%	123
Providence Centralia Hospital[2]	Centralia	99%	105
Providence Holy Family Hospital	Spokane	99%	214
Swedish Edmonds Hospital	Edmonds	99%	158
Valley Hospital	Spokane	99%	135
Yakima Valley Memorial Hospital	Yakima	99%	158
Cascade Valley Hospital	Arlington	98%	41
Harborview Medical Center	Seattle	98%	64
Highline Medical Center	Burien	98%	189
Legacy Salmon Creek Medical Center	Vancouver	98%	125
Peacehealth United General Medical Center	Sedro Woolley	98%	50
Seattle VA Med Ctr-VA Pugit Sound	Seattle	98%	55
Sunnyside Community Hospital[2]	Sunnyside	98%	47
University of Washington Medical Center	Seattle	98%	40
Central Washington Hospital	Wenatchee	97%	112
Deaconess Hospital	Spokane	97%	104
Peacehealth Saint Joseph Medical Center	Bellingham	97%	227
Providence Saint Peter Hospital	Olympia	97%	243
Saint Anthony Hospital[2]	Gig Harbor	97%	110
Saint Clare Hospital[2]	Lakewood	97%	113
Skagit Valley Hospital[2]	Mount Vernon	97%	116
Swedish Medical Center	Seattle	97%	144
Tacoma General Allenmore Hospital[2]	Tacoma	97%	191
Walla Walla General Hospital	Walla Walla	97%	31
Whitman Hospital & Medical Center	Colfax	97%	29
Harrison Memorial Center[2]	Bremerton	96%	68
Mid Valley Hospital	Omak	96%	27
Multicare Good Samaritan Hospital[2]	Puyallup	96%	114
Yakima Regional Medical & Cardiac Center	Yakima	96%	91
Evergreen Hospital Medical Center	Kirkland	95%	144
Peacehealth Southwest Medical Center[2]	Vancouver	95%	80
Providence Reg Med Ctr Everett[2]	Everett	95%	151
Multicare Auburn Medical Center[2]	Auburn	94%	81
Olympic Medical Center	Port Angeles	94%	99
Providence Mount Carmel Hospital	Colville	94%	47
Saint Joseph Medical Center[2]	Tacoma	94%	119
Swedish Issaquah	Issaquah	94%	49
Valley General Hospital	Monroe	94%	36
Virginia Mason Medical Center[2]	Seattle	94%	138
Whidbey General Hospital	Coupeville	94%	69
Mason General Hospital	Shelton	93%	60
Tri - State Memorial Hospital	Clarkston	93%	46
Providence Sacred Heart Medical Center	Spokane	92%	194
Saint Elizabeth Hospital[2]	Enumclaw	92%	40
Island Hospital	Anacortes	91%	69
Capital Medical Center	Olympia	88%	41
Jefferson Healthcare Hospital[2]	Port Townsend	84%	31
Willapa Harbor Hospital[2]	South Bend	84%	44
Grays Harbor Community Hospital	Aberdeen	82%	125
Pullman Regional Hospital	Pullman	81%	31

Blood Culture Timing

Hospital Name	City	Rate	Cases
Deaconess Hospital	Spokane	100%	142
Harrison Memorial Center[2]	Bremerton	100%	109
Kennewick General Hospital	Kennewick	100%	47
Kittitas Valley Community Hospital[3]	Ellensburg	100%	36
Mid Valley Hospital	Omak	100%	40
Overlake Hospital Medical Center	Bellevue	100%	140
Providence Mount Carmel Hospital	Colville	100%	69
Saint Elizabeth Hospital[2]	Enumclaw	100%	61
Samaritan Hospital[2]	Moses Lake	100%	61
Skagit Valley Hospital[2]	Mount Vernon	100%	195
Spokane VA Medical Center	Spokane	100%	38
Tri - State Memorial Hospital	Clarkston	100%	81
Valley General Hospital	Monroe	100%	74
Kadlec Regional Medical Center[2]	Richland	99%	168
Northwest Hospital[2]	Seattle	99%	155
Olympic Medical Center	Port Angeles	99%	130
Providence Centralia Hospital[2]	Centralia	99%	131
Providence Saint Peter Hospital	Olympia	99%	304
Saint Anthony Hospital[2]	Gig Harbor	99%	208
Saint Clare Hospital[2]	Lakewood	99%	208
Seattle VA Med Ctr-VA Pugit Sound	Seattle	99%	95
Swedish Issaquah	Issaquah	99%	69
Toppenish Community Hospital	Toppenish	99%	76
Valley Hospital	Spokane	99%	195
Cascade Valley Hospital	Arlington	98%	58
Central Washington Hospital	Wenatchee	98%	161
Evergreen Hospital Medical Center	Kirkland	98%	242
Highline Medical Center	Burien	98%	332
Jefferson Healthcare Hospital[2]	Port Townsend	98%	43
Legacy Salmon Creek Medical Center[2]	Vancouver	98%	260
Multicare Auburn Medical Center[2]	Auburn	98%	128
Multicare Good Samaritan Hospital[2]	Puyallup	98%	171
Providence Holy Family Hospital	Spokane	98%	276
Providence Saint Mary Medical Center	Walla Walla	98%	92

NOTE: Hospital profiles are in alphabetical order by state, then city, then hospital within the city; Rankings exclude hospitals with less than 25 cases except for patient surveys which excludes hospitals with less than 100 cases; (a) 100-299 cases; (1) The number of cases/patients is too few to report; (2) Data submitted were based on a sample of cases/patients; (3) Results are based on a shorter time period than required; (4) Data suppressed by CMS for one or more quarters; (5) Results are not available for this reporting period; (6) Fewer than 100 patients completed the HCAHPS survey; (7) No cases met the criteria for this measure; (8) The lower limit of the confidence interval cannot be calculated if the number of observed infections equals zero; (9) No data are available from the state/territory for this reporting period; (10) The scores shown reflect fewer than 50 completed surveys; (11) There were discrepancies in the data collection process; (12) This measure does not apply to this hospital for this reporting period; (13) Results cannot be calculated for this reporting period; (14) The results for this state are combined with nearby states to protect confidentiality; Please refer to the User's Guide for a full explanation of data.

Saint Francis Community Hospital[2]	Federal Way	98%	197
Walla Walla General Hospital	Walla Walla	98%	55
Capital Medical Center	Olympia	97%	66
Providence Sacred Heart Medical Center	Spokane	97%	290
Pullman Regional Hospital	Pullman	97%	34
Saint Joseph Medical Center[2]	Tacoma	97%	196
Swedish Medical Center	Seattle	97%	272
Swedish Medical Center - Cherry Hill	Seattle	97%	30
Valley Medical Center[2]	Renton	97%	146
Virginia Mason Medical Center[2]	Seattle	97%	193
Yakima Regional Medical & Cardiac Center	Yakima	97%	119
Yakima Valley Memorial Hospital	Yakima	97%	322
Harborview Medical Center	Seattle	96%	167
Providence Reg Med Ctr Everett[2]	Everett	96%	258
Tacoma General Allenmore Hospital[2]	Tacoma	96%	291
Whidbey General Hospital	Coupeville	96%	84
Peacehealth Southwest Medical Center[2]	Vancouver	95%	195
Peachealth Saint John Medical Center	Longview	95%	296
Swedish Edmonds Hospital	Edmonds	95%	216
University of Washington Medical Center	Seattle	95%	129
Island Hospital	Anacortes	94%	110
Peacehealth Saint Joseph Medical Center	Bellingham	94%	362
Lourdes Medical Center	Pasco	93%	27
Peacehealth United General Medical Center	Sedro Woolley	93%	57
Sunnyside Community Hospital[2]	Sunnyside	93%	73
Grays Harbor Community Hospital	Aberdeen	92%	145
Mason General Hospital	Shelton	92%	71
Willapa Harbor Hospital[2]	South Bend	89%	38

Pregnancy and Delivery Care

Newborns whose Deliveries were Scheduled Early

Hospital Name	City	Rate	Cases
Central Washington Hospital	Wenatchee	0%	142
Group Health Central Hospital[2]	Seattle	0%	27
Highline Medical Center	Burien	0%	152
Kennewick General Hospital[2]	Kennewick	0%	29
Legacy Salmon Creek Medical Center[2]	Vancouver	0%	43
Overlake Hospital Medical Center	Bellevue	0%	398
Providence Centralia Hospital[2]	Centralia	0%	32
Providence Reg Med Ctr Everett	Everett	0%	338
Providence Sacred Heart Medical Center[2]	Spokane	0%	29
Saint Elizabeth Hospital	Enumclaw	0%	25
Skagit Valley Hospital	Mount Vernon	0%	113
Valley Hospital[2]	Spokane	0%	44
Multicare Good Samaritan Hospital	Puyallup	1%	196
Peacehealth Saint Joseph Medical Center	Bellingham	1%	131
Providence Saint Peter Hospital	Olympia	1%	138
Saint Francis Community Hospital	Federal Way	1%	72
Samaritan Hospital	Moses Lake	1%	81
Swedish Edmonds Hospital	Edmonds	1%	91
Swedish Issaquah	Issaquah	1%	78
Tacoma General Allenmore Hospital	Tacoma	1%	203
Yakima Valley Memorial Hospital[2]	Yakima	1%	211
Evergreen Hospital Medical Center	Kirkland	2%	331
Multicare Auburn Medical Center[2]	Auburn	2%	44
Peacehealth Southwest Medical Center	Vancouver	2%	225
Providence Saint Mary Medical Center[2]	Walla Walla	2%	45
Saint Joseph Medical Center	Tacoma	2%	303
Sunnyside Community Hospital[2,3]	Sunnyside	2%	64
Swedish Medical Center	Seattle	2%	377
Valley Medical Center	Renton	2%	382
Peachealth Saint John Medical Center	Longview	3%	74
Deaconess Hospital[2]	Spokane	4%	25
Kadlec Regional Medical Center[2]	Richland	4%	91
Olympic Medical Center	Port Angeles	4%	46
Toppenish Community Hospital	Toppenish	4%	48
Grays Harbor Community Hospital	Aberdeen	5%	60
Harrison Memorial Center	Bremerton	5%	142
Cascade Valley Hospital	Arlington	9%	47
Island Hospital	Anacortes	12%	33

Preventive Care

Immunization for Influenza

Hospital Name	City	Rate	Cases
Skagit Valley Hospital[2]	Mount Vernon	100%	519
Kadlec Regional Medical Center[2]	Richland	99%	504
Kittitas Valley Community Hospital[2,3]	Ellensburg	99%	112
Confluence Hlth-Wenatchee Valley Hosp	Wenatchee	98%	246
Deaconess Hospital[2]	Spokane	98%	606
Island Hospital[2]	Anacortes	98%	307
Overlake Hospital Medical Center[2]	Bellevue	98%	524
Providence Holy Family Hospital[2]	Spokane	98%	508
Providence Mount Carmel Hospital[2]	Colville	98%	253
Swedish Medical Center - Cherry Hill[2]	Seattle	98%	602
University of Washington Medical Center[2]	Seattle	98%	542
Virginia Mason Medical Center[2]	Seattle	98%	590
Capital Medical Center[2]	Olympia	97%	421
Northwest Hospital[2]	Seattle	97%	515
Valley Hospital[2]	Spokane	97%	613
Kennewick General Hospital[2]	Kennewick	96%	467
Providence Saint Joseph Hospital	Chewelah	96%	160
Cascade Valley Hospital[2]	Arlington	95%	261
Olympic Medical Center[2]	Port Angeles	95%	394
Peachealth Saint John Medical Center[2]	Longview	95%	568
Saint Anthony Hospital[2]	Gig Harbor	95%	528
Swedish Issaquah[2]	Issaquah	95%	505
Multicare Good Samaritan Hospital[2]	Puyallup	94%	548
Providence Sacred Heart Medical Center[2]	Spokane	94%	522
Skyline Hospital[2]	White Salmon	94%	31
Harrison Memorial Center[2]	Bremerton	93%	589
Saint Joseph Medical Center[2]	Tacoma	93%	571
Toppenish Community Hospital[2]	Toppenish	93%	348
Walla Walla General Hospital[2]	Walla Walla	93%	241
Swedish Medical Center[2]	Seattle	92%	879
Valley General Hospital[2]	Monroe	92%	287
Harborview Medical Center[2]	Seattle	91%	584
Saint Clare Hospital[2]	Lakewood	91%	619
Evergreen Hospital Medical Center[2]	Kirkland	90%	604
Highline Medical Center[2]	Burien	90%	507
Providence Saint Mary Medical Center[2]	Walla Walla	90%	386
Saint Francis Community Hospital[2]	Federal Way	90%	569
Swedish Edmonds Hospital[2]	Edmonds	90%	519
Yakima Regional Medical & Cardiac Center[2]	Yakima	90%	571
Peacehealth Saint Joseph Medical Center[2]	Bellingham	89%	516
Legacy Salmon Creek Medical Center[2]	Vancouver	88%	520
Tacoma General Allenmore Hospital[2]	Tacoma	88%	890
Central Washington Hospital[2]	Wenatchee	87%	567
Providence Centralia Hospital[2]	Centralia	86%	486
Providence Saint Peter Hospital[2]	Olympia	86%	527
Grays Harbor Community Hospital[2]	Aberdeen	84%	505
Group Health Central Hospital[2]	Seattle	84%	313
Samaritan Hospital[2]	Moses Lake	83%	341
Klickitat Valley Hospital[3]	Goldendale	82%	44
Peacehealth Southwest Medical Center[2]	Vancouver	81%	566
Multicare Auburn Medical Center[2]	Auburn	80%	569
Saint Elizabeth Hospital[2]	Enumclaw	79%	261
Providence Reg Med Ctr Everett[2]	Everett	71%	526
Yakima Valley Memorial Hospital[2]	Yakima	63%	489
Valley Medical Center[2]	Renton	62%	470

Immunization for Pneumonia

Hospital Name	City	Rate	Cases
Lake Chelan Community Hospital	Chelan	100%	43
Skagit Valley Hospital[2]	Mount Vernon	100%	623
Deaconess Hospital[2]	Spokane	99%	714
Kadlec Regional Medical Center[2]	Richland	99%	566
University of Washington Medical Center[2]	Seattle	99%	512
Swedish Issaquah[2]	Issaquah	98%	441
Island Hospital[2]	Anacortes	97%	426
Kennewick General Hospital[2]	Kennewick	97%	474
Providence Mount Carmel Hospital[2]	Colville	97%	305
Skyline Hospital[2]	White Salmon	97%	63
Valley Hospital[2]	Spokane	97%	739
Capital Medical Center[2]	Olympia	96%	477
Northwest Hospital[2]	Seattle	96%	609
Harrison Memorial Center[2]	Bremerton	95%	679
Overlake Hospital Medical Center[2]	Bellevue	95%	512
Peachealth Saint John Medical Center[2]	Longview	95%	740
Providence Saint Joseph Hospital	Chewelah	95%	239
Saint Anthony Hospital[2]	Gig Harbor	95%	743
Grays Harbor Community Hospital[2]	Aberdeen	94%	591
Highline Medical Center[2]	Burien	94%	612
Kittitas Valley Community Hospital[2,3]	Ellensburg	94%	173
Providence Holy Family Hospital[2]	Spokane	94%	597
Cascade Valley Hospital[2]	Arlington	93%	276
Multicare Good Samaritan Hospital[2]	Puyallup	93%	674
Toppenish Community Hospital[2]	Toppenish	93%	306
Evergreen Hospital Medical Center[2]	Kirkland	92%	515
Harborview Medical Center[2]	Seattle	92%	501
Swedish Medical Center - Cherry Hill[2]	Seattle	92%	826
Central Washington Hospital[2]	Wenatchee	91%	727
Confluence Hlth-Wenatchee Valley Hosp	Wenatchee	91%	266
Legacy Salmon Creek Medical Center[2]	Vancouver	91%	510
Peacehealth Saint Joseph Medical Center[2]	Bellingham	91%	598
Saint Clare Hospital[2]	Lakewood	91%	825
Valley General Hospital[2]	Monroe	91%	345
Walla Walla General Hospital[2]	Walla Walla	91%	275
Providence Sacred Heart Medical Center[2]	Spokane	90%	525
Saint Francis Community Hospital[2]	Federal Way	90%	627
Saint Joseph Medical Center[2]	Tacoma	90%	595
Virginia Mason Medical Center[2]	Seattle	90%	840
Providence Centralia Hospital[2]	Centralia	89%	654
Providence Saint Peter Hospital[2]	Olympia	89%	625
Tacoma General Allenmore Hospital[2]	Tacoma	89%	1093
Yakima Regional Medical & Cardiac Center[2]	Yakima	89%	788
Providence Saint Mary Medical Center[2]	Walla Walla	88%	444
Swedish Edmonds Hospital[2]	Edmonds	88%	601
Swedish Medical Center[2]	Seattle	87%	686
Olympic Medical Center[2]	Port Angeles	86%	534
Peacehealth Southwest Medical Center[2]	Vancouver	85%	705
Saint Elizabeth Hospital[2]	Enumclaw	83%	287
Yakima Valley Memorial Hospital[2]	Yakima	81%	476
Multicare Auburn Medical Center[2]	Auburn	80%	731
Klickitat Valley Hospital[2,3]	Goldendale	79%	76
Samaritan Hospital[2]	Moses Lake	79%	276
Valley Medical Center[2]	Renton	75%	460
Providence Reg Med Ctr Everett[2]	Everett	74%	604
Group Health Central Hospital[2]	Seattle	31%	26

Stroke Care

Anticoagulation Therapy for Atrial Fibrillation

Hospital Name	City	Rate	Cases
Evergreen Hospital Medical Center	Kirkland	100%	32
Harrison Memorial Center	Bremerton	100%	36
Multicare Good Samaritan Hospital[2]	Puyallup	100%	32
Overlake Hospital Medical Center	Bellevue	100%	36
Peacehealth Southwest Medical Center	Vancouver	100%	51
Providence Sacred Heart Medical Center	Spokane	96%	72
Providence Saint Peter Hospital	Olympia	95%	55
Saint Joseph Medical Center	Tacoma	91%	34

Antithrombotic Therapy Timing

Hospital Name	City	Rate	Cases
Island Hospital	Anacortes	100%	28
Kennewick General Hospital	Kennewick	100%	31
Legacy Salmon Creek Medical Center	Vancouver	100%	64
Multicare Good Samaritan Hospital[2]	Puyallup	100%	155
Northwest Hospital[2]	Seattle	100%	99
Overlake Hospital Medical Center	Bellevue	100%	123
Peachealth Saint John Medical Center	Longview	100%	61
Providence Centralia Hospital	Centralia	100%	63
Providence Reg Med Ctr Everett	Everett	100%	277
Providence Saint Mary Medical Center[2]	Walla Walla	100%	37
Saint Anthony Hospital	Gig Harbor	100%	49
Saint Clare Hospital	Lakewood	100%	34
Saint Francis Community Hospital	Federal Way	100%	74
Skagit Valley Hospital	Mount Vernon	100%	65
Tacoma General Allenmore Hospital[2]	Tacoma	100%	103
University of Washington Medical Center	Seattle	100%	38
Valley Hospital	Spokane	100%	25
Yakima Valley Memorial Hospital	Yakima	100%	82
Central Washington Hospital	Wenatchee	99%	107
Harborview Medical Center	Seattle	99%	111
Providence Holy Family Hospital	Spokane	99%	99
Saint Joseph Medical Center	Tacoma	99%	211
Swedish Edmonds Hospital	Edmonds	99%	108
Valley Medical Center[2]	Renton	99%	75
Deaconess Hospital	Spokane	98%	65
Evergreen Hospital Medical Center	Kirkland	98%	135
Harrison Memorial Center	Bremerton	98%	170
Highline Medical Center	Burien	98%	95
Providence Sacred Heart Medical Center	Spokane	98%	268
Providence Saint Peter Hospital	Olympia	98%	154
Swedish Medical Center - Cherry Hill	Seattle	98%	93
Virginia Mason Medical Center	Seattle	98%	123
Yakima Regional Medical & Cardiac Center	Yakima	98%	52
Kadlec Regional Medical Center	Richland	97%	157
Multicare Auburn Medical Center	Auburn	97%	38
Peacehealth Southwest Medical Center	Vancouver	97%	266
Swedish Issaquah	Issaquah	97%	38
Peacehealth Saint Joseph Medical Center[2]	Bellingham	93%	61
Walla Walla General Hospital[2]	Walla Walla	93%	27
Grays Harbor Community Hospital	Aberdeen	89%	46
Olympic Medical Center	Port Angeles	85%	55

Assessed for Rehabilitation

Hospital Name	City	Rate	Cases
Central Washington Hospital	Wenatchee	100%	152
Evergreen Hospital Medical Center	Kirkland	100%	186
Harrison Memorial Center	Bremerton	100%	178
Legacy Salmon Creek Medical Center	Vancouver	100%	84
Multicare Auburn Medical Center	Auburn	100%	44
Peachealth Saint John Medical Center	Longview	100%	69
Providence Reg Med Ctr Everett	Everett	100%	380
Providence Saint Mary Medical Center[2]	Walla Walla	100%	57
Saint Francis Community Hospital	Federal Way	100%	75
Skagit Valley Hospital	Mount Vernon	100%	74
Swedish Edmonds Hospital	Edmonds	100%	123
University of Washington Medical Center	Seattle	100%	46
Valley Hospital	Spokane	100%	29
Harborview Medical Center	Seattle	99%	367
Kadlec Regional Medical Center	Richland	99%	213
Northwest Hospital[2]	Seattle	99%	125
Overlake Hospital Medical Center	Bellevue	99%	172
Providence Holy Family Hospital	Spokane	99%	116
Providence Sacred Heart Medical Center	Spokane	99%	405
Valley Medical Center[2]	Renton	99%	96

NOTE: Hospital profiles are in alphabetical order by state, then city, then hospital within the city; Rankings exclude hospitals with less than 25 cases except for patient surveys which excludes hospitals with less than 100 cases; (a) 100-299 cases; (1) The number of cases/patients is too few to report; (2) Data submitted were based on a sample of cases/patients; (3) Results are based on a shorter time period than required; (4) Data suppressed by CMS for one or more quarters; (5) Results are not available for this reporting period; (6) Fewer than 100 patients completed the HCAHPS survey; (7) No cases met the criteria for this measure; (8) The lower limit of the confidence interval cannot be calculated if the number of observed infections equals zero; (9) No data are available from the state/territory for this reporting period; (10) The scores shown reflect fewer than 50 completed surveys; (11) There were discrepancies in the data collection process; (12) This measure does not apply to this hospital for this reporting period; (13) Results cannot be calculated for this reporting period; (14) The results for this state are combined with nearby states to protect confidentiality; Please refer to the User's Guide for a full explanation of data.

Hospital Name	City	Rate	Cases
Virginia Mason Medical Center	Seattle	99%	187
Yakima Valley Memorial Hospital	Yakima	99%	107
Deaconess Hospital	Spokane	98%	91
Highline Medical Center	Burien	98%	115
Multicare Good Samaritan Hospital[2]	Puyallup	98%	192
Peacehealth Southwest Medical Center	Vancouver	98%	373
Swedish Medical Center - Cherry Hill	Seattle	98%	242
Peacehealth Saint Joseph Medical Center[2]	Bellingham	97%	91
Swedish Medical Center	Seattle	97%	31
Tacoma General Allenmore Hospital[2]	Tacoma	97%	149
Walla Walla General Hospital[2]	Walla Walla	97%	32
Grays Harbor Community Hospital	Aberdeen	96%	51
Olympic Medical Center	Port Angeles	96%	69
Swedish Issaquah	Issaquah	96%	56
Kennewick General Hospital	Kennewick	95%	41
Providence Centralia Hospital	Centralia	95%	76
Saint Clare Hospital	Lakewood	95%	40
Providence Saint Peter Hospital	Olympia	94%	283
Saint Anthony Hospital	Gig Harbor	93%	54
Saint Joseph Medical Center	Tacoma	93%	319
Island Hospital	Anacortes	86%	37
Yakima Regional Medical & Cardiac Center	Yakima	85%	62

Discharged on Antithrombotic Therapy

Hospital Name	City	Rate	Cases
Central Washington Hospital	Wenatchee	100%	145
Deaconess Hospital	Spokane	100%	77
Evergreen Hospital Medical Center	Kirkland	100%	169
Harborview Medical Center	Seattle	100%	148
Harrison Memorial Center	Bremerton	100%	176
Island Hospital	Anacortes	100%	36
Kadlec Regional Medical Center	Richland	100%	178
Kennewick General Hospital	Kennewick	100%	40
Legacy Salmon Creek Medical Center	Vancouver	100%	77
Multicare Auburn Medical Center	Auburn	100%	43
Overlake Hospital Medical Center	Bellevue	100%	155
Peacehealth Southwest Medical Center	Vancouver	100%	330
Peacehealth Saint John Medical Center	Longview	100%	64
Providence Centralia Hospital	Centralia	100%	76
Providence Holy Family Hospital	Spokane	100%	109
Providence Reg Med Ctr Everett	Everett	100%	352
Providence Sacred Heart Medical Center	Spokane	100%	336
Providence Saint Mary Medical Center[2]	Walla Walla	100%	51
Providence Saint Peter Hospital	Olympia	100%	235
Saint Anthony Hospital	Gig Harbor	100%	54
Saint Clare Hospital	Lakewood	100%	40
Saint Francis Community Hospital	Federal Way	100%	72
Skagit Valley Hospital	Mount Vernon	100%	70
Swedish Medical Center	Seattle	100%	30
University of Washington Medical Center	Seattle	100%	44
Valley Hospital	Spokane	100%	28
Valley Medical Center[2]	Renton	100%	85
Virginia Mason Medical Center	Seattle	100%	157
Yakima Valley Memorial Hospital	Yakima	100%	103
Multicare Good Samaritan Hospital[2]	Puyallup	99%	186
Northwest Hospital[2]	Seattle	99%	113
Peacehealth Saint Joseph Medical Center[2]	Bellingham	99%	75
Saint Joseph Medical Center	Tacoma	99%	254
Swedish Edmonds Hospital	Edmonds	99%	122
Swedish Medical Center - Cherry Hill	Seattle	99%	159
Tacoma General Allenmore Hospital[2]	Tacoma	99%	127
Highline Medical Center	Burien	98%	97
Swedish Issaquah	Issaquah	98%	54
Olympic Medical Center	Port Angeles	97%	67
Walla Walla General Hospital[2]	Walla Walla	97%	32
Yakima Regional Medical & Cardiac Center	Yakima	89%	56
Grays Harbor Community Hospital	Aberdeen	79%	48

Discharged on Statin Medication

Hospital Name	City	Rate	Cases
Deaconess Hospital	Spokane	100%	64
Legacy Salmon Creek Medical Center	Vancouver	100%	65
Overlake Hospital Medical Center	Bellevue	100%	111
Providence Sacred Heart Medical Center	Spokane	100%	255
Skagit Valley Hospital	Mount Vernon	100%	63
Valley Medical Center[2]	Renton	100%	68
Central Washington Hospital	Wenatchee	99%	110
Harrison Memorial Center	Bremerton	99%	148
Kadlec Regional Medical Center	Richland	99%	135
Providence Reg Med Ctr Everett	Everett	99%	274
Evergreen Hospital Medical Center	Kirkland	98%	121
Multicare Good Samaritan Hospital[2]	Puyallup	98%	151
Swedish Medical Center - Cherry Hill	Seattle	98%	117
Highline Medical Center	Burien	97%	74
Multicare Auburn Medical Center	Auburn	97%	33
Peacehealth Southwest Medical Center	Vancouver	97%	243
Saint Clare Hospital	Lakewood	97%	33
Swedish Edmonds Hospital	Edmonds	97%	87
Yakima Valley Memorial Hospital	Yakima	97%	88
Peacehealth Saint John Medical Center	Longview	96%	50
Providence Saint Peter Hospital	Olympia	96%	193
Swedish Medical Center	Seattle	96%	27
Tacoma General Allenmore Hospital[2]	Tacoma	96%	102
Saint Joseph Medical Center	Tacoma	95%	210
Saint Francis Community Hospital	Federal Way	94%	62
Harborview Medical Center	Seattle	93%	108
Northwest Hospital[2]	Seattle	92%	76
Providence Holy Family Hospital	Spokane	92%	75
University of Washington Medical Center	Seattle	92%	37
Virginia Mason Medical Center	Seattle	92%	119
Kennewick General Hospital	Kennewick	91%	34
Peacehealth Saint Joseph Medical Center[2]	Bellingham	91%	66
Providence Centralia Hospital	Centralia	91%	65
Saint Anthony Hospital	Gig Harbor	91%	47
Swedish Issaquah	Issaquah	91%	43
Providence Saint Mary Medical Center[2]	Walla Walla	90%	39
Island Hospital	Anacortes	89%	28
Olympic Medical Center	Port Angeles	87%	52
Grays Harbor Community Hospital	Aberdeen	85%	41
Yakima Regional Medical & Cardiac Center	Yakima	80%	45

Thrombolytic Therapy Timing

Hospital Name	City	Rate	Cases
Providence Sacred Heart Medical Center	Spokane	93%	27
Saint Joseph Medical Center	Tacoma	92%	26
Peacehealth Southwest Medical Center	Vancouver	85%	33
Providence Saint Peter Hospital	Olympia	75%	32
Overlake Hospital Medical Center	Bellevue	29%	38

Venous Thromboembolism (VTE) Prophylaxis

Hospital Name	City	Rate	Cases
Multicare Auburn Medical Center	Auburn	100%	42
Deaconess Hospital	Spokane	99%	85
Evergreen Hospital Medical Center	Kirkland	99%	170
Harrison Memorial Center	Bremerton	99%	171
Kadlec Regional Medical Center	Richland	99%	212
Skagit Valley Hospital	Mount Vernon	99%	68
Central Washington Hospital	Wenatchee	98%	132
Northwest Hospital[2]	Seattle	98%	130
Providence Reg Med Ctr Everett	Everett	98%	332
Providence Sacred Heart Medical Center	Spokane	98%	403
Swedish Medical Center - Cherry Hill	Seattle	98%	252
Highline Medical Center	Burien	97%	118
Legacy Salmon Creek Medical Center	Vancouver	97%	78
Peacehealth Southwest Medical Center	Vancouver	97%	364
Overlake Hospital Medical Center	Bellevue	96%	152
Providence Saint Peter Hospital	Olympia	96%	269
Saint Anthony Hospital	Gig Harbor	96%	47
Saint Francis Community Hospital	Federal Way	96%	75
Valley Hospital	Spokane	96%	25
Yakima Valley Memorial Hospital	Yakima	96%	106
Tacoma General Allenmore Hospital[2]	Tacoma	95%	139
Virginia Mason Medical Center	Seattle	95%	177
Multicare Good Samaritan Hospital[2]	Puyallup	94%	170
Providence Saint Mary Medical Center[2]	Walla Walla	94%	51
Harborview Medical Center	Seattle	93%	400
Providence Holy Family Hospital	Spokane	93%	104
Valley Medical Center[2]	Renton	93%	105
Kennewick General Hospital	Kennewick	92%	39
Saint Clare Hospital	Lakewood	92%	39
Saint Joseph Medical Center	Tacoma	92%	345
Olympic Medical Center	Port Angeles	90%	68
Swedish Edmonds Hospital	Edmonds	90%	116
University of Washington Medical Center	Seattle	90%	42
Island Hospital	Anacortes	86%	28
Peacehealth Saint Joseph Medical Center[2]	Bellingham	85%	88
Swedish Medical Center	Seattle	85%	26
Grays Harbor Community Hospital	Aberdeen	84%	50
Peacehealth Saint John Medical Center	Longview	82%	65
Providence Centralia Hospital	Centralia	80%	56
Swedish Issaquah	Issaquah	80%	41
Yakima Regional Medical & Cardiac Center	Yakima	58%	60

Written Stroke Educational Materials Given

Hospital Name	City	Rate	Cases
Island Hospital	Anacortes	100%	25
Kadlec Regional Medical Center	Richland	100%	116
Virginia Mason Medical Center	Seattle	99%	97
Legacy Salmon Creek Medical Center	Vancouver	98%	50
Multicare Good Samaritan Hospital[2]	Puyallup	98%	133
Providence Reg Med Ctr Everett	Everett	98%	219
Skagit Valley Hospital	Mount Vernon	98%	48
Yakima Valley Memorial Hospital	Yakima	98%	58
Highline Medical Center	Burien	97%	66
Deaconess Hospital	Spokane	95%	58
Harrison Memorial Center	Bremerton	95%	83
Northwest Hospital[2]	Seattle	95%	66
Providence Saint Peter Hospital	Olympia	95%	113
Providence Holy Family Hospital	Spokane	93%	72
Tacoma General Allenmore Hospital[2]	Tacoma	92%	86
Overlake Hospital Medical Center	Bellevue	91%	79
Central Washington Hospital	Wenatchee	90%	93
Providence Sacred Heart Medical Center	Spokane	90%	193
Evergreen Hospital Medical Center	Kirkland	89%	112
Swedish Edmonds Hospital	Edmonds	89%	79
Valley Medical Center[2]	Renton	89%	64
Harborview Medical Center	Seattle	87%	184
Swedish Medical Center - Cherry Hill	Seattle	86%	111
Providence Saint Mary Medical Center[2]	Walla Walla	85%	27
Peacehealth Saint Joseph Medical Center[2]	Bellingham	83%	54
Peachealth Saint John Medical Center	Longview	83%	47
Grays Harbor Community Hospital	Aberdeen	81%	27
Multicare Auburn Medical Center	Auburn	81%	26
Peacehealth Southwest Medical Center	Vancouver	78%	218
Saint Joseph Medical Center	Tacoma	77%	166
Swedish Issaquah	Issaquah	69%	32
Yakima Regional Medical & Cardiac Center	Yakima	67%	27
University of Washington Medical Center	Seattle	59%	27
Saint Anthony Hospital	Gig Harbor	51%	39
Saint Clare Hospital	Lakewood	48%	27
Saint Francis Community Hospital	Federal Way	47%	49
Olympic Medical Center	Port Angeles	36%	39
Providence Centralia Hospital	Centralia	20%	51

Surgical Care Improvement Project

Appropriate Beta Blocker Usage

Hospital Name	City	Rate	Cases
Capital Medical Center[2]	Olympia	100%	93
Central Washington Hospital	Wenatchee	100%	400
Confluence Hlth-Wenatchee Valley Hosp	Wenatchee	100%	29
Harborview Medical Center[2]	Seattle	100%	60
Kadlec Regional Medical Center[2]	Richland	100%	206
Legacy Salmon Creek Medical Center[2]	Vancouver	100%	105
Mason General Hospital	Shelton	100%	27
Providence Holy Family Hospital[2]	Spokane	100%	69
Providence Saint Mary Medical Center	Walla Walla	100%	127
Swedish Medical Center[2]	Seattle	100%	203
Swedish Medical Center - Cherry Hill[2]	Seattle	100%	171
Valley Hospital	Spokane	100%	145
Virginia Mason Medical Center[2]	Seattle	100%	318
Whidbey General Hospital	Coupeville	100%	33
Deaconess Hospital	Spokane	99%	285
Lourdes Medical Center	Pasco	99%	141
Olympic Medical Center	Port Angeles	99%	121
Overlake Hospital Medical Center[2]	Bellevue	99%	198
Peacehealth Southwest Medical Center[2]	Vancouver	99%	213
Peacehealth Saint John Medical Center	Longview	99%	214
Providence Reg Med Ctr Everett[2]	Everett	99%	236
Providence Sacred Heart Medical Center[2]	Spokane	99%	162
Saint Anthony Hospital[2]	Gig Harbor	99%	83
Saint Joseph Medical Center[2]	Tacoma	99%	356
Skagit Valley Hospital[2]	Mount Vernon	99%	122
Tacoma General Allenmore Hospital[2]	Tacoma	99%	315
University of Washington Medical Center[2]	Seattle	99%	157
Harrison Memorial Center[2]	Bremerton	98%	283
Highline Medical Center	Burien	98%	120
Peacehealth Saint Joseph Medical Center[2]	Bellingham	98%	218
Providence Saint Peter Hospital[2]	Olympia	98%	203
Swedish Issaquah[2]	Issaquah	98%	65
Yakima Regional Medical & Cardiac Center	Yakima	98%	172
Yakima Valley Memorial Hospital[2]	Yakima	98%	197
Multicare Good Samaritan Hospital[2]	Puyallup	97%	89
Saint Clare Hospital[2]	Lakewood	97%	101
Saint Francis Community Hospital[2]	Federal Way	97%	117
Valley Medical Center[2]	Renton	97%	73
Island Hospital	Anacortes	96%	112
Kennewick General Hospital[2]	Kennewick	96%	46
Cascade Valley Hospital	Arlington	95%	43
Multicare Auburn Medical Center[2]	Auburn	95%	61
Northwest Hospital[2]	Seattle	95%	126
Providence Centralia Hospital[2]	Centralia	95%	78
Swedish Edmonds Hospital	Edmonds	95%	140
Evergreen Hospital Medical Center[2]	Kirkland	94%	97
Walla Walla General Hospital[2]	Walla Walla	93%	29
Seattle VA Med Ctr-VA Pugit Sound[2]	Seattle	92%	172
Samaritan Hospital	Moses Lake	91%	56
Grays Harbor Community Hospital	Aberdeen	89%	57
Saint Elizabeth Hospital[2]	Enumclaw	89%	37

Appropriate VTP Within 24 Hours

Hospital Name	City	Rate	Cases
Deaconess Hospital	Spokane	100%	906
Harrison Memorial Center[2]	Bremerton	100%	353
Highline Medical Center	Burien	100%	390
Jefferson Healthcare Hospital	Port Townsend	100%	68
Mid Valley Hospital	Omak	100%	30
Peachealth Saint John Medical Center	Longview	100%	558
Prosser Memorial Hospital	Prosser	100%	29
Providence Reg Med Ctr Everett[2]	Everett	100%	335

NOTE: Hospital profiles are in alphabetical order by state, then city, then hospital within the city; Rankings exclude hospitals with less than 25 cases except for patient surveys which excludes hospitals with less than 100 cases; (a) 100-299 cases; (1) The number of cases/patients is too few to report; (2) Data submitted were based on a sample of cases/patients; (3) Results are based on a shorter time period than required; (4) Data suppressed by CMS for one or more quarters; (5) Results are not available for this reporting period; (6) Fewer than 100 patients completed the HCAHPS survey; (7) No cases met the criteria for this measure; (8) The lower limit of the confidence interval cannot be calculated if the number of observed infections equals zero; (9) No data are available from the state/territory for this reporting period; (10) The scores shown reflect fewer than 50 completed surveys; (11) There were discrepancies in the data collection process; (12) This measure does not apply to this hospital for this reporting period; (13) Results cannot be calculated for this reporting period; (14) The results for this state are combined with nearby states to protect confidentiality; Please refer to the User's Guide for a full explanation of data.

Providence Sacred Heart Medical Center[2]	Spokane	100%	330
Providence Saint Mary Medical Center	Walla Walla	100%	428
Swedish Medical Center - Cherry Hill[2]	Seattle	100%	118
Virginia Mason Medical Center[2]	Seattle	100%	417
Central Washington Hospital	Wenatchee	99%	959
Confluence Hlth-Wenatchee Valley Hosp	Wenatchee	99%	123
Harborview Medical Center[2]	Seattle	99%	158
Lourdes Medical Center	Pasco	99%	580
Multicare Good Samaritan Hospital[2]	Puyallup	99%	408
Overlake Hospital Medical Center[2]	Bellevue	99%	465
Peacehealth Saint Joseph Medical Center[2]	Bellingham	99%	315
Saint Joseph Medical Center[2]	Tacoma	99%	456
Seattle VA Med Ctr-VA Pugit Sound[2]	Seattle	99%	350
Skagit Valley Hospital[2]	Mount Vernon	99%	362
Swedish Medical Center[2]	Seattle	99%	763
Tri - State Memorial Hospital[2]	Clarkston	99%	164
Valley General Hospital	Monroe	99%	89
Valley Hospital	Spokane	99%	593
Valley Medical Center[2]	Renton	99%	281
Capital Medical Center[2]	Olympia	98%	349
Legacy Salmon Creek Medical Center[2]	Vancouver	98%	364
Multicare Auburn Medical Center[2]	Auburn	98%	248
Peacehealth Southwest Medical Center[2]	Vancouver	98%	390
Providence Holy Family Hospital[2]	Spokane	98%	287
Providence Saint Peter Hospital[2]	Olympia	98%	302
Saint Anthony Hospital[2]	Gig Harbor	98%	300
Swedish Issaquah[2]	Issaquah	98%	287
Tacoma General Allenmore Hospital[2]	Tacoma	98%	677
University of Washington Medical Center[2]	Seattle	98%	332
Yakima Valley Memorial Hospital[2]	Yakima	98%	751
Cascade Valley Hospital	Arlington	97%	116
Kadlec Regional Medical Center[2]	Richland	97%	438
Kittitas Valley Community Hospital[3]	Ellensburg	97%	93
Mason General Hospital	Shelton	97%	87
Northwest Hospital[2]	Seattle	97%	354
Olympic Medical Center	Port Angeles	97%	391
Pullman Regional Hospital	Pullman	97%	177
Saint Clare Hospital[2]	Lakewood	97%	312
Sunnyside Community Hospital	Sunnyside	97%	30
Swedish Edmonds Hospital	Edmonds	97%	527
Island Hospital	Anacortes	96%	328
Kennewick General Hospital[2]	Kennewick	96%	214
Providence Centralia Hospital[2]	Centralia	96%	306
Saint Elizabeth Hospital[2]	Enumclaw	96%	123
Saint Francis Community Hospital[2]	Federal Way	95%	280
Walla Walla General Hospital[2]	Walla Walla	95%	118
Yakima Regional Medical & Cardiac Center	Yakima	95%	297
Evergreen Hospital Medical Center[2]	Kirkland	94%	309
Whitman Hospital & Medical Center	Colfax	94%	51
Providence Mount Carmel Hospital[2]	Colville	93%	41
Samaritan Hospital	Moses Lake	92%	194
Whidbey General Hospital	Coupeville	92%	126
Grays Harbor Community Hospital	Aberdeen	89%	195

Controlled Postoperative Blood Glucose

Hospital Name	City	Rate	Cases
Central Washington Hospital	Wenatchee	100%	145
Kadlec Regional Medical Center[2]	Richland	99%	148
Peacehealth Saint Joseph Medical Center[2]	Bellingham	99%	147
Peacehealth Southwest Medical Center[2]	Vancouver	99%	152
Providence Reg Med Ctr Everett[2]	Everett	99%	152
Harrison Memorial Center[2]	Bremerton	98%	214
Northwest Hospital[2]	Seattle	98%	65
Providence Sacred Heart Medical Center[2]	Spokane	98%	131
Seattle VA Med Ctr-VA Pugit Sound[2]	Seattle	98%	47
University of Washington Medical Center[2]	Seattle	98%	143
Overlake Hospital Medical Center[2]	Bellevue	97%	121
Providence Saint Peter Hospital[2]	Olympia	97%	159
Saint Joseph Medical Center[2]	Tacoma	97%	306
Swedish Medical Center - Cherry Hill[2]	Seattle	97%	226
Deaconess Hospital	Spokane	94%	116
Tacoma General Allenmore Hospital[2]	Tacoma	94%	200
Yakima Regional Medical & Cardiac Center	Yakima	94%	154
Virginia Mason Medical Center[2]	Seattle	91%	332

Perioperative Temperature Management

Hospital Name	City	Rate	Cases
Capital Medical Center[2]	Olympia	100%	478
Central Washington Hospital	Wenatchee	100%	1181
Confluence Hlth-Wenatchee Valley Hosp	Wenatchee	100%	224
Deaconess Hospital	Spokane	100%	1037
Evergreen Hospital Medical Center[2]	Kirkland	100%	492
Harborview Medical Center[2]	Seattle	100%	253
Harrison Memorial Center[2]	Bremerton	100%	485
Highline Medical Center	Burien	100%	463
Island Hospital	Anacortes	100%	396
Jefferson Healthcare Hospital	Port Townsend	100%	72
Kadlec Regional Medical Center[2]	Richland	100%	590
Kennewick General Hospital[2]	Kennewick	100%	242
Kittitas Valley Community Hospital[3]	Ellensburg	100%	110
Legacy Salmon Creek Medical Center[2]	Vancouver	100%	477
Lourdes Medical Center	Pasco	100%	631
Mason General Hospital	Shelton	100%	104
Mid Valley Hospital	Omak	100%	32
Multicare Good Samaritan Hospital[2]	Puyallup	100%	450
Northwest Hospital[2]	Seattle	100%	412
Olympic Medical Center	Port Angeles	100%	439
Overlake Hospital Medical Center[2]	Bellevue	100%	577
Peacehealth Saint Joseph Medical Center[2]	Bellingham	100%	433
Peacehealth Southwest Medical Center[2]	Vancouver	100%	531
Peachealth Saint John Medical Center	Longview	100%	750
Prosser Memorial Hospital	Prosser	100%	33
Providence Centralia Hospital[2]	Centralia	100%	348
Providence Holy Family Hospital[2]	Spokane	100%	336
Providence Mount Carmel Hospital[2]	Colville	100%	44
Providence Reg Med Ctr Everett[2]	Everett	100%	494
Providence Sacred Heart Medical Center[2]	Spokane	100%	469
Providence Saint Mary Medical Center	Walla Walla	100%	508
Providence Saint Peter Hospital[2]	Olympia	100%	500
Saint Anthony Hospital[2]	Gig Harbor	100%	328
Saint Clare Hospital[2]	Lakewood	100%	350
Saint Elizabeth Hospital[2]	Enumclaw	100%	130
Saint Francis Community Hospital[2]	Federal Way	100%	380
Saint Joseph Medical Center[2]	Tacoma	100%	557
Skagit Valley Hospital[2]	Mount Vernon	100%	438
Sunnyside Community Hospital	Sunnyside	100%	39
Swedish Edmonds Hospital	Edmonds	100%	652
Swedish Issaquah[2]	Issaquah	100%	380
Swedish Medical Center[2]	Seattle	100%	1053
Swedish Medical Center - Cherry Hill[2]	Seattle	100%	283
Tacoma General Allenmore Hospital[2]	Tacoma	100%	837
University of Washington Medical Center[2]	Seattle	100%	402
Valley Hospital	Spokane	100%	680
Valley Medical Center[2]	Renton	100%	376
Virginia Mason Medical Center[2]	Seattle	100%	521
Walla Walla General Hospital[2]	Walla Walla	100%	164
Yakima Regional Medical & Cardiac Center	Yakima	100%	406
Yakima Valley Memorial Hospital[2]	Yakima	100%	888
Cascade Valley Hospital	Arlington	99%	153
Multicare Auburn Medical Center[2]	Auburn	99%	290
Pullman Regional Hospital	Pullman	99%	190
Tri - State Memorial Hospital[2]	Clarkston	99%	188
Valley General Hospital	Monroe	99%	115
Whidbey General Hospital	Coupeville	99%	155
Seattle VA Med Ctr-VA Pugit Sound[2]	Seattle	98%	453
Whitman Hospital & Medical Center	Colfax	98%	57
Samaritan Hospital	Moses Lake	97%	256
Grays Harbor Community Hospital	Aberdeen	93%	229

Prophylactic Antibiotic Selection

Hospital Name	City	Rate	Cases
Cascade Valley Hospital	Arlington	100%	105
Central Washington Hospital	Wenatchee	100%	918
Confluence Hlth-Wenatchee Valley Hosp	Wenatchee	100%	112
Harborview Medical Center[2]	Seattle	100%	98
Harrison Memorial Center[2]	Bremerton	100%	506
Highline Medical Center	Burien	100%	246
Jefferson Healthcare Hospital	Port Townsend	100%	62
Kennewick General Hospital[2]	Kennewick	100%	148
Multicare Auburn Medical Center[2]	Auburn	100%	180
Multicare Good Samaritan Hospital[2]	Puyallup	100%	282
Peacehealth Southwest Medical Center[2]	Vancouver	100%	501
Peachealth Saint John Medical Center	Longview	100%	529
Providence Mount Carmel Hospital[2]	Colville	100%	25
Saint Anthony Hospital[2]	Gig Harbor	100%	217
Saint Clare Hospital[2]	Lakewood	100%	217
Saint Elizabeth Hospital[2]	Enumclaw	100%	93
Saint Joseph Medical Center[2]	Tacoma	100%	644
Samaritan Hospital	Moses Lake	100%	211
Skagit Valley Hospital[2]	Mount Vernon	100%	287
Swedish Issaquah[2]	Issaquah	100%	254
Swedish Medical Center - Cherry Hill[2]	Seattle	100%	240
Valley Hospital	Spokane	100%	519
Virginia Mason Medical Center[2]	Seattle	100%	613
Whitman Hospital & Medical Center	Colfax	100%	48
Yakima Valley Memorial Hospital[2]	Yakima	100%	695
Capital Medical Center[2]	Olympia	99%	345
Deaconess Hospital	Spokane	99%	571
Kittitas Valley Community Hospital[3]	Ellensburg	99%	92
Legacy Salmon Creek Medical Center[2]	Vancouver	99%	340
Lourdes Medical Center	Pasco	99%	528
Olympic Medical Center	Port Angeles	99%	335
Overlake Hospital Medical Center[2]	Bellevue	99%	521
Peacehealth Saint Joseph Medical Center[2]	Bellingham	99%	398
Providence Holy Family Hospital[2]	Spokane	99%	222
Providence Reg Med Ctr Everett[2]	Everett	99%	479
Providence Sacred Heart Medical Center[2]	Spokane	99%	409
Providence Saint Mary Medical Center	Walla Walla	99%	396
Saint Francis Community Hospital[2]	Federal Way	99%	226
Seattle VA Med Ctr-VA Pugit Sound	Seattle	99%	368
Swedish Medical Center[2]	Seattle	99%	763
Tacoma General Allenmore Hospital[2]	Tacoma	99%	669
University of Washington Medical Center[2]	Seattle	99%	334
Yakima Regional Medical & Cardiac Center	Yakima	99%	345
Evergreen Hospital Medical Center[2]	Kirkland	98%	345
Island Hospital	Anacortes	98%	278
Kadlec Regional Medical Center[2]	Richland	98%	578
Mason General Hospital	Shelton	98%	62
Northwest Hospital[2]	Seattle	98%	328
Providence Saint Peter Hospital[2]	Olympia	98%	451
Swedish Edmonds Hospital	Edmonds	98%	371
Tri - State Memorial Hospital[2]	Clarkston	98%	132
Valley General Hospital	Monroe	98%	65
Walla Walla General Hospital[2]	Walla Walla	98%	113
Valley Medical Center[2]	Renton	97%	275
Whidbey General Hospital	Coupeville	97%	129
Prosser Memorial Hospital	Prosser	96%	28
Providence Centralia Hospital[2]	Centralia	96%	241
Pullman Regional Hospital	Pullman	96%	141
Grays Harbor Community Hospital	Aberdeen	94%	147

Prophylactic Antibiotic Selection (Outpatient)

Hospital Name	City	Rate	Cases
Saint Anthony Hospital	Gig Harbor	100%	43
Swedish Issaquah	Issaquah	100%	200
Swedish Medical Center - Cherry Hill	Seattle	100%	388
Capital Medical Center	Olympia	99%	141
Harborview Medical Center	Seattle	99%	225
Harrison Memorial Center	Bremerton	99%	387
Kadlec Regional Medical Center	Richland	99%	582
Legacy Salmon Creek Medical Center	Vancouver	99%	284
Multicare Good Samaritan Hospital	Puyallup	99%	452
Northwest Hospital	Seattle	99%	337
Peacehealth Saint Joseph Medical Center	Bellingham	99%	282
Peachealth Saint John Medical Center	Longview	99%	110
Providence Saint Mary Medical Center	Walla Walla	99%	177
Saint Francis Community Hospital	Federal Way	99%	215
Saint Joseph Medical Center	Tacoma	99%	744
Skagit Valley Hospital	Mount Vernon	99%	366
University of Washington Medical Center	Seattle	99%	552
Valley Medical Center	Renton	99%	334
Virginia Mason Medical Center	Seattle	99%	828
Central Washington Hospital	Wenatchee	98%	289
Confluence Hlth-Wenatchee Valley Hosp	Wenatchee	98%	681
Deaconess Hospital	Spokane	98%	515
Evergreen Hospital Medical Center	Kirkland	98%	638
Group Health Central Hospital	Seattle	98%	126
Kennewick General Hospital	Kennewick	98%	176
Overlake Hospital Medical Center	Bellevue	98%	490
Peacehealth Southwest Medical Center	Vancouver	98%	529
Providence Holy Family Hospital	Spokane	98%	231
Providence Reg Med Ctr Everett	Everett	98%	560
Providence Sacred Heart Medical Center	Spokane	98%	789
Swedish Medical Center	Seattle	98%	504
Valley Hospital	Spokane	98%	106
Highline Medical Center	Burien	97%	100
Olympic Medical Center	Port Angeles	97%	110
Saint Clare Hospital	Lakewood	97%	58
Samaritan Hospital	Moses Lake	97%	35
Yakima Regional Medical & Cardiac Center	Yakima	97%	117
Providence Saint Peter Hospital	Olympia	96%	284
Swedish Edmonds Hospital	Edmonds	96%	146
Tacoma General Allenmore Hospital	Tacoma	96%	823
Providence Mount Carmel Hospital	Colville	95%	37
Yakima Valley Memorial Hospital	Yakima	95%	335
Island Hospital	Anacortes	94%	48
Tri - State Memorial Hospital	Clarkston	94%	82
Multicare Auburn Medical Center	Auburn	90%	41

Prophylactic Antibiotic Stopped

Hospital Name	City	Rate	Cases
Central Washington Hospital	Wenatchee	100%	903
Confluence Hlth-Wenatchee Valley Hosp	Wenatchee	100%	110
Mason General Hospital	Shelton	100%	61
Northwest Hospital[2]	Seattle	100%	320
Overlake Hospital Medical Center[2]	Bellevue	100%	513
Peacehealth Southwest Medical Center[2]	Vancouver	100%	487
Peachealth Saint John Medical Center	Longview	100%	514
Prosser Memorial Hospital	Prosser	100%	28
Providence Reg Med Ctr Everett[2]	Everett	100%	465
Providence Saint Mary Medical Center	Walla Walla	100%	396
Pullman Regional Hospital	Pullman	100%	141
Saint Clare Hospital[2]	Lakewood	100%	203
Saint Elizabeth Hospital[2]	Enumclaw	100%	92
Swedish Medical Center - Cherry Hill[2]	Seattle	100%	236
Valley Hospital	Spokane	100%	510
Valley Medical Center[2]	Renton	100%	273
Harrison Memorial Center[2]	Bremerton	99%	495
Highline Medical Center	Burien	99%	238
Kittitas Valley Community Hospital[3]	Ellensburg	99%	90
Legacy Salmon Creek Medical Center[2]	Vancouver	99%	335

NOTE: Hospital profiles are in alphabetical order by state, then city, then hospital within the city; Rankings exclude hospitals with less than 25 cases except for patient surveys which excludes hospitals with less than 100 cases; (a) 100-299 cases; (1) The number of cases/patients is too few to report; (2) Data submitted were based on a sample of cases/patients; (3) Results are based on a shorter time period than required; (4) Data suppressed by CMS for one or more quarters; (5) Results are not available for this reporting period; (6) Fewer than 100 patients completed the HCAHPS survey; (7) No cases met the criteria for this measure; (8) The lower limit of the confidence interval cannot be calculated if the number of observed infections equals zero; (9) No data are available from the state/territory for this reporting period; (10) The scores shown reflect fewer than 50 completed surveys; (11) There were discrepancies in the data collection process; (12) This measure does not apply to this hospital for this reporting period; (13) Results cannot be calculated for this reporting period; (14) The results for this state are combined with nearby states to protect confidentiality; Please refer to the User's Guide for a full explanation of data.

Hospital Name	City	Rate	Cases
Multicare Good Samaritan Hospital[2]	Puyallup	99%	278
Providence Holy Family Hospital[2]	Spokane	99%	213
Providence Sacred Heart Medical Center[2]	Spokane	99%	401
Saint Anthony Hospital[2]	Gig Harbor	99%	213
Saint Francis Community Hospital[2]	Federal Way	99%	218
Saint Joseph Medical Center[2]	Tacoma	99%	624
Samaritan Hospital	Moses Lake	99%	211
Skagit Valley Hospital[2]	Mount Vernon	99%	280
Swedish Medical Center[2]	Seattle	99%	745
Tacoma General Allenmore Hospital[2]	Tacoma	99%	661
Tri - State Memorial Hospital[2]	Clarkston	99%	132
Whidbey General Hospital	Coupeville	99%	125
Capital Medical Center[2]	Olympia	98%	343
Deaconess Hospital	Spokane	98%	527
Evergreen Hospital Medical Center[2]	Kirkland	98%	339
Jefferson Healthcare Hospital	Port Townsend	98%	62
Kennewick General Hospital[2]	Kennewick	98%	146
Olympic Medical Center	Port Angeles	98%	329
Peacehealth Saint Joseph Medical Center[2]	Bellingham	98%	394
Swedish Issaquah[2]	Issaquah	98%	248
University of Washington Medical Center[2]	Seattle	98%	317
Valley General Hospital	Monroe	98%	65
Virginia Mason Medical Center[2]	Seattle	98%	597
Walla Walla General Hospital[2]	Walla Walla	98%	110
Yakima Valley Memorial Hospital[2]	Yakima	98%	684
Cascade Valley Hospital	Arlington	97%	102
Harborview Medical Center[2]	Seattle	97%	94
Island Hospital	Anacortes	97%	272
Kadlec Regional Medical Center[2]	Richland	97%	556
Lourdes Medical Center	Pasco	97%	525
Providence Centralia Hospital[2]	Centralia	97%	239
Providence Saint Peter Hospital[2]	Olympia	97%	447
Seattle VA Med Ctr-VA Pugit Sound	Seattle	97%	365
Swedish Edmonds Hospital	Edmonds	96%	365
Whitman Hospital & Medical Center	Colfax	96%	47
Yakima Regional Medical & Cardiac Center	Yakima	96%	334
Multicare Auburn Medical Center[2]	Auburn	94%	178
Grays Harbor Community Hospital	Aberdeen	92%	144

Prophylactic Antibiotic Timing

Hospital Name	City	Rate	Cases
Confluence Hlth-Wenatchee Valley Hosp	Wenatchee	100%	112
Highline Medical Center	Burien	100%	246
Kittitas Valley Community Hospital[3]	Ellensburg	100%	92
Overlake Hospital Medical Center[2]	Bellevue	100%	522
Peacehealth Southwest Medical Center[2]	Vancouver	100%	504
Prosser Memorial Hospital	Prosser	100%	28
Providence Holy Family Hospital[2]	Spokane	100%	222
Providence Reg Med Ctr Everett[2]	Everett	100%	479
Providence Saint Mary Medical Center	Walla Walla	100%	396
Skagit Valley Hospital[2]	Mount Vernon	100%	287
Valley General Hospital	Monroe	100%	65
Valley Hospital	Spokane	100%	519
Cascade Valley Hospital	Arlington	99%	105
Central Washington Hospital	Wenatchee	99%	918
Deaconess Hospital	Spokane	99%	571
Evergreen Hospital Medical Center[2]	Kirkland	99%	345
Harborview Medical Center[2]	Seattle	99%	99
Harrison Memorial Center[2]	Bremerton	99%	508
Kadlec Regional Medical Center[2]	Richland	99%	579
Kennewick General Hospital[2]	Kennewick	99%	148
Legacy Salmon Creek Medical Center[2]	Vancouver	99%	340
Multicare Good Samaritan Hospital[2]	Puyallup	99%	283
Peacehealth Saint Joseph Medical Center[2]	Bellingham	99%	398
Peachealth Saint John Medical Center	Longview	99%	529
Providence Sacred Heart Medical Center[2]	Spokane	99%	409
Pullman Regional Hospital	Pullman	99%	141
Saint Elizabeth Hospital[2]	Enumclaw	99%	93
Saint Joseph Medical Center[2]	Tacoma	99%	646
Swedish Edmonds Hospital	Edmonds	99%	371
Swedish Medical Center[2]	Seattle	99%	763
University of Washington Medical Center[2]	Seattle	99%	336
Virginia Mason Medical Center[2]	Seattle	99%	613
Walla Walla General Hospital[2]	Walla Walla	99%	113
Whidbey General Hospital	Coupeville	99%	129
Yakima Valley Memorial Hospital[2]	Yakima	99%	695
Lourdes Medical Center	Pasco	98%	528
Northwest Hospital[2]	Seattle	98%	329
Providence Centralia Hospital[2]	Centralia	98%	241
Saint Anthony Hospital[2]	Gig Harbor	98%	218
Saint Francis Community Hospital[2]	Federal Way	98%	226
Seattle VA Med Ctr-VA Pugit Sound	Seattle	98%	368
Swedish Issaquah[2]	Issaquah	98%	256
Tacoma General Allenmore Hospital[2]	Tacoma	98%	670
Tri - State Memorial Hospital[2]	Clarkston	98%	133
Valley Medical Center[2]	Renton	98%	275
Capital Medical Center[2]	Olympia	97%	345
Island Hospital	Anacortes	97%	279
Jefferson Healthcare Hospital	Port Townsend	97%	62
Providence Saint Peter Hospital[2]	Olympia	97%	455
Saint Clare Hospital[2]	Lakewood	97%	217
Swedish Medical Center - Cherry Hill[2]	Seattle	97%	241
Yakima Regional Medical & Cardiac Center	Yakima	97%	348
Olympic Medical Center	Port Angeles	95%	337
Multicare Auburn Medical Center[2]	Auburn	94%	180
Samaritan Hospital	Moses Lake	94%	211
Whitman Hospital & Medical Center	Colfax	94%	48
Mason General Hospital	Shelton	92%	62
Providence Mount Carmel Hospital[2]	Colville	92%	25
Grays Harbor Community Hospital	Aberdeen	90%	147

Prophylactic Antibiotic Timing (Outpatient)

Hospital Name	City	Rate	Cases
Harborview Medical Center	Seattle	100%	189
Legacy Salmon Creek Medical Center	Vancouver	100%	284
Peacehealth Saint Joseph Medical Center	Bellingham	100%	281
Saint Anthony Hospital	Gig Harbor	100%	43
Skagit Valley Hospital	Mount Vernon	100%	367
Capital Medical Center	Olympia	99%	143
Deaconess Hospital	Spokane	99%	515
Harrison Memorial Center	Bremerton	99%	388
Multicare Good Samaritan Hospital	Puyallup	99%	454
Overlake Hospital Medical Center	Bellevue	99%	491
Peacehealth Southwest Medical Center	Vancouver	99%	531
Peacehealth Saint John Medical Center	Longview	99%	96
Saint Joseph Medical Center	Tacoma	99%	748
Swedish Issaquah	Issaquah	99%	200
Swedish Medical Center	Seattle	99%	507
Swedish Medical Center - Cherry Hill	Seattle	99%	389
Tacoma General Allenmore Hospital	Tacoma	99%	826
Yakima Valley Memorial Hospital	Yakima	99%	338
Highline Medical Center	Burien	98%	100
Island Hospital	Anacortes	98%	49
Kadlec Regional Medical Center	Richland	98%	585
Kennewick General Hospital	Kennewick	98%	177
Northwest Hospital	Seattle	98%	339
Providence Reg Med Ctr Everett	Everett	98%	561
Providence Sacred Heart Medical Center	Spokane	98%	790
Providence Saint Mary Medical Center	Walla Walla	98%	177
Saint Clare Hospital	Lakewood	98%	59
Tri - State Memorial Hospital	Clarkston	98%	84
Valley Hospital	Spokane	98%	106
Yakima Regional Medical & Cardiac Center	Yakima	98%	118
Confluence Hlth-Wenatchee Valley Hosp	Wenatchee	97%	352
Evergreen Hospital Medical Center	Kirkland	97%	643
Providence Holy Family Hospital	Spokane	97%	234
Samaritan Hospital	Moses Lake	97%	36
Swedish Edmonds Hospital	Edmonds	97%	147
Valley Medical Center	Renton	97%	338
Virginia Mason Medical Center	Seattle	97%	621
Central Washington Hospital	Wenatchee	96%	295
Olympic Medical Center	Port Angeles	96%	98
Saint Francis Community Hospital	Federal Way	96%	216
Group Health Central Hospital	Seattle	94%	127
Providence Saint Peter Hospital	Olympia	92%	288
University of Washington Medical Center	Seattle	91%	392
Multicare Auburn Medical Center	Auburn	86%	44

Urinary Catheter Removal

Hospital Name	City	Rate	Cases
Cascade Valley Hospital	Arlington	100%	79
Harborview Medical Center[2]	Seattle	100%	88
Jefferson Healthcare Hospital	Port Townsend	100%	65
Kittitas Valley Community Hospital[3]	Ellensburg	100%	84
Legacy Salmon Creek Medical Center[2]	Vancouver	100%	299
Mason General Hospital	Shelton	100%	60
Mid Valley Hospital	Omak	100%	31
Peachealth Saint John Medical Center	Longview	100%	453
Seattle VA Med Ctr-VA Pugit Sound[2]	Seattle	100%	306
Swedish Issaquah[2]	Issaquah	100%	172
Swedish Medical Center[2]	Seattle	100%	492
Swedish Medical Center - Cherry Hill[2]	Seattle	100%	300
Whidbey General Hospital	Coupeville	100%	119
Whitman Hospital & Medical Center	Colfax	100%	50
Deaconess Hospital	Spokane	99%	578
Kennewick General Hospital[2]	Kennewick	99%	147
Overlake Hospital Medical Center[2]	Bellevue	99%	305
Peacehealth Southwest Medical Center[2]	Vancouver	99%	441
Providence Holy Family Hospital[2]	Spokane	99%	128
Providence Sacred Heart Medical Center[2]	Spokane	99%	370
Pullman Regional Hospital	Pullman	99%	115
Valley Hospital	Spokane	99%	538
Capital Medical Center[2]	Olympia	98%	225
Harrison Memorial Center[2]	Bremerton	98%	256
Lourdes Medical Center	Pasco	98%	133
Multicare Good Samaritan Hospital[2]	Puyallup	98%	283
Northwest Hospital[2]	Seattle	98%	313
Providence Reg Med Ctr Everett[2]	Everett	98%	409
Providence Saint Mary Medical Center	Walla Walla	98%	186
University of Washington Medical Center[2]	Seattle	98%	273
Valley Medical Center[2]	Renton	98%	231
Yakima Valley Memorial Hospital[2]	Yakima	98%	654
Confluence Hlth-Wenatchee Valley Hosp	Wenatchee	97%	86
Island Hospital	Anacortes	97%	295
Olympic Medical Center	Port Angeles	97%	327
Peacehealth Saint Joseph Medical Center[2]	Bellingham	97%	246
Samaritan Hospital	Moses Lake	97%	196
Skagit Valley Hospital[2]	Mount Vernon	97%	252
Tri - State Memorial Hospital[2]	Clarkston	97%	152
Valley General Hospital	Monroe	97%	92
Central Washington Hospital	Wenatchee	96%	983
Virginia Mason Medical Center[2]	Seattle	96%	434
Highline Medical Center	Burien	95%	244
Kadlec Regional Medical Center[2]	Richland	95%	480
Swedish Edmonds Hospital	Edmonds	95%	350
Walla Walla General Hospital[2]	Walla Walla	95%	55
Evergreen Hospital Medical Center[2]	Kirkland	94%	160
Grays Harbor Community Hospital	Aberdeen	94%	172
Providence Centralia Hospital[2]	Centralia	93%	214
Saint Elizabeth Hospital[2]	Enumclaw	93%	27
Saint Joseph Medical Center[2]	Tacoma	93%	288
Yakima Regional Medical & Cardiac Center	Yakima	92%	234
Multicare Auburn Medical Center[2]	Auburn	91%	202
Tacoma General Allenmore Hospital[2]	Tacoma	91%	394
Providence Saint Peter Hospital[2]	Olympia	90%	227
Saint Francis Community Hospital[2]	Federal Way	90%	219
Saint Clare Hospital[2]	Lakewood	82%	71
Saint Anthony Hospital[2]	Gig Harbor	75%	68

Survey of Patients' Hospital Experiences

Area Around Room 'Always' Quiet at Night

Hospital Name	City	Rate	Cases
Whitman Hospital & Medical Center	Colfax	71%	(a)
Legacy Salmon Creek Medical Center	Vancouver	69%	300+
Group Health Central Hospital	Seattle	66%	300+
Kittitas Valley Community Hospital	Ellensburg	66%	(a)
Evergreen Hospital Medical Center	Kirkland	65%	300+
Providence Mount Carmel Hospital	Colville	65%	(a)
Walla Walla General Hospital	Walla Walla	64%	(a)
Othello Community Hospital	Othello	63%	(a)
Peacehealth United General Medical Center	Sedro Woolley	63%	(a)
Kadlec Regional Medical Center[11]	Richland	62%	300+
Pullman Regional Hospital	Pullman	61%	300+
Swedish Issaquah	Issaquah	61%	300+
Saint Anthony Hospital	Gig Harbor	60%	300+
Island Hospital	Anacortes	59%	300+
Samaritan Hospital	Moses Lake	59%	300+
Toppenish Community Hospital	Toppenish	59%	(a)
Central Washington Hospital	Wenatchee	58%	300+
Confluence Hlth-Wenatchee Valley Hosp	Wenatchee	58%	(a)
Deaconess Hospital	Spokane	58%	300+
Providence Saint Mary Medical Center	Walla Walla	58%	300+
Saint Elizabeth Hospital	Enumclaw	58%	(a)
Overlake Hospital Medical Center	Bellevue	57%	300+
Multicare Good Samaritan Hospital	Puyallup	56%	300+
Peacehealth Southwest Medical Center	Vancouver	56%	300+
University of Washington Medical Center	Seattle	55%	300+
Valley Medical Center	Renton	55%	300+
Prosser Memorial Hospital	Prosser	54%	(a)
Providence Centralia Hospital	Centralia	54%	300+
Providence Saint Peter Hospital	Olympia	54%	300+
Swedish Medical Center	Seattle	54%	300+
Capital Medical Center	Olympia	53%	300+
Kennewick General Hospital	Kennewick	52%	300+
Saint Clare Hospital	Lakewood	52%	300+
Lincoln Hospital	Davenport	51%	(a)
Providence Reg Med Ctr Everett	Everett	51%	300+
Tacoma General Allenmore Hospital	Tacoma	51%	300+
Grays Harbor Community Hospital	Aberdeen	50%	300+
Highline Medical Center	Burien	50%	300+
Providence Sacred Heart Medical Center	Spokane	50%	300+
Cascade Valley Hospital[3]	Arlington	49%	(a)
Tri - State Memorial Hospital	Clarkston	49%	300+
Valley Hospital	Spokane	49%	300+
Yakima Valley Memorial Hospital	Yakima	49%	300+
Northwest Hospital	Seattle	48%	300+
Saint Francis Community Hospital	Federal Way	48%	300+
Swedish Edmonds Hospital	Edmonds	48%	300+
Yakima Regional Medical & Cardiac Center	Yakima	48%	300+
Providence Holy Family Hospital	Spokane	46%	300+
Saint Joseph Medical Center	Tacoma	46%	300+
Skagit Valley Hospital	Mount Vernon	46%	300+
Olympic Medical Center	Port Angeles	45%	300+
Peachealth Saint John Medical Center	Longview	45%	300+
Whidbey General Hospital	Coupeville	45%	300+
Harborview Medical Center	Seattle	44%	300+
Sunnyside Community Hospital	Sunnyside	44%	(a)
Swedish Medical Center - Cherry Hill	Seattle	44%	300+
Virginia Mason Medical Center	Seattle	44%	300+
Multicare Auburn Medical Center	Auburn	43%	300+

NOTE: Hospital profiles are in alphabetical order by state, then city, then hospital within the city; Rankings exclude hospitals with less than 25 cases except for patient surveys which excludes hospitals with less than 100 cases; (a) 100-299 cases; (1) The number of cases/patients is too few to report; (2) Data submitted were based on a sample of cases/patients; (3) Results are based on a shorter time period than required; (4) Data suppressed by CMS for one or more quarters; (5) Results are not available for this reporting period; (6) Fewer than 100 patients completed the HCAHPS survey; (7) No cases met the criteria for this measure; (8) The lower limit of the confidence interval cannot be calculated if the number of observed infections equals zero; (9) No data are available from the state/territory for this reporting period; (10) The scores shown reflect fewer than 50 completed surveys; (11) There were discrepancies in the data collection process; (12) This measure does not apply to this hospital for this reporting period; (13) Results cannot be calculated for this reporting period; (14) The results for this state are combined with nearby states to protect confidentiality; Please refer to the User's Guide for a full explanation of data.

Peacehealth Saint Joseph Medical Center	Bellingham	43%	300+
Harrison Memorial Center	Bremerton	41%	300+
Valley General Hospital	Monroe	41%	(a)

Doctors 'Always' Communicated Well

Hospital Name	City	Rate	Cases
Whitman Hospital & Medical Center	Colfax	91%	(a)
Confluence Hlth-Wenatchee Valley Hosp	Wenatchee	89%	(a)
Lincoln Hospital	Davenport	86%	(a)
Saint Elizabeth Hospital	Enumclaw	86%	(a)
Central Washington Hospital	Wenatchee	85%	300+
Providence Saint Mary Medical Center	Walla Walla	85%	300+
Providence Mount Carmel Hospital	Colville	84%	(a)
Pullman Regional Hospital	Pullman	84%	300+
Toppenish Community Hospital	Toppenish	84%	(a)
Virginia Mason Medical Center	Seattle	84%	300+
Cascade Valley Hospital[3]	Arlington	83%	(a)
Capital Medical Center	Olympia	82%	300+
Evergreen Hospital Medical Center	Kirkland	82%	300+
Island Hospital	Anacortes	82%	300+
Kittitas Valley Community Hospital	Ellensburg	82%	(a)
Northwest Hospital	Seattle	82%	300+
Overlake Hospital Medical Center	Bellevue	82%	300+
Swedish Issaquah	Issaquah	82%	300+
Deaconess Hospital	Spokane	81%	300+
Legacy Salmon Creek Medical Center	Vancouver	81%	300+
Olympic Medical Center	Port Angeles	81%	300+
Peacehealth Southwest Medical Center	Vancouver	81%	300+
Providence Saint Peter Hospital	Olympia	81%	300+
Swedish Medical Center	Seattle	81%	300+
Kennewick General Hospital	Kennewick	80%	300+
Othello Community Hospital	Othello	80%	(a)
Peacehealth Saint Joseph Medical Center	Bellingham	80%	300+
Peacehealth United General Medical Center	Sedro Woolley	80%	(a)
Swedish Medical Center - Cherry Hill	Seattle	80%	300+
University of Washington Medical Center	Seattle	80%	300+
Grays Harbor Community Hospital	Aberdeen	79%	300+
Group Health Central Hospital	Seattle	79%	300+
Harrison Memorial Center	Bremerton	79%	300+
Kadlec Regional Medical Center[11]	Richland	79%	300+
Providence Reg Med Ctr Everett	Everett	79%	300+
Providence Sacred Heart Medical Center	Spokane	79%	300+
Samaritan Hospital	Moses Lake	79%	300+
Tri - State Memorial Hospital	Clarkston	79%	300+
Valley Hospital	Spokane	79%	300+
Valley Medical Center	Renton	79%	300+
Walla Walla General Hospital	Walla Walla	79%	(a)
Peacehealth Saint John Medical Center	Longview	78%	300+
Prosser Memorial Hospital	Prosser	78%	(a)
Providence Centralia Hospital	Centralia	78%	300+
Whidbey General Hospital	Coupeville	78%	300+
Yakima Valley Memorial Hospital	Yakima	78%	300+
Providence Holy Family Hospital	Spokane	77%	300+
Saint Anthony Hospital	Gig Harbor	77%	300+
Saint Joseph Medical Center	Tacoma	77%	300+
Swedish Edmonds Hospital	Edmonds	77%	300+
Yakima Regional Medical & Cardiac Center	Yakima	77%	300+
Highline Medical Center	Burien	76%	300+
Multicare Good Samaritan Hospital	Puyallup	76%	300+
Skagit Valley Hospital	Mount Vernon	76%	300+
Saint Clare Hospital	Lakewood	75%	300+
Saint Francis Community Hospital	Federal Way	75%	300+
Tacoma General Allenmore Hospital	Tacoma	75%	300+
Valley General Hospital	Monroe	75%	(a)
Harborview Medical Center	Seattle	74%	300+
Sunnyside Community Hospital	Sunnyside	74%	(a)
Multicare Auburn Medical Center	Auburn	70%	300+

Home Recovery Information Given

Hospital Name	City	Rate	Cases
Whitman Hospital & Medical Center	Colfax	93%	(a)
Confluence Hlth-Wenatchee Valley Hosp	Wenatchee	91%	(a)
Kittitas Valley Community Hospital	Ellensburg	91%	(a)
Pullman Regional Hospital	Pullman	91%	300+
Saint Elizabeth Hospital	Enumclaw	91%	(a)
Toppenish Community Hospital	Toppenish	91%	(a)
Peacehealth Saint Joseph Medical Center	Bellingham	90%	300+
University of Washington Medical Center	Seattle	90%	300+
Valley General Hospital	Monroe	90%	(a)
Valley Hospital	Spokane	90%	300+
Central Washington Hospital	Wenatchee	89%	300+
Group Health Central Hospital	Seattle	89%	300+
Legacy Salmon Creek Medical Center	Vancouver	89%	300+
Peacehealth Saint John Medical Center	Longview	89%	300+
Saint Joseph Medical Center	Tacoma	89%	300+
Virginia Mason Medical Center	Seattle	89%	300+
Capital Medical Center	Olympia	88%	300+
Deaconess Hospital	Spokane	88%	300+
Grays Harbor Community Hospital	Aberdeen	88%	300+
Overlake Hospital Medical Center	Bellevue	88%	300+
Saint Anthony Hospital	Gig Harbor	88%	300+
Saint Clare Hospital	Lakewood	88%	300+
Yakima Regional Medical & Cardiac Center	Yakima	88%	300+
Harborview Medical Center	Seattle	87%	300+
Kadlec Regional Medical Center[11]	Richland	87%	300+
Kennewick General Hospital	Kennewick	87%	300+
Multicare Good Samaritan Hospital	Puyallup	87%	300+
Providence Centralia Hospital	Centralia	87%	300+
Providence Reg Med Ctr Everett	Everett	87%	300+
Providence Sacred Heart Medical Center	Spokane	87%	300+
Providence Saint Peter Hospital	Olympia	87%	300+
Tri - State Memorial Hospital	Clarkston	87%	300+
Walla Walla General Hospital	Walla Walla	87%	(a)
Evergreen Hospital Medical Center	Kirkland	86%	300+
Harrison Memorial Center	Bremerton	86%	300+
Island Hospital	Anacortes	86%	300+
Northwest Hospital	Seattle	86%	300+
Peacehealth United General Medical Center	Sedro Woolley	86%	(a)
Prosser Memorial Hospital	Prosser	86%	(a)
Saint Francis Community Hospital	Federal Way	86%	300+
Samaritan Hospital	Moses Lake	86%	300+
Valley Medical Center	Renton	86%	300+
Yakima Valley Memorial Hospital	Yakima	86%	300+
Cascade Valley Hospital[3]	Arlington	85%	(a)
Multicare Auburn Medical Center	Auburn	85%	300+
Peacehealth Southwest Medical Center	Vancouver	85%	300+
Providence Mount Carmel Hospital	Colville	85%	(a)
Providence Saint Mary Medical Center	Walla Walla	85%	300+
Tacoma General Allenmore Hospital	Tacoma	85%	300+
Highline Medical Center	Burien	84%	300+
Olympic Medical Center	Port Angeles	84%	300+
Othello Community Hospital	Othello	84%	(a)
Providence Holy Family Hospital	Spokane	84%	300+
Swedish Edmonds Hospital	Edmonds	84%	300+
Swedish Issaquah	Issaquah	84%	300+
Swedish Medical Center - Cherry Hill	Seattle	84%	300+
Whidbey General Hospital	Coupeville	84%	300+
Skagit Valley Hospital	Mount Vernon	83%	300+
Swedish Medical Center	Seattle	83%	300+
Lincoln Hospital	Davenport	79%	(a)
Sunnyside Community Hospital	Sunnyside	79%	(a)

Hospital Given 9 or 10 on 10 Point Scale

Hospital Name	City	Rate	Cases
Whitman Hospital & Medical Center	Colfax	90%	(a)
Pullman Regional Hospital	Pullman	83%	300+
Saint Elizabeth Hospital	Enumclaw	82%	(a)
Confluence Hlth-Wenatchee Valley Hosp	Wenatchee	80%	(a)
Providence Mount Carmel Hospital	Colville	80%	(a)
University of Washington Medical Center	Seattle	79%	300+
Virginia Mason Medical Center	Seattle	79%	300+
Evergreen Hospital Medical Center	Kirkland	78%	300+
Island Hospital	Anacortes	78%	300+
Legacy Salmon Creek Medical Center	Vancouver	78%	300+
Swedish Issaquah	Issaquah	78%	300+
Providence Saint Peter Hospital	Olympia	77%	300+
Central Washington Hospital	Wenatchee	76%	300+
Kittitas Valley Community Hospital	Ellensburg	76%	(a)
Lincoln Hospital	Davenport	76%	(a)
Providence Saint Mary Medical Center	Walla Walla	76%	300+
Tri - State Memorial Hospital	Clarkston	74%	300+
Northwest Hospital	Seattle	72%	300+
Overlake Hospital Medical Center	Bellevue	72%	300+
Peacehealth United General Medical Center	Sedro Woolley	72%	(a)
Providence Reg Med Ctr Everett	Everett	72%	300+
Providence Sacred Heart Medical Center	Spokane	72%	300+
Swedish Medical Center - Cherry Hill	Seattle	72%	300+
Kadlec Regional Medical Center[11]	Richland	71%	300+
Peacehealth Southwest Medical Center	Vancouver	71%	300+
Saint Anthony Hospital	Gig Harbor	71%	300+
Swedish Medical Center	Seattle	71%	300+
Toppenish Community Hospital	Toppenish	71%	(a)
Valley Medical Center	Renton	71%	300+
Walla Walla General Hospital	Walla Walla	71%	(a)
Prosser Memorial Hospital	Prosser	70%	(a)
Capital Medical Center	Olympia	69%	300+
Cascade Valley Hospital[3]	Arlington	69%	(a)
Harborview Medical Center	Seattle	69%	300+
Kennewick General Hospital	Kennewick	69%	300+
Multicare Good Samaritan Hospital	Puyallup	69%	300+
Othello Community Hospital	Othello	69%	(a)
Deaconess Hospital	Spokane	68%	300+
Group Health Central Hospital	Seattle	68%	300+
Providence Holy Family Hospital	Spokane	68%	300+
Saint Francis Community Hospital	Federal Way	68%	300+
Valley Hospital	Spokane	68%	300+
Olympic Medical Center	Port Angeles	67%	300+
Peacehealth Saint Joseph Medical Center	Bellingham	67%	300+
Providence Centralia Hospital	Centralia	67%	300+
Harrison Memorial Center	Bremerton	66%	300+
Saint Clare Hospital	Lakewood	66%	300+
Saint Joseph Medical Center	Tacoma	66%	300+
Grays Harbor Community Hospital	Aberdeen	65%	300+
Yakima Valley Memorial Hospital	Yakima	65%	300+
Peacehealth Saint John Medical Center	Longview	64%	300+
Skagit Valley Hospital	Mount Vernon	64%	300+
Tacoma General Allenmore Hospital	Tacoma	64%	300+
Highline Medical Center	Burien	63%	300+
Samaritan Hospital	Moses Lake	63%	300+
Whidbey General Hospital	Coupeville	61%	300+
Sunnyside Community Hospital	Sunnyside	59%	(a)
Swedish Edmonds Hospital	Edmonds	59%	300+
Valley General Hospital	Monroe	58%	(a)
Yakima Regional Medical & Cardiac Center	Yakima	55%	300+
Multicare Auburn Medical Center	Auburn	42%	300+

Meds 'Always' Explained Before Given

Hospital Name	City	Rate	Cases
Confluence Hlth-Wenatchee Valley Hosp	Wenatchee	73%	(a)
Whitman Hospital & Medical Center	Colfax	73%	(a)
Saint Elizabeth Hospital	Enumclaw	72%	(a)
Providence Mount Carmel Hospital	Colville	69%	(a)
Pullman Regional Hospital	Pullman	69%	300+
Central Washington Hospital	Wenatchee	68%	300+
Group Health Central Hospital	Seattle	68%	300+
Island Hospital	Anacortes	68%	300+
Providence Saint Mary Medical Center	Walla Walla	68%	300+
Toppenish Community Hospital	Toppenish	68%	(a)
University of Washington Medical Center	Seattle	68%	300+
Walla Walla General Hospital	Walla Walla	68%	(a)
Kennewick General Hospital	Kennewick	66%	300+
Legacy Salmon Creek Medical Center	Vancouver	66%	300+
Tri - State Memorial Hospital	Clarkston	66%	300+
Capital Medical Center	Olympia	65%	300+
Deaconess Hospital	Spokane	65%	300+
Kittitas Valley Community Hospital	Ellensburg	65%	(a)
Overlake Hospital Medical Center	Bellevue	65%	300+
Peacehealth Saint John Medical Center	Longview	65%	300+
Virginia Mason Medical Center	Seattle	65%	300+
Kadlec Regional Medical Center[11]	Richland	64%	300+
Olympic Medical Center	Port Angeles	64%	300+
Peacehealth Southwest Medical Center	Vancouver	64%	300+
Whidbey General Hospital	Coupeville	64%	300+
Peacehealth United General Medical Center	Sedro Woolley	63%	(a)
Prosser Memorial Hospital	Prosser	63%	(a)
Providence Centralia Hospital	Centralia	63%	300+
Swedish Issaquah	Issaquah	63%	300+
Valley Hospital	Spokane	63%	300+
Evergreen Hospital Medical Center	Kirkland	62%	300+
Peacehealth Saint Joseph Medical Center	Bellingham	62%	300+
Providence Reg Med Ctr Everett	Everett	62%	300+
Providence Saint Peter Hospital	Olympia	62%	300+
Saint Francis Community Hospital	Federal Way	62%	300+
Valley General Hospital	Monroe	62%	(a)
Valley Medical Center	Renton	62%	300+
Grays Harbor Community Hospital	Aberdeen	61%	300+
Providence Holy Family Hospital	Spokane	61%	300+
Providence Sacred Heart Medical Center	Spokane	61%	300+
Saint Anthony Hospital	Gig Harbor	61%	300+
Saint Joseph Medical Center	Tacoma	61%	300+
Samaritan Hospital	Moses Lake	61%	300+
Swedish Edmonds Hospital	Edmonds	61%	300+
Swedish Medical Center - Cherry Hill	Seattle	61%	300+
Harborview Medical Center	Seattle	60%	300+
Lincoln Hospital	Davenport	60%	(a)
Northwest Hospital	Seattle	60%	300+
Sunnyside Community Hospital	Sunnyside	60%	(a)
Swedish Medical Center	Seattle	60%	300+
Yakima Valley Memorial Hospital	Yakima	60%	300+
Harrison Memorial Center	Bremerton	59%	300+
Multicare Good Samaritan Hospital	Puyallup	59%	300+
Othello Community Hospital	Othello	59%	(a)
Saint Clare Hospital	Lakewood	59%	300+
Highline Medical Center	Burien	58%	300+
Skagit Valley Hospital	Mount Vernon	57%	300+
Cascade Valley Hospital[3]	Arlington	56%	(a)
Tacoma General Allenmore Hospital	Tacoma	56%	300+
Yakima Regional Medical & Cardiac Center	Yakima	55%	300+
Multicare Auburn Medical Center	Auburn	51%	300+

Nurses 'Always' Communicated Well

Hospital Name	City	Rate	Cases
Whitman Hospital & Medical Center	Colfax	89%	(a)
Confluence Hlth-Wenatchee Valley Hosp	Wenatchee	85%	(a)
Lincoln Hospital	Davenport	83%	(a)
Pullman Regional Hospital	Pullman	83%	300+
Island Hospital	Anacortes	81%	300+
Providence Mount Carmel Hospital	Colville	81%	(a)
Kennewick General Hospital	Kennewick	80%	300+
Providence Saint Mary Medical Center	Walla Walla	80%	300+
Saint Elizabeth Hospital	Enumclaw	80%	(a)

NOTE: Hospital profiles are in alphabetical order by state, then city, then hospital within the city; Rankings exclude hospitals with less than 25 cases except for patient surveys which excludes hospitals with less than 100 cases; (a) 100-299 cases; (1) The number of cases/patients is too few to report; (2) Data submitted were based on a sample of cases/patients; (3) Results are based on a shorter time period than required; (4) Data suppressed by CMS for one or more quarters; (5) Results are not available for this reporting period; (6) Fewer than 100 patients completed the HCAHPS survey; (7) No cases met the criteria for this measure; (8) The lower limit of the confidence interval cannot be calculated if the number of observed infections equals zero; (9) No data are available from the state/territory for this reporting period; (10) The scores shown reflect fewer than 50 completed surveys; (11) There were discrepancies in the data collection process; (12) This measure does not apply to this hospital for this reporting period; (13) Results cannot be calculated for this reporting period; (14) The results for this state are combined with nearby states to protect confidentiality; Please refer to the User's Guide for a full explanation of data.

Walla Walla General Hospital	Walla Walla	80%	(a)
Kadlec Regional Medical Center[11]	Richland	79%	300+
Kittitas Valley Community Hospital	Ellensburg	79%	(a)
Legacy Salmon Creek Medical Center	Vancouver	79%	300+
Peacehealth United General Medical Center	Sedro Woolley	79%	(a)
Peacehealth Saint John Medical Center	Longview	79%	300+
Providence Saint Peter Hospital	Olympia	79%	300+
Toppenish Community Hospital	Toppenish	79%	(a)
University of Washington Medical Center	Seattle	79%	300+
Virginia Mason Medical Center	Seattle	79%	300+
Central Washington Hospital	Wenatchee	78%	300+
Group Health Central Hospital	Seattle	78%	300+
Othello Community Hospital	Othello	78%	(a)
Peacehealth Saint Joseph Medical Center	Bellingham	78%	300+
Peacehealth Southwest Medical Center	Vancouver	78%	300+
Providence Centralia Hospital	Centralia	78%	300+
Tri - State Memorial Hospital	Clarkston	78%	300+
Capital Medical Center	Olympia	77%	300+
Grays Harbor Community Hospital	Aberdeen	77%	300+
Olympic Medical Center	Port Angeles	77%	300+
Providence Holy Family Hospital	Spokane	77%	300+
Providence Sacred Heart Medical Center	Spokane	77%	300+
Saint Joseph Medical Center	Tacoma	77%	300+
Harrison Memorial Center	Bremerton	76%	300+
Overlake Hospital Medical Center	Bellevue	76%	300+
Providence Reg Med Ctr Everett	Everett	76%	300+
Swedish Issaquah	Issaquah	76%	300+
Swedish Medical Center - Cherry Hill	Seattle	76%	300+
Whidbey General Hospital	Coupeville	76%	300+
Cascade Valley Hospital[3]	Arlington	75%	(a)
Deaconess Hospital	Spokane	75%	300+
Multicare Good Samaritan Hospital	Puyallup	75%	300+
Northwest Hospital	Seattle	75%	300+
Samaritan Hospital	Moses Lake	75%	300+
Swedish Medical Center	Seattle	75%	300+
Valley Hospital	Spokane	75%	300+
Harborview Medical Center	Seattle	74%	300+
Sunnyside Community Hospital	Sunnyside	74%	(a)
Evergreen Hospital Medical Center	Kirkland	73%	300+
Prosser Memorial Hospital	Prosser	73%	(a)
Saint Anthony Hospital	Gig Harbor	73%	300+
Saint Clare Hospital	Lakewood	73%	300+
Saint Francis Community Hospital	Federal Way	73%	300+
Tacoma General Allenmore Hospital	Tacoma	73%	300+
Valley Medical Center	Renton	73%	300+
Yakima Valley Memorial Hospital	Yakima	73%	300+
Skagit Valley Hospital	Mount Vernon	72%	300+
Swedish Edmonds Hospital	Edmonds	72%	300+
Valley General Hospital	Monroe	72%	(a)
Highline Medical Center	Burien	70%	300+
Yakima Regional Medical & Cardiac Center	Yakima	70%	300+
Multicare Auburn Medical Center	Auburn	62%	300+

Pain 'Always' Well Controlled

Hospital Name	City	Rate	Cases
Lincoln Hospital	Davenport	82%	(a)
Whitman Hospital & Medical Center	Colfax	79%	(a)
Confluence Hlth-Wenatchee Valley Hosp	Wenatchee	77%	(a)
Pullman Regional Hospital	Pullman	77%	300+
Peacehealth United General Medical Center	Sedro Woolley	76%	(a)
Island Hospital	Anacortes	75%	300+
Kennewick General Hospital	Kennewick	74%	300+
Othello Community Hospital	Othello	73%	(a)
Overlake Hospital Medical Center	Bellevue	73%	300+
Legacy Salmon Creek Medical Center	Vancouver	72%	300+
Providence Mount Carmel Hospital	Colville	72%	(a)
Providence Saint Mary Medical Center	Walla Walla	72%	300+
Toppenish Community Hospital	Toppenish	72%	(a)
Tri - State Memorial Hospital	Clarkston	72%	300+
University of Washington Medical Center	Seattle	72%	300+
Capital Medical Center	Olympia	71%	300+
Central Washington Hospital	Wenatchee	71%	300+
Peacehealth Saint Joseph Medical Center	Bellingham	71%	300+
Providence Sacred Heart Medical Center	Spokane	71%	300+
Samaritan Hospital	Moses Lake	71%	300+
Swedish Medical Center - Cherry Hill	Seattle	71%	300+
Valley General Hospital	Monroe	71%	(a)
Valley Hospital	Spokane	71%	300+
Cascade Valley Hospital[3]	Arlington	70%	(a)
Deaconess Hospital	Spokane	70%	300+
Kittitas Valley Community Hospital	Ellensburg	70%	(a)
Northwest Hospital	Seattle	70%	300+
Peacehealth Saint John Medical Center	Longview	70%	300+
Providence Centralia Hospital	Centralia	70%	300+
Providence Reg Med Ctr Everett	Everett	70%	300+
Providence Saint Peter Hospital	Olympia	70%	300+
Saint Joseph Medical Center	Tacoma	70%	300+
Swedish Issaquah	Issaquah	70%	300+
Virginia Mason Medical Center	Seattle	70%	300+
Grays Harbor Community Hospital	Aberdeen	69%	300+
Peacehealth Southwest Medical Center	Vancouver	69%	300+
Providence Holy Family Hospital	Spokane	69%	300+
Swedish Medical Center	Seattle	69%	300+
Walla Walla General Hospital	Walla Walla	69%	(a)
Group Health Central Hospital	Seattle	68%	300+
Evergreen Hospital Medical Center	Kirkland	67%	300+
Highline Medical Center	Burien	67%	300+
Multicare Good Samaritan Hospital	Puyallup	67%	300+
Olympic Medical Center	Port Angeles	67%	300+
Skagit Valley Hospital	Mount Vernon	67%	300+
Swedish Edmonds Hospital	Edmonds	67%	300+
Valley Medical Center	Renton	67%	300+
Whidbey General Hospital	Coupeville	67%	300+
Harborview Medical Center	Seattle	66%	300+
Kadlec Regional Medical Center[11]	Richland	66%	300+
Prosser Memorial Hospital	Prosser	66%	(a)
Saint Francis Community Hospital	Federal Way	66%	300+
Harrison Memorial Center	Bremerton	65%	300+
Saint Anthony Hospital	Gig Harbor	65%	300+
Saint Clare Hospital	Lakewood	65%	300+
Saint Elizabeth Hospital	Enumclaw	65%	(a)
Tacoma General Allenmore Hospital	Tacoma	64%	300+
Yakima Valley Memorial Hospital	Yakima	64%	300+
Yakima Regional Medical & Cardiac Center	Yakima	60%	300+
Multicare Auburn Medical Center	Auburn	59%	300+
Sunnyside Community Hospital	Sunnyside	59%	(a)

Room and Bathroom 'Always' Clean

Hospital Name	City	Rate	Cases
Providence Mount Carmel Hospital	Colville	87%	(a)
Peacehealth United General Medical Center	Sedro Woolley	85%	(a)
Lincoln Hospital	Davenport	84%	(a)
Whitman Hospital & Medical Center	Colfax	84%	(a)
Island Hospital	Anacortes	83%	300+
Cascade Valley Hospital[3]	Arlington	79%	(a)
Confluence Hlth-Wenatchee Valley Hosp	Wenatchee	78%	(a)
Kennewick General Hospital	Kennewick	78%	300+
Pullman Regional Hospital	Pullman	78%	300+
Saint Elizabeth Hospital	Enumclaw	78%	(a)
Tri - State Memorial Hospital	Clarkston	78%	300+
Central Washington Hospital	Wenatchee	77%	300+
Group Health Central Hospital	Seattle	76%	300+
Kittitas Valley Community Hospital	Ellensburg	76%	(a)
Kadlec Regional Medical Center[11]	Richland	75%	300+
Providence Saint Mary Medical Center	Walla Walla	75%	300+
Harborview Medical Center	Seattle	74%	300+
Providence Centralia Hospital	Centralia	74%	300+
Providence Holy Family Hospital	Spokane	74%	300+
Sunnyside Community Hospital	Sunnyside	74%	(a)
Toppenish Community Hospital	Toppenish	74%	(a)
Overlake Hospital Medical Center	Bellevue	73%	300+
Providence Saint Peter Hospital	Olympia	73%	300+
Skagit Valley Hospital	Mount Vernon	73%	300+
Virginia Mason Medical Center	Seattle	73%	300+
Walla Walla General Hospital	Walla Walla	73%	(a)
Whidbey General Hospital	Coupeville	73%	300+
Multicare Good Samaritan Hospital	Puyallup	72%	300+
Olympic Medical Center	Port Angeles	72%	300+
Peacehealth Saint John Medical Center	Longview	72%	300+
Providence Sacred Heart Medical Center	Spokane	72%	300+
Samaritan Hospital	Moses Lake	72%	300+
Swedish Issaquah	Issaquah	72%	300+
University of Washington Medical Center	Seattle	72%	300+
Grays Harbor Community Hospital	Aberdeen	71%	300+
Legacy Salmon Creek Medical Center	Vancouver	71%	300+
Northwest Hospital	Seattle	71%	300+
Peacehealth Saint Joseph Medical Center	Bellingham	71%	300+
Yakima Valley Memorial Hospital	Yakima	71%	300+
Evergreen Hospital Medical Center	Kirkland	70%	300+
Othello Community Hospital	Othello	70%	(a)
Prosser Memorial Hospital	Prosser	70%	(a)
Providence Reg Med Ctr Everett	Everett	70%	300+
Saint Anthony Hospital	Gig Harbor	70%	300+
Saint Joseph Medical Center	Tacoma	70%	300+
Swedish Medical Center - Cherry Hill	Seattle	70%	300+
Capital Medical Center	Olympia	69%	300+
Peacehealth Southwest Medical Center	Vancouver	69%	300+
Valley Hospital	Spokane	69%	300+
Valley Medical Center	Renton	69%	300+
Highline Medical Center	Burien	68%	300+
Swedish Medical Center	Seattle	68%	300+
Tacoma General Allenmore Hospital	Tacoma	68%	300+
Valley General Hospital	Monroe	68%	(a)
Saint Clare Hospital	Lakewood	67%	300+
Saint Francis Community Hospital	Federal Way	67%	300+
Yakima Regional Medical & Cardiac Center	Yakima	66%	300+
Swedish Edmonds Hospital	Edmonds	65%	300+
Harrison Memorial Center	Bremerton	64%	300+
Deaconess Hospital	Spokane	63%	300+
Multicare Auburn Medical Center	Auburn	58%	300+

Timely Help 'Always' Received

Hospital Name	City	Rate	Cases
Whitman Hospital & Medical Center	Colfax	86%	(a)
Peacehealth United General Medical Center	Sedro Woolley	79%	(a)
Pullman Regional Hospital	Pullman	79%	300+
Confluence Hlth-Wenatchee Valley Hosp	Wenatchee	78%	(a)
Kittitas Valley Community Hospital	Ellensburg	75%	(a)
Lincoln Hospital	Davenport	75%	(a)
Tri - State Memorial Hospital	Clarkston	75%	300+
Cascade Valley Hospital[3]	Arlington	74%	(a)
Island Hospital	Anacortes	73%	300+
Providence Mount Carmel Hospital	Colville	72%	(a)
Olympic Medical Center	Port Angeles	71%	300+
Samaritan Hospital	Moses Lake	71%	300+
Legacy Salmon Creek Medical Center	Vancouver	70%	300+
Providence Saint Mary Medical Center	Walla Walla	70%	300+
Walla Walla General Hospital	Walla Walla	70%	(a)
Swedish Issaquah	Issaquah	69%	300+
Toppenish Community Hospital	Toppenish	68%	(a)
Central Washington Hospital	Wenatchee	67%	300+
Grays Harbor Community Hospital	Aberdeen	67%	300+
Kennewick General Hospital	Kennewick	67%	300+
Providence Centralia Hospital	Centralia	67%	300+
Virginia Mason Medical Center	Seattle	67%	300+
Providence Sacred Heart Medical Center	Spokane	66%	300+
Providence Saint Peter Hospital	Olympia	66%	300+
Northwest Hospital	Seattle	65%	300+
Saint Elizabeth Hospital	Enumclaw	65%	(a)
Evergreen Hospital Medical Center	Kirkland	64%	300+
Harrison Memorial Center	Bremerton	64%	300+
Kadlec Regional Medical Center[11]	Richland	64%	300+
University of Washington Medical Center	Seattle	64%	300+
Whidbey General Hospital	Coupeville	64%	300+
Group Health Central Hospital	Seattle	63%	300+
Providence Reg Med Ctr Everett	Everett	63%	300+
Valley General Hospital	Monroe	63%	(a)
Capital Medical Center	Olympia	62%	300+
Peacehealth Saint Joseph Medical Center	Bellingham	62%	300+
Swedish Medical Center - Cherry Hill	Seattle	62%	300+
Othello Community Hospital	Othello	61%	(a)
Overlake Hospital Medical Center	Bellevue	61%	300+
Peacehealth Southwest Medical Center	Vancouver	61%	300+
Providence Holy Family Hospital	Spokane	61%	300+
Skagit Valley Hospital	Mount Vernon	61%	300+
Sunnyside Community Hospital	Sunnyside	61%	(a)
Swedish Medical Center	Seattle	61%	300+
Valley Hospital	Spokane	61%	300+
Prosser Memorial Hospital	Prosser	60%	(a)
Saint Anthony Hospital	Gig Harbor	60%	300+
Saint Joseph Medical Center	Tacoma	60%	300+
Valley Medical Center	Renton	60%	300+
Yakima Valley Memorial Hospital	Yakima	60%	300+
Deaconess Hospital	Spokane	59%	300+
Harborview Medical Center	Seattle	59%	300+
Multicare Good Samaritan Hospital	Puyallup	59%	300+
Saint Francis Community Hospital	Federal Way	57%	300+
Swedish Edmonds Hospital	Edmonds	57%	300+
Highline Medical Center	Burien	56%	300+
Peacehealth Saint John Medical Center	Longview	55%	300+
Yakima Regional Medical & Cardiac Center	Yakima	54%	300+
Tacoma General Allenmore Hospital	Tacoma	53%	300+
Saint Clare Hospital	Lakewood	52%	300+
Multicare Auburn Medical Center	Auburn	39%	300+

Would Definitely Recommend Hospital

Hospital Name	City	Rate	Cases
Pullman Regional Hospital	Pullman	88%	300+
Whitman Hospital & Medical Center	Colfax	88%	(a)
Island Hospital	Anacortes	84%	300+
University of Washington Medical Center	Seattle	83%	300+
Virginia Mason Medical Center	Seattle	83%	300+
Legacy Salmon Creek Medical Center	Vancouver	82%	300+
Saint Elizabeth Hospital	Enumclaw	82%	(a)
Swedish Issaquah	Issaquah	82%	300+
Central Washington Hospital	Wenatchee	81%	300+
Evergreen Hospital Medical Center	Kirkland	81%	300+
Kadlec Regional Medical Center[11]	Richland	81%	300+
Providence Saint Peter Hospital	Olympia	81%	300+
Providence Saint Mary Medical Center	Walla Walla	80%	300+
Providence Mount Carmel Hospital	Colville	79%	(a)
Providence Sacred Heart Medical Center	Spokane	79%	300+
Tri - State Memorial Hospital	Clarkston	79%	300+
Confluence Hlth-Wenatchee Valley Hosp	Wenatchee	78%	(a)
Lincoln Hospital	Davenport	78%	(a)
Northwest Hospital	Seattle	78%	300+
Providence Reg Med Ctr Everett	Everett	78%	300+
Swedish Medical Center	Seattle	78%	300+
Swedish Medical Center - Cherry Hill	Seattle	78%	300+
Peacehealth United General Medical Center	Sedro Woolley	77%	(a)
Saint Anthony Hospital	Gig Harbor	77%	300+

NOTE: Hospital profiles are in alphabetical order by state, then city, then hospital within the city; Rankings exclude hospitals with less than 25 cases except for patient surveys which excludes hospitals with less than 100 cases; (a) 100-299 cases; (1) The number of cases/patients is too few to report; (2) Data submitted were based on a sample of cases/patients; (3) Results are based on a shorter time period than required; (4) Data suppressed by CMS for one or more quarters; (5) Results are not available for this reporting period; (6) Fewer than 100 patients completed the HCAHPS survey; (7) No cases met the criteria for this measure; (8) The lower limit of the confidence interval cannot be calculated if the number of observed infections equals zero; (9) No data are available from the state/territory for this reporting period; (10) The scores shown reflect fewer than 50 completed surveys; (11) There were discrepancies in the data collection process; (12) This measure does not apply to this hospital for this reporting period; (13) Results cannot be calculated for this reporting period; (14) The results for this state are combined with nearby states to protect confidentiality; Please refer to the User's Guide for a full explanation of data.

Overlake Hospital Medical Center	Bellevue	76%	300+
Peacehealth Southwest Medical Center	Vancouver	76%	300+
Peacehealth Saint Joseph Medical Center	Bellingham	75%	300+
Walla Walla General Hospital	Walla Walla	75%	(a)
Harborview Medical Center	Seattle	74%	300+
Saint Joseph Medical Center	Tacoma	74%	300+
Group Health Central Hospital	Seattle	73%	300+
Kennewick General Hospital	Kennewick	73%	300+
Kittitas Valley Community Hospital	Ellensburg	73%	(a)
Providence Holy Family Hospital	Spokane	73%	300+
Valley Medical Center	Renton	73%	300+
Olympic Medical Center	Port Angeles	72%	300+
Othello Community Hospital	Othello	72%	(a)
Tacoma General Allenmore Hospital	Tacoma	72%	300+
Capital Medical Center	Olympia	71%	300+
Cascade Valley Hospital[3]	Arlington	71%	(a)
Saint Francis Community Hospital	Federal Way	71%	300+
Valley Hospital	Spokane	71%	300+
Yakima Valley Memorial Hospital	Yakima	71%	300+
Deaconess Hospital	Spokane	70%	300+
Harrison Memorial Center	Bremerton	70%	300+
Multicare Good Samaritan Hospital	Puyallup	70%	300+
Highline Medical Center	Burien	67%	300+
Skagit Valley Hospital	Mount Vernon	66%	300+
Grays Harbor Community Hospital	Aberdeen	65%	300+
Toppenish Community Hospital	Toppenish	65%	(a)
Whidbey General Hospital	Coupeville	65%	300+
Prosser Memorial Hospital	Prosser	64%	(a)
Providence Centralia Hospital	Centralia	64%	300+
Saint Clare Hospital	Lakewood	64%	300+
Swedish Edmonds Hospital	Edmonds	63%	300+
Sunnyside Community Hospital	Sunnyside	61%	(a)
Peachealth Saint John Medical Center	Longview	60%	300+
Valley General Hospital	Monroe	60%	(a)
Yakima Regional Medical & Cardiac Center	Yakima	60%	300+
Samaritan Hospital	Moses Lake	58%	300+
Multicare Auburn Medical Center	Auburn	42%	300+

Use of Medical Imaging

Cardiac Imaging Stress Test before OP Surgery

Hospital Name	City	Rate	Cases
Providence Mount Carmel Hospital	Colville	0.0%	55
Mid Valley Hospital	Omak	1.7%	58
Kittitas Valley Community Hospital	Ellensburg	2.2%	90
Tacoma General Allenmore Hospital	Tacoma	2.2%	316
Kennewick General Hospital	Kennewick	2.5%	240
Saint Anthony Hospital	Gig Harbor	2.7%	148
Harrison Memorial Center	Bremerton	2.8%	217
Confluence Hlth-Wenatchee Valley Hosp	Wenatchee	2.9%	727
Peacehealth Saint Joseph Medical Center	Bellingham	3.1%	1014
Yakima Valley Memorial Hospital	Yakima	3.1%	671
Deaconess Hospital	Spokane	3.2%	1185
Grays Harbor Community Hospital	Aberdeen	3.2%	506
Multicare Auburn Medical Center	Auburn	3.6%	195
Northwest Hospital	Seattle	3.6%	887
Providence Saint Peter Hospital	Olympia	3.7%	747
Skagit Valley Hospital	Mount Vernon	3.8%	494
Valley Medical Center	Renton	3.8%	53
Legacy Salmon Creek Medical Center	Vancouver	4.1%	145
Saint Elizabeth Hospital	Enumclaw	4.1%	49
Swedish Medical Center - Cherry Hill	Seattle	4.1%	1327
Providence Sacred Heart Medical Center	Spokane	4.2%	1143
Swedish Edmonds Hospital	Edmonds	4.2%	544
Evergreen Hospital Medical Center	Kirkland	4.3%	1354
Kadlec Regional Medical Center	Richland	4.3%	531
Peachealth Saint John Medical Center	Longview	4.3%	232
Yakima Regional Medical & Cardiac Center	Yakima	4.3%	116
Providence Saint Mary Medical Center	Walla Walla	4.4%	274
Harborview Medical Center	Seattle	4.5%	176
Overlake Hospital Medical Center	Bellevue	4.5%	1323
Providence Centralia Hospital	Centralia	4.5%	200
Central Washington Hospital	Wenatchee	4.6%	87
Walla Walla General Hospital	Walla Walla	4.8%	146
University of Washington Medical Center	Seattle	4.9%	555
Valley Hospital	Spokane	5.1%	178
Olympic Medical Center	Port Angeles	5.2%	572
Providence Reg Med Ctr Everett	Everett	5.6%	372
Saint Joseph Medical Center	Tacoma	5.9%	404
Peacehealth Southwest Medical Center	Vancouver	6.2%	451
Cascade Valley Hospital	Arlington	6.3%	95
Providence Holy Family Hospital	Spokane	6.3%	79
Saint Francis Community Hospital	Federal Way	6.3%	80
Swedish Issaquah	Issaquah	6.3%	255
Island Hospital	Anacortes	7.4%	162
Virginia Mason Medical Center	Seattle	7.8%	796
Multicare Good Samaritan Hospital	Puyallup	8.7%	196

Combination Abdominal CT Scan

Hospital Name	City	Rate	Cases
Toppenish Community Hospital	Toppenish	0.0%	100
Valley Hospital	Spokane	0.0%	505
Providence Sacred Heart Medical Center	Spokane	0.2%	489
Providence Holy Family Hospital	Spokane	0.3%	634
Deaconess Hospital	Spokane	0.6%	338
Peacehealth Saint Joseph Medical Center	Bellingham	0.8%	639
Providence Saint Joseph Hospital	Chewelah	1.4%	212
Multicare Good Samaritan Hospital	Puyallup	1.6%	642
Valley Medical Center	Renton	1.6%	806
Evergreen Hospital Medical Center	Kirkland	1.7%	813
Othello Community Hospital	Othello	1.7%	58
Yakima Regional Medical & Cardiac Center	Yakima	1.7%	461
Olympic Medical Center	Port Angeles	1.8%	1306
Yakima Valley Memorial Hospital	Yakima	1.9%	1387
Ferry County Memorial Hospital	Republic	2.0%	51
Skyline Hospital	White Salmon	2.1%	94
Providence Reg Med Ctr Everett	Everett	2.4%	904
Saint Elizabeth Hospital	Enumclaw	2.5%	364
Multicare Auburn Medical Center	Auburn	2.6%	313
Kittitas Valley Community Hospital	Ellensburg	2.8%	397
Cascade Valley Hospital	Arlington	3.2%	216
Swedish Edmonds Hospital	Edmonds	3.2%	603
Walla Walla General Hospital	Walla Walla	3.3%	245
Willapa Harbor Hospital	South Bend	3.3%	180
Saint Anthony Hospital	Gig Harbor	3.4%	557
Summit Pacific Medical Center	Elma	3.4%	117
Central Washington Hospital	Wenatchee	3.5%	401
Saint Francis Community Hospital	Federal Way	3.6%	607
Harrison Memorial Center	Bremerton	3.7%	615
Lincoln Hospital	Davenport	3.7%	108
Morton Swing Bed	Morton	3.7%	109
Legacy Salmon Creek Medical Center	Vancouver	3.9%	484
Klickitat Valley Hospital	Goldendale	4.5%	132
Providence Saint Peter Hospital	Olympia	4.5%	717
Swedish Medical Center - Cherry Hill	Seattle	4.6%	350
Peachealth Saint John Medical Center	Longview	4.8%	624
Saint Joseph Medical Center	Tacoma	4.9%	761
Peacehealth United General Medical Center	Sedro Woolley	5.2%	404
Kennewick General Hospital	Kennewick	5.3%	589
Sunnyside Community Hospital	Sunnyside	5.4%	278
Samaritan Hospital	Moses Lake	5.5%	271
Valley General Hospital	Monroe	5.7%	158
Peacehealth Southwest Medical Center	Vancouver	5.8%	891
Newport Community Hospital	Newport	6.0%	150
Saint Clare Hospital	Lakewood	6.1%	586
Coulee Community Hospital	Grand Coulee	6.2%	81
Highline Medical Center	Burien	6.5%	541
Providence Centralia Hospital	Centralia	6.6%	828
Capital Medical Center	Olympia	6.9%	449
Tacoma General Allenmore Hospital	Tacoma	7.3%	1946
Providence Saint Mary Medical Center	Walla Walla	7.5%	493
Skagit Valley Hospital	Mount Vernon	7.6%	834
Swedish Medical Center	Seattle	7.6%	1072
Jefferson Healthcare Hospital	Port Townsend	7.8%	473
Providence Mount Carmel Hospital	Colville	7.8%	293
Overlake Hospital Medical Center	Bellevue	8.5%	832
Harborview Medical Center	Seattle	8.6%	419
University of Washington Medical Center	Seattle	9.0%	1142
Kadlec Regional Medical Center	Richland	9.1%	1318
Tri - State Memorial Hospital	Clarkston	9.3%	496
Swedish Issaquah	Issaquah	9.5%	379
Island Hospital	Anacortes	9.6%	436
Grays Harbor Community Hospital	Aberdeen	10.3%	682
Northwest Hospital	Seattle	11.0%	783
North Valley Hospital	Tonasket	11.4%	132
Virginia Mason Medical Center	Seattle	15.2%	1404
Mid Valley Hospital	Omak	17.8%	366
Lake Chelan Community Hospital	Chelan	28.9%	76
Confluence Hlth-Wenatchee Valley Hosp	Wenatchee	57.3%	881
Columbia Basin Hospital	Ephrata	63.9%	61

Combination Brain/Sinus CT Scan

Hospital Name	City	Rate	Cases
Ferry County Memorial Hospital	Republic	0.0%	35
Othello Community Hospital	Othello	0.0%	74
Skyline Hospital	White Salmon	0.0%	126
Central Washington Hospital	Wenatchee	0.2%	559
Providence Saint Mary Medical Center	Walla Walla	0.3%	328
Harborview Medical Center	Seattle	0.4%	509
University of Washington Medical Center	Seattle	0.5%	430
Newport Community Hospital	Newport	0.6%	163
Highline Medical Center	Burien	0.7%	546
Legacy Salmon Creek Medical Center	Vancouver	0.8%	491
Providence Mount Carmel Hospital	Colville	0.9%	229
Swedish Issaquah	Issaquah	1.0%	397
Swedish Medical Center - Cherry Hill	Seattle	1.1%	614
Tri - State Memorial Hospital	Clarkston	1.1%	349
Jefferson Healthcare Hospital	Port Townsend	1.2%	419
Skagit Valley Hospital	Mount Vernon	1.2%	486
Island Hospital	Anacortes	1.3%	318
Yakima Valley Memorial Hospital	Yakima	1.3%	865
Kadlec Regional Medical Center	Richland	1.4%	1036
Harrison Memorial Center	Bremerton	1.6%	980
Valley Medical Center	Renton	1.7%	895
Peachealth Saint John Medical Center	Longview	1.8%	622
Swedish Edmonds Hospital	Edmonds	1.8%	609
Olympic Medical Center	Port Angeles	1.9%	720
Providence Saint Peter Hospital	Olympia	1.9%	959
Overlake Hospital Medical Center	Bellevue	2.1%	969
Peacehealth Saint Joseph Medical Center	Bellingham	2.1%	745
Providence Centralia Hospital	Centralia	2.2%	505
Saint Joseph Medical Center	Tacoma	2.3%	657
Yakima Regional Medical & Cardiac Center	Yakima	2.3%	526
Evergreen Hospital Medical Center	Kirkland	2.4%	664
Multicare Good Samaritan Hospital	Puyallup	2.6%	700
Tacoma General Allenmore Hospital	Tacoma	2.7%	1158
Peacehealth Southwest Medical Center	Vancouver	2.8%	779
Providence Reg Med Ctr Everett	Everett	2.8%	926
Grays Harbor Community Hospital	Aberdeen	2.9%	782
Northwest Hospital	Seattle	3.6%	718
Providence Sacred Heart Medical Center	Spokane	4.2%	715
Saint Anthony Hospital	Gig Harbor	4.3%	442
Swedish Medical Center	Seattle	4.3%	805
Kennewick General Hospital	Kennewick	4.8%	621
Providence Saint Joseph Hospital	Chewelah	5.9%	188
Valley Hospital	Spokane	5.9%	355
Providence Holy Family Hospital	Spokane	6.1%	705
Deaconess Hospital	Spokane	6.7%	357

Combination Chest CT Scan

Hospital Name	City	Rate	Cases
Capital Medical Center	Olympia	0.0%	224
Cascade Valley Hospital	Arlington	0.0%	134
Central Washington Hospital	Wenatchee	0.0%	114
Coulee Community Hospital	Grand Coulee	0.0%	56
Deaconess Hospital	Spokane	0.0%	75
Harborview Medical Center	Seattle	0.0%	328
Harrison Memorial Center	Bremerton	0.0%	101
Highline Medical Center	Burien	0.0%	239
Island Hospital	Anacortes	0.0%	334
Kittitas Valley Community Hospital	Ellensburg	0.0%	186
Lake Chelan Community Hospital	Chelan	0.0%	54
Legacy Salmon Creek Medical Center	Vancouver	0.0%	141
Mid Valley Hospital	Omak	0.0%	330
Multicare Auburn Medical Center	Auburn	0.0%	205
Newport Community Hospital	Newport	0.0%	94
Peacehealth United General Medical Center	Sedro Woolley	0.0%	283
Peachealth Saint John Medical Center	Longview	0.0%	376
Providence Holy Family Hospital	Spokane	0.0%	63
Providence Sacred Heart Medical Center	Spokane	0.0%	121
Providence Saint Joseph Hospital	Chewelah	0.0%	126
Providence Saint Peter Hospital	Olympia	0.0%	188
Toppenish Community Hospital	Toppenish	0.0%	52
Valley General Hospital	Monroe	0.0%	79
Valley Hospital	Spokane	0.0%	122
Yakima Regional Medical & Cardiac Center	Yakima	0.0%	152
Yakima Valley Memorial Hospital	Yakima	0.0%	1053
Olympic Medical Center	Port Angeles	0.1%	1009
University of Washington Medical Center	Seattle	0.1%	1239
Northwest Hospital	Seattle	0.2%	549
Saint Joseph Medical Center	Tacoma	0.2%	415
Grays Harbor Community Hospital	Aberdeen	0.3%	394
Saint Francis Community Hospital	Federal Way	0.3%	326
Skagit Valley Hospital	Mount Vernon	0.3%	578
Swedish Medical Center	Seattle	0.3%	397
Valley Medical Center	Renton	0.3%	350
Peacehealth Southwest Medical Center	Vancouver	0.4%	549
Swedish Issaquah	Issaquah	0.4%	228
Providence Reg Med Ctr Everett	Everett	0.5%	438
Saint Clare Hospital	Lakewood	0.5%	215
Evergreen Hospital Medical Center	Kirkland	0.6%	649
Overlake Hospital Medical Center	Bellevue	0.6%	644
Providence Mount Carmel Hospital	Colville	0.6%	181
Virginia Mason Medical Center	Seattle	0.7%	1380
Providence Centralia Hospital	Centralia	0.8%	591
Swedish Edmonds Hospital	Edmonds	0.9%	345
Peacehealth Saint Joseph Medical Center	Bellingham	1.0%	102
Jefferson Healthcare Hospital	Port Townsend	1.1%	276
Tri - State Memorial Hospital	Clarkston	1.1%	282
Providence Saint Mary Medical Center	Walla Walla	1.2%	582
Kadlec Regional Medical Center	Richland	1.3%	1047
Saint Anthony Hospital	Gig Harbor	1.3%	398
Tacoma General Allenmore Hospital	Tacoma	1.4%	1506
Multicare Good Samaritan Hospital	Puyallup	1.8%	113
Swedish Medical Center - Cherry Hill	Seattle	1.8%	169
Skyline Hospital	White Salmon	1.9%	54
Saint Elizabeth Hospital	Enumclaw	2.5%	197
Kennewick General Hospital	Kennewick	2.7%	513
Willapa Harbor Hospital	South Bend	2.8%	107

NOTE: Hospital profiles are in alphabetical order by state, then city, then hospital within the city; Rankings exclude hospitals with less than 25 cases except for patient surveys which excludes hospitals with less than 100 cases; (a) 100-299 cases; (1) The number of cases/patients is too few to report; (2) Data submitted were based on a sample of cases/patients; (3) Results are based on a shorter time period than required; (4) Data suppressed by CMS for one or more quarters; (5) Results are not available for this reporting period; (6) Fewer than 100 patients completed the HCAHPS survey; (7) No cases met the criteria for this measure; (8) The lower limit of the confidence interval cannot be calculated if the number of observed infections equals zero; (9) No data are available from the state/territory for this reporting period; (10) The scores shown reflect fewer than 50 completed surveys; (11) There were discrepancies in the data collection process; (12) This measure does not apply to this hospital for this reporting period; (13) Results cannot be calculated for this reporting period; (14) The results for this state are combined with nearby states to protect confidentiality; Please refer to the User's Guide for a full explanation of data.

Hospital Name	City	Rate	Cases
Walla Walla General Hospital	Walla Walla	2.9%	140
Confluence Hlth-Wenatchee Valley Hosp	Wenatchee	3.6%	1125
Summit Pacific Medical Center	Elma	4.0%	50
Morton Swing Bed	Morton	5.3%	57
Klickitat Valley Hospital	Goldendale	5.8%	86
Samaritan Hospital	Moses Lake	9.6%	177
North Valley Hospital	Tonasket	13.3%	83
Sunnyside Community Hospital	Sunnyside	14.2%	134

Follow-up Mammogram/Ultrasound

A follow-up rate near zero may indicate missed cancer; a rate higher than 14% may mean there is unnecessary follow up.

Hospital Name	City	Rate	Cases
Providence Centralia Hospital	Centralia	3.3%	962
Coulee Community Hospital	Grand Coulee	3.6%	138
Summit Pacific Medical Center	Elma	3.6%	169
Northwest Hospital	Seattle	4.1%	2600
North Valley Hospital	Tonasket	4.8%	231
Peachealth Saint John Medical Center	Longview	5.6%	2040
Lincoln Hospital	Davenport	5.7%	211
Capital Medical Center	Olympia	5.9%	897
Lake Chelan Community Hospital	Chelan	6.3%	143
Walla Walla General Hospital	Walla Walla	6.3%	537
Central Washington Hospital	Wenatchee	6.4%	629
Kennewick General Hospital	Kennewick	6.4%	827
Sunnyside Community Hospital	Sunnyside	6.6%	395
Morton Swing Bed	Morton	6.7%	134
Columbia Basin Hospital	Ephrata	7.2%	111
Othello Community Hospital	Othello	7.3%	96
Providence Reg Med Ctr Everett	Everett	7.4%	1514
University of Washington Medical Center	Seattle	7.5%	891
Legacy Salmon Creek Medical Center	Vancouver	7.6%	471
Valley General Hospital	Monroe	7.6%	236
Island Hospital	Anacortes	7.7%	956
Peacehealth Southwest Medical Center	Vancouver	7.8%	960
Valley Medical Center	Renton	7.8%	2524
Tacoma General Allenmore Hospital	Tacoma	7.9%	1627
Yakima Regional Medical & Cardiac Center	Yakima	8.3%	470
Providence Saint Mary Medical Center	Walla Walla	8.4%	818
Virginia Mason Medical Center	Seattle	8.4%	1365
Yakima Valley Memorial Hospital	Yakima	8.4%	2659
Swedish Edmonds Hospital	Edmonds	8.6%	1350
Saint Anthony Hospital	Gig Harbor	9.0%	613
Peacehealth United General Medical Center	Sedro Woolley	9.1%	536
Kadlec Regional Medical Center	Richland	9.3%	2557
Kittitas Valley Community Hospital	Ellensburg	9.3%	601
Samaritan Hospital	Moses Lake	9.4%	171
Overlake Hospital Medical Center	Bellevue	9.7%	3126
Toppenish Community Hospital	Toppenish	10.1%	189
Newport Community Hospital	Newport	10.2%	284
Cascade Valley Hospital	Arlington	10.4%	270
Swedish Medical Center	Seattle	10.6%	4203
Olympic Medical Center	Port Angeles	10.9%	2853
Deaconess Hospital	Spokane	11.2%	562
Saint Francis Community Hospital	Federal Way	11.3%	733
Willapa Harbor Hospital	South Bend	12.3%	179
Klickitat Valley Hospital	Goldendale	12.5%	192
Providence Saint Joseph Hospital	Chewelah	12.6%	103
Evergreen Hospital Medical Center	Kirkland	13.5%	2154
Multicare Auburn Medical Center	Auburn	13.6%	242
Group Health Central Hospital	Seattle	13.9%	72
Tri - State Memorial Hospital	Clarkston	14.7%	992
Saint Elizabeth Hospital	Enumclaw	14.9%	355
Providence Mount Carmel Hospital	Colville	15.0%	347
Mid Valley Hospital	Omak	15.9%	182
Skyline Hospital	White Salmon	16.0%	131
Swedish Issaquah	Issaquah	16.5%	387
Jefferson Healthcare Hospital	Port Townsend	17.9%	773

Lumbar Spine MRI for Low Back Pain

Hospital Name	City	Rate	Cases
Olympic Medical Center	Port Angeles	26.7%	344
Skagit Valley Hospital	Mount Vernon	26.8%	179
Virginia Mason Medical Center	Seattle	28.0%	93
Saint Joseph Medical Center	Tacoma	29.3%	99
Kadlec Regional Medical Center	Richland	31.3%	319
Jefferson Healthcare Hospital	Port Townsend	31.4%	51
University of Washington Medical Center	Seattle	31.8%	132
Swedish Medical Center - Cherry Hill	Seattle	32.0%	103
Providence Saint Peter Hospital	Olympia	32.3%	93
Peachealth Saint John Medical Center	Longview	34.0%	144
Capital Medical Center	Olympia	34.4%	64
Peacehealth Southwest Medical Center	Vancouver	34.8%	115
Yakima Valley Memorial Hospital	Yakima	35.0%	408
Overlake Hospital Medical Center	Bellevue	35.3%	136
Legacy Salmon Creek Medical Center	Vancouver	35.6%	59
Peacehealth United General Medical Center	Sedro Woolley	35.8%	53
Saint Anthony Hospital	Gig Harbor	36.5%	74
Yakima Regional Medical & Cardiac Center	Yakima	36.8%	106
Providence Reg Med Ctr Everett	Everett	37.3%	110
Central Washington Hospital	Wenatchee	37.8%	143
Kennewick General Hospital	Kennewick	38.1%	84
Island Hospital	Anacortes	38.4%	99
Providence Saint Mary Medical Center	Walla Walla	39.3%	183
Saint Clare Hospital	Lakewood	39.7%	58
Swedish Issaquah	Issaquah	41.4%	87
Northwest Hospital	Seattle	42.0%	88
Highline Medical Center	Burien	42.5%	40
Tri - State Memorial Hospital	Clarkston	42.6%	94
Tacoma General Allenmore Hospital	Tacoma	43.4%	235
Kittitas Valley Community Hospital	Ellensburg	43.5%	62
Harborview Medical Center	Seattle	43.8%	80
Providence Centralia Hospital	Centralia	44.0%	84
Swedish Medical Center	Seattle	45.4%	108
Saint Francis Community Hospital	Federal Way	46.7%	60
Walla Walla General Hospital	Walla Walla	48.7%	39
Valley Medical Center	Renton	50.0%	38
Newport Community Hospital	Newport	52.6%	38
Providence Mount Carmel Hospital	Colville	55.3%	47
Mid Valley Hospital	Omak	64.6%	82

NOTE: Hospital profiles are in alphabetical order by state, then city, then hospital within the city; Rankings exclude hospitals with less than 25 cases except for patient surveys which excludes hospitals with less than 100 cases; (a) 100-299 cases; (1) The number of cases/patients is too few to report; (2) Data submitted were based on a sample of cases/patients; (3) Results are based on a shorter time period than required; (4) Data suppressed by CMS for one or more quarters; (5) Results are not available for this reporting period; (6) Fewer than 100 patients completed the HCAHPS survey; (7) No cases met the criteria for this measure; (8) The lower limit of the confidence interval cannot be calculated if the number of observed infections equals zero; (9) No data are available from the state/territory for this reporting period; (10) The scores shown reflect fewer than 50 completed surveys; (11) There were discrepancies in the data collection process; (12) This measure does not apply to this hospital for this reporting period; (13) Results cannot be calculated for this reporting period; (14) The results for this state are combined with nearby states to protect confidentiality; Please refer to the User's Guide for a full explanation of data.

Grays Harbor Community Hospital

915 Anderson Drive Phone: 360-532-8330
Aberdeen, WA 98520 Fax: 360-537-5039
URL: www.ghchwa.org
Type: Acute Care Hospitals Emergency Services: Yes
Ownership: Voluntary non-profit - Private Beds: 200

Key Personnel:
Quality Assurance . . . . Linda Bluhm
Chief of Medical Staff . . . . Sally Bohlmann-Nicho, MD
Infection Control . . . . Lin Boulay, RN
Operating Room. . . . . Mike Huelsman, RN
CEO . . . . Tom Jensen
Pediatric Ambulatory Care . . . . . . Jane Rudd, MD
Pediatric In-Patient Care . . . . Jane Rudd, MD
Radiology. . . . . Joseph Stengel, MD

Measure	Cases	This Hosp.	State Avg.	U.S. Avg.
Blood Clot Prevention and Treatment				
Anticoagulation Overlap Therapy[2]	23	96%	97%	93%
ICU Venous Thromboembolism Prophylaxis[2]	242	86%	92%	92%
Incidence of Potentially Preventable VTE[1,2]	-	-	9%	10%
UFH with Dosages/Platelet Monitoring[2]	14	100%	99%	97%
Venous Thromboembolism Prophylaxis[2]	1,181	78%	86%	85%
Warfarin Therapy Discharge Instructions[2]	18	94%	74%	75%
Chest Pain/Possible Heart Attack Care				
Aspirin Given Within 24 Hours of Arrival	50	94%	97%	96%
Fibrinolytic Meds Within 30 Min. of Arrival	14	29%	51%	58%
Average Time to ECG (minutes)	59	15	9	7
Average Time to Transfer (minutes)[1]	-	-	54	60
Children's Asthma Care				
Received Home Management Plan of Care	-	-	-	88%
Received Reliever Medication	-	-	-	100%
Received Systemic Corticosteroids	-	-	-	100%
Emergency Department				
Admittance Decision Time (minutes)[2]	434	92	96	98
Head CT Results Within 45 Min. of Arrival	25	84%	63%	57%
Patients Who Left ER Before Being Seen	31,869	2%	2%	2%
Time from ER Arrival to Admit. (minutes)[2]	502	248	259	274
Time from ER Arrival to Discharge (minutes)	553	125	135	134
Time in ER Before Being Evaluated (minutes)	636	22	22	26
Time to Pain Meds for Fractures (minutes)	163	74	52	57
Heart Attack Care				
Aspirin Given at Discharge	14	93%	99%	99%
Fibrinolytic Meds Within 30 Min. of Arrival[7]	-	-	62%	54%
PCI Within 90 Minutes of Arrival[7]	-	-	97%	96%
Statin Prescribed at Discharge	12	67%	98%	98%
Heart Failure Care				
ACE Inhibitor or ARB for LVSD	59	83%	97%	97%
Discharge Instructions Given	147	93%	93%	94%
Evaluation of LVS Function	188	98%	99%	99%
Medicare Spending				
Medicare Spending per Patient (ratio)	-	0.91	0.91	0.98
Pneumonia Care				
Appropriate Initial Antibiotic Given	125	82%	96%	95%
Blood Culture Timing	145	92%	97%	98%
Pregnancy and Delivery Care				
Newborn Deliveries Scheduled Early	60	5%	2%	6%
Preventive Care				
Immunization for Influenza[2]	505	84%	91%	90%
Immunization for Pneumonia[2]	591	94%	91%	92%
Stroke Care				
Anticoagulation Therapy for Atrial Fibrillation[1]	-	-	94%	95%
Antithrombotic Therapy Timing	46	89%	98%	98%
Assessed for Rehabilitation	51	96%	98%	97%
Discharged on Antithrombotic Therapy	48	79%	99%	99%
Discharged on Statin Medication	41	85%	96%	94%
Thrombolytic Therapy Timing[1]	-	-	73%	66%
Venous Thromboembolism Prophylaxis	50	84%	94%	94%
Written Stroke Educational Materials Given	27	81%	86%	88%
Surgical Care Improvement Project				
Appropriate Beta Blocker Usage	57	89%	98%	98%
Appropriate VTP Within 24 Hours	195	89%	98%	98%
Controlled Postoperative Blood Glucose[7]	-	-	97%	97%
Perioperative Temperature Management	229	93%	100%	100%
Prophylactic Antibiotic Selection	147	94%	99%	99%
Prophylactic Antibiotic Selection (Outpatient)	19	37%	98%	98%
Prophylactic Antibiotic Stopped	144	92%	99%	98%
Prophylactic Antibiotic Timing	147	90%	98%	99%
Prophylactic Antibiotic Timing (Outpatient)	22	82%	98%	98%
Urinary Catheter Removal	172	94%	97%	97%
Survey of Patients' Hospital Experiences				
Area Around Room 'Always' Quiet at Night	300+	50%	54%	61%
Doctors 'Always' Communicated Well	300+	79%	81%	82%
Home Recovery Information Given	300+	88%	87%	85%
Hospital Given 9 or 10 on 10 Point Scale	300+	65%	70%	71%
Meds 'Always' Explained Before Given	300+	61%	64%	64%
Nurses 'Always' Communicated Well	300+	77%	77%	79%
Pain 'Always' Well Controlled	300+	69%	70%	71%
Room and Bathroom 'Always' Clean	300+	71%	73%	73%
Timely Help 'Always' Received	300+	67%	65%	68%
Would Definitely Recommend Hospital	300+	65%	73%	71%
Use of Medical Imaging				
Cardiac Imaging Stress Test before Surgery	506	3.2%	4.3%	5.3%
Combination Abdominal CT Scan	682	10.3%	6.9%	10.5%
Combination Brain/Sinus CT Scan	782	2.9%	2.3%	2.7%
Combination Chest CT Scan	394	0.3%	1.1%	2.7%
Follow-up Mammogram/Ultrasound[7]	-	-	9.1%	8.8%
Lumbar Spine MRI for Low Back Pain[1]	-	-	37.9%	37.2%

Island Hospital

1211 24th Street Phone: 360-299-1300
Anacortes, WA 98221 Fax: 360-299-1384
URL: www.islandhospital.org
Type: Acute Care Hospitals Emergency Services: Yes
Ownership: Govt - Hospital Dist/Auth Beds: 43

Key Personnel:
Cardiac Laboratory. . . . . Richard E Gubner
Quality Assurance . . . . Carolyn Kozik
Operating Room. . . . . Bojan Kuure, RN
CEO/President. . . . . Vincent C Oliver
Intensive Care Unit. . . . . Lois Pate
Infection Control. . . . . Gary Preston
Patient Relations . . . . Barbara Ringhouse, RN
Chief of Medical Staff. . . . . Judy Tempelton

Measure	Cases	This Hosp.	State Avg.	U.S. Avg.
Blood Clot Prevention and Treatment				
Anticoagulation Overlap Therapy[2]	23	78%	97%	93%
ICU Venous Thromboembolism Prophylaxis[2]	43	81%	92%	92%
Incidence of Potentially Preventable VTE[1,2]	-	-	9%	10%
UFH with Dosages/Platelet Monitoring[1,2]	-	-	99%	97%
Venous Thromboembolism Prophylaxis[2]	246	74%	86%	85%
Warfarin Therapy Discharge Instructions[2]	21	52%	74%	75%
Chest Pain/Possible Heart Attack Care				
Aspirin Given Within 24 Hours of Arrival	69	97%	97%	96%
Fibrinolytic Meds Within 30 Min. of Arrival[1]	-	-	51%	58%
Average Time to ECG (minutes)	69	13	9	7
Average Time to Transfer (minutes)[1]	-	-	54	60
Children's Asthma Care				
Received Home Management Plan of Care	-	-	-	88%
Received Reliever Medication	-	-	-	100%
Received Systemic Corticosteroids	-	-	-	100%
Emergency Department				
Admittance Decision Time (minutes)[2]	319	65	96	98
Head CT Results Within 45 Min. of Arrival	15	60%	63%	57%
Patients Who Left ER Before Being Seen	12,324	1%	2%	2%
Time from ER Arrival to Admit. (minutes)[2]	374	186	259	274
Time from ER Arrival to Discharge (minutes)	466	112	135	134
Time in ER Before Being Evaluated (minutes)	416	17	22	26
Time to Pain Meds for Fractures (minutes)	80	54	52	57
Heart Attack Care				
Aspirin Given at Discharge	13	100%	99%	99%
Fibrinolytic Meds Within 30 Min. of Arrival[7]	-	-	62%	54%
PCI Within 90 Minutes of Arrival[7]	-	-	97%	96%
Statin Prescribed at Discharge	16	81%	98%	98%
Heart Failure Care				
ACE Inhibitor or ARB for LVSD	23	74%	97%	97%
Discharge Instructions Given	29	93%	93%	94%
Evaluation of LVS Function	41	100%	99%	99%
Medicare Spending				
Medicare Spending per Patient (ratio)	-	0.93	0.91	0.98
Pneumonia Care				
Appropriate Initial Antibiotic Given	69	91%	96%	95%
Blood Culture Timing	110	94%	97%	98%
Pregnancy and Delivery Care				
Newborn Deliveries Scheduled Early	33	12%	2%	6%
Preventive Care				
Immunization for Influenza[2]	307	98%	91%	90%
Immunization for Pneumonia[2]	426	97%	91%	92%
Stroke Care				
Anticoagulation Therapy for Atrial Fibrillation[1]	-	-	94%	95%
Antithrombotic Therapy Timing	28	100%	98%	98%
Assessed for Rehabilitation	37	86%	98%	97%
Discharged on Antithrombotic Therapy	36	100%	99%	99%
Discharged on Statin Medication	28	89%	96%	94%
Thrombolytic Therapy Timing[1]	-	-	73%	66%
Venous Thromboembolism Prophylaxis	28	86%	94%	94%
Written Stroke Educational Materials Given	25	100%	86%	88%
Surgical Care Improvement Project				
Appropriate Beta Blocker Usage	112	96%	98%	98%
Appropriate VTP Within 24 Hours	328	96%	98%	98%
Controlled Postoperative Blood Glucose[7]	-	-	97%	97%
Perioperative Temperature Management	396	100%	100%	100%
Prophylactic Antibiotic Selection	278	98%	99%	99%
Prophylactic Antibiotic Selection (Outpatient)	48	94%	98%	98%
Prophylactic Antibiotic Stopped	272	97%	99%	98%
Prophylactic Antibiotic Timing	279	97%	98%	99%
Prophylactic Antibiotic Timing (Outpatient)	49	98%	98%	98%
Urinary Catheter Removal	295	97%	97%	97%
Survey of Patients' Hospital Experiences				
Area Around Room 'Always' Quiet at Night	300+	59%	54%	61%
Doctors 'Always' Communicated Well	300+	82%	81%	82%
Home Recovery Information Given	300+	86%	87%	85%
Hospital Given 9 or 10 on 10 Point Scale	300+	78%	70%	71%
Meds 'Always' Explained Before Given	300+	68%	64%	64%
Nurses 'Always' Communicated Well	300+	81%	77%	79%
Pain 'Always' Well Controlled	300+	75%	70%	71%
Room and Bathroom 'Always' Clean	300+	83%	73%	73%
Timely Help 'Always' Received	300+	73%	65%	68%
Would Definitely Recommend Hospital	300+	84%	73%	71%
Use of Medical Imaging				
Cardiac Imaging Stress Test before Surgery	162	7.4%	4.3%	5.3%
Combination Abdominal CT Scan	436	9.6%	6.9%	10.5%
Combination Brain/Sinus CT Scan	318	1.3%	2.3%	2.7%
Combination Chest CT Scan	334	0.0%	1.1%	2.7%
Follow-up Mammogram/Ultrasound	956	7.7%	9.1%	8.8%
Lumbar Spine MRI for Low Back Pain	99	38.4%	37.9%	37.2%

Cascade Valley Hospital

330 S Stillaguamish Ave Phone: 360-435-2133
Arlington, WA 98223 Fax: 360-435-0513
URL: www.cascadevalley.org/hospital
Type: Acute Care Hospitals Emergency Services: Yes
Ownership: Govt - Hospital Dist/Auth Beds: 48

Key Personnel:
Quality Assurance . . . . Connie Digregorio
Chief of Medical Staff . . . . Roff Hartling
Radiology. . . . . Ross P Hartling
Emergency Room . . . . Gerald Hook

Measure	Cases	This Hosp.	State Avg.	U.S. Avg.
Blood Clot Prevention and Treatment				
Anticoagulation Overlap Therapy[2]	13	100%	97%	93%
ICU Venous Thromboembolism Prophylaxis[2]	27	96%	92%	92%
Incidence of Potentially Preventable VTE[2,7]	-	-	9%	10%
UFH with Dosages/Platelet Monitoring[1,2]	-	-	99%	97%
Venous Thromboembolism Prophylaxis[2]	117	95%	86%	85%
Warfarin Therapy Discharge Instructions[2]	13	92%	74%	75%
Chest Pain/Possible Heart Attack Care				
Aspirin Given Within 24 Hours of Arrival	37	100%	97%	96%
Fibrinolytic Meds Within 30 Min. of Arrival[7]	-	-	51%	58%
Average Time to ECG (minutes)	37	11	9	7
Average Time to Transfer (minutes)[1]	-	-	54	60
Children's Asthma Care				

NOTE: Hospital profiles are in alphabetical order by state, then city, then hospital within the city; Rankings exclude hospitals with less than 25 cases except for patient surveys which excludes hospitals with less than 100 cases; (a) 100-299 cases; (1) The number of cases/patients is too few to report; (2) Data submitted were based on a sample of cases/patients; (3) Results are based on a shorter time period than required; (4) Data suppressed by CMS for one or more quarters; (5) Results are not available for this reporting period; (6) Fewer than 100 patients completed the HCAHPS survey; (7) No cases met the criteria for this measure; (8) The lower limit of the confidence interval cannot be calculated if the number of observed infections equals zero; (9) No data are available from the state/territory for this reporting period; (10) The scores shown reflect fewer than 50 completed surveys; (11) There were discrepancies in the data collection process; (12) This measure does not apply to this hospital for this reporting period; (13) Results cannot be calculated for this reporting period; (14) The results for this state are combined with nearby states to protect confidentiality; Please refer to the User's Guide for a full explanation of data.

Received Home Management Plan of Care	-	-	-	88%
Received Reliever Medication	-	-	-	100%
Received Systemic Corticosteroids	-	-	-	100%
Emergency Department				
Admittance Decision Time (minutes)[2]	288	72	96	98
Head CT Results Within 45 Min. of Arrival[1]	-	-	63%	57%
Patients Who Left ER Before Being Seen	19,575	0%	2%	2%
Time from ER Arrival to Admit. (minutes)[2]	325	236	259	274
Time from ER Arrival to Discharge (minutes)	401	90	135	134
Time in ER Before Being Evaluated (minutes)	424	22	22	26
Time to Pain Meds for Fractures (minutes)	74	57	52	57
Heart Attack Care				
Aspirin Given at Discharge[1]	-	-	99%	99%
Fibrinolytic Meds Within 30 Min. of Arrival[7]	-	-	62%	54%
PCI Within 90 Minutes of Arrival[7]	-	-	97%	96%
Statin Prescribed at Discharge[1]	-	-	98%	98%
Heart Failure Care				
ACE Inhibitor or ARB for LVSD[1]	-	-	97%	97%
Discharge Instructions Given	34	97%	93%	94%
Evaluation of LVS Function	38	100%	99%	99%
Medicare Spending				
Medicare Spending per Patient (ratio)	-	0.93	0.91	0.98
Pneumonia Care				
Appropriate Initial Antibiotic Given	41	98%	96%	95%
Blood Culture Timing	58	98%	97%	98%
Pregnancy and Delivery Care				
Newborn Deliveries Scheduled Early	47	9%	2%	6%
Preventive Care				
Immunization for Influenza[2]	261	95%	91%	90%
Immunization for Pneumonia[2]	276	93%	91%	92%
Stroke Care				
Anticoagulation Therapy for Atrial Fibrillation[1]	-	-	94%	95%
Antithrombotic Therapy Timing	16	100%	98%	98%
Assessed for Rehabilitation	15	100%	98%	97%
Discharged on Antithrombotic Therapy	15	100%	99%	99%
Discharged on Statin Medication	14	93%	96%	94%
Thrombolytic Therapy Timing[7]	-	-	73%	66%
Venous Thromboembolism Prophylaxis	15	93%	94%	94%
Written Stroke Educational Materials Given[1]	-	-	86%	88%
Surgical Care Improvement Project				
Appropriate Beta Blocker Usage	43	95%	98%	98%
Appropriate VTP Within 24 Hours	116	97%	98%	98%
Controlled Postoperative Blood Glucose[7]	-	-	97%	97%
Perioperative Temperature Management	153	99%	100%	100%
Prophylactic Antibiotic Selection	105	100%	99%	99%
Prophylactic Antibiotic Selection (Outpatient)[3]	12	100%	98%	98%
Prophylactic Antibiotic Stopped	102	97%	99%	98%
Prophylactic Antibiotic Timing	105	99%	98%	99%
Prophylactic Antibiotic Timing (Outpatient)[3]	12	100%	98%	98%
Urinary Catheter Removal	79	100%	97%	97%
Survey of Patients' Hospital Experiences				
Area Around Room 'Always' Quiet at Night[3]	(a)	49%	54%	61%
Doctors 'Always' Communicated Well[3]	(a)	83%	81%	82%
Home Recovery Information Given[3]	(a)	85%	87%	85%
Hospital Given 9 or 10 on 10 Point Scale[3]	(a)	69%	70%	71%
Meds 'Always' Explained Before Given[3]	(a)	56%	64%	64%
Nurses 'Always' Communicated Well[3]	(a)	75%	77%	79%
Pain 'Always' Well Controlled[3]	(a)	70%	70%	71%
Room and Bathroom 'Always' Clean[3]	(a)	79%	73%	73%
Timely Help 'Always' Received[3]	(a)	74%	65%	68%
Would Definitely Recommend Hospital[3]	(a)	71%	73%	71%
Use of Medical Imaging				
Cardiac Imaging Stress Test before Surgery	95	6.3%	4.3%	5.3%
Combination Abdominal CT Scan	216	3.2%	6.9%	10.5%
Combination Brain/Sinus CT Scan[1]	-	-	2.3%	2.7%
Combination Chest CT Scan	134	0.0%	1.1%	2.7%
Follow-up Mammogram/Ultrasound	270	10.4%	9.1%	8.8%
Lumbar Spine MRI for Low Back Pain[1]	-	-	37.9%	37.2%

Multicare Auburn Medical Center

202 North Division Street Plaza One
Auburn, WA 98001
Phone: 253-833-7711
Fax: 253-939-2376
E-mail: armcuhs@hotmail.com
URL: www.armcuhs.com/p1.html
Type: Acute Care Hospitals
Emergency Services: Yes
Ownership: Voluntary non-profit - Private
Beds: 149

Key Personnel:
Operating Room. . . . . Andrew Bair
Quality Assurance . . . . Mary Lindsay
CEO/President. . . . . William G. Robertson
Infection Control. . . . . Beth Scott
Emergency Room . . . . Vicki Seaman
Patient Relations . . . . Anne Urlie

Measure	Cases	This Hosp.	State Avg.	U.S. Avg.
Blood Clot Prevention and Treatment				
Anticoagulation Overlap Therapy[2]	59	98%	97%	93%
ICU Venous Thromboembolism Prophylaxis[2]	73	100%	92%	92%
Incidence of Potentially Preventable VTE[1,2]	-	-	9%	10%
UFH with Dosages/Platelet Monitoring[2]	38	100%	99%	97%
Venous Thromboembolism Prophylaxis[2]	339	98%	86%	85%
Warfarin Therapy Discharge Instructions[2]	44	89%	74%	75%
Chest Pain/Possible Heart Attack Care				
Aspirin Given Within 24 Hours of Arrival[1,3]	-	-	97%	96%
Fibrinolytic Meds Within 30 Min. of Arrival[3,7]	-	-	51%	58%
Average Time to ECG (minutes)[1,3]	-	-	9	7
Average Time to Transfer (minutes)[3,7]	-	-	54	60
Children's Asthma Care				
Received Home Management Plan of Care	-	-	-	88%
Received Reliever Medication	-	-	-	100%
Received Systemic Corticosteroids	-	-	-	100%
Emergency Department				
Admittance Decision Time (minutes)[2]	725	106	96	98
Head CT Results Within 45 Min. of Arrival	26	62%	63%	57%
Patients Who Left ER Before Being Seen[5]	-	-	2%	2%
Time from ER Arrival to Admit. (minutes)[2]	758	298	259	274
Time from ER Arrival to Discharge (minutes)	385	160	135	134
Time in ER Before Being Evaluated (minutes)	296	36	22	26
Time to Pain Meds for Fractures (minutes)	126	59	52	57
Heart Attack Care				
Aspirin Given at Discharge	116	99%	99%	99%
Fibrinolytic Meds Within 30 Min. of Arrival[7]	-	-	62%	54%
PCI Within 90 Minutes of Arrival	36	100%	97%	96%
Statin Prescribed at Discharge	118	100%	98%	98%
Heart Failure Care				
ACE Inhibitor or ARB for LVSD[2]	80	94%	97%	97%
Discharge Instructions Given[2]	206	79%	93%	94%
Evaluation of LVS Function[2]	240	99%	99%	99%
Medicare Spending				
Medicare Spending per Patient (ratio)	-	1.00	0.91	0.98
Pneumonia Care				
Appropriate Initial Antibiotic Given[2]	81	94%	96%	95%
Blood Culture Timing[2]	128	98%	97%	98%
Pregnancy and Delivery Care				
Newborn Deliveries Scheduled Early[2]	44	2%	2%	6%
Preventive Care				
Immunization for Influenza[2]	569	80%	91%	90%
Immunization for Pneumonia[2]	731	80%	91%	92%
Stroke Care				
Anticoagulation Therapy for Atrial Fibrillation[1]	-	-	94%	95%
Antithrombotic Therapy Timing	38	97%	98%	98%
Assessed for Rehabilitation	44	100%	98%	97%
Discharged on Antithrombotic Therapy	43	100%	99%	99%
Discharged on Statin Medication	33	97%	96%	94%
Thrombolytic Therapy Timing[1]	-	-	73%	66%
Venous Thromboembolism Prophylaxis	42	100%	94%	94%
Written Stroke Educational Materials Given	26	81%	86%	88%
Surgical Care Improvement Project				
Appropriate Beta Blocker Usage[2]	61	95%	98%	98%
Appropriate VTP Within 24 Hours[2]	248	98%	98%	98%
Controlled Postoperative Blood Glucose[2,7]	-	-	97%	97%
Perioperative Temperature Management[2]	290	99%	100%	100%
Prophylactic Antibiotic Selection[2]	180	100%	99%	99%
Prophylactic Antibiotic Selection (Outpatient)	41	90%	98%	98%
Prophylactic Antibiotic Stopped[2]	178	94%	99%	98%
Prophylactic Antibiotic Timing[2]	180	94%	98%	99%
Prophylactic Antibiotic Timing (Outpatient)	44	86%	98%	98%
Urinary Catheter Removal[2]	202	91%	97%	97%
Survey of Patients' Hospital Experiences				
Area Around Room 'Always' Quiet at Night	300+	43%	54%	61%
Doctors 'Always' Communicated Well	300+	70%	81%	82%
Home Recovery Information Given	300+	85%	87%	85%
Hospital Given 9 or 10 on 10 Point Scale	300+	42%	70%	71%
Meds 'Always' Explained Before Given	300+	51%	64%	64%
Nurses 'Always' Communicated Well	300+	62%	77%	79%
Pain 'Always' Well Controlled	300+	59%	70%	71%
Room and Bathroom 'Always' Clean	300+	58%	73%	73%
Timely Help 'Always' Received	300+	39%	65%	68%
Would Definitely Recommend Hospital	300+	42%	73%	71%
Use of Medical Imaging				
Cardiac Imaging Stress Test before Surgery	195	3.6%	4.3%	5.3%
Combination Abdominal CT Scan	313	2.6%	6.9%	10.5%
Combination Brain/Sinus CT Scan[1]	-	-	2.3%	2.7%
Combination Chest CT Scan	205	0.0%	1.1%	2.7%
Follow-up Mammogram/Ultrasound	242	13.6%	9.1%	8.8%
Lumbar Spine MRI for Low Back Pain[1]	-	-	37.9%	37.2%

Overlake Hospital Medical Center

1035-116th Ave Ne
Bellevue, WA 98004
Phone: 425-688-5000
Fax: 425-688-5959
URL: www.overlakehospital.org
Type: Acute Care Hospitals
Emergency Services: Yes
Ownership: Voluntary non-profit - Other
Beds: 337

Key Personnel:
Quality Assurance . . . . Richard Bryan
Radiology. . . . . Bill Crenshaw, MD
Coronary Care . . . . Joseph Doucette, MD
Pediatric In-Patient Care . . . . Otero Flowers, MD
Infection Control. . . . . Peter Hashisaki, MD
Cardiology . . . . James Leggett, MD
CEO/President. . . . . J. Michael Marsh
Chief of Medical Staff . . . . Tom Miller, MD

Measure	Cases	This Hosp.	State Avg.	U.S. Avg.
Blood Clot Prevention and Treatment				
Anticoagulation Overlap Therapy[2]	105	93%	97%	93%
ICU Venous Thromboembolism Prophylaxis[2]	54	89%	92%	92%
Incidence of Potentially Preventable VTE[2]	15	7%	9%	10%
UFH with Dosages/Platelet Monitoring[2]	56	100%	99%	97%
Venous Thromboembolism Prophylaxis[2]	259	85%	86%	85%
Warfarin Therapy Discharge Instructions[2]	91	74%	74%	75%
Chest Pain/Possible Heart Attack Care				
Aspirin Given Within 24 Hours of Arrival[1,3]	-	-	97%	96%
Fibrinolytic Meds Within 30 Min. of Arrival[5]	-	-	51%	58%
Average Time to ECG (minutes)[1,3]	-	-	9	7
Average Time to Transfer (minutes)[5]	-	-	54	60
Children's Asthma Care				
Received Home Management Plan of Care	-	-	-	88%
Received Reliever Medication	-	-	-	100%
Received Systemic Corticosteroids	-	-	-	100%
Emergency Department				
Admittance Decision Time (minutes)[2]	381	140	96	98
Head CT Results Within 45 Min. of Arrival[1]	-	-	63%	57%
Patients Who Left ER Before Being Seen	43,750	1%	2%	2%
Time from ER Arrival to Admit. (minutes)[2]	408	251	259	274
Time from ER Arrival to Discharge (minutes)	377	161	135	134
Time in ER Before Being Evaluated (minutes)	298	20	22	26
Time to Pain Meds for Fractures (minutes)	354	46	52	57
Heart Attack Care				
Aspirin Given at Discharge	246	100%	99%	99%
Fibrinolytic Meds Within 30 Min. of Arrival[7]	-	-	62%	54%
PCI Within 90 Minutes of Arrival	58	98%	97%	96%
Statin Prescribed at Discharge	246	99%	98%	98%
Heart Failure Care				
ACE Inhibitor or ARB for LVSD	82	100%	97%	97%
Discharge Instructions Given	273	94%	93%	94%
Evaluation of LVS Function	331	100%	99%	99%
Medicare Spending				
Medicare Spending per Patient (ratio)	-	0.94	0.91	0.98

NOTE: Hospital profiles are in alphabetical order by state, then city, then hospital within the city; Rankings exclude hospitals with less than 25 cases except for patient surveys which excludes hospitals with less than 100 cases; (a) 100-299 cases; (1) The number of cases/patients is too few to report; (2) Data submitted were based on a sample of cases/patients; (3) Results are based on a shorter time period than required; (4) Data suppressed by CMS for one or more quarters; (5) Results are not available for this reporting period; (6) Fewer than 100 patients completed the HCAHPS survey; (7) No cases met the criteria for this measure; (8) The lower limit of the confidence interval cannot be calculated if the number of observed infections equals zero; (9) No data are available from the state/territory for this reporting period; (10) The scores shown reflect fewer than 50 completed surveys; (11) There were discrepancies in the data collection process; (12) This measure does not apply to this hospital for this reporting period; (13) Results cannot be calculated for this reporting period; (14) The results for this state are combined with nearby states to protect confidentiality; Please refer to the User's Guide for a full explanation of data.

Measure	Cases	This Hosp.	State Avg.	U.S. Avg.
Pneumonia Care				
Appropriate Initial Antibiotic Given	123	99%	96%	95%
Blood Culture Timing	140	100%	97%	98%
Pregnancy and Delivery Care				
Newborn Deliveries Scheduled Early	398	0%	2%	6%
Preventive Care				
Immunization for Influenza[2]	524	98%	91%	90%
Immunization for Pneumonia[2]	512	95%	91%	92%
Stroke Care				
Anticoagulation Therapy for Atrial Fibrillation	36	100%	94%	95%
Antithrombotic Therapy Timing	123	100%	98%	98%
Assessed for Rehabilitation	172	99%	98%	97%
Discharged on Antithrombotic Therapy	155	100%	99%	99%
Discharged on Statin Medication	111	100%	96%	94%
Thrombolytic Therapy Timing	38	29%	73%	66%
Venous Thromboembolism Prophylaxis	152	96%	94%	94%
Written Stroke Educational Materials Given	79	91%	86%	88%
Surgical Care Improvement Project				
Appropriate Beta Blocker Usage[2]	198	99%	98%	98%
Appropriate VTP Within 24 Hours[2]	465	99%	98%	98%
Controlled Postoperative Blood Glucose[2]	121	97%	97%	97%
Perioperative Temperature Management[2]	577	100%	100%	100%
Prophylactic Antibiotic Selection[2]	521	99%	99%	99%
Prophylactic Antibiotic Selection (Outpatient)	490	98%	98%	98%
Prophylactic Antibiotic Stopped[2]	513	100%	99%	98%
Prophylactic Antibiotic Timing[2]	522	100%	98%	99%
Prophylactic Antibiotic Timing (Outpatient)	491	99%	98%	98%
Urinary Catheter Removal[2]	305	99%	97%	97%
Survey of Patients' Hospital Experiences				
Area Around Room 'Always' Quiet at Night	300+	57%	54%	61%
Doctors 'Always' Communicated Well	300+	82%	81%	82%
Home Recovery Information Given	300+	88%	87%	85%
Hospital Given 9 or 10 on 10 Point Scale	300+	72%	70%	71%
Meds 'Always' Explained Before Given	300+	65%	64%	64%
Nurses 'Always' Communicated Well	300+	76%	77%	79%
Pain 'Always' Well Controlled	300+	73%	70%	71%
Room and Bathroom 'Always' Clean	300+	73%	73%	73%
Timely Help 'Always' Received	300+	61%	65%	68%
Would Definitely Recommend Hospital	300+	76%	73%	71%
Use of Medical Imaging				
Cardiac Imaging Stress Test before Surgery	1,323	4.5%	4.3%	5.3%
Combination Abdominal CT Scan	832	8.5%	6.9%	10.5%
Combination Brain/Sinus CT Scan	969	2.1%	2.3%	2.7%
Combination Chest CT Scan	644	0.6%	1.1%	2.7%
Follow-up Mammogram/Ultrasound	3,126	9.7%	9.1%	8.8%
Lumbar Spine MRI for Low Back Pain	136	35.3%	37.9%	37.2%

Peacehealth Saint Joseph Medical Center

2901 Squalicum Parkway
Bellingham, WA 98225
URL: www.peacehealth.org
Type: Acute Care Hospitals
Ownership: Voluntary non-profit - Other
Phone: 360-734-5400
Fax: 360-738-6393
Emergency Services: Yes
Beds: 253

Key Personnel:
CEO .... Josiah SY Johnson
Chief of Medical Staff .... Berle Stratton, MD
President .... Alan Yordy

Measure	Cases	This Hosp.	State Avg.	U.S. Avg.
Blood Clot Prevention and Treatment				
Anticoagulation Overlap Therapy[2]	89	98%	97%	93%
ICU Venous Thromboembolism Prophylaxis[2]	82	88%	92%	92%
Incidence of Potentially Preventable VTE[2]	12	17%	9%	10%
UFH with Dosages/Platelet Monitoring[2]	82	99%	99%	97%
Venous Thromboembolism Prophylaxis[2]	289	76%	86%	85%
Warfarin Therapy Discharge Instructions[2]	69	74%	74%	75%
Chest Pain/Possible Heart Attack Care				
Aspirin Given Within 24 Hours of Arrival[5]	-	-	97%	96%
Fibrinolytic Meds Within 30 Min. of Arrival[5]	-	-	51%	58%
Average Time to ECG (minutes)[5]	-	-	9	7
Average Time to Transfer (minutes)[5]	-	-	54	60
Children's Asthma Care				
Received Home Management Plan of Care	-	-	-	88%
Received Reliever Medication	-	-	-	100%
Received Systemic Corticosteroids	-	-	-	100%
Emergency Department				
Admittance Decision Time (minutes)[2]	565	139	96	98
Head CT Results Within 45 Min. of Arrival[1]	-	-	63%	57%
Patients Who Left ER Before Being Seen	57,109	3%	2%	2%
Time from ER Arrival to Admit. (minutes)[2]	566	286	259	274
Time from ER Arrival to Discharge (minutes)	332	164	135	134
Time in ER Before Being Evaluated (minutes)	384	36	22	26
Time to Pain Meds for Fractures (minutes)	263	73	52	57
Heart Attack Care				
Aspirin Given at Discharge	347	99%	99%	99%
Fibrinolytic Meds Within 30 Min. of Arrival[7]	-	-	62%	54%
PCI Within 90 Minutes of Arrival	73	92%	97%	96%
Statin Prescribed at Discharge	333	95%	98%	98%
Heart Failure Care				
ACE Inhibitor or ARB for LVSD	87	90%	97%	97%
Discharge Instructions Given	274	90%	93%	94%
Evaluation of LVS Function	337	99%	99%	99%
Medicare Spending				
Medicare Spending per Patient (ratio)	-	0.92	0.91	0.98
Pneumonia Care				
Appropriate Initial Antibiotic Given	227	97%	96%	95%
Blood Culture Timing	362	94%	97%	98%
Pregnancy and Delivery Care				
Newborn Deliveries Scheduled Early	131	1%	2%	6%
Preventive Care				
Immunization for Influenza[2]	516	89%	91%	90%
Immunization for Pneumonia[2]	598	91%	91%	92%
Stroke Care				
Anticoagulation Therapy for Atrial Fibrillation[2]	17	100%	94%	95%
Antithrombotic Therapy Timing[2]	61	93%	98%	98%
Assessed for Rehabilitation[2]	91	97%	98%	97%
Discharged on Antithrombotic Therapy[2]	75	99%	99%	99%
Discharged on Statin Medication[2]	66	91%	96%	94%
Thrombolytic Therapy Timing[2]	13	46%	73%	66%
Venous Thromboembolism Prophylaxis[2]	88	85%	94%	94%
Written Stroke Educational Materials Given[2]	54	83%	86%	88%
Surgical Care Improvement Project				
Appropriate Beta Blocker Usage[2]	218	98%	98%	98%
Appropriate VTP Within 24 Hours[2]	315	99%	98%	98%
Controlled Postoperative Blood Glucose[2]	147	99%	97%	97%
Perioperative Temperature Management[2]	433	100%	100%	100%
Prophylactic Antibiotic Selection[2]	398	99%	99%	99%
Prophylactic Antibiotic Selection (Outpatient)	282	99%	98%	98%
Prophylactic Antibiotic Stopped[2]	394	98%	99%	98%
Prophylactic Antibiotic Timing[2]	398	99%	98%	99%
Prophylactic Antibiotic Timing (Outpatient)	281	100%	98%	98%
Urinary Catheter Removal[2]	246	97%	97%	97%
Survey of Patients' Hospital Experiences				
Area Around Room 'Always' Quiet at Night	300+	43%	54%	61%
Doctors 'Always' Communicated Well	300+	80%	81%	82%
Home Recovery Information Given	300+	90%	87%	85%
Hospital Given 9 or 10 on 10 Point Scale	300+	67%	70%	71%
Meds 'Always' Explained Before Given	300+	62%	64%	64%
Nurses 'Always' Communicated Well	300+	78%	77%	79%
Pain 'Always' Well Controlled	300+	71%	70%	71%
Room and Bathroom 'Always' Clean	300+	71%	73%	73%
Timely Help 'Always' Received	300+	62%	65%	68%
Would Definitely Recommend Hospital	300+	75%	73%	71%
Use of Medical Imaging				
Cardiac Imaging Stress Test before Surgery	1,014	3.1%	4.3%	5.3%
Combination Abdominal CT Scan	639	0.8%	6.9%	10.5%
Combination Brain/Sinus CT Scan	745	2.1%	2.3%	2.7%
Combination Chest CT Scan	102	1.0%	1.1%	2.7%
Follow-up Mammogram/Ultrasound[7]	-	-	9.1%	8.8%
Lumbar Spine MRI for Low Back Pain[1]	-	-	37.9%	37.2%

Harrison Memorial Center

2520 Cherry Avenue
Bremerton, WA 98310
E-mail: juli.may@harrisonmedical.org
URL: www.harrisonmedical.org
Type: Acute Care Hospitals
Ownership: Voluntary non-profit - Private
Phone: 360-377-3911
Fax: 360-792-6515
Emergency Services: Yes
Beds: 297

Key Personnel:
Quality Assurance .... Judy Anderson
CEO/President .... Scott Bosch
Radiology .... Redge Campbell
Chair/CEO .... James T. Civilla
Chief of Medical Staff .... Gordon Cromwell, MD
Operating Room .... Kim Raney, RN
Pediatric Ambulatory Care ...... Shara Summers
Pediatric In-Patient Care .... Shara Summers

Measure	Cases	This Hosp.	State Avg.	U.S. Avg.
Blood Clot Prevention and Treatment				
Anticoagulation Overlap Therapy[2]	138	98%	97%	93%
ICU Venous Thromboembolism Prophylaxis[2]	58	95%	92%	92%
Incidence of Potentially Preventable VTE[2]	11	9%	9%	10%
UFH with Dosages/Platelet Monitoring[2]	114	100%	99%	97%
Venous Thromboembolism Prophylaxis[2]	314	91%	86%	85%
Warfarin Therapy Discharge Instructions[2]	114	70%	74%	75%
Chest Pain/Possible Heart Attack Care				
Aspirin Given Within 24 Hours of Arrival[5]	-	-	97%	96%
Fibrinolytic Meds Within 30 Min. of Arrival[5]	-	-	51%	58%
Average Time to ECG (minutes)[5]	-	-	9	7
Average Time to Transfer (minutes)[5]	-	-	54	60
Children's Asthma Care				
Received Home Management Plan of Care	-	-	-	88%
Received Reliever Medication	-	-	-	100%
Received Systemic Corticosteroids	-	-	-	100%
Emergency Department				
Admittance Decision Time (minutes)[2]	546	103	96	98
Head CT Results Within 45 Min. of Arrival	20	45%	63%	57%
Patients Who Left ER Before Being Seen	71,744	2%	2%	2%
Time from ER Arrival to Admit. (minutes)[2]	605	262	259	274
Time from ER Arrival to Discharge (minutes)	375	152	135	134
Time in ER Before Being Evaluated (minutes)	415	25	22	26
Time to Pain Meds for Fractures (minutes)	167	52	52	57
Heart Attack Care				
Aspirin Given at Discharge	360	99%	99%	99%
Fibrinolytic Meds Within 30 Min. of Arrival[1]	-	-	62%	54%
PCI Within 90 Minutes of Arrival	60	100%	97%	96%
Statin Prescribed at Discharge	347	99%	98%	98%
Heart Failure Care				
ACE Inhibitor or ARB for LVSD	115	97%	97%	97%
Discharge Instructions Given	265	88%	93%	94%
Evaluation of LVS Function	361	100%	99%	99%
Medicare Spending				
Medicare Spending per Patient (ratio)	-	0.96	0.91	0.98
Pneumonia Care				
Appropriate Initial Antibiotic Given[2]	68	96%	96%	95%
Blood Culture Timing[2]	109	100%	97%	98%
Pregnancy and Delivery Care				
Newborn Deliveries Scheduled Early	142	5%	2%	6%
Preventive Care				
Immunization for Influenza[2]	589	93%	91%	90%
Immunization for Pneumonia[2]	679	95%	91%	92%
Stroke Care				
Anticoagulation Therapy for Atrial Fibrillation	36	100%	94%	95%
Antithrombotic Therapy Timing	170	98%	98%	98%
Assessed for Rehabilitation	178	100%	98%	97%
Discharged on Antithrombotic Therapy	176	100%	99%	99%
Discharged on Statin Medication	148	99%	96%	94%
Thrombolytic Therapy Timing	17	88%	73%	66%
Venous Thromboembolism Prophylaxis	171	99%	94%	94%
Written Stroke Educational Materials Given	83	95%	86%	88%
Surgical Care Improvement Project				
Appropriate Beta Blocker Usage[2]	283	98%	98%	98%
Appropriate VTP Within 24 Hours[2]	353	100%	98%	98%
Controlled Postoperative Blood Glucose[2]	214	98%	97%	97%
Perioperative Temperature Management[2]	485	100%	100%	100%

NOTE: Hospital profiles are in alphabetical order by state, then city, then hospital within the city; Rankings exclude hospitals with less than 25 cases except for patient surveys which excludes hospitals with less than 100 cases; (a) 100-299 cases; (1) The number of cases/patients is too few to report; (2) Data submitted were based on a sample of cases/patients; (3) Results are based on a shorter time period than required; (4) Data suppressed by CMS for one or more quarters; (5) Results are not available for this reporting period; (6) Fewer than 100 patients completed the HCAHPS survey; (7) No cases met the criteria for this measure; (8) The lower limit of the confidence interval cannot be calculated if the number of observed infections equals zero; (9) No data are available from the state/territory for this reporting period; (10) The scores shown reflect fewer than 50 completed surveys; (11) There were discrepancies in the data collection process; (12) This measure does not apply to this hospital for this reporting period; (13) Results cannot be calculated for this reporting period; (14) The results for this state are combined with nearby states to protect confidentiality; Please refer to the User's Guide for a full explanation of data.

Measure	Cases	This Hosp.	State Avg.	U.S. Avg.
Prophylactic Antibiotic Selection[2]	506	100%	99%	99%
Prophylactic Antibiotic Selection (Outpatient)	387	99%	98%	98%
Prophylactic Antibiotic Stopped[2]	495	99%	99%	98%
Prophylactic Antibiotic Timing[2]	508	99%	98%	99%
Prophylactic Antibiotic Timing (Outpatient)	388	99%	98%	98%
Urinary Catheter Removal[2]	256	98%	97%	97%
Survey of Patients' Hospital Experiences				
Area Around Room 'Always' Quiet at Night	300+	41%	54%	61%
Doctors 'Always' Communicated Well	300+	79%	81%	82%
Home Recovery Information Given	300+	86%	87%	85%
Hospital Given 9 or 10 on 10 Point Scale	300+	66%	70%	71%
Meds 'Always' Explained Before Given	300+	59%	64%	64%
Nurses 'Always' Communicated Well	300+	76%	77%	79%
Pain 'Always' Well Controlled	300+	65%	70%	71%
Room and Bathroom 'Always' Clean	300+	64%	73%	73%
Timely Help 'Always' Received	300+	64%	65%	68%
Would Definitely Recommend Hospital	300+	70%	73%	71%
Use of Medical Imaging				
Cardiac Imaging Stress Test before Surgery	217	2.8%	4.3%	5.3%
Combination Abdominal CT Scan	615	3.7%	6.9%	10.5%
Combination Brain/Sinus CT Scan	980	1.6%	2.3%	2.7%
Combination Chest CT Scan	101	0.0%	1.1%	2.7%
Follow-up Mammogram/Ultrasound[7]	-	-	9.1%	8.8%
Lumbar Spine MRI for Low Back Pain[1]	-	-	37.9%	37.2%

Three Rivers Hospital

507 Hospital Way
Brewster, WA 98812
Phone: 509-689-2517
Type: Critical Access Hospitals
Emergency Services: Yes
Ownership: Govt - Hospital Dist/Auth

Measure	Cases	This Hosp.	State Avg.	U.S. Avg.
Blood Clot Prevention and Treatment				
Anticoagulation Overlap Therapy[5]	-	-	97%	93%
ICU Venous Thromboembolism Prophylaxis[5]	-	-	92%	92%
Incidence of Potentially Preventable VTE[5]	-	-	9%	10%
UFH with Dosages/Platelet Monitoring[5]	-	-	99%	97%
Venous Thromboembolism Prophylaxis[5]	-	-	86%	85%
Warfarin Therapy Discharge Instructions[5]	-	-	74%	75%
Chest Pain/Possible Heart Attack Care				
Aspirin Given Within 24 Hours of Arrival	-	-	97%	96%
Fibrinolytic Meds Within 30 Min. of Arrival	-	-	51%	58%
Average Time to ECG (minutes)	-	-	9	7
Average Time to Transfer (minutes)	-	-	54	60
Children's Asthma Care				
Received Home Management Plan of Care	-	-	-	88%
Received Reliever Medication	-	-	-	100%
Received Systemic Corticosteroids	-	-	-	100%
Emergency Department				
Admittance Decision Time (minutes)[5]	-	-	96	98
Head CT Results Within 45 Min. of Arrival	-	-	63%	57%
Patients Who Left ER Before Being Seen	-	-	2%	2%
Time from ER Arrival to Admit. (minutes)[5]	-	-	259	274
Time from ER Arrival to Discharge (minutes)	-	-	135	134
Time in ER Before Being Evaluated (minutes)	-	-	22	26
Time to Pain Meds for Fractures (minutes)	-	-	52	57
Heart Attack Care				
Aspirin Given at Discharge[5]	-	-	99%	99%
Fibrinolytic Meds Within 30 Min. of Arrival[5]	-	-	62%	54%
PCI Within 90 Minutes of Arrival[5]	-	-	97%	96%
Statin Prescribed at Discharge[5]	-	-	98%	98%
Heart Failure Care				
ACE Inhibitor or ARB for LVSD[1,3]	-	-	97%	97%
Discharge Instructions Given[1,3]	-	-	93%	94%
Evaluation of LVS Function[1,3]	-	-	99%	99%
Medicare Spending				
Medicare Spending per Patient (ratio)	-	-	0.91	0.98
Pneumonia Care				
Appropriate Initial Antibiotic Given[1]	-	-	96%	95%
Blood Culture Timing[1]	-	-	97%	98%
Pregnancy and Delivery Care				
Newborn Deliveries Scheduled Early[5]	-	-	2%	6%
Preventive Care				
Immunization for Influenza[5]	-	-	91%	90%
Immunization for Pneumonia[5]	-	-	91%	92%
Stroke Care				
Anticoagulation Therapy for Atrial Fibrillation[5]	-	-	94%	95%
Antithrombotic Therapy Timing[5]	-	-	98%	98%
Assessed for Rehabilitation[5]	-	-	98%	97%
Discharged on Antithrombotic Therapy[5]	-	-	99%	99%
Discharged on Statin Medication[5]	-	-	96%	94%
Thrombolytic Therapy Timing[5]	-	-	73%	66%
Venous Thromboembolism Prophylaxis[5]	-	-	94%	94%
Written Stroke Educational Materials Given[5]	-	-	86%	88%
Surgical Care Improvement Project				
Appropriate Beta Blocker Usage[1]	-	-	98%	98%
Appropriate VTP Within 24 Hours	19	53%	98%	98%
Controlled Postoperative Blood Glucose[7]	-	-	97%	97%
Perioperative Temperature Management	22	73%	100%	100%
Prophylactic Antibiotic Selection	18	94%	99%	99%
Prophylactic Antibiotic Selection (Outpatient)	-	-	98%	98%
Prophylactic Antibiotic Stopped	18	100%	99%	98%
Prophylactic Antibiotic Timing	18	94%	98%	99%
Prophylactic Antibiotic Timing (Outpatient)	-	-	98%	98%
Urinary Catheter Removal	14	93%	97%	97%
Survey of Patients' Hospital Experiences				
Area Around Room 'Always' Quiet at Night[5]	-	-	54%	61%
Doctors 'Always' Communicated Well[5]	-	-	81%	82%
Home Recovery Information Given[5]	-	-	87%	85%
Hospital Given 9 or 10 on 10 Point Scale[5]	-	-	70%	71%
Meds 'Always' Explained Before Given[5]	-	-	64%	64%
Nurses 'Always' Communicated Well[5]	-	-	77%	79%
Pain 'Always' Well Controlled[5]	-	-	70%	71%
Room and Bathroom 'Always' Clean[5]	-	-	73%	73%
Timely Help 'Always' Received[5]	-	-	65%	68%
Would Definitely Recommend Hospital[5]	-	-	73%	71%
Use of Medical Imaging				
Cardiac Imaging Stress Test before Surgery	-	-	4.3%	5.3%
Combination Abdominal CT Scan	-	-	6.9%	10.5%
Combination Brain/Sinus CT Scan	-	-	2.3%	2.7%
Combination Chest CT Scan	-	-	1.1%	2.7%
Follow-up Mammogram/Ultrasound	-	-	9.1%	8.8%
Lumbar Spine MRI for Low Back Pain	-	-	37.9%	37.2%

Highline Medical Center

16251 Sylvester Road Sw
Burien, WA 98166
Phone: 206-244-9970
Fax: 206-246-5385
E-mail: commrelations@highlinemedical.org
URL: www.hchnet.org
Type: Acute Care Hospitals
Emergency Services: Yes
Ownership: Voluntary non-profit - Private
Beds: 207
Key Personnel:
CEO/President. . . . . Mark Benedum
Chief of Medical Staff. . . . . Jeffrey Frankel, MD
Radiology. . . . . Rachel Gerson
Infection Control. . . . . Bevelrly Haggan
Pediatric In-Patient Care . . . . Ritchie Kindred, MD
Operating Room. . . . . Marco Sobrino
Quality Assurance . . . . Pat Tennent

Measure	Cases	This Hosp.	State Avg.	U.S. Avg.
Blood Clot Prevention and Treatment				
Anticoagulation Overlap Therapy[2]	52	100%	97%	93%
ICU Venous Thromboembolism Prophylaxis[2]	47	83%	92%	92%
Incidence of Potentially Preventable VTE[1,2]	-	-	9%	10%
UFH with Dosages/Platelet Monitoring[2]	45	100%	99%	97%
Venous Thromboembolism Prophylaxis[2]	332	86%	86%	85%
Warfarin Therapy Discharge Instructions[2]	45	40%	74%	75%
Chest Pain/Possible Heart Attack Care				
Aspirin Given Within 24 Hours of Arrival	20	90%	97%	96%
Fibrinolytic Meds Within 30 Min. of Arrival[3,7]	-	-	51%	58%
Average Time to ECG (minutes)	21	0	9	7
Average Time to Transfer (minutes)[3,7]	-	-	54	60
Children's Asthma Care				
Received Home Management Plan of Care	-	-	-	88%
Received Reliever Medication	-	-	-	100%
Received Systemic Corticosteroids	-	-	-	100%
Emergency Department				
Admittance Decision Time (minutes)[2]	692	132	96	98
Head CT Results Within 45 Min. of Arrival[1]	-	-	63%	57%
Patients Who Left ER Before Being Seen	58,095	1%	2%	2%
Time from ER Arrival to Admit. (minutes)[2]	695	264	259	274
Time from ER Arrival to Discharge (minutes)	360	109	135	134
Time in ER Before Being Evaluated (minutes)	382	20	22	26
Time to Pain Meds for Fractures (minutes)	136	47	52	57
Heart Attack Care				
Aspirin Given at Discharge	131	97%	99%	99%
Fibrinolytic Meds Within 30 Min. of Arrival[7]	-	-	62%	54%
PCI Within 90 Minutes of Arrival	28	96%	97%	96%
Statin Prescribed at Discharge	119	97%	98%	98%
Heart Failure Care				
ACE Inhibitor or ARB for LVSD	47	100%	97%	97%
Discharge Instructions Given	134	98%	93%	94%
Evaluation of LVS Function	170	100%	99%	99%
Medicare Spending				
Medicare Spending per Patient (ratio)	-	0.95	0.91	0.98
Pneumonia Care				
Appropriate Initial Antibiotic Given	189	98%	96%	95%
Blood Culture Timing	332	98%	97%	98%
Pregnancy and Delivery Care				
Newborn Deliveries Scheduled Early	152	0%	2%	6%
Preventive Care				
Immunization for Influenza[2]	507	90%	91%	90%
Immunization for Pneumonia[2]	612	94%	91%	92%
Stroke Care				
Anticoagulation Therapy for Atrial Fibrillation	21	100%	94%	95%
Antithrombotic Therapy Timing	95	98%	98%	98%
Assessed for Rehabilitation	115	98%	98%	97%
Discharged on Antithrombotic Therapy	97	98%	99%	99%
Discharged on Statin Medication	74	97%	96%	94%
Thrombolytic Therapy Timing[1]	-	-	73%	66%
Venous Thromboembolism Prophylaxis	118	97%	94%	94%
Written Stroke Educational Materials Given	66	97%	86%	88%
Surgical Care Improvement Project				
Appropriate Beta Blocker Usage	120	98%	98%	98%
Appropriate VTP Within 24 Hours	390	100%	98%	98%
Controlled Postoperative Blood Glucose[7]	-	-	97%	97%
Perioperative Temperature Management	463	100%	100%	100%
Prophylactic Antibiotic Selection	246	100%	99%	99%
Prophylactic Antibiotic Selection (Outpatient)	100	97%	98%	98%
Prophylactic Antibiotic Stopped	238	99%	99%	98%
Prophylactic Antibiotic Timing	246	100%	98%	99%
Prophylactic Antibiotic Timing (Outpatient)	100	98%	98%	98%
Urinary Catheter Removal	244	95%	97%	97%
Survey of Patients' Hospital Experiences				
Area Around Room 'Always' Quiet at Night	300+	50%	54%	61%
Doctors 'Always' Communicated Well	300+	76%	81%	82%
Home Recovery Information Given	300+	84%	87%	85%
Hospital Given 9 or 10 on 10 Point Scale	300+	63%	70%	71%
Meds 'Always' Explained Before Given	300+	58%	64%	64%
Nurses 'Always' Communicated Well	300+	70%	77%	79%
Pain 'Always' Well Controlled	300+	67%	70%	71%
Room and Bathroom 'Always' Clean	300+	68%	73%	73%
Timely Help 'Always' Received	300+	56%	65%	68%
Would Definitely Recommend Hospital	300+	67%	73%	71%
Use of Medical Imaging				
Cardiac Imaging Stress Test before Surgery[1]	-	-	4.3%	5.3%
Combination Abdominal CT Scan	541	6.5%	6.9%	10.5%
Combination Brain/Sinus CT Scan	546	0.7%	2.3%	2.7%
Combination Chest CT Scan	239	0.0%	1.1%	2.7%
Follow-up Mammogram/Ultrasound[7]	-	-	9.1%	8.8%
Lumbar Spine MRI for Low Back Pain	40	42.5%	37.9%	37.2%

Providence Centralia Hospital

914 S Scheuber Road
Centralia, WA 98531
Phone: 360-736-2803
Fax: 360-330-8576
E-mail: chris.thomas@providence.org
URL: www.providence.org/swsa
Type: Acute Care Hospitals
Emergency Services: Yes
Ownership: Voluntary non-profit - Other
Beds: 191
Key Personnel:
CEO/President. . . . . Scott Bondn

NOTE: Hospital profiles are in alphabetical order by state, then city, then hospital within the city; Rankings exclude hospitals with less than 25 cases except for patient surveys which excludes hospitals with less than 100 cases; (a) 100-299 cases; (1) The number of cases/patients is too few to report; (2) Data submitted were based on a sample of cases/patients; (3) Results are based on a shorter time period than required; (4) Data suppressed by CMS for one or more quarters; (5) Results are not available for this reporting period; (6) Fewer than 100 patients completed the HCAHPS survey; (7) No cases met the criteria for this measure; (8) The lower limit of the confidence interval cannot be calculated if the number of observed infections equals zero; (9) No data are available from the state/territory for this reporting period; (10) The scores shown reflect fewer than 50 completed surveys; (11) There were discrepancies in the data collection process; (12) This measure does not apply to this hospital for this reporting period; (13) Results cannot be calculated for this reporting period; (14) The results for this state are combined with nearby states to protect confidentiality; Please refer to the User's Guide for a full explanation of data.

Coronary Care . . . . Iva Fulmer, RN
Chief of Medical Staff . . . . Renae Hamshar
Emergency Room . . . . Doug Hayden
Operating Room. . . . . Stephen D Hennessey, RN
Radiology. . . . . Peter Ping Hu, RN
Quality Assurance . . . . Jeanell Rasmussen
Infection Control. . . . . Barbara Wagner

Measure	Cases	This Hosp.	State Avg.	U.S. Avg.
Blood Clot Prevention and Treatment				
Anticoagulation Overlap Therapy[2]	31	94%	97%	93%
ICU Venous Thromboembolism Prophylaxis[2]	46	93%	92%	92%
Incidence of Potentially Preventable VTE[1,2]	-	-	9%	10%
UFH with Dosages/Platelet Monitoring[1,2]	-	-	99%	97%
Venous Thromboembolism Prophylaxis[2]	313	82%	86%	85%
Warfarin Therapy Discharge Instructions[2]	31	61%	74%	75%
Chest Pain/Possible Heart Attack Care				
Aspirin Given Within 24 Hours of Arrival	103	92%	97%	96%
Fibrinolytic Meds Within 30 Min. of Arrival[7]	-	-	51%	58%
Average Time to ECG (minutes)	109	9	9	7
Average Time to Transfer (minutes)	28	54	54	60
Children's Asthma Care				
Received Home Management Plan of Care	-	-	-	88%
Received Reliever Medication	-	-	-	100%
Received Systemic Corticosteroids	-	-	-	100%
Emergency Department				
Admittance Decision Time (minutes)[2]	731	103	96	98
Head CT Results Within 45 Min. of Arrival	23	83%	63%	57%
Patients Who Left ER Before Being Seen	30,424	4%	2%	2%
Time from ER Arrival to Admit. (minutes)[2]	734	281	259	274
Time from ER Arrival to Discharge (minutes)	353	162	135	134
Time in ER Before Being Evaluated (minutes)	284	45	22	26
Time to Pain Meds for Fractures (minutes)	144	58	52	57
Heart Attack Care				
Aspirin Given at Discharge	23	100%	99%	99%
Fibrinolytic Meds Within 30 Min. of Arrival[7]	-	-	62%	54%
PCI Within 90 Minutes of Arrival[7]	-	-	97%	96%
Statin Prescribed at Discharge	20	95%	98%	98%
Heart Failure Care				
ACE Inhibitor or ARB for LVSD[2]	59	97%	97%	97%
Discharge Instructions Given[2]	153	95%	93%	94%
Evaluation of LVS Function[2]	179	99%	99%	99%
Medicare Spending				
Medicare Spending per Patient (ratio)	-	0.90	0.91	0.98
Pneumonia Care				
Appropriate Initial Antibiotic Given[2]	105	99%	96%	95%
Blood Culture Timing[2]	131	99%	97%	98%
Pregnancy and Delivery Care				
Newborn Deliveries Scheduled Early[2]	32	0%	2%	6%
Preventive Care				
Immunization for Influenza[2]	486	86%	91%	90%
Immunization for Pneumonia[2]	654	89%	91%	92%
Stroke Care				
Anticoagulation Therapy for Atrial Fibrillation	22	86%	94%	95%
Antithrombotic Therapy Timing	63	100%	98%	98%
Assessed for Rehabilitation	76	95%	98%	97%
Discharged on Antithrombotic Therapy	76	100%	99%	99%
Discharged on Statin Medication	65	91%	96%	94%
Thrombolytic Therapy Timing[1]	-	-	73%	66%
Venous Thromboembolism Prophylaxis	56	80%	94%	94%
Written Stroke Educational Materials Given	51	20%	86%	88%
Surgical Care Improvement Project				
Appropriate Beta Blocker Usage[2]	78	95%	98%	98%
Appropriate VTP Within 24 Hours[2]	306	96%	98%	98%
Controlled Postoperative Blood Glucose[2,7]	-	-	97%	97%
Perioperative Temperature Management[2]	348	100%	100%	100%
Prophylactic Antibiotic Selection[2]	241	96%	99%	99%
Prophylactic Antibiotic Selection (Outpatient)	21	100%	98%	98%
Prophylactic Antibiotic Stopped[2]	239	97%	99%	98%
Prophylactic Antibiotic Timing[2]	241	98%	98%	99%
Prophylactic Antibiotic Timing (Outpatient)	22	95%	98%	98%
Urinary Catheter Removal[2]	214	93%	97%	97%
Survey of Patients' Hospital Experiences				
Area Around Room 'Always' Quiet at Night	300+	54%	54%	61%
Doctors 'Always' Communicated Well	300+	78%	81%	82%
Home Recovery Information Given	300+	87%	87%	85%
Hospital Given 9 or 10 on 10 Point Scale	300+	67%	70%	71%
Meds 'Always' Explained Before Given	300+	63%	64%	64%
Nurses 'Always' Communicated Well	300+	78%	77%	79%
Pain 'Always' Well Controlled	300+	70%	70%	71%
Room and Bathroom 'Always' Clean	300+	74%	73%	73%
Timely Help 'Always' Received	300+	67%	65%	68%
Would Definitely Recommend Hospital	300+	64%	73%	71%
Use of Medical Imaging				
Cardiac Imaging Stress Test before Surgery	200	4.5%	4.3%	5.3%
Combination Abdominal CT Scan	828	6.6%	6.9%	10.5%
Combination Brain/Sinus CT Scan	505	2.2%	2.3%	2.7%
Combination Chest CT Scan	591	0.8%	1.1%	2.7%
Follow-up Mammogram/Ultrasound	962	3.3%	9.1%	8.8%
Lumbar Spine MRI for Low Back Pain	84	44.0%	37.9%	37.2%

Lake Chelan Community Hospital

503 East Highland
Chelan, WA 98816
Phone: 509-682-3300
Fax: 509-682-3475
E-mail: info@lakechelancommunityhospital.com
URL: www.lakechelancommunityhospital.com
Type: Critical Access Hospitals
Emergency Services: Yes
Ownership: Govt - Hospital Dist/Auth
Beds: 34

Key Personnel:
CEO . . . . Kevin Abel
Chief of Medical Staff . . . . Bill Cagoe
Emergency Room . . . . Karl Jonasson
Quality Assurance . . . . Pat Lemonidis
Infection Control. . . . . Lee Tinsley, RN
Anesthesiology. . . . . Mary Ann Walter

Measure	Cases	This Hosp.	State Avg.	U.S. Avg.
Blood Clot Prevention and Treatment				
Anticoagulation Overlap Therapy[7]	-	-	97%	93%
ICU Venous Thromboembolism Prophylaxis[7]	-	-	92%	92%
Incidence of Potentially Preventable VTE[7]	-	-	9%	10%
UFH with Dosages/Platelet Monitoring[7]	-	-	99%	97%
Venous Thromboembolism Prophylaxis	20	95%	86%	85%
Warfarin Therapy Discharge Instructions[7]	-	-	74%	75%
Chest Pain/Possible Heart Attack Care				
Aspirin Given Within 24 Hours of Arrival[1,3]	-	-	97%	96%
Fibrinolytic Meds Within 30 Min. of Arrival[1,3]	-	-	51%	58%
Average Time to ECG (minutes)[1,3]	-	-	9	7
Average Time to Transfer (minutes)[3,7]	-	-	54	60
Children's Asthma Care				
Received Home Management Plan of Care	-	-	-	88%
Received Reliever Medication	-	-	-	100%
Received Systemic Corticosteroids	-	-	-	100%
Emergency Department				
Admittance Decision Time (minutes)	21	24	96	98
Head CT Results Within 45 Min. of Arrival[1]	-	-	63%	57%
Patients Who Left ER Before Being Seen[5]	-	-	2%	2%
Time from ER Arrival to Admit. (minutes)	21	186	259	274
Time from ER Arrival to Discharge (minutes)[7]	-	-	135	134
Time in ER Before Being Evaluated (minutes)	90	11	22	26
Time to Pain Meds for Fractures (minutes)[1]	-	-	52	57
Heart Attack Care				
Aspirin Given at Discharge[5]	-	-	99%	99%
Fibrinolytic Meds Within 30 Min. of Arrival[5]	-	-	62%	54%
PCI Within 90 Minutes of Arrival[5]	-	-	97%	96%
Statin Prescribed at Discharge[5]	-	-	98%	98%
Heart Failure Care				
ACE Inhibitor or ARB for LVSD[3,7]	-	-	97%	97%
Discharge Instructions Given[3,7]	-	-	93%	94%
Evaluation of LVS Function[3,7]	-	-	99%	99%
Medicare Spending				
Medicare Spending per Patient (ratio)	-	-	0.91	0.98
Pneumonia Care				
Appropriate Initial Antibiotic Given[7]	-	-	96%	95%
Blood Culture Timing[7]	-	-	97%	98%
Pregnancy and Delivery Care				
Newborn Deliveries Scheduled Early[3]	13	0%	2%	6%
Preventive Care				
Immunization for Influenza	23	91%	91%	90%
Immunization for Pneumonia	43	100%	91%	92%
Stroke Care				
Anticoagulation Therapy for Atrial Fibrillation[3,7]	-	-	94%	95%
Antithrombotic Therapy Timing[3,7]	-	-	98%	98%
Assessed for Rehabilitation[1,3]	-	-	98%	97%
Discharged on Antithrombotic Therapy[1,3]	-	-	99%	99%
Discharged on Statin Medication[1,3]	-	-	96%	94%
Thrombolytic Therapy Timing[3,7]	-	-	73%	66%
Venous Thromboembolism Prophylaxis[1,3]	-	-	94%	94%
Written Stroke Educational Materials Given[1,3]	-	-	86%	88%
Surgical Care Improvement Project				
Appropriate Beta Blocker Usage[1,3]	-	-	98%	98%
Appropriate VTP Within 24 Hours[1,3]	-	-	98%	98%
Controlled Postoperative Blood Glucose[3,7]	-	-	97%	97%
Perioperative Temperature Management[3,7]	-	-	100%	100%
Prophylactic Antibiotic Selection[1,3]	-	-	99%	99%
Prophylactic Antibiotic Selection (Outpatient)[1,3]	-	-	98%	98%
Prophylactic Antibiotic Stopped[1,3]	-	-	99%	98%
Prophylactic Antibiotic Timing[1,3]	-	-	98%	99%
Prophylactic Antibiotic Timing (Outpatient)[1,3]	-	-	98%	98%
Urinary Catheter Removal[1,3]	-	-	97%	97%
Survey of Patients' Hospital Experiences				
Area Around Room 'Always' Quiet at Night[6]	<100	43%	54%	61%
Doctors 'Always' Communicated Well[6]	<100	85%	81%	82%
Home Recovery Information Given[6]	<100	91%	87%	85%
Hospital Given 9 or 10 on 10 Point Scale[6]	<100	63%	70%	71%
Meds 'Always' Explained Before Given[6]	<100	57%	64%	64%
Nurses 'Always' Communicated Well[6]	<100	79%	77%	79%
Pain 'Always' Well Controlled[6]	<100	70%	70%	71%
Room and Bathroom 'Always' Clean[6]	<100	58%	73%	73%
Timely Help 'Always' Received[6]	<100	68%	65%	68%
Would Definitely Recommend Hospital[6]	<100	68%	73%	71%
Use of Medical Imaging				
Cardiac Imaging Stress Test before Surgery[7]	-	-	4.3%	5.3%
Combination Abdominal CT Scan	76	28.9%	6.9%	10.5%
Combination Brain/Sinus CT Scan[1]	-	-	2.3%	2.7%
Combination Chest CT Scan	54	0.0%	1.1%	2.7%
Follow-up Mammogram/Ultrasound	143	6.3%	9.1%	8.8%
Lumbar Spine MRI for Low Back Pain[1]	-	-	37.9%	37.2%

Providence Saint Joseph Hospital

500 East Webster
Chewelah, WA 99109
Phone: 509-935-8211
Fax: 509-935-5257
URL: www.sjhospital.org
Type: Critical Access Hospitals
Emergency Services: Yes
Ownership: Voluntary non-profit - Church
Beds: 65

Key Personnel:
Operating Room. . . . . Diana Bryant
Quality Assurance . . . . Susan Burmeister
CEO/President. . . . . Robert Campbell
Chair/CEO . . . . Gary Livingston, MD
Infection Control. . . . . Becky Miner
Chief of Medical Staff . . . . Kirk Rowbotham, MD

Measure	Cases	This Hosp.	State Avg.	U.S. Avg.
Blood Clot Prevention and Treatment				
Anticoagulation Overlap Therapy[5]	-	-	97%	93%
ICU Venous Thromboembolism Prophylaxis[5]	-	-	92%	92%
Incidence of Potentially Preventable VTE[5]	-	-	9%	10%
UFH with Dosages/Platelet Monitoring[5]	-	-	99%	97%
Venous Thromboembolism Prophylaxis[5]	-	-	86%	85%
Warfarin Therapy Discharge Instructions[5]	-	-	74%	75%
Chest Pain/Possible Heart Attack Care				
Aspirin Given Within 24 Hours of Arrival	16	100%	97%	96%
Fibrinolytic Meds Within 30 Min. of Arrival[1]	-	-	51%	58%
Average Time to ECG (minutes)	16	8	9	7
Average Time to Transfer (minutes)[1]	-	-	54	60
Children's Asthma Care				
Received Home Management Plan of Care	-	-	-	88%
Received Reliever Medication	-	-	-	100%
Received Systemic Corticosteroids	-	-	-	100%
Emergency Department				
Admittance Decision Time (minutes)	180	36	96	98
Head CT Results Within 45 Min. of Arrival[1]	-	-	63%	57%
Patients Who Left ER Before Being Seen[5]	-	-	2%	2%

NOTE: Hospital profiles are in alphabetical order by state, then city, then hospital within the city; Rankings exclude hospitals with less than 25 cases except for patient surveys which excludes hospitals with less than 100 cases; (a) 100-299 cases; (1) The number of cases/patients is too few to report; (2) Data submitted were based on a sample of cases/patients; (3) Results are based on a shorter time period than required; (4) Data suppressed by CMS for one or more quarters; (5) Results are not available for this reporting period; (6) Fewer than 100 patients completed the HCAHPS survey; (7) No cases met the criteria for this measure; (8) The lower limit of the confidence interval cannot be calculated if the number of observed infections equals zero; (9) No data are available from the state/territory for this reporting period; (10) The scores shown reflect fewer than 50 completed surveys; (11) There were discrepancies in the data collection process; (12) This measure does not apply to this hospital for this reporting period; (13) Results cannot be calculated for this reporting period; (14) The results for this state are combined with nearby states to protect confidentiality; Please refer to the User's Guide for a full explanation of data.

Measure	Cases	This Hosp.	State Avg.	U.S. Avg.
Time from ER Arrival to Admit. (minutes)	205	158	259	274
Time from ER Arrival to Discharge (minutes)	299	114	135	134
Time in ER Before Being Evaluated (minutes)	288	29	22	26
Time to Pain Meds for Fractures (minutes)	26	44	52	57
Heart Attack Care				
Aspirin Given at Discharge[3,7]	-	-	99%	99%
Fibrinolytic Meds Within 30 Min. of Arrival[3,7]	-	-	62%	54%
PCI Within 90 Minutes of Arrival[3,7]	-	-	97%	96%
Statin Prescribed at Discharge[3,7]	-	-	98%	98%
Heart Failure Care				
ACE Inhibitor or ARB for LVSD[1]	-	-	97%	97%
Discharge Instructions Given[1]	-	-	93%	94%
Evaluation of LVS Function[1]	-	-	99%	99%
Medicare Spending				
Medicare Spending per Patient (ratio)	-	-	0.91	0.98
Pneumonia Care				
Appropriate Initial Antibiotic Given	21	95%	96%	95%
Blood Culture Timing	23	100%	97%	98%
Pregnancy and Delivery Care				
Newborn Deliveries Scheduled Early[5]	-	-	2%	6%
Preventive Care				
Immunization for Influenza	160	96%	91%	90%
Immunization for Pneumonia	239	95%	91%	92%
Stroke Care				
Anticoagulation Therapy for Atrial Fibrillation[5]	-	-	94%	95%
Antithrombotic Therapy Timing[5]	-	-	98%	98%
Assessed for Rehabilitation[5]	-	-	98%	97%
Discharged on Antithrombotic Therapy[5]	-	-	99%	99%
Discharged on Statin Medication[5]	-	-	96%	94%
Thrombolytic Therapy Timing[5]	-	-	73%	66%
Venous Thromboembolism Prophylaxis[5]	-	-	94%	94%
Written Stroke Educational Materials Given[5]	-	-	86%	88%
Surgical Care Improvement Project				
Appropriate Beta Blocker Usage[5]	-	-	98%	98%
Appropriate VTP Within 24 Hours[5]	-	-	98%	98%
Controlled Postoperative Blood Glucose[5]	-	-	97%	97%
Perioperative Temperature Management[5]	-	-	100%	100%
Prophylactic Antibiotic Selection[5]	-	-	99%	99%
Prophylactic Antibiotic Selection (Outpatient)[1]	-	-	98%	98%
Prophylactic Antibiotic Stopped[5]	-	-	99%	98%
Prophylactic Antibiotic Timing[5]	-	-	98%	99%
Prophylactic Antibiotic Timing (Outpatient)[1]	-	-	98%	98%
Urinary Catheter Removal[5]	-	-	97%	97%
Survey of Patients' Hospital Experiences				
Area Around Room 'Always' Quiet at Night[6]	<100	60%	54%	61%
Doctors 'Always' Communicated Well[6]	<100	87%	81%	82%
Home Recovery Information Given[6]	<100	90%	87%	85%
Hospital Given 9 or 10 on 10 Point Scale[6]	<100	76%	70%	71%
Meds 'Always' Explained Before Given[6]	<100	72%	64%	64%
Nurses 'Always' Communicated Well[6]	<100	82%	77%	79%
Pain 'Always' Well Controlled[6]	<100	78%	70%	71%
Room and Bathroom 'Always' Clean[6]	<100	72%	73%	73%
Timely Help 'Always' Received[6]	<100	73%	65%	68%
Would Definitely Recommend Hospital[6]	<100	74%	73%	71%
Use of Medical Imaging				
Cardiac Imaging Stress Test before Surgery[7]	-	-	4.3%	5.3%
Combination Abdominal CT Scan	212	1.4%	6.9%	10.5%
Combination Brain/Sinus CT Scan	188	5.9%	2.3%	2.7%
Combination Chest CT Scan	126	0.0%	1.1%	2.7%
Follow-up Mammogram/Ultrasound	103	12.6%	9.1%	8.8%
Lumbar Spine MRI for Low Back Pain[1]	-	-	37.9%	37.2%

Tri - State Memorial Hospital

1221 Highland Avenue — Phone: 509-758-5511
Clarkston, WA 99403 — Fax: 509-758-3566
E-mail: triadmin@clarkston.com
URL: www.tristatehospital.org
Type: Critical Access Hospitals — Emergency Services: Yes
Ownership: Voluntary non-profit - Private — Beds: 25

Key Personnel:
Quality Assurance . . . . Sharon Cooper
Intensive Care Unit. . . . . Kalene Gatz, RN
Operating Room. . . . . Diane Loseth
Infection Control. . . . . Tenna Pennick-Sutton
Radiology. . . . . Gary Pritchett
CEO/President. . . . . Donald J Wee
Chief of Medical Staff. . . . . Kim Wilson, MD

Measure	Cases	This Hosp.	State Avg.	U.S. Avg.
Blood Clot Prevention and Treatment				
Anticoagulation Overlap Therapy[5]	-	-	97%	93%
ICU Venous Thromboembolism Prophylaxis[5]	-	-	92%	92%
Incidence of Potentially Preventable VTE[5]	-	-	9%	10%
UFH with Dosages/Platelet Monitoring[5]	-	-	99%	97%
Venous Thromboembolism Prophylaxis[5]	-	-	86%	85%
Warfarin Therapy Discharge Instructions[5]	-	-	74%	75%
Chest Pain/Possible Heart Attack Care				
Aspirin Given Within 24 Hours of Arrival	41	98%	97%	96%
Fibrinolytic Meds Within 30 Min. of Arrival[1]	-	-	51%	58%
Average Time to ECG (minutes)	45	3	9	7
Average Time to Transfer (minutes)[1]	-	-	54	60
Children's Asthma Care				
Received Home Management Plan of Care	-	-	-	88%
Received Reliever Medication	-	-	-	100%
Received Systemic Corticosteroids	-	-	-	100%
Emergency Department				
Admittance Decision Time (minutes)[5]	-	-	96	98
Head CT Results Within 45 Min. of Arrival[5]	-	-	63%	57%
Patients Who Left ER Before Being Seen[5]	-	-	2%	2%
Time from ER Arrival to Admit. (minutes)[5]	-	-	259	274
Time from ER Arrival to Discharge (minutes)[5]	-	-	135	134
Time in ER Before Being Evaluated (minutes)[5]	-	-	22	26
Time to Pain Meds for Fractures (minutes)[5]	-	-	52	57
Heart Attack Care				
Aspirin Given at Discharge[3,7]	-	-	99%	99%
Fibrinolytic Meds Within 30 Min. of Arrival[3,7]	-	-	62%	54%
PCI Within 90 Minutes of Arrival[3,7]	-	-	97%	96%
Statin Prescribed at Discharge[3,7]	-	-	98%	98%
Heart Failure Care				
ACE Inhibitor or ARB for LVSD	12	83%	97%	97%
Discharge Instructions Given	25	88%	93%	94%
Evaluation of LVS Function	38	92%	99%	99%
Medicare Spending				
Medicare Spending per Patient (ratio)	-	-	0.91	0.98
Pneumonia Care				
Appropriate Initial Antibiotic Given	46	93%	96%	95%
Blood Culture Timing	81	100%	97%	98%
Pregnancy and Delivery Care				
Newborn Deliveries Scheduled Early[5]	-	-	2%	6%
Preventive Care				
Immunization for Influenza[5]	-	-	91%	90%
Immunization for Pneumonia[5]	-	-	91%	92%
Stroke Care				
Anticoagulation Therapy for Atrial Fibrillation[5]	-	-	94%	95%
Antithrombotic Therapy Timing[5]	-	-	98%	98%
Assessed for Rehabilitation[5]	-	-	98%	97%
Discharged on Antithrombotic Therapy[5]	-	-	99%	99%
Discharged on Statin Medication[5]	-	-	96%	94%
Thrombolytic Therapy Timing[5]	-	-	73%	66%
Venous Thromboembolism Prophylaxis[5]	-	-	94%	94%
Written Stroke Educational Materials Given[5]	-	-	86%	88%
Surgical Care Improvement Project				
Appropriate Beta Blocker Usage[2]	16	100%	98%	98%
Appropriate VTP Within 24 Hours[2]	164	99%	98%	98%
Controlled Postoperative Blood Glucose[2,7]	-	-	97%	97%
Perioperative Temperature Management[2]	188	99%	100%	100%
Prophylactic Antibiotic Selection[2]	132	98%	99%	99%
Prophylactic Antibiotic Selection (Outpatient)	82	94%	98%	98%
Prophylactic Antibiotic Stopped[2]	132	99%	99%	98%
Prophylactic Antibiotic Timing[2]	133	98%	98%	99%
Prophylactic Antibiotic Timing (Outpatient)	84	98%	98%	98%
Urinary Catheter Removal[2]	152	97%	97%	97%
Survey of Patients' Hospital Experiences				
Area Around Room 'Always' Quiet at Night	300+	49%	54%	61%
Doctors 'Always' Communicated Well	300+	79%	81%	82%
Home Recovery Information Given	300+	87%	87%	85%
Hospital Given 9 or 10 on 10 Point Scale	300+	74%	70%	71%
Meds 'Always' Explained Before Given	300+	66%	64%	64%
Nurses 'Always' Communicated Well	300+	78%	77%	79%
Pain 'Always' Well Controlled	300+	72%	70%	71%
Room and Bathroom 'Always' Clean	300+	78%	73%	73%
Timely Help 'Always' Received	300+	75%	65%	68%
Would Definitely Recommend Hospital	300+	79%	73%	71%
Use of Medical Imaging				
Cardiac Imaging Stress Test before Surgery[7]	-	-	4.3%	5.3%
Combination Abdominal CT Scan	496	9.3%	6.9%	10.5%
Combination Brain/Sinus CT Scan	349	1.1%	2.3%	2.7%
Combination Chest CT Scan	282	1.1%	1.1%	2.7%
Follow-up Mammogram/Ultrasound	992	14.7%	9.1%	8.8%
Lumbar Spine MRI for Low Back Pain	94	42.6%	37.9%	37.2%

Whitman Hospital & Medical Center

1200 West Fairview — Phone: 509-397-3435
Colfax, WA 99111
URL: www.whitmanhospital.com
Type: Critical Access Hospitals — Emergency Services: Yes
Ownership: Physician

Measure	Cases	This Hosp.	State Avg.	U.S. Avg.
Blood Clot Prevention and Treatment				
Anticoagulation Overlap Therapy[5]	-	-	97%	93%
ICU Venous Thromboembolism Prophylaxis[5]	-	-	92%	92%
Incidence of Potentially Preventable VTE[5]	-	-	9%	10%
UFH with Dosages/Platelet Monitoring[5]	-	-	99%	97%
Venous Thromboembolism Prophylaxis[5]	-	-	86%	85%
Warfarin Therapy Discharge Instructions[5]	-	-	74%	75%
Chest Pain/Possible Heart Attack Care				
Aspirin Given Within 24 Hours of Arrival	-	-	97%	96%
Fibrinolytic Meds Within 30 Min. of Arrival	-	-	51%	58%
Average Time to ECG (minutes)	-	-	9	7
Average Time to Transfer (minutes)	-	-	54	60
Children's Asthma Care				
Received Home Management Plan of Care	-	-	-	88%
Received Reliever Medication	-	-	-	100%
Received Systemic Corticosteroids	-	-	-	100%
Emergency Department				
Admittance Decision Time (minutes)[5]	-	-	96	98
Head CT Results Within 45 Min. of Arrival	-	-	63%	57%
Patients Who Left ER Before Being Seen	-	-	2%	2%
Time from ER Arrival to Admit. (minutes)[5]	-	-	259	274
Time from ER Arrival to Discharge (minutes)	-	-	135	134
Time in ER Before Being Evaluated (minutes)	-	-	22	26
Time to Pain Meds for Fractures (minutes)	-	-	52	57
Heart Attack Care				
Aspirin Given at Discharge[3,7]	-	-	99%	99%
Fibrinolytic Meds Within 30 Min. of Arrival[3,7]	-	-	62%	54%
PCI Within 90 Minutes of Arrival[3,7]	-	-	97%	96%
Statin Prescribed at Discharge[1,3]	-	-	98%	98%
Heart Failure Care				
ACE Inhibitor or ARB for LVSD[1]	-	-	97%	97%
Discharge Instructions Given[1]	-	-	93%	94%
Evaluation of LVS Function[1]	-	-	99%	99%
Medicare Spending				
Medicare Spending per Patient (ratio)	-	-	0.91	0.98
Pneumonia Care				
Appropriate Initial Antibiotic Given	29	97%	96%	95%
Blood Culture Timing	18	100%	97%	98%
Pregnancy and Delivery Care				
Newborn Deliveries Scheduled Early[5]	-	-	2%	6%
Preventive Care				
Immunization for Influenza[5]	-	-	91%	90%
Immunization for Pneumonia[5]	-	-	91%	92%
Stroke Care				
Anticoagulation Therapy for Atrial Fibrillation[5]	-	-	94%	95%
Antithrombotic Therapy Timing[5]	-	-	98%	98%
Assessed for Rehabilitation[5]	-	-	98%	97%
Discharged on Antithrombotic Therapy[5]	-	-	99%	99%
Discharged on Statin Medication[5]	-	-	96%	94%
Thrombolytic Therapy Timing[5]	-	-	73%	66%
Venous Thromboembolism Prophylaxis[5]	-	-	94%	94%
Written Stroke Educational Materials Given[5]	-	-	86%	88%

NOTE: Hospital profiles are in alphabetical order by state, then city, then hospital within the city; Rankings exclude hospitals with less than 25 cases except for patient surveys which excludes hospitals with less than 100 cases; (a) 100-299 cases; (1) The number of cases/patients is too few to report; (2) Data submitted were based on a sample of cases/patients; (3) Results are based on a shorter time period than required; (4) Data suppressed by CMS for one or more quarters; (5) Results are not available for this reporting period; (6) Fewer than 100 patients completed the HCAHPS survey; (7) No cases met the criteria for this measure; (8) The lower limit of the confidence interval cannot be calculated if the number of observed infections equals zero; (9) No data are available from the state/territory for this reporting period; (10) The scores shown reflect fewer than 50 completed surveys; (11) There were discrepancies in the data collection process; (12) This measure does not apply to this hospital for this reporting period; (13) Results cannot be calculated for this reporting period; (14) The results for this state are combined with nearby states to protect confidentiality; Please refer to the User's Guide for a full explanation of data.

Measure	Cases	This Hosp.	State Avg.	U.S. Avg.
Surgical Care Improvement Project				
Appropriate Beta Blocker Usage	18	83%	98%	98%
Appropriate VTP Within 24 Hours	51	94%	98%	98%
Controlled Postoperative Blood Glucose[7]	-	-	97%	97%
Perioperative Temperature Management	57	98%	100%	100%
Prophylactic Antibiotic Selection	48	100%	99%	99%
Prophylactic Antibiotic Selection (Outpatient)	-	-	98%	98%
Prophylactic Antibiotic Stopped	47	96%	99%	98%
Prophylactic Antibiotic Timing	48	94%	98%	99%
Prophylactic Antibiotic Timing (Outpatient)	-	-	98%	98%
Urinary Catheter Removal	50	100%	97%	97%
Survey of Patients' Hospital Experiences				
Area Around Room 'Always' Quiet at Night	(a)	71%	54%	61%
Doctors 'Always' Communicated Well	(a)	91%	81%	82%
Home Recovery Information Given	(a)	93%	87%	85%
Hospital Given 9 or 10 on 10 Point Scale	(a)	90%	70%	71%
Meds 'Always' Explained Before Given	(a)	73%	64%	64%
Nurses 'Always' Communicated Well	(a)	89%	77%	79%
Pain 'Always' Well Controlled	(a)	79%	70%	71%
Room and Bathroom 'Always' Clean	(a)	84%	73%	73%
Timely Help 'Always' Received	(a)	86%	65%	68%
Would Definitely Recommend Hospital	(a)	88%	73%	71%
Use of Medical Imaging				
Cardiac Imaging Stress Test before Surgery	-	-	4.3%	5.3%
Combination Abdominal CT Scan	-	-	6.9%	10.5%
Combination Brain/Sinus CT Scan	-	-	2.3%	2.7%
Combination Chest CT Scan	-	-	1.1%	2.7%
Follow-up Mammogram/Ultrasound	-	-	9.1%	8.8%
Lumbar Spine MRI for Low Back Pain	-	-	37.9%	37.2%

Providence Mount Carmel Hospital

982 East Columbia Phone: 509-684-2561
Colville, WA 99114 Fax: 509-685-2492
URL: www.mtcarmelhospital.org
Type: Critical Access Hospitals Emergency Services: Yes
Ownership: Voluntary non-profit - Church Beds: 25

Key Personnel:
Emergency Room . . . . Lisa Barber
Quality Assurance . . . . Patty Gardener
Infection Control. . . . . Ellen Imsland
Radiology. . . . . Vivienne M Kezuka
Anesthesiology. . . . . Robin Marsh Carna
CEO/President. . . . . Gordon Mc Lean
Chief of Medical Staff. . . . . Kathleen Schuerman, DO

Measure	Cases	This Hosp.	State Avg.	U.S. Avg.
Blood Clot Prevention and Treatment				
Anticoagulation Overlap Therapy[5]	-	-	97%	93%
ICU Venous Thromboembolism Prophylaxis[5]	-	-	92%	92%
Incidence of Potentially Preventable VTE[5]	-	-	9%	10%
UFH with Dosages/Platelet Monitoring[5]	-	-	99%	97%
Venous Thromboembolism Prophylaxis[5]	-	-	86%	85%
Warfarin Therapy Discharge Instructions[5]	-	-	74%	75%
Chest Pain/Possible Heart Attack Care				
Aspirin Given Within 24 Hours of Arrival	41	100%	97%	96%
Fibrinolytic Meds Within 30 Min. of Arrival[1]	-	-	51%	58%
Average Time to ECG (minutes)	46	3	9	7
Average Time to Transfer (minutes)[1]	-	-	54	60
Children's Asthma Care				
Received Home Management Plan of Care	-	-	-	88%
Received Reliever Medication	-	-	-	100%
Received Systemic Corticosteroids	-	-	-	100%
Emergency Department				
Admittance Decision Time (minutes)[2]	253	43	96	98
Head CT Results Within 45 Min. of Arrival[1]	-	-	63%	57%
Patients Who Left ER Before Being Seen[5]	-	-	2%	2%
Time from ER Arrival to Admit. (minutes)[2]	263	186	259	274
Time from ER Arrival to Discharge (minutes)	329	127	135	134
Time in ER Before Being Evaluated (minutes)	364	13	22	26
Time to Pain Meds for Fractures (minutes)	54	47	52	57
Heart Attack Care				
Aspirin Given at Discharge[1]	-	-	99%	99%
Fibrinolytic Meds Within 30 Min. of Arrival[7]	-	-	62%	54%
PCI Within 90 Minutes of Arrival[7]	-	-	97%	96%
Statin Prescribed at Discharge[1]	-	-	98%	98%

Measure	Cases	This Hosp.	State Avg.	U.S. Avg.
Heart Failure Care				
ACE Inhibitor or ARB for LVSD	11	82%	97%	97%
Discharge Instructions Given	27	93%	93%	94%
Evaluation of LVS Function	34	100%	99%	99%
Medicare Spending				
Medicare Spending per Patient (ratio)	-	-	0.91	0.98
Pneumonia Care				
Appropriate Initial Antibiotic Given	47	94%	96%	95%
Blood Culture Timing	69	100%	97%	98%
Pregnancy and Delivery Care				
Newborn Deliveries Scheduled Early[5]	-	-	2%	6%
Preventive Care				
Immunization for Influenza[2]	253	98%	91%	90%
Immunization for Pneumonia[2]	305	97%	91%	92%
Stroke Care				
Anticoagulation Therapy for Atrial Fibrillation[5]	-	-	94%	95%
Antithrombotic Therapy Timing[5]	-	-	98%	98%
Assessed for Rehabilitation[5]	-	-	98%	97%
Discharged on Antithrombotic Therapy[5]	-	-	99%	99%
Discharged on Statin Medication[5]	-	-	96%	94%
Thrombolytic Therapy Timing[5]	-	-	73%	66%
Venous Thromboembolism Prophylaxis[5]	-	-	94%	94%
Written Stroke Educational Materials Given[5]	-	-	86%	88%
Surgical Care Improvement Project				
Appropriate Beta Blocker Usage[1,2]	-	-	98%	98%
Appropriate VTP Within 24 Hours[2]	41	93%	98%	98%
Controlled Postoperative Blood Glucose[2,7]	-	-	97%	97%
Perioperative Temperature Management[2]	44	100%	100%	100%
Prophylactic Antibiotic Selection[2]	25	100%	99%	99%
Prophylactic Antibiotic Selection (Outpatient)	37	95%	98%	98%
Prophylactic Antibiotic Stopped[2]	22	95%	99%	98%
Prophylactic Antibiotic Timing[2]	25	92%	98%	99%
Prophylactic Antibiotic Timing (Outpatient)	13	92%	98%	98%
Urinary Catheter Removal[2]	24	92%	97%	97%
Survey of Patients' Hospital Experiences				
Area Around Room 'Always' Quiet at Night	(a)	65%	54%	61%
Doctors 'Always' Communicated Well	(a)	84%	81%	82%
Home Recovery Information Given	(a)	85%	87%	85%
Hospital Given 9 or 10 on 10 Point Scale	(a)	80%	70%	71%
Meds 'Always' Explained Before Given	(a)	69%	64%	64%
Nurses 'Always' Communicated Well	(a)	81%	77%	79%
Pain 'Always' Well Controlled	(a)	72%	70%	71%
Room and Bathroom 'Always' Clean	(a)	87%	73%	73%
Timely Help 'Always' Received	(a)	72%	65%	68%
Would Definitely Recommend Hospital	(a)	79%	73%	71%
Use of Medical Imaging				
Cardiac Imaging Stress Test before Surgery	55	0.0%	4.3%	5.3%
Combination Abdominal CT Scan	293	7.8%	6.9%	10.5%
Combination Brain/Sinus CT Scan	229	0.9%	2.3%	2.7%
Combination Chest CT Scan	181	0.6%	1.1%	2.7%
Follow-up Mammogram/Ultrasound	347	15.0%	9.1%	8.8%
Lumbar Spine MRI for Low Back Pain	47	55.3%	37.9%	37.2%

Whidbey General Hospital

101 North Main Street Phone: 360-678-5151
Coupeville, WA 98239 Fax: 360-678-0945
E-mail: rhines@whidbeygen.com
URL: www.whidbeygen.org
Type: Critical Access Hospitals Emergency Services: Yes
Ownership: Govt - Hospital Dist/Auth Beds: 101

Key Personnel:
Cardiology . . . . Sujata T. Agnani, MD
Pediatrics. . . . . Gabriel W. Barrio, MD
Pediatrics. . . . . John R. Beumer, MD
Emergency Room . . . . Samir Bishai
Operating Room. . . . . Katie Carr
Radiology. . . . . Robert Hawkins
Chief of Medical Staff. . . . . D Terry Lee
CEO/President. . . . . Tom Tomasino

Measure	Cases	This Hosp.	State Avg.	U.S. Avg.
Blood Clot Prevention and Treatment				
Anticoagulation Overlap Therapy[1,2]	-	-	97%	93%
ICU Venous Thromboembolism Prophylaxis[2]	48	92%	92%	92%
Incidence of Potentially Preventable VTE[2,7]	-	-	9%	10%
UFH with Dosages/Platelet Monitoring[1,2]	-	-	99%	97%
Venous Thromboembolism Prophylaxis[2]	131	95%	86%	85%
Warfarin Therapy Discharge Instructions[1,2]	-	-	74%	75%
Chest Pain/Possible Heart Attack Care				
Aspirin Given Within 24 Hours of Arrival	-	-	97%	96%
Fibrinolytic Meds Within 30 Min. of Arrival	-	-	51%	58%
Average Time to ECG (minutes)	-	-	9	7
Average Time to Transfer (minutes)	-	-	54	60
Children's Asthma Care				
Received Home Management Plan of Care	-	-	-	88%
Received Reliever Medication	-	-	-	100%
Received Systemic Corticosteroids	-	-	-	100%
Emergency Department				
Admittance Decision Time (minutes)[2]	429	81	96	98
Head CT Results Within 45 Min. of Arrival	-	-	63%	57%
Patients Who Left ER Before Being Seen	-	-	2%	2%
Time from ER Arrival to Admit. (minutes)[2]	475	252	259	274
Time from ER Arrival to Discharge (minutes)	-	-	135	134
Time in ER Before Being Evaluated (minutes)	-	-	22	26
Time to Pain Meds for Fractures (minutes)	-	-	52	57
Heart Attack Care				
Aspirin Given at Discharge[1]	-	-	99%	99%
Fibrinolytic Meds Within 30 Min. of Arrival[7]	-	-	62%	54%
PCI Within 90 Minutes of Arrival[7]	-	-	97%	96%
Statin Prescribed at Discharge[1]	-	-	98%	98%
Heart Failure Care				
ACE Inhibitor or ARB for LVSD	13	100%	97%	97%
Discharge Instructions Given	39	79%	93%	94%
Evaluation of LVS Function	50	92%	99%	99%
Medicare Spending				
Medicare Spending per Patient (ratio)	-	-	0.91	0.98
Pneumonia Care				
Appropriate Initial Antibiotic Given	69	94%	96%	95%
Blood Culture Timing	84	96%	97%	98%
Pregnancy and Delivery Care				
Newborn Deliveries Scheduled Early[1,2]	-	-	2%	6%
Preventive Care				
Immunization for Influenza[5]	-	-	91%	90%
Immunization for Pneumonia[5]	-	-	91%	92%
Stroke Care				
Anticoagulation Therapy for Atrial Fibrillation[1]	-	-	94%	95%
Antithrombotic Therapy Timing	22	100%	98%	98%
Assessed for Rehabilitation	17	94%	98%	97%
Discharged on Antithrombotic Therapy	16	100%	99%	99%
Discharged on Statin Medication	15	87%	96%	94%
Thrombolytic Therapy Timing[7]	-	-	73%	66%
Venous Thromboembolism Prophylaxis	20	95%	94%	94%
Written Stroke Educational Materials Given[1]	-	-	86%	88%
Surgical Care Improvement Project				
Appropriate Beta Blocker Usage	33	100%	98%	98%
Appropriate VTP Within 24 Hours	126	92%	98%	98%
Controlled Postoperative Blood Glucose[7]	-	-	97%	97%
Perioperative Temperature Management	155	99%	100%	100%
Prophylactic Antibiotic Selection	129	97%	99%	99%
Prophylactic Antibiotic Selection (Outpatient)	-	-	98%	98%
Prophylactic Antibiotic Stopped	125	99%	99%	98%
Prophylactic Antibiotic Timing	129	99%	98%	99%
Prophylactic Antibiotic Timing (Outpatient)	-	-	98%	98%
Urinary Catheter Removal	119	100%	97%	97%
Survey of Patients' Hospital Experiences				
Area Around Room 'Always' Quiet at Night	300+	45%	54%	61%
Doctors 'Always' Communicated Well	300+	78%	81%	82%
Home Recovery Information Given	300+	84%	87%	85%
Hospital Given 9 or 10 on 10 Point Scale	300+	61%	70%	71%
Meds 'Always' Explained Before Given	300+	64%	64%	64%
Nurses 'Always' Communicated Well	300+	76%	77%	79%
Pain 'Always' Well Controlled	300+	67%	70%	71%
Room and Bathroom 'Always' Clean	300+	73%	73%	73%
Timely Help 'Always' Received	300+	64%	65%	68%
Would Definitely Recommend Hospital	300+	65%	73%	71%
Use of Medical Imaging				
Cardiac Imaging Stress Test before Surgery	-	-	4.3%	5.3%

NOTE: Hospital profiles are in alphabetical order by state, then city, then hospital within the city; Rankings exclude hospitals with less than 25 cases except for patient surveys which excludes hospitals with less than 100 cases; (a) 100-299 cases; (1) The number of cases/patients is too few to report; (2) Data submitted were based on a sample of cases/patients; (3) Results are based on a shorter time period than required; (4) Data suppressed by CMS for one or more quarters; (5) Results are not available for this reporting period; (6) Fewer than 100 patients completed the HCAHPS survey; (7) No cases met the criteria for this measure; (8) The lower limit of the confidence interval cannot be calculated if the number of observed infections equals zero; (9) No data are available from the state/territory for this reporting period; (10) The scores shown reflect fewer than 50 completed surveys; (11) There were discrepancies in the data collection process; (12) This measure does not apply to this hospital for this reporting period; (13) Results cannot be calculated for this reporting period; (14) The results for this state are combined with nearby states to protect confidentiality; Please refer to the User's Guide for a full explanation of data.

Measure	Cases	This Hosp.	State Avg.	U.S. Avg.
Combination Abdominal CT Scan	-	-	6.9%	10.5%
Combination Brain/Sinus CT Scan	-	-	2.3%	2.7%
Combination Chest CT Scan	-	-	1.1%	2.7%
Follow-up Mammogram/Ultrasound	-	-	9.1%	8.8%
Lumbar Spine MRI for Low Back Pain	-	-	37.9%	37.2%

Lincoln Hospital

10 Nichols Street
Davenport, WA 99122
Phone: 509-725-7101
Fax: 509-725-2112
E-mail: tmsrtin@fanrc.org
URL: www.lincolnhospital.org

Type: Critical Access Hospitals
Emergency Services: Yes
Ownership: Govt - Hospital Dist/Auth
Beds: 88

Key Personnel:

Anesthesiology. . . . . Steve Beckstrom
Infection Control. . . . . Cindy McCall
Operating Room. . . . . Cindy McCall
Emergency Room . . . . Jodie Perry, RN
Chief of Medical Staff. . . . . Frederick Reed, MD
Radiology. . . . . Jean Riendeau
Quality Assurance . . . . Marilynn Snider

Measure	Cases	This Hosp.	State Avg.	U.S. Avg.
Blood Clot Prevention and Treatment				
Anticoagulation Overlap Therapy[5]	-	-	97%	93%
ICU Venous Thromboembolism Prophylaxis[5]	-	-	92%	92%
Incidence of Potentially Preventable VTE[5]	-	-	9%	10%
UFH with Dosages/Platelet Monitoring[5]	-	-	99%	97%
Venous Thromboembolism Prophylaxis[5]	-	-	86%	85%
Warfarin Therapy Discharge Instructions[5]	-	-	74%	75%
Chest Pain/Possible Heart Attack Care				
Aspirin Given Within 24 Hours of Arrival[1,3]	-	-	97%	96%
Fibrinolytic Meds Within 30 Min. of Arrival[1,3]	-	-	51%	58%
Average Time to ECG (minutes)[1,3]	-	-	9	7
Average Time to Transfer (minutes)[1,3]	-	-	54	60
Children's Asthma Care				
Received Home Management Plan of Care	-	-	-	88%
Received Reliever Medication	-	-	-	100%
Received Systemic Corticosteroids	-	-	-	100%
Emergency Department				
Admittance Decision Time (minutes)[5]	-	-	96	98
Head CT Results Within 45 Min. of Arrival[5]	-	-	63%	57%
Patients Who Left ER Before Being Seen[5]	-	-	2%	2%
Time from ER Arrival to Admit. (minutes)[5]	-	-	259	274
Time from ER Arrival to Discharge (minutes)[5]	-	-	135	134
Time in ER Before Being Evaluated (minutes)[5]	-	-	22	26
Time to Pain Meds for Fractures (minutes)[5]	-	-	52	57
Heart Attack Care				
Aspirin Given at Discharge[3,7]	-	-	99%	99%
Fibrinolytic Meds Within 30 Min. of Arrival[3,7]	-	-	62%	54%
PCI Within 90 Minutes of Arrival[3,7]	-	-	97%	96%
Statin Prescribed at Discharge[3,7]	-	-	98%	98%
Heart Failure Care				
ACE Inhibitor or ARB for LVSD[1]	-	-	97%	97%
Discharge Instructions Given[1]	-	-	93%	94%
Evaluation of LVS Function	13	100%	99%	99%
Medicare Spending				
Medicare Spending per Patient (ratio)	-	-	0.91	0.98
Pneumonia Care				
Appropriate Initial Antibiotic Given	24	96%	96%	95%
Blood Culture Timing[1]	-	-	97%	98%
Pregnancy and Delivery Care				
Newborn Deliveries Scheduled Early[5]	-	-	2%	6%
Preventive Care				
Immunization for Influenza[5]	-	-	91%	90%
Immunization for Pneumonia[5]	-	-	91%	92%
Stroke Care				
Anticoagulation Therapy for Atrial Fibrillation[5]	-	-	94%	95%
Antithrombotic Therapy Timing[5]	-	-	98%	98%
Assessed for Rehabilitation[5]	-	-	98%	97%
Discharged on Antithrombotic Therapy[5]	-	-	99%	99%
Discharged on Statin Medication[5]	-	-	96%	94%
Thrombolytic Therapy Timing[5]	-	-	73%	66%
Venous Thromboembolism Prophylaxis[5]	-	-	94%	94%
Written Stroke Educational Materials Given[5]	-	-	86%	88%
Surgical Care Improvement Project				
Appropriate Beta Blocker Usage[1]	-	-	98%	98%
Appropriate VTP Within 24 Hours	14	100%	98%	98%
Controlled Postoperative Blood Glucose[3,7]	-	-	97%	97%
Perioperative Temperature Management	15	100%	100%	100%
Prophylactic Antibiotic Selection	12	92%	99%	99%
Prophylactic Antibiotic Selection (Outpatient)[5]	-	-	98%	98%
Prophylactic Antibiotic Stopped	12	100%	99%	98%
Prophylactic Antibiotic Timing	12	100%	98%	99%
Prophylactic Antibiotic Timing (Outpatient)[5]	-	-	98%	98%
Urinary Catheter Removal[1]	-	-	97%	97%
Survey of Patients' Hospital Experiences				
Area Around Room 'Always' Quiet at Night	(a)	51%	54%	61%
Doctors 'Always' Communicated Well	(a)	86%	81%	82%
Home Recovery Information Given	(a)	79%	87%	85%
Hospital Given 9 or 10 on 10 Point Scale	(a)	76%	70%	71%
Meds 'Always' Explained Before Given	(a)	60%	64%	64%
Nurses 'Always' Communicated Well	(a)	83%	77%	79%
Pain 'Always' Well Controlled	(a)	82%	70%	71%
Room and Bathroom 'Always' Clean	(a)	84%	73%	73%
Timely Help 'Always' Received	(a)	75%	65%	68%
Would Definitely Recommend Hospital	(a)	78%	73%	71%
Use of Medical Imaging				
Cardiac Imaging Stress Test before Surgery[7]	-	-	4.3%	5.3%
Combination Abdominal CT Scan	108	3.7%	6.9%	10.5%
Combination Brain/Sinus CT Scan[1]	-	-	2.3%	2.7%
Combination Chest CT Scan[1]	-	-	1.1%	2.7%
Follow-up Mammogram/Ultrasound	211	5.7%	9.1%	8.8%
Lumbar Spine MRI for Low Back Pain[1]	-	-	37.9%	37.2%

Dayton General Hospital

1012 South 3rd Street
Dayton, WA 99328
Phone: 509-382-2531

Type: Critical Access Hospitals
Emergency Services: Yes
Ownership: Govt - Hospital Dist/Auth

Measure	Cases	This Hosp.	State Avg.	U.S. Avg.
Blood Clot Prevention and Treatment				
Anticoagulation Overlap Therapy[5]	-	-	97%	93%
ICU Venous Thromboembolism Prophylaxis[5]	-	-	92%	92%
Incidence of Potentially Preventable VTE[5]	-	-	9%	10%
UFH with Dosages/Platelet Monitoring[5]	-	-	99%	97%
Venous Thromboembolism Prophylaxis[5]	-	-	86%	85%
Warfarin Therapy Discharge Instructions[5]	-	-	74%	75%
Chest Pain/Possible Heart Attack Care				
Aspirin Given Within 24 Hours of Arrival[1,3]	-	-	97%	96%
Fibrinolytic Meds Within 30 Min. of Arrival[3,7]	-	-	51%	58%
Average Time to ECG (minutes)[1,3]	-	-	9	7
Average Time to Transfer (minutes)[1,3]	-	-	54	60
Children's Asthma Care				
Received Home Management Plan of Care	-	-	-	88%
Received Reliever Medication	-	-	-	100%
Received Systemic Corticosteroids	-	-	-	100%
Emergency Department				
Admittance Decision Time (minutes)[5]	-	-	96	98
Head CT Results Within 45 Min. of Arrival[5]	-	-	63%	57%
Patients Who Left ER Before Being Seen[5]	-	-	2%	2%
Time from ER Arrival to Admit. (minutes)[5]	-	-	259	274
Time from ER Arrival to Discharge (minutes)[5]	-	-	135	134
Time in ER Before Being Evaluated (minutes)[5]	-	-	22	26
Time to Pain Meds for Fractures (minutes)[5]	-	-	52	57
Heart Attack Care				
Aspirin Given at Discharge[5]	-	-	99%	99%
Fibrinolytic Meds Within 30 Min. of Arrival[5]	-	-	62%	54%
PCI Within 90 Minutes of Arrival[5]	-	-	97%	96%
Statin Prescribed at Discharge[5]	-	-	98%	98%
Heart Failure Care				
ACE Inhibitor or ARB for LVSD[7]	-	-	97%	97%
Discharge Instructions Given[1]	-	-	93%	94%
Evaluation of LVS Function[1]	-	-	99%	99%
Medicare Spending				
Medicare Spending per Patient (ratio)	-	-	0.91	0.98
Pneumonia Care				
Appropriate Initial Antibiotic Given[1,3]	-	-	96%	95%
Blood Culture Timing[1,3]	-	-	97%	98%
Pregnancy and Delivery Care				
Newborn Deliveries Scheduled Early[5]	-	-	2%	6%
Preventive Care				
Immunization for Influenza[5]	-	-	91%	90%
Immunization for Pneumonia[5]	-	-	91%	92%
Stroke Care				
Anticoagulation Therapy for Atrial Fibrillation[5]	-	-	94%	95%
Antithrombotic Therapy Timing[5]	-	-	98%	98%
Assessed for Rehabilitation[5]	-	-	98%	97%
Discharged on Antithrombotic Therapy[5]	-	-	99%	99%
Discharged on Statin Medication[5]	-	-	96%	94%
Thrombolytic Therapy Timing[5]	-	-	73%	66%
Venous Thromboembolism Prophylaxis[5]	-	-	94%	94%
Written Stroke Educational Materials Given[5]	-	-	86%	88%
Surgical Care Improvement Project				
Appropriate Beta Blocker Usage[5]	-	-	98%	98%
Appropriate VTP Within 24 Hours[5]	-	-	98%	98%
Controlled Postoperative Blood Glucose[5]	-	-	97%	97%
Perioperative Temperature Management[5]	-	-	100%	100%
Prophylactic Antibiotic Selection[5]	-	-	99%	99%
Prophylactic Antibiotic Selection (Outpatient)[5]	-	-	98%	98%
Prophylactic Antibiotic Stopped[5]	-	-	99%	98%
Prophylactic Antibiotic Timing[5]	-	-	98%	99%
Prophylactic Antibiotic Timing (Outpatient)[5]	-	-	98%	98%
Urinary Catheter Removal[5]	-	-	97%	97%
Survey of Patients' Hospital Experiences				
Area Around Room 'Always' Quiet at Night[10]	<100	54%	54%	61%
Doctors 'Always' Communicated Well[10]	<100	91%	81%	82%
Home Recovery Information Given[10]	<100	89%	87%	85%
Hospital Given 9 or 10 on 10 Point Scale[10]	<100	70%	70%	71%
Meds 'Always' Explained Before Given[10]	<100	92%	64%	64%
Nurses 'Always' Communicated Well[10]	<100	85%	77%	79%
Pain 'Always' Well Controlled[10]	<100	78%	70%	71%
Room and Bathroom 'Always' Clean[10]	<100	75%	73%	73%
Timely Help 'Always' Received[10]	<100	80%	65%	68%
Would Definitely Recommend Hospital[10]	<100	78%	73%	71%
Use of Medical Imaging				
Cardiac Imaging Stress Test before Surgery[7]	-	-	4.3%	5.3%
Combination Abdominal CT Scan[1]	-	-	6.9%	10.5%
Combination Brain/Sinus CT Scan[1]	-	-	2.3%	2.7%
Combination Chest CT Scan[1]	-	-	1.1%	2.7%
Follow-up Mammogram/Ultrasound[7]	-	-	9.1%	8.8%
Lumbar Spine MRI for Low Back Pain[1]	-	-	37.9%	37.2%

Swedish Edmonds Hospital

21601 76th Avenue West
Edmonds, WA 98026
Phone: 425-640-4000
Fax: 425-640-4010
URL: www.stevenshealthcare.org

Type: Acute Care Hospitals
Emergency Services: Yes
Ownership: Voluntary non-profit - Private
Beds: 217

Key Personnel:

Radiology. . . . . Jane Barry
Pediatric Ambulatory Care . . . . . . T Ray Cardwell, MD
Pediatric In-Patient Care . . . . T Ray Cardwell, MD
CEO/President. . . . . Michael C Carter, MD
Operating Room. . . . . Sheri Grigg, RN
Quality Assurance . . . . Lorie Kelly
Chief of Medical Staff. . . . . Timothy Roddy, MD

Measure	Cases	This Hosp.	State Avg.	U.S. Avg.
Blood Clot Prevention and Treatment				
Anticoagulation Overlap Therapy[2]	64	95%	97%	93%
ICU Venous Thromboembolism Prophylaxis[2]	45	89%	92%	92%
Incidence of Potentially Preventable VTE[1,2]	-	-	9%	10%
UFH with Dosages/Platelet Monitoring[2]	38	100%	99%	97%
Venous Thromboembolism Prophylaxis[2]	296	87%	86%	85%
Warfarin Therapy Discharge Instructions[2]	53	0%	74%	75%
Chest Pain/Possible Heart Attack Care				
Aspirin Given Within 24 Hours of Arrival	18	94%	97%	96%
Fibrinolytic Meds Within 30 Min. of Arrival[3,7]	-	-	51%	58%
Average Time to ECG (minutes)	18	7	9	7
Average Time to Transfer (minutes)[3,7]	-	-	54	60
Children's Asthma Care				

NOTE: *Hospital profiles are in alphabetical order by state, then city, then hospital within the city; Rankings exclude hospitals with less than 25 cases except for patient surveys which excludes hospitals with less than 100 cases; (a) 100-299 cases; (1) The number of cases/patients is too few to report; (2) Data submitted were based on a sample of cases/patients; (3) Results are based on a shorter time period than required; (4) Data suppressed by CMS for one or more quarters; (5) Results are not available for this reporting period; (6) Fewer than 100 patients completed the HCAHPS survey; (7) No cases met the criteria for this measure; (8) The lower limit of the confidence interval cannot be calculated if the number of observed infections equals zero; (9) No data are available from the state/territory for this reporting period; (10) The scores shown reflect fewer than 50 completed surveys; (11) There were discrepancies in the data collection process; (12) This measure does not apply to this hospital for this reporting period; (13) Results cannot be calculated for this reporting period; (14) The results for this state are combined with nearby states to protect confidentiality; Please refer to the User's Guide for a full explanation of data.*

Measure	Cases	This Hosp.	State Avg.	U.S. Avg.
Received Home Management Plan of Care	-	-	-	88%
Received Reliever Medication	-	-	-	100%
Received Systemic Corticosteroids	-	-	-	100%
Emergency Department				
Admittance Decision Time (minutes)[2]	548	129	96	98
Head CT Results Within 45 Min. of Arrival	18	67%	63%	57%
Patients Who Left ER Before Being Seen	41,092	1%	2%	2%
Time from ER Arrival to Admit. (minutes)[2]	549	287	259	274
Time from ER Arrival to Discharge (minutes)	371	138	135	134
Time in ER Before Being Evaluated (minutes)	279	11	22	26
Time to Pain Meds for Fractures (minutes)	167	34	52	57
Heart Attack Care				
Aspirin Given at Discharge	182	95%	99%	99%
Fibrinolytic Meds Within 30 Min. of Arrival[7]	-	-	62%	54%
PCI Within 90 Minutes of Arrival	58	95%	97%	96%
Statin Prescribed at Discharge	175	93%	98%	98%
Heart Failure Care				
ACE Inhibitor or ARB for LVSD	77	97%	97%	97%
Discharge Instructions Given	147	82%	93%	94%
Evaluation of LVS Function	170	100%	99%	99%
Medicare Spending				
Medicare Spending per Patient (ratio)	-	0.98	0.91	0.98
Pneumonia Care				
Appropriate Initial Antibiotic Given	158	99%	96%	95%
Blood Culture Timing	216	95%	97%	98%
Pregnancy and Delivery Care				
Newborn Deliveries Scheduled Early	91	1%	2%	6%
Preventive Care				
Immunization for Influenza[2]	519	90%	91%	90%
Immunization for Pneumonia[2]	601	88%	91%	92%
Stroke Care				
Anticoagulation Therapy for Atrial Fibrillation	18	100%	94%	95%
Antithrombotic Therapy Timing	108	99%	98%	98%
Assessed for Rehabilitation	123	100%	98%	97%
Discharged on Antithrombotic Therapy	122	99%	99%	99%
Discharged on Statin Medication	87	97%	96%	94%
Thrombolytic Therapy Timing	11	100%	73%	66%
Venous Thromboembolism Prophylaxis	116	90%	94%	94%
Written Stroke Educational Materials Given	79	89%	86%	88%
Surgical Care Improvement Project				
Appropriate Beta Blocker Usage	140	95%	98%	98%
Appropriate VTP Within 24 Hours	527	97%	98%	98%
Controlled Postoperative Blood Glucose[7]	-	-	97%	97%
Perioperative Temperature Management	652	100%	100%	100%
Prophylactic Antibiotic Selection	371	98%	99%	99%
Prophylactic Antibiotic Selection (Outpatient)	146	96%	98%	98%
Prophylactic Antibiotic Stopped	365	96%	99%	98%
Prophylactic Antibiotic Timing	371	99%	98%	99%
Prophylactic Antibiotic Timing (Outpatient)	147	97%	98%	98%
Urinary Catheter Removal	350	95%	97%	97%
Survey of Patients' Hospital Experiences				
Area Around Room 'Always' Quiet at Night	300+	48%	54%	61%
Doctors 'Always' Communicated Well	300+	77%	81%	82%
Home Recovery Information Given	300+	84%	87%	85%
Hospital Given 9 or 10 on 10 Point Scale	300+	59%	70%	71%
Meds 'Always' Explained Before Given	300+	61%	64%	64%
Nurses 'Always' Communicated Well	300+	72%	77%	79%
Pain 'Always' Well Controlled	300+	67%	70%	71%
Room and Bathroom 'Always' Clean	300+	65%	73%	73%
Timely Help 'Always' Received	300+	57%	65%	68%
Would Definitely Recommend Hospital	300+	63%	73%	71%
Use of Medical Imaging				
Cardiac Imaging Stress Test before Surgery	544	4.2%	4.3%	5.3%
Combination Abdominal CT Scan	603	3.2%	6.9%	10.5%
Combination Brain/Sinus CT Scan	609	1.8%	2.3%	2.7%
Combination Chest CT Scan	345	0.9%	1.1%	2.7%
Follow-up Mammogram/Ultrasound	1,350	8.6%	9.1%	8.8%
Lumbar Spine MRI for Low Back Pain[1]	-	-	37.9%	37.2%

Kittitas Valley Community Hospital

603 South Chestnut
Ellensburg, WA 98926
URL: www.kvch.com
Type: Critical Access Hospitals
Ownership: Govt - Hospital Dist/Auth
Phone: 509-962-9841
Fax: 509-925-8485
Emergency Services: Yes
Beds: 25

Key Personnel:
Radiology.................. Sharon Davis
Patient Relations .... Rhonda Holden
Emergency Room .... Jack Horsley
Chief of Medical Staff.......... Robert G Johnson Jr, MD
Intensive Care Unit............ Vicki Machorro
CEO .... Paul Nurick
Quality Assurance .... Andrea Sciaudone
Operating Room.............. Lois Welke, RN

Measure	Cases	This Hosp.	State Avg.	U.S. Avg.
Blood Clot Prevention and Treatment				
Anticoagulation Overlap Therapy[1,2]	-	-	97%	93%
ICU Venous Thromboembolism Prophylaxis[2]	23	96%	92%	92%
Incidence of Potentially Preventable VTE[2,7]	-	-	9%	10%
UFH with Dosages/Platelet Monitoring[1,2]	-	-	99%	97%
Venous Thromboembolism Prophylaxis[2]	170	90%	86%	85%
Warfarin Therapy Discharge Instructions[1,2]	-	-	74%	75%
Chest Pain/Possible Heart Attack Care				
Aspirin Given Within 24 Hours of Arrival	34	100%	97%	96%
Fibrinolytic Meds Within 30 Min. of Arrival[7]	-	-	51%	58%
Average Time to ECG (minutes)	37	3	9	7
Average Time to Transfer (minutes)[1]	-	-	54	60
Children's Asthma Care				
Received Home Management Plan of Care	-	-	-	88%
Received Reliever Medication	-	-	-	100%
Received Systemic Corticosteroids	-	-	-	100%
Emergency Department				
Admittance Decision Time (minutes)[5]	-	-	96	98
Head CT Results Within 45 Min. of Arrival	14	100%	63%	57%
Patients Who Left ER Before Being Seen	11,935	1%	2%	2%
Time from ER Arrival to Admit. (minutes)[5]	-	-	259	274
Time from ER Arrival to Discharge (minutes)[5]	-	-	135	134
Time in ER Before Being Evaluated (minutes)[5]	-	-	22	26
Time to Pain Meds for Fractures (minutes)	73	44	52	57
Heart Attack Care				
Aspirin Given at Discharge[1,3]	-	-	99%	99%
Fibrinolytic Meds Within 30 Min. of Arrival[3,7]	-	-	62%	54%
PCI Within 90 Minutes of Arrival[3,7]	-	-	97%	96%
Statin Prescribed at Discharge[1,3]	-	-	98%	98%
Heart Failure Care				
ACE Inhibitor or ARB for LVSD[1,3]	-	-	97%	97%
Discharge Instructions Given[3]	12	100%	93%	94%
Evaluation of LVS Function[3]	13	100%	99%	99%
Medicare Spending				
Medicare Spending per Patient (ratio)	-	-	0.91	0.98
Pneumonia Care				
Appropriate Initial Antibiotic Given[3]	14	100%	96%	95%
Blood Culture Timing[3]	36	100%	97%	98%
Pregnancy and Delivery Care				
Newborn Deliveries Scheduled Early[5]	-	-	2%	6%
Preventive Care				
Immunization for Influenza[2,3]	112	99%	91%	90%
Immunization for Pneumonia[2,3]	173	94%	91%	92%
Stroke Care				
Anticoagulation Therapy for Atrial Fibrillation[1,3]	-	-	94%	95%
Antithrombotic Therapy Timing[1,3]	-	-	98%	98%
Assessed for Rehabilitation[1,3]	-	-	98%	97%
Discharged on Antithrombotic Therapy[1,3]	-	-	99%	99%
Discharged on Statin Medication[1,3]	-	-	96%	94%
Thrombolytic Therapy Timing[3,7]	-	-	73%	66%
Venous Thromboembolism Prophylaxis[1,3]	-	-	94%	94%
Written Stroke Educational Materials Given[1,3]	-	-	86%	88%
Surgical Care Improvement Project				
Appropriate Beta Blocker Usage[3]	23	100%	98%	98%
Appropriate VTP Within 24 Hours[3]	93	97%	98%	98%
Controlled Postoperative Blood Glucose[3,7]	-	-	97%	97%
Perioperative Temperature Management[3]	110	100%	100%	100%
Prophylactic Antibiotic Selection[3]	92	99%	99%	99%
Prophylactic Antibiotic Selection (Outpatient)[1]	-	-	98%	98%
Prophylactic Antibiotic Stopped[3]	90	99%	99%	98%
Prophylactic Antibiotic Timing[3]	92	100%	98%	99%
Prophylactic Antibiotic Timing (Outpatient)[1]	-	-	98%	98%
Urinary Catheter Removal[3]	84	100%	97%	97%
Survey of Patients' Hospital Experiences				
Area Around Room 'Always' Quiet at Night	(a)	66%	54%	61%
Doctors 'Always' Communicated Well	(a)	82%	81%	82%
Home Recovery Information Given	(a)	91%	87%	85%
Hospital Given 9 or 10 on 10 Point Scale	(a)	76%	70%	71%
Meds 'Always' Explained Before Given	(a)	65%	64%	64%
Nurses 'Always' Communicated Well	(a)	79%	77%	79%
Pain 'Always' Well Controlled	(a)	70%	70%	71%
Room and Bathroom 'Always' Clean	(a)	76%	73%	73%
Timely Help 'Always' Received	(a)	75%	65%	68%
Would Definitely Recommend Hospital	(a)	73%	73%	71%
Use of Medical Imaging				
Cardiac Imaging Stress Test before Surgery	90	2.2%	4.3%	5.3%
Combination Abdominal CT Scan	397	2.8%	6.9%	10.5%
Combination Brain/Sinus CT Scan[1]	-	-	2.3%	2.7%
Combination Chest CT Scan	186	0.0%	1.1%	2.7%
Follow-up Mammogram/Ultrasound	601	9.3%	9.1%	8.8%
Lumbar Spine MRI for Low Back Pain	62	43.5%	37.9%	37.2%

Summit Pacific Medical Center

600 East Main Street
Elma, WA 98541
Type: Critical Access Hospitals
Ownership: Govt - Hospital Dist/Auth
Phone: 360-346-2222
Fax: 360-495-4566
Emergency Services: Yes
Beds: 24

Key Personnel:
Emergency Room .... Robert Billings, MD
CEO/President.............. Georgett Hiles
Chief of Medical Staff.......... Edward Macke, MD

Measure	Cases	This Hosp.	State Avg.	U.S. Avg.
Blood Clot Prevention and Treatment				
Anticoagulation Overlap Therapy[5]	-	-	97%	93%
ICU Venous Thromboembolism Prophylaxis[5]	-	-	92%	92%
Incidence of Potentially Preventable VTE[5]	-	-	9%	10%
UFH with Dosages/Platelet Monitoring[5]	-	-	99%	97%
Venous Thromboembolism Prophylaxis[5]	-	-	86%	85%
Warfarin Therapy Discharge Instructions[5]	-	-	74%	75%
Chest Pain/Possible Heart Attack Care				
Aspirin Given Within 24 Hours of Arrival[3]	11	100%	97%	96%
Fibrinolytic Meds Within 30 Min. of Arrival[5]	-	-	51%	58%
Average Time to ECG (minutes)[3]	11	6	9	7
Average Time to Transfer (minutes)[5]	-	-	54	60
Children's Asthma Care				
Received Home Management Plan of Care	-	-	-	88%
Received Reliever Medication	-	-	-	100%
Received Systemic Corticosteroids	-	-	-	100%
Emergency Department				
Admittance Decision Time (minutes)[5]	-	-	96	98
Head CT Results Within 45 Min. of Arrival[1,3]	-	-	63%	57%
Patients Who Left ER Before Being Seen[5]	-	-	2%	2%
Time from ER Arrival to Admit. (minutes)[5]	-	-	259	274
Time from ER Arrival to Discharge (minutes)[5]	-	-	135	134
Time in ER Before Being Evaluated (minutes)[5]	-	-	22	26
Time to Pain Meds for Fractures (minutes)[5]	-	-	52	57
Heart Attack Care				
Aspirin Given at Discharge[5]	-	-	99%	99%
Fibrinolytic Meds Within 30 Min. of Arrival[5]	-	-	62%	54%
PCI Within 90 Minutes of Arrival[5]	-	-	97%	96%
Statin Prescribed at Discharge[5]	-	-	98%	98%
Heart Failure Care				
ACE Inhibitor or ARB for LVSD[3,7]	-	-	97%	97%
Discharge Instructions Given[1,3]	-	-	93%	94%
Evaluation of LVS Function[1,3]	-	-	99%	99%
Medicare Spending				
Medicare Spending per Patient (ratio)	-	-	0.91	0.98
Pneumonia Care				
Appropriate Initial Antibiotic Given[1]	-	-	96%	95%
Blood Culture Timing[1]	-	-	97%	98%
Pregnancy and Delivery Care				

NOTE: Hospital profiles are in alphabetical order by state, then city, then hospital within the city; Rankings exclude hospitals with less than 25 cases except for patient surveys which excludes hospitals with less than 100 cases; (a) 100-299 cases; (1) The number of cases/patients is too few to report; (2) Data submitted were based on a sample of cases/patients; (3) Results are based on a shorter time period than required; (4) Data suppressed by CMS for one or more quarters; (5) Results are not available for this reporting period; (6) Fewer than 100 patients completed the HCAHPS survey; (7) No cases met the criteria for this measure; (8) The lower limit of the confidence interval cannot be calculated if the number of observed infections equals zero; (9) No data are available from the state/territory for this reporting period; (10) The scores shown reflect fewer than 50 completed surveys; (11) There were discrepancies in the data collection process; (12) This measure does not apply to this hospital for this reporting period; (13) Results cannot be calculated for this reporting period; (14) The results for this state are combined with nearby states to protect confidentiality; Please refer to the User's Guide for a full explanation of data.

Newborn Deliveries Scheduled Early[5]	-	-	2%	6%
Preventive Care				
Immunization for Influenza[5]	-	-	91%	90%
Immunization for Pneumonia[5]	-	-	91%	92%
Stroke Care				
Anticoagulation Therapy for Atrial Fibrillation[5]	-	-	94%	95%
Antithrombotic Therapy Timing[5]	-	-	98%	98%
Assessed for Rehabilitation[5]	-	-	98%	97%
Discharged on Antithrombotic Therapy[5]	-	-	99%	99%
Discharged on Statin Medication[5]	-	-	96%	94%
Thrombolytic Therapy Timing[5]	-	-	73%	66%
Venous Thromboembolism Prophylaxis[5]	-	-	94%	94%
Written Stroke Educational Materials Given[5]	-	-	86%	88%
Surgical Care Improvement Project				
Appropriate Beta Blocker Usage[5]	-	-	98%	98%
Appropriate VTP Within 24 Hours[5]	-	-	98%	98%
Controlled Postoperative Blood Glucose[5]	-	-	97%	97%
Perioperative Temperature Management[5]	-	-	100%	100%
Prophylactic Antibiotic Selection[5]	-	-	99%	99%
Prophylactic Antibiotic Selection (Outpatient)[5]	-	-	98%	98%
Prophylactic Antibiotic Stopped[5]	-	-	99%	98%
Prophylactic Antibiotic Timing[5]	-	-	98%	99%
Prophylactic Antibiotic Timing (Outpatient)[5]	-	-	98%	98%
Urinary Catheter Removal[5]	-	-	97%	97%
Survey of Patients' Hospital Experiences				
Area Around Room 'Always' Quiet at Night[5]	-	-	54%	61%
Doctors 'Always' Communicated Well[5]	-	-	81%	82%
Home Recovery Information Given[5]	-	-	87%	85%
Hospital Given 9 or 10 on 10 Point Scale[5]	-	-	70%	71%
Meds 'Always' Explained Before Given[5]	-	-	64%	64%
Nurses 'Always' Communicated Well[5]	-	-	77%	79%
Pain 'Always' Well Controlled[5]	-	-	70%	71%
Room and Bathroom 'Always' Clean[5]	-	-	73%	73%
Timely Help 'Always' Received[5]	-	-	65%	68%
Would Definitely Recommend Hospital[5]	-	-	73%	71%
Use of Medical Imaging				
Cardiac Imaging Stress Test before Surgery[7]	-	-	4.3%	5.3%
Combination Abdominal CT Scan	117	3.4%	6.9%	10.5%
Combination Brain/Sinus CT Scan[1]	-	-	2.3%	2.7%
Combination Chest CT Scan	50	4.0%	1.1%	2.7%
Follow-up Mammogram/Ultrasound	169	3.6%	9.1%	8.8%
Lumbar Spine MRI for Low Back Pain[1]	-	-	37.9%	37.2%

Saint Elizabeth Hospital

1450 Battersby Avenue Phone: 360-825-2505
Enumclaw, WA 98022 Fax: 360-802-3274
URL: www.enumclawhospital.org
Type: Critical Access Hospitals Emergency Services: Yes
Ownership: Voluntary non-profit - Private Beds: 38

Key Personnel:
Quality Assurance . . . . Nancy Caldwell
Operating Room. . . . . Samuel Cargill
Emergency Room . . . . Richard Dickson
Radiology. . . . . Lon Hayne
Chief of Medical Staff. . . . . Everett W Newcomb III, MD
CEO/President. . . . . Sue Reiter, RN

Measure	Cases	This Hosp.	State Avg.	U.S. Avg.
Blood Clot Prevention and Treatment				
Anticoagulation Overlap Therapy[2]	15	100%	97%	93%
ICU Venous Thromboembolism Prophylaxis[2]	22	91%	92%	92%
Incidence of Potentially Preventable VTE[2,7]	-	-	9%	10%
UFH with Dosages/Platelet Monitoring[1,2]	-	-	99%	97%
Venous Thromboembolism Prophylaxis[2]	101	84%	86%	85%
Warfarin Therapy Discharge Instructions[1,2]	-	-	74%	75%
Chest Pain/Possible Heart Attack Care				
Aspirin Given Within 24 Hours of Arrival	40	98%	97%	96%
Fibrinolytic Meds Within 30 Min. of Arrival[1]	-	-	51%	58%
Average Time to ECG (minutes)	40	12	9	7
Average Time to Transfer (minutes)[1]	-	-	54	60
Children's Asthma Care				
Received Home Management Plan of Care	-	-	-	88%
Received Reliever Medication	-	-	-	100%
Received Systemic Corticosteroids	-	-	-	100%
Emergency Department				
Admittance Decision Time (minutes)[2]	286	75	96	98
Head CT Results Within 45 Min. of Arrival[1]	-	-	63%	57%
Patients Who Left ER Before Being Seen	13,730	0%	2%	2%
Time from ER Arrival to Admit. (minutes)[2]	332	235	259	274
Time from ER Arrival to Discharge (minutes)	407	127	135	134
Time in ER Before Being Evaluated (minutes)	428	13	22	26
Time to Pain Meds for Fractures (minutes)	93	38	52	57
Heart Attack Care				
Aspirin Given at Discharge[1,2]	-	-	99%	99%
Fibrinolytic Meds Within 30 Min. of Arrival[2,7]	-	-	62%	54%
PCI Within 90 Minutes of Arrival[2,7]	-	-	97%	96%
Statin Prescribed at Discharge[1,2]	-	-	98%	98%
Heart Failure Care				
ACE Inhibitor or ARB for LVSD[2]	17	100%	97%	97%
Discharge Instructions Given[2]	34	85%	93%	94%
Evaluation of LVS Function[2]	43	100%	99%	99%
Medicare Spending				
Medicare Spending per Patient (ratio)	-	-	0.91	0.98
Pneumonia Care				
Appropriate Initial Antibiotic Given[2]	40	92%	96%	95%
Blood Culture Timing[2]	61	100%	97%	98%
Pregnancy and Delivery Care				
Newborn Deliveries Scheduled Early	25	0%	2%	6%
Preventive Care				
Immunization for Influenza[2]	261	79%	91%	90%
Immunization for Pneumonia[2]	287	83%	91%	92%
Stroke Care				
Anticoagulation Therapy for Atrial Fibrillation[1]	-	-	94%	95%
Antithrombotic Therapy Timing	13	92%	98%	98%
Assessed for Rehabilitation	12	92%	98%	97%
Discharged on Antithrombotic Therapy	12	100%	99%	99%
Discharged on Statin Medication	11	91%	96%	94%
Thrombolytic Therapy Timing[7]	-	-	73%	66%
Venous Thromboembolism Prophylaxis	14	86%	94%	94%
Written Stroke Educational Materials Given	11	45%	86%	88%
Surgical Care Improvement Project				
Appropriate Beta Blocker Usage[2]	37	89%	98%	98%
Appropriate VTP Within 24 Hours[2]	123	96%	98%	98%
Controlled Postoperative Blood Glucose[2,3]	-	-	97%	97%
Perioperative Temperature Management[2]	130	100%	100%	100%
Prophylactic Antibiotic Selection[2]	93	100%	99%	99%
Prophylactic Antibiotic Selection (Outpatient)[1,3]	-	-	98%	98%
Prophylactic Antibiotic Stopped[2]	92	100%	99%	98%
Prophylactic Antibiotic Timing[2]	93	99%	98%	99%
Prophylactic Antibiotic Timing (Outpatient)[1,3]	-	-	98%	98%
Urinary Catheter Removal[2]	27	93%	97%	97%
Survey of Patients' Hospital Experiences				
Area Around Room 'Always' Quiet at Night	(a)	58%	54%	61%
Doctors 'Always' Communicated Well	(a)	86%	81%	82%
Home Recovery Information Given	(a)	91%	87%	85%
Hospital Given 9 or 10 on 10 Point Scale	(a)	82%	70%	71%
Meds 'Always' Explained Before Given	(a)	72%	64%	64%
Nurses 'Always' Communicated Well	(a)	80%	77%	79%
Pain 'Always' Well Controlled	(a)	65%	70%	71%
Room and Bathroom 'Always' Clean	(a)	78%	73%	73%
Timely Help 'Always' Received	(a)	65%	65%	68%
Would Definitely Recommend Hospital	(a)	82%	73%	71%
Use of Medical Imaging				
Cardiac Imaging Stress Test before Surgery	49	4.1%	4.3%	5.3%
Combination Abdominal CT Scan	364	2.5%	6.9%	10.5%
Combination Brain/Sinus CT Scan[1]	-	-	2.3%	2.7%
Combination Chest CT Scan	197	2.5%	1.1%	2.7%
Follow-up Mammogram/Ultrasound	355	14.9%	9.1%	8.8%
Lumbar Spine MRI for Low Back Pain[1]	-	-	37.9%	37.2%

Columbia Basin Hospital

200 Nat Washington Way Phone: 509-754-4631
Ephrata, WA 98823
Type: Critical Access Hospitals Emergency Services: Yes
Ownership: Govt - Hospital Dist/Auth

Measure	Cases	This Hosp.	State Avg.	U.S. Avg.
Blood Clot Prevention and Treatment				
Anticoagulation Overlap Therapy[5]	-	-	97%	93%
ICU Venous Thromboembolism Prophylaxis[5]	-	-	92%	92%
Incidence of Potentially Preventable VTE[5]	-	-	9%	10%
UFH with Dosages/Platelet Monitoring[5]	-	-	99%	97%
Venous Thromboembolism Prophylaxis[5]	-	-	86%	85%
Warfarin Therapy Discharge Instructions[5]	-	-	74%	75%
Chest Pain/Possible Heart Attack Care				
Aspirin Given Within 24 Hours of Arrival[1,3]	-	-	97%	96%
Fibrinolytic Meds Within 30 Min. of Arrival[1,3]	-	-	51%	58%
Average Time to ECG (minutes)[3]	11	4	9	7
Average Time to Transfer (minutes)[1,3]	-	-	54	60
Children's Asthma Care				
Received Home Management Plan of Care	-	-	-	88%
Received Reliever Medication	-	-	-	100%
Received Systemic Corticosteroids	-	-	-	100%
Emergency Department				
Admittance Decision Time (minutes)[5]	-	-	96	98
Head CT Results Within 45 Min. of Arrival[5]	-	-	63%	57%
Patients Who Left ER Before Being Seen[5]	-	-	2%	2%
Time from ER Arrival to Admit. (minutes)[5]	-	-	259	274
Time from ER Arrival to Discharge (minutes)[5]	-	-	135	134
Time in ER Before Being Evaluated (minutes)[5]	-	-	22	26
Time to Pain Meds for Fractures (minutes)[5]	-	-	52	57
Heart Attack Care				
Aspirin Given at Discharge[5]	-	-	99%	99%
Fibrinolytic Meds Within 30 Min. of Arrival[5]	-	-	62%	54%
PCI Within 90 Minutes of Arrival[5]	-	-	97%	96%
Statin Prescribed at Discharge[5]	-	-	98%	98%
Heart Failure Care				
ACE Inhibitor or ARB for LVSD[1]	-	-	97%	97%
Discharge Instructions Given[1]	-	-	93%	94%
Evaluation of LVS Function[1]	-	-	99%	99%
Medicare Spending				
Medicare Spending per Patient (ratio)	-	-	0.91	0.98
Pneumonia Care				
Appropriate Initial Antibiotic Given[1]	-	-	96%	95%
Blood Culture Timing[1]	-	-	97%	98%
Pregnancy and Delivery Care				
Newborn Deliveries Scheduled Early[5]	-	-	2%	6%
Preventive Care				
Immunization for Influenza[5]	-	-	91%	90%
Immunization for Pneumonia[5]	-	-	91%	92%
Stroke Care				
Anticoagulation Therapy for Atrial Fibrillation[5]	-	-	94%	95%
Antithrombotic Therapy Timing[5]	-	-	98%	98%
Assessed for Rehabilitation[5]	-	-	98%	97%
Discharged on Antithrombotic Therapy[5]	-	-	99%	99%
Discharged on Statin Medication[5]	-	-	96%	94%
Thrombolytic Therapy Timing[5]	-	-	73%	66%
Venous Thromboembolism Prophylaxis[5]	-	-	94%	94%
Written Stroke Educational Materials Given[5]	-	-	86%	88%
Surgical Care Improvement Project				
Appropriate Beta Blocker Usage[5]	-	-	98%	98%
Appropriate VTP Within 24 Hours[5]	-	-	98%	98%
Controlled Postoperative Blood Glucose[5]	-	-	97%	97%
Perioperative Temperature Management[5]	-	-	100%	100%
Prophylactic Antibiotic Selection[5]	-	-	99%	99%
Prophylactic Antibiotic Selection (Outpatient)[5]	-	-	98%	98%
Prophylactic Antibiotic Stopped[5]	-	-	99%	98%
Prophylactic Antibiotic Timing[5]	-	-	98%	99%
Prophylactic Antibiotic Timing (Outpatient)[5]	-	-	98%	98%
Urinary Catheter Removal[5]	-	-	97%	97%
Survey of Patients' Hospital Experiences				
Area Around Room 'Always' Quiet at Night[5]	-	-	54%	61%
Doctors 'Always' Communicated Well[5]	-	-	81%	82%
Home Recovery Information Given[5]	-	-	87%	85%
Hospital Given 9 or 10 on 10 Point Scale[5]	-	-	70%	71%
Meds 'Always' Explained Before Given[5]	-	-	64%	64%
Nurses 'Always' Communicated Well[5]	-	-	77%	79%
Pain 'Always' Well Controlled[5]	-	-	70%	71%
Room and Bathroom 'Always' Clean[5]	-	-	73%	73%
Timely Help 'Always' Received[5]	-	-	65%	68%

NOTE: Hospital profiles are in alphabetical order by state, then city, then hospital within the city; Rankings exclude hospitals with less than 25 cases except for patient surveys which excludes hospitals with less than 100 cases; (a) 100-299 cases; (1) The number of cases/patients is too few to report; (2) Data submitted were based on a sample of cases/patients; (3) Results are based on a shorter time period than required; (4) Data suppressed by CMS for one or more quarters; (5) Results are not available for this reporting period; (6) Fewer than 100 patients completed the HCAHPS survey; (7) No cases met the criteria for this measure; (8) The lower limit of the confidence interval cannot be calculated if the number of observed infections equals zero; (9) No data are available from the state/territory for this reporting period; (10) The scores shown reflect fewer than 50 completed surveys; (11) There were discrepancies in the data collection process; (12) This measure does not apply to this hospital for this reporting period; (13) Results cannot be calculated for this reporting period; (14) The results for this state are combined with nearby states to protect confidentiality; Please refer to the User's Guide for a full explanation of data.

Measure	Cases	This Hosp.	State Avg.	U.S. Avg.
Would Definitely Recommend Hospital[5]	-	-	73%	71%
Use of Medical Imaging				
Cardiac Imaging Stress Test before Surgery[7]	-	-	4.3%	5.3%
Combination Abdominal CT Scan	61	63.9%	6.9%	10.5%
Combination Brain/Sinus CT Scan[1]	-	-	2.3%	2.7%
Combination Chest CT Scan[1]	-	-	1.1%	2.7%
Follow-up Mammogram/Ultrasound	111	7.2%	9.1%	8.8%
Lumbar Spine MRI for Low Back Pain[1]	-	-	37.9%	37.2%

Providence Regional Medical Center Everett

1321 Colby Avenue — Phone: 425-261-2000
Everett, WA 98201 — Fax: 425-261-4051
URL: www.providence.org
Type: Acute Care Hospitals — Emergency Services: Yes
Ownership: Voluntary non-profit - Church — Beds: 362

Key Personnel:
Chief of Medical Staff . . . . Clinton Anderson
CEO/President. . . . . John Koster

Measure	Cases	This Hosp.	State Avg.	U.S. Avg.
Blood Clot Prevention and Treatment				
Anticoagulation Overlap Therapy[2]	235	99%	97%	93%
ICU Venous Thromboembolism Prophylaxis[2]	50	94%	92%	92%
Incidence of Potentially Preventable VTE[2]	14	7%	9%	10%
UFH with Dosages/Platelet Monitoring[2]	133	100%	99%	97%
Venous Thromboembolism Prophylaxis[2]	296	98%	86%	85%
Warfarin Therapy Discharge Instructions[2]	196	86%	74%	75%
Chest Pain/Possible Heart Attack Care				
Aspirin Given Within 24 Hours of Arrival[5]	-	-	97%	96%
Fibrinolytic Meds Within 30 Min. of Arrival[5]	-	-	51%	58%
Average Time to ECG (minutes)[5]	-	-	9	7
Average Time to Transfer (minutes)[5]	-	-	54	60
Children's Asthma Care				
Received Home Management Plan of Care	-	-	-	88%
Received Reliever Medication	-	-	-	100%
Received Systemic Corticosteroids	-	-	-	100%
Emergency Department				
Admittance Decision Time (minutes)[2]	593	105	96	98
Head CT Results Within 45 Min. of Arrival	32	34%	63%	57%
Patients Who Left ER Before Being Seen	92,075	1%	2%	2%
Time from ER Arrival to Admit. (minutes)[2]	593	307	259	274
Time from ER Arrival to Discharge (minutes)	398	186	135	134
Time in ER Before Being Evaluated (minutes)	430	23	22	26
Time to Pain Meds for Fractures (minutes)	387	62	52	57
Heart Attack Care				
Aspirin Given at Discharge[2]	348	99%	99%	99%
Fibrinolytic Meds Within 30 Min. of Arrival[2,7]	-	-	62%	54%
PCI Within 90 Minutes of Arrival[2]	61	100%	97%	96%
Statin Prescribed at Discharge[2]	333	98%	98%	98%
Heart Failure Care				
ACE Inhibitor or ARB for LVSD[2]	105	100%	97%	97%
Discharge Instructions Given[2]	279	89%	93%	94%
Evaluation of LVS Function[2]	343	100%	99%	99%
Medicare Spending				
Medicare Spending per Patient (ratio)	-	0.93	0.91	0.98
Pneumonia Care				
Appropriate Initial Antibiotic Given[2]	151	95%	96%	95%
Blood Culture Timing[2]	258	96%	97%	98%
Pregnancy and Delivery Care				
Newborn Deliveries Scheduled Early	338	0%	2%	6%
Preventive Care				
Immunization for Influenza[2]	526	71%	91%	90%
Immunization for Pneumonia[2]	604	74%	91%	92%
Stroke Care				
Anticoagulation Therapy for Atrial Fibrillation	19	100%	94%	95%
Antithrombotic Therapy Timing	277	100%	98%	98%
Assessed for Rehabilitation	380	100%	98%	97%
Discharged on Antithrombotic Therapy	352	100%	99%	99%
Discharged on Statin Medication	274	99%	96%	94%
Thrombolytic Therapy Timing	20	95%	73%	66%
Venous Thromboembolism Prophylaxis	332	98%	94%	94%
Written Stroke Educational Materials Given	219	98%	86%	88%
Surgical Care Improvement Project				
Appropriate Beta Blocker Usage[2]	236	99%	98%	98%
Appropriate VTP Within 24 Hours[2]	335	100%	98%	98%
Controlled Postoperative Blood Glucose[2]	152	99%	97%	97%
Perioperative Temperature Management[2]	494	100%	100%	100%
Prophylactic Antibiotic Selection[2]	479	99%	99%	99%
Prophylactic Antibiotic Selection (Outpatient)	560	98%	98%	98%
Prophylactic Antibiotic Stopped[2]	465	100%	99%	98%
Prophylactic Antibiotic Timing[2]	479	100%	98%	99%
Prophylactic Antibiotic Timing (Outpatient)	561	98%	98%	98%
Urinary Catheter Removal[2]	409	98%	97%	97%
Survey of Patients' Hospital Experiences				
Area Around Room 'Always' Quiet at Night	300+	51%	54%	61%
Doctors 'Always' Communicated Well	300+	79%	81%	82%
Home Recovery Information Given	300+	87%	87%	85%
Hospital Given 9 or 10 on 10 Point Scale	300+	72%	70%	71%
Meds 'Always' Explained Before Given	300+	62%	64%	64%
Nurses 'Always' Communicated Well	300+	76%	77%	79%
Pain 'Always' Well Controlled	300+	70%	70%	71%
Room and Bathroom 'Always' Clean	300+	70%	73%	73%
Timely Help 'Always' Received	300+	63%	65%	68%
Would Definitely Recommend Hospital	300+	78%	73%	71%
Use of Medical Imaging				
Cardiac Imaging Stress Test before Surgery	372	5.6%	4.3%	5.3%
Combination Abdominal CT Scan	904	2.4%	6.9%	10.5%
Combination Brain/Sinus CT Scan	926	2.8%	2.3%	2.7%
Combination Chest CT Scan	438	0.5%	1.1%	2.7%
Follow-up Mammogram/Ultrasound	1,514	7.4%	9.1%	8.8%
Lumbar Spine MRI for Low Back Pain	110	37.3%	37.9%	37.2%

Saint Francis Community Hospital

34515 9th Avenue South — Phone: 253-944-8100
Federal Way, WA 98003 — Fax: 253-952-7988
URL: www.fhshealth.org
Type: Acute Care Hospitals — Emergency Services: Yes
Ownership: Voluntary non-profit - Church — Beds: 110

Key Personnel:
CEO . . . . Mark Benedum
President/CEO. . . . . Scott W. Bosch
Quality Assurance . . . . Julie Burns
Radiology. . . . . Stanley G Cheng
Emergency Room . . . . Bif Fink
Intensive Care Unit. . . . . Susan Merian-Tresch
Chief of Medical Staff . . . . Frank Senecal, MD
CEO . . . . Joseph Wilczek

Measure	Cases	This Hosp.	State Avg.	U.S. Avg.
Blood Clot Prevention and Treatment				
Anticoagulation Overlap Therapy[2]	69	91%	97%	93%
ICU Venous Thromboembolism Prophylaxis[2]	38	87%	92%	92%
Incidence of Potentially Preventable VTE[1,2]	-	-	9%	10%
UFH with Dosages/Platelet Monitoring[2]	55	100%	99%	97%
Venous Thromboembolism Prophylaxis[2]	326	88%	86%	85%
Warfarin Therapy Discharge Instructions[2]	52	83%	74%	75%
Chest Pain/Possible Heart Attack Care				
Aspirin Given Within 24 Hours of Arrival	13	100%	97%	96%
Fibrinolytic Meds Within 30 Min. of Arrival[3,7]	-	-	51%	58%
Average Time to ECG (minutes)	13	6	9	7
Average Time to Transfer (minutes)[3,7]	-	-	54	60
Children's Asthma Care				
Received Home Management Plan of Care	-	-	-	88%
Received Reliever Medication	-	-	-	100%
Received Systemic Corticosteroids	-	-	-	100%
Emergency Department				
Admittance Decision Time (minutes)[2]	683	147	96	98
Head CT Results Within 45 Min. of Arrival	41	78%	63%	57%
Patients Who Left ER Before Being Seen	47,896	1%	2%	2%
Time from ER Arrival to Admit. (minutes)[2]	708	328	259	274
Time from ER Arrival to Discharge (minutes)	400	150	135	134
Time in ER Before Being Evaluated (minutes)	438	25	22	26
Time to Pain Meds for Fractures (minutes)	188	54	52	57
Heart Attack Care				
Aspirin Given at Discharge	148	99%	99%	99%
Fibrinolytic Meds Within 30 Min. of Arrival[1]	-	-	62%	54%
PCI Within 90 Minutes of Arrival	26	96%	97%	96%
Statin Prescribed at Discharge	145	99%	98%	98%
Heart Failure Care				
ACE Inhibitor or ARB for LVSD	72	99%	97%	97%
Discharge Instructions Given	163	88%	93%	94%
Evaluation of LVS Function	185	99%	99%	99%
Medicare Spending				
Medicare Spending per Patient (ratio)	-	0.99	0.91	0.98
Pneumonia Care				
Appropriate Initial Antibiotic Given[2]	114	100%	96%	95%
Blood Culture Timing[2]	197	98%	97%	98%
Pregnancy and Delivery Care				
Newborn Deliveries Scheduled Early	72	1%	2%	6%
Preventive Care				
Immunization for Influenza[2]	569	90%	91%	90%
Immunization for Pneumonia[2]	627	90%	91%	92%
Stroke Care				
Anticoagulation Therapy for Atrial Fibrillation	15	87%	94%	95%
Antithrombotic Therapy Timing	74	100%	98%	98%
Assessed for Rehabilitation	75	100%	98%	97%
Discharged on Antithrombotic Therapy	72	100%	99%	99%
Discharged on Statin Medication	62	94%	96%	94%
Thrombolytic Therapy Timing[1]	-	-	73%	66%
Venous Thromboembolism Prophylaxis	75	96%	94%	94%
Written Stroke Educational Materials Given	49	47%	86%	88%
Surgical Care Improvement Project				
Appropriate Beta Blocker Usage[2]	117	97%	98%	98%
Appropriate VTP Within 24 Hours[2]	280	95%	98%	98%
Controlled Postoperative Blood Glucose[2,7]	-	-	97%	97%
Perioperative Temperature Management[2]	380	100%	100%	100%
Prophylactic Antibiotic Selection[2]	226	99%	99%	99%
Prophylactic Antibiotic Selection (Outpatient)	215	99%	98%	98%
Prophylactic Antibiotic Stopped[2]	218	99%	99%	98%
Prophylactic Antibiotic Timing[2]	226	98%	98%	99%
Prophylactic Antibiotic Timing (Outpatient)	216	96%	98%	98%
Urinary Catheter Removal[2]	219	90%	97%	97%
Survey of Patients' Hospital Experiences				
Area Around Room 'Always' Quiet at Night	300+	48%	54%	61%
Doctors 'Always' Communicated Well	300+	75%	81%	82%
Home Recovery Information Given	300+	86%	87%	85%
Hospital Given 9 or 10 on 10 Point Scale	300+	68%	70%	71%
Meds 'Always' Explained Before Given	300+	62%	64%	64%
Nurses 'Always' Communicated Well	300+	73%	77%	79%
Pain 'Always' Well Controlled	300+	66%	70%	71%
Room and Bathroom 'Always' Clean	300+	67%	73%	73%
Timely Help 'Always' Received	300+	57%	65%	68%
Would Definitely Recommend Hospital	300+	71%	73%	71%
Use of Medical Imaging				
Cardiac Imaging Stress Test before Surgery	80	6.3%	4.3%	5.3%
Combination Abdominal CT Scan	607	3.6%	6.9%	10.5%
Combination Brain/Sinus CT Scan[1]	-	-	2.3%	2.7%
Combination Chest CT Scan	326	0.3%	1.1%	2.7%
Follow-up Mammogram/Ultrasound	733	11.3%	9.1%	8.8%
Lumbar Spine MRI for Low Back Pain	60	46.7%	37.9%	37.2%

Forks Community Hospital

530 Bogachiel Way — Phone: 360-374-6271
Forks, WA 98331
Type: Critical Access Hospitals — Emergency Services: Yes
Ownership: Govt - Hospital Dist/Auth

Measure	Cases	This Hosp.	State Avg.	U.S. Avg.
Blood Clot Prevention and Treatment				
Anticoagulation Overlap Therapy[5]	-	-	97%	93%
ICU Venous Thromboembolism Prophylaxis[5]	-	-	92%	92%
Incidence of Potentially Preventable VTE[5]	-	-	9%	10%
UFH with Dosages/Platelet Monitoring[5]	-	-	99%	97%
Venous Thromboembolism Prophylaxis[5]	-	-	86%	85%
Warfarin Therapy Discharge Instructions[5]	-	-	74%	75%
Chest Pain/Possible Heart Attack Care				
Aspirin Given Within 24 Hours of Arrival	-	-	97%	96%
Fibrinolytic Meds Within 30 Min. of Arrival	-	-	51%	58%
Average Time to ECG (minutes)	-	-	9	7
Average Time to Transfer (minutes)	-	-	54	60
Children's Asthma Care				
Received Home Management Plan of Care	-	-	-	88%

NOTE: Hospital profiles are in alphabetical order by state, then city, then hospital within the city; Rankings exclude hospitals with less than 25 cases except for patient surveys which excludes hospitals with less than 100 cases; (a) 100-299 cases; (1) The number of cases/patients is too few to report; (2) Data submitted were based on a sample of cases/patients; (3) Results are based on a shorter time period than required; (4) Data suppressed by CMS for one or more quarters; (5) Results are not available for this reporting period; (6) Fewer than 100 patients completed the HCAHPS survey; (7) No cases met the criteria for this measure; (8) The lower limit of the confidence interval cannot be calculated if the number of observed infections equals zero; (9) No data are available from the state/territory for this reporting period; (10) The scores shown reflect fewer than 50 completed surveys; (11) There were discrepancies in the data collection process; (12) This measure does not apply to this hospital for this reporting period; (13) Results cannot be calculated for this reporting period; (14) The results for this state are combined with nearby states to protect confidentiality; Please refer to the User's Guide for a full explanation of data.

Measure	Cases	This Hosp.	State Avg.	U.S. Avg.
Received Reliever Medication	-	-	-	100%
Received Systemic Corticosteroids	-	-	-	100%
Emergency Department				
Admittance Decision Time (minutes)[5]	-	-	96	98
Head CT Results Within 45 Min. of Arrival	-	-	63%	57%
Patients Who Left ER Before Being Seen	-	-	2%	2%
Time from ER Arrival to Admit. (minutes)[5]	-	-	259	274
Time from ER Arrival to Discharge (minutes)	-	-	135	134
Time in ER Before Being Evaluated (minutes)	-	-	22	26
Time to Pain Meds for Fractures (minutes)	-	-	52	57
Heart Attack Care				
Aspirin Given at Discharge[5]	-	-	99%	99%
Fibrinolytic Meds Within 30 Min. of Arrival[5]	-	-	62%	54%
PCI Within 90 Minutes of Arrival[5]	-	-	97%	96%
Statin Prescribed at Discharge[5]	-	-	98%	98%
Heart Failure Care				
ACE Inhibitor or ARB for LVSD[1,3]	-	-	97%	97%
Discharge Instructions Given[1,3]	-	-	93%	94%
Evaluation of LVS Function[1,3]	-	-	99%	99%
Medicare Spending				
Medicare Spending per Patient (ratio)	-	-	0.91	0.98
Pneumonia Care				
Appropriate Initial Antibiotic Given[1,3]	-	-	96%	95%
Blood Culture Timing[1,3]	-	-	97%	98%
Pregnancy and Delivery Care				
Newborn Deliveries Scheduled Early[5]	-	-	2%	6%
Preventive Care				
Immunization for Influenza[5]	-	-	91%	90%
Immunization for Pneumonia[5]	-	-	91%	92%
Stroke Care				
Anticoagulation Therapy for Atrial Fibrillation[5]	-	-	94%	95%
Antithrombotic Therapy Timing[5]	-	-	98%	98%
Assessed for Rehabilitation[5]	-	-	98%	97%
Discharged on Antithrombotic Therapy[5]	-	-	99%	99%
Discharged on Statin Medication[5]	-	-	96%	94%
Thrombolytic Therapy Timing[5]	-	-	73%	66%
Venous Thromboembolism Prophylaxis[5]	-	-	94%	94%
Written Stroke Educational Materials Given[5]	-	-	86%	88%
Surgical Care Improvement Project				
Appropriate Beta Blocker Usage[5]	-	-	98%	98%
Appropriate VTP Within 24 Hours[5]	-	-	98%	98%
Controlled Postoperative Blood Glucose[5]	-	-	97%	97%
Perioperative Temperature Management[5]	-	-	100%	100%
Prophylactic Antibiotic Selection[5]	-	-	99%	99%
Prophylactic Antibiotic Selection (Outpatient)	-	-	98%	98%
Prophylactic Antibiotic Stopped[5]	-	-	99%	98%
Prophylactic Antibiotic Timing[5]	-	-	98%	99%
Prophylactic Antibiotic Timing (Outpatient)	-	-	98%	98%
Urinary Catheter Removal[5]	-	-	97%	97%
Survey of Patients' Hospital Experiences				
Area Around Room 'Always' Quiet at Night[5]	-	-	54%	61%
Doctors 'Always' Communicated Well[5]	-	-	81%	82%
Home Recovery Information Given[5]	-	-	87%	85%
Hospital Given 9 or 10 on 10 Point Scale[5]	-	-	70%	71%
Meds 'Always' Explained Before Given[5]	-	-	64%	64%
Nurses 'Always' Communicated Well[5]	-	-	77%	79%
Pain 'Always' Well Controlled[5]	-	-	70%	71%
Room and Bathroom 'Always' Clean[5]	-	-	73%	73%
Timely Help 'Always' Received[5]	-	-	65%	68%
Would Definitely Recommend Hospital[5]	-	-	73%	71%
Use of Medical Imaging				
Cardiac Imaging Stress Test before Surgery	-	-	4.3%	5.3%
Combination Abdominal CT Scan	-	-	6.9%	10.5%
Combination Brain/Sinus CT Scan	-	-	2.3%	2.7%
Combination Chest CT Scan	-	-	1.1%	2.7%
Follow-up Mammogram/Ultrasound	-	-	9.1%	8.8%
Lumbar Spine MRI for Low Back Pain	-	-	37.9%	37.2%

Peacehealth Peace Island Medical Center

1117 Spring Street Phone: 360-378-2141
Friday Harbor, WA 98250
Type: Critical Access Hospitals Emergency Services: Yes
Ownership: Voluntary non-profit - Private

Measure	Cases	This Hosp.	State Avg.	U.S. Avg.
Blood Clot Prevention and Treatment				
Anticoagulation Overlap Therapy[3,7]	-	-	97%	93%
ICU Venous Thromboembolism Prophylaxis[3,7]	-	-	92%	92%
Incidence of Potentially Preventable VTE[3,7]	-	-	9%	10%
UFH with Dosages/Platelet Monitoring[3,7]	-	-	99%	97%
Venous Thromboembolism Prophylaxis[3]	18	28%	86%	85%
Warfarin Therapy Discharge Instructions[3,7]	-	-	74%	75%
Chest Pain/Possible Heart Attack Care				
Aspirin Given Within 24 Hours of Arrival[1,3]	-	-	97%	96%
Fibrinolytic Meds Within 30 Min. of Arrival[3,7]	-	-	51%	58%
Average Time to ECG (minutes)[1,3]	-	-	9	7
Average Time to Transfer (minutes)[3,7]	-	-	54	60
Children's Asthma Care				
Received Home Management Plan of Care	-	-	-	88%
Received Reliever Medication	-	-	-	100%
Received Systemic Corticosteroids	-	-	-	100%
Emergency Department				
Admittance Decision Time (minutes)[2,3]	21	46	96	98
Head CT Results Within 45 Min. of Arrival[1,3]	-	-	63%	57%
Patients Who Left ER Before Being Seen[5]	-	-	2%	2%
Time from ER Arrival to Admit. (minutes)[2,3]	22	208	259	274
Time from ER Arrival to Discharge (minutes)[3]	68	91	135	134
Time in ER Before Being Evaluated (minutes)[3]	84	12	22	26
Time to Pain Meds for Fractures (minutes)[3]	12	34	52	57
Heart Attack Care				
Aspirin Given at Discharge[5]	-	-	99%	99%
Fibrinolytic Meds Within 30 Min. of Arrival[5]	-	-	62%	54%
PCI Within 90 Minutes of Arrival[5]	-	-	97%	96%
Statin Prescribed at Discharge[5]	-	-	98%	98%
Heart Failure Care				
ACE Inhibitor or ARB for LVSD[5]	-	-	97%	97%
Discharge Instructions Given[5]	-	-	93%	94%
Evaluation of LVS Function[5]	-	-	99%	99%
Medicare Spending				
Medicare Spending per Patient (ratio)	-	-	0.91	0.98
Pneumonia Care				
Appropriate Initial Antibiotic Given[1,3]	-	-	96%	95%
Blood Culture Timing[1,3]	-	-	97%	98%
Pregnancy and Delivery Care				
Newborn Deliveries Scheduled Early[3,7]	-	-	2%	6%
Preventive Care				
Immunization for Influenza[5]	-	-	91%	90%
Immunization for Pneumonia[2,3]	17	76%	91%	92%
Stroke Care				
Anticoagulation Therapy for Atrial Fibrillation[5]	-	-	94%	95%
Antithrombotic Therapy Timing[5]	-	-	98%	98%
Assessed for Rehabilitation[5]	-	-	98%	97%
Discharged on Antithrombotic Therapy[5]	-	-	99%	99%
Discharged on Statin Medication[5]	-	-	96%	94%
Thrombolytic Therapy Timing[5]	-	-	73%	66%
Venous Thromboembolism Prophylaxis[5]	-	-	94%	94%
Written Stroke Educational Materials Given[5]	-	-	86%	88%
Surgical Care Improvement Project				
Appropriate Beta Blocker Usage[5]	-	-	98%	98%
Appropriate VTP Within 24 Hours[5]	-	-	98%	98%
Controlled Postoperative Blood Glucose[5]	-	-	97%	97%
Perioperative Temperature Management[5]	-	-	100%	100%
Prophylactic Antibiotic Selection[5]	-	-	99%	99%
Prophylactic Antibiotic Selection (Outpatient)[5]	-	-	98%	98%
Prophylactic Antibiotic Stopped[5]	-	-	99%	98%
Prophylactic Antibiotic Timing[5]	-	-	98%	99%
Prophylactic Antibiotic Timing (Outpatient)[5]	-	-	98%	98%
Urinary Catheter Removal[5]	-	-	97%	97%
Survey of Patients' Hospital Experiences				
Area Around Room 'Always' Quiet at Night[5]	-	-	54%	61%
Doctors 'Always' Communicated Well[5]	-	-	81%	82%
Home Recovery Information Given[5]	-	-	87%	85%
Hospital Given 9 or 10 on 10 Point Scale[5]	-	-	70%	71%
Meds 'Always' Explained Before Given[5]	-	-	64%	64%
Nurses 'Always' Communicated Well[5]	-	-	77%	79%
Pain 'Always' Well Controlled[5]	-	-	70%	71%
Room and Bathroom 'Always' Clean[5]	-	-	73%	73%
Timely Help 'Always' Received[5]	-	-	65%	68%
Would Definitely Recommend Hospital[5]	-	-	73%	71%
Use of Medical Imaging				
Cardiac Imaging Stress Test before Surgery[7]	-	-	4.3%	5.3%
Combination Abdominal CT Scan[7]	-	-	6.9%	10.5%
Combination Brain/Sinus CT Scan[7]	-	-	2.3%	2.7%
Combination Chest CT Scan[7]	-	-	1.1%	2.7%
Follow-up Mammogram/Ultrasound[7]	-	-	9.1%	8.8%
Lumbar Spine MRI for Low Back Pain[7]	-	-	37.9%	37.2%

Saint Anthony Hospital

11567 Canterwood Boulevard Nw Phone: 253-530-2050
Gig Harbor, WA 98332
URL: www.fhshealth.org
Type: Acute Care Hospitals Emergency Services: Yes
Ownership: Voluntary non-profit - Church Beds: 80
Key Personnel:
CEO .... Joseph Wilczek

Measure	Cases	This Hosp.	State Avg.	U.S. Avg.
Blood Clot Prevention and Treatment				
Anticoagulation Overlap Therapy[2]	52	92%	97%	93%
ICU Venous Thromboembolism Prophylaxis[2]	24	96%	92%	92%
Incidence of Potentially Preventable VTE[1,2]	-	-	9%	10%
UFH with Dosages/Platelet Monitoring[2]	51	100%	99%	97%
Venous Thromboembolism Prophylaxis[2]	336	91%	86%	85%
Warfarin Therapy Discharge Instructions[2]	40	70%	74%	75%
Chest Pain/Possible Heart Attack Care				
Aspirin Given Within 24 Hours of Arrival	31	100%	97%	96%
Fibrinolytic Meds Within 30 Min. of Arrival[7]	-	-	51%	58%
Average Time to ECG (minutes)	31	6	9	7
Average Time to Transfer (minutes)[7]	-	-	54	60
Children's Asthma Care				
Received Home Management Plan of Care	-	-	-	88%
Received Reliever Medication	-	-	-	100%
Received Systemic Corticosteroids	-	-	-	100%
Emergency Department				
Admittance Decision Time (minutes)[2]	766	140	96	98
Head CT Results Within 45 Min. of Arrival[1]	-	-	63%	57%
Patients Who Left ER Before Being Seen	22,418	0%	2%	2%
Time from ER Arrival to Admit. (minutes)[2]	782	298	259	274
Time from ER Arrival to Discharge (minutes)	376	165	135	134
Time in ER Before Being Evaluated (minutes)	424	8	22	26
Time to Pain Meds for Fractures (minutes)	107	28	52	57
Heart Attack Care				
Aspirin Given at Discharge	49	100%	99%	99%
Fibrinolytic Meds Within 30 Min. of Arrival[7]	-	-	62%	54%
PCI Within 90 Minutes of Arrival	14	100%	97%	96%
Statin Prescribed at Discharge	45	98%	98%	98%
Heart Failure Care				
ACE Inhibitor or ARB for LVSD	42	95%	97%	97%
Discharge Instructions Given	118	87%	93%	94%
Evaluation of LVS Function	134	100%	99%	99%
Medicare Spending				
Medicare Spending per Patient (ratio)	-	0.97	0.91	0.98
Pneumonia Care				
Appropriate Initial Antibiotic Given[2]	110	97%	96%	95%
Blood Culture Timing[2]	208	99%	97%	98%
Pregnancy and Delivery Care				
Newborn Deliveries Scheduled Early[7]	-	-	2%	6%
Preventive Care				
Immunization for Influenza[2]	528	95%	91%	90%
Immunization for Pneumonia[2]	743	95%	91%	92%
Stroke Care				
Anticoagulation Therapy for Atrial Fibrillation[1]	-	-	94%	95%
Antithrombotic Therapy Timing	49	100%	98%	98%
Assessed for Rehabilitation	54	93%	98%	97%
Discharged on Antithrombotic Therapy	54	100%	99%	99%

NOTE: Hospital profiles are in alphabetical order by state, then city, then hospital within the city; Rankings exclude hospitals with less than 25 cases except for patient surveys which excludes hospitals with less than 100 cases; (a) 100-299 cases; (1) The number of cases/patients is too few to report; (2) Data submitted were based on a sample of cases/patients; (3) Results are based on a shorter time period than required; (4) Data suppressed by CMS for one or more quarters; (5) Results are not available for this reporting period; (6) Fewer than 100 patients completed the HCAHPS survey; (7) No cases met the criteria for this measure; (8) The lower limit of the confidence interval cannot be calculated if the number of observed infections equals zero; (9) No data are available from the state/territory for this reporting period; (10) The scores shown reflect fewer than 50 completed surveys; (11) There were discrepancies in the data collection process; (12) This measure does not apply to this hospital for this reporting period; (13) Results cannot be calculated for this reporting period; (14) The results for this state are combined with nearby states to protect confidentiality; Please refer to the User's Guide for a full explanation of data.

Measure	Cases	This Hosp.	State Avg.	U.S. Avg.
Discharged on Statin Medication	47	91%	96%	94%
Thrombolytic Therapy Timing[1]	-	-	73%	66%
Venous Thromboembolism Prophylaxis	47	96%	94%	94%
Written Stroke Educational Materials Given	39	51%	86%	88%
Surgical Care Improvement Project				
Appropriate Beta Blocker Usage[2]	83	99%	98%	98%
Appropriate VTP Within 24 Hours[2]	300	98%	98%	98%
Controlled Postoperative Blood Glucose[2,7]	-	-	97%	97%
Perioperative Temperature Management[2]	328	100%	100%	100%
Prophylactic Antibiotic Selection[2]	217	100%	99%	99%
Prophylactic Antibiotic Selection (Outpatient)	43	100%	98%	98%
Prophylactic Antibiotic Stopped[2]	213	99%	99%	98%
Prophylactic Antibiotic Timing[2]	218	98%	98%	99%
Prophylactic Antibiotic Timing (Outpatient)	43	100%	98%	98%
Urinary Catheter Removal[2]	68	75%	97%	97%
Survey of Patients' Hospital Experiences				
Area Around Room 'Always' Quiet at Night	300+	60%	54%	61%
Doctors 'Always' Communicated Well	300+	77%	81%	82%
Home Recovery Information Given	300+	88%	87%	85%
Hospital Given 9 or 10 on 10 Point Scale	300+	71%	70%	71%
Meds 'Always' Explained Before Given	300+	61%	64%	64%
Nurses 'Always' Communicated Well	300+	73%	77%	79%
Pain 'Always' Well Controlled	300+	65%	70%	71%
Room and Bathroom 'Always' Clean	300+	70%	73%	73%
Timely Help 'Always' Received	300+	60%	65%	68%
Would Definitely Recommend Hospital	300+	77%	73%	71%
Use of Medical Imaging				
Cardiac Imaging Stress Test before Surgery	148	2.7%	4.3%	5.3%
Combination Abdominal CT Scan	557	3.4%	6.9%	10.5%
Combination Brain/Sinus CT Scan	442	4.3%	2.3%	2.7%
Combination Chest CT Scan	398	1.3%	1.1%	2.7%
Follow-up Mammogram/Ultrasound	613	9.0%	9.1%	8.8%
Lumbar Spine MRI for Low Back Pain	74	36.5%	37.9%	37.2%

Klickitat Valley Hospital

310 South Roosevelt
Goldendale, WA 98620
Phone: 509-773-4022
Fax: 509-773-4543
E-mail: kvh@gorge.net
URL: www.kvhs.net
Type: Critical Access Hospitals
Emergency Services: Yes
Ownership: Govt - Hospital Dist/Auth
Beds: 25

Key Personnel:
CEO . . . . Leslie Hiebert
Operating Room. . . . . Jeffrey Mathisen
Chief of Medical Staff. . . . . Ahn Nguyen, MD
Radiology. . . . . Sandy Rorabaugh
Patient Relations . . . . Peggy Skeahon
Anesthesiology. . . . . Michael Steinbock
Infection Control. . . . . Donna Tuning

Measure	Cases	This Hosp.	State Avg.	U.S. Avg.
Blood Clot Prevention and Treatment				
Anticoagulation Overlap Therapy[1]	-	-	97%	93%
ICU Venous Thromboembolism Prophylaxis[7]	-	-	92%	92%
Incidence of Potentially Preventable VTE[7]	-	-	9%	10%
UFH with Dosages/Platelet Monitoring[1]	-	-	99%	97%
Venous Thromboembolism Prophylaxis	80	12%	86%	85%
Warfarin Therapy Discharge Instructions[1]	-	-	74%	75%
Chest Pain/Possible Heart Attack Care				
Aspirin Given Within 24 Hours of Arrival[1,3]	-	-	97%	96%
Fibrinolytic Meds Within 30 Min. of Arrival[3,7]	-	-	51%	58%
Average Time to ECG (minutes)[1,3]	-	-	9	7
Average Time to Transfer (minutes)[3,7]	-	-	54	60
Children's Asthma Care				
Received Home Management Plan of Care	-	-	-	88%
Received Reliever Medication	-	-	-	100%
Received Systemic Corticosteroids	-	-	-	100%
Emergency Department				
Admittance Decision Time (minutes)[3]	50	59	96	98
Head CT Results Within 45 Min. of Arrival[1,3]	-	-	63%	57%
Patients Who Left ER Before Being Seen[5]	-	-	2%	2%
Time from ER Arrival to Admit. (minutes)[3]	76	259	259	274
Time from ER Arrival to Discharge (minutes)[3]	169	93	135	134
Time in ER Before Being Evaluated (minutes)[3]	98	17	22	26
Time to Pain Meds for Fractures (minutes)[1,3]	-	-	52	57
Heart Attack Care				
Aspirin Given at Discharge[3,7]	-	-	99%	99%
Fibrinolytic Meds Within 30 Min. of Arrival[3,7]	-	-	62%	54%
PCI Within 90 Minutes of Arrival[3,7]	-	-	97%	96%
Statin Prescribed at Discharge[3,7]	-	-	98%	98%
Heart Failure Care				
ACE Inhibitor or ARB for LVSD[3,7]	-	-	97%	97%
Discharge Instructions Given[1,3]	-	-	93%	94%
Evaluation of LVS Function[1,3]	-	-	99%	99%
Medicare Spending				
Medicare Spending per Patient (ratio)	-	-	0.91	0.98
Pneumonia Care				
Appropriate Initial Antibiotic Given[1,3]	-	-	96%	95%
Blood Culture Timing[1,3]	-	-	97%	98%
Pregnancy and Delivery Care				
Newborn Deliveries Scheduled Early[5]	-	-	2%	6%
Preventive Care				
Immunization for Influenza[3]	44	82%	91%	90%
Immunization for Pneumonia[2,3]	76	79%	91%	92%
Stroke Care				
Anticoagulation Therapy for Atrial Fibrillation[7]	-	-	94%	95%
Antithrombotic Therapy Timing[1]	-	-	98%	98%
Assessed for Rehabilitation[1]	-	-	98%	97%
Discharged on Antithrombotic Therapy[1]	-	-	99%	99%
Discharged on Statin Medication[1]	-	-	96%	94%
Thrombolytic Therapy Timing[1]	-	-	73%	66%
Venous Thromboembolism Prophylaxis[1]	-	-	94%	94%
Written Stroke Educational Materials Given[7]	-	-	86%	88%
Surgical Care Improvement Project				
Appropriate Beta Blocker Usage[3,7]	-	-	98%	98%
Appropriate VTP Within 24 Hours[1,3]	-	-	98%	98%
Controlled Postoperative Blood Glucose[3,7]	-	-	97%	97%
Perioperative Temperature Management[1,3]	-	-	100%	100%
Prophylactic Antibiotic Selection[3,7]	-	-	99%	99%
Prophylactic Antibiotic Selection (Outpatient)[5]	-	-	98%	98%
Prophylactic Antibiotic Stopped[3,7]	-	-	99%	98%
Prophylactic Antibiotic Timing[3,7]	-	-	98%	99%
Prophylactic Antibiotic Timing (Outpatient)[5]	-	-	98%	98%
Urinary Catheter Removal[3,7]	-	-	97%	97%
Survey of Patients' Hospital Experiences				
Area Around Room 'Always' Quiet at Night[6]	<100	42%	54%	61%
Doctors 'Always' Communicated Well[6]	<100	76%	81%	82%
Home Recovery Information Given[6]	<100	76%	87%	85%
Hospital Given 9 or 10 on 10 Point Scale[6]	<100	45%	70%	71%
Meds 'Always' Explained Before Given[6]	<100	48%	64%	64%
Nurses 'Always' Communicated Well[6]	<100	65%	77%	79%
Pain 'Always' Well Controlled[6]	<100	53%	70%	71%
Room and Bathroom 'Always' Clean[6]	<100	64%	73%	73%
Timely Help 'Always' Received[6]	<100	60%	65%	68%
Would Definitely Recommend Hospital[6]	<100	45%	73%	71%
Use of Medical Imaging				
Cardiac Imaging Stress Test before Surgery[7]	-	-	4.3%	5.3%
Combination Abdominal CT Scan	132	4.5%	6.9%	10.5%
Combination Brain/Sinus CT Scan[1]	-	-	2.3%	2.7%
Combination Chest CT Scan	86	5.8%	1.1%	2.7%
Follow-up Mammogram/Ultrasound	192	12.5%	9.1%	8.8%
Lumbar Spine MRI for Low Back Pain[1]	-	-	37.9%	37.2%

Coulee Community Hospital

411 Fortuyn Road
Grand Coulee, WA 99133
Phone: 509-633-1753
Fax: 509-633-0295
URL: www.couleecommhosp.org
Type: Critical Access Hospitals
Emergency Services: Yes
Ownership: Govt - Hospital Dist/Auth
Beds: 25

Key Personnel:
Chief of Medical Staff. . . . . Andrew Castrodale
CEO/President. . . . . Jerry Lane

Measure	Cases	This Hosp.	State Avg.	U.S. Avg.
Blood Clot Prevention and Treatment				
Anticoagulation Overlap Therapy[5]	-	-	97%	93%
ICU Venous Thromboembolism Prophylaxis[5]	-	-	92%	92%
Incidence of Potentially Preventable VTE[5]	-	-	9%	10%
UFH with Dosages/Platelet Monitoring[5]	-	-	99%	97%
Venous Thromboembolism Prophylaxis[5]	-	-	86%	85%
Warfarin Therapy Discharge Instructions[5]	-	-	74%	75%
Chest Pain/Possible Heart Attack Care				
Aspirin Given Within 24 Hours of Arrival[1,3]	-	-	97%	96%
Fibrinolytic Meds Within 30 Min. of Arrival[3,7]	-	-	51%	58%
Average Time to ECG (minutes)[1,3]	-	-	9	7
Average Time to Transfer (minutes)[3,7]	-	-	54	60
Children's Asthma Care				
Received Home Management Plan of Care	-	-	-	88%
Received Reliever Medication	-	-	-	100%
Received Systemic Corticosteroids	-	-	-	100%
Emergency Department				
Admittance Decision Time (minutes)[5]	-	-	96	98
Head CT Results Within 45 Min. of Arrival[5]	-	-	63%	57%
Patients Who Left ER Before Being Seen[5]	-	-	2%	2%
Time from ER Arrival to Admit. (minutes)[5]	-	-	259	274
Time from ER Arrival to Discharge (minutes)[5]	-	-	135	134
Time in ER Before Being Evaluated (minutes)[5]	-	-	22	26
Time to Pain Meds for Fractures (minutes)[5]	-	-	52	57
Heart Attack Care				
Aspirin Given at Discharge[5]	-	-	99%	99%
Fibrinolytic Meds Within 30 Min. of Arrival[5]	-	-	62%	54%
PCI Within 90 Minutes of Arrival[5]	-	-	97%	96%
Statin Prescribed at Discharge[5]	-	-	98%	98%
Heart Failure Care				
ACE Inhibitor or ARB for LVSD[1]	-	-	97%	97%
Discharge Instructions Given[1]	-	-	93%	94%
Evaluation of LVS Function	13	46%	99%	99%
Medicare Spending				
Medicare Spending per Patient (ratio)	-	-	0.91	0.98
Pneumonia Care				
Appropriate Initial Antibiotic Given[7]	-	-	96%	95%
Blood Culture Timing[1]	-	-	97%	98%
Pregnancy and Delivery Care				
Newborn Deliveries Scheduled Early[5]	-	-	2%	6%
Preventive Care				
Immunization for Influenza[5]	-	-	91%	90%
Immunization for Pneumonia[5]	-	-	91%	92%
Stroke Care				
Anticoagulation Therapy for Atrial Fibrillation[5]	-	-	94%	95%
Antithrombotic Therapy Timing[5]	-	-	98%	98%
Assessed for Rehabilitation[5]	-	-	98%	97%
Discharged on Antithrombotic Therapy[5]	-	-	99%	99%
Discharged on Statin Medication[5]	-	-	96%	94%
Thrombolytic Therapy Timing[5]	-	-	73%	66%
Venous Thromboembolism Prophylaxis[5]	-	-	94%	94%
Written Stroke Educational Materials Given[5]	-	-	86%	88%
Surgical Care Improvement Project				
Appropriate Beta Blocker Usage[5]	-	-	98%	98%
Appropriate VTP Within 24 Hours[5]	-	-	98%	98%
Controlled Postoperative Blood Glucose[5]	-	-	97%	97%
Perioperative Temperature Management[5]	-	-	100%	100%
Prophylactic Antibiotic Selection[5]	-	-	99%	99%
Prophylactic Antibiotic Selection (Outpatient)[5]	-	-	98%	98%
Prophylactic Antibiotic Stopped[5]	-	-	99%	98%
Prophylactic Antibiotic Timing[5]	-	-	98%	99%
Prophylactic Antibiotic Timing (Outpatient)[5]	-	-	98%	98%
Urinary Catheter Removal[5]	-	-	97%	97%
Survey of Patients' Hospital Experiences				
Area Around Room 'Always' Quiet at Night[6]	<100	65%	54%	61%
Doctors 'Always' Communicated Well[6]	<100	89%	81%	82%
Home Recovery Information Given[6]	<100	91%	87%	85%
Hospital Given 9 or 10 on 10 Point Scale[6]	<100	72%	70%	71%
Meds 'Always' Explained Before Given[6]	<100	69%	64%	64%
Nurses 'Always' Communicated Well[6]	<100	82%	77%	79%
Pain 'Always' Well Controlled[6]	<100	81%	70%	71%
Room and Bathroom 'Always' Clean[6]	<100	72%	73%	73%
Timely Help 'Always' Received[6]	<100	72%	65%	68%
Would Definitely Recommend Hospital[6]	<100	68%	73%	71%
Use of Medical Imaging				
Cardiac Imaging Stress Test before Surgery[7]	-	-	4.3%	5.3%
Combination Abdominal CT Scan	81	6.2%	6.9%	10.5%

NOTE: Hospital profiles are in alphabetical order by state, then city, then hospital within the city; Rankings exclude hospitals with less than 25 cases except for patient surveys which excludes hospitals with less than 100 cases; (a) 100-299 cases; (1) The number of cases/patients is too few to report; (2) Data submitted were based on a sample of cases/patients; (3) Results are based on a shorter time period than required; (4) Data suppressed by CMS for one or more quarters; (5) Results are not available for this reporting period; (6) Fewer than 100 patients completed the HCAHPS survey; (7) No cases met the criteria for this measure; (8) The lower limit of the confidence interval cannot be calculated if the number of observed infections equals zero; (9) No data are available from the state/territory for this reporting period; (10) The scores shown reflect fewer than 50 completed surveys; (11) There were discrepancies in the data collection process; (12) This measure does not apply to this hospital for this reporting period; (13) Results cannot be calculated for this reporting period; (14) The results for this state are combined with nearby states to protect confidentiality; Please refer to the User's Guide for a full explanation of data.

Combination Brain/Sinus CT Scan[1]	-	-	2.3%	2.7%
Combination Chest CT Scan	56	0.0%	1.1%	2.7%
Follow-up Mammogram/Ultrasound	138	3.6%	9.1%	8.8%
Lumbar Spine MRI for Low Back Pain[1]	-	-	37.9%	37.2%

Ocean Beach Hospital

174 First Avenue North Phone: 360-642-3181
Ilwaco, WA 98624 Fax: 360-642-8070
Type: Critical Access Hospitals Emergency Services: Yes
Ownership: Govt - Hospital Dist/Auth Beds: 25

Key Personnel:
Chief of Medical Staff.......... Randy Ensminger
Quality Assurance .... Julie Oakes
CEO/President............... Kendall Sawa

Measure	Cases	This Hosp.	State Avg.	U.S. Avg.
Blood Clot Prevention and Treatment				
Anticoagulation Overlap Therapy[5]	-	-	97%	93%
ICU Venous Thromboembolism Prophylaxis[5]	-	-	92%	92%
Incidence of Potentially Preventable VTE[5]	-	-	9%	10%
UFH with Dosages/Platelet Monitoring[5]	-	-	99%	97%
Venous Thromboembolism Prophylaxis[5]	-	-	86%	85%
Warfarin Therapy Discharge Instructions[5]	-	-	74%	75%
Chest Pain/Possible Heart Attack Care				
Aspirin Given Within 24 Hours of Arrival	-	-	97%	96%
Fibrinolytic Meds Within 30 Min. of Arrival	-	-	51%	58%
Average Time to ECG (minutes)	-	-	9	7
Average Time to Transfer (minutes)	-	-	54	60
Children's Asthma Care				
Received Home Management Plan of Care	-	-	-	88%
Received Reliever Medication	-	-	-	100%
Received Systemic Corticosteroids	-	-	-	100%
Emergency Department				
Admittance Decision Time (minutes)[5]	-	-	96	98
Head CT Results Within 45 Min. of Arrival	-	-	63%	57%
Patients Who Left ER Before Being Seen	-	-	2%	2%
Time from ER Arrival to Admit. (minutes)[5]	-	-	259	274
Time from ER Arrival to Discharge (minutes)	-	-	135	134
Time in ER Before Being Evaluated (minutes)	-	-	22	26
Time to Pain Meds for Fractures (minutes)	-	-	52	57
Heart Attack Care				
Aspirin Given at Discharge[5]	-	-	99%	99%
Fibrinolytic Meds Within 30 Min. of Arrival[5]	-	-	62%	54%
PCI Within 90 Minutes of Arrival[5]	-	-	97%	96%
Statin Prescribed at Discharge[5]	-	-	98%	98%
Heart Failure Care				
ACE Inhibitor or ARB for LVSD[1,3]	-	-	97%	97%
Discharge Instructions Given[1,3]	-	-	93%	94%
Evaluation of LVS Function[3]	11	100%	99%	99%
Medicare Spending				
Medicare Spending per Patient (ratio)	-	-	0.91	0.98
Pneumonia Care				
Appropriate Initial Antibiotic Given[2]	12	75%	96%	95%
Blood Culture Timing[2]	14	100%	97%	98%
Pregnancy and Delivery Care				
Newborn Deliveries Scheduled Early[5]	-	-	2%	6%
Preventive Care				
Immunization for Influenza[5]	-	-	91%	90%
Immunization for Pneumonia[5]	-	-	91%	92%
Stroke Care				
Anticoagulation Therapy for Atrial Fibrillation[5]	-	-	94%	95%
Antithrombotic Therapy Timing[5]	-	-	98%	98%
Assessed for Rehabilitation[5]	-	-	98%	97%
Discharged on Antithrombotic Therapy[5]	-	-	99%	99%
Discharged on Statin Medication[5]	-	-	96%	94%
Thrombolytic Therapy Timing[5]	-	-	73%	66%
Venous Thromboembolism Prophylaxis[5]	-	-	94%	94%
Written Stroke Educational Materials Given[5]	-	-	86%	88%
Surgical Care Improvement Project				
Appropriate Beta Blocker Usage[1,3]	-	-	98%	98%
Appropriate VTP Within 24 Hours[1,3]	-	-	98%	98%
Controlled Postoperative Blood Glucose[3,7]	-	-	97%	97%
Perioperative Temperature Management[3]	12	100%	100%	100%
Prophylactic Antibiotic Selection[3]	12	100%	99%	99%
Prophylactic Antibiotic Selection (Outpatient)	-	-	98%	98%
Prophylactic Antibiotic Stopped[3]	12	100%	99%	98%
Prophylactic Antibiotic Timing[3]	12	83%	98%	99%
Prophylactic Antibiotic Timing (Outpatient)	-	-	98%	98%
Urinary Catheter Removal[3,7]	-	-	97%	97%
Survey of Patients' Hospital Experiences				
Area Around Room 'Always' Quiet at Night[5]	-	-	54%	61%
Doctors 'Always' Communicated Well[5]	-	-	81%	82%
Home Recovery Information Given[5]	-	-	87%	85%
Hospital Given 9 or 10 on 10 Point Scale[5]	-	-	70%	71%
Meds 'Always' Explained Before Given[5]	-	-	64%	64%
Nurses 'Always' Communicated Well[5]	-	-	77%	79%
Pain 'Always' Well Controlled[5]	-	-	70%	71%
Room and Bathroom 'Always' Clean[5]	-	-	73%	73%
Timely Help 'Always' Received[5]	-	-	65%	68%
Would Definitely Recommend Hospital[5]	-	-	73%	71%
Use of Medical Imaging				
Cardiac Imaging Stress Test before Surgery	-	-	4.3%	5.3%
Combination Abdominal CT Scan	-	-	6.9%	10.5%
Combination Brain/Sinus CT Scan	-	-	2.3%	2.7%
Combination Chest CT Scan	-	-	1.1%	2.7%
Follow-up Mammogram/Ultrasound	-	-	9.1%	8.8%
Lumbar Spine MRI for Low Back Pain	-	-	37.9%	37.2%

Swedish Issaquah

751 Ne Blakely Dr Phone: 425-313-4000
Issaquah, WA 98029
URL: www.swedish.org/locations/issaquah-campus
Type: Acute Care Hospitals Emergency Services: Yes
Ownership: Voluntary non-profit - Private

Measure	Cases	This Hosp.	State Avg.	U.S. Avg.
Blood Clot Prevention and Treatment				
Anticoagulation Overlap Therapy[2]	28	100%	97%	93%
ICU Venous Thromboembolism Prophylaxis[2]	37	86%	92%	92%
Incidence of Potentially Preventable VTE[1,2]	-	-	9%	10%
UFH with Dosages/Platelet Monitoring[2]	11	100%	99%	97%
Venous Thromboembolism Prophylaxis[2]	227	93%	86%	85%
Warfarin Therapy Discharge Instructions[2]	22	82%	74%	75%
Chest Pain/Possible Heart Attack Care				
Aspirin Given Within 24 Hours of Arrival[1,3]	-	-	97%	96%
Fibrinolytic Meds Within 30 Min. of Arrival[3,7]	-	-	51%	58%
Average Time to ECG (minutes)[1,3]	-	-	9	7
Average Time to Transfer (minutes)[3,7]	-	-	54	60
Children's Asthma Care				
Received Home Management Plan of Care	-	-	-	88%
Received Reliever Medication	-	-	-	100%
Received Systemic Corticosteroids	-	-	-	100%
Emergency Department				
Admittance Decision Time (minutes)[2]	490	72	96	98
Head CT Results Within 45 Min. of Arrival[1]	-	-	63%	57%
Patients Who Left ER Before Being Seen	22,789	0%	2%	2%
Time from ER Arrival to Admit. (minutes)[2]	490	154	259	274
Time from ER Arrival to Discharge (minutes)	406	86	135	134
Time in ER Before Being Evaluated (minutes)	412	7	22	26
Time to Pain Meds for Fractures (minutes)	111	38	52	57
Heart Attack Care				
Aspirin Given at Discharge	67	100%	99%	99%
Fibrinolytic Meds Within 30 Min. of Arrival[7]	-	-	62%	54%
PCI Within 90 Minutes of Arrival	24	96%	97%	96%
Statin Prescribed at Discharge	63	97%	98%	98%
Heart Failure Care				
ACE Inhibitor or ARB for LVSD	24	100%	97%	97%
Discharge Instructions Given	67	99%	93%	94%
Evaluation of LVS Function	81	100%	99%	99%
Medicare Spending				
Medicare Spending per Patient (ratio)	-	0.92	0.91	0.98
Pneumonia Care				
Appropriate Initial Antibiotic Given	49	94%	96%	95%
Blood Culture Timing	69	99%	97%	98%
Pregnancy and Delivery Care				
Newborn Deliveries Scheduled Early	78	1%	2%	6%
Preventive Care				
Immunization for Influenza[2]	505	95%	91%	90%
Immunization for Pneumonia[2]	441	98%	91%	92%
Stroke Care				
Anticoagulation Therapy for Atrial Fibrillation[1]	-	-	94%	95%
Antithrombotic Therapy Timing	38	97%	98%	98%
Assessed for Rehabilitation	56	96%	98%	97%
Discharged on Antithrombotic Therapy	54	98%	99%	99%
Discharged on Statin Medication	43	91%	96%	94%
Thrombolytic Therapy Timing[1]	-	-	73%	66%
Venous Thromboembolism Prophylaxis	41	80%	94%	94%
Written Stroke Educational Materials Given	32	69%	86%	88%
Surgical Care Improvement Project				
Appropriate Beta Blocker Usage[2]	65	98%	98%	98%
Appropriate VTP Within 24 Hours[2]	287	98%	98%	98%
Controlled Postoperative Blood Glucose[2,7]	-	-	97%	97%
Perioperative Temperature Management[2]	380	100%	100%	100%
Prophylactic Antibiotic Selection[2]	254	100%	99%	99%
Prophylactic Antibiotic Selection (Outpatient)	200	100%	98%	98%
Prophylactic Antibiotic Stopped[2]	248	98%	99%	98%
Prophylactic Antibiotic Timing[2]	256	98%	98%	99%
Prophylactic Antibiotic Timing (Outpatient)	200	99%	98%	98%
Urinary Catheter Removal[2]	172	100%	97%	97%
Survey of Patients' Hospital Experiences				
Area Around Room 'Always' Quiet at Night	300+	61%	54%	61%
Doctors 'Always' Communicated Well	300+	82%	81%	82%
Home Recovery Information Given	300+	84%	87%	85%
Hospital Given 9 or 10 on 10 Point Scale	300+	78%	70%	71%
Meds 'Always' Explained Before Given	300+	63%	64%	64%
Nurses 'Always' Communicated Well	300+	76%	77%	79%
Pain 'Always' Well Controlled	300+	70%	70%	71%
Room and Bathroom 'Always' Clean	300+	72%	73%	73%
Timely Help 'Always' Received	300+	69%	65%	68%
Would Definitely Recommend Hospital	300+	82%	73%	71%
Use of Medical Imaging				
Cardiac Imaging Stress Test before Surgery	255	6.3%	4.3%	5.3%
Combination Abdominal CT Scan	379	9.5%	6.9%	10.5%
Combination Brain/Sinus CT Scan	397	1.0%	2.3%	2.7%
Combination Chest CT Scan	228	0.4%	1.1%	2.7%
Follow-up Mammogram/Ultrasound	387	16.5%	9.1%	8.8%
Lumbar Spine MRI for Low Back Pain	87	41.4%	37.9%	37.2%

Kennewick General Hospital

900 South Auburn Street Phone: 509-586-6111
Kennewick, WA 99336
URL: www.kennewickgeneral.com
Type: Acute Care Hospitals Emergency Services: Yes
Ownership: Govt - Hospital Dist/Auth Beds: 101

Key Personnel:
CEO/President............... Glen Marshall
Radiology................... Richard Rhee

Measure	Cases	This Hosp.	State Avg.	U.S. Avg.
Blood Clot Prevention and Treatment				
Anticoagulation Overlap Therapy[2]	27	100%	97%	93%
ICU Venous Thromboembolism Prophylaxis[2]	48	98%	92%	92%
Incidence of Potentially Preventable VTE[1,2]	-	-	9%	10%
UFH with Dosages/Platelet Monitoring[2]	15	100%	99%	97%
Venous Thromboembolism Prophylaxis[2]	343	88%	86%	85%
Warfarin Therapy Discharge Instructions[2]	22	91%	74%	75%
Chest Pain/Possible Heart Attack Care				
Aspirin Given Within 24 Hours of Arrival	33	100%	97%	96%
Fibrinolytic Meds Within 30 Min. of Arrival[7]	-	-	51%	58%
Average Time to ECG (minutes)	34	11	9	7
Average Time to Transfer (minutes)	11	35	54	60
Children's Asthma Care				
Received Home Management Plan of Care	-	-	-	88%
Received Reliever Medication	-	-	-	100%
Received Systemic Corticosteroids	-	-	-	100%
Emergency Department				
Admittance Decision Time (minutes)[2]	487	100	96	98
Head CT Results Within 45 Min. of Arrival	11	73%	63%	57%
Patients Who Left ER Before Being Seen	32,458	2%	2%	2%
Time from ER Arrival to Admit. (minutes)[2]	526	232	259	274
Time from ER Arrival to Discharge (minutes)	358	114	135	134

NOTE: Hospital profiles are in alphabetical order by state, then city, then hospital within the city; Rankings exclude hospitals with less than 25 cases except for patient surveys which excludes hospitals with less than 100 cases; (a) 100-299 cases; (1) The number of cases/patients is too few to report; (2) Data submitted were based on a sample of cases/patients; (3) Results are based on a shorter time period than required; (4) Data suppressed by CMS for one or more quarters; (5) Results are not available for this reporting period; (6) Fewer than 100 patients completed the HCAHPS survey; (7) No cases met the criteria for this measure; (8) The lower limit of the confidence interval cannot be calculated if the number of observed infections equals zero; (9) No data are available from the state/territory for this reporting period; (10) The scores shown reflect fewer than 50 completed surveys; (11) There were discrepancies in the data collection process; (12) This measure does not apply to this hospital for this reporting period; (13) Results cannot be calculated for this reporting period; (14) The results for this state are combined with nearby states to protect confidentiality; Please refer to the User's Guide for a full explanation of data.

Time in ER Before Being Evaluated (minutes)	378	30	22	26
Time to Pain Meds for Fractures (minutes)	97	35	52	57
Heart Attack Care				
Aspirin Given at Discharge[1]	-	-	99%	99%
Fibrinolytic Meds Within 30 Min. of Arrival[7]	-	-	62%	54%
PCI Within 90 Minutes of Arrival[7]	-	-	97%	96%
Statin Prescribed at Discharge[1]	-	-	98%	98%
Heart Failure Care				
ACE Inhibitor or ARB for LVSD	43	98%	97%	97%
Discharge Instructions Given	153	100%	93%	94%
Evaluation of LVS Function	180	96%	99%	99%
Medicare Spending				
Medicare Spending per Patient (ratio)	-	0.93	0.91	0.98
Pneumonia Care				
Appropriate Initial Antibiotic Given	64	100%	96%	95%
Blood Culture Timing	47	100%	97%	98%
Pregnancy and Delivery Care				
Newborn Deliveries Scheduled Early[2]	29	0%	2%	6%
Preventive Care				
Immunization for Influenza[2]	467	96%	91%	90%
Immunization for Pneumonia[2]	474	97%	91%	92%
Stroke Care				
Anticoagulation Therapy for Atrial Fibrillation[1]	-	-	94%	95%
Antithrombotic Therapy Timing	31	100%	98%	98%
Assessed for Rehabilitation	41	95%	98%	97%
Discharged on Antithrombotic Therapy	40	100%	99%	99%
Discharged on Statin Medication	34	91%	96%	94%
Thrombolytic Therapy Timing[1]	-	-	73%	66%
Venous Thromboembolism Prophylaxis	39	92%	94%	94%
Written Stroke Educational Materials Given	21	71%	86%	88%
Surgical Care Improvement Project				
Appropriate Beta Blocker Usage[2]	46	96%	98%	98%
Appropriate VTP Within 24 Hours[2]	214	96%	98%	98%
Controlled Postoperative Blood Glucose[2,7]	-	-	97%	97%
Perioperative Temperature Management[2]	242	100%	100%	100%
Prophylactic Antibiotic Selection[2]	148	100%	99%	99%
Prophylactic Antibiotic Selection (Outpatient)	176	98%	98%	98%
Prophylactic Antibiotic Stopped[2]	146	98%	99%	98%
Prophylactic Antibiotic Timing[2]	148	99%	98%	99%
Prophylactic Antibiotic Timing (Outpatient)	177	98%	98%	98%
Urinary Catheter Removal[2]	147	99%	97%	97%
Survey of Patients' Hospital Experiences				
Area Around Room 'Always' Quiet at Night	300+	52%	54%	61%
Doctors 'Always' Communicated Well	300+	80%	81%	82%
Home Recovery Information Given	300+	87%	87%	85%
Hospital Given 9 or 10 on 10 Point Scale	300+	69%	70%	71%
Meds 'Always' Explained Before Given	300+	66%	64%	64%
Nurses 'Always' Communicated Well	300+	80%	77%	79%
Pain 'Always' Well Controlled	300+	74%	70%	71%
Room and Bathroom 'Always' Clean	300+	78%	73%	73%
Timely Help 'Always' Received	300+	67%	65%	68%
Would Definitely Recommend Hospital	300+	73%	73%	71%
Use of Medical Imaging				
Cardiac Imaging Stress Test before Surgery	240	2.5%	4.3%	5.3%
Combination Abdominal CT Scan	589	5.3%	6.9%	10.5%
Combination Brain/Sinus CT Scan	621	4.8%	2.3%	2.7%
Combination Chest CT Scan	513	2.7%	1.1%	2.7%
Follow-up Mammogram/Ultrasound	827	6.4%	9.1%	8.8%
Lumbar Spine MRI for Low Back Pain	84	38.1%	37.9%	37.2%

Evergreen Hospital Medical Center

12040 Ne 128th Street Phone: 425-899-1000
Kirkland, WA 98034 Fax: 425-899-2759
E-mail: info@evergreenhealthcare.org
URL: www.evergreenhospital.org
Type: Acute Care Hospitals Emergency Services: Yes
Ownership: Govt - Hospital Dist/Auth Beds: 275

Key Personnel:
Coronary Care . . . . James Brown, MD
Surgery . . . . Kelly Clinch, MD
Emergency Room . . . . Kevin Hanson, MD
Patient Relations . . . . Mary Jim Montgomery, RN
Anesthesiology. . . . . Steven Sasaki, MD
Pediatrics. . . . . Steve Schiebel, MD
Chief of Medical Staff. . . . . Jeff Tomlin, MD
Cardiology . . . . Rachael Wyman, MD

Measure	Cases	This Hosp.	State Avg.	U.S. Avg.
Blood Clot Prevention and Treatment				
Anticoagulation Overlap Therapy[2]	130	100%	97%	93%
ICU Venous Thromboembolism Prophylaxis[2]	69	88%	92%	92%
Incidence of Potentially Preventable VTE[1,2]	-	-	9%	10%
UFH with Dosages/Platelet Monitoring[2]	84	100%	99%	97%
Venous Thromboembolism Prophylaxis[2]	312	85%	86%	85%
Warfarin Therapy Discharge Instructions[2]	100	91%	74%	75%
Chest Pain/Possible Heart Attack Care				
Aspirin Given Within 24 Hours of Arrival	18	94%	97%	96%
Fibrinolytic Meds Within 30 Min. of Arrival[3,7]	-	-	51%	58%
Average Time to ECG (minutes)	19	6	9	7
Average Time to Transfer (minutes)[3,7]	-	-	54	60
Children's Asthma Care				
Received Home Management Plan of Care	-	-	-	88%
Received Reliever Medication	-	-	-	100%
Received Systemic Corticosteroids	-	-	-	100%
Emergency Department				
Admittance Decision Time (minutes)[2]	564	105	96	98
Head CT Results Within 45 Min. of Arrival	12	83%	63%	57%
Patients Who Left ER Before Being Seen	44,797	1%	2%	2%
Time from ER Arrival to Admit. (minutes)[2]	568	256	259	274
Time from ER Arrival to Discharge (minutes)	385	139	135	134
Time in ER Before Being Evaluated (minutes)	282	19	22	26
Time to Pain Meds for Fractures (minutes)	269	47	52	57
Heart Attack Care				
Aspirin Given at Discharge	217	100%	99%	99%
Fibrinolytic Meds Within 30 Min. of Arrival[7]	-	-	62%	54%
PCI Within 90 Minutes of Arrival	63	97%	97%	96%
Statin Prescribed at Discharge	205	98%	98%	98%
Heart Failure Care				
ACE Inhibitor or ARB for LVSD	51	100%	97%	97%
Discharge Instructions Given	202	99%	93%	94%
Evaluation of LVS Function	248	100%	99%	99%
Medicare Spending				
Medicare Spending per Patient (ratio)	-	0.93	0.91	0.98
Pneumonia Care				
Appropriate Initial Antibiotic Given	144	95%	96%	95%
Blood Culture Timing	242	98%	97%	98%
Pregnancy and Delivery Care				
Newborn Deliveries Scheduled Early	331	2%	2%	6%
Preventive Care				
Immunization for Influenza[2]	604	90%	91%	90%
Immunization for Pneumonia[2]	515	92%	91%	92%
Stroke Care				
Anticoagulation Therapy for Atrial Fibrillation	32	100%	94%	95%
Antithrombotic Therapy Timing	135	98%	98%	98%
Assessed for Rehabilitation	186	100%	98%	97%
Discharged on Antithrombotic Therapy	169	100%	99%	99%
Discharged on Statin Medication	121	98%	96%	94%
Thrombolytic Therapy Timing	14	93%	73%	66%
Venous Thromboembolism Prophylaxis	170	99%	94%	94%
Written Stroke Educational Materials Given	112	89%	86%	88%
Surgical Care Improvement Project				
Appropriate Beta Blocker Usage[2]	97	94%	98%	98%
Appropriate VTP Within 24 Hours[2]	309	94%	98%	98%
Controlled Postoperative Blood Glucose[2,7]	-	-	97%	97%
Perioperative Temperature Management[2]	492	100%	100%	100%
Prophylactic Antibiotic Selection[2]	345	98%	99%	99%
Prophylactic Antibiotic Selection (Outpatient)	638	98%	98%	98%
Prophylactic Antibiotic Stopped[2]	339	98%	99%	98%
Prophylactic Antibiotic Timing[2]	345	99%	98%	99%
Prophylactic Antibiotic Timing (Outpatient)	643	97%	98%	98%
Urinary Catheter Removal[2]	160	94%	97%	97%
Survey of Patients' Hospital Experiences				
Area Around Room 'Always' Quiet at Night	300+	65%	54%	61%
Doctors 'Always' Communicated Well	300+	82%	81%	82%
Home Recovery Information Given	300+	86%	87%	85%
Hospital Given 9 or 10 on 10 Point Scale	300+	78%	70%	71%
Meds 'Always' Explained Before Given	300+	62%	64%	64%
Nurses 'Always' Communicated Well	300+	73%	77%	79%
Pain 'Always' Well Controlled	300+	67%	70%	71%
Room and Bathroom 'Always' Clean	300+	70%	73%	73%
Timely Help 'Always' Received	300+	64%	65%	68%
Would Definitely Recommend Hospital	300+	81%	73%	71%
Use of Medical Imaging				
Cardiac Imaging Stress Test before Surgery	1,354	4.3%	4.3%	5.3%
Combination Abdominal CT Scan	813	1.7%	6.9%	10.5%
Combination Brain/Sinus CT Scan	664	2.4%	2.3%	2.7%
Combination Chest CT Scan	649	0.6%	1.1%	2.7%
Follow-up Mammogram/Ultrasound	2,154	13.5%	9.1%	8.8%
Lumbar Spine MRI for Low Back Pain[1]	-	-	37.9%	37.2%

Saint Clare Hospital

11315 Bridgeport Way S W Phone: 253-588-1711
Lakewood, WA 98499 Fax: 253-512-2708
URL: www.fhshealth.org
Type: Acute Care Hospitals Emergency Services: Yes
Ownership: Voluntary non-profit - Church Beds: 106

Key Personnel:
CEO . . . . Mark Benedum
President/CEO. . . . . Scott W. Bosch
Radiology. . . . . Alison Reinbold-Carter
Quality Assurance . . . . Ricki Strader
CEO . . . . Joseph Wilczek

Measure	Cases	This Hosp.	State Avg.	U.S. Avg.
Blood Clot Prevention and Treatment				
Anticoagulation Overlap Therapy[2]	52	92%	97%	93%
ICU Venous Thromboembolism Prophylaxis[2]	27	93%	92%	92%
Incidence of Potentially Preventable VTE[1,2]	-	-	9%	10%
UFH with Dosages/Platelet Monitoring[2]	47	100%	99%	97%
Venous Thromboembolism Prophylaxis[2]	324	92%	86%	85%
Warfarin Therapy Discharge Instructions[2]	41	61%	74%	75%
Chest Pain/Possible Heart Attack Care				
Aspirin Given Within 24 Hours of Arrival	63	98%	97%	96%
Fibrinolytic Meds Within 30 Min. of Arrival[7]	-	-	51%	58%
Average Time to ECG (minutes)	63	12	9	7
Average Time to Transfer (minutes)	18	58	54	60
Children's Asthma Care				
Received Home Management Plan of Care	-	-	-	88%
Received Reliever Medication	-	-	-	100%
Received Systemic Corticosteroids	-	-	-	100%
Emergency Department				
Admittance Decision Time (minutes)[2]	945	151	96	98
Head CT Results Within 45 Min. of Arrival	13	38%	63%	57%
Patients Who Left ER Before Being Seen	46,048	2%	2%	2%
Time from ER Arrival to Admit. (minutes)[2]	966	330	259	274
Time from ER Arrival to Discharge (minutes)	380	165	135	134
Time in ER Before Being Evaluated (minutes)	410	22	22	26
Time to Pain Meds for Fractures (minutes)	81	47	52	57
Heart Attack Care				
Aspirin Given at Discharge[1]	-	-	99%	99%
Fibrinolytic Meds Within 30 Min. of Arrival[7]	-	-	62%	54%
PCI Within 90 Minutes of Arrival[7]	-	-	97%	96%
Statin Prescribed at Discharge[1]	-	-	98%	98%
Heart Failure Care				
ACE Inhibitor or ARB for LVSD	66	100%	97%	97%
Discharge Instructions Given	145	94%	93%	94%
Evaluation of LVS Function	174	100%	99%	99%
Medicare Spending				
Medicare Spending per Patient (ratio)	-	0.95	0.91	0.98
Pneumonia Care				
Appropriate Initial Antibiotic Given[2]	113	97%	96%	95%
Blood Culture Timing[2]	208	99%	97%	98%
Pregnancy and Delivery Care				
Newborn Deliveries Scheduled Early[7]	-	-	2%	6%
Preventive Care				
Immunization for Influenza[2]	619	91%	91%	90%
Immunization for Pneumonia[2]	825	91%	91%	92%
Stroke Care				
Anticoagulation Therapy for Atrial Fibrillation[1]	-	-	94%	95%
Antithrombotic Therapy Timing	34	100%	98%	98%
Assessed for Rehabilitation	40	95%	98%	97%
Discharged on Antithrombotic Therapy	40	100%	99%	99%
Discharged on Statin Medication	33	97%	96%	94%
Thrombolytic Therapy Timing[7]	-	-	73%	66%

NOTE: Hospital profiles are in alphabetical order by state, then city, then hospital within the city; Rankings exclude hospitals with less than 25 cases except for patient surveys which excludes hospitals with less than 100 cases; (a) 100-299 cases; (1) The number of cases/patients is too few to report; (2) Data submitted were based on a sample of cases/patients; (3) Results are based on a shorter time period than required; (4) Data suppressed by CMS for one or more quarters; (5) Results are not available for this reporting period; (6) Fewer than 100 patients completed the HCAHPS survey; (7) No cases met the criteria for this measure; (8) The lower limit of the confidence interval cannot be calculated if the number of observed infections equals zero; (9) No data are available from the state/territory for this reporting period; (10) The scores shown reflect fewer than 50 completed surveys; (11) There were discrepancies in the data collection process; (12) This measure does not apply to this hospital for this reporting period; (13) Results cannot be calculated for this reporting period; (14) The results for this state are combined with nearby states to protect confidentiality; Please refer to the User's Guide for a full explanation of data.

Measure	Cases	This Hosp.	State Avg.	U.S. Avg.
Venous Thromboembolism Prophylaxis	39	92%	94%	94%
Written Stroke Educational Materials Given	27	48%	86%	88%
Surgical Care Improvement Project				
Appropriate Beta Blocker Usage[2]	101	97%	98%	98%
Appropriate VTP Within 24 Hours[2]	312	97%	98%	98%
Controlled Postoperative Blood Glucose[2,7]	-	-	97%	97%
Perioperative Temperature Management[2]	350	100%	100%	100%
Prophylactic Antibiotic Selection[2]	217	100%	99%	99%
Prophylactic Antibiotic Selection (Outpatient)	58	97%	98%	98%
Prophylactic Antibiotic Stopped[2]	203	100%	99%	98%
Prophylactic Antibiotic Timing[2]	217	97%	98%	99%
Prophylactic Antibiotic Timing (Outpatient)	59	98%	98%	98%
Urinary Catheter Removal[2]	71	82%	97%	97%
Survey of Patients' Hospital Experiences				
Area Around Room 'Always' Quiet at Night	300+	52%	54%	61%
Doctors 'Always' Communicated Well	300+	75%	81%	82%
Home Recovery Information Given	300+	88%	87%	85%
Hospital Given 9 or 10 on 10 Point Scale	300+	66%	70%	71%
Meds 'Always' Explained Before Given	300+	59%	64%	64%
Nurses 'Always' Communicated Well	300+	73%	77%	79%
Pain 'Always' Well Controlled	300+	65%	70%	71%
Room and Bathroom 'Always' Clean	300+	67%	73%	73%
Timely Help 'Always' Received	300+	52%	65%	68%
Would Definitely Recommend Hospital	300+	64%	73%	71%
Use of Medical Imaging				
Cardiac Imaging Stress Test before Surgery[1]	-	-	4.3%	5.3%
Combination Abdominal CT Scan	586	6.1%	6.9%	10.5%
Combination Brain/Sinus CT Scan[1]	-	-	2.3%	2.7%
Combination Chest CT Scan	215	0.5%	1.1%	2.7%
Follow-up Mammogram/Ultrasound[7]	-	-	9.1%	8.8%
Lumbar Spine MRI for Low Back Pain	58	39.7%	37.9%	37.2%

Cascade Medical Center

817 Commercial Street
Leavenworth, WA 98826
Phone: 509-548-5815
Type: Critical Access Hospitals
Emergency Services: Yes
Ownership: Govt - Hospital Dist/Auth

Measure	Cases	This Hosp.	State Avg.	U.S. Avg.
Blood Clot Prevention and Treatment				
Anticoagulation Overlap Therapy[5]	-	-	97%	93%
ICU Venous Thromboembolism Prophylaxis[5]	-	-	92%	92%
Incidence of Potentially Preventable VTE[5]	-	-	9%	10%
UFH with Dosages/Platelet Monitoring[5]	-	-	99%	97%
Venous Thromboembolism Prophylaxis[5]	-	-	86%	85%
Warfarin Therapy Discharge Instructions[5]	-	-	74%	75%
Chest Pain/Possible Heart Attack Care				
Aspirin Given Within 24 Hours of Arrival	-	-	97%	96%
Fibrinolytic Meds Within 30 Min. of Arrival	-	-	51%	58%
Average Time to ECG (minutes)	-	-	9	7
Average Time to Transfer (minutes)	-	-	54	60
Children's Asthma Care				
Received Home Management Plan of Care	-	-	-	88%
Received Reliever Medication	-	-	-	100%
Received Systemic Corticosteroids	-	-	-	100%
Emergency Department				
Admittance Decision Time (minutes)[5]	-	-	96	98
Head CT Results Within 45 Min. of Arrival	-	-	63%	57%
Patients Who Left ER Before Being Seen	-	-	2%	2%
Time from ER Arrival to Admit. (minutes)[5]	-	-	259	274
Time from ER Arrival to Discharge (minutes)	-	-	135	134
Time in ER Before Being Evaluated (minutes)	-	-	22	26
Time to Pain Meds for Fractures (minutes)	-	-	52	57
Heart Attack Care				
Aspirin Given at Discharge[5]	-	-	99%	99%
Fibrinolytic Meds Within 30 Min. of Arrival[5]	-	-	62%	54%
PCI Within 90 Minutes of Arrival[5]	-	-	97%	96%
Statin Prescribed at Discharge[5]	-	-	98%	98%
Heart Failure Care				
ACE Inhibitor or ARB for LVSD[1,3]	-	-	97%	97%
Discharge Instructions Given[1,3]	-	-	93%	94%
Evaluation of LVS Function[1,3]	-	-	99%	99%
Medicare Spending				
Medicare Spending per Patient (ratio)	-	-	0.91	0.98
Pneumonia Care				
Appropriate Initial Antibiotic Given[1,3]	-	-	96%	95%
Blood Culture Timing[3,7]	-	-	97%	98%
Pregnancy and Delivery Care				
Newborn Deliveries Scheduled Early[5]	-	-	2%	6%
Preventive Care				
Immunization for Influenza[5]	-	-	91%	90%
Immunization for Pneumonia[5]	-	-	91%	92%
Stroke Care				
Anticoagulation Therapy for Atrial Fibrillation[5]	-	-	94%	95%
Antithrombotic Therapy Timing[5]	-	-	98%	98%
Assessed for Rehabilitation[5]	-	-	98%	97%
Discharged on Antithrombotic Therapy[5]	-	-	99%	99%
Discharged on Statin Medication[5]	-	-	96%	94%
Thrombolytic Therapy Timing[5]	-	-	73%	66%
Venous Thromboembolism Prophylaxis[5]	-	-	94%	94%
Written Stroke Educational Materials Given[5]	-	-	86%	88%
Surgical Care Improvement Project				
Appropriate Beta Blocker Usage[5]	-	-	98%	98%
Appropriate VTP Within 24 Hours[5]	-	-	98%	98%
Controlled Postoperative Blood Glucose[5]	-	-	97%	97%
Perioperative Temperature Management[5]	-	-	100%	100%
Prophylactic Antibiotic Selection[5]	-	-	99%	99%
Prophylactic Antibiotic Selection (Outpatient)	-	-	98%	98%
Prophylactic Antibiotic Stopped[5]	-	-	99%	98%
Prophylactic Antibiotic Timing[5]	-	-	98%	99%
Prophylactic Antibiotic Timing (Outpatient)	-	-	98%	98%
Urinary Catheter Removal[5]	-	-	97%	97%
Survey of Patients' Hospital Experiences				
Area Around Room 'Always' Quiet at Night[5]	-	-	54%	61%
Doctors 'Always' Communicated Well[5]	-	-	81%	82%
Home Recovery Information Given[5]	-	-	87%	85%
Hospital Given 9 or 10 on 10 Point Scale[5]	-	-	70%	71%
Meds 'Always' Explained Before Given[5]	-	-	64%	64%
Nurses 'Always' Communicated Well[5]	-	-	77%	79%
Pain 'Always' Well Controlled[5]	-	-	70%	71%
Room and Bathroom 'Always' Clean[5]	-	-	73%	73%
Timely Help 'Always' Received[5]	-	-	65%	68%
Would Definitely Recommend Hospital[5]	-	-	73%	71%
Use of Medical Imaging				
Cardiac Imaging Stress Test before Surgery	-	-	4.3%	5.3%
Combination Abdominal CT Scan	-	-	6.9%	10.5%
Combination Brain/Sinus CT Scan	-	-	2.3%	2.7%
Combination Chest CT Scan	-	-	1.1%	2.7%
Follow-up Mammogram/Ultrasound	-	-	9.1%	8.8%
Lumbar Spine MRI for Low Back Pain	-	-	37.9%	37.2%

Peachealth Saint John Medical Center

1615 Delaware Street
Longview, WA 98632
Phone: 360-414-2000
Fax: 360-414-7243
URL: www.peacehealth.org
Type: Acute Care Hospitals
Emergency Services: Yes
Ownership: Voluntary non-profit - Church
Beds: 193

Key Personnel:

Chief of Medical Staff. . . . . Steven X Cabrales, MD
CEO . . . . Howard Graman, MD
Ambulatory Care . . . . Randy Ross
Quality Assurance . . . . Sharon Warning
President/CEO. . . . . Alan Yordy

Measure	Cases	This Hosp.	State Avg.	U.S. Avg.
Blood Clot Prevention and Treatment				
Anticoagulation Overlap Therapy[2]	60	95%	97%	93%
ICU Venous Thromboembolism Prophylaxis[2]	90	98%	92%	92%
Incidence of Potentially Preventable VTE[1,2]	-	-	9%	10%
UFH with Dosages/Platelet Monitoring[2]	28	100%	99%	97%
Venous Thromboembolism Prophylaxis[2]	329	84%	86%	85%
Warfarin Therapy Discharge Instructions[2]	47	83%	74%	75%
Chest Pain/Possible Heart Attack Care				
Aspirin Given Within 24 Hours of Arrival	148	98%	97%	96%
Fibrinolytic Meds Within 30 Min. of Arrival	12	83%	51%	58%
Average Time to ECG (minutes)	156	6	9	7
Average Time to Transfer (minutes)	15	43	54	60
Children's Asthma Care				
Received Home Management Plan of Care	-	-	-	88%
Received Reliever Medication	-	-	-	100%
Received Systemic Corticosteroids	-	-	-	100%
Emergency Department				
Admittance Decision Time (minutes)[2]	704	85	96	98
Head CT Results Within 45 Min. of Arrival	40	88%	63%	57%
Patients Who Left ER Before Being Seen	50,432	2%	2%	2%
Time from ER Arrival to Admit. (minutes)[2]	713	231	259	274
Time from ER Arrival to Discharge (minutes)	399	126	135	134
Time in ER Before Being Evaluated (minutes)	398	31	22	26
Time to Pain Meds for Fractures (minutes)	189	53	52	57
Heart Attack Care				
Aspirin Given at Discharge	144	99%	99%	99%
Fibrinolytic Meds Within 30 Min. of Arrival[7]	-	-	62%	54%
PCI Within 90 Minutes of Arrival	11	91%	97%	96%
Statin Prescribed at Discharge	148	95%	98%	98%
Heart Failure Care				
ACE Inhibitor or ARB for LVSD	77	95%	97%	97%
Discharge Instructions Given	177	94%	93%	94%
Evaluation of LVS Function	198	100%	99%	99%
Medicare Spending				
Medicare Spending per Patient (ratio)	-	0.91	0.91	0.98
Pneumonia Care				
Appropriate Initial Antibiotic Given	152	100%	96%	95%
Blood Culture Timing	296	95%	97%	98%
Pregnancy and Delivery Care				
Newborn Deliveries Scheduled Early	74	3%	2%	6%
Preventive Care				
Immunization for Influenza[2]	568	95%	91%	90%
Immunization for Pneumonia[2]	740	95%	91%	92%
Stroke Care				
Anticoagulation Therapy for Atrial Fibrillation	15	93%	94%	95%
Antithrombotic Therapy Timing	61	100%	98%	98%
Assessed for Rehabilitation	69	100%	98%	97%
Discharged on Antithrombotic Therapy	64	100%	99%	99%
Discharged on Statin Medication	50	96%	96%	94%
Thrombolytic Therapy Timing[7]	-	-	73%	66%
Venous Thromboembolism Prophylaxis	65	82%	94%	94%
Written Stroke Educational Materials Given	47	83%	86%	88%
Surgical Care Improvement Project				
Appropriate Beta Blocker Usage	214	99%	98%	98%
Appropriate VTP Within 24 Hours	558	100%	98%	98%
Controlled Postoperative Blood Glucose[7]	-	-	97%	97%
Perioperative Temperature Management	750	100%	100%	100%
Prophylactic Antibiotic Selection	529	100%	99%	99%
Prophylactic Antibiotic Selection (Outpatient)	110	99%	98%	98%
Prophylactic Antibiotic Stopped	514	100%	99%	98%
Prophylactic Antibiotic Timing	529	99%	98%	99%
Prophylactic Antibiotic Timing (Outpatient)	96	99%	98%	98%
Urinary Catheter Removal	453	100%	97%	97%
Survey of Patients' Hospital Experiences				
Area Around Room 'Always' Quiet at Night	300+	45%	54%	61%
Doctors 'Always' Communicated Well	300+	78%	81%	82%
Home Recovery Information Given	300+	89%	87%	85%
Hospital Given 9 or 10 on 10 Point Scale	300+	64%	70%	71%
Meds 'Always' Explained Before Given	300+	65%	64%	64%
Nurses 'Always' Communicated Well	300+	79%	77%	79%
Pain 'Always' Well Controlled	300+	70%	70%	71%
Room and Bathroom 'Always' Clean	300+	72%	73%	73%
Timely Help 'Always' Received	300+	55%	65%	68%
Would Definitely Recommend Hospital	300+	60%	73%	71%
Use of Medical Imaging				
Cardiac Imaging Stress Test before Surgery	232	4.3%	4.3%	5.3%
Combination Abdominal CT Scan	624	4.8%	6.9%	10.5%
Combination Brain/Sinus CT Scan	622	1.8%	2.3%	2.7%
Combination Chest CT Scan	376	0.0%	1.1%	2.7%
Follow-up Mammogram/Ultrasound	2,040	5.6%	9.1%	8.8%
Lumbar Spine MRI for Low Back Pain	144	34.0%	37.9%	37.2%

NOTE: Hospital profiles are in alphabetical order by state, then city, then hospital within the city; Rankings exclude hospitals with less than 25 cases except for patient surveys which excludes hospitals with less than 100 cases; (a) 100-299 cases; (1) The number of cases/patients is too few to report; (2) Data submitted were based on a sample of cases/patients; (3) Results are based on a shorter time period than required; (4) Data suppressed by CMS for one or more quarters; (5) Results are not available for this reporting period; (6) Fewer than 100 patients completed the HCAHPS survey; (7) No cases met the criteria for this measure; (8) The lower limit of the confidence interval cannot be calculated if the number of observed infections equals zero; (9) No data are available from the state/territory for this reporting period; (10) The scores shown reflect fewer than 50 completed surveys; (11) There were discrepancies in the data collection process; (12) This measure does not apply to this hospital for this reporting period; (13) Results cannot be calculated for this reporting period; (14) The results for this state are combined with nearby states to protect confidentiality; Please refer to the User's Guide for a full explanation of data.

Valley General Hospital

14701 179th Se
Monroe, WA 98272
Phone: 360-794-7497
Fax: 360-794-1486
URL: www.valleygeneral.com
Type: Acute Care Hospitals
Emergency Services: Yes
Ownership: Govt - Hospital Dist/Auth
Beds: 72

Key Personnel:
Radiology. . . . . Larry Anderson
Chief of Medical Staff . . . . Victoria Baker-Hall, MD
Emergency Room . . . . Eric M Fields, DO
CEO . . . . Eric P Jensen, FACHE
Quality Assurance . . . . Dana Martinson, RN
Infection Control. . . . . Gary Preston, MD
Operating Room. . . . . James Swenson, RN

Measure	Cases	This Hosp.	State Avg.	U.S. Avg.
Blood Clot Prevention and Treatment				
Anticoagulation Overlap Therapy[2]	14	100%	97%	93%
ICU Venous Thromboembolism Prophylaxis[2]	23	87%	92%	92%
Incidence of Potentially Preventable VTE[2,7]	-	-	9%	10%
UFH with Dosages/Platelet Monitoring[1,2]	-	-	99%	97%
Venous Thromboembolism Prophylaxis[2]	80	85%	86%	85%
Warfarin Therapy Discharge Instructions[2]	13	100%	74%	75%
Chest Pain/Possible Heart Attack Care				
Aspirin Given Within 24 Hours of Arrival	36	100%	97%	96%
Fibrinolytic Meds Within 30 Min. of Arrival[7]	-	-	51%	58%
Average Time to ECG (minutes)	41	12	9	7
Average Time to Transfer (minutes)[1]	-	-	54	60
Children's Asthma Care				
Received Home Management Plan of Care	-	-	-	88%
Received Reliever Medication	-	-	-	100%
Received Systemic Corticosteroids	-	-	-	100%
Emergency Department				
Admittance Decision Time (minutes)[2]	426	50	96	98
Head CT Results Within 45 Min. of Arrival	16	62%	63%	57%
Patients Who Left ER Before Being Seen	15,017	1%	2%	2%
Time from ER Arrival to Admit. (minutes)[2]	465	236	259	274
Time from ER Arrival to Discharge (minutes)	350	142	135	134
Time in ER Before Being Evaluated (minutes)	353	27	22	26
Time to Pain Meds for Fractures (minutes)	46	46	52	57
Heart Attack Care				
Aspirin Given at Discharge[1,3]	-	-	99%	99%
Fibrinolytic Meds Within 30 Min. of Arrival[3,7]	-	-	62%	54%
PCI Within 90 Minutes of Arrival[3,7]	-	-	97%	96%
Statin Prescribed at Discharge[1,3]	-	-	98%	98%
Heart Failure Care				
ACE Inhibitor or ARB for LVSD[1]	-	-	97%	97%
Discharge Instructions Given	22	86%	93%	94%
Evaluation of LVS Function	25	88%	99%	99%
Medicare Spending				
Medicare Spending per Patient (ratio)	-	0.82	0.91	0.98
Pneumonia Care				
Appropriate Initial Antibiotic Given	36	94%	96%	95%
Blood Culture Timing	74	100%	97%	98%
Pregnancy and Delivery Care				
Newborn Deliveries Scheduled Early[7]	-	-	2%	6%
Preventive Care				
Immunization for Influenza[2]	287	92%	91%	90%
Immunization for Pneumonia[2]	345	91%	91%	92%
Stroke Care				
Anticoagulation Therapy for Atrial Fibrillation[1]	-	-	94%	95%
Antithrombotic Therapy Timing[1]	-	-	98%	98%
Assessed for Rehabilitation	16	100%	98%	97%
Discharged on Antithrombotic Therapy	12	100%	99%	99%
Discharged on Statin Medication	14	93%	96%	94%
Thrombolytic Therapy Timing[1]	-	-	73%	66%
Venous Thromboembolism Prophylaxis	12	67%	94%	94%
Written Stroke Educational Materials Given	12	92%	86%	88%
Surgical Care Improvement Project				
Appropriate Beta Blocker Usage	17	100%	98%	98%
Appropriate VTP Within 24 Hours	89	99%	98%	98%
Controlled Postoperative Blood Glucose[7]	-	-	97%	97%
Perioperative Temperature Management	115	99%	100%	100%
Prophylactic Antibiotic Selection	65	98%	99%	99%
Prophylactic Antibiotic Selection (Outpatient)[1,3]	-	-	98%	98%
Prophylactic Antibiotic Stopped	65	98%	99%	98%
Prophylactic Antibiotic Timing	65	100%	98%	99%
Prophylactic Antibiotic Timing (Outpatient)[1,3]	-	-	98%	98%
Urinary Catheter Removal	92	97%	97%	97%
Survey of Patients' Hospital Experiences				
Area Around Room 'Always' Quiet at Night	(a)	41%	54%	61%
Doctors 'Always' Communicated Well	(a)	75%	81%	82%
Home Recovery Information Given	(a)	90%	87%	85%
Hospital Given 9 or 10 on 10 Point Scale	(a)	58%	70%	71%
Meds 'Always' Explained Before Given	(a)	62%	64%	64%
Nurses 'Always' Communicated Well	(a)	72%	77%	79%
Pain 'Always' Well Controlled	(a)	71%	70%	71%
Room and Bathroom 'Always' Clean	(a)	68%	73%	73%
Timely Help 'Always' Received	(a)	63%	65%	68%
Would Definitely Recommend Hospital	(a)	60%	73%	71%
Use of Medical Imaging				
Cardiac Imaging Stress Test before Surgery[1]	-	-	4.3%	5.3%
Combination Abdominal CT Scan	158	5.7%	6.9%	10.5%
Combination Brain/Sinus CT Scan[1]	-	-	2.3%	2.7%
Combination Chest CT Scan	79	0.0%	1.1%	2.7%
Follow-up Mammogram/Ultrasound	236	7.6%	9.1%	8.8%
Lumbar Spine MRI for Low Back Pain[1]	-	-	37.9%	37.2%

Morton Swing Bed

521 Adams Street
Morton, WA 98356
Phone: 360-496-5112
Type: Critical Access Hospitals
Emergency Services: Yes
Ownership: Govt - Hospital Dist/Auth

Measure	Cases	This Hosp.	State Avg.	U.S. Avg.
Blood Clot Prevention and Treatment				
Anticoagulation Overlap Therapy[5]	-	-	97%	93%
ICU Venous Thromboembolism Prophylaxis[5]	-	-	92%	92%
Incidence of Potentially Preventable VTE[5]	-	-	9%	10%
UFH with Dosages/Platelet Monitoring[5]	-	-	99%	97%
Venous Thromboembolism Prophylaxis[5]	-	-	86%	85%
Warfarin Therapy Discharge Instructions[5]	-	-	74%	75%
Chest Pain/Possible Heart Attack Care				
Aspirin Given Within 24 Hours of Arrival	17	94%	97%	96%
Fibrinolytic Meds Within 30 Min. of Arrival[1]	-	-	51%	58%
Average Time to ECG (minutes)	18	6	9	7
Average Time to Transfer (minutes)[7]	-	-	54	60
Children's Asthma Care				
Received Home Management Plan of Care	-	-	-	88%
Received Reliever Medication	-	-	-	100%
Received Systemic Corticosteroids	-	-	-	100%
Emergency Department				
Admittance Decision Time (minutes)[5]	-	-	96	98
Head CT Results Within 45 Min. of Arrival[5]	-	-	63%	57%
Patients Who Left ER Before Being Seen[5]	-	-	2%	2%
Time from ER Arrival to Admit. (minutes)[5]	-	-	259	274
Time from ER Arrival to Discharge (minutes)[5]	-	-	135	134
Time in ER Before Being Evaluated (minutes)[5]	-	-	22	26
Time to Pain Meds for Fractures (minutes)[5]	-	-	52	57
Heart Attack Care				
Aspirin Given at Discharge[1,3]	-	-	99%	99%
Fibrinolytic Meds Within 30 Min. of Arrival[3,7]	-	-	62%	54%
PCI Within 90 Minutes of Arrival[5]	-	-	97%	96%
Statin Prescribed at Discharge[1,3]	-	-	98%	98%
Heart Failure Care				
ACE Inhibitor or ARB for LVSD[1]	-	-	97%	97%
Discharge Instructions Given[1]	-	-	93%	94%
Evaluation of LVS Function[1]	-	-	99%	99%
Medicare Spending				
Medicare Spending per Patient (ratio)	-	-	0.91	0.98
Pneumonia Care				
Appropriate Initial Antibiotic Given[1]	-	-	96%	95%
Blood Culture Timing	14	86%	97%	98%
Pregnancy and Delivery Care				
Newborn Deliveries Scheduled Early[5]	-	-	2%	6%
Preventive Care				
Immunization for Influenza[5]	-	-	91%	90%
Immunization for Pneumonia[5]	-	-	91%	92%
Stroke Care				
Anticoagulation Therapy for Atrial Fibrillation[5]	-	-	94%	95%
Antithrombotic Therapy Timing[5]	-	-	98%	98%
Assessed for Rehabilitation[5]	-	-	98%	97%
Discharged on Antithrombotic Therapy[5]	-	-	99%	99%
Discharged on Statin Medication[5]	-	-	96%	94%
Thrombolytic Therapy Timing[5]	-	-	73%	66%
Venous Thromboembolism Prophylaxis[5]	-	-	94%	94%
Written Stroke Educational Materials Given[5]	-	-	86%	88%
Surgical Care Improvement Project				
Appropriate Beta Blocker Usage[1]	-	-	98%	98%
Appropriate VTP Within 24 Hours[1]	-	-	98%	98%
Controlled Postoperative Blood Glucose[3,7]	-	-	97%	97%
Perioperative Temperature Management	15	100%	100%	100%
Prophylactic Antibiotic Selection	11	100%	99%	99%
Prophylactic Antibiotic Selection (Outpatient)[5]	-	-	98%	98%
Prophylactic Antibiotic Stopped[1]	-	-	99%	98%
Prophylactic Antibiotic Timing	11	100%	98%	99%
Prophylactic Antibiotic Timing (Outpatient)[5]	-	-	98%	98%
Urinary Catheter Removal[1]	-	-	97%	97%
Survey of Patients' Hospital Experiences				
Area Around Room 'Always' Quiet at Night[5]	-	-	54%	61%
Doctors 'Always' Communicated Well[5]	-	-	81%	82%
Home Recovery Information Given[5]	-	-	87%	85%
Hospital Given 9 or 10 on 10 Point Scale[5]	-	-	70%	71%
Meds 'Always' Explained Before Given[5]	-	-	64%	64%
Nurses 'Always' Communicated Well[5]	-	-	77%	79%
Pain 'Always' Well Controlled[5]	-	-	70%	71%
Room and Bathroom 'Always' Clean[5]	-	-	73%	73%
Timely Help 'Always' Received[5]	-	-	65%	68%
Would Definitely Recommend Hospital[5]	-	-	73%	71%
Use of Medical Imaging				
Cardiac Imaging Stress Test before Surgery[1]	-	-	4.3%	5.3%
Combination Abdominal CT Scan	109	3.7%	6.9%	10.5%
Combination Brain/Sinus CT Scan[1]	-	-	2.3%	2.7%
Combination Chest CT Scan	57	5.3%	1.1%	2.7%
Follow-up Mammogram/Ultrasound	134	6.7%	9.1%	8.8%
Lumbar Spine MRI for Low Back Pain[1]	-	-	37.9%	37.2%

Samaritan Hospital

801 East Wheeler Road
Moses Lake, WA 98837
Phone: 509-765-5606
Fax: 509-764-6507
URL: www.samaritanhealthcare.com
Type: Acute Care Hospitals
Emergency Services: Yes
Ownership: Govt - Hospital Dist/Auth
Beds: 50

Key Personnel:
Infection Control. . . . . Pat Harrington
Operating Room. . . . . James Irwin
Chief of Medical Staff . . . . James R. Irwin, MD
Radiology. . . . . Vivienne Kezuka
Intensive Care Unit. . . . . Maureen King
Emergency Room . . . . Steve Rusnock
Quality Assurance . . . . Glen Stambaugh
CEO/President. . . . . John White

Measure	Cases	This Hosp.	State Avg.	U.S. Avg.
Blood Clot Prevention and Treatment				
Anticoagulation Overlap Therapy[2]	24	83%	97%	93%
ICU Venous Thromboembolism Prophylaxis[2]	16	94%	92%	92%
Incidence of Potentially Preventable VTE[1,2]	-	-	9%	10%
UFH with Dosages/Platelet Monitoring[2]	14	14%	99%	97%
Venous Thromboembolism Prophylaxis[2]	102	81%	86%	85%
Warfarin Therapy Discharge Instructions[2]	20	85%	74%	75%
Chest Pain/Possible Heart Attack Care				
Aspirin Given Within 24 Hours of Arrival	135	97%	97%	96%
Fibrinolytic Meds Within 30 Min. of Arrival	13	23%	51%	58%
Average Time to ECG (minutes)	140	15	9	7
Average Time to Transfer (minutes)[1]	-	-	54	60
Children's Asthma Care				
Received Home Management Plan of Care	-	-	-	88%
Received Reliever Medication	-	-	-	100%
Received Systemic Corticosteroids	-	-	-	100%
Emergency Department				
Admittance Decision Time (minutes)[2]	269	65	96	98
Head CT Results Within 45 Min. of Arrival[1,3]	-	-	63%	57%

NOTE: Hospital profiles are in alphabetical order by state, then city, then hospital within the city; Rankings exclude hospitals with less than 25 cases except for patient surveys which excludes hospitals with less than 100 cases; (a) 100-299 cases; (1) The number of cases/patients is too few to report; (2) Data submitted were based on a sample of cases/patients; (3) Results are based on a shorter time period than required; (4) Data suppressed by CMS for one or more quarters; (5) Results are not available for this reporting period; (6) Fewer than 100 patients completed the HCAHPS survey; (7) No cases met the criteria for this measure; (8) The lower limit of the confidence interval cannot be calculated if the number of observed infections equals zero; (9) No data are available from the state/territory for this reporting period; (10) The scores shown reflect fewer than 50 completed surveys; (11) There were discrepancies in the data collection process; (12) This measure does not apply to this hospital for this reporting period; (13) Results cannot be calculated for this reporting period; (14) The results for this state are combined with nearby states to protect confidentiality; Please refer to the User's Guide for a full explanation of data.

Measure	Cases	This Hosp.	State Avg.	U.S. Avg.
Patients Who Left ER Before Being Seen	13,032	2%	2%	2%
Time from ER Arrival to Admit. (minutes)[2]	285	236	259	274
Time from ER Arrival to Discharge (minutes)	426	136	135	134
Time in ER Before Being Evaluated (minutes)	451	29	22	26
Time to Pain Meds for Fractures (minutes)	82	53	52	57
Heart Attack Care				
Aspirin Given at Discharge[1,2]	-	-	99%	99%
Fibrinolytic Meds Within 30 Min. of Arrival[2,7]	-	-	62%	54%
PCI Within 90 Minutes of Arrival[2,7]	-	-	97%	96%
Statin Prescribed at Discharge[1,2]	-	-	98%	98%
Heart Failure Care				
ACE Inhibitor or ARB for LVSD[1,2]	-	-	97%	97%
Discharge Instructions Given[2]	31	90%	93%	94%
Evaluation of LVS Function[2]	40	95%	99%	99%
Medicare Spending				
Medicare Spending per Patient (ratio)	-	0.85	0.91	0.98
Pneumonia Care				
Appropriate Initial Antibiotic Given[2]	45	100%	96%	95%
Blood Culture Timing[2]	61	100%	97%	98%
Pregnancy and Delivery Care				
Newborn Deliveries Scheduled Early	81	1%	2%	6%
Preventive Care				
Immunization for Influenza[2]	341	83%	91%	90%
Immunization for Pneumonia[2]	276	79%	91%	92%
Stroke Care				
Anticoagulation Therapy for Atrial Fibrillation[1]	-	-	94%	95%
Antithrombotic Therapy Timing	20	95%	98%	98%
Assessed for Rehabilitation	22	100%	98%	97%
Discharged on Antithrombotic Therapy	22	95%	99%	99%
Discharged on Statin Medication	17	88%	96%	94%
Thrombolytic Therapy Timing[1]	-	-	73%	66%
Venous Thromboembolism Prophylaxis	21	86%	94%	94%
Written Stroke Educational Materials Given	15	100%	86%	88%
Surgical Care Improvement Project				
Appropriate Beta Blocker Usage	56	91%	98%	98%
Appropriate VTP Within 24 Hours	194	92%	98%	98%
Controlled Postoperative Blood Glucose[7]	-	-	97%	97%
Perioperative Temperature Management	256	97%	100%	100%
Prophylactic Antibiotic Selection	211	100%	99%	99%
Prophylactic Antibiotic Selection (Outpatient)	35	97%	98%	98%
Prophylactic Antibiotic Stopped	211	99%	99%	98%
Prophylactic Antibiotic Timing	211	94%	98%	99%
Prophylactic Antibiotic Timing (Outpatient)	36	97%	98%	98%
Urinary Catheter Removal	196	97%	97%	97%
Survey of Patients' Hospital Experiences				
Area Around Room 'Always' Quiet at Night	300+	59%	54%	61%
Doctors 'Always' Communicated Well	300+	79%	81%	82%
Home Recovery Information Given	300+	86%	87%	85%
Hospital Given 9 or 10 on 10 Point Scale	300+	63%	70%	71%
Meds 'Always' Explained Before Given	300+	61%	64%	64%
Nurses 'Always' Communicated Well	300+	75%	77%	79%
Pain 'Always' Well Controlled	300+	71%	70%	71%
Room and Bathroom 'Always' Clean	300+	72%	73%	73%
Timely Help 'Always' Received	300+	71%	65%	68%
Would Definitely Recommend Hospital	300+	58%	73%	71%
Use of Medical Imaging				
Cardiac Imaging Stress Test before Surgery[1]	-	-	4.3%	5.3%
Combination Abdominal CT Scan	271	5.5%	6.9%	10.5%
Combination Brain/Sinus CT Scan[1]	-	-	2.3%	2.7%
Combination Chest CT Scan	177	9.6%	1.1%	2.7%
Follow-up Mammogram/Ultrasound	171	9.4%	9.1%	8.8%
Lumbar Spine MRI for Low Back Pain[1]	-	-	37.9%	37.2%

Skagit Valley Hospital

1415 Kincaid Street
Mount Vernon, WA 98274
Phone: 360-424-4111
Fax: 360-428-2416
E-mail: kranten@skagitvalleyhospital.org
URL: www.skagitvalleyhospital.org
Type: Acute Care Hospitals
Emergency Services: Yes
Ownership: Govt - Hospital Dist/Auth
Beds: 115

Key Personnel:
Radiology. . . . . Lori A Ahrens
CEO/President. . . . . Gregg Davidson, FACHE
Chief of Medical Staff. . . . . Connie Davis, MD
Administrator . . . . Jane Root

Measure	Cases	This Hosp.	State Avg.	U.S. Avg.
Blood Clot Prevention and Treatment				
Anticoagulation Overlap Therapy[2]	39	97%	97%	93%
ICU Venous Thromboembolism Prophylaxis[2]	64	91%	92%	92%
Incidence of Potentially Preventable VTE[1,2]	-	-	9%	10%
UFH with Dosages/Platelet Monitoring[2]	29	100%	99%	97%
Venous Thromboembolism Prophylaxis[2]	336	98%	86%	85%
Warfarin Therapy Discharge Instructions[2]	31	87%	74%	75%
Chest Pain/Possible Heart Attack Care				
Aspirin Given Within 24 Hours of Arrival[1]	-	-	97%	96%
Fibrinolytic Meds Within 30 Min. of Arrival[3,7]	-	-	51%	58%
Average Time to ECG (minutes)[1]	-	-	9	7
Average Time to Transfer (minutes)[3,7]	-	-	54	60
Children's Asthma Care				
Received Home Management Plan of Care	-	-	-	88%
Received Reliever Medication	-	-	-	100%
Received Systemic Corticosteroids	-	-	-	100%
Emergency Department				
Admittance Decision Time (minutes)[2]	358	78	96	98
Head CT Results Within 45 Min. of Arrival	19	84%	63%	57%
Patients Who Left ER Before Being Seen	29,720	2%	2%	2%
Time from ER Arrival to Admit. (minutes)[2]	563	258	259	274
Time from ER Arrival to Discharge (minutes)	361	159	135	134
Time in ER Before Being Evaluated (minutes)	358	34	22	26
Time to Pain Meds for Fractures (minutes)	125	51	52	57
Heart Attack Care				
Aspirin Given at Discharge	195	99%	99%	99%
Fibrinolytic Meds Within 30 Min. of Arrival[7]	-	-	62%	54%
PCI Within 90 Minutes of Arrival	39	97%	97%	96%
Statin Prescribed at Discharge	184	99%	98%	98%
Heart Failure Care				
ACE Inhibitor or ARB for LVSD	55	100%	97%	97%
Discharge Instructions Given	138	97%	93%	94%
Evaluation of LVS Function	165	100%	99%	99%
Medicare Spending				
Medicare Spending per Patient (ratio)	-	0.96	0.91	0.98
Pneumonia Care				
Appropriate Initial Antibiotic Given[2]	116	97%	96%	95%
Blood Culture Timing[2]	195	100%	97%	98%
Pregnancy and Delivery Care				
Newborn Deliveries Scheduled Early	113	0%	2%	6%
Preventive Care				
Immunization for Influenza[2]	519	100%	91%	90%
Immunization for Pneumonia[2]	623	100%	91%	92%
Stroke Care				
Anticoagulation Therapy for Atrial Fibrillation	14	100%	94%	95%
Antithrombotic Therapy Timing	65	100%	98%	98%
Assessed for Rehabilitation	74	100%	98%	97%
Discharged on Antithrombotic Therapy	70	100%	99%	99%
Discharged on Statin Medication	63	100%	96%	94%
Thrombolytic Therapy Timing[1]	-	-	73%	66%
Venous Thromboembolism Prophylaxis	68	99%	94%	94%
Written Stroke Educational Materials Given	48	98%	86%	88%
Surgical Care Improvement Project				
Appropriate Beta Blocker Usage[2]	122	99%	98%	98%
Appropriate VTP Within 24 Hours[2]	362	99%	98%	98%
Controlled Postoperative Blood Glucose[2,7]	-	-	97%	97%
Perioperative Temperature Management[2]	438	100%	100%	100%
Prophylactic Antibiotic Selection[2]	287	100%	99%	99%
Prophylactic Antibiotic Selection (Outpatient)	366	99%	98%	98%
Prophylactic Antibiotic Stopped[2]	280	99%	99%	98%
Prophylactic Antibiotic Timing[2]	287	100%	98%	99%
Prophylactic Antibiotic Timing (Outpatient)	367	100%	98%	98%
Urinary Catheter Removal[2]	252	97%	97%	97%
Survey of Patients' Hospital Experiences				
Area Around Room 'Always' Quiet at Night	300+	46%	54%	61%
Doctors 'Always' Communicated Well	300+	76%	81%	82%
Home Recovery Information Given	300+	83%	87%	85%
Hospital Given 9 or 10 on 10 Point Scale	300+	64%	70%	71%
Meds 'Always' Explained Before Given	300+	57%	64%	64%
Nurses 'Always' Communicated Well	300+	72%	77%	79%
Pain 'Always' Well Controlled	300+	67%	70%	71%
Room and Bathroom 'Always' Clean	300+	73%	73%	73%
Timely Help 'Always' Received	300+	61%	65%	68%
Would Definitely Recommend Hospital	300+	66%	73%	71%
Use of Medical Imaging				
Cardiac Imaging Stress Test before Surgery	494	3.8%	4.3%	5.3%
Combination Abdominal CT Scan	834	7.6%	6.9%	10.5%
Combination Brain/Sinus CT Scan	486	1.2%	2.3%	2.7%
Combination Chest CT Scan	578	0.3%	1.1%	2.7%
Follow-up Mammogram/Ultrasound[7]	-	-	9.1%	8.8%
Lumbar Spine MRI for Low Back Pain	179	26.8%	37.9%	37.2%

Newport Community Hospital

714 West Pine Street
Phone: 509-447-2441
Newport, WA 99156
Type: Critical Access Hospitals
Emergency Services: Yes
Ownership: Govt - Hospital Dist/Auth

Measure	Cases	This Hosp.	State Avg.	U.S. Avg.
Blood Clot Prevention and Treatment				
Anticoagulation Overlap Therapy[5]	-	-	97%	93%
ICU Venous Thromboembolism Prophylaxis[5]	-	-	92%	92%
Incidence of Potentially Preventable VTE[5]	-	-	9%	10%
UFH with Dosages/Platelet Monitoring[5]	-	-	99%	97%
Venous Thromboembolism Prophylaxis[5]	-	-	86%	85%
Warfarin Therapy Discharge Instructions[5]	-	-	74%	75%
Chest Pain/Possible Heart Attack Care				
Aspirin Given Within 24 Hours of Arrival	23	96%	97%	96%
Fibrinolytic Meds Within 30 Min. of Arrival[7]	-	-	51%	58%
Average Time to ECG (minutes)	24	4	9	7
Average Time to Transfer (minutes)[1]	-	-	54	60
Children's Asthma Care				
Received Home Management Plan of Care	-	-	-	88%
Received Reliever Medication	-	-	-	100%
Received Systemic Corticosteroids	-	-	-	100%
Emergency Department				
Admittance Decision Time (minutes)[5]	-	-	96	98
Head CT Results Within 45 Min. of Arrival[5]	-	-	63%	57%
Patients Who Left ER Before Being Seen[5]	-	-	2%	2%
Time from ER Arrival to Admit. (minutes)[5]	-	-	259	274
Time from ER Arrival to Discharge (minutes)[5]	-	-	135	134
Time in ER Before Being Evaluated (minutes)[5]	-	-	22	26
Time to Pain Meds for Fractures (minutes)[5]	-	-	52	57
Heart Attack Care				
Aspirin Given at Discharge[5]	-	-	99%	99%
Fibrinolytic Meds Within 30 Min. of Arrival[5]	-	-	62%	54%
PCI Within 90 Minutes of Arrival[5]	-	-	97%	96%
Statin Prescribed at Discharge[5]	-	-	98%	98%
Heart Failure Care				
ACE Inhibitor or ARB for LVSD[1,3]	-	-	97%	97%
Discharge Instructions Given[1,3]	-	-	93%	94%
Evaluation of LVS Function[1,3]	-	-	99%	99%
Medicare Spending				
Medicare Spending per Patient (ratio)	-	-	0.91	0.98
Pneumonia Care				
Appropriate Initial Antibiotic Given	19	42%	96%	95%
Blood Culture Timing[1]	-	-	97%	98%
Pregnancy and Delivery Care				
Newborn Deliveries Scheduled Early[5]	-	-	2%	6%
Preventive Care				
Immunization for Influenza[5]	-	-	91%	90%
Immunization for Pneumonia[5]	-	-	91%	92%
Stroke Care				
Anticoagulation Therapy for Atrial Fibrillation[5]	-	-	94%	95%
Antithrombotic Therapy Timing[5]	-	-	98%	98%
Assessed for Rehabilitation[5]	-	-	98%	97%
Discharged on Antithrombotic Therapy[5]	-	-	99%	99%
Discharged on Statin Medication[5]	-	-	96%	94%
Thrombolytic Therapy Timing[5]	-	-	73%	66%
Venous Thromboembolism Prophylaxis[5]	-	-	94%	94%
Written Stroke Educational Materials Given[5]	-	-	86%	88%
Surgical Care Improvement Project				
Appropriate Beta Blocker Usage[5]	-	-	98%	98%
Appropriate VTP Within 24 Hours[5]	-	-	98%	98%

NOTE: Hospital profiles are in alphabetical order by state, then city, then hospital within the city; Rankings exclude hospitals with less than 25 cases except for patient surveys which excludes hospitals with less than 100 cases; (a) 100-299 cases; (1) The number of cases/patients is too few to report; (2) Data submitted were based on a sample of cases/patients; (3) Results are based on a shorter time period than required; (4) Data suppressed by CMS for one or more quarters; (5) Results are not available for this reporting period; (6) Fewer than 100 patients completed the HCAHPS survey; (7) No cases met the criteria for this measure; (8) The lower limit of the confidence interval cannot be calculated if the number of observed infections equals zero; (9) No data are available from the state/territory for this reporting period; (10) The scores shown reflect fewer than 50 completed surveys; (11) There were discrepancies in the data collection process; (12) This measure does not apply to this hospital for this reporting period; (13) Results cannot be calculated for this reporting period; (14) The results for this state are combined with nearby states to protect confidentiality; Please refer to the User's Guide for a full explanation of data.

Measure	Cases	This Hosp.	State Avg.	U.S. Avg.
Controlled Postoperative Blood Glucose[5]	-	-	97%	97%
Perioperative Temperature Management[5]	-	-	100%	100%
Prophylactic Antibiotic Selection[5]	-	-	99%	99%
Prophylactic Antibiotic Selection (Outpatient)[5]	-	-	98%	98%
Prophylactic Antibiotic Stopped[5]	-	-	99%	98%
Prophylactic Antibiotic Timing[5]	-	-	98%	99%
Prophylactic Antibiotic Timing (Outpatient)[5]	-	-	98%	98%
Urinary Catheter Removal[5]	-	-	97%	97%
Survey of Patients' Hospital Experiences				
Area Around Room 'Always' Quiet at Night[6]	<100	46%	54%	61%
Doctors 'Always' Communicated Well[6]	<100	86%	81%	82%
Home Recovery Information Given[6]	<100	90%	87%	85%
Hospital Given 9 or 10 on 10 Point Scale[6]	<100	71%	70%	71%
Meds 'Always' Explained Before Given[6]	<100	71%	64%	64%
Nurses 'Always' Communicated Well[6]	<100	77%	77%	79%
Pain 'Always' Well Controlled[6]	<100	67%	70%	71%
Room and Bathroom 'Always' Clean[6]	<100	81%	73%	73%
Timely Help 'Always' Received[6]	<100	63%	65%	68%
Would Definitely Recommend Hospital[6]	<100	76%	73%	71%
Use of Medical Imaging				
Cardiac Imaging Stress Test before Surgery[7]	-	-	4.3%	5.3%
Combination Abdominal CT Scan	150	6.0%	6.9%	10.5%
Combination Brain/Sinus CT Scan	163	0.6%	2.3%	2.7%
Combination Chest CT Scan	94	0.0%	1.1%	2.7%
Follow-up Mammogram/Ultrasound	284	10.2%	9.1%	8.8%
Lumbar Spine MRI for Low Back Pain	38	52.6%	37.9%	37.2%

Odessa Memorial Healthcare Center

502 E Amende Drive
Odessa, WA 99159
Phone: 509-982-2611
Type: Critical Access Hospitals
Emergency Services: Yes
Ownership: Govt - Hospital Dist/Auth

Measure	Cases	This Hosp.	State Avg.	U.S. Avg.
Blood Clot Prevention and Treatment				
Anticoagulation Overlap Therapy[5]	-	-	97%	93%
ICU Venous Thromboembolism Prophylaxis[5]	-	-	92%	92%
Incidence of Potentially Preventable VTE[5]	-	-	9%	10%
UFH with Dosages/Platelet Monitoring[5]	-	-	99%	97%
Venous Thromboembolism Prophylaxis[5]	-	-	86%	85%
Warfarin Therapy Discharge Instructions[5]	-	-	74%	75%
Chest Pain/Possible Heart Attack Care				
Aspirin Given Within 24 Hours of Arrival	-	-	97%	96%
Fibrinolytic Meds Within 30 Min. of Arrival	-	-	51%	58%
Average Time to ECG (minutes)	-	-	9	7
Average Time to Transfer (minutes)	-	-	54	60
Children's Asthma Care				
Received Home Management Plan of Care	-	-	-	88%
Received Reliever Medication	-	-	-	100%
Received Systemic Corticosteroids	-	-	-	100%
Emergency Department				
Admittance Decision Time (minutes)[5]	-	-	96	98
Head CT Results Within 45 Min. of Arrival	-	-	63%	57%
Patients Who Left ER Before Being Seen	-	-	2%	2%
Time from ER Arrival to Admit. (minutes)[5]	-	-	259	274
Time from ER Arrival to Discharge (minutes)	-	-	135	134
Time in ER Before Being Evaluated (minutes)	-	-	22	26
Time to Pain Meds for Fractures (minutes)	-	-	52	57
Heart Attack Care				
Aspirin Given at Discharge[5]	-	-	99%	99%
Fibrinolytic Meds Within 30 Min. of Arrival[5]	-	-	62%	54%
PCI Within 90 Minutes of Arrival[5]	-	-	97%	96%
Statin Prescribed at Discharge[5]	-	-	98%	98%
Heart Failure Care				
ACE Inhibitor or ARB for LVSD[5]	-	-	97%	97%
Discharge Instructions Given[5]	-	-	93%	94%
Evaluation of LVS Function[5]	-	-	99%	99%
Medicare Spending				
Medicare Spending per Patient (ratio)	-	-	0.91	0.98
Pneumonia Care				
Appropriate Initial Antibiotic Given[3,7]	-	-	96%	95%
Blood Culture Timing[3,7]	-	-	97%	98%
Pregnancy and Delivery Care				
Newborn Deliveries Scheduled Early[5]	-	-	2%	6%
Preventive Care				
Immunization for Influenza[5]	-	-	91%	90%
Immunization for Pneumonia[5]	-	-	91%	92%
Stroke Care				
Anticoagulation Therapy for Atrial Fibrillation[5]	-	-	94%	95%
Antithrombotic Therapy Timing[5]	-	-	98%	98%
Assessed for Rehabilitation[5]	-	-	98%	97%
Discharged on Antithrombotic Therapy[5]	-	-	99%	99%
Discharged on Statin Medication[5]	-	-	96%	94%
Thrombolytic Therapy Timing[5]	-	-	73%	66%
Venous Thromboembolism Prophylaxis[5]	-	-	94%	94%
Written Stroke Educational Materials Given[5]	-	-	86%	88%
Surgical Care Improvement Project				
Appropriate Beta Blocker Usage[5]	-	-	98%	98%
Appropriate VTP Within 24 Hours[5]	-	-	98%	98%
Controlled Postoperative Blood Glucose[5]	-	-	97%	97%
Perioperative Temperature Management[5]	-	-	100%	100%
Prophylactic Antibiotic Selection[5]	-	-	99%	99%
Prophylactic Antibiotic Selection (Outpatient)	-	-	98%	98%
Prophylactic Antibiotic Stopped[5]	-	-	99%	98%
Prophylactic Antibiotic Timing[5]	-	-	98%	99%
Prophylactic Antibiotic Timing (Outpatient)	-	-	98%	98%
Urinary Catheter Removal[5]	-	-	97%	97%
Survey of Patients' Hospital Experiences				
Area Around Room 'Always' Quiet at Night[5]	-	-	54%	61%
Doctors 'Always' Communicated Well[5]	-	-	81%	82%
Home Recovery Information Given[5]	-	-	87%	85%
Hospital Given 9 or 10 on 10 Point Scale[5]	-	-	70%	71%
Meds 'Always' Explained Before Given[5]	-	-	64%	64%
Nurses 'Always' Communicated Well[5]	-	-	77%	79%
Pain 'Always' Well Controlled[5]	-	-	70%	71%
Room and Bathroom 'Always' Clean[5]	-	-	73%	73%
Timely Help 'Always' Received[5]	-	-	65%	68%
Would Definitely Recommend Hospital[5]	-	-	73%	71%
Use of Medical Imaging				
Cardiac Imaging Stress Test before Surgery	-	-	4.3%	5.3%
Combination Abdominal CT Scan	-	-	6.9%	10.5%
Combination Brain/Sinus CT Scan	-	-	2.3%	2.7%
Combination Chest CT Scan	-	-	1.1%	2.7%
Follow-up Mammogram/Ultrasound	-	-	9.1%	8.8%
Lumbar Spine MRI for Low Back Pain	-	-	37.9%	37.2%

Capital Medical Center

3900 Capital Mall Dr Sw
Olympia, WA 98502
Phone: 360-754-5858
Fax: 360-956-2574
URL: www.capitalmedical.com
Type: Acute Care Hospitals
Emergency Services: Yes
Ownership: Voluntary non-profit - Private
Beds: 119

Key Personnel:

Radiology. . . . . Lawrence N Bennett
Operating Room. . . . . David M Deitz
Quality Assurance . . . . Eleanor Jones
Intensive Care Unit. . . . . Dona Kravis
CEO/President. . . . . Mike Motte
Chief of Medical Staff. . . . . Marnee Obendorf
Infection Control. . . . . Ira Rice, RN
Emergency Room . . . . Cynthia Wolfe, MD

Measure	Cases	This Hosp.	State Avg.	U.S. Avg.
Blood Clot Prevention and Treatment				
Anticoagulation Overlap Therapy[2]	23	91%	97%	93%
ICU Venous Thromboembolism Prophylaxis[2]	74	100%	92%	92%
Incidence of Potentially Preventable VTE[1,2]	-	-	9%	10%
UFH with Dosages/Platelet Monitoring[1,2]	-	-	99%	97%
Venous Thromboembolism Prophylaxis[2]	240	97%	86%	85%
Warfarin Therapy Discharge Instructions[2]	16	100%	74%	75%
Chest Pain/Possible Heart Attack Care				
Aspirin Given Within 24 Hours of Arrival[1]	-	-	97%	96%
Fibrinolytic Meds Within 30 Min. of Arrival[3,7]	-	-	51%	58%
Average Time to ECG (minutes)[1]	-	-	9	7
Average Time to Transfer (minutes)[3,7]	-	-	54	60
Children's Asthma Care				
Received Home Management Plan of Care	-	-	-	88%
Received Reliever Medication	-	-	-	100%
Received Systemic Corticosteroids	-	-	-	100%
Emergency Department				
Admittance Decision Time (minutes)[2]	288	76	96	98
Head CT Results Within 45 Min. of Arrival[1,3]	-	-	63%	57%
Patients Who Left ER Before Being Seen	17,286	2%	2%	2%
Time from ER Arrival to Admit. (minutes)[2]	291	252	259	274
Time from ER Arrival to Discharge (minutes)	474	155	135	134
Time in ER Before Being Evaluated (minutes)	497	22	22	26
Time to Pain Meds for Fractures (minutes)	44	55	52	57
Heart Attack Care				
Aspirin Given at Discharge	75	100%	99%	99%
Fibrinolytic Meds Within 30 Min. of Arrival[7]	-	-	62%	54%
PCI Within 90 Minutes of Arrival	12	67%	97%	96%
Statin Prescribed at Discharge	69	96%	98%	98%
Heart Failure Care				
ACE Inhibitor or ARB for LVSD	24	96%	97%	97%
Discharge Instructions Given	64	88%	93%	94%
Evaluation of LVS Function	82	100%	99%	99%
Medicare Spending				
Medicare Spending per Patient (ratio)	-	0.96	0.91	0.98
Pneumonia Care				
Appropriate Initial Antibiotic Given	41	88%	96%	95%
Blood Culture Timing	66	97%	97%	98%
Pregnancy and Delivery Care				
Newborn Deliveries Scheduled Early[2]	22	9%	2%	6%
Preventive Care				
Immunization for Influenza[2]	421	97%	91%	90%
Immunization for Pneumonia[2]	477	96%	91%	92%
Stroke Care				
Anticoagulation Therapy for Atrial Fibrillation[1]	-	-	94%	95%
Antithrombotic Therapy Timing	17	100%	98%	98%
Assessed for Rehabilitation	20	100%	98%	97%
Discharged on Antithrombotic Therapy	20	100%	99%	99%
Discharged on Statin Medication	18	83%	96%	94%
Thrombolytic Therapy Timing[1]	-	-	73%	66%
Venous Thromboembolism Prophylaxis	19	100%	94%	94%
Written Stroke Educational Materials Given	13	85%	86%	88%
Surgical Care Improvement Project				
Appropriate Beta Blocker Usage[2]	93	100%	98%	98%
Appropriate VTP Within 24 Hours[2]	349	98%	98%	98%
Controlled Postoperative Blood Glucose[2,7]	-	-	97%	97%
Perioperative Temperature Management[2]	478	100%	100%	100%
Prophylactic Antibiotic Selection[2]	345	99%	99%	99%
Prophylactic Antibiotic Selection (Outpatient)	141	99%	98%	98%
Prophylactic Antibiotic Stopped[2]	343	98%	99%	98%
Prophylactic Antibiotic Timing[2]	345	97%	98%	99%
Prophylactic Antibiotic Timing (Outpatient)	143	99%	98%	98%
Urinary Catheter Removal[2]	225	98%	97%	97%
Survey of Patients' Hospital Experiences				
Area Around Room 'Always' Quiet at Night	300+	53%	54%	61%
Doctors 'Always' Communicated Well	300+	82%	81%	82%
Home Recovery Information Given	300+	88%	87%	85%
Hospital Given 9 or 10 on 10 Point Scale	300+	69%	70%	71%
Meds 'Always' Explained Before Given	300+	65%	64%	64%
Nurses 'Always' Communicated Well	300+	77%	77%	79%
Pain 'Always' Well Controlled	300+	71%	70%	71%
Room and Bathroom 'Always' Clean	300+	69%	73%	73%
Timely Help 'Always' Received	300+	62%	65%	68%
Would Definitely Recommend Hospital	300+	71%	73%	71%
Use of Medical Imaging				
Cardiac Imaging Stress Test before Surgery[1]	-	-	4.3%	5.3%
Combination Abdominal CT Scan	449	6.9%	6.9%	10.5%
Combination Brain/Sinus CT Scan[1]	-	-	2.3%	2.7%
Combination Chest CT Scan	224	0.0%	1.1%	2.7%
Follow-up Mammogram/Ultrasound	897	5.9%	9.1%	8.8%
Lumbar Spine MRI for Low Back Pain	64	34.4%	37.9%	37.2%

NOTE: Hospital profiles are in alphabetical order by state, then city, then hospital within the city; Rankings exclude hospitals with less than 25 cases except for patient surveys which excludes hospitals with less than 100 cases; (a) 100-299 cases; (1) The number of cases/patients is too few to report; (2) Data submitted were based on a sample of cases/patients; (3) Results are based on a shorter time period than required; (4) Data suppressed by CMS for one or more quarters; (5) Results are not available for this reporting period; (6) Fewer than 100 patients completed the HCAHPS survey; (7) No cases met the criteria for this measure; (8) The lower limit of the confidence interval cannot be calculated if the number of observed infections equals zero; (9) No data are available from the state/territory for this reporting period; (10) The scores shown reflect fewer than 50 completed surveys; (11) There were discrepancies in the data collection process; (12) This measure does not apply to this hospital for this reporting period; (13) Results cannot be calculated for this reporting period; (14) The results for this state are combined with nearby states to protect confidentiality; Please refer to the User's Guide for a full explanation of data.

Providence Saint Peter Hospital

413 Lilly Road Ne Phone: 360-491-9480
Olympia, WA 98506 Fax: 360-493-7268
URL: www.providence.org/swsa
Type: Acute Care Hospitals Emergency Services: Yes
Ownership: Voluntary non-profit - Church Beds: 390

Key Personnel:
CEO/President. . . . . Scott Bond
Radiology. Karen Charter
Coronary Care . . . . Cheryl Hartsook
Infection Control. . . . . Lou Hilken
Quality Assurance . . . . Karen Lindsay
Operating Room. . . . . Pam Massey
Chief of Medical Staff . . . . Mike Matiock, MD
Pediatric Ambulatory Care . . . . . . Eileen Mellett

Measure	Cases	This Hosp.	State Avg.	U.S. Avg.
Blood Clot Prevention and Treatment				
Anticoagulation Overlap Therapy[2]	141	96%	97%	93%
ICU Venous Thromboembolism Prophylaxis[2]	45	96%	92%	92%
Incidence of Potentially Preventable VTE[2]	17	12%	9%	10%
UFH with Dosages/Platelet Monitoring[2]	48	100%	99%	97%
Venous Thromboembolism Prophylaxis[2]	262	85%	86%	85%
Warfarin Therapy Discharge Instructions[2]	116	25%	74%	75%
Chest Pain/Possible Heart Attack Care				
Aspirin Given Within 24 Hours of Arrival[1,3]	-	-	97%	96%
Fibrinolytic Meds Within 30 Min. of Arrival[5]	-	-	51%	58%
Average Time to ECG (minutes)[1,3]	-	-	9	7
Average Time to Transfer (minutes)[5]	-	-	54	60
Children's Asthma Care				
Received Home Management Plan of Care	33	76%	-	88%
Received Reliever Medication	37	100%	-	100%
Received Systemic Corticosteroids	37	97%	-	100%
Emergency Department				
Admittance Decision Time (minutes)[2]	552	100	96	98
Head CT Results Within 45 Min. of Arrival	12	25%	63%	57%
Patients Who Left ER Before Being Seen	66,867	2%	2%	2%
Time from ER Arrival to Admit. (minutes)[2]	578	263	259	274
Time from ER Arrival to Discharge (minutes)	357	166	135	134
Time in ER Before Being Evaluated (minutes)	99	64	22	26
Time to Pain Meds for Fractures (minutes)	234	66	52	57
Heart Attack Care				
Aspirin Given at Discharge	564	99%	99%	99%
Fibrinolytic Meds Within 30 Min. of Arrival[7]	-	-	62%	54%
PCI Within 90 Minutes of Arrival	79	99%	97%	96%
Statin Prescribed at Discharge	547	99%	98%	98%
Heart Failure Care				
ACE Inhibitor or ARB for LVSD	154	97%	97%	97%
Discharge Instructions Given	382	95%	93%	94%
Evaluation of LVS Function	483	100%	99%	99%
Medicare Spending				
Medicare Spending per Patient (ratio)	-	0.91	0.91	0.98
Pneumonia Care				
Appropriate Initial Antibiotic Given	243	97%	96%	95%
Blood Culture Timing	304	99%	97%	98%
Pregnancy and Delivery Care				
Newborn Deliveries Scheduled Early	138	1%	2%	6%
Preventive Care				
Immunization for Influenza[2]	527	86%	91%	90%
Immunization for Pneumonia[2]	625	89%	91%	92%
Stroke Care				
Anticoagulation Therapy for Atrial Fibrillation	55	95%	94%	95%
Antithrombotic Therapy Timing	154	98%	98%	98%
Assessed for Rehabilitation	283	94%	98%	97%
Discharged on Antithrombotic Therapy	235	100%	99%	99%
Discharged on Statin Medication	193	96%	96%	94%
Thrombolytic Therapy Timing	32	75%	73%	66%
Venous Thromboembolism Prophylaxis	269	96%	94%	94%
Written Stroke Educational Materials Given	113	95%	86%	88%
Surgical Care Improvement Project				
Appropriate Beta Blocker Usage[2]	203	98%	98%	98%
Appropriate VTP Within 24 Hours[2]	302	98%	98%	98%
Controlled Postoperative Blood Glucose[2]	159	97%	97%	97%
Perioperative Temperature Management[2]	500	100%	100%	100%
Prophylactic Antibiotic Selection[2]	451	98%	99%	99%
Prophylactic Antibiotic Selection (Outpatient)	284	96%	98%	98%
Prophylactic Antibiotic Stopped[2]	447	97%	99%	98%
Prophylactic Antibiotic Timing[2]	455	97%	98%	99%
Prophylactic Antibiotic Timing (Outpatient)	288	92%	98%	98%
Urinary Catheter Removal[2]	227	90%	97%	97%
Survey of Patients' Hospital Experiences				
Area Around Room 'Always' Quiet at Night	300+	54%	54%	61%
Doctors 'Always' Communicated Well	300+	81%	81%	82%
Home Recovery Information Given	300+	87%	87%	85%
Hospital Given 9 or 10 on 10 Point Scale	300+	77%	70%	71%
Meds 'Always' Explained Before Given	300+	62%	64%	64%
Nurses 'Always' Communicated Well	300+	79%	77%	79%
Pain 'Always' Well Controlled	300+	70%	70%	71%
Room and Bathroom 'Always' Clean	300+	73%	73%	73%
Timely Help 'Always' Received	300+	66%	65%	68%
Would Definitely Recommend Hospital	300+	81%	73%	71%
Use of Medical Imaging				
Cardiac Imaging Stress Test before Surgery	747	3.7%	4.3%	5.3%
Combination Abdominal CT Scan	717	4.5%	6.9%	10.5%
Combination Brain/Sinus CT Scan	959	1.9%	2.3%	2.7%
Combination Chest CT Scan	188	0.0%	1.1%	2.7%
Follow-up Mammogram/Ultrasound[7]	-	-	9.1%	8.8%
Lumbar Spine MRI for Low Back Pain	93	32.3%	37.9%	37.2%

Mid Valley Hospital

810 Jasmine Street Phone: 509-826-1760
Omak, WA 98841
Type: Critical Access Hospitals Emergency Services: Yes
Ownership: Govt - Hospital Dist/Auth

Measure	Cases	This Hosp.	State Avg.	U.S. Avg.
Blood Clot Prevention and Treatment				
Anticoagulation Overlap Therapy[5]	-	-	97%	93%
ICU Venous Thromboembolism Prophylaxis[5]	-	-	92%	92%
Incidence of Potentially Preventable VTE[5]	-	-	9%	10%
UFH with Dosages/Platelet Monitoring[5]	-	-	99%	97%
Venous Thromboembolism Prophylaxis[5]	-	-	86%	85%
Warfarin Therapy Discharge Instructions[5]	-	-	74%	75%
Chest Pain/Possible Heart Attack Care				
Aspirin Given Within 24 Hours of Arrival	28	96%	97%	96%
Fibrinolytic Meds Within 30 Min. of Arrival[1]	-	-	51%	58%
Average Time to ECG (minutes)	31	15	9	7
Average Time to Transfer (minutes)[7]	-	-	54	60
Children's Asthma Care				
Received Home Management Plan of Care	-	-	-	88%
Received Reliever Medication	-	-	-	100%
Received Systemic Corticosteroids	-	-	-	100%
Emergency Department				
Admittance Decision Time (minutes)[5]	-	-	96	98
Head CT Results Within 45 Min. of Arrival[5]	-	-	63%	57%
Patients Who Left ER Before Being Seen[5]	-	-	2%	2%
Time from ER Arrival to Admit. (minutes)[5]	-	-	259	274
Time from ER Arrival to Discharge (minutes)[5]	-	-	135	134
Time in ER Before Being Evaluated (minutes)[5]	-	-	22	26
Time to Pain Meds for Fractures (minutes)[5]	-	-	52	57
Heart Attack Care				
Aspirin Given at Discharge[5]	-	-	99%	99%
Fibrinolytic Meds Within 30 Min. of Arrival[5]	-	-	62%	54%
PCI Within 90 Minutes of Arrival[5]	-	-	97%	96%
Statin Prescribed at Discharge[5]	-	-	98%	98%
Heart Failure Care				
ACE Inhibitor or ARB for LVSD[7]	-	-	97%	97%
Discharge Instructions Given[1]	-	-	93%	94%
Evaluation of LVS Function	11	64%	99%	99%
Medicare Spending				
Medicare Spending per Patient (ratio)	-	-	0.91	0.98
Pneumonia Care				
Appropriate Initial Antibiotic Given	27	96%	96%	95%
Blood Culture Timing	40	100%	97%	98%
Pregnancy and Delivery Care				
Newborn Deliveries Scheduled Early[5]	-	-	2%	6%
Preventive Care				
Immunization for Influenza[5]	-	-	91%	90%
Immunization for Pneumonia[5]	-	-	91%	92%
Stroke Care				
Anticoagulation Therapy for Atrial Fibrillation[5]	-	-	94%	95%
Antithrombotic Therapy Timing[5]	-	-	98%	98%
Assessed for Rehabilitation[5]	-	-	98%	97%
Discharged on Antithrombotic Therapy[5]	-	-	99%	99%
Discharged on Statin Medication[5]	-	-	96%	94%
Thrombolytic Therapy Timing[5]	-	-	73%	66%
Venous Thromboembolism Prophylaxis[5]	-	-	94%	94%
Written Stroke Educational Materials Given[5]	-	-	86%	88%
Surgical Care Improvement Project				
Appropriate Beta Blocker Usage[1]	-	-	98%	98%
Appropriate VTP Within 24 Hours	30	100%	98%	98%
Controlled Postoperative Blood Glucose[7]	-	-	97%	97%
Perioperative Temperature Management	32	100%	100%	100%
Prophylactic Antibiotic Selection	22	91%	99%	99%
Prophylactic Antibiotic Selection (Outpatient)[5]	-	-	98%	98%
Prophylactic Antibiotic Stopped	22	95%	99%	98%
Prophylactic Antibiotic Timing	22	95%	98%	99%
Prophylactic Antibiotic Timing (Outpatient)[5]	-	-	98%	98%
Urinary Catheter Removal	31	100%	97%	97%
Survey of Patients' Hospital Experiences				
Area Around Room 'Always' Quiet at Night[5]	-	-	54%	61%
Doctors 'Always' Communicated Well[5]	-	-	81%	82%
Home Recovery Information Given[5]	-	-	87%	85%
Hospital Given 9 or 10 on 10 Point Scale[5]	-	-	70%	71%
Meds 'Always' Explained Before Given[5]	-	-	64%	64%
Nurses 'Always' Communicated Well[5]	-	-	77%	79%
Pain 'Always' Well Controlled[5]	-	-	70%	71%
Room and Bathroom 'Always' Clean[5]	-	-	73%	73%
Timely Help 'Always' Received[5]	-	-	65%	68%
Would Definitely Recommend Hospital[5]	-	-	73%	71%
Use of Medical Imaging				
Cardiac Imaging Stress Test before Surgery	58	1.7%	4.3%	5.3%
Combination Abdominal CT Scan	366	17.8%	6.9%	10.5%
Combination Brain/Sinus CT Scan[1]	-	-	2.3%	2.7%
Combination Chest CT Scan	330	0.0%	1.1%	2.7%
Follow-up Mammogram/Ultrasound	182	15.9%	9.1%	8.8%
Lumbar Spine MRI for Low Back Pain	82	64.6%	37.9%	37.2%

Othello Community Hospital

315 North 14th Avenue Phone: 509-488-2636
Othello, WA 99344 Fax: 509-488-3857
URL: www.othellocommunityhospital.org
Type: Critical Access Hospitals Emergency Services: Yes
Ownership: Govt - Hospital Dist/Auth Beds: 49

Key Personnel:
Chief of Medical Staff . . . . Fay Coats
CEO/President. . . . . Larry McCourtie
President . . . . Shirley McCullough
Operating Room. . . . . Mary McCurtie
Intensive Care Unit. . . . . Kathi Trussell

Measure	Cases	This Hosp.	State Avg.	U.S. Avg.
Blood Clot Prevention and Treatment				
Anticoagulation Overlap Therapy[5]	-	-	97%	93%
ICU Venous Thromboembolism Prophylaxis[5]	-	-	92%	92%
Incidence of Potentially Preventable VTE[5]	-	-	9%	10%
UFH with Dosages/Platelet Monitoring[5]	-	-	99%	97%
Venous Thromboembolism Prophylaxis[5]	-	-	86%	85%
Warfarin Therapy Discharge Instructions[5]	-	-	74%	75%
Chest Pain/Possible Heart Attack Care				
Aspirin Given Within 24 Hours of Arrival[1,3]	-	-	97%	96%
Fibrinolytic Meds Within 30 Min. of Arrival[3,7]	-	-	51%	58%
Average Time to ECG (minutes)[1,3]	-	-	9	7
Average Time to Transfer (minutes)[1,3]	-	-	54	60
Children's Asthma Care				
Received Home Management Plan of Care	-	-	-	88%
Received Reliever Medication	-	-	-	100%
Received Systemic Corticosteroids	-	-	-	100%
Emergency Department				
Admittance Decision Time (minutes)[5]	-	-	96	98
Head CT Results Within 45 Min. of Arrival[3,7]	-	-	63%	57%
Patients Who Left ER Before Being Seen[5]	-	-	2%	2%

NOTE: Hospital profiles are in alphabetical order by state, then city, then hospital within the city; Rankings exclude hospitals with less than 25 cases except for patient surveys which excludes hospitals with less than 100 cases; (a) 100-299 cases; (1) The number of cases/patients is too few to report; (2) Data submitted were based on a sample of cases/patients; (3) Results are based on a shorter time period than required; (4) Data suppressed by CMS for one or more quarters; (5) Results are not available for this reporting period; (6) Fewer than 100 patients completed the HCAHPS survey; (7) No cases met the criteria for this measure; (8) The lower limit of the confidence interval cannot be calculated if the number of observed infections equals zero; (9) No data are available from the state/territory for this reporting period; (10) The scores shown reflect fewer than 50 completed surveys; (11) There were discrepancies in the data collection process; (12) This measure does not apply to this hospital for this reporting period; (13) Results cannot be calculated for this reporting period; (14) The results for this state are combined with nearby states to protect confidentiality; Please refer to the User's Guide for a full explanation of data.

Measure	Cases	This Hosp.	State Avg.	U.S. Avg.
Time from ER Arrival to Admit. (minutes)[5]	-	-	259	274
Time from ER Arrival to Discharge (minutes)[5]	-	-	135	134
Time in ER Before Being Evaluated (minutes)[5]	-	-	22	26
Time to Pain Meds for Fractures (minutes)[5]	-	-	52	57
Heart Attack Care				
Aspirin Given at Discharge[5]	-	-	99%	99%
Fibrinolytic Meds Within 30 Min. of Arrival[5]	-	-	62%	54%
PCI Within 90 Minutes of Arrival[5]	-	-	97%	96%
Statin Prescribed at Discharge[5]	-	-	98%	98%
Heart Failure Care				
ACE Inhibitor or ARB for LVSD[1,3]	-	-	97%	97%
Discharge Instructions Given[1,3]	-	-	93%	94%
Evaluation of LVS Function[1,3]	-	-	99%	99%
Medicare Spending				
Medicare Spending per Patient (ratio)	-	-	0.91	0.98
Pneumonia Care				
Appropriate Initial Antibiotic Given[1,3]	-	-	96%	95%
Blood Culture Timing[1,3]	-	-	97%	98%
Pregnancy and Delivery Care				
Newborn Deliveries Scheduled Early[5]	-	-	2%	6%
Preventive Care				
Immunization for Influenza[5]	-	-	91%	90%
Immunization for Pneumonia[5]	-	-	91%	92%
Stroke Care				
Anticoagulation Therapy for Atrial Fibrillation[3,7]	-	-	94%	95%
Antithrombotic Therapy Timing[3,7]	-	-	98%	98%
Assessed for Rehabilitation[1,3]	-	-	98%	97%
Discharged on Antithrombotic Therapy[1,3]	-	-	99%	99%
Discharged on Statin Medication[1,3]	-	-	96%	94%
Thrombolytic Therapy Timing[3,7]	-	-	73%	66%
Venous Thromboembolism Prophylaxis[1,3]	-	-	94%	94%
Written Stroke Educational Materials Given[3,7]	-	-	86%	88%
Surgical Care Improvement Project				
Appropriate Beta Blocker Usage[3,7]	-	-	98%	98%
Appropriate VTP Within 24 Hours[1,3]	-	-	98%	98%
Controlled Postoperative Blood Glucose[3,7]	-	-	97%	97%
Perioperative Temperature Management[1,3]	-	-	100%	100%
Prophylactic Antibiotic Selection[1,3]	-	-	99%	99%
Prophylactic Antibiotic Selection (Outpatient)[1,3]	-	-	98%	98%
Prophylactic Antibiotic Stopped[1,3]	-	-	99%	98%
Prophylactic Antibiotic Timing[1,3]	-	-	98%	99%
Prophylactic Antibiotic Timing (Outpatient)[1,3]	-	-	98%	98%
Urinary Catheter Removal[3,7]	-	-	97%	97%
Survey of Patients' Hospital Experiences				
Area Around Room 'Always' Quiet at Night	(a)	63%	54%	61%
Doctors 'Always' Communicated Well	(a)	80%	81%	82%
Home Recovery Information Given	(a)	84%	87%	85%
Hospital Given 9 or 10 on 10 Point Scale	(a)	69%	70%	71%
Meds 'Always' Explained Before Given	(a)	59%	64%	64%
Nurses 'Always' Communicated Well	(a)	78%	77%	79%
Pain 'Always' Well Controlled	(a)	73%	70%	71%
Room and Bathroom 'Always' Clean	(a)	70%	73%	73%
Timely Help 'Always' Received	(a)	61%	65%	68%
Would Definitely Recommend Hospital	(a)	72%	73%	71%
Use of Medical Imaging				
Cardiac Imaging Stress Test before Surgery[7]	-	-	4.3%	5.3%
Combination Abdominal CT Scan	58	1.7%	6.9%	10.5%
Combination Brain/Sinus CT Scan	74	0.0%	2.3%	2.7%
Combination Chest CT Scan[1]	-	-	1.1%	2.7%
Follow-up Mammogram/Ultrasound	96	7.3%	9.1%	8.8%
Lumbar Spine MRI for Low Back Pain[1]	-	-	37.9%	37.2%

Lourdes Medical Center

520 N Fourth Avenue
Pasco, WA 99301
Phone: 509-546-2278
Fax: 509-546-2291
URL: www.lourdesonline.org
Type: Critical Access Hospitals
Emergency Services: Yes
Ownership: Voluntary non-profit - Church
Beds: 95

Key Personnel:

Infection Control. . . . . Joanne Dixon
Operating Room. . . . . Barbara Edwards
Emergency Room . . . . Bev Harn
Pediatric In-Patient Care . . . . Dee Hazel
Intensive Care Unit. . . . . Dee Huzel
Quality Assurance . . . . Anita Kongslie
CEO/President. . . . . John Serle
Chief of Medical Staff . . . . Richard Shallman

Measure	Cases	This Hosp.	State Avg.	U.S. Avg.
Blood Clot Prevention and Treatment				
Anticoagulation Overlap Therapy[2]	12	100%	97%	93%
ICU Venous Thromboembolism Prophylaxis[2]	14	86%	92%	92%
Incidence of Potentially Preventable VTE[1,2]	-	-	9%	10%
UFH with Dosages/Platelet Monitoring[1,2]	-	-	99%	97%
Venous Thromboembolism Prophylaxis[2]	65	83%	86%	85%
Warfarin Therapy Discharge Instructions[1,2]	-	-	74%	75%
Chest Pain/Possible Heart Attack Care				
Aspirin Given Within 24 Hours of Arrival	-	-	97%	96%
Fibrinolytic Meds Within 30 Min. of Arrival	-	-	51%	58%
Average Time to ECG (minutes)	-	-	9	7
Average Time to Transfer (minutes)	-	-	54	60
Children's Asthma Care				
Received Home Management Plan of Care	-	-	-	88%
Received Reliever Medication	-	-	-	100%
Received Systemic Corticosteroids	-	-	-	100%
Emergency Department				
Admittance Decision Time (minutes)[5]	-	-	96	98
Head CT Results Within 45 Min. of Arrival	-	-	63%	57%
Patients Who Left ER Before Being Seen	-	-	2%	2%
Time from ER Arrival to Admit. (minutes)[5]	-	-	259	274
Time from ER Arrival to Discharge (minutes)	-	-	135	134
Time in ER Before Being Evaluated (minutes)	-	-	22	26
Time to Pain Meds for Fractures (minutes)	-	-	52	57
Heart Attack Care				
Aspirin Given at Discharge[1]	-	-	99%	99%
Fibrinolytic Meds Within 30 Min. of Arrival[7]	-	-	62%	54%
PCI Within 90 Minutes of Arrival[7]	-	-	97%	96%
Statin Prescribed at Discharge[1]	-	-	98%	98%
Heart Failure Care				
ACE Inhibitor or ARB for LVSD[1,3]	-	-	97%	97%
Discharge Instructions Given[3]	13	77%	93%	94%
Evaluation of LVS Function[3]	14	100%	99%	99%
Medicare Spending				
Medicare Spending per Patient (ratio)	-	-	0.91	0.98
Pneumonia Care				
Appropriate Initial Antibiotic Given	15	80%	96%	95%
Blood Culture Timing	27	93%	97%	98%
Pregnancy and Delivery Care				
Newborn Deliveries Scheduled Early[5]	-	-	2%	6%
Preventive Care				
Immunization for Influenza[5]	-	-	91%	90%
Immunization for Pneumonia[5]	-	-	91%	92%
Stroke Care				
Anticoagulation Therapy for Atrial Fibrillation[1]	-	-	94%	95%
Antithrombotic Therapy Timing[1]	-	-	98%	98%
Assessed for Rehabilitation[1]	-	-	98%	97%
Discharged on Antithrombotic Therapy[1]	-	-	99%	99%
Discharged on Statin Medication[1]	-	-	96%	94%
Thrombolytic Therapy Timing[7]	-	-	73%	66%
Venous Thromboembolism Prophylaxis[1]	-	-	94%	94%
Written Stroke Educational Materials Given[1]	-	-	86%	88%
Surgical Care Improvement Project				
Appropriate Beta Blocker Usage	141	99%	98%	98%
Appropriate VTP Within 24 Hours	580	99%	98%	98%
Controlled Postoperative Blood Glucose[7]	-	-	97%	97%
Perioperative Temperature Management	631	100%	100%	100%
Prophylactic Antibiotic Selection	528	99%	99%	99%
Prophylactic Antibiotic Selection (Outpatient)	-	-	98%	98%
Prophylactic Antibiotic Stopped	525	97%	99%	98%
Prophylactic Antibiotic Timing	528	98%	98%	99%
Prophylactic Antibiotic Timing (Outpatient)	-	-	98%	98%
Urinary Catheter Removal	133	98%	97%	97%
Survey of Patients' Hospital Experiences				
Area Around Room 'Always' Quiet at Night[5]	-	-	54%	61%
Doctors 'Always' Communicated Well[5]	-	-	81%	82%
Home Recovery Information Given[5]	-	-	87%	85%
Hospital Given 9 or 10 on 10 Point Scale[5]	-	-	70%	71%
Meds 'Always' Explained Before Given[5]	-	-	64%	64%
Nurses 'Always' Communicated Well[5]	-	-	77%	79%
Pain 'Always' Well Controlled[5]	-	-	70%	71%
Room and Bathroom 'Always' Clean[5]	-	-	73%	73%
Timely Help 'Always' Received[5]	-	-	65%	68%
Would Definitely Recommend Hospital[5]	-	-	73%	71%
Use of Medical Imaging				
Cardiac Imaging Stress Test before Surgery	-	-	4.3%	5.3%
Combination Abdominal CT Scan	-	-	6.9%	10.5%
Combination Brain/Sinus CT Scan	-	-	2.3%	2.7%
Combination Chest CT Scan	-	-	1.1%	2.7%
Follow-up Mammogram/Ultrasound	-	-	9.1%	8.8%
Lumbar Spine MRI for Low Back Pain	-	-	37.9%	37.2%

Garfield County Memorial Hospital

66 North Sixth Street
Phone: 509-843-1591
Pomeroy, WA 99347
Type: Critical Access Hospitals
Emergency Services: Yes
Ownership: Govt - Hospital Dist/Auth

Measure	Cases	This Hosp.	State Avg.	U.S. Avg.
Blood Clot Prevention and Treatment				
Anticoagulation Overlap Therapy[5]	-	-	97%	93%
ICU Venous Thromboembolism Prophylaxis[5]	-	-	92%	92%
Incidence of Potentially Preventable VTE[5]	-	-	9%	10%
UFH with Dosages/Platelet Monitoring[5]	-	-	99%	97%
Venous Thromboembolism Prophylaxis[5]	-	-	86%	85%
Warfarin Therapy Discharge Instructions[5]	-	-	74%	75%
Chest Pain/Possible Heart Attack Care				
Aspirin Given Within 24 Hours of Arrival[1,3]	-	-	97%	96%
Fibrinolytic Meds Within 30 Min. of Arrival[3,7]	-	-	51%	58%
Average Time to ECG (minutes)[1,3]	-	-	9	7
Average Time to Transfer (minutes)[1,3]	-	-	54	60
Children's Asthma Care				
Received Home Management Plan of Care	-	-	-	88%
Received Reliever Medication	-	-	-	100%
Received Systemic Corticosteroids	-	-	-	100%
Emergency Department				
Admittance Decision Time (minutes)[5]	-	-	96	98
Head CT Results Within 45 Min. of Arrival[5]	-	-	63%	57%
Patients Who Left ER Before Being Seen[5]	-	-	2%	2%
Time from ER Arrival to Admit. (minutes)[5]	-	-	259	274
Time from ER Arrival to Discharge (minutes)[5]	-	-	135	134
Time in ER Before Being Evaluated (minutes)[5]	-	-	22	26
Time to Pain Meds for Fractures (minutes)[5]	-	-	52	57
Heart Attack Care				
Aspirin Given at Discharge[5]	-	-	99%	99%
Fibrinolytic Meds Within 30 Min. of Arrival[5]	-	-	62%	54%
PCI Within 90 Minutes of Arrival[5]	-	-	97%	96%
Statin Prescribed at Discharge[5]	-	-	98%	98%
Heart Failure Care				
ACE Inhibitor or ARB for LVSD[5]	-	-	97%	97%
Discharge Instructions Given[5]	-	-	93%	94%
Evaluation of LVS Function[5]	-	-	99%	99%
Medicare Spending				
Medicare Spending per Patient (ratio)	-	-	0.91	0.98
Pneumonia Care				
Appropriate Initial Antibiotic Given[5]	-	-	96%	95%
Blood Culture Timing[5]	-	-	97%	98%
Pregnancy and Delivery Care				
Newborn Deliveries Scheduled Early[5]	-	-	2%	6%
Preventive Care				
Immunization for Influenza[5]	-	-	91%	90%
Immunization for Pneumonia[5]	-	-	91%	92%
Stroke Care				
Anticoagulation Therapy for Atrial Fibrillation[5]	-	-	94%	95%
Antithrombotic Therapy Timing[5]	-	-	98%	98%
Assessed for Rehabilitation[5]	-	-	98%	97%
Discharged on Antithrombotic Therapy[5]	-	-	99%	99%
Discharged on Statin Medication[5]	-	-	96%	94%
Thrombolytic Therapy Timing[5]	-	-	73%	66%
Venous Thromboembolism Prophylaxis[5]	-	-	94%	94%
Written Stroke Educational Materials Given[5]	-	-	86%	88%
Surgical Care Improvement Project				

NOTE: Hospital profiles are in alphabetical order by state, then city, then hospital within the city; Rankings exclude hospitals with less than 25 cases except for patient surveys which excludes hospitals with less than 100 cases; (a) 100-299 cases; (1) The number of cases/patients is too few to report; (2) Data submitted were based on a sample of cases/patients; (3) Results are based on a shorter time period than required; (4) Data suppressed by CMS for one or more quarters; (5) Results are not available for this reporting period; (6) Fewer than 100 patients completed the HCAHPS survey; (7) No cases met the criteria for this measure; (8) The lower limit of the confidence interval cannot be calculated if the number of observed infections equals zero; (9) No data are available from the state/territory for this reporting period; (10) The scores shown reflect fewer than 50 completed surveys; (11) There were discrepancies in the data collection process; (12) This measure does not apply to this hospital for this reporting period; (13) Results cannot be calculated for this reporting period; (14) The results for this state are combined with nearby states to protect confidentiality; Please refer to the User's Guide for a full explanation of data.

Measure	Cases	This Hosp.	State Avg.	U.S. Avg.
Appropriate Beta Blocker Usage[5]	-	-	98%	98%
Appropriate VTP Within 24 Hours[5]	-	-	98%	98%
Controlled Postoperative Blood Glucose[5]	-	-	97%	97%
Perioperative Temperature Management[5]	-	-	100%	100%
Prophylactic Antibiotic Selection[5]	-	-	99%	99%
Prophylactic Antibiotic Selection (Outpatient)[5]	-	-	98%	98%
Prophylactic Antibiotic Stopped[5]	-	-	99%	98%
Prophylactic Antibiotic Timing[5]	-	-	98%	99%
Prophylactic Antibiotic Timing (Outpatient)[5]	-	-	98%	98%
Urinary Catheter Removal[5]	-	-	97%	97%
Survey of Patients' Hospital Experiences				
Area Around Room 'Always' Quiet at Night[5]	-	-	54%	61%
Doctors 'Always' Communicated Well[5]	-	-	81%	82%
Home Recovery Information Given[5]	-	-	87%	85%
Hospital Given 9 or 10 on 10 Point Scale[5]	-	-	70%	71%
Meds 'Always' Explained Before Given[5]	-	-	64%	64%
Nurses 'Always' Communicated Well[5]	-	-	77%	79%
Pain 'Always' Well Controlled[5]	-	-	70%	71%
Room and Bathroom 'Always' Clean[5]	-	-	73%	73%
Timely Help 'Always' Received[5]	-	-	65%	68%
Would Definitely Recommend Hospital[5]	-	-	73%	71%
Use of Medical Imaging				
Cardiac Imaging Stress Test before Surgery[7]	-	-	4.3%	5.3%
Combination Abdominal CT Scan[7]	-	-	6.9%	10.5%
Combination Brain/Sinus CT Scan[7]	-	-	2.3%	2.7%
Combination Chest CT Scan[7]	-	-	1.1%	2.7%
Follow-up Mammogram/Ultrasound[7]	-	-	9.1%	8.8%
Lumbar Spine MRI for Low Back Pain[7]	-	-	37.9%	37.2%

Olympic Medical Center

939 Caroline St
Port Angeles, WA 98362
Phone: 360-417-7000
Fax: 360-417-7307
URL: www.olympicmedical.org
Type: Acute Care Hospitals
Emergency Services: Yes
Ownership: Government - Local
Beds: 126

Key Personnel:
Radiology. . . . . Richard Clark
Chief of Medical Staff . . . . Scott Kennedy, MD
CEO . . . . Eric Lewis
Anesthesiology. . . . . Mary Romstadt, RN

Measure	Cases	This Hosp.	State Avg.	U.S. Avg.
Blood Clot Prevention and Treatment				
Anticoagulation Overlap Therapy[2]	22	100%	97%	93%
ICU Venous Thromboembolism Prophylaxis[2]	75	93%	92%	92%
Incidence of Potentially Preventable VTE[1,2]	-	-	9%	10%
UFH with Dosages/Platelet Monitoring[2]	13	85%	99%	97%
Venous Thromboembolism Prophylaxis[2]	287	88%	86%	85%
Warfarin Therapy Discharge Instructions[2]	15	7%	74%	75%
Chest Pain/Possible Heart Attack Care				
Aspirin Given Within 24 Hours of Arrival	100	98%	97%	96%
Fibrinolytic Meds Within 30 Min. of Arrival[1]	-	-	51%	58%
Average Time to ECG (minutes)	100	2	9	7
Average Time to Transfer (minutes)[7]	-	-	54	60
Children's Asthma Care				
Received Home Management Plan of Care	-	-	-	88%
Received Reliever Medication	-	-	-	100%
Received Systemic Corticosteroids	-	-	-	100%
Emergency Department				
Admittance Decision Time (minutes)[2]	514	75	96	98
Head CT Results Within 45 Min. of Arrival	11	55%	63%	57%
Patients Who Left ER Before Being Seen	22,633	2%	2%	2%
Time from ER Arrival to Admit. (minutes)[2]	554	239	259	274
Time from ER Arrival to Discharge (minutes)	449	150	135	134
Time in ER Before Being Evaluated (minutes)	408	43	22	26
Time to Pain Meds for Fractures (minutes)	81	68	52	57
Heart Attack Care				
Aspirin Given at Discharge	22	100%	99%	99%
Fibrinolytic Meds Within 30 Min. of Arrival[1]	-	-	62%	54%
PCI Within 90 Minutes of Arrival[7]	-	-	97%	96%
Statin Prescribed at Discharge	21	95%	98%	98%
Heart Failure Care				
ACE Inhibitor or ARB for LVSD	43	98%	97%	97%
Discharge Instructions Given	102	91%	93%	94%
Evaluation of LVS Function	122	99%	99%	99%
Medicare Spending				
Medicare Spending per Patient (ratio)	-	0.97	0.91	0.98
Pneumonia Care				
Appropriate Initial Antibiotic Given	99	94%	96%	95%
Blood Culture Timing	130	99%	97%	98%
Pregnancy and Delivery Care				
Newborn Deliveries Scheduled Early	46	4%	2%	6%
Preventive Care				
Immunization for Influenza[2]	394	95%	91%	90%
Immunization for Pneumonia[2]	534	86%	91%	92%
Stroke Care				
Anticoagulation Therapy for Atrial Fibrillation[1]	-	-	94%	95%
Antithrombotic Therapy Timing	55	85%	98%	98%
Assessed for Rehabilitation	69	96%	98%	97%
Discharged on Antithrombotic Therapy	67	97%	99%	99%
Discharged on Statin Medication	52	87%	96%	94%
Thrombolytic Therapy Timing[1]	-	-	73%	66%
Venous Thromboembolism Prophylaxis	68	90%	94%	94%
Written Stroke Educational Materials Given	39	36%	86%	88%
Surgical Care Improvement Project				
Appropriate Beta Blocker Usage	121	99%	98%	98%
Appropriate VTP Within 24 Hours	391	97%	98%	98%
Controlled Postoperative Blood Glucose[7]	-	-	97%	97%
Perioperative Temperature Management	439	100%	100%	100%
Prophylactic Antibiotic Selection	335	99%	99%	99%
Prophylactic Antibiotic Selection (Outpatient)	110	97%	98%	98%
Prophylactic Antibiotic Stopped	329	98%	99%	98%
Prophylactic Antibiotic Timing	337	95%	98%	99%
Prophylactic Antibiotic Timing (Outpatient)	98	96%	98%	98%
Urinary Catheter Removal	327	97%	97%	97%
Survey of Patients' Hospital Experiences				
Area Around Room 'Always' Quiet at Night	300+	45%	54%	61%
Doctors 'Always' Communicated Well	300+	81%	81%	82%
Home Recovery Information Given	300+	84%	87%	85%
Hospital Given 9 or 10 on 10 Point Scale	300+	67%	70%	71%
Meds 'Always' Explained Before Given	300+	64%	64%	64%
Nurses 'Always' Communicated Well	300+	77%	77%	79%
Pain 'Always' Well Controlled	300+	67%	70%	71%
Room and Bathroom 'Always' Clean	300+	72%	73%	73%
Timely Help 'Always' Received	300+	71%	65%	68%
Would Definitely Recommend Hospital	300+	72%	73%	71%
Use of Medical Imaging				
Cardiac Imaging Stress Test before Surgery	572	5.2%	4.3%	5.3%
Combination Abdominal CT Scan	1,306	1.8%	6.9%	10.5%
Combination Brain/Sinus CT Scan	720	1.9%	2.3%	2.7%
Combination Chest CT Scan	1,009	0.1%	1.1%	2.7%
Follow-up Mammogram/Ultrasound	2,853	10.9%	9.1%	8.8%
Lumbar Spine MRI for Low Back Pain	344	26.7%	37.9%	37.2%

Jefferson Healthcare Hospital

834 Sheridan Street
Port Townsend, WA 98368
Phone: 360-385-2200
Fax: 360-379-2242
URL: www.jgh.org
Type: Critical Access Hospitals
Emergency Services: Yes
Ownership: Govt - Hospital Dist/Auth
Beds: 25

Key Personnel:
Infection Control. . . . . Joanne Clyde
Emergency Room . . . . Jim DeCianne
CEO . . . . Mike Glenn
Chief of Medical Staff. . . . . Dr. Joe Mattern
Quality Assurance . . . . Sharon Wagner

Measure	Cases	This Hosp.	State Avg.	U.S. Avg.
Blood Clot Prevention and Treatment				
Anticoagulation Overlap Therapy[5]	-	-	97%	93%
ICU Venous Thromboembolism Prophylaxis[5]	-	-	92%	92%
Incidence of Potentially Preventable VTE[5]	-	-	9%	10%
UFH with Dosages/Platelet Monitoring[5]	-	-	99%	97%
Venous Thromboembolism Prophylaxis[5]	-	-	86%	85%
Warfarin Therapy Discharge Instructions[5]	-	-	74%	75%
Chest Pain/Possible Heart Attack Care				
Aspirin Given Within 24 Hours of Arrival[3]	28	96%	97%	96%
Fibrinolytic Meds Within 30 Min. of Arrival[1,3]	-	-	51%	58%
Average Time to ECG (minutes)[3]	32	7	9	7
Average Time to Transfer (minutes)[1,3]	-	-	54	60
Children's Asthma Care				
Received Home Management Plan of Care	-	-	-	88%
Received Reliever Medication	-	-	-	100%
Received Systemic Corticosteroids	-	-	-	100%
Emergency Department				
Admittance Decision Time (minutes)[5]	-	-	96	98
Head CT Results Within 45 Min. of Arrival[5]	-	-	63%	57%
Patients Who Left ER Before Being Seen[5]	-	-	2%	2%
Time from ER Arrival to Admit. (minutes)[5]	-	-	259	274
Time from ER Arrival to Discharge (minutes)[5]	-	-	135	134
Time in ER Before Being Evaluated (minutes)[5]	-	-	22	26
Time to Pain Meds for Fractures (minutes)[5]	-	-	52	57
Heart Attack Care				
Aspirin Given at Discharge[1]	-	-	99%	99%
Fibrinolytic Meds Within 30 Min. of Arrival[7]	-	-	62%	54%
PCI Within 90 Minutes of Arrival[7]	-	-	97%	96%
Statin Prescribed at Discharge[1]	-	-	98%	98%
Heart Failure Care				
ACE Inhibitor or ARB for LVSD[1]	-	-	97%	97%
Discharge Instructions Given	25	76%	93%	94%
Evaluation of LVS Function	27	100%	99%	99%
Medicare Spending				
Medicare Spending per Patient (ratio)	-	-	0.91	0.98
Pneumonia Care				
Appropriate Initial Antibiotic Given[2]	31	84%	96%	95%
Blood Culture Timing[2]	43	98%	97%	98%
Pregnancy and Delivery Care				
Newborn Deliveries Scheduled Early[5]	-	-	2%	6%
Preventive Care				
Immunization for Influenza[5]	-	-	91%	90%
Immunization for Pneumonia[5]	-	-	91%	92%
Stroke Care				
Anticoagulation Therapy for Atrial Fibrillation[7]	-	-	94%	95%
Antithrombotic Therapy Timing[1]	-	-	98%	98%
Assessed for Rehabilitation[1]	-	-	98%	97%
Discharged on Antithrombotic Therapy[1]	-	-	99%	99%
Discharged on Statin Medication[1]	-	-	96%	94%
Thrombolytic Therapy Timing[1]	-	-	73%	66%
Venous Thromboembolism Prophylaxis[1]	-	-	94%	94%
Written Stroke Educational Materials Given[1]	-	-	86%	88%
Surgical Care Improvement Project				
Appropriate Beta Blocker Usage	14	93%	98%	98%
Appropriate VTP Within 24 Hours	68	100%	98%	98%
Controlled Postoperative Blood Glucose[3,7]	-	-	97%	97%
Perioperative Temperature Management	72	100%	100%	100%
Prophylactic Antibiotic Selection	62	100%	99%	99%
Prophylactic Antibiotic Selection (Outpatient)[5]	-	-	98%	98%
Prophylactic Antibiotic Stopped	62	98%	99%	98%
Prophylactic Antibiotic Timing	62	97%	98%	99%
Prophylactic Antibiotic Timing (Outpatient)[5]	-	-	98%	98%
Urinary Catheter Removal	65	100%	97%	97%
Survey of Patients' Hospital Experiences				
Area Around Room 'Always' Quiet at Night[5]	-	-	54%	61%
Doctors 'Always' Communicated Well[5]	-	-	81%	82%
Home Recovery Information Given[5]	-	-	87%	85%
Hospital Given 9 or 10 on 10 Point Scale[5]	-	-	70%	71%
Meds 'Always' Explained Before Given[5]	-	-	64%	64%
Nurses 'Always' Communicated Well[5]	-	-	77%	79%
Pain 'Always' Well Controlled[5]	-	-	70%	71%
Room and Bathroom 'Always' Clean[5]	-	-	73%	73%
Timely Help 'Always' Received[5]	-	-	65%	68%
Would Definitely Recommend Hospital[5]	-	-	73%	71%
Use of Medical Imaging				
Cardiac Imaging Stress Test before Surgery[1]	-	-	4.3%	5.3%
Combination Abdominal CT Scan	473	7.8%	6.9%	10.5%
Combination Brain/Sinus CT Scan	419	1.2%	2.3%	2.7%
Combination Chest CT Scan	276	1.1%	1.1%	2.7%
Follow-up Mammogram/Ultrasound	773	17.9%	9.1%	8.8%
Lumbar Spine MRI for Low Back Pain	51	31.4%	37.9%	37.2%

NOTE: Hospital profiles are in alphabetical order by state, then city, then hospital within the city; Rankings exclude hospitals with less than 25 cases except for patient surveys which excludes hospitals with less than 100 cases; (a) 100-299 cases; (1) The number of cases/patients is too few to report; (2) Data submitted were based on a sample of cases/patients; (3) Results are based on a shorter time period than required; (4) Data suppressed by CMS for one or more quarters; (5) Results are not available for this reporting period; (6) Fewer than 100 patients completed the HCAHPS survey; (7) No cases met the criteria for this measure; (8) The lower limit of the confidence interval cannot be calculated if the number of observed infections equals zero; (9) No data are available from the state/territory for this reporting period; (10) The scores shown reflect fewer than 50 completed surveys; (11) There were discrepancies in the data collection process; (12) This measure does not apply to this hospital for this reporting period; (13) Results cannot be calculated for this reporting period; (14) The results for this state are combined with nearby states to protect confidentiality; Please refer to the User's Guide for a full explanation of data.

Prosser Memorial Hospital

723 Memorial Street
Prosser, WA 99350
Phone: 509-786-2222
Fax: 509-786-6683
E-mail: administration@pphdwa.org
URL: www.prosserhospital.com
Type: Critical Access Hospitals
Emergency Services: Yes
Ownership: Voluntary non-profit - Other
Beds: 26

Key Personnel:
Patient Relations . . . . Leann Anderson
Quality Assurance . . . . Leann Anderson
Emergency Room . . . . Ember Christensen
Infection Control. . . . . Susan Flory
Operating Room. . . . . Susan Flory
CEO/President. . . . . Julie Petersen
Chief of Medical Staff . . . . Ben Sonnichsen
Anesthesiology. . . . . Alan Steen

Measure	Cases	This Hosp.	State Avg.	U.S. Avg.
Blood Clot Prevention and Treatment				
Anticoagulation Overlap Therapy[5]	-	-	97%	93%
ICU Venous Thromboembolism Prophylaxis[5]	-	-	92%	92%
Incidence of Potentially Preventable VTE[5]	-	-	9%	10%
UFH with Dosages/Platelet Monitoring[5]	-	-	99%	97%
Venous Thromboembolism Prophylaxis[5]	-	-	86%	85%
Warfarin Therapy Discharge Instructions[5]	-	-	74%	75%
Chest Pain/Possible Heart Attack Care				
Aspirin Given Within 24 Hours of Arrival	-	-	97%	96%
Fibrinolytic Meds Within 30 Min. of Arrival	-	-	51%	58%
Average Time to ECG (minutes)	-	-	9	7
Average Time to Transfer (minutes)	-	-	54	60
Children's Asthma Care				
Received Home Management Plan of Care	-	-	-	88%
Received Reliever Medication	-	-	-	100%
Received Systemic Corticosteroids	-	-	-	100%
Emergency Department				
Admittance Decision Time (minutes)[5]	-	-	96	98
Head CT Results Within 45 Min. of Arrival	-	-	63%	57%
Patients Who Left ER Before Being Seen	-	-	2%	2%
Time from ER Arrival to Admit. (minutes)[5]	-	-	259	274
Time from ER Arrival to Discharge (minutes)	-	-	135	134
Time in ER Before Being Evaluated (minutes)	-	-	22	26
Time to Pain Meds for Fractures (minutes)	-	-	52	57
Heart Attack Care				
Aspirin Given at Discharge[3,7]	-	-	99%	99%
Fibrinolytic Meds Within 30 Min. of Arrival[3,7]	-	-	62%	54%
PCI Within 90 Minutes of Arrival[3,7]	-	-	97%	96%
Statin Prescribed at Discharge[3,7]	-	-	98%	98%
Heart Failure Care				
ACE Inhibitor or ARB for LVSD[1,3]	-	-	97%	97%
Discharge Instructions Given[1,3]	-	-	93%	94%
Evaluation of LVS Function[1,3]	-	-	99%	99%
Medicare Spending				
Medicare Spending per Patient (ratio)	-	-	0.91	0.98
Pneumonia Care				
Appropriate Initial Antibiotic Given[1]	-	-	96%	95%
Blood Culture Timing	15	93%	97%	98%
Pregnancy and Delivery Care				
Newborn Deliveries Scheduled Early[5]	-	-	2%	6%
Preventive Care				
Immunization for Influenza[1]	-	-	91%	90%
Immunization for Pneumonia[1,3]	-	-	91%	92%
Stroke Care				
Anticoagulation Therapy for Atrial Fibrillation[3,7]	-	-	94%	95%
Antithrombotic Therapy Timing[1,3]	-	-	98%	98%
Assessed for Rehabilitation[1,3]	-	-	98%	97%
Discharged on Antithrombotic Therapy[1,3]	-	-	99%	99%
Discharged on Statin Medication[1,3]	-	-	96%	94%
Thrombolytic Therapy Timing[3,7]	-	-	73%	66%
Venous Thromboembolism Prophylaxis[1,3]	-	-	94%	94%
Written Stroke Educational Materials Given[1,3]	-	-	86%	88%
Surgical Care Improvement Project				
Appropriate Beta Blocker Usage[1]	-	-	98%	98%
Appropriate VTP Within 24 Hours	29	100%	98%	98%
Controlled Postoperative Blood Glucose[3,7]	-	-	97%	97%
Perioperative Temperature Management	33	100%	100%	100%
Prophylactic Antibiotic Selection	28	96%	99%	99%
Prophylactic Antibiotic Selection (Outpatient)	-	-	98%	98%
Prophylactic Antibiotic Stopped	28	100%	99%	98%
Prophylactic Antibiotic Timing	28	100%	98%	99%
Prophylactic Antibiotic Timing (Outpatient)	-	-	98%	98%
Urinary Catheter Removal	14	100%	97%	97%
Survey of Patients' Hospital Experiences				
Area Around Room 'Always' Quiet at Night	(a)	54%	54%	61%
Doctors 'Always' Communicated Well	(a)	78%	81%	82%
Home Recovery Information Given	(a)	86%	87%	85%
Hospital Given 9 or 10 on 10 Point Scale	(a)	70%	70%	71%
Meds 'Always' Explained Before Given	(a)	63%	64%	64%
Nurses 'Always' Communicated Well	(a)	73%	77%	79%
Pain 'Always' Well Controlled	(a)	66%	70%	71%
Room and Bathroom 'Always' Clean	(a)	70%	73%	73%
Timely Help 'Always' Received	(a)	60%	65%	68%
Would Definitely Recommend Hospital	(a)	64%	73%	71%
Use of Medical Imaging				
Cardiac Imaging Stress Test before Surgery	-	-	4.3%	5.3%
Combination Abdominal CT Scan	-	-	6.9%	10.5%
Combination Brain/Sinus CT Scan	-	-	2.3%	2.7%
Combination Chest CT Scan	-	-	1.1%	2.7%
Follow-up Mammogram/Ultrasound	-	-	9.1%	8.8%
Lumbar Spine MRI for Low Back Pain	-	-	37.9%	37.2%

Pullman Regional Hospital

835 S Bishop Blvd
Pullman, WA 99163
Phone: 509-332-2541
Fax: 509-332-6767
E-mail: sadams@complete.bbs.com
URL: www.pullmanhospital.org
Type: Critical Access Hospitals
Emergency Services: Yes
Ownership: Govt - Hospital Dist/Auth
Beds: 25

Key Personnel:
Chief of Medical Staff. . . . . Stephen C Bergmann
Infection Control. . . . . Karen Cannon
Pediatric In-Patient Care . . . . Alvin Frosted, MD
Quality Assurance . . . . Dorcas Hirzel
Intensive Care Unit. . . . . Laurie Larsen
CEO/President. . . . . Joe Pitzer
Radiology. . . . . Roderick Saxey
Operating Room. . . . . John Visger

Measure	Cases	This Hosp.	State Avg.	U.S. Avg.
Blood Clot Prevention and Treatment				
Anticoagulation Overlap Therapy[5]	-	-	97%	93%
ICU Venous Thromboembolism Prophylaxis[5]	-	-	92%	92%
Incidence of Potentially Preventable VTE[5]	-	-	9%	10%
UFH with Dosages/Platelet Monitoring[5]	-	-	99%	97%
Venous Thromboembolism Prophylaxis[5]	-	-	86%	85%
Warfarin Therapy Discharge Instructions[5]	-	-	74%	75%
Chest Pain/Possible Heart Attack Care				
Aspirin Given Within 24 Hours of Arrival	-	-	97%	96%
Fibrinolytic Meds Within 30 Min. of Arrival	-	-	51%	58%
Average Time to ECG (minutes)	-	-	9	7
Average Time to Transfer (minutes)	-	-	54	60
Children's Asthma Care				
Received Home Management Plan of Care	-	-	-	88%
Received Reliever Medication	-	-	-	100%
Received Systemic Corticosteroids	-	-	-	100%
Emergency Department				
Admittance Decision Time (minutes)[5]	-	-	96	98
Head CT Results Within 45 Min. of Arrival	-	-	63%	57%
Patients Who Left ER Before Being Seen	-	-	2%	2%
Time from ER Arrival to Admit. (minutes)[5]	-	-	259	274
Time from ER Arrival to Discharge (minutes)	-	-	135	134
Time in ER Before Being Evaluated (minutes)	-	-	22	26
Time to Pain Meds for Fractures (minutes)	-	-	52	57
Heart Attack Care				
Aspirin Given at Discharge[5]	-	-	99%	99%
Fibrinolytic Meds Within 30 Min. of Arrival[5]	-	-	62%	54%
PCI Within 90 Minutes of Arrival[5]	-	-	97%	96%
Statin Prescribed at Discharge[5]	-	-	98%	98%
Heart Failure Care				
ACE Inhibitor or ARB for LVSD[5]	-	-	97%	97%
Discharge Instructions Given[5]	-	-	93%	94%
Evaluation of LVS Function[5]	-	-	99%	99%
Medicare Spending				
Medicare Spending per Patient (ratio)	-	-	0.91	0.98
Pneumonia Care				
Appropriate Initial Antibiotic Given	31	81%	96%	95%
Blood Culture Timing	34	97%	97%	98%
Pregnancy and Delivery Care				
Newborn Deliveries Scheduled Early[5]	-	-	2%	6%
Preventive Care				
Immunization for Influenza[5]	-	-	91%	90%
Immunization for Pneumonia[5]	-	-	91%	92%
Stroke Care				
Anticoagulation Therapy for Atrial Fibrillation[5]	-	-	94%	95%
Antithrombotic Therapy Timing[5]	-	-	98%	98%
Assessed for Rehabilitation[5]	-	-	98%	97%
Discharged on Antithrombotic Therapy[5]	-	-	99%	99%
Discharged on Statin Medication[5]	-	-	96%	94%
Thrombolytic Therapy Timing[5]	-	-	73%	66%
Venous Thromboembolism Prophylaxis[5]	-	-	94%	94%
Written Stroke Educational Materials Given[5]	-	-	86%	88%
Surgical Care Improvement Project				
Appropriate Beta Blocker Usage	21	100%	98%	98%
Appropriate VTP Within 24 Hours	177	97%	98%	98%
Controlled Postoperative Blood Glucose[7]	-	-	97%	97%
Perioperative Temperature Management	190	99%	100%	100%
Prophylactic Antibiotic Selection	141	96%	99%	99%
Prophylactic Antibiotic Selection (Outpatient)	-	-	98%	98%
Prophylactic Antibiotic Stopped	141	100%	99%	98%
Prophylactic Antibiotic Timing	141	99%	98%	99%
Prophylactic Antibiotic Timing (Outpatient)	-	-	98%	98%
Urinary Catheter Removal	115	99%	97%	97%
Survey of Patients' Hospital Experiences				
Area Around Room 'Always' Quiet at Night	300+	61%	54%	61%
Doctors 'Always' Communicated Well	300+	84%	81%	82%
Home Recovery Information Given	300+	91%	87%	85%
Hospital Given 9 or 10 on 10 Point Scale	300+	83%	70%	71%
Meds 'Always' Explained Before Given	300+	69%	64%	64%
Nurses 'Always' Communicated Well	300+	83%	77%	79%
Pain 'Always' Well Controlled	300+	77%	70%	71%
Room and Bathroom 'Always' Clean	300+	78%	73%	73%
Timely Help 'Always' Received	300+	79%	65%	68%
Would Definitely Recommend Hospital	300+	88%	73%	71%
Use of Medical Imaging				
Cardiac Imaging Stress Test before Surgery	-	-	4.3%	5.3%
Combination Abdominal CT Scan	-	-	6.9%	10.5%
Combination Brain/Sinus CT Scan	-	-	2.3%	2.7%
Combination Chest CT Scan	-	-	1.1%	2.7%
Follow-up Mammogram/Ultrasound	-	-	9.1%	8.8%
Lumbar Spine MRI for Low Back Pain	-	-	37.9%	37.2%

Multicare Good Samaritan Hospital

401 15th Avenue Se
Puyallup, WA 98372
Phone: 253-697-2102
URL: www.multicare.org/goodsam
Type: Acute Care Hospitals
Emergency Services: Yes
Ownership: Voluntary non-profit - Private

Key Personnel:
CEO/President. . . . . William G. Robertson

Measure	Cases	This Hosp.	State Avg.	U.S. Avg.
Blood Clot Prevention and Treatment				
Anticoagulation Overlap Therapy[2]	123	99%	97%	93%
ICU Venous Thromboembolism Prophylaxis[2]	32	94%	92%	92%
Incidence of Potentially Preventable VTE[2]	23	13%	9%	10%
UFH with Dosages/Platelet Monitoring[2]	98	100%	99%	97%
Venous Thromboembolism Prophylaxis[2]	383	87%	86%	85%
Warfarin Therapy Discharge Instructions[2]	100	96%	74%	75%
Chest Pain/Possible Heart Attack Care				
Aspirin Given Within 24 Hours of Arrival	22	95%	97%	96%
Fibrinolytic Meds Within 30 Min. of Arrival[3,7]	-	-	51%	58%
Average Time to ECG (minutes)	25	0	9	7
Average Time to Transfer (minutes)[3,7]	-	-	54	60
Children's Asthma Care				
Received Home Management Plan of Care	22	95%	-	88%

NOTE: Hospital profiles are in alphabetical order by state, then city, then hospital within the city; Rankings exclude hospitals with less than 25 cases except for patient surveys which excludes hospitals with less than 100 cases; (a) 100-299 cases; (1) The number of cases/patients is too few to report; (2) Data submitted were based on a sample of cases/patients; (3) Results are based on a shorter time period than required; (4) Data suppressed by CMS for one or more quarters; (5) Results are not available for this reporting period; (6) Fewer than 100 patients completed the HCAHPS survey; (7) No cases met the criteria for this measure; (8) The lower limit of the confidence interval cannot be calculated if the number of observed infections equals zero; (9) No data are available from the state/territory for this reporting period; (10) The scores shown reflect fewer than 50 completed surveys; (11) There were discrepancies in the data collection process; (12) This measure does not apply to this hospital for this reporting period; (13) Results cannot be calculated for this reporting period; (14) The results for this state are combined with nearby states to protect confidentiality; Please refer to the User's Guide for a full explanation of data.

Measure	Cases	This Hosp.	State Avg.	U.S. Avg.
Received Reliever Medication	22	100%	-	100%
Received Systemic Corticosteroids	22	100%	-	100%
Emergency Department				
Admittance Decision Time (minutes)[2]	712	118	96	98
Head CT Results Within 45 Min. of Arrival	11	91%	63%	57%
Patients Who Left ER Before Being Seen	68,228	1%	2%	2%
Time from ER Arrival to Admit. (minutes)[2]	749	300	259	274
Time from ER Arrival to Discharge (minutes)	382	185	135	134
Time in ER Before Being Evaluated (minutes)	94	62	22	26
Time to Pain Meds for Fractures (minutes)	231	92	52	57
Heart Attack Care				
Aspirin Given at Discharge	280	99%	99%	99%
Fibrinolytic Meds Within 30 Min. of Arrival[7]	-	-	62%	54%
PCI Within 90 Minutes of Arrival	70	100%	97%	96%
Statin Prescribed at Discharge	272	100%	98%	98%
Heart Failure Care				
ACE Inhibitor or ARB for LVSD[2]	103	100%	97%	97%
Discharge Instructions Given[2]	274	99%	93%	94%
Evaluation of LVS Function[2]	315	100%	99%	99%
Medicare Spending				
Medicare Spending per Patient (ratio)	-	0.92	0.91	0.98
Pneumonia Care				
Appropriate Initial Antibiotic Given[2]	114	96%	96%	95%
Blood Culture Timing[2]	171	98%	97%	98%
Pregnancy and Delivery Care				
Newborn Deliveries Scheduled Early	196	1%	2%	6%
Preventive Care				
Immunization for Influenza[2]	548	94%	91%	90%
Immunization for Pneumonia[2]	674	93%	91%	92%
Stroke Care				
Anticoagulation Therapy for Atrial Fibrillation[2]	32	100%	94%	95%
Antithrombotic Therapy Timing[2]	155	100%	98%	98%
Assessed for Rehabilitation[2]	192	98%	98%	97%
Discharged on Antithrombotic Therapy[2]	186	99%	99%	99%
Discharged on Statin Medication[2]	151	98%	96%	94%
Thrombolytic Therapy Timing[1,2]	-	-	73%	66%
Venous Thromboembolism Prophylaxis[2]	170	94%	94%	94%
Written Stroke Educational Materials Given[2]	133	98%	86%	88%
Surgical Care Improvement Project				
Appropriate Beta Blocker Usage[2]	89	97%	98%	98%
Appropriate VTP Within 24 Hours[2]	408	99%	98%	98%
Controlled Postoperative Blood Glucose[2,7]	-	-	97%	97%
Perioperative Temperature Management[2]	450	100%	100%	100%
Prophylactic Antibiotic Selection[2]	282	100%	99%	99%
Prophylactic Antibiotic Selection (Outpatient)	452	99%	98%	98%
Prophylactic Antibiotic Stopped[2]	278	99%	99%	98%
Prophylactic Antibiotic Timing[2]	283	99%	98%	99%
Prophylactic Antibiotic Timing (Outpatient)	454	99%	98%	98%
Urinary Catheter Removal[2]	283	98%	97%	97%
Survey of Patients' Hospital Experiences				
Area Around Room 'Always' Quiet at Night	300+	56%	54%	61%
Doctors 'Always' Communicated Well	300+	76%	81%	82%
Home Recovery Information Given	300+	87%	87%	85%
Hospital Given 9 or 10 on 10 Point Scale	300+	69%	70%	71%
Meds 'Always' Explained Before Given	300+	59%	64%	64%
Nurses 'Always' Communicated Well	300+	75%	77%	79%
Pain 'Always' Well Controlled	300+	67%	70%	71%
Room and Bathroom 'Always' Clean	300+	72%	73%	73%
Timely Help 'Always' Received	300+	59%	65%	68%
Would Definitely Recommend Hospital	300+	70%	73%	71%
Use of Medical Imaging				
Cardiac Imaging Stress Test before Surgery	196	8.7%	4.3%	5.3%
Combination Abdominal CT Scan	642	1.6%	6.9%	10.5%
Combination Brain/Sinus CT Scan	700	2.6%	2.3%	2.7%
Combination Chest CT Scan	113	1.8%	1.1%	2.7%
Follow-up Mammogram/Ultrasound[7]	-	-	9.1%	8.8%
Lumbar Spine MRI for Low Back Pain[1]	-	-	37.9%	37.2%

Quincy Valley Hospital

908 10th Avenue Southwest — Phone: 509-787-3531
Quincy, WA 98848
Type: Critical Access Hospitals — Emergency Services: Yes
Ownership: Govt - Hospital Dist/Auth

Measure	Cases	This Hosp.	State Avg.	U.S. Avg.
Blood Clot Prevention and Treatment				
Anticoagulation Overlap Therapy[3,7]	-	-	97%	93%
ICU Venous Thromboembolism Prophylaxis[3,7]	-	-	92%	92%
Incidence of Potentially Preventable VTE[3,7]	-	-	9%	10%
UFH with Dosages/Platelet Monitoring[3,7]	-	-	99%	97%
Venous Thromboembolism Prophylaxis[3,7]	-	-	86%	85%
Warfarin Therapy Discharge Instructions[3,7]	-	-	74%	75%
Chest Pain/Possible Heart Attack Care				
Aspirin Given Within 24 Hours of Arrival[1]	-	-	97%	96%
Fibrinolytic Meds Within 30 Min. of Arrival[1,3]	-	-	51%	58%
Average Time to ECG (minutes)[1]	-	-	9	7
Average Time to Transfer (minutes)[3,7]	-	-	54	60
Children's Asthma Care				
Received Home Management Plan of Care	-	-	-	88%
Received Reliever Medication	-	-	-	100%
Received Systemic Corticosteroids	-	-	-	100%
Emergency Department				
Admittance Decision Time (minutes)[5]	-	-	96	98
Head CT Results Within 45 Min. of Arrival[3,7]	-	-	63%	57%
Patients Who Left ER Before Being Seen[5]	-	-	2%	2%
Time from ER Arrival to Admit. (minutes)[5]	-	-	259	274
Time from ER Arrival to Discharge (minutes)[5]	-	-	135	134
Time in ER Before Being Evaluated (minutes)[5]	-	-	22	26
Time to Pain Meds for Fractures (minutes)[3]	24	42	52	57
Heart Attack Care				
Aspirin Given at Discharge[5]	-	-	99%	99%
Fibrinolytic Meds Within 30 Min. of Arrival[5]	-	-	62%	54%
PCI Within 90 Minutes of Arrival[5]	-	-	97%	96%
Statin Prescribed at Discharge[5]	-	-	98%	98%
Heart Failure Care				
ACE Inhibitor or ARB for LVSD[3,7]	-	-	97%	97%
Discharge Instructions Given[1,3]	-	-	93%	94%
Evaluation of LVS Function[1,3]	-	-	99%	99%
Medicare Spending				
Medicare Spending per Patient (ratio)	-	-	0.91	0.98
Pneumonia Care				
Appropriate Initial Antibiotic Given[1]	-	-	96%	95%
Blood Culture Timing[1]	-	-	97%	98%
Pregnancy and Delivery Care				
Newborn Deliveries Scheduled Early[5]	-	-	2%	6%
Preventive Care				
Immunization for Influenza[3]	14	79%	91%	90%
Immunization for Pneumonia[3]	11	64%	91%	92%
Stroke Care				
Anticoagulation Therapy for Atrial Fibrillation[5]	-	-	94%	95%
Antithrombotic Therapy Timing[5]	-	-	98%	98%
Assessed for Rehabilitation[5]	-	-	98%	97%
Discharged on Antithrombotic Therapy[5]	-	-	99%	99%
Discharged on Statin Medication[5]	-	-	96%	94%
Thrombolytic Therapy Timing[5]	-	-	73%	66%
Venous Thromboembolism Prophylaxis[5]	-	-	94%	94%
Written Stroke Educational Materials Given[5]	-	-	86%	88%
Surgical Care Improvement Project				
Appropriate Beta Blocker Usage[5]	-	-	98%	98%
Appropriate VTP Within 24 Hours[5]	-	-	98%	98%
Controlled Postoperative Blood Glucose[5]	-	-	97%	97%
Perioperative Temperature Management[5]	-	-	100%	100%
Prophylactic Antibiotic Selection[5]	-	-	99%	99%
Prophylactic Antibiotic Selection (Outpatient)[5]	-	-	98%	98%
Prophylactic Antibiotic Stopped[5]	-	-	99%	98%
Prophylactic Antibiotic Timing[5]	-	-	98%	99%
Prophylactic Antibiotic Timing (Outpatient)[5]	-	-	98%	98%
Urinary Catheter Removal[5]	-	-	97%	97%
Survey of Patients' Hospital Experiences				
Area Around Room 'Always' Quiet at Night[5]	-	-	54%	61%
Doctors 'Always' Communicated Well[5]	-	-	81%	82%
Home Recovery Information Given[5]	-	-	87%	85%
Hospital Given 9 or 10 on 10 Point Scale[5]	-	-	70%	71%
Meds 'Always' Explained Before Given[5]	-	-	64%	64%
Nurses 'Always' Communicated Well[5]	-	-	77%	79%
Pain 'Always' Well Controlled[5]	-	-	70%	71%
Room and Bathroom 'Always' Clean[5]	-	-	73%	73%
Timely Help 'Always' Received[5]	-	-	65%	68%
Would Definitely Recommend Hospital[5]	-	-	73%	71%
Use of Medical Imaging				
Cardiac Imaging Stress Test before Surgery[7]	-	-	4.3%	5.3%
Combination Abdominal CT Scan[1]	-	-	6.9%	10.5%
Combination Brain/Sinus CT Scan[1]	-	-	2.3%	2.7%
Combination Chest CT Scan[1]	-	-	1.1%	2.7%
Follow-up Mammogram/Ultrasound[7]	-	-	9.1%	8.8%
Lumbar Spine MRI for Low Back Pain[1]	-	-	37.9%	37.2%

Valley Medical Center

400 S 43rd St — Phone: 425-228-3450
Renton, WA 98055 — Fax: 425-656-4202
URL: www.valleymed.org
Type: Acute Care Hospitals — Emergency Services: Yes
Ownership: Govt - Hospital Dist/Auth — Beds: 303

Key Personnel:
Patient Relations . . . . Helen Adams, RN
Emergency Room . . . . Kayett Asuquo, RN
Chair/CEO . . . . Lisa Jenson
Quality Assurance . . . . Elaine Lobdell, RN
Chief of Medical Staff . . . . Tori McFall, MD
Radiology. . . . . Marcus Neeley
CEO/President. . . . . Richard D Roodman
Intensive Care Unit. . . . . Mary Van Hoomissen

Measure	Cases	This Hosp.	State Avg.	U.S. Avg.
Blood Clot Prevention and Treatment				
Anticoagulation Overlap Therapy[2]	104	99%	97%	93%
ICU Venous Thromboembolism Prophylaxis[2]	51	90%	92%	92%
Incidence of Potentially Preventable VTE[1,2]	-	-	9%	10%
UFH with Dosages/Platelet Monitoring[2]	49	100%	99%	97%
Venous Thromboembolism Prophylaxis[2]	292	89%	86%	85%
Warfarin Therapy Discharge Instructions[2]	83	87%	74%	75%
Chest Pain/Possible Heart Attack Care				
Aspirin Given Within 24 Hours of Arrival[1,3]	-	-	97%	96%
Fibrinolytic Meds Within 30 Min. of Arrival[5]	-	-	51%	58%
Average Time to ECG (minutes)[1,3]	-	-	9	7
Average Time to Transfer (minutes)[5]	-	-	54	60
Children's Asthma Care				
Received Home Management Plan of Care	-	-	-	88%
Received Reliever Medication	-	-	-	100%
Received Systemic Corticosteroids	-	-	-	100%
Emergency Department				
Admittance Decision Time (minutes)[2]	501	93	96	98
Head CT Results Within 45 Min. of Arrival	17	59%	63%	57%
Patients Who Left ER Before Being Seen	76,771	1%	2%	2%
Time from ER Arrival to Admit. (minutes)[2]	501	303	259	274
Time from ER Arrival to Discharge (minutes)	360	156	135	134
Time in ER Before Being Evaluated (minutes)	363	23	22	26
Time to Pain Meds for Fractures (minutes)	212	54	52	57
Heart Attack Care				
Aspirin Given at Discharge	249	99%	99%	99%
Fibrinolytic Meds Within 30 Min. of Arrival[7]	-	-	62%	54%
PCI Within 90 Minutes of Arrival	55	96%	97%	96%
Statin Prescribed at Discharge	242	98%	98%	98%
Heart Failure Care				
ACE Inhibitor or ARB for LVSD[2]	106	100%	97%	97%
Discharge Instructions Given[2]	225	87%	93%	94%
Evaluation of LVS Function[2]	283	99%	99%	99%
Medicare Spending				
Medicare Spending per Patient (ratio)	-	0.95	0.91	0.98
Pneumonia Care				
Appropriate Initial Antibiotic Given[2]	98	100%	96%	95%
Blood Culture Timing[2]	146	97%	97%	98%
Pregnancy and Delivery Care				
Newborn Deliveries Scheduled Early	382	2%	2%	6%
Preventive Care				
Immunization for Influenza[2]	470	62%	91%	90%

NOTE: Hospital profiles are in alphabetical order by state, then city, then hospital within the city; Rankings exclude hospitals with less than 25 cases except for patient surveys which excludes hospitals with less than 100 cases; (a) 100-299 cases; (1) The number of cases/patients is too few to report; (2) Data submitted were based on a sample of cases/patients; (3) Results are based on a shorter time period than required; (4) Data suppressed by CMS for one or more quarters; (5) Results are not available for this reporting period; (6) Fewer than 100 patients completed the HCAHPS survey; (7) No cases met the criteria for this measure; (8) The lower limit of the confidence interval cannot be calculated if the number of observed infections equals zero; (9) No data are available from the state/territory for this reporting period; (10) The scores shown reflect fewer than 50 completed surveys; (11) There were discrepancies in the data collection process; (12) This measure does not apply to this hospital for this reporting period; (13) Results cannot be calculated for this reporting period; (14) The results for this state are combined with nearby states to protect confidentiality; Please refer to the User's Guide for a full explanation of data.

Immunization for Pneumonia[2]	460	75%	91%	92%
Stroke Care				
Anticoagulation Therapy for Atrial Fibrillation[2]	15	93%	94%	95%
Antithrombotic Therapy Timing[2]	75	99%	98%	98%
Assessed for Rehabilitation[2]	96	99%	98%	97%
Discharged on Antithrombotic Therapy[2]	85	100%	99%	99%
Discharged on Statin Medication[2]	68	100%	96%	94%
Thrombolytic Therapy Timing[2]	16	81%	73%	66%
Venous Thromboembolism Prophylaxis[2]	105	93%	94%	94%
Written Stroke Educational Materials Given[2]	64	89%	86%	88%
Surgical Care Improvement Project				
Appropriate Beta Blocker Usage[2]	73	97%	98%	98%
Appropriate VTP Within 24 Hours[2]	281	99%	98%	98%
Controlled Postoperative Blood Glucose[2,7]	-	-	97%	97%
Perioperative Temperature Management[2]	376	100%	100%	100%
Prophylactic Antibiotic Selection[2]	275	97%	99%	99%
Prophylactic Antibiotic Selection (Outpatient)	334	99%	98%	98%
Prophylactic Antibiotic Stopped[2]	273	100%	99%	98%
Prophylactic Antibiotic Timing[2]	275	98%	98%	99%
Prophylactic Antibiotic Timing (Outpatient)	338	97%	98%	98%
Urinary Catheter Removal[2]	231	98%	97%	97%
Survey of Patients' Hospital Experiences				
Area Around Room 'Always' Quiet at Night	300+	55%	54%	61%
Doctors 'Always' Communicated Well	300+	79%	81%	82%
Home Recovery Information Given	300+	86%	87%	85%
Hospital Given 9 or 10 on 10 Point Scale	300+	71%	70%	71%
Meds 'Always' Explained Before Given	300+	62%	64%	64%
Nurses 'Always' Communicated Well	300+	73%	77%	79%
Pain 'Always' Well Controlled	300+	67%	70%	71%
Room and Bathroom 'Always' Clean	300+	69%	73%	73%
Timely Help 'Always' Received	300+	60%	65%	68%
Would Definitely Recommend Hospital	300+	73%	73%	71%
Use of Medical Imaging				
Cardiac Imaging Stress Test before Surgery	53	3.8%	4.3%	5.3%
Combination Abdominal CT Scan	806	1.6%	6.9%	10.5%
Combination Brain/Sinus CT Scan	895	1.7%	2.3%	2.7%
Combination Chest CT Scan	350	0.3%	1.1%	2.7%
Follow-up Mammogram/Ultrasound	2,524	7.8%	9.1%	8.8%
Lumbar Spine MRI for Low Back Pain	38	50.0%	37.9%	37.2%

Ferry County Memorial Hospital

36 Klondike Road — Phone: 509-775-3333
Republic, WA 99166
Type: Critical Access Hospitals — Emergency Services: Yes
Ownership: Govt - Hospital Dist/Auth

Measure	Cases	This Hosp.	State Avg.	U.S. Avg.
Blood Clot Prevention and Treatment				
Anticoagulation Overlap Therapy[5]	-	-	97%	93%
ICU Venous Thromboembolism Prophylaxis[5]	-	-	92%	92%
Incidence of Potentially Preventable VTE[5]	-	-	9%	10%
UFH with Dosages/Platelet Monitoring[5]	-	-	99%	97%
Venous Thromboembolism Prophylaxis[5]	-	-	86%	85%
Warfarin Therapy Discharge Instructions[5]	-	-	74%	75%
Chest Pain/Possible Heart Attack Care				
Aspirin Given Within 24 Hours of Arrival[1,3]	-	-	97%	96%
Fibrinolytic Meds Within 30 Min. of Arrival[5]	-	-	51%	58%
Average Time to ECG (minutes)[1,3]	-	-	9	7
Average Time to Transfer (minutes)[5]	-	-	54	60
Children's Asthma Care				
Received Home Management Plan of Care	-	-	-	88%
Received Reliever Medication	-	-	-	100%
Received Systemic Corticosteroids	-	-	-	100%
Emergency Department				
Admittance Decision Time (minutes)[5]	-	-	96	98
Head CT Results Within 45 Min. of Arrival[5]	-	-	63%	57%
Patients Who Left ER Before Being Seen[5]	-	-	2%	2%
Time from ER Arrival to Admit. (minutes)[5]	-	-	259	274
Time from ER Arrival to Discharge (minutes)[5]	-	-	135	134
Time in ER Before Being Evaluated (minutes)[5]	-	-	22	26
Time to Pain Meds for Fractures (minutes)[5]	-	-	52	57
Heart Attack Care				
Aspirin Given at Discharge[5]	-	-	99%	99%
Fibrinolytic Meds Within 30 Min. of Arrival[5]	-	-	62%	54%
PCI Within 90 Minutes of Arrival[5]	-	-	97%	96%
Statin Prescribed at Discharge[5]	-	-	98%	98%
Heart Failure Care				
ACE Inhibitor or ARB for LVSD[3,7]	-	-	97%	97%
Discharge Instructions Given[3,7]	-	-	93%	94%
Evaluation of LVS Function[1,3]	-	-	99%	99%
Medicare Spending				
Medicare Spending per Patient (ratio)	-	-	0.91	0.98
Pneumonia Care				
Appropriate Initial Antibiotic Given	11	82%	96%	95%
Blood Culture Timing[1]	-	-	97%	98%
Pregnancy and Delivery Care				
Newborn Deliveries Scheduled Early[5]	-	-	2%	6%
Preventive Care				
Immunization for Influenza[5]	-	-	91%	90%
Immunization for Pneumonia[5]	-	-	91%	92%
Stroke Care				
Anticoagulation Therapy for Atrial Fibrillation[5]	-	-	94%	95%
Antithrombotic Therapy Timing[5]	-	-	98%	98%
Assessed for Rehabilitation[5]	-	-	98%	97%
Discharged on Antithrombotic Therapy[5]	-	-	99%	99%
Discharged on Statin Medication[5]	-	-	96%	94%
Thrombolytic Therapy Timing[5]	-	-	73%	66%
Venous Thromboembolism Prophylaxis[5]	-	-	94%	94%
Written Stroke Educational Materials Given[5]	-	-	86%	88%
Surgical Care Improvement Project				
Appropriate Beta Blocker Usage[5]	-	-	98%	98%
Appropriate VTP Within 24 Hours[5]	-	-	98%	98%
Controlled Postoperative Blood Glucose[5]	-	-	97%	97%
Perioperative Temperature Management[5]	-	-	100%	100%
Prophylactic Antibiotic Selection[5]	-	-	99%	99%
Prophylactic Antibiotic Selection (Outpatient)[5]	-	-	98%	98%
Prophylactic Antibiotic Stopped[5]	-	-	99%	98%
Prophylactic Antibiotic Timing[5]	-	-	98%	99%
Prophylactic Antibiotic Timing (Outpatient)[5]	-	-	98%	98%
Urinary Catheter Removal[5]	-	-	97%	97%
Survey of Patients' Hospital Experiences				
Area Around Room 'Always' Quiet at Night[5]	-	-	54%	61%
Doctors 'Always' Communicated Well[5]	-	-	81%	82%
Home Recovery Information Given[5]	-	-	87%	85%
Hospital Given 9 or 10 on 10 Point Scale[5]	-	-	70%	71%
Meds 'Always' Explained Before Given[5]	-	-	64%	64%
Nurses 'Always' Communicated Well[5]	-	-	77%	79%
Pain 'Always' Well Controlled[5]	-	-	70%	71%
Room and Bathroom 'Always' Clean[5]	-	-	73%	73%
Timely Help 'Always' Received[5]	-	-	65%	68%
Would Definitely Recommend Hospital[5]	-	-	73%	71%
Use of Medical Imaging				
Cardiac Imaging Stress Test before Surgery[7]	-	-	4.3%	5.3%
Combination Abdominal CT Scan	51	2.0%	6.9%	10.5%
Combination Brain/Sinus CT Scan	35	0.0%	2.3%	2.7%
Combination Chest CT Scan[1]	-	-	1.1%	2.7%
Follow-up Mammogram/Ultrasound[7]	-	-	9.1%	8.8%
Lumbar Spine MRI for Low Back Pain[1]	-	-	37.9%	37.2%

Kadlec Regional Medical Center

888 Swift Blvd — Phone: 509-946-4611
Richland, WA 99352 — Fax: 509-942-2634
URL: www.kadlecmed.org
Type: Acute Care Hospitals — Emergency Services: Yes
Ownership: Voluntary non-profit - Private — Beds: 168

Key Personnel:
Emergency Room .... Jeffrey Allgaier
Chief of Medical Staff .... Fredrick Bowers, MD
Radiology .... Dwane Brittain, Jr
CEO/President .... Julie Meek
Cardiac Laboratory .... Brent O'Brian

Measure	Cases	This Hosp.	State Avg.	U.S. Avg.
Blood Clot Prevention and Treatment				
Anticoagulation Overlap Therapy[2]	117	99%	97%	93%
ICU Venous Thromboembolism Prophylaxis[2]	101	80%	92%	92%
Incidence of Potentially Preventable VTE[2]	13	0%	9%	10%
UFH with Dosages/Platelet Monitoring[2]	90	100%	99%	97%
Venous Thromboembolism Prophylaxis[2]	414	94%	86%	85%
Warfarin Therapy Discharge Instructions[2]	106	100%	74%	75%
Chest Pain/Possible Heart Attack Care				
Aspirin Given Within 24 Hours of Arrival[1,3]	-	-	97%	96%
Fibrinolytic Meds Within 30 Min. of Arrival[3,7]	-	-	51%	58%
Average Time to ECG (minutes)[1,3]	-	-	9	7
Average Time to Transfer (minutes)[3,7]	-	-	54	60
Children's Asthma Care				
Received Home Management Plan of Care	-	-	-	88%
Received Reliever Medication	-	-	-	100%
Received Systemic Corticosteroids	-	-	-	100%
Emergency Department				
Admittance Decision Time (minutes)[2]	421	142	96	98
Head CT Results Within 45 Min. of Arrival[1]	-	-	63%	57%
Patients Who Left ER Before Being Seen	59,572	1%	2%	2%
Time from ER Arrival to Admit. (minutes)[2]	437	291	259	274
Time from ER Arrival to Discharge (minutes)	365	133	135	134
Time in ER Before Being Evaluated (minutes)	343	22	22	26
Time to Pain Meds for Fractures (minutes)	273	43	52	57
Heart Attack Care				
Aspirin Given at Discharge	412	99%	99%	99%
Fibrinolytic Meds Within 30 Min. of Arrival[7]	-	-	62%	54%
PCI Within 90 Minutes of Arrival	60	100%	97%	96%
Statin Prescribed at Discharge	393	99%	98%	98%
Heart Failure Care				
ACE Inhibitor or ARB for LVSD	88	99%	97%	97%
Discharge Instructions Given	246	99%	93%	94%
Evaluation of LVS Function	300	100%	99%	99%
Medicare Spending				
Medicare Spending per Patient (ratio)	-	0.98	0.91	0.98
Pneumonia Care				
Appropriate Initial Antibiotic Given[2]	79	100%	96%	95%
Blood Culture Timing[2]	168	99%	97%	98%
Pregnancy and Delivery Care				
Newborn Deliveries Scheduled Early[2]	91	4%	2%	6%
Preventive Care				
Immunization for Influenza[2]	504	99%	91%	90%
Immunization for Pneumonia[2]	566	99%	91%	92%
Stroke Care				
Anticoagulation Therapy for Atrial Fibrillation	22	100%	94%	95%
Antithrombotic Therapy Timing	157	97%	98%	98%
Assessed for Rehabilitation	213	99%	98%	97%
Discharged on Antithrombotic Therapy	178	100%	99%	99%
Discharged on Statin Medication	135	99%	96%	94%
Thrombolytic Therapy Timing[1]	-	-	73%	66%
Venous Thromboembolism Prophylaxis	212	99%	94%	94%
Written Stroke Educational Materials Given	116	100%	86%	88%
Surgical Care Improvement Project				
Appropriate Beta Blocker Usage[2]	206	100%	98%	98%
Appropriate VTP Within 24 Hours[2]	438	97%	98%	98%
Controlled Postoperative Blood Glucose[2]	148	99%	97%	97%
Perioperative Temperature Management[2]	590	100%	100%	100%
Prophylactic Antibiotic Selection[2]	578	98%	99%	99%
Prophylactic Antibiotic Selection (Outpatient)	582	99%	98%	98%
Prophylactic Antibiotic Stopped[2]	556	97%	99%	98%
Prophylactic Antibiotic Timing[2]	579	99%	98%	99%
Prophylactic Antibiotic Timing (Outpatient)	585	98%	98%	98%
Urinary Catheter Removal[2]	480	95%	97%	97%
Survey of Patients' Hospital Experiences				
Area Around Room 'Always' Quiet at Night[11]	300+	62%	54%	61%
Doctors 'Always' Communicated Well[11]	300+	79%	81%	82%
Home Recovery Information Given[11]	300+	87%	87%	85%
Hospital Given 9 or 10 on 10 Point Scale[11]	300+	71%	70%	71%
Meds 'Always' Explained Before Given[11]	300+	64%	64%	64%
Nurses 'Always' Communicated Well[11]	300+	79%	77%	79%
Pain 'Always' Well Controlled[11]	300+	66%	70%	71%
Room and Bathroom 'Always' Clean[11]	300+	75%	73%	73%
Timely Help 'Always' Received[11]	300+	64%	65%	68%
Would Definitely Recommend Hospital[11]	300+	81%	73%	71%
Use of Medical Imaging				
Cardiac Imaging Stress Test before Surgery	531	4.3%	4.3%	5.3%

NOTE: Hospital profiles are in alphabetical order by state, then city, then hospital within the city; Rankings exclude hospitals with less than 25 cases except for patient surveys which excludes hospitals with less than 100 cases; (a) 100-299 cases; (1) The number of cases/patients is too few to report; (2) Data submitted were based on a sample of cases/patients; (3) Results are based on a shorter time period than required; (4) Data suppressed by CMS for one or more quarters; (5) Results are not available for this reporting period; (6) Fewer than 100 patients completed the HCAHPS survey; (7) No cases met the criteria for this measure; (8) The lower limit of the confidence interval cannot be calculated if the number of observed infections equals zero; (9) No data are available from the state/territory for this reporting period; (10) The scores shown reflect fewer than 50 completed surveys; (11) There were discrepancies in the data collection process; (12) This measure does not apply to this hospital for this reporting period; (13) Results cannot be calculated for this reporting period; (14) The results for this state are combined with nearby states to protect confidentiality; Please refer to the User's Guide for a full explanation of data.

Measure	Cases	This Hosp.	State Avg.	U.S. Avg.
Combination Abdominal CT Scan	1,318	9.1%	6.9%	10.5%
Combination Brain/Sinus CT Scan	1,036	1.4%	2.3%	2.7%
Combination Chest CT Scan	1,047	1.3%	1.1%	2.7%
Follow-up Mammogram/Ultrasound	2,557	9.3%	9.1%	8.8%
Lumbar Spine MRI for Low Back Pain	319	31.3%	37.9%	37.2%

East Adams Rural Hospital

903 South Adams — Phone: 509-659-1200
Ritzville, WA 99169
Type: Critical Access Hospitals — Emergency Services: Yes
Ownership: Govt - Hospital Dist/Auth

Measure	Cases	This Hosp.	State Avg.	U.S. Avg.
Blood Clot Prevention and Treatment				
Anticoagulation Overlap Therapy[5]	-	-	97%	93%
ICU Venous Thromboembolism Prophylaxis[5]	-	-	92%	92%
Incidence of Potentially Preventable VTE[5]	-	-	9%	10%
UFH with Dosages/Platelet Monitoring[5]	-	-	99%	97%
Venous Thromboembolism Prophylaxis[5]	-	-	86%	85%
Warfarin Therapy Discharge Instructions[5]	-	-	74%	75%
Chest Pain/Possible Heart Attack Care				
Aspirin Given Within 24 Hours of Arrival[5]	-	-	97%	96%
Fibrinolytic Meds Within 30 Min. of Arrival[5]	-	-	51%	58%
Average Time to ECG (minutes)[5]	-	-	9	7
Average Time to Transfer (minutes)[5]	-	-	54	60
Children's Asthma Care				
Received Home Management Plan of Care	-	-	-	88%
Received Reliever Medication	-	-	-	100%
Received Systemic Corticosteroids	-	-	-	100%
Emergency Department				
Admittance Decision Time (minutes)[5]	-	-	96	98
Head CT Results Within 45 Min. of Arrival[5]	-	-	63%	57%
Patients Who Left ER Before Being Seen[5]	-	-	2%	2%
Time from ER Arrival to Admit. (minutes)[5]	-	-	259	274
Time from ER Arrival to Discharge (minutes)[5]	-	-	135	134
Time in ER Before Being Evaluated (minutes)[5]	-	-	22	26
Time to Pain Meds for Fractures (minutes)[5]	-	-	52	57
Heart Attack Care				
Aspirin Given at Discharge[5]	-	-	99%	99%
Fibrinolytic Meds Within 30 Min. of Arrival[5]	-	-	62%	54%
PCI Within 90 Minutes of Arrival[5]	-	-	97%	96%
Statin Prescribed at Discharge[5]	-	-	98%	98%
Heart Failure Care				
ACE Inhibitor or ARB for LVSD[5]	-	-	97%	97%
Discharge Instructions Given[5]	-	-	93%	94%
Evaluation of LVS Function[5]	-	-	99%	99%
Medicare Spending				
Medicare Spending per Patient (ratio)	-	-	0.91	0.98
Pneumonia Care				
Appropriate Initial Antibiotic Given[1,3]	-	-	96%	95%
Blood Culture Timing[1,3]	-	-	97%	98%
Pregnancy and Delivery Care				
Newborn Deliveries Scheduled Early[5]	-	-	2%	6%
Preventive Care				
Immunization for Influenza[5]	-	-	91%	90%
Immunization for Pneumonia[5]	-	-	91%	92%
Stroke Care				
Anticoagulation Therapy for Atrial Fibrillation[5]	-	-	94%	95%
Antithrombotic Therapy Timing[5]	-	-	98%	98%
Assessed for Rehabilitation[5]	-	-	98%	97%
Discharged on Antithrombotic Therapy[5]	-	-	99%	99%
Discharged on Statin Medication[5]	-	-	96%	94%
Thrombolytic Therapy Timing[5]	-	-	73%	66%
Venous Thromboembolism Prophylaxis[5]	-	-	94%	94%
Written Stroke Educational Materials Given[5]	-	-	86%	88%
Surgical Care Improvement Project				
Appropriate Beta Blocker Usage[5]	-	-	98%	98%
Appropriate VTP Within 24 Hours[5]	-	-	98%	98%
Controlled Postoperative Blood Glucose[5]	-	-	97%	97%
Perioperative Temperature Management[5]	-	-	100%	100%
Prophylactic Antibiotic Selection[5]	-	-	99%	99%
Prophylactic Antibiotic Selection (Outpatient)[5]	-	-	98%	98%
Prophylactic Antibiotic Stopped[5]	-	-	99%	98%
Prophylactic Antibiotic Timing[5]	-	-	98%	99%
Prophylactic Antibiotic Timing (Outpatient)[5]	-	-	98%	98%
Urinary Catheter Removal[5]	-	-	97%	97%
Survey of Patients' Hospital Experiences				
Area Around Room 'Always' Quiet at Night[5]	-	-	54%	61%
Doctors 'Always' Communicated Well[5]	-	-	81%	82%
Home Recovery Information Given[5]	-	-	87%	85%
Hospital Given 9 or 10 on 10 Point Scale[5]	-	-	70%	71%
Meds 'Always' Explained Before Given[5]	-	-	64%	64%
Nurses 'Always' Communicated Well[5]	-	-	77%	79%
Pain 'Always' Well Controlled[5]	-	-	70%	71%
Room and Bathroom 'Always' Clean[5]	-	-	73%	73%
Timely Help 'Always' Received[5]	-	-	65%	68%
Would Definitely Recommend Hospital[5]	-	-	73%	71%
Use of Medical Imaging				
Cardiac Imaging Stress Test before Surgery[7]	-	-	4.3%	5.3%
Combination Abdominal CT Scan[1]	-	-	6.9%	10.5%
Combination Brain/Sinus CT Scan[1]	-	-	2.3%	2.7%
Combination Chest CT Scan[1]	-	-	1.1%	2.7%
Follow-up Mammogram/Ultrasound[7]	-	-	9.1%	8.8%
Lumbar Spine MRI for Low Back Pain[1]	-	-	37.9%	37.2%

Group Health Central Hospital

201 - 16th Avenue East — Phone: 206-326-3000
Seattle, WA 98112 — Fax: 206-326-3436
URL: www.ghc.org
Type: Acute Care Hospitals — Emergency Services: Yes
Ownership: Voluntary non-profit - Other — Beds: 326

Key Personnel:
CEO/President . . . . Scott E Armstrong
Chair/CEO . . . . Porsche Everson
Quality Assurance . . . . James Hereford
Chief of Medical Staff . . . . Stephen Tarnoff, MD

Measure	Cases	This Hosp.	State Avg.	U.S. Avg.
Blood Clot Prevention and Treatment				
Anticoagulation Overlap Therapy[7]	-	-	97%	93%
ICU Venous Thromboembolism Prophylaxis[7]	-	-	92%	92%
Incidence of Potentially Preventable VTE[1]	-	-	9%	10%
UFH with Dosages/Platelet Monitoring[7]	-	-	99%	97%
Venous Thromboembolism Prophylaxis[1]	-	-	86%	85%
Warfarin Therapy Discharge Instructions[7]	-	-	74%	75%
Chest Pain/Possible Heart Attack Care				
Aspirin Given Within 24 Hours of Arrival[5]	-	-	97%	96%
Fibrinolytic Meds Within 30 Min. of Arrival[5]	-	-	51%	58%
Average Time to ECG (minutes)[5]	-	-	9	7
Average Time to Transfer (minutes)[5]	-	-	54	60
Children's Asthma Care				
Received Home Management Plan of Care	-	-	-	88%
Received Reliever Medication	-	-	-	100%
Received Systemic Corticosteroids	-	-	-	100%
Emergency Department				
Admittance Decision Time (minutes)[2,7]	-	-	96	98
Head CT Results Within 45 Min. of Arrival[5]	-	-	63%	57%
Patients Who Left ER Before Being Seen[5]	-	-	2%	2%
Time from ER Arrival to Admit. (minutes)[2,7]	-	-	259	274
Time from ER Arrival to Discharge (minutes)[5]	-	-	135	134
Time in ER Before Being Evaluated (minutes)[5]	-	-	22	26
Time to Pain Meds for Fractures (minutes)[5]	-	-	52	57
Heart Attack Care				
Aspirin Given at Discharge[5]	-	-	99%	99%
Fibrinolytic Meds Within 30 Min. of Arrival[5]	-	-	62%	54%
PCI Within 90 Minutes of Arrival[5]	-	-	97%	96%
Statin Prescribed at Discharge[5]	-	-	98%	98%
Heart Failure Care				
ACE Inhibitor or ARB for LVSD[5]	-	-	97%	97%
Discharge Instructions Given[5]	-	-	93%	94%
Evaluation of LVS Function[5]	-	-	99%	99%
Medicare Spending				
Medicare Spending per Patient (ratio)[1]	-	-	0.91	0.98
Pneumonia Care				
Appropriate Initial Antibiotic Given[5]	-	-	96%	95%
Blood Culture Timing[5]	-	-	97%	98%
Pregnancy and Delivery Care				
Newborn Deliveries Scheduled Early[2]	27	0%	2%	6%
Preventive Care				
Immunization for Influenza[2]	313	84%	91%	90%
Immunization for Pneumonia[2]	26	31%	91%	92%
Stroke Care				
Anticoagulation Therapy for Atrial Fibrillation[5]	-	-	94%	95%
Antithrombotic Therapy Timing[5]	-	-	98%	98%
Assessed for Rehabilitation[5]	-	-	98%	97%
Discharged on Antithrombotic Therapy[5]	-	-	99%	99%
Discharged on Statin Medication[5]	-	-	96%	94%
Thrombolytic Therapy Timing[5]	-	-	73%	66%
Venous Thromboembolism Prophylaxis[5]	-	-	94%	94%
Written Stroke Educational Materials Given[5]	-	-	86%	88%
Surgical Care Improvement Project				
Appropriate Beta Blocker Usage[5]	-	-	98%	98%
Appropriate VTP Within 24 Hours[5]	-	-	98%	98%
Controlled Postoperative Blood Glucose[5]	-	-	97%	97%
Perioperative Temperature Management[5]	-	-	100%	100%
Prophylactic Antibiotic Selection[5]	-	-	99%	99%
Prophylactic Antibiotic Selection (Outpatient)	126	98%	98%	98%
Prophylactic Antibiotic Stopped[5]	-	-	99%	98%
Prophylactic Antibiotic Timing[5]	-	-	98%	99%
Prophylactic Antibiotic Timing (Outpatient)	127	94%	98%	98%
Urinary Catheter Removal[5]	-	-	97%	97%
Survey of Patients' Hospital Experiences				
Area Around Room 'Always' Quiet at Night	300+	66%	54%	61%
Doctors 'Always' Communicated Well	300+	79%	81%	82%
Home Recovery Information Given	300+	89%	87%	85%
Hospital Given 9 or 10 on 10 Point Scale	300+	68%	70%	71%
Meds 'Always' Explained Before Given	300+	68%	64%	64%
Nurses 'Always' Communicated Well	300+	78%	77%	79%
Pain 'Always' Well Controlled	300+	68%	70%	71%
Room and Bathroom 'Always' Clean	300+	76%	73%	73%
Timely Help 'Always' Received	300+	63%	65%	68%
Would Definitely Recommend Hospital	300+	73%	73%	71%
Use of Medical Imaging				
Cardiac Imaging Stress Test before Surgery[1]	-	-	4.3%	5.3%
Combination Abdominal CT Scan[1]	-	-	6.9%	10.5%
Combination Brain/Sinus CT Scan[1]	-	-	2.3%	2.7%
Combination Chest CT Scan[1]	-	-	1.1%	2.7%
Follow-up Mammogram/Ultrasound	72	13.9%	9.1%	8.8%
Lumbar Spine MRI for Low Back Pain[1]	-	-	37.9%	37.2%

Harborview Medical Center

325 9th Avenue — Phone: 206-731-3000
Seattle, WA 98104 — Fax: 206-731-8551
URL: www.harborview.org
Type: Acute Care Hospitals — Emergency Services: Yes
Ownership: Government - Local — Beds: 411

Key Personnel:
Pediatric Ambulatory Care . . . . . . Abraham Bergman, MD
Pediatric In-Patient Care . . . . Abraham Bergman, MD
Quality Assurance . . . . John Culver, MD
Chief of Medical Staff . . . . J. Richard Goss, MD
CEO/President . . . . David Jaffe
Infection Control . . . . Walter Stamm, MD
Operating Room . . . . Mary Sweeney, RN
Radiology . . . . Lee Talner, MD

Measure	Cases	This Hosp.	State Avg.	U.S. Avg.
Blood Clot Prevention and Treatment				
Anticoagulation Overlap Therapy[2]	93	96%	97%	93%
ICU Venous Thromboembolism Prophylaxis[2]	184	98%	92%	92%
Incidence of Potentially Preventable VTE[2]	58	0%	9%	10%
UFH with Dosages/Platelet Monitoring[2]	78	100%	99%	97%
Venous Thromboembolism Prophylaxis[2]	223	91%	86%	85%
Warfarin Therapy Discharge Instructions[2]	51	90%	74%	75%
Chest Pain/Possible Heart Attack Care				
Aspirin Given Within 24 Hours of Arrival[5]	-	-	97%	96%
Fibrinolytic Meds Within 30 Min. of Arrival[5]	-	-	51%	58%
Average Time to ECG (minutes)[5]	-	-	9	7
Average Time to Transfer (minutes)[5]	-	-	54	60
Children's Asthma Care				
Received Home Management Plan of Care	-	-	-	88%
Received Reliever Medication	-	-	-	100%

NOTE: Hospital profiles are in alphabetical order by state, then city, then hospital within the city; Rankings exclude hospitals with less than 25 cases except for patient surveys which excludes hospitals with less than 100 cases; (a) 100-299 cases; (1) The number of cases/patients is too few to report; (2) Data submitted were based on a sample of cases/patients; (3) Results are based on a shorter time period than required; (4) Data suppressed by CMS for one or more quarters; (5) Results are not available for this reporting period; (6) Fewer than 100 patients completed the HCAHPS survey; (7) No cases met the criteria for this measure; (8) The lower limit of the confidence interval cannot be calculated if the number of observed infections equals zero; (9) No data are available from the state/territory for this reporting period; (10) The scores shown reflect fewer than 50 completed surveys; (11) There were discrepancies in the data collection process; (12) This measure does not apply to this hospital for this reporting period; (13) Results cannot be calculated for this reporting period; (14) The results for this state are combined with nearby states to protect confidentiality; Please refer to the User's Guide for a full explanation of data.

Measure	Cases	This Hosp.	State Avg.	U.S. Avg.
Received Systemic Corticosteroids	-	-	-	100%
Emergency Department				
Admittance Decision Time (minutes)[2]	199	229	96	98
Head CT Results Within 45 Min. of Arrival[3,7]	-	-	63%	57%
Patients Who Left ER Before Being Seen	68,534	5%	2%	2%
Time from ER Arrival to Admit. (minutes)[2]	564	402	259	274
Time from ER Arrival to Discharge (minutes)	297	222	135	134
Time in ER Before Being Evaluated (minutes)	375	27	22	26
Time to Pain Meds for Fractures (minutes)	79	61	52	57
Heart Attack Care				
Aspirin Given at Discharge	73	100%	99%	99%
Fibrinolytic Meds Within 30 Min. of Arrival[7]	-	-	62%	54%
PCI Within 90 Minutes of Arrival	16	94%	97%	96%
Statin Prescribed at Discharge	70	100%	98%	98%
Heart Failure Care				
ACE Inhibitor or ARB for LVSD	72	100%	97%	97%
Discharge Instructions Given	120	97%	93%	94%
Evaluation of LVS Function	144	100%	99%	99%
Medicare Spending				
Medicare Spending per Patient (ratio)	-	0.97	0.91	0.98
Pneumonia Care				
Appropriate Initial Antibiotic Given	64	98%	96%	95%
Blood Culture Timing	167	96%	97%	98%
Pregnancy and Delivery Care				
Newborn Deliveries Scheduled Early[7]	-	-	2%	6%
Preventive Care				
Immunization for Influenza[2]	584	91%	91%	90%
Immunization for Pneumonia[2]	501	92%	91%	92%
Stroke Care				
Anticoagulation Therapy for Atrial Fibrillation	21	95%	94%	95%
Antithrombotic Therapy Timing	111	99%	98%	98%
Assessed for Rehabilitation	367	99%	98%	97%
Discharged on Antithrombotic Therapy	148	100%	99%	99%
Discharged on Statin Medication	108	93%	96%	94%
Thrombolytic Therapy Timing[1]	-	-	73%	66%
Venous Thromboembolism Prophylaxis	400	93%	94%	94%
Written Stroke Educational Materials Given	184	87%	86%	88%
Surgical Care Improvement Project				
Appropriate Beta Blocker Usage[2]	60	100%	98%	98%
Appropriate VTP Within 24 Hours[2]	158	99%	98%	98%
Controlled Postoperative Blood Glucose[2,7]	-	-	97%	97%
Perioperative Temperature Management[2]	253	100%	100%	100%
Prophylactic Antibiotic Selection[2]	98	100%	99%	99%
Prophylactic Antibiotic Selection (Outpatient)	225	99%	98%	98%
Prophylactic Antibiotic Stopped[2]	94	97%	99%	98%
Prophylactic Antibiotic Timing[2]	99	99%	98%	99%
Prophylactic Antibiotic Timing (Outpatient)	189	100%	98%	98%
Urinary Catheter Removal[2]	88	100%	97%	97%
Survey of Patients' Hospital Experiences				
Area Around Room 'Always' Quiet at Night	300+	44%	54%	61%
Doctors 'Always' Communicated Well	300+	74%	81%	82%
Home Recovery Information Given	300+	87%	87%	85%
Hospital Given 9 or 10 on 10 Point Scale	300+	69%	70%	71%
Meds 'Always' Explained Before Given	300+	60%	64%	64%
Nurses 'Always' Communicated Well	300+	74%	77%	79%
Pain 'Always' Well Controlled	300+	66%	70%	71%
Room and Bathroom 'Always' Clean	300+	74%	73%	73%
Timely Help 'Always' Received	300+	59%	65%	68%
Would Definitely Recommend Hospital	300+	74%	73%	71%
Use of Medical Imaging				
Cardiac Imaging Stress Test before Surgery	176	4.5%	4.3%	5.3%
Combination Abdominal CT Scan	419	8.6%	6.9%	10.5%
Combination Brain/Sinus CT Scan	509	0.4%	2.3%	2.7%
Combination Chest CT Scan	328	0.0%	1.1%	2.7%
Follow-up Mammogram/Ultrasound[7]	-	-	9.1%	8.8%
Lumbar Spine MRI for Low Back Pain	80	43.8%	37.9%	37.2%

Northwest Hospital

1550 North 115th Street | Phone: 206-364-0500
Seattle, WA 98133 | Fax: 206-368-1990
URL: www.nwhospital.org
Type: Acute Care Hospitals | Emergency Services: Yes
Ownership: Voluntary non-profit - Other | Beds: 345

Key Personnel:
Anesthesiology. . . . . Ronald Abrams, MD
Quality Assurance . . . . William Braswell
Chairman/CEO . . . . Peter Evans
Emergency Room . . . . Warren Fisher, MD
Radiology. . . . . Thaddeus Paprocki, MD
Operating Room. . . . . Stuart Schrader
CEO/President. . . . . Will Sthenider

Measure	Cases	This Hosp.	State Avg.	U.S. Avg.
Blood Clot Prevention and Treatment				
Anticoagulation Overlap Therapy[2]	73	100%	97%	93%
ICU Venous Thromboembolism Prophylaxis[2]	63	87%	92%	92%
Incidence of Potentially Preventable VTE[2]	16	0%	9%	10%
UFH with Dosages/Platelet Monitoring[2]	31	100%	99%	97%
Venous Thromboembolism Prophylaxis[2]	296	91%	86%	85%
Warfarin Therapy Discharge Instructions[2]	51	90%	74%	75%
Chest Pain/Possible Heart Attack Care				
Aspirin Given Within 24 Hours of Arrival[3,7]	-	-	97%	96%
Fibrinolytic Meds Within 30 Min. of Arrival[5]	-	-	51%	58%
Average Time to ECG (minutes)[3,7]	-	-	9	7
Average Time to Transfer (minutes)[5]	-	-	54	60
Children's Asthma Care				
Received Home Management Plan of Care	-	-	-	88%
Received Reliever Medication	-	-	-	100%
Received Systemic Corticosteroids	-	-	-	100%
Emergency Department				
Admittance Decision Time (minutes)[2]	591	102	96	98
Head CT Results Within 45 Min. of Arrival[1]	-	-	63%	57%
Patients Who Left ER Before Being Seen	34,150	1%	2%	2%
Time from ER Arrival to Admit. (minutes)[2]	591	265	259	274
Time from ER Arrival to Discharge (minutes)	379	151	135	134
Time in ER Before Being Evaluated (minutes)	408	30	22	26
Time to Pain Meds for Fractures (minutes)	100	59	52	57
Heart Attack Care				
Aspirin Given at Discharge	156	99%	99%	99%
Fibrinolytic Meds Within 30 Min. of Arrival[7]	-	-	62%	54%
PCI Within 90 Minutes of Arrival	44	100%	97%	96%
Statin Prescribed at Discharge	150	96%	98%	98%
Heart Failure Care				
ACE Inhibitor or ARB for LVSD	63	95%	97%	97%
Discharge Instructions Given	147	96%	93%	94%
Evaluation of LVS Function	201	100%	99%	99%
Medicare Spending				
Medicare Spending per Patient (ratio)	-	0.95	0.91	0.98
Pneumonia Care				
Appropriate Initial Antibiotic Given[2]	77	100%	96%	95%
Blood Culture Timing[2]	155	99%	97%	98%
Pregnancy and Delivery Care				
Newborn Deliveries Scheduled Early[2]	12	0%	2%	6%
Preventive Care				
Immunization for Influenza[2]	515	97%	91%	90%
Immunization for Pneumonia[2]	609	96%	91%	92%
Stroke Care				
Anticoagulation Therapy for Atrial Fibrillation[2]	14	93%	94%	95%
Antithrombotic Therapy Timing[2]	99	100%	98%	98%
Assessed for Rehabilitation[2]	125	99%	98%	97%
Discharged on Antithrombotic Therapy[2]	113	99%	99%	99%
Discharged on Statin Medication[2]	76	92%	96%	94%
Thrombolytic Therapy Timing[2]	12	83%	73%	66%
Venous Thromboembolism Prophylaxis[2]	130	98%	94%	94%
Written Stroke Educational Materials Given[2]	66	95%	86%	88%
Surgical Care Improvement Project				
Appropriate Beta Blocker Usage[2]	126	95%	98%	98%
Appropriate VTP Within 24 Hours[2]	354	97%	98%	98%
Controlled Postoperative Blood Glucose[2]	65	98%	97%	97%
Perioperative Temperature Management[2]	412	100%	100%	100%
Prophylactic Antibiotic Selection[2]	328	98%	99%	99%
Prophylactic Antibiotic Selection (Outpatient)	337	99%	98%	98%
Prophylactic Antibiotic Stopped[2]	320	100%	99%	98%
Prophylactic Antibiotic Timing[2]	329	98%	98%	99%
Prophylactic Antibiotic Timing (Outpatient)	339	98%	98%	98%
Urinary Catheter Removal[2]	313	98%	97%	97%
Survey of Patients' Hospital Experiences				
Area Around Room 'Always' Quiet at Night	300+	48%	54%	61%
Doctors 'Always' Communicated Well	300+	82%	81%	82%
Home Recovery Information Given	300+	86%	87%	85%
Hospital Given 9 or 10 on 10 Point Scale	300+	72%	70%	71%
Meds 'Always' Explained Before Given	300+	60%	64%	64%
Nurses 'Always' Communicated Well	300+	75%	77%	79%
Pain 'Always' Well Controlled	300+	70%	70%	71%
Room and Bathroom 'Always' Clean	300+	71%	73%	73%
Timely Help 'Always' Received	300+	65%	65%	68%
Would Definitely Recommend Hospital	300+	78%	73%	71%
Use of Medical Imaging				
Cardiac Imaging Stress Test before Surgery	887	3.6%	4.3%	5.3%
Combination Abdominal CT Scan	783	11.0%	6.9%	10.5%
Combination Brain/Sinus CT Scan	718	3.6%	2.3%	2.7%
Combination Chest CT Scan	549	0.2%	1.1%	2.7%
Follow-up Mammogram/Ultrasound	2,600	4.1%	9.1%	8.8%
Lumbar Spine MRI for Low Back Pain	88	42.0%	37.9%	37.2%

Seattle Children's Hospital

4800 Sand Point Way Ne, PO Box C-5371 | Phone: 206-987-2000
Seattle, WA 98105 | Fax: 206-987-5022
E-mail: ehealth@seattlechildrens.org
URL: www.seattlechildrens.org
Type: Childrens | Emergency Services: Yes
Ownership: Voluntary non-profit - Private

Key Personnel:
Radiology. . . . . Puneet Bhargava
Ambulatory Care . . . . Cindy Evans
Chief of Medical Staff . . . . Patrick J Hagan, MD
CEO/President. . . . . Thomas N Hansen, MD
Operating Room. . . . . Robert S Sawin, MD
Pediatric Ambulatory Care . . . . . . F Bruder Stapleton, MD

Measure	Cases	This Hosp.	State Avg.	U.S. Avg.
Blood Clot Prevention and Treatment				
Anticoagulation Overlap Therapy[5]	-	-	97%	93%
ICU Venous Thromboembolism Prophylaxis[5]	-	-	92%	92%
Incidence of Potentially Preventable VTE[5]	-	-	9%	10%
UFH with Dosages/Platelet Monitoring[5]	-	-	99%	97%
Venous Thromboembolism Prophylaxis[5]	-	-	86%	85%
Warfarin Therapy Discharge Instructions[5]	-	-	74%	75%
Chest Pain/Possible Heart Attack Care				
Aspirin Given Within 24 Hours of Arrival	-	-	97%	96%
Fibrinolytic Meds Within 30 Min. of Arrival	-	-	51%	58%
Average Time to ECG (minutes)	-	-	9	7
Average Time to Transfer (minutes)	-	-	54	60
Children's Asthma Care				
Received Home Management Plan of Care	-	-	-	88%
Received Reliever Medication	-	-	-	100%
Received Systemic Corticosteroids	-	-	-	100%
Emergency Department				
Admittance Decision Time (minutes)[5]	-	-	96	98
Head CT Results Within 45 Min. of Arrival	-	-	63%	57%
Patients Who Left ER Before Being Seen	-	-	2%	2%
Time from ER Arrival to Admit. (minutes)[5]	-	-	259	274
Time from ER Arrival to Discharge (minutes)	-	-	135	134
Time in ER Before Being Evaluated (minutes)	-	-	22	26
Time to Pain Meds for Fractures (minutes)	-	-	52	57
Heart Attack Care				
Aspirin Given at Discharge[5]	-	-	99%	99%
Fibrinolytic Meds Within 30 Min. of Arrival[5]	-	-	62%	54%
PCI Within 90 Minutes of Arrival[5]	-	-	97%	96%
Statin Prescribed at Discharge[5]	-	-	98%	98%
Heart Failure Care				
ACE Inhibitor or ARB for LVSD[5]	-	-	97%	97%
Discharge Instructions Given[5]	-	-	93%	94%
Evaluation of LVS Function[5]	-	-	99%	99%
Medicare Spending				
Medicare Spending per Patient (ratio)	-	-	0.91	0.98
Pneumonia Care				

NOTE: Hospital profiles are in alphabetical order by state, then city, then hospital within the city; Rankings exclude hospitals with less than 25 cases except for patient surveys which excludes hospitals with less than 100 cases; (a) 100-299 cases; (1) The number of cases/patients is too few to report; (2) Data submitted were based on a sample of cases/patients; (3) Results are based on a shorter time period than required; (4) Data suppressed by CMS for one or more quarters; (5) Results are not available for this reporting period; (6) Fewer than 100 patients completed the HCAHPS survey; (7) No cases met the criteria for this measure; (8) The lower limit of the confidence interval cannot be calculated if the number of observed infections equals zero; (9) No data are available from the state/territory for this reporting period; (10) The scores shown reflect fewer than 50 completed surveys; (11) There were discrepancies in the data collection process; (12) This measure does not apply to this hospital for this reporting period; (13) Results cannot be calculated for this reporting period; (14) The results for this state are combined with nearby states to protect confidentiality; Please refer to the User's Guide for a full explanation of data.

Measure	Cases	This Hosp.	State Avg.	U.S. Avg.
Appropriate Initial Antibiotic Given[5]	-	-	96%	95%
Blood Culture Timing[5]	-	-	97%	98%
Pregnancy and Delivery Care				
Newborn Deliveries Scheduled Early[5]	-	-	2%	6%
Preventive Care				
Immunization for Influenza[5]	-	-	91%	90%
Immunization for Pneumonia[5]	-	-	91%	92%
Stroke Care				
Anticoagulation Therapy for Atrial Fibrillation[5]	-	-	94%	95%
Antithrombotic Therapy Timing[5]	-	-	98%	98%
Assessed for Rehabilitation[5]	-	-	98%	97%
Discharged on Antithrombotic Therapy[5]	-	-	99%	99%
Discharged on Statin Medication[5]	-	-	96%	94%
Thrombolytic Therapy Timing[5]	-	-	73%	66%
Venous Thromboembolism Prophylaxis[5]	-	-	94%	94%
Written Stroke Educational Materials Given[5]	-	-	86%	88%
Surgical Care Improvement Project				
Appropriate Beta Blocker Usage[5]	-	-	98%	98%
Appropriate VTP Within 24 Hours[5]	-	-	98%	98%
Controlled Postoperative Blood Glucose[5]	-	-	97%	97%
Perioperative Temperature Management[5]	-	-	100%	100%
Prophylactic Antibiotic Selection[5]	-	-	99%	99%
Prophylactic Antibiotic Selection (Outpatient)	-	-	98%	98%
Prophylactic Antibiotic Stopped[5]	-	-	99%	98%
Prophylactic Antibiotic Timing[5]	-	-	98%	99%
Prophylactic Antibiotic Timing (Outpatient)	-	-	98%	98%
Urinary Catheter Removal[5]	-	-	97%	97%
Survey of Patients' Hospital Experiences				
Area Around Room 'Always' Quiet at Night[5]	-	-	54%	61%
Doctors 'Always' Communicated Well[5]	-	-	81%	82%
Home Recovery Information Given[5]	-	-	87%	85%
Hospital Given 9 or 10 on 10 Point Scale[5]	-	-	70%	71%
Meds 'Always' Explained Before Given[5]	-	-	64%	64%
Nurses 'Always' Communicated Well[5]	-	-	77%	79%
Pain 'Always' Well Controlled[5]	-	-	70%	71%
Room and Bathroom 'Always' Clean[5]	-	-	73%	73%
Timely Help 'Always' Received[5]	-	-	65%	68%
Would Definitely Recommend Hospital[5]	-	-	73%	71%
Use of Medical Imaging				
Cardiac Imaging Stress Test before Surgery	-	-	4.3%	5.3%
Combination Abdominal CT Scan	-	-	6.9%	10.5%
Combination Brain/Sinus CT Scan	-	-	2.3%	2.7%
Combination Chest CT Scan	-	-	1.1%	2.7%
Follow-up Mammogram/Ultrasound	-	-	9.1%	8.8%
Lumbar Spine MRI for Low Back Pain	-	-	37.9%	37.2%

Seattle VA Medical Center - VA Pugit Sound

1660 S. Columbian Way
Seattle, WA 98108
Phone: 206-764-2299
Fax: 206-764-2250
URL: www.va.gov/pugetsound
Type: Acute Care - VA
Emergency Services: No
Ownership: Government Federal
Beds: 474

Key Personnel:
Quality Assurance .... Robins S Cook, RN
CEO/President............... Stan Johnson
Radiology.................... Joseph Rajendran, MD
Chief of Medical Staff.......... Gordon Starkenbaum, MD

Measure	Cases	This Hosp.	State Avg.	U.S. Avg.
Blood Clot Prevention and Treatment				
Anticoagulation Overlap Therapy	-	-	97%	93%
ICU Venous Thromboembolism Prophylaxis	-	-	92%	92%
Incidence of Potentially Preventable VTE	-	-	9%	10%
UFH with Dosages/Platelet Monitoring	-	-	99%	97%
Venous Thromboembolism Prophylaxis	-	-	86%	85%
Warfarin Therapy Discharge Instructions	-	-	74%	75%
Chest Pain/Possible Heart Attack Care				
Aspirin Given Within 24 Hours of Arrival	-	-	97%	96%
Fibrinolytic Meds Within 30 Min. of Arrival	-	-	51%	58%
Average Time to ECG (minutes)	-	-	9	7
Average Time to Transfer (minutes)	-	-	54	60
Children's Asthma Care				
Received Home Management Plan of Care	-	-	-	88%
Received Reliever Medication	-	-	-	100%
Received Systemic Corticosteroids	-	-	-	100%
Emergency Department				
Admittance Decision Time (minutes)	-	-	96	98
Head CT Results Within 45 Min. of Arrival	-	-	63%	57%
Patients Who Left ER Before Being Seen	-	-	2%	2%
Time from ER Arrival to Admit. (minutes)	-	-	259	274
Time from ER Arrival to Discharge (minutes)	-	-	135	134
Time in ER Before Being Evaluated (minutes)	-	-	22	26
Time to Pain Meds for Fractures (minutes)	-	-	52	57
Heart Attack Care				
Aspirin Given at Discharge	64	100%	99%	99%
Fibrinolytic Meds Within 30 Min. of Arrival[5]	-	-	62%	54%
PCI Within 90 Minutes of Arrival[5]	-	-	97%	96%
Statin Prescribed at Discharge	64	97%	98%	98%
Heart Failure Care				
ACE Inhibitor or ARB for LVSD	55	100%	97%	97%
Discharge Instructions Given	153	97%	93%	94%
Evaluation of LVS Function	181	100%	99%	99%
Medicare Spending				
Medicare Spending per Patient (ratio)	-	-	0.91	0.98
Pneumonia Care				
Appropriate Initial Antibiotic Given	55	98%	96%	95%
Blood Culture Timing	95	99%	97%	98%
Pregnancy and Delivery Care				
Newborn Deliveries Scheduled Early	-	-	2%	6%
Preventive Care				
Immunization for Influenza[5]	-	-	91%	90%
Immunization for Pneumonia[5]	-	-	91%	92%
Stroke Care				
Anticoagulation Therapy for Atrial Fibrillation	-	-	94%	95%
Antithrombotic Therapy Timing	-	-	98%	98%
Assessed for Rehabilitation	-	-	98%	97%
Discharged on Antithrombotic Therapy	-	-	99%	99%
Discharged on Statin Medication	-	-	96%	94%
Thrombolytic Therapy Timing	-	-	73%	66%
Venous Thromboembolism Prophylaxis	-	-	94%	94%
Written Stroke Educational Materials Given	-	-	86%	88%
Surgical Care Improvement Project				
Appropriate Beta Blocker Usage[2]	172	92%	98%	98%
Appropriate VTP Within 24 Hours[2]	350	99%	98%	98%
Controlled Postoperative Blood Glucose[2]	47	98%	97%	97%
Perioperative Temperature Management[2]	453	98%	100%	100%
Prophylactic Antibiotic Selection	368	99%	99%	99%
Prophylactic Antibiotic Selection (Outpatient)	-	-	98%	98%
Prophylactic Antibiotic Stopped	365	97%	99%	98%
Prophylactic Antibiotic Timing	368	98%	98%	99%
Prophylactic Antibiotic Timing (Outpatient)	-	-	98%	98%
Urinary Catheter Removal[2]	306	100%	97%	97%
Survey of Patients' Hospital Experiences				
Area Around Room 'Always' Quiet at Night	-	-	54%	61%
Doctors 'Always' Communicated Well	-	-	81%	82%
Home Recovery Information Given	-	-	87%	85%
Hospital Given 9 or 10 on 10 Point Scale	-	-	70%	71%
Meds 'Always' Explained Before Given	-	-	64%	64%
Nurses 'Always' Communicated Well	-	-	77%	79%
Pain 'Always' Well Controlled	-	-	70%	71%
Room and Bathroom 'Always' Clean	-	-	73%	73%
Timely Help 'Always' Received	-	-	65%	68%
Would Definitely Recommend Hospital	-	-	73%	71%
Use of Medical Imaging				
Cardiac Imaging Stress Test before Surgery	-	-	4.3%	5.3%
Combination Abdominal CT Scan	-	-	6.9%	10.5%
Combination Brain/Sinus CT Scan	-	-	2.3%	2.7%
Combination Chest CT Scan	-	-	1.1%	2.7%
Follow-up Mammogram/Ultrasound	-	-	9.1%	8.8%
Lumbar Spine MRI for Low Back Pain	-	-	37.9%	37.2%

Swedish Medical Center

747 Broadway
Seattle, WA 98122
Phone: 206-386-6000
Fax: 206-386-6138
URL: www.swedish.org
Type: Acute Care Hospitals
Emergency Services: Yes
Ownership: Voluntary non-profit - Private
Beds: 697

Key Personnel:
CEO .... Anthony Armada, FACHE
Chief of Medical Staff.......... Nancy J Auer, MD
CEO/President............... Rodney F Hochman, MD
Radiology................... Timothy Larson, MD
Quality Assurance .... Judy C Morton, PhD
Pediatric Ambulatory Care ...... Brent Oldham, MD
Pediatric In-Patient Care .... Brent Oldham, MD
Infection Control............. Will Shelton

Measure	Cases	This Hosp.	State Avg.	U.S. Avg.
Blood Clot Prevention and Treatment				
Anticoagulation Overlap Therapy[2]	87	98%	97%	93%
ICU Venous Thromboembolism Prophylaxis[2]	61	100%	92%	92%
Incidence of Potentially Preventable VTE[2]	22	9%	9%	10%
UFH with Dosages/Platelet Monitoring[2]	53	100%	99%	97%
Venous Thromboembolism Prophylaxis[2]	400	80%	86%	85%
Warfarin Therapy Discharge Instructions[2]	63	11%	74%	75%
Chest Pain/Possible Heart Attack Care				
Aspirin Given Within 24 Hours of Arrival	181	94%	97%	96%
Fibrinolytic Meds Within 30 Min. of Arrival[7]	-	-	51%	58%
Average Time to ECG (minutes)	190	9	9	7
Average Time to Transfer (minutes)	27	39	54	60
Children's Asthma Care				
Received Home Management Plan of Care	-	-	-	88%
Received Reliever Medication	-	-	-	100%
Received Systemic Corticosteroids	-	-	-	100%
Emergency Department				
Admittance Decision Time (minutes)[2]	438	79	96	98
Head CT Results Within 45 Min. of Arrival	15	73%	63%	57%
Patients Who Left ER Before Being Seen	96,621	0%	2%	2%
Time from ER Arrival to Admit. (minutes)[2]	440	211	259	274
Time from ER Arrival to Discharge (minutes)	1,572	92	135	134
Time in ER Before Being Evaluated (minutes)	1,659	8	22	26
Time to Pain Meds for Fractures (minutes)	284	34	52	57
Heart Attack Care				
Aspirin Given at Discharge	14	100%	99%	99%
Fibrinolytic Meds Within 30 Min. of Arrival[7]	-	-	62%	54%
PCI Within 90 Minutes of Arrival[7]	-	-	97%	96%
Statin Prescribed at Discharge	16	94%	98%	98%
Heart Failure Care				
ACE Inhibitor or ARB for LVSD	47	100%	97%	97%
Discharge Instructions Given	167	95%	93%	94%
Evaluation of LVS Function	227	100%	99%	99%
Medicare Spending				
Medicare Spending per Patient (ratio)	-	0.91	0.91	0.98
Pneumonia Care				
Appropriate Initial Antibiotic Given	144	97%	96%	95%
Blood Culture Timing	272	97%	97%	98%
Pregnancy and Delivery Care				
Newborn Deliveries Scheduled Early	377	2%	2%	6%
Preventive Care				
Immunization for Influenza[2]	879	92%	91%	90%
Immunization for Pneumonia[2]	686	87%	91%	92%
Stroke Care				
Anticoagulation Therapy for Atrial Fibrillation[1]	-	-	94%	95%
Antithrombotic Therapy Timing	24	100%	98%	98%
Assessed for Rehabilitation	31	97%	98%	97%
Discharged on Antithrombotic Therapy	30	100%	99%	99%
Discharged on Statin Medication	27	96%	96%	94%
Thrombolytic Therapy Timing[1]	-	-	73%	66%
Venous Thromboembolism Prophylaxis	26	85%	94%	94%
Written Stroke Educational Materials Given	23	87%	86%	88%
Surgical Care Improvement Project				
Appropriate Beta Blocker Usage[2]	203	100%	98%	98%
Appropriate VTP Within 24 Hours[2]	763	99%	98%	98%
Controlled Postoperative Blood Glucose[2,7]	-	-	97%	97%
Perioperative Temperature Management[2]	1,053	100%	100%	100%
Prophylactic Antibiotic Selection[2]	763	99%	99%	99%

NOTE: Hospital profiles are in alphabetical order by state, then city, then hospital within the city; Rankings exclude hospitals with less than 25 cases except for patient surveys which excludes hospitals with less than 100 cases; (a) 100-299 cases; (1) The number of cases/patients is too few to report; (2) Data submitted were based on a sample of cases/patients; (3) Results are based on a shorter time period than required; (4) Data suppressed by CMS for one or more quarters; (5) Results are not available for this reporting period; (6) Fewer than 100 patients completed the HCAHPS survey; (7) No cases met the criteria for this measure; (8) The lower limit of the confidence interval cannot be calculated if the number of observed infections equals zero; (9) No data are available from the state/territory for this reporting period; (10) The scores shown reflect fewer than 50 completed surveys; (11) There were discrepancies in the data collection process; (12) This measure does not apply to this hospital for this reporting period; (13) Results cannot be calculated for this reporting period; (14) The results for this state are combined with nearby states to protect confidentiality; Please refer to the User's Guide for a full explanation of data.

Prophylactic Antibiotic Selection (Outpatient)	504	98%	98%	98%
Prophylactic Antibiotic Stopped[2]	745	99%	99%	98%
Prophylactic Antibiotic Timing[2]	763	99%	98%	99%
Prophylactic Antibiotic Timing (Outpatient)	507	99%	98%	98%
Urinary Catheter Removal[2]	492	100%	97%	97%
Survey of Patients' Hospital Experiences				
Area Around Room 'Always' Quiet at Night	300+	54%	54%	61%
Doctors 'Always' Communicated Well	300+	81%	81%	82%
Home Recovery Information Given	300+	83%	87%	85%
Hospital Given 9 or 10 on 10 Point Scale	300+	71%	70%	71%
Meds 'Always' Explained Before Given	300+	60%	64%	64%
Nurses 'Always' Communicated Well	300+	75%	77%	79%
Pain 'Always' Well Controlled	300+	69%	70%	71%
Room and Bathroom 'Always' Clean	300+	68%	73%	73%
Timely Help 'Always' Received	300+	61%	65%	68%
Would Definitely Recommend Hospital	300+	78%	73%	71%
Use of Medical Imaging				
Cardiac Imaging Stress Test before Surgery[1]	-	-	4.3%	5.3%
Combination Abdominal CT Scan	1,072	7.6%	6.9%	10.5%
Combination Brain/Sinus CT Scan	805	4.3%	2.3%	2.7%
Combination Chest CT Scan	397	0.3%	1.1%	2.7%
Follow-up Mammogram/Ultrasound	4,203	10.6%	9.1%	8.8%
Lumbar Spine MRI for Low Back Pain	108	45.4%	37.9%	37.2%

Swedish Medical Center - Cherry Hill

500 17th Avenue Phone: 206-320-2000
Seattle, WA 98122
URL: www.swedish.org
Type: Acute Care Hospitals Emergency Services: Yes
Ownership: Voluntary non-profit - Church Beds: 224

Measure	Cases	This Hosp.	State Avg.	U.S. Avg.
Blood Clot Prevention and Treatment				
Anticoagulation Overlap Therapy[2]	45	96%	97%	93%
ICU Venous Thromboembolism Prophylaxis[2]	153	97%	92%	92%
Incidence of Potentially Preventable VTE[2]	15	0%	9%	10%
UFH with Dosages/Platelet Monitoring[2]	38	100%	99%	97%
Venous Thromboembolism Prophylaxis[2]	211	83%	86%	85%
Warfarin Therapy Discharge Instructions[2]	25	24%	74%	75%
Chest Pain/Possible Heart Attack Care				
Aspirin Given Within 24 Hours of Arrival[1]	-	-	97%	96%
Fibrinolytic Meds Within 30 Min. of Arrival[3,7]	-	-	51%	58%
Average Time to ECG (minutes)[1]	-	-	9	7
Average Time to Transfer (minutes)[3,7]	-	-	54	60
Children's Asthma Care				
Received Home Management Plan of Care	-	-	-	88%
Received Reliever Medication	-	-	-	100%
Received Systemic Corticosteroids	-	-	-	100%
Emergency Department				
Admittance Decision Time (minutes)[2]	332	79	96	98
Head CT Results Within 45 Min. of Arrival[7]	-	-	63%	57%
Patients Who Left ER Before Being Seen	18,916	0%	2%	2%
Time from ER Arrival to Admit. (minutes)[2]	334	186	259	274
Time from ER Arrival to Discharge (minutes)	346	130	135	134
Time in ER Before Being Evaluated (minutes)	416	11	22	26
Time to Pain Meds for Fractures (minutes)	40	55	52	57
Heart Attack Care				
Aspirin Given at Discharge	359	99%	99%	99%
Fibrinolytic Meds Within 30 Min. of Arrival[7]	-	-	62%	54%
PCI Within 90 Minutes of Arrival	60	100%	97%	96%
Statin Prescribed at Discharge	357	97%	98%	98%
Heart Failure Care				
ACE Inhibitor or ARB for LVSD	128	96%	97%	97%
Discharge Instructions Given	290	100%	93%	94%
Evaluation of LVS Function	344	100%	99%	99%
Medicare Spending				
Medicare Spending per Patient (ratio)	-	0.98	0.91	0.98
Pneumonia Care				
Appropriate Initial Antibiotic Given[1]	-	-	96%	95%
Blood Culture Timing	30	97%	97%	98%
Pregnancy and Delivery Care				
Newborn Deliveries Scheduled Early[7]	-	-	2%	6%
Preventive Care				
Immunization for Influenza[2]	602	98%	91%	90%
Immunization for Pneumonia[2]	826	92%	91%	92%
Stroke Care				
Anticoagulation Therapy for Atrial Fibrillation	24	83%	94%	95%
Antithrombotic Therapy Timing	93	98%	98%	98%
Assessed for Rehabilitation	242	98%	98%	97%
Discharged on Antithrombotic Therapy	159	99%	99%	99%
Discharged on Statin Medication	117	98%	96%	94%
Thrombolytic Therapy Timing	18	89%	73%	66%
Venous Thromboembolism Prophylaxis	252	98%	94%	94%
Written Stroke Educational Materials Given	111	86%	86%	88%
Surgical Care Improvement Project				
Appropriate Beta Blocker Usage[2]	171	100%	98%	98%
Appropriate VTP Within 24 Hours[2]	118	100%	98%	98%
Controlled Postoperative Blood Glucose[2]	226	97%	97%	97%
Perioperative Temperature Management[2]	283	100%	100%	100%
Prophylactic Antibiotic Selection[2]	240	100%	99%	99%
Prophylactic Antibiotic Selection (Outpatient)	388	100%	98%	98%
Prophylactic Antibiotic Stopped[2]	236	100%	99%	98%
Prophylactic Antibiotic Timing[2]	241	97%	98%	99%
Prophylactic Antibiotic Timing (Outpatient)	389	99%	98%	98%
Urinary Catheter Removal[2]	300	100%	97%	97%
Survey of Patients' Hospital Experiences				
Area Around Room 'Always' Quiet at Night	300+	44%	54%	61%
Doctors 'Always' Communicated Well	300+	80%	81%	82%
Home Recovery Information Given	300+	84%	87%	85%
Hospital Given 9 or 10 on 10 Point Scale	300+	72%	70%	71%
Meds 'Always' Explained Before Given	300+	61%	64%	64%
Nurses 'Always' Communicated Well	300+	76%	77%	79%
Pain 'Always' Well Controlled	300+	71%	70%	71%
Room and Bathroom 'Always' Clean	300+	70%	73%	73%
Timely Help 'Always' Received	300+	62%	65%	68%
Would Definitely Recommend Hospital	300+	78%	73%	71%
Use of Medical Imaging				
Cardiac Imaging Stress Test before Surgery	1,327	4.1%	4.3%	5.3%
Combination Abdominal CT Scan	350	4.6%	6.9%	10.5%
Combination Brain/Sinus CT Scan	614	1.1%	2.3%	2.7%
Combination Chest CT Scan	169	1.8%	1.1%	2.7%
Follow-up Mammogram/Ultrasound[7]	-	-	9.1%	8.8%
Lumbar Spine MRI for Low Back Pain	103	32.0%	37.9%	37.2%

University of Washington Medical Center

1959 Ne Pacific Saint Box 356151 Phone: 206-598-3300
Seattle, WA 98195 Fax: 206-547-4937
URL: www.washington.edu/medical/uwmc
Type: Acute Care Hospitals Emergency Services: Yes
Ownership: Government - State Beds: 396

Key Personnel:
Cardiac Laboratory. . . . . Larry Dean, MD
Coronary Care . . . . Susan Grant
Radiology. . . . . Lynn Pappas
Pediatric Ambulatory Care . . . . . . Jane Schultz
CEO/President. . . . . Larry H Shapiro, MD
Operating Room. . . . . Barbara Zuelzke

Measure	Cases	This Hosp.	State Avg.	U.S. Avg.
Blood Clot Prevention and Treatment				
Anticoagulation Overlap Therapy[2]	51	100%	97%	93%
ICU Venous Thromboembolism Prophylaxis[2]	102	98%	92%	92%
Incidence of Potentially Preventable VTE[2]	34	18%	9%	10%
UFH with Dosages/Platelet Monitoring[2]	69	100%	99%	97%
Venous Thromboembolism Prophylaxis[2]	350	80%	86%	85%
Warfarin Therapy Discharge Instructions[2]	40	38%	74%	75%
Chest Pain/Possible Heart Attack Care				
Aspirin Given Within 24 Hours of Arrival[3,7]	-	-	97%	96%
Fibrinolytic Meds Within 30 Min. of Arrival[3,7]	-	-	51%	58%
Average Time to ECG (minutes)[1,3]	-	-	9	7
Average Time to Transfer (minutes)[3,7]	-	-	54	60
Children's Asthma Care				
Received Home Management Plan of Care	-	-	-	88%
Received Reliever Medication	-	-	-	100%
Received Systemic Corticosteroids	-	-	-	100%
Emergency Department				
Admittance Decision Time (minutes)[2]	277	176	96	98
Head CT Results Within 45 Min. of Arrival	11	36%	63%	57%
Patients Who Left ER Before Being Seen	24,221	3%	2%	2%
Time from ER Arrival to Admit. (minutes)[2]	285	423	259	274
Time from ER Arrival to Discharge (minutes)	357	231	135	134
Time in ER Before Being Evaluated (minutes)	402	24	22	26
Time to Pain Meds for Fractures (minutes)	61	65	52	57
Heart Attack Care				
Aspirin Given at Discharge	107	100%	99%	99%
Fibrinolytic Meds Within 30 Min. of Arrival[7]	-	-	62%	54%
PCI Within 90 Minutes of Arrival	13	100%	97%	96%
Statin Prescribed at Discharge	108	99%	98%	98%
Heart Failure Care				
ACE Inhibitor or ARB for LVSD	148	100%	97%	97%
Discharge Instructions Given	260	99%	93%	94%
Evaluation of LVS Function	297	100%	99%	99%
Medicare Spending				
Medicare Spending per Patient (ratio)	-	0.95	0.91	0.98
Pneumonia Care				
Appropriate Initial Antibiotic Given	40	98%	96%	95%
Blood Culture Timing	129	95%	97%	98%
Pregnancy and Delivery Care				
Newborn Deliveries Scheduled Early[2]	15	7%	2%	6%
Preventive Care				
Immunization for Influenza[2]	542	98%	91%	90%
Immunization for Pneumonia[2]	512	99%	91%	92%
Stroke Care				
Anticoagulation Therapy for Atrial Fibrillation[1]	-	-	94%	95%
Antithrombotic Therapy Timing	38	100%	98%	98%
Assessed for Rehabilitation	46	100%	98%	97%
Discharged on Antithrombotic Therapy	44	100%	99%	99%
Discharged on Statin Medication	37	92%	96%	94%
Thrombolytic Therapy Timing[1]	-	-	73%	66%
Venous Thromboembolism Prophylaxis	42	90%	94%	94%
Written Stroke Educational Materials Given	27	59%	86%	88%
Surgical Care Improvement Project				
Appropriate Beta Blocker Usage[2]	157	99%	98%	98%
Appropriate VTP Within 24 Hours[2]	332	98%	98%	98%
Controlled Postoperative Blood Glucose[2]	143	98%	97%	97%
Perioperative Temperature Management[2]	402	100%	100%	100%
Prophylactic Antibiotic Selection[2]	334	99%	99%	99%
Prophylactic Antibiotic Selection (Outpatient)	552	99%	98%	98%
Prophylactic Antibiotic Stopped[2]	317	98%	99%	98%
Prophylactic Antibiotic Timing[2]	336	99%	98%	99%
Prophylactic Antibiotic Timing (Outpatient)	392	91%	98%	98%
Urinary Catheter Removal[2]	273	98%	97%	97%
Survey of Patients' Hospital Experiences				
Area Around Room 'Always' Quiet at Night	300+	55%	54%	61%
Doctors 'Always' Communicated Well	300+	80%	81%	82%
Home Recovery Information Given	300+	90%	87%	85%
Hospital Given 9 or 10 on 10 Point Scale	300+	79%	70%	71%
Meds 'Always' Explained Before Given	300+	68%	64%	64%
Nurses 'Always' Communicated Well	300+	79%	77%	79%
Pain 'Always' Well Controlled	300+	72%	70%	71%
Room and Bathroom 'Always' Clean	300+	72%	73%	73%
Timely Help 'Always' Received	300+	64%	65%	68%
Would Definitely Recommend Hospital	300+	83%	73%	71%
Use of Medical Imaging				
Cardiac Imaging Stress Test before Surgery	555	4.9%	4.3%	5.3%
Combination Abdominal CT Scan	1,142	9.0%	6.9%	10.5%
Combination Brain/Sinus CT Scan	430	0.5%	2.3%	2.7%
Combination Chest CT Scan	1,239	0.1%	1.1%	2.7%
Follow-up Mammogram/Ultrasound	891	7.5%	9.1%	8.8%
Lumbar Spine MRI for Low Back Pain	132	31.8%	37.9%	37.2%

Virginia Mason Medical Center

1100 Ninth Avenue (po Box 900) Phone: 206-223-6600
Seattle, WA 98111 Fax: 206-341-0596
URL: www.vmmc.org
Type: Acute Care Hospitals Emergency Services: Yes
Ownership: Voluntary non-profit - Private Beds: 336

Key Personnel:
Anesthesiology. . . . . Peter Ackerman, MD
Quality Assurance . . . . Gerry Ellis
Cardiac Laboratory. . . . . Christopher Fellows
Emergency Room . . . . Michael Glenn

NOTE: Hospital profiles are in alphabetical order by state, then city, then hospital within the city; Rankings exclude hospitals with less than 25 cases except for patient surveys which excludes hospitals with less than 100 cases; (a) 100-299 cases; (1) The number of cases/patients is too few to report; (2) Data submitted were based on a sample of cases/patients; (3) Results are based on a shorter time period than required; (4) Data suppressed by CMS for one or more quarters; (5) Results are not available for this reporting period; (6) Fewer than 100 patients completed the HCAHPS survey; (7) No cases met the criteria for this measure; (8) The lower limit of the confidence interval cannot be calculated if the number of observed infections equals zero; (9) No data are available from the state/territory for this reporting period; (10) The scores shown reflect fewer than 50 completed surveys; (11) There were discrepancies in the data collection process; (12) This measure does not apply to this hospital for this reporting period; (13) Results cannot be calculated for this reporting period; (14) The results for this state are combined with nearby states to protect confidentiality; Please refer to the User's Guide for a full explanation of data.

CEO/President. . . . . Gary S Kaplan, MD, FACP, FACMP
Infection Control. . . . . Uma Malhotria, MD
Chief of Medical Staff . . . . Daniel Paull

Measure	Cases	This Hosp.	State Avg.	U.S. Avg.
Blood Clot Prevention and Treatment				
Anticoagulation Overlap Therapy[2]	131	96%	97%	93%
ICU Venous Thromboembolism Prophylaxis[2]	71	97%	92%	92%
Incidence of Potentially Preventable VTE[2]	51	2%	9%	10%
UFH with Dosages/Platelet Monitoring[2]	115	100%	99%	97%
Venous Thromboembolism Prophylaxis[2]	294	94%	86%	85%
Warfarin Therapy Discharge Instructions[2]	111	86%	74%	75%
Chest Pain/Possible Heart Attack Care				
Aspirin Given Within 24 Hours of Arrival[1,3]	-	-	97%	96%
Fibrinolytic Meds Within 30 Min. of Arrival[5]	-	-	51%	58%
Average Time to ECG (minutes)[1,3]	-	-	9	7
Average Time to Transfer (minutes)[5]	-	-	54	60
Children's Asthma Care				
Received Home Management Plan of Care	-	-	-	88%
Received Reliever Medication	-	-	-	100%
Received Systemic Corticosteroids	-	-	-	100%
Emergency Department				
Admittance Decision Time (minutes)[2]	317	91	96	98
Head CT Results Within 45 Min. of Arrival[1]	-	-	63%	57%
Patients Who Left ER Before Being Seen	22,978	2%	2%	2%
Time from ER Arrival to Admit. (minutes)[2]	322	246	259	274
Time from ER Arrival to Discharge (minutes)	410	156	135	134
Time in ER Before Being Evaluated (minutes)	129	27	22	26
Time to Pain Meds for Fractures (minutes)	121	61	52	57
Heart Attack Care				
Aspirin Given at Discharge	225	100%	99%	99%
Fibrinolytic Meds Within 30 Min. of Arrival[7]	-	-	62%	54%
PCI Within 90 Minutes of Arrival	29	93%	97%	96%
Statin Prescribed at Discharge	230	100%	98%	98%
Heart Failure Care				
ACE Inhibitor or ARB for LVSD	79	99%	97%	97%
Discharge Instructions Given	306	97%	93%	94%
Evaluation of LVS Function	398	100%	99%	99%
Medicare Spending				
Medicare Spending per Patient (ratio)	-	0.94	0.91	0.98
Pneumonia Care				
Appropriate Initial Antibiotic Given[2]	138	94%	96%	95%
Blood Culture Timing[2]	193	97%	97%	98%
Pregnancy and Delivery Care				
Newborn Deliveries Scheduled Early[7]	-	-	2%	6%
Preventive Care				
Immunization for Influenza[2]	590	98%	91%	90%
Immunization for Pneumonia[2]	840	90%	91%	92%
Stroke Care				
Anticoagulation Therapy for Atrial Fibrillation	12	100%	94%	95%
Antithrombotic Therapy Timing	123	98%	98%	98%
Assessed for Rehabilitation	187	99%	98%	97%
Discharged on Antithrombotic Therapy	157	100%	99%	99%
Discharged on Statin Medication	119	92%	96%	94%
Thrombolytic Therapy Timing[1]	-	-	73%	66%
Venous Thromboembolism Prophylaxis	177	95%	94%	94%
Written Stroke Educational Materials Given	97	99%	86%	88%
Surgical Care Improvement Project				
Appropriate Beta Blocker Usage[2]	318	100%	98%	98%
Appropriate VTP Within 24 Hours[2]	417	100%	98%	98%
Controlled Postoperative Blood Glucose[2]	332	91%	97%	97%
Perioperative Temperature Management[2]	521	100%	100%	100%
Prophylactic Antibiotic Selection[2]	613	100%	99%	99%
Prophylactic Antibiotic Selection (Outpatient)	828	99%	98%	98%
Prophylactic Antibiotic Stopped[2]	597	98%	99%	98%
Prophylactic Antibiotic Timing[2]	613	99%	98%	99%
Prophylactic Antibiotic Timing (Outpatient)	621	97%	98%	98%
Urinary Catheter Removal[2]	434	96%	97%	97%
Survey of Patients' Hospital Experiences				
Area Around Room 'Always' Quiet at Night	300+	44%	54%	61%
Doctors 'Always' Communicated Well	300+	84%	81%	82%
Home Recovery Information Given	300+	89%	87%	85%
Hospital Given 9 or 10 on 10 Point Scale	300+	79%	70%	71%
Meds 'Always' Explained Before Given	300+	65%	64%	64%
Nurses 'Always' Communicated Well	300+	79%	77%	79%
Pain 'Always' Well Controlled	300+	70%	70%	71%
Room and Bathroom 'Always' Clean	300+	73%	73%	73%
Timely Help 'Always' Received	300+	67%	65%	68%
Would Definitely Recommend Hospital	300+	83%	73%	71%
Use of Medical Imaging				
Cardiac Imaging Stress Test before Surgery	796	7.8%	4.3%	5.3%
Combination Abdominal CT Scan	1,404	15.2%	6.9%	10.5%
Combination Brain/Sinus CT Scan[1]	-	-	2.3%	2.7%
Combination Chest CT Scan	1,380	0.7%	1.1%	2.7%
Follow-up Mammogram/Ultrasound	1,365	8.4%	9.1%	8.8%
Lumbar Spine MRI for Low Back Pain	93	28.0%	37.9%	37.2%

Peacehealth United General Medical Center

2000 Hospital Drive
Sedro Woolley, WA 98284
Phone: 360-856-6021
URL: www.unitedgeneral.org
Type: Critical Access Hospitals
Emergency Services: Yes
Ownership: Govt - Hospital Dist/Auth
Key Personnel:
Radiology. . . . . Nicholas Muff
CEO/President. . . . . Greg Reed

Measure	Cases	This Hosp.	State Avg.	U.S. Avg.
Blood Clot Prevention and Treatment				
Anticoagulation Overlap Therapy[5]	-	-	97%	93%
ICU Venous Thromboembolism Prophylaxis[5]	-	-	92%	92%
Incidence of Potentially Preventable VTE[5]	-	-	9%	10%
UFH with Dosages/Platelet Monitoring[5]	-	-	99%	97%
Venous Thromboembolism Prophylaxis[5]	-	-	86%	85%
Warfarin Therapy Discharge Instructions[5]	-	-	74%	75%
Chest Pain/Possible Heart Attack Care				
Aspirin Given Within 24 Hours of Arrival	91	100%	97%	96%
Fibrinolytic Meds Within 30 Min. of Arrival[7]	-	-	51%	58%
Average Time to ECG (minutes)	92	10	9	7
Average Time to Transfer (minutes)	37	196	54	60
Children's Asthma Care				
Received Home Management Plan of Care	-	-	-	88%
Received Reliever Medication	-	-	-	100%
Received Systemic Corticosteroids	-	-	-	100%
Emergency Department				
Admittance Decision Time (minutes)[5]	-	-	96	98
Head CT Results Within 45 Min. of Arrival[5]	-	-	63%	57%
Patients Who Left ER Before Being Seen[5]	-	-	2%	2%
Time from ER Arrival to Admit. (minutes)[5]	-	-	259	274
Time from ER Arrival to Discharge (minutes)[5]	-	-	135	134
Time in ER Before Being Evaluated (minutes)[5]	-	-	22	26
Time to Pain Meds for Fractures (minutes)[5]	-	-	52	57
Heart Attack Care				
Aspirin Given at Discharge[3,7]	-	-	99%	99%
Fibrinolytic Meds Within 30 Min. of Arrival[3,7]	-	-	62%	54%
PCI Within 90 Minutes of Arrival[3,7]	-	-	97%	96%
Statin Prescribed at Discharge[3,7]	-	-	98%	98%
Heart Failure Care				
ACE Inhibitor or ARB for LVSD[1]	-	-	97%	97%
Discharge Instructions Given	12	92%	93%	94%
Evaluation of LVS Function	18	100%	99%	99%
Medicare Spending				
Medicare Spending per Patient (ratio)	-	-	0.91	0.98
Pneumonia Care				
Appropriate Initial Antibiotic Given	50	98%	96%	95%
Blood Culture Timing	57	93%	97%	98%
Pregnancy and Delivery Care				
Newborn Deliveries Scheduled Early[5]	-	-	2%	6%
Preventive Care				
Immunization for Influenza[5]	-	-	91%	90%
Immunization for Pneumonia[5]	-	-	91%	92%
Stroke Care				
Anticoagulation Therapy for Atrial Fibrillation[5]	-	-	94%	95%
Antithrombotic Therapy Timing[5]	-	-	98%	98%
Assessed for Rehabilitation[5]	-	-	98%	97%
Discharged on Antithrombotic Therapy[5]	-	-	99%	99%
Discharged on Statin Medication[5]	-	-	96%	94%
Thrombolytic Therapy Timing[5]	-	-	73%	66%
Venous Thromboembolism Prophylaxis[5]	-	-	94%	94%
Written Stroke Educational Materials Given[5]	-	-	86%	88%
Surgical Care Improvement Project				
Appropriate Beta Blocker Usage[1]	-	-	98%	98%
Appropriate VTP Within 24 Hours	15	93%	98%	98%
Controlled Postoperative Blood Glucose[7]	-	-	97%	97%
Perioperative Temperature Management	16	100%	100%	100%
Prophylactic Antibiotic Selection[1]	-	-	99%	99%
Prophylactic Antibiotic Selection (Outpatient)[1,3]	-	-	98%	98%
Prophylactic Antibiotic Stopped[1]	-	-	99%	98%
Prophylactic Antibiotic Timing[1]	-	-	98%	99%
Prophylactic Antibiotic Timing (Outpatient)[1,3]	-	-	98%	98%
Urinary Catheter Removal	13	77%	97%	97%
Survey of Patients' Hospital Experiences				
Area Around Room 'Always' Quiet at Night	(a)	63%	54%	61%
Doctors 'Always' Communicated Well	(a)	80%	81%	82%
Home Recovery Information Given	(a)	86%	87%	85%
Hospital Given 9 or 10 on 10 Point Scale	(a)	72%	70%	71%
Meds 'Always' Explained Before Given	(a)	63%	64%	64%
Nurses 'Always' Communicated Well	(a)	79%	77%	79%
Pain 'Always' Well Controlled	(a)	76%	70%	71%
Room and Bathroom 'Always' Clean	(a)	85%	73%	73%
Timely Help 'Always' Received	(a)	79%	65%	68%
Would Definitely Recommend Hospital	(a)	77%	73%	71%
Use of Medical Imaging				
Cardiac Imaging Stress Test before Surgery[1]	-	-	4.3%	5.3%
Combination Abdominal CT Scan	404	5.2%	6.9%	10.5%
Combination Brain/Sinus CT Scan[1]	-	-	2.3%	2.7%
Combination Chest CT Scan	283	0.0%	1.1%	2.7%
Follow-up Mammogram/Ultrasound	536	9.1%	9.1%	8.8%
Lumbar Spine MRI for Low Back Pain	53	35.8%	37.9%	37.2%

Mason General Hospital & Family of Clinics

901 Mt View Drive
Shelton, WA 98584
Phone: 360-426-1611
Fax: 360-427-3603
URL: www.masongeneral.com
Type: Critical Access Hospitals
Emergency Services: Yes
Ownership: Govt - Hospital Dist/Auth
Beds: 68
Key Personnel:
Chief of Medical Staff . . . . Bonnie J Davis
Radiology. . . . . David Luethekhans
President . . . . Don Wilson

Measure	Cases	This Hosp.	State Avg.	U.S. Avg.
Blood Clot Prevention and Treatment				
Anticoagulation Overlap Therapy[5]	-	-	97%	93%
ICU Venous Thromboembolism Prophylaxis[5]	-	-	92%	92%
Incidence of Potentially Preventable VTE[5]	-	-	9%	10%
UFH with Dosages/Platelet Monitoring[5]	-	-	99%	97%
Venous Thromboembolism Prophylaxis[5]	-	-	86%	85%
Warfarin Therapy Discharge Instructions[5]	-	-	74%	75%
Chest Pain/Possible Heart Attack Care				
Aspirin Given Within 24 Hours of Arrival	-	-	97%	96%
Fibrinolytic Meds Within 30 Min. of Arrival	-	-	51%	58%
Average Time to ECG (minutes)	-	-	9	7
Average Time to Transfer (minutes)	-	-	54	60
Children's Asthma Care				
Received Home Management Plan of Care	-	-	-	88%
Received Reliever Medication	-	-	-	100%
Received Systemic Corticosteroids	-	-	-	100%
Emergency Department				
Admittance Decision Time (minutes)[5]	-	-	96	98
Head CT Results Within 45 Min. of Arrival	-	-	63%	57%
Patients Who Left ER Before Being Seen	-	-	2%	2%
Time from ER Arrival to Admit. (minutes)[5]	-	-	259	274
Time from ER Arrival to Discharge (minutes)	-	-	135	134
Time in ER Before Being Evaluated (minutes)	-	-	22	26
Time to Pain Meds for Fractures (minutes)	-	-	52	57
Heart Attack Care				
Aspirin Given at Discharge[1,3]	-	-	99%	99%
Fibrinolytic Meds Within 30 Min. of Arrival[3,7]	-	-	62%	54%
PCI Within 90 Minutes of Arrival[3,7]	-	-	97%	96%

NOTE: Hospital profiles are in alphabetical order by state, then city, then hospital within the city; Rankings exclude hospitals with less than 25 cases except for patient surveys which excludes hospitals with less than 100 cases; (a) 100-299 cases; (1) The number of cases/patients is too few to report; (2) Data submitted were based on a sample of cases/patients; (3) Results are based on a shorter time period than required; (4) Data suppressed by CMS for one or more quarters; (5) Results are not available for this reporting period; (6) Fewer than 100 patients completed the HCAHPS survey; (7) No cases met the criteria for this measure; (8) The lower limit of the confidence interval cannot be calculated if the number of observed infections equals zero; (9) No data are available from the state/territory for this reporting period; (10) The scores shown reflect fewer than 50 completed surveys; (11) There were discrepancies in the data collection process; (12) This measure does not apply to this hospital for this reporting period; (13) Results cannot be calculated for this reporting period; (14) The results for this state are combined with nearby states to protect confidentiality; Please refer to the User's Guide for a full explanation of data.

Measure	Cases	This Hosp.	State Avg.	U.S. Avg.
Statin Prescribed at Discharge[1,3]	-	-	98%	98%
Heart Failure Care				
ACE Inhibitor or ARB for LVSD	14	100%	97%	97%
Discharge Instructions Given	39	100%	93%	94%
Evaluation of LVS Function	52	100%	99%	99%
Medicare Spending				
Medicare Spending per Patient (ratio)		-	0.91	0.98
Pneumonia Care				
Appropriate Initial Antibiotic Given	60	93%	96%	95%
Blood Culture Timing	71	92%	97%	98%
Pregnancy and Delivery Care				
Newborn Deliveries Scheduled Early[5]	-	-	2%	6%
Preventive Care				
Immunization for Influenza[5]	-	-	91%	90%
Immunization for Pneumonia[5]	-	-	91%	92%
Stroke Care				
Anticoagulation Therapy for Atrial Fibrillation[5]	-	-	94%	95%
Antithrombotic Therapy Timing[5]	-	-	98%	98%
Assessed for Rehabilitation[5]	-	-	98%	97%
Discharged on Antithrombotic Therapy[5]	-	-	99%	99%
Discharged on Statin Medication[5]	-	-	96%	94%
Thrombolytic Therapy Timing[5]	-	-	73%	66%
Venous Thromboembolism Prophylaxis[5]	-	-	94%	94%
Written Stroke Educational Materials Given[5]	-	-	86%	88%
Surgical Care Improvement Project				
Appropriate Beta Blocker Usage	27	100%	98%	98%
Appropriate VTP Within 24 Hours	87	97%	98%	98%
Controlled Postoperative Blood Glucose[7]	-	-	97%	97%
Perioperative Temperature Management	104	100%	100%	100%
Prophylactic Antibiotic Selection	62	98%	99%	99%
Prophylactic Antibiotic Selection (Outpatient)	-	-	98%	98%
Prophylactic Antibiotic Stopped	61	100%	99%	98%
Prophylactic Antibiotic Timing	62	92%	98%	99%
Prophylactic Antibiotic Timing (Outpatient)	-	-	98%	98%
Urinary Catheter Removal	60	100%	97%	97%
Survey of Patients' Hospital Experiences				
Area Around Room 'Always' Quiet at Night[5]	-	-	54%	61%
Doctors 'Always' Communicated Well[5]	-	-	81%	82%
Home Recovery Information Given[5]	-	-	87%	85%
Hospital Given 9 or 10 on 10 Point Scale[5]	-	-	70%	71%
Meds 'Always' Explained Before Given[5]	-	-	64%	64%
Nurses 'Always' Communicated Well[5]	-	-	77%	79%
Pain 'Always' Well Controlled[5]	-	-	70%	71%
Room and Bathroom 'Always' Clean[5]	-	-	73%	73%
Timely Help 'Always' Received[5]	-	-	65%	68%
Would Definitely Recommend Hospital[5]	-	-	73%	71%
Use of Medical Imaging				
Cardiac Imaging Stress Test before Surgery	-	-	4.3%	5.3%
Combination Abdominal CT Scan	-	-	6.9%	10.5%
Combination Brain/Sinus CT Scan	-	-	2.3%	2.7%
Combination Chest CT Scan	-	-	1.1%	2.7%
Follow-up Mammogram/Ultrasound	-	-	9.1%	8.8%
Lumbar Spine MRI for Low Back Pain	-	-	37.9%	37.2%

Snoqualmie Valley Hospital

9575 Ethan Wade Way Se Phone: 425-831-2300
Snoqualmie, WA 98065
URL: www.snoqualmiehospital.org
Type: Critical Access Hospitals Emergency Services: Yes
Ownership: Govt - Hospital Dist/Auth Beds: 18
Key Personnel:
CEO . . . . Rodger McCollum

Measure	Cases	This Hosp.	State Avg.	U.S. Avg.
Blood Clot Prevention and Treatment				
Anticoagulation Overlap Therapy[5]	-	-	97%	93%
ICU Venous Thromboembolism Prophylaxis[5]	-	-	92%	92%
Incidence of Potentially Preventable VTE[5]	-	-	9%	10%
UFH with Dosages/Platelet Monitoring[5]	-	-	99%	97%
Venous Thromboembolism Prophylaxis[5]	-	-	86%	85%
Warfarin Therapy Discharge Instructions[5]	-	-	74%	75%
Chest Pain/Possible Heart Attack Care				
Aspirin Given Within 24 Hours of Arrival[1,3]	-	-	97%	96%
Fibrinolytic Meds Within 30 Min. of Arrival[3,7]	-	-	51%	58%
Average Time to ECG (minutes)[1,3]	-	-	9	7
Average Time to Transfer (minutes)[3,7]	-	-	54	60
Children's Asthma Care				
Received Home Management Plan of Care	-	-	-	88%
Received Reliever Medication	-	-	-	100%
Received Systemic Corticosteroids	-	-	-	100%
Emergency Department				
Admittance Decision Time (minutes)[5]	-	-	96	98
Head CT Results Within 45 Min. of Arrival[5]	-	-	63%	57%
Patients Who Left ER Before Being Seen[5]	-	-	2%	2%
Time from ER Arrival to Admit. (minutes)[5]	-	-	259	274
Time from ER Arrival to Discharge (minutes)[5]	-	-	135	134
Time in ER Before Being Evaluated (minutes)[5]	-	-	22	26
Time to Pain Meds for Fractures (minutes)[5]	-	-	52	57
Heart Attack Care				
Aspirin Given at Discharge[5]	-	-	99%	99%
Fibrinolytic Meds Within 30 Min. of Arrival[5]	-	-	62%	54%
PCI Within 90 Minutes of Arrival[5]	-	-	97%	96%
Statin Prescribed at Discharge[5]	-	-	98%	98%
Heart Failure Care				
ACE Inhibitor or ARB for LVSD[3,7]	-	-	97%	97%
Discharge Instructions Given[1,3]	-	-	93%	94%
Evaluation of LVS Function[1,3]	-	-	99%	99%
Medicare Spending				
Medicare Spending per Patient (ratio)		-	0.91	0.98
Pneumonia Care				
Appropriate Initial Antibiotic Given[1,3]	-	-	96%	95%
Blood Culture Timing[1,3]	-	-	97%	98%
Pregnancy and Delivery Care				
Newborn Deliveries Scheduled Early[5]	-	-	2%	6%
Preventive Care				
Immunization for Influenza[5]	-	-	91%	90%
Immunization for Pneumonia[5]	-	-	91%	92%
Stroke Care				
Anticoagulation Therapy for Atrial Fibrillation[5]	-	-	94%	95%
Antithrombotic Therapy Timing[5]	-	-	98%	98%
Assessed for Rehabilitation[5]	-	-	98%	97%
Discharged on Antithrombotic Therapy[5]	-	-	99%	99%
Discharged on Statin Medication[5]	-	-	96%	94%
Thrombolytic Therapy Timing[5]	-	-	73%	66%
Venous Thromboembolism Prophylaxis[5]	-	-	94%	94%
Written Stroke Educational Materials Given[5]	-	-	86%	88%
Surgical Care Improvement Project				
Appropriate Beta Blocker Usage[5]	-	-	98%	98%
Appropriate VTP Within 24 Hours[5]	-	-	98%	98%
Controlled Postoperative Blood Glucose[5]	-	-	97%	97%
Perioperative Temperature Management[5]	-	-	100%	100%
Prophylactic Antibiotic Selection[5]	-	-	99%	99%
Prophylactic Antibiotic Selection (Outpatient)[5]	-	-	98%	98%
Prophylactic Antibiotic Stopped[5]	-	-	99%	98%
Prophylactic Antibiotic Timing[5]	-	-	98%	99%
Prophylactic Antibiotic Timing (Outpatient)[5]	-	-	98%	98%
Urinary Catheter Removal[5]	-	-	97%	97%
Survey of Patients' Hospital Experiences				
Area Around Room 'Always' Quiet at Night[5]	-	-	54%	61%
Doctors 'Always' Communicated Well[5]	-	-	81%	82%
Home Recovery Information Given[5]	-	-	87%	85%
Hospital Given 9 or 10 on 10 Point Scale[5]	-	-	70%	71%
Meds 'Always' Explained Before Given[5]	-	-	64%	64%
Nurses 'Always' Communicated Well[5]	-	-	77%	79%
Pain 'Always' Well Controlled[5]	-	-	70%	71%
Room and Bathroom 'Always' Clean[5]	-	-	73%	73%
Timely Help 'Always' Received[5]	-	-	65%	68%
Would Definitely Recommend Hospital[5]	-	-	73%	71%
Use of Medical Imaging				
Cardiac Imaging Stress Test before Surgery[7]	-	-	4.3%	5.3%
Combination Abdominal CT Scan[1]	-	-	6.9%	10.5%
Combination Brain/Sinus CT Scan[1]	-	-	2.3%	2.7%
Combination Chest CT Scan[1]	-	-	1.1%	2.7%
Follow-up Mammogram/Ultrasound[7]	-	-	9.1%	8.8%
Lumbar Spine MRI for Low Back Pain[1]	-	-	37.9%	37.2%

Willapa Harbor Hospital

800 Alder Street Phone: 360-875-5526
South Bend, WA 98586
Type: Critical Access Hospitals Emergency Services: Yes
Ownership: Government - Local

Measure	Cases	This Hosp.	State Avg.	U.S. Avg.
Blood Clot Prevention and Treatment				
Anticoagulation Overlap Therapy[5]	-	-	97%	93%
ICU Venous Thromboembolism Prophylaxis[5]	-	-	92%	92%
Incidence of Potentially Preventable VTE[5]	-	-	9%	10%
UFH with Dosages/Platelet Monitoring[5]	-	-	99%	97%
Venous Thromboembolism Prophylaxis[5]	-	-	86%	85%
Warfarin Therapy Discharge Instructions[5]	-	-	74%	75%
Chest Pain/Possible Heart Attack Care				
Aspirin Given Within 24 Hours of Arrival[1,3]	-	-	97%	96%
Fibrinolytic Meds Within 30 Min. of Arrival[1,3]	-	-	51%	58%
Average Time to ECG (minutes)[1,3]	-	-	9	7
Average Time to Transfer (minutes)[3,7]	-	-	54	60
Children's Asthma Care				
Received Home Management Plan of Care	-	-	-	88%
Received Reliever Medication	-	-	-	100%
Received Systemic Corticosteroids	-	-	-	100%
Emergency Department				
Admittance Decision Time (minutes)[5]	-	-	96	98
Head CT Results Within 45 Min. of Arrival[5]	-	-	63%	57%
Patients Who Left ER Before Being Seen[5]	-	-	2%	2%
Time from ER Arrival to Admit. (minutes)[5]	-	-	259	274
Time from ER Arrival to Discharge (minutes)[5]	-	-	135	134
Time in ER Before Being Evaluated (minutes)[5]	-	-	22	26
Time to Pain Meds for Fractures (minutes)[5]	-	-	52	57
Heart Attack Care				
Aspirin Given at Discharge[5]	-	-	99%	99%
Fibrinolytic Meds Within 30 Min. of Arrival[5]	-	-	62%	54%
PCI Within 90 Minutes of Arrival[5]	-	-	97%	96%
Statin Prescribed at Discharge[5]	-	-	98%	98%
Heart Failure Care				
ACE Inhibitor or ARB for LVSD[1,2]	-	-	97%	97%
Discharge Instructions Given[1,2]	-	-	93%	94%
Evaluation of LVS Function[1,2]	-	-	99%	99%
Medicare Spending				
Medicare Spending per Patient (ratio)		-	0.91	0.98
Pneumonia Care				
Appropriate Initial Antibiotic Given[2]	44	84%	96%	95%
Blood Culture Timing[2]	38	89%	97%	98%
Pregnancy and Delivery Care				
Newborn Deliveries Scheduled Early[5]	-	-	2%	6%
Preventive Care				
Immunization for Influenza[5]	-	-	91%	90%
Immunization for Pneumonia[5]	-	-	91%	92%
Stroke Care				
Anticoagulation Therapy for Atrial Fibrillation[5]	-	-	94%	95%
Antithrombotic Therapy Timing[5]	-	-	98%	98%
Assessed for Rehabilitation[5]	-	-	98%	97%
Discharged on Antithrombotic Therapy[5]	-	-	99%	99%
Discharged on Statin Medication[5]	-	-	96%	94%
Thrombolytic Therapy Timing[5]	-	-	73%	66%
Venous Thromboembolism Prophylaxis[5]	-	-	94%	94%
Written Stroke Educational Materials Given[5]	-	-	86%	88%
Surgical Care Improvement Project				
Appropriate Beta Blocker Usage[2,3]	-	-	98%	98%
Appropriate VTP Within 24 Hours[1,2]	-	-	98%	98%
Controlled Postoperative Blood Glucose[2,3]	-	-	97%	97%
Perioperative Temperature Management[1,2]	-	-	100%	100%
Prophylactic Antibiotic Selection[1,2]	-	-	99%	99%
Prophylactic Antibiotic Selection (Outpatient)[5]	-	-	98%	98%
Prophylactic Antibiotic Stopped[1,2]	-	-	99%	98%
Prophylactic Antibiotic Timing[1,2]	-	-	98%	99%
Prophylactic Antibiotic Timing (Outpatient)[5]	-	-	98%	98%
Urinary Catheter Removal[1,2]	-	-	97%	97%
Survey of Patients' Hospital Experiences				
Area Around Room 'Always' Quiet at Night[5]	-	-	54%	61%
Doctors 'Always' Communicated Well[5]	-	-	81%	82%

NOTE: Hospital profiles are in alphabetical order by state, then city, then hospital within the city; Rankings exclude hospitals with less than 25 cases except for patient surveys which excludes hospitals with less than 100 cases; (a) 100-299 cases; (1) The number of cases/patients is too few to report; (2) Data submitted were based on a sample of cases/patients; (3) Results are based on a shorter time period than required; (4) Data suppressed by CMS for one or more quarters; (5) Results are not available for this reporting period; (6) Fewer than 100 patients completed the HCAHPS survey; (7) No cases met the criteria for this measure; (8) The lower limit of the confidence interval cannot be calculated if the number of observed infections equals zero; (9) No data are available from the state/territory for this reporting period; (10) The scores shown reflect fewer than 50 completed surveys; (11) There were discrepancies in the data collection process; (12) This measure does not apply to this hospital for this reporting period; (13) Results cannot be calculated for this reporting period; (14) The results for this state are combined with nearby states to protect confidentiality; Please refer to the User's Guide for a full explanation of data.

Measure	Cases	This Hosp.	State Avg.	U.S. Avg.
Home Recovery Information Given[5]	-	-	87%	85%
Hospital Given 9 or 10 on 10 Point Scale[5]	-	-	70%	71%
Meds 'Always' Explained Before Given[5]	-	-	64%	64%
Nurses 'Always' Communicated Well[5]	-	-	77%	79%
Pain 'Always' Well Controlled[5]	-	-	70%	71%
Room and Bathroom 'Always' Clean[5]	-	-	73%	73%
Timely Help 'Always' Received[5]	-	-	65%	68%
Would Definitely Recommend Hospital[5]	-	-	73%	71%
Use of Medical Imaging				
Cardiac Imaging Stress Test before Surgery[1]	-	-	4.3%	5.3%
Combination Abdominal CT Scan	180	3.3%	6.9%	10.5%
Combination Brain/Sinus CT Scan[1]	-	-	2.3%	2.7%
Combination Chest CT Scan	107	2.8%	1.1%	2.7%
Follow-up Mammogram/Ultrasound	179	12.3%	9.1%	8.8%
Lumbar Spine MRI for Low Back Pain[1]	-	-	37.9%	37.2%

Deaconess Hospital

W 800 Fifth Avenue Phone: 509-473-5800
Spokane, WA 99210 Fax: 509-473-7684
E-mail: deaconess@empirehealth.org
URL: www.deaconessmedicalcenter.org
Type: Acute Care Hospitals Emergency Services: Yes
Ownership: Voluntary non-profit - Private Beds: 388

Key Personnel:
Infection Control. . . . . Margaret Christian
Quality Assurance . . . . Dave Martin
Operating Room. . . . . Carol Messoramith
Intensive Care Unit. . . . . Sherry Nosh
Chief of Medical Staff . . . . Angie O'Brien
Pediatric In-Patient Care . . . . Frank Reynolds, MD
CEO/President. . . . . Thomas White
Emergency Room . . . . Pat Yost

Measure	Cases	This Hosp.	State Avg.	U.S. Avg.
Blood Clot Prevention and Treatment				
Anticoagulation Overlap Therapy[2]	63	98%	97%	93%
ICU Venous Thromboembolism Prophylaxis[2]	76	96%	92%	92%
Incidence of Potentially Preventable VTE[1,2]	-	-	9%	10%
UFH with Dosages/Platelet Monitoring[2]	46	100%	99%	97%
Venous Thromboembolism Prophylaxis[2]	372	96%	86%	85%
Warfarin Therapy Discharge Instructions[2]	51	90%	74%	75%
Chest Pain/Possible Heart Attack Care				
Aspirin Given Within 24 Hours of Arrival[1,3]	-	-	97%	96%
Fibrinolytic Meds Within 30 Min. of Arrival[5]	-	-	51%	58%
Average Time to ECG (minutes)[1,3]	-	-	9	7
Average Time to Transfer (minutes)[5]	-	-	54	60
Children's Asthma Care				
Received Home Management Plan of Care	-	-	-	88%
Received Reliever Medication	-	-	-	100%
Received Systemic Corticosteroids	-	-	-	100%
Emergency Department				
Admittance Decision Time (minutes)[2]	377	61	96	98
Head CT Results Within 45 Min. of Arrival[1]	-	-	63%	57%
Patients Who Left ER Before Being Seen	25,694	2%	2%	2%
Time from ER Arrival to Admit. (minutes)[2]	495	222	259	274
Time from ER Arrival to Discharge (minutes)	388	140	135	134
Time in ER Before Being Evaluated (minutes)	369	26	22	26
Time to Pain Meds for Fractures (minutes)	49	52	52	57
Heart Attack Care				
Aspirin Given at Discharge	246	100%	99%	99%
Fibrinolytic Meds Within 30 Min. of Arrival[7]	-	-	62%	54%
PCI Within 90 Minutes of Arrival	20	100%	97%	96%
Statin Prescribed at Discharge	235	100%	98%	98%
Heart Failure Care				
ACE Inhibitor or ARB for LVSD	87	99%	97%	97%
Discharge Instructions Given	187	96%	93%	94%
Evaluation of LVS Function	224	100%	99%	99%
Medicare Spending				
Medicare Spending per Patient (ratio)	-	0.99	0.91	0.98
Pneumonia Care				
Appropriate Initial Antibiotic Given	104	97%	96%	95%
Blood Culture Timing	142	100%	97%	98%
Pregnancy and Delivery Care				
Newborn Deliveries Scheduled Early[2]	25	4%	2%	6%
Preventive Care				
Immunization for Influenza[2]	606	98%	91%	90%
Immunization for Pneumonia[2]	714	99%	91%	92%
Stroke Care				
Anticoagulation Therapy for Atrial Fibrillation	13	100%	94%	95%
Antithrombotic Therapy Timing	65	98%	98%	98%
Assessed for Rehabilitation	91	98%	98%	97%
Discharged on Antithrombotic Therapy	77	100%	99%	99%
Discharged on Statin Medication	64	100%	96%	94%
Thrombolytic Therapy Timing[1]	-	-	73%	66%
Venous Thromboembolism Prophylaxis	85	99%	94%	94%
Written Stroke Educational Materials Given	58	95%	86%	88%
Surgical Care Improvement Project				
Appropriate Beta Blocker Usage	285	99%	98%	98%
Appropriate VTP Within 24 Hours	906	100%	98%	98%
Controlled Postoperative Blood Glucose	116	94%	97%	97%
Perioperative Temperature Management	1,037	100%	100%	100%
Prophylactic Antibiotic Selection	571	99%	99%	99%
Prophylactic Antibiotic Selection (Outpatient)	515	98%	98%	98%
Prophylactic Antibiotic Stopped	527	98%	99%	98%
Prophylactic Antibiotic Timing	571	99%	98%	99%
Prophylactic Antibiotic Timing (Outpatient)	515	99%	98%	98%
Urinary Catheter Removal	578	99%	97%	97%
Survey of Patients' Hospital Experiences				
Area Around Room 'Always' Quiet at Night	300+	58%	54%	61%
Doctors 'Always' Communicated Well	300+	81%	81%	82%
Home Recovery Information Given	300+	88%	87%	85%
Hospital Given 9 or 10 on 10 Point Scale	300+	68%	70%	71%
Meds 'Always' Explained Before Given	300+	65%	64%	64%
Nurses 'Always' Communicated Well	300+	75%	77%	79%
Pain 'Always' Well Controlled	300+	70%	70%	71%
Room and Bathroom 'Always' Clean	300+	63%	73%	73%
Timely Help 'Always' Received	300+	59%	65%	68%
Would Definitely Recommend Hospital	300+	70%	73%	71%
Use of Medical Imaging				
Cardiac Imaging Stress Test before Surgery	1,185	3.2%	4.3%	5.3%
Combination Abdominal CT Scan	338	0.6%	6.9%	10.5%
Combination Brain/Sinus CT Scan	357	6.7%	2.3%	2.7%
Combination Chest CT Scan	75	0.0%	1.1%	2.7%
Follow-up Mammogram/Ultrasound	562	11.2%	9.1%	8.8%
Lumbar Spine MRI for Low Back Pain[1]	-	-	37.9%	37.2%

Providence Holy Family Hospital

5633 North Lidgerwood Phone: 509-482-2450
Spokane, WA 99208 Fax: 509-482-2587
E-mail: crabtrl@holy-family.org
URL: www.holy-family.org
Type: Acute Care Hospitals Emergency Services: Yes
Ownership: Voluntary non-profit - Church Beds: 272

Key Personnel:
Hemotology Center . . . . Marna Bateman
Intensive Care Unit. . . . . Kay Ely
CEO/President. . . . . Alex Jackson
Pediatric In-Patient Care . . . . Mary McCarthy
Infection Control. . . . . Kim Richardson
Quality Assurance . . . . Janis Simpson
Emergency Room . . . . Robbie Thorn
Radiology. . . . . Al Wichtendahl

Measure	Cases	This Hosp.	State Avg.	U.S. Avg.
Blood Clot Prevention and Treatment				
Anticoagulation Overlap Therapy[2]	96	99%	97%	93%
ICU Venous Thromboembolism Prophylaxis[2]	56	96%	92%	92%
Incidence of Potentially Preventable VTE[1,2]	-	-	9%	10%
UFH with Dosages/Platelet Monitoring[2]	86	100%	99%	97%
Venous Thromboembolism Prophylaxis[2]	291	89%	86%	85%
Warfarin Therapy Discharge Instructions[2]	79	75%	74%	75%
Chest Pain/Possible Heart Attack Care				
Aspirin Given Within 24 Hours of Arrival	104	93%	97%	96%
Fibrinolytic Meds Within 30 Min. of Arrival[7]	-	-	51%	58%
Average Time to ECG (minutes)	110	12	9	7
Average Time to Transfer (minutes)	25	47	54	60
Children's Asthma Care				
Received Home Management Plan of Care	-	-	-	88%
Received Reliever Medication	-	-	-	100%
Received Systemic Corticosteroids	-	-	-	100%
Emergency Department				
Admittance Decision Time (minutes)[2]	593	129	96	98
Head CT Results Within 45 Min. of Arrival[1]	-	-	63%	57%
Patients Who Left ER Before Being Seen	64,776	3%	2%	2%
Time from ER Arrival to Admit. (minutes)[2]	646	323	259	274
Time from ER Arrival to Discharge (minutes)	366	152	135	134
Time in ER Before Being Evaluated (minutes)	383	31	22	26
Time to Pain Meds for Fractures (minutes)	193	67	52	57
Heart Attack Care				
Aspirin Given at Discharge	28	100%	99%	99%
Fibrinolytic Meds Within 30 Min. of Arrival[7]	-	-	62%	54%
PCI Within 90 Minutes of Arrival[7]	-	-	97%	96%
Statin Prescribed at Discharge	28	89%	98%	98%
Heart Failure Care				
ACE Inhibitor or ARB for LVSD	54	93%	97%	97%
Discharge Instructions Given	130	92%	93%	94%
Evaluation of LVS Function	169	99%	99%	99%
Medicare Spending				
Medicare Spending per Patient (ratio)	-	0.97	0.91	0.98
Pneumonia Care				
Appropriate Initial Antibiotic Given	214	99%	96%	95%
Blood Culture Timing	276	98%	97%	98%
Pregnancy and Delivery Care				
Newborn Deliveries Scheduled Early[2]	17	0%	2%	6%
Preventive Care				
Immunization for Influenza[2]	508	98%	91%	90%
Immunization for Pneumonia[2]	597	94%	91%	92%
Stroke Care				
Anticoagulation Therapy for Atrial Fibrillation	18	72%	94%	95%
Antithrombotic Therapy Timing	99	99%	98%	98%
Assessed for Rehabilitation	116	99%	98%	97%
Discharged on Antithrombotic Therapy	109	100%	99%	99%
Discharged on Statin Medication	75	92%	96%	94%
Thrombolytic Therapy Timing	13	54%	73%	66%
Venous Thromboembolism Prophylaxis	104	93%	94%	94%
Written Stroke Educational Materials Given	72	93%	86%	88%
Surgical Care Improvement Project				
Appropriate Beta Blocker Usage[2]	69	100%	98%	98%
Appropriate VTP Within 24 Hours[2]	287	98%	98%	98%
Controlled Postoperative Blood Glucose[2,7]	-	-	97%	97%
Perioperative Temperature Management[2]	336	100%	100%	100%
Prophylactic Antibiotic Selection[2]	222	99%	99%	99%
Prophylactic Antibiotic Selection (Outpatient)	231	98%	98%	98%
Prophylactic Antibiotic Stopped[2]	213	99%	99%	98%
Prophylactic Antibiotic Timing[2]	222	100%	98%	99%
Prophylactic Antibiotic Timing (Outpatient)	234	97%	98%	98%
Urinary Catheter Removal[2]	128	99%	97%	97%
Survey of Patients' Hospital Experiences				
Area Around Room 'Always' Quiet at Night	300+	46%	54%	61%
Doctors 'Always' Communicated Well	300+	77%	81%	82%
Home Recovery Information Given	300+	84%	87%	85%
Hospital Given 9 or 10 on 10 Point Scale	300+	68%	70%	71%
Meds 'Always' Explained Before Given	300+	61%	64%	64%
Nurses 'Always' Communicated Well	300+	77%	77%	79%
Pain 'Always' Well Controlled	300+	69%	70%	71%
Room and Bathroom 'Always' Clean	300+	74%	73%	73%
Timely Help 'Always' Received	300+	61%	65%	68%
Would Definitely Recommend Hospital	300+	73%	73%	71%
Use of Medical Imaging				
Cardiac Imaging Stress Test before Surgery	79	6.3%	4.3%	5.3%
Combination Abdominal CT Scan	634	0.3%	6.9%	10.5%
Combination Brain/Sinus CT Scan	705	6.1%	2.3%	2.7%
Combination Chest CT Scan	63	0.0%	1.1%	2.7%
Follow-up Mammogram/Ultrasound[7]	-	-	9.1%	8.8%
Lumbar Spine MRI for Low Back Pain[1]	-	-	37.9%	37.2%

NOTE: Hospital profiles are in alphabetical order by state, then city, then hospital within the city; Rankings exclude hospitals with less than 25 cases except for patient surveys which excludes hospitals with less than 100 cases; (a) 100-299 cases; (1) The number of cases/patients is too few to report; (2) Data submitted were based on a sample of cases/patients; (3) Results are based on a shorter time period than required; (4) Data suppressed by CMS for one or more quarters; (5) Results are not available for this reporting period; (6) Fewer than 100 patients completed the HCAHPS survey; (7) No cases met the criteria for this measure; (8) The lower limit of the confidence interval cannot be calculated if the number of observed infections equals zero; (9) No data are available from the state/territory for this reporting period; (10) The scores shown reflect fewer than 50 completed surveys; (11) There were discrepancies in the data collection process; (12) This measure does not apply to this hospital for this reporting period; (13) Results cannot be calculated for this reporting period; (14) The results for this state are combined with nearby states to protect confidentiality; Please refer to the User's Guide for a full explanation of data.

Providence Sacred Heart Medical Center

101 West 8th Avenue Phone: 509-474-3040
Spokane, WA 99204 Fax: 509-474-3153
E-mail: pr@shmc.org
URL: www.shmc.org
Type: Acute Care Hospitals Emergency Services: Yes
Ownership: Voluntary non-profit - Church Beds: 623

Key Personnel:
Radiology. . . . . Gerry Altermatt
Operating Room. . . . . Marilyn Bash
Patient Relations . . . . Brenda Gramling
CEO/President. . . . . Alex Jackson
Chief of Medical Staff. . . . . G Thomas Miller, MD

Measure	Cases	This Hosp.	State Avg.	U.S. Avg.
Blood Clot Prevention and Treatment				
Anticoagulation Overlap Therapy[2]	119	99%	97%	93%
ICU Venous Thromboembolism Prophylaxis[2]	103	94%	92%	92%
Incidence of Potentially Preventable VTE[2]	14	0%	9%	10%
UFH with Dosages/Platelet Monitoring[2]	110	99%	99%	97%
Venous Thromboembolism Prophylaxis[2]	264	84%	86%	85%
Warfarin Therapy Discharge Instructions[2]	92	91%	74%	75%
Chest Pain/Possible Heart Attack Care				
Aspirin Given Within 24 Hours of Arrival[1,3]	-	-	97%	96%
Fibrinolytic Meds Within 30 Min. of Arrival[3,7]	-	-	51%	58%
Average Time to ECG (minutes)[1,3]	-	-	9	7
Average Time to Transfer (minutes)[3,7]	-	-	54	60
Children's Asthma Care				
Received Home Management Plan of Care	48	65%	-	88%
Received Reliever Medication	48	100%	-	100%
Received Systemic Corticosteroids	48	100%	-	100%
Emergency Department				
Admittance Decision Time (minutes)[2]	293	53	96	98
Head CT Results Within 45 Min. of Arrival[1]	-	-	63%	57%
Patients Who Left ER Before Being Seen	71,543	3%	2%	2%
Time from ER Arrival to Admit. (minutes)[2]	422	211	259	274
Time from ER Arrival to Discharge (minutes)	328	176	135	134
Time in ER Before Being Evaluated (minutes)	260	54	22	26
Time to Pain Meds for Fractures (minutes)	204	48	52	57
Heart Attack Care				
Aspirin Given at Discharge	674	100%	99%	99%
Fibrinolytic Meds Within 30 Min. of Arrival[7]	-	-	62%	54%
PCI Within 90 Minutes of Arrival	92	98%	97%	96%
Statin Prescribed at Discharge	649	100%	98%	98%
Heart Failure Care				
ACE Inhibitor or ARB for LVSD	160	97%	97%	97%
Discharge Instructions Given	342	92%	93%	94%
Evaluation of LVS Function	426	100%	99%	99%
Medicare Spending				
Medicare Spending per Patient (ratio)	-	0.94	0.91	0.98
Pneumonia Care				
Appropriate Initial Antibiotic Given	194	92%	96%	95%
Blood Culture Timing	290	97%	97%	98%
Pregnancy and Delivery Care				
Newborn Deliveries Scheduled Early[2]	29	0%	2%	6%
Preventive Care				
Immunization for Influenza[2]	522	94%	91%	90%
Immunization for Pneumonia[2]	525	90%	91%	92%
Stroke Care				
Anticoagulation Therapy for Atrial Fibrillation	72	96%	94%	95%
Antithrombotic Therapy Timing	268	98%	98%	98%
Assessed for Rehabilitation	405	99%	98%	97%
Discharged on Antithrombotic Therapy	336	100%	99%	99%
Discharged on Statin Medication	255	100%	96%	94%
Thrombolytic Therapy Timing	27	93%	73%	66%
Venous Thromboembolism Prophylaxis	403	98%	94%	94%
Written Stroke Educational Materials Given	193	90%	86%	88%
Surgical Care Improvement Project				
Appropriate Beta Blocker Usage[2]	162	99%	98%	98%
Appropriate VTP Within 24 Hours[2]	330	100%	98%	98%
Controlled Postoperative Blood Glucose[2]	131	98%	97%	97%
Perioperative Temperature Management[2]	469	100%	100%	100%
Prophylactic Antibiotic Selection[2]	409	99%	99%	99%
Prophylactic Antibiotic Selection (Outpatient)	789	98%	98%	98%
Prophylactic Antibiotic Stopped[2]	401	99%	99%	98%
Prophylactic Antibiotic Timing[2]	409	99%	98%	99%
Prophylactic Antibiotic Timing (Outpatient)	790	98%	98%	98%
Urinary Catheter Removal[2]	370	99%	97%	97%
Survey of Patients' Hospital Experiences				
Area Around Room 'Always' Quiet at Night	300+	50%	54%	61%
Doctors 'Always' Communicated Well	300+	79%	81%	82%
Home Recovery Information Given	300+	87%	87%	85%
Hospital Given 9 or 10 on 10 Point Scale	300+	72%	70%	71%
Meds 'Always' Explained Before Given	300+	61%	64%	64%
Nurses 'Always' Communicated Well	300+	77%	77%	79%
Pain 'Always' Well Controlled	300+	71%	70%	71%
Room and Bathroom 'Always' Clean	300+	72%	73%	73%
Timely Help 'Always' Received	300+	66%	65%	68%
Would Definitely Recommend Hospital	300+	79%	73%	71%
Use of Medical Imaging				
Cardiac Imaging Stress Test before Surgery	1,143	4.2%	4.3%	5.3%
Combination Abdominal CT Scan	489	0.2%	6.9%	10.5%
Combination Brain/Sinus CT Scan	715	4.2%	2.3%	2.7%
Combination Chest CT Scan	121	0.0%	1.1%	2.7%
Follow-up Mammogram/Ultrasound[7]	-	-	9.1%	8.8%
Lumbar Spine MRI for Low Back Pain[1]	-	-	37.9%	37.2%

Spokane VA Medical Center

4815 N. Assembly Street Phone: 509-434-7000
Spokane, WA 99205 Fax: 509-434-7119
URL: www.spokane.med.va.gov
Type: Acute Care - VA Emergency Services: No
Ownership: Government Federal Beds: 88

Key Personnel:
CEO/President. . . . . Hal Blair
Quality Assurance . . . . Thom John
Hemotology Center . . . . Hakan Kaya, MD
Operating Room. . . . . Doug Koch, RN
Chief of Medical Staff. . . . . Nirmala Rozario, MD

Measure	Cases	This Hosp.	State Avg.	U.S. Avg.
Blood Clot Prevention and Treatment				
Anticoagulation Overlap Therapy	-	-	97%	93%
ICU Venous Thromboembolism Prophylaxis	-	-	92%	92%
Incidence of Potentially Preventable VTE	-	-	9%	10%
UFH with Dosages/Platelet Monitoring	-	-	99%	97%
Venous Thromboembolism Prophylaxis	-	-	86%	85%
Warfarin Therapy Discharge Instructions	-	-	74%	75%
Chest Pain/Possible Heart Attack Care				
Aspirin Given Within 24 Hours of Arrival	-	-	97%	96%
Fibrinolytic Meds Within 30 Min. of Arrival	-	-	51%	58%
Average Time to ECG (minutes)	-	-	9	7
Average Time to Transfer (minutes)	-	-	54	60
Children's Asthma Care				
Received Home Management Plan of Care	-	-	-	88%
Received Reliever Medication	-	-	-	100%
Received Systemic Corticosteroids	-	-	-	100%
Emergency Department				
Admittance Decision Time (minutes)	-	-	96	98
Head CT Results Within 45 Min. of Arrival	-	-	63%	57%
Patients Who Left ER Before Being Seen	-	-	2%	2%
Time from ER Arrival to Admit. (minutes)	-	-	259	274
Time from ER Arrival to Discharge (minutes)	-	-	135	134
Time in ER Before Being Evaluated (minutes)	-	-	22	26
Time to Pain Meds for Fractures (minutes)	-	-	52	57
Heart Attack Care				
Aspirin Given at Discharge[1]	-	-	99%	99%
Fibrinolytic Meds Within 30 Min. of Arrival[5]	-	-	62%	54%
PCI Within 90 Minutes of Arrival[5]	-	-	97%	96%
Statin Prescribed at Discharge[1]	-	-	98%	98%
Heart Failure Care				
ACE Inhibitor or ARB for LVSD[1]	-	-	97%	97%
Discharge Instructions Given	36	86%	93%	94%
Evaluation of LVS Function	39	100%	99%	99%
Medicare Spending				
Medicare Spending per Patient (ratio)	-	-	0.91	0.98
Pneumonia Care				
Appropriate Initial Antibiotic Given	27	100%	96%	95%
Blood Culture Timing	38	100%	97%	98%
Pregnancy and Delivery Care				
Newborn Deliveries Scheduled Early	-	-	2%	6%
Preventive Care				
Immunization for Influenza[5]	-	-	91%	90%
Immunization for Pneumonia[5]	-	-	91%	92%
Stroke Care				
Anticoagulation Therapy for Atrial Fibrillation	-	-	94%	95%
Antithrombotic Therapy Timing	-	-	98%	98%
Assessed for Rehabilitation	-	-	98%	97%
Discharged on Antithrombotic Therapy	-	-	99%	99%
Discharged on Statin Medication	-	-	96%	94%
Thrombolytic Therapy Timing	-	-	73%	66%
Venous Thromboembolism Prophylaxis	-	-	94%	94%
Written Stroke Educational Materials Given	-	-	86%	88%
Surgical Care Improvement Project				
Appropriate Beta Blocker Usage[5]	-	-	98%	98%
Appropriate VTP Within 24 Hours[5]	-	-	98%	98%
Controlled Postoperative Blood Glucose[5]	-	-	97%	97%
Perioperative Temperature Management[5]	-	-	100%	100%
Prophylactic Antibiotic Selection[5]	-	-	99%	99%
Prophylactic Antibiotic Selection (Outpatient)	-	-	98%	98%
Prophylactic Antibiotic Stopped[5]	-	-	99%	98%
Prophylactic Antibiotic Timing[5]	-	-	98%	99%
Prophylactic Antibiotic Timing (Outpatient)	-	-	98%	98%
Urinary Catheter Removal[5]	-	-	97%	97%
Survey of Patients' Hospital Experiences				
Area Around Room 'Always' Quiet at Night	-	-	54%	61%
Doctors 'Always' Communicated Well	-	-	81%	82%
Home Recovery Information Given	-	-	87%	85%
Hospital Given 9 or 10 on 10 Point Scale	-	-	70%	71%
Meds 'Always' Explained Before Given	-	-	64%	64%
Nurses 'Always' Communicated Well	-	-	77%	79%
Pain 'Always' Well Controlled	-	-	70%	71%
Room and Bathroom 'Always' Clean	-	-	73%	73%
Timely Help 'Always' Received	-	-	65%	68%
Would Definitely Recommend Hospital	-	-	73%	71%
Use of Medical Imaging				
Cardiac Imaging Stress Test before Surgery	-	-	4.3%	5.3%
Combination Abdominal CT Scan	-	-	6.9%	10.5%
Combination Brain/Sinus CT Scan	-	-	2.3%	2.7%
Combination Chest CT Scan	-	-	1.1%	2.7%
Follow-up Mammogram/Ultrasound	-	-	9.1%	8.8%
Lumbar Spine MRI for Low Back Pain	-	-	37.9%	37.2%

Valley Hospital

12606 East Mission Avenue Phone: 509-924-6650
Spokane, WA 99216 Fax: 509-473-7684
URL: www.valleyhospital.org
Type: Acute Care Hospitals Emergency Services: Yes
Ownership: Voluntary non-profit - Private Beds: 123

Key Personnel:
Operating Room. . . . . Rana N Ahmad
Radiology. . . . . David A Atkins
Emergency Room . . . . T Brodie, MD
Infection Control. . . . . Margaret Christian
Chief of Medical Staff. . . . . Robert Hartman
Quality Assurance . . . . Dave Martin
Intensive Care Unit. . . . . Merriee Moshier
CEO/President. . . . . Jeff Nelson

Measure	Cases	This Hosp.	State Avg.	U.S. Avg.
Blood Clot Prevention and Treatment				
Anticoagulation Overlap Therapy[2]	60	100%	97%	93%
ICU Venous Thromboembolism Prophylaxis[2]	62	100%	92%	92%
Incidence of Potentially Preventable VTE[1,2]	-	-	9%	10%
UFH with Dosages/Platelet Monitoring[2]	50	100%	99%	97%
Venous Thromboembolism Prophylaxis[2]	317	95%	86%	85%
Warfarin Therapy Discharge Instructions[2]	58	91%	74%	75%
Chest Pain/Possible Heart Attack Care				
Aspirin Given Within 24 Hours of Arrival	107	100%	97%	96%
Fibrinolytic Meds Within 30 Min. of Arrival[7]	-	-	51%	58%
Average Time to ECG (minutes)	108	5	9	7
Average Time to Transfer (minutes)	17	47	54	60
Children's Asthma Care				
Received Home Management Plan of Care	-	-	-	88%
Received Reliever Medication	-	-	-	100%

NOTE: Hospital profiles are in alphabetical order by state, then city, then hospital within the city; Rankings exclude hospitals with less than 25 cases except for patient surveys which excludes hospitals with less than 100 cases; (a) 100-299 cases; (1) The number of cases/patients is too few to report; (2) Data submitted were based on a sample of cases/patients; (3) Results are based on a shorter time period than required; (4) Data suppressed by CMS for one or more quarters; (5) Results are not available for this reporting period; (6) Fewer than 100 patients completed the HCAHPS survey; (7) No cases met the criteria for this measure; (8) The lower limit of the confidence interval cannot be calculated if the number of observed infections equals zero; (9) No data are available from the state/territory for this reporting period; (10) The scores shown reflect fewer than 50 completed surveys; (11) There were discrepancies in the data collection process; (12) This measure does not apply to this hospital for this reporting period; (13) Results cannot be calculated for this reporting period; (14) The results for this state are combined with nearby states to protect confidentiality; Please refer to the User's Guide for a full explanation of data.

Measure	Cases	This Hosp.	State Avg.	U.S. Avg.
Received Systemic Corticosteroids	-	-	-	100%
Emergency Department				
Admittance Decision Time (minutes)[2]	686	102	96	98
Head CT Results Within 45 Min. of Arrival[1]	-	-	63%	57%
Patients Who Left ER Before Being Seen	41,280	2%	2%	2%
Time from ER Arrival to Admit. (minutes)[2]	767	275	259	274
Time from ER Arrival to Discharge (minutes)	366	159	135	134
Time in ER Before Being Evaluated (minutes)	293	41	22	26
Time to Pain Meds for Fractures (minutes)	145	50	52	57
Heart Attack Care				
Aspirin Given at Discharge[1]	-	-	99%	99%
Fibrinolytic Meds Within 30 Min. of Arrival[7]	-	-	62%	54%
PCI Within 90 Minutes of Arrival[7]	-	-	97%	96%
Statin Prescribed at Discharge[1]	-	-	98%	98%
Heart Failure Care				
ACE Inhibitor or ARB for LVSD	26	100%	97%	97%
Discharge Instructions Given	92	90%	93%	94%
Evaluation of LVS Function	109	100%	99%	99%
Medicare Spending				
Medicare Spending per Patient (ratio)	-	0.99	0.91	0.98
Pneumonia Care				
Appropriate Initial Antibiotic Given	135	99%	96%	95%
Blood Culture Timing	195	99%	97%	98%
Pregnancy and Delivery Care				
Newborn Deliveries Scheduled Early[2]	44	0%	2%	6%
Preventive Care				
Immunization for Influenza[2]	613	97%	91%	90%
Immunization for Pneumonia[2]	739	97%	91%	92%
Stroke Care				
Anticoagulation Therapy for Atrial Fibrillation[1]	-	-	94%	95%
Antithrombotic Therapy Timing	25	100%	98%	98%
Assessed for Rehabilitation	29	100%	98%	97%
Discharged on Antithrombotic Therapy	28	100%	99%	99%
Discharged on Statin Medication	19	100%	96%	94%
Thrombolytic Therapy Timing[7]	-	-	73%	66%
Venous Thromboembolism Prophylaxis	25	96%	94%	94%
Written Stroke Educational Materials Given	15	80%	86%	88%
Surgical Care Improvement Project				
Appropriate Beta Blocker Usage	145	100%	98%	98%
Appropriate VTP Within 24 Hours	593	99%	98%	98%
Controlled Postoperative Blood Glucose[7]	-	-	97%	97%
Perioperative Temperature Management	680	100%	100%	100%
Prophylactic Antibiotic Selection	519	100%	99%	99%
Prophylactic Antibiotic Selection (Outpatient)	106	98%	98%	98%
Prophylactic Antibiotic Stopped	510	100%	99%	98%
Prophylactic Antibiotic Timing	519	100%	98%	99%
Prophylactic Antibiotic Timing (Outpatient)	106	98%	98%	98%
Urinary Catheter Removal	538	99%	97%	97%
Survey of Patients' Hospital Experiences				
Area Around Room 'Always' Quiet at Night	300+	49%	54%	61%
Doctors 'Always' Communicated Well	300+	79%	81%	82%
Home Recovery Information Given	300+	90%	87%	85%
Hospital Given 9 or 10 on 10 Point Scale	300+	68%	70%	71%
Meds 'Always' Explained Before Given	300+	63%	64%	64%
Nurses 'Always' Communicated Well	300+	75%	77%	79%
Pain 'Always' Well Controlled	300+	71%	70%	71%
Room and Bathroom 'Always' Clean	300+	69%	73%	73%
Timely Help 'Always' Received	300+	61%	65%	68%
Would Definitely Recommend Hospital	300+	71%	73%	71%
Use of Medical Imaging				
Cardiac Imaging Stress Test before Surgery	178	5.1%	4.3%	5.3%
Combination Abdominal CT Scan	505	0.0%	6.9%	10.5%
Combination Brain/Sinus CT Scan	355	5.9%	2.3%	2.7%
Combination Chest CT Scan	122	0.0%	1.1%	2.7%
Follow-up Mammogram/Ultrasound[1]	-	-	9.1%	8.8%
Lumbar Spine MRI for Low Back Pain[1]	-	-	37.9%	37.2%

Sunnyside Community Hospital

1016 Tacoma Avenue
Sunnyside, WA 98944
Phone: 509-837-1500
Fax: 509-837-1740
URL: www.sunnysidehospital.com
Type: Critical Access Hospitals
Emergency Services: Yes
Ownership: Voluntary non-profit - Private
Beds: 25

Key Personnel:

Radiology. . . . . Robert Coleman, DO
Emergency Room . . . . David W Johnson, DO
Anesthesiology. . . . . Chas Leonard
Operating Room. . . . . Debbie Mains, RN
Pediatric In-Patient Care . . . . Anne M Nealen, MD
Infection Control. . . . . S Robinson, RN
CEO/President. . . . . Jon D Smiley
Chief of Medical Staff . . . . Coke R Smith, MD

Measure	Cases	This Hosp.	State Avg.	U.S. Avg.
Blood Clot Prevention and Treatment				
Anticoagulation Overlap Therapy[5]	-	-	97%	93%
ICU Venous Thromboembolism Prophylaxis[5]	-	-	92%	92%
Incidence of Potentially Preventable VTE[5]	-	-	9%	10%
UFH with Dosages/Platelet Monitoring[5]	-	-	99%	97%
Venous Thromboembolism Prophylaxis[5]	-	-	86%	85%
Warfarin Therapy Discharge Instructions[5]	-	-	74%	75%
Chest Pain/Possible Heart Attack Care				
Aspirin Given Within 24 Hours of Arrival	22	95%	97%	96%
Fibrinolytic Meds Within 30 Min. of Arrival[7]	-	-	51%	58%
Average Time to ECG (minutes)	27	14	9	7
Average Time to Transfer (minutes)	11	60	54	60
Children's Asthma Care				
Received Home Management Plan of Care	-	-	-	88%
Received Reliever Medication	-	-	-	100%
Received Systemic Corticosteroids	-	-	-	100%
Emergency Department				
Admittance Decision Time (minutes)[5]	-	-	96	98
Head CT Results Within 45 Min. of Arrival[5]	-	-	63%	57%
Patients Who Left ER Before Being Seen[5]	-	-	2%	2%
Time from ER Arrival to Admit. (minutes)[5]	-	-	259	274
Time from ER Arrival to Discharge (minutes)[5]	-	-	135	134
Time in ER Before Being Evaluated (minutes)[5]	-	-	22	26
Time to Pain Meds for Fractures (minutes)[5]	-	-	52	57
Heart Attack Care				
Aspirin Given at Discharge[5]	-	-	99%	99%
Fibrinolytic Meds Within 30 Min. of Arrival[5]	-	-	62%	54%
PCI Within 90 Minutes of Arrival[5]	-	-	97%	96%
Statin Prescribed at Discharge[5]	-	-	98%	98%
Heart Failure Care				
ACE Inhibitor or ARB for LVSD[2]	18	89%	97%	97%
Discharge Instructions Given[2]	43	81%	93%	94%
Evaluation of LVS Function[2]	61	95%	99%	99%
Medicare Spending				
Medicare Spending per Patient (ratio)	-	-	0.91	0.98
Pneumonia Care				
Appropriate Initial Antibiotic Given[2]	47	98%	96%	95%
Blood Culture Timing[2]	73	93%	97%	98%
Pregnancy and Delivery Care				
Newborn Deliveries Scheduled Early[2,3]	64	2%	2%	6%
Preventive Care				
Immunization for Influenza[5]	-	-	91%	90%
Immunization for Pneumonia[5]	-	-	91%	92%
Stroke Care				
Anticoagulation Therapy for Atrial Fibrillation[5]	-	-	94%	95%
Antithrombotic Therapy Timing[5]	-	-	98%	98%
Assessed for Rehabilitation[5]	-	-	98%	97%
Discharged on Antithrombotic Therapy[5]	-	-	99%	99%
Discharged on Statin Medication[5]	-	-	96%	94%
Thrombolytic Therapy Timing[5]	-	-	73%	66%
Venous Thromboembolism Prophylaxis[5]	-	-	94%	94%
Written Stroke Educational Materials Given[5]	-	-	86%	88%
Surgical Care Improvement Project				
Appropriate Beta Blocker Usage	11	73%	98%	98%
Appropriate VTP Within 24 Hours	30	97%	98%	98%
Controlled Postoperative Blood Glucose[7]	-	-	97%	97%
Perioperative Temperature Management	39	100%	100%	100%
Prophylactic Antibiotic Selection	20	100%	99%	99%
Prophylactic Antibiotic Selection (Outpatient)[5]	-	-	98%	98%
Prophylactic Antibiotic Stopped	19	95%	99%	98%
Prophylactic Antibiotic Timing	20	75%	98%	99%
Prophylactic Antibiotic Timing (Outpatient)[5]	-	-	98%	98%
Urinary Catheter Removal	13	92%	97%	97%
Survey of Patients' Hospital Experiences				
Area Around Room 'Always' Quiet at Night	(a)	44%	54%	61%
Doctors 'Always' Communicated Well	(a)	74%	81%	82%
Home Recovery Information Given	(a)	79%	87%	85%
Hospital Given 9 or 10 on 10 Point Scale	(a)	59%	70%	71%
Meds 'Always' Explained Before Given	(a)	60%	64%	64%
Nurses 'Always' Communicated Well	(a)	74%	77%	79%
Pain 'Always' Well Controlled	(a)	59%	70%	71%
Room and Bathroom 'Always' Clean	(a)	74%	73%	73%
Timely Help 'Always' Received	(a)	61%	65%	68%
Would Definitely Recommend Hospital	(a)	61%	73%	71%
Use of Medical Imaging				
Cardiac Imaging Stress Test before Surgery[1]	-	-	4.3%	5.3%
Combination Abdominal CT Scan	278	5.4%	6.9%	10.5%
Combination Brain/Sinus CT Scan[1]	-	-	2.3%	2.7%
Combination Chest CT Scan	134	14.2%	1.1%	2.7%
Follow-up Mammogram/Ultrasound	395	6.6%	9.1%	8.8%
Lumbar Spine MRI for Low Back Pain[1]	-	-	37.9%	37.2%

Saint Joseph Medical Center

1717 South J Street
Tacoma, WA 98405
Phone: 253-627-4101
Fax: 253-426-6880
URL: www.fhshealth.org
Type: Acute Care Hospitals
Emergency Services: Yes
Ownership: Voluntary non-profit - Church
Beds: 320

Key Personnel:

Chief of Medical Staff . . . . Mark Adams, MD
CEO/President. . . . . Syd Bersante
Radiology. . . . . Stanley Cheng

Measure	Cases	This Hosp.	State Avg.	U.S. Avg.
Blood Clot Prevention and Treatment				
Anticoagulation Overlap Therapy[2]	138	93%	97%	93%
ICU Venous Thromboembolism Prophylaxis[2]	53	98%	92%	92%
Incidence of Potentially Preventable VTE[2]	25	8%	9%	10%
UFH with Dosages/Platelet Monitoring[2]	126	100%	99%	97%
Venous Thromboembolism Prophylaxis[2]	314	90%	86%	85%
Warfarin Therapy Discharge Instructions[2]	116	69%	74%	75%
Chest Pain/Possible Heart Attack Care				
Aspirin Given Within 24 Hours of Arrival[1]	-	-	97%	96%
Fibrinolytic Meds Within 30 Min. of Arrival[3,7]	-	-	51%	58%
Average Time to ECG (minutes)[1]	-	-	9	7
Average Time to Transfer (minutes)[1,3]	-	-	54	60
Children's Asthma Care				
Received Home Management Plan of Care	-	-	-	88%
Received Reliever Medication	-	-	-	100%
Received Systemic Corticosteroids	-	-	-	100%
Emergency Department				
Admittance Decision Time (minutes)[2]	365	168	96	98
Head CT Results Within 45 Min. of Arrival[1]	-	-	63%	57%
Patients Who Left ER Before Being Seen	53,136	1%	2%	2%
Time from ER Arrival to Admit. (minutes)[2]	387	330	259	274
Time from ER Arrival to Discharge (minutes)	347	151	135	134
Time in ER Before Being Evaluated (minutes)	407	29	22	26
Time to Pain Meds for Fractures (minutes)	66	48	52	57
Heart Attack Care				
Aspirin Given at Discharge[2]	452	100%	99%	99%
Fibrinolytic Meds Within 30 Min. of Arrival[2,7]	-	-	62%	54%
PCI Within 90 Minutes of Arrival[2]	59	95%	97%	96%
Statin Prescribed at Discharge[2]	451	99%	98%	98%
Heart Failure Care				
ACE Inhibitor or ARB for LVSD[2]	136	99%	97%	97%
Discharge Instructions Given[2]	330	85%	93%	94%
Evaluation of LVS Function[2]	382	100%	99%	99%
Medicare Spending				
Medicare Spending per Patient (ratio)	-	0.97	0.91	0.98
Pneumonia Care				
Appropriate Initial Antibiotic Given[2]	119	94%	96%	95%
Blood Culture Timing[2]	196	97%	97%	98%

NOTE: Hospital profiles are in alphabetical order by state, then city, then hospital within the city; Rankings exclude hospitals with less than 25 cases except for patient surveys which excludes hospitals with less than 100 cases; (a) 100-299 cases; (1) The number of cases/patients is too few to report; (2) Data submitted were based on a sample of cases/patients; (3) Results are based on a shorter time period than required; (4) Data suppressed by CMS for one or more quarters; (5) Results are not available for this reporting period; (6) Fewer than 100 patients completed the HCAHPS survey; (7) No cases met the criteria for this measure; (8) The lower limit of the confidence interval cannot be calculated if the number of observed infections equals zero; (9) No data are available from the state/territory for this reporting period; (10) The scores shown reflect fewer than 50 completed surveys; (11) There were discrepancies in the data collection process; (12) This measure does not apply to this hospital for this reporting period; (13) Results cannot be calculated for this reporting period; (14) The results for this state are combined with nearby states to protect confidentiality; Please refer to the User's Guide for a full explanation of data.

Pregnancy and Delivery Care				
Newborn Deliveries Scheduled Early	303	2%	2%	6%
Preventive Care				
Immunization for Influenza[2]	571	93%	91%	90%
Immunization for Pneumonia[2]	595	90%	91%	92%
Stroke Care				
Anticoagulation Therapy for Atrial Fibrillation	34	91%	94%	95%
Antithrombotic Therapy Timing	211	99%	98%	98%
Assessed for Rehabilitation	319	93%	98%	97%
Discharged on Antithrombotic Therapy	254	99%	99%	99%
Discharged on Statin Medication	210	95%	96%	94%
Thrombolytic Therapy Timing	26	92%	73%	66%
Venous Thromboembolism Prophylaxis	345	92%	94%	94%
Written Stroke Educational Materials Given	166	77%	86%	88%
Surgical Care Improvement Project				
Appropriate Beta Blocker Usage[2]	356	99%	98%	98%
Appropriate VTP Within 24 Hours[2]	456	99%	98%	98%
Controlled Postoperative Blood Glucose[2]	306	97%	97%	97%
Perioperative Temperature Management[2]	557	100%	100%	100%
Prophylactic Antibiotic Selection[2]	644	100%	99%	99%
Prophylactic Antibiotic Selection (Outpatient)	744	99%	98%	98%
Prophylactic Antibiotic Stopped[2]	624	99%	99%	98%
Prophylactic Antibiotic Timing[2]	646	99%	98%	99%
Prophylactic Antibiotic Timing (Outpatient)	748	99%	98%	98%
Urinary Catheter Removal[2]	288	93%	97%	97%
Survey of Patients' Hospital Experiences				
Area Around Room 'Always' Quiet at Night	300+	46%	54%	61%
Doctors 'Always' Communicated Well	300+	77%	81%	82%
Home Recovery Information Given	300+	89%	87%	85%
Hospital Given 9 or 10 on 10 Point Scale	300+	66%	70%	71%
Meds 'Always' Explained Before Given	300+	61%	64%	64%
Nurses 'Always' Communicated Well	300+	77%	77%	79%
Pain 'Always' Well Controlled	300+	70%	70%	71%
Room and Bathroom 'Always' Clean	300+	70%	73%	73%
Timely Help 'Always' Received	300+	60%	65%	68%
Would Definitely Recommend Hospital	300+	74%	73%	71%
Use of Medical Imaging				
Cardiac Imaging Stress Test before Surgery	404	5.9%	4.3%	5.3%
Combination Abdominal CT Scan	761	4.9%	6.9%	10.5%
Combination Brain/Sinus CT Scan	657	2.3%	2.3%	2.7%
Combination Chest CT Scan	415	0.2%	1.1%	2.7%
Follow-up Mammogram/Ultrasound[7]	-	-	9.1%	8.8%
Lumbar Spine MRI for Low Back Pain	99	29.3%	37.9%	37.2%

Tacoma General Allenmore Hospital

315 S Mlk Jr Way Phone: 253-403-1000
Tacoma, WA 98415 Fax: 253-403-1180
E-mail: hrweb@multicare.org
URL: www.multicare.org
Type: Acute Care Hospitals Emergency Services: Yes
Ownership: Voluntary non-profit - Private Beds: 593

Key Personnel:

CEO/President. . . . . Diane Cecchettini
Infection Control. . . . . Christi McCarren
Operating Room. . . . . Shelly Mullin
Radiology. . . . . Nina Noldon
Pediatric Ambulatory Care . . . . . . Gary Park, MD
Pediatric In-Patient Care . . . . Gary Park, MD
Quality Assurance . . . . Erik Rasmussen
Chief of Medical Staff. . . . . Richard Stubbs, MD

Measure	Cases	This Hosp.	State Avg.	U.S. Avg.
Blood Clot Prevention and Treatment				
Anticoagulation Overlap Therapy[2]	131	100%	97%	93%
ICU Venous Thromboembolism Prophylaxis[2]	122	97%	92%	92%
Incidence of Potentially Preventable VTE[2]	30	10%	9%	10%
UFH with Dosages/Platelet Monitoring[2]	77	100%	99%	97%
Venous Thromboembolism Prophylaxis[2]	628	89%	86%	85%
Warfarin Therapy Discharge Instructions[2]	96	94%	74%	75%
Chest Pain/Possible Heart Attack Care				
Aspirin Given Within 24 Hours of Arrival	59	98%	97%	96%
Fibrinolytic Meds Within 30 Min. of Arrival[7]	-	-	51%	58%
Average Time to ECG (minutes)	63	8	9	7
Average Time to Transfer (minutes)[1]	-	-	54	60
Children's Asthma Care				
Received Home Management Plan of Care	-	-	-	88%
Received Reliever Medication	-	-	-	100%
Received Systemic Corticosteroids	-	-	-	100%
Emergency Department				
Admittance Decision Time (minutes)[2]	1,037	86	96	98
Head CT Results Within 45 Min. of Arrival[1,3]	-	-	63%	57%
Patients Who Left ER Before Being Seen	78,161	1%	2%	2%
Time from ER Arrival to Admit. (minutes)[2]	1,046	294	259	274
Time from ER Arrival to Discharge (minutes)	1,225	177	135	134
Time in ER Before Being Evaluated (minutes)	459	46	22	26
Time to Pain Meds for Fractures (minutes)	172	62	52	57
Heart Attack Care				
Aspirin Given at Discharge	322	100%	99%	99%
Fibrinolytic Meds Within 30 Min. of Arrival[7]	-	-	62%	54%
PCI Within 90 Minutes of Arrival	36	100%	97%	96%
Statin Prescribed at Discharge	300	100%	98%	98%
Heart Failure Care				
ACE Inhibitor or ARB for LVSD[2]	102	100%	97%	97%
Discharge Instructions Given[2]	345	97%	93%	94%
Evaluation of LVS Function[2]	402	100%	99%	99%
Medicare Spending				
Medicare Spending per Patient (ratio)	-	0.93	0.91	0.98
Pneumonia Care				
Appropriate Initial Antibiotic Given[2]	191	97%	96%	95%
Blood Culture Timing[2]	291	96%	97%	98%
Pregnancy and Delivery Care				
Newborn Deliveries Scheduled Early	203	1%	2%	6%
Preventive Care				
Immunization for Influenza[2]	890	88%	91%	90%
Immunization for Pneumonia[2]	1,093	89%	91%	92%
Stroke Care				
Anticoagulation Therapy for Atrial Fibrillation[2]	22	100%	94%	95%
Antithrombotic Therapy Timing[2]	103	100%	98%	98%
Assessed for Rehabilitation[2]	149	97%	98%	97%
Discharged on Antithrombotic Therapy[2]	127	99%	99%	99%
Discharged on Statin Medication[2]	102	96%	96%	94%
Thrombolytic Therapy Timing[1,2]	-	-	73%	66%
Venous Thromboembolism Prophylaxis[2]	139	95%	94%	94%
Written Stroke Educational Materials Given[2]	86	92%	86%	88%
Surgical Care Improvement Project				
Appropriate Beta Blocker Usage[2]	315	99%	98%	98%
Appropriate VTP Within 24 Hours[2]	677	98%	98%	98%
Controlled Postoperative Blood Glucose[2]	200	94%	97%	97%
Perioperative Temperature Management[2]	837	100%	100%	100%
Prophylactic Antibiotic Selection[2]	669	99%	99%	99%
Prophylactic Antibiotic Selection (Outpatient)	823	96%	98%	98%
Prophylactic Antibiotic Stopped[2]	661	99%	99%	98%
Prophylactic Antibiotic Timing[2]	670	98%	98%	99%
Prophylactic Antibiotic Timing (Outpatient)	826	99%	98%	98%
Urinary Catheter Removal[2]	394	91%	97%	97%
Survey of Patients' Hospital Experiences				
Area Around Room 'Always' Quiet at Night	300+	51%	54%	61%
Doctors 'Always' Communicated Well	300+	75%	81%	82%
Home Recovery Information Given	300+	85%	87%	85%
Hospital Given 9 or 10 on 10 Point Scale	300+	64%	70%	71%
Meds 'Always' Explained Before Given	300+	56%	64%	64%
Nurses 'Always' Communicated Well	300+	73%	77%	79%
Pain 'Always' Well Controlled	300+	64%	70%	71%
Room and Bathroom 'Always' Clean	300+	68%	73%	73%
Timely Help 'Always' Received	300+	53%	65%	68%
Would Definitely Recommend Hospital	300+	72%	73%	71%
Use of Medical Imaging				
Cardiac Imaging Stress Test before Surgery	316	2.2%	4.3%	5.3%
Combination Abdominal CT Scan	1,946	7.3%	6.9%	10.5%
Combination Brain/Sinus CT Scan	1,158	2.7%	2.3%	2.7%
Combination Chest CT Scan	1,506	1.4%	1.1%	2.7%
Follow-up Mammogram/Ultrasound	1,627	7.9%	9.1%	8.8%
Lumbar Spine MRI for Low Back Pain	235	43.4%	37.9%	37.2%

North Valley Hospital

203 South Western Phone: 509-486-2151
Tonasket, WA 98855
Type: Critical Access Hospitals Emergency Services: Yes
Ownership: Govt - Hospital Dist/Auth

Measure	Cases	This Hosp.	State Avg.	U.S. Avg.
Blood Clot Prevention and Treatment				
Anticoagulation Overlap Therapy[5]	-	-	97%	93%
ICU Venous Thromboembolism Prophylaxis[5]	-	-	92%	92%
Incidence of Potentially Preventable VTE[5]	-	-	9%	10%
UFH with Dosages/Platelet Monitoring[5]	-	-	99%	97%
Venous Thromboembolism Prophylaxis[5]	-	-	86%	85%
Warfarin Therapy Discharge Instructions[5]	-	-	74%	75%
Chest Pain/Possible Heart Attack Care				
Aspirin Given Within 24 Hours of Arrival	26	100%	97%	96%
Fibrinolytic Meds Within 30 Min. of Arrival[1]	-	-	51%	58%
Average Time to ECG (minutes)	28	5	9	7
Average Time to Transfer (minutes)[1]	-	-	54	60
Children's Asthma Care				
Received Home Management Plan of Care	-	-	-	88%
Received Reliever Medication	-	-	-	100%
Received Systemic Corticosteroids	-	-	-	100%
Emergency Department				
Admittance Decision Time (minutes)[5]	-	-	96	98
Head CT Results Within 45 Min. of Arrival[5]	-	-	63%	57%
Patients Who Left ER Before Being Seen[5]	-	-	2%	2%
Time from ER Arrival to Admit. (minutes)[5]	-	-	259	274
Time from ER Arrival to Discharge (minutes)[5]	-	-	135	134
Time in ER Before Being Evaluated (minutes)[5]	-	-	22	26
Time to Pain Meds for Fractures (minutes)[5]	-	-	52	57
Heart Attack Care				
Aspirin Given at Discharge[5]	-	-	99%	99%
Fibrinolytic Meds Within 30 Min. of Arrival[5]	-	-	62%	54%
PCI Within 90 Minutes of Arrival[5]	-	-	97%	96%
Statin Prescribed at Discharge[5]	-	-	98%	98%
Heart Failure Care				
ACE Inhibitor or ARB for LVSD[1]	-	-	97%	97%
Discharge Instructions Given[1]	-	-	93%	94%
Evaluation of LVS Function[1]	-	-	99%	99%
Medicare Spending				
Medicare Spending per Patient (ratio)	-	-	0.91	0.98
Pneumonia Care				
Appropriate Initial Antibiotic Given[1,2]	-	-	96%	95%
Blood Culture Timing[2]	12	75%	97%	98%
Pregnancy and Delivery Care				
Newborn Deliveries Scheduled Early[5]	-	-	2%	6%
Preventive Care				
Immunization for Influenza[5]	-	-	91%	90%
Immunization for Pneumonia[5]	-	-	91%	92%
Stroke Care				
Anticoagulation Therapy for Atrial Fibrillation[5]	-	-	94%	95%
Antithrombotic Therapy Timing[5]	-	-	98%	98%
Assessed for Rehabilitation[5]	-	-	98%	97%
Discharged on Antithrombotic Therapy[5]	-	-	99%	99%
Discharged on Statin Medication[5]	-	-	96%	94%
Thrombolytic Therapy Timing[5]	-	-	73%	66%
Venous Thromboembolism Prophylaxis[5]	-	-	94%	94%
Written Stroke Educational Materials Given[5]	-	-	86%	88%
Surgical Care Improvement Project				
Appropriate Beta Blocker Usage[5]	-	-	98%	98%
Appropriate VTP Within 24 Hours[5]	-	-	98%	98%
Controlled Postoperative Blood Glucose[5]	-	-	97%	97%
Perioperative Temperature Management[5]	-	-	100%	100%
Prophylactic Antibiotic Selection[5]	-	-	99%	99%
Prophylactic Antibiotic Selection (Outpatient)[5]	-	-	98%	98%
Prophylactic Antibiotic Stopped[5]	-	-	99%	98%
Prophylactic Antibiotic Timing[5]	-	-	98%	99%
Prophylactic Antibiotic Timing (Outpatient)[5]	-	-	98%	98%
Urinary Catheter Removal[5]	-	-	97%	97%
Survey of Patients' Hospital Experiences				
Area Around Room 'Always' Quiet at Night[5]	-	-	54%	61%
Doctors 'Always' Communicated Well[5]	-	-	81%	82%

NOTE: Hospital profiles are in alphabetical order by state, then city, then hospital within the city; Rankings exclude hospitals with less than 25 cases except for patient surveys which excludes hospitals with less than 100 cases; (a) 100-299 cases; (1) The number of cases/patients is too few to report; (2) Data submitted were based on a sample of cases/patients; (3) Results are based on a shorter time period than required; (4) Data suppressed by CMS for one or more quarters; (5) Results are not available for this reporting period; (6) Fewer than 100 patients completed the HCAHPS survey; (7) No cases met the criteria for this measure; (8) The lower limit of the confidence interval cannot be calculated if the number of observed infections equals zero; (9) No data are available from the state/territory for this reporting period; (10) The scores shown reflect fewer than 50 completed surveys; (11) There were discrepancies in the data collection process; (12) This measure does not apply to this hospital for this reporting period; (13) Results cannot be calculated for this reporting period; (14) The results for this state are combined with nearby states to protect confidentiality; Please refer to the User's Guide for a full explanation of data.

Measure	Cases	This Hosp.	State Avg.	U.S. Avg.
Home Recovery Information Given[5]	-	-	87%	85%
Hospital Given 9 or 10 on 10 Point Scale[5]	-	-	70%	71%
Meds 'Always' Explained Before Given[5]	-	-	64%	64%
Nurses 'Always' Communicated Well[5]	-	-	77%	79%
Pain 'Always' Well Controlled[5]	-	-	70%	71%
Room and Bathroom 'Always' Clean[5]	-	-	73%	73%
Timely Help 'Always' Received[5]	-	-	65%	68%
Would Definitely Recommend Hospital[5]	-	-	73%	71%
Use of Medical Imaging				
Cardiac Imaging Stress Test before Surgery[7]	-	-	4.3%	5.3%
Combination Abdominal CT Scan	132	11.4%	6.9%	10.5%
Combination Brain/Sinus CT Scan[1]	-	-	2.3%	2.7%
Combination Chest CT Scan	83	13.3%	1.1%	2.7%
Follow-up Mammogram/Ultrasound	231	4.8%	9.1%	8.8%
Lumbar Spine MRI for Low Back Pain[1]	-	-	37.9%	37.2%

Toppenish Community Hospital

502 W Fourth Ave Phone: 509-865-1520
Toppenish, WA 98948 Fax: 509-865-1519
URL: www.hma-corp.com
Type: Acute Care Hospitals Emergency Services: Yes
Ownership: Proprietary Beds: 63
Key Personnel:
Radiology. . . . . William C Feldmann
CEO/President. . . . . Perry Gay
Emergency Room . . . . Linn Walker
Quality Assurance . . . . Kathy Whitner

Measure	Cases	This Hosp.	State Avg.	U.S. Avg.
Blood Clot Prevention and Treatment				
Anticoagulation Overlap Therapy[1,2]	-	-	97%	93%
ICU Venous Thromboembolism Prophylaxis[2]	40	72%	92%	92%
Incidence of Potentially Preventable VTE[1,2]	-	-	9%	10%
UFH with Dosages/Platelet Monitoring[1,2]	-	-	99%	97%
Venous Thromboembolism Prophylaxis[2]	145	74%	86%	85%
Warfarin Therapy Discharge Instructions[1,2]	-	-	74%	75%
Chest Pain/Possible Heart Attack Care				
Aspirin Given Within 24 Hours of Arrival	34	97%	97%	96%
Fibrinolytic Meds Within 30 Min. of Arrival[7]	-	-	51%	58%
Average Time to ECG (minutes)	37	9	9	7
Average Time to Transfer (minutes)[1]	-	-	54	60
Children's Asthma Care				
Received Home Management Plan of Care	-	-	-	88%
Received Reliever Medication	-	-	-	100%
Received Systemic Corticosteroids	-	-	-	100%
Emergency Department				
Admittance Decision Time (minutes)[2]	420	63	96	98
Head CT Results Within 45 Min. of Arrival	12	83%	63%	57%
Patients Who Left ER Before Being Seen	17,320	0%	2%	2%
Time from ER Arrival to Admit. (minutes)[2]	420	188	259	274
Time from ER Arrival to Discharge (minutes)	915	83	135	134
Time in ER Before Being Evaluated (minutes)	958	13	22	26
Time to Pain Meds for Fractures (minutes)	91	48	52	57
Heart Attack Care				
Aspirin Given at Discharge[1]	-	-	99%	99%
Fibrinolytic Meds Within 30 Min. of Arrival[7]	-	-	62%	54%
PCI Within 90 Minutes of Arrival[7]	-	-	97%	96%
Statin Prescribed at Discharge[1]	-	-	98%	98%
Heart Failure Care				
ACE Inhibitor or ARB for LVSD	20	90%	97%	97%
Discharge Instructions Given	37	97%	93%	94%
Evaluation of LVS Function	42	100%	99%	99%
Medicare Spending				
Medicare Spending per Patient (ratio)	-	0.86	0.91	0.98
Pneumonia Care				
Appropriate Initial Antibiotic Given	43	100%	96%	95%
Blood Culture Timing	76	99%	97%	98%
Pregnancy and Delivery Care				
Newborn Deliveries Scheduled Early	48	4%	2%	6%
Preventive Care				
Immunization for Influenza[2]	348	93%	91%	90%
Immunization for Pneumonia[2]	306	93%	91%	92%
Stroke Care				
Anticoagulation Therapy for Atrial Fibrillation[1]	-	-	94%	95%
Antithrombotic Therapy Timing[1]	-	-	98%	98%
Assessed for Rehabilitation	17	100%	98%	97%
Discharged on Antithrombotic Therapy	16	100%	99%	99%
Discharged on Statin Medication[1]	-	-	96%	94%
Thrombolytic Therapy Timing[7]	-	-	73%	66%
Venous Thromboembolism Prophylaxis[1]	-	-	94%	94%
Written Stroke Educational Materials Given	12	33%	86%	88%
Surgical Care Improvement Project				
Appropriate Beta Blocker Usage[1]	-	-	98%	98%
Appropriate VTP Within 24 Hours	19	100%	98%	98%
Controlled Postoperative Blood Glucose[7]	-	-	97%	97%
Perioperative Temperature Management	22	100%	100%	100%
Prophylactic Antibiotic Selection	15	100%	99%	99%
Prophylactic Antibiotic Selection (Outpatient)[1,3]	-	-	98%	98%
Prophylactic Antibiotic Stopped	15	100%	99%	98%
Prophylactic Antibiotic Timing	14	100%	98%	99%
Prophylactic Antibiotic Timing (Outpatient)[1,3]	-	-	98%	98%
Urinary Catheter Removal[1]	-	-	97%	97%
Survey of Patients' Hospital Experiences				
Area Around Room 'Always' Quiet at Night	(a)	59%	54%	61%
Doctors 'Always' Communicated Well	(a)	84%	81%	82%
Home Recovery Information Given	(a)	91%	87%	85%
Hospital Given 9 or 10 on 10 Point Scale	(a)	71%	70%	71%
Meds 'Always' Explained Before Given	(a)	68%	64%	64%
Nurses 'Always' Communicated Well	(a)	79%	77%	79%
Pain 'Always' Well Controlled	(a)	72%	70%	71%
Room and Bathroom 'Always' Clean	(a)	74%	73%	73%
Timely Help 'Always' Received	(a)	68%	65%	68%
Would Definitely Recommend Hospital	(a)	65%	73%	71%
Use of Medical Imaging				
Cardiac Imaging Stress Test before Surgery[7]	-	-	4.3%	5.3%
Combination Abdominal CT Scan	100	0.0%	6.9%	10.5%
Combination Brain/Sinus CT Scan[1]	-	-	2.3%	2.7%
Combination Chest CT Scan	52	0.0%	1.1%	2.7%
Follow-up Mammogram/Ultrasound	189	10.1%	9.1%	8.8%
Lumbar Spine MRI for Low Back Pain[7]	-	-	37.9%	37.2%

Legacy Salmon Creek Medical Center

2211 Ne 139th Street Phone: 360-487-1000
Vancouver, WA 98686
Type: Acute Care Hospitals Emergency Services: Yes
Ownership: Voluntary non-profit - Private
Key Personnel:
CEO/President. . . . . Lee Domanico
Chief of Medical Staff. . . . . Eve Logsdon
Anesthesiology. . . . . Deborah McKissack

Measure	Cases	This Hosp.	State Avg.	U.S. Avg.
Blood Clot Prevention and Treatment				
Anticoagulation Overlap Therapy[2]	62	100%	97%	93%
ICU Venous Thromboembolism Prophylaxis[2]	68	96%	92%	92%
Incidence of Potentially Preventable VTE[1,2]	-	-	9%	10%
UFH with Dosages/Platelet Monitoring[2]	31	100%	99%	97%
Venous Thromboembolism Prophylaxis[2]	239	97%	86%	85%
Warfarin Therapy Discharge Instructions[2]	52	90%	74%	75%
Chest Pain/Possible Heart Attack Care				
Aspirin Given Within 24 Hours of Arrival	79	99%	97%	96%
Fibrinolytic Meds Within 30 Min. of Arrival[7]	-	-	51%	58%
Average Time to ECG (minutes)	79	13	9	7
Average Time to Transfer (minutes)	26	45	54	60
Children's Asthma Care				
Received Home Management Plan of Care	-	-	-	88%
Received Reliever Medication	-	-	-	100%
Received Systemic Corticosteroids	-	-	-	100%
Emergency Department				
Admittance Decision Time (minutes)[2]	572	92	96	98
Head CT Results Within 45 Min. of Arrival[1]	-	-	63%	57%
Patients Who Left ER Before Being Seen	50,602	1%	2%	2%
Time from ER Arrival to Admit. (minutes)[2]	572	250	259	274
Time from ER Arrival to Discharge (minutes)	359	157	135	134
Time in ER Before Being Evaluated (minutes)	388	30	22	26
Time to Pain Meds for Fractures (minutes)	230	41	52	57
Heart Attack Care				
Aspirin Given at Discharge	34	100%	99%	99%
Fibrinolytic Meds Within 30 Min. of Arrival[7]	-	-	62%	54%
PCI Within 90 Minutes of Arrival[7]	-	-	97%	96%
Statin Prescribed at Discharge	30	100%	98%	98%
Heart Failure Care				
ACE Inhibitor or ARB for LVSD	65	100%	97%	97%
Discharge Instructions Given	180	98%	93%	94%
Evaluation of LVS Function	213	100%	99%	99%
Medicare Spending				
Medicare Spending per Patient (ratio)	-	0.89	0.91	0.98
Pneumonia Care				
Appropriate Initial Antibiotic Given	125	98%	96%	95%
Blood Culture Timing	260	98%	97%	98%
Pregnancy and Delivery Care				
Newborn Deliveries Scheduled Early[2]	43	0%	2%	6%
Preventive Care				
Immunization for Influenza[2]	520	88%	91%	90%
Immunization for Pneumonia[2]	510	91%	91%	92%
Stroke Care				
Anticoagulation Therapy for Atrial Fibrillation	15	100%	94%	95%
Antithrombotic Therapy Timing	64	100%	98%	98%
Assessed for Rehabilitation	84	100%	98%	97%
Discharged on Antithrombotic Therapy	77	100%	99%	99%
Discharged on Statin Medication	65	100%	96%	94%
Thrombolytic Therapy Timing[1]	-	-	73%	66%
Venous Thromboembolism Prophylaxis	78	97%	94%	94%
Written Stroke Educational Materials Given	50	98%	86%	88%
Surgical Care Improvement Project				
Appropriate Beta Blocker Usage[2]	105	100%	98%	98%
Appropriate VTP Within 24 Hours[2]	364	98%	98%	98%
Controlled Postoperative Blood Glucose[2,7]	-	-	97%	97%
Perioperative Temperature Management[2]	477	100%	100%	100%
Prophylactic Antibiotic Selection[2]	340	99%	99%	99%
Prophylactic Antibiotic Selection (Outpatient)	284	99%	98%	98%
Prophylactic Antibiotic Stopped[2]	335	99%	99%	98%
Prophylactic Antibiotic Timing[2]	340	99%	98%	99%
Prophylactic Antibiotic Timing (Outpatient)	284	100%	98%	98%
Urinary Catheter Removal[2]	299	100%	97%	97%
Survey of Patients' Hospital Experiences				
Area Around Room 'Always' Quiet at Night	300+	69%	54%	61%
Doctors 'Always' Communicated Well	300+	81%	81%	82%
Home Recovery Information Given	300+	89%	87%	85%
Hospital Given 9 or 10 on 10 Point Scale	300+	78%	70%	71%
Meds 'Always' Explained Before Given	300+	66%	64%	64%
Nurses 'Always' Communicated Well	300+	79%	77%	79%
Pain 'Always' Well Controlled	300+	72%	70%	71%
Room and Bathroom 'Always' Clean	300+	71%	73%	73%
Timely Help 'Always' Received	300+	70%	65%	68%
Would Definitely Recommend Hospital	300+	82%	73%	71%
Use of Medical Imaging				
Cardiac Imaging Stress Test before Surgery	145	4.1%	4.3%	5.3%
Combination Abdominal CT Scan	484	3.9%	6.9%	10.5%
Combination Brain/Sinus CT Scan	491	0.8%	2.3%	2.7%
Combination Chest CT Scan	141	0.0%	1.1%	2.7%
Follow-up Mammogram/Ultrasound	471	7.6%	9.1%	8.8%
Lumbar Spine MRI for Low Back Pain	59	35.6%	37.9%	37.2%

Peacehealth Southwest Medical Center

400 Ne Mother Joseph Place Phone: 360-256-2000
Vancouver, WA 98668 Fax: 360-514-2267
URL: www.swmedicalcenter.org
Type: Acute Care Hospitals Emergency Services: Yes
Ownership: Voluntary non-profit - Private Beds: 442
Key Personnel:
Infection Control. . . . . Lucinda Eling
Radiology. . . . . Mario A Fabris
Operating Room. . . . . Carol Hammes
CEO/President. . . . . Joseph M Kortum
Chief of Medical Staff . . . . Alden Roberts, MD

Measure	Cases	This Hosp.	State Avg.	U.S. Avg.
Blood Clot Prevention and Treatment				
Anticoagulation Overlap Therapy[2]	161	100%	97%	93%
ICU Venous Thromboembolism Prophylaxis[2]	104	98%	92%	92%
Incidence of Potentially Preventable VTE[2]	23	4%	9%	10%

NOTE: Hospital profiles are in alphabetical order by state, then city, then hospital within the city; Rankings exclude hospitals with less than 25 cases except for patient surveys which excludes hospitals with less than 100 cases; (a) 100-299 cases; (1) The number of cases/patients is too few to report; (2) Data submitted were based on a sample of cases/patients; (3) Results are based on a shorter time period than required; (4) Data suppressed by CMS for one or more quarters; (5) Results are not available for this reporting period; (6) Fewer than 100 patients completed the HCAHPS survey; (7) No cases met the criteria for this measure; (8) The lower limit of the confidence interval cannot be calculated if the number of observed infections equals zero; (9) No data are available from the state/territory for this reporting period; (10) The scores shown reflect fewer than 50 completed surveys; (11) There were discrepancies in the data collection process; (12) This measure does not apply to this hospital for this reporting period; (13) Results cannot be calculated for this reporting period; (14) The results for this state are combined with nearby states to protect confidentiality; Please refer to the User's Guide for a full explanation of data.

Measure	Cases	This Hosp.	State Avg.	U.S. Avg.
UFH with Dosages/Platelet Monitoring[2]	141	100%	99%	97%
Venous Thromboembolism Prophylaxis[2]	310	94%	86%	85%
Warfarin Therapy Discharge Instructions[2]	134	57%	74%	75%
Chest Pain/Possible Heart Attack Care				
Aspirin Given Within 24 Hours of Arrival[1,3]	-	-	97%	96%
Fibrinolytic Meds Within 30 Min. of Arrival[5]	-	-	51%	58%
Average Time to ECG (minutes)[1,3]	-	-	9	7
Average Time to Transfer (minutes)[5]	-	-	54	60
Children's Asthma Care				
Received Home Management Plan of Care	-	-	-	88%
Received Reliever Medication	-	-	-	100%
Received Systemic Corticosteroids	-	-	-	100%
Emergency Department				
Admittance Decision Time (minutes)[2]	689	85	96	98
Head CT Results Within 45 Min. of Arrival[1]	-	-	63%	57%
Patients Who Left ER Before Being Seen	79,277	2%	2%	2%
Time from ER Arrival to Admit. (minutes)[2]	701	230	259	274
Time from ER Arrival to Discharge (minutes)	353	156	135	134
Time in ER Before Being Evaluated (minutes)	395	45	22	26
Time to Pain Meds for Fractures (minutes)	202	58	52	57
Heart Attack Care				
Aspirin Given at Discharge	565	99%	99%	99%
Fibrinolytic Meds Within 30 Min. of Arrival[1]	-	-	62%	54%
PCI Within 90 Minutes of Arrival	78	90%	97%	96%
Statin Prescribed at Discharge	540	99%	98%	98%
Heart Failure Care				
ACE Inhibitor or ARB for LVSD	195	96%	97%	97%
Discharge Instructions Given	587	97%	93%	94%
Evaluation of LVS Function	716	100%	99%	99%
Medicare Spending				
Medicare Spending per Patient (ratio)	-	0.88	0.91	0.98
Pneumonia Care				
Appropriate Initial Antibiotic Given[2]	80	95%	96%	95%
Blood Culture Timing[2]	195	95%	97%	98%
Pregnancy and Delivery Care				
Newborn Deliveries Scheduled Early	225	2%	2%	6%
Preventive Care				
Immunization for Influenza[2]	566	81%	91%	90%
Immunization for Pneumonia[2]	705	85%	91%	92%
Stroke Care				
Anticoagulation Therapy for Atrial Fibrillation	51	100%	94%	95%
Antithrombotic Therapy Timing	266	97%	98%	98%
Assessed for Rehabilitation	373	98%	98%	97%
Discharged on Antithrombotic Therapy	330	100%	99%	99%
Discharged on Statin Medication	243	97%	96%	94%
Thrombolytic Therapy Timing	33	85%	73%	66%
Venous Thromboembolism Prophylaxis	364	97%	94%	94%
Written Stroke Educational Materials Given	218	78%	86%	88%
Surgical Care Improvement Project				
Appropriate Beta Blocker Usage[2]	213	99%	98%	98%
Appropriate VTP Within 24 Hours[2]	390	98%	98%	98%
Controlled Postoperative Blood Glucose[2]	152	99%	97%	97%
Perioperative Temperature Management[2]	531	100%	100%	100%
Prophylactic Antibiotic Selection[2]	501	100%	99%	99%
Prophylactic Antibiotic Selection (Outpatient)	529	98%	98%	98%
Prophylactic Antibiotic Stopped[2]	487	100%	99%	98%
Prophylactic Antibiotic Timing[2]	504	100%	98%	99%
Prophylactic Antibiotic Timing (Outpatient)	531	99%	98%	98%
Urinary Catheter Removal[2]	441	99%	97%	97%
Survey of Patients' Hospital Experiences				
Area Around Room 'Always' Quiet at Night	300+	56%	54%	61%
Doctors 'Always' Communicated Well	300+	81%	81%	82%
Home Recovery Information Given	300+	85%	87%	85%
Hospital Given 9 or 10 on 10 Point Scale	300+	71%	70%	71%
Meds 'Always' Explained Before Given	300+	64%	64%	64%
Nurses 'Always' Communicated Well	300+	78%	77%	79%
Pain 'Always' Well Controlled	300+	69%	70%	71%
Room and Bathroom 'Always' Clean	300+	69%	73%	73%
Timely Help 'Always' Received	300+	61%	65%	68%
Would Definitely Recommend Hospital	300+	76%	73%	71%
Use of Medical Imaging				
Cardiac Imaging Stress Test before Surgery	451	6.2%	4.3%	5.3%
Combination Abdominal CT Scan	891	5.8%	6.9%	10.5%
Combination Brain/Sinus CT Scan	779	2.8%	2.3%	2.7%
Combination Chest CT Scan	549	0.4%	1.1%	2.7%
Follow-up Mammogram/Ultrasound	960	7.8%	9.1%	8.8%
Lumbar Spine MRI for Low Back Pain	115	34.8%	37.9%	37.2%

Providence Saint Mary Medical Center

401 W Poplar St
Walla Walla, WA 99362
Phone: 509-522-5900
Fax: 509-522-5950
E-mail: schima@smmc.com
URL: www.smmc.com
Type: Acute Care Hospitals
Emergency Services: Yes
Ownership: Voluntary non-profit - Private
Beds: 142
Key Personnel:
Pulmonology . . . . Michael Bernstein, MD
CEO/President. . . . . John A Isely
Emergency Room . . . . Thomas Moroldo
Chief of Medical Staff. . . . . Lester Joseph Wojek

Measure	Cases	This Hosp.	State Avg.	U.S. Avg.
Blood Clot Prevention and Treatment				
Anticoagulation Overlap Therapy[2]	22	100%	97%	93%
ICU Venous Thromboembolism Prophylaxis[2]	44	91%	92%	92%
Incidence of Potentially Preventable VTE[1,2]	-	-	9%	10%
UFH with Dosages/Platelet Monitoring[1,2]	-	-	99%	97%
Venous Thromboembolism Prophylaxis[2]	235	83%	86%	85%
Warfarin Therapy Discharge Instructions[2]	18	100%	74%	75%
Chest Pain/Possible Heart Attack Care				
Aspirin Given Within 24 Hours of Arrival	45	100%	97%	96%
Fibrinolytic Meds Within 30 Min. of Arrival[1]	-	-	51%	58%
Average Time to ECG (minutes)	46	9	9	7
Average Time to Transfer (minutes)[1]	-	-	54	60
Children's Asthma Care				
Received Home Management Plan of Care	-	-	-	88%
Received Reliever Medication	-	-	-	100%
Received Systemic Corticosteroids	-	-	-	100%
Emergency Department				
Admittance Decision Time (minutes)[2]	428	51	96	98
Head CT Results Within 45 Min. of Arrival[1,3]	-	-	63%	57%
Patients Who Left ER Before Being Seen	19,814	1%	2%	2%
Time from ER Arrival to Admit. (minutes)[2]	429	249	259	274
Time from ER Arrival to Discharge (minutes)	357	95	135	134
Time in ER Before Being Evaluated (minutes)	379	21	22	26
Time to Pain Meds for Fractures (minutes)	88	42	52	57
Heart Attack Care				
Aspirin Given at Discharge	30	100%	99%	99%
Fibrinolytic Meds Within 30 Min. of Arrival[7]	-	-	62%	54%
PCI Within 90 Minutes of Arrival[7]	-	-	97%	96%
Statin Prescribed at Discharge	27	100%	98%	98%
Heart Failure Care				
ACE Inhibitor or ARB for LVSD	22	100%	97%	97%
Discharge Instructions Given	74	100%	93%	94%
Evaluation of LVS Function	99	98%	99%	99%
Medicare Spending				
Medicare Spending per Patient (ratio)	-	0.94	0.91	0.98
Pneumonia Care				
Appropriate Initial Antibiotic Given	54	100%	96%	95%
Blood Culture Timing	92	98%	97%	98%
Pregnancy and Delivery Care				
Newborn Deliveries Scheduled Early[2]	45	2%	2%	6%
Preventive Care				
Immunization for Influenza[2]	386	90%	91%	90%
Immunization for Pneumonia[2]	444	88%	91%	92%
Stroke Care				
Anticoagulation Therapy for Atrial Fibrillation[1,2]	-	-	94%	95%
Antithrombotic Therapy Timing[2]	37	100%	98%	98%
Assessed for Rehabilitation[2]	57	100%	98%	97%
Discharged on Antithrombotic Therapy[2]	51	100%	99%	99%
Discharged on Statin Medication[2]	39	90%	96%	94%
Thrombolytic Therapy Timing[1,2]	-	-	73%	66%
Venous Thromboembolism Prophylaxis[2]	51	94%	94%	94%
Written Stroke Educational Materials Given[2]	27	85%	86%	88%
Surgical Care Improvement Project				
Appropriate Beta Blocker Usage	127	100%	98%	98%
Appropriate VTP Within 24 Hours	428	100%	98%	98%
Controlled Postoperative Blood Glucose[7]	-	-	97%	97%
Perioperative Temperature Management	508	100%	100%	100%
Prophylactic Antibiotic Selection	396	99%	99%	99%
Prophylactic Antibiotic Selection (Outpatient)	177	99%	98%	98%
Prophylactic Antibiotic Stopped	396	100%	99%	98%
Prophylactic Antibiotic Timing	396	100%	98%	99%
Prophylactic Antibiotic Timing (Outpatient)	177	98%	98%	98%
Urinary Catheter Removal	186	98%	97%	97%
Survey of Patients' Hospital Experiences				
Area Around Room 'Always' Quiet at Night	300+	58%	54%	61%
Doctors 'Always' Communicated Well	300+	85%	81%	82%
Home Recovery Information Given	300+	85%	87%	85%
Hospital Given 9 or 10 on 10 Point Scale	300+	76%	70%	71%
Meds 'Always' Explained Before Given	300+	68%	64%	64%
Nurses 'Always' Communicated Well	300+	80%	77%	79%
Pain 'Always' Well Controlled	300+	72%	70%	71%
Room and Bathroom 'Always' Clean	300+	75%	73%	73%
Timely Help 'Always' Received	300+	70%	65%	68%
Would Definitely Recommend Hospital	300+	80%	73%	71%
Use of Medical Imaging				
Cardiac Imaging Stress Test before Surgery	274	4.4%	4.3%	5.3%
Combination Abdominal CT Scan	493	7.5%	6.9%	10.5%
Combination Brain/Sinus CT Scan	328	0.3%	2.3%	2.7%
Combination Chest CT Scan	582	1.2%	1.1%	2.7%
Follow-up Mammogram/Ultrasound	818	8.4%	9.1%	8.8%
Lumbar Spine MRI for Low Back Pain	183	39.3%	37.9%	37.2%

Walla Walla General Hospital

1025 S Second Ave
Walla Walla, WA 99362
Phone: 509-525-0480
Fax: 509-527-8258
URL: www.wwgh.com
Type: Acute Care Hospitals
Emergency Services: Yes
Ownership: Voluntary non-profit - Church
Beds: 72
Key Personnel:
Coronary Care . . . . Jan Huntsman
CEO/President. . . . . Monty E Knittel
Quality Assurance . . . . Peggy LaDuke
Anesthesiology. . . . . Gary Reiber
Emergency Room . . . . Adrian Selfa
Infection Control. . . . . Doris Tucker

Measure	Cases	This Hosp.	State Avg.	U.S. Avg.
Blood Clot Prevention and Treatment				
Anticoagulation Overlap Therapy[2]	18	83%	97%	93%
ICU Venous Thromboembolism Prophylaxis[2]	21	95%	92%	92%
Incidence of Potentially Preventable VTE[1,2]	-	-	9%	10%
UFH with Dosages/Platelet Monitoring[1,2]	-	-	99%	97%
Venous Thromboembolism Prophylaxis[2]	64	95%	86%	85%
Warfarin Therapy Discharge Instructions[2]	14	100%	74%	75%
Chest Pain/Possible Heart Attack Care				
Aspirin Given Within 24 Hours of Arrival[1]	-	-	97%	96%
Fibrinolytic Meds Within 30 Min. of Arrival[3,7]	-	-	51%	58%
Average Time to ECG (minutes)[1]	-	-	9	7
Average Time to Transfer (minutes)[3,7]	-	-	54	60
Children's Asthma Care				
Received Home Management Plan of Care	-	-	-	88%
Received Reliever Medication	-	-	-	100%
Received Systemic Corticosteroids	-	-	-	100%
Emergency Department				
Admittance Decision Time (minutes)[2]	126	62	96	98
Head CT Results Within 45 Min. of Arrival[1]	-	-	63%	57%
Patients Who Left ER Before Being Seen	10,711	0%	2%	2%
Time from ER Arrival to Admit. (minutes)[2]	178	194	259	274
Time from ER Arrival to Discharge (minutes)	353	100	135	134
Time in ER Before Being Evaluated (minutes)	381	15	22	26
Time to Pain Meds for Fractures (minutes)	36	37	52	57
Heart Attack Care				
Aspirin Given at Discharge	30	100%	99%	99%
Fibrinolytic Meds Within 30 Min. of Arrival[7]	-	-	62%	54%
PCI Within 90 Minutes of Arrival[1]	-	-	97%	96%
Statin Prescribed at Discharge	28	100%	98%	98%
Heart Failure Care				
ACE Inhibitor or ARB for LVSD	14	100%	97%	97%
Discharge Instructions Given	40	98%	93%	94%
Evaluation of LVS Function	54	100%	99%	99%

NOTE: Hospital profiles are in alphabetical order by state, then city, then hospital within the city; Rankings exclude hospitals with less than 25 cases except for patient surveys which excludes hospitals with less than 100 cases; (a) 100-299 cases; (1) The number of cases/patients is too few to report; (2) Data submitted were based on a sample of cases/patients; (3) Results are based on a shorter time period than required; (4) Data suppressed by CMS for one or more quarters; (5) Results are not available for this reporting period; (6) Fewer than 100 patients completed the HCAHPS survey; (7) No cases met the criteria for this measure; (8) The lower limit of the confidence interval cannot be calculated if the number of observed infections equals zero; (9) No data are available from the state/territory for this reporting period; (10) The scores shown reflect fewer than 50 completed surveys; (11) There were discrepancies in the data collection process; (12) This measure does not apply to this hospital for this reporting period; (13) Results cannot be calculated for this reporting period; (14) The results for this state are combined with nearby states to protect confidentiality; Please refer to the User's Guide for a full explanation of data.

Measure	Cases	This Hosp.	State Avg.	U.S. Avg.
Medicare Spending				
Medicare Spending per Patient (ratio)	-	0.89	0.91	0.98
Pneumonia Care				
Appropriate Initial Antibiotic Given	31	97%	96%	95%
Blood Culture Timing	55	98%	97%	98%
Pregnancy and Delivery Care				
Newborn Deliveries Scheduled Early[2]	18	0%	2%	6%
Preventive Care				
Immunization for Influenza[2]	241	93%	91%	90%
Immunization for Pneumonia[2]	275	91%	91%	92%
Stroke Care				
Anticoagulation Therapy for Atrial Fibrillation[1,2]	-	-	94%	95%
Antithrombotic Therapy Timing[2]	27	93%	98%	98%
Assessed for Rehabilitation[2]	32	97%	98%	97%
Discharged on Antithrombotic Therapy[2]	32	97%	99%	99%
Discharged on Statin Medication[2]	23	87%	96%	94%
Thrombolytic Therapy Timing[1,2]	-	-	73%	66%
Venous Thromboembolism Prophylaxis[2]	22	91%	94%	94%
Written Stroke Educational Materials Given[2]	15	87%	86%	88%
Surgical Care Improvement Project				
Appropriate Beta Blocker Usage[2]	29	93%	98%	98%
Appropriate VTP Within 24 Hours[2]	118	95%	98%	98%
Controlled Postoperative Blood Glucose[2,7]	-	-	97%	97%
Perioperative Temperature Management[2]	164	100%	100%	100%
Prophylactic Antibiotic Selection[2]	113	98%	99%	99%
Prophylactic Antibiotic Selection (Outpatient)	22	100%	98%	98%
Prophylactic Antibiotic Stopped[2]	110	98%	99%	98%
Prophylactic Antibiotic Timing[2]	113	99%	98%	99%
Prophylactic Antibiotic Timing (Outpatient)	23	87%	98%	98%
Urinary Catheter Removal[2]	55	95%	97%	97%
Survey of Patients' Hospital Experiences				
Area Around Room 'Always' Quiet at Night	(a)	64%	54%	61%
Doctors 'Always' Communicated Well	(a)	79%	81%	82%
Home Recovery Information Given	(a)	87%	87%	85%
Hospital Given 9 or 10 on 10 Point Scale	(a)	71%	70%	71%
Meds 'Always' Explained Before Given	(a)	68%	64%	64%
Nurses 'Always' Communicated Well	(a)	80%	77%	79%
Pain 'Always' Well Controlled	(a)	69%	70%	71%
Room and Bathroom 'Always' Clean	(a)	73%	73%	73%
Timely Help 'Always' Received	(a)	70%	65%	68%
Would Definitely Recommend Hospital	(a)	75%	73%	71%
Use of Medical Imaging				
Cardiac Imaging Stress Test before Surgery	146	4.8%	4.3%	5.3%
Combination Abdominal CT Scan	245	3.3%	6.9%	10.5%
Combination Brain/Sinus CT Scan[1]	-	-	2.3%	2.7%
Combination Chest CT Scan	140	2.9%	1.1%	2.7%
Follow-up Mammogram/Ultrasound	537	6.3%	9.1%	8.8%
Lumbar Spine MRI for Low Back Pain	39	48.7%	37.9%	37.2%

Walla Walla VA Medical Center

77 Wainwright Drive
Walla Walla, WA 99362
Phone: 509-527-3450
Fax: 509-527-3463
Type: Acute Care - VA
Emergency Services: No
Ownership: Government Federal

Key Personnel:
Chief of Medical Staff.......... Delwyn Baker
Quality Assurance .... Steve Bird
Infection Control.............. Bonny Weed

Measure	Cases	This Hosp.	State Avg.	U.S. Avg.
Blood Clot Prevention and Treatment				
Anticoagulation Overlap Therapy	-	-	97%	93%
ICU Venous Thromboembolism Prophylaxis	-	-	92%	92%
Incidence of Potentially Preventable VTE	-	-	9%	10%
UFH with Dosages/Platelet Monitoring	-	-	99%	97%
Venous Thromboembolism Prophylaxis	-	-	86%	85%
Warfarin Therapy Discharge Instructions	-	-	74%	75%
Chest Pain/Possible Heart Attack Care				
Aspirin Given Within 24 Hours of Arrival	-	-	97%	96%
Fibrinolytic Meds Within 30 Min. of Arrival	-	-	51%	58%
Average Time to ECG (minutes)	-	-	9	7
Average Time to Transfer (minutes)	-	-	54	60
Children's Asthma Care				
Received Home Management Plan of Care	-	-	-	88%
Received Reliever Medication	-	-	-	100%
Received Systemic Corticosteroids	-	-	-	100%
Emergency Department				
Admittance Decision Time (minutes)	-	-	96	98
Head CT Results Within 45 Min. of Arrival	-	-	63%	57%
Patients Who Left ER Before Being Seen	-	-	2%	2%
Time from ER Arrival to Admit. (minutes)	-	-	259	274
Time from ER Arrival to Discharge (minutes)	-	-	135	134
Time in ER Before Being Evaluated (minutes)	-	-	22	26
Time to Pain Meds for Fractures (minutes)	-	-	52	57
Heart Attack Care				
Aspirin Given at Discharge[5]	-	-	99%	99%
Fibrinolytic Meds Within 30 Min. of Arrival[5]	-	-	62%	54%
PCI Within 90 Minutes of Arrival[5]	-	-	97%	96%
Statin Prescribed at Discharge[5]	-	-	98%	98%
Heart Failure Care				
ACE Inhibitor or ARB for LVSD[5]	-	-	97%	97%
Discharge Instructions Given[5]	-	-	93%	94%
Evaluation of LVS Function[5]	-	-	99%	99%
Medicare Spending				
Medicare Spending per Patient (ratio)	-	-	0.91	0.98
Pneumonia Care				
Appropriate Initial Antibiotic Given[5]	-	-	96%	95%
Blood Culture Timing[5]	-	-	97%	98%
Pregnancy and Delivery Care				
Newborn Deliveries Scheduled Early	-	-	2%	6%
Preventive Care				
Immunization for Influenza[5]	-	-	91%	90%
Immunization for Pneumonia[5]	-	-	91%	92%
Stroke Care				
Anticoagulation Therapy for Atrial Fibrillation	-	-	94%	95%
Antithrombotic Therapy Timing	-	-	98%	98%
Assessed for Rehabilitation	-	-	98%	97%
Discharged on Antithrombotic Therapy	-	-	99%	99%
Discharged on Statin Medication	-	-	96%	94%
Thrombolytic Therapy Timing	-	-	73%	66%
Venous Thromboembolism Prophylaxis	-	-	94%	94%
Written Stroke Educational Materials Given	-	-	86%	88%
Surgical Care Improvement Project				
Appropriate Beta Blocker Usage[5]	-	-	98%	98%
Appropriate VTP Within 24 Hours[5]	-	-	98%	98%
Controlled Postoperative Blood Glucose[5]	-	-	97%	97%
Perioperative Temperature Management[5]	-	-	100%	100%
Prophylactic Antibiotic Selection[5]	-	-	99%	99%
Prophylactic Antibiotic Selection (Outpatient)	-	-	98%	98%
Prophylactic Antibiotic Stopped[5]	-	-	99%	98%
Prophylactic Antibiotic Timing[5]	-	-	98%	99%
Prophylactic Antibiotic Timing (Outpatient)	-	-	98%	98%
Urinary Catheter Removal[5]	-	-	97%	97%
Survey of Patients' Hospital Experiences				
Area Around Room 'Always' Quiet at Night	-	-	54%	61%
Doctors 'Always' Communicated Well	-	-	81%	82%
Home Recovery Information Given	-	-	87%	85%
Hospital Given 9 or 10 on 10 Point Scale	-	-	70%	71%
Meds 'Always' Explained Before Given	-	-	64%	64%
Nurses 'Always' Communicated Well	-	-	77%	79%
Pain 'Always' Well Controlled	-	-	70%	71%
Room and Bathroom 'Always' Clean	-	-	73%	73%
Timely Help 'Always' Received	-	-	65%	68%
Would Definitely Recommend Hospital	-	-	73%	71%
Use of Medical Imaging				
Cardiac Imaging Stress Test before Surgery	-	-	4.3%	5.3%
Combination Abdominal CT Scan	-	-	6.9%	10.5%
Combination Brain/Sinus CT Scan	-	-	2.3%	2.7%
Combination Chest CT Scan	-	-	1.1%	2.7%
Follow-up Mammogram/Ultrasound	-	-	9.1%	8.8%
Lumbar Spine MRI for Low Back Pain	-	-	37.9%	37.2%

Central Washington Hospital

1201 South Miller Street
Wenatchee, WA 98807
Phone: 509-662-1511
Fax: 509-662-6770
E-mail: contactus@cwhs.com
URL: www.cwhs.com
Type: Acute Care Hospitals
Emergency Services: Yes
Ownership: Voluntary non-profit - Private
Beds: 210

Key Personnel:
Hemotology Center .... Jeanine Allen
Intensive Care Unit............ Mike Brendal
Chief of Medical Staff.......... Stuart Freed, MD
Emergency Room .... Vickie Hammond
Quality Assurance .... Darlene Holt
Patient Relations .... Tracey Kasnic
CEO .... Peter Rutherford, MD

Measure	Cases	This Hosp.	State Avg.	U.S. Avg.
Blood Clot Prevention and Treatment				
Anticoagulation Overlap Therapy[2]	54	100%	97%	93%
ICU Venous Thromboembolism Prophylaxis[2]	89	89%	92%	92%
Incidence of Potentially Preventable VTE[1,2]	-	-	9%	10%
UFH with Dosages/Platelet Monitoring[2]	46	100%	99%	97%
Venous Thromboembolism Prophylaxis[2]	267	81%	86%	85%
Warfarin Therapy Discharge Instructions[2]	40	68%	74%	75%
Chest Pain/Possible Heart Attack Care				
Aspirin Given Within 24 Hours of Arrival[5]	-	-	97%	96%
Fibrinolytic Meds Within 30 Min. of Arrival[5]	-	-	51%	58%
Average Time to ECG (minutes)[5]	-	-	9	7
Average Time to Transfer (minutes)[5]	-	-	54	60
Children's Asthma Care				
Received Home Management Plan of Care	-	-	-	88%
Received Reliever Medication	-	-	-	100%
Received Systemic Corticosteroids	-	-	-	100%
Emergency Department				
Admittance Decision Time (minutes)[2]	355	76	96	98
Head CT Results Within 45 Min. of Arrival[1]	-	-	63%	57%
Patients Who Left ER Before Being Seen	26,513	1%	2%	2%
Time from ER Arrival to Admit. (minutes)[2]	359	227	259	274
Time from ER Arrival to Discharge (minutes)	877	134	135	134
Time in ER Before Being Evaluated (minutes)	441	36	22	26
Time to Pain Meds for Fractures (minutes)	148	50	52	57
Heart Attack Care				
Aspirin Given at Discharge	323	100%	99%	99%
Fibrinolytic Meds Within 30 Min. of Arrival[7]	-	-	62%	54%
PCI Within 90 Minutes of Arrival	19	89%	97%	96%
Statin Prescribed at Discharge	317	99%	98%	98%
Heart Failure Care				
ACE Inhibitor or ARB for LVSD	62	98%	97%	97%
Discharge Instructions Given	201	85%	93%	94%
Evaluation of LVS Function	219	100%	99%	99%
Medicare Spending				
Medicare Spending per Patient (ratio)	-	0.89	0.91	0.98
Pneumonia Care				
Appropriate Initial Antibiotic Given	112	97%	96%	95%
Blood Culture Timing	161	98%	97%	98%
Pregnancy and Delivery Care				
Newborn Deliveries Scheduled Early	142	0%	2%	6%
Preventive Care				
Immunization for Influenza[2]	567	87%	91%	90%
Immunization for Pneumonia[2]	727	91%	91%	92%
Stroke Care				
Anticoagulation Therapy for Atrial Fibrillation	23	91%	94%	95%
Antithrombotic Therapy Timing	107	99%	98%	98%
Assessed for Rehabilitation	152	100%	98%	97%
Discharged on Antithrombotic Therapy	145	100%	99%	99%
Discharged on Statin Medication	110	99%	96%	94%
Thrombolytic Therapy Timing	13	92%	73%	66%
Venous Thromboembolism Prophylaxis	132	98%	94%	94%
Written Stroke Educational Materials Given	93	90%	86%	88%
Surgical Care Improvement Project				
Appropriate Beta Blocker Usage	400	100%	98%	98%
Appropriate VTP Within 24 Hours	959	99%	98%	98%
Controlled Postoperative Blood Glucose	145	100%	97%	97%
Perioperative Temperature Management	1,181	100%	100%	100%
Prophylactic Antibiotic Selection	918	100%	99%	99%

NOTE: Hospital profiles are in alphabetical order by state, then city, then hospital within the city; Rankings exclude hospitals with less than 25 cases except for patient surveys which excludes hospitals with less than 100 cases; (a) 100-299 cases; (1) The number of cases/patients is too few to report; (2) Data submitted were based on a sample of cases/patients; (3) Results are based on a shorter time period than required; (4) Data suppressed by CMS for one or more quarters; (5) Results are not available for this reporting period; (6) Fewer than 100 patients completed the HCAHPS survey; (7) No cases met the criteria for this measure; (8) The lower limit of the confidence interval cannot be calculated if the number of observed infections equals zero; (9) No data are available from the state/territory for this reporting period; (10) The scores shown reflect fewer than 50 completed surveys; (11) There were discrepancies in the data collection process; (12) This measure does not apply to this hospital for this reporting period; (13) Results cannot be calculated for this reporting period; (14) The results for this state are combined with nearby states to protect confidentiality; Please refer to the User's Guide for a full explanation of data.

Measure	Cases	This Hosp.	State Avg.	U.S. Avg.
Prophylactic Antibiotic Selection (Outpatient)	289	98%	98%	98%
Prophylactic Antibiotic Stopped	903	100%	99%	98%
Prophylactic Antibiotic Timing	918	99%	98%	99%
Prophylactic Antibiotic Timing (Outpatient)	295	96%	98%	98%
Urinary Catheter Removal	983	96%	97%	97%
Survey of Patients' Hospital Experiences				
Area Around Room 'Always' Quiet at Night	300+	58%	54%	61%
Doctors 'Always' Communicated Well	300+	85%	81%	82%
Home Recovery Information Given	300+	89%	87%	85%
Hospital Given 9 or 10 on 10 Point Scale	300+	76%	70%	71%
Meds 'Always' Explained Before Given	300+	68%	64%	64%
Nurses 'Always' Communicated Well	300+	78%	77%	79%
Pain 'Always' Well Controlled	300+	71%	70%	71%
Room and Bathroom 'Always' Clean	300+	77%	73%	73%
Timely Help 'Always' Received	300+	67%	65%	68%
Would Definitely Recommend Hospital	300+	81%	73%	71%
Use of Medical Imaging				
Cardiac Imaging Stress Test before Surgery	87	4.6%	4.3%	5.3%
Combination Abdominal CT Scan	401	3.5%	6.9%	10.5%
Combination Brain/Sinus CT Scan	559	0.2%	2.3%	2.7%
Combination Chest CT Scan	114	0.0%	1.1%	2.7%
Follow-up Mammogram/Ultrasound	629	6.4%	9.1%	8.8%
Lumbar Spine MRI for Low Back Pain	143	37.8%	37.9%	37.2%

Confluence Health-Wenatchee Valley Hospital & Clinics

820 North Chelan Avenue
Wenatchee, WA 98801
Phone: 509-663-8711
Fax: 509-665-5864
URL: www.wvmedical.com
Type: Acute Care Hospitals
Emergency Services: No
Ownership: Proprietary
Beds: 20
Key Personnel:
Chief of Medical Staff.......... Stuart Freed
CEO/President............... Shaun Koos

Measure	Cases	This Hosp.	State Avg.	U.S. Avg.
Blood Clot Prevention and Treatment				
Anticoagulation Overlap Therapy[1]	-	-	97%	93%
ICU Venous Thromboembolism Prophylaxis[7]	-	-	92%	92%
Incidence of Potentially Preventable VTE[1]	-	-	9%	10%
UFH with Dosages/Platelet Monitoring[7]	-	-	99%	97%
Venous Thromboembolism Prophylaxis	74	46%	86%	85%
Warfarin Therapy Discharge Instructions[1]	-	-	74%	75%
Chest Pain/Possible Heart Attack Care				
Aspirin Given Within 24 Hours of Arrival[5]	-	-	97%	96%
Fibrinolytic Meds Within 30 Min. of Arrival[5]	-	-	51%	58%
Average Time to ECG (minutes)[5]	-	-	9	7
Average Time to Transfer (minutes)[5]	-	-	54	60
Children's Asthma Care				
Received Home Management Plan of Care	-	-	-	88%
Received Reliever Medication	-	-	-	100%
Received Systemic Corticosteroids	-	-	-	100%
Emergency Department				
Admittance Decision Time (minutes)[7]	-	-	96	98
Head CT Results Within 45 Min. of Arrival[5]	-	-	63%	57%
Patients Who Left ER Before Being Seen	8,747	1%	2%	2%
Time from ER Arrival to Admit. (minutes)[7]	-	-	259	274
Time from ER Arrival to Discharge (minutes)[5]	-	-	135	134
Time in ER Before Being Evaluated (minutes)[5]	-	-	22	26
Time to Pain Meds for Fractures (minutes)[5]	-	-	52	57
Heart Attack Care				
Aspirin Given at Discharge[5]	-	-	99%	99%
Fibrinolytic Meds Within 30 Min. of Arrival[5]	-	-	62%	54%
PCI Within 90 Minutes of Arrival[5]	-	-	97%	96%
Statin Prescribed at Discharge[5]	-	-	98%	98%
Heart Failure Care				
ACE Inhibitor or ARB for LVSD[5]	-	-	97%	97%
Discharge Instructions Given[5]	-	-	93%	94%
Evaluation of LVS Function[5]	-	-	99%	99%
Medicare Spending				
Medicare Spending per Patient (ratio)	-	0.82	0.91	0.98
Pneumonia Care				
Appropriate Initial Antibiotic Given[1,3]	-	-	96%	95%
Blood Culture Timing[3,7]	-	-	97%	98%
Pregnancy and Delivery Care				
Newborn Deliveries Scheduled Early[7]	-	-	2%	6%
Preventive Care				
Immunization for Influenza	246	98%	91%	90%
Immunization for Pneumonia	266	91%	91%	92%
Stroke Care				
Anticoagulation Therapy for Atrial Fibrillation[5]	-	-	94%	95%
Antithrombotic Therapy Timing[5]	-	-	98%	98%
Assessed for Rehabilitation[5]	-	-	98%	97%
Discharged on Antithrombotic Therapy[5]	-	-	99%	99%
Discharged on Statin Medication[5]	-	-	96%	94%
Thrombolytic Therapy Timing[5]	-	-	73%	66%
Venous Thromboembolism Prophylaxis[5]	-	-	94%	94%
Written Stroke Educational Materials Given[5]	-	-	86%	88%
Surgical Care Improvement Project				
Appropriate Beta Blocker Usage	29	100%	98%	98%
Appropriate VTP Within 24 Hours	123	99%	98%	98%
Controlled Postoperative Blood Glucose[7]	-	-	97%	97%
Perioperative Temperature Management	224	100%	100%	100%
Prophylactic Antibiotic Selection	112	100%	99%	99%
Prophylactic Antibiotic Selection (Outpatient)	681	98%	98%	98%
Prophylactic Antibiotic Stopped	110	100%	99%	98%
Prophylactic Antibiotic Timing	112	100%	98%	99%
Prophylactic Antibiotic Timing (Outpatient)	352	97%	98%	98%
Urinary Catheter Removal	86	97%	97%	97%
Survey of Patients' Hospital Experiences				
Area Around Room 'Always' Quiet at Night	(a)	58%	54%	61%
Doctors 'Always' Communicated Well	(a)	89%	81%	82%
Home Recovery Information Given	(a)	91%	87%	85%
Hospital Given 9 or 10 on 10 Point Scale	(a)	80%	70%	71%
Meds 'Always' Explained Before Given	(a)	73%	64%	64%
Nurses 'Always' Communicated Well	(a)	85%	77%	79%
Pain 'Always' Well Controlled	(a)	77%	70%	71%
Room and Bathroom 'Always' Clean	(a)	78%	73%	73%
Timely Help 'Always' Received	(a)	78%	65%	68%
Would Definitely Recommend Hospital	(a)	78%	73%	71%
Use of Medical Imaging				
Cardiac Imaging Stress Test before Surgery	727	2.9%	4.3%	5.3%
Combination Abdominal CT Scan	881	57.3%	6.9%	10.5%
Combination Brain/Sinus CT Scan[1]	-	-	2.3%	2.7%
Combination Chest CT Scan	1,125	3.6%	1.1%	2.7%
Follow-up Mammogram/Ultrasound[7]	-	-	9.1%	8.8%
Lumbar Spine MRI for Low Back Pain[7]	-	-	37.9%	37.2%

Skyline Hospital

211 Skyline Drive
White Salmon, WA 98672
Phone: 509-491-1101
Fax: 509-493-5114
URL: www.skylinehospital.com
Type: Critical Access Hospitals
Emergency Services: Yes
Ownership: Govt - Hospital Dist/Auth
Beds: 32
Key Personnel:
Emergency Room .... Donna Clack
Radiology.................... James Cogswell
Operating Room.............. Michael Hauty
Chief of Medical Staff.......... James Janney, MD
CEO .... Robb Kimmes
Quality Assurance .... Robin Loamis
Hemotology Center .... Linda Pickens
Infection Control.............. Beth Robinson

Measure	Cases	This Hosp.	State Avg.	U.S. Avg.
Blood Clot Prevention and Treatment				
Anticoagulation Overlap Therapy[3,7]	-	-	97%	93%
ICU Venous Thromboembolism Prophylaxis[3,7]	-	-	92%	92%
Incidence of Potentially Preventable VTE[3,7]	-	-	9%	10%
UFH with Dosages/Platelet Monitoring[3,7]	-	-	99%	97%
Venous Thromboembolism Prophylaxis[3]	28	89%	86%	85%
Warfarin Therapy Discharge Instructions[3,7]	-	-	74%	75%
Chest Pain/Possible Heart Attack Care				
Aspirin Given Within 24 Hours of Arrival	11	91%	97%	96%
Fibrinolytic Meds Within 30 Min. of Arrival[7]	-	-	51%	58%
Average Time to ECG (minutes)	11	3	9	7
Average Time to Transfer (minutes)[7]	-	-	54	60
Children's Asthma Care				
Received Home Management Plan of Care	-	-	-	88%
Received Reliever Medication	-	-	-	100%
Received Systemic Corticosteroids	-	-	-	100%
Emergency Department				
Admittance Decision Time (minutes)[3]	28	8	96	98
Head CT Results Within 45 Min. of Arrival[1]	-	-	63%	57%
Patients Who Left ER Before Being Seen[5]	-	-	2%	2%
Time from ER Arrival to Admit. (minutes)[3]	41	204	259	274
Time from ER Arrival to Discharge (minutes)	70	158	135	134
Time in ER Before Being Evaluated (minutes)	78	23	22	26
Time to Pain Meds for Fractures (minutes)	27	41	52	57
Heart Attack Care				
Aspirin Given at Discharge[5]	-	-	99%	99%
Fibrinolytic Meds Within 30 Min. of Arrival[5]	-	-	62%	54%
PCI Within 90 Minutes of Arrival[5]	-	-	97%	96%
Statin Prescribed at Discharge[5]	-	-	98%	98%
Heart Failure Care				
ACE Inhibitor or ARB for LVSD[1]	-	-	97%	97%
Discharge Instructions Given[1]	-	-	93%	94%
Evaluation of LVS Function	13	100%	99%	99%
Medicare Spending				
Medicare Spending per Patient (ratio)	-	-	0.91	0.98
Pneumonia Care				
Appropriate Initial Antibiotic Given	18	89%	96%	95%
Blood Culture Timing	16	100%	97%	98%
Pregnancy and Delivery Care				
Newborn Deliveries Scheduled Early[5]	-	-	2%	6%
Preventive Care				
Immunization for Influenza[2]	31	94%	91%	90%
Immunization for Pneumonia[2]	63	97%	91%	92%
Stroke Care				
Anticoagulation Therapy for Atrial Fibrillation[5]	-	-	94%	95%
Antithrombotic Therapy Timing[5]	-	-	98%	98%
Assessed for Rehabilitation[5]	-	-	98%	97%
Discharged on Antithrombotic Therapy[5]	-	-	99%	99%
Discharged on Statin Medication[5]	-	-	96%	94%
Thrombolytic Therapy Timing[5]	-	-	73%	66%
Venous Thromboembolism Prophylaxis[5]	-	-	94%	94%
Written Stroke Educational Materials Given[5]	-	-	86%	88%
Surgical Care Improvement Project				
Appropriate Beta Blocker Usage[5]	-	-	98%	98%
Appropriate VTP Within 24 Hours[5]	-	-	98%	98%
Controlled Postoperative Blood Glucose[5]	-	-	97%	97%
Perioperative Temperature Management[5]	-	-	100%	100%
Prophylactic Antibiotic Selection[5]	-	-	99%	99%
Prophylactic Antibiotic Selection (Outpatient)[1,3]	-	-	98%	98%
Prophylactic Antibiotic Stopped[5]	-	-	99%	98%
Prophylactic Antibiotic Timing[5]	-	-	98%	99%
Prophylactic Antibiotic Timing (Outpatient)[1,3]	-	-	98%	98%
Urinary Catheter Removal[5]	-	-	97%	97%
Survey of Patients' Hospital Experiences				
Area Around Room 'Always' Quiet at Night[6]	<100	70%	54%	61%
Doctors 'Always' Communicated Well[6]	<100	91%	81%	82%
Home Recovery Information Given[6]	<100	87%	87%	85%
Hospital Given 9 or 10 on 10 Point Scale[6]	<100	81%	70%	71%
Meds 'Always' Explained Before Given[6]	<100	73%	64%	64%
Nurses 'Always' Communicated Well[6]	<100	88%	77%	79%
Pain 'Always' Well Controlled[6]	<100	79%	70%	71%
Room and Bathroom 'Always' Clean[6]	<100	88%	73%	73%
Timely Help 'Always' Received[6]	<100	82%	65%	68%
Would Definitely Recommend Hospital[6]	<100	69%	73%	71%
Use of Medical Imaging				
Cardiac Imaging Stress Test before Surgery[7]	-	-	4.3%	5.3%
Combination Abdominal CT Scan	94	2.1%	6.9%	10.5%
Combination Brain/Sinus CT Scan	126	0.0%	2.3%	2.7%
Combination Chest CT Scan	54	1.9%	1.1%	2.7%
Follow-up Mammogram/Ultrasound	131	16.0%	9.1%	8.8%
Lumbar Spine MRI for Low Back Pain[1]	-	-	37.9%	37.2%

NOTE: Hospital profiles are in alphabetical order by state, then city, then hospital within the city; Rankings exclude hospitals with less than 25 cases except for patient surveys which excludes hospitals with less than 100 cases; (a) 100-299 cases; (1) The number of cases/patients is too few to report; (2) Data submitted were based on a sample of cases/patients; (3) Results are based on a shorter time period than required; (4) Data suppressed by CMS for one or more quarters; (5) Results are not available for this reporting period; (6) Fewer than 100 patients completed the HCAHPS survey; (7) No cases met the criteria for this measure; (8) The lower limit of the confidence interval cannot be calculated if the number of observed infections equals zero; (9) No data are available from the state/territory for this reporting period; (10) The scores shown reflect fewer than 50 completed surveys; (11) There were discrepancies in the data collection process; (12) This measure does not apply to this hospital for this reporting period; (13) Results cannot be calculated for this reporting period; (14) The results for this state are combined with nearby states to protect confidentiality; Please refer to the User's Guide for a full explanation of data.

Yakima Regional Medical & Cardiac Center

110 South Ninth Ave Phone: 509-575-5102
Yakima, WA 98902 Fax: 509-454-6193
URL: www.yakimaregional.org
Type: Acute Care Hospitals Emergency Services: Yes
Ownership: Proprietary Beds: 169

Key Personnel:

Operating Room. . . . . Barry D Bernfeld
CEO/President. . . . . Monte Bostwick
Radiology. . . . . William C Feldmann
Chief of Medical Staff. . . . . Ron Fought
Pediatric In-Patient Care . . . . Sheila Leman
Coronary Care . . . . Maureen Ritter
Infection Control. . . . . Debi Westland
Quality Assurance . . . . Kathy Whitener

Measure	Cases	This Hosp.	State Avg.	U.S. Avg.
Blood Clot Prevention and Treatment				
Anticoagulation Overlap Therapy[2]	42	81%	97%	93%
ICU Venous Thromboembolism Prophylaxis[2]	69	65%	92%	92%
Incidence of Potentially Preventable VTE[1,2]	-	-	9%	10%
UFH with Dosages/Platelet Monitoring[2]	44	100%	99%	97%
Venous Thromboembolism Prophylaxis[2]	296	61%	86%	85%
Warfarin Therapy Discharge Instructions[2]	35	40%	74%	75%
Chest Pain/Possible Heart Attack Care				
Aspirin Given Within 24 Hours of Arrival[1,3]	-	-	97%	96%
Fibrinolytic Meds Within 30 Min. of Arrival[5]	-	-	51%	58%
Average Time to ECG (minutes)[1,3]	-	-	9	7
Average Time to Transfer (minutes)[5]	-	-	54	60
Children's Asthma Care				
Received Home Management Plan of Care	-	-	-	88%
Received Reliever Medication	-	-	-	100%
Received Systemic Corticosteroids	-	-	-	100%
Emergency Department				
Admittance Decision Time (minutes)[2]	554	108	96	98
Head CT Results Within 45 Min. of Arrival[1,3]	-	-	63%	57%
Patients Who Left ER Before Being Seen	31,900	2%	2%	2%
Time from ER Arrival to Admit. (minutes)[2]	626	244	259	274
Time from ER Arrival to Discharge (minutes)	351	127	135	134
Time in ER Before Being Evaluated (minutes)	397	26	22	26
Time to Pain Meds for Fractures (minutes)	72	52	52	57
Heart Attack Care				
Aspirin Given at Discharge	265	99%	99%	99%
Fibrinolytic Meds Within 30 Min. of Arrival[7]	-	-	62%	54%
PCI Within 90 Minutes of Arrival	25	100%	97%	96%
Statin Prescribed at Discharge	257	98%	98%	98%
Heart Failure Care				
ACE Inhibitor or ARB for LVSD	80	98%	97%	97%
Discharge Instructions Given	156	93%	93%	94%
Evaluation of LVS Function	193	99%	99%	99%
Medicare Spending				
Medicare Spending per Patient (ratio)	-	0.97	0.91	0.98
Pneumonia Care				
Appropriate Initial Antibiotic Given	91	96%	96%	95%
Blood Culture Timing	119	97%	97%	98%
Pregnancy and Delivery Care				
Newborn Deliveries Scheduled Early[7]	-	-	2%	6%
Preventive Care				
Immunization for Influenza[2]	571	90%	91%	90%
Immunization for Pneumonia[2]	788	89%	91%	92%
Stroke Care				
Anticoagulation Therapy for Atrial Fibrillation[1]	-	-	94%	95%
Antithrombotic Therapy Timing	52	98%	98%	98%
Assessed for Rehabilitation	62	85%	98%	97%
Discharged on Antithrombotic Therapy	56	89%	99%	99%
Discharged on Statin Medication	45	80%	96%	94%
Thrombolytic Therapy Timing[1]	-	-	73%	66%
Venous Thromboembolism Prophylaxis	60	58%	94%	94%
Written Stroke Educational Materials Given	27	67%	86%	88%
Surgical Care Improvement Project				
Appropriate Beta Blocker Usage	172	98%	98%	98%
Appropriate VTP Within 24 Hours	297	95%	98%	98%
Controlled Postoperative Blood Glucose	154	94%	97%	97%
Perioperative Temperature Management	406	100%	100%	100%
Prophylactic Antibiotic Selection	345	99%	99%	99%
Prophylactic Antibiotic Selection (Outpatient)	117	97%	98%	98%
Prophylactic Antibiotic Stopped	334	96%	99%	98%
Prophylactic Antibiotic Timing	348	97%	98%	99%
Prophylactic Antibiotic Timing (Outpatient)	118	98%	98%	98%
Urinary Catheter Removal	234	92%	97%	97%
Survey of Patients' Hospital Experiences				
Area Around Room 'Always' Quiet at Night	300+	48%	54%	61%
Doctors 'Always' Communicated Well	300+	77%	81%	82%
Home Recovery Information Given	300+	88%	87%	85%
Hospital Given 9 or 10 on 10 Point Scale	300+	55%	70%	71%
Meds 'Always' Explained Before Given	300+	55%	64%	64%
Nurses 'Always' Communicated Well	300+	70%	77%	79%
Pain 'Always' Well Controlled	300+	60%	70%	71%
Room and Bathroom 'Always' Clean	300+	66%	73%	73%
Timely Help 'Always' Received	300+	54%	65%	68%
Would Definitely Recommend Hospital	300+	60%	73%	71%
Use of Medical Imaging				
Cardiac Imaging Stress Test before Surgery	116	4.3%	4.3%	5.3%
Combination Abdominal CT Scan	461	1.7%	6.9%	10.5%
Combination Brain/Sinus CT Scan	526	2.3%	2.3%	2.7%
Combination Chest CT Scan	152	0.0%	1.1%	2.7%
Follow-up Mammogram/Ultrasound	470	8.3%	9.1%	8.8%
Lumbar Spine MRI for Low Back Pain	106	36.8%	37.9%	37.2%

Yakima Valley Memorial Hospital

2811 Tieton Drive Phone: 509-575-8000
Yakima, WA 98902 Fax: 509-576-5772
URL: www.yakimamemorialhospital.org
Type: Acute Care Hospitals Emergency Services: Yes
Ownership: Voluntary non-profit - Private Beds: 218

Key Personnel:

Operating Room. . . . . Barry Bernfeld
Radiology. . . . . William Feldmann
Chief of Medical Staff. . . . . Esther Hunte
President/CEO. . . . . Russ Myers
Infection Control. . . . . Gay Scott

Measure	Cases	This Hosp.	State Avg.	U.S. Avg.
Blood Clot Prevention and Treatment				
Anticoagulation Overlap Therapy[2]	63	94%	97%	93%
ICU Venous Thromboembolism Prophylaxis[2]	51	80%	92%	92%
Incidence of Potentially Preventable VTE[2]	12	17%	9%	10%
UFH with Dosages/Platelet Monitoring[2]	57	100%	99%	97%
Venous Thromboembolism Prophylaxis[2]	310	72%	86%	85%
Warfarin Therapy Discharge Instructions[2]	51	82%	74%	75%
Chest Pain/Possible Heart Attack Care				
Aspirin Given Within 24 Hours of Arrival[1,3]	-	-	97%	96%
Fibrinolytic Meds Within 30 Min. of Arrival[5]	-	-	51%	58%
Average Time to ECG (minutes)[1,3]	-	-	9	7
Average Time to Transfer (minutes)[5]	-	-	54	60
Children's Asthma Care				
Received Home Management Plan of Care	-	-	-	88%
Received Reliever Medication	-	-	-	100%
Received Systemic Corticosteroids	-	-	-	100%
Emergency Department				
Admittance Decision Time (minutes)[2]	516	74	96	98
Head CT Results Within 45 Min. of Arrival[1]	-	-	63%	57%
Patients Who Left ER Before Being Seen	69,471	1%	2%	2%
Time from ER Arrival to Admit. (minutes)[2]	516	203	259	274
Time from ER Arrival to Discharge (minutes)	386	93	135	134
Time in ER Before Being Evaluated (minutes)	408	21	22	26
Time to Pain Meds for Fractures (minutes)	249	44	52	57
Heart Attack Care				
Aspirin Given at Discharge	163	100%	99%	99%
Fibrinolytic Meds Within 30 Min. of Arrival[7]	-	-	62%	54%
PCI Within 90 Minutes of Arrival	21	100%	97%	96%
Statin Prescribed at Discharge	164	100%	98%	98%
Heart Failure Care				
ACE Inhibitor or ARB for LVSD	53	100%	97%	97%
Discharge Instructions Given	203	98%	93%	94%
Evaluation of LVS Function	274	100%	99%	99%
Medicare Spending				
Medicare Spending per Patient (ratio)	-	0.90	0.91	0.98
Pneumonia Care				
Appropriate Initial Antibiotic Given	158	99%	96%	95%
Blood Culture Timing	322	97%	97%	98%
Pregnancy and Delivery Care				
Newborn Deliveries Scheduled Early[2]	211	1%	2%	6%
Preventive Care				
Immunization for Influenza[2]	489	63%	91%	90%
Immunization for Pneumonia[2]	476	81%	91%	92%
Stroke Care				
Anticoagulation Therapy for Atrial Fibrillation	17	100%	94%	95%
Antithrombotic Therapy Timing	82	100%	98%	98%
Assessed for Rehabilitation	107	99%	98%	97%
Discharged on Antithrombotic Therapy	103	100%	99%	99%
Discharged on Statin Medication	88	97%	96%	94%
Thrombolytic Therapy Timing	14	86%	73%	66%
Venous Thromboembolism Prophylaxis	106	96%	94%	94%
Written Stroke Educational Materials Given	58	98%	86%	88%
Surgical Care Improvement Project				
Appropriate Beta Blocker Usage[2]	197	98%	98%	98%
Appropriate VTP Within 24 Hours[2]	751	98%	98%	98%
Controlled Postoperative Blood Glucose[2,7]	-	-	97%	97%
Perioperative Temperature Management[2]	888	100%	100%	100%
Prophylactic Antibiotic Selection[2]	695	100%	99%	99%
Prophylactic Antibiotic Selection (Outpatient)	335	95%	98%	98%
Prophylactic Antibiotic Stopped[2]	684	98%	99%	98%
Prophylactic Antibiotic Timing[2]	695	99%	98%	99%
Prophylactic Antibiotic Timing (Outpatient)	338	99%	98%	98%
Urinary Catheter Removal[2]	654	98%	97%	97%
Survey of Patients' Hospital Experiences				
Area Around Room 'Always' Quiet at Night	300+	49%	54%	61%
Doctors 'Always' Communicated Well	300+	78%	81%	82%
Home Recovery Information Given	300+	86%	87%	85%
Hospital Given 9 or 10 on 10 Point Scale	300+	65%	70%	71%
Meds 'Always' Explained Before Given	300+	60%	64%	64%
Nurses 'Always' Communicated Well	300+	73%	77%	79%
Pain 'Always' Well Controlled	300+	64%	70%	71%
Room and Bathroom 'Always' Clean	300+	71%	73%	73%
Timely Help 'Always' Received	300+	60%	65%	68%
Would Definitely Recommend Hospital	300+	71%	73%	71%
Use of Medical Imaging				
Cardiac Imaging Stress Test before Surgery	671	3.1%	4.3%	5.3%
Combination Abdominal CT Scan	1,387	1.9%	6.9%	10.5%
Combination Brain/Sinus CT Scan	865	1.3%	2.3%	2.7%
Combination Chest CT Scan	1,053	0.0%	1.1%	2.7%
Follow-up Mammogram/Ultrasound	2,659	8.4%	9.1%	8.8%
Lumbar Spine MRI for Low Back Pain	408	35.0%	37.9%	37.2%

NOTE: Hospital profiles are in alphabetical order by state, then city, then hospital within the city; Rankings exclude hospitals with less than 25 cases except for patient surveys which excludes hospitals with less than 100 cases; (a) 100-299 cases; (1) The number of cases/patients is too few to report; (2) Data submitted were based on a sample of cases/patients; (3) Results are based on a shorter time period than required; (4) Data suppressed by CMS for one or more quarters; (5) Results are not available for this reporting period; (6) Fewer than 100 patients completed the HCAHPS survey; (7) No cases met the criteria for this measure; (8) The lower limit of the confidence interval cannot be calculated if the number of observed infections equals zero; (9) No data are available from the state/territory for this reporting period; (10) The scores shown reflect fewer than 50 completed surveys; (11) There were discrepancies in the data collection process; (12) This measure does not apply to this hospital for this reporting period; (13) Results cannot be calculated for this reporting period; (14) The results for this state are combined with nearby states to protect confidentiality; Please refer to the User's Guide for a full explanation of data.

Blood Clot Prevention and Treatment

Anticoagulation Overlap Therapy

Hospital Name	City	Rate	Cases
Wyoming Medical Center[2]	Casper	100%	36
Cheyenne Regional Medical Center[2]	Cheyenne	88%	60

ICU Venous Thromboembolism Prophylaxis

Hospital Name	City	Rate	Cases
Saint Johns Medical Center[2]	Jackson	100%	51
Sagewest Health Care[2]	Riverton	97%	33
Wyoming Medical Center[2]	Casper	97%	37
Sheridan Memorial Hospital[2]	Sheridan	94%	33
Cheyenne Regional Medical Center[2]	Cheyenne	90%	59
Lander Regional Hospital[2]	Lander	86%	42
Campbell County Memorial Hospital[2]	Gillette	71%	55

UFH with Dosages/Platelet Count Monitoring

Hospital Name	City	Rate	Cases
Wyoming Medical Center[2]	Casper	100%	37
Cheyenne Regional Medical Center[2]	Cheyenne	88%	26

Venous Thromboembolism Prophylaxis

Hospital Name	City	Rate	Cases
Evanston Regional Hospital[2]	Evanston	100%	135
Wyoming Medical Center[2]	Casper	99%	333
Saint Johns Medical Center[2]	Jackson	96%	122
Mountain View Regional Hospital[2]	Casper	94%	203
Sagewest Health Care[2]	Riverton	94%	102
Cheyenne Regional Medical Center[2]	Cheyenne	85%	282
Ivinson Memorial Hospital[2]	Laramie	85%	96
South Lincoln Medical Center	Kemmerer	85%	33
Memorial Hospital Sweetwater County[2]	Rock Springs	83%	101
Sheridan Memorial Hospital[2]	Sheridan	77%	112
Lander Regional Hospital[2]	Lander	76%	89
West Park Hospital District[2]	Cody	74%	47
Campbell County Memorial Hospital[2]	Gillette	69%	118
Star Valley Medical Center[2,3]	Afton	56%	91

Warfarin Therapy Discharge Instructions

Hospital Name	City	Rate	Cases
Wyoming Medical Center[2]	Casper	97%	30
Campbell County Memorial Hospital[2]	Gillette	84%	25
Cheyenne Regional Medical Center[2]	Cheyenne	13%	61

Chest Pain/Possible Heart Attack Care

Aspirin Given Within 24 Hours of Arrival

Hospital Name	City	Rate	Cases
Campbell County Memorial Hospital	Gillette	100%	84
Evanston Regional Hospital	Evanston	100%	27
Sagewest Health Care	Riverton	100%	42
Community Hospital	Torrington	97%	29
Memorial Hospital Sweetwater County	Rock Springs	97%	74
Memorial Hospital of Carbon County	Rawlins	96%	25
Saint Johns Medical Center	Jackson	96%	27
Ivinson Memorial Hospital	Laramie	95%	43
Lander Regional Hospital	Lander	95%	39

Average Time to ECG (minutes)

Hospital Name	City	Min.	Cases
Lander Regional Hospital	Lander	0	41
Evanston Regional Hospital	Evanston	1	28
Campbell County Memorial Hospital	Gillette	5	88
Saint Johns Medical Center	Jackson	5	27
Ivinson Memorial Hospital	Laramie	6	41
Sagewest Health Care	Riverton	6	44
Community Hospital	Torrington	7	29
Memorial Hospital Sweetwater County	Rock Springs	10	77

Children's Asthma Care

No hospitals met the 25 case threshold.

Emergency Department

Admittance Decision Time (minutes)

Hospital Name	City	Min.	Cases
Mountain View Regional Hospital[2]	Casper	34	49
Evanston Regional Hospital[2]	Evanston	35	290
Star Valley Medical Center[2]	Afton	40	63
Saint Johns Medical Center[2]	Jackson	42	119
Campbell County Memorial Hospital[2]	Gillette	53	276
Sheridan Memorial Hospital[2]	Sheridan	56	60
Sagewest Health Care[2]	Riverton	64	332
Lander Regional Hospital[2]	Lander	67	185
Ivinson Memorial Hospital[2]	Laramie	70	174
Cheyenne Regional Medical Center[2]	Cheyenne	74	526
Memorial Hospital Sweetwater County[2]	Rock Springs	105	289
Wyoming Medical Center[2]	Casper	123	511

Patients Who Left ER Before Being Seen

Hospital Name	City	Rate	Cases
Evanston Regional Hospital	Evanston	0%	8577
Memorial Hospital of Carbon County	Rawlins	0%	7531
Platte County Memorial Hospital	Wheatland	0%	3765
Saint Johns Medical Center	Jackson	0%	8395
Sheridan Memorial Hospital	Sheridan	0%	8607
South Lincoln Medical Center	Kemmerer	0%	2143
Washakie Medical Center	Worland	0%	4866
West Park Hospital District	Cody	0%	6455
Campbell County Memorial Hospital	Gillette	1%	20677
Community Hospital	Torrington	1%	4202
Ivinson Memorial Hospital	Laramie	1%	12510
Lander Regional Hospital	Lander	1%	11546
Mountain View Regional Hospital	Casper	1%	5001
Memorial Hospital Sweetwater County	Rock Springs	2%	19161
Wyoming Medical Center	Casper	2%	38006
Cheyenne Regional Medical Center	Cheyenne	3%	39723
Sagewest Health Care	Riverton	3%	11928

Time from ER Arrival to Being Admitted (minutes)

Hospital Name	City	Min.	Cases
Evanston Regional Hospital[2]	Evanston	159	292
Sheridan Memorial Hospital[2]	Sheridan	166	74
Star Valley Medical Center[2]	Afton	172	78
Saint Johns Medical Center[2]	Jackson	178	140
Mountain View Regional Hospital[2]	Casper	192	52
Lander Regional Hospital[2]	Lander	193	203
Campbell County Memorial Hospital[2]	Gillette	200	278
Sagewest Health Care[2]	Riverton	202	332
Ivinson Memorial Hospital[2]	Laramie	227	252
Cheyenne Regional Medical Center[2]	Cheyenne	244	560
Wyoming Medical Center[2]	Casper	248	548
Memorial Hospital Sweetwater County[2]	Rock Springs	256	289
West Park Hospital District[2]	Cody	261	221

Time from ER Arrival to Discharge (minutes)

Hospital Name	City	Min.	Cases
Evanston Regional Hospital	Evanston	73	389
South Lincoln Medical Center[3]	Kemmerer	80	118
Lander Regional Hospital	Lander	82	396
Saint Johns Medical Center	Jackson	93	357
Sagewest Health Care	Riverton	101	371
Sheridan Memorial Hospital	Sheridan	101	259
Mountain View Regional Hospital	Casper	120	401
Memorial Hospital Sweetwater County	Rock Springs	129	350
Campbell County Memorial Hospital	Gillette	137	415
Star Valley Medical Center	Afton	137	247
Ivinson Memorial Hospital	Laramie	141	380
Cheyenne Regional Medical Center	Cheyenne	162	383
Wyoming Medical Center	Casper	176	364

Time in ER Before Being Evaluated (minutes)

Hospital Name	City	Min.	Cases
Star Valley Medical Center	Afton	4	280
Lander Regional Hospital	Lander	7	433
Ivinson Memorial Hospital	Laramie	8	317
Sagewest Health Care	Riverton	8	430
Evanston Regional Hospital	Evanston	9	421
Saint Johns Medical Center	Jackson	14	348
South Lincoln Medical Center[3]	Kemmerer	16	135
Cheyenne Regional Medical Center	Cheyenne	17	365
Sheridan Memorial Hospital	Sheridan	26	203
Mountain View Regional Hospital	Casper	27	395
Wyoming Medical Center	Casper	30	409
Memorial Hospital Sweetwater County	Rock Springs	37	373
Campbell County Memorial Hospital	Gillette	41	429

Time to Pain Meds for Bone Fractures (minutes)

Hospital Name	City	Min.	Cases
Evanston Regional Hospital	Evanston	19	68
Star Valley Medical Center	Afton	20	36
Saint Johns Medical Center	Jackson	30	53
Sagewest Health Care	Riverton	34	72
Lander Regional Hospital	Lander	35	31
Sheridan Memorial Hospital	Sheridan	44	55
Campbell County Memorial Hospital	Gillette	48	105
Wyoming Medical Center	Casper	51	139
Cheyenne Regional Medical Center	Cheyenne	58	212
Memorial Hospital Sweetwater County	Rock Springs	58	90
Ivinson Memorial Hospital	Laramie	59	99

Heart Attack Care

Aspirin Given at Discharge

Hospital Name	City	Rate	Cases
Wyoming Medical Center	Casper	100%	335
Cheyenne Regional Medical Center	Cheyenne	98%	181

PCI Within 90 Minutes of Arrival

Hospital Name	City	Rate	Cases
Cheyenne Regional Medical Center	Cheyenne	100%	29
Wyoming Medical Center	Casper	100%	47

Statin Prescribed at Discharge

Hospital Name	City	Rate	Cases
Wyoming Medical Center	Casper	100%	329
Cheyenne Regional Medical Center	Cheyenne	99%	171

Heart Failure Care

ACE Inhibitor or ARB for LVSD

Hospital Name	City	Rate	Cases
Cheyenne Regional Medical Center	Cheyenne	100%	33
Wyoming Medical Center	Casper	100%	52

Discharge Instructions Given

Hospital Name	City	Rate	Cases
Wyoming Medical Center	Casper	98%	174
Sagewest Health Care	Riverton	97%	32
Cheyenne Regional Medical Center	Cheyenne	95%	92
Campbell County Memorial Hospital	Gillette	88%	34
Memorial Hospital Sweetwater County	Rock Springs	41%	29

Evaluation of LVS Function

Hospital Name	City	Rate	Cases
Campbell County Memorial Hospital	Gillette	100%	41
Sagewest Health Care	Riverton	100%	36
Sheridan Memorial Hospital[2]	Sheridan	100%	28
Wyoming Medical Center	Casper	100%	212
Cheyenne Regional Medical Center	Cheyenne	97%	119
Ivinson Memorial Hospital	Laramie	96%	28
Memorial Hospital Sweetwater County	Rock Springs	86%	37

Medicare Spending

Medicare Spending per Patient (ratio)

Hospital Name	City	Ratio	Cases
Evanston Regional Hospital	Evanston	0.86	-
Ivinson Memorial Hospital	Laramie	0.87	-
Saint Johns Medical Center	Jackson	0.87	-
Lander Regional Hospital	Lander	0.89	-
Campbell County Memorial Hospital	Gillette	0.90	-
Memorial Hospital Sweetwater County	Rock Springs	0.90	-
Sheridan Memorial Hospital	Sheridan	0.94	-
Sagewest Health Care	Riverton	0.95	-
Wyoming Medical Center	Casper	1.01	-
Cheyenne Regional Medical Center	Cheyenne	1.03	-
Mountain View Regional Hospital	Casper	1.03	-

Pneumonia Care

Appropriate Initial Antibiotic Given

Hospital Name	City	Rate	Cases
Cheyenne Regional Medical Center	Cheyenne	98%	146
Wyoming Medical Center	Casper	98%	144
Lander Regional Hospital	Lander	97%	36
Ivinson Memorial Hospital	Laramie	94%	49
Sagewest Health Care	Riverton	94%	36
Sheridan Memorial Hospital[2]	Sheridan	94%	47
Campbell County Memorial Hospital	Gillette	93%	44
Memorial Hospital Sweetwater County	Rock Springs	93%	29
Evanston Regional Hospital	Evanston	91%	32
West Park Hospital District	Cody	87%	30
North Big Horn Hospital District	Lovell	85%	26
Saint Johns Medical Center	Jackson	85%	27

Blood Culture Timing

Hospital Name	City	Rate	Cases
Evanston Regional Hospital	Evanston	100%	28
Ivinson Memorial Hospital	Laramie	100%	80
Memorial Hospital of Converse County	Douglas	100%	29
Saint Johns Medical Center	Jackson	100%	30
Campbell County Memorial Hospital	Gillette	99%	70
Cheyenne Regional Medical Center	Cheyenne	99%	154
Wyoming Medical Center	Casper	99%	206
Lander Regional Hospital	Lander	98%	47
Sagewest Health Care	Riverton	98%	48

NOTE: Hospital profiles are in alphabetical order by state, then city, then hospital within the city; Rankings exclude hospitals with less than 25 cases except for patient surveys which excludes hospitals with less than 100 cases; (a) 100-299 cases; (1) The number of cases/patients is too few to report; (2) Data submitted were based on a sample of cases/patients; (3) Results are based on a shorter time period than required; (4) Data suppressed by CMS for one or more quarters; (5) Results are not available for this reporting period; (6) Fewer than 100 patients completed the HCAHPS survey; (7) No cases met the criteria for this measure; (8) The lower limit of the confidence interval cannot be calculated if the number of observed infections equals zero; (9) No data are available from the state/territory for this reporting period; (10) The scores shown reflect fewer than 50 completed surveys; (11) There were discrepancies in the data collection process; (12) This measure does not apply to this hospital for this reporting period; (13) Results cannot be calculated for this reporting period; (14) The results for this state are combined with nearby states to protect confidentiality; Please refer to the User's Guide for a full explanation of data.

Hospital Name	City	Rate	Cases
Sheridan Memorial Hospital[2]	Sheridan	98%	47
Memorial Hospital Sweetwater County	Rock Springs	97%	37
Washakie Medical Center	Worland	97%	30
West Park Hospital District	Cody	89%	35

Pregnancy and Delivery Care

Newborns whose Deliveries were Scheduled Early

Hospital Name	City	Rate	Cases
Evanston Regional Hospital[2]	Evanston	0%	29
Sagewest Health Care[2]	Riverton	3%	29
Wyoming Medical Center	Casper	3%	87
Campbell County Memorial Hospital	Gillette	6%	84
Lander Regional Hospital[2]	Lander	10%	39
Cheyenne Regional Medical Center[2]	Cheyenne	11%	27
Memorial Hospital Sweetwater County[2]	Rock Springs	11%	28
Saint Johns Medical Center[2]	Jackson	14%	37
Ivinson Memorial Hospital[2]	Laramie	15%	34

Preventive Care

Immunization for Influenza

Hospital Name	City	Rate	Cases
Evanston Regional Hospital[2]	Evanston	99%	262
Sagewest Health Care[2]	Riverton	96%	271
Campbell County Memorial Hospital[2]	Gillette	95%	248
Saint Johns Medical Center[2]	Jackson	95%	233
Star Valley Medical Center	Afton	92%	51
Mountain View Regional Hospital[2]	Casper	90%	337
Wyoming Medical Center[2]	Casper	90%	556
Cheyenne Regional Medical Center[2]	Cheyenne	88%	542
Memorial Hospital of Carbon County[2]	Rawlins	85%	39
Sheridan VA Medical Center[2,3]	Sheridan	85%	139
Cheyenne VA Medical Center[2,3]	Cheyenne	84%	139
Sheridan Memorial Hospital[2]	Sheridan	84%	259
Ivinson Memorial Hospital[2]	Laramie	81%	263
Lander Regional Hospital[2]	Lander	80%	246
Memorial Hospital Sweetwater County[2]	Rock Springs	68%	242
West Park Hospital District[2]	Cody	64%	261

Immunization for Pneumonia

Hospital Name	City	Rate	Cases
Evanston Regional Hospital[2]	Evanston	99%	209
Sagewest Health Care[2]	Riverton	97%	250
South Lincoln Medical Center[2]	Kemmerer	97%	32
Wyoming Medical Center[2]	Casper	96%	590
Saint Johns Medical Center[2]	Jackson	95%	173
Cheyenne VA Medical Center[2,3]	Cheyenne	94%	310
Mountain View Regional Hospital[2]	Casper	94%	387
Lander Regional Hospital[2]	Lander	93%	215
Sheridan VA Medical Center[2,3]	Sheridan	93%	195
Star Valley Medical Center	Afton	92%	137
Memorial Hospital of Carbon County[2,3]	Rawlins	91%	34
West Park Hospital District[2]	Cody	91%	246
Ivinson Memorial Hospital[2]	Laramie	87%	247
Campbell County Memorial Hospital[2]	Gillette	80%	204
Memorial Hospital Sweetwater County[2]	Rock Springs	75%	199
Sheridan Memorial Hospital[2]	Sheridan	74%	253
Cheyenne Regional Medical Center[2]	Cheyenne	73%	530

Stroke Care

Antithrombotic Therapy Timing

Hospital Name	City	Rate	Cases
Campbell County Memorial Hospital	Gillette	100%	25
Cheyenne Regional Medical Center	Cheyenne	96%	57
Wyoming Medical Center	Casper	96%	55

Assessed for Rehabilitation

Hospital Name	City	Rate	Cases
Wyoming Medical Center	Casper	100%	89
Cheyenne Regional Medical Center	Cheyenne	93%	70
Campbell County Memorial Hospital	Gillette	88%	26

Discharged on Antithrombotic Therapy

Hospital Name	City	Rate	Cases
Campbell County Memorial Hospital	Gillette	100%	25
Wyoming Medical Center	Casper	100%	75
Cheyenne Regional Medical Center	Cheyenne	95%	63

Discharged on Statin Medication

Hospital Name	City	Rate	Cases
Wyoming Medical Center	Casper	98%	48
Cheyenne Regional Medical Center	Cheyenne	72%	50

Thrombolytic Therapy Timing

Hospital Name	City	Rate	Cases
Cheyenne Regional Medical Center	Cheyenne	26%	27

Venous Thromboembolism (VTE) Prophylaxis

Hospital Name	City	Rate	Cases
Wyoming Medical Center	Casper	93%	85
Cheyenne Regional Medical Center	Cheyenne	85%	72

Written Stroke Educational Materials Given

Hospital Name	City	Rate	Cases
Wyoming Medical Center	Casper	98%	46
Cheyenne Regional Medical Center	Cheyenne	31%	36

Surgical Care Improvement Project

Appropriate Beta Blocker Usage

Hospital Name	City	Rate	Cases
Wyoming Medical Center[2]	Casper	99%	166
Saint Johns Medical Center[2]	Jackson	97%	37
Cheyenne Regional Medical Center	Cheyenne	96%	186
Ivinson Memorial Hospital	Laramie	91%	57
Sheridan Memorial Hospital[2]	Sheridan	90%	48
West Park Hospital District[2]	Cody	81%	90

Appropriate VTP Within 24 Hours

Hospital Name	City	Rate	Cases
Evanston Regional Hospital	Evanston	100%	55
Memorial Hospital of Converse County	Douglas	100%	102
Powell Valley Hospital	Powell	100%	38
Star Valley Medical Center	Afton	100%	62
Washakie Medical Center	Worland	100%	40
Saint Johns Medical Center[2]	Jackson	99%	219
Cheyenne Regional Medical Center	Cheyenne	98%	440
West Park Hospital District[2]	Cody	98%	269
Sagewest Health Care	Riverton	96%	49
Wyoming Medical Center[2]	Casper	96%	423
Ivinson Memorial Hospital	Laramie	93%	123
Lander Regional Hospital	Lander	93%	72
Sheridan Memorial Hospital[2]	Sheridan	93%	205
Memorial Hospital Sweetwater County	Rock Springs	87%	61
Mountain View Regional Hospital[2]	Casper	87%	121
Campbell County Memorial Hospital	Gillette	82%	130

Controlled Postoperative Blood Glucose

Hospital Name	City	Rate	Cases
Cheyenne Regional Medical Center	Cheyenne	99%	69
Wyoming Medical Center[2]	Casper	99%	113

Perioperative Temperature Management

Hospital Name	City	Rate	Cases
Cheyenne Regional Medical Center	Cheyenne	100%	590
Evanston Regional Hospital	Evanston	100%	66
Lander Regional Hospital	Lander	100%	103
Memorial Hospital of Converse County	Douglas	100%	114
Memorial Hospital Sweetwater County	Rock Springs	100%	75
Powell Valley Hospital	Powell	100%	46
Sagewest Health Care	Riverton	100%	58
Saint Johns Medical Center[2]	Jackson	100%	239
Star Valley Medical Center	Afton	100%	73
Washakie Medical Center	Worland	100%	42
West Park Hospital District[2]	Cody	100%	308
Campbell County Memorial Hospital	Gillette	99%	139
Ivinson Memorial Hospital	Laramie	99%	278
Mountain View Regional Hospital[2]	Casper	99%	135
Sheridan Memorial Hospital[2]	Sheridan	99%	270
Wyoming Medical Center[2]	Casper	99%	554

Prophylactic Antibiotic Selection

Hospital Name	City	Rate	Cases
Cheyenne Regional Medical Center	Cheyenne	100%	434
Evanston Regional Hospital	Evanston	100%	47
Memorial Hospital of Converse County	Douglas	100%	101
Sagewest Health Care	Riverton	100%	40
Star Valley Medical Center	Afton	100%	60
Washakie Medical Center	Worland	100%	28
Lander Regional Hospital	Lander	99%	81
Saint Johns Medical Center[2]	Jackson	99%	180
Sheridan Memorial Hospital[2]	Sheridan	99%	202
West Park Hospital District[2]	Cody	99%	254
Wyoming Medical Center[2]	Casper	99%	491
Ivinson Memorial Hospital	Laramie	98%	224
Mountain View Regional Hospital[2]	Casper	97%	94
Powell Valley Hospital	Powell	97%	34
Campbell County Memorial Hospital	Gillette	95%	107
Memorial Hospital Sweetwater County	Rock Springs	95%	42

Prophylactic Antibiotic Selection (Outpatient)

Hospital Name	City	Rate	Cases
Memorial Hospital of Converse County	Douglas	100%	67
Mountain View Regional Hospital	Casper	100%	95
Sheridan Memorial Hospital	Sheridan	100%	92
Lander Regional Hospital	Lander	97%	29
Campbell County Memorial Hospital	Gillette	96%	90
Ivinson Memorial Hospital	Laramie	96%	114
Saint Johns Medical Center	Jackson	95%	74
Wyoming Medical Center	Casper	94%	221
Cheyenne Regional Medical Center	Cheyenne	93%	236
Star Valley Medical Center	Afton	93%	27

Prophylactic Antibiotic Stopped

Hospital Name	City	Rate	Cases
Campbell County Memorial Hospital	Gillette	100%	107
Powell Valley Hospital	Powell	100%	34
Sagewest Health Care	Riverton	100%	39
Star Valley Medical Center	Afton	100%	60
Washakie Medical Center	Worland	100%	28
Wyoming Medical Center[2]	Casper	100%	481
Cheyenne Regional Medical Center	Cheyenne	99%	429
Lander Regional Hospital	Lander	99%	79
Saint Johns Medical Center[2]	Jackson	99%	179
Evanston Regional Hospital	Evanston	98%	47
Ivinson Memorial Hospital	Laramie	98%	223
Memorial Hospital of Converse County	Douglas	98%	100
Sheridan Memorial Hospital[2]	Sheridan	96%	199
Mountain View Regional Hospital[2]	Casper	94%	93
Memorial Hospital Sweetwater County	Rock Springs	90%	40
West Park Hospital District[2]	Cody	83%	247

Prophylactic Antibiotic Timing

Hospital Name	City	Rate	Cases
Campbell County Memorial Hospital	Gillette	100%	107
Cheyenne Regional Medical Center	Cheyenne	100%	435
Evanston Regional Hospital	Evanston	100%	48
Sagewest Health Care	Riverton	100%	40
Star Valley Medical Center	Afton	100%	60
Washakie Medical Center	Worland	100%	28
Mountain View Regional Hospital[2]	Casper	99%	94
Wyoming Medical Center[2]	Casper	99%	493
Memorial Hospital of Converse County	Douglas	98%	101
Saint Johns Medical Center[2]	Jackson	98%	181
Sheridan Memorial Hospital[2]	Sheridan	98%	203
West Park Hospital District[2]	Cody	98%	254
Ivinson Memorial Hospital	Laramie	97%	224
Lander Regional Hospital	Lander	96%	82
Memorial Hospital Sweetwater County	Rock Springs	93%	42
Powell Valley Hospital	Powell	91%	34

Prophylactic Antibiotic Timing (Outpatient)

Hospital Name	City	Rate	Cases
Campbell County Memorial Hospital	Gillette	100%	90
Lander Regional Hospital	Lander	100%	29
Memorial Hospital of Converse County	Douglas	100%	67
Mountain View Regional Hospital	Casper	99%	95
Ivinson Memorial Hospital	Laramie	98%	116
Wyoming Medical Center	Casper	98%	221
Star Valley Medical Center	Afton	96%	28
Saint Johns Medical Center	Jackson	95%	76
Sheridan Memorial Hospital	Sheridan	94%	94
Cheyenne Regional Medical Center	Cheyenne	92%	247

Urinary Catheter Removal

Hospital Name	City	Rate	Cases
Memorial Hospital of Converse County	Douglas	99%	107
Saint Johns Medical Center[2]	Jackson	98%	187
Star Valley Medical Center	Afton	98%	60
Wyoming Medical Center[2]	Casper	98%	347
Ivinson Memorial Hospital	Laramie	97%	217
Powell Valley Hospital	Powell	97%	30
Cheyenne Regional Medical Center	Cheyenne	95%	183
West Park Hospital District[2]	Cody	95%	190
Campbell County Memorial Hospital	Gillette	93%	56
Sheridan Memorial Hospital[2]	Sheridan	92%	159
Evanston Regional Hospital	Evanston	91%	34
Memorial Hospital Sweetwater County	Rock Springs	85%	27
Mountain View Regional Hospital[2]	Casper	82%	104

Survey of Patients' Hospital Experiences

Area Around Room 'Always' Quiet at Night

Hospital Name	City	Rate	Cases
Washakie Medical Center[11]	Worland	71%	(a)
Memorial Hospital of Converse County	Douglas	70%	(a)
Memorial Hospital of Carbon County	Rawlins	68%	(a)
Mountain View Regional Hospital	Casper	67%	300+

NOTE: Hospital profiles are in alphabetical order by state, then city, then hospital within the city; Rankings exclude hospitals with less than 25 cases except for patient surveys which excludes hospitals with less than 100 cases; (a) 100-299 cases; (1) The number of cases/patients is too few to report; (2) Data submitted were based on a sample of cases/patients; (3) Results are based on a shorter time period than required; (4) Data suppressed by CMS for one or more quarters; (5) Results are not available for this reporting period; (6) Fewer than 100 patients completed the HCAHPS survey; (7) No cases met the criteria for this measure; (8) The lower limit of the confidence interval cannot be calculated if the number of observed infections equals zero; (9) No data are available from the state/territory for this reporting period; (10) The scores shown reflect fewer than 50 completed surveys; (11) There were discrepancies in the data collection process; (12) This measure does not apply to this hospital for this reporting period; (13) Results cannot be calculated for this reporting period; (14) The results for this state are combined with nearby states to protect confidentiality; Please refer to the User's Guide for a full explanation of data.

Community Hospital[11]	Torrington	66%	(a)
Campbell County Memorial Hospital	Gillette	62%	300+
Evanston Regional Hospital	Evanston	62%	(a)
Memorial Hospital Sweetwater County	Rock Springs	62%	300+
Saint Johns Medical Center	Jackson	60%	300+
Sheridan Memorial Hospital	Sheridan	59%	300+
West Park Hospital District	Cody	58%	300+
Ivinson Memorial Hospital	Laramie	56%	300+
Cheyenne Regional Medical Center	Cheyenne	55%	300+
Lander Regional Hospital	Lander	55%	300+
Sagewest Health Care	Riverton	52%	(a)
Wyoming Medical Center	Casper	44%	300+
Hot Springs County Memorial Hospital	Thermopolis	43%	(a)

Doctors 'Always' Communicated Well

Hospital Name	City	Rate	Cases
Community Hospital[11]	Torrington	90%	(a)
West Park Hospital District	Cody	85%	300+
Hot Springs County Memorial Hospital	Thermopolis	83%	(a)
Lander Regional Hospital	Lander	83%	300+
Washakie Medical Center[11]	Worland	83%	(a)
Evanston Regional Hospital	Evanston	82%	(a)
Mountain View Regional Hospital	Casper	82%	300+
Ivinson Memorial Hospital	Laramie	81%	300+
Memorial Hospital of Converse County	Douglas	81%	(a)
Saint Johns Medical Center	Jackson	81%	300+
Memorial Hospital of Carbon County	Rawlins	80%	(a)
Sheridan Memorial Hospital	Sheridan	80%	300+
Cheyenne Regional Medical Center	Cheyenne	78%	300+
Campbell County Memorial Hospital	Gillette	77%	300+
Memorial Hospital Sweetwater County	Rock Springs	77%	300+
Wyoming Medical Center	Casper	76%	300+
Sagewest Health Care	Riverton	75%	(a)

Home Recovery Information Given

Hospital Name	City	Rate	Cases
Washakie Medical Center[11]	Worland	94%	(a)
Community Hospital[11]	Torrington	93%	(a)
Ivinson Memorial Hospital	Laramie	92%	300+
West Park Hospital District	Cody	91%	300+
Memorial Hospital of Converse County	Douglas	90%	(a)
Mountain View Regional Hospital	Casper	90%	300+
Campbell County Memorial Hospital	Gillette	88%	300+
Evanston Regional Hospital	Evanston	88%	(a)
Sheridan Memorial Hospital	Sheridan	88%	300+
Hot Springs County Memorial Hospital	Thermopolis	87%	(a)
Lander Regional Hospital	Lander	87%	300+
Memorial Hospital Sweetwater County	Rock Springs	87%	300+
Saint Johns Medical Center	Jackson	86%	300+
Sagewest Health Care	Riverton	85%	(a)
Wyoming Medical Center	Casper	85%	300+
Cheyenne Regional Medical Center	Cheyenne	84%	300+
Memorial Hospital of Carbon County	Rawlins	76%	(a)

Hospital Given 9 or 10 on 10 Point Scale

Hospital Name	City	Rate	Cases
Mountain View Regional Hospital	Casper	86%	300+
Community Hospital[11]	Torrington	84%	(a)
Washakie Medical Center[11]	Worland	78%	(a)
Saint Johns Medical Center	Jackson	76%	300+
Memorial Hospital of Converse County	Douglas	70%	(a)
Ivinson Memorial Hospital	Laramie	69%	300+
Sheridan Memorial Hospital	Sheridan	69%	300+
West Park Hospital District	Cody	69%	300+
Lander Regional Hospital	Lander	66%	300+
Campbell County Memorial Hospital	Gillette	63%	300+
Cheyenne Regional Medical Center	Cheyenne	63%	300+
Evanston Regional Hospital	Evanston	62%	(a)
Memorial Hospital Sweetwater County	Rock Springs	60%	300+
Wyoming Medical Center	Casper	59%	300+
Hot Springs County Memorial Hospital	Thermopolis	58%	(a)
Memorial Hospital of Carbon County	Rawlins	50%	(a)
Sagewest Health Care	Riverton	49%	(a)

Meds 'Always' Explained Before Given

Hospital Name	City	Rate	Cases
Washakie Medical Center[11]	Worland	82%	(a)
Community Hospital[11]	Torrington	78%	(a)
Mountain View Regional Hospital	Casper	73%	300+
Ivinson Memorial Hospital	Laramie	69%	300+
Memorial Hospital of Converse County	Douglas	69%	(a)
Evanston Regional Hospital	Evanston	68%	(a)
Hot Springs County Memorial Hospital	Thermopolis	68%	(a)
Memorial Hospital of Carbon County	Rawlins	67%	(a)
West Park Hospital District	Cody	67%	300+
Campbell County Memorial Hospital	Gillette	66%	300+
Memorial Hospital Sweetwater County	Rock Springs	66%	300+
Saint Johns Medical Center	Jackson	65%	300+
Lander Regional Hospital	Lander	64%	300+
Cheyenne Regional Medical Center	Cheyenne	61%	300+
Sagewest Health Care	Riverton	61%	(a)
Sheridan Memorial Hospital	Sheridan	60%	300+
Wyoming Medical Center	Casper	58%	300+

Nurses 'Always' Communicated Well

Hospital Name	City	Rate	Cases
Washakie Medical Center[11]	Worland	85%	(a)
Mountain View Regional Hospital	Casper	84%	300+
Community Hospital[11]	Torrington	83%	(a)
Memorial Hospital of Converse County	Douglas	80%	(a)
Ivinson Memorial Hospital	Laramie	79%	300+
Saint Johns Medical Center	Jackson	79%	300+
Cheyenne Regional Medical Center	Cheyenne	77%	300+
Memorial Hospital of Carbon County	Rawlins	77%	(a)
West Park Hospital District	Cody	77%	300+
Memorial Hospital Sweetwater County	Rock Springs	76%	300+
Campbell County Memorial Hospital	Gillette	75%	300+
Evanston Regional Hospital	Evanston	75%	(a)
Hot Springs County Memorial Hospital	Thermopolis	75%	(a)
Sheridan Memorial Hospital	Sheridan	75%	300+
Lander Regional Hospital	Lander	74%	300+
Wyoming Medical Center	Casper	73%	300+
Sagewest Health Care	Riverton	68%	(a)

Pain 'Always' Well Controlled

Hospital Name	City	Rate	Cases
Community Hospital[11]	Torrington	76%	(a)
Washakie Medical Center[11]	Worland	76%	(a)
Mountain View Regional Hospital	Casper	75%	300+
Memorial Hospital of Carbon County	Rawlins	72%	(a)
Evanston Regional Hospital	Evanston	70%	(a)
Ivinson Memorial Hospital	Laramie	70%	300+
Memorial Hospital Sweetwater County	Rock Springs	70%	300+
Saint Johns Medical Center	Jackson	70%	300+
West Park Hospital District	Cody	70%	300+
Cheyenne Regional Medical Center	Cheyenne	68%	300+
Memorial Hospital of Converse County	Douglas	68%	(a)
Campbell County Memorial Hospital	Gillette	67%	300+
Sheridan Memorial Hospital	Sheridan	67%	300+
Lander Regional Hospital	Lander	63%	300+
Sagewest Health Care	Riverton	63%	(a)
Wyoming Medical Center	Casper	63%	300+
Hot Springs County Memorial Hospital	Thermopolis	60%	(a)

Room and Bathroom 'Always' Clean

Hospital Name	City	Rate	Cases
Community Hospital[11]	Torrington	87%	(a)
Memorial Hospital of Converse County	Douglas	84%	(a)
Washakie Medical Center[11]	Worland	84%	(a)
Mountain View Regional Hospital	Casper	83%	300+
Ivinson Memorial Hospital	Laramie	80%	300+
Saint Johns Medical Center	Jackson	78%	300+
Cheyenne Regional Medical Center	Cheyenne	76%	300+
Sheridan Memorial Hospital	Sheridan	73%	300+
West Park Hospital District	Cody	72%	300+
Memorial Hospital of Carbon County	Rawlins	70%	(a)
Memorial Hospital Sweetwater County	Rock Springs	70%	300+
Campbell County Memorial Hospital	Gillette	67%	300+
Wyoming Medical Center	Casper	67%	300+
Evanston Regional Hospital	Evanston	64%	(a)
Hot Springs County Memorial Hospital	Thermopolis	63%	(a)
Sagewest Health Care	Riverton	60%	(a)
Lander Regional Hospital	Lander	58%	300+

Timely Help 'Always' Received

Hospital Name	City	Rate	Cases
Community Hospital[11]	Torrington	83%	(a)
Memorial Hospital of Carbon County	Rawlins	82%	(a)
Mountain View Regional Hospital	Casper	82%	300+
Memorial Hospital of Converse County	Douglas	78%	(a)
Ivinson Memorial Hospital	Laramie	76%	300+
Washakie Medical Center[11]	Worland	75%	(a)
Saint Johns Medical Center	Jackson	72%	300+
Sheridan Memorial Hospital	Sheridan	72%	300+
Evanston Regional Hospital	Evanston	69%	(a)
Campbell County Memorial Hospital	Gillette	68%	300+
Memorial Hospital Sweetwater County	Rock Springs	67%	300+
West Park Hospital District	Cody	67%	300+
Lander Regional Hospital	Lander	64%	300+
Hot Springs County Memorial Hospital	Thermopolis	62%	(a)
Cheyenne Regional Medical Center	Cheyenne	60%	300+
Sagewest Health Care	Riverton	55%	(a)
Wyoming Medical Center	Casper	55%	300+

Would Definitely Recommend Hospital

Hospital Name	City	Rate	Cases
Mountain View Regional Hospital	Casper	90%	300+
Saint Johns Medical Center	Jackson	77%	300+
Memorial Hospital of Converse County	Douglas	76%	(a)
Washakie Medical Center[11]	Worland	76%	(a)
Ivinson Memorial Hospital	Laramie	72%	300+
West Park Hospital District	Cody	72%	300+
Community Hospital[11]	Torrington	71%	(a)
Sheridan Memorial Hospital	Sheridan	66%	300+
Lander Regional Hospital	Lander	64%	300+
Hot Springs County Memorial Hospital	Thermopolis	63%	(a)
Cheyenne Regional Medical Center	Cheyenne	62%	300+
Wyoming Medical Center	Casper	62%	300+
Evanston Regional Hospital	Evanston	58%	(a)
Campbell County Memorial Hospital	Gillette	56%	300+
Memorial Hospital of Carbon County	Rawlins	53%	(a)
Memorial Hospital Sweetwater County	Rock Springs	52%	300+
Sagewest Health Care	Riverton	43%	(a)

Use of Medical Imaging

Cardiac Imaging Stress Test before OP Surgery

Hospital Name	City	Rate	Cases
Sagewest Health Care	Riverton	2.1%	48
Cheyenne Regional Medical Center	Cheyenne	3.5%	664
Hot Springs County Memorial Hospital	Thermopolis	3.8%	53
Saint Johns Medical Center	Jackson	4.8%	104
Ivinson Memorial Hospital	Laramie	4.9%	123
Memorial Hospital Sweetwater County	Rock Springs	4.9%	123
West Park Hospital District	Cody	4.9%	103
Sheridan Memorial Hospital	Sheridan	6.5%	170
Campbell County Memorial Hospital	Gillette	6.7%	89
Wyoming Medical Center	Casper	9.8%	102

Combination Abdominal CT Scan

Hospital Name	City	Rate	Cases
West Park Hospital District	Cody	0.2%	421
Wyoming Medical Center	Casper	0.8%	524
Saint Johns Medical Center	Jackson	1.3%	228
Memorial Hospital of Carbon County	Rawlins	5.2%	96
Lander Regional Hospital	Lander	6.5%	200
Cheyenne Regional Medical Center	Cheyenne	7.8%	612
Star Valley Medical Center	Afton	8.5%	106
Hot Springs County Memorial Hospital	Thermopolis	11.7%	111
Washakie Medical Center	Worland	12.3%	162
Platte County Memorial Hospital	Wheatland	13.1%	107
Memorial Hospital Sweetwater County	Rock Springs	15.7%	185
Community Hospital	Torrington	15.9%	138
Evanston Regional Hospital	Evanston	16.7%	84
Memorial Hospital of Converse County	Douglas	17.0%	94
Ivinson Memorial Hospital	Laramie	19.0%	306
Campbell County Memorial Hospital	Gillette	27.3%	256
Sagewest Health Care	Riverton	50.7%	203
Sheridan Memorial Hospital	Sheridan	74.8%	107

Combination Brain/Sinus CT Scan

Hospital Name	City	Rate	Cases
Hot Springs County Memorial Hospital	Thermopolis	0.0%	67
West Park Hospital District	Cody	0.8%	254
Cheyenne Regional Medical Center	Cheyenne	1.6%	687
Sagewest Health Care	Riverton	5.9%	136

Combination Chest CT Scan

Hospital Name	City	Rate	Cases
Evanston Regional Hospital	Evanston	0.0%	78
Hot Springs County Memorial Hospital	Thermopolis	0.0%	61
Lander Regional Hospital	Lander	0.0%	110
Saint Johns Medical Center	Jackson	0.0%	179
West Park Hospital District	Cody	0.0%	363
Wyoming Medical Center	Casper	0.0%	308
Sagewest Health Care	Riverton	1.3%	158
Washakie Medical Center	Worland	1.5%	66
Campbell County Memorial Hospital	Gillette	3.7%	243
Cheyenne Regional Medical Center	Cheyenne	4.3%	282
Memorial Hospital Sweetwater County	Rock Springs	5.8%	103
Ivinson Memorial Hospital	Laramie	9.8%	174

Follow-up Mammogram/Ultrasound

A follow-up rate near zero may indicate missed cancer; a rate higher than 14% may mean there is unnecessary follow up.

Hospital Name	City	Rate	Cases
Lander Regional Hospital	Lander	2.7%	332
Memorial Hospital of Carbon County	Rawlins	3.2%	157
Sagewest Health Care	Riverton	3.7%	297
Washakie Medical Center	Worland	3.7%	161
Saint Johns Medical Center	Jackson	4.6%	417
Memorial Hospital of Converse County	Douglas	5.5%	183
Hot Springs County Memorial Hospital	Thermopolis	6.3%	174
Star Valley Medical Center	Afton	8.1%	210
Community Hospital	Torrington	8.5%	270
Sheridan Memorial Hospital	Sheridan	8.8%	646

NOTE: Hospital profiles are in alphabetical order by state, then city, then hospital within the city; Rankings exclude hospitals with less than 25 cases except for patient surveys which excludes hospitals with less than 100 cases; (a) 100-299 cases; (1) The number of cases/patients is too few to report; (2) Data submitted were based on a sample of cases/patients; (3) Results are based on a shorter time period than required; (4) Data suppressed by CMS for one or more quarters; (5) Results are not available for this reporting period; (6) Fewer than 100 patients completed the HCAHPS survey; (7) No cases met the criteria for this measure; (8) The lower limit of the confidence interval cannot be calculated if the number of observed infections equals zero; (9) No data are available from the state/territory for this reporting period; (10) The scores shown reflect fewer than 50 completed surveys; (11) There were discrepancies in the data collection process; (12) This measure does not apply to this hospital for this reporting period; (13) Results cannot be calculated for this reporting period; (14) The results for this state are combined with nearby states to protect confidentiality; Please refer to the User's Guide for a full explanation of data.

Campbell County Memorial Hospital	Gillette	9.3%	259
Platte County Memorial Hospital	Wheatland	12.1%	239
Ivinson Memorial Hospital	Laramie	12.5%	506
Evanston Regional Hospital	Evanston	12.6%	190
Memorial Hospital Sweetwater County	Rock Springs	16.7%	359
West Park Hospital District	Cody	17.5%	607

Lumbar Spine MRI for Low Back Pain

Hospital Name	City	Rate	Cases
Cheyenne Regional Medical Center	Cheyenne	34.8%	69
West Park Hospital District	Cody	36.8%	68
Lander Regional Hospital	Lander	44.7%	47
Campbell County Memorial Hospital	Gillette	45.2%	62
Star Valley Medical Center	Afton	47.4%	38
Saint Johns Medical Center	Jackson	51.1%	94
Memorial Hospital Sweetwater County	Rock Springs	55.3%	47

NOTE: Hospital profiles are in alphabetical order by state, then city, then hospital within the city; Rankings exclude hospitals with less than 25 cases except for patient surveys which excludes hospitals with less than 100 cases; (a) 100-299 cases; (1) The number of cases/patients is too few to report; (2) Data submitted were based on a sample of cases/patients; (3) Results are based on a shorter time period than required; (4) Data suppressed by CMS for one or more quarters; (5) Results are not available for this reporting period; (6) Fewer than 100 patients completed the HCAHPS survey; (7) No cases met the criteria for this measure; (8) The lower limit of the confidence interval cannot be calculated if the number of observed infections equals zero; (9) No data are available from the state/territory for this reporting period; (10) The scores shown reflect fewer than 50 completed surveys; (11) There were discrepancies in the data collection process; (12) This measure does not apply to this hospital for this reporting period; (13) Results cannot be calculated for this reporting period; (14) The results for this state are combined with nearby states to protect confidentiality; Please refer to the User's Guide for a full explanation of data.

Star Valley Medical Center

901 Adams Street
Afton, WY 83110
Phone: 307-885-5800
Fax: 307-885-5889
E-mail: sperry@svmcwy.org
URL: www.svmcwy.org
Type: Critical Access Hospitals
Emergency Services: Yes
Ownership: Govt - Hospital Dist/Auth
Beds: 24

Key Personnel:
Infection Control. . . . . Amy Johnson
Quality Assurance . . . . Amy Johnson
Operating Room. . . . . Lori Johnson, LPN
Radiology. . . . . Terry Lemon
CEO/President. . . . . J Steve Perry
Pediatric In-Patient Care . . . . Jean Pinter
Chief of Medical Staff . . . . David L Schrader

Measure	Cases	This Hosp.	State Avg.	U.S. Avg.
Blood Clot Prevention and Treatment				
Anticoagulation Overlap Therapy[1,2]	-	-	90%	93%
ICU Venous Thromboembolism Prophylaxis[2,3]	-	-	90%	92%
Incidence of Potentially Preventable VTE[2,3]	-	-	12%	10%
UFH with Dosages/Platelet Monitoring[2,3]	-	-	97%	97%
Venous Thromboembolism Prophylaxis[2,3]	91	56%	86%	85%
Warfarin Therapy Discharge Instructions[1,2]	-	-	62%	75%
Chest Pain/Possible Heart Attack Care				
Aspirin Given Within 24 Hours of Arrival	22	100%	97%	96%
Fibrinolytic Meds Within 30 Min. of Arrival[1]	-	-	69%	58%
Average Time to ECG (minutes)	23	10	6	7
Average Time to Transfer (minutes)[7]	-	-	163	60
Children's Asthma Care				
Received Home Management Plan of Care	-	-	-	88%
Received Reliever Medication	-	-	-	100%
Received Systemic Corticosteroids	-	-	-	100%
Emergency Department				
Admittance Decision Time (minutes)[2]	63	40	70	98
Head CT Results Within 45 Min. of Arrival[1]	-	-	36%	57%
Patients Who Left ER Before Being Seen[5]	-	-	2%	2%
Time from ER Arrival to Admit. (minutes)[2]	78	172	218	274
Time from ER Arrival to Discharge (minutes)	247	137	116	134
Time in ER Before Being Evaluated (minutes)	280	4	16	26
Time to Pain Meds for Fractures (minutes)	36	20	46	57
Heart Attack Care				
Aspirin Given at Discharge[1]	-	-	99%	99%
Fibrinolytic Meds Within 30 Min. of Arrival[7]	-	-	100%	54%
PCI Within 90 Minutes of Arrival[7]	-	-	99%	96%
Statin Prescribed at Discharge[1]	-	-	97%	98%
Heart Failure Care				
ACE Inhibitor or ARB for LVSD[1]	-	-	95%	97%
Discharge Instructions Given	11	82%	86%	94%
Evaluation of LVS Function	15	60%	94%	99%
Medicare Spending				
Medicare Spending per Patient (ratio)	-	-	0.93	0.98
Pneumonia Care				
Appropriate Initial Antibiotic Given[1]	-	-	94%	95%
Blood Culture Timing[1]	-	-	97%	98%
Pregnancy and Delivery Care				
Newborn Deliveries Scheduled Early[5]	-	-	7%	6%
Preventive Care				
Immunization for Influenza	51	92%	86%	90%
Immunization for Pneumonia	137	92%	88%	92%
Stroke Care				
Anticoagulation Therapy for Atrial Fibrillation[1,3]	-	-	93%	95%
Antithrombotic Therapy Timing[1,3]	-	-	95%	98%
Assessed for Rehabilitation[1,3]	-	-	94%	97%
Discharged on Antithrombotic Therapy[1,3]	-	-	97%	99%
Discharged on Statin Medication[1,3]	-	-	89%	94%
Thrombolytic Therapy Timing[3,7]	-	-	42%	66%
Venous Thromboembolism Prophylaxis[1,3]	-	-	87%	94%
Written Stroke Educational Materials Given[3,7]	-	-	68%	88%
Surgical Care Improvement Project				
Appropriate Beta Blocker Usage	15	100%	94%	98%
Appropriate VTP Within 24 Hours	62	100%	95%	98%
Controlled Postoperative Blood Glucose[7]	-	-	99%	97%
Perioperative Temperature Management	73	100%	99%	100%
Prophylactic Antibiotic Selection	60	100%	99%	99%
Prophylactic Antibiotic Selection (Outpatient)	27	93%	95%	98%
Prophylactic Antibiotic Stopped	60	100%	97%	98%
Prophylactic Antibiotic Timing	60	100%	98%	99%
Prophylactic Antibiotic Timing (Outpatient)	28	96%	96%	98%
Urinary Catheter Removal	60	98%	95%	97%
Survey of Patients' Hospital Experiences				
Area Around Room 'Always' Quiet at Night[6]	<100	73%	61%	61%
Doctors 'Always' Communicated Well[6]	<100	86%	82%	82%
Home Recovery Information Given[6]	<100	92%	88%	85%
Hospital Given 9 or 10 on 10 Point Scale[6]	<100	77%	68%	71%
Meds 'Always' Explained Before Given[6]	<100	72%	66%	64%
Nurses 'Always' Communicated Well[6]	<100	82%	78%	79%
Pain 'Always' Well Controlled[6]	<100	78%	69%	71%
Room and Bathroom 'Always' Clean[6]	<100	80%	74%	73%
Timely Help 'Always' Received[6]	<100	77%	70%	68%
Would Definitely Recommend Hospital[6]	<100	77%	67%	71%
Use of Medical Imaging				
Cardiac Imaging Stress Test before Surgery[1]	-	-	4.8%	5.3%
Combination Abdominal CT Scan	106	8.5%	13.1%	10.5%
Combination Brain/Sinus CT Scan[1]	-	-	2.1%	2.7%
Combination Chest CT Scan[1]	-	-	3.8%	2.7%
Follow-up Mammogram/Ultrasound	210	8.1%	9.7%	8.8%
Lumbar Spine MRI for Low Back Pain	38	47.4%	46.1%	37.2%

South Big Horn County Critical Access Hospital

388 Us Highway 20 South
Basin, WY 82410
Phone: 307-568-3311
Type: Critical Access Hospitals
Emergency Services: Yes
Ownership: Govt - Hospital Dist/Auth
Beds: 43

Key Personnel:
Radiology. . . . . Trish Brown
CEO/President. . . . . Jackie Claudson

Measure	Cases	This Hosp.	State Avg.	U.S. Avg.
Blood Clot Prevention and Treatment				
Anticoagulation Overlap Therapy[3,7]	-	-	90%	93%
ICU Venous Thromboembolism Prophylaxis[3,7]	-	-	90%	92%
Incidence of Potentially Preventable VTE[3,7]	-	-	12%	10%
UFH with Dosages/Platelet Monitoring[3,7]	-	-	97%	97%
Venous Thromboembolism Prophylaxis[1,3]	-	-	86%	85%
Warfarin Therapy Discharge Instructions[3,7]	-	-	62%	75%
Chest Pain/Possible Heart Attack Care				
Aspirin Given Within 24 Hours of Arrival	-	-	97%	96%
Fibrinolytic Meds Within 30 Min. of Arrival	-	-	69%	58%
Average Time to ECG (minutes)	-	-	6	7
Average Time to Transfer (minutes)	-	-	163	60
Children's Asthma Care				
Received Home Management Plan of Care	-	-	-	88%
Received Reliever Medication	-	-	-	100%
Received Systemic Corticosteroids	-	-	-	100%
Emergency Department				
Admittance Decision Time (minutes)[5]	-	-	70	98
Head CT Results Within 45 Min. of Arrival	-	-	36%	57%
Patients Who Left ER Before Being Seen	-	-	2%	2%
Time from ER Arrival to Admit. (minutes)[5]	-	-	218	274
Time from ER Arrival to Discharge (minutes)	-	-	116	134
Time in ER Before Being Evaluated (minutes)	-	-	16	26
Time to Pain Meds for Fractures (minutes)	-	-	46	57
Heart Attack Care				
Aspirin Given at Discharge[5]	-	-	99%	99%
Fibrinolytic Meds Within 30 Min. of Arrival[5]	-	-	100%	54%
PCI Within 90 Minutes of Arrival[5]	-	-	99%	96%
Statin Prescribed at Discharge[5]	-	-	97%	98%
Heart Failure Care				
ACE Inhibitor or ARB for LVSD[3,7]	-	-	95%	97%
Discharge Instructions Given[1,3]	-	-	86%	94%
Evaluation of LVS Function[1,3]	-	-	94%	99%
Medicare Spending				
Medicare Spending per Patient (ratio)	-	-	0.93	0.98
Pneumonia Care				
Appropriate Initial Antibiotic Given[1,3]	-	-	94%	95%
Blood Culture Timing[1,3]	-	-	97%	98%
Pregnancy and Delivery Care				
Newborn Deliveries Scheduled Early[5]	-	-	7%	6%
Preventive Care				
Immunization for Influenza[5]	-	-	86%	90%
Immunization for Pneumonia[5]	-	-	88%	92%
Stroke Care				
Anticoagulation Therapy for Atrial Fibrillation[3,7]	-	-	93%	95%
Antithrombotic Therapy Timing[3,7]	-	-	95%	98%
Assessed for Rehabilitation[1,3]	-	-	94%	97%
Discharged on Antithrombotic Therapy[1,3]	-	-	97%	99%
Discharged on Statin Medication[1,3]	-	-	89%	94%
Thrombolytic Therapy Timing[3,7]	-	-	42%	66%
Venous Thromboembolism Prophylaxis[3,7]	-	-	87%	94%
Written Stroke Educational Materials Given[1,3]	-	-	68%	88%
Surgical Care Improvement Project				
Appropriate Beta Blocker Usage[5]	-	-	94%	98%
Appropriate VTP Within 24 Hours[5]	-	-	95%	98%
Controlled Postoperative Blood Glucose[5]	-	-	99%	97%
Perioperative Temperature Management[5]	-	-	99%	100%
Prophylactic Antibiotic Selection[5]	-	-	99%	99%
Prophylactic Antibiotic Selection (Outpatient)	-	-	95%	98%
Prophylactic Antibiotic Stopped[5]	-	-	97%	98%
Prophylactic Antibiotic Timing[5]	-	-	98%	99%
Prophylactic Antibiotic Timing (Outpatient)	-	-	96%	98%
Urinary Catheter Removal[5]	-	-	95%	97%
Survey of Patients' Hospital Experiences				
Area Around Room 'Always' Quiet at Night[5]	-	-	61%	61%
Doctors 'Always' Communicated Well[5]	-	-	82%	82%
Home Recovery Information Given[5]	-	-	88%	85%
Hospital Given 9 or 10 on 10 Point Scale[5]	-	-	68%	71%
Meds 'Always' Explained Before Given[5]	-	-	66%	64%
Nurses 'Always' Communicated Well[5]	-	-	78%	79%
Pain 'Always' Well Controlled[5]	-	-	69%	71%
Room and Bathroom 'Always' Clean[5]	-	-	74%	73%
Timely Help 'Always' Received[5]	-	-	70%	68%
Would Definitely Recommend Hospital[5]	-	-	67%	71%
Use of Medical Imaging				
Cardiac Imaging Stress Test before Surgery	-	-	4.8%	5.3%
Combination Abdominal CT Scan	-	-	13.1%	10.5%
Combination Brain/Sinus CT Scan	-	-	2.1%	2.7%
Combination Chest CT Scan	-	-	3.8%	2.7%
Follow-up Mammogram/Ultrasound	-	-	9.7%	8.8%
Lumbar Spine MRI for Low Back Pain	-	-	46.1%	37.2%

Johnson County Healthcare Center

497 West Lott
Buffalo, WY 82834
Phone: 307-684-5521
URL: www.buffalohealthcare.vcn.com
Type: Critical Access Hospitals
Emergency Services: Yes
Ownership: Government - Local

Key Personnel:
Radiology. . . . . Tom Greet, RT
Operating Room. . . . . Blaine Ruby, MD

Measure	Cases	This Hosp.	State Avg.	U.S. Avg.
Blood Clot Prevention and Treatment				
Anticoagulation Overlap Therapy[5]	-	-	90%	93%
ICU Venous Thromboembolism Prophylaxis[5]	-	-	90%	92%
Incidence of Potentially Preventable VTE[5]	-	-	12%	10%
UFH with Dosages/Platelet Monitoring[5]	-	-	97%	97%
Venous Thromboembolism Prophylaxis[5]	-	-	86%	85%
Warfarin Therapy Discharge Instructions[5]	-	-	62%	75%
Chest Pain/Possible Heart Attack Care				
Aspirin Given Within 24 Hours of Arrival	-	-	97%	96%
Fibrinolytic Meds Within 30 Min. of Arrival	-	-	69%	58%
Average Time to ECG (minutes)	-	-	6	7
Average Time to Transfer (minutes)	-	-	163	60
Children's Asthma Care				
Received Home Management Plan of Care	-	-	-	88%
Received Reliever Medication	-	-	-	100%
Received Systemic Corticosteroids	-	-	-	100%
Emergency Department				
Admittance Decision Time (minutes)[5]	-	-	70	98
Head CT Results Within 45 Min. of Arrival	-	-	36%	57%
Patients Who Left ER Before Being Seen	-	-	2%	2%
Time from ER Arrival to Admit. (minutes)[5]	-	-	218	274

NOTE: Hospital profiles are in alphabetical order by state, then city, then hospital within the city; Rankings exclude hospitals with less than 25 cases except for patient surveys which excludes hospitals with less than 100 cases; (a) 100-299 cases; (1) The number of cases/patients is too few to report; (2) Data submitted were based on a sample of cases/patients; (3) Results are based on a shorter time period than required; (4) Data suppressed by CMS for one or more quarters; (5) Results are not available for this reporting period; (6) Fewer than 100 patients completed the HCAHPS survey; (7) No cases met the criteria for this measure; (8) The lower limit of the confidence interval cannot be calculated if the number of observed infections equals zero; (9) No data are available from the state/territory for this reporting period; (10) The scores shown reflect fewer than 50 completed surveys; (11) There were discrepancies in the data collection process; (12) This measure does not apply to this hospital for this reporting period; (13) Results cannot be calculated for this reporting period; (14) The results for this state are combined with nearby states to protect confidentiality; Please refer to the User's Guide for a full explanation of data.

Measure	Cases	This Hosp.	State Avg.	U.S. Avg.
Time from ER Arrival to Discharge (minutes)	-	-	116	134
Time in ER Before Being Evaluated (minutes)	-	-	16	26
Time to Pain Meds for Fractures (minutes)	-	-	46	57
Heart Attack Care				
Aspirin Given at Discharge[5]	-	-	99%	99%
Fibrinolytic Meds Within 30 Min. of Arrival[5]	-	-	100%	54%
PCI Within 90 Minutes of Arrival[5]	-	-	99%	96%
Statin Prescribed at Discharge[5]	-	-	97%	98%
Heart Failure Care				
ACE Inhibitor or ARB for LVSD[3,7]	-	-	95%	97%
Discharge Instructions Given[1,3]	-	-	86%	94%
Evaluation of LVS Function[1,3]	-	-	94%	99%
Medicare Spending				
Medicare Spending per Patient (ratio)	-	-	0.93	0.98
Pneumonia Care				
Appropriate Initial Antibiotic Given	16	88%	94%	95%
Blood Culture Timing[1]	-	-	97%	98%
Pregnancy and Delivery Care				
Newborn Deliveries Scheduled Early[5]	-	-	7%	6%
Preventive Care				
Immunization for Influenza[5]	-	-	86%	90%
Immunization for Pneumonia[5]	-	-	88%	92%
Stroke Care				
Anticoagulation Therapy for Atrial Fibrillation[5]	-	-	93%	95%
Antithrombotic Therapy Timing[5]	-	-	95%	98%
Assessed for Rehabilitation[5]	-	-	94%	97%
Discharged on Antithrombotic Therapy[5]	-	-	97%	99%
Discharged on Statin Medication[5]	-	-	89%	94%
Thrombolytic Therapy Timing[5]	-	-	42%	66%
Venous Thromboembolism Prophylaxis[5]	-	-	87%	94%
Written Stroke Educational Materials Given[5]	-	-	68%	88%
Surgical Care Improvement Project				
Appropriate Beta Blocker Usage[5]	-	-	94%	98%
Appropriate VTP Within 24 Hours[5]	-	-	95%	98%
Controlled Postoperative Blood Glucose[5]	-	-	99%	97%
Perioperative Temperature Management[5]	-	-	99%	100%
Prophylactic Antibiotic Selection[5]	-	-	99%	99%
Prophylactic Antibiotic Selection (Outpatient)	-	-	95%	98%
Prophylactic Antibiotic Stopped[5]	-	-	97%	98%
Prophylactic Antibiotic Timing[5]	-	-	98%	99%
Prophylactic Antibiotic Timing (Outpatient)	-	-	96%	98%
Urinary Catheter Removal[5]	-	-	95%	97%
Survey of Patients' Hospital Experiences				
Area Around Room 'Always' Quiet at Night[5]	-	-	61%	61%
Doctors 'Always' Communicated Well[5]	-	-	82%	82%
Home Recovery Information Given[5]	-	-	88%	85%
Hospital Given 9 or 10 on 10 Point Scale[5]	-	-	68%	71%
Meds 'Always' Explained Before Given[5]	-	-	66%	64%
Nurses 'Always' Communicated Well[5]	-	-	78%	79%
Pain 'Always' Well Controlled[5]	-	-	69%	71%
Room and Bathroom 'Always' Clean[5]	-	-	74%	73%
Timely Help 'Always' Received[5]	-	-	70%	68%
Would Definitely Recommend Hospital[5]	-	-	67%	71%
Use of Medical Imaging				
Cardiac Imaging Stress Test before Surgery	-	-	4.8%	5.3%
Combination Abdominal CT Scan	-	-	13.1%	10.5%
Combination Brain/Sinus CT Scan	-	-	2.1%	2.7%
Combination Chest CT Scan	-	-	3.8%	2.7%
Follow-up Mammogram/Ultrasound	-	-	9.7%	8.8%
Lumbar Spine MRI for Low Back Pain	-	-	46.1%	37.2%

Mountain View Regional Hospital

6550 East 2nd Street
Casper, WY 82605
Phone: 307-995-8100
URL: www.monroehospital.com
Type: Acute Care Hospitals
Emergency Services: Yes
Ownership: Proprietary
Beds: 168
Key Personnel:
CEO . . . . Jeff VanHorn

Measure	Cases	This Hosp.	State Avg.	U.S. Avg.
Blood Clot Prevention and Treatment				
Anticoagulation Overlap Therapy[1,2]	-	-	90%	93%
ICU Venous Thromboembolism Prophylaxis[2]	19	84%	90%	92%
Incidence of Potentially Preventable VTE[2,7]	-	-	12%	10%
UFH with Dosages/Platelet Monitoring[1,2]	-	-	97%	97%
Venous Thromboembolism Prophylaxis[2]	203	94%	86%	85%
Warfarin Therapy Discharge Instructions[1,2]	-	-	62%	75%
Chest Pain/Possible Heart Attack Care				
Aspirin Given Within 24 Hours of Arrival[5]	-	-	97%	96%
Fibrinolytic Meds Within 30 Min. of Arrival[5]	-	-	69%	58%
Average Time to ECG (minutes)[5]	-	-	6	7
Average Time to Transfer (minutes)[5]	-	-	163	60
Children's Asthma Care				
Received Home Management Plan of Care	-	-	-	88%
Received Reliever Medication	-	-	-	100%
Received Systemic Corticosteroids	-	-	-	100%
Emergency Department				
Admittance Decision Time (minutes)[2]	49	34	70	98
Head CT Results Within 45 Min. of Arrival[1,3]	-	-	36%	57%
Patients Who Left ER Before Being Seen	5,001	1%	2%	2%
Time from ER Arrival to Admit. (minutes)[2]	52	192	218	274
Time from ER Arrival to Discharge (minutes)	401	120	116	134
Time in ER Before Being Evaluated (minutes)	395	27	16	26
Time to Pain Meds for Fractures (minutes)[1,3]	-	-	46	57
Heart Attack Care				
Aspirin Given at Discharge[5]	-	-	99%	99%
Fibrinolytic Meds Within 30 Min. of Arrival[5]	-	-	100%	54%
PCI Within 90 Minutes of Arrival[5]	-	-	99%	96%
Statin Prescribed at Discharge[5]	-	-	97%	98%
Heart Failure Care				
ACE Inhibitor or ARB for LVSD[2,3]	-	-	95%	97%
Discharge Instructions Given[1,2]	-	-	86%	94%
Evaluation of LVS Function[1,2]	-	-	94%	99%
Medicare Spending				
Medicare Spending per Patient (ratio)	-	1.03	0.93	0.98
Pneumonia Care				
Appropriate Initial Antibiotic Given[1,2]	-	-	94%	95%
Blood Culture Timing[1,2]	-	-	97%	98%
Pregnancy and Delivery Care				
Newborn Deliveries Scheduled Early[2,7]	-	-	7%	6%
Preventive Care				
Immunization for Influenza[2]	337	90%	86%	90%
Immunization for Pneumonia[2]	387	94%	88%	92%
Stroke Care				
Anticoagulation Therapy for Atrial Fibrillation[2,3]	-	-	93%	95%
Antithrombotic Therapy Timing[2,3]	-	-	95%	98%
Assessed for Rehabilitation[2,3]	-	-	94%	97%
Discharged on Antithrombotic Therapy[2,3]	-	-	97%	99%
Discharged on Statin Medication[2,3]	-	-	89%	94%
Thrombolytic Therapy Timing[2,3]	-	-	42%	66%
Venous Thromboembolism Prophylaxis[2,3]	-	-	87%	94%
Written Stroke Educational Materials Given[2,3]	-	-	68%	88%
Surgical Care Improvement Project				
Appropriate Beta Blocker Usage[2]	18	89%	94%	98%
Appropriate VTP Within 24 Hours[2]	121	87%	95%	98%
Controlled Postoperative Blood Glucose[2,7]	-	-	99%	97%
Perioperative Temperature Management[2]	135	99%	99%	100%
Prophylactic Antibiotic Selection[2]	94	97%	99%	99%
Prophylactic Antibiotic Selection (Outpatient)	95	100%	95%	98%
Prophylactic Antibiotic Stopped[2]	93	94%	97%	98%
Prophylactic Antibiotic Timing[2]	94	99%	98%	99%
Prophylactic Antibiotic Timing (Outpatient)	95	99%	96%	98%
Urinary Catheter Removal[2]	104	82%	95%	97%
Survey of Patients' Hospital Experiences				
Area Around Room 'Always' Quiet at Night	300+	67%	61%	61%
Doctors 'Always' Communicated Well	300+	82%	82%	82%
Home Recovery Information Given	300+	90%	88%	85%
Hospital Given 9 or 10 on 10 Point Scale	300+	86%	68%	71%
Meds 'Always' Explained Before Given	300+	73%	66%	64%
Nurses 'Always' Communicated Well	300+	84%	78%	79%
Pain 'Always' Well Controlled	300+	75%	69%	71%
Room and Bathroom 'Always' Clean	300+	83%	74%	73%
Timely Help 'Always' Received	300+	82%	70%	68%
Would Definitely Recommend Hospital	300+	90%	67%	71%
Use of Medical Imaging				
Cardiac Imaging Stress Test before Surgery[7]	-	-	4.8%	5.3%
Combination Abdominal CT Scan[1]	-	-	13.1%	10.5%
Combination Brain/Sinus CT Scan[1]	-	-	2.1%	2.7%
Combination Chest CT Scan[1]	-	-	3.8%	2.7%
Follow-up Mammogram/Ultrasound[7]	-	-	9.7%	8.8%
Lumbar Spine MRI for Low Back Pain[1]	-	-	46.1%	37.2%

Wyoming Medical Center

1233 East 2nd St
Casper, WY 82601
Phone: 307-577-7201
Fax: 307-237-1703
E-mail: info@wmcnet.org
URL: www.wyomingmedicalcenter.com
Type: Acute Care Hospitals
Emergency Services: Yes
Ownership: Govt - Hospital Dist/Auth
Beds: 282
Key Personnel:
CEO/President. . . . . Vickie Diamond
Patient Relations . . . . Vickie Diamond
Emergency Room . . . . Becky Hansen, RN
Radiology. . . . . Steve Horn
Cardiac Laboratory. . . . . Carol Nelson
Chief of Medical Staff . . . . Carol Solie, MD
Operating Room. . . . . Debra Weaver
Quality Assurance . . . . Dick Williams

Measure	Cases	This Hosp.	State Avg.	U.S. Avg.
Blood Clot Prevention and Treatment				
Anticoagulation Overlap Therapy[2]	36	100%	90%	93%
ICU Venous Thromboembolism Prophylaxis[2]	37	97%	90%	92%
Incidence of Potentially Preventable VTE[1,2]	-	-	12%	10%
UFH with Dosages/Platelet Monitoring[2]	37	100%	97%	97%
Venous Thromboembolism Prophylaxis[2]	333	99%	86%	85%
Warfarin Therapy Discharge Instructions[2]	30	97%	62%	75%
Chest Pain/Possible Heart Attack Care				
Aspirin Given Within 24 Hours of Arrival[5]	-	-	97%	96%
Fibrinolytic Meds Within 30 Min. of Arrival[5]	-	-	69%	58%
Average Time to ECG (minutes)[5]	-	-	6	7
Average Time to Transfer (minutes)[5]	-	-	163	60
Children's Asthma Care				
Received Home Management Plan of Care	-	-	-	88%
Received Reliever Medication	-	-	-	100%
Received Systemic Corticosteroids	-	-	-	100%
Emergency Department				
Admittance Decision Time (minutes)[2]	511	123	70	98
Head CT Results Within 45 Min. of Arrival[1]	-	-	36%	57%
Patients Who Left ER Before Being Seen	38,006	2%	2%	2%
Time from ER Arrival to Admit. (minutes)[2]	548	248	218	274
Time from ER Arrival to Discharge (minutes)	364	176	116	134
Time in ER Before Being Evaluated (minutes)	409	30	16	26
Time to Pain Meds for Fractures (minutes)	139	51	46	57
Heart Attack Care				
Aspirin Given at Discharge	335	100%	99%	99%
Fibrinolytic Meds Within 30 Min. of Arrival[7]	-	-	100%	54%
PCI Within 90 Minutes of Arrival	47	100%	99%	96%
Statin Prescribed at Discharge	329	100%	97%	98%
Heart Failure Care				
ACE Inhibitor or ARB for LVSD	52	100%	95%	97%
Discharge Instructions Given	174	98%	86%	94%
Evaluation of LVS Function	212	100%	94%	99%
Medicare Spending				
Medicare Spending per Patient (ratio)	-	1.01	0.93	0.98
Pneumonia Care				
Appropriate Initial Antibiotic Given	144	98%	94%	95%
Blood Culture Timing	206	99%	97%	98%
Pregnancy and Delivery Care				
Newborn Deliveries Scheduled Early	87	3%	7%	6%
Preventive Care				
Immunization for Influenza[2]	556	90%	86%	90%
Immunization for Pneumonia[2]	590	96%	88%	92%
Stroke Care				
Anticoagulation Therapy for Atrial Fibrillation	14	100%	93%	95%
Antithrombotic Therapy Timing	55	96%	95%	98%
Assessed for Rehabilitation	89	100%	94%	97%
Discharged on Antithrombotic Therapy	75	100%	97%	99%
Discharged on Statin Medication	48	98%	89%	94%
Thrombolytic Therapy Timing	11	91%	42%	66%

NOTE: Hospital profiles are in alphabetical order by state, then city, then hospital within the city; Rankings exclude hospitals with less than 25 cases except for patient surveys which excludes hospitals with less than 100 cases; (a) 100-299 cases; (1) The number of cases/patients is too few to report; (2) Data submitted were based on a sample of cases/patients; (3) Results are based on a shorter time period than required; (4) Data suppressed by CMS for one or more quarters; (5) Results are not available for this reporting period; (6) Fewer than 100 patients completed the HCAHPS survey; (7) No cases met the criteria for this measure; (8) The lower limit of the confidence interval cannot be calculated if the number of observed infections equals zero; (9) No data are available from the state/territory for this reporting period; (10) The scores shown reflect fewer than 50 completed surveys; (11) There were discrepancies in the data collection process; (12) This measure does not apply to this hospital for this reporting period; (13) Results cannot be calculated for this reporting period; (14) The results for this state are combined with nearby states to protect confidentiality; Please refer to the User's Guide for a full explanation of data.

Measure	Cases	This Hosp.	State Avg.	U.S. Avg.
Venous Thromboembolism Prophylaxis	85	93%	87%	94%
Written Stroke Educational Materials Given	46	98%	68%	88%
Surgical Care Improvement Project				
Appropriate Beta Blocker Usage[2]	166	99%	94%	98%
Appropriate VTP Within 24 Hours[2]	423	96%	95%	98%
Controlled Postoperative Blood Glucose[2]	113	99%	99%	97%
Perioperative Temperature Management[2]	554	99%	99%	100%
Prophylactic Antibiotic Selection[2]	491	99%	99%	99%
Prophylactic Antibiotic Selection (Outpatient)	221	94%	95%	98%
Prophylactic Antibiotic Stopped[2]	481	100%	97%	98%
Prophylactic Antibiotic Timing[2]	493	99%	98%	99%
Prophylactic Antibiotic Timing (Outpatient)	221	98%	96%	98%
Urinary Catheter Removal[2]	347	98%	95%	97%
Survey of Patients' Hospital Experiences				
Area Around Room 'Always' Quiet at Night	300+	44%	61%	61%
Doctors 'Always' Communicated Well	300+	76%	82%	82%
Home Recovery Information Given	300+	85%	88%	85%
Hospital Given 9 or 10 on 10 Point Scale	300+	59%	68%	71%
Meds 'Always' Explained Before Given	300+	58%	66%	64%
Nurses 'Always' Communicated Well	300+	73%	78%	79%
Pain 'Always' Well Controlled	300+	63%	69%	71%
Room and Bathroom 'Always' Clean	300+	67%	74%	73%
Timely Help 'Always' Received	300+	55%	70%	68%
Would Definitely Recommend Hospital	300+	62%	67%	71%
Use of Medical Imaging				
Cardiac Imaging Stress Test before Surgery	102	9.8%	4.8%	5.3%
Combination Abdominal CT Scan	524	0.8%	13.1%	10.5%
Combination Brain/Sinus CT Scan[1]	-	-	2.1%	2.7%
Combination Chest CT Scan	308	0.0%	3.8%	2.7%
Follow-up Mammogram/Ultrasound[7]	-	-	9.7%	8.8%
Lumbar Spine MRI for Low Back Pain[7]	-	-	46.1%	37.2%

Cheyenne Regional Medical Center

214 East 23rd Street
Cheyenne, WY 82001
Phone: 307-634-2273
Fax: 307-633-7600
URL: www.crmcwy.org
Type: Acute Care Hospitals
Emergency Services: Yes
Ownership: Voluntary non-profit - Other
Beds: 218

Key Personnel:
Cardiac Laboratory. . . . . Heather Bagget
Pediatric In-Patient Care . . . . Cheryl Crumpton, RN
Quality Assurance . . . . Joanny Davison
Operating Room. . . . . Richard A Fermelia, RN
Infection Control. . . . . Jay Jones
CEO . . . . Margo Karsten, Ph.D.
Chief of Medical Staff. . . . . David Lind, MD
Radiology. . . . . Michael L Sloan

Measure	Cases	This Hosp.	State Avg.	U.S. Avg.
Blood Clot Prevention and Treatment				
Anticoagulation Overlap Therapy[2]	60	88%	90%	93%
ICU Venous Thromboembolism Prophylaxis[2]	59	90%	90%	92%
Incidence of Potentially Preventable VTE[1,2]	-	-	12%	10%
UFH with Dosages/Platelet Monitoring[2]	26	88%	97%	97%
Venous Thromboembolism Prophylaxis[2]	282	85%	86%	85%
Warfarin Therapy Discharge Instructions[2]	61	13%	62%	75%
Chest Pain/Possible Heart Attack Care				
Aspirin Given Within 24 Hours of Arrival[1,3]	-	-	97%	96%
Fibrinolytic Meds Within 30 Min. of Arrival[3,7]	-	-	69%	58%
Average Time to ECG (minutes)[1,3]	-	-	6	7
Average Time to Transfer (minutes)[3,7]	-	-	163	60
Children's Asthma Care				
Received Home Management Plan of Care	-	-	-	88%
Received Reliever Medication	-	-	-	100%
Received Systemic Corticosteroids	-	-	-	100%
Emergency Department				
Admittance Decision Time (minutes)[2]	526	74	70	98
Head CT Results Within 45 Min. of Arrival	13	23%	36%	57%
Patients Who Left ER Before Being Seen	39,723	3%	2%	2%
Time from ER Arrival to Admit. (minutes)[2]	560	244	218	274
Time from ER Arrival to Discharge (minutes)	383	162	116	134
Time in ER Before Being Evaluated (minutes)	365	17	16	26
Time to Pain Meds for Fractures (minutes)	212	58	46	57
Heart Attack Care				
Aspirin Given at Discharge	181	98%	99%	99%
Fibrinolytic Meds Within 30 Min. of Arrival[7]	-	-	100%	54%
PCI Within 90 Minutes of Arrival	29	100%	99%	96%
Statin Prescribed at Discharge	171	99%	97%	98%
Heart Failure Care				
ACE Inhibitor or ARB for LVSD	33	100%	95%	97%
Discharge Instructions Given	92	95%	86%	94%
Evaluation of LVS Function	119	97%	94%	99%
Medicare Spending				
Medicare Spending per Patient (ratio)	-	1.03	0.93	0.98
Pneumonia Care				
Appropriate Initial Antibiotic Given	146	98%	94%	95%
Blood Culture Timing	154	99%	97%	98%
Pregnancy and Delivery Care				
Newborn Deliveries Scheduled Early[2]	27	11%	7%	6%
Preventive Care				
Immunization for Influenza[2]	542	88%	86%	90%
Immunization for Pneumonia[2]	530	73%	88%	92%
Stroke Care				
Anticoagulation Therapy for Atrial Fibrillation[1]	-	-	93%	95%
Antithrombotic Therapy Timing	57	96%	95%	98%
Assessed for Rehabilitation	70	93%	94%	97%
Discharged on Antithrombotic Therapy	63	95%	97%	99%
Discharged on Statin Medication	50	72%	89%	94%
Thrombolytic Therapy Timing	27	26%	42%	66%
Venous Thromboembolism Prophylaxis	72	85%	87%	94%
Written Stroke Educational Materials Given	36	31%	68%	88%
Surgical Care Improvement Project				
Appropriate Beta Blocker Usage	186	96%	94%	98%
Appropriate VTP Within 24 Hours	440	98%	95%	98%
Controlled Postoperative Blood Glucose	69	99%	99%	97%
Perioperative Temperature Management	590	100%	99%	100%
Prophylactic Antibiotic Selection	434	100%	99%	99%
Prophylactic Antibiotic Selection (Outpatient)	236	93%	95%	98%
Prophylactic Antibiotic Stopped	429	99%	97%	98%
Prophylactic Antibiotic Timing	435	100%	98%	99%
Prophylactic Antibiotic Timing (Outpatient)	247	92%	96%	98%
Urinary Catheter Removal	183	95%	95%	97%
Survey of Patients' Hospital Experiences				
Area Around Room 'Always' Quiet at Night	300+	55%	61%	61%
Doctors 'Always' Communicated Well	300+	78%	82%	82%
Home Recovery Information Given	300+	84%	88%	85%
Hospital Given 9 or 10 on 10 Point Scale	300+	63%	68%	71%
Meds 'Always' Explained Before Given	300+	61%	66%	64%
Nurses 'Always' Communicated Well	300+	77%	78%	79%
Pain 'Always' Well Controlled	300+	68%	69%	71%
Room and Bathroom 'Always' Clean	300+	76%	74%	73%
Timely Help 'Always' Received	300+	60%	70%	68%
Would Definitely Recommend Hospital	300+	62%	67%	71%
Use of Medical Imaging				
Cardiac Imaging Stress Test before Surgery	664	3.5%	4.8%	5.3%
Combination Abdominal CT Scan	612	7.8%	13.1%	10.5%
Combination Brain/Sinus CT Scan	687	1.6%	2.1%	2.7%
Combination Chest CT Scan	282	4.3%	3.8%	2.7%
Follow-up Mammogram/Ultrasound[7]	-	-	9.7%	8.8%
Lumbar Spine MRI for Low Back Pain	69	34.8%	46.1%	37.2%

Cheyenne VA Medical Center

2360 E. Pershing Blvd.
Cheyenne, WY 82001
Phone: 307-778-7300
Fax: 307-778-7336
URL: www.va.gov/visn19/cheyenne.htm
Type: Acute Care - VA
Emergency Services: No
Ownership: Government Federal

Key Personnel:
Patient Relations . . . . Dick Hennebry
Chief of Medical Staff . . . . Roger M Johnson
Operating Room. . . . . Patricia Stepp

Measure	Cases	This Hosp.	State Avg.	U.S. Avg.
Blood Clot Prevention and Treatment				
Anticoagulation Overlap Therapy	-	-	90%	93%
ICU Venous Thromboembolism Prophylaxis	-	-	90%	92%
Incidence of Potentially Preventable VTE	-	-	12%	10%
UFH with Dosages/Platelet Monitoring	-	-	97%	97%
Venous Thromboembolism Prophylaxis	-	-	86%	85%
Warfarin Therapy Discharge Instructions	-	-	62%	75%
Chest Pain/Possible Heart Attack Care				
Aspirin Given Within 24 Hours of Arrival	-	-	97%	96%
Fibrinolytic Meds Within 30 Min. of Arrival	-	-	69%	58%
Average Time to ECG (minutes)	-	-	6	7
Average Time to Transfer (minutes)	-	-	163	60
Children's Asthma Care				
Received Home Management Plan of Care	-	-	-	88%
Received Reliever Medication	-	-	-	100%
Received Systemic Corticosteroids	-	-	-	100%
Emergency Department				
Admittance Decision Time (minutes)	-	-	70	98
Head CT Results Within 45 Min. of Arrival	-	-	36%	57%
Patients Who Left ER Before Being Seen	-	-	2%	2%
Time from ER Arrival to Admit. (minutes)	-	-	218	274
Time from ER Arrival to Discharge (minutes)	-	-	116	134
Time in ER Before Being Evaluated (minutes)	-	-	16	26
Time to Pain Meds for Fractures (minutes)	-	-	46	57
Heart Attack Care				
Aspirin Given at Discharge[5]	-	-	99%	99%
Fibrinolytic Meds Within 30 Min. of Arrival[5]	-	-	100%	54%
PCI Within 90 Minutes of Arrival[5]	-	-	99%	96%
Statin Prescribed at Discharge[5]	-	-	97%	98%
Heart Failure Care				
ACE Inhibitor or ARB for LVSD[5]	-	-	95%	97%
Discharge Instructions Given[5]	-	-	86%	94%
Evaluation of LVS Function[5]	-	-	94%	99%
Medicare Spending				
Medicare Spending per Patient (ratio)	-	-	0.93	0.98
Pneumonia Care				
Appropriate Initial Antibiotic Given[5]	-	-	94%	95%
Blood Culture Timing[5]	-	-	97%	98%
Pregnancy and Delivery Care				
Newborn Deliveries Scheduled Early	-	-	7%	6%
Preventive Care				
Immunization for Influenza[2,3]	139	84%	86%	90%
Immunization for Pneumonia[2,3]	310	94%	88%	92%
Stroke Care				
Anticoagulation Therapy for Atrial Fibrillation	-	-	93%	95%
Antithrombotic Therapy Timing	-	-	95%	98%
Assessed for Rehabilitation	-	-	94%	97%
Discharged on Antithrombotic Therapy	-	-	97%	99%
Discharged on Statin Medication	-	-	89%	94%
Thrombolytic Therapy Timing	-	-	42%	66%
Venous Thromboembolism Prophylaxis	-	-	87%	94%
Written Stroke Educational Materials Given	-	-	68%	88%
Surgical Care Improvement Project				
Appropriate Beta Blocker Usage[5]	-	-	94%	98%
Appropriate VTP Within 24 Hours[5]	-	-	95%	98%
Controlled Postoperative Blood Glucose[5]	-	-	99%	97%
Perioperative Temperature Management[5]	-	-	99%	100%
Prophylactic Antibiotic Selection[5]	-	-	99%	99%
Prophylactic Antibiotic Selection (Outpatient)	-	-	95%	98%
Prophylactic Antibiotic Stopped[5]	-	-	97%	98%
Prophylactic Antibiotic Timing[5]	-	-	98%	99%
Prophylactic Antibiotic Timing (Outpatient)	-	-	96%	98%
Urinary Catheter Removal[5]	-	-	95%	97%
Survey of Patients' Hospital Experiences				
Area Around Room 'Always' Quiet at Night	-	-	61%	61%
Doctors 'Always' Communicated Well	-	-	82%	82%
Home Recovery Information Given	-	-	88%	85%
Hospital Given 9 or 10 on 10 Point Scale	-	-	68%	71%
Meds 'Always' Explained Before Given	-	-	66%	64%
Nurses 'Always' Communicated Well	-	-	78%	79%
Pain 'Always' Well Controlled	-	-	69%	71%
Room and Bathroom 'Always' Clean	-	-	74%	73%
Timely Help 'Always' Received	-	-	70%	68%
Would Definitely Recommend Hospital	-	-	67%	71%
Use of Medical Imaging				
Cardiac Imaging Stress Test before Surgery	-	-	4.8%	5.3%
Combination Abdominal CT Scan	-	-	13.1%	10.5%
Combination Brain/Sinus CT Scan	-	-	2.1%	2.7%

NOTE: Hospital profiles are in alphabetical order by state, then city, then hospital within the city; Rankings exclude hospitals with less than 25 cases except for patient surveys which excludes hospitals with less than 100 cases; (a) 100-299 cases; (1) The number of cases/patients is too few to report; (2) Data submitted were based on a sample of cases/patients; (3) Results are based on a shorter time period than required; (4) Data suppressed by CMS for one or more quarters; (5) Results are not available for this reporting period; (6) Fewer than 100 patients completed the HCAHPS survey; (7) No cases met the criteria for this measure; (8) The lower limit of the confidence interval cannot be calculated if the number of observed infections equals zero; (9) No data are available from the state/territory for this reporting period; (10) The scores shown reflect fewer than 50 completed surveys; (11) There were discrepancies in the data collection process; (12) This measure does not apply to this hospital for this reporting period; (13) Results cannot be calculated for this reporting period; (14) The results for this state are combined with nearby states to protect confidentiality; Please refer to the User's Guide for a full explanation of data.

Measure	Cases	This Hosp.	State Avg.	U.S. Avg.
Combination Chest CT Scan	-	-	3.8%	2.7%
Follow-up Mammogram/Ultrasound	-	-	9.7%	8.8%
Lumbar Spine MRI for Low Back Pain	-	-	46.1%	37.2%

West Park Hospital District

707 Sheridan Avenue Phone: 307-578-2488
Cody, WY 82414 Fax: 307-578-2485
URL: www.westparkhospital.org
Type: Critical Access Hospitals Emergency Services: Yes
Ownership: Govt - Hospital Dist/Auth Beds: 173

Key Personnel:
Radiology. . . . . Karen Beemer
Quality Assurance . . . . Vicki Carrasa
Operating Room. . . . . Lille Ennist
Chief of Medical Staff . . . . Sue Foor
Coronary Care . . . . Jeanne Kaiser
CEO . . . . Doug McMillan
Emergency Room . . . . Kathy Williams
Patient Relations . . . . Carol Wolf

Measure	Cases	This Hosp.	State Avg.	U.S. Avg.
Blood Clot Prevention and Treatment				
Anticoagulation Overlap Therapy[2]	11	82%	90%	93%
ICU Venous Thromboembolism Prophylaxis[1,2]	-	-	90%	92%
Incidence of Potentially Preventable VTE[2,7]	-	-	12%	10%
UFH with Dosages/Platelet Monitoring[1,2]	-	-	97%	97%
Venous Thromboembolism Prophylaxis[2]	47	74%	86%	85%
Warfarin Therapy Discharge Instructions[1,2]	-	-	62%	75%
Chest Pain/Possible Heart Attack Care				
Aspirin Given Within 24 Hours of Arrival	23	96%	97%	96%
Fibrinolytic Meds Within 30 Min. of Arrival[1]	-	-	69%	58%
Average Time to ECG (minutes)	22	12	6	7
Average Time to Transfer (minutes)[7]	-	-	163	60
Children's Asthma Care				
Received Home Management Plan of Care	-	-	-	88%
Received Reliever Medication	-	-	-	100%
Received Systemic Corticosteroids	-	-	-	100%
Emergency Department				
Admittance Decision Time (minutes)[2,7]	-	-	70	98
Head CT Results Within 45 Min. of Arrival[5]	-	-	36%	57%
Patients Who Left ER Before Being Seen	6,455	0%	2%	2%
Time from ER Arrival to Admit. (minutes)[2]	221	261	218	274
Time from ER Arrival to Discharge (minutes)[5]	-	-	116	134
Time in ER Before Being Evaluated (minutes)[5]	-	-	16	26
Time to Pain Meds for Fractures (minutes)[5]	-	-	46	57
Heart Attack Care				
Aspirin Given at Discharge[1]	-	-	99%	99%
Fibrinolytic Meds Within 30 Min. of Arrival[7]	-	-	100%	54%
PCI Within 90 Minutes of Arrival[7]	-	-	99%	96%
Statin Prescribed at Discharge[1]	-	-	97%	98%
Heart Failure Care				
ACE Inhibitor or ARB for LVSD[1]	-	-	95%	97%
Discharge Instructions Given	21	67%	86%	94%
Evaluation of LVS Function	24	88%	94%	99%
Medicare Spending				
Medicare Spending per Patient (ratio)	-	-	0.93	0.98
Pneumonia Care				
Appropriate Initial Antibiotic Given	30	87%	94%	95%
Blood Culture Timing	35	89%	97%	98%
Pregnancy and Delivery Care				
Newborn Deliveries Scheduled Early[5]	-	-	7%	6%
Preventive Care				
Immunization for Influenza[2]	261	64%	86%	90%
Immunization for Pneumonia[2]	246	91%	88%	92%
Stroke Care				
Anticoagulation Therapy for Atrial Fibrillation[1]	-	-	93%	95%
Antithrombotic Therapy Timing[1]	-	-	95%	98%
Assessed for Rehabilitation	14	79%	94%	97%
Discharged on Antithrombotic Therapy	13	92%	97%	99%
Discharged on Statin Medication	12	83%	89%	94%
Thrombolytic Therapy Timing[1]	-	-	42%	66%
Venous Thromboembolism Prophylaxis[1]	-	-	87%	94%
Written Stroke Educational Materials Given[1]	-	-	68%	88%
Surgical Care Improvement Project				
Appropriate Beta Blocker Usage[2]	90	81%	94%	98%
Appropriate VTP Within 24 Hours[2]	269	98%	95%	98%
Controlled Postoperative Blood Glucose[2,7]	-	-	99%	97%
Perioperative Temperature Management[2]	308	100%	99%	100%
Prophylactic Antibiotic Selection[2]	254	99%	99%	99%
Prophylactic Antibiotic Selection (Outpatient)	15	100%	95%	98%
Prophylactic Antibiotic Stopped[2]	247	83%	97%	98%
Prophylactic Antibiotic Timing[2]	254	98%	98%	99%
Prophylactic Antibiotic Timing (Outpatient)	17	82%	96%	98%
Urinary Catheter Removal[2]	190	95%	95%	97%
Survey of Patients' Hospital Experiences				
Area Around Room 'Always' Quiet at Night	300+	58%	61%	61%
Doctors 'Always' Communicated Well	300+	85%	82%	82%
Home Recovery Information Given	300+	91%	88%	85%
Hospital Given 9 or 10 on 10 Point Scale	300+	69%	68%	71%
Meds 'Always' Explained Before Given	300+	67%	66%	64%
Nurses 'Always' Communicated Well	300+	77%	78%	79%
Pain 'Always' Well Controlled	300+	70%	69%	71%
Room and Bathroom 'Always' Clean	300+	72%	74%	73%
Timely Help 'Always' Received	300+	67%	70%	68%
Would Definitely Recommend Hospital	300+	72%	67%	71%
Use of Medical Imaging				
Cardiac Imaging Stress Test before Surgery	103	4.9%	4.8%	5.3%
Combination Abdominal CT Scan	421	0.2%	13.1%	10.5%
Combination Brain/Sinus CT Scan	254	0.8%	2.1%	2.7%
Combination Chest CT Scan	363	0.0%	3.8%	2.7%
Follow-up Mammogram/Ultrasound	607	17.5%	9.7%	8.8%
Lumbar Spine MRI for Low Back Pain	68	36.8%	46.1%	37.2%

Memorial Hospital of Converse County

111 South 5th Street Phone: 307-358-2122
Douglas, WY 82633 Fax: 307-358-3630
E-mail: info@mhccwyo.org
URL: www.conversehospital.com
Type: Critical Access Hospitals Emergency Services: Yes
Ownership: Voluntary non-profit - Other Beds: 15

Key Personnel:
Quality Assurance . . . . Billie Engleman
Emergency Room . . . . Tracy Forward, RN
Radiology. . . . . Linda Holden
Chief of Medical Staff . . . . Kirby C Kirkland, MD
Infection Control . . . . Kirby C Kirkland, MD
Pediatric In-Patient Care . . . . James F Morgan, MD
CEO . . . . Ryan Smith
Operating Room. . . . . William White

Measure	Cases	This Hosp.	State Avg.	U.S. Avg.
Blood Clot Prevention and Treatment				
Anticoagulation Overlap Therapy[5]	-	-	90%	93%
ICU Venous Thromboembolism Prophylaxis[5]	-	-	90%	92%
Incidence of Potentially Preventable VTE[5]	-	-	12%	10%
UFH with Dosages/Platelet Monitoring[5]	-	-	97%	97%
Venous Thromboembolism Prophylaxis[5]	-	-	86%	85%
Warfarin Therapy Discharge Instructions[5]	-	-	62%	75%
Chest Pain/Possible Heart Attack Care				
Aspirin Given Within 24 Hours of Arrival	11	100%	97%	96%
Fibrinolytic Meds Within 30 Min. of Arrival[1]	-	-	69%	58%
Average Time to ECG (minutes)	12	5	6	7
Average Time to Transfer (minutes)[7]	-	-	163	60
Children's Asthma Care				
Received Home Management Plan of Care	-	-	-	88%
Received Reliever Medication	-	-	-	100%
Received Systemic Corticosteroids	-	-	-	100%
Emergency Department				
Admittance Decision Time (minutes)[5]	-	-	70	98
Head CT Results Within 45 Min. of Arrival[5]	-	-	36%	57%
Patients Who Left ER Before Being Seen[5]	-	-	2%	2%
Time from ER Arrival to Admit. (minutes)[5]	-	-	218	274
Time from ER Arrival to Discharge (minutes)[5]	-	-	116	134
Time in ER Before Being Evaluated (minutes)[5]	-	-	16	26
Time to Pain Meds for Fractures (minutes)[5]	-	-	46	57
Heart Attack Care				
Aspirin Given at Discharge[1]	-	-	99%	99%
Fibrinolytic Meds Within 30 Min. of Arrival[7]	-	-	100%	54%
PCI Within 90 Minutes of Arrival[7]	-	-	99%	96%
Statin Prescribed at Discharge[1]	-	-	97%	98%
Heart Failure Care				
ACE Inhibitor or ARB for LVSD[7]	-	-	95%	97%
Discharge Instructions Given[1]	-	-	86%	94%
Evaluation of LVS Function[1]	-	-	94%	99%
Medicare Spending				
Medicare Spending per Patient (ratio)	-	-	0.93	0.98
Pneumonia Care				
Appropriate Initial Antibiotic Given	16	100%	94%	95%
Blood Culture Timing	29	100%	97%	98%
Pregnancy and Delivery Care				
Newborn Deliveries Scheduled Early[5]	-	-	7%	6%
Preventive Care				
Immunization for Influenza[5]	-	-	86%	90%
Immunization for Pneumonia[5]	-	-	88%	92%
Stroke Care				
Anticoagulation Therapy for Atrial Fibrillation[5]	-	-	93%	95%
Antithrombotic Therapy Timing[5]	-	-	95%	98%
Assessed for Rehabilitation[5]	-	-	94%	97%
Discharged on Antithrombotic Therapy[5]	-	-	97%	99%
Discharged on Statin Medication[5]	-	-	89%	94%
Thrombolytic Therapy Timing[5]	-	-	42%	66%
Venous Thromboembolism Prophylaxis[5]	-	-	87%	94%
Written Stroke Educational Materials Given[5]	-	-	68%	88%
Surgical Care Improvement Project				
Appropriate Beta Blocker Usage	19	100%	94%	98%
Appropriate VTP Within 24 Hours	102	100%	95%	98%
Controlled Postoperative Blood Glucose[7]	-	-	99%	97%
Perioperative Temperature Management	114	100%	99%	100%
Prophylactic Antibiotic Selection	101	100%	99%	99%
Prophylactic Antibiotic Selection (Outpatient)	67	100%	95%	98%
Prophylactic Antibiotic Stopped	100	98%	97%	98%
Prophylactic Antibiotic Timing	101	98%	98%	99%
Prophylactic Antibiotic Timing (Outpatient)	67	100%	96%	98%
Urinary Catheter Removal	107	99%	95%	97%
Survey of Patients' Hospital Experiences				
Area Around Room 'Always' Quiet at Night	(a)	70%	61%	61%
Doctors 'Always' Communicated Well	(a)	81%	82%	82%
Home Recovery Information Given	(a)	90%	88%	85%
Hospital Given 9 or 10 on 10 Point Scale	(a)	70%	68%	71%
Meds 'Always' Explained Before Given	(a)	69%	66%	64%
Nurses 'Always' Communicated Well	(a)	80%	78%	79%
Pain 'Always' Well Controlled	(a)	68%	69%	71%
Room and Bathroom 'Always' Clean	(a)	84%	74%	73%
Timely Help 'Always' Received	(a)	78%	70%	68%
Would Definitely Recommend Hospital	(a)	76%	67%	71%
Use of Medical Imaging				
Cardiac Imaging Stress Test before Surgery[1]	-	-	4.8%	5.3%
Combination Abdominal CT Scan	94	17.0%	13.1%	10.5%
Combination Brain/Sinus CT Scan[1]	-	-	2.1%	2.7%
Combination Chest CT Scan[1]	-	-	3.8%	2.7%
Follow-up Mammogram/Ultrasound	183	5.5%	9.7%	8.8%
Lumbar Spine MRI for Low Back Pain[7]	-	-	46.1%	37.2%

Evanston Regional Hospital

190 Arrowhead Dr Phone: 307-789-3636
Evanston, WY 82930 Fax: 307-783-8237
URL: www.evanstonregionalhospital.com
Type: Acute Care Hospitals Emergency Services: Yes
Ownership: Proprietary Beds: 42

Key Personnel:
Quality Assurance . . . . Yvonne Adams
Emergency Room . . . . Kevin O'Meara
CEO/President. . . . . Chris Parj
Chief of Medical Staff . . . . Mike Stellers

Measure	Cases	This Hosp.	State Avg.	U.S. Avg.
Blood Clot Prevention and Treatment				
Anticoagulation Overlap Therapy[2]	15	73%	90%	93%
ICU Venous Thromboembolism Prophylaxis[2]	16	100%	90%	92%
Incidence of Potentially Preventable VTE[1,2]	-	-	12%	10%
UFH with Dosages/Platelet Monitoring[2]	15	100%	97%	97%
Venous Thromboembolism Prophylaxis[2]	135	100%	86%	85%
Warfarin Therapy Discharge Instructions[2]	13	100%	62%	75%
Chest Pain/Possible Heart Attack Care				

NOTE: Hospital profiles are in alphabetical order by state, then city, then hospital within the city; Rankings exclude hospitals with less than 25 cases except for patient surveys which excludes hospitals with less than 100 cases; (a) 100-299 cases; (1) The number of cases/patients is too few to report; (2) Data submitted were based on a sample of cases/patients; (3) Results are based on a shorter time period than required; (4) Data suppressed by CMS for one or more quarters; (5) Results are not available for this reporting period; (6) Fewer than 100 patients completed the HCAHPS survey; (7) No cases met the criteria for this measure; (8) The lower limit of the confidence interval cannot be calculated if the number of observed infections equals zero; (9) No data are available from the state/territory for this reporting period; (10) The scores shown reflect fewer than 50 completed surveys; (11) There were discrepancies in the data collection process; (12) This measure does not apply to this hospital for this reporting period; (13) Results cannot be calculated for this reporting period; (14) The results for this state are combined with nearby states to protect confidentiality; Please refer to the User's Guide for a full explanation of data.

Measure	Cases	This Hosp.	State Avg.	U.S. Avg.
Aspirin Given Within 24 Hours of Arrival	27	100%	97%	96%
Fibrinolytic Meds Within 30 Min. of Arrival[1]	-	-	69%	58%
Average Time to ECG (minutes)	28	1	6	7
Average Time to Transfer (minutes)[1]	-	-	163	60
Children's Asthma Care				
Received Home Management Plan of Care	-	-	-	88%
Received Reliever Medication	-	-	-	100%
Received Systemic Corticosteroids	-	-	-	100%
Emergency Department				
Admittance Decision Time (minutes)[2]	290	35	70	98
Head CT Results Within 45 Min. of Arrival[1]	-	-	36%	57%
Patients Who Left ER Before Being Seen	8,577	0%	2%	2%
Time from ER Arrival to Admit. (minutes)[2]	292	159	218	274
Time from ER Arrival to Discharge (minutes)	389	73	116	134
Time in ER Before Being Evaluated (minutes)	421	9	16	26
Time to Pain Meds for Fractures (minutes)	68	19	46	57
Heart Attack Care				
Aspirin Given at Discharge[3,7]	-	-	99%	99%
Fibrinolytic Meds Within 30 Min. of Arrival[3,7]	-	-	100%	54%
PCI Within 90 Minutes of Arrival[3,7]	-	-	99%	96%
Statin Prescribed at Discharge[3,7]	-	-	97%	98%
Heart Failure Care				
ACE Inhibitor or ARB for LVSD[1]	-	-	95%	97%
Discharge Instructions Given[1]	-	-	86%	94%
Evaluation of LVS Function	11	82%	94%	99%
Medicare Spending				
Medicare Spending per Patient (ratio)	-	0.86	0.93	0.98
Pneumonia Care				
Appropriate Initial Antibiotic Given	32	91%	94%	95%
Blood Culture Timing	28	100%	97%	98%
Pregnancy and Delivery Care				
Newborn Deliveries Scheduled Early[2]	29	0%	7%	6%
Preventive Care				
Immunization for Influenza[2]	262	99%	86%	90%
Immunization for Pneumonia[2]	209	99%	88%	92%
Stroke Care				
Anticoagulation Therapy for Atrial Fibrillation[7]	-	-	93%	95%
Antithrombotic Therapy Timing[1]	-	-	95%	98%
Assessed for Rehabilitation[1]	-	-	94%	97%
Discharged on Antithrombotic Therapy[1]	-	-	97%	99%
Discharged on Statin Medication[1]	-	-	89%	94%
Thrombolytic Therapy Timing[7]	-	-	42%	66%
Venous Thromboembolism Prophylaxis[1]	-	-	87%	94%
Written Stroke Educational Materials Given[1]	-	-	68%	88%
Surgical Care Improvement Project				
Appropriate Beta Blocker Usage	11	100%	94%	98%
Appropriate VTP Within 24 Hours	55	100%	95%	98%
Controlled Postoperative Blood Glucose[7]	-	-	99%	97%
Perioperative Temperature Management	66	100%	99%	100%
Prophylactic Antibiotic Selection	47	100%	99%	99%
Prophylactic Antibiotic Selection (Outpatient)	19	100%	95%	98%
Prophylactic Antibiotic Stopped	47	98%	97%	98%
Prophylactic Antibiotic Timing	48	100%	98%	99%
Prophylactic Antibiotic Timing (Outpatient)	11	100%	96%	98%
Urinary Catheter Removal	34	91%	95%	97%
Survey of Patients' Hospital Experiences				
Area Around Room 'Always' Quiet at Night	(a)	62%	61%	61%
Doctors 'Always' Communicated Well	(a)	82%	82%	82%
Home Recovery Information Given	(a)	88%	88%	85%
Hospital Given 9 or 10 on 10 Point Scale	(a)	62%	68%	71%
Meds 'Always' Explained Before Given	(a)	68%	66%	64%
Nurses 'Always' Communicated Well	(a)	75%	78%	79%
Pain 'Always' Well Controlled	(a)	70%	69%	71%
Room and Bathroom 'Always' Clean	(a)	64%	74%	73%
Timely Help 'Always' Received	(a)	69%	70%	68%
Would Definitely Recommend Hospital	(a)	58%	67%	71%
Use of Medical Imaging				
Cardiac Imaging Stress Test before Surgery[1]	-	-	4.8%	5.3%
Combination Abdominal CT Scan	84	16.7%	13.1%	10.5%
Combination Brain/Sinus CT Scan[1]	-	-	2.1%	2.7%
Combination Chest CT Scan	78	0.0%	3.8%	2.7%
Follow-up Mammogram/Ultrasound	190	12.6%	9.7%	8.8%
Lumbar Spine MRI for Low Back Pain[1]	-	-	46.1%	37.2%

Campbell County Memorial Hospital

501 South Burma Avenue | Phone: 307-688-1551
Gillette, WY 82716 | Fax: 307-688-1515
URL: www.ccmh.net
Type: Acute Care Hospitals | Emergency Services: Yes
Ownership: Govt - Hospital Dist/Auth | Beds: 90

Key Personnel:
Intensive Care Unit. . . . . Bette Amith
Patient Relations . . . . Mary Barks
Operating Room. . . . . Rodney Biggs
Chief of Medical Staff. . . . . Larry Long, MD
Hemotology Center . . . . Philip McMahill
CEO/President. . . . . Bob Morasko
Radiology. . . . . John Stamato
Quality Assurance . . . . Sue Ullrich

Measure	Cases	This Hosp.	State Avg.	U.S. Avg.
Blood Clot Prevention and Treatment				
Anticoagulation Overlap Therapy[2]	24	92%	90%	93%
ICU Venous Thromboembolism Prophylaxis[2]	55	71%	90%	92%
Incidence of Potentially Preventable VTE[1,2]	-	-	12%	10%
UFH with Dosages/Platelet Monitoring[1,2]	-	-	97%	97%
Venous Thromboembolism Prophylaxis[2]	118	69%	86%	85%
Warfarin Therapy Discharge Instructions[2]	25	84%	62%	75%
Chest Pain/Possible Heart Attack Care				
Aspirin Given Within 24 Hours of Arrival	84	100%	97%	96%
Fibrinolytic Meds Within 30 Min. of Arrival	18	89%	69%	58%
Average Time to ECG (minutes)	88	5	6	7
Average Time to Transfer (minutes)[1]	-	-	163	60
Children's Asthma Care				
Received Home Management Plan of Care	-	-	-	88%
Received Reliever Medication	-	-	-	100%
Received Systemic Corticosteroids	-	-	-	100%
Emergency Department				
Admittance Decision Time (minutes)[2]	276	53	70	98
Head CT Results Within 45 Min. of Arrival[1]	-	-	36%	57%
Patients Who Left ER Before Being Seen	20,677	1%	2%	2%
Time from ER Arrival to Admit. (minutes)[2]	278	200	218	274
Time from ER Arrival to Discharge (minutes)	415	137	116	134
Time in ER Before Being Evaluated (minutes)	429	41	16	26
Time to Pain Meds for Fractures (minutes)	105	48	46	57
Heart Attack Care				
Aspirin Given at Discharge[1,3]	-	-	99%	99%
Fibrinolytic Meds Within 30 Min. of Arrival[3,7]	-	-	100%	54%
PCI Within 90 Minutes of Arrival[3,7]	-	-	99%	96%
Statin Prescribed at Discharge[1,3]	-	-	97%	98%
Heart Failure Care				
ACE Inhibitor or ARB for LVSD	19	89%	95%	97%
Discharge Instructions Given	34	88%	86%	94%
Evaluation of LVS Function	41	100%	94%	99%
Medicare Spending				
Medicare Spending per Patient (ratio)	-	0.90	0.93	0.98
Pneumonia Care				
Appropriate Initial Antibiotic Given	44	93%	94%	95%
Blood Culture Timing	70	99%	97%	98%
Pregnancy and Delivery Care				
Newborn Deliveries Scheduled Early	84	6%	7%	6%
Preventive Care				
Immunization for Influenza[2]	248	95%	86%	90%
Immunization for Pneumonia[2]	204	80%	88%	92%
Stroke Care				
Anticoagulation Therapy for Atrial Fibrillation[1]	-	-	93%	95%
Antithrombotic Therapy Timing	25	100%	95%	98%
Assessed for Rehabilitation	26	88%	94%	97%
Discharged on Antithrombotic Therapy	25	100%	97%	99%
Discharged on Statin Medication	20	95%	89%	94%
Thrombolytic Therapy Timing[7]	-	-	42%	66%
Venous Thromboembolism Prophylaxis	22	77%	87%	94%
Written Stroke Educational Materials Given	13	69%	68%	88%
Surgical Care Improvement Project				
Appropriate Beta Blocker Usage	17	94%	94%	98%
Appropriate VTP Within 24 Hours	130	82%	95%	98%
Controlled Postoperative Blood Glucose[7]	-	-	99%	97%
Perioperative Temperature Management	139	99%	99%	100%
Prophylactic Antibiotic Selection	107	95%	99%	99%
Prophylactic Antibiotic Selection (Outpatient)	90	96%	95%	98%
Prophylactic Antibiotic Stopped	107	100%	97%	98%
Prophylactic Antibiotic Timing	107	100%	98%	99%
Prophylactic Antibiotic Timing (Outpatient)	90	100%	96%	98%
Urinary Catheter Removal	56	93%	95%	97%
Survey of Patients' Hospital Experiences				
Area Around Room 'Always' Quiet at Night	300+	62%	61%	61%
Doctors 'Always' Communicated Well	300+	77%	82%	82%
Home Recovery Information Given	300+	88%	88%	85%
Hospital Given 9 or 10 on 10 Point Scale	300+	63%	68%	71%
Meds 'Always' Explained Before Given	300+	66%	66%	64%
Nurses 'Always' Communicated Well	300+	75%	78%	79%
Pain 'Always' Well Controlled	300+	67%	69%	71%
Room and Bathroom 'Always' Clean	300+	67%	74%	73%
Timely Help 'Always' Received	300+	68%	70%	68%
Would Definitely Recommend Hospital	300+	56%	67%	71%
Use of Medical Imaging				
Cardiac Imaging Stress Test before Surgery	89	6.7%	4.8%	5.3%
Combination Abdominal CT Scan	256	27.3%	13.1%	10.5%
Combination Brain/Sinus CT Scan[1]	-	-	2.1%	2.7%
Combination Chest CT Scan	243	3.7%	3.8%	2.7%
Follow-up Mammogram/Ultrasound	259	9.3%	9.7%	8.8%
Lumbar Spine MRI for Low Back Pain	62	45.2%	46.1%	37.2%

Saint Johns Medical Center

625 East Broadway | Phone: 307-733-3636
Jackson, WY 83001 | Fax: 307-739-7522
URL: www.tetonhospital.org
Type: Acute Care Hospitals | Emergency Services: Yes
Ownership: Govt - Hospital Dist/Auth | Beds: 117

Key Personnel:
Hemotology Center . . . . Judy Basye, RN
Radiology. . . . . Robert Berlin
Chief of Medical Staff . . . . Dennis Butcher, MDS
CEO . . . . Louis I. Hochheiser, MD
Operating Room. . . . . Heidi Jost, RN
Emergency Room . . . . Karen Petrozella, RN
CEO/President. . . . . Jim Schuessler
Chair/CEO . . . . Michael Tennican

Measure	Cases	This Hosp.	State Avg.	U.S. Avg.
Blood Clot Prevention and Treatment				
Anticoagulation Overlap Therapy[2]	11	100%	90%	93%
ICU Venous Thromboembolism Prophylaxis[2]	51	100%	90%	92%
Incidence of Potentially Preventable VTE[1,2]	-	-	12%	10%
UFH with Dosages/Platelet Monitoring[2,7]	-	-	97%	97%
Venous Thromboembolism Prophylaxis[2]	122	96%	86%	85%
Warfarin Therapy Discharge Instructions[1,2]	-	-	62%	75%
Chest Pain/Possible Heart Attack Care				
Aspirin Given Within 24 Hours of Arrival	27	96%	97%	96%
Fibrinolytic Meds Within 30 Min. of Arrival[1,3]	-	-	69%	58%
Average Time to ECG (minutes)	27	5	6	7
Average Time to Transfer (minutes)[3,7]	-	-	163	60
Children's Asthma Care				
Received Home Management Plan of Care	-	-	-	88%
Received Reliever Medication	-	-	-	100%
Received Systemic Corticosteroids	-	-	-	100%
Emergency Department				
Admittance Decision Time (minutes)[2]	119	42	70	98
Head CT Results Within 45 Min. of Arrival[1]	-	-	36%	57%
Patients Who Left ER Before Being Seen	8,395	0%	2%	2%
Time from ER Arrival to Admit. (minutes)[2]	140	178	218	274
Time from ER Arrival to Discharge (minutes)	357	93	116	134
Time in ER Before Being Evaluated (minutes)	348	14	16	26
Time to Pain Meds for Fractures (minutes)	53	30	46	57
Heart Attack Care				
Aspirin Given at Discharge[1,3]	-	-	99%	99%
Fibrinolytic Meds Within 30 Min. of Arrival[3,7]	-	-	100%	54%
PCI Within 90 Minutes of Arrival[3,7]	-	-	99%	96%
Statin Prescribed at Discharge[1,3]	-	-	97%	98%
Heart Failure Care				
ACE Inhibitor or ARB for LVSD[1]	-	-	95%	97%
Discharge Instructions Given	19	89%	86%	94%

NOTE: Hospital profiles are in alphabetical order by state, then city, then hospital within the city; Rankings exclude hospitals with less than 25 cases except for patient surveys which excludes hospitals with less than 100 cases; (a) 100-299 cases; (1) The number of cases/patients is too few to report; (2) Data submitted were based on a sample of cases/patients; (3) Results are based on a shorter time period than required; (4) Data suppressed by CMS for one or more quarters; (5) Results are not available for this reporting period; (6) Fewer than 100 patients completed the HCAHPS survey; (7) No cases met the criteria for this measure; (8) The lower limit of the confidence interval cannot be calculated if the number of observed infections equals zero; (9) No data are available from the state/territory for this reporting period; (10) The scores shown reflect fewer than 50 completed surveys; (11) There were discrepancies in the data collection process; (12) This measure does not apply to this hospital for this reporting period; (13) Results cannot be calculated for this reporting period; (14) The results for this state are combined with nearby states to protect confidentiality; Please refer to the User's Guide for a full explanation of data.

Evaluation of LVS Function	18	100%	94%	99%
Medicare Spending				
Medicare Spending per Patient (ratio)	-	0.87	0.93	0.98
Pneumonia Care				
Appropriate Initial Antibiotic Given	27	85%	94%	95%
Blood Culture Timing	30	100%	97%	98%
Pregnancy and Delivery Care				
Newborn Deliveries Scheduled Early[2]	37	14%	7%	6%
Preventive Care				
Immunization for Influenza[2]	233	95%	86%	90%
Immunization for Pneumonia[2]	173	95%	88%	92%
Stroke Care				
Anticoagulation Therapy for Atrial Fibrillation[1,2]	-	-	93%	95%
Antithrombotic Therapy Timing[1,2]	-	-	95%	98%
Assessed for Rehabilitation[1,2]	-	-	94%	97%
Discharged on Antithrombotic Therapy[1,2]	-	-	97%	99%
Discharged on Statin Medication[1,2]	-	-	89%	94%
Thrombolytic Therapy Timing[1,2]	-	-	42%	66%
Venous Thromboembolism Prophylaxis[1,2]	-	-	87%	94%
Written Stroke Educational Materials Given[1,2]	-	-	68%	88%
Surgical Care Improvement Project				
Appropriate Beta Blocker Usage[2]	37	97%	94%	98%
Appropriate VTP Within 24 Hours[2]	219	99%	95%	98%
Controlled Postoperative Blood Glucose[2,7]	-	-	99%	97%
Perioperative Temperature Management[2]	239	100%	99%	100%
Prophylactic Antibiotic Selection[2]	180	99%	99%	99%
Prophylactic Antibiotic Selection (Outpatient)	74	95%	95%	98%
Prophylactic Antibiotic Stopped[2]	179	99%	97%	98%
Prophylactic Antibiotic Timing[2]	181	98%	98%	99%
Prophylactic Antibiotic Timing (Outpatient)	76	95%	96%	98%
Urinary Catheter Removal[2]	187	98%	95%	97%
Survey of Patients' Hospital Experiences				
Area Around Room 'Always' Quiet at Night	300+	60%	61%	61%
Doctors 'Always' Communicated Well	300+	81%	82%	82%
Home Recovery Information Given	300+	86%	88%	85%
Hospital Given 9 or 10 on 10 Point Scale	300+	76%	68%	71%
Meds 'Always' Explained Before Given	300+	65%	66%	64%
Nurses 'Always' Communicated Well	300+	79%	78%	79%
Pain 'Always' Well Controlled	300+	70%	69%	71%
Room and Bathroom 'Always' Clean	300+	78%	74%	73%
Timely Help 'Always' Received	300+	72%	70%	68%
Would Definitely Recommend Hospital	300+	77%	67%	71%
Use of Medical Imaging				
Cardiac Imaging Stress Test before Surgery	104	4.8%	4.8%	5.3%
Combination Abdominal CT Scan	228	1.3%	13.1%	10.5%
Combination Brain/Sinus CT Scan[1]	-	-	2.1%	2.7%
Combination Chest CT Scan	179	0.0%	3.8%	2.7%
Follow-up Mammogram/Ultrasound	417	4.6%	9.7%	8.8%
Lumbar Spine MRI for Low Back Pain	94	51.1%	46.1%	37.2%

South Lincoln Medical Center

PO Box 390 Phone: 307-877-4401
Kemmerer, WY 83101 Fax: 307-877-3236
E-mail: ms@allwest.net
URL: www.southlincolnmedical.com
Type: Critical Access Hospitals Emergency Services: Yes
Ownership: Govt - Hospital Dist/Auth Beds: 16

Key Personnel:
CEO . . . . Eric Boley
Cardiology . . . . Ronald Brown

Measure	Cases	This Hosp.	State Avg.	U.S. Avg.
Blood Clot Prevention and Treatment				
Anticoagulation Overlap Therapy[1]	-	-	90%	93%
ICU Venous Thromboembolism Prophylaxis[7]	-	-	90%	92%
Incidence of Potentially Preventable VTE[7]	-	-	12%	10%
UFH with Dosages/Platelet Monitoring[7]	-	-	97%	97%
Venous Thromboembolism Prophylaxis	33	85%	86%	85%
Warfarin Therapy Discharge Instructions[1]	-	-	62%	75%
Chest Pain/Possible Heart Attack Care				
Aspirin Given Within 24 Hours of Arrival[1,3]	-	-	97%	96%
Fibrinolytic Meds Within 30 Min. of Arrival[1,3]	-	-	69%	58%
Average Time to ECG (minutes)[1,3]	-	-	6	7
Average Time to Transfer (minutes)[3,7]	-	-	163	60
Children's Asthma Care				
Received Home Management Plan of Care	-	-	-	88%
Received Reliever Medication	-	-	-	100%
Received Systemic Corticosteroids	-	-	-	100%
Emergency Department				
Admittance Decision Time (minutes)[5]	-	-	70	98
Head CT Results Within 45 Min. of Arrival[3,7]	-	-	36%	57%
Patients Who Left ER Before Being Seen	2,143	0%	2%	2%
Time from ER Arrival to Admit. (minutes)[5]	-	-	218	274
Time from ER Arrival to Discharge (minutes)[3]	118	80	116	134
Time in ER Before Being Evaluated (minutes)[3]	135	16	16	26
Time to Pain Meds for Fractures (minutes)[3]	11	30	46	57
Heart Attack Care				
Aspirin Given at Discharge[5]	-	-	99%	99%
Fibrinolytic Meds Within 30 Min. of Arrival[5]	-	-	100%	54%
PCI Within 90 Minutes of Arrival[5]	-	-	99%	96%
Statin Prescribed at Discharge[5]	-	-	97%	98%
Heart Failure Care				
ACE Inhibitor or ARB for LVSD[3,7]	-	-	95%	97%
Discharge Instructions Given[3,7]	-	-	86%	94%
Evaluation of LVS Function[1,3]	-	-	94%	99%
Medicare Spending				
Medicare Spending per Patient (ratio)	-	-	0.93	0.98
Pneumonia Care				
Appropriate Initial Antibiotic Given[2]	11	91%	94%	95%
Blood Culture Timing[1,2]	-	-	97%	98%
Pregnancy and Delivery Care				
Newborn Deliveries Scheduled Early[5]	-	-	7%	6%
Preventive Care				
Immunization for Influenza[2]	17	71%	86%	90%
Immunization for Pneumonia[2]	32	97%	88%	92%
Stroke Care				
Anticoagulation Therapy for Atrial Fibrillation[3,7]	-	-	93%	95%
Antithrombotic Therapy Timing[1,3]	-	-	95%	98%
Assessed for Rehabilitation[1,3]	-	-	94%	97%
Discharged on Antithrombotic Therapy[1,3]	-	-	97%	99%
Discharged on Statin Medication[1,3]	-	-	89%	94%
Thrombolytic Therapy Timing[3,7]	-	-	42%	66%
Venous Thromboembolism Prophylaxis[1,3]	-	-	87%	94%
Written Stroke Educational Materials Given[1,3]	-	-	68%	88%
Surgical Care Improvement Project				
Appropriate Beta Blocker Usage[2,7]	-	-	94%	98%
Appropriate VTP Within 24 Hours[1,2]	-	-	95%	98%
Controlled Postoperative Blood Glucose[2,7]	-	-	99%	97%
Perioperative Temperature Management[2]	12	100%	99%	100%
Prophylactic Antibiotic Selection[2]	12	100%	99%	99%
Prophylactic Antibiotic Selection (Outpatient)[1,3]	-	-	95%	98%
Prophylactic Antibiotic Stopped[2]	12	100%	97%	98%
Prophylactic Antibiotic Timing[2]	12	92%	98%	99%
Prophylactic Antibiotic Timing (Outpatient)[1,3]	-	-	96%	98%
Urinary Catheter Removal[1,2]	-	-	95%	97%
Survey of Patients' Hospital Experiences				
Area Around Room 'Always' Quiet at Night[10]	<100	64%	61%	61%
Doctors 'Always' Communicated Well[10]	<100	86%	82%	82%
Home Recovery Information Given[10]	<100	91%	88%	85%
Hospital Given 9 or 10 on 10 Point Scale[10]	<100	78%	68%	71%
Meds 'Always' Explained Before Given[10]	<100	58%	66%	64%
Nurses 'Always' Communicated Well[10]	<100	85%	78%	79%
Pain 'Always' Well Controlled[10]	<100	53%	69%	71%
Room and Bathroom 'Always' Clean[10]	<100	77%	74%	73%
Timely Help 'Always' Received[10]	<100	66%	70%	68%
Would Definitely Recommend Hospital[10]	<100	78%	67%	71%
Use of Medical Imaging				
Cardiac Imaging Stress Test before Surgery[7]	-	-	4.8%	5.3%
Combination Abdominal CT Scan[1]	-	-	13.1%	10.5%
Combination Brain/Sinus CT Scan[1]	-	-	2.1%	2.7%
Combination Chest CT Scan[1]	-	-	3.8%	2.7%
Follow-up Mammogram/Ultrasound[1]	-	-	9.7%	8.8%
Lumbar Spine MRI for Low Back Pain[1]	-	-	46.1%	37.2%

Lander Regional Hospital

1320 Bishop Randall Dr Phone: 307-332-4420
Lander, WY 82520 Fax: 307-332-3548
URL: www.landerhospital.com
Type: Acute Care Hospitals Emergency Services: Yes
Ownership: Proprietary Beds: 81

Key Personnel:
Pediatrics. . . . . Ryan G Firth
Pediatrics. . . . . Michael Fisher
Anesthesiology. . . . . Edward J Frink
Anesthesiology. . . . . Emiley M Horne
Pediatrics. . . . . Tara Mercer
CEO/President. . . . . Phil Paton

Measure	Cases	This Hosp.	State Avg.	U.S. Avg.
Blood Clot Prevention and Treatment				
Anticoagulation Overlap Therapy[1,2]	-	-	90%	93%
ICU Venous Thromboembolism Prophylaxis[2]	42	86%	90%	92%
Incidence of Potentially Preventable VTE[1,2]	-	-	12%	10%
UFH with Dosages/Platelet Monitoring[1,2]	-	-	97%	97%
Venous Thromboembolism Prophylaxis[2]	89	76%	86%	85%
Warfarin Therapy Discharge Instructions[1,2]	-	-	62%	75%
Chest Pain/Possible Heart Attack Care				
Aspirin Given Within 24 Hours of Arrival	39	95%	97%	96%
Fibrinolytic Meds Within 30 Min. of Arrival[1]	-	-	69%	58%
Average Time to ECG (minutes)	41	0	6	7
Average Time to Transfer (minutes)[7]	-	-	163	60
Children's Asthma Care				
Received Home Management Plan of Care	-	-	-	88%
Received Reliever Medication	-	-	-	100%
Received Systemic Corticosteroids	-	-	-	100%
Emergency Department				
Admittance Decision Time (minutes)[2]	185	67	70	98
Head CT Results Within 45 Min. of Arrival[1,3]	-	-	36%	57%
Patients Who Left ER Before Being Seen	11,546	1%	2%	2%
Time from ER Arrival to Admit. (minutes)[2]	203	193	218	274
Time from ER Arrival to Discharge (minutes)	396	82	116	134
Time in ER Before Being Evaluated (minutes)	433	7	16	26
Time to Pain Meds for Fractures (minutes)	31	35	46	57
Heart Attack Care				
Aspirin Given at Discharge[1,3]	-	-	99%	99%
Fibrinolytic Meds Within 30 Min. of Arrival[3,7]	-	-	100%	54%
PCI Within 90 Minutes of Arrival[3,7]	-	-	99%	96%
Statin Prescribed at Discharge[1,3]	-	-	97%	98%
Heart Failure Care				
ACE Inhibitor or ARB for LVSD[1]	-	-	95%	97%
Discharge Instructions Given	19	95%	86%	94%
Evaluation of LVS Function	21	100%	94%	99%
Medicare Spending				
Medicare Spending per Patient (ratio)	-	0.89	0.93	0.98
Pneumonia Care				
Appropriate Initial Antibiotic Given	36	97%	94%	95%
Blood Culture Timing	47	98%	97%	98%
Pregnancy and Delivery Care				
Newborn Deliveries Scheduled Early[2]	39	10%	7%	6%
Preventive Care				
Immunization for Influenza[2]	246	80%	86%	90%
Immunization for Pneumonia[2]	215	93%	88%	92%
Stroke Care				
Anticoagulation Therapy for Atrial Fibrillation[1]	-	-	93%	95%
Antithrombotic Therapy Timing[1]	-	-	95%	98%
Assessed for Rehabilitation[1]	-	-	94%	97%
Discharged on Antithrombotic Therapy[1]	-	-	97%	99%
Discharged on Statin Medication[1]	-	-	89%	94%
Thrombolytic Therapy Timing[1]	-	-	42%	66%
Venous Thromboembolism Prophylaxis[1]	-	-	87%	94%
Written Stroke Educational Materials Given[1]	-	-	68%	88%
Surgical Care Improvement Project				
Appropriate Beta Blocker Usage	15	100%	94%	98%
Appropriate VTP Within 24 Hours	72	93%	95%	98%
Controlled Postoperative Blood Glucose[7]	-	-	99%	97%
Perioperative Temperature Management	103	100%	99%	100%
Prophylactic Antibiotic Selection	81	99%	99%	99%
Prophylactic Antibiotic Selection (Outpatient)	29	97%	95%	98%
Prophylactic Antibiotic Stopped	79	99%	97%	98%

NOTE: Hospital profiles are in alphabetical order by state, then city, then hospital within the city; Rankings exclude hospitals with less than 25 cases except for patient surveys which excludes hospitals with less than 100 cases; (a) 100-299 cases; (1) The number of cases/patients is too few to report; (2) Data submitted were based on a sample of cases/patients; (3) Results are based on a shorter time period than required; (4) Data suppressed by CMS for one or more quarters; (5) Results are not available for this reporting period; (6) Fewer than 100 patients completed the HCAHPS survey; (7) No cases met the criteria for this measure; (8) The lower limit of the confidence interval cannot be calculated if the number of observed infections equals zero; (9) No data are available from the state/territory for this reporting period; (10) The scores shown reflect fewer than 50 completed surveys; (11) There were discrepancies in the data collection process; (12) This measure does not apply to this hospital for this reporting period; (13) Results cannot be calculated for this reporting period; (14) The results for this state are combined with nearby states to protect confidentiality; Please refer to the User's Guide for a full explanation of data.

Measure	Cases	This Hosp.	State Avg.	U.S. Avg.
Prophylactic Antibiotic Timing	82	96%	98%	99%
Prophylactic Antibiotic Timing (Outpatient)	29	100%	96%	98%
Urinary Catheter Removal[1]	-	-	95%	97%
Survey of Patients' Hospital Experiences				
Area Around Room 'Always' Quiet at Night	300+	55%	61%	61%
Doctors 'Always' Communicated Well	300+	83%	82%	82%
Home Recovery Information Given	300+	87%	88%	85%
Hospital Given 9 or 10 on 10 Point Scale	300+	66%	68%	71%
Meds 'Always' Explained Before Given	300+	64%	66%	64%
Nurses 'Always' Communicated Well	300+	74%	78%	79%
Pain 'Always' Well Controlled	300+	63%	69%	71%
Room and Bathroom 'Always' Clean	300+	58%	74%	73%
Timely Help 'Always' Received	300+	64%	70%	68%
Would Definitely Recommend Hospital	300+	64%	67%	71%
Use of Medical Imaging				
Cardiac Imaging Stress Test before Surgery[1]	-	-	4.8%	5.3%
Combination Abdominal CT Scan	200	6.5%	13.1%	10.5%
Combination Brain/Sinus CT Scan[1]	-	-	2.1%	2.7%
Combination Chest CT Scan	110	0.0%	3.8%	2.7%
Follow-up Mammogram/Ultrasound	332	2.7%	9.7%	8.8%
Lumbar Spine MRI for Low Back Pain	47	44.7%	46.1%	37.2%

Ivinson Memorial Hospital

255 N 30th Phone: 307-742-2141
Laramie, WY 82072 Fax: 307-742-2150
URL: www.ivinsonhospital.org
Type: Acute Care Hospitals Emergency Services: Yes
Ownership: Govt - Hospital Dist/Auth Beds: 99

Key Personnel:
Emergency Room . . . . Charles Ballard, MD
Chair/CEO . . . . Dona Cofey
Anesthesiology. . . . . Al Jones, MD
CEO/President. . . . . Nelson Toebbe
Chief of Medical Staff. . . . . Thomas Vienz

Measure	Cases	This Hosp.	State Avg.	U.S. Avg.
Blood Clot Prevention and Treatment				
Anticoagulation Overlap Therapy[2]	19	95%	90%	93%
ICU Venous Thromboembolism Prophylaxis[2]	23	96%	90%	92%
Incidence of Potentially Preventable VTE[1,2]	-	-	12%	10%
UFH with Dosages/Platelet Monitoring[2,7]	-	-	97%	97%
Venous Thromboembolism Prophylaxis[2]	96	85%	86%	85%
Warfarin Therapy Discharge Instructions[2]	16	75%	62%	75%
Chest Pain/Possible Heart Attack Care				
Aspirin Given Within 24 Hours of Arrival	43	95%	97%	96%
Fibrinolytic Meds Within 30 Min. of Arrival[1]	-	-	69%	58%
Average Time to ECG (minutes)	41	6	6	7
Average Time to Transfer (minutes)[1]	-	-	163	60
Children's Asthma Care				
Received Home Management Plan of Care	-	-	-	88%
Received Reliever Medication	-	-	-	100%
Received Systemic Corticosteroids	-	-	-	100%
Emergency Department				
Admittance Decision Time (minutes)[2]	174	70	70	98
Head CT Results Within 45 Min. of Arrival[1]	-	-	36%	57%
Patients Who Left ER Before Being Seen	12,510	1%	2%	2%
Time from ER Arrival to Admit. (minutes)[2]	252	227	218	274
Time from ER Arrival to Discharge (minutes)	380	141	116	134
Time in ER Before Being Evaluated (minutes)	317	8	16	26
Time to Pain Meds for Fractures (minutes)	99	59	46	57
Heart Attack Care				
Aspirin Given at Discharge[1]	-	-	99%	99%
Fibrinolytic Meds Within 30 Min. of Arrival[7]	-	-	100%	54%
PCI Within 90 Minutes of Arrival[7]	-	-	99%	96%
Statin Prescribed at Discharge[1]	-	-	97%	98%
Heart Failure Care				
ACE Inhibitor or ARB for LVSD[1]	-	-	95%	97%
Discharge Instructions Given	23	83%	86%	94%
Evaluation of LVS Function	28	96%	94%	99%
Medicare Spending				
Medicare Spending per Patient (ratio)	-	0.87	0.93	0.98
Pneumonia Care				
Appropriate Initial Antibiotic Given	49	94%	94%	95%
Blood Culture Timing	80	100%	97%	98%
Pregnancy and Delivery Care				
Newborn Deliveries Scheduled Early[2]	34	15%	7%	6%
Preventive Care				
Immunization for Influenza[2]	263	81%	86%	90%
Immunization for Pneumonia[2]	247	87%	88%	92%
Stroke Care				
Anticoagulation Therapy for Atrial Fibrillation[1]	-	-	93%	95%
Antithrombotic Therapy Timing[1]	-	-	95%	98%
Assessed for Rehabilitation[1]	-	-	94%	97%
Discharged on Antithrombotic Therapy[1]	-	-	97%	99%
Discharged on Statin Medication[1]	-	-	89%	94%
Thrombolytic Therapy Timing[1]	-	-	42%	66%
Venous Thromboembolism Prophylaxis[1]	-	-	87%	94%
Written Stroke Educational Materials Given[1]	-	-	68%	88%
Surgical Care Improvement Project				
Appropriate Beta Blocker Usage	57	91%	94%	98%
Appropriate VTP Within 24 Hours	123	93%	95%	98%
Controlled Postoperative Blood Glucose[7]	-	-	99%	97%
Perioperative Temperature Management	278	99%	99%	100%
Prophylactic Antibiotic Selection	224	98%	99%	99%
Prophylactic Antibiotic Selection (Outpatient)	114	96%	95%	98%
Prophylactic Antibiotic Stopped	223	98%	97%	98%
Prophylactic Antibiotic Timing	224	97%	98%	99%
Prophylactic Antibiotic Timing (Outpatient)	116	98%	96%	98%
Urinary Catheter Removal	217	97%	95%	97%
Survey of Patients' Hospital Experiences				
Area Around Room 'Always' Quiet at Night	300+	56%	61%	61%
Doctors 'Always' Communicated Well	300+	81%	82%	82%
Home Recovery Information Given	300+	92%	88%	85%
Hospital Given 9 or 10 on 10 Point Scale	300+	69%	68%	71%
Meds 'Always' Explained Before Given	300+	69%	66%	64%
Nurses 'Always' Communicated Well	300+	79%	78%	79%
Pain 'Always' Well Controlled	300+	70%	69%	71%
Room and Bathroom 'Always' Clean	300+	80%	74%	73%
Timely Help 'Always' Received	300+	76%	70%	68%
Would Definitely Recommend Hospital	300+	72%	67%	71%
Use of Medical Imaging				
Cardiac Imaging Stress Test before Surgery	123	4.9%	4.8%	5.3%
Combination Abdominal CT Scan	306	19.0%	13.1%	10.5%
Combination Brain/Sinus CT Scan[1]	-	-	2.1%	2.7%
Combination Chest CT Scan	174	9.8%	3.8%	2.7%
Follow-up Mammogram/Ultrasound	506	12.5%	9.7%	8.8%
Lumbar Spine MRI for Low Back Pain[1]	-	-	46.1%	37.2%

North Big Horn Hospital District

1115 Lane 12 Phone: 307-548-5200
Lovell, WY 82431 Fax: 307-548-5205
URL: www.nbhh.com
Type: Critical Access Hospitals Emergency Services: Yes
Ownership: Govt - Hospital Dist/Auth Beds: 15

Key Personnel:
Cardiology . . . . Lael Beachler, DPM
Infection Control. . . . . Jacqueline Bischoff, RN
Operating Room. . . . . Jaqueline Bischoff, RN
Chief of Medical Staff . . . . David Hoffman, MD
Ambulatory Care . . . . Trish Mangus, RN, DON
Cardiac Laboratory. . . . . Jodi McLure
CEO . . . . Rick Schroeder

Measure	Cases	This Hosp.	State Avg.	U.S. Avg.
Blood Clot Prevention and Treatment				
Anticoagulation Overlap Therapy[5]	-	-	90%	93%
ICU Venous Thromboembolism Prophylaxis[5]	-	-	90%	92%
Incidence of Potentially Preventable VTE[5]	-	-	12%	10%
UFH with Dosages/Platelet Monitoring[5]	-	-	97%	97%
Venous Thromboembolism Prophylaxis[5]	-	-	86%	85%
Warfarin Therapy Discharge Instructions[5]	-	-	62%	75%
Chest Pain/Possible Heart Attack Care				
Aspirin Given Within 24 Hours of Arrival	-	-	97%	96%
Fibrinolytic Meds Within 30 Min. of Arrival	-	-	69%	58%
Average Time to ECG (minutes)	-	-	6	7
Average Time to Transfer (minutes)	-	-	163	60
Children's Asthma Care				
Received Home Management Plan of Care	-	-	-	88%
Received Reliever Medication	-	-	-	100%
Received Systemic Corticosteroids	-	-	-	100%
Emergency Department				
Admittance Decision Time (minutes)[5]	-	-	70	98
Head CT Results Within 45 Min. of Arrival	-	-	36%	57%
Patients Who Left ER Before Being Seen	-	-	2%	2%
Time from ER Arrival to Admit. (minutes)[5]	-	-	218	274
Time from ER Arrival to Discharge (minutes)	-	-	116	134
Time in ER Before Being Evaluated (minutes)	-	-	16	26
Time to Pain Meds for Fractures (minutes)	-	-	46	57
Heart Attack Care				
Aspirin Given at Discharge[1,3]	-	-	99%	99%
Fibrinolytic Meds Within 30 Min. of Arrival[3,7]	-	-	100%	54%
PCI Within 90 Minutes of Arrival[3,7]	-	-	99%	96%
Statin Prescribed at Discharge[1,3]	-	-	97%	98%
Heart Failure Care				
ACE Inhibitor or ARB for LVSD[1]	-	-	95%	97%
Discharge Instructions Given[1]	-	-	86%	94%
Evaluation of LVS Function	13	85%	94%	99%
Medicare Spending				
Medicare Spending per Patient (ratio)	-	-	0.93	0.98
Pneumonia Care				
Appropriate Initial Antibiotic Given	26	85%	94%	95%
Blood Culture Timing[1]	-	-	97%	98%
Pregnancy and Delivery Care				
Newborn Deliveries Scheduled Early[5]	-	-	7%	6%
Preventive Care				
Immunization for Influenza[5]	-	-	86%	90%
Immunization for Pneumonia[5]	-	-	88%	92%
Stroke Care				
Anticoagulation Therapy for Atrial Fibrillation[5]	-	-	93%	95%
Antithrombotic Therapy Timing[5]	-	-	95%	98%
Assessed for Rehabilitation[5]	-	-	94%	97%
Discharged on Antithrombotic Therapy[5]	-	-	97%	99%
Discharged on Statin Medication[5]	-	-	89%	94%
Thrombolytic Therapy Timing[5]	-	-	42%	66%
Venous Thromboembolism Prophylaxis[5]	-	-	87%	94%
Written Stroke Educational Materials Given[5]	-	-	68%	88%
Surgical Care Improvement Project				
Appropriate Beta Blocker Usage[5]	-	-	94%	98%
Appropriate VTP Within 24 Hours[5]	-	-	95%	98%
Controlled Postoperative Blood Glucose[5]	-	-	99%	97%
Perioperative Temperature Management[5]	-	-	99%	100%
Prophylactic Antibiotic Selection[5]	-	-	99%	99%
Prophylactic Antibiotic Selection (Outpatient)	-	-	95%	98%
Prophylactic Antibiotic Stopped[5]	-	-	97%	98%
Prophylactic Antibiotic Timing[5]	-	-	98%	99%
Prophylactic Antibiotic Timing (Outpatient)	-	-	96%	98%
Urinary Catheter Removal[5]	-	-	95%	97%
Survey of Patients' Hospital Experiences				
Area Around Room 'Always' Quiet at Night[10]	<100	69%	61%	61%
Doctors 'Always' Communicated Well[10]	<100	85%	82%	82%
Home Recovery Information Given[10]	<100	94%	88%	85%
Hospital Given 9 or 10 on 10 Point Scale[10]	<100	66%	68%	71%
Meds 'Always' Explained Before Given[10]	<100	61%	66%	64%
Nurses 'Always' Communicated Well[10]	<100	87%	78%	79%
Pain 'Always' Well Controlled[10]	<100	74%	69%	71%
Room and Bathroom 'Always' Clean[10]	<100	90%	74%	73%
Timely Help 'Always' Received[10]	<100	80%	70%	68%
Would Definitely Recommend Hospital[10]	<100	65%	67%	71%
Use of Medical Imaging				
Cardiac Imaging Stress Test before Surgery	-	-	4.8%	5.3%
Combination Abdominal CT Scan	-	-	13.1%	10.5%
Combination Brain/Sinus CT Scan	-	-	2.1%	2.7%
Combination Chest CT Scan	-	-	3.8%	2.7%
Follow-up Mammogram/Ultrasound	-	-	9.7%	8.8%
Lumbar Spine MRI for Low Back Pain	-	-	46.1%	37.2%

NOTE: Hospital profiles are in alphabetical order by state, then city, then hospital within the city; Rankings exclude hospitals with less than 25 cases except for patient surveys which excludes hospitals with less than 100 cases; (a) 100-299 cases; (1) The number of cases/patients is too few to report; (2) Data submitted were based on a sample of cases/patients; (3) Results are based on a shorter time period than required; (4) Data suppressed by CMS for one or more quarters; (5) Results are not available for this reporting period; (6) Fewer than 100 patients completed the HCAHPS survey; (7) No cases met the criteria for this measure; (8) The lower limit of the confidence interval cannot be calculated if the number of observed infections equals zero; (9) No data are available from the state/territory for this reporting period; (10) The scores shown reflect fewer than 50 completed surveys; (11) There were discrepancies in the data collection process; (12) This measure does not apply to this hospital for this reporting period; (13) Results cannot be calculated for this reporting period; (14) The results for this state are combined with nearby states to protect confidentiality; Please refer to the User's Guide for a full explanation of data.

Niobrara Health & Life Center

921 South Ballancee Avenue
Lusk, WY 82225
URL: www.niobrarahospital.com
Type: Critical Access Hospitals
Ownership: Govt - Hospital Dist/Auth

Phone: 307-334-4000
Fax: 307-334-4059
Emergency Services: Yes
Beds: 25

Measure	Cases	This Hosp.	State Avg.	U.S. Avg.
Blood Clot Prevention and Treatment				
Anticoagulation Overlap Therapy[5]	-	-	90%	93%
ICU Venous Thromboembolism Prophylaxis[5]	-	-	90%	92%
Incidence of Potentially Preventable VTE[5]	-	-	12%	10%
UFH with Dosages/Platelet Monitoring[5]	-	-	97%	97%
Venous Thromboembolism Prophylaxis[5]	-	-	86%	85%
Warfarin Therapy Discharge Instructions[5]	-	-	62%	75%
Chest Pain/Possible Heart Attack Care				
Aspirin Given Within 24 Hours of Arrival	-	-	97%	96%
Fibrinolytic Meds Within 30 Min. of Arrival	-	-	69%	58%
Average Time to ECG (minutes)	-	-	6	7
Average Time to Transfer (minutes)	-	-	163	60
Children's Asthma Care				
Received Home Management Plan of Care	-	-	-	88%
Received Reliever Medication	-	-	-	100%
Received Systemic Corticosteroids	-	-	-	100%
Emergency Department				
Admittance Decision Time (minutes)[5]	-	-	70	98
Head CT Results Within 45 Min. of Arrival	-	-	36%	57%
Patients Who Left ER Before Being Seen	-	-	2%	2%
Time from ER Arrival to Admit. (minutes)[5]	-	-	218	274
Time from ER Arrival to Discharge (minutes)	-	-	116	134
Time in ER Before Being Evaluated (minutes)	-	-	16	26
Time to Pain Meds for Fractures (minutes)	-	-	46	57
Heart Attack Care				
Aspirin Given at Discharge[5]	-	-	99%	99%
Fibrinolytic Meds Within 30 Min. of Arrival[5]	-	-	100%	54%
PCI Within 90 Minutes of Arrival[5]	-	-	99%	96%
Statin Prescribed at Discharge[5]	-	-	97%	98%
Heart Failure Care				
ACE Inhibitor or ARB for LVSD[3,7]	-	-	95%	97%
Discharge Instructions Given[1,3]	-	-	86%	94%
Evaluation of LVS Function[1,3]	-	-	94%	99%
Medicare Spending				
Medicare Spending per Patient (ratio)	-	-	0.93	0.98
Pneumonia Care				
Appropriate Initial Antibiotic Given[1,3]	-	-	94%	95%
Blood Culture Timing[1,3]	-	-	97%	98%
Pregnancy and Delivery Care				
Newborn Deliveries Scheduled Early[5]	-	-	7%	6%
Preventive Care				
Immunization for Influenza[5]	-	-	86%	90%
Immunization for Pneumonia[5]	-	-	88%	92%
Stroke Care				
Anticoagulation Therapy for Atrial Fibrillation[5]	-	-	93%	95%
Antithrombotic Therapy Timing[5]	-	-	95%	98%
Assessed for Rehabilitation[5]	-	-	94%	97%
Discharged on Antithrombotic Therapy[5]	-	-	97%	99%
Discharged on Statin Medication[5]	-	-	89%	94%
Thrombolytic Therapy Timing[5]	-	-	42%	66%
Venous Thromboembolism Prophylaxis[5]	-	-	87%	94%
Written Stroke Educational Materials Given[5]	-	-	68%	88%
Surgical Care Improvement Project				
Appropriate Beta Blocker Usage[5]	-	-	94%	98%
Appropriate VTP Within 24 Hours[5]	-	-	95%	98%
Controlled Postoperative Blood Glucose[5]	-	-	99%	97%
Perioperative Temperature Management[5]	-	-	99%	100%
Prophylactic Antibiotic Selection[5]	-	-	99%	99%
Prophylactic Antibiotic Selection (Outpatient)	-	-	95%	98%
Prophylactic Antibiotic Stopped[5]	-	-	97%	98%
Prophylactic Antibiotic Timing[5]	-	-	98%	99%
Prophylactic Antibiotic Timing (Outpatient)	-	-	96%	98%
Urinary Catheter Removal[5]	-	-	95%	97%
Survey of Patients' Hospital Experiences				
Area Around Room 'Always' Quiet at Night[5]	-	-	61%	61%
Doctors 'Always' Communicated Well[5]	-	-	82%	82%
Home Recovery Information Given[5]	-	-	88%	85%
Hospital Given 9 or 10 on 10 Point Scale[5]	-	-	68%	71%
Meds 'Always' Explained Before Given[5]	-	-	66%	64%
Nurses 'Always' Communicated Well[5]	-	-	78%	79%
Pain 'Always' Well Controlled[5]	-	-	69%	71%
Room and Bathroom 'Always' Clean[5]	-	-	74%	73%
Timely Help 'Always' Received[5]	-	-	70%	68%
Would Definitely Recommend Hospital[5]	-	-	67%	71%
Use of Medical Imaging				
Cardiac Imaging Stress Test before Surgery	-	-	4.8%	5.3%
Combination Abdominal CT Scan	-	-	13.1%	10.5%
Combination Brain/Sinus CT Scan	-	-	2.1%	2.7%
Combination Chest CT Scan	-	-	3.8%	2.7%
Follow-up Mammogram/Ultrasound	-	-	9.7%	8.8%
Lumbar Spine MRI for Low Back Pain	-	-	46.1%	37.2%

Weston County Health Services

1124 Washington Boulevard
Newcastle, WY 82701
Type: Critical Access Hospitals
Ownership: Govt - Hospital Dist/Auth

Phone: 307-746-4491
Fax: 307-746-4579
Emergency Services: Yes
Beds: 21

Key Personnel:
Infection Control . . . . Donalda Bennett
CEO/President. . . . . Kay Garcia
Chief of Medical Staff . . . . Piper Orsborn
Quality Assurance . . . . Piper Orsborn

Measure	Cases	This Hosp.	State Avg.	U.S. Avg.
Blood Clot Prevention and Treatment				
Anticoagulation Overlap Therapy[5]	-	-	90%	93%
ICU Venous Thromboembolism Prophylaxis[5]	-	-	90%	92%
Incidence of Potentially Preventable VTE[5]	-	-	12%	10%
UFH with Dosages/Platelet Monitoring[5]	-	-	97%	97%
Venous Thromboembolism Prophylaxis[5]	-	-	86%	85%
Warfarin Therapy Discharge Instructions[5]	-	-	62%	75%
Chest Pain/Possible Heart Attack Care				
Aspirin Given Within 24 Hours of Arrival	-	-	97%	96%
Fibrinolytic Meds Within 30 Min. of Arrival	-	-	69%	58%
Average Time to ECG (minutes)	-	-	6	7
Average Time to Transfer (minutes)	-	-	163	60
Children's Asthma Care				
Received Home Management Plan of Care	-	-	-	88%
Received Reliever Medication	-	-	-	100%
Received Systemic Corticosteroids	-	-	-	100%
Emergency Department				
Admittance Decision Time (minutes)[5]	-	-	70	98
Head CT Results Within 45 Min. of Arrival	-	-	36%	57%
Patients Who Left ER Before Being Seen	-	-	2%	2%
Time from ER Arrival to Admit. (minutes)[5]	-	-	218	274
Time from ER Arrival to Discharge (minutes)	-	-	116	134
Time in ER Before Being Evaluated (minutes)	-	-	16	26
Time to Pain Meds for Fractures (minutes)	-	-	46	57
Heart Attack Care				
Aspirin Given at Discharge[5]	-	-	99%	99%
Fibrinolytic Meds Within 30 Min. of Arrival[5]	-	-	100%	54%
PCI Within 90 Minutes of Arrival[5]	-	-	99%	96%
Statin Prescribed at Discharge[5]	-	-	97%	98%
Heart Failure Care				
ACE Inhibitor or ARB for LVSD[7]	-	-	95%	97%
Discharge Instructions Given[1]	-	-	86%	94%
Evaluation of LVS Function[1]	-	-	94%	99%
Medicare Spending				
Medicare Spending per Patient (ratio)	-	-	0.93	0.98
Pneumonia Care				
Appropriate Initial Antibiotic Given[1,3]	-	-	94%	95%
Blood Culture Timing[1,3]	-	-	97%	98%
Pregnancy and Delivery Care				
Newborn Deliveries Scheduled Early[5]	-	-	7%	6%
Preventive Care				
Immunization for Influenza[5]	-	-	86%	90%
Immunization for Pneumonia[5]	-	-	88%	92%
Stroke Care				
Anticoagulation Therapy for Atrial Fibrillation[5]	-	-	93%	95%
Antithrombotic Therapy Timing[5]	-	-	95%	98%
Assessed for Rehabilitation[5]	-	-	94%	97%
Discharged on Antithrombotic Therapy[5]	-	-	97%	99%
Discharged on Statin Medication[5]	-	-	89%	94%
Thrombolytic Therapy Timing[5]	-	-	42%	66%
Venous Thromboembolism Prophylaxis[5]	-	-	87%	94%
Written Stroke Educational Materials Given[5]	-	-	68%	88%
Surgical Care Improvement Project				
Appropriate Beta Blocker Usage[5]	-	-	94%	98%
Appropriate VTP Within 24 Hours[5]	-	-	95%	98%
Controlled Postoperative Blood Glucose[5]	-	-	99%	97%
Perioperative Temperature Management[5]	-	-	99%	100%
Prophylactic Antibiotic Selection[5]	-	-	99%	99%
Prophylactic Antibiotic Selection (Outpatient)	-	-	95%	98%
Prophylactic Antibiotic Stopped[5]	-	-	97%	98%
Prophylactic Antibiotic Timing[5]	-	-	98%	99%
Prophylactic Antibiotic Timing (Outpatient)	-	-	96%	98%
Urinary Catheter Removal[5]	-	-	95%	97%
Survey of Patients' Hospital Experiences				
Area Around Room 'Always' Quiet at Night[5]	-	-	61%	61%
Doctors 'Always' Communicated Well[5]	-	-	82%	82%
Home Recovery Information Given[5]	-	-	88%	85%
Hospital Given 9 or 10 on 10 Point Scale[5]	-	-	68%	71%
Meds 'Always' Explained Before Given[5]	-	-	66%	64%
Nurses 'Always' Communicated Well[5]	-	-	78%	79%
Pain 'Always' Well Controlled[5]	-	-	69%	71%
Room and Bathroom 'Always' Clean[5]	-	-	74%	73%
Timely Help 'Always' Received[5]	-	-	70%	68%
Would Definitely Recommend Hospital[5]	-	-	67%	71%
Use of Medical Imaging				
Cardiac Imaging Stress Test before Surgery	-	-	4.8%	5.3%
Combination Abdominal CT Scan	-	-	13.1%	10.5%
Combination Brain/Sinus CT Scan	-	-	2.1%	2.7%
Combination Chest CT Scan	-	-	3.8%	2.7%
Follow-up Mammogram/Ultrasound	-	-	9.7%	8.8%
Lumbar Spine MRI for Low Back Pain	-	-	46.1%	37.2%

Powell Valley Hospital

777 Avenue H
Powell, WY 82435
URL: www.pvhc.org
Type: Critical Access Hospitals
Ownership: Voluntary non-profit - Private

Phone: 307-754-2267
Fax: 307-754-3176
Emergency Services: Yes
Beds: 25

Key Personnel:
Operating Room. . . . . Krista Blough, RN
Intensive Care Unit. . . . . Cathy Campbell, RN
Chief of Medical Staff . . . . Robert Chandler, MD
Infection Control. . . . . Carole Genz-Mould, RN
Patient Relations . . . . Faith Jones
CEO . . . . Bill Patten
Quality Assurance . . . . Robin Roling, RN
Radiology. . . . . Jeffrey Zuckerman

Measure	Cases	This Hosp.	State Avg.	U.S. Avg.
Blood Clot Prevention and Treatment				
Anticoagulation Overlap Therapy[5]	-	-	90%	93%
ICU Venous Thromboembolism Prophylaxis[5]	-	-	90%	92%
Incidence of Potentially Preventable VTE[5]	-	-	12%	10%
UFH with Dosages/Platelet Monitoring[5]	-	-	97%	97%
Venous Thromboembolism Prophylaxis[5]	-	-	86%	85%
Warfarin Therapy Discharge Instructions[5]	-	-	62%	75%
Chest Pain/Possible Heart Attack Care				
Aspirin Given Within 24 Hours of Arrival	-	-	97%	96%
Fibrinolytic Meds Within 30 Min. of Arrival	-	-	69%	58%
Average Time to ECG (minutes)	-	-	6	7
Average Time to Transfer (minutes)	-	-	163	60
Children's Asthma Care				
Received Home Management Plan of Care	-	-	-	88%
Received Reliever Medication	-	-	-	100%
Received Systemic Corticosteroids	-	-	-	100%
Emergency Department				
Admittance Decision Time (minutes)[5]	-	-	70	98
Head CT Results Within 45 Min. of Arrival	-	-	36%	57%
Patients Who Left ER Before Being Seen	-	-	2%	2%
Time from ER Arrival to Admit. (minutes)[5]	-	-	218	274

NOTE: Hospital profiles are in alphabetical order by state, then city, then hospital within the city; Rankings exclude hospitals with less than 25 cases except for patient surveys which excludes hospitals with less than 100 cases; (a) 100-299 cases; (1) The number of cases/patients is too few to report; (2) Data submitted were based on a sample of cases/patients; (3) Results are based on a shorter time period than required; (4) Data suppressed by CMS for one or more quarters; (5) Results are not available for this reporting period; (6) Fewer than 100 patients completed the HCAHPS survey; (7) No cases met the criteria for this measure; (8) The lower limit of the confidence interval cannot be calculated if the number of observed infections equals zero; (9) No data are available from the state/territory for this reporting period; (10) The scores shown reflect fewer than 50 completed surveys; (11) There were discrepancies in the data collection process; (12) This measure does not apply to this hospital for this reporting period; (13) Results cannot be calculated for this reporting period; (14) The results for this state are combined with nearby states to protect confidentiality; Please refer to the User's Guide for a full explanation of data.

Measure	Cases	This Hosp.	State Avg.	U.S. Avg.
Time from ER Arrival to Discharge (minutes)	-	-	116	134
Time in ER Before Being Evaluated (minutes)	-	-	16	26
Time to Pain Meds for Fractures (minutes)	-	-	46	57
Heart Attack Care				
Aspirin Given at Discharge[5]	-	-	99%	99%
Fibrinolytic Meds Within 30 Min. of Arrival[5]	-	-	100%	54%
PCI Within 90 Minutes of Arrival[5]	-	-	99%	96%
Statin Prescribed at Discharge[5]	-	-	97%	98%
Heart Failure Care				
ACE Inhibitor or ARB for LVSD[1]	-	-	95%	97%
Discharge Instructions Given	17	59%	86%	94%
Evaluation of LVS Function	20	95%	94%	99%
Medicare Spending				
Medicare Spending per Patient (ratio)	-	-	0.93	0.98
Pneumonia Care				
Appropriate Initial Antibiotic Given[1]	-	-	94%	95%
Blood Culture Timing	11	82%	97%	98%
Pregnancy and Delivery Care				
Newborn Deliveries Scheduled Early[5]	-	-	7%	6%
Preventive Care				
Immunization for Influenza[5]	-	-	86%	90%
Immunization for Pneumonia[5]	-	-	88%	92%
Stroke Care				
Anticoagulation Therapy for Atrial Fibrillation[5]	-	-	93%	95%
Antithrombotic Therapy Timing[5]	-	-	95%	98%
Assessed for Rehabilitation[5]	-	-	94%	97%
Discharged on Antithrombotic Therapy[5]	-	-	97%	99%
Discharged on Statin Medication[5]	-	-	89%	94%
Thrombolytic Therapy Timing[5]	-	-	42%	66%
Venous Thromboembolism Prophylaxis[5]	-	-	87%	94%
Written Stroke Educational Materials Given[5]	-	-	68%	88%
Surgical Care Improvement Project				
Appropriate Beta Blocker Usage	14	100%	94%	98%
Appropriate VTP Within 24 Hours	38	100%	95%	98%
Controlled Postoperative Blood Glucose[3,7]	-	-	99%	97%
Perioperative Temperature Management	46	100%	99%	100%
Prophylactic Antibiotic Selection	34	97%	99%	99%
Prophylactic Antibiotic Selection (Outpatient)	-	-	95%	98%
Prophylactic Antibiotic Stopped	34	100%	97%	98%
Prophylactic Antibiotic Timing	34	91%	98%	99%
Prophylactic Antibiotic Timing (Outpatient)	-	-	96%	98%
Urinary Catheter Removal	30	97%	95%	97%
Survey of Patients' Hospital Experiences				
Area Around Room 'Always' Quiet at Night[3,6,11]	<100	59%	61%	61%
Doctors 'Always' Communicated Well[3,6,11]	<100	76%	82%	82%
Home Recovery Information Given[3,6,11]	<100	79%	88%	85%
Hospital Given 9 or 10 on 10 Point Scale[3,6,11]	<100	58%	68%	71%
Meds 'Always' Explained Before Given[3,6,11]	<100	53%	66%	64%
Nurses 'Always' Communicated Well[3,6,11]	<100	71%	78%	79%
Pain 'Always' Well Controlled[3,6,11]	<100	70%	69%	71%
Room and Bathroom 'Always' Clean[3,6,11]	<100	66%	74%	73%
Timely Help 'Always' Received[3,6,11]	<100	59%	70%	68%
Would Definitely Recommend Hospital[3,6,11]	<100	62%	67%	71%
Use of Medical Imaging				
Cardiac Imaging Stress Test before Surgery	-	-	4.8%	5.3%
Combination Abdominal CT Scan	-	-	13.1%	10.5%
Combination Brain/Sinus CT Scan	-	-	2.1%	2.7%
Combination Chest CT Scan	-	-	3.8%	2.7%
Follow-up Mammogram/Ultrasound	-	-	9.7%	8.8%
Lumbar Spine MRI for Low Back Pain	-	-	46.1%	37.2%

Memorial Hospital of Carbon County

2221 West Elm Street
Rawlins, WY 82301
Phone: 307-324-2221
Type: Critical Access Hospitals
Emergency Services: Yes
Ownership: Government - Local

Measure	Cases	This Hosp.	State Avg.	U.S. Avg.
Blood Clot Prevention and Treatment				
Anticoagulation Overlap Therapy[3,7]	-	-	90%	93%
ICU Venous Thromboembolism Prophylaxis[1,3]	-	-	90%	92%
Incidence of Potentially Preventable VTE[3,7]	-	-	12%	10%
UFH with Dosages/Platelet Monitoring[3,7]	-	-	97%	97%
Venous Thromboembolism Prophylaxis[3]	21	38%	86%	85%
Warfarin Therapy Discharge Instructions[3,7]	-	-	62%	75%
Chest Pain/Possible Heart Attack Care				
Aspirin Given Within 24 Hours of Arrival	25	96%	97%	96%
Fibrinolytic Meds Within 30 Min. of Arrival[3]	11	27%	69%	58%
Average Time to ECG (minutes)	24	12	6	7
Average Time to Transfer (minutes)[1,3]	-	-	163	60
Children's Asthma Care				
Received Home Management Plan of Care	-	-	-	88%
Received Reliever Medication	-	-	-	100%
Received Systemic Corticosteroids	-	-	-	100%
Emergency Department				
Admittance Decision Time (minutes)[5]	-	-	70	98
Head CT Results Within 45 Min. of Arrival[1,3]	-	-	36%	57%
Patients Who Left ER Before Being Seen	7,531	0%	2%	2%
Time from ER Arrival to Admit. (minutes)[5]	-	-	218	274
Time from ER Arrival to Discharge (minutes)[5]	-	-	116	134
Time in ER Before Being Evaluated (minutes)[5]	-	-	16	26
Time to Pain Meds for Fractures (minutes)[5]	-	-	46	57
Heart Attack Care				
Aspirin Given at Discharge[1,3]	-	-	99%	99%
Fibrinolytic Meds Within 30 Min. of Arrival[3,7]	-	-	100%	54%
PCI Within 90 Minutes of Arrival[3,7]	-	-	99%	96%
Statin Prescribed at Discharge[1,3]	-	-	97%	98%
Heart Failure Care				
ACE Inhibitor or ARB for LVSD[1]	-	-	95%	97%
Discharge Instructions Given	14	71%	86%	94%
Evaluation of LVS Function	17	53%	94%	99%
Medicare Spending				
Medicare Spending per Patient (ratio)	-	-	0.93	0.98
Pneumonia Care				
Appropriate Initial Antibiotic Given[1,2]	-	-	94%	95%
Blood Culture Timing[2]	13	85%	97%	98%
Pregnancy and Delivery Care				
Newborn Deliveries Scheduled Early[5]	-	-	7%	6%
Preventive Care				
Immunization for Influenza[2]	39	85%	86%	90%
Immunization for Pneumonia[2,3]	34	91%	88%	92%
Stroke Care				
Anticoagulation Therapy for Atrial Fibrillation[3,7]	-	-	93%	95%
Antithrombotic Therapy Timing[1,3]	-	-	95%	98%
Assessed for Rehabilitation[1,3]	-	-	94%	97%
Discharged on Antithrombotic Therapy[1,3]	-	-	97%	99%
Discharged on Statin Medication[3,7]	-	-	89%	94%
Thrombolytic Therapy Timing[3,7]	-	-	42%	66%
Venous Thromboembolism Prophylaxis[1,3]	-	-	87%	94%
Written Stroke Educational Materials Given[3,7]	-	-	68%	88%
Surgical Care Improvement Project				
Appropriate Beta Blocker Usage[1,3]	-	-	94%	98%
Appropriate VTP Within 24 Hours[3]	11	45%	95%	98%
Controlled Postoperative Blood Glucose[3,7]	-	-	99%	97%
Perioperative Temperature Management[1,3]	-	-	99%	100%
Prophylactic Antibiotic Selection[1,3]	-	-	99%	99%
Prophylactic Antibiotic Selection (Outpatient)[5]	-	-	95%	98%
Prophylactic Antibiotic Stopped[1,3]	-	-	97%	98%
Prophylactic Antibiotic Timing[1,3]	-	-	98%	99%
Prophylactic Antibiotic Timing (Outpatient)[5]	-	-	96%	98%
Urinary Catheter Removal[1,3]	-	-	95%	97%
Survey of Patients' Hospital Experiences				
Area Around Room 'Always' Quiet at Night	(a)	68%	61%	61%
Doctors 'Always' Communicated Well	(a)	80%	82%	82%
Home Recovery Information Given	(a)	76%	88%	85%
Hospital Given 9 or 10 on 10 Point Scale	(a)	50%	68%	71%
Meds 'Always' Explained Before Given	(a)	67%	66%	64%
Nurses 'Always' Communicated Well	(a)	77%	78%	79%
Pain 'Always' Well Controlled	(a)	72%	69%	71%
Room and Bathroom 'Always' Clean	(a)	70%	74%	73%
Timely Help 'Always' Received	(a)	82%	70%	68%
Would Definitely Recommend Hospital	(a)	53%	67%	71%
Use of Medical Imaging				
Cardiac Imaging Stress Test before Surgery[1]	-	-	4.8%	5.3%
Combination Abdominal CT Scan	96	5.2%	13.1%	10.5%
Combination Brain/Sinus CT Scan[1]	-	-	2.1%	2.7%
Combination Chest CT Scan[1]	-	-	3.8%	2.7%
Follow-up Mammogram/Ultrasound	157	3.2%	9.7%	8.8%
Lumbar Spine MRI for Low Back Pain[1]	-	-	46.1%	37.2%

Sagewest Health Care

2100 W Sunset Dr
Riverton, WY 82501
Phone: 307-856-4161
Fax: 307-857-3571
E-mail: rebecca.smith@lpnt.net
URL: www.riverton-hospital.com
Type: Acute Care Hospitals
Emergency Services: Yes
Ownership: Proprietary
Beds: 70

Key Personnel:

Pediatric In-Patient Care . . . . Michael Fisher, MD
Operating Room. . . . . Dennis Lewis, RN
Quality Assurance . . . . Debbie McClure
Infection Control. . . . . Clare Miller
Chief of Medical Staff . . . . John Reckling, MD
CEO/President. . . . . Chris Smolik
Radiology. . . . . James Taylor, MD

Measure	Cases	This Hosp.	State Avg.	U.S. Avg.
Blood Clot Prevention and Treatment				
Anticoagulation Overlap Therapy[1,2]	-	-	90%	93%
ICU Venous Thromboembolism Prophylaxis[2]	33	97%	90%	92%
Incidence of Potentially Preventable VTE[2,7]	-	-	12%	10%
UFH with Dosages/Platelet Monitoring[1,2]	-	-	97%	97%
Venous Thromboembolism Prophylaxis[2]	102	94%	86%	85%
Warfarin Therapy Discharge Instructions[1,2]	-	-	62%	75%
Chest Pain/Possible Heart Attack Care				
Aspirin Given Within 24 Hours of Arrival	42	100%	97%	96%
Fibrinolytic Meds Within 30 Min. of Arrival[1]	-	-	69%	58%
Average Time to ECG (minutes)	44	6	6	7
Average Time to Transfer (minutes)[1]	-	-	163	60
Children's Asthma Care				
Received Home Management Plan of Care	-	-	-	88%
Received Reliever Medication	-	-	-	100%
Received Systemic Corticosteroids	-	-	-	100%
Emergency Department				
Admittance Decision Time (minutes)[2]	332	64	70	98
Head CT Results Within 45 Min. of Arrival[1]	-	-	36%	57%
Patients Who Left ER Before Being Seen	11,928	3%	2%	2%
Time from ER Arrival to Admit. (minutes)[2]	332	202	218	274
Time from ER Arrival to Discharge (minutes)	371	101	116	134
Time in ER Before Being Evaluated (minutes)	430	8	16	26
Time to Pain Meds for Fractures (minutes)	72	34	46	57
Heart Attack Care				
Aspirin Given at Discharge[1]	-	-	99%	99%
Fibrinolytic Meds Within 30 Min. of Arrival[7]	-	-	100%	54%
PCI Within 90 Minutes of Arrival[7]	-	-	99%	96%
Statin Prescribed at Discharge[1]	-	-	97%	98%
Heart Failure Care				
ACE Inhibitor or ARB for LVSD[1]	-	-	95%	97%
Discharge Instructions Given	32	97%	86%	94%
Evaluation of LVS Function	36	100%	94%	99%
Medicare Spending				
Medicare Spending per Patient (ratio)	-	0.95	0.93	0.98
Pneumonia Care				
Appropriate Initial Antibiotic Given	36	94%	94%	95%
Blood Culture Timing	48	98%	97%	98%
Pregnancy and Delivery Care				
Newborn Deliveries Scheduled Early[2]	29	3%	7%	6%
Preventive Care				
Immunization for Influenza[2]	271	96%	86%	90%
Immunization for Pneumonia[2]	250	97%	88%	92%
Stroke Care				
Anticoagulation Therapy for Atrial Fibrillation[3,7]	-	-	93%	95%
Antithrombotic Therapy Timing[1,3]	-	-	95%	98%
Assessed for Rehabilitation[1,3]	-	-	94%	97%
Discharged on Antithrombotic Therapy[1,3]	-	-	97%	99%
Discharged on Statin Medication[1,3]	-	-	89%	94%
Thrombolytic Therapy Timing[3,7]	-	-	42%	66%
Venous Thromboembolism Prophylaxis[1,3]	-	-	87%	94%
Written Stroke Educational Materials Given[1,3]	-	-	68%	88%

NOTE: Hospital profiles are in alphabetical order by state, then city, then hospital within the city; Rankings exclude hospitals with less than 25 cases except for patient surveys which excludes hospitals with less than 100 cases; (a) 100-299 cases; (1) The number of cases/patients is too few to report; (2) Data submitted were based on a sample of cases/patients; (3) Results are based on a shorter time period than required; (4) Data suppressed by CMS for one or more quarters; (5) Results are not available for this reporting period; (6) Fewer than 100 patients completed the HCAHPS survey; (7) No cases met the criteria for this measure; (8) The lower limit of the confidence interval cannot be calculated if the number of observed infections equals zero; (9) No data are available from the state/territory for this reporting period; (10) The scores shown reflect fewer than 50 completed surveys; (11) There were discrepancies in the data collection process; (12) This measure does not apply to this hospital for this reporting period; (13) Results cannot be calculated for this reporting period; (14) The results for this state are combined with nearby states to protect confidentiality; Please refer to the User's Guide for a full explanation of data.

Surgical Care Improvement Project				
Appropriate Beta Blocker Usage	12	92%	94%	98%
Appropriate VTP Within 24 Hours	49	96%	95%	98%
Controlled Postoperative Blood Glucose[7]	-	-	99%	97%
Perioperative Temperature Management	58	100%	99%	100%
Prophylactic Antibiotic Selection	40	100%	99%	99%
Prophylactic Antibiotic Selection (Outpatient)	15	93%	95%	98%
Prophylactic Antibiotic Stopped	39	100%	97%	98%
Prophylactic Antibiotic Timing	40	100%	98%	99%
Prophylactic Antibiotic Timing (Outpatient)	15	87%	96%	98%
Urinary Catheter Removal	21	90%	95%	97%
Survey of Patients' Hospital Experiences				
Area Around Room 'Always' Quiet at Night	(a)	52%	61%	61%
Doctors 'Always' Communicated Well	(a)	75%	82%	82%
Home Recovery Information Given	(a)	85%	88%	85%
Hospital Given 9 or 10 on 10 Point Scale	(a)	49%	68%	71%
Meds 'Always' Explained Before Given	(a)	61%	66%	64%
Nurses 'Always' Communicated Well	(a)	68%	78%	79%
Pain 'Always' Well Controlled	(a)	63%	69%	71%
Room and Bathroom 'Always' Clean	(a)	60%	74%	73%
Timely Help 'Always' Received	(a)	55%	70%	68%
Would Definitely Recommend Hospital	(a)	43%	67%	71%
Use of Medical Imaging				
Cardiac Imaging Stress Test before Surgery	48	2.1%	4.8%	5.3%
Combination Abdominal CT Scan	203	50.7%	13.1%	10.5%
Combination Brain/Sinus CT Scan	136	5.9%	2.1%	2.7%
Combination Chest CT Scan	158	1.3%	3.8%	2.7%
Follow-up Mammogram/Ultrasound	297	3.7%	9.7%	8.8%
Lumbar Spine MRI for Low Back Pain[7]	-	-	46.1%	37.2%

Memorial Hospital Sweetwater County

1200 College Drive
Rock Springs, WY 82901
Phone: 307-362-3711
Fax: 307-362-8391
E-mail: mhschr@minershospital.com
URL: www.minershospital.com
Type: Acute Care Hospitals
Emergency Services: Yes
Ownership: Government - Local
Beds: 99

Key Personnel:

Chief of Medical Staff. . . . . Kirk Brownell, MD
Emergency Room . . . . Tracy Culver
CEO/President. . . . . Kevin Hawk
Operating Room. . . . . John Iliya
Radiology. . . . . Frederick Matti
Infection Control. . . . . Madlyna Rowland
Intensive Care Unit. . . . . Barbara Walker
Quality Assurance . . . . Jackson Waters

Measure	Cases	This Hosp.	State Avg.	U.S. Avg.
Blood Clot Prevention and Treatment				
Anticoagulation Overlap Therapy[2]	23	87%	90%	93%
ICU Venous Thromboembolism Prophylaxis[2]	16	94%	90%	92%
Incidence of Potentially Preventable VTE[1,2]	-	-	12%	10%
UFH with Dosages/Platelet Monitoring[1,2]	-	-	97%	97%
Venous Thromboembolism Prophylaxis[2]	101	83%	86%	85%
Warfarin Therapy Discharge Instructions[2]	15	40%	62%	75%
Chest Pain/Possible Heart Attack Care				
Aspirin Given Within 24 Hours of Arrival	74	97%	97%	96%
Fibrinolytic Meds Within 30 Min. of Arrival[1]	-	-	69%	58%
Average Time to ECG (minutes)	77	10	6	7
Average Time to Transfer (minutes)[1]	-	-	163	60
Children's Asthma Care				
Received Home Management Plan of Care	-	-	-	88%
Received Reliever Medication	-	-	-	100%
Received Systemic Corticosteroids	-	-	-	100%
Emergency Department				
Admittance Decision Time (minutes)[2]	289	105	70	98
Head CT Results Within 45 Min. of Arrival[1]	-	-	36%	57%
Patients Who Left ER Before Being Seen	19,161	2%	2%	2%
Time from ER Arrival to Admit. (minutes)[2]	289	256	218	274
Time from ER Arrival to Discharge (minutes)	350	129	116	134
Time in ER Before Being Evaluated (minutes)	373	37	16	26
Time to Pain Meds for Fractures (minutes)	90	58	46	57
Heart Attack Care				
Aspirin Given at Discharge[1]	-	-	99%	99%
Fibrinolytic Meds Within 30 Min. of Arrival[7]	-	-	100%	54%
PCI Within 90 Minutes of Arrival[7]	-	-	99%	96%
Statin Prescribed at Discharge[1]	-	-	97%	98%
Heart Failure Care				
ACE Inhibitor or ARB for LVSD[1]	-	-	95%	97%
Discharge Instructions Given	29	41%	86%	94%
Evaluation of LVS Function	37	86%	94%	99%
Medicare Spending				
Medicare Spending per Patient (ratio)	-	0.90	0.93	0.98
Pneumonia Care				
Appropriate Initial Antibiotic Given	29	93%	94%	95%
Blood Culture Timing	37	97%	97%	98%
Pregnancy and Delivery Care				
Newborn Deliveries Scheduled Early[2]	28	11%	7%	6%
Preventive Care				
Immunization for Influenza[2]	242	68%	86%	90%
Immunization for Pneumonia[2]	199	75%	88%	92%
Stroke Care				
Anticoagulation Therapy for Atrial Fibrillation[1]	-	-	93%	95%
Antithrombotic Therapy Timing[1]	-	-	95%	98%
Assessed for Rehabilitation[1]	-	-	94%	97%
Discharged on Antithrombotic Therapy[1]	-	-	97%	99%
Discharged on Statin Medication[1]	-	-	89%	94%
Thrombolytic Therapy Timing[7]	-	-	42%	66%
Venous Thromboembolism Prophylaxis[1]	-	-	87%	94%
Written Stroke Educational Materials Given[1]	-	-	68%	88%
Surgical Care Improvement Project				
Appropriate Beta Blocker Usage[1]	-	-	94%	98%
Appropriate VTP Within 24 Hours	61	87%	95%	98%
Controlled Postoperative Blood Glucose[7]	-	-	99%	97%
Perioperative Temperature Management	75	100%	99%	100%
Prophylactic Antibiotic Selection	42	95%	99%	99%
Prophylactic Antibiotic Selection (Outpatient)	14	50%	95%	98%
Prophylactic Antibiotic Stopped	40	90%	97%	98%
Prophylactic Antibiotic Timing	42	93%	98%	99%
Prophylactic Antibiotic Timing (Outpatient)	14	86%	96%	98%
Urinary Catheter Removal	27	85%	95%	97%
Survey of Patients' Hospital Experiences				
Area Around Room 'Always' Quiet at Night	300+	62%	61%	61%
Doctors 'Always' Communicated Well	300+	77%	82%	82%
Home Recovery Information Given	300+	87%	88%	85%
Hospital Given 9 or 10 on 10 Point Scale	300+	60%	68%	71%
Meds 'Always' Explained Before Given	300+	66%	66%	64%
Nurses 'Always' Communicated Well	300+	76%	78%	79%
Pain 'Always' Well Controlled	300+	70%	69%	71%
Room and Bathroom 'Always' Clean	300+	70%	74%	73%
Timely Help 'Always' Received	300+	67%	70%	68%
Would Definitely Recommend Hospital	300+	52%	67%	71%
Use of Medical Imaging				
Cardiac Imaging Stress Test before Surgery	123	4.9%	4.8%	5.3%
Combination Abdominal CT Scan	185	15.7%	13.1%	10.5%
Combination Brain/Sinus CT Scan[1]	-	-	2.1%	2.7%
Combination Chest CT Scan	103	5.8%	3.8%	2.7%
Follow-up Mammogram/Ultrasound	359	16.7%	9.7%	8.8%
Lumbar Spine MRI for Low Back Pain	47	55.3%	46.1%	37.2%

Sheridan Memorial Hospital

1401 W 5th St
Sheridan, WY 82801
Phone: 307-672-1000
Fax: 307-672-1153
E-mail: mhscmk@sheridanhospital.org
URL: www.sheridanhospital.org
Type: Acute Care Hospitals
Emergency Services: Yes
Ownership: Government - Local
Beds: 66

Key Personnel:

Radiology. . . . . Daniel R Alzheimer
Chief of Medical Staff . . . . Lawrence Gill
CEO/President. . . . . Ken Huey
Quality Assurance . . . . Tom Mc Lain
Hemotology Center . . . . John Stamato, MD
Emergency Room . . . . Thomas L Walsh, MD

Measure	Cases	This Hosp.	State Avg.	U.S. Avg.
Blood Clot Prevention and Treatment				
Anticoagulation Overlap Therapy[2]	13	69%	90%	93%
ICU Venous Thromboembolism Prophylaxis[2]	33	94%	90%	92%
Incidence of Potentially Preventable VTE[1,2]	-	-	12%	10%
UFH with Dosages/Platelet Monitoring[1,2]	-	-	97%	97%
Venous Thromboembolism Prophylaxis[2]	112	77%	86%	85%
Warfarin Therapy Discharge Instructions[1,2]	-	-	62%	75%
Chest Pain/Possible Heart Attack Care				
Aspirin Given Within 24 Hours of Arrival	21	90%	97%	96%
Fibrinolytic Meds Within 30 Min. of Arrival[1]	-	-	69%	58%
Average Time to ECG (minutes)	21	3	6	7
Average Time to Transfer (minutes)[7]	-	-	163	60
Children's Asthma Care				
Received Home Management Plan of Care	-	-	-	88%
Received Reliever Medication	-	-	-	100%
Received Systemic Corticosteroids	-	-	-	100%
Emergency Department				
Admittance Decision Time (minutes)[2]	60	56	70	98
Head CT Results Within 45 Min. of Arrival[1]	-	-	36%	57%
Patients Who Left ER Before Being Seen	8,607	0%	2%	2%
Time from ER Arrival to Admit. (minutes)[2]	74	166	218	274
Time from ER Arrival to Discharge (minutes)	259	101	116	134
Time in ER Before Being Evaluated (minutes)	203	26	16	26
Time to Pain Meds for Fractures (minutes)	55	44	46	57
Heart Attack Care				
Aspirin Given at Discharge[2]	21	86%	99%	99%
Fibrinolytic Meds Within 30 Min. of Arrival[1,2]	-	-	100%	54%
PCI Within 90 Minutes of Arrival[1,2]	-	-	99%	96%
Statin Prescribed at Discharge[2]	21	95%	97%	98%
Heart Failure Care				
ACE Inhibitor or ARB for LVSD[2]	13	77%	95%	97%
Discharge Instructions Given[2]	20	60%	86%	94%
Evaluation of LVS Function[2]	28	100%	94%	99%
Medicare Spending				
Medicare Spending per Patient (ratio)	-	0.94	0.93	0.98
Pneumonia Care				
Appropriate Initial Antibiotic Given[2]	47	94%	94%	95%
Blood Culture Timing[2]	47	98%	97%	98%
Pregnancy and Delivery Care				
Newborn Deliveries Scheduled Early[2]	17	0%	7%	6%
Preventive Care				
Immunization for Influenza[2]	259	84%	86%	90%
Immunization for Pneumonia[2]	253	74%	88%	92%
Stroke Care				
Anticoagulation Therapy for Atrial Fibrillation[2,7]	-	-	93%	95%
Antithrombotic Therapy Timing[2]	17	100%	95%	98%
Assessed for Rehabilitation[2]	18	89%	94%	97%
Discharged on Antithrombotic Therapy[2]	14	100%	97%	99%
Discharged on Statin Medication[2]	13	100%	89%	94%
Thrombolytic Therapy Timing[2,7]	-	-	42%	66%
Venous Thromboembolism Prophylaxis[2]	19	84%	87%	94%
Written Stroke Educational Materials Given[2]	13	77%	68%	88%
Surgical Care Improvement Project				
Appropriate Beta Blocker Usage[2]	48	90%	94%	98%
Appropriate VTP Within 24 Hours[2]	205	93%	95%	98%
Controlled Postoperative Blood Glucose[2,7]	-	-	99%	97%
Perioperative Temperature Management[2]	270	99%	99%	100%
Prophylactic Antibiotic Selection[2]	202	99%	99%	99%
Prophylactic Antibiotic Selection (Outpatient)	92	100%	95%	98%
Prophylactic Antibiotic Stopped[2]	199	96%	97%	98%
Prophylactic Antibiotic Timing[2]	203	98%	98%	99%
Prophylactic Antibiotic Timing (Outpatient)	94	94%	96%	98%
Urinary Catheter Removal[2]	159	92%	95%	97%
Survey of Patients' Hospital Experiences				
Area Around Room 'Always' Quiet at Night	300+	59%	61%	61%
Doctors 'Always' Communicated Well	300+	80%	82%	82%
Home Recovery Information Given	300+	88%	88%	85%
Hospital Given 9 or 10 on 10 Point Scale	300+	69%	68%	71%
Meds 'Always' Explained Before Given	300+	60%	66%	64%
Nurses 'Always' Communicated Well	300+	75%	78%	79%
Pain 'Always' Well Controlled	300+	67%	69%	71%
Room and Bathroom 'Always' Clean	300+	73%	74%	73%
Timely Help 'Always' Received	300+	72%	70%	68%
Would Definitely Recommend Hospital	300+	66%	67%	71%
Use of Medical Imaging				
Cardiac Imaging Stress Test before Surgery	170	6.5%	4.8%	5.3%

NOTE: Hospital profiles are in alphabetical order by state, then city, then hospital within the city; Rankings exclude hospitals with less than 25 cases except for patient surveys which excludes hospitals with less than 100 cases; (a) 100-299 cases; (1) The number of cases/patients is too few to report; (2) Data submitted were based on a sample of cases/patients; (3) Results are based on a shorter time period than required; (4) Data suppressed by CMS for one or more quarters; (5) Results are not available for this reporting period; (6) Fewer than 100 patients completed the HCAHPS survey; (7) No cases met the criteria for this measure; (8) The lower limit of the confidence interval cannot be calculated if the number of observed infections equals zero; (9) No data are available from the state/territory for this reporting period; (10) The scores shown reflect fewer than 50 completed surveys; (11) There were discrepancies in the data collection process; (12) This measure does not apply to this hospital for this reporting period; (13) Results cannot be calculated for this reporting period; (14) The results for this state are combined with nearby states to protect confidentiality; Please refer to the User's Guide for a full explanation of data.

Combination Abdominal CT Scan	107	74.8%	13.1%	10.5%
Combination Brain/Sinus CT Scan[1]	-	-	2.1%	2.7%
Combination Chest CT Scan[1]	-	-	3.8%	2.7%
Follow-up Mammogram/Ultrasound	646	8.8%	9.7%	8.8%
Lumbar Spine MRI for Low Back Pain[1]	-	-	46.1%	37.2%

Sheridan VA Medical Center

1898 Fort Road Phone: 307-672-1675
Sheridan, WY 82801 Fax: 307-672-1900
URL: www.sheridan.va.gov
Type: Acute Care - VA Emergency Services: No
Ownership: Government Federal Beds: 199
Key Personnel:
Patient Relations . . . . Travis Jones
Quality Assurance . . . . Deb Nicholas-Olson
Chief of Medical Staff . . . . Wendell Robinson, MD
Operating Room. . . . . Wendell Robinson, MD

Measure	Cases	This Hosp.	State Avg.	U.S. Avg.
Blood Clot Prevention and Treatment				
Anticoagulation Overlap Therapy	-	-	90%	93%
ICU Venous Thromboembolism Prophylaxis	-	-	90%	92%
Incidence of Potentially Preventable VTE	-	-	12%	10%
UFH with Dosages/Platelet Monitoring	-	-	97%	97%
Venous Thromboembolism Prophylaxis	-	-	86%	85%
Warfarin Therapy Discharge Instructions	-	-	62%	75%
Chest Pain/Possible Heart Attack Care				
Aspirin Given Within 24 Hours of Arrival	-	-	97%	96%
Fibrinolytic Meds Within 30 Min. of Arrival	-	-	69%	58%
Average Time to ECG (minutes)	-	-	6	7
Average Time to Transfer (minutes)	-	-	163	60
Children's Asthma Care				
Received Home Management Plan of Care	-	-	-	88%
Received Reliever Medication	-	-	-	100%
Received Systemic Corticosteroids	-	-	-	100%
Emergency Department				
Admittance Decision Time (minutes)	-	-	70	98
Head CT Results Within 45 Min. of Arrival	-	-	36%	57%
Patients Who Left ER Before Being Seen	-	-	2%	2%
Time from ER Arrival to Admit. (minutes)	-	-	218	274
Time from ER Arrival to Discharge (minutes)	-	-	116	134
Time in ER Before Being Evaluated (minutes)	-	-	16	26
Time to Pain Meds for Fractures (minutes)	-	-	46	57
Heart Attack Care				
Aspirin Given at Discharge[5]	-	-	99%	99%
Fibrinolytic Meds Within 30 Min. of Arrival[5]	-	-	100%	54%
PCI Within 90 Minutes of Arrival[5]	-	-	99%	96%
Statin Prescribed at Discharge[5]	-	-	97%	98%
Heart Failure Care				
ACE Inhibitor or ARB for LVSD[5]	-	-	95%	97%
Discharge Instructions Given[5]	-	-	86%	94%
Evaluation of LVS Function[5]	-	-	94%	99%
Medicare Spending				
Medicare Spending per Patient (ratio)	-	-	0.93	0.98
Pneumonia Care				
Appropriate Initial Antibiotic Given[1]	-	-	94%	95%
Blood Culture Timing[1]	-	-	97%	98%
Pregnancy and Delivery Care				
Newborn Deliveries Scheduled Early	-	-	7%	6%
Preventive Care				
Immunization for Influenza[2,3]	139	85%	86%	90%
Immunization for Pneumonia[2,3]	195	93%	88%	92%
Stroke Care				
Anticoagulation Therapy for Atrial Fibrillation	-	-	93%	95%
Antithrombotic Therapy Timing	-	-	95%	98%
Assessed for Rehabilitation	-	-	94%	97%
Discharged on Antithrombotic Therapy	-	-	97%	99%
Discharged on Statin Medication	-	-	89%	94%
Thrombolytic Therapy Timing	-	-	42%	66%
Venous Thromboembolism Prophylaxis	-	-	87%	94%
Written Stroke Educational Materials Given	-	-	68%	88%
Surgical Care Improvement Project				
Appropriate Beta Blocker Usage[5]	-	-	94%	98%
Appropriate VTP Within 24 Hours[5]	-	-	95%	98%
Controlled Postoperative Blood Glucose[5]	-	-	99%	97%
Perioperative Temperature Management[5]	-	-	99%	100%
Prophylactic Antibiotic Selection[5]	-	-	99%	99%
Prophylactic Antibiotic Selection (Outpatient)	-	-	95%	98%
Prophylactic Antibiotic Stopped[5]	-	-	97%	98%
Prophylactic Antibiotic Timing[5]	-	-	98%	99%
Prophylactic Antibiotic Timing (Outpatient)	-	-	96%	98%
Urinary Catheter Removal[5]	-	-	95%	97%
Survey of Patients' Hospital Experiences				
Area Around Room 'Always' Quiet at Night	-	-	61%	61%
Doctors 'Always' Communicated Well	-	-	82%	82%
Home Recovery Information Given	-	-	88%	85%
Hospital Given 9 or 10 on 10 Point Scale	-	-	68%	71%
Meds 'Always' Explained Before Given	-	-	66%	64%
Nurses 'Always' Communicated Well	-	-	78%	79%
Pain 'Always' Well Controlled	-	-	69%	71%
Room and Bathroom 'Always' Clean	-	-	74%	73%
Timely Help 'Always' Received	-	-	70%	68%
Would Definitely Recommend Hospital	-	-	67%	71%
Use of Medical Imaging				
Cardiac Imaging Stress Test before Surgery	-	-	4.8%	5.3%
Combination Abdominal CT Scan	-	-	13.1%	10.5%
Combination Brain/Sinus CT Scan	-	-	2.1%	2.7%
Combination Chest CT Scan	-	-	3.8%	2.7%
Follow-up Mammogram/Ultrasound	-	-	9.7%	8.8%
Lumbar Spine MRI for Low Back Pain	-	-	46.1%	37.2%

Crook County Memorial Hospital

713 Oak Street Phone: 307-283-3501
Sundance, WY 82729
URL: www.crookcountymedical.com
Type: Critical Access Hospitals Emergency Services: Yes
Ownership: Govt - Hospital Dist/Auth Beds: 32
Key Personnel:
CEO/President. . . . . Doris Brown

Measure	Cases	This Hosp.	State Avg.	U.S. Avg.
Blood Clot Prevention and Treatment				
Anticoagulation Overlap Therapy[5]	-	-	90%	93%
ICU Venous Thromboembolism Prophylaxis[5]	-	-	90%	92%
Incidence of Potentially Preventable VTE[5]	-	-	12%	10%
UFH with Dosages/Platelet Monitoring[5]	-	-	97%	97%
Venous Thromboembolism Prophylaxis[5]	-	-	86%	85%
Warfarin Therapy Discharge Instructions[5]	-	-	62%	75%
Chest Pain/Possible Heart Attack Care				
Aspirin Given Within 24 Hours of Arrival	-	-	97%	96%
Fibrinolytic Meds Within 30 Min. of Arrival	-	-	69%	58%
Average Time to ECG (minutes)	-	-	6	7
Average Time to Transfer (minutes)	-	-	163	60
Children's Asthma Care				
Received Home Management Plan of Care	-	-	-	88%
Received Reliever Medication	-	-	-	100%
Received Systemic Corticosteroids	-	-	-	100%
Emergency Department				
Admittance Decision Time (minutes)[5]	-	-	70	98
Head CT Results Within 45 Min. of Arrival	-	-	36%	57%
Patients Who Left ER Before Being Seen	-	-	2%	2%
Time from ER Arrival to Admit. (minutes)[5]	-	-	218	274
Time from ER Arrival to Discharge (minutes)	-	-	116	134
Time in ER Before Being Evaluated (minutes)	-	-	16	26
Time to Pain Meds for Fractures (minutes)	-	-	46	57
Heart Attack Care				
Aspirin Given at Discharge[5]	-	-	99%	99%
Fibrinolytic Meds Within 30 Min. of Arrival[5]	-	-	100%	54%
PCI Within 90 Minutes of Arrival[5]	-	-	99%	96%
Statin Prescribed at Discharge[5]	-	-	97%	98%
Heart Failure Care				
ACE Inhibitor or ARB for LVSD[3,7]	-	-	95%	97%
Discharge Instructions Given[1,3]	-	-	86%	94%
Evaluation of LVS Function[1,3]	-	-	94%	99%
Medicare Spending				
Medicare Spending per Patient (ratio)	-	-	0.93	0.98
Pneumonia Care				
Appropriate Initial Antibiotic Given[7]	-	-	94%	95%
Blood Culture Timing[7]	-	-	97%	98%
Pregnancy and Delivery Care				
Newborn Deliveries Scheduled Early[5]	-	-	7%	6%
Preventive Care				
Immunization for Influenza[5]	-	-	86%	90%
Immunization for Pneumonia[5]	-	-	88%	92%
Stroke Care				
Anticoagulation Therapy for Atrial Fibrillation[5]	-	-	93%	95%
Antithrombotic Therapy Timing[5]	-	-	95%	98%
Assessed for Rehabilitation[5]	-	-	94%	97%
Discharged on Antithrombotic Therapy[5]	-	-	97%	99%
Discharged on Statin Medication[5]	-	-	89%	94%
Thrombolytic Therapy Timing[5]	-	-	42%	66%
Venous Thromboembolism Prophylaxis[5]	-	-	87%	94%
Written Stroke Educational Materials Given[5]	-	-	68%	88%
Surgical Care Improvement Project				
Appropriate Beta Blocker Usage[5]	-	-	94%	98%
Appropriate VTP Within 24 Hours[5]	-	-	95%	98%
Controlled Postoperative Blood Glucose[5]	-	-	99%	97%
Perioperative Temperature Management[5]	-	-	99%	100%
Prophylactic Antibiotic Selection[5]	-	-	99%	99%
Prophylactic Antibiotic Selection (Outpatient)	-	-	95%	98%
Prophylactic Antibiotic Stopped[5]	-	-	97%	98%
Prophylactic Antibiotic Timing[5]	-	-	98%	99%
Prophylactic Antibiotic Timing (Outpatient)	-	-	96%	98%
Urinary Catheter Removal[5]	-	-	95%	97%
Survey of Patients' Hospital Experiences				
Area Around Room 'Always' Quiet at Night[5]	-	-	61%	61%
Doctors 'Always' Communicated Well[5]	-	-	82%	82%
Home Recovery Information Given[5]	-	-	88%	85%
Hospital Given 9 or 10 on 10 Point Scale[5]	-	-	68%	71%
Meds 'Always' Explained Before Given[5]	-	-	66%	64%
Nurses 'Always' Communicated Well[5]	-	-	78%	79%
Pain 'Always' Well Controlled[5]	-	-	69%	71%
Room and Bathroom 'Always' Clean[5]	-	-	74%	73%
Timely Help 'Always' Received[5]	-	-	70%	68%
Would Definitely Recommend Hospital[5]	-	-	67%	71%
Use of Medical Imaging				
Cardiac Imaging Stress Test before Surgery	-	-	4.8%	5.3%
Combination Abdominal CT Scan	-	-	13.1%	10.5%
Combination Brain/Sinus CT Scan	-	-	2.1%	2.7%
Combination Chest CT Scan	-	-	3.8%	2.7%
Follow-up Mammogram/Ultrasound	-	-	9.7%	8.8%
Lumbar Spine MRI for Low Back Pain	-	-	46.1%	37.2%

Hot Springs County Memorial Hospital

150 East Arapahoe Phone: 307-864-3121
Thermopolis, WY 82443 Fax: 307-864-5050
E-mail: tim.knight@hscmh.org
URL: www.hscmh.org
Type: Critical Access Hospitals Emergency Services: Yes
Ownership: Government - Local Beds: 25
Key Personnel:
Ambulatory Care . . . . Robin Griffin
Emergency Room . . . . Robin Griffin
Operating Room. . . . . Robin Griffin
Quality Assurance . . . . Sheila Lutz
Radiology. . . . . Daryl Mathern
Chief of Medical Staff . . . . V W Miller, MD
CEO/President. . . . . Charles P Myers, FACHE
Anesthesiology. . . . . Chris Paris

Measure	Cases	This Hosp.	State Avg.	U.S. Avg.
Blood Clot Prevention and Treatment				
Anticoagulation Overlap Therapy[5]	-	-	90%	93%
ICU Venous Thromboembolism Prophylaxis[5]	-	-	90%	92%
Incidence of Potentially Preventable VTE[5]	-	-	12%	10%
UFH with Dosages/Platelet Monitoring[5]	-	-	97%	97%
Venous Thromboembolism Prophylaxis[5]	-	-	86%	85%
Warfarin Therapy Discharge Instructions[5]	-	-	62%	75%
Chest Pain/Possible Heart Attack Care				
Aspirin Given Within 24 Hours of Arrival[1,3]	-	-	97%	96%
Fibrinolytic Meds Within 30 Min. of Arrival[1,3]	-	-	69%	58%
Average Time to ECG (minutes)[1,3]	-	-	6	7
Average Time to Transfer (minutes)[3,7]	-	-	163	60

NOTE: Hospital profiles are in alphabetical order by state, then city, then hospital within the city; Rankings exclude hospitals with less than 25 cases except for patient surveys which excludes hospitals with less than 100 cases; (a) 100-299 cases; (1) The number of cases/patients is too few to report; (2) Data submitted were based on a sample of cases/patients; (3) Results are based on a shorter time period than required; (4) Data suppressed by CMS for one or more quarters; (5) Results are not available for this reporting period; (6) Fewer than 100 patients completed the HCAHPS survey; (7) No cases met the criteria for this measure; (8) The lower limit of the confidence interval cannot be calculated if the number of observed infections equals zero; (9) No data are available from the state/territory for this reporting period; (10) The scores shown reflect fewer than 50 completed surveys; (11) There were discrepancies in the data collection process; (12) This measure does not apply to this hospital for this reporting period; (13) Results cannot be calculated for this reporting period; (14) The results for this state are combined with nearby states to protect confidentiality; Please refer to the User's Guide for a full explanation of data.

Children's Asthma Care				
Received Home Management Plan of Care	-	-	-	88%
Received Reliever Medication	-	-	-	100%
Received Systemic Corticosteroids	-	-	-	100%
Emergency Department				
Admittance Decision Time (minutes)[5]	-	-	70	98
Head CT Results Within 45 Min. of Arrival[5]	-	-	36%	57%
Patients Who Left ER Before Being Seen[5]	-	-	2%	2%
Time from ER Arrival to Admit. (minutes)[5]	-	-	218	274
Time from ER Arrival to Discharge (minutes)[5]	-	-	116	134
Time in ER Before Being Evaluated (minutes)[5]	-	-	16	26
Time to Pain Meds for Fractures (minutes)[5]	-	-	46	57
Heart Attack Care				
Aspirin Given at Discharge[1,3]	-	-	99%	99%
Fibrinolytic Meds Within 30 Min. of Arrival[3,7]	-	-	100%	54%
PCI Within 90 Minutes of Arrival[3,7]	-	-	99%	96%
Statin Prescribed at Discharge[1,3]	-	-	97%	98%
Heart Failure Care				
ACE Inhibitor or ARB for LVSD[1]	-	-	95%	97%
Discharge Instructions Given	15	87%	86%	94%
Evaluation of LVS Function	21	100%	94%	99%
Medicare Spending				
Medicare Spending per Patient (ratio)	-	-	0.93	0.98
Pneumonia Care				
Appropriate Initial Antibiotic Given	11	100%	94%	95%
Blood Culture Timing	20	95%	97%	98%
Pregnancy and Delivery Care				
Newborn Deliveries Scheduled Early[5]	-	-	7%	6%
Preventive Care				
Immunization for Influenza[5]	-	-	86%	90%
Immunization for Pneumonia[5]	-	-	88%	92%
Stroke Care				
Anticoagulation Therapy for Atrial Fibrillation[5]	-	-	93%	95%
Antithrombotic Therapy Timing[5]	-	-	95%	98%
Assessed for Rehabilitation[5]	-	-	94%	97%
Discharged on Antithrombotic Therapy[5]	-	-	97%	99%
Discharged on Statin Medication[5]	-	-	89%	94%
Thrombolytic Therapy Timing[5]	-	-	42%	66%
Venous Thromboembolism Prophylaxis[5]	-	-	87%	94%
Written Stroke Educational Materials Given[5]	-	-	68%	88%
Surgical Care Improvement Project				
Appropriate Beta Blocker Usage[1,3]	-	-	94%	98%
Appropriate VTP Within 24 Hours[3]	13	100%	95%	98%
Controlled Postoperative Blood Glucose[3,7]	-	-	99%	97%
Perioperative Temperature Management[3]	15	100%	99%	100%
Prophylactic Antibiotic Selection[1,3]	-	-	99%	99%
Prophylactic Antibiotic Selection (Outpatient)[5]	-	-	95%	98%
Prophylactic Antibiotic Stopped[1,3]	-	-	97%	98%
Prophylactic Antibiotic Timing[1,3]	-	-	98%	99%
Prophylactic Antibiotic Timing (Outpatient)[5]	-	-	96%	98%
Urinary Catheter Removal[3]	12	92%	95%	97%
Survey of Patients' Hospital Experiences				
Area Around Room 'Always' Quiet at Night	(a)	43%	61%	61%
Doctors 'Always' Communicated Well	(a)	83%	82%	82%
Home Recovery Information Given	(a)	87%	88%	85%
Hospital Given 9 or 10 on 10 Point Scale	(a)	58%	68%	71%
Meds 'Always' Explained Before Given	(a)	68%	66%	64%
Nurses 'Always' Communicated Well	(a)	75%	78%	79%
Pain 'Always' Well Controlled	(a)	60%	69%	71%
Room and Bathroom 'Always' Clean	(a)	63%	74%	73%
Timely Help 'Always' Received	(a)	62%	70%	68%
Would Definitely Recommend Hospital	(a)	63%	67%	71%
Use of Medical Imaging				
Cardiac Imaging Stress Test before Surgery	53	3.8%	4.8%	5.3%
Combination Abdominal CT Scan	111	11.7%	13.1%	10.5%
Combination Brain/Sinus CT Scan	67	0.0%	2.1%	2.7%
Combination Chest CT Scan	61	0.0%	3.8%	2.7%
Follow-up Mammogram/Ultrasound	174	6.3%	9.7%	8.8%
Lumbar Spine MRI for Low Back Pain[1]	-	-	46.1%	37.2%

Community Hospital

2000 Campbell Drive
Torrington, WY 82240
URL: www.bannerhealth.com
Phone: 307-532-4181
Fax: 307-532-3783
Type: Critical Access Hospitals
Emergency Services: Yes
Ownership: Voluntary non-profit - Private
Beds: 25

Key Personnel:

Chief of Medical Staff. . . . . Richard Cambell
Emergency Room . . . . Tedd Church
Operating Room. . . . . Sharon Hickman
Infection Control . . . . Julia Kimsey
CEO/President. . . . . Brenda Strum

Measure	Cases	This Hosp.	State Avg.	U.S. Avg.
Blood Clot Prevention and Treatment				
Anticoagulation Overlap Therapy[5]	-	-	90%	93%
ICU Venous Thromboembolism Prophylaxis[5]	-	-	90%	92%
Incidence of Potentially Preventable VTE[5]	-	-	12%	10%
UFH with Dosages/Platelet Monitoring[5]	-	-	97%	97%
Venous Thromboembolism Prophylaxis[5]	-	-	86%	85%
Warfarin Therapy Discharge Instructions[5]	-	-	62%	75%
Chest Pain/Possible Heart Attack Care				
Aspirin Given Within 24 Hours of Arrival	29	97%	97%	96%
Fibrinolytic Meds Within 30 Min. of Arrival[1]	-	-	69%	58%
Average Time to ECG (minutes)	29	7	6	7
Average Time to Transfer (minutes)[1]	-	-	163	60
Children's Asthma Care				
Received Home Management Plan of Care	-	-	-	88%
Received Reliever Medication	-	-	-	100%
Received Systemic Corticosteroids	-	-	-	100%
Emergency Department				
Admittance Decision Time (minutes)[5]	-	-	70	98
Head CT Results Within 45 Min. of Arrival[5]	-	-	36%	57%
Patients Who Left ER Before Being Seen	4,202	1%	2%	2%
Time from ER Arrival to Admit. (minutes)[5]	-	-	218	274
Time from ER Arrival to Discharge (minutes)[5]	-	-	116	134
Time in ER Before Being Evaluated (minutes)[5]	-	-	16	26
Time to Pain Meds for Fractures (minutes)[5]	-	-	46	57
Heart Attack Care				
Aspirin Given at Discharge[1,3]	-	-	99%	99%
Fibrinolytic Meds Within 30 Min. of Arrival[3,7]	-	-	100%	54%
PCI Within 90 Minutes of Arrival[3,7]	-	-	99%	96%
Statin Prescribed at Discharge[1,3]	-	-	97%	98%
Heart Failure Care				
ACE Inhibitor or ARB for LVSD[1]	-	-	95%	97%
Discharge Instructions Given[1]	-	-	86%	94%
Evaluation of LVS Function	12	100%	94%	99%
Medicare Spending				
Medicare Spending per Patient (ratio)	-	-	0.93	0.98
Pneumonia Care				
Appropriate Initial Antibiotic Given	17	100%	94%	95%
Blood Culture Timing	12	100%	97%	98%
Pregnancy and Delivery Care				
Newborn Deliveries Scheduled Early[3,7]	-	-	7%	6%
Preventive Care				
Immunization for Influenza[5]	-	-	86%	90%
Immunization for Pneumonia[5]	-	-	88%	92%
Stroke Care				
Anticoagulation Therapy for Atrial Fibrillation[5]	-	-	93%	95%
Antithrombotic Therapy Timing[5]	-	-	95%	98%
Assessed for Rehabilitation[5]	-	-	94%	97%
Discharged on Antithrombotic Therapy[5]	-	-	97%	99%
Discharged on Statin Medication[5]	-	-	89%	94%
Thrombolytic Therapy Timing[5]	-	-	42%	66%
Venous Thromboembolism Prophylaxis[5]	-	-	87%	94%
Written Stroke Educational Materials Given[5]	-	-	68%	88%
Surgical Care Improvement Project				
Appropriate Beta Blocker Usage[3,7]	-	-	94%	98%
Appropriate VTP Within 24 Hours[1,3]	-	-	95%	98%
Controlled Postoperative Blood Glucose[3,7]	-	-	99%	97%
Perioperative Temperature Management[1,3]	-	-	99%	100%
Prophylactic Antibiotic Selection[1,3]	-	-	99%	99%
Prophylactic Antibiotic Selection (Outpatient)[1,3]	-	-	95%	98%
Prophylactic Antibiotic Stopped[1,3]	-	-	97%	98%
Prophylactic Antibiotic Timing[1,3]	-	-	98%	99%
Prophylactic Antibiotic Timing (Outpatient)[1,3]	-	-	96%	98%
Urinary Catheter Removal[1,3]	-	-	95%	97%
Survey of Patients' Hospital Experiences				
Area Around Room 'Always' Quiet at Night[11]	(a)	66%	61%	61%
Doctors 'Always' Communicated Well[11]	(a)	90%	82%	82%
Home Recovery Information Given[11]	(a)	93%	88%	85%
Hospital Given 9 or 10 on 10 Point Scale[11]	(a)	84%	68%	71%
Meds 'Always' Explained Before Given[11]	(a)	78%	66%	64%
Nurses 'Always' Communicated Well[11]	(a)	83%	78%	79%
Pain 'Always' Well Controlled[11]	(a)	76%	69%	71%
Room and Bathroom 'Always' Clean[11]	(a)	87%	74%	73%
Timely Help 'Always' Received[11]	(a)	83%	70%	68%
Would Definitely Recommend Hospital[11]	(a)	71%	67%	71%
Use of Medical Imaging				
Cardiac Imaging Stress Test before Surgery[1]	-	-	4.8%	5.3%
Combination Abdominal CT Scan	138	15.9%	13.1%	10.5%
Combination Brain/Sinus CT Scan[1]	-	-	2.1%	2.7%
Combination Chest CT Scan[1]	-	-	3.8%	2.7%
Follow-up Mammogram/Ultrasound	270	8.5%	9.7%	8.8%
Lumbar Spine MRI for Low Back Pain[1]	-	-	46.1%	37.2%

Platte County Memorial Hospital

201 14th Street
Wheatland, WY 82201
URL: www.bannerhealth.com/plattecounty
Phone: 307-322-3636
Fax: 307-322-3690
Type: Critical Access Hospitals
Emergency Services: Yes
Ownership: Govt - Hospital Dist/Auth
Beds: 25

Key Personnel:

Infection Control. . . . . Peggy Anderson
Radiology. . . . . Randy Blackman
Patient Relations . . . . Connie Britton
CEO/President. . . . . Mark Leonard
Chief of Medical Staff . . . . Bernie Sergent, MD
Emergency Room . . . . Shawn Smith, MD
Quality Assurance . . . . Cindy Woods, RN

Measure	Cases	This Hosp.	State Avg.	U.S. Avg.
Blood Clot Prevention and Treatment				
Anticoagulation Overlap Therapy[5]	-	-	90%	93%
ICU Venous Thromboembolism Prophylaxis[5]	-	-	90%	92%
Incidence of Potentially Preventable VTE[5]	-	-	12%	10%
UFH with Dosages/Platelet Monitoring[5]	-	-	97%	97%
Venous Thromboembolism Prophylaxis[5]	-	-	86%	85%
Warfarin Therapy Discharge Instructions[5]	-	-	62%	75%
Chest Pain/Possible Heart Attack Care				
Aspirin Given Within 24 Hours of Arrival	16	100%	97%	96%
Fibrinolytic Meds Within 30 Min. of Arrival[7]	-	-	69%	58%
Average Time to ECG (minutes)	16	6	6	7
Average Time to Transfer (minutes)[1]	-	-	163	60
Children's Asthma Care				
Received Home Management Plan of Care	-	-	-	88%
Received Reliever Medication	-	-	-	100%
Received Systemic Corticosteroids	-	-	-	100%
Emergency Department				
Admittance Decision Time (minutes)[5]	-	-	70	98
Head CT Results Within 45 Min. of Arrival[5]	-	-	36%	57%
Patients Who Left ER Before Being Seen	3,765	0%	2%	2%
Time from ER Arrival to Admit. (minutes)[5]	-	-	218	274
Time from ER Arrival to Discharge (minutes)[5]	-	-	116	134
Time in ER Before Being Evaluated (minutes)[5]	-	-	16	26
Time to Pain Meds for Fractures (minutes)[5]	-	-	46	57
Heart Attack Care				
Aspirin Given at Discharge[1,3]	-	-	99%	99%
Fibrinolytic Meds Within 30 Min. of Arrival[3,7]	-	-	100%	54%
PCI Within 90 Minutes of Arrival[3,7]	-	-	99%	96%
Statin Prescribed at Discharge[1,3]	-	-	97%	98%
Heart Failure Care				
ACE Inhibitor or ARB for LVSD[1]	-	-	95%	97%
Discharge Instructions Given[1]	-	-	86%	94%
Evaluation of LVS Function[1]	-	-	94%	99%
Medicare Spending				
Medicare Spending per Patient (ratio)	-	-	0.93	0.98
Pneumonia Care				
Appropriate Initial Antibiotic Given	14	100%	94%	95%

NOTE: Hospital profiles are in alphabetical order by state, then city, then hospital within the city; Rankings exclude hospitals with less than 25 cases except for patient surveys which excludes hospitals with less than 100 cases; (a) 100-299 cases; (1) The number of cases/patients is too few to report; (2) Data submitted were based on a sample of cases/patients; (3) Results are based on a shorter time period than required; (4) Data suppressed by CMS for one or more quarters; (5) Results are not available for this reporting period; (6) Fewer than 100 patients completed the HCAHPS survey; (7) No cases met the criteria for this measure; (8) The lower limit of the confidence interval cannot be calculated if the number of observed infections equals zero; (9) No data are available from the state/territory for this reporting period; (10) The scores shown reflect fewer than 50 completed surveys; (11) There were discrepancies in the data collection process; (12) This measure does not apply to this hospital for this reporting period; (13) Results cannot be calculated for this reporting period; (14) The results for this state are combined with nearby states to protect confidentiality; Please refer to the User's Guide for a full explanation of data.

Measure	Cases	This Hosp.	State Avg.	U.S. Avg.
Blood Culture Timing[1]	-	-	97%	98%
Pregnancy and Delivery Care				
Newborn Deliveries Scheduled Early[3,7]	-	-	7%	6%
Preventive Care				
Immunization for Influenza[5]	-	-	86%	90%
Immunization for Pneumonia[5]	-	-	88%	92%
Stroke Care				
Anticoagulation Therapy for Atrial Fibrillation[5]	-	-	93%	95%
Antithrombotic Therapy Timing[5]	-	-	95%	98%
Assessed for Rehabilitation[5]	-	-	94%	97%
Discharged on Antithrombotic Therapy[5]	-	-	97%	99%
Discharged on Statin Medication[5]	-	-	89%	94%
Thrombolytic Therapy Timing[5]	-	-	42%	66%
Venous Thromboembolism Prophylaxis[5]	-	-	87%	94%
Written Stroke Educational Materials Given[5]	-	-	68%	88%
Surgical Care Improvement Project				
Appropriate Beta Blocker Usage[1]	-	-	94%	98%
Appropriate VTP Within 24 Hours[1]	-	-	95%	98%
Controlled Postoperative Blood Glucose[7]	-	-	99%	97%
Perioperative Temperature Management[1]	-	-	99%	100%
Prophylactic Antibiotic Selection[1]	-	-	99%	99%
Prophylactic Antibiotic Selection (Outpatient)[1,3]	-	-	95%	98%
Prophylactic Antibiotic Stopped[1]	-	-	97%	98%
Prophylactic Antibiotic Timing[1]	-	-	98%	99%
Prophylactic Antibiotic Timing (Outpatient)[1,3]	-	-	96%	98%
Urinary Catheter Removal[7]	-	-	95%	97%
Survey of Patients' Hospital Experiences				
Area Around Room 'Always' Quiet at Night[6,11]	<100	73%	61%	61%
Doctors 'Always' Communicated Well[6,11]	<100	89%	82%	82%
Home Recovery Information Given[6,11]	<100	90%	88%	85%
Hospital Given 9 or 10 on 10 Point Scale[6,11]	<100	76%	68%	71%
Meds 'Always' Explained Before Given[6,11]	<100	66%	66%	64%
Nurses 'Always' Communicated Well[6,11]	<100	86%	78%	79%
Pain 'Always' Well Controlled[6,11]	<100	71%	69%	71%
Room and Bathroom 'Always' Clean[6,11]	<100	75%	74%	73%
Timely Help 'Always' Received[6,11]	<100	76%	70%	68%
Would Definitely Recommend Hospital[6,11]	<100	72%	67%	71%
Use of Medical Imaging				
Cardiac Imaging Stress Test before Surgery[1]	-	-	4.8%	5.3%
Combination Abdominal CT Scan	107	13.1%	13.1%	10.5%
Combination Brain/Sinus CT Scan[1]	-	-	2.1%	2.7%
Combination Chest CT Scan[1]	-	-	3.8%	2.7%
Follow-up Mammogram/Ultrasound	239	12.1%	9.7%	8.8%
Lumbar Spine MRI for Low Back Pain[1]	-	-	46.1%	37.2%

Washakie Medical Center

400 South 15th Street
Worland, WY 82401
Phone: 307-347-3221
Fax: 307-347-6995
URL: www.washakiemedicalcenter.com
Type: Critical Access Hospitals
Emergency Services: Yes
Ownership: Voluntary non-profit - Other
Beds: 30

Key Personnel:

Pediatric Ambulatory Care . . . . . . Terri Dankelmar
Infection Control. . . . . Maryjo Hake
Quality Assurance . . . . Dianne Martinson
Radiology. . . . . Thomas McCallum
CEO/President. . . . . Margie Molitor
Intensive Care Unit. . . . . Roy Peahoby
Chief of Medical Staff . . . . James Randolph

Measure	Cases	This Hosp.	State Avg.	U.S. Avg.
Blood Clot Prevention and Treatment				
Anticoagulation Overlap Therapy[5]	-	-	90%	93%
ICU Venous Thromboembolism Prophylaxis[5]	-	-	90%	92%
Incidence of Potentially Preventable VTE[5]	-	-	12%	10%
UFH with Dosages/Platelet Monitoring[5]	-	-	97%	97%
Venous Thromboembolism Prophylaxis[5]	-	-	86%	85%
Warfarin Therapy Discharge Instructions[5]	-	-	62%	75%
Chest Pain/Possible Heart Attack Care				
Aspirin Given Within 24 Hours of Arrival[1]	-	-	97%	96%
Fibrinolytic Meds Within 30 Min. of Arrival[1,3]	-	-	69%	58%
Average Time to ECG (minutes)[1]	-	-	6	7
Average Time to Transfer (minutes)[3,7]	-	-	163	60
Children's Asthma Care				
Received Home Management Plan of Care	-	-	-	88%
Received Reliever Medication	-	-	-	100%
Received Systemic Corticosteroids	-	-	-	100%
Emergency Department				
Admittance Decision Time (minutes)[5]	-	-	70	98
Head CT Results Within 45 Min. of Arrival[5]	-	-	36%	57%
Patients Who Left ER Before Being Seen	4,866	0%	2%	2%
Time from ER Arrival to Admit. (minutes)[5]	-	-	218	274
Time from ER Arrival to Discharge (minutes)[5]	-	-	116	134
Time in ER Before Being Evaluated (minutes)[5]	-	-	16	26
Time to Pain Meds for Fractures (minutes)[5]	-	-	46	57
Heart Attack Care				
Aspirin Given at Discharge[3,7]	-	-	99%	99%
Fibrinolytic Meds Within 30 Min. of Arrival[3,7]	-	-	100%	54%
PCI Within 90 Minutes of Arrival[3,7]	-	-	99%	96%
Statin Prescribed at Discharge[3,7]	-	-	97%	98%
Heart Failure Care				
ACE Inhibitor or ARB for LVSD[1]	-	-	95%	97%
Discharge Instructions Given	16	88%	86%	94%
Evaluation of LVS Function	17	100%	94%	99%
Medicare Spending				
Medicare Spending per Patient (ratio)	-	-	0.93	0.98
Pneumonia Care				
Appropriate Initial Antibiotic Given	20	100%	94%	95%
Blood Culture Timing	30	97%	97%	98%
Pregnancy and Delivery Care				
Newborn Deliveries Scheduled Early[3,7]	-	-	7%	6%
Preventive Care				
Immunization for Influenza[5]	-	-	86%	90%
Immunization for Pneumonia[5]	-	-	88%	92%
Stroke Care				
Anticoagulation Therapy for Atrial Fibrillation[5]	-	-	93%	95%
Antithrombotic Therapy Timing[5]	-	-	95%	98%
Assessed for Rehabilitation[5]	-	-	94%	97%
Discharged on Antithrombotic Therapy[5]	-	-	97%	99%
Discharged on Statin Medication[5]	-	-	89%	94%
Thrombolytic Therapy Timing[5]	-	-	42%	66%
Venous Thromboembolism Prophylaxis[5]	-	-	87%	94%
Written Stroke Educational Materials Given[5]	-	-	68%	88%
Surgical Care Improvement Project				
Appropriate Beta Blocker Usage[1]	-	-	94%	98%
Appropriate VTP Within 24 Hours	40	100%	95%	98%
Controlled Postoperative Blood Glucose[7]	-	-	99%	97%
Perioperative Temperature Management	42	100%	99%	100%
Prophylactic Antibiotic Selection	28	100%	99%	99%
Prophylactic Antibiotic Selection (Outpatient)[1,3]	-	-	95%	98%
Prophylactic Antibiotic Stopped	28	100%	97%	98%
Prophylactic Antibiotic Timing	28	100%	98%	99%
Prophylactic Antibiotic Timing (Outpatient)[3,7]	-	-	96%	98%
Urinary Catheter Removal	15	100%	95%	97%
Survey of Patients' Hospital Experiences				
Area Around Room 'Always' Quiet at Night[11]	(a)	71%	61%	61%
Doctors 'Always' Communicated Well[11]	(a)	83%	82%	82%
Home Recovery Information Given[11]	(a)	94%	88%	85%
Hospital Given 9 or 10 on 10 Point Scale[11]	(a)	78%	68%	71%
Meds 'Always' Explained Before Given[11]	(a)	82%	66%	64%
Nurses 'Always' Communicated Well[11]	(a)	85%	78%	79%
Pain 'Always' Well Controlled[11]	(a)	76%	69%	71%
Room and Bathroom 'Always' Clean[11]	(a)	84%	74%	73%
Timely Help 'Always' Received[11]	(a)	75%	70%	68%
Would Definitely Recommend Hospital[11]	(a)	76%	67%	71%
Use of Medical Imaging				
Cardiac Imaging Stress Test before Surgery[7]	-	-	4.8%	5.3%
Combination Abdominal CT Scan	162	12.3%	13.1%	10.5%
Combination Brain/Sinus CT Scan[1]	-	-	2.1%	2.7%
Combination Chest CT Scan	66	1.5%	3.8%	2.7%
Follow-up Mammogram/Ultrasound	161	3.7%	9.7%	8.8%
Lumbar Spine MRI for Low Back Pain[1]	-	-	46.1%	37.2%

NOTE: Hospital profiles are in alphabetical order by state, then city, then hospital within the city; Rankings exclude hospitals with less than 25 cases except for patient surveys which excludes hospitals with less than 100 cases; (a) 100-299 cases; (1) The number of cases/patients is too few to report; (2) Data submitted were based on a sample of cases/patients; (3) Results are based on a shorter time period than required; (4) Data suppressed by CMS for one or more quarters; (5) Results are not available for this reporting period; (6) Fewer than 100 patients completed the HCAHPS survey; (7) No cases met the criteria for this measure; (8) The lower limit of the confidence interval cannot be calculated if the number of observed infections equals zero; (9) No data are available from the state/territory for this reporting period; (10) The scores shown reflect fewer than 50 completed surveys; (11) There were discrepancies in the data collection process; (12) This measure does not apply to this hospital for this reporting period; (13) Results cannot be calculated for this reporting period; (14) The results for this state are combined with nearby states to protect confidentiality; Please refer to the User's Guide for a full explanation of data.

Appendix A: 30-Day Death (Mortality) Rates

What Do These Mortality Categories Show?

These categories show how hospitals' risk-adjusted 30-day death (mortality) rates for heart attack, heart failure, and pneumonia compare to the rate across the U.S., after making adjustments for how sick patients were before they were admitted to the hospital and taking into account differences in death rates that might be due to chance.

This first part of this appendix shows hospitals with 30-day risk-adjusted death (mortality) rates that are lower (better) or higher (worse) than the national rate for all three categories. Hospitals are shown to be better or worse than the U.S. national rate only if the data shows with 95% certainty, that the difference between their surgical complication rates and the U.S. national rate is not due to chance.

The second part of this appendix contains state and national summaries with the following column headers:

- **Better Than U.S. National Rate.** Hospitals in the Better Than U.S. National Rate category have risk-adjusted 30-day death (mortality) rates that are lower than the U.S. National Rate, with 95% certainty that this difference is not due to chance.
- **Worse Than U.S. National Rate.** Hospitals in the Worse Than U.S. National Rate category have risk-adjusted 30-day death (mortality) rates that are higher than the U.S. National Rate, with 95% certainty that this difference is not due to chance.
- **No Different Than U.S. National Rate.** Many hospitals in the No Different Than U.S. National Rate category have risk-adjusted 30-day death (mortality) rates that are about the same as the U.S. National Rate. Other hospitals in this category have rates that are higher or lower than the U.S. National Rate, without 95% certainty that these differences are not due to chance.
- **Number of Cases Too Small.** The number of cases is too small to classify the hospital.

Why are Death Rates for Individual Hospitals Not Shown?

Comparisons based on estimated death (mortality) rates alone can be misleading. Risk-adjusted death (mortality) rates are estimated for individual hospitals based on information taken from a particular time period. If a slightly different time period had been chosen, chances are that each hospital's results would have been somewhat different.

A range ("confidence interval" or in this case an "interval estimate") around estimates show how much variation might be due to this kind of chance. In this case, researchers are 95% confident that a hospital's death (mortality) rate fell somewhere within this specified range. The smaller the range, the more precise the estimate.

When hospitals treat a very large number of patients, chance differences will not have much effect on the overall rates. The range will be small, and the estimated death (mortality) rates will be more precise. In hospitals that treat smaller numbers of patients, however, even small chance differences could have a big impact on death (mortality) rates. The 95% confidence interval, or range, will be large, and the estimated death (mortality) rates will be less precise.

Because the number of patients treated at U.S. hospitals varies widely, the precision of hospitals' estimated death (mortality) rates also varies.

Calculation of 30-Day Risk-Standardized Mortality Rates

The 30-day death (mortality) measures are estimates of deaths from any cause within 30 days of a hospital admission, for patients hospitalized with one of several primary diagnoses. Deaths can be counted in the measures regardless of whether the patient dies while still in the hospital or after discharge. Using deaths within 30 days instead of inpatient deaths show a more consistent measurement time window because length of hospital stay varies across patients and hospitals. Also, mortality over longer time periods (such as 90 days) may have less to do with the care received in the hospital and more to do with other complicating illnesses, patients' own behavior, or care provided to patients after hospital discharge. *The Comparative Guide to American Hospitals* reports on the following 30-day mortality measures:

- 30-day death rate for heart attack (acute myocardial infarction [AMI]) patients
- 30-day death rate for heart failure (HF) patients
- 30-day death rate for pneumonia patients

Which Patients are Included

The 30-day death (mortality) measures include hospitalizations for Medicare beneficiaries aged 65 or older who were enrolled in Original Medicare (traditional fee-for-service Medicare) for the entire 12 months prior to their hospital admission. The AMI, heart failure, and pneumonia (death) mortality measures also include patients aged 65 or older who were admitted to Veteran's Health Administration (VA) hospitals. Beneficiaries enrolled in Medicare managed care plans are not included.

Where the Information Comes From

The Centers for Medicare & Medicaid Services (CMS) calculates hospital-specific 30-day mortality rates using Medicare claims and eligibility information. The AMI, HF, and pneumonia mortality measures are also calculated using VA administrative data. Using administrative data makes it possible to calculate mortality rates without having to do medical chart reviews or requiring hospitals to report additional information to CMS. Research conducted during development of the AMI, HF, and pneumonia death (mortality) measures showed that statistical models based on claims data performed well in estimating hospital mortality rates compared to models that are based on information from medical chart reviews.

Risk Adjustment

To make comparison of hospital performance equitable, the 30-day (death) mortality measures adjust for patient characteristics that may make death more likely, even if the hospital provided higher quality of care. These characteristics include the patient's age, past medical history, and other diseases or conditions (comorbidities) the patient had when admitted that are known to increase the patient's risk of dying.

Significance Testing

The statistical model used to calculate 30-day (death) mortality measures also determines how precise the estimates are, and provides the upper and lower bounds of the 95% interval estimates for each hospital's risk-adjusted mortality rates. Interval estimates, which are like confidence intervals, describe the level of uncertainty around the estimated mortality rates.

Comparing Individual Hospital Rates to the U.S. National Rate

To assign hospitals to performance categories, the hospital's interval estimate is compared to the U.S. national 30-day observed (death) mortality rate. If the 95% interval estimate includes the national observed rate for that measure, the hospital's performance is in the "No Different than U.S. National Rate" category. If the entire 95% interval estimate is below the national observed rate for that measure, then the hospital is performing "Better Than U.S. National Rate." If the entire 95% interval estimate is above the national observed rate for that measure, its performance is "WorseTthan U.S. National Rate." Hospitals with fewer than 25 eligible cases are placed into a separate category that indicates that the hospital did not have enough cases to reliably tell how well the hospital is performing.

Additional Information

For more detail on how the 30-day (death) mortality rates are calculated, visit QualityNet—Mortality Measures at www.qualitynet.org.

Hospitals whose Acute Myocardial Infarction (Heart Attack) 30-Day Mortality Rate is Better (Lower) than the U.S. National Rate

Hospital	City	State	Phone	Web Site
Advocate Lutheran General Hospital	Park Ridge	Illinois	847-723-2210	www.advocatehealth.com
Alexian Brothers Medical Center	Elk Grove Village	Illinois	847-437-5500	www.alexian.org
Arkansas Heart Hospital	Little Rock	Arkansas	501-219-7000	www.arheart.com
The Aroostook Medical Center	Presque Isle	Maine	207-768-4000	www.tamc.org
Avera Heart Hospital of South Dakota	Sioux Falls	South Dakota	605-977-7000	www.avera.org/heart-hospital
Baptist Memorial Hospital	Memphis	Tennessee	901-226-5000	www.bmhcc.org
Baptist Saint Anthony's Hospital	Amarillo	Texas	806-212-2000	www.bsahs.com
Beebe Medical Center	Lewes	Delaware	302-645-3300	www.beebemed.org
Beth Israel Deaconess Medical Center	Boston	Massachusetts	617-667-7000	www.bidmc.harvard.edu
Boca Raton Regional Hospital	Boca Raton	Florida	561-362-5002	www.brrh.com
Boone Hospital Center	Columbia	Missouri	573-815-8000	www.boone.org
Catholic Medical Center	Manchester	New Hampshire	603-668-3545	www.catholicmedicalcenter.org
Cedars - Sinai Medical Center	Los Angeles	California	310-423-5000	www.cedars-sinai.edu
Centegra Health System - Woodstock Hospital	Woodstock	Illinois	815-788-5823	www.centegra.org
Centinela Hospital Medical Center	Inglewood	California	310-673-4660	www.centinelafreeman.com
Chambersburg Hospital	Chambersburg	Pennsylvania	717-267-3000	www.summithealth.org
Champlain Valley Physicians Hospital Medical Center	Plattsburgh	New York	518-561-2000	www.cvph.org
Cypress Fairbanks Medical Center	Houston	Texas	281-897-3100	www.cyfairhospital.com
Doylestown Hospital	Doylestown	Pennsylvania	215-345-2200	www.dh.org
East Orange General Hospital	East Orange	New Jersey	973-266-4401	www.evh.org
Englewood Hospital & Medical Center	Englewood	New Jersey	201-894-3000	www.englewoodhospital.com
Evangelical Community Hospital	Lewisburg	Pennsylvania	570-522-2200	www.evanhospital.com
Firsthealth Moore Regional Hospital	Pinehurst	North Carolina	910-715-1000	www.firsthealth.org
French Hospital Medical Center	San Luis Obispo	California	805-543-5353	www.frenchmedicalcenter.org
Glendale Adventist Medical Center	Glendale	California	818-409-8202	www.glendaleadventist.com
Good Samaritan Hospital	Dayton	Ohio	937-278-2612	www.goodsamdayton.org
Hackensack University Medical Center	Hackensack	New Jersey	201-996-2000	www.humed.com
Hays Medical Center	Hays	Kansas	785-623-5000	www.haysmed.com
Henry Ford Hospital	Detroit	Michigan	313-916-2600	www.henryfordhospital.com
Holy Cross Hospital	Silver Spring	Maryland	301-754-7000	www.holycrosshealth.org
Holy Name Medical Center	Teaneck	New Jersey	201-833-3000	www.holyname.org
John T Mather Memorial Hospital of Port Jefferson	Port Jefferson	New York	631-473-1320	www.matherhospital.com
Lawrence Hospital Center	Bronxville	New York	914-787-1000	www.lawrencehealth.org
Lehigh Valley Hospital	Allentown	Pennsylvania	610-402-2273	www.lvhhn.org
Lehigh Valley Hospital - Hazleton	Hazleton	Pennsylvania	570-501-4000	www.ghha.org
Loyola Gottlieb Memorial Hospital	Melrose Park	Illinois	708-450-4924	www.gottliebhospital.org
Maimonides Medical Center	Brooklyn	New York	718-283-6000	www.maimonidesmed.org
Massachusetts General Hospital	Boston	Massachusetts	617-726-2000	www.massgeneral.org
Minneapolis VA Medical Center	Minneapolis	Minnesota	612-725-2000	www1.va.gov/minneapolis
Miriam Hospital	Providence	Rhode Island	401-793-2500	www.lifespan.org/partners/tmh
Missouri Baptist Medical Center	Town & Country	Missouri	314-996-5000	www.missouribaptistmedicalcenter.org
Montefiore Medical Center	Bronx	New York	718-920-4321	www.montefiore.org
Morristown Medical Center	Morristown	New Jersey	973-971-5450	www.morristownmemorialhospital.org
Mount Sinai Medical Center	Miami Beach	Florida	305-674-2121	www.msmc.com
Munson Medical Center	Traverse City	Michigan	231-935-5000	www.munsonhealthcare.org
New York - Presbyterian Hospital	New York	New York	212-746-4189	www.nyp.org
North Shore University Hospital	Manhasset	New York	516-562-0100	www.northshorelij.com
Northwestern Memorial Hospital	Chicago	Illinois	312-926-2000	www.nmh.org
NYU Hospitals Center	New York	New York	212-263-7300	www.med.nyu.edu
Oakwood Hospital - Dearborn	Dearborn	Michigan	313-593-7125	www.oakwood.org
Olympia Medical Center	Los Angeles	California	310-657-5900	www.olympiamc.com
Overlook Medical Center	Summit	New Jersey	908-522-2000	www.atlantichealth.org
Palisades Medical Center	North Bergen	New Jersey	201-854-5000	www.palisadesmedical.org
Presence Saint Joseph Hospital - Chicago	Chicago	Illinois	773-665-3000	www.res-health.org
Presence Saint Joseph Medical Center	Joliet	Illinois	815-725-7133	www.provena.org/stjoes
Providence Hospital & Medical Centers	Southfield	Michigan	248-849-3011	www.stjohn.org/providence
Rhode Island Hospital	Providence	Rhode Island	401-444-4000	www.rhodeislandhospital.org
Sarasota Memorial Hospital	Sarasota	Florida	941-917-9000	www.smh.com
Sherman Oaks Hospital	Sherman Oaks	California	818-981-7111	www.shermanoakshospital.com
Southcoast Hospital Group	Fall River	Massachusetts	508-679-3131	www.southcoast.org/charlton
Southside Hospital	Bay Shore	New York	631-968-3000	www.northshorelij.com
Saint Francis Hospital - Roslyn	Roslyn	New York	516-562-6000	www.stfrancisheartcenter.com
Saint Joseph Mercy Hospital	Ann Arbor	Michigan	734-712-3791	www.stjoesannarbor.or
Saint Luke's Hospital Bethlehem	Bethlehem	Pennsylvania	610-954-4000	www.slhn-lehighvalley.org
Saint Luke's Hospital	Chesterfield	Missouri	314-434-1500	www.goodhealthmatters.com

Hospital	City	State	Phone	Web Site
Saint Luke's Hospital of Kansas City	Kansas City	Missouri	816-932-2000	www.staintlukeshealthsystem.org
Saint Mary's Medical Center	Huntington	West Virginia	304-526-1234	www.st-marys.org
Saint Vincent Heart Center of Indiana	Indianapolis	Indiana	317-583-5000	www.theheartcenter.com
Trinity Rock Island	Rock Island	Illinois	309-779-5000	www.trinityqc.com
University of California Davis Medical Center	Sacramento	California	916-734-2011	www.ucdmc.ucdavis.edu
Valley Hospital	Ridgewood	New Jersey	201-447-8000	www.valleyhealth.com
Wakemed - Cary Hospital	Cary	North Carolina	919-350-2550	www.wakemed.org
Waterbury Hospital	Waterbury	Connecticut	203-573-6000	www.waterburyhospital.org
William Beaumont Hospital - Troy	Troy	Michigan	248-964-8800	www.beaumonthospitals.com
Winchester Hospital	Winchester	Massachusetts	781-729-9000	www.winchesterhospital.org
Yale-New Haven Hospital	New Haven	Connecticut	203-688-4242	www.ynhh.org
Yuma Regional Medical Center	Yuma	Arizona	928-336-7275	www.yumaregional.org

Note: Table shows hospitals nationwide whose acute myocardial infarction 30-day risk-adjusted mortality rate is better (lower) than U.S. rate of 15.2%

Hospitals whose Acute Myocardial Infarction (Heart Attack) 30-Day Mortality Rate is Worse (Higher) than the U.S. National Rate

Hospital	City	State	Phone	Web Site
Altru Hospital	Grand Forks	North Dakota	701-780-5000	www.altru.org
Baptist Health Corbin	Corbin	Kentucky	606-528-1212	www.baptistregional.com
Bronson Battle Creek Hospital	Battle Creek	Michigan	269-966-8000	www.bchealth.com
Dallas Regional Medical Center	Mesquite	Texas	214-320-7000	www.dallasregionalmedicalcenter.com
Desert Springs Hospital	Las Vegas	Nevada	702-369-7600	www.desertspringshospital.net/p12.html
Hurley Medical Center	Flint	Michigan	810-257-9000	www.hurleymc.com
Kaweah Delta Medical Center	Visalia	California	559-624-2000	www.kaweahdelta.org
Lafayette General Medical Center	Lafayette	Louisiana	337-289-7991	www.lafayettegeneral.org
Lakes Region General Hospital	Laconia	New Hampshire	603-524-3211	www.lrgh.org
Laredo Medical Center	Laredo	Texas	956-796-5000	www.laredomedical.com
Mclaren Bay Region	Bay City	Michigan	989-894-3000	www.baymed.org
National Park Medical Center	Hot Springs	Arkansas	501-321-1000	www.nationalparkmedical.com
North Hills Hospital	North Richland Hills	Texas	817-255-1000	www.northhillshospital.com
Penobscot Valley Hospital	Lincoln	Maine	207-794-3321	www.pvhhealthcare.org
Robert Wood Johnson University Hospital at Rahway	Rahway	New Jersey	732-381-4200	www.rwjuhr.com/about/history.html
Schuylkill Medical Center - East Norwegian Street	Pottsville	Pennsylvania	570-621-4000	www.schuylkillhealth.com
Saint Marys Regional Medical Center	Russellville	Arkansas	479-968-2841	www.saintmarysregional.com
University Hospital SUNY Health Science Center	Syracuse	New York	315-473-4240	www.upstate.edu
Winter Haven Hospital	Winter Haven	Florida	863-293-1121	www.winterhavenhospital.com

Note: Table shows hospitals nationwide whose acute myocardial infarction 30-day risk-adjusted mortality rate is worse (higher) than U.S. rate of 15.2%

Hospitals whose Heart Failure 30-Day Mortality Rate is Better (Lower) than the U.S. National Rate

Hospital	City	State	Phone	Web Site
Abbott Northwestern Hospital	Minneapolis	Minnesota	612-863-4509	www.abbottnorthwestern.com
Advocate Trinity Hospital	Chicago	Illinois	773-967-2000	www.advocatehealth.com/trin
Alexian Brothers Medical Center	Elk Grove Village	Illinois	847-437-5500	www.alexian.org
Atlanticare Regional Medical Center	Atlantic City	New Jersey	609-441-8020	www.atlanticare.org/acmc/index.html
Aurora Saint Lukes Medical Center	Milwaukee	Wisconsin	414-649-6000	www.aurorahealthcare.org
Banner Thunderbird Medical Center	Glendale	Arizona	602-588-5555	www.bannerhealth.com
Baptist Medical Center	San Antonio	Texas	210-297-1020	www.baptisthealthsystem.org
Bay Medical Center Sacred Heart Health System	Panama City	Florida	850-769-1511	www.baymedical.org
Bayhealth - Kent General Hospital	Dover	Delaware	302-744-7001	www.bayhealth.org/about/kent.asp
Beaumont Health System	Royal Oak	Michigan	248-898-5000	www.beaumonthospitals.com
Beth Israel Deaconess Medical Center	Boston	Massachusetts	617-667-7000	www.bidmc.harvard.edu
Beverly Hospital	Montebello	California	323-726-1222	www.beverly.org
Birmingham VA Medical Center	Birmingham	Alabama	205-933-4515	www.birmingham.va.gov
Boston Medical Center Corporation	Boston	Massachusetts	617-638-8000	www.bmc.org
Brigham & Women's Hospital	Boston	Massachusetts	617-732-5500	www.brighamandwomens.org
California Hospital Medical Center Los Angeles	Los Angeles	California	213-748-2411	www.chmcla.org
Cedars - Sinai Medical Center	Los Angeles	California	310-423-5000	www.cedars-sinai.edu
Centinela Hospital Medical Center	Inglewood	California	310-673-4660	www.centinelafreeman.com
Centrastate Medical Center	Freehold	New Jersey	732-431-2000	www.centrastate.com
Champlain Valley Physicians Hospital Medical Center	Plattsburgh	New York	518-561-2000	www.cvph.org
Charleston Area Medical Center	Charleston	West Virginia	304-388-6203	www.camc.org
Clara Maass Medical Center	Belleville	New Jersey	973-450-2002	www.sbhcs.com/hospitals
Cleveland - Wade Park VA Medical Center	Cleveland	Ohio	216-791-3800	www.cleveland.va.gov
Community Hospital	Munster	Indiana	219-836-1600	www.comhs.org/community
Conemaugh Valley Memorial Hospital	Johnstown	Pennsylvania	814-534-9000	www.conemaugh.org
Desert Valley Hospital	Victorville	California	760-241-8000	www.dvmc.com
East Orange General Hospital	East Orange	New Jersey	973-266-4401	www.evh.org
Edward Hospital	Naperville	Illinois	630-527-3000	www.edward.org
Emory University Hospital Midtown	Atlanta	Georgia	404-686-4411	www.emoryhealthcare.org
Essentia Health Saint Joseph's Medical Center	Brainerd	Minnesota	218-829-2861	www.sjmcmn.org
Excela Health Frick Hospital	Mount Pleasant	Pennsylvania	724-547-1500	www.excelahealth.org
Fairview Hospital	Cleveland	Ohio	216-476-7000	www.fairviewhospital.org
Falmouth Hospital	Falmouth	Massachusetts	508-548-5300	www.capecodhealth.com
Fawcett Memorial Hospital	Port Charlotte	Florida	941-629-1181	www.fawcetthospital.com
Firsthealth Moore Regional Hospital	Pinehurst	North Carolina	910-715-1000	www.firsthealth.org
Flagler Hospital	Saint Augustine	Florida	904-819-4426	www.flaglerhospital.com
Florida Hospital Heartland Medical Center	Sebring	Florida	863-314-4466	www.fhhd.org
Forbes Regional Hospital	Monroeville	Pennsylvania	412-858-2000	www.wpahs.org
Fort Duncan Medical Center	Eagle Pass	Texas	830-773-5321	www.fortduncanmedicalcenter.com
Fountain Valley Regional Hospital & Medical Center	Fountain Valley	California	714-966-7200	www.fountainvalleyhospital.com
Franciscan Saint James Health	Olympia Fields	Illinois	708-747-4000	www.franciscanalliance.org
Franciscan Saint Margaret Health - Hammond	Hammond	Indiana	219-932-2300	www.smmhc.com
Frederick Memorial Hospital	Frederick	Maryland	240-566-3300	www.fmh.org
Genesys Regional Medical Center - Health Park	Grand Blanc	Michigan	810-606-5000	www.genesys.org
Glendale Adventist Medical Center	Glendale	California	818-409-8202	www.glendaleadventist.com
Glendale Memorial Hospital & Health Center	Glendale	California	818-502-1900	www.glendalememorialhospital.org
Good Samaritan Hospital	Los Angeles	California	213-977-2121	www.goodsam.org
Good Shepherd Medical Center	Longview	Texas	903-315-2000	www.goodshepherdhealth.org
Grand View Hospital	Sellersville	Pennsylvania	215-453-4615	www.gvh.org
Hahnemann University Hospital	Philadelphia	Pennsylvania	215-762-7000	www.hahnemannhospital.com
Harper University Hospital	Detroit	Michigan	313-745-6211	www.harperhospital.org
Henry Ford Hospital	Detroit	Michigan	313-916-2600	www.henryfordhospital.com
Henry Ford Wyandotte Hospital	Wyandotte	Michigan	734-246-6000	www.henryfordwyandotte.com
Hillcrest Hospital	Mayfield Heights	Ohio	440-312-4500	www.hillcresthospital.org
Hollywood Presbyterian Medical Center	Los Angeles	California	213-413-3000	www.qahpmc.com
Holy Name Medical Center	Teaneck	New Jersey	201-833-3000	www.holyname.org
Houston VA Medical Center	Houston	Texas	713-794-7100	www.houston.med.va.gov
Howard County General Hospital	Columbia	Maryland	410-740-7890	www.hcgh.org
Huntington Beach Hospital	Huntington Beach	California	714-843-5000	www.hbhospital.com
Huron Valley - Sinai Hospital	Commerce Township	Michigan	248-937-3370	www.hvsh.org
Ingalls Memorial Hospital	Harvey	Illinois	708-333-2300	www.ingalls.org
Inova Fairfax Hospital	Falls Church	Virginia	703-776-3332	www.inova.org
Jersey Shore University Medical Center	Neptune	New Jersey	732-776-4900	www.meridianhealth.com
Jesse Brown VA Medical Center - VA Chicago	Chicago	Illinois	312-569-8387	www.va.gov
Kingsbrook Jewish Medical Center	Brooklyn	New York	718-604-5789	www.kingsbrook.org

Hospital	City	State	Phone	Web Site
Lawrence General Hospital	Lawrence	Massachusetts	978-683-4000	www.lawrencegeneral.org
Lehigh Valley Hospital	Allentown	Pennsylvania	610-402-2273	www.lvhhn.org
Lehigh Valley Hospital - Hazleton	Hazleton	Pennsylvania	570-501-4000	www.ghha.org
Lenox Hill Hospital	New York	New York	212-439-2345	www.lenoxhillhospital.org
Libertyhealth - Jersey City Medical Center Campus	Jersey City	New Jersey	201-915-2000	www.libertyhcs.org
Long Beach Memorial Medical Center	Long Beach	California	562-933-2000	www.memorialcare.com/long_beach
Louis A Weiss Memorial Hospital	Chicago	Illinois	773-878-8700	www.weisshospital.org
Maimonides Medical Center	Brooklyn	New York	718-283-6000	www.maimonidesmed.org
Main Line Hospital Bryn Mawr Campus	Bryn Mawr	Pennsylvania	610-526-3000	www.mainlinehealth.org
Main Line Hospital Lankenau	Wynnewood	Pennsylvania	610-645-2000	www.mainlinehealth.org/lh
Marymount Hospital	Garfield Heights	Ohio	216-581-0500	www.marymount.org
Mclaren Flint	Flint	Michigan	810-342-2000	www.mclaren.org
Medical Center of Southeastern Oklahoma	Durant	Oklahoma	405-924-3080	www.mcsohealth.com
Medstar Franklin Square Medical Center	Baltimore	Maryland	443-777-7850	www.franklinsquare.org
Medstar Good Samaritan Hospital	Baltimore	Maryland	443-444-3902	www.goodsam-md.org
Medstar Washington Hospital Center	Washington	District of Columbia	202-877-7000	www.whcenter.org
Mercy Fitzgerald Hospital	Darby	Pennsylvania	215-237-4000	www.mercyhealth.org
Mercy Hospital & Medical Center	Chicago	Illinois	312-567-2000	www.mercy-chicago.org
Mercy Medical Center	Springfield	Massachusetts	413-748-9000	www.mercycares.com
Mercy Saint Vincent Medical Center	Toledo	Ohio	419-251-3232	www.mhsnr.org
The Methodist Hospital	Houston	Texas	713-790-2221	www.methodisthealth.com
Mission Hospital Regional Medical Center	Mission Viejo	California	949-364-1400	www.mission4health.com
Missouri Baptist Medical Center	Town & Country	Missouri	314-996-5000	www.missouribaptistmedicalcenter.org
Montefiore Medical Center	Bronx	New York	718-920-4321	www.montefiore.org
Morristown Medical Center	Morristown	New Jersey	973-971-5450	www.morristownmemorialhospital.org
Mount Sinai Hospital	New York	New York	212-241-7981	www.mountsinai.org
Mountainview Hospital	Las Vegas	Nevada	702-255-5065	www.mountainview-hospital.com
New York Hospital Medical Center of Queens	Flushing	New York	718-670-1231	www.nyhq.org
New York - Presbyterian Hospital	New York	New York	212-746-4189	www.nyp.org
Newark Beth Israel Medical Center	Newark	New Jersey	973-926-7850	www.sbhcs.com
Newton - Wellesley Hospital	Newton	Massachusetts	617-243-6000	www.nwh.org
North Florida Regional Medical Center	Gainesville	Florida	352-333-4100	www.nfrmc.com
North Shore Medical Center	Salem	Massachusetts	978-741-1215	www.nsmc.partners.org
Northridge Hospital Medical Center	Northridge	California	818-885-8500	www.northridgehospital.org
Northwestern Memorial Hospital	Chicago	Illinois	312-926-2000	www.nmh.org
NYU Hospitals Center	New York	New York	212-263-7300	www.med.nyu.edu
Oakwood Hospital - Dearborn	Dearborn	Michigan	313-593-7125	www.oakwood.org
Oklahoma Heart Hospital South	Oklahoma City	Oklahoma	405-628-6000	www.okheart.com/south-campus
Olympia Medical Center	Los Angeles	California	310-657-5900	www.olympiamc.com
Oroville Hospital	Oroville	California	530-533-8500	www.orovillehospital.com
Palm Beach Gardens Medical Center	Palm Beach Gardens	Florida	561-622-1411	www.pbgmc.com
Palmetto Health Richland	Columbia	South Carolina	803-296-5678	www.palmettohealth.org
Paradise Valley Hospital	National City	California	619-470-4321	www.paradisevalleyhospital.org
Penn Presbyterian Medical Center	Philadelphia	Pennsylvania	215-662-8000	www.pennhealth.com
Pennsylvania Hospital of the Univ of PA Health Sys	Philadelphia	Pennsylvania	215-829-3000	www.pennmedicine.org/pahosp
Philadelphia VA Medical Center	Philadelphia	Pennsylvania	215-823-5857	www.philadelphia.va.gov
Portland VA Medical Center	Portland	Oregon	503-220-8262	www.va.gov/portland/index.asp
Presence Saint Joseph Hospital - Chicago	Chicago	Illinois	773-665-3000	www.res-health.org
Presence Saint Joseph Medical Center	Joliet	Illinois	815-725-7133	www.provena.org/stjoes
Presence Saints Mary & Elizabeth Medical Center	Chicago	Illinois	312-770-2000	www.reshealth.org
Providence Holy Cross Medical Center	Mission Hills	California	818-365-8051	www.providence.org
Providence Hospital	Washington	District of Columbia	202-269-7000	www.provhosp.org
Providence Hospital & Medical Centers	Southfield	Michigan	248-849-3011	www.stjohn.org/providence
Providence Little Co of Mary Medical Center Torrance	Torrance	California	310-540-7676	www.lcmhs.org
Providence Tarzana Medical Center	Tarzana	California	818-881-0800	www.encino-tarzana.com
Raritan Bay Medical Center	Perth Amboy	New Jersey	732-442-3700	www.rbmc.org
Regional Medical Center of San Jose	San Jose	California	408-259-5000	www.regionalmedicalsanjose.com
Rex Hospital	Raleigh	North Carolina	919-784-3100	www.rexhealth.com
Rio Grande Regional Hospital	Mcallen	Texas	956-632-6000	www.riohealth.com
Ronald Reagan UCLA Medical Center	Los Angeles	California	310-825-6301	www.uclahealth.org
Rush Oak Park Hospital	Oak Park	Illinois	708-383-9300	www.oakparkhospital.org
Rush University Medical Center	Chicago	Illinois	312-942-5000	www.ruch.edu
Saint Agnes Hospital	Baltimore	Maryland	410-368-2101	www.stagnes.org
Saint Francis Medical Center	Lynwood	California	310-900-8900	www.stfrancis.dochs.org
Saint Michael's Medical Center	Newark	New Jersey	973-877-5350	www.cathedralhealth.org
Saint Vincent Medical Center	Los Angeles	California	213-484-7111	www.stvincent.dochs.org
Santa Monica - UCLA Medical Center & Orthopaedic Hospital	Santa Monica	California	310-319-4000	www.healthcare.ucla.edu

Hospital	City	State	Phone	Web Site
Scottsdale Healthcare - Shea Medical Center	Scottsdale	Arizona	480-323-3009	www.shc.org
Scripps Green Hospital	La Jolla	California	858-554-3600	www.scrippshealth.org
Scripps Mercy Hospital	San Diego	California	619-294-8111	www.scrippshealth.org
Shore Medical Center	Somers Point	New Jersey	609-653-3545	www.shorememorial.org
Sinai Hospital of Baltimore	Baltimore	Maryland	410-601-5131	www.sinai-balt.com
Sinai - Grace Hospital	Detroit	Michigan	313-966-3300	www.sinaigrace.org
South Pointe Hospital	Warrensville Heights	Ohio	216-491-6000	www.southpointehospital.org
South Texas Health System	Edinburg	Texas	956-632-4000	www.edinburgregional.com
Southcoast Hospital Group	Fall River	Massachusetts	508-679-3131	www.southcoast.org/charlton
Southeastern Regional Medical Center	Lumberton	North Carolina	910-671-5000	www.srmc.org
SSM Saint Marys Health Center	Richmond Heights	Missouri	314-768-8000	www.ssmhealth.com/stmarys
Saint Alexius Medical Center	Hoffman Estates	Illinois	847-843-2000	www.alexianbrothershealth.org
Saint Catherine Hospital	East Chicago	Indiana	219-392-7004	www.comhs.org/stcatherine
Saint Elizabeth's Medical Center	Brighton	Massachusetts	617-789-3000	www.semc.org
Saint Francis Hospital & Medical Center	Hartford	Connecticut	860-714-4000	www.saintfranciscare.com
Saint Francis Hospital - Roslyn	Roslyn	New York	516-562-6000	www.stfrancisheartcenter.com
Saint John Hospital & Medical Center	Detroit	Michigan	313-343-4000	www.stjohnprovidence.org
Saint Luke's Hospital	Chesterfield	Missouri	314-434-1500	www.goodhealthmatters.com
Saint Luke's Hospital of Kansas City	Kansas City	Missouri	816-932-2000	www.staintlukeshealthsystem.org
Saint Vincent's Medical Center Southside	Jacksonville	Florida	904-296-3700	www.jaxhealth.com
Thomas Jefferson University Hospital	Philadelphia	Pennsylvania	215-955-6000	www.jeffersonhospital.org
Touro Infirmary	New Orleans	Louisiana	504-897-7011	www.touro.com
Tufts Medical Center	Boston	Massachusetts	617-636-5000	www.tuftsmedicalcenter.org
University Hospital of Brooklyn - Downstate Medical Center	Brooklyn	New York	718-270-1000	www.downstate.edu
University of Maryland Charles Regional Medical Center	La Plata	Maryland	301-609-4265	www.civista.org
University of Miami Hospital	Miami	Florida	305-325-5511	www.cedarsmedicalcenter.com
UPMC Mckeesport	Mc Keesport	Pennsylvania	412-664-2000	www.selectmedicalcorp.com
UPMC Passavant	Pittsburgh	Pennsylvania	412-367-6700	www.passavant.upmc.com
UT Southwestern University Hospital	Dallas	Texas	214-879-3758	www.utsouthwestern.edu
VA Boston Healthcare System - Jamaica Plain	Jamaica Plain	Massachusetts	617-232-9500	www.vaww.visn1.med.va.gov/boston
VA Greater Los Angeles Healthcare System	West Los Angeles	California	310-478-3711	www1.va.gov
VA New York Harbor Healthcare System	New York	New York	212-686-7500	www.nyharbor.va.gov
Valley Hospital	Ridgewood	New Jersey	201-447-8000	www.valleyhealth.com
Valley Presbyterian Hospital	Van Nuys	California	818-902-3906	www.valleypres.org
Wakemed - Raleigh Campus	Raleigh	North Carolina	919-350-8000	www.wakemed.org
Washington Adventist Hospital	Takoma Park	Maryland	301-891-5651	www.adventisthealthcare.com/wah
Waukesha Memorial Hospital	Waukesha	Wisconsin	262-928-1000	www.waukeshamemorial.org
West Haven VA Medical Center	West Haven	Connecticut	203-932-5711	www.visn1.med.va.gov/vact
Wheaton Franciscan Healthcare Saint Francis	Milwaukee	Wisconsin	414-647-5000	www.mywheaton.org
White Memorial Medical Center	Los Angeles	California	323-268-5000	www.whitememorial.com
William Beaumont Hospital - Troy	Troy	Michigan	248-964-8800	www.beaumonthospitals.com
Willis Knighton Medical Center	Shreveport	Louisiana	318-212-4000	www.wkhs.com//locations/medicalcenter.aspx
Winchester Hospital	Winchester	Massachusetts	781-729-9000	www.winchesterhospital.org
Wing Memorial Hospital & Medical Center	Palmer	Massachusetts	413-283-7651	www.winghealth.org
Yale-New Haven Hospital	New Haven	Connecticut	203-688-4242	www.ynhh.org

Note: Table shows hospitals nationwide whose heart failure 30-day risk-adjusted mortality rate is better (lower) than U.S. rate of 11.7%

Hospitals whose Heart Failure 30-Day Mortality Rate is Worse (Higher) than the U.S. National Rate

Hospital	City	State	Phone	Web Site
Abbeville General Hospital	Abbeville	Louisiana	337-893-5466	www.abgen.net
Abrom Kaplan Memorial Hospital	Kaplan	Louisiana	337-643-8300	www.compasshealthcare.com/site78.php
Albany Memorial Hospital	Albany	New York	518-471-3221	www.nehealth.com
Alegent Creighton Health Immanuel Medical Center	Omaha	Nebraska	402-572-2121	www.alegent.com
Anne Arundel Medical Center	Annapolis	Maryland	443-481-1307	www.aahs.org
Appleton Medical Center	Appleton	Wisconsin	920-731-4101	www.thedacare.org
Arkansas Methodist Medical Center	Paragould	Arkansas	870-239-7000	www.arkansasmethodist.org
Baptist Health Medical Center - North Little Rock	North Little Rock	Arkansas	501-202-3000	www.baptist-health.org
Baptist Memorial Hospital/Golden Triangle	Columbus	Mississippi	662-244-1500	www.bmhcc.org/facilities/goldentriangle
Baxter Regional Medical Center	Mountain Home	Arkansas	870-508-1000	www.baxterregional.org
Blanchard Valley Hospital	Findlay	Ohio	419-423-4500	www.bvha.org
Bolivar Medical Center	Cleveland	Mississippi	662-846-2551	www.bolivarmedical.com
Brattleboro Memorial Hospital	Brattleboro	Vermont	802-257-0341	www.bmhvt.org
Bronson Methodist Hospital	Kalamazoo	Michigan	269-341-6000	www.bronsonhealth.com
Capital Region Medical Center	Jefferson City	Missouri	573-632-5000	www.crmc.org
Carilion Roanoke Memorial Hospital	Roanoke	Virginia	540-981-7000	www.carilion.com/crmh
Carolinas Medical Center/Behaviorial Health	Charlotte	North Carolina	704-355-2000	www.carolinasmedicalcenter.org
Carroll Hospital Center	Westminster	Maryland	410-848-3000	www.carrollhospitalcenter.org
Carson Tahoe Regional Medical Center	Carson City	Nevada	775-445-8000	www.carsontahoehospital.com
Cayuga Medical Center at Ithaca	Ithaca	New York	607-274-4401	www.cayugamed.org
Central Maine Medical Center	Lewiston	Maine	207-795-0111	www.cmmc.org
Central Washington Hospital	Wenatchee	Washington	509-662-1511	www.cwhs.com
Cherokee Regional Medical Center	Cherokee	Iowa	712-225-5101	www.cherokeermc.org
Chicot Memorial Medical Center	Lake Village	Arkansas	870-265-5351	www.chicotmemorial.com
Christus Hospital	Beaumont	Texas	409-892-7171	www.christushealth.org
Citizens Baptist Medical Center	Talladega	Alabama	256-761-4542	www.bhsala.com
Citrus Memorial Hospital	Inverness	Florida	352-726-1551	www.citrusmh.com
Clarion Hospital	Clarion	Pennsylvania	814-226-9500	www.clarionhospital.org
Clovis Community Medical Center	Clovis	California	559-324-4000	www.communitymedical.org
Columbia Saint Marys Hospital Ozaukee	Mequon	Wisconsin	262-243-7300	www.columbia-stmarys.org
Community Hospital North	Indianapolis	Indiana	317-621-5335	www.ecommunity.com/north
Conway Regional Medical Center	Conway	Arkansas	501-329-3831	www.conwayregional.org
Copley Memorial Hospital	Aurora	Illinois	630-978-6200	www.rushcopley.com
Coshocton County Memorial Hospital	Coshocton	Ohio	740-622-6411	www.ccmh.com
Dekalb Regional Medical Center	Fort Payne	Alabama	256-845-3150	www.baptistmedical.org
Dominican Hospital	Santa Cruz	California	831-462-7700	www.dominicanhospital.org
Edward W Sparrow Hospital	Lansing	Michigan	517-364-1000	www.sparrow.org
Emerson Hospital	W Concord	Massachusetts	978-369-1400	www.emersonhospital.org
Fletcher Allen Hospital of Vermont	Burlington	Vermont	802-847-0000	www.fletcherallen.org
Floyd Medical Center	Rome	Georgia	706-509-6900	www.floydmed.org
Geisinger Medical Center	Danville	Pennsylvania	570-271-6211	www.geisinger.org
Geneva General Hospital	Geneva	New York	315-787-4175	www.flhealth.org
GHS Greenville Memorial Medical Center	Greenville	South Carolina	864-455-7000	www.ghs.org
Good Samaritan Hospital	Lebanon	Pennsylvania	717-270-7500	www.gshleb.org
Grossmont Hospital	La Mesa	California	619-465-0711	www.sharp.com
Hendrick Medical Center	Abilene	Texas	325-670-2000	www.ehendrick.org
Highland Hospital	Rochester	New York	585-473-2200	www.urmc.rochester.edu
Hilton Head Regional Medical Center	Hilton Head Island	South Carolina	843-681-6122	www.hiltonheadmedctr.com
Hopkins County Memorial Hospital	Sulphur Springs	Texas	903-885-7671	www.hcmh.com
Hutchinson Regional Medical Center	Hutchinson	Kansas	620-665-2001	www.hutchinsonhospital.com
Iberia General Hospital & Medical Center	New Iberia	Louisiana	337-364-0441	www.iberiamedicalcenter.com
Indiana University Health La Porte Hospital	La Porte	Indiana	219-326-1234	www.laportehealth.org
Integris Grove Hospital	Grove	Oklahoma	918-786-2243	www.integris-health.com
IU Health Goshen Hospital	Goshen	Indiana	574-364-1000	www.goshenhosp.com
Jane Phillips Medical Center	Bartlesville	Oklahoma	918-333-7200	www.jpmc.org
JFK Medical Center - A M Yelencsics Comm Hospital	Edison	New Jersey	732-321-7000	www.jfkmc.org
Johnson Memorial Hospital	Franklin	Indiana	317-736-3300	www.johnsonmemorial.org
Kadlec Regional Medical Center	Richland	Washington	509-946-4611	www.kadlecmed.org
Kootenai Medical Center	Coeur D'alene	Idaho	208-625-4001	www.kootenaihealth.org
Lake Cumberland Regional Hospital	Somerset	Kentucky	606-679-7441	www.lakecumberlandhospital.com
Lake Granbury Medical Center	Granbury	Texas	817-573-2683	www.lakegranburymedicalcenter.com
Lawrence & Memorial Hospital	New London	Connecticut	860-442-0711	www.lmhospital.org
Los Alamitos Medical Center	Los Alamitos	California	562-799-3220	www.losalamitosmedctr.com
Manatee Memorial Hospital	Bradenton	Florida	941-746-5111	www.manateememorial.com
Manchester Memorial Hospital	Manchester	Connecticut	860-647-4780	www.echn.org

Hospital	City	State	Phone	Web Site
Maury Regional Hospital	Columbia	Tennessee	931-381-1111	www.maurgregional.com
Mclaren - Greater Lansing	Lansing	Michigan	517-975-6000	www.mclaren.org
Meadville Medical Center	Meadville	Pennsylvania	814-333-5000	www.mmchs.org
Medcentral Health System Mansfield Hospital	Mansfield	Ohio	419-526-8000	www.medcentral.org
Memorial Hospital of South Bend	South Bend	Indiana	574-647-1000	www.qualityoflife.org
Mercy Health System Corp	Janesville	Wisconsin	608-756-6080	www.mercyhealthsystem.org
Mercy Hospital Springfield	Springfield	Missouri	417-820-2000	www.stjohns.com
Mercy Medical Center - Redding	Redding	California	530-225-6102	www.redding.mercy.org
Mercy Medical Center - North Iowa	Mason City	Iowa	641-428-7000	www.mercynorthiowa.com
Mountain View Regional Medical Center	Las Cruces	New Mexico	575-556-7600	www.mountainviewregional.com
Nathan Littauer Hospital	Gloversville	New York	518-725-8621	www.nlh.org
Nea Baptist Memorial Hospital	Jonesboro	Arkansas	870-972-7000	www.baptistonline.com
New Hanover Regional Medical Center	Wilmington	North Carolina	910-343-7000	www.nhrmc.org
New Milford Hospital	New Milford	Connecticut	860-355-2611	www.newmilfordhospital.org
Norman Regional Health System	Norman	Oklahoma	405-321-1700	www.normanregional.com
North Mississippi Medical Center	Tupelo	Mississippi	662-377-3000	www.nmhs.net/nmmc
North Shore University Hospital	Manhasset	New York	516-562-0100	www.northshorelij.com
Northwest Community Hospital	Arlington Heights	Illinois	847-618-1000	www.nch.org
Northwest Hospital	Seattle	Washington	206-364-0500	www.nwhospital.org
O'Connor Hospital	San Jose	California	408-947-2500	www.oconnorhospital.org
Olympic Medical Center	Port Angeles	Washington	360-417-7000	www.olympicmedical.org
Our Lady of the Lake Regional Medical Center	Baton Rouge	Louisiana	225-765-6565	www.ololrmc.com
Overton Brooks VA Medical Center - Shreveport	Shreveport	Louisiana	318-424-6037	www.va.gov/sta/guide/home.asp
Pinnacle Health Hospitals	Harrisburg	Pennsylvania	717-782-5181	www.pinnaclehealth.org
Poplar Bluff Regional Medical Center	Poplar Bluff	Missouri	573-785-7721	www.poplarbluffregional.com
Porter Regional Hospital	Valparaiso	Indiana	219-983-8300	www.portermemorial.org
Providence Alaska Medical Center	Anchorage	Alaska	907-261-3675	www.providence.org
Providence Sacred Heart Medical Center	Spokane	Washington	509-474-3040	www.shmc.org
Rideout Memorial Hospital	Marysville	California	530-749-4300	www.frhg.org
Riverview Hospital Assoc	Wisconsin Rapids	Wisconsin	715-423-6060	www.riverviewhospital.net
Sacred Heart Medical Center - Riverbend	Springfield	Oregon	541-222-7300	www.peacehealth.org/sacred-heart-riverbend
Saint Anthony Medical Center	Rockford	Illinois	815-226-2000	www.osfhealth.com
Saint Francis Medical Center	Peoria	Illinois	309-655-2000	www.osfsaintfrancis.org
Salem Hospital	Salem	Oregon	503-561-5200	www.salemhospital.org
Saline Memorial Hospital	Benton	Arkansas	501-776-6000	www.salinememorial.org
San Juan Regional Medical Center	Farmington	New Mexico	505-609-2000	www.sanjuanregional.com
Sanford Usd Medical Center	Sioux Falls	South Dakota	605-333-1000	www.sanfordhealth.org
Santa Rosa Memorial Hospital	Santa Rosa	California	707-525-5300	www.stjosephhealth.org
Sarasota Memorial Hospital	Sarasota	Florida	941-917-9000	www.smh.com
Scenic Mountain Medical Center	Big Spring	Texas	432-263-1211	www.smmccares.com
Sentara Obici Hospital	Suffolk	Virginia	757-934-4000	www.sentara.com
Saint Anthony's Hospital	Saint Petersburg	Florida	727-825-1100	www.stanthonys.com
Saint Bernards Medical Center	Jonesboro	Arkansas	870-972-4100	www.sbrmc.com
Saint Francis - Downtown	Greenville	South Carolina	864-255-1000	www.stfrancishealth.org
Saint Johns Hospital	Springfield	Illinois	217-544-6464	www.st-johns.org
Saint Joseph Regional Health Center	Bryan	Texas	979-776-3912	www.st-joseph.org/sjrhc
Saint Joseph's Mercy Health Center	Hot Springs	Arkansas	501-622-1000	www.saintjosephs.com
Saint Lucie Medical Center	Port Saint Lucie	Florida	772-335-4000	www.stluciemed.com
Saint Marys Hospital Medical Center	Green Bay	Wisconsin	920-498-4200	www.stmgb.org
Saint Marys Regional Medical Center	Russellville	Arkansas	479-968-2841	www.saintmarysregional.com
Saint Nicholas Hospital	Sheboygan	Wisconsin	920-459-8300	www.stnicholashospital.org
Saint Rose Dominican Hospitals - Rose De Lima Campus	Henderson	Nevada	702-616-5000	www.dignityhealth.org/las-vegas
Starr Regional Medical Center Athens	Athens	Tennessee	423-745-1411	www.athensrmc.com
Swedish Edmonds Hospital	Edmonds	Washington	425-640-4000	www.stevenshealthcare.org
Texas Health Harris Methodist Fort Worth	Fort Worth	Texas	817-250-2100	www.texashealth.org
The Nebraska Medical Center	Omaha	Nebraska	402-552-2040	www.nebraskamed.com
Theda Clark Medical Center	Neenah	Wisconsin	920-729-3100	www.thedacare.org
Thibodaux Regional Medical Center	Thibodaux	Louisiana	985-447-5500	www.thibodaux.com
Tulare Regional Medical Center	Tulare	California	559-688-0821	www.tdhs.org
Ukiah Valley Medical Center	Ukiah	California	707-462-3111	www.uvmc.org
Union General Hospital	Blairsville	Georgia	706-745-2111	www.uniongeneralhospital.com
United Health Services Hospitals	Johnson City	New York	607-763-6000	www.vhs.ent
United Regional Health Care System	Wichita Falls	Texas	940-764-3055	www.urhcs.org
University of Missouri Health Care	Columbia	Missouri	573-882-4141	www.missouri.edu
Utah Valley Regional Medical Center	Provo	Utah	801-373-7850	www.intermountainhealthcare.org/hospitals/uvrmc
VA Southern Arizona Healthcare System	Tucson	Arizona	520-629-1821	www.va.gov/sta/guide/home.asp
Valley Hospital	Spokane	Washington	509-924-6650	www.valleyhospital.org

Hospital	City	State	Phone	Web Site
Western Missouri Medical Center	Warrensburg	Missouri	660-747-2500	www.wmmc.com
White County Medical Center	Searcy	Arkansas	501-278-3100	www.centralarkhospital.com
Wilkes-Barre General Hospital	Wilkes-Barre	Pennsylvania	570-829-8111	www.wvhcs.org
Wyoming Medical Center	Casper	Wyoming	307-577-7201	www.wyomingmedicalcenter.com

Note: Table shows hospitals nationwide whose heart failure 30-day risk-adjusted mortality rate is worse (higher) than U.S. rate of 11.7%

Hospitals whose Pneumonia 30-Day Mortality Rate is Better (Lower) than the U.S. National Rate

Hospital	City	State	Phone	Web Site
Adventist La Grange Memorial Hospital	La Grange	Illinois	708-352-1200	www.keepingyouwell.com
Ahmc Anaheim Regional Medical Center	Anaheim	California	714-774-1450	www.memorialcare.org/anaheim
Akron General Medical Center	Akron	Ohio	330-344-6000	www.akrongeneral.org
Alhambra Hospital Medical Center	Alhambra	California	626-570-1606	www.alhambrahospital.com
Arnot Ogden Medical Center	Elmira	New York	607-737-4100	www.arnothealth.org
Augusta Health	Fishersville	Virginia	540-932-4000	www.augustamed.com
Aurora Saint Lukes Medical Center	Milwaukee	Wisconsin	414-649-6000	www.aurorahealthcare.org
Aventura Hospital & Medical Center	Aventura	Florida	305-682-7000	www.aventurahospital.com
Banner Thunderbird Medical Center	Glendale	Arizona	602-588-5555	www.bannerhealth.com
Baptist Hospital of Miami	Miami	Florida	786-596-1960	www.baptisthealth.net
Barnes-Jewish Saint Peters Hospital	Saint Peters	Missouri	636-916-9000	www.bjsph.org
Bay Medical Center Sacred Heart Health System	Panama City	Florida	850-769-1511	www.baymedical.org
Baylor Regional Medical Center at Grapevine	Grapevine	Texas	817-481-1588	www.baylorhealth.com
Beaumont Health System	Grosse Pointe	Michigan	313-343-1000	www.beaumonthospitals.com
Beaumont Health System	Royal Oak	Michigan	248-898-5000	www.beaumonthospitals.com
Benefis Hospitals	Great Falls	Montana	406-455-5000	www.benefis.org
Berkshire Medical Center	Pittsfield	Massachusetts	413-447-2000	www.berkshirehealthsystems.org
Beth Israel Deaconess Medical Center	Boston	Massachusetts	617-667-7000	www.bidmc.harvard.edu
Betsy Johnson Regional Hospital	Dunn	North Carolina	910-892-7161	www.bjrh.org
Cape Cod Hospital	Hyannis	Massachusetts	508-771-1800	www.capecodhealth.org
Casey County Hospital	Liberty	Kentucky	606-787-6275	
Cedars - Sinai Medical Center	Los Angeles	California	310-423-5000	www.cedars-sinai.edu
Centinela Hospital Medical Center	Inglewood	California	310-673-4660	www.centinelafreeman.com
Centura Health - Littleton Adventist Hospital	Littleton	Colorado	303-730-5888	www.littletonhosp.org
Christ Hospital	Cincinnati	Ohio	513-585-2000	www.thechristhospital.com
Cobre Valley Regional Medical Center	Globe	Arizona	928-425-3261	www.cvchospital.com
Community Medical Center	Toms River	New Jersey	732-557-8000	www.sbhcs.com
Corning Hospital	Corning	New York	607-937-7200	www.corninghospital.org
Cox Medical Center Branson	Branson	Missouri	417-335-7000	www.skaggs.net
Delray Medical Center	Delray Beach	Florida	561-498-4440	www.delraymedicalctr.com
Desert Valley Hospital	Victorville	California	760-241-8000	www.dvmc.com
Doctors Hospital at Renaissance	Edinburg	Texas	956-362-8677	www.dhr-rgv.com
Duke University Hospital	Durham	North Carolina	919-684-8111	www.dukehealth.org
East Valley Hospital Medical Center	Glendora	California	626-335-0231	www.eastvalleyhospital.org
Edward Hospital	Naperville	Illinois	630-527-3000	www.edward.org
Eisenhower Medical Center	Rancho Mirage	California	760-340-3911	www.emc.org
Elmhurst Memorial Hospital	Elmhurst	Illinois	630-833-1400	www.emhc.org
Englewood Hospital & Medical Center	Englewood	New Jersey	201-894-3000	www.englewoodhospital.com
Evanston Hospital	Evanston	Illinois	847-432-8000	www.enh.org
Evergreen Hospital Medical Center	Kirkland	Washington	425-899-1000	www.evergreenhospital.org
Exempla Lutheran Medical Center	Wheat Ridge	Colorado	303-425-4500	www.exemlpa.org
Falmouth Hospital	Falmouth	Massachusetts	508-548-5300	www.capecodhealth.com
Firsthealth Moore Regional Hospital	Pinehurst	North Carolina	910-715-1000	www.firsthealth.org
Flagler Hospital	Saint Augustine	Florida	904-819-4426	www.flaglerhospital.com
Forbes Regional Hospital	Monroeville	Pennsylvania	412-858-2000	www.wpahs.org
Fountain Valley Regional Hospital & Medical Center	Fountain Valley	California	714-966-7200	www.fountainvalleyhospital.com
Franklin Woods Community Hospital	Johnson City	Tennessee	423-302-1120	www.msha.com
Frederick Memorial Hospital	Frederick	Maryland	240-566-3300	www.fmh.org
Frisbie Memorial Hospital	Rochester	New Hampshire	603-332-5211	www.frisbiehospital.com
Garden Grove Hospital & Medical Center	Garden Grove	California	714-537-5160	www.gardengrovehospital.com
Garfield Medical Center	Monterey Park	California	626-573-2222	www.garfieldmedicalcenter.com
Geisinger - Bloomsburg Hospital	Bloomsburg	Pennsylvania	570-387-2100	www.tbhonline.org
Genesis Healthcare System	Zanesville	Ohio	740-454-5000	www.genesishcs.org
Genesys Regional Medical Center - Health Park	Grand Blanc	Michigan	810-606-5000	www.genesys.org
Glendale Adventist Medical Center	Glendale	California	818-409-8202	www.glendaleadventist.com
Grandview Hospital & Medical Center	Dayton	Ohio	937-723-3312	www.kmcnetwork.org
Greater Baltimore Medical Center	Baltimore	Maryland	443-849-2000	www.gbmc.org
Harper University Hospital	Detroit	Michigan	313-745-6211	www.harperhospital.org
Heartland Regional Medical Center	Saint Joseph	Missouri	816-271-6000	www.heartland-health.com
Henry Ford Macomb Hospital	Clinton Township	Michigan	586-263-2300	www.stjoe-macomb.com
Hillcrest Hospital	Mayfield Heights	Ohio	440-312-4500	www.hillcresthospital.org
Hinsdale Hospital	Hinsdale	Illinois	630-856-9000	www.keepingyouwell.com
Hollywood Presbyterian Medical Center	Los Angeles	California	213-413-3000	www.qahpmc.com
Holy Name Medical Center	Teaneck	New Jersey	201-833-3000	www.holyname.org
The Hospital of Central Connecticut	New Britain	Connecticut	860-224-5011	www.thocc.org

Hospital	City	State	Phone	Web Site
Huntington Beach Hospital	Huntington Beach	California	714-843-5000	www.hbhospital.com
Huntington Memorial Hospital	Pasadena	California	626-397-5000	www.huntingtonhospital.com
Indiana University Health	Indianapolis	Indiana	317-962-5900	www.iuhealth.org
Ingalls Memorial Hospital	Harvey	Illinois	708-333-2300	www.ingalls.org
Inova Loudoun Hospital	Leesburg	Virginia	703-858-6600	www.loudounhealthcare.org
Jersey Shore University Medical Center	Neptune	New Jersey	732-776-4900	www.meridianhealth.com
Jupiter Medical Center	Jupiter	Florida	561-747-2234	www.jupitermed.com
Kane Community Hospital	Kane	Pennsylvania	814-837-8585	www.kanehosp.com
Kingsbrook Jewish Medical Center	Brooklyn	New York	718-604-5789	www.kingsbrook.org
Lehigh Valley Hospital	Allentown	Pennsylvania	610-402-2273	www.lvhhn.org
Lehigh Valley Hospital - Hazleton	Hazleton	Pennsylvania	570-501-4000	www.ghha.org
Lehigh Valley Hospital - Muhlenberg	Bethlehem	Pennsylvania	610-402-2273	www.lvhn.org
Liberty Hospital	Liberty	Missouri	816-781-7200	www.libertyhospital.org
Los Angeles Community Hospital	Los Angeles	California	323-267-0477	www.altacorp.com
Los Robles Hospital & Medical Center	Thousand Oaks	California	805-497-2727	www.losrobleshospital.com
Maimonides Medical Center	Brooklyn	New York	718-283-6000	www.maimonidesmed.org
Mary Greeley Medical Center	Ames	Iowa	515-239-2011	www.mgmc.org
Mayo Clinic Hospital	Phoenix	Arizona	480-342-2000	www.mayoclinic.org
Medical Center of Southeastern Oklahoma	Durant	Oklahoma	405-924-3080	www.mcsohealth.com
Medical City Dallas Hospital	Dallas	Texas	972-566-6222	www.medicalcityhospital.com
Medstar Franklin Square Medical Center	Baltimore	Maryland	443-777-7850	www.franklinsquare.org
Medstar Good Samaritan Hospital	Baltimore	Maryland	443-444-3902	www.goodsam-md.org
Medstar Harbor Hospital	Baltimore	Maryland	410-350-3201	www.harborhospital.org
Memorial Mission Hospital & Asheville Surgery Center	Asheville	North Carolina	828-213-1111	www.missionhospitals.org
Mercy Memorial Hospital System	Monroe	Michigan	734-240-8400	www.mercymemorial.org
The Methodist Hospital	Houston	Texas	713-790-2221	www.methodisthealth.com
Methodist Sugar Land Hospital	Sugar Land	Texas	281-274-8000	www.methodisthealth.com/sugarland
Milford Regional Medical Center	Milford	Massachusetts	508-473-1190	www.milfordregional.org
Missouri Baptist Medical Center	Town & Country	Missouri	314-996-5000	www.missouribaptistmedicalcenter.org
Monmouth Medical Center - Southern Campus	Lakewood	New Jersey	732-363-1900	www.sbhcs.com
Montefiore Medical Center	Bronx	New York	718-920-4321	www.montefiore.org
Morristown Medical Center	Morristown	New Jersey	973-971-5450	www.morristownmemorialhospital.org
Mount Auburn Hospital	Cambridge	Massachusetts	617-492-3500	www.mountauburnhospital.org
Mount Sinai Hospital	New York	New York	212-241-7981	www.mountsinai.org
Mount Sinai Medical Center	Miami Beach	Florida	305-674-2121	www.msmc.com
New York - Presbyterian Hospital	New York	New York	212-746-4189	www.nyp.org
Newton Memorial Hospital	Newton	New Jersey	973-383-2121	www.itsyourlife.com
North Shore Medical Center	Salem	Massachusetts	978-741-1215	www.nsmc.partners.org
North Shore University Hospital	Manhasset	New York	516-562-0100	www.northshorelij.com
Northern Westchester Hospital	Mount Kisco	New York	914-666-1200	www.nwhc.net
Northwestern Memorial Hospital	Chicago	Illinois	312-926-2000	www.nmh.org
Norton Community Hospital	Norton	Virginia	703-679-8865	www.nchosp.org
NYU Hospitals Center	New York	New York	212-263-7300	www.med.nyu.edu
Oakwood Hospital - Dearborn	Dearborn	Michigan	313-593-7125	www.oakwood.org
Olympia Medical Center	Los Angeles	California	310-657-5900	www.olympiamc.com
Oroville Hospital	Oroville	California	530-533-8500	www.orovillehospital.com
Our Lady of Lourdes Medical Center	Camden	New Jersey	856-757-3500	www.lourdesnet.org
Overlook Medical Center	Summit	New Jersey	908-522-2000	www.atlantichealth.org
Owensboro Health Regional Hospital	Owensboro	Kentucky	270-688-2000	www.omhs.org
Palos Community Hospital	Palos Heights	Illinois	708-923-4000	www.paloshospital.org
Paradise Valley Hospital	National City	California	619-470-4321	www.paradisevalleyhospital.org
Park Plaza Hospital	Houston	Texas	713-527-5019	www.parkplazahospital.com
Parkland Health Center	Farmington	Missouri	573-431-6005	www.bjc.org
Piedmont Hospital	Atlanta	Georgia	404-605-5000	www.piedmonthospital.org
Portland VA Medical Center	Portland	Oregon	503-220-8262	www.va.gov/portland/index.asp
Presbyterian Intercommunity Hospital	Whittier	California	526-698-0811	www.whittierpres.com
Presence Resurrection Medical Center	Chicago	Illinois	773-774-8000	www.reshealthcare.org
Presence Saint Joseph Hospital - Chicago	Chicago	Illinois	773-665-3000	www.res-health.org
Presence Saint Joseph Medical Center	Joliet	Illinois	815-725-7133	www.provena.org/stjoes
Presence Saint Marys Hospital	Kankakee	Illinois	815-937-2490	www.provenastmarys.com
Providence Hospital & Medical Centers	Southfield	Michigan	248-849-3011	www.stjohn.org/providence
Providence Little Co of Mary Medical Center Torrance	Torrance	California	310-540-7676	www.lcmhs.org
Providence Saint Joseph Medical Center	Burbank	California	818-843-5111	www.providence.org/losangeles
Providence Tarzana Medical Center	Tarzana	California	818-881-0800	www.encino-tarzana.com
Randolph Hospital	Asheboro	North Carolina	336-625-5151	www.randolphhospital.org
Raritan Bay Medical Center	Perth Amboy	New Jersey	732-442-3700	www.rbmc.org
Reading Hospital	Reading	Pennsylvania	610-988-8000	www.readinghospital.org

Hospital	City	State	Phone	Web Site
Rex Hospital	Raleigh	North Carolina	919-784-3100	www.rexhealth.com
Rhode Island Hospital	Providence	Rhode Island	401-444-4000	www.rhodeislandhospital.org
Rio Grande Regional Hospital	Mcallen	Texas	956-632-6000	www.riohealth.com
Riverside Medical Center	Kankakee	Illinois	815-933-1671	www.riversidehealthcare.org
Riverview Medical Center	Red Bank	New Jersey	732-741-2700	www.meridianhealth.com
Robert Wood Johnson University Hospital	New Brunswick	New Jersey	732-937-8900	www.rwjuh.edu
Rockingham Memorial Hospital	Harrisonburg	Virginia	540-689-1000	www.rmhonline.com
Ronald Reagan UCLA Medical Center	Los Angeles	California	310-825-6301	www.uclahealth.org
Saint Clare's Hospital	Denville	New Jersey	973-625-6000	www.saintclares.org
Saint Francis Hospital	Tulsa	Oklahoma	918-494-2200	www.saintfrancis.com
Saint Vincent Medical Center	Los Angeles	California	213-484-7111	www.stvincent.dochs.org
San Francisco VA Medical Center	San Francisco	California	415-221-4810	www.sanfrancisco.va.gov
San Gabriel Valley Medical Center	San Gabriel	California	626-289-5454	www.sangabrielvalleymedctr.org
Santa Monica - UCLA Medical Center & Orthopaedic Hospital	Santa Monica	California	310-319-4000	www.healthcare.ucla.edu
Scott & White Hospital - Round Rock	Round Rock	Texas	512-509-0100	www.sw.org
Scott & White Memorial Hospital	Temple	Texas	254-724-2111	www.sw.org
Scripps Memorial Hospital La Jolla	La Jolla	California	858-626-4123	www.scrippshealth.org
Scripps Mercy Hospital	San Diego	California	619-294-8111	www.scrippshealth.org
Sharon Regional Health System	Sharon	Pennsylvania	724-983-3800	www.sharonregional.com
Sinai Hospital of Baltimore	Baltimore	Maryland	410-601-5131	www.sinai-balt.com
South Pointe Hospital	Warrensville Heights	Ohio	216-491-6000	www.southpointehospital.org
Southampton Hospital	Southampton	New York	516-726-8200	www.southamptonhospital.org
Southcoast Hospital Group	Fall River	Massachusetts	508-679-3131	www.southcoast.org/charlton
Southwest General Health Center	Middleburg Heights	Ohio	440-816-8000	www.swgeneral.com
Spartanburg Regional Medical Center	Spartanburg	South Carolina	864-560-6000	www.srhs.com
Spring Valley Hospital Medical Center	Las Vegas	Nevada	702-853-3000	www.springvalleyhospital.com
Saint Alexius Medical Center	Hoffman Estates	Illinois	847-843-2000	www.alexianbrothershealth.org
Saint Anthony Community Hospital	Warwick	New York	845-986-2276	www.stanthonycommunityhosp.org
Saint Luke's Hospital Bethlehem	Bethlehem	Pennsylvania	610-954-4000	www.slhn-lehighvalley.org
Saint Luke's Roosevelt Hospital	New York	New York	212-523-4000	www.wehealny.org
Saint Luke's Episcopal Hospital	Houston	Texas	832-355-1000	www.sleh.com
Saint Luke's Hospital	Cedar Rapids	Iowa	319-369-7211	www.crstlukes.com
Saint Luke's Hospital	Chesterfield	Missouri	314-434-1500	www.goodhealthmatters.com
Saint Marys Hospital	Madison	Wisconsin	608-251-6100	www.stmarysmadison.com
Saint Peter's Hospital	Albany	New York	518-525-1550	www.stpetershealthcare.org
Stafford Hospital	Stafford	Virginia	540-741-9000	www.marywashingtonhealthcare.com
Swedish Covenant Hospital	Chicago	Illinois	773-878-8200	www.swedishcovenant.org
Tomball Regional Medical Center	Tomball	Texas	281-351-1623	www.tomballhospital.org
Tri Valley Health System	Cambridge	Nebraska	308-697-3329	www.trivalleyhealth.com
Tri - City Regional Medical Center	Hawaiian Gardens	California	562-860-0401	www.tri-cityrmc.org
Trumbull Memorial Hospital	Warren	Ohio	330-841-9011	www.trumhosp.org
Tufts Medical Center	Boston	Massachusetts	617-636-5000	www.tuftsmedicalcenter.org
United Regional Medical Center	Manchester	Tennessee	931-728-3586	www.urmchealthcare.com
University Medical Center of Princeton at Plainsboro	Plainsboro	New Jersey	866-460-4776	www.princetonhcs.org
University Hospitals - Elyria Medical Center	Elyria	Ohio	440-329-7500	www.emh-healthcare.org
University of California San Diego Medical Center	San Diego	California	619-543-6222	www.health.ucsd.edu
University of Maryland Shore Medical Center at Easton	Easton	Maryland	410-822-1000	www.shorehealth.org
University of Michigan Health System	Ann Arbor	Michigan	734-764-1505	www.med.umich.edu
University of Texas Health Science Center at Tyler	Tyler	Texas	903-877-7777	www.uthct.edu
UPMC Mckeesport	Mc Keesport	Pennsylvania	412-664-2000	www.selectmedicalcorp.com
VA Boston Healthcare System - Jamaica Plain	Jamaica Plain	Massachusetts	617-232-9500	www.vaww.visn1.med.va.gov/boston
VA North Florida/South Georgia Healthcare System	Gainesville	Florida	352-376-1611	www.northflorida.va.gov
VA Sierra Nevada Healthcare System	Reno	Nevada	775-328-1263	www.reno.va.gov
Valley Hospital	Ridgewood	New Jersey	201-447-8000	www.valleyhealth.com
VHS Harlingen Hospital Company	Harlingen	Texas	956-389-1100	www.vbmc.org
Virginia Mason Medical Center	Seattle	Washington	206-223-6600	www.vmmc.org
W Palm Beach VA Medical Center	West Palm Beach	Florida	561-422-8600	www.va.gov
Waukesha Memorial Hospital	Waukesha	Wisconsin	262-928-1000	www.waukeshamemorial.org
Weirton Medical Center	Weirton	West Virginia	304-797-6000	www.weirtonmedical.com
West Anaheim Medical Center	Anaheim	California	714-827-3000	www.wamc.phcs.us
West Haven VA Medical Center	West Haven	Connecticut	203-932-5711	www.visn1.med.va.gov/vact
Wheaton Franciscan Healthcare Saint Francis	Milwaukee	Wisconsin	414-647-5000	www.mywheaton.org
White Memorial Medical Center	Los Angeles	California	323-268-5000	www.whitememorial.com
William Beaumont Hospital - Troy	Troy	Michigan	248-964-8800	www.beaumonthospitals.com
Willis Knighton Medical Center	Shreveport	Louisiana	318-212-4000	www.wkhs.com//locations/medicalcenter.aspx
Yale-New Haven Hospital	New Haven	Connecticut	203-688-4242	www.ynhh.org

Note: Table shows hospitals nationwide whose pneumonia 30-day risk-adjusted mortality rate is better (lower) than U.S. rate of 11.9%

Hospitals whose Pneumonia 30-Day Mortality Rate is Worse (Higher) than the U.S. National Rate

Hospital	City	State	Phone	Web Site
Abilene Regional Medical Center	Abilene	Texas	325-428-1000	www.abileneregional.com
Acmh Hospital	Kittanning	Pennsylvania	724-543-8404	www.acmh.org
Albemarle Hospital Authority	Elizabeth City	North Carolina	252-335-0531	www.albemarlehealth.org
Antelope Valley Hospital	Lancaster	California	661-949-5000	www.avhospital.org
Aspirus Grand View Hospital	Ironwood	Michigan	906-932-2525	www.gvhs.org
Augusta VA Medical Center	Augusta	Georgia	706-823-2201	www.va.gov
Auxilio Mutuo Hospital	Hato Rey	Puerto Rico	787-758-2000	www.auxiliopr.com
Avera Sacred Heart Hospital	Yankton	South Dakota	605-668-8000	www.avera.org/sacred-heart
Bacon County Hospital	Alma	Georgia	912-632-8961	www.baconcountyhospital.com
Baptist Memorial Hospital/Golden Triangle	Columbus	Mississippi	662-244-1500	www.bmhcc.org/facilities/goldentriangle
Baptist Memorial Hospital Union City	Union City	Tennessee	731-885-2410	www.bmhcc.org
Baxter Regional Medical Center	Mountain Home	Arkansas	870-508-1000	www.baxterregional.org
Bay Area Hospital	Coos Bay	Oregon	541-269-8111	www.bayareahospital.org
Bolivar Medical Center	Cleveland	Mississippi	662-846-2551	www.bolivarmedical.com
Bon Secours Maryview Medical Center	Portsmouth	Virginia	757-398-2200	www.bonsecourshamptonroads.com
Caldwell Medical Center	Princeton	Kentucky	270-365-0300	www.caldwellhosp.org
Cameron Regional Medical Center	Cameron	Missouri	816-632-2101	www.cameronregional.org
Carilion Roanoke Memorial Hospital	Roanoke	Virginia	540-981-7000	www.carilion.com/crmh
Carondelet Saint Joseph's Hospital	Tucson	Arizona	520-873-3000	www.carondelet.org
Carson Tahoe Regional Medical Center	Carson City	Nevada	775-445-8000	www.carsontahoehospital.com
Catawba Valley Medical Center	Hickory	North Carolina	828-326-3809	www.catawbavalleymc.org
Central Carolina Hospital	Sanford	North Carolina	919-774-2100	www.centralcarolinahosp.com
Citizens Memorial Hospital	Bolivar	Missouri	417-326-6000	www.citizensmemorial.com
Cleveland Regional Medical Center	Shelby	North Carolina	704-487-3000	www.clevelandregional.org
Community Hospital East	Indianapolis	Indiana	317-355-5411	www.ecommunity.com
Conway Regional Medical Center	Conway	Arkansas	501-329-3831	www.conwayregional.org
Coshocton County Memorial Hospital	Coshocton	Ohio	740-622-6411	www.ccmh.com
Dallas County Medical Center	Fordyce	Arkansas	870-352-6300	www.dallascountymedicalcenter.com
Dekalb Regional Medical Center	Fort Payne	Alabama	256-845-3150	www.baptistmedical.org
Delano Regional Medical Center	Delano	California	661-725-4800	www.drmc.com
Desert Springs Hospital	Las Vegas	Nevada	702-369-7600	www.desertspringshospital.net/p12.html
Doctors Medical Center	Modesto	California	209-578-1211	www.dmc-modesto.com
East Georgia Regional Medical Center	Statesboro	Georgia	912-486-1500	www.egrmc.com
East Liverpool City Hospital	East Liverpool	Ohio	330-385-7200	www.elch.org
Eastern Niagara Hospital	Lockport	New York	716-514-5700	www.enhs.org
El Centro Regional Medical Center	El Centro	California	760-339-7100	www.ecrmc.org
Eliza Coffee Memorial Hospital	Florence	Alabama	256-768-8400	www.chgroup.org
Erlanger Medical Center	Chattanooga	Tennessee	423-778-7000	www.erlanger.org
Essentia Health Saint Mary's Medical Center	Duluth	Minnesota	218-786-4000	www.smdc.org
Florida Hospital Deland	Deland	Florida	386-943-4772	www.fhdeland.org
Floyd County Memorial Hospital	Charles City	Iowa	641-228-6830	www.fcmc.us.com
Franklin General Hospital	Hampton	Iowa	641-456-5000	www.franklingeneral.com
Franklin Medical Center	Winnsboro	Louisiana	318-435-9411	www.fmc-cares.com
Fremont Area Medical Center	Fremont	Nebraska	402-721-1610	www.famc.org
Frye Regional Medical Center	Hickory	North Carolina	828-322-6070	www.fryemedctr.com
Fulton County Hospital	Salem	Arkansas	870-895-2691	www.fultoncountyhospital.org
GV (Sonny) Montgomery VA Medical Center Jackson	Jackson	Mississippi	601-362-4471	www.visn16.med.va.gov
Gadsden Regional Medical Center	Gadsden	Alabama	256-494-4000	www.gadsdenregional.com
Galesburg Cottage Hospital	Galesburg	Illinois	309-345-4555	www.cottagehospital.com
Gateway Medical Center	Clarksville	Tennessee	931-502-1000	www.todaysgateway.com
GHS Laurens County Memorial Hospital	Clinton	South Carolina	864-833-9100	www.lchcs.org
Glenwood Regional Medical Center	West Monroe	Louisiana	318-329-4600	www.grmc.com
Good Samaritan Hospital	Kearney	Nebraska	308-865-7100	www.gshs.org
Good Samaritan Hospital	Lebanon	Pennsylvania	717-270-7500	www.gshleb.org
Greenview Regional Hospital	Bowling Green	Kentucky	270-793-1000	www.greenviewhospital.com
Grossmont Hospital	La Mesa	California	619-465-0711	www.sharp.com
Halifax Health Medical Center	Daytona Beach	Florida	386-254-4000	www.halifax.org
Hammond Henry Hospital	Geneseo	Illinois	309-944-6431	www.hammondhenry.com
Harrison County Hospital	Corydon	Indiana	812-738-4251	www.hchin.org
Harrison Memorial Hospital	Cynthiana	Kentucky	859-234-2300	www.harrisonmemhosp.com
Harton Regional Medical Center	Tullahoma	Tennessee	931-393-3000	www.hartonmedicalcenter.com
Helen Keller Memorial Hospital	Sheffield	Alabama	256-386-4556	www.helenkeller.com
Helena Regional Medical Center	Helena	Arkansas	870-338-5800	www.helenaregionalmedicalcenter.com
Hemet Valley Medical Center	Hemet	California	951-652-2811	www.valleyhealthsystem.com/hemmain
Highland Hospital	Rochester	New York	585-473-2200	www.urmc.rochester.edu

Hospital	City	State	Phone	Web Site
Highlands Regional Medical Center	Sebring	Florida	863-385-6101	www.highlandsregional.com
Highline Medical Center	Burien	Washington	206-244-9970	www.hchnet.org
Hospital Pavia Santurce	Fernandez Juncos	Puerto Rico	787-727-6060	www.paviahospitalsanturce.com
Howard Memorial Hospital	Nashville	Arkansas	870-845-4400	www.howardmemorial.com
Hutchinson Regional Medical Center	Hutchinson	Kansas	620-665-2001	www.hutchinsonhospital.com
Iberia General Hospital & Medical Center	New Iberia	Louisiana	337-364-0441	www.iberiamedicalcenter.com
Indiana University Health Bloomington Hospital	Bloomington	Indiana	812-353-9555	www.bloomingtonhospital.org
Indiana University Health La Porte Hospital	La Porte	Indiana	219-326-1234	www.laportehealth.org
Inspira Medical Center Vineland	Vineland	New Jersey	856-641-6610	www.sjhs.com
Integris Grove Hospital	Grove	Oklahoma	918-786-2243	www.integris-health.com
IU Health Goshen Hospital	Goshen	Indiana	574-364-1000	www.goshenhosp.com
Jackson Hospital & Clinic	Montgomery	Alabama	334-293-8000	www.jackson.org
Jackson Memorial Hospital	Miami	Florida	305-585-1111	www.jhsmiami.org
Jacksonville Medical Center	Jacksonville	Alabama	256-782-4538	www.jmchealth.com
Jane Phillips Medical Center	Bartlesville	Oklahoma	918-333-7200	www.jpmc.org
Jeff Davis Hospital	Hazlehurst	Georgia	912-375-7781	www.jeffdavishospital.org
Jennie Stuart Medical Center	Hopkinsville	Kentucky	270-887-0100	www.jsmc.org
JFK Medical Center - A M Yelencsics Comm Hospital	Edison	New Jersey	732-321-7000	www.jfkmc.org
Keokuk Area Hospital	Keokuk	Iowa	319-524-7150	www.keokukhealthsystems.org
Lafayette General Medical Center	Lafayette	Louisiana	337-289-7991	www.lafayettegeneral.org
Lake Charles Memorial Hospital	Lake Charles	Louisiana	337-494-3200	www.lcmh.com
Lake Cumberland Regional Hospital	Somerset	Kentucky	606-679-7441	www.lakecumberlandhospital.com
Lake Granbury Medical Center	Granbury	Texas	817-573-2683	www.lakegranburymedicalcenter.com
Lexington Medical Center	West Columbia	South Carolina	803-791-2000	www.lexmed.com
Lexington VA Medical Center	Lexington	Kentucky	859-233-4511	www.lexington.va.gov
Livingston Regional Hospital	Livingston	Tennessee	931-823-5611	www.livingstonregionalhospital.com
Lompoc Valley Medical Center	Lompoc	California	805-737-3300	www.lompochospital.org
Louisville VA Medical Center	Louisville	Kentucky	502-287-4000	www.va.gov/603louisville
Madera Community Hospital	Madera	California	559-675-5555	www.maderahospital.org
Mahaska Health Partnership	Oskaloosa	Iowa	641-672-3100	www.mahaskahospital.com
Margaret Mary Community Hospital	Batesville	Indiana	812-934-6624	www.mmch.org
Marion General Hospital	Columbia	Mississippi	601-736-6303	
Marshall Medical Center South	Boaz	Alabama	256-593-8310	www.mmcenters.com/mmcsouth.php
McGehee Hospital	Mcgehee	Arkansas	870-222-5600	
Medical Center Hospital	Odessa	Texas	432-640-4000	www.mchodessa.com
Memorial Medical Center	Modesto	California	209-526-4500	www.memorialmedicalcenter.org
Memorial Healthcare	Owosso	Michigan	989-723-5211	www.memorialhealthcare.org
Memorial Hospital & Manor	Bainbridge	Georgia	229-246-3500	www.mh-m.org
Memorial Hospital of Martinsville & Henry County	Martinsville	Virginia	276-666-7200	www.martinsvillehospital.com
Memorial Hospital of South Bend	South Bend	Indiana	574-647-1000	www.qualityoflife.org
Memorial Medical Center of East Texas	Lufkin	Texas	936-634-8111	www.mymemorialhealth.org
Mercy Health - West Hospital	Cincinnati	Ohio	513-215-5000	www.e-mercy.com/west-hospital.aspx
Mercy Hospital Oklahoma City	Oklahoma City	Oklahoma	405-752-3754	www.mercyok.net/mhc
Mercy Hospital Springfield	Springfield	Missouri	417-820-2000	www.stjohns.com
Mercy Medical Center	Merced	California	209-564-5000	www.mercymercedcares.org
Mercy Medical Center	Rockville Centre	New York	516-705-2525	www.mercymedicalcenter.info
Mercy Medical Center - Mount Shasta	Mount Shasta	California	530-926-6111	www.mercymtshasta.org
Mercy Memorial Health Center	Ardmore	Oklahoma	405-223-5400	www.mercyok.com/mmhc
Methodist Healthcare Memphis Hospitals	Memphis	Tennessee	901-516-8274	www.methodisthealth.org
Mid Coast Hospital	Brunswick	Maine	207-729-0181	www.midcoasthealth.com
Midtown Medical Center	Columbus	Georgia	706-571-1000	www.columbusregional.com
Milford Hospital	Milford	Connecticut	203-876-4000	www.milfordhospital.org
Mississippi Baptist Medical Center	Jackson	Mississippi	601-968-1000	www.mbmc.org
Mizell Memorial Hospital	Opp	Alabama	334-493-3541	www.mizellmh.com
Mobile Infirmary	Mobile	Alabama	251-435-4700	www.mimc.com
Morris Hospital & Healthcare Centers	Morris	Illinois	815-942-2932	www.morrishospital.org
Mount Carmel West	Columbus	Ohio	614-234-5000	www.mountcarmelhealth.com
Multicare Good Samaritan Hospital	Puyallup	Washington	253-697-2102	www.multicare.org/goodsam
Neshoba County General Hospital	Philadelphia	Mississippi	601-663-1200	www.neshobageneral.com
New London Family Medical Center	New London	Wisconsin	920-531-2000	www.thedacare.org
North Mississippi Medical Center	Tupelo	Mississippi	662-377-3000	www.nmhs.net/nmmc
North Valley Hospital	Whitefish	Montana	406-863-3550	www.nvhosp.org
Northern Louisiana Medical Center	Ruston	Louisiana	318-254-2100	www.lincolnhealth.com
Novant Health Rowan Medical Center	Salisbury	North Carolina	704-210-5000	www.rowan.org
Novant Health Thomasville Medical Center	Thomasville	North Carolina	336-472-2000	www.thomasvillemedicalcenter.org
Och Regional Medical Center	Starkville	Mississippi	662-323-4320	www.och.org
Ohio Valley General Hospital	Mckees Rocks	Pennsylvania	412-777-6161	www.ohiovalleyhospital.org

Hospital	City	State	Phone	Web Site
Olympic Medical Center	Port Angeles	Washington	360-417-7000	www.olympicmedical.org
Orange Park Medical Center	Orange Park	Florida	904-276-8500	www.opmedical.com
Paris Regional Medical Center	Paris	Texas	903-785-4521	www.parisregional.com
Passavant Area Hospital	Jacksonville	Illinois	217-245-9551	www.passavanthospital.com
Petaluma Valley Hospital	Petaluma	California	707-778-1111	www.stjosephhealth.org
Peterson Regional Medical Center	Kerrville	Texas	830-896-4200	www.petersonrmc.com
Piedmont Medical Center	Rock Hill	South Carolina	803-329-1234	www.piedmontmedicalcenter.com
Pike Community Hospital	Waverly	Ohio	740-947-2186	www.adena.org
Pinnacle Health Hospitals	Harrisburg	Pennsylvania	717-782-5181	www.pinnaclehealth.org
Pottstown Memorial Medical Center	Pottstown	Pennsylvania	610-327-7000	www.pmmctr.org
Rappahannock General Hospital	Kilmarnock	Virginia	804-435-8000	www.rgh-hospital.com
Redlands Community Hospital	Redlands	California	909-335-5500	www.redlandshospital.com
River Parishes Hospital	Laplace	Louisiana	985-652-7000	www.riverparisheshospital.com
River Valley Medical Center	Dardanelle	Arkansas	479-229-4677	
Rockcastle County Hospital	Mount Vernon	Kentucky	606-256-2195	www.rockcastlehospital.com
Rush Foundation Hospital	Meridian	Mississippi	601-483-0011	www.rushhealthsystems.org
Rush Memorial Hospital	Rushville	Indiana	765-932-7513	www.rushmemorial.com
Russell Hospital	Alexander City	Alabama	256-329-7100	www.russellmedcenter.com
Saint Joseph Mount Sterling	Mount Sterling	Kentucky	859-498-1220	www.marychiles.org
San Gorgonio Memorial Hospital	Banning	California	951-769-2101	www.sgmh.org
San Juan VA Medical Center	San Juan	Puerto Rico	800-449-8729	www.visn8.med.va.gov/caribbean
Sentara Careplex Hospital	Hampton	Virginia	757-736-1000	www.sentara.com
Sentara Leigh Hospital	Norfolk	Virginia	757-261-6601	www.sentara.com
Sentara Obici Hospital	Suffolk	Virginia	757-934-4000	www.sentara.com
Seven Rivers Regional Medical Center	Crystal River	Florida	352-795-6560	www.srrmc.com
Shands Live Oak Regional Medical Center	Live Oak	Florida	904-362-1413	www.shands.org
Sierra View District Hospital	Porterville	California	559-784-1110	www.sierra-view.com
Skyridge Medical Center	Cleveland	Tennessee	423-339-4132	www.skyridgemedcenter.com
Somerset Medical Center	Somerville	New Jersey	908-685-2200	www.somersetmedicalcenter.com
South Central Regional Medical Center	Laurel	Mississippi	601-649-4000	www.scrmc.com
South Shore Hospital	South Weymouth	Massachusetts	781-340-8000	www.southshorehospital.org
Southampton Memorial Hospital	Franklin	Virginia	757-569-6100	www.smhfranklin.com
Southern Virginia Regional Medical Center	Emporia	Virginia	434-348-4400	www.svrmc.com
Spectrum Health - Reed City Campus	Reed City	Michigan	231-832-3271	www.spectrum-health.org
Spencer Municipal Hospital	Spencer	Iowa	712-264-8300	www.spencerhospital.org
Springfield Regional Medical Center	Springfield	Ohio	937-523-1000	www.communityhospital.com
Springs Memorial Hospital	Lancaster	South Carolina	803-286-1481	www.springsmemorial.com
Saint Anthony Regional Hospital & Nursing Home	Carroll	Iowa	712-792-3581	www.stanthonyhospital.org
Saint Anthony Shawnee Hospital	Shawnee	Oklahoma	405-273-2270	www.unityhealthcenter.com
Saint Catherine Hospital	Garden City	Kansas	620-272-2561	www.stcath-hosp.org
Saint Francis Community Hospital	Federal Way	Washington	253-944-8100	www.fhshealth.org
Saint Francis Hospital	Litchfield	Illinois	217-324-2191	www.stfrancis-litchfield.org
Saint Francis Hospital	Memphis	Tennessee	901-765-1000	www.saintfrancishosp.com
Saint Francis Hospital	Columbus	Georgia	706-596-4020	www.wecareforlife.com
Saint Francis - Downtown	Greenville	South Carolina	864-255-1000	www.stfrancishealth.org
Saint Joseph Hospital	Orange	California	714-633-9111	www.sjo.org
Saint Joseph Hospital & Health Center	Kokomo	Indiana	765-456-5300	www.stvincent.org
Saint Joseph's Hospital - Savannah	Savannah	Georgia	912-819-4100	www.sjchs.org
Saint Joseph's Medical Center of Stockton	Stockton	California	209-943-2000	www.stjospehscares.org
Saint Peter's Hospital	Helena	Montana	406-442-2480	www.stpetes.org
Saint Vincent Dunn Hospital	Bedford	Indiana	812-275-3331	www.stvincent.org/St-Vincent-Dunn
Saint Vincent's East	Birmingham	Alabama	205-838-3122	www.nolandhealth.com
Starr Regional Medical Center Athens	Athens	Tennessee	423-745-1411	www.athensrmc.com
Sumner Regional Medical Center	Gallatin	Tennessee	615-452-4210	www.mysumnermedical.com
Sunbury Community Hospital	Sunbury	Pennsylvania	570-286-3333	www.schopc.org
Sunrise Hospital & Medical Center	Las Vegas	Nevada	702-731-8000	www.sunrisehospital.com
Teche Regional Medical Center	Morgan City	Louisiana	985-384-2200	www.techeregional.com
Terrebonne General Medical Center	Houma	Louisiana	985-873-4141	www.tgmc.com
Texoma Medical Center	Denison	Texas	903-416-4000	www.texomamedicalcenter.net
Thibodaux Regional Medical Center	Thibodaux	Louisiana	985-447-5500	www.thibodaux.com
Thomas Memorial Hospital	South Charleston	West Virginia	304-766-3600	www.thomaswv.org
Trinity Medical Center	Birmingham	Alabama	205-592-1000	www.bhsala.com/montclair
Trinity Rock Island	Rock Island	Illinois	309-779-5000	www.trinityqc.com
Tuality Community Hospital	Hillsboro	Oregon	503-681-1111	www.tuality.com
Twin County Regional Hospital	Galax	Virginia	276-236-8181	www.tcrh.org
Union General Hospital	Farmerville	Louisiana	318-368-9751	www.uniongen.org
United Health Services Hospitals	Johnson City	New York	607-763-6000	www.vhs.ent

Hospital	City	State	Phone	Web Site
University Mcduffie County Regional Medical Center	Thomson	Georgia	706-595-1411	www.mrmc.org
University of Missouri Health Care	Columbia	Missouri	573-882-4141	www.missouri.edu
Upson Regional Medical Center	Thomaston	Georgia	706-647-8111	www.urmc.org
Upstate New York VA Healthcare System - Western NY	Buffalo	New York	716-862-3611	www.buffalo.va.gov
Utah Valley Regional Medical Center	Provo	Utah	801-373-7850	www.intermountainhealthcare.org/hospitals/uvrmc
VA Middle Tennessee Healthcare System	Nashville	Tennessee	615-327-5332	www.tennesseevalley.va.gov
VA Salt Lake City Healthcare - George E. Wahlen VA	Salt Lake City	Utah	801-584-1211	www1.va.gov/directory/guide/facility.asp?
Vidant Edgecombe Hospital	Tarboro	North Carolina	252-641-7700	www.vidanthealth.com/edgecombe
Vista Medical Center East	Waukegan	Illinois	847-360-4000	www.vistahealth.com
Western Plains Medical Complex	Dodge City	Kansas	620-225-8400	www.westernplainsmc.com
Wilkes-Barre General Hospital	Wilkes-Barre	Pennsylvania	570-829-8111	www.wvhcs.org
Wilson Medical Center	Wilson	North Carolina	252-399-8040	www.wilmed.org/contact.asp
Wise Regional Health System	Decatur	Texas	940-627-5921	www.wiseregional.com
Woodland Heights Medical Center	Lufkin	Texas	936-634-8311	www.woodlandheights.net
Woodland Memorial Hospital	Woodland	California	530-662-3961	www.woodlandhealthcare.org
Yakima Valley Memorial Hospital	Yakima	Washington	509-575-8000	www.yakimamemorialhospital.org
Yuma Regional Medical Center	Yuma	Arizona	928-336-7275	www.yumaregional.org

Note: Table shows hospitals nationwide whose pneumonia 30-day risk-adjusted mortality rate is worse (higher) than U.S. rate of 11.9%

Hospital Mortality from Heart Attack: State and National Summary

Area	Number of Hospitals			
	Better than U.S. National Rate[1]	Worse than U.S. National Rate[2]	No Different than U.S. National Rate[3]	Number of Cases Too Small[4]
U.S. and Territories	77	19	2579	1889
Alabama	0	0	50	50
Alaska	0	0	5	15
American Samoa	0	0	0	1
Arizona	1	0	49	19
Arkansas	1	2	30	40
California	7	1	219	103
Colorado	0	0	33	35
Connecticut	2	0	28	1
Delaware	1	0	5	1
District of Columbia	0	0	6	2
Florida	3	1	157	22
Georgia	0	0	74	65
Guam	0	0	1	0
Hawaii	0	0	12	4
Idaho	0	0	10	23
Illinois	8	0	112	61
Indiana	1	0	68	49
Iowa	0	0	35	81
Kansas	1	0	29	91
Kentucky	0	1	51	43
Louisiana	0	1	49	52
Maine	1	1	30	5
Maryland	1	0	40	6
Massachusetts	4	0	54	6
Michigan	6	3	72	49
Minnesota	1	0	36	85
Mississippi	0	0	34	50
Missouri	4	0	57	54
Montana	0	0	8	39
N. Mariana Islands	0	0	0	1
Nebraska	0	0	20	56
Nevada	0	1	18	13
New Hampshire	1	1	17	6
New Jersey	8	1	54	3
New Mexico	0	0	13	26
New York	10	1	141	31
North Carolina	2	0	83	24
North Dakota	0	1	8	32
Ohio	1	0	112	47
Oklahoma	0	0	35	71
Oregon	0	0	29	31
Pennsylvania	6	1	122	33
Puerto Rico	0	0	21	24
Rhode Island	2	0	9	0
South Carolina	0	0	42	20
South Dakota	1	0	10	40
Tennessee	1	0	66	46
Texas	2	3	189	149
Utah	0	0	16	19
Vermont	0	0	10	5
Virgin Islands	0	0	1	1
Virginia	0	0	73	9
Washington	0	0	44	40
West Virginia	1	0	29	24
Wisconsin	0	0	60	62
Wyoming	0	0	3	24

Note: (1) 30-day risk-adjusted mortality rate is better (lower) than U.S. rate of 15.2%; (2) 30-day risk-adjusted mortality rate is worse (higher) than U.S. rate of 15.2%; (3) 30-day risk-adjusted mortality rate is about the same as U.S. rate of 15.2%; (4) The number of cases is too small to classify the hospital

Hospital Mortality from Heart Failure: State and National Summary

Area	Number of Hospitals			
	Better than U.S. National Rate[1]	Worse than U.S. National Rate[2]	No Different than U.S. National Rate[3]	Number of Cases Too Small[4]
U.S. and Territories	181	139	3732	725
Alabama	1	2	89	8
Alaska	0	1	9	12
American Samoa	0	0	0	1
Arizona	2	1	57	17
Arkansas	0	11	59	7
California	30	10	246	51
Colorado	0	0	55	19
Connecticut	4	3	24	1
Delaware	1	0	6	0
District of Columbia	2	0	6	0
Florida	8	5	166	8
Georgia	1	2	126	15
Guam	0	0	1	0
Hawaii	0	0	14	5
Idaho	0	1	21	15
Illinois	16	5	156	7
Indiana	3	7	108	2
Iowa	0	2	95	21
Kansas	0	1	83	49
Kentucky	0	1	92	3
Louisiana	2	6	82	19
Maine	0	1	34	2
Maryland	9	2	35	1
Massachusetts	14	1	47	2
Michigan	12	3	106	14
Minnesota	2	0	81	48
Mississippi	0	3	77	18
Missouri	4	5	96	11
Montana	0	0	26	35
N. Mariana Islands	0	0	0	1
Nebraska	0	2	48	35
Nevada	1	2	27	5
New Hampshire	0	0	25	1
New Jersey	13	1	52	0
New Mexico	0	2	30	9
New York	13	7	156	7
North Carolina	4	3	97	8
North Dakota	0	0	24	20
Ohio	6	3	144	13
Oklahoma	2	3	84	29
Oregon	1	2	49	8
Pennsylvania	16	6	136	6
Puerto Rico	0	0	28	21
Rhode Island	0	0	11	1
South Carolina	1	3	57	2
South Dakota	0	1	26	26
Tennessee	0	2	107	7
Texas	8	8	294	62
Utah	0	1	24	17
Vermont	0	2	12	1
Virgin Islands	0	0	2	0
Virginia	1	2	79	2
Washington	0	7	58	24
West Virginia	1	0	47	6
Wisconsin	3	8	101	12
Wyoming	0	1	17	11

Note: (1) 30-day risk-adjusted mortality rate is better (lower) than U.S. rate of 11.7%; (2) 30-day risk-adjusted mortality rate is worse (higher) than U.S. rate of 11.7%; (3) 30-day risk-adjusted mortality rate is about the same as U.S. rate of 11.7%; (4) The number of cases is too small to classify the hospital

Hospital Mortality from Pneumonia: State and National Summary

Area	Number of Hospitals			
	Better than U.S. National Rate[1]	Worse than U.S. National Rate[2]	No Different than U.S. National Rate[3]	Number of Cases Too Small[4]
U.S. and Territories	203	223	4014	377
Alabama	0	13	84	4
Alaska	0	0	15	7
American Samoa	0	0	1	0
Arizona	3	2	66	10
Arkansas	0	8	66	3
California	34	19	244	45
Colorado	2	0	60	13
Connecticut	4	1	27	0
Delaware	0	0	7	0
District of Columbia	0	0	8	0
Florida	9	7	167	5
Georgia	1	11	128	3
Guam	0	0	1	0
Hawaii	0	0	14	8
Idaho	0	0	33	6
Illinois	16	7	157	4
Indiana	1	10	107	2
Iowa	2	6	105	5
Kansas	0	3	116	13
Kentucky	2	9	85	0
Louisiana	1	11	86	14
Maine	0	1	35	1
Maryland	8	0	37	1
Massachusetts	10	1	51	3
Michigan	10	3	116	6
Minnesota	1	1	112	17
Mississippi	0	10	78	10
Missouri	7	4	101	5
Montana	1	2	39	20
N. Mariana Islands	0	0	1	0
Nebraska	1	2	70	13
Nevada	3	3	24	6
New Hampshire	1	0	25	0
New Jersey	15	3	48	0
New Mexico	0	0	38	4
New York	14	6	161	4
North Carolina	6	9	94	4
North Dakota	0	0	39	5
Ohio	9	6	146	4
Oklahoma	2	5	101	11
Oregon	1	2	54	3
Pennsylvania	10	7	143	5
Puerto Rico	0	3	26	21
Rhode Island	1	0	10	1
South Carolina	1	5	55	2
South Dakota	0	1	49	6
Tennessee	2	13	96	5
Texas	13	10	306	48
Utah	0	2	33	7
Vermont	0	0	15	0
Virgin Islands	0	0	2	0
Virginia	5	10	67	5
Washington	2	5	73	9
West Virginia	1	1	51	1
Wisconsin	4	1	115	5
Wyoming	0	0	26	3

Note: (1) 30-day risk-adjusted mortality rate is better (lower) than U.S. rate of 11.9%; (2) 30-day risk-adjusted mortality rate is worse (higher) than U.S. rate of 11.9%; (3) 30-day risk-adjusted mortality rate is about the same as U.S. rate of 11.9%; (4) The number of cases is too small to classify the hospital

Appendix B: 30-Day Readmission Rates

What Do These Readmission Categories Show?

"Readmission" is when patients who have had a recent stay in the hospital go back into a hospital again. The information shows how often patients are readmitted within 30 days of discharge from a previous hospital stay for heart attack, heart failure, or pneumonia. Patients may have been readmitted back to the same hospital or to a different hospital or acute care facility. They may have been readmitted for the same condition as their recent hospital stay, or for a different reason.

This first part of this appendix shows hospitals with risk-adjusted 30-day unplanned readmission rates that are lower (better) or higher (worse) than the national rate for all three categories. Hospitals are shown to be better or worse than the U.S. national rate only if the data shows with 95% certainty, that the difference between their surgical complication rates and the U.S. national rate is not due to chance.

The second part of this appendix contains state and national summaries with the following column headers:

- **Better Than U.S. National Rate.** Hospitals in the Better Than U.S. National Rate category have risk-adjusted 30-day unplanned readmission rates that are lower than the U.S. National Rate, and with 95% certainty that this difference is not due to chance.
- **Worse Than U.S. National Rate.** Hospitals in the Worse Than U.S. National Rate category have risk-adjusted 30-day unplanned readmission rates that are higher than the U.S. National Rate, and with 95% certainty that this difference is not due to chance.
- **No Different Than U.S. National Rate.** Many hospitals in the No Different Than U.S. National Rate category have risk-adjusted 30-day unplanned readmission rates that are about the same as the U.S. National Rate. Other hospitals in this category have rates that are higher or lower than the U.S. National Rate, but without 95% certainty that these differences are not due to chance.
- **Number of Cases Too Small.** The number of cases is too small to classify the hospital..

Why are Readmission Rates for Individual Hospitals Not Shown?

Comparisons based on estimated readmission rates alone can be misleading. Risk-adjusted readmission rates are estimated for individual hospitals based on information taken from a particular time period. If a slightly different time period had been chosen, chances are that each hospital's results would have been somewhat different.

A range ("confidence interval" or in this case an "interval estimate") around estimates show how much variation might be due to this kind of chance. In this case, researchers are 95% confident that a hospital's readmission rate fell somewhere within this specified range. The smaller the range, the more precise the estimate.

When hospitals treat a very large number of patients, chance differences will not have much effect on the overall rates. The range will be small, and the estimated readmission rates will be more precise. In hospitals that treat smaller numbers of patients, however, even small chance differences could have a big impact on readmission rates. The 95% confidence interval, or range, will be large, and the estimated readmission rates will be less precise.

Because the number of patients treated at U.S. hospitals varies widely, the precision of hospitals' estimated readmission rates also varies.

Calculation of 30-Day Risk-Standardized Rates of Readmission

The 30-day readmission measures are estimates of unplanned readmission for any cause to any acute care hospital within 30 days of discharge from a hospitalization. Using unplanned readmissions within 30 days instead of over longer time periods (such as 90 days) eliminate factors outside hospitals' control such as other complicating illnesses, patients' own behavior, or care provided to patients after discharge. *The Comparative Guide to American Hospitals* reports the following 30-day readmission measures:

- 30-day unplanned readmission for heart attack (AMI) patients
- 30-day unplanned readmission for heart failure (HF) patients
- 30-day unplanned readmission for pneumonia patients
- 30-day unplanned readmission for hip/knee replacement patients
- 30-day overall rate of unplanned readmission after discharge from the hospital (hospital-wide readmission). Note: This measure includes patients admitted for internal medicine, surgery/gynecology, cardiorespiratory, cardiovascular, and neurology services. It is not a composite measure.

Which Patients are Included

The 30-day unplanned readmission measures include hospitalizations for Medicare beneficiaries aged 65 or older who were enrolled in Original Medicare (traditional fee-for-service Medicare) for the entire 12 months prior to their hospital admission (and for readmissions, for 30 days after their original admission). The AMI, heart failure, and pneumonia unplanned readmission measures also include patients aged 65 or older who were admitted to Veteran's Health Administration (VA) hospitals. Beneficiaries enrolled in Medicare managed care plans are not included. The unplanned readmission measures do not include patients who died during the index admission, or who left the hospital against medical advice.

Where the Information Comes From

The Centers for Medicare & Medicaid Services (CMS) calculates hospital-specific 30-day readmission rates using Medicare claims and eligibility information. The AMI, HF, and pneumonia readmission measures are also calculated using VA administrative data. Using administrative data makes it possible to calculate readmission rates without having to do medical chart reviews or requiring hospitals to report additional information to CMS.

Risk Adjustment

To make comparison of hospital performance equitable, the 30-day unplanned readmission measures adjust for patient characteristics that may make unplanned readmission more likely, even if the hospital provided higher quality of care. These characteristics include the patient's age, past medical history, and other diseases or conditions (comorbidities) the patient had when admitted that are known to increase the patient's risk of having an unplanned readmission.

Significance Testing

The statistical model used to calculate 30-day unplanned readmission measures also determines how precise the estimates are, and provides the upper and lower bounds of the 95% interval estimates for each hospital's readmission rates. Interval estimates, which are like confidence intervals, describe the level of uncertainty around the estimated readmission rates.

Comparing Individual Hospital Rates to the U.S. National Rate

To assign hospitals to performance categories, the hospital's interval estimate is compared to the U.S. national 30-day observed unplanned readmission rate. If the 95% interval estimate includes the national observed rate for that measure, the hospital's performance is in the "No Different than U.S. National Rate" category. If the entire 95% interval estimate is below the national observed rate for that measure, then the hospital is performing "Better Than U.S. National Rate." If the entire 95% interval estimate is above the national observed rate for that measure, its performance is "Worse Than U.S. National Rate." Hospitals with fewer than 25 eligible cases are placed into a separate category that indicates that the hospital did not have enough cases to reliably tell how well the hospital is performing.

Additional information

For more detail on how the 30-day unplanned readmission rates are calculated, please visit QualityNet—Readmission Measures at www.qualitynet.org.

Hospitals whose Acute Myocardial Infarction (Heart Attack) 30-Day Readmission Rate is Better (Lower) than the U.S. National Rate

Hospital	City	State	Phone	Web Site
Asante Rogue Regional Medical Center	Medford	Oregon	541-789-7000	www.asante.org
Aspirus Wausau Hospital	Wausau	Wisconsin	715-847-2121	www.aspirus.org
Aurora Saint Lukes Medical Center	Milwaukee	Wisconsin	414-649-6000	www.aurorahealthcare.org
Baylor Heart & Vascular Hospital	Dallas	Texas	214-820-0670	www.baylorhearthospital.com
Bellin Memorial Hospital	Green Bay	Wisconsin	920-433-3500	www.bellin.org
Central Washington Hospital	Wenatchee	Washington	509-662-1511	www.cwhs.com
Frye Regional Medical Center	Hickory	North Carolina	828-322-6070	www.fryemedctr.com
GHS Greenville Memorial Medical Center	Greenville	South Carolina	864-455-7000	www.ghs.org
Lancaster General Hospital	Lancaster	Pennsylvania	717-299-5511	www.lancastergeneral.org
Lovelace Medical Center	Albuquerque	New Mexico	505-727-8000	www.lovelace.com
Maine Medical Center	Portland	Maine	207-662-0111	www.mmc.org
Mercy Health Partners - Mercy Campus	Muskegon	Michigan	231-672-3901	www.mghp.com
Munroe Regional Medical Center	Ocala	Florida	352-351-7200	www.munroeregional.com
Parkview Regional Medical Center	Fort Wayne	Indiana	260-266-1000	www.parkview.com
Providence Sacred Heart Medical Center	Spokane	Washington	509-474-3040	www.shmc.org
Saint Joseph's Hospital of Atlanta	Atlanta	Georgia	678-843-5720	www.stjosephsatlanta.org
Sanford Medical Center Fargo	Fargo	North Dakota	701-234-2000	www.meritcare.com
Sarasota Memorial Hospital	Sarasota	Florida	941-917-9000	www.smh.com
Saint Luke's Episcopal Hospital	Houston	Texas	832-355-1000	www.sleh.com
Saint Vincent Heart Center of Indiana	Indianapolis	Indiana	317-583-5000	www.theheartcenter.com
Sutter Roseville Medical Center	Roseville	California	916-781-1000	www.sutterroseville.org
University Colo Health Memorial Hospital Central	Colorado Springs	Colorado	719-365-5000	www.memorialhospital.com
Venice Regional Medical Center - Bayfront Health	Venice	Florida	941-485-7711	www.veniceregional.com

Note: Table shows hospitals nationwide whose acute myocardial infarction 30-day readmission rate is better (lower) than U.S. rate of 18.3%

Hospitals whose Acute Myocardial Infarction (Heart Attack) 30-Day Readmission Rate is Worse (Higher) than the U.S. National Rate

Hospital	City	State	Phone	Web Site
Baxter Regional Medical Center	Mountain Home	Arkansas	870-508-1000	www.baxterregional.org
Boston Medical Center Corporation	Boston	Massachusetts	617-638-8000	www.bmc.org
Carolinas Hospital System	Florence	South Carolina	843-674-2500	www.carolinashospital.com
Centra Health	Lynchburg	Virginia	434-200-4789	www.centrahealth.com
Community Medical Center	Toms River	New Jersey	732-557-8000	www.sbhcs.com
Florida Hospital	Orlando	Florida	407-303-1976	www.floridahospital.com
Good Samaritan Regional Health Center	Mount Vernon	Illinois	618-899-1469	www.smgsi.com
Hillcrest Medical Center	Tulsa	Oklahoma	918-579-1000	www.hillcrest.com
Ingalls Memorial Hospital	Harvey	Illinois	708-333-2300	www.ingalls.org
Johnson City Medical Center	Johnson City	Tennessee	423-431-6111	www.msha.com
Kaleida Health	Buffalo	New York	716-859-8620	www.kaleidahealth.org
Lewisgale Medical Center	Salem	Virginia	540-776-4000	www.lewis-gale.com
Mercy Hospital & Medical Center	Chicago	Illinois	312-567-2000	www.mercy-chicago.org
Montefiore Medical Center	Bronx	New York	718-920-4321	www.montefiore.org
Newark Beth Israel Medical Center	Newark	New Jersey	973-926-7850	www.sbhcs.com
North Shore University Hospital	Manhasset	New York	516-562-0100	www.northshorelij.com
Northside Hospital	Saint Petersburg	Florida	813-521-5000	www.northsidehospital.com
Northwest Community Hospital	Arlington Heights	Illinois	847-618-1000	www.nch.org
Olympia Medical Center	Los Angeles	California	310-657-5900	www.olympiamc.com
Presence Saint Joseph Medical Center	Joliet	Illinois	815-725-7133	www.provena.org/stjoes
Raleigh General Hospital	Beckley	West Virginia	304-256-4100	www.raleighgeneral.com
Saint Clare's Hospital	Denville	New Jersey	973-625-6000	www.saintclares.org
Saint Michael's Medical Center	Newark	New Jersey	973-877-5350	www.cathedralhealth.org
San Juan VA Medical Center	San Juan	Puerto Rico	800-449-8729	www.visn8.med.va.gov/caribbean
Saint Joseph's Regional Medical Center	Paterson	New Jersey	973-754-2010	www.sjhmc.org
Saint Vincent's Medical Center	Bridgeport	Connecticut	203-576-5551	www.stvincents.org
Tampa VA Medical Center	Tampa	Florida	813-972-2000	www.tampa.va.gov
University Hospital - Stony Brook	Stony Brook	New York	631-444-4000	www.stonybrookmedicalcenter.org
Vidant Medical Center	Greenville	North Carolina	252-847-4100	www.uhseast.com

Note: Table shows hospitals nationwide whose acute myocardial infarction 30-day readmission rate is worse (higher) than U.S. rate of 18.3%

Hospitals whose Heart Failure 30-Day Readmission Rate is Better (Lower) than the U.S. National Rate

Hospital	City	State	Phone	Web Site
Abilene Regional Medical Center	Abilene	Texas	325-428-1000	www.abileneregional.com
Alegent Creighton Health Bergan Mercy Medical Center	Omaha	Nebraska	402-398-6060	www.alegent.com
Alpena Regional Medical Center	Alpena	Michigan	989-356-7390	www.agh.org
Asante Rogue Regional Medical Center	Medford	Oregon	541-789-7000	www.asante.org
Audrain Medical Center	Mexico	Missouri	573-582-5000	www.audrainmedicalcenter.com
Aurora Sheboygan Memorial Medical Center	Sheboygan	Wisconsin	920-451-5000	www.aurorahealthcare.org/facilities
Banner Boswell Medical Center	Sun City	Arizona	623-977-7211	www.bannerhealth.com
Banner Good Samaritan Medical Center	Phoenix	Arizona	602-239-2000	www.bannerhealth.com
Baptist Memorial Hospital	Memphis	Tennessee	901-226-5000	www.bmhcc.org
Baptist Saint Anthony's Hospital	Amarillo	Texas	806-212-2000	www.bsahs.com
Bay Medical Center Sacred Heart Health System	Panama City	Florida	850-769-1511	www.baymedical.org
Baylor All Saints Medical Center at FW	Fort Worth	Texas	817-926-2544	www.baylorhealth.com/locations/allsaints
Baylor Medical Center at Garland	Garland	Texas	972-487-5000	www.baylorhealth.com
Baylor University Medical Center	Dallas	Texas	214-820-0111	www.baylorhealth.com
Bellin Memorial Hospital	Green Bay	Wisconsin	920-433-3500	www.bellin.org
Billings Clinic Hospital	Billings	Montana	406-657-4000	www.billingsclinic.com
Boca Raton Regional Hospital	Boca Raton	Florida	561-362-5002	www.brrh.com
Boone Hospital Center	Columbia	Missouri	573-815-8000	www.boone.org
Boulder Community Hospital	Boulder	Colorado	303-440-2273	www.bch.org
Bronson Methodist Hospital	Kalamazoo	Michigan	269-341-6000	www.bronsonhealth.com
Bryan Medical Center	Lincoln	Nebraska	402-481-1111	www.bryan.org
Carolinas Medical Center/Behaviorial Health	Charlotte	North Carolina	704-355-2000	www.carolinasmedicalcenter.org
Carondelet Saint Marys Hospital	Tucson	Arizona	520-872-3000	www.carondelet.org
Catawba Valley Medical Center	Hickory	North Carolina	828-326-3809	www.catawbavalleymc.org
Cedars - Sinai Medical Center	Los Angeles	California	310-423-5000	www.cedars-sinai.edu
Central Maine Medical Center	Lewiston	Maine	207-795-0111	www.cmmc.org
Central Washington Hospital	Wenatchee	Washington	509-662-1511	www.cwhs.com
Chester County Hospital	West Chester	Pennsylvania	610-431-5000	www.cchosp.com
Christus Santa Rosa Hospital	San Antonio	Texas	210-704-2011	www.christussantarosa.org
Citrus Memorial Hospital	Inverness	Florida	352-726-1551	www.citrusmh.com
Columbia Saint Marys Hospital Ozaukee	Mequon	Wisconsin	262-243-7300	www.columbia-stmarys.org
Columbus Regional Hospital	Columbus	Indiana	812-379-4441	www.crh.org
Community Hospital of the Monterey Peninsula	Monterey	California	831-624-5311	www.chomp.org
Cox Medical Center	Springfield	Missouri	417-269-6000	www.coxhealth.com
Decatur Morgan Hospital - Decatur Campus	Decatur	Alabama	256-341-2000	www.decaturgeneral.org
Dixie Regional Medical Center	Saint George	Utah	435-251-2100	www.intermountainhealthcare.org
Dominican Hospital	Santa Cruz	California	831-462-7700	www.dominicanhospital.org
East Jefferson General Hospital	Metairie	Louisiana	504-454-4000	www.eastjeffhospital.org
Eisenhower Medical Center	Rancho Mirage	California	760-340-3911	www.emc.org
Eliza Coffee Memorial Hospital	Florence	Alabama	256-768-8400	www.chgroup.org
Elmhurst Memorial Hospital	Elmhurst	Illinois	630-833-1400	www.emhc.org
Emory University Hospital	Atlanta	Georgia	404-686-8500	www.emoryhealthcare.org
Exempla Lutheran Medical Center	Wheat Ridge	Colorado	303-425-4500	www.exemlpa.org
Fargo VA Medical Center	Fargo	North Dakota	701-232-3241	www.fargo.va.gov
Fremont Area Medical Center	Fremont	Nebraska	402-721-1610	www.famc.org
Frye Regional Medical Center	Hickory	North Carolina	828-322-6070	www.fryemedctr.com
Genesis Medical Center - Davenport	Davenport	Iowa	563-421-1000	www.genesishealth.com
GHS Greenville Memorial Medical Center	Greenville	South Carolina	864-455-7000	www.ghs.org
Hartford Hospital	Hartford	Connecticut	860-545-5000	www.harthosp.org
Hutchinson Regional Medical Center	Hutchinson	Kansas	620-665-2001	www.hutchinsonhospital.com
Integris Baptist Medical Center	Oklahoma City	Oklahoma	405-951-8110	www.integris-health.com
Intermountain Medical Center	Murray	Utah	801-507-7000	www.intermountainhealthcare.org
Iowa Methodist Medical Center	Des Moines	Iowa	515-241-6212	www.iowahealth.org
John D Archbold Memorial Hospital	Thomasville	Georgia	229-228-2880	www.archbold.org
John Muir Medical Center - Concord Campus	Concord	California	925-674-2002	www.johnmuirhealth.com
John Muir Medical Center - Walnut Creek Campus	Walnut Creek	California	925-939-3000	www.jmmdhs.com
Lancaster General Hospital	Lancaster	Pennsylvania	717-299-5511	www.lancastergeneral.org
Licking Memorial Hospital	Newark	Ohio	740-348-4000	www.lmhealth.org
Lima Memorial Health System	Lima	Ohio	419-998-4731	www.limamemorial.org
Maine Medical Center	Portland	Maine	207-662-0111	www.mmc.org
Marshalltown Medical & Surgical Center	Marshalltown	Iowa	641-754-5151	www.everydaychampions.org
Mary Hitchcock Memorial Hospital	Lebanon	New Hampshire	603-650-5000	www.dhmc.org
Mayo Clinic Health System - Eau Claire Hospital	Eau Claire	Wisconsin	715-838-3311	www.luthermidelfort.org
McKay Dee Hospital	Ogden	Utah	801-387-2800	www.intermountainhealthcare.org
Mclaren Bay Region	Bay City	Michigan	989-894-3000	www.baymed.org

Hospital	City	State	Phone	Web Site
Memorial Healthcare System	Chattanooga	Tennessee	423-495-2525	www.memorial.org
Memorial Hermann Hospital System	Houston	Texas	713-448-6796	www.memorialhermann.org
Memorial Hermann Memorial City Medical Center	Houston	Texas	713-242-3000	www.mhhs.org
Memorial Hospital of South Bend	South Bend	Indiana	574-647-1000	www.qualityoflife.org
Memorial Mission Hospital & Asheville Surgery Center	Asheville	North Carolina	828-213-1111	www.missionhospitals.org
Mercy Health Partners - Mercy Campus	Muskegon	Michigan	231-672-3901	www.mghp.com
Mercy Hospital Springfield	Springfield	Missouri	417-820-2000	www.stjohns.com
Mercy Medical Center - Redding	Redding	California	530-225-6102	www.redding.mercy.org
Methodist Charlton Medical Center	Dallas	Texas	214-947-7777	www.methodisthealthsystem.org
Methodist Hospital	San Antonio	Texas	210-575-4000	www.mh.sahealth.com
The Methodist Hospital	Houston	Texas	713-790-2221	www.methodisthealth.com
Morristown Medical Center	Morristown	New Jersey	973-971-5450	www.morristownmemorialhospital.org
Morton Plant Hospital	Clearwater	Florida	727-462-7000	www.measehospitals.com
Munson Medical Center	Traverse City	Michigan	231-935-5000	www.munsonhealthcare.org
Naples Community Hospital	Naples	Florida	239-436-5000	www.nchmd.org
New Hanover Regional Medical Center	Wilmington	North Carolina	910-343-7000	www.nhrmc.org
North Shore Medical Center	Salem	Massachusetts	978-741-1215	www.nsmc.partners.org
Northeast Georgia Medical Center	Gainesville	Georgia	770-535-3553	www.nghs.com
Oklahoma Heart Hospital	Oklahoma City	Oklahoma	405-608-3200	www.okheart.com
Owensboro Health Regional Hospital	Owensboro	Kentucky	270-688-2000	www.omhs.org
Parkview Regional Medical Center	Fort Wayne	Indiana	260-266-1000	www.parkview.com
Penn Highlands Dubois	Dubois	Pennsylvania	814-371-2200	www.drmc.org
Penn Presbyterian Medical Center	Philadelphia	Pennsylvania	215-662-8000	www.pennhealth.com
Pocono Medical Center	East Stroudsburg	Pennsylvania	570-476-3348	www.poconohealthsystem.org
Portneuf Medical Center	Pocatello	Idaho	208-239-1000	www.portmed.org
Providence Saint Peter Hospital	Olympia	Washington	360-491-9480	www.providence.org/swsa
Providence Saint Vincent Medical Center	Portland	Oregon	503-216-1234	www.providence.org
Reading Hospital	Reading	Pennsylvania	610-988-8000	www.readinghospital.org
Rex Hospital	Raleigh	North Carolina	919-784-3100	www.rexhealth.com
Roper Hospital	Charleston	South Carolina	843-724-2800	www.ropersaintfrancis.com
Sacred Heart Medical Center - Riverbend	Springfield	Oregon	541-222-7300	www.peacehealth.org/sacred-heart-riverbend
Saint Vincent Hospital	Erie	Pennsylvania	814-452-5000	www.svhs.org
Santa Rosa Memorial Hospital	Santa Rosa	California	707-525-5300	www.stjosephhealth.org
Sarasota Memorial Hospital	Sarasota	Florida	941-917-9000	www.smh.com
Scripps Green Hospital	La Jolla	California	858-554-3600	www.scrippshealth.org
Sisters of Charity Providence Hospitals	Columbia	South Carolina	803-256-5300	www.providencehospitals.com
Spartanburg Regional Medical Center	Spartanburg	South Carolina	864-560-6000	www.srhs.com
Spectrum Health - Butterworth Campus	Grand Rapids	Michigan	616-391-1774	www.spectrum-health.org
Saint Charles Medical Center - Bend	Bend	Oregon	541-382-4321	www.scmc.org
Saint Francis - Downtown	Greenville	South Carolina	864-255-1000	www.stfrancishealth.org
Saint Joseph's Hospital	Saint Paul	Minnesota	651-232-7707	www.stjosephs-stpaul.org
Saint Luke's Regional Medical Center	Boise	Idaho	208-381-2222	www.slrmc.org
Saint Vincent Hospital	Santa Fe	New Mexico	505-913-5201	www.stvin.org
Sutter Roseville Medical Center	Roseville	California	916-781-1000	www.sutterroseville.org
Tallahassee Memorial Hospital	Tallahassee	Florida	850-431-1155	www.tmh.org
Tennova Healthcare	Knoxville	Tennessee	865-545-8000	www.stmaryshealth.com
The Queens Medical Center	Honolulu	Hawaii	808-538-9011	www.queens.org
Trident Medical Center	Charleston	South Carolina	843-797-8800	www.tridenthealthsystem.com
University Colo Health Memorial Hospital Central	Colorado Springs	Colorado	719-365-5000	www.memorialhospital.com
UPMC Hamot	Erie	Pennsylvania	814-877-6000	www.hamot.org
Venice Regional Medical Center - Bayfront Health	Venice	Florida	941-485-7711	www.veniceregional.com
Virginia Hospital Center	Arlington	Virginia	703-558-5000	www.virginiahospitalcenter.com
Wesley Medical Center	Wichita	Kansas	316-962-2000	www.wesleymc.com
Williamsport Regional Medical Center	Williamsport	Pennsylvania	570-321-1000	www.susquehannahealth.org
Willis Knighton Medical Center	Shreveport	Louisiana	318-212-4000	www.wkhs.com//locations/medicalcenter.aspx

Note: Table shows hospitals nationwide whose heart failure 30-day readmission rate is better (lower) than U.S. rate of 23.0%

Hospitals whose Heart Failure 30-Day Readmission Rate is Worse (Higher) than the U.S. National Rate

Hospital	City	State	Phone	Web Site
Abbeville General Hospital	Abbeville	Louisiana	337-893-5466	www.abgen.net
Advocate Trinity Hospital	Chicago	Illinois	773-967-2000	www.advocatehealth.com/trin
Banner Baywood Medical Center	Mesa	Arizona	480-321-2000	www.bannerhealth.com
Baptist Health Medical Center - North Little Rock	North Little Rock	Arkansas	501-202-3000	www.baptist-health.org
Barnes-Jewish Hospital	Saint Louis	Missouri	314-747-3000	www.barnesjewish.org
Beaumont Health System	Royal Oak	Michigan	248-898-5000	www.beaumonthospitals.com
Beckley ARH Hospital	Beckley	West Virginia	304-255-3456	www.arh.org/beckley
Beth Israel Medical Center	New York	New York	212-420-2000	www.wehealny.org
Bolivar Medical Center	Cleveland	Mississippi	662-846-2551	www.bolivarmedical.com
Brookhaven Memorial Hospital Medical Center	Patchogue	New York	631-654-7100	www.brookhavenhospitalorg
Camden Clark Medical Center	Parkersburg	West Virginia	304-424-2111	www.ccmh.org
Capital Health System - Fuld Campus	Trenton	New Jersey	609-394-6000	www.capitalhealth.org
Capital Regional Medical Center	Tallahassee	Florida	850-656-5000	www.capitalregionalmedicalcenter.com
Carepoint Health - Bayonne Hospital Center	Bayonne	New Jersey	201-858-5000	www.bayonnemedicalcenter.org
Carepoint Health - Christ Hospital	Jersey City	New Jersey	201-795-8200	www.christhospital.org
Carepoint Health - Hoboken UMC	Hoboken	New Jersey	201-418-1004	www.bonsecoursnj.com
Carolinas Hospital System	Florence	South Carolina	843-674-2500	www.carolinashospital.com
Centegra Health System - Mc Henry Hospital	Mchenry	Illinois	815-344-5000	www.centegra.org
Chicot Memorial Medical Center	Lake Village	Arkansas	870-265-5351	www.chicotmemorial.com
Cincinnati VA Medical Center	Cincinnati	Ohio	513-861-3100	www.cincinnati.va.gov
Clinch Valley Medical Center	Richlands	Virginia	276-596-6000	www.clinchvalleymedicalcenter.com
Community Medical Center	Toms River	New Jersey	732-557-8000	www.sbhcs.com
Coney Island Hospital	Brooklyn	New York	718-616-3000	www.coneyislandhospital.com
Covenant Medical Center	Saginaw	Michigan	989-583-4000	www.covenanthealthcare.com
Crozer Chester Medical Center	Upland	Pennsylvania	610-447-2000	www.crozer.org
Culpeper Regional Hospital	Culpeper	Virginia	540-829-4100	www.culpeperhospital.com
Dallas VA Medical Center - VA North Texas	Dallas	Texas	214-742-8387	www.north-texas.med.va.gov
Danville Regional Medical Center	Danville	Virginia	434-799-2100	www.danvilleregional.org
Davis Memorial Hospital	Elkins	West Virginia	304-636-3300	www.davishealthcare.org
Detroit Receiving Hospital & University Health Center	Detroit	Michigan	313-745-3104	www.drhuhc.org
Doctors Hospital of Manteca	Manteca	California	209-823-3111	www.doctorsmanteca.com
East Georgia Regional Medical Center	Statesboro	Georgia	912-486-1500	www.egrmc.com
East Orange General Hospital	East Orange	New Jersey	973-266-4401	www.evh.org
Etmc Henderson	Henderson	Texas	903-657-7541	www.hmhtx.org
Florida Hospital	Orlando	Florida	407-303-1976	www.floridahospital.com
Flushing Hospital Medical Center	Flushing	New York	718-670-5000	www.flushinghospital.org
Forrest General Hospital	Hattiesburg	Mississippi	601-288-7000	www.forrestgeneral.com
Fountain Valley Regional Hospital & Medical Center	Fountain Valley	California	714-966-7200	www.fountainvalleyhospital.com
Franciscan Saint James Health	Olympia Fields	Illinois	708-747-4000	www.franciscanalliance.org
GV (Sonny) Montgomery VA Medical Center Jackson	Jackson	Mississippi	601-362-4471	www.visn16.med.va.gov
Georgetown Memorial Hospital	Georgetown	South Carolina	843-527-7000	www.gmhsc.com
Glenwood Regional Medical Center	West Monroe	Louisiana	318-329-4600	www.grmc.com
Griffin Hospital	Derby	Connecticut	203-732-7500	www.griffinhealth.org
Harlan Appalachian Regional Healthcare Hospital	Harlan	Kentucky	606-573-8100	www.arh.org
Harmon Memorial Hospital	Hollis	Oklahoma	580-688-3363	
Hazard ARH Regional Medical Center	Hazard	Kentucky	606-439-6600	www.arh.org/hazard
Henry Ford Hospital	Detroit	Michigan	313-916-2600	www.henryfordhospital.com
Hialeah Hospital	Hialeah	Florida	305-693-6100	www.hialeahhosp.com
Highlands Regional Medical Center	Prestonsburg	Kentucky	606-886-8511	www.hrmc.org
Hines VA Medical Center	Hines	Illinois	708-202-8387	www.visn12.med.va.gov/hines
Holy Name Medical Center	Teaneck	New Jersey	201-833-3000	www.holyname.org
Holzer Medical Center	Gallipolis	Ohio	740-446-5000	www.holzer.org
Howard University Hospital	Washington	District of Columbia	202-745-6100	www.huhosp.org
Huntington VA Medical Center	Huntington	West Virginia	304-429-0241	www.huntington.med.gov
Inspira Medical Center Woodbury	Woodbury	New Jersey	856-845-0100	www.umhospital.org
Interfaith Medical Center	Brooklyn	New York	718-613-4000	www.interfaithmedical.com
Jackson Memorial Hospital	Miami	Florida	305-585-1111	www.jhsmiami.org
Jamestown Regional Medical Center	Jamestown	Tennessee	931-879-3352	www.jamestownregional.org
Jefferson Regional Medical Center	Pittsburgh	Pennsylvania	412-469-5000	www.jeffersonregional.com
Jennings American Legion Hospital	Jennings	Louisiana	337-616-7000	www.jalh.com
Jesse Brown VA Medical Center - VA Chicago	Chicago	Illinois	312-569-8387	www.va.gov
JFK Medical Center	Atlantis	Florida	561-965-7300	www.jfkmc.com
Johns Hopkins Bayview Medical Center	Baltimore	Maryland	410-550-0123	www.hopkinsbayview.org
Jordan Hospital	Plymouth	Massachusetts	508-746-2000	www.jordanhospital.org
Kennedy University Hospital - Stratford Div	Stratford	New Jersey	856-346-6000	www.kennedyhealth.org

Hospital	City	State	Phone	Web Site
King's Daughters' Medical Center	Ashland	Kentucky	606-408-4000	www.kdmc.com
Leesburg Regional Medical Center	Leesburg	Florida	352-323-5762	www.leesburgregional.org
Lewisgale Hospital Pulaski	Pulaski	Virginia	540-994-8100	www.lewisgale.com
Libertyhealth - Jersey City Medical Center Campus	Jersey City	New Jersey	201-915-2000	www.libertyhcs.org
Lutheran Medical Center	Brooklyn	New York	718-630-8000	www.lmcmc.com
Madison River Oaks Medical Center	Canton	Mississippi	601-855-5323	www.madisonriveroaks.com
Mayo Clinic Health System - Fairmont	Fairmont	Minnesota	507-238-8101	www.fairmontmedicalcenter.org
Medical Center of Southeastern Oklahoma	Durant	Oklahoma	405-924-3080	www.mcsohealth.com
Medical Center of Trinity	Trinity	Florida	727-848-1733	www.communityhospitalnpr.com
Medstar Harbor Hospital	Baltimore	Maryland	410-350-3201	www.harborhospital.org
Memorial Hospital of Rhode Island	Pawtucket	Rhode Island	401-729-2000	www.mhriweb.org
Memorial Regional Hospital	Hollywood	Florida	954-987-2000	www.memorialregional.com
Mercy Fitzgerald Hospital	Darby	Pennsylvania	215-237-4000	www.mercyhealth.org
Mercy Hospital Saint Louis	Saint Louis	Missouri	314-569-6000	www.stjohnsmercy.org
Methodist Healthcare Memphis Hospitals	Memphis	Tennessee	901-516-8274	www.methodisthealth.org
Methodist Hospitals	Gary	Indiana	219-886-4642	www.methodisthospital.org
Metrosouth Medical Center	Blue Island	Illinois	708-597-2000	www.stfrancisblueisland.com
Midwest Regional Medical Center	Midwest City	Oklahoma	405-610-8530	www.midwestregional.com
Monmouth Medical Center - Southern Campus	Lakewood	New Jersey	732-363-1900	www.sbhcs.com
Montefiore Medical Center	Bronx	New York	718-920-4321	www.montefiore.org
Montefiore New Rochelle Hospital	New Rochelle	New York	914-632-5000	www.ssmc.org
Morton Hospital	Taunton	Massachusetts	508-828-7000	www.mortonhospital.org
Multicare Auburn Medical Center	Auburn	Washington	253-833-7711	www.armcuhs.com/p1.html
Nassau University Medical Center	East Meadow	New York	516-572-0123	www.numc.edu
New York Community Hospital of Brooklyn	Brooklyn	New York	718-692-5302	www.nych.com
New York Methodist Hospital	Brooklyn	New York	718-780-3000	www.nym.org
New York - Presbyterian Hospital	New York	New York	212-746-4189	www.nyp.org
North Carolina Baptist Hospital	Winston-Salem	North Carolina	336-716-2011	www.wfubmc.edu
North Shore Medical Center	Miami	Florida	305-835-6000	www.northshoremedical.com
North Shore University Hospital	Manhasset	New York	516-562-0100	www.northshorelij.com
Northwest Hospital Center	Randallstown	Maryland	410-521-5995	www.lifebridgehealth.org
Northwest Mississippi Regional Medical Center	Clarksdale	Mississippi	662-627-3211	www.nwmsregionalmedcenter.com
Oakwood Hospital - Dearborn	Dearborn	Michigan	313-593-7125	www.oakwood.org
Ochsner Medical Center	New Orleans	Louisiana	504-842-3000	www.ochsner.org
Olympia Medical Center	Los Angeles	California	310-657-5900	www.olympiamc.com
Orange Regional Medical Center	Middletown	New York	845-343-2424	www.ormc.org
Palisades Medical Center	North Bergen	New Jersey	201-854-5000	www.palisadesmedical.org
Palm Springs General Hospital	Hialeah	Florida	305-558-2500	www.psghosp.com
Pineville Community Hospital	Pineville	Kentucky	606-337-3051	www.pinevillehospital.com
Poplar Bluff VA Medical Center	Poplar Bluff	Missouri	573-686-4151	www.poplarbluff.va.gov
Port Huron Hospital	Port Huron	Michigan	810-987-5000	www.porthuronhospital.org
Presence Saint Joseph Medical Center	Joliet	Illinois	815-725-7133	www.provena.org/stjoes
Presence United Samaritans Medical Center	Danville	Illinois	217-443-5000	www.provena.org/usmc
Prince Georges Hospital Center	Cheverly	Maryland	301-618-2000	www.princegeorgeshospital.org
Providence VA Medical Center	Providence	Rhode Island	401-457-3042	www.visn1.med.va.gov/providence
Raritan Bay Medical Center	Perth Amboy	New Jersey	732-442-3700	www.rbmc.org
Riverview Regional Medical Center	Gadsden	Alabama	256-543-5200	www.riverviewregional.com
San Antonio VA Medical Center	San Antonio	Texas	210-617-5300	www.vasthcs.med.va.gov
San Juan VA Medical Center	San Juan	Puerto Rico	800-449-8729	www.visn8.med.va.gov/caribbean
Schuylkill Medical Center - East Norwegian Street	Pottsville	Pennsylvania	570-621-4000	www.schuylkillhealth.com
Sinai - Grace Hospital	Detroit	Michigan	313-966-3300	www.sinaigrace.org
Singing River Hospital	Pascagoula	Mississippi	228-809-5000	www.srhshealth.com
Skyridge Medical Center	Cleveland	Tennessee	423-339-4132	www.skyridgemedcenter.com
Somerset Medical Center	Somerville	New Jersey	908-685-2200	www.somersetmedicalcenter.com
South Nassau Communities Hospital	Oceanside	New York	516-632-3000	www.southnassau.org
Southcoast Hospital Group	Fall River	Massachusetts	508-679-3131	www.southcoast.org/charlton
Southeastern Regional Medical Center	Lumberton	North Carolina	910-671-5000	www.srmc.org
Southern Tennessee Medical Center	Winchester	Tennessee	931-967-8295	www.southerntennessee.com
Southside Regional Medical Center	Petersburg	Virginia	804-765-5000	www.srmconline.com
SSM Depaul Health Center	Bridgeton	Missouri	314-344-6000	www.ssmdepaul.com
SSM Saint Marys Health Center	Richmond Heights	Missouri	314-768-8000	www.ssmhealth.com/stmarys
Saint Catherine of Siena Hospital	Smithtown	New York	631-862-3000	www.stcatherines.chsli.org
Saint Francis Medical Center	Monroe	Louisiana	318-966-4000	www.stfran.com
Saint John Hospital & Medical Center	Detroit	Michigan	313-343-4000	www.stjohnprovidence.org
Saint John's Episcopal Hospital at South Shore	Far Rockaway	New York	718-869-7000	www.ehs.org
Saint John's Riverside Hospital	Yonkers	New York	914-964-4444	www.riversidehealth.org
Saint Joseph's Hospital	Tampa	Florida	813-870-4398	www.stjosephstampa.org

Hospital	City	State	Phone	Web Site
Saint Joseph's Regional Medical Center	Paterson	New Jersey	973-754-2010	www.sjhmc.org
Saint Louis - John Cochran VA Medical Center	Saint Louis	Missouri	314-652-4100	www.stlouis.va.gov
Saint Luke's Hospital Bethlehem	Bethlehem	Pennsylvania	610-954-4000	www.slhn-lehighvalley.org
Saint Luke's Roosevelt Hospital	New York	New York	212-523-4000	www.wehealny.org
Saint Mary Mercy Hospital	Livonia	Michigan	734-655-4800	www.stmarymercy.org
Saint Marys Hospital	Centralia	Illinois	618-436-6519	www.stmarys-goodsamaritan.com
Swedish Covenant Hospital	Chicago	Illinois	773-878-8200	www.swedishcovenant.org
Tampa VA Medical Center	Tampa	Florida	813-972-2000	www.tampa.va.gov
Univerity of MD Balto Washington Medical Center	Glen Burnie	Maryland	410-595-1967	www.bwmc.umms.org
University Hospital of Brooklyn - Downstate Medical Center	Brooklyn	New York	718-270-1000	www.downstate.edu
University of Miami Hospital	Miami	Florida	305-325-5511	www.cedarsmedicalcenter.com
VA Middle Tennessee Healthcare System	Nashville	Tennessee	615-327-5332	www.tennesseevalley.va.gov
VA New York Harbor Healthcare System	New York	New York	212-686-7500	www.nyharbor.va.gov
VA North Florida/South Georgia Healthcare System	Gainesville	Florida	352-376-1611	www.northflorida.va.gov
Valley Hospital	Ridgewood	New Jersey	201-447-8000	www.valleyhealth.com
W Palm Beach VA Medical Center	West Palm Beach	Florida	561-422-8600	www.va.gov
Wellmont Bristol Regional Medical Center	Bristol	Tennessee	423-844-1121	www.wellmont.org
Western Maryland Regional Medical Center	Cumberland	Maryland	240-964-8001	www.wmhs.com
Westlake Regional Hospital	Columbia	Kentucky	270-384-4753	www.westlake-healthcare.org
Whitesburg ARH Hospital	Whitesburg	Kentucky	606-633-3500	www.arh.org/whitesburg
William Beaumont Hospital - Troy	Troy	Michigan	248-964-8800	www.beaumonthospitals.com
Williamson ARH Hospital	South Williamson	Kentucky	606-237-1700	www.arh.org
Wuesthoff Medical Center Rockledge	Rockledge	Florida	321-637-2603	www.wuesthoff.org
Wyckoff Heights Medical Center	Brooklyn	New York	718-963-7272	www.wyckoffhospital.org

Note: Table shows hospitals nationwide whose heart failure 30-day readmission rate is worse (higher) than U.S. rate of 23.0%

Hospitals whose Pneumonia 30-Day Readmission Rate is Better (Lower) than the U.S. National Rate

Hospital	City	State	Phone	Web Site
Bay Medical Center Sacred Heart Health System	Panama City	Florida	850-769-1511	www.baymedical.org
Boca Raton Regional Hospital	Boca Raton	Florida	561-362-5002	www.brrh.com
Bronson Methodist Hospital	Kalamazoo	Michigan	269-341-6000	www.bronsonhealth.com
Cayuga Medical Center at Ithaca	Ithaca	New York	607-274-4401	www.cayugamed.org
Citrus Memorial Hospital	Inverness	Florida	352-726-1551	www.citrusmh.com
Eisenhower Medical Center	Rancho Mirage	California	760-340-3911	www.emc.org
Evergreen Hospital Medical Center	Kirkland	Washington	425-899-1000	www.evergreenhospital.org
Florida Hospital Waterman	Tavares	Florida	352-253-3300	www.fhwat.org
Freeman Health System - Freeman West	Joplin	Missouri	417-347-1111	www.freemanhealth.com
Kalispell Regional Medical Center	Kalispell	Montana	406-752-5111	www.krmc.org
Lake Regional Health System	Osage Beach	Missouri	573-348-8000	www.lakeregional.com
Memorial Healthcare System	Chattanooga	Tennessee	423-495-2525	www.memorial.org
Memorial Hermann Hospital System	Houston	Texas	713-448-6796	www.memorialhermann.org
Memorial Hermann Memorial City Medical Center	Houston	Texas	713-242-3000	www.mhhs.org
Memorial Medical Center of West Michigan	Ludington	Michigan	231-843-2591	www.mmcwm.com
Mercy Medical Center - Redding	Redding	California	530-225-6102	www.redding.mercy.org
Owensboro Health Regional Hospital	Owensboro	Kentucky	270-688-2000	www.omhs.org
Parkview Medical Center	Pueblo	Colorado	719-584-4000	www.parkviewmc.com
Parkview Regional Medical Center	Fort Wayne	Indiana	260-266-1000	www.parkview.com
Providence Saint Vincent Medical Center	Portland	Oregon	503-216-1234	www.providence.org
Rex Hospital	Raleigh	North Carolina	919-784-3100	www.rexhealth.com
Saint Joseph Regional Medical Center	Mishawaka	Indiana	574-335-5000	www.sjmed.com
Saint Joseph's Hospital of Atlanta	Atlanta	Georgia	678-843-5720	www.stjosephsatlanta.org
Salem Regional Medical Center	Salem	Ohio	330-332-1551	www.salemhosp.com
San Antonio Community Hospital	Upland	California	714-985-2811	www.sach.org
Sarasota Memorial Hospital	Sarasota	Florida	941-917-9000	www.smh.com
South Texas Health System	Edinburg	Texas	956-632-4000	www.edinburgregional.com
Spartanburg Regional Medical Center	Spartanburg	South Carolina	864-560-6000	www.srhs.com
Saint Edward Mercy Medical Center	Fort Smith	Arkansas	479-314-6000	www.stedwardmercy.com
Saint Francis Hospital - Roslyn	Roslyn	New York	516-562-6000	www.stfrancisheartcenter.com
Saint Francis - Downtown	Greenville	South Carolina	864-255-1000	www.stfrancishealth.org
Saint Mary's Regional Medical Center	Enid	Oklahoma	580-233-6100	www.stmarysregional.com
Saint Patrick Hospital	Missoula	Montana	406-543-7271	www.saintpatrick.org
Stormont - Vail Healthcare	Topeka	Kansas	785-354-6121	www.stormontvail.org
Virtua Memorial Hospital of Burlington County	Mount Holly	New Jersey	609-914-6200	www.virtua.org
Williamsport Regional Medical Center	Williamsport	Pennsylvania	570-321-1000	www.susquehannahealth.org
Willis Knighton Medical Center	Shreveport	Louisiana	318-212-4000	www.wkhs.com//locations/medicalcenter.aspx

Note: Table shows hospitals nationwide whose pneumonia 30-day readmission rate is better (lower) than U.S. rate of 17.6%

Hospitals whose Pneumonia 30-Day Readmission Rate is Worse (Higher) than the U.S. National Rate

Hospital	City	State	Phone	Web Site
Adena Regional Medical Center	Chillicothe	Ohio	740-779-7500	www.adena.org
Advocate Lutheran General Hospital	Park Ridge	Illinois	847-723-2210	www.advocatehealth.com
Advocate South Suburban Hospital	Hazel Crest	Illinois	708-799-8000	www.advocatehealth.com
Arnot Ogden Medical Center	Elmira	New York	607-737-4100	www.arnothealth.org
Baptist Memorial Hospital Desoto	Southaven	Mississippi	662-772-4000	www.bmhcc.org/facilities/desoto
Barnes-Jewish Hospital	Saint Louis	Missouri	314-747-3000	www.barnesjewish.org
Baxter Regional Medical Center	Mountain Home	Arkansas	870-508-1000	www.baxterregional.org
Bay Area Hospital	Coos Bay	Oregon	541-269-8111	www.bayareahospital.org
Bay Pines VA Medical Center	Bay Pines	Florida	727-398-6661	www.baypines.va.gov
Bayfront Health Punta Gorda	Punta Gorda	Florida	941-639-3131	www.charlotteregional.com
Beaumont Health System	Royal Oak	Michigan	248-898-5000	www.beaumonthospitals.com
Beckley VA Medical Center	Beckley	West Virginia	304-255-2121	www.beckley.va.gov
Beth Israel Medical Center	New York	New York	212-420-2000	www.wehealny.org
Blount Memorial Hospital	Maryville	Tennessee	865-983-7211	www.blountmemorial.org
Brandon Regional Hospital	Brandon	Florida	813-681-5551	www.brandonregionalhospital.com
Bronx VA Medical Center	Bronx	New York	718-584-9000	www.med.va.gov
Bronx - Lebanon Hospital Center	Bronx	New York	212-588-7000	www.bronx-leb.org
Brookhaven Memorial Hospital Medical Center	Patchogue	New York	631-654-7100	www.brookhavenhospitalorg
Cape Fear Valley Medical Center	Fayetteville	North Carolina	910-609-4000	www.capefearvalley.com
Casey County Hospital	Liberty	Kentucky	606-787-6275	
Chambers Memorial Hospital	Danville	Arkansas	479-495-2241	www.chambershospital.com
Cleveland Clinic	Cleveland	Ohio	216-444-2200	www.clevelandclinic.org
Cleveland - Wade Park VA Medical Center	Cleveland	Ohio	216-791-3800	www.cleveland.va.gov
Columbia MO VA Medical Center	Columbia	Missouri	573-814-6000	www.columbiamo.vc.gov
Community Hospital	Munster	Indiana	219-836-1600	www.comhs.org/community
Dallas VA Medical Center - VA North Texas	Dallas	Texas	214-742-8387	www.north-texas.med.va.gov
Davis Regional Medical Center	Statesville	North Carolina	704-873-0281	www.davisregional.com
Doctors' Community Hospital	Lanham	Maryland	301-552-8085	www.dchweb.org
East Orange General Hospital	East Orange	New Jersey	973-266-4401	www.evh.org
Florida Hospital	Orlando	Florida	407-303-1976	www.floridahospital.com
Florida Hospital Tampa	Tampa	Florida	813-615-7200	www.uch.org
Forest Hills Hospital	Forest Hills	New York	718-830-4000	www.northshorelij.com
Franklin Medical Center	Winnsboro	Louisiana	318-435-9411	www.fmc-cares.com
Garden City Hospital	Garden City	Michigan	734-421-3300	www.gchosp.org
Great River Medical Center	Blytheville	Arkansas	870-838-7300	www.greatrivermc.com
Harlan Appalachian Regional Healthcare Hospital	Harlan	Kentucky	606-573-8100	www.arh.org
Hazard ARH Regional Medical Center	Hazard	Kentucky	606-439-6600	www.arh.org/hazard
Heartland Regional Medical Center	Marion	Illinois	618-998-7000	www.heartlandregional.com
Henry Ford Hospital	Detroit	Michigan	313-916-2600	www.henryfordhospital.com
Highlands Regional Medical Center	Sebring	Florida	863-385-6101	www.highlandsregional.com
Hillcrest Hospital	Mayfield Heights	Ohio	440-312-4500	www.hillcresthospital.org
Hines VA Medical Center	Hines	Illinois	708-202-8387	www.visn12.med.va.gov/hines
Holzer Medical Center	Gallipolis	Ohio	740-446-5000	www.holzer.org
Houston VA Medical Center	Houston	Texas	713-794-7100	www.houston.med.va.gov
Howard County General Hospital	Columbia	Maryland	410-740-7890	www.hcgh.org
Huntington Hospital	Huntington	New York	631-351-2000	www.hunthosp.org
Huntington VA Medical Center	Huntington	West Virginia	304-429-0241	www.huntington.med.gov
Jackson Parish Hospital	Jonesboro	Louisiana	318-259-4435	www.jacksonparishhospital.com
Jewish Hospital & Saint Mary's Healthcare	Louisville	Kentucky	502-587-4011	www.jhhs.org
Johns Hopkins Bayview Medical Center	Baltimore	Maryland	410-550-0123	www.hopkinsbayview.org
Kennedy University Hospital - Stratford Div	Stratford	New Jersey	856-346-6000	www.kennedyhealth.org
King's Daughters' Medical Center	Ashland	Kentucky	606-408-4000	www.kdmc.com
Lake City Medical Center	Lake City	Florida	386-719-9000	www.lakecitymedical.com
Lake Health	Concord	Ohio	440-953-9600	www.lakehealth.org
Lehigh Valley Hospital - Hazleton	Hazleton	Pennsylvania	570-501-4000	www.ghha.org
Lenox Hill Hospital	New York	New York	212-439-2345	www.lenoxhillhospital.org
Little Company of Mary Hospital	Evergreen Park	Illinois	708-422-6200	www.lcmh.org
Livingston Regional Hospital	Livingston	Tennessee	931-823-5611	www.livingstonregionalhospital.com
Logan Regional Medical Center	Logan	West Virginia	304-831-1350	www.loganregionalmedicalcenter.com
Marymount Hospital	Garfield Heights	Ohio	216-581-0500	www.marymount.org
Medical Center of Southeastern Oklahoma	Durant	Oklahoma	405-924-3080	www.mcsohealth.com
Medstar Good Samaritan Hospital	Baltimore	Maryland	443-444-3902	www.goodsam-md.org
Memorial Hospital	Manchester	Kentucky	606-598-5104	www.manchestermemorial.com
Mercy Memorial Health Center	Ardmore	Oklahoma	405-223-5400	www.mercyok.com/mmhc
Metrosouth Medical Center	Blue Island	Illinois	708-597-2000	www.stfrancisblueisland.com

Hospital	City	State	Phone	Web Site
Mississippi Baptist Medical Center	Jackson	Mississippi	601-968-1000	www.mbmc.org
Monroe County Medical Center	Tompkinsville	Kentucky	270-487-9231	www.mcmccares.com
Mount Sinai Hospital	New York	New York	212-241-7981	www.mountsinai.org
Muskogee VA Medical Center	Muskogee	Oklahoma	918-577-3000	www.visn16.med.va.gov/muskogee.asp
Nassau University Medical Center	East Meadow	New York	516-572-0123	www.numc.edu
New York Hospital Medical Center of Queens	Flushing	New York	718-670-1231	www.nyhq.org
New York Methodist Hospital	Brooklyn	New York	718-780-3000	www.nym.org
North Carolina Baptist Hospital	Winston-Salem	North Carolina	336-716-2011	www.wfubmc.edu
North Oaks Medical Center	Hammond	Louisiana	985-345-2700	www.northoaks.org
Northern Westchester Hospital	Mount Kisco	New York	914-666-1200	www.nwhc.net
Northwest Hospital Center	Randallstown	Maryland	410-521-5995	www.lifebridgehealth.org
Northwestern Memorial Hospital	Chicago	Illinois	312-926-2000	www.nmh.org
Oakwood Hospital - Wayne	Wayne	Michigan	734-467-4175	www.oakwood.org
Orange Regional Medical Center	Middletown	New York	845-343-2424	www.ormc.org
Oroville Hospital	Oroville	California	530-533-8500	www.orovillehospital.com
Palos Community Hospital	Palos Heights	Illinois	708-923-4000	www.paloshospital.org
Piedmont Medical Center	Rock Hill	South Carolina	803-329-1234	www.piedmontmedicalcenter.com
Pineville Community Hospital	Pineville	Kentucky	606-337-3051	www.pinevillehospital.com
Presence United Samaritans Medical Center	Danville	Illinois	217-443-5000	www.provena.org/usmc
Princeton Community Hospital	Princeton	West Virginia	304-487-7260	www.pchonline.org
Raleigh General Hospital	Beckley	West Virginia	304-256-4100	www.raleighgeneral.com
Richmond VA Medical Center	Richmond	Virginia	804-675-5000	www.med.va.gov
Robert Packer Hospital	Sayre	Pennsylvania	570-888-6666	www.guthrie.org
Russell County Medical Center	Lebanon	Virginia	276-883-8100	www.msha.com
Saint Anne's Hospital	Fall River	Massachusetts	508-674-5600	www.saintanneshospital.org
Saint Thomas Rutherford Hospital	Murfreesboro	Tennessee	615-396-4100	www.mtmc.org
San Gabriel Valley Medical Center	San Gabriel	California	626-289-5454	www.sangabrielvalleymedctr.org
San Juan VA Medical Center	San Juan	Puerto Rico	800-449-8729	www.visn8.med.va.gov/caribbean
Santa Monica - UCLA Medical Center & Orthopaedic Hospital	Santa Monica	California	310-319-4000	www.healthcare.ucla.edu
Sentara Careplex Hospital	Hampton	Virginia	757-736-1000	www.sentara.com
Silver Cross Hospital & Medical Centers	New Lenox	Illinois	815-300-1100	www.silvercross.org
Sinai Hospital of Baltimore	Baltimore	Maryland	410-601-5131	www.sinai-balt.com
Singing River Hospital	Pascagoula	Mississippi	228-809-5000	www.srhshealth.com
Springfield Regional Medical Center	Springfield	Ohio	937-523-1000	www.communityhospital.com
Saint Anthony's Medical Center	Saint Louis	Missouri	314-525-1000	www.samcstl.org
Saint Bernard Hospital	Chicago	Illinois	773-962-3900	www.stbernardhospital.com
Saint Catherine of Siena Hospital	Smithtown	New York	631-862-3000	www.stcatherines.chsli.org
Saint Francis Hospital	Poughkeepsie	New York	845-483-5000	www.sfhhc.org
Saint Joseph's Hospital Health Center	Syracuse	New York	315-448-5111	www.sjhsyr.org
Saint Luke's Roosevelt Hospital	New York	New York	212-523-4000	www.wehealny.org
Saint Rose Dominican Hospitals - Rose De Lima Campus	Henderson	Nevada	702-616-5000	www.dignityhealth.org/las-vegas
Sumner Regional Medical Center	Gallatin	Tennessee	615-452-4210	www.mysumnermedical.com
Syracuse VA Medical Center	Syracuse	New York	315-425-4400	www1.va.gov/visns/visn02
Tampa VA Medical Center	Tampa	Florida	813-972-2000	www.tampa.va.gov
Univerity of MD Balto Washington Medical Center	Glen Burnie	Maryland	410-595-1967	www.bwmc.umms.org
University Hospital - Stony Brook	Stony Brook	New York	631-444-4000	www.stonybrookmedicalcenter.org
University Hospitals - Elyria Medical Center	Elyria	Ohio	440-329-7500	www.emh-healthcare.org
University of Alabama Hospital	Birmingham	Alabama	205-934-4011	www.health.uab.edu
University of Maryland Medical Center	Baltimore	Maryland	410-328-8667	www.umm.edu
University of Maryland Charles Regional Medical Center	La Plata	Maryland	301-609-4265	www.civista.org
Upper Valley Medical Center	Troy	Ohio	937-440-7853	www.uvmc.com
Upstate New York VA Healthcare System - Western NY	Buffalo	New York	716-862-3611	www.buffalo.va.gov
VA Central Arkansas Veterans Healthcare System	Little Rock	Arkansas	501-257-1000	www.visn16.med.va.gov
VA Maryland Healthcare System - Baltimore	Baltimore	Maryland	410-605-7016	www.maryland.va.gov
VA Middle Tennessee Healthcare System	Nashville	Tennessee	615-327-5332	www.tennesseevalley.va.gov
VA Pittsburgh Healthcare System	Pittsburgh	Pennsylvania	412-688-6100	www.pittsburg.va.gov
Vassar Brothers Medical Center	Poughkeepsie	New York	845-454-8500	www.vasserbrothers.org
Wadley Regional Medical Center	Texarkana	Texas	903-798-8000	www.wadleyhealth.com
Washington Hospital	Fremont	California	510-797-1111	www.whhs.com
Wayne Memorial Hospital	Goldsboro	North Carolina	919-736-1110	www.waynehealth.org
White County Medical Center	Searcy	Arkansas	501-278-3100	www.centralarkhospital.com
White Plains Hospital Center	White Plains	New York	914-681-0600	www.wphospital.org
William Beaumont Hospital - Troy	Troy	Michigan	248-964-8800	www.beaumonthospitals.com
Wing Memorial Hospital & Medical Center	Palmer	Massachusetts	413-283-7651	www.winghealth.org
Wyckoff Heights Medical Center	Brooklyn	New York	718-963-7272	www.wyckoffhospital.org

Note: Table shows hospitals nationwide whose pneumonia 30-day readmission rate is worse (higher) than U.S. rate of 17.6%

Hospitals whose Rate of Readmission After Hip/Knee Surgery is Better (Lower) than the U.S. National Rate

Hospital	City	State	Phone	Web Site
Arkansas Surgical Hospital	No Little Rock	Arkansas	501-748-8000	www.arksurgicalhospital.com
Blake Medical Center	Bradenton	Florida	941-792-6611	www.blakemedicalcenter.com
Boca Raton Regional Hospital	Boca Raton	Florida	561-362-5002	www.brrh.com
Christus Santa Rosa Hospital	San Antonio	Texas	210-704-2011	www.christussantarosa.org
Community Memorial Hospital	Hamilton	New York	315-824-1100	www.communitymemorial.org
Eisenhower Medical Center	Rancho Mirage	California	760-340-3911	www.emc.org
Elkhart General Hospital	Elkhart	Indiana	574-294-2621	www.egh.org
Emory University Hospital	Atlanta	Georgia	404-686-8500	www.emoryhealthcare.org
Evanston Hospital	Evanston	Illinois	847-432-8000	www.enh.org
Grace Medical Center	Lubbock	Texas	806-788-4100	www.highlandcommunityhospital.com
Heart of Florida Regional Medical Center	Davenport	Florida	863-422-4971	www.heartofflorida.com
Heartland Regional Medical Center	Saint Joseph	Missouri	816-271-6000	www.heartland-health.com
Hoag Orthopedic Institute	Irvine	California	949-727-5000	www.orthopedichospital.com
Holy Cross Hospital	Fort Lauderdale	Florida	954-771-8000	www.holy-cross.com
Hospital For Special Surgery	New York	New York	212-606-1000	www.hss.edu
Inova Mount Vernon Hospital	Alexandria	Virginia	703-664-7000	www.inova.com/inovapublic.srt/imvh/index.jsp
Kalispell Regional Medical Center	Kalispell	Montana	406-752-5111	www.krmc.org
Kansas Medical Center	Andover	Kansas	316-300-4000	www.ksmedcenter.com
Kettering Medical Center	Kettering	Ohio	937-298-4331	www.khnetwork.org
Maine Medical Center	Portland	Maine	207-662-0111	www.mmc.org
Meadville Medical Center	Meadville	Pennsylvania	814-333-5000	www.mmchs.org
Memorial Healthcare System	Chattanooga	Tennessee	423-495-2525	www.memorial.org
Memorial Mission Hospital & Asheville Surgery Center	Asheville	North Carolina	828-213-1111	www.missionhospitals.org
Mercy Medical Center - Cedar Rapids	Cedar Rapids	Iowa	319-398-6011	www.mercycare.org
Mercy Medical Center - Redding	Redding	California	530-225-6102	www.redding.mercy.org
New England Baptist Hospital	Boston	Massachusetts	617-754-5800	www.nebh.caregroup.org
Ocala Regional Medical Center	Ocala	Florida	352-401-1000	www.ocalaregional.com
Oklahoma Surgical Hospital	Tulsa	Oklahoma	918-477-5000	www.oklahomasurgicalhospital.com
Orthopaedic Hospital at Parkview North	Fort Wayne	Indiana	260-672-4050	www.parkview.com
Orthopaedic Hospital of Wisconsin	Glendale	Wisconsin	414-961-6800	www.ohow.org
Poudre Valley Hospital	Fort Collins	Colorado	970-495-7000	www.pvhs.org
Presbyterian Hospital	Albuquerque	New Mexico	505-724-8386	www.phs.org
Providence Saint John's Health Center	Santa Monica	California	310-829-5511	www.stjohns.org
Reading Hospital	Reading	Pennsylvania	610-988-8000	www.readinghospital.org
Sacred Heart Medical Center - Riverbend	Springfield	Oregon	541-222-7300	www.peacehealth.org/sacred-heart-riverbend
Saint Elizabeth Regional Medical Center	Lincoln	Nebraska	402-219-7700	www.stelizabethonline.com
Saint Joseph's Hospital of Atlanta	Atlanta	Georgia	678-843-5720	www.stjosephsatlanta.org
Saint Thomas West Hospital	Nashville	Tennessee	615-222-2111	www.stthomas.org
Salinas Valley Memorial Hospital	Salinas	California	831-757-4333	www.svmh.com
Samaritan Regional Health System	Ashland	Ohio	419-289-0491	www.samho.org
Sanford Medical Center Fargo	Fargo	North Dakota	701-234-2000	www.meritcare.com
Scottsdale Healthcare - Shea Medical Center	Scottsdale	Arizona	480-323-3009	www.shc.org
Sentara Leigh Hospital	Norfolk	Virginia	757-261-6601	www.sentara.com
Saint Joseph Hospital	Orange	California	714-633-9111	www.sjo.org
Saint Joseph Mercy Oakland	Pontiac	Michigan	248-858-3000	www.stjoesoakland.org
Sutter General Hospital	Sacramento	California	916-733-8999	www.suttermedicalcenter.org
The Orthopaedic Hospital of Lutheran Health Network	Fort Wayne	Indiana	260-435-2999	www.lutheranhealth.net
United Health Services Hospitals	Johnson City	New York	607-763-6000	www.vhs.ent
VHS Harlingen Hospital Company	Harlingen	Texas	956-389-1100	www.vbmc.org
Washington Hospital	Fremont	California	510-797-1111	www.whhs.com
Wythe County Community Hospital	Wytheville	Virginia	276-228-0200	www.wcch.org

Note: Table shows hospitals nationwide whose rate of readmission after hip/knee surgery is better (lower) than U.S. rate of 5.4%

Hospitals whose Rate of Readmission After Hip/Knee Surgery is Worse (Higher) than the U.S. National Rate

Hospital	City	State	Phone	Web Site
Abington Memorial Hospital	Abington	Pennsylvania	215-481-2000	www.amh.org
Advocate Christ Hospital & Medical Center	Oak Lawn	Illinois	708-684-8000	www.advocatehealth.com
Advocate Good Samaritan Hospital	Downers Grove	Illinois	630-275-5900	www.advocatehealth.com/gsam
Bayfront Health - Saint Petersburg	Saint Petersburg	Florida	727-823-1234	www.bayfront.org
Beaufort County Memorial Hospital	Beaufort	South Carolina	843-522-5200	www.bmhsc.org
Beaumont Health System	Royal Oak	Michigan	248-898-5000	www.beaumonthospitals.com
Centrastate Medical Center	Freehold	New Jersey	732-431-2000	www.centrastate.com
Christus Saint Michael Health System	Texarkana	Texas	903-614-1000	www.christusstmichael.org
Des Peres Hospital	Saint Louis	Missouri	314-966-9100	www.despereshospital.com
Doctors' Community Hospital	Lanham	Maryland	301-552-8085	www.dchweb.org
Enloe Medical Center	Chico	California	530-332-7300	www.enloe.org
Froedtert Memorial Lutheran Hospital	Milwaukee	Wisconsin	414-805-3000	www.froedtert.com
Galesburg Cottage Hospital	Galesburg	Illinois	309-345-4555	www.cottagehospital.com
Grant Medical Center	Columbus	Ohio	614-566-9978	www.ohiohealth.com
Jackson County Memorial Hospital	Altus	Oklahoma	580-379-5000	www.jcmh.com
Leesburg Regional Medical Center	Leesburg	Florida	352-323-5762	www.leesburgregional.org
Mercy Hospital Saint Louis	Saint Louis	Missouri	314-569-6000	www.stjohnsmercy.org
Mercy Saint Anne Hospital	Toledo	Ohio	419-407-2663	www.mercyweb.org
Minden Medical Center	Minden	Louisiana	318-377-2321	www.mindenmedicalcenter.com
Northwestern Memorial Hospital	Chicago	Illinois	312-926-2000	www.nmh.org
Orlando Health	Orlando	Florida	321-841-5111	www.orlandoregionalmedicalcenter.org
Parkwest Medical Center	Knoxville	Tennessee	865-970-9800	www.yesparkwest.com
Penn Presbyterian Medical Center	Philadelphia	Pennsylvania	215-662-8000	www.pennhealth.com
Pennsylvania Hospital of the Univ of PA Health Sys	Philadelphia	Pennsylvania	215-829-3000	www.pennmedicine.org/pahosp
Peterson Regional Medical Center	Kerrville	Texas	830-896-4200	www.petersonrmc.com
Providence Hospital	Washington	District of Columbia	202-269-7000	www.provhosp.org
Reston Hospital Center	Reston	Virginia	703-689-9000	www.restonhospital.com
Saint Agnes Hospital	Baltimore	Maryland	410-368-2101	www.stagnes.org
Saline Memorial Hospital	Benton	Arkansas	501-776-6000	www.salinememorial.org
Shannon Medical Center	San Angelo	Texas	325-653-6741	www.shannonhealth.com
Sinai Hospital of Baltimore	Baltimore	Maryland	410-601-5131	www.sinai-balt.com
Southside Regional Medical Center	Petersburg	Virginia	804-765-5000	www.srmconline.com
Saint Joseph Regional Health Center	Bryan	Texas	979-776-3912	www.st-joseph.org/sjrhc
Saint Joseph's Hospital	Tampa	Florida	813-870-4398	www.stjosephstampa.org
Thomas Jefferson University Hospital	Philadelphia	Pennsylvania	215-955-6000	www.jeffersonhospital.org
Wellmont Holston Valley Medical Center	Kingsport	Tennessee	423-224-4000	www.wellmont.org
Woodland Heights Medical Center	Lufkin	Texas	936-634-8311	www.woodlandheights.net

Note: Table shows hospitals nationwide whose rate of readmission after hip/knee surgery is better (lower) than U.S. rate of 5.4%

Hospitals whose Rate of Readmission After Discharge From Hospital (Hospital-wide) is Better (Lower) than the U.S. National Rate

Hospital	City	State	Phone	Web Site
Abbott Northwestern Hospital	Minneapolis	Minnesota	612-863-4509	www.abbottnorthwestern.com
Alegent Creighton Health Bergan Mercy Medical Center	Omaha	Nebraska	402-398-6060	www.alegent.com
Alexian Brothers Medical Center	Elk Grove Village	Illinois	847-437-5500	www.alexian.org
Alpena Regional Medical Center	Alpena	Michigan	989-356-7390	www.agh.org
Alta Bates Summit Medical Center	Oakland	California	510-655-4000	www.altabates.com
American Fork Hospital	American Fork	Utah	801-855-3305	www.ihc.com/facility/facilityresults.jsp
Anderson Regional Medical Center	Meridian	Mississippi	601-553-6000	www.jarmc.org
Appleton Medical Center	Appleton	Wisconsin	920-731-4101	www.thedacare.org
Arkansas Surgical Hospital	No Little Rock	Arkansas	501-748-8000	www.arksurgicalhospital.com
Asante Rogue Regional Medical Center	Medford	Oregon	541-789-7000	www.asante.org
Aspirus Wausau Hospital	Wausau	Wisconsin	715-847-2121	www.aspirus.org
Athens Regional Medical Center	Athens	Georgia	706-475-7000	www.armc.org
Augusta Health	Fishersville	Virginia	540-932-4000	www.augustamed.com
Aurora Lakeland Medical Center	Elkhorn	Wisconsin	262-741-2000	www.aurorahealthcare.org/facilities
Aurora Medical Center Manitowoc County	Two Rivers	Wisconsin	920-794-5000	www.aurorahealthcare.org
Aurora Medical Center Washington County	Hartford	Wisconsin	262-673-2300	www.aurorahealthcare.org
Aurora Saint Lukes Medical Center	Milwaukee	Wisconsin	414-649-6000	www.aurorahealthcare.org
Aurora West Allis Medical Center	West Allis	Wisconsin	414-328-6000	www.aurorahealthcare.org
Avera Mckennan Hospital & University Health Center	Sioux Falls	South Dakota	605-322-8000	www.mckennan.org
Avera Queen of Peace	Mitchell	South Dakota	605-995-2000	www.averaqueenofpeace.org
Avera Saint Lukes	Aberdeen	South Dakota	605-622-5000	www.averastlukes.org
Banner Good Samaritan Medical Center	Phoenix	Arizona	602-239-2000	www.bannerhealth.com
Baptist Health Louisville	Louisville	Kentucky	502-897-8100	www.baptisteast.com
Baptist Medical Center	San Antonio	Texas	210-297-1020	www.baptisthealthsystem.org
Baptist Memorial Hospital	Memphis	Tennessee	901-226-5000	www.bmhcc.org
Baptist Saint Anthony's Hospital	Amarillo	Texas	806-212-2000	www.bsahs.com
Baylor All Saints Medical Center at FW	Fort Worth	Texas	817-926-2544	www.baylorhealth.com/locations/allsaints
Baylor Medical Center at Garland	Garland	Texas	972-487-5000	www.baylorhealth.com
Baylor Medical Center at Irving	Irving	Texas	972-579-8100	www.baylorhealth.com
Baylor Regional Medical Center at Grapevine	Grapevine	Texas	817-481-1588	www.baylorhealth.com
Baylor University Medical Center	Dallas	Texas	214-820-0111	www.baylorhealth.com
Baystate Medical Center	Springfield	Massachusetts	413-794-0000	www.baystatehealth.com
Bellin Memorial Hospital	Green Bay	Wisconsin	920-433-3500	www.bellin.org
Billings Clinic Hospital	Billings	Montana	406-657-4000	www.billingsclinic.com
Blanchard Valley Hospital	Findlay	Ohio	419-423-4500	www.bvha.org
Bon Secours Maryview Medical Center	Portsmouth	Virginia	757-398-2200	www.bonsecourshamptonroads.com
Boone Hospital Center	Columbia	Missouri	573-815-8000	www.boone.org
Borgess Medical Center	Kalamazoo	Michigan	269-226-7000	www.borgess.com
Boulder Community Hospital	Boulder	Colorado	303-440-2273	www.bch.org
Bronson Methodist Hospital	Kalamazoo	Michigan	269-341-6000	www.bronsonhealth.com
Bryan Medical Center	Lincoln	Nebraska	402-481-1111	www.bryan.org
Caldwell Memorial Hospital	Lenoir	North Carolina	828-757-5100	www.caldwellmemorial.org
California Pacific Medical Center - Pacific Campus Hospital	San Francisco	California	415-600-6000	www.cpmc.org
Cape Cod Hospital	Hyannis	Massachusetts	508-771-1800	www.capecodhealth.org
Carolinas Medical Center - Pineville	Charlotte	North Carolina	704-379-5000	www.carolinashealthcare.org
Carondelet Saint Marys Hospital	Tucson	Arizona	520-872-3000	www.carondelet.org
Carondelet Saint Joseph's Hospital	Tucson	Arizona	520-873-3000	www.carondelet.org
Carteret General Hospital	Morehead City	North Carolina	252-808-6000	www.ccgh.org
Catawba Valley Medical Center	Hickory	North Carolina	828-326-3809	www.catawbavalleymc.org
Central Dupage Hospital	Winfield	Illinois	630-682-1600	www.cdh.org
Central Vermont Medical Center	Barre	Vermont	802-371-4100	www.cvmc.hitchcock.org
Central Washington Hospital	Wenatchee	Washington	509-662-1511	www.cwhs.com
Centura Health - Penrose Saint Francis Health Services	Colorado Springs	Colorado	719-776-5000	www.centurahealth.com
Centura Health - Saint Mary Corwin Medical Center	Pueblo	Colorado	719-557-4000	www.stmarycorwin.org
Chandler Regional Medical Center	Chandler	Arizona	480-963-4561	www.chandlerregional.com
Charlotte Hungerford Hospital	Torrington	Connecticut	860-496-6666	www.charlottesweb.hungerford.org
Cheyenne Regional Medical Center	Cheyenne	Wyoming	307-634-2273	www.crmcwy.org
Christus Health Shreveport - Bossier	Shreveport	Louisiana	318-681-5000	www.christusschumpert.org
Citizens Medical Center	Victoria	Texas	361-572-5113	www.citizensmedicalcenter.org
Citrus Memorial Hospital	Inverness	Florida	352-726-1551	www.citrusmh.com
CMC - Blue Ridge	Morganton	North Carolina	828-580-5000	www.gracehcs.org
Comanche County Memorial Hospital	Lawton	Oklahoma	580-355-8620	www.memorialhealthsource.org
Community Hospital of the Monterey Peninsula	Monterey	California	831-624-5311	www.chomp.org
Community Memorial Hospital San Buenaventura	Ventura	California	805-652-5011	www.cmhhospital.org
The Corpus Christi Medical Center	Corpus Christi	Texas	361-761-1501	www.ccmedicalcenter.com

Hospital	City	State	Phone	Web Site
Covenant Medical Center	Lubbock	Texas	806-725-6000	www.covenanthealth.org
Deaconess Hospital	Oklahoma City	Oklahoma	405-604-6109	www.deaconessokc.com
Dixie Regional Medical Center	Saint George	Utah	435-251-2100	www.intermountainhealthcare.org
Doctors Hospital of Sarasota	Sarasota	Florida	941-342-1100	www.doctorsofsarasota.com
Dominican Hospital	Santa Cruz	California	831-462-7700	www.dominicanhospital.org
East Jefferson General Hospital	Metairie	Louisiana	504-454-4000	www.eastjeffhospital.org
Eastern Idaho Regional Medical Center	Idaho Falls	Idaho	208-529-6111	www.eirmc.org
Eisenhower Medical Center	Rancho Mirage	California	760-340-3911	www.emc.org
Englewood Community Hospital	Englewood	Florida	941-475-6571	www.englewoodcommunityhospital.com
Ephrata Community Hospital	Ephrata	Pennsylvania	717-733-0311	www.ephratahospital.org
Evergreen Hospital Medical Center	Kirkland	Washington	425-899-1000	www.evergreenhospital.org
Exempla Lutheran Medical Center	Wheat Ridge	Colorado	303-425-4500	www.exemlpa.org
Fairview Southdale Hospital	Edina	Minnesota	952-924-5000	www.fairview.org
Falmouth Hospital	Falmouth	Massachusetts	508-548-5300	www.capecodhealth.com
Flagler Hospital	Saint Augustine	Florida	904-819-4426	www.flaglerhospital.com
Flagstaff Medical Center	Flagstaff	Arizona	928-773-2009	www.nahealth.com
Franciscan Saint Elizabeth Health - Lafayette East	Lafayette	Indiana	765-502-4334	www.ste.org
Freeman Health System - Freeman West	Joplin	Missouri	417-347-1111	www.freemanhealth.com
Genesis Medical Center - Davenport	Davenport	Iowa	563-421-1000	www.genesishealth.com
GHS Greenville Memorial Medical Center	Greenville	South Carolina	864-455-7000	www.ghs.org
Grand View Hospital	Sellersville	Pennsylvania	215-453-4615	www.gvh.org
Greater Baltimore Medical Center	Baltimore	Maryland	443-849-2000	www.gbmc.org
Gundersen Lutheran Medical Center	La Crosse	Wisconsin	608-782-7300	www.gundluth.org
Gwinnett Medical Center	Lawrenceville	Georgia	678-312-1000	www.gwinnettmedicalcenter.org
Harlingen Medical Center	Harlingen	Texas	956-365-1000	www.harlingenmedicalcenter.com
Harrison Memorial Center	Bremerton	Washington	360-377-3911	www.harrisonmedical.org
Hill Country Memorial Hospital	Fredericksburg	Texas	830-997-4353	www.hcmbs.org
Hinsdale Hospital	Hinsdale	Illinois	630-856-9000	www.keepingyouwell.com
Hoag Memorial Hospital Presbyterian	Newport Beach	California	949-645-8600	www.hoaghospital.org
Hoag Orthopedic Institute	Irvine	California	949-727-5000	www.orthopedichospital.com
Hospital For Special Surgery	New York	New York	212-606-1000	www.hss.edu
Huguley Memorial Medical Center	Burleson	Texas	817-568-5317	www.huguley.org
Huntington Memorial Hospital	Pasadena	California	626-397-5000	www.huntingtonhospital.com
Hutchinson Regional Medical Center	Hutchinson	Kansas	620-665-2001	www.hutchinsonhospital.com
Indian River Medical Center	Vero Beach	Florida	772-567-4311	www.irmh.com
Indiana University Health Ball Memorial Hospital	Muncie	Indiana	765-747-3111	www.accesschs.org/baal-memorial-l
Indiana University Health North Hospital	Carmel	Indiana	317-688-2000	www.iuhealth.org/north
Integris Baptist Medical Center	Oklahoma City	Oklahoma	405-951-8110	www.integris-health.com
Intermountain Medical Center	Murray	Utah	801-507-7000	www.intermountainhealthcare.org
Iowa Lutheran Hospital	Des Moines	Iowa	515-263-5612	www.ihsdesmoines.org
Iowa Methodist Medical Center	Des Moines	Iowa	515-241-6212	www.iowahealth.org
IU Health West Hospital	Avon	Indiana	317-217-3000	www.iuhealth.org/west
Jane Phillips Medical Center	Bartlesville	Oklahoma	918-333-7200	www.jpmc.org
John Muir Medical Center - Walnut Creek Campus	Walnut Creek	California	925-939-3000	www.jmmdhs.com
Kalispell Regional Medical Center	Kalispell	Montana	406-752-5111	www.krmc.org
Kaweah Delta Medical Center	Visalia	California	559-624-2000	www.kaweahdelta.org
Kenmore Mercy Hospital	Kenmore	New York	716-447-6100	www.chsbuffalo.org
Kettering Medical Center	Kettering	Ohio	937-298-4331	www.khnetwork.org
Kootenai Medical Center	Coeur D'alene	Idaho	208-625-4001	www.kootenaihealth.org
Lakeview Memorial Hospital	Stillwater	Minnesota	651-439-5330	www.lakeview.org
Lancaster General Hospital	Lancaster	Pennsylvania	717-299-5511	www.lancastergeneral.org
Lawrence & Memorial Hospital	New London	Connecticut	860-442-0711	www.lmhospital.org
Lawrence Memorial Hospital	Lawrence	Kansas	785-505-6100	www.lmh.org
Lehigh Valley Hospital	Allentown	Pennsylvania	610-402-2273	www.lvhhn.org
Lexington Medical Center	West Columbia	South Carolina	803-791-2000	www.lexmed.com
Lovelace Medical Center	Albuquerque	New Mexico	505-727-8000	www.lovelace.com
Mainegeneral Medical Center	Augusta	Maine	207-872-1000	www.mainegeneral.org
Margaret R Pardee Memorial Hospital	Hendersonville	North Carolina	828-696-1000	www.pardeehospital.org
Marian Regional Medical Center	Santa Maria	California	805-739-3000	www.marinmedicalcenter.org
Marion General Hospital	Marion	Indiana	765-660-6000	www.mgh.net
Marquette General Hospital	Marquette	Michigan	906-228-9440	www.mgh.org
Marshalltown Medical & Surgical Center	Marshalltown	Iowa	641-754-5151	www.everydaychampions.org
Mary Lanning Healthcare	Hastings	Nebraska	402-463-4521	www.marylanning.org
Maui Memorial Medical Center	Wailuku	Hawaii	808-442-5101	www.mauimemorialmedical.org
Mayo Clinic Health System - Eau Claire Hospital	Eau Claire	Wisconsin	715-838-3311	www.luthermidelfort.org
Mayo Clinic Hospital	Phoenix	Arizona	480-342-2000	www.mayoclinic.org
McBride Clinic Orthopedic Hospital	Oklahoma City	Oklahoma	405-478-1717	www.mcbrideclinic.com

Hospital	City	State	Phone	Web Site
McKay Dee Hospital	Ogden	Utah	801-387-2800	www.intermountainhealthcare.org
Mclaren - Northern Michigan	Petoskey	Michigan	231-487-4000	www.northernhealth.org
The Medical Center of Aurora	Aurora	Colorado	303-695-2600	www.auroramed.com
Medical City Dallas Hospital	Dallas	Texas	972-566-6222	www.medicalcityhospital.com
Medwest Haywood	Clyde	North Carolina	828-456-7311	www.haymed.org
Memorial Healthcare System	Chattanooga	Tennessee	423-495-2525	www.memorial.org
Memorial Hermann Hospital System	Houston	Texas	713-448-6796	www.memorialhermann.org
Memorial Hermann Memorial City Medical Center	Houston	Texas	713-242-3000	www.mhhs.org
Memorial Hospital & Health Care Center	Jasper	Indiana	812-996-2345	www.mhhcc.org
Memorial Hospital of South Bend	South Bend	Indiana	574-647-1000	www.qualityoflife.org
Memorial Medical Center of West Michigan	Ludington	Michigan	231-843-2591	www.mmcwm.com
Memorial Mission Hospital & Asheville Surgery Center	Asheville	North Carolina	828-213-1111	www.missionhospitals.org
Mercy General Hospital	Sacramento	California	916-453-4545	www.mercygeneral.org
Mercy Health Partners - Mercy Campus	Muskegon	Michigan	231-672-3901	www.mghp.com
Mercy Hospital	Iowa City	Iowa	319-339-0300	www.mercyiowacity.org
Mercy Hospital	Portland	Maine	207-879-3000	www.mercyhospital.com
Mercy Hospital	Buffalo	New York	716-826-7000	www.chsbuffalo.org
Mercy Hospital - Grayling	Grayling	Michigan	989-348-5461	www.mercygrayling.munsonhealthcare.org
Mercy Hospital Northwest Arkansas	Rogers	Arkansas	479-338-8000	www.mercy4u.com
Mercy Hospital Springfield	Springfield	Missouri	417-820-2000	www.stjohns.com
Mercy Medical Center	Canton	Ohio	330-489-1001	www.thequalityhospital.com
Mercy Medical Center	Roseburg	Oregon	541-673-0611	www.mercyrose.org
Mercy Medical Center - Redding	Redding	California	530-225-6102	www.redding.mercy.org
Mercy Medical Center - Des Moines	Des Moines	Iowa	515-247-3121	www.mercydesmoines.org
Meriter Hospital	Madison	Wisconsin	608-417-6000	www.meriter.com
Methodist Hospital	San Antonio	Texas	210-575-4000	www.mh.sahealth.com
Methodist Stone Oak Hospital	San Antonio	Texas	210-638-2100	www.stoneoakhealth.com
Methodist Sugar Land Hospital	Sugar Land	Texas	281-274-8000	www.methodisthealth.com/sugarland
Midland Memorial Hospital	Midland	Texas	432-685-1111	www.midland-memorial.com
Mills - Peninsula Medical Center	Burlingame	California	650-696-5270	www.mills-peninsula.org
Morristown Medical Center	Morristown	New Jersey	973-971-5450	www.morristownmemorialhospital.org
Morton Plant Hospital	Clearwater	Florida	727-462-7000	www.measehospitals.com
The Moses H Cone Memorial Hospital	Greensboro	North Carolina	336-832-7000	www.mosescone.com
Mother Frances Hospital	Tyler	Texas	903-593-8441	www.tmfhs.org
Munroe Regional Medical Center	Ocala	Florida	352-351-7200	www.munroeregional.com
Munson Medical Center	Traverse City	Michigan	231-935-5000	www.munsonhealthcare.org
Naples Community Hospital	Naples	Florida	239-436-5000	www.nchmd.org
Nebraska Heart Hospital	Lincoln	Nebraska	402-328-3000	www.neheart.com
New England Baptist Hospital	Boston	Massachusetts	617-754-5800	www.nebh.caregroup.org
New Hanover Regional Medical Center	Wilmington	North Carolina	910-343-7000	www.nhrmc.org
Newton Medical Center	Newton	Kansas	316-804-6001	www.newtonmedicalcenter.com
Norman Regional Health System	Norman	Oklahoma	405-321-1700	www.normanregional.com
North Memorial Medical Center	Robbinsdale	Minnesota	763-520-5200	www.northmemorial.com
North Shore Medical Center	Salem	Massachusetts	978-741-1215	www.nsmc.partners.org
Northside Hospital	Atlanta	Georgia	404-851-8000	www.northside.com
Northwest Community Hospital	Arlington Heights	Illinois	847-618-1000	www.nch.org
Northwest Hospital	Seattle	Washington	206-364-0500	www.nwhospital.org
Northwest Texas Hospital	Amarillo	Texas	806-354-1110	www.nxtexashealthcare.com
Novant Health Huntersville Medical Center	Huntersville	North Carolina	704-316-4000	www.presbyterian.org
Oklahoma Heart Hospital	Oklahoma City	Oklahoma	405-608-3200	www.okheart.com
Oklahoma Surgical Hospital	Tulsa	Oklahoma	918-477-5000	www.oklahomasurgicalhospital.com
Olympic Medical Center	Port Angeles	Washington	360-417-7000	www.olympicmedical.org
Our Lady of the Lake Regional Medical Center	Baton Rouge	Louisiana	225-765-6565	www.ololrmc.com
Overlake Hospital Medical Center	Bellevue	Washington	425-688-5000	www.overlakehospital.org
Owensboro Health Regional Hospital	Owensboro	Kentucky	270-688-2000	www.omhs.org
Palmetto Health Baptist	Columbia	South Carolina	803-296-5678	www.palmettohealth.org
Palmetto Health Richland	Columbia	South Carolina	803-296-5678	www.palmettohealth.org
Park Nicollet Methodist Hospital	Saint Louis Park	Minnesota	952-993-5000	www.parknicollet.com/methodist
Parkview Medical Center	Pueblo	Colorado	719-584-4000	www.parkviewmc.com
Parkview Regional Medical Center	Fort Wayne	Indiana	260-266-1000	www.parkview.com
Peacehealth Saint Joseph Medical Center	Bellingham	Washington	360-734-5400	www.peacehealth.org
Peninsula Regional Medical Center	Salisbury	Maryland	410-543-7111	www.peninsula.org
Penn Highlands Dubois	Dubois	Pennsylvania	814-371-2200	www.drmc.org
Petaluma Valley Hospital	Petaluma	California	707-778-1111	www.stjosephhealth.org
Phelps County Regional Medical Center	Rolla	Missouri	573-458-8899	www.rollanet.org/~pcrmc
Piedmont Fayette Hospital	Fayetteville	Georgia	770-719-7071	www.fayettehospital.org
Piedmont Hospital	Atlanta	Georgia	404-605-5000	www.piedmonthospital.org

Hospital	City	State	Phone	Web Site
Plaza Medical Center of Fort Worth	Fort Worth	Texas	817-336-2100	www.plazamedicalcenter.com
Porter Regional Hospital	Valparaiso	Indiana	219-983-8300	www.portermemorial.org
Portneuf Medical Center	Pocatello	Idaho	208-239-1000	www.portmed.org
Presbyterian Hospital	Albuquerque	New Mexico	505-724-8386	www.phs.org
Presbyterian Hospital Matthews	Matthews	North Carolina	704-384-6500	www.presbyterian.org
Providence Alaska Medical Center	Anchorage	Alaska	907-261-3675	www.providence.org
Providence Holy Family Hospital	Spokane	Washington	509-482-2450	www.holy-family.org
Providence Hospital	Mobile	Alabama	251-633-1000	www.providencehospital.org
Providence Regional Medical Center Everett	Everett	Washington	425-261-2000	www.providence.org
Providence Sacred Heart Medical Center	Spokane	Washington	509-474-3040	www.shmc.org
Providence Saint John's Health Center	Santa Monica	California	310-829-5511	www.stjohns.org
Providence Saint Mary Medical Center	Walla Walla	Washington	509-522-5900	www.smmc.com
Providence Saint Peter Hospital	Olympia	Washington	360-491-9480	www.providence.org/swsa
Providence Saint Vincent Medical Center	Portland	Oregon	503-216-1234	www.providence.org
Rapid City Regional Hospital	Rapid City	South Dakota	605-719-1000	www.rcrh.org
Reading Hospital	Reading	Pennsylvania	610-988-8000	www.readinghospital.org
Reid Hospital & Health Care Services	Richmond	Indiana	765-983-3000	www.reidhosp.com
Rex Hospital	Raleigh	North Carolina	919-784-3100	www.rexhealth.com
Roper Hospital	Charleston	South Carolina	843-724-2800	www.ropersaintfrancis.com
Sacred Heart Medical Center - Riverbend	Springfield	Oregon	541-222-7300	www.peacehealth.org/sacred-heart-riverbend
Saddleback Memorial Medical Center	Laguna Hills	California	949-837-4500	www.memorialcare.org/saddleback
Saint Barnabas Medical Center	Livingston	New Jersey	973-322-5000	www.saintbarnabas.com
Saint Elizabeth Regional Medical Center	Lincoln	Nebraska	402-219-7700	www.stelizabethonline.com
Saint Joseph Regional Medical Center	Mishawaka	Indiana	574-335-5000	www.sjmed.com
Saint Joseph's Hospital of Atlanta	Atlanta	Georgia	678-843-5720	www.stjosephsatlanta.org
Saint Mary's Health Care	Grand Rapids	Michigan	616-685-5000	www.smhealthcare.org
Saint Thomas West Hospital	Nashville	Tennessee	615-222-2111	www.stthomas.org
Saint Vincent Hospital	Erie	Pennsylvania	814-452-5000	www.svhs.org
Salem Hospital	Salem	Oregon	503-561-5200	www.salemhospital.org
Salem Regional Medical Center	Salem	Ohio	330-332-1551	www.salemhosp.com
Salina Regional Health Center	Salina	Kansas	785-452-7000	www.srhc.com
Salinas Valley Memorial Hospital	Salinas	California	831-757-4333	www.svmh.com
Samaritan Albany General Hospital	Albany	Oregon	541-812-4000	www.samhealth.org/shs_facilities
Sampson Regional Medical Center	Clinton	North Carolina	910-592-8511	www.sampsonrmc.org
San Jacinto Methodist Hospital	Baytown	Texas	281-420-8600	www.methodisthealth.com/sanjacinto
Sanford Bemidji Medical Center	Bemidji	Minnesota	218-751-5430	www.nchs.com
Sanford Medical Center Fargo	Fargo	North Dakota	701-234-2000	www.meritcare.com
Sanford Usd Medical Center	Sioux Falls	South Dakota	605-333-1000	www.sanfordhealth.org
Santa Barbara Cottage Hospital	Santa Barbara	California	805-682-7111	www.cottagehealthsystem.org
Santa Rosa Memorial Hospital	Santa Rosa	California	707-525-5300	www.stjosephhealth.org
Sarasota Memorial Hospital	Sarasota	Florida	941-917-9000	www.smh.com
Saratoga Hospital	Saratoga Springs	New York	518-587-3222	www.saratogacare.org
Scottsdale Healthcare Osborn Medical Center	Scottsdale	Arizona	480-882-4000	www.shc.org
Scottsdale Healthcare - Shea Medical Center	Scottsdale	Arizona	480-323-3009	www.shc.org
Scottsdale Healthcare - Thompson Peak Hospital	Scottsdale	Arizona	480-324-7004	www.shc.org
Scripps Memorial Hospital - Encinitas	Encinitas	California	760-753-6501	www.scripps.org
Sentara Williamsburg Regional Medical Center	Williamsburg	Virginia	757-984-6000	www.sentara.com
Sequoia Hospital	Redwood City	California	650-367-5551	www.sequoiahospital.org
Seven Rivers Regional Medical Center	Crystal River	Florida	352-795-6560	www.srrmc.com
Sisters of Charity Providence Hospitals	Columbia	South Carolina	803-256-5300	www.providencehospitals.com
Sky Lakes Medical Center	Klamath Falls	Oregon	541-274-6150	www.skylakes.org
Sky Ridge Medical Center	Lone Tree	Colorado	720-225-1000	www.skyridgemedcenter.com
Sonoma Valley Hospital	Sonoma	California	707-935-5000	www.svh.com
Sonora Regional Medical Center	Sonora	California	209-532-3161	www.sonorahospital.org
South Lake Hospital	Clermont	Florida	352-394-4071	www.southlakehospital.com
Spartanburg Regional Medical Center	Spartanburg	South Carolina	864-560-6000	www.srhs.com
Spectrum Health - Butterworth Campus	Grand Rapids	Michigan	616-391-1774	www.spectrum-health.org
Saint Agnes Hospital	Fond Du Lac	Wisconsin	920-929-2300	www.agnesian.com
Saint Alexius Medical Center	Bismarck	North Dakota	701-530-7000	www.st.alexius.org
Saint Alphonsus Regional Medical Center	Boise	Idaho	208-367-2121	www.saintalphonsus.org
Saint Bernardine Medical Center	San Bernardino	California	909-881-4440	www.stbernardinemedicalcenter.com
Saint Charles Medical Center - Bend	Bend	Oregon	541-382-4321	www.scmc.org
Saint David's Medical Center	Austin	Texas	512-476-7111	www.stdavidsrehab.com
Saint Edward Mercy Medical Center	Fort Smith	Arkansas	479-314-6000	www.stedwardmercy.com
Saint Francis Hospital	Columbus	Georgia	706-596-4020	www.wecareforlife.com
Saint Francis Hospital - Roslyn	Roslyn	New York	516-562-6000	www.stfrancisheartcenter.com
Saint Francis Medical Center	Grand Island	Nebraska	308-384-4600	www.saintfrancisgi.org

Hospital	City	State	Phone	Web Site
Saint Francis - Downtown	Greenville	South Carolina	864-255-1000	www.stfrancishealth.org
Saint Joseph Hospital	Eureka	California	707-445-8121	www.stjosepheureka.org
Saint Joseph Hospital & Health Center	Kokomo	Indiana	765-456-5300	www.stvincent.org
Saint Joseph Medical Center	Reading	Pennsylvania	610-378-2300	www.sjmcberks.org
Saint Joseph Regional Medical Center	Lewiston	Idaho	208-743-2511	www.sjrmc.org
Saint Luke's Regional Medical Center	Boise	Idaho	208-381-2222	www.slrmc.org
Saint Luke's Hospital	Cedar Rapids	Iowa	319-369-7211	www.crstlukes.com
Saint Luke's Hospital	Duluth	Minnesota	218-249-5555	www.slhduluth.com
Saint Marks Hospital	Salt Lake City	Utah	801-268-7700	www.stmarkshospital.com
Saint Mary's Regional Medical Center	Enid	Oklahoma	580-233-6100	www.stmarysregional.com
Saint Marys Hospital	Madison	Wisconsin	608-251-6100	www.stmarysmadison.com
Saint Marys Hospital & Medical Center	Grand Junction	Colorado	970-298-1950	www.stmarygj.org
Saint Marys Regional Medical Center	Lewiston	Maine	207-777-8100	www.stmarysmaine.com
Saint Patrick Hospital	Missoula	Montana	406-543-7271	www.saintpatrick.org
Saint Peter's Hospital	Albany	New York	518-525-1550	www.stpetershealthcare.org
Saint Rose Dominican Hospitals - Siena Campus	Henderson	Nevada	702-616-5000	www.strosehospitals.org
Saint Vincent Heart Center of Indiana	Indianapolis	Indiana	317-583-5000	www.theheartcenter.com
Saint Vincent Hospital	Green Bay	Wisconsin	920-433-0111	www.stvincenthospital.org
Saint Vincent Hospital & Health Services	Indianapolis	Indiana	317-338-7000	www.indianapolis.stvincent.org
Sutter Auburn Faith Hospital	Auburn	California	530-888-4500	www.sutterauburnfaith.org
Sutter Roseville Medical Center	Roseville	California	916-781-1000	www.sutterroseville.org
Tallahassee Memorial Hospital	Tallahassee	Florida	850-431-1155	www.tmh.org
Tennova Healthcare	Knoxville	Tennessee	865-545-8000	www.stmaryshealth.com
Texas Health Harris Methodist Fort Worth	Fort Worth	Texas	817-250-2100	www.texashealth.org
Texas Health Presbyterian Hospital Plano	Plano	Texas	972-981-8000	www.presbyplano.org
Texas Health Presbyterian Hospital - WNJ	Sherman	Texas	903-870-4611	www.wnj.org
Texas Orthopedic Hospital	Houston	Texas	713-799-8600	www.texasorthopedic.com
The Queens Medical Center	Honolulu	Hawaii	808-538-9011	www.queens.org
The Toledo Hospital	Toledo	Ohio	419-291-7463	www.promedica.org
Touro Infirmary	New Orleans	Louisiana	504-897-7011	www.touro.com
United Hospital	Saint Paul	Minnesota	651-241-8802	www.allinahealth.org/ahs/united.nsf
University Colo Health Memorial Hospital Central	Colorado Springs	Colorado	719-365-5000	www.memorialhospital.com
University of Wisconsin Hospitals & Clinics Authority	Madison	Wisconsin	608-263-8991	www.uwhealth.org
UPMC Altoona	Altoona	Pennsylvania	814-889-2011	www.altoonaregional.org
UPMC Hamot	Erie	Pennsylvania	814-877-6000	www.hamot.org
Utah Valley Regional Medical Center	Provo	Utah	801-373-7850	www.intermountainhealthcare.org/hospitals/uvrmc
Venice Regional Medical Center - Bayfront Health	Venice	Florida	941-485-7711	www.veniceregional.com
VHS Harlingen Hospital Company	Harlingen	Texas	956-389-1100	www.vbmc.org
Via Christi Hospital Pittsburg	Pittsburg	Kansas	620-231-6100	www.via-christi.org
Via Christi Hospitals Wichita	Wichita	Kansas	316-268-5000	www.via-christi.org
Wakemed - Raleigh Campus	Raleigh	North Carolina	919-350-8000	www.wakemed.org
Wentworth - Douglass Hospital	Dover	New Hampshire	603-740-2580	www.wdhospital.com
Wesley Medical Center	Wichita	Kansas	316-962-2000	www.wesleymc.com
West Calcasieu Cameron Hospital	Sulphur	Louisiana	337-527-7034	www.wcch.com
West Shore Medical Center	Manistee	Michigan	231-398-1000	www.westshoremedcenter.org
Williamsport Regional Medical Center	Williamsport	Pennsylvania	570-321-1000	www.susquehannahealth.org
Willis Knighton Medical Center	Shreveport	Louisiana	318-212-4000	www.wkhs.com//locations/medicalcenter.aspx
Woodland Heights Medical Center	Lufkin	Texas	936-634-8311	www.woodlandheights.net
Wooster Community Hospital	Wooster	Ohio	330-263-8100	www.woosterhospital.org

Note: Table shows hospitals nationwide whose rate of readmission after discharge from hospital (hospital-wide) is better (lower) than U.S. rate of 16.0%

Hospitals whose Rate of Readmission After Discharge From Hospital (Hospital-wide) is Worse (Higher) than the U.S. National Rate

Hospital	City	State	Phone	Web Site
Adena Regional Medical Center	Chillicothe	Ohio	740-779-7500	www.adena.org
Advocate Christ Hospital & Medical Center	Oak Lawn	Illinois	708-684-8000	www.advocatehealth.com
Advocate Illinois Masonic Medical Center	Chicago	Illinois	773-975-1600	www.advocatehealth.com/immc
Advocate Trinity Hospital	Chicago	Illinois	773-967-2000	www.advocatehealth.com/trin
Albert Einstein Medical Center	Philadelphia	Pennsylvania	215-456-6090	www.einstein.edu
Anne Arundel Medical Center	Annapolis	Maryland	443-481-1307	www.aahs.org
Aria Health	Philadelphia	Pennsylvania	215-612-4129	www.ariahealth.com
Arkansas Methodist Medical Center	Paragould	Arkansas	870-239-7000	www.arkansasmethodist.org
Atlanticare Regional Medical Center	Atlantic City	New Jersey	609-441-8020	www.atlanticare.org/acmc/index.html
Aventura Hospital & Medical Center	Aventura	Florida	305-682-7000	www.aventurahospital.com
B R F Hospital Holdings	Shreveport	Louisiana	318-675-5000	www.lsumc.edu
Banner Desert Medical Center	Mesa	Arizona	480-412-3000	www.bannerhealth.com
Baptist Beaumont Hospital	Beaumont	Texas	409-212-5012	www.mhbh.org
Baptist Memorial Hospital Desoto	Southaven	Mississippi	662-772-4000	www.bmhcc.org/facilities/desoto
Barnes-Jewish Hospital	Saint Louis	Missouri	314-747-3000	www.barnesjewish.org
Baxter Regional Medical Center	Mountain Home	Arkansas	870-508-1000	www.baxterregional.org
Beaumont Health System	Grosse Pointe	Michigan	313-343-1000	www.beaumonthospitals.com
Beaumont Health System	Royal Oak	Michigan	248-898-5000	www.beaumonthospitals.com
Beckley ARH Hospital	Beckley	West Virginia	304-255-3456	www.arh.org/beckley
Bellevue Hospital Center	New York	New York	212-561-4132	www.nyc.gov/html/hhc/html/facilities/bellevue.shtml
Beth Israel Deaconess Hospital - Milton	Milton	Massachusetts	617-696-4600	www.miltonhosital.org
Beth Israel Deaconess Medical Center	Boston	Massachusetts	617-667-7000	www.bidmc.harvard.edu
Beth Israel Medical Center	New York	New York	212-420-2000	www.wehealny.org
Bluefield Regional Medical Center	Bluefield	West Virginia	304-327-1100	www.bluefield.org
Bolivar Medical Center	Cleveland	Mississippi	662-846-2551	www.bolivarmedical.com
Boston Medical Center Corporation	Boston	Massachusetts	617-638-8000	www.bmc.org
Botsford Hospital	Farmington Hills	Michigan	248-471-8000	www.botsfordsystem.org
Bridgeport Hospital	Bridgeport	Connecticut	203-384-3000	www.bridgeporthospital.com
Brigham & Women's Faulkner Hospital	Boston	Massachusetts	617-983-7000	www.brighamandwomensfaulkner.org
Brigham & Women's Hospital	Boston	Massachusetts	617-732-5500	www.brighamandwomens.org
Bronx - Lebanon Hospital Center	Bronx	New York	212-588-7000	www.bronx-leb.org
Brookdale Hospital Medical Center	Brooklyn	New York	718-240-5966	www.brookdalehospital.org
Brookhaven Memorial Hospital Medical Center	Patchogue	New York	631-654-7100	www.brookhavenhospitalorg
Brooklyn Hospital Center at Downtown Campus	Brooklyn	New York	718-250-8000	www.tbh.org
Byrd Regional Hospital	Leesville	Louisiana	337-239-9041	www.chs.net
California Hospital Medical Center Los Angeles	Los Angeles	California	213-748-2411	www.chmcla.org
Camden Clark Medical Center	Parkersburg	West Virginia	304-424-2111	www.ccmh.org
Capital Health System - Fuld Campus	Trenton	New Jersey	609-394-6000	www.capitalhealth.org
Capital Regional Medical Center	Tallahassee	Florida	850-656-5000	www.capitalregionalmedicalcenter.com
Carepoint Health - Christ Hospital	Jersey City	New Jersey	201-795-8200	www.christhospital.org
Carepoint Health - Hoboken UMC	Hoboken	New Jersey	201-418-1004	www.bonsecoursnj.com
Carolinas Hospital System	Florence	South Carolina	843-674-2500	www.carolinashospital.com
Casey County Hospital	Liberty	Kentucky	606-787-6275	
Catskill Regional Medical Center	Harris	New York	845-794-3300	www.crmcny.org
Chambers Memorial Hospital	Danville	Arkansas	479-495-2241	www.chambershospital.com
Chesapeake General Hospital	Chesapeake	Virginia	757-312-8121	www.chesapeakehealth.com
Clay County Hospital	Flora	Illinois	618-662-2131	www.claycountyhospital.org
Cleveland Clinic	Cleveland	Ohio	216-444-2200	www.clevelandclinic.org
Cleveland Clinic Hospital	Weston	Florida	954-689-5000	www.clevelandclinic.org
Clinch Valley Medical Center	Richlands	Virginia	276-596-6000	www.clinchvalleymedicalcenter.com
Coffee Regional Medical Center	Douglas	Georgia	229-384-1900	www.coffeeregional.org
Coliseum Medical Center	Macon	Georgia	478-765-4100	www.coliseumhealthsystem.com
Community Regional Medical Center	Fresno	California	559-459-6000	www.communitymedical.org
Conemaugh Valley Memorial Hospital	Johnstown	Pennsylvania	814-534-9000	www.conemaugh.org
Coney Island Hospital	Brooklyn	New York	718-616-3000	www.coneyislandhospital.com
Cooper University Hospital	Camden	New Jersey	856-342-2000	www.cooperhealth.org
Covenant Medical Center	Saginaw	Michigan	989-583-4000	www.covenanthealthcare.com
Crittenden Health System	Marion	Kentucky	270-965-5281	www.crittenden-health.org
Danville Regional Medical Center	Danville	Virginia	434-799-2100	www.danvilleregional.org
Davis Memorial Hospital	Elkins	West Virginia	304-636-3300	www.davishealthcare.org
Desert Valley Hospital	Victorville	California	760-241-8000	www.dvmc.com
Desoto Memorial Hospital	Arcadia	Florida	863-494-3535	www.dmh.org
Detroit Receiving Hospital & University Health Center	Detroit	Michigan	313-745-3104	www.drhuhc.org
Doctors Hospital	Columbus	Ohio	614-544-1000	www.columbusregional.com
Doctors Hospital of Manteca	Manteca	California	209-823-3111	www.doctorsmanteca.com

Hospital	City	State	Phone	Web Site
Drew Memorial Hospital	Monticello	Arkansas	870-367-2411	www.drewmemorial.org
Duke University Hospital	Durham	North Carolina	919-684-8111	www.dukehealth.org
Dyersburg Regional Medical Center	Dyersburg	Tennessee	731-285-2410	www.dyersburgregionalmc.com
East Georgia Regional Medical Center	Statesboro	Georgia	912-486-1500	www.egrmc.com
East Ohio Regional Hospital	Martins Ferry	Ohio	740-633-4151	www.eastohioregionalhospital.com
East Orange General Hospital	East Orange	New Jersey	973-266-4401	www.evh.org
Eastern Niagara Hospital	Lockport	New York	716-514-5700	www.enhs.org
Eastern State Hospital	Williamsburg	Virginia	757-253-5161	www.ehs.dmhmrsas.virginia.gov
Easton Hospital	Easton	Pennsylvania	610-250-4076	www.easton-hospital.com
Elmhurst Hospital Center	Elmhurst	New York	718-334-1141	www.nyc.gov
Emanuel Medical Center	Turlock	California	209-667-4200	www.emanuelmedicalcenter.org
Excela Health Frick Hospital	Mount Pleasant	Pennsylvania	724-547-1500	www.excelahealth.org
Fauquier Hospital	Warrenton	Virginia	540-316-5000	www.fauquierhospital.org
Fayette County Hospital	Vandalia	Illinois	618-283-1231	www.fayettecountyhospital.org
Fitzgibbon Hospital	Marshall	Missouri	660-886-7431	www.fitzgibbon.org
Florida Hospital	Orlando	Florida	407-303-1976	www.floridahospital.com
Flushing Hospital Medical Center	Flushing	New York	718-670-5000	www.flushinghospital.org
Forest Hills Hospital	Forest Hills	New York	718-830-4000	www.northshorelij.com
Franciscan Saint James Health	Olympia Fields	Illinois	708-747-4000	www.franciscanalliance.org
Franciscan Saint Margaret Health - Hammond	Hammond	Indiana	219-932-2300	www.smmhc.com
Franklin Hospital	Valley Stream	New York	516-256-6000	www.northshorelij.com
Frederick Memorial Hospital	Frederick	Maryland	240-566-3300	www.fmh.org
Garden City Hospital	Garden City	Michigan	734-421-3300	www.gchosp.org
Gateway Medical Center	Clarksville	Tennessee	931-502-1000	www.todaysgateway.com
Genesis Healthcare System	Zanesville	Ohio	740-454-5000	www.genesishcs.org
George Washington Univ Hospital	Washington	District of Columbia	202-716-4605	www.gwhospital.com
Glenwood Regional Medical Center	West Monroe	Louisiana	318-329-4600	www.grmc.com
Good Samaritan Hospital of Suffern	Suffern	New York	914-368-5000	www.goodsamhosp.org
Grant Medical Center	Columbus	Ohio	614-566-9978	www.ohiohealth.com
Great River Medical Center	Blytheville	Arkansas	870-838-7300	www.greatrivermc.com
Harlan Appalachian Regional Healthcare Hospital	Harlan	Kentucky	606-573-8100	www.arh.org
Harlem Hospital Center	New York	New York	212-491-8400	www.nyc.gov/hhc
Harper University Hospital	Detroit	Michigan	313-745-6211	www.harperhospital.org
Harris Hospital	Newport	Arkansas	870-523-8911	www.harrishospital.com
Harton Regional Medical Center	Tullahoma	Tennessee	931-393-3000	www.hartonmedicalcenter.com
Hazard ARH Regional Medical Center	Hazard	Kentucky	606-439-6600	www.arh.org/hazard
Health Alliance Hospital Broadway Campus	Kingston	New York	914-331-3131	www.kingstonregionalhealth.org
Henry Ford Hospital	Detroit	Michigan	313-916-2600	www.henryfordhospital.com
Hialeah Hospital	Hialeah	Florida	305-693-6100	www.hialeahhosp.com
Highlands Regional Medical Center	Prestonsburg	Kentucky	606-886-8511	www.hrmc.org
Hollywood Presbyterian Medical Center	Los Angeles	California	213-413-3000	www.qahpmc.com
Holy Cross Hospital	Chicago	Illinois	773-471-8000	www.holycrosshospital.org
Holzer Medical Center	Gallipolis	Ohio	740-446-5000	www.holzer.org
Hospital of Univ of Pennsylvania	Philadelphia	Pennsylvania	215-662-3227	www.upenn.edu
Howard University Hospital	Washington	District of Columbia	202-745-6100	www.huhosp.org
Hudson Valley Hospital Center	Cortlandt Manor	New York	914-734-3611	www.hvhc.org
Illinois Valley Community Hospital	Peru	Illinois	815-223-3300	www.ivch.org
Ingalls Memorial Hospital	Harvey	Illinois	708-333-2300	www.ingalls.org
Jackson Memorial Hospital	Miami	Florida	305-585-1111	www.jhsmiami.org
Jackson Parish Hospital	Jonesboro	Louisiana	318-259-4435	www.jacksonparishhospital.com
Jackson Park Hospital	Chicago	Illinois	773-947-7500	www.jacksonparkhospital.org
Jacobi Medical Center	Bronx	New York	718-918-5000	www.ci.nyc.ny.us/html/hhc
Jamaica Hospital Medical Center	Jamaica	New York	718-262-6000	www.jamaicahospital.org
Jane Todd Crawford Hospital	Greensburg	Kentucky	270-932-4211	
Jeanes Hospital	Philadelphia	Pennsylvania	215-728-2000	www.jeanes.com
Jennie Stuart Medical Center	Hopkinsville	Kentucky	270-887-0100	www.jsmc.org
Jennings American Legion Hospital	Jennings	Louisiana	337-616-7000	www.jalh.com
JFK Medical Center	Atlantis	Florida	561-965-7300	www.jfkmc.com
JFK Medical Center - A M Yelencsics Comm Hospital	Edison	New Jersey	732-321-7000	www.jfkmc.org
John H Stroger Jr Hospital	Chicago	Illinois	312-864-6000	www.cookcountygov.com
Johns Hopkins Bayview Medical Center	Baltimore	Maryland	410-550-0123	www.hopkinsbayview.org
The Johns Hopkins Hospital	Baltimore	Maryland	410-955-9540	www.jhmi.edu
Johnson City Medical Center	Johnson City	Tennessee	423-431-6111	www.msha.com
Kendall Regional Medical Center	Miami	Florida	305-223-3000	www.kendallmed.com
Kennedy University Hospital - Stratford Div	Stratford	New Jersey	856-346-6000	www.kennedyhealth.org
Kent County Memorial Hospital	Warwick	Rhode Island	401-737-7000	www.kentri.org
Kentucky River Medical Center	Jackson	Kentucky	606-666-6000	www.kentuckyrivermc.com

Hospital	City	State	Phone	Web Site
King's Daughters' Medical Center	Ashland	Kentucky	606-408-4000	www.kdmc.com
Kings County Hospital Center	Brooklyn	New York	718-245-3901	www.nyc.gov/html/hhc/html/facilities/kings.shtml
Kingsbrook Jewish Medical Center	Brooklyn	New York	718-604-5789	www.kingsbrook.org
Knox County Hospital	Barbourville	Kentucky	606-546-4175	www.knoxcohospital.com
Lahey Hospital & Medical Center - Burlington	Burlington	Massachusetts	781-744-5100	www.lahey.org
Lake Pointe Medical Center	Rowlett	Texas	972-412-2273	www.lakepointemedical.com
Lake Wales Medical Center	Lake Wales	Florida	863-676-1433	www.lakewalesmedicalcenter.com
Larkin Community Hospital	South Miami	Florida	305-284-7500	www.larkinhospital.com
Laurel Regional Medical Center	Laurel	Maryland	301-725-4300	www.laurelregionalhospital.org
Lawrence Hospital Center	Bronxville	New York	914-787-1000	www.lawrencehealth.org
Leesburg Regional Medical Center	Leesburg	Florida	352-323-5762	www.leesburgregional.org
Lenox Hill Hospital	New York	New York	212-439-2345	www.lenoxhillhospital.org
Lewisgale Hospital Pulaski	Pulaski	Virginia	540-994-8100	www.lewisgale.com
Libertyhealth - Jersey City Medical Center Campus	Jersey City	New Jersey	201-915-2000	www.libertyhcs.org
Lincoln Medical & Mental Health Center	Bronx	New York	718-579-5000	www.nyc.gov/html/hhc/lincoln
Little Company of Mary Hospital	Evergreen Park	Illinois	708-422-6200	www.lcmh.org
Long Island Jewish Medical Center	New Hyde Park	New York	718-470-7000	www.northshorelij.com
Lowell General Hospital	Lowell	Massachusetts	978-937-6000	www.lowellgeneral.org
Loyola University Medical Center	Maywood	Illinois	708-216-9000	www.lumc.edu
Lutheran Medical Center	Brooklyn	New York	718-630-8000	www.lmcmc.com
Maimonides Medical Center	Brooklyn	New York	718-283-6000	www.maimonidesmed.org
Mary Immaculate Hospital	Newport News	Virginia	757-886-6000	www.bonsecourshamptonroad.com
Medical Center of Southeastern Oklahoma	Durant	Oklahoma	405-924-3080	www.mcsohealth.com
Medical College of Georgia Hospitals & Clinics	Augusta	Georgia	706-721-6569	www.mcghealth.org
Medical College of Virginia Hospitals	Richmond	Virginia	804-828-0938	www.vcuhealth.org
Medstar Good Samaritan Hospital	Baltimore	Maryland	443-444-3902	www.goodsam-md.org
Medstar Montgomery Medical Center	Olney	Maryland	301-774-8882	www.montgomerygeneral.com
Memorial Hospital	Manchester	Kentucky	606-598-5104	www.manchestermemorial.com
Memorial Hospital	Nacogdoches	Texas	936-564-4611	www.nacmem.org
Memorial Hospital of Gardena	Gardena	California	310-532-4200	www.avantihospitals.com
Memorial Hospital of Salem County	Salem	New Jersey	856-935-1000	www.mhshealth.com
Memorial Hospital of Stilwell	Stilwell	Oklahoma	918-696-3101	www.stilwellmemorialhospital.com
Memorial Regional Hospital	Hollywood	Florida	954-987-2000	www.memorialregional.com
Mercy Fitzgerald Hospital	Darby	Pennsylvania	215-237-4000	www.mercyhealth.org
Mercy Hospital & Medical Center	Chicago	Illinois	312-567-2000	www.mercy-chicago.org
Mercy Hospital Anderson	Cincinnati	Ohio	513-624-4006	www.e-mercy.com/mercy-hospital-anderson.aspx
Mercy Hospital Fairfield	Fairfield	Ohio	513-870-7197	www.e-mercy.com/mercy-hospital-fairfield.aspx
Mercy Hospital Jefferson	Crystal City	Missouri	636-933-1000	www.jeffersonmemorial.org
Mercy Medical Center	Baltimore	Maryland	410-332-9237	www.mdmercy.com
Mercy Regional Medical Center	Ville Platte	Louisiana	337-363-5684	www.vpmc.com
Methodist Hospital	Henderson	Kentucky	270-827-7700	www.methodisthospital.net
Methodist Hospitals	Gary	Indiana	219-886-4642	www.methodisthospital.org
Metrosouth Medical Center	Blue Island	Illinois	708-597-2000	www.stfrancisblueisland.com
Middlesboro Appalachian Regional Healthcare Hospital	Middlesboro	Kentucky	606-242-1101	www.arh.org/middlesboro
Midwest Regional Medical Center	Midwest City	Oklahoma	405-610-8530	www.midwestregional.com
Milford Regional Medical Center	Milford	Massachusetts	508-473-1190	www.milfordregional.org
Miriam Hospital	Providence	Rhode Island	401-793-2500	www.lifespan.org/partners/tmh
Mission Regional Medical Center	Mission	Texas	956-323-9000	www.missionhospital.org
Monmouth Medical Center - Southern Campus	Lakewood	New Jersey	732-363-1900	www.sbhcs.com
Monroe County Medical Center	Tompkinsville	Kentucky	270-487-9231	www.mcmccares.com
Montefiore Medical Center	Bronx	New York	718-920-4321	www.montefiore.org
Montefiore New Rochelle Hospital	New Rochelle	New York	914-632-5000	www.ssmc.org
Morgan County ARH Hospital	West Liberty	Kentucky	606-743-3186	www.arh.org/morgan
Morton Hospital	Taunton	Massachusetts	508-828-7000	www.mortonhospital.org
Mountainview Hospital	Las Vegas	Nevada	702-255-5065	www.mountainview-hospital.com
Musc Medical Center	Charleston	South Carolina	843-792-2300	www.musc.edu
Nacogdoches Medical Center	Nacogdoches	Texas	936-569-9481	www.nacmedicalcenter.com
Nassau University Medical Center	East Meadow	New York	516-572-0123	www.numc.edu
Natchez Community Hospital	Natchez	Mississippi	601-445-6205	www.natchezcommunityhospital.com
Nazareth Hospital	Philadelphia	Pennsylvania	215-335-6000	www.nazarethhospital.org
New York Community Hospital of Brooklyn	Brooklyn	New York	718-692-5302	www.nych.com
New York Hospital Medical Center of Queens	Flushing	New York	718-670-1231	www.nyhq.org
New York Methodist Hospital	Brooklyn	New York	718-780-3000	www.nym.org
New York - Presbyterian Hospital	New York	New York	212-746-4189	www.nyp.org
Newark Beth Israel Medical Center	Newark	New Jersey	973-926-7850	www.sbhcs.com
North Oaks Medical Center	Hammond	Louisiana	985-345-2700	www.northoaks.org
North Shore University Hospital	Manhasset	New York	516-562-0100	www.northshorelij.com

Hospital	City	State	Phone	Web Site
Northside Hospital	Saint Petersburg	Florida	813-521-5000	www.northsidehospital.com
Northwest Hospital Center	Randallstown	Maryland	410-521-5995	www.lifebridgehealth.org
Northwest Mississippi Regional Medical Center	Clarksdale	Mississippi	662-627-3211	www.nwmsregionalmedcenter.com
Northwestern Memorial Hospital	Chicago	Illinois	312-926-2000	www.nmh.org
Norwegian - American Hospital	Chicago	Illinois	773-292-8200	www.nahospital.org
Nyack Hospital	Nyack	New York	845-348-2000	www.nyackhospital.org
NYU Hospitals Center	New York	New York	212-263-7300	www.med.nyu.edu
Oakwood Hospital - Dearborn	Dearborn	Michigan	313-593-7125	www.oakwood.org
Oakwood Hospital - Taylor	Taylor	Michigan	313-295-5253	www.oakwod.org
Oakwood Hospital - Wayne	Wayne	Michigan	734-467-4175	www.oakwood.org
Ohio State University Hospitals	Columbus	Ohio	614-293-9700	www.jamesline.com
Olympia Medical Center	Los Angeles	California	310-657-5900	www.olympiamc.com
Orange Regional Medical Center	Middletown	New York	845-343-2424	www.ormc.org
Oroville Hospital	Oroville	California	530-533-8500	www.orovillehospital.com
Osceola Regional Medical Center	Kissimmee	Florida	407-846-2266	www.osceolaregional.com
Pacifica Hospital of the Valley	Sun Valley	California	818-767-3310	www.pacificahospital.com
Palisades Medical Center	North Bergen	New Jersey	201-854-5000	www.palisadesmedical.org
Palm Springs General Hospital	Hialeah	Florida	305-558-2500	www.psghosp.com
Palmetto General Hospital	Hialeah	Florida	305-823-5000	www.palmettogeneral.com
Palms West Hospital	Loxahatchee	Florida	561-753-4245	www.palmswesthospital.com
Peacehealth Southwest Medical Center	Vancouver	Washington	360-256-2000	www.swmedicalcenter.org
Peconic Bay Medical Center	Riverhead	New York	631-548-6000	www.pbmedicalcenter.org
Pekin Memorial Hospital	Pekin	Illinois	309-347-1151	www.pekinhospital.org
Pennsylvania Hospital of the Univ of PA Health Sys	Philadelphia	Pennsylvania	215-829-3000	www.pennmedicine.org/pahosp
Perry Community Hospital	Linden	Tennessee	931-589-2121	www.perryhealth.org
Pineville Community Hospital	Pineville	Kentucky	606-337-3051	www.pinevillehospital.com
Poplar Bluff Regional Medical Center	Poplar Bluff	Missouri	573-785-7721	www.poplarbluffregional.com
Pottstown Memorial Medical Center	Pottstown	Pennsylvania	610-327-7000	www.pmmctr.org
Presence Saint Francis Hospital	Evanston	Illinois	847-316-4000	www.reshealth.org
Presence Saint Joseph Hospital - Chicago	Chicago	Illinois	773-665-3000	www.res-health.org
Presence Saint Joseph Medical Center	Joliet	Illinois	815-725-7133	www.provena.org/stjoes
Presence Saints Mary & Elizabeth Medical Center	Chicago	Illinois	312-770-2000	www.reshealth.org
Presence Saint Marys Hospital	Kankakee	Illinois	815-937-2490	www.provenastmarys.com
Presence United Samaritans Medical Center	Danville	Illinois	217-443-5000	www.provena.org/usmc
Providence Hospital	Washington	District of Columbia	202-269-7000	www.provhosp.org
Providence Hospital & Medical Centers	Southfield	Michigan	248-849-3011	www.stjohn.org/providence
Queens Hospital Center	Jamaica	New York	718-883-3000	www.nyc.gov/html/hhc/qhn/home.html
Raleigh General Hospital	Beckley	West Virginia	304-256-4100	www.raleighgeneral.com
Raritan Bay Medical Center	Perth Amboy	New Jersey	732-442-3700	www.rbmc.org
Reston Hospital Center	Reston	Virginia	703-689-9000	www.restonhospital.com
Rhode Island Hospital	Providence	Rhode Island	401-444-4000	www.rhodeislandhospital.org
Richmond University Medical Center	Staten Island	New York	718-818-1234	www.rumcsi.org
Riverside Methodist Hospital	Columbus	Ohio	614-566-5000	www.ohiohealth.com
Robert Packer Hospital	Sayre	Pennsylvania	570-888-6666	www.guthrie.org
Robert Wood Johnson University Hospital	New Brunswick	New Jersey	732-937-8900	www.rwjuh.edu
Ronald Reagan UCLA Medical Center	Los Angeles	California	310-825-6301	www.uclahealth.org
Roseland Community Hospital	Chicago	Illinois	773-995-3000	www.roselandhospital.org
Roxborough Memorial Hospital	Philadelphia	Pennsylvania	215-483-9900	www.roxboroughmemorial.com
Rush University Medical Center	Chicago	Illinois	312-942-5000	www.ruch.edu
Saint Francis Hospital	Tulsa	Oklahoma	918-494-2200	www.saintfrancis.com
Saint Francis Medical Center	Peoria	Illinois	309-655-2000	www.osfsaintfrancis.org
Saint Michael's Medical Center	Newark	New Jersey	973-877-5350	www.cathedralhealth.org
Saint Peter's University Hospital	New Brunswick	New Jersey	732-745-8600	www.saintpetersuh.com
Saint Thomas Rutherford Hospital	Murfreesboro	Tennessee	615-396-4100	www.mtmc.org
Saline Memorial Hospital	Benton	Arkansas	501-776-6000	www.salinememorial.org
San Joaquin Community Hospital	Bakersfield	California	661-395-3000	www.sanjoaquinhospital.org
San Luke's Memorial Hospital	Ponce	Puerto Rico	787-844-2080	www.ssepr.com/hospital_sanlucas.html
Sandhills Regional Medical Center	Hamlet	North Carolina	910-958-2361	www.hma-corp.com
Santa Monica - UCLA Medical Center & Orthopaedic Hospital	Santa Monica	California	310-319-4000	www.healthcare.ucla.edu
Scotland Memorial Hospital	Laurinburg	North Carolina	910-291-7000	www.scotlandhealth.org
Silver Cross Hospital & Medical Centers	New Lenox	Illinois	815-300-1100	www.silvercross.org
Sinai Hospital of Baltimore	Baltimore	Maryland	410-601-5131	www.sinai-balt.com
Sinai - Grace Hospital	Detroit	Michigan	313-966-3300	www.sinaigrace.org
Singing River Hospital	Pascagoula	Mississippi	228-809-5000	www.srhshealth.com
South Nassau Communities Hospital	Oceanside	New York	516-632-3000	www.southnassau.org
South Shore Hospital	Chicago	Illinois	773-768-0810	www.southshorehospital.com
Southern Tennessee Medical Center	Winchester	Tennessee	931-967-8295	www.southerntennessee.com

Hospital	City	State	Phone	Web Site
Southern Virginia Regional Medical Center	Emporia	Virginia	434-348-4400	www.svrmc.com
Southwest Healthcare System	Murrieta	California	951-696-6000	www.ivrmc-rsmc.com
Saint Anthony's Medical Center	Saint Louis	Missouri	314-525-1000	www.samcstl.org
Saint Barnabas Hospital	Bronx	New York	212-960-9000	www.stbarnabashospital.org
Saint Bernard Hospital	Chicago	Illinois	773-962-3900	www.stbernardhospital.com
Saint Catherine of Siena Hospital	Smithtown	New York	631-862-3000	www.stcatherines.chsli.org
Saint Claire Regional Medical Center	Morehead	Kentucky	606-783-6500	www.st-claire.org
Saint Elizabeth Hospital	Belleville	Illinois	618-234-2120	www.steliz.org
Saint Elizabeth's Medical Center	Brighton	Massachusetts	617-789-3000	www.semc.org
Saint Francis Hospital	Poughkeepsie	New York	845-483-5000	www.sfhhc.org
Saint John Hospital & Medical Center	Detroit	Michigan	313-343-4000	www.stjohnprovidence.org
Saint John Macomb - Oakland Hospital - Macomb Center	Warren	Michigan	586-573-5000	www.stjohn.org
Saint John's Episcopal Hospital at South Shore	Far Rockaway	New York	718-869-7000	www.ehs.org
Saint John's Riverside Hospital	Yonkers	New York	914-964-4444	www.riversidehealth.org
Saint Joseph Health Services of RI	North Providence	Rhode Island	401-456-3000	www.fatimahospital.com
Saint Joseph Mercy Oakland	Pontiac	Michigan	248-858-3000	www.stjoesoakland.org
Saint Joseph Regional Health Center	Bryan	Texas	979-776-3912	www.st-joseph.org/sjrhc
Saint Joseph's Hospital	Philadelphia	Pennsylvania	215-787-2000	www.nphs.com
Saint Joseph's Medical Center	Yonkers	New York	914-378-7000	www.saintjosephs.org
Saint Joseph's Regional Medical Center	Paterson	New Jersey	973-754-2010	www.sjhmc.org
Saint Louis University Hospital	Saint Louis	Missouri	314-577-8000	www.slucare.edu/clinical
Saint Luke's Roosevelt Hospital	New York	New York	212-523-4000	www.wehealny.org
Saint Luke's Episcopal Hospital	Houston	Texas	832-355-1000	www.sleh.com
Saint Mary Medical Center	Hobart	Indiana	219-942-0551	www.comhs.org/stmary
Saint Mary Mercy Hospital	Livonia	Michigan	734-655-4800	www.stmarymercy.org
Saint Mary's of Michigan Medical Center	Saginaw	Michigan	989-776-8000	www.stmarysofmichigan.org
Saint Marys Hospital	Centralia	Illinois	618-436-6519	www.stmarys-goodsamaritan.com
Saint Rose Hospital	Hayward	California	510-782-6200	www.strosehospital.org
Saint Vincent Hospital	Worcester	Massachusetts	508-363-5000	www.stvincenthospital.com
Saint Vincent's Medical Center	Bridgeport	Connecticut	203-576-5551	www.stvincents.org
Saint Vincent's Medical Center	Jacksonville	Florida	904-308-7300	www.jaxhealth.com
Staten Island University Hospital	Staten Island	New York	718-226-9000	www.siuh.edu
Stephens County Hospital	Toccoa	Georgia	706-282-4250	www.stephenscountyhospital.com
Strong Memorial Hospital	Rochester	New York	585-275-2121	www.urmc.rochester.edu
Summa Health System Barberton Hospital	Barberton	Ohio	330-615-3000	www.barbhosp.com
Sumner Regional Medical Center	Gallatin	Tennessee	615-452-4210	www.mysumnermedical.com
Sunrise Hospital & Medical Center	Las Vegas	Nevada	702-731-8000	www.sunrisehospital.com
Swedish Covenant Hospital	Chicago	Illinois	773-878-8200	www.swedishcovenant.org
Temple University Hospital	Philadelphia	Pennsylvania	215-707-2000	www.tuh.templehealth.org
The University of Chicago Medical Center	Chicago	Illinois	773-702-1000	www.uchospitals.edu
Thomas Jefferson University Hospital	Philadelphia	Pennsylvania	215-955-6000	www.jeffersonhospital.org
Thorek Memorial Hospital	Chicago	Illinois	312-525-6780	www.thorek.org
Trinitas Regional Medical Center	Elizabeth	New Jersey	908-994-5000	www.trinitashospital.org
Tristar Summit Medical Center	Hermitage	Tennessee	615-316-3000	www.summitmedctr.com
Tufts Medical Center	Boston	Massachusetts	617-636-5000	www.tuftsmedicalcenter.org
Tulane Medical Center	New Orleans	Louisiana	504-988-1900	www.tuhc.com
UAMS Medical Center	Little Rock	Arkansas	501-686-5000	www.uams.edu/medcenter
UF Health Shands Hospital	Gainesville	Florida	352-265-8000	www.shands.org
Umass Memorial Medical Center	Worcester	Massachusetts	508-334-1000	www.umassmemorial.org
Union Hospital	Terre Haute	Indiana	812-238-7606	www.uhhg.org
University Health Care/University Hospitals & Clinics	Salt Lake City	Utah	801-581-2121	www.healthcare.utah.edu
University Hospital	Newark	New Jersey	973-972-5658	www.theuniversityhospital.com
University Hospital - Stony Brook	Stony Brook	New York	631-444-4000	www.stonybrookmedicalcenter.org
University Hospital of Brooklyn - Downstate Medical Center	Brooklyn	New York	718-270-1000	www.downstate.edu
University Hospitals - Elyria Medical Center	Elyria	Ohio	440-329-7500	www.emh-healthcare.org
University Hospitals Ahuja Medical Center	Beachwood	Ohio	216-767-8793	www.uhhospitals.org/ahuja
University Hospitals Case Medical Center	Cleveland	Ohio	216-844-1000	www.uhhs.com
University of Alabama Hospital	Birmingham	Alabama	205-934-4011	www.health.uab.edu
University of Arizona Medical Center	Tucson	Arizona	520-694-0111	www.azumc.com
University of Cincinnati Medical Center	Cincinnati	Ohio	513-584-1000	www.universityhospitalcincinnati.com
University of Illinois Hospital	Chicago	Illinois	312-996-3900	www.uic.edu
University of Iowa Hospital & Clinics	Iowa City	Iowa	319-356-1616	www.uihealthcare.com
University of Kentucky Hospital	Lexington	Kentucky	859-323-5000	www.uhealthcare.uky.edu
University of Louisville Hospital	Louisville	Kentucky	502-562-3000	www.uoflhealthcare.org
University of Maryland Medical Center	Baltimore	Maryland	410-328-8667	www.umm.edu
University of Maryland Medical Center Midtown Campus	Baltimore	Maryland	410-225-8996	www.marylandgeneral.org
University of Miami Hospital	Miami	Florida	305-325-5511	www.cedarsmedicalcenter.com

Hospital	City	State	Phone	Web Site
University of Michigan Health System	Ann Arbor	Michigan	734-764-1505	www.med.umich.edu
University of North Carolina Hospital	Chapel Hill	North Carolina	919-966-4131	www.unchealthcare.org
University of Texas Medical Branch Galveston	Galveston	Texas	409-772-1011	www.utmb.edu
University of Virginia Medical Center	Charlottesville	Virginia	800-251-3627	www.uvahealth.com
UPMC Presbyterian Shadyside	Pittsburgh	Pennsylvania	412-647-8788	www.upmc.edu
Valley Hospital	Ridgewood	New Jersey	201-447-8000	www.valleyhealth.com
Valley Hospital Medical Center	Las Vegas	Nevada	702-388-4000	www.valleyhealthsystem.org
Vanderbilt University Hospital	Nashville	Tennessee	615-322-3454	www.mc.vanderbilt.edu
Vassar Brothers Medical Center	Poughkeepsie	New York	845-454-8500	www.vasserbrothers.org
Vidant Medical Center	Greenville	North Carolina	252-847-4100	www.uhseast.com
Vidant Roanoke Chowan Hospital	Ahoskie	North Carolina	252-209-3000	www.uhseast.com
Washington Hospital	Fremont	California	510-797-1111	www.whhs.com
Wellmont Bristol Regional Medical Center	Bristol	Tennessee	423-844-1121	www.wellmont.org
Wellmont Holston Valley Medical Center	Kingsport	Tennessee	423-224-4000	www.wellmont.org
Wesley Medical Center	Hattiesburg	Mississippi	601-268-8000	www.wesley.com
West Chester Hospital	West Chester	Ohio	513-298-3000	www.westchesterhospital.uchealth.com
West River Regional Medical Center	Hettinger	North Dakota	701-567-4561	www.wrhs.com
West Virginia University Hospitals	Morgantown	West Virginia	304-598-4000	www.wvuh.com
Westchester General Hospital	Miami	Florida	305-263-9270	www.westchestergeneralhospital.com
Westchester Medical Center	Valhalla	New York	914-285-7017	www.wcmc.com
Western Arizona Regional Medical Center	Bullhead City	Arizona	928-763-2273	www.warmc.com
Western Maryland Regional Medical Center	Cumberland	Maryland	240-964-8001	www.wmhs.com
White County Medical Center	Searcy	Arkansas	501-278-3100	www.centralarkhospital.com
White River Medical Center	Batesville	Arkansas	870-262-1200	www.wrmc.com
William Beaumont Hospital - Troy	Troy	Michigan	248-964-8800	www.beaumonthospitals.com
Williamson ARH Hospital	South Williamson	Kentucky	606-237-1700	www.arh.org
Williamson Memorial Hospital	Williamson	West Virginia	304-235-2500	www.hmawmh.com
Winter Haven Hospital	Winter Haven	Florida	863-293-1121	www.winterhavenhospital.com
Wyckoff Heights Medical Center	Brooklyn	New York	718-963-7272	www.wyckoffhospital.org
Yale-New Haven Hospital	New Haven	Connecticut	203-688-4242	www.ynhh.org

Note: Table shows hospitals nationwide whose rate of readmission after discharge from hospital (hospital-wide) is better (lower) than U.S. rate of 16.0%

Hospital Heart Attack Readmission Rates: State and National Summary

Area	Number of Hospitals			
	Better than U.S. National Rate[1]	Worse than U.S. National Rate[2]	No Different than U.S. National Rate[3]	Number of Cases Too Small[4]
U.S. and Territories	23	29	2327	2085
Alabama	0	0	39	58
Alaska	0	0	5	14
American Samoa	0	0	0	1
Arizona	0	0	47	21
Arkansas	0	1	27	46
California	1	1	201	122
Colorado	1	0	32	33
Connecticut	0	1	27	3
Delaware	0	0	6	1
District of Columbia	0	0	6	2
Florida	3	3	144	32
Georgia	1	0	64	72
Guam	0	0	1	0
Hawaii	0	0	11	5
Idaho	0	0	9	23
Illinois	0	5	103	71
Indiana	2	0	61	54
Iowa	0	0	27	82
Kansas	0	0	27	82
Kentucky	0	0	40	55
Louisiana	0	0	44	56
Maine	1	0	21	15
Maryland	0	0	39	7
Massachusetts	0	1	52	10
Michigan	1	0	76	51
Minnesota	0	0	31	89
Mississippi	0	0	30	49
Missouri	0	0	53	59
Montana	0	0	8	35
N. Mariana Islands	0	0	1	0
Nebraska	0	0	19	53
Nevada	0	0	18	14
New Hampshire	0	0	15	10
New Jersey	0	5	55	6
New Mexico	1	0	11	26
New York	0	4	132	45
North Carolina	1	1	67	40
North Dakota	1	0	7	33
Ohio	0	0	96	61
Oklahoma	0	1	31	67
Oregon	1	0	23	36
Pennsylvania	1	0	120	41
Puerto Rico	0	1	12	32
Rhode Island	0	0	11	0
South Carolina	1	1	36	22
South Dakota	0	0	9	38
Tennessee	0	1	56	55
Texas	2	0	176	153
Utah	0	0	14	20
Vermont	0	0	8	7
Virgin Islands	0	0	1	1
Virginia	0	2	62	17
Washington	2	0	40	40
West Virginia	0	1	24	28
Wisconsin	3	0	50	68
Wyoming	0	0	2	24

Note: (1) 30-day readmission rate is better (lower) than U.S. rate of 18.3%; (2) 30-day readmission rate is worse (higher) than U.S. rate of 18.3%; (3) 30-day readmission rate is about the same as U.S. rate of 18.3%; (4) The number of cases is too small to classify the hospital

Hospital Heart Failure Readmission Rates: State and National Summary

Area	Number of Hospitals			
	Better than U.S. National Rate[1]	Worse than U.S. National Rate[2]	No Different than U.S. National Rate[3]	Number of Cases Too Small[4]
U.S. and Territories	120	159	3876	631
Alabama	2	1	92	6
Alaska	0	0	12	10
American Samoa	0	0	0	1
Arizona	3	1	60	14
Arkansas	0	3	71	3
California	10	3	280	46
Colorado	3	0	54	17
Connecticut	1	2	29	0
Delaware	0	0	7	0
District of Columbia	0	1	7	0
Florida	8	16	157	6
Georgia	3	1	129	11
Guam	0	0	1	0
Hawaii	1	0	13	5
Idaho	2	0	20	16
Illinois	1	10	168	5
Indiana	3	1	113	3
Iowa	3	0	97	18
Kansas	2	0	85	46
Kentucky	1	8	86	1
Louisiana	2	5	86	16
Maine	2	0	33	2
Maryland	0	6	40	1
Massachusetts	1	3	59	1
Michigan	6	10	108	11
Minnesota	1	1	86	43
Mississippi	0	6	77	13
Missouri	4	6	101	6
Montana	1	0	30	29
N. Mariana Islands	0	0	0	1
Nebraska	3	0	47	35
Nevada	0	0	30	5
New Hampshire	1	0	24	1
New Jersey	1	16	49	1
New Mexico	1	0	32	9
New York	0	22	156	5
North Carolina	6	2	97	8
North Dakota	1	0	24	19
Ohio	2	2	153	10
Oklahoma	2	3	87	25
Oregon	4	0	51	5
Pennsylvania	9	5	144	6
Puerto Rico	0	1	28	20
Rhode Island	0	2	9	1
South Carolina	6	2	53	2
South Dakota	0	0	29	26
Tennessee	3	6	102	4
Texas	11	3	308	52
Utah	3	0	22	17
Vermont	0	0	14	1
Virgin Islands	0	0	2	0
Virginia	1	5	76	2
Washington	2	1	64	21
West Virginia	0	5	45	4
Wisconsin	4	0	111	10
Wyoming	0	0	18	11

Note: (1) 30-day readmission rate is better (lower) than U.S. rate of 23.0%; (2) 30-day readmission rate is worse (higher) than U.S. rate of 23.0%; (3) 30-day readmission rate is about the same as U.S. rate of 23.0%; (4) The number of cases is too small to classify the hospital

Hospital Pneumonia Readmission Rates: State and National Summary

Area	Number of Hospitals			
	Better than U.S. National Rate[1]	Worse than U.S. National Rate[2]	No Different than U.S. National Rate[3]	Number of Cases Too Small[4]
U.S. and Territories	37	135	4285	376
Alabama	0	1	96	5
Alaska	0	0	15	6
American Samoa	0	0	1	0
Arizona	0	0	72	9
Arkansas	1	5	68	3
California	3	5	290	46
Colorado	1	0	62	12
Connecticut	0	1	31	0
Delaware	0	0	7	0
District of Columbia	0	0	8	0
Florida	5	8	170	5
Georgia	1	0	138	4
Guam	0	0	1	0
Hawaii	0	0	14	8
Idaho	0	0	33	7
Illinois	0	11	169	5
Indiana	2	1	115	2
Iowa	0	0	113	5
Kansas	1	0	118	13
Kentucky	1	8	87	0
Louisiana	1	3	95	13
Maine	0	0	36	1
Maryland	0	11	34	1
Massachusetts	0	2	62	1
Michigan	2	5	122	6
Minnesota	0	0	112	19
Mississippi	0	3	87	8
Missouri	2	3	107	6
Montana	2	0	40	20
N. Mariana Islands	0	0	1	0
Nebraska	0	0	77	9
Nevada	0	1	29	6
New Hampshire	0	0	26	0
New Jersey	1	2	63	2
New Mexico	0	0	39	3
New York	2	24	154	5
North Carolina	1	4	104	5
North Dakota	0	0	40	4
Ohio	1	11	149	6
Oklahoma	1	3	103	12
Oregon	1	1	55	3
Pennsylvania	1	3	157	4
Puerto Rico	0	1	26	23
Rhode Island	0	0	11	1
South Carolina	2	1	58	2
South Dakota	0	0	51	5
Tennessee	1	5	105	5
Texas	3	4	325	49
Utah	0	0	37	5
Vermont	0	0	15	0
Virgin Islands	0	0	2	0
Virginia	0	3	79	7
Washington	1	0	81	7
West Virginia	0	5	48	1
Wisconsin	0	0	120	5
Wyoming	0	0	27	2

Note: (1) 30-day readmission rate is better (lower) than U.S. rate of 17.6%; (2) 30-day readmission rate is worse (higher) than U.S. rate of 17.6%; (3) 30-day readmission rate is about the same as U.S. rate of 17.6%; (4) The number of cases is too small to classify the hospital

Hospital Readmission Rate After Hip/Knee Surgery: State and National Summary

Area	Number of Hospitals			
	Better than U.S. National Rate[1]	Worse than U.S. National Rate[2]	No Different than U.S. National Rate[3]	Number of Cases Too Small[4]
U.S. and Territories	51	38	2738	665
Alabama	0	0	52	9
Alaska	0	0	8	0
American Samoa	0	0	0	0
Arizona	1	0	48	7
Arkansas	1	1	28	7
California	8	1	199	90
Colorado	1	0	49	6
Connecticut	0	1	28	0
Delaware	0	0	5	1
District of Columbia	0	1	4	2
Florida	5	4	138	15
Georgia	2	0	77	15
Guam	0	0	0	0
Hawaii	0	0	8	6
Idaho	0	0	23	5
Illinois	1	4	110	24
Indiana	3	0	78	29
Iowa	1	0	47	17
Kansas	1	0	42	12
Kentucky	0	0	42	19
Louisiana	0	1	59	15
Maine	1	0	25	6
Maryland	0	3	40	2
Massachusetts	1	0	55	5
Michigan	1	1	96	18
Minnesota	0	0	67	16
Mississippi	0	0	29	7
Missouri	1	2	64	13
Montana	1	0	19	6
N. Mariana Islands	0	0	0	0
Nebraska	1	0	31	13
Nevada	0	0	23	2
New Hampshire	0	0	22	4
New Jersey	0	1	54	7
New Mexico	1	0	21	3
New York	3	0	119	30
North Carolina	1	0	82	6
North Dakota	1	0	7	1
Ohio	2	2	133	20
Oklahoma	1	1	45	19
Oregon	1	0	39	10
Pennsylvania	2	4	123	29
Puerto Rico	0	0	8	28
Rhode Island	0	0	9	1
South Carolina	0	1	40	13
South Dakota	0	0	17	1
Tennessee	2	2	53	19
Texas	3	5	204	51
Utah	0	0	26	6
Vermont	0	0	12	1
Virgin Islands	0	0	1	0
Virginia	3	2	55	9
Washington	0	0	53	9
West Virginia	0	0	26	6
Wisconsin	1	1	82	21
Wyoming	0	0	13	4

Note: (1) 30-day readmission rate is better (lower) than U.S. rate of 5.4%; (2) 30-day readmission rate is worse (higher) than U.S. rate of 5.4%; (3) 30-day readmission rate is about the same as U.S. rate of 5.4%; (4) The number of cases is too small to classify the hospital

Hospital Readmission Rate After Discharge From Hospital (Hospital-wide): State and National Summary

Area	Number of Hospitals			
	Better than U.S. National Rate[1]	Worse than U.S. National Rate[2]	No Different than U.S. National Rate[3]	Number of Cases Too Small[4]
U.S. and Territories	316	369	3966	158
Alabama	1	1	92	3
Alaska	1	0	20	1
American Samoa	0	0	1	0
Arizona	9	3	64	5
Arkansas	3	11	60	0
California	29	17	283	10
Colorado	9	0	63	3
Connecticut	2	4	25	0
Delaware	0	0	6	0
District of Columbia	0	3	4	0
Florida	13	23	143	2
Georgia	7	5	129	1
Guam	0	0	1	0
Hawaii	2	0	13	6
Idaho	6	0	32	2
Illinois	4	37	137	1
Indiana	14	4	104	2
Iowa	7	1	106	2
Kansas	7	0	125	6
Kentucky	2	20	72	0
Louisiana	6	8	102	9
Maine	3	0	32	1
Maryland	3	14	28	0
Massachusetts	5	13	46	0
Michigan	12	20	93	6
Minnesota	8	0	119	4
Mississippi	1	6	86	5
Missouri	4	6	100	2
Montana	3	0	50	8
N. Mariana Islands	0	0	0	1
Nebraska	6	0	79	4
Nevada	1	3	28	3
New Hampshire	1	0	25	0
New Jersey	2	21	41	0
New Mexico	2	0	38	2
New York	6	57	110	4
North Carolina	15	6	88	2
North Dakota	2	1	38	2
Ohio	6	17	141	7
Oklahoma	9	4	106	6
Oregon	8	0	48	2
Pennsylvania	11	17	134	7
Puerto Rico	0	1	47	4
Rhode Island	0	4	7	0
South Carolina	8	2	52	0
South Dakota	5	0	52	2
Tennessee	4	12	96	1
Texas	31	8	341	20
Utah	6	1	34	2
Vermont	1	0	13	0
Virgin Islands	0	0	2	0
Virginia	3	11	66	4
Washington	12	1	71	2
West Virginia	0	7	42	1
Wisconsin	15	0	107	1
Wyoming	1	0	24	2

Note: (1) 30-day readmission rate is better (lower) than U.S. rate of 16.0%; (2) 30-day readmission rate is worse (higher) than U.S. rate of 16.0%; (3) 30-day readmission rate is about the same as U.S. rate of 16.0%; (4) The number of cases is too small to classify the hospital

Appendix C: Surgical Complication Rates

What Do These Surgical Complication Measures Show?

This appendix shows how hospitals' surgical complication rates compare to the rate across the U.S. The categories are:

- A Wound That Splits Open After Surgery on the Abdomen or Pelvis
- Accidental Cuts and Tears From Medical Treatment
- Collapsed Lung Due to Medical Treatment
- Deaths Among Patients With Serious Treatable Complications After Surgery
- Rate of Complications for Hip/Knee Replacement Patients
- Serious Blood Clots After Surgery
- Serious Complications (see below for details)

This first part of this appendix shows hospitals with surgical complication rates that are lower (better) or higher (worse) than the national rate for all categories. Hospitals are shown to be better or worse than the U.S. national rate only if the data shows with 95% certainty, the difference between their surgical complication rates and the U.S. national rate is not due to chance.

The second part of this appendix contains state and national summaries with the following column headers:

- **Better Than U.S. National Rate.** Hospitals in the Better Than U.S. National Rate category have surgical complication rates that are lower than the U.S. National Rate, with 95% certainty that this difference is not due to chance.
- **Worse Than U.S. National Rate.** Hospitals in the Worse Than U.S. National Rate category have surgical complication rates that are higher than the U.S. National Rate, with 95% certainty that this difference is not due to chance.
- **No Different Than U.S. National Rate.** Many hospitals in the No Different Than U.S. National Rate category have surgical complication rates that are about the same as the U.S. National Rate. Other hospitals in this category have rates that are higher or lower than the U.S. National Rate, without 95% certainty that these differences are not due to chance.
- **Number of Cases Too Small.** The number of cases is too small to classify the hospital.

Serious Complications

Measures of serious complications are drawn from the Agency for Healthcare Research and Quality (AHRQ) Patient Safety Indicators (PSIs). The overall score for serious complications is based on how often adult patients had certain serious, but potentially preventable, complications related to medical or surgical inpatient hospital care. This composite or summary measure is based on the following measures:

- Collapsed lung that results from medical treatment (Iatrogenic pneumothorax, adult)
- Blood clots, in the lung or a large vein, after surgery (Postoperative Pulmonary Embolism or Deep Vein Thrombosis Rate)
- A wound that splits open after surgery (Postoperative wound dehiscence)
- Accidental cuts and tears (Accidental puncture or laceration)
- Pressure sores (Pressure ulcers)
- Infections from a large venous catheters (Central venous catheter-related blood stream infection rate)
- Broken hip from a fall after surgery (Postoperative hip fracture rate)
- Blood stream infection after surgery (Postoperative sepsis)

Which Patients are Included

The Serious Complications measure applies only to Medicare beneficiaries enrolled in Original Medicare (traditional fee-for-service (FFS) Medicare) who were discharged from a hospital that was paid through the inpatient prospective payment system (IPPS) after the beneficiary had an inpatient stay. Non-Medicare patients and beneficiaries enrolled in Medicare managed care plans are also excluded from the data.

Where the Information Comes From

The Centers for Medicare & Medicaid Services (CMS) calculates the indicators of patient safety data from the claims hospitals submit for Medicare beneficiaries enrolled in Original Medicare(traditional FFS Medicare). The rate for each PSI is calculated by dividing the actual number of outcomes at each hospital by the number of eligible discharges for that measure at each hospital, multiplied by 1,000. The composite value reported on Hospital Compare is the weighted averages of the component indicators. PSI data are only calculated for hospitals that are paid through the IPPS, which excludes Critical Access hospitals (CAHs), long-term care hospitals (LTCHs), Maryland waiver hospitals, cancer hospitals, children's inpatient facilities, rural health clinics, federally qualified health centers, inpatient psychiatric hospitals, inpatient rehabilitation facilities, Veterans Administration/ Department of Defense hospitals, and religious, non-medical health care institutions.

Risk Adjustment

The measures of serious complications reported are risk adjusted to account for differences in hospital patients' characteristics. In addition, the rates reported are "smoothed" to reflect the fact that measures for small hospitals are measured less accurately (i.e., are less reliable) than for larger hospitals.

Comparing Individual Hospital Rates to Benchmarks

For the composite measure, CMS assigns comparative performance categories. If the interval estimate includes and/or overlaps with the national composite value, the hospital's performance is in the "no different than U.S. national rate" category. If the entire interval estimate is below the national composite value, then the hospital is performing "better than U.S. national rate." If the entire interval estimate is above the national composite value, it is "worse than U.S. national rate."

Additional Information

For more detail on Serious Complications measures (AHRQ Patient Safety Indicators) visit the Agency for Healthcare Research and Quality (AHRQ) Patient Safety Indicator Resources Web site at www.qualityindicators.ahrq.gov.

Hospitals whose Surgical Complication Rate is Better (Lower) than the U.S. National Rate

Measure: A Wound That Splits Open After Surgery on the Abdomen or Pelvis

Hospital	City	State	Phone	Web Site
No hospitals met this criteria.				

Note: Table shows hospitals nationwide whose surgical complication rate is better (lower) than U.S. rate of 0.92%

Hospitals whose Surgical Complication Rate is Worse (Higher) than the U.S. National Rate

Measure: A Wound That Splits Open After Surgery on the Abdomen or Pelvis

Hospital	City	State	Phone	Web Site
Aurora Lakeland Medical Center	Elkhorn	Wisconsin	262-741-2000	www.aurorahealthcare.org/facilities
Banner Thunderbird Medical Center	Glendale	Arizona	602-588-5555	www.bannerhealth.com
Beaumont Health System	Royal Oak	Michigan	248-898-5000	www.beaumonthospitals.com
Bronson Methodist Hospital	Kalamazoo	Michigan	269-341-6000	www.bronsonhealth.com
Central Carolina Hospital	Sanford	North Carolina	919-774-2100	www.centralcarolinahosp.com
Cjw Medical Center	Richmond	Virginia	804-330-2001	www.hcavirginia.com
Eastern Idaho Regional Medical Center	Idaho Falls	Idaho	208-529-6111	www.eirmc.org
Erlanger Medical Center	Chattanooga	Tennessee	423-778-7000	www.erlanger.org
Exeter Hospital	Exeter	New Hampshire	603-778-7311	www.exeterhospital.com
Fairfield Medical Center	Lancaster	Ohio	740-687-8009	www.fmchealth.org
Florida Hospital Deland	Deland	Florida	386-943-4772	www.fhdeland.org
Florida Hospital Fish Memorial	Orange City	Florida	386-917-5000	www.fhfishmemorial.org
Frye Regional Medical Center	Hickory	North Carolina	828-322-6070	www.fryemedctr.com
Genesys Regional Medical Center - Health Park	Grand Blanc	Michigan	810-606-5000	www.genesys.org
Good Samaritan Hospital	San Jose	California	408-559-2011	www.goodsamsj.org
Health Alliance Hospital Broadway Campus	Kingston	New York	914-331-3131	www.kingstonregionalhealth.org
Inspira Medical Center Woodbury	Woodbury	New Jersey	856-845-0100	www.umhospital.org
Lake Cumberland Regional Hospital	Somerset	Kentucky	606-679-7441	www.lakecumberlandhospital.com
Lake Regional Health System	Osage Beach	Missouri	573-348-8000	www.lakeregional.com
Lakeland Hospital - Saint Joseph	Saint Joseph	Michigan	269-983-8300	www.lakelandhealth.org
Longmont United Hospital	Longmont	Colorado	303-651-5111	www.luhcares.org
Maine Medical Center	Portland	Maine	207-662-0111	www.mmc.org
Mayo Clinic Hospital Rochester	Rochester	Minnesota	507-255-5123	www.mayoclinic.org/saintmaryshospital
The Medical Center of Aurora	Aurora	Colorado	303-695-2600	www.auroramed.com
Medstar Washington Hospital Center	Washington	District of Columbia	202-877-7000	www.whcenter.org
Memorial Health Univ Medical Center	Savannah	Georgia	912-350-8000	www.memorialhealth.com
Mercy Saint Anne Hospital	Toledo	Ohio	419-407-2663	www.mercyweb.org
Miami Valley Hospital	Dayton	Ohio	937-208-8000	www.miamivalleyhospital.com
Mountainview Hospital	Las Vegas	Nevada	702-255-5065	www.mountainview-hospital.com
Norton Hospitals	Louisville	Kentucky	502-629-6560	www.nortonhealthcare.com
Pali Momi Medical Center	Aiea	Hawaii	808-486-6000	www.kapiolani.org
Pottstown Memorial Medical Center	Pottstown	Pennsylvania	610-327-7000	www.pmmctr.org
Robert Wood Johnson University Hospital at Rahway	Rahway	New Jersey	732-381-4200	www.rwjuhr.com/about/history.html
Southeast Georgia Health System - Brunswick Campus	Brunswick	Georgia	912-466-7000	www.sghs.org
Spring Valley Hospital Medical Center	Las Vegas	Nevada	702-853-3000	www.springvalleyhospital.com
Saint Joseph Regional Health Center	Bryan	Texas	979-776-3912	www.st-joseph.org/sjrhc
Saint Luke's Episcopal Hospital	Houston	Texas	832-355-1000	www.sleh.com
Touro Infirmary	New Orleans	Louisiana	504-897-7011	www.touro.com
University of Wisconsin Hospitals & Clinics Authority	Madison	Wisconsin	608-263-8991	www.uwhealth.org
UNM Hospital	Albuquerque	New Mexico	505-272-2111	www.hospitals.unm.edu/unmh
Wayne Memorial Hospital	Honesdale	Pennsylvania	570-253-8100	www.wmh.org

Note: Table shows hospitals nationwide whose surgical complication rate is worse (higher) than U.S. rate of 0.92%

Hospitals whose Surgical Complication Rate is Better (Lower) than the U.S. National Rate

Measure: Accidental Cuts and Tears From Medical Treatment

Hospital	City	State	Phone	Web Site
Advocate Christ Hospital & Medical Center	Oak Lawn	Illinois	708-684-8000	www.advocatehealth.com
Advocate Good Samaritan Hospital	Downers Grove	Illinois	630-275-5900	www.advocatehealth.com/gsam
Advocate Lutheran General Hospital	Park Ridge	Illinois	847-723-2210	www.advocatehealth.com
Arkansas Heart Hospital	Little Rock	Arkansas	501-219-7000	www.arheart.com
Asante Rogue Regional Medical Center	Medford	Oregon	541-789-7000	www.asante.org
Atlanticare Regional Medical Center	Atlantic City	New Jersey	609-441-8020	www.atlanticare.org/acmc/index.html
Aventura Hospital & Medical Center	Aventura	Florida	305-682-7000	www.aventurahospital.com
Baptist Beaumont Hospital	Beaumont	Texas	409-212-5012	www.mhbh.org
Baystate Medical Center	Springfield	Massachusetts	413-794-0000	www.baystatehealth.com
Bethesda Hospital East	Boynton Beach	Florida	561-737-7733	www.bethesdahealthcare.com
Cape Regional Medical Center	Cape May Ct House	New Jersey	609-463-2000	www.caperegional.com
Cedars - Sinai Medical Center	Los Angeles	California	310-423-5000	www.cedars-sinai.edu
Central Dupage Hospital	Winfield	Illinois	630-682-1600	www.cdh.org
Christiana Care Health Services	Newark	Delaware	302-733-1000	www.christianacare.org
Christus Spohn Hospital Corpus Christi	Corpus Christi	Texas	361-902-4103	www.christusspohn.org
Clear Lake Regional Medical Center	Webster	Texas	281-332-2511	www.clearlakermc.com
Community Medical Center	Toms River	New Jersey	732-557-8000	www.sbhcs.com
Delray Medical Center	Delray Beach	Florida	561-498-4440	www.delraymedicalctr.com
Duke University Hospital	Durham	North Carolina	919-684-8111	www.dukehealth.org
Englewood Hospital & Medical Center	Englewood	New Jersey	201-894-3000	www.englewoodhospital.com
Florida Hospital	Orlando	Florida	407-303-1976	www.floridahospital.com
Floyd Medical Center	Rome	Georgia	706-509-6900	www.floydmed.org
Glendale Adventist Medical Center	Glendale	California	818-409-8202	www.glendaleadventist.com
Good Samaritan Hospital Medical Center	West Islip	New York	631-376-3000	www.good-samaritan-hospital.org
Good Samaritan Medical Center	Brockton	Massachusetts	508-427-3000	www.goodsamaritanmedical.org
Indiana University Health	Indianapolis	Indiana	317-962-5900	www.iuhealth.org
Integris Baptist Medical Center	Oklahoma City	Oklahoma	405-951-8110	www.integris-health.com
Integris Southwest Medical Center	Oklahoma City	Oklahoma	405-636-7000	www.integris-health.com
Jackson - Madison County General Hospital	Jackson	Tennessee	731-541-5000	www.wth.org
Lakeland Regional Medical Center	Lakeland	Florida	863-687-1100	www.lrmc.com
Laredo Medical Center	Laredo	Texas	956-796-5000	www.laredomedical.com
Lovelace Medical Center	Albuquerque	New Mexico	505-727-8000	www.lovelace.com
Marietta Memorial Hospital	Marietta	Ohio	740-374-1400	www.mmhospital.org
Marion General Hospital	Marion	Ohio	740-383-8400	www.mariongeneral.com
Mayo Clinic	Jacksonville	Florida	904-953-2000	www.mayoclinic.org/jacksonville
Mayo Clinic Hospital	Phoenix	Arizona	480-342-2000	www.mayoclinic.org
Mayo Clinic Hospital Rochester	Rochester	Minnesota	507-255-5123	www.mayoclinic.org/saintmaryshospital
Mayo Clinic Methodist- Hospital	Rochester	Minnesota	507-266-7890	www.mayoclinic.org/methodisthospital
Mclaren Bay Region	Bay City	Michigan	989-894-3000	www.baymed.org
Memorial Healthcare System	Chattanooga	Tennessee	423-495-2525	www.memorial.org
Memorial Hermann Hospital System	Houston	Texas	713-448-6796	www.memorialhermann.org
Memorial Hermann Memorial City Medical Center	Houston	Texas	713-242-3000	www.mhhs.org
Memorial Hermann Texas Medical Center	Houston	Texas	713-704-3700	www.mhhs.org
Memorial Hospital	Belleville	Illinois	618-233-7750	www.memhosp.com
Memorial Regional Hospital	Hollywood	Florida	954-987-2000	www.memorialregional.com
Mercy Hospital Fairfield	Fairfield	Ohio	513-870-7197	www.e-mercy.com/mercy-hospital-fairfield.aspx
Methodist Hospital	San Antonio	Texas	210-575-4000	www.mh.sahealth.com
The Methodist Hospital	Houston	Texas	713-790-2221	www.methodisthealth.com
Methodist Willowbrook Hospital	Houston	Texas	281-477-1000	www.houstonmethodist.org/willowbrook-hospital
Mississippi Baptist Medical Center	Jackson	Mississippi	601-968-1000	www.mbmc.org
Munroe Regional Medical Center	Ocala	Florida	352-351-7200	www.munroeregional.com
North Florida Regional Medical Center	Gainesville	Florida	352-333-4100	www.nfrmc.com
Northwestern Memorial Hospital	Chicago	Illinois	312-926-2000	www.nmh.org
Ocala Regional Medical Center	Ocala	Florida	352-401-1000	www.ocalaregional.com
Our Lady of Lourdes Medical Center	Camden	New Jersey	856-757-3500	www.lourdesnet.org
Overlook Medical Center	Summit	New Jersey	908-522-2000	www.atlantichealth.org
Palos Community Hospital	Palos Heights	Illinois	708-923-4000	www.paloshospital.org
Presence Resurrection Medical Center	Chicago	Illinois	773-774-8000	www.reshealthcare.org
Presence Saint Joseph Medical Center	Joliet	Illinois	815-725-7133	www.provena.org/stjoes
Providence Little Co of Mary Medical Center Torrance	Torrance	California	310-540-7676	www.lcmhs.org
Providence Tarzana Medical Center	Tarzana	California	818-881-0800	www.encino-tarzana.com
Roper Hospital	Charleston	South Carolina	843-724-2800	www.ropersaintfrancis.com
Saint Thomas West Hospital	Nashville	Tennessee	615-222-2111	www.stthomas.org
Scripps Memorial Hospital La Jolla	La Jolla	California	858-626-4123	www.scrippshealth.org

Hospital	City	State	Phone	Web Site
Sentara Careplex Hospital	Hampton	Virginia	757-736-1000	www.sentara.com
Sentara Leigh Hospital	Norfolk	Virginia	757-261-6601	www.sentara.com
Sentara Norfolk General Hospital	Norfolk	Virginia	757-388-3000	www.sentara.com
Sentara Virginia Beach General Hospital	Virginia Beach	Virginia	757-395-8000	www.sentara.com
Shasta Regional Medical Center	Redding	California	530-244-5454	www.shastaregional.com
South Shore Hospital	South Weymouth	Massachusetts	781-340-8000	www.southshorehospital.org
Saint Francis Hospital	Columbus	Georgia	706-596-4020	www.wecareforlife.com
Saint Francis Hospital - Roslyn	Roslyn	New York	516-562-6000	www.stfrancisheartcenter.com
Saint John Medical Center	Tulsa	Oklahoma	918-744-3606	www.sjmc.org
Saint John's Riverside Hospital	Yonkers	New York	914-964-4444	www.riversidehealth.org
Saint Luke's Episcopal Hospital	Houston	Texas	832-355-1000	www.sleh.com
Saint Mary Medical Center	Langhorne	Pennsylvania	215-750-2003	www.stmaryhealthcare.org
Saint Mary Mercy Hospital	Livonia	Michigan	734-655-4800	www.stmarymercy.org
Saint Vincent Heart Center of Indiana	Indianapolis	Indiana	317-583-5000	www.theheartcenter.com
Staten Island University Hospital	Staten Island	New York	718-226-9000	www.siuh.edu
Sutter General Hospital	Sacramento	California	916-733-8999	www.suttermedicalcenter.org
Swedish Covenant Hospital	Chicago	Illinois	773-878-8200	www.swedishcovenant.org
Tennova Healthcare	Knoxville	Tennessee	865-545-8000	www.stmaryshealth.com
The Nebraska Medical Center	Omaha	Nebraska	402-552-2040	www.nebraskamed.com
Tuomey Healthcare System	Sumter	South Carolina	803-774-8900	www.tuomey.com
UF Health Shands Hospital	Gainesville	Florida	352-265-8000	www.shands.org
United Hospital Center	Bridgeport	West Virginia	681-342-1000	www.uhcwv.org
University of Kentucky Hospital	Lexington	Kentucky	859-323-5000	www.uhealthcare.uky.edu
University of Michigan Health System	Ann Arbor	Michigan	734-764-1505	www.med.umich.edu
Valley Hospital	Ridgewood	New Jersey	201-447-8000	www.valleyhealth.com
Vanderbilt University Hospital	Nashville	Tennessee	615-322-3454	www.mc.vanderbilt.edu
Virtua West Jersey Hospitals Berlin	Berlin	New Jersey	856-322-3200	www.virtua.org
Williamsport Regional Medical Center	Williamsport	Pennsylvania	570-321-1000	www.susquehannahealth.org
Winchester Medical Center	Winchester	Virginia	540-536-8000	www.valleyhealthlink.com
Winthrop - University Hospital	Mineola	New York	516-663-0333	www.winthrop.org

Note: Table shows hospitals nationwide whose surgical complication rate is better (lower) than U.S. rate of 1.83%

Hospitals whose Surgical Complication Rate is Worse (Higher) than the U.S. National Rate

Measure: Accidental Cuts and Tears From Medical Treatment

Hospital	City	State	Phone	Web Site
Adena Regional Medical Center	Chillicothe	Ohio	740-779-7500	www.adena.org
Adirondack Medical Center	Saranac Lake	New York	518-891-4141	www.amccares.org
Aiken Regional Medical Center	Aiken	South Carolina	803-641-5900	www.aikenregional.com
Alaska Native Medical Center	Anchorage	Alaska	907-563-2662	www.anmc.org
Appleton Medical Center	Appleton	Wisconsin	920-731-4101	www.thedacare.org
Atlanta Medical Center	Atlanta	Georgia	404-265-4000	www.atlantamedcenter.com
B R F Hospital Holdings	Shreveport	Louisiana	318-675-5000	www.lsumc.edu
Baptist Saint Anthony's Hospital	Amarillo	Texas	806-212-2000	www.bsahs.com
Barnes-Jewish Hospital	Saint Louis	Missouri	314-747-3000	www.barnesjewish.org
Baylor University Medical Center	Dallas	Texas	214-820-0111	www.baylorhealth.com
Beth Israel Deaconess Medical Center	Boston	Massachusetts	617-667-7000	www.bidmc.harvard.edu
Blessing Hospital	Quincy	Illinois	217-223-5811	www.blessinghealthsystem.org
Borgess Medical Center	Kalamazoo	Michigan	269-226-7000	www.borgess.com
Boston Medical Center Corporation	Boston	Massachusetts	617-638-8000	www.bmc.org
Bridgeport Hospital	Bridgeport	Connecticut	203-384-3000	www.bridgeporthospital.com
Carney Hospital	Boston	Massachusetts	617-506-2000	www.caritascarney.org
Caromont Regional Medical Center	Gastonia	North Carolina	704-834-4891	www.caromont.org
Catholic Medical Center	Manchester	New Hampshire	603-668-3545	www.catholicmedicalcenter.org
Centra Health	Lynchburg	Virginia	434-200-4789	www.centrahealth.com
Central Texas Medical Center	San Marcos	Texas	512-753-3690	www.ctmc.org
Centrastate Medical Center	Freehold	New Jersey	732-431-2000	www.centrastate.com
Cheshire Medical Center	Keene	New Hampshire	603-354-5400	www.cheshire-med.com
Chilton Medical Center	Pompton Plains	New Jersey	973-831-5000	www.chiltonmemorial.org
Clearview Regional Medical Center	Monroe	Georgia	770-267-1792	www.clearviewregionalmedicalcenter.com
Cleveland Clinic	Cleveland	Ohio	216-444-2200	www.clevelandclinic.org
Clovis Community Medical Center	Clovis	California	559-324-4000	www.communitymedical.org
Community Regional Medical Center	Fresno	California	559-459-6000	www.communitymedical.org
Covenant Hospital Plainview	Plainview	Texas	806-296-5531	www.covenantplainview.org
Crestwood Medical Center	Huntsville	Alabama	256-882-3100	www.crestwoodmedcenter.com
Crossgates River Oaks Hospital	Brandon	Mississippi	601-825-2811	www.rankinmedcenter.com
Crouse Hospital	Syracuse	New York	315-470-7449	www.crouse.org
Dameron Hospital	Stockton	California	209-944-5550	www.dameronhospital.org
Deaconess Hospital	Spokane	Washington	509-473-5800	www.deaconessmedicalcenter.org
Deaconess Hospital	Evansville	Indiana	812-450-5000	www.deaconess.com
Desert Regional Medical Center	Palm Springs	California	760-323-6511	www.desertmedctr.com
Eisenhower Medical Center	Rancho Mirage	California	760-340-3911	www.emc.org
El Camino Hospital	Mountain View	California	650-940-7000	www.elcaminohospital.org
Eliza Coffee Memorial Hospital	Florence	Alabama	256-768-8400	www.chgroup.org
Emory University Hospital Midtown	Atlanta	Georgia	404-686-4411	www.emoryhealthcare.org
Faith Regional Health Services	Norfolk	Nebraska	402-371-4880	www.frhs.org
Firsthealth Moore Regional Hospital	Pinehurst	North Carolina	910-715-1000	www.firsthealth.org
Geisinger Medical Center	Danville	Pennsylvania	570-271-6211	www.geisinger.org
Geisinger Wyoming Valley Medical Center	Wilkes Barre	Pennsylvania	570-826-7300	www.geisinger.org
Gila Regional Medical Center	Silver City	New Mexico	575-538-4000	www.grmc.org
Good Samaritan Hospital	San Jose	California	408-559-2011	www.goodsamsj.org
Good Samaritan Hospital	Dayton	Ohio	937-278-2612	www.goodsamdayton.org
Good Shepherd Medical Center Marshall	Marshall	Texas	903-927-6712	www.marshallregional.org
Grady Memorial Hospital	Atlanta	Georgia	404-616-4252	www.gradyhealthsystem.org
Grinnell Regional Medical Center	Grinnell	Iowa	641-236-7511	www.grmc.us
Grossmont Hospital	La Mesa	California	619-465-0711	www.sharp.com
Harborview Medical Center	Seattle	Washington	206-731-3000	www.harborview.org
Hennepin County Medical Center	Minneapolis	Minnesota	612-873-3000	www.hcmc.org
Henrico Doctors' Hospital	Richmond	Virginia	804-289-4500	www.henricodoctors.com
Heritage Valley Beaver	Beaver	Pennsylvania	412-728-7000	www.heritagevalley.org
The Indiana Heart Hospital	Indianapolis	Indiana	317-621-8063	www.hearthospital.com
Inspira Medical Center Vineland	Vineland	New Jersey	856-641-6610	www.sjhs.com
Intermountain Medical Center	Murray	Utah	801-507-7000	www.intermountainhealthcare.org
Jewish Hospital & Saint Mary's Healthcare	Louisville	Kentucky	502-587-4011	www.jhhs.org
John Dempsey Hospital	Farmington	Connecticut	860-679-1145	www.uconnhealth.orgorwww.uchc.edu
JPS Health Network	Fort Worth	Texas	817-921-3431	www.jpshealthnet.org
Jupiter Medical Center	Jupiter	Florida	561-747-2234	www.jupitermed.com
Kadlec Regional Medical Center	Richland	Washington	509-946-4611	www.kadlecmed.org
Kaiser Foundation Hospital - Fontana	Fontana	California	909-427-5500	www.kaiserpermanente.com
Kaweah Delta Medical Center	Visalia	California	559-624-2000	www.kaweahdelta.org

Hospital	City	State	Phone	Web Site
Keck Hospital of USC	Los Angeles	California	323-442-8656	www.uscuh.com
Kingman Regional Medical Center	Kingman	Arizona	928-757-2101	www.azkrmc.com
Kuakini Medical Center	Honolulu	Hawaii	808-536-2236	www.kuakini.org
LDS Hospital	Salt Lake City	Utah	801-408-1100	www.intermountainhealthcare.org
Lourdes Hospital	Paducah	Kentucky	270-444-2444	www.ehealthconnection.com
Magee Womens Hospital of UPMC Health System	Pittsburgh	Pennsylvania	412-641-4010	www.magee.edu
Maine Medical Center	Portland	Maine	207-662-0111	www.mmc.org
Manchester Memorial Hospital	Manchester	Connecticut	860-647-4780	www.echn.org
Marin General Hospital	Greenbrae	California	415-925-7900	www.maringeneral.com
Mary Hitchcock Memorial Hospital	Lebanon	New Hampshire	603-650-5000	www.dhmc.org
Mat-Su Regional Medical Center	Palmer	Alaska	907-746-8600	www.matsuregional.com
Mayo Clinic Health System - Mankato	Mankato	Minnesota	507-625-4031	www.isj-mhs.org
Mayo Clinic Health System - Eau Claire Hospital	Eau Claire	Wisconsin	715-838-3311	www.luthermidelfort.org
McKay Dee Hospital	Ogden	Utah	801-387-2800	www.intermountainhealthcare.org
Medical College of Virginia Hospitals	Richmond	Virginia	804-828-0938	www.vcuhealth.org
Medical West	Bessemer	Alabama	205-481-7000	www.uab.edu
Medstar Washington Hospital Center	Washington	District of Columbia	202-877-7000	www.whcenter.org
Memorial Medical Center	Modesto	California	209-526-4500	www.memorialmedicalcenter.org
Memorial Health Univ Medical Center	Savannah	Georgia	912-350-8000	www.memorialhealth.com
Memorial Hospital	York	Pennsylvania	717-843-8623	www.mhyork.org
Memorial Hospital & Health Care Center	Jasper	Indiana	812-996-2345	www.mhhcc.org
Memorial Hospital of Carbondale	Carbondale	Illinois	618-549-0721	www.sih.net
Memorial Medical Center	Springfield	Illinois	217-788-3000	www.memorialmedical.com
Mercy General Hospital	Sacramento	California	916-453-4545	www.mercygeneral.org
Mercy Health Hackley Campus	Muskegon	Michigan	231-726-3511	www.hackley.org
Mercy Hospital - Cadillac	Cadillac	Michigan	231-876-7200	www.mercycadillac.munsonhealthcare.org
Mercy Medical Center - Des Moines	Des Moines	Iowa	515-247-3121	www.mercydesmoines.org
Mercy Memorial Health Center	Ardmore	Oklahoma	405-223-5400	www.mercyok.com/mmhc
Methodist Hospital of Sacramento	Sacramento	California	916-423-6010	www.methodistsacramento.org
Methodist Jennie Edmundson	Council Bluffs	Iowa	712-396-6000	www.bestcare.org
Metro Health Hospital	Wyoming	Michigan	616-252-7200	www.metrohealth.net
Metrohealth System	Cleveland	Ohio	216-778-7089	www.metrohealth.org
Miami Valley Hospital	Dayton	Ohio	937-208-8000	www.miamivalleyhospital.com
Milton S Hershey Medical Center	Hershey	Pennsylvania	717-531-8521	www.hmc.psu.edu
Montrose Memorial Hospital	Montrose	Colorado	970-249-2211	www.montrosehospital.com
Morton Plant Hospital	Clearwater	Florida	727-462-7000	www.measehospitals.com
Mount Sinai Hospital	New York	New York	212-241-7981	www.mountsinai.org
Muhlenberg Community Hospital	Greenville	Kentucky	270-338-8000	www.mchky.org
Multicare Good Samaritan Hospital	Puyallup	Washington	253-697-2102	www.multicare.org/goodsam
Musc Medical Center	Charleston	South Carolina	843-792-2300	www.musc.edu
Nash General Hospital	Rocky Mount	North Carolina	252-443-8000	www.nhcs.org
New Hanover Regional Medical Center	Wilmington	North Carolina	910-343-7000	www.nhrmc.org
Newport Hospital	Newport	Rhode Island	401-846-6400	www.newporthospital.org
Northwest Medical Center	Tucson	Arizona	520-742-9000	www.northwestmedicalcenter.com
Novant Health Presbyterian Medical Center	Charlotte	North Carolina	704-384-4000	www.presbyterian.org
O U Medical Center	Oklahoma City	Oklahoma	405-271-5911	www.oumedcenter.com
OHSU Hospital & Clinics	Portland	Oregon	503-494-4036	www.ohsu.edu
Oklahoma State University Medical Center	Tulsa	Oklahoma	918-587-2561	www.tulsaregional.com
Our Lady of the Lake Regional Medical Center	Baton Rouge	Louisiana	225-765-6565	www.ololrmc.com
Overland Park Regional Medical Center	Overland Park	Kansas	913-541-5301	www.oprmc.com
Parkview Medical Center	Pueblo	Colorado	719-584-4000	www.parkviewmc.com
Peacehealth Saint Joseph Medical Center	Bellingham	Washington	360-734-5400	www.peacehealth.org
Phelps County Regional Medical Center	Rolla	Missouri	573-458-8899	www.rollanet.org/~pcrmc
Physicians Regional Medical Center - Pine Ridge	Naples	Florida	239-348-4000	www.physiciansregional.com
Pinnacle Health Hospitals	Harrisburg	Pennsylvania	717-782-5181	www.pinnaclehealth.org
Providence Holy Cross Medical Center	Mission Hills	California	818-365-8051	www.providence.org
Providence Sacred Heart Medical Center	Spokane	Washington	509-474-3040	www.shmc.org
Rhode Island Hospital	Providence	Rhode Island	401-444-4000	www.rhodeislandhospital.org
Ridgeview Medical Center	Waconia	Minnesota	952-442-2191	www.ridgeviewmedical.org
Riverview Hospital Assoc	Wisconsin Rapids	Wisconsin	715-423-6060	www.riverviewhospital.net
Ronald Reagan UCLA Medical Center	Los Angeles	California	310-825-6301	www.uclahealth.org
Rush University Medical Center	Chicago	Illinois	312-942-5000	www.ruch.edu
Russellville Hospital	Russellville	Alabama	256-332-1611	www.russellvillehospital.com
Sacred Heart Hospital	Eau Claire	Wisconsin	715-717-4121	www.sacredhearteauclaire.org
Saint Anthony Medical Center	Rockford	Illinois	815-226-2000	www.osfhealth.com
Saint Francis Medical Center	Peoria	Illinois	309-655-2000	www.osfsaintfrancis.org
Saint Joseph's Hospital of Atlanta	Atlanta	Georgia	678-843-5720	www.stjosephsatlanta.org

Hospital	City	State	Phone	Web Site
Saint Mary's Health Care	Grand Rapids	Michigan	616-685-5000	www.smhealthcare.org
Saint Mary's Regional Medical Center	Reno	Nevada	775-770-3000	www.saintmarysreno.com
Salem Hospital	Salem	Oregon	503-561-5200	www.salemhospital.org
Salina Regional Health Center	Salina	Kansas	785-452-7000	www.srhc.com
Sanford Usd Medical Center	Sioux Falls	South Dakota	605-333-1000	www.sanfordhealth.org
Santiam Memorial Hospital	Stayton	Oregon	503-769-2175	www.santiamhospital.com
Sarasota Memorial Hospital	Sarasota	Florida	941-917-9000	www.smh.com
Seton Medical Center Austin	Austin	Texas	512-324-1000	www.seton.net
Sharp Memorial Hospital	San Diego	California	858-939-3400	www.sharp.com/memorial
Sky Ridge Medical Center	Lone Tree	Colorado	720-225-1000	www.skyridgemedcenter.com
Slidell Memorial Hospital	Slidell	Louisiana	985-643-2200	www.sliddelmemorial.org
Southeast Alabama Medical Center	Dothan	Alabama	334-793-8701	www.samc.org
Southwestern Vermont Medical Center	Bennington	Vermont	802-442-6361	www.svhealthcare.org
Spectrum Health - Butterworth Campus	Grand Rapids	Michigan	616-391-1774	www.spectrum-health.org
Springhill Medical Center	Mobile	Alabama	251-344-9630	www.springhillmedicalcenter.com
Saint Elizabeth Health Center	Youngstown	Ohio	330-746-7211	www.hmhs.org
Saint Elizabeth Medical Center	Utica	New York	315-798-8100	www.stemc.org
Saint Francis Health Center	Topeka	Kansas	785-295-8000	www.stfrancistopeka.org
Saint Francis - Downtown	Greenville	South Carolina	864-255-1000	www.stfrancishealth.org
Saint Helena Hospital	Saint Helena	California	707-963-3611	www.sthelenahospital.org
Saint Joseph Medical Center	Tacoma	Washington	253-627-4101	www.fhshealth.org
Saint Joseph Mercy Hospital	Ann Arbor	Michigan	734-712-3791	www.stjoesannarbor.or
Saint Joseph's Hospital & Medical Center	Phoenix	Arizona	602-406-3000	www.stjosephs-phx.org
Saint Louis University Hospital	Saint Louis	Missouri	314-577-8000	www.slucare.edu/clinical
Saint Luke's Hospital Bethlehem	Bethlehem	Pennsylvania	610-954-4000	www.slhn-lehighvalley.org
Saint Luke's Hospital	Chesterfield	Missouri	314-434-1500	www.goodhealthmatters.com
Saint Luke's Hospital of Kansas City	Kansas City	Missouri	816-932-2000	www.staintlukeshealthsystem.org
Saint Marys Hospital	Madison	Wisconsin	608-251-6100	www.stmarysmadison.com
Stanford Hospital	Stanford	California	650-723-5708	www.stanfordhospital.com
Swedish Medical Center	Seattle	Washington	206-386-6000	www.swedish.org
Swedish Medical Center - Cherry Hill	Seattle	Washington	206-320-2000	www.swedish.org
Tacoma General Allenmore Hospital	Tacoma	Washington	253-403-1000	www.multicare.org
Tampa General Hospital	Tampa	Florida	813-844-7000	www.tgh.org
Heart Hospital Baylor Plano	Plano	Texas	469-814-3278	www.thehearthospitalbaylor.com
Theda Clark Medical Center	Neenah	Wisconsin	920-729-3100	www.thedacare.org
Thomas Hospital	Fairhope	Alabama	251-928-2375	www.thomashospital.com
Town & Country Hospital	Tampa	Florida	813-882-7159	www.townandcountryhospital.com
Trinity Hospitals	Minot	North Dakota	701-857-5000	www.trinityhealth.org
Trinity Medical Center	Birmingham	Alabama	205-592-1000	www.bhsala.com/montclair
Trinity Rock Island	Rock Island	Illinois	309-779-5000	www.trinityqc.com
Trumbull Memorial Hospital	Warren	Ohio	330-841-9011	www.trumhosp.org
Tulane Medical Center	New Orleans	Louisiana	504-988-1900	www.tuhc.com
UF Health Jacksonville	Jacksonville	Florida	904-244-0411	www.shandsjacksonville.org
UMC of Southern Nevada	Las Vegas	Nevada	702-383-2000	www.umc-cares.org
University Colo Health Memorial Hospital Central	Colorado Springs	Colorado	719-365-5000	www.memorialhospital.com
University Health Care/University Hospitals & Clinics	Salt Lake City	Utah	801-581-2121	www.healthcare.utah.edu
University Health System	San Antonio	Texas	210-358-4000	www.universityhealthsystem.com
University of California Davis Medical Center	Sacramento	California	916-734-2011	www.ucdmc.ucdavis.edu
University of Cincinnati Medical Center	Cincinnati	Ohio	513-584-1000	www.universityhospitalcincinnati.com
University of Colorado Hospital	Aurora	Colorado	720-848-0000	www.uch.edu
University of Kansas Hospital	Kansas City	Kansas	913-588-7332	www.kumc.edu
University of Miami Hospital	Miami	Florida	305-325-5511	www.cedarsmedicalcenter.com
University of Minnesota Medical Center - Fairview	Minneapolis	Minnesota	612-273-3000	www.uofmmedicalcenter.org
University of Toledo Medical Center	Toledo	Ohio	419-383-3407	www.utmc.utoledo.edu
University of Wisconsin Hospitals & Clinics Authority	Madison	Wisconsin	608-263-8991	www.uwhealth.org
UPMC Hamot	Erie	Pennsylvania	814-877-6000	www.hamot.org
UPMC Passavant	Pittsburgh	Pennsylvania	412-367-6700	www.passavant.upmc.com
UPMC Presbyterian Shadyside	Pittsburgh	Pennsylvania	412-647-8788	www.upmc.edu
UT Southwestern University Hospital	Dallas	Texas	214-879-3758	www.utsouthwestern.edu
Utah Valley Regional Medical Center	Provo	Utah	801-373-7850	www.intermountainhealthcare.org/hospitals/uvrmc
Ventura County Medical Center	Ventura	California	805-652-6075	www.vchca.org
Vidant Medical Center	Greenville	North Carolina	252-847-4100	www.uhseast.com
Virginia Mason Medical Center	Seattle	Washington	206-223-6600	www.vmmc.org
Waukesha Memorial Hospital	Waukesha	Wisconsin	262-928-1000	www.waukeshamemorial.org
Wesley Medical Center	Hattiesburg	Mississippi	601-268-8000	www.wesley.com
West Virginia University Hospitals	Morgantown	West Virginia	304-598-4000	www.wvuh.com
Wheaton Franciscan Saint Joseph	Milwaukee	Wisconsin	414-447-2000	www.wfhealthcare.org

Hospital	City	State	Phone	Web Site
Winchester Hospital	Winchester	Massachusetts	781-729-9000	www.winchesterhospital.org
Women & Infants Hospital of Rhode Island	Providence	Rhode Island	401-274-1100	www.womenandinfants.com
The Women's Hospital	Newburgh	Indiana	812-842-4200	www.deaconess.com
Yavapai Regional Medical Center	Prescott	Arizona	928-771-5676	www.yrmc.org

Note: Table shows hospitals nationwide whose surgical complication rate is worse (higher) than U.S. rate of 1.83%

Hospitals whose Surgical Complication Rate is Better (Lower) than the U.S. National Rate

Measure: Collapsed Lung Due to Medical Treatment

Hospital	City	State	Phone	Web Site
Centinela Hospital Medical Center	Inglewood	California	310-673-4660	www.centinelafreeman.com
Centra Health	Lynchburg	Virginia	434-200-4789	www.centrahealth.com
Community Medical Center	Toms River	New Jersey	732-557-8000	www.sbhcs.com
Evanston Hospital	Evanston	Illinois	847-432-8000	www.enh.org
New York - Presbyterian Hospital	New York	New York	212-746-4189	www.nyp.org
Norton Hospitals	Louisville	Kentucky	502-629-6560	www.nortonhealthcare.com
Spectrum Health - Butterworth Campus	Grand Rapids	Michigan	616-391-1774	www.spectrum-health.org
Virtua West Jersey Hospitals Berlin	Berlin	New Jersey	856-322-3200	www.virtua.org
Willis Knighton Medical Center	Shreveport	Louisiana	318-212-4000	www.wkhs.com//locations/medicalcenter.aspx

Note: Table shows hospitals nationwide whose surgical complication rate is better (lower) than U.S. rate of 0.32%

Hospitals whose Surgical Complication Rate is Worse (Higher) than the U.S. National Rate

Measure: Collapsed Lung Due to Medical Treatment

Hospital	City	State	Phone	Web Site
Abilene Regional Medical Center	Abilene	Texas	325-428-1000	www.abileneregional.com
Banner Heart Hospital	Mesa	Arizona	480-854-5050	www.bannerhealth.com
Baylor Medical Center at Garland	Garland	Texas	972-487-5000	www.baylorhealth.com
Baylor Regional Medical Center at Grapevine	Grapevine	Texas	817-481-1588	www.baylorhealth.com
Bert Fish Medical Center	New Smyrna Beach	Florida	386-424-5000	www.bertfish.com
Beth Israel Deaconess Medical Center	Boston	Massachusetts	617-667-7000	www.bidmc.harvard.edu
Bryan Medical Center	Lincoln	Nebraska	402-481-1111	www.bryan.org
Capital Region Medical Center	Jefferson City	Missouri	573-632-5000	www.crmc.org
Carolinas Medical Center - Union	Monroe	North Carolina	704-283-3100	www.carolinashealthcare.org/cmc-union
Champlain Valley Physicians Hospital Medical Center	Plattsburgh	New York	518-561-2000	www.cvph.org
Community Regional Medical Center	Fresno	California	559-459-6000	www.communitymedical.org
Des Peres Hospital	Saint Louis	Missouri	314-966-9100	www.despereshospital.com
Feather River Hospital	Paradise	California	530-877-9361	www.frhosp.org
Florida Hospital	Orlando	Florida	407-303-1976	www.floridahospital.com
Hays Medical Center	Hays	Kansas	785-623-5000	www.haysmed.com
Inova Fairfax Hospital	Falls Church	Virginia	703-776-3332	www.inova.org
Kansas Medical Center	Andover	Kansas	316-300-4000	www.ksmedcenter.com
Largo Medical Center	Largo	Florida	727-588-5200	www.largomedical.com
Lawrence Memorial Hospital	Lawrence	Kansas	785-505-6100	www.lmh.org
Loma Linda University Medical Center	Loma Linda	California	909-558-4000	www.llumc.edu
Madera Community Hospital	Madera	California	559-675-5555	www.maderahospital.org
Maine Medical Center	Portland	Maine	207-662-0111	www.mmc.org
Massachusetts General Hospital	Boston	Massachusetts	617-726-2000	www.massgeneral.org
Mclaren - Northern Michigan	Petoskey	Michigan	231-487-4000	www.northernhealth.org
Medical West	Bessemer	Alabama	205-481-7000	www.uab.edu
Midmichigan Medical Center - Midland	Midland	Michigan	989-839-3000	www.midmichigan.org
Mills - Peninsula Medical Center	Burlingame	California	650-696-5270	www.mills-peninsula.org
Norman Regional Health System	Norman	Oklahoma	405-321-1700	www.normanregional.com
Northwest Texas Hospital	Amarillo	Texas	806-354-1110	www.nxtexashealthcare.com
NYU Hospitals Center	New York	New York	212-263-7300	www.med.nyu.edu
Orange Regional Medical Center	Middletown	New York	845-343-2424	www.ormc.org
Orlando Health	Orlando	Florida	321-841-5111	www.orlandoregionalmedicalcenter.org
Parkridge Medical Center	Chattanooga	Tennessee	423-894-4220	www.tristarhealth.com
Piedmont Hospital	Atlanta	Georgia	404-605-5000	www.piedmonthospital.org
Pikeville Medical Center	Pikeville	Kentucky	606-218-3500	www.pikevillehospital.org
Providence Health Center	Waco	Texas	254-751-4000	www.providence.net
Providence Saint Vincent Medical Center	Portland	Oregon	503-216-1234	www.providence.org
Ronald Reagan UCLA Medical Center	Los Angeles	California	310-825-6301	www.uclahealth.org
Saint Francis Medical Center	Peoria	Illinois	309-655-2000	www.osfsaintfrancis.org
Saint Joseph Hospital	Lexington	Kentucky	859-313-1000	www.sjhlex.org
Saint Joseph's Hospital of Atlanta	Atlanta	Georgia	678-843-5720	www.stjosephsatlanta.org
Sanford Medical Center Fargo	Fargo	North Dakota	701-234-2000	www.meritcare.com
Self Regional Healthcare	Greenwood	South Carolina	864-227-4111	www.selfregional.org
Sentara Norfolk General Hospital	Norfolk	Virginia	757-388-3000	www.sentara.com
Sharp Memorial Hospital	San Diego	California	858-939-3400	www.sharp.com/memorial
Silver Cross Hospital & Medical Centers	New Lenox	Illinois	815-300-1100	www.silvercross.org
SSM Depaul Health Center	Bridgeton	Missouri	314-344-6000	www.ssmdepaul.com
Saint Bernards Medical Center	Jonesboro	Arkansas	870-972-4100	www.sbrmc.com
Saint John Medical Center	Tulsa	Oklahoma	918-744-3606	www.sjmc.org
Saint John's Episcopal Hospital at South Shore	Far Rockaway	New York	718-869-7000	www.ehs.org
Saint Luke's Hospital of Kansas City	Kansas City	Missouri	816-932-2000	www.staintlukeshealthsystem.org
Saint Tammany Parish Hospital	Covington	Louisiana	985-898-4000	www.stph.org
Sturdy Memorial Hospital	Attleboro	Massachusetts	508-222-5200	www.sturdymemorial.org
Theda Clark Medical Center	Neenah	Wisconsin	920-729-3100	www.thedacare.org
UMC of Southern Nevada	Las Vegas	Nevada	702-383-2000	www.umc-cares.org
University Medical Center of El Paso	El Paso	Texas	915-521-7602	www.thomasoncares.org
University of Alabama Hospital	Birmingham	Alabama	205-934-4011	www.health.uab.edu
University of Toledo Medical Center	Toledo	Ohio	419-383-3407	www.utmc.utoledo.edu
UPMC Presbyterian Shadyside	Pittsburgh	Pennsylvania	412-647-8788	www.upmc.edu
Williamsport Regional Medical Center	Williamsport	Pennsylvania	570-321-1000	www.susquehannahealth.org

Note: Table shows hospitals nationwide whose surgical complication rate is worse (higher) than U.S. rate of 0.32%

Hospitals whose Surgical Complication Rate is Better (Lower) than the U.S. National Rate

Measure: Deaths Among Patients With Serious Treatable Complications After Surgery

Hospital	City	State	Phone	Web Site
Advocate Lutheran General Hospital	Park Ridge	Illinois	847-723-2210	www.advocatehealth.com
Alexian Brothers Medical Center	Elk Grove Village	Illinois	847-437-5500	www.alexian.org
Aurora West Allis Medical Center	West Allis	Wisconsin	414-328-6000	www.aurorahealthcare.org
Banner Thunderbird Medical Center	Glendale	Arizona	602-588-5555	www.bannerhealth.com
Baptist Saint Anthony's Hospital	Amarillo	Texas	806-212-2000	www.bsahs.com
Bayfront Health Punta Gorda	Punta Gorda	Florida	941-639-3131	www.charlotteregional.com
Delray Medical Center	Delray Beach	Florida	561-498-4440	www.delraymedicalctr.com
Emory University Hospital	Atlanta	Georgia	404-686-8500	www.emoryhealthcare.org
Evanston Hospital	Evanston	Illinois	847-432-8000	www.enh.org
Fawcett Memorial Hospital	Port Charlotte	Florida	941-629-1181	www.fawcetthospital.com
Franciscan Saint Francis Health - Indianapolis	Indianapolis	Indiana	317-865-5001	www.stfrancishospitals.org
Gwinnett Medical Center	Lawrenceville	Georgia	678-312-1000	www.gwinnettmedicalcenter.org
Hackensack University Medical Center	Hackensack	New Jersey	201-996-2000	www.humed.com
Henry Ford Wyandotte Hospital	Wyandotte	Michigan	734-246-6000	www.henryfordwyandotte.com
Hinsdale Hospital	Hinsdale	Illinois	630-856-9000	www.keepingyouwell.com
Hospital For Special Surgery	New York	New York	212-606-1000	www.hss.edu
JFK Medical Center	Atlantis	Florida	561-965-7300	www.jfkmc.com
JFK Medical Center - A M Yelencsics Comm Hospital	Edison	New Jersey	732-321-7000	www.jfkmc.org
Los Robles Hospital & Medical Center	Thousand Oaks	California	805-497-2727	www.losrobleshospital.com
Martin Medical Center	Stuart	Florida	772-287-5200	www.mmhs.com
Mayo Clinic Hospital	Phoenix	Arizona	480-342-2000	www.mayoclinic.org
Mayo Clinic Methodist- Hospital	Rochester	Minnesota	507-266-7890	www.mayoclinic.org/methodisthospital
Mclaren Flint	Flint	Michigan	810-342-2000	www.mclaren.org
Memorial Hermann Memorial City Medical Center	Houston	Texas	713-242-3000	www.mhhs.org
Missouri Baptist Medical Center	Town & Country	Missouri	314-996-5000	www.missouribaptistmedicalcenter.org
Mother Frances Hospital	Tyler	Texas	903-593-8441	www.tmfhs.org
North Colorado Medical Center	Greeley	Colorado	970-352-4121	www.bannerhealth.com
North Kansas City Hospital	North Kansas City	Missouri	816-691-2000	www.nkch.org
Northwestern Memorial Hospital	Chicago	Illinois	312-926-2000	www.nmh.org
NYU Hospitals Center	New York	New York	212-263-7300	www.med.nyu.edu
OHSU Hospital & Clinics	Portland	Oregon	503-494-4036	www.ohsu.edu
Palm Beach Gardens Medical Center	Palm Beach Gardens	Florida	561-622-1411	www.pbgmc.com
Palos Community Hospital	Palos Heights	Illinois	708-923-4000	www.paloshospital.org
Providence Hospital & Medical Centers	Southfield	Michigan	248-849-3011	www.stjohn.org/providence
Saint Alexius Medical Center	Hoffman Estates	Illinois	847-843-2000	www.alexianbrothershealth.org
Saint Alexius Medical Center	Bismarck	North Dakota	701-530-7000	www.st.alexius.org
Saint David's Medical Center	Austin	Texas	512-476-7111	www.stdavidsrehab.com
Saint Elizabeth Health Center	Youngstown	Ohio	330-746-7211	www.hmhs.org
Saint John Macomb - Oakland Hospital - Macomb Center	Warren	Michigan	586-573-5000	www.stjohn.org
Saint Joseph's Hospital & Medical Center	Phoenix	Arizona	602-406-3000	www.stjosephs-phx.org
Saint Luke's Hospital	Cedar Rapids	Iowa	319-369-7211	www.crstlukes.com
Heart Hospital Baylor Plano	Plano	Texas	469-814-3278	www.thehearthospitalbaylor.com
University of Wisconsin Hospitals & Clinics Authority	Madison	Wisconsin	608-263-8991	www.uwhealth.org

Note: Table shows hospitals nationwide whose surgical complication rate is better (lower) than U.S. rate of 110.25%

Hospitals whose Surgical Complication Rate is Worse (Higher) than the U.S. National Rate

Measure: Deaths Among Patients With Serious Treatable Complications After Surgery

Hospital	City	State	Phone	Web Site
Baptist Health Medical Center - Little Rock	Little Rock	Arkansas	501-202-2000	www.baptist-health.com
Baptist Medical Center	San Antonio	Texas	210-297-1020	www.baptisthealthsystem.org
Carolinas Hospital System	Florence	South Carolina	843-674-2500	www.carolinashospital.com
Carolinas Medical Center/Behaviorial Health	Charlotte	North Carolina	704-355-2000	www.carolinasmedicalcenter.org
Christian Hospital Northeast - Northwest	Saint Louis	Missouri	314-653-5000	www.christianhospital.org
Christiana Care Health Services	Newark	Delaware	302-733-1000	www.christianacare.org
Community Regional Medical Center	Fresno	California	559-459-6000	www.communitymedical.org
Conway Medical Center	Conway	South Carolina	843-347-8037	www.conwayhospital.com
Cooper University Hospital	Camden	New Jersey	856-342-2000	www.cooperhealth.org
Cullman Regional Medical Center	Cullman	Alabama	256-737-2000	www.crmchospital.com
Doctors Hospital	Augusta	Georgia	706-651-6008	www.doctors-hospital.net
Doctors Medical Center	Modesto	California	209-578-1211	www.dmc-modesto.com
Duke University Hospital	Durham	North Carolina	919-684-8111	www.dukehealth.org
East Texas Medical Center	Tyler	Texas	903-597-0351	www.etmc.org
Erlanger Medical Center	Chattanooga	Tennessee	423-778-7000	www.erlanger.org
Fairbanks Memorial Hospital	Fairbanks	Alaska	907-452-8181	www.bannerhealth.com
Fletcher Allen Hospital of Vermont	Burlington	Vermont	802-847-0000	www.fletcherallen.org
Florida Hospital Tampa	Tampa	Florida	813-615-7200	www.uch.org
Good Samaritan Hospital Medical Center	West Islip	New York	631-376-3000	www.good-samaritan-hospital.org
Halifax Health Medical Center	Daytona Beach	Florida	386-254-4000	www.halifax.org
Health Alliance Hospital Broadway Campus	Kingston	New York	914-331-3131	www.kingstonregionalhealth.org
Hillcrest Medical Center	Tulsa	Oklahoma	918-579-1000	www.hillcrest.com
Integris Baptist Medical Center	Oklahoma City	Oklahoma	405-951-8110	www.integris-health.com
Jewish Hospital & Saint Mary's Healthcare	Louisville	Kentucky	502-587-4011	www.jhhs.org
Kaleida Health	Buffalo	New York	716-859-8620	www.kaleidahealth.org
Lake Cumberland Regional Hospital	Somerset	Kentucky	606-679-7441	www.lakecumberlandhospital.com
Lakeland Regional Medical Center	Lakeland	Florida	863-687-1100	www.lrmc.com
Magnolia Regional Health Center	Corinth	Mississippi	662-293-7660	www.mrhc.org
Marian Regional Medical Center	Santa Maria	California	805-739-3000	www.marinmedicalcenter.org
Mary Hitchcock Memorial Hospital	Lebanon	New Hampshire	603-650-5000	www.dhmc.org
Medical Center of Central Georgia	Macon	Georgia	478-633-6805	www.mccg.org
Medical Center of Plano	Plano	Texas	972-596-6800	www.medicalcenterofplano.com
Medical College of Georgia Hospitals & Clinics	Augusta	Georgia	706-721-6569	www.mcghealth.org
Methodist Healthcare Memphis Hospitals	Memphis	Tennessee	901-516-8274	www.methodisthealth.org
Milton S Hershey Medical Center	Hershey	Pennsylvania	717-531-8521	www.hmc.psu.edu
Mobile Infirmary	Mobile	Alabama	251-435-4700	www.mimc.com
Nazareth Hospital	Philadelphia	Pennsylvania	215-335-6000	www.nazarethhospital.org
North Carolina Baptist Hospital	Winston-Salem	North Carolina	336-716-2011	www.wfubmc.edu
North Mississippi Medical Center	Tupelo	Mississippi	662-377-3000	www.nmhs.net/nmmc
Northeast Alabama Regional Medical Center	Anniston	Alabama	256-235-5121	www.rmccares.org
Oklahoma State University Medical Center	Tulsa	Oklahoma	918-587-2561	www.tulsaregional.com
Phoebe Putney Memorial Hospital	Albany	Georgia	229-312-4068	www.phoebeputney.com
Renown Regional Medical Center	Reno	Nevada	775-982-4100	www.renown.org
Riverside Methodist Hospital	Columbus	Ohio	614-566-5000	www.ohiohealth.com
Robert Wood Johnson University Hospital	New Brunswick	New Jersey	732-937-8900	www.rwjuh.edu
Robert Wood Johnson University Hospital - Hamilton	Hamilton	New Jersey	609-586-7900	www.rwjhamilton.org
Saint Francis Medical Center	Peoria	Illinois	309-655-2000	www.osfsaintfrancis.org
Sentara Norfolk General Hospital	Norfolk	Virginia	757-388-3000	www.sentara.com
Saint John Medical Center	Tulsa	Oklahoma	918-744-3606	www.sjmc.org
Saint Joseph's Hospital - Savannah	Savannah	Georgia	912-819-4100	www.sjchs.org
Saint Luke's Episcopal Hospital	Houston	Texas	832-355-1000	www.sleh.com
Saint Mary's Medical Center	Huntington	West Virginia	304-526-1234	www.st-marys.org
Saint Vincent's East	Birmingham	Alabama	205-838-3122	www.nolandhealth.com
Strong Memorial Hospital	Rochester	New York	585-275-2121	www.urmc.rochester.edu
Sunrise Hospital & Medical Center	Las Vegas	Nevada	702-731-8000	www.sunrisehospital.com
Tampa General Hospital	Tampa	Florida	813-844-7000	www.tgh.org
Trident Medical Center	Charleston	South Carolina	843-797-8800	www.tridenthealthsystem.com
UF Health Shands Hospital	Gainesville	Florida	352-265-8000	www.shands.org
Umass Memorial Medical Center	Worcester	Massachusetts	508-334-1000	www.umassmemorial.org
University Hospital	Newark	New Jersey	973-972-5658	www.theuniversityhospital.com
University Medical Center	Lubbock	Texas	806-775-8200	www.teamumc.org
University of Alabama Hospital	Birmingham	Alabama	205-934-4011	www.health.uab.edu
University of Kentucky Hospital	Lexington	Kentucky	859-323-5000	www.uhealthcare.uky.edu
University of Mississippi Medical Center	Jackson	Mississippi	601-984-4100	www.umc.edu

Hospital	City	State	Phone	Web Site
University of South Alabama Medical Center	Mobile	Alabama	251-471-7110	www.southalabama.edu/usamc
Vidant Medical Center	Greenville	North Carolina	252-847-4100	www.uhseast.com
Virtua West Jersey Hospitals Berlin	Berlin	New Jersey	856-322-3200	www.virtua.org

Note: Table shows hospitals nationwide whose surgical complication rate is worse (higher) than U.S. rate of 110.25%

Hospitals whose Surgical Complication Rate is Better (Lower) than the U.S. National Rate

Measure: Rate of Complications for Hip/Knee Replacement Patients

Hospital	City	State	Phone	Web Site
Arkansas Surgical Hospital	No Little Rock	Arkansas	501-748-8000	www.arksurgicalhospital.com
Baptist Health Louisville	Louisville	Kentucky	502-897-8100	www.baptisteast.com
Barnes-Jewish Hospital	Saint Louis	Missouri	314-747-3000	www.barnesjewish.org
Beaumont Health System	Royal Oak	Michigan	248-898-5000	www.beaumonthospitals.com
Boone Hospital Center	Columbia	Missouri	573-815-8000	www.boone.org
Bronson Methodist Hospital	Kalamazoo	Michigan	269-341-6000	www.bronsonhealth.com
Cape Cod Hospital	Hyannis	Massachusetts	508-771-1800	www.capecodhealth.org
Carilion Roanoke Memorial Hospital	Roanoke	Virginia	540-981-7000	www.carilion.com/crmh
Covenant Medical Center	Lubbock	Texas	806-725-6000	www.covenanthealth.org
Crittenton Hospital Medical Center	Rochester	Michigan	248-652-5000	www.crittenton.com
Delray Medical Center	Delray Beach	Florida	561-498-4440	www.delraymedicalctr.com
Doctors Hospital at Renaissance	Edinburg	Texas	956-362-8677	www.dhr-rgv.com
Florida Hospital Memorial Medical Center	Daytona Beach	Florida	386-676-6000	www.fhmd.com
Franciscan Saint Elizabeth Health - Lafayette East	Lafayette	Indiana	765-502-4334	www.ste.org
Heart of Florida Regional Medical Center	Davenport	Florida	863-422-4971	www.heartofflorida.com
Heartland Regional Medical Center	Saint Joseph	Missouri	816-271-6000	www.heartland-health.com
Hoag Orthopedic Institute	Irvine	California	949-727-5000	www.orthopedichospital.com
Holy Cross Hospital	Fort Lauderdale	Florida	954-771-8000	www.holy-cross.com
Hospital For Special Surgery	New York	New York	212-606-1000	www.hss.edu
Indian River Medical Center	Vero Beach	Florida	772-567-4311	www.irmh.com
Indiana Orthopaedic Hospital	Indianapolis	Indiana	317-956-1000	www.indianaorthopaedichospital.com
Jupiter Medical Center	Jupiter	Florida	561-747-2234	www.jupitermed.com
Kansas Medical Center	Andover	Kansas	316-300-4000	www.ksmedcenter.com
Kansas Surgery & Recovery Center	Wichita	Kansas	316-634-0090	www.ksrc.org
Maine Medical Center	Portland	Maine	207-662-0111	www.mmc.org
Mayo Clinic Methodist- Hospital	Rochester	Minnesota	507-266-7890	www.mayoclinic.org/methodisthospital
Mclaren - Greater Lansing	Lansing	Michigan	517-975-6000	www.mclaren.org
Memorial Healthcare System	Chattanooga	Tennessee	423-495-2525	www.memorial.org
Memorial Mission Hospital & Asheville Surgery Center	Asheville	North Carolina	828-213-1111	www.missionhospitals.org
Mississippi Baptist Medical Center	Jackson	Mississippi	601-968-1000	www.mbmc.org
Nebraska Orthopaedic Hospital	Omaha	Nebraska	402-609-1600	www.neorthohospital.com
New England Baptist Hospital	Boston	Massachusetts	617-754-5800	www.nebh.caregroup.org
North Mississippi Medical Center	Tupelo	Mississippi	662-377-3000	www.nmhs.net/nmmc
Ocala Regional Medical Center	Ocala	Florida	352-401-1000	www.ocalaregional.com
Oklahoma Surgical Hospital	Tulsa	Oklahoma	918-477-5000	www.oklahomasurgicalhospital.com
Olathe Medical Center	Olathe	Kansas	913-791-4200	www.ohsi.com
Orthopaedic Hospital at Parkview North	Fort Wayne	Indiana	260-672-4050	www.parkview.com
Plaza Medical Center of Fort Worth	Fort Worth	Texas	817-336-2100	www.plazamedicalcenter.com
Poudre Valley Hospital	Fort Collins	Colorado	970-495-7000	www.pvhs.org
Proctor Hospital	Peoria	Illinois	309-691-1000	www.proctor.org
Providence Saint John's Health Center	Santa Monica	California	310-829-5511	www.stjohns.org
Quail Creek Surgical Hospital	Amarillo	Texas	806-354-6100	www.physurg.com
Riverside Medical Center	Kankakee	Illinois	815-933-1671	www.riversidehealthcare.org
Roper Hospital	Charleston	South Carolina	843-724-2800	www.ropersaintfrancis.com
Sacred Heart Hospital	Pensacola	Florida	850-416-7000	www.sacred-heart.org
Saint Elizabeth Regional Medical Center	Lincoln	Nebraska	402-219-7700	www.stelizabethonline.com
Saint Joseph Regional Medical Center	Mishawaka	Indiana	574-335-5000	www.sjmed.com
Saint Joseph's Hospital of Atlanta	Atlanta	Georgia	678-843-5720	www.stjosephsatlanta.org
Saint Thomas Midtown Hospital	Nashville	Tennessee	615-284-5555	www.baptisthospital.com
Samaritan Regional Health System	Ashland	Ohio	419-289-0491	www.samho.org
Sanford Medical Center Bismarck	Bismarck	North Dakota	701-323-6000	www.medcenterone.com
Sentara Leigh Hospital	Norfolk	Virginia	757-261-6601	www.sentara.com
Seton Medical Center Austin	Austin	Texas	512-324-1000	www.seton.net
South Nassau Communities Hospital	Oceanside	New York	516-632-3000	www.southnassau.org
Southside Hospital	Bay Shore	New York	631-968-3000	www.northshorelij.com
Southwest General Health Center	Middleburg Heights	Ohio	440-816-8000	www.swgeneral.com
Saint Francis Hospital & Medical Center	Hartford	Connecticut	860-714-4000	www.saintfranciscare.com
Saint Helena Hospital	Saint Helena	California	707-963-3611	www.sthelenahospital.org
Saint Joseph Hospital	Orange	California	714-633-9111	www.sjo.org
Saint Joseph Mercy Oakland	Pontiac	Michigan	248-858-3000	www.stjoesoakland.org
Saint Joseph's Hospital - Savannah	Savannah	Georgia	912-819-4100	www.sjchs.org
Saint Peter's Hospital	Albany	New York	518-525-1550	www.stpetershealthcare.org
Saint Vincent's Medical Center	Jacksonville	Florida	904-308-7300	www.jaxhealth.com
Sutter General Hospital	Sacramento	California	916-733-8999	www.suttermedicalcenter.org

Hospital	City	State	Phone	Web Site
Tampa General Hospital	Tampa	Florida	813-844-7000	www.tgh.org
Texas Health Presbyterian Hospital Dallas	Dallas	Texas	214-345-6789	www.texashealth.org
Torrance Memorial Medical Center	Torrance	California	310-325-9110	www.torrancememorial.org
Valley Medical Center	Renton	Washington	425-228-3450	www.valleymed.org
VHS Harlingen Hospital Company	Harlingen	Texas	956-389-1100	www.vbmc.org
Washington Hospital	Fremont	California	510-797-1111	www.whhs.com
Western Maryland Regional Medical Center	Cumberland	Maryland	240-964-8001	www.wmhs.com
William Beaumont Hospital - Troy	Troy	Michigan	248-964-8800	www.beaumonthospitals.com
Yavapai Regional Medical Center	Prescott	Arizona	928-771-5676	www.yrmc.org

Note: Table shows hospitals nationwide whose surgical complication rate is better (lower) than U.S. rate of 3.4%

Hospitals whose Surgical Complication Rate is Worse (Higher) than the U.S. National Rate

Measure: Rate of Complications for Hip/Knee Replacement Patients

Hospital	City	State	Phone	Web Site
Alegent Health Mercy Hospital	Council Bluffs	Iowa	712-328-5000	www.alegent.com/mercy
Atrium Medical Center	Franklin	Ohio	513-420-5102	www.atriummedcenter.org
Baptist Memorial Hospital	Memphis	Tennessee	901-226-5000	www.bmhcc.org
Baptist Saint Anthony's Hospital	Amarillo	Texas	806-212-2000	www.bsahs.com
Beaumont Health System	Grosse Pointe	Michigan	313-343-1000	www.beaumonthospitals.com
Bridgeport Hospital	Bridgeport	Connecticut	203-384-3000	www.bridgeporthospital.com
Carolinas Medical Center - Northeast	Concord	North Carolina	704-783-3000	www.northeastmedical.org
Central Maine Medical Center	Lewiston	Maine	207-795-0111	www.cmmc.org
Community Memorial Hospital San Buenaventura	Ventura	California	805-652-5011	www.cmhhospital.org
D C H Regional Medical Center	Tuscaloosa	Alabama	205-759-7111	www.dchsystem.com
Decatur Morgan Hospital - Decatur Campus	Decatur	Alabama	256-341-2000	www.decaturgeneral.org
Defiance Regional Medical Center	Defiance	Ohio	419-783-6955	www.promedica.org/defiance
Doctors Medical Center	Modesto	California	209-578-1211	www.dmc-modesto.com
East Ohio Regional Hospital	Martins Ferry	Ohio	740-633-4151	www.eastohioregionalhospital.com
Floyd Medical Center	Rome	Georgia	706-509-6900	www.floydmed.org
Froedtert Memorial Lutheran Hospital	Milwaukee	Wisconsin	414-805-3000	www.froedtert.com
Gadsden Regional Medical Center	Gadsden	Alabama	256-494-4000	www.gadsdenregional.com
Genesis Medical Center - Davenport	Davenport	Iowa	563-421-1000	www.genesishealth.com
Genesys Regional Medical Center - Health Park	Grand Blanc	Michigan	810-606-5000	www.genesys.org
Grant Medical Center	Columbus	Ohio	614-566-9978	www.ohiohealth.com
Henry County Medical Center	Paris	Tennessee	731-642-1220	www.hcmc-tn.org
Houston Orthopedic & Spine Hospital	Bellaire	Texas	713-622-2262	www.foundationsurgicalhospital.com
Johnson City Medical Center	Johnson City	Tennessee	423-431-6111	www.msha.com
Lancaster General Hospital	Lancaster	Pennsylvania	717-299-5511	www.lancastergeneral.org
Louis A Weiss Memorial Hospital	Chicago	Illinois	773-878-8700	www.weisshospital.org
The Medical Center of Aurora	Aurora	Colorado	303-695-2600	www.auroramed.com
Mercy Health System Corp	Janesville	Wisconsin	608-756-6080	www.mercyhealthsystem.org
Mercy Saint Anne Hospital	Toledo	Ohio	419-407-2663	www.mercyweb.org
Mountain View Hospital	Payson	Utah	801-465-7100	www.mvhpayson.com
North Colorado Medical Center	Greeley	Colorado	970-352-4121	www.bannerhealth.com
North Kansas City Hospital	North Kansas City	Missouri	816-691-2000	www.nkch.org
Northwestern Memorial Hospital	Chicago	Illinois	312-926-2000	www.nmh.org
Novant Health Rowan Medical Center	Salisbury	North Carolina	704-210-5000	www.rowan.org
NYU Hospitals Center	New York	New York	212-263-7300	www.med.nyu.edu
Onslow Memorial Hospital	Jacksonville	North Carolina	910-577-2345	www.onslowmemorial.org
Overland Park Regional Medical Center	Overland Park	Kansas	913-541-5301	www.oprmc.com
Park Ridge Health	Hendersonville	North Carolina	828-684-8501	www.parkridgehospital.org
Pennsylvania Hospital of the Univ of PA Health Sys	Philadelphia	Pennsylvania	215-829-3000	www.pennmedicine.org/pahosp
Peterson Regional Medical Center	Kerrville	Texas	830-896-4200	www.petersonrmc.com
Pinnacle Health Hospitals	Harrisburg	Pennsylvania	717-782-5181	www.pinnaclehealth.org
Poplar Bluff Regional Medical Center	Poplar Bluff	Missouri	573-785-7721	www.poplarbluffregional.com
Reston Hospital Center	Reston	Virginia	703-689-9000	www.restonhospital.com
Riddle Memorial Hospital	Media	Pennsylvania	610-566-9400	www.riddlehospital.org
Saint Michael's Medical Center	Newark	New Jersey	973-877-5350	www.cathedralhealth.org
Shady Grove Adventist Hospital	Rockville	Maryland	240-826-6517	www.adventisthealthcare.com/sgah
Shannon Medical Center	San Angelo	Texas	325-653-6741	www.shannonhealth.com
South Central Regional Medical Center	Laurel	Mississippi	601-649-4000	www.scrmc.com
South Lake Hospital	Clermont	Florida	352-394-4071	www.southlakehospital.com
Southside Regional Medical Center	Petersburg	Virginia	804-765-5000	www.srmconline.com
Spring Valley Hospital Medical Center	Las Vegas	Nevada	702-853-3000	www.springvalleyhospital.com
Saint Alexius Medical Center	Hoffman Estates	Illinois	847-843-2000	www.alexianbrothershealth.org
Saint Anthony Hospital	Oklahoma City	Oklahoma	405-272-7000	www.saintsok.com
Saint Catherine of Siena Hospital	Smithtown	New York	631-862-3000	www.stcatherines.chsli.org
Saint Clair Memorial Hospital	Pittsburgh	Pennsylvania	412-942-6209	www.stclair.org
Saint Elizabeth Hospital	Appleton	Wisconsin	920-738-2000	www.affinityhealth.org
Saint Luke's Hospital Bethlehem	Bethlehem	Pennsylvania	610-954-4000	www.slhn-lehighvalley.org
Saint Marys Hospital	Madison	Wisconsin	608-251-6100	www.stmarysmadison.com
Saint Vincent Anderson Regional Hospital	Anderson	Indiana	765-646-8373	www.stjohnshealthsystem.org
Saint Vincent Healthcare	Billings	Montana	406-657-7000	www.svh-mt.org
Saint Vincent's Medical Center	Bridgeport	Connecticut	203-576-5551	www.stvincents.org
Sutter Auburn Faith Hospital	Auburn	California	530-888-4500	www.sutterauburnfaith.org
Sutter Solano Medical Center	Vallejo	California	707-554-5280	www.suttersolano.org
Swedish Medical Center	Englewood	Colorado	303-788-5000	www.swedishhospital.com/default.asp
Trinity Medical Center	Birmingham	Alabama	205-592-1000	www.bhsala.com/montclair

Hospital	City	State	Phone	Web Site
University of Kansas Hospital	Kansas City	Kansas	913-588-7332	www.kumc.edu
University of Toledo Medical Center	Toledo	Ohio	419-383-3407	www.utmc.utoledo.edu
Wentworth - Douglass Hospital	Dover	New Hampshire	603-740-2580	www.wdhospital.com
White River Medical Center	Batesville	Arkansas	870-262-1200	www.wrmc.com

Note: Table shows hospitals nationwide whose surgical complication rate is worse (higher) than U.S. rate of 3.4%

Hospitals whose Surgical Complication Rate is Better (Lower) than the U.S. National Rate

Measure: Serious Blood Clots After Surgery

Hospital	City	State	Phone	Web Site
Abbott Northwestern Hospital	Minneapolis	Minnesota	612-863-4509	www.abbottnorthwestern.com
Advocate Condell Medical Center	Libertyville	Illinois	847-990-5200	www.condell.org
Allegiance Health	Jackson	Michigan	517-788-4800	www.footehealth.org
Arkansas Heart Hospital	Little Rock	Arkansas	501-219-7000	www.arheart.com
Asante Rogue Regional Medical Center	Medford	Oregon	541-789-7000	www.asante.org
Aurora Saint Lukes Medical Center	Milwaukee	Wisconsin	414-649-6000	www.aurorahealthcare.org
Avera Mckennan Hospital & University Health Center	Sioux Falls	South Dakota	605-322-8000	www.mckennan.org
Avera Saint Lukes	Aberdeen	South Dakota	605-622-5000	www.averastlukes.org
Bakersfield Memorial Hospital	Bakersfield	California	661-327-1792	www.bakersfieldmemorial.org
Banner Baywood Medical Center	Mesa	Arizona	480-321-2000	www.bannerhealth.com
Banner Good Samaritan Medical Center	Phoenix	Arizona	602-239-2000	www.bannerhealth.com
Baptist Beaumont Hospital	Beaumont	Texas	409-212-5012	www.mhbh.org
Baptist Health Lexington	Lexington	Kentucky	859-260-6104	www.centralbap.com
Baptist Health Louisville	Louisville	Kentucky	502-897-8100	www.baptisteast.com
Baptist Health Medical Center - Little Rock	Little Rock	Arkansas	501-202-2000	www.baptist-health.com
Baystate Medical Center	Springfield	Massachusetts	413-794-0000	www.baystatehealth.com
Benefis Hospitals	Great Falls	Montana	406-455-5000	www.benefis.org
Berkshire Medical Center	Pittsfield	Massachusetts	413-447-2000	www.berkshirehealthsystems.org
Billings Clinic Hospital	Billings	Montana	406-657-4000	www.billngsclinic.com
Camden Clark Medical Center	Parkersburg	West Virginia	304-424-2111	www.ccmh.org
Cape Cod Hospital	Hyannis	Massachusetts	508-771-1800	www.capecodhealth.org
Carilion New River Valley Medical Center	Christiansburg	Virginia	540-731-2000	www.carilion.com
Carolinas Medical Center/Behaviorial Health	Charlotte	North Carolina	704-355-2000	www.carolinasmedicalcenter.org
Caromont Regional Medical Center	Gastonia	North Carolina	704-834-4891	www.caromont.org
Carson Tahoe Regional Medical Center	Carson City	Nevada	775-445-8000	www.carsontahoehospital.com
Centra Health	Lynchburg	Virginia	434-200-4789	www.centrahealth.com
Central Maine Medical Center	Lewiston	Maine	207-795-0111	www.cmmc.org
Charlotte Hungerford Hospital	Torrington	Connecticut	860-496-6666	www.charlottesweb.hungerford.org
Comanche County Memorial Hospital	Lawton	Oklahoma	580-355-8620	www.memorialhealthsource.org
Community Hospital North	Indianapolis	Indiana	317-621-5335	www.ecommunity.com/north
Community Medical Center	Toms River	New Jersey	732-557-8000	www.sbhcs.com
Cox Medical Center	Springfield	Missouri	417-269-6000	www.coxhealth.com
Doctors Hospital of Sarasota	Sarasota	Florida	941-342-1100	www.doctorsofsarasota.com
Duke University Hospital	Durham	North Carolina	919-684-8111	www.dukehealth.org
Eastern Idaho Regional Medical Center	Idaho Falls	Idaho	208-529-6111	www.eirmc.org
Eisenhower Medical Center	Rancho Mirage	California	760-340-3911	www.emc.org
El Camino Hospital	Mountain View	California	650-940-7000	www.elcaminohospital.org
Elkhart General Hospital	Elkhart	Indiana	574-294-2621	www.egh.org
Essentia Health - Fargo	Fargo	North Dakota	701-364-8000	www.dakotaclinic.com
Exeter Hospital	Exeter	New Hampshire	603-778-7311	www.exeterhospital.com
Flagstaff Medical Center	Flagstaff	Arizona	928-773-2009	www.nahealth.com
Fort Sanders Regional Medical Center	Knoxville	Tennessee	865-541-1101	www.fsregional.com
Franciscan Saint Elizabeth Health - Lafayette East	Lafayette	Indiana	765-502-4334	www.ste.org
Geisinger - Community Medical Center	Scranton	Pennsylvania	570-969-8240	www.cmchealthsys.org
Genesis Medical Center - Davenport	Davenport	Iowa	563-421-1000	www.genesishealth.com
Glens Falls Hospital	Glens Falls	New York	518-926-1000	www.glensfallshospital.org
Good Samaritan Regional Medical Center	Corvallis	Oregon	541-768-5111	www.samhealth.org/shs_facilities
Gundersen Lutheran Medical Center	La Crosse	Wisconsin	608-782-7300	www.gundluth.org
Harrison Memorial Center	Bremerton	Washington	360-377-3911	www.harrisonmedical.org
Hays Medical Center	Hays	Kansas	785-623-5000	www.haysmed.com
Heartland Regional Medical Center	Saint Joseph	Missouri	816-271-6000	www.heartland-health.com
Hendrick Medical Center	Abilene	Texas	325-670-2000	www.ehendrick.org
Holy Cross Hospital	Fort Lauderdale	Florida	954-771-8000	www.holy-cross.com
Indiana University Health Bloomington Hospital	Bloomington	Indiana	812-353-9555	www.bloomingtonhospital.org
Indiana University Health North Hospital	Carmel	Indiana	317-688-2000	www.iuhealth.org/north
Inova Mount Vernon Hospital	Alexandria	Virginia	703-664-7000	www.inova.com/inovapublic.srt/imvh/index.jsp
Integris Baptist Medical Center	Oklahoma City	Oklahoma	405-951-8110	www.integris-health.com
Jackson Hospital & Clinic	Montgomery	Alabama	334-293-8000	www.jackson.org
Jackson - Madison County General Hospital	Jackson	Tennessee	731-541-5000	www.wth.org
John Muir Medical Center - Concord Campus	Concord	California	925-674-2002	www.johnmuirhealth.com
John Muir Medical Center - Walnut Creek Campus	Walnut Creek	California	925-939-3000	www.jmmdhs.com
Kalispell Regional Medical Center	Kalispell	Montana	406-752-5111	www.krmc.org
Kootenai Medical Center	Coeur D'alene	Idaho	208-625-4001	www.kootenaihealth.org
Lakeland Hospital - Saint Joseph	Saint Joseph	Michigan	269-983-8300	www.lakelandhealth.org

Hospital	City	State	Phone	Web Site
Marian Regional Medical Center	Santa Maria	California	805-739-3000	www.marinmedicalcenter.org
Mary Washington Hospital	Fredericksburg	Virginia	540-741-1100	www.medicorp.org
Maury Regional Hospital	Columbia	Tennessee	931-381-1111	www.maurgregional.com
Mayo Clinic Methodist- Hospital	Rochester	Minnesota	507-266-7890	www.mayoclinic.org/methodisthospital
Mcleod Regional Medical Center - Pee Dee	Florence	South Carolina	843-777-2900	www.mcleodhealth.org
Medical Center of Central Georgia	Macon	Georgia	478-633-6805	www.mccg.org
Memorial Healthcare System	Chattanooga	Tennessee	423-495-2525	www.memorial.org
Memorial Hospital at Gulfport	Gulfport	Mississippi	228-867-4000	www.gulfportmemorial.com
Memorial Hospital of Carbondale	Carbondale	Illinois	618-549-0721	www.sih.net
Memorial Mission Hospital & Asheville Surgery Center	Asheville	North Carolina	828-213-1111	www.missionhospitals.org
Mercy Hospital	Coon Rapids	Minnesota	763-236-8205	www.allinamercy.org
Mercy Medical Center - Cedar Rapids	Cedar Rapids	Iowa	319-398-6011	www.mercycare.org
Mercy Medical Center - Redding	Redding	California	530-225-6102	www.redding.mercy.org
Mercy Medical Center - North Iowa	Mason City	Iowa	641-428-7000	www.mercynorthiowa.com
Methodist Hospital	San Antonio	Texas	210-575-4000	www.mh.sahealth.com
Methodist Medical Center of Oak Ridge	Oak Ridge	Tennessee	865-835-1000	www.mmcoakridge.com
Mother Frances Hospital	Tyler	Texas	903-593-8441	www.tmfhs.org
Munson Medical Center	Traverse City	Michigan	231-935-5000	www.munsonhealthcare.org
New England Baptist Hospital	Boston	Massachusetts	617-754-5800	www.nebh.caregroup.org
Novant Health Charlotte Orthopedic Hospital	Charlotte	North Carolina	704-316-2000	www.presbyterian.org
NW Arkansas Hospitals	Springdale	Arkansas	479-751-5711	www.northwesthealth.org
Ochsner Medical Center	New Orleans	Louisiana	504-842-3000	www.ochsner.org
Oklahoma Heart Hospital	Oklahoma City	Oklahoma	405-608-3200	www.okheart.com
Olathe Medical Center	Olathe	Kansas	913-791-4200	www.ohsi.com
Parker Adventist Hospital	Parker	Colorado	303-269-4000	www.parkerhospital.org
Parkview Medical Center	Pueblo	Colorado	719-584-4000	www.parkviewmc.com
Parkview Regional Medical Center	Fort Wayne	Indiana	260-266-1000	www.parkview.com
Parkwest Medical Center	Knoxville	Tennessee	865-970-9800	www.yesparkwest.com
Peacehealth Saint Joseph Medical Center	Bellingham	Washington	360-734-5400	www.peacehealth.org
Peconic Bay Medical Center	Riverhead	New York	631-548-6000	www.pbmedicalcenter.org
Presence Covenant Medical Center	Urbana	Illinois	217-337-2000	www.provena.org/covenant
Providence Sacred Heart Medical Center	Spokane	Washington	509-474-3040	www.shmc.org
Providence Saint John's Health Center	Santa Monica	California	310-829-5511	www.stjohns.org
Providence Saint Joseph Medical Center	Burbank	California	818-843-5111	www.providence.org/losangeles
Regional Medical Center Bayonet Point	Hudson	Florida	727-819-2929	www.mchealth.comorwww.heartoftampa.com
Riverview Medical Center	Red Bank	New Jersey	732-741-2700	www.meridianhealth.com
Sacred Heart Medical Center - Riverbend	Springfield	Oregon	541-222-7300	www.peacehealth.org/sacred-heart-riverbend
Saint Francis Medical Center	Cape Girardeau	Missouri	573-331-3000	www.sfmc.net
Saint Joseph Hospital	Lexington	Kentucky	859-313-1000	www.sjhlex.org
Saint Joseph Regional Medical Center	Mishawaka	Indiana	574-335-5000	www.sjmed.com
Saint Mary's Health Care	Grand Rapids	Michigan	616-685-5000	www.smhealthcare.org
Saint Thomas West Hospital	Nashville	Tennessee	615-222-2111	www.stthomas.org
Salinas Valley Memorial Hospital	Salinas	California	831-757-4333	www.svmh.com
San Jacinto Methodist Hospital	Baytown	Texas	281-420-8600	www.methodisthealth.com/sanjacinto
Sanford Medical Center Fargo	Fargo	North Dakota	701-234-2000	www.meritcare.com
Sanford Usd Medical Center	Sioux Falls	South Dakota	605-333-1000	www.sanfordhealth.org
Sarasota Memorial Hospital	Sarasota	Florida	941-917-9000	www.smh.com
Scott & White Memorial Hospital	Temple	Texas	254-724-2111	www.sw.org
Seton Medical Center Austin	Austin	Texas	512-324-1000	www.seton.net
Shannon Medical Center	San Angelo	Texas	325-653-6741	www.shannonhealth.com
Shasta Regional Medical Center	Redding	California	530-244-5454	www.shastaregional.com
South Georgia Medical Center	Valdosta	Georgia	229-333-1020	www.sgmc.org
Saint Charles Medical Center - Bend	Bend	Oregon	541-382-4321	www.scmc.org
Saint Cloud Hospital	Saint Cloud	Minnesota	320-251-2700	www.centracare.com
Saint David's Medical Center	Austin	Texas	512-476-7111	www.stdavidsrehab.com
Saint Elizabeth Medical Center	Lakeside Park	Kentucky	859-292-2000	www.stelizabeth.com
Saint Helena Hospital	Saint Helena	California	707-963-3611	www.sthelenahospital.org
Saint Joseph Hospital	Orange	California	714-633-9111	www.sjo.org
Saint Joseph Mercy Oakland	Pontiac	Michigan	248-858-3000	www.stjoesoakland.org
Saint Joseph's Hospital Health Center	Syracuse	New York	315-448-5111	www.sjhsyr.org
Saint Joseph's Medical Center of Stockton	Stockton	California	209-943-2000	www.stjospehscares.org
Saint Luke's Hospital	Cedar Rapids	Iowa	319-369-7211	www.crstlukes.com
Saint Mary's Regional Medical Center	Enid	Oklahoma	580-233-6100	www.stmarysregional.com
Saint Marys Hospital	Madison	Wisconsin	608-251-6100	www.stmarysmadison.com
Saint Patrick Hospital	Missoula	Montana	406-543-7271	www.saintpatrick.org
Saint Vincent Healthcare	Billings	Montana	406-657-7000	www.svh-mt.org
Saint Vincent Hospital	Santa Fe	New Mexico	505-913-5201	www.stvin.org

Hospital	City	State	Phone	Web Site
Saint Vincent Hospital & Health Services	Indianapolis	Indiana	317-338-7000	www.indianapolis.stvincent.org
Saint Vincent's Medical Center	Jacksonville	Florida	904-308-7300	www.jaxhealth.com
Sutter General Hospital	Sacramento	California	916-733-8999	www.suttermedicalcenter.org
Swedish American Hospital	Rockford	Illinois	815-968-4400	www.swedishamerican.org
Swedish Medical Center	Seattle	Washington	206-386-6000	www.swedish.org
Tallahassee Memorial Hospital	Tallahassee	Florida	850-431-1155	www.tmh.org
Texas Health Harris Methodist Hurst - Euless - Bedford	Bedford	Texas	817-848-4000	www.texashealth.org
Thibodaux Regional Medical Center	Thibodaux	Louisiana	985-447-5500	www.thibodaux.com
Trinity Rock Island	Rock Island	Illinois	309-779-5000	www.trinityqc.com
United Regional Health Care System	Wichita Falls	Texas	940-764-3055	www.urhcs.org
University Health Care/University Hospitals & Clinics	Salt Lake City	Utah	801-581-2121	www.healthcare.utah.edu
University Medical Center	Lubbock	Texas	806-775-8200	www.teamumc.org
University of Washington Medical Center	Seattle	Washington	206-598-3300	www.washington.edu/medical/uwmc
Vanderbilt University Hospital	Nashville	Tennessee	615-322-3454	www.mc.vanderbilt.edu
VHS Harlingen Hospital Company	Harlingen	Texas	956-389-1100	www.vbmc.org
Via Christi Hospitals Wichita	Wichita	Kansas	316-268-5000	www.via-christi.org
Virginia Mason Medical Center	Seattle	Washington	206-223-6600	www.vmmc.org
Wakemed - Raleigh Campus	Raleigh	North Carolina	919-350-8000	www.wakemed.org
Washington Hospital	Fremont	California	510-797-1111	www.whhs.com
Wesley Medical Center	Wichita	Kansas	316-962-2000	www.wesleymc.com
Winchester Medical Center	Winchester	Virginia	540-536-8000	www.valleyhealthlink.com
Winter Haven Hospital	Winter Haven	Florida	863-293-1121	www.winterhavenhospital.com
Wyoming Medical Center	Casper	Wyoming	307-577-7201	www.wyomingmedicalcenter.com
Yakima Valley Memorial Hospital	Yakima	Washington	509-575-8000	www.yakimamemorialhospital.org

Note: Table shows hospitals nationwide whose surgical complication rate is better (lower) than U.S. rate of 4.14%

Hospitals whose Surgical Complication Rate is Worse (Higher) than the U.S. National Rate

Measure: Serious Blood Clots After Surgery

Hospital	City	State	Phone	Web Site
Advocate Good Samaritan Hospital	Downers Grove	Illinois	630-275-5900	www.advocatehealth.com/gsam
Advocate Illinois Masonic Medical Center	Chicago	Illinois	773-975-1600	www.advocatehealth.com/immc
Advocate Lutheran General Hospital	Park Ridge	Illinois	847-723-2210	www.advocatehealth.com
Albert Einstein Medical Center	Philadelphia	Pennsylvania	215-456-6090	www.einstein.edu
Alegent Health Mercy Hospital	Council Bluffs	Iowa	712-328-5000	www.alegent.com/mercy
Alexian Brothers Medical Center	Elk Grove Village	Illinois	847-437-5500	www.alexian.org
Aultman Hospital	Canton	Ohio	330-452-9911	www.aultman.com
B R F Hospital Holdings	Shreveport	Louisiana	318-675-5000	www.lsumc.edu
Baptist Memorial Hospital Desoto	Southaven	Mississippi	662-772-4000	www.bmhcc.org/facilities/desoto
Barnes-Jewish Hospital	Saint Louis	Missouri	314-747-3000	www.barnesjewish.org
Beaumont Health System	Grosse Pointe	Michigan	313-343-1000	www.beaumonthospitals.com
Beaumont Health System	Royal Oak	Michigan	248-898-5000	www.beaumonthospitals.com
Bon Secours Saint Francis Medical Center	Midlothian	Virginia	804-594-7400	www.richmond.bonsecours.com
Bridgeport Hospital	Bridgeport	Connecticut	203-384-3000	www.bridgeporthospital.com
Brigham & Women's Hospital	Boston	Massachusetts	617-732-5500	www.brighamandwomens.org
Brookdale Hospital Medical Center	Brooklyn	New York	718-240-5966	www.brookdalehospital.org
Brookwood Medical Center	Birmingham	Alabama	205-877-1000	www.bwmc.com
Cape Coral Hospital	Cape Coral	Florida	239-574-2323	www.leememorial.org
Carilion Roanoke Memorial Hospital	Roanoke	Virginia	540-981-7000	www.carilion.com/crmh
Cedars - Sinai Medical Center	Los Angeles	California	310-423-5000	www.cedars-sinai.edu
Centennial Medical Center	Frisco	Texas	972-963-3333	www.centennialmedcenter.com
Charleston Area Medical Center	Charleston	West Virginia	304-388-6203	www.camc.org
Christian Hospital Northeast - Northwest	Saint Louis	Missouri	314-653-5000	www.christianhospital.org
Christiana Care Health Services	Newark	Delaware	302-733-1000	www.christianacare.org
Christus Saint Frances Cabrini Hospital	Alexandria	Louisiana	318-487-1122	www.cabrini.org
Christus Saint Michael Health System	Texarkana	Texas	903-614-1000	www.christusstmichael.org
Cleveland Clinic	Cleveland	Ohio	216-444-2200	www.clevelandclinic.org
Conemaugh Valley Memorial Hospital	Johnstown	Pennsylvania	814-534-9000	www.conemaugh.org
Coney Island Hospital	Brooklyn	New York	718-616-3000	www.coneyislandhospital.com
Cooper University Hospital	Camden	New Jersey	856-342-2000	www.cooperhealth.org
Crouse Hospital	Syracuse	New York	315-470-7449	www.crouse.org
D C H Regional Medical Center	Tuscaloosa	Alabama	205-759-7111	www.dchsystem.com
Danbury Hospital	Danbury	Connecticut	203-797-7000	www.danburyhospital.com
Delnor Community Hospital	Geneva	Illinois	630-208-3000	www.delnor.com
Doctors Hospital	Augusta	Georgia	706-651-6008	www.doctors-hospital.net
Doctors Hospital	Coral Gables	Florida	305-666-2111	www.baptisthealth.net
Edward Hospital	Naperville	Illinois	630-527-3000	www.edward.org
El Paso Specialty Hospital	El Paso	Texas	915-544-3636	www.elpasospecialtyhospital.com
Emory University Hospital Midtown	Atlanta	Georgia	404-686-4411	www.emoryhealthcare.org
Evanston Hospital	Evanston	Illinois	847-432-8000	www.enh.org
Flagler Hospital	Saint Augustine	Florida	904-819-4426	www.flaglerhospital.com
Florida Hospital	Orlando	Florida	407-303-1976	www.floridahospital.com
Franciscan Saint Margaret Health - Hammond	Hammond	Indiana	219-932-2300	www.smmhc.com
Geisinger Medical Center	Danville	Pennsylvania	570-271-6211	www.geisinger.org
Genesys Regional Medical Center - Health Park	Grand Blanc	Michigan	810-606-5000	www.genesys.org
Glen Cove Hospital	Glen Cove	New York	516-674-7300	www.northshorelij.com
Grady Memorial Hospital	Atlanta	Georgia	404-616-4252	www.gradyhealthsystem.org
Grand View Hospital	Sellersville	Pennsylvania	215-453-4615	www.gvh.org
Gulf Coast Medical Center Lee Memorial Health System	Fort Myers	Florida	239-768-5000	www.leememorial.org
Hackensack University Medical Center	Hackensack	New Jersey	201-996-2000	www.humed.com
Hackettstown Regional Medical Center	Hackettstown	New Jersey	908-852-5100	www.hrmcnj.org
Hahnemann University Hospital	Philadelphia	Pennsylvania	215-762-7000	www.hahnemannhospital.com
Harris Health System	Houston	Texas	713-566-6417	www.hchdonline.com
Hartford Hospital	Hartford	Connecticut	860-545-5000	www.harthosp.org
Henry Ford Hospital	Detroit	Michigan	313-916-2600	www.henryfordhospital.com
Henry Ford West Bloomfield Hospital	W Bloomfield	Michigan	248-325-1000	www.henryford.com
Henry Ford Wyandotte Hospital	Wyandotte	Michigan	734-246-6000	www.henryfordwyandotte.com
Heritage Valley Beaver	Beaver	Pennsylvania	412-728-7000	www.heritagevalley.org
Heritage Valley Sewickley	Sewickley	Pennsylvania	412-741-6600	www.heritagevalley.org
Hillcrest Hospital	Mayfield Heights	Ohio	440-312-4500	www.hillcresthospital.org
Holmes Regional Medical Center	Melbourne	Florida	321-434-7000	www.healthfirst.org
Holy Name Medical Center	Teaneck	New Jersey	201-833-3000	www.holyname.org
Hospital of Univ of Pennsylvania	Philadelphia	Pennsylvania	215-662-3227	www.upenn.edu
Huntington Memorial Hospital	Pasadena	California	626-397-5000	www.huntingtonhospital.com

Hospital	City	State	Phone	Web Site
Hurley Medical Center	Flint	Michigan	810-257-9000	www.hurleymc.com
Ingalls Memorial Hospital	Harvey	Illinois	708-333-2300	www.ingalls.org
Intermountain Medical Center	Murray	Utah	801-507-7000	www.intermountainhealthcare.org
Jackson Memorial Hospital	Miami	Florida	305-585-1111	www.jhsmiami.org
Jeanes Hospital	Philadelphia	Pennsylvania	215-728-2000	www.jeanes.com
JFK Medical Center	Atlantis	Florida	561-965-7300	www.jfkmc.com
JFK Medical Center - A M Yelencsics Comm Hospital	Edison	New Jersey	732-321-7000	www.jfkmc.org
John H Stroger Jr Hospital	Chicago	Illinois	312-864-6000	www.cookcountygov.com
JPS Health Network	Fort Worth	Texas	817-921-3431	www.jpshealthnet.org
Jupiter Medical Center	Jupiter	Florida	561-747-2234	www.jupitermed.com
Lancaster General Hospital	Lancaster	Pennsylvania	717-299-5511	www.lancastergeneral.org
Lee Memorial Hospital	Fort Myers	Florida	239-332-1111	www.leememorial.org
Legacy Emanuel Medical Center	Portland	Oregon	503-413-2200	www.legacyhealth.org
Lehigh Valley Hospital	Allentown	Pennsylvania	610-402-2273	www.lvhhn.org
Lehigh Valley Hospital - Muhlenberg	Bethlehem	Pennsylvania	610-402-2273	www.lvhn.org
Lenox Hill Hospital	New York	New York	212-439-2345	www.lenoxhillhospital.org
Little Company of Mary Hospital	Evergreen Park	Illinois	708-422-6200	www.lcmh.org
Louis A Weiss Memorial Hospital	Chicago	Illinois	773-878-8700	www.weisshospital.org
Lourdes Hospital	Paducah	Kentucky	270-444-2444	www.ehealthconnection.com
Lovelace Medical Center	Albuquerque	New Mexico	505-727-8000	www.lovelace.com
Loyola University Medical Center	Maywood	Illinois	708-216-9000	www.lumc.edu
Magee Womens Hospital of UPMC Health System	Pittsburgh	Pennsylvania	412-641-4010	www.magee.edu
Maimonides Medical Center	Brooklyn	New York	718-283-6000	www.maimonidesmed.org
Marin General Hospital	Greenbrae	California	415-925-7900	www.maringeneral.com
Mary Hitchcock Memorial Hospital	Lebanon	New Hampshire	603-650-5000	www.dhmc.org
Marymount Hospital	Garfield Heights	Ohio	216-581-0500	www.marymount.org
Mclaren Flint	Flint	Michigan	810-342-2000	www.mclaren.org
The Medical Center of Aurora	Aurora	Colorado	303-695-2600	www.auroramed.com
Medical Center of Mckinney	Mckinney	Texas	972-547-8000	www.medicalcenterofmckinney.com
Medical Center of Plano	Plano	Texas	972-596-6800	www.medicalcenterofplano.com
Medstar Georgetown University Hospital	Washington	District of Columbia	202-784-3000	www.georgetownuniversityhospital.org
Memorial Healthcare	Owosso	Michigan	989-723-5211	www.memorialhealthcare.org
Memorial Hermann Texas Medical Center	Houston	Texas	713-704-3700	www.mhhs.org
Memorial Hospital Jacksonville	Jacksonville	Florida	904-399-6111	www.memorialhospitaljax.com
Memorial Medical Center	Las Cruces	New Mexico	575-522-8641	www.mmclc.org
Menorah Medical Center	Overland Park	Kansas	913-498-6773	www.menorahmedicalcenter.com
Mercy Fitzgerald Hospital	Darby	Pennsylvania	215-237-4000	www.mercyhealth.org
Mercy Hospital Springfield	Springfield	Missouri	417-820-2000	www.stjohns.com
Mercy Saint Vincent Medical Center	Toledo	Ohio	419-251-3232	www.mhsnr.org
Miami Valley Hospital	Dayton	Ohio	937-208-8000	www.miamivalleyhospital.com
Midwest Orthopedic Specialty Hospital	Franklin	Wisconsin	414-817-5800	www.mymosh.com
Milton S Hershey Medical Center	Hershey	Pennsylvania	717-531-8521	www.hmc.psu.edu
Ministry Saint Josephs Hospital	Marshfield	Wisconsin	715-387-7850	www.stjosephs-marshfield.org
Mobile Infirmary	Mobile	Alabama	251-435-4700	www.mimc.com
Montefiore Medical Center	Bronx	New York	718-920-4321	www.montefiore.org
Morristown Medical Center	Morristown	New Jersey	973-971-5450	www.morristownmemorialhospital.org
Naples Community Hospital	Naples	Florida	239-436-5000	www.nchmd.org
Nason Hospital	Roaring Spring	Pennsylvania	814-224-2141	www.nasonhospital.com
Nathan Littauer Hospital	Gloversville	New York	518-725-8621	www.nlh.org
Newark Beth Israel Medical Center	Newark	New Jersey	973-926-7850	www.sbhcs.com
North Shore University Hospital	Manhasset	New York	516-562-0100	www.northshorelij.com
North Suburban Medical Center	Thornton	Colorado	303-451-7800	www.northsuburban.com
Northside Hospital	Atlanta	Georgia	404-851-8000	www.northside.com
Northwestern Memorial Hospital	Chicago	Illinois	312-926-2000	www.nmh.org
Novant Health Rowan Medical Center	Salisbury	North Carolina	704-210-5000	www.rowan.org
NYU Hospitals Center	New York	New York	212-263-7300	www.med.nyu.edu
O U Medical Center	Oklahoma City	Oklahoma	405-271-5911	www.oumedcenter.com
Oakwood Hospital - Southshore	Trenton	Michigan	734-671-3800	www.oakwood.org/oakwood-hospital-southshore
Och Regional Medical Center	Starkville	Mississippi	662-323-4320	www.och.org
OHSU Hospital & Clinics	Portland	Oregon	503-494-4036	www.ohsu.edu
Orlando Health	Orlando	Florida	321-841-5111	www.orlandoregionalmedicalcenter.org
Our Lady of the Lake Regional Medical Center	Baton Rouge	Louisiana	225-765-6565	www.ololrmc.com
Overlook Medical Center	Summit	New Jersey	908-522-2000	www.atlantichealth.org
Owensboro Health Regional Hospital	Owensboro	Kentucky	270-688-2000	www.omhs.org
Palmetto General Hospital	Hialeah	Florida	305-823-5000	www.palmettogeneral.com
Parkland Health & Hospital System	Dallas	Texas	214-590-8000	www.parklandhospital.com
Pennsylvania Hospital of the Univ of PA Health Sys	Philadelphia	Pennsylvania	215-829-3000	www.pennmedicine.org/pahosp
Piedmont Hospital	Atlanta	Georgia	404-605-5000	www.piedmonthospital.org

Hospital	City	State	Phone	Web Site
Pinnacle Health Hospitals	Harrisburg	Pennsylvania	717-782-5181	www.pinnaclehealth.org
Plainview Hospital	Plainview	New York	516-719-3000	www.nslij.com
Pratt Regional Medical Center	Pratt	Kansas	620-450-1160	www.prmc.org
Proctor Hospital	Peoria	Illinois	309-691-1000	www.proctor.org
Providence Hospital & Medical Centers	Southfield	Michigan	248-849-3011	www.stjohn.org/providence
Providence Memorial Hospital	El Paso	Texas	915-577-6011	www.sphn.com
Raleigh General Hospital	Beckley	West Virginia	304-256-4100	www.raleighgeneral.com
Regional Medical Center at Memphis	Memphis	Tennessee	901-545-7928	www.the-med.org
Riddle Memorial Hospital	Media	Pennsylvania	610-566-9400	www.riddlehospital.org
Robert Wood Johnson University Hospital	New Brunswick	New Jersey	732-937-8900	www.rwjuh.edu
Rose Medical Center	Denver	Colorado	303-320-2121	www.rosemed.com
Saint Barnabas Medical Center	Livingston	New Jersey	973-322-5000	www.saintbarnabas.com
Saint Peter's University Hospital	New Brunswick	New Jersey	732-745-8600	www.saintpetersuh.com
Saratoga Hospital	Saratoga Springs	New York	518-587-3222	www.saratogacare.org
Scripps Memorial Hospital La Jolla	La Jolla	California	858-626-4123	www.scrippshealth.org
Scripps Mercy Hospital	San Diego	California	619-294-8111	www.scrippshealth.org
Sentara Norfolk General Hospital	Norfolk	Virginia	757-388-3000	www.sentara.com
Sharp Memorial Hospital	San Diego	California	858-939-3400	www.sharp.com/memorial
Sierra Medical Center	El Paso	Texas	915-747-4000	www.sphn.com
Sinai - Grace Hospital	Detroit	Michigan	313-966-3300	www.sinaigrace.org
Somerset Medical Center	Somerville	New Jersey	908-685-2200	www.somersetmedicalcenter.com
South Lake Hospital	Clermont	Florida	352-394-4071	www.southlakehospital.com
Saint Alphonsus Regional Medical Center	Boise	Idaho	208-367-2121	www.saintalphonsus.org
Saint Anthonys Memorial Hospital	Effingham	Illinois	217-342-2121	www.stanthonyshospital.org
Saint Catherine of Siena Hospital	Smithtown	New York	631-862-3000	www.stcatherines.chsli.org
Saint Clare Hospital	Lakewood	Washington	253-588-1711	www.fhshealth.org
Saint Elizabeth Hospital	Belleville	Illinois	618-234-2120	www.steliz.org
Saint John's Episcopal Hospital at South Shore	Far Rockaway	New York	718-869-7000	www.ehs.org
Saint Joseph Hospital	Nashua	New Hampshire	603-882-3000	www.stjosephhospital.com
Saint Joseph Medical Center	Tacoma	Washington	253-627-4101	www.fhshealth.org
Saint Louis University Hospital	Saint Louis	Missouri	314-577-8000	www.slucare.edu/clinical
Saint Luke's Hospital Bethlehem	Bethlehem	Pennsylvania	610-954-4000	www.slhn-lehighvalley.org
Saint Luke's Roosevelt Hospital	New York	New York	212-523-4000	www.wehealny.org
Saint Luke's Warren Hospital	Phillipsburg	New Jersey	908-859-6700	www.warrenhospital.org
Saint Luke's Episcopal Hospital	Houston	Texas	832-355-1000	www.sleh.com
Saint Luke's Hospital	Chesterfield	Missouri	314-434-1500	www.goodhealthmatters.com
Saint Mary's Medical Center	West Palm Beach	Florida	561-840-6202	www.stmarysmc.com
Saint Mary's of Michigan Medical Center	Saginaw	Michigan	989-776-8000	www.stmarysofmichigan.org
Saint Vincent Hospital	Worcester	Massachusetts	508-363-5000	www.stvincenthospital.com
Staten Island University Hospital	Staten Island	New York	718-226-9000	www.siuh.edu
Summa Health Systems Hospitals	Akron	Ohio	330-375-3000	www.summahealth.org
Swedish Medical Center	Englewood	Colorado	303-788-5000	www.swedishhospital.com/default.asp
Tampa General Hospital	Tampa	Florida	813-844-7000	www.tgh.org
Temple University Hospital	Philadelphia	Pennsylvania	215-707-2000	www.tuh.templehealth.org
Carle Foundation Hospital	Urbana	Illinois	217-383-3311	www.carle.com
The University of Chicago Medical Center	Chicago	Illinois	773-702-1000	www.uchospitals.edu
Thomas Jefferson University Hospital	Philadelphia	Pennsylvania	215-955-6000	www.jeffersonhospital.org
Tri - City Medical Center	Oceanside	California	760-724-8411	www.tricitymed.org
Tucson Medical Center	Tucson	Arizona	520-327-5461	www.tmcaz.com
University Hospital	Augusta	Georgia	706-722-9011	www.universityhealth.org
University Hospital	Newark	New Jersey	973-972-5658	www.theuniversityhospital.com
University Hospital - Stony Brook	Stony Brook	New York	631-444-4000	www.stonybrookmedicalcenter.org
University Hospital SUNY Health Science Center	Syracuse	New York	315-473-4240	www.upstate.edu
University of California Davis Medical Center	Sacramento	California	916-734-2011	www.ucdmc.ucdavis.edu
University of Cincinnati Medical Center	Cincinnati	Ohio	513-584-1000	www.universityhospitalcincinnati.com
University of Illinois Hospital	Chicago	Illinois	312-996-3900	www.uic.edu
University of Miami Hospital	Miami	Florida	305-325-5511	www.cedarsmedicalcenter.com
University of Mississippi Medical Center	Jackson	Mississippi	601-984-4100	www.umc.edu
University of North Carolina Hospital	Chapel Hill	North Carolina	919-966-4131	www.unchealthcare.org
University of Tn Memorial Hospital	Knoxville	Tennessee	865-544-9000	www.utmedicalcenter.org
University of Toledo Medical Center	Toledo	Ohio	419-383-3407	www.utmc.utoledo.edu
University of Virginia Medical Center	Charlottesville	Virginia	800-251-3627	www.uvahealth.com
UPMC Presbyterian Shadyside	Pittsburgh	Pennsylvania	412-647-8788	www.upmc.edu
Valley Hospital	Ridgewood	New Jersey	201-447-8000	www.valleyhealth.com
Westchester Medical Center	Valhalla	New York	914-285-7017	www.wcmc.com
Wyckoff Heights Medical Center	Brooklyn	New York	718-963-7272	www.wyckoffhospital.org
Yale-New Haven Hospital	New Haven	Connecticut	203-688-4242	www.ynhh.org

Note: Table shows hospitals nationwide whose surgical complication rate is worse (higher) than U.S. rate of 4.14%

Hospitals whose Surgical Complication Rate is Better (Lower) than the U.S. National Rate

Measure: Serious Complications

Hospital	City	State	Phone	Web Site
Advocate Christ Hospital & Medical Center	Oak Lawn	Illinois	708-684-8000	www.advocatehealth.com
Allegiance Health	Jackson	Michigan	517-788-4800	www.footehealth.org
Anmed Health	Anderson	South Carolina	864-261-1109	www.anmed.com
Arkansas Heart Hospital	Little Rock	Arkansas	501-219-7000	www.arheart.com
Asante Rogue Regional Medical Center	Medford	Oregon	541-789-7000	www.asante.org
Atlanticare Regional Medical Center	Atlantic City	New Jersey	609-441-8020	www.atlanticare.org/acmc/index.html
Avera Mckennan Hospital & University Health Center	Sioux Falls	South Dakota	605-322-8000	www.mckennan.org
Baptist Beaumont Hospital	Beaumont	Texas	409-212-5012	www.mhbh.org
Baptist Health Lexington	Lexington	Kentucky	859-260-6104	www.centralbap.com
Baptist Health Louisville	Louisville	Kentucky	502-897-8100	www.baptisteast.com
Baystate Medical Center	Springfield	Massachusetts	413-794-0000	www.baystatehealth.com
Bethesda Hospital East	Boynton Beach	Florida	561-737-7733	www.bethesdahealthcare.com
Bethesda North	Cincinnati	Ohio	513-865-1241	www.trihealth.com
Billings Clinic Hospital	Billings	Montana	406-657-4000	www.billingsclinic.com
Carolina East Medical Center	New Bern	North Carolina	252-633-8640	www.cravenhealthcare.org
Carson Tahoe Regional Medical Center	Carson City	Nevada	775-445-8000	www.carsontahoehospital.com
Centinela Hospital Medical Center	Inglewood	California	310-673-4660	www.centinelafreeman.com
Central Dupage Hospital	Winfield	Illinois	630-682-1600	www.cdh.org
Christus Hospital	Beaumont	Texas	409-892-7171	www.christushealth.org
Christus Spohn Hospital Corpus Christi	Corpus Christi	Texas	361-902-4103	www.christusspohn.org
Community Hospital	Munster	Indiana	219-836-1600	www.comhs.org/community
Community Medical Center	Toms River	New Jersey	732-557-8000	www.sbhcs.com
Conway Regional Medical Center	Conway	Arkansas	501-329-3831	www.conwayregional.org
Cox Medical Center	Springfield	Missouri	417-269-6000	www.coxhealth.com
Delray Medical Center	Delray Beach	Florida	561-498-4440	www.delraymedicalctr.com
Duke University Hospital	Durham	North Carolina	919-684-8111	www.dukehealth.org
East Texas Medical Center	Tyler	Texas	903-597-0351	www.etmc.org
Englewood Hospital & Medical Center	Englewood	New Jersey	201-894-3000	www.englewoodhospital.com
Exeter Hospital	Exeter	New Hampshire	603-778-7311	www.exeterhospital.com
Floyd Medical Center	Rome	Georgia	706-509-6900	www.floydmed.org
Floyd Memorial Hospital & Health Services	New Albany	Indiana	812-949-5500	www.floydmedical.org
Genesis Medical Center - Davenport	Davenport	Iowa	563-421-1000	www.genesishealth.com
Glens Falls Hospital	Glens Falls	New York	518-926-1000	www.glensfallshospital.org
Heartland Regional Medical Center	Saint Joseph	Missouri	816-271-6000	www.heartland-health.com
Holy Cross Hospital	Fort Lauderdale	Florida	954-771-8000	www.holy-cross.com
Indiana University Health	Indianapolis	Indiana	317-962-5900	www.iuhealth.org
Indiana University Health Arnett Hospital	Lafayette	Indiana	765-448-8000	www.iuhealth.org/arnett
Integris Baptist Medical Center	Oklahoma City	Oklahoma	405-951-8110	www.integris-health.com
Integris Southwest Medical Center	Oklahoma City	Oklahoma	405-636-7000	www.integris-health.com
Jackson - Madison County General Hospital	Jackson	Tennessee	731-541-5000	www.wth.org
John Muir Medical Center - Concord Campus	Concord	California	925-674-2002	www.johnmuirhealth.com
Lakeland Hospital - Saint Joseph	Saint Joseph	Michigan	269-983-8300	www.lakelandhealth.org
Laredo Medical Center	Laredo	Texas	956-796-5000	www.laredomedical.com
Lehigh Valley Hospital - Hazleton	Hazleton	Pennsylvania	570-501-4000	www.ghha.org
Marietta Memorial Hospital	Marietta	Ohio	740-374-1400	www.mmhospital.org
Mary Washington Hospital	Fredericksburg	Virginia	540-741-1100	www.medicorp.org
Mayo Clinic	Jacksonville	Florida	904-953-2000	www.mayoclinic.org/jacksonville
Mayo Clinic Hospital	Phoenix	Arizona	480-342-2000	www.mayoclinic.org
Mayo Clinic Methodist- Hospital	Rochester	Minnesota	507-266-7890	www.mayoclinic.org/methodisthospital
Mclaren Bay Region	Bay City	Michigan	989-894-3000	www.baymed.org
Mcleod Regional Medical Center - Pee Dee	Florence	South Carolina	843-777-2900	www.mcleodhealth.org
Medcentral Health System Mansfield Hospital	Mansfield	Ohio	419-526-8000	www.medcentral.org
Memorial Healthcare System	Chattanooga	Tennessee	423-495-2525	www.memorial.org
Memorial Hermann Hospital System	Houston	Texas	713-448-6796	www.memorialhermann.org
Memorial Mission Hospital & Asheville Surgery Center	Asheville	North Carolina	828-213-1111	www.missionhospitals.org
Mercy Medical Center - Cedar Rapids	Cedar Rapids	Iowa	319-398-6011	www.mercycare.org
Methodist Hospital	San Antonio	Texas	210-575-4000	www.mh.sahealth.com
Methodist Medical Center of Illinois	Peoria	Illinois	309-672-5522	www.mmci.org
Methodist Willowbrook Hospital	Houston	Texas	281-477-1000	www.houstonmethodist.org/willowbrook-hospital
Metrowest Medical Center	Framingham	Massachusetts	508-383-1000	www.mwmc.com
Mississippi Baptist Medical Center	Jackson	Mississippi	601-968-1000	www.mbmc.org
Monongalia County General Hospital	Morgantown	West Virginia	304-598-1200	www.mongeneral.com
Mother Frances Hospital	Tyler	Texas	903-593-8441	www.tmfhs.org
Munroe Regional Medical Center	Ocala	Florida	352-351-7200	www.munroeregional.com

Hospital	City	State	Phone	Web Site
Munson Medical Center	Traverse City	Michigan	231-935-5000	www.munsonhealthcare.org
Nebraska Heart Hospital	Lincoln	Nebraska	402-328-3000	www.neheart.com
New York Community Hospital of Brooklyn	Brooklyn	New York	718-692-5302	www.nych.com
North Mississippi Medical Center	Tupelo	Mississippi	662-377-3000	www.nmhs.net/nmmc
Oklahoma Heart Hospital	Oklahoma City	Oklahoma	405-608-3200	www.okheart.com
Our Lady of Lourdes Medical Center	Camden	New Jersey	856-757-3500	www.lourdesnet.org
Palos Community Hospital	Palos Heights	Illinois	708-923-4000	www.paloshospital.org
Parkview Regional Medical Center	Fort Wayne	Indiana	260-266-1000	www.parkview.com
Parkwest Medical Center	Knoxville	Tennessee	865-970-9800	www.yesparkwest.com
Pomona Valley Hospital Medical Center	Pomona	California	909-865-9500	www.pvhmc.com
Presence Saint Joseph Medical Center	Joliet	Illinois	815-725-7133	www.provena.org/stjoes
Providence Little Co of Mary Medical Center Torrance	Torrance	California	310-540-7676	www.lcmhs.org
Providence Saint Joseph Medical Center	Burbank	California	818-843-5111	www.providence.org/losangeles
Redmond Regional Medical Center	Rome	Georgia	706-802-3012	www.redmondregional.com
Regional Medical Center Bayonet Point	Hudson	Florida	727-819-2929	www.mchealth.comorwww.heartoftampa.com
Roper Hospital	Charleston	South Carolina	843-724-2800	www.ropersaintfrancis.com
Saint Thomas West Hospital	Nashville	Tennessee	615-222-2111	www.stthomas.org
Sentara Careplex Hospital	Hampton	Virginia	757-736-1000	www.sentara.com
Sentara Leigh Hospital	Norfolk	Virginia	757-261-6601	www.sentara.com
Shasta Regional Medical Center	Redding	California	530-244-5454	www.shastaregional.com
Southcoast Hospital Group	Fall River	Massachusetts	508-679-3131	www.southcoast.org/charlton
Saint Elizabeth Medical Center	Lakeside Park	Kentucky	859-292-2000	www.stelizabeth.com
Saint Francis Hospital	Columbus	Georgia	706-596-4020	www.wecareforlife.com
Saint Francis Hospital - Roslyn	Roslyn	New York	516-562-6000	www.stfrancisheartcenter.com
Saint Luke's Hospital	Cedar Rapids	Iowa	319-369-7211	www.crstlukes.com
Saint Mary Medical Center	Langhorne	Pennsylvania	215-750-2003	www.stmaryhealthcare.org
Saint Mary Mercy Hospital	Livonia	Michigan	734-655-4800	www.stmarymercy.org
Saint Vincent Heart Center of Indiana	Indianapolis	Indiana	317-583-5000	www.theheartcenter.com
Saint Vincent Hospital & Health Services	Indianapolis	Indiana	317-338-7000	www.indianapolis.stvincent.org
Saint Vincent's Medical Center	Jacksonville	Florida	904-308-7300	www.jaxhealth.com
Sutter General Hospital	Sacramento	California	916-733-8999	www.suttermedicalcenter.org
Texas Health Harris Methodist Hurst - Euless - Bedford	Bedford	Texas	817-848-4000	www.texashealth.org
Thibodaux Regional Medical Center	Thibodaux	Louisiana	985-447-5500	www.thibodaux.com
Tuomey Healthcare System	Sumter	South Carolina	803-774-8900	www.tuomey.com
United Hospital Center	Bridgeport	West Virginia	681-342-1000	www.uhcwv.org
University Hospitals - Elyria Medical Center	Elyria	Ohio	440-329-7500	www.emh-healthcare.org
University of Michigan Health System	Ann Arbor	Michigan	734-764-1505	www.med.umich.edu
UPMC Altoona	Altoona	Pennsylvania	814-889-2011	www.altoonaregional.org
Vanderbilt University Hospital	Nashville	Tennessee	615-322-3454	www.mc.vanderbilt.edu
Virtua West Jersey Hospitals Berlin	Berlin	New Jersey	856-322-3200	www.virtua.org
Washington Hospital	Fremont	California	510-797-1111	www.whhs.com
Williamsport Regional Medical Center	Williamsport	Pennsylvania	570-321-1000	www.susquehannahealth.org
Willis Knighton Bossier Health Center	Bossier City	Louisiana	318-212-7000	www.wkhs.com/locations/bossier.aspx
Winchester Medical Center	Winchester	Virginia	540-536-8000	www.valleyhealthlink.com

Note: Table shows hospitals nationwide whose surgical complication rate is better (lower) than U.S. rate of 0.61%

Hospitals whose Surgical Complication Rate is Worse (Higher) than the U.S. National Rate

Measure: Serious Complications

Hospital	City	State	Phone	Web Site
Adirondack Medical Center	Saranac Lake	New York	518-891-4141	www.amccares.org
Appleton Medical Center	Appleton	Wisconsin	920-731-4101	www.thedacare.org
Aurora Medical Center Kenosha	Kenosha	Wisconsin	262-948-5600	www.aurorahealthcare.org
B R F Hospital Holdings	Shreveport	Louisiana	318-675-5000	www.lsumc.edu
Baptist Memorial Hospital Desoto	Southaven	Mississippi	662-772-4000	www.bmhcc.org/facilities/desoto
Baptist Saint Anthony's Hospital	Amarillo	Texas	806-212-2000	www.bsahs.com
Barnes-Jewish Hospital	Saint Louis	Missouri	314-747-3000	www.barnesjewish.org
Baylor University Medical Center	Dallas	Texas	214-820-0111	www.baylorhealth.com
Beaumont Health System	Royal Oak	Michigan	248-898-5000	www.beaumonthospitals.com
Beth Israel Deaconess Medical Center	Boston	Massachusetts	617-667-7000	www.bidmc.harvard.edu
Blessing Hospital	Quincy	Illinois	217-223-5811	www.blessinghealthsystem.org
Boston Medical Center Corporation	Boston	Massachusetts	617-638-8000	www.bmc.org
Bridgeport Hospital	Bridgeport	Connecticut	203-384-3000	www.bridgeporthospital.com
Brigham & Women's Hospital	Boston	Massachusetts	617-732-5500	www.brighamandwomens.org
Cape Coral Hospital	Cape Coral	Florida	239-574-2323	www.leememorial.org
Carilion Roanoke Memorial Hospital	Roanoke	Virginia	540-981-7000	www.carilion.com/crmh
Centennial Medical Center	Frisco	Texas	972-963-3333	www.centennialmedcenter.com
Central Texas Medical Center	San Marcos	Texas	512-753-3690	www.ctmc.org
Charleston Area Medical Center	Charleston	West Virginia	304-388-6203	www.camc.org
Chilton Medical Center	Pompton Plains	New Jersey	973-831-5000	www.chiltonmemorial.org
Christus Saint Frances Cabrini Hospital	Alexandria	Louisiana	318-487-1122	www.cabrini.org
Clearview Regional Medical Center	Monroe	Georgia	770-267-1792	www.clearviewregionalmedicalcenter.com
Cleveland Clinic	Cleveland	Ohio	216-444-2200	www.clevelandclinic.org
Clovis Community Medical Center	Clovis	California	559-324-4000	www.communitymedical.org
Community Regional Medical Center	Fresno	California	559-459-6000	www.communitymedical.org
Conemaugh Valley Memorial Hospital	Johnstown	Pennsylvania	814-534-9000	www.conemaugh.org
Cooper University Hospital	Camden	New Jersey	856-342-2000	www.cooperhealth.org
Crouse Hospital	Syracuse	New York	315-470-7449	www.crouse.org
Dameron Hospital	Stockton	California	209-944-5550	www.dameronhospital.org
Deaconess Hospital	Spokane	Washington	509-473-5800	www.deaconessmedicalcenter.org
Emory University Hospital Midtown	Atlanta	Georgia	404-686-4411	www.emoryhealthcare.org
Evanston Hospital	Evanston	Illinois	847-432-8000	www.enh.org
Firsthealth Moore Regional Hospital	Pinehurst	North Carolina	910-715-1000	www.firsthealth.org
Geisinger Medical Center	Danville	Pennsylvania	570-271-6211	www.geisinger.org
Geisinger Wyoming Valley Medical Center	Wilkes Barre	Pennsylvania	570-826-7300	www.geisinger.org
Genesys Regional Medical Center - Health Park	Grand Blanc	Michigan	810-606-5000	www.genesys.org
Gila Regional Medical Center	Silver City	New Mexico	575-538-4000	www.grmc.org
Good Samaritan Hospital	San Jose	California	408-559-2011	www.goodsamsj.org
Good Shepherd Medical Center Marshall	Marshall	Texas	903-927-6712	www.marshallregional.org
Grady Memorial Hospital	Atlanta	Georgia	404-616-4252	www.gradyhealthsystem.org
Grand View Hospital	Sellersville	Pennsylvania	215-453-4615	www.gvh.org
Grossmont Hospital	La Mesa	California	619-465-0711	www.sharp.com
Gulf Coast Medical Center Lee Memorial Health System	Fort Myers	Florida	239-768-5000	www.leememorial.org
Hackettstown Regional Medical Center	Hackettstown	New Jersey	908-852-5100	www.hrmcnj.org
Hahnemann University Hospital	Philadelphia	Pennsylvania	215-762-7000	www.hahnemannhospital.com
Harborview Medical Center	Seattle	Washington	206-731-3000	www.harborview.org
Hartford Hospital	Hartford	Connecticut	860-545-5000	www.harthosp.org
Hennepin County Medical Center	Minneapolis	Minnesota	612-873-3000	www.hcmc.org
Henry Ford Hospital	Detroit	Michigan	313-916-2600	www.henryfordhospital.com
Henry Ford West Bloomfield Hospital	W Bloomfield	Michigan	248-325-1000	www.henryford.com
Heritage Valley Beaver	Beaver	Pennsylvania	412-728-7000	www.heritagevalley.org
Holy Cross Hospital	Taos	New Mexico	575-758-8883	www.taoshospital.org
Hospital of Univ of Pennsylvania	Philadelphia	Pennsylvania	215-662-3227	www.upenn.edu
Huntington Memorial Hospital	Pasadena	California	626-397-5000	www.huntingtonhospital.com
Inova Fairfax Hospital	Falls Church	Virginia	703-776-3332	www.inova.org
Inspira Medical Center Vineland	Vineland	New Jersey	856-641-6610	www.sjhs.com
Intermountain Medical Center	Murray	Utah	801-507-7000	www.intermountainhealthcare.org
Jackson Memorial Hospital	Miami	Florida	305-585-1111	www.jhsmiami.org
JFK Medical Center - A M Yelencsics Comm Hospital	Edison	New Jersey	732-321-7000	www.jfkmc.org
John Dempsey Hospital	Farmington	Connecticut	860-679-1145	www.uconnhealth.orgorwww.uchc.edu
JPS Health Network	Fort Worth	Texas	817-921-3431	www.jpshealthnet.org
Kaweah Delta Medical Center	Visalia	California	559-624-2000	www.kaweahdelta.org
Keck Hospital of USC	Los Angeles	California	323-442-8656	www.uscuh.com
Lancaster General Hospital	Lancaster	Pennsylvania	717-299-5511	www.lancastergeneral.org

Hospital	City	State	Phone	Web Site
LDS Hospital	Salt Lake City	Utah	801-408-1100	www.intermountainhealthcare.org
Lee Memorial Hospital	Fort Myers	Florida	239-332-1111	www.leememorial.org
Lenox Hill Hospital	New York	New York	212-439-2345	www.lenoxhillhospital.org
Lourdes Hospital	Paducah	Kentucky	270-444-2444	www.ehealthconnection.com
Lower Keys Medical Center	Key West	Florida	305-294-5531	www.lkmc.com
Loyola University Medical Center	Maywood	Illinois	708-216-9000	www.lumc.edu
Magee Womens Hospital of UPMC Health System	Pittsburgh	Pennsylvania	412-641-4010	www.magee.edu
Maine Medical Center	Portland	Maine	207-662-0111	www.mmc.org
Marin General Hospital	Greenbrae	California	415-925-7900	www.maringeneral.com
Mary Hitchcock Memorial Hospital	Lebanon	New Hampshire	603-650-5000	www.dhmc.org
Mayo Clinic Health System - Mankato	Mankato	Minnesota	507-625-4031	www.isj-mhs.org
McKay Dee Hospital	Ogden	Utah	801-387-2800	www.intermountainhealthcare.org
The Medical Center of Aurora	Aurora	Colorado	303-695-2600	www.auroramed.com
Medical Center of Plano	Plano	Texas	972-596-6800	www.medicalcenterofplano.com
Medical College of Virginia Hospitals	Richmond	Virginia	804-828-0938	www.vcuhealth.org
Medical West	Bessemer	Alabama	205-481-7000	www.uab.edu
Medstar Georgetown University Hospital	Washington	District of Columbia	202-784-3000	www.georgetownuniversityhospital.org
Medstar Washington Hospital Center	Washington	District of Columbia	202-877-7000	www.whcenter.org
Memorial Medical Center	Modesto	California	209-526-4500	www.memorialmedicalcenter.org
Memorial Hospital Jacksonville	Jacksonville	Florida	904-399-6111	www.memorialhospitaljax.com
Memorial Medical Center	Springfield	Illinois	217-788-3000	www.memorialmedical.com
Menorah Medical Center	Overland Park	Kansas	913-498-6773	www.menorahmedicalcenter.com
Mercy Hospital - Cadillac	Cadillac	Michigan	231-876-7200	www.mercycadillac.munsonhealthcare.org
Mercy Memorial Health Center	Ardmore	Oklahoma	405-223-5400	www.mercyok.com/mmhc
Mercy Saint Vincent Medical Center	Toledo	Ohio	419-251-3232	www.mhsnr.org
Metrohealth System	Cleveland	Ohio	216-778-7089	www.metrohealth.org
Miami Valley Hospital	Dayton	Ohio	937-208-8000	www.miamivalleyhospital.com
Milton S Hershey Medical Center	Hershey	Pennsylvania	717-531-8521	www.hmc.psu.edu
Ministry Saint Josephs Hospital	Marshfield	Wisconsin	715-387-7850	www.stjosephs-marshfield.org
Montefiore Medical Center	Bronx	New York	718-920-4321	www.montefiore.org
Newark Beth Israel Medical Center	Newark	New Jersey	973-926-7850	www.sbhcs.com
North Shore University Hospital	Manhasset	New York	516-562-0100	www.northshorelij.com
North Suburban Medical Center	Thornton	Colorado	303-451-7800	www.northsuburban.com
Novant Health Presbyterian Medical Center	Charlotte	North Carolina	704-384-4000	www.presbyterian.org
NYU Hospitals Center	New York	New York	212-263-7300	www.med.nyu.edu
O U Medical Center	Oklahoma City	Oklahoma	405-271-5911	www.oumedcenter.com
OHSU Hospital & Clinics	Portland	Oregon	503-494-4036	www.ohsu.edu
Our Lady of the Lake Regional Medical Center	Baton Rouge	Louisiana	225-765-6565	www.ololrmc.com
Overland Park Regional Medical Center	Overland Park	Kansas	913-541-5301	www.oprmc.com
Parkland Health & Hospital System	Dallas	Texas	214-590-8000	www.parklandhospital.com
Parkview Medical Center	Pueblo	Colorado	719-584-4000	www.parkviewmc.com
Piedmont Hospital	Atlanta	Georgia	404-605-5000	www.piedmonthospital.org
Pinnacle Health Hospitals	Harrisburg	Pennsylvania	717-782-5181	www.pinnaclehealth.org
Plainview Hospital	Plainview	New York	516-719-3000	www.nslij.com
Providence Holy Cross Medical Center	Mission Hills	California	818-365-8051	www.providence.org
Providence Sacred Heart Medical Center	Spokane	Washington	509-474-3040	www.shmc.org
Rhode Island Hospital	Providence	Rhode Island	401-444-4000	www.rhodeislandhospital.org
Ridgeview Medical Center	Waconia	Minnesota	952-442-2191	www.ridgeviewmedical.org
Robert Wood Johnson University Hospital	New Brunswick	New Jersey	732-937-8900	www.rwjuh.edu
Ronald Reagan UCLA Medical Center	Los Angeles	California	310-825-6301	www.uclahealth.org
Rose Medical Center	Denver	Colorado	303-320-2121	www.rosemed.com
Rush University Medical Center	Chicago	Illinois	312-942-5000	www.ruch.edu
Sacred Heart Hospital	Eau Claire	Wisconsin	715-717-4121	www.sacredhearteauclaire.org
Saint Anthony Medical Center	Rockford	Illinois	815-226-2000	www.osfhealth.com
Saint Barnabas Medical Center	Livingston	New Jersey	973-322-5000	www.saintbarnabas.com
Saint Francis Medical Center	Peoria	Illinois	309-655-2000	www.osfsaintfrancis.org
Saint Mary's Health Care	Grand Rapids	Michigan	616-685-5000	www.smhealthcare.org
Santa Clara Valley Medical Center	San Jose	California	408-885-5000	www.sccgov.org
Saratoga Hospital	Saratoga Springs	New York	518-587-3222	www.saratogacare.org
Sentara Norfolk General Hospital	Norfolk	Virginia	757-388-3000	www.sentara.com
Sharp Memorial Hospital	San Diego	California	858-939-3400	www.sharp.com/memorial
Sierra Medical Center	El Paso	Texas	915-747-4000	www.sphn.com
Sinai - Grace Hospital	Detroit	Michigan	313-966-3300	www.sinaigrace.org
Somerset Medical Center	Somerville	New Jersey	908-685-2200	www.somersetmedicalcenter.com
Springhill Medical Center	Mobile	Alabama	251-344-9630	www.springhillmedicalcenter.com
Saint Alphonsus Regional Medical Center	Boise	Idaho	208-367-2121	www.saintalphonsus.org
Saint Clare Hospital	Lakewood	Washington	253-588-1711	www.fhshealth.org

Hospital	City	State	Phone	Web Site
Saint Elizabeth Health Center	Youngstown	Ohio	330-746-7211	www.hmhs.org
Saint Joseph Medical Center	Tacoma	Washington	253-627-4101	www.fhshealth.org
Saint Joseph Mercy Hospital	Ann Arbor	Michigan	734-712-3791	www.stjoesannarbor.or
Saint Joseph's Hospital & Medical Center	Phoenix	Arizona	602-406-3000	www.stjosephs-phx.org
Saint Louis University Hospital	Saint Louis	Missouri	314-577-8000	www.slucare.edu/clinical
Saint Luke's Hospital Bethlehem	Bethlehem	Pennsylvania	610-954-4000	www.slhn-lehighvalley.org
Saint Luke's Episcopal Hospital	Houston	Texas	832-355-1000	www.sleh.com
Saint Luke's Hospital	Chesterfield	Missouri	314-434-1500	www.goodhealthmatters.com
Saint Luke's Hospital of Kansas City	Kansas City	Missouri	816-932-2000	www.staintlukeshealthsystem.org
Stamford Hospital	Stamford	Connecticut	203-276-1000	www.stamhealth.org
Summa Health Systems Hospitals	Akron	Ohio	330-375-3000	www.summahealth.org
Sunrise Hospital & Medical Center	Las Vegas	Nevada	702-731-8000	www.sunrisehospital.com
Swedish Medical Center	Englewood	Colorado	303-788-5000	www.swedishhospital.com/default.asp
Swedish Medical Center - Cherry Hill	Seattle	Washington	206-320-2000	www.swedish.org
Tampa General Hospital	Tampa	Florida	813-844-7000	www.tgh.org
The University of Chicago Medical Center	Chicago	Illinois	773-702-1000	www.uchospitals.edu
Theda Clark Medical Center	Neenah	Wisconsin	920-729-3100	www.thedacare.org
Thomas Hospital	Fairhope	Alabama	251-928-2375	www.thomashospital.com
Thomas Jefferson University Hospital	Philadelphia	Pennsylvania	215-955-6000	www.jeffersonhospital.org
Trinity Hospitals	Minot	North Dakota	701-857-5000	www.trinityhealth.org
Trinity Medical Center	Birmingham	Alabama	205-592-1000	www.bhsala.com/montclair
Tucson Medical Center	Tucson	Arizona	520-327-5461	www.tmcaz.com
Tulane Medical Center	New Orleans	Louisiana	504-988-1900	www.tuhc.com
UF Health Jacksonville	Jacksonville	Florida	904-244-0411	www.shandsjacksonville.org
UMC of Southern Nevada	Las Vegas	Nevada	702-383-2000	www.umc-cares.org
University Colo Health Memorial Hospital Central	Colorado Springs	Colorado	719-365-5000	www.memorialhospital.com
University Health System	San Antonio	Texas	210-358-4000	www.universityhealthsystem.com
University Hospital - Stony Brook	Stony Brook	New York	631-444-4000	www.stonybrookmedicalcenter.org
University Hospital SUNY Health Science Center	Syracuse	New York	315-473-4240	www.upstate.edu
University Medical Center of El Paso	El Paso	Texas	915-521-7602	www.thomasoncares.org
University of Alabama Hospital	Birmingham	Alabama	205-934-4011	www.health.uab.edu
University of California Davis Medical Center	Sacramento	California	916-734-2011	www.ucdmc.ucdavis.edu
University of Cincinnati Medical Center	Cincinnati	Ohio	513-584-1000	www.universityhospitalcincinnati.com
University of Illinois Hospital	Chicago	Illinois	312-996-3900	www.uic.edu
University of Kansas Hospital	Kansas City	Kansas	913-588-7332	www.kumc.edu
University of Miami Hospital	Miami	Florida	305-325-5511	www.cedarsmedicalcenter.com
University of Mississippi Medical Center	Jackson	Mississippi	601-984-4100	www.umc.edu
University of Toledo Medical Center	Toledo	Ohio	419-383-3407	www.utmc.utoledo.edu
UPMC Hamot	Erie	Pennsylvania	814-877-6000	www.hamot.org
UPMC Passavant	Pittsburgh	Pennsylvania	412-367-6700	www.passavant.upmc.com
UPMC Presbyterian Shadyside	Pittsburgh	Pennsylvania	412-647-8788	www.upmc.edu
UT Southwestern University Hospital	Dallas	Texas	214-879-3758	www.utsouthwestern.edu
Utah Valley Regional Medical Center	Provo	Utah	801-373-7850	www.intermountainhealthcare.org/hospitals/uvrmc
Valley Hospital	Ridgewood	New Jersey	201-447-8000	www.valleyhealth.com
Vidant Medical Center	Greenville	North Carolina	252-847-4100	www.uhseast.com
Waukesha Memorial Hospital	Waukesha	Wisconsin	262-928-1000	www.waukeshamemorial.org
Wesley Medical Center	Hattiesburg	Mississippi	601-268-8000	www.wesley.com
West Virginia University Hospitals	Morgantown	West Virginia	304-598-4000	www.wvuh.com
Wheaton Franciscan Saint Joseph	Milwaukee	Wisconsin	414-447-2000	www.wfhealthcare.org
Yale-New Haven Hospital	New Haven	Connecticut	203-688-4242	www.ynhh.org

Note: Table shows hospitals nationwide whose surgical complication rate is worse (higher) than U.S. rate of 0.61%

Surgical Complication Rate: State and National Summary

Measure: A Wound That Splits Open After Surgery on the Abdomen or Pelvis

Area	Number of Hospitals			
	Better than U.S. National Rate[1]	Worse than U.S. National Rate[2]	No Different than U.S. National Rate[3]	Number of Cases Too Small[4]
U.S. and Territories	0	42	2703	391
Alabama	0	0	58	18
Alaska	0	0	8	0
American Samoa	n/a	n/a	n/a	n/a
Arizona	0	1	49	9
Arkansas	0	0	35	9
California	0	2	245	49
Colorado	0	2	37	4
Connecticut	0	0	29	0
Delaware	0	0	6	0
District of Columbia	0	1	6	0
Florida	0	2	157	3
Georgia	0	2	83	15
Guam	n/a	n/a	n/a	n/a
Hawaii	0	1	11	2
Idaho	0	1	10	1
Illinois	0	0	122	3
Indiana	0	0	72	11
Iowa	0	0	30	4
Kansas	0	0	39	11
Kentucky	0	2	51	10
Louisiana	0	1	62	17
Maine	0	1	18	1
Maryland	n/a	n/a	n/a	n/a
Massachusetts	0	0	57	1
Michigan	0	4	80	6
Minnesota	0	1	40	9
Mississippi	0	0	37	7
Missouri	0	1	61	10
Montana	0	0	11	1
N. Mariana Islands	n/a	n/a	n/a	n/a
Nebraska	0	0	19	0
Nevada	0	2	19	0
New Hampshire	0	1	12	0
New Jersey	0	2	59	3
New Mexico	0	1	22	3
New York	0	1	146	9
North Carolina	0	2	79	4
North Dakota	0	0	6	0
Ohio	0	3	117	7
Oklahoma	0	0	47	21
Oregon	0	0	32	0
Pennsylvania	0	2	128	14
Puerto Rico	n/a	n/a	n/a	n/a
Rhode Island	0	0	11	0
South Carolina	0	0	49	4
South Dakota	0	0	10	7
Tennessee	0	1	66	22
Texas	0	2	205	55
Utah	0	0	23	4
Vermont	0	0	6	0
Virgin Islands	n/a	n/a	n/a	n/a
Virginia	0	1	64	7
Washington	0	0	46	2
West Virginia	0	0	28	3
Wisconsin	0	2	58	4
Wyoming	0	0	9	2

Note: (1) Surgical complication rate is better (lower) than U.S. rate of 0.92%; (2) Surgical complication rate is worse (higher) than U.S. rate of 0.92%; (3) Surgical complication rate is about the same as U.S. rate of 0.92%; (4) The number of cases is too small to classify the hospital; n/a not available

Surgical Complication Rate: State and National Summary

Measure: Accidental Cuts and Tears From Medical Treatment

Area	Number of Hospitals			
	Better than U.S. National Rate[1]	Worse than U.S. National Rate[2]	No Different than U.S. National Rate[3]	Number of Cases Too Small[4]
U.S. and Territories	95	203	3133	42
Alabama	0	8	89	0
Alaska	0	2	7	0
American Samoa	n/a	n/a	n/a	n/a
Arizona	1	4	61	1
Arkansas	1	0	45	0
California	7	22	280	1
Colorado	0	5	40	1
Connecticut	0	4	27	1
Delaware	1	0	5	0
District of Columbia	0	1	6	0
Florida	11	8	151	1
Georgia	2	6	100	0
Guam	n/a	n/a	n/a	n/a
Hawaii	0	1	13	0
Idaho	0	0	13	1
Illinois	10	7	111	1
Indiana	2	4	83	1
Iowa	0	3	31	0
Kansas	0	4	52	0
Kentucky	1	3	61	0
Louisiana	0	4	88	6
Maine	0	1	19	0
Maryland	n/a	n/a	n/a	n/a
Massachusetts	3	4	54	0
Michigan	3	7	85	0
Minnesota	2	4	46	0
Mississippi	1	2	61	3
Missouri	0	5	71	2
Montana	0	0	13	0
N. Mariana Islands	n/a	n/a	n/a	n/a
Nebraska	1	1	21	1
Nevada	0	2	22	0
New Hampshire	0	3	10	0
New Jersey	8	3	54	1
New Mexico	1	1	31	0
New York	5	4	158	2
North Carolina	1	6	82	0
North Dakota	0	1	6	0
Ohio	3	9	126	3
Oklahoma	3	3	83	2
Oregon	1	3	29	0
Pennsylvania	2	11	140	3
Puerto Rico	n/a	n/a	n/a	n/a
Rhode Island	0	3	8	0
South Carolina	2	3	52	0
South Dakota	0	1	20	0
Tennessee	5	0	92	0
Texas	11	10	301	7
Utah	0	5	26	1
Vermont	0	1	5	0
Virgin Islands	n/a	n/a	n/a	n/a
Virginia	5	3	70	2
Washington	0	11	37	0
West Virginia	1	1	29	0
Wisconsin	0	9	57	0
Wyoming	0	0	11	0

Note: (1) Surgical complication rate is better (lower) than U.S. rate of 1.83%; (2) Surgical complication rate is worse (higher) than U.S. rate of 1.83%; (3) Surgical complication rate is about the same as U.S. rate of 1.83%; (4) The number of cases is too small to classify the hospital; n/a not available

Surgical Complication Rate: State and National Summary

Measure: Collapsed Lung Due to Medical Treatment

Area	Number of Hospitals			
	Better than U.S. National Rate[1]	Worse than U.S. National Rate[2]	No Different than U.S. National Rate[3]	Number of Cases Too Small[4]
U.S. and Territories	9	60	3366	38
Alabama	0	2	95	0
Alaska	0	0	9	0
American Samoa	n/a	n/a	n/a	n/a
Arizona	0	1	65	1
Arkansas	0	1	45	0
California	1	7	302	0
Colorado	0	0	45	1
Connecticut	0	0	31	1
Delaware	0	0	6	0
District of Columbia	0	0	7	0
Florida	0	4	166	1
Georgia	0	2	106	0
Guam	n/a	n/a	n/a	n/a
Hawaii	0	0	14	0
Idaho	0	0	13	1
Illinois	1	2	125	1
Indiana	0	0	89	1
Iowa	0	0	34	0
Kansas	0	3	52	1
Kentucky	1	2	62	0
Louisiana	1	1	92	4
Maine	0	1	19	0
Maryland	n/a	n/a	n/a	n/a
Massachusetts	0	3	58	0
Michigan	1	2	92	0
Minnesota	0	0	52	0
Mississippi	0	0	64	3
Missouri	0	4	72	2
Montana	0	0	13	0
N. Mariana Islands	n/a	n/a	n/a	n/a
Nebraska	0	1	23	0
Nevada	0	1	23	0
New Hampshire	0	0	13	0
New Jersey	2	0	63	1
New Mexico	0	0	33	0
New York	1	4	162	2
North Carolina	0	1	88	0
North Dakota	0	1	6	0
Ohio	0	1	136	4
Oklahoma	0	2	88	1
Oregon	0	1	32	0
Pennsylvania	0	2	152	2
Puerto Rico	n/a	n/a	n/a	n/a
Rhode Island	0	0	11	0
South Carolina	0	1	56	0
South Dakota	0	0	21	0
Tennessee	0	1	96	0
Texas	0	6	316	7
Utah	0	0	31	1
Vermont	0	0	6	0
Virgin Islands	n/a	n/a	n/a	n/a
Virginia	1	2	75	2
Washington	0	0	48	0
West Virginia	0	0	31	0
Wisconsin	0	1	65	0
Wyoming	0	0	11	0

Note: (1) Surgical complication rate is better (lower) than U.S. rate of 0.32%; (2) Surgical complication rate is worse (higher) than U.S. rate of 0.32%; (3) Surgical complication rate is about the same as U.S. rate of 0.32%; (4) The number of cases is too small to classify the hospital; n/a not available

Surgical Complication Rate: State and National Summary

Measure: Deaths Among Patients With Serious Treatable Complications After Surgery

Area	Number of Hospitals			
	Better than U.S. National Rate[1]	Worse than U.S. National Rate[2]	No Different than U.S. National Rate[3]	Number of Cases Too Small[4]
U.S. and Territories	43	70	1831	1058
Alabama	0	6	33	29
Alaska	0	1	4	3
American Samoa	n/a	n/a	n/a	n/a
Arizona	3	0	39	15
Arkansas	0	1	20	17
California	1	3	164	116
Colorado	1	0	27	14
Connecticut	0	0	22	7
Delaware	0	1	4	1
District of Columbia	0	0	6	1
Florida	6	5	124	26
Georgia	2	5	50	41
Guam	n/a	n/a	n/a	n/a
Hawaii	0	0	5	9
Idaho	0	0	8	4
Illinois	7	1	87	29
Indiana	1	0	54	29
Iowa	1	0	22	10
Kansas	0	0	25	23
Kentucky	0	3	31	25
Louisiana	0	0	38	28
Maine	0	0	9	11
Maryland	n/a	n/a	n/a	n/a
Massachusetts	0	1	42	15
Michigan	4	0	56	28
Minnesota	1	0	23	24
Mississippi	0	3	20	16
Missouri	2	1	44	23
Montana	0	0	9	2
N. Mariana Islands	n/a	n/a	n/a	n/a
Nebraska	0	0	17	5
Nevada	0	2	14	5
New Hampshire	0	1	10	2
New Jersey	2	5	50	7
New Mexico	0	0	10	14
New York	2	4	91	58
North Carolina	0	4	57	25
North Dakota	1	0	5	0
Ohio	1	1	84	37
Oklahoma	0	4	27	27
Oregon	1	0	17	14
Pennsylvania	0	2	80	60
Puerto Rico	n/a	n/a	n/a	n/a
Rhode Island	0	0	7	4
South Carolina	0	3	29	21
South Dakota	0	0	6	9
Tennessee	0	2	45	30
Texas	5	5	147	81
Utah	0	0	16	11
Vermont	0	1	3	2
Virgin Islands	n/a	n/a	n/a	n/a
Virginia	0	1	46	21
Washington	0	0	40	6
West Virginia	0	1	19	8
Wisconsin	2	0	39	25
Wyoming	0	0	2	9

Note: (1) Surgical complication rate is better (lower) than U.S. rate of 110.25%; (2) Surgical complication rate is worse (higher) than U.S. rate of 110.25%; (3) Surgical complication rate is about the same as U.S. rate of 110.25%; (4) The number of cases is too small to classify the hospital; n/a not available

Surgical Complication Rate: State and National Summary

Measure: Rate of Complications for Hip/Knee Replacement Patients

Area	Number of Hospitals			
	Better than U.S. National Rate[1]	Worse than U.S. National Rate[2]	No Different than U.S. National Rate[3]	Number of Cases Too Small[4]
U.S. and Territories	75	68	2655	687
Alabama	0	4	46	11
Alaska	0	0	7	1
American Samoa	0	0	0	0
Arizona	1	0	48	6
Arkansas	1	1	28	7
California	7	4	196	89
Colorado	1	3	46	6
Connecticut	1	2	26	0
Delaware	0	0	5	1
District of Columbia	0	0	5	2
Florida	11	1	134	16
Georgia	2	1	76	15
Guam	0	0	0	0
Hawaii	0	0	8	6
Idaho	0	0	23	5
Illinois	2	3	108	25
Indiana	4	1	73	32
Iowa	0	2	46	17
Kansas	3	2	37	13
Kentucky	1	0	41	19
Louisiana	0	0	59	16
Maine	1	1	24	5
Maryland	2	1	41	1
Massachusetts	2	0	54	5
Michigan	6	2	88	20
Minnesota	1	0	65	17
Mississippi	2	1	24	9
Missouri	3	2	61	14
Montana	0	1	19	6
N. Mariana Islands	0	0	0	0
Nebraska	2	0	30	13
Nevada	0	1	22	2
New Hampshire	0	1	21	4
New Jersey	0	1	53	9
New Mexico	0	0	22	2
New York	4	2	116	30
North Carolina	1	4	77	8
North Dakota	1	0	7	1
Ohio	2	6	128	21
Oklahoma	1	1	46	18
Oregon	0	0	40	10
Pennsylvania	0	6	123	27
Puerto Rico	0	0	8	27
Rhode Island	0	0	9	1
South Carolina	1	0	39	14
South Dakota	0	0	16	2
Tennessee	2	3	50	21
Texas	7	4	198	54
Utah	0	1	25	6
Vermont	0	0	12	1
Virgin Islands	0	0	1	0
Virginia	2	2	54	11
Washington	1	0	52	9
West Virginia	0	0	26	6
Wisconsin	0	4	79	22
Wyoming	0	0	13	4

Note: (1) Surgical complication rate is better (lower) than U.S. rate of 3.4%; (2) Surgical complication rate is worse (higher) than U.S. rate of 3.4%; (3) Surgical complication rate is about the same as U.S. rate of 3.4%; (4) The number of cases is too small to classify the hospital; n/a not available

Surgical Complication Rate: State and National Summary

Measure: Serious Blood Clots After Surgery

Area	Number of Hospitals			
	Better than U.S. National Rate[1]	Worse than U.S. National Rate[2]	No Different than U.S. National Rate[3]	Number of Cases Too Small[4]
U.S. and Territories	155	203	2846	114
Alabama	1	3	72	5
Alaska	0	0	8	1
American Samoa	n/a	n/a	n/a	n/a
Arizona	3	1	58	1
Arkansas	3	0	41	2
California	16	8	274	5
Colorado	2	4	38	0
Connecticut	1	5	23	0
Delaware	0	1	5	0
District of Columbia	0	1	6	0
Florida	7	18	138	2
Georgia	2	6	92	4
Guam	n/a	n/a	n/a	n/a
Hawaii	0	0	14	0
Idaho	2	1	10	1
Illinois	5	20	100	2
Indiana	8	1	79	1
Iowa	4	1	29	0
Kansas	4	2	46	3
Kentucky	4	2	57	2
Louisiana	2	3	80	7
Maine	1	0	19	0
Maryland	n/a	n/a	n/a	n/a
Massachusetts	4	2	52	2
Michigan	5	13	74	0
Minnesota	4	0	47	0
Mississippi	1	3	39	9
Missouri	3	5	62	5
Montana	5	0	7	1
N. Mariana Islands	n/a	n/a	n/a	n/a
Nebraska	0	0	23	0
Nevada	1	0	20	0
New Hampshire	1	2	10	0
New Jersey	2	15	47	1
New Mexico	1	2	23	3
New York	3	21	133	5
North Carolina	6	2	79	0
North Dakota	2	0	4	0
Ohio	0	9	122	4
Oklahoma	4	1	68	11
Oregon	4	2	26	1
Pennsylvania	1	23	127	2
Puerto Rico	n/a	n/a	n/a	n/a
Rhode Island	0	0	11	0
South Carolina	1	0	54	2
South Dakota	3	0	15	1
Tennessee	8	2	77	5
Texas	13	12	257	23
Utah	1	1	27	1
Vermont	0	0	6	0
Virgin Islands	n/a	n/a	n/a	n/a
Virginia	5	4	62	1
Washington	7	2	39	0
West Virginia	1	2	28	0
Wisconsin	3	2	61	0
Wyoming	1	0	10	0

Note: (1) Surgical complication rate is better (lower) than U.S. rate of 4.14%; (2) Surgical complication rate is worse (higher) than U.S. rate of 4.14%; (3) Surgical complication rate is about the same as U.S. rate of 4.14%; (4) The number of cases is too small to classify the hospital; n/a not available

Surgical Complication Rate: State and National Summary

Measure: Serious Complications

Area	Number of Hospitals			
	Better than U.S. National Rate[1]	Worse than U.S. National Rate[2]	No Different than U.S. National Rate[3]	Number of Cases Too Small[4]
U.S. and Territories	108	182	3184	0
Alabama	0	5	92	0
Alaska	0	0	9	0
American Samoa	n/a	n/a	n/a	n/a
Arizona	1	2	64	0
Arkansas	2	0	44	0
California	8	15	287	0
Colorado	0	6	40	0
Connecticut	0	6	26	0
Delaware	0	0	6	0
District of Columbia	0	2	5	0
Florida	7	9	155	0
Georgia	3	4	101	0
Guam	n/a	n/a	n/a	n/a
Hawaii	0	0	14	0
Idaho	0	1	13	0
Illinois	5	9	115	0
Indiana	7	0	83	0
Iowa	3	0	31	0
Kansas	0	3	53	0
Kentucky	3	1	61	0
Louisiana	2	4	92	0
Maine	0	1	19	0
Maryland	n/a	n/a	n/a	n/a
Massachusetts	3	3	55	0
Michigan	6	8	81	0
Minnesota	1	3	48	0
Mississippi	2	3	62	0
Missouri	2	4	72	0
Montana	1	0	12	0
N. Mariana Islands	n/a	n/a	n/a	n/a
Nebraska	1	0	23	0
Nevada	1	2	21	0
New Hampshire	1	1	11	0
New Jersey	5	10	51	0
New Mexico	0	2	31	0
New York	3	10	157	0
North Carolina	3	3	83	0
North Dakota	0	1	6	0
Ohio	4	8	129	0
Oklahoma	3	2	86	0
Oregon	1	1	31	0
Pennsylvania	4	16	136	0
Puerto Rico	n/a	n/a	n/a	n/a
Rhode Island	0	1	10	0
South Carolina	4	0	53	0
South Dakota	1	0	20	0
Tennessee	5	0	92	0
Texas	10	13	306	0
Utah	0	4	28	0
Vermont	0	0	6	0
Virgin Islands	n/a	n/a	n/a	n/a
Virginia	4	4	72	0
Washington	0	6	42	0
West Virginia	2	2	27	0
Wisconsin	0	7	59	0
Wyoming	0	0	11	0

Note: (1) Surgical complication rate is better (lower) than U.S. rate of 0.61%; (2) Surgical complication rate is worse (higher) than U.S. rate of 0.61%; (3) Surgical complication rate is about the same as U.S. rate of 0.61%; (4) The number of cases is too small to classify the hospital; n/a not available

Appendix D: Best Hospitals by Selected Category

What Do These Tables Show?

This appendix shows the best hospitals nationwide based on their average scores in 11 categories. The categories are:

- Blood Clot Prevention and Treatment
- Children's Asthma Care
- Emergency Department Care
- Heart Care
- Pneumonia Care
- Preventative Care
- Stroke Care
- Surgical Care
- Patient's Hospital Experiences
- Use of Medical Imaging
- Lowest Medicare Spending per Beneficiary

How Were the Hospitals Selected?

Hospitals were selected for inclusion in three ways:

- Hospitals that achieved a perfect 100% average score in all qualified measures in a given category.
- Hospitals that were in the top 5% of hospitals based on their average score in a given category.
- Hospitals whose Medicare spending ratios fell below a certain threshold.

How Were Average Scores Calculated?

The average score for any given category was calculated by averaging the scores of the individual measures that made up that category. In some instances, not all measures were included in the average score calculation. A meaure was omitted if: 1) data was not available 2) the measure did not meet the 25 case threshold for inclusion (except Patient's Hospital Experiences in which the threshold was 100 or more completed surveys). Note that the Pregnancy Care category did not have enough information available to calculate an average score.

Best Hospitals for Blood Clot Prevention and Treatment

Hospital	City	State	Phone	Web Site
Baptist Hospital of Miami	Miami	Florida	786-596-1960	www.baptisthealth.net
Berkshire Medical Center	Pittsfield	Massachusetts	413-447-2000	www.berkshirehealthsystems.org
Blanchard Valley Hospital	Findlay	Ohio	419-423-4500	www.bvha.org
Boca Raton Regional Hospital	Boca Raton	Florida	561-362-5002	www.brrh.com
Brandon Regional Hospital	Brandon	Florida	813-681-5551	www.brandonregionalhospital.com
Capital Regional Medical Center	Tallahassee	Florida	850-656-5000	www.capitalregionalmedicalcenter.com
Centerpoint Medical Center	Independence	Missouri	816-698-7000	www.centerpointmedical.com
Community Hospital of the Monterey Peninsula	Monterey	California	831-624-5311	www.chomp.org
Delray Medical Center	Delray Beach	Florida	561-498-4440	www.delraymedicalctr.com
Doctors' Community Hospital	Lanham	Maryland	301-552-8085	www.dchweb.org
Fairview Southdale Hospital	Edina	Minnesota	952-924-5000	www.fairview.org
Flushing Hospital Medical Center	Flushing	New York	718-670-5000	www.flushinghospital.org
Fort Sanders Regional Medical Center	Knoxville	Tennessee	865-541-1101	www.fsregional.com
Henrico Doctors' Hospital	Richmond	Virginia	804-289-4500	www.henricodoctors.com
Heritage Valley Beaver	Beaver	Pennsylvania	412-728-7000	www.heritagevalley.org
Heritage Valley Sewickley	Sewickley	Pennsylvania	412-741-6600	www.heritagevalley.org
John Randolph Medical Center	Hopewell	Virginia	804-541-1600	www.johnrandolphmed.com
Kaiser Foundation Hospital - Roseville	Roseville	California	916-784-4000	www.kaiserpermanente.org/roseville
Kendall Regional Medical Center	Miami	Florida	305-223-3000	www.kendallmed.com
Lewisgale Medical Center	Salem	Virginia	540-776-4000	www.lewis-gale.com
Lovelace Medical Center	Albuquerque	New Mexico	505-727-8000	www.lovelace.com
Mclaren Lapeer Region	Lapeer	Michigan	810-667-5500	www.lapeerregional.org
The Medical Center of Aurora	Aurora	Colorado	303-695-2600	www.auroramed.com
Medical Center of Plano	Plano	Texas	972-596-6800	www.medicalcenterofplano.com
Memorial Hospital Pembroke	Pembroke Pines	Florida	954-962-9650	www.memorialpembroke.com\
Memorial Hospital West	Pembroke Pines	Florida	954-436-5000	www.memorialwest.com
Memorial Regional Hospital	Hollywood	Florida	954-987-2000	www.memorialregional.com
Mercy Hospital of Folsom	Folsom	California	916-983-7400	www.mercyfolsom.org
Mercy Memorial Hospital System	Monroe	Michigan	734-240-8400	www.mercymemorial.org
Methodist Dallas Medical Center	Dallas	Texas	214-947-2879	www.mhd.com
Mountain View Regional Medical Center	Las Cruces	New Mexico	575-556-7600	www.mountainviewregional.com
Nazareth Hospital	Philadelphia	Pennsylvania	215-335-6000	www.nazarethhospital.org
North Florida Regional Medical Center	Gainesville	Florida	352-333-4100	www.nfrmc.com
Northside Hospital	Atlanta	Georgia	404-851-8000	www.northside.com
Northside Hospital Cherokee	Canton	Georgia	770-720-5298	www.northside.com/cherokee
Northside Hospital Forsyth	Cumming	Georgia	404-851-8700	www.gbhcs.org
Novant Health Forsyth Medical Center	Winston-Salem	North Carolina	336-718-5000	www.forsythmedicalcenter.org
Oak Hill Hospital	Brooksville	Florida	352-596-6632	www.oakhillhospital.com
Orange Park Medical Center	Orange Park	Florida	904-276-8500	www.opmedical.com
Overland Park Regional Medical Center	Overland Park	Kansas	913-541-5301	www.oprmc.com
Rapides Regional Medical Center	Alexandria	Louisiana	318-769-3000	www.rapidesregional.com
Regional Medical Center Bayonet Point	Hudson	Florida	727-819-2929	www.mchealth.comorwww.heartoftampa.com
Riverside Medical Center	Kankakee	Illinois	815-933-1671	www.riversidehealthcare.org
Rockdale Medical Center	Conyers	Georgia	770-918-3000	www.rockdalehospital.org
Rose Medical Center	Denver	Colorado	303-320-2121	www.rosemed.com
Saint Clares Hospital of Weston	Weston	Wisconsin	715-393-3000	www.ministryhealth.org
Saint Lucie Medical Center	Port Saint Lucie	Florida	772-335-4000	www.stluciemed.com
Saint Mary Medical Center	Hobart	Indiana	219-942-0551	www.comhs.org/stmary
Saint Mary's Medical Center	West Palm Beach	Florida	561-840-6202	www.stmarysmc.com
Saint Mary's Medical Center	Blue Springs	Missouri	816-228-5900	www.stmaryskc.com
Saint Vincent's Medical Center Southside	Jacksonville	Florida	904-296-3700	www.jaxhealth.com
Sisters of Charity Hospital	Buffalo	New York	716-862-1000	www.chsbuffalo.org
South Miami Hospital	South Miami	Florida	786-662-4000	www.baptisthealth.net
Southern Hills Hospital & Medical Center	Las Vegas	Nevada	702-880-2100	www.southernhillshospital.com
Springs Memorial Hospital	Lancaster	South Carolina	803-286-1481	www.springsmemorial.com
Summa Western Reserve Hospital	Cuyahoga Falls	Ohio	330-971-7000	www.westernreservehospital.org
Texoma Medical Center	Denison	Texas	903-416-4000	www.texomamedicalcenter.net
Trinity Medical Center	Birmingham	Alabama	205-592-1000	www.bhsala.com/montclair
Tulane Medical Center	New Orleans	Louisiana	504-988-1900	www.tuhc.com
United Hospital Center	Bridgeport	West Virginia	681-342-1000	www.uhcwv.org
University Medical Center of El Paso	El Paso	Texas	915-521-7602	www.thomasoncares.org
UPMC Horizon	Greenville	Pennsylvania	724-588-2100	www.upmc.com
UPMC Mckeesport	Mc Keesport	Pennsylvania	412-664-2000	www.selectmedicalcorp.com
Venice Regional Medical Center - Bayfront Health	Venice	Florida	941-485-7711	www.veniceregional.com
Vista Medical Center East	Waukegan	Illinois	847-360-4000	www.vistahealth.com

Hospital	City	State	Phone	Web Site
Wesley Medical Center	Wichita	Kansas	316-962-2000	www.wesleymc.com
West Georgia Medical Center	Lagrange	Georgia	706-882-1411	www.wghealth.org
West Virginia University Hospitals	Morgantown	West Virginia	304-598-4000	www.wvuh.com

Note: The hospitals shown above represent the top 5% of the 1,268 hospitals nationwide for which an average score was calculated. Average scores were calculated for hospitals with qualifying data (25 cases or more) in at least 5 of 6 measures in the Blood Clot Prevention and Treatment category.

Best Hospitals for Children's Asthma Care

Hospital	City	State	Phone	Web Site
Carroll Hospital Center	Westminster	Maryland	410-848-3000	www.carrollhospitalcenter.org
Cleveland Clinic	Cleveland	Ohio	216-444-2200	www.clevelandclinic.org
Lawnwood Regional Medical Center & Heart Institute	Fort Pierce	Florida	772-461-4000	www.lawnwoodmed.com
Memorial Regional Hospital	Hollywood	Florida	954-987-2000	www.memorialregional.com
Renown Regional Medical Center	Reno	Nevada	775-982-4100	www.renown.org

Note: The hospitals shown above represent the top 5% of the 90 hospitals nationwide for which an average score was calculated. Average scores were calculated for hospitals with qualifying data (25 cases or more) in all three measures in the Children's Asthma category.

Best Hospitals for Emergency Department Care

Hospital	City	State	Phone	Web Site
Abraham Lincoln Memorial Hospital	Lincoln	Illinois	217-732-2161	www.almh.org
Albemarle Hospital Authority	Elizabeth City	North Carolina	252-335-0531	www.albemarlehealth.org
Alliance Community Hospital	Alliance	Ohio	330-596-7527	www.achosp.org
Ashtabula County Medical Center	Ashtabula	Ohio	440-997-2262	www.acmchealth.org
Aspirus Wausau Hospital	Wausau	Wisconsin	715-847-2121	www.aspirus.org
Aurora Medical Center	Summit	Wisconsin	262-434-1000	www.aurorahealthcare.org
Avera Sacred Heart Hospital	Yankton	South Dakota	605-668-8000	www.avera.org/sacred-heart
Avera Saint Mary's Hospital	Pierre	South Dakota	605-224-3100	www.st-marys.com
Avoyelles Hospital	Marksville	Louisiana	318-253-8611	www.avoyelleshospital.com
Bates County Memorial Hospital	Butler	Missouri	660-200-7000	www.bcmhospital.com
Bear River Valley Hospital	Tremonton	Utah	435-207-4708	www.intermountainhealthcare.org
Bellevue Hospital	Bellevue	Ohio	419-483-4040	www.bellevuehospital.com
Bluffton Hospital	Bluffton	Ohio	419-358-9010	www.bvhealthsystem.org
Bourbon Community Hospital	Paris	Kentucky	859-987-3600	www.bourbonhospital.com
Brigham City Community Hospital	Brigham City	Utah	435-734-9471	www.brighamcityhospital.com
Brookings Hospital	Brookings	South Dakota	605-696-7701	www.brookingshospital.org
Cache Valley Speciality Hospital	North Logan	Utah	435-713-9700	www.cachevalleyhospital.com
Cameron Regional Medical Center	Cameron	Missouri	816-632-2101	www.cameronregional.org
Carson City Hospital	Carson City	Michigan	989-584-3131	www.carsoncityhospital.com
Cogdell Memorial Hospital	Snyder	Texas	325-574-7437	www.cogdellhospital.com
Colorado Plains Medical Center	Fort Morgan	Colorado	970-867-3391	www.coloradoplainsmedicalcenter.com
Crossroads Community Hospital	Mount Vernon	Illinois	618-244-5500	www.crossroadscommnityhospital.com
Custer Regional Hospital	Custer	South Dakota	605-673-2229	www.rcrh.org/facilities
Dauterive Hospital	New Iberia	Louisiana	337-365-7311	www.dauterivehospital.com
Daviess Community Hospital	Washington	Indiana	812-254-2760	www.dchosp.org
Decatur County Memorial Hospital	Greensburg	Indiana	812-663-4331	www.dcmh.net
Detroit Receiving Hospital & University Health Center	Detroit	Michigan	313-745-3104	www.drhuhc.org
Dupont Hospital	Fort Wayne	Indiana	260-416-3000	www.theduponthospital.com
East Cooper Medical Center	Mount Pleasant	South Carolina	843-881-0100	www.eastcoopermedctr.com
El Paso Specialty Hospital	El Paso	Texas	915-544-3636	www.elpasospecialtyhospital.com
Encino Hospital Medical Center	Encino	California	818-995-5000	www.encino-tarzana.com
Englewood Community Hospital	Englewood	Florida	941-475-6571	www.englewoodcommunityhospital.com
Evanston Regional Hospital	Evanston	Wyoming	307-789-3636	www.evanstonregionalhospital.com
Excela Health Frick Hospital	Mount Pleasant	Pennsylvania	724-547-1500	www.excelahealth.org
Fairmont General Hospital	Fairmont	West Virginia	304-367-7100	www.fghi.com
Fort Hamilton Hughes Memorial Hospital	Hamilton	Ohio	513-867-2000	www.forthamiltonhospital.com
Fremont Area Medical Center	Fremont	Nebraska	402-721-1610	www.famc.org
Genesis Medical Center - Dewitt	Dewitt	Iowa	563-659-4200	www.genesishealth.com
Good Samaritan Health Center	Merrill	Wisconsin	715-536-5511	www.ministryhealth.org/GSHC/home.nws
Good Samaritan Hospital	Kearney	Nebraska	308-865-7100	www.gshs.org
Graham Hospital Association	Canton	Illinois	309-647-5240	www.grahamhospital.org
Great Bend Regional Hospital	Great Bend	Kansas	620-792-8833	www.greatbendsurgical.com
Grove City Medical Center	Grove City	Pennsylvania	724-450-7000	www.uchpa.org
Hamilton General Hospital	Hamilton	Texas	254-386-3151	www.hamiltonhospital.org
Harrington Memorial Hospital	Southbridge	Massachusetts	508-765-9771	www.harringtonhospital.org
Harris Hospital	Newport	Arkansas	870-523-8911	www.harrishospital.com
Heber Valley Medical Center	Heber City	Utah	435-654-2500	www.intermountainhealthcare.org
Henderson County Community Hospital	Lexington	Tennessee	731-968-1801	www.hendersoncchospital.com
Hill Regional Hospital	Hillsboro	Texas	254-580-8500	www.hillregionalhospital.com
Hillside Hospital	Pulaski	Tennessee	931-363-7531	www.hillsidehospital.com
Holdenville Hospital Authority	Holdenville	Oklahoma	405-379-4200	
The Hospital at Westlake Medical Center	Austin	Texas	512-327-0000	www.westlakemedical.com
Hutchinson Health	Hutchinson	Minnesota	320-234-5000	www.hahc-hmc.com
Illinois Valley Community Hospital	Peru	Illinois	815-223-3300	www.ivch.org
Integris Blackwell Regional Hospital	Blackwell	Oklahoma	580-363-2311	www.integrisblackwell.com
Integris Health Edmond	Edmond	Oklahoma	405-657-3000	www.integrisok.com/integris-health-edmond-ok
Integris Marshall County Medical Center	Madill	Oklahoma	580-795-3384	www.integris-health.com/integris
Iroquois Memorial Hospital	Watseka	Illinois	815-432-5201	www.iroquoismemorial.com
Kansas Medical Center	Andover	Kansas	316-300-4000	www.ksmedcenter.com
Lafayette Regional Health Center	Lexington	Missouri	660-259-2203	www.lafayetteregionalhealthcenter.com
Lake Region Healthcare Corporation	Fergus Falls	Minnesota	218-736-8000	www.lrhc.org
Lakeland Community Hospital	Haleyville	Alabama	205-485-7117	www.lifepointhospitals.com
Lakeland Regional Medical Center	Lakeland	Florida	863-687-1100	www.lrmc.com
Lander Regional Hospital	Lander	Wyoming	307-332-4420	www.landerhospital.com
Lawrence Medical Center	Moulton	Alabama	256-974-2200	www.lawrencemedicalcenter.com

Hospital	City	State	Phone	Web Site
Livingston Regional Hospital	Livingston	Tennessee	931-823-5611	www.livingstonregionalhospital.com
Madison Memorial Hospital	Rexburg	Idaho	208-359-6900	www.madisonhospital.org
Maple Grove Hospital	Maple Grove	Minnesota	763-581-1000	www.maplegrove.org
Mary Greeley Medical Center	Ames	Iowa	515-239-2011	www.mgmc.org
Mary Lanning Healthcare	Hastings	Nebraska	402-463-4521	www.marylanning.org
Mayo Clinic Health System - Fairmont	Fairmont	Minnesota	507-238-8101	www.fairmontmedicalcenter.org
McBride Clinic Orthopedic Hospital	Oklahoma City	Oklahoma	405-478-1717	www.mcbrideclinic.com
McCullough - Hyde Memorial Hospital	Oxford	Ohio	513-523-2111	www.mhmh.org
McDonough District Hospital	Macomb	Illinois	309-833-4101	www.mdh.org
Mercer County Joint Township Community Hospital	Coldwater	Ohio	419-678-4843	www.mercer-health.com
Mercy Health System Corp	Janesville	Wisconsin	608-756-6080	www.mercyhealthsystem.org
Mercy Medical Center	Roseburg	Oregon	541-673-0611	www.mercyrose.org
Mercy Medical Center - Dubuque	Dubuque	Iowa	563-589-8000	www.mercydubuque.com
Mercy Regional Medical Center	Ville Platte	Louisiana	337-363-5684	www.vpmc.com
Meriter Hospital	Madison	Wisconsin	608-417-6000	www.meriter.com
Mesa View Regional Hospital	Mesquite	Nevada	702-346-8040	www.mesaviewhospital.com
Minden Medical Center	Minden	Louisiana	318-377-2321	www.mindenmedicalcenter.com
Ministry Saint Michaels Hospital of Stevens Point	Stevens Point	Wisconsin	715-346-5000	www.saintmichaelshospital.org
Moore County Hospital District	Dumas	Texas	806-935-7171	www.mchd.net
Mount Pleasant Hospital	Mount Pleasant	South Carolina	843-724-2954	www.rsfh.com
Mountain View Hospital	Payson	Utah	801-465-7100	www.mvhpayson.com
Neshoba County General Hospital	Philadelphia	Mississippi	601-663-1200	www.neshobageneral.com
Nevada Regional Medical Center	Nevada	Missouri	417-667-3355	www.nrmchealth.com
Ottawa Regional Hospital & Healthcare Center	Ottawa	Illinois	815-433-3100	www.community-hospital.org
Park City Medical Center	Park City	Utah	435-658-7000	www.intermountainhealthcare.org
Parkview Lagrange Hospital	Lagrange	Indiana	260-463-9000	www.parkview.com
Ponca City Medical Center	Ponca City	Oklahoma	580-765-3321	www.poncamedcenter.com
Portage Health	Hancock	Michigan	906-483-1000	www.portagehealth.org
Prairie Lakes Hospital	Watertown	South Dakota	605-882-7000	www.prairielakes.com
Presbyterian Saint Lukes Medical Center	Denver	Colorado	303-839-6000	www.pslmc.com
Proctor Hospital	Peoria	Illinois	309-691-1000	www.proctor.org
Providence Seaside Hospital	Seaside	Oregon	503-717-7000	www.providence.org/northcoast
Pushmataha County - Town of Antlers Hospital Authority	Antlers	Oklahoma	580-298-3341	www.pushhospital.com
Riverview Regional Medical Center	Carthage	Tennessee	615-735-9815	www.sumner.org
Rockcastle County Hospital	Mount Vernon	Kentucky	606-256-2195	www.rockcastlehospital.com
Sagewest Health Care	Riverton	Wyoming	307-856-4161	www.riverton-hospital.com
Saint Charles Parish Hospital	Luling	Louisiana	985-785-6242	www.stch.net
Saint Clare Hospital Health Services	Baraboo	Wisconsin	608-356-1400	www.stclare.com
Saint Elizabeth Grant	Williamstown	Kentucky	859-824-8240	www.stelizabeth.com
Saint Elizabeth Hospital	Appleton	Wisconsin	920-738-2000	www.affinityhealth.org
Saint James Healthcare	Butte	Montana	406-723-2500	www.stjameshealthcare.org
Saint James Hospital	Pontiac	Illinois	815-842-2828	www.osfsaintjames.org
Saint John Hospital	Leavenworth	Kansas	913-596-3930	www.providence-health.org
Saint Johns Medical Center	Jackson	Wyoming	307-733-3636	www.tetonhospital.org
Saint Margarets Hospital	Spring Valley	Illinois	815-664-1176	www.aboutsmh.org
Saint Marys Hospital	Madison	Wisconsin	608-251-6100	www.stmarysmadison.com
Saint Marys Hospital Superior	Superior	Wisconsin	715-817-7000	www.smdc.org
Saint Marys Janesville Hospital	Janesville	Wisconsin	608-373-8000	www.stmarysjanesville.com
Samaritan Albany General Hospital	Albany	Oregon	541-812-4000	www.samhealth.org/shs_facilities
Sanford Medical Center Bismarck	Bismarck	North Dakota	701-323-6000	www.medcenterone.com
Sanford Worthington Medical Center	Worthington	Minnesota	507-372-2941	www.worthingtonhospital.com
Santa Ynez Valley Cottage Hospital	Solvang	California	805-688-6431	www.cottagehealthsystem.org
Seton Smithville Regional Hospital	Smithville	Texas	512-237-3214	www.srhnet.com
Share Memorial Hospital	Alva	Oklahoma	580-327-2800	www.smcok.com
Shelby Memorial Hospital	Shelbyville	Illinois	217-774-3961	www.mysmh.org
Silverton Hospital	Silverton	Oregon	503-873-1500	www.silvertonhospital.org
Smyth County Community Hospital	Marion	Virginia	276-378-1000	www.scchosp.org
South Central Kansas Medical Center	Arkansas City	Kansas	620-442-2500	www.sckrmc.com
Spearfish Regional Hospital	Spearfish	South Dakota	605-644-4000	www.rcrh.org
Spencer Municipal Hospital	Spencer	Iowa	712-264-8300	www.spencerhospital.org
Springhill Medical Center	Springhill	Louisiana	318-539-1000	www.smccare.com
Stephens Memorial Hospital	Breckenridge	Texas	254-559-2241	www.smhtx.com
Stonewall Jackson Memorial Hospital	Weston	West Virginia	304-269-8080	www.stonewallhospital.com
Swedish Issaquah	Issaquah	Washington	425-313-4000	www.swedish.org/locations/issaquah-campus
Swedish Medical Center	Seattle	Washington	206-386-6000	www.swedish.org
Taylorville Memorial Hospital	Taylorville	Illinois	217-824-3331	www.svmh.org
Toppenish Community Hospital	Toppenish	Washington	509-865-1520	www.hma-corp.com

Hospital	City	State	Phone	Web Site
Tristar Ashland City Medical Center	Ashland City	Tennessee	615-792-3030	www.centennialashlandcity.com
UPMC Bedford Memorial	Everett	Pennsylvania	814-623-6161	www.upmc.com
UPMC Northwest	Seneca	Pennsylvania	814-676-7600	www.northwest.upmc.com
Valley West Community Hospital	Sandwich	Illinois	815-786-8484	www.snd.softfarm.com/sandhosp
Via Christi Hospital Wichita Saint Teresa	Wichita	Kansas	316-796-7800	www.via-christi.org
Walla Walla General Hospital	Walla Walla	Washington	509-525-0480	www.wwgh.com
Winn Parish Medical Center	Winnfield	Louisiana	318-648-3000	www.winnparishmedical.com
Winona Health Services	Winona	Minnesota	507-454-3650	www.winonahealth.org
Woodward Regional Hospital	Woodward	Oklahoma	580-254-8492	www.woodwardhospital.com
Yampa Valley Medical Center	Steamboat Springs	Colorado	970-879-1322	www.yvmc.org
York Hospital	York	Maine	207-363-4321	www.yorkhospital.com

Note: The hospitals shown above represent the top 5% of the 2,872 hospitals nationwide for which an average score was calculated. Average scores were calculated for hospitals with qualifying data (25 cases or more) in at least 6 of 7 measures in the Emergency Department Care category.

Best Hospitals for Heart Care

Hospital	City	State	Phone	Web Site
Advocate Good Shepherd Hospital	Barrington	Illinois	847-381-9600	www.advocatehealth.com
Advocate Illinois Masonic Medical Center	Chicago	Illinois	773-975-1600	www.advocatehealth.com/immc
Alegent Creighton Health Immanuel Medical Center	Omaha	Nebraska	402-572-2121	www.alegent.com
Arkansas Heart Hospital	Little Rock	Arkansas	501-219-7000	www.arheart.com
Baptist Hospital of Miami	Miami	Florida	786-596-1960	www.baptisthealth.net
Baylor Heart & Vascular Hospital	Dallas	Texas	214-820-0670	www.baylorhearthospital.com
Beaumont Health System	Grosse Pointe	Michigan	313-343-1000	www.beaumonthospitals.com
Blanchard Valley Hospital	Findlay	Ohio	419-423-4500	www.bvha.org
Boca Raton Regional Hospital	Boca Raton	Florida	561-362-5002	www.brrh.com
Brooklyn Hospital Center at Downtown Campus	Brooklyn	New York	718-250-8000	www.tbh.org
Broward Health North	Pompano Beach	Florida	954-786-6950	www.browardhealth.org
Calvert Memorial Hospital	Prince Frederick	Maryland	410-535-8239	www.calverthospital.com
Carepoint Health - Bayonne Hospital Center	Bayonne	New Jersey	201-858-5000	www.bayonnemedicalcenter.org
Cedars - Sinai Medical Center	Los Angeles	California	310-423-5000	www.cedars-sinai.edu
Centinela Hospital Medical Center	Inglewood	California	310-673-4660	www.centinelafreeman.com
Decatur Memorial Hospital	Decatur	Illinois	217-877-8121	www.dmhcares.org
Dekalb Regional Medical Center	Fort Payne	Alabama	256-845-3150	www.baptistmedical.org
Delray Medical Center	Delray Beach	Florida	561-498-4440	www.delraymedicalctr.com
Doctors Hospital	Augusta	Georgia	706-651-6008	www.doctors-hospital.net
Doctors Hospital	Columbus	Ohio	614-544-1000	www.columbusregional.com
Eastern Idaho Regional Medical Center	Idaho Falls	Idaho	208-529-6111	www.eirmc.org
Fairview Southdale Hospital	Edina	Minnesota	952-924-5000	www.fairview.org
Florida Hospital North Pinellas	Tarpon Springs	Florida	727-942-5000	www.hemh.com
Fort Sanders Regional Medical Center	Knoxville	Tennessee	865-541-1101	www.fsregional.com
Gateway Regional Medical Center	Granite City	Illinois	618-798-3175	www.sehs.com
Good Samaritan Hospital Medical Center	West Islip	New York	631-376-3000	www.good-samaritan-hospital.org
Good Samaritan Hospital of Suffern	Suffern	New York	914-368-5000	www.goodsamhosp.org
Hackettstown Regional Medical Center	Hackettstown	New Jersey	908-852-5100	www.hrmcnj.org
Health Central	Ocoee	Florida	407-296-1820	www.health-central.org
High Point Regional Hospital	High Point	North Carolina	336-878-6000	www.highpointregional.com
Holy Name Medical Center	Teaneck	New Jersey	201-833-3000	www.holyname.org
Homestead Hospital	Homestead	Florida	786-243-8000	www.baptisthealth.net
Hospital De La Concepcion	San German	Puerto Rico	787-892-1860	www.hospitalconcepcion.org
Hospital of Univ of Pennsylvania	Philadelphia	Pennsylvania	215-662-3227	www.upenn.edu
Hudson Valley Hospital Center	Cortlandt Manor	New York	914-734-3611	www.hvhc.org
Indiana University Health Bloomington Hospital	Bloomington	Indiana	812-353-9555	www.bloomingtonhospital.org
Ingalls Memorial Hospital	Harvey	Illinois	708-333-2300	www.ingalls.org
Jamaica Hospital Medical Center	Jamaica	New York	718-262-6000	www.jamaicahospital.org
JFK Medical Center	Atlantis	Florida	561-965-7300	www.jfkmc.com
John Dempsey Hospital	Farmington	Connecticut	860-679-1145	www.uconnhealth.orgorwww.uchc.edu
Kaiser Foundation Hospital	Honolulu	Hawaii	808-432-0000	www.kaiserpermanente.com
Kaiser Foundation Hospital - Fremont/Hayward	Hayward	California	510-784-4000	www.kaiserpermanente.org
Kaiser Foundation Hospital - Manteca	Manteca	California	209-825-3700	www.healthy.kaiserpermanente.org
Kaiser Foundation Hospital - Orange Co-Anaheim	Anaheim	California	714-644-2000	www.healthy.kaiserpermanente.org
Kaiser Foundation Hospital - Redwood City	Redwood City	California	650-299-2000	www.seiu-uhw.org/aboutuhw
Kaiser Foundation Hospital - Sacramento	Sacramento	California	916-973-5000	www.kaiserpermanente.org
Kaiser Foundation Hospital - Santa Clara	Santa Clara	California	408-236-6400	www.members.kaiserpermanente.org
Kaiser Foundation Hospital - South Bay	Harbor City	California	310-517-6441	www.kaiserpermanente.org
Kaiser Foundation Hospital - South San Francisco	South San Francisco	California	650-742-3200	www.healthy.kaiserpermanente.org
Kaiser Foundation Hospital South Sacramento	Sacramento	California	916-688-2000	www.mydoctor.kaiserpermanente.org
Kansas Medical Center	Andover	Kansas	316-300-4000	www.ksmedcenter.com
Keck Hospital of USC	Los Angeles	California	323-442-8656	www.uscuh.com
La Palma Intercommunity Hospital	La Palma	California	714-670-7400	www.lapalmaintercommunityhospital.com
Lakeview Hospital	Bountiful	Utah	801-299-2211	www.lakeviewhospital.com
Lakeview Regional Medical Center	Covington	Louisiana	985-867-4443	www.lakeviewregional.com
Laredo Medical Center	Laredo	Texas	956-796-5000	www.laredomedical.com
Las Colinas Medical Center	Irving	Texas	972-969-2000	www.lascolinas.com
Lawnwood Regional Medical Center & Heart Institute	Fort Pierce	Florida	772-461-4000	www.lawnwoodmed.com
Lawrence Memorial Hospital	Lawrence	Kansas	785-505-6100	www.lmh.org
Lewisgale Medical Center	Salem	Virginia	540-776-4000	www.lewis-gale.com
Loyola University Medical Center	Maywood	Illinois	708-216-9000	www.lumc.edu
Manatee Memorial Hospital	Bradenton	Florida	941-746-5111	www.manateememorial.com
Mary Greeley Medical Center	Ames	Iowa	515-239-2011	www.mgmc.org
Medical Center of Arlington	Arlington	Texas	817-465-3241	www.medicalcenterarlington.com
Medical Center of Trinity	Trinity	Florida	727-848-1733	www.communityhospitalnpr.com

Hospital	City	State	Phone	Web Site
Memorial Regional Hospital	Hollywood	Florida	954-987-2000	www.memorialregional.com
Mercy Fitzgerald Hospital	Darby	Pennsylvania	215-237-4000	www.mercyhealth.org
Methodist Mansfield Medical Center	Mansfield	Texas	682-622-2059	www.methodisthealthsystem.com
Methodist Sugar Land Hospital	Sugar Land	Texas	281-274-8000	www.methodisthealth.com/sugarland
Metropolitan Hospital of Miami	Miami	Florida	305-264-1000	www.pahnet.org
Mid Coast Hospital	Brunswick	Maine	207-729-0181	www.midcoasthealth.com
Newark Beth Israel Medical Center	Newark	New Jersey	973-926-7850	www.sbhcs.com
North Florida Regional Medical Center	Gainesville	Florida	352-333-4100	www.nfrmc.com
North Hills Hospital	North Richland Hills	Texas	817-255-1000	www.northhillshospital.com
North Okaloosa Medical Center	Crestview	Florida	850-689-8100	www.northokaloosa.com
North Suburban Medical Center	Thornton	Colorado	303-451-7800	www.northsuburban.com
Novant Health Forsyth Medical Center	Winston-Salem	North Carolina	336-718-5000	www.forsythmedicalcenter.org
NYU Hospitals Center	New York	New York	212-263-7300	www.med.nyu.edu
Ocala Regional Medical Center	Ocala	Florida	352-401-1000	www.ocalaregional.com
Orange Park Medical Center	Orange Park	Florida	904-276-8500	www.opmedical.com
Palms West Hospital	Loxahatchee	Florida	561-753-4245	www.palmswesthospital.com
Paradise Valley Hospital	Phoenix	Arizona	602-923-5000	www.paradisevalleyhospital.com
Paradise Valley Hospital	National City	California	619-470-4321	www.paradisevalleyhospital.org
Parma Community General Hospital	Parma	Ohio	440-743-3000	www.parmahopsital.org
Penn Presbyterian Medical Center	Philadelphia	Pennsylvania	215-662-8000	www.pennhealth.com
Phelps Memorial Hospital Assn	Sleepy Hollow	New York	914-366-3000	www.phelpshospital.org
Pikeville Medical Center	Pikeville	Kentucky	606-218-3500	www.pikevillehospital.org
Plaza Medical Center of Fort Worth	Fort Worth	Texas	817-336-2100	www.plazamedicalcenter.com
Porter Regional Hospital	Valparaiso	Indiana	219-983-8300	www.portermemorial.org
Portsmouth Regional Hospital	Portsmouth	New Hampshire	603-436-5110	www.portsmouthhospital.com
Presbyterian Community Hospital	San Juan	Puerto Rico	787-721-2160	www.presbypr.com
Providence Memorial Hospital	El Paso	Texas	915-577-6011	www.sphn.com
Riverside Community Hospital	Riverside	California	951-788-3000	www.rchc.org
Riverside Methodist Hospital	Columbus	Ohio	614-566-5000	www.ohiohealth.com
Riverview Regional Medical Center	Gadsden	Alabama	256-543-5200	www.riverviewregional.com
Roper Hospital	Charleston	South Carolina	843-724-2800	www.ropersaintfrancis.com
Rose Medical Center	Denver	Colorado	303-320-2121	www.rosemed.com
Round Rock Medical Center	Round Rock	Texas	512-341-1000	www.roundrockmedicalcenter.com
Saint Anthony Hospital	Oklahoma City	Oklahoma	405-272-7000	www.saintsok.com
Saint John's Riverside Hospital	Yonkers	New York	914-964-4444	www.riversidehealth.org
Saint Luke's Magic Valley Rmc	Twin Falls	Idaho	208-814-1000	www.stlukesonline.org/magic_valley
Saint Mary Medical Center	Hobart	Indiana	219-942-0551	www.comhs.org/stmary
Saint Mary Medical Center	Langhorne	Pennsylvania	215-750-2003	www.stmaryhealthcare.org
Saint Mary's Health Center	Jefferson City	Missouri	573-761-7000	www.stmarys-jeffcity.com
Saint Mary's Hospital - Passaic	Passaic	New Jersey	973-365-4300	www.smh-nj.com
Sanford Medical Center Bismarck	Bismarck	North Dakota	701-323-6000	www.medcenterone.com
Scripps Green Hospital	La Jolla	California	858-554-3600	www.scrippshealth.org
Scripps Memorial Hospital La Jolla	La Jolla	California	858-626-4123	www.scrippshealth.org
Sebastian River Medical Center	Sebastian	Florida	772-589-3187	www.srmcenter.com
Sentara Norfolk General Hospital	Norfolk	Virginia	757-388-3000	www.sentara.com
Shady Grove Adventist Hospital	Rockville	Maryland	240-826-6517	www.adventisthealthcare.com/sgah
Sistema Integrados De Salud Del Sur Oeste	Mayaguez	Puerto Rico	787-652-9200	
Southern Hills Hospital & Medical Center	Las Vegas	Nevada	702-880-2100	www.southernhillshospital.com
Spotsylvania Regional Medical Center	Fredericksburg	Virginia	540-498-4000	www.spotsrmc.com
SSM Depaul Health Center	Bridgeton	Missouri	314-344-6000	www.ssmdepaul.com
SSM Saint Marys Health Center	Richmond Heights	Missouri	314-768-8000	www.ssmhealth.com/stmarys
Sutter Medical Center of Santa Rosa	Santa Rosa	California	707-576-4000	www.suttersantarosa.org
University Hospital	Newark	New Jersey	973-972-5658	www.theuniversityhospital.com
University of South Alabama Medical Center	Mobile	Alabama	251-471-7110	www.southalabama.edu/usamc
Venice Regional Medical Center - Bayfront Health	Venice	Florida	941-485-7711	www.veniceregional.com
Vista Medical Center East	Waukegan	Illinois	847-360-4000	www.vistahealth.com
Walker Baptist Medical Center	Jasper	Alabama	205-387-4000	www.bhsala.com/walker
Wellmont Bristol Regional Medical Center	Bristol	Tennessee	423-844-1121	www.wellmont.org
Wesley Medical Center	Wichita	Kansas	316-962-2000	www.wesleymc.com
West Florida Hospital	Pensacola	Florida	850-494-4000	www.westfloridahospital.com
West Virginia University Hospitals	Morgantown	West Virginia	304-598-4000	www.wvuh.com
Wichita VA Medical Center	Wichita	Kansas	316-685-2221	www.wichita.va.gov

Note: The 127 hospitals shown above all achieved a perfect 100% average score. Average scores were calculated for hospitals with qualifying data (25 cases or more) in at least 5 of 11 measures in the following categories: Chest Pain/Possible Heart Attack; Heart Attack; Heart Failure. A total of 2,234 hospitals nationwide were considered.

Best Hospitals for Pneumonia Care

Hospital	City	State	Phone	Web Site
Abilene Regional Medical Center	Abilene	Texas	325-428-1000	www.abileneregional.com
Advocate Christ Hospital & Medical Center	Oak Lawn	Illinois	708-684-8000	www.advocatehealth.com
Advocate Illinois Masonic Medical Center	Chicago	Illinois	773-975-1600	www.advocatehealth.com/immc
Alaska Regional Hospital	Anchorage	Alaska	907-276-1131	www.alaskaregional.com
Alegent Creighton Health Creighton University Med	Omaha	Nebraska	402-449-4000	www.creightonhospital.com
Alegent Creighton Health Midlands Hospital	Papillion	Nebraska	402-593-3000	www.alegent.com
Allegheny General Hospital	Pittsburgh	Pennsylvania	412-359-3131	www.allhealth.edu
Asante Ashland Community Hospital	Ashland	Oregon	541-201-4001	www.ashlandhospital.org
Asante Rogue Regional Medical Center	Medford	Oregon	541-789-7000	www.asante.org
Ashtabula County Medical Center	Ashtabula	Ohio	440-997-2262	www.acmchealth.org
Aurora Baycare Medical Center	Green Bay	Wisconsin	920-288-8000	www.aurorabaycare.com
Aurora West Allis Medical Center	West Allis	Wisconsin	414-328-6000	www.aurorahealthcare.org
Aventura Hospital & Medical Center	Aventura	Florida	305-682-7000	www.aventurahospital.com
Avera Marshall Regional Medical Center	Marshall	Minnesota	507-537-9661	www.averamarshall.org
Baptist Hospital of Miami	Miami	Florida	786-596-1960	www.baptisthealth.net
Baptist Memorial Hospital Huntingdon	Huntingdon	Tennessee	731-986-4461	www.bmhcc.org
Baptist Memorial Hospital North Mississippi	Oxford	Mississippi	662-232-8100	www.baptistonline.org/facilities/oxford
Baptist Memorial Hospital Union City	Union City	Tennessee	731-885-2410	www.bmhcc.org
Beaumont Health System	Grosse Pointe	Michigan	313-343-1000	www.beaumonthospitals.com
Bellevue Medical Center	Bellevue	Nebraska	402-763-3600	www.bellevuemed.com
Berkshire Medical Center	Pittsfield	Massachusetts	413-447-2000	www.berkshirehealthsystems.org
Big Bend Regional Medical Center	Alpine	Texas	432-837-3447	www.bigbendhealthcare.com
Bolivar Medical Center	Cleveland	Mississippi	662-846-2551	www.bolivarmedical.com
Bon Secours Memorial Regional Medical Center	Mechanicsville	Virginia	804-764-6000	www.bonsecours.com
Bonner General Hospital	Sandpoint	Idaho	208-263-1441	www.bonnergeneral.org
Brigham & Women's Faulkner Hospital	Boston	Massachusetts	617-983-7000	www.brighamandwomensfaulkner.org
Broadlawns Medical Center	Des Moines	Iowa	515-282-2200	www.broadlawns.org
Brookings Hospital	Brookings	South Dakota	605-696-7701	www.brookingshospital.org
Broward Health North	Pompano Beach	Florida	954-786-6950	www.browardhealth.org
Buchanan General Hospital	Grundy	Virginia	276-935-1000	www.bgh.org
Bucyrus Community Hospital	Bucyrus	Ohio	419-562-4677	www.bchonline.org
California Pacific Medical Center - Pacific Campus Hospital	San Francisco	California	415-600-6000	www.cpmc.org
California Pacific Medical Center - Saint Luke's Campus	San Francisco	California	415-641-6562	www.stlukes.sf.org
Carepoint Health - Bayonne Hospital Center	Bayonne	New Jersey	201-858-5000	www.bayonnemedicalcenter.org
Carney Hospital	Boston	Massachusetts	617-506-2000	www.caritascarney.org
Carolinas Hospital System	Florence	South Carolina	843-674-2500	www.carolinashospital.com
Centinela Hospital Medical Center	Inglewood	California	310-673-4660	www.centinelafreeman.com
Central Peninsula General Hospital	Soldotna	Alaska	907-262-4404	www.cpgh.org
Chatuge Regional Hospital	Hiawassee	Georgia	706-896-2222	www.chatugeregionalhospital.org
Coffee Regional Medical Center	Douglas	Georgia	229-384-1900	www.coffeeregional.org
Conroe Regional Medical Center	Conroe	Texas	936-539-1111	www.conroeregional.com
Coosa Valley Medical Center	Sylacauga	Alabama	256-249-5000	www.cvhealth.net
Coral Gables Hospital	Coral Gables	Florida	305-445-8461	www.coralgableshospital.com
The Corpus Christi Medical Center	Corpus Christi	Texas	361-761-1501	www.ccmedicalcenter.com
Davis Hospital & Medical Center	Layton	Utah	801-807-1000	www.davishospital.com
Delray Medical Center	Delray Beach	Florida	561-498-4440	www.delraymedicalctr.com
Detar Hospital Navarro	Victoria	Texas	361-575-7441	www.detar.com
Detroit (John D. Dingell) VA Medical Center	Detroit	Michigan	313-576-1000	www.detroit.va.gov
Doctors Hospital	Augusta	Georgia	706-651-6008	www.doctors-hospital.net
Dominican Hospital	Santa Cruz	California	831-462-7700	www.dominicanhospital.org
Down East Community Hospital	Machias	Maine	207-255-3356	www.dech.org
Dupont Hospital	Fort Wayne	Indiana	260-416-3000	www.theduponthospital.com
East Texas Medical Center - Gilmer	Gilmer	Texas	903-841-7100	www.etmc.org
Eastern Idaho Regional Medical Center	Idaho Falls	Idaho	208-529-6111	www.eirmc.org
El Camino Hospital	Mountain View	California	650-940-7000	www.elcaminohospital.org
Encino Hospital Medical Center	Encino	California	818-995-5000	www.encino-tarzana.com
Englewood Community Hospital	Englewood	Florida	941-475-6571	www.englewoodcommunityhospital.com
Excela Health Latrobe Hospital	Latrobe	Pennsylvania	724-537-1000	www.excelahealth.org
Faith Regional Health Services	Norfolk	Nebraska	402-371-4880	www.frhs.org
Falmouth Hospital	Falmouth	Massachusetts	508-548-5300	www.capecodhealth.com
Fannin Regional Hospital	Blue Ridge	Georgia	706-632-3711	www.fanninregionalhospital.com
Fawcett Memorial Hospital	Port Charlotte	Florida	941-629-1181	www.fawcetthospital.com
Florida Hospital North Pinellas	Tarpon Springs	Florida	727-942-5000	www.hemh.com
Flowers Hospital	Dothan	Alabama	334-793-5000	www.flowershospital.com
Forest Hills Hospital	Forest Hills	New York	718-830-4000	www.northshorelij.com

Hospital	City	State	Phone	Web Site
Fostoria Community Hospital	Fostoria	Ohio	419-435-7734	www.promedica.org
Franciscan Saint Anthony Health - Michigan City	Michigan City	Indiana	219-879-8511	www.samhc.org
Franciscan Saint Elizabeth Health - Lafayette East	Lafayette	Indiana	765-502-4334	www.ste.org
Frankfort Regional Medical Center	Frankfort	Kentucky	502-875-5240	www.frankfortregional.com
Garden Grove Hospital & Medical Center	Garden Grove	California	714-537-5160	www.gardengrovehospital.com
Garden Park Medical Center	Gulfport	Mississippi	228-575-7000	www.gardenparkmedical.com
Genesis Medical Center - Davenport	Davenport	Iowa	563-421-1000	www.genesishealth.com
Georgetown Memorial Hospital	Georgetown	South Carolina	843-527-7000	www.gmhsc.com
Good Samaritan Hospital Medical Center	West Islip	New York	631-376-3000	www.good-samaritan-hospital.org
Greene Memorial Hospital	Xenia	Ohio	937-352-2000	www.ketteringhealth.org/greene
Hackensack - Umc Mountainside	Montclair	New Jersey	973-429-6000	www.mountainsidenow.org
Hackettstown Regional Medical Center	Hackettstown	New Jersey	908-852-5100	www.hrmcnj.org
Hammond Henry Hospital	Geneseo	Illinois	309-944-6431	www.hammondhenry.com
Hardin Memorial Hospital	Kenton	Ohio	419-673-0761	www.hardinmemorial.org
Harlingen Medical Center	Harlingen	Texas	956-365-1000	www.harlingenmedicalcenter.com
Heart of Lancaster Regional Medical Center	Lititz	Pennsylvania	717-625-5000	www.heartoflancaster.com
Helena Regional Medical Center	Helena	Arkansas	870-338-5800	www.helenaregionalmedicalcenter.com
Henderson County Community Hospital	Lexington	Tennessee	731-968-1801	www.hendersonchospital.com
Holy Family Memorial	Manitowoc	Wisconsin	920-320-2011	www.hfmhealth.org
Hospital Pavia Santurce	Fernandez Juncos	Puerto Rico	787-727-6060	www.paviahospitalsanturce.com
Howard Memorial Hospital	Nashville	Arkansas	870-845-4400	www.howardmemorial.com
Huntington Beach Hospital	Huntington Beach	California	714-843-5000	www.hbhospital.com
Hutchinson Health	Hutchinson	Minnesota	320-234-5000	www.hahc-hmc.com
Ingalls Memorial Hospital	Harvey	Illinois	708-333-2300	www.ingalls.org
Intermountain Medical Center	Murray	Utah	801-507-7000	www.intermountainhealthcare.org
Jackson Hospital & Clinic	Montgomery	Alabama	334-293-8000	www.jackson.org
Jamaica Hospital Medical Center	Jamaica	New York	718-262-6000	www.jamaicahospital.org
Jay Hospital	Jay	Florida	850-675-4532	www.bhcpns.org
Jefferson Medical Center	Ranson	West Virginia	304-728-1600	www.jeffmem.com
Jennings American Legion Hospital	Jennings	Louisiana	337-616-7000	www.jalh.com
JFK Medical Center	Atlantis	Florida	561-965-7300	www.jfkmc.com
The Johns Hopkins Hospital	Baltimore	Maryland	410-955-9540	www.jhmi.edu
Kaiser Foundation Hospital - Orange Co-Anaheim	Anaheim	California	714-644-2000	www.healthy.kaiserpermanente.org
Kaiser Foundation Hospital - San Jose	San Jose	California	408-972-7000	www.mydoctor.kaiserpermanente.org
Kaiser Foundation Hospital - Santa Clara	Santa Clara	California	408-236-6400	www.members.kaiserpermanente.org
Kendall Regional Medical Center	Miami	Florida	305-223-3000	www.kendallmed.com
Kenmore Mercy Hospital	Kenmore	New York	716-447-6100	www.chsbuffalo.org
Kennewick General Hospital	Kennewick	Washington	509-586-6111	www.kennewickgeneral.com
Lake City Medical Center	Lake City	Florida	386-719-9000	www.lakecitymedical.com
Lake Forest Hospital	Lake Forest	Illinois	847-234-5600	www.lakeforesthospital.com
Lake Wales Medical Center	Lake Wales	Florida	863-676-1433	www.lakewalesmedicalcenter.com
Lakeview Medical Center	Rice Lake	Wisconsin	715-234-1515	www.lakeviewmedical.com
Lakeview Regional Medical Center	Covington	Louisiana	985-867-4443	www.lakeviewregional.com
Lancaster Regional Medical Center	Lancaster	Pennsylvania	717-291-8123	www.lancasterregional.com
Laredo Medical Center	Laredo	Texas	956-796-5000	www.laredomedical.com
Largo Medical Center	Largo	Florida	727-588-5200	www.largomedical.com
Las Colinas Medical Center	Irving	Texas	972-969-2000	www.lascolinas.com
Lawnwood Regional Medical Center & Heart Institute	Fort Pierce	Florida	772-461-4000	www.lawnwoodmed.com
Lawrence Memorial Hospital	Walnut Ridge	Arkansas	870-886-1200	www.lawrencehealth.net
Lee's Summit Medical Center	Lees Summit	Missouri	816-282-5000	www.leessummithospital.com
Lehigh Regional Medical Center	Lehigh Acres	Florida	239-369-2101	www.lehighregional.com
Lewisgale Hospital Montgomery	Blacksburg	Virginia	540-951-1111	www.mrhospital.com
Lewisgale Medical Center	Salem	Virginia	540-776-4000	www.lewis-gale.com
Libertyhealth - Jersey City Medical Center Campus	Jersey City	New Jersey	201-915-2000	www.libertyhcs.org
Little Company of Mary Hospital	Evergreen Park	Illinois	708-422-6200	www.lcmh.org
Littleton Regional Healthcare	Littleton	New Hampshire	603-444-9000	www.littletonhospital.org
Lock Haven Hospital	Lock Haven	Pennsylvania	570-893-5000	www.lockhavenhospital.com
Lucas County Health Center	Chariton	Iowa	641-774-3000	www.lchcia.com
Marin General Hospital	Greenbrae	California	415-925-7900	www.maringeneral.com
Mary Greeley Medical Center	Ames	Iowa	515-239-2011	www.mgmc.org
Maryvale Hospital	Phoenix	Arizona	623-848-5000	www.maryvalehospital.com
Mat-Su Regional Medical Center	Palmer	Alaska	907-746-8600	www.matsuregional.com
Mayo Clinic Health System - Fairmont	Fairmont	Minnesota	507-238-8101	www.fairmontmedicalcenter.org
Mayo Clinic Health System - Northland	Barron	Wisconsin	715-537-3186	www.luthermidelfortnorthland.org
McKenzie Regional Hospital	Mc Kenzie	Tennessee	731-352-5344	www.mckenzieregionalhospital.com
Mease Hospital Dunedin	Dunedin	Florida	727-733-1111	www.measehospitals.com
Medical Center of Arlington	Arlington	Texas	817-465-3241	www.medicalcenterarlington.com

Hospital	City	State	Phone	Web Site
Medical Center of Trinity	Trinity	Florida	727-848-1733	www.communityhospitalnpr.com
Medical City Dallas Hospital	Dallas	Texas	972-566-6222	www.medicalcityhospital.com
Medwest Swain	Bryson City	North Carolina	828-488-2155	www.westcarehealth.org
Memorial Healthcare System	Chattanooga	Tennessee	423-495-2525	www.memorial.org
Memorial Hospital Los Banos	Los Banos	California	209-826-0591	www.memoriallosbanos.org
Memorial Hospital Pembroke	Pembroke Pines	Florida	954-962-9650	www.memorialpembroke.com\
Memorial Hospital West	Pembroke Pines	Florida	954-436-5000	www.memorialwest.com
Memorial Regional Hospital	Hollywood	Florida	954-987-2000	www.memorialregional.com
Menorah Medical Center	Overland Park	Kansas	913-498-6773	www.menorahmedicalcenter.com
Mercy General Hospital	Sacramento	California	916-453-4545	www.mercygeneral.org
Mercy Hospital - Fort Scott	Fort Scott	Kansas	620-223-7057	www.mercy.net
Mercy Hospital of Defiance	Defiance	Ohio	419-782-8444	www.mercyweb.org/mercy_defiance.aspx
Mercy Medical Center	Springfield	Massachusetts	413-748-9000	www.mercycares.com
Mercy Regional Health Center	Manhattan	Kansas	785-776-2831	www.mercyregional.org
Methodist Medical Center of Oak Ridge	Oak Ridge	Tennessee	865-835-1000	www.mmcoakridge.com
Methodist Richardson Medical Center	Richardson	Texas	972-498-4000	www.richardsonregional.com
Metroplex Hospital	Killeen	Texas	254-526-7523	www.mplex.org
Minden Medical Center	Minden	Louisiana	318-377-2321	www.mindenmedicalcenter.com
Ministry Sacred Heart Hospital	Tomahawk	Wisconsin	715-453-7700	www.ministryhealth.org
Ministry Saint Marys Hospital	Rhinelander	Wisconsin	715-361-2000	www.ministryhealth.org
Ministry Saint Michaels Hospital of Stevens Point	Stevens Point	Wisconsin	715-346-5000	www.saintmichaelshospital.org
Moberly Regional Medical Center	Moberly	Missouri	660-263-8400	www.moberlyhospital.com
Monmouth Medical Center - Southern Campus	Lakewood	New Jersey	732-363-1900	www.sbhcs.com
Mount Pleasant Hospital	Mount Pleasant	South Carolina	843-724-2954	www.rsfh.com
Mountain Home VA Medical Center	Mountain Home	Tennessee	423-926-1171	www.mountainhome.va.gov
Mountain View Hospital	Payson	Utah	801-465-7100	www.mvhpayson.com
Mountain View Regional Medical Center	Las Cruces	New Mexico	575-556-7600	www.mountainviewregional.com
Myrtue Medical Center	Harlan	Iowa	712-755-5161	www.shelbycohealth.com
New Ulm Medical Center	New Ulm	Minnesota	507-233-1000	www.newulmmedicalcenter.com
New York Community Hospital of Brooklyn	Brooklyn	New York	718-692-5302	www.nych.com
Noble Hospital	Westfield	Massachusetts	413-568-2811	www.noblehospital.org
North Austin Medical Center	Austin	Texas	512-901-1000	www.cornerstonehealthcaregroup.com
North Florida Regional Medical Center	Gainesville	Florida	352-333-4100	www.nfrmc.com
North Shore Medical Center	Miami	Florida	305-835-6000	www.northshoremedical.com
North Suburban Medical Center	Thornton	Colorado	303-451-7800	www.northsuburban.com
Northeast Regional Medical Center	Kirksville	Missouri	660-785-1000	www.nermc.com
Northern Westchester Hospital	Mount Kisco	New York	914-666-1200	www.nwhc.net
Northside Hospital	Saint Petersburg	Florida	813-521-5000	www.northsidehospital.com
Northside Hospital	Atlanta	Georgia	404-851-8000	www.northside.com
Northside Hospital Cherokee	Canton	Georgia	770-720-5298	www.northside.com/cherokee
Norwalk Hospital Association	Norwalk	Connecticut	203-852-2000	www.norwalkhosp.org
Novant Health Forsyth Medical Center	Winston-Salem	North Carolina	336-718-5000	www.forsythmedicalcenter.org
Novant Health Franklin Medical Center	Louisburg	North Carolina	919-496-5131	www.franklinregionalmedicalctr.com
Novant Health Huntersville Medical Center	Huntersville	North Carolina	704-316-4000	www.presbyterian.org
Novant Health Thomasville Medical Center	Thomasville	North Carolina	336-472-2000	www.thomasvillemedicalcenter.org
Oak Hill Hospital	Brooksville	Florida	352-596-6632	www.oakhillhospital.com
Oaklawn Hospital	Marshall	Michigan	269-781-4271	www.oaklawnhospital.org
OHSU Hospital & Clinics	Portland	Oregon	503-494-4036	www.ohsu.edu
Oklahoma State University Medical Center	Tulsa	Oklahoma	918-587-2561	www.tulsaregional.com
Orange Park Medical Center	Orange Park	Florida	904-276-8500	www.opmedical.com
Overton Brooks VA Medical Center - Shreveport	Shreveport	Louisiana	318-424-6037	www.va.gov/sta/guide/home.asp
Palm Bay Hospital	Palm Bay	Florida	321-434-8000	www.health-first.org
Parkway Regional Hospital	Fulton	Kentucky	270-472-2522	www.parkwayregionalhospital.com
Piggott Community Hospital	Piggott	Arkansas	870-598-3881	www.piggottcommunityhospital.com
Plateau Medical Center	Oak Hill	West Virginia	304-469-8600	www.plateaumedicalcenter.com
Pleasant Valley Hospital	Point Pleasant	West Virginia	304-675-4340	www.pvalley.org
Pomerene Hospital	Millersburg	Ohio	330-674-1015	www.pomerenehospital.org
Portsmouth Regional Hospital	Portsmouth	New Hampshire	603-436-5110	www.portsmouthhospital.com
Promedica Herrick Hospital	Tecumseh	Michigan	517-424-3000	www.promedica.org/herrick
Putnam General Hospital	Eatonton	Georgia	706-485-2711	www.putnamgeneral.com
Rapides Regional Medical Center	Alexandria	Louisiana	318-769-3000	www.rapidesregional.com
Raulerson Hospital	Okeechobee	Florida	863-763-2151	www.raulersonhospital.com
Regional Hospital of Jackson	Jackson	Tennessee	731-661-2000	www.regionalhospitaljackson.com
Regional Medical Center of San Jose	San Jose	California	408-259-5000	www.regionalmedicalsanjose.com
Renown South Meadows Medical Center	Reno	Nevada	775-982-7000	www.renown.org
River Parishes Hospital	Laplace	Louisiana	985-652-7000	www.riverparisheshospital.com
Riverview Medical Center	Red Bank	New Jersey	732-741-2700	www.meridianhealth.com

Hospital	City	State	Phone	Web Site
Rockford Memorial Hospital	Rockford	Illinois	815-968-6861	www.rhsnet.org
Roper Hospital	Charleston	South Carolina	843-724-2800	www.ropersaintfrancis.com
Rose Medical Center	Denver	Colorado	303-320-2121	www.rosemed.com
Roxborough Memorial Hospital	Philadelphia	Pennsylvania	215-483-9900	www.roxboroughmemorial.com
Saint Anthony Hospital	Chicago	Illinois	773-521-1710	www.cath-health.org
Saint Anthony Shawnee Hospital	Shawnee	Oklahoma	405-273-2270	www.unityhealthcenter.com
Saint Anthony's Health Center	Alton	Illinois	618-465-2571	www.sahc.org
Saint Barnabas Medical Center	Livingston	New Jersey	973-322-5000	www.saintbarnabas.com
Saint Catherine Hospital	East Chicago	Indiana	219-392-7004	www.comhs.org/stcatherine
Saint Clare Hospital Health Services	Baraboo	Wisconsin	608-356-1400	www.stclare.com
Saint Clares Hospital of Weston	Weston	Wisconsin	715-393-3000	www.ministryhealth.org
Saint Francis Hospital	Escanaba	Michigan	906-786-3311	www.osfstfrancis.or
Saint Francis Medical Center	Trenton	New Jersey	609-599-5000	www.stfrancismedical.com
Saint James Hospital	Pontiac	Illinois	815-842-2828	www.osfsaintjames.org
Saint Joseph Hospital	Fort Wayne	Indiana	260-425-3000	www.stjoehospital.com
Saint Joseph Hospital & Health Center	Kokomo	Indiana	765-456-5300	www.stvincent.org
Saint Joseph Mercy Port Huron	Port Huron	Michigan	810-985-1510	www.mercyporthuron.com
Saint Joseph Regional Medical Center - Plymouth	Plymouth	Indiana	574-948-4000	www.sjmed.com
Saint Joseph's Hospital	Breese	Illinois	618-526-4511	www.stjoebreese.com
Saint Joseph's Mercy Health Center	Hot Springs	Arkansas	501-622-1000	www.saintjosephs.com
Saint Louise Regional Hospital	Gilroy	California	408-848-2000	www.saintlouiseregionalhospital.org
Saint Lucie Medical Center	Port Saint Lucie	Florida	772-335-4000	www.stluciemed.com
Saint Luke's Magic Valley Rmc	Twin Falls	Idaho	208-814-1000	www.stlukesonline.org/magic_valley
Saint Luke's Quakertown Hospital	Quakertown	Pennsylvania	215-538-4500	www.slhn-lehighvalley.com
Saint Margarets Hospital	Spring Valley	Illinois	815-664-1176	www.aboutsmh.org
Saint Mary Medical Center	Hobart	Indiana	219-942-0551	www.comhs.org/stmary
Saint Mary's Good Samaritan Hospital	Greensboro	Georgia	706-453-7331	www.stmarysgoodsam.org
Saint Vincent Anderson Regional Hospital	Anderson	Indiana	765-646-8373	www.stjohnshealthsystem.org
Saint Vincent's Birmingham	Birmingham	Alabama	205-939-7000	www.stv.org
Saint Vincent's East	Birmingham	Alabama	205-838-3122	www.nolandhealth.com
Saint Vincent's Medical Center Southside	Jacksonville	Florida	904-296-3700	www.jaxhealth.com
Samaritan Hospital	Moses Lake	Washington	509-765-5606	www.samaritanhealthcare.com
San Angelo Community Medical Center	San Angelo	Texas	325-949-9511	www.sacmc.com
Scripps Mercy Hospital	San Diego	California	619-294-8111	www.scrippshealth.org
Sebastian River Medical Center	Sebastian	Florida	772-589-3187	www.srmcenter.com
Seton Highland Lakes	Burnet	Texas	512-715-3000	www.seton.net
Shands Lake Shore Regional Medical Center	Lake City	Florida	386-292-8000	www.shands.org
Sharp Coronado Hospital & Healthcare Center	Coronado	California	619-435-6251	www.sharp.com/coronado
Shasta Regional Medical Center	Redding	California	530-244-5454	www.shastaregional.com
Sibley Memorial Hospital	Washington	District of Columbia	202-537-4680	www.sibley.org
Signature Healthcare Brockton Hospital	Brockton	Massachusetts	508-941-7000	www.brocktonhospital.com
Silverton Hospital	Silverton	Oregon	503-873-1500	www.silvertonhospital.org
Singing River Hospital	Pascagoula	Mississippi	228-809-5000	www.srhshealth.com
Sisters of Charity Hospital	Buffalo	New York	716-862-1000	www.chsbuffalo.org
South Miami Hospital	South Miami	Florida	786-662-4000	www.baptisthealth.net
Southern Nh Medical Center	Nashua	New Hampshire	603-577-2000	www.snhmc.org
Sparks Regional Medical Center	Fort Smith	Arkansas	501-441-4000	www.sparks.org
Spokane VA Medical Center	Spokane	Washington	509-434-7000	www.spokane.med.va.gov
Spotsylvania Regional Medical Center	Fredericksburg	Virginia	540-498-4000	www.spotsrmc.com
Stafford Hospital	Stafford	Virginia	540-741-9000	www.marywashingtonhealthcare.com
Staten Island University Hospital	Staten Island	New York	718-226-9000	www.siuh.edu
Summit Medical Center	Van Buren	Arkansas	479-471-4300	www.summitmc.net
Sutter Medical Center of Santa Rosa	Santa Rosa	California	707-576-4000	www.suttersantarosa.org
Sycamore Medical Center	Miamisburg	Ohio	937-384-8776	www.khnetwork.org/sycamore
Takoma Regional Hospital	Greeneville	Tennessee	423-639-3151	www.takoma.org
Texas Health Arlington Memorial Hospital	Arlington	Texas	817-548-6100	www.texashealth.org
Texas Health Harris Methodist Hospital Alliance	Fort Worth	Texas	682-212-2004	www.texashealth.org/alliance
Texoma Medical Center	Denison	Texas	903-416-4000	www.texomamedicalcenter.net
Thorek Memorial Hospital	Chicago	Illinois	312-525-6780	www.thorek.org
Three Rivers Medical Center	Louisa	Kentucky	606-638-9451	www.threeriversmedicalcenter.com
Togus VA Medical Center	Augusta	Maine	207-623-8411	www.maine.va.gov
Transylvania Regional Hospital	Brevard	North Carolina	828-883-5302	www.tchospital.org
Trinity Medical Center	Birmingham	Alabama	205-592-1000	www.bhsala.com/montclair
Tristar Hendersonville Medical Center	Hendersonville	Tennessee	615-338-1000	www.hendersonvillemedicalcenter.com
Tristar Southern Hills Medical Center	Nashville	Tennessee	615-781-4000	www.southernhills.com
Tristar Stonecrest Medical Center	Smyrna	Tennessee	615-768-2000	www.stonecrestmedical.com
Tucson Medical Center	Tucson	Arizona	520-327-5461	www.tmcaz.com

Hospital	City	State	Phone	Web Site
Twin Cities Hospital	Niceville	Florida	850-678-4131	www.tchealthcare.com
UH Geauga Medical Center	Chardon	Ohio	440-269-6000	www.uhgeauga.org
UHHS Memorial Hospital of Geneva	Geneva	Ohio	440-466-1141	www.uhhospitals.org/geneva
University of Maryland Medical Center	Baltimore	Maryland	410-328-8667	www.umm.edu
University of Miami Hospital	Miami	Florida	305-325-5511	www.cedarsmedicalcenter.com
UPMC Mckeesport	Mc Keesport	Pennsylvania	412-664-2000	www.selectmedicalcorp.com
VA Pittsburgh Healthcare System	Pittsburgh	Pennsylvania	412-688-6100	www.pittsburg.va.gov
Valley West Community Hospital	Sandwich	Illinois	815-786-8484	www.snd.softfarm.com/sandhosp
Venice Regional Medical Center - Bayfront Health	Venice	Florida	941-485-7711	www.veniceregional.com
Viera Hospital	Melbourne	Florida	321-434-9000	www.health-first.org
Waupun Memorial Hospital	Waupun	Wisconsin	920-324-6530	www.agnesian.com
Wayne County Hospital	Monticello	Kentucky	606-348-9343	www.waynehospital.org
Weatherford Regional Medical Center	Weatherford	Texas	817-599-1190	www.campbellhealth.com
Wesley Medical Center	Wichita	Kansas	316-962-2000	www.wesleymc.com
West Palm Hospital	West Palm Beach	Florida	561-844-6141	www.columbiahospital.com
Western Pennsylvania Hospital	Pittsburgh	Pennsylvania	412-578-5000	www.wpahs.org/wph/contact/index.html
White County Medical Center	Searcy	Arkansas	501-278-3100	www.centralarkhospital.com
Wichita VA Medical Center	Wichita	Kansas	316-685-2221	www.wichita.va.gov
Wilcox Memorial Hospital	Lihue	Hawaii	808-245-1103	www.wilcoxhealth.org
William Beaumont Hospital - Troy	Troy	Michigan	248-964-8800	www.beaumonthospitals.com
Williamsport Regional Medical Center	Williamsport	Pennsylvania	570-321-1000	www.susquehannahealth.org
Woodward Regional Hospital	Woodward	Oklahoma	580-254-8492	www.woodwardhospital.com

Note: The 288 hospitals shown above all achieved a perfect 100% average score. Average scores were calculated for hospitals with qualifying data (25 cases or more) in both measures in the Pneumonia Care category. A total of 3,347 hospitals nationwide were considered.

Best Hospitals for Preventative Care

Hospital	City	State	Phone	Web Site
Abilene Regional Medical Center	Abilene	Texas	325-428-1000	www.abileneregional.com
Adena Regional Medical Center	Chillicothe	Ohio	740-779-7500	www.adena.org
Alton Memorial Hospital	Alton	Illinois	618-463-7300	www.altonmemorialhospital.org
Arizona Spine & Joint Hospital	Mesa	Arizona	480-832-4770	www.azspineandjoint.com
Atrium Medical Center	Franklin	Ohio	513-420-5102	www.atriummedcenter.org
Avera Heart Hospital of South Dakota	Sioux Falls	South Dakota	605-977-7000	www.avera.org/heart-hospital
Bailey Medical Center	Owasso	Oklahoma	918-376-8000	www.baileymedicalcenter.com
Baptist Hospital of Miami	Miami	Florida	786-596-1960	www.baptisthealth.net
Baptist Memorial Hospital Huntingdon	Huntingdon	Tennessee	731-986-4461	www.bmhcc.org
Barstow Community Hospital	Barstow	California	760-256-1761	www.barstowhospital.com
Belton Regional Medical Center	Belton	Missouri	816-348-1236	www.beltonregionalmedicalcenter.com
Biloxi Regional Medical Center	Biloxi	Mississippi	228-436-1104	www.hmabrmc.com
Broward Health North	Pompano Beach	Florida	954-786-6950	www.browardhealth.org
Byrd Regional Hospital	Leesville	Louisiana	337-239-9041	www.chs.net
Calhoun Health Services	Calhoun City	Mississippi	662-628-6611	www.nmhs.net
Carepoint Health - Bayonne Hospital Center	Bayonne	New Jersey	201-858-5000	www.bayonnemedicalcenter.org
Carrington Health Center	Carrington	North Dakota	701-652-3141	www.carringtonhealthcenter.net
Centerpoint Medical Center	Independence	Missouri	816-698-7000	www.centerpointmedical.com
Centinela Hospital Medical Center	Inglewood	California	310-673-4660	www.centinelafreeman.com
Central Mississippi Medical Center	Jackson	Mississippi	601-376-1000	www.centralmississippimedicalcenter.com
Chesterfield General Hospital	Cheraw	South Carolina	843-537-7881	www.chesterfieldgeneral.com
Clay County Hospital	Flora	Illinois	618-662-2131	www.claycountyhospital.org
Coosa Valley Medical Center	Sylacauga	Alabama	256-249-5000	www.cvhealth.net
Coral Gables Hospital	Coral Gables	Florida	305-445-8461	www.coralgableshospital.com
The Corpus Christi Medical Center	Corpus Christi	Texas	361-761-1501	www.ccmedicalcenter.com
Cypress Pointe Hospital East	Slidell	Louisiana	504-690-8200	
Delray Medical Center	Delray Beach	Florida	561-498-4440	www.delraymedicalctr.com
Detar Hospital Navarro	Victoria	Texas	361-575-7441	www.detar.com
Dyersburg Regional Medical Center	Dyersburg	Tennessee	731-285-2410	www.dyersburgregionalmc.com
Encino Hospital Medical Center	Encino	California	818-995-5000	www.encino-tarzana.com
Fannin Regional Hospital	Blue Ridge	Georgia	706-632-3711	www.fanninregionalhospital.com
Flowers Hospital	Dothan	Alabama	334-793-5000	www.flowershospital.com
Garden Grove Hospital & Medical Center	Garden Grove	California	714-537-5160	www.gardengrovehospital.com
Garden Park Medical Center	Gulfport	Mississippi	228-575-7000	www.gardenparkmedical.com
Greenbrier Valley Medical Center	Ronceverte	West Virginia	304-647-4411	www.gvmc.com
Hedrick Medical Center	Chillicothe	Missouri	660-646-1480	www.saintlukeshealthsystem.org
Helena Regional Medical Center	Helena	Arkansas	870-338-5800	www.helenaregionalmedicalcenter.com
Henderson County Community Hospital	Lexington	Tennessee	731-968-1801	www.hendersoncchospital.com
Henry County Memorial Hospital	New Castle	Indiana	765-521-0890	www.hcmhcares.org
Heritage Medical Center	Shelbyville	Tennessee	931-685-5433	www.heritagemedicalcenter.com
Highlands Regional Medical Center	Sebring	Florida	863-385-6101	www.highlandsregional.com
Holy Name Medical Center	Teaneck	New Jersey	201-833-3000	www.holyname.org
The Hospital at Westlake Medical Center	Austin	Texas	512-327-0000	www.westlakemedical.com
Huntington Beach Hospital	Huntington Beach	California	714-843-5000	www.hbhospital.com
Indiana University Health Blackford Hospital	Hartford City	Indiana	765-348-0300	www.accesschs.org
Ingalls Memorial Hospital	Harvey	Illinois	708-333-2300	www.ingalls.org
Integris Mayes County Medical Center	Pryor	Oklahoma	918-825-1600	www.integris-health.com
Jeff Davis Hospital	Hazlehurst	Georgia	912-375-7781	www.jeffdavishospital.org
JFK Medical Center	Atlantis	Florida	561-965-7300	www.jfkmc.com
John Randolph Medical Center	Hopewell	Virginia	804-541-1600	www.johnrandolphmed.com
Kansas Medical Center	Andover	Kansas	316-300-4000	www.ksmedcenter.com
Kentucky River Medical Center	Jackson	Kentucky	606-666-6000	www.kentuckyrivermc.com
L V Stabler Memorial Hospital	Greenville	Alabama	334-382-2200	www.lvstabler.com
Lafayette Regional Health Center	Lexington	Missouri	660-259-2203	www.lafayetteregionalhealthcenter.com
Lakeview Regional Medical Center	Covington	Louisiana	985-867-4443	www.lakeviewregional.com
Laredo Medical Center	Laredo	Texas	956-796-5000	www.laredomedical.com
Lawnwood Regional Medical Center & Heart Institute	Fort Pierce	Florida	772-461-4000	www.lawnwoodmed.com
Lehigh Regional Medical Center	Lehigh Acres	Florida	239-369-2101	www.lehighregional.com
Lehigh Valley Hospital - Hazleton	Hazleton	Pennsylvania	570-501-4000	www.ghha.org
Lewisgale Medical Center	Salem	Virginia	540-776-4000	www.lewis-gale.com
Livingston Regional Hospital	Livingston	Tennessee	931-823-5611	www.livingstonregionalhospital.com
Logan Regional Medical Center	Logan	West Virginia	304-831-1350	www.loganregionalmedicalcenter.com
McNairy Regional Hospital	Selmer	Tennessee	731-645-3221	www.mcnairyregionalhospital.com
Medical Center of Plano	Plano	Texas	972-596-6800	www.medicalcenterofplano.com
Medical Center of Southeastern Oklahoma	Durant	Oklahoma	405-924-3080	www.mcsohealth.com

Hospital	City	State	Phone	Web Site
Medical Center South Arkansas	El Dorado	Arkansas	870-863-2000	www.themedcenter.net
Memorial Hospital Los Banos	Los Banos	California	209-826-0591	www.memoriallosbanos.org
Memorial Hospital Pembroke	Pembroke Pines	Florida	954-962-9650	www.memorialpembroke.com\
Memorial Hospital West	Pembroke Pines	Florida	954-436-5000	www.memorialwest.com
Menorah Medical Center	Overland Park	Kansas	913-498-6773	www.menorahmedicalcenter.com
Methodist Stone Oak Hospital	San Antonio	Texas	210-638-2100	www.stoneoakhealth.com
Mills - Peninsula Medical Center	Burlingame	California	650-696-5270	www.mills-peninsula.org
Mimbres Memorial Hospital	Deming	New Mexico	575-546-5803	www.mimbresmemorial.com
Minden Medical Center	Minden	Louisiana	318-377-2321	www.mindenmedicalcenter.com
Moberly Regional Medical Center	Moberly	Missouri	660-263-8400	www.moberlyhospital.com
Mount Desert Island Hospital	Bar Harbor	Maine	207-288-5081	www.mdihospital.com
Mountain View Hospital	Idaho Falls	Idaho	208-557-2899	www.mountainviewhospital.org
Mountain View Regional Medical Center	Las Cruces	New Mexico	575-556-7600	www.mountainviewregional.com
Newberry County Memorial Hospital	Newberry	South Carolina	803-405-7145	www.newberryhospital.org
North Carolina Specialty Hospital	Durham	North Carolina	919-956-9300	www.ncspecialty.com
Northeast Regional Medical Center	Kirksville	Missouri	660-785-1000	www.nermc.com
Northern Louisiana Medical Center	Ruston	Louisiana	318-254-2100	www.lincolnhealth.com
Northern Maine Medical Center	Fort Kent	Maine	207-834-3195	www.nmmc.org
Ocala Regional Medical Center	Ocala	Florida	352-401-1000	www.ocalaregional.com
Oconee Regional Medical Center	Milledgeville	Georgia	478-454-3550	www.oconeeregional.com
Oklahoma Heart Hospital South	Oklahoma City	Oklahoma	405-628-6000	www.okheart.com/south-campus
Oklahoma Surgical Hospital	Tulsa	Oklahoma	918-477-5000	www.oklahomasurgicalhospital.com
Orange Park Medical Center	Orange Park	Florida	904-276-8500	www.opmedical.com
Palm Springs General Hospital	Hialeah	Florida	305-558-2500	www.psghosp.com
Pampa Regional Medical Center	Pampa	Texas	806-665-3721	www.prmctx.com
Parkway Regional Hospital	Fulton	Kentucky	270-472-2522	www.parkwayregionalhospital.com
Person Memorial Hospital	Roxboro	North Carolina	336-599-2121	www.personhospital.com
Ponca City Medical Center	Ponca City	Oklahoma	580-765-3321	www.poncamedcenter.com
Rapides Regional Medical Center	Alexandria	Louisiana	318-769-3000	www.rapidesregional.com
Raulerson Hospital	Okeechobee	Florida	863-763-2151	www.raulersonhospital.com
Regional Hospital of Jackson	Jackson	Tennessee	731-661-2000	www.regionalhospitaljackson.com
Regional Medical Center Bayonet Point	Hudson	Florida	727-819-2929	www.mchealth.comorwww.heartoftampa.com
The Regional Medical Center of Acadiana	Lafayette	Louisiana	337-981-2949	www.medicalcentersw.com
Renown South Meadows Medical Center	Reno	Nevada	775-982-7000	www.renown.org
Research Medical Center	Kansas City	Missouri	816-276-4000	www.researchmedicalcenter.com
Riverview Medical Center	Red Bank	New Jersey	732-741-2700	www.meridianhealth.com
Riverview Regional Medical Center	Gadsden	Alabama	256-543-5200	www.riverviewregional.com
Rolling Plains Memorial Hospital	Sweetwater	Texas	325-235-1701	www.rpmh.net
Rush University Medical Center	Chicago	Illinois	312-942-5000	www.ruch.edu
Russellville Hospital	Russellville	Alabama	256-332-1611	www.russellvillehospital.com
Saint Elizabeth Florence	Florence	Kentucky	859-212-5220	www.stlukehospitals.com
Saint Elizabeth Ft Thomas	Fort Thomas	Kentucky	859-572-3100	www.cardinalhill.org
Saint Elizabeth Grant	Williamstown	Kentucky	859-824-8240	www.stelizabeth.com
Saint Elizabeth Medical Center	Lakeside Park	Kentucky	859-292-2000	www.stelizabeth.com
Saint James Mercy Hospital	Hornell	New York	607-324-8000	www.stjamesmercy.org
Saint Joseph Hospital & Health Center	Kokomo	Indiana	765-456-5300	www.stvincent.org
Saint Luke's Miners Memorial Hospital	Coaldale	Pennsylvania	570-645-2131	www.slhn-lehighvalley.org
Saint Mary's Health Center	Jefferson City	Missouri	573-761-7000	www.stmarys-jeffcity.com
Sebastian River Medical Center	Sebastian	Florida	772-589-3187	www.srmcenter.com
Sherman Oaks Hospital	Sherman Oaks	California	818-981-7111	www.shermanoakshospital.com
Skagit Valley Hospital	Mount Vernon	Washington	360-424-4111	www.skagitvalleyhospital.org
Sonoma Developmental Center	Eldridge	California	707-938-6393	www.dds.ca.gov/sonoma/index.cfm
South Baldwin Regional Medical Center	Foley	Alabama	251-949-3400	www.southbaldwinrmc.com
South Bay Hospital	Sun City Center	Florida	813-634-3301	www.southbayhospital.com
Southwest General Hospital	San Antonio	Texas	210-921-2000	www.swgeneralhospital.com
Stones River Hospital & Dekalb Community Hospital	Smithville	Tennessee	615-215-5000	www.dekalb-hospital.com
Stormont - Vail Healthcare	Topeka	Kansas	785-354-6121	www.stormontvail.org
Temple Community Hospital	Los Angeles	California	213-382-7252	www.templecommunityhospital.com
Terre Haute Regional Hospital	Terre Haute	Indiana	812-232-0021	www.regionalhospital.com
Texas Health Harris Methodist Hospital Azle	Azle	Texas	817-444-8700	www.hmhs.org
Tomah Memorial Hospital	Tomah	Wisconsin	608-372-2181	www.tomahhospital.org
Trinity Hospital of Augusta	Augusta	Georgia	706-481-7000	www.trinityofaugusta.com
Trinity Medical Center	Birmingham	Alabama	205-592-1000	www.bhsala.com/montclair
Twin Cities Hospital	Niceville	Florida	850-678-4131	www.tchealthcare.com
Tyrone Hospital	Tyrone	Pennsylvania	814-684-1255	www.tyronehospital.org
UPMC East	Monroeville	Pennsylvania	412-357-3000	www.upmc.com
Valley West Community Hospital	Sandwich	Illinois	815-786-8484	www.snd.softfarm.com/sandhosp

Hospital	City	State	Phone	Web Site
Vaughan Regional Medical Center Parkway Campus	Selma	Alabama	334-418-4100	www.vaughanregional.com
Vista Medical Center East	Waukegan	Illinois	847-360-4000	www.vistahealth.com
Walker Baptist Medical Center	Jasper	Alabama	205-387-4000	www.bhsala.com/walker
Weatherford Regional Medical Center	Weatherford	Texas	817-599-1190	www.campbellhealth.com
West Anaheim Medical Center	Anaheim	California	714-827-3000	www.wamc.phcs.us
West Kendall Baptist Hospital	Miami	Florida	786-467-2011	www.baptisthealth.net
West Palm Hospital	West Palm Beach	Florida	561-844-6141	www.columbiahospital.com
West Virginia University Hospitals	Morgantown	West Virginia	304-598-4000	www.wvuh.com
Western Arizona Regional Medical Center	Bullhead City	Arizona	928-763-2273	www.warmc.com
Westside Regional Medical Center	Plantation	Florida	954-473-6600	www.westsidehospital.com
Woodland Heights Medical Center	Lufkin	Texas	936-634-8311	www.woodlandheights.net
Woodward Regional Hospital	Woodward	Oklahoma	580-254-8492	www.woodwardhospital.com

Note: The 144 hospitals shown above all achieved a perfect 100% average score. Average scores were calculated for hospitals with qualifying data (25 cases or more) in both measures in the Preventative Care category. A total of 3,674 hospitals nationwide were considered.

Best Hospitals for Stroke Care

Hospital	City	State	Phone	Web Site
Baptist Hospital of Miami	Miami	Florida	786-596-1960	www.baptisthealth.net
Bellevue Medical Center	Bellevue	Nebraska	402-763-3600	www.bellevuemed.com
Blanchard Valley Hospital	Findlay	Ohio	419-423-4500	www.bvha.org
Boca Raton Regional Hospital	Boca Raton	Florida	561-362-5002	www.brrh.com
Bronx - Lebanon Hospital Center	Bronx	New York	212-588-7000	www.bronx-leb.org
Brookdale Hospital Medical Center	Brooklyn	New York	718-240-5966	www.brookdalehospital.org
Cabell Huntington Hospital	Huntington	West Virginia	304-526-2000	www.cabellhuntington.org
Capital Health Medical Center - Hopewell	Pennington	New Jersey	609-303-4000	www.capitalhealth.org
Capital Regional Medical Center	Tallahassee	Florida	850-656-5000	www.capitalregionalmedicalcenter.com
Caromont Regional Medical Center	Gastonia	North Carolina	704-834-4891	www.caromont.org
Catawba Valley Medical Center	Hickory	North Carolina	828-326-3809	www.catawbavalleymc.org
Central Carolina Hospital	Sanford	North Carolina	919-774-2100	www.centralcarolinahosp.com
Cjw Medical Center	Richmond	Virginia	804-330-2001	www.hcavirginia.com
Cleveland Clinic Hospital	Weston	Florida	954-689-5000	www.clevelandclinic.org
Cox Medical Center Branson	Branson	Missouri	417-335-7000	www.skaggs.net
Delray Medical Center	Delray Beach	Florida	561-498-4440	www.delraymedicalctr.com
Detar Hospital Navarro	Victoria	Texas	361-575-7441	www.detar.com
Doctors Hospital	Augusta	Georgia	706-651-6008	www.doctors-hospital.net
Falmouth Hospital	Falmouth	Massachusetts	508-548-5300	www.capecodhealth.com
Fawcett Memorial Hospital	Port Charlotte	Florida	941-629-1181	www.fawcetthospital.com
Forest Hills Hospital	Forest Hills	New York	718-830-4000	www.northshorelij.com
Fort Walton Beach Medical Center	Fort Walton Beach	Florida	850-862-1111	www.fwbmedicalcenter.com
Good Samaritan Hospital Medical Center	West Islip	New York	631-376-3000	www.good-samaritan-hospital.org
Grant Medical Center	Columbus	Ohio	614-566-9978	www.ohiohealth.com
Heartland Regional Medical Center	Saint Joseph	Missouri	816-271-6000	www.heartland-health.com
Holland Community Hospital	Holland	Michigan	616-392-5141	www.hoho.org
Homestead Hospital	Homestead	Florida	786-243-8000	www.baptisthealth.net
John Randolph Medical Center	Hopewell	Virginia	804-541-1600	www.johnrandolphmed.com
Kaiser Foundation Hospital - Redwood City	Redwood City	California	650-299-2000	www.seiu-uhw.org/aboutuhw
Kaiser Foundation Hospital - San Diego	San Diego	California	619-528-5000	www.members.kaiserpermanente.org
Kaiser Foundation Hospital - South Bay	Harbor City	California	310-517-6441	www.kaiserpermanente.org
Kaiser Foundation Hospital - South San Francisco	South San Francisco	California	650-742-3200	www.healthy.kaiserpermanente.org
Lake Pointe Medical Center	Rowlett	Texas	972-412-2273	www.lakepointemedical.com
Lakeview Regional Medical Center	Covington	Louisiana	985-867-4443	www.lakeviewregional.com
Lawnwood Regional Medical Center & Heart Institute	Fort Pierce	Florida	772-461-4000	www.lawnwoodmed.com
Lewisgale Medical Center	Salem	Virginia	540-776-4000	www.lewis-gale.com
Libertyhealth - Jersey City Medical Center Campus	Jersey City	New Jersey	201-915-2000	www.libertyhcs.org
Los Alamitos Medical Center	Los Alamitos	California	562-799-3220	www.losalamitosmedctr.com
Lovelace Medical Center	Albuquerque	New Mexico	505-727-8000	www.lovelace.com
Main Line Hospital Paoli	Paoli	Pennsylvania	610-648-1000	www.mainlinehealth.org
Marshall Medical Center	Placerville	California	530-622-1441	www.marshallmedical.org
Mary Immaculate Hospital	Newport News	Virginia	757-886-6000	www.bonsecourshamptonroad.com
Maui Memorial Medical Center	Wailuku	Hawaii	808-442-5101	www.mauimemorialmedical.org
Memorial Hospital Pembroke	Pembroke Pines	Florida	954-962-9650	www.memorialpembroke.com\
Memorial Hospital West	Pembroke Pines	Florida	954-436-5000	www.memorialwest.com
Mercy Hospital	Bakersfield	California	661-632-5000	www.mercybakersfield.org
Methodist Dallas Medical Center	Dallas	Texas	214-947-2879	www.mhd.com
Methodist Hospital of Southern California	Arcadia	California	626-445-4441	www.methodisthospital.org
Methodist Mansfield Medical Center	Mansfield	Texas	682-622-2059	www.methodisthealthsystem.com
Methodist Medical Center of Oak Ridge	Oak Ridge	Tennessee	865-835-1000	www.mmcoakridge.com
Methodist Richardson Medical Center	Richardson	Texas	972-498-4000	www.richardsonregional.com
Methodist Stone Oak Hospital	San Antonio	Texas	210-638-2100	www.stoneoakhealth.com
Metroplex Hospital	Killeen	Texas	254-526-7523	www.mplex.org
Mills - Peninsula Medical Center	Burlingame	California	650-696-5270	www.mills-peninsula.org
Monmouth Medical Center - Southern Campus	Lakewood	New Jersey	732-363-1900	www.sbhcs.com
Morristown Hamblen Hospital Association	Morristown	Tennessee	423-586-4231	www.mhhs1.org
Newton - Wellesley Hospital	Newton	Massachusetts	617-243-6000	www.nwh.org
North Austin Medical Center	Austin	Texas	512-901-1000	www.cornerstonehealthcaregroup.com
North Cypress Medical Center	Cypress	Texas	281-890-0203	www.ncmc-hospital.com
North Hills Hospital	North Richland Hills	Texas	817-255-1000	www.northhillshospital.com
Northside Hospital	Saint Petersburg	Florida	813-521-5000	www.northsidehospital.com
Northwest Community Hospital	Arlington Heights	Illinois	847-618-1000	www.nch.org
Novant Health Forsyth Medical Center	Winston-Salem	North Carolina	336-718-5000	www.forsythmedicalcenter.org
Novant Health Thomasville Medical Center	Thomasville	North Carolina	336-472-2000	www.thomasvillemedicalcenter.org
Oak Hill Hospital	Brooksville	Florida	352-596-6632	www.oakhillhospital.com

Hospital	City	State	Phone	Web Site
Pali Momi Medical Center	Aiea	Hawaii	808-486-6000	www.kapiolani.org
Palms of Pasadena Hospital	Saint Petersburg	Florida	727-381-1000	www.palmspasadena.com
Pikeville Medical Center	Pikeville	Kentucky	606-218-3500	www.pikevillehospital.org
Portsmouth Regional Hospital	Portsmouth	New Hampshire	603-436-5110	www.portsmouthhospital.com
Presence Saints Mary & Elizabeth Medical Center	Chicago	Illinois	312-770-2000	www.reshealth.org
Reston Hospital Center	Reston	Virginia	703-689-9000	www.restonhospital.com
Richmond University Medical Center	Staten Island	New York	718-818-1234	www.rumcsi.org
Saint Catherine of Siena Hospital	Smithtown	New York	631-862-3000	www.stcatherines.chsli.org
Saint Clair Memorial Hospital	Pittsburgh	Pennsylvania	412-942-6209	www.stclair.org
Saint Joseph Medical Center	Kansas City	Missouri	816-942-4000	www.stjosehkc.com
Saint Mary's Medical Center	San Francisco	California	415-668-1000	www.stmarysmedicalcenter.org
Salinas Valley Memorial Hospital	Salinas	California	831-757-4333	www.svmh.com
San Gabriel Valley Medical Center	San Gabriel	California	626-289-5454	www.sangabrielvalleymedctr.org
San Ramon Regional Medical Center	San Ramon	California	925-275-9200	www.sanramonmedctr.com
Scripps Memorial Hospital La Jolla	La Jolla	California	858-626-4123	www.scrippshealth.org
Sebastian River Medical Center	Sebastian	Florida	772-589-3187	www.srmcenter.com
Shasta Regional Medical Center	Redding	California	530-244-5454	www.shastaregional.com
Sherman Hospital	Elgin	Illinois	847-742-9800	www.shermanhealth.com
Sierra Nevada Memorial Hospital	Grass Valley	California	530-274-6000	www.snmh.org
South Baldwin Regional Medical Center	Foley	Alabama	251-949-3400	www.southbaldwinrmc.com
South Bay Hospital	Sun City Center	Florida	813-634-3301	www.southbayhospital.com
South Miami Hospital	South Miami	Florida	786-662-4000	www.baptisthealth.net
South Pointe Hospital	Warrensville Heights	Ohio	216-491-6000	www.southpointehospital.org
Southern Nh Medical Center	Nashua	New Hampshire	603-577-2000	www.snhmc.org
Sparks Regional Medical Center	Fort Smith	Arkansas	501-441-4000	www.sparks.org
Springs Memorial Hospital	Lancaster	South Carolina	803-286-1481	www.springsmemorial.com
Sunrise Hospital & Medical Center	Las Vegas	Nevada	702-731-8000	www.sunrisehospital.com
Sutter Auburn Faith Hospital	Auburn	California	530-888-4500	www.sutterauburnfaith.org
Temple Community Hospital	Los Angeles	California	213-382-7252	www.templecommunityhospital.com
Texas Health Harris Methodist Hurst - Euless - Bedford	Bedford	Texas	817-848-4000	www.texashealth.org
Texas Health Presbyterian Hospital Plano	Plano	Texas	972-981-8000	www.presbyplano.org
Texoma Medical Center	Denison	Texas	903-416-4000	www.texomamedicalcenter.net
Thibodaux Regional Medical Center	Thibodaux	Louisiana	985-447-5500	www.thibodaux.com
Trinity Medical Center	Birmingham	Alabama	205-592-1000	www.bhsala.com/montclair
University Hospitals Case Medical Center	Cleveland	Ohio	216-844-1000	www.uhhs.com
University of Kentucky Hospital	Lexington	Kentucky	859-323-5000	www.uhealthcare.uky.edu
UPMC East	Monroeville	Pennsylvania	412-357-3000	www.upmc.com
Vaughan Regional Medical Center Parkway Campus	Selma	Alabama	334-418-4100	www.vaughanregional.com
Vista Medical Center East	Waukegan	Illinois	847-360-4000	www.vistahealth.com
Wellmont Bristol Regional Medical Center	Bristol	Tennessee	423-844-1121	www.wellmont.org
Wesley Medical Center	Wichita	Kansas	316-962-2000	www.wesleymc.com
West Florida Hospital	Pensacola	Florida	850-494-4000	www.westfloridahospital.com
West Houston Medical Center	Houston	Texas	281-588-8080	www.westhoustonmedical.com
Wilcox Memorial Hospital	Lihue	Hawaii	808-245-1103	www.wilcoxhealth.org

Note: The hospitals shown above represent the top 5% of the 1,762 hospitals nationwide for which an average score was calculated. Average scores were calculated for hospitals with qualifying data (25 cases or more) in at least 6 of 11 measures in the Stroke Care category.

Best Hospitals for Surgical Care

Hospital	City	State	Phone	Web Site
Arizona Orthopedic & Surgical Speciality Hospital	Chandler	Arizona	480-603-9000	www.azosh.com
Avera Queen of Peace	Mitchell	South Dakota	605-995-2000	www.averaqueenofpeace.org
Baptist Health Corbin	Corbin	Kentucky	606-528-1212	www.baptistregional.com
Baptist Memorial Hospital Union City	Union City	Tennessee	731-885-2410	www.bmhcc.org
Baptist Memorial Hospital Union County	New Albany	Mississippi	662-538-7631	www.baptistonline.org
Baylor Medical Center at Uptown	Dallas	Texas	214-443-3000	www.bmcuptown.com
Baylor Regional Medical Center at Plano	Plano	Texas	469-814-2000	www.baylorhealth.com
Belton Regional Medical Center	Belton	Missouri	816-348-1236	www.beltonregionalmedicalcenter.com
Boca Raton Regional Hospital	Boca Raton	Florida	561-362-5002	www.brrh.com
Broward Health Coral Springs	Coral Springs	Florida	954-344-3000	www.coralspringsmedicalcenter.org
Broward Health Imperial Point	Fort Lauderdale	Florida	954-776-8500	www.nbhd.org
Broward Health Medical Center	Fort Lauderdale	Florida	954-355-4400	www.browardhealth.org
Carolinas Medical Center - Pineville	Charlotte	North Carolina	704-379-5000	www.carolinashealthcare.org
Caromont Regional Medical Center	Gastonia	North Carolina	704-834-4891	www.caromont.org
Dauterive Hospital	New Iberia	Louisiana	337-365-7311	www.dauterivehospital.com
Doctors Hospital	Augusta	Georgia	706-651-6008	www.doctors-hospital.net
Dupont Hospital	Fort Wayne	Indiana	260-416-3000	www.theduponthospital.com
East Alabama Medical Center	Opelika	Alabama	334-749-3411	www.eamc.org
Englewood Community Hospital	Englewood	Florida	941-475-6571	www.englewoodcommunityhospital.com
Exempla Good Samaritan Medical Center	Lafayette	Colorado	303-689-4000	www.exempla.org
Fairview Park Hospital	Dublin	Georgia	478-274-3100	www.fairviewparkhospital.com
Fannin Regional Hospital	Blue Ridge	Georgia	706-632-3711	www.fanninregionalhospital.com
Flowers Hospital	Dothan	Alabama	334-793-5000	www.flowershospital.com
Fort Walton Beach Medical Center	Fort Walton Beach	Florida	850-862-1111	www.fwbmedicalcenter.com
Garden Park Medical Center	Gulfport	Mississippi	228-575-7000	www.gardenparkmedical.com
GHS Patewood Memorial Hospital	Greenville	South Carolina	864-797-1000	www.ghs.org
Holland Community Hospital	Holland	Michigan	616-392-5141	www.hoho.org
Ingalls Memorial Hospital	Harvey	Illinois	708-333-2300	www.ingalls.org
Institute For Orthopaedic Surgery	Lima	Ohio	419-224-7586	www.ioshospital.com
Jefferson Regional Medical Center	Pine Bluff	Arkansas	870-541-7100	www.jrmc.org
JFK Medical Center	Atlantis	Florida	561-965-7300	www.jfkmc.com
Jupiter Medical Center	Jupiter	Florida	561-747-2234	www.jupitermed.com
Kansas Medical Center	Andover	Kansas	316-300-4000	www.ksmedcenter.com
Lake City Medical Center	Lake City	Florida	386-719-9000	www.lakecitymedical.com
Lawnwood Regional Medical Center & Heart Institute	Fort Pierce	Florida	772-461-4000	www.lawnwoodmed.com
Lee's Summit Medical Center	Lees Summit	Missouri	816-282-5000	www.leessummithospital.com
Lewisgale Hospital Montgomery	Blacksburg	Virginia	540-951-1111	www.mrhospital.com
Magee Womens Hospital of UPMC Health System	Pittsburgh	Pennsylvania	412-641-4010	www.magee.edu
Margaret R Pardee Memorial Hospital	Hendersonville	North Carolina	828-696-1000	www.pardeehospital.org
Marion General Hospital	Marion	Ohio	740-383-8400	www.mariongeneral.com
Mary Greeley Medical Center	Ames	Iowa	515-239-2011	www.mgmc.org
McKenzie - Willamette Medical Center	Springfield	Oregon	541-726-4400	www.mckweb.com
Medical Center Enterprise	Enterprise	Alabama	334-347-0584	www.mcehospital.com
Memorial Hospital Pembroke	Pembroke Pines	Florida	954-962-9650	www.memorialpembroke.com\
Memorial Hospital West	Pembroke Pines	Florida	954-436-5000	www.memorialwest.com
Memorial Regional Hospital	Hollywood	Florida	954-987-2000	www.memorialregional.com
Mercy Medical Center	Roseburg	Oregon	541-673-0611	www.mercyrose.org
Methodist Dallas Medical Center	Dallas	Texas	214-947-2879	www.mhd.com
Methodist Mansfield Medical Center	Mansfield	Texas	682-622-2059	www.methodisthealthsystem.com
Mountain View Regional Medical Center	Las Cruces	New Mexico	575-556-7600	www.mountainviewregional.com
Mountainview Hospital	Las Vegas	Nevada	702-255-5065	www.mountainview-hospital.com
North Carolina Specialty Hospital	Durham	North Carolina	919-956-9300	www.ncspecialty.com
North Central Surgical Center	Dallas	Texas	214-265-2810	www.northcentral-sc.com
North Florida Regional Medical Center	Gainesville	Florida	352-333-4100	www.nfrmc.com
North Mississippi Medical Center	Tupelo	Mississippi	662-377-3000	www.nmhs.net/nmmc
North Suburban Medical Center	Thornton	Colorado	303-451-7800	www.northsuburban.com
Northern Westchester Hospital	Mount Kisco	New York	914-666-1200	www.nwhc.net
Northside Hospital	Atlanta	Georgia	404-851-8000	www.northside.com
Northside Hospital Cherokee	Canton	Georgia	770-720-5298	www.northside.com/cherokee
Northside Hospital Forsyth	Cumming	Georgia	404-851-8700	www.gbhcs.org
Northwest Medical Center	Margate	Florida	954-974-0400	www.northwestmed.com
Novant Health Charlotte Orthopedic Hospital	Charlotte	North Carolina	704-316-2000	www.presbyterian.org
Novant Health Forsyth Medical Center	Winston-Salem	North Carolina	336-718-5000	www.forsythmedicalcenter.org
Novant Health Park Hospital	Winston-Salem	North Carolina	336-718-0600	www.novanthealth.org
Novant Health Rowan Medical Center	Salisbury	North Carolina	704-210-5000	www.rowan.org

Hospital	City	State	Phone	Web Site
Ocala Regional Medical Center	Ocala	Florida	352-401-1000	www.ocalaregional.com
Oklahoma Surgical Hospital	Tulsa	Oklahoma	918-477-5000	www.oklahomasurgicalhospital.com
Orange Park Medical Center	Orange Park	Florida	904-276-8500	www.opmedical.com
The Orthopaedic Hospital of Lutheran Health Network	Fort Wayne	Indiana	260-435-2999	www.lutheranhealth.net
Orthopaedic Hospital of Wisconsin	Glendale	Wisconsin	414-961-6800	www.ohow.org
Oss Orthopaedic Hospital	York	Pennsylvania	717-718-2000	www.osshealth.com
Pinnacle Health Hospitals	Harrisburg	Pennsylvania	717-782-5181	www.pinnaclehealth.org
Portsmouth Regional Hospital	Portsmouth	New Hampshire	603-436-5110	www.portsmouthhospital.com
Quail Creek Surgical Hospital	Amarillo	Texas	806-354-6100	www.physurg.com
Rapides Regional Medical Center	Alexandria	Louisiana	318-769-3000	www.rapidesregional.com
Raulerson Hospital	Okeechobee	Florida	863-763-2151	www.raulersonhospital.com
Regional Hospital of Jackson	Jackson	Tennessee	731-661-2000	www.regionalhospitaljackson.com
The Regional Medical Center of Acadiana	Lafayette	Louisiana	337-981-2949	www.medicalcentersw.com
Renown South Meadows Medical Center	Reno	Nevada	775-982-7000	www.renown.org
Reston Hospital Center	Reston	Virginia	703-689-9000	www.restonhospital.com
River Oaks Hospital	Flowood	Mississippi	601-936-2390	www.riveroakshospital.org
Rose Medical Center	Denver	Colorado	303-320-2121	www.rosemed.com
Saint Anthony's Health Center	Alton	Illinois	618-465-2571	www.sahc.org
Saint Charles Hospital	Port Jefferson	New York	631-474-6000	www.stcharles.org
Saint Elizabeth Florence	Florence	Kentucky	859-212-5220	www.stlukehospitals.com
Saint Elizabeth Medical Center	Lakeside Park	Kentucky	859-292-2000	www.stelizabeth.com
Saint Francis Regional Medical Center	Shakopee	Minnesota	952-403-3000	www.stfrancis-shakopee.com
Saint Lucie Medical Center	Port Saint Lucie	Florida	772-335-4000	www.stluciemed.com
Saint Luke's Lakeside Hospital	The Woodlands	Texas	936-266-4055	www.stlukeslakeside.com
Saint Luke's South Hospital	Overland Park	Kansas	913-317-7904	www.saintlukeshealthsystem.org
Saint Mary Medical Center	Hobart	Indiana	219-942-0551	www.comhs.org/stmary
Saint Vincent Healthcare	Billings	Montana	406-657-7000	www.svh-mt.org
Saint Vincent's Medical Center Southside	Jacksonville	Florida	904-296-3700	www.jaxhealth.com
San Angelo Community Medical Center	San Angelo	Texas	325-949-9511	www.sacmc.com
Scripps Green Hospital	La Jolla	California	858-554-3600	www.scrippshealth.org
Scripps Memorial Hospital - Encinitas	Encinitas	California	760-753-6501	www.scripps.org
Sebastian River Medical Center	Sebastian	Florida	772-589-3187	www.srmcenter.com
South Baldwin Regional Medical Center	Foley	Alabama	251-949-3400	www.southbaldwinrmc.com
South Miami Hospital	South Miami	Florida	786-662-4000	www.baptisthealth.net
South Nassau Communities Hospital	Oceanside	New York	516-632-3000	www.southnassau.org
Sparks Regional Medical Center	Fort Smith	Arkansas	501-441-4000	www.sparks.org
Springs Memorial Hospital	Lancaster	South Carolina	803-286-1481	www.springsmemorial.com
Strong Memorial Hospital	Rochester	New York	585-275-2121	www.urmc.rochester.edu
Tanner Medical Center - Carrollton	Carrollton	Georgia	770-836-9580	www.tanner.org
Texas Health Harris Methodist Hospital Southlake	Southlake	Texas	817-748-8700	www.texashealthsouthlake.com
Texas Orthopedic Hospital	Houston	Texas	713-799-8600	www.texasorthopedic.com
Trinity Medical Center	Birmingham	Alabama	205-592-1000	www.bhsala.com/montclair
Twin Cities Hospital	Niceville	Florida	850-678-4131	www.tchealthcare.com
UH Geauga Medical Center	Chardon	Ohio	440-269-6000	www.uhgeauga.org
UPMC East	Monroeville	Pennsylvania	412-357-3000	www.upmc.com
Venice Regional Medical Center - Bayfront Health	Venice	Florida	941-485-7711	www.veniceregional.com
Walker Baptist Medical Center	Jasper	Alabama	205-387-4000	www.bhsala.com/walker
West Florida Hospital	Pensacola	Florida	850-494-4000	www.westfloridahospital.com
West Georgia Medical Center	Lagrange	Georgia	706-882-1411	www.wghealth.org
West Kendall Baptist Hospital	Miami	Florida	786-467-2011	www.baptisthealth.net
West Palm Hospital	West Palm Beach	Florida	561-844-6141	www.columbiahospital.com

Note: The hospitals shown above represent the top 5% of the 2,338 hospitals nationwide for which an average score was calculated. Average scores were calculated for hospitals with qualifying data (25 cases or more) in at least 9 of 10 measures in the Surgical Care Improvment Project category.

Best Hospitals in Terms of Patient's Hospital Experiences

Hospital	City	State	Phone	Web Site
Abbeville Area Medical Center	Abbeville	South Carolina	864-366-5011	www.abbevilleareamc.com
Advanced Surgical Hospital	Washington	Pennsylvania	724-884-0710	www.ashospital.net
Animas Surgical Hospital	Durango	Colorado	970-247-3537	www.animassorgical.com
Arizona Orthopedic & Surgical Speciality Hospital	Chandler	Arizona	480-603-9000	www.azosh.com
Arkansas Heart Hospital	Little Rock	Arkansas	501-219-7000	www.arheart.com
Arkansas Surgical Hospital	No Little Rock	Arkansas	501-748-8000	www.arksurgicalhospital.com
Avera Heart Hospital of South Dakota	Sioux Falls	South Dakota	605-977-7000	www.avera.org/heart-hospital
Avera Saint Anthony's Hospital	O' Neill	Nebraska	402-336-2611	www.avera-sta.org
Baptist Emergency Hospital	San Antonio	Texas	210-402-4092	www.baptistemergencyhospital.com
Barton County Memorial Hospital	Lamar	Missouri	417-682-6081	www.bcmh.net
Baylor Heart & Vascular Hospital	Dallas	Texas	214-820-0670	www.baylorhearthospital.com
Baylor Medical Center at Frisco	Frisco	Texas	214-618-2000	www.bmcf.com
Baylor Medical Center at Trophy Club	Trophy Club	Texas	817-837-4600	www.tc-mc.com
Baylor Medical Center at Uptown	Dallas	Texas	214-443-3000	www.bmcuptown.com
Baylor Orthopedic & Spine Hospital at Arlington	Arlington	Texas	817-549-2364	www.baylorarlington.com
Baylor Surgical Hospital at Las Colinas	Irving	Texas	972-868-4000	www.ic-sh.com
Bear River Valley Hospital	Tremonton	Utah	435-207-4708	www.intermountainhealthcare.org
Bigfork Valley Hospital	Bigfork	Minnesota	218-743-3177	www.bigforkvalley.org
Black Hills Surgical Hospital	Rapid City	South Dakota	605-721-4700	www.bhsh.com
Black River Memorial Hospital	Black River Falls	Wisconsin	715-284-5361	www.brmh.net
Blue Hill Memorial Hospital	Blue Hill	Maine	207-374-2836	www.bhmh.org/default.html
Bluffton Hospital	Bluffton	Ohio	419-358-9010	www.bvhealthsystem.org
Boone County Health Center	Albion	Nebraska	402-395-2191	www.boonecohealth.org
Brodstone Memorial Hospital	Superior	Nebraska	402-879-3281	www.brodstonehospital.org
Bucks County Specialty Hospital	Bensalem	Pennsylvania	215-244-7400	www.bcshospital.com
Caldwell Memorial Hospital	Columbia	Louisiana	318-649-6111	
Central Louisiana Surgical Hospital	Alexandria	Louisiana	318-449-6400	www.clshospital.com
Chickasaw Nation Medical Center	Ada	Oklahoma	580-436-3980	www.chickasaw.net
Choctaw Nation Healthcare	Talihina	Oklahoma	918-567-7000	www.choctawnationhealth.com
Citizens Medical Center	Columbia	Louisiana	318-649-6106	www.citizensmedcenter.com
Clinton County Hospital	Albany	Kentucky	606-387-6421	www.clintoncountyhospital.com
Columbia Center	Mequon	Wisconsin	262-243-7408	www.columbiacenter.org
Community Hospital	Torrington	Wyoming	307-532-4181	www.bannerhealth.com
Community Medical Center	Falls City	Nebraska	402-245-2428	www.hhs.state.ne.us/index.htm
Community Memorial Hospital	Hicksville	Ohio	419-542-6692	www.cmhosp.com
Coordinated Health Orthopedic Hospital	Bethlehem	Pennsylvania	610-691-4300	www.coordinatedhealth.com
Cypress Pointe Surgical Hospital	Hammond	Louisiana	985-510-6200	www.cpsh.org
Dakota Plains Surgical Center	Aberdeen	South Dakota	605-225-3300	www.orthopediccenterofthedakotas.com
Doctors Hospital at Deer Creek	Leesville	Louisiana	337-392-5088	www.dhdc.md
East Texas Medical Center - Gilmer	Gilmer	Texas	903-841-7100	www.etmc.org
East Texas Medical Center Pittsburg	Pittsburg	Texas	903-856-4520	www.etmc.org
Electra Memorial Hospital	Electra	Texas	940-495-3981	www.electrahospital.com
Fairview Hospital	Great Barrington	Massachusetts	413-528-0790	www.berkshirehealthsystems.com
Fairway Medical Center	Covington	Louisiana	985-801-3010	www.fairwaymedical.com
Fayette Medical Center	Fayette	Alabama	205-932-5966	www.dchsystem.com
First Care Health Center	Park River	North Dakota	701-284-7500	www.firstcarehc.com
Floyd County Memorial Hospital	Charles City	Iowa	641-228-6830	www.fcmc.us.com
Fostoria Community Hospital	Fostoria	Ohio	419-435-7734	www.promedica.org
Foundation Surgical Hospital of San Antonio	San Antonio	Texas	210-478-5400	www.fshsanantonio.com
Fresno Surgical Hospital	Fresno	California	559-431-8000	www.fresnosurgerycenter.com
GHS Patewood Memorial Hospital	Greenville	South Carolina	864-797-1000	www.ghs.org
Glacial Ridge Hospital	Glenwood	Minnesota	320-634-2208	www.glacialridge.org
Grant Regional Health Center	Lancaster	Wisconsin	608-723-2143	www.grantregional.com
Great Falls Clinic Medical Center	Great Falls	Montana	406-216-8000	www.gfclinic.com
Green Clinic Surgical Hospital	Ruston	Louisiana	318-232-7700	www.green-clinic.com
Grundy County Memorial Hospital	Grundy Center	Iowa	319-824-5421	www.grundyhospital.com
H B Magruder Memorial Hospital	Port Clinton	Ohio	419-734-3131	www.magruderhospital.com
Heart Hospital Baylor Plano	Plano	Texas	469-814-3278	www.thehearthospitalbaylor.com
Heart Hospital of Lafayette	Lafayette	Louisiana	337-521-1000	www.hearthospitaloflafayette.com
Heritage Park Surgical Hospital	Sherman	Texas	903-813-3728	www.heritageparksurgicalhospital.com
Hill Country Memorial Hospital	Fredericksburg	Texas	830-997-4353	www.hcmbs.org
Hillsboro Area Hospital	Hillsboro	Illinois	217-532-6111	www.hillsboroareahospital.org
Hoag Orthopedic Institute	Irvine	California	949-727-5000	www.orthopedichospital.com
Houston Orthopedic & Spine Hospital	Bellaire	Texas	713-622-2262	www.foundationsurgicalhospital.com
Houston Physicians' Hospital	Webster	Texas	281-335-1700	www.houstonphysicianshospital.com

Hospital	City	State	Phone	Web Site
Indiana Orthopaedic Hospital	Indianapolis	Indiana	317-956-1000	www.indianaorthopaedichospital.com
Institute For Orthopaedic Surgery	Lima	Ohio	419-224-7586	www.ioshospital.com
Integris Health Edmond	Edmond	Oklahoma	405-657-3000	www.integrisok.com/integris-health-edmond-ok
Jefferson County Health Center	Fairfield	Iowa	641-472-4111	www.jchospital.org
Kansas City Orthopaedic Institute	Leawood	Kansas	913-319-7633	www.kcoi.com
Kentuckiana Medical Center	Clarksville	Indiana	812-280-3300	www.kentuckianamedcen.com
King's Daughters Medical Center - Brookhaven	Brookhaven	Mississippi	601-833-6011	www.kdmc.org
Lady of the Sea General Hospital	Cut Off	Louisiana	985-632-6401	www.losgh.org
Lafayette Surgical Specialty Hospital	Lafayette	Louisiana	337-769-4100	www.lafayettesurgical.com
Lakeview Memorial Hospital	Stillwater	Minnesota	651-439-5330	www.lakeview.org
Lawrence County Hospital	Monticello	Mississippi	601-587-4051	www.smrmc.com/index.php
Lincoln Surgical Hospital	Lincoln	Nebraska	402-484-9090	www.lincolnsurgery.com
Mackinac Straits Hospital & Health Center	Saint Ignace	Michigan	906-643-8585	www.mackinacstraitshealth.org
Manhattan Surgical Hospital	Manhattan	Kansas	785-776-5100	www.manhattansurgical.com
Mariners Hospital	Tavernier	Florida	305-434-3000	www.baptisthealth.net
Marion Regional Medical Center	Hamilton	Alabama	205-921-6200	www.nmhs.net
Mayo Clinic Hospital	Phoenix	Arizona	480-342-2000	www.mayoclinic.org
McBride Clinic Orthopedic Hospital	Oklahoma City	Oklahoma	405-478-1717	www.mcbrideclinic.com
Menlo Park Surgical Hospital	Menlo Park	California	650-324-8500	www.pamf.org/mpsh
Mercy Willard Hospital	Willard	Ohio	419-964-5000	www.mercyweb.org/mercy_willard.aspx
Miami County Medical Center	Paola	Kansas	913-557-4385	www.olathehealth.org
Mid - Valley Hospital	Peckville	Pennsylvania	570-383-5000	
Midwest Orthopedic Specialty Hospital	Franklin	Wisconsin	414-817-5800	www.mymosh.com
Midwest Surgical Hospital	Omaha	Nebraska	402-399-1900	www.mwsurgicalhospital.com
Millinocket Regional Hospital	Millinocket	Maine	207-723-5161	www.mrhme.org
Ministry Door County Medical Center	Sturgeon Bay	Wisconsin	920-743-5566	www.doorcountymemorial.org
Mount Carmel New Albany Surgical Hospital	New Albany	Ohio	614-775-6600	www.mountcarmelhealth.com
Mount Desert Island Hospital	Bar Harbor	Maine	207-288-5081	www.mdihospital.com
Mountain View Regional Hospital	Casper	Wyoming	307-995-8100	www.monroehospital.com
Nebraska Orthopaedic Hospital	Omaha	Nebraska	402-609-1600	www.neorthohospital.com
The Neuromedical Center Hospital	Baton Rouge	Louisiana	225-763-9900	www.theneuromedicalcenter.com
North Carolina Specialty Hospital	Durham	North Carolina	919-956-9300	www.ncspecialty.com
North Central Surgical Center	Dallas	Texas	214-265-2810	www.northcentral-sc.com
Northside Medical Center	Columbus	Georgia	706-494-2100	www.hughstonsports.com
Northwest Hills Surgical Hospital	Austin	Texas	512-346-1994	www.scasurgery.com
Northwest Specialty Hospital	Post Falls	Idaho	208-262-2300	www.northwestspecialtyhospital.com
Northwest Surgical Hospital	Oklahoma City	Oklahoma	404-848-1918	www.nwsurgicalokc.com
Oak Leaf Surgical Hospital	Eau Claire	Wisconsin	715-831-8130	www.oakleafsurgical.com
Ogallala Community Hospital	Ogallala	Nebraska	308-284-4011	www.bannerhealth.com
Oklahoma Center for Orthopaedic & Multi-Spec	Oklahoma City	Oklahoma	405-602-6500	www.ocomhospital.com
Oklahoma Heart Hospital	Oklahoma City	Oklahoma	405-608-3200	www.okheart.com
Oklahoma Heart Hospital South	Oklahoma City	Oklahoma	405-628-6000	www.okheart.com/south-campus
Oklahoma Spine Hospital	Oklahoma City	Oklahoma	405-749-2700	www.oklahomaspine.com
Oklahoma Surgical Hospital	Tulsa	Oklahoma	918-477-5000	www.oklahomasurgicalhospital.com
Orange City Area Health System	Orange City	Iowa	712-737-4984	www.ochealthsystem.org
Orthopaedic Hospital of Wisconsin	Glendale	Wisconsin	414-961-6800	www.ohow.org
OSF Holy Family Medical Center	Monmouth	Illinois	309-734-3141	www.cmchospital.com
Oss Orthopaedic Hospital	York	Pennsylvania	717-718-2000	www.osshealth.com
Ouachita Community Hospital	West Monroe	Louisiana	318-322-1339	www.ouachitahospital.com
P & S Surgical Hospital	Monroe	Louisiana	318-388-4040	www.pssurgery.com
Patients' Hospital of Redding	Redding	California	530-225-8700	www.patientshospital.com
Pella Regional Health Center	Pella	Iowa	641-628-3150	www.pellahealth.org
Pender Community Hospital	Pender	Nebraska	402-385-3083	www.pendercommunityhospital.com
Physician's Care Surgical Hospital	Royersford	Pennsylvania	610-495-4793	www.phycarehospital.com
The Physicians Centre	Bryan	Texas	979-731-3100	www.thephysicianscentre.com
Physicians Medical Center	Houma	Louisiana	985-853-1390	www.physicianshouma.com
Physicians' Medical Center	New Albany	Indiana	812-206-7660	www.pmcdev.interactivemedialab.com
Physicians' Specialty Hospital	Fayetteville	Arkansas	479-571-7002	www.pshfay.com
Quail Creek Surgical Hospital	Amarillo	Texas	806-354-6100	www.physurg.com
Richland Parish Hospital - Delhi	Delhi	Louisiana	318-878-5171	www.delhihospital.com
River Falls Area Hospital	River Falls	Wisconsin	715-307-6000	www.allina.com
Rochelle Community Hospital	Rochelle	Illinois	815-562-2181	www.rcha.net
Rockcastle County Hospital	Mount Vernon	Kentucky	606-256-2195	www.rockcastlehospital.com
Rollins Brook Community Hospital	Lampasas	Texas	512-556-3682	www.mplex.org
Sacred Heart Hospital on the Gulf	Port Saint Joe	Florida	850-229-5600	www.sacred-heart.org/gulf
Saint Joseph Memorial Hospital	Murphysboro	Illinois	618-684-3156	www.sih.net
Saint Joseph's Hospital	Breese	Illinois	618-526-4511	www.stjoebreese.com

Hospital	City	State	Phone	Web Site
Saint Luke's Lakeside Hospital	The Woodlands	Texas	936-266-4055	www.stlukeslakeside.com
Saint Luke's Wood River Medical Center	Ketchum	Idaho	208-727-8800	www.stlukesonline.org/wood_river
Saint Thomas Hospital for Spinal Surgery	Nashville	Tennessee	615-515-8200	www.hospitalforspinalsurgery.com
Salina Surgical Hospital	Salina	Kansas	785-827-0610	www.salinasurgical.com
Sanford Luverne Medical Center	Luverne	Minnesota	507-283-2321	www.sanfordluverne.org
Sauk Prairie Hospital	Prairie Du Sac	Wisconsin	608-643-3311	www.spmh.org
Sharp Coronado Hospital & Healthcare Center	Coronado	California	619-435-6251	www.sharp.com/coronado
Sioux Falls Specialty Hospital	Sioux Falls	South Dakota	605-334-6730	www.sfsurgical.com
Siouxland Surgery Center	Dakota Dunes	South Dakota	605-232-3332	www.siouxlandsurg.com
South Texas Spine & Surgical Hospital	San Antonio	Texas	210-404-0800	www.southtexassurgical.com
South Texas Surgical Hospital	Corpus Christi	Texas	361-993-2000	www.nshinc.com
Southern Surgical Hospital	Slidell	Louisiana	985-641-0600	www.sshla.com
Southwestern Regional Medical Center	Tulsa	Oklahoma	918-496-5000	www.cancercenter.com/southwestern
Specialists Hospital Shreveport	Shreveport	Louisiana	318-213-3800	www.specialistshospitalshreveport.com
Stanislaus Surgical Hospital	Modesto	California	209-572-2700	www.stanislaussurgical.com
Stewart Memorial Community Hospital	Lake City	Iowa	712-464-3171	www.stewartmemorial.org
Stoughton Hospital	Stoughton	Wisconsin	608-873-6611	www.stoughtonhospital.com
Sugar Land Surgical Hospital	Sugar Land	Texas	281-243-1000	www.sugarlandsurgicalhospital.com
Surgical Hospital at Southwoods	Youngstown	Ohio	330-758-1954	www.surgeryatsouthwoods.com
Surgical Institute of Reading	Wyomissing	Pennsylvania	717-999-9999	www.sireading.com
Surgical Specialty Center at Coordinated Health	Allentown	Pennsylvania	610-871-9110	www.coordinatedhealth.com
Surgical Specialty Center of Baton Rouge	Baton Rouge	Louisiana	225-408-5730	www.sscbr.com
Sutter Surgical Hospital - North Valley	Yuba City	California	530-749-5700	www.suttersurgicalhospitalnorthvalley.org
Texas Health Center for Diagnostics & Surgery	Plano	Texas	972-403-2700	www.ppcds.com
Texas Health Harris Methodist Hospital Southlake	Southlake	Texas	817-748-8700	www.texashealthsouthlake.com
Texas Institute for Surgery at Presbyterian Hospital	Dallas	Texas	214-647-5300	www.texasinstituteforsurgery.org
Texas Spine & Joint Hospital	Tyler	Texas	903-525-3300	www.tsjh.org
Tishomingo Health Services	Iuka	Mississippi	662-423-6051	www.nmhs.net/iuka
Tops Surgical Specialty Hospital	Houston	Texas	281-539-2900	www.tops-hospital.com
Treasure Valley Hospital	Boise	Idaho	208-373-5000	www.treasurevalleyhospital.com
Tulsa Spine & Specialty Hospital	Tulsa	Oklahoma	918-388-5701	www.tulsaspinehospital.com
United Regional Medical Center	Manchester	Tennessee	931-728-3586	www.urmchealthcare.com
University Hospitals Conneaut Medical Center	Conneaut	Ohio	440-593-1131	www.uhhospitals.org/conneaut
Upland Hills Health	Dodgeville	Wisconsin	608-930-8000	www.uplandhillshealth.org
USMD Hospital at Arlington	Arlington	Texas	817-472-3400	www.usmdhospital.com
USMD Hospital at Fort Worth	Fort Worth	Texas	817-433-9100	www.usmdfortworth.com
Vernon Memorial Hospital	Viroqua	Wisconsin	608-637-2101	www.vmh.org
Vidant Bertie Hospital	Windsor	North Carolina	252-794-6600	www.vidanthealth.com/bertie
W J Mangold Memorial Hospital	Lockney	Texas	806-652-3373	www.mangoldmemorial.org
Wellspan Surgery & Rehabilitation Hospital	York	Pennsylvania	717-812-6100	www.wellspan.org
West Kendall Baptist Hospital	Miami	Florida	786-467-2011	www.baptisthealth.net
Westlake Regional Hospital	Columbia	Kentucky	270-384-4753	www.westlake-healthcare.org
Whitman Hospital & Medical Center	Colfax	Washington	509-397-3435	www.whitmanhospital.com
Wright Memorial Hospital	Trenton	Missouri	660-359-5621	www.saintlukeshealthsystem.org
York Hospital	York	Maine	207-363-4321	www.yorkhospital.com

Note: The hospitals shown above represent the top 5% of the 3,591 hospitals nationwide for which an average score was calculated. Average scores were calculated for hospitals with qualifying data (100 completed surveys or more) in all ten measures in the Survey of Patient's Hospital Experiences category.

Best Hospitals in Terms of Use of Medical Imaging

Hospital	City	State	Phone	Web Site
Alameda Hospital	Alameda	California	510-522-3700	www.alamedahospital.org
Bartlett Regional Hospital	Juneau	Alaska	907-796-8900	www.bartletthospital.org
Caldwell Memorial Hospital	Lenoir	North Carolina	828-757-5100	www.caldwellmemorial.org
Capital Regional Medical Center	Tallahassee	Florida	850-656-5000	www.capitalregionalmedicalcenter.com
Carroll County Memorial Hospital	Carrollton	Kentucky	502-732-4321	www.ccmhosp.com
Centrastate Medical Center	Freehold	New Jersey	732-431-2000	www.centrastate.com
Chandler Regional Medical Center	Chandler	Arizona	480-963-4561	www.chandlerregional.com
Chinese Hospital	San Francisco	California	415-982-2400	www.chinesehospital-sf.org
Community Regional Medical Center	Fresno	California	559-459-6000	www.communitymedical.org
Conemaugh Valley Memorial Hospital	Johnstown	Pennsylvania	814-534-9000	www.conemaugh.org
Deaconess Hospital	Spokane	Washington	509-473-5800	www.deaconessmedicalcenter.org
Doctors Medical Center	Modesto	California	209-578-1211	www.dmc-modesto.com
Doctors Medical Center - San Pablo	San Pablo	California	510-970-5000	www.doctorsmedicalcenter.org
Dominican Hospital	Santa Cruz	California	831-462-7700	www.dominicanhospital.org
Emanuel Medical Center	Turlock	California	209-667-4200	www.emanuelmedicalcenter.org
Enloe Medical Center	Chico	California	530-332-7300	www.enloe.org
Evergreen Hospital Medical Center	Kirkland	Washington	425-899-1000	www.evergreenhospital.org
Exempla Saint Joseph Hospital	Denver	Colorado	303-837-7111	www.exempla.org
Fairview Hospital	Cleveland	Ohio	216-476-7000	www.fairviewhospital.org
Fairview Park Hospital	Dublin	Georgia	478-274-3100	www.fairviewparkhospital.com
Glens Falls Hospital	Glens Falls	New York	518-926-1000	www.glensfallshospital.org
Good Samaritan Hospital	San Jose	California	408-559-2011	www.goodsamsj.org
Halifax Health Medical Center	Daytona Beach	Florida	386-254-4000	www.halifax.org
Harrison Memorial Center	Bremerton	Washington	360-377-3911	www.harrisonmedical.org
Hartford Hospital	Hartford	Connecticut	860-545-5000	www.harthosp.org
Healthalliance Hospitals	Leominster	Massachusetts	978-466-2000	www.healthalliance.com
Heart Hospital Baylor Plano	Plano	Texas	469-814-3278	www.thehearthospitalbaylor.com
Holy Redeemer Hospital & Medical Center	Meadowbrook	Pennsylvania	215-947-3000	www.holyredeemer.com
Huntington Hospital	Huntington	New York	631-351-2000	www.hunthosp.org
Huntington Memorial Hospital	Pasadena	California	626-397-5000	www.huntingtonhospital.com
Indiana University Health White Memorial Hospital	Monticello	Indiana	574-583-7111	www.whitecmh.org
Inova Fairfax Hospital	Falls Church	Virginia	703-776-3332	www.inova.org
Jefferson Medical Center	Ranson	West Virginia	304-728-1600	www.jeffmem.com
Johnson Memorial Hospital	Stafford Springs	Connecticut	860-684-4251	www.johnsonhealthnetwork.com
Lake City Medical Center	Lake City	Florida	386-719-9000	www.lakecitymedical.com
Lake Regional Health System	Osage Beach	Missouri	573-348-8000	www.lakeregional.com
Lakewood Regional Medical Center	Lakewood	California	562-602-6751	www.lakewoodregional.com
Lasalle General Hospital	Jena	Louisiana	318-992-9200	www.lasallegeneralhospital.com
Little Falls Hospital	Little Falls	New York	315-823-5261	www.lfhny.org
Long Island Jewish Medical Center	New Hyde Park	New York	718-470-7000	www.northshorelij.com
Lourdes Medical Center of Burlington County	Willingboro	New Jersey	609-835-2900	www.lourdesnet.org/lourdes
Lovelace Medical Center	Albuquerque	New Mexico	505-727-8000	www.lovelace.com
Lowell General Hospital	Lowell	Massachusetts	978-937-6000	www.lowellgeneral.org
Mainegeneral Medical Center	Augusta	Maine	207-872-1000	www.mainegeneral.org
Maria Parham Medical Center	Henderson	North Carolina	252-438-4143	www.mphosp.org
Marin General Hospital	Greenbrae	California	415-925-7900	www.maringeneral.com
Mary Greeley Medical Center	Ames	Iowa	515-239-2011	www.mgmc.org
Mary Washington Hospital	Fredericksburg	Virginia	540-741-1100	www.medicorp.org
Maui Memorial Medical Center	Wailuku	Hawaii	808-442-5101	www.mauimemorialmedical.org
Mayo Clinic Health System - Albert Lea	Albert Lea	Minnesota	507-373-2384	www.mayoclinichealthsystem.org
McKenzie - Willamette Medical Center	Springfield	Oregon	541-726-4400	www.mckweb.com
Medstar Franklin Square Medical Center	Baltimore	Maryland	443-777-7850	www.franklinsquare.org
Medstar Southern Maryland Hospital Center	Clinton	Maryland	301-868-8000	www.medstarhealth.org
Memorial Medical Center	Modesto	California	209-526-4500	www.memorialmedicalcenter.org
Mercy General Hospital	Sacramento	California	916-453-4545	www.mercygeneral.org
Mercy Gilbert Medical Center	Gilbert	Arizona	480-728-8327	www.dignityhealth.org/mercygilbert
Mercy Hospital	Coon Rapids	Minnesota	763-236-8205	www.allinamercy.org
Mercy Medical Center - Clinton	Clinton	Iowa	563-244-5555	www.mercyclinton.com
Mercy Medical Center - Redding	Redding	California	530-225-6102	www.redding.mercy.org
Mercy San Juan Medical Center	Carmichael	California	916-537-5000	www.mercysanjuan.org
Mercy Willard Hospital	Willard	Ohio	419-964-5000	www.mercyweb.org/mercy_willard.aspx
Methodist Hospital of Sacramento	Sacramento	California	916-423-6010	www.methodistsacramento.org
Methodist Hospital of Southern California	Arcadia	California	626-445-4441	www.methodisthospital.org
Metrosouth Medical Center	Blue Island	Illinois	708-597-2000	www.stfrancisblueisland.com
Miriam Hospital	Providence	Rhode Island	401-793-2500	www.lifespan.org/partners/tmh

Hospital	City	State	Phone	Web Site
Nashoba Valley Medical Center	Ayer	Massachusetts	978-784-9000	www.nashobamed.com
Newton Memorial Hospital	Newton	New Jersey	973-383-2121	www.itsyourlife.com
North Florida Regional Medical Center	Gainesville	Florida	352-333-4100	www.nfrmc.com
Northbay Medical Center	Fairfield	California	707-646-5000	www.northbay.org
Ocala Regional Medical Center	Ocala	Florida	352-401-1000	www.ocalaregional.com
Page Memorial Hospital	Luray	Virginia	540-743-4561	www.pagememorialhospital.org
Palomar Health Downtown Campus	Escondido	California	760-739-3000	www.pph.org
Paris Regional Medical Center	Paris	Texas	903-785-4521	www.parisregional.com
Peacehealth Saint Joseph Medical Center	Bellingham	Washington	360-734-5400	www.peacehealth.org
Penobscot Bay Medical Center	Rockport	Maine	207-596-8000	www.nehealth.org
PIH Hospital - Downey	Downey	California	526-904-5000	www.drmci.org
Pomerado Hospital	Poway	California	858-485-6511	www.pph.org
Providence Sacred Heart Medical Center	Spokane	Washington	509-474-3040	www.shmc.org
Regional Medical Center of San Jose	San Jose	California	408-259-5000	www.regionalmedicalsanjose.com
Riverview Hospital Assoc	Wisconsin Rapids	Wisconsin	715-423-6060	www.riverviewhospital.net
Robert Wood Johnson University Hospital	New Brunswick	New Jersey	732-937-8900	www.rwjuh.edu
Saint Alphonsus Medical Center - Ontario	Ontario	Oregon	541-881-7000	www.holyrosary-ontario.org
Saint Alphonsus Regional Medical Center	Boise	Idaho	208-367-2121	www.saintalphonsus.org
Saint David's Medical Center	Austin	Texas	512-476-7111	www.stdavidsrehab.com
Saint Joseph Mercy Port Huron	Port Huron	Michigan	810-985-1510	www.mercyporthuron.com
Saint Joseph's Hospital Health Center	Syracuse	New York	315-448-5111	www.sjhsyr.org
Saint Mary's Hospital - Troy	Troy	New York	518-272-5000	www.setonhealth.org
Saint Marys Hospital	Waterbury	Connecticut	203-574-6000	www.stmh.org
Saint Thomas Rutherford Hospital	Murfreesboro	Tennessee	615-396-4100	www.mtmc.org
Salinas Valley Memorial Hospital	Salinas	California	831-757-4333	www.svmh.com
Santa Rosa Memorial Hospital	Santa Rosa	California	707-525-5300	www.stjosephhealth.org
Santiam Memorial Hospital	Stayton	Oregon	503-769-2175	www.santiamhospital.com
Scottsdale Healthcare - Thompson Peak Hospital	Scottsdale	Arizona	480-324-7004	www.shc.org
Scottsdale Healthcare Osborn Medical Center	Scottsdale	Arizona	480-882-4000	www.shc.org
Shady Grove Adventist Hospital	Rockville	Maryland	240-826-6517	www.adventisthealthcare.com/sgah
Sharp Chula Vista Medical Center	Chula Vista	California	619-502-5800	www.sharp.com
Southwest Regional Medical Center	Georgetown	Ohio	513-378-7800	www.browncountygeneralhospital.com
Stafford Hospital	Stafford	Virginia	540-741-9000	www.marywashingtonhealthcare.com
Sutter Delta Medical Center	Antioch	California	925-779-7200	www.sutterdelta.org
Sutter General Hospital	Sacramento	California	916-733-8999	www.suttermedicalcenter.org
Sutter Roseville Medical Center	Roseville	California	916-781-1000	www.sutterroseville.org
Swedish Edmonds Hospital	Edmonds	Washington	425-640-4000	www.stevenshealthcare.org
Tallahassee Memorial Hospital	Tallahassee	Florida	850-431-1155	www.tmh.org
Texas Health Presbyterian Hospital Dallas	Dallas	Texas	214-345-6789	www.texashealth.org
Trinity Rock Island	Rock Island	Illinois	309-779-5000	www.trinityqc.com
Union Hospital Clinton	Clinton	Indiana	765-832-1234	www.unionhospitalhealthgroup.org/wcch
University Medical Center at Brackenridge	Austin	Texas	512-324-7000	www.seton.net/locations/brackenridge
University Medical Center of Princeton at Plainsboro	Plainsboro	New Jersey	866-460-4776	www.princetonhcs.org
Valley Hospital	Spokane	Washington	509-924-6650	www.valleyhospital.org
Vidant Duplin Hospital	Kenansville	North Carolina	910-296-0941	www.dgh.org
Virtua Memorial Hospital of Burlington County	Mount Holly	New Jersey	609-914-6200	www.virtua.org
Warren Memorial Hospital	Front Royal	Virginia	703-636-0300	www.valleyhealthlink.com
Waterbury Hospital	Waterbury	Connecticut	203-573-6000	www.waterburyhospital.org
Watsonville Community Hospital	Watsonville	California	831-724-4741	www.watsonvillehospital.com
West Hills Hospital & Medical Center	West Hills	California	818-676-4100	www.westhillshospital.com
West Valley Medical Center	Caldwell	Idaho	208-459-4641	www.westvalleymedctr.com
Wooster Community Hospital	Wooster	Ohio	330-263-8100	www.woosterhospital.org

Note: The hospitals shown above represent the top 5% of the 2,308 hospitals nationwide for which an average score was calculated. Average scores were calculated for hospitals with qualifying data (25 cases or more) in at least 4 of 5 measures in the Use of Medical Imaging category. The measure, Follow-up Mammogram/Ultrasound, was not included in the average score.

Hospitals with the Lowest Medicare Spending per Beneficiary

Hospital	City	State	Phone	Web Site
Basin Healthcare Center	Odessa	Texas	432-425-9510	www.bhcodessa.com
Beaver Valley Hospital	Beaver	Utah	435-438-7102	
Bob Wilson Memorial Grant County Hospital	Ulysses	Kansas	620-356-1266	www.bwmgch.com
Brighton Hospital	Brighton	Michigan	810-227-1211	www.stjohn.org/brighton
Cherokee Indian Hospital Authority	Cherokee	North Carolina	704-497-9163	
Chinle Comprehensive Health Care Facility	Chinle	Arizona	928-674-7001	
Crownpoint Healthcare Facility	Crownpoint	New Mexico	505-786-5291	www.ihs.gov
Dhhs Usphs Indian Health Services	San Fidel	New Mexico	505-552-5300	www.ihs.gov
Eastern State Hospital	Williamsburg	Virginia	757-253-5161	www.ehs.dmhmrsas.virginia.gov
Epic Medical Center	Eufaula	Oklahoma	918-689-2535	
Fort Defiance Indian Hospital	Fort Defiance	Arizona	928-729-8000	www.home.navajo.his.gov
Gallup Indian Medical Center	Gallup	New Mexico	505-722-1000	www.ihs.gov/facilitiesservices
Guadalupe County Hospital	Santa Rosa	New Mexico	575-472-3417	
Harmon Memorial Hospital	Hollis	Oklahoma	580-688-3363	
Ira Davenport Memorial Hospital	Bath	New York	607-776-8500	www.davenportandtaylor.org
Kaiser Foundation Hospital - Antioch	Antioch	California	925-813-6500	www.kaiserpermanente.org
Kaiser Foundation Hospital - Fresno	Fresno	California	559-448-4500	www.kaiserpermanente.org
Kaiser Foundation Hospital - San Diego	San Diego	California	619-528-5000	www.members.kaiserpermanente.org
Kaiser Foundation Hospital - San Francisco	San Francisco	California	415-833-2646	www.permanente.net
Kaiser Foundation Hospital - South San Francisco	South San Francisco	California	650-742-3200	www.healthy.kaiserpermanente.org
Kaiser Foundation Hospital - Vacaville	Vacaville	California	707-624-4000	www.kaiserpermanente.org
Kaiser Sunnyside Medical Center	Clackamas	Oregon	503-571-2880	www.members.kaiserpermanente.org
Keefe Memorial Hospital	Cheyenne Wells	Colorado	719-767-5661	
Laguna Honda Hospital & Rehabilitation Center	San Francisco	California	415-759-2300	www.dph.sf.ca.us/chn/lagunahondahosp
Lewis County General Hospital	Lowville	New York	315-376-5200	www.lcgh.net
Memorial Hospital of Texas County	Guymon	Oklahoma	580-338-6515	www.mhtcguymon.org
Morton County Hospital	Elkhart	Kansas	620-697-2141	www.mchswecare.com
Mount Edgecumbe Hospital	Sitka	Alaska	907-966-2411	www.searhc.org
Newman Memorial Hospital	Shattuck	Oklahoma	580-938-2551	
P H S Indian Hospital at Belcourt - Quentin N Burdick	Belcourt	North Dakota	701-477-6111	
P H S Indian Hospital at Browning - Blackfeet	Browning	Montana	406-338-6157	www.ihs.gov
Phoenix Indian Medical Center	Phoenix	Arizona	602-263-1200	www.ihs.gov
PHS Indian Hospital at Pine Ridge	Pine Ridge	South Dakota	605-867-5131	www.ihs.gov
PHS Indian Hospital at Rosebud	Rosebud	South Dakota	605-747-2231	www.ihs.gov
Provident Hospital of Chicago	Chicago	Illinois	312-572-2000	www.providentfoundation.org
Red Lake Hospital	Redlake	Minnesota	218-679-3912	
Sacred Heart University District	Eugene	Oregon	541-686-7300	www.peacehealth.org
Sonoma Developmental Center	Eldridge	California	707-938-6393	www.dds.ca.gov/sonoma/index.cfm
South Lyon Medical Center	Yerington	Nevada	775-781-3761	
Tuba City Regional Health Care Corporation	Tuba City	Arizona	928-283-2501	www.tcrhcc.org
USPHS Lawton Indian Hospital	Lawton	Oklahoma	580-354-5000	
Valley Forge Medical Center & Hospital	Norristown	Pennsylvania	215-539-8500	www.vfmc.net
Wayne Medical Center	Waynesboro	Tennessee	931-722-5411	
Whiteriver PHS Indian Hospital	Whiteriver	Arizona	928-338-4911	
Whitfield Medical Surgical Hospital	Whitfield	Mississippi	601-351-8001	
Yalobusha General Hospital	Water Valley	Mississippi	662-473-1411	
Yukon Kuskokwim Delta Regional Hospital	Bethel	Alaska	907-543-6300	www.ykhc.org
Zuni Comprehensive Community Health Center	Zuni	New Mexico	505-782-4431	www.ihs.gov

Note: These 48 hospitals had an average ratio of 0.75 or less in the Medicare Spending per Beneficiary category. A total of 3,229 hospitals had medicare spending data available.

Appendix E: Glossary

Accreditation
An evaluative process in which a healthcare organization undergoes an examination of its policies, procedures and performance by an external private sector organization ("accrediting body") to ensure that it is meeting predetermined criteria. It usually involves both on- and off-site surveys. Also see the terms American Osteopathic Association, The Joint Commission, and Medicare-Certified Hospitals.

Acute Care—VA Medical Center
The Veterans Health Administration (VA) Medical Centers deliver inpatient hospital care and related services for surgery and short-term health conditions, as well as comprehensive primary, specialty and long-term care. The VA's medical benefits package is available to Veterans (including Reservists and National Guard) who served on active duty and meet eligibility requirements. Other groups can also be eligible. For more information, visit the U.S. Department of Veterans Affairs.

Acute care hospital
A hospital that provides inpatient medical care and other related services for surgery, acute medical conditions or injuries (usually for a short-term illness or condition).

Acute myocardial infarction (AMI)
See Heart Attack.

American Hospital Association (AHA)
The national organization that represents and serves all types of hospitals, health care networks, and their patients and communities. AHA takes part in national health policy development, legislative and regulatory debates, and legal matters. It also provides education for health care leaders and is a source of information on health care issues and trends.

American Osteopathic Association (AOA)
A member association representing approximately 52,000 osteopathic physicians (D.O.s). The AOA serves as the primary certifying body for D.O.s, and is the accrediting agency for all osteopathic medical colleges and health care facilities. The AOA writes a performance report on each hospital that it checks. You can call or write to AOA to find out a hospital's level of accreditation.

Angioplasty
In angioplasty, a catheter is used to insert a balloon that is inflated to open a blocked blood vessel. Percutaneous transluminal coronary angioplasty (PTCA) is one of several procedures used to open a blocked blood vessel, known collectively as a percutaneous coronary intervention (PCI).

Angiotensin converting enzyme (ACE) inhibitor
A drug used to treat heart attacks, heart failure, or a decreased function of the left heart. It stops production of a hormone that can narrow blood vessels, which helps reduce the pressure in the heart and lower blood pressure.

Angiotensin receptor blocker (ARB)
A drug used to treat patients with heart failure and a decreased function of the left heart. ARBs block the action of a hormone that can narrow blood vessels. This helps reduce the pressure in the heart and lower blood pressure.

Antibiotic
Drugs used to fight bacteria in the body.

ASA Physical Status Classification
Assessment by the anesthesiologist of the patient's preoperative physical condition using the American Society of Anesthesiologists' (ASA) Classification of Physical Status.

Asthma
A chronic lung condition that causes problems getting air in and out of the lungs. Children with asthma may experience wheezing, coughing, chest tightness and trouble breathing.

Atherectomy
A procedure where a blade or laser on a catheter cuts through and removes blockages in blood vessels. It is one of several procedures used to open a blocked blood vessel (known as a Percutaneous Coronary Intervention or PCI).

Beta blocker
A type of drug that is used to lower blood pressure, treat chest pain (angina) and heart failure, and to help prevent a heart attack. Beta blockers relieve the stress on the heart by slowing the heart rate and reducing the force with which the heart muscles contract to pump blood. They also help keep blood vessels from constricting in the heart, brain, and body.

Blood clot
Blood clots are clumps that occur when blood hardens from a liquid to a solid. A blood clot can partly or completely block the flow of blood in a blood vessel.

Blood culture
A blood test that shows if there are bacteria in the blood and what type of bacteria exist. It helps your doctor decide which antibiotic to use to treat a bacterial infection.

Blood thinners
Blood thinners reduce the risk of heart attack and stroke by reducing the formation of blood clots in arteries and veins. There are two main types of blood thinners-anticoagulants, such as heparin or warfarin (also called Coumadin) and antiplatelet drugs, such as aspirin.

Cardiac surgery registry
A registry collects and analyzes information on certain medical topics, conditions, or procedures for hospitals or other providers. The registry then provides the hospitals or providers with information to help them improve the care they provide. A cardiac surgery registry is one example of a registry in which hospitals or providers that perform cardiac surgery can participate.

Centers for Medicare & Medicaid Services (CMS)
The federal agency that runs the Medicare program for the elderly aged and disabled. In addition, CMS works with the states to run the Medicaid program for low-income individuals. CMS works to make sure that the people in these programs are able to get high quality health care.

Centers for Medicare & Medicaid Services (CMS) National Surgical Quality Pilot
In September of 2011, CMS engaged the American College of Surgeons (ACS) to publically report surgical outcome measures on the Hospital Compare website. Hospitals volunteering in this multispecialty surgical registry are provided with nationally validated, risk-adjusted, outcomes-based surgical quality measures. Hospitals report for one or any combination of three surgical measures—elderly surgical outcomes, colectomy outcomes, and lower-extremity bypass outcomes—collected through participation in the American College of Surgeons National Surgical Quality Improvement Program (ACS NSQIP®), a nationally validated, risk-adjusted, outcomes-based program to measure and improve the quality of surgical care in the private sector.

Certification (Medicare-certified)
State government agencies inspect health care providers, including hospitals, nursing homes, dialysis facilities and home health agencies, as well as other health care providers. These providers are certified if they pass inspection. Being certified is not the same as being accredited. Medicare or Medicaid only pays for care provided by certified or accredited providers.

Cesarean section (C-section)
A cesarean section (C-section) is the delivery of a baby through a surgical opening in the mother's lower belly area. A C-section delivery is done when it is not possible or safe for the mother to deliver the baby through the vagina.

Children's hospital
A hospital with a majority of its inpatients under the age of 18, which participates and is paid in the Medicare program as a children's hospital.

Chronic illness
An illness that persists over a long period of time.

Comorbidities
Two or more diseases that are present at the same time.

Critical access hospital (CAH)
A small facility that provides outpatient services, as well as inpatient services on a limited basis, to people in rural areas.

Computerized tomography (CT) scan
An imaging test that uses multiple x-rays to produce detailed pictures of the inside of the body (bones, organs, and other body parts).

Department of Health And Human Services (DHHS)
A federal agency that administers programs for protecting the health of all Americans, including Medicare, Medicaid, and the Children's Health Insurance Program (CHIP).

Diastolic pressure
The lowest pressure in the artery, occurring when the heart is filling with blood. In a blood pressure reading, the diastolic pressure is the second number recorded.

Elective delivery
An elective delivery is a delivery performed for a nonmedical reason. Some nonmedical reasons include wanting to schedule the birth of the baby on a specific date, living far away from the hospital, or discomfort in the last weeks of pregnancy.

Fibrinolysis, fibrinolytic drugs
Fibrinolytic drugs are "clot-busting" drugs that can help dissolve blood clots in blood vessels and improve blood flow to your heart. They are important for treating heart attacks. If you have a heart attack, your doctor may give you a fibrinolytic drug, perform a percutaneous coronary intervention (PCI), or both.

Heart attack
A heart attack, also called an acute myocardial infarction (AMI), happens when one of the heart's arteries becomes blocked and the supply of blood and oxygen to part of the heart muscle is slowed or stopped. When the heart muscle doesn't get the oxygen and nutrients it needs, the affected heart tissue may die.

Heart failure
In heart failure, the heart cannot pump enough blood through the body. The heart cannot fill with enough blood or pump with enough force, or both. Heart failure develops over time as the pumping action of the heart gets weaker. It can affect the right, the left, or both sides of the heart. Heart failure does not mean that the heart has stopped working or is about to stop working.

Hemorrhagic stroke
A hemorrhagic stroke occurs when a blood vessel in part of the brain becomes weak and bursts open, causing blood to leak into the brain. Some people have defects in the blood vessels of the brain that make this more likely.

Heparin injection
Heparin is a type of anticoagulant or "blood thinner," and is used to prevent blood clots from forming in people who have certain medical conditions or who are undergoing certain medical procedures that increase the chance that clots will form. Heparin is also used to stop the growth of clots that have already formed in the blood vessels.

Index admission
An index admission is the admission with a principal diagnosis of a specified condition that meets the inclusion and exclusion criteria for the measure.

Influenza
A serious and sometimes deadly lung infection that can spread quickly in a community. Symptoms include fever-often a high temperature of more than 102° Fahrenheit (38.9° Celsius), headache, muscle aches and pains, chills, cough and chest pain when you take a breath ("pleuritic chest pain"). Although most people recover from the illness, the Centers for Disease Control and Prevention (the CDC) estimates that in the United States more than 200,000 people are hospitalized and about 36,000 people die from the flu and its complications every year.

Influenza vaccination ("Flu Shot")
The main way to keep from getting flu is to get a yearly flu vaccination. Learn more about the flu from the Centers for Disease Control and Prevention (CDC). Hospitals should check to make sure that pneumonia patients get a flu shot during flu season to protect them from another lung infection and to help prevent the spread of influenza in the community.

Inpatient hospital services
Services you get when you're admitted to a hospital, including bed and board, nursing services, diagnostic or therapeutic services, and medical or surgical services.

International Classification of Diseases, Ninth Revision, Clinical Modification (ICD-9-CM)
The classification used to code and classify mortality data from death certificates.

Ischemic stroke
Ischemic stroke occurs when a blood vessel that supplies blood to the brain is blocked by a blood clot. Ischemic strokes may be caused by clogged arteries. Fat, cholesterol, and other substances collect on the artery walls, forming a sticky substance called plaque.

Left ventricular function assessment
A test to check how well the heart is pumping.

Long-term care hospital
Acute care hospitals that provide treatment for patients who stay, on average, more than 25 days. Most patients are transferred from an intensive or critical care unit. These hospitals provide services like comprehensive rehabilitation, respiratory therapy, head trauma treatment, and pain management.

Magnetic resonance imaging (MRI)
An imaging test that uses powerful magnets and radio waves to create pictures of the body. It does not use radiation (x-rays).

Measurement
The process of collecting data to assess performance conducted at a single point in time or repeated over time.

Medicaid
A joint federal and state program that helps with medical costs for some people with low incomes and limited resources. Medicaid programs vary from state to state, but most health care costs are covered if you qualify for both Medicare and Medicaid.

Medical imaging
Tests that create images of various parts of the body to screen for or diagnose medical conditions. Examples of medical imaging include CT Scans, MRIs, and mammograms.

Medicare Advantage Plan (Part C)
A type of Medicare health plan offered by a private company that contracts with Medicare to provide you with all your Part A and Part B benefits. Medicare Advantage Plans include Health Maintenance Organizations (HMOs), Preferred Provider Organizations (PPOs), Private Fee-for-Service Plans, Special Needs Plans, and Medicare Medical Savings Account Plans. If you're enrolled in a Medicare Advantage Plan, Medicare services are covered through the plan and aren't paid for under Original Medicare. Most Medicare Advantage Plans offer prescription drug coverage.

Medicare health plan
A plan offered by a private company that contracts with Medicare to provide Part A and Part B benefits to people with Medicare who enroll in the plan. Medicare health plans include all Medicare Advantage Plans, Medicare Cost Plans, Demonstration/Pilot Programs, and Programs of All-inclusive Care for the Elderly (PACE).

Medicare Severity-Diagnosis Related Group (MS-DRG)
The Medicare Severity - Diagnosis Related Groups (MS-DRGs) are payment groups designed for the Medicare population. Patients who have similar clinical characteristics and similar costs are assigned to an MS-DRG. The MS-DRG will be linked to a fixed payment amount based on the average cost of patients in the group. Patients can be assigned to an MS-DRG based on their diagnosis, surgical procedures, age and other information. Hospitals provide this information on their bills and Medicare uses this information to decide how much the hospitals should be paid. There may be some groups of MS-DRGs that are based on complications or comorbidities (CCs) or major complications or comorbidities (MCCs). Complications are new problems that are the result of a procedure, treatment, or illness.

Medicare-certified hospital
In order to receive any payment from either the Medicare or Medicaid programs, a hospital must meet a set of basic standards for quality of care, called "conditions of participation." Medicare-certified hospitals are reviewed periodically (every three years), either by their State Survey Agency or a CMS-approved national accreditation organization, to assure that they are continuing to provide services of acceptable quality. Accreditation is optional, but most short-term acute hospitals in the United States choose to be Medicare-certified based on accreditation by a CMS approved national accreditation organization. There are currently three CMS-approved national hospital accreditation organizations: the American Osteopathic Association/health care Facilities Accreditation Program (AOA/HFAP), Det Norske Veritas Healthcare (DNV Healthcare), and The Joint Commission (TJC).

Number of completed surveys
The "number of completed surveys" is the total number of patients who completed a survey. When at least 300 patients have completed the survey for a hospital, we can be more confident that the survey results are fully representative of patients' experiences at that hospital and are reliable for assessing the hospital's performance. However, smaller hospitals could sample all of their HCAHPS-eligible discharges but, because of their small size, still have fewer than 300 completed surveys.

Original Medicare
Original Medicare is fee-for-service coverage under which the government pays your health care providers directly for your Part A and/or Part B benefits.

Osteopathic doctor
A licensed physician who can do surgery and prescribe drugs who has training in manipulative therapy. Also called a Doctor of Osteopathy (DO).

Outpatient hospital care
Medical or surgical care you get from a hospital when your doctor hasn't written an order to admit you to the hospital as an inpatient. Outpatient hospital care may include emergency department services, observation services, outpatient surgery, lab tests, or X-rays. Your care may be considered outpatient hospital care even if you spend the night at the hospital.

Outpatient Prospective Payment System (OPPS)
Under the Outpatient Prospective Payment System (OPPS), hospitals are paid a set amount of money (called the payment rate) to provide certain outpatient services to people with Medicare.

Oxygenation assessment
Test that measures the amount of oxygen in your blood to see if you need oxygen therapy.

Patient discharge
Patients are considered "discharged" from a hospital when they are released to go home or to another health care setting, or when they die during the hospital stay.

Percutaneous coronary interventions (PCI)
The procedures called percutaneous coronary interventions (PCI), such as angioplasty and atherectomy are among those that are the most effective for opening blocked blood vessels that cause heart attacks. Doctors may perform a PCI, or give certain drugs to open the blockage, and in some cases, they may do both.

Plan of care
A written plan of care created with your physician and hospital staff. It tells what services you will get to reach and keep your best physical, mental, and social wellbeing. The hospital staff keeps your doctor up-to-date on how you are doing and updates your care plan as needed.

Pneumonia
An inflammation of the lungs caused by a viral or bacterial infection. This fills your lungs with mucus and lowers the oxygen level in your blood. Symptoms can include fever, fatigue, difficulty breathing, chills, a "wet" cough, and chest pain. For more on pneumonia, visit MedlinePlus

Pneumonia (pneumococcal) vaccination
Vaccine given to prevent pneumonia, estimated to protect against 80% of bacteria causing pneumonia.

Provider
A doctor, hospital, health care professional or health care facility.

Psychiatric hospital
A facility that provides inpatient psychiatric services for the diagnosis and treatment of mental illness on a 24-hour basis, by or under the supervision of a physician.

Quality
Quality health care is how well a doctor, hospital, health plan, or other provider of health care, keeps its patients healthy or treats them when they are sick. Good quality health care means doing the right thing at the right time, in the right way, for the right person and getting the best possible results.

Quality assurance
The process of looking at how well a medical service is provided. The process may include formally reviewing health care given to a person, or group of persons, locating the problem, correcting the problem, and then checking to see if what was done worked.

Quality Improvement Organizations (QIOs)
A group of practicing doctors and other health care experts paid by the federal government to check and improve the care given to people with Medicare.

Ratio
The amount of one thing compared to the amount of another, such as the number of combination CT scans done compared to the number of all CT scans done.

Readmissions
Patients who are admitted to the hospital for treatment of medical problems sometimes get other serious injuries, complications, or conditions, and may even die. Some patients may experience problems soon after they are discharged and need to be admitted to the hospital again. These events can often be prevented if hospitals follow best practices for treating patients.

Registry
A registry collects and analyzes information on certain medical topics, conditions, or procedures for hospitals or other providers. The registry then provides the hospitals or providers with information to help them improve the care they provide. Examples of registries in which hospitals can participate include: a multispecialty surgical registry , a nursing care registry, and a stroke care registry.

Rehabilitation hospital
A hospital that specializes in improving or restoring a patient's functional ability through therapies. Sometimes called a post-acute hospital.

Reliever medications
Relievers are medications that relax the bands of muscle surrounding the airways and are used to quickly make breathing easier.

Risk-adjusted
"Risk-adjusted" means that the measure calculations take into account how sick patients were when they went in for their initial hospital stay. When rates are risk-adjusted, it means that hospitals that usually take care of sicker patients won't have a worse rate just because their patients were sicker when they arrived at the hospital. When rates are risk-adjusted, it helps make comparisons fair and meaningful.

Risk-adjusted 30-day death (mortality) rates
The 30-day Risk-Adjusted Death (Mortality) Rates are produced using a complex statistical model, that relies on Medicare claims and enrollment information. The model predicts patient deaths for any cause within 30 days of hospital admission for heart attack or heart failure, whether the patients die while still in the hospital or after discharge. Thirty-day mortality is used because this is the time period when deaths are most likely to be related to the care patients received in the hospital. Deaths that occur outside the hospital within 30 days are included along with deaths that occur in the hospital, because some hospitals discharge patients sooner than others.

Screening mammogram
A medical procedure to check for breast cancer before you or a doctor may be able to find it manually.

Stent
A small wire tube inserted in a blood vessel by a catheter to hold open a blocked blood vessel. This is one of several procedures called a percutaneous coronary intervention (PCI) that are used to open a blocked blood vessel.

Structural measures
A structural measure reflects the environment in which providers care for patients, such as whether or not a hospital uses an electronic health record.

Survey of patients' experiences
A national, standardized survey of hospital patients about their experiences during a recent inpatient hospital stay. This is also referred to as HCAHPS (Hospital Consumer Assessment of Healthcare Providers and Systems).

Survey response rate
Tells what percentage of patients who were asked to complete the survey actually did complete it. In general, the higher this response rate percentage, the more confident we can be that the survey results for a hospital are representative of patients' experiences at that hospital and are reliable for assessing the hospital's performance.

Systemic corticosteroid
Inflammation-reducing, anti-allergic medications that affect the body as a whole.

Teaching hospital
Hospitals that train residents in approved medical, osteopathic, dental or podiatry residency programs.

The Joint Commission (JC)
An independent, not-for-profit organization that accredits and certifies a large number of health care organizations and programs in the United States. The Joint Commission's hospital accreditation program has held deeming authority since the inception of the Medicare program in 1965. The Joint Commission's mission is to continuously improve health care for the public, in collaboration with other stakeholders, by evaluating health care organizations and inspiring them to excel in providing safe and effective care of the highest quality and value.

Thrombolytic therapy
Thrombolytic therapy is the use of drugs to break up or dissolve blood clots, which are the main cause of both heart attacks and stroke.

Treatment
Something done to help with a health problem. For example, giving certain drugs and performing surgery are treatments.

Treatment options
The choices you have when there is more than one way to treat your health problem.

Venous thromboembolism (VTE)
Venous thromboembolism (VTE) is a term that includes both deep vein thrombosis and pulmonary embolism. A deep vein thrombosis (DVT) is a blood clot that forms in a vein deep in the body. A pulmonary embolism (PE) is a loose blood clot that travels to an artery in the lungs and can block blood flow.

Warfarin
A medication used to prevent blood clots from forming or growing larger in your blood and blood vessels.

Source: Medicare.gov

Regional Hospital Profile Index

National Hospital Profile Index

2014 Title List

Visit **www.SalemPress.com** for Product Information, Table of Contents and Sample Pages

Literature

American Ethnic Writers
Critical Insights: Authors
Critical Insights: New Literary Collection Bundles
Critical Insights: Themes
Critical Insights: Works
Critical Survey of Drama
Critical Survey of Graphic Novels: Heroes & Super Heroes
Critical Survey of Graphic Novels: History, Theme & Technique
Critical Survey of Graphic Novels: Independents & Underground Classics
Critical Survey of Graphic Novels: Manga
Critical Survey of Long Fiction
Critical Survey of Mystery & Detective Fiction
Critical Survey of Mythology and Folklore: Heroes and Heroines
Critical Survey of Mythology and Folklore: Love, Sexuality & Desire
Critical Survey of Mythology and Folklore: World Mythology
Critical Survey of Poetry
Critical Survey of Poetry: American Poetry
Critical Survey of Poetry: British, Irish & Commonwealth Poets
Critical Survey of Poetry: European Poets
Critical Survey of Poetry: European Poets
Critical Survey of Poetry: Topical Essays
Critical Survey of Poetry: World Poets
Critical Survey of Science Fiction & Fantasy Literature
Critical Survey of Shakespeare's Sonnets
Critical Survey of Short Fiction
Critical Survey of Short Fiction: American Writers
Critical Survey of Short Fiction: British, Irish & Commonwealth Poets
Critical Survey of Short Fiction: European Writers
Critical Survey of Short Fiction: Topical Essays
Critical Survey of Short Fiction: World Writers
Cyclopedia of Literary Characters
Introduction to Literary Context: American Post-Modernist Novels
Introduction to Literary Context: American Short Fiction
Introduction to Literary Context: English Literature
Introduction to Literary Context: World Literature
Magill's Literary Annual 2014
Magill's Survey of American Literature
Magill's Survey of World Literature
Masterplots
Masterplots II: African American Literature
Masterplots II: Christian Literature
Masterplots II: Drama Series
Masterplots II: Short Story Series
Notable African American Writers
Notable American Novelists
Notable Playwrights
Short Story Writers

Science, Careers & Mathematics

Applied Science
Applied Science: Engineering & Mathematics
Applied Science: Science & Medicine
Applied Science: Technology
Biomes and Ecosystems
Careers in Chemistry
Careers in Communications & Media
Careers in Healthcare
Careers in Hospitality & Tourism
Careers in Law & Criminology
Careers in Physics
Computer Technology Inventors
Contemporary Biographies in Chemistry
Contemporary Biographies in Communications & Media
Contemporary Biographies in Healthcare
Contemporary Biographies in Hospitality & Tourism
Contemporary Biographies in Law & Criminology
Contemporary Biographies in Physics
Earth Science
Earth Science: Earth Materials & Resources
Earth Science: Earth's Surface and History
Earth Science: Physics & Chemistry of the Earth
Earth Science: Weather, Water & Atmosphere
Encyclopedia of Energy
Encyclopedia of Environmental Issues
Encyclopedia of Global Resources
Encyclopedia of Global Warming
Encyclopedia of Mathematics and Society
Encyclopedia of the Ancient World
Forensic Science
Internet Innovators
Introduction to Chemistry
Magill's Encyclopedia of Science: Animal Life
Magill's Encyclopedia of Science: Plant life
Magill's Medical Guide
Notable Natural Disasters
Solar System

Health

Addictions & Substance Abuse
Cancer
Complementary & Alternative Medicine
Genetics & Inherited Conditions
Infectious Diseases & Conditions
Magill's Medical Guide
Psychology & Mental Health
Psychology Basics

SALEM PRESS

SALEM PRESS

2014 Title List

Visit **www.SalemPress.com** for Product Information, Table of Contents and Sample Pages

History and Social Science

A 2000s in America
50 States
African American History
Agriculture in History (check)
American First Ladies
American Heroes
American Indian Tribes
American Presidents
American Villains
Ancient Greece
Bill of Rights, The
Cold War, The
Defining Documents: American Revolution 1754-1805
Defining Documents: Civil War 1860-1865
Defining Documents: Emergence of Modern America, 1868-1918
Defining Documents: Exploration & Colonial America 1492-1755
Defining Documents: Manifest Destiny 1803-1860
Defining Documents: Reconstruction, 1865-1880
Defining Documents: The 1920s
Defining Documents: The 1930s
Defining Documents: World War I
Eighties in America
Encyclopedia of American Immigration
Fifties in America
Forties in America
Great Athletes
Great Events from History: 17th Century
Great Events from History: 18th Century
Great Events from History: 19th Century
Great Events from History: 20th Century, 1901-1940
Great Events from History: 20th Century, 1941-1970
Great Events from History: 20th Century, 1971-200
Great Events from History: Ancient World
Great Events from History: Middle Ages
Great Events from History: Modern Scandals
Great Events from History: Renaissance & Early Modern Era
Great Lives from History: 17th Century
Great Lives from History: 18th Century
Great Lives from History: 19th Century
Great Lives from History: 20th Century
Great Lives from History: African Americans
Great Lives from History: Ancient World
Great Lives from History: Asian & Pacific Islander Americans
Great Lives from History: Incredibly Wealthy
Great Lives from History: Inventors & Inventions
Great Lives from History: Jewish Americans
Great Lives from History: Latinos
Great Lives from History: Middle Ages
Great Lives from History: Notorious Lives
Great Lives from History: Renaissance & Early Modern Era
Great Lives from History: Scientists & Science
Historical Encyclopedia of American Business
Immigration in U.S. History
Magill's Guide to Military History
Milestone Documents in African American History
Milestone Documents in American History
Milestone Documents in World History
Milestone Documents of American Leaders
Milestone Documents of World Religions
Musicians & Composers 20th Century
Nineties in America
Seventies in America
Sixties in America
Survey of American Industry and Careers
Thirties in America
Twenties in America
U.S. Court Cases
U.S. Laws, Acts, and Treaties
U.S. Legal System
U.S. Supreme Court
United States at War
USA in Space
Weapons and Warfare
World Conflicts: Asia and the Middle East

Grey House Publishing | Salem Press | H.W. Wilson
4919 Route, 22 PO Box 56, Amenia NY 12501-0056

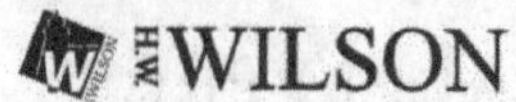

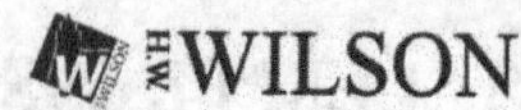

2014 Title List

Visit **www.HwWilsonInPrint.com** for Product Information, Table of Contents and Sample Pages

Current Biography
Current Biography Cumulative Index 1946-2013
Current Biography Magazine
Current Biography Yearbook-2004
Current Biography Yearbook-2005
Current Biography Yearbook-2006
Current Biography Yearbook-2007
Current Biography Yearbook-2008
Current Biography Yearbook-2009
Current Biography Yearbook-2010
Current Biography Yearbook-2011
Current Biography Yearbook-2012
Current Biography Yearbook-2013
Current Biography Yearbook-2014

Core Collections
Senior High Core Collection
Middle & Junior High School Core
Children's Core Collection
Fiction Core Collection
Public Library Core Collection: Nonfiction

Sears List
Sears List of Subject Headings
Sears: Lista de Encabezamientos de Materia

The Reference Shelf
Aging in America
Revisiting Gender
The U.S. National Debate Topic, 2014/2015
Embracing New Paradigms in education
Marijuana Reform
Representative American Speeches 2013-2014
Reality Television
The Business of Food
The Future of U.S. Economic Relations: Mexico, Cuba, and Venezuela
Sports in America
Global Climate Change
Representative American Speeches, 2012-2013
Conspiracy Theories
The Arab Spring
U.S. National Debate Topic: Transportation Infrastructure
Families: Traditional and New Structures
Faith & Science
Representative American Speeches 2011-2012
Social Networking
Dinosaurs
Space Exploration & Development
U.S. Infrastructure
Politics of the Ocean
Representative American Speeches 2010-2011
Robotics
The News and its Future
American Military Presence Overseas
Russia
Graphic Novels and Comic Books
Representative American Speeches 2009-2010

Readers' Guide
Readers Guide to Periodicals Literature
Abridged Readers' Guide to Periodical Literature
Short Story Index

Indexes
Short Story Index
Index to Legal Periodicals & Books

Facts About Series
Facts About the Presidents, Eighth Edition
Facts About China
Facts About the 20th Century
Facts About American Immigration
Facts About World's Languages

Nobel Prize Winners
Nobel Prize Winners, 2002-2013

World Authors
World Authors 2000-2005
World Authors 2006-2013

Famous First Facts
Famous First Facts, Seventh Edition
Famous First Facts About American Politics
Famous First Facts About Sports
Famous First Facts About the Environment
Famous First Facts, International Edition

American Book of Days
The American Book of Days, Fifth Edition
The International Book of Days

Junior Authors & Illustrators
Tenth Book of Junior Authors & Illustrations

Monographs
The Barnhart Dictionary of Etymology
Celebrate the World
Indexing from A to Z
Radical Change: Books for Youth in a Digital Age
The Poetry Break
Guide to the Ancient World

Wilson Chronology
Wilson Chronology of Asia and the Pacific
Wilson Chronology of Human Rights
Wilson Chronology of Ideas
Wilson Chronology of the Arts
Wilson Chronology of the World's Religions
Wilson Chronology of Women's Achievements

Book Review Digest
Book Review Digest, 2014

Grey House Publishing | Salem Press | H.W. Wilson
4919 Route, 22 PO Box 56, Amenia NY 12501-0056

LINDENHURST MEMORIAL LIBRARY
3 1801 00550 8522